尼尔森儿科学
Nelson
TEXTBOOK OF
PEDIATRICS

KLIEGMAN | ST GEME
BLUM | SHAH | TASKER | WILSON

第21版（影印中文导读版）

编译委员会名誉主任委员　张金哲

编译委员会主任委员　王天有

中册

EDITION
21
VOLUME 2

ELSEVIER　CTS | K 湖南科学技术出版社

Contents 目 录

PART III

Behavioral and Psychiatric Disorders
第三部分 行为和精神障碍

PART IV

Learning and Developmental Disorders
第四部分 学习及发育障碍

PART V

Nutrition
第五部分　营养

PART VI

Fluid and Electrolyte Disorders
第六部分　水和电解质紊乱

PART VII

Pediatric Drug Therapy
第七部分　儿科药物治疗

PART VIII
Emergency Medicine and Critical Care
第八部分　急危重症

PART IX
Human Genetics
第九部分　人类遗传学

Volume 2
中　册

PART XIV

Allergic Disorders
第十四部分　过敏性疾病

PART **XVII**

The Digestive System
第十七部分　消化系统

---

†Deceased.

Volume 3
下　册

PART **XIX**
The Cardiovascular System
第十九部分　心血管系统

Section **1** DEVELOPMENTAL BIOLOGY OF THE CARDIOVASCULAR SYSTEM
第一篇　心血管系统发育生理学

PART **XX**

Diseases of the Blood
第二十部分 血液系统疾病

PART XXV

The Endocrine System
第二十五部分　内分泌系统

Section 1 DISORDERS OF THE HYPOTHALAMUS AND PITUITARY GLAND
第一篇　下丘脑垂体疾病

Section 2 DISORDERS OF THE THYROID GLAND
第二篇　甲状腺疾病

Section 3 DISORDERS OF THE PARATHYROID GLAND
第三篇　甲状旁腺疾病

Section 4 DISORDERS OF THE ADRENAL GLAND
第四篇　肾上腺疾病

PART XXIX
The Ear
第二十九部分　耳部疾病

PART XXX
The Skin
第三十部分　皮肤病

PART **XXXII**

Rehabilitation Medicine
第三十二部分　康复医学

PART **XXXIII**

Environmental Health
第三十三部分 环境卫生

Allergic Disorders
过敏性疾病

Chapter 166

Allergy and the Immunologic Basis of Atopic Disease

Cezmi A. Akdis and Scott H. Sicherer

第一百六十六章
特应性疾病的过敏和免疫学基础

中文导读

本章主要介绍了过敏性疾病的基础免疫学机制。具体阐述了参与过敏性疾病发病过程的关键免疫细胞和免疫组分，描述了过敏原及其分子结构和理化特征对抗原递呈以及穿透胞膜的重要性；T细胞的各亚型包括Th2细胞及其细胞因子在过敏免疫反应速发炎症进程中的重要作用；上皮细胞在呼吸道暴露变应原后的免疫炎症反应过程。对Th17和Th22细胞在组织炎症中所起作用进行了说明。详述了调节性T细胞（Treg）介导过敏免疫耐受机制，先天淋巴细胞（ILCs）在无抗原和变应原暴露下与上皮细胞间作用参与过敏炎症。重点阐述了DCs在成熟阶段的表面分子特点及其经历的表型和功能变化。对IgE及其受体在急性过敏炎症反应的作用以及在严重过敏反应机制

的差异性进行说明，并描述IgE合成的双信号机制。讲述了嗜酸性粒细胞及其脱颗粒产生的炎症蛋白类等促进局部组织过敏炎症作用，突出强调了嗜酸性粒细胞等多种细胞在趋化因子作用下主要参与的迟发相炎症反应。描述了免疫系统来源的2型免疫反应在过敏性疾病包括哮喘为主的普遍机制，和以上皮细胞为主的组织细胞及其细胞因子激活的过敏炎症。进一步阐述了过敏免疫炎症反应在组织重构和过敏性疾病慢性化中的作用。对特应性遗传基础的阐述具体介绍了调节特应性的系统性基因表达和屏障功能相关基因以及模式识别受体相关基因、调控细胞因子合成基因等。解释了5q23-25区域拥有一系列在过敏性疾病发生中起作用的基因包括IL-4和IL-13相关的调控基因。

Allergic or atopic patients have an altered state of reactivity to common environmental and food antigens that do not cause clinical reactions in unaffected people. Patients with clinical allergy usually produce immunoglobulin E (IgE) antibodies to the antigens that trigger their illness. The term *allergy* represents the clinical expression of IgE-mediated allergic diseases that have a familial predisposition and that manifest as

hyperresponsiveness in target organs such as the lung, skin, gastrointestinal (GI) tract, and nose. The significant increase in the prevalence of allergic diseases in the last few decades is attributed to changes in environmental factors such as exposure to tobacco smoke, air pollution, indoor and outdoor allergens, respiratory viruses, obesity, and perhaps a decline in certain infectious diseases (hygiene hypothesis).

KEY ELEMENTS OF ALLERGIC DISEASES
Allergens

Allergens are almost always *proteins,* but not all proteins are allergens. For a protein antigen to display allergenic activity, it must induce IgE production, which must lead to a type 1 hypersensitivity response on subsequent exposure to the same protein. Biochemical properties of the allergen; stimulating factors of the innate immune response around the allergen substances at the time of exposure; stability of the allergen in the tissues, digestive system, skin, or mucosa; and the dose and time of stay in lymphatic organs during the interaction with the immune system are factors that may cause an antigen to become an allergen. This is distinguished from general antigen responses, which induce a state of immune responsiveness without associated IgE production.

Most allergens are proteins with molecular weight of 10-70 kDa. Molecules <10 kDa do not bridge adjacent IgE antibody molecules on the surfaces of mast cells or basophils. Most molecules >70 kDa do not pass through mucosal surfaces, a feature needed to reach **antigen-presenting cells (APCs)** for stimulation of the immune system. Allergens frequently contain **proteases**, which promote skin and mucosal epithelial barrier dysfunction and increase allergen penetration into host tissues. Low-molecular-weight moieties, such as drugs, can become allergens by reacting with serum proteins or cell membrane proteins to be recognized by the immune system. Carbohydrate structures can also be allergens and are most relevant with the increasing use of *biologics* in clinical practice; patients with cetuximab-induced anaphylaxis have IgE antibodies specific for galactose-α-1,3-galactose.

T Cells

Everyone is exposed to potential allergens. Atopic individuals respond to allergen exposure with rapid expansion of **T-helper type 2 (Th2)** cells that secrete cytokines, such as interleukin (IL)-4, IL-5, and IL-13, favoring IgE synthesis and eosinophilia. Allergen-specific IgE antibodies associated with atopic response are detectable by serum testing or positive immediate reactions to allergen extracts on skin-prick testing. The Th2 cytokines IL-4 and IL-13 play a key role in immunoglobulin isotype switching to IgE (Fig. 166.1). IL-5 and IL-9 are important in differentiation and development of eosinophils. The combination of IL-3, IL-4, and IL-9 contributes to mast cell activation. IL-9 is responsible for mucus production. Th2 cytokines are important effector molecules in the pathogenesis of asthma and allergic diseases; acute allergic reactions are characterized by infiltration of Th2 cells into affected tissues. In addition, IL-25, IL-33, and **thymic stromal lymphopoietin (TSLP)** secreted from epithelial cells on exposure to allergens and respiratory viruses contribute to Th2 response and eosinophilia.

A fraction of the immune response to allergen results in proliferation of **T-helper type 1 (Th1)** cells. Th1 cells are typically involved in the eradication of intracellular organisms, such as mycobacteria, because of the ability of Th1 cytokines to activate phagocytes and promote the production of opsonizing and complement-fixing antibodies. The Th1 component of allergen-specific immune response contributes to chronicity and the effector phase in allergic disease. Activation and apoptosis of epithelial cells induced by Th1 cell–secreted interferon-γ (IFN-γ), tumor necrosis factor (TNF)-α, and Fas ligand constitute an essential pathogenetic event for the formation of eczematous lesions in atopic dermatitis and bronchial epithelial cell shedding in asthma.

Chronic lesions of allergic reactions are characterized by infiltration of Th1 and **Th17 cells**. This is important because Th1 cytokines such as IFN-γ can potentiate the function of allergic inflammatory effector cells such as eosinophils and thereby contribute to disease severity. Th17 and Th22 cells link the immune response to tissue inflammation; IL-17A and IL-17F and IL-22 are their respective prototype cytokines. Although both T-helper cell subsets play roles in immune defense to extracellular bacteria, IL-17 augments inflammation, whereas IL-22 plays a tissue-protective role. Cytokines in the IL-17 family act on multiple cell types, including epithelial cells and APCs, to cause the release of chemokines, antimicrobial peptides, and proinflammatory cytokines to enhance inflammation and antimicrobial responses. In addition, Th9 cells produce IL-9, but not other typical Th1, Th2, and

Th17 cytokines, and constitute a distinct population of effector T cells that promotes tissue inflammation. Fig. 166.2 depicts the complex cytokine cascades involving Th1, Th2, Th9, Th17, and Th22 cells.

T-regulatory (or regulatory T) **cells (Tregs)** are a subset of T cells thought to play a critical role in expression of allergic and autoimmune diseases. These cells have the ability to suppress effector T cells of Th1, Th2, Th9, Th17, and Th22 phenotypes (Fig. 166.3). Tregs express CD4⁺CD25⁺ surface molecules and immunosuppressive cytokines such as IL-10 and transforming growth factor-β (TGF-β₁). The forkhead box/winged-helix transcription factor gene *FOXP3* is expressed specifically by CD4⁺CD25⁺ Tregs and programs their development and function. Adoptive transfer of Tregs inhibits the development of airway eosinophilia and protects against airway hyperreactivity in animal models of asthma. T-cell response to allergens in healthy individuals shows a wide range, from no detectable response to involvement of active peripheral tolerance mechanisms mediated by different subsets of Tregs. Individuals who are not allergic even though they are exposed to high doses of allergens, such as beekeepers and cat owners, show a detectable allergen-specific IgG4 response accompanied by IL-10–producing Tregs. It is thought that CD4⁺CD25⁺ Tregs play an important role in mitigating the allergic immune response, and that the lack of such cells may predispose to the development of allergic diseases. Patients with mutations in the human *FOXP3* gene lack CD4⁺CD25⁺ Tregs and develop severe immune dysregulation, with polyendocrinopathy, food allergy, and high serum IgE levels (XLAAD/IPEX disease) (see Chapter 152). In addition to Treg cells, IL-10–secreting and allergen-specific Breg cells increase during allergen-specific immunotherapy and may play a role in allergen tolerance.

Innate Lymphoid Cells

Immune responses in populations of lymphoid cells that lack rearranged T- and B-cell antigen receptors and surface markers for myeloid and lymphoid lineages, such as T, B, and natural killer (NK) cells, show

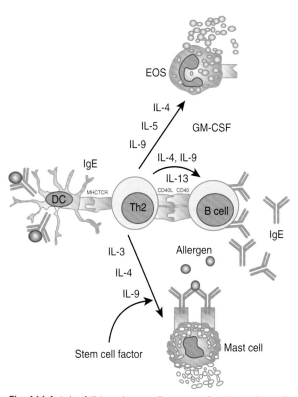

Fig. 166.1 Role of Th2 cytokines in allergic cascade. *DC,* Dendritic cell; *EOS,* eosinophil; *GM-CSF,* granulocyte-macrophage colony-stimulating factor; *IL,* interleukin; *Th2,* T-helper type 2 cell.

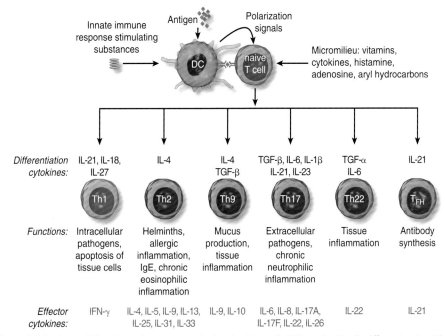

Fig. 166.2 Effector T-cell subsets. Following antigen presentation by dendritic cells (DCs), naïve T cells differentiate into Th1, Th2, Th9, Th17, Th22, and follicular helper (TFH) effector subsets. Their differentiation requires cytokines and other cofactors that are released from DCs and also expressed in the micromilieu. T-cell activation in the presence of interleukin-4 (IL-4) enhances differentiation and clonal expansion of Th2 cells, perpetuating the allergic response. IFN-γ, Interferon-γ; TGF-β, transforming growth factor-β. *(From Akdis M, Palomares O, van de Veen W, et al: TH17 and TH22 cells: a confusion of antimicrobial response with tissue inflammation versus protection,* J Allergy Clin Immunol *129:1438–1449, 2012.)*

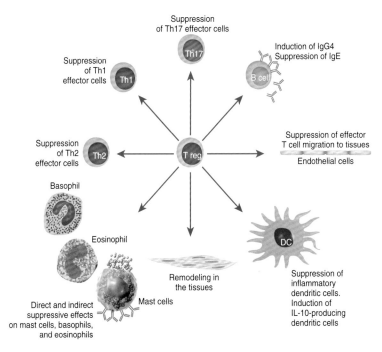

Fig. 166.3 Control of allergen-specific immune responses. FoxP3⁺, CD4⁺, CD25⁺, and Tr1 cells contribute to the control of allergen-specific immune responses in several major ways: Suppression of dendritic cells (DCs) that support the generation of effector T cells; suppression of Th1, Th2, and Th17 cells; suppression of allergen-specific IgE, and induction of IgG₄ and/or IgA; suppression of mast cells, basophils, and eosinophils; interaction with resident tissue cells and remodeling, and suppression of effector T-cell migration to tissues. IL-10, Interleukin-10. *(From Akdis CA, Akdis M: Mechanisms and treatment of allergic disease in the big picture of regulatory T cells,* J Allergy Clin Immunol *123:735–746, 2009.)*

similarities to Th1, Th2, and Th17/Th22 types of immune responses. These latter cells are defined as the innate lymphoid cells **ILC1s, ILC2s,** and **ILC3s,** respectively, based on their transcription factors and cytokine production patterns. ILC1s mainly produce IFN-γ; ILC2s produce IL-5, IL-9, and IL-13; and ILC3s produce IL-17 and IL-22 without any need of antigen/allergen exposure. Strong evidence indicates that ILCs play substantial roles in protection against infection and the pathogenesis

of inflammatory diseases, such as asthma, allergic diseases, and autoimmune diseases. ILCs control the mucosal environment through close interaction with epithelial cells and other tissue cells, cytokine production, and induction of chemokines that recruit suitable cell populations to initiate and promote distinct types of immune response development and tissue inflammation. ILC2s are likely involved in the induction of asthma, allergic rhinitis, eosinophilic esophagitis, and atopic dermatitis through activation by epithelium-derived cytokines (e.g., IL-33, IL-25, TSLP) and interaction with other immune cells.

Antigen-Presenting Cells

Dendritic cells (DCs), Langerhans cells, monocytes, and macrophages have the ability to present allergens to T cells and thereby modulate allergic inflammation by controlling the type of T-cell development. APCs are a heterogeneous group of cells that share the property of antigen presentation in the context of the major histocompatibility complex (MHC) and are found primarily in lymphoid organs and the skin. DCs and Langerhans cells are unique in their ability to prime naïve T cells and are responsible for the primary immune response, or the **sensitization phase** of allergy. Monocytes and macrophages are thought to contribute to activating memory T-cell responses on reexposure to allergen, which characterizes the **elicitation phase** of allergy.

Peripheral DCs residing in sites such as the skin, intestinal lamina propria, and lung are relatively immature. These immature DCs take up antigens in tissues and then migrate to the T-cell areas in locally draining lymph nodes. The DCs undergo phenotypic and functional changes during migration, characterized by increased expression of MHC class I, MHC class II, and co-stimulatory molecules that react with CD28 expressed on T cells. In the lymph nodes, they directly present processed antigens to resting T cells to induce their proliferation and differentiation.

Mature DCs have been designated as **myeloid** or **plasmacytoid** on the basis of their ability to favor Th1 or Th2 differentiation, respectively. The critical factor for polarization to Th1 cells is the level of IL-12 produced by myeloid DC. By contrast, plasmacytoid DCs have low levels of IL-12. Plasmacytoid DC particularly play a role in antiviral immunity by rapid production of high amounts of IFN-α and also help B cells for antibody production. There is considerable interest in the role of TSLP, which is overexpressed in the mucosal surfaces and skin of atopic individuals. TSLP enhances Th2 differentiation by inducing expression of OX40L on immature myeloid DCs in the absence of IL-12 production.

Presence of allergen-specific IgE on the cell surfaces of APCs is a unique feature of atopy. Importantly, the formation of high-affinity IgE receptor I (**FcεRI**)/IgE/allergen complexes on APC surfaces greatly facilitates allergen uptake and presentation. The clinical importance of this phenomenon is supported by the observation that FcεRI-positive Langerhans cells bearing IgE molecules are a prerequisite for skin-applied, aeroallergen provocation of eczematous lesions in patients with atopic dermatitis. The role of the low-affinity IgE receptor II (**FcεRII, CD23**) on monocytes/macrophages is less clear, although under certain conditions it apparently can also facilitate antigen capture. Cross-linking of FcεRII, as well as FcεRI, on monocytes/macrophages leads to the release of inflammatory mediators. There is a critical role for DCs in induction of oral tolerance; tolerogenic DCs are compartmentalized within the mucosa and present antigen through a mechanism designed to produce a Th1/Treg-suppressive response that ablates allergen-specific T cells.

Immunoglobulin E and Its Receptors

The acute allergic response depends on IgE and its ability to bind selectively to the α chain of the high-affinity FcεRI or the low-affinity FcεRII (CD23). Cross-linking of receptor-bound IgE molecules by allergen initiates a complex intracellular signaling cascade, followed by the release of various mediators of allergic inflammation from mast cells and basophils. The FcεRI molecule is also found on the surface of antigen-presenting DCs (e.g., Langerhans cells), but differs from the structure found on mast cells/basophils in that the FcεRI molecule found on DCs lacks the β chain. CD23 is found on B cells, eosinophils, platelets, and DCs. Cross-linking and FcεRI aggregation on mast cells and basophils can also lead to anaphylaxis (see Chapter 174). Differential expression of tyrosine kinases responsible for positive and negative regulation of mast cell/basophil degranulation are thought to be responsible for this aberrant allergic response.

The induction of IgE synthesis requires 2 major signals. The 1st signal (signal 1) initiates IL-4 or IL-13 activation of germline transcription at the ε Ig locus, which dictates isotype specificity. The 2nd signal (signal

2) involves the engagement of CD40 on B cells by CD40 ligand expressed on T cells. This engagement results in activation of the recombination machinery, resulting in DNA switch recombination. Interactions between several co-stimulatory molecule pairs (CD28 and B7; lymphocyte function–associated antigen-1 and intercellular adhesion molecule-1; CD2 and CD58) can further amplify signal 1 and signal 2 to enhance IgE synthesis. Factors that inhibit IgE synthesis include Th1-type cytokines (IL-12, IFN-α, IFN-γ), IL-10 from Tregs, Breg cells, as well as regulatory DCs and microbial DNA containing CpG (cytosine-phosphate-guanine) repeats.

Eosinophils

Allergic diseases are characterized by peripheral blood and tissue eosinophilia. Eosinophils participate in both innate and adaptive immune responses and, like mast cells, contain dense intracellular granules that are sources of inflammatory proteins (see Fig. 155.1). These granule proteins include major basic protein, eosinophil-derived neurotoxin, peroxidase, and cationic protein. Eosinophil granule proteins damage epithelial cells, induce airway hyperresponsiveness, and cause degranulation of basophils and mast cells. Major basic protein released from eosinophils can bind to an acidic moiety on the M2 muscarinic receptor and block its function, thereby leading to increased acetylcholine levels and the development of increased airway hyperreactivity. Eosinophils are also a rich source of prostaglandins and leukotrienes; in particular, cysteinyl leukotriene C4 contracts airway smooth muscle and increases vascular permeability. Other secretory products of eosinophils include cytokines (IL-4, IL-5, TNF-α), proteolytic enzymes, and reactive oxygen intermediates, all of which significantly enhance allergic tissue inflammation.

Several cytokines regulate the function of eosinophils in allergic disease. Eosinophils develop and mature in the bone marrow from myeloid precursor cells activated by IL-3, IL-5, and granulocyte-macrophage colony-stimulating factor (GM-CSF). Allergen exposure of allergic patients causes resident hematopoietic CD34 cells to express the IL-5 receptor. The IL-5 receptor activation induces eosinophil maturation, causing eosinophils to synthesize granule proteins, prolonging their survival, potentiating degranulation of eosinophils, and stimulating release of eosinophils from the bone marrow. GM-CSF also enhances proliferation, cell survival, cytokine production, and degranulation of eosinophils. Certain chemokines, such as RANTES (regulated on activation, normal T-cell expressed and secreted), macrophage inflammatory protein-1α (MIP-1α), and eotaxins, are important for recruiting eosinophils into local allergic tissue inflammatory reactions. Eotaxins mobilize IL-5–dependent eosinophil colony–forming progenitor cells from the bone marrow. These progenitors are rapidly cleared from the blood and either return to the bone marrow or are recruited to inflamed tissue sites.

Mast Cells

Mast cells are derived from CD34 hematopoietic progenitor cells that arise in bone marrow. On entering the circulation, they travel to peripheral tissue, where they undergo tissue-specific maturation. Mast cell development and survival relies on interactions between the tyrosine kinase receptor c-kit expressed on the surface of mast cells and the fibroblast-derived c-kit ligand, the stem cell factor. Unlike mature basophils, mature mast cells do not typically circulate in the blood. They are instead widely distributed throughout connective tissues, where they often lie adjacent to blood vessels and beneath epithelial surfaces that are exposed to the external environment, such as the respiratory tract, gastrointestinal (GI) tract, and skin. So placed, mast cells are positioned anatomically to participate in allergic reactions. At least 2 subpopulations of human mast cells are recognized: mast cells with tryptase and mast cells with both tryptase and chymase. Mast cells with tryptase are the predominant type found in the lung and small intestinal mucosa, whereas mast cells with both tryptase and chymase are the predominant type found in skin, the GI submucosa, and blood vessels.

Mast cells contain, or produce on appropriate stimulation, a diverse array of mediators that have different effects on allergic inflammation and organ function. They include preformed granule-associated mediators (histamine, serine proteases, proteoglycans) and membrane-derived lipid, cytokine, and chemokine mediators arising from de novo synthesis and release. The most important mast cell–derived lipid mediators are the **cyclooxygenase** and **lipoxygenase** metabolites of arachidonic acid, which have potent inflammatory activities. The major cyclooxygenase product of mast cells is **prostaglandin D$_2$**, and the major lipoxygenase products are the sulfidopeptide **leukotrienes** (LTs): LTC$_4$ and its peptidolytic derivatives LTD$_4$ and LTE$_4$. Mast cells also can produce cytokines that promote Th2-type responses (IL-4, IL-13, GM-CSF) and inflammation (TNF-α, IL-6) and regulate tissue remodeling (TGF, vascular endothelial cell growth factor). Immunologic activation of mast cells and basophils typically begins with cross-linkage of IgE bound to the FcεRI with multivalent allergen. Mast cell surface FcεRI is increased by IL-4 and IgE. Surface levels of FcεRI decrease in patients receiving treatment with anti-IgE antibody that lowers serum IgE, which is of potential therapeutic interest.

MECHANISMS OF ALLERGIC TISSUE INFLAMMATION

IgE-mediated immune responses can be classified chronologically according to 3 reaction patterns. The **early-phase response** is the immediate response after allergen is introduced into target organs. This response is characterized by mast cell degranulation and release of preformed mediators, occurring within an immediate time frame of 1-30 min after allergen exposure and resolving within 1-3 hr. Acute reactions are associated with increased local vascular permeability, which leads to leakage of plasma proteins, tissue swelling, and increased blood flow, as well as itching, sneezing, wheezing, and acute abdominal cramps in the skin, nose, lung, and GI tract, respectively, depending on the targeted organ.

A 2nd, **late-phase response** can occur within hours of allergen exposure, reaching a maximum at 6-12 hr and resolving by 24 hr. Late-phase responses are characterized in the skin by edema, redness, and induration; in the nose by sustained nasal blockage; and in the lung by airway obstruction and persistent wheezing. In general, late-phase responses are associated with early infiltration of neutrophils and eosinophils, followed by basophils, monocytes, macrophages, and Th2-type cells. Recruitment of inflammatory cells from the circulation requires increased expression of adhesion molecules on their cell surfaces and expression of their ligand on endothelial cells, which are under the control of cytokines. Several hours after allergen exposure, TNF-α released by activated mast cells induces the vascular endothelial expression of cell adhesion molecules, and this change leads to transendothelial migration of various inflammatory cells. Preferential accumulation of eosinophils occurs through interactions between selective adhesion molecules on the eosinophil cell surface (e.g., α$_4$β$_1$ integrin or very late antigen-4); vascular cell adhesion molecule-1 surface expression can be enhanced by IL-4 and IL-13 on endothelial cells. ILC2s receive signals from the epithelial cells, such as IL-33, TSLP, and IL-25, and are activated and start to release their cytokines IL-5 and IL-13 to initiate a type 2 immune response.

Chemokines are chemotactic cytokines that play a central role in tissue-directed migration of inflammatory cells. RANTES, MIP-1α, monocyte chemotactic protein (MCP)-3, and MCP-4 are chemoattractants for eosinophils and mononuclear cells, whereas eotaxins are relatively selective for eosinophils. These chemoattractants have been detected in epithelium, macrophages, lymphocytes, and eosinophils at sites of late-phase responses and allergic tissue inflammation. Blockade of these chemokines leads to significant reduction in tissue-directed migration of allergic effector cells.

In the 3rd reaction pattern, **chronic allergic disease**, tissue inflammation can persist for days to years. Several factors contribute to persistent tissue inflammation, including recurrent exposure to allergens and microbial agents. The repeated stimulation of allergic effector cells such as mast cells, basophils, eosinophils, and Th2 cells contributes to unresolved inflammatory conditions. Additionally, Th2-type cytokines (IL-3, IL-5, GM-CSF) secreted during allergic reactions can prolong survival of allergic effector cells by delaying apoptosis. Local differentiation of tissue-infiltrating eosinophil precursors induced by IL-5 results in self-generation of eosinophils, further sustaining damage

of local tissue. Tissue remodeling leading to irreversible changes in target organs is also a feature of chronic allergic disease. In asthma, **remodeling** involves thickening of the airway walls and submucosal tissue, as well as smooth muscle hypertrophy and hyperplasia, which are associated with a decline in lung function. This is an unexpected role for eosinophils in airway remodeling as well as chronic inflammation. In atopic dermatitis, lichenification is an obvious manifestation of skin remodeling.

Generally, it is considered that a type 2 immune response underlines a majority of asthma cases, atopic dermatitis, chronic rhinosinusitis, and allergic rhinitis as a general characteristic of an immune/inflammatory response. Type 2 immune response involves Th2 cells, type 2 B cells, ILC2, IL-4 secreting NK T cells, basophils, eosinophils and mast cells and their major cytokines. From a complex network of cytokines, IL-4, IL-5, IL-9, and IL-13 are mainly secreted from the immune system cells, and IL-25, IL-31, IL-33, and TSLP from tissue cells, particularly epithelial cells. Many asthma-related antigens, such as protease allergens, fungal extracts, and viral infection, trigger IL-33, TSLP, and IL-25 production from epithelial cells and various immune cells and induce eosinophilic asthma–like airway inflammation through activation of lung ILC2s.

IL-31, on the other hand, plays a role in pruritus in atopic dermatitis. Th2 cytokines do not only maintain allergic inflammation but also influence tissue remodeling by activating resident cells in target organs; IL-4, IL-9, and IL-13 induce mucus hypersecretion and metaplasia of mucus cells; IL-4 and IL-13 stimulate fibroblast growth and synthesis of extracellular matrix proteins; and IL-5 and IL-9 increase subepithelial fibrosis. TGF-β produced by eosinophils and fibroblasts can also enhance subepithelial fibrosis. IL-11 expressed by eosinophils and epithelial cells contributes to subepithelial fibrosis, in addition to enhancing deposition of collagen and the accumulation of fibroblasts. The resulting tissue injury amplifies further epithelial injury through proinflammatory cytokine release, extracellular matrix deposition in target organs, and angiogenesis. Genetic predisposition to aberrant injury-repair responses may contribute to chronicity of illness. Once the allergic immune response is established, it can be self-perpetuating due to a general type 2 immune response and can lead to chronic disease in genetically predisposed individuals. The subsequent infiltration of Th1 cells and Th17 cells enhances the inflammatory potential of allergic effector cells and contributes to chronic tissue inflammatory responses through the release of proinflammatory cytokines and chemokines. In addition, an autoimmune response might be playing a causative role in allergic inflammation resulting from possible mechanisms through IgE autoantibodies, IgG autoantibodies, and Th1-cell and Th17-cell autoreactivity.

GENETIC BASIS OF ATOPY

Allergic diseases are complex genetic conditions susceptible to environmental triggers. Several major groups of genes are associated with allergic diseases: genes that regulate systemic expression of atopy (increased IgE synthesis, eosinophilia, mast cell responses) and that are usually expressed among various allergic diseases, genes that control barrier function in specific target organs (e.g., skin in atopic dermatitis, lung in asthma, GI tract in food allergy), and genes encoding pattern-recognition receptors of the innate immune system that engage microbial pathogens and influence adaptive immune responses. Once allergic responses have been initiated, a genetic predisposition to chronic allergic inflammation and aberrant injury-repair responses contribute to tissue remodeling and persistent disease.

Atopic diseases have a strong familial predisposition, with approximately 60% heritability found in twin studies of asthma and atopic dermatitis. The 5q23-35 region comprises several genes implicated in allergic disease pathogenesis, including genes coding for Th2 cytokines (IL-3, IL-4, IL-5, IL-9, IL-13, GM-CSF). Among these, *IL4* is a well-studied potential candidate gene. A nucleotide change at position 589 of the *IL4* promoter region is associated with the formation of a unique binding site for NF-AT (**n**uclear **f**actor for **a**ctivated **T** cells) transcription factor, increased IL-4 gene transcription, higher NF-AT binding affinity, and increased IgE production. Similarly, *IL13* coding region variants have been associated with asthma and atopic dermatitis. An association has been found between atopy and a gain-of-function polymorphism on chromosome 16, which codes for the α subunit of the IL-4R. This finding is consistent with the important role of IL-4, IL-13, and their receptors in the immunopathogenesis of allergic diseases.

Genome-wide searches have also linked atopy to chromosome region 11q13. The gene encoding the β subunit of FcεRI-β has been proposed to be the candidate gene in this region. The β subunit gene modifies the FcεRI activity on mast cells, and several genetic variants of FcεRI-β are associated with asthma and atopic dermatitis. Chromosome 6 contains genes coding for human leukocyte antigen class I and class II molecules, which regulate the specificity and intensity of the immune responses to specific allergens. IgE responses to specific allergens, such as ragweed antigen Amb a V and mite allergen Der p I, have been linked to specific MHC class II loci. TNF-α, a key cytokine that contributes to the influx of inflammatory cells, is also located on chromosome 6. TNF-α polymorphisms are associated with asthma. A recent genome-wide association study showed that genetic polymorphisms in the gene encoding IL-33, which is a major activator of ILC2s, and its receptor IL-1RL1 (ST2) are strongly linked to asthma development.

Barrier dysfunction has a key role in the pathogenesis of allergic diseases. Genetic linkage studies of atopic dermatitis have demonstrated the importance of chromosome 1q21, which contains a cluster of genes involved in epidermal differentiation. **Filaggrin** is a protein that is essential in the formation of the stratum corneum. Null mutations of the filaggrin gene are strongly associated with early onset and severe atopic dermatitis. Mutations in the gene encoding the serine protease inhibitor SPINK5 has been shown to cause **Netherton disease**, a single-gene disorder associated with erythroderma, food allergy, and high serum IgE levels. A common polymorphism in SPINK5 (in particular, Glu420Lys) increases the risk of developing atopic dermatitis and asthma. SPINK5 is expressed in the outer epidermis and is thought to be critical to neutralizing the proteolytic activity of *Staphylococcus aureus* and common allergens such as *Der p* I, which use these proteases to penetrate the skin to induce allergic responses. Barrier dysfunction is involved in other allergic diseases, such as asthma and rhinosinusitis, but likely involves other barrier genes, such as those encoding gap junctions.

Candidate genes associated with asthma susceptibility have been identified by positional cloning: *GPRA* (G-protein coupled receptor for asthma susceptibility on chromosome 7p14), *ADAM-33* (a disintegrin and metalloproteinase 33 on chromosome 20p), and *DPP10* (dipeptidyl peptidase 10 on chromosome 2q14). The functions of these genes do not fit into classical pathways of atopy and therefore provide new insights into asthma pathogenesis. *GPRA* encodes a G-protein coupled receptor, with isoforms expressed in bronchial epithelial cells and smooth muscle in asthmatic persons, suggesting an important role for these tissues in asthma. *ADAM-33* is expressed in bronchial smooth muscle and has been linked to bronchial hyperresponsiveness. *DPP10* encodes a dipeptidyl dipeptidase that can remove the terminal 2 peptides from certain proinflammatory chemokines, a change that may modulate allergic inflammation.

Pattern-recognition receptors of the innate immune system, which are expressed by epithelial cells and DCs, are associated with disease susceptibility. These receptors recognize specific microbial components. Polymorphisms in CD14 (engages endotoxin), Toll-like receptor 2 (which engages *S. aureus*), and T-cell immunoglobulin domain and mucin domain (which engage hepatitis A virus) correlate with asthma and/or atopic dermatitis susceptibility. Dysregulation of these frontline immune defense systems would permit abnormal response to common environmental allergens.

Bibliography is available at Expert Consult.

Chapter **167**

Diagnosis of Allergic Disease

Supinda Bunyavanich, Jacob Kattan, and Scott H. Sicherer

第一百六十七章
过敏性疾病诊断学

中文导读

　　本章主要介绍了过敏性疾病的诊断方法，包括采集过敏史、体格检查、体外检测、体内检测。具体描述了如何采集完整的病史、过敏儿童中常出现的典型行为、发病时间和症状进展之间的关系、气传变应原、室内变应原、年龄对于诊断的意义、食物过敏以及环境调查的重要性；具体描述了哮喘、过敏性结膜炎、变应性鼻炎、特应性皮炎患儿查体的注意事项，包括监测身高、血压、心率，过敏性暗影及Dennie-Morgan褶皱等特异性体征，哮喘急性发作时的重点体征，皮肤湿疹及干燥情况等；具体描述了嗜酸性粒细胞与过敏性疾病的关系以及T–IgE和sIgE的检测手段和价值；阐述了变应原皮肤点刺的原理、方法和结果解读；介绍了乙酰甲胆碱激发试验以及口服食物激发试验的原理、方法和意义。

ALLERGY HISTORY

Obtaining a complete history from the allergic patient involves eliciting a description of all symptoms along with their timing and duration, exposure to common allergens, and responses to previous therapies. Because patients often suffer from more than one allergic disease, the presence or absence of other allergic diseases, including allergic rhinoconjunctivitis, asthma, food allergy, eosinophilic esophagitis, atopic dermatitis, and drug allergy, should be determined. A family history of allergic disease is common and is one of the most important factors predisposing a child to the development of allergies. The risk of allergic disease in a child approaches 50% when 1 parent is allergic and 66% when both parents are allergic, with maternal history of atopy having a greater effect than paternal history.

Several characteristic behaviors are often seen in allergic children. Because of nasal pruritus and rhinorrhea, children with allergic rhinitis often perform the **allergic salute** by rubbing their nose upward with the palm of their hand. This repeated maneuver may give rise to the **nasal crease**, a horizontal wrinkle over the bridge of the nose. Characteristic vigorous **grinding** of the eyes with the thumb and side of the fist is frequently observed in children with allergic conjunctivitis. The **allergic cluck** is produced when the tongue is placed against the roof of the mouth to form a seal and withdrawn rapidly in an effort to scratch the palate. The presence of other symptoms, such as fever, unilateral nasal obstruction, and purulent nasal discharge, suggests other diagnoses.

The timing of onset and the progression of symptoms are relevant. The onset of recurrent or persistent nasal symptoms coinciding with placement in a daycare center might suggest recurrent infection rather than allergy. When patients present with a history of episodic acute symptoms, it is important to review the setting in which symptoms occur as well as the activities and exposures that immediately precede their onset. Symptoms associated with lawn mowing suggest allergy to grass pollen or fungi, whereas if symptoms occur in homes with pets, animal dander sensitivity is an obvious consideration. Reproducible reactions after ingestion of a specific food raise the possibility of food allergy. When symptoms wax and wane but evolve gradually and are more chronic in duration, a closer look at whether the timing and progression of symptoms correlate with exposure to a seasonal aeroallergen is warranted.

Aeroallergens, such as pollens and fungal spores, are prominent causes of allergic disease. The concentrations of these allergens in outdoor air fluctuate seasonally. Correlating symptoms with seasonal pollination patterns of geographically relevant plants and trees along with information provided by local pollen counts can aid in identifying the allergen. Throughout most of the United States, trees pollinate in the early spring, grasses pollinate in the late spring and early summer, and weeds pollinate in late summer through the fall. The presence of fungal spores in the atmosphere follows a seasonal pattern in the northern United States, with spore counts rising with the onset of warmer weather and peaking in late summer months, only to recede again with the first frost through the winter. In warmer regions of the southern United States, fungal spores and grass pollens may cause symptoms on a perennial basis.

Rather than experiencing seasonal symptoms, some patients suffer allergic symptoms year-round. In these patients, sensitization to perennial allergens usually found indoors, such as dust mites, animal dander, cockroaches, and fungi, warrants consideration. Species of certain fungi, such as *Aspergillus* and *Penicillium,* are found indoors, whereas *Alternaria* is found in both indoor and outdoor environments. Cockroach and rodent allergens are often problematic in inner-city environments. Patients sensitive to perennial allergens often also become sensitized to seasonal allergens and experience baseline symptoms year-round with worsening during the pollen seasons.

The age of the patient is an important consideration in identifying potential allergens. Infants and young children are first sensitized to allergens that are in their environment on a continuous basis, such as dust mites, animal dander, and fungi. Sensitization to seasonal allergens usually takes several seasons of exposure to develop and is thus unlikely to be a significant trigger of symptoms in infants and toddlers.

Food allergies are more common in infants and young children, resulting primarily in cutaneous, gastrointestinal, and, less frequently, respiratory and cardiovascular symptoms. Symptoms of immediate or IgE-mediated hypersensitivity food reactions develop within minutes to 2 hr after ingestion of the offending food. Symptoms of non–IgE-mediated food allergies are often delayed or chronic (see Chapter 176).

Complete information from previous evaluations and prior treatments for allergic disease should be reviewed, including impact of changes in local environment (e.g., home vs school), response to medications, elimination diets, and duration and impact of allergen immunotherapy (if applicable). Improvement in symptoms with medications or avoidance strategies used to treat allergic disease provides additional evidence for an allergic process.

A thorough environmental survey should be performed, focusing on potential sources of allergen and/or irritant exposure, particularly when respiratory symptoms (upper/lower) are reported. The age and type of the dwelling, how it is heated and cooled, the use of humidifiers or air filtration units, and any history of water damage should be noted. Forced air heating may stir up dust mite, fungi, and animal allergens. The irritant effects of wood-burning stoves, fireplaces, and kerosene heaters may provoke respiratory symptoms. Increased humidity or water damage in the home is often associated with greater exposure to dust mites and fungi. Carpeting serves as a reservoir for dust mites, fungi, and animal dander. The number of domestic pets and their movements about the house should be ascertained. Special attention should be focused on the bedroom, where a child spends a significant proportion of time. The age and type of bedding, the use of dust mite covers on pillows and mattresses, the number of stuffed animals, type of window treatments, and the accessibility of pets to the room should be reviewed. The number of smokers in the home, and what and where they smoke is useful information. Activities that might result in exposure to allergens or respiratory irritants such as paint fumes, cleansers, sawdust, or glues should be identified. Similar information should be obtained in other environments where the child spends long periods, such as a relative's home or school setting.

PHYSICAL EXAMINATION

In patients with **asthma**, *spirometry* should be performed. If **respiratory distress** is observed, *pulse oximetry* should be performed.

The child presenting with a chief complaint of rhinitis or rhinoconjunctivitis should be observed for mouth breathing, paroxysms of sneezing, sniffing/snorting, throat clearing, and rubbing of the nose and eyes (representing pruritus). Infants should be observed during feeding for nasal obstruction severe enough to interfere with feeding or for more obvious signs of aspiration or gastroesophageal reflux. The frequency and nature of coughing that occurs during the interview and any positional change in coughing or wheezing should be noted. Children with asthma should be observed for congested or wet cough, tachypnea at rest, retractions, and audible wheezes, which may worsen with crying. Patients with atopic dermatitis should be monitored for repetitive scratching and the extent of skin involvement.

Because children with severe asthma as well as those receiving chronic or frequent oral corticosteroids may experience growth suppression, an accurate height should be plotted at regular intervals. Long-term follow-up studies suggest that use of inhaled glucocorticoids in prepubertal children is associated with a small initial decrease in attained height (1 cm) that may persist as a reduction in adult height. Poor weight gain in a child with chronic chest symptoms should prompt consideration of cystic fibrosis. Anthropometric measures are also important to monitor in those on restricted diets because of multiple food allergies or eosinophilic esophagitis. Blood pressure should be measured to evaluate for steroid-induced hypertension. The patient with acute asthma may present with **pulsus paradoxus**, defined as a drop in systolic blood pressure during inspiration >10 mm Hg. Moderate to severe airway obstruction is indicated by a decrease of >20 mm Hg. An increased heart rate may be the result of an asthma flare or the use of a β-agonist or decongestant. Fever is not caused by allergy alone and should prompt consideration of an infectious process, which may exacerbate asthma.

Parents are often concerned about blue-gray to purple discolorations beneath their child's lower eyelids, which can be attributed to venous stasis and are referred to as **allergic shiners** (Fig. 167.1). They are found in up to 60% of allergic patients and almost 40% of patients *without* allergic disease. Thus, "shiners" may suggest, but are not diagnostic of, allergic disease. In contrast, the **Dennie-Morgan folds** (Dennie lines) are a feature of atopic dermatitis (Fig. 167.1). These are prominent infraorbital skin folds that extend in an arc from the inner canthus beneath and parallel to the lower lid margin.

In patients with **allergic conjunctivitis**, involvement of the eyes is typically bilateral. Examination of the conjunctiva reveals varying degrees of lacrimation, conjunctival injection, and edema. In severe cases, periorbital edema involving primarily the lower eyelids or **chemosis** (conjunctival edema that is gelatinous in appearance) may be observed. The classic discharge associated with allergic conjunctivitis is usually described as "stringy" or "ropy." In children with vernal conjunctivitis, a more severe, chronic phenotype, examination of the tarsal conjunctiva may reveal cobblestoning. **Keratoconus**, or protrusion of the cornea, may occur in patients with vernal conjunctivitis or periorbital atopic dermatitis as a result of repeated trauma produced by persistent rubbing of the eyes. Children treated with high-dose or chronic corticosteroids are at risk for development of posterior subcapsular cataracts.

The external ear should be examined for eczematous changes in patients with atopic dermatitis, including the postauricular area and base of the earlobe. Because otitis media with effusion is common in children with allergic rhinitis, pneumatic otoscopy should be performed to evaluate for the presence of fluid in the middle ear and to exclude infection.

Examination of the nose in allergic patients may reveal the presence of a nasal crease. Nasal patency should be assessed, and the nose examined for structural abnormalities affecting nasal airflow, such as septal deviation, turbinate hypertrophy, and nasal polyps. Decrease or absence of the sense of smell should raise concern about chronic sinusitis or nasal polyps. Nasal polyps in children should raise concerns of cystic fibrosis. The nasal mucosa in allergic rhinitis is classically described as pale to purple compared with the beefy-red mucosa of patients with nonallergic rhinitis. Allergic nasal secretions are typically thin and clear. Purulent secretions suggest another cause of rhinitis. The frontal and maxillary sinuses should be palpated to identify tenderness to pressure that might be associated with acute sinusitis.

Examination of the lips may reveal cheilitis caused by drying of the lips from continuous mouth breathing or repeated licking of the lips in an attempt to replenish moisture and relieve discomfort (**lip licker's dermatitis**). Tonsillar and adenoidal hypertrophy along with a history of impressive snoring raises the possibility of obstructive sleep apnea. The posterior pharynx should be examined for the presence of postnasal drip and posterior pharyngeal lymphoid hyperplasia ("cobblestoning").

Chest findings in asthmatic children vary significantly and may depend on disease duration, severity, and activity. In a child with well-controlled asthma, the chest should appear entirely normal on examination between asthma exacerbations. Examination of the same child during an acute

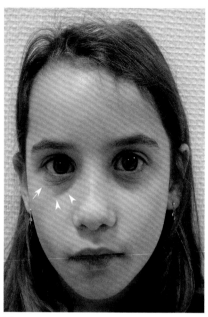

Fig. 167.1 Bilateral Dennie-Morgan folds. Several linear wrinkles beneath the lower eyelashes *(white arrow)* associated with bilateral allergic shiners: dark circles beneath the lower eyelid *(arrowheads)*. *(From Blanc S, Bourrier T, Albertini M, et al: Dennie-Morgan fold plus dark circles: suspect atopy at first sight, J Pediatr 166:1541, 2015.)*

episode of asthma may reveal hyperinflation, tachypnea, use of accessory muscles (retractions), wheezing, and decreased air exchange with a prolonged expiratory time. Tachycardia may be caused by the asthma exacerbation or accompanied by jitteriness after treatment with β-agonists. Decreased airflow or rhonchi and wheezes over the right chest may be noted in children with mucus plugging and right middle lobe atelectasis. The presence of cyanosis indicates severe respiratory compromise. Unilateral wheezing after an episode of coughing and choking in a small child without a history of previous respiratory illness suggests **foreign body aspiration**. Wheezing limited to the larynx in association with inspiratory stridor may be seen in older children and adolescents with **vocal cord dysfunction**. Digital clubbing is rarely seen in patients with uncomplicated asthma and should prompt further evaluation to rule out other potential chronic diagnoses, such as cystic fibrosis.

The skin of the allergic patient should be examined for evidence of urticaria/angioedema or atopic dermatitis. **Xerosis**, or dry skin, is the most common skin abnormality of allergic children. **Keratosis pilaris**, often found on facial cheeks and extensor surfaces of the upper arms and thighs, is a benign condition characterized by skin-colored or slightly pink papules caused by keratin plugs lodged in the openings of hair follicles. Examination of the skin of the palms and soles may reveal thickened skin and exaggerated palmar and plantar creases (**hyperlinearity**) in children with moderate to severe atopic dermatitis.

DIAGNOSTIC TESTING
In Vitro Tests
Allergic diseases are often associated with increased numbers of eosinophils circulating in the peripheral blood and invading the tissues and secretions of target organs. **Eosinophilia**, defined as the presence of >500 eosinophils/μL in peripheral blood, is the most common hematologic abnormality of allergic patients. Seasonal increases in the number of circulating eosinophils may be observed in sensitized patients after exposure to allergens such as tree, grass, and weed pollens. The number of circulating eosinophils can be suppressed by certain infections and systemic corticosteroids. In certain pathologic conditions, such as

drug reactions, eosinophilic pneumonias, and eosinophilic esophagitis, significantly increased numbers of eosinophils may be present in the target organ in the absence of peripheral blood eosinophilia. Increased numbers of eosinophils are observed in a wide variety of disorders in addition to allergy; eosinophil counts >1500 without an identifiable etiology should suggest 1 of the 2 hypereosinophilic syndromes (Table 167.1; see Chapter 155).

Nasal and bronchial secretions may be examined for the presence of eosinophils. The presence of eosinophils in the sputum of asthmatic patients is classic. An increased number of eosinophils in a smear of nasal mucus with Hansel stain is a more sensitive indicator of nasal allergies than peripheral blood eosinophilia and can aid in distinguishing allergic rhinitis from other causes of rhinitis. An elevated IgE value is often found in the serum of allergic patients, because IgE is the primary antibody associated with immediate hypersensitivity reactions. IgE values are measured in international units (IU), with 1 IU equal to 2.4 ng of IgE. Maternal IgE (unlike IgG) does not cross the placenta. Serum IgE levels gradually rise over the first years of life to peak in the teen years and decrease steadily thereafter. Additional factors, such as genetic influences, race, gender, certain diseases, and exposure to cigarette smoke and allergens, also affect serum IgE levels. Total serum IgE levels may increase 2- to 4-fold during and immediately after the pollen season and then gradually decline until the next pollen season. Comparison of total IgE levels among patients with allergic diseases reveals that those with atopic dermatitis tend to have the highest levels, whereas patients with allergic asthma generally have higher levels than those with allergic rhinitis. Although average total IgE levels are higher in populations of allergic patients than in comparable populations without allergic disease, the overlap in levels is such that the diagnostic value of a total IgE level is poor. Approximately half of patients with allergic disease have total IgE levels in the normal range. However, measurement of total IgE is indicated when the diagnosis of **allergic bronchopul-monary aspergillosis** is suspected because total serum IgE concentration >1,000 ng/mL is a criterion for diagnosis of this disorder (see Chapter 264.1). Total serum IgE may also be elevated in several nonallergic diseases (Table 167.2; see Chapter 152).

The presence of IgE specific for a particular allergen can be documented in vivo by skin testing or in vitro by the measurement of **allergen-specific IgE (sIgE)** levels in the serum (Table 167.3). The first test for documenting the presence of sIgE was called the radioallergosorbent test (RAST) because it used a radiolabeled anti-IgE antibody. The RAST has been replaced by an improved generation of automated enzymatic sIgE immunoassays. These assays use solid-phase supports to which allergens of an individual allergen extract are bound. A small amount of the patient's serum is incubated with the allergen-coated support. The allergen-coated support bound to the patient's sIgE is then incubated with enzyme-conjugated antihuman IgE. Incubation of this sIgE–antihuman IgE complex with a fluorescent substrate of the conjugated enzyme results in the generation of fluorescence that is proportional to the amount of sIgE in the serum sample. The amount of sIgE is calculated by interpolation from a standard calibration curve and reported in arbitrary mass units (kilo-IU of allergen-specific antibody per unit volume of sample, kU_A/L). Laboratory reports may specify classes, counts, or units, but quantification of results in kU_A/L is most useful. The 3 commercial detection systems approved by the U.S. Food and Drug Administration have excellent performance characteristics, but the individual systems do not measure sIgE antibodies with comparable efficiencies and thus are not interchangeable. **Component testing** refers to diagnostic tests where sIgE is measured to specific proteins that comprise allergens (e.g., Ara h 2 from peanut, Bet v 1 from birch pollen), rather than to a mixture of the allergens extracted from the source. Testing sIgE to component allergens may add additional diagnostic value by differentiating immune responses that are directed toward clinically relevant allergenic proteins.

Table 167.1	Differential Diagnosis of Childhood Eosinophilia

PHYSIOLOGIC
Prematurity
Infants receiving hyperalimentation
Hereditary

INFECTIOUS
Parasitic (with tissue-invasive helminths, e.g., trichinosis, strongyloidiasis, pneumocystosis, filariasis, cysticercosis, cutaneous and visceral larva migrans, echinococcosis)
Bacterial (brucellosis, tularemia, cat-scratch disease, *Chlamydia*)
Fungal (histoplasmosis, blastomycosis, coccidioidomycosis, allergic bronchopulmonary aspergillosis)
Mycobacterial (tuberculosis, leprosy)
Viral (HIV-1, HTLV-1, hepatitis A, hepatitis B, hepatitis C, Epstein-Barr virus)

PULMONARY
Allergic (rhinitis, asthma)
Eosinophilic granulomatosis with polyangiitis (Churg-Strauss syndrome)
Loeffler syndrome
Hypersensitivity pneumonitis
Eosinophilic pneumonia (chronic, acute)
Pulmonary interstitial eosinophilia

DERMATOLOGIC
Atopic dermatitis
Pemphigus
Dermatitis herpetiformis
Infantile eosinophilic pustular folliculitis
Eosinophilic fasciitis (Schulman syndrome)
Eosinophilic cellulitis (Wells syndrome)
Kimura disease (angiolymphoid hyperplasia with eosinophilia)

HEMATOLOGIC/ONCOLOGIC
Neoplasm (lung, gastrointestinal, uterine)
Leukemia/lymphoma
Myelofibrosis
Myeloproliferative (FIP1L1-PDGFRA–positive) hypereosinophilic syndrome
Lymphatic hypereosinophilic syndrome
Systemic mastocytosis

IMMUNOLOGIC
T-cell immunodeficiencies
Hyper-IgE (Job) syndrome
Wiskott-Aldrich syndrome
Graft-versus-host disease
Drug hypersensitivity
Postirradiation
Postsplenectomy

ENDOCRINE
Addison disease
Hypopituitarism

CARDIOVASCULAR
Loeffler disease (fibroplastic endocarditis)
Congenital heart disease
Hypersensitivity vasculitis
Eosinophilic myocarditis

GASTROINTESTINAL
Benign proctocolitis
Inflammatory bowel disease
Eosinophilic gastrointestinal diseases (EGID)

FIP1L1-PDGFRA, FIP1-like 1–platelet-derived growth factor receptor α.

Table 167.2	Nonallergic Diseases Associated With Increased Serum IgE Concentrations

PARASITIC INFESTATIONS
Ascariasis
Capillariasis
Echinococcosis
Fascioliasis
Filariasis
Hookworm
Onchocerciasis
Malaria
Paragonimiasis
Schistosomiasis
Strongyloidiasis
Trichinosis
Visceral larva migrans

INFECTIONS
Allergic bronchopulmonary aspergillosis
Candidiasis, systemic
Coccidioidomycosis
Cytomegalovirus mononucleosis
HIV type 1 infections
Infectious mononucleosis (Epstein-Barr virus)
Leprosy
Pertussis
Viral respiratory infections

IMMUNODEFICIENCY
Autosomal dominant hyper-IgE syndrome (*STAT3* mutations)
Autosomal recessive hyper-IgE syndrome (*DOCK8, TYK2* mutations)
IgA deficiency, selective
Nezelof syndrome (cellular immunodeficiency with immunoglobulins)
Thymic hypoplasia (DiGeorge anomaly)
Wiskott-Aldrich syndrome

NEOPLASTIC DISEASES
Hodgkin disease
IgE myeloma
Bronchial carcinoma

OTHER DISEASES AND DISORDERS
Alopecia areata
Bone marrow transplantation
Burns
Cystic fibrosis
Dermatitis, chronic acral
Erythema nodosum, streptococcal infection
Guillain-Barré syndrome
Kawasaki disease
Liver disease
Medication related
Nephritis, drug-induced interstitial
Nephrotic syndrome
Pemphigus, bullous
Polyarteritis nodosa, infantile
Primary pulmonary hemosiderosis
Juvenile idiopathic arthritis

Table 167.3	Determination of Allergen-Specific IgE by Skin Testing vs In Vitro Testing

VARIABLE	SKIN TEST*	sIgE ASSAY
Risk of allergic reaction	Yes (especially ID)	No
Relative sensitivity	High	High
Affected by antihistamines	Yes	No
Affected by corticosteroids	Usually not	No
Affected by extensive dermatitis or dermographism	Yes	No
Broad selection of antigens	Fewer	Yes
Immediate results	Yes	No
Expensive	No	Yes
Lability of allergens	Yes	No
Results evident to patient	Yes	No

*Skin testing may be the prick test or intradermal (ID) injection.

In Vivo Tests

Allergen skin testing is the primary in vivo procedure for the diagnosis of allergic disease. Mast cells with sIgE antibodies attached to high-affinity receptors on their surface reside in the skin of allergic patients. The introduction of minute amounts of an allergen into the skin of the sensitized patient results in cross-linking of IgE antibodies on the mast cell surface, thereby triggering local mast cell activation. Once activated, these mast cells release a variety of preformed and newly generated mediators that act on surrounding tissues. **Histamine** is the mediator most responsible for the immediate **wheal and flare reactions** observed in skin testing. Examination of the site of a positive skin test result

reveals a pruritic wheal surrounded by erythema. The time course of these reactions is rapid in onset, reaching a peak within 10-20 min and usually resolving over the next 30 min.

Skin testing is performed using the **prick/puncture technique.** With this technique, a small drop of allergen is applied to the skin surface, and a tiny amount is introduced into the epidermis by lightly pricking or puncturing the outer layer of skin through the drop of extract with a small needle or other device. When the **skin-prick test (SPT)** result is negative but the history suggestive, selective skin testing (for vaccines, venom, drugs, and aeroallergens) using the **intradermal technique** may be performed. This technique involves using a 26-gauge needle to inject 0.01-0.02 mL of an allergen extract diluted 1,000- to 10-fold into the dermis of the arm. Intradermal skin tests are *not recommended for use with food allergens* because of the risk of triggering anaphylaxis. Irritant rather than allergic reactions can occur with intradermal skin testing if higher concentrations of extracts are used. Although skin-prick testing is less sensitive than intradermal skin testing, positive SPT results tend to correlate better with clinical symptoms.

The number of skin tests performed should be individualized, with the allergens suggested by the history. A positive and negative control SPT, using histamine and saline, respectively, is performed with each set of skin tests. A negative control is necessary to assess for **dermatographism**, in which reactions are caused merely by applying pressure to overly sensitive skin. A positive control is necessary to establish the presence of a cutaneous response to histamine. Medications with antihistaminic properties, in addition to adrenergic agents such as ephedrine and epinephrine, suppress skin test responses and should be avoided for appropriate intervals (approximately 5 half-lives) before skin testing. Prolonged courses of systemic corticosteroids may suppress cutaneous reactivity by decreasing the number of tissue mast cells as well as their ability to release mediators.

Whether identified via serologic or skin testing, detection of sIgE denotes a sensitized state (i.e., atopy or a tendency toward development of allergic disease) but is not equivalent to a clinically relevant allergic diagnosis. *Many children with positive tests have no clinical symptoms on exposure to the allergen.* Increasingly strong test results (higher serum sIgE results or larger SPT wheal sizes) generally correlate with increasing likelihood of clinical reactivity (but not severity). Neither serologic testing nor skin testing for allergy is predictive of reaction severity or threshold of reactivity, and these tests will be negative when the allergy is not IgE mediated, such as in food protein–induced enterocolitis syndrome. The limitations of these test modalities underscore the need for a detailed medical history that can guide the selection and interpretation of test results. Large panels of indiscriminately performed screening tests may provide misleading information and are not recommended.

Both serum sIgE tests and SPT are sensitive and have similar diagnostic properties. The benefits of the serologic immunoassays are that performance is not limited by presence of skin disease (i.e., active atopic dermatitis) or medication use (i.e., antihistamines). Advantages of skin testing are that they provide rapid results to the patient/family during the clinic visit, do not require venipuncture, and are less costly.

Under certain circumstances, **provocation testing** is performed to examine the association between allergen exposure and the development of symptoms. The bronchial provocation test most frequently performed clinically is the **methacholine challenge,** which causes potent bronchoconstriction of asthmatic but not of normal airways; it is performed to document the presence and degree of bronchial hyperreactivity in a patient with suspected asthma. After baseline spirometry values are obtained, increasing concentrations of nebulized methacholine are inhaled until a drop occurs in lung function, specifically a 20% decrease in FEV_1 (forced expiratory volume in 1st second of expiration), or the patient is able to tolerate the inhalation of a set concentration of methacholine, typically 25 mg/mL.

Oral **food challenges** are performed to determine whether a specific food causes symptoms or whether a suspected food can be added to the diet. Food challenges are performed when the history and results of skin tests and immunoassays for sIgE fail to clarify the diagnosis of an allergy. These challenges may be performed in an open single-blind, double-blind, or double-blind placebo-controlled manner and involve the ingestion of gradually increasing amounts of the suspected food at set intervals until the patient either experiences a reaction or tolerates a normal portion (i.e., 1 serving size) of the food openly. Although the double-blind placebo-controlled food challenge is currently the gold standard test for diagnosing food allergy, it is typically only performed in research studies due to the time and labor-intensive nature of this method. Because of the potential for significant allergic reactions, oral food challenges should be performed only in an appropriately equipped facility with personnel experienced in the performance of food challenges and the treatment of anaphylaxis, including cardiopulmonary resuscitation.

Upper gastrointestinal **endoscopy** is required to confirm the diagnosis of eosinophilic esophagitis. One or more biopsy specimens from the proximal and distal esophagus must show eosinophil-predominant inflammation. With few exceptions, 15 eosinophils/hpf (high-power field) (peak value) is considered a minimum threshold for the diagnosis.

Bibliography is available at Expert Consult.

Chapter **168**
Allergic Rhinitis
Henry Milgrom and Scott H. Sicherer
第一百六十八章
变应性鼻炎

中文导读

本章主要介绍了变应性鼻炎的定义、病因学及分类、发病机制、临床特征、鉴别诊断、并发症、实验室检测、治疗及展望。具体描述了儿童变应性鼻炎的发病情况及危险因素；主要介绍了基于症状及吸入变应原致敏引起的变应性鼻炎种类；描述了各种炎症细胞及炎症介质在迟发及速发型超敏反应中的作用；变应性鼻炎的临床特征包括症状、体征及病史；变应性鼻炎合并症包括鼻窦炎、哮喘以及造成儿童情绪心理方面的异常；变应性鼻炎的实验室检测主要包括皮肤变应原测试及血清免疫学测试；变应性鼻炎的治疗包括多种不同的用药方案及免疫治疗。

Allergic rhinitis (AR) is a common chronic disease affecting 20–30% of children. AR is an inflammatory disorder of the nasal mucosa marked by nasal congestion, rhinorrhea, and itching, often accompanied by sneezing and conjunctival inflammation. Its recognition as a major chronic respiratory disease of children derives from its high prevalence, detrimental effects on quality of life and school performance, and comorbidities. Children with AR often have related conjunctivitis, sinusitis, otitis media, serous otitis, hypertrophic tonsils and adenoids, and eczema. Childhood AR is associated with a 3-fold increase in risk for asthma at an older age. Over the past 50 yr an upsurge in AR has been observed throughout the world, with some symptom surveys reporting incidence rates approaching 40%. Heritability of allergic conditions attests to genetic factors, but the increase stems from changes in the environment, diet, and the microbiome. The symptoms may appear in infancy; with the diagnosis generally established by the time the child reaches age 6 yr. The prevalence peaks late in childhood.

Risk factors include family history of atopy and serum IgE higher than 100 IU/mL before age 6 yr. Early life exposures and/or their absence have a profound influence on the development of the allergic phenotype. The risk increases in children whose mothers smoke heavily, even before delivery and above all before the infants reach 1 yr, and those with heavy exposure to indoor allergens. A critical period exists early in infancy when the genetically susceptible child is at greatest risk of sensitization. Delivery by cesarean section is associated with AR and atopy in children with a parental history of asthma or allergies. This association may be explained by the lack of exposure to the maternal microbiota through fecal/vaginal flora during delivery.

Children between 2 and 3 yr old who have elevated anticockroach and antimouse IgE are at increased risk of wheezing, AR, and atopic dermatitis. The occurrence of 3 or more episodes of rhinorrhea in the 1st yr of life is associated with AR at age 7 yr. Favorably, the exposure to dogs, cats, and endotoxin early in childhood protects against the development of atopy. Prolonged breastfeeding, not necessarily exclusive, is beneficial. There is also a decreased risk of asthma, AR, and atopic sensitization with early introduction to wheat, rye, oats, barley, fish, and eggs. However, reduced diversity of the intestinal microbiota during infancy is associated with increased risk of allergic disease at school age.

ETIOLOGY AND CLASSIFICATION

Two factors necessary for expression of AR are sensitivity to an allergen and the presence of the allergen in the environment. AR classification as **seasonal** or **perennial** is giving way to the designations **intermittent** and **persistent**. The 2 sets of terms are based on different suppositions, but inhalant allergens are the main cause of all forms of AR irrespective of terminology. AR may also be categorized as **mild-intermittent, moderate-severe intermittent, mild-persistent,** and **moderate-severe persistent** (Fig. 168.1). The symptoms of intermittent AR occur on <4 days per week or for <4 consecutive weeks. In persistent AR, symptoms occur on >4 days per week and/or for >4 consecutive weeks. The symptoms are considered mild when they are not troublesome, the sleep is normal, there is no impairment in daily activities, and there is no incapacity at work or school. Severe symptoms result in sleep disturbance and impairment in daily activities and school performance.

In temperate climates, airborne pollen responsible for exacerbation of intermittent AR appear in distinct phases: trees pollinate in the spring, grasses in the early summer, and weeds in the late summer. In temperate climates, mold spores persist outdoors only in the summer, but in warm climates they persist throughout the year. Symptoms of intermittent AR typically cease with the appearance of frost. Knowledge of the time of symptom occurrence, the regional patterns of pollination and mold sporulation, and the patient's allergen-specific IgE (**sIgE**) is necessary to recognize the cause of intermittent AR. Persistent AR is most often associated with the indoor allergens: house dust mites, animal danders, mice, and cockroaches. Cat and dog allergies are of major importance in the United States. The allergens from saliva and sebaceous secretions may remain airborne for a prolonged time. The ubiquitous major cat allergen, Fel d 1, may be carried on cat owners' clothing into such "cat-free" settings as schools and hospitals.

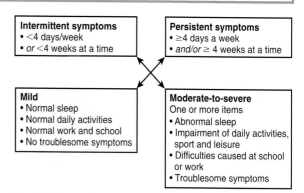

Fig. 168.1 ARIA classification of allergic rhinitis. Every box can be subclassified further into seasonal or perennial on the basis of timing of symptoms or when causative and allergen therapeutic factors are considered. For example, a UK patient with grass pollen allergy might have moderate-severe persistent seasonal rhinitis in June and July and may be suitable for specific allergen immunotherapy. ARIA, Global Allergic Rhinitis and its Impact on Asthma. *(From Scadding GK, Durham SR, Mirakian R, et al: BASCI guidelines for the management of allergic and non-allergic rhinitis, Clin Exp Allergy 38:19–42, 2008.)*

PATHOGENESIS

The exposure of an atopic host to an allergen leads to the production of sIgE, which is strongly associated with eczema throughout childhood and with asthma and rhinitis after age 4 yr. The clinical reactions on reexposure to the allergen have been designated as *early-phase* and *late-phase* allergic responses. Bridging of the IgE molecules on the surface of mast cells by allergen initiates the early-phase allergic response, characterized by degranulation of mast cells and release of preformed and newly generated inflammatory mediators, including histamine, prostaglandin 2, and the cysteinyl leukotrienes. The late-phase allergic response appears 4-8 hr following allergen exposure. Inflammatory cells, including basophils, eosinophils, neutrophils, mast cells, and mononuclear cells, infiltrate the nasal mucosa. Eosinophils release proinflammatory mediators, including cysteinyl leukotrienes, cationic proteins, eosinophil peroxidase, and major basic protein, and serve as a source of interleukin-3 (IL-3), IL-5, granulocyte-macrophage colony-stimulating factor, and IL-13. Repeated intranasal introduction of allergens causes "priming"—a more brisk response even with a lesser provocation. Over the course of an allergy season, a multifold increase in submucosal mast cells takes place. These cells, once thought to have a role exclusively in the early-phase allergic response, have an important function in sustaining chronic allergic disease.

CLINICAL MANIFESTATIONS

Symptoms of AR may be ignored or mistakenly attributed to a respiratory infection. Older children blow their noses, but younger children tend to sniff and snort. Nasal itching brings on grimacing, twitching, and picking of the nose that may result in epistaxis. Children with AR often perform the **allergic salute**, an upward rubbing of the nose with an open palm or extended index finger. This maneuver relieves itching and briefly unblocks the nasal airway. It also gives rise to the **nasal crease**, a horizontal skin fold over the bridge of the nose. The diagnosis of AR is based on symptoms in the absence of an upper respiratory tract infection and structural abnormalities. Typical complaints include intermittent nasal congestion, itching, sneezing, clear rhinorrhea, and conjunctival irritation. Symptoms increase with greater exposure to the responsible allergen. The patients may lose their sense of smell and taste. Some experience headaches, wheezing, and coughing. Preschoolers with chronic wheezing and rhinitis experience more severe wheezing than children without rhinitis. Nasal congestion is often more severe at night, inducing mouth breathing and snoring, interfering with sleep, and rousing irritability.

Signs on physical examination include abnormalities of facial development, dental malocclusion, the **allergic gape** (continuous open-mouth breathing), chapped lips, **allergic shiners** (dark circles under the eyes; see Fig. 167.1), and the transverse nasal crease. Conjunctival edema, itching, tearing, and hyperemia are frequent findings. A nasal exam performed with a source of light and a speculum may reveal clear nasal secretions; edematous, boggy, and bluish mucus membranes with little or no erythema; and swollen turbinates that may block the nasal airway. It may be necessary to use a topical decongestant to perform an adequate examination. Thick, purulent nasal secretions indicate the presence of infection.

DIFFERENTIAL DIAGNOSIS

Evaluation of AR entails a thorough history, including details of the patient's environment and diet and a family history of allergic conditions (e.g., eczema, asthma, AR), physical examination, and laboratory evaluation. The history and laboratory findings provide clues to the provoking factors. Symptoms such as sneezing, rhinorrhea, nasal itching, and congestion and lab findings of elevated IgE, sIgE antibodies, and positive allergy skin test results typify AR. Intermittent AR differs from persistent AR by history and skin test results. **Nonallergic rhinitides** give rise to sporadic symptoms; their causes are often unknown. Nonallergic inflammatory rhinitis with eosinophils imitates AR in presentation and response to treatment, but without elevated IgE antibodies. **Vasomotor rhinitis** is characterized by excessive responsiveness of the nasal mucosa to physical stimuli. Other nonallergic conditions, such as infectious rhinitis, structural problems (e.g., nasal polyps, septal deviation), **rhinitis medicamentosa** (caused by overuse of topical vasoconstrictors), hormonal rhinitis associated with pregnancy or hypothyroidism, neoplasms, vasculitides, and granulomatous disorders may mimic AR (Table 168.1 and Fig. 168.2). Occupational risks for rhinitis include exposure to allergens (grain dust, insects, latex, enzymes) and irritants (wood dust, paint, solvents, smoke, cold air).

COMPLICATIONS

AR is associated with complications and comorbid conditions. Undertreated AR detracts from the quality of life, aggravates asthma, and enhances its progression. Children with AR experience frustration over their appearance. Allergic conjunctivitis, characterized by itching, redness, and swelling of the conjunctivae, has been reported in at least 20% of the population and >70% of patients with AR, most frequently in older children and young adults. The 2 conditions share pathophysiologic mechanisms and epidemiologic characteristics (see Chapter 172). Chronic sinusitis is a common complication of AR, sometimes associated with purulent infection, but most patients have negative bacterial cultures despite marked mucosal thickening, and sinus opacification. The inflammatory process is characterized by marked eosinophilia.

Allergens, possibly fungal, are the inciting agents. The sinusitis of **triad asthma** (asthma, sinusitis with nasal polyposis, and aspirin sensitivity) often responds poorly to therapy. Patients who undergo repeated endoscopic surgery derive diminishing benefit with each successive procedure.

Rhinitis that coexists with asthma may be taken too lightly or completely overlooked. Up to 78% of patients with asthma have AR, and 38% of patients with AR have asthma. Aggravation of AR coincides with exacerbation of asthma, and treatment of nasal inflammation reduces bronchospasm, asthma-related emergency department visits, and hospitalizations. Postnasal drip associated with AR commonly causes persistent or recurrent cough. Eustachian tube obstruction and middle ear effusion are frequent complications. Chronic allergic inflammation causes hypertrophy of adenoids and tonsils that may be associated with eustachian tube obstruction, serous effusion, otitis media, and obstructive sleep apnea. AR is linked to snoring in children. The association between rhinitis and sleep abnormalities and subsequent daytime fatigue is well documented and may require multidisciplinary intervention.

The Pediatric Rhinoconjunctivitis Quality of Life Questionnaire (PRQLQ) is suitable for children 6-12 yr old, and the Adolescent Rhinoconjunctivitis Quality of Life Questionnaire (ARQLQ) is appropriate for patients 12-17 yr. Children with rhinitis have anxiety and physical, social, and emotional issues that affect learning and the ability to integrate with peers. The disorder contributes to headaches and fatigue, limits

Table 168.1	Causes of Rhinitis

ALLERGIC RHINITIS
Seasonal
Perennial
Perennial with seasonal exacerbations

NONALLERGIC RHINITIS
Structural/Mechanical Factors
Deviated septum/septal wall anomalies
Hypertrophic turbinates
Adenoidal hypertrophy
Foreign bodies
Nasal tumors
   Benign
   Malignant
Choanal atresia

Infectious
Acute infections
Chronic infections

Inflammatory/Immunologic
Granulomatosis with polyangiitis
Sarcoidosis
Midline granuloma
Systemic lupus erythematosus
Sjögren syndrome
Nasal polyposis

Physiologic
Ciliary dyskinesia syndrome
Atrophic rhinitis
Hormonally induced
   Hypothyroidism
   Pregnancy
   Oral contraceptives
   Menstrual cycle
   Exercise
   Atrophic
Drug induced
   Rhinitis medicamentosa
   Oral contraceptives
   Antihypertensive therapy
   Aspirin
   Nonsteroidal antiinflammatory drugs
Reflex induced
   Gustatory rhinitis
   Chemical or irritant induced
   Posture reflexes
   Nasal cycle
Environmental factors
   Odors
   Temperature
   Weather/barometric pressure
   Occupational

NONALLERGIC RHINITIS WITH EOSINOPHILIA SYNDROME

PERENNIAL NONALLERGIC RHINITIS (VASOMOTOR RHINITIS)

EMOTIONAL FACTORS

From Skoner DP: Allergic rhinitis: definition, epidemiology, pathophysiology, detection, and diagnosis, *J Allergy Clin Immunol* 108(1 Suppl);108:S2–S8, 2001 (original source).

daily activities, and interferes with sleep. There is evidence of impaired cognitive functioning and learning that may be exacerbated by the adverse effects of sedating medications. AR causes an estimated 824,000 missed school days and 4,230,000 days of decline in quality-of-life activities. Patients with AR report an impairment in the activities of daily living similar to patients with moderate to severe asthma. Some (but not many) patients improve during their teenage years, only to

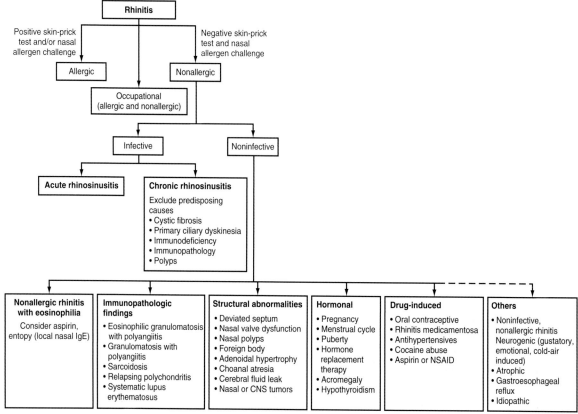

Fig. 168.2 Diagnostic algorithm for rhinitis. Nasal allergen challenge is a research procedure and is not undertaken routinely. CNS, Central nervous system; NSAID, nonsteroidal antiinflammatory drug. (*From Greiner AN, Hellings PW, Rotiroti G, Scadding GK: Allergic rhinitis*, Lancet *378:2112–2120, 2011.*)

develop symptoms again as young adults. Symptoms often abate in the 5th decade of life.

LABORATORY FINDINGS

Epicutaneous skin tests provide the best method for detection of sIgE, with a positive predictive value (PPV) of 48.7% for epidemiologic diagnosis of AR. Skin tests are inexpensive and sensitive, and the risks and discomfort are minimal. Responses to seasonal respiratory allergens are rare before 2 seasons of exposure, and children <1 yr old seldom display positive skin test responses to these allergens. To avoid false-negative results, montelukast should be withheld for 1 day, most sedating antihistamine preparations for 3-4 days, and nonsedating antihistamines for 5-7 days. Serum immunoassays for sIgE provide a suitable alternative (PPV of 43.5%) for patients with dermatographism or extensive dermatitis, those taking medications that interfere with mast cell degranulation, others at high risk for anaphylaxis, and some who cannot cooperate with the procedure. Presence of eosinophils in the nasal smear supports the diagnosis of AR, and neutrophils suggest infectious rhinitis. Eosinophilia and measurements of total serum IgE concentrations have relatively low sensitivity.

TREATMENT

Guideline-directed management has been shown to improve disease control. **Global Allergic Rhinitis and its Impact on Asthma (ARIA)** provides an evidence-based approach to treatment and includes quality-of-life measures useful for the evaluation of symptoms and the assessment of the response to therapy. Safe effective prevention and relief of symptoms are the current goals of treatment. *Specific measures to limit indoor allergen exposure may reduce the risk of sensitization and symptoms of allergic respiratory disease.* Sealing the patient's mattress, pillow, and

covers in allergen-proof encasings reduces the exposure to mite allergen. Bed linen and blankets should be washed every week in hot water (>54.4°C [130°F]). The only effective measure for avoiding animal allergens in the home is the removal of the pet. Avoidance of pollen and outdoor molds can be accomplished by staying in a controlled environment. Air conditioning allows for keeping windows and doors closed, reducing the pollen exposure. High-efficiency particulate air (HEPA) filters lower the counts of airborne mold spores.

Oral antihistamines help reduce sneezing, rhinorrhea, and ocular symptoms. Administered as needed, antihistamines provide acceptable treatment for mild-intermittent disease. Antihistamines have been classified as **first generation** (relatively sedating) or **second generation** (relatively nonsedating). Antihistamines usually are administered by mouth but are also available for topical ophthalmic and intranasal use. Both first- and second-generation antihistamines are available as nonprescription drugs. *Second-generation antihistamines are preferred because they cause less sedation.* Preparations containing **pseudoephedrine**, typically in combination with other agents, are used for relief of nasal and sinus congestion and pressure and other symptoms such as rhinorrhea, sneezing, lacrimation, itching eyes, oronasopharyngeal itching, and cough. Pseudoephedrine is available without prescription (generally in fixed combination with other agents such as first-generation antihistamines: brompheniramine, chlorpheniramine, triprolidine; second-generation antihistamines: desloratadine, fexofenadine, loratadine; antipyretics: acetaminophen, ibuprofen; antitussives: guaifenesin, dextromethorphan; anticholinergic: methscopolamine). Pseudoephedrine is an oral vasoconstrictor distrusted for causing irritability and insomnia and for its association with infant mortality. Because younger children (2-3 yr) are at increased risk of overdosage and toxicity, some manufacturers of oral nonprescription cough and cold preparations have voluntarily revised their product labeling to warn against the use of preparations containing pseudoephedrine for children <4 yr old. Pseudoephedrine is misused as a starting material for the synthesis of methamphetamine and methcathinone. Tables 168.2, 168.3, and 168.4 provide examples of prescription, nonprescription, and combined oral agents, respectively, for treatment of AR.

The anticholinergic **nasal spray** ipratropium bromide is effective for the treatment of *serous* rhinorrhea (Table 168.5). **Intranasal decongestants** (oxymetazoline and phenylephrine) should be used for <5 days and should not to be repeated more than once a month to avoid rebound nasal congestion. Sodium cromoglycate (available as nonprescription drug) is effective but requires frequent administration, every 4 hr. Leukotriene-modifying agents have a modest effect on rhinorrhea and nasal blockage (see Chapter 169 for additional indications and side effects). Nasal saline irrigation is a good adjunctive option with all other treatments of AR. Patients with more persistent, severe symptoms require **intranasal corticosteroids**, the most effective therapy for AR, which may also be beneficial for concomitant allergic conjunctivitis (Table 168.6). These agents reduce the symptoms of AR with eosinophilic inflammation, but not those of rhinitis associated with neutrophils or free of inflammation. Beclomethasone, triamcinolone, and flunisolide are absorbed from the gastrointestinal tract, as well as from the respiratory tract; budesonide, fluticasone, mometasone, and ciclesonide offer greater topical activity with lower systemic exposure. More severely affected patients may benefit from simultaneous treatment with oral antihistamines and intranasal corticosteroids.

Allergen-specific immunotherapy is a well-defined treatment for IgE-mediated allergic disease. It may be administered by subcutaneous or sublingual routes. **Sublingual immunotherapy** (SLIT) has been used successfully in Europe and South America and is now approved by the U.S. Food and Drug Administration. **Allergy immunotherapy** (AIT) is an effective treatment for AR and allergic conjunctivitis. In addition to reducing symptoms, it may change the course of allergic disease and induce allergen-specific immune tolerance. Immunotherapy should be considered for children in whom IgE-mediated allergic symptoms cannot be adequately controlled by avoidance and medication, especially in the presence of comorbid conditions. Immunotherapy for AR prevents the onset of asthma. Moreover, progress in molecular characterization of allergens raises the possibility of defined vaccines for allergen immunotherapy. Omalizumab (anti-IgE antibody) is effective for difficult-to-control asthma and is likely to have a beneficial effect on coexisting AR.

Table 168.2	Oral Allergic Rhinitis Treatments (Prescription, Examples)		
GENERIC/BRAND	**STRENGTH**	**FORMULATIONS**	**DOSING**
SECOND-GENERATION ANTIHISTAMINES			
Desloratadine			Children 6-11 mo of age: 1 mg once daily
Clarinex Reditabs*	2.5 mg, 5 mg	Orally disintegrating tablet	Children 12 mo-5 yr: 1.25 mg once daily
Clarinex Tablets	5 mg	Tabs	Children 6-11 yr: 2.5 mg once daily
Clarinex Syrup	0.5 mg/mL	Syrup	Adults and adolescents ≥12 yr: 5 mg once daily
Levocetirizine dihydrochloride			
Xyzal Oral Solution	0.5 mg/mL	Solution	6 mo-5 yr: max 1.25 mg once daily in the PM
			6-11 yr: max 2.5 mg once daily in the PM
LEUKOTRIENE ANTAGONIST			
Montelukast			6 mo-5 yr: 4 mg daily
Singulair	10 mg	Tablets	6-14 yr: 5 mg daily
Singulair Chewables*	4 mg, 5 mg	Chewable tablets	>14 yr: 10 mg daily
Singulair Oral Granules	4 mg/packet	Oral granules	

*Contains phenylalanine.

Dosing recommendations taken in part from Engorn B, Flerlage J, for the Johns Hopkins Hospital: *The Harriet Lane Handbook*, ed 20, Philadelphia, 2015, Elsevier/Saunders.

Table 168.3	Oral Allergic Rhinitis Treatments (Nonprescription, Examples)		
GENERIC/BRAND	**STRENGTH**	**FORMULATIONS**	**DOSING**
FIRST-GENERATION H$_1$ ANTAGONISTS			
Chlorpheniramine maleate			2-5 yr: 1 mg every 4-6 hr (max 6 mg/day)
Chlor-Trimeton	4 mg	Tablets	6-11 yr: 2 mg every 4-6 hr (max 12 mg/day)
OTC (over the counter)			>12 yr: 4 mg every 4-6 hr (max 24 mg/day)
Chlor-Trimeton Syrup	2 mg/5 mL	Syrup	
OTC			
SECOND-GENERATION H$_1$ ANTAGONISTS			
Cetirizine			6-12 mo: 2.5 mg once daily
Children's Zyrtec Allergy Syrup	1 mg/mL	Syrup	12-23 mo: initial: 2.5 mg once daily; dosage may be
OTC			increased to 2.5 mg twice daily
Children's Zyrtec	5 mg, 10 mg	Chewable tablets	2-5 yr: 2.5 mg/day; may be increased to max of 5 mg/day
Chewable			given either as a single dose or divided into 2 doses
OTC			
Zyrtec tablets	5 mg, 10 mg	Tablets	
OTC			

Continued

Table 168.3	Oral Allergic Rhinitis Treatments (Nonprescription, Examples)—cont'd		
GENERIC/BRAND	**STRENGTH**	**FORMULATIONS**	**DOSING**
Zyrtec Liquid Gels OTC	10 mg	Liquid-filled gels	≥6 yr: 5-10 mg/day as a single dose or divided into 2 doses
Levocetirizine Xyzal	5 mg 0.5 mg/mL	Tablet Oral solution	2-5 yr: 1.25 mg once daily in the evening 6-11 yr: 2.5 mg orally once daily in the evening ≥12 yr: 5 mg orally once daily in the evening
Desloratadine Clarinex	0.5 mg/mL	Oral solution	6-11 mo: 2 mL once daily 12 mo-5 yr: 2.5 mL once daily 6-11 yr: 5 mL once daily
Desloratadine Clarinex	5 mg	Tablet	12-adult: 5 mg once daily
Fexofenadine HCl OTC	30 mg, 60 mg, 180 mg	Tablet	6-11 yr: 30 mg twice daily 12-adult: 60 mg twice daily; 180 mg once daily
Children's Claritin OTC	5 mg/5 mL	Syrup	2-5 yr: 5 mg once daily 6-adult: 10 mg once daily
Children's Allegra OTC ODT*	30 mg	Orally disintegrating tablets	6-11 yr: 30 mg twice daily
Children's Allegra Oral Suspension OTC	30 mg/5 mL	Suspension	>2-11 yr: 30 mg every 12 hr
Allegra OTC Loratadine	Tabs 30, 60, 180 mg	Tablet	>12 yr-adult: 60 mg every 12 hr; 180 mg once daily
Alavert OTC ODT*	10 mg 10 mg 10 mg 5 mg 1 mg/mL	Orally disintegrating tablets Tablets Liquid-filled caps Chewable tablets Syrup	2-5 yr: 5 mg once daily >6 yr: 10 mg once daily or 5 mg twice daily

*Contains phenylalanine.
Dosing recommendations taken in part from Engorn B, Flerlage J, for the Johns Hopkins Hospital: *The Harriet Lane Handbook*, ed 20. Philadelphia, 2015 Elsevier/Saunders.

Table 168.4	Combined Antihistamine + Sympathomimetic (Examples)		
GENERIC	**STRENGTH**	**FORMULATIONS**	**DOSING**
Chlorpheniramine maleate Phenylephrine HCl Sudafed Sinus & Allergy	4 mg 10 mg	Tablets	>12 yr: 1 tablet every 4 hr, not to exceed 6 tablets per day
Cetirizine + pseudoephedrine Zyrtec-D 12 hour	5 mg cetirizine + 120 mg pseudoephedrine	Extended-release tablet	>12 yr: 1 tablet every 12 hr

Dosing recommendations taken in part from Engorn B, MD, Flerlage J for the Johns Hopkins Hospital: *The Harriet Lane Handbook*, ed 20. Philadelphia, 2015 Elsevier/Saunders.

Table 168.5	Miscellaneous Intranasal Sprays	
DRUG	**INDICATIONS (I), MECHANISM(s) OF ACTION (M), AND DOSING**	**COMMENTS, CAUTIONS, ADVERSE EVENTS, AND MONITORING**
Ipratropium bromide: Atrovent nasal spray (0.06%)	I: Symptomatic relief of rhinorrhea M: Anticholinergic Colds (symptomatic relief of rhinorrhea): 5-12 yr: 2 sprays in each nostril tid ≥12 yr and adults: 2 sprays in each nostril tid-qid	Atrovent inhalation aerosol is contraindicated in patients with hypersensitivity to soy lecithin. Safety and efficacy of use beyond 4 days in patients with the common cold have not been established. *Adverse effects:* Epistaxis, nasal dryness, nausea
Azelastine: Astelin	I: Treatment of rhinorrhea, sneezing, and nasal pruritus M: Antagonism of histamine H_1 receptor 6-12 yr: 1 spray bid >12 yr: 1-2 sprays bid	May cause drowsiness *Adverse effects:* Headache, somnolence, bitter taste
Cromolyn sodium: NasalCrom	I: AR. M: Inhibition of mast cell degranulation >2 yr: 1 spray tid-qid; max 6 times daily	Not effective immediately; requires frequent administration

Continued

Table 168.5	Miscellaneous Intranasal Sprays—cont'd

DRUG	INDICATIONS (I), MECHANISM(s) OF ACTION (M), AND DOSING	COMMENTS, CAUTIONS, ADVERSE EVENTS, AND MONITORING
Oxymetazoline: Afrin Nostrilla	*I:* Symptomatic relief of nasal mucosal congestion *M:* Adrenergic agonist, vasoconstricting agent 0.05% solution: instill 2-3 sprays into each nostril bid; therapy should not exceed 3 days.	Excessive dosage may cause profound central nervous system (CNS) depression. Use in excess of 3 days may result in severe rebound nasal congestion. Do not repeat more than once a month. Use with caution in patients with hyperthyroidism, heart disease, hypertension, or diabetes. *Adverse effects:* Hypertension, palpitations, reflex bradycardia, nervousness, dizziness, insomnia, headache, CNS depression, convulsions, hallucinations, nausea, vomiting, mydriasis, elevated intraocular pressure, blurred vision
Phenylephrine: Neo-Synephrine	*I:* Symptomatic relief of nasal mucosal congestion *M:* Adrenergic, vasoconstricting agent 2-6 yr: 1 drop every 2-4 hr of 0.125% solution as needed. *Note:* Therapy should not exceed 3 continuous days. 6-12 yr: 1-2 sprays or 1-2 drops every 4 hr of 0.25% solution as needed. *Note:* Therapy should not exceed 3 continuous days. >12 yr: 1-2 sprays or 1-2 drops every 4 hr of 0.25% to 0.5% solution as needed; 1% solution may be used in adults with extreme nasal congestion. *Note:* Therapy should not exceed 3 continuous days.	Use in excess of 3 days may result in severe rebound nasal congestion. Do not repeat more than once a month. 0.16% and 0.125% solutions are not commercially available. *Adverse effects:* Reflex bradycardia, excitability, headache, anxiety, dizziness

bid, 2 times daily; tid, 3 times daily; qid, 4 times daily.

Table 168.6	Intranasal Inhaled Corticosteroids

DRUG	INDICATIONS (I), MECHANISM(s) OF ACTION (M), AND DOSING	COMMENTS, CAUTIONS, ADVERSE EVENTS, AND MONITORING
Beclomethasone: OTC (over the counter) Beconase AQ (42 µg/spray) Qnasl (80 µg/spray) OTC	*I:* AR *M:* Antiinflammatory, immune modulator 6-12 yr: 1 spray in each nostril bid; may increase if needed to 2 sprays in each nostril bid >12 yr: 1 or 2 sprays in each nostril bid	Shake container before use; blow nose; occlude 1 nostril, administer dose to the other nostril. *Adverse effects:* Burning and irritation of nasal mucosa, epistaxis Monitor growth.
Flunisolide OTC	6-14 yr: 1 spray each nostril tid *or* 2 sprays in each nostril bid; not to exceed 4 sprays/day in each nostril ≥15 yr: 2 sprays each nostril bid (morning and evening); may increase to 2 sprays tid; maximum dose: 8 sprays/day in each nostril (400 µg/day)	Shake container before use; blow nose; occlude 1 nostril, administer dose to the other nostril. *Adverse effects:* Burning and irritation of nasal mucosa, epistaxis Monitor growth.
Triamcinolone Nasacort AQ (55 µg/spray) OTC Fluticasone propionate (available as generic preparation): OTC	*I:* AR *M:* Antiinflammatory, immune modulator 2-6 yr: 1 spray in each nostril qd 6-12 yr: 1-2 sprays in each nostril qd ≥12 yr: 2 sprays in each nostril qd *I:* AR *M:* Antiinflammatory, immune modulator	Shake container before use; blow nose; occlude 1 nostril, administer dose to the other nostril. *Adverse effects:* Burning and irritation of nasal mucosa, epistaxis Monitor growth. Shake container before use; blow nose; occlude 1 nostril, administer dose to the other nostril. Ritonavir significantly increases fluticasone serum concentrations and may result in systemic corticosteroid effects. Use fluticasone with caution in patients receiving ketoconazole or other potent cytochrome P450 3A4 isoenzyme inhibitor. *Adverse effects:* Burning and irritation of nasal mucosa, epistaxis Monitor growth.
Flonase (50 µg/spray) OTC	≥4 yr: 1-2 sprays in each nostril qd	

Continued

Table 168.6	Intranasal Inhaled Corticosteroids—cont'd	
DRUG	**INDICATIONS (I), MECHANISM(s) OF ACTION (M), AND DOSING**	**COMMENTS, CAUTIONS, ADVERSE EVENTS, AND MONITORING**
Fluticasone furoate: Veramyst (27.5 µg/spray)	2-12 yr: Initial dose: 1 spray (27.5 µg/spray) per nostril qd (55 µg/day) Patients who do not show adequate response may use 2 sprays per nostril qd (110 µg/day) Once symptoms are controlled, dosage may be reduced to 55 µg qd Total daily dosage should not exceed 2 sprays in each nostril (110 µg)/day ≥12 yr and adolescents: Initial dose: 2 sprays (27.5 µg/spray) per nostril qd (110 µg/day) Once symptoms are controlled, dosage may be reduced to 1 spray per nostril qd (55 µg/day). Total daily dosage should not exceed 2 sprays in each nostril (110 µg)/day.	
Mometasone: Nasonex (50 µg/spray)	I: AR M: Antiinflammatory, immune modulator 2-12 yr: 1 spray in each nostril qd >12 yr: 2 sprays in each nostril qd	Mometasone and its major metabolites are undetectable in plasma after nasal administration of recommended doses. Preventive treatment of seasonal AR should begin 2-4 wk prior to pollen season. Shake container before use; blow nose; occlude 1 nostril, administer dose to the other nostril. *Adverse effects:* Burning and irritation of nasal mucosa, epistaxis Monitor growth.
Budesonide: OTC Rhinocort Aqua (32 µg/spray) OTC	I: AR M: Antiinflammatory, immune modulator 6-12 yr: 2 sprays in each nostril qd >12 yr: up to 4 sprays in each nostril qd (max dose)	Shake container before use; blow nose; occlude 1 nostril, administer dose to the other nostril. *Adverse effects:* Burning and irritation of nasal mucosa, epistaxis Monitor growth.
Ciclesonide: Omnaris Zetonna (50 µg/spray)	I: AR M: Antiinflammatory, immune modulator 2-12 yr: 1-2 sprays in each nostril qd >12 yr: 2 sprays in each nostril qd	Prior to initial use, gently shake, then prime the pump by actuating 8 times. If the product is not used for 4 consecutive days, gently shake and reprime with 1 spray or until a fine mist appears.
Azelastine/fluticasone (137 µg azelastine/50 µg fluticasone) Dymista	>12 yr: 1 spray in each nostril bid	Shake bottle gently before using. Blow nose to clear nostrils. Keep head tilted downward when spraying. Insert applicator tip ¼ to ½ inch into nostril, keeping bottle upright, and close off the other nostril. Breathe in through nose. While inhaling, press pump to release spray.

qd, Once daily; bid, 2 times daily; tid, 3 times daily.

Typically, treatment of AR with oral antihistamines and nasal corticosteroids provides sufficient relief for most patients with coexisting **allergic conjunctivitis**. If it fails, additional therapies directed primarily at allergic conjunctivitis may be added (see Chapter 172). Intranasal corticosteroids are of some value for the treatment of ocular symptoms, but ophthalmic corticosteroids remain the most potent pharmacologic agents for ocular allergy, although they carry the risk of adverse effects such as delayed wound healing, secondary infection, elevated intraocular pressure, and formation of cataracts. Ophthalmic corticosteroids are only suited for the treatment of allergic conjunctivitis that does not respond to the medications previously discussed. Sound practice calls for the assistance of an ophthalmologist.

PROGNOSIS

Therapy with nonsedating antihistamines and topical corticosteroids, when taken appropriately, improves health-related quality-of-life measures in patients with allergic rhinitis. The reported rates of remission among children are 10–23%. Pharmacotherapy that will target cells and cytokines involved in inflammation and treat allergy as a systemic process is on the horizon, and more selective targeting of drugs based on the development of specific biomarkers and genetic profiling may soon be realized.

Bibliography is available at Expert Consult.

Chapter **169**
Childhood Asthma

Andrew H. Liu, Joseph D. Spahn,
and Scott H. Sicherer

第一百六十九章
儿童哮喘

中文导读

本章主要介绍了儿童哮喘的病因学、流行病学、发病机制、临床表现及诊断、鉴别诊断、实验室检查、治疗、预后和预防。具体描述了遗传学和环境因素；重点阐述了诊断、鉴别诊断、实验室检查；实验室检查具体描述了肺功能测定、呼出气一氧化氮，以及影像学检查的意义。治疗与管理方面具体描述了哮喘的定期评估和监测、患者教育、影响哮喘严重程度的因素以及如何控制；详细阐述了哮喘药物治疗原则、长期控制药物、快速缓解药物、吸入装置和吸入技术、哮喘急性发作及其治疗、哮喘急性发作的家庭管理、急诊处理、医院管理和特殊情况管理，其中特殊情况管理又包括婴幼儿管理和术中哮喘的处理。

Asthma is a chronic inflammatory condition of the lung airways resulting in episodic airflow obstruction. This chronic inflammation heightens the twitchiness of the airways—**airways hyperresponsiveness (AHR)**—to common provocative exposures. Asthma management is aimed at reducing airways inflammation by minimizing proinflammatory environmental exposures, using daily controller antiinflammatory medications, and controlling comorbid conditions that can worsen asthma. Less inflammation typically leads to better asthma control, with fewer exacerbations and decreased need for quick-reliever asthma medications. Nevertheless, exacerbations can still occur. Early intervention with systemic corticosteroids greatly reduces the severity of such episodes. Advances in asthma management and especially pharmacotherapy enable all but the uncommon child with difficult asthma to live normally.

ETIOLOGY

Although the cause of childhood asthma has not been determined, a combination of environmental exposures and inherent biologic and genetic susceptibilities has been implicated (Fig. 169.1). In the susceptible host, immune responses to common airways exposures (e.g., respiratory viruses, allergens, tobacco smoke, air pollutants) can stimulate prolonged, pathogenic inflammation and aberrant repair of injured airways tissues (Fig. 169.2). Lung dysfunction (AHR, reduced airflow) and airway remodeling develop. These pathogenic processes in the growing lung during early life adversely affect airways growth and differentiation, leading to altered airways at mature ages. Once asthma has developed, ongoing inflammatory exposures appear to worsen it, driving disease persistence and increasing the risk of severe exacerbations.

Genetics

To date, more than 100 genetic loci have been linked to asthma, although relatively few have consistently been linked to asthma in different study cohorts. Consistent loci include genetic variants that underlie susceptibility to common exposures such as respiratory viruses and air pollutants.

Environment

Recurrent wheezing episodes in early childhood are associated with common respiratory viruses, especially rhinoviruses, respiratory syncytial virus (RSV), influenza virus, adenovirus, parainfluenza virus, and human metapneumovirus. This association implies that host features affecting immunologic host defense, inflammation, and the extent of airways injury from ubiquitous viral pathogens underlie susceptibility to recurrent wheezing in early childhood. Other airways exposures can also exacerbate ongoing airways inflammation, increase disease severity, and drive asthma persistence. Home allergen exposures in sensitized individuals can initiate airways inflammation and hypersensitivity to other irritant exposures and are causally linked to disease severity, exacerbations, and persistence. Consequently, eliminating the offending allergen(s) can lead to resolution of asthma symptoms and can sometimes cure asthma. Environmental tobacco smoke and common air pollutants can aggravate airways inflammation and increase asthma severity. Cold, dry air, hyperventilation from physical play or exercise, and strong odors can trigger bronchoconstriction. Although many exposures that trigger and aggravate asthma are well recognized, the causal environmental features underlying the development of host susceptibilities to the various common airway exposures are not as well defined. Living in rural or

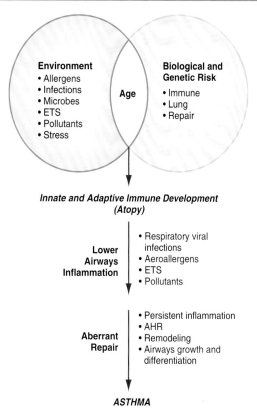

Fig. 169.1 Etiology and pathogenesis of asthma. A combination of environmental and genetic factors in early life shape how the immune system develops and responds to ubiquitous environmental exposures. Respiratory microbes, inhaled allergens, and pollutants that can inflame the lower airways target the disease process to the lungs. Aberrant immune and repair responses to airways injury underlie persistent disease. AHR, Airways hyperresponsiveness; ETS, environmental tobacco smoke.

farming communities may be a protective environmental factor.

EPIDEMIOLOGY

Asthma is a common chronic disease, causing considerable morbidity. In 2011, >10 million children (14% of U.S. children) had ever been diagnosed with asthma, with 70% of this group reporting current asthma. Male gender and living in poverty are demographic risk factors for having childhood asthma in the United States. About 15% of boys vs 13% of girls have had asthma; and 18% of all children living in poor families (income <$25,000/yr), vs 12% of children in families not classified as poor, have had asthma.

Childhood asthma is among the most common causes of childhood emergency department visits, hospitalizations, and missed school days. In the United States in 2006, childhood asthma accounted for 593,000 emergency department (ED) visits, 155,000 hospitalizations, and 167 deaths. A disparity in asthma outcomes links high rates of asthma hospitalization and death with poverty, ethnic minorities, and urban living. In the past 2 decades, black children have had 2-7 times more ED visits, hospitalizations, and deaths as a result of asthma than nonblack children. Although current asthma prevalence is higher in black than in nonblack U.S. children (in 2011, 16.5% vs 8.1% for white and 9.8% for Latino children), prevalence differences cannot fully account for this disparity in asthma outcomes.

Worldwide, childhood asthma appears to be increasing in prevalence, despite considerable improvements in our management and pharmacopeia to treat asthma. Although childhood asthma may have plateaued in the United States after 2008, numerous studies conducted in other countries have reported an increase in asthma prevalence of

approximately 50% per decade. Globally, childhood asthma prevalence varies widely in different locales. A study of childhood asthma prevalence in 233 centers in 97 countries (International Study of Asthma and Allergies in Childhood, Phase 3) found a wide range in the prevalence of current wheeze in 6-7 yr (2.4–37.6%) and 13-14 yr old children (0.8–32.6%). Asthma prevalence correlated well with reported allergic rhinoconjunctivitis and atopic eczema prevalence. Childhood asthma seems more prevalent in modern metropolitan locales and more affluent nations, and is strongly linked with other allergic conditions. In contrast, children living in rural areas of developing countries and farming communities with domestic animals are less likely to experience asthma and allergy.

Approximately 80% of all asthmatic patients report disease onset prior to 6 yr of age. However, of all young children who experience recurrent wheezing, only a minority go on to have persistent asthma in later childhood. Early childhood risk factors for persistent asthma have been identified (Table 169.1) and have been described as major (parent asthma, eczema, inhalant allergen sensitization) and minor (allergic rhinitis, wheezing apart from colds, ≥4% peripheral blood eosinophils, food allergen sensitization) risk factors. *Allergy in young children with recurrent cough and/or wheeze* is the strongest identifiable factor for the persistence of childhood asthma.

Types of Childhood Asthma

There are 2 common types of childhood asthma based on different natural courses: (1) **recurrent wheezing** in *early* childhood, primarily triggered by common respiratory viral infections, usually resolves during the preschool/lower school years; and (2) **chronic asthma** associated with *allergy* that persists into later childhood and often adulthood (Table 169.2). School-age children with mild-moderate persistent asthma generally improve as teenagers, with some (about 40%) developing intermittent disease. Milder disease is more likely to remit. Inhaled corticosteroid controller therapy for children with persistent asthma does not alter the likelihood of outgrowing asthma in later childhood; however, because children with asthma generally improve with age, their need for controller therapy subsequently lessens and often resolves. Reduced growth and progressive decline in lung function can be features of persistent, problematic disease.

Asthma is also classified by **disease severity** (e.g., intermittent or persistent [mild, moderate, or severe]) or **control** (e.g., well, not well, or very poorly controlled), especially for asthma management purposes. Because most children with asthma can be well controlled with conventional management guidelines, children with asthma can also be characterized according to treatment response and medication requirements as being (1) **easy to control**: well controlled with low levels of controller therapy; (2) **difficult to control**: not as well controlled with multiple and/or high levels of controller therapies; (3) **exacerbators**: despite being controlled, continue to have severe exacerbations; and (4) **refractory asthma**: continue to have poorly controlled asthma despite multiple and high levels of controller therapies (Table 169.2). Different airways pathologic processes, causing airways inflammation, AHR, and airways congestion and blockage, are believed to underlie these different types of asthma.

PATHOGENESIS

Airflow obstruction in asthma is the result of numerous pathologic processes. In the small airways, airflow is regulated by smooth muscle encircling the airway lumen; bronchoconstriction of these bronchiolar muscular bands restricts or blocks airflow. A cellular inflammatory infiltrate and exudates distinguished by eosinophils, but also including other inflammatory cell types (neutrophils, monocytes, lymphocytes, mast cells, basophils), can fill and obstruct the airways and induce epithelial damage and desquamation into the airways lumen. Helper T lymphocytes and other immune cells that produce proallergic, proinflammatory cytokines (interleukin [IL]-4, IL-5, IL-13), and chemokines (eotaxins) mediate this inflammatory process (see Fig. 169.2). Pathogenic immune responses and inflammation may also result from a breach in normal immune regulatory processes (e.g., regulatory T lymphocytes that produce IL-10 and transforming growth factor-β) that

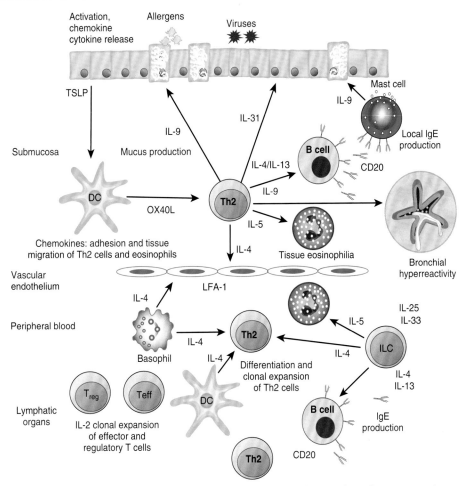

Fig. 169.2 Asthmatic inflammation (effector phase). Epithelial cell activation with production of proinflammatory cytokines and chemokines induces inflammation and contributes to a T-helper cell type 2 (Th2) response with tumor necrosis factor (TNF)-α, interleukin (IL)-13, thymic stromal lymphopoietin (TSLP), IL-25, IL-31, and IL-33. Migration of inflammatory cells to asthmatic tissues is regulated by chemokines. Th2 and eosinophil migration are induced by eotaxin, monocyte-derived chemokine (MDC), and activation-regulated chemokine (TARC). Epithelial apoptosis and shedding is observed, mainly mediated by interferon (IFN)-γ and TNF-α. The adaptive Th2 response includes the production of IL-4, IL-5, IL-9, and IL-13. Innate lymphoid cells, particularly ILC2, also secrete IL-5 and IL-13. Tissue eosinophilia is regulated by IL-5, IL-25, and IL-33. Local and systemic IgE production is observed in bronchial mucosa. Cross-linking of IgE receptor FcεRI on the surface of mast cells and basophils and their degranulation take place on allergen challenge. (*From Leung DYM, Szefler SJ, Bonilla FA, et al, editors: Pediatric allergy principles and practice, ed 3, Philadelphia, 2016, Elsevier, p 260*).

dampen effector immunity and inflammation when they are no longer needed. Hypersensitivity or susceptibility to a variety of provocative exposures or triggers (Table 169.3) can lead to airways inflammation, AHR, edema, basement membrane thickening, subepithelial collagen deposition, smooth muscle and mucous gland hypertrophy, and mucus hypersecretion—all processes that contribute to airflow obstruction.

CLINICAL MANIFESTATIONS AND DIAGNOSIS

Intermittent dry coughing and expiratory wheezing are the most common chronic symptoms of asthma. Older children and adults report associated shortness of breath and chest congestion and tightness; younger children are more likely to report intermittent, nonfocal chest pain. Respiratory symptoms can be worse at night, associated with sleep, especially during prolonged exacerbations triggered by respiratory infections or inhalant allergens. Daytime symptoms, often linked with physical activities (exercise-induced) or play, are reported with greatest frequency in children. Other asthma symptoms in children can be subtle and non-specific, including self-imposed limitation of physical activities, general fatigue (possibly resulting from sleep disturbance), and difficulty keeping up with peers in physical activities. Asking about previous experience

Table 169.1	Early Childhood Risk Factors for Persistent Asthma

Parental asthma*
Allergy:
• Atopic dermatitis (eczema)*
• Allergic rhinitis
• Food allergy
• Inhalant allergen sensitization*
• Food allergen sensitization
Severe lower respiratory tract infection:
• Pneumonia
• Bronchiolitis requiring hospitalization
Wheezing apart from colds
Male gender
Low birthweight
Environmental tobacco smoke exposure
Reduced lung function at birth
Formula feeding rather than breastfeeding

*Major risk factors.

with asthma medications (bronchodilators) may provide a history of symptomatic improvement with treatment that supports the diagnosis of asthma. Lack of improvement with bronchodilator and corticosteroid therapy is inconsistent with underlying asthma and should prompt more vigorous consideration of asthma-masquerading conditions.

Asthma symptoms can be triggered by numerous common events or exposures: physical exertion and hyperventilation (laughing), cold or dry air, and airways irritants (see Table 169.3). Exposures that induce airways

inflammation, such as infections with common respiratory pathogens (rhinovirus, RSV, metapneumovirus, parainfluenza virus, influenza virus, adenovirus, *Mycoplasma pneumoniae, Chlamydia pneumoniae*), and inhaled allergens in sensitized children, also increase AHR to dry, cold air and irritant exposures. An environmental history is essential for optimal asthma management.

The presence of risk factors, such as a history of other allergic conditions (allergic rhinitis, allergic conjunctivitis, atopic dermatitis, food allergies), parental asthma, and/or symptoms apart from colds, supports the diagnosis of asthma. During routine clinic visits, children with asthma typically present without abnormal signs, emphasizing the importance of the medical history in diagnosing asthma. Some may exhibit a dry, persistent cough. The chest findings are often normal. Deeper breaths can sometimes elicit otherwise undetectable wheezing. In clinic, quick resolution (within 10 min) or convincing improvement in symptoms and signs of asthma with administration of an **inhaled short-acting β-agonist** (**SABA**; e.g., albuterol) is supportive of the diagnosis of asthma.

Asthma exacerbations can be classified by their severity based on symptoms, signs, and functional impairment (Table 169.4). Expiratory wheezing and a prolonged exhalation phase can usually be appreciated by auscultation. Decreased breath sounds in some of the lung fields,

---

Table 169.2	Asthma Patterns in Childhood, Based on Natural History and Asthma Management

TRANSIENT NONATOPIC WHEEZING
Common in early preschool years
Recurrent cough/wheeze, primarily triggered by common respiratory viral infections
Usually resolves during the preschool and lower school years, without increased risk for asthma in later life
Reduced airflow at birth, suggestive of relatively narrow airways; AHR near birth; improves by school age

PERSISTENT ATOPY-ASSOCIATED ASTHMA
Begins in early preschool years
Associated with atopy in early preschool years:
• Clinical (e.g., atopic dermatitis in infancy, allergic rhinitis, food allergy)
• Biologic (e.g., early inhalant allergen sensitization, increased serum IgE, increased blood eosinophils)
• Highest risk for persistence into later childhood and adulthood
Lung function abnormalities:
• Those with onset before 3 yr of age acquire reduced airflow by school age.
• Those with later onset of symptoms, or with later onset of allergen sensitization, are less likely to experience airflow limitation in childhood.

ASTHMA WITH DECLINING LUNG FUNCTION
Children with asthma with progressive increase in airflow limitation
Associated with hyperinflation in childhood, male gender

ASTHMA MANAGEMENT TYPES
(From national and international asthma management guidelines)

*Severity Classification**
• Intrinsic disease severity while not taking asthma medications
Intermittent
Persistent:
• Mild
• Moderate
• Severe

*Control Classification**
• Clinical assessment while asthma being managed and treated
Well controlled
Not well controlled
Very poorly controlled

Management Patterns
• **Easy-to-control:** well controlled with low levels of daily controller therapy
• **Difficult-to-control:** well controlled with multiple and/or high levels of controller therapies
• **Exacerbators:** despite being well controlled, continue to have severe exacerbations
• **Refractory:** continue to have poorly controlled asthma despite multiple and high levels of controller therapies

*From National Asthma Education and Prevention Program Expert Panel Report 3 (EPR3): *Guideline for the diagnosis and management of asthma*, NIH Pub No 07-4051, Bethesda, MD, 2007, US Department of Health and Human Services; National Institutes of Health; National Heart, Lung, and Blood Institute; National Asthma Education and Prevention Program. https://www.nhlbi.nih.gov/health-pro/guidelines/current/asthma-guidelines/full-report.
AHR, Airways hyperresponsiveness.

Table 169.3	Asthma Triggers

COMMON VIRAL INFECTIONS OF RESPIRATORY TRACT

AEROALLERGENS IN SENSITIZED ASTHMATIC PATIENTS
Indoor Allergens
• Animal dander
• Dust mites
• Cockroaches
• Molds

Seasonal Aeroallergens
• Pollens (trees, grasses, weeds)
• Seasonal molds

AIR POLLUTANTS
• Environmental tobacco smoke
• Ozone
• Nitrogen dioxide
• Sulfur dioxide
• Particulate matter
• Wood- or coal-burning smoke
• Mycotoxins
• Endotoxin
• Dust

STRONG OR NOXIOUS ODORS OR FUMES
• Perfumes, hairsprays
• Cleaning agents

OCCUPATIONAL EXPOSURES
• Farm and barn exposures
• Formaldehydes, cedar, paint fumes

COLD DRY AIR

EXERCISE

CRYING, LAUGHTER, HYPERVENTILATION

COMORBID CONDITIONS
• Rhinitis
• Sinusitis
• Gastroesophageal reflux

DRUGS
• Aspirin and other nonsteroidal antiinflammatory drugs
• β-Blocking agents

| Table 169.4 | Formal Evaluation of Asthma Exacerbation Severity in the Urgent or Emergency Care Setting* |

	MILD	MODERATE	SEVERE	SUBSET: RESPIRATORY ARREST IMMINENT
SYMPTOMS				
Breathlessness	While walking	While at rest (infant—softer, shorter cry, difficulty feeding)	While at rest (infant— stops feeding)	Extreme dyspnea Anxiety
	Can lie down	Prefers sitting	Sits upright	Upright, leaning forward
Talks in...	Sentences	Phrases	Words	Unable to talk
Alertness	May be agitated	Usually agitated	Usually agitated	Drowsy or confused
SIGNS				
Respiratory rate†	Increased	Increased	Often >30 breaths/min	
Use of accessory muscles; suprasternal retractions	Usually not	Commonly	Usually	Paradoxical thoracoabdominal movement
Wheeze	Moderate; often only end-expiratory	Loud; throughout exhalation	Usually loud; throughout inhalation and exhalation	Absence of wheeze
Pulse rate (beats/min)‡	<100	100-120	>120	Bradycardia
Pulsus paradoxus	Absent <10 mm Hg	May be present 10-25 mm Hg	Often present >25 mm Hg (adult) 20-40 mm Hg (child)	Absence suggests respiratory muscle fatigue
FUNCTIONAL ASSESSMENT				
Peak expiratory flow (value predicted or personal best)	≥70%	Approx. 40–69% or response lasts <2 hr	<40%	<25%§
PaO_2 (breathing air)	Normal (test not usually necessary)	≥60 mm Hg (test not usually necessary)	<60 mm Hg; possible cyanosis	
and/or				
PCO_2	<42 mm Hg (test not usually necessary)	<42 mm Hg (test not usually necessary)	≥42 mm Hg; possible respiratory failure	
SaO_2 (breathing air) at sea level	>95% (test not usually necessary)	90–95% (test not usually necessary)	<90%	Hypoxia despite oxygen therapy
		Hypercapnia (hypoventilation) develops more readily in young children than in adults and adolescents.		

*Notes:
- The presence of several parameters, but not necessarily all, indicates the general classification of the exacerbation.
- Many of these parameters have not been systematically studied, especially as they correlate with each other; thus they serve only as general guides.
- The emotional impact of asthma symptoms on the patient and family is variable but must be recognized and addressed and can affect approaches to treatment and follow-up.

†Normal breathing rates in awake children by age: <2 mo, <60 breaths/min; 2-12 mo, <50 breaths/min; 1-5 yr, <40 breaths/min; 6-8 yr, <30 breaths/min.
‡Normal pulse rates in children by age: 2-12 mo, <160 beats/min; 1-2 yr, <120 beats/min; 2-8 yr, <110 beats/min.
§Peak expiratory flow testing may not be needed in very severe attacks.

Adapted from National Asthma Education and Prevention Program Expert Panel Report 3 (EPR3): *Guideline for the diagnosis and management of asthma*, NIH Pub No 07-4051, Bethesda, MD, 2007, US Department of Health and Human Services; National Institutes of Health; National Heart, Lung, and Blood Institute; National Asthma Education and Prevention Program. https://www.nhlbi.nih.gov/health-pro/guidelines/current/asthma-guidelines/full-report.

commonly the right lower posterior lung field, are consistent with regional hypoventilation caused by airways obstruction. **Rhonchi** and **crackles (or rales)** can sometimes be heard, resulting from excess mucus production and inflammatory exudate in the airways. The combination of segmental crackles and poor breath sounds can indicate lung segmental atelectasis that is difficult to distinguish from bronchial pneumonia and can complicate acute asthma management. In severe exacerbations the greater extent of airways obstruction causes labored breathing and respiratory distress, which manifests as inspiratory and expiratory wheezing, increased prolongation of exhalation, poor air entry, suprasternal and intercostal retractions, nasal flaring, and accessory respiratory muscle use. In extremis, airflow may be so limited that wheezing cannot be heard (**silent chest**).

DIFFERENTIAL DIAGNOSIS

Many childhood respiratory conditions can present with symptoms and signs similar to those of asthma (Table 169.5). Besides asthma, other common causes of chronic, intermittent coughing include gastroesophageal reflux (GER) and rhinosinusitis. Both GER and chronic sinusitis can be challeng spirometric lung function testing to diagnose in children. Often, GER is clinically silent in children, and children with chronic sinusitis do not report sinusitis-specific symptoms, such as localized sinus pressure and tenderness. In addition, both GER and rhinosinusitis are often comorbid with childhood asthma and, if not specifically treated, may make asthma difficult to manage.

In early life, chronic coughing and wheezing can indicate recurrent aspiration, **tracheobronchomalacia** (congenital anatomic abnormality of airways), foreign body aspiration, cystic fibrosis, or bronchopulmonary dysplasia.

In older children and adolescents, **vocal cord dysfunction (VCD)** can manifest as intermittent daytime wheezing. The vocal cords involuntarily close inappropriately during inspiration and sometimes exhalation, producing shortness of breath, coughing, throat tightness, and often audible laryngeal wheezing and/or stridor. In most cases of VCD, spirometric lung function testing reveals truncated and inconsistent inspiratory and expiratory flow-volume loops, a pattern that differs from the reproducible pattern of airflow limitation in asthma that improves with bronchodilators. VCD can coexist with asthma. Hypercarbia and severe hypoxia are uncommon in VCD. Flexible rhinolaryngoscopy in the patient with symptomatic VCD can reveal paradoxical vocal cord movements with anatomically normal vocal cords. Prior to the diagnosis, patients with VCD are often treated unsuccessfully with multiple different classes of asthma medications. This condition can be well managed with specialized speech therapy training in the relaxation and control of vocal cord movement. Furthermore, treatment of underlying causes of vocal cord irritability (e.g., high GER/aspiration, allergic rhinitis, rhinosinusitis, asthma) can improve VCD. During acute VCD exacerbations, relaxation breathing techniques in conjunction with inhalation of heliox (a mixture of 70% helium and 30% oxygen) can relieve vocal cord spasm and VCD symptoms.

Table 169.5	Differential Diagnosis of Childhood Asthma

UPPER RESPIRATORY TRACT CONDITIONS
Allergic rhinitis*
Chronic rhinitis*
Sinusitis*
Adenoidal or tonsillar hypertrophy
Nasal foreign body

MIDDLE RESPIRATORY TRACT CONDITIONS
Laryngotracheobronchomalacia*
Laryngotracheobronchitis (e.g., pertussis)*
Laryngeal web, cyst, or stenosis
Exercise-induced laryngeal obstruction
Vocal cord dysfunction*
Vocal cord paralysis
Tracheoesophageal fistula
Vascular ring, sling, or external mass compressing on the airway (e.g., tumor)
Endobronchial tumor
Foreign body aspiration*
Chronic bronchitis from environmental tobacco smoke exposure*
Repaired tracheoesophageal fistula
Toxic inhalations

LOWER RESPIRATORY TRACT CONDITIONS
Bronchopulmonary dysplasia (chronic lung disease of preterm infants)
Viral bronchiolitis*
Gastroesophageal reflux*
Causes of bronchiectasis:
- Cystic fibrosis
- Immunodeficiency
- Allergic bronchopulmonary mycoses (e.g., aspergillosis)
- Chronic aspiration
Primary ciliary dyskinesia, immotile cilia syndrome
Bronchiolitis obliterans
Interstitial lung diseases
Hypersensitivity pneumonitis
Eosinophilic granulomatosis with angiitis
Eosinophilic pneumonia
Pulmonary hemosiderosis
Tuberculosis
Pneumonia
Pulmonary edema (e.g., congestive heart failure)
Vasculitis
Sarcoidosis
Medications associated with chronic cough:
- Acetylcholinesterase inhibitors
- β-Adrenergic antagonists
- Angiotensin-converting enzyme inhibitors

*More common asthma masqueraders.

In some locales, hypersensitivity pneumonitis (farming communities, homes of bird owners), pulmonary parasitic infestations (rural areas of developing countries), or tuberculosis may be common causes of chronic coughing and/or wheezing. Rare mimics of asthma in childhood are noted in Table 169.5. Chronic pulmonary diseases often produce clubbing, but clubbing is a very unusual finding in childhood asthma.

LABORATORY FINDINGS
Lung function tests can help to confirm the diagnosis of asthma and to determine disease severity.

Pulmonary Function Testing
Forced expiratory airflow measures are helpful in diagnosing and monitoring asthma and in assessing efficacy of therapy. Lung function testing is particularly helpful in children with asthma who are poor perceivers of airflow obstruction, or when physical signs of asthma do not occur until airflow obstruction is severe.

Many asthma guidelines promote spirometric measures of airflow and lung volumes during forced expiratory maneuvers as standard for asthma assessment. **Spirometry** is a helpful objective measure of airflow limitation (Fig. 169.3). Spirometry is an essential assessment tool in children who are at risk for severe asthma exacerbations and those who have poor perception of asthma symptoms. Valid spirometric measures depend on a patient's ability to properly perform a full, forceful, and prolonged expiratory maneuver, usually feasible in children >6 yr old (with some younger exceptions).

In asthma, airways blockage results in reduced airflow with forced exhalation (see Fig. 169.3). Because asthmatic patients typically have hyperinflated lungs, forced expiratory volume in 1 sec (FEV_1) can be simply adjusted for full expiratory lung volume—the forced vital capacity (FVC)—with an FEV_1/FVC ratio. Generally, an FEV_1/FVC ratio <0.80 indicates airflow obstruction (Table 169.6). Normative values for FEV_1 have been determined for children by height, gender, and ethnicity. Abnormally low FEV_1 as a percentage of predicted norms is 1 of 6 criteria used to determine asthma severity and control in asthma management guidelines sponsored by the U.S. National Institutes of Health (NIH) and the **Global Initiative for Asthma (GINA)**.

Such measures of airflow alone are not diagnostic of asthma, because numerous other conditions can cause airflow limitation. In addition, approximately 50% of children with mild-moderate persistent asthma will have normal spirometric values when well. **Bronchodilator response** to an inhaled β-agonist (e.g., albuterol) is greater in asthmatic patients than nonasthmatic persons; an improvement in FEV_1 ≥12% is consistent with asthma. **Bronchoprovocation challenges** can be helpful in diagnosing asthma and optimizing asthma management. Asthmatic airways are hyperresponsive and therefore more sensitive to inhaled methacholine, mannitol, and cold or dry air. The degree of AHR to these exposures correlates to some extent with asthma severity and airways inflammation. Although bronchoprovocation challenges are carefully dosed and monitored in an investigational setting, their use is rarely practical in general practice. **Exercise challenges** (aerobic exertion or "running" for 6-8 min) can help to identify children with exercise-induced bronchospasm. Although the airflow response of nonasthmatic persons to exercise is to increase functional lung volumes and improve FEV_1 slightly (5–10%), exercise often provokes airflow obstruction in persons with inadequately treated asthma. Accordingly, in asthmatic patients, FEV_1 typically decreases during or after exercise by >15% (see Table 169.6). The onset of exercise-induced bronchospasm usually begins within 5 min, reaching a peak at 15 min following vigorous exercise, and often spontaneously resolves within 30-60 min. Studies of exercise challenges in school-age children typically identify an additional 5–10% with exercise-induced bronchospasm and previously unrecognized asthma. There are 2 caveats regarding exercise challenges: (1) treadmill challenges in the clinic are not completely reliable and can miss exertional asthma that can be demonstrated on the playing field; and (2) exercise challenges can induce severe exacerbations in at-risk patients. Careful patient selection for exercise challenges and preparedness for severe asthma exacerbations are required.

Peak expiratory flow (PEF) monitoring devices provide simple and inexpensive home-use tools to measure airflow and can be helpful in a number of circumstances (Fig. 169.4). Similar to spirometry in clinics, poor perceivers of asthma may benefit by monitoring PEFs at home to assess their airflow as an indicator of asthma control or problems. PEF devices vary in the ability to detect airflow obstruction; they are less sensitive and reliable than spirometry to detect airflow obstruction, such that, in some patients, PEF values decline only when airflow obstruction is severe. Therefore, PEF monitoring should be started by measuring morning and evening PEFs (best of 3 attempts) for several

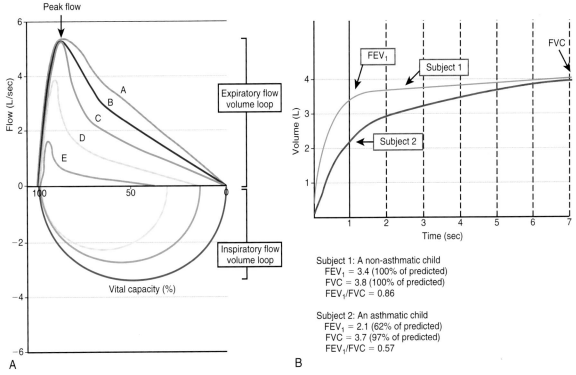

Fig. 169.3 Spirometry. **A,** Spirometric flow-volume loops. Loop A is an expiratory flow-volume loop of a nonasthmatic person without airflow limitation. B through E are expiratory flow-volume loops in asthmatic patients with increasing degrees of airflow limitation (B is mild; E is severe). Note the "scooped" or concave appearance of the asthmatic expiratory flow-volume loops; with increasing obstruction, there is greater "scooping." **B,** Spirometric volume-time curves. Subject 1 is a nonasthmatic person; subject 2 is an asthmatic patient. Note how the FEV_1 and FVC lung volumes are obtained. The FEV_1 is the volume of air exhaled in the 1st sec of a forced expiratory effort. The FVC is the total volume of air exhaled during a forced expiratory effort, or forced vital capacity. Note that subject 2's FEV_1 and FEV_1:FVC ratio are smaller than subject 1's, demonstrating airflow limitation. Also, subject 2's FVC is very close to what is expected.

weeks for patients to practice the technique, to determine diurnal variation and a "personal best," and to correlate PEF values with symptoms (and ideally spirometry). Diurnal variation in PEF >20% is consistent with asthma (see Fig. 169.4 and Table 169.6).

Exhaled Nitric Oxide (FeNO)

Exhaled nitric oxide is a noninvasive measure of allergic airways inflammation used in clinical settings. Nitric oxide (NO) is a marker of allergic/eosinophilic inflammation that is easily and quickly measured in exhaled breath. Children as young as 5 yr can perform this test. FeNO can be used to distinguish asthma from other airways diseases that are mediated by nonallergic/noneosinophilic inflammation, such as GER, VCD, and cystic fibrosis. FeNO can substantiate the diagnosis of asthma, complement the assessment of asthma control, predict response to inhaled corticosteroid (ICS) therapy, assess adherence with ICS therapy, predict loss of control with ICS tapering, and predict future asthma exacerbations.

Radiology

The findings of chest radiographs (posteroanterior and lateral views) in children with asthma often appear to be normal, aside from subtle and nonspecific findings of hyperinflation (e.g., flattening of the diaphragms) and peribronchial thickening (Fig. 169.5). Chest radiographs can help identify abnormalities that are hallmarks of asthma mimics (aspiration pneumonitis, hyperlucent lung fields in bronchiolitis obliterans) and complications during asthma exacerbations (atelectasis, pneumomediastinum, pneumothorax). Some lung abnormalities can be better appreciated with high-resolution, thin-section chest CT scans. **Bronchiectasis,** which is sometimes difficult to appreciate on chest

Table 169.6	Lung Function Abnormalities in Asthma and Assessment of Airway Inflammation

Spirometry (in clinic)[‡†]:
  Airflow limitation:
  • Low FEV_1 (relative to percentage of predicted norms)
  • FEV_1/FVC ratio <0.80
Bronchodilator response (to inhaled β-agonist) assesses *reversibility* of airflow limitation.
  Reversibility is determined by an increase in either FEV_1 >12% or predicted FEV_1 >10% after inhalation of a short-acting β-agonist (SABA)*
Exercise challenge:
  • Worsening in FEV_1 ≥15%*
Daily peak expiratory flow (PEF)[‡] or FEV_1 monitoring: day-to-day and/or AM-to-PM variation ≥20%*
Exhaled nitric oxide (FeNO)
  • A value of >20 ppb supports the clinical diagnosis of asthma in children
  • FeNO can be used to predict response to ICS therapy:
    • <20 ppb: Unlikely to respond to ICS because eosinophilic inflammation unlikely
    • 20-35 ppb: Intermediate, may respond to ICS
    • >35 ppb: Likely to respond to ICS because eosinophilic inflammation is likely

*Main criteria consistent with asthma.
[†]Of note, >50%of children with mild to moderate asthma will have a normal FEV_1 and will not have a significant bronchodilator response.
[‡]PEF variability is insensitive, while being highly specific for asthma.
FEV_1, forced expiratory volume in 1 sec; FVC, forced vital capacity; ICS, inhaled corticosteroid; ppb, parts per billion.

radiograph but is clearly seen on CT scan, implicates an asthma mimic such as cystic fibrosis, allergic bronchopulmonary mycoses (aspergillosis), ciliary dyskinesias, or immune deficiencies.

Other tests, such as allergy testing to assess sensitization to inhalant allergens, help with the management and prognosis of asthma. In a comprehensive U.S. study of 5-12 yr old asthmatic children, the **Childhood Asthma Management Program (CAMP)**, 88% of patients had inhalant allergen sensitization according to results of allergy skin-prick testing.

TREATMENT

The NIH-sponsored **National Asthma Education and Prevention Program's Expert Panel Report 3 (EPR3)**, *Guidelines for the Diagnosis and Management of Asthma 2007,* is available online.* Similar guidelines from GINA, *Global Strategy for Asthma Management and Prevention, 2016,* are also available (www.ginasthma.org). The key components to optimal asthma management are specified (Fig. 169.6). Management of asthma should have the following components: (1) assessment and monitoring of disease activity; (2) education to enhance patient and family knowledge and skills for self-management; (3) identification and management of precipitating factors and comorbid conditions that worsen asthma; and (4) appropriate selection of medications to address the patient's needs. The long-term goal of asthma management is attainment of optimal asthma control.

Component 1: Regular Assessment and Monitoring

Regular assessment and monitoring are based on the concepts of asthma severity, asthma control, and responsiveness to therapy. **Asthma severity** is the intrinsic intensity of disease, and assessment is generally most accurate in patients not receiving controller therapy. Therefore, assessing asthma severity directs the initial level of therapy. The 2 general categories are **intermittent** asthma and **persistent** asthma, the latter being further subdivided into **mild, moderate,** and **severe.** In contrast, **asthma control** is dynamic and refers to the day-to-day variability of an asthmatic patient. In children receiving controller therapy, assessment of asthma control is important in adjusting therapy and is categorized in 3 levels: well controlled, not well controlled, and very poorly controlled. **Responsiveness to therapy** is the ease or difficulty with which asthma control is attained by treatment.

Classification of asthma severity and control is based on the domains of **impairment** and **risk**. These domains do not necessarily correlate with each other and may respond differently to treatment. Childhood asthma is characterized by minimal day-to-day impairment, with the potential for frequent, severe exacerbations most often triggered by viral infections, whereas adults with asthma have greater impairment with less potential for risk. The NIH guidelines have distinct criteria for 3 childhood age groups—0-4 yr, 5-11 yr, and ≥12 yr—for the evaluation of both severity (Table 169.7) and control (Table 169.8). The level of asthma severity or control is based on the most severe impairment or risk category. In assessing asthma severity, **impairment** consists of an assessment of the patient's recent symptom frequency (daytime and nighttime, with subtle differences in numeric cutoffs between the 3 age-groups), SABA use for quick relief, ability to engage in normal or desired activities, and airflow compromise evaluated by spirometry in children ≥5 yr. **Risk** refers to the likelihood of developing severe asthma exacerbations. Of note, even in the absence of frequent symptoms, persistent asthma can be diagnosed and long-term controller therapy initiated. For children ≥5 yr, 2 exacerbations requiring oral corticosteroids in 1 yr, and for infants and preschool-aged children who have risk factors for asthma (see earlier) and 4 or more episodes of wheezing over the past year that lasted longer than 1 day and affected sleep, or 2 or more exacerbations in 6 mo requiring systemic corticosteroids, qualifies them as having persistent asthma.

Asthma management can be optimized through regular clinic visits every 2-6 wk until good asthma control is achieved. For children on controller medication therapy, management is tailored to the child's level of control. The NIH guidelines provide tables for evaluating asthma control for the 3 age-groups (see Table 169.8). In evaluation of asthma control, as in severity assessment, impairment includes an assessment of the patient's symptom frequency (daytime and nighttime), SABA use for quick relief, ability to engage in normal or desired activities, and for older children, airflow measurements. Validated asthma control questionnaires such as the **Asthma Control Test** (ACT, for adults and children ≥12 yr) and the Childhood ACT (C-ACT, for children 4-11 yr) can also be used to assess level of control. An ACT score of ≥20 indicates a child with **well-controlled** asthma, a value of 16-19 indicates **not well-controlled** asthma, and ≤15 indicates **very poorly controlled** asthma. For the C-ACT, a score ≥20 indicates *well controlled,* 13-19 indicates *not well controlled;* and ≤12 indicates *very poorly controlled.*

Assessment of risk, in addition to considering severity and frequency of exacerbations requiring systemic corticosteroids, includes tracking the lung growth of older children, in an attempt to identify those with reduced and/or progressive loss of lung function, and monitoring adverse effects of medications. The degree of impairment and presence of risk are used to determine the patient's level of asthma control as well controlled, not well controlled, or very poorly controlled. Children with

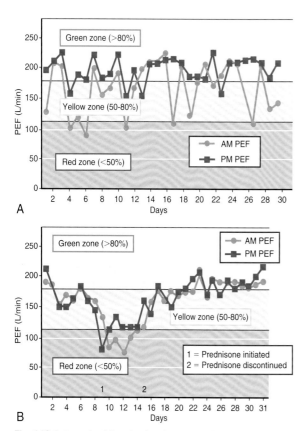

Fig. 169.4 Example of the role of peak expiratory flow (PEF) monitoring in childhood asthma. **A,** PEFs performed and recorded twice daily, in the morning (AM) and evening (PM), over 1 mo in an asthmatic child. This child's "personal best" PEF value is 220 L/min; therefore the *green* zone (>80–100% of best) is 175-220 L/min; the *yellow* zone (50–80%) is 110-175 L/min; and the *red* zone (<50%) is <110 L/min. Note that this child's PM PEF values are almost always in the *green* zone, whereas his AM PEFs are often in the *yellow* or *red* zone. This pattern illustrates the typical diurnal AM-to-PM variation of inadequately controlled asthma. **B,** PEFs performed twice daily, in the morning (AM) and evening (PM), over 1 mo in an asthmatic child in whom an asthma exacerbation developed from a viral respiratory tract infection. Note that the child's PEF values were initially in the *green* zone. A viral respiratory tract infection led to asthma worsening, with a decline in PEF to the *yellow* zone that continued to worsen until PEF values were in the *red* zone. At that point, a 4-day prednisone course was administered, followed by improvement in PEF back to the *green* zone.

*https://www.nhlbi.nih.gov/health-pro/guidelines/current/asthma-guidelines/full-report.

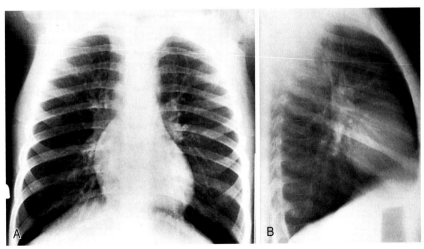

Fig. 169.5 A 4-year-old boy with asthma. Frontal (**A**) and lateral (**B**) radiographs show pulmonary hyperinflation, flattening of the diaphragms, and minimal peribronchial thickening. No asthmatic complication is apparent.

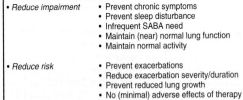

Recurrent/chronic cough, wheeze, chest tightness and/or shortness of breath

Diagnosis
- Symptoms
- Exacerbations
- Risk factors (Tables 169.1, 169.2)
- Triggers (Table 169.3)
- Lung function (Figs. 169.2, 169.3; Table 169.6)
- Differential diagnosis (Table 169.5)

Asthma

Management

- *Assessment and monitoring*
  - Assess severity (Tables 169.4, 169.7)
  - Monitor control (Table 169.8)
  - Med adverse effects (Table 169.14)

- *Education*
  - Key elements (Table 169.9)

- *Contol environmental factors and co-morbid conditions*
  - Environmental controls (Table 169.10)
  - Co-morbidities (Table 169.10)

- *Medications*
  - Long-term controllers (Tables 169.11 to 169.13)
  - Quick relievers (Table 169.11)

- *Exacerbations*
  - Assessment (Table 169.4)
  - Management (Table 169.15)
  - High-risk features (Table 169.16)
  - Home asthma action plan

Optimal goal: Well controlled asthma

- *Reduce impairment*
  - Prevent chronic symptoms
  - Prevent sleep disturbance
  - Infrequent SABA need
  - Maintain (near) normal lung function
  - Maintain normal activity

- *Reduce risk*
  - Prevent exacerbations
  - Reduce exacerbation severity/duration
  - Prevent reduced lung growth
  - No (minimal) adverse effects of therapy

Fig. 169.6 The key elements to optimal asthma management. SABA, Short-acting β-agonist.

well-controlled asthma have daytime symptoms ≤2 days/wk and need a rescue bronchodilator ≤2 days/wk; an FEV_1 of >80% of predicted (and FEV_1/FVC ratio >80% for children 5-11 yr); no interference with normal activity; and <2 exacerbations in the past year and an ACT score of ≥20. The impairment criteria vary slightly depending on age-group. Children whose status does not meet all the criteria of well-controlled asthma are determined to have either *not well-controlled* or *very poorly controlled* asthma, which is determined by the single criterion with the poorest rating.

Two to four asthma checkups per year are recommended for reassessing and maintaining good asthma control. Lung function testing (spirometry) is recommended at least annually and more often if asthma is poorly perceived, is inadequately controlled, and/or lung function is abnormally low. PEF monitoring at home can be helpful in the assessment of asthmatic children with poor symptom perception, moderate to severe asthma, or a history of severe asthma exacerbations. PEF monitoring is feasible in children as young as 4 yr who are able to master this skill. Use of a **stoplight zone system** tailored to each child's "personal best" PEF values can optimize effectiveness and interest (see Fig. 169.4): The green zone (80–100% of personal best) indicates good control; the yellow zone (50–80%) indicates less-than-optimal control and necessitates increased awareness and treatment; and the red zone (<50%) indicates poor control and greater likelihood of an exacerbation, requiring immediate intervention. In actuality, these ranges are approximate and may need to be adjusted for many asthmatic children by raising the ranges that indicate inadequate control (e.g., yellow zone, 70–90% in children with poor perception and those with lung hyperinflation). Once-daily PEF monitoring is preferable in the morning when peak flows are typically lower. Adherence to PEF monitoring is difficult, results may be variable and PEF monitoring alone is not more effective than symptoms monitoring on influencing asthma outcomes. Therefore, although PEF may be helpful in some circumstances to monitor those who are poor perceivers of airway obstruction, PEF monitoring is no longer generally recommended.

Component 2: Patient Education

Specific educational elements in the clinical care of children with asthma are believed to make an important difference in home management and in adherence of families to an optimal plan of care, eventually impacting patient outcomes (Table 169.9). Every visit presents an important opportunity to educate the child and family, allowing them to become knowledgeable partners in asthma management, because optimal management depends on their daily assessments and implementation of any management plan. Effective communications take into account sociocultural and ethnic factors of children and their families, provide an open forum for concerns about asthma and its treatment to be raised and addressed, and include patients and families as active participants in the development of treatment goals and selection of medications. Self-management skills should be reevaluated regularly (e.g., inhaler medication technique).

During initial patient visits, a basic understanding of the pathogenesis of asthma (chronic inflammation and AHR underlying a clinically intermittent presentation) can help children with asthma and their parents understand the importance of recommendations aimed at

Table 169.7	Assessing Asthma Severity and Initiating Treatment for Patients Who Are Not Currently Taking Long-Term Control Medications*

		CLASSIFICATION OF ASTHMA SEVERITY		
			PERSISTENT	
	INTERMITTENT	Mild	Moderate	Severe
COMPONENTS OF SEVERITY				
Impairment				
Daytime symptoms	≤2 days/wk	>2 days/wk but not daily	Daily	Throughout the day
Nighttime awakenings:				
Age 0-4 yr	0	1-2×/mo	3-4×/mo	>1×/wk
Age ≥5 yr	≤2×/mo	3-4×/mo	>1×/wk but not nightly	Often 7×/wk
Short-acting β₂-agonist use for symptoms (not for EIB prevention)	≤2 days/wk	>2 days/wk but not daily, and not more than 1× on any day	Daily	Several times per day
Interference with normal activity	None	Minor limitation	Some limitation	Extreme limitation
Lung function:				
FEV₁ % predicted, age ≥5 yr	Normal FEV₁ between exacerbations >80% predicted	≥80% predicted	60–80% predicted	<60% predicted
FEV₁/FVC ratio†:				
Age 5-11 yr	>85%	>80%	75-80%	<75%
Age ≥12 yr	Normal	Normal	Reduced 5%	Reduced >5%
Risk				
Exacerbations requiring systemic corticosteroids:				
Age 0-4 yr	0-1/yr (see notes)	≥2 exacerbations in 6 mo requiring systemic CS *or* ≥4 wheezing episodes/yr lasting >1 day *and* risk factors for persistent asthma		
Age ≥ 5 yr	0-1/yr (see notes)	≥2/yr (see notes)	≥2/yr (see notes)	≥2/yr (see notes)

Consider severity and interval since last exacerbation.
Frequency and severity may fluctuate over time for patients in any severity category.
Relative annual risk of exacerbations may be related to FEV₁.

RECOMMENDED STEP FOR INITIATING THERAPY
(See Table 169.11 for treatment steps.)
The stepwise approach is meant to assist, not replace, the clinical decision-making required to meet individual patient needs.

All ages	Step 1	Step 2		
Age 0-4 yr			Step 3 and consider a short course of systemic CS	Step 3 and consider a short course of systemic CS
Age 5-11 yr			Step 3: medium-dose ICS option and consider a short course of systemic CS	Step 3: medium-dose ICS option *or* Step 4 and consider a short course of CS

In 2-6 wk, depending on severity, evaluate level of asthma control that is achieved.
- Children 0-4 yr old: If no clear benefit is observed in 4-6 wk, stop treatment and consider alternative diagnoses or adjusting therapy accordingly.
- Children 5-11 yr old: Adjust therapy accordingly.

*Notes:
- Level of severity is determined by both impairment and risk. Assess impairment domain by patient's/caregiver's recall of previous 2-4 wk. Symptom assessment for longer periods should reflect a global assessment, such as inquiring whether a patient's asthma is better or worse since the last visit. Assign severity to the most severe category in which any feature occurs.
- At present, there are inadequate data to correspond frequencies of exacerbations with different levels of asthma severity. For treatment purposes, patients who had ≥2 exacerbations requiring oral systemic corticosteroids in the past 6 mo, or ≥4 wheezing episodes in the past year, and who have risk factors for persistent asthma, may be considered the same as patients who have persistent asthma, even in the absence of impairment levels consistent with persistent asthma.
†Normal FEV₁/FVC: 8-19 yr, 85%; 20-39 yr, 80%.

FEV₁, Forced expiratory volume in 1 sec; FVC, forced vital capacity; CS corticosteroid; ICS, inhaled corticosteroid: EIB, exercise-induced bronchospasm.

Adapted from the National Asthma Education and Prevention Program Expert Panel Report 3 (EPR3): Guidelines for the diagnosis and management of asthma—summary report 2007, *J Allergy Clin Immunol* 120(Suppl):S94–S138, 2007.

reducing airways inflammation to achieve and maintain good asthma control. It is helpful to specify the expectations of good asthma control resulting from optimal asthma management (see Fig. 169.6). Addressing concerns about potential adverse effects of asthma pharmacotherapeutic agents, especially their risks relative to their benefits, is essential in achieving long-term adherence with asthma pharmacotherapy and environmental control measures.

All children with asthma should benefit from a written Asthma Action Plan (Fig. 169.7). This plan has two main components: (1) a daily "routine" management plan describing regular asthma medication use and other measures to keep asthma under good control; and (2) an action plan

to manage worsening asthma, describing indicators of impending exacerbations, identifying what medications to take, and specifying when and how to contact the regular physician and/or obtain urgent/emergency medical care.

Regular follow-up visits are recommended to help to maintain optimal asthma control. In addition to determining disease control level, revising PEF values daily and exacerbation management plans accordingly, follow-up visits are important teaching opportunities to encourage open communication of concerns with asthma management recommendations (e.g., daily administration of controller medications). Reassessing patients' and parents' understanding of the role of different medications in asthma

| Table 169.8 | Assessing Asthma Control and Adjusting Therapy in Children* |

CLASSIFICATION OF ASTHMA CONTROL

	Well-Controlled	Not Well-Controlled	Very Poorly Controlled
COMPONENTS OF CONTROL			
Impairment			
Symptoms	≤2 days/wk but not more than once on each day	>2 days/wk or multiple times on ≤2 days/wk	Throughout the day
Nighttime awakenings:			
Age 0-4 yr	≤1×/mo	>1×/mo	>1×/wk
Age 5-11 yr	≤1×/mo	≥2×/mo	≥2×/wk
Age ≥12 yr	≤2×/mo	1-3×/wk	≥4×/wk
Short-acting β_2-agonist use for symptoms (not for EIB pretreatment)	≤2 days/wk	>2 days/wk	Several times per day
Interference with normal activity	None	Some limitation	Extremely limited
Lung function:			
Age 5-11 yr:			
FEV_1 (% predicted or peak flow)	>80% predicted or personal best	60-80% predicted or personal best	<60% predicted or personal best
FEV_1/FVC:	>80%	75-80%	<75%
Age ≥12 yr:			
FEV_1 (% predicted or peak flow)	>80% predicted or personal best	60-80% predicted or personal best	<60% predicted or personal best
Validated questionnaires[†]:			
Age ≥12 yr:			
ATAQ	0	1-2	3-4
ACQ	≤0.75	≤1.5	N/A
ACT	≥20	16-19	≤15
Risk			
Exacerbations requiring systemic corticosteroids:			
Age 0-4 yr	0-1/yr	2-3/yr	>3/yr
Age ≥5 yr	0-1/yr	≥2/yr (see notes)	
Consider severity and interval since last exacerbation.			
Treatment-related adverse effects	Medication side effects can vary in intensity from none to very troublesome and worrisome. The level of intensity does not correlate to specific levels of control but should be considered in the overall assessment of risk.		
Reduction in lung growth *or* progressive loss of lung function	Evaluation requires long-term follow-up care.		
RECOMMENDED ACTION FOR TREATMENT			
	Maintain current step. Regular follow-up every 1-6 mo to maintain control. Consider step down if well controlled for at least 3 mo.	Step up[‡] (1 step) and reevaluate in 2-6 wk. If no clear benefit in 4-6 wk, consider alternative diagnoses or adjusting therapy. For side effects, consider alternative options.	Consider short course of oral corticosteroids. Step up[§] (1-2 steps) and reevaluate in 2 wk. If no clear benefit in 4-6 wk, consider alternative diagnoses or adjusting therapy. For side effects, consider alternative options.

*Notes:
- The stepwise approach is meant to assist, not replace, the clinical decision making required to meet individual patient needs.
- The level of control is based on the most severe impairment or risk category. Assess impairment domain by caregiver's recall of previous 2-4 wk. Symptom assessment for longer periods should reflect a global assessment, such as inquiring whether the patient's asthma is better or worse since the last visit.
- At present, there are inadequate data to correspond frequencies of exacerbations with different levels of asthma control. In general, more frequent and intense exacerbations (e.g., requiring urgent, unscheduled care, hospitalization, or intensive care unit admission) indicate poorer disease control. For treatment purposes, patients who had ≥2 exacerbations requiring oral systemic corticosteroids in the past year may be considered the same as patients who have not-well-controlled asthma, even in the absence of impairment levels consistent with not-well-controlled asthma.

[†]Validated questionnaires for the impairment domain (the questionnaires do not assess lung function or the risk domain) and definition of minimal important difference (MID) for each:
- ATAQ, Asthma Therapy Assessment Questionnaire; MID = 1.0.
- ACQ, Asthma Control Questionnaire; MID = 0.5.
- ACT, Asthma Control Test; MID not determined.

[‡]ACQ values of 0.76-1.40 are indeterminate regarding well-controlled asthma.

[§]Before step-up therapy: (a) review adherence to medications, inhaler technique, and environmental control; (b) if alternative treatment option was used in a step, discontinue it and use preferred treatment for that step.

FEV_1, Forced expiratory volume in 1 sec; FVC, forced vital capacity; EIB, exercise-induced bronchospasm; N/A, not available.

Adapted from the National Asthma Education and Prevention Program Expert Panel Report 3 (EPR 3): Guidelines for the diagnosis and management of asthma—summary report 2007, *J Allergy Clin Immunol* 120(Suppl):S94–S138, 2007.

management and control, and their technique in using inhaled medications, can be insightful and can help guide teaching to improve adherence to a management plan that might not have been adequately or properly implemented.

Adherence

Asthma is a chronic condition that is usually best managed with daily controller medication. However, symptoms wax and wane, severe exacerbations are infrequent, and when asthma is asymptomatic, a natural tendency is to reduce or discontinue daily controller therapies. As such, adherence to a daily controller regimen is frequently suboptimal; ICSs are underused 60% of the time. In one study, children with asthma who required an oral corticosteroid course for an asthma exacerbation had used their daily controller ICS 15% of the time. Misconceptions about controller medication time to onset, efficacy, and safety often underlie poor adherence and can be addressed by asking about such concerns at each visit.

Component 3: Control of Factors Contributing to Asthma Severity

Controllable factors that can worsen asthma can be generally grouped as (1) environmental exposures and (2) comorbid conditions (Table 169.10).

Eliminating and Reducing Problematic Environmental Exposures

Most children with asthma have an **allergic component** to their disease; steps should be taken to investigate and minimize allergen exposures in sensitized asthmatic patients. The medical history should identify exposure to smoke, pollutant, and potential allergen triggers (see later), especially in the patient's home. Since often patients have chronic symptoms and cannot identify potential triggers, **allergy testing** should be considered for at least those with persistent asthma. For asthmatic patients who are allergic to allergens in their homes and/or schools or daycare centers, reducing or eliminating these indoor allergen exposures can reduce asthma symptoms, medication requirements, AHR, severe exacerbations, and disease persistence. Common home, school, and daycare allergen exposures include furred or feathered animals as pets (cats, dogs, rodents, birds) or as pests (mice, rats, cockroaches), and occult indoor allergens such as dust mites and molds. Although removing or eradicating these exposures from the home, school, and daycare setting of sensitized asthmatic patients is the most effective means of greatly reducing problematic allergen exposures, it can take ≥6 mo for the levels of these indoor allergens to drop significantly. Dust mite allergen exposure can be reduced by

(1) encasing bedding and pillows in allergen-impermeable covers; (2) washing bedding weekly in hot water (> 130°F); (3) removing wall-to-wall carpeting and upholstered furniture; and (4) reducing and maintaining indoor humidity <50%.

Tobacco, wood and coal smoke, dusts, strong odors, and noxious air pollutants (e.g., nitrogen dioxide from inadequately vented gas stoves and furnaces) can aggravate asthma. These airway irritants should be eliminated from or reduced in the homes, schools/daycare centers, and automobiles/school transportation used by children with asthma. Annual influenza vaccination continues to be recommended for all children with asthma to reduce the risk of severe complications, although influenza is not responsible for the large majority of virus-induced asthma exacerbations experienced by children.

Treating Comorbid Conditions

Rhinitis, sinusitis, and GER often accompany asthma and worsen disease severity. They can also mimic asthma symptoms and lead to misclassification of asthma severity and control. Indeed, these conditions, along with asthma are the most common causes of chronic cough. Effective management of these comorbid conditions may improve asthma symptoms and disease severity, such that less asthma medication is needed to achieve good asthma control.

Gastroesophageal reflux is common in children with persistent asthma (see Chapter 349). GER may worsen asthma through 2 postulated mechanisms: (1) aspiration of refluxed gastric contents (micro- or macro-aspiration); and (2) vagally mediated reflex bronchospasm. Occult GER should be suspected in individuals with difficult-to-control asthma, especially patients who have prominent nocturnal asthma symptoms or who prop themselves up in bed to reduce nocturnal symptoms. GER can be demonstrated by reflux of barium into the esophagus during a barium swallow procedure or by esophageal probe monitoring. Because radiographic studies lack sufficient sensitivity and specificity, extended esophageal monitoring is the method of choice for diagnosing GER. If significant GER is noted, reflux precautions should be instituted (no food 2 hr before bedtime, head of bed elevated 6 inches, avoidance of caffeinated beverages), and medications such as proton pump inhibitors (omeprazole, lansoprazole) or H₂-receptor antagonists (cimetidine, ranitidine) administered for 8-12 wk. Of note, proton pump inhibition did not improve asthma control in a study of children with persistent, poorly controlled asthma and GER.

Rhinitis is usually comorbid with asthma, detected in about 90% of children with asthma. Rhinitis can be seasonal and/or perennial, with allergic and nonallergic components. Rhinitis complicates and worsens asthma via numerous direct and indirect mechanisms. Nasal breathing

Table 169.9	Key Elements of Productive Clinic Visits for Asthma

Standardize assessment of asthma control (e.g., Asthma Control Test, exacerbations in past 12 mo)
Specify goals of asthma management
Explain basic facts about asthma:
- Contrast normal vs asthmatic airways.
- Link airways inflammation, "twitchiness," and bronchoconstriction.
- Long-term-control and quick-relief medications
- Address concerns about potential adverse effects of asthma pharmacotherapy.

Teach, demonstrate, and have patient show proper technique for:
- Inhaled medication use (spacer use with metered-dose inhaler)

Investigate and manage factors that contribute to asthma severity:
- Environmental exposures
- Comorbid conditions

Create written 2-part Asthma Action Plan (see Fig. 169.7):
- Daily management
- Action plan for asthma exacerbations

Regular follow-up visits:
- Twice yearly (more often if asthma not well controlled)
- Monitor lung function at least annually

Table 169.10	Control of Factors Contributing to Asthma Severity

ELIMINATE OR REDUCE PROBLEMATIC ENVIRONMENTAL EXPOSURES

Environmental tobacco smoke elimination or reduction in home and automobiles
Allergen exposure elimination or reduction in sensitized asthmatic patients:
- Animal danders: pets (cats, dogs, rodents, birds)
- Pests (mice, rats)
- Dust mites
- Cockroaches
- Molds

Other airway irritants:
- Wood- or coal-burning smoke
- Strong chemical odors and perfumes (e.g., household cleaners)
- Dusts

TREAT COMORBID CONDITIONS
- Rhinitis
- Sinusitis
- Gastroesophageal reflux

Asthma Action Plan

For: _____ Doctor: _____ Date: _____

Doctor's Phone Number_____ Hospital/Emergency Department Phone Number _____

GREEN ZONE

Doing Well

- No cough, wheeze, chest tightness, or shortness of breath during the day or night
- Can do usual activities

And, if a peak flow meter is used,

Peak flow: more than _____
(80 percent or more of my best peak flow)

My best peak flow is: _____

Before exercise

Take these long-term control medicines each day (include an anti-inflammatory).

Medicine	How much to take	When to take it
_____	_____	_____
_____	_____	_____
_____	_____	_____
_____	_____	_____

☐ _____ ☐ 2 or ☐ 4 puffs_____ 5 minutes before exercise

YELLOW ZONE

Asthma Is Getting Worse

- Cough, wheeze, chest tightness, or shortness of breath, or
- Waking at night due to asthma, or
- Can do some, but not all, usual activities

-Or-

Peak flow: _____ to _____
(50 to 79 percent of my best peak flow)

First Add: quick-relief medicine—and keep taking your GREEN ZONE medicine.

_____ ☐ 2 or ☐ 4 puffs, every 20 minutes for up to 1 hour
(short-acting beta$_2$-agonist) ☐ Nebulizer, once

Second **If your symptoms (and peak flow, if used) return to GREEN ZONE after 1 hour of above treatment:**
☐ Continue monitoring to be sure you stay in the green zone.

-Or-

If your symptoms (and peak flow, if used) do not return to GREEN ZONE after 1 hour of above treatment:
☐ Take: _____ ☐ 2 or ☐ 4 puffs or ☐ Nebulizer
(short-acting beta$_2$-agonist)

☐ Add: _____ mg per day For _____(3–10) days
(oral steroid)

☐ Call the doctor ☐ before/ ☐ within_____ hours after taking the oral steroid.

RED ZONE

Medical Alert!

- Very short of breath, or
- Quick-relief medicines have not helped, or
- Cannot do usual activities, or
- Symptoms are same or get worse after 24 hours in Yellow Zone

-Or-

Peak flow: less than _____
(50 percent of my best peak flow)

Take this medicine:

☐ _____ ☐ 4 or ☐ 6 puffs or ☐ Nebulizer
(short-acting beta$_2$-agonist)

☐ _____ mg
(oral steroid)

Then call your doctor NOW. Go to the hospital or call an ambulance if:
- You are still in the red zone after 15 minutes AND
- You have not reached your doctor.

DANGER SIGNS ■ Trouble walking and talking due to shortness of breath ■ Take ☐ 4 or ☐ 6 puffs of your quick-relief medicine AND

■ Lips or fingernails are blue ■ Go to the hospital or call for an ambulance _____ NOW!
(phone)

See the reverse side for things you can do to avoid your asthma triggers.

How To Control Things That Make Your Asthma Worse

This guide suggests things you can do to avoid your asthma triggers. Put a check next to the triggers that you know make your asthma worse and ask your doctor to help you find out if you have other triggers as well. Then decide with your doctor what steps you will take.

Allergens

☐ **Animal Dander**
Some people are allergic to the flakes of skin or dried saliva from animals with fur or feathers.
The best thing to do:
- Keep furred or feathered pets out of your home.
If you can't keep the pet outdoors, then:
- Keep the pet out of your bedroom and other sleeping areas at all times, and keep the door closed.
- Remove carpets and furniture covered with cloth from your home. If that is not possible, keep the pet away from fabric-covered furniture and carpets.

☐ **Dust Mites**
Many people with asthma are allergic to dust mites. Dust mites are tiny bugs that are found in every home—in mattresses, pillows, carpets, upholstered furniture, bedcovers, clothes, stuffed toys, and fabric or other fabric-covered items.
Things that can help:
- Encase your mattress in a special dust-proof cover.
- Encase your pillow in a special dust-proof cover or wash the pillow each week in hot water. Water must be hotter than 130° F to kill the mites. Cold or warm water used with detergent and bleach can also be effective.
- Wash the sheets and blankets on your bed each week in hot water.
- Reduce indoor humidity to below 60 percent (ideally between 30—50 percent). Dehumidifiers or central air conditioners can do this.
- Try not to sleep or lie on cloth-covered cushions.
- Remove carpets from your bedroom and those laid on concrete, if you can.
- Keep stuffed toys out of the bed or wash the toys weekly in hot water or cooler water with detergent and bleach.

☐ **Cockroaches**
Many people with asthma are allergic to the dried droppings and remains of cockroaches.
The best thing to do:
- Keep food and garbage in closed containers. Never leave food out.
- Use poison baits, powders, gels, or paste (for example, boric acid). You can also use traps.
- If a spray is used to kill roaches, stay out of the room until the odor goes away.

☐ **Indoor Mold**
- Fix leaky faucets, pipes, or other sources of water that have mold around them.
- Clean moldy surfaces with a cleaner that has bleach in it.

☐ **Pollen and Outdoor Mold**
What to do during your allergy season (when pollen or mold spore counts are high):
- Try to keep your windows closed.
- Stay indoors with windows closed from late morning to afternoon, if you can. Pollen and some mold spore counts are highest at that time.
- Ask your doctor whether you need to take or increase anti-inflammatory medicine before your allergy season starts.

Irritants

☐ **Tobacco Smoke**
- If you smoke, ask your doctor for ways to help you quit. Ask family members to quit smoking, too.
- Do not allow smoking in your home or car.

☐ **Smoke, Strong Odors, and Sprays**
- If possible, do not use a wood-burning stove, kerosene heater, or fireplace.
- Try to stay away from strong odors and sprays, such as perfume, talcum powder, hair spray, and paints.

Other things that bring on asthma symptoms in some people include:

☐ **Vacuum Cleaning**
- Try to get someone else to vacuum for you once or twice a week, if you can. Stay out of rooms while they are being vacuumed and for a short while afterward.
- If you vacuum, use a dust mask (from a hardware store), a double-layered or microfilter vacuum cleaner bag, or a vacuum cleaner with a HEPA filter.

☐ **Other Things That Can Make Asthma Worse**
- Sulfites in foods and beverages: Do not drink beer or wine or eat dried fruit, processed potatoes, or shrimp if they cause asthma symptoms.
- Cold air: Cover your nose and mouth with a scarf on cold or windy days.
- Other medicines: Tell your doctor about all the medicines you take. Include cold medicines, aspirin, vitamins and other supplements, and nonselective beta-blockers (including those in eye drops).

U.S. Department of Health and Human Services
National Institutes of Health

National Heart
Lung and Blood Institute

For More Information, go to: www.nhlbi.nih.gov

NIH Publication No. 07-5251
April 2007

Fig. 169.7 **Asthma action plan for home use.** This plan has two main components: (1) a daily management plan to keep asthma in good control; and (2) an action plan to recognize and manage worsening asthma. (*From US Department of Health and Human Services, National Institutes of Health, National Heart, Lung, and Blood Institute, NIH Pub No 07-5251, April 2007. https://www.nhlbi.nih.gov/health/resources/lung/asthma-action-plan*).

may improve asthma and reduce exercise-induced bronchospasm by humidifying and warming inspired air and filtering out allergens and irritants that can trigger asthma and worsen airway inflammation. Reduction of nasal congestion and obstruction can help the nose to perform these humidifying, warming, and filtering functions. In asthmatic patients, improvement in rhinitis is also associated with modest reductions in AHR, airways inflammation, asthma symptoms, and asthma medication use. Optimal rhinitis management in children is similar to asthma management in regard to the importance of interventions to reduce nasal inflammation (see Chapter 168).

Radiographic evidence for **sinus disease** is common in patients with asthma. There is usually significant improvement in asthma control in patients diagnosed and treated for sinus disease. A coronal, "screening" or "limited" CT scan of the sinuses is the gold standard test for sinus disease and can be helpful if recurrent sinusitis has been suspected and repeatedly treated without such evidence. In comparison, sinus radiographs are inaccurate and should be avoided. If the patient with asthma has clinical and radiographic evidence for sinusitis, topical therapy to include nasal saline irrigations, intranasal corticosteroids, and a 2-3 wk course of antibiotics should be considered.

Component 4: Principles of Asthma Pharmacotherapy

The current version of NIH asthma guidelines (2007) provides treatment recommendations that vary by level of asthma severity and age-groups (Table 169.11). There are 6 treatment steps. Patients at **Treatment Step 1** have intermittent asthma. Children with mild persistent asthma are at **Treatment Step 2**. Children with moderate persistent asthma can be at **Treatment Step 3 or 4**. Children with severe persistent asthma are at **Treatment Steps 5 and 6**. The goals of therapy are to achieve a well-controlled state by reducing the components of both impairment (e.g., preventing or minimizing symptoms, infrequently needing quick-reliever medications, maintaining "normal" lung function and normal activity levels) and risk (e.g., preventing recurrent exacerbations, reduced lung growth, and medication adverse effects). The recommendations for initial therapy are based on assessment of asthma severity, while level of control determines any modifications of treatment in children who are already using controller therapy. A major objective of this approach is to identify and treat all "persistent" and inadequately controlled asthma with antiinflammatory controller medication. Management of Treatment Step 1 (intermittent asthma) is simply the use of a SABA as needed for symptoms and for pretreatment in those with exercise-induced bronchospasm (see Table 169.11).

The preferred treatment for all patients with persistent asthma is ICS therapy, as monotherapy or in combination with adjunctive therapy. The type(s) and amount(s) of daily controller medications to be used are determined by the asthma severity and control rating.

Low-dose ICS therapy is the treatment of choice for all children at Treatment Step 2 (mild persistent asthma). Alternative medications include a leukotriene-modifying agent (montelukast), nonsteroidal antiinflammatory drugs (cromolyn, nedocromil), and theophylline. There are 4 co-equal choices for the treatment of school-aged children at Treatment Step 3 (moderate persistent asthma): medium-dose ICS, combination low-dose ICS and **inhaled long-acting β$_2$-agonist (LABA)**, a **leukotriene receptor antagonist (LTRA)**, or theophylline. In a study of children with uncontrolled asthma receiving low-dose ICS, the addition of LABA provided greater improvement than either adding an **LTRA** or increasing ICS dosage. However, some children had a good response to medium-dose ICS or the addition of an LTRA, justifying them as step-up controller therapy options. The preferred therapy for children at Treatment Step 4 (also moderate persistent asthma) is medium-dose ICS/LABA combination. Alternatives include medium-dose ICS with either theophylline or an LTRA. For young children (≤4 yr) at Treatment Step 3, medium-dose ICS is recommended, while medium-dose ICS plus either a LABA or an LTRA are recommended for preschool-age children at Treatment Step 4.

Children with severe persistent asthma (Treatment Steps 5 and 6) should receive combination high-dose ICS plus LABA. Long-term administration of oral corticosteroids as controller therapy is effective but is rarely required.

In addition, omalizumab can be used in children ≥6 yr old with severe allergic asthma, while mepolizumab is approved for children ≥12 yr with severe asthma eosinophilic asthma. A rescue course of systemic corticosteroids may be necessary at any step for very poorly controlled asthma. For children age ≥5 yr with allergic asthma requiring Treatment Steps 2-4 care, allergen immunotherapy can also be considered.

"Step-Up, Step-Down" Approach

The NIH guidelines emphasize initiating higher-level controller therapy at the outset to establish prompt control, with measures to "step-down" therapy once good asthma control is achieved. Initially, airflow limitation and the pathology of asthma may limit the delivery and efficacy of ICS such that stepping up to higher doses and/or combination therapy may be needed to gain asthma control. Furthermore, ICS requires weeks to months of daily administration for optimal efficacy to occur. Combination pharmacotherapy can achieve relatively immediate improvement while also providing daily ICS to improve long-term control and reduce exacerbation risk.

Asthma therapy can be stepped down after good asthma control has been achieved and maintained for at least 3 mo. By determining the lowest number or dose of daily controller medications that can maintain good control, the potential for medication adverse effects is reduced. Regular follow-up is still emphasized because the variability of asthma's course is well recognized. When asthma is not well controlled, therapy should be escalated by increasing controller treatment step by 1 level and closely monitoring for clinical improvement. For a child with very poorly controlled asthma, the recommendations are to consider a short course of prednisone, or to increase therapy by 2 steps, with reevaluation in 2 wk. If step-up therapy is being considered, it is important to check inhaler technique and adherence, implement environmental control measures, and identify and treat comorbid conditions.

Referral to Asthma Specialist

Referral to an asthma specialist for consultation or co-management is recommended if there are difficulties in achieving or maintaining good asthma control. For children <4 yr, referral is recommended if the patient requires at least Treatment Step 3 care, and should be considered if the patient requires Treatment Step 2 care. For children ≥5 yr, consultation with a specialist is recommended if the patient requires Treatment Step 4 care or higher, and should be considered if Treatment Step 3 is required. Referral is also recommended if allergen immunotherapy or biologic therapy is being considered.

Long-Term Controller Medications

All levels of persistent asthma should be treated with ICS therapy to reduce airway inflammation and improve long-term control (see Table 169.11). Other long-term controller medications include LABAs, leukotriene modifiers, cromolyn, sustained-release theophylline, and tiotropium in adolescents. Omalizumab (Xolair) and mepolizumab (Nucala) are approved by the U.S. Food and Drug Administration (FDA) for use as an add-on therapy in children ≥6 yr and ≥12 yr who have severe allergic asthma or eosinophilic asthma, respectively, that remains difficult to control. Corticosteroids are the most potent and most effective medications used to treat both the acute (administered systemically) and the chronic (administered by inhalation) manifestations of asthma. They are available in inhaled, oral, and parenteral forms (Tables 169.12 and 169.13).

Inhaled Corticosteroids

ICS therapy improves lung function; reduces asthma symptoms, AHR, and use of "rescue" medications; improves quality of life; and most importantly reduces the need for prednisone, urgent care visits, and hospitalizations by approximately 50%. Epidemiologic studies have also shown that ICS therapy substantially lowers the risk of death attributable to asthma if used regularly. Because ICS therapy can achieve all the goals of asthma management, it is viewed as first-line treatment for persistent asthma.

Seven ICSs are FDA approved for use in children. The NIH and GINA guidelines provide equivalence classifications (see Table 169.13),

Table 169.11 | Stepwise Approach for Managing Asthma in Children*

AGE	THERAPY[†]	INTERMITTENT ASTHMA	PERSISTENT ASTHMA: DAILY MEDICATION				

←── STEP DOWN if possible (and asthma is well controlled at least 3 months)   ASSESS CONTROL   STEP UP if needed (first check inhaler technique, adherence, environmental control, and comorbid condition) ──→

AGE	THERAPY[†]	Step 1	Step 2	Step 3	Step 4	Step 5	Step 6
0-4 yr	Preferred	SABA prn	Low-dose ICS	Medium-dose ICS	Medium-dose ICS + *either* LABA *or* LTRA	High-dose ICS + *either* LABA *or* LTRA	High-dose ICS + *either* LABA *or* LTRA *and* OCS
	Alternative		Cromolyn or montelukast				
5-11 yr	Preferred	SABA prn	Low-dose ICS	*Either* low-dose ICS ± LABA, LTRA, or theophylline *or* Medium-dose ICS	Medium-dose ICS + LABA	High-dose ICS + LABA	High-dose ICS + LABA *and* OCS
	Alternative		Cromolyn, LTRA, nedocromil, or theophylline		Medium-dose ICS + *either* LTRA *or* Theophylline	High-dose ICS + *either* LTRA *or* Theophylline	High-dose ICS + *either* LTRA *or* Theophylline *and* OCS
≥12 yr	Preferred	SABA prn	Low-dose ICS	Low-dose ICS + LABA *or* Medium-dose ICS	Medium-dose ICS + LABA	High-dose ICS + LABA *and* Consider omalizumab for patients with allergies	High-dose ICS + LABA + OCS *and* Consider mepolizumab for patients with eosinophilic asthma Consider omalizumab for patients with allergies
	Alternative		Cromolyn, LTRA, nedocromil, or theophylline	Low-dose ICS + LTRA, theophylline, or zileuton	Medium-dose ICS + LTRA, theophylline, or zileuton		

Each step: Patient education, environmental control, and management of comorbidities.
Age ≥5 yr: Steps 2-4: Consider subcutaneous allergen immunotherapy for patients who have allergic asthma.
QUICK-RELIEF MEDICATION FOR ALL PATIENTS
SABA as needed for symptoms. Intensity of treatment depends on severity of symptoms: up to 3 treatments at 20-min intervals as needed. Short course of oral systemic corticosteroids may be needed.
Caution: Use of SABA >2 days/wk for symptom relief (not prevention of exercise-induced bronchospasm) generally indicates inadequate control and the need to step up treatment.
For ages 0-4 yr: With viral respiratory infection: SABA q4-6h up to 24 hr (longer with physician consult). Consider short course of systemic corticosteroids if exacerbation is severe or patient has history of previous severe exacerbations.

*Notes:
• The stepwise approach is meant to assist, not replace, the clinical decision making required to meet individual patient needs.
• If alternative treatment is used and response is inadequate, discontinue it and use the preferred treatment before stepping up.
• If clear benefit is not observed within 4-6 wk and patient/family medication technique and adherence are satisfactory, consider adjusting therapy or alternative diagnosis.
• Studies on children age 0-4 yr are limited.
• Clinicians who administer immunotherapy or omalizumab should be prepared and equipped to identify and treat anaphylaxis that may occur.
• Theophylline is a less desirable alternative because of the need to monitor serum concentration levels. The 2016 GINA guidelines do not recommend the use of theophylline as a controller medication and in IV forms to treat status asthmaticus due to its severe adverse effects profile.
• Zileuton is less desirable alternative because of limited studies as adjunctive therapy and the need to monitor liver function.
[†]Alphabetical order is used when more than 1 treatment option is listed within *either* preferred or alternative therapy.
ICS, Inhaled corticosteroid; LABA, inhaled long-acting β₂-agonist; LTRA, leukotriene receptor antagonist; OCS, oral corticosteroid; prn, as needed; SABA, inhaled short-acting β₂-agonist.
Adapted from the National Asthma Education and Prevention Program Expert Panel Report 3 (EPR3): Guidelines for the diagnosis and management of asthma—summary report 2007, *J Allergy Clin Immunol* 120(Suppl):S94–S138, 2007.

Table 169.12	Usual Dosages for Long-Term Control Medications		
	AGE		
MEDICATION	**0-4 yr**	**5-11 yr**	**≥12 yr**
INHALED CORTICOSTEROIDS (see Table 169.13)			
Methylprednisolone: 2, 4, 8, 16, 32 mg tablets Prednisolone: 5 mg tablets; 5 mg/5 mL, 15 mg/5 mL Prednisone: 1, 2.5, 5, 10, 20, 50 mg tablets; 5 mg/mL, 5 mg/5 mL	0.25-2 mg/kg daily in single dose in AM or qod as needed for control Short-course "burst": 1-2 mg/kg/day; maximum 30 mg/day for 3-10 days	0.25-2 mg/kg daily in single dose in AM or qod as needed for control Short-course "burst": 1-2 mg/kg/day; maximum 60 mg/day for 3-10 days	7.5-60 mg daily in a single dose in AM or qod as needed for control Short-course "burst" to achieve control: 40-60 mg/day as single or 2 divided doses for 3-10 days
Fluticasone/salmeterol (Advair): DPI: 100, 250, or 500 µg/50 µg	N/A	1 inhalation bid; dose depends on level of severity or control (the 100/50 dosage is indicated in children ≥4 yr)	1 inhalation bid; dose depends on level of severity or control
HFA: 45 µg/21 µg, 115 µg/21 µg, 230 µg/21 µg			2 inhalations bid; dose depends on level of severity or control
Budesonide/formoterol (Symbicort): HFA: 80 µg/4.5 µg, 160 µg/4.5 µg	N/A		2 inhalations bid; dose depends on level of severity or control
Mometasone/formoterol (Dulera): HFA: 100 µg/5 µg, 200 µg/5 µg			2 inhalations bid; dose depends on level of severity or control
Leukotriene receptor antagonists: Montelukast (Singulair): 4 or 5 mg chewable tablet 4 mg granule packets 10 mg tablet	4 mg qhs (1-5 yr of age)	5 mg qhs (6-14 yr)	10 mg qhs (indicated in children ≥15 yr)
Zafirlukast (Accolate): 10 or 20 mg tablet	N/A	10 mg bid (7-11 yr)	40 mg daily (20 mg tablet bid)
5-Lipoxygenase inhibitor: (Zileuton CR): 600 mg tablet	N/A	N/A	1,200 mg bid (give 2 tablets bid)
Immunomodulators: Omalizumab (anti-IgE; Xolair): SC injection, 150 mg/1.2 mL after reconstitution with 1.4 mL sterile water for injection	N/A	N/A	150-375 mg SC q 2-4 wk, depending on body weight and pretreatment serum IgE level
Mepolizumab (anti–IL-5; Nucala): SC injection, 100 mg after reconstitution with 1.2 mL sterile water for injection	N/A	N/A	100 mg SC q 4 wk

bid, 2 times daily; DPI, dry powder inhaler; HFA, hydrofluoroalkane; MDI, metered-dose inhaler; q, every; qhs, every night; qid, 4 times daily; qod, every other day; SC, subcutaneous(ly).

although direct comparisons of efficacy and safety outcomes are lacking. ICSs are available in metered-dose inhalers (MDIs) using hydrofluoroalkane (HFA) as their propellant, in dry powder inhalers (DPIs), or in suspension for nebulization. Fluticasone propionate, fluticasone furoate, mometasone furoate, ciclesonide, and to a lesser extent budesonide are considered "second-generation" ICSs, in that they have greater antiinflammatory potency and less *systemic* bioavailability (and thus potential for systemic adverse effects) because of their extensive first-pass hepatic metabolism. The selection of the initial ICS dose is based on the determination of disease severity.

Even though ICSs can be very effective, there has been some reluctance to treat children with ICSs due to parental and occasionally physician concerns regarding their potential for adverse effects with chronic use. The adverse effects that occur with long-term systemic corticosteroid therapy have not been seen or have only rarely been reported in children receiving ICSs in recommended doses. The risk of adverse effects from ICS therapy is related to the dose and frequency of administration (Table 169.14). High doses (≥1,000 µg/day in children) and frequent administration (4 times/day) are more likely to have both local and systemic adverse effects. Children who receive maintenance therapy with higher ICS doses are also likely to require frequent systemic corticosteroid courses for asthma exacerbations, further increasing their risk of corticosteroid adverse effects.

The most commonly encountered ICS adverse effects are local: oral **candidiasis** (thrush) and **dysphonia** (hoarse voice). Thrush results from propellant-induced mucosal irritation and local immunosuppression, and dysphonia is the result of vocal cord myopathy. These effects are dose dependent and are most common in individuals receiving high-dose ICS or oral corticosteroid therapy. The incidence of these local effects can be greatly minimized by using a spacer with an MDI with the ICS, because spacers reduce oropharyngeal deposition of the drug and propellant. Mouth rinsing using a "swish and spit" technique after ICS use is also recommended.

The potential for growth suppression and osteoporosis with long-term ICS use had been an unanswered concern. However, a long-term, prospective NIH-sponsored study (CAMP) followed the growth and bone mineral density (BMD) of >1,000 children (age 6-12 yr at entry) with mild to moderate asthma until they reached adulthood and found slight growth suppression and osteopenia in some children who received long-term ICS therapy. A small (1.1 cm), limited (1 year) growth suppressive effect was noted in children receiving budesonide, 200 µg twice daily, after 5 yr of therapy. Height was then followed until all children had reached adulthood (mean age 25 yr). Those who received ICS therapy remained approximately 1 cm shorter than those who received placebo. Thus, children treated with long-term ICS therapy are likely to be about 1 cm shorter than expected as an adult, which is of little clinical

Table 169.13	Estimated Comparative Inhaled Corticosteroid Doses		
GLUCOCORTICOID	**LOW DAILY DOSE**	**MEDIUM DAILY DOSE**	**HIGH DAILY DOSE**
Beclomethasone (Qvar) MDI: 40 or 80 μg (Approved for children ≥5 yr)	80-160 μg	160-320 μg	>320 μg
Budesonide (Pulmicort Flexhaler) DPI: 90, 180 μg (Approved for children ≥6 yr)	200 μg	200-400 μg	>400 μg
Budesonide suspension for nebulization (Generic and Pulmicort Respules) 0.25 mg, 0.5 mg, 1 mg (Approved for children 1-8 yr)	0.5 mg	1.0 mg	2.0 mg
Ciclesonide (Alvesco) MDI: 80, 160 μg (Approved for children ≥12 yr)	80 μg	80-160 μg	160 μg
Flunisolide (Aerospan) MDI: 80 μg/puff (Approved for children ≥6 yr)	80 μg	80-160 μg	160 μg
Fluticasone propionate (Flovent, Flovent Diskus) MDI: 44, 110, 220 μg DPI: 50, 100, 250 μg (44 and 50 μg approved for children ≥4 yr)	88-176 μg 100-200 μg	176-440 μg 200-500 μg	>440 μg >500 μg
Fluticasone furoate (Arnuity Ellipta) DPI: 100, 200 μg (Approved for children ≥12 yr)	100 μg	100-200 μg	200 μg
Mometasone Furoate (Asmanex, Asmanex Twisthaler) MDI: 100, 200 μg DPI: 110, 220 μg (Approved for children ≥4 yr)	110 μg 100 μg	110 μg 100 μg	110 μg 100 μg

DPI, Dry powder inhaler; MDI, metered-dose inhaler.

Adapted from National Asthma Education and Prevention Program Expert Panel Report 3 (EPR3): Guidelines for the diagnosis and management of asthma—summary report 2007, *J Allergy Clin Immunol* 120(Suppl):S94–S138, 2007.

significance. BMD was no different in those receiving budesonide vs placebo during the duration of the study, while a follow-up study after a mean of 7 years found a slight dose-dependent effect of ICS therapy on bone mineral accretion only among males. A much greater effect on BMD was observed with increasing numbers of oral corticosteroid bursts for acute asthma, as well as an increase in risk for osteopenia, which was again limited to males. These findings were with use of low-dose budesonide; higher ICS doses, especially of agents with increased potency, have a greater potential for adverse effects. Thus, corticosteroid adverse effects screening and osteoporosis prevention measures are recommended for patients receiving higher ICS doses, since these patients are also likely to require systemic courses for exacerbations (see Table 169.14).

Systemic Corticosteroids

The development of second-generation ICSs, especially when used in combination with a LABA in a single device, have allowed the vast majority of children with asthma to achieve and maintain good control without need for maintenance oral corticosteroid (OCS) therapy. Thus, OCSs are used primarily to treat asthma exacerbations and, rarely, in children with very severe disease. In these patients, every attempt should be made to exclude comorbid conditions and to keep the OCS dose at ≤20 mg every other day. Doses exceeding this amount are associated with numerous adverse effects (see Chapter 593). To determine the need for continued OCS therapy, tapering of the OCS dose over several weeks should be attempted, with close monitoring of the patient's symptoms and lung function.

Prednisone, prednisolone, and methylprednisolone are rapidly and completely absorbed, with peak plasma concentrations occurring within 1-2 hr. Prednisone is an inactive prodrug that requires biotransformation via first-pass hepatic metabolism to prednisolone, its active form.

Corticosteroids are metabolized in the liver into inactive compounds, with the rate of metabolism influenced by drug interactions and disease states. Anticonvulsants (phenytoin, phenobarbital, carbamazepine) increase the metabolism of prednisolone, methylprednisolone, and dexamethasone, with methylprednisolone most significantly affected. Rifampin also enhances the clearance of corticosteroids and can result in diminished therapeutic effect. Other medications (ketoconazole, oral contraceptives) can significantly delay corticosteroid metabolism. Some macrolide antibiotics, such as erythromycin and clarithromycin, delay the clearance of only methylprednisolone.

Long-term OCS therapy can result in a number of adverse effects over time (see Chapter 595). Some occur immediately (metabolic effects), whereas others can develop insidiously over several months to years (growth suppression, osteoporosis, cataracts). Most adverse effects occur in a cumulative dose- and duration-dependent manner. Children who require routine or frequent short courses of OCSs, especially with concurrent high-dose ICSs, should receive corticosteroid adverse effects screening (see Table 169.14) and osteoporosis preventive measures (see Chapter 726).

Long-Acting Inhaled β-Agonists

Although considered daily controller medications, *LABAs (salmeterol, formoterol) are not intended for use as monotherapy for persistent asthma because they can increase the risk for serious asthma exacerbations (ICU admission, endotracheal intubation) and asthma-related deaths when used without an ICS.* The likely mechanism involves the ability of LABAs to "mask" worsening asthma inflammation and asthma severity, leading to a delay in seeking urgent care and increased risk of a life-threatening exacerbation. Although both salmeterol and formoterol have a prolonged duration of effect (≥12 hr), salmeterol has a prolonged onset of effect (60 min), while formoterol's onset of effect is rapid (5-10 min) after

Table 169.14	Risk Assessment for Corticosteroid Adverse Effects	
	CONDITIONS	**RECOMMENDATIONS**
Low risk	(≤1 risk factor*) Low- to medium-dose ICS (see Table 169.13)	Monitor blood pressure and weight with each physician visit. Measure height annually (stadiometry); monitor periodically for declining growth rate and pubertal developmental delay. Encourage regular physical exercise. Ensure adequate dietary calcium and vitamin D with additional supplements for daily calcium if needed. Avoid smoking and alcohol. Ensure TSH status if patient has history of thyroid abnormality.
Medium risk	(If >1 risk factor,* consider evaluating as high risk) High-dose ICS (see Table 169.13) At least 4 courses of OCS/yr	As above, *plus*: Yearly ophthalmologic evaluations to monitor for cataracts or glaucoma Baseline bone densitometry (DEXA scan) Consider patient at increased risk for adrenal insufficiency, especially with physiologic stressors (e.g., surgery, accident, significant illness).
High risk	Chronic systemic corticosteroids (>7.5 mg daily or equivalent for >1 mo) ≥7 OCS burst treatments/year Very-high-dose ICS (e.g., fluticasone propionate ≥800 µg/day)	As above, *plus*: DEXA scan: if DEXA z score ≤1.0, recommend close monitoring (every 12 mo) Consider referral to a bone or endocrine specialist. Bone age assessment Complete blood count Serum calcium, phosphorus, and alkaline phosphatase determinations Urine calcium and creatinine measurements Measurements of testosterone in males, estradiol in amenorrheic premenopausal women, vitamin D (25-OH and 1,25-OH vitamin D), parathyroid hormone, and osteocalcin Urine telopeptides for those receiving long-term systemic or frequent OCS treatment Assume adrenal insufficiency for physiologic stressors (e.g., surgery, accident, significant illness).

*Risk factors for osteoporosis: presence of other chronic illness(es), medications (corticosteroids, anticonvulsants, heparin, diuretics), low body weight, family history of osteoporosis, significant fracture history disproportionate to trauma, recurrent falls, impaired vision, low dietary calcium and vitamin D intake, and lifestyle factors (decreased physical activity, smoking, alcohol intake).

DEXA, Dual-energy x-ray absorptiometry; ICS, inhaled corticosteroid; OCS, oral corticosteroid; TSH, thyroid-stimulating hormone.

administration. Given their long duration of action, LABAs are well suited for patients with nocturnal asthma and for individuals who require frequent use of SABA inhalations during the day to prevent exercise-induced bronchospasm (EIB), but only in combination with ICSs. Of note, the FDA requires all LABA-containing medications to be labeled with a warning of an increase in severe asthma episodes associated with these agents. In addition, the FDA recommends that once a patient is well controlled on combination ICS/LABA therapy, the LABA component should be discontinued while continuing treatment with the ICS.

Combination ICS/LABA Therapy
Combination ICS/LABA therapy is recommended for patients who are suboptimally controlled with ICS therapy alone and those with moderate or severe persistent asthma. In those inadequately controlled with ICS alone, combination ICS/LABA therapy is superior to add-on therapy with either an LTRA or theophylline or doubling the ICS dose. Benefits include improvement in baseline lung function, less need for rescue SABA therapy, improved quality of life, and fewer asthma exacerbations. A large study by the NIH-sponsored CARE Network found that in children inadequately controlled with low-dose ICS therapy, combination low-dose fluticasone/salmeterol (100 µg/21 µg) twice daily was almost twice as effective as other step-up regimens, including fluticasone (250 µg) twice daily or low-dose fluticasone (100 µg twice daily) plus montelukast once daily, with the greatest improvement in reducing exacerbations requiring prednisone and study withdrawals due to poorly controlled asthma. In addition, combination fluticasone/salmeterol was as effective as medium-dose fluticasone and was superior to combination fluticasone/montelukast therapy in black children, arguing against the notion that black children are more prone to serious asthma exacerbations than white children when treated with combination ICS/LABA therapy.

Despite their efficacy and widespread use, the long-term safety of LABAs, even when used in combination with ICS in a single inhaler, has

been questioned. To address this concern of rare, severe asthma-related events with LABA/ICS use, large randomized controlled trials (RCTs) compared the safety of combination ICS/LABA vs ICS monotherapy. Two studies of >23,000 adults and adolescents ≥12 yr old with various levels of asthma severity were randomized to receive ICS (low or medium dose) monotherapy vs equivalent ICS/LABA (fluticasone vs fluticasone/salmeterol; budesonide vs budesonide/formoterol) over 26 weeks to determine if small but significant differences might occur in asthma hospitalization, intubation, or death attributable to ICS/LABA. No intubations or asthma deaths occurred during the study, and no differences in asthma hospitalizations between treatment groups were observed. The similar pediatric study enrolled >6,000 children age 4-11 yr with various levels of asthma severity to receive either fluticasone (low or medium dose) or equivalent fluticasone/salmeterol dose over 26 weeks, with similar findings of no significant differences in severe asthma-related events between treatment groups. *These results strongly suggest that the use of combination ICS/LABA products in children and adults with moderate to severe persistent asthma is both effective and safe.*

Leukotriene-Modifying Agents
Leukotrienes are potent proinflammatory mediators that can induce bronchospasm, mucus secretion, and airways edema. Two classes of leukotriene modifiers have been developed: inhibitors of leukotriene synthesis and leukotriene receptor antagonists (LTRAs). Zileuton, the only synthesis inhibitor, is not approved for use in children <12 yr. Because zileuton can result in elevated liver function enzyme values in 2–4% of patients, and interacts with medications metabolized via the cytochrome P450 system, it is rarely prescribed for children with asthma.

LTRAs have bronchodilator and targeted antiinflammatory properties and reduce exercise-, aspirin-, and allergen-induced bronchoconstriction. LTRAs are recommended as an alternative treatment for mild persistent asthma and as an add-on medication with ICS for moderate persistent asthma. Two LTRAs with FDA-approved use in children are montelukast and zafirlukast. Both medications improve asthma symptoms, decrease the need for rescue β-agonist use, and modestly improve lung function. **Montelukast** is approved for use in children ≥1 yr of age and is administered once daily, whereas **zafirlukast** is approved in children ≥5 yr and is given twice daily. LTRAs are less effective than ICSs in patients with mild persistent asthma (e.g., ICSs improve baseline lung function 5–15%, whereas LTRAs improve lung function 2.5–7.5%). LTRAs have few, if any, significant adverse effects, although case reports have described mood changes and suicidality in adolescents soon after instituting montelukast. When initially prescribing montelukast, a precaution is to inform the child and family that, if mood changes are noted after starting montelukast, they should discontinue its use and contact their physician.

Nonsteroidal Antiinflammatory Agents

Cromolyn and **nedocromil** are considered nonsteroidal antiinflammatory drugs (NSAIDs), although they have little efficacy as a long-term controller for asthma. They can block EIB and bronchospasm caused by allergen challenge. Although both drugs are considered alternative controller agents for children with mild persistent asthma, *the 2016 GINA guidelines no longer recommend cromolyn or nedocromil.* Because they inhibit EIB and allergen-triggered responses, cromolyn (nedocromil is no longer available in the United States) can be used as an alternative or add-on to SABAs for these specific circumstances.

Theophylline is a phosphodiesterase inhibitor with bronchodilator and antiinflammatory effects that can reduce asthma symptoms and rescue SABA use. Although the National Heart, Lung, and Blood Institute (NHLBI) guidelines continue to include theophylline as an add-on agent to ICS in school-age children at Treatment Step 3 and beyond, it is rarely used in children today because of its potential toxicity. Theophylline has a narrow therapeutic window, with overdosage associated with headaches, vomiting, cardiac arrhythmias, seizures, and death. Therefore, when used, serum theophylline levels need to be carefully and routinely monitored, especially if the patient has a viral illness associated with a fever or is concomitantly taking a medication known to delay theophylline clearance. As a result, *the 2016 GINA guidelines no longer recommend theophylline* at any level of asthma severity or control.

Long-Acting Inhaled Anticholinergics

Tiotropium is a long-acting anticholinergic agent (24-hr duration of action) that is FDA approved for use in children with asthma ≥12 yr old. Studies in adults and adolescents have found tiotropium to be equivalent to a LABA when used in combination with an ICS. It has also been found to reduce exacerbations and improve lung function in patients with inadequately controlled asthma despite treatment with combination ICS/LABA products.

Allergen Immunotherapy

Allergen immunotherapy (**AIT**) involves administering gradually increasing doses of allergens to a person with allergic disease to reduce or eliminate the patient's allergic response to those allergens, including allergic rhinoconjunctivitis and asthma. When properly administered to an appropriate candidate, AIT is a safe, effective therapy capable not only of reducing or preventing symptoms, but also of potentially altering the natural history of the disease by minimizing disease duration and preventing disease progression. Conventional AIT is given subcutaneously (subcutaneous immunotherapy, **SCIT**) under the direction of an experienced allergist. Sublingual immunotherapy (**SLIT**) is less potent but can still be effective, and has less potential for severe allergic adverse reactions.

The goal of SCIT or SLIT is to increase the dose of allergen extract administered in order to reach a therapeutic maintenance dose of each major allergen, in a manner that minimizes the likelihood of systemic allergic reactions. For SCIT, allergen extracts are formulated for each patient based on documented allergen sensitizations and problematic exposures. Maintenance doses are generally given monthly for SCIT or daily for SLIT, to complete a 3-5 yr course. Most of the controlled trials examining AIT efficacy on seasonal or perennial allergic asthma are favorable. A meta-analysis of 20 trials examining the effects of SCIT on allergic asthma revealed significant improvement with fewer symptoms, improved lung function, less need for medication, and AHR reduction.

Although AIT is regarded as safe, the potential for **anaphylaxis** always exists when patients receive extracts containing allergens to which they are sensitized. Local transient allergic reactions are common (SCIT: injection site allergic reaction; SLIT: mild oral itching). Systemic allergic reactions have been very rarely reported with SLIT, such that it is typically administered at home. In comparison, systemic allergic reactions occur more often with SCIT, with fatal anaphylaxis occurring in approximately 1 per 2 million injections. Because of the risks of systemic allergic reactions to SCIT, standard precautions include administering SCIT in medical settings where a physician with access to emergency equipment and medications required for the treatment of anaphylaxis is available (see Chapter 174). Patients should be observed in the office for 30 min after each injection because most systemic reactions to SCIT begin within this time frame. *SCIT should never be given at home or by untrained personnel.* Because of the complexities and risks of administration, SCIT should only be administered by an experienced allergist.

AIT should be discontinued in patients who have not shown improvement after 1 yr of receiving maintenance doses of an appropriate allergen extract(s), or who have a serious systemic allergic or adverse reaction.

Biologic Therapies

Biologic therapies are genetically engineered proteins derived from human genes and designed to inhibit specific immune mediators of disease. Several are FDA approved as add-on controller therapies (i.e., in addition to conventional controller therapies) for severe asthma in adults and children.

Omalizumab (Anti-IgE Antibody). Omalizumab is a humanized monoclonal antibody (mAb) that binds IgE and prevents its binding to the high-affinity IgE receptor, thereby blocking IgE-mediated allergic responses and inflammation. It is FDA approved for patients >6 yr old with severe allergic asthma who continue to have inadequate disease control despite treatment with high-dose ICS and/or OCS. Omalizumab is given every 2-4 wk subcutaneously, with the dosage based on body weight and serum IgE levels. Omalizumab can improve asthma control while allowing ICS and/or OCS dose reduction. Omalizumab has been studied in inner-city children with exacerbation-prone asthma. When added to guideline-based controller management, omalizumab reduced exacerbations (50%) that peak in the spring and fall seasons. A follow-up prospective preseasonal treatment study confirmed the effect on fall seasonal exacerbations and demonstrated how omalizumab restores antiviral (IFN-α) immune responses to rhinovirus (the most common infectious trigger of exacerbations) that are impaired by IgE-mediated mechanisms. Omalizumab is well tolerated, although local injection site reactions can occur. Hypersensitivity reactions (including anaphylaxis) have been reported following approximately 0.1% of injections. As a result, omalizumab has an FDA black box warning of potentially serious and life-threatening anaphylactic adverse reactions.

Mepolizumab (Anti–IL-5 Antibody). Mepolizumab, an anti–IL-5 antibody that blocks IL-5-mediated eosinophilopoiesis, reduces severe asthma exacerbations and lowers sputum and blood eosinophils while allowing for a significant reduction in OCS dose in adults with severe exacerbation-prone eosinophilic asthma. It is administered subcutaneously every 4 wk and is FDA approved for severe eosinophilic asthmatic children ≥12 yr old. **Reslizumab**, another anti–IL-5 antibody therapeutic, is administered intravenously and is FDA approved for severe asthmatics ≥18 yr old (i.e., not currently approved for use in children).

Dupilumab (Anti–IL-4 Receptor α Antibody). Dupilumab, an anti–IL-4 receptor antibody that inhibits both IL-4 and IL-13 production (both cytokines share the same IL-4 receptor) and atopic immune responses, reduces exacerbations and symptoms and improves lung function in moderate to severe asthmatic patients with persistent eosinophilia. Although not yet FDA approved, studies are ongoing in both children and adults.

Quick-Reliever Medications

Quick-reliever or "rescue" medications (SABAs, inhaled anticholinergics, and short-course systemic corticosteroids) are used in the management of acute asthma symptoms (Table 169.15).

Short-Acting Inhaled β-Agonists

Given their rapid onset of action, effectiveness, and 4-6 hr duration of action, SABAs (albuterol, levalbuterol, terbutaline, pirbuterol) are the drugs of choice for acute asthma symptoms ("rescue" medication) and for preventing EIB. β-Adrenergic agonists cause bronchodilation by inducing airway smooth muscle relaxation, reducing vascular permeability and airways edema, and improving mucociliary clearance. Levalbuterol, the R-isomer of albuterol, is associated with less tachycardia and tremor, which can be bothersome to some asthmatic patients. Overuse of β-agonists is associated with an increased risk of death or near-death episodes from asthma. This is a major concern for some patients with asthma who rely on the frequent use of SABAs as a "quick fix" for their asthma, rather than using controller medications in a preventive manner. It is helpful to monitor the frequency of SABA use, in that use of at least 1 MDI/mo or at least 3 MDIs/year (200 inhalations/MDI) indicates inadequate asthma control and necessitates improving other aspects of asthma therapy and management.

Anticholinergic Agents

As bronchodilators, the anticholinergic agents (e.g., ipratropium bromide) are less potent than the β-agonists. Inhaled ipratropium is used primarily in the treatment of acute severe asthma. When used in combination with albuterol, ipratropium can improve lung function and reduce the rate of hospitalization in children who present to the ED with acute asthma. Ipratropium has few central nervous system adverse effects and is available in both MDI and nebulizer formulations. Although widely used in all children with asthma exacerbations, it is FDA approved for use in children >12 yr old. A combination ipratropium/albuterol product is also available in both nebulized (generic and Duoneb) and mist formulations (Combivent Respimat).

Delivery Devices and Inhalation Technique

Inhaled medications are delivered in aerosolized form in a MDI, as a DPI formulation, or in a suspension form delivered via a nebulizer. **Spacer devices**, recommended for the administration of all MDI medications, are simple and inexpensive tools that (1) decrease the coordination required to use MDIs, especially in young children; (2) improve the delivery of inhaled drug to the lower airways; and (3) minimize the risk of drug and propellant-mediated oropharyngeal adverse effects (dysphonia and thrush). Optimal inhalation technique for each puff of MDI-delivered medication is a slow (5 sec) inhalation, then a 5-10 sec breathhold. No waiting time is required between puffs of medication. Preschool-age children cannot perform this inhalation technique. As a result, MDI medications in this age-group are delivered with a spacer and mask, using a different technique: Each puff is administered with regular breathing for about 30 sec or 5-10 breaths; a tight seal must be maintained; and talking, coughing, or crying will blow the medication out of the spacer. This technique will not deliver as much medication per puff as the optimal MDI technique used by older children and adults.

Dry powder inhaler devices (e.g., Diskus, Flexhaler, Autohaler, Twisthaler, Aerolizer, Ellipta) are popular because of their simplicity of use, although adequate inspiratory flow is needed. DPIs are breath-actuated devices (the drug comes out only as it is breathed in), and spacers are not needed. Mouth rinsing is recommended after ICS use to remove ICS deposited on the oral mucosa and reduce the swallowed ICS and the risk of thrush.

Nebulizers are the mainstay of aerosol treatment for infants and young children. An advantage of using nebulizers is the simple technique required of relaxed breathing. The preferential nasal breathing, small airways, low tidal volume, and high respiratory rate of infants greatly increase the difficulty of inhaled drug therapy targeting the lung airways. Disadvantages of nebulizers include need for a power source, inconvenience in that treatments take about 5 min, expense, and potential for bacterial contamination.

Asthma Exacerbations and Their Management

Asthma exacerbations are acute or subacute episodes of progressively worsening symptoms and airflow obstruction. Airflow obstruction during exacerbations can become extensive, resulting in life-threatening respiratory insufficiency. Often, asthma exacerbations worsen during sleep (between midnight and 8 AM), when airways inflammation and hyperresponsiveness are at their peak. Importantly, SABAs, which are first-line therapy for asthma symptoms and exacerbations, increase pulmonary blood flow through obstructed, unoxygenated areas of the lungs with increasing dosage and frequency. When airways obstruction is not resolved with SABA use, ventilation/perfusion mismatching can cause hypoxemia, which can perpetuate bronchoconstriction and further worsen the condition. Severe, progressive asthma exacerbations need to be managed in a medical setting, with administration of supplemental oxygen as first-line therapy and close monitoring for potential worsening. Complications that can occur during severe exacerbations include atelectasis (common) and air leaks in the chest (pneumomediastinum, pneumothorax; rare).

A severe exacerbation of asthma that does not improve with standard therapy is termed **status asthmaticus**. Immediate management of an asthma exacerbation involves a rapid evaluation of the severity of obstruction and assessment of risk for further clinical deterioration (Fig. 169.8; see Tables 169.14 and 169.15). For most patients, exacerbations improve with frequent bronchodilator treatments and a course of systemic (oral or intravenous) corticosteroid. However, the optimal management of a child with an asthma exacerbation should include a more comprehensive assessment of the events leading up to the exacerbation and the underlying disease severity. Indeed, the frequency and severity of asthma exacerbations help define the severity of a patient's asthma. Whereas most children who experience life-threatening asthma episodes have moderate to severe asthma by other criteria, some children with asthma appear to have mild disease except when they have severe, even near-fatal exacerbations. The biologic, environmental, economic, and psychosocial risk factors associated with asthma morbidity and death can further guide this assessment (Table 169.16).

Asthma exacerbations characteristically vary among individuals but tend to be similar in the same patient. Severe asthma exacerbations, resulting in respiratory distress, hypoxia, hospitalization, and respiratory failure, are the best predictors of future life-threatening exacerbations or a fatal asthma episode. In addition to distinguishing such high-risk children, some experience exacerbations that develop over days, with airflow obstruction resulting from progressive inflammation, epithelial sloughing, and cast impaction of small airways. When such a process is extreme, respiratory failure as a result of fatigue can ensue, necessitating mechanical ventilation for numerous days. In contrast, some children experience abrupt-onset exacerbations that may result from extreme AHR and physiologic susceptibility to airways closure. Such exacerbations, when extreme, are asphyxial in nature, often occur outside medical settings, are initially associated with very high arterial partial pressure of carbon dioxide (PCO_2) levels, and tend to require only brief periods of supportive ventilation. Recognizing the characteristic differences in asthma exacerbations is important for optimizing their early management.

Home Management of Asthma Exacerbations

Families of all children with asthma should have a **written Asthma Action Plan** (see Fig. 169.7) to guide their recognition and management of exacerbations, along with the necessary medications and tools to manage them. Early recognition of asthma exacerbations in order to intensify treatment early can often prevent further worsening and keep exacerbations from becoming severe. A written home action plan can reduce the risk of asthma death by 70%. The NIH guidelines recommend immediate treatment with "rescue" medication (inhaled SABA, up to 3 treatments in 1 hr). A good response is characterized by resolution of symptoms within 1 hr, no further symptoms over the next 4 hr, and improvement in PEF value to at least 80% of personal best. The child's physician should be contacted for follow-up, especially if bronchodilators are required

Table 169.15	Management of Asthma Exacerbation (Status Asthmaticus)

RISK ASSESSMENT ON ADMISSION

Focused history	Onset of current exacerbation
	Frequency and severity of daytime and nighttime symptoms and activity limitation
	Frequency of rescue bronchodilator use
	Current medications and allergies
	Potential triggers
	History of systemic steroid courses, emergency department visits, hospitalization, intubation, or life-threatening episodes
Clinical assessment	Physical examination findings: vital signs, breathlessness, air movement, use of accessory muscles, retractions, anxiety level, alteration in mental status
	Pulse oximetry
	Lung function (defer in patients with moderate to severe distress or history of labile disease)
Risk factors for asthma morbidity and death	See Table 169.16.

TREATMENT

Drug and Trade Name	Mechanisms of Action and Dosing	Cautions and Adverse Effects
Oxygen (mask or nasal cannula)	Treats hypoxia	Monitor pulse oximetry to maintain O_2 saturation >92% Cardiorespiratory monitoring
Inhaled short-acting β-agonists:	Bronchodilator	During exacerbations, frequent or continuous doses can cause pulmonary vasodilation, $\dot{V}/\dot{Q}$ mismatch, and hypoxemia. Adverse effects: palpitations, tachycardia, arrhythmias, tremor, hypoxemia
Albuterol nebulizer solution (5 mg/mL concentrate; 2.5 mg/3 mL, 1.25 mg/3 mL, 0.63 mg/3 mL)	Nebulizer: 0.15 mg/kg (minimum 2.5 mg) as often as every 20 min for 3 doses as needed, then 0.15-0.3 mg/kg up to 10 mg every 1-4 hr as needed, or up to 0.5 mg/kg/hr by continuous nebulization	Nebulizer: when giving concentrated forms, dilute with saline to 3 mL total nebulized volume.
Albuterol MDI (90 μg/puff)	2-8 puffs up to every 20 min for 3 doses as needed, then every 1-4 hr as needed	For MDI: use spacer/holding chamber
Levalbuterol (Xopenex) nebulizer solution (1.25 mg/0.5 mL concentrate; 0.31 mg/3 mL, 0.63 mg/3 mL, 1.25 mg/3 mL)	0.075 mg/kg (minimum 1.25 mg) every 20 min for 3 doses, then 0.075-0.15 mg/kg up to 5 mg every 1-4 hr as needed, or 0.25 mg/kg/hr by continuous nebulization	Levalbuterol 0.63 mg is equivalent to 1.25 mg of standard albuterol for both efficacy and side effects.
Systemic corticosteroids:	Antiinflammatory	If patient has been exposed to chickenpox or measles, consider passive immunoglobulin prophylaxis; also, risk of complications with herpes simplex and tuberculosis. For daily dosing, 8 AM administration minimizes adrenal suppression. Children may benefit from dosage tapering if course exceeds 7 days. Adverse effects monitoring: frequent therapy bursts risk numerous corticosteroid adverse effects (see Chapter 595); see Table 169.14 for adverse effects screening recommendations.
Prednisone: 1, 2.5, 5, 10, 20, 50 mg tablets Methylprednisolone (Medrol): 2, 4, 8, 16, 24, 32 mg tablets Prednisolone: 5 mg tablets; 5 mg/5 mL and 15 mg/5 mL solution	0.5-1 mg/kg every 6-12 hr for 48 hr, then 1-2 mg/kg/day bid (maximum 60 mg/day)	
Depo-Medrol (IM); Solu-Medrol (IV)	Short-course "burst" for exacerbation: 1-2 mg/kg/day qd or bid for 3-7 days	
Dexamethasone	See text	See text
Anticholinergics:	Mucolytic/bronchodilator	Should not be used as first-line therapy; added to β₂-agonist therapy
Ipratropium: Atrovent (nebulizer solution 0.5 mg/2.5 mL; MDI 18 μg/inhalation)	Nebulizer: 0.5 mg q6-8h (tid-qid) as needed MDI: 2 puffs qid	
Ipratropium with albuterol: DuoNeb nebulizer solution (0.5 mg ipratropium + 2.5 mg albuterol/3 mL vial)	1 vial by nebulizer qid	Nebulizer: may mix ipratropium with albuterol
Injectable sympathomimetic epinephrine:	Bronchodilator	For extreme circumstances (e.g., impending respiratory failure despite high-dose inhaled SABA, respiratory failure)
Adrenalin 1 mg/mL (1:1000) EpiPen autoinjection device (0.3 mg; EpiPen Jr 0.15 mg)	SC or IM: 0.01 mg/kg (max dose 0.5 mg); may repeat after 15-30 min	

Continued

Table 169.15	Management of Asthma Exacerbation (Status Asthmaticus)—cont'd	
Terbutaline:		Terbutaline is β-agonist–selective relative to epinephrine. Monitoring with continuous infusion: cardiorespiratory monitor, pulse oximetry, blood pressure, serum potassium Adverse effects: tremor, tachycardia, palpitations, arrhythmia, hypertension, headaches, nervousness, nausea, vomiting, hypoxemia
Brethine 1 mg/mL	Continuous IV infusion (terbutaline only): 2-10 µg/kg loading dose, followed by 0.1-0.4 µg/kg/min Titrate in 0.1-0.2 µg/kg/min increments every 30 min, depending on clinical response.	
RISK ASSESSMENT FOR DISCHARGE		
Medical stability	Discharge home if there has been sustained improvement in symptoms and bronchodilator treatments are at least 3 hr apart, physical findings are normal, PEF >70% of predicted or personal best, and oxygen saturation >92% when breathing room air.	
Home supervision	Capability to administer intervention and to observe and respond appropriately to clinical deterioration	
Asthma education	See Table 169.8.	

IM, Intramuscular; MDI, metered-dose inhaler; PEF, peak expiratory flow; SABA, short-acting β-agonist; SC, subcutaneous; V̇/Q̇, ventilation/perfusion; bid, 2 times daily; tid, 3 times daily; qid; 4 times daily; qd, every day.

repeatedly over the next 24-48 hr. If the child has an incomplete response to initial treatment with rescue medication (persistent symptoms and/or PEF <80% of personal best), a short course of OCS therapy (prednisone, 1-2 mg/kg/day [not to exceed 60 mg/day] for 4 days) should be instituted, in addition to inhaled β-agonist therapy. The physician should also be contacted for further instructions. Immediate medical attention should be sought for severe exacerbations, persistent signs of respiratory distress, lack of expected response or sustained improvement after initial treatment, further deterioration, or high-risk factors for asthma morbidity or mortality (e.g., previous history of severe exacerbations). For patients with severe asthma and/or a history of life-threatening episodes, especially if abrupt in onset, an epinephrine autoinjector and perhaps portable oxygen at home can be considered. Use of either of these extreme measures for home management of asthma exacerbations would be an indication to call 911 for emergency support services.

Emergency Department Management of Asthma Exacerbations

In the ED, the primary goals of asthma management include correction of hypoxemia, rapid improvement of airflow obstruction, and prevention of progression or recurrence of symptoms. Interventions are based on clinical severity on arrival, response to initial therapy, and presence of risk factors associated with asthma morbidity and mortality (see Table 169.16). Indications of a severe exacerbation include breathlessness, dyspnea, retractions, accessory muscle use, tachypnea or labored breathing, cyanosis, mental status changes, a silent chest with poor air exchange, and severe airflow limitation (PEF or FEV_1 value <50% of personal best or predicted values). Initial treatment includes supplemental oxygen, inhaled β-agonist therapy every 20 min for 1 hr, and, if necessary, oral or intravenous (IV) systemic corticosteroids (see Table 169.15 and Fig. 169.8). In the ED, single oral, intravenous, or intramuscular (IM) dose dexamethasone (0.6 mg/kg, maximum 16 mg) has been found to be an effective alternative to prednisone and with a lower incidence of emesis. In addition, a second dose of dexamethasone should be given the next day whether discharged or admitted to the hospital. Inhaled ipratropium may be added to the β-agonist treatment if no significant response is seen with the 1st inhaled β-agonist treatment. An IM injection of epinephrine or other β-agonist may be administered in severe cases. Oxygen should be administered and continued for at least 20 min after

Table 169.16	Risk Factors for Asthma Morbidity and Mortality

BIOLOGIC
Previous severe asthma exacerbation (intensive care unit admission, intubation for asthma)
Sudden asphyxia episodes (respiratory failure, arrest)
Two or more hospitalizations for asthma in past year
Three or more emergency department visits for asthma in past year
Increasing and large diurnal variation in peak flows
Use of >2 canisters of short-acting β-agonists per month
Poor response to systemic corticosteroid therapy
Male gender
Low birthweight
Nonwhite (especially black) ethnicity
Sensitivity to *Alternaria*

ENVIRONMENTAL
Allergen exposure
Environmental tobacco smoke exposure
Air pollution exposure
Urban environment

ECONOMIC AND PSYCHOSOCIAL
Poverty
Crowding
Mother <20 yr old
Mother with less than high school education
Inadequate medical care:
    Inaccessible
    Unaffordable
    No regular medical care (only emergency)
    Lack of written Asthma Action Plan
    No care sought for chronic asthma symptoms
    Delay in care of asthma exacerbations
    Inadequate hospital care for asthma exacerbation
Psychopathology in the parent or child
Poor perception of asthma symptoms or severity
Alcohol or substance abuse

Follow this plan for After Hours patients only. Nurse may decide not to follow this home management plan if:
- Parent does not seem comfortable with or capable of following plan
- Nurse is not comfortable with this plan, based on situation and judgment
- Nurse's time does not allow for callbacks

In all cases, tell parent to call 9-1-1 if signs of respiratory distress occur during the episode
NOTE: If action plan has already been attempted without success, go to "RED ZONE — poor response" or "YELLOW ZONE — incomplete response" as symptoms indicate.

Assess symptoms/peak flow

YELLOW ZONE
Mild-to-moderate exacerbation
PEF 50–80% predicted or personal best
or
Signs and symptoms
- Coughing, shortness of breath or chest tightness (correlate imperfectly with severity of exacerbation), or
- Unable to sleep at night due to asthma, or
- Decreased ability to perform usual activities
- With or without wheezing

RED ZONE
Severe exacerbation
PEF < 50% predicted or personal best or
Signs and symptoms
- Very hard time breathing; constant coughing
- Trouble walking or talking due to asthma (unable to complete sentences; only using 2- to 3-word phrases)
- Nails blue
- Suprasternal or supraclavicular retractions
- Albuterol not relieving symptoms within 10–15 minutes
- With or without wheezing

Instructions to patient
Inhaled short-acting β_2-agonist:
- 2–4 puffs of inhaler or nebulizer treatment every 20 minutes up to 3 times in 1 hour
- Assess asthma symptoms and/or peak flow 15–20 minutes after each treatment
- Nurse to call family after 1 hour
- If patient worsens during treatment, have parent call back immediately or call 9-1-1

GREEN ZONE — Good response
Mild exacerbation
PEF > 80% predicted or personal best
or
Signs and symptoms
- No wheezing, shortness of breath, cough or chest tightness, and
- Response to β_2-agonist sustained for 4 hours

YELLOW ZONE — Incomplete response
Moderate exacerbation PEF 50–80% predicted or personal best
or
Signs and symptoms
- Persistent wheezing, shortness of breath, cough or chest tightness

RED ZONE — Poor response
Severe exacerbation
PEF < 50% predicted or personal best
or
Signs and symptoms
- Marked wheezing, shortness of breath, cough, or chest tightness
- Distress is severe and nonresponsive
- Response to β_2-agonist last < 2 hours
Instructions to patient
- Proceed to ED, or call ambulance or 9-1-1 and repeat treatment while waiting

Instructions to patient
- May continue 2–4 puffs (or nebulizer) β_2-agonist every 3–4 hours for 24–28 hours prn
- For patients on inhaled steroids, double dose for 7–10 days
- Contact PCP within 48 hours for instructions

Instructions to patient
- Take 2–4 puffs (or nebulizer) β_2-agonist every 2–4 hours for 24–48 hours prn
- Add oral steroid* (see contraindications below)
- Contact PCP urgently (within 24 hours) for instructions

Instructions to patient
IMMEDIATELY:
- Take 4-6 puffs (or nebulizer) β_2-agonist
- Start oral steroids* if available (see contraindications below)
- Instruct parent to call back in 5 minutes after treatment finished
- If still in **RED ZONE** proceed to ED, or call ambulance or 9-1-1 and repeat treatment while waiting
- If in **YELLOW ZONE**, move to **YELLOW ZONE** protocol (top left box)

Documentation faxed or given to PCP within 24 hours; phone or verbal contact sooner as indicated.
* Ask patient about preexisting conditions that may be contraindications to oral steroids (including type 1 diabetes, active chicken pox, chicken pox exposure or varicella vaccine within 21 days, MMR within 14 days). If so, nurse to contact PCP before initiating steroids. Oral steroid dosages: Child: 2 mg/kg/day, maximum 60 mg/day, for 5 days.

Date: _____

Signature _____

Fig. 169.8 Algorithm for treatment of acute asthma symptoms. PEF, Peak expiratory flow; ED, emergency department; PCP, primary care physician. *(Courtesy of BJC Healthcare/Washington University School of Medicine, Community Asthma Program, January 2000.)*

SABA administration to compensate for possible ventilation/perfusion abnormalities caused by SABAs.

Close monitoring of clinical status, hydration, and oxygenation are essential elements of immediate management. A poor response to intensified treatment in the 1st hr suggests that the exacerbation will not remit quickly. The patient may be discharged home if there is sustained improvement in symptoms, normal physical findings, PEF >70% of predicted or personal best, and oxygen saturation >92% while the patient is breathing room air for 4 hr. Discharge medications include administration of an inhaled β-agonist up to every 3-4 hr plus a 3-7 day course of an OCS. Optimizing controller therapy before discharge is also recommended. The addition of ICS to a course of OCS in the ED setting reduces the risk of exacerbation recurrence over the subsequent month.

Hospital Management of Asthma Exacerbations

For patients with severe exacerbations that do not adequately improve within 1-2 hr of intensive treatment, observation and/or admission to the hospital, at least overnight, is likely to be needed. Other indications for hospital admission include high-risk features for asthma morbidity or death (see Table 169.16). Admission to an intensive care unit (ICU) is indicated for patients with severe respiratory distress, poor response to therapy, and concern for potential respiratory failure and arrest.

Supplemental oxygen, frequent or continuous administration of an inhaled bronchodilator, and systemic corticosteroid therapy are the conventional interventions for children admitted to the hospital for status asthmaticus (see Table 169.15). Supplemental oxygen is administered because many children hospitalized with acute asthma have or eventually have hypoxemia, especially at night and with increasing SABA administration. SABAs can be delivered frequently (every 20 min to 1 hr) or continuously (at 5-15 mg/hr). When administered continuously, significant systemic absorption of β-agonist occurs, and thus continuous nebulization can obviate the need for IV β-agonist therapy. Adverse effects of frequently administered β-agonist therapy include tremor, irritability, tachycardia, and hypokalemia; lactic acidosis is an uncommon complication. Patients requiring frequent or continuous nebulized β-agonist therapy should have ongoing cardiac monitoring. Because frequent β-agonist therapy can cause ventilation/perfusion mismatch and hypoxemia, oximetry is also indicated. Inhaled ipratropium is often added to albuterol every 6 hr if patients do not show a remarkable improvement, although there is little evidence to support its use in hospitalized children receiving aggressive inhaled β-agonist therapy and systemic corticosteroids. In addition to its potential to provide a synergistic effect with a β-agonist agent in relieving severe bronchospasm, ipratropium may be beneficial in patients who have mucus hypersecretion or who are receiving β-blockers.

Short-course systemic corticosteroid therapy is recommended for use in moderate to severe asthma exacerbations to hasten recovery and prevent recurrence of symptoms. Corticosteroids are effective as single doses administered in the ED, short courses in the clinic setting, and both oral and IV formulations in hospitalized children. Studies in children hospitalized with acute asthma have found corticosteroids administered orally to be as effective as IV corticosteroids. Accordingly, OCS therapy can often be used, although children with sustained respiratory distress and those unable to tolerate oral preparations or liquids are obvious candidates for IV corticosteroid therapy.

Patients with persistent severe dyspnea and high-flow oxygen requirements require additional evaluation, such as complete blood count, arterial blood gases, serum electrolytes, and chest radiograph, to monitor for respiratory insufficiency, comorbidities, infection, and dehydration. Hydration status monitoring is especially important in infants and young children, whose increased respiratory rate (insensible losses) and decreased oral intake put them at higher risk for dehydration. Further complicating this situation is the association of increased antidiuretic hormone secretion with status asthmaticus. Administration of fluids at or slightly below maintenance fluid requirements is recommended. Chest physical therapy, incentive spirometry, and mucolytics are not recommended during the early acute period of asthma exacerbations because they can trigger severe bronchoconstriction.

Despite intensive therapy, some asthmatic children remain critically ill and at risk for respiratory failure, intubation, and mechanical ventilation. Complications (e.g., air leaks) related to asthma exacerbations increase with intubation and assisted ventilation, so every effort should be made to relieve bronchospasm and prevent respiratory failure. Several therapies, including parenteral β-agonists, magnesium sulfate (25-75 mg/kg, maximum dose 2.5 g, given intravenously over 20 min) and inhaled heliox (helium and oxygen mixture) have demonstrated some benefit as adjunctive therapies in patients with severe status asthmaticus. Administration of magnesium sulfate requires monitoring of serum levels and cardiovascular status. Parenteral (SC, IM, or IV) epinephrine or terbutaline sulfate may be effective in patients with life-threatening obstruction that is not responding to high doses of inhaled β-agonists, because inhaled medication may not reach the lower airway in such patients.

Rarely, a severe asthma exacerbation in a child results in respiratory failure, and intubation and mechanical ventilation become necessary. **Mechanical ventilation** in severe asthma exacerbations requires the careful balance of enough pressure to overcome airways obstruction while reducing hyperinflation, air trapping, and the likelihood of barotrauma (pneumothorax, pneumomediastinum) (see Chapter 439). To minimize the likelihood of such complications, mechanical ventilation should be anticipated, and asthmatic children at risk for the development of respiratory failure should be managed in a pediatric ICU. Elective tracheal intubation with rapid-induction sedatives and paralytic agents is safer than emergency intubation. Mechanical ventilation aims to achieve adequate oxygenation while tolerating mild to moderate hypercapnia (PCO_2 50-70 mm Hg) to minimize barotrauma. Volume-cycled ventilators, using short inspiratory and long expiratory times, 10-15 mL/kg tidal volume, 8-15 breaths/min, peak pressures <60 cm H_2O, and without positive end-expiratory pressure are starting mechanical ventilation parameters that can achieve these goals. As measures to relieve mucus plugs, chest percussion and airways lavage are not recommended because they can induce further bronchospasm. One must consider the nature of asthma exacerbations leading to respiratory failure; those of rapid or abrupt onset tend to resolve quickly (hours to 2 days), whereas those that progress gradually to respiratory failure can require days to weeks of mechanical ventilation. Such prolonged cases are further complicated by corticosteroid-induced myopathy, which can lead to severe muscle weakness requiring prolonged rehabilitation.

In children, management of severe exacerbations in medical centers is usually successful, even when extreme measures are required. Consequently, asthma deaths in children rarely occur in medical centers; most occur at home or in community settings before lifesaving medical care can be administered. This point highlights the importance of home and community management of asthma exacerbations, early intervention measures to keep exacerbations from becoming severe, and steps to reduce asthma severity. A follow-up appointment within 1-2 wk of a child's discharge from the hospital after resolution of an asthma exacerbation should be used to monitor clinical improvement and to reinforce key educational elements, including action plans and controller medications.

Special Management Circumstances
Management of Infants and Young Children

Recurrent wheezing episodes in preschool-age children are common, occurring in as much as one third of this population. Of these, most improve and even become asymptomatic during the prepubescent school-age years, whereas others have lifelong persistent asthma. All require management of their recurrent wheezing problems (see Tables 169.5, 169.6, and 169.11). The NIH guidelines recommend risk assessment to identify preschool-age children who are likely to have persistent asthma. One implication of this recommendation is that these at-risk children may be candidates for conventional asthma management, including daily controller therapy and early intervention with exacerbations (see Tables 169.7, 169.8, and 169.11). For young children with a history of moderate to severe exacerbations, nebulized budesonide is FDA approved, and its use as a controller medication could prevent subsequent exacerbations.

Using aerosol therapy in infants and young children with asthma presents unique challenges. There are 2 delivery systems for inhaled medications for this age-group: the nebulizer and the MDI with spacer/holding chamber and face mask. Multiple studies demonstrate the effectiveness of both nebulized albuterol in acute episodes and nebulized budesonide in the treatment of recurrent wheezing in infants and young children. In such young children, inhaled medications administered via MDI with spacer and face mask may be acceptable, although perhaps not preferred because of limited published information and lack of FDA approval for children <4 yr of age.

Asthma Management During Surgery

Patients with asthma are at risk from disease-related complications from surgery, such as bronchoconstriction and asthma exacerbation, atelectasis, impaired coughing, respiratory infection, and latex exposure, which may induce asthma complications in patients with latex allergy. All patients with asthma should be evaluated before surgery, and those who are inadequately controlled should allow time for intensified treatment to improve asthma stability before surgery, if possible. A systemic corticosteroid course may be indicated for the patient who is having symptoms and/or FEV_1 or PEF values <80% of the patient's personal best. In addition, patients who have received >2 wk of systemic corticosteroid and/or moderate- to high-dose ICS therapy may be at risk for intraoperative adrenal insufficiency. For these patients, anesthesia services should be alerted to provide "stress" replacement doses of systemic corticosteroid for the surgical procedure and possibly the postoperative period.

PROGNOSIS

Recurrent coughing and wheezing occurs in 35% of preschool-age children. Of these, approximately one third continue to have persistent asthma into later childhood, and approximately two thirds improve on their own through their teen years. Asthma severity by ages 7-10 yr is predictive of asthma persistence in adulthood. Children with moderate to severe asthma and with lower lung function measures are likely to have persistent asthma as adults. Children with milder asthma and normal lung function are likely to improve over time, with some becoming periodically asthmatic (disease-free for months to years); however, complete remission for 5 yr in childhood is uncommon.

PREVENTION

Although chronic airways inflammation may result in pathologic remodeling of lung airways, conventional antiinflammatory interventions—the cornerstone of asthma control—do not help children outgrow their asthma. Although controller medications reduce asthma morbidities, most children with moderate to severe asthma continue to have symptoms into young adulthood. Investigations into the environmental and lifestyle factors responsible for the lower prevalence of childhood asthma in rural areas and farming communities suggest that early immunomodulatory intervention might prevent asthma development. A *hygiene hypothesis* purports that naturally occurring microbial exposures in early life might drive early immune development away from allergic sensitization, persistent airways inflammation, and remodeling through early microbiome and innate immune development. If these natural microbial exposures truly have an asthma-protective effect, without significant adverse health consequences, these findings may foster new strategies for asthma prevention.

Several nonpharmacotherapeutic measures with numerous positive health attributes—avoidance of environmental tobacco smoke (beginning prenatally), prolonged breastfeeding (>4 mo), an active lifestyle, and a healthy diet—might reduce the likelihood of asthma development. Immunizations are currently not considered to increase the likelihood of development of asthma; therefore all standard childhood immunizations are recommended for children with asthma, including varicella and annual influenza vaccines.

Bibliography is available at Expert Consult.

Chapter **170**
Atopic Dermatitis (Atopic Eczema)
Donald Y.M. Leung and Scott H. Sicherer

第一百七十章
特应性皮炎（特应性湿疹）

中文导读

　　本章主要介绍了特应性皮炎的发病率、病因、病理、发病机制、临床表现、实验室检查、诊断与鉴别诊断、治疗、避免触发因素、并发症、目前的研究进展概述以及预防。具体描述了遗传因素和皮肤屏障的作用；阐述了急性期皮肤损伤的病理表现；发病机制方面介绍了主要细胞和细胞因子的变化，FLG基因突变对于皮肤屏障功能损伤的作用；描述了诱发因素、不同类型特应性皮炎的临床表现；实验室检查方面介绍了有价值的辅助检查。介绍了常见的鉴别诊断；治疗上具体描述了水化、局部抗炎以及目前一些未经证实的方法；阐述了可能诱发疾病的常见触发因素如刺激物、食物、空气变应原；介绍了剥脱性皮炎和眼疾病等；具体描述了特应性皮炎随年龄的进展变化；预防方面介绍了母乳喂养、益生菌、消除触发因素、皮肤保湿等。

Atopic dermatitis (AD), or eczema, is the most common chronic relapsing skin disease seen in infancy and childhood. It affects 10–30% of children worldwide and frequently occurs in families with other atopic diseases. Infants with AD are predisposed to development of food allergy, allergic rhinitis, and asthma later in childhood, a process called *the atopic march.*

ETIOLOGY

AD is a complex genetic disorder that results in a defective skin barrier, reduced skin innate immune responses, and polarized adaptive immune responses to environmental allergens and microbes that lead to chronic skin inflammation.

PATHOLOGY

Acute AD skin lesions are characterized by **spongiosis**, or marked intercellular edema, of the epidermis. In AD, dendritic antigen-presenting cells (APCs) in the epidermis, such as Langerhans cells, exhibit surface-bound IgE molecules with cell processes that reach into upper epidermis to sense allergens and pathogens. These APCs play an important role in cutaneous responses to type 2 immune responses (see Chapter 166). There is marked perivenular T-cell and inflammatory monocyte-macrophage infiltration in acute AD lesions. Chronic, lichenified AD is characterized by a hyperplastic epidermis with hyperkeratosis and minimal spongiosis. There are predominantly IgE-bearing Langerhans cells in the epidermis, and macrophages in the dermal mononuclear cell infiltrate. Mast cell and eosinophil numbers are increased, contributing to skin inflammation.

PATHOGENESIS

AD is associated with multiple phenotypes and endotypes that have overlapping clinical presentations. **Atopic eczema** is associated with IgE-mediated sensitization (at onset or during the course of eczema) and occurs in 70–80% of patients with AD. **Nonatopic eczema** is not associated with IgE-mediated sensitization and is seen in 20–30% of patients with AD. Both forms of AD are associated with eosinophilia. In atopic eczema, circulating T cells expressing the skin homing receptor **cutaneous lymphocyte-associated antigen** produce increased levels of T-helper type 2 (Th2) cytokines, including interleukin (IL)-4 and IL-13, which induce isotype switching to IgE synthesis. Another cytokine, IL-5, plays an important role in eosinophil development and survival. Nonatopic eczema is associated with lower IL-4 and IL-13 but increased IL-17 and IL-23 production than in atopic eczema. Age and race have also been found to affect the immune profile in AD.

Compared with the skin of healthy individuals, both unaffected skin and acute skin lesions of patients with AD have an increased number of cells expressing IL-4 and IL-13. Chronic AD skin lesions, by contrast, have fewer cells that express IL-4 and IL-13, but increased numbers of cells that express IL-5, granulocyte-macrophage colony-stimulating factor, IL-12, and interferon (IFN)-γ than acute AD lesions. Despite increased type 1 and type 17 immune responses in chronic AD, IL-4 and IL-13 as well as other type 2 cytokines (e.g. TSLP, IL-31, IL-33) predominate and reflect increased numbers of Type 2 innate lymphoid cells and Th2 cells. The infiltration of IL-22–expressing T cells correlates with severity of AD, blocks keratinocyte differentiation, and induces epidermal hyperplasia. The importance of IL-4 and IL-13 in driving severe persistent AD has been validated by multiple clinical trials now demonstrating that biologics blocking IL-4 and IL-13 action lead to clinical improvement in moderate to severe AD.

In healthy people the skin acts as a protective barrier against external irritants, moisture loss, and infection. Proper function of the skin depends on adequate moisture and lipid content, functional immune responses, and structural integrity. *Severely dry skin is a hallmark of AD.* This results from compromise of the epidermal barrier, which leads to excess transepidermal water loss, allergen penetration, and microbial colonization. **Filaggrin**, a structural protein in the epidermis, and its breakdown products are critical to skin barrier function, including moisturization of the skin. Genetic mutations in the filaggrin gene *(FLG)* family have been identified in patients with ichthyosis vulgaris (dry skin, palmar hyperlinearity) and in up to 50% of patients with severe AD. *FLG* mutation is strongly associated with development of food allergy and eczema herpeticum. Nonetheless, up to 60% of carriers of a *FLG* mutation do not develop atopic diseases. Cytokines found in allergic inflammation, such as IL-4, IL-13, IL-22, IL-25, and tumor necrosis factor, can also reduce filaggrin and other epidermal proteins and lipids. AD patients are at increased risk of bacterial, viral, and fungal infection related to impairment of innate immunity, disturbances in the microbiome, skin epithelial dysfunction, and overexpression of polarized immune pathways, which dampen host antimicrobial responses.

CLINICAL MANIFESTATIONS

AD typically begins in infancy. Approximately 50% of patients experience symptoms in the 1st yr of life, and an additional 30% are diagnosed between 1 and 5 yr of age. Intense **pruritus**, especially at night, and **cutaneous reactivity** are the cardinal features of AD. Scratching and excoriation cause increased skin inflammation that contributes to the development of more pronounced eczematous skin lesions. Foods (cow's milk, egg, peanut, tree nuts, soy, wheat, fish, shellfish), aeroallergens (pollen, grass, animal dander, dust mites), infection (*Staphylococcus aureus*, herpes simplex, coxsackievirus, molluscum), reduced humidity,

Table 170.1	Clinical Features of Atopic Dermatitis

MAJOR FEATURES
Pruritus
Facial and extensor eczema in infants and children
Flexural eczema in adolescents
Chronic or relapsing dermatitis
Personal or family history of atopic disease

ASSOCIATED FEATURES
Xerosis
Cutaneous infections (*Staphylococcus aureus*, group A streptococcus, herpes simplex, coxsackievirus, vaccinia, molluscum, warts)
Nonspecific dermatitis of the hands or feet
Ichthyosis, palmar hyperlinearity, keratosis pilaris
Nipple eczema
White dermatographism and delayed blanch response
Anterior subcapsular cataracts, keratoconus
Elevated serum IgE levels
Positive results of immediate-type allergy skin tests
Early age at onset
Dennie lines (Dennie-Morgan infraorbital folds)
Facial erythema or pallor
Course influenced by environmental and/or emotional factors

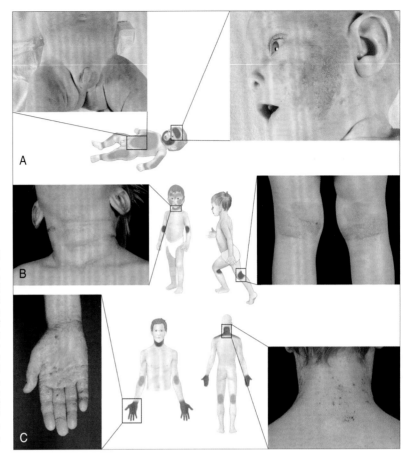

Fig. 170.1 Typical clinical appearance and locations of atopic dermatitis at different ages. **Top row,** In infants, atopic dermatitis is generally acute, with lesions mainly on the face and the extensor surfaces of the limbs. The trunk might be affected, but the napkin area is typically spared. **Middle row,** From age 1-2 yr onward, polymorphous manifestations with different types of skin lesions are seen, particularly in flexural folds. **Bottom row,** Adolescents and adults often present lichenified and excoriated plaques at flexures, wrists, ankles, and eyelids; in the head and neck type, the upper trunk, shoulders, and scalp are involved. Adults might have only chronic hand eczema or present with prurigo-like lesions. *(From Weidinger S, Novak N: Atopic dermatitis, Lancet 387:1111, 2016.)*

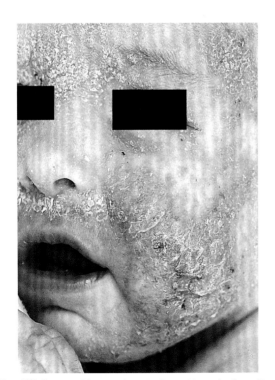

Fig. 170.2 Crusted lesions of atopic dermatitis on the face. *(From Eichenfield LF, Friedan IJ, Esterly NB: Textbook of neonatal dermatology, Philadelphia, 2001, Saunders, p 242.)*

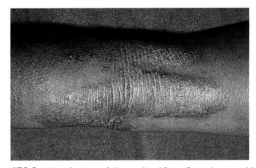

Fig. 170.3 Lichenification of the popliteal fossa from chronic rubbing of the skin in atopic dermatitis. *(From Weston WL, Lane AT, Morelli JG: Color textbook of pediatric dermatology, ed 2, St Louis, 1996, Mosby, p 33.)*

excessive sweating, and irritants (wool, acrylic, soaps, toiletries, fragrances, detergents) can trigger pruritus and scratching.

Acute AD skin lesions are intensely pruritic with erythematous papules (Figs. 170.1 and 170.2). Subacute dermatitis manifests as erythematous, excoriated, scaling papules. In contrast, chronic AD is characterized by **lichenification** (Fig. 170.3), or thickening of the skin with accentuated surface markings, and **fibrotic papules**. In chronic AD, all 3 types of skin reactions may coexist in the same individual. Most patients with AD have dry, lackluster skin regardless of their stage of illness. Skin reaction pattern and distribution vary with the patient's age and disease activity. AD is generally more acute in infancy and involves the face, scalp, and extensor surfaces of the extremities. The diaper area is usually spared. Older children and children with chronic AD have lichenification and localization of the rash to the flexural folds of the extremities. AD can go into remission as the patient grows older, however, many children with AD have persistent eczema as an adult (Fig. 170.1C).

LABORATORY FINDINGS

There are no specific laboratory tests to diagnose AD. Many patients have peripheral blood eosinophilia and increased serum IgE levels. Serum IgE measurement or skin-prick testing can identify the allergens (foods, inhalant/microbial allergens) to which patients are sensitized. The diagnosis of clinical allergy to these allergens requires confirmation by history and environmental challenges.

DIAGNOSIS AND DIFFERENTIAL DIAGNOSIS

AD is diagnosed on the basis of 3 major features: pruritus, an eczematous dermatitis that fits into a typical pattern of skin inflammation, and a chronic or chronically relapsing course (Table 170.1). Associated features,

such as a family history of asthma, hay fever, elevated IgE, and immediate skin test reactivity, reinforce the diagnosis of AD.

Many inflammatory skin diseases, immunodeficiencies, skin malignancies, genetic disorders, infectious diseases, and infestations share symptoms with AD and should be considered and excluded before a diagnosis of AD is established (Tables 170.2 and 170.3). Severe combined immunodeficiency (see Chapter 152.1) should be considered for infants presenting in the first yr of life with diarrhea, failure to thrive, generalized scaling rash, and recurrent cutaneous and/or systemic infection. Histiocytosis should be excluded in any infant with AD and failure to thrive (see Chapter 534). Wiskott-Aldrich syndrome, an X-linked recessive disorder associated with thrombocytopenia, immune defects, and recurrent severe bacterial infections, is characterized by a rash almost indistinguishable from that in AD (see Chapter 152.2). One of the hyper-IgE syndromes is characterized by markedly elevated serum IgE values, recurrent deep-seated bacterial infections, chronic

Table 170.2	Differential Diagnosis of Atopic Dermatitis (AD)		
	MAIN AGE GROUP AFFECTED	FREQUENCY*	CHARACTERISTICS AND CLINICAL FEATURES
OTHER TYPES OF DERMATITIS			
Seborrheic dermatitis	Infants	Common	Salmon-red greasy scaly lesions, often on the scalp (cradle cap) and napkin area; generally presents in the 1st 6 wk of life; typically clears within weeks
Seborrheic dermatitis	Adults	Common	Erythematous patches with yellow, white, or grayish scales in seborrheic areas, particularly the scalp, central face, and anterior chest
Nummular dermatitis	Children and adults	Common	Coin-shaped scaly patches, mostly on legs and buttocks; usually no itch
Irritant contact dermatitis	Children and adults	Common	Acute to chronic eczematous lesions, mostly confined to the site of exposure; history of locally applied irritants is a risk factor; might coexist with AD
Allergic contact dermatitis	Children and adults	Common	Eczematous rash with maximum expression at sites of direct exposure but might spread; history of locally applied irritants is a risk factor; might coexist with AD
Lichen simplex chronicus	Adults	Uncommon	One or more localized, circumscribed, lichenified plaques that result from repetitive scratching or rubbing because of intense itch
Asteatotic eczema	Adults	Common	Scaly, fissured patches of dermatitis overlying dry skin, most often on lower legs
INFECTIOUS SKIN DISEASES			
Dermatophyte infection	Children and adults	Common	One or more demarcated scaly plaques with central clearing and slightly raised reddened edge; variable itch
Impetigo	Children	Common	Demarcated erythematous patches with blisters or honey-yellow crusting
Scabies	Children	Common†	Itchy superficial burrows and pustules on palms and soles, between fingers, and on genitalia; might produce secondary eczematous changes
HIV	Children and adults	Uncommon	Seborrhea-like rash
CONGENITAL IMMUNODEFICIENCIES (see Table 170.3)			
Keratinization Disorders			
Ichthyosis vulgaris	Infants and adults	Uncommon	Dry skin with fine scaling, particularly on the lower abdomen and extensor areas; perifollicular skin roughening; palmar hyperlinearity; full form (i.e., 2 *FLG* mutations) is uncommon; often coexists with AD
NUTRITIONAL DEFICIENCY–METABOLIC DISORDERS			
Zinc deficiency (acrodermatitis enteropathica)	Children	Uncommon	Erythematous scaly patches and plaques, most often around the mouth and anus; rare congenital form accompanied by diarrhea and alopecia
Biotin deficiency (nutritional or biotinidase deficiency)	Infants	Uncommon	Scaly periorofacial dermatitis, alopecia, conjunctivitis, lethargy, hypotonia
Pellagra (niacin deficiency)	All ages	Uncommon	Scaly crusted epidermis, desquamation, sun-exposed areas, diarrhea
Kwashiorkor	Infants and children	Geographic dependent	Flaky scaly dermatitis, swollen limbs with cracked peeling patches
Phenylketonuria	Infants	Uncommon	Eczematous rash, hypopigmentation, blonde hair, developmental delay
NEOPLASTIC DISEASE			
Cutaneous T-cell lymphoma	Adults	Uncommon	Erythematous pink-brown macules and plaques with a fine scale; poorly responsive to topical corticosteroids; variable itch (in early stages)
Langerhans cell histiocytosis	Infants	Uncommon	Scaly and purpuric dermatosis, hepatosplenomegaly, cytopenias

*Common = approximately 1 in 10 to 1 in 100; uncommon = 1 in 100 to 1 in 1000; rare = 1 in 1000 to 1 in 10,000; very rare = <1 in 10,000.
†Especially in developing countries.
FLG, filaggrin gene.

dermatitis, and refractory dermatophytosis. Many of these patients have disease as a result of autosomal dominant *STAT3* mutations. In contrast, some patients with hyper-IgE syndrome present with increased susceptibility to viral infections and an autosomal recessive pattern of disease inheritance. These patients may have a *DOCK8* (dedicator of cytokinesis 8 gene) mutation. This diagnosis should be considered in young children with severe eczema, food allergy, and disseminated skin viral infections.

Adolescents who present with an eczematous dermatitis but no history of childhood eczema, respiratory allergy, or atopic family history may have allergic **contact dermatitis** (see Chapter 674.1). A contact allergen may be the problem in any patient whose AD does not respond to appropriate therapy. Sensitizing chemicals, such as parabens and lanolin, can be irritants for patients with AD and are commonly found as vehicles in therapeutic topical agents. Topical glucocorticoid contact allergy has been reported in patients with chronic dermatitis receiving topical corticosteroid therapy. Eczematous dermatitis has also been reported with HIV infection as well as with a variety of infestations such as scabies. Other conditions that can be confused with AD include psoriasis, ichthyosis, and seborrheic dermatitis.

TREATMENT

The treatment of AD requires a systematic, multifaceted approach that incorporates skin moisturization, topical antiinflammatory therapy, identification and elimination of flare factors (Table 170.4), and, if necessary, systemic therapy. Assessment of the severity also helps direct therapy (Table 170.5).

Cutaneous Hydration

Because patients with AD have impaired skin barrier function from reduced filaggrin and skin lipid levels, they present with diffuse, abnormally dry skin, or **xerosis**. *Moisturizers are first-line therapy.*

Table 170.3	Features of Primary Immunodeficiencies Associated With Eczematous Dermatitis			
DISEASE	**GENE**	**INHERITANCE**	**CLINICAL FEATURES**	**LAB ABNORMALITIES**
AD-HIES	*STAT3*	AD, less commonly sporadic	Cold abscesses Recurrent sinopulmonary infections Mucocutaneous candidiasis Coarse facies Minimal trauma fractures Scoliosis Joint hyperextensibility Retained primary teeth Coronary artery tortuosity or dilation Lymphoma	High IgE (>2000 IU/µL) Eosinophilia
DOCK8 deficiency	*DOCK8*	AR	Severe mucocutaneous viral infections Mucocutaneous candidiasis Atopic features (asthma, allergies) Squamous cell carcinoma Lymphoma	High IgE Eosinophilia With or without decreased IgM
PGM3 deficiency	*PGM3*	AR	Neurologic abnormalities Leukocytoclastic vasculitis Atopic features (asthma, allergies) Sinopulmonary infections Mucocutaneous viral infections	High IgE Eosinophilia
WAS	*WASP*	XLR	Hepatosplenomegaly Lymphadenopathy Atopic diathesis Autoimmune conditions (especially hemolytic anemia) Lymphoreticular malignancies	Thrombocytopenia (<80,000/µL) Low mean platelet volume Eosinophilia is common Lymphopenia Low IgM, variable IgG
SCID	Variable, depends on type	XLR and AR most common	Recurrent, severe infections Failure to thrive Persistent diarrhea Recalcitrant oral candidiasis Omenn syndrome: lymphadenopathy, hepatosplenomegaly, erythroderma	Lymphopenia common Variable patterns of reduced lymphocyte subsets (T, B, natural killer cells) Omenn syndrome: high lymphocytes, eosinophilia, high IgE
IPEX	*FOXP3*	XLR	Severe diarrhea (autoimmune enteropathy) Various autoimmune endocrinopathies (especially diabetes mellitus, thyroiditis) Food allergies	High IgE Eosinophilia Various autoantibodies
Netherton syndrome	*SPINK5*	AR	Hair shaft abnormalities Erythroderma Ichthyosis linearis circumflexa Food allergies Recurrent gastroenteritis Neonatal hypernatremic dehydration Upper and lower respiratory infections	High IgE Eosinophilia

AD, Autosomal dominant; AD-HIES, autosomal-dominant hyper-IgE syndrome; AR, autosomal recessive; *DOCK8*, dedicator of cytokinesis 8 gene; IPEX, immune dysregulation, polyendocrinopathy, enteropathy, X-linked syndrome; PGM3, phosphoglucomutase 3; SCID, severe combined immunodeficiency; WAS, Wiskott-Aldrich syndrome.

From Kliegman RM, Bordini BJ, editors: *Undiagnosed and Rare Diseases in Children* 64(1):41–42, 2017.

Table 170.4	Counseling and Aggravating Factors for Patients With Atopic Dermatitis (AD)

Maintain cool temperature in bedroom, and avoid too many bed covers.

Increase emollient use with cold weather.

Avoid exposure to herpes sores; urgent visit if flare of unusual aspect.

Clothing: Avoid skin contact with irritating fibers (wool, large-fiber textiles).

  Do not use tight and too-warm clothing, to avoid excessive sweating.

  New, nonirritating clothing designed for AD children is being evaluated.

Tobacco: Avoid exposure.

Vaccines: Normal schedule in noninvolved skin, including egg-allergic patients (see text).

Sun exposure: No specific restriction.

  Usually helpful because of improvement of epidermal barrier.

  Encourage summer holidays in altitude or at beach resorts.

Physical exercise, sports: no restriction.

  If sweating induces flares of AD, progressive adaptation to exercise.

  Shower and emollients after swimming pool.

Food allergens:

  Maintain breastfeeding exclusively to 4-6 mo if possible.

  Consider evaluation for early introduction of allergens (see Chapter 176).

  Otherwise normal diet, unless an allergy workup has proved the need to exclude a specific food.

Indoor aeroallergens: House dust mites

  Use adequate ventilation of housing; keep the rooms well aerated even in winter.

  Avoid wall-to-wall carpeting.

  Remove dust with a wet sponge.

  Vacuum floors and upholstery with an adequately filtered cleaner once a week.

  Avoid soft toys in bed (cradle), except washable ones.

  Wash bedsheets at a temperature higher than 55°C (131°F) every 10 days.

  Use bed and pillow encasings made of Gore-Tex or similar material.

Furred pets: Advise to avoid. If allergy is demonstrated, be firm on avoidance measures, such as pet removal.

Pollen: Close windows during peak pollen season on warm and dry weather days, and restrict, if possible, time outdoors.

  Windows may be open at night and early in the morning or during rainy weather.

  Avoid exposure to risk situations (lawn mowing).

  Use pollen filters in motor vehicles.

  Clothes and pets can vectorize aeroallergens, including pollen.

Adapted from Darsow U, Wollenberg A, Simon D, et al: ETFAD/EADV Eczema Task Force 2009 position paper on diagnosis and treatment of atopic dermatitis, *J Eur Acad Dermatol Venereol* 24:321, 2010.

Table 170.5	Categorization of Physical Severity of Atopic Eczema

Clear—Normal skin, with no evidence of atopic eczema

Mild—Areas of dry skin, infrequent itching (with or without small areas of redness)

Moderate—Areas of dry skin, frequent itching, redness (with or without excoriation and localized skin thickening)

Severe—Widespread areas of dry skin, incessant itching, redness (with or without excoriation, extensive skin thickening, bleeding, oozing, cracking, and alteration of pigmentation)

From Lewis-Jones S, Mugglestone MA; Guideline Development Group: Management of atopic eczema in children aged up to 12 years: summary of NICE guidance, *BMJ* 335:1263–1264, 2007.

Lukewarm soaking baths or showers for 15-20 min followed by the application of an occlusive emollient to retain moisture provide symptomatic relief. Hydrophilic ointments of varying degrees of viscosity can be used according to the patient's preference. Occlusive ointments are sometimes not well tolerated because of interference with the function of the eccrine sweat ducts and may induce the development of folliculitis. In these patients, less occlusive agents should be used. Several prescription (classified as a medical device) "therapeutic moisturizers" or "barrier creams" are available, containing components such as ceramides and filaggrin acid metabolites intended to improve skin barrier function. There are minimal data demonstrating their efficacy over standard emollients.

Hydration by baths or wet dressings promotes transepidermal penetration of topical glucocorticoids. Dressings may also serve as effective barriers against persistent scratching, in turn promoting healing of excoriated lesions. Wet dressings are recommended for use on severely affected or chronically involved areas of dermatitis refractory to skin care. It is critical that wet dressing therapy be followed by topical emollient application to avoid potential drying and fissuring from the therapy. Wet dressing therapy can be complicated by maceration and secondary infection and should be closely monitored by a physician.

Topical Corticosteroids

Topical corticosteroids are the cornerstone of antiinflammatory treatment for acute exacerbations of AD. Patients should be carefully instructed on their use of topical glucocorticoids to avoid potential adverse effects. There are 7 classes of topical glucocorticoids, ranked according to their potency, as determined by vasoconstrictor assays (Table 170.6). Because of their potential adverse effects, the ultrahigh-potency glucocorticoids

Table 170.6	Selected Topical Corticosteroid Preparations*

GROUP 1

Clobetasol propionate (Temovate) 0.05% ointment/cream
Betamethasone dipropionate (Diprolene) 0.05% ointment/lotion/gel
Fluocinonide (Vanos) 0.1% cream

GROUP 2

Mometasone furoate (Elocon) 0.1% ointment
Halcinonide (Halog) 0.1% cream
Fluocinonide (Lidex) 0.05% ointment/cream
Desoximetasone (Topicort) 0.25% ointment/cream
Betamethasone dipropionate (Diprolene) 0.05% cream

GROUP 3

Fluticasone propionate (Cutivate) 0.005% ointment
Halcinonide (Halog) 0.1% ointment
Betamethasone valerate (Valisone) 0.1% ointment

GROUP 4

Mometasone furoate (Elocon) 0.1% cream
Triamcinolone acetonide (Kenalog) 0.1% ointment/cream
Fluocinolone acetonide (Synalar) 0.025% ointment

GROUP 5

Fluocinolone acetonide (Synalar) 0.025% cream
Hydrocortisone valerate (Westcort) 0.2% ointment

GROUP 6

Desonide (DesOwen) 05% ointment/cream/lotion
Alclometasone dipropionate (Aclovate) 0.05% ointment/cream

GROUP 7

Hydrocortisone (Hytone) 2.5%, 1%, 0.5% ointment/cream/lotion

*Representative corticosteroids are listed by group from 1 (superpotent) through 7 (least potent).

Adapted from Stoughton RB: Vasoconstrictor assay-specific applications. In Malbach HI, Surber C, editors: *Topical corticosteroids*, Basel, Switzerland, 1992, Karger, pp 42–53.

should not be used on the face or intertriginous areas and should be used only for very short periods on the trunk and extremities. Mid-potency glucocorticoids can be used for longer periods to treat chronic AD involving the trunk and extremities. Long-term control can be maintained with twice-weekly applications of topical fluticasone or mometasone to areas that have healed but are prone to relapse, once control of AD is achieved after a daily regimen of topical corticosteroids. Compared with creams, ointments have a greater potential to occlude the epidermis, resulting in enhanced systemic absorption.

Adverse effects of topical glucocorticoids can be divided into local adverse effects and systemic adverse effects, the latter resulting from suppression of the hypothalamic-pituitary-adrenal axis. *Local* adverse effects include the development of striae and skin atrophy. *Systemic* adverse effects are related to the potency of the topical corticosteroid, site of application, occlusiveness of the preparation, percentage of the body surface area covered, and length of use. The potential for adrenal suppression from potent topical corticosteroids is greatest in infants and young children with severe AD requiring intensive therapy.

Topical Calcineurin Inhibitors

The nonsteroidal topical calcineurin inhibitors are effective in reducing AD skin inflammation. Pimecrolimus cream 1% (Elidel) is indicated for mild to moderate AD. Tacrolimus ointment 0.1% and 0.03% (Protopic) is indicated for moderate to severe AD. Both are approved for short-term or intermittent long-term treatment of AD in patients ≥2 yr whose disease is unresponsive to or who are intolerant of other conventional therapies or for whom these therapies are inadvisable because of potential risks. Topical calcineurin inhibitors may be better than topical corticosteroids in the treatment of patients whose AD is poorly responsive to topical steroids, patients with steroid phobia, and those with face and neck dermatitis, in whom ineffective, low-potency topical corticosteroids are typically used because of fears of steroid-induced skin atrophy.

Phosphodiesterase Inhibitor

Crisaborole (Eucrisa) is an approved nonsteroidal topical antiinflammatory phosphodiesterase-4 (PDE-4) inhibitor indicated for the treatment of mild to moderate AD down to age 2 yr. It may be used as an alternative to topical corticosteroids or calcineurin inhibitors.

Tar Preparations

Coal tar preparations have antipruritic and antiinflammatory effects on the skin; however, their antiinflammatory effects are usually not as pronounced as those of topical glucocorticoids or calcineurin inhibitors. Therefore, topical tar preparations are not a preferred approach for management of AD. Tar shampoos can be particularly beneficial for scalp dermatitis. Adverse effects associated with tar preparations include skin irritation, folliculitis, and photosensitivity.

Antihistamines

Systemic antihistamines act primarily by blocking the histamine H_1 receptors in the dermis, thereby reducing histamine-induced pruritus. Histamine is only one of many mediators that induce pruritus of the skin, so patients may derive minimal benefit from antihistaminic therapy. Because pruritus is usually worse at night, sedating antihistamines (hydroxyzine, diphenhydramine) may offer an advantage with their soporific side effects when used at bedtime. Doxepin hydrochloride has both tricyclic antidepressant and H_1- and H_2-receptor blocking effects. Short-term use of a sedative to allow adequate rest may be appropriate in cases of severe nocturnal pruritus. Studies of newer, nonsedating antihistamines have shown variable effectiveness in controlling pruritus in AD, although they may be useful in the small subset of patients with AD and concomitant urticaria. For children, melatonin may be effective in promoting sleep because production is deficient in AD.

Systemic Corticosteroids

Systemic corticosteroids are rarely indicated in the treatment of chronic AD. The dramatic clinical improvement that may occur with systemic corticosteroids is frequently associated with a severe rebound flare of AD after therapy discontinuation. Short courses of oral corticosteroids may be appropriate for an acute exacerbation of AD while other treatment measures are being instituted in parallel. If a short course of oral corticosteroids is given, as during an asthma exacerbation, it is important to taper the dosage and begin intensified skin care, particularly with topical corticosteroids, and frequent bathing, followed by application of emollients or proactive topical corticosteroids, to prevent rebound flaring of AD.

Cyclosporine

Cyclosporine is a potent immunosuppressive drug that acts primarily on T cells by suppressing cytokine gene transcription and has been shown to be effective in the control of severe AD. Cyclosporin forms a complex with an intracellular protein, cyclophilin, and this complex in turn inhibits calcineurin, a phosphatase required for activation of NFAT (nuclear factor of activated T cells), a transcription factor necessary for cytokine gene transcription. Cyclosporine (5 mg/kg/day) for short-term and long-term (1 yr) use has been beneficial for children with severe, refractory AD. Possible adverse effects include renal impairment and hypertension.

Dupilumab

A monoclonal antibody that binds to the IL-4 receptor α subunit, dupilumab (Dupixent) inhibits the signaling of IL-4 and IL-13, cytokines associated with AD. In adults with moderate to severe AD not controlled by standard topical therapy, dupilumab reduces pruritus and improves skin clearing.

Antimetabolites

Mycophenolate mofetil is a purine biosynthesis inhibitor used as an immunosuppressant in organ transplantation that has been used for treatment of refractory AD. Aside from immunosuppression, herpes simplex retinitis and dose-related bone marrow suppression have been reported with its use. Of note, not all patients benefit from treatment. Therefore, mycophenolate mofetil should be discontinued if the disease does not respond within 4-8 wk.

Methotrexate is an antimetabolite with potent inhibitory effects on inflammatory cytokine synthesis and cell chemotaxis. Methotrexate has been used for patients with recalcitrant AD. In AD, dosing is more frequent than the weekly dosing used for psoriasis.

Azathioprine is a purine analog with antiinflammatory and antiproliferative effects that has been used for severe AD. Myelosuppression is a significant adverse effect, and thiopurine methyltransferase levels may identify individuals at risk.

Before any of these drugs is used, patients should be referred to an AD specialist who is familiar with treatment of severe AD to weigh relative benefits of alternative therapies.

Phototherapy

Natural sunlight is often beneficial to patients with AD as long as sunburn and excessive sweating are avoided. Many phototherapy modalities are effective for AD, including ultraviolet A-1, ultraviolet B, narrow-band ultraviolet B, and psoralen plus ultraviolet A. Phototherapy is generally reserved for patients in whom standard treatments fail. Maintenance treatments are usually required for phototherapy to be effective. Short-term adverse effects with phototherapy include erythema, skin pain, pruritus, and pigmentation. Long-term adverse effects include predisposition to cutaneous malignancies.

Unproven Therapies

Other therapies may be considered in patients with refractory AD.

Interferon-γ

IFN-γ is known to suppress Th2-cell function. Several studies, including a multicenter, double-blind, placebo-controlled trial and several open trials, have demonstrated that treatment with recombinant human IFN-γ results in clinical improvement of AD. Reduction in clinical severity of AD correlated with the ability of IFN-γ to decrease total circulating eosinophil counts. Influenza-like symptoms are common side effects during the treatment course.

Omalizumab

Treatment of patients who have severe AD and elevated serum IgE values with monoclonal anti-IgE may be considered in those with allergen-induced flares of AD. However, there have been no published double-blind, placebo-controlled trials of omalizumab's use. Most reports have been case studies and show inconsistent responses to anti-IgE.

Allergen Immunotherapy

In contrast to its acceptance for treatment of allergic rhinitis and extrinsic asthma, immunotherapy with aeroallergens in the treatment of AD is controversial. There are reports of both disease exacerbation and improvement. Studies suggest that specific immunotherapy in patients with AD sensitized to dust mite allergen showed improvement in severity of skin disease, as well as reduction in topical corticosteroid use.

Probiotics

Perinatal administration of the probiotic *Lactobacillus rhamnosus* strain GG has been shown to reduce the incidence of AD in at-risk children during the 1st 2 yr of life. The treatment response has been found to be more pronounced in patients with positive skin-prick test results and elevated IgE values. Other studies have not demonstrated a benefit.

Chinese Herbal Medications

Several placebo-controlled clinical trials have suggested that patients with severe AD may benefit from treatment with traditional Chinese herbal therapy. The patients had significantly reduced skin disease and decreased pruritus. The beneficial response of Chinese herbal therapy is often temporary, and effectiveness may wear off despite continued treatment. The possibility of hepatic toxicity, cardiac side effects, or idiosyncratic reactions remains a concern. The specific ingredients of the herbs also remain to be elucidated, and some preparations have been found to be contaminated with corticosteroids. At present, Chinese herbal therapy for AD is considered investigational.

Vitamin D

Vitamin D deficiency often accompanies severe AD. Vitamin D enhances skin barrier function, reduces corticosteroid requirements to control inflammation, and augments skin antimicrobial function. Several small clinical studies suggest vitamin D can enhance antimicrobial peptide expression in the skin and reduce severity of skin disease, especially in patients with low baseline vitamin D, as during winter, when exacerbation of AD often occurs. Patients with AD might benefit from supplementation with vitamin D, particularly if they have a documented low level or low vitamin D intake.

AVOIDING TRIGGERS

It is essential to identify and eliminate triggering factors for AD, both during the period of acute symptoms and on a long-term basis to prevent recurrences (see Table 170.4).

Irritants

Patients with AD have a low threshold response to irritants that trigger their itch-scratch cycle. Soaps or detergents, chemicals, smoke, abrasive clothing, and exposure to extremes of temperature and humidity are common triggers. *Patients with AD should use soaps with minimal defatting properties and a neutral pH.* New clothing should be laundered before wearing to decrease levels of formaldehyde and other chemicals. Residual laundry detergent in clothing may trigger the itch-scratch cycle; using a liquid rather than powder detergent and adding a 2nd rinse cycle facilitates removal of the detergent.

Every attempt should be made to allow children with AD to be as normally active as possible. A sport such as swimming may be better tolerated than others that involve intense perspiration, physical contact, or heavy clothing and equipment. Rinsing off chlorine immediately and lubricating the skin after swimming are important. Although ultraviolet light may be beneficial to some patients with AD, high–sun protection factor (SPF) sunscreens should be used to avoid sunburn.

Foods

Food allergy is comorbid in approximately 40% of infants and young children with moderate to severe AD (see Chapter 176). Undiagnosed food allergies in patients with AD may induce eczematous dermatitis in some patients and urticarial reactions, wheezing, or nasal congestion in others. Increased severity of AD symptoms and younger age correlate directly with the presence of food allergy. Removal of food allergens from the diet leads to significant clinical improvement but requires much education, because most common allergens (egg, milk, peanut, wheat, soy) contaminate many foods and are difficult to avoid.

Potential allergens can be identified by a careful history and performing selective skin-prick tests or in vitro blood testing for allergen-specific IgE. Negative skin and blood test results for allergen-specific IgE have a high predictive value for excluding suspected allergens. Positive results of skin or blood tests using foods often do not correlate with clinical symptoms and should be confirmed with controlled food challenges and elimination diets. Extensive elimination diets, which can be nutritionally deficient, are rarely required. Even with multiple positive skin test results, the majority of patients react to fewer than 3 foods under controlled challenge conditions.

Aeroallergens

In older children, AD flares can occur after intranasal or epicutaneous exposure to aeroallergens such as fungi, animal dander, grass, and ragweed pollen. Avoiding aeroallergens, particularly dust mites, can result in clinical improvement of AD. Avoidance measures for dust mite–allergic patients include using dust mite–proof encasings on pillows, mattresses, and box springs; washing bedding in hot water weekly; removing bedroom carpeting; and decreasing indoor humidity levels with air conditioning.

Infections

Patients with AD have increased susceptibility to bacterial, viral, and fungal skin infections. Antistaphylococcal antibiotics are very helpful for treating patients who are heavily colonized or infected with *Staphylococcus aureus*. Erythromycin and azithromycin are usually beneficial for patients who are not colonized with a resistant *S. aureus* strain; a first-generation cephalosporin (cephalexin) is recommended for macrolide-resistant *S. aureus*. Topical mupirocin is useful in the treatment of localized impetiginous lesions, with systemic clindamycin or trimethoprim/sulfamethoxazole needed for methicillin-resistant *S. aureus* (MRSA). Cytokine-mediated skin inflammation contributes to skin colonization with *S. aureus*. This finding supports the importance of combining effective antiinflammatory therapy with antibiotics for treating moderate to severe AD to avoid the need for repeated courses of antibiotics, which can lead to the emergence of antibiotic-resistant strains of *S. aureus*. Dilute bleach baths ($\frac{1}{2}$ cup of bleach in 40 gallons of water) twice weekly may be also considered to reduce *S. aureus* colonization. In one randomized trial, the group who received the bleach baths plus intranasal mupirocin (5 days/mo) had significantly decreased severity of AD at 1 and 3 mo compared with placebo. Patients rinse off after the soaking. Bleach baths may not only reduce *S. aureus* abundance on the skin but also have antiinflammatory effects.

Herpes simplex virus (HSV) can provoke recurrent dermatitis and may be misdiagnosed as *S. aureus* infection (Fig. 170.4). The presence of punched-out erosions, vesicles, and infected skin lesions that fail to respond to oral antibiotics suggests HSV infection, which can be diagnosed by a Giemsa-stained Tzanck smear of cells scraped from the vesicle base or by viral polymerase chain reaction or culture. Topical corticosteroids should be temporarily discontinued if HSV infection is suspected. Reports of life-threatening dissemination of HSV infections in patients with AD who have widespread disease mandate antiviral treatment. Persons with AD are also susceptible to **eczema vaccinatum**, which is similar in appearance to eczema herpeticum and historically follows smallpox (vaccinia virus) vaccination.

Cutaneous warts, coxsackievirus, and molluscum contagiosum are additional viral infections affecting children with AD.

Dermatophyte infections can also contribute to exacerbation of AD. Patients with AD have been found to have a greater susceptibility to

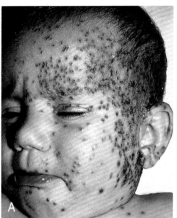 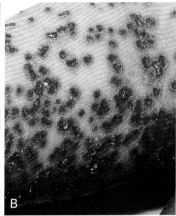

Fig. 170.4 Eczema herpeticum infection in a patient with atopic dermatitis. *Numerous punched-out vesicles and erosions involving the face* (**A**) *and extremities* (**B**). (From Papulosquamous eruptions. In Cohen BA, editor: Pediatric dermatology, Philadelphia,2013, Saunders, pp 68–103.)

Trichophyton rubrum fungal infections than nonatopic controls. There has been particular interest in the role of *Malassezia furfur* (formerly known as *Pityrosporum ovale*) in AD because it is a lipophilic yeast commonly present in the seborrheic areas of the skin. IgE antibodies against *M. furfur* have been found in patients with head and neck dermatitis. A reduction of AD severity has been observed in these patients after treatment with antifungal agents.

COMPLICATIONS
Exfoliative dermatitis may develop in patients with extensive skin involvement. It is associated with generalized redness, scaling, weeping, crusting, systemic toxicity, lymphadenopathy, and fever and is usually caused by superinfection (e.g., with toxin-producing *S. aureus* or HSV infection) or inappropriate therapy. In some cases the withdrawal of systemic glucocorticoids used to control severe AD precipitates exfoliative erythroderma.

Eyelid dermatitis and chronic blepharitis may result in visual impairment from corneal scarring. **Atopic keratoconjunctivitis** is usually bilateral and can have disabling symptoms that include itching, burning, tearing, and copious mucoid discharge. Vernal conjunctivitis is associated with papillary hypertrophy or cobblestoning of the upper eyelid conjunctiva. It typically occurs in younger patients and has a marked seasonal incidence with spring exacerbations. **Keratoconus** is a conical deformity of the cornea believed to result from chronic rubbing of the eyes in patients with AD. Cataracts may be a primary manifestation of AD or from extensive use of systemic and topical glucocorticoids, particularly around the eyes.

PROGNOSIS
AD generally tends to be more severe and persistent in young children, particularly if they have null mutations in their filaggrin genes. Periods of remission occur more frequently as patients grow older. Spontaneous resolution of AD has been reported to occur after age 5 yr in 40–60% of patients affected during infancy, particularly for mild disease. Earlier studies suggested that approximately 84% of children outgrow their AD by adolescence; however, later studies reported that AD resolves in approximately 20% of children monitored from infancy until adolescence and becomes less severe in 65%. Of those adolescents treated for mild dermatitis, >50% may experience a relapse of disease as adults, which frequently manifests as *hand dermatitis*, especially if daily activities require repeated hand wetting. Predictive factors of a poor prognosis for AD include widespread AD in childhood, *FLG* null mutations, concomitant allergic rhinitis and asthma, family history of AD in parents or siblings, early age at onset of AD, being an only child, and very high serum IgE levels.

PREVENTION
Breastfeeding may be beneficial. Probiotics and prebiotics may also reduce the incidence or severity of AD, but this approach is unproven. If an infant with AD is diagnosed with food allergy, the breastfeeding mother may need to eliminate the implicated food allergen from her diet. For infants with severe eczema, introduction of infant-safe forms of peanut as early as 4-6 mo, after other solids are tolerated, is recommended after consultation with the child's pediatrician and/or allergist for allergy testing. This approach may prevent peanut allergy (see Chapter 176). Identification and elimination of triggering factors are the mainstay for prevention of flares as well as for the long-term treatment of AD.

Emollient therapy applied to the whole body for the 1st few mo of life may enhance the cutaneous barrier and reduce the risk of eczema.

Bibliography is available at Expert Consult.

Chapter **171**
Insect Allergy
Julie Wang and Scott H. Sicherer

第一百七十一章
昆虫过敏

中文导读

　　本章主要介绍了昆虫过敏的病因、发病机制、临床表现、诊断、治疗及预防。具体介绍了不同种类昆虫引起的过敏反应具有不同的发病率及临床表现；昆虫过敏可表现为局限性反应、大范围的局部反应、全身皮肤反应、全身反应、毒性反应和延迟/迟发反应，强调了昆虫过敏的诊断包括接触史、典型症状和体格检查。皮肤点刺试验或体外鉴定毒液特异性IgE测试具有一定的参考价值；昆虫过敏的治疗主要分为对症治疗，毒液免疫疗法及吸入性变应原的规避；最后强调了昆虫过敏反应的预防策略。

Allergic responses to stinging or, more rarely, biting insects vary from localized cutaneous reactions to systemic anaphylaxis. **Allergic reactions** caused by inhalation of airborne particles of insect origin result in acute and chronic respiratory symptoms of seasonal or perennial rhinitis, conjunctivitis, and asthma.

ETIOLOGY

Most reactions to stinging and biting insects, such as those induced by wasps, mosquitoes, flies, and fleas, are limited to a primary lesion isolated to the area of the sting or bite and do not represent an allergic response. Occasionally, insect stings or bites induce pronounced localized reactions or systemic reactions that may be based on immediate or delayed hypersensitivity reactions. Systemic allergic responses to insects are usually attributed to IgE antibody–mediated responses, which are caused primarily by stings from venomous insects of the order **Hymenoptera** and more rarely from ticks, spiders, scorpions, and *Triatoma* (kissing bug). Members of the order Hymenoptera include *apids* (honeybee, bumblebee), *vespids* (yellow jacket, wasp, hornet), and *formicids* (fire and harvester ants) (Fig. 171.1). Among winged stinging insects, yellow jackets are the most notorious for stinging because they are aggressive and ground dwelling, and they linger near activities involving food. Hornets nest in trees, whereas wasps build honeycomb nests in dark areas such as under porches; both are aggressive if disturbed. Honeybees are less aggressive and nest in tree hollows; unlike the stings of other flying Hymenoptera, honeybee stings almost always leave a barbed stinger with venom sac.

In the United States, fire ants are found increasingly in the Southeast, living in large mounds of soil. When disturbed, the ants attack in large numbers, anchor themselves to the skin by their mandibles, and sting multiple times in a circular pattern. Sterile pseudopustules form at the sting sites. Systemic reactions to stinging insects occur in 0.4–0.8% of

children and 3% of adults and account for approximately 40 deaths each year in the United States.

Although reactions to insect bites are common, IgE-mediated reactions are infrequently reported and anaphylaxis is rare. The *Triatoma* (kissing bug) bite causes an erythematous plaque that is painless. Mosquito bites generally result in local reactions that are pruritic. Large, local reactions to mosquito bites can occur in some young children; this is known as **skeeter syndrome** and is often misdiagnosed as cellulitis. The *tabanid*

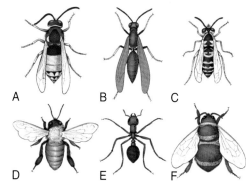

Fig. 171.1 Representative venomous Hymenoptera. **A,** Hornet (*Vespula maculata*). **B,** Wasp (*Chlorion ichneumerea*). **C,** Yellowjacket (*Vespula maculiforma*). **D,** Honeybee (*Apis mellifera*). **E,** Fire ant (*Solenopsis invicta*). **F,** Bumblebee (*Bombus species*). (From Erickson TB, Marquez A: Arthropod envenomation and parasitism. In Auerbach PS, Cushing TA, Harris NS (eds): *Auerbach's wilderness medicine, ed 7,* Philadelphia, 2017, Elsevier, Fig 41-1, p 937.)

species (horsefly, deerfly), typically found in rural and suburban areas, are large flies that induce painful bites.

IgE antibody–mediated allergic responses to airborne particulate matter carrying insect emanations contribute to seasonal and perennial symptoms affecting the upper and lower airways. Seasonal allergy is attributed to exposures to a variety of insects, particularly aquatic insects such as the caddis fly and midge, or lake fly, at a time when larvae pupate and adult flies are airborne. **Perennial allergy** is attributed to sensitization to insects such as cockroaches and ladybugs, as well as house dust mite, which is phylogenetically related to spiders rather than insects and has 8 rather than 6 legs.

PATHOGENESIS

Hymenoptera venoms contain numerous components with toxic and pharmacologic activity and with allergenic potential. These constituents include vasoactive substances such as histamine, acetylcholine, and kinins; enzymes such as phospholipase and hyaluronidase; apamin; melittin; and formic acid. The majority of patients who experience systemic reactions after Hymenoptera stings have IgE-mediated sensitivity to antigenic substances in the venom. Some venom allergens are homologous among members of the Hymenoptera order; others are family specific. There is substantial cross-reactivity among vespid venoms, but these venom allergies are distinct from honeybee venom allergies.

Localized skin responses to biting insects are caused primarily by vasoactive or irritant materials derived from insect saliva; they rarely occur from IgE-associated responses. Systemic IgE-mediated allergic reactions to salivary proteins of biting insects such as mosquitoes are reported but uncommon.

A variety of proteins derived from insects can become airborne and induce IgE-mediated respiratory responses, causing inhalant allergies. The primary allergen from the caddis fly is a hemocyanin-like protein, and that from the midge fly is derived from hemoglobin. Allergens from the cockroach are the best studied and are derived from cockroach saliva, secretions, fecal material, and debris from skin casts.

CLINICAL MANIFESTATIONS

Clinical reactions to stinging venomous insects are categorized as local, large local, generalized cutaneous, systemic, toxic, and delayed/late. Simple **local reactions** involve limited swelling and pain and generally last <24 hr. **Large local reactions** develop over hours and days, involve swelling of extensive areas (>10 cm) that are contiguous with the sting site, and may last for days. **Generalized cutaneous reactions** typically progress within minutes and include cutaneous symptoms of urticaria, angioedema, and pruritus beyond the site of the sting. **Systemic reactions** are identical to anaphylaxis from other triggers and may include symptoms of generalized urticaria, laryngeal edema, bronchospasm, and hypotension. Stings from a large number of insects at once may result in **toxic reactions** of fever, malaise, emesis, and nausea because of the chemical properties of the venom in large doses. Serum sickness, nephrotic syndrome, vasculitis, neuritis, or encephalopathy may occur as **delayed/late reactions** to stinging insects.

Insect bites are usually urticarial but may be papular or vesicular. **Papular urticaria** affecting the lower extremities in children is usually caused by multiple bites. Occasionally, individuals have large, local reactions. IgE antibody–associated immediate- and late-phase allergic responses to mosquito bites sometimes mimic cellulitis.

Inhalant allergy caused by insects results in clinical disease similar to that induced by other inhalant allergens such as pollens. Depending on individual sensitivity and exposure, reactions may result in seasonal or perennial rhinitis, conjunctivitis, or asthma.

DIAGNOSIS

The diagnosis of allergy from stinging and biting insects is generally evident from the history of exposure, typical symptoms, and physical findings. The diagnosis of Hymenoptera allergy rests in part on the identification of venom-specific IgE by skin-prick testing or in vitro testing. The primary reasons to pursue testing are to confirm reactivity when venom immunotherapy (**VIT**) is being considered or when it is clinically necessary to confirm venom hypersensitivity as a cause of a

reaction. Venoms of 5 Hymenoptera (honeybee, yellow jacket, yellow hornet, white-faced hornet, and wasp), as well as the jack jumper ant in Australia and whole body extract of fire ant, are available for skin testing. Although skin tests are considered to be the most sensitive modality for detection of venom-specific IgE, additional evaluation with an in vitro serum assay for venom-specific IgE is recommended if skin test results are negative in the presence of a convincing history of a severe systemic reaction. In vitro tests have a 20% incidence of both false-positive and false-negative results, so it is not appropriate to exclude venom hypersensitivity based on this test alone. If initial skin-prick and in vitro test results are negative in the context of a convincing history of a severe reaction, repeat testing is recommended before concluding that allergy is unlikely. Skin tests are usually accurate within 1 wk of a sting reaction, but occasionally a refractory period is observed that warrants retesting after 4-6 wk if the initial results are negative.

An elevated **basal tryptase** level is associated with more severe reactions to venom stings. Therefore, basal tryptase should be measured if there is a history of severe reaction to a sting, hypotensive reaction, lack of urticaria in a systemic sting reaction, or negative venom IgE in a patient who has a history of systemic reaction to a sting. As many as 40% of skin test–positive patients may not experience anaphylaxis on sting challenge, so testing without an appropriate clinical history is potentially misleading.

The diagnosis of inhalant insect allergy may be evident from a history of typical symptoms. A chronic respiratory symptom during long-term exposure, as may occur with cockroach allergy, is less amenable to identification by history alone. Skin-prick or in vitro immunoassay tests for specific IgE to the insect are used to confirm inhalant insect allergy. Allergy tests may be particularly warranted for potential cockroach allergy in patients with persistent asthma and known cockroach exposure.

TREATMENT

For local cutaneous reactions caused by insect stings and bites, treatment with cold compresses, topical medications to relieve itching, and occasionally a systemic antihistamine and oral analgesic are appropriate. Stingers should be removed promptly by scraping, with caution not to squeeze the venom sac because doing so could inject more venom. Sting sites rarely become infected, possibly because of the antibacterial actions of venom constituents. Vesicles left by fire ant stings that are scratched open should be cleansed to prevent secondary infection.

Anaphylactic reactions after a Hymenoptera sting are treated the same as anaphylaxis from any cause; *epinephrine is the drug of choice.* Adjunctive treatment includes antihistamines, corticosteroids, intravenous fluids, oxygen, and transport to the emergency department (see Chapter 174). Referral to an allergist-immunologist should be considered for patients who have experienced a generalized cutaneous or systemic reaction to an insect sting, who need education about avoidance and emergency treatment, who may be candidates for VIT, or who have a condition that may complicate management of anaphylaxis (e.g., use of β-blockers).

Venom Immunotherapy

Hymenoptera VIT is highly effective (95–97%) in decreasing the risk for **severe anaphylaxis**. The selection of patients for VIT depends on several factors (Table 171.1). Individuals with local reactions, regardless of age, are not at increased risk for severe systemic reactions on a subsequent sting and are not candidates for VIT. The risk of a systemic reaction for those who experienced a large, local reaction is approximately 7%; testing or VIT is usually not recommended, and prescription of self-injectable epinephrine is considered optional but usually not necessary. There is growing evidence that VIT can reduce the size and duration of large, local reactions, and therefore VIT may be considered for those with frequent or unavoidable large, local reactions. *Those who experience severe systemic reactions, such as airway involvement or hypotension, and who have specific IgE to venom allergens should receive immunotherapy.* Immunotherapy against winged Hymenoptera is generally not required when stings have caused only generalized urticaria or angioedema,

Table 171.1	Indications for Venom Immunotherapy (VIT) Against Winged Hymenoptera			
SYMPTOMS	SKIN TEST/IN VITRO TEST	RISK OF SYSTEMIC REACTION IF UNTREATED*		VIT RECOMMENDED
Large local reaction	Usually not indicated	~7%		Usually not indicated
Generalized cutaneous reaction	Usually not indicated	10%		Usually not indicated
Systemic reaction	Positive result	Child: 40% Adult: 30–60%		Yes
	Negative result	—		Usually not indicated

*Risks generally decrease after 10 yr.

because the risk for a systemic reaction after a subsequent sting is approximately 10% and the chance of a more severe reaction is <3%. VIT may be considered if there are potential high-risk cofactors such as comorbid cardiovascular disease or use of specific cardiovascular medications (e.g., ACE inhibitors, β-blockers), elevated basal tryptase level, or high likelihood of future stings. VIT is usually not indicated if there is no evidence of IgE to venom.

The incidence of adverse effects in the course of treatment is not trivial in adults; 50% experience large, local reactions, and about 10% experience systemic reactions. The incidence of both local and systemic reactions is much lower in children. Patients treated with honeybee venom are at higher risk for systemic reactions to VIT than those receiving treatment with vespid venom. Individuals with mast cell disorders are at increased risk for severe anaphylaxis and more frequent systemic reactions with VIT; thus some experts recommend basal tryptase level for risk assessment purposes.

It is uncertain how long immunotherapy with Hymenoptera venom should continue. In general, treatment duration of 3-5 yr is recommended because >80% of adults who have received 5 yr of therapy tolerate challenge stings without systemic reactions for 5-10 yr after completion of treatment. Long-term responses to treatment are even better for children. Follow-up over a mean of 18 yr of children with moderate to severe insect sting reactions who received VIT for a mean of 3-5 yr and were stung again showed a reaction rate of only 5%; untreated children experienced a reaction rate of 32%. Whereas duration of therapy with VIT may be individualized, it is clear that a significant number of untreated children retain their allergy. Extended or lifelong treatment may be considered for those who have had life-threatening anaphylaxis with insect stings, those with honeybee allergy, and those with occupational exposures to Hymenoptera. Lifelong VIT should also be considered for patients with mast cell disorders because they have a higher rate of failure of VIT and relapse when VIT is discontinued.

Less is known about the natural history of fire ant hypersensitivity and efficacy of immunotherapy for this allergy. The criteria for starting immunotherapy are similar to those for hypersensitivities to other Hymenoptera, but there is stronger consideration to treat patients who have only cutaneous systemic reactions with VIT. Only whole body fire ant extract is commercially available for diagnostic skin testing and immunotherapy.

Inhalant Allergy
The symptoms of inhalant allergy caused by insects are managed as for other causes of seasonal or perennial rhinitis (see Chapter 168), conjunctivitis (Chapter 172), and asthma (Chapter 169).

PREVENTION
Avoidance of stings and bites is essential. To reduce the risk of stings, sensitized individuals should have known or suspected nests near the home removed by trained professionals, should wear gloves when gardening, should wear long pants and shoes with socks when walking in the grass or through fields, and should avoid or be cautious about eating or drinking outdoors. Typical insect repellents do not guard against Hymenoptera.

Individuals who are at high risk for future severe reactions to Hymenoptera stings should have immediate access to self-injectable epinephrine. High-risk individuals include those who have a history of severe reactions, are prescribed angiotensin-converting enzyme (ACE) inhibitors or β-adrenergic blockers, or have elevated basal tryptase level. Adults responsible for allergic children and older patients who can self-treat must be carefully taught the indications and technique of administration for this medication. Particular attention is necessary for children in out-of-home daycare centers, at school, or attending camps, to ensure that an emergency action plan is in place. The individual at risk for anaphylaxis from an insect sting should also wear an identification bracelet indicating the allergy.

Avoidance of the insect is the preferred management of inhalant allergy. This can prove difficult, particularly for those living in apartments, where eradication of cockroaches may be problematic. Immunotherapy for dust mites is effective and should be considered in conjunction with avoidance measures. In contrast, there is limited data regarding the efficacy of cockroach immunotherapy.

Bibliography is available at Expert Consult.

Chapter **172**
Ocular Allergies
Christine B. Cho, Mark Boguniewicz,
and Scott H. Sicherer
第一百七十二章
眼部过敏

中 文 导 读

　　本章主要介绍了眼部过敏的临床表现、诊断及治疗。具体描述了眼部过敏包括过敏性结膜炎、春季角膜结膜炎、特应性角膜结膜炎、巨乳头结膜炎、接触性过敏；眼部过敏的诊断需综合考虑病因、症状及鉴别诊断；眼部过敏的主要治疗方法包括规避变应原、眼部冷敷和润滑。二级治疗方案包括口服或局部使用抗组胺药，必要时使用局部减充血剂、肥大细胞稳定剂和抗炎药。

The **eye** is a common target of allergic disorders because of its marked vascularity and direct contact with allergens in the environment. The **conjunctiva** is the most immunologically active tissue of the external eye. Ocular allergies can occur as isolated target organ disease or more often in conjunction with nasal allergies. Ocular symptoms can significantly affect quality of life.

CLINICAL MANIFESTATIONS

There are a few distinct entities that constitute allergic eye disease, all of which have bilateral involvement. Sensitization is necessary for all these except giant papillary conjunctivitis. Vernal and atopic keratoconjunctivitis are potentially sight threatening (see Chapter 652).

Allergic Conjunctivitis

Allergic conjunctivitis is the most common hypersensitivity response of the eye, affecting approximately 25% of the general population and 30% of children with atopy. It is caused by direct exposure of the mucosal surfaces of the eye to environmental allergens. Patients complain of variable ocular itching, rather than pain, with increased tearing. Clinical signs include bilateral injected conjunctivae with vascular congestion that may progress to *chemosis,* or conjunctival swelling, and a watery discharge (Fig. 172.1).

Allergic conjunctivitis occurs in a seasonal or, less frequently, perennial form. **Seasonal allergic conjunctivitis** is typically associated with allergic rhinitis (see Chapter 168) and is most commonly triggered by pollens. Major pollen groups in the temperate zones include trees (late winter to early spring), grasses (late spring to early summer), and weeds (late summer to early fall), but seasons can vary significantly in different parts of the United States. Mold spores can also cause seasonal allergy symptoms, principally in the summer and fall. Seasonal allergy symptoms may be aggravated by coincident exposure to perennial allergens.

Perennial allergic conjunctivitis is triggered by allergens such as animal danders or dust mites that are present throughout the year. Symptoms are usually less severe than with seasonal allergic conjunctivitis. Because pollens and soil molds may be present intermittently by season, and exposure to allergens such as furred animals may be perennial, classification as intermittent (symptoms present <4 days/wk or for <4 wk) and persistent (symptoms present >4 days/wk and for >4 wk) has been proposed.

Vernal Keratoconjunctivitis

Vernal keratoconjunctivitis is a severe bilateral chronic inflammatory process of the upper tarsal conjunctival surface that occurs in a limbal or palpebral form. It may threaten eyesight if there is corneal involvement. Although vernal keratoconjunctivitis is not IgE mediated, it occurs most frequently in children with seasonal allergies, asthma, or atopic dermatitis. Vernal keratoconjunctivitis affects boys twice as often as girls and is more common in persons of Asian and African descent. It affects primarily children in temperate areas, with exacerbations in the spring and summer, but can occur throughout the year. Symptoms include severe ocular itching exacerbated by exposure to irritants, light, or perspiration. In addition, patients may complain of severe photophobia, foreign body sensation, and lacrimation. Giant papillae occur predominantly on the upper tarsal plate and are typically described as *cobblestoning* (Fig. 172.2). Other signs include a stringy or thick, ropey discharge, cobblestone papillae, transient yellow-white points in the limbus (*Trantas dots*) and conjunctiva (*Horner points*), corneal "shield" ulcers, and Dennie lines (Dennie-Morgan folds), which are prominent symmetric skin folds that extend in an arc from the inner canthus beneath and parallel to the lower lid margin. Children with vernal keratoconjunctivitis have measurably longer eyelashes, which may represent a reaction to ocular inflammation.

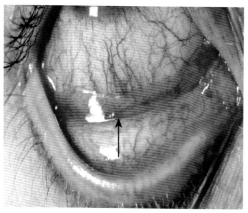

Fig. 172.1 Allergic conjunctivitis. *Arrow* indicates area of chemosis in the conjunctivitis. *(From Adkinson NF Jr, Bochner BS, Burks AW, et al, editors: Middleton's allergy: principles & practice, ed 8, vol 1, St Louis, Mosby/Elsevier, 2014, p 619.)*

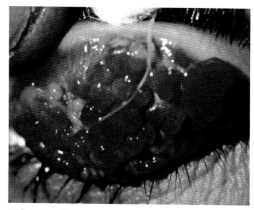

Fig. 172.2 Vernal keratoconjunctivitis. Cobblestone papillae and ropey discharge are seen on the underside (tarsal conjunctiva) of the upper eyelid. *(From Adkinson NF Jr, Bochner BS, Burks AW, et al, editors: Middleton's allergy: principles & practice, ed 8, vol 1, St Louis, Mosby/Elsevier, 2014, p 627.)*

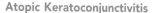

Atopic Keratoconjunctivitis

Atopic keratoconjunctivitis is a chronic inflammatory ocular disorder most often involving the lower tarsal conjunctiva. It may threaten eyesight if there is corneal involvement. Almost all patients have atopic dermatitis, and a significant number have asthma. Atopic keratoconjunctivitis rarely presents before late adolescence. Symptoms include severe bilateral ocular itching, burning, photophobia, and tearing with a mucoid discharge that are much more severe than in allergic conjunctivitis and persist throughout the year. The bulbar conjunctiva is injected and chemotic; cataracts may occur. Trantas dots or giant papillae may also be present. Eyelid eczema can extend to the periorbital skin and cheeks with erythema and thick, dry scaling. Secondary staphylococcal blepharitis is common because of eyelid induration and maceration. Chronic eye rubbing associated with vernal and atopic keratoconjunctivitis can lead to **keratoconus**, a noninflammatory cone-shaped corneal ectasia. This may lead to corneal thinning and perforation.

Giant Papillary Conjunctivitis

Giant papillary conjunctivitis has been linked to chronic exposure to foreign bodies, such as contact lenses, both hard and soft, ocular prostheses, and sutures. Symptoms and signs include mild bilateral ocular itching, tearing, a foreign body sensation, and excessive ocular discomfort with mild mucoid discharge with white or clear exudate on awakening, which may become thick and stringy. Trantas dots, limbal infiltration, bulbar conjunctival hyperemia, and edema may develop.

Contact Allergy

Contact allergy typically involves the eyelids but can also involve the conjunctivae. It is being recognized more frequently in association with increased exposure to topical medications, contact lens solutions, and preservatives.

DIAGNOSIS

Nonallergic conjunctivitis can be viral, bacterial, or chlamydial in origin. It is typically unilateral but can be bilateral with symptoms initially developing in 1 eye (see Chapter 644). Symptoms include stinging or burning rather than itching and often a foreign body sensation. Ocular discharge can be watery, mucoid, or purulent. Masqueraders of ocular allergy also include nasolacrimal duct obstruction, foreign body, blepharoconjunctivitis, dry eye, uveitis, and trauma.

TREATMENT

Primary treatment of ocular allergies includes avoidance of allergens, cold compresses, and lubrication. **Secondary treatment** regimens include the use of oral or topical antihistamines and, if necessary, topical decongestants, mast cell stabilizers, and antiinflammatory agents (Table 172.1). Drugs with dual antihistamine and mast cell–blocking activities provide the most advantageous approach in treating allergic conjunctivitis, with both fast-acting symptomatic relief and disease-modifying action. Children often complain of stinging or burning with use of topical ophthalmic preparations and usually prefer oral antihistamines for allergic conjunctivitis. It is important not to contaminate topical ocular medications by allowing the applicator tip to contact the eye or eyelid. Using refrigerated medications may decrease some of the discomfort associated with their use. Topical decongestants act as vasoconstrictors, reducing erythema, vascular congestion, and eyelid edema, but do not diminish the allergic response. Adverse effects of topical vasoconstrictors include burning or stinging and rebound hyperemia or conjunctivitis medicamentosa with chronic use. Combined use of an antihistamine and a vasoconstrictor is more effective than use of either agent alone. Use of topical nasal corticosteroids for allergic rhinoconjunctivitis decreases ocular symptoms, presumably through a nasoocular reflex.

Tertiary treatment of ocular allergy includes topical (or rarely oral) corticosteroids and should be conducted in conjunction with an ophthalmologist. Local administration of topical corticosteroids may be associated with increased intraocular pressure, viral infections, and cataract formation. Other immunomodulatory medications, such as topical tacrolimus or topical cyclosporine, are used as steroid-sparing agents by ophthalmologists. Allergen immunotherapy can be very effective in seasonal and perennial allergic conjunctivitis, especially when associated with rhinitis, and can decrease the need for oral or topical medications to control allergy symptoms.

Because vernal and atopic keratoconjunctivitis can be associated with visual morbidity, if these diagnoses are suspected, the patient should be referred to an ophthalmologist. *Symptoms that should prompt referral to an ophthalmologist include unilateral red eye with pain, photophobia, change in vision, refractory dry eyes, or corneal abnormality.*

Bibliography is available at Expert Consult.

| Table 172.1 | Topical Ophthalmic Medications for Allergic Conjunctivitis |

DRUG AND TRADE NAMES	MECHANISM OF ACTION AND DOSING	CAUTIONS AND ADVERSE EVENTS
Azelastine hydrochloride 0.05% Optivar	Antihistamine Children ≥3 yr: 1 gtt bid	Not for treatment of contact lens–related irritation; the preservative may be absorbed by soft contact lenses. Wait at least 10 min after administration before inserting soft contact lenses.
Emedastine difumarate 0.05% Emadine	Antihistamine Children ≥3 yr: 1 gtt qid	Soft contact lenses should not be worn if the eye is red. Wait at least 10 min after administration before inserting soft contact lenses.
Levocabastine hydrochloride 0.05% Livostin	Antihistamine Children ≥12 yr: 1 gtt bid-qid up to 2 wk	Not for use in patients wearing soft contact lenses during treatment.
Pheniramine maleate	Antihistamine/vasoconstrictor	Avoid prolonged use (>3-4 days) to avoid rebound symptoms. Not for use with contact lenses.
0.3% Naphazoline hydrochloride 0.025% Naphcon-A, Opcon-A	Children >6 yr: 1-2 gtt qid	
Cromolyn sodium 4% Crolom, Opticrom	Mast cell stabilizer Children >4 yr: 1-2 gtt q4-6h	Can be used to treat giant papillary conjunctivitis and vernal keratitis. Not for use with contact lenses.
Lodoxamide tromethamine 0.1% Alomide	Mast cell stabilizer Children ≥2 yr: 1-2 gtt qid up to 3 mo	Can be used to treat vernal keratoconjunctivitis. Not for use in patients wearing soft contact lenses during treatment.
Nedocromil sodium 2% Alocril	Mast cell stabilizer Children ≥3 yr: 1-2 gtt bid	Avoid wearing contact lenses while exhibiting the signs and symptoms of allergic conjunctivitis.
Pemirolast potassium 0.1% Alamast	Mast cell stabilizer Children >3 yr: 1-2 gtt qid	Not for treatment of contact lens–related irritation; the preservative may be absorbed by soft contact lenses. Wait at least 10 min after administration before inserting soft contact lenses.
Epinastine hydrochloride 0.05% Elestat	Antihistamine/mast cell stabilizer Children ≥3 yr: 1 gtt bid	Contact lenses should be removed before use. Wait at least 15 min after administration before inserting soft contact lenses. Not for the treatment of contact lens irritation.
Ketotifen fumarate 0.025% Zaditor	Antihistamine/mast cell stabilizer Children ≥3 yr: 1 gtt bid q8-12h	Not for treatment of contact lens–related irritation; the preservative may be absorbed by soft contact lenses. Wait at least 10 min after administration before inserting soft contact lenses.
Olopatadine hydrochloride 0.1%, 0.2%, 0.7% Patanol Pataday Pazeo	Antihistamine/mast cell stabilizer Children ≥3 yr: 1 gtt bid (8 hr apart) Children ≥2 yr: 1 gtt qd	Not for treatment of contact lens–related irritation; the preservative may be absorbed by soft contact lenses. Wait at least 10 min after administration before inserting soft contact lenses.
Alcaftadine, 0.25% Lastacaft	Antihistamine/mast cell stabilizer Children > 2 yr: 1 gtt bid q8-12h	Contact lenses should be removed before application; may be inserted after 10 min. Not for the treatment of contact lens irritation.
Bepotastine besilate 1.5% Bepreve	Antihistamine/mast cell stabilizer Children >2 yr: 1 gtt bid q8-12h	Contact lenses should be removed before application, may be inserted after 10 min. Not for the treatment of contact lens irritation.
Ketorolac tromethamine 0.5% Acular	NSAID Children ≥3 yr: 1 gtt qid	Avoid with aspirin or NSAID sensitivity. Use ocular product with caution in patients with complicated ocular surgeries, corneal denervation or epithelial defects, ocular surface diseases (e.g., dry eye syndrome), repeated ocular surgeries within a short period, diabetes mellitus, or rheumatoid arthritis; these patients may be at risk for corneal adverse events that may be sight threatening. *Do not use while wearing contact lenses.*
Fluorometholone 0.1%, 0.25% suspension (0.1%, 0.25%) and ointment (0.1%) FML, FML Forte, Flarex	Fluorinated corticosteroid Children ≥2 yr, 1 gtt into conjunctival sac of affected eye(s) bid-qid. During initial 24-48 hr, dosage may be increased to 1 gtt q4h. Ointment (~1.3 cm in length) into conjunctival sac of affected eye(s) 1-3 times daily. May be applied q4h during initial 24-48 hr of therapy.	If improvement does not occur after 2 days, patient should be reevaluated. Patient should remove soft contact lenses before administering (contains benzalkonium chloride) and delay reinsertion of lenses for ≥15 min after administration. Close monitoring for development of glaucoma and cataracts.

NSAID, Nonsteroidal antiinflammatory drug; bid, 2 times daily; gtt, drops; qid, 4 times daily; q4-6h; every 4-6 hr; qd, every day.

Chapter **173**

Urticaria (Hives) and Angioedema

*Amy P. Stallings, Stephen C. Dreskin,
Michael M. Frank, and Scott H. Sicherer*

第一百七十三章

荨麻疹（风团）和血管性水肿

中文导读

　　本章主要介绍了荨麻疹和血管性水肿的病因和发病机制、不同类型的荨麻疹、诊断、治疗、遗传性血管性水肿的并发症以及治疗等。具体描述了触发因素、典型的皮疹表现；具体阐述了不同类型的荨麻疹，包括物理性荨麻疹、胆碱能性荨麻疹、皮肤划痕症、压力相关性荨麻疹和血管性水肿、日光性荨麻疹、慢性特发性荨麻疹等；讲述了急慢性荨麻疹的常见原因；治疗方面避免触发因素的重要性；具体描述了遗传性血管性水肿的临床表现，喉头水肿的治疗，补体C1抑制物（C1-INH）的药理学机制。

Urticaria and angioedema affect 20% of individuals at some point in their life. Episodes of hives that last for <6 wk are considered *acute*, whereas those that occur on most days of the week for >6 wk are designated *chronic*. The distinction is important, because the causes and mechanisms of urticaria formation and the therapeutic approaches are different in each instance.

ETIOLOGY AND PATHOGENESIS

Acute urticaria and angioedema are often caused by an allergic IgE–mediated reaction (Table 173.1). This form of urticaria is a self-limited process that occurs when an allergen activates mast cells in the skin. Common causes of acute generalized urticaria include foods, drugs (particularly antibiotics), and stinging-insect venoms. If an allergen (latex, animal dander) penetrates the skin locally, hives often can develop at the site of exposure. Acute urticaria can also result from non–IgE–mediated stimulation of mast cells, caused by radiocontrast agents, viral agents (including hepatitis B and Epstein-Barr virus), opiates, and nonsteroidal antiinflammatory drugs (NSAIDs). The diagnosis of **chronic urticaria** is established when lesions occur on most days of the week for >6 wk and are not physical urticaria or recurrent acute urticaria with repeated exposures to a specific agent (Tables 173.2 and 173.3). In about half the cases, chronic urticaria is accompanied by angioedema. Rarely, angioedema occurs without urticaria. Angioedema without urticaria is often a result of allergy, but recurrent angioedema suggests other diagnoses.

A typical **hive** is an erythematous, pruritic, raised wheal that blanches with pressure, is transient, and resolves without residual lesions, unless the area was intensely scratched. In contrast, urticaria associated with

Table 173.1	Etiology of Acute Urticaria
Foods	Egg, milk, wheat, peanuts, tree nuts, soy, shellfish, fish, (direct mast cell degranulation)
Medications	Suspect all medications, even nonprescription or homeopathic
Insect stings	Hymenoptera (honeybee, yellow jacket, hornets, wasp, fire ants), biting insects (papular urticaria)
Infections	**Bacterial** (streptococcal pharyngitis, *Mycoplasma*, sinusitis); viral (hepatitis, mononucleosis [Epstein-Barr virus], coxsackieviruses A and B); **Parasitic** (*Ascaris, Ancylostoma, Echinococcus, Fasciola, Filaria, Schistosoma, Strongyloides, Toxocara, Trichinella*); **Fungal** (dermatophytes, *Candida*)
Contact allergy	Latex, pollen, animal saliva, nettle plants, caterpillars
Transfusion reactions	Blood, blood products, or IV immune globulin administration

From Lasley MV, Kennedy MS, Altman LC: Urticaria and angioedema. In Altman LC, Becker JW, Williams PV, editors: *Allergy in primary care*, Philadelphia, 2000, Saunders, p 232.

Table 173.2	Etiology of Chronic Urticaria
Idiopathic/autoimmune	Approximately 30% of chronic urticaria cases are physical urticaria, and 60–70% are idiopathic. Of the idiopathic cases approximately 35–40% have anti-IgE or anti-FcεRI (high-affinity IgE receptor α chain) autoantibodies (autoimmune chronic urticaria)
Physical	Dermatographism Cholinergic urticaria Cold urticaria (see Table 173.5) Delayed pressure urticaria Solar urticaria Vibratory urticaria Aquagenic urticaria
Autoimmune diseases	Systemic lupus erythematosus Juvenile idiopathic arthritis Thyroid disease (Graves, Hashimoto) Celiac disease Inflammatory bowel disease Leukocytoclastic vasculitis
Autoinflammatory/periodic fever syndromes	See Tables 173.3 and 173.5.
Neoplastic	Lymphoma Mastocytosis Leukemia
Angioedema	Hereditary angioedema (autosomal dominant inherited deficiency of C1-esterase inhibitor) Acquired angioedema Angiotensin-converting enzyme inhibitors

From Lasley MV, Kennedy MS, Altman LC: Urticaria and angioedema. In Altman LC, Becker JW, Williams PV, editors: *Allergy in primary care*, Philadelphia, 2000, Saunders, p 234.

serum sickness reactions, systemic lupus erythematosus (SLE), or other vasculitides in which a skin biopsy reveals a small-vessel vasculitis, often have distinguishing clinical features. Lesions that burn more than itch, last >24 hr, do not blanch, blister, heal with scarring, or that are associated with bleeding into the skin (purpura) suggest urticarial vasculitis. Atypical aspects of the gross appearance of the hives or associated symptoms should heighten concern that the urticaria or angioedema may be the manifestation of a systemic disease process (Table 173.4).

PHYSICAL URTICARIA
Physically induced urticaria and angioedema share the common property of being induced by an environmental stimulus, such as a change in temperature or direct stimulation of the skin with pressure, stroking, vibration, or light (see Table 173.2).

Cold-Dependent Disorders
Cold urticaria is characterized by the development of localized pruritus, erythema, and urticaria/angioedema after exposure to a cold stimulus. Total body exposure, as seen with swimming in cold water, can cause massive release of vasoactive mediators, resulting in hypotension, loss of consciousness, and even death if not promptly treated. The diagnosis is confirmed by challenge testing for an *isomorphic cold reaction* by holding an ice cube in place on the patient's skin for 5 min. In patients with cold urticaria, an urticarial lesion develops about 10 min after removal of the ice cube and on rewarming of the chilled skin. Cold urticaria can be associated with the presence of **cryoproteins** such as cold agglutinins, cryoglobulins, cryofibrinogen, and the Donath-Landsteiner antibody seen in secondary syphilis (paroxysmal cold hemoglobinuria). In patients with cryoglobulins the isolated proteins appear to transfer cold sensitivity and activate the complement cascade on in vitro incubation with normal

plasma. The term **idiopathic cold urticaria** generally applies to patients without abnormal circulating plasma proteins such as cryoglobulins. Cold urticaria has also been reported after viral infections. Cold urticaria must be distinguished from the **familial cold autoinflammatory syndrome** (see later, Diagnosis) (Table 173.5; see also Table 173.3 and Chapter 188).

Cholinergic Urticaria
Cholinergic urticaria is characterized by the onset of small, punctate pruritic wheals surrounded by a prominent erythematous flare and associated with exercise, hot showers, and sweating. Once the patient cools down, the rash usually subsides in 30-60 min. Occasionally, symptoms of more generalized cholinergic stimulation, such as lacrimation, wheezing, salivation, and syncope, are observed. These symptoms are mediated by cholinergic nerve fibers that innervate the musculature via parasympathetic neurons and innervate the sweat glands by cholinergic fibers that travel with the sympathetic nerves. Elevated plasma histamine values parallel the onset of urticaria triggered by changes in body temperature.

Dermatographism
The ability to write on skin, dermatographism (also called *dermographism* or *urticaria factitia*) may occur as an isolated disorder or may accompany chronic urticaria or other physical urticaria. It can be diagnosed by observing the skin after stroking it with a tongue depressor. In patients with dermatographism, a linear response occurs secondary to reflex vasoconstriction, followed by pruritus, erythema, and a linear flare caused by secondary dilation of the vessel and extravasation of plasma.

Pressure-Induced Urticaria and Angioedema
Pressure-induced urticaria differs from most types of urticaria or angioedema in that symptoms typically occur 4-6 hr after pressure has been applied. The disorder is clinically heterogeneous. Some patients may complain of swelling, with or without pruritus, secondary to pressure, with normal-appearing skin (no urticaria), so the term *angioedema* is more appropriate. Other lesions are predominantly urticarial and may or may not be associated with significant swelling. When urticaria is present, an infiltrative skin lesion is seen, characterized by a perivascular mononuclear cell infiltrate and dermal edema similar to that seen in chronic idiopathic urticaria. Symptoms occur at sites of tight clothing; foot swelling is common after walking; and buttock swelling may be prominent after sitting for a few hours. This condition can coexist with chronic idiopathic urticaria or can occur separately. The diagnosis is confirmed by challenge testing in which pressure is applied perpendicular to the skin. This is often done with a sling attached to a 10 lb weight that is placed over the patient's arm for 20 min.

Solar Urticaria
Solar urticaria is a rare disorder in which urticaria develops within minutes of direct sun exposure. Typically, pruritus occurs first, in approximately 30 sec, followed by edema confined to the light-exposed area and surrounded by a prominent erythematous zone. The lesions usually disappear within 1-3 hr after cessation of sun exposure. When large areas of the body are exposed, systemic symptoms may occur, including hypotension and wheezing. Solar urticaria has been classified into 6 types, depending on the wavelength of light that induces skin lesions and the ability or inability to transfer the disorder passively with serum IgE. The rare inborn error of metabolism **erythropoietic protoporphyria** can be confused with solar urticaria because of the development of itching and burning of exposed skin immediately after sun exposure. In erythropoietic protoporphyria, fluorescence of ultraviolet-irradiated red blood cells can be demonstrated, and protoporphyrins are found in the urine.

Aquagenic Urticaria
Patients with aquagenic urticaria demonstrate small wheals after contact with water, regardless of its temperature, and are thereby distinguishable from patients with cold urticaria or cholinergic urticaria. Direct

Table 173.3	Febrile Autoinflammatory Diseases Causing Urticaria in Children					
DISEASE	**GENE (PROTEIN)**	**INHERITANCE**	**ATTACK LENGTH**	**TIMING OF ONSET**	**CUTANEOUS FEATURES**	**EXTRACUTANEOUS CLINICAL FEATURES**
FCAS	*NLRP3* (cryopyrin)	AD	Brief; minutes to 3 days	Neonatal or infantile	Cold-induced urticaria	Arthralgia Conjunctivitis Headache
Muckle-Wells syndrome	*NLRP3* (cryopyrin)	AD	1-3 days	Neonatal, infantile, childhood (can be later)	Widespread urticaria	Arthralgia/arthritis Sensorineural hearing loss Conjunctivitis/episcleritis Headache Amyloidosis
Chronic infantile neurologic cutaneous articular syndrome; neonatal-onset multisystem inflammatory disease	*NLRP3* (cryopyrin)	AD	Continuous flares	Neonatal or infantile	Widespread urticaria	Deforming osteoarthropathy, epiphyseal overgrowth Sensorineural hearing loss Dysmorphic facies Chronic aseptic meningitis, headaches, papilledema, seizures Conjunctivitis/uveitis, optic atrophy Growth retardation Developmental delay Amyloidosis
HIDS	*MVK* (mevalonate kinase)	AR	3-7 days	Infancy (<2 yr)	Intermittent morbilliform or urticarial rash Aphthous mucosal ulcers Erythema nodosum	Arthralgia/arthritis Cervical lymphadenopathy Severe abdominal pain Diarrhea/vomiting Headache Elevated IgD and IgA antibody levels Elevated urine mevalonic acid during attacks
Tumor necrosis factor receptor–associated periodic syndrome	*TNFRSF1A* (TNFR1)	AD	>7 days	Childhood	Intermittent migratory erythematous macules and edematous plaques overlying areas of myalgia, often on limbs Periorbital edema	Migratory myalgia Conjunctivitis Serositis Amyloidosis
Systemic-onset juvenile idiopathic arthritis (SoJIA)	Polygenic	Varies	Daily (quotidian)	Peak onset at 1-6 yr	Nonfixed erythematous rash; may be urticarial With or without dermatographism With or without periorbital edema	Polyarthritis Myalgia Hepatosplenomegaly Lymphadenopathy Serositis
PLAID	*PLCG2*	AD	N/A	Infancy	Urticaria induced by evaporative cooling Ulcers in cold-exposed areas	Allergies Autoimmune disease Recurrent sinopulmonary infections Elevated IgE antibody levels Decreased IgA and IgM antibody levels Often elevated antinuclear antibody titers

AD, Autosomal dominant; AR, autosomal recessive; HIDS, hyperimmunoglobulinemia D syndrome; FCAS, familial cold-induced autoinflammatory syndrome; N/A, not available; PLAID, PLCγ2-associated antibody deficiency and immune dysregulation.

From Youseff MJ, Chiu YE: Eczema and urticaria as manifestations of undiagnosed and rare diseases, *Pediatr Clin North Am* 64:39–56, 2017 (Table 2, pp 49–50).

application of a compress of water to the skin is used to test for the presence of aquagenic urticaria. Rarely, chlorine or other trace contaminants may be responsible for the reaction.

CHRONIC IDIOPATHIC URTICARIA AND ANGIOEDEMA

A common disorder of unknown origin, chronic idiopathic urticaria and angioedema is often associated with normal routine laboratory values and no evidence of systemic disease. Chronic urticaria does

not appear to result from an allergic reaction. It differs from allergen-induced skin reactions and from physically induced urticaria in that histologic studies reveal cellular infiltrate predominantly around small venules. Skin examination reveals infiltrative hives with palpably elevated borders, sometimes varying greatly in size and shape but generally being rounded.

Biopsy of a typical lesion reveals nonnecrotizing, perivascular, mononuclear cellular infiltration. Varying histopathologic processes can occur in the skin and manifest as urticaria. Patients with **hypocomplementemia** and **cutaneous vasculitis** can have urticaria and/or angioedema. Biopsy of these lesions in patients with urticaria, arthralgias, myalgias, and an elevated erythrocyte sedimentation rate (ESR) as manifestations of necrotizing venulitis can reveal fibrinoid necrosis with a predominantly neutrophilic infiltrate. However, the urticarial lesions may be clinically indistinguishable from those seen in the more typical, nonvasculitic cases.

Chronic urticaria is increasingly associated with the presence of antithyroid antibodies. Affected patients generally have antibodies to thyroglobulin or a microsomally derived antigen (peroxidase), even if they are euthyroid. The incidence of elevated thyroid antibodies in patients with chronic urticaria is approximately 12%, compared with 3–6% in the general population. Although some patients show clinical reduction of the urticaria with thyroid replacement therapy, others do not. The role of thyroid autoantibodies in chronic urticaria is uncertain; their presence may reflect a tendency of the patient to develop autoantibodies, but they may not play a direct role in chronic urticaria. Of patients with chronic urticaria, 35–40% have a positive **autologous serum skin test** result: If serum from these patients is intradermally injected into their skin, a significant wheal and flare reaction develops. Such patients frequently have a complement-activating IgG antibody directed against the α subunit of the IgE receptor that can cross-link

the IgE receptor (α subunit) and degranulate mast cells and basophils. An additional 5–10% of patients with chronic urticaria have anti-IgE antibodies rather than an anti–IgE receptor antibody.

Diagnosis

The diagnosis of both acute and chronic urticaria is primarily clinical and requires that the physician be aware of the various forms of urticaria.

Urticaria is transient, pruritic, erythematous, raised wheals that may become tense and painful. The lesions may coalesce and form

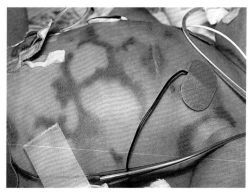

Fig. 173.1 Polycyclic lesions of urticaria associated with prostaglandin E₂ infusion. *(From Eichenfield LF, Friedan IJ, Esterly NB: Textbook of neonatal dermatology, Philadelphia, 2001, WB Saunders, p. 300.)*

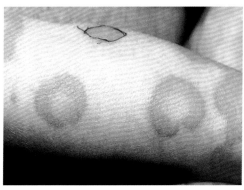

Fig. 173.2 Annular urticaria of unknown etiology. *(From Eichenfield LF, Friedan IJ, Esterly NB: Textbook of neonatal dermatology, Philadelphia, 2001, WB Saunders, p. 301.)*

Table 173.4	Distinguishing Features Between Urticaria and Systemic Urticarial Syndromes
COMMON URTICARIA	**URTICARIAL SYNDROMES (≥1 of following)**
Only typical wheals: Erythematous edematous lesions Transient (<24-36 hr) Asymmetric distribution Resolution without signs No associated different elementary lesions (papules, vesicles, purpura, crustae) Pruritic (rarely stinging/burning) Possibly associated with angioedema No associated systemic symptoms	Atypical "wheals": Infiltrated plaques Persistent (>24-36 hr) Symmetric distribution Resolution with signs (hypo/hyperpigmentation, bruising, or scarring) Associated different elementary lesions (papules, vesicles, purpura, scaling, crustae) Not pruritic; rather painful or burning Usually no associated angioedema Often associated with systemic symptoms (fever, malaise, arthralgia, abdominal pain, weight loss, acral circulatory abnormalities, neurologic signs

From Peroni A, Colato C, Zanoni G, Girolomoni G: Urticarial lesions: if not urticaria, what else? The differential diagnosis of urticaria, *J Am Acad Dermatol* 62(4):559, 2009.

Table 173.5	Hereditary Diseases With Cold-Induced Urticaria	
	EPISODIC SYMPTOMS	**SUSTAINED/PROGRESSIVE SYMPTOMS**
CAPS FCAS	Urticarial rash, arthralgia, myalgia, chills, fever, swelling of extremities	Renal amyloidosis
MWS	Urticarial rash, arthralgia, chills, fever	Sensorineural deafness, renal amyloidosis
CINCA	Fever	Rash, arthritis, chronic meningitis, visual defect, deafness, growth retardation, renal amyloidosis
NAPS12 (FCAS2)	Fever, arthralgia, myalgia, urticaria, abdominal pain, aphthous ulcers, lymphadenopathy	Sensorineural deafness
PLAID (FCAS3)	Urticaria induced by evaporative cooling, sinopulmonary infections	Serum low IgM and IgA levels; high IgE levels; decreased B and NK cells; granulomata; antinuclear antibodies

CAPS, Cryopyrin-associated periodic syndromes; FCAS, familial cold-induced autoinflammatory syndrome; MWS, Muckle-Wells syndrome; CINCA, chronic infantile neurologic cutaneous articular syndrome; NAPS, NLRP-12–associated periodic syndrome; PLAID, PLCG2-associated antibody deficiency and immune dysregulation.
From Kanazawa N: Hereditary disorders presenting with urticaria, *Immunol Allergy Clin NORTH Am* 34:169–179, 2014 (Table 4, p 176).

polymorphous, serpiginous, or annular lesions (Figs. 173.1 and 173.2). Individual lesions usually last 20 min to 3 hr and rarely more than 24 hr. The lesions often disappear, only to reappear at another site. **Angioedema** involves the deeper subcutaneous tissues in locations such as the eyelids, lips, tongue, genitals, dorsum of the hands or feet, or wall of the gastrointestinal (GI) tract.

Drugs and foods are the most common causes of acute urticaria. In children, viral infections also frequently trigger hives. Allergy skin testing for foods can be helpful in sorting out causes of acute urticaria, especially when supported by historical evidence. The role of an offending food can then be proved by elimination and careful challenge in a controlled setting, when needed. In the absence of information implicating an ingestant cause, skin testing for foods and implementation of elimination diets are generally not useful for either acute or chronic urticaria. Patients with delayed urticaria 3-6 hr after a meal consisting of mammalian meat should be evaluated for IgE to galactose-α-1,3-galactose ("alpha-gal"), a carbohydrate allergen. Alpha-gal has been identified as a trigger in this circumstance, with sensitization apparently linked to tick bites in specific geographic regions, such as the mid-Atlantic area of the United States. Skin testing for aeroallergens is not indicated unless there is a concern about contact urticaria (animal dander or grass pollen). Dermatographism is common in patients with urticaria and can complicate allergy skin testing by causing false-positive reactions, but this distinction is usually discernible.

Autoimmune diseases are rare causes of chronic urticarial or angioedema. In vitro testing for serum-derived activity that activates basophils involves detection of the expression of the surface marker CD63 or CD203c by donor basophils after incubation with patient serum. The clinical applicability and significance of these tests remains debated. The **differential diagnosis** of chronic urticaria includes cutaneous or systemic mastocytosis, complement-mediated mast cell degranulation as may occur with circulating immune complexes, malignancies, mixed connective tissue diseases, and cutaneous blistering disorders (e.g., bullous pemphigoid; see Table 173.2). In general, laboratory testing should be limited to a complete blood cell count with differential, ESR determination, urinalysis, thyroid autoantibody testing, and liver function tests. Further studies are warranted if the patient has fever, arthralgias, or elevated ESR (Table 173.6; see also Table 173.4). Testing for antibodies directed at the high-affinity IgE receptor may be warranted in patients with intractable urticaria. **Hereditary angioedema** is potentially life threatening, usually associated with deficient C1 inhibitor activity, and the most important familial form of angioedema (see Chapter 160.3), but it is not associated with typical urticaria. In patients with eosinophilia, stools should be obtained for ova and parasite testing, because infection with helminthic parasites has been associated with urticaria. A syndrome of episodic angioedema/urticaria and fever with associated **eosinophilia** has been described in both adults and children. In contrast to other hypereosinophilic syndromes, this entity has a benign course.

Skin biopsy for diagnosis of possible **urticarial vasculitis** is recommended for urticarial lesions that persist at the same location for >24 hr, those with pigmented or purpuric components, and those that burn more than itch. Collagen vascular diseases such as SLE may manifest urticarial vasculitis as a presenting feature. The skin biopsy in urticarial vasculitis typically shows endothelial cell swelling of postcapillary venules with necrosis of the vessel wall, perivenular neutrophil infiltrate, diapedesis of red blood cells, and fibrin deposition associated with deposition of immune complexes.

Mastocytosis is characterized by mast cell hyperplasia in the bone marrow, liver, spleen, lymph nodes, and skin. Clinical effects of mast cell activation are common, including pruritus, flushing, urtication, abdominal pain, nausea, and vomiting. The diagnosis is confirmed by a bone marrow biopsy showing increased numbers of spindle-shaped mast cells that express CD2 and CD25. **Urticaria pigmentosa** is the most common skin manifestation of mastocytosis and may occur as an isolated skin finding. It appears as small, yellow-tan to reddish brown macules or raised papules that urticate on scratching (**Darier sign**). This sign can be masked by antihistamines. The diagnosis is confirmed by a skin biopsy that shows increased numbers of dermal mast cells.

Table 173.6	Diagnostic Testing for Urticaria and Angioedema
DIAGNOSIS	**DIAGNOSTIC TESTING**
Food and drug reactions	Elimination of offending agent, skin testing, and challenge with suspected foods
Autoimmune urticaria	Autologous serum skin test; antithyroid antibodies; antibodies against the high-affinity IgE receptor
Thyroiditis	Thyroid-stimulating hormone; antithyroid antibodies
Infections	Appropriate cultures or serology
Collagen vascular diseases and cutaneous vasculitis	Skin biopsy, CH_{50}, C1q, C4, C3, factor B, immunofluorescence of tissues, antinuclear antibodies, cryoglobulins
Malignancy with angioedema	CH_{50}, C1q, C4, C1-INH determinations
Cold urticaria	Ice cube test usually positive but may be negative in some familial autoinflammatory disorders
Solar urticaria	Exposure to defined wavelengths of light, red blood cell protoporphyrin, fecal protoporphyrin, and coproporphyrin
Dermatographism	Stroking with narrow object (e.g., tongue blade, fingernail)
Pressure urticaria	Application of pressure for defined time and intensity
Vibratory urticaria	Vibration for 4 min
Aquagenic urticaria	Challenge with tap water at various temperatures
Urticaria pigmentosa	Skin biopsy, test for dermatographism
Hereditary angioedema	C4, C2, CH_{50}, C1-INH testing by protein and function
Familial cold urticaria	Challenge by cold exposure, measurement of temperature, white blood cell count, erythrocyte sedimentation rate, skin biopsy
C3b inactivator deficiency	C3, factor B, C3b inactivator determinations
Chronic idiopathic urticaria	Skin biopsy, immunofluorescence (negative result), autologous skin test

Physical urticaria should be considered in any patient with chronic urticaria and a suggestive history (see Table 173.2). Papular urticaria often occurs in small children, generally on the extremities. It manifests as grouped or linear, highly pruritic wheals or papules mainly on exposed skin at the sites of insect bites.

Exercise-induced anaphylaxis manifests as varying combinations of pruritus, urticaria, angioedema, wheezing, laryngeal obstruction, or hypotension after exercise (see Chapter 174). Cholinergic urticaria is differentiated by positive results of heat challenge tests and the rare occurrence of anaphylactic shock. The combination of ingestion of various food allergens and postprandial exercise has been associated with urticaria/angioedema and anaphylaxis. In patients with this combination disorder, food or exercise alone does not produce the reaction.

Muckle-Wells syndrome and familial cold autoinflammatory syndrome are rare, dominantly inherited conditions associated with recurrent urticaria-like lesions. **Muckle-Wells syndrome** is characterized by arthritis and joint pain that usually appears in adolescence. It is associated with progressive nerve deafness, recurrent fever, elevated ESR (see Tables 173.3 and 173.5), hypergammaglobulinemia, renal amyloidosis, and a poor prognosis. **Familial cold autoinflammatory syndrome** is characterized by a cold-induced rash that has urticarial features but is rarely pruritic. Cold exposure leads to additional symptoms such as conjunctivitis, sweating, headache, and nausea. Patient longevity is usually normal.

TREATMENT

Acute urticaria is a self-limited illness requiring little treatment other than antihistamines and avoidance of any identified trigger. Hydroxyzine and diphenhydramine are sedating but are effective and frequently used for treatment of urticaria. Loratadine, fexofenadine, and cetirizine are also effective and are preferable because of reduced frequency of drowsiness and longer duration of action (Table 173.7). Epinephrine 1:1,000, 0.01 mL/kg (maximum 0.3 mL) intramuscularly, usually provides rapid relief of acute, severe urticaria/angioedema but is seldom required. A short course of oral corticosteroids should be given only for severe episodes of urticaria and angioedema that are unresponsive to antihistamines.

The best treatment of physical urticaria is avoidance of the stimulus. Antihistamines are also helpful. Cyproheptadine in divided doses is the drug of choice for cold-induced urticaria. Treatment of dermatographism consists of local skin care and antihistamines; for severe symptoms, high doses may be needed. The initial objective of therapy is to decrease pruritus so that the stimulation for scratching is diminished. A combination of antihistamines, sunscreens, and avoidance of sunlight is helpful for most patients.

Chronic urticaria only rarely responds favorably to dietary manipulation. The mainstay of therapy is the use of nonsedating or low-sedating H_1 antihistamines. In those patients not showing response to standard doses, pushing the H_1 blockade with higher than the usual recommended doses of these agents is a common next approach. The 3-drug combination of H_1 and H_2 antihistamine with a leukotriene receptor antagonist (montelukast) is helpful for many patients. If hives persist after maximal H_1- and/or H_2-receptor blockade has been achieved, a brief course of oral corticosteroids may be considered, but long-term steroid use is best avoided. The monoclonal antibody omalizumab (anti-IgE) is FDA approved for the treatment of chronic urticaria in children 12 years and older. Other agents that have been used for chronic urticaria but are not approved by the U.S. Food and Drug Administration (FDA) for this condition include cyclosporine, hydroxychloroquine, sulfasalazine, colchicine, dapsone, mycophenolate, intravenous immune globulin (IVIG), and plasmapheresis.

HEREDITARY ANGIOEDEMA

Hereditary angioedema (**HAE**, types 1 and 2) is an inherited autosomal dominant disease caused by low functional levels of the plasma protein **C1 inhibitor (C1-INH)** (see Chapter 160.3). Patients typically report episodic attacks of angioedema or deep localized swelling, most often on a hand or foot, that begin during childhood and become much more severe during adolescence. Cutaneous nonpitting and nonpruritic edema not associated with urticaria is the most common symptom. The swelling usually becomes more severe over about 1.5 days and then resolves over about the same period. However, the duration of attacks can be quite variable. In some patients, attacks are preceded by the development of a rash, **erythema marginatum**, that is erythematous, not raised, and not pruritic. A 2nd major symptom complex noted by patients is attacks of severe abdominal pain caused by edema of the mucosa of any portion of the GI tract. The intensity of the pain can approximate that of an acute abdomen, often resulting in unnecessary surgery. Either constipation or diarrhea during these attacks can be noted. The GI edema generally follows the same time course to resolution as the cutaneous attacks and often does not occur at the same time as the peripheral edema. Patients usually have a *prodrome,* a tightness or tingling in the area that will swell, usually lasting several hours, followed by the development of angioedema.

Laryngeal edema, the most feared complication of HAE, can cause complete respiratory obstruction. Although life-threatening attacks are infrequent, more than half of patients with HAE experience laryngeal involvement at some time during their lives. Dental work with the

Table 173.7	Treatment of Urticaria and Angioedema	
CLASS/DRUG	**DOSE**	**FREQUENCY**
ANTIHISTAMINES, TYPE H₁ (SECOND GENERATION)		
Fexofenadine	6-11 yr: 30 mg	Twice daily
	>12 yr: 60 mg	
	Adult: 180 mg	Once daily
Loratadine	2-5 yr: 5 mg	Once daily
	>6 yr: 10 mg	
Desloratadine	6-11 mo: 1 mg	Once daily
	12 mo-5 yr: 1.25 mg	
	6-11 yr: 2.5 mg	
	>12 yr: 5 mg	
Cetirizine	6-23 mo: 2.5 mg	Once daily
	2-6 yr: 2.5-5 mg	
	>6 yr: 5-10 mg	
Levocetirizine	6 mo-5 yr: 1.25 mg	Once daily
	6-11 yr: 2.5 mg	Once daily
	>12 yr: 5 mg	Once daily
ANTIHISTAMINES, TYPE H₂		
Cimetidine	Infants: 10-20 mg/kg/day	Divided q6-12h
	Children: 20-40 mg/kg/day	
Ranitidine	1 mo-16 yr: 5-10 mg/kg/day	Divided q12h
Famotidine	3-12 mo: 1 mg/kg/day	Divided q12h
	1-16 yr: 1-2 mg/kg/day	
LEUKOTRIENE PATHWAY MODIFIERS		
Montelukast	12 mo-5 yr: 4 mg	Once daily
	6-14 yr: 5 mg	
	>14 yr: 10 mg	
Zafirlukast	5-11 yr: 10 mg	Twice daily
IMMUNOMODULATORY DRUGS		
Omalizumab (anti IgE)	>11 yr: 150 mg or 300 mg	Every 28 days
Cyclosporine	3-4 mg/kg/day	Divided q12h*
Sulfasalazine	>6 yr: 30 mg/kg/day	Divided q6h†
Intravenous immune globulin (IVIG)	400 mg/kg/day	5 consecutive days

*Monitor blood pressure and serum creatinine, potassium, and magnesium levels monthly.
†Monitor complete blood count and liver function tests at baseline, every 2 wk for 3 mo, and then every 1-3 mo.

injection of procaine hydrochloride (Novocain) into the gums is a common precipitant, but laryngeal edema can be spontaneous. The clinical condition may deteriorate rapidly, progressing through mild discomfort to complete airway obstruction over hours. Soft tissue edema can be readily seen when the disease involves the throat and uvula. If this edema progresses to difficulty swallowing secretions or a change in the tone of the voice, the patient may require emergency intubation or even tracheostomy to ensure an adequate airway. Other presentations are less common. These patients typically do not respond well to treatment with epinephrine, antihistamines, or glucocorticoids.

In most cases the cause of the attack is unknown, but in some patients, trauma or emotional stress clearly precipitates attacks. Drugs such as angiotensin-converting enzyme (ACE) inhibitors that inhibit the degradation of bradykinin make the disease strikingly worse, and estrogens also make attacks more severe. In some females, menstruation also regularly induces attacks. The frequency of attacks varies greatly among affected individuals and at different times in the same individual. Some individuals experience weekly episodes, whereas others may go years between attacks. Episodes can start at any age.

C1-INH is a member of the serpin family of proteases, similar to α-antitrypsin, antithrombin III, and angiotensinogen. These proteins stoichiometrically inactivate their target proteases by forming stable, 1:1 complexes with the protein to be inhibited. Synthesized primarily by hepatocytes, C1-INH is also synthesized by monocytes. The regulation of the protein production is not completely understood, but it is believed that androgens may stimulate C1-INH synthesis, because patients with

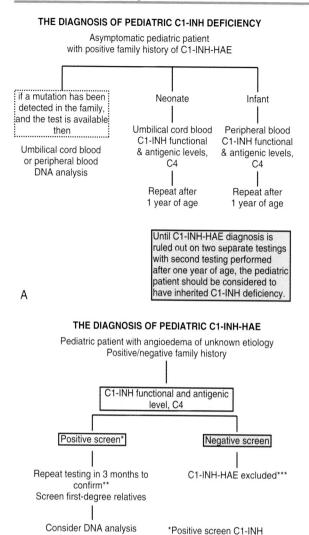

THE DIAGNOSIS OF PEDIATRIC C1-INH DEFICIENCY

Asymptomatic pediatric patient
with positive family history of C1-INH-HAE

if a mutation has been
detected in the family,
and the test is available
then

Umbilical cord blood
or peripheral blood
DNA analysis

Neonate

Umbilical cord blood
C1-INH functional
& antigenic levels,
C4

Repeat after
1 year of age

Infant

Peripheral blood
C1-INH functional
& antigenic levels,
C4

Repeat after
1 year of age

Until C1-INH-HAE diagnosis is
ruled out on two separate testings
with second testing performed
after one year of age, the pediatric
patient should be considered to
have inherited C1-INH deficiency.

A

THE DIAGNOSIS OF PEDIATRIC C1-INH-HAE

Pediatric patient with angioedema of unknown etiology
Positive/negative family history

C1-INH functional and antigenic
level, C4

Positive screen*

Repeat testing in 3 months to
confirm**
Screen first-degree relatives

Consider DNA analysis

Negative screen

C1-INH-HAE excluded***

*Positive screen C1-INH
functional level and C4 are
low, accompanied by a low
C1-INH antigenic level in
HAE type 1
**Repeated after 1 year of age
***Angioedema with acquired
C1-INH deficiency is also
excluded, but HAE with normal
C1-INH function, which is very
rare in pediatric patients, is not
ruled out

B

Fig. 173.3 A, Diagnosis of C1-INH deficiency in families with known C1-INH-HAE. **B,** Diagnosis of C1-INH-HAE in pediatric patients with angioedema of unknown etiology. *(From Farkas H, Martinez-Saguer I, Bork K, et al: International consensus on the diagnosis and management of pediatric patients with hereditary angioedema with C1 inhibitor deficiency. Eur J Allergy Clin Immunol 72:300-313, 2017, Fig.1, p. 304.)*

the disorder respond clinically to androgen therapy with elevated serum C1-INH levels. C1-INH deficiency is an autosomal dominant disease, with as many as 25% of patients giving no family history. Because all C1-INH–deficient patients are heterozygous for this gene defect, it is believed that half the normal level of C1-INH is not sufficient to prevent attacks. Fig. 173.3 shows the diagnostic approach.

Although named for its action on the 1st component of complement (C1 esterase), C1-INH also inhibits components of the fibrinolytic, clotting, and kinin pathways. Specifically, C1-INH inactivates plasmin-activated Hageman factor (factor XII), activated factor XI, plasma thromboplastin antecedent, and kallikrein. Within the complement system, C1-INH blocks the activation of C1 and the rest of the classical complement pathway by binding to C1r and C1s. Without adequate C1-INH, unchecked activation of C1 causes cleavage of C4 and C2, the proteins following in the complement cascade. Levels of C3 are normal. C1-INH also inhibits serine proteases associated with activation of the lectin activation pathway. The major factor responsible for the edema formation is bradykinin, an important nonapeptide mediator that can induce leakage of postcapillary venules. Bradykinin is derived from cleavage of the circulating protein high-molecular-weight kininogen by the plasma enzyme kallikrein.

Two major genetic types of C1-INH deficiency are described that result in essentially the same phenotypic expression. The C1-INH gene is located on chromosome 11 in the p11-q13 region. The inheritance is autosomal dominant with incomplete penetrance. Persons inheriting the abnormal gene can have a clinical spectrum ranging from asymptomatic to severely affected. **Type 1** HAE is the most common form, accounting for approximately 85% of cases. Synthesis of C1-INH is blocked at the site of the faulty allele, or the protein is not secreted normally because of faulty protein processing, but secretion occurs at the normal allele. The result is secretion of the normal protein, yielding quantitative serum concentrations of C1-INH approximately 20–40% of normal. **Type 2** HAE accounts for approximately 15% of cases. Mutations of 1 of the amino acids near the active site of the inhibitor lead to synthesis of nonfunctional C1-INH protein and again less than half of the normal functioning protein. Patients with type 2 HAE have either normal or increased concentrations of the protein but low values in assays of C1-INH function.

A clinical syndrome resembling HAE termed **HAE with normal C1-INH** has been described that affects mostly women, with a tendency to cause fewer abdominal attacks and more upper airway attacks. In this condition, no abnormalities of complement or of C1-INH have been described. Approximately 20% of affected patients have been found to have a gain-of-function abnormality of clotting factor XII, but the fundamental cause is of this syndrome still unknown.

The FDA has approved purified C1-INH for prophylaxis to prevent attacks. **Androgens** like the gonadotropin inhibitor danazol were previously used to prevent attacks. Weak androgens have many side effects that preclude their use in some patients. Their use in children is problematic because of the possibility of premature closure of the epiphyses, and these agents are not used in pregnant women. The fibrinolysis inhibitor ε-aminocaproic acid (**EACA**) is also effective in preventing attacks and has been used in children, but its use is attended by the development of severe fatigue and muscle weakness over time. A cyclized analog of EACA, **tranexamic acid**, has been used extensively in Europe; because of limited availability, it has been used less extensively in the United States. Tranexamic acid is believed to be more effective than EACA and has lower toxicity, but there have been few direct studies. Its mechanism of action is not clearly defined, and not all patients respond to this agent.

In 2008 the FDA approved, for adolescents and older patients, the use of purified C1-INH (Cinryze), prepared from human plasma and given intravenously, for *prophylaxis* of this disease. The half-life of this plasma protein is relatively short, about 40 hr, and the approved regimen is 1,000 units twice a week. In 2009 a similar purified C1-inhibitor product, Berinert, administered as 20 U/kg intravenously, was approved for the *treatment* of acute attacks. A recombinant C1-INH product has been FDA approved for *treatment* of acute attacks (and in Europe). In 2009 the FDA approved a kallikrein inhibitor, **ecallantide**, given subcutaneously, for *acute treatment* in patients age 16 yr and older. This 60–amino acid peptide causes anaphylaxis rarely and is approved only for administration by medical personnel. In 2010 a bradykinin type 2 receptor antagonist, **icatibant**, was approved for *acute treatment* in patients age 18 yr and older and in summer 2016 was approved for the treatment of all children. All treatments are most effective when given early in an attack and begin to have noticeable effect about 1-4 hr after treatment.

Bibliography is available at Expert Consult.

Chapter **174**
Anaphylaxis
Hugh A. Sampson, Julie Wang, and Scott H. Sicherer

第一百七十四章
严重过敏反应

中文导读

　　本章主要介绍了严重过敏反应的定义，阐述了儿科常见病因之一为医院外发生的食物过敏反应和医院内发生的乳胶过敏反应。列举了严重过敏反应在美国的年发生率估计为42例／100000人，年总病例数＞150000例病例。解读了危险因素包括患有哮喘和肥大细胞增生症，发病机制包括IgE介导和非IgE介导。叙述了临床表现有赖于病因而不同。简述严重过敏反应的实验室检查主要是发现变应原IgE抗体增高或类胰蛋白酶增高。采用流程图的方式介绍了严重过敏反应的诊断和鉴别诊断。急诊医疗以肌内注射肾上腺素作为一线治疗。并简介了难治性低血压的病例需要替代肾上腺素的其他血管加压药物。阐述了对双相严重过敏反应发生的监测与管理。强调了对规避变应原、识别早期症状体征、急救用肾上腺素自行注射器和书面的急救计划在预防中的重要作用。

Anaphylaxis is defined as a serious allergic reaction that is rapid in onset and may cause death. Anaphylaxis in children, particularly infants, is underdiagnosed. Anaphylaxis occurs when there is a sudden release of potent, biologically active mediators from mast cells and basophils, leading to cutaneous (urticaria, angioedema, flushing), respiratory (bronchospasm, laryngeal edema), cardiovascular (hypotension, dysrhythmias, myocardial ischemia), and gastrointestinal (nausea, colicky abdominal pain, vomiting, diarrhea) symptoms (Table 174.1 and Fig. 174.1).

ETIOLOGY

The most common causes of anaphylaxis in children are different for hospital and community settings. Anaphylaxis occurring in the hospital results primarily from allergic reactions to medications and latex. **Food allergy** is the most common cause of anaphylaxis occurring outside the hospital, accounting for about half the anaphylactic reactions reported in pediatric surveys from the United States, Italy, and South Australia (Table 174.2). **Peanut allergy** is an important cause of food-induced anaphylaxis, accounting for the majority of fatal and near-fatal reactions. In the hospital, latex is a particular problem for children undergoing multiple operations, such as patients with spina bifida and urologic disorders, and has prompted many hospitals to switch to latex-free products. Patients with **latex allergy** may also experience food-allergic reactions from homologous proteins in foods such as bananas, kiwi, avocado, chestnut, and passion fruit. Anaphylaxis to galactose-α-1,3-galactose has been reported 3-6 hr after eating red meat.

EPIDEMIOLOGY

The overall annual incidence of anaphylaxis in the United States is estimated at 42 cases per 100,000 person-years, totaling >150,000 cases/yr. Food allergens are the most common trigger in children, with an incidence rate of approximately 20 per 100,000 person-years. An Australian parental survey found that 0.59% of children 3-17 yr of age had experienced at least 1 anaphylactic event. Having asthma and the severity of asthma are important anaphylaxis risk factors (Table 174.3). In addition, patients with systemic mastocytosis or monoclonal mast cell–activating syndrome are at increased risk for anaphylaxis, as are patients with an elevated baseline serum tryptase level.

PATHOGENESIS

Principal pathologic features in fatal anaphylaxis include acute bronchial obstruction with pulmonary hyperinflation, pulmonary edema, intraalveolar hemorrhaging, visceral congestion, laryngeal edema, and urticaria and angioedema. Acute hypotension is attributed to vasomotor dilation and cardiac dysrhythmias.

　　Most cases of anaphylaxis are believed to be the result of activation of mast cells and basophils via cell-bound allergen-specific IgE molecules (see Fig. 174.1). Patients initially must be exposed to the responsible allergen to generate allergen-specific antibodies. In many cases the child and the parent are unaware of the initial exposure, which may be from passage of food proteins in maternal breast milk or exposure to inflamed skin (e.g., eczematous lesions). When the child is reexposed to the sensitizing allergen, mast cells and basophils, and possibly other cells

Table 174.1	Symptoms and Signs of Anaphylaxis in Infants	
ANAPHYLAXIS SYMPTOMS THAT INFANTS CANNOT DESCRIBE	**ANAPHYLAXIS SIGNS THAT MAY BE DIFFICULT TO INTERPRET/UNHELPFUL IN INFANTS, AND WHY**	**ANAPHYLAXIS SIGNS IN INFANTS**
GENERAL		
Feeling of warmth, weakness, anxiety, apprehension, impending doom	Nonspecific behavioral changes such as persistent crying, fussing, irritability, fright, suddenly becoming quiet	
SKIN/MUCOUS MEMBRANES		
Itching of lips, tongue, palate, uvula, ears, throat, nose, eyes, etc.; mouth-tingling or metallic taste	Flushing (may also occur with fever, hyperthermia, or crying spells)	Rapid onset of hives (potentially difficult to discern in infants with acute atopic dermatitis; scratching and excoriations will be absent in young infants); angioedema (face, tongue, oropharynx)
RESPIRATORY SYSTEM		
Nasal congestion, throat tightness; chest tightness; shortness of breath	Hoarseness, dysphonia (common after a crying spell); drooling or increased secretions (common in infants)	Rapid onset of coughing, choking, stridor, wheezing, dyspnea, apnea, cyanosis
GASTROINTESTINAL SYSTEM		
Dysphagia, nausea, abdominal pain/cramping	Spitting up/regurgitation (common after feeds), loose stools (normal in infants, especially if breastfed); colicky abdominal pain	Sudden, profuse vomiting
CARDIOVASCULAR SYSTEM		
Feeling faint, presyncope, dizziness, confusion, blurred vision, difficulty in hearing	Hypotension (need appropriate-size blood pressure cuff; low systolic blood pressure for children is defined as <70 mm Hg from 1 mo to 1 yr, and less than (70 mm Hg + [2 × age in yr]) from 1-10 yr; tachycardia, defined as >140 beats/min from 3 mo to 2 yr, inclusive; loss of bowel and bladder control (ubiquitous in infants)	Weak pulse, arrhythmia, diaphoresis/sweating, collapse/unconsciousness
CENTRAL NERVOUS SYSTEM		
Headache	Drowsiness, somnolence (common in infants after feeds)	Rapid onset of unresponsiveness, lethargy, or hypotonia; seizures

Adapted from Simons FER: Anaphylaxis in infants: can recognition and management be improved? *J Allergy Clin Immunol* 120:537–540, 2007.

such as macrophages, release a variety of mediators (histamine, tryptase) and cytokines that can produce allergic symptoms in any or all target organs. Clinical anaphylaxis may also be caused by mechanisms other than IgE-mediated reactions, including direct release of mediators from mast cells by medications and physical factors (morphine, exercise, cold), disturbances of leukotriene metabolism (aspirin and nonsteroidal antiinflammatory drugs), immune aggregates and complement activation (blood products), probable complement activation (radiocontrast dyes, dialysis membranes), and IgG-mediated reactions (high-molecular-weight dextran, chimeric or humanized monoclonal antibodies) (see Table 174.2).

Idiopathic anaphylaxis is a diagnosis of exclusion when no inciting agent is identified and other disorders have been excluded (see Chapter 678.1). Symptoms are similar to IgE mediated causes of anaphylaxis; episodes often recur.

CLINICAL MANIFESTATIONS
The onset of symptoms may vary depending on the cause of the reaction. Reactions from ingested allergens (foods, medications) are delayed in onset (minutes to 2 hr) compared with those from injected allergens (insect sting, medications) and tend to have more gastrointestinal (GI) symptoms. Initial symptoms may include any of the following constellation of symptoms: pruritus about the mouth and face; flushing, urticaria and angioedema, oral or cutaneous pruritus; a sensation of warmth, weakness, and apprehension (sense of doom); tightness in the throat, dry staccato cough and hoarseness, periocular pruritus, nasal congestion, sneezing, dyspnea, deep cough and wheezing; nausea, abdominal cramping, and vomiting, especially with ingested allergens; uterine contractions (manifesting as lower back pain); and faintness and loss of consciousness in severe cases. Some degree of obstructive laryngeal edema is typically encountered with severe reactions. Cutaneous symptoms may be absent in up to 10% of cases, and the *acute* onset of severe bronchospasm in a previously well person with asthma should

suggest the diagnosis of anaphylaxis. Sudden collapse in the absence of cutaneous symptoms should also raise suspicion of vasovagal collapse, myocardial infarction, aspiration, pulmonary embolism, or seizure disorder. Laryngeal edema, especially with abdominal pain, may also be a result of hereditary angioedema (see Chapter 173). Symptoms in infants may not be easy to identify (see Table 174.1).

LABORATORY FINDINGS
Laboratory studies may indicate the presence of IgE antibodies to a suspected causative agent, but this result is not definitive. Plasma histamine is elevated for a brief period but is unstable and difficult to measure in a clinical setting. **Plasma tryptase** is more stable and remains elevated for several hours but often is not elevated, especially in food-induced anaphylactic reactions.

DIAGNOSIS
A National Institutes of Health (NIH)–sponsored expert panel has recommended an approach to the diagnosis of anaphylaxis (Table 174.4). The differential diagnosis includes other forms of shock (hemorrhagic, cardiogenic, septic); vasopressor reactions, including flushing syndromes (e.g., carcinoid syndrome); ingestion of monosodium glutamate; scombroidosis; and hereditary angioedema. In addition, panic attack, vocal cord dysfunction, pheochromocytoma, and red man syndrome (caused by vancomycin) should be considered.

TREATMENT
Anaphylaxis is a medical emergency requiring aggressive management with intramuscular (IM, first line) or intravenous (IV) epinephrine, IM or IV H$_1$ and H$_2$ antihistamine antagonists, oxygen, IV fluids, inhaled β-agonists, and corticosteroids (Table 174.5 and Fig. 174.2). The initial assessment should ensure an adequate airway with effective respiration, circulation, and perfusion. **Epinephrine** is the most important medication, and there should be no delay in its administration.

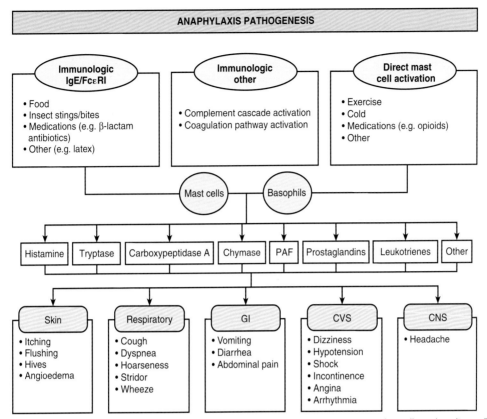

Fig. 174.1 Summary of the pathogenesis of anaphylaxis. See text for details about mechanisms, triggers, key cells, and mediators. Two or more target organ systems are typically involved in anaphylaxis. CNS, Central nervous system; CVS, cardiovascular system; GI, gastrointestinal; PAF, platelet-activating factor. (*From Leung DYM, Szefler SJ, Bonilla FA Akdis CA, Sampson HA, editors: Pediatric allergy principles and practice, ed 3, Philadelphia, 2016, Elsevier, p 525.*)

Table 174.2	Anaphylaxis Triggers in the Community*	

ALLERGEN TRIGGERS (IgE-DEPENDENT IMMUNOLOGIC MECHANISM)*	Inhalants (rare) (e.g., horse or hamster dander, grass pollen)
Foods (e.g., peanut, tree nuts, shellfish, fish, milk, egg, wheat, soy, sesame, meat [galactose-α-1,3-galactose])	Previously unrecognized allergens (foods, venoms, biting insect saliva, medications, biologic agents)
Food additives (e.g., spices, colorants, vegetable gums, contaminants)	**OTHER IMMUNE MECHANISMS (IgE INDEPENDENT)**
Stinging insects: Hymenoptera species (e.g., bees, yellow jackets, wasps, hornets, fire ants)	IgG mediated (infliximab, high-molecular-weight dextrans)
Medications (e.g., β-lactam antibiotics, ibuprofen)	Immune aggregates (IVIG)
Biologic agents (e.g., monoclonal antibodies [infliximab, omalizumab] and allergens [challenge tests, specific immunotherapy])	Drugs (aspirin, NSAID, opiates, contrast material, ethylene oxide/dialysis tubing)
Natural rubber latex	Complement activation
Vaccines	Physical factors (e.g., exercise,† cold, heat, sunlight/ultraviolet radiation)
	Ethanol
	Idiopathic*

*In the pediatric population, some anaphylaxis triggers, such as hormones (progesterone), seminal fluid, and occupational allergens, are uncommon, as is idiopathic anaphylaxis.
†Exercise with or without a co-trigger, such as a food or medication, cold air, or cold water.
IVIG, Intravenous immune globulin; NSAID, nonsteroidal antiinflammatory drug.
Adapted from Leung DYM, Sampson HA, Geha RS, et al: *Pediatric allergy principles and practice*, Philadelphia, 2010, Elsevier, p 652.

Epinephrine should be given by the IM route to the lateral thigh (1:1000 dilution, 0.01 mg/kg; maximum 0.5 mg). For children ≥12 yr, many recommend the 0.5 mg IM dose. The IM dose can be repeated at intervals of 5-15 min if symptoms persist or worsen. If there is no response to multiple doses of epinephrine, IV epinephrine using the 1:10,000 dilution may be needed. If IV access is not readily available, epinephrine can be administered via the endotracheal or intraosseous routes.

For refractory hypotension, other vasopressors may be used as alternative agents to epinephrine. Anaphylaxis refractory to repeated doses of epinephrine in a patient receiving β-adrenergic blockers has anecdotally been treated with glucagon. The patient should be placed in a supine position when there is concern for hemodynamic compromise. Fluids are also important in patients with shock. Other drugs (antihistamines, glucocorticosteroids) have a secondary role in the management of anaphylaxis.

Table 174.3	Patient Risk Factors for Anaphylaxis

AGE-RELATED FACTORS

Infants: anaphylaxis can be difficult to recognize, especially if the first episode; patients cannot describe symptoms.

Adolescents and young adults: increased risk-taking behaviors, such as failure to avoid known triggers and to carry an epinephrine autoinjector consistently

Pregnancy: risk of iatrogenic anaphylaxis, as from β lactam antibiotics to prevent neonatal group B streptococcal infection, agents used perioperatively during caesarean sections, and natural rubber latex

Older people: increased risk of death because of concomitant disease and drugs

CONCOMITANT DISEASES

Asthma and other chronic respiratory diseases
Cardiovascular diseases
Systemic mastocytosis or monoclonal mast cell–activating syndrome
Allergic rhinitis and eczema*
Depression, cognitive dysfunction, substance misuse

DRUGS

β-Adrenergic blockers[†]
Angiotensin-converting enzyme (ACE) inhibitors[†]
Sedatives, antidepressants, narcotics, recreational drugs, and alcohol may decrease the patient's ability to recognize triggers and symptoms.

FACTORS THAT MAY INCREASE RISK FOR ANAPHYLAXIS OR MAKE IT MORE DIFFICULT TO TREAT

Age
Asthma
Atopy
Drugs
Alcohol
Other cofactors such as exercise, infection, menses

*Atopic diseases are a risk factor for anaphylaxis triggered by food, latex, and exercise, but not for anaphylaxis triggered by most drugs or by insect stings.
[†]Patients taking β-blockers or ACE inhibitors seem to be at increased risk for severe anaphylaxis. In addition, those taking β-blockers may not respond optimally to epinephrine treatment and may need glucagon, a polypeptide with non–catecholamine-dependent inotropic and chronotropic cardiac effects, atropine for persistent bradycardia, or ipratropium for persistent bronchospasm.
Adapted from Lieberman P, Nicklas RA, Randolph C, et al: Anaphylaxis—a practice parameter update 2015, *Ann Allergy Asthma Immunol* 115(5):341–384, 2015, Table I-9.

Patients may experience **biphasic anaphylaxis**, which occurs when anaphylactic symptoms recur after apparent resolution. The mechanism of this phenomenon is unknown, but it appears to be more common when therapy is initiated late and symptoms at presentation are more severe. It does not appear to be affected by the administration of corticosteroids during the initial therapy. More than 90% of biphasic responses occur within 4 hr, so patients should be observed for at least 4 hr before being discharged from the emergency department. Referrals should be made to appropriate specialists for further evaluation and follow-up.

PREVENTION

For patients experiencing anaphylactic reactions, the triggering agent should be avoided, and education regarding early recognition of anaphylactic symptoms and administration of emergency medications should be provided. Patients with food allergies must be educated in allergen avoidance, including active reading of food ingredient labels and knowledge of potential contamination and high-risk situations. Any child with food allergy and a history of asthma, peanut, tree nut, fish, or shellfish allergy or a previous systemic reaction should be given

Table 174.4	Diagnosis of Anaphylaxis

Anaphylaxis is **highly likely** when *any 1 of the following 3 criteria* is fulfilled:

1. Acute onset of an illness (minutes to several hours) with involvement of the skin and/or mucosal tissue (e.g., *generalized* hives, pruritus or flushing, swollen lips/tongue/uvula) AND *at least 1 of the following*:
   a. Respiratory compromise (e.g., dyspnea, wheeze/bronchospasm, stridor, reduced peak PEF, hypoxemia)
   b. Reduced BP or associated symptoms of end-organ dysfunction (e.g., hypotonia [collapse], syncope, incontinence)

2. *Two or more of the following* that occur rapidly after exposure **to a likely allergen for that patient** (minutes to several hours):
   a. Involvement of the skin/mucosal tissue (e.g., *generalized* hives, itch/flush, swollen lips/tongue/uvula)
   b. Respiratory compromise (e.g., dyspnea, wheeze/bronchospasm, stridor, reduced PEF, hypoxemia)
   c. Reduced BP or associated symptoms (e.g., hypotonia [collapse], syncope, incontinence)
   d. **Persistent** gastrointestinal symptoms (e.g., crampy abdominal pain, vomiting)

3. Reduced BP following exposure to **known allergen for that patient** (minutes to several hours):
   a. Infants and children: low systolic BP (age specific) or >30% drop in systolic BP
   b. Adults: systolic BP <90 mm Hg or >30% drop from patient's baseline

BP, Blood pressure; PEF, peak expiratory flow.
Adapted from Sampson HA, Muñoz-Furlong A, Campbell RL, et al: Second Symposium on the Definition and Management of Anaphylaxis: summary report, Second National Institute of Allergy and Infectious Disease/Food Allergy and Anaphylaxis Network Symposium, *J Allergy Clin Immunol* 117: 391–397, 2006.

an epinephrine autoinjector. The expert panel also indicates that epinephrine autoinjectors should be considered for any patient with IgE-mediated food allergy. In addition, liquid cetirizine (or alternatively, diphenhydramine) and a written emergency plan should also be provided in case of accidental ingestion or allergic reaction. A form can be downloaded from the American Academy of Pediatrics (www.aap.org) or Food Allergy Research & Education (www.foodallergy.org).

In cases of food-associated exercise-induced anaphylaxis, children must not exercise within 2-3 hr of ingesting the triggering food and, as in children with exercise-induced anaphylaxis, should exercise with a friend, learn to recognize the early signs of anaphylaxis (sensation of warmth, facial pruritus), stop exercising, and seek help immediately if symptoms develop. Children experiencing a systemic anaphylactic reaction, including respiratory symptoms, to an insect sting should be evaluated and treated with immunotherapy, which is >90% protective. Reactions to medications can be reduced and minimized by using oral medications instead of injected forms and avoiding cross-reacting medications. Low-osmolarity radiocontrast dyes and pretreatment can be used in patients with suspected reactions to previous radiocontrast dye. Nonlatex gloves and materials should be used in children undergoing multiple operations.

Any child at risk for anaphylaxis should receive emergency medications (including epinephrine autoinjector), education on identification of signs and symptoms of anaphylaxis and proper administration of medications (Table 174.6), and a written emergency plan in case of accidental exposure. They should be encouraged to wear medical identification jewelry.

Bibliography is available at Expert Consult.

Table 174.5 | Management of a Patient With Anaphylaxis

TREATMENT	MECHANISM(S) OF EFFECT	DOSAGE(S)	COMMENTS; ADVERSE REACTIONS
PATIENT EMERGENCY MANAGEMENT (dependent on severity of symptoms)			
Epinephrine (adrenaline)	α_1-, β_1-, β_2-Adrenergic effects	0.01 mg/kg, up to 0.5 mg IM in lateral thigh Adrenaclick, Auvi-Q, EpiPen Jr/EpiPen: 0.15 mg IM for 8-25 kg 0.3 mg IM for 25 kg or more Epinephrine autoinjector: 0.1 mg for 7.5-15 kg 0.15 mg for 15 to 25 kg 0.3 mg for 25 kg or more	Tachycardia, hypertension, nervousness, headache, nausea, irritability, tremor
Cetirizine (liquid)	Antihistamine (competitive of H_1 receptor)	Cetirizine liquid: 5 mg/5 mL 0.25 mg/kg, up to 10 mg PO	Hypotension, tachycardia, somnolence
Alternative: Diphenhydramine	Antihistamine (competitive of H_1 receptor)	1.25 mg/kg up to 50 mg PO or IM	Hypotension, tachycardia, somnolence, paradoxical excitement
Transport to an emergency facility			
EMERGENCY PERSONNEL MANAGEMENT (dependent on severity of symptoms)			
Epinephrine (adrenaline)	α_1-, β_1-, β_2-Adrenergic effects	0.01 mg/kg, up to 0.5 mg IM in lateral thigh Epinephrine autoinjector: 0.1 mg for 7.5-15 kg 0.15 mg for 15 to 25 kg 0.3 mg for 25 kg or more 0.01 mL/kg/dose of 1:1,000 (vial) solution, up to 0.5 mL IM May repeat every 10-15 min For severe hypotension: 0.01 mL/kg/dose of 1:10,000 slow IV push	Tachycardia, hypertension, nervousness, headache, nausea, irritability, tremor
Supplemental oxygen and airway management			
Volume Expanders			
Crystalloids (normal saline or Ringer lactate)		30 mL/kg in 1st hr	Rate titrated against BP response If tolerated, place patient supine with legs raised.
Colloids (hydroxyethyl starch)		10 mL/kg rapidly followed by slow infusion	Rate titrated against BP response If tolerated, place patient supine with legs raised.
Antihistamines			
Cetirizine (liquid)	Antihistamine (competitive of H_1 receptor)	Cetirizine liquid: 5 mg/5 mL 0.25 mg/kg, up to 10 mg PO	Hypotension, tachycardia, somnolence
Alternative: Diphenhydramine	Antihistamine (competitive of H_1 receptor)	1.25 mg/kg, up to 50 mg PO, IM, or IV	Hypotension, tachycardia, somnolence, paradoxical excitement
Ranitidine	Antihistamine (competitive of H_2 receptor)	1 mg/kg, up to 50 mg IV Should be administered slowly	Headache, mental confusion
Alternative: Cimetidine	Antihistamine (competitive of H_2 receptor)	4 mg/kg, up to 200 mg IV Should be administered slowly	Headache, mental confusion
Corticosteroids			
Methylprednisolone	Antiinflammatory	Solu-Medrol (IV): 1-2 mg/kg, up to 125 mg IV Depo-Medrol (IM): 1 mg/kg, up to 80 mg IM	Hypertension, edema, nervousness, agitation
Prednisone	Antiinflammatory	1 mg/kg up, to 75 mg PO	Hypertension, edema, nervousness, agitation
Nebulized albuterol	β-Agonist	0.83 mg/mL (3 mL) via mask with O_2	Palpitations, nervousness, CNS stimulation, tachycardia; use to supplement epinephrine when bronchospasm appears unresponsive; may repeat
POSTEMERGENCY MANAGEMENT			
Antihistamine		Cetirizine (5-10 mg qd) or loratadine (5-10 mg qd) for 3 days	
Corticosteroids		*Optional:* Oral prednisone (1 mg/kg up to 75 mg) daily for 3 days	

Preventive Treatment
Prescription for epinephrine autoinjector and antihistamine
Provide written plan outlining patient emergency management (may download form from http://www.aap.org or http://www.foodallergy.org)
Follow-up evaluation to determine/confirm etiology
Immunotherapy for insect sting allergy

Patient Education
Instruction on avoidance of causative agent
Information on recognizing early signs of anaphylaxis
Stress early treatment of allergic symptoms to avoid systemic anaphylaxis
Encourage wearing medical identification jewelry

BP, Blood pressure; CNS, central nervous system; IM, Intramuscularly; IV, intravenously; PO, orally; qd, every day.

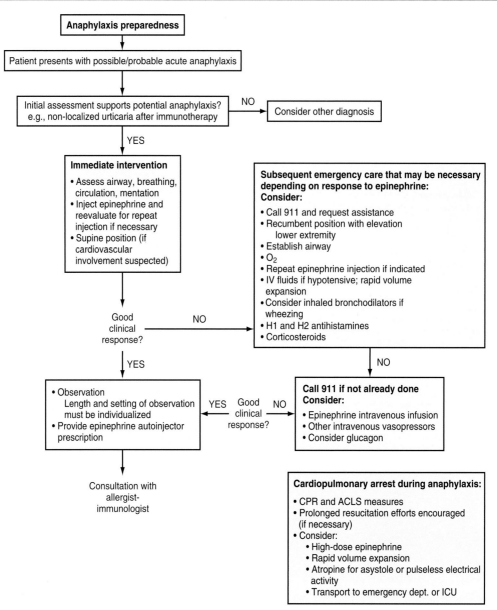

Fig. 174.2 Algorithm for treatment of anaphylactic event in outpatient setting. ACLS, Advance cardiac life support; CPR, cardiopulmonary resuscitation; ICU, intensive care unit; IV, intravenous. *(From Lieberman P, Nicklas RA, Oppenheimer J, et al: The diagnosis and management of anaphylaxis practice parameter: 2010 update, J Allergy Clin Immunol 126:477–480 e471–442, 2010.)*

Table 174.6	Considerations With Epinephrine Injection for Anaphylaxis

Why Healthcare Professionals Fail to Inject Epinephrine Promptly
- Lack of recognition of anaphylaxis symptoms; failure to diagnose anaphylaxis
- Episode appears mild, or there is a history of previous mild episode(s)*
- Inappropriate concern about transient mild pharmacologic effects of epinephrine (e.g., tremor)
- Lack of awareness that serious adverse effects are almost always attributable to epinephrine overdose or IV administration, especially IV bolus, rapid IV infusion, or IV infusion of a 1:1,000 epinephrine solution instead of an appropriately diluted solution (1:10,000 or 1:100,000 concentration)

Why Patients and Caregivers Fail to Inject Epinephrine Promptly
- Lack of recognition of anaphylaxis symptoms; failure to diagnose anaphylaxis
- Episode appears mild, or there is a history of previous mild episode(s)*
- H₁ antihistamine or asthma puffer is used initially instead, relieving early warning signs such as itch or cough, respectively.
- Prescription for epinephrine autoinjectors (EAIs) is not provided by physician.
- Prescription for EAIs is provided but not filled at pharmacy (e.g., not affordable).
- Patients do not carry EAIs consistently (due to size and bulk, or "don't think they'll need it").
- Patients and caregivers are afraid to use EAIs (concern about making an error when giving the injection or about a bad outcome).

- Patients and caregivers are concerned about injury from EAIs.
- Competence in using EAIs is associated with regular allergy clinic visits; it decreases as time elapses from first EAI instruction; regular retraining is needed.
- Difficulty in understanding how to use EAIs (15% of mothers with no EAI experience could not fire an EAI immediately after a one-on-one demonstration)
- Errors in EAI use can occur despite education, possibly related to the design of some EAIs.

Why Patients Occasionally Fail to Respond to Epinephrine Injection
- Delayed recognition of anaphylaxis symptoms; delayed diagnosis
- Error in diagnosis: problem being treated (e.g., foreign body inhalation) is not anaphylaxis.
- Rapid progression of anaphylaxis†
  Epinephrine†:
  - Injected too late; dose too low on mg/kg basis; dose too low because epinephrine solution has degraded (e.g., past the expiration date, stored in a hot place)
  - Injection route or site not optimal; dose took too long to be absorbed.
  - Patient suddenly sits up or walks or runs, leading to the empty ventricle syndrome.
  - Concurrent use of certain medications (e.g., β-adrenergic blockers)

*Subsequent anaphylaxis episodes can be more severe, less severe, or similar in severity.
†Median times to respiratory or cardiac arrest are 5 min in iatrogenic anaphylaxis, 15 min in stinging-insect venom anaphylaxis, and 30 min in food anaphylaxis; however, regardless of the trigger, respiratory or cardiac arrest can occur within 1 min in anaphylaxis.
Adapted from Leung DYM, Szefler SJ, Bonilla FA Akdis CA, Sampson HA, editors: *Pediatric allergy principles and practice*, Philadelphia, 2016, Elsevier, p 531.

Chapter **175**
Serum Sickness
Anna Nowak-Węgrzyn and Scott H. Sicherer

第一百七十五章
血清病

中文导读

　　本章主要介绍了血清病的定义、病因学、发病机制、临床表现、鉴别诊断、诊断、治疗与预防。具体描述了引起血清病的潜在致病因素及抗原–抗体复合物的形成和补体激活在血清病中的作用；介绍了血清病的症状出现和消失时间、常见临床表现、皮疹特点和罕见并发症，亦需要与多种其他疾病相鉴别；血清病的诊断上是基于临床病史，描述了有助于诊断的辅助检查；在治疗方面无基于指南的推荐治疗方案，主要为对症支持治疗；最后强调了血清病的预防主要是积极寻找替代治疗。

Serum sickness is a systemic, immune complex–mediated hypersensitivity vasculitis classically attributed to the therapeutic administration of foreign serum proteins or other medications (Table 175.1).

ETIOLOGY

Immune complexes involving heterologous (animal) serum proteins and complement activation are important pathogenic mechanisms in serum sickness. Antibody therapies derived from the horse, sheep, or rabbit are available for treatment of envenomation by the black widow spider and a variety of snakes, for treatment of botulism, and for immunosuppression (**antithymocyte globulin**, ATG). The availability of alternative medical therapies, modified or bioengineered antibodies, and biologics of human origin have supplanted the use of nonhuman antisera, reducing the risk of serum sickness. However, rabbit-generated ATGs, which target human T cells, continue to be widely used as immunosuppressive agents during treatment of kidney allograft recipients; serum sickness is associated with a late graft loss in kidney transplant recipients. A **serum sickness–like reaction** may be attributed to drug allergy, triggered by antibiotics (particularly cefaclor). In contrast to a true serum sickness, serum sickness–like reactions do not exhibit the immune complexes, hypocomplementemia, vasculitis, and renal lesions that are seen in serum sickness reactions.

PATHOGENESIS

Serum sickness is a classic example of a type III hypersensitivity reaction caused by antigen-antibody complexes. In the rabbit model using bovine serum albumin as the antigen, symptoms develop with the appearance of antibody against the injected antigen. As free antigen concentration falls and antibody production increases over days, antigen-antibody complexes of various sizes develop in a manner analogous to a precipitin curve. Whereas small complexes usually circulate harmlessly and large

Table 175.1	Proteins and Medications That Cause Serum Sickness*

PROTEINS FROM OTHER SPECIES
Antibotulinum globulin
Antithymocyte globulin
Antitetanus toxoid
Antivenin (Crotalidae) polyvalent (horse serum based)
Crotalidae polyvalent immune Fab (ovine serum based)
Antirabies globulin
Infliximab
Rituximab
Etanercept
Anti-HIV antibodies ([PE]HRG214)
Hymenoptera stings
Streptokinase
H1N1 influenza vaccine

DRUGS
Antibiotics
Cefaclor
Penicillins
Trimethoprim sulfate
Minocycline
Meropenem

Neurologic
Bupropion
Carbamazepine
Phenytoin
Sulfonamides
Barbiturates

*Based on review of most current literature. Other medications that are not listed might also cause serum sickness.
   HIV, Human immunodeficiency virus.
   From Aceves SS: Serum sickness. In Burg FD, Ingelfinger JR, Polin RA, Gershon AA, editors: *Current pediatric therapy*, ed 18, Philadelphia, 2006, Elsevier, p 1138.

complexes are cleared by the reticuloendothelial system, intermediate-sized complexes that develop at the point of slight antigen excess may deposit in blood vessel walls and tissues. There the immune microprecipitates induce vascular (leukocytoclastic vasculitis with immune complex deposition) and tissue damage through activation of complement and granulocytes.

Complement activation (C3a, C5a) promotes chemotaxis and adherence of neutrophils to the site of immune complex deposition. The processes of immune complex deposition and of neutrophil accumulation may be facilitated by increased vascular permeability, because of the release of vasoactive amines from tissue mast cells. Mast cells may be activated by binding of antigen to IgE or through contact with anaphylatoxins (C3a). Tissue injury results from the liberation of proteolytic enzymes and oxygen radicals from the neutrophils.

CLINICAL MANIFESTATIONS

The symptoms of serum sickness generally begin 7-12 days after injection of the foreign material, but may appear as late as 3 wk afterward. The onset of symptoms may be accelerated if there has been earlier exposure or previous allergic reaction to the same antigen. A few days before the onset of generalized symptoms, the site of injection may become edematous and erythematous. Symptoms usually include fever, malaise, and rashes. Urticaria and morbilliform rashes are the predominant types of skin eruptions (Fig. 175.1). In a prospective study of serum sickness induced by administration of equine ATG, an initial rash was noted in most patients. It began as a thin, serpiginous band of erythema along the sides of the hands, fingers, feet, and toes at the junction of the palmar or plantar skin with the skin of the dorsolateral surface. In most patients the band of erythema was replaced by petechiae or purpura, presumably because of low platelet counts or local damage to small blood vessels. Additional symptoms include edema, myalgia, lymphadenopathy, symmetric arthralgia or arthritis involving multiple joints, and gastrointestinal complaints, including pain, nausea, diarrhea, and melena. Symptoms typically resolve within 2 wk of removal of the offending agent, although in unusual cases, symptoms can persist for as long as 2-3 mo.

Carditis, glomerulonephritis, Guillain-Barré syndrome, and peripheral neuritis are rare complications. Serum sickness–like reactions from drugs are characterized by fever, pruritus, urticaria, and arthralgias that usually begin 1-3 wk after drug exposure. The urticarial skin eruption becomes increasingly erythematous as the reaction progresses and can evolve into dusky centers with round plaques.

DIFFERENTIAL DIAGNOSIS

The differential diagnosis of serum sickness and serum sickness–like reactions includes viral illnesses with exanthems, hypersensitivity vasculitis, Kawasaki disease, acute rheumatic fever, acute meningococcal or gonococcal infection, endocarditis, systemic-onset juvenile idiopathic

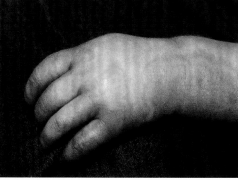

Fig. 175.1 Serum sickness–like reaction (SSLR). Note the swollen hand and large urticarial wheals in this girl with SSLR and arthralgias. *(From Paller AS, Mancini AJ, editors: Hurwitz clinical pediatric dermatology, ed 5, Philadelphia, 2016, Elsevier, p 476.)*

arthritis (Still disease), Lyme disease, hepatitis, and other types of drug reactions (see Chapter 177).

DIAGNOSIS

In most patients the diagnosis of serum sickness is made clinically based on the characteristic pattern of acute or subacute onset of a rash, fever, and severe arthralgia and myalgia disproportionate to the degree of swelling, occurring after exposure to a potential culprit. Patients who appear moderately or severely ill, or who are not taking a medication that can be readily identified as the culprit, should be evaluated with the following laboratory tests:

- Complete blood count and differential; thrombocytopenia is often present.
- Erythrocyte sedimentation rate (ESR) and C-reactive protein; ESR is usually elevated.
- Urinalysis; mild proteinuria, hemoglobinuria, and microscopic hematuria may be seen.
- Serum chemistries, including blood urea nitrogen, creatinine, and liver function tests.
- Complement studies, including CH_{50}, C3, and C4; serum complement levels (C3 and C4) are generally decreased and reach a nadir at about day 10. C3a anaphylatoxin may be increased.
- Testing for specific infectious diseases, if indicated by the history or physical examination.
- Appropriate viral or bacterial cultures if an infection is suspected.

Skin biopsies are not usually necessary for confirming the diagnosis, because the findings are variable and not specific for serum sickness. Direct immunofluorescence studies of skin lesions often reveal immune deposits of IgM, IgA, IgE, or C3.

TREATMENT

There are no evidence-based guidelines or controlled trials on which to base therapy recommendations. Treatment is primarily supportive, consisting of discontinuation of the offending agent, antihistamines for pruritus, and nonsteroidal antiinflammatory drugs and analgesics for low-grade fever and mild arthralgia. When the symptoms are especially severe, for example, fever >38.5°C (101.3°F), severe arthralgia or myalgia, or renal dysfunction, systemic corticosteroids can be used. Prednisone (1-2 mg/kg/day; maximum 60 mg/day) for 1-2 wk is usually sufficient. Once the offending agent is discontinued and depending on its half-life, symptoms resolve spontaneously in 1-4 wk. Symptoms lasting longer suggest another diagnosis.

PREVENTION

The primary mode of prevention of serum sickness is to seek alternative therapies. In some cases, non–animal-derived formulations may be available (human-derived botulinum immune globulin). Other alternatives are partially digested antibodies of animal origin and engineered (humanized) antibodies. The potential of these therapies to elicit serum sickness–like disease appears low. When only animal-derived antitoxin/antivenom is available, skin tests should be performed before administration of serum, but this procedure indicates the risk only of anaphylaxis, not of serum sickness. For patients who have evidence of anaphylactic sensitivity to horse serum, a risk/benefit assessment must be made to determine the need to proceed with treatment. If needed, the serum can usually be successfully administered by a process of rapid desensitization using protocols of gradual administration outlined by the manufacturers. Serum sickness is not prevented by desensitization or by pretreatment with corticosteroids.

Bibliography is available at Expert Consult.

Chapter **176**

Food Allergy and Adverse Reactions to Foods

Anna Nowak-Węgrzyn, Hugh A. Sampson, and Scott H. Sicherer

第一百七十六章

食物过敏和食物不良反应

中文导读

　　本章主要介绍了食物不良反应的定义及食物过敏的发病率、遗传学、发病机制、临床表现、诊断、治疗、预防。具体描述了食物不耐受与食物过敏的区别、常见食物过敏的发生率及与食物过敏相关的候选基因；阐述了食物过敏的发病机制为免疫介导（分为IgE介导、非IgE介导、混合机制的IgE/非IgE介导）；具体描述了食物过敏累及不同靶器官的相应表现（胃肠道表现、皮肤表现、呼吸道表现、严重过敏反应）；食物过敏的诊断上强调必须全面了解病史，结合有诊断价值的辅助检查（皮肤点刺试验、体外试验、口服食物激发试验）；膳食回避是目前治疗食物过敏唯一有效的方法，食物过敏随时间推移会发生改变，因此需定期专科随诊评估；最后介绍了食物过敏的预防策

略（高危过敏婴儿的早期花生引入、生后早期采取改善婴儿皮肤屏障功能的措施）。

Adverse reactions to foods consist of any untoward reaction following the ingestion of a food or food additive and are classically divided into **food intolerances** (e.g., **lactose intolerance**), which are adverse *physiologic* responses, and **food allergies,** which are adverse *immunologic* responses and can be IgE mediated or non–IgE mediated (Tables 176.1 and 176.2). As with other atopic disorders, food allergies appear to have increased over the past 3 decades, primarily in countries with a Western lifestyle. Worldwide, estimates of food allergy prevalence range from 1–10%; food allergies affect an estimated 3.5% of the U.S. population. Up to 6% of children experience food allergic reactions in the 1st 3 yr of life, including approximately 2.5% with cow's milk allergy, 2% with egg allergy, and 2–3% with peanut allergy. **Peanut allergy** prevalence tripled over the past decade. Most children "outgrow" milk and egg allergies, with approximately 50% doing so by school-age. In contrast, 80–90% of children with peanut, tree nut, or seafood allergy retain their allergy for life.

GENETICS

Genetic factors play an important role in the development of food allergy. Family and twin studies show that family history confers a 2-10–fold increased risk, depending on the study setting, population, specific food, and diagnostic test. Candidate gene studies suggest that genetic variants in the HLA-DQ locus (HLA-DQB1*02 and DQB1*06:03P), filaggrin, interleukin-10, *STAT6*, and *FOXP3* genes are associated with food allergy, although the results are inconsistent across different populations. In a genome-wide association study, differential methylation at the HLA-DR and -DQ regions was associated with food allergy. Epigenetic studies implicate DNA methylation effects on interleukins 4, 5, and 10 and interferon (IFN)-γ genes and in the mitogen-activated protein kinase (MAPK) pathway.

PATHOGENESIS

Food intolerances are the result of a variety of mechanisms, whereas food allergy is predominantly caused by IgE-mediated and cell-mediated immune mechanisms. In susceptible individuals exposed to certain allergens, food-specific IgE antibodies are formed that bind to Fcε receptors on mast cells, basophils, macrophages, and dendritic cells. When food allergens penetrate mucosal barriers and reach cell-bound IgE antibodies, mediators are released that induce vasodilation, smooth muscle contraction, and mucus secretion, which result in symptoms of immediate hypersensitivity (allergy). Activated mast cells and macrophages may release several cytokines that attract and activate other cells, such as eosinophils and lymphocytes, leading to prolonged inflammation. Symptoms elicited during acute IgE-mediated reactions can affect the skin (urticaria, angioedema, flushing), gastrointestinal (GI) tract (oral pruritus, angioedema, nausea, abdominal pain, vomiting, diarrhea), respiratory tract (nasal congestion, rhinorrhea, nasal pruritus, sneezing, laryngeal edema, dyspnea, wheezing), and cardiovascular system (dysrhythmias, hypotension, loss of consciousness). In non-IgE food allergies, lymphocytes, primarily food allergen–specific T cells, secrete excessive amounts of various cytokines that lead to a "delayed," more chronic inflammatory process affecting the skin (pruritus, erythematous rash), GI tract (failure to thrive, early satiety, abdominal pain, vomiting, diarrhea), and respiratory tract (food-induced pulmonary hemosiderosis). Mixed IgE and cellular responses to food allergens can also lead to chronic disorders, such as atopic dermatitis, asthma, eosinophilic esophagitis, and gastroenteritis.

Children who develop IgE-mediated food allergies may be sensitized by food allergens penetrating the GI barrier, referred to as **class 1 food**

Table 176.1	Adverse Food Reactions

FOOD INTOLERANCE (non–immune system mediated, nontoxic, noninfectious)
Host Factors
Enzyme deficiencies—lactase (primary or secondary), sucrase/isomaltase, hereditary fructose intolerance, galactosemia
Gastrointestinal disorders—inflammatory bowel disease, irritable bowel syndrome, pseudoobstruction, colic
Idiosyncratic reactions—caffeine in soft drinks ("hyperactivity")
Psychologic—food phobias, obsessive/compulsive disorder
Migraines (rare)

Food Factors (Toxic or Infectious or Pharmacologic)
Infectious organisms—*Escherichia coli, Staphylococcus aureus, Clostridium perfringens, Shigella,* botulism, *Salmonella, Yersinia, Campylobacter*
Toxins—histamine (scombroid poisoning), saxitoxin (shellfish)
Pharmacologic agents—caffeine, theobromine (chocolate, tea), tryptamine (tomatoes), tyramine (cheese), benzoic acid in citrus fruits (perioral flare)
Contaminants—heavy metals, pesticides, antibiotics

FOOD ALLERGY
IgE Mediated
Cutaneous—urticaria, angioedema, morbilliform rashes, flushing, contact urticarial
Gastrointestinal—oral allergy syndrome, gastrointestinal anaphylaxis
Respiratory—acute rhinoconjunctivitis, bronchospasm
Generalized—anaphylactic shock, exercise-induced anaphylaxis

Mixed IgE Mediated and Non–IgE Mediated
Cutaneous—atopic dermatitis, contact dermatitis
Gastrointestinal—allergic eosinophilic esophagitis and gastroenteritis
Respiratory—asthma

Non–IgE Mediated
Cutaneous—contact dermatitis, dermatitis herpetiformis (celiac disease)
Gastrointestinal—food protein–induced enterocolitis, proctocolitis, and enteropathy syndromes, celiac disease
Respiratory—food-induced pulmonary hemosiderosis (Heiner syndrome)
Unclassified

IgE, Immunoglobulin E.

allergens, or by food allergens that are partially homologous to plant pollens penetrating the respiratory tract, referred to as **class 2 food allergens.** Any food may serve as a class 1 food allergen, but *egg, milk, peanuts, tree nuts, fish, soy,* and *wheat* account for 90% of food allergies during childhood. Many of the major allergenic proteins of these foods have been characterized. There is variable but significant cross-reactivity with other proteins within an individual food group. Exposure and sensitization to these proteins often occur very early in life. Virtually all milk allergies develop by 12 mo of age and all egg allergies by 18 mo, and the median age of 1st peanut allergic reactions is 14 mo. Class 2 food allergens are typically vegetable, fruit, or nut proteins that are partially homologous with pollen proteins (Table 176.3). With the development of seasonal allergic rhinitis from birch, grass, or ragweed pollens, subsequent ingestion of certain uncooked fruits or vegetables provokes the **oral allergy syndrome**. *Intermittent ingestion* of allergenic foods may lead to acute symptoms such as urticaria or anaphylaxis, whereas *prolonged exposure* may lead to chronic disorders such as atopic dermatitis and asthma. Cell-mediated sensitivity typically develops to class 1 allergens.

Table 176.2	Differential Diagnosis of Adverse Food Reactions

GASTROINTESTINAL DISORDERS (with vomiting and/or diarrhea)
Structural abnormalities (pyloric stenosis, Hirschsprung disease, reflux)
Enzyme deficiencies (primary or secondary):
  Disaccharidase deficiency—lactase, fructase, sucrase-isomaltase
  Galactosemia
Malignancy with obstruction
Other: pancreatic insufficiency (cystic fibrosis), peptic disease

CONTAMINANTS AND ADDITIVES
Flavorings and preservatives—rarely cause symptoms:
  Sodium metabisulfite, monosodium glutamate, nitrites
Dyes and colorings—very rarely cause symptoms (urticaria, eczema):
  Tartrazine
Toxins:
  Bacterial, fungal (aflatoxin), fish related (scombroid, ciguatera)
Infectious organisms:
  Bacteria (*Salmonella, Escherichia coli, Shigella*)
  Virus (rotavirus, enterovirus)
  Parasites (*Giardia, Akis simplex* [in fish])
Accidental contaminants:
  Heavy metals, pesticides
Pharmacologic agents:
  Caffeine, glycosidal alkaloid solanine (potato spuds), histamine (fish), serotonin (banana, tomato), tryptamine (tomato), tyramine (cheese)

PSYCHOLOGIC REACTIONS
Food phobias

CLINICAL MANIFESTATIONS

From a clinical and diagnostic standpoint, it is most useful to subdivide food hypersensitivity disorders according to the predominant target organ (Table 176.4) and immune mechanism (see Table 176.1).

Gastrointestinal Manifestations

GI food allergies are often the 1st form of allergy to affect infants and young children and typically manifest as irritability, vomiting or "spitting-up," diarrhea, and poor weight gain. Cell-mediated hypersensitivities without IgE involvement predominate, making standard allergy tests such as skin-prick tests and in vitro tests for food-specific IgE antibodies of little diagnostic value.

Food protein–induced enterocolitis syndrome (FPIES) typically manifests in the 1st several mo of life as irritability, intermittent vomiting, and protracted diarrhea and may result in dehydration (Table 176.5). Vomiting generally occurs 1-4 hr after feeding, and continued exposure may result in abdominal distention, bloody diarrhea, anemia, and failure to thrive. Symptoms are most often provoked by cow's milk or soy protein–based formulas. A similar enterocolitis syndrome occurs in older infants and children from rice, oat, wheat, egg, peanut, nut, chicken, turkey, or fish. Hypotension occurs in approximately 15% of patients after allergen ingestion and may initially be thought to be caused by sepsis. FPIES usually resolves by age 3-5 yr.

Food protein–induced allergic proctocolitis (FPIAP) presents in the 1st few mo of life as blood-streaked stools in otherwise healthy infants (Table 176.5). Approximately 60% of cases occur among breastfed infants, with the remainder largely among infants fed cow's milk or soy protein–based formula. Blood loss is typically modest but can occasionally produce anemia.

Food protein–induced enteropathy (FPE) often manifests in the 1st several mo of life as diarrhea, often with steatorrhea and poor weight gain (Table 176.5). Symptoms include protracted diarrhea, vomiting in up to 65% of cases, failure to thrive, abdominal distention, early satiety, and malabsorption. Anemia, edema, and hypoproteinemia occur occasionally. **Cow's milk sensitivity** is the most common cause of FPE in young infants, but it has also been associated with sensitivity to soy, egg, wheat, rice, chicken, and fish in older children. **Celiac disease**, the most severe form of FPE, occurs in about 1 per 100 U.S. population, although it may be "silent" in many patients (see Chapter 364.2). The

Table 176.3	Natural History of Food Allergy and Cross-Reactivity Between Common Food Allergies		
FOOD	**USUAL AGE AT ONSET OF ALLERGY**	**CROSS REACTIVITY**	**USUAL AGE AT RESOLUTION**
Hen's egg white	0-1 yr	Other avian eggs	7 yr (75% of cases resolve)*
Cow's milk	0-1 yr	Goat's milk, sheep's milk, buffalo milk	5 yr (76% of cases resolve)*
Peanuts	1-2 yr	Other legumes, peas, lentils; coreactivity with tree nuts	Persistent (20% of cases resolve)
Tree nuts	1-2 yr; in adults, onset occurs after cross reactivity to birch pollen	Other tree nuts; co-reactivity with peanuts	Persistent (9% of cases resolve)
Fish	Late childhood and adulthood	Other fish (low cross-reactivity with tuna and swordfish)	Persistent†
Shellfish	Adulthood (in 60% of patients with this allergy)	Other shellfish	Persistent
Wheat*	6-24 mo	Other grains containing gluten (rye, barley)	5 yr (80% of cases resolve)
Soybeans*	6-24 mo	Other legumes	2 yr (67% of cases resolve)
Kiwi	Any age	Banana, avocado, latex	Unknown
Apples, carrots, and peaches§	Late childhood and adulthood	Birch pollen, other fruits, nuts	Unknown

*Recent studies suggest that resolution may occur at a later age, especially in children with multiple food allergies and lifetime peak food-specific IgE >50 kU$_A$/L.
†Fish allergy that is acquired in childhood can resolve.
§Allergy to fresh apples, carrots, and peaches (**oral allergy syndrome**) is typically caused by heat-labile proteins. Fresh fruit causes oral pruritus, but cooked fruit is tolerated. There is generally no risk of anaphylaxis, although in rare cases, allergies to cross-reactive lipid transfer protein can cause anaphylaxis after ingestion of fruits (e.g., peach) and vegetables.
Adapted from Lack G: Food allergy, *N Engl J Med* 359:1252–1260, 2008.

Table 176.4	Symptoms of Food-Induced Allergic Reactions	
TARGET ORGAN	**IMMEDIATE SYMPTOMS**	**DELAYED SYMPTOMS**
Cutaneous	Erythema Pruritus Urticaria Morbilliform eruption Angioedema	Erythema Flushing Pruritus Morbilliform eruption Angioedema Eczematous rash
Ocular	Pruritus Conjunctival erythema Tearing Periorbital edema	Pruritus Conjunctival erythema Tearing Periorbital edema
Upper respiratory	Nasal congestion Pruritus Rhinorrhea Sneezing Laryngeal edema Hoarseness Dry staccato cough	
Lower respiratory	Cough Chest tightness Dyspnea Wheezing Intercostal retractions Accessory muscle use	Cough, dyspnea, wheezing
Gastrointestinal (oral)	Angioedema of the lips, tongue, or palate Oral pruritus Tongue swelling	
Gastrointestinal (lower)	Nausea Colicky abdominal pain Reflux Vomiting Diarrhea	Nausea Abdominal pain Reflux Vomiting Diarrhea Hematochezia Irritability and food refusal with weight loss (young children)
Cardiovascular	Tachycardia (occasionally bradycardia in anaphylaxis) Hypotension Dizziness Fainting Loss of consciousness	
Miscellaneous	Uterine contractions Sense of "impending doom"	

From Boyce JA, Assa'ad A, Burks AW, et al: Guideline for the diagnosis and management of food allergy in the United States: report of the NIAID-sponsored expert panel, *J Allergy Clin Immunol* 126(6):S1–S58, 2010 (Table IV, p S19).

full-blown form is characterized by extensive loss of absorptive villi and hyperplasia of the crypts, leading to malabsorption, chronic diarrhea, steatorrhea, abdominal distention, flatulence, and weight loss or failure to thrive. Oral ulcers and other extraintestinal symptoms secondary to malabsorption may occur. Genetically susceptible individuals (HLA-DQ2 or HLA-DQ8) demonstrate a cell-mediated response to tissue trans-glutaminase deamidated gliadin (a fraction of gluten), which is found in wheat, rye, and barley.

Eosinophilic esophagitis (EoE) may appear from infancy through adolescence, more frequently in boys (see Chapter 350). In young children, EoE is primarily cell mediated and manifests as chronic gastroesophageal reflux (GER), intermittent emesis, food refusal,

abdominal pain, dysphagia, irritability, sleep disturbance, and failure to respond to conventional GER medications. EoE is a clinicopathologic diagnosis. The diagnosis is confirmed when 15 eosinophils per high-power field are seen on esophageal biopsy following treatment with proton pump inhibitors. **Eosinophilic gastroenteritis** occurs at any age and causes symptoms similar to those of EoE, as well as prominent weight loss or failure to thrive, both of which are the hallmarks of this disorder. More than 50% of patients with this disorder are atopic; however, food-induced IgE-mediated reactions have been implicated only in a minority of patients. Generalized edema secondary to hypo-albuminemia may occur in some infants with marked protein-losing enteropathy.

Oral allergy syndrome (pollen-associated food allergy syndrome) is an IgE-mediated hypersensitivity that occurs in many older children with birch and ragweed pollen–induced allergic rhinitis. Symptoms are usually confined to the oropharynx and consist of the rapid onset of oral pruritus; tingling and angioedema of the lips, tongue, palate, and throat; and occasionally a sensation of pruritus in the ears and tightness in the throat. Symptoms are generally short lived and are caused by local mast cell activation following contact with fresh raw fruit and vegetable proteins that cross-react with birch pollen (apple, carrot, potato, celery, hazel nuts, peanuts, kiwi, cherry, pear), grass pollen (potato, tomato, watermelon, kiwi), and ragweed pollen (banana, melons such as watermelon and cantaloupe).

Acute gastrointestinal allergy generally manifests as acute abdominal pain, vomiting, or diarrhea that accompanies IgE-mediated allergic symptoms in other target organs.

Skin Manifestations

Cutaneous food allergies are also common in infants and young children.

Atopic dermatitis is a form of eczema that generally begins in early infancy and is characterized by pruritus, a chronically relapsing course, and association with asthma and allergic rhinitis (see Chapter 170). Although not often apparent from history, at least 30% of children with moderate to severe atopic dermatitis have food allergies. The younger the child and the more severe the eczema, the more likely food allergy is playing a pathogenic role in the disorder.

Acute urticaria and angioedema are among the most common symptoms of food allergic reactions (see Chapter 173). The onset of symptoms may be very rapid, within minutes after ingestion of the responsible allergen. Symptoms result from activation of IgE-bearing mast cells by food allergens that are absorbed and circulated rapidly throughout the body. Foods most commonly incriminated in children include egg, milk, peanuts, and nuts, although reactions to various seeds (sesame, poppy) and fruits (kiwi) are becoming more common. Chronic urticaria and angioedema are rarely caused by food allergies.

Perioral dermatitis is often a contact dermatitis caused by substances in toothpaste, gums, lipstick, or medications. **Perioral flushing** is often noted in infants fed citrus fruits and may be caused by benzoic acid in the food. It may also occur during nursing. In both situations the effect is benign. Flushing may also be caused by auriculotemporal nerve (Frey) syndrome (familial, forceps delivery), which resolves spontaneously.

Respiratory Manifestations

Respiratory food allergies are uncommon as isolated symptoms. Although many parents believe that nasal congestion in infants is often caused by milk allergy, studies show this not to be the case. **Food-induced rhinoconjunctivitis** symptoms typically accompany allergic symptoms in other target organs, such as skin, and consist of typical allergic rhinitis symptoms (periocular pruritus and tearing, nasal congestion and pruritus, sneezing, rhinorrhea). Wheezing occurs in approximately 25% of IgE-mediated food allergic reactions, but only 10% of asthmatic patients have food-induced respiratory symptoms.

Anaphylaxis

Anaphylaxis is defined as a serious, multisystem allergic reaction that is rapid in onset and potentially fatal. Food allergic reactions are the

Table 176.5 | Food Protein–Induced Gastrointestinal Syndromes

	FPIES	PROCTOCOLITIS	ENTEROPATHY	EOSINOPHILIC GASTROENTEROPATHIES*
Age at onset	1 day–1 year	1 day–6 months	Dependent of age of exposure to antigen, cow's milk and soy up to 2 yr	Infant to adolescent
Food proteins implicated				
Most common	Cow's milk, soy	Cow's milk, soy	Cow's milk, soy	Cow's milk, soy, egg white, wheat, peanut
Less common	Rice, chicken, turkey, fish, pea	Egg, corn, chocolate	Wheat, egg	Meats, corn, rice, fruits, vegetables, fish
Multiple food hypersensitivities	>50% both cow's milk and soy	40% both cow's milk and soy	Rare	Common
Feeding at the time of onset	Formula	>50% exclusive breastfeeding	Formula	Formula
Atopic background				
Family history of atopy	40–70%	25%	Unknown	~50% (often history of eosinophilic esophagitis)
Personal history of atopy	30%	22%	22%	~50%
Symptoms				
Emesis	Prominent	No	Intermittent	Intermittent
Diarrhea	Severe	No	Moderate	Moderate
Bloody stools	Severe	Moderate	Rare	Moderate
Edema	Acute, severe	No	Moderate	Moderate
Shock	15%	No	No	No
Failure to thrive	Moderate	No	Moderate	Moderate
Laboratory findings				
Anemia	Moderate	Mild	Moderate	Mild-moderate
Hypoalbuminemia	Acute	Rare	Moderate	Mild-severe
Methemoglobinemia	May be present	No	No	No
Allergy evaluation				
Food skin-prick test	Negative[†]	Negative	Negative	Positive in ~50%
Serum food allergen IgE	Negative[†]	Negative	Negative	Positive in ~50%
Total IgE	Normal	Negative	Normal	Normal to elevated
Peripheral blood eosinophilia	No	Occasional	No	Present in <50%
Biopsy findings				
Colitis	Prominent	Focal	No	May be present
Lymph nodular hyperplasia	No	Common	No	Yes
Eosinophils	Prominent	Prominent	Few	Prominent; also neutrophilic infiltrates, papillary elongation, and basal zone hyperplasia
Food challenge	Vomiting in 1-4 hr; diarrhea in 5-8 hr	Rectal bleeding in 6-72 hr	Vomiting, diarrhea, or both in 40-72 hr	Vomiting and diarrhea in hours to days
Treatment	Protein elimination, 80% respond to casein hydrolysate and symptoms clear in 3-10 days; rechallenge under supervision in 1.5-2 yr	Protein elimination, symptoms clear in 3 days with casein hydrolysate; resume/continue breastfeeding on maternal antigen-restricted diet; reintroduce at home after 9-12 mo of age	Protein elimination, symptoms clear in 1-3 wk; rechallenge and biopsy in 1-2 yr	Protein elimination, good response to casein hydrolysate, excellent response to elemental diet; symptoms clear in 2-3 wk, excellent acute response to steroids; rechallenge by introducing food at home and biopsy in 1-2 yr
Natural history	Cow's milk: 60% resolved by 2 yr Soy: 25% resolved by 2 yr	Resolved by 9-12 mo	Most cases resolve in 2-3 yr	Typically a prolonged, relapsing course
Reintroduction of the food	Supervised food challenge	At home, gradually advancing from 1 oz to full feedings over 2 wk	Home, gradually advancing	Home, gradually advancing

*Eosinophilic gastroenteropathies encompass esophagitis, gastritis, and gastroenterocolitis.
[†]If positive, may be a risk factor for persistent disease.
FPIES, Food protein–induced enterocolitis syndrome.
From Nowak-Węgrzyn A, Muraro A: Food protein-induced enterocolitis syndrome, *Curr Opin Allergy Immunol* 9:371–377, 2009 (Table 1, p 372).

most common cause of anaphylaxis seen in U.S. hospital emergency departments. In addition to the rapid onset of cutaneous, respiratory, and GI symptoms, patients may demonstrate cardiovascular symptoms, including hypotension, vascular collapse, and cardiac dysrhythmias, which are presumably caused by massive mast cell–mediator release. **Food-dependent exercise-induced anaphylaxis** occurs more frequently among teenage athletes, especially females (see Chapter 174).

DIAGNOSIS

A thorough medical history is necessary to determine whether a patient's symptomatology represents an adverse food reaction (see Table 176.2), whether it is an intolerance or food allergic reaction, and if the latter, whether it is likely to be an IgE-mediated or a cell-mediated response (Fig. 176.1). The following facts should be established: (1) the food suspected of provoking the reaction and the quantity ingested, (2) the interval between ingestion and the development of symptoms, (3) the types of symptoms elicited by the ingestion, (4) whether ingesting the suspected food produced similar symptoms on other occasions, (5) whether other inciting factors, such as exercise, are necessary, and (6) the interval from the last reaction to the food.

Skin-prick tests and in vitro laboratory tests are useful for demonstrating *IgE sensitization,* defined as presence of food-specific IgE antibodies. Many fruits and vegetables require skin-prick testing with fresh produce because labile proteins are destroyed during commercial preparation.

A negative skin test result virtually excludes an IgE-mediated form of food allergy. Conversely, most children with positive skin test responses to a food do not react when the food is ingested, so more definitive tests, such as quantitative IgE tests or food elimination and challenge, are often necessary to establish a diagnosis of food allergy. Serum food-specific IgE levels ≥ 15 kU$_A$/L for milk (≥ 5 kU$_A$/L for children ≤ 1 yr), ≥ 7 kU$_A$/L for egg (≥ 2 kU$_A$/L for children <2 yr), and ≥ 14 kU$_A$/L for peanut are associated with a >95% likelihood of clinical reactivity to these foods in children with suspected reactivity. In the absence of a clear history of reactivity to a food and evidence of food-specific IgE antibodies, definitive studies must be performed before recommendations are made for avoidance or the use of highly restrictive diets that may be nutritionally deficient, logistically impractical, disruptive to the family, expensive, or a potential source of future feeding disorders. IgE-mediated food allergic reactions are generally very food specific, so the use of broad exclusionary diets, such as avoidance of all legumes, cereal grains, or animal products, is not warranted (Table 176.6; see also Table 176.3).

There are no laboratory studies to help identify foods responsible for cell-mediated reactions. Consequently, *elimination diets followed by oral food challenges* are the only way to establish the diagnosis. Allergists experienced in dealing with food allergic reactions and able to treat anaphylaxis should perform food challenges. Before a food challenge is initiated, the suspected food should be eliminated from the diet for 10-14 days for IgE-mediated food allergy and up to 8 wk for some

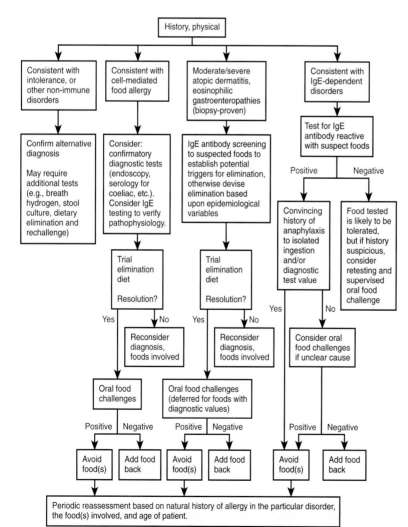

Fig. 176.1 General scheme for diagnosis of food allergy. *(From Sicherer SH: Food allergy, Lancet 360:701–710, 2002.)*

Table 176.6 | Clinical Implications of Cross-Reactive Proteins in IgE-Mediated Allergy

FOOD FAMILY	RISK OF ALLERGY TO ≥1 MEMBER (%; approximate)	FEATURE(S)
Legumes	5	Main causes of reactions are peanut, soybean, lentil, lupine, and garbanzo (chickpea).
Tree nuts (e.g., almond, cashew, hazelnut, walnut, brazil)	35	Reactions are often severe.
Fish	50	Reactions can be severe.
Shellfish	75	Reactions can be severe.
Grains	20	
Mammalian milks	90	Cow's milk is highly cross-reactive with goat's or sheep's milk (92%) but not with mare's milk (4%).
Rosaceae (pitted fruits)	55	Risk of reactions to >3 related foods is very low (<10%); symptoms are usually mild (oral allergy syndrome).
Latex-food	35	For individuals allergic to latex, banana, kiwi, fig, chestnut, and avocado are the main causes of reactions.
Food-latex	11	Individuals allergic to banana, kiwi, fig, chestnut, and avocado may be at an increased risk of reactions to latex.

Modified from Sicherer SH: Food allergy, *Lancet* 360:701–710, 2002.

cell-mediated disorders, such as EoE. Some children with cell-mediated reactions to cow's milk do not tolerate hydrolysate formulas and must receive amino acid–derived formulas. If symptoms remain unchanged despite appropriate elimination diets, it is unlikely that food allergy is responsible for the child's disorder.

TREATMENT
Appropriate identification and elimination of foods responsible for food hypersensitivity reactions are the only validated treatments for food allergies. Complete elimination of common foods (milk, egg, soy, wheat, rice, chicken, fish, peanut, nuts) is very difficult because of their widespread use in a variety of processed foods. The lay organization **Food Allergy Research and Education (FARE, www.foodallergy.org)** provides excellent information to help parents deal with both the practical and emotional issues surrounding these diets. Validated educational materials are also available through the **Consortium of Food Allergy Research** (www.cofargroup.org).

Children with asthma and IgE-mediated food allergy, peanut or nut allergy, or a history of a previous severe reaction should be given self-injectable epinephrine and a written emergency plan in case of accidental ingestion (see Chapter 174). Because many food allergies are outgrown, children should be reevaluated periodically by an allergist to determine whether they have lost their clinical reactivity. A number of clinical trials are evaluating the efficacy of oral, sublingual, and epicutaneous (patch) immunotherapy for the treatment of IgE-mediated food allergies (milk, egg, peanut). Combining oral immunotherapy with anti-IgE treatment (omalizumab) may improve safety compared to oral immunotherapy alone. Furthermore, extensively heated milk or egg in baked products are tolerated by the majority of milk and egg–allergic children. Regular ingestion of baked products with milk and egg appears to accelerate resolution of milk and egg allergy. Table 176.7 provides vaccination recommendations for egg-allergic children who require immunization.

PREVENTION
It was once thought that avoidance of allergenic foods and delayed introduction to the diet would prevent allergy, but the opposite is probably true; *delayed introduction of these foods may increase the risk of allergy,* especially in children with atopic dermatitis. A trial of early introduction of dietary peanut randomized 640 infants age 4-11 mo with severe eczema, egg allergy, or both to consume or avoid peanut until age 60 mo. The early introduction of peanut dramatically decreased the development of peanut allergy among children at high risk for this allergy. A theory behind this approach is that early oral introduction of peanut induces oral tolerance that precedes the potential sensitization to peanut via the disrupted skin barrier. Infants with early-onset atopic disease (e.g., severe eczema) or egg allergy in the 1st 4 to 6 mo of life might benefit from evaluation by an allergist or physician trained in management of allergic diseases to diagnose any food allergy and assist in implementing appropriate early peanut introduction. The clinician can perform an observed peanut challenge for those with evidence of a positive peanut skin test response or serum peanut-specific IgE >0.35 kU_A/L to determine whether they are clinically reactive before initiating at-home introduction of infant-safe forms of peanut. Additional details for the early introduction of peanut are available from the National Institute of Allergy and Infectious Diseases (NIAID).[*]

There is no compelling evidence to support the practice of restricting the maternal diet during pregnancy or while breastfeeding, or of delaying introduction of various allergenic foods to infants from atopic families (Table 176.8). Exclusive breastfeeding for the 1st 4-6 mo of life may reduce allergic disorders in the 1st few yr of life in infants at high risk for development of allergic disease. Potentially allergenic foods (eggs, milk, wheat, soy, peanut/tree nut products, fish) should be introduced after this period of exclusive breastfeeding and may prevent the development of allergies later in life. Use of hydrolyzed formulas may be beneficial if breastfeeding cannot be continued for 4-6 mo or after weaning, especially to prevent eczema in high-risk families, but this approach remains controversial. **Probiotic supplements** may also reduce the incidence and severity of eczema. Because some **skin preparations** contain peanut oil, which may sensitize young infants, especially those with cutaneous inflammation, such preparations should be avoided. Since inflamed/disrupted skin barrier is a risk factor for food allergy, trials are underway to enhance the skin barrier from birth, using emollients and decreasing bathing frequency, to reduce the incidence of atopic dermatitis in high-risk neonates.

Bibliography is available at Expert Consult.

---

[*]https://www.niaid.nih.gov/diseases-conditions/guidelines-clinicians-and-patients-food-allergy.

Table 176.7	ACIP and AAP Recommendations for Administering Vaccines to Patients With Egg Allergy	
VACCINE	**ACIP, CDC, 2016**	**AAP, 2016**
MMR/MMRV	May be used	May be used
Influenza	Receive with no special precautions*	Receive with no special precautions*
Rabies	Use caution	No specific recommendation
Yellow fever	Contraindicated, but desensitization protocols may be followed to administer vaccine if necessary (citing PI)	Contraindicated, but desensitization protocols may be followed to administer vaccine if necessary (citing PI)

ACIP, Advisory Committee on Immunization Practices, Centers for Disease Control and Prevention; AAP, American Academy of Pediatrics; PI, product insert.

From Boyce JA, Assa'ad A, Burks AW, et al: Guideline for the diagnosis and management of food allergy in the United States: report of the NIAID-sponsored expert panel, *J Allergy Clin Immunol* 126(6):S1–S58, 2010 (Table V, p S31).

*In 2016, recommendations changed to suggest all children with any severity of egg allergy receive the injectable influenza vaccine as appropriate for age in a medical setting without any special testing and with the same precautions as those suggested for other vaccinations, including a 15 minute observation period and being in a setting where personnel and equipment are available to recognize and treat allergic reactions and anaphylaxis.

Table 176.8	Prevention of Food Allergy

Breastfeed exclusively for 4-6 mo.
Introduce solid (complementary) foods after 4-6 mo of exclusive breastfeeding.
Introduce low-risk complementary foods 1 at a time.
Introduce potentially highly allergenic foods (fish, eggs, peanut, milk, wheat) soon after the lower-risk foods (no need to avoid or delay).
    Infants with early-onset atopic disease (e.g., severe eczema) or egg allergy in the 1st 4-6 mo of life.
Do not avoid allergenic foods during pregnancy or nursing.
Soy-based formulas do not prevent allergic disease.

Chapter **177**

Adverse Reactions to Drugs

Christine B. Cho, Mark Boguniewicz, and Scott H. Sicherer

第一百七十七章
药物不良反应

中文导读

　　本章主要介绍了药物不良反应的定义、流行病学、发病机制及临床表现、诊断、治疗。具体介绍了药物不良反应的分类及其特点；描述了药物不良反应的发病情况、药疹常见类型及常见致敏药物；阐述了药物不良反应分型、药物与免疫受体的药理相互作用（p-i概念）、药物代谢与药物不良反应及引起药物过敏反应的危险因素；在诊断方面首先是准确了解临床病史，识别可疑药物，及一些相关检测（皮肤试验、血清类胰蛋白酶、斑贴试验、分级激发）支持诊断。治疗上具体描述了不同类药物所致的药疹类型及相应治疗措施。

Adverse drug reactions can be divided into predictable (type A) and unpredictable (type B) reactions. **Predictable drug reactions**, including drug toxicity, drug interactions, and adverse effects, are dose dependent, can be related to known pharmacologic actions of the drug, and occur in patients without any unique susceptibility. **Unpredictable drug reactions** are dose independent, often are not related to the pharmacologic actions of the drug, and occur in patients who are genetically predisposed. These include idiosyncratic reactions, allergic (hypersensitivity) reactions, and pseudoallergic reactions. **Allergic reactions** require prior sensitization, manifest as signs or symptoms characteristic of an underlying allergic mechanism, such as anaphylaxis or urticaria, and occur in genetically susceptible individuals. They can occur at doses significantly below the therapeutic range. **Pseudoallergic reactions** resemble allergic reactions but are caused by non–IgE-mediated release of mediators from mast cells and basophils. Drug-independent cross-reactive antigens can induce sensitization manifesting as drug allergy. Patients with cetuximab-induced anaphylaxis have IgE antibodies in pretreatment samples specific for galactose-α-1,3-galactose. This antigen is present on the antigen-binding portion of the cetuximab heavy chain and is similar to structures in the ABO blood group. Sensitization to galactose-α-1,3-galactose may occur from tick bites caused by cross-reactive tick salivary antigens.

EPIDEMIOLOGY

The incidence of adverse drug reactions (ADRs) in the general as well as pediatric populations remains unknown, although data from hospitalized patients show it to be 6.7%, with a 0.32% incidence of fatal ADRs. Databases such as the U.S. Food and Drug Administration (FDA) MedWatch program (http://www.fda.gov/medwatch/index.html) likely suffer from underreporting. Cutaneous reactions are the most common form of ADRs, with ampicillin, amoxicillin, penicillin, and trimethoprim/sulfamethoxazole (TMP/SMX) being the most frequently implicated drugs (Tables 177.1 and 177.2). Although the majority of ADRs do not appear to be allergic in nature, 6–10% can be attributed to an allergic or immunologic mechanism. Importantly, given the high probability of recurrence of allergic reactions, these reactions should be preventable, and information technology–based interventions may be especially useful to reduce risk of reexposure.

PATHOGENESIS AND CLINICAL MANIFESTATIONS

Immunologically mediated ADRs have been classified according to the Gell and Coombs classification: immediate hypersensitivity reactions (**type I**), cytotoxic antibody reactions (**type II**), immune complex reactions (**type III**), and delayed-type hypersensitivity reactions (**type IV**). **Immediate hypersensitivity reactions** occur when a drug or drug metabolite interacts with preformed drug-specific IgE antibodies that are bound to the surfaces of tissue mast cells and/or circulating basophils. The cross-linking of adjacent receptor-bound IgE by antigen causes the release of preformed and newly synthesized mediators, such as histamine and leukotrienes, that contribute to the clinical development of urticaria, bronchospasm, or anaphylaxis. **Cytotoxic antibody reactions** involve IgG or IgM antibodies that recognize drug antigen on the cell membrane. In the presence of serum complement, the antibody-coated cell is either cleared by the monocyte-macrophage system or is destroyed. Examples are drug-induced hemolytic anemia and thrombocytopenia. **Immune complex reactions** are caused by soluble complexes of drug or metabolite

Table 177.1	Heterogeneity of Drug-Induced Allergic Reactions	
ORGAN-SPECIFIC REACTIONS	**CLINICAL FEATURES**	**EXAMPLES OF CAUSATIVE AGENTS**
CUTANEOUS		
Exanthems	Diffuse fine macules and papules evolve over days after drug initiation Delayed-type hypersensitivity	Allopurinol, aminopenicillins, cephalosporins, antiepileptic agents, and antibacterial sulfonamides
Urticaria, angioedema	Onset within minutes of drug initiation Potential for anaphylaxis Often IgE mediated	IgE mediated: β-lactam antibiotics Bradykinin mediated: ACEI
Fixed drug eruption	Hyperpigmented plaques Recur at same skin or mucosal site	Tetracycline, sulfonamides, NSAIDs, and carbamazepine
Pustules	Acneiform Acute generalized exanthematous pustulosis (AGEP)	Acneiform: corticosteroids, sirolimus AGEP: antibiotics, calcium-channel blockers
Bullous	Tense blisters Flaccid blisters	Furosemide, vancomycin Captopril, penicillamine
SJS	Fever, erosive stomatitis, ocular involvement, purpuric macules on face and trunk with <10% epidermal detachment	Antibacterial sulfonamides, anticonvulsants, oxicam NSAIDs, and allopurinol
TEN	Similar features as SJS but >30% epidermal detachment Mortality as high as 50%	Same as SJS
Cutaneous lupus	Erythematous/scaly plaques in photodistribution	Hydrochlorothiazide, calcium channel blockers, ACEIs
Hematologic	Hemolytic anemia, thrombocytopenia, granulocytopenia	Penicillin, quinine, sulfonamides
Hepatic	Hepatitis, cholestatic jaundice	Paraaminosalicylic acid, sulfonamides, phenothiazines
Pulmonary	Pneumonitis, fibrosis	Nitrofurantoin, bleomycin, methotrexate
Renal	Interstitial nephritis, membranous glomerulonephritis	Penicillin, sulfonamides, gold, penicillamine, allopurinol
MULTIORGAN REACTIONS		
Anaphylaxis	Urticaria/angioedema, bronchospasm, gastrointestinal symptoms, hypotension IgE- and non–IgE-dependent reactions	β-Lactam antibiotics, monoclonal antibodies
DRESS	Cutaneous eruption, fever, eosinophilia, hepatic dysfunction, lymphadenopathy	Anticonvulsants, sulfonamides, minocycline, allopurinol
Serum sickness	Urticaria, arthralgias, fever	Heterologous antibodies, infliximab
Systemic lupus erythematosus	Arthralgias, myalgias, fever, malaise	Hydralazine, procainamide, isoniazid
Vasculitis	Cutaneous or visceral vasculitis	Hydralazine, penicillamine, propylthiouracil

ACEI, Angiotensin-converting enzyme inhibitor; DRESS, drug rash with eosinophilia and systemic symptoms; NSAID, nonsteroidal antiinflammatory drug; SJS, Stevens-Johnson syndrome; TEN, toxic epidermal necrolysis.
From Khan DA, Solensky R: Drug allergy, *J Allergy Clin Immunol* 125:S126–S137, 2010 (Table 1, p S127).

Table 177.2	Delayed Hypersensitivity Drug Rashes by Category

MACULOPAPULAR EXANTHEMS—ANY DRUG CAN PRODUCE A RASH 7-10 DAYS AFTER THE FIRST DOSE

Allopurinol
Antibiotics: penicillin, sulfonamides
Antiepileptics: phenytoin, phenobarbital
Antihypertensives: captopril, thiazide diuretics
Contrast dye: iodine
Gold salts
Hypoglycemic drugs
Meprobamate
Phenothiazines
Quinine

DRUG RASH WITH EOSINOPHILIA AND SYSTEMIC SYMPTOMS (DRESS)

Anticonvulsants: phenytoin, phenobarbital, valproate, lamotrigine
Antibiotics: sulfonamides, minocycline, dapsone, ampicillin, ethambutol, isoniazid, linezolid, metronidazole, rifampin, streptomycin, vancomycin
Antihypertensives: amlodipine, captopril
Antidepressants: bupropion, fluoxetine
Allopurinol
Celecoxib
Ibuprofen
Phenothiazines

ERYTHEMA MULTIFORME/STEVENS-JOHNSON SYNDROME

Sulfonamides, phenytoin, barbiturates, carbamazepine, allopurinol, amikacin, phenothiazines
Toxic epidermal necrolysis: same as for erythema multiforme but also acetazolamide, gold, nitrofurantoin, pentazocine, tetracycline, quinidine

ACUTE GENERALIZED EXANTHEMIC PUSTULOSIS

Antibiotics: penicillins, macrolides, cephalosporins, clindamycin, imipenem, fluoroquinolones, isoniazid, vancomycin, minocycline, doxycycline, linezolid
Antimalarials: chloroquine, hydroxychloroquine
Antifungals: terbinafine, nystatin
Anticonvulsants: carbamazepine
Calcium-channel blockers
Furosemide
Systemic corticosteroids
Protease inhibitors

COLLAGEN VASCULAR OR LUPUS-LIKE REACTIONS

Procainamide, hydralazine, phenytoin, penicillamine, trimethadione, methyldopa, carbamazepine, griseofulvin, nalidixic acid, oral contraceptives, propranolol

ERYTHEMA NODOSUM

Oral contraceptives, penicillin, sulfonamides, diuretics, gold, clonidine, propranolol, opiates

FIXED DRUG REACTIONS

Phenolphthalein, barbiturates, gold, sulfonamides, meprobamate, penicillin, tetracycline, analgesics

See Chapter 664 and Table 664.3.
From Duvic M: Urticaria, drug hypersensitivity rashes, nodules and tumors, and atrophic diseases. In Goldman L, Schafer AI, editors: Goldman-Cecil medicine, ed 25, Philadelphia, 2016, Elsevier, Table 440.3.

in slight antigen excess with IgG or IgM antibodies. The immune complex is deposited in blood vessel walls and causes injury by activating the complement cascade, as seen in serum sickness. Clinical manifestations include fever, urticaria, rash, lymphadenopathy, and arthralgias. Symptoms typically appear 1-3 wk after the last dose of an offending drug and subside when the drug and/or its metabolite is cleared from the body. **Delayed-type hypersensitivity reactions** are mediated by drug-specific T lymphocytes. Sensitization usually occurs by the topical route

of administration, resulting in allergic contact dermatitis. Commonly implicated drugs include neomycin and local anesthetics in topical formulations.

Certain ADRs, including drug fever and the morbilliform rash seen with use of ampicillin or amoxicillin in the setting of Epstein-Barr virus (EBV) infection, are not easily classified. Studies point to the role of T cells and eosinophils in delayed maculopapular reactions to a number of antibiotics. The mechanisms of T-cell–mediated drug hypersensitivity are not well understood. A novel hypothesis, the **p-i concept**, suggests pharmacologic interactions of drugs with immune receptors as another class of drug hypersensitivity. In T-cell–mediated allergic drug reactions, the specificity of the T-cell receptor (TCR) that is stimulated by the drug may be directed to a cross-reactive major histocompatibility complex (MHC)–peptide compound. This information suggests that even poorly reactive native drugs are capable of transmitting a stimulatory signal through the TCR, which activates T cells and results in proliferation, cytokine production, and cytotoxicity. Previous contact with the causative drug is not obligatory, and an immune mechanism should be considered as the cause of hypersensitivity, even in reactions that occur with first exposure. Such reactions have been described for radiocontrast media and neuromuscular blocking agents.

Drug Metabolism and Adverse Reactions

Most drugs and their metabolites are not immunologically detectable until they have become covalently attached to a macromolecule. This multivalent hapten-protein complex forms a new immunogenic epitope that can elicit T- and B-lymphocyte responses. The penicillins and related β-lactam antibiotics are highly reactive with proteins and can directly haptenate protein carriers, possibly accounting for the frequency of immune-mediated hypersensitivity reactions with this class of antibiotics.

Incomplete or delayed metabolism of some drugs can give rise to toxic metabolites. Hydroxylamine, a reactive metabolite produced by cytochrome P450 oxidative metabolism, may mediate adverse reactions to sulfonamides. Patients who are *slow acetylators* appear to be at increased risk (see Chapter 72). In addition, cutaneous reactions in patients with AIDS treated with TMP/SMX, rifampin, or other drugs may be caused by glutathione deficiency resulting in toxic metabolites. Serum sickness–like reactions in which immune complexes have not been documented, which occur most often with cefaclor, may result from an inherited propensity for hepatic biotransformation of drugs into toxic or immunogenic metabolites.

Risk Factors for Hypersensitivity Reactions

Risk factors for ADRs include prior exposure, previous reactions, age (20-49 yr), route of administration (parenteral or topical), dose (high), and dosing schedule (intermittent), as well as genetic predisposition (slow acetylators). Atopy does not appear to predispose patients to allergic reactions to low-molecular-weight compounds, but atopic patients in whom an allergic reaction develops have a significantly increased risk of serious reaction. Atopic patients also appear to be at greater risk for pseudoallergic reactions induced by radiocontrast media. Pharmacogenomics has an important role in identifying individuals at risk for certain drug reactions (see Chapter 72).

DIAGNOSIS

An accurate medical history is an important first step in evaluating a patient with a possible ADR. Suspected drugs need to be identified, along with dosages, route of administration, previous exposures, and dates of administration. In addition, underlying hepatic or renal disease may influence drug metabolism. A detailed description of past reactions may yield clues to the nature of the ADR. The propensity for a particular drug to cause the suspected reaction can be checked with information in *Physicians' Desk Reference, Drug Eruption Reference Manual,* or directly from the drug manufacturer. It is important to remember, however, that the history may be unreliable, and many patients are inappropriately labeled as being "drug allergic." This label can result in inappropriate withholding of a needed drug or class of drugs. In addition, relying solely on the history can lead to overuse of drugs reserved for special indications, such as vancomycin in patients in whom penicillin allergy is suspected. *Approximately 90% of patients with a clinical history of penicillin allergy do not have evidence of penicillin-specific IgE antibodies on testing.*

Skin testing is the most rapid and sensitive method of demonstrating the presence of *IgE antibodies* to a specific allergen. It can be performed with high-molecular-weight compounds, such as foreign antisera, hormones, enzymes, and toxoids. Reliable skin testing can also be performed with penicillin, but not with most other antibiotics. Most immunologically mediated ADRs are caused by metabolites rather than by parent compounds, and the metabolites for most drugs other than penicillin have not been defined. In addition, many metabolites are unstable or must combine with larger proteins to be useful for diagnosis. Testing with nonstandardized reagents requires caution in interpretation of both positive and negative results, because some drugs can induce nonspecific irritant reactions. Whereas a wheal and flare reaction is suggestive of drug-specific IgE antibodies, a negative skin test result does not exclude the presence of such antibodies because the relevant immunogen may not have been used as the testing reagent.

A positive skin test response to the major or minor determinants of penicillin has a 60% positive predictive value (PPV) for an immediate hypersensitivity reaction to penicillin. In patients in whom skin test responses to the major and minor determinants of penicillin are negative, 97–99% (depending on the reagents used) tolerate the drug without an immediate reaction. At present, the major determinant of penicillin testing reagent benzylpenicilloyl polylysine (Pre-Pen) in the United States is available, but the minor determinant mixture has not been FDA approved as a testing reagent. Limited studies utilizing serum tests for IgE to β-lactams suggest high specificity (97–100%) but low sensitivity (29–68%). The PPV and negative predictive value (NPV) of skin testing for antibiotics other than penicillin are not well established. Nevertheless, positive immediate hypersensitivity skin test responses to nonirritant concentrations of nonpenicillin antibiotics may be interpreted as a presumptive risk of an immediate reaction to such agents.

Results of direct and indirect Coombs tests are often positive in drug-induced hemolytic anemia. Assays for specific IgG and IgM have been shown to correlate with a drug reaction in immune cytopenia, but in most other reactions, such assays are not diagnostic. In general, many more patients express humoral or T-cell immune responses to drug determinants than express clinical disease. Serum **tryptase** is elevated with systemic mast cell degranulation and can be seen with drug-associated mast cell activation, although it is not pathognomonic for drug hypersensitivity, and nonelevated tryptase values can be seen in well-defined anaphylaxis. **Patch testing** is the most reliable technique for diagnosis of contact dermatitis caused by topically applied drugs. **Graded challenge** is the administration of a drug under medical supervision in an incremental fashion dosed faster than used for desensitization (see later) until a therapeutic dose is achieved. This can be attempted when the risk of reactions are judged to be low, and is a means to prove that the drug is tolerated or to identify an adverse or allergic reaction.

TREATMENT

Specific **desensitization**, which involves the progressive administration of an allergen to render effector cells less reactive, is reserved for patients with IgE antibodies to a particular drug for whom an alternative drug is not available or appropriate. Specific protocols for many different drugs have been developed. Desensitization should be performed in a hospital setting, usually in consultation with an allergist and with resuscitation equipment available at all times. Although mild complications, such as pruritus and rash, are fairly common and often respond to adjustments in the drug dose or dosing intervals and medications to relieve symptoms, more severe systemic reactions can occur. Oral desensitization may be less likely to induce anaphylaxis than parenteral administration. Protocols for gradual exposure are also used for adverse reaction to drugs that are not IgE mediated, for example for aspirin- or nonsteroidal antiinflammatory drug (NSAID)–intolerant patients, particularly those with respiratory reactions and those with mild rashes from TMP/SMX. Pretreatment with antihistamines or corticosteroids is not usually recommended. It is important to recognize that desensitization to a drug is effective only while the drug continues to be admin-

istered, and that after a period of interruption or discontinuation, hypersensitivity can recur. Patients with severe non–IgE-mediated hypersensitivity reactions should not receive the predisposing agents even in the small amounts used for skin testing (see Table 177.2).

β-Lactam Hypersensitivity

Penicillin is a frequent cause of anaphylaxis and is responsible for the majority of all drug-mediated anaphylactic deaths in the United States. If a patient requires penicillin and has a previous history suggestive of penicillin allergy, it is necessary to perform skin tests on the patient for the presence of penicillin-specific IgE, ideally with both the major and minor determinants of penicillin. Skin tests for minor determinants of penicillin are important because approximately 20% of patients with documented anaphylaxis do not demonstrate skin reactivity to the major determinant. The major determinant is commercially available (Pre-Pen). The minor determinant mixture is currently not licensed and is synthesized as a nonstandardized testing reagent at select academic centers. Penicillin G is often used as a substitute for the minor determinant mixture and may have NPV similar to testing with major and minor determinants. Patients should be referred to an allergist capable of performing appropriate testing. If the skin test response is positive to either major or minor determinants of penicillin, the patient should receive an alternative non–cross-reacting antibiotic. If administration of penicillin is deemed necessary, desensitization can be performed by an allergist in an appropriate medical setting. Skin testing for penicillin-specific IgE is not predictive for delayed-onset cutaneous, bullous, or immune complex reactions. In addition, penicillin skin testing does not appear to resensitize the patient.

Other β-lactam antibiotics, including semisynthetic penicillins, cephalosporins, carbacephems, and carbapenems, share the β-lactam ring structure. Patients with late-onset morbilliform rashes with amoxicillin are not considered to be at risk for IgE-mediated reactions to penicillin and do not require skin testing before penicillin administration. Many patients with EBV infections treated with ampicillin or amoxicillin can experience a nonpruritic rash. Similar reactions occur in patients who receive allopurinol as treatment for elevated uric acid or have chronic lymphocytic leukemia. If the rash to ampicillin or amoxicillin is urticarial or systemic or the history is unclear, the patient should undergo penicillin skin testing if a penicillin is needed. There have been reports of antibodies specific for semisynthetic penicillin side chains in the absence of β-lactam ring–specific antibodies, although the clinical significance of such side chain–specific antibodies is unclear.

Varying degrees of in vitro cross-reactivity have been documented between *cephalosporins* and penicillins. Although the risk of allergic reactions to cephalosporins in patients with positive skin test responses to penicillin appears to be low (<2%), anaphylactic reactions have occurred after administration of cephalosporins in patients with a history of penicillin anaphylaxis. If a patient has a history of penicillin allergy and requires a cephalosporin, skin testing for major and minor determinants of penicillin should preferably be performed to determine whether the patient has penicillin-specific IgE antibodies. If skin test results are negative, the patient can receive a cephalosporin with no greater risk than found in the general population. If skin test results are positive for penicillin, recommendations may include administration of an alternative antibiotic; cautious graded challenge with appropriate monitoring, with the recognition that there is a 2% chance of inducing an anaphylactic reaction; and desensitization to the required cephalosporin. Cross-reactivity is most likely when the cephalosporin shares the same side chain as the penicillin (Table 177.3).

Conversely, patients who require penicillin and have a history of an IgE-mediated reaction to a cephalosporin should also undergo penicillin skin testing. Patients with a negative result can receive penicillin. Patients with a positive result should either receive an alternative medication or undergo desensitization to penicillin. In patients with a history of allergic reaction to one cephalosporin who require another cephalosporin, skin testing with the required cephalosporin can be performed, with the recognition that the NPV of such testing is unknown. If the skin test response to the cephalosporin is positive, the significance of the test should be checked further in controls to determine whether the

Table 177.3	Groups of β-Lactam Antibiotics That Share Identical R1-Group Side Chains*				
Amoxicillin	Ampicillin	Ceftriaxone	Cefoxitin	Cefamandole	Ceftazidime
Cefadroxil	Cefaclor	Cefotaxime	Cephaloridine	Cefonicid	Aztreonam
Cefprozil	Cephalexin	Cefpodoxime	Cephalothin		
Cefatrizine	Cephradine	Cefditoren			
	Cephaloglycin	Ceftizoxime			
	Loracarbef	Cefmenoxime			

*Each column represents a group with identical R1 side chains.
From Solensky R, Khan DA: Drug allergy: an updated practice parameter, *Ann Allergy Asthma Immunol* 105:273e1–273e78, 2010 (Table 16, p 273e49).

positive response is IgE mediated or an irritant response. The drug can then be administered by graded challenge or desensitization.

Carbapenems (imipenem, meropenem) represent another class of β-lactam antibiotics with a bicyclic nucleus that demonstrate a high degree of cross-reactivity with penicillins, although prospective studies suggest incidence of cross-reactivity on skin testing of approximately 1%. In contrast to β-lactam antibiotics, *monobactams* (aztreonam) have a monocyclic ring structure. Aztreonam-specific antibodies have been shown to be predominantly side chain-specific; data suggest that aztreonam can be safely administered to most penicillin-allergic patients. On the other hand, administration of aztreonam to a patient with ceftazidime allergy may be associated with increased risk of allergic reaction because of the similarity of side chains.

Sulfonamides

The most common type of reaction to sulfonamides is a maculopapular eruption often associated with fever that occurs after 7-12 days of therapy. Immediate reactions, including anaphylaxis, as well as other immunologic reactions, have also been suggested. Hypersensitivity reactions to sulfonamides occur with much greater frequency in HIV-infected individuals. For patients in whom maculopapular rashes develop after sulfonamide administration, both graded challenge and desensitization protocols have been shown to be effective. These regimens should not be used in individuals with a history of Stevens-Johnson syndrome (SJS) or toxic epidermal necrolysis (TEN). Hypersensitivity reactions to *sulfasalazine* used for treatment of inflammatory bowel disease appear to result from the sulfapyridine moiety. Slow desensitization over about 1 mo permits tolerance of the drug in many patients. In addition, oral and enema forms of 5-aminosalicylic acid, thought to be the pharmacologically active agent in sulfasalazine, are effective alternative therapies.

Stevens-Johnson Syndrome and Toxic Epidermal Necrolysis

Blistering mucocutaneous disorders induced by drugs encompass a spectrum of reactions, including SJS and TEN (see Chapters 673.2 and 673.3). While their pathophysiology remains incompletely understood, HLA associations including HLA-B*1502 with carbamazepine-induced TEN have been recognized, and the pathogenic roles of drug-specific cytotoxic T cells and granulysin have been reported. Epidermal detachment of <10% is suggestive of SJS, 30% detachment suggests TEN, and 10–30% detachment suggests overlap of the 2 syndromes. The features of SJS include confluent purpuric macules on face and trunk and severe, explosive mucosal erosions, usually at more than 1 mucosal surface, accompanied by fever and constitutional symptoms. Ocular involvement may be particularly severe, and the liver, kidneys, and lungs may also be involved. TEN, which appears to be related to keratinocyte apoptosis, manifests as widespread areas of confluent erythema followed by epidermal necrosis and detachment with severe mucosal involvement. Skin biopsy differentiates subepidermal cleavage characteristic of TEN from intraepidermal cleavage characteristic of the scalded-skin syndrome induced by staphylococcal toxins. The risks of infection and mortality remain high, but improved outcomes have been demonstrated by immediate withdrawal of the implicated drug, early transfer to an intensive care or burn unit, and aggressive supportive care. Additional management is reviewed in Chapter 673.3.

Hypersensitivity to Antiretroviral Agents

A growing number of ADRs have been observed with antiretroviral agents, including reverse-transcriptase inhibitors, protease inhibitors, and fusion inhibitors. Hypersensitivity to abacavir is a well-recognized, multiorgan, potentially life-threatening reaction that occurs in HIV-infected children. The reaction is independent of dose, with onset generally within 9-11 days of initiation of drug therapy. Rechallenge can be accompanied by significant hypotension and potential mortality (rate of 0.03%), and thus hypersensitivity to abacavir is an absolute contraindication for any subsequent use. Prophylaxis with prednisolone does not appear to prevent hypersensitivity reactions to abacavir. Importantly, genetic susceptibility appears to be conferred by the HLA-B*5701 allele, with a PPV >70% and NPV of 95–98%. Genetic screening would be cost-effective in white populations but not in populations of African or Asian descent, in which HLA-B*5701 allele frequency is <1%.

Chemotherapeutic Agents

Hypersensitivity reactions to chemotherapeutic drugs have been described, including to monoclonal antibodies. Rapid desensitization to a variety of unrelated agents, including carboplatin, paclitaxel, and rituximab, can be safely achieved in a 12-step protocol. Of note, this approach appears to be successful in both IgE-mediated and non–IgE-mediated reactions.

Biologics

An increasing number of biologic agents have become available for the treatment of autoimmune, allergic, cardiovascular, infectious, and neoplastic diseases. Their use may be associated with a variety of ADRs, including hypersensitivity reactions. Given the occurrence of anaphylaxis, including cases with delayed onset and protracted progression in spontaneous postmarketing adverse event reports, the FDA issued a black box warning regarding risk of anaphylaxis and need for patient monitoring with use of omalizumab (see Chapter 169).

Vaccines

Allergy to vaccines may occur from reactivity to various vaccine components. Measles-mumps-rubella (MMR) vaccine has been shown to be safe in egg-allergic patients (although rare reactions to gelatin or neomycin can occur). The ovalbumin content in influenza vaccine is extremely low. Skin testing with the influenza vaccine is not recommended for egg-allergic patients but may be helpful if allergy to the vaccine itself is suspected. Egg-allergic patients do not appear to be at higher risk of reacting to the influenza vaccine than those without egg allergy, and they may receive it in the usual manner with the same 15-min waiting period suggested for other vaccinations and in a medical setting prepared to treat anaphylaxis.

Perioperative Agents

Anaphylactoid (non–IgE-mediated anaphylaxis) reactions occurring during general anesthesia may be caused by induction agents (thiopental) or muscle-relaxing agents (succinylcholine, pancuronium). Quaternary ammonium muscle relaxants (succinylcholine) can act as bivalent antigens in IgE-mediated reactions. Negative skin test results do not necessarily predict that a drug will be tolerated. Latex allergy should always be considered in the differential diagnosis of a perioperative reaction.

Local Anesthetics

ADRs associated with local anesthetic agents are primarily toxic reactions resulting from rapid drug absorption, inadvertent intravenous (IV) injection, or overdose. Local anesthetics are classified as esters of benzoic acid (group I) or amides (group II). Group I includes benzocaine and procaine; group II includes lidocaine, bupivacaine, and mepivacaine. In suspected local anesthetic allergy, skin testing followed by a graded challenge can be performed or an anesthetic agent from a different group can be used.

Insulin

Insulin use has been associated with a spectrum of ADRs, including local and systemic IgE-mediated reactions, hemolytic anemia, serum sickness reactions, and delayed-type hypersensitivity. In general, human insulin is less allergenic than porcine insulin, which is less allergenic than bovine insulin, but for individual patients, porcine or bovine insulin may be the least allergenic. Patients treated with nonhuman insulin have had systemic reactions to recombinant human insulin even on the first exposure. More than 50% of patients who receive insulin develop antibodies against the insulin preparation, although there may not be any clinical manifestations. Local cutaneous reactions usually do not require treatment and resolve with continued insulin administration, possibly because of IgG-blocking antibodies. More severe local reactions can be treated with antihistamines or by splitting the insulin dose between separate administration sites. Local reactions to the protamine component of neutral protamine Hagedorn insulin may be avoided by switching to Lente insulin. Immediate-type reactions to insulin, including urticaria and anaphylactic shock, are unusual and almost always occur after reinstitution of insulin therapy in sensitized patients.

Insulin therapy should not be interrupted if a systemic reaction to insulin occurs, and continued insulin therapy is essential. Skin testing may identify a less antigenic insulin preparation. The dose following a systemic reaction is usually reduced to one-third, and successive doses are increased in 2-5 unit increments until the dose resulting in glucose control is attained. Insulin skin testing and desensitization are required if insulin treatment is subsequently interrupted for >24-48 hr.

Immunologic resistance usually occurs when high titers of predominantly IgG antibodies to insulin develop. A rare form of insulin resistance caused by circulating antibodies to tissue insulin receptors is associated with acanthosis nigricans and lipodystrophy. Coexisting insulin allergy may be present in up to one third of patients with insulin resistance. Approximately half of affected patients benefit from substitution with a less reactive insulin preparation, based on skin testing.

Drug-Induced Hypersensitivity Syndrome

Drug-induced hypersensitivity syndrome, or **DRESS** (drug rash with eosinophilia and systemic symptoms) syndrome, is a potentially life-threatening syndrome that has been described primarily with anticonvulsants, although many other medications have been implicated (see Tables 177.1 and 177.2). It is characterized by fever, maculopapular rash, facial edema, eosinophilia, generalized lymphadenopathy, and potentially life-threatening damage of one or more organs, usually renal or hepatic. Onset is delayed, usually weeks after initiation of the medication. It has been associated with reactivation of human herpesvirus 6. Treatment is withdrawal of the medication, systemic steroids, and supportive care, but symptoms can worsen or persist for weeks to months after the drug has been discontinued.

Red Man Syndrome

Red man syndrome is caused by nonspecific histamine release and is most often described with administration of IV vancomycin. It can be prevented by slowing the vancomycin infusion rate or by preadministration of H_1-receptor blockers.

Radiocontrast Media

Anaphylactoid reactions to radiocontrast media or dye can occur after intravascular administration and during myelograms or retrograde pyelograms. No single pathogenic mechanism has been defined, but it is likely that mast cell activation accounts for the majority of these reactions. Complement activation has also been described. There is no evidence that sensitivity to seafood or iodine predisposes to radiocontrast media reactions. Predictive tests are not available. Patients who have atopic profiles, who are taking β-blockers, and who have had prior anaphylactoid reactions are at increased risk. Other diagnostic alternatives should be considered, or patients can be given low-osmolality radiocontrast media with a pretreatment regimen including oral prednisone, diphenhydramine, and albuterol, with or without cimetidine or ranitidine.

Narcotic Analgesics

Opiates such as morphine and related narcotics can induce direct mast cell degranulation. Patients may experience generalized pruritus, urticaria, and occasionally, wheezing. If there is a suggestive history and analgesia is required, a nonnarcotic medication should be considered. If this intervention does not control pain, graded challenge with an alternative opiate is an option.

Aspirin and Nonsteroidal Antiinflammatory Drugs

Aspirin and NSAIDs can cause anaphylactoid reactions or urticaria and angioedema in children and, rarely, asthma with or without rhinoconjunctivitis in adolescents. There is no skin or in vitro test to identify patients who may react to aspirin or other NSAIDs. Once aspirin or NSAID intolerance has been established, options include avoidance and pharmacologic desensitization and subsequent continued treatment with aspirin or NSAIDs, if indicated. A number of studies suggest that cyclooxygenase-2 inhibitors are tolerated by the majority of patients with NSAID-induced adverse reactions.

Bibliography is available at Expert Consult.

Rheumatic Diseases of Childhood (Connective Tissue Disease, Collagen Vascular Diseases)

PART XV

儿童风湿性疾病（结缔组织病–胶原血管病）

第十五部分

Chapter 178
Evaluation of Suspected Rheumatic Disease

C. Egla Rabinovich

第一百七十八章
疑似风湿性疾病的评估

中文导读

本章主要介绍了风湿性疾病的症状、提示风湿性疾病的体征、实验室检查和影像学检查。其中风湿性疾病的症状主要包括发热、关节痛、虚弱、胸痛、背痛和疲劳等；风湿性疾病的体征主要包括颧部红斑、口腔溃疡、紫癜样皮疹、高春征、关节炎等；实验室检查包括自身抗体检测、全血细胞计数、类风湿因子、炎性标志物（红细胞沉降率、C反应蛋白）、肌酶（天冬氨酸氨基转移酶、门冬氨酸氨基转移酶、肌酸激酶、醛缩酶和乳酸脱氢酶）；影像学检查主要包括平片、放射性骨扫描和磁共振检查。

Rheumatic diseases are defined by the constellation of results of the physical examination, autoimmune marker and other serologic tests, tissue pathology, and imaging. Defined diagnostic criteria exist for most rheumatic diseases. Recognition of clinical patterns remains essential for diagnosis because there is no single diagnostic test, and results may be positive in the absence of disease. Further complicating the diagnosis, children sometimes present with partial criteria that evolve over time or with features of more than one rheumatic disease (**overlap syndromes**). The primary mimics of rheumatic diseases are **infection** and **malignancy** but also include metabolic, orthopedic, immune deficiencies, autoinflammatory diseases, and chronic pain conditions. Exclusion of possible mimicking disorders is essential before initiation of treatment for a presumptive diagnosis, especially corticosteroids.

After careful evaluation has excluded nonrheumatic causes, referral to a pediatric rheumatologist for confirmation of the diagnosis and treatment should be considered.

SYMPTOMS SUGGESTIVE OF RHEUMATIC DISEASE
There are no classic symptoms of a rheumatic disease, but common symptoms include joint pain, fever, fatigue, and rash. Presenting signs and symptoms help direct the evaluation and limit unnecessary testing. Once a differential diagnosis is developed on the basis of history and physical findings, a directed assessment assists in determining the diagnosis.

Arthralgias are common in childhood and are a frequent reason for referral to pediatric rheumatologists. Arthralgias without physical findings for arthritis suggest infection, malignancy, orthopedic conditions, benign syndromes, or pain syndromes such as fibromyalgia (Table 178.1). Although rheumatic diseases may manifest as arthralgias, **arthritis** is a stronger predictor of the presence of rheumatic disease and a reason for referral to a pediatric rheumatologist. The timing of joint pain along with associated symptoms, including poor sleep and interference with normal activities, provides important clues. Poor sleep, debilitating generalized joint pain that worsens with activity, school absences, and normal physical and laboratory findings in an adolescent suggest a **pain syndrome** (e.g., fibromyalgia). If arthralgia is accompanied by a history of dry skin, hair loss, fatigue, growth disturbance, or cold intolerance, testing for **thyroid disease** is merited. Nighttime awakenings because of severe pain along with decreased platelet or white blood cell count or, alternatively, a very high WBC count, may lead to the diagnosis of malignancy, especially marrow-occupying lesions such as **acute lymphocytic leukemia** and **neuroblastoma**. Pain with physical activity suggests a mechanical problem such as an overuse syndrome or orthopedic condition. An adolescent girl presenting with knee pain aggravated by walking up stairs and on patellar distraction likely has **patellofemoral syndrome**. Children age 3-10 yr who have a history of episodic pain that occurs at night after increased daytime physical activity that is relieved by rubbing, but who have no limp or complaints in the morning, likely have **growing pains**. There is often a positive family history for growing pains, which may aid in this diagnosis. Intermittent pain in a child, especially a girl 3-10 yr old, that is increased with activity and is associated with hyperextensible joints on examination, is likely **benign hypermobility syndrome**. Many febrile illnesses cause arthralgias that improve when the temperature normalizes, and arthralgias are part of the diagnostic criteria for **acute rheumatic fever** (**ARF**; see Chapter 210.1).

Arthralgia may also be a presenting symptom of pediatric **systemic lupus erythematosus** (**SLE**) and chronic childhood arthritis such as **juvenile idiopathic arthritis** (**JIA**). Interestingly, many children with JIA do not complain of joint symptoms at presentation. Other symptoms more suggestive of arthritis include morning stiffness, joint swelling, limited range of motion, pain with joint motion, gait disturbance, fever, and fatigue or stiffness after physical inactivity (*gelling phenomenon*). A diagnosis of JIA cannot be made without the finding of arthritis on physical examination (see Chapters 180 and 181). No laboratory test is diagnostic of JIA or any other chronic inflammatory arthritis in childhood.

Fatigue is a nonspecific symptom that may point to the presence of a rheumatic disease but is also common in nonrheumatic causes, such as viral infections, pain syndromes, depression, and malignancy. Fatigue, rather than the specific complaints of muscle weakness, is a common presenting complaint in **juvenile dermatomyositis** (**JDM**). It is also frequently present in SLE, vasculitis, and the chronic childhood arthritides. Overwhelming fatigue with inability to attend school is more suggestive of chronic fatigue syndrome, pediatric fibromyalgia, or other amplified pain syndrome.

SIGNS SUGGESTIVE OF RHEUMATIC DISEASE

A complete physical examination is mandated in any child with suspected rheumatic disease, because many diseases have associated subtle physical findings that will further refine the differential diagnosis. In addition, many rheumatic diseases have multisystem effects, and a stepped assessment should focus on delineating the extent of organ system involvement (e.g., skin, joints, muscle, hepatic, renal, cardiopulmonary).

Presence of a **photosensitive malar rash** that spares the nasolabial folds is suggestive of SLE (Table 178.2; see Fig. 183.1*A*), especially in an adolescent girl. Diffuse facial rash is more indicative of JDM. A hyperkeratotic rash on the face or around the ears of an adolescent black girl may represent discoid lupus (see Fig. 183.1*D*). A palpable purpuric rash on the extensor surfaces of the lower extremities points to **Henoch-Schönlein purpura** (see Fig. 192.2*A*). Less localized purpuric rashes and petechiae are present in systemic vasculitis or blood dyscrasias, including coagulopathies. Nonblanching erythematous papules on the palms are seen in vasculitis and SLE as well as endocarditis. Gottron papules (see Fig. 184.2) and heliotrope rashes (see Fig. 184.1) along with erythematous rashes on the elbows and knees are pathognomonic of JDM. Dilated capillary loops in the nail beds (periungual telangiectasias; see Fig. 184.3) are common in JDM, scleroderma, and secondary Raynaud phenomenon. An evanescent macular rash associated with fever is part of the diagnostic criteria for systemic-onset arthritis (see Fig. 180.12). Sun sensitivity or photosensitive rashes are indicative of SLE or JDM but can also be caused by antibiotics.

Mouth ulcers are part of the diagnostic criteria for SLE and Behçet disease (see Fig. 183.1*C*); painless nasal ulcers and erythematous macules on the hard palate are also common in SLE. Cartilage loss in the nose, causing a saddle nose deformity, is classically present in granulomatosis with polyangiitis (formally Wegener granulomatosis; see Fig. 192.8) but is also seen in relapsing polychondritis and syphilis. Alopecia can be associated with SLE but is also found in localized scleroderma (see Fig. 185.4) and JDM. **Raynaud phenomenon** may be a primary benign idiopathic disorder or can be a presenting complaint in the child with scleroderma, lupus, mixed connective tissue disease (MCTD), or an overlap syndrome. Diffuse lymphadenopathy is present in many rheumatic diseases, including SLE, polyarticular JIA, and systemic JIA. Irregular pupils may represent the insidious and unrecognized onset of **uveitis** associated with JIA. Erythematous conjunctivae may be a result of uveitis or episcleritis associated with JIA, SLE, sarcoidosis, spondyloarthropathies, or vasculitis.

A pericardial rub and orthopnea are suggestive of **pericarditis**, often seen in systemic JIA, SLE, and sarcoid. Coronary artery dilation is strongly suggestive of Kawasaki disease but may also be a finding in systemic

Table 178.1	Symptoms Suggestive of Rheumatic Disease	
SYMPTOM	**RHEUMATIC DISEASE(S)**	**POSSIBLE NONRHEUMATIC DISEASES CAUSING SIMILAR SYMPTOMS**
Fevers	Systemic JIA, SLE, vasculitis, acute rheumatic fever, sarcoidosis, MCTD	Malignancies, infections and postinfectious syndromes, inflammatory bowel disease, periodic fever (autoinflammatory) syndromes, Kawasaki disease, HSP
Arthralgias	JIA, SLE, rheumatic fever, JDM, vasculitis, scleroderma, sarcoidosis	Hypothyroidism, trauma, endocarditis, other infections, pain syndromes, growing pains, malignancies, overuse syndromes
Weakness	JDM, myositis secondary to SLE, MCTD, and deep localized scleroderma	Muscular dystrophies, metabolic and other myopathies, hypothyroidism
Chest pain	Juvenile idiopathic arthritis, SLE (with associated pericarditis or costochondritis)	Costochondritis (isolated), rib fracture, viral pericarditis, panic attack, hyperventilation
Back pain	Enthesitis-related arthritis, juvenile ankylosing spondylitis	Vertebral compression fracture, diskitis, intraspinal tumor, spondylolysis, spondylolisthesis, bone marrow–occupying malignancy, pain syndromes, osteomyelitis, muscle spasm, injury
Fatigue	SLE, JDM, MCTD, vasculitis, JIA	Pain syndromes, chronic infections, chronic fatigue syndrome, depression

HSP, Henoch-Schönlein purpura; JDM, juvenile dermatomyositis; JIA, juvenile idiopathic arthritis; MCTD, mixed connective tissue disease; SLE, systemic lupus erythematosus.

Table 178.2	Signs Suggestive of Rheumatic Disease		
SIGN	**RHEUMATIC DISEASES**	**COMMENTS**	**NONRHEUMATIC CAUSES**
Malar rash	SLE, JDM	SLE classically spares nasolabial folds	Sunburn, parvovirus B19 (fifth disease), Kawasaki disease
Oral ulcers	SLE, Behçet disease	Behçet disease also associated with genital ulcers	HSV infection, PFAPA syndrome
Purpuric rash	Vasculitis, e.g., ANCA-associated vasculitis, HSP	HSP typically starts as small lesions on lower extremities and buttocks that coalesce	Meningococcemia, thrombocytopenia, clotting disorders
Gottron papules	JDM	Look for associated heliotrope rash, periungual telangiectasias	Psoriasis, eczema
Arthritis	Juvenile idiopathic arthritis, SLE, vasculitis, HSP, MCTD, scleroderma, acute rheumatic fever, reactive arthritis	Chronic joint swelling (>6 wk) required for diagnosis of chronic arthritis of childhood; MCTD associated with diffuse puffiness of hands	Postviral arthritis, reactive arthritis, trauma, infection, Lyme disease, Kawasaki disease, malignancy, overuse syndromes

ANCA, Antineutrophil cytoplasmic antibody; HSP, Henoch-Schönlein purpura; HSV, herpes simplex virus; JDM, juvenile dermatomyositis; MCTD, mixed connective tissue disease; PFAPA, periodic fever, aphthous stomatitis, pharyngitis, and adenitis; SLE, systemic lupus erythematosus.

arthritis and other forms of systemic vasculitis. Interstitial lung disease, suggested by dyspnea on exertion or the finding of basilar rales with decreased carbon monoxide diffusion capacity, occurs in SLE, MCTD, and systemic sclerosis. Signs consistent with pulmonary hemorrhage points to granulomatosis with polyangiitis, microscopic angiitis, or SLE. Pulmonary vascular aneurysms are indicative of Behçet disease.

Arthritis is defined by the presence of intraarticular swelling or 2 or more of the following findings on joint examination: pain on motion, loss of motion, erythema, and heat. Arthritis is present in all the chronic childhood arthritis syndromes, along with SLE, JDM, vasculitis, Behçet disease, sarcoidosis, Kawasaki disease, and Henoch-Schönlein purpura. Nonrheumatic causes of arthritis include malignancy, septic arthritis, Lyme disease, osteomyelitis, viral infections (e.g., rubella, hepatitis B, parvovirus B19, chikungunya), and postinfectious etiologies such as Epstein-Barr virus (EBV), ARF, and reactive arthritis. ARF typically involves a migratory (lasting hours to days), painful arthritis. Pain on palpation of long bones is suggestive of malignancy. Specific muscle testing for weakness should be performed in a child presenting with fatigue or difficulty with daily tasks, because both these symptoms may be manifestations of muscle inflammation.

LABORATORY TESTING

There are no specific screening tests for rheumatologic disease. Once a differential diagnosis is determined, appropriate testing can be performed (Tables 178.3 and 178.4). Initial studies are generally performed in standard local laboratories. Screening for specific autoantibodies can be performed in commercial laboratories, but confirmation of results in a tertiary care center immunology laboratory is often necessary.

One essential laboratory test for rheumatic disease assessment is the *complete blood count* (CBC), since it yields many diagnostic clues. Elevated WBC count is compatible with malignancy, infection, systemic JIA, and vasculitis. Leukopenia can be postinfectious, especially viral, or caused by SLE or malignancy. Lymphopenia is more specific for SLE than is leukopenia. Platelets are acute-phase reactants and are therefore elevated with inflammatory markers. Exceptions are a bone marrow–occupying malignancy, such as leukemia or neuroblastoma, SLE, and early Kawasaki disease. **Anemia** is nonspecific and may be caused by any chronic illness, but hemolytic anemia (positive Coombs test result) may point to SLE or MCTD. Rheumatoid factor (RF) is present in <10% of children with JIA and thus has poor sensitivity as a diagnostic tool; RF may be elevated by infections such as endocarditis, tuberculosis, syphilis, and viruses (parvovirus B19, hepatitides B and C, mycoplasma), as well as primary biliary cirrhosis and malignancies. In a child with chronic arthritis, RF serves as a prognostic indicator.

Inflammatory markers (erythrocyte sedimentation rate, C-reactive protein) are nonspecific and are elevated in infections and malignancies as well as rheumatic diseases (Tables 178.5 and 178.6). Their levels may also be normal in rheumatic diseases such as arthritis, scleroderma, and dermatomyositis. Inflammatory marker measurements are more useful in rheumatic diseases for following response to treatment than as diagnostic tests. Muscle enzymes include aspartate transaminase (AST), alanine transaminase (ALT), creatinine phosphokinase (CPK), aldolase, and lactate dehydrogenase (LDH), any of which may be elevated in JDM as well as in other diseases causing muscle breakdown. Muscle-building supplements, medications, and extreme physical activity may also cause muscle breakdown and enzyme elevations. AST, ALT, and aldolase are also elevated secondary to liver disease, and a γ-glutamyltransferase (GGT) measurement may help differentiate whether the source is muscle or liver.

The use of an antinuclear antibody (ANA) measurement as a screening test is *not* recommended because it has low specificity. A positive ANA test result may be induced by infection, especially EBV infection, endocarditis, and parvovirus B19 infection. The ANA test result is also positive in up to 30% of normal children, and ANA level is increased in those with a first-degree relative with a known rheumatic disease. In the majority of children with a positive ANA test result without signs of a rheumatic disease on initial evaluation, autoimmune disease does not develop over time, so this finding does not necessitate referral to a pediatric rheumatologist. A positive ANA test result is found in many rheumatic diseases, including JIA, in which it serves as a predictor of the risk for inflammatory eye disease (Table 178.7). Once a positive ANA test result is discovered in a child, the need for specific autoantibody testing is directed by the presence of clinical signs and symptoms (see Table 178.3).

IMAGING STUDIES

Plain radiographs are useful in evaluation of arthralgias and arthritis, as they offer reassurance in benign pain syndromes and their findings may be abnormal in malignancies, osteomyelitis, and long-standing chronic juvenile arthritis. Radionucleotide bone scans help localize areas of abnormality in the patient with diffuse pains caused by osteomyelitis, neuroblastoma, chronic multifocal osteomyelitis, and systemic arthritis. MRI findings are abnormal in inflammatory myositis and suggest the optimal site for biopsy. *MRI is more sensitive than plain radiographs in detecting the presence of early erosive arthritis and demonstrates increased joint fluid, synovial enhancement, and sequela of trauma with internal joint derangement.* MRI is also helpful in ruling out infection or malignancy. Cardiopulmonary evaluation is suggested for diseases commonly affecting the heart and lung, including SLE, systemic scleroderma, MCTD, JDM, and sarcoid, as clinical manifestations may be subtle. This evaluation, which may include echocardiogram, pulmonary function tests, and high-resolution CT of the lungs along with consideration of bronchoalveolar lavage, is generally performed by a pediatric rheumatologist to whom the patient is referred (see Table 178.4).

Bibliography is available at Expert Consult.

Table 178.3	Autoantibody Specificity and Disease Associations		
ANTIBODY	**DISEASE**	**PREVALENCE (%)**	**SPECIFICITY**
Antinuclear antibody (ANA)	SLE, juvenile rheumatoid arthritis, dermatomyositis, scleroderma, psoriatic arthritis, MCTD	—	Associated with increased risk of uveitis in JIA and psoriatic arthritis Up to 30% of children testing positive for ANAs have no underlying rheumatic disease
Double-stranded DNA (dsDNA)	SLE	60-70	High specificity for SLE; associated with lupus nephritis
Smith (Sm)	SLE	20-30	Highly specific for SLE; associated with lupus nephritis
Smooth muscle (Sm)	Autoimmune hepatitis	—	—
Pm-Scl (polymyositis-scleroderma)	Sclerodermatomyositis	—	—
SSA (Ro)	SLE, Sjögren syndrome	25-30	Associated with neonatal lupus syndrome, subacute cutaneous lupus, thrombocytopenia
SSB (La)	SLE, Sjögren syndrome	25-30	Usually coexists with anti-SSA antibody
Ribonuclease protein (RNP)	MCTD, SLE	30-40	Suggestive of MCTD unless meets criteria for SLE
Histone	Drug-induced lupus, SLE	—	—
Centromere	Limited cutaneous systemic sclerosis	70	Nonspecific for systemic sclerosis
Topoisomerase I (Scl-70)	Systemic sclerosis	—	Rare in childhood
Antineutrophil cytoplasmic antibodies (ANCAs)	Vasculitis	—	—
Cytoplasmic (cANCAs)/PR3-ANCA		—	cANCAs associated with granulomatosis with polyangiitis (Wegener), cystic fibrosis
Perinuclear (pANCAs)/MPO-ANCA		—	pANCAs associated with microscopic polyangiitis, polyarteritis nodosa, SLE, inflammatory bowel disease, cystic fibrosis, primary sclerosing cholangitis, Henoch-Schönlein purpura, Kawasaki disease, Churg-Strauss syndrome
Anticitrullinated protein (ACPA); also called anti–cyclic citrullinated protein (anti-CCP)	RF-positive JIA	50-90	Specific for JIA (RF+), may be positive before RF

MCTD, Mixed connective tissue disease; MPO-ANCA, antimyeloperoxidase; PR3-ANCA, antiproteinase 3; RF, rheumatoid factor; SLE, systemic lupus erythematosus.
Adapted from Aggerwal A: Clinical application of tests used in rheumatology, *Indian J Pediatr* 69:889–892, 2002.

Table 178.4	Evaluation Based on Suspected Diagnosis of Rheumatic Disease		
SUSPECTED RHEUMATIC DISEASE(S)	**INITIAL EVALUATION**	**FURTHER EVALUATION**	**SUBSPECIALTY EVALUATION**
Systemic lupus erythematosus (SLE) Mixed connective tissue disease (MCTD)	CBC, ESR, ANA, ALT, AST, CPK, creatinine, albumin, total protein, urinalysis, BP, thyroid profile	If ANA test result is positive: anti-SSA (Ro), anti-SSB (La), anti-Smith, and anti-RNP Abs; anti-dsDNA Ab, C3, C4, Coombs, spot urine protein/creatinine ratio, CXR	Antiphospholipid Abs, lupus anticoagulant, anti-β$_2$-glycoprotein, echocardiogram; consider renal biopsy, PFTs, bronchoscopy with lavage, HRCT of chest; consider lung biopsy
Juvenile dermatomyositis (JDM)	CBC, CPK, ALT, AST, LDH, aldolase, ANA; check gag reflex	Consider MRI of muscle	Consider electromyography and possible muscle biopsy, PFTs, swallowing study, serum neopterin
Juvenile idiopathic arthritis (JIA)	CBC, ESR, creatinine, ALT, AST, consider anti–streptolysin O/anti–DNAase B for streptococcus-induced arthritis, Epstein-Barr virus titers, Lyme titer, parvovirus B19 titer, plain radiograph of joints	Consider Ab titers to unusual infectious agents, purified protein derivative, RF, ANA, HLA-B27, anti-CCP	MRI
Granulomatosis with polyangiitis (Wegener granulomatosis)	CBC, ANCA, AST, ALT, albumin, creatinine, ESR, urinalysis, CXR, BP	Spot urine protein/creatinine ratio, anti–myeloperoxidase and anti–proteinase-3 Abs, PFTs	Bronchoscopy with lavage, HRCT chest; consider lung and kidney biopsies
Sarcoidosis	CBC, electrolytes, AST, ALT, albumin, creatinine, calcium, phosphorous, ACE, BP	CXR, PFTs	Consider testing for Blau syndrome in infants (see Chapter 184); HRCT of chest; consider renal and lung biopsy

Continued

Table 178.4	Evaluation Based on Suspected Diagnosis of Rheumatic Disease—cont'd		
SUSPECTED RHEUMATIC DISEASE(S)	**INITIAL EVALUATION**	**FURTHER EVALUATION**	**SUBSPECIALTY EVALUATION**
Localized scleroderma	Skin biopsy, CBC, ESR		Serum IgG, ANA, RF, single-stranded DNA Ab, antihistone Ab, CPK
Systemic scleroderma	ANA, CBC, ESR, BP, AST, ALT, CPK, creatinine, CXR	Anti-Scl70, PFTs	HRCT of chest, echocardiogram, upper GI radiography series

Ab, Antibody; ACE, angiotensin-converting enzyme (normally elevated in childhood; interpret with caution); ALT, alanine transaminase; ANA, antinuclear antibody; anti-dsDNA Ab, anti–double-stranded DNA antibody; AST, aspartate transaminase; BP, blood pressure; CBCD, complete blood count with differential; CCP, cyclic citrullinated protein; CPK, creatine phosphokinase; CXR, chest radiograph; ESR, erythrocyte sedimentation rate; GI, gastrointestinal; HRCT, high-resolution CT; LDH, lactate dehydrogenase; PFTs, pulmonary function tests; RF, rheumatoid factor; RNP, ribonucleoprotein.

Table 178.5	Comparison of Erythrocyte Sedimentation Rate and C-Reactive Protein	
	ERYTHROCYTE SEDIMENTATION RATE	**C-REACTIVE PROTEIN**
Advantages	Much clinical information in the literature May reflect overall health status	Rapid response to inflammatory stimuli Wide range of clinically relevant values are detectable Unaffected by age and gender Reflects value of a single acute-phase protein Can be measured on stored sera Quantitation is precise and reproducible
Disadvantages	Affected by red blood cell morphology Affected by anemia and polycythemia Reflects levels of many plasma proteins, not all of which are acute-phase proteins Responds slowly to inflammatory stimuli Requires fresh sample May be affected by drugs (IVIG)	Not sensitive to changes in SLE disease activity

IVIG, Intravenous immune globulin; SLE, systemic lupus erythematosus.
From Firestein GS, Budd RC, Gabriel SE, et al, editors: *Kelley & Firestein's textbook of rheumatology*, ed 10, Philadelphia, 2017, Elsevier (Table 57.3, p 849).

Table 178.6	Conditions Associated With Elevated C-Reactive Protein Levels

NORMAL OR MINOR ELEVATION (<1 mg/dL)
1. Vigorous exercise
2. Common cold
3. Pregnancy
4. Gingivitis
5. Seizures
6. Depression
7. Insulin resistance and diabetes
8. Several genetic polymorphisms
9. Obesity

MODERATE ELEVATION (1-10 mg/dL)
1. Myocardial infarction
2. Malignancies
3. Pancreatitis
4. Mucosal infection (bronchitis, cystitis)
5. Most systemic autoimmune diseases
6. Rheumatoid arthritis

MARKED ELEVATION (>10 mg/dL)
1. Acute bacterial infection (80–85%)
2. Major trauma, surgery
3. Systemic vasculitis

From Firestein GS, Budd RC, Gabriel SE, et al, editors: *Kelley & Firestein's textbook of rheumatology*, ed 10, Philadelphia, 2017, Elsevier (Table 57-4, p 849).

Table 178.7	Other Nonrheumatic Conditions With Elevated Acute Phase Responses

NEUROENDOCRINE CHANGES
Fever, somnolence, and anorexia
Increased secretion of corticotropin-releasing hormone, corticotropin, and cortisol
Increased secretion of arginine vasopressin
Decreased production of insulin-like growth factor I
Increased adrenal secretion of catecholamines

HEMATOPOIETIC CHANGES
Anemia of chronic disease
Leukocytosis
Thrombocytosis

METABOLIC CHANGES
Loss of muscle and negative nitrogen balance
Decreased gluconeogenesis

Osteoporosis
Increased hepatic lipogenesis
Increased lipolysis in adipose tissue
Decreased lipoprotein lipase activity in muscle and adipose tissue
Cachexia

HEPATIC CHANGES
Increased metallothionein, inducible nitric oxide synthase, heme oxygenase, manganese superoxide dismutase, and tissue inhibitor of metalloproteinase 1
Decreased phosphoenolpyruvate carboxykinase activity

CHANGES IN NONPROTEIN PLASMA CONSTITUENTS
Hypozincemia, hypoferremia, and hypercupremia
Increased plasma retinol and glutathione concentrations

From Gabay C, Kushner I: Acute-phase proteins and other systemic responses to inflammation, *N Engl J Med* 340:448–454, 1999.

Chapter **179**

Treatment of Rheumatic Diseases

Jeffrey A. Dvergsten, Esi Morgan, and C. Egla Rabinovich

第一百七十九章
风湿性疾病的治疗

中文导读

　　本章主要介绍了建立多学科儿科风湿病团队以及风湿性疾病的治疗。具体描述了非甾体抗炎药、非生物改善病情抗风湿药、生物制剂、细胞毒性药物以及其他药物治疗。其中非生物改善病情抗风湿药包括甲氨蝶呤、羟氯喹、来氟米特、柳氮磺胺吡啶、吗替麦考酚酯和糖皮质激素。生物制剂包括肿瘤坏死因子-α拮抗药、T细胞活化调节剂、B细胞耗竭治疗、白细胞介素-1拮抗药、白细胞介素-6受体拮抗药以及静脉注射免疫球蛋白。细胞毒性药物包括环磷酰胺，其他药物主要包括硫唑嘌呤等。

Nonpharmacologic as well as pharmacologic interventions are often necessary to meet the desired goals of disease management. Optimal disease management requires family-centered care delivered by a multidisciplinary team of healthcare professionals providing medical, psychological, social, and school support. Rheumatologic conditions most often follow a course marked by flares and periods of remission, although some children have unremitting disease. The goals of treatment are to control disease, relieve discomfort, avoid or limit drug toxicity, prevent or reduce organ damage, and maximize the physical function and quality of life of affected children. Nonpharmacologic therapy is an important adjunct to medical management of rheumatic diseases (see Chapter 76). A key predictor of long-term outcome is early recognition and referral to a rheumatology team experienced in the specialized care of children with rheumatic diseases. Significant differences in outcome are seen 10 yr after disease onset in patients with **juvenile idiopathic arthritis (JIA)** depending on whether referral to a pediatric rheumatology center was accomplished within 6 mo of onset.

PEDIATRIC RHEUMATOLOGY TEAMS AND PRIMARY CARE PHYSICIANS

The **multidisciplinary pediatric rheumatology team** offers coordinated services for children and their families (Table 179.1). General principles of treatment include: early recognition of signs and symptoms of rheumatic disease with timely referral to rheumatology for prompt initiation of treatment; monitoring for disease complications and adverse effects of treatment; coordination of subspecialty care and rehabilitation services with communication of clinical information; and child- and family-centered chronic illness care, including self-management support, alliance with community resources, partnership with schools, resources for dealing with the financial burdens of disease, and connection with advocacy groups. Planning for transition to adult care providers needs to start in adolescence. Central to effective care is partnership with the primary care provider, who helps coordinate care, monitor compliance with treatment plans, ensure appropriate immunization, monitor for medication toxicities, and identify disease exacerbations and concomitant infections. Communication between the primary care provider and subspecialty team permits timely intervention when needed.

THERAPEUTICS

A key principle of pharmacologic management of rheumatic diseases is that early disease control, striving for induction of remission, leads to less tissue and organ damage with improved short- and long-term outcomes. Medications are chosen from broad therapeutic classes on the basis of diagnosis, disease severity, anthropometrics, and adverse effect profile. Many drug therapies used do not have U.S. Food and Drug Administration (FDA) indications for pediatric rheumatic diseases given the relative rarity of these conditions. The evidence base may be limited to case series, uncontrolled studies, or extrapolation from use in adults. The exception is JIA, for which there is a growing body of randomized controlled trial (RCT) evidence, particularly for newer therapeutics. Therapeutic agents used for treatment of childhood rheumatic diseases have various mechanisms of action, but all suppress inflammation (Table 179.2). *Both biologic and nonbiologic disease-modifying antirheumatic drugs (DMARDs) directly affect the immune system.* DMARDs should be prescribed by specialists. Live vaccines are contraindicated in patients taking immunosuppressive glucocorticoids or DMARDs. A negative test result for tuberculosis (purified protein derivative and/or QuantiFERON-TB Gold) should be verified and the patient's immunization status updated, if possible, before such treatment is initiated. Killed vaccines are not contraindicated, and annual injectable influenza vaccine is recommended.

Nonsteroidal Antiinflammatory Drugs

NSAIDs are prescribed to decrease both the pain and the acute and chronic inflammation associated with arthritis, pleuritis, pericarditis, uveitis, and cutaneous vasculitis, but they are not disease modifying. NSAID antiinflammatory effects require regular administration at adequate doses based on weight (mg/kg) or body surface area (mg/m²), for longer periods than needed for analgesia alone. The mean time to achieve antiinflammatory effect in JIA is 4-6 wk of consistent administration. NSAIDs work primarily by inhibiting the enzyme cyclooxygenase (COX), which is critical in the production of **prostaglandins**, a family of substances that promote inflammation. Two types of COX receptors have been demonstrated; **selective** COX-2 inhibitors such as *celecoxib* and *meloxicam* inhibit receptors responsible for promoting inflammation, with potential for fewer gastrointestinal (GI) adverse effects. Clinical trials in children with JIA found that celecoxib and meloxicam were similar in effectiveness and tolerability to the **nonselective** NSAID *naproxen*.

The most frequent adverse effects of NSAIDs in children are nausea, decreased appetite, and abdominal pain. Gastritis or ulceration occurs less frequently in children. Less common adverse effects (≤5% of children

Table 179.1	Multidisciplinary Treatment of Rheumatic Diseases in Childhood
Accurate diagnosis and education of family	Pediatric rheumatologist Pediatrician Nurse: • Disease-related education • Medication administration (injection teaching) • Safety monitoring Social worker: • Facilitation of school services • Resource identification (community, government, financial, advocacy groups, vocational rehabilitation)
Physical medicine and rehabilitation	Physical therapy: • Addressing deficits in joint or muscle mobility, limb length discrepancies, gait abnormalities, and weakness Occupational therapy: • Splinting to reduce joint contractures/deformities and lessen stress on joints; adaptive devices for activities of daily living
Consultant team	Ophthalmology: • Eye screening for uveitis (see Table 180.4) • Screening for medication-related ocular toxicity (hydroxychloroquine, glucocorticoids) Nephrology Orthopedics Dermatology Gastroenterology
Physical and psychosocial growth and development	Nutrition: • Addressing undernourishment from systemic illness and obesity/overnourishment from glucocorticoids School integration: • Individualized educational plan (IEP) or 504 plan Peer-group relationships Individual and family counseling
Coordination of care	Involvement of patient and family as active team members Communication among healthcare providers Involvement of school (school nurse) and community (social worker) resources

undergoing long-term NSAID therapy), include mood change, concentration difficulty that can simulate attention deficit disorder, sleepiness, irritability, headache, tinnitus, alopecia, anemia, elevated liver enzyme values, proteinuria, and hematuria. Certain agents (indomethacin) have a higher risk of toxicity than others (ibuprofen); naproxen has an intermediate risk. These NSAID-associated adverse effects reverse quickly once the medication is stopped. Additional rare NSAID-specific adverse reactions may also occur. Aseptic meningitis has been associated with ibuprofen, primarily in patients with lupus. Naproxen is more likely than other NSAIDs to cause a unique skin reaction called **pseudoporphyria**, which is characterized by small, hypopigmented depressed scars occurring in areas of minor skin trauma, such as fingernail scratches. Pseudoporphyria is more likely to occur in fair-skinned individuals and on sun-exposed areas. If pseudoporphyria develops, the inciting NSAID should be discontinued because scars can persist for years or may be permanent. NSAIDs should be used cautiously in patients with dermatomyositis or systemic vasculitis because of an increased frequency of GI ulceration with these disorders. *Salicylates have been supplanted by other NSAIDs because of the relative frequency of salicylate hepatotoxicity and the association with Reye syndrome.*

Table 179.2	Therapeutics for Childhood Rheumatic Diseases*				
CLASSIFICATION	THERAPEUTIC[†]	DOSE	INDICATION[†]	ADVERSE REACTIONS	MONITORING
Nonsteroidal antiinflammatory drugs (NSAIDs)[‡]	Etodolac[a]	PO once-daily dose: 20-30 kg: 400 mg 31-45 kg: 600 mg 46-60 kg: 800 mg >60 kg: 1,000 mg	JIA Spondyloarthropathy Pain Serositis Cutaneous vasculitis Uveitis	GI intolerance (abdominal pain, nausea), gastritis, hepatitis, tinnitus, anemia, pseudoporphyria, aseptic meningitis, headache, renal disease	CBC, LFTs, BUN/creatinine, urinalysis at baseline, then every 6-12 mo
	Ibuprofen[a]	40 mg/kg/day PO in 3 divided doses Max: 2400 mg/day			
	Naproxen[a]	15 mg/kg/day PO in 2 divided doses Max 1,000 mg/day			
	Celecoxib[a]	10-25 kg: 50 mg PO bid >25 kg: 100 mg PO bid			
	Meloxicam[a]	0.125 mg/kg PO qd Max 7.5 mg			
Disease-modifying antirheumatic drugs (DMARDs)	Methotrexate[a]	10-20 mg/m^2/wk (0.35-0.65 mg/kg/wk) PO 20-30 mg/m^2/wk (0.65-1 mg/kg/wk) SC; higher doses better absorbed by SC injection	JIA Uveitis	GI intolerance (nausea, vomiting), hepatitis, myelosuppression, mucositis, teratogenesis, lymphoma, interstitial pneumonitis	CBC, LFTs at baseline, monthly ×3, then every 8-12 wk
	Leflunomide	PO once daily: 10 to <20 kg: 10 mg 20-40 kg: 15 mg >40 kg: 20 mg	JIA	Hepatitis, hepatic necrosis, cytopenias, mucositis, teratogenesis, peripheral neuropathy	CBC, LFTs, at baseline, monthly ×6, then every 8-12 wk
	Hydroxychloroquine	5 mg/kg PO qd; do not exceed 5 mg/kg/daily Max 400 mg daily	SLE JDMS Antiphospholipid antibody syndrome	Retinal toxicity, GI intolerance, rash, skin discoloration, anemia, cytopenias, myopathy, CNS stimulation, death (overdose)	Ophthalmologic screening every 6-12 mo
	Sulfasalazine[a]	30-50 mg/kg/day in 2 divided doses Adult max 3 g/day	Spondyloarthropathy, JIA	GI intolerance, rash, hypersensitivity reactions, Stevens-Johnson syndrome, cytopenias, hepatitis, headache	CBC, LFTs, BUN/creatinine, urinalysis at baseline, every other wk ×3 mo, monthly ×3, then every 3 mo
Tumor necrosis factor (TNF)-α antagonists	Adalimumab[a]	SC once every other wk: 10 to <15 kg: 10 mg 15 to <30 kg: 20 mg ≥30 kg: 40 mg	JIA Spondyloarthropathy Psoriatic arthritis Uveitis	Injection site reaction, infection, rash, cytopenias, lupus-like syndrome, potential increased malignancy risk	TB test; anti-dsDNA, CBC
	Etanercept[a]	0.8 mg/kg SC once weekly (max 50 mg/dose) or 0.4 mg/kg SC twice weekly (max 25 mg/dose)	JIA	Injection site reactions, infections, rash, demyelinating disorders, cytopenias, potential increased malignancy risk	TB test; CBC
	Infliximab	5-10 mg/kg IV every 4-8 wk	JIA Spondyloarthropathy Uveitis Sarcoidosis	Infusion reactions, hepatitis, potential increased malignancy risk	TB test; anti-dsDNA, LFTs
Modulate T-cell activation	Abatacept[a]	IV every 2 wk ×3 doses, then monthly for ≥6 yr of age: <75 kg: 10 mg/kg 75-100 kg: 750 mg >100 kg: 1,000 mg SC once weekly: 10 to <25 kg: 50 mg ≥25 to <50 kg: 87.5 mg ≥50 kg: 125 mg	JIA	Infection, headache, potential increased malignancy risk	
Anti-CD20 (B-cell) antibody	Rituximab	575 mg/m^2, max 1,000 mg, IV on days 1 and 15	SLE	Infusion reactions, lymphopenia, reactivation hepatitis B, rash, serum sickness, arthritis, PML	CBC, BMP; consider monitoring quantitative IgG

Continued

Table 179.2 | Therapeutics for Childhood Rheumatic Diseases—cont'd

CLASSIFICATION	THERAPEUTIC[†]	DOSE	INDICATION[†]	ADVERSE REACTIONS	MONITORING
Anti-BLyS antibody	Belimumab[e]	10 mg/kg IV every 2 wk ×3 doses, then every 4 wk	SLE	Infusion reactions, infection, depression	
Interleukin (IL)-1 antagonist	Anakinra	1-2 mg/kg/daily Adult max 100 mg	Systemic JIA CAPS	Injection site reactions, infection	CBC
	Canakinumab[b]	Given SC every 8 wk (CAPS) every 4 wk (systemic JIA): 15-40 kg: 2 mg/kg (up to 3 mg/kg if needed) >40 kg: 150 mg	CAPS Systemic JIA	Injection site reaction, infection, diarrhea, nausea, vertigo, headache	
		IV: <30 kg: 10 mg/kg/dose every 4 wk ≥30 kg: 8 mg/kg/dose every 4 wk; maximum dose: 800 mg/dose SC: <30 kg: 162 mg/dose once every 3 wk ≥30 kg: 162 mg/dose once every 2 wk	Polyarticular JIA		
IL-6 antagonist	Tocilizumab[a]	≥2 yr and ≥30 kg: 8 mg/kg/dose every 2 wk ≥2 yr and ≤30 kg: 12 mg/kg/dose every 2 wk	Systemic JIA	Infusion reactions, elevated LFTs, elevated lipids, thrombocytopenia, infections	CBC, LFTs, platelet count, serum lipid profile
Intravenous immune globulin	IVIG[c]	1,000-2,000 mg/kg IV infusion For JDMS, give monthly	Kawasaki disease JDMS SLE	Infusion reaction, aseptic meningitis, renal failure	Serum creatinine, BUN, IgG level
Cytotoxic	Cyclophosphamide	0.5-1 g/m² IV (max 1.5 g) monthly for 6 mo induction, then every 2-3 mo Oral regimen: 1-2 mg/kg/daily; max 150 mg/daily	SLE Vasculitis JDMS Pulmonary hemorrhage	Nausea, vomiting, myelosuppression, mucositis, hyponatremia, alopecia, hemorrhagic cystitis, gonadal failure, teratogenesis, secondary malignancy	CBC
Immunosuppressive	Mycophenolate mofetil	Oral suspension: max 1,200 mg/m²/day PO (up to 2 g/day) divided bid Capsules: max 1,500 mg/day PO for BSA 1.25-1.5 m², 2 g/day PO for BSA >1.5 m² divided bid	SLE Uveitis	GI intolerance (diarrhea, nausea, vomiting), renal impairment, neutropenia, teratogenesis, secondary malignancy, PML	CBC, BMP
Glucocorticoids	Prednisone[a,d-f]	0.05-2 mg/kg/day PO given in 1-4 divided doses; max varies by individual (80 mg/daily) Adverse effects are dose dependent; lowest effective dose should be used	SLE JDMS Vasculitis JIA Uveitis Sarcoidosis	Cushing syndrome, osteoporosis, increased appetite, weight gain, striae, hypertension, adrenal suppression, hyperglycemia, infection, avascular necrosis	Blood glucose, potassium Blood pressure
	Methylprednisolone[a,d-g]	0.5-1.7 mg/kg/day or 5-25 mg/m²/day IM/IV in divided doses every 6-12 hr For severe manifestations: 30 mg/kg/dose (max 1 g) daily for 1-5 days	SLE JDMS Vasculitis Sarcoidosis Localized scleroderma		
	Intraarticular	Dose varies by joint and formulation	JIA	Subcutaneous atrophy, skin hypopigmentation, calcification, infection	
	Prednisolone ophthalmic suspension	1-2 drops into eye up to every hr while awake Needs monitoring by ophthalmologist	Uveitis	Ocular hypertension, glaucoma, nerve damage, cataract, infection	Ophthalmologic exam

qd, Once daily; bid, twice daily; Blys, B-lymphocyte stimulator; BMP, basic metabolic panel; BSA, body surface area; BUN, blood urea nitrogen; CAPS, cryopyrin-associated periodic syndrome; CBC, complete blood count; CNS, central nervous system; dsDNA, double-stranded DNA; GI, gastrointestinal; IM, intramuscular(ly); IV, intravenous(ly); IVIG, intravenous immune globulin; JDMS, juvenile dermatomyositis; JIA, juvenile idiopathic arthritis; LFTs, liver function tests; PML, progressive multifocal leukoencephalopathy; PO, by mouth; SC, subcutaneous(ly); SLE, systemic lupus erythematosus; TB, tuberculosis.

*Consult a clinical pharmacology reference for current dosing and monitoring guidelines, and complete list of known adverse effects.

[†]Therapeutics used in practice may not have a FDA-approved indication. Individual therapeutics annotated with FDA-approved indication as follows: a, JIA; b, CAPS; c, Kawasaki disease; d, sarcoidosis; e, SLE; f, uveitis; g, dermatomyositis.

[‡]Many more products available in this class.

The response to NSAIDs varies greatly among individual patients, but overall, 40–60% of children with JIA experience improvement in their arthritis with NSAID therapy. Patients may try several different NSAIDs for 6 wk trials before finding one that demonstrates clinical benefit. NSAIDs with longer half-lives or sustained-release formulations allow for once- or twice-daily dosing and improve compliance. Laboratory monitoring for toxicity includes a complete blood count (CBC), serum creatinine, liver function tests (LFTs), and urinalysis every 6-12 mo, although guidelines for frequency of testing are not established.

Nonbiologic Disease-Modifying Antirheumatic Drugs
Methotrexate
Methotrexate (MTX), an antimetabolite, is a cornerstone of therapy in pediatric rheumatology because of its sustained effectiveness and relative low toxicity over prolonged periods of treatment. The mechanism of action low-dose MTX in arthritis is complex but is believed to result from the inhibition of folate-dependent processes by MTX polyglutamates, primarily their effect on the enzyme 5-aminoimidazole-4-carboxamide ribonucleotide (AICAR) transformylase, leading to an increase of extracellular adenosine and consequently, cyclic adenosine monophosphate (cAMP), which inhibits the production of proinflammatory cytokines such as tumor necrosis factor (TNF)-α and interleukin (IL)-1β and their downstream effects on lymphocyte activation and proliferation.

MTX has a central role in the treatment of arthritis, especially in children with polyarticular JIA. The response to oral MTX (10 mg/m^2 once a week) is better than the response to placebo (63% vs 36%). Children who show no response to standard doses of MTX often do show response to higher doses (15 or 30 mg/m^2/wk). Subcutaneous (SC) administration of MTX is similar in absorption and pharmacokinetic properties to intramuscular (IM) injection, with less pain. MTX is typically used in treatment of juvenile dermatomyositis as a steroid-sparing agent, with efficacy in 70% of patients. It has also been used successfully at a dosage of 10-20 mg/m^2/wk in patients with systemic lupus erythematosus (SLE) to treat arthritis, serositis, and rash.

Because of the lower dose used in treating rheumatic diseases, MTX is well tolerated by children, with toxicity being milder and qualitatively different from that observed with treatment of neoplasms. Adverse effects include elevated liver enzyme values (15%), GI toxicity (13%), stomatitis (3%), headache (1–2%), and leukopenia, interstitial pneumonitis, rash, and alopecia (<1%). Hepatotoxicity observed among adults with rheumatoid arthritis (RA) treated with MTX has raised concern about similar problems in children. Analysis of liver biopsy specimens in children with JIA undergoing long-term MTX treatment has revealed occasional mild fibrosis but no evidence of even moderate liver damage. Children receiving MTX should be counseled to avoid alcohol, smoking, and pregnancy. *Folic acid* (1 mg daily) is given as an adjunct to minimize adverse effects. Lymphoproliferative disorders have been reported in adults treated with MTX, primarily in association with Epstein-Barr virus (EBV) infection. Regression of lymphoma may follow withdrawal of MTX.

Monitoring laboratory tests for MTX toxicity include CBC and LFTs at regular intervals, initially every 4 wk for the 1st 3 mo of treatment, then every 8-12 wk, with more frequent intervals after dosing adjustments or in response to abnormal values.

Hydroxychloroquine
Hydroxychloroquine sulfate is an antimalarial drug important in the treatment of SLE and dermatomyositis, particularly cutaneous manifestations of disease and to reduce lupus flares. It is not indicated to treat JIA because of lack of efficacy. The most significant potential adverse effect is retinal toxicity, which occurs rarely but results in irreversible color blindness or loss of central vision. Complete ophthalmologic examinations, including assessment of peripheral vision and color fields, are conducted at baseline and every 6-12 mo to screen for retinal toxicity. Retinal toxicity is rare (1/5,000 patients) and is associated with weight-based dosing exceeding 6.5 mg/kg/day; therefore recommended dosing is <6.5 mg/kg/day, not to exceed 400 mg/day. Other potential adverse effects include rash, skin discoloration, gastric irritation, bone marrow suppression, central nervous system (CNS) stimulation, and myositis.

Leflunomide
Leflunomide is a DMARD approved for treatment of RA that offers an alternative to MTX for treatment of JIA. MTX outperformed leflunomide for treatment of JIA in a randomized trial (at 16 wk, 89% of patients receiving MTX achieved a 30% response rate vs 68% of those receiving leflunomide), although both drugs were effective. Dosing is oral, once daily, and weight based: 10 mg for children 10 to <20 kg, 15 mg for children 20-40 kg, and 20 mg for children >40 kg. Adverse reactions include paresthesias and peripheral neuropathy, GI intolerance, elevated liver transaminases and hepatic failure, cytopenias, alopecia, and teratogenesis. Leflunomide has a long half-life, and in cases in which discontinuation of the agent is required, a drug elimination protocol with cholestyramine may be indicated. Avoidance of pregnancy is essential. Laboratory tests (e.g., CBC, LFTs) are monitored every 4 wk for the 1st 6 mo of treatment, then every 8-12 wk.

Sulfasalazine
Sulfasalazine is used to treat children with polyarticular JIA, oligoarticular JIA, and the peripheral arthritis and enthesitis associated with **juvenile ankylosing spondylitis**. In JIA, sulfasalazine, 50 mg/kg/day (adult maximum: 3,000 mg/day), achieves greater improvement in joint inflammation, global assessment parameters, and laboratory parameters than placebo. More than 30% of sulfasalazine-treated patients withdraw from the treatment because of adverse effects, primarily GI irritation and skin rashes. Sulfasalazine is associated with severe systemic hypersensitivity reactions, including Stevens-Johnson syndrome. Sulfasalazine is generally considered contraindicated in children with active systemic JIA because of increased hypersensitivity reactions. Sulfasalazine should not be used in patients with sulfa or salicylate hypersensitivity or porphyria.

Monitoring laboratory tests for sulfasalazine toxicity include CBC, LFTs, serum creatinine/blood urea nitrogen (BUN), and urinalysis, every other week for the 1st 3 mo of treatment, monthly for 3 mo, every 3 mo for 1 yr, then every 6 mo.

Mycophenolate Mofetil
Mycophenolate mofetil (MMF) is an immunosuppressive drug approved by the FDA for organ transplant rejection. In rheumatology, MMF is used primarily for treatment of lupus, uveitis, and autoimmune skin manifestations. In adult clinical trials, MMF was noninferior to cyclophosphamide for induction therapy of lupus nephritis, with a potential for less adverse effects (infection, gonadal toxicity). Dosing is based on body surface area (BSA): 600 mg/m^2 orally twice daily, with maximum dosage limits varying by formulation and BSA. The most common adverse reaction is GI intolerance; infections, cytopenias, and secondary malignancies are also reported.

Glucocorticoids
Glucocorticoids are given through oral, intravenous (IV), ocular, topical, and intraarticular administration as part of treatment of rheumatic disease. **Oral** corticosteroids are foundational treatment for moderate to severe lupus, dermatomyositis, and most forms of vasculitis; their long-term use is associated with many well-described, dose-dependent complications, including linear growth suppression, Cushingoid features, osteoporosis, avascular necrosis, hypertension, impaired glucose tolerance, mood disturbance, and increased infection risk. Glucocorticoids should be tapered to the lowest effective dose over time and DMARDs introduced as steroid-sparing agents.

Intravenous corticosteroids have been used to treat severe, acute manifestations of systemic rheumatic diseases such as SLE, dermatomyositis, and vasculitis. The IV route allows for higher doses to obtain an immediate, profound antiinflammatory effect. *Methylprednisolone*, 10-30 mg/kg/dose up to a maximum of 1 g, given over 1 hr daily for 1-5 days, is the IV preparation of choice. Although generally associated with fewer adverse effects than oral corticosteroids, IV steroids are associated with significant and occasionally life-threatening toxicities, such as cardiac arrhythmia, acute hypertension, hypotension, hyperglycemia, shock, pancreatitis, and avascular necrosis.

Ocular corticosteroids are prescribed by ophthalmologists as ophthalmologic drops or injections into the soft tissue surrounding the globe (sub–Tenon capsule injection) for active **uveitis**. Long-term ocular corticosteroid use leads to cataract formation and glaucoma. Current ophthalmologic management has significantly decreased the frequency of blindness as a complication of JIA-associated uveitis.

Intraarticular corticosteroids are being used with increasing frequency as initial therapy for children with oligoarticular JIA or as bridge therapy while awaiting efficacy of a DMARD in polyarticular disease. Most patients have significant clinical improvement within 3 days. Duration of response depends on steroid preparation used, joint affected, and arthritis subtype; the anticipated response rate to knee injection is 60–80% at 6 mo. Intraarticular administration may result in subcutaneous atrophy and hypopigmentation of the skin at the injection site, as well as subcutaneous calcifications along the needle track.

Biologic Agents

Biologic agents are proteins that have been engineered to target and modulate specific components of the immune system, with the goal of decreasing the inflammatory response. Antibodies have been developed to target specific cytokines such as IL-1 and IL-6 or to interfere with specific immune cell function through depletion of B cells or suppression of T-cell activation (Table 179.3). The availability of biologic agents has dramatically increased the therapeutic options for treating rheumatic disease recalcitrant to nonbiologic therapies, and in some cases biologics are becoming first-line interventions. A primary concern is the increased risk of malignancy when biologics are combined with other immunosuppressants.

Tumor Necrosis Factor-α Antagonists

Two TNF antagonists have an FDA indication for treatment of children with moderate to severe polyarticular JIA (etanercept and adalimumab). *Etanercept* is a genetically engineered fusion protein consisting of 2 identical chains of the recombinant extracellular TNF receptor monomer fused with the Fc domain of human immunoglobulin G_1. Etanercept binds both TNF-α and lymphotoxin-α (formerly called TNF-β) and inhibits their activity. Three fourths of children with active polyarticular JIA that fails to respond to MTX demonstrate response to etanercept after 3 mo of therapy. Dosing is 0.8 mg/kg subcutaneously weekly (max 50 mg/dose) or 0.4 mg/kg SC twice weekly (max 25 mg/dose). *Adalimumab* is a fully human anti-TNF monoclonal antibody (mAb) used alone or in combination with MTX. In a placebo-controlled withdrawal-design study, children continuing to receive adalimumab were less likely to experience disease flares (43% vs. 71%) even if they were also taking MTX (37% vs 65%). Adalimumab is administered subcutaneously every other week at a dose of 10 mg for children weighing 10 to <15 kg, 20 mg for children weighing 15 to <30 kg and 40 mg for those weighing ≥30 kg.

Infliximab, a chimeric mouse-human mAb, was tested in an RCT for use in JIA but did not achieve study end-points. However, it is FDA approved for pediatric inflammatory bowel disease and has been used "off label" for treatment of polyarticular JIA, uveitis, Behçet syndrome, and sarcoidosis. Two additional anti-TNF agents—*golimumab,* a human mAb against TNF, and *certolizumab pegol,* a pegylated humanized antibody against TNF—have been approved by the FDA for RA in adults and are currently in pediatric trials.

The most common adverse effects are injection site reactions that diminish over time. TNF blockade is associated with an increased frequency of serious systemic infections, including sepsis, dissemination of latent tuberculosis (TB), and invasive fungal infections in endemic areas. TNF blockade should not be initiated in patients with a history of chronic or frequent recurrent infections. TB testing should be done before initiation of therapy with TNF antagonists. If test results are positive, antitubercular treatment must be administered before anti-TNF treatment can be started. Theoretically, risk of malignancy increases with TNF-α antagonists. Case reports describe the development of lupus-like syndromes, leukocytoclastic vasculitis, interstitial lung disease, demyelinating syndromes, antibody formation to the drug, rashes, cytopenias, anaphylaxis, serum sickness, and other reactions. The benefit/risk profile appears favorable after a decade of experience with this therapeutic class; the safety of longer-term suppression of TNF function is unknown.

Modulator of T-Cell Activation

Abatacept is a selective inhibitor of T-cell co-stimulation resulting in T-cell anergy. It is FDA approved for treatment of moderate to severe polyarticular JIA. In a double-blind withdrawal RCT in children whose disease had not responded to DMARDs, 53% of placebo-treated patients vs 20% of abatacept-treated patients experienced disease flares during the withdrawal period. The frequency of adverse events did not differ between the groups. Abatacept is administered IV every other week for 3 doses (<75 kg: 10 mg/kg/dose; 75-100 kg: 750 mg/dose; >100 kg: 1,000 mg/dose; maximum 1,000 mg/dose at 0, 2, and 4 wk) and then monthly thereafter. Abatacept administered by SC injection was given FDA approval in March 2017 for children ≥4 yr old for treatment of polyarticular JIA, at doses given weekly: 50 mg for 10-25 kg, 87.5 mg for ≥25 to <50 kg, and 125 mg for ≥50 kg.

B-Cell Depletion

Rituximab is a chimeric mAb to the antigen CD20, a transmembrane protein on the surface of B-cell precursors and mature B lymphocytes. This antibody induces B-cell apoptosis and causes depletion of circulating and tissue-based B cells. Antibody production is not completely abrogated because plasma cells are not removed. Rituximab is licensed for treatment of B-cell non-Hodgkin lymphoma and is FDA approved for use in adult RA and idiopathic thrombocytopenic purpura but does not have a pediatric indication. Rituximab may also have a role in treatment of SLE, particularly its hematologic manifestations. Adverse events include serious infusion reactions, cytopenias, hepatitis B virus reactivation, hypogammaglobulinemia, infections, serum sickness, vasculitis, and a rare but fatal side effect, **progressive multifocal leukoencephalopathy**. Resistance to rituximab may develop over time in patients being treated for lymphoma.

Belimumab is a human mAb to B-lymphocyte stimulator that negatively affects B-cell proliferation, differentiation, and long-term survival. It is approved for treatment of SLE in adults, and studies of long-term safety and efficacy are ongoing. Belimumab is *not* FDA approved for use in pediatric SLE.

Interleukin-1 Antagonists

Anakinra, a recombinant form of the human IL-1 receptor antagonist, competitively inhibits binding of IL-1α and IL-1β to the natural receptor,

Table 179.3	Method of Action of Biologic Therapies Studied in Juvenile Idiopathic Arthritis
DRUG	**METHOD OF ACTION**
Etanercept	Soluble TNF p75 receptor fusion protein that binds to and inactivates TNF-α
Infliximab	Chimeric human/mouse monoclonal antibody that binds to soluble TNF-α and its membrane-bound precursor, neutralizing its action
Adalimumab	A humanized IgG_1 monoclonal antibody that binds to TNF-α
Abatacept	Soluble, fully human fusion protein of the extracellular domain of (CTLA-4, linked to a modified Fc portion of the human IgG_1. It acts as a co-stimulatory signal inhibitor by binding competitively to CD80 or CD86, where it selectively inhibits T-cell activation
Tocilizumab	A humanized anti–human IL-6 receptor monoclonal antibody
Anakinra	An IL-1 receptor antagonist (IL-1RA)

CTLA, Cytotoxic T lymphocyte–associated antigen; IL, interleukin; TNF, tumor necrosis factor.

From Beresford MW, Baildam EM: New advances in the management of juvenile idiopathic arthritis. Part 2. The era of biologicals, *Arch Dis Child Educ Pract Ed* 94:151–156, 2009.

interrupting the cytokine proinflammatory cascade. Anakinra has been approved for RA in adults. In meta-analyses of treatments for RA, anakinra was outperformed by TNF-α antagonists but has a special niche in pediatric rheumatology for treatment of **systemic JIA (sJIA)** and other autoinflammatory syndromes, such as **cryopyrin-associated periodic syndrome (CAPS)**. The medication is dosed SC, 1-2 mg/kg, once daily. An IL-1β mAb, *canakinumab,* is FDA approved for use in CAPS, dosed SC every 8 wk, and sJIA, dosed SC every 4 wk. Adverse reactions include significant injection site reactions and increased bacterial infections.

Interleukin-6 Receptor Antagonist

Tocilizumab is an anti–IL-6 receptor antibody binding to both soluble as well as membrane-associated receptors. Tocilizumab has FDA approval for treatment of sJIA and polyarticular JIA. Adverse reactions include transaminase and lipid elevations. Tocilizumab is given as an IV infusion every 2 wk (sJIA) to 4 wk (polyarticular JIA), and SC for polyarticular JIA 162 mg every 3 wk for those <30 kg and every 2 wk for ≥30 kg.

Intravenous Immune Globulin

IVIG is thought to be beneficial in various clinical conditions. IVIG significantly improves the short- and long-term natural history of **Kawasaki disease**. Open studies have supported benefit for juvenile dermatomyositis, lupus-associated thrombocytopenia, and polyarticular JIA. IVIG is given as 1-2 g/kg/dose, administered once monthly. It has been occasionally associated with severe, systemic allergy–like reactions and postinfusion aseptic meningitis (headache, stiff neck).

Cytotoxics
Cyclophosphamide

Cyclophosphamide requires metabolic conversion in the liver to its active metabolites, which alkylate the guanine in DNA, leading to immunosuppression by inhibition of the S2 phase of mitosis. The subsequent decrease in numbers of T and B lymphocytes results in

diminished humoral and cellular immune responses. Cyclophosphamide infusions (500-1,000 mg/m^2) given monthly for 6 mo, then every 3 mo for 12-18 mo, have been shown to reduce the frequency of renal failure in patients with lupus and diffuse proliferative glomerulonephritis. Open trials suggest efficacy in severe CNS lupus. Oral cyclophosphamide (1-2 mg/kg/day) is effective as induction treatment of severe antineutrophilic cytoplasmic antibody (ANCA)–associated vasculitis and other forms of systemic vasculitis, as well as interstitial lung disease or pulmonary hemorrhage associated with rheumatic disease.

Cyclophosphamide is a potent cytotoxic drug associated with significant toxicities. Potential short-term adverse effects include nausea, vomiting, anorexia, alopecia, mucositis, hemorrhagic cystitis, and bone marrow suppression. Long-term complications include an increased risk for sterility and cancer, especially leukemia, lymphoma, and bladder cancer. In adult women with lupus treated with IV cyclophosphamide, 30–40% become infertile; the risk of ovarian failure appears to be significantly lower in adolescent and premenarchal girls. Ovarian suppression with an inhibitor of gonadotropin-releasing hormone to preserve fertility is currently being studied.

Other Drugs

Azathioprine is sometimes used to treat ANCA-associated vasculitis following induction therapy or to treat SLE. *Cyclosporine* has been used occasionally in the treatment of dermatomyositis on the basis of uncontrolled studies and is helpful in the treatment of macrophage activation syndrome complicating sJIA (see Chapter 155). Case reports describe the successful use of *thalidomide*, or its analog *lenalidomide,* as treatment for sJIA, inflammatory skin disorders, and Behçet disease.

Several drugs commonly used in the past to treat arthritis are no longer part of standard treatment, including salicylates, gold compounds, and D-penicillamine.

Bibliography is available at Expert Consult.

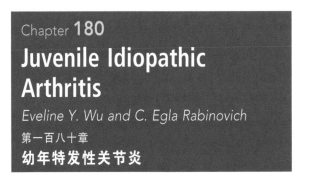

Chapter **180**
Juvenile Idiopathic Arthritis
Eveline Y. Wu and C. Egla Rabinovich

第一百八十章
幼年特发性关节炎

中文导读

　　本章主要介绍了幼年特发性关节炎的流行病学、病因、发病机制、临床表现、诊断、鉴别诊断、实验室检查、治疗以及预后。流行病学中描述了本病不同亚型、年龄、性别的患病差异；病因中描述了免疫遗传易感性和外部触发因素；临床表现中描述了七种亚型及其对应的临床表现；诊断中明确幼年特发性关节炎为临床诊断；鉴别诊断中阐述了与其他导致关节炎和四肢疼痛的疾病鉴别诊断、鉴别要点；治疗中详细讲述了幼年特发性关节炎的治疗目标以及针对不同亚型关节炎的预后及影响预后的因素等。
型的药物治疗、剂量和副作用；预后中描述了不同亚

Juvenile idiopathic arthritis (JIA) is the most common rheumatic disease in children and one of the more common chronic illnesses of childhood. JIA represents a heterogeneous group of disorders sharing the clinical manifestation of arthritis. The etiology and pathogenesis of JIA are largely unknown, and the genetic component is complex, making clear distinction among various subtypes difficult. As a result, several classification schemes exist, each with its own limitations. The former classification of the **American College of Rheumatology (ACR)** uses the term *juvenile rheumatoid arthritis* and categorizes the disease into 3 onset types (Table 180.1). Attempting to standardize nomenclature, the **International League of Associations for Rheumatology (ILAR)** proposed a different classification using the term *juvenile idiopathic arthritis* (Table 180.2), inclusive of all subtypes of chronic juvenile arthritis. We refer to the ILAR classification criteria; see Chapter 181 for enthesitis-related arthritis (ERA) and psoriatic JIA (Tables 180.3 and 180.4).

EPIDEMIOLOGY

The worldwide incidence of JIA ranges from 0.8-22.6 per 100,000 children per year, with prevalence ranges from 7-401 per 100,000. These wide-ranging numbers reflect population differences, particularly environmental exposure and immunogenetic susceptibility, along with variations in diagnostic criteria, difficulty in case ascertainment, and lack of population-based data. An estimated 300,000 U.S. children have arthritis, including 100,000 with a form of JIA. **Oligoarthritis** is the most common subtype (40–50%), followed by **polyarthritis** (25–30%) and **systemic JIA** (5–15%) (see Table 180.4). There is no sex predominance in systemic JIA (**sJIA**), but more girls than boys are affected in both oligoarticular (3 : 1) and polyarticular (5 : 1) JIA. The peak age at onset is 2-4 yr for oligoarticular disease. Age of onset has a bimodal distribution in polyarthritis, with peaks at 2-4 yr and 10-14 yr. sJIA occurs throughout childhood, with a peak at 1-5 yr.

ETIOLOGY

The etiology and pathogenesis of JIA are not completely understood, although both immunogenetic susceptibility and an external trigger are considered necessary. Twin and family studies suggest a substantial role for **genetic** factors. JIA is a complex genetic trait in which multiple genes may affect disease susceptibility. Variants in major histocompatibility complex (MHC) class I and class II regions have indisputably been associated with different JIA subtypes. Non-HLA candidate loci are also associated with JIA, including polymorphisms in the genes encoding protein tyrosine phosphatase nonreceptor 22 (PTPN22), tumor necrosis factor (TNF)-α, macrophage inhibitory factor, interleukin (IL)-6 and its receptor, and IL-1α. Possible **nongenetic** triggers include bacterial and viral infections, enhanced immune responses to bacterial or mycobacterial heat shock proteins, abnormal reproductive hormone levels, and joint trauma.

PATHOGENESIS

JIA is an autoimmune disease associated with alterations in both humoral and cell-mediated immunity. T lymphocytes have a central role, releasing proinflammatory cytokines favoring a type 1 helper T lymphocyte response. Studies of T-cell receptor expression confirm recruitment of T lymphocytes specific for synovial non–self-antigens. B-cell activation, immune complex formation, and complement activation also promote inflammation. Inheritance of specific cytokine alleles may predispose to upregulation of inflammatory networks, resulting in systemic disease or more severe articular disease.

Systemic JIA is characterized by dysregulation of the innate immune system with a lack of autoreactive T cells and autoantibodies. It therefore may be more accurately classified as an **autoinflammatory disorder**, more like familial Mediterranean fever, than the other subtypes of JIA. This theory is also supported by work demonstrating similar expression patterns of a phagocytic protein (S100A12) in sJIA and familial Mediterranean fever, as well as the same marked responsiveness to IL-1 inhibitors.

All these immunologic abnormalities cause inflammatory synovitis, characterized pathologically by villous hypertrophy and hyperplasia with hyperemia and edema of the synovial tissue. Vascular endothelial hyperplasia is prominent and is characterized by infiltration of mononuclear and plasma cells with a predominance of T lymphocytes (Fig. 180.1). Advanced and uncontrolled disease leads to pannus formation and progressive erosion of articular cartilage and contiguous bone (Figs. 180.2 and 180.3).

CLINICAL MANIFESTATIONS

Arthritis must be present ≥6 wk to make a diagnosis of any JIA subtype. Arthritis is defined by intraarticular swelling or the presence of ≥2 of the following signs: limitation in range of motion (ROM), tenderness or pain on motion, and warmth. Initial symptoms may be subtle or acute and often include morning stiffness with a limp or gelling after inactivity. Easy fatigability and poor sleep quality may be present. Involved joints are often swollen, warm to touch, and uncomfortable on movement or palpation with reduced ROM, but usually are not erythematous. Arthritis in large joints, especially knees, initially accelerates linear growth and causes the affected limb to be longer, resulting in a discrepancy in limb lengths. Continued inflammation stimulates rapid and premature closure of the growth plate, resulting in shortened bones.

Oligoarthritis is defined as involving ≤4 joints within the 1st 6 mo of disease onset, and often only a single joint is involved (see Table 180.4). It predominantly affects the large joints of the lower extremities, such as the knees and ankles (Fig. 180.4). Isolated involvement of upper-extremity large joints is less common. Those in whom disease never develops in >4 joints are regarded as having **persistent oligoarticular JIA**, whereas evolution of disease in >4 joints after 6 mo changes the classification to **extended oligoarticular JIA** and is associated with a worse prognosis. Isolated involvement of the hip is *almost never* a presenting sign and suggests ERA (see Chapter 181) or a nonrheumatic cause. The presence of a positive antinuclear antibody (ANA) test confers increased risk for asymptomatic anterior uveitis, requiring periodic

Table 180.1	Criteria for the Classification of Juvenile Rheumatoid Arthritis

Age at onset: <16 yr
Arthritis (swelling or effusion, or the presence of ≥2 of the following signs: limitation of range of motion, tenderness or pain on motion, increased heat) in ≥1 joint
Duration of disease: ≥6 wk
Onset type defined by type of articular involvement in the 1st 6 mo after onset:
    Polyarthritis: ≥5 inflamed joints
    Oligoarthritis: ≤4 inflamed joints
    Systemic-onset disease: arthritis with rash and a characteristic quotidian fever
Exclusion of other forms of juvenile arthritis

Adapted from Cassidy JT, Levison JE, Bass JC, et al: A study of classification criteria for a diagnosis of juvenile rheumatoid arthritis, *Arthritis Rheum* 29:174–181, 1986.

Table 180.2	International League of Associations for Rheumatology Classification of Juvenile Idiopathic Arthritis (JIA)	
CATEGORY	**DEFINITION**	**EXCLUSIONS**
Systemic JIA	Arthritis in ≥1 joint with, or preceded by, fever of at least 2 wk in duration that is documented to be daily (quotidian*) for at least 3 days and accompanied by ≥1 of the following: 1. Evanescent (nonfixed) erythematous rash 2. Generalized lymph node enlargement 3. Hepatomegaly or splenomegaly or both 4. Serositis†	a. Psoriasis or a history of psoriasis in patient or first-degree relative b. Arthritis in an HLA-B27–positive boy beginning after 6th birthday c. Ankylosing spondylitis, enthesitis-related arthritis, sacroiliitis with IBD, Reiter syndrome, or acute anterior uveitis, or history of 1 of these disorders in first-degree relative d. Presence of IgM RF on at least 2 occasions at least 3 mo apart
Oligoarthritis	Arthritis affecting 1-4 joints during 1st 6 mo of disease; 2 subcategories are recognized: 1. Persistent oligoarthritis—affecting ≤4 joints throughout the disease course 2. Extended oligoarthritis—affecting >4 joints after 1st 6 mo of disease	a, b, c, d (above) *plus* e. Presence of systemic JIA in the patient
Polyarthritis (RF negative)	Arthritis affecting ≥5 joints during 1st 6 mo of disease; a test for RF is negative	a, b, c, d, e
Polyarthritis (RF positive)	Arthritis affecting ≥5 joints during 1st 6 mo of disease; ≥2 tests for RF at least 3 mo apart during 1st 6 mo of disease are positive	a, b, c, e
Psoriatic arthritis	Arthritis and psoriasis, or arthritis and at least 2 of the following: 1. Dactylitis‡ 2. Nail pitting§ and onycholysis 3. Psoriasis in first-degree relative	b, c, d, e
Enthesitis-related arthritis	Arthritis and enthesitis,‖ or arthritis or enthesitis with at least 2 of the following: 1. Presence of or history of sacroiliac joint tenderness or inflammatory lumbosacral pain, or both¶ 2. Presence of HLA-B27 antigen 3. Onset of arthritis in a male >6 yr old 4. Acute (symptomatic) anterior uveitis 5. History of ankylosing spondylitis, enthesitis-related arthritis, sacroiliitis with IBD, Reiter syndrome, or acute anterior uveitis in first-degree relative	a, d, e
Undifferentiated arthritis	Arthritis that fulfills criteria in no category or in ≥2 of the above categories.	

*Quotidian fever is defined as a fever that rises to 39°C (102.2°F) once daily and returns to 37°C (98.6°F) between fever peaks.
†Serositis refers to pericarditis, pleuritis, or peritonitis, or some combination of the 3.
‡Dactylitis is swelling of ≥1 digit(s), usually in an asymmetric distribution, that extends beyond the joint margin.
§A minimum of 2 pits on any 1 or more nails at any time.
‖Enthesitis is defined as tenderness at the insertion of a tendon, ligament, joint capsule, or fascia to bone.
¶Inflammatory lumbosacral pain refers to lumbosacral pain at rest with morning stiffness that improves on movement.
IBD, Inflammatory bowel disease; RF, rheumatoid factor.
From Firestein GS, Budd RC, Harris ED Jr, et al, editors: *Kelley's textbook of rheumatology*, ed 8, Philadelphia, 2009, Saunders.

Table 180.3	Characteristics of ACR and ILAR Classifications of Childhood Chronic Arthritis	
PARAMETER	**ACR (1977)**	**ILAR (1997)**
Term	Juvenile rheumatoid arthritis (JRA)	Juvenile idiopathic arthritis (JIA)
Minimum duration	≥6 wk	≥6 wk
Age at onset	<16 yr	<16 yr
≤4 joints in 1st 6 mo after presentation	Pauciarticular	Oligoarthritis: Persistent: <4 joints for course of disease Extended: >4 joints after 6 mo
>4 joints in 1st 6 mo after presentation	Polyarticular	Polyarthritis, RF negative Polyarthritis, RF positive
Fever, rash, arthritis	Systemic onset	Systemic
Other categories included	Exclusion of other forms	Psoriatic arthritis Enthesitis-related arthritis Undifferentiated: Fits no other category Fits >1 category
Inclusion of psoriatic arthritis, inflammatory bowel disease, ankylosing spondylitis	No (see Chapter 181)	Yes

ACR, American College of Rheumatology; ILAR, International League of Associations for Rheumatology; RF, rheumatoid factor.

| Table 180.4 | Overview of Main Features of Subtypes of Juvenile Idiopathic Arthritis (JIA) |

ILAR SUBTYPE	PEAK AGE at ONSET (yr)	FEMALE:MALE RATIO	% of ALL JIA CASES	ARTHRITIS PATTERN	EXTRAARTICULAR FEATURES	LABORATORY INVESTIGATIONS	NOTES ON THERAPY
Systemic arthritis	1-5	1:1	5-15	Polyarticular, often affecting knees, wrists, and ankles; also fingers, neck, and hips	Daily fever; evanescent rash; pericarditis; pleuritis	Anemia; WBC ↑↑; ESR ↑↑; CRP ↑↑; ferritin ↑; platelets ↑↑ (normal or ↓ in MAS)	Less responsive to standard treatment with MTX and anti-TNF agents; consider IL-1 or IL-6 inhibitors in resistant cases or as first-line therapy
Oligoarthritis	2-4	3:1	40-50 (but ethnic variation)	Knees ++; ankles, fingers +	Uveitis in 30% of cases	ANA positive in 60%; other test results usually normal; may have mildly ↑ ESR/CRP	NSAIDs and intraarticular corticosteroids; MTX occasionally required
Polyarthritis: RF negative	2-4 and 10-14	3:1 and 10:1	20-35	Symmetric or asymmetric; small and large joints; cervical spine; temporomandibular joint	Uveitis in 10%	ANA positive in 40%; RF negative; ESR ↑ or ↑↑; CRP ↑ or normal; mild anemia	Standard therapy with MTX and NSAIDs; then, if nonresponsive, anti-TNF agents or other biologics, including abatacept, indicated as first-line therapy
RF positive	9-12	9:1	<10	Aggressive symmetric polyarthritis	Rheumatoid nodules in 10%; low-grade fever	RF positive; ESR ↑↑; CRP ↑/normal; mild anemia	Long-term remission unlikely; early aggressive therapy is warranted
Psoriatic arthritis	2-4 and 9-11	2:1	5-10	Asymmetric arthritis of small or medium-sized joints	Uveitis in 10%; psoriasis in 50%	ANA positive in 50%; ESR ↑; CRP ↑ or normal; mild anemia	NSAIDs and intraarticular corticosteroids; MTX, anti-TNF agents
Enthesitis-related arthritis	9-12	1:7	5-10	Predominantly lower limb joints affected; sometimes axial skeleton (but less than in adult, ankylosing spondylitis)	Acute anterior uveitis; association with reactive arthritis and inflammatory bowel disease	80% of patients positive for HLA-B27	NSAIDs and intraarticular corticosteroids; consider sulfasalazine as alternative to MTX; anti-TNF agents

ILAR, International League of Associations for Rheumatology; ANA, antinuclear antibody; CRP, C-reactive protein; ESR, erythrocyte sedimentation rate; MAS, macrophage activation syndrome; MTX, methotrexate; NSAIDs, nonsteroidal antiinflammatory drugs; RF, rheumatoid factor; TNF, tumor necrosis factor; WBC, white blood cell count.
From Firestein GS, Budd RC, Harris ED Jr, et al, editors: Kelley's textbook of rheumatology, ed 8, Philadelphia, 2009, Saunders.

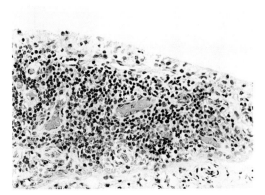

Fig. 180.1 Synovial biopsy specimen from a 10 yr old child with oligoarticular juvenile idiopathic arthritis. There is a dense infiltration of lymphocytes and plasma cells in the synovium.

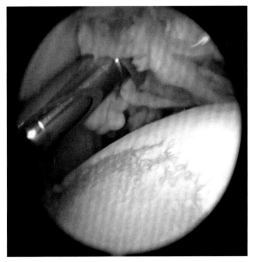

Fig. 180.2 Arthroscopy in the shoulder of a child with juvenile idiopathic arthritis showing pannus formation and cartilage erosions. *(Courtesy of Dr. Alison Toth.)*

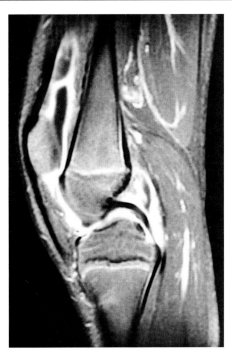

Fig. 180.3 MRI with gadolinium of a 10 yr old child with juvenile idiopathic arthritis (same patient as in Fig. 180.1). The dense white signal in the synovium near the distal femur, proximal tibia, and patella reflects inflammation. MRI of the knee is useful to exclude ligamentous injury, chondromalacia of the patella, and tumor.

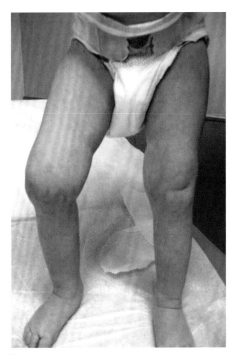

Fig. 180.4 Oligoarticular juvenile idiopathic arthritis with swelling and flexion contracture of the right knee.

slit-lamp examination (Table 180.5). ANA positivity may also be correlated with younger age at disease onset, female sex, asymmetric arthritis, and fewer involved joints over time.

Polyarthritis is characterized by inflammation of ≥5 joints in both upper and lower extremities (Figs. 180.5 and 180.6). Rheumatoid factor (RF)–positive polyarthritis resembles the characteristic symmetric presentation of adult rheumatoid arthritis. **Rheumatoid nodules** on the extensor surfaces of the elbows, spine, and over the Achilles tendons, although unusual, are associated with a more severe course and almost exclusively occur in RF-positive individuals (Fig. 180.7). **Micrognathia** reflects chronic temporomandibular joint disease (Fig. 180.8). Cervical spine involvement (Fig. 180.9), manifesting as decreased neck extension, occurs with a risk of atlantoaxial subluxation and neurologic sequelae. Hip disease may be subtle, with findings of decreased or painful ROM on examination (Fig. 180.10).

Systemic JIA is characterized by arthritis, fever, rash, and prominent visceral involvement, including hepatosplenomegaly, lymphadenopathy, and serositis (pericarditis). The characteristic fever, defined as spiking temperatures to ≥39°C (102.2°F), occurs on a daily or twice-daily basis for at least 2 wk, with a rapid return to normal or subnormal temperatures (Fig. 180.11). The fever is often present in the evening and is frequently accompanied by a characteristic faint, erythematous, macular rash. The evanescent **salmon-colored lesions,** classic for sJIA, are linear or circular and are usually distributed over the trunk and proximal extremities (Fig. 180.12). The classic rash is nonpruritic and migratory with lesions

lasting <1 hr. **Koebner phenomenon,** a cutaneous hypersensitivity in which classic lesions are brought on by superficial trauma, is often present. Heat can also evoke rash. Fever, rash, hepatosplenomegaly, and lymphadenopathy are present in >70% of affected children. Without arthritis, the **differential diagnosis** includes the episodic fever

Table 180.5	Frequency of Ophthalmologic Examination in Patients With Juvenile Idiopathic Arthritis

REFERRAL

- Patients should be referred at time of diagnosis, or suspicion, of JIA

INITIAL SCREENING EXAMINATION

- Should occur as soon as possible and no later than 6 wk from referral
- Symptomatic ocular patients should be seen within a week of referral

ONGOING SCREENING

- Screening at two monthly intervals from onset of arthritis for 6 mo
- Followed by 3-4 monthly screening for time outlined below

OLIGOARTICULAR JIA, PSORIATIC ARTHRITIS, AND ENTHESITIS-RELATED ARTHRITIS IRRESPECTIVE OF ANA STATUS, ONSET UNDER 11 YR

AGE AT ONSET (YR)	LENGTH OF SCREENING (YR)
<3	8
3-4	6
5-8	3
9-10	1

POLYARTICULAR, ANA-POSITIVE JIA, ONSET <10 YR

AGE AT ONSET (YR)	LENGTH OF SCREENING (YR)
<6	5
6-9	2

- Polyarticular, ANA-negative JIA, onset <7 yr
- 5-yr screening for all children
- Systemic JIA and rheumatoid factor–positive polyarticular JIA
  Uveitis risk very low; however, diagnostic uncertainty in the early stages and overlap of symptoms may mean initial screening is indicated
- All categories, onset >11 yr
  1-yr screening for all children
- After stopping immunosuppression (eg, methotrexate)
  Two monthly screening for 6 mo, then revert to previous screening frequency as above
- After discharge from screening
  Patients should receive advice about regular self-monitoring by checking vision uniocularly once weekly and when to seek medical advice
  Screening may need to continue indefinitely in situations where a young person may be unable to detect a change in vision or be unwilling to seek re-referral
  Annual check by optometrist as a useful adjunct

From Clarke SLN, Sen ES, Ramanan AV: Juvenile idiopathic arthritis-associated uveitis. *Pediatr Rheumatol* 14:27, 2016. p. 3.

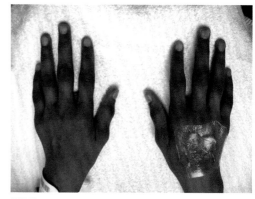

Fig. 180.5 Hands and wrists of a girl with polyarticular juvenile idiopathic arthritis, rheumatoid factor negative. Notice the symmetric involvement of the wrists, metacarpophalangeal joints, and proximal and distal interphalangeal joints. In this photograph, there is cream with occlusive dressing on the patient's right hand in preparation for placement of an intravenous line for administration of a biologic agent.

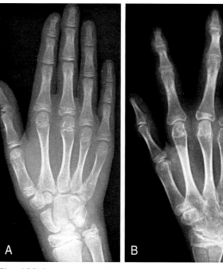

Fig. 180.6 Progression of joint destruction in a girl with polyarticular juvenile idiopathic arthritis, rheumatoid factor positive, despite doses of corticosteroids sufficient to suppress symptoms in the interval between the radiographs shown in **A** and **B. A,** Radiograph of the hand at onset. **B,** Radiograph taken 4 yr later, showing a loss of articular cartilage and destructive changes in the distal and proximal interphalangeal and metacarpophalangeal joints as well as destruction and fusion of wrist bones.

(autoinflammatory) syndromes (see Chapter 188), infection (endocarditis, rheumatic fever, brucellosis), other rheumatic disorders (SLE, vasculitis syndromes, serum sickness, Kawasaki disease, sarcoidosis, Castleman disease), inflammatory bowel disease, hemophagocytic syndromes, and malignancy. Some children initially present with only systemic features and evolve over time, but definitive diagnosis requires presence of arthritis. Arthritis may affect any number of joints, but the course is classically polyarticular, may be very destructive, and can include hip, cervical spine, and temporomandibular joint involvement.

Macrophage activation syndrome (MAS) is a rare but potentially fatal complication of sJIA that can occur at any time (onset, medication change, active or remission) during the disease course. It is also referred to as *secondary hemophagocytic syndrome* or *hemophagocytic lymphohistiocytosis* (HLH) (see Chapter 534.2). There is increasing evidence that sJIA/MAS and HLH share similar functional defects in granule-dependent cytotoxic lymphocyte activity. In addition, sJIA-associated

MAS and HLH share genetic variants in approximately 35% of patients with sJIA/MAS. MAS classically manifests as acute onset of high-spiking fevers, lymphadenopathy, hepatosplenomegaly, and encephalopathy. Laboratory evaluation shows thrombocytopenia and leukopenia with elevated liver enzymes, lactate dehydrogenase, ferritin, and triglycerides. Patients may have purpura and mucosal bleeding, as well as elevated fibrin split product values and prolonged prothrombin and partial prothromboplastin times. The erythrocyte sedimentation rate (ESR) falls because of hypofibrinogenemia and hepatic dysfunction, a feature useful in distinguishing MAS from a flare of systemic disease (Table 180.6). An international consensus panel developed a set of classification criteria for sJIA-associated MAS, including hyperferritinemia (>684 ng/mL) and any 2 of the following: thrombocytopenia (≤181 × 10^9/L), elevated liver enzymes (aspartate transaminase >48 U/L), hypertriglyceridemia (>156 mg/dL), and hypofibrinogenemia (≤360 mg/dL) (Table 180.6). These criteria apply to a febrile patient suspected of sJIA *and*

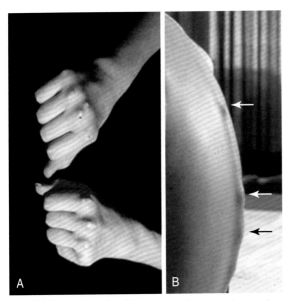

Fig. 180.7 Rheumatoid nodules overlying bony prominences in an adolescent with rheumatoid factor–positive polyarthritis. *(From Rosenberg AM, Oen KG: Polyarthritis. In Cassiday JT, Petty RE, Laxer RM, et al, editors: Textbook of pediatric rheumatology, ed 6, Philadelphia, 2011, Saunders Elsevier, Fig 15-5, p 257.)*

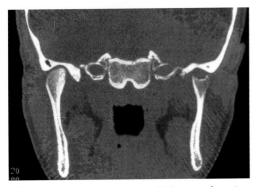

Fig. 180.8 CT scan of the temporomandibular joint of a patient with juvenile idiopathic arthritis exhibiting destruction on the right.

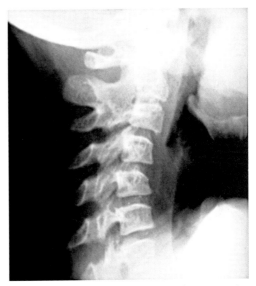

Fig. 180.9 Radiograph of the cervical spine of a patient with active juvenile idiopathic arthritis, showing fusion of the neural arch between joints C2 and C3, narrowing and erosion of the remaining neural arch joints, obliteration of the apophyseal space, and loss of the normal lordosis.

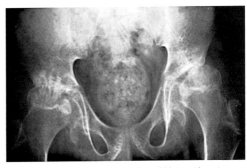

Fig. 180.10 Severe hip disease in 13 yr old boy with active systemic juvenile idiopathic arthritis. Radiograph shows destruction of the femoral head and acetabula, joint space narrowing, and subluxation of left hip. The patient had received corticosteroids systemically for 9 yr.

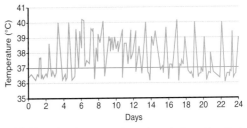

Fig. 180.11 High-spiking intermittent fever in 3 yr old patient with systemic juvenile idiopathic arthritis. *(From Ravelli A, Martini A: Juvenile idiopathic arthritis, Lancet 369:767–778, 2007.)*

in the absence of disorders such as immune-mediated thrombocytopenia, infectious hepatitis, familial hypertriglyceridemia or visceral leishmaniasis. *A relative change in laboratory values is likely more relevant in making an early diagnosis than are absolute normal values.* A bone marrow aspiration and biopsy may be helpful in diagnosis, but evidence of hemophagocytosis is not always evident. Emergency treatment with high-dose intravenous methylprednisolone, cyclosporine, or anakinra may be effective. Severe cases may require therapy similar to that for primary HLH (see Chapter 534.2).

Bone mineral metabolism and skeletal maturation are adversely affected in children with JIA, regardless of subtype. Children with JIA have decreased bone mass (osteopenia), which appears to be associated with increased disease activity. Increased levels of cytokines such as TNF-α and IL-6, both key regulators in bone metabolism, have deleterious effects on bone within the joint as well as systemically in the axial and appendicular bones. Abnormalities of skeletal maturation become most prominent during the pubertal growth spurt.

DIAGNOSIS

JIA is a clinical diagnosis without any diagnostic laboratory tests. The meticulous clinical exclusion of other diseases and many mimics is

therefore essential. Laboratory studies, including tests for ANA and RF, are only supportive or prognostic, and their results may be normal in patients with JIA (see Tables 180.1, 180.3, and 180.4).

DIFFERENTIAL DIAGNOSIS

The differential diagnosis for arthritis is broad and a careful, thorough investigation for other underlying etiology is imperative (Table 180.7). History, physical examination, laboratory tests, and radiography may

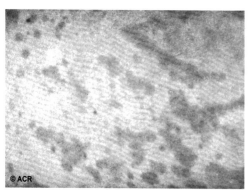

Fig. 180.12 The rash of systemic juvenile idiopathic arthritis is salmon-colored, macular, and nonpruritic. Individual lesions are transient and occur in crops over the trunk and extremities. *(Reprinted from the American College of Rheumatology: Clinical slide collection on the rheumatic diseases, Atlanta, copyright 1991, 1995, 1997, ACR. Used with permission of the American College of Rheumatology.)*

Table 180.6	Macrophage Activation Syndrome (MAS)

LABORATORY FEATURES*
1. Cytopenias
2. Abnormal liver function tests
3. Coagulopathy (hypofibrinogenemia)
4. Decreased erythrocyte sedimentation rate
5. Hypertriglyceridemia
6. Hyponatremia
7. Hypoalbuminemia
8. Hyperferritinemia
9. Elevated sCD25 and sCD163

CLINICAL FEATURES*
1. Nonremitting fever
2. Hepatomegaly
3. Splenomegaly
4. Lymphadenopathy
5. Hemorrhages
6. Central nervous system dysfunction (headache, seizures, lethargy, coma, disorientation)

HISTOPATHOLOGIC FEATURES*
1. Macrophage hemophagocytosis in the bone marrow aspirate
2. Increased CD163 staining of the bone marrow

PROPOSED CRITERIA FOR MAS IN SJIA†
- Serum ferritin >684 ng/mL *and*
- Any 2 of the following:
  - Thrombocytopenia (≤181 × 10⁹/L)
  - Elevated liver enzymes (aspartate transaminase >48 U/L)
  - Hypertriglyceridemia (>156 mg/dL)
  - Hypofibrinogenemia (≤360 mg/dL)

*From Ravelli A, Grom A, Behrens E, Cron R: Macrophage activation syndrome as part of systemic juvenile idiopathic arthritis: diagnosis, genetics, pathophysiology and treatment, *Genes Immun* 13:289–298, 2012.
†From Ravelli A, Minoia F, Davì S, et al: 2016 Classification criteria for macrophage activation syndrome complicating systemic juvenile idiopathic arthritis: a European League Against Rheumatism/American College of Rheumatology/Paediatric Rheumatology International Trials Organisation collaborative initiative, *Arthritis Rheumatol* 68:566-576, 2016.

help exclude other possible causes. Arthritis can be a presenting manifestation for any of the multisystem rheumatic diseases of childhood, including systemic lupus erythematosus (see Chapter 183), juvenile dermatomyositis (see Chapter 184), sarcoidosis (see Chapter 190), and the vasculitic syndromes (see Chapter 192). In scleroderma (see Chapter 185), limited ROM caused by sclerotic skin overlying a joint may be confused with sequelae from chronic inflammatory arthritis. **Acute**

rheumatic fever is characterized by exquisite joint pain and tenderness, remittent fever, and migratory polyarthritis. **Autoimmune hepatitis** can also be associated with an acute arthritis.

Many infections are associated with arthritis, and a recent history of infectious symptoms may help make a distinction. Viruses, including parvovirus B19, rubella, Epstein-Barr virus, hepatitis B virus, and HIV, can induce a transient arthritis. Arthritis may follow enteric infections (see Chapter 182). **Lyme disease** should be considered in children with oligoarthritis living in or visiting endemic areas (see Chapter 249). Although a history of tick exposure, preceding flulike illness, and subsequent rash should be sought, these are not always present. Monoarticular arthritis unresponsive to antiinflammatory treatment may be the result of chronic mycobacterial or other infection, such as *Kingella kingae*, and the diagnosis is established by synovial fluid analysis (PCR) or biopsy. Acute onset of fever and a painful, erythematous, hot joint suggests septic arthritis (see Chapter 705). Isolated hip pain with limited ROM suggests suppurative arthritis, osteomyelitis (see Chapter 704), toxic synovitis, Legg-Calvé-Perthes disease, slipped capital femoral epiphysis, and chondrolysis of the hip (see Chapter 698).

Lower-extremity arthritis and tenderness over insertion of ligaments and tendons, especially in a boy, suggests ERA (see Chapter 181). **Psoriatic arthritis** can manifest as limited joint involvement in an unusual distribution (e.g., small joints of hand and ankle) years before onset of cutaneous disease. **Inflammatory bowel disease** may manifest as oligoarthritis, usually affecting joints in the lower extremities, as well as gastrointestinal symptoms, elevations in ESR, and microcytic anemia.

Many conditions present solely with arthralgia (i.e., joint pain). Hypermobility may cause joint pain, especially in the lower extremities. Growing pains should be suspected in a child age 4-12 yr complaining of leg pain in the evening with normal investigative studies and no morning symptoms. Nocturnal pain that awakens the child also alerts to the possibility of a malignancy. An adolescent with missed school days may suggest a diagnosis of fibromyalgia (see Chapter 193).

Children with **leukemia** or **neuroblastoma** may have joint or bone pain resulting from malignant infiltration of the bone, synovium, or more often the bone marrow, sometimes months before demonstrating lymphoblasts on peripheral blood smear. Physical examination may reveal no tenderness, a deeper pain with palpation of the bone, or pain out of proportion to exam findings. Malignant pain often awakens the child from sleep and may cause cytopenias. Because platelets are an acute-phase reactant, a high ESR with leukopenia and a low normal platelet count may also be a clue to underlying leukemia. In addition, the characteristic quotidian fever of sJIA is absent in malignancy. Bone marrow examination is necessary for diagnosis. Some diseases, such as cystic fibrosis, diabetes mellitus, and the glycogen storage diseases, have associated arthropathies (see Chapter 194). Swelling that extends beyond the joint can be a sign of lymphedema or Henoch-Schönlein purpura (see Chapter 192.1). A peripheral arthritis indistinguishable from JIA occurs in the humoral immunodeficiencies (see Chapter 150), such as common variable immunodeficiency and X-linked agammaglobulinemia. Skeletal dysplasias associated with a degenerative arthropathy are diagnosed from their characteristic radiologic abnormalities.

Systemic onset of JIA often presents as a fever of unknown origin (see Chapter 204). Important considerations in the differential diagnosis include infections (endocarditis, brucellosis, cat scratch disease, Q fever, mononucleosis), autoinflammatory disease (see Chapter 188) malignancy (leukemia, lymphoma, neuroblastoma) and HLH (see Chapter 534.2).

LABORATORY FINDINGS

Hematologic abnormalities often reflect the degree of systemic or articular inflammation, with elevated white blood cell (WBC) and platelet counts and a microcytic anemia. Inflammation may also cause elevations in ESR and C-reactive protein, although it is not unusual for both to be normal in children with JIA.

Elevated ANA titers are present in 40–85% of children with oligoarticular or polyarticular JIA, but are rare with sJIA. ANA seropositivity is associated with increased risk of **chronic uveitis** in JIA. Approximately 5–15% of patients with polyarticular JIA are seropositive for RF. Anti–cyclic citrullinated peptide antibody, as with RF, is a marker of

Table 180.7	Conditions Causing Arthritis or Extremity Pain

RHEUMATIC AND INFLAMMATORY DISEASES
Juvenile idiopathic arthritis
Systemic lupus erythematosus
Juvenile dermatomyositis
Polyarteritis nodosa
Scleroderma
Sjögren syndrome
Behçet disease
Overlap syndromes
Antineutrophilic cytoplasmic antibody (ANCA)–associated vasculitis
Sarcoidosis
Kawasaki syndrome
Henoch-Schönlein purpura
Chronic recurrent multifocal osteomyelitis

SERONEGATIVE SPONDYLOARTHROPATHIES
Juvenile ankylosing spondylitis
Inflammatory bowel disease
Psoriatic arthritis
Reactive arthritis associated with urethritis, iridocyclitis, and mucocutaneous lesions

INFECTIOUS ILLNESSES
Bacterial arthritis (septic arthritis, *Staphylococcus aureus*, *Kingella kingae*, pneumococcal, gonococcal, *Haemophilus influenzae*)
Lyme disease
Viral illness (parvovirus, rubella, mumps, Epstein-Barr, hepatitis B, chikungunya)
Fungal arthritis
Mycobacterial infection
Spirochetal infection
Endocarditis

REACTIVE ARTHRITIS
Acute rheumatic fever
Reactive arthritis (postinfectious caused by *Shigella*, *Salmonella*, *Yersinia*, *Chlamydia*, or meningococcus)
Serum sickness
Toxic synovitis of the hip
Postimmunization

IMMUNODEFICIENCIES
Hypogammaglobulinemia
Immunoglobulin A deficiency
Common variable immunodeficiency disease (CVID)
Human immunodeficiency virus (HIV)

CONGENITAL AND METABOLIC DISORDERS
Gout
Pseudogout
Mucopolysaccharidoses
Thyroid disease (hypothyroidism, hyperthyroidism)
Hyperparathyroidism

Vitamin C deficiency (scurvy)
Hereditary connective tissue disease (Marfan syndrome, Ehlers-Danlos syndrome)
Fabry disease
Farber disease
Amyloidosis (familial Mediterranean fever)

BONE AND CARTILAGE DISORDERS
Trauma
Patellofemoral syndrome
Hypermobility syndromes
Osteochondritis dissecans
Avascular necrosis (including Legg-Calvé-Perthes disease)
Hypertrophic osteoarthropathy
Slipped capital femoral epiphysis
Osteolysis
Benign bone tumors (including osteoid osteoma)
Langerhans cell histiocytosis
Rickets

NEUROPATHIC DISORDERS
Peripheral neuropathies
Carpal tunnel syndrome
Charcot joints

NEOPLASTIC DISORDERS
Leukemia
Neuroblastoma
Lymphoma
Bone tumors (osteosarcoma, Ewing sarcoma)
Histiocytic syndromes
Synovial tumors

HEMATOLOGIC DISORDERS
Hemophilia
Hemoglobinopathies (including sickle cell disease)

MISCELLANEOUS DISORDERS
Autoinflammatory diseases
Recurrent multifocal osteomyelitis
Pigmented villonodular synovitis
Plant-thorn synovitis (foreign body arthritis)
Myositis ossificans
Eosinophilic fasciitis
Tendinitis (overuse injury)
Raynaud phenomenon
Hemophagocytic syndromes

PAIN SYNDROMES
Fibromyalgia
Growing pains
Depression (with somatization)
Complex regional pain syndrome

more aggressive disease. Both ANA and RF seropositivity can occur in association with transient events, such as viral infection.

Children with sJIA usually have striking elevations in inflammatory markers and WBC and platelet counts. Hemoglobin levels are low, typically 7-10 g/dL, with indices consistent with anemia of chronic disease. The ESR is usually high, except in MAS. Although immunoglobulin levels tend to be high, ANA and RF are uncommon. Ferritin values are typically elevated and can be markedly increased in MAS (>10,000 ng/mL). In the setting of MAS, all cell lines have the potential to decline precipitously because of the consumptive process. A low or normal WBC count and/or platelet count in a child with active sJIA should raise concerns for MAS.

Early radiographic changes of arthritis include soft tissue swelling, periarticular osteopenia, and periosteal new-bone apposition around affected joints (Fig. 180.13). Continued active disease may lead to subchondral erosions, loss of cartilage, with varying degrees of bony

destruction, and fusion. Characteristic radiographic changes in cervical spine, most frequently in the neural arch joints at C2-C3 (see Fig. 180.9), may progress to atlantoaxial subluxation. MRI is more sensitive than radiography to detect early changes (Fig. 180.14).

TREATMENT

The goals of treatment are to achieve disease remission, prevent or halt joint damage, and foster normal growth and development. All children with JIA need individualized treatment plans, and management is tailored according to disease subtype and severity, presence of poor prognostic indicators, and response to medications. Disease management also requires monitoring for potential medication toxicities (see Chapter 179).

Children with oligoarthritis often show partial response to nonsteroidal antiinflammatory drugs (NSAIDs), with improvement in inflammation and pain (Table 180.8). Those who have no or partial response after 4-6 wk of treatment with NSAIDs, or who have functional limitations such as joint contracture or leg-length discrepancy, benefit from injection of intraarticular corticosteroids. *Triamcinolone hexacetonide* is a long-lasting preparation that provides a prolonged response. A substantial fraction of patients with oligoarthritis show no response to NSAIDs and injections, and therefore require treatment with disease-modifying antirheumatic drugs (DMARDs), including methotrexate, and, if no response, TNF inhibitors.

NSAIDs alone rarely induce remission in children with polyarthritis or sJIA. *Methotrexate* is the oldest and least toxic of the DMARDs available for adjunctive therapy. It may take 6-12 wk to see the effects of methotrexate. Failure of methotrexate monotherapy warrants the

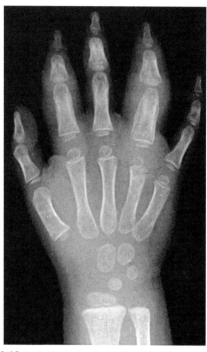

Fig. 180.13 Early (6 mo duration) radiographic changes of juvenile idiopathic arthritis. Soft-tissue swelling and periosteal new bone formation appear adjacent to the 2nd and 4th proximal interphalangeal joints.

addition of a biologic DMARD. Biologic medications that inhibit proinflammatory cytokines, such as TNF-α, IL-1, and IL-6, demonstrated excellent disease control. TNF-α antagonists (e.g., *etanercept, adalimumab*) are used to treat children with an inadequate response to methotrexate, with poor prognostic factors, or with severe disease onset. Early aggressive therapy with a combination of methotrexate and a TNF-α antagonist may result in earlier achievement of clinically inactive disease. *Abatacept,* a selective inhibitor of T-cell activation, and *tocilizumab,* an IL-6 receptor antagonist, have demonstrated efficacy in and are approved for treatment of polyarticular JIA (Table 180.8).

TNF inhibition is not as effective for the systemic symptoms found in sJIA. When systemic symptoms dominate, systemic corticosteroids are started followed by the initiation of IL-1 or IL-6 antagonist therapy, which often induces a dramatic and rapid response. Patients with severe disease activity may go directly to anakinra. *Canakinumab,* an IL-1β inhibitor, and tocilizumab are FDA-approved treatments for sJIA in children older than 2 yr (Table 180.8). Standardized consensus treatment plans to guide therapy for sJIA outline 4 treatment plans based on glucocorticoids, methotrexate, anakinra, or tocilizumab, with optional glucocorticoid use in the latter 3 plans as clinically indicated.

With the advent of newer DMARDs, the use of systemic corticosteroids can often be avoided or minimized. Systemic corticosteroids are recommended only for management of severe systemic illness, for *bridge therapy* during the wait for therapeutic response to a DMARD, and for control of uveitis. Steroids impose risks of severe toxicities, including Cushing syndrome, growth retardation, and osteopenia, and they do not prevent joint destruction.

Oral Janus kinase (JAK) inhibitors (tofacitinib, ruxolitinib) inhibit JAK signaling pathways involved in immune activation and inflammation. *Tofacitinib* is FDA approved for adults with rheumatoid arthritis.

Management of JIA must include periodic slit-lamp ophthalmologic examinations to monitor for asymptomatic uveitis (Figs. 180.15 and 180.16; see Table 180.4). Optimal treatment of uveitis requires collaboration between the ophthalmologist and rheumatologist; initial management may include mydriatics and corticosteroids used topically, systemically, or through periocular injection. DMARDs allow for a decrease in exposure to steroids, and methotrexate and TNF-α inhibitors (adalimumab and infliximab) are effective in treating severe uveitis.

Dietary evaluation and counseling to ensure appropriate calcium, vitamin D, protein, and caloric intake are important for children with JIA. Physical therapy and occupational therapy are invaluable adjuncts to any treatment program. A social worker and nurse clinician can be important resources for families, to recognize stresses imposed by a

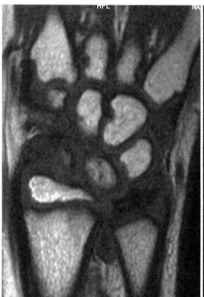
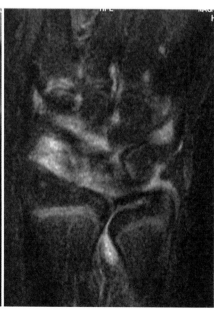

Fig. 180.14 MRI of the wrist in a child with wrist arthritis. *Left,* Image shows multiple erosions of carpal bones. *Right,* Image obtained after administration of gadolinium contrast agent reveals uptake consistent with active synovitis.

Table 180.8	Pharmacologic Treatment of Juvenile Idiopathic Arthritis (JIA)		
TYPICAL MEDICATIONS	**TYPICAL DOSES**	**JIA SUBTYPE**	**SIDE EFFECT(S)**
NONSTEROIDAL ANTIINFLAMMATORY DRUGS			
Naproxen	15 mg/kg/day PO divided bid (maximum dose 500 mg bid)	Polyarthritis Systemic Oligoarthritis	Gastritis, renal and hepatic toxicity, pseudoporphyria
Ibuprofen	40 mg/kg/day PO divided tid (maximum dose 800 mg tid)	Same as above	Same as above
Meloxicam	0.125 mg/kg PO once daily (maximum dose 15 mg daily)	Same as above	Same as above
DISEASE-MODIFYING ANTIRHEUMATIC DRUGS			
Methotrexate	0.5-1 mg/kg PO or SC weekly (maximum dose 25 mg/wk)	Polyarthritis Systemic Persistent or extended oligoarthritis	Nausea, vomiting, oral ulcerations, hepatic toxicity, blood count dyscrasias, immunosuppression, teratogenicity
Sulfasalazine	Initial 12.5 mg/kg PO daily; increase by 10 mg/kg/day Maintenance: 40-50 mg/kg divided bid (maximum dose 2 g/day)	Polyarthritis	GI upset, allergic reaction, pancytopenia, renal and hepatic toxicity, Stevens-Johnson syndrome
Leflunomide*	10-20 mg PO daily	Polyarthritis	GI upset, hepatic toxicity, allergic rash, alopecia (reversible), teratogenicity (needs washout with cholestyramine)
BIOLOGIC AGENTS			
Anti–Tumor Necrosis Factor-α			
Etanercept	0.8 mg/kg SC weekly or 0.4 mg/kg SC twice weekly (maximum dose 50 mg/wk)	Polyarthritis Systemic Persistent or extended oligoarthritis	Immunosuppressant, concern for malignancy, demyelinating disease, lupus-like reaction, injection site reaction
Infliximab*	3-10 mg/kg IV q4-8 wk	Same as above	Same as above, infusion reaction
Adalimumab	10 to <15 kg: 10 mg SC every other week 15 to <30 kg: 20 mg SC every other week >30 kg: 40 mg SC every other week	Same as above	Same as above
Anticytotoxic T-Lymphocyte–Associated Antigen-4 Immunoglobulin			
Abatacept	<75 kg: 10 mg/kg/dose IV q4wk 75-100 kg: 750 mg/dose IV q4wk >100 kg: 1,000 mg/dose IV q4wk SC once weekly: 10 to <25 kg: 50 mg ≥25 to <50 kg: 87.5 mg ≥50 kg: 125 mg	Polyarthritis	Immunosuppressant, concern for malignancy, infusion reaction
Anti-CD20			
Rituximab*	750 mg/m² IV 2 wk × 2 (maximum dose 1,000 mg)	Polyarthritis	Immunosuppressant, infusion reaction, progressive multifocal encephalopathy
Interleukin-1 Inhibitors			
Anakinra*	1-2 mg/kg SC daily (maximum dose 100 mg/day)	Systemic	Immunosuppressant, GI upset, injection site reaction
Canakinumab	15-40 kg: 2 mg/kg/dose SC q8wk >40 kg: 150 mg SC q8wk	Systemic	Immunosuppressant, headache, GI upset, injection site reaction
Rilonacept*	2.2 mg/kg/dose SC weekly (maximum dose 160 mg)	Systemic	Immunosuppressant, allergic reaction, dyslipidemia, injection site reaction
Interleukin-6 Receptor Antagonist			
Tocilizumab	IV q2 wk: <30 kg: 12 mg/kg/dose q2wk >30 kg: 8 mg/kg/dose q2wk (maximum dose 800 mg) SC: <30 kg: 162 mg/dose q3wk ≥30 kg: 162 mg/dose q2wk	Systemic Polyarthritis Polyarthritis	Immunosuppressant, hepatic toxicity, dyslipidemia, cytopenias, GI upset, infusion reaction

bid, Twice daily; GI, gastrointestinal; IV, intravenous; PO, oral; q, every; SC, subcutaneous; tid, 3 times daily.
*Not indicated by the U.S. Food and Drug Administration for use in JIA as of 2018.

chronic illness, to identify appropriate community resources, and to aid compliance with the treatment protocol.

PROGNOSIS

Although the course of JIA in an individual child is unpredictable, some prognostic generalizations can be made on the basis of disease type and course. Studies analyzing management of JIA in the pre–TNF-α era indicate that up to 50% of patients with JIA have active disease persisting into early adulthood, often with severe limitations of physical function.

Children with persistent oligoarticular disease fare well, with a majority achieving disease remission. Those with extended oligoarticular disease have a poorer prognosis. Children with oligoarthritis, particularly girls who are ANA positive and with onset of arthritis before 6 yr of age, are at greatest risk for development of chronic uveitis. There is no association between the activity or severity of arthritis and uveitis. Persistent, uncontrolled anterior uveitis (see Fig. 180.15) can cause posterior synechiae, cataracts, glaucoma, and band keratopathy, with resultant blindness. Morbidity can be averted with early diagnosis and

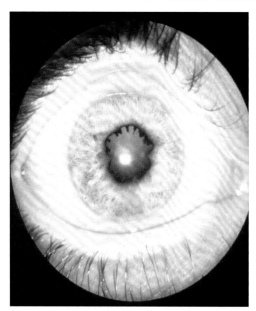

Fig. 180.15 Chronic anterior uveitis demonstrating posterior synechiae and absence of significant scleral inflammation. *(From Firestein GS, Budd RC, Gabriel SE, et al, editors: Kelley & Firestein's textbook of rheumatology, ed 10, Philadelphia, 2017, Elsevier, Fig 107-5, p 1838.)*

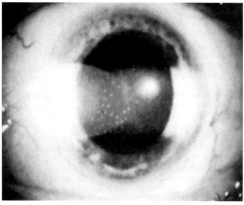

Fig. 180.16 Slit-lamp examination shows "flare" in the fluid of the anterior chamber (caused by increased protein content) and keratic precipitates on the posterior surface of the cornea, representing small collections of inflammatory cells. *(Courtesy of Dr. H.J. Kaplan. From Petty RE, Rosenbaum JT: Uveitis in juvenile idiopathic arthritis. In Cassidy JT, Petty RE, Laxer RM, et al, editors, Textbook of pediatric rheumatology, ed 6, Philadelphia, 2011, Saunders, Fig 20-3, p 309.)*

implementation of systemic therapy.

The child with polyarticular JIA often has a more prolonged course of active joint inflammation and requires early and aggressive therapy. Predictors of severe and persistent disease include young age at onset, RF seropositivity or rheumatoid nodules, presence of anti–cyclic citrullinated peptide antibodies, and many affected joints. Disease involving the hip and hand/wrist is also associated with a poorer prognosis and may lead to significant functional impairment.

Systemic JIA is often the most difficult to control in terms of both articular inflammation and systemic manifestations. Poorer prognosis is related to polyarticular distribution of arthritis, fever lasting >3 mo, and increased inflammatory markers, such as platelet count and ESR, for >6 mo. IL-1 and IL-6 inhibitors have changed the management and improved the outcomes for children with severe and prolonged systemic disease.

Orthopedic complications include leg length discrepancy and flexion contractures, particularly of the knees, hips, and wrists. Discrepancies in leg length can be managed with a shoe lift on the shorter side to prevent secondary scoliosis. Joint contractures require aggressive medical control of arthritis, often in conjunction with intraarticular corticosteroid injections, appropriate splinting, and stretching of the affected tendons. Popliteal cysts may require no treatment if they are small or respond to intraarticular corticosteroids in the anterior knee.

Psychosocial adaptation may be affected by JIA. Studies indicate that, compared with controls, a significant number of children with JIA have problems with lifetime adjustment and employment. Disability not directly associated with arthritis may continue into young adulthood in as many as 20% of patients, together with continuing chronic pain syndromes at a similar frequency. Psychological complications, including problems with school attendance and socialization, may respond to counseling by mental health professionals.

Bibliography is available at Expert Consult.

Chapter **181**
Ankylosing Spondylitis and Other Spondyloarthritides

Pamela F. Weiss and Robert A. Colbert

第一百八十一章
强直性脊柱炎和其他脊柱关节病

中文导读

本章主要介绍了幼年强直性脊柱炎和其他脊柱关节病的流行病学、病因和发病机制、临床表现和诊断、实验室检查、治疗及预后。流行病学描述了不同性别、种族患病差异及家族特点；病因中描述了有关遗传基因位点及可能的发病机制；临床表现中详细阐述了附着点相关的关节炎、银屑病关节炎、幼年强直性脊柱炎、炎性肠病性关节炎的临床表现；实验室检查中重点讲述了疾病的影像学表现；治疗中具体描述了治疗目标，非甾体抗炎药、改善病情抗风湿药和生物制剂等的使用策略以及理疗和低强度运动在治疗计划中的必要性；预后中详细阐述了病情缓解率、疾病进展相关因素以及与成人预后的对比。

The diseases collectively referred to as *spondyloarthritides* include **ankylosing spondylitis (AS)**, arthritis associated with inflammatory bowel disease (IBD) or psoriasis, and reactive arthritis following gastrointestinal (GI) or genitourinary (GU) infections (Table 181.1 and Table 181.2). **Spondyloarthritis** is more common in adults, but all forms can present during childhood with varying symptoms and signs. Many children with spondyloarthritis are classified in the **juvenile idiopathic arthritis (JIA)** categories of **enthesitis-related arthritis (ERA)** or psoriatic arthritis. Children and adolescents with spondyloarthritis who may not meet JIA criteria include arthritis associated with IBD, juvenile ankylosing spondylitis (JAS), and reactive arthritis.

EPIDEMIOLOGY

JIA is diagnosed in 90 per 100,000 U.S. children every year (see Chapter 180). ERA accounts for 10–20% of JIA, and has a mean age at onset of 12 yr. In India, ERA is the most common category of JIA, accounting for 35% of cases. Unlike other JIA categories, males are affected more often than females, accounting for 60% of ERA cases. AS occurs in 0.2–0.5% of adults, with approximately 15% of cases beginning in childhood. These disorders can be familial, largely as a result of the influence of human leukocyte antigen (**HLA**)-**B27**, which is found in 90% of JAS and 50% of ERA patients compared to 7% of healthy individuals. Approximately 20% of children with ERA have a family history of HLA-B27–associated disease, such as reactive arthritis, AS, or IBD with sacroiliitis.

ETIOLOGY AND PATHOGENESIS

Spondyloarthritides are complex diseases in which susceptibility is largely genetically determined. Only 30% of heritability has been defined, with HLA-B27 responsible for two thirds of the total, and >100 additional genetic loci accounting for only one third. Genes that influence interleukin (IL)-23 responses (e.g., *CARD9, IL23R, JAK2, TYK2, STAT3*) and the function of HLA-B27 *(ERAP1)* are particularly important. Unusual properties of HLA-B27, such as its tendency to misfold and form abnormal cell surface structures, may have a role. Infection with certain GI or GU pathogens can trigger reactive arthritis (see Table 181.2 and Chapter 182). Altered gut microbiota and an abnormal immune response to normal microbiota may also play a role in pathogenesis. Inflamed joints and entheses in spondyloarthritis contain T and B cells, macrophages, osteoclasts, proliferating fibroblasts, and osteoblasts, with activation of the IL-23/IL-17 pathway. Bone loss and osteoproliferation in and around vertebral bodies and facet joints in long-standing AS contribute to significant morbidity.

CLINICAL MANIFESTATIONS AND DIAGNOSIS

Clinical manifestations that help distinguish spondyloarthritis from other forms of juvenile arthritis include arthritis of the axial skeleton (sacroiliac joints) and hips, enthesitis (inflammation at the site of tendon, ligament, or joint capsule attachment to bone), symptomatic eye inflammation (acute anterior uveitis), and GI inflammation (even in the absence of IBD) (Tables 181.1 and 181.3).

Table 181.1	Overlapping Characteristics of the Spondyloarthritides*			
CHARACTERISTIC	**JUVENILE ANKYLOSING SPONDYLITIS**	**JUVENILE PSORIATIC ARTHRITIS**	**INFLAMMATORY BOWEL DISEASE**	**REACTIVE ARTHRITIS**
Enthesitis	+++	+	+	++
Axial arthritis	+++	++	++	+
Peripheral arthritis	+++	+++	+++	+++
HLA-B27 positive	+++	+	++	+++
Antinuclear antibody positive	–	++	–	–
Rheumatoid factor positive	–	–	–	–
SYSTEMIC DISEASE:				
Eyes	+	+	+	+
Skin	–	+++	+	+
Mucous membranes	–	–	+	+
Gastrointestinal tract	–	–	++++	+++

*Frequency of characteristics: –, absent; +, <25%; ++, 25–50%; +++, 50–75%; ++++, ≥75%.
From Cassidy JT, Petty RE: *Textbook of pediatric rheumatology*, ed 6, Philadelphia, 2011, Elsevier/Saunders.

Table 181.2	Etiologic Microorganisms of Reactive Arthritis

PROBABLE	POSSIBLE
Chlamydia trachomatis	*Neisseria gonorrhoeae*
Shigella species	*Mycoplasma fermentans*
Salmonella enteritidis	*Mycoplasma genitalium*
Salmonella typhimurium	*Ureaplasma urealyticum*
Yersinia enterocolitica	*Escherichia coli*
Yersinia pseudotuberculosis	*Cryptosporidium*
Campylobacter jejuni and *coli*	*Entamoeba histolytica*
	Giardia lamblia
	Brucella abortus
	Clostridium difficile
	Streptococcus pyogenes
	Chlamydia pneumoniae
	Chlamydia psittaci

From Kim PS, Klausmeier TL, Orr DP: Reactive arthritis: a review, *J Adolesc Health* 44:309–315, 2009 (Table 2, p 311).

Enthesitis-Related Arthritis

Children have ERA if they have *either* arthritis and enthesitis *or* arthritis or enthesitis, with at least 2 of the following characteristics: (1) sacroiliac joint tenderness or inflammatory lumbosacral pain, (2) presence of HLA-B27, (3) onset of arthritis in a male older than 6 yr, (4) acute anterior uveitis, and (5) a family history of an HLA-B27–associated disease (ERA, sacroiliitis with IBD, reactive arthritis, or acute anterior uveitis) in a first-degree relative. Patients with psoriasis (or a family history of psoriasis in a first-degree relative), a positive–rheumatoid factor (RF) test result, or systemic arthritis are excluded from this group. During the 1st 6 mo of disease the arthritis is typically asymmetric and involves ≤4 joints. most frequently the knees, ankles, and hips. Inflammation of the small joints of the foot, or *tarsitis*, is highly suggestive of ERA. Enthesitis is typically symmetric and typically affects the lower limbs. Up to 40% of children develop clinical or radiographic evidence of sacroiliac joint arthritis as part of their disease; approximately 20% have evidence of sacroiliac joint arthritis at diagnosis. When the sacroiliac or other axial joints are involved, children may experience **inflammatory back pain** (Table 181.4), hip pain, and alternating buttock pain. Patients may also experience pain with palpation of the lower back or with pelvic compression. The risk of sacroiliac joint arthritis is highest in children who are HLA-B27 positive and have an elevated C-reactive protein (CRP). Untreated sacroiliitis may, but does not always, evolve into AS; additional risk factors for progression are unclear.

Psoriatic Arthritis

Psoriatic arthritis accounts for approximately 5% of JIA. Common clinical features of psoriatic arthritis are nail pitting (Fig. 181.1), onycholysis, and dactylitis (sausage-like swelling of fingers or toes).

Children have psoriatic arthritis if they have arthritis and psoriasis *or* arthritis and at least 2 of the following: (1) dactylitis, (2) nail pitting or onycholysis, and (3) psoriasis in a first-degree relative. The presence of psoriasis aids in diagnosis but is not required. Disease onset peaks during the preschool and early adolescent years. Children with onset during the preschool years are more often female, antinuclear antibody (ANA) positive, and at risk for asymptomatic ocular inflammation. Disease onset during adolescence is equally common among males and females. In the majority of children the arthritis is asymmetric and affects ≤4 joints at presentation. Large (knees and ankles) and small (fingers and toes) joints may be involved. Although distal interphalangeal joint involvement is uncommon, it is highly suggestive of the diagnosis. Enthesitis is detectable in 20–60% of patients and seems to be more frequent in those who present at an older age. Axial (sacroiliac) and root (hip) joints may be affected in up to 30% of children; the risk of axial arthritis is highest in those who are HLA-B27 positive.

Juvenile Ankylosing Spondylitis

JAS frequently begins with oligoarthritis and enthesitis. The arthritis occurs predominantly in the lower extremities and often involves the hips. In comparison to adult-onset AS, axial disease and inflammatory back pain are less frequent at disease onset, whereas enthesitis and peripheral arthritis are more common. AS is diagnosed according to the modified New York (NY) criteria if there is sufficient radiographic evidence of sacroiliitis (sacroiliitis of grade 2 or greater bilaterally or at least grade 3 unilaterally) and if the patient meets at least 1 clinical criterion involving inflammatory back pain, limitation of motion in the lumbar spine (Fig. 181.2), or limitation of chest expansion. JAS is present if the patient is <16 yr old. Juvenile-*onset* AS is frequently used to describe adult AS when the symptoms began before 16 yr of age, but full criteria were not met until later.

To fulfill the modified NY criteria for AS, patients must have radiographic changes in the sacroiliac joints as well as clinical sequelae of axial disease. Because radiographic sacroiliitis can take many years to develop in adults and even longer in children, and clinical sequelae may lag further behind, criteria to identify preradiographic axial spondyloarthritis were developed by the **Assessment of SpondyloArthritis International Society**. To meet criteria for axial spondyloarthritis (SpA), patients must have at least 3 mo of back pain and sacroiliitis on imaging (acute inflammation on MRI or definite radiographic sacroiliitis by NY criteria) plus 1 feature of SpA (inflammatory back pain, arthritis, enthesitis [heel], uveitis, dactylitis, psoriasis, Crohn disease/ulcerative colitis, good response to nonsteroidal antiinflammatory drugs [NSAIDs], family history for SpA,

Table 181.3	Assessment in Spondyloarthritis International Society (ASAS) Classification Criteria for Spondyloarthritis (SpA)

AXIAL SpA		PERIPHERAL SpA
In patients with ≥3 mo back pain and age at onset <45 yr		In patients with peripheral symptoms ONLY
Sacroiliitis on imaging* *plus* ≥1 SpA feature(s) *or* HLA-B27 *plus* ≥2 other SpA features		Arthritis *or* enthesitis *or* dactylitis *plus*
SpA features • Inflammatory back pain (IBP) • Arthritis • Enthesitis (heel) • Uveitis • Dactylitis • Psoriasis • Crohn disease/ulcerative colitis • Good response to NSAIDs • Family history for SpA • HLA-B27 • Elevated CRP		≥1 SpA feature(s) • Uveitis • Psoriasis • Crohn disease/ulcerative colitis • Preceding infection • HLA-B27 • Sacroiliitis on imaging* *or* ≥2 other SpA features • Arthritis • Enthesitis • Dactylitis • IBP ever • Family history for SpA

*Active (acute) inflammation on MRI highly suggestive of sacroiliitis associated with SpA. Definite radiographic sacroiliitis according to modified NY criteria.
  CRP, C-reactive protein; NSAIDs, nonsteroidal antiinflammatory drugs.
  Adapted from Rudwaleit M, van der Heijde D, Landewé R, et al: The development of Assessment of Spondyloarthritis International Society classification criteria for axial spondyloarthritis. Part II. Validation and final selection, Ann Rheum Dis 68(6):777–783, 2009; and The Assessment of Spondyloarthritis International Society classification criteria for peripheral spondyloarthritis and for spondyloarthritis in general, Ann Rheum Dis 70(1):25–31, 2011.

Table 181.4	Symptoms Characteristic of Inflammatory Back Pain

Pain at night with morning stiffness (and improvement on arising)
No improvement with rest
Improvement with exercise
Insidious onset
Good response to nonsteroidal antiinflammatory drugs

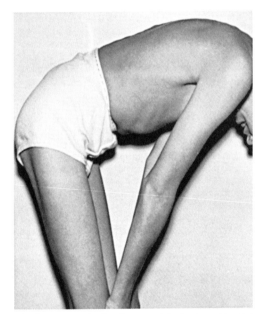

Fig. 181.2 Loss of lumbodorsal spine mobility in a boy with ankylosing spondylitis. The lower spine remains straight when the patient bends forward.

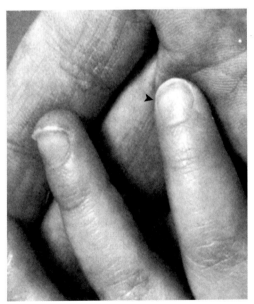

Fig. 181.1 Nail pitting *(arrowhead)* and "sausage digit" (dactylitis) of the left index finger of a girl with juvenile psoriatic arthritis. *(From Petty RE, Malleson P: Spondyloarthropathies of childhood, Pediatr Clin North Am 33:1079–1096, 1986.)*

HLA-B27, or elevated C-reactive protein). Alternatively, patients can fulfill axial SpA criteria if they are HLA-B27 positive and have at least 2 SpA features. These criteria have low sensitivity and specificity in the pediatric population but, in the absence of alternate pediatric criteria, may be useful as a guide to evaluating preradiographic axial SpA.

Arthritis With Inflammatory Bowel Disease
The presence of erythema nodosum, pyoderma gangrenosum, oral ulcers, abdominal pain, diarrhea, fever, weight loss, or anorexia in a child with chronic arthritis should raise suspicion of IBD. Two patterns of arthritis complicate IBD. **Polyarthritis** affecting large and small joints is most common and often reflects the activity of the intestinal inflammation. Less frequently, **arthritis of the axial skeleton**, including the sacroiliac joints, occurs. As with psoriatic arthritis, the presence of HLA-B27 is

a risk factor for the development of axial disease. The severity of axial involvement is independent of the activity of the GI inflammation.

LABORATORY FINDINGS

Laboratory evidence of systemic inflammation with elevation of the erythrocyte sedimentation rate (ESR) and/or CRP value is variable in most spondyloarthritides and may or may not be present at the onset of disease. RF and ANAs are absent, except in children with psoriatic arthritis, as many as 50% of whom are ANA positive. HLA-B27 is present in approximately 90% of children with JAS, compared with 7% of healthy individuals, but is less frequent in ERA and other SpA types.

Imaging

Conventional radiographs detect chronic bony changes and damage but not active inflammation. Early radiographic changes in the sacroiliac joints include indistinct margins and erosions that can result in joint space widening. **Sclerosis** typically starts on the iliac side of the joint (Fig. 181.3). Peripheral joints may exhibit periarticular **osteoporosis**, with loss of sharp cortical margins in areas of enthesitis, which may eventually show erosions or bony spurs (enthesophytes). Squaring of the corners of the vertebral bodies and syndesmophyte formation resulting in the classic "bamboo spine" characteristic of advanced AS is rare in early disease, particularly in childhood. CT, like radiographs, can detect chronic bony changes but not active inflammation and has the disadvantage of more radiation exposure. The gold standard for early visualization of sacroiliitis is evidence of bone marrow edema adjacent to the joint on MRI with fluid-sensitive sequences such as short-T1 inversion recovery (STIR). Gadolinium does not add value to the study of the sacroiliac joints if STIR is used. MRI will reveal abnormalities before the plain radiograph. Whole body MRI is also used to evaluate the axial skeleton in adults with early disease because it can detect vertebral lesions in addition to sacroiliac changes.

DIFFERENTIAL DIAGNOSIS

The onset of arthritis following a recent history of diarrhea or symptoms of urethritis or conjunctivitis may suggest **reactive arthritis** (see Chapter 182). Lower back pain can be caused by suppurative arthritis of the sacroiliac joint, osteomyelitis of the pelvis or spine, osteoid osteoma of the posterior elements of the spine, pelvic muscle pyomyositis, or malignancies. In addition, mechanical conditions such as spondylolysis, spondylolisthesis, and Scheuermann disease should be considered. Back pain secondary to **fibromyalgia** usually affects the soft tissues of the upper back in a symmetric pattern and is associated with well-localized tender points and sleep disturbance (see Chapter 193.3). Legg-Calvé-Perthes disease (avascular necrosis of the femoral head), slipped capital femoral epiphysis, and chondrolysis may also manifest as pain over the inguinal ligament and loss of internal rotation of the hip joint, but without other SpA features, such as involvement of other entheses and/or joints. Radiography or MRI is critical for distinguishing these conditions.

TREATMENT

The goals of therapy are to control inflammation, minimize pain, preserve function, and prevent ankylosis (fusion of adjacent bones) using a combination of antiinflammatory medications, physical therapy, and education. Treatment regimens for SpA include monotherapy or combination therapy with NSAIDs, disease-modifying antirheumatic drugs (DMARDs), or biologic agents. NSAIDs, such as naproxen (15-20 mg/kg/day), are frequently used initially and may slow the progression of

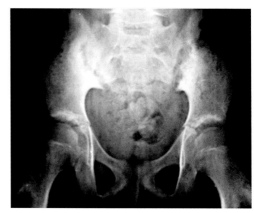

Fig. 181.3 Well-developed sacroiliitis in a boy with ankylosing spondylitis. Both sacroiliac joints show extensive sclerosis, erosion of joint margins, and apparent widening of the joint space.

structural damage (syndesmophyte formation and growth) if used continually. With relatively mild disease, intraarticular corticosteroids (e.g., triamcinolone acetonide/hexacetonide) may also help to control peripheral joint inflammation. However, for moderate disease and JAS, it is typically necessary to add a second-line agent. DMARDs such as sulfasalazine (up to 50 mg/kg/day; maximum 3 g/day) or methotrexate (10 mg/m^2) may be beneficial for peripheral arthritis, but these medications have not been shown to improve axial disease in adults. Tumor necrosis factor (TNF) inhibitors (e.g., etanercept, infliximab, adalimumab) have been efficacious in reducing symptoms and improving function in adults with AS, and there is evidence that similar responses are seen in children. It remains unclear whether TNF inhibitors have an impact on structural damage in established AS, underscoring the need for earlier recognition and better therapies. Drugs that target IL-17 and IL-23/IL-12 (secukinumab and ustekinumab, respectively) also reduce clinical disease activity in adults with AS, but have not been studied in children.

Physical therapy and low-impact exercise should be included in the treatment program for all children with spondyloarthritis. Exercise to maintain range of motion in the back, thorax, and affected joints should be instituted early in the disease course. Custom-fitted insoles and heel cups are particularly useful in management of painful entheses around the feet, and the use of pillows to position the lower extremities while the child is in bed can be helpful.

PROGNOSIS

Observational studies suggest that ongoing disease activity for >5 yr in juvenile spondyloarthritis predicts disability. Disease remission occurs in <20% of children with spondyloarthritis 5 yr after diagnosis. Factors associated with disease progression include tarsitis, HLA-B27 positivity, hip arthritis within the 1st 6 mo, and disease onset after age 8. Important questions, such as which patients with ERA will go on to have JAS/AS, have yet to be addressed. Outcomes for JAS compared with adult-onset AS suggest that hip disease requiring replacement is more common in children but axial disease is more severe in adults.

Bibliography is available at Expert Consult.

Chapter **182**

Reactive and Postinfectious Arthritis

Pamela F. Weiss and Robert A. Colbert

第一百八十二章

反应性和感染后关节炎

中文导读

本章主要介绍了反应性和感染后关节炎的发病机制、临床表现和鉴别诊断、诊断、治疗及并发症和预后。发病机制中描述了常见病原体及HLA-B27在疾病易感性中的影响；临床表现和鉴别诊断中描述了不同病因所致的反应性和感染后关节炎的临床特点；诊断中描述了不同临床表现、实验室检查、影像学检查指向或排除的诊断；治疗中描述了各类反应性和感染后关节炎在治疗过程中非甾体抗炎药、糖皮质激素、改善病情的抗风湿药及物理治疗等的使用策略；并发症和预后中描述了常见并发症及影响预后的因素。

In addition to causing arthritis by means of direct microbial infection (i.e., septic arthritis; see Chapter 705), microbes activate innate and adaptive immune responses, which can lead to the generation and deposition of immune complexes as well as antibody or T cell–mediated cross-reactivity with self. In addition, microbes may influence the immune system in ways that promote immune-mediated inflammatory diseases such as systemic lupus erythematosus (SLE), inflammatory bowel disease (IBD), juvenile idiopathic arthritis (JIA), and spondyloarthritis. **Reactive arthritis** and **postinfectious arthritis** are defined as joint inflammation caused by a sterile inflammatory reaction following a recent infection. We use *reactive arthritis* to refer to arthritis that occurs following enteropathic or urogenital infections and *postinfectious arthritis* to describe arthritis that occurs after infectious illnesses not classically considered in the reactive arthritis group, such as infection with group A streptococcus or viruses. In some patients, nonviable components of the initiating organism have been demonstrated in affected joints, and the presence of viable, yet nonculturable, bacteria within the joint remains an area of investigation.

The course of reactive arthritis is variable and may remit or progress to a chronic spondyloarthritis, including ankylosing spondylitis (see Chapter 181). In postinfectious arthritis the pain or joint swelling is usually transient, lasting <6 wk, and does not necessarily share the typical spondyloarthritis pattern of joint involvement. The distinction between postinfectious arthritis and reactive arthritis is not always clear, either clinically or pathophysiologically.

PATHOGENESIS

Reactive arthritis typically follows enteric infection with *Salmonella* species, *Shigella flexneri*, *Yersinia enterocolitica*, *Campylobacter jejuni*, or genitourinary (GU) tract infection with *Chlamydia trachomatis*. *Escherichia coli* and *Clostridium difficile* are also causative enteric agents, although less common (see Table 181.2). Acute **rheumatic fever** caused by group A streptococcus (see Chapters 182 and 210.1), arthritis associated with infective endocarditis (see Chapter 464), and the tenosynovitis associated with *Neisseria gonorrhoeae* are similar in some respects to reactive arthritis.

Approximately 75% of patients with reactive arthritis are HLA-B27 positive. Incomplete elimination of bacteria and bacterial products, such as DNA, has been proposed as a factor in reactive arthritis. A relationship with clinical characteristics of specific infectious disorders is not present. In postinfectious arthritis, several viruses (rubella, varicella-zoster, herpes simplex, cytomegalovirus) have been isolated from the joints of patients. Antigens from other viruses (e.g., hepatitis B, adenovirus) have been identified in immune complexes from joint tissue.

Patients with reactive arthritis who are HLA-B27 positive have an increased frequency of acute and symptomatic uveitis and other extraarticular features. In addition, HLA-B27 is a risk factor for persistent gastrointestinal (GI) inflammation following enteric infections, even after resolution of the initial infection, and significantly increases the risk that the individual will develop chronic spondyloarthritis. Nevertheless, reactive arthritis also occurs in HLA-B27–negative patients, emphasizing the importance of other genes in disease susceptibility.

CLINICAL MANIFESTATIONS AND DIFFERENTIAL DIAGNOSIS

Symptoms of reactive arthritis begin approximately 3 days to 6 wk following infection. The classic triad of arthritis, urethritis, and con-

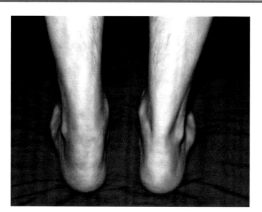

Fig. 182.1 Enthesitis—swelling of the posterior aspect of the left heel and lateral aspect of the ankle. *(Courtesy of Nora Singer, Case Western Reserve University and Rainbow Babies' Hospital.)*

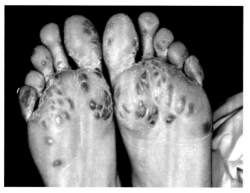

Fig. 182.2 Keratoderma blennorrhagica. *(Courtesy of Dr. M.F. Rein and Centers for Disease Control and Prevention Public Health Image Library, 1976. Image #6950.)*

Table 182.1	Viruses Associated With Arthritis
TOGAVIRUSES	**HERPESVIRUSES**
	Epstein-Barr
RUBIVIRUS	Cytomegalovirus
Rubella	Varicella-zoster
	Herpes simplex
ALPHAVIRUSES	
Ross River	**PARAMYXOVIRUSES**
Chikungunya	Mumps
O'nyong-nyong	
Mayaro	**FLAVIVIRUS**
Sindbis	Zika virus
Ockelbo	
Pogosta	**HEPADNAVIRUS**
	Hepatitis B
ORTHOPOXVIRUSES	
Variola virus (smallpox)	**ENTEROVIRUSES**
Vaccinia virus	Echovirus
Parvoviruses	Coxsackievirus B
ADENOVIRUSES	
Adenovirus 7	

Adapted from Infectious arthritis and osteomyelitis. In Petty RE, Laxer R, Lindsley CB, et al: *Textbook of pediatric rheumatology,* ed 7, Philadelphia, 2015, Saunders Elsevier.

junctivitis is relatively uncommon in children. The arthritis is typically asymmetric, oligoarticular, with a predilection for lower extremities. Dactylitis may occur, and enthesitis is common, affecting as many as 90% of patients (Fig. 182.1). Cutaneous manifestations can occur and may include circinate balanitis, ulcerative vulvitis, erythematous oral macules or plaques or erosions, erythema nodosum, paronychia, painful erosions or pustules on fingertips, and keratoderma blennorrhagica, which is similar in appearance to pustular psoriasis (Fig. 182.2). Systemic symptoms may include fever, malaise, and fatigue. Less common features may include conjunctivitis, optic neuritis, aortic valve involvement, sterile pyuria, and polyneuropathy. Early in the disease course, markers of inflammation—erythrocyte sedimentation rate (ESR), C-reactive protein, and platelets—may be greatly elevated. The clinical manifestations may last for weeks to months.

Familiarity with other causes of postinfectious arthritis is vital when a diagnosis of reactive arthritis is being considered. Numerous viruses are associated with postinfectious arthritis and may result in particular patterns of joint involvement (Table 182.1). Rubella and hepatitis B virus typically affect the small joints, whereas mumps and varicella often involve large joints, especially the knees. The **hepatitis B arthritis–dermatitis syndrome** is characterized by urticarial rash and a symmetric migratory polyarthritis resembling that of serum sickness. Rubella-associated arthropathy may follow natural rubella infection and, infrequently, rubella immunization. It typically occurs in young women, with an increased frequency with advancing age, and is uncommon in preadolescent children and in males. Arthralgia of the knees and hands usually begins within 7 days of onset of the rash or 10-28 days after immunization. Parvovirus B19, which is responsible for erythema infectiosum (fifth disease), can cause arthralgia, symmetric joint swelling, and morning stiffness, particularly in adult women and less frequently in children. Arthritis occurs occasionally during cytomegalovirus infection and may occur during varicella infections but is rare after Epstein-Barr virus infection. Varicella may also be complicated by suppurative arthritis, usually secondary to group A streptococcus infection. HIV is associated with an arthritis that resembles psoriatic arthritis more than JIA (see Chapter 180).

Poststreptococcal arthritis may follow infection with either group A or group G streptococcus. It is typically oligoarticular, affecting lower-extremity joints, and mild symptoms can persist for months. Poststreptococcal arthritis differs from rheumatic fever, which typically manifests with painful migratory polyarthritis of brief duration. Because valvular lesions have occasionally been documented by echocardiography after the acute illness, some clinicians consider poststreptococcal arthritis to be an incomplete form of acute rheumatic fever (see Chapter 210.1). Certain HLA-DRB1 types may predispose children to development of either poststreptococcal arthritis (HLA-DRB1*01) or acute rheumatic fever (HLA-DRB1*16).

Transient synovitis (toxic synovitis), another form of postinfectious arthritis, typically affects the hip, often after an upper respiratory tract infection (see Chapter 698.2). Boys 3-10 yr of age are most often affected and have acute onset of severe pain in the hip (groin), with referred pain to the thigh or knee, lasting approximately 1 wk. ESR and white blood cell count are usually normal. Radiologic or ultrasound examination may confirm widening of the joint space secondary to an effusion. Aspiration of joint fluid is often necessary to exclude septic arthritis and typically results in dramatic clinical improvement. The trigger is presumed to be viral, although responsible microbes have not been identified.

Nonsuppurative arthritis has been reported in children, usually adolescent boys, in association with severe truncal acne. Patients often have fever and persistent infection of the pustular lesions. **Pyogenic (sterile) arthritis, pyoderma gangrenosum, and acne (cystic) syndrome**, an autosomal dominant disorder caused by a mutation in the *PSTPIP1* gene, is a difficult-to-treat but rare autoinflammatory disorder that has responded to anakinra or anti–tumor necrosis factor antibody therapy in a few patients. Recurrent episodes of erosive arthritis begin in childhood; cystic acne and the painful ulcerating lesions of pyoderma gangrenosum begin during adolescence. Recurrent episodes may also be associated with a sterile myopathy and may last for several months.

Infective endocarditis can be associated with arthralgia, arthritis, or signs suggestive of vasculitis, such as Osler nodes, Janeway lesions, and Roth spots. Postinfectious arthritis, perhaps because of immune complexes, also occurs in children with *N. gonorrhoeae, Neisseria meningitidis, Haemophilus influenzae* type b, and *Mycoplasma pneumoniae* infections.

DIAGNOSIS

A recent GU or GI infection may suggest the diagnosis of reactive arthritis, but there is no diagnostic test. A complete blood count, acute-phase reactants, complete metabolic panel, and urinalysis may be helpful to exclude other etiologies. Although stool or urogenital tract cultures can be performed in an attempt to isolate it, the triggering organism is not typically found at the time arthritis presents. Imaging findings are nonspecific or normal. Documenting previous streptococcal infection with antibody testing (anti-streptolysin O and anti-DNAse B) may help to diagnose postinfectious arthritis. Serum sickness associated with the antibiotic treatment of preceding infection must be excluded.

Because the preceding infection can be remote or mild and often not recalled by the patient, it is also important to rule out other causes of arthritis. Acute and painful arthritis affecting a single joint suggests septic arthritis, mandating joint aspiration. Osteomyelitis may cause pain and an effusion in an adjacent joint but is more often associated with focal bone pain and tenderness at the site of infection. Arthritis affecting a single joint, particularly the knee, may also be secondary to Lyme disease in endemic areas. The diagnosis of postinfectious arthritis is often established by exclusion and after the arthritis has resolved. Arthritis associated with GI symptoms or abnormal liver function test results may be triggered by infectious or autoimmune hepatitis. Arthritis or spondyloarthritis may occur in children with IBD, such as Crohn disease or ulcerative colitis (see Chapter 362.1). Parvovirus infection, macrophage activation (hemophagocytic) syndrome, and leukemia should be strongly considered when 2 or more blood cell lines are low or progressively decrease in a child with arthritis. Persistent arthritis (>6 wk) suggests the possibility of a chronic rheumatic disease, including JIA (see Chapters 180) and systemic lupus erythematosus (see Chapter 183).

TREATMENT

Specific treatment is unnecessary for most cases of reactive or postinfectious arthritis. Nonsteroidal antiinflammatory drugs (NSAIDs) are often needed for management of pain and functional limitation. Unless ongoing *Chlamydia* infection is suspected, attempts to treat the offending organism are not warranted. If swelling or arthralgia recurs, further evaluation may be necessary to exclude active infection or evolving rheumatic disease. Intraarticular corticosteroid injections may be given for refractory or severely involved joints once acute infection has been ruled out. Systemic corticosteroids or disease-modifying antirheumatic drugs (DMARDs) are rarely indicated but may be considered for chronic disease. Participation in physical activity should be encouraged, and physical therapy may be needed to maintain normal function and prevent muscle atrophy. For postinfectious arthritis caused by streptococcal disease, current recommendations include penicillin prophylaxis for at least 1 yr. Long-term prophylaxis is often recommended, but the duration is controversial and may need to be individualized.

COMPLICATIONS AND PROGNOSIS

Postinfectious arthritis following viral infections usually resolves without complications unless it is associated with involvement of other organs, such as **encephalomyelitis**. Children with reactive arthritis after enteric infections occasionally experience IBD months to years after onset. Both **uveitis** and **carditis** have been reported in children diagnosed with reactive arthritis. Reactive arthritis, especially after bacterial enteric infection or GU tract infection with *C. trachomatis,* has the potential for evolving to chronic arthritis, particularly spondyloarthritis (see Chapter 181). The presence of HLA-B27 or significant systemic features increases the risk of chronic disease.

Bibliography is available at Expert Consult.

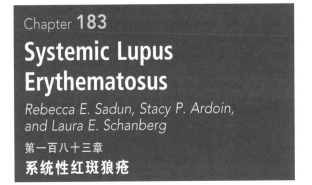

Chapter **183**
Systemic Lupus Erythematosus
Rebecca E. Sadun, Stacy P. Ardoin, and Laura E. Schanberg

第一百八十三章
系统性红斑狼疮

中文导读

　　本章主要介绍了系统性红斑狼疮的病因、流行病学、病理、发病机制、临床表现、诊断、鉴别诊断、实验室检查、治疗、并发症、预后及新生儿狼疮综合征。病因及发病机制中分析了遗传、激素和环境因素的作用；流行病学中描述了发病率、不同人种及性别的患病差异；病理中描述了肾脏及皮肤病理特点；

临床表现中描述了各系统症状特点；诊断及鉴别诊断中描述了ACR、SLICC分类标准、鉴别要点及药物性狼疮；实验室检查中描述了各免疫指标的特点；治疗中描述了羟氯喹、糖皮质激素等的疗效；并描述了新生儿狼疮的发病机制、临床表现和治疗等。

Systemic lupus erythematosus (SLE) is a chronic autoimmune disease characterized by multisystem inflammation and the presence of circulating autoantibodies directed against self-antigens. SLE occurs in both children and adults, disproportionately affecting females of reproductive age. Although nearly every organ may be affected, most frequently involved are the skin, joints, kidneys, blood-forming cells, blood vessels, and central nervous system. Systemic signs of inflammation such as fever and lymphadenopathy can also be seen. Compared with adults, children and adolescents with SLE have more severe disease and more widespread organ involvement.

ETIOLOGY

The pathogenesis of SLE remains largely unknown, but several factors likely influence risk and severity of disease, including genetics, hormonal milieu, and environmental exposures. A genetic predisposition to SLE is suggested by the association with specific genetic abnormalities, including congenital deficiencies of C1q, C2, and C4, as well as several polymorphisms (e.g., interferon regulatory factor 5, protein tyrosine phosphatase N22), and familial clustering of SLE or other autoimmune disease. In addition, certain human leukocyte antigen (HLA) types (including HLA-B8, HLA-DR2, and HLA-DR3) occur with increased frequency in patients with SLE. Although SLE clearly has a genetic component, its occurrence is sporadic in families and its concordance incomplete (estimated at 2–5% among dizygotic twins and 25–60% among monozygotic twins), suggesting **nonmendelian genetics** as well as involvement of epigenetic and environmental factors. Patients with SLE often have family members, especially mothers and sisters, with SLE or other autoimmune diseases.

Because SLE preferentially affects females, especially during their reproductive years, it is suspected that hormonal factors are important in pathogenesis. Of individuals with SLE, 90% are female, making **female sex** the strongest risk factor for SLE. Estrogens are likely to play a role in SLE, and both in vitro and animal model studies suggest that estrogen exposure promotes B-cell autoreactivity. Estrogen-containing oral contraceptives do not appear to induce flares in quiescent SLE, although the risk of flares may be increased in postmenopausal women receiving hormone replacement therapy.

Environmental exposures that may trigger the development of SLE remain largely unknown; certain viral infections, including Epstein-Barr virus (EBV), may play a role in susceptible individuals, and ultraviolet light exposure is known to trigger SLE disease activity. Environmental influences also may induce epigenetic modifications to DNA, increasing the risk of SLE and drug-induced lupus. In mouse models, drugs such as procainamide and hydralazine can promote lymphocyte hypomethylation, causing a lupus-like syndrome.

EPIDEMIOLOGY

The reported prevalence of SLE in children and adolescents (1-6/100,000) is lower than that in adults (20-70/100,000). Prevalence of SLE is highest among blacks, Asians, Hispanics, Native Americans, and Pacific Islanders for both adult and pediatric populations. SLE predominantly affects females, with reported 2-5:1 ratio before puberty, 9:1 ratio during reproductive years, and return to near-prepubertal ratios in the postmenopausal period. Childhood SLE is rare before 5 yr of age and is usually diagnosed in adolescence, with a median age at diagnosis of 11-12 yr. Up to 20% of all individuals with SLE are diagnosed before age 16 yr. Some define pediatric-onset lupus as onset of symptoms before age 16, and others as onset before age 18.

PATHOLOGY

Histologic features most suggestive of SLE include findings in the kidney and skin. Renal manifestations of SLE are classified histologically according to the criteria of the International Society of Nephrology (see Chapter 538.2). The finding of diffuse proliferative glomerulonephritis (class IV) significantly increases risk for renal morbidity. Renal biopsies are helpful to establish the diagnosis of SLE and to stage disease. Immune complexes are typically found with "full house" deposition of immunoglobulin and complement.

The characteristic **discoid rash** depicted in Figure 183.1*D* is characterized on biopsy by hyperkeratosis, follicular plugging, and infiltration of mononuclear cells into the dermal-epidermal junction (DEJ). The histopathology of photosensitive rashes can be nonspecific, but immunofluorescence examination of both affected and nonaffected skin may reveal deposition of immune complexes within the DEJ. This finding is called the **lupus band test**, which is specific for SLE.

PATHOGENESIS

A hallmark of SLE is the generation of **autoantibodies** directed against self-antigens, particularly nucleic acids. These intracellular antigens are ubiquitously expressed but are usually inaccessible and cloistered within

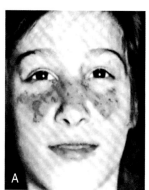 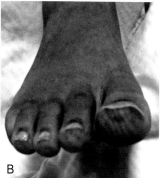 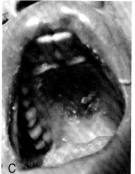 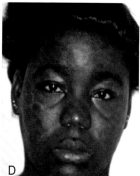

Fig. 183.1 Mucocutaneous manifestations of SLE. **A,** Malar rash; **B,** vasculitic rash on toes; **C,** oral mucosal ulcers; **D,** discoid rash in malar distribution.

the cell. During cell necrosis or apoptosis, the antigens are released. SLE skin cells are highly susceptible to damage from ultraviolet (UV) light, and the resulting cell death leads to release of cell contents, including nucleic antigens. Individuals with SLE may have greatly increased levels of apoptosis or significantly impaired ability to clear cell debris, causing prolonged exposure to nucleic antigens in the bloodstream and increased opportunity for recognition by immune cells, leading to B-cell stimulation and autoantibody production. Circulating autoantibodies form immune complexes and deposit in tissues, leading to local complement activation, initiation of a proinflammatory cascade, and, ultimately, tissue damage. Antibodies to **double-stranded (ds) DNA** can form immune complexes, deposit in glomeruli, and initiate inflammation leading to glomerulonephritis. However, many individuals with SLE have circulating antibodies to dsDNA but do not have nephritis, suggesting that autoantibodies are not the only pathway leading to end-organ damage in SLE.

Both the innate and the adaptive arms of the immune system have been implicated in the dysregulation of the immune system seen in SLE. High levels of interferon (IFN)-α production by plasmacytoid dendritic cells (DCs) promote expression of other proinflammatory cytokines and chemokines, maturation of monocytes into myeloid DCs, promotion of autoreactive B and T cells, and loss of self-tolerance. Almost 85% of patients with SLE exhibit this cytokine profile, known as the **type I interferon signature**. Other cytokines with increased expression in SLE include interleukin (IL)-1, IL-2, IL-6, IL-10, IL-12, IL-17, IL-21, anti–tumor necrosis factor-α, and IFN-γ, and B-lymphocyte stimulator (**BLyS**), also known as B-cell activating factor (**BAFF**). Both B and T cells demonstrate functional impairments in SLE. In active SLE, B-cell populations have impaired tolerance and increased autoreactivity, enhancing their ability to produce autoantibodies after exposure to self-antigen. In addition, cytokines such as BLyS/BAFF may promote abnormal B-cell number and function. T-cell abnormalities in SLE include increased numbers of memory T cells and decreased number and function of T-regulatory cells. SLE T cells display aberrant signaling and increased autoreactivity. As a result, they are resistant to attrition by normal apoptosis pathways. In addition, a neutrophil signature can be identified in 65% of adult SLE patients and has recently been recognized as a potential biomarker for active lupus nephritis.

CLINICAL MANIFESTATIONS

Any organ system can be involved in SLE, so the potential clinical manifestations are myriad (Tables 183.1 and 183.2). The presentation of SLE in childhood or adolescence differs somewhat from that seen in adults. The most common presenting complaints of children with SLE include fever, fatigue, hematologic abnormalities, arthralgia, and arthritis. Arthritis is usually present in the 1st yr of diagnosis; arthritis may be painful or painless swelling, often with stiffness in the morning, and is usually a **symmetric polyarthritis** affecting large and small joints. Tenosynovitis is often present, but joint erosions or other radiographic changes are rare.

Renal disease in SLE is often asymptomatic, underscoring the need for careful monitoring of blood pressure and urinalyses; in adolescents, SLE can present with **nephrotic syndrome** and/or **renal failure** with the predominant symptoms being edema, fatigue, changes in urine color, and nausea/vomiting. Because SLE symptoms and findings may develop serially over several years, and not all may be present simultaneously, the diagnosis may require longitudinal follow up. SLE is often characterized by periods of flare and disease quiescence but may follow a more smoldering disease course. The **neuropsychiatric complications** of SLE may occur with or without apparently active SLE, posing a particularly difficult diagnostic challenge in adolescents, who are already at high risk for mood disorders (Fig. 183.2). Long-term complications of SLE and its therapy, including accelerated atherosclerosis and osteoporosis, become clinically evident in young to middle adulthood. SLE is a disease that evolves over time in each affected individual, and new manifestations arise even many years after diagnosis.

DIAGNOSIS

The diagnosis of SLE requires a comprehensive clinical and laboratory assessment revealing characteristic multisystem disease and excluding

Table 183.1	Potential Clinical Manifestations of Systemic Lupus Erythematosus
TARGET ORGAN	**POTENTIAL CLINICAL MANIFESTATIONS**
Constitutional	Fatigue, anorexia, weight loss, fever, lymphadenopathy
Musculoskeletal	Arthritis, myositis, tendonitis, arthralgias, myalgias, avascular necrosis, osteoporosis
Skin	Malar rash, discoid (annular) rash, photosensitive rash, cutaneous vasculitis (petechiae, palpable purpura, digit ulcers, gangrene, urticaria), livedo reticularis, periungual capillary abnormalities, Raynaud phenomenon, alopecia, oral and nasal ulcers, panniculitis, chilblains, alopecia
Renal	Hypertension, proteinuria, hematuria, edema, nephrotic syndrome, renal failure
Cardiovascular	Pericarditis, myocarditis, conduction system abnormalities, Libman-Sacks endocarditis
Neuropsychiatric	Seizures, psychosis, cerebritis, stroke, transverse myelitis, depression, cognitive impairment, headaches, migraines, pseudotumor, peripheral neuropathy (mononeuritis multiplex), polyneuropathy, myasthenia gravis, chorea, optic neuritis, cranial nerve palsies, plexopathy, acute confusional states, dural sinus thrombosis, aseptic meningitis, depression, psychosis, anxiety disorder
Pulmonary	Pleuritis, interstitial lung disease, pulmonary hemorrhage, pulmonary hypertension, pulmonary embolism
Hematologic	Immune-mediated cytopenias (hemolytic anemia, thrombocytopenia or leukopenia), anemia of chronic inflammation, hypercoagulability, thrombocytopenic thrombotic microangiopathy
Gastroenterology	Hepatosplenomegaly, pancreatitis, vasculitis affecting bowel, protein-losing enteropathy, peritonitis
Ocular	Retinal vasculitis, scleritis, episcleritis, papilledema, dry eyes, optic neuritis
Other	Macrophage activation syndrome

other etiologies, including infection and malignancy. Presence of 4 of the 11 **American College of Rheumatology (ACR)** 1997 revised classification criteria for SLE simultaneously or cumulatively over time establishes the diagnosis (Table 183.3). Of note, although a positive antinuclear antibody (ANA) test result is not required for the diagnosis of SLE, ANA-negative lupus is extremely rare. ANA is very sensitive for SLE (95–99%), but it is not very specific (50%). The ANA may be positive many years before a diagnosis of SLE is established. However, most asymptomatic, ANA-positive patients do not have SLE or other autoimmune disease.

Antibodies against dsDNA and **anti-Smith** are specific for SLE (98%) but not as sensitive (40–65%). **Hypocomplementemia**, although common in SLE, is not one of the ACR classification criteria; however, hypocomplementemia has been added to updated criteria validated by the **Systemic Lupus International Collaborating Clinics (SLICC)** in 2012 (Table 183.4). Other differences in the SLICC criteria include the addition of nonscarring alopecia, additional cutaneous and neurologic manifestations of lupus, and a positive direct Coombs test in the absence of hemolytic anemia. The SLICC criteria have been validated in pediatric SLE and have been shown to have higher sensitivity (93% vs 77%) but lower specificity (85% vs 99%) than the ACR criteria.

Table 183.2	Frequency of Clinical Features of Children and Adolescents With Systemic Lupus Erythematosus	
CLINICAL FEATURE*	**WITHIN 1 YR OF DIAGNOSIS (%)**	**ANY TIME (%)**
Fever	35-90	37-100
Lymphadenopathy	11-45	13-45
Hepatosplenomegaly	16-42	19-43
Weight loss	20-30	21-32
Arthritis	60-88	60-90
Myositis	<5	<5
Any skin involvement	60-80	60-90
Malar rash	22-68	30-80
Discoid rash	<5	<5
Photosensitivity	12-45	17-58
Mucosal ulceration	25-32	30-40
Alopecia	10-30	15-35
Other rashes	40-52	42-55
Nephritis	20-80	48-100
Neuropsychiatric disease	5-30[†]	15-95[‡]
Psychosis	5-12	8-18
Seizures	5-15	5-47
Headache	5-22	10-95
Cognitive dysfunction	6-15	12-55
Acute confusional state	5-15	8-35
Peripheral nerve involvement	<5	<5
Cardiovascular disease	5-30	25-60
Pericarditis	12-20	20-30

*Not all reports commented on all features or incidence in 1st yr.
[†]Had highest prevalence of central nervous system disease but did not describe incidence in 1st yr.
[‡]Headache reported in 95% of patients.
From Petty RE, Laxer RM, Lindsley CB, Wedderburn LR, editors: *Textbook of pediatric rheumatology*, ed 7, Philadelphia, 2016, Elsevier (Table 23.5, p 291).

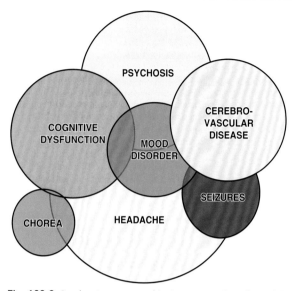

Fig. 183.2 Overlapping neuropsychiatric symptoms in pediatric SLE. Patients with pediatric SLE typically have >1 neuropsychiatric symptom—in particular for seizures. *(From Silverman E, Eddy A: Systemic lupus erythematosus. In Cassidy JT, Petty RE, Laxer RM, et al, editors, Textbook of pediatric rheumatology, ed 6, Philadelphia, 2011, Saunders Elsevier, Fig 21-17, p 329.)*

Table 183.3	American College of Rheumatology (ACR) 1997 Revised Classification Criteria for Systemic Lupus Erythematosus*

Malar rash
Discoid rash
Photosensitivity
Oral or nasal ulcers
Arthritis
　Nonerosive, ≥2 joints
Serositis
　Pleuritis, pericarditis, or peritonitis
Renal manifestations[†]
　Consistent renal biopsy
　Persistent proteinuria or renal casts
Seizure or psychosis
Hematologic manifestations[†]
　Hemolytic anemia
　Leukopenia (<4,000 leukocytes/mm³)
　Lymphopenia (<1,500 leukocytes/mm³)
　Thrombocytopenia (<100,000 thrombocytes/mm³)
Immunologic abnormalities[†]
　Positive anti–double-stranded DNA or anti-Smith antibody
　False-positive rapid plasma reagin test result, positive lupus
　　anticoagulant test result, or elevated anticardiolipin IgG or
　　IgM antibody
Positive antinuclear antibody test result

*The presence of 4 of 11 criteria establishes the diagnosis of SLE. These criteria were developed for classification in clinical trials and not for clinical diagnosis.
[†]Each of these criteria counts as a single criterion whether 1 or more definitions are satisfied.
Adapted from Hochberg MC: Updating the American College of Rheumatology revised criteria for the classification of systemic lupus erythematosus, *Arthritis Rheum* 40:1725, 1997.

DIFFERENTIAL DIAGNOSIS

Multiorgan disease is the hallmark of SLE. Given its wide array of potential clinical manifestations, SLE is in the differential diagnosis of many clinical scenarios, including unexplained fevers, joint pain or arthritis, rash, cytopenias, nephritis, nephrotic syndrome, pleural or pericardial effusions or other cardiopulmonary abnormalities, and new-onset psychosis, movement disorders, or seizures. For patients ultimately diagnosed with pediatric SLE, the initial differential diagnosis often includes infections (sepsis, EBV, parvovirus B19, endocarditis), malignancies (leukemia, lymphoma), poststreptococcal glomerulonephritis, other rheumatologic conditions (juvenile idiopathic arthritis, vasculitides), and drug-induced lupus.

Drug-induced lupus refers to the presence of SLE manifestations triggered by exposure to specific medications, including hydralazine, minocycline, many anticonvulsants, sulfonamides, and antiarrhythmic agents (Table 183.5). In individuals prone to SLE, these agents may act as a trigger for true SLE, but more often these agents provoke a reversible lupus-like syndrome. Unlike SLE, drug-induced lupus affects males and females equally. A genetic predisposition toward slow drug acetylation may increase the risk of drug-induced lupus. Circulating **antihistone antibodies** are often present in drug-induced SLE; these antibodies are only detected in up to 20% of individuals with SLE. Hepatitis, which is rare in SLE, is more common in drug-induced lupus. Individuals

with drug-induced lupus are less likely to demonstrate antibodies to dsDNA, hypocomplementemia, and significant renal or neurologic disease. In contrast to SLE, manifestations of drug-induced lupus typically resolve after withdrawal of the offending medication; however, complete recovery may take several months to years, requiring treatment with hydroxychloroquine, NSAIDs, and/or corticosteroids.

Table 183.4	Systemic Lupus International Collaborating Clinics (SLICC) Classification Criteria for Systemic Lupus Erythematosus*

CLINICAL CRITERIA

Acute cutaneous lupus
Malar rash, bullous lupus, toxic epidermal necrolysis variant of SLE, maculopapular lupus rash, photosensitive lupus rash, or subacute cutaneous lupus

Chronic cutaneous lupus
Classic discoid rash, lupus panniculitis, mucosal lupus, lupus erythematous tumidus, chilblains lupus, discoid lupus/lichen planus overlap

Oral or nasal ulcers

Nonscarring alopecia

Synovitis (≥2 joints)

Serositis
Pleurisy or pericardial pain ≥1 day, pleural effusion or rub, pericardial effusion or rub, ECG evidence of pericarditis

Renal
Presence of red blood cell casts or urine protein/creatinine ratio representing >500 mg protein/24 hr

Neurologic
Seizures, psychosis, mononeuritis multiplex, myelitis, peripheral or cranial neuropathy, or acute confusional state

Hemolytic anemia

Leukopenia (<4,000/mm^3) or lymphopenia (<1,000/mm^3)

Thrombocytopenia (<100,000/mm^3)

IMMUNOLOGIC CRITERIA

Positive antinuclear antibody

Positive double-stranded DNA antibody

Positive anti-Smith antibody

Antiphospholipid antibody positivity
Positive lupus anticoagulant, false-positive test for rapid plasma regain, medium- to high-titer anticardiolipin antibody level (IgA, IgG, IgM), or positive anti–β$_2$-glycoprotein-1 antibody (IgA, IgG, IgM)

Low complement
Low C3, C4, or CH$_{50}$ level

Positive direct Coombs test

*The presence of 4 criteria (including at least 1 clinical and 1 immunologic criterion) establishes the diagnosis of SLE. Biopsy-proven lupus nephritis with positive ANA or anti–double-stranded DNA also satisfies the diagnosis of SLE. These criteria were developed for classification in clinical trials and not for clinical diagnosis.

Adapted from Petri M: Derivation and validation of the Systemic Lupus International Collaborating Clinics classification criteria for systemic lupus erythematosus, *Arthritis Rheum* 64(8):2677–2686, 2012.

Table 183.5	Medications Associated With Drug-Induced Lupus

DEFINITE ASSOCIATION

Minocycline, procainamide, hydralazine, isoniazid, penicillamine, diltiazem, interferon-α, methyldopa, chlorpromazine, etanercept, infliximab, adalimumab

PROBABLE ASSOCIATION

Phenytoin, ethosuximide, carbamazepine, sulfasalazine, amiodarone, quinidine, rifampin, nitrofurantoin, β-blockers, lithium, captopril, interferon-γ, hydrochlorothiazide, glyburide, docetaxel, penicillin, tetracycline, statins, gold, valproate, griseofulvin, gemfibrozil, propylthiouracil

LABORATORY FINDINGS

A positive ANA test is present in 95–99% of SLE patients. ANA has poor specificity for SLE, however, because up to 20% of healthy individuals also have a positive ANA test result, making the ANA a poor screen for SLE when used in isolation. High titers are more suggestive of

Table 183.6	Autoantibodies Typically Associated With Systemic Lupus Erythematosus
ANTIBODY	**CLINICAL ASSOCIATION**
Anti–double-stranded DNA	Specific for the diagnosis of SLE Correlates with disease activity, especially nephritis, in some with SLE
Anti-Smith antibody	Specific for the diagnosis of SLE
Antiribonucleoprotein (anti-RNP) antibody	Increased risk for Raynaud phenomenon, intersitial lung disease, and pulmonary hypertension
Anti-Ro antibody (anti-SSA antibody) Anti-La antibody (anti-SSB antibody)	Associated with sicca syndrome May suggest diagnosis of Sjögren syndrome Increased risk of neonatal lupus in offspring (congenital heart block) May be associated with cutaneous and pulmonary manifestations of SLE May be associated with isolated discoid lupus
Antiphospholipid antibodies (including anticardiolipin antibodies)	Increased risk for venous and arterial thrombotic events
Antihistone antibodies	Present in a majority of patients with drug-induced lupus May be present in SLE

underlying autoimmune disease, but ANA titers do not correlate with disease activity, so repeating ANA titers after diagnosis is not helpful. Antibodies to dsDNA are specific for SLE, and in many individuals, anti-dsDNA levels correlate with disease activity, particularly in those with significant nephritis. Anti-Smith antibody, although found specifically in patients with SLE, does not correlate with disease activity. Serum levels of total hemolytic complement (CH$_{50}$), C3, and C4 are typically decreased in active disease and often improve with treatment. Table 183.6 lists autoantibodies found in SLE along with their clinical associations. Hypergammaglobulinemia is a common but nonspecific finding. Inflammatory markers, particularly erythrocyte sedimentation rate, are often elevated in active disease. C-reactive protein (CRP) correlates less well with disease activity; significantly elevated CRP values often reflect infection, whereas chronic mild elevation may indicate increased cardiovascular risk.

Antiphospholipid antibodies, which increase clotting risk, can be found in up to 66% of children and adolescents with SLE. Antiphospholipid laboratory findings include the presence of anticardiolipin or anti–β$_2$-glycoprotein antibodies, prolonged phospholipid-dependent coagulation test results (partial thromboplastin time, dilute Russell viper-venom time), and circulating **lupus anticoagulant** (which confirms that a prolonged PPT is not corrected with mixing studies). When an arterial or venous clotting event occurs in the presence of an antiphospholipid antibody, **antiphospholipid antibody syndrome** is diagnosed, which can occur in the context of SLE (secondary) or independent of SLE (primary) (see Chapter 479).

TREATMENT

Treatment of SLE is tailored to the individual and is based on specific disease manifestations and medication tolerability. For all patients, sunscreen and avoidance of prolonged direct sun exposure and other UV light may help control disease and should be reinforced at every visit with the patient. *Hydroxychloroquine* is recommended for all individuals with SLE when tolerated. In addition to treating mild SLE manifestations such as rash and mild arthritis, hydroxychloroquine prevents SLE flares, improves lipid profiles, and may improve mortality and renal outcomes. Potential toxicities include retinal deposition and subsequent vision impairment; therefore, annual ophthalmology exams are recommended for patients taking hydroxychloroquine, including automated visual field testing as well as spectral-domain optical coherence tomography (SD-OCT). Given that risk factors for ocular toxicity include duration of use and dose, hydroxychloroquine in SLE should never be prescribed at doses >6.5 mg/kg (maximum 400 mg daily), and newer ophthalmology guidelines recommend limiting maintenance dosing to 4-5 mg/kg.

Corticosteroids are a treatment mainstay for significant manifestations of SLE and work quickly to improve acute deterioration; side effects often limit patient adherence, especially in adolescence, and potential toxicities are worrisome. It is important to limit dose and length of exposure to corticosteroids whenever possible. Potential consequences of corticosteroid therapy include growth disturbance, weight gain, striae, acne, hyperglycemia, hypertension, cataracts, avascular necrosis, and osteoporosis. The optimal dosing of corticosteroids in children and adolescents with SLE remains unknown; severe disease is often treated with high doses of intravenous (IV) methylprednisolone (e.g., 30 mg/kg/day to a maximum of 1,000 mg/day for 3 days, sometimes followed by a period of weekly pulses) and/or high doses of oral prednisone (1-2 mg/kg/day). As disease manifestations improve, corticosteroid dosages are gradually tapered over months. For most patients it is necessary to introduce a steroid-sparing immunosuppressive medication to limit cumulative steroid exposure.

Steroid-sparing immunosuppressive agents for the treatment of pediatric SLE include methotrexate, leflunomide, azathioprine, mycophenolate mofetil (MMF), tacrolimus, cyclophosphamide, rituximab, and belimumab. Methotrexate, leflunomide, and azathioprine are often used to treat persistent moderate disease, including arthritis, significant cutaneous or hematologic involvement, and pleural disease. Cyclophosphamide, MMF, and azathioprine are appropriate for the treatment of lupus nephritis, whereas MMF and rituximab are often used for significant hematologic manifestations, including severe leukopenia, hemolytic anemia, or thrombocytopenia.

Cyclophosphamide, usually administered intravenously, is reserved for the most severe, potentially life-threatening SLE manifestations, such as renal, neurologic, and cardiopulmonary disease. Although cyclophosphamide is highly effective in controlling disease, the potential toxicities are significant, including cytopenias, infection, hemorrhagic cystitis, premature gonadal failure, and increased risk of future malignancy. Attention to adequate hydration can attenuate the risk of hemorrhagic cystitis. Fortunately, young girls are at much lower risk of gonadal failure than older women, and the use of gonadotropin-releasing hormone agonists, such as leuprolide acetate, may help prevent gonadal failure.

The **Childhood Arthritis Rheumatology Research Alliance (CARRA)** consensus treatment plan for induction therapy of newly diagnosed **proliferative lupus nephritis** (class IV) is specific to the pediatric SLE population. The treatment is considered necessary for class IV lupus nephritis but also appropriate for certain patients with class III, V, or VI lupus nephritis. The CARRA treatment plans advise 6 mo of induction therapy with either cyclophosphamide (given per NIH Protocol as 500-1000 mg/m² IV monthly) or MMF (600 mg/m², up to 1500 mg, twice daily), used in combination with 1 of 3 standardized glucocorticoid regimens. For patients who fail to achieve a partial response in 6 mo, it is appropriate to switch agents. For adult-weight adolescents, the cyclophosphamide dosing regimen used in the **Euro-Lupus Nephritis Trial** can be considered instead of the above 6 mo therapy to reduce toxicity from cyclophosphamide exposure. Per this protocol, a fixed dose of 500 mg is given every 2 wk for 3 mo; this regimen is thought to reduce adverse effects while maintaining comparable efficacy for lupus nephritis in adults, but has not been studied specifically in pediatric lupus. Oral medication adherence is very poor in pediatric SLE, which must be considered when weighing the benefits of an IV infusion vs a twice-daily oral medication such as MMF. Maintenance therapy of lupus nephritis consists of cyclophosphamide every 3 mo, or MMF, or azathioprine, typically for 36 mo after completion of induction therapy.

Clinical trial data on the use of *rituximab* in SLE with treatment-resistant glomerulonephritis has been largely disappointing, but results from the LUNAR study suggest a possible benefit for subpopulations of SLE patients. The U.S. Food and Drug Administration (FDA) has approved the use of *belimumab*, a monoclonal antibody against BLyS/BAFF, for the treatment of lupus in adults; when added to standard SLE therapy, belimumab improves multiple markers of disease severity. Other therapies being studied for treatment of lupus include rigerimod (a polypeptide corresponding to a sequence of the snRNP protein) and anifrolumab (monoclonal antibody to IFN-α receptor), all with encouraging phase II results.

Given the lifelong nature of SLE, optimal care of children and adolescents with this disease also involves preventive practices. Because of the enhanced risk of atherosclerosis in SLE, attention to cholesterol levels, smoking status, body mass index, blood pressure, and other traditional cardiovascular risk factors is warranted. Even though the **Atherosclerosis Prevention in Pediatric Lupus Erythematosus (APPLE)** study failed to support placing all children with SLE on a statin, post hoc analyses suggest that statins should be considered for primary prevention of atherosclerotic disease in certain clinical circumstances, particularly pubertal patients with an elevated CRP.

SLE patients with antiphospholipid antibody syndrome (antiphospholipid antibodies *and* a history of clot) are treated with long-term anticoagulation to prevent thrombotic events. For SLE patients who are antiphospholipid antibody positive without a history of clot, many pediatric rheumatologists prescribe aspirin (81 mg daily).

For all SLE patients, adequate intake of calcium and vitamin D is necessary to prevent future osteoporosis, particularly as vitamin D levels are lower in pediatric SLE patients compared to age-matched healthy controls. Studies suggest a link between hypovitaminosis D and SLE susceptibility, with a possible emerging role for vitamin D in immunomodulation.

Infections, particularly pneumococcal disease, frequently complicate SLE, so routine immunization is recommended, including the annual influenza vaccination. In addition, pediatric SLE patients age 6 or older should receive an additional pneumococcal 13 vaccination, followed by the pneumococcal 23 vaccination at least 2 mo later. It is important to note that many of the immunosuppressants used in SLE contraindicate live vaccines. Prompt attention to febrile episodes should include an evaluation for serious infections. Because pediatric SLE patients are at high risk for developing anxiety and depression, screening for depression is also essential. Peer support and cognitive-behavioral therapy interventions reduce pain and enhance resilience in pediatric SLE.

It should be remembered that pregnancy can worsen SLE, and obstetric complications are common. In addition, many medications used to treat SLE are teratogenic, so it is important to counsel adolescent girls about these risks and facilitate access to appropriate contraceptive options. Hydroxychloroquine is recommended throughout the pregnancy of all SLE patients, and other medications may need to be adjusted.

COMPLICATIONS

Within the first several years of diagnosis, the most common causes of death in SLE patients are infection and complications of glomerulonephritis and neuropsychiatric disease (Table 183.7). Over the long-term, the most common causes of mortality are complications of atherosclerosis and malignancy. The increased risk of premature atherosclerosis in SLE is not explained by traditional risk factors and is partly a result of the chronic immune dysregulation and inflammation associated with SLE. Increased malignancy rates may be caused by immune dysregulation as well as exposure to medications with carcinogenic potential.

PROGNOSIS

The severity of pediatric SLE is notably worse than the typical course for adult-onset SLE. However, because of advances in the diagnosis and treatment of SLE, survival has improved dramatically over the past 50 yr. Currently, the 5 yr survival rate for pediatric SLE is approximately 95%, although the 10 yr survival rate remains 80–90%. Given their long burden of disease, children and adolescents with SLE face high risks of future morbidity and mortality from the disease and its complications, as well as medication side effects (see Table 183.7). Given the complex and chronic nature of SLE, it is optimal for children and adolescents

Table 183.7	Morbidity in Childhood Lupus
SYSTEM	**MORBIDITY**
Renal	Hypertension, dialysis, transplantation
Central nervous	Organic brain syndrome, seizures, psychosis, neurocognitive dysfunction
Cardiovascular	Atherosclerosis, myocardial infarction, cardiomyopathy, valvular disease
Immune	Recurrent infection, functional asplenia, malignancy
Musculoskeletal	Osteopenia, compression fractures, avascular necrosis
Ocular	Cataracts, glaucoma, retinal detachment, blindness
Endocrine	Diabetes, obesity, growth failure, infertility, fetal wastage

From Cassidy JT, Petty RE: *Textbook of pediatric rheumatology, ed 6,* Philadelphia, 2011, Elsevier Saunders.

with SLE to be treated by pediatric rheumatologists in a multidisciplinary clinic with access to a full complement of pediatric subspecialists.

Bibliography is available at Expert Consult.

183.1 Neonatal Lupus

Deborah M. Friedman, Jill P. Buyon, Rebecca E. Sadun, Stacy P. Ardoin, and Laura E. Schanberg

Neonatal lupus erythematosus (NLE), an entity distinct from SLE, is one of the few rheumatic disorders manifesting in the neonate. NLE is not an autoimmune disease of the fetus but instead results from passively acquired autoimmunity, when maternal immunoglobulin G autoantibodies cross the placenta and enter the fetal circulation. In contrast to SLE, neonatal lupus is not characterized by ongoing immune dysregulation, although infants with neonatal lupus may be at some increased risk for development of future autoimmune disease. The vast majority of NLE cases are associated with maternal **anti-Ro** (also known as anti-SSA), **anti-La** antibodies (also known as anti-SSB), or **anti-RNP** (antiribonucleoprotein) autoantibodies. Despite the clear association with maternal autoantibodies, their presence alone is not sufficient to cause disease, because only 2% of offspring born to mothers with anti-Ro and anti-La antibodies develop neonatal lupus. Siblings of infants with NLE have a 15–20% chance of developing NLE. Neonatal lupus seems to be independent of maternal health since many mothers are asymptomatic and only identified to have anti-Ro/anti-La antibodies subsequent to the diagnosis of NLE. Half the infants with NLE are born to the mothers with a defined rheumatic disease, such as Sjögren syndrome or SLE.

Clinical manifestations of neonatal lupus include a characteristic annular or macular rash typically affecting the face (especially the periorbital area), trunk, and scalp (Fig. 183.3). The rash can be present at birth but more often appears within the first 6-8 wk of life, after exposure to UV light, and typically lasts 3-4 mo. Infants may also have cytopenias and hepatitis, each occurring in approximately 25% of cases, but the most feared complication is **congenital heart block**.

Conduction system abnormalities range from prolongation of the PR interval to complete heart block, with development of progressive cardiomyopathy in the most severe cases. The noncardiac manifestations of NLE are usually reversible, whereas third-degree congenital heart block is permanent. Conduction system abnormalities can be detected in utero by fetal echocardiogram beginning at 16 wk gestational age. Neonatal lupus cardiac disease has a mortality rate of approximately 20%. Cardiac NLE can manifest as heart block, cardiomyopathy, valvular

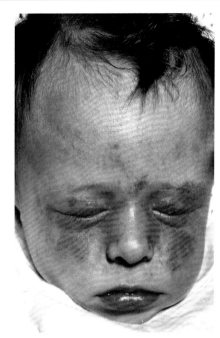

Fig. 183.3 Neonatal lupus syndrome. Typical rash, often photosensitive with a malar distribution, appearing as plaques with erythema and scaling. *(Reproduced, with written parental permission, from Pain C, Beresford MW: Neonatal lupus syndrome, Paediatr Child Health 17:223–227, 2007.)*

dysfunction, and endocardial fibroelastosis. Fetal bradycardia from heart block can lead to **hydrops fetalis**.

In vitro studies suggest that during cardiac development via apoptosis, Ro and La antigens may be exposed on the surface of cardiac cells in the proximity of the atrioventricular node, making the antigens accessible to maternal autoantibodies. Binding incites a local immune response, resulting in fibrosis within the conduction system as well as more extensive disease in fatal cases. In the skin, exposure to ultraviolet light results in cell damage and the subsequent exposure of Ro and La antigens, inducing a similar local inflammatory response that produces the characteristic rash.

Although the scant clinical trial data have been mixed, fluorinated corticosteroids (dexamethasone or betamethasone), intravenous immune globulin (IVIG) at 1–2 g/kg maternal weight, plasmapheresis, hydroxychloroquine, and terbutaline (combined with steroids) have been used in pregnant women with anti-Ro or anti-La antibodies to prevent occurrence or progression of fetal cardiac abnormalities.

Most encouraging are retrospective cohort studies suggesting maternal treatment with *hydroxychloroquine* may reduce the frequency and recurrence of congenital heart block. In a case control study of women with lupus and known anti-Ro autoantibodies, maternal use of hydroxychloroquine decreased the rate of cardiac disease (odds ratio 0.28). This was confirmed in an expanded international study in which the recurrence rate of cardiac disease was 64% lower in pregnant women given hydroxychloroquine than controls (7.5% vs 21.2%). All clinical data on the use of hydroxychloroquine in pregnancy point to safety; prospective clinical studies are examining efficacy in the prevention of recurrent congenital heart block in pregnant women known to be anti-Ro and/or anti-La positive.

In utero, fluorinated corticosteroids seem to improve cases of hydrops fetalis. Furthermore, the addition of β-agonist therapy to increase fetal heart rate, used in combination with corticosteroids or IVIG, may help prevent hydrops in cases of severe fetal heart block. However, recent data from the **Research Registry for Neonatal Lupus** suggest that dexamethasone is not efficacious in preventing progression of isolated third-degree block, influencing the need for pacing after birth, or overall survival.

Management of the Anti-Ro ± Anti-La Pregnancy

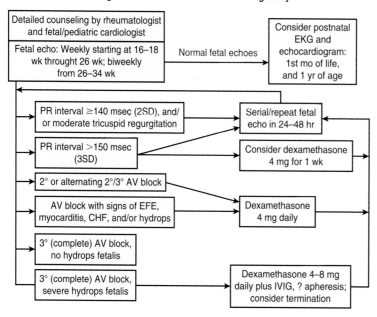

Fig. 183.4 Algorithm for the management of the anti-Ro ± anti-La pregnancy. All such pregnancies should include counseling and serial fetal echocardiograms. AV, Atrioventricular; CHF, congestive heart failure; EFE, endocardial fibroelastosis; SD, standard deviations.

Significant conduction system abnormalities after birth are treated with cardiac pacing and occasionally IVIG and corticosteroids, whereas severe cardiomyopathy may require cardiac transplantation. If the conduction defect is not addressed, affected children are at risk for exercise intolerance, arrhythmias, and death. With cardiac pacing, children with conduction system disease in the absence of cardiomyopathy have an excellent prognosis.

Noncardiac manifestations are typically transient and are conservatively managed, often with supportive care alone. Topical corticosteroids can be used to treat moderate to severe NLE rash. Cytopenias may improve over time, but severe cases occasionally require IVIG. Supportive care is usually appropriate for hepatic and neurologic manifestation. As the neonate clears maternal autoantibodies over the 1st 6 mo of life, these inflammatory manifestations gradually resolve.

Because maternal autoantibodies gain access to the fetus through the placenta via FcRn at about 12 wk of gestation, all pregnant women with circulating anti-Ro and/or anti-La antibodies, or those with a history of offspring with NLE or congenital heart block, are monitored by a pediatric cardiologist, with screening fetal echocardiography performed weekly from 16-26 wk of gestation and then biweekly through 34 wk. The period of greatest vulnerability is usually 18-24 wk. If fetal bradycardia is found during in utero monitoring, and if fetal echocardiography confirms a conduction defect, screening for maternal anti-Ro and anti-La antibodies is warranted. Figure 183.4 presents a proposed management algorithm.

Bibliography is available at Expert Consult.

Chapter **184**
Juvenile Dermatomyositis
Angela Byun Robinson and Ann M. Reed

第一百八十四章
幼年皮肌炎

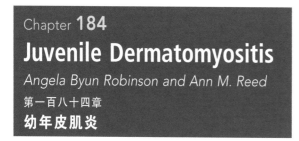

中文导读

　　本章主要介绍了幼年皮肌炎的病因、流行病学、发病机制、临床表现、诊断、鉴别诊断、实验室检查、治疗、并发症和预后。病因及发病机制中描述了易感因素及炎症级联反应等机制；流行病学中描述了发病率、性别及种族的患病差异；临床表现中描述了可能出现的症状及不同肌肉受累的临床特点；诊断及鉴别诊断中描述了诊断标准和不同情况下的鉴别要点；实验室检查中描述了不同指标的评估的作用；治

疗中描述了糖皮质激素等治疗手段的使用策略及疗效；并发症中描述了常见的并发症及其特点；预后中描述了长期预后及可能改善预后的方法。

Juvenile dermatomyositis (JDM) is the most common inflammatory myositis in children, distinguished by proximal muscle weakness and a characteristic rash. Inflammatory cell infiltrates result in *vascular inflammation,* the underlying pathology in this disorder.

ETIOLOGY

Evidence suggests that the etiology of JDM is multifactorial, based on genetic predisposition and an unknown environmental trigger. Human leukocyte antigen (HLA) alleles such as B8, DRB1*0301, DQA1*0501, and DQA1*0301 are associated with increased susceptibility to JDM in selected populations. Maternal microchimerism may play a part in the etiology of JDM by causing graft-versus-host disease (GVHD) or autoimmune phenomena. Persistent maternal cells have been found in blood and tissue samples of children with JDM. An increased number of these maternal cells are positive for HLA-DQA1*0501, which may assist with transfer or persistence of chimeric cells. Specific cytokine polymorphisms in tumor necrosis factor (TNF)-α promoter and variable-number tandem repeats of the interleukin (IL)-1 receptor antagonist may increase genetic susceptibility. These polymorphisms are common in the general population. A history of infection in the 3 mo before disease onset is usually reported; multiple studies have failed to produce a causative organism. Constitutional signs and upper respiratory symptoms predominate, but one third of patients report preceding gastrointestinal (GI) symptoms. Group A streptococcus, upper respiratory infections, GI infections, coxsackievirus B, toxoplasma, enteroviruses, parvovirus B19, and multiple other organisms have been postulated as possible pathogens in the etiology of JDM. Despite these concerns, results of serum antibody testing and polymerase chain reaction amplification of the blood and muscle tissue for multiple infectious diseases have not been revealing. Environmental factors may also play a contributing role, with geographic and seasonal clustering reported. Short-term increases in UV index prior to onset of disease have been reported; however, no clear theory of etiology has emerged.

EPIDEMIOLOGY

The incidence of JDM is approximately 3 cases/1 million children/yr, without racial predilection. Peak age of onset is 4-10 yr. A 2nd peak of dermatomyositis onset occurs in late adulthood (45-64 yr), but adult-onset dermatomyositis appears to be a distinctly separate entity in prognosis and etiology. In the United States the ratio of girls to boys with JDM is 2:1. Multiple cases of myositis in a single family are rare, but familial autoimmune disease may be increased in families with children who have JDM than in families of healthy children. Reports of seasonal association have not been confirmed, although clusters of cases may occur.

PATHOGENESIS

Interferon (IFN) upregulates genes critical in immunoregulation and major histocompatibility complex (MHC) class I expression, activates natural killer (NK) cells, and supports dendritic cell (DC) maturation. Upregulation of gene products controlled by type I IFNs occurs in patients with dermatomyositis, potentially correlating with disease activity and holding promise as clinical biomarkers.

It appears that children with genetic susceptibility to JDM (HLA-DQA1*0501, HLA-DRB*0301) may have prolonged exposure to maternal chimeric cells and/or an unknown environmental trigger. Once triggered, an inflammatory cascade with type I IFN response leads to upregulation

of MHC class I expression and maturation of DCs. Overexpression of MHC class I upregulates adhesion molecules, which influence migration of lymphocytes, leading to inflammatory infiltration of muscle. In an autoregulatory feedback loop, muscle inflammation increases the type I IFN response, regenerating the cycle of inflammation. Cells involved in the inflammatory cascade include NK cells (CD56), T-cell subsets (CD4, CD8, Th17), monocytes/macrophages (CD14), and plasmacytoid DCs. Neopterin, IFN-inducible protein 10, monocyte chemoattractant protein, myxovirus resistance protein, and von Willebrand factor products, as well as other markers of vascular inflammation, may be elevated in patients with JDM who have active inflammation.

CLINICAL MANIFESTATIONS

Children with JDM present with either rash, insidious onset of weakness, or both. Fevers, dysphagia or dysphonia, arthritis, muscle tenderness, and fatigue are also commonly reported at diagnosis (Tables 184.1 and 184.2).

Rash develops as the first symptom in 50% of patients and appears concomitant with weakness only 25% of the time. Children often exhibit extreme photosensitivity to ultraviolet (UV) light exposure with generalized erythema in sun-exposed areas. If seen over the chest and neck, this erythema is known as the **shawl sign.** Erythema is also commonly seen over the knees and elbows. The characteristic **heliotrope rash** is a blue-violet discoloration of the eyelids that may be associated with periorbital edema (Fig. 184.1). Facial erythema crossing the nasolabial folds is also common, in contrast to the malar rash without nasolabial involvement typical of systemic lupus erythematosus (SLE). Classic **Gottron papules** are bright-pink or pale, shiny, thickened or atrophic plaques over the proximal interphalangeal joints and distal interphalangeal joints and occasionally on the knees, elbows, small joints of the toes, and ankle malleoli (Fig. 184.2). The rash of JDM is sometimes mistaken for eczema or psoriasis. Rarely, a thickened erythematous and scaly rash develops in children over the palms (known as **mechanic's hands**) and soles along the flexor tendons, which is associated with anti–Jo-1 antibodies.

Table 184.1	Diagnostic Criteria for Juvenile Dermatomyositis
Classic rash	Heliotrope rash of the eyelids
	Gottron papules
Plus 3 of the following:	
Weakness	Symmetric
	Proximal
Muscle enzyme elevation (≥1)	Creatine kinase
	Aspartate transaminase
	Lactate dehydrogenase
	Aldolase
Electromyographic changes	Short, small polyphasic motor unit potentials
	Fibrillations
	Positive sharp waves
	Insertional irritability
	Bizarre, high-frequency repetitive discharges
Muscle biopsy	Necrosis
	Inflammation

Data from Bohan A, Peter JB: Polymyositis and dermatomyositis (2nd of 2 parts), *N Engl J Med* 292:403–407, 1975.

Table 184.2	Clinical Features of Juvenile Dermatomyositis During Disease Course	
FEATURE		**%**
Muscle weakness		90-100
Dysphagia or dysphonia		13-40
Muscle atrophy		10
Muscle pain and tenderness		30-75
Skin lesions		85-100
Heliotrope rash of eyelids		66-95
Gottron papules		57-95
Erythematous rash of malar/facial area		42-100
Periungual (nail fold) capillary changes		80-90
Photosensitive rash		5-42
Ulcerations		22-30
Calcinosis		12-30
Lipodystrophy		11-14
Raynaud phenomenon		2-15
Arthritis and arthralgia		22-58
Joint contractures		26-27
Fever		16-65
Gastrointestinal signs and symptoms		8-37
Restrictive pulmonary disease		4-32
Interstitial lung disease		1-7
Cardiac involvement		0-3

From Rider LG, Lindsley CB, Cassidy JT: Juvenile dermatomyositis. In Cassidy JT, Petty RE, Laxer RM, et al, editors: *Textbook of pediatric rheumatology*, ed 6, Philadelphia, 2011, Saunders (Table 24.20, p 410).

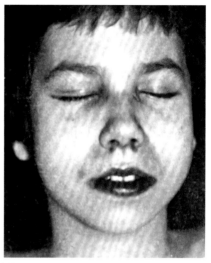

Fig. 184.1 The facial rash of juvenile dermatomyositis. There is erythema over the bridge of the nose and malar areas with violaceous (heliotropic) discolorations of the upper eyelids.

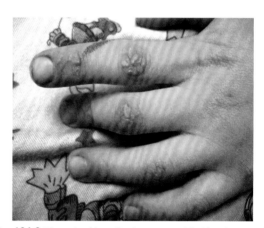

Fig. 184.2 The rash of juvenile dermatomyositis. The skin over the metacarpal and proximal interphalangeal joints may be hypertrophic and pale red (Gottron papules).

Evidence of small-vessel inflammation is often visible in the nail folds and gums as individual capillary loops that are thickened, tortuous, or absent (Fig. 184.3C). Telangiectasias may be visible to the naked eye but are more easily visualized under capillaroscopy or with a magnifier (e.g., ophthalmoscope). Severe vascular inflammation causes cutaneous ulcers on toes, fingers, axillae, or epicanthal folds.

Weakness associated with JDM is often insidious and difficult to differentiate from fatigue at onset. It is typically symmetric, affecting proximal muscles such as the neck flexors, shoulder girdle, and hip flexors. Parents may report difficulty climbing stairs, combing hair, and getting out of bed. Examination reveals inability to perform a sit-up, head lag in a child after infancy, and **Gower sign** (use of hands on thighs to stand from a sitting position). Patients with JDM may roll to the side rather than sit straight up from lying to compensate for truncal weakness. Approximately half of children exhibit muscle tenderness as a result of muscle inflammation.

Esophageal and respiratory muscles are also affected, resulting in aspiration or respiratory failure. It is essential to assess for dysphonia or nasal speech, palatal elevation with gag, dysphagia, and gastroesophageal reflux by means of history, physical examination, and swallow study, if symptoms are present. Respiratory muscle weakness can be a medical emergency and lead to respiratory failure. Children with respiratory muscle weakness do *not* manifest typical symptoms of impending respiratory failure with increased work of breathing, instead demonstrating **hypercarbia** rather than hypoxemia.

DIAGNOSIS

Diagnosis of dermatomyositis requires the presence of characteristic rash as well as at least 3 signs of muscle inflammation and weakness (see Table 184.1). Diagnostic criteria developed in 1975 predate the use

of MRI and have not been validated in children. Diagnosis is often delayed because of the insidious nature of disease onset.

Electromyography (EMG) shows signs of myopathy (increased insertional activity, fibrillations, sharp waves) as well as muscle fiber necrosis (decreased action potential amplitude and duration). Nerve conduction studies are typically normal unless severe muscle necrosis and atrophy are present. It is important that EMG be performed in a center with experience in pediatric EMG and its interpretation. Muscle biopsy is typically indicated when diagnosis is in doubt or for grading disease severity (Fig. 184.3A). Biopsy of involved muscle reveals focal necrosis and phagocytosis of muscle fibers, fiber regeneration, endomysial proliferation, inflammatory cell infiltrates and vasculitis, and tubuloreticular inclusion bodies within endothelial cells. Findings of lymphoid structures and vasculopathy may portend more severe disease.

Some children present with classic rash but no apparent muscle weakness or inflammation; this variation is called **amyopathic JDM** or **dermatomyositis sine myositis**. It is unclear whether these children have isolated skin disease or mild undetected muscle inflammation, risking progression to more severe muscle involvement with long-term sequelae such as calcinosis and lipodystrophy if untreated.

DIFFERENTIAL DIAGNOSIS

Differential diagnosis depends on the presenting symptoms. If the presenting complaint is solely weakness without rash or atypical disease, other causes of myopathy should be considered, including polymyositis, infection-related myositis (influenza A and B, coxsackievirus B, and other viral illnesses), muscular dystrophies (e.g., Duchenne, Becker), myasthenia gravis, Guillain-Barré syndrome, endocrinopathies (hyperthyroidism, hypothyroidism, Cushing syndrome, Addison disease, parathyroid disorders), mitochondrial myopathies, TNF receptor–associated periodic syndrome (TRAPS), and metabolic disorders (glycogen and lipid storage diseases). Infections associated with prominent muscular symptoms include trichinosis, *Bartonella* infection, toxoplasmosis, and staphylococcal pyomyositis. Blunt trauma and crush injuries may lead to transient rhabdomyolysis with myoglobinuria. Myositis in children may also be associated with vaccinations, drugs, growth hormone, and GVHD. The rash of JDM may be confused with eczema, dyshidrosis, psoriasis, erythema nodosa, malar rash from SLE, capillary telangiectasias from Raynaud phenomenon, and other rheumatic diseases. Muscle inflammation is also seen in children with SLE, juvenile idiopathic arthritis, mixed connective tissue disease, inflammatory bowel disease, and antineutrophil cytoplasmic antibody–positive vasculitides. Necrotizing immune-mediated myopathies are characterized by muscle necrosis without lymphocytic infiltration. Antibodies to signal recognition particle (SRP) or 3-hydroxy-3-methylglutaryl-coenzyme A (HMG-CoA) distinguish two types from each other and from JDM. Table 184.3 compares other juvenile idiopathic inflammatory myositis disorders: JDM, juvenile polymyositis, and juvenile connective tissue myositis.

LABORATORY FINDINGS

Elevated serum levels of muscle-derived enzymes (creatine kinase [CK], aldolase, aspartate transaminase, alanine transaminase [ALT], lactate dehydrogenase) reflect muscle inflammation. Not all enzyme levels rise with inflammation in a specific individual; ALT is usually elevated on initial presentation, whereas CK level may be normal. The erythrocyte sedimentation rate (ESR) is often normal, and the rheumatoid factor (RF) test result is typically negative. There may be anemia consistent with chronic disease. Antinuclear antibody (ANA) is present in >80% of children with JDM. Serologic testing results are divided into 2 groups:

myositis-associated antibodies (MAAs) and myositis-specific antibodies (MSAs). MAAs are associated with JDM, but are not specific and can be seen in both overlap conditions and other rheumatic diseases. MSAs are specific for myositis. Presence of MAAs such as SSA, SSB, Sm, ribonucleoprotein (RNP), and double-stranded (ds) DNA may increase the likelihood of overlap disease or connective tissue myositis. Antibodies to Pm/Scl identify a small, distinct subgroup of myopathies with a protracted disease course, often complicated by pulmonary interstitial fibrosis and cardiac involvement. Similar to what is seen in adults, the presence of MSAs in JDM such as anti–Jo-1, anti–Mi-2, anti-p155/140, anti-NXP2, and other myositis-specific autoantibodies help define distinct clinical subsets and may predict the development of complications, although differences remain in certain aspects such as malignancy between adults and children. Anti-p155/140 antibodies also known as TIF-1-γ are reported in 23–30% of children with JDM and are associated with photosensitive rashes, ulceration, and lipodystrophy. Unlike in adults, this antibody is not associated with malignancy in children with JDM. Anti-MJ antibodies, also known as NXP2, are reported in 12–23% of children with JDM and are associated with cramps, muscle atrophy, contractures, and dysphonia. Anti-MDA5 antibodies have been recently reported in 7–33% of children with JDM, and are concerning for development of interstitial lung disease.

Radiographic studies aid both diagnosis and medical management. MRI using T2-weighted images and fat suppression (Fig. 184.3*B*) identifies active sites of disease, reducing sampling error and increasing the sensitivity of muscle biopsy and EMG, results of which are nondiagnostic in 20% of cases if the procedures are not directed by MRI. Extensive rash and abnormal MRI findings may be found despite normal serum levels of muscle-derived enzymes. Muscle biopsy often demonstrates evidence of disease activity and chronicity that is not suspected from the levels of the serum enzymes alone.

A contrast swallow study may document palatal dysfunction and risk of aspiration. Pulmonary function testing detects a restrictive defect consistent with respiratory weakness and reduced diffusion capacity of carbon monoxide from alveolar fibrosis associated with other connective tissue diseases. Serial measurement of vital capacity or negative inspiratory force can document changes in respiratory weakness, especially in an inpatient setting. **Calcinosis** is seen easily on radiographs, along the

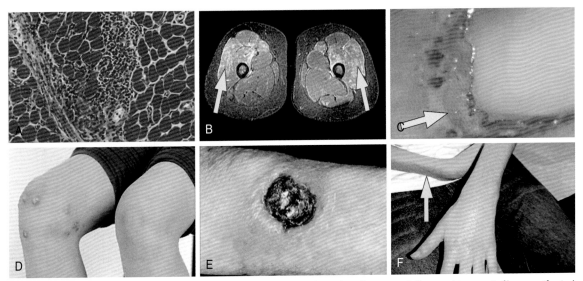

Fig. 184.3 Features of juvenile dermatomyositis. **A,** Perivascular and perifascicular inflammatory infiltrates with necrotic fibers, perifascicular atrophy, and regeneration in a muscle biopsy. **B,** MRI is a sensitive indicator of myositis. Inflamed areas appear bright on short-tau inversion recovery–weighted images *(arrows)*. **C,** Capillaries are most often abnormal when viewed at the nail fold. Typical changes of dilation with adjacent dropout *(arrow)* is seen. **D,** About 30% of juvenile dermatomyositis (JDM) patients have dystrophic calcinosis. **E,** Cutaneous ulceration with central necrosis, crust, and surrounding erythema at the elbow of 10-year-old boy with severe JDM. **F,** Lipoatrophy of the forearm *(arrow)* in a boy with JDM. *(From Feldman BM, Rider LG, Reed AM, Pachman LM: Juvenile dermatomyositis and other idiopathic inflammatory myopathies of childhood, Lancet 371:2201–2212, 2008, Fig 3, p 2205.)*

| Table 184.3 | Frequency of Manifestations of Juvenile Dermatomyositis, Juvenile Polymyositis, and Overlap Myositis |

Manifestation	FREQUENCY AT ONSET (%)		
	JDM	JPM	Overlap Myositis
Progressive proximal muscle weakness	82-100	100	100
Easy fatigue	80-100	85	84
Gottron papules	57-91	0	74-80
Heliotrope rash	66-87	0	40-59
Erythematous rash of malar/facial area	42-100	0-6	20-51
Periungual nailfold capillary changes	35-91	33	67-80
Muscle pain or tenderness	25-83	61-66	55
Weight loss	33-36	52	53
Falling episodes	40	59	29
Arthritis	10-65	0-45	69-80
Fever	16-65	0-41	0-49
Lymphadenopathy	8-75	0-12	20-22
Dysphagia or dysphonia	15-44	39	40
Joint contractures	9-55	17-42	57-60
V- or shawl-sign rashes	19-29	3-6	8-14
Dyspnea on exertion	5-43	17-42	40
Gastrointestinal symptoms	5-37	9-33	6-53
Photosensitive rashes	5-51	0-6	22-40
Raynaud phenomenon	9-28	0-24	41-60
Edema	11-34	15	20
Gingivitis	6-30	9	0-37
Cutaneous ulceration	5-30	3	20-22
Calcinosis	3-34	6	24
Cardiac involvement	2-13	36	19
Interstitial lung disease	5	15	26
Lipodystrophy	4-14	3	0-6
Gastrointestinal bleeding or ulceration	3-4	3	4-10

JDM, Juvenile dermatomyositis; JPM, juvenile polymyositis.
From Rider LG, Lindsley CB, Miller FW: Juvenile Dermatomyositis. IN Petty RE, Laxer RM, Lindsley CB, Wedderburn L, editors: *Textbook of pediatric rheumatology*, ed 7, Philadelphia, 2016, Elsevier, Table 26.4.

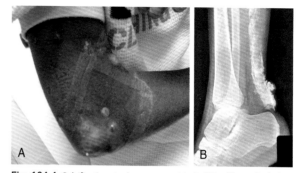

Fig. 184.4 Calcifications in dermatomyositis. **A,** Skin effects of calcification. **B,** Radiographic evidence of calcification.

fascial planes and within muscles (Figs. 184.3*D, E* and 184.4).

TREATMENT

The aid of an experienced pediatric rheumatologist is invaluable in outlining an appropriate course of treatment for a child with JDM. Before the advent of corticosteroids, one third of patients spontaneously improved, a third had a chronic, lingering course, and a third died from the disease. Corticosteroids have altered the course of disease, lowering morbidity and mortality. *Methotrexate* decreases the length of treatment with corticosteroids, thereby reducing morbidity from steroid toxicity. Intravenous (IV) gamma globulin is frequently used as an adjunct for treatment of severe disease and can be given at 2 g/kg (maximum 70 g) every 2 wk for 3 doses, then every 4 wk as needed. Consensus treatment plans for guiding treatment of North American children with JDM are available from the **Childhood Arthritis and Rheumatology Research Alliance** online through PubMed.

Corticosteroids are still the mainstay of treatment. In a clinically stable child without debilitating weakness, oral prednisone at 2 mg/kg/day (maximum 60 mg daily) is usually started. Children with GI involvement have decreased absorption of oral corticosteroids and require IV administration. In more severe cases with respiratory or oropharyngeal weakness, high-dose pulse methylprednisolone is used (30 mg/kg/day for 3 days, maximum dose 1 g/day) with ongoing weekly or monthly IV dosing along with daily oral corticosteroids as needed. Corticosteroid dosage is slowly tapered over 12 mo, after indicators of inflammation (muscle enzymes) normalize and strength improves.

Weekly oral, IV, or subcutaneous methotrexate (the lesser of 1 mg/kg or 15 mg/m², maximum 40 mg) is often used as a steroid-sparing agent in JDM. The concomitant use of methotrexate halves the cumulative dosage of steroids needed for disease control. Risks of methotrexate include immunosuppression, blood count dyscrasias, chemical hepatitis, pulmonary toxicity, nausea/vomiting, and teratogenicity. Folic acid is typically given with methotrexate starting at a dose of 1 mg daily to reduce toxicity and side effects of folate inhibition (oral ulcers, nausea, anemia). Children who are taking immunosuppressive medications such as methotrexate should avoid live-virus vaccination, although inactivated influenza vaccination is recommended yearly. An international trial found the combination of methotrexate plus corticosteroids to perform better than corticosteroids alone and with fewer side effects than corticosteroids plus cyclosporine A.

Hydroxychloroquine has little toxicity risk and is used as a secondary disease-modifying agent to reduce rash and maintain remission. Typically, it is administered at doses of 4-6 mg/kg/day orally in either tablet or liquid form. Ophthalmologic follow-up 1-2 times per year to monitor for rare retinal toxicity is recommended. Other side effects include hemolysis in patients with glucose-6-phosphate deficiency, GI intolerance, and skin/hair discoloration.

The use of *rituximab* in a trial of steroid-dependent patients with resistant inflammatory myopathies, including JDM, did not meet the primary study end-point showing a difference in time to improvement between individuals given rituximab at baseline or at 8 wk, but overall, 83% of all patients met the definition of improvement in the trial. Reports of the use of other biologic agents are based on case reports with mixed results.

Other medications for severe unresponsive disease include intravenous immune globulin, mycophenolate mofetil, cyclosporine, and cyclophosphamide. Children with pharyngeal weakness may need nasogastric or gastrostomy feedings to avoid aspiration, whereas those with GI vasculitis require full bowel rest. Rarely, children with severe respiratory weakness require ventilator therapy and even tracheostomy until the respiratory weakness improves.

Physical therapy and **occupational therapy** are integral parts of the treatment program, initially for passive stretching early in the disease course and then for direct reconditioning of muscles to regain strength and range of motion. Therapy may improve strength muscle measures and cardiovascular fitness. Bed rest is not indicated, because weight bearing improves bone density and prevents contractures. Social work and psychology services may facilitate adjustment to the frustration of physical impairment in a previously active child and aid with sleep disturbances associated with rheumatic disease.

All children with JDM should avoid sun exposure and apply high-SPF (sun protection factor) sunscreen daily, even in winter and on cloudy days. Vitamin D and calcium supplements are indicated for all children undergoing long-term corticosteroid therapy to reduce drug-induced osteopenia and osteoporosis.

COMPLICATIONS

Most complications from JDM are related to prolonged and severe weakness from muscle atrophy to cutaneous calcifications and scarring or atrophy to lipodystrophy. Secondary complications from medical treatments are also common. Children with acute and severe weakness are at risk for aspiration pneumonia and respiratory failure and occasionally require nasogastric feeding and mechanical ventilation until weakness improves. Rarely, **vasculitis** of the GI tract develops in children with severe JDM. Crampy abdominal pain and occult GI bleeding may indicate bowel wall vasculitis and lead to ischemia, GI bleeding, and perforation if not treated with complete bowel rest and aggressive treatment for the underlying inflammation. Surgery should be avoided if possible, because the GI vasculitis is diffuse and not easily amenable to surgical intervention. Contrast-enhanced CT may show dilation or thickening of the bowel wall, intraluminal air, or evidence of bowel necrosis.

Involvement of the cardiac muscle with pericarditis, myocarditis, and conduction defects with arrhythmias has been reported, as well as reduced diastolic and systolic function related to ongoing disease activity.

Lipodystrophy and **calcinosis** are thought to be associated with long-standing or undertreated disease (Fig. 184.3, *D-F*). Dystrophic deposition of calcium phosphate, hydroxyapatite, or fluoroapatite crystals occurs in subcutaneous plaques or nodules, resulting in painful ulceration of the skin with extrusion of crystals or calcific liquid. Calcification is found in up to 40% of large cohorts of children with JDM. Pathologic calcifications may be related to severity of disease and prolonged delay to treatment and potentially to genetic polymorphisms of TNF-α-308. Calcium deposits tend to form in subcutaneous tissue and along muscle. Some ulcerate through the skin and drain a soft calcific liquid, and others manifest as hard nodules along extensor surfaces or embedded along muscle. Draining lesions serve as a nidus for cellulitis or

osteomyelitis. Nodules cause skin inflammation that may mimic cellulitis. Spontaneous regression of calcium deposits may occur, but there is no evidence-based recommendation for treatment of calcinosis. Some experts recommend aggressive treatment of underlying myositis. Others have recommended bisphosphonates, TNF inhibitors, and sodium thiosulfate, but no evidence-based trials have been conducted for this condition.

Lipodystrophy manifests in 10–40% of patients with JDM and can be difficult to recognize. Lipodystrophy results in progressive loss of subcutaneous and visceral fat, typically over the face and upper body, and may be associated with a metabolic syndrome similar to polycystic ovarian syndrome with insulin resistance, hirsutism, acanthosis, hypertriglyceridemia, and abnormal glucose tolerance. Lipodystrophy may be generalized or localized.

Children receiving prolonged corticosteroid therapy are prone to complications such as cessation of linear growth, weight gain, hirsutism, adrenal suppression, immunosuppression, striae, cushingoid fat deposition, mood changes, osteoporosis, cataracts, avascular necrosis, and steroid myopathy. Families should be counseled on the effects of corticosteroids and advised to use medical alert identification and to consult a nutritionist regarding a low-salt, low-fat diet with adequate vitamin D and calcium supplementation.

An association with malignancy at disease onset is observed in adults with dermatomyositis but very rarely in children.

PROGNOSIS

The mortality rate in JDM has decreased since the advent of corticosteroids, from 33% to currently approximately 1%; little is known about the long-term consequences of persistent vascular inflammation. The period of active symptoms has decreased from about 3.5 yr to <1.5 yr with more aggressive immunosuppressive therapy; the vascular, skin, and muscle symptoms of children with JDM generally respond well to therapy. At 7 yr of follow-up, 75% of patients have little to no residual disability, but 25% continue to have chronic weakness and 40% have chronic rash. Up to one-third may need long-term medications to control their disease. Children with JDM appear able to repair inflammatory damage to vasculature and muscle, but there is some emerging concern about long-term effects on cardiovascular risk.

Bibliography is available at Expert Consult.

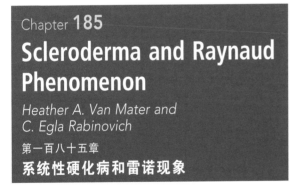

Chapter **185**

Scleroderma and Raynaud Phenomenon

Heather A. Van Mater and
C. Egla Rabinovich

第一百八十五章
系统性硬化病和雷诺现象

中文导读

本章主要介绍了系统性硬化病和雷诺现象的病因　　和发病机制、分类、流行病学、临床表现、诊断、鉴别诊断、实验室检查、治疗和预后。病因和发病机制中分析了血管病变、自身免疫和免疫激活的影像；分类中描述了不同亚型及各亚型的共存情况；流行病学中描述了不同年龄、性别及各亚型的患病差异；临床表现中描述了局限性系统性硬化病、系统性硬化症及

雷诺现象的症状特点；诊断及鉴别诊断中描述了诊断标准及鉴别要点；实验室检查中描述了各种辅助检查的作用；治疗中描述了糖皮质激素等的使用策略及疗效；预后中描述了硬皮病可能的结局及远期生存率。

Juvenile scleroderma encompasses a range of conditions unified by the presence of fibrosis of the skin. Juvenile scleroderma is divided into 2 major categories, **juvenile localized scleroderma** (JLS, also known as **morphea**), which is largely limited to the skin, and **juvenile systemic sclerosis** (JSSc), with multisystem organ involvement. Localized disease is the predominant type seen in pediatric populations (>95%), but systemic sclerosis is associated with mortality and severe multiorgan morbidity.

ETIOLOGY AND PATHOGENESIS

The etiology of scleroderma is unknown, but the mechanism of disease appears to be a combination of a vasculopathy, autoimmunity, immune activation, and fibrosis. Triggers, including trauma, infection, and, possibly, subclinical graft-versus-host reaction from persistent maternal cells (*microchimerism*), injure vascular endothelial cells, resulting in increased expression of adhesion molecules. These molecules entrap platelets and inflammatory cells, resulting in vascular changes with manifestations such as Raynaud phenomenon and pulmonary hypertension. Inflammatory cells infiltrate the area of initial vascular damage, causing further vascular damage and resulting in thickened artery walls and reduction in capillary numbers. Macrophages and other inflammatory cells then migrate into affected tissues and secrete cytokines that induce fibroblasts to reproduce and synthesize excessive amounts of collagen,

resulting in fibrosis and subsequent lipoatrophy, dermal fibrosis, with loss of sweat glands and hair follicles. In late stages the entire dermis may be replaced by compact collagen fibers.

Autoimmunity is believed to be a key process in the pathogenesis of both localized and systemic scleroderma, given the high percentage of affected children with autoantibodies. Children with localized disease often have a positive antinuclear antibody (ANA) test result (42%), and 47% of this subgroup have antihistone antibodies. Children with JSSc have higher rates of ANA positivity (80.7%) and may have anti–Scl-70 antibody (34%, antitopoisomerase I). The relationship between specific autoantibodies and the various forms of scleroderma is not well understood, and all antibody test results may be negative, especially in JLS.

CLASSIFICATION

Localized scleroderma is distinct from systemic scleroderma and rarely progresses to systemic disease. The category of JLS includes several subtypes differentiated by both the distribution of the lesions and the depth of involvement (Tables 185.1 and 185.2). Up to 15% of children have a combination of 2 or more subtypes.

EPIDEMIOLOGY

Juvenile scleroderma is rare, with an estimated prevalence of 1 in 100,000 children. LS is much more common than SSc in children, by a 10:1

Table 185.1	Classification of Pediatric Scleroderma (Morphea)

LOCALIZED SCLERODERMA

Plaque Morphea
Confined to dermis, occasionally superficial panniculus
Well-circumscribed circular area of induration, often a central waxy, ivory-colored area surrounded by a violaceous halo; unilateral

Generalized Morphea
Involves dermis primarily, occasionally panniculus
Defined as confluence of individual morphea plaques or lesions in ≥3 anatomic sites; more likely to be bilateral

Bullous Morphea
Bullous lesions that can occur with any of the subtypes of morphea

Linear Scleroderma
Linear lesions can extend through the dermis, subcutaneous tissue, and muscle to underlying bone; more likely unilateral
Limbs/trunk:
 One or more linear streaks of the extremities or trunk
 Flexion contracture occurs when lesion extends over a joint; limb length discrepancies
En coup de sabre:
 Involves the scalp and/or face; lesions can extend into the central nervous system, resulting in neurologic sequelae, most commonly seizures and headaches
Parry-Romberg syndrome:
 Hemifacial atrophy without a clearly definable en coup de sabre lesion; can also have neurologic involvement

Deep Morphea
Involves deeper layers, including panniculus, fascia, and muscle; more likely to be bilateral
Subcutaneous morphea:
 Primarily involves the panniculus or subcutaneous tissue
 Plaques are hyperpigmented and symmetric
Eosinophilic fasciitis:
 Fasciitis with marked blood eosinophilia
 Fascia is the primary site of involvement; typically involves extremities
 Classic description is "peau d'orange" or orange peel texture, but early disease manifests as edema (see Fig. 185.2)
Morphea profunda:
 Deep lesion extending to fascia and sometimes muscle, but may be limited to a single plaque, often on trunk
Disabling pansclerotic morphea of childhood:
 Generalized full-thickness involvement of skin on the trunk, face and extremities, sparing fingertips and toes

SYSTEMIC SCLEROSIS
Diffuse
Most common type in childhood
Symmetric thickening and hardening of the skin (sclerosis) with fibrous and degenerative changes of viscera

Limited
Rare in childhood
Previously known as CREST (calcinosis cutis, Raynaud phenomenon, esophageal dysfunction, sclerodactyly, and telangiectasia) syndrome

Table 185.2	Provisional Criteria for Classification of Juvenile Systemic Sclerosis (JSSc)

MAJOR CRITERION (REQUIRED)*
Proximal skin sclerosis/induration of the skin proximal to metacarpophalangeal or metatarsophalangeal joints

MINOR CRITERIA (AT LEAST 2 REQUIRED)
Cutaneous: Sclerodactyly
Peripheral vascular: Raynaud phenomenon, nail fold capillary abnormalities (telangiectasias), digital tip ulcers
Gastrointestinal: Dysphagia, gastroesophageal reflux
Cardiac: Arrhythmias, heart failure
Renal: Renal crisis, new-onset arterial hypertension
Respiratory: Pulmonary fibrosis (high-resolution CT/radiography), decreased diffusing capacity for carbon monoxide, pulmonary arterial hypertension
Neurologic: Neuropathy, carpal tunnel syndrome
Musculoskeletal: Tendon friction rubs, arthritis, myositis
Serologic: Antinuclear antibodies—SSc-selective autoantibodies (anticentromere, antitopoisomerase I [Scl-70], antifibrillarin, anti-PM/Scl, antifibrillin, or anti-RNA polymerase I or III

*Diagnosis requires at least 1 major and at least 2 minor criteria.
From Zulian F, Woo P, Athreya BH, et al: The Pediatric Rheumatology European Society/American College of Rheumatology/European League against Rheumatism provisional classification criteria for juvenile systemic sclerosis, *Arthritis Rheum* 57:203–212, 2007.

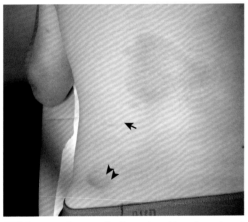

Fig. 185.1 Boy with generalized morphea. Note the active circular lesion *(arrowheads)* with a surrounding rim of erythema. The largest lesion has areas of postinflammatory hyperpigmentation and depression with an area of erythema on the right. The small lesion *(arrow)* demonstrates depression caused by lipoatrophy.

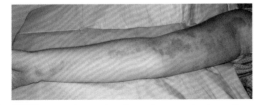

Fig. 185.2 Inactive linear scleroderma demonstrating hyperpigmented lesion with areas of normal skin (skip lesions).

ratio, with **linear scleroderma** being the most common subtype. LS is predominantly a pediatric condition, with 65% of patients diagnosed before age 18 yr. After age 8 yr the female/male ratio for both LS and SSc is approximately 3 : 1, whereas in patients younger than 8 yr, there is no sex predilection.

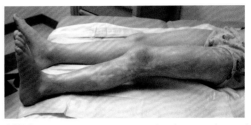

Fig. 185.3 Child with untreated linear scleroderma resulting in knee contracture, immobility of ankle, chronic skin breakdown of scar on the lateral knee, and areas of hypopigmentation and hyperpigmentation. The affected leg is 1 cm shorter.

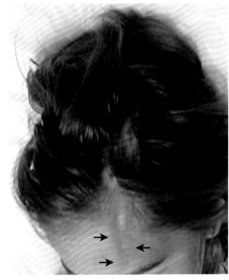

Fig. 185.4 Child with en coup de sabre lesion on scalp extending down to forehead. Before treatment, the skin on the scalp was bound down with chronic skin breakdown. Note the area of hypopigmentation extending down the forehead *(arrows)*.

CLINICAL MANIFESTATIONS
Localized Scleroderma
The onset of scleroderma is generally insidious, and manifestations vary according to disease subtype. The initial skin manifestations of localized disease usually include erythema or a bluish hue seen around an area of waxy induration; subtle erythema may be the only presenting sign (Fig. 185.1). Edema and erythema are followed by indurated, hypopigmented or hyperpigmented atrophic lesions (Fig. 185.2). LS varies in size from a few centimeters to the entire length of the extremity, with varying depth. Patients may present with arthralgias, synovitis, or flexion contractures (Fig. 185.3). Children also experience limb length discrepancies as a result of growth impairment caused by involvement of muscle and bone. Children with **en coup de sabre** may have symptoms unique to central nervous system (CNS) involvement, such as seizures, hemifacial atrophy, ipsilateral uveitis, and learning/behavioral changes (Fig. 185.4). Up to 25% of children with LS have extracutaneous manifestations, most frequently arthritis (47%) and neurologic symptoms (17%) associated with en coup de sabre.

Systemic Scleroderma
SSc also has an insidious onset with a prolonged course characterized by periods of remission and exacerbation, ending in either remission or, more often, chronic disability and death.

The **skin manifestations** of SSc include an early phase of edema that spreads proximally from the dorsum of the hands and fingers and includes the face. An eventual decrease in edema is followed by induration and fibrosis of skin, ultimately resulting in loss of subcutaneous fat, sweat glands, and hair follicles. Later, atrophic skin becomes shiny and waxy in appearance. As lesions spread proximally, flexion contractures develop at the elbows, hips, and knees associated with secondary muscle weakness and atrophy. In the face, this process results in a small oral stoma with decreased mouth aperture. Skin ulceration over pressure points, such as the elbows, may be associated with subcutaneous calcifications. Severe **Raynaud phenomenon** causes ulceration of the fingertips with subsequent loss of tissue pulp and tapered fingers (**sclerodactyly**) (Fig. 185.5). Resorption of the distal tufts of the distal phalanges may occur (**acrosteolysis**). Hyperpigmented postinflammatory changes surrounded by atrophic depigmentation gives a salt-and-pepper appearance to skin.

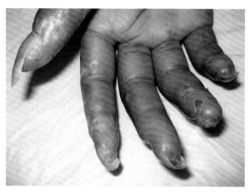

Fig. 185.5 Sclerodactyly and finger ulcerations in a patient with systemic sclerosis who is poorly compliant with treatment.

Over years, remodeling of lesions sometimes results in focal improvement in skin thickening.

Pulmonary disease is the most common visceral manifestation of SSc and includes both arterial and interstitial involvement (alveolitis). Symptoms range from asymptomatic disease to exercise intolerance, dyspnea at rest, and right-sided heart failure. **Pulmonary arterial hypertension** is a poor prognostic sign, developing because of lung disease or independently as part of the vasculopathy. Clinical manifestations of pulmonary arterial hypertension in children appear late in the course, are subtle, and include cough and dyspnea on exertion. Pulmonary evaluation should include pulmonary function tests (PFTs) such as diffusion capacity of carbon monoxide (DLCO), bronchoalveolar lavage (BAL), and high-resolution chest computed tomography (HRCT). PFTs reveal decreased vital capacity and decreased DLCO, whereas neutrophilia or eosinophilia on BAL suggest active alveolitis. Chest CT is much more sensitive than chest radiographs, which are often normal, showing typical basilar ground-glass abnormalities, reticular linear opacities, nodules, honeycombing, and mediastinal adenopathy.

Gastrointestinal tract disease is seen in 25% of children with SSc. Common manifestations include esophageal and intestinal dysmotility resulting in dysphagia, reflux, dyspepsia, gastroparesis, bacterial overgrowth, dilated bowel loops and pseudoobstruction, and dental caries, as well as malabsorption and failure to thrive. **Renal** arterial disease can cause chronic or severe episodic hypertension; unlike adult disease, renal crisis is rare. **Cardiac** fibrosis is associated with arrhythmias, ventricular hypertrophy, and decreased cardiac function. Mortality from JSSc is usually a result of cardiopulmonary disease. A scoring system helps identify the severity of the multiorgan involvement (Table 185.3).

Raynaud Phenomenon

Raynaud phenomenon (RP) is the most frequent initial symptom in pediatric systemic sclerosis, present in 70% of affected children months

Table 185.3	Medsger Systemic Sclerosis Severity Scale*				
ORGAN SYSTEM	**0 (NORMAL)**	**1 (MILD)**	**2 (MODERATE)**	**3 (SEVERE)**	**4 (END STAGE)**
General	Wt loss <5% Hct 37%+ Hb 12.3+ g/dL	Wt loss 5–10% Hct 33–37% Hb 11.0-12.2 g/dL	Wt loss 10–15% Hct 29–33% Hb 9.7-10.9 g/dL	Wt loss 15–20% Hct 25–29% Hb 8.3-9.6 g/dL	Wt loss 20%+ Hct 25% Hb <8.3 g/dL
Peripheral vascular	No RP; RP not requiring vasodilators	RP requiring vasodilators	Digital pitting scars	Digital tip ulcerations	Digital gangrene
Skin	TSS 0	TSS 1-14	TSS 15-29	TSS 30-39	TSS 40+
Joint/tendon	FTP 0-0.9 cm	FTP 1.0-1.9 cm	FTP 2.0-3.9 cm	FTP 4.0-4.9 cm	FTP 5.0+ cm
Muscle	Normal proximal muscle strength	Proximal weakness, mild	Proximal weakness, moderate	Proximal weakness, severe	Ambulation aids required
Gastrointestinal tract	Normal esophagogram; normal small bowel series	Distal esophageal hypoperistalsis; small bowel series abnormal	Antibiotics required for bacterial overgrowth	Malabsorption syndrome; episodes of pseudoobstruction	Hyperalimentation required
Lung	DLCO 80%+ FVC 80%+ No fibrosis on radiograph sPAP <35 mm Hg	DLCO 70–79% FVC 70–79% Basilar rales; fibrosis on radiograph sPAP 35-49 mm Hg	DLCO 50–69% FVC 50–69% sPAP 50-64 mm Hg	DLCO <50% FVC <50% sPAP 65+ mm Hg	Oxygen required
Heart	ECG normal LVEF 50%+	ECG conduction defect LVEF 45–49%	ECG arrhythmia LVEF 40–44%	ECG arrhythmia requiring therapy LVEF 30–40%	CHF LVEF <30%
Kidney	No history of SRC with serum creatinine <1.3 mg/dL	History of SRC with serum creatinine <1.5 mg/dL	History of SRC with serum creatinine 1.5-2.4 mg/dL	History of SRC with serum creatinine 2.5-5.0 mg/dL	History of SRC with serum creatinine >5.0 mg/dL or dialysis required

CHF, Congestive heart failure; DLCO, diffusing capacity for carbon monoxide, % predicted; ECG, electrocardiogram; FTP, fingertip-to-palm distance in flexion; FVC, forced vital capacity, % predicted; Hb, hemoglobin; Hct, hematocrit; LVEF, left ventricular ejection fraction; RP, Raynaud phenomenon; sPAP, estimated pulmonary artery pressure by Doppler echo; SRC, scleroderma renal crisis; TSS, total skin score; Wt, weight.

*If 2 items are included for a severity grade, only 1 is required for the patient to be scored as having disease of that severity level.

Modified from Medsger TA Jr, Bombardieri S, Czirjak L, et al: Assessment of disease severity and prognosis, *Clin Exp Rheumatol* 21(3 Suppl 29):S51, 2003 (Table 1, p S-43).

to years before other manifestations. RP refers to the classic triphasic sequence of blanching, cyanosis, and erythema of the digits induced by cold exposure and/or emotional stress. RP is typically independent of an underlying rheumatic disease (Raynaud disease) but can result from rheumatic diseases such as scleroderma, systemic lupus erythematosus (SLE), and mixed connective tissue disease (Fig. 185.6). The color changes are brought about by (1) initial arterial vasoconstriction, resulting in hypoperfusion and pallor (blanching), (2) venous stasis (cyanosis), and (3) reflex vasodilation caused by the factors released from the ischemic phase (erythema). The color change is classically reproduced by immersing the hands in iced water and reversed by warming. During the blanching phase, there is inadequate tissue perfusion in the affected area, associated with pain and paresthesias and resulting in ischemic damage only when associated with a rheumatic disease. The blanching usually affects the distal fingers but may also involve thumbs, toes, ears, and tip of the nose. The affected area is usually well demarcated and uniformly white. *Digital ulcers* associated with RP are indicative of underlying rheumatic disease.

Raynaud disease often begins in adolescence and is characterized by symmetric occurrence, the absence of tissue necrosis and gangrene, and the lack of manifestations of an underlying rheumatic disease. Children have normal nail fold capillaries (absence of periungual telangiectasias). RP should be distinguished from acrocyanosis and chilblains. **Acrocyanosis** is a vasospastic disorder resulting in cool, painless, bluish discoloration in the hands and sometimes feet despite normal tissue perfusion. It may be exacerbated by stimulant medications used to treat attention-deficit disorder. **Chilblains** is a condition with episodic color changes and the development of nodules related to severe cold exposure and spasm-induced vessel and tissue damage; it has been associated with SLE.

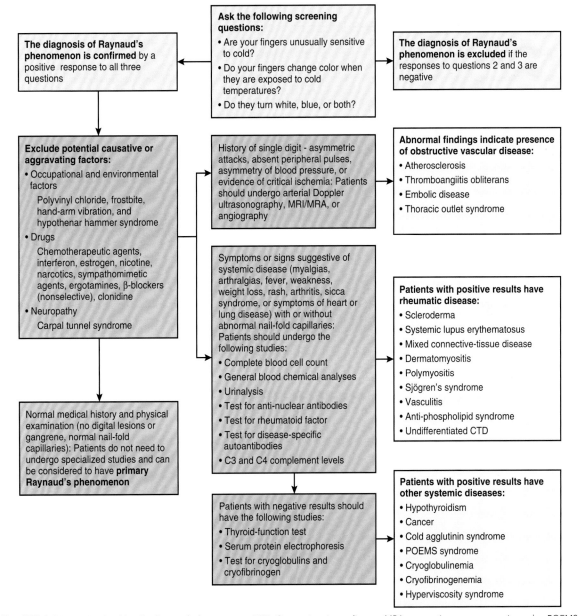

Fig. 185.6 Diagnostic algorithm for Raynaud phenomenon. CTD, Connective tissue disease; MRA, magnetic resonance angiography; POEMS, polyneuropathy, organomegaly, endocrinopathy, monoclonal gammopathy, and skin changes. *(From Firestein GS, Budd, RC, Gabriel SE, et al, editors: Kelley & Firestein's textbook of rheumatology, ed 10, Philadelphia, 2016, Elsevier, Fig 84-3.)*

DIAGNOSIS

The diagnosis of JLS is based on the distribution and depth of characteristic lesions. Biopsy is helpful to confirm the diagnosis. The diagnosis of JSSc requires proximal sclerosis/induration of the skin as well as the presence of 2 of 20 minor criteria (see Table 185.2).

DIFFERENTIAL DIAGNOSIS

The most important condition to differentiate from JLS is JSSc. Contractures and synovitis from juvenile arthritis can be differentiated from those caused by linear scleroderma by the absence of skin changes. Other conditions to consider include chemically induced scleroderma-like disease, diabetic cheiroarthropathy, pseudoscleroderma, and scleredema. **Pseudoscleroderma** comprises a group of unrelated diseases characterized by patchy or diffuse cutaneous fibrosis without the other manifestations of scleroderma. These include phenylketonuria, syndromes of premature aging, and localized idiopathic fibrosis. **Scleredema** is a transient, self-limited disease of both children and adults that has sudden onset after a febrile illness (especially streptococcal infections) and is characterized by patchy sclerodermatous lesions on the neck and shoulders and extending to the face, trunk, and arms.

LABORATORY FINDINGS

No laboratory studies are diagnostic of either localized or systemic scleroderma. Although the results of complete blood counts, serum chemistry analyses, and urinalysis are normal, children may have elevated erythrocyte sedimentation rate, eosinophilia, or hypergammaglobulinemia, all of which normalize with treatment. Elevations of muscle enzymes, particularly aldolase, can be seen with muscle involvement. Patients with JSSc may have anemia, leukocytosis, and eosinophilia and autoantibodies (ANA, anti–Scl-70). Imaging studies delineate the affected area and can be used to follow disease progression. MRI is useful in en coup de sabre and Parry-Romberg syndrome (facial hemiatrophy) for determination of CNS or orbital involvement. Infrared thermography uses the temperature variation between areas of active and inactive cutaneous disease to help differentiate active disease from damage. The role of ultrasound to examine lesion activity is evolving. HRCT, PFTs, echocardiography, and manometry are useful tools for diagnosing and monitoring visceral involvement in JSSc.

TREATMENT

Treatment for scleroderma varies according to the subtype and severity. Superficial morphea may benefit from topical corticosteroids or ultraviolet therapy. For lesions involving deeper structures, systemic therapy is recommended. A combination of *methotrexate* and *corticosteroids* is effective in treating **JLS** by preventing lesion extension and resulting in significant skin softening and improved range of motion of affected joints. The treatment plan for JLS includes (1) weekly subcutaneous (SC) methotrexate at 1 mg/kg (maximum dose 25 mg); (2) weekly SC methotrexate (1 mg/kg; max 25 mg) *plus* either 3 mo of high-dose intravenous (IV) corticosteroids (30 mg/kg; max 1,000 mg) for 3 consecutive days a month *or* weekly corticosteroids at the same dose for 3 mo; or (3) high-dose daily oral corticosteroids (2 mg/kg/day, max 60 mg) with a slow taper over 48 wk. *Mycophenolate mofetil* (MMF) is a second-line agent for recalcitrant disease. Physical and occupational therapy are important adjuncts to pharmacologic treatment. Eosinophilic fasciitis often responds well to corticosteroids and methotrexate.

Treatments for **JSSc** target specific disease manifestations. **RP** is treated with cold avoidance, and pharmacologic interventions are reserved for severe disease. Calcium channel blockers (nifedipine, 30-60 mg sustained-release form daily; amlodipine, 2.5-10 mg daily) are the most common pharmacologic interventions. Additional potential therapies for RP include losartan, prazosin, bosentan, and sildenafil. Angiotensin-converting enzyme (ACE) inhibitors (captopril, enalapril) are recommended for hypertension associated with renal disease. Methotrexate or MMF may be beneficial for skin manifestations. Cyclophosphamide and MMF are used to treat pulmonary alveolitis and prevent fibrosis. Corticosteroids should be used cautiously in SSc because of an association with renal crisis. Adults with SSc have been successfully treated with high-dose cyclophosphamide, antithymocyte globulin, and autologous stem cell transplantation.

The treatment of **RP** begins with avoiding cold stimuli, using hand and foot warmers, and avoiding carrying bags by their handles (impairs circulation). Nifedipine (10-20 mg 3 times daily adult dose) reduces but does not eliminate the number and severity of episodes. Side effects include headache, flushing, and hypotension. Topical nitrates may result in digital vasodilation and may reduce the severity of an episode.

PROGNOSIS

JLS is generally self-limited, with initial inflammatory stage followed by a period of stabilization and then softening, for an average disease duration of 3-5 yr, although there are reports of active disease lasting up to 20 yr. Prolonged disease activity is associated primarily with linear and deep disease subtypes. JLS, especially linear and deep subtypes, can result in significant morbidity, disfigurement, and disability as a result of joint contractures, muscle atrophy, limb shortening, facial asymmetry, and hyper- and hypopigmentation. Death from a en coup de sabre lesion with progressive neurologic decline has been reported.

JSSc has a more variable prognosis. Although many children have a slow, insidious course, others demonstrate a rapidly progressive form with early organ failure and death. Skin manifestations reportedly soften years after disease onset. Overall, the prognosis of JSSc is better than that of the adult form, with 5-, 10-, and 15-year survival rates, respectively, in children of 89%, 80–87%, and 74–87%. The most common cause of death is heart failure caused by myocardial and pulmonary fibrosis.

Bibliography is available at Expert Consult.

Chapter 186
Behçet Disease
Seza Özen

第一百八十六章
白塞综合征

中文导读

本章主要介绍了白塞综合征的流行病学、病因与发病机制、临床表现与诊断、治疗与预后。流行病学中描述了不同种族、性别的患病率及家族特点；病因与发病机制中分析了基因位点、炎症反应及病毒感染因素；临床表现与诊断中描述了疾病的临床特点及各个系统受累的临床表现；治疗可使用咪唑硫嘌呤、阿普斯特、秋水仙碱、抗TNF-α，白塞综合征患者死亡率很低，早期诊断和有效治疗可提高预后。

Behçet disease (BD) is classified as a primary *variable vessel vasculitis*, emphasizing the involvement of any size and type (arterial, venous) of blood vessel. BD is also recognized as an autoinflammatory disease. Originally described with recurrent oral ulcerations, uveitis, and skin abnormalities, the BD spectrum is much broader.

EPIDEMIOLOGY
Behçet disease has a high prevalence in countries along the *Silk Road,* extending from Japan to the eastern Mediterranean. It is increasingly recognized among people of European ancestry. BD has a prevalence of 5-7 per 100,000 adults, which makes it more frequent than the other vasculitides such as granulomatosis polyangiitis (Wegener disease). The increased disease recognition might have had a role in the rising prevalence of BD as well as the immigrations of the 20th century. Prevalence in children is probably not more than 10% of the adult counterparts in eastern Mediterranean countries; boys and girls are equally affected. Family history of BD is present in approximately 20% of the cases. Onset in children is 8-12 yr of age. Newborns of affected mothers have demonstrated symptoms of BD.

ETIOLOGY AND PATHOGENESIS
Behçet disease is a polygenic autoinflammatory disorder. Genetic contribution to BD is evident through the well-known association with HLA-B5101, the familial cases, the sibling and twin recurrence rate, the specific frequency of the disease among people along the Silk Road, evidence for genetic anticipation, and genome-wide analysis. Genome wide analysis studies among Turkish and Japanese BD patients confirm the marked association with HLA-B5101. Other significant associations include interleukin (IL)-10 and IL-23R/IL-12Rβ_2 genes. Other possible susceptibility loci in a Turkish cohort demonstrate associations with *STAT4* (a transcription factor in a signaling pathway related to cytokines such as IL-12, type I interferons, and IL-23) and *ERAP1* (an endoplasmic reticulum–expressed aminopeptidase that functions in processing of peptides onto major histocompatibility complex class I).

The autoinflammatory nature of BD is suggested by its episodic nature, the prominent innate immune system activation, the absence of identifiable autoantibodies, and the co-association with the *MEFV* (Mediterranean fever) gene. An infectious agent may be responsible for inducing the aberrant innate immune system attacks in the genetically predisposed host. A number of infectious agents have been implicated and include streptococci, herpes simplex virus type 1, and parvovirus B19.

CLINICAL MANIFESTATIONS AND DIAGNOSIS
The course of BD is characterized by exacerbations and remissions. There is also marked heterogeneity in disease manifestation (Table 186.1).

The mean age of the first symptom is between 8 and 12 yr. The most frequent initial symptom is a painful **oral ulcer** (Fig. 186.1). The oral

Table 186.1	Consensus Classification of Pediatric Behçet Disease
ITEM	**DESCRIPTION**
Recurrent oral aphthosis	At least three attacks/year
Genital ulceration or aphthosis	Typically with scar
Skin involvement	Necrotic folliculitis, acneiform lesions, erythema nodosum
Ocular involvement	Anterior uveitis, posterior uveitis, retinal vasculitis
Neurologic signs	With the exception of isolated headaches
Vascular signs	Venous thrombosis, arterial thrombosis, arterial aneurysm

From Koné-Paut I, Shahram F, Darce-Bello M, et al, for PEDBD group: Consensus classification criteria for paediatric Behçet's disease from a prospective observational cohort: PEDBD, *Ann Rheum Dis* 75:958–964, 2016.

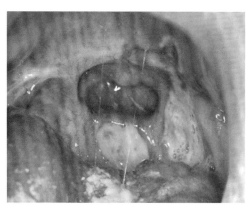

Fig. 186.1 A major aphthous ulcer in a patient with Behçet disease. *(From Summers SA, Tilakaratne WM, Fortune F, Ashman N: Renal disease and the mouth. Am J Med 120:568-573, 2007.)*

ulcers are often recurrent, may be single or multiple, range from 2-10 mm, and may be in any location in the oral cavity. They are often very painful. The oral ulcers last 3-10 days and heal without scarring. In contrast, the genital ulcers heal with scars. Genital scars are noted in 60–85% of the patients, usually occur after puberty, and are seen on the labia, scrotum, penis, or the anal area.

Another key feature of BD that has significant morbidity is bilateral eye involvement seen in 30–60% of pediatric patients. The main symptoms of **anterior uveitis** are blurred vision, redness, periorbital or global pain, and photophobia. Although it is often in the form of panuveitis, anterior uveitis may be seen in females. Uveitis in general is more common in males. Vitreitis and retinal vasculitis are the most prominent features of posterior involvement. Complications of uveitis include blindness (unusual with treatment), glaucoma, and cataracts. Retinal vasculitis, retinal detachment, and retrobulbar neuritis (optic neuritis) are less common eye manifestations of BD.

The **skin lesions** of BD range from erythema nodosum (seen in approximately 50% of patients) to papulopustular acneiform lesions (85%), folliculitis, purpura, and ulcers. **Pathergy** (seen in 50%) is another skin feature associated with BD and is a pustular reaction occurring 24-48 hr after a sterile needle puncture or saline injection; it is not pathognomonic of BD.

The **vasculitis** of BD involves both arteries and veins, thrombosis and aneurysm formation, occlusions, or stenosis in arteries of any size. In children, deep venous thrombosis of the lower limbs is the most frequent vasculitic feature. If the hepatic vein is thrombosed, Budd-Chiari syndrome may occur. Pulmonary aneurysms are the most severe feature of pediatric BD, associated with the highest mortality. Coronary artery aneurysms may confuse BD with Kawasaki disease. Microvascular involvement may be noted in the nail bed capillaries.

Central nervous system (CNS) manifestations (approximately 10%) in children include meningoencephalitis (headache, meningismus, cerebrospinal fluid pleocytosis), encephalomyelitis, pseudotumor cerebri, dural sinus thrombosis, and organic psychiatric disorders (psychosis, depression, dementia). **Dural sinus thrombosis** is the most common CNS manifestation in children.

Gastrointestinal (GI) involvement (seen in 10–30%) manifests with abdominal pain, diarrhea, and intestinal ulcerations, most often in the ileocecal region. Gastrointestinal BD may be difficult to distinguish from inflammatory bowel disease. Oligoarticular **arthritis/arthralgia** is present in >50% of patients and can be recurrent, but is nondeforming. Other rare manifestations include orchitis, renal vasculitis, glomerulonephritis, or amyloidosis and cardiac involvement.

The **International Study Group for Behçet Disease** (ISG) criteria are most widely used and require the presence of oral ulcers (at least 3 times per year) along with 2 other major features, including genital ulcers, a positive pathergy test, uveitis, and the characteristic skin lesions (see Table 186.1). If only 1 of the criteria is present along with oral ulcerations, the term *incomplete* or *partial Behçet disease* is applied.

Classification criteria for children have been suggested by the use of an international prospective observational cohort. According to these criteria, BD is diagnosed when 3 of the following criteria are present: recurrent oral aphthosis, genital ulcers, skin involvement (necrotic folliculitis, acneiform lesions, erythema nodosum), ocular involvement, neurologic involvement, and vascular involvement (venous thrombosis, arterial thrombosis, arterial aneurysm). These criteria performed better than the ISG criteria in the pediatric cohort.

There are no specific laboratory tests. Acute-phase reactants are often mildly elevated. The diagnosis relies on the constellation of symptoms and excluding other causes.

TREATMENT AND PROGNOSIS

Azathioprine is highly recommended to treat inflammatory eye disease. Anti–tumor necrosis factor (TNF) treatment and interferon (IFN)-α should be considered for refractory eye disease. For oral and genital ulcers, topical treatment is recommended (sucralfate, corticosteroids). A placebo-controlled study has shown that *apremilast*, an oral phosphodiesterase-4 inhibitor, is effective in treating the oral ulcers of Behçet disease. *Colchicine* is recommended for erythema nodosum or arthritis in males and females and for genital ulcers in females. There is no evidence-based treatment for GI disease, but thalidomide, sulfasalazine, corticosteroids, azathioprine, and anti-TNF agents have been recommended. For CNS disease and vasculitis, corticosteroids, azathioprine, cyclophosphamide, and IFN-α are recommended, and in unresponsive CNS disease, anti-TNF agents. There is no consensus about the benefit of anticoagulation in the management of vein thrombosis in BD.

In patients without major organ involvement, colchicine significantly improves oral and genital ulcers, skin features, and disease activity. In pediatric patients with vascular involvement with venous thrombosis, corticosteroids and azathioprine have been used. In patients with pulmonary arterial or cardiac involvement, cyclophosphamide is typically used initially. Patients treated with anti-TNF drugs have had persistent responses in 90%, 89%, 100%, and 91% of patients with resistant mucocutaneous, ocular, GI, and CNS involvement, respectively.

Mortality in children with BD is low except for the pulmonary aneurysms. However, BD is a chronic disease associated with significant morbidity. Early diagnosis and effective treatment improve the outcome of BD.

Bibliography is available at Expert Consult.

Chapter **187**
Sjögren Syndrome
C. Egla Rabinovich

第一百八十七章
干燥综合征

中文导读

本章主要介绍了干燥综合征的流行病学、病因和发病机制、临床表现、诊断、鉴别诊断、治疗及并发症与预后。流行病学中描述了不同种族、性别的患病率；病因和发病机制分析了遗传易感及感染触发因素；临床表现中描述了外分泌腺体受累及非外分泌腺表现；诊断中具体描述了基于临床表现、病理及其他辅助检查的诊断价值；治疗上阐述了对症治疗策略及包括糖皮质激素、非甾体抗炎药和羟氯喹在内的治疗；并发症与预后上，本病进展缓慢，可能并发黏膜相关淋巴瘤。

Sjögren syndrome is a chronic, inflammatory, autoimmune disease characterized by progressive lymphocytic and plasma cell infiltration of the exocrine glands, especially salivary and lacrimal, with potential for systemic manifestations. It is rare in children and predominantly affects middle-age women with classic symptoms of dry eyes (**keratoconjunctivitis sicca**) and dry mouth (**xerostomia**).

EPIDEMIOLOGY
Sjögren syndrome typically manifests at 35-45 yr of age, with 90% of cases among women, but it is underrecognized in children because symptoms often start in childhood. The mean age at diagnosis in children is 9-10 yr; 75% are girls. The disease can occur as an isolated disorder, referred to as **primary** Sjögren syndrome (**sicca complex**), or as a **secondary** Sjögren syndrome in association with other rheumatic disorders, such as systemic lupus erythematosus (SLE), scleroderma, or mixed connective tissue disease, which usually precedes the associated autoimmune disease by years.

ETIOLOGY AND PATHOGENESIS
The etiology of Sjögren syndrome is complex and includes genetic predisposition and possibly an infectious trigger. Lymphocytes and plasma cells infiltrate salivary glands, forming distinct periductal and periacinar foci that become confluent and may replace epithelial structure. Several genes regulating apoptosis influence the chronicity of lymphocytic infiltration.

CLINICAL MANIFESTATIONS
International classification criteria have been developed for the diagnosis of Sjögren syndrome in adult patients, but these criteria apply poorly to children. Although diagnostic criteria in children have been proposed, they have not been validated (Table 187.1). Recurrent parotid gland

Table 187.1	Proposed Criteria for Pediatric Sjögren Syndrome*

I. CLINICAL SYMPTOMS
 1. Oral: recurrent parotitis or enlargement of parotid gland, dry mouth (xerostomia)
 2. Ocular: dry eyes (xerophthalmia) recurrent conjunctivitis without obvious allergic or infectious etiology, keratoconjunctivitis sicca
 3. Other mucosal: recurrent vaginitis
 4. Systemic: fever, noninflammatory arthralgias, hypokalemic paralysis, abdominal pain
II. IMMUNOLOGIC ABNORMALITIES
 Presence of at least 1 of the following antibodies: anti-SSA, anti-SSB, high-titer antinuclear antibody, rheumatoid factor
III. OTHER ABNORMALITIES OR INVESTIGATIONS
 1. Biochemical: elevated serum amylase
 2. Hematologic: leukopenia, high erythrocyte sedimentation rate
 3. Immunologic: polyclonal hyperimmunoglobulinemia
 4. Renal: renal tubular acidosis
 5. Histologic proof of lymphocytic infiltration of salivary glands or other organs (i.e., liver)
 6. Objective documentation of ocular dryness (rose bengal staining or Schirmer test)
 7. Positive findings of parotid gland scintigraphy
IV. Exclusion of all other autoimmune diseases

*Diagnosis requires ≥4 criteria.
 From Bartunkova J. Primary Sjögren syndrome in children and adolescents: proposal for diagnostic criteria, *Clin Exp Rheumatol* 17:381–386, 1999.

enlargement and parotitis are the most common manifestations in children (>70%), whereas **sicca syndrome** (dry mouth, painful mucosa, sensitivity to spicy foods, halitosis, widespread dental caries) predominates in adults. In a cross-sectional study of children with Sjögren syndrome, manifestations included recurrent parotitis (72%), sicca symptoms (38%), polyarthritis (18%), vulvovaginitis (12%), hepatitis (10%), Raynaud phenomenon (10%), fever (8%), renal tubular acidosis (9%), lymphadenopathy (8%), and central nervous system (CNS) involvement (5%).

Subjective symptoms of xerostomia complaints are relatively rare in juvenile cases, perhaps indicating that Sjögren syndrome is a slowly progressive disease; however, increased dental caries is seen clinically in children. Serologic markers (antinuclear antibodies [ANAs], antibodies to Ro [SSA] and La [SSB]) and articular manifestations are significantly more common in adults. Reported frequencies of ANAs and SSA and SSB antibodies in children are 78%, 75%, and 65%, respectively, with rheumatoid factor present in 67%. Additional clinical manifestations from a variety of organ involvement patterns include a decreased sense of smell, hoarseness, chronic otitis media, leukocytoclastic vasculitis (purpura), and internal organ exocrine disease involving the lungs (diffuse interstitial lymphocytosis), pancreas, hepatobiliary system, gastrointestinal tract, kidneys (renal tubular acidosis), musculoskeletal (arthritis and arthralgia), hematologic (cytopenias), peripheral nervous system (sensory and autonomic neuropathy), and CNS (optic neuritis, transverse myelitis, meningoencephalitis).

Nonexocrine disease manifestations of Sjögren syndrome may be related to inflammatory vascular disease (skin, muscle and joints, serosal surfaces, CNS, peripheral nervous system), noninflammatory vascular disease (Raynaud phenomenon), mediator-induced disease (hematologic cytopenias, fatigue, fever), and autoimmune endocrinopathy (thyroiditis).

DIAGNOSIS

Clinical presentation of recurrent **parotitis** and or recurrent parotid gland swelling in a child or adolescent is characteristic and should raise the suspicion for Sjögren syndrome. The diagnosis is based on clinical features supported by biopsy of salivary or parotid glands demonstrating foci of lymphocytic infiltration, the current gold standard for diagnosis. Children are more likely to have normal minor salivary gland but abnormal parotid gland biopsies. Supporting laboratory abnormalities include cryoglobulinemia, elevated erythrocyte sedimentation rate, hypergammaglobulinemia, positive rheumatoid factor, and detection of SSA and SSB antibodies. Anti–β-fodrin autoantibodies, directed against an apoptotic cleavage product of α-fodrin, are a useful diagnostic marker for juvenile Sjögren syndrome. The **Schirmer test** detects abnormal tear production (≤5 mm of wetting of filter paper strip in 5 min). **Rose bengal staining** detects damaged ocular epithelial conjunctival and corneal cells. Imaging studies, including MRI, technetium (^{99m}Tc) scintigraphy, and sialography, are useful in the diagnostic evaluation for Sjögren syndrome (Fig. 187.1).

DIFFERENTIAL DIAGNOSIS

The differential diagnosis of Sjögren syndrome in children includes **juvenile recurrent parotitis**, characterized by intermittent unilateral parotid swelling typically lasting only a few days. It is frequently associated with fever and may undergo remission with puberty. Unlike in Sjögren syndrome, there is a male predominance, juvenile recurrent parotitis is seen in the younger children (3-6 yr), and there is a lack of focal lymphocytic infiltrates on biopsy. Other conditions in the

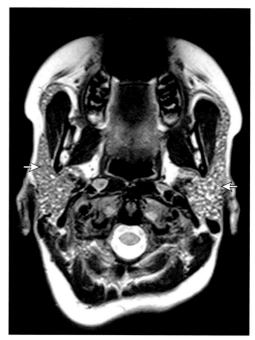

Fig. 187.1 T2-weighted MRI of child with Sjögren syndrome showing parotitis *(arrows)*.

differential diagnosis include eating disorders, infectious parotitis (mumps, streptococcal and staphylococcal infections, Epstein-Barr virus, cytomegalovirus, HIV, parainfluenza, influenza enterovirus), and local trauma to the buccal mucosa. Rarely, polycystic parotid disease, tumors, and sarcoidosis may present with recurrent parotid swelling. In these conditions, sicca complex, rash, arthralgia, and ANAs are usually absent.

TREATMENT

Symptomatic treatment of Sjögren syndrome includes the use of artificial tears, massage of the parotids, oral lozenges, and fluids to limit the damaging effects of decreased secretions. Corticosteroids, nonsteroidal antiinflammatory drugs, and hydroxychloroquine are among the more commonly used agents for treatment, with reports of methotrexate and etanercept used for treatment of arthritis. Stronger immunosuppressive agents, such as cyclosporine and cyclophosphamide, are reserved for severe functional disorders and life-threatening complications.

COMPLICATIONS AND PROGNOSIS

The symptoms of Sjögren syndrome develop and progress slowly. Diminished salivary flow typically remains constant for years. Because monoclonal B-lymphocyte disease originates chiefly from lymphocytic foci within salivary glands or from parenchymal internal organs, there is increased risk for mucosa-associated lymphoid tissue lymphoma. Maternal Sjögren syndrome can be an antecedent to the **neonatal lupus** syndrome (see Chapter 183.1).

Bibliography is available at Expert Consult.

Chapter 188

Hereditary Periodic Fever Syndromes and Other Systemic Autoinflammatory Diseases

James W. Verbsky

第一百八十八章

遗传性周期性发热综合征和其他系统性自身炎症性疾病

中文导读

本章主要介绍了自身炎症性疾病的分类、伴有周期性或明显发热的自身炎症性疾病、其他符合孟德尔遗传规律的自身炎症性疾病、复杂遗传性自身炎症性疾病。伴有周期性或明显发热的自身炎症性疾病具体描述了家族性地中海热（FMF）、高IgD综合征（HIDS）、肿瘤坏死因子受体相关周期性发热综合征（TRAPS）、冷吡啉相关的周期性综合征（CAPS）。其他符合孟德尔遗传自身炎症性疾病中描述了伴有坏疽性脓皮病和痤疮的化脓性关节炎综合征（PAPA综合征）、IL-1受体拮抗剂缺陷病（DIRA）、Blau综合征、

自身炎症–磷脂酶Cγ2缺陷与免疫失调（APLAID）、腺苷脱氨酶2缺乏症（DADA2）、铁幼粒细胞贫血–免疫缺陷–发热和发育延迟综合征（SIFD）、IL-36受体拮抗剂缺陷病（DITRA）、家族性寒冷型自身炎症综合征2型（FCAS2）、自体炎症伴小肠结肠炎、Majeed综合征、干扰素病、非典型慢性中性粒细胞与脂肪代谢障碍性皮肤病和高体温综合征（CANDLE）、婴儿起病的STING相关血管炎（SAVI）。复杂遗传性自身炎症性疾病中描述了周期热–阿弗他口炎–咽炎–淋巴结炎（PFAPA）、慢性复发性多灶性骨髓炎（CRMO）。

The hereditary periodic fever syndromes are a group of monogenic diseases that present with recurrent bouts of fever and associated pleural and/or peritoneal inflammation, arthritis, and various types of skin rash. A number of identifiable disorders present with recurrent episodes of inflammation, although fevers may not be common feature. Therefore the term **systemic autoinflammatory diseases** is used to include all diseases that present with seemingly unprovoked episodes of inflammation, without the high-titer autoantibodies or antigen-specific T cells typically seen in autoimmune diseases. Whereas the autoimmune diseases are disorders of the *adaptive* immune system, driven by B and T lymphocyte effector cells, autoinflammatory diseases largely represent

disorders of the phylogenetically more primitive *innate* immune system, mediated by myeloid effector cells and germline-encoded receptors. Autoinflammatory diseases exhibit episodic or persistent inflammation characterized by an acute-phase response with elevation of the erythrocyte sedimentation rate (ESR), C-reactive protein (CRP), and serum amyloid A (AA). In some patients, untreated autoinflammatory disorders over time will lead to AA amyloidosis (see Chapter 189).

It is important to note that autoinflammatory disorders are rare, whereas fever in childhood caused by innocuous illness is very common. The approach to a child with fevers should include a detailed history, physical examination, and limited laboratory investigations to rule out other conditions that lead to fevers, including autoimmune disorders and malignancies (Table 188.1). If there is evidence of recurrent infections with fevers, an immune deficiency could be considered and evaluated. If the workup is reassuring, the inflammatory episodes resolve, and the child is otherwise well without unusual physical findings, observance is often warranted because these episodes are likely to resolve as the child's immune system matures.

CLASSIFICATION OF AUTOINFLAMMATORY DISORDERS

Because of the rapidly expanding number of autoinflammatory disorders and their varied clinical presentation, it can be difficult to group these disorders in a meaningful manner. Some autoinflammatory disorders present with prominent fevers and are known as **hereditary periodic fever syndromes**. These include 2 disorders with an *autosomal recessive* mode of inheritance, familial Mediterranean fever (**FMF**; MIM249100) and the hyperimmunoglobulinemia D (hyper-IgD) with periodic fever syndrome (**HIDS**; MIM260920). Hereditary periodic fever syndromes with an *autosomal dominant* mode of inheritance include the tumor necrosis factor (TNF) receptor–associated periodic syndrome (**TRAPS**; MIM191190) and a spectrum of disorders known as the cryopyrin-associated periodic syndromes (**CAPS**), or cryopyrinopathies. From mildest to most severe, CAPS include the familial cold autoinflammatory syndrome (**FCAS1**; MIM120100), Muckle-Wells syndrome (**MWS**; MIM191100), and neonatal-onset multisystem inflammatory disease (**NOMID**; MIM607115) (also known as chronic infantile neurologic cutaneous and articular syndrome, **CINCA**) (Table 188.2).

A variety of mendelian *autoinflammatory disorders* may or may not exhibit prominent fevers and are not considered periodic fever syndromes, but do have continuous or repeated episodes of spontaneous inflammation with unique clinical characteristics. These include the syndrome of pyogenic arthritis with pyoderma gangrenosum and acne (**PAPA**; MIM604416), deficiency of the interleukin-1 (IL-1) receptor antagonist (**DIRA**; MIM612852), **Blau syndrome** caused by mutations in *NOD2*

(also known as *early-onset sarcoidosis*; MIM186580), autoinflammation with phospholipase Cγ₂-associated antibody deficiency and immune dysregulation (**APLAID**; MIM614878), and deficiency of adenosine deaminase-2 (**DADA2**). Other disorders include congenital sideroblastic anemia with B-cell immunodeficiency, periodic fevers, and developmental delay (**SIFD**) caused by biallelic mutations of the *TRNT1* gene (MIM616084), autoinflammation with infantile enterocolitis caused by mutations in *NLRC4* (**AIFEC**; MIM616060), familial cold autoinflammatory syndrome type 2 caused by mutations in *NLRP12* (**FCAS2**; MIM611762), **CARD14** (MIM607211), and deficiency in IL-36 receptor antagonist (**DITRA**; 614204).

In addition to the previous autoinflammatory disorders, a variety of disorders are characterized by inappropriate *interferon expression*, the **interferonopathies**. Type 1 interferons (e.g., IFN-α, IFN-β) are cytokines expressed by many cells in response to viral infections. Disorders that result in spontaneous interferon production and inflammatory manifestations include STING-associated vasculopathy of infancy (**SAVI**; MIM615934) and chronic atypical neutrophilic dermatosis with lipodystrophy and elevated temperature (**CANDLE**; MIM256040).

There are also a number of autoinflammatory disorders with a complex mode of inheritance. These include the syndrome of periodic fever with aphthous stomatitis, pharyngitis, and adenitis (**PFAPA**) and chronic recurrent multifocal osteomyelitis (**CRMO**; MIM259680). Other genetically complex disorders that are sometimes considered autoinflammatory include **systemic-onset juvenile idiopathic arthritis** (see Chapter 180), **Behçet disease** (see Chapter 186), and **Crohn disease** (see Chapter 362.2).

Distinguishing autoinflammatory disorders from one another can be difficult because their presentations can vary, and many display similarities. Some disorders have characteristic fever patterns (Fig. 188.1), whereas others have characteristic skin findings that can aid in a diagnosis (Table 188.3). Others can have characteristic physical features or organ involvement. Some of these disorders have bone involvement (Table 188.4). Other clinical features can also be helpful, such as ethnicity, age of onset, triggers, laboratory testing, and response to therapies (Table 188.5). Genetic panels are increasingly being used to screen for most if not all of these defects in a single test, rather than individual genetic assessment based on clinical findings.

AUTOINFLAMMATORY DISEASES WITH PERIODIC OR PROMINENT FEVERS

The first descriptions of autoinflammatory disorders focused on genetic diseases that presented with prominent fevers, the periodic fever syndromes. As new autoinflammatory diseases were discovered, it was clear that a variety of inflammatory disorders can occur in the absence of fever.

Familial Mediterranean Fever

FMF is a recessively inherited autoinflammatory disease usually characterized by recurrent, short-lived (1-3 days), self-limited episodes of fever, serositis, mono- or pauciarticular arthritis, or an erysipeloid rash, sometimes complicated by AA amyloidosis. Most patients with FMF present with symptoms in childhood, with 90% presenting before age 20. Clinical features of FMF may include fever, serositis presenting as pleuritic chest pain or severe abdominal pain, arthritis, and rash. The pleural pain is typically unilateral, whereas the abdominal pain (sterile peritonitis) can be generalized or localized to 1 quadrant, similar to other forms of peritonitis. FMF-associated arthritis occurs primarily in the large joints, may be accompanied by large, neutrophil-rich effusions, and is usually nonerosive and nondestructive. The hallmark cutaneous finding is an erysipeloid erythematous rash that overlies the ankle or dorsum of the foot (Fig. 188.2). Other clinical findings include scrotal pain caused by inflammation of the tunica vaginalis testis, febrile myalgia, exercise-induced myalgia (particularly common in children), and an association with various forms of vasculitis, including Henoch-Schönlein purpura, in as many as 5% of pediatric patients. FMF episodes may be triggered by stress, menses, or infections. Between flares, patients are generally symptom free but may have persistent elevation of their inflammatory markers. The attack frequency can vary from weekly to 1-2 flares per year. Table 188.6 lists diagnostic criteria for FMF.

Table 188.1	Differential Diagnosis of Periodic Fever

HEREDITARY
See Table 188.2.

NONHEREDITARY
A. Infectious
  1. Hidden infectious focus (e.g., aortoenteric fistula, lung sequestration)
  2. Recurrent infection/reinfection (e.g., chronic meningococcemia, immune deficiency)
  3. Specific infection (e.g., Whipple disease, malaria)
B. Noninfectious inflammatory disorder:
  1. Adult-onset Still disease
  2. Systemic-onset juvenile idiopathic arthritis
  3. Periodic fever, aphthous stomatitis, pharyngitis, and adenitis
  4. Schnitzler syndrome
  5. Behçet syndrome
  6. Crohn disease
  7. Sarcoidosis
C. Neoplastic
  1. Lymphoma (e.g., Hodgkin disease, angioimmunoblastic lymphoma)
  2. Solid tumor (e.g., pheochromocytoma, myxoma, colon carcinoma)
  3. Histiocytic disorders
D. Vascular (e.g., recurrent pulmonary embolism)
E. Hypothalamic
F. Psychogenic periodic fever
G. Factitious or fraudulent

Adapted from Simon A, van der Meer JWM, Drenth JPH: Familial autoinflammatory syndromes. In Firestein GS, Budd RC, Gabriel SE, et al, editors: *Kelley's textbook of rheumatology*, ed 9, Philadelphia, 2012, Saunders (Table 97-2).

Table 188.2 Autoinflammatory Disorders

DISEASE	GENETIC DEFECT/PRESUMED PATHOGENESIS	INHERITANCE	AFFECTED CELLS	FUNCTIONAL DEFECTS	ASSOCIATED FEATURES
Familial Mediterranean fever	Mutations of *MEFV* (lead to gain of pyrin function, resulting in inappropriate IL-1β release)	AR	Mature granulocytes, cytokine-activated monocytes	Decreased production of pyrin permits ASC-induced IL-1 processing and inflammation following subclinical serosal injury; macrophage apoptosis decreased	Recurrent fever, serositis, and inflammation responsive to colchicine. Predisposes to vasculitis and inflammatory bowel disease
Mevalonate kinase deficiency (hyper IgD syndrome)	Mutations of *MVK* (lead to a block in the mevalonate pathway). Interleukin-1β mediates the inflammatory phenotype	AR		Affecting cholesterol synthesis; pathogenesis of disease is unclear	Periodic fever and leukocytosis with high IgD levels
Muckle–Wells syndrome	Mutations of *NLRP3* (also called *PYPAF1* or *NALP3*) lead to constitutive activation of the NLRP3 inflammasome	AD	PMNs, monocytes	Defect in cryopyrin, involved in leukocyte apoptosis and NF-κB signaling and IL-1 processing	Urticaria, SNHL, amyloidosis
Familial cold autoinflammatory syndrome	Mutations of *NLRP3* (see above) Mutations of *NLRP12*	AD	PMNs, monocytes	Same as above	Nonpruritic urticaria, arthritis, chills, fever, and leukocytosis after cold exposure
Neonatal-onset multisystem inflammatory disease (NOMID) or chronic infantile neurologic cutaneous and articular syndrome (CINCA)	Mutations of *NLRP3* (see above)	AD	PMNs, chondrocytes	Same as above	Neonatal-onset rash, chronic meningitis, and arthropathy with fever and inflammation
TNF receptor–associated periodic syndrome (TRAPS)	Mutations of *TNFRSF1A* (resulting in increased TNF inflammatory signaling)	AD	PMNs, monocytes	Mutations of 55-kDa TNF receptor leading to intracellular receptor retention or diminished soluble cytokine receptor available to bind TNF	Recurrent fever, serositis, rash, and ocular or joint inflammation
Pyogenic sterile arthritis, pyoderma gangrenosum, acne (PAPA) syndrome	Mutations of *PSTPIP1* (also called *C2BP1*) (affects both pyrin and protein tyrosine phosphatase to regulate innate and adaptive immune responses)	AD	Hematopoietic tissues, upregulated in activated T cells	Disordered actin reorganization leading to compromised physiologic signaling during inflammatory response	Destructive arthritis, inflammatory skin rash, myositis
Blau syndrome	Mutations of *NOD2* (also called *CARD15*) (involved in various inflammatory processes)	AD	Monocytes	Mutations in nucleotide binding site of CARD15, possibly disrupting interactions with lipopolysaccharides and NF-κB signaling	Uveitis, granulomatous synovitis, campodactyly, rash, and cranial neuropaties, 30% develop Crohn disease
Chronic recurrent multifocal osteomyelitis and congenital dyserythropoietic anemia (Majeed syndrome)	Mutations of *LPIN2* (increased expression of the proinflammatory genes)	AR	Neutrophils, bone marrow cells	Undefined	Chronic recurrent multifocal osteomyelitis, transfusion-dependent anemia, cutaneous inflammatory disorders
Early-onset inflammatory bowel disease	Mutations in *IL-10* (results in increase of many proinflammatory cytokines)	AR	Monocyte/macrophage, activated T cells	IL-10 deficiency leads to increase of TNFγ and other proinflammatory cytokines	Enterocolitis, enteric fistulas, perianal abscesses, chronic folliculitis
Early-onset inflammatory bowel disease	Mutations in *IL-10RA* (see above)	AR	Monocyte/macrophage, activated T cells	Mutation in IL-10 receptor alpha leads to increase of TNFγ and other proinflammatory cytokines	Enterocolitis, enteric fistulas, perianal abscesses, chronic folliculitis
Early-onset inflammatory bowel disease	Mutations in *IL-10RB* (see above)	AR	Monocyte/macrophage, activated T cells	Mutation in IL-10 receptor beta leads to increase of TNFγ and other proinflammatory cytokines	Enterocolitis, enteric fistulas, perianal abscesses, chronic folliculitis

AD, autosomal dominant; AR, autosomal recessive; Ig, immunoglobulin; IL, interleukin; NF-κB, nuclear factor-κB; PMN, polymorphonuclear neutrophil; SNHL, sensorineural hearing loss; TNF, tumor necrosis factor.

From Verbsky JW, Routes JR: Recurrent fever, infections, immune disorders, and autoinflammatory diseases. In Kliegman RM, Lyse PS, Bordini BJ, et al, editors: Nelson pediatric symptom-based diagnosis. Philadelphia, 2018, Elsevier, Table 41-5.

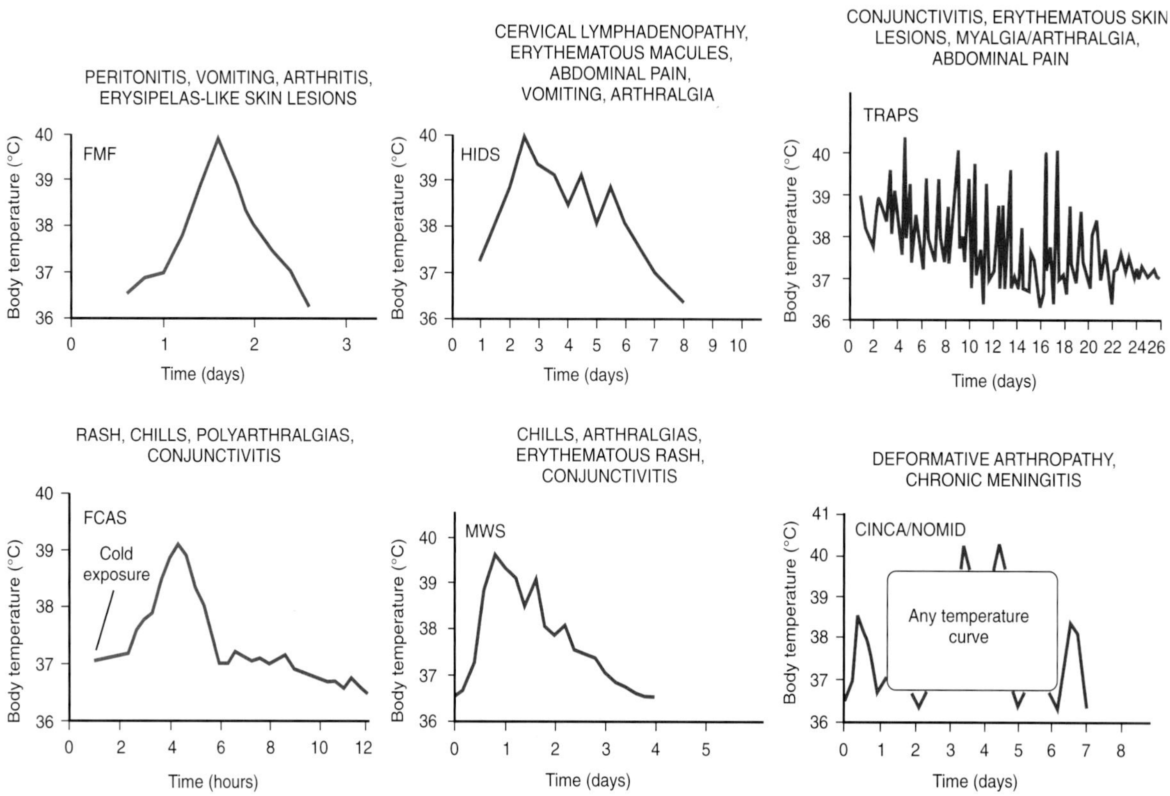

Fig. 188.1 Characteristic patterns of body temperature during inflammatory attacks in the familial autoinflammatory syndromes. Interindividual variability for each syndrome is considerable, and even for the individual patient, the fever pattern may vary greatly from episode to episode. Note the different time scales on the x axes. CINCA/NOMID, Chronic infantile neurologic cutaneous and articular syndrome/neonatal-onset multisystemic inflammatory disease; FCAS, familial cold autoinflammatory syndrome; HIDS, hyper-IgD syndrome; MWS, Muckle-Wells syndrome; TRAPS, tumor necrosis factor receptor–associated periodic syndrome. *(From Simon A, van der Meer JWM, Drenth JPH: Familial autoinflammatory syndromes. In Firestein GS, Budd RC, Gabriel SE, et al, editors: Kelley's textbook of rheumatology, ed 9, Philadelphia, 2012, Saunders, Fig 97-1.)*

Table 188.3	Clinical Grouping of Autoinflammatory Diseases by Skin Manifestations

1. Neutrophilic urticaria (the cryopyrinopathies)
   Recurrent fever attacks of short duration (typically <24 hr)
   • CAPS/FCAS: familial cold autoinflammatory syndrome
   • CAPS/MWS: Muckle-Wells syndrome
   • FCAS2/NLRP12
   Continuous low-grade fever
   • CAPS/NOMID: neonatal-onset multisystem inflammatory disease (NOMID)/chronic infantile neurologic cutaneous and articular syndrome (CINCA)
2. Granulomatous skin lesions and minimal or low-grade fever attacks
   • Blau syndrome/early-onset sarcoidosis (pediatric granulomatous arthritis)
3. Pustular skin rashes and fever
   With inflammatory bone disease
   • DIRA: deficiency of interleukin-1 receptor agonist
   • Majeed syndrome

With pyogenic arthritis
   • PAPA: pyogenic arthritis, pyoderma gangrenosum, and acne syndrome
Without other organ involvement
   • DITRA: deficiency of interleukin-36 receptor antagonist
   • CAMPS: CARD14-mediated psoriasis
4. Atypical neutrophilic dermatosis with histiocytic-like infiltrate
   • CANDLE: proteasome associated autoinflammatory syndromes
5. Livedo reticularis, vasculopathy with ulcerations
   • SAVI; STING associated vasculopathy, infantile onset
6. Livedo racemosa, vasculitis with ulcerations
   • ADA2; adenosine deaminase-2 deficiency

CAPS, Cryopyrin-associated periodic syndromes.
Modified from Almeida de Jesus A, Goldbach-Mansky R: Monogenic autoinflammatory diseases: concept and clinical manifestations, *Clin Immunol* 147:155–174, 2013 (Table 1).

FMF is caused by autosomal recessive mutations in *MEFV*, a gene encoding a 781 amino acid protein denoted *pyrin* (Greek for "fever"). Pyrin is expressed in granulocytes, monocytes, and dendritic cells (DCs) and in peritoneal, synovial, and dermal fibroblasts. The N-terminal approximately 90 amino acids of pyrin are the prototype for a motif (the PYRIN domain) that mediates protein-protein interactions and is found in >20 different human proteins that regulate inflammation and apoptosis. Many of the FMF-associated mutations in pyrin are found at the C-terminal B30.2 domain of pyrin, encoded by exon 10 of *MEFV*. More than 50 such FMF mutations are listed in an online database (http://fmf.igh.cnrs.fr/ISSAID/infevers/), almost all of which are missense substitutions. Homozygosity for the M694V mutation may be associated

Table 188.4	Autoinflammatory Bone Disorders				
	CRMO	**MAJEED SYNDROME**	**DIRA**	**CHERUBISM**	**CMO AND LUPO MICE**
Ethnicity	Worldwide, but mostly European	Arabic	European, Puerto Rican, Arabic	Worldwide	Occurs in various backgrounds
Fever	Uncommon	Common	Uncommon	No	Not assessed
Sites of osseous involvement	Metaphyses of long bones > vertebrae, clavicle, sternum, pelvis, others	Similar to CRMO	Anterior rib ends, metaphyses of long bones, vertebrae, others	Mandible > maxilla Rarely ribs	Vertebrae hind > forefeet
Extraosseous manifestations	PPP, psoriasis, IBD, others	Dyserythropoietic anemia, Sweet syndrome, HSM, growth failure	Generalized pustulosis, nail changes, lung disease, vasculitis	Cervical lymphadenopathy	Dermatitis, extramedullary hematopoiesis, splenomegaly
Family history of inflammatory disorders	Psoriasis, PPP, arthritis, IBD, others	Psoriasis in some obligate carriers	No known associations	No known associations	Heterozygotes normal
Inheritance	Not clear	Autosomal recessive	Autosomal recessive	Autosomal dominant; incomplete penetrance	Autosomal recessive
Gene defect	Unknown	*LPIN2*	*IL1RN*	*SH3BP2 >> PTPN11*	*Pstpip2*
Protein name	?	Lipin2	IL-1Ra	SH3BP2	PSTPIP2 (MAYP)
Protein function	?	Fat metabolism: (PAP enzyme activity), ↑ message to oxidative stress, ? role in mitosis	Antagonist of IL-1 receptor	↑ Myeloid cell response to M-CSF and RANKL, ↑ TNF-α expression in macrophages	Macrophage proliferation, macrophage recruitment to sites of inflammation, cytoskeletal function
Cytokine abnormalities	↑ serum TNF-α	Not tested	↑ IL-1α, IL-1β, MIP-1α, TNF-α, IL-8, IL-6 ex vivo monocyte assay; skin reveals ↑ IL-17 staining	↑ serum TNF-α in mouse model	cmo: ↑ serum IL-6, MIP-1α, TNF-α, CSF-1, IP-10 Lupo: ↑ serum MIP-1α, IL-4, RANTES, TGF-β

CRMO, Chronic recurrent multifocal osteomyelitis; CSF, colony-stimulating factor; DIRA, deficiency of interleukin-1 receptor antagonist; HSM, hepatosplenomegaly; IBD, inflammatory bowel disease; IL, interleukin; IL-1Ra, interleukin-1 receptor antagonist; IP-10, interferon-inducible protein-10; M-CSF, macrophage colony-stimulating factor; MIP-1α, macrophage inflammatory protein-1α; PAP, phosphatidate phosphatase; PPP, palmar-plantar pustulosis; PSTPIP2, proline-serine-threonine phosphatase interacting protein; RANKL, receptor activator of nuclear factor-κB ligand; RANTES, regulated on activation, normal T cell expressed and secreted; SH3BP2, SH3 binding protein 2; TGF, transforming growth factor; TNF-α, tumor necrosis factor alpha.

From Ferguson PJ, Laxer RM: Autoinflammatory bone disorders. In Cassidy JT, Petty RE, Laxer RM, et al, editors: *Textbook of pediatric rheumatology*, ed 6, Philadelphia, 2010, Saunders (Table 44-2).

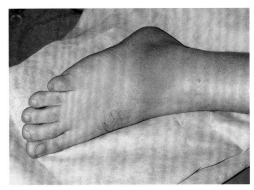

Fig. 188.2 Characteristic erysipeloid erythema associated with familial Mediterranean fever. This rash appears during a flare and overlies the ankle or dorsum of the foot.

with an earlier age of onset, arthritis, and an increased risk of amyloidosis. The substitution of glutamine for glutamic acid at residue 148 (E148Q) is considered either a mild mutation or a functional polymorphism in the pyrin protein. The carrier frequency of FMF mutations among several Mediterranean populations is very high, suggesting the possibility of a heterozygote advantage.

FMF occurs primarily among ethnic groups of Mediterranean ancestry, most frequently Jews, Turks, Armenians, Arabs, and Italians. Because of a higher frequency of the M694V mutation, FMF is more severe and more readily recognized in the Sephardic (North African) than the Ashkenazi (East European) Jewish population. With the advent of genetic testing, mutation-positive FMF has been documented worldwide, although at lower frequency than in the Mediterranean basin and Middle East.

Through PYRIN-domain interactions, pyrin can activate **caspase-1**, the enzyme that converts the 31 kDa pro–IL-1β molecule into the biologically active 17 kDa IL-1β, which is a major mediator of fever and inflammation. FMF mutations lead to a gain-of-function activation of caspase-1 and IL-1β–dependent inflammation, with a gene-dosage effect. These results may explain why as many as 30% of heterozygous carriers of FMF mutations have biochemical evidence of inflammation.

Prophylactic daily oral colchicine decreases the frequency, duration, and intensity of FMF flares. This regimen also prevents the development of systemic AA amyloidosis. Colchicine is generally well tolerated and safe in children, with the most common side effects being diarrhea and other gastrointestinal (GI) complaints. Some patients develop lactose intolerance while taking colchicine. GI side effects can be minimized by initiating therapy at a low dose (for young children, 0.3 mg/day) and slowly titrating upward. A dose-related transaminitis may also be observed; bone marrow suppression is rarely seen at the dosages prescribed for FMF. Pediatric patients may require doses of colchicine similar to those needed in adults (1-2 mg/day), reflecting that children

Table 188.5	Clues That May Assist in Diagnosis of Autoinflammatory Syndromes

AGE OF ONSET

At birth	NOMID, DIRA, MWS
Infancy and 1st yr of life	HIDS, FCAS, NLRP12
Toddler	PFAPA
Late childhood	PAPA
Most common of autoinflammatory syndromes to have onset in adulthood	TRAPS, DITRA
Variable (mostly in childhood)	All others

ETHNICITY AND GEOGRAPHY

Armenians, Turks, Italian, Sephardic Jews	FMF
Arabs	FMF, DITRA (Arab Tunisian)
Dutch, French, German, Western Europe	HIDS, MWS, NLRP12
United States	FCAS
Can occur in blacks (West Africa origin)	TRAPS
Eastern Canada, Puerto Rico	DIRA
Worldwide	All others

TRIGGERS

Vaccines	HIDS
Cold exposure	FCAS, NLRP12
Stress, menses	FMF, TRAPS, MWS, PAPA, DITRA
Minor trauma	PAPA, MWS, TRAPS, HIDS
Exercise	FMF, TRAPS
Pregnancy	DITRA
Infections	All, especially DITRA

ATTACK DURATION

<24 hr	FCAS, FMF
1-3 days	FMF, MWS, DITRA (fever)
3-7 days	HIDS, PFAPA
>7 days	TRAPS, PAPA
Almost always "in attack"	NOMID, DIRA

INTERVAL BETWEEN ATTACKS

3-6 wk	PFAPA, HIDS
>6 wk	TRAPS
Mostly unpredictable	All others
Truly periodic	PFAPA, cyclic neutropenia

USEFUL LABORATORY TESTS

Acute-phase reactants must be normal between attacks	PFAPA
Urine mevalonic acid in attack	HIDS
IgD > 100 mg/dL	HIDS
Proteinuria (amyloidosis)	FMF, TRAPS, MWS, NOMID

RESPONSE TO THERAPY

Corticosteroid dramatic	PFAPA
Corticosteroid partial	TRAPS, FCAS, MWS, NOMID, PAPA*
Colchicine	FMF, PFAPA (30% effective)
Cimetidine	PFAPA (30% effective)
Etanercept	TRAPS, FMF arthritis
Anti–IL-1 dramatic	DIRA (anakinra), FCAS, MWS, NOMID, PFAPA
Anti–IL-1 mostly	TRAPS, FMF
Anti–IL-1 partial	HIDS, PAPA

DIRA, Deficiency of IL-1 receptor antagonist; DITRA, deficiency of IL-36 receptor antagonist (generalized pustular psoriasis); FCAS, familial cold autoinflammatory syndrome; FMF, familial Mediterranean fever; HIDS, hyper-IgD syndrome; IL, interleukin; MWS, Muckle-Wells syndrome; NLRP, nucleotide oligomerization domain–like receptor family, pyrin domain; NOMID, neonatal-onset multisystem inflammatory disorder; PAPA, pyogenic sterile arthritis, pyoderma gangrenosum, acne syndrome; PFAPA, periodic fever, aphthous stomatitis, pharyngitis, adenitis; TRAPS, tumor necrosis factor receptor–associated periodic syndrome.

*For intraarticular corticosteroids.

From Hashkes PJ, Toker O: Autoinflammatory syndromes, *Pediatr Clin North Am* 59:447–470, 2012 (Table 2).

Table 188.6	Diagnostic Criteria for Familial Mediterranean Fever (FMF)*

MAJOR CRITERIA

1. Typical attacks[†] with peritonitis (generalized)
2. Typical attacks with pleuritis (unilateral) or pericarditis
3. Typical attacks with monoarthritis (hip, knee, ankle)
4. Typical attacks with fever alone
5. Incomplete abdominal attack

MINOR CRITERIA

1. Incomplete attacks[‡] involving chest pain
2. Incomplete attacks involving monoarthritis
3. Exertional leg pain
4. Favorable response to colchicine

*Requirements for diagnosis of FMF are ≥1 major criteria or ≥2 minor criteria.
  [†]Typical attacks are defined as recurrent (≥3 of the same type), febrile (≥38°C), and short (lasting between 12 hr and 3 days).
  [‡]Incomplete attacks are defined as painful and recurrent attacks not fulfilling the criteria for a typical attack.
  From Livneh A, Langevitz P, Zemer D, et al: Criteria for the diagnosis of familial Mediterranean fever, *Arthritis Rheum* 40:1879–1885, 1997.

metabolize the drug more rapidly than adults. It is not always possible to find a tolerated dose of colchicine at which all symptoms are suppressed, but approximately 90% of patients have a marked improvement in disease-related symptoms. A small percentage of FMF patients are either unresponsive to or intolerant of therapeutic doses of colchicine. Based on the role of pyrin in IL-1β activation, a trial demonstrated the safety and effectiveness of *rilonacept*, an IL-1 inhibitor, in FMF; there are case reports of the effectiveness of *anakinra*, a recombinant interleukin-1 receptor (IL-1R) antagonist.

Amyloidosis is the most serious complication of FMF, and in its absence FMF patients may live a normal life span. Amyloidosis may develop when serum AA, an acute-phase reactant found at extremely high levels in the blood during FMF attacks, is cleaved to produce a 76–amino acid fragment that misfolds and deposits ectopically, usually in the kidneys, GI tract, spleen, lungs, testes, thyroid, and adrenals. Rarely, cardiac amyloidosis may develop; macroglossia and amyloid neuropathy are generally not seen with the amyloidosis of FMF. The most common presenting sign of AA amyloidosis is proteinuria. The diagnosis is then usually confirmed by rectal or renal biopsy. In a small number of case reports, mostly from the Middle East, amyloidosis may actually precede overt FMF attacks, presumably because of subclinical inflammation. Risk factors for the development of amyloidosis in FMF include homozygosity for the M694V *MEFV* mutation, polymorphisms of the serum AA gene (encoding AA), noncompliance with colchicine treatment, male gender, and a positive family history of AA amyloid. For unclear reasons, country of origin is also a major risk factor for amyloidosis in FMF, with patients raised in the Middle East having a much higher risk than genotypically identical patients raised in the West. Aggressive lifelong suppression of the acute-phase reactants should be the goal in patients with FMF amyloidosis, and documented cases show this may result in resorption of amyloid deposits. The natural history of untreated amyloidosis in FMF is the inexorable progression to renal failure, often within 3-5 yr.

Hyperimmunoglobulinemia D With Periodic Fever Syndrome

HIDS, also known as **mevalonate kinase deficiency**, was initially described in a cohort of Dutch patients and occurs primarily in patients of Northern European descent. HIDS is recessively inherited and caused by mutations of *MVK*, a gene that encodes mevalonate kinase (MK). The clinical features of HIDS generally appear within the 1st 6 mo of life. Febrile attacks last 3-7 days, with abdominal pain often accompanied by diarrhea, nausea, and vomiting. Other clinical manifestations include cervical lymphadenopathy, diffuse macular rash, aphthous ulcers, headaches, and occasional splenomegaly (Figs. 188.3 to 188.5). Arthritis or arthralgia can be present in an oligoarticular or polyarticular pattern.

Inflammatory disease–like illness and Kawasaki disease–like presentation have also been reported. Attacks are often precipitated by intercurrent illness, immunizations, and surgery. Families frequently recount flares around the time of birthdays, holidays, and family vacations. The symptoms of HIDS may persist for years but tend to become less prominent in adulthood. Patients with HIDS usually have a normal life span. Unlike FMF and TRAPS, the incidence of AA amyloidosis is quite low. Complete MK deficiency results in mevalonic aciduria that presents with severe mental retardation, ataxia, myopathy, cataracts, and failure to thrive (see Chapter 103).

MK is expressed in multiple tissues and catalyzes the conversion of mevalonic acid to 5-phosphomevalonic acid in the biosynthesis of cholesterol and nonsterol isoprenoids. Patients with HIDS-associated mutations have greatly reduced, but not absent, MK enzymatic activity. HIDS patients usually have low-normal serum cholesterol levels, but the deficiency of isoprenoids may cause increased IL-1β production by aberrant activation of the small guanosine triphosphatase Rac1. Temperature elevation may further exacerbate this process by more complete inhibition of MK activity, leading to a possible positive feedback loop.

The diagnosis of HIDS may be confirmed either by 2 mutations in *MVK* (approximately 10% of patients with seemingly typical disease have only a single identifiable mutation) or by elevated levels of mevalonate in the urine during acute attacks. HIDS-associated mutations are distributed throughout the MK protein, but the 2 most common mutations are the substitution of isoleucine for valine at residue 377 (V377I), a variant that is quite common in the Dutch population, and the substitution of threonine for isoleucine at residue 268 (I268T). The eponymous elevation in serum IgD levels is not universally present, especially in young children; IgA levels can also be elevated. Conversely, serum IgD levels may be increased in other autoinflammatory disorders as well as in some chronic infections. During attacks, leukocytosis and increased serum levels of acute-phase reactants and proinflammatory cytokines are frequently present. Table 188.7 lists diagnostic criteria for HIDS.

Standards for the **treatment** of HIDS are evolving. Very few patients respond to colchicine, and milder disease courses may respond to nonsteroidal antiinflammatory drugs (NSAIDs). Corticosteroids are of limited utility. Small trials of both etanercept and either intermittent or daily anakinra in HIDS are promising.

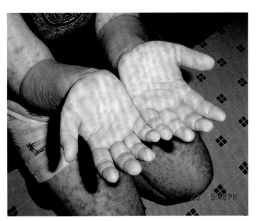

Fig. 188.3 Polymorphic rash on the hands, arms, and legs of a patient with hyper-IgD syndrome (HIDS). *(From Takada K, Aksentijevich I, Mahadevan V, et al. Favorable preliminary experience with etanercept in two patients with the hyperimmunoglobulinemia D and periodic fever syndrome, Arthritis Rheum 48:2646, 2003.)*

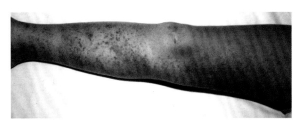

Fig. 188.4 Petechiae on the leg of a hyper-IgD syndrome patient during a febrile attack. *(From Simon A, van der Meer JWM, Drenth JPH: Familial autoinflammatory syndromes. In Firestein GS, Budd RC, Gabriel SE, et al, editors: Kelley's textbook of rheumatology, ed 9, Philadelphia, 2012, Saunders, Fig 97-7.)*

Tumor Necrosis Factor Receptor–Associated Periodic Syndrome

TRAPS is characterized by recurrent fevers and localized inflammation and is inherited in an autosomal dominant manner. TRAPS has a number of distinguishing clinical and immunologic features. TRAPS was first recognized in patients of Irish descent and denoted *familial Hibernian fever* to draw a contrast with FMF, but the current nomenclature was

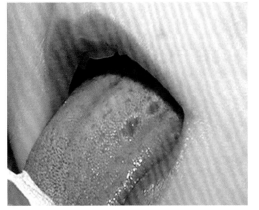

Fig. 188.5 Aphthous ulceration detected on the tongue of a patient with hyper-IgD syndrome. *(Courtesy Dr. K. Antila, North Carelian Central Hospital, Joensuu, Finland; from Simon A, van der Meer JWM, Drenth JPH: Familial autoinflammatory syndromes. In Firestein GS, Budd RC, Gabriel SE, et al, editors: Kelley's textbook of rheumatology, ed 9, Philadelphia, 2012, Saunders, Fig 97-8.)*

Table 188.7	Diagnostic Indicators of Hyper-IgD Syndrome

AT TIME OF ATTACKS
1. Elevated erythrocyte sedimentation rate and leukocytosis
2. Abrupt onset of fever (≥38.5°C)
3. Recurrent attacks
4. Lymphadenopathy (especially cervical)
5. Abdominal distress (e.g., vomiting, diarrhea, pain)
6. Skin manifestations (e.g., erythematous macules and papules)
7. Arthralgias and arthritis
8. Splenomegaly

CONSTANTLY PRESENT
1. Elevated IgD (above upper limit of normal) measured on 2 occasions at least 1 mo apart*
2. Elevated IgA (≥2.6 g/L)

SPECIFIC FEATURES
1. Mutations in mevalonate kinase gene
2. Decreased mevalonate kinase enzyme activity

*Extremely high serum concentrations of IgD are characteristic but not obligatory.
From Firestein GS, Budd RC, Gabriel SE, et al, editors: *Kelly & Firestein's textbook of rheumatology*, ed 10, Philadelphia, 2016, Elsevier (Table 97-4, p 1674).

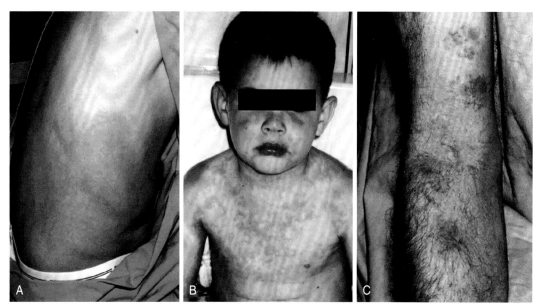

Fig. 188.6 Cutaneous manifestations of tumor necrosis factor receptor–associated periodic syndrome. **A,** Right flank of a patient with the T50M mutation. **B,** Serpiginous rash involving the face, neck, torso, and upper extremities of a child with the C30S mutation. **C,** Erythematous, macular patches with crusting on the flexor surface of the right arm of a patient with the T50M mutation. *(From Hull KM, Drewe, Aksentijevich I, et al: The TNF receptor-associated periodic syndrome [TRAPS]: emerging concepts of an autoinflammatory syndrome, Medicine (Baltimore) 81:349–368, 2002.)*

Table 188.8	Diagnostic Indicators of Tumor Necrosis Factor Receptor–Associated Periodic Syndrome (TRAPS)

1. Recurrent episodes of inflammatory symptoms spanning >6 mo duration (several symptoms generally occur simultaneously)
   a. Fever
   b. Abdominal pain
   c. Myalgia (migratory)
   d. Rash (erythematous macular rash occurs with myalgia)
   e. Conjunctivitis or periorbital edema
   f. Chest pain
   g. Arthralgia or monoarticular synovitis
2. Episodes last >5 days on average (although variable)
3. Responsive to glucocorticosteroids but not colchicine
4. Affects family members in autosomal dominant pattern (although may not always be present)
5. Any ethnicity may be affected

From Hull KM, Drewe E, Aksentijevich I, et al: The TNF receptor-associated periodic syndrome (TRAPS): emerging concepts of an autoinflammatory disorder, *Medicine (Baltimore)* 81:349–368, 2002.

proposed when mutations in *TNFRSF1A* were discovered not only in the original Irish family, but in families from a number of other ethnic backgrounds. *TNFRSF1A* encodes the 55 kDa receptor (denoted p55, TNFR1, or CD120a) for TNF-α that is widely expressed on a number of cell types. A 2nd 75 kDa receptor is largely restricted to leukocytes.

Patients with TRAPS typically present within the 1st decade of life with flares that occur with variable frequency but of often substantially longer duration than FMF or HIDS flares. The febrile episodes of TRAPS last at least 3 days and can persist for weeks. There may be pleural and peritoneal involvement. At times, patients present with signs of an acute abdomen; on exploration such patients have *sterile peritonitis*, sometimes with adhesions from previous episodes. Patients may also have nausea and frequently report constipation at the onset of flares that progresses to diarrhea by the conclusion. Ocular signs include periorbital edema and conjunctivitis. TRAPS patients may also experience severe myalgia and on imaging, the muscle groups may have focal areas of edema.

Many rashes can be seen in TRAPS patients, but the most common is an erythematous macular rash that on biopsy contains superficial and deep perivascular infiltrates of mononuclear cells. Patients often report that the rash migrates distally on a limb during its course with an underlying myalgia and can resemble cellulitis. Other rashes include erythematous annular patches as well as a serpiginous rash (Fig. 188.6). Approximately 10–15% of patients with TRAPS may develop AA amyloidosis; the presence of cysteine mutations and a positive family history are risk factors for this complication. If amyloidosis does not develop, TRAPS patients have a normal life expectancy. Table 188.8 lists diagnostic criteria.

Almost all the TRAPS-associated mutations are in the extracellular domain of the TNFR1 protein, with about one-third involving the substitution of another amino acid for a highly conserved cysteine residue, thus disrupting disulfide bonds and leading to protein misfolding. A number of other missense mutations not involving cysteine residues have been shown to have a similar effect on TNFR1 protein folding. Misfolded TNFR1 aggregates intracellularly and leads to constitutive signaling through mitogen-activated protein kinases or nuclear factor (NF)-κB, resulting in the release of proinflammatory cytokines such as IL-6, IL-1β and TNF-α. The substitution of glutamine for arginine at residue 92 (R92Q) and the substitution of leucine for proline at residue 46 (P46L) are seen in >1% of the white and black population, respectively. These variants do not lead to the same biochemical or signaling abnormalities seen with more-severe TRAPS mutations, and as with E148Q in FMF, debate surrounds whether they are mild mutations or functional polymorphisms.

Colchicine is generally not effective in TRAPS. For relatively mild disease, NSAIDs may suffice. For more severe disease with infrequent attacks, corticosteroids at the time of an attack may be effective, but it is not unusual for steroid requirements to increase over time. Etanercept is often effective in reducing the severity and frequency of flares, but longitudinal follow-up of TRAPS patients treated with etanercept indicates waning efficacy with time. Of note, treatment of TRAPS with anti-TNF-α monoclonal antibodies has sometimes led to a paradoxical worsening of disease. Clinical responses to anakinra, *canakinumab*, a monoclonal anti–IL-1β antibody, and *tocilizumab*, a monoclonal anti-IL6 antibody, has been favorable in TRAPS patients.

Cryopyrin-Associated Periodic Fever Syndromes

CAPS represent a spectrum of clinical disorders, including **familial cold autoinflammatory syndrome** (FCAS), **Muckle-Wells syndrome** (MWS), and **neonatal-onset multisystem inflammatory disorder** (NOMID). Although 3 separate clinical diagnoses have been defined, it should be emphasized that the **cryopyrinopathies** are really a continuum of disease severity. This spectrum of illness is caused by mutations in *NLRP3* (formerly known as *CIAS1*), which encodes a protein called **cryopyrin**; >100 disease-associated *NLRP3* mutations have been enumerated on the *Infevers* online database. Advances in next-generation sequencing have also permitted the identification of symptomatic individuals with somatic *NLRP3* mosaicism.

NLRP3 is a PYRIN domain-containing protein that is strongly expressed in myeloid cells and to a lesser degree in other tissues. It is a part of a macromolecular complex termed the *NLRP3 inflammasome* that activates pro–IL-1β to its mature form in response to a variety of endogenous danger-associated molecular patterns and pathogen-associated molecular patterns. Patients with cryopyrinopathies have *gain-of-function mutations* in *NLRP3* that result in constitutive or easily-triggered activation of the NLRP3 inflammasome.

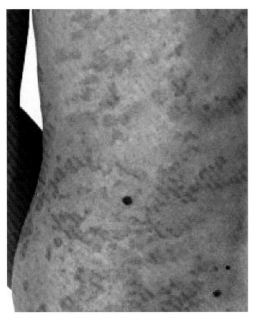

Fig. 188.7 Urticarial-like rash. Inflammatory clinical manifestations and organ damage in the IL-1–mediated diseases; in neonatal-onset multisystem inflammatory disease (NOMID), which is the severe form of cryopyrin-associated periodic syndromes (CAPS); and deficiency of IL-1 receptor antagonist (DIRA). This rash is not truly urticarial and occurs due to neutrophil infiltrates into the skin. *(From Jesus AA, Goldbach-Mansky R: IL-1 blockade in autoinflammatory syndromes. Annu Rev Med 65:223–244, 2014, Fig. 2.)*

Table 188.9	Diagnostic Criteria for Familial Cold Autoinflammatory Syndrome (FCAS)

1. Recurrent intermittent episodes of fever and rash that primarily follow generalized cold exposures
2. Autosomal dominant pattern of disease inheritance
3. Age of onset <6 mo
4. Duration of most attacks <24 hr
5. Presence of conjunctivitis associated with attacks
6. Absence of deafness, periorbital edema, lymphadenopathy, and serositis

From Hoffman HM, Wanderer AA, Broide DH: Familial cold autoinflammatory syndrome: phenotype and genotype of an autosomal dominant periodic fever, J Allergy Clin Immunol 108:615–620, 2001.

The cryopyrinopathies are characterized by recurrent fevers and an urticaria-like rash that develops early in infancy (Fig. 188.7). Histopathologic examination reveals a perivascular neutrophilic infiltrate without the mast cells or mast cell degranulation seen with true urticaria. In patients with FCAS, febrile attacks generally begin 1-3 hr after generalized cold exposure. FCAS patients also experience polyarthralgia of the hands, knees, and ankles, and conjunctivitis may also develop during attacks. FCAS episodes are self-limited and generally resolve within 24 hr. AA amyloidosis rarely occurs in FCAS. Table 188.9 lists diagnostic criteria for FCAS.

In contrast to FCAS, the febrile episodes of **MWS** are not cold induced but are characterized by the same urticarial-like rash seen in FCAS (Fig. 188.8). Many MWS patients also develop progressive sensorineural hearing loss, and untreated, approximately 30% of MWS patients develop AA amyloidosis. **NOMID** patients present in the neonatal period with a diffuse, urticarial rash, daily fevers, and dysmorphic features (Fig. 188.9). Significant joint deformities, particularly of the knees, may develop because of bony overgrowth of the epiphyses of the long bones (Fig. 188.10). NOMID patients also develop chronic aseptic meningitis, leading to increased intracranial pressure, optic disc edema, visual impairment, progressive sensorineural hearing loss, and intellectual disability (Fig. 188.11).

Targeted therapy with anakinra (recombinant IL-1R antagonist) has been life changing for NOMID patients, not only controlling fever and rash, but also preventing end-organ damage. Anakinra, rilonocept, and canakinumab are all effective in both FCAS and MWS; they are approved by the U.S. Food and Drug Administration (FDA) for both conditions. Aggressive IL-1 blockade has resulted in attenuation of amyloidosis in the cryopyrinopathies.

OTHER MENDELIAN AUTOINFLAMMATORY DISEASES

Syndrome of Pyogenic Arthritis With Pyoderma Gangrenosum and Acne

PAPA syndrome is a rare autosomal dominant disorder caused by mutations in *PSTPIP1*, a gene that encodes the cytoskeletal proline serine threonine phosphatase–interacting protein-1 (PSTPIP). The PSTPIP1 protein interacts with a number of immunologically important molecules, including CD2, the Wiskott-Aldrich syndrome protein (WASP), and pyrin. PAPA-associated *PSTPIP1* mutations greatly increase its affinity to pyrin and cause increased IL-1β production.

Clinical manifestations of PAPA syndrome begin in early childhood with recurrent episodes of sterile, pyogenic arthritis that leads to erosions and joint destruction, and appears to develop spontaneously or after minor trauma. Fever is not a dominant feature. Cutaneous manifestations tend to develop in adolescence, at which time patients are prone to developing severe cystic acne. Additionally, PAPA patients commonly

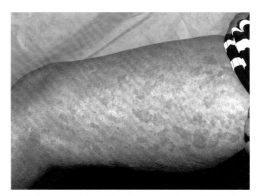

Fig. 188.8 Urticarial-like skin rash in a patient with Muckle-Wells syndrome. *(Courtesy Dr. D. L. Kastner, National Institutes of Health, Bethesda, Maryland; from Simon A, van der Meer JWM, Drenth JPH: Familial autoinflammatory syndromes. In Firestein GS, Budd RC, Gabriel SE, et al, editors: Kelley's textbook of rheumatology, ed 9, Philadelphia, 2012, Saunders, Fig 97-14.)*

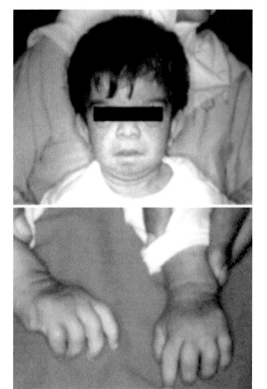

Fig. 188.9 A 3 yr old girl with NOMID/CINCA disease. Note the markedly deformed hands, rash, frontal bossing, and large head. (*From Padeh S: Periodic fever syndromes, Pediatr Clin North Am 52:577–560, 2005.*)

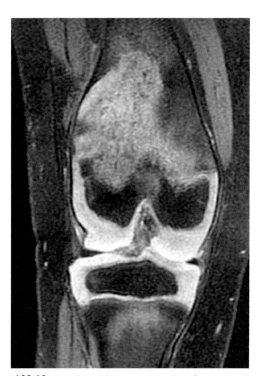

Fig. 188.10 Metaphyseal bone overgrowth. Inflammatory clinical manifestations and organ damage in the IL-1–mediated diseases; in NOMID, the severe form of CAPS; and DIRA. (*From Jesus AA, Goldbach-Mansky R: IL-1 blockade in autoinflammatory syndromes. Annu Rev Med 65:223–244, 2014, Fig 2.*)

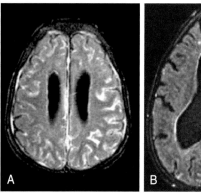

Fig. 188.11 A, Leptomeningeal enhancement; **B,** hydrocephalus and cerebral atrophy. Inflammatory clinical manifestations and organ damage in the IL-1–mediated diseases, NOMID (severe form of CAPS), and DIRA. (*From Jesus AA, Goldbach-Mansky R: IL-1 blockade in autoinflammatory syndromes,* Annu Rev Med 65:223–244, 2014, Fig 2.)

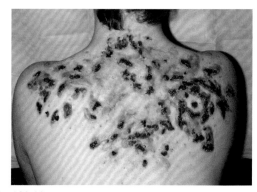

Fig. 188.12 Pyoderma gangrenosum lesions in a patient with PAPA syndrome and the A230T mutation in *PSTPIP1*. Note the diffuse scarring indicative of prior lesions on his upper back.

develop ulcerating pyoderma gangrenosum lesions (Fig. 188.12), and some develop pathergy reactions.

The treatment of PAPA syndrome may involve the use of corticosteroids, IL-1 antagonists, and TNF-α inhibitors, sometimes in combination. The joint manifestations of PAPA appear to respond to IL-1 blockade, whereas the cutaneous manifestations seem to respond more favorably to TNF-α blockade. Local measures, such as joint aspiration and drainage and intensive wound care, are also important in the care of PAPA patients, as is pain management for cutaneous disease. Caution should be taken when prescribing sulfonamides because some PAPA patients develop pancytopenia.

Deficiency of Interleukin-1 Receptor Antagonist

DIRA is an autosomal recessive autoinflammatory disease that is distinct from the cryopyrinopathies. DIRA typically presents in the neonatal period with systemic inflammation and a neutrophilic pustulosis, sterile multifocal osteomyelitis, widening of the anterior ends of the ribs, periostitis, and osteopenia (Figs. 188.13 and 188.14). Although fever is not a prominent clinical feature, patients do have greatly elevated acute-phase reactants. Multiorgan failure and pulmonary interstitial fibrosis can occur and can be fatal.

DIRA is caused by loss-of-function mutations in *IL1RN*, encoding the IL-1R antagonist. Because of the lack of antagonistic activity, the cells are hyperresponsive to IL-1β stimulation. Numerous treatments for DIRA have been tried, including NSAIDs, glucocorticoids, intravenous immune globulin (IVIG), methotrexate, cyclosporine, and etanercept. However, *anakinra is the treatment of choice,* essentially replacing the lost protein and resulting in a rapid clinical response. Anakinra is dosed daily, with the dose titrated to achieve a normal CRP. There are now longer-acting anti-IL-1 agents, canakinumab and rilonacept, which are effective and require less frequent dosing than anakinra.

Blau Syndrome

Blau syndrome is a rare autosomal dominant disorder that manifests as early-onset (<5 yr of age) granulomatous arthritis, uveitis, and rash. The arthritis may affect the ankles and wrists and may lead to flexion contractures of the fingers and toes (camptodactyly). **Early-onset sarcoidosis** presents with a similar clinical picture, sometimes with visceral involvement, and both conditions are caused by mutations in the caspase recruitment domain protein 15 (CARD15), also known as nucleotide-binding oligomerization domain-2 protein (NOD2). NOD2 is an intracellular sensor of bacterial products in DCs, myelomonocytic cells, and Paneth cells. Mutations in the NACHT oligomerization domain of this protein cause Blau syndrome/early-onset sarcoidosis, whereas

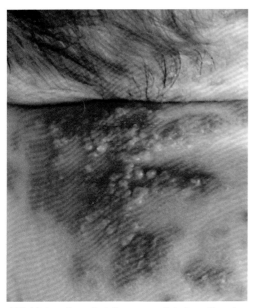

Fig. 188.13 Pustular rash. Inflammatory clinical manifestations and organ damage in the IL-1–mediated diseases, NOMID (severe form of CAPS), and DIRA. This can also be seen in deficiency of IL-36 receptor antagonist (DITRA). *(From Jesus AA, Goldbach-Mansky R: IL-1 blockade in autoinflammatory syndromes, Annu Rev Med 65:223–244, 2014, Fig 2.)*

variants primarily in the leucine-rich repeat domain are associated with susceptibility to **Crohn disease**. Corticosteroids have been the mainstay of therapy for Blau syndrome. There are a number of case reports of the beneficial effects of TNF-α inhibitors in Blau syndrome.

Autoinflammation With Phospholipase Cγ2–Associated Antibody Deficiency and Immune Dysregulation

APLAID is a dominantly inherited disorder characterized by recurrent blistering skin lesions, bronchiolitis, arthralgia, ocular inflammation, enterocolitis, absence of autoantibodies, and mild immunodeficiency. Rash is the first manifestation of APLAID, which is described as a full-body epidermolysis bullosa–like eruption. Over time, this rash changes to recurrent plaques and vesiculopustular lesions that are triggered by heat and sunlight. Colitis also presents in childhood before age 5 yr. Ocular manifestations begin before age 1 yr and include corneal ulcerations and erosions as well as cataracts. Immune manifestations include markedly decreased class-switched memory B cells, resulting in low IgM and IgA.

Patients with APLAID show a gain-of-function missense mutation in the autoinhibitory region of phospholipase Cγ2 (PLCγ2), leading to increased activity of downstream mediators and stimulation of lymphocytes. Despite the enhanced signaling, the resulting populations of immune cells have poor function. Interestingly, a different mutation in the PLCγ2 complex leads to a syndrome known as **PLCγ2-associated antibody deficiency and immune dysregulation (PLAID)**, characterized by cold-induced urticaria, hypogammaglobulinemia with resulting susceptibility to infection, and autoimmunity.

Because of the low number of affected patients described, there are no agreed treatment regimens for APLAID. Patients have been treated with NSAIDs, and corticosteroids can be effective, but side effects limit their long term use. TNF-α inhibitors and IL-1 inhibitors have been used with some success.

Deficiency of Adenosine Deaminase 2

DADA2 is an autoinflammatory disorder caused by loss-of-function mutations in *CECR1*, encoding adenosine deaminase 2. DADA2 presents with recurrent fevers and a spectrum of vascular manifestations that includes livedo racemosa, early-onset ischemic lacunar strokes, and systemic vasculitis of medium side vessels similar to **polyarteritis nodosa**. The lacunar strokes, typically affecting the deep brain nuclei and the brainstem, transpire before age 5 yr and typically occur during inflammatory episodes. The livedoid rash is also a prominent feature during inflammatory episodes, and biopsies demonstrate a predominance of neutrophils and macrophages as well as vasculitis in medium-sized vessels. Acute-phase reactants are typically elevated. Other features include ophthalmologic involvement, various degrees of lymphopenia, hypogammaglobulinemia (usually IgM), hepatosplenomegaly, portal

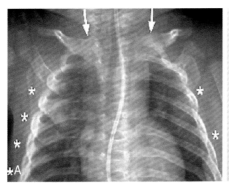
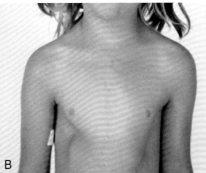

Fig. 188.14 A, Widening of multiple ribs (*) and clavicles *(arrows)* in DIRA osteomyelitis; **B,** chest deformity. Inflammatory clinical manifestations and organ damage in the IL-1-mediated diseases, NOMID, and DIRA. *(From Jesus AA, Goldbach-Mansky R: IL-1 blockade in autoinflammatory syndromes, Annu Rev Med 65:223–244, 2014, Fig 2.)*

hypertension, and neutropenia. Patients may meet criteria for polyarteritis nodosa and can exhibit digit necrosis and Raynaud phenomenon.

ADA2 is produced primarily by monocytes and macrophages, is found in plasma, and appears to act as a growth and differentiation factor for a subset of inflammatory macrophages. Numerous antiinflammatories have been tried in patients with DAD2, including glucocorticoids and cyclophosphamide. TNF-α inhibitors (etanercept or adalimumab) are the mainstay of treatment, and anecdotal reports have shown a benefit of anakinra. Macrophages and monocytes are the main sources of ADA2, raising the possibility of bone marrow transplant to achieve a permanent cure.

Sideroblastic Anemia With Immunodeficiency, Fevers, and Development Delay

SIFD is a syndrome characterized by systemic inflammation, fevers, enteritis, and sideroblastic anemia and caused by biallelic mutations in *TRNT1*. SIFD presents in infancy with fever, elevated inflammatory markers, gastroenteritis, and anemia. Bone marrow biopsies demonstrate ringed sideroblasts. Other features include hypogammaglobulinemia, B-cell lymphopenia, developmental delay, and variable neurodevelopmental degeneration, seizures, and sensorineural hearing loss. Brain imaging was notable for cerebellar atrophy, delayed white matter myelination, and decreased perfusion. Other, isolated clinical features include nephrocalcinosis, aminoaciduria, ichthyotic skin, cardiomyopathy, and retinitis pigmentosa. TRNT1 is an RNA polymerase that is necessary for maturation of cytosolic and mitochondrial transfer RNAs, by the addition of 2 cytosines and 1 adenosine to the tRNA ends.

Symptomatic treatment with regular blood transfusions and immunoglobulin replacement therapy is the mainstay of SIFD therapy. Iron overload from the transfusion often requires chelation therapy. Anakinra relieved the febrile episodes in one patient but did not alter the other clinical manifestations. Patients with SIFD have a high mortality rate. One patient underwent hematopoietic bone marrow transplantation at 9 mo of age that resulted in correction of the hematologic and immunologic abnormalities.

Deficiency of Interleukin-36 Receptor Antagonist (DITRA)

DITRA is characterized by episodes of diffuse erythematous pustular rash (generalized pustular psoriasis), fevers, general malaise, and systemic inflammation. Attacks can be triggered by events such as infections, pregnancy, or menstruation or can occur randomly. The underlying genetic etiology has been determined to be autosomal recessive mutations in the *IL36RN* gene, which encodes an IL-36R antagonist. IL-36 is related to and acts similarly to IL1R antagonist, preventing production of inflammatory cytokines such as IL-8. Interestingly, the rash of DITRA is similar to the rash of DIRA (IL-1R deficiency; see earlier), but DITRA is largely skin limited. DITRA has been treated with various modalities, including vitamin A analogs, cyclosporine, methotrexate, and TNF-α inhibitors. The use of anakinra has been described in case reports and results in alleviation of the symptoms.

Familial Cold Autoinflammatory Syndrome Type 2

Mutations in *NLRP12* lead to a periodic fever syndrome characterized by fevers >40°C, arthralgias, and myalgias lasting from 2-10 days. This disorder is named FCAS2 because these episodes can be precipitated by cold. Clinical findings may include an urticarial-like rash, abdominal pain and vomiting, aphthous ulcers, and lymphadenopathy. As with Muckle-Wells syndrome, sensorineural hearing loss and optic neuritis have been described. NALP12 is a member of the CATERPILLAR family of proteins, which are important in innate immunity. Similar to Toll-like receptors (TLRs) that act to recognize pathogen-associated molecular patterns (PAMPs), NLRP12 also senses PAMPs and can lead to the activation of the inflammasome and generation of IL-1β. Treatment of *NALP12* mutations was difficult until the advent of anti–IL-1 agents (e.g., anakinra), which are the preferred treatment for FCAS2 and result in remarkable resolution of symptoms. Colchicine can be partially effective, and systemic glucocorticoids can reduce the duration of the attacks.

Autoinflammation With Enterocolitis

A disorder caused by mutations in *NLRC4* was described with neonatal-onset enterocolitis, fever, and autoinflammatory episodes. Inflammatory markers are typically elevated, including CRP and ferritin. **Macrophage activation syndrome**, characterized by pancytopenia, hypertriglyceridemia, and coagulopathies, is common during acute flares, which can be precipitated by emotional and physical stress. Recurrent myalgias with febrile episodes often occur as well. This disorder is caused by gain-of-function missense mutations in NOD-like receptor C4 (NLRC4), which normally aids in the activation of the inflammasome. The resulting protein leads to constitutive production of IL-1. The mainstay of treatment is anti-IL-1 agents such as anakinra, canakinumab, and rilonacept. Before their diagnosis, patients with *NLRC4* mutations had been treated with colchicine and oral glucocorticoids, with varying success.

Majeed Syndrome

Majeed syndrome is an autosomal recessive disorder caused by mutations in the *LPIN2* gene (see Table 188.4). The clinical manifestation of Majeed syndrome begin in childhood with recurrent fevers, sterile osteomyelitis, congenital dyserythropoietic anemia (CDA), neutrophilic dermatosis, failure to thrive, and hepatomegaly. Treatment of Majeed syndrome has included NSAIDs, corticosteroids, and IL-1R antagonist. How mutations in *LPIN2* lead to an autoinflammatory disorder is not known.

Interferonopathies

Type 1 interferons (IFN-α and IFN-β) are the first line of defense against viral infections and are produced by a variety of cell types. During viral infections, a variety of products are made by the virus, including ssRNA, dsRNA, and CpG-containing DNA, and are recognized by intracellular sensors. These sensors then induce type 1 IFN production that activates IFN receptors and activates IFN-responsive genes to help control the spread of the virus until the adaptive immune system can be activated to clear the virus. Inappropriate activation of these pathways leads to IFN production and interferonopathies.

Chronic Atypical Neutrophilic Dermatosis With Lipodystrophy and Elevated Temperature

CANDLE syndrome, also known as **proteasome-associated autoinflammatory syndrome (PRAAS)** or **joint contractures, muscular atrophy, panniculitis-induced lipodystrophy (JMP) syndrome**, is an autosomal recessive disease. Patients present early in life with recurrent fevers and systemic inflammation; skin involvement, including annular erythema, erythema nodosum–like panniculitis, or neutrophilic dermatosis; small joint contractures; lipodystrophy; muscle atrophy or myositis; violaceous eyelid swelling; and anemia. Conjunctivitis, aseptic meningitis, and organomegaly are common. Acute-phase reactants and platelet counts are elevated. Autoimmunity can occur, including Coombs-positive hemolytic anemia and hypothyroidism. Intelligence and development are typically spared, although mild developmental delays have been reported. CANDLE is caused by loss-of-function mutations in *PSMB8*, the gene that encodes the β5i subunit of the proteasome. Proteosomes are important in the degradation of ubiquinated proteins to ensure proper protein homeostasis, and defects in proteasomes result in cellular stress and inflammatory cytokine release, including type 1 interferons.

There is no established treatment for CANDLE, although multiple treatment modalities have been attempted, including colchicine, dapsone, cyclosporine, infliximab, and etanercept, all with minimal success. Glucocorticoids and methotrexate have provided slight improvement in symptoms. Anakinra has not proved successful, whereas IL-6–blocking agents have shown some benefit. Since interferon receptors use the JAK/STAT pathway to signal, JAK inhibitors (tofacitinib, ruxolitinib, and baricitinib) show promise.

STING-Associated Vasculopathy With Onset in Infancy

SAVI is a rare disorder that presents in infancy. It is caused by mutations in the *TMEM173* gene, which encodes for the stimulator of interferon genes (STING). Systemic inflammation is an early manifestation, with fever and elevated inflammatory markers. Skin involvement includes a neutrophilic rash as well as violaceous lesions of fingers, toes, nose, cheeks, and ears. These lesions worsen over time and can become necrotic with vascular occlusion. Histology of the lesions reveals dermal inflammation with leukocytoclastic vasculitis and microthrombotic angiopathy. Since STING is also expressed in pulmonary epithelium, SAVI patients also developed pulmonary complications, including paratracheal adenopathy, interstitial lung disease, and fibrosis.

STING is an adapter protein of the intracellular DNA sensing machinery and mediates the production of interferon-β (IFN-β). The IFN-β then signals through the IFN receptor by activating the JAK/STAT signaling pathway and downstream IFN-responsive genes, including IL-6 and TNF-α. Mutations in STING that cause SAVI are de novo gain-of-function mutations that activate spontaneous IFN-β production.

Treatment options for patients with SAVI are limited at this time, although recent data with JAK inhibitors (tofacitinib, ruxolitinib, and baricitinib) have shown promise in blocking IFN-β receptor signaling and the activation of IFN-response genes.

GENETICALLY COMPLEX AUTOINFLAMMATORY DISEASES
Periodic Fever, Aphthous Stomatitis, Pharyngitis, and Adenitis

PFAPA is the most common recurrent fever syndrome in children. It usually presents between ages 2 and 5 yr with recurring episodes of fever, malaise, exudative-appearing tonsillitis with negative throat cultures, cervical lymphadenopathy, oral aphthae, and less often headache, abdominal pain, and arthralgia. The episodes last 4-6 days, regardless of antipyretic or antibiotic treatment, and often occur with clock-like regularity on 3-6 wk cycles. Findings during the episodes may include mild hepatosplenomegaly, mild leukocytosis, and elevated acute-phase reactants. Both the frequency and the intensity of the episodes diminish with increasing age. The etiology and pathogenesis of PFAPA remain unknown.

Most patients show dramatic response to a single oral dose of prednisone (0.6-2.0 mg/kg), although this approach does not prevent recurrence and may actually shorten the interval between flares. Cimetidine at 20-40 mg/kg/day is effective at preventing recurrences in approximately one third of cases. Small series have shown that anakinra may be effective during a flare, but because corticosteroids are effective, this may not be a cost-effective approach. Colchicine may extend the time between flares. Complete resolution has been reported after tonsillectomy, although medical management should be the first approach.

Chronic Recurrent Multifocal Osteomyelitis

CRMO is a form of inflammatory bone disease most frequently seen in children (see Table 188.4). Histologically and radiologically, CRMO is virtually indistinguishable from infectious osteomyelitis (Fig. 188.15). Patients typically present with bone pain and may also have fever, soft

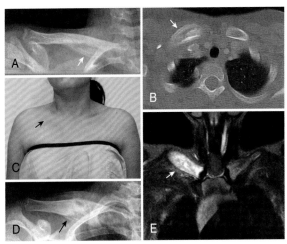

Fig. 188.15 Clavicular involvement in chronic recurrent multifocal osteomyelitis. Adolescent female with unilateral clavicular involvement. **A,** Plain radiograph of the right clavicle at presentation reveals widening of the medial two thirds, with associated periosteal reaction. **B,** Corresponding CT scan of the right clavicle demonstrates expansion of the medial right clavicle with areas of increased sclerosis accompanied by a surrounding periosteal reaction (*arrow*). **C,** Flare of disease 18 months later showing further clavicular enlargement (clinical photo). **D,** Plain radiograph of the right clavicle at that time demonstrates marked interval sclerosis and thickening. **E,** MRI at the same time shows increased signal intensity on fat-suppressed contrast-enhanced T1-weighted images of the right medial clavicle consistent with continued inflammation. (*Images courtesy Dr. Paul Babyn, University of Saskatchewan and Saskatchewan Health Authority, Saskatchewan, Canada.*)

tissue swelling, and elevated acute-phase reactants. Cultures are sterile. Typically involved bones include the distal femur, proximal tibia or fibula, spine, and pelvis. Both metaphyseal and epiphyseal lesions may occur; premature physeal closure may develop. Less frequently involved bones include the clavicle and mandible. The differential diagnosis includes infectious osteomyelitis, histiocytosis, and malignancy (neuroblastoma, lymphoma, leukemia, Ewing sarcoma). **SAPHO** (synovitis, acne, pustulosis, hyperostosis, and osteitis) may be an adult equivalent to CRMO. The etiology of sporadic CRMO is unknown. CRMO is seen in Majeed syndrome (see earlier), in association with inflammatory bowel disease, and inflammatory skin disease such as palmoplantar pustulosis. Initial therapy includes NSAIDs. Second-line treatments include corticosteroids, TNF inhibitors, and bisphosphonates.

Bibliography is available at Expert Consult.

Chapter 189

Amyloidosis
Karyl S. Barron and Amanda K. Ombrello

第一百八十九章
淀粉样变性

中文导读

　　本章主要介绍了淀粉样变性的病因、流行病学、发病机制、临床表现、诊断、实验室诊断、治疗、预后和预防。病因上分为遗传性淀粉样变性、再生障碍性淀粉样变性；流行病学中描述了不同类型淀粉样变性在不同风湿性疾病中的患病差异；描述了不同类型的淀粉样变性可能的发病机制；描述了不同受累部位的临床表现；诊断需对病变组织进行活检；实验室检查表现为炎性反应物升高及免疫球蛋白升高；治疗中描述了不同类型淀粉样变性的治疗措施及疗效；预后中描述了本病的死亡原因及预后影响因素。

Amyloidosis comprises a group of diseases characterized by extracellular deposition of insoluble, fibrous amyloid proteins in various body tissues.

ETIOLOGY

Amyloidosis is a disease caused by protein misfolding. These misfolded proteins infiltrate, aggregate, and form insoluble fibrils that can affect the normal function of a number of vital organs.

In the amyloidosis nomenclature, a distinction is made between amyloidosis that develops from mutations in the *amyloid fibril protein itself* and amyloidosis associated with genetic mutation in nonamyloid proteins. The former are referred to as **hereditary amyloidoses**; examples include mutations in the genes for transthyretin and apolipoprotein A, both of which are uncommon in young children. This is in contrast to **amyloid A (AA) amyloidosis**, which develops in patients with chronic inflammatory states. It is estimated that, worldwide, approximately 45% of all amyloid cases are AA amyloidosis. In the past, chronic infectious diseases such as tuberculosis, malaria, leprosy, and chronic osteomyelitis accounted for most cases of AA amyloidosis. With effective treatment for these infections, other causes of AA have become more common. A number of chronic inflammatory rheumatic diseases, such as **rheumatoid arthritis (RA)**, **juvenile idiopathic arthritis (JIA)**, and **ankylosing spondylitis**, as well as hereditary autoinflammatory diseases, have an increased risk for the development of AA amyloidosis. AA amyloidosis has also been associated with granulomatous diseases such as sarcoidosis, cystic fibrosis, Crohn disease, malignancies such as mesothelioma and Hodgkin diseases, intravenous drug abuse, and other infections, such as bronchiectasis and HIV. Approximately 6% of AA amyloidosis cases have no identified disease association. **AL amyloidosis** (formerly known as *idiopathic amyloidosis* or *myeloma-associated amyloidosis*) is extremely rare in children, occurring in middle-aged or older individuals.

EPIDEMIOLOGY

Only AA amyloidosis affects children in appreciable numbers. The factors that determine the risk for amyloidosis as a complication of inflammation are not clear, because many individuals with long-standing inflammatory disease do not demonstrate tissue amyloid deposition, whereas some children with relatively recent onset of disease may develop amyloid. In developed countries, before the initiation of therapy with disease-modifying antirheumatic drugs (DMARDs) and biologic agents, RA was the most common inflammatory disease associated with AA amyloidosis. Patients who had a long history of poorly controlled severe disease with extraarticular manifestations were the most at risk for developing amyloidosis, and the median time from first symptoms of their rheumatic condition to the diagnosis of amyloidosis was 212 mo. The full effect of DMARD and biologic therapy in RA-associated amyloidosis has yet to be fully appreciated, but studies are showing a sustained decline in the number of new cases.

JIA is another rheumatic disease associated with development of AA amyloidosis, with the highest prevalence in patients with systemic JIA, followed by those with polyarticular disease (see Chapter 180). In the pre-DMARDs and prebiologics era, the prevalence of AA amyloidosis in JIA patients ranged from 1–10%. Higher prevalence was seen in Northern European patients, especially Polish patients, who had a prevalence of 10.6%; lower prevalence was observed in North America. The reasons for this discrepancy are not completely understood, although it is speculated that selection bias, genetic background, and tendency toward earlier, more aggressive therapy in North Americans may have played a role. AA amyloidosis has been observed in JIA patients as early as 1 yr after diagnosis. Similar to RA, the occurrence of new amyloid cases has significantly decreased in the past 20 yr because of the increased efficacy of treatment with DMARDs and biologics.

The **hereditary autoinflammatory diseases** define a group of illnesses characterized by attacks of seemingly unprovoked recurrent inflammation without significant levels of either autoantibodies or antigen-specific T cells, which are typically found in patients with autoimmune diseases (see Chapter 188). Although seemingly unprovoked, these attacks are often initiated by stress, immunization, or trauma, suggesting that gene-environment interactions play an important role in pathogenesis. Although there is some variability among the autoinflammatory diseases, common findings include fevers, cutaneous rashes, arthritis, serositis, and ocular involvement. The inflammatory attacks are accompanied by intense acute-phase responses (erythrocyte sedimentation rate and C-reactive protein) and high levels of serum amyloid A (SAA). Amyloidosis AA is associated with some but not all the hereditary autoinflammatory diseases.

Familial Mediterranean fever (FMF) is the most common of the mendelian autoinflammatory diseases and is seen most frequently in the Armenian, Arab, Turkish, and Sephardi Jewish populations. FMF is an autosomal recessive disease that results from mutations in the *MEFV* gene, which encodes the pyrin/marenostrin protein. *MEFV* mutations affecting the M680 and M694 amino acid residues are associated with early onset of FMF, severe disease, and an increased risk of AA amyloidosis. Patients residing in Armenia, Turkey, and Arabian countries have an increased risk of developing AA amyloidosis compared to patients with the same mutations of *MEFV* living in North America. While one may assume that FMF patients who have frequent, severe attacks would be at the most risk for the development of AA amyloidosis, this is not always the case. Some patients have had a history of frequent attacks and never develop amyloidosis, and others develop amyloidosis at an early age. There is also a subset of FMF patients referred to as **phenotype II**. These patients present with AA amyloidosis before their first FMF attack. In this group the distribution of the common *MEFV* mutation is similar to that found in FMF patients with typical symptoms.

Tumor necrosis factor receptor–associated periodic syndrome (TRAPS) is associated with mutations in the *TNFRSF1A* gene, which encodes the 55 kDa tumor necrosis factor (TNF) receptor protein (TNFR1). It is estimated that 14-25% of patients with TRAPS develop AA amyloidosis. Patients with mutations in *TNFRSF1A* that affect cysteine residues have the highest risk of developing AA amyloidosis. It is thought that these cysteine residues participate in assembly of disulfide bonds important for TNFR1 folding, and that disruption of these bonds affects protein folding.

Mutations in the *NLRP3* gene (also known as *CIAS1*, cold-induced autoinflammatory syndrome 1) cause 3 clinically distinct diseases: **familial cold autoinflammatory syndrome (FCAS), Muckle-Wells syndrome (MWS),** and **neonatal-onset multisystem inflammatory disease (NOMID)**, also known as **chronic infantile neurologic cutaneous and articular (CINCA) syndrome**. Mutations in *NLRP3* are inherited in an autosomal dominant fashion or as de novo mutations in patients with the most severe disease. A smaller portion of patients have been found to carry somatic mutations in *NLRP3*.

FCAS is generally the least severe of the cryopyrinopathies and is rarely associated with AA amyloidosis. MWS presents with fevers, myalgias, arthralgias, urticarial-like rash, and progressive sensorineural hearing loss. AA amyloidosis is quite common in MWS, affecting up to one third of the patients. NOMID/CINCA is the most severe cryopyrinopathy. Historically, 20% of patients died before reaching adulthood, but with current therapies, many are living longer lives. Some NOMID patients develop AA amyloidosis as they get older, although not as often as MWS patients, possibly because of a shortened life span in these patients.

Hyper-IgD syndrome (HIDS) is another autoinflammatory disease that presents in early childhood with chills, high fevers, abdominal pain, lymphadenopathy, and occasional rash. HIDS is an autosomal recessive disease that involves loss-of-function mutations in the *MVK* gene that encodes the mevalonate kinase enzyme. Severe *MVK* mutations that completely abolish enzyme activity are identified in patients with **mevalonic aciduria**, who present with recurrent fevers, dysmorphic features, and developmental delays. HIDS-associated mutations are milder loss-of-function mutations. Inflammatory markers, including

SAA, are high during attacks and may remain elevated in the intercurrent period. AA amyloidosis is rare in HIDS but has been reported.

Although seen less frequently than in the hereditary periodic fever syndromes, the risk of AA amyloidosis has been well established in patients with Crohn disease. AA amyloidosis occurs in an estimated 1% of U.S. patients and up to 3% in Northern European patients. Conversely, AA amyloidosis presenting in patients with ulcerative colitis is extremely rare, with estimated prevalence of 0.07%. The patients have a long-standing history of aggressive, poorly controlled disease, although there are reports of amyloidosis in patients with well-controlled inflammatory markers.

Transthyretin-related hereditary amyloidosis is an autosomal dominant disorder with variable penetrance and onset in the 2nd to 3rd decade of life. More than 120 single or double mutations in the *TTR* gene are responsible for disease. Manifestations include neuropathy (familial amyloidotic polyneuropathy: motor, sensory, autonomic), familial amyloid cardiomyopathy, nephropathy, and ocular disease.

PATHOGENESIS

The deposition of AA amyloid fibrils is a result of a prolonged inflammatory state that leads to misfolding of the AA amyloid protein and deposition into tissues. The precursor protein of the fibrils in AA amyloidosis is an apolipoprotein called *serum amyloid A* (SAA). SAA is expressed by 3 different genes that are localized on chromosome p15.1. SAA1 and SAA2 are 2 isoforms that are acute-phase reactants synthesized by the liver that can form amyloid. SAA is produced in response to proinflammatory cytokines such as interleukin (IL)-1, IL-6, and TNF-α and can increase >1,000-fold during inflammation. It has been speculated that SAA has a role as a chemoattractant and in lipid metabolism. Supporting this theory is the finding that amyloid deposition occurs initially in organs that are major sites of lipid and cholesterol metabolism, such as the kidney, liver, and spleen. Approximately 80% of secreted SAA1 and SAA2 are bound to lipoprotein.

Under normal circumstances, SAA secreted by the liver is completely degraded by macrophages. The secreted SAA protein is 104 amino acids in length and is primarily secreted in an α-helix structure. For reasons not completely understood, patients with AA amyloidosis have a flaw resulting in incomplete degradation and accumulation of intermediate SAA products. In these patients, SAA is transferred to the lysosome, where the c-terminal portion of the SAA protein is cleaved, allowing the remaining protein to fold into a β-pleated sheet configuration. Deposited amyloid contains only 66-76 amino acids, compared to the 104 in secreted SAA. These cleaved fragments polymerize and form fibrils that are deposited in the extracellular space and bind proteoglycans and other proteins such as serum amyloid P. These fibrils then become resistant to proteolysis and deposit in organ tissues.

Development of AA amyloid may be associated with a number of risk factors. The gene encoding SAA1 has polymorphisms that, when present, carry a 3-7–fold increased risk for the development of AA amyloidosis. Caucasian patients with RA, JIA, or autoinflammatory diseases who have the SAAα/α (alpha/alpha) genotype have an increased risk of amyloidosis. In that group of patients, the SSA1γ (gamma) allele is associated with a decreased risk of amyloidosis. Interestingly, the risk in Japanese patients is reversed, with SAAα/α genotype is associated with a decreased susceptibility to amyloidosis development but the SAA1γ genotype carries an increased risk.

CLINICAL MANIFESTATIONS

Although organ involvement may vary, AA amyloidosis most frequently affects the kidneys; 90% of patients have some degree of renal involvement. Unexplained proteinuria may be the presenting feature in some patients. Nephrotic syndrome and renal failure may develop if the underlying inflammatory condition is not controlled or if diagnosis is delayed. Median survival after diagnosis has been reported to be 133 mo; patients with higher SAA levels had significantly higher risk of death than those with lower SAA levels. Gastrointestinal involvement is seen in approximately 20% of patients and usually manifests as chronic diarrhea, GI bleeding, abdominal pain, and malabsorption. When biopsied, the testes are frequently involved (87%). Relatively uncommon findings associated with AA amyloidosis include anemia, amyloid goiter, hepatomegaly, splenomegaly, adrenal involvement, and pulmonary involvement. Tissues, such as the heart, tongue, and skin, are rarely involved.

DIAGNOSIS

The diagnosis of amyloidosis is established by biopsy demonstrating amyloid fibril proteins in affected tissues. The tissues tested include kidney, rectum, abdominal fat pad, and gingiva. Amyloid deposits are composed of seemingly homogeneous eosinophilic material that stains with Congo red dye and demonstrates the pathognomonic "apple-green birefringence" in polarized light. Tissue and genetic testing is useful for transthyretin amyloidosis.

LABORATORY FINDINGS

Patients with AA amyloidosis usually show elevated acute-phase reactants and high levels of immunoglobulins. In the United States, specific laboratory testing is not commercially available for AA amyloid, but in other countries, SAA levels can be monitored and used to guide response to treatment.

TREATMENT

There is no established therapy for AA amyloidosis, and thus the primary approach is aggressive management of the underlying inflammatory or infectious disease, which decreases levels of SAA protein. As newer therapies are developed to treat the underlying condition, emerging evidence shows that the incidence of AA amyloidosis is decreasing. *Colchicine* is effective not only in controlling the attacks of FMF but also in preventing the development of amyloidosis associated with FMF. Children with FMF who are homozygous for the M694V mutation in *MEFV* are at greater risk for development of amyloidosis and should be monitored closely.

Unlike AA amyloidosis associated with FMF, AA amyloidosis associated with other autoinflammatory diseases (including TRAPS, cryopyrin-associated periodic syndrome, and rarely HIDS) and chronic rheumatic diseases (JIA, RA, and ankylosing spondylitis) does not respond to colchicine. Although AA amyloidosis associated with JIA may respond to *chlorambucil*, this drug is associated with chromosome breakage and a risk of subsequent malignancy.

Increasing use of biologic medicines (**biologics**) against proinflammatory cytokines to treat RA, JIA, spondyloarthropathies, and the hereditary autoinflammatory diseases seems to impact risk factors for the development of AA amyloidosis. The class of medications referred to as the *anti–TNF-α drugs* have been paramount in the management of RA and other autoimmune disease. In both autoimmune and auto-inflammatory conditions with accompanying AA amyloidosis, there are reports documenting the effectiveness of anti-TNF agents in blunting the progression of amyloidosis. Adverse effects of anti-TNF medications include reactivation of tuberculosis and hepatitis B, and thus careful screening should be performed before instituting therapy. Additionally, the development of various antibodies, autoantibodies, and autoimmune disease has been noted in patients taking anti-TNF agents. Extreme caution should be used in prescribing anti-TNF agents to patients with a history of heart failure or demyelinating disease, because use can cause exacerbations in their underlying cardiac and neurologic diseases.

The IL-1 pathway is the target of multiple biologic medications used in autoimmune and autoinflammatory diseases. The 3 available IL-1 antagonists are *anakinra* (IL-1 receptor antagonist), *rilonacept* (soluble IL-1 receptor decoy), and *canakinumab* (long-acting fully humanized IgG$_1$ anti–IL-1β monoclonal antibody). The various IL-1 inhibitors have been successful at slowing the progression of AA amyloidosis, and in some cases treatment results in regression of amyloid-associated proteinuria.

Tocilizumab, an anti–IL-6 receptor antibody, has been shown to attenuate experimental AA amyloid and to reverse AA amyloidosis complicating FMF, JIA, and RA. A recent trial using *eprodisate disodium* in AA amyloid patients failed to meet its primary end-point of reducing progression to end-stage renal disease.

Transthyretin amyloidosis has been treated with liver transplantation and transthyretin-stabilizing agents.

PROGNOSIS

End-stage renal failure is the underlying cause of death in 40–60% of patients with amyloidosis, with a median survival time from diagnosis of 2-10 yr. According to a large-scale study of 374 patients with AA amyloidosis, the factors associated with a poor prognosis include older age, a lower albumin serum level, end-stage renal disease at baseline, and prolonged serum elevation of SAA. An elevated SAA value was the most powerful risk factor for end-stage renal disease and death from AA amyloidosis.

PREVENTION

The primary means of preventing AA amyloidosis is treatment of the underlying inflammatory or infectious disease, resulting in decreases in the level of SAA protein and the risk of amyloid deposition. Although the period of latency between the onset of inflammation (of the underlying disease) and the initial clinical signs of AA amyloidosis may vary and is often prolonged, progression of the amyloid depositions can be rapid.

Bibliography is available at Expert Consult.

Chapter **190**
Sarcoidosis

Eveline Y. Wu

第一百九十章
结节病

中文导读

本章主要介绍了结节病的病因学、流行病学、病理学及病理、临床表现、实验室检查、诊断、鉴别诊断、治疗及预后。病因及病理中分析了遗传易感性、环境及职业接触等因素；流行病学中描述了不同年龄、种族发病的差异；病理学上描述了肉芽肿病变的病理特点及高钙血症、高钙尿症的病理；临床表现上具体阐述了全身各个部位受累的临床表现；实验室检查描述了各辅助检查特点；诊断性检查具体包括活检、胸片、肝肾功能、裂隙灯及支气管镜等检查；鉴别诊断包括肉芽肿性炎症、肉芽肿性病变相关的免疫缺陷病、淋巴瘤及结节性关节炎等；治疗中描述了皮质类固醇、免疫抑制剂及生物制剂治疗及疗效；预后中主要描述了不受累部位及程度相应预后。

Sarcoidosis is a rare multisystem granulomatous disease of unknown etiology. The name is derived from a Greek word meaning "flesh-like condition," in reference to the characteristic skin lesions. There appear to be 2 distinct, age-dependent patterns of disease among children with sarcoidosis. The clinical features in older children are similar to those in adults (pediatric-onset adult sarcoidosis), with frequent systemic features (fever, weight loss, malaise), pulmonary involvement, and lymphadenopathy. In contrast, early-onset sarcoidosis manifesting in children <4 yr of age is characterized by the triad of rash, uveitis, and polyarthritis.

ETIOLOGY

The etiology of sarcoidosis remains obscure but likely results from exposure of a genetically susceptible individual to 1 or more unidentified antigens. This exposure initiates an exaggerated immunologic response that ultimately leads to the formation of granulomas. The human major histocompatibility complex is located on chromosome 6, and specific human leukocyte antigen (HLA) class I and class II alleles are associated with disease phenotype. Genetic polymorphisms involving various cytokines and chemokines may also have a role in development of sarcoidosis. Familial clustering supports the contribution of genetic factors to sarcoidosis susceptibility. Environmental and occupational exposures are also associated with disease risk. There are positive associations between sarcoidosis and agricultural employment, occupational exposure to insecticides, and moldy environments typically associated with microbial bioaerosols.

Blau syndrome is an autosomal dominant, familial form of sarcoidosis and is typified by the early onset of granulomatous inflammation involving the skin, eyes, and joints. Missense mutations in the *CARD15/NOD2* gene on chromosome 16 have been found in affected family members and appear to be associated with development of sarcoidosis. The 2 most common amino acid substitutions are R334W (arginine to glutamine) and R334Q (arginine to tryptophan). Similar genetic mutations also have been found in individuals with a sporadic **early-onset sarcoidosis (EOS)** (rash, uveitis, arthritis), suggesting that this nonfamilial form and Blau syndrome are genetically and phenotypically identical (see Chapter 188).

EPIDEMIOLOGY

A nationwide patient registry of childhood sarcoidosis in Denmark estimated the annual incidence to be 0.22-0.27 per 100,000 children. The incidence increases with age, and peak onset occurs at 20-39 yr. The most common age of reported childhood cases is 13-15 yr. Annual incidence is about 11 per 100,000 in adult white Americans and is 3 times higher in blacks. There is no clear sex predominance in childhood sarcoidosis. The majority of U.S. childhood sarcoidosis cases are reported in the southeastern and south-central states.

An international registry and Spanish cohort of Blau syndrome and EOS reported the mean age of disease onset as 30 mo and 36 mo, respectively. All but 3 of these young patients presented before 5 yr of age. There does not appear to be a sex predilection in either condition.

PATHOLOGY AND PATHOGENESIS

Noncaseating, epithelioid granulomatous lesions are a cardinal feature of sarcoidosis. Activated macrophages, epithelioid cells, and multinucleated giant cells as well as CD4$^+$ T lymphocytes accumulate and become tightly packed in the center of the granuloma. The causative agent that initiates this inflammatory process is not known. The periphery of the granuloma contains a loose collection of monocytes, CD4$^+$ and CD8$^+$ T lymphocytes, and fibroblasts. The interaction between the macrophages and CD4$^+$ T lymphocytes is important in the formation and maintenance of the granuloma. The activated macrophages secrete high levels of tumor necrosis factor (TNF)-α and other proinflammatory mediators. The CD4$^+$ T lymphocytes differentiate into type 1 helper T cells and release interleukin (IL)-2 and interferon (IFN)-γ, promoting proliferation of lymphocytes. Granulomas may heal or resolve with complete preservation of the parenchyma. In approximately 20% of the lesions, the fibroblasts in the periphery proliferate and produce fibrotic scar tissue, leading to significant and irreversible organ dysfunction.

The sarcoid macrophage is able to produce and secrete 1,25-(OH)$_2$-vitamin D or *calcitriol*, an active form of vitamin D typically produced in the kidneys. The hormone's natural functions are to increase intestinal absorption of calcium and bone resorption and decrease renal excretion of calcium and phosphate. An excess of calcitriol may result in hypercalcemia and hypercalciuria in patients with sarcoidosis.

CLINICAL MANIFESTATIONS

Sarcoidosis is a multisystem disease, and granulomatous lesions may occur in any organ of the body. The clinical manifestations depend on the extent and degree of granulomatous inflammation and are extremely variable. Children may present with nonspecific symptoms, such as fever, weight loss, and general malaise. In adults and older children, pulmonary involvement is most frequent, with infiltration of the thoracic lymph nodes and lung parenchyma. Isolated bilateral hilar adenopathy on chest radiograph is the most common finding (Fig. 190.1), but parenchymal infiltrates and miliary nodules may also be seen (Figs. 190.2 and 190.3). Patients with lung involvement are usually found to have restrictive changes on pulmonary function testing. Symptoms of pulmonary disease are seldom severe and generally consist of a dry, persistent cough.

Extrathoracic lymphadenopathy and infiltration of the liver, spleen, and bone marrow also occur often (Table 190.1). Infiltration of the liver and spleen typically leads to isolated hepatomegaly and splenomegaly, respectively, but actual organ dysfunction is rare. Cutaneous disease, such as plaques, nodules, erythema nodosum in acute disease, or lupus pernio in chronic sarcoidosis, appears in one quarter of cases and is usually present at onset. Red-brown to purple maculopapular lesions <1 cm on the face, neck, upper back, and extremities are the most common skin finding (Fig. 190.4). Ocular involvement is frequent and has variable manifestations, including anterior or posterior uveitis, conjunctival granulomas, eyelid inflammation, and orbital or lacrimal gland infiltration. The arthritis in sarcoidosis can be confused with **juvenile idiopathic arthritis** (JIA). Central nervous system (CNS) involvement is rare in early childhood but may manifest as seizures, cranial nerve involvement, intracranial mass lesions, and hypothalamic dysfunction (Fig. 190.5). Kidney disease occurs infrequently in children but typically manifests as renal insufficiency, proteinuria, transient pyuria, or microscopic hematuria caused by early monocellular infiltration or granuloma formation in kidney tissue. Only a small fraction of children have hypercalcemia or hypercalciuria, which is therefore an infrequent cause of kidney disease. Sarcoid granulomas can also infiltrate the heart and lead to cardiac arrhythmias and, rarely, sudden death. Other rare sites of disease involvement include blood vessels of any size, the gastrointestinal tract, parotid gland, muscles, bones, and testes.

In contrast to the variable clinical presentation of sarcoidosis in older children, **Blau syndrome and EOS** (NOD2-associated sarcoidosis) classically manifests as the triad of uveitis, arthritis, and rash. These classic manifestations do not always occur simultaneously. Skin disease usually develops before 1 yr, arthritis at 2-4 yr, and uveitis before 4 yr. Pulmonary disease and lymphadenopathy are less common. The arthritis is polyarticular and symmetric, with large, boggy effusions. Large and small joints are involved. Tenosynovitis is an associated finding. Joints are stiff and moderately tender. The rash may wax and wane and is diffuse (mostly truncal), erythematous or tan, macular-papular, and often desquamates, at times being confused with eczema or ichthyosis

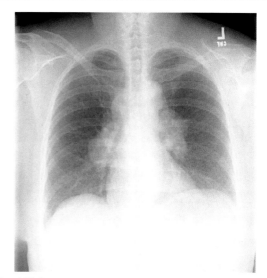

Fig. 190.1 Sarcoidosis. Chest radiograph demonstrating a stage I disease with enlarged mediastinal and hilar lymph nodes. *(From Iannuzzi M: Sarcoidosis. In Goldman L, Schafer AI, editors,* Goldman's Cecil medicine, *ed 24, Philadelphia, 2012, Saunders, Fig 95-1, p 582.)*

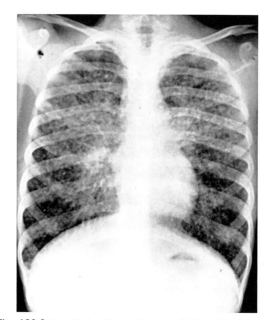

Fig. 190.2 Sarcoidosis. Chest radiograph of 10 yr old girl showing widely disseminated peribronchial infiltrates, multiple small nodular densities, hyperaeration of the lungs, and hilar lymphadenopathy.

vulgaris. Tender subcutaneous nodules resembling erythema nodosum may be seen on the legs. Noncaseating granulomas are demonstrated on biopsy of the skin or joint synovium. Insidious granulomatous iridocyclitis and posterior uveitis are often bilateral and may progress to **panuveitis**, which has a high risk for vision loss. Iris nodules, photophobia, erythema, cataracts, or glaucoma may be present or develop over time.

Most patients with Blau syndrome and EOS display this more restricted phenotype and develop all or some combination of the rash, arthritis, and uveitis. Many, however, also have an extended phenotype. Additional disease manifestations include fever, hepatosplenomegaly, lymphadenopathy, and lung, kidney, and CNS involvement.

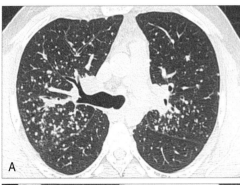

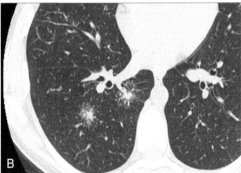

Fig. 190.3 Typical features of lung sarcoidosis on CT. **A,** Usual perilymphatic distribution of micronodules with fissural spreading. **B,** Typical nodules with irregular margins and satellite micronodules known as the *galaxy sign. (From Valerye D, Prasse A, Nunes H, et al: Sarcoidosis, Lancet 383:1155–1167, 2014, Fig 2, p 1158).*

Infantile-onset panniculitis with uveitis and systemic granulomatosis is an uncommon manifestation of sarcoidosis. Sarcoidosis has also been reported in adults treated with type 1 interferons for hepatitis or multiple sclerosis.

LABORATORY FINDINGS

There is no single standard laboratory test diagnostic of sarcoidosis. Anemia, leukopenia, and eosinophilia may be seen. Other nonspecific findings include hypergammaglobulinemia and elevations in acute-phase reactants, including erythrocyte sedimentation rate and C-reactive protein value. Hypercalcemia and/or hypercalciuria occur in only a small proportion of children with sarcoidosis. Angiotensin-converting enzyme (ACE) is produced by the epithelioid cells of the granuloma, and its serum value may be elevated, but this finding lacks diagnostic

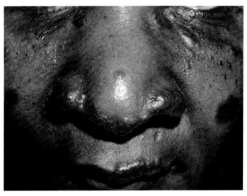

Fig. 190.4 Sarcoidosis nodules on the face. *(From Shah BR, Laude TA: Atlas of pediatric clinical diagnosis, Philadelphia, 2000, Saunders.)*

Table 190.1	Sarcoidosis: Extrapulmonary Localizations
	SYMPTOMS
Skin	Papules, nodules, plaques, scar sarcoidosis, lupus pernio, subcutaneous sarcoidosis
Peripheral lymphadenopathy	Mostly cervical or supraclavicular; inguinal, axillary, epitrochlear, or submandibular lymph node sites also possible; painless and mobile
Eye	Anterior, intermediate, or posterior uveitis; retinal vascular change; conjunctival nodules; lacrimal gland enlargement
Liver	Often symptom free; abnormal liver function tests in 20–30% of patients; hepatomegaly; rarely hepatic insufficiency, chronic intrahepatic cholestasis, or portal hypertension
Spleen	Splenomegaly; rarely, pain or pancytopenia; very rarely, splenic rupture
Heart	Atrioventricular or bundle branch block; ventricular tachycardia or fibrillation; congestive heart failure; pericarditis; impairment of sympathetic nerve activity; sudden death
Nervous system	Facial nerve palsy, optic neuritis, leptomeningitis, diabetes insipidus, hypopituitarism, seizures, cognitive dysfunction, deficits, hydrocephalus, psychiatric manifestations, spinal cord disease, polyneuropathy, small-fiber neuropathy
Kidney	Rare symptoms; increased creatininemia sometimes associated with hypercalcemia; nephrocalcinosis; kidney stones
Parotitis	Symmetric parotid swelling; Heerfordt syndrome when associated with uveitis, fever, and facial palsy
Nose	Nasal stuffiness, nasal bleeding, crusting, anosmia
Larynx	Hoarseness, breathlessness, stridor, dysphagia
Bones	Often asymptomatic; hands and feet classically most involved, also large bones and axial skeleton
Skeletal muscles	Proximal muscle weakness, amyotrophy, myalgia, intramuscular nodules
Genitourinary tract	All organs can be involved, including breast, uterus, epididymis, and testicle
Gastrointestinal tract	Most often symptom free, but the esophagus, stomach, small intestine, and colon can be involved

Adapted from Valerye D, Prasse A, Nunes H, et al: Sarcoidosis, *Lancet* 383:1155–1167, 2014 (Table 1, p 1159).

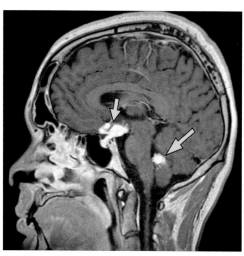

Fig. 190.5 Neurologic involvement in sarcoidosis. Typical involvement of hypothalamus, pituitary gland, and optic chiasm seen on a sagittal gadolinium-enhanced T1-weighted sequence MRI (small arrow). Abnormal nodular enhancement of the 4th ventricle is seen (large arrow). (Modified from Valerye D, Prasse A, Nunes H, et al: Sarcoidosis, Lancet 383:1155–1167, 2014, Fig 3d, p 1160.)

sensitivity and specificity. ACE levels are estimated to be elevated in >50% of children with sarcoidosis. In addition, ACE values may be difficult to interpret because reference values for serum ACE are age dependent. Fluorodeoxyglucose F 18 positron emission tomography can help identify nonpulmonary sites for a diagnostic biopsy.

DIAGNOSIS
Definitive diagnosis ultimately requires demonstration of the characteristic noncaseating granulomatous lesions in a biopsy specimen (usually taken from the most readily available affected organ) and exclusion of other known causes of granulomatous inflammation. Skin and transbronchial lung biopsies have higher yield, greater specificity, and fewer associated adverse events than biopsy of mediastinal lymph nodes or liver. Additional diagnostic testing should include chest radiography, pulmonary function testing with measurement of diffusion capacity, hepatic enzyme measurements, and renal function assessment. Ophthalmologic slit-lamp examination is essential because ocular inflammation is frequently present and may be asymptomatic in sarcoidosis, and vision loss is a sequela of untreated disease.

Bronchoalveolar lavage may be used to assess for disease activity, and the fluid typically reveals an excess of lymphocytes with an increased $CD4^+/CD8^+$ ratio of 2-13:1. In addition to flexible bronchoscopy with transbronchial biopsy, endosonographic-guided intrathoracic node aspiration has been valuable in obtaining tissue to assess for noncaseating granulomas.

DIFFERENTIAL DIAGNOSIS
Because of its protean manifestations, the differential diagnosis of sarcoidosis is extremely broad and depends largely on the initial clinical manifestations. **Granulomatous infections**, including tuberculosis, cryptococcosis, pulmonary mycoses (histoplasmosis, blastomycosis, coccidioidomycosis), brucellosis, tularemia, and toxoplasmosis, must be excluded. Other causes of granulomatous inflammation are granulomatosis with polyangiitis (formerly Wegener granulomatosis), hypersensitivity pneumonia, chronic berylliosis, and other occupational exposures to metals. Localized granulomatous lesions of the head and neck may be due to **orofacial granulomatosis.** Immunodeficiencies

that may manifest with granulomatous lesions include common variable immunodeficiency, selective IgA deficiency, chronic granulomatous disease, ataxia telangiectasia, and severe combined immunodeficiency. Granulomas of the lung, skin, or lymph nodes have been reported in patients treated with anti-TNF agents. Lymphoma should be ruled out in cases of hilar or other lymphadenopathy. Sarcoid arthritis may mimic JIA. Evaluation for endocrine disorders is needed in the setting of hypercalcemia or hypercalciuria.

TREATMENT
Treatment should be based on disease severity as well as the number and type of organs involved. *Corticosteroids are the mainstay of treatment for most acute and chronic disease manifestations.* The optimal dose and duration of corticosteroid therapy in children have not been established. Induction treatment typically begins with oral prednisone or prednisolone (1-2 mg/kg/day up to 40 mg daily) for 8-12 wk until manifestations improve. Corticosteroid dosage is then gradually decreased over 6-12 mo to the minimal effective maintenance dose (e.g., 5-10 mg/day) that controls symptoms, or discontinued if symptoms resolve. *Methotrexate or leflunomide* may be effective as a corticosteroid-sparing agent. On the basis of the role of TNF-α in the formation of granulomas, there is rationale for use of TNF-α antagonists. Results of small clinical trials showed modest effects with *infliximab* and *adalimumab* treatment of selected disease manifestations (CNS, lupus pernio, pulmonary, ocular), whereas etanercept does not appear to be particularly effective. Other therapeutics used for sarcoidosis manifestations include topical corticosteroids (eye), inhaled corticosteroids (lung), azathioprine (CNS), cyclophosphamide (cardiac, CNS), hydroxychloroquine (skin), mycophenolate mofetil (CNS, skin), thalidomide or its analogs (skin), and nonsteroidal antiinflammatory drugs (joints).

With regard to treatment of Blau syndrome and EOS, there are few case reports and series on the successful use of corticosteroids, methotrexate, thalidomide, and TNF-α antagonists adalimumab and infliximab. Findings of elevated IL-1 levels and response to human IL-1 receptor antagonist (anakinra) have been inconsistent.

PROGNOSIS
The prognosis of childhood sarcoidosis is not well defined. The disease may be self-limited with complete recovery or may persist with a progressive or relapsing course. Outcome is worse in the setting of multiorgan or CNS involvement. Most children requiring treatment experience considerable improvement with corticosteroids, although a significant number have morbid sequelae, mainly involving the lungs and eyes. Children with EOS have a poorer prognosis and generally experience a more chronic, progressive disease course. The greatest morbidity is associated with ocular involvement, including cataract formation, development of synechiae, and loss of visual acuity or blindness. Long-term systemic treatment may be required for the eye disease. Progressive polyarthritis may result in joint destruction. The overall mortality rate in childhood sarcoidosis is low.

Serial pulmonary function tests and chest radiographs are useful in following the course of lung involvement. Monitoring for other organ involvement should also include electrocardiogram with consideration of an echocardiogram, urinalysis, renal function tests, and measurements of hepatic enzymes and serum calcium. Other potential indicators of disease activity include inflammatory markers and serum ACE, although changes in ACE level do not always correlate with other indicators of disease status. Given the frequency of asymptomatic eye disease and the ocular morbidity associated with pediatric sarcoidosis, all patients should have an ophthalmologic examination at presentation with monitoring at regular intervals, perhaps every 3-6 mo, as recommended in children with JIA.

Bibliography is available at Expert Consult.

Chapter **191**
Kawasaki Disease
Mary Beth F. Son and Jane W. Newburger

第一百九十一章
川崎病

中文导读

本章主要介绍了川崎病的病因、流行病学、病理、临床表现、实验室和影像学检查、诊断、鉴别诊断、治疗、并发症及预后。病因及病理中分析了感染、遗传等因素，描述了血管受累的病理表现；流行病学中描述了不同年龄、种族的发病差异；临床表现中描述了不同系统受累特征及病程分期；实验室和影像学检查中描述了各辅助检查特点；诊断及鉴别诊断中描述了诊断标准及鉴别要点；治疗中描述了静脉注射丙种球蛋白等的使用策略及疗效；并发症中描述了常见的并发症及抗凝治疗；预后中主要描述了不同冠状动脉受累程度下的长期预后。

Kawasaki disease (KD), formerly known as *mucocutaneous lymph node syndrome* and *infantile polyarteritis nodosa*, is an acute febrile illness of childhood seen worldwide, with the highest incidence occurring in Asian children. KD is a systemic inflammatory disorder manifesting as a vasculitis with a predilection for the coronary arteries. Approximately 20–25% of untreated children develop **coronary artery abnormalities (CAA)** including aneurysms, whereas <5% of children treated with intravenous immune globulin (IVIG) develop CAA. Nonetheless, KD is the leading cause of acquired heart disease in children in most developed countries, including the United States and Japan.

ETIOLOGY

The cause of KD remains unknown. Certain epidemiologic and clinical features support an infectious origin, including the young age-group affected, epidemics with wavelike geographic spread of illness, the self-limited nature of the acute febrile illness, and the clinical features of fever, rash, enanthem, conjunctival injection, and cervical lymphadenopathy. Further evidence of an infectious trigger includes the infrequent occurrence of the illness in infants <3 mo old, possibly the result of maternal antibodies, and the rarity of cases in adults, possibly the result of prior exposures with subsequent immunity. However, there are features that are not consistent with an infectious origin. For example, it is unusual to have multiple cases present at the same time within a family or daycare center. Furthermore, no single infectious etiologic agent has been successfully identified, despite a comprehensive search.

A genetic role in the pathogenesis of KD seems likely, as evidenced by the higher risk of KD in Asian children regardless of country of residence and in siblings and children of individuals with a history of KD. Furthermore, linkage studies and genome-wide association studies (GWAS) have identified significant potential associations between polymorphisms in the *ITPKC* gene, a T-cell regulator, with increased susceptibility to KD and more severe disease. Other candidate genes for KD identified by GWAS include *CASP3, BLK,* and *FCGR2A.* Lastly, associations of single nucleotide polymorphisms (SNPs) in the human leukocyte antigen class II region (HLA-DQB2 and HLA-DOB) with KD have been reported. The concordance rate among identical twins, however, is approximately 13%.

EPIDEMIOLOGY

For the majority of patients, KD is a disease of early childhood, and nearly all epidemiologic studies show a higher susceptibility to KD in boys. Data from the Kids Inpatient Database to study trends in KD hospitalizations in 2003, 2006, 2009, and 2012 reported that U.S. hospitalizations for KD seemed to decline significantly over the study period, with 6.68 per 100,000 children hospitalized for KD in 2006 vs 6.11 per 100,000 in 2012. Children age <5 yr had the highest annual hospitalization rates, and children of Asian and Pacific Islander ancestry had the highest rates among all racial groups. In other countries, such as the United Kingdom, South Korea, and Japan, the rate of KD seems to be increasing.

In Japan, nationwide surveys have been administered every 2 yr to monitor trends in KD incidence. In 2012 the highest recorded rate thus far of 264.8 per 100,000 children ages 0-4 yr was described, with the highest rate in young children ages 9-11 mo. Fortunately, the proportion of Japanese patients with coronary aneurysm and myocardial infarction has decreased over time, at 2.8% in the most recent survey.

Several risk stratification models have been constructed to determine which patients with KD are at highest risk for CAA. Predictors of poor outcome across several studies include young age, male gender, persistent fever, poor response to IVIG, and laboratory abnormalities, including neutrophilia, thrombocytopenia, transaminitis, hyponatremia, hypoalbuminemia, elevated levels of N-terminal–brain natriuretic protein and elevated C-reactive protein (CRP) levels. Asian and Pacific Islander race and Hispanic ethnicity are also risk factors for CAA. Three specific risk scores have been constructed by Japanese researchers; of these, the **Kobayashi score** is the most widely used and has high sensitivity and specificity. Unfortunately, application of these risk scores in non-Japanese populations does not appear to accurately identify all children at risk for IVIG resistance and CAA. Body surface area (BSA)–adjusted coronary artery dimensions on baseline echocardiography in the 1st 10 days of illness appear to be good predictors of involvement during follow-up. Accordingly, baseline z scores may provide a useful imaging biomarker.

PATHOLOGY

KD is a vasculitis that predominantly affects the medium-size arteries. The coronary arteries are most often involved, although other arteries (e.g., axillary, subclavian, femoral, popliteal, brachial) can also develop dilation. A 3-phase process to the arteriopathy of KD has been described. The 1st phase is a neutrophilic necrotizing arteritis occurring in the 1st 2 wk of illness that begins in the endothelium and moves through the coronary wall. Saccular aneurysms may form from this arteritis. The 2nd phase is a subacute/chronic vasculitis driven by lymphocytes, plasma cells, and eosinophils, which may last weeks to years and results in fusiform aneurysms. The vessels affected by the subacute/chronic vasculitis then develop smooth muscle cell myofibroblasts, which cause progressive stenosis in the 3rd phase. Thrombi may form in the lumen and obstruct blood flow (Fig. 191.1).

CLINICAL MANIFESTATIONS

Fever is characteristically high spiking (≥38.3°C [101°F]), remitting, and unresponsive to antipyretics. The duration of fever without treatment is generally 1-2 wk but may be as short as 5 days or may persist for

3-4 wk. In addition to fever, the **5 principal clinical criteria** of KD are (1) bilateral *nonexudative* conjunctival injection with limbal sparing; (2) erythema of the oral and pharyngeal mucosa with strawberry tongue and red, cracked lips; (3) edema (induration) and erythema of the hands and feet; (4) rash of various forms (maculopapular, erythema multiforme, scarlatiniform or less often psoriatic-like, urticarial or micropustular); and (5) nonsuppurative cervical lymphadenopathy, usually unilateral, with node size >1.5 cm (Table 191.1 and Figs. 191.2 to 191.5). Perineal desquamation is common in the acute phase. Periungual desquamation of the fingers and toes begins 2-3 wk after the onset of illness and may progress to involve the entire hand and foot (Fig. 191.6).

Symptoms other than the principal clinical criteria are common in the 10 days before diagnosis of KD, which may be explained in part by the finding that up to a third of patients with KD have confirmed, concurrent infections. Gastrointestinal (GI) symptoms (vomiting, diarrhea, or abdominal pain) occur in >60% of patients, and at least 1 respiratory symptom (rhinorrhea or cough) occurs in 35%. Other clinical findings include significant irritability that is especially prominent in infants and likely caused by aseptic meningitis, mild hepatitis, hydrops of the gallbladder, urethritis and meatitis with sterile pyuria, and arthritis. Arthritis may occur early in the illness or may develop in the 2nd or 3rd wk. Small or large joints may be affected, and the arthralgias may persist for several weeks. Clinical features that are *not consistent* with KD include exudative conjunctivitis, exudative pharyngitis, generalized lymphadenopathy, discrete oral lesions (ulceration or exudative pharyngitis), splenomegaly, and bullous, petechial, or vesicular rashes.

Cardiac involvement is the most important manifestation of KD. Myocarditis occurs in most patients with acute KD and manifests as tachycardia disproportionate to fever, along with diminished left ventricular systolic function. Occasionally, patients with KD present

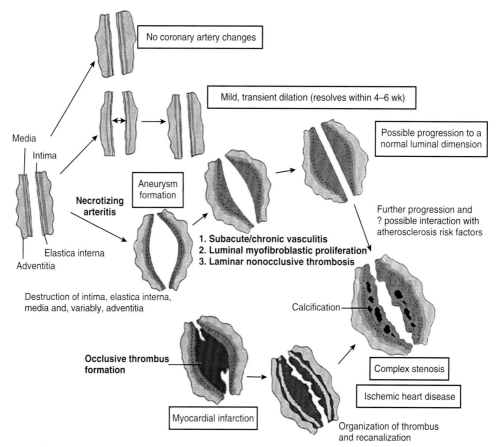

Fig. 191.1 Natural history of coronary artery abnormalities. *(Modified from Kato H: Cardiovascular complications in Kawasaki disease: coronary artery lumen and long-term consequences, Prog Pediatr Cardiol 19:137–145, 2004.)*

Table 191.1	Clinical and Laboratory Features of Kawasaki Disease

EPIDEMIOLOGIC CASE DEFINITION (CLASSIC CLINICAL CRITERIA)*

Fever persisting at least 5 days[†]

Presence of at least 4 principal features:

Changes in extremities
- Acute: erythema of palms, soles; edema of hands, feet
- Subacute: periungual peeling of fingers, toes in wk 2 and 3

Polymorphous exanthem

Bilateral bulbar conjunctival injection without exudate

Erythema and cracking of lips, strawberry tongue, and/or erythema of oral and pharyngeal mucosa

Cervical lymphadenopathy (>1.5 cm diameter), usually unilateral

Exclusion of other diseases with similar findings[‡]

These features do not have to occur concurrently.

OTHER CLINICAL AND LABORATORY FINDINGS

Cardiovascular System

Myocarditis, pericarditis, valvular regurgitation, shock

Coronary artery abnormalities

Aneurysms of medium-sized noncoronary arteries

Peripheral gangrene

Aortic root enlargement

Respiratory System

Peribronchial and interstitial infiltrates on chest radiograph

Pulmonary nodules

Musculoskeletal System

Arthritis, arthralgias (pleocytosis of synovial fluid)

Gastrointestinal Tract

Diarrhea, vomiting, abdominal pain

Hepatitis, jaundice

Hydrops of gallbladder

Pancreatitis

Central Nervous System

Extreme irritability

Aseptic meningitis (pleocytosis of cerebrospinal fluid)

Facial nerve palsy

Sensorineural hearing loss

Genitourinary System

Urethritis/meatitis, hydrocele

Other Findings

Desquamating rash in groin

Retropharyngeal phlegmon

Anterior uveitis by slit-lamp examination

Erythema, induration at bacille Calmette-Guérin inoculation site

LABORATORY FINDINGS IN ACUTE KAWASAKI DISEASE

Leukocytosis with neutrophilia and immature forms

Elevated erythrocyte sedimentation rate

Elevated C-reactive protein

Anemia

Abnormal plasma lipids

Hypoalbuminemia

Hyponatremia

Thrombocytosis after wk 1[§]

Sterile pyuria

Elevated serum transaminases

Elevated serum γ-glutamyl transpeptidase

Pleocytosis of cerebrospinal fluid

Leukocytosis in synovial fluid

*Patients with fever at least 5 days and <4 principal criteria can be diagnosed with Kawasaki disease when coronary artery abnormalities are detected by 2-dimensional echocardiography or angiography.

[†]In the presence of ≥4 principal criteria, particularly when redness and swelling of the hands and feet are present, Kawasaki disease diagnosis can be made on day 4 of illness. Experienced clinicians who have treated many patients with Kawasaki disease may establish diagnosis before day 4 in rare cases.

[§]Some infants present with thrombocytopenia and disseminated intravascular coagulation.

[‡]See differential diagnosis (Table 191.2).

From McCrindle BW, Rowley A, Newburger JW et al: Diagnosis, treatment, and long-term management of Kawasaki disease: a scientific statement for health professionals from the American Heart Association, Circulation 135(17):e927–e999, 2017.)

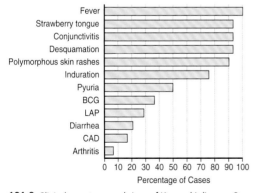

Fig. 191.2 Clinical symptoms and signs of Kawasaki disease. Summary of clinical features from 110 cases of Kawasaki disease seen in Kaohsiung, Taiwan. *LAP,* Lymphadenopathy in head and neck area; *BCG,* reactivation of bacille Calmette-Guérin inoculation site; *CAD,* coronary artery *dilation,* defined by an internal diameter >3 mm. *(From Wang CL, Wu YT, Liu CA, et al: Kawasaki disease: infection, immunity and genetics, Pediatr Infect Dis J 24:998–1004, 2005.)*

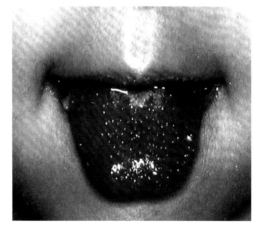

Fig. 191.3 Kawasaki disease. Strawberry tongue in patient with mucocutaneous lymph node syndrome. *(Courtesy of Tomisaku Kawasaki, MD. From Hurwitz S: Clinical pediatric dermatology, ed 2, Philadelphia, 1993, Saunders.)*

in cardiogenic shock (**KD shock syndrome**), with greatly diminished left ventricular function. Case series of KD shock syndrome indicate that these patients may be at higher risk for coronary artery dilation. Pericarditis with a small pericardial effusion can also occur during the acute illness. Mitral regurgitation of at least mild severity is evident on

echocardiography in 10–25% of patients at presentation but diminishes over time, except among rare patients with coronary aneurysms and ischemic heart disease. Up to 25% of untreated patients develop CAA in the 2nd to 3rd week of illness; initially these are usually asymptomatic and detected by echocardiography. Almost all the morbidity and mortality in

KD occur in patients with **large or giant coronary artery aneurysms**, defined by the 2017 American Heart Association (AHA) scientific statement on the diagnosis and treatment of KD as having a z score ≥ 10 or an absolute dimension of ≥ 8 mm. Specifically, large or giant aneurysms are associated with the greatest risk of thrombosis or stenosis, angina, and myocardial infarction (Figs. 191.7 and 191.8*A*). Rupture of a giant aneurysm is a rare complication that generally occurs in the 1st months after illness onset and may present as hemopericardium with tamponade. Axillary, popliteal, iliac, or other arteries may also become aneurysmal, but always in the setting of giant coronary aneurysms (Fig. 191.8*B*).

Occasionally KD initially presents with only fever and lymphadenopathy (**node-first KD**). This presentation may be confused with bacterial or viral cervical lymphadenopathy or lymphadenitis and may delay the diagnosis of KD. Persistence of high fever, lack of response to antibiotics, and subsequent development of other signs of KD suggest the diagnosis. Children with node-first KD tend to be older (4 vs 2 yr) and have more days of fever and higher CRP levels. In addition to cervical adenopathy, many had retropharyngeal and peritonsillar inflammation on CT scans (Fig. 191.9).

KD can be divided into 3 clinical phases. The **acute febrile phase** is characterized by fever and the other acute signs of illness and usually lasts 1-2 wk. The **subacute phase** is associated with desquamation, thrombocytosis, development of CAA, and the highest risk of sudden death in patients who develop aneurysms; it generally lasts 3 wk. The **convalescent phase** begins when all clinical signs of illness have disappeared and continues until the erythrocyte sedimentation rate (ESR) returns to normal, typically 6-8 wk after the onset of illness.

LABORATORY AND RADIOLOGY FINDINGS

There is no diagnostic test for KD, but patients usually have characteristic laboratory findings. The leukocyte count is often elevated, with a predominance of neutrophils and immature forms. Normocytic, normochromic anemia is common. The platelet count is generally normal in the 1st wk of illness and rapidly increases by the 2nd to 3rd wk of illness, sometimes exceeding 1 million/mm³. An elevated ESR or CRP value is universally present in the acute phase of illness. The ESR may remain elevated for weeks, in part from the effect of IVIG. Sterile pyuria, mild elevations of the hepatic transaminases, hyperbilirubinemia, and cerebrospinal fluid pleocytosis may also be present. KD is unlikely if the ESR, CRP, and platelet counts are normal after 7 days of fever.

Two-dimensional echocardiography is the most useful test to monitor for development of CAA. Although frank aneurysms are rarely detected in the 1st week of illness, coronary arteries are commonly ectatic. Moreover, coronary artery dimensions, adjusted for BSA (z scores), may be increased in the 1st 5 wk after presentation, and as previously noted, baseline z scores may offer prognostic information regarding

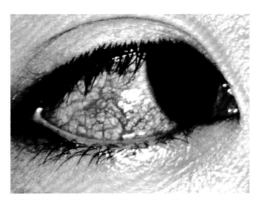

Fig. 191.4 Kawasaki disease. Congestion of bulbar conjunctiva in a patient with mucocutaneous lymph node syndrome. *(Courtesy of Tomisaku Kawasaki, MD. From Hurwitz S: Clinical pediatric dermatology, ed 2, Philadelphia, 1993, Saunders.)*

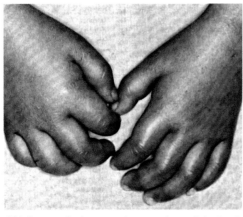

Fig. 191.5 Kawasaki disease. Indurative edema of the hands in a patient with mucocutaneous lymph node syndrome. *(Courtesy of Tomisaku Kawasaki, MD. From Hurwitz S: Clinical pediatric dermatology, ed 2, Philadelphia, 1993, Saunders.)*

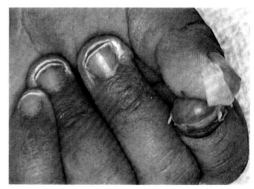

Fig. 191.6 Kawasaki disease. Desquamation of the fingers in a patient with mucocutaneous lymph node syndrome. *(Courtesy of Tomisaku Kawasaki, MD. From Hurwitz S: Clinical pediatric dermatology, ed 2, Philadelphia, 1993, Saunders.)*

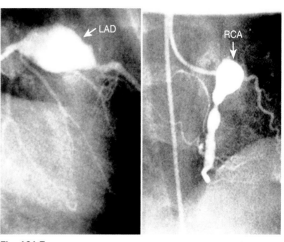

Fig. 191.7 Coronary angiograms in 6 yr old boy with Kawasaki disease. *Left,* Giant aneurysm of the left anterior descending coronary artery (LAD) with obstruction. *Right,* Giant aneurysm of the right coronary artery (RCA) with an area of severe narrowing. *(From Newburger JW, Takahashi M, Gerber MA, et al: Diagnosis, treatment, and long-term management of Kawasaki disease, Pediatrics 114:1708–1733, 2004.)*

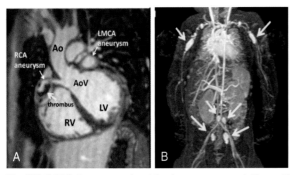

Fig. 191.8 MRI of coronary and peripheral artery aneurysms in Kawasaki disease. **A,** Image of left ventricular outflow tract showing a giant right coronary artery (RCA) aneurysm with nonocclusive thrombus (*yellow arrow*) and a giant left main coronary artery (LMCA) aneurysm. Ao, Aorta; AoV, aortic valve; LV, left ventricle; RV, right ventricle. **B,** Aneurysms in the axillary and subclavian arteries and the iliac and femoral arteries (*yellow arrows*). (*From McCrindle BW, Rowley A, Newburger JW et al: Diagnosis, treatment, and long-term management of Kawasaki disease: a scientific statement for health professionals from the American Heart Association, Circulation 135(17):e927-e999, 2017, Fig 2GH, p e935.*)

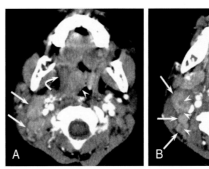

Fig. 191.9 Contrast-enhanced CT in 3 yr old boy with Kawasaki disease. **A,** Right-sided cervical lymphadenopathy (*arrows*), peritonsillar hypodense area (*curved arrow*), and swelling of right palatine tonsil (*arrowhead*). **B,** Right-sided cervical lymphadenopathy with perinodal infiltration (*arrows*) and intranodal focal low attenuation (*arrowheads*). (*From Kato H, Kanematsu M, Kato Z, et al: Computed tomographic findings of Kawasaki disease with cervical lymphadenopathy, J Comput Assist Tomogr 36(1):138–142, 2012, Fig 1, p 139.*)

ultimate coronary artery dimensions. Children with non-KD febrile illnesses also have mildly increased z scores compared with nonfebrile controls, but not to the same degree as patients with KD. Aneurysms have been defined with use of absolute dimensions by the Japanese Ministry of Health and are classified as small (≤4 mm internal diameter [ID]), medium (>4 to ≤8 mm ID), or giant (>8 mm ID). Some experts believe that a z-score–based system for classification of aneurysm size may be more discriminating, because it adjusts the coronary dimension for BSA. The AHA z-score classification system is as follows:

1. No involvement: always <2
2. Dilation only: 2 to <2.5; or if initially <2, a decrease in z score during follow-up ≥1
3. Small aneurysm: ≥2.5 to <5
4. Medium aneurysm: ≥5 to <10, and absolute dimension <8 mm
5. Large or giant aneurysm: ≥10, or absolute dimension ≥8 mm

Echocardiography should be performed at diagnosis and again after 1-2 wk of illness. If the results are normal, a repeat study should be performed 6-8 wk after onset of illness. If results of either of the initial studies are abnormal or the patient has recurrent fever or symptoms, more frequent echocardiography or other studies may be necessary. In patients without CCA at any time during the illness, echocardiography and a lipid profile are recommended 1 yr later. After this time, periodic evaluation for preventive cardiology counseling is warranted, and some experts recommend cardiologic follow-up every 5 yr. For patients with CAA, the type of testing and the frequency of cardiology follow-up visits are tailored to the patient's coronary status.

DIAGNOSIS

The diagnosis of KD is based on the presence of characteristic clinical signs. For **classic KD** the diagnostic criteria require the presence of fever for at least 4 days and at least 4 of 5 of the other principal characteristics of the illness (see Table 191.1). The diagnosis of KD should be made within 10 days, and ideally within 7 days, of fever onset to improve coronary artery outcomes. In **atypical or incomplete KD**, patients have persistent fever but <4 of the 5 characteristic clinical signs. In these patients, laboratory and echocardiographic data can assist in the diagnosis (Fig. 191.10). Incomplete cases occur most frequently in infants, who also have the highest likelihood of development of CAA. Ambiguous cases should be referred to a center with experience in the diagnosis of KD. Establishing the diagnosis with prompt institution of treatment is essential to prevent potentially devastating coronary artery disease. For this reason, *it is recommended that any infant age ≤6 mo with fever for ≥7 days without explanation undergo echocardiography to assess the coronary arteries.*

DIFFERENTIAL DIAGNOSIS

Adenovirus, measles, and scarlet fever lead the list of common childhood infections that mimic KD (Table 191.2). Children with **adenovirus** typically have exudative pharyngitis and exudative conjunctivitis, allowing differentiation from KD. A common clinical problem is the differentiation of **scarlet fever** from KD in a child who is a group A streptococcal carrier. Patients with scarlet fever typically have a rapid clinical response to appropriate antibiotic therapy. Such treatment for 24-48 hr with clinical reassessment generally clarifies the diagnosis. Furthermore, ocular findings are quite rare in group A streptococcal pharyngitis and may assist in the diagnosis of KD.

Features of **measles** that distinguish it from KD include exudative conjunctivitis, Koplik spots, rash that begins on the face and hairline and behind the ears, and leukopenia. **Cervical lymphadenitis** can be the initial diagnosis in children who are ultimately recognized to have KD. Less common infections such as Rocky Mountain spotted fever and leptospirosis are occasionally confused with KD. **Rocky Mountain spotted fever** is a potentially lethal bacterial infection, and appropriate antibiotics should not be withheld if the diagnosis is under consideration. Its distinguishing features include pronounced myalgias and headache at onset, centripedal rash, and petechiae on the palms and soles. **Leptospirosis** can also be an illness of considerable severity. Risk factors include exposure to water contaminated with urine from infected animals. The classic description of leptospirosis is of a biphasic illness with a few asymptomatic days between an initial period of fever and headache and a late phase with renal and hepatic failure. In contrast, patients with KD have consecutive days of fever at diagnosis and rarely have renal or hepatic failure.

Children with KD and pronounced myocarditis may demonstrate hypotension with a clinical picture similar to that of toxic shock syndrome. Features of **toxic shock syndrome** that are not usually seen in KD include renal insufficiency, coagulopathy, pancytopenia, and myositis. Drug hypersensitivity reactions, including Stevens-Johnson syndrome, share some characteristics with KD. Drug reaction features such as the presence of periorbital edema, oral ulcerations, and a normal or minimally elevated ESR are not seen in KD. Systemic-onset **juvenile idiopathic arthritis** (sJIA) is also characterized by fever and rash, but physical findings include diffuse lymphadenopathy and hepatosplenomegaly. Arthritis is required to develop at some point in the disease course to make the diagnosis, but may not be present in the 1st few wk of illness. Laboratory findings may include coagulopathy, elevated fibrin degradation product values, and hyperferritinemia. Interestingly, there are reports of children with sJIA who have echocardiographic evidence of CAA. Coronary aneurysms have also been reported in Behçet disease, primary cytomegalovirus infection, and meningococcemia.

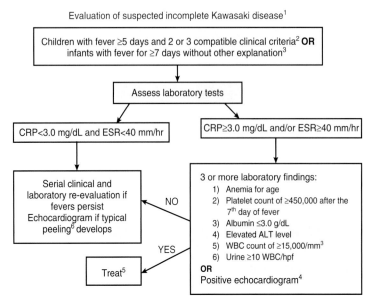

Evaluation of suspected incomplete Kawasaki disease[1]

Children with fever ≥5 days and 2 or 3 compatible clinical criteria[2] **OR** infants with fever for ≥7 days without other explanation[3]

Assess laboratory tests

CRP<3.0 mg/dL and ESR<40 mm/hr

CRP≥3.0 mg/dL and/or ESR≥40 mm/hr

Serial clinical and laboratory re-evaluation if fevers persist Echocardiogram if typical peeling[6] develops

NO

3 or more laboratory findings:
1) Anemia for age
2) Platelet count of ≥450,000 after the 7th day of fever
3) Albumin ≤3.0 g/dL
4) Elevated ALT level
5) WBC count of ≥15,000/mm[3]
6) Urine ≥10 WBC/hpf
OR
Positive echocardiogram[4]

YES

Treat[5]

Fig. 191.10 Evaluation of suspected incomplete Kawasaki disease (KD). [1]In the absence of a gold standard for diagnosis of KD, this algorithm cannot be evidence based but rather represents the informed opinion of the expert committee. Consultation with an expert should be sought any time assistance is needed. [2]Clinical findings of KD are listed in Table 191.1. Characteristics suggesting that another diagnosis should be considered include exudative conjunctivitis, exudative pharyngitis, ulcerative intraoral lesions, bullous or vesicular rash, generalized adenopathy, and splenomegaly. [3]Infants ≤6 mo of age are most likely to develop prolonged fever without other clinical criteria for KD; these infants are at particularly high risk of developing coronary artery abnormalities. [4]Echocardiography is considered positive for purposes of this algorithm if any of 3 conditions are met: z score of left anterior descending coronary artery or right coronary artery ≥2.5; coronary artery aneurysm is observed; or ≥3 other suggestive features exist, including decreased left ventricular function, mitral regurgitation, pericardial effusion, or z scores in left anterior descending coronary artery or right coronary artery of 2-2.5. [5]If the echocardiogram is positive, treatment should be given within 10 days of fever onset or after the 10th day of fever in the presence of clinical and laboratory signs (C-reactive protein [CRP], erythrocyte sedimentation rate [ESR]) of ongoing inflammation. [6]Typical peeling begins under the nail beds of fingers and toes. ALT, Alanine transaminase; WBC, white blood cell. *(From McCrindle BW, Rowley A, Newburger JW et al: Diagnosis, treatment, and long-term management of Kawasaki disease: a scientific statement for health professionals from the American Heart Association, Circulation 135(17):e927–e999, 2017, Fig 2, p e937.)*

TREATMENT

Patients with acute KD should be treated with 2 g/kg of IVIG as a single infusion, usually administered over 10-12 hr within 10 days of disease onset, and ideally as soon as possible after diagnosis (Table 191.3). In addition, moderate (30-50 mg/kg/day divided every 6 hr) to high-dose aspirin (80-100 mg/kg/day divided every 6 hr) should be administered until the patient is afebrile, then lowered to antiplatelet doses. Other NSAIDs should not be given during therapy with aspirin because they may block the action of aspirin. The mechanism of action of IVIG in KD is unknown, but treatment results in defervescence and resolution of clinical signs of illness in approximately 85% of patients. The prevalence of coronary disease, in 20–25% in children treated with aspirin alone, is <5% in those treated with IVIG and aspirin within the 1st 10 days of illness. Strong consideration should be given to treating patients with persistent fever, abnormal dimensions of the coronary arteries, or signs of systemic inflammation who are diagnosed after the 10th day of fever. The dose of aspirin is usually decreased from antiinflammatory to antithrombotic doses (3-5 mg/kg/day as a single dose) after the patient has been afebrile for 48 hr. Aspirin is continued for its antithrombotic effect until 6-8 wk after illness onset and is then discontinued in patients who have had normal echocardiography findings throughout the course of their illness. Patients with CAA continue with aspirin therapy and may require anticoagulation, depending on the degree of coronary dilation (see later).

Corticosteroids have been used as primary therapy with the 1st dose of IVIG in hopes of improving coronary outcomes. A North American trial using a single pulse dose of intravenous methylprednisolone (30 mg/kg) with IVIG as primary therapy did not improve coronary outcomes. However, a trial in Japan utilizing the Kobayashi score to identify high-risk children demonstrated improved coronary outcomes with a regimen of prednisolone (2 mg/kg) plus IVIG as primary therapy. Furthermore,

a systematic review and meta-analysis of 16 comparative studies demonstrated that early treatment with corticosteroids improved coronary artery outcomes in children with KD. Despite these promising results, administration of corticosteroids as primary therapy to all children with KD awaits the development of a risk score that identifies high-risk children in a multiracial population.

IVIG-resistant KD occurs in approximately 15% of patients and is defined by persistent or recrudescent fever 36 hr after completion of the initial IVIG infusion. Patients with IVIG resistance are at increased risk for CAA. Therapeutic options for the child with IVIG resistance include a 2nd dose of IVIG (2 g/kg), a tapering course of corticosteroids, and/or infliximab (Table 191.4). For the most severely affected patients with enlarging coronary aneurysms, additional therapies such as cyclosporine or cyclophosphamide may be administered, with consultation from specialists in pediatric rheumatology and cardiology.

COMPLICATIONS

Patients with KD and aneurysms may experience myocardial infarction, angina, and sudden death. For this reason, antithrombotic medications are the cornerstone of therapy for the child with coronary disease. Aspirin is continued indefinitely in children with coronary aneurysms. When aneurysms are moderate sized, dual-antiplatelet therapy is sometimes administered. For those with large or giant aneurysms, anticoagulation with warfarin or low-molecular-weight heparin is added to aspirin. For acute thrombosis that occasionally occurs in an aneurysmal or stenotic coronary artery, thrombolytic therapy may be lifesaving.

Long-term follow-up of patients with coronary artery aneurysms is tailored to the past (i.e., worst-ever) and current coronary status, with a schedule of testing recommended in the 2017 AHA scientific statement on KD. Testing may include echocardiography, assessment for inducible ischemia, advanced imaging (CT, MRI, or invasive angiography), physical activity counseling, and cardiovascular risk factor assessment and management. Patients with coronary artery stenosis and inducible ischemia may be managed with coronary artery bypass grafting (CABG) or catheter interventions, including percutaneous transluminal coronary rotational ablation, directional coronary atherectomy, and stent implantation.

Patients undergoing long-term aspirin therapy should receive annual influenza vaccination to reduce the risk of Reye syndrome. A different antiplatelet agent can be substituted for aspirin during the 6 wk after varicella vaccination. IVIG may interfere with the immune response to live-virus vaccines as a result of specific antiviral antibody, so the measles-mumps-rubella and varicella vaccinations should generally be deferred until 11 mo after IVIG administration. Nonlive vaccinations do not need to be delayed.

Table 191.2	Differential Diagnosis of Kawasaki Disease

VIRAL INFECTIONS*
Adenovirus
Enterovirus
Measles
Epstein-Barr virus
Cytomegalovirus

BACTERIAL INFECTIONS
Scarlet fever
Rocky Mountain spotted fever
Leptospirosis
Bacterial cervical lymphadenitis ± retropharyngeal phlegmon
Meningococcemia
Urinary tract infection

RHEUMATOLOGIC DISEASE
Systemic-onset juvenile idiopathic arthritis
Behçet disease
Rheumatic fever

OTHER
Toxic shock syndromes
Serum sickness
Staphylococcal scalded skin syndrome
Macrophage activation syndrome
Drug hypersensitivity reactions
Stevens-Johnson syndrome
Aseptic meningitis

*Detection of a virus does not exclude Kawasaki disease in the presence of the principal clinical features (see Table 191.1).

PROGNOSIS

The vast majority of patients with KD return to normal health; timely treatment reduces the risk of coronary aneurysms to <5%. Acute KD recurs in 1–3% of cases. The prognosis for patients with CCA depends on the severity of coronary disease; therefore, recommendations for follow-up and management are stratified according to coronary artery status. Published fatality rates are very low, generally <1.0%. Overall, 50% of coronary artery aneurysms regress to normal lumen diameter by 1-2 yr after the illness, with smaller aneurysms being more likely to regress. Intravascular ultrasonography has demonstrated that regressed aneurysms are associated with marked myointimal thickening and abnormal functional behavior of the vessel wall. Giant aneurysms are less likely to regress to normal lumen diameter and are most likely to lead to thrombosis or stenosis. CABG may be required if there is inducible ischemia; it is best accomplished with the use of arterial grafts, which grow with the child and are more likely than venous grafts to remain patent over the long-term. Heart transplantation has been required in rare cases where revascularization is not feasible because of distal coronary stenoses, distal aneurysms, or severe ischemic cardiomyopathy. A study from Japan reported outcomes in adult patients with a history of KD and giant aneurysms. These patients required multiple cardiac and surgical procedures, but the 30-yr survival rate approached 90%.

Table 191.3	Treatment of Kawasaki Disease

ACUTE STAGE
Intravenous immune globulin 2 g/kg over 10-12 hr
   and
Aspirin 30-50 mg/kg/day or 80-100 mg/kg/day divided every 6 hr
   orally until patient is afebrile for at least 48 hr

CONVALESCENT STAGE
Aspirin 3-5 mg/kg once daily orally until 6-8 wk after illness onset if
   normal coronary findings throughout course

LONG-TERM THERAPY FOR PATIENTS WITH CORONARY ABNORMALITIES
Aspirin 3-5 mg/kg once daily orally
Clopidogrel 1 mg/kg/day (maximum 75 mg/day)
Most experts add warfarin or low-molecular-weight heparin for
   those patients at particularly high risk of thrombosis

ACUTE CORONARY THROMBOSIS
Prompt fibrinolytic therapy with tissue plasminogen activator or
   other thrombolytic agent under supervision of a pediatric
   cardiologist

Table 191.4	Treatment Options for IVIG-Resistant Patients With Kawasaki Disease*		
AGENT	**DESCRIPTION**		**DOSE**
MOST FREQUENTLY ADMINISTERED			
IVIG: 2nd infusion	Pooled polyclonal IG		2 g/kg IV
IVIG + prednisolone	IVIG + corticosteroid		IVIG: 2 g/kg IV + prednisolone 2 mg·kg⁻¹·d⁻¹ IV divided every 8 hr until afebrile, then prednisone orally until CRP normalized, then taper over 2-3 wk
Infliximab	Monoclonal antibody against TNF-α		Single infusion: 5 mg/kg IV given over 2 hr
ALTERNATIVE TREATMENTS			
Cyclosporine	Inhibitor of calcineurin-NFAT pathway		IV: 3 mg·kg⁻¹·d⁻¹ divided every 12 hr PO: 4-8 mg·kg⁻¹·d⁻¹ divided every 12 hr Adjust dose to achieve trough 50-150 ng/mL; 2 hr peak level 300-600 ng/mL
Anakinra	Recombinant IL-1β receptor antagonist		2-6 mg·kg⁻¹·d⁻¹ given by subcutaneous injection
Cyclophosphamide	Alkylating agent blocks DNA replication		2 mg·kg⁻¹·d⁻¹ IV
Plasma exchange	Replaces plasma with albumin		Not applicable

*IVIG resistance is defined as persistent or recrudescent fever at least 36 hours and <7 days after completion of 1st IVIG infusion. The top 3 treatments have been most frequently used, although no comparative effectiveness trial has been performed. Pulsed high-dose corticosteroid treatment is not recommended. The alternative treatments have been used in a limited number of patients with KD.

  CRP, C-reactive protein; IG, immunoglobulin; IL, interleukin; IV, intravenous(ly); IVIG, intravenous immune globulin; NFAT, nuclear factor of activated T cells; PO, oral; TNF, tumor necrosis factor.

Whether children who have had KD and normal echocardiography findings throughout their course are at higher risk for the development of atherosclerotic heart disease in adulthood remains unclear. Studies of endothelial dysfunction in children with a history of KD and normal coronary dimensions have produced conflicting results. However, reassuring data suggest that the standardized mortality ratio among adults in Japan who had KD in childhood without aneurysms is indistinguishable from that of the general population. All children with a history of KD should be counseled regarding a heart-healthy diet, adequate amounts of exercise, tobacco avoidance, and intermittent lipid monitoring. Among children with coronary aneurysms, the AHA recommends treatment thresholds for risk factors for atherosclerotic heart disease that are lower than those for the normal population.

Bibliography is available at Expert Consult.

Chapter 192
Vasculitis Syndromes
Vidya Sivaraman, Edward C. Fels, and Stacy P. Ardoin

第一百九十二章
血管炎综合征

中文导读

本章主要介绍了儿童血管炎的分类、血管炎综合征的临床特点、儿童血管炎的临床病例特点，并分别介绍了过敏性紫癜、多发性大动脉炎、结节性多动脉炎和皮肤结节性多动脉炎、ANCA相关性血管炎及其他血管炎综合征。具体描述了过敏性紫癜、多发性大动脉炎、结节性多动脉炎和皮肤结节性多动脉炎、ANCA相关性血管炎的流行病学、病理、发病机制、临床表现、诊断、实验室检查、治疗、并发症及预后；描述了其他血管炎综合征的临床表现、诊断方法及治疗。

Childhood vasculitis encompasses a broad spectrum of diseases that share inflammation of the blood vessels as the central pathophysiology. The pathogenesis of the vasculitides is generally idiopathic. Some forms of vasculitis are associated with infectious agents and medications, whereas others may occur in the setting of preexisting autoimmune disease. The pattern of vessel injury provides insight into the form of vasculitis and serves as a framework to delineate the different vasculitic syndromes. The distribution of vascular injury includes *small vessels* (capillaries, arterioles, and postcapillary venules), *medium vessels* (renal arteries, mesenteric vasculature, and coronary arteries), and *large vessels* (the aorta and its proximal branches) (Fig. 192.1). Additionally, some forms of small vessel vasculitis are characterized by the presence of **antineutrophil cytoplasmic antibodies (ANCAs)**, whereas others are associated with **immune complex** deposition in affected tissues. A combination of clinical features, histologic appearance of involved vessels, and laboratory data is used to classify vasculitis (Tables 192.1 to 192.3). A nomenclature system from the 2012 International Chapel Hill Consensus Conference has proposed using the pathologic diagnosis rather than eponyms for vasculitis nomenclature. For example, Henoch-Schönlein purpura would be referred to as IgA vasculitis. Additionally, the classification criteria endorsed by the European League Against Rheumatism, Pediatric Rheumatology International Trial Organization, and Pediatric Rheumatology European Society (EULAR/ PRINTO/PRES) have been validated in childhood vasculitis. (Table 192.1).

Childhood vasculitis varies from a relatively benign and self-limited disease such as Henoch-Schönlein purpura to catastrophic disease with end-organ damage, as seen in granulomatosis with polyangiitis (formerly Wegener granulomatosis). Vasculitis generally manifests as a heterogeneous multisystem disease. Although some features, such as purpura, are easily identifiable, others, such as hypertension secondary to renal artery occlusion or glomerulonephritis, can be subtler. Ultimately, the key to recognizing vasculitis relies heavily on *pattern recognition*. Demonstration of vessel injury and inflammation on biopsy or vascular imaging is required to confirm a diagnosis of vasculitis.

Bibliography is available at Expert Consult.

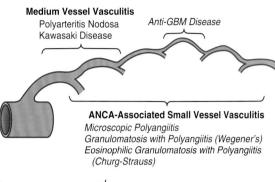

Immune Complex Small Vessel Vasculitis
Cryoglobulinemic Vasculitis
IgA Vasculitis (Henoch-Schönlein)
Hypocomplementemic Urticarial Vasculitis
(Anti-C1q Vasculitis)

Medium Vessel Vasculitis
Polyarteritis Nodosa   *Anti-GBM Disease*
Kawasaki Disease

ANCA-Associated Small Vessel Vasculitis
Microscopic Polyangiitis
Granulomatosis with Polyangiitis (Wegener's)
Eosinophilic Granulomatosis with Polyangiitis
(Churg-Strauss)

Large Vessel Vasculitis
Takayasu Arteritis
Giant Cell Arteritis

Fig. 192.1 Distribution of vessel involvement in large, medium, and small vessel vasculitis. There is substantial overlap with respect to arterial involvement, and all 3 major categories of vasculitis can affect any-size artery. Large vessel vasculitis affects large arteries more often than other vasculitides. Medium vessel vasculitis predominantly affects medium arteries. Small vessel vasculitis predominantly affects small vessels, but medium arteries and veins may be affected, although immune complex small vessel vasculitis rarely affects arteries. Not shown is *variable vessel vasculitis*, which can affect any type of vessel, from aorta to veins. The diagram depicts (from *left* to *right*) aorta, large artery, medium artery, small artery/arteriole, capillary, venule, and vein. ANCA, Antineutrophil cytoplasmic antibody; GBM, glomerular basement membrane. (*From Jennette JC, Falk RJ, Bacon PA, et al: 2012 Revised International Chapel Hill Consensus Conference Nomenclature of Vasculitides*, Arthritis Rheum 65(1):1–11, 2013, Fig 2, p 4.)

Table 192.1	Classification of Childhood Vasculitis

2012 CHAPEL HILL CONSENSUS CONFERENCE NOMENCLATURE OF VASCULITIDES	EUROPEAN LEAGUE AGAINST RHEUMATISM/PEDIATRIC RHEUMATOLOGY EUROPEAN SOCIETY CLASSIFICATION OF CHILDHOOD VASCULITIS
I. Large vessel vasculitis 　Takayasu arteritis 　Giant cell arteritis II. Medium vessel vasculitis 　Polyarteritis nodosa 　Kawasaki disease III. Small vessel vasculitis 　Antineutrophil cytoplasmic antibody (ANCA)–associated vasculitis 　　• Microscopic polyangiitis 　　• Granulomatosis with polyangiitis 　　• Eosinophilic granulomatosis with polyangiitis 　Immune complex small vessel vasculitis 　　• Anti–glomerular basement membrane (anti-GBM) disease 　　• IgA vasculitis (Henoch-Schönlein purpura) 　　• Hypocomplementemic urticarial vasculitis IV. Variable vessel vasculitis 　Behçet disease 　Cogan syndrome V. Single-organ vasculitis 　Cutaneous leukocytoclastic vasculitis 　Cutaneous arteritis 　Primary central nervous system vasculitis 　Isolated aortitis 　Others VI. Vasculitis associated with systemic disease 　Lupus vasculitis 　Rheumatoid vasculitis 　Sarcoid vasculitis 　Others VII. Vasculitis associated with probable etiology 　Hepatitis C virus–associated cryoglobulinemic vasculitis 　Hepatitis B virus–associated vasculitis 　Syphilis-associated aortitis 　Drug-associated immune complex vasculitis 　Drug-associated ANCA-associated vasculitis 　Cancer-associated vasculitis 　Others	Predominantly large vessel vasculitis 　Takayasu arteritis Predominantly medium vessel vasculitis 　Childhood polyarteritis nodosa 　Cutaneous polyarteritis nodosa 　Kawasaki disease Predominantly small vessel vasculitis 　Granulomatous: 　　• Granulomatosis with polyangiitis (Wegener granulomatosis)* 　　• Eosinophilic granulomatosis with polyangiitis (Churg-Strauss syndrome)* 　Nongranulomatous: 　　• Microscopic polyangiitis* 　　• Henoch-Schönlein purpura (IgA vasculitis) 　　• Isolated cutaneous leukocytoclastic vasculitis 　　• Hypocomplementemic urticarial vasculitis Other vasculitides 　Behçet disease 　Vasculitis secondary to infection (including hepatitis B–associated polyarteritis nodosa), malignancies, and drugs (including hypersensitivity vasculitis) 　Vasculitis associated with connective tissue disease 　Isolated vasculitis of central nervous system 　Cogan syndrome 　Unclassified

*Associated with antineutrophil cytoplasmic antibody.
　Adapted from Jennette JC, Falk RJ, Bacon PA, et al: 2012 Revised International Chapel Hill Consensus Conference nomenclature of vasculitides, *Arthritis Rheum* 65:1–11; 2013; and Ozen S, Pistorio A, Iusan SM, et al: EULAR/PRINTO/PRES criteria for Henoch-Schönlein purpura, childhood polyarteritis nodosa, childhood Wegener granulomatosis and childhood Takayasu arteritis: Ankara 2008. Part II. Final classification criteria, *Ann Rheum Dis* 69:798–806; 2010.

Table 192.2	Features That Suggest a Vasculitic Syndrome

CLINICAL FEATURES	LABORATORY FEATURES
Fever, weight loss, fatigue of unknown origin Skin lesions (palpable purpura, fixed urticaria, livedo reticularis, nodules, ulcers) Neurologic lesions (headache, mononeuritis multiplex, focal central nervous system lesions) Arthralgia or arthritis, myalgia, or myositis, serositis Hypertension, hematuria, renal failure Pulmonary infiltrates or hemorrhage Myocardial ischemia, arrhythmias	Increased erythrocytes sedimentation rate or C-reactive protein level Leukocytosis, anemia, thrombocytosis Eosinophilia Antineutrophil cytoplasmic antibodies Elevated factor VIII–related antigen (von Willebrand factor) Cryoglobulinemia Circulating immune complexes Hematuria

From Petty RE, Laxer RM, Lindsley CB, Wedderburn LR: *Textbook of pediatric rheumatology*, ed 7, Philadelphia, 2016, Elsevier Saunders.

Table 192.3	Clinicopathologic Characteristics of Vasculitides in Childhood

SYNDROME	FREQUENCY	VESSELS AFFECTED	CHARACTERISTIC PATHOLOGY
POLYARTERITIS			
Polyarteritis nodosa	Rare	Medium-size and small muscular arteries and sometimes arterioles	Focal segmental (often near bifurcations); fibrinoid necrosis; gastrointestinal, renal microaneurysms; lesions at various stages of evolution
Kawasaki disease	Common	Coronary and other muscular arteries	Thrombosis, fibrosis, aneurysms, especially of coronary vessels
LEUKOCYTOCLASTIC VASCULITIS			
Henoch-Schönlein purpura (IgA vasculitis)	Common	Arterioles and venules, often small arteries and veins	Leukocytoclasis; mixed cells, eosinophils, IgA deposits in affected vessels
Hypersensitivity angitis	Rare	Arterioles and venules	Leukocytoclastic or lymphocytic, varying eosinophils, occasionally granulomatous; widespread lesions at same stage of evolution
GRANULOMATOUS VASCULITIS			
Granulomatosis with polyangiitis (Wegener granulomatosis)	Rare	Small arteries and veins, occasionally larger vessels	Upper and lower respiratory tract, necrotizing granulomata glomerulonephritis
Eosinophilic granulomatosis with polyangiitis (Churg-Strauss syndrome)	Rare	Small arteries and veins, often arterioles and venules	Necrotizing extravascular granulomata; lung involvement; eosinophilia
GIANT CELL ARTERITIS			
Takayasu arteries	Uncommon	Large arteries	Granulomatous inflammation, giant cells; aneurysms, dissection
Temporal arteritis	Rare	Medium-size and large arteries	Granulomatous inflammation, giant cell arteries

Adapted from Cassidy JT, Petty RE: *Textbook of pediatric rheumatology*, ed 6, Philadelphia, 2011, Elsevier Saunders.

192.1 Henoch-Schönlein Purpura

Vidya Sivaraman, Edward C. Fels, and Stacy P. Ardoin

Henoch-Schönlein purpura (**HSP**) is the most common vasculitis of childhood and is characterized by leukocytoclastic vasculitis and immunoglobulin A deposition in the small vessels in the skin, joints, gastrointestinal tract, and kidney. According to the 2012 International Chapel Hill Consensus Conference nomenclature, HSP is also referred to as **IgA vasculitis**, based on the presence of vasculitis with predominance of IgA deposits affecting small vessels.

EPIDEMIOLOGY

HSP occurs worldwide and affects all ethnic groups but is more common in white and Asian populations. The incidence of HSP is estimated at 14-20 per 100,000 children per year and affects males more than females, with a 1.2-1.8 : 1 male/female ratio. Approximately 90% of HSP cases occur in children, usually between ages 3 and 10 yr. HSP is distinctly less common in adults, who often have severe and chronic complications. HSP is more common in the winter and spring and is unusual in summer

months. Many cases of HSP follow a documented upper respiratory infection.

PATHOLOGY

Skin biopsies demonstrate **leukocytoclastic vasculitis** of the dermal capillaries and postcapillary venules. The inflammatory infiltrate includes neutrophils and monocytes. Renal histopathology typically shows endocapillary proliferative glomerulonephritis, ranging from a focal segmental process to extensive crescentic involvement. In all tissues, immunofluorescence identifies IgA deposition in walls of small vessels (Fig. 192.2), accompanied to a lesser extent by deposition of C3, fibrin, and IgM.

PATHOGENESIS

The exact pathogenesis of HSP remains unknown. Given the seasonality of HSP and the frequency of preceding upper respiratory infections, infectious triggers such as group A β-hemolytic streptococcus, *Staphylococcus aureus*, mycoplasma, and adenovirus have been suspected. The common finding of deposition of IgA, specifically IgA_1, suggests that HSP is a disease mediated by IgA and IgA immune complexes. HSP occasionally clusters in families, suggesting a genetic component.

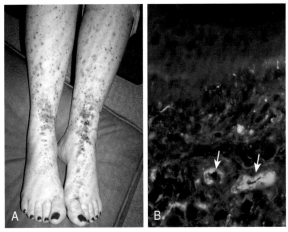

Fig. 192.2 Girl with Henoch-Schönlein purpura. **A,** Typical palpable purpura in lower extremities. **B,** Skin biopsy of lesion shows direct immunofluorescence of IgA *(arrows)* within the walls of dermal capillaries.

HLA-B34 and HLA-DRB1*01 alleles have been linked to HSP nephritis. Patients with familial Mediterranean fever, hereditary periodic fever syndromes, and complement deficiencies are at increased risk for developing HSP, suggesting that genetically determined immune dysregulation may contribute.

CLINICAL MANIFESTATIONS

The hallmark of HSP is its **rash**: palpable purpura starting as pink macules or wheals and developing into petechiae, raised purpura, or larger ecchymoses. Occasionally, bullae and ulcerations develop. The skin lesions are usually symmetric and occur in gravity-dependent areas (lower extremities), extensor aspect of the upper extremities or on pressure points (buttocks) (Figs. 192.2 and 192.3). The skin lesions often evolve in groups, typically lasting 3-10 days, and may recur up to 4 mo after initial presentation. Subcutaneous edema localized to the dorsa of hands and feet, periorbital area, lips, scrotum, or scalp is also common.

Musculoskeletal involvement, including arthritis and arthralgias, is common, occurring in up to 75% of children with HSP. The arthritis tends to be self-limited and oligoarticular, with a predilection for large joints such as the knees and ankles, and does not lead to deformities. Periarticular swelling and tenderness without erythema or effusions are common. The arthritis usually resolves within 2 wk but can recur.

Gastrointestinal (GI) manifestations occur in up to 80% of children with HSP and include abdominal pain, vomiting, diarrhea, paralytic ileus, and melena. Intussusception, mesenteric ischemia, and intestinal perforation are rare but serious complications. Endoscopic evaluation is usually not needed but may identify vasculitis of the intestinal tract.

Renal involvement occurs in up to 30% of children with HSP, manifesting as microscopic hematuria, proteinuria, hypertension, frank nephritis, nephrotic syndrome, and acute or chronic renal failure. However, progression to end-stage renal disease (ESRD) is uncommon in children (1–2%) (see Chapter 538.3). Renal manifestations can be delayed for several months after the initial illness, so close follow-up with serial urinalyses and blood pressure monitoring is necessary.

Neurologic manifestations of HSP, caused by hypertension (posterior reversible encephalopathy syndrome) or central nervous system (CNS) vasculitis, may also occur, including intracerebral hemorrhage, seizures, headaches, depressed level of consciousness, cranial or peripheral neuropathies, and behavior changes. Other, less common potential manifestations of HSP are inflammatory eye disease, carditis, pulmonary hemorrhage, orchitis, and testicular torsion.

DIAGNOSIS

The diagnosis of HSP is clinical and often straightforward when the typical rash is present. However, in at least 25% of cases, the rash appears

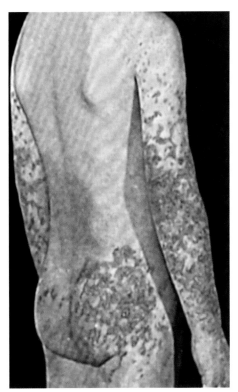

Fig. 192.3 Henoch-Schönlein purpura. *(From Korting GW: Hautkrankheiten bei Kindern und Jungendlichen, ed 3, Stuttgart, 1982, FK Schattaur Verlag.)*

Table 192.4	Classification Criteria for Henoch-Schönlein Purpura*

EUROPEAN LEAGUE AGAINST RHEUMATISM/PEDIATRIC RHEUMATOLOGY EUROPEAN SOCIETY CRITERIA†
Palpable purpura (in absence of coagulopathy or thrombocytopenia) and 1 or more of the following criteria must be present:
- Abdominal pain (acute, diffuse, colicky pain)
- Arthritis or arthralgia
- Biopsy of affected tissue demonstrating predominant IgA deposition
- Renal involvement (proteinuria >3 g/24 hr), hematuria or red cell casts

*Classification criteria are developed for use in research and not validated for clinical diagnosis.
†Developed for use in pediatric populations only.
Adapted from Ozen S, Pistorio A, Iusan SM, et al: EULAR/PRINTO/PRES criteria for Henoch-Schönlein purpura, childhood polyarteritis nodosa, childhood Wegener granulomatosis and childhood Takayasu arteritis: Ankara 2008. Part II. Final classification criteria, *Ann Rheum Dis* 69:798–806; 2010.

after other manifestations, making early diagnosis challenging. Table 192.4 summarizes the EULAR/PRES classification criteria for HSP. Most patients are afebrile.

The **differential diagnosis** for HSP depends on specific organ involvement but usually includes other small vessel vasculitides, infections, acute poststreptococcal glomerulonephritis, hemolytic-uremic syndrome, coagulopathies, and other acute intraabdominal processes. Additional disorders in the differential include papular-purpuric glove and sock syndrome, systemic lupus erythematosus (SLE), other vasculitides (urticarial, hypersensitivity), and thrombocytopenia.

Infantile acute hemorrhagic edema (AHE), an isolated cutaneous leukocytoclastic vasculitis that affects infants <2 yr of age, resembles

HSP clinically. AHE manifests as fever; tender edema of the face, scrotum, hands, and feet; and ecchymosis (usually larger than the purpura of HSP) on the face and extremities (Fig. 192.4). The trunk is spared, but petechiae may be seen in mucous membranes. The patient usually appears well except for the rash. The platelet count is normal or elevated, and the urinalysis results are normal. The younger age, the nature of the lesions, absence of other organ involvement, and a biopsy may help distinguish infantile AHE from HSP.

LABORATORY FINDINGS
No laboratory finding is diagnostic of HSP. Common but nonspecific findings include leukocytosis, thrombocytosis, mild anemia, and elevations of erythrocyte sedimentation rate (ESR) and C-reactive protein (CRP). *The platelet count is normal in HSP.* Occult blood is frequently found in stool specimens. Serum albumin levels may be low because of renal or intestinal protein loss. Autoantibody testing such as antinuclear antibody (ANA) is not useful diagnostically except to exclude other diseases. Serum IgA values are often elevated but are not routinely measured. Assessment of renal involvement with blood pressure, urinalysis, and serum creatinine is necessary.

Ultrasound is often used in the setting of GI complaints to look for bowel wall edema or the rare occurrence of an associated intussusception. Barium enema can also be used to both diagnose and treat intussusception. Although often unnecessary in typical HSP, biopsies of skin and kidney can provide important diagnostic information, particularly in atypical or severe cases, and characteristically show leukocytoclastic vasculitis with IgA deposition in affected tissues.

TREATMENT
Treatment for mild and self-limited HSP is *supportive,* with an emphasis on ensuring adequate hydration, nutrition, and analgesia. Corticosteroids are most often used to treat significant GI involvement or other life-threatening manifestations. Glucocorticoids such as oral prednisone (1-2 mg/kg/day), or in severe cases, intravenous (IV) methylprednisolone for 1-2 wk, followed by taper, reduce abdominal and joint pain but do not alter overall prognosis. Corticosteroids are not routinely recommended for prevention of complications such as nephritis. Rapid tapering

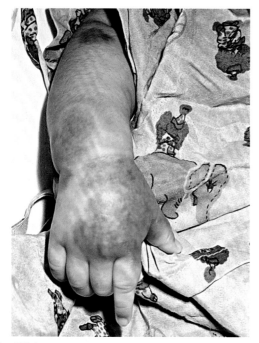

Fig. 192.4 Infantile acute hemorrhagic edema. Typical lesions on the arm of an infant. *(From Eichenfield LF, Frieden IJ, Esterly NB: Textbook of neonatal dermatology, Philadelphia, 2001, WB Saunders.)*

of corticosteroids may lead to a flare of HSP symptoms. Although few data are available to demonstrate efficacy, intravenous immune globulin (IVIG) and plasma exchange are sometimes used for severe disease. In some patients, chronic HSP renal disease is managed with a variety of immunosuppressants, including azathioprine, cyclophosphamide, cyclosporine, and mycophenolate mofetil. ESRD develops in <5% of children with HSP nephritis.

COMPLICATIONS
Acutely, serious GI involvement, including intussusception and intestinal perforation, imparts significant morbidity and mortality. Renal disease is the major long-term complication, occurring in 1–2% of children with HSP. Renal disease can develop up to 6 mo after diagnosis but rarely does so if the initial urinalysis findings are normal. Therefore, it is recommended that children with HSP undergo serial monitoring of blood pressure and urinalysis for at least 6 mo after diagnosis to monitor for development of nephritis.

PROGNOSIS
Overall, the prognosis for childhood HSP is excellent, and most children experience an acute, self-limited course lasting on average 4 wk. However, 15–60% of children with HSP experience 1 or more recurrences, typically within 4-6 mo of diagnosis. With each relapse, symptoms are usually milder than at presentation. Children with a more severe initial course are at higher risk for relapse. The long-term prognosis usually depends on the severity and duration of GI or renal involvement. Chronic renal disease develops in 1–2% of children with HSP, and <5% of those with HSP nephritis go on to have ESRD. The risk of HSP recurrence and graft loss following renal transplantation is estimated at 7.5% after 10 yr.

Bibliography is available at Expert Consult.

192.2 Takayasu Arteritis
*Vidya Sivaraman, Edward C. Fels,
and Stacy P. Ardoin*

Takayasu arteritis (**TA**), also known as **pulseless disease**, is a chronic large vessel vasculitis of unknown etiology that predominantly involves the aorta and its major branches.

EPIDEMIOLOGY
Although TA occurs worldwide and can affect all ethnic groups, the disease is most common in Asians. Age of onset is typically between 10 and 40 yr. Most children are diagnosed as adolescents, on average at age 13 yr. Up to 20% of individuals with TA are diagnosed before 19 yr. Younger children may be affected, but diagnosis in infancy is rare. TA preferentially affects females, with a reported 2-4:1 female/male ratio in children and adolescents and a 9:1 ratio among adults. Occlusive complications are more common in the United States, Western Europe, and Japan, whereas aneurysms predominate in Southeast Asia and Africa.

PATHOLOGY
TA is characterized by inflammation of the vessel wall, starting in the vasa vasorum. Involved vessels are infiltrated by T cells, natural killer cells, plasma cells, and macrophages. Giant cells and granulomatous inflammation develop in the media. Persistent inflammation damages the elastic lamina and muscular media, leading to blood vessel dilation and the formation of aneurysms. Progressive scarring and intimal proliferation can result in stenotic or occluded vessels. The subclavian, renal, and carotid arteries are the most commonly involved aortic branches; pulmonary, coronary, and vertebral arteries may also be affected.

PATHOGENESIS
The etiology of TA remains unknown. The presence of abundant T cells with a restricted repertoire of T-cell receptors in TA vascular lesions

points to the importance of cellular immunity and suggests the existence of a specific but unknown aortic tissue antigen. Expression of interleukin (IL)-1, IL-6, and tumor necrosis factor (TNF)-α is reported to be higher in patients with active TA than in patients with inactive TA and in healthy controls. In some patient populations, IL-1 genetic polymorphisms are linked to TA. Some individuals with TA have elevated serum values of antiendothelial antibodies. The increased prevalence of TA in certain ethnic populations and its occasional occurrence in monozygotic twins and families suggest a genetic predisposition to the disease.

CLINICAL MANIFESTATIONS

The diagnosis of TA is challenging, because early disease manifestations are often nonspecific. As a result, diagnosis can be delayed for several months, and the time to diagnosis is usually longer in children than in adults. Fever, malaise, weight loss, headache, hypertension, myalgias, arthralgias, dizziness, and abdominal pain are common early complaints in the *pre-pulseless* phase of the disease. Among children, hypertension and headache are particularly common presenting manifestations and should prompt consideration of TA when present without alternative explanation. Some individuals with TA report no systemic symptoms and instead present with vascular complications. It is only after substantial vascular injury that evidence of hypoperfusion becomes clinically evident. Later manifestations of disease include diminished pulse, asymmetric blood pressure, claudication, Raynaud phenomenon, renal failure, and symptoms of pulmonary or cardiac ischemia. Inflammation can extend to the aortic valve, resulting in valvular insufficiency. Other findings may include pericardial effusion, pericarditis, pleuritis, splenomegaly, and arthritis.

Supradiaphragmatic (aortic arch) disease often manifests with CNS (stroke, transient ischemic attack) and cardiac (heart failure, palpitations) symptoms. **Infradiaphragmatic** (mid-aortic syndrome) disease may produce hypertension, abdominal bruits, and pain. Most patients have involvement in both areas.

DIAGNOSIS

Specific pediatric criteria for TA have been proposed (Table 192.5). *Radiographic demonstration of large vessel vasculitis is necessary.* A thorough physical examination is required to detect an aortic murmur, diminished or asymmetric pulses, and vascular bruits. Four extremity blood pressures should be measured; >10 mm Hg asymmetry in systolic pressure is indicative of disease.

DIFFERENTIAL DIAGNOSIS

In the early phase of TA, when nonspecific symptoms predominate, the differential diagnosis includes a wide array of systemic infections, autoimmune conditions, and malignancies. Although **giant cell arteritis**, also known as *temporal arteritis*, is a common large vessel vasculitis in older adults, this entity is rare in childhood. Noninflammatory conditions that can cause large vessel compromise include fibromuscular dysplasia, Marfan syndrome, and Ehlers-Danlos syndrome.

LABORATORY FINDINGS

The laboratory findings in TA are nonspecific, and there is no specific diagnostic laboratory test. ESR and CRP value are typically elevated, and other nonspecific markers of chronic inflammation may include leukocytosis, thrombocytosis, anemia of chronic inflammation, and hypergammaglobulinemia. Autoantibodies, including ANA and ANCA, are not useful in diagnosing TA except to help exclude other autoimmune diseases.

Radiographic assessment is essential to establish large vessel arterial involvement. Conventional arteriography of the aorta and major branches, including carotid, subclavian, pulmonary, renal, and mesenteric branches, can identify luminal defects, including dilation, aneurysms, and stenoses, even in smaller vessels such as the mesenteric arteries. Fig. 192.5 shows a conventional arteriogram in a child with TA. Although not yet thoroughly validated in TA, magnetic resonance angiography (MRA) and computed tomography angiography (CTA) also provide important information about vessel wall thickness and enhancement, although they may not image smaller vessels as well as conventional angiography.

Table 192.5	Proposed Classification Criteria for Pediatric-Onset Takayasu Arteritis

Angiographic abnormalities (conventional, CT, or magnetic resonance angiography) of the aorta or its main branches and at least 1 of the following criteria:
- Decreased peripheral artery pulse(s) and/or claudication of extremities
- Blood pressure difference between arms or legs of >10 mm Hg
- Bruits over the aorta and/or its major branches
- Hypertension (defined by childhood normative data)
- Elevated acute-phase reactant (erythrocyte sedimentation rate or C-reactive protein)

Adapted from Ozen S, Pistorio A, Iusan SM, et al: EULAR/PRINTO/PRES criteria for Henoch-Schönlein purpura, childhood polyarteritis nodosa, childhood Wegener granulomatosis and childhood Takayasu arteritis: Ankara 2008. Part II. Final classification criteria, *Ann Rheum Dis* 69:798–806; 2010.

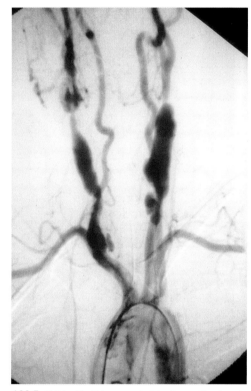

Fig. 192.5 Child with Takayasu arteritis. Conventional angiogram shows massive bilateral carotid dilation, stenosis, and poststenotic dilation.

Positron emission tomography (PET) may detect vessel wall inflammation but has not been studied extensively. Ultrasound with duplex color flow Doppler imaging may identify vessel wall thickening and assesses arterial flow. Echocardiography is recommended to assess for aortic valvular involvement. Serial vascular imaging is usually necessary to assess response to treatment and to detect progressive vascular damage.

TREATMENT

Glucocorticoids are the mainstay of therapy, typically starting with high doses (1-2 mg/kg/day of prednisone or methylprednisolone IV) followed by gradual dosage tapering. When TA progresses or recurs, steroid-sparing therapy is often required, usually involving methotrexate or azathioprine. *Cyclophosphamide* is reserved for severe or refractory disease. Results of small case series also suggest that *mycophenolate mofetil* or anti–TNF-α therapy may be beneficial in select patients. Anti–IL-6 therapy with tocilizumab has shown promising results in a small case series of children with TA. Antihypertensive medications are often necessary to control blood pressure caused by renovascular disease.

COMPLICATIONS
Progressive vascular damage can result in arterial stenoses, aneurysms, and occlusions, which produce ischemic symptoms and can be organ or life threatening. Potential ischemic complications include stroke, renal impairment or failure, myocardial infarction, mesenteric ischemia, and limb-threatening arterial disease. When these complications occur or are imminent, intervention with surgical vascular grafting or catheter-based angioplasty and stent placement may be necessary to restore adequate blood flow. A high rate of recurrent stenosis has been reported after angioplasty and stent placement. Aortic valve replacement may be required if significant aortic insufficiency develops.

PROGNOSIS
Although up to 20% of individuals with TA have a monophasic course and achieve sustained remission, most suffer relapses. Survival for individuals with TA has improved considerably over the decades, although higher mortality rates are reported in children and adolescents. The overall estimated survival for individuals with TA is 93% at 5 yr and 87% at 10 yr. However, morbidity from vascular complications remains high, particularly when there is evidence of ongoing active inflammation as detected by elevated CRP or ESR. Given the chronic endothelial insult and inflammation, children and adolescents with TA are probably at high risk for accelerated atherosclerosis. Early detection and treatment are critical to optimizing outcome in TA.

Bibliography is available at Expert Consult.

192.3 Polyarteritis Nodosa and Cutaneous Polyarteritis Nodosa
Vidya Sivaraman, Edward C. Fels, and Stacy P. Ardoin

Polyarteritis nodosa (**PAN**) is a systemic necrotizing vasculitis affecting small and medium-size arteries. Aneurysms and stenoses form at irregular intervals throughout affected arteries. Cutaneous PAN is limited to the skin.

EPIDEMIOLOGY
PAN is rare in childhood. Boys and girls are equally affected, and the mean age at presentation is 9 yr. The cause is unknown, but the development of PAN following infections, including group A streptococcus and chronic hepatitis B, suggests that PAN may represent a postinfectious autoimmune response. Infections with other organisms, including Epstein-Barr virus, *Mycobacterium tuberculosis*, cytomegalovirus, parvovirus B19, and hepatitis C virus, have also been associated with PAN. There is a possible association between PAN and familial Mediterranean fever.

PATHOLOGY
Biopsies show **necrotizing vasculitis** with granulocytes and monocytes infiltrating the walls of small and medium-size arteries (Fig. 192.6). Involvement is usually segmental and tends to occur at vessel bifurcations. Granulomatous inflammation is not present, and deposition of complement and immune complexes is rarely observed. Different stages of inflammation are found, ranging from mild inflammatory changes to panmural fibrinoid necrosis associated with aneurysm formation, thrombosis, and vascular occlusion.

PATHOGENESIS
Immune complexes are believed to be pathogenic, but the mechanism is poorly understood. It is not known why PAN has a predilection for

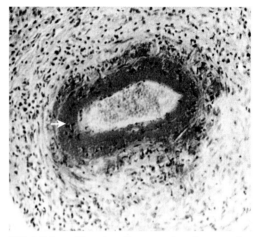

Fig. 192.6 Polyarteritis nodosa. Biopsy specimen from a medium-size muscular artery that exhibits marked fibrinoid necrosis of the vessel wall *(arrow). (From Cassidy JT, Petty RE: Polyarteritis and related vasculitides.* In Textbook of pediatric rheumatology, *ed 5, Philadelphia, 2005, Elsevier/ Saunders.)*

small and medium-size blood vessels. The inflamed vessel wall becomes thickened and narrowed, impeding blood flow and contributing to end-organ damage characteristic of this disease. Although there is no clear genetic association with PAN, PAN-like vasculitis is a component of 3 recently described monogenic autoinflammatory conditions.

Deficiency in **adenosine deaminase 2 (DADA2)**, caused by mutations in the *CECR1* gene, causes a familial form of vasculitis in Georgian Jewish patients with an autosomal recessive inheritance (see Chapter 188).

CLINICAL MANIFESTATIONS
The clinical presentation of PAN is variable but generally reflects the distribution of inflamed vessels. Constitutional symptoms are present in most children at disease onset. Weight loss and severe abdominal pain suggest mesenteric arterial inflammation and ischemia. Renovascular arteritis can cause hypertension, hematuria, or proteinuria, although glomerulonephritis is not typical. Cutaneous manifestations include purpura, livedo reticularis, ulcerations, digital ischemia, and painful nodules. Arteritis affecting the nervous system can result in cerebrovascular accidents, transient ischemic attacks, psychosis, and ischemic motor or sensory peripheral neuropathy (**mononeuritis multiplex**). Myocarditis or coronary arteritis can lead to heart failure and myocardial ischemia; pericarditis and arrhythmias have also been reported. Arthralgias, arthritis, or myalgias are frequently present. Less common symptoms include testicular pain that mimics testicular torsion, bone pain, and vision loss as a result of retinal arteritis. The pulmonary vasculature is usually spared in PAN.

DIAGNOSIS
The diagnosis of PAN requires demonstration of vessel involvement on biopsy or angiography (Table 192.6). Biopsy of cutaneous lesions shows small or medium vessel vasculitis (see Fig. 192.6). Kidney biopsy in patients with renal manifestations may show necrotizing arteritis. Electromyography in children with peripheral neuropathy identifies affected nerves, and sural nerve biopsy may reveal vasculitis. Conventional arteriography is the gold standard diagnostic imaging study for PAN and reveals areas of aneurysmal dilation and segmental stenosis, the classic "beads on a string" appearance (Fig. 192.7). MRA and CTA, less invasive imaging alternatives, are gaining acceptance, but may not be as effective in identifying small vessel disease or in younger children.

DIFFERENTIAL DIAGNOSIS
Early skin lesions may resemble those of HSP, although the finding of nodular lesions and presence of systemic features help distinguish PAN.

Table 192.6	Proposed Classification Criteria for Pediatric-Onset Polyarteritis Nodosa*
CRITERION	**FINDINGS**
Histopathology	Necrotizing vasculitis in medium or small arteries
Angiographic abnormalities	Angiography showing aneurysm, stenosis, or occlusion of medium or small artery not from noninflammatory cause
Cutaneous findings	Livedo reticularis, tender subcutaneous nodules, superficial skin ulcers, deep skin ulcers, digital necrosis, nail bed infarctions, or splinter hemorrhages
Muscle involvement	Myalgia or muscle tenderness
Hypertension	Systolic or diastolic blood pressure >95th percentile for height
Peripheral neuropathy	Sensory peripheral neuropathy, motor mononeuritis multiplex
Renal involvement	Proteinuria (>300 mg/24 hr equivalent), hematuria or red blood cell casts, impaired renal function (glomerular filtration rate <50% normal)

*The presence of 5 criteria provides 89.6% sensitivity and 99.6% specificity for the diagnosis of childhood-onset polyarteritis nodosa.

Adapted from Ozen S, Pistorio A, Iusan SM, et al: EULAR/PRINTO/PRES criteria for Henoch-Schönlein purpura, childhood polyarteritis nodosa, childhood Wegener granulomatosis and childhood Takayasu arteritis: Ankara 2008. Part II. Final classification criteria, *Ann Rheum Dis* 69:798–806; 2010.

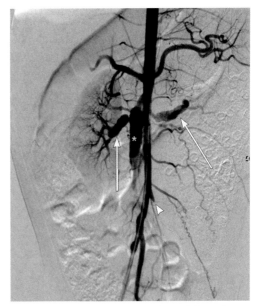

Fig. 192.7 Child with polyarteritis nodosa. Abdominal aortogram shows bilateral renal artery aneurysms *(arrows)*, superior mesenteric artery aneurysm *(asterisk)*, and left common iliac artery occlusion *(arrowhead)*. *(Courtesy of Dr. M. Hogan.)*

Because pulmonary vascular involvement is very rare in PAN, pulmonary lesions suggest ANCA-associated vasculitis or Goodpasture disease. Other rheumatic diseases, including SLE, have characteristic target-organ involvement and associated autoantibodies distinguishing them from PAN. Prolonged fever and weight loss should also prompt consideration of inflammatory bowel disease or malignancy.

LABORATORY FINDINGS

Nonspecific laboratory findings include elevations of ESR and CRP, anemia, leukocytosis, and hypergammaglobulinemia. Abnormal urine sediment, proteinuria, and hematuria indicate renal disease. Laboratory findings may be normal in cutaneous PAN or similar to those of systemic PAN. Elevated hepatic enzyme values may suggest hepatitis B or C infection. Serologic tests for hepatitis (hepatitis B surface antigen and hepatitis C antibody) should be performed in all patients.

TREATMENT

Oral *prednisone* (1-2 mg/kg/day) or IV pulse *methylprednisolone* (30 mg/kg/day) are the mainstay of therapy. Oral or IV cyclophosphamide are often used as adjunctive therapy, and plasma exchange may be warranted for life-threatening disease. If hepatitis B is identified, appropriate antiviral therapy should be initiated (see Chapter 385). Most cases of cutaneous PAN can be treated with less intense therapy such as corticosteroids alone, nonsteroidal antiinflammatory drugs (NSAIDs), and methotrexate. Azathioprine, mycophenolate mofetil, IVIG, thalidomide, cyclosporine, and anti-TNF agents such as infliximab have all been reported as successful in treatment of refractory cutaneous or systemic PAN, although clinical trials are lacking. If an infectious trigger for PAN is identified, antibiotic prophylaxis can be considered.

COMPLICATIONS

Cutaneous nodules may ulcerate and become infected. Hypertension and chronic renal disease may develop from renovascular involvement in PAN. Cardiac involvement may lead to decreased cardiac function or coronary artery disease. Mesenteric vasculitis can predispose to bowel infarction, rupture, and malabsorption. Stroke and rupture of hepatic arterial aneurysm are uncommon complications of this disorder.

PROGNOSIS

The course of PAN varies from mild disease with few complications to a severe, multiorgan disease with high morbidity and mortality. Poor prognostic factors in PAN include elevated serum creatinine, proteinuria, severe GI involvement, cardiomyopathy, and CNS involvement. Early and aggressive immunosuppressive therapy increases the likelihood of clinical remission. Compared with disease in adults, childhood PAN is associated with less mortality. Cutaneous PAN is unlikely to transition to systemic disease. Early recognition and treatment of the disease are important to minimizing potential long-term vascular complications.

Bibliography is available at Expert Consult.

192.4 Antineutrophilic Cytoplasmic Antibody–Associated Vasculitis

Vidya Sivaraman, Edward C. Fels and Stacy P. Ardoin

The ANCA-associated vasculitides are characterized by small vessel involvement, circulating ANCAs, and paucity of immune complex deposition in affected tissues, thus the term **pauci-immune vasculitis**. ANCA-associated vasculitis is categorized into 3 distinct forms: **granulomatosis with polyangiitis (GPA)**, formerly Wegener granulomatosis; **microscopic polyangiitis (MPA)**; and **eosinophilic granulomatosis with polyangiitis**, formerly Churg-Strauss syndrome (**CSS**) (see Table 192.1).

EPIDEMIOLOGY

GPA is a necrotizing granulomatous small and medium vessel vasculitis that occurs at all ages and targets the upper and lower respiratory tracts and the kidneys. Although most cases of GPA occur in adults, the disease also occurs in children with a mean age at diagnosis of 14 yr. There is a female predominance of 3-4:1, and pediatric GPA is most prevalent in Caucasians.

MPA is a small vessel necrotizing vasculitis with clinical features similar to those of GPA, but without granulomas and upper airway involvement. CSS is a small vessel necrotizing granulomatous (allergic granulomatosis) vasculitis associated with a history of refractory asthma and peripheral eosinophilia. MPA and CSS are rare in children, and there does not appear to be a gender predilection in either disease.

PATHOLOGY

Necrotizing vasculitis is the cardinal histologic feature in both GPA and MPA. Kidney biopsies typically demonstrate crescentic glomerulonephritis with little or no immune complex deposition ("pauci-immune"), in contrast to biopsies from patients with SLE. Although granulomatous inflammation is common in GPA and CSS, it is typically not present in MPA. Biopsies showing perivascular eosinophilic infiltrates distinguish CSS syndrome from both MPA and GPA (Table 192.7).

PATHOGENESIS

The etiology of ANCA-associated vasculitis remains unknown, although neutrophils, monocytes, and endothelial cells are involved in disease pathogenesis. Neutrophils and monocytes are activated by ANCAs, specifically by the ANCA-associated antigens proteinase-3 (PR3) and myeloperoxidase (MPO), and release proinflammatory cytokines such as TNF-α and IL-8. Localization of these inflammatory cells to the endothelium results in vascular damage characteristic of the ANCA vasculitides. Why the respiratory tract and kidneys are preferential targets in GPA and MPA is unknown.

CLINICAL MANIFESTATIONS

Early disease course is characterized by nonspecific constitutional symptoms, including fever, malaise, weight loss, myalgias, and arthralgias.

In GPA, upper airway involvement can manifest as sinusitis, nasal ulceration, epistaxis, otitis media, and hearing loss. Lower respiratory tract symptoms in GPA include cough, wheezing, dyspnea, and hemoptysis. Pulmonary hemorrhage can cause rapid respiratory failure. Compared with adults, childhood GPA is more frequently complicated by subglottic stenosis (Fig. 192.8). Inflammation-induced damage to the nasal cartilage can produce a saddle nose deformity (Fig. 192.8). Ophthalmic involvement includes conjunctivitis, scleritis, uveitis, optic neuritis, and invasive orbital pseudotumor (causing proptosis). Perineural vasculitis or direct compression on nerves by granulomatous lesions can cause cranial and peripheral neuropathies. Hematuria, proteinuria, and hypertension in GPA signal renal disease. Cutaneous lesions include palpable purpura and ulcers. Venous thromboembolism is a rare but potentially fatal complication of GPA. The frequencies of organ system involvement throughout the disease course in GPA follow: respiratory tract, 74%; kidneys, 83%; joints, 65%; eyes, 43%; skin, 47%; sinuses, 70%; and nervous system, 20%. Table 192.8 lists the classification criteria for pediatric-onset GPA.

The clinical presentation of MPA closely resembles that of GPA, although sinus disease is less common; systemic features of fever, malaise, weight loss, myalgias, and arthralgias may be dominant. MPA predominantly affects the kidney and lungs; other organ systems include skin, CNS, muscle, heart, and eyes.

CSS frequently causes inflammation of the upper and lower respiratory tracts, but cartilage destruction is rare. CSS may initially demonstrate chronic or recurrent rhinitis/sinusitis, nasal polyposis, nonfixed

Table 192.7	Differential Diagnostic Features of Small Vessel Vasculitis				
FEATURE	**HENOCH-SCHÖNLEIN PURPURA**	**GRANULOMATOSIS WITH POLYANGIITIS**	**CHURG-STRAUSS SYNDROME***	**MICROSCOPIC POLYANGIITIS**
Signs and symptoms of small vessel vasculitis[†]	+	+	+	+
IgA-dominant immune deposits	+	−	−	−
Circulating antineutrophil cytoplasmic antibodies	−	+ (PR3)	+ (MPO > PR3)	+ (MPO)
Necrotizing vasculitis	−	+	+	+
Granulomatous inflammation	−	+	+	−
Asthma and eosinophilia	−	−	+	−

*Eosinophilic granulomatosis with polyangiitis.
[†]Signs and symptoms of small vessel vasculitis include purpura, other rash, arthralgias, arthritis, and constitutional symptoms.
MPO, Myeloperoxidase-reactive antibodies; PR3, proteinase-3–reactive antibodies; +, present; −, absent.
Adapted from Jeannett JC, Falk RJ: Small-vessel vasculitis, *N Engl J Med* 337:1512–1523, 1997.

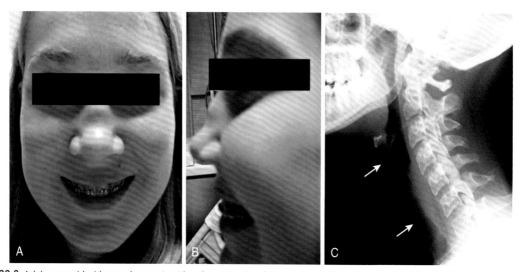

Fig. 192.8 Adolescent girl with granulomatosis with polyangiitis. **A** and **B**, Anterior and lateral views of saddle nose deformity. **C**, Segment of subglottic posterior tracheal irregularity (between *arrows*) on lateral neck radiograph.

pulmonary lesions, and difficult-to-treat asthma. Eosinophilia (>10% of leukocytes) with pulmonary infiltrates may precede a vasculitic phase. Other organ involvement includes skin, cardiac, peripheral neuropathy, GI tract, and muscle. Renal involvement in CSS is uncommon.

DIAGNOSIS

GPA should be considered in children who have recalcitrant sinusitis, pulmonary infiltrates, and evidence of nephritis. Chest radiography often fails to detect pulmonary lesions, and chest CT may show nodules, ground-glass opacities, mediastinal lymphadenopathy, and cavitary lesions (Fig. 192.9). The diagnosis is confirmed by the presence of c-ANCA with anti-PR3 specificity (PR3-ANCAs) and the finding of necrotizing granulomatous vasculitis on pulmonary, sinus, or renal biopsy. The ANCA test result is positive in approximately 90% of children with GPA, and the presence of anti-PR3 increases the specificity of the test.

In MPA, ANCAs are also frequently present (70% of patients) but are usually p-ANCA with reactivity to MPO (MPO-ANCAs). MPA can be distinguished from PAN by the presence of ANCAs and the tendency for small vessel involvement. The ANCA test result is positive in 50–70% of cases of CSS, and MPO-ANCAs are more common than PR3-ANCAs. In addition, the presence of chronic asthma and peripheral eosinophilia suggests the diagnosis of CSS.

DIFFERENTIAL DIAGNOSIS

ANCAs are absent in other granulomatous diseases, such as sarcoidosis and tuberculosis. **Goodpasture syndrome** is characterized by antibodies to glomerular basement membrane. Medications such as propylthiouracil, hydralazine, and minocycline are associated with drug-induced ANCA

Table 192.8	EULAR/PReS Classification Criteria for Pediatric-Onset Granulomatosis with Polyangiitis*

Histopathology showing granulomatous inflammation
Upper airway involvement
Laryngeal, tracheal or bronchial involvement
Antineutrophil cytoplasmic antibody (ANCA) positivity
Renal involvement
Proteinuria, hematuria, red blood cell casts, necrotizing pauci-
immune glomerulonephritis

*Diagnosis requires 3 of 6 criteria.
  Adapted from: Ozen S, Pistorio A, Iusan SM, et al: EULAR/PRINTO/PRES criteria for Henoch-Schönlein purpura, childhood polyarteritis nodosa, childhood Wegener granulomatosis and childhood Takayasu arteritis: Ankara 2008. Part II. Final classification criteria, *Ann Rheum Dis* 69:798–806; 2010.

(usually perinuclear ANCA) vasculitis. SLE and HSP can manifest as pulmonary hemorrhage and nephritis.

LABORATORY FINDINGS

Nonspecific laboratory abnormalities include elevated ESR and CRP values, leukocytosis, and thrombocytosis, which are present in most patients with an ANCA-associated vasculitis but are nonspecific. Anemia may be caused by chronic inflammation or pulmonary hemorrhage. ANCA antibodies show 2 distinct immunofluorescence patterns: *perinuclear* (p-ANCA) and *cytoplasmic* (c-ANCA). In addition, ANCAs can also be defined by their specificity for PR3 or MPO antigen. GPA is strongly associated with c-ANCAs/anti-PR3 antibodies, whereas 75% of patients with MPA have a positive p-ANCA (see Table 192.7). There is no clear correlation between ANCA titers and disease activity or relapse.

TREATMENT

When the lower respiratory tract or kidneys are significantly involved, initial induction therapy usually consists of prednisone (oral 2 mg/kg/day oral or IV methylprednisolone 30 mg/kg/day × 3 days) in conjunction with daily oral or monthly IV cyclophosphamide. *Rituximab*, a monoclonal antibody to CD20 on activated B cells, is an option for induction therapy in ANCA-positive vasculitides, although it has been studied primarily in adults. *Plasmapheresis* in conjunction with methylprednisolone has a role in the therapy of patients with severe disease manifestations such as pulmonary hemorrhage or ESRD, with the potential for reducing dialysis dependency. Patients are transitioned to a less toxic maintenance medication (usually methotrexate, azathioprine, or mycophenolate mofetil) within 3-6 mo once remission is achieved. Trimethoprim-sulfamethoxazole (one 180 mg/800 mg tablet 3 days/wk) is often prescribed both for prophylaxis against *Pneumocystis jiroveci* infection and to reduce upper respiratory bacterial colonization with *S. aureus*, which may trigger disease activity. If disease is limited to the upper respiratory tract, corticosteroids (1-2 mg/kg/day) and methotrexate (0.5-1.0 mg/kg/wk) may be first-line treatment.

Mepolizumab, an anti–IL-5 monoclonal antibody, may have a role in the treatment of eosinophilic granulomatosis with polyangiitis (CSS).

COMPLICATIONS

Upper respiratory tract lesions can invade the orbit and threaten the optic nerve, and lesions in the ear can cause permanent hearing loss. Respiratory complications include potentially life-threatening pulmonary hemorrhage and upper airway obstruction caused by subglottic stenosis. Chronic lung disease secondary to granulomatous inflammation, cavitary lesions, and scarring can predispose to infectious complications. Chronic

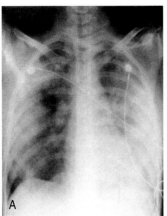 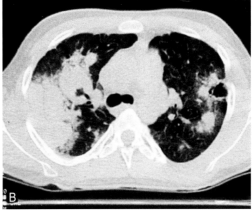

Fig. 192.9 Radiographs of lower respiratory tract disease in granulomatosis with polyangiitis (GPA). **A,** Chest radiograph of 14 yr old girl with GPA and pulmonary hemorrhage. Extensive bilateral, fluffy infiltrates are visualized. **B,** Chest CT scan in 17 yr old boy with GPA. Air space consolidation, septal thickening, and a single cavitary lesion are present. (**A** from Cassidy JT, Petty RE: Granulomatous vasculitis, giant cell arteritis and sarcoidosis. In Textbook of pediatric rheumatology, ed 3, Philadelphia, 1995, Saunders; **B** from Kuhn JP, Slovis TL, Haller JO: Caffey's pediatric diagnostic imaging, ed 10, vol 1, Philadelphia, 2004, Mosby.)

glomerulonephritis may progress to ESRD in a subset of patients with advanced or undertreated disease.

PROGNOSIS

The course is variable, but disease relapse occurs in up to 60% of patients. Mortality has been reduced with the introduction of cyclophosphamide and other immunosuppressive agents. Compared with adults, children are more likely to develop multiorgan involvement, renal involvement, and subglottic stenosis.

Bibliography is available at Expert Consult.

192.5 Other Vasculitis Syndromes

*Vidya Sivaraman, Edward C. Fels,
and Stacy P. Ardoin*

Other vasculitic conditions can occur in childhood; the most common is **Kawasaki disease** (see Chapter 191). **Behçet disease** is a rare form of vasculitis seen in children of Turkish and Mediterranean descent, characterized by the triad of recurrent aphthous stomatitis, genital ulcers, and uveitis (see Chapter 186).

Hypersensitivity vasculitis is a cutaneous vasculitis triggered by medication or toxin exposure. The rash consists of palpable purpura or other, nonspecific rash. Skin biopsies reveal characteristic changes of **leukocytoclastic vasculitis** (small vessels with neutrophilic perivascular or extravascular neutrophilic infiltration) (Table 192.9). **Hypocomplementemic urticarial vasculitis** involves small vessels and manifests as recurrent urticaria that resolves over several days but leaves residual hyperpigmentation. This condition is associated with low levels of complement component C1q and systemic findings that include fever, GI symptoms, arthritis, and glomerulonephritis. Some patients with urticarial vasculitis have normal complement levels. **Cryoglobulinemic vasculitis** can complicate mixed essential cryoglobulinemia and is a small vessel vasculitis affecting skin, joints, kidneys, and lungs.

Primary angiitis of the central nervous system represents vasculitis confined to the CNS and requires exclusion of other systemic vasculitides. **Large vessel disease** (angiography positive) may be progressive or nonprogressive and may manifest with focal deficits similar to an occlusive stroke, with hemiparesis, focal gross or fine motor deficits, language disorders, or cranial nerve deficits. Diffuse cognitive, memory, and concentration deficits as well as behavioral disorders are seen in 30–40% of patients. **Small vessel disease** (angiography negative, biopsy positive) more often results in language problems and diffuse deficits,

Table 192.9	Criteria for Diagnosis of Hypersensitivity Vasculitis*
CRITERION	**DEFINITION**
Age at onset >16 yr	Development of symptoms after 16 yr of age
Medication at disease onset	Medication that may have been a precipitating factor was taken at the onset of symptoms
Palpable purpura	Slightly elevated purpuric rash over 1 or more areas; does not blanch with pressure and is not related to thrombocytopenia
Maculopapular rash	Flat and raised lesions of various sizes over 1 or more areas of the skin
Biopsy, including arteriole and venule	Histologic changes showing granulocytes in a perivascular or extravascular location

*For purposes of classification, a patient is said to have hypersensitivity vasculitis if at least 3 of these criteria are present. The presence of ≥3 criteria has a diagnostic sensitivity of 71.0% and specificity of 83.9%. The age criterion is not applicable for children.
Adapted from Calabrese LH, Michel BA, Bloch DA, et al: The American College of Rheumatology 1990 criteria for the classification of hypersensitivity vasculitis, *Arthritis Rheum* 33:1108–1113, 1990 (Table 2, p 1110); and *Textbook of pediatric rheumatology*, ed 7, Philadelphia, 2016, Elsevier (Table 38.2, p 511).

Table 192.10	Differential Diagnosis of Small Vessel Primary Central Nervous System (CNS) Vasculitis in Children
CNS VASCULITIS COMPLICATING OTHER DISEASES *Infections* • Bacterial: *Mycobacterium tuberculosis, Mycoplasma pneumoniae, Streptococcus pneumoniae* • Viral: Epstein-Barr virus, cytomegalovirus, enterovirus, varicella-zoster virus, hepatitis C virus, parvovirus B19, West Nile virus • Fungal: *Candida albicans, Actinomyces, Aspergillus* • Spirochetal: *Borrelia burgdorferi, Treponema pallidum* *Rheumatic and Inflammatory Diseases* • Systemic vasculitis such as granulomatosis with polyangiitis, microscopic polyangiitis, Henoch-Schönlein purpura, Kawasaki disease, polyarteritis nodosa, Behçet disease • Systemic lupus erythematosus, juvenile dermatomyositis, morphea • Inflammatory bowel disease • Autoinflammatory syndromes • Hemophagocytic lymphohistiocytosis • Neurosarcoidosis • Adenosine deaminase-2 deficiency *Other* • Drug-induced vasculitis • Malignancy-associated vasculitis	**NONVASCULITIS INFLAMMATORY BRAIN DISEASES** *Demyelinating Diseases* • Multiple sclerosis, acute demyelinating encephalomyelitis (ADEM), optic neuritis, transverse myelitis *Antibody-Mediated Inflammatory Brain Disease* • Anti–NMDA receptor encephalitis, neuromyelitis optica (NMO), antibody-associated limbic encephalitis (antibodies against LGI, AMP, AMP-binding protein), Hashimoto encephalopathy, celiac disease, pediatric autoimmune neuropsychiatric disorders associated with streptococcal infections (PANDAS) *T-Cell–Associated Inflammatory Brain Disease* • Rasmussen encephalitis *Other* • Febrile infection-related epilepsy syndrome (FIRES) **NONINFLAMMATORY VASCULOPATHIES** • Hemoglobinopathies (sickle cell disease), thromboembolic disease • Radiation vasculopathy, graft-versus-host disease • Metabolic and genetic diseases such as cerebral autosomal dominant arteriopathy with subcortical infarcts and leukoencephalopathy (CADASIL), mitochondrial encephalopathy lactic acidosis and stroke-like episodes (MELAS), CARASIL (cerebral autosomal recessive arteriopathy with subcortical infarcts and leukoencephalopathy), moyamoya disease, Fabray disease • Malignancy (lymphoma)

Modified from Gowdie P, Twilt M, Benseler SM: Primary and secondary central nervous system vasculitis. *J Child Neurol* 27:1448–1459, 2012.

such as cognitive, memory, behavior, and concentration problems, as well as focal seizures. In both types of cerebral angiitis, patients may have an elevated ESR or CRP and abnormal CSF findings (increased protein, pleocytosis), although these are not consistent findings in all patients. Diagnosis remains a challenge, and brain biopsy is often indicated to confirm the diagnosis and exclude vasculitis mimics such as infections that could worsen with immunosuppressive therapy (Table 192.10).

Nonprogressive angiography-positive CNS vasculitis, also known as *transient CNS angiopathy,* represents a more benign variant and can be seen in children after varicella infection. **Cogan syndrome** is rare in children; its potential clinical manifestations include constitutional symptoms; inflammatory eye disease such as uveitis, episcleritis, or interstitial keratitis; vestibuloauditory dysfunction (vertigo, hearing loss, tinnitus); arthritis; and large vessel vasculitis or aortitis. Cerebral autosomal **dominant** arteriopathy with subcortical infarcts and leuko-encephalopathy (**CADASIL**) is caused by mutations in the *NOTCH3* gene and manifests with stroke, mood changes, cognitive decline, and migraines; it is a vasculitis mimic and demonstrates osmophilic granules in cerebral arteries. **CARASIL** (cerebral autosomal **recessive** arteriopathy with subcortical infarcts and leukoencephalopathy) is another mimic of angiitis caused by mutations in the *HTRA1* gene. It manifests with early-onset hair loss, spasticity, stroke, memory loss, and personality changes.

Identification of these vasculitis syndromes requires a comprehensive history and physical examination. Table 192.11 outlines other diagnostic considerations. Although tailored to disease severity, treatment generally includes prednisone (up to 2 mg/kg/day). Potent immunosuppressive medications, such as cyclophosphamide, are often indicated, particularly in primary angiitis of the CNS to prevent rapid neurologic decline. For hypersensitivity vasculitis, withdrawal of the triggering medication or toxin is indicated if possible.

Bibliography is available at Expert Consult.

Table 192.11	Diagnostic Considerations for Other Vasculitis Syndromes
VASCULITIS SYNDROME	**APPROACH TO DIAGNOSIS**
Hypersensitivity vasculitis	Skin biopsy demonstrating leukocytoclastic vasculitis
Hypocomplementemic urticarial vasculitis	Biopsy of affected tissue demonstrating small vessel vasculitis Low levels of circulating C1q
Cryoglobulinemic vasculitis	Biopsy of affected tissue demonstrating small vessel vasculitis Measurement of serum cryoglobulins Exclusion of hepatitides B and C infections
Primary angiitis of CNS	Conventional, CT, or MRA evidence of CNS vasculitis Consideration of dura or brain biopsy
Nonprogressive angiography-positive CNS vasculitis	Conventional, CT, or MRA evidence of CNS vasculitis
Cogan syndrome	Ophthalmology and audiology evaluations Conventional, CT, or MRA evidence of CNS or aortic vasculitis

CNS, Central nervous system; CT, computed tomography; MRA, magnetic resonance angiography.

Chapter 193

Musculoskeletal Pain Syndromes

Kelly K. Anthony and Laura E. Schanberg

第一百九十三章

肌肉骨骼疼痛综合征

中文导读

　　本章主要介绍了肌肉骨骼疼痛综合征的临床表现、诊断及鉴别诊断、治疗、并发症及预后，并介绍了生长痛、小纤维多神经病、纤维肌痛症、复杂区域疼痛综合征、红斑肢痛症。并具体描述了生长痛、小纤维多神经病、纤维肌痛症、复杂区域疼痛综合征、红斑肢痛症的可能的病因、临床特点、治疗及诊断与鉴别诊断。

Musculoskeletal pain is a frequent complaint of children presenting to general pediatricians and is the most common presenting problem of children referred to pediatric rheumatology clinics. Prevalence estimates of persistent musculoskeletal pain in community samples range from 10–30%. Although diseases such as juvenile idiopathic arthritis (JIA) and systemic lupus erythematosus (SLE) may manifest as persistent musculoskeletal pain, the majority of musculoskeletal pain complaints in children are benign in nature and attributable to trauma, overuse, and normal skeletal growth variations. In a subset of children, chronic pain complaints develop in the absence of physical or laboratory abnormalities. Children with idiopathic musculoskeletal pain syndromes also typically develop marked subjective distress and functional impairment. Therefore the treatment of children with musculoskeletal pain syndromes optimally includes both pharmacologic and nonpharmacologic interventions.

CLINICAL MANIFESTATIONS
Chronic musculoskeletal pain syndromes involve pain complaints at least 3 mo in duration in the absence of objective abnormalities on physical examination or laboratory screening. Additionally, children and adolescents with musculoskeletal pain syndromes often complain of persistent pain despite previous treatment with nonsteroidal antiinflammatory drugs (NSAIDs) and analgesic agents. The location varies, with pain complaints either localized to a single extremity or more diffuse and involving multiple extremities. The pain may start in a single area of the body before intensifying and radiating to other areas over time. The prevalence of musculoskeletal pain syndromes increases with age and is higher in females, thus rendering adolescent girls at highest risk.

The somatic complaints of children and adolescents with musculoskeletal pain syndromes are typically accompanied by psychological distress, sleep difficulties, and functional impairment across home, school, and peer domains. **Psychological distress** may include symptoms of anxiety and depression, such as frequent crying spells, fatigue, sleep disturbance, feelings of worthlessness, poor concentration, and frequent worry. Indeed, a substantial number of children with musculoskeletal pain syndromes display the full range of psychological symptoms, warranting an additional diagnosis of a comorbid mood or anxiety disorder (e.g., major depressive episode, generalized anxiety disorder). **Sleep disturbance** in children with musculoskeletal pain syndromes may include difficulty falling asleep, multiple night awakenings, disrupted sleep–wake cycles with increased daytime sleeping, nonrestorative sleep, and fatigue.

For children and adolescents with musculoskeletal pain syndromes, the constellation of pain, psychological distress, and sleep disturbance

often leads to a high degree of functional impairment. Poor school attendance is common, and children may struggle to complete other daily activities relating to self-care and participation in household chores. Decreased physical fitness can also occur, as well as changes in gait and posture, as children avoid contact with or use of the body area affected by pain. Peer relationships may also be disrupted by decreased opportunities for social interaction because of pain. As such, children and adolescents with musculoskeletal pain syndromes often report loneliness and social isolation characterized by few friends and lack of participation in extracurricular activities.

DIAGNOSIS AND DIFFERENTIAL DIAGNOSIS
The diagnosis of a musculoskeletal pain syndrome is typically one of exclusion when careful, repeated physical examinations and laboratory testing do not reveal an etiology. At initial presentation, children with pain complaints require a thorough clinical history and a complete physical examination to look for an obvious etiology (sprains, strains, or fractures), characteristics of the pain (localized or diffuse), and evidence of systemic involvement. A comprehensive history can be particularly useful in providing clues to the possibility of underlying illness or systemic disease. The presence of current or recent fever can be indicative of an inflammatory or neoplastic process if the pain is also accompanied by worsening symptoms over time or weight loss.

Subsequent, *repeated* physical examinations of children with musculoskeletal pain complaints may reveal eventual development and manifestations of rheumatic or other diseases. The need for additional testing should be individualized, depending on the specific symptoms and physical findings. Laboratory screening and radiography should be pursued if there is suspicion of certain underlying disease processes. Possible indicators of a serious, vs a benign, cause of musculoskeletal pain include pain present at rest, pain that may be relieved by activity, objective joint swelling on physical examination, stiffness or limited range of motion in joints, bony tenderness, muscle weakness, poor growth and/or weight loss, and constitutional symptoms (e.g., fever, malaise) (Table 193.1). In the case of laboratory screenings, a complete blood count (CBC) and erythrocyte sedimentation rate (ESR) are likely to be abnormal in children whose pain is secondary to a bone or joint infection, SLE, or a malignancy. Bone tumors, fractures, and other focal pathology resulting from infection, malignancy, or trauma can often be identified through imaging studies, including plain radiographs, MRI, and less often technetium-99m bone scans.

The presence of persistent pain, accompanied by psychological distress, sleep disturbance, and/or functional impairment, in the absence of objective laboratory or physical examination abnormalities, suggests

Table 193.1	Potential Indicators of Benign vs Serious Causes of Musculoskeletal Pain	
CLINICAL FINDING	**BENIGN CAUSE**	**SERIOUS CAUSE**
Effects of rest vs activity on pain	Relieved by rest and worsened by activity	Present at rest and may be relieved by activity
Time of day pain occurs	End of the day and nights	Morning*
Objective joint swelling	No	Yes
Joint characteristics	Hypermobile/normal	Stiffness, limited range of motion
Bony tenderness	No	Yes
Muscle strength	Normal	Muscle weakness
Gait	Normal	Limp or refusal to walk
Growth	Normal growth pattern or weight gain	Poor growth and/or weight loss
Constitutional symptoms (e.g., fever, malaise)	Fatigue without other constitutional symptoms	Yes
Lab findings	Normal CBC, ESR, CRP	Abnormal CBC, raised ESR and CRP
Imaging findings	Normal	Effusion, osteopenia, radiolucent metaphyseal lines, joint space loss, bony destruction

*Cancer pain is often severe and worst at night.
CBC, Complete blood count; CRP, C-reactive protein level; ESR, erythrocyte sedimentation rate.
Adapted from Malleson PN, Beauchamp RD: Diagnosing musculoskeletal pain in children, *CMAJ* 165:183–188, 2001.

the diagnosis of an **idiopathic** musculoskeletal pain syndrome. All pediatric musculoskeletal pain syndromes share this general constellation of symptoms at presentation. Several more specific pain syndromes routinely seen by pediatric practitioners can be differentiated by anatomic region and associated symptoms. Table 193.2 outlines pediatric musculoskeletal pain syndromes, including growing pains (see Chapter 193.1), fibromyalgia (Chapter 193.3), complex regional pain syndrome (Chapter 193.4), localized pain syndromes, low back pain, and chronic sports-related pain syndromes (e.g., Osgood-Schlatter disease).

TREATMENT
The primary goal of treatment for pediatric musculoskeletal pain syndromes is to improve function rather than relieve pain, and these 2 desirable outcomes may not occur simultaneously. Indeed, it is common for children with musculoskeletal pain syndromes to continue complaining of pain even as they resume normal function (e.g., increased school attendance and participation in extracurricular activities). For all children and adolescents with pediatric musculoskeletal pain syndromes, regular school attendance is crucial, because this is a hallmark of normal functioning in this age-group. The dual nature of treatment, targeting both *function* and *pain,* needs to be clearly explained to children and their families to outline better the goals by which treatment success will be measured. Indeed, children and families need to be supported in disengaging from the sole pursuit of pain relief and embracing broader treatment goals of improved functioning.

Recommended treatment modalities typically include physical and/or occupational therapy, pharmacologic interventions, and cognitive-behavioral and/or other psychotherapeutic interventions. The overarching goal of **physical therapy** is to improve children's physical function and should emphasize participation in aggressive but graduated aerobic exercise. **Pharmacologic** interventions should be used judiciously. Low-dose tricyclic antidepressants (amitriptyline, 10-50 mg orally 30 min before bedtime) are indicated for treatment of sleep disturbance; selective serotonin reuptake inhibitors (sertraline, 10-20 mg daily) may prove useful in treating symptoms of depression and anxiety if present. Referral for psychological evaluation is warranted if these symptoms do not resolve with initial treatment efforts or if suicidal ideation is present. **Cognitive-behavioral therapy (CBT)** and/or other **psychotherapeutic** interventions are typically designed to teach children and adolescents coping skills for controlling the behavioral, cognitive, and physiologic responses to pain. Specific components often include cognitive restructuring, relaxation, distraction, and problem-solving skills; additional targets of therapy include sleep hygiene and activity scheduling, all with the goal of restoring normal sleep patterns and activities of daily living. Parent education and involvement in the psychological intervention is important to ensure maintenance of progress. More intensive family-based approaches are warranted if barriers to treatment success are identified at the family level. These could include parenting strategies or family dynamics that serve to maintain children's pain complaints, such as overly solicitous responses to the child's pain and maladaptive models for pain coping.

COMPLICATIONS AND PROGNOSIS
Musculoskeletal pain syndromes can negatively affect the child's development and future role functioning. Worsening pain and the associated symptoms of depression and anxiety can lead to substantial school absences, peer isolation, and developmental delays later in adolescence and early adulthood. Specifically, adolescents with musculoskeletal pain syndromes may fail to achieve the level of autonomy and independence necessary for age-appropriate activities, such as attending college, living away from home, and maintaining a job. Fortunately, not all children and adolescents with musculoskeletal pain syndromes experience this degree of impairment, but many children experience pain that persists for 1 yr or more. Factors that contribute to the persistence of pain are increasingly understood and include female gender, pubertal stage at pain onset, older age of pain onset, increased psychological distress associated with the pain, joint hypermobility, and greater functional impairment. The likelihood of positive health outcomes is increased with multidisciplinary treatment.

Bibliography is available at Expert Consult.

Table 193.2	Common Musculoskeletal Pain Syndromes in Children by Anatomic Region	
ANATOMIC REGION	**PAIN SYNDROMES**	
Shoulder	Impingement syndrome	
Elbow	"Little League elbow" Avulsion fractures Osteochondritis dissecans	Tennis elbow Panner disease
Arm	Localized hypermobility syndrome Complex regional pain syndrome	
Pelvis and hip	Avulsion injuries Legg-Calvé-Perthes syndrome	Slipped capital femoral epiphysis Congenital hip dysplasia
Knee	Osteochondritis dissecans Osgood-Schlatter disease Sinding-Larsen syndrome	Patellofemoral syndrome Malalignment syndromes
Leg	Growing pains Complex regional pain syndrome Localized hypermobility syndrome	Shin splints Stress fractures Compartment syndromes
Foot	Plantar fasciitis Tarsal coalition Stress fractures	Achilles tendonitis Juvenile bunion
Spine	Musculoskeletal strain Spondylolisthesis Spondylolysis	Scoliosis Scheuermann disease (kyphosis) Low back pain
Generalized	Hypermobility syndrome Juvenile fibromyalgia Generalized pain syndrome	

Adapted from Anthony KK, Schanberg LE: Assessment and management of pain syndromes and arthritis pain in children and adolescents, *Rheum Dis Clin North Am* 33:625–660, 2007 (Box 1).

193.1 Growing Pains

Kelly K. Anthony and Laura E. Schanberg

More appropriately termed **benign nocturnal pains of childhood**, growing pains affect 10–20% of children, with peak incidence between age 4 and 12 yr. Pain does not occur during periods of rapid growth or at growth sites. The most common cause of recurrent musculoskeletal pain in children, growing pains are intermittent and bilateral, predominantly affecting the anterior thigh, shin, and calf, but not joints. Occasionally, bilateral upper extremity pain may be associated with leg pain; isolated upper extremity pain does not occur. Children typically describe cramping or aching that occurs in the late afternoon or evening. Pain may wake the child from sleep and may last a few minutes to hours, but resolves quickly with massage or analgesics; pain is never present the following morning (Table 193.3). Pain often follows a day with exercise or other physical activities. Physical findings are normal, and gait is not impaired.

Although growing pains are generally considered a benign, time-limited condition, evidence suggests they represent a **pain amplification syndrome**. Indeed, growing pains persist in a significant percentage of children, with some children developing other pain syndromes such as abdominal pain and headaches. Growing pains are more likely to persist in children with a parent who has a history of a pain syndrome and in children who have lower pain thresholds not just at the site of pain, but throughout their body. Disordered somatosensory testing, lower bone strength, and lower calcium intake have also been shown to be present in children with growing pains.

Treatment should also focus on reassurance, education, and healthy sleep hygiene. Massage during the episode is very effective, and physical therapy and muscle stretching may also be important parts of treatment. NSAIDs agents may be useful for frequent episodes. CBT may be indicated if the pain persists.

Restless legs syndrome (**RLS**, Willis-Ekbom disease), seen more frequently among adolescents and adults, is a sensorimotor disturbance that may be confused with growing pains (see Chapter 31). Often familial, RLS is a difficult-to-control *urge* to move the leg that is exacerbated during rest and at night and is relieved by movement (Table 193.3). There is significant overlap in the diagnostic features of growing pains and RLS, leading to diagnostic confusion. Moreover, these conditions can be comorbid, and there is a high incidence of RLS in the parents of children with growing pains. RLS appears to be best distinguished from growing pains by the *urge* to move the legs, associated uncomfortable leg sensations that may not be described as painful; the worsening with periods of rest; and relief through movement. Iron supplementation may benefit pediatric patients with RLS.

Bibliography is available at Expert Consult.

193.2 Small Fiber Polyneuropathy

Kelly K. Anthony and Laura E. Schanberg

Many patients with juvenile-onset widespread pain syndromes, as well as patients with pediatric fibromyalgia (Chapter 193.3), complex regional pain syndrome type I (Chapter 193.4), and erythromelalgia (Chapter 193.5), have evidence of a small fiber polyneuropathy causing dysfunctional or degeneration of small-diameter unmyelinated C fibers and thinly myelinated A delta fibers that mediate nociception and the autonomic nervous system. Fibromyalgia includes **chronic widespread pain**, defined as ≥3 mo duration of axial pain that is often bilateral and that also affects the upper and lower extremities. In addition, many patients have associated chronic cardiovascular (dizziness, postural orthostasis syndrome) symptoms, as well as chronic abdominal pain and ileus, headaches, fatigue, and erythromelalgia, suggestive of **dysautonomia**.

There are no typical findings on physical examination or standard laboratory tests. The diagnosis of small fiber polyneuropathy requires distal leg immunolabeled skin biopsy to identify epidermal nociceptive fibers and autonomic function testing to examine cardiovagal, adrenergic, and sudomotor small fiber function.

Treatment of patients with small fiber polyneuropathy and isolated juvenile-onset widespread pain syndrome, or those subsets of patients with small fiber polyneuropathy and fibromyalgia, complex regional pain syndrome, or erythromelalgia, is evolving and has included prednisone or intravenous immune globulin.

Bibliography is available at Expert Consult.

Table 193.3	Inclusion and Exclusion Criteria for Growing Pains Including Features of Restless Leg Syndromes (RLS)		
	INCLUSIONS	**EXCLUSIONS**	**RLS FEATURES**
Nature of pain	Intermittent; some pain-free days and nights, deep aching, cramping	Persistent; increasing intensity, pain during the day	Urge to move legs often accompanied by unpleasant sensations in legs, but may not be painful
Unilateral or bilateral	Bilateral	Unilateral	
Location of pain	Anterior thigh, calf, posterior knee—in muscles not the joints	Articular, back, or groin pain	Urge to move and discomfort throughout leg
Onset of pain	Late afternoon or evening	Pain still present next morning	Worse later in day or night but also present at periods of rest or inactivity throughout the day
Physical findings	Normal	Swelling, erythema, tenderness; local trauma or infection; reduced joint range of motion; limping, fever, weight loss, mass	
Laboratory findings	Normal	Objective evidence of abnormalities; increased erythrocyte sedimentation rate or C-reactive protein; abnormal complete blood count, radiography, bone scan, or MRI	

Adapted from Evans AM, Scutter SD: Prevalence of "growing pains" in young children, *J Pediatr* 145:255–258, 2004; and Walters AS, Gabelia D, Frauscher B: Restless legs syndrome (Willis-Ekbom disease) and growing pains: are they the same thing? A side-by-side comparison of the diagnostic criteria for both and recommendations for future research, *Sleep Med* 14:1247–1252, 2013.

193.3 Fibromyalgia

Kelly K. Anthony and Laura E. Schanberg

Juvenile primary fibromyalgia syndrome (JPFS) is a common pediatric musculoskeletal pain syndrome. Approximately 25–40% of children with chronic pain syndromes can be diagnosed with JPFS. Although specific diagnostic criteria for JPFS have not been determined, the adult criteria set forth by the American College of Rheumatology (ACR) in 2010 have been shown to have a high degree of sensitivity and specificity in the diagnosis of JPFS (Fig. 193.1 and Table 193.4). Previous studies describing children and adolescents with JPFS noted diffuse, multifocal, waxing and waning, and at times migratory musculoskeletal pain in at least 3 areas of the body persisting for at least 3 mo in the absence of an underlying condition. Results of laboratory tests were normal, and physical examination revealed at least 5 well-defined tender points (Fig. 193.2). There is considerable overlap among symptoms associated with JPFS and complaints associated with other **functional disorders** (e.g., irritable bowel disease, migraines, temporomandibular joint disorder, premenstrual syndrome, mood and anxiety disorders, chronic fatigue syndrome), suggesting that these disorders may be part of a larger spectrum of related syndromes.

Although the precise cause of JPFS is unknown, there is an emerging understanding that the development and maintenance of JPFS are related both to biologic and psychological factors. JPFS is an abnormality of central pain processing characterized by disordered sleep physiology, enhanced pain perception with abnormal levels of substance P in cerebrospinal fluid, disordered mood, and dysregulation of hypothalamic-pituitary-adrenal and other neuroendocrine axes, resulting in lower tender-point pain thresholds and increased pain sensitivity. Evolving

Table 193.4	American College of Rheumatology Fibromyalgia Diagnostic Criteria

The following 3 conditions must be met:
1. Widespread pain index (WPI) ≥7 and symptom severity (SS) scale score ≥5 *or* WPI 3-6 and SS scale score ≥9.
2. Symptoms have been present at a similar level for at least 3 mo.
3. The patient does not have a disorder that would otherwise explain the pain.

ASCERTAINMENT OF WPI

The WPI is the number of areas in which a patient has had pain over the last week. The score will be between 0 and 19: left shoulder girdle left, right shoulder girdle, left upper arm, right upper arm, left lower arm, right lower arm, left hip (buttock, trochanter), right hip (buttock, trochanter), left upper leg, right upper leg, left lower leg, right lower leg, left jaw, right jaw, chest, abdomen, upper back, lower back, and neck.

ASCERTAINMENT OF SS SCALE SCORE

The SS scale score is the sum of the severity of 3 symptoms (fatigue, waking unrefreshed, and cognitive symptoms) *plus* the severity of somatic symptoms in general. The final score is between 0 and 12.
- For each of the 3 symptoms, the level of severity over the past week is rated using the following scale:
  0 = No problem
  1 = Slight or mild problems, generally mild or intermittent
  2 = Moderate, considerable problems, often present and/or at a moderate level
  3 = Severe: pervasive, continuous, life-disturbing problems
- Considering somatic symptoms in general, the following scale is used to indicated the number of symptoms:
  0 = No symptoms
  1 = Few symptoms
  2 = Moderate number of symptoms
  3 = Great deal of symptoms
- Somatic symptoms that can be considered include muscle pain, irritable bowel syndrome, fatigue, thinking problems, muscle weakness, headache, abdominal pain, numbness/tingling, dizziness, insomnia, depression, constipation, pain in the upper abdomen, nausea, nervousness, chest pain, blurred vision, fever, diarrhea, dry mouth, itching, wheezing, Raynaud phenomenon, hives/welts, ringing in ears, vomiting, heartburn, oral ulcers, loss of/change in taste, seizures, dry eyes, shortness of breath, loss of appetite, rash, sun sensitivity, hearing difficulties, easy bruising, hair loss, frequent urination, painful urination, and bladder spasms.

Adapted from Wolfe F, Clauw DJ, Fitzcharles MA, et al: The American College of Rheumatology preliminary diagnostic criteria for fibromyalgia and measurement of symptom severity, *Arthritis Care Res* 62: 600–610, 2010.

WIDESPREAD PAIN INDEX (WPI)
A. Have you had pain in the following location(s) in the last week?

Shoulder, right	Shoulder, left	Upper arm, right	Upper arm, left
Lower arm, right	Lower arm, left	Hip (buttock), right	Hip (buttock), left
Upper leg, right	Upper leg, left	Lower leg, right	Lower leg, left
Jaw, right	Jaw, left	Chest	Abdomen
Upper back	Lower back	Neck	

Part A score = Total number of areas marked yes

SYMPTOM SEVERITY (SS)
B. How much of a problem have the following been for you during the past week?

	No problem	Slight/mild problem, generally mild or intermittent	Moderate, considerable problem, often present	Severe, pervasive, continuous, life disturbing problem
Fatigue	0	1	2	3
Waking still feeling tired	0	1	2	3
Concentration or memory problems	0	1	2	3

Part B score: Total of all domains

C. Have you had problems with any of the following during the past three months?

Muscle pain	Headache	Sun sensitivity	Chest pain
Muscle weakness	Dizziness	Blurred vision	Hair loss
Numbness/tingling	Shortness of breath	Loss/changes in taste	Fever
IBS	Nervousness	Hearing difficulties	Thinking problem
Abdominal pain/cramps	Depression	Ringing in ears	Dry mouth
Diarrhea	Fatigue/tiredness	Easy bruising	Dry eyes
Constipation	Insomnia	Frequent urination	Itching
Heartburn	Loss of appetite	Bladder spasms	Wheezing
Vomiting	Rash	Painful urination	Oral ulcers
Nausea	Hives/welts	Seizures	Raynaud's

Part C score: 0 = No symptoms, 1 = Few symptoms, 2 = Moderate number of symptoms, 3 = A great deal of symptoms

WPI = A score
SS = B score + C score
Fibromyalgia if: WPI ≥ 7 *and* SS ≥ 5 OR WPI 3-6 *and* SS ≥ 9

Fig. 193.1 Fibromyalgia questionnaire. American College of Rheumatology criteria. IBS, Irritable bowel syndrome. *(Adapted from Wolfe F, Clauw DJ, Fitzcharles MA, et al. The American College of Rheumatology preliminary diagnostic criteria for fibromyalgia and measurement of symptom severity.* Arthritis Care Res *62:600–610, 2010.)*

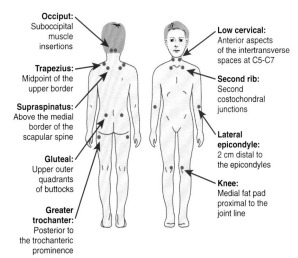

Occiput: Suboccipital muscle insertions

Trapezius: Midpoint of the upper border

Supraspinatus: Above the medial border of the scapular spine

Gluteal: Upper outer quadrants of buttocks

Greater trochanter: Posterior to the trochanteric prominence

Low cervical: Anterior aspects of the intertransverse spaces at C5-C7

Second rib: Second costochondral junctions

Lateral epicondyle: 2 cm distal to the epicondyles

Knee: Medial fat pad proximal to the joint line

Fig. 193.2 Fibromyalgia tender points.

evidence also suggests that up to 50% of patients with fibromyalgia may have a small fiber polyneuropathy (see Chapter 193.2), and that patients with JPFS may also have chronotropic incompetence (inability to increase heart rate commensurate with activity) and autonomic dysfunction at diagnosis. Children and adolescents with fibromyalgia often find themselves in a vicious cycle of pain, where symptoms build on one another and contribute to the onset and maintenance of new symptoms (Fig. 193.3).

JPFS has a chronic course that can detrimentally affect child health and development. Adolescents with JPFS who do not receive treatment or who are inadequately treated may withdraw from school and the social milieu, complicating their transition to adulthood. **Treatment** of JPFS generally follows consensus statements of the American Pain Society. The major goals are to restore function and alleviate pain, as well as improve comorbid mood and sleep disorders. Treatment strategies include parent/child education, pharmacologic interventions, exercise-based interventions, and psychological interventions. Graduated aerobic exercise is the recommended exercise-based intervention, whereas psychological interventions should include training in pain coping skills, stress management skills, emotional support, and sleep hygiene. CBT is particularly effective in reducing symptoms of depression in children and adolescents with JPFS and also helps to reduce functional disability.

Drug therapies, although largely unsuccessful in isolation, may include tricyclic antidepressants (amitriptyline, 10-50 mg orally 30 min before bedtime), selective serotonin reuptake inhibitors (sertraline, 10-20 mg daily), and anticonvulsants. Pregabalin and duloxetine hydrochloride are approved by the U.S. Food and Drug Administration (FDA) for treatment of fibromyalgia in adults (≥18 yr of age). The safety and efficacy of *pregabalin* in adolescents age 12-17 yr was recently demonstrated in a 15 wk randomized controlled trial and 6 mo open-label study. Safety was consistent with that shown in adults, with preliminary evidence for improvement in secondary pain outcomes, impressions of change, and better sleep. *Duloxetine* has not been studied in children with JPFS. Muscle relaxants are generally not used in children because they affect school performance.

Bibliography is available at Expert Consult.

193.4 Complex Regional Pain Syndrome
Kelly K. Anthony and Laura E. Schanberg

Complex regional pain syndrome (CRPS) is characterized by ongoing burning limb pain subsequent to an injury, immobilization, or another noxious event affecting the extremity. **CRPS1**, formerly called *reflex sympathetic dystrophy*, has no evidence of nerve injury, whereas **CRPS2**, formerly called *causalgia*, follows a prior nerve injury. Key associated features are pain disproportionate to the inciting event, persisting **allodynia** (a heightened pain response to normally nonnoxious stimuli), **hyperalgesia** (exaggerated pain reactivity to noxious stimuli), swelling of distal extremities, and indicators of **autonomic dysfunction** (cyanosis, mottling, hyperhidrosis).

There are currently no gold standard diagnostic criteria for pediatric CPRS; although in adults, the **Budapest criteria** have been shown to be more sensitive and specific than previous diagnostic guidelines (Table 193.5). The diagnosis requires an initiating noxious event or immobilization; continued pain, allodynia, and hyperalgesia out of proportion to the inciting event; evidence of edema, skin blood flow abnormalities, or sudomotor activity; and exclusion of other disorders. Associated features include atrophy of hair or nails; altered hair growth; loss of joint mobility; weakness, tremor, dystonia; and sympathetically maintained pain.

Although the majority of pediatric patients with CRPS present with a history of minor trauma or repeated stress injury (e.g., caused by competitive sports), a sizable proportion are unable to identify a precipitating event. Usual age of onset is between 8 and 16 yr, and girls outnumber boys with the disease by as much as 6 : 1. Childhood CRPS differs from the adult form in that lower extremities, rather than upper extremities, are most often affected. The incidence of CRPS in children is unknown, largely because it is often undiagnosed or diagnosed late, with the diagnosis frequently delayed by almost 1 yr. Left untreated, CRPS can have severe consequences for children, including bone demineralization, muscle wasting, and joint contractures.

An evidence-based approach to the **treatment** of CRPS continues to suggest a multistage approach. Aggressive *physical therapy* (PT) should be initiated as soon as the diagnosis is made and CBT added as needed. PT is recommended 3-4 times/wk, and children may need analgesic premedication at the onset, particularly before PT sessions. PT is initially limited to desensitization and then moves to weight-bearing, range-of-motion, and other functional activities. CBT used as an adjunctive

Table 193.5	Budapest Clinical Diagnostic Criteria for Complex Regional Pain Syndrome

All the following criteria must be met:
1. Continuing pain, which is disproportionate to any inciting event
2. Must report at least 1 symptom in each of the following 4 categories:
   - *Sensory*: Hyperesthesia and/or allodynia
   - *Vasomotor*: Temperature asymmetry, skin color changes, and/or skin color asymmetry
   - *Sudomotor/edema*: Edema, sweating changes, and/or sweating asymmetry
   - *Motor/trophic*: Decreased range of motion, motor dysfunction (tremor, weakness, dystonia) and/or trophic changes (hair, nail, skin)
3. Must display at least 1 sign at time of evaluation in ≥2 of the following 4 categories:
   - *Sensory*: Evidence of hyperesthesia (to pin prick) and/or allodynia (to light touch, temperature sensation, deep somatic pressure, and/or joint movement)
   - *Vasomotor*: Evidence of temperature asymmetry (>1°C), skin color changes, and/or skin color asymmetry
   - *Sudomotor/edema*: Edema, sweating changes, and/or sweating asymmetry
   - *Motor/trophic*: Decreased range of motion, motor dysfunction (tremor, weakness, dystonia) and/or trophic changes (hair, nail, skin)
4. There is no other diagnosis that better explains the signs and symptoms.

Adapted from Harden RN, Bruel S, Stanton-Hicks, et al: Proposed new diagnostic criteria for complex regional pain syndrome, Pain Med 8:326–331, 2007.

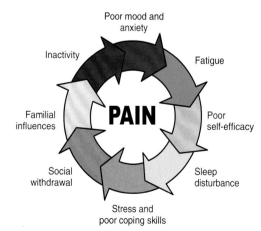

Fig. 193.3 Juvenile primary fibromyalgia syndrome. Vicious cycle promoting symptom maintenance. (*Adapted from Anthony KK, Schanberg LE: Juvenile primary fibromyalgia syndrome, Curr Rheumatol Rep 3:167–171, 2001, Fig. 1.*)

therapy targets psychosocial obstacles to fully participating in PT and provides pain-coping skills training. Sympathetic and epidural *nerve blocks* should be attempted only under the auspices of a pediatric pain specialist. The goal of both pharmacologic and adjunctive treatments for CRPS is to provide sufficient pain relief to allow the child to participate in aggressive physical rehabilitation. If CRPS is identified and treated early, the majority of children and adolescents can be treated successfully with low-dose *amitriptyline* (10-50 mg orally 30 min before bedtime), aggressive PT, and CBT interventions. Opioids and anticonvulsants such as gabapentin can also be helpful. Notably, multiple studies have shown that noninvasive treatments, particularly PT and CBT, are at least as efficacious as nerve blocks in helping children with CRPS achieve resolution of their symptoms.

There is growing evidence that some patients with CRPS I have a small fiber polyneuropathy (see Chapter 193.2).

Bibliography is available at Expert Consult.

193.5 Erythromelalgia

Laura E. Schanberg

Children with **erythromelalgia** experience episodes of intense pain, erythema, and heat in their hands and feet (Fig. 193.4). Less frequently involved are the face, ears, or knees. Symptoms may be triggered by exercise and exposure to heat, lasting for hours and occasionally for days. It is more common in girls and in the teenage years, and diagnosis is often delayed for years. Although most cases are sporadic, an autosomal dominant hereditary form results from mutations of the *SCN9A* gene on chromosome 2q31-32, causing a painful channelopathy. **Secondary** erythromelalgia is associated with an array of disorders, including myeloproliferative diseases, peripheral neuropathy, frostbite, hypertension, and rheumatic disease. Treatment includes avoidance of heat exposure and other precipitating situations and utilization of cooling techniques

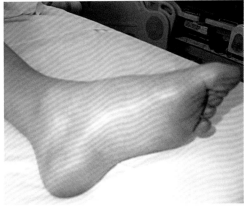

Fig. 193.4 **Erythromelalgia.** Typical redness and edema of the foot. *(From Pfund Z, Stankovics J, Decsi T, Illes Z: Childhood steroid-responsive acute erythromelalgia with axonal neuropathy of large myelinated fibers: a dysimmune neuropathy? Neuromuscul Disord 19:49–52, 2009, Fig 1A, p 50.)*

that do not cause tissue damage during attacks. NSAIDs, narcotics, anesthetic agents (lidocaine patch), anticonvulsants (oxcarbazepine, carbamazepine, gabapentin), and antidepressants, as well as biofeedback and hypnosis, may help manage pain. Drugs acting on the vascular system (aspirin, sodium nitroprusside, magnesium, misoprostol) may also be somewhat effective. However, a reliably efficacious treatment is not available, resulting in substantial negative impact on physical and mental health.

There is growing evidence that some patients with erythromelalgia have a small fiber polyneuropathy (see Chapter 193.2).

Bibliography is available at Expert Consult.

Chapter 194

Miscellaneous Conditions Associated With Arthritis

Angela Byun Robinson and C. Egla Rabinovich

第一百九十四章

与关节炎相关的其他疾病

中文导读

本章主要介绍了复发性多软骨炎、Mucha-Habermann病/急性痘疮样苔藓样糠疹、Sweet综合征/急性发热性中性粒细胞性皮肤病、肥厚性骨关节病、植物刺性滑膜炎、色素沉着绒毛结节性滑膜炎。并具体描述了复发性多软骨炎的临床特点、诊断与鉴别诊断和治疗；描述了急性痘疮样苔藓样糠疹临床特点、流行病学、病理和治疗；描述了Sweet综合征的临床特点、诊断标准和治疗；描述了原发性和继发性肥厚性骨关节病；

描述了植物刺性滑膜炎的临床特点及诊断；描述了色素沉着绒毛结节性滑膜炎组织学特点、诊断和治疗。

RELAPSING POLYCHONDRITIS

Relapsing polychondritis (RP) is a rare condition characterized by episodic chondritis causing cartilage destruction and deformation of the ears (sparing the earlobes), nose, larynx, and tracheobronchial tree. Antibodies to matrillin-1 and collagen (type II, IX and XI) are present in approximately 60% of patients with RP, suggesting an autoimmune pathogenesis. Patients may experience arthritis, uveitis, and hearing loss resulting from inflammation near the auditory and vestibular nerves. Children may initially relate episodes of intense erythema over the outer ears. Other dermatologic manifestations may include erythema nodosum, maculopapular rash, and purpura. Cardiac involvement, including conduction defects and coronary vasculitis, has been reported. Severe, progressive, and potentially fatal disease resulting from destruction of the tracheobronchial tree and airway obstruction is unusual in childhood. **Diagnostic criteria** established for adults are useful guidelines for evaluating children with suggestive symptoms (Table 194.1). The clinical course of RP is variable; flares of disease are often associated with elevations of acute-phase reactants and may remit spontaneously. Although seen more often in the adult population, RP may coexist with other rheumatic disease (e.g., systemic lupus erythematosus, Sjögren syndrome, Henoch-Schönlein purpura) in up to 30% of patients. The differential diagnosis includes **ANCA-associated vasculitis** (granulomatosis with polyangiitis) (see Chapter 192.4) and **Cogan syndrome**, which is characterized by auditory nerve inflammation and keratitis but not chondritis. Many children respond to nonsteroidal antiinflammatory drugs, but some require corticosteroids or other immunosuppressive agents (azathioprine, methotrexate, hydroxychloroquine, colchicine, cyclophosphamide, cyclosporine, and anti–tumor necrosis factor [TNF] agents), as reported in small series and case reports.

MUCHA-HABERMANN DISEASE/PITYRIASIS LICHENOIDES ET VARIOLIFORMIS ACUTA

Pityriasis lichenoides et varioliformis acuta (**PLEVA**) is a benign, self-limited cutaneous vasculitis characterized by episodes of macules, papules, and papulovesicular lesions that can develop central ulceration, necrosis, and crusting (Fig. 194.1). Different stages of development are usually seen at once. **PLEVA fulminans** or febrile ulceronecrotic Mucha-Habermann disease (**FUMHD**) is the severe, life threatening form of PLEVA. Large, coalescing, ulceronecrotic lesions are seen, accompanied by high fever and elevated erythrocyte sedimentation rate (ESR). Systemic manifestations can include interstitial pneumonitis, abdominal pain, malabsorption, arthritis, and neurologic manifestations. PLEVA has a male predominance and occurs more frequently in childhood. The diagnosis is confirmed by biopsy of skin lesions, which reveals perivascular and intramural lymphocytic inflammation affecting capillaries and venules in the upper dermis that may lead to keratinocyte necrosis. When disease is severe, corticosteroids have been used with questionable effect, and methotrexate has been reported to induce rapid remission in resistant cases. Cyclosporine and anti-TNF agents have also been efficacious in case reports.

SWEET SYNDROME

Sweet syndrome, or **acute febrile neutrophilic dermatosis**, is a rare entity in children. It is characterized by fever, elevated neutrophil count, and raised, tender erythematous plaques and nodules over the face, extremities, and trunk. Skin biopsy reveals neutrophilic perivascular infiltration in the upper dermis. Female predominance is seen in the adult population, whereas gender distribution is equal in children. Established criteria are useful for diagnosis (Table 194.2). Children can also have arthritis, sterile osteomyelitis, myositis, and other extracutaneous manifestations. Sweet

Table 194.1	Suggested Criteria for Relapsing Polychondritis*

MAJOR
Typical inflammatory episodes of ear cartilage
Typical inflammatory episodes of nose cartilage
Typical inflammatory episodes of laryngotracheal cartilage

MINOR
Eye inflammation (conjunctivitis, keratitis, episcleritis, uveitis)
Hearing loss
Vestibular dysfunction
Seronegative inflammatory arthritis

*The diagnosis is established by the presence of 2 major or 1 major and 2 minor criteria. Histologic examination of affected cartilage is required when the presentation is atypical.
Data from Michet CJ Jr, McKenna CH, Luthra HS, et al: Relapsing polychondritis: survival and predictive role of early disease manifestations, *Ann Intern Med* 104:74-78, 1986.

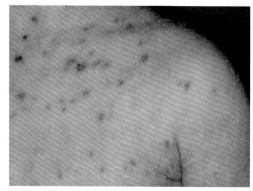

Fig. 194.1 Pityriasis lichenoides et varioliformis acuta (PLEVA). Symmetric, oval and round, reddish brown macular, popular, necrotic, and crusted lesions on chest of 9 yr old boy. (*From Paller AS, Mancini AJ, editors: Hurwitz clinical pediatric dermatology, ed 5, Philadelphia, 2016, Elsevier, Fig 4-33, p 87.*)

syndrome may be idiopathic or secondary to malignancy (particularly acute myelogenous leukemia), drugs (granulocyte colony-stimulating factor, tretinoin or trimethoprim-sulfamethoxazole), or rheumatic diseases (Behçet disease, antiphospholipid antibody syndrome, systemic lupus erythematosus). The condition usually responds to treatment with corticosteroids, treatment of underlying disease, or removal of associated medication.

HYPERTROPHIC OSTEOARTHROPATHY

Children with chronic disease, especially pulmonary or cardiac disease, can demonstrate clubbing of the terminal phalanges and have associated periosteal reaction and arthritis. These findings characterize the classic presentation of hypertrophic osteoarthropathy. HOA can be **primary** (idiopathic) or secondary. Although rare, **secondary** HOA is more common in children and is seen in those with chronic pulmonary disease (cystic fibrosis), congenital heart disease, gastrointestinal disease (malabsorption syndromes, biliary atresia, inflammatory bowel disease), and malignancy (nasopharyngeal sarcoma, osteosarcoma, Hodgkin disease). It may precede diagnosis of cardiopulmonary disease or

Table 194.2	Diagnostic Criteria for Classic Sweet Syndrome*

MAJOR CRITERIA

Abrupt onset of painful erythematous plaques or nodules
Histopathologic evidence of dense neutrophilic infiltrate without evidence of leukocytoclastic vasculitis

MINOR CRITERIA

Pyrexia >38°C
Association with underlying hematologic or visceral malignancy, inflammatory disease or pregnancy, *or* preceded by an upper respiratory or gastrointestinal infection or vaccination
Excellent response to systemic corticosteroids or potassium iodide
Abnormal laboratory values at presentation (3 of 4):
 Erythrocyte sedimentation rate >20 mm/hr
 Positive C-reactive protein test result
 >8,000 leukocytes/mm^3
 >70% neutrophils/mm^3

*The diagnosis is established by the presence of 2 major criteria *plus* 2 of the 4 minor criteria.
 Adapted from Walker DC, Cohen PR: Trimethoprim-sulfamethoxazole-associated acute febrile neutrophilic dermatosis: case report and review of drug induced Sweet's syndrome. *J Am Acad Dermatol* 34:918–923, 1996.

malignancy. The pathogenesis of secondary HOA is unknown; symptoms often improve if the underlying condition is treated successfully. HOA-related pain can be disabling; in adults, management with bisphosphonates has been reported. Evaluation of children presenting with HOA should include a chest radiograph to evaluate for pulmonary disease or intrathoracic mass. Autosomal recessive mutations in prostaglandin pathway genes have recently been described in primary HOA, also described as **pachydermoperiostosis**.

PLANT THORN SYNOVITIS

A diagnosis of plant thorn synovitis should be considered in children with monoarticular arthritis nonresponsive to antiinflammatory therapy. Acute or chronic arthritis can occur after a plant thorn or other foreign object penetrates a joint. Unlike septic arthritis, children with plant thorn synovitis are usually afebrile. The most common organism seen with plant thorn synovitis is *Pantoea agglomerans*, although cultures are often negative. The initial injury may be unknown or forgotten, making diagnosis difficult. Ultrasound or MRI can be useful in identifying the foreign body. Removal of the foreign body using arthroscopy, followed by an antibiotic course, is the accepted therapy.

PIGMENTED VILLONODULAR SYNOVITIS

Proliferation of synovial tissue is seen in pigmented villonodular synovitis (PVNS). This proliferation is localized or diffuse and can affect the joint, tendon sheath, or bursa. Macrophages and multinucleated giant cells with brownish hemosiderin are present histologically. It is unclear if the etiology of PVNS is inflammatory or neoplastic in nature. Although findings are not pathognomonic, MRI with contrast is a useful diagnostic tool by which PVNS can be seen as a mass or bone erosion. Brown or bloody synovial fluid is seen with arthrocentesis, but the diagnosis is made by tissue biopsy. Surgical removal of the affected tissue is the therapeutic modality, and with diffuse disease, a total synovectomy is recommended.

Bibliography is available at Expert Consult.

Infectious Diseases
感染性疾病

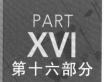

Section 1
General Considerations
第一篇
总论

Chapter **195**
Diagnostic Microbiology
Carey-Ann D. Burnham
and Gregory A. Storch
第一百九十五章
诊断微生物学

中文导读

　　本章主要介绍了标本采集、细菌和真菌感染的实验室诊断、抗生素药敏试验、即时诊断、寄生虫感染实验室检测、血清学诊断和病毒感染的实验室诊断。在细菌和真菌感染的实验室诊断中具体描述了显微镜检查和病原的分离与鉴定。在病毒感染的实验室诊断中详细介绍了样本采集、抗原检测试验、病毒培养和分子诊断。其中，在病原体分离和鉴定中详细阐述了血培养、脑脊液培养、尿培养、生殖道培养、咽喉和呼吸道培养、肠道病原体检测、其他体液和组织培养、筛查培养或监测培养等内容。

Laboratory evidence to support the diagnosis of an infectious disease may be based on one or more of the following: direct examination of specimens using microscopic or antigen detection techniques, isolation of microorganisms in culture, serologic testing, host gene expression patterns, or molecular detection of an organism, resistance determinant, or virulence factor. Some additional roles of the clinical microbiology laboratory include performing antimicrobial susceptibility testing and supporting hospital infection prevention in the detection and characterization of pathogens associated with nosocomial infections.

SPECIMEN COLLECTION
The success of a diagnostic microbiology assay, that is, detection of a pathogen if present, is directly linked to specimen collection techniques. In general, this means collecting the correct specimen type for the disease or condition in question and promptly transporting the specimen to the laboratory for analysis. Although **swab specimens** may be necessary for some conditions, in general a swab is a suboptimal specimen. A swab is only able to hold a very small amount of specimen (approximately 100 μL), and, using a traditional swab, only a small fraction of organisms that are absorbed onto a swab will be released back into the culture. **Flocked swabs** coupled with transport medium improve organism recovery. However, when possible, fluid or tissue should be submitted to the laboratory for analysis. If anaerobic infection is suspected, the sample should be transported in appropriate medium to preserve viability of anaerobic bacteria. For the recovery of some organism types, such as viruses and *Neisseria gonorrhoeae*, specific transport media may be required. Considerations specific to the collection of blood cultures are addressed in the blood culture section.

Table 195.1	Stains Used for Microscopic Examination

TYPE OF STAIN	CLINICAL USE
Gram stain	Stains bacteria (with differentiation of gram-positive and gram-negative organisms), fungi, leukocytes, and epithelial cells.
Potassium hydroxide (KOH)	A 10% solution dissolves cellular and organic debris and facilitates detection of fungal elements in clinical specimens.
Calcofluor white stain	Nonspecific fluorochrome that binds to cellulose and chitin in fungal cell walls, can be combined with 10% KOH to dissolve cellular material.
Ziehl-Neelsen and Kinyoun stains	Acid-fast stains, using basic carbolfuchsin, followed by acid-alcohol decolorization and methylene blue counterstaining. Acid-fast organisms (e.g., *Mycobacterium*) resist decolorization and stain pink. A weaker decolorizing agent is used for partially acid-fast organisms (e.g., *Nocardia, Cryptosporidium, Cyclospora, Isospora*).
Auramine-rhodamine stain	Acid-fast stain using fluorochromes that bind to mycolic acid in mycobacterial cell walls and resist acid-alcohol decolorization; usually performed directly on clinical specimens. Acid-fast organisms stain orange-yellow against a black background.
Acridine orange stain	Fluorescent dye that intercalates into DNA, used to aid in differentiation of organisms from debris during direct specimen examination, and also for detection of organisms that are not visible with Gram stain. Bacteria and fungi stain orange, and background cellular material stains green.
Lugol iodine stain	Added to wet preparations of fecal specimens for ova and parasites to enhance contrast of the internal structures (nuclei, glycogen vacuoles).
Wright and Giemsa stains	Primarily for detecting blood parasites (*Plasmodium, Babesia,* and *Leishmania*), detection of amoeba in preparations of cerebrospinal fluid, and fungi in tissues (yeasts, *Histoplasma*)
Trichrome stain	Stains stool specimens for identification of protozoa.
Direct fluorescent-antibody stain	Used for direct detection of a variety of organisms in clinical specimens by using specific fluorescein-labeled antibodies (e.g., *Pneumocystis jiroveci,* many viruses).

LABORATORY DIAGNOSIS OF BACTERIAL AND FUNGAL INFECTIONS

Although the scope and availability of molecular methods for detection of bacterial and fungal pathogens have increased rapidly, the diagnosis of many of these infections depends on microscopic detection of organisms or cultivation of organisms on **culture media**.

Microscopy

The **Gram stain** is an extremely valuable diagnostic technique to provide rapid and inexpensive information regarding the absence or presence of inflammatory cells and organisms in clinical specimens. For some specimen types, the presence of inflammatory and epithelial cells is used to judge the suitability of a specimen for culture. For example, the presence of >10 epithelial cells per low-power field in a sputum specimen is highly suggestive of a specimen contaminated with oral secretions. In addition, a preliminary assessment of the etiologic agent can be made based on the morphology (e.g., cocci vs rods) and stain reaction (e.g., gram-positive isolates are purple; gram-negative isolates are red) of the microorganisms. However, a negative Gram stain does not rule out infection, since 10^4 to 10^5 microorganisms per milliliter (mL) in the specimen are required for detection by this method.

In addition to the Gram stain, many other stains are used in microbiology, both to detect organisms and to help infer their identity (Table 195.1).

Isolation and Identification

The approach to isolation of microorganisms in a clinical specimen will vary depending on the body site and pathogen suspected. For body sites that are usually sterile, such as cerebrospinal fluid, **nutrient-rich media** such as sheep blood agar and chocolate agar are used to aid in the recovery of fastidious pathogens. In contrast, stool specimens contain abundant amounts of commensal bacteria, and thus to isolate pathogens, selective and differential media must be used. **Selective media** will inhibit the growth of some organisms to aid in isolation of suspect pathogens; **differential media** rely on growth characteristics or carbohydrate assimilation characteristics to impart a growth pattern that differentiates organisms. MacConkey agar supports growth of gram-

negative rods while suppressing gram-positive organisms, and a color change in the media from clear to pink distinguishes lactose-fermenting organisms from other gram-negative rods. Special media, such as Sabouraud dextrose agar and inhibitory mold agar, are used to recover fungi in clinical specimens. Many pathogens, including *Bartonella, Bordetella pertussis, Legionella, Mycoplasma,* some *Vibrio* spp., and certain fungal pathogens such as *Malassezia furfur,* require specialized growth media or incubation conditions. Consultation with the laboratory is advised when these pathogens are suspected.

Once an organism is recovered in culture, additional testing is performed to identify the isolate. Confirmation of microbial identity has classically been performed using tests that rely on the phenotypic properties of an isolate; examples include coagulase activity, carbohydrate assimilation patterns, indole production, and motility. However, phenotypic methods are not able to resolve all organisms to species level, and they require incubation time. In some instances, sequence-based identification may be necessary. For bacteria, this is usually based on sequence analysis of the bacterial 16S rRNA gene. This gene is a molecular chronometer that is highly conserved within a species but variable between species; as such, it is an excellent resource for organism identification.

Matrix-assisted laser desorption-ionization time-of-flight mass spectrometry (**MALDI-TOF MS**) is a rapid and accurate technique that is based on generating a protein fingerprint of an organism and comparing that fingerprint to a library of known organisms to produce an identification. This method can identify bacteria or yeast that have been recovered in culture within minutes, and the consumable costs for these analyses are minimal. However, this methodology currently lacks the ability to resolve polymicrobial samples, and the biomass required for successful MALDI-TOF MS analysis generally precludes analysis directly from clinical specimens.

Blood Culture

The detection of microbes in blood culture specimens of patients with bloodstream infection is one of the most important functions of the clinical microbiology laboratory. Most blood cultures are performed by collecting blood into bottles of nutrient-rich broth to facilitate the growth of bacteria or yeast. Blood cultures are frequently submitted as a set that includes an aerobic and an anaerobic bottle, although in children, especially neonates, typically only an aerobic bottle is used. Some blood culture media contain resins or other agents to help neutralize antibiotics that may be present in the patients' blood. Blood culture bottles are then placed into an automated blood culture incubator that will monitor the blood culture bottle at regular intervals for evidence of growth. Once the instrument detects evidence of microbial growth, an alarm alerts the laboratory. Approximately 80% of blood cultures that will ultimately be positive are identified within the 1st 24 hr of incubation. A portion of broth from a blood culture bottle that has signaled positive is then gram-stained and subsequently inoculated onto appropriate growth media so that the organism can be isolated and identified. Numerous preanalytical variables can influence the accuracy of blood culture results. To facilitate accurate interpretation of a positive blood culture, a minimum of 2 blood cultures drawn from different sites should be collected whenever possible. Growth of an organism that is part of the normal skin flora from a single blood culture raises concern that the isolate resulted from contamination of the culture.

To maximize detection of bloodstream infection, up to 4 blood cultures should be collected over 24 hr. Proper skin antisepsis is essential before blood collection. Chlorhexidine is frequently used for this purpose, but alcohol is also used. If blood is collected through an indwelling line, proper antisepsis before collection is also important. The practice of obtaining blood for culture from intravascular catheters without accompanying peripheral venous blood cultures should be discouraged, because it is difficult to determine the significance of coagulase-negative staphylococci and other skin flora or environmental organisms isolated from blood obtained from line cultures. Differential time to positivity of 2 hr or more between paired blood cultures drawn simultaneously from a catheter and peripheral vein has been cited as an indicator of catheter-related bloodstream infection.

The volume of blood collected is also an important factor in the recovery of bloodstream pathogens, especially as the number of organisms per milliliter of blood in sepsis may be low (<10 colony-forming units/mL). The optimal amount of blood to collect from a pediatric patient varies depending on the weight of the child. The **Clinical and Laboratory Standards Institute** (CLSI) and Cumitech provide guidance on the amount of blood that is safe to collect from children of different sizes. For children from 3 to <12 kg, 3-5 mL is suggested; from 12 to <36 kg, 5-10 mL; from 36-50 kg, 10-15 mL, and >50 kg, 20 mL.

A number of **rapid diagnostic assays** can be performed directly on positive blood culture broth to identify pathogens frequently associated with bacteremia and some antimicrobial resistance determinants. Most of these rapid diagnostic assays are based on nucleic acid detection techniques. For example, the Verigene system can identify staphylococcal, streptococcal, and enterococcal species, as well as *mecA* and *vanA* genes, in positive blood culture broth in approximately 2 hr using the gram-positive blood culture panel. After specimen preparation to concentrate microorganisms and remove residual broth and blood from the blood culture specimen, MALDI-TOF MS can also be performed on blood culture broth that is positive for growth of microorganisms. These assays can help shorten the interval between a positive blood culture and definitive organism identification, with the goal of early optimization of antimicrobial therapy.

Detection of mycobacteria and some filamentous fungi (e.g., *Histoplasma capsulatum*) from the bloodstream is maximized using lysis-centrifugation techniques, such as the Isolator system (Wampole, Cranbury, NJ).

Cerebrospinal Fluid Culture

Cerebrospinal fluid (CSF) should be transported quickly to the laboratory and then cytocentrifuged to concentrate organisms for microscopic examination. CSF is routinely cultured on blood agar and chocolate agar, which support the growth of common pathogens causing meningitis. If tuberculosis is suspected, cultures for mycobacteria should be specifically requested. Culture of larger volumes of CSF (>10 mL) significantly improves yield of mycobacteria.

Historically, rapid antigen detection tests for bacterial pathogens such as *Haemophilus influenzae* type b and *Streptococcus pneumoniae* were used to attempt to detect organisms in CSF without the need for culture. These techniques lack sensitivity and in some cases specificity. A cytospin Gram stain is as sensitive as bacterial antigen tests for detection of microorganisms in CSF. In contrast, the cryptococcal antigen test can be useful when cryptococcal meningitis is suspected. Historically, India ink preparations were used to detect *Cryptococcus* in CSF, but this method is insensitive compared with the antigen detection assay.

In the postvaccine era, the epidemiology of infectious meningitis is rapidly changing, and acute bacterial meningitis is now a relatively infrequent event in North America. Many CSF infections are associated with shunts or other hardware, and *Propionibacterium* and coagulase-negative staphylococci are the organisms most frequently isolated from shunt infections. The laboratory should include media to facilitate the growth of *Propionibacterium* in CSF specimens received from neurosurgery patients.

Urine Culture

Urine for culture (including colony count) can be obtained by collecting clean-voided midstream specimens, by catheterization, or by suprapubic aspiration. Urine samples collected by placing bags on the perineum are unacceptable for culture because samples are often contaminated. Rapid transport of unpreserved urine to the laboratory (<2 hr) is imperative, and delay in transport or plating of specimens renders colony counts unreliable. Refrigeration or urine transport devices with boric acid preservative may be used when delay is unavoidable.

The specific colony counts used to define growth in a urine culture as *significant* are somewhat controversial and vary by laboratory. Urine obtained by suprapubic aspirate is normally sterile, and thus any organism growth is typically considered significant. Urine collected by catheterization is likely to reflect infection if there are $\geq 10^3$ to 10^4 organisms/mL. In general, clean-voided urine is considered abnormal if $\geq 10^4$ to 10^5 organisms/mL are present, although culture interpretation can be variable depending on the patient's age and the clinical setting.

Genital Culture

Neisseria gonorrhoeae is a fragile organism, and collection and transport in special medium are essential for efficient recovery. Selective agar, such as modified Thayer-Martin medium, should be used to enhance recovery of *N. gonorrhoeae* in clinical specimens, such as genital, anorectal, and pharyngeal swabs. Antimicrobial resistance is increasing in *N. gonorrhoeae* and is cited as an Urgent Threat by the U.S. Centers for Disease Control and Prevention (CDC), although few clinical laboratories have the ability to perform antimicrobial susceptibility testing for this organism. In pediatric patients, the identification of an organism as *N. gonorrhoeae* should be confirmed using 2 independent methods.

Specimens for **Chlamydia trachomatis** culture are obtained by cotton-tipped, aluminum-shafted urethral swabs. Endocervical specimens, using swabs with aluminum or plastic shafts, should be collected by rubbing the swab vigorously against the endocervical wall to obtain as much cellular material as possible. *C. trachomatis* is an obligate intracellular organism and is cultured by inoculation into cell culture systems, followed by immunofluorescent staining with monoclonal antibody against the organism. Nonculture methods such as DNA amplification methods are widely used and are more cost-effective than culture.

Although **nucleic acid amplification test (NAAT)** assays for *N. gonorrhoeae* and *C. trachomatis* are not approved by the U.S. Food and Drug Administration (FDA) for use in children, these assays are frequently used in this population to detect these organisms in urine specimens, endocervical and vaginal swabs, and penile swabs. The NAAT assays exhibit superior sensitivity compared to culture-based techniques. Some laboratories take the approach of confirming all NAAT-positive specimens with an alternative NAAT test that detects an alternative genetic target.

Throat and Respiratory Culture

Streptococcal pharyngitis and tonsillitis is a common diagnosis in pediatric patients; vigorous swabbing of the tonsillar area and posterior pharynx can be done to obtain a specimen for detection of group A streptococcus *(Streptococcus pyogenes)*. Rapid antigen detection assays or rapid nucleic acid detection assays are frequently used when group A streptococcus pharyngitis is suspected. Negative rapid antigen assays should be confirmed using culture-based techniques. Rapid NAAT assays for detection of group A streptococcus are also being used with increasing frequency. These assays have increased sensitivity, but clinical experience with them is still limited and there are not yet recommendations regarding whether backup culture is required. Most laboratories screen throat cultures exclusively for the presence of group A streptococci. However, large colony variants of group C and group G streptococci *(Streptococcus dysgalactiae)* have also been associated with pharyngitis but are not associated with the same postinfectious sequelae attributed to group A streptococcus; laboratory practices for detecting and reporting group C and group G streptococci are variable and an area of controversy.

In addition to the detection of pathogenic streptococci, the clinical laboratory may query for diphtheria, gonococcal pharyngitis, or infection with *Arcanobacterium haemolyticum* in pharyngeal specimens. The laboratory should be notified if any of these pathogens is suspected, to ensure that appropriate methods are used to recover these organisms if present.

Cultures for *Bordetella pertussis* can be obtained by aspiration or swabbing of the nasopharynx using a Dacron or calcium alginate swab. The aspirate or swab is inoculated onto special charcoal-blood (Regan-Lowe) or Bordet-Gengou media, although molecular assays are now frequently used for detection of *B. pertussis* in these specimens.

The cause of lower respiratory tract disease in children is frequently difficult to confirm microbiologically because of the challenge of obtaining adequate sputum specimens. Gram-stained smears of specimens should be performed to assess the adequacy of sputum samples; specimens with large numbers of epithelial cells (>10 per high-power field) or with few neutrophils are unsuitable for culture, because correlation is lacking between upper respiratory tract flora and organisms causing lower respiratory tract disease. For patients with **cystic fibrosis**, special media should be used to detect pathogens important in cystic fibrosis, such as *Burkholderia cepacia* complex.

Endotracheal aspirates from intubated patients may be useful if the Gram stain shows abundant neutrophils and bacteria, although pathogens recovered from such specimens might still reflect only contamination from the endotracheal tube or upper airway. Quantitative cultures of bronchoalveolar lavage fluid may be valuable for distinguishing upper respiratory tract contamination from lower respiratory disease.

If infection with *Legionella* is suspected, the laboratory should be alerted so that the specimen can be inoculated to special media (e.g., buffered charcoal–yeast extract agar) to facilitate the recovery of this pathogen. The *Legionella* urinary antigen test is a noninvasive, sensitive and specific method for rapid detection of *L. pneumophila* serogroup 1.

The diagnosis of pulmonary **tuberculosis** in young children is best made by culture of early-morning gastric aspirates, obtained on 3 consecutive days. Sputum induction for obtaining specimens for mycobacterial culture has also proved useful in young children but requires skilled personnel and containment facilities to prevent exposure of healthcare workers. Cultures for *Mycobacterium tuberculosis* should be processed only in laboratories equipped with appropriate biologic safety cabinets and containment facilities. NAATs for detection of *M. tuberculosis* in respiratory specimens (e.g., Cepheid Xpert MTB assay) are becoming widely available and have very high sensitivity when performed on smear-positive sputum specimens.

Detection of Enteric Pathogens

In pediatric patients with diarrheal illnesses, culture of stool for enteric pathogens may be requested. A fresh stool specimen is preferred but is not always possible to obtain. If there is an unavoidable delay in specimen transport, the specimens should be placed in an appropriate transport medium, such as Cary-Blair. Rectal swabs for enteric culture are also acceptable specimens if the swab is visibly soiled. In general, enteric cultures should be performed on specimens from outpatients or patients who have been hospitalized for <3 days, since nosocomial acquisition of an enteric pathogen is extremely uncommon.

Stool specimens are typically plated on a series of selective and differential media to decrease the overgrowth of normal flora and recover pathogenic organisms if present. The specific pathogens queried vary by laboratory. Most laboratories in North America will routinely culture for *Salmonella, Shigella, Campylobacter,* and Shiga toxin–producing strains of *Escherichia coli*. The CDC recommends that all laboratories use an agar-based medium for recovery of *E. coli* O157 in addition to an assay for detection of Shiga toxin production (e.g., immunoassay to detect Shiga toxin(s), nucleic acid detection assay for stx1/stx2). Practices surrounding the routine culture for *Yersinia enterocolitica, Vibrio cholerae, Edwardsiella, Aeromonas,* and *Plesiomonas* will vary with local epidemiology, and the laboratory should always be notified if one of these pathogens is specifically suspected.

Clostridium difficile is an important cause of antibiotic-associated diarrhea. *C. difficile* was long characterized as a nosocomial pathogen of older adults, but community-associated disease is emerging, and the incidence and severity of *C. difficile* infection in children are increasing. The optimal method for detection of *C. difficile* in fecal specimens is highly controversial; in general, however, detection of *C. difficile* toxin in fecal specimens has higher clinical specificity than toxigenic culture or nucleic acid detection methods. Testing for *C. difficile* in children <1 yr old should be discouraged because of the high incidence of colonization in this patient population.

Viruses are an important cause of **gastroenteritis** in pediatric patients. Methods for viral detection will vary but may include antigen detection (e.g., for rotavirus or adenovirus 40/41) or nucleic acid detection methods (e.g., for norovirus). In North America the burden of *parasitic* gastroenteritis is low. Complete microscopic exams for ova and parasite detection in stool samples is usually of low yield, and antigen detection assays for *Cryptosporidium* and *Giardia*, the most commonly encountered agents, are a sensitive and cost-effective method for detection of these pathogens.

Multiplex nucleic acid detection tests for simultaneous detection of a dozen or more enteric pathogens, including bacteria, viruses, and parasites, have been FDA-cleared and are available for clinical use. The deployment of these assays in clinical laboratories is variable, and the results of this testing can be difficult to interpret, especially when multiple targets are detected in a specimen (e.g., co-detection of *C. difficile* and an enteric bacterial pathogen in a young child).Culture-independent diagnostics may also challenge the public health response if bacterial isolates are not available for epidemiologic analysis. Although these assays have great promise to expedite the detection of the causative agent of diarrhea in children, laboratories and clinicians are still in the learning phase of how best to deploy this testing.

Culture of Other Fluids and Tissues

Abscesses, wounds, pleural fluid, peritoneal fluid, joint fluid, and other purulent fluids are cultured onto solid agar and, in some cases, broth media. Whenever possible, fluid and/or tissue rather than swabs from infected sites should be sent to the laboratory, because culture of a larger volume of fluid can detect organisms present in low concentration. **Anaerobic** organisms are involved in many abdominal and wound abscesses. These specimens should be collected and transported to the laboratory rapidly in anaerobic transport medium.

Although *Staphylococcus aureus* is the most common cause of bone and joint infections, *Kingella kingae* is an important cause of **septic arthritis** in children, especially in children <4 yr old. The detection of *K. kingae* is maximized by inoculation of synovial fluid into blood culture broth in addition to plating on solid medium. A number of studies suggest that molecular detection of *K. kingae* in specimens from young patients with suspected septic arthritis may be the most sensitive way to make this diagnosis.

Screening/Surveillance Cultures

Clinical laboratories may perform surveillance cultures for specific pathogens either to assist infection control in identifying patients requiring contact isolation or for outbreak investigation. Screening cultures for detection of methicillin-resistant *S. aureus* in the anterior nares or vancomycin-resistant enterococci in fecal specimens or rectal swabs may be routinely performed in certain patient populations. In addition, hospitals with carbapenem-resistant *Enterobacteriaceae* or a high prevalence of extended-spectrum β-lactamase–producing *Enterobacteriaceae* (ESBLs) may screen patients for fecal carriage of these organisms. Chromogenic media are frequently used for this purpose. These media contain proprietary compounds to select for the resistant organisms and result in growth of colored colonies to assist in the identification of the microbe of interest.

ANTIMICROBIAL SUSCEPTIBILITY TESTING

Antimicrobial susceptibility tests are generally performed on organisms of clinical significance for which standards and interpretive criteria for susceptibility testing exist. In North America, most laboratories use commercial, automated systems for susceptibility testing. The output from these systems is a *minimum inhibitory concentration* (MIC) value and interpretation of that value as susceptible, intermediate, or resistant. The next most common technique is Kirby-Bauer **disk diffusion**, in which a standardized inoculum of the organism is seeded onto an agar plate. Antibiotic-impregnated filter paper disks are then placed on the agar surface. After overnight incubation, the zone of inhibition of bacterial growth around each disk is measured and compared with nationally determined standards for susceptibility or resistance.

A less common technique is **broth or microbroth dilution** testing. A standard concentration of a microorganism is inoculated into serially diluted concentrations of antibiotic, and the MIC in μg/mL, the lowest concentration of antibiotic required to inhibit growth of the microorganism, is determined. The **gradient diffusion** method such as E-test is a hybrid of disk diffusion and broth dilution and can be used to determine the MIC of individual antibiotics on an agar plate. It uses a paper strip impregnated with a known continuous concentration gradient of antibiotic that diffuses across the agar surface, inhibiting microbial growth in an elliptical zone. The MIC is read off the printed strip at the point at which the zone intersects the strip. Major advantages of the gradient diffusion method are reliable interpretation, reproducibility, and applicability to organisms that require special media or growth conditions.

In addition to providing data to guide the treatment of individual patients, laboratories use aggregate susceptibility testing data to generate institution-specific **antibiogram** reports. These reports summarize susceptibility trends for common organisms and can be used to guide empirical therapy before the availability of specific susceptibility testing results.

Antimicrobial susceptibility patterns are rapidly changing as microbes evolve new resistance mechanisms. Recommendations for performance standards for antimicrobial susceptibility tests and their interpretation are regularly updated by groups such as the CLSI and **European Committee on Antimicrobial Susceptibility Testing** (EUCAST).

Fungal Cultures

Special growth media is used to recover fungi, both yeasts and molds, in clinical specimens. Since most fungi prefer reduced growth temperatures and some species grow slowly, fungal cultures are incubated at 30°C (86°F) for 4 wk. All manipulations of filamentous fungi should take place in the biologic safety cabinet to avoid infecting laboratory personnel and prevent laboratory contamination.

Most yeasts are identified using methods similar to those used for bacteria. In contrast, the standard of care for identification of filamentous fungi has not changed in nearly a century. The laboratory takes into consideration the growth rate, color, and colony characteristics of an isolate and then prepares the specimen in lactophenol alanine blue for microscopic evaluation. These features in aggregate are used to identify the isolate. In some cases, DNA sequencing is used for fungal identification, and MALDI-TOF MS is also emerging for identification of filamentous fungi. Antigen detection assays are also available for some fungal pathogens such as *Cryptococcus neoformans* and *Histoplasma capsulatum*. Assays to detect galactomannan, a molecule found in the cell wall of *Aspergillus* (in addition to some other filamentous fungi), are commercially available and increasingly used to assist in making the diagnosis of invasive aspergillosis in immunocompromised populations.

POINT-OF-CARE DIAGNOSTICS

Some assays to detect infections may be performed in the office setting, provided the site is certified as meeting appropriate quality assurance standards specified by the **Clinical Laboratory Improvement Amendments** (CLIA) of 1988. These include procedures listed under the category of *provider-performed microscopy* such as wet mounts, potassium hydroxide preparations, pinworm examinations, and urinalysis.

Many pediatric offices perform rapid antigen and CLIA-waived nucleic acid detection assays for detection of group A streptococcal pharyngitis and common respiratory viruses such as influenza. The sensitivity of point-of-care testing depends on specimen collection technique, the type of kit used, and the concentration of target analyte present in the sample. In addition, some antigen detection assays for influenza lack sensitivity. Providers using point-of-care diagnostics should familiarize themselves with the analytical performance characteristics of these tests and seek alternative testing methods when clinically indicated.

Office laboratories licensed to perform waived tests are limited to performing these tests and avoid having to undergo inspections and proficiency testing, although they are still subject to CLIA certification requirements specific to these tests. Gram staining, culture inoculation, and isolation of bacteria are considered moderately to highly complex tests under CLIA specifications. Any office laboratory performing Gram stains or cultures must comply with the same requirements and inspections for quality assurance, proficiency testing, and personnel requirements as fully licensed microbiology laboratories.

LABORATORY DETECTION OF PARASITIC INFECTIONS

Most parasites are detected by microscopic examination of clinical specimens. *Plasmodium* and *Babesia* can be detected in stained blood smears, *Leishmania* can be detected in stained bone marrow smears, and helminth eggs, *Entamoeba histolytica,* and *Giardia lamblia* can be detected in stained fecal smears (see Table 195.1). Serologic tests are important in documenting exposure to certain parasites that are not typically found in stool or blood, and thus are difficult to demonstrate in clinical specimens, such as *Trichinella.*

Pinworm is a relatively common parasitic infection in pediatric patients. A diagnosis of pinworm can be made by evaluating a pinworm prep. The best time to obtain this specimen is first thing in the morning, before the patient has bathed or had a bowel movement. A piece of clear tape is pressed onto the perianal region of the patient and then applied to a clear microscope slide. The slide is examined for recovery of pinworm eggs or worms.

Fecal specimens should not be contaminated with water or urine, because water can contain free-living organisms that can be confused with human parasites, and urine can destroy motile organisms. Mineral oil, barium, and bismuth interfere with the detection of parasites, and specimen collection should be delayed for 7-10 days after ingestion of these substances. Because *Giardia* and many worm eggs are shed intermittently into feces, a minimum of 3 specimens on nonconsecutive days are recommended to exclude the diagnosis of an enteric parasite. Because many protozoan parasites are easily destroyed, collection kits with appropriate stool preservatives should be used if a delay is anticipated between time of specimen collection and transport to the laboratory.

Ova and parasite examination of fecal specimens includes a wet mount (to detect motile organisms if fresh stool is received), concentration (to improve yield), and permanent staining (e.g., trichrome) for microscopic examination. *Cryptosporidium, Cyclospora,* and *Isospora* are detected by modified acid-fast stain, and microsporidia are detected by a modification of the trichrome stain. In addition, *Cyclospora* and *Isospora* autofluoresce under ultraviolet (UV) microscopy. The laboratory should be alerted if these parasites are suspected. Detection of certain intestinal parasites, especially *Giardia* and *Cryptosporidium,* can be simplified by using antigen detection tests (immunoassays or direct fluorescent-antibody assays). In addition, *Giardia* and/or *Cryptosporidium* spp. may be targets included on multiplex molecular panels for detection of pathogens causing diarrhea.

Amebic encephalitis, caused by *Acanthamoeba*, *Balamuthia*, or *Naegleria*, is a rare but devastating and rapidly progressive disease. Special laboratory stains and procedures are required to detect these organisms. The laboratory should be notified if this infection is suspected.

Rapid antigen detection tests for *Plasmodium* spp. are available. The sensitivity and specificity of these tests vary depending on the burden of parasite in the sample and the specific *Plasmodium* species. In general, these tests are most sensitive for detecting *P. falciparum* and least sensitive for detecting *P. malariae*. These tests are particularly useful for laboratories lacking personnel trained in evaluation of thick and thin smears for malaria, or to provide a rapid preliminary result while awaiting microscopy. All positive and negative rapid malaria assays should be confirmed with blood smear analysis.

Trichomonas vaginalis is a sexually transmitted protozoan parasite that can also be transmitted on household fomites. Infected individuals may be asymptomatic or may have mild inflammation or severe inflammation and discomfort. *Trichomonas* may be detected using a wet mount, but this method is insensitive. Rapid antigen assays and culture-based methods are available. NAATs are a rapid and sensitive way to detect *Trichomonas*.

SEROLOGIC DIAGNOSIS

Serologic tests are primarily used in the diagnosis of infectious agents that are difficult to culture in vitro or detect by direct examination, such as *Bartonella*, *Francisella*, *Legionella*, *Borrelia* (Lyme disease), *Treponema pallidum*, *Mycoplasma*, *Rickettsia*, some viruses (HIV, Epstein-Barr, hepatitis A), and some parasites (*Toxoplasma*, *Trichinella*).

Antibody tests may be specific for immunoglobulin (Ig) G or IgM or can measure antibody response regardless of immunoglobulin class. In very general terms, the IgM response occurs earlier in the illness, generally peaking at 7-10 days after infection, and usually disappears within a few weeks, but for some infections (e.g., hepatitis A, West Nile) it can persist for months. The IgG response peaks at 4-6 wk and often persists for life. Because the IgM response is transient, the presence of IgM antibody in most cases correlates with recent infection. Methods for IgM antibody detection are difficult to standardize, however, and false-positive results typically occur with some IgM assays. The presence of IgG antibody can indicate new seroconversion or past exposure to the pathogen. To confirm a new infection using IgG testing, it is essential to demonstrate either seroconversion or a rising IgG titer. A 4-fold increase in a convalescent titer obtained 3-4 wk after the acute titer is considered diagnostic in most situations. In neonates, interpretation of serologic tests is difficult because of passive transfer of maternal IgG that can persist for 6-18 mo after birth.

Context is extremely important in the interpretation of serologic findings. Important considerations are the ability of the host to mount an immune response, the background rate of seropositivity (especially for IgG detection assays), and for some diseases the antibody titer. In addition, interpretation of some serologic assays, such as those used to diagnose **Lyme disease**, are problematic because of lack of specificity of the immunoassays. A confirmatory immunoblot (Western blot) is required for all positive and equivocal enzyme immunoassay (EIA) results for Lyme disease.

LABORATORY DIAGNOSIS OF VIRAL INFECTIONS

Viral diseases are extremely important in pediatrics, and **diagnostic virology** has long been important to pediatric practice, especially in the inpatient setting.

Specimens

Specimens for viral diagnosis are selected on the basis of knowledge of the site that is most likely to yield the suspected pathogen. When evaluating patients with acute viral infections, specimens should be collected early in the course of infection, when viral shedding tends to be maximal. Swabs should be rubbed vigorously against mucosal or skin surfaces to obtain as much cellular material as possible and sent in viral transport media that contain antibiotics to inhibit bacterial growth. Rectal swabs should contain visible fecal material. Flocked swabs have been shown to provide more material for the laboratory with consequent improvement in the performance of diagnostic tests. Fluids and respiratory secretions should be collected in sterile containers and promptly delivered to the laboratory. All specimens should be transported on ice if delay is anticipated. Freezing specimens, especially at −20°C (−4°F), can result in a significant decrease in culture sensitivity. Consultation with the laboratory is recommended, because some commercial diagnostic test kits used by laboratories may require specific collection devices.

Laboratory diagnosis of viral infections may be by electron microscopy, antigen detection, virus isolation in culture, serologic testing, or molecular techniques to detect viral nucleic acids. In the past few years, **molecular tests** have emerged as the primary means for detecting viral infections, with some virology laboratories abandoning the use of viral culture altogether. An exciting development is the availability of FDA-cleared multiplex assays that simultaneously detect multiple viruses as well as nonviral agents. Serologic testing still has an important role, especially for arboviral infections such as West Nile, Zika, chikungunya, and dengue; acute Epstein-Barr virus (EBV) infections; HIV; hepatitis A to E, and diseases of childhood such as measles, rubella, and mumps. Serology is also uniquely useful for defining immunity to specific viral infections.

Antigen Detection Tests

Immunofluorescent antibody (IFA) techniques or other methods, such as EIA, were the mainstay of the diagnosis of respiratory viral infections but are now being replaced by molecular tests. IFA assays of cellular material from respiratory secretions can identify the antigens of respiratory syncytial virus (RSV), adenovirus, influenza A and B viruses, parainfluenza virus types 1-3, and human metapneumovirus within 2-3 hr after the specimen is received. The sensitivity of IFA staining for RSV exceeds that of culture in many laboratories but is less than that of molecular tests. Sensitive IFA staining techniques are also commercially available for identifying varicella-zoster virus and herpes simplex virus. A method for detecting cytomegalovirus (CMV) pp65 antigen in blood of immunocompromised patients is also available but has been largely replaced by molecular testing. IFA is not useful for detecting viruses in specimens that do not contain an adequate number of infected cells.

Rapid antigen tests are usually based on lateral flow immunochromatography (similar to rapid tests for group A streptococcus) and have been approved by the FDA for detection of influenza A and B and RSV. Recent modifications that increase sensitivity include fluorescent labels and instrumented readers. Some rapid antigen tests have waived status under CLIA, meaning that they can be performed by personnel who are not trained laboratory technologists, with relatively little formal quality control other than controls that are incorporated into the test devices. Some require only 10 min to perform. Consequently, these tests can be performed in a physician's office or an emergency department. Sensitivity in children is 50–80%, generally higher for children than for adults. Rapid antigen tests can be useful in managing patients with acute respiratory infections, provided the caregiver keeps in mind that a negative test does not rule out the diagnosis of influenza or RSV. Positive tests that are properly read tend to be reliable, but the presence of a virus such as influenza or RSV does not rule out the presence of concomitant bacterial infection.

In addition to their role in respiratory virus infections, antigen detection EIA tests are often used for the diagnosis of viruses that are difficult to culture, such as rotavirus, enteric adenovirus, and hepatitis B virus. The detection of the p24 antigen of HIV along with HIV antibodies is included in fourth-generation EIA tests used in the diagnostic algorithm for HIV.

Viral Culture

Viruses require living cells for propagation; the cells used most often are human- or animal-derived tissue culture monolayers, such as human embryonic lung fibroblasts or monkey kidney cells. Historically, in vivo methods such as inoculation of suckling mice were also used but are rarely used today. Viral growth in susceptible cell culture is usually accomplished by detecting characteristic cytopathic effect that is visible by light microscopy under low magnification in the cultured cells. The most reliable confirmatory method for viral detection in cell culture involves fluorescein- or enzyme-labeled monoclonal antibody staining of infected cell monolayers. An important technical improvement in respiratory viral cultures is the development of cell culture systems that include more than 1 type of cell (R-Mix, Diagnostic Hybrids/Quidel, San Diego, CA) and employ IFA staining for virus detection. This system provides results in 16-40 hr from the time the specimen is received in the laboratory, compared to 2-10 days for conventional cultures. Cell culture methods are now being steadily replaced by molecular tests, which are faster, may be more sensitive, and have the potential to detect viruses that do not grow readily in cell cultures.

Molecular Diagnostics

Molecular tests to detect viruses use the polymerase chain reaction (PCR) and other comparable nucleic acid amplification methods. FDA-cleared multiplex tests have become available for the diagnosis of respiratory, gastrointestinal, and central nervous system (CNS) infections. Some of these tests detect 20 or more different agents at the same time and may require only about 65 min to perform. The infectious agents detected by multiplex panels may include bacteria, fungi, and parasites as well as viruses (Table 195.2).

Herpes simplex virus (HSV) PCR of CSF was the first PCR-based test to become widely accepted dating to the mid-1990s. The first FDA-cleared test for this purpose was approved in 2014. Some laboratories still use laboratory-developed tests for which performance characteristics must be validated as specified by CLIA, resulting in testing that is not standardized and performance characteristics (sensitivity, specificity) that may vary from laboratory to laboratory. Well-performing CSF PCR assays for HSV have sensitivity and specificity exceeding 95% for the diagnosis of HSV encephalitis. PCR is also increasingly used to diagnose mucocutaneous HSV and varicella-zoster virus infections. Molecular testing is more sensitive than virus culture and provides a more rapid turnaround time. Because molecular tests detect nonviable as well as

viable virus, they may detect virus from the healing phase of the illness, when cultures would be negative.

An FDA-cleared test for enterovirus in CSF (GeneXpert, Cepheid, Sunnyvale, CA) provides sensitive detection of enteroviruses in approximately 3 hr. Because this testing is simple, some hospital laboratories are able to perform testing around the clock, thus maximizing the clinical utility of the test. The **parechoviruses**, which may cause illnesses similar to those caused by enteroviruses, especially in infants <6 mo of age, must be detected by separate molecular assays.

Respiratory viruses detected by multiplex panels include influenza A and B, RSV, parainfluenza 1-4, human metapneumovirus, rhinovirus/ enterovirus, coronaviruses OC43, 229E, NL63, and HKU1, and adenoviruses (Table 195.2). The specific viruses (and nonviral agents) included differ among tests produced by different manufacturers. In addition, rapid CLIA-waived molecular tests are available for the simultaneous detection of influenza A and B and the trio of influenza A/B and RSV. These tests are similar to cleared CLIA-waived molecular tests for group A streptococcus and have the potential to make sensitive molecular diagnosis available in emergency departments, urgent care centers, and physician offices. Molecular tests are more expensive than antigen-based tests, and studies of clinical utility and cost-effectiveness are not yet available.

Gastrointestinal multiplex panels recently FDA-approved may include tests for group A rotaviruses, noroviruses GI and GII, enteric adenoviruses (group F, serotypes 40 and 41), astrovirus, and sapovirus, but not all are included in each manufacturer's test. Tests for bacterial and parasitic causes are also included. For clinicians, these tests provide information about the presence of potential etiologic agents not previously available. Numerous questions arise about whether detected pathogens are actually clinically significant and how to sort out the detection of >1 pathogen in the same sample. For laboratories, these tests raise questions about whether they can replace previously used techniques such as bacterial culture. The clinical utility and cost-effectiveness of using these tests have not been determined.

A multiplex panel for viral and bacterial and 1 fungal agent of CNS infection was cleared by the FDA. This test provides information about

Table 195.2	Multiplex Molecular Assays for Viral Diagnosis

TEST	MANUFACTURER	PATHOGENS DETECTED*
RESPIRATORY		
NxTag	Luminex, Austin, TX	Flu A, AH1, AH3, Flu B, RSV A/B, PIV 1-4, HMPV, RV/EV,[†] HCoV OC43/229E/NL63/HKU1, AdV, human bocavirus, *Mycoplasma pneumoniae, Chlamydophila pneumoniae*
Verigene	Luminex, Austin, TX	Flu A, AH1, AH3, Flu B, RSV A/B, PIV 1-4, HMPV, RV, AdV, *Bordetella pertussis, B. parapertussis/ bronchiseptica, B. holmesii*
FilmArray	BioFire, Salt Lake City, UT	Flu A, AH1, AH1(2009), AH3, Flu B, RSV, PIV 1-4, HMPV, RV/EV,[†] CoV OC43/229E/ NL63/HKU1, AdV, *Mycoplasma pneumoniae, Chlamydophila pneumoniae, Bordetella pertussis*
ePlex	GenMark	Flu A, AH1, AH1(2009), AH3, Flu B, RSV, PIV 1-4, HMPV, RV, AdV B/C/E
GASTROINTESTINAL		
NxTag	Luminex, Austin, TX	Rotavirus A, norovirus GI/GII, AdV 40/41, *Campylobacter, Clostridium difficile* toxin A/B, *Escherichia coli* O157, enterotoxigenic *E. coli*, LT/ST, Shiga-like toxin–producing *E. coli* (stx1/2), *Salmonella, Shigella, Vibrio cholerae, Yersinia enterocolitica, Cryptosporidium, Entamoeba histolytica, Giardia*
Verigene	Luminex, Austin, TX	Rotavirus, norovirus, *Campylobacter, Salmonella, Shigella, Vibrio, Yersinia,* stx1/2
FilmArray	BioFire, Salt Lake City, UT	Rotavirus A, norovirus GI/GII, AdV 40/41, astrovirus, sapovirus I, II, IV, V, *Campylobacter, C. difficile* toxin A/B, *Plesiomonas shigelloides, Salmonella, Y. enterocolitica, Vibrio,* enteroaggregative *E. coli,* enteropathogenic *E. coli,* enterotoxigenic *E. coli,* Shiga-like toxin–producing *E. coli* (stx1/2)/*E. coli* O157, *Shigella*/enteroinvasive *E. coli, Cryptosporidium, Cyclospora cayetanensis, E. histolytica, Giardia lamblia*
CENTRAL NERVOUS SYSTEM		
FilmArray	BioFire, Salt Lake City, UT	HSV-1, HSV-2, VZV, CMV, HHV-6, enterovirus, parechovirus, *E. coli* K1, *Haemophilus influenzae, Listeria monocytogenes, Neisseria meningitidis, Streptococcus agalactiae, Streptococcus pneumoniae, Cryptococcus neoformans/gattii*

*Cleared by the U.S. Food and Drug Administration (FDA) as of March 2017. Other versions that detect additional viruses are available outside the United States.
[†]Detects rhinoviruses and enteroviruses but does not distinguish between them.

AdV, Adenovirus; AH1, influenza A, hemagglutinin type 1; AH3, influenza A, hemagglutinin type 3; CMV, cytomegalovirus; CoV, coronavirus; EV, enterovirus; flu A, influenza A; flu B, influenza B; HHV, human herpesvirus; HMPV, human metapneumovirus; HSV, herpes simplex virus; LT/ST, heat-labile; heat-stable toxins; PIV, parainfluenza virus; RSV, respiratory syncytial virus; RV, rhinovirus; VZV, varicella-zoster virus.

the presence of diverse etiologic agents that challenged many laboratories in the past. As for the other multiplex molecular panels, clinical utility and cost-effectiveness remain to be determined. Susceptibility to contamination during performance of the assay has been a concern not yet fully resolved.

Another important area of application of molecular testing is the detection of viruses in the blood. FDA-approved assays to detect HIV RNA and hepatitis C RNA are essential for the management of these infections, including the prevention of transmission from mother to infant. Hepatitis B molecular testing is also increasingly used. In addition, molecular testing is now widely used for viruses that cause systemic disease in immunocompromised patients, especially CMV, EBV, HSV, the BK polyomavirus, and adenovirus. BK virus is often tested for in urine samples as well as in blood. For these viruses, as well as for HIV and the hepatitis viruses, quantitative testing is required. An FDA-approved PCR assay for the quantitative measurement of CMV DNA in plasma is now available. In addition, international standards for CMV, EBV, and BK virus have been developed. This is important because their utilization improves the comparability of viral levels measured in different laboratories.

Laboratory-developed PCR and other molecular assays are used by some laboratories for numerous other viruses, including parvovirus B19, human herpesvirus 6, human papillomavirus, mumps, measles, rubella, and the JC polyomavirus. **Host gene expression** patterns in whole blood have been used to attempt to differentiate viral from bacterial infections. This approach may rapidly identify a viral or bacterial profile of host gene expression reprise, thus greatly shortening the time to diagnosis and potentially avoiding inappropriate treatment while suggesting indicated therapies. Implementation in the clinic awaits development of rapid tests that incorporate this information.

Bibliography is available at Expert Consult.

Chapter **196**
The Microbiome and Pediatric Health

Patrick C. Seed

第一百九十六章
微生物与儿童健康

中文导读

本章主要介绍了微生物检测、儿童发育早期的微生物、微生物和生理发育、微生物对疾病的影响和微生物治疗措施。在微生物和生理发育中具体描述了微生物与代谢、微生物与炎症和免疫、微生物与神经生物学的关系。在微生物对疾病的影响中详细介绍了微生物对疾病的影响、坏死性小肠结肠炎微生物的变化、微生物与过敏性疾病、囊性纤维化与气道微生物、抗生素相关性腹泻和艰难梭菌结肠炎与微生物、炎性肠病与微生物的关系、肥胖与微生物、营养不良与微生物。

From the time of birth, the human infant is exposed to a myriad of microbes found on the mother and in the surrounding environment. Microbes rapidly form assemblages across exposed areas of the body, including the skin and enteral tract. The microbial communities are called the **microbiota** and make a substantial impact on short- and long-term physiology, including immunologic and metabolic development and function. Together the number of body-associated bacterial cells is estimated to be 10 times greater than the number of human cells in the body. In aggregate, the totality of the microbes, including their microbial genes and environmental interactions, constitute the **microbiome**, and the microbial genes in the human microbiome are estimated to exceed the number of human genes by at least 100-fold, together making a macroorganism with an inseparable collective physiology. Current evidence indicates that the microbiome evolves over the life span to influence health and disease.

MEASURING THE MICROBIOME

Prior knowledge of microbes on and around the human body was based on specific methods to cultivate organisms. Molecular technologies have revolutionized the identification of poorly cultivatable microbes, rare microbes, and microbes in complex communities such as those associated with the human body (Fig. 196.1). The development of the

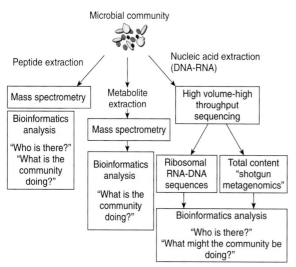

Fig. 196.1 Common molecular methodologies for identifying the components and the functions of complex microbial communities.

polymerase chain reaction (PCR) and the availability of modern nucleic acid sequencing have improved the sensitivity of detection of many organisms and have resulted in the discovery of new organisms. Modern sequencing technologies, called **next-generation sequencing** platforms, allow sequencing in high volume and depth, with millions of sequences obtained from a single biologic sample. Three major approaches utilize next-generation sequencing to understand the composition, diversity, and activity of the microbiome: (1) sequencing species-specific regions of genomes such as ribosomal RNA–encoding tracks and intergenic regions termed **metagenomics**, (2) total DNA sequencing from a sample (e.g., feces, saliva) and assembly of the sequence fragments into large genome pieces termed **shotgun metagenomics**, and (3) RNA transcript sequencing to decipher the composition and, as a surrogate for functional activity, the transcriptional activity of a microbiome termed **metatranscriptomics**. Massive computational power and new bioinformatics tools have allowed the analysis and comparison of the large datasets arising from these methods.

Two additional approaches to measure the microbiome phenotype have rapidly developed as well. First, large-scale measurements of the peptide composition of the microbiota, called **proteomics**, have been increasingly used to describe the activity of a microbiome sample, as peptides provide information about the composition and function of a microbiome. Second, in a complementary approach called **metabolomics**, microbiome-derived metabolites are measured using advanced gas chromatography and mass spectrometry techniques. Together, proteomics and metabolomics better describe the activity of a microbiome than the nucleotide-sequencing approaches; however, at this point, they provide less depth of resolution and specificity relative to the composition and phenotype of a microbiome.

Despite the power of these methodologies to interrogate the microbiome, they do not yet replace cultivation of microbes in many clinical circumstances. *Cultivation of organisms still represents the most practical means to differentiate potential pathogenic species from more benign species* and to provide clinically actionable information such as susceptibility to a range of antimicrobials.

EARLY CHILDHOOD DEVELOPMENT OF THE MICROBIOME

Emerging studies suggest that the placenta and fetus are exposed to microbes in utero, but the effect of such an exposure remains to be fully appreciated. **Prematurity** as a complication of an infection of the fetal membranes and either subclinical or clinical **chorioamnionitis** may alter the in utero exposure to microbes. The rupture of the fetal membranes and subsequent delivery provide substantial exposure to new maternal and environmental microbes that will assume common

places in the developing microbiota. Mode of delivery has a major influence on the early life microbiome, with vaginally delivered infants becoming acutely colonized with intestinal organisms that reflect the mother's vaginal tract and infants delivered by cesarean section becoming colonized with organisms reflective of maternal skin and oral cavity, including staphylococci and streptococci, as well as the surrounding environment.

In the term infant delivered vaginally, the first intestinal microbes, so-called pioneering organisms, include *Escherichia* and other Enterobacteriaceae, *Bacteroides*, and *Parabacteroides*. Exclusive breastfeeding has been reported to result in high levels of bifidobacteria and *Lactobacillus* in the week following the start of feeding. These probiotic organisms have unique capacities to exclude would-be pathogens from colonization by sequestering nutrients and producing antimicrobial factors while stimulating the intestinal epithelium to tighten cellular junctions and express antimicrobial peptides. However, these genera have been notably deficient from some breastfed infant cohorts, particularly in the United States.

The premature infant is more likely to be delivered by cesarean section and thus is more abundantly colonized with skin-related organisms such as coagulase-negative staphylococci, similar to the term infant delivered by cesarean section. However, the premature infant may fail to progress through the same stages of expansion and diversification of the microbiome over the 1st week to month of life as the term infant. The factors related to the delayed maturation are not fully clear but are predictably related to delayed or limited enteral feeding, normal environmental exposure to the household environment, and exposure to medical interventions such as antimicrobial therapy.

The most significant shift in the intestinal microbiota appears to occur after weaning and the introduction of solid foods. As the infant transitions from breast milk to a solid-food diet containing complex plant-derived polysaccharides, the microbiota begins to reshape progressively into a more mature composition beginning to resemble the adult microbiota. At the same time, the metabolic potential of the microbiome shifts to accommodate the changing diet, with the newborn microbiome enriched with phosphotransferase system (PTS) genes and then shifting to increasing abundance of lactose transporter genes by 4 mo of age, reflecting milk intake, and further shifting to a high abundance of genes such as β-glucoside transporters and enzymes necessary to break down complex carbohydrates by age 12 mo. The maturation of the childhood microbiome after the early years to adulthood is less well understood, and more studies are required in large numbers of children to understand fully the developmental stages of maturation and similarity to the mature, healthy adult state.

The oral microbiota of the newborn is of maternal origin, with vaginally born infants having predominantly *Lactobacillus*, *Prevotella*, and *Sneathia*, whereas cesarean-born infants have more maternal skin organisms, including *Staphylococcus*, *Corynebacterium*, and *Propionobacterium*. Within the 1st day of life, Firmucutes dominate the oral cavity, including *Streptococcus* and *Staphylococcus*. Formula-fed babies acquire more Bacteroidetes, whereas breast-fed babies have more bacteria of the phyla Proteobacteria and Actinobacteria. With the eruption of first teeth, new environmental niches are formed to foster microbial communities. Although cariogenic bacteria such as *Streptococcus mutans* were thought to be acquired after dentition, recent data demonstrate the presence of these organisms prior to tooth eruption in a soft tissue reservoir, highlighting the importance of good infant oral care even before primary dentition.

By age 3 yr, the childhood oral and salivary microbiome is complex but less diverse than the adult microbiome. The composition of the microbiota within the oral cavity in the presence of full adult dentition has an estimated 1,000 bacterial species. Even with oral health, the diversity in the gingiva of different types of teeth (**geodiversity**) is substantial, and the diversity changes dramatically with the development of oral disease such as periodontitis. How the microbiota evolves between preschool and adulthood remains a topic for future study. Furthermore, the placement and removal of oral hardware for orthodontics is common in childhood and may produce significant alterations in the microbiome of the oral cavity.

During the 1st yr of life, the infant skin microbiome increases in diversity, including species richness and evenness. The skin of the younger infant is relatively undifferentiated between body sites, with more shared species among different body sites such as arms, forehead, and buttocks than the older infant when the microbial communities at each site undergo differentiation. As with the early infancy oral microbiota, skin of the young infant skin is predominantly colonized by Firmicutes, including Streptococcaceae and Staphylococcaceae, with the inclusion of bacteria from other phyla such as Actinobacteria, Proteobacteria, and Bacteroidetes as the skin matures. The adult skin microbiome displays a high degree of geodiversity—differences in composition depending on site and local physiology, with major differences in dry and wet skin sites. However, the linkage between skin development in childhood and maturation of the skin microbiome remains a subject of ongoing studies.

Social structure and family interactions likely play a significant role in the development of the early life microbiome. Breast milk feeding provides a microbiologic link between mothers and infants, including transmission of probiotic-like organisms such as lactobacilli and bifidobacteria, each of which may have some protective effects, including protection against diarrheal diseases and atopy. Pediatricians have long been aware of the infectious disease risks and benefits of daycare attendance, with examples of shared pneumococcal strains producing otitis media and outbreaks of respiratory syncytial virus infection and associations with reduced atopy, allergy, and possibly asthma. Family contacts are risks for acquisition of methicillin-resistant *Staphylococcus aureus* and subsequent disease. Studies also demonstrate transmission of parts of the human microbiome between household individuals and domesticated pets such as dogs and cats. For example, family members share the same strains of *Escherichia coli* known to produce urinary tract infections in one of the household members. There may be differences in the oral microbiota among infants for whom the parents did and did not use the practice of pacifier sucking for cleaning. In rural settings, microbiome sharing extends to livestock, household surfaces, and household members. Thus, development of the microbiome during childhood with environmental interactions is a complicated process that continues to be explored.

THE MICROBIOME AND PHYSIOLOGIC DEVELOPMENT

Increasingly complex roles are being identified for the microbiome in the development of mammalian physiology (Fig. 196.2). These roles include the development of the enteral tract, respiratory tract, immune system, hematologic system, metabolic-endocrine system, and neurologic system. The details of how the microbiome contributes to these developmental processes in humans are still under intense investigation; however, modeling in other mammalian systems predicts that the microbiome will have a critical role across species.

Microbiome and Metabolism

Soon after entry into the physical world, the mammalian *enteral tract* is colonized, and the interaction of early pioneering microbes in the enteral tract stimulates the development of the intestinal mucosa. In neonatal and juvenile animal models, delayed or absent intestinal colonization results in incomplete development of the epithelium, flattening of the intestinal crypts, loss of vasculature, and severely reduced enzymatic function, including alkaline phosphatase and glucosidases.

The enteric microbiota has a large number of roles in the physiology of the *intestinal tract*. It stimulates mucosal and systemic immune development, development and regeneration of the epithelium and endothelium, and the maturation and maintenance of metabolism. The latter includes the digestion of otherwise indigestible plant polysaccharides; (2) production of vitamins and cofactors; (3) metabolism of xenobiotics, including clinically relevant drugs; and (4) stimulation of local and systemic metabolism, including lipid storage. Germ-free animals lacking the enteric microbiota have limited nutrient extraction and have a failure-to-thrive phenotype.

Germ-free mice born into a sterile environment serve as a model to understand the role of the microbiome in health. Germ-free mice are humanized through selective colonization with human fecal microbial communities. Similar to weaning to solid-food transition, feeding the humanized mice diets with and without polysaccharides results in dramatic alterations in central metabolites. Humanized mice transitioned from a polysaccharide-rich, low-fat diet to a more Westernized diet high in fat and monosaccharides undergo a blossoming of the phyla Actinobacteria and Firmicutes in the enteric microbiota, with a commensurate reduction in Bacteroidetes, similar to observations of increased Firmicutes and reduced Bacteroidetes in human obesity.

Common patterns of mature enteric microbiota community composition and its predicted function may exist among humans. Sequencing of the fecal microbes from adults across multiple nations revealed 3 common patterns of microbial community compositions, called **biotypes**. High proportions of *Bacteroides, Prevotella,* and *Ruminococcus* in unique biotypes serve as sentinels for each different biotype, and biotypes vary in individuals from different continents, including North America, Europe, and Asia, largely reflecting cultural and dietary variances. The infant microbiome varies considerably; mature, stable biotypes form in the early postweaning period and after infancy. Breast milk and formula feeding biotypes have been described, with notable enrichment of enteric gram-negative bacteria such as *E. coli* and anaerobic *Clostridia* spp. among the formula-fed infants. The vaginal biotypes of young and aging women are well described and vary by age, race, and ethnicity.

Microbiome, Inflammation, and Immunity

The organisms that compose the microbiome are critical for early immune programming, the development of immune tolerance, and overall maintenance of immune set points. Cells produce a variety of receptors to recognize microbial ligands in a process called **pattern recognition**. In turn, microbes produce intentional and unintentional stimulation of those cellular receptors to activate and repress inflammatory pathways. Classic examples of such regulatory interactions include peptidoglycan on bacteria binding to Toll-like receptor 2 (TLR-2, in complex with TLR-3 and TLR-6), lipopolysaccharide of gram-negative bacteria binding to TLR-4, and glucans of fungi binding to the dectin receptor. The results of these receptor interactions include the production of chemokines and cytokines, cell differentiation and development, alteration in metabolism, and stimulation of cell death and survival programs, all contingent on the type of cell, state of the cell, and magnitude of stimulation.

Microbial stimulation of these microbial recognition systems is so critical in development that animals raised in the absence of microbes have diminished innate immune responses such as antimicrobial peptides

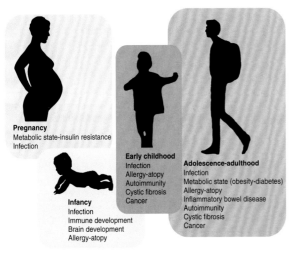

Fig. 196.2 Physiologic and pathologic roles of the microbiome relevant to pediatrics. The human microbiome has an impact on health and development from pregnancy through adulthood, including infection and non–infection-related processes.

at mucosal surfaces, dysregulated proinflammatory and immunologic tolerance responses, and reduced T- and B-cell populations. Following the restoration of normal enteric tract colonization weeks after being sterile, animals retain long-term aberrant cytokine responses with hyperactive proinflammatory responses to stimuli, demonstrating the persistent consequences of altering early microbial acquisition. Different early life colonization patterns also correlate with long-term immune development. In a Scandinavian study, children with persistent early life *E. coli* colonization had higher sustained memory B-cell (CD3+CD20+CD27+) levels by 1.5 yr old than children with lower levels of *E. coli* colonization, even despite abundant colonization with the prototypical probiotic bacteria *Lactobacillus*.

Microbiome-Neurobiologic Connections

Emerging studies are demonstrating a gut-brain axis that may be altered by the composition and activity of the enteric microbiome. Investigations in animal models have shown that the microbiome alters the hypothalamic-pituitary-adrenal system. Germ-free mice have exaggerated stress-anxiety behavior accompanied by elevated corticosterone and adrenocorticotropin levels compared with conventionally colonized, pathogen-free mice. *Neuroplasticity* including neurogenesis and microglia activation are regulated by the microbiota. Functional MRI has shown that the ingestion of 5 strains of probiotic-like bacteria alters brain activity in humans, resulting in decreased brain responses to emotional attention tasks in sensory and emotional input regions of the brain. Although the mechanism underlying these changes can only be inferred, the tractus solitarius and thus the vagus nerve appear to mediate the enteral tract–brain connection.

Another mechanism through which the enteric microbiome may alter brain activity is by the metabolites it produces. Administration of fermented milk with probiotic-like organisms, most notably *Bifidobacterium animalis* subsp. *lactis*, to monozygotic human twins and mice did not dramatically change the intestinal microbiome composition but did alter its transcriptional profiles, with a shift to increased carbohydrate fermentation to fatty acids, thought to attenuate sad emotional behavior in humans.

CONTRIBUTIONS OF MICROBIOME TO DISEASE

Studies demonstrate that some microbial communities may act in concert to exert negative health effects, whereas other communities may be restorative or resistant to disease. Some examples of this concept of altered microbial communities, also termed **dysbiosis**, are provided in the following sections.

Microbiome of Premature Birth

Although the etiology of premature birth is multifactorial, inflammatory conditions such as subclinical and clinically overt infections of the mother and fetus instigate premature birth. Inflammatory biomarker profiling highlights this point, because women who proceed to preterm birth have increased angiotensin, interleukin-8, and tumor necrosis factor receptor 1, along with race-specific alterations in additional cytokines and chemokines. Prior work reported that women experiencing preterm birth have increased vaginal colonization with *Gardnerella* spp. and *Lactobacillus crispatus*. Diversity of the microbiota of the posterior vaginal fornix of women experiencing preterm birth is lower compared to women delivering at term. A meta-analysis of early treatment of vaginosis with clindamycin before 22 wk of pregnancy demonstrated a reduction in spontaneous preterm birth at <37 wk, consistent with an association between dysbiosis of the pregnancy-associated microbiota and preterm birth.

Traditionally, the amniotic cavity and the fetus have been presumed to be sterile before the rupture of the fetal membranes and birth. However, several reports identify evidence for bacterial DNA in meconium with 2 predominant meconium types regardless of the mode of delivery: (1) dominated by Enterobacteriaceae and (2) dominated by Leuconostocaceae, Enterococcaceae, and Streptococcaceae. Furthermore, data indicate that the amniotic fluid in subclinical and clinically apparent chorioamnionitis has evidence of vaginal-derived microbes present, including poorly or noncultivatable organisms such as *Mycoplasma* spp., *Ureaplasma*

spp., *Bacteroides* spp., *Fusobacterium, Sneathia sanguinegens,* and *Leptotrichia amnionii*. A correlation exists between the burden of intraamniotic organisms and the degree of prematurity. Microbial invasion of the amniotic space may lead to induction of inflammatory pathways through innate immune microbial pattern recognition receptors such as the TLRs. The result may be the induction of labor and physiologic stress on the fetus and mother. Exposure to microbial factors may have consequences on lung and intestinal development, setting the stage for postnatal pathology, including necrotizing enterocolitis. Beyond the acute threat to the maternal-fetal dyad, chorioamnionitis may not produce the long-term neurodevelopmental consequences it once was thought to cause, with formerly premature infants born to women with chorioamnionitis having similar cognitive and neuropsychiatric outcomes, even to age 18 yr, as infants not exposed to chorioamnionitis.

Changes in the Microbiome With Necrotizing Enterocolitis

Necrotizing enterocolitis (NEC) is a devastating disease of the neonatal intestine that disproportionately affects severely premature infants who weigh <1,500 g at birth. The pathologic steps in NEC include intestinal inflammation with loss of barrier function, microbial invasion of the bowel, and eventual death of the affected bowel. Years of research implicated specific organisms as the cause of NEC in case series; however, none of the proposed specific etiologies proved to be common to all cases of NEC and, instead, appeared to be the emergent organisms after serious intestinal pathology had ensued.

Currently, a model of dysbiosis of the early life intestinal microbiome has been favored in the pathogenesis of NEC. Epidemiologic studies in very-low-birthweight infants have demonstrated an association of cephalosporins and duration of antibiotic exposure with the development of NEC, consistent with the idea that shifts in the microbiota predispose to or incite NEC. Studies demonstrate decreased diversity of the microbiota preceding and during NEC. The NEC microbiota at the time of clinical symptoms resembles the microbiota 72 hr before onset, but not the microbiota 1 wk before onset of symptoms, suggesting that a shift in the intestinal microbiota begins well in advance of the appearance of NEC. Some differences in early colonization after birth may portend an increased risk for NEC.

Microbiome and Allergic Disorders

Given the role of the microbiome in the development and modulation of innate and adaptive immune responses, considerable interest surrounds its role in the development and exacerbation of allergic conditions such as **atopic dermatitis**. The microbiome of the skin has been studied before, during, and after treatment of flares of atopic dermatitis. Flares result in the loss of diversity of bacteria on the affected area, and treatment introduces new diversity. *Staphylococus aureus* and *S. epidermidis* increase before and during atopic flares, whereas *Streptococcus* and *Corynebacterium* spp. increase immediately preceding and during clinical improvement. In mice, oral treatment of infant animals with nonabsorbable antibiotics increases serum immunoglobulin (Ig) E, increases clinical symptoms such as itching, and produces atopic-like features. These data suggest that atopic dermatitis is influenced by the local skin microbiome and more distant microbiomes such as in the intestinal tract, also suggesting why the administration of oral probiotics such as *Lactobacillus* spp. may decrease atopic dermatitis with an accompanying shift in the T-helper cell (Th1/Th2) balance and increased interferon-γ, which are part of immune tolerance.

The respiratory tract is a common site of allergic disease, and infections have long been associated with allergic exacerbations of the respiratory tract. Traditional teaching is that the lower respiratory tree is sterile; however, studies of the airway microbiome in healthy and asthmatic children and adults indicate that this teaching is incorrect. Measured through careful bronchoscopic sampling and cytology brushings, the airways have a diverse microbiota during good health.

Measurement of the microbiota in the lower respiratory tract of healthy and asthmatic children indicates significant differences. Past culture-based studies indicate that early life colonization of the neonatal respiratory tree by *Haemophilus influenzae, Moraxella catarrhalis,* and *Streptococcus pneumoniae* is associated with an increased risk for childhood asthma. These same organisms also are closely associated with exacerbations of asthma. In a mouse model, early life colonization of the neonatal nasopharynx with *H. influenzae* results in reduced airway-associated regulatory T cells, and colonized animals have enhanced airway hyperresponsiveness following allergen sensitization and inhalation challenge. *Mycoplasma pneumoniae* has been proposed as a major bacterial inducer of childhood asthma exacerbations when infection is identified. The employment of culture-independent measurements of lower airway microbiota composition (see Fig. 196.1) indicates that children with asthma are more likely to have higher levels of Proteobacteria, including *H. influenzae*, as well as Firmicutes such as *Staphylococcus* and *Streptococcus* spp. Remarkably, healthy children are more likely than age-matched asthmatic children to have lower airway Bacteroidetes, particularly *Prevotella* spp., a group of anaerobic bacteria. The association of healthy airways with an anaerobic lower respiratory tree bacterial population is unexpected because the high–oxygen tension environment was previously assumed to be toxic to anaerobes. This study indicates that the airway environment is significantly different than previously understood, and the potentially protective attributes of a native health-associated microbiota need to be studied to determine if these associations are also causal.

Airway Microbiome of Cystic Fibrosis

Cystic fibrosis (CF) is characterized by progressive airway disease and inflammation with acute exacerbations accompanied by loss of pulmonary function. An age-dependent change in lower airway colonization occurs among CF patients, which starts in early childhood with *S. aureus* and *H. influenzae* and progressively shifts toward more intrinsically multidrug-resistant organisms, including the notoriously persistent and treatment-refractory bacteria *Pseudomonas aeruginosa* and *Burkholderia cepacia* complex. Culture-independent molecular analysis of the lung-associated microbiota in CF has revealed much more complex microbial communities than previously expected and has demonstrated an association between patient age and disease severity. In addition to the presence of a variety of previously unexpected airway organisms such as anaerobes and mycobacteria, disease severity is inversely related to the lower airway microbial community diversity, with less advanced disease associated with greater species richness and evenness. In contrast, the loss of diversity, including the shift from less complex microbial communities to those dominated by *P. aeruginosa*, is strongly correlated with disease severity, and levels of *H. influenzae*, the early childhood colonizer, have a negative correlation with disease severity. Although antibiotics decrease the rate of progressive lung function deterioration, they also decrease the community diversity, thus suggesting a balance between a diverse microbiota and reducing the dominance of certain organisms such as *P. aeruginosa*.

Microbiome During Antibiotic-Associated Diarrhea and *Clostridium difficile* Colitis

Treatment with oral and parenteral antibiotics results in a rapid and significant alteration of the intestinal microbiota. Healthy study participants taking **ciprofloxacin** experience dramatic but individualized microbiome changes in response to the antibiotic, with significant reductions in bacteria outside its expected spectrum, emphasizing the interdependence of microbial community members on one another for their stability in the community as a whole. Furthermore, the response to ciprofloxacin among participants varied by individual, suggesting different degrees of stability of the microbiota and resilience under stress such as antibiotics. In general, except for some rare members, the community was largely restored within 4 wk after completion of the antibiotic course.

Some antibiotics, such as amoxicillin-clavulanate, for which antibiotic-associated diarrhea is a well-known adverse event, produce a loss of *Clostridium* and *Bacteroides*, known to be important in the production of short-chain fatty acids (SCFAs) and the metabolism of otherwise undigestible carbohydrates. Together, their loss may decrease the metabolic integrity of the intestinal epithelium that uses SCFAs for energy, while resulting in a high-osmotic environment in which fluid is drawn into the intestinal lumen. Antibiotic-associated diarrhea may result from these combined effects.

One of the most severe complications from antibiotic exposure is the development of ***Clostridium difficile*–associated diarrhea (CDAD)**, which has high associated morbidity and even mortality. Microbiologic surveys suggest that *C. difficile* is a common constituent of the developing microbiota early in life, with less prevalence over the life span. More than 30% of infants are colonized with *C. difficile* in the 1st month of life, continuing until approximately 6 mo. By 1 yr of age, colonization ranges between approximately 15% and 70% and then declines through to adulthood, when carriage is estimated to be <3%. Although *C. difficile* has been found within the vaginal microbiota of pregnant women, vaginal delivery has not been associated with increased rates of neonatal *C. difficile* colonization, with vaginal and cesarean delivery having rates of colonization at 30% and 37%, respectively. CDAD has been reported to result in 35-45 hospitalizations per 10,000 pediatric admissions among children 1-9 yr old.

Although the studies have not yet determined the natural history of the intestinal microbiome preceding, during, and with the resolution of CDAD in children, molecular studies of the intestinal microbiota in adults provide some details of the consequences of CDAD on the intestinal microbiota. Studies employing deep sequencing of stool from individuals with CDAD and *C. difficile* colonization without disease have revealed depletion of certain bacterial genera accompanying the presence of *C. difficile* colonization. These genera include *Blautia, Pseudobutyrivibrio, Roseburia, Faecalibacterium, Anaerostipes, Subdoligranulum, Ruminococcus, Streptococcus, Dorea,* and *Coprococcus.* The causal relationship of microbiome changes and the events triggering the transition from colonization to symptomatic disease remain unknown, but presumably relate to depletion of competitive species to *C. difficile*. Similar to the studies of antibiotic-associated diarrhea, these studies also demonstrate a reduction in butyrate-producing *Clostridium* spp., which are proposed to be important for producing butyrate as an energy sources for the intestinal epithelium and its robust integrity.

Although antibiotics such as metronidazole and vancomycin have been employed to treat CDAD, traditional treatment does not eliminate recurrent CDAD to the extent that might be expected. To address this problem, **fecal transplantation**, or administration of feces from healthy donors to CDAD recipients, is cost-effective treatment and superior to antibiotics in reducing the likelihood of recurrent disease. Accompanying clinical resolution is repletion of Bacteroidetes and *Clostridium* clusters IV and XIVa with a matched decrease in Proteobacteria. A recent study of children with CDAD demonstrated 94%, 75%, and 54% successful resolution following intragastric-administered fecal transplant from a donor stool bank in previously healthy children, medically complex children, and children with IBD, respectively.

Microbiome and Association With Inflammatory Bowel Disease

Crohn disease and **ulcerative colitis** are chronic inflammatory diseases of the enteric tract and are believed to be the result of the intersection of host susceptibility and a dysbiosis, an alteration in the intestinal microbiota. Twin-twin studies indicate concordance rates in monozygotic twins of 10–15% in ulcerative colitis and 30–35% in Crohn disease, thus demonstrating a genetic component for each disease while highlighting environmental factors that likely induce and drive disease progression. More than 150 single nucleotide polymorphisms (SNPs) are associated with the diseases, revealing potential defects in handling microbes, including those involved in barrier function, innate immunity, autophagy, adaptive immunity, and metabolism and cellular homeostasis.

In inflammatory bowel disease (IBD), the microbiota undergoes a shift in association with the disease throughout the intestinal tract. Although considerable heterogeneity has been described, IBD is often demonstrated to be accompanied by a decrease in bacteroides, clostridia, bifidobacteria, and Firmicutes. Reciprocally, outgrowths of *E. coli* and other Enterobacteriaceae are described. Increased sulfur-metabolizers have been described with IBD as well. Antibiotics along with biologic therapies such as antibodies directed at neutralizing tumor necrosis factor have been employed to manage the IBD dysbiosis and inflammatory reaction. Trials of fecal transplantation are underway to determine if a noninflammatory microbiota from a healthy donor may mitigate IBD symptoms and progression.

Microbiome of Obesity

Obesity and the metabolic syndrome are associated with notable changes in the intestinal microbiome regarding composition and metabolic function, ultimately resulting in greater energy extraction from the diet. Although a highly cited early study on the microbiome in obesity observed an increase in the ratio of the phyla Firmicutes:Bacteroidetes, debate continues about obesity-specific changes in the microbiome. Multiple studies have demonstrated decreased Firmicutes:Bacteroidetes ratios in the fecal microbiota from obese individuals compared to lean controls. Further studies show that proportions of phyla-level groups may be less important than changes in Firmicutes subgroups that produce **butyrate**, a known fatty acid substrate easily acquired and utilized by the intestinal epithelium, and thus ready calories for the host.

The intestinal microbiome benefits the host in meaningful ways, including enhancing caloric extraction from indigestible substrates such as polysaccharides in the diet. The microbiome produces degradative enzymes to break down these substrates where enzymes with comparable functions, such as some glycosyl hydrolases, are not encoded in the human genome. Molecular studies indicate that the intestinal microbiome may also interact with the intestinal epithelium in such a way as to alter general energy homeostasis and fat storage. For instance, the intestinal microbiome may produce SCFAs, which in turn alter endocrine peptide expression such as glucagon-like peptide 1 and peptide YY, which alter glucose homeostasis and satiety, respectively. Furthermore, through the production of SCFAs and ketones, the microbiota may alter sympathetic tone. Specific microbiomes are known to suppress others to induce fastening-induced **adipose factor** (also called angiopoietin-like protein 4), a lipoprotein lipase inhibitor of intestinal, hepatic, and adipose origins. Colonization with a diverse microbiota suppresses fastening-induced adipose factor expression, and dietary supplementation of a Western diet with *Lactobacillus paracasei* further suppressed otherwise high fastening-induced adipose factor expression. Mice fed a Western diet developed adiposity, which was transferrable to recipient lean mice following transplantation with the obese mice microbiota. Reciprocally, obese mice treated with antibiotics experienced less insulin resistance, lower fasting glycemic indices, and improved glucose tolerance compared to untreated counterparts, further implicating the microbiome in these physiologic changes.

Microbiome During Malnutrition

Malnutrition is a leading cause of morbidity and mortality across the world. In its most severe form, malnutrition may result in **kwashiorkor**, which is characterized by generalized edema, anorexia, enlarged fatty liver, skin ulcerations, and irritability. Ready-to-use foods are distributed to restore nutrition in areas with severe food restrictions. Monozygotic and dizygotic twins in Malawi were studied for the alterations in the microbiome in association with moderate to severe malnutrition, including kwashiorkor. Among the twins with discordant degrees of malnutrition on food supplements, the twins with mild preexisting malnutrition had intestinal microbiota that changed significantly over the course of supplementation. In contrast, the twins with preexisting kwashiorkor had microbiota with poor to no change in response to nutritional supplementation. These findings were recapitulated to some extent following transplantation of the twins' microbiota into previous sterile mice. Those mice receiving the microbiota of Malawian twins with kwashiorkor experienced more dramatic weight loss on a Malawian-type diet and more rapid loss of their weight gain once off ready-to-use food supplements than did mice transplanted with the feces of more healthy twins. The mice with the transplanted kwashiorkor microbiota had sustained problems with carbohydrate, lipid, and amino acid metabolism despite nutritional supplementation of the Malawian diet. Together these data indicate that severe malnutrition results from the combination of nutritional deficits and a microbiome with altered metabolic capabilities that are not readily restored with contemporary nutritional supplementation treatments.

THERAPEUTIC MANIPULATION OF THE MICROBIOME

Therapeutic manipulation of the microbiome falls into 6 general categories: antimicrobials, prebiotics, probiotics, synbiotics, postbiotics, and fecal transplantation (see CDAD and IBD earlier). **Postbiotics** are nonviable microbial components or metabolites that may alter the microbiota or produce physiologic changes in the host. Insufficient data exist to warrant a discussion of postbiotic therapeutics here.

Prebiotics

Prebiotic is defined as "nondigestible food components that beneficially affect the host by selectively stimulating the growth and/or activity of one or a limited number of bacteria in the colon and thereby improving host health." Whereas antimicrobials deplete portions of the microbiota, prebiotics aim to promote the growth of beneficial organisms such as bifidobacteria and lactobacteria. Typically, prebiotics are carbohydrates such as oligosaccharides that may be selectively metabolized by constituents of the microbiota. They may not only stimulate outgrowth of desirable organisms but also may be catabolized to beneficial end products such as SCFAs, which in turn may be utilized as energy substrates by the intestinal epithelium. Prebiotic oligosaccharides are naturally found in breast milk and have been used as supplements to human breast milk and formula.

Administration of prebiotics to term infants has demonstrated the expected outgrowth of bacteria; however, clinically significant benefits from prebiotic supplementation have not been clearly established. Treatment of term infants with fructooligosaccharides increases fecal bifidobacteria but without a change in infant growth, despite some infants having increased SCFAs in the fecal mass. A systematic review of the topic provided a similar conclusion.

Preterm infants have low to absent levels of bifidobacteria and lactobacilli in their intestinal tracts, despite full breast milk nutrition. Prebiotic supplementation has been proposed to increase these bacterial populations in the preterm infant intestinal tract. Among the proposed benefits may be a decrease in NEC. However, appropriately powered, randomized trials have not been performed to demonstrate the validity of this hypothesis.

Probiotics

Probiotics are viable organisms that have health benefits after administration. Almost all probiotics are isolates from the human microbiota, although they may not necessarily reside in the individual taking them for therapeutic purposes. Alternatively, probiotics may be administered to increase the levels of an organism already present within the microbiota. Generally, probiotics have been administered orally or as vaginal suppositories.

Multiple bacterial and fungal genera and species have been studied for probiotic effects. Common bacterial genera include bifidobacteria, lactobacilli, streptococci, enterococci, and *E. coli*. Fewer nonbacterial organisms have been studied for probiotic effects. *Saccharomyces boulardii* is related to baker's yeast (*Saccharomyces cerevisiae*) but was isolated for specific beneficial effects.

These probiotic organisms should not be confused with more pathogenic strains within their genera and species. Most probiotics have been isolated on the basis of being associated with healthy states. Bifidobacteria and lactobacilli are common to breast milk and stool among infants with low rates of diarrheal diseases and allergy. With the exception of individuals with significant immunodeficiency, severely compromised mucosal barriers, or central line catheters, where many of these organisms may adhere to the plastic with otherwise benign, transient translocation from the intestinal tract, these bacterial probiotics have proved to be relatively safe even with the administration of billions of colony-forming units. The most common adverse events associated with probiotics include abdominal cramping, nausea, fever, soft stools, flatulence, and taste disturbance.

Although bacterial probiotics have been administered widely to humans, evidence for their efficacy is limited to a small number of conditions. Probiotics have consistently shown efficacy for specific conditions, including antibiotic-associated diarrhea, prevention and reduction of atopy in high-risk children, and reductions in duration and recurrence of *C. difficile* infection. Trials indicate a reduction in NEC among preterm infants. Probiotics may reduce the risk for respiratory infections and recurrent urinary tract infection while reducing the symptoms and frequency of flares in IBD.

Antibiotic-associated diarrhea is reduced in frequency and duration. Meta-analysis indicated a relative risk (RR) of antibiotic-associated diarrhea with probiotic administration of 0.58 (95% confidence interval [CI], 0.05-0.68) among combined studies using *Lactobacillus*, *Bifidobacterium*, *Saccharomyces*, *Streptococcus*, *Enterococcus*, and/or *Bacillus*. Administration of combinations of organisms has not generally resulted in greater efficacy.

Meta-analysis specifically for the efficacy of probiotics in decreasing the incidence of CDAD demonstrated moderate evidence for the practice. In an analysis of >1,800 trials, including many in the pediatric population, probiotics reduced CDAD by 64% with RR of 0.36 (95% CI, 0.26-0.51). A pediatric subgroup was analyzed across relevant studies, revealing benefit in pediatric patients and a well-child subgroup (RR, 0.37; 95%

CI, 0.23-0.60). A number of probiotics were used, including different *Lactobacillus* strains and *S. boulardii*.

More than 15 trials have been performed to study the effect of probiotic administration during pregnancy and to infants to prevent atopic dermatitis. Meta-analysis suggests a modest benefit from probiotic administration to prevent the development of atopic dermatitis. Trials have primarily involved the administration of *Lactobacillus rhamnosus*. Studies included administration to the pregnant mother, or the infant, or both. The overall RR of 0.79 (95% CI, 0.71-0.88) was generally consistent regardless of the treatment of the mother, child, or both. The duration was generally >6 mo; apparently, however, duration did not significantly alter the effect. The RR was similar for the prevention of IgE- and non–IgE-associated atopic dermatitis.

Synbiotics are combinations of a probiotic and a prebiotic that is specifically used by the probiotic. A large, double-blind placebo-controlled trial of >4,500 infants in India demonstrated that a daily oral symbiotic preparation of *Lactobacillus plantarum* and fructooligosaccharide given through the neonatal period produced significant reductions in sepsis, pneumonia, skin infections, and all-cause mortality.

Bibliography is available at Expert Consult.

Section **2**
Preventive Measures

第二篇
预防措施

Chapter **197**
Immunization Practices

Henry H. Bernstein, Alexandra Kilinsky, and Walter A. Orenstein

第一百九十七章
免疫接种实践

中文导读

　　本章主要介绍了被动免疫、主动免疫、美国的疫苗接种系统、免疫接种时间表推荐、特殊情况的接种疫苗推荐、预防措施和禁忌证、医学豁免、提高免疫接种的覆盖和疫苗犹豫。在被动免疫中具体描述了肌肉的免疫球蛋白、静脉的免疫球蛋白、皮下的免疫球蛋白、高免动物血清制剂和单克隆抗体。在美国的疫苗接种系统中详细阐述了疫苗生产、疫苗政策、疫苗筹资、疫苗安全性监测和疫苗传递等内容。

Immunization is one of the most beneficial and cost-effective disease-prevention measures available. As a result of effective and safe vaccines, smallpox has been eradicated, polio is close to worldwide eradication, and measles and rubella are no longer endemic in the United States. However, cases of vaccine-preventable diseases, including measles, mumps, and pertussis, continue to occur in the United States. Incidence of most vaccine-preventable diseases of childhood has been reduced by ≥99% from representative 20th century annual morbidity, usually before development of the corresponding vaccines (Table 197.1a), with most of the newer vaccines not achieving quite the same percentage decrease (Table 197.1b). An analysis of effective prevention measures recommended for widespread use by the U.S. Preventive Services Task Force (USPSTF) reported that childhood immunization received a perfect score based on clinically preventable disease burden and cost-effectiveness.

Immunization is the process of inducing immunity against a specific disease. Immunity can be induced either passively or actively. **Passive immunity** is generated through administration of an antibody-containing preparation. **Active immunity** is achieved by administering a vaccine or toxoid to stimulate the immune system to produce a prolonged humoral and/or cellular immune response. As of 2019, infants, children, and adolescents in the United States are recommended to be routinely immunized against **16 pathogens**: *Corynebacterium diphtheriae, Clostridium tetani, Bordetella pertusis,* polio virus, *Haemophilus influenzae* type b (**Hib**), hepatitis A, hepatitis B, measles virus, mumps virus, rubella virus, rotavirus, varicella zoster virus, pneumococcus, meningococcus, influenza virus, and human papillomavirus (**HPV**).

PASSIVE IMMUNITY

Rather than producing antibodies through the body's own immune system, passive immunity is achieved by administration of preformed antibodies. Protection is immediate, yet transient, lasting weeks to months. Products used include:

* Immunoglobulin administered intramuscularly (**IGIM**), intravenously (**IGIV**), or subcutaneously (**IGSC**)
* Specific or hyperimmune immunoglobulin preparations administered IM or IV
* Antibodies of animal origin
* Monoclonal antibodies

Passive immunity also can be induced naturally through transplacental transfer of maternal antibodies (IgG) during gestation. This transfer can provide protection during an infant's 1st few mo of life; other antibodies (IgA) are transferred to the infant during breastfeeding. Protection for some diseases can persist for as long as 1 yr after birth, depending on the quantity of antibody transferred and the time until levels fall below those considered protective.

The major indications for inducing passive immunity are immuno-deficiencies in children with B-lymphocyte defects who have difficulty making antibodies (e.g., hypogammaglobulinemia, secondary immunodeficiencies), who have exposure to infectious diseases or to imminent risk of exposure when there is inadequate time for them to develop an active immune response to a vaccine (e.g., newborn exposed to maternal hepatitis B), and who have infectious diseases that require antibody administration as part of the specific therapy (Table 197.2).

Intramuscular Immunoglobulin

Immunoglobulin is a sterile antibody-containing solution, usually derived through cold ethanol fractionation of large pools of human plasma from adults. Antibody concentrations reflect the infectious disease exposure and immunization experience of plasma donors. Intramuscular immunoglobulin (IGIM) contains 15–18% protein and is predominantly IgG. Intravenous use of human IGIM is contraindicated. Immunoglobulin is not known to transmit infectious agents, including viral hepatitis and HIV. The major indications for immunoglobulin are:

* Replacement therapy for children with antibody deficiency disorders
* Measles prophylaxis
* Hepatitis A prophylaxis

For **replacement therapy**, the usual dose of IGIM is 100 mg/kg (equivalent to 0.66 mL/kg) monthly. The usual interval between doses is 2-4 wk depending on trough IgG serum concentrations and clinical response. In practice, IGIV has replaced IGIM for replacement therapy.

Table 197.1a	Comparison of 20th Century Annual Morbidity and Current Morbidity: Vaccine-Preventable Diseases

DISEASE	20TH CENTURY ANNUAL MORBIDITY*	2016 REPORTED CASES[†]	PERCENT DECREASE
Smallpox	29,005	0	100%
Diphtheria	21,053	0	100%
Measles	530,217	122	>99%
Mumps	162,344	5,629	96%
Pertussis	200,752	15,808	92%
Polio (paralytic)	16,316	0	100%
Rubella	47,745	9	>99%
Congenital rubella syndrome	152	2	99%
Tetanus	580	31	95%
Haemophilus influenzae type b (Hib)	20,000	22[‡]	>99%

*Data from Roush SW, Murphy TV, Vaccine-Preventable Disease Table Working Group: Historical comparisons of morbidity and mortality for vaccine-preventable diseases in the United States, *JAMA* 298(18):2155–2163, 2007.
[†]Data from Centers for Disease Control and Prevention: Notifiable diseases and mortality tables, *MMWR* 66(52):ND-924–ND-941, 2018.
[‡]Hib <5 yr of age. An additional 237 cases of *Haemophilus influenzae* (<5 yr of age) have been reported with unknown serotype.

Table 197.1b	Comparison of Pre–Vaccine Era Estimated Annual Morbidity With Current Estimate: Vaccine-Preventable Diseases

DISEASE	PRE–VACCINE ERA ANNUAL ESTIMATE*	2016 ESTIMATE (UNLESS OTHERWISE SPECIFIED)	PERCENT DECREASE
Hepatitis A	117,333*	4,000[†]	97%
Hepatitis B (acute)	66,232*	20,900[†]	68%
Pneumococcus (invasive)			
All ages	63,067*	30,400[§]	52%
<5 yr of age	16,069*	1,700[§]	89%
Rotavirus (hospitalizations, <3 yr of age)	62,500[‡]	30,625[‖]	51%
Varicella	4,085,120*	102,128[¶]	98%

*Data from Roush SW, Murphy TV; Vaccine-Preventable Disease Table Working Group: Historical comparisons of morbidity and mortality for vaccine-preventable diseases in the United States, *JAMA* 298(18):2155–2163, 2007.
[†]Data from Centers for Disease Control and Prevention: Viral hepatitis surveillance—United States, 2016.
[‡]Data from Centers for Disease Control and Prevention: Prevention of rotavirus gastroenteritis among infants and children: recommendations of the Advisory Committee on Immunization Practices, *MMWR Recomm Rep* 58(RR-2):1–25, 2009.
[§]Data from Centers for Disease Controls and Prevention: Active bacterial core surveillance, 2016 (unpublished).
[‖]Data from New Vaccine Surveillance Network 2017 data: U.S. rotavirus disease now has biennial pattern (unpublished).
[¶]Data from Centers for Disease Control and Prevention: Varicella Program, 2017 (unpublished).

Table 197.2	Immunoglobulin and Animal Antisera Preparations
PRODUCT	**MAJOR INDICATIONS**
Immune globulin intramuscular (IGIM)	Replacement therapy in antibody-deficiency disorders Hepatitis A prophylaxis Measles prophylaxis Rubella prophylaxis (pregnant women)
Immune globulin intravenous (IGIV)	Replacement therapy in antibody-deficiency disorders Kawasaki disease Pediatric HIV infection Hypogammaglobulinemia in chronic B-lymphocyte lymphocytic leukemia Varicella postexposure prophylaxis Guillain-Barré syndrome and chronic inflammatory demyelinating polyneuropathy and multifocal motor neuropathy Toxic shock syndrome May be useful in a variety of other conditions
Immune globulin subcutaneous (IGSC)	Treatment of patients with primary immunodeficiencies
Hepatitis B immunoglobulin (IM)	Postexposure prophylaxis Prevention of perinatal infection in infants born to hepatitis B surface antigen–positive mothers
Rabies immunoglobulin (IM)	Postexposure prophylaxis
Tetanus immunoglobulin (IM)	Wound prophylaxis Treatment of tetanus
Varicella-zoster immunoglobulin (VariZIG, IM)	Postexposure prophylaxis of susceptible people at high risk for complications from varicella
Cytomegalovirus (IV)	Prophylaxis of disease in seronegative transplant recipients
Vaccinia immunoglobulin (IV)	Reserved for certain complications of smallpox immunization and has no role in treatment of smallpox
Human botulism (IV), BabyBIG	Treatment of infant botulism
Diphtheria antitoxin, equine	Treatment of diphtheria
Heptavalent botulinum antitoxin against all 7 (A-G) botulinum toxin types (BAT)	Treatment of noninfant food and wound botulism
Palivizumab (monoclonal antibody), humanized mouse (IM)	Prophylaxis for infants against respiratory syncytial virus (see Chapter 287)

Data from American Academy of Pediatrics: Passive immunization. In Kimberlin DW, Brady MT, Jackson MA, Long SS, editors: *Red Book 2018: Report of the Committee on Infectious Diseases*, ed 31, Elk Grove Village, IL, 2018, American Academy of Pediatrics. (Recommendations for use of specific immune globulins are located in the sections for specific diseases in Section 3 of *Red Book*.)

IGIM can be used to prevent or modify **measles** if administered to susceptible children within 6 days of exposure (usual dose: 0.5 mL/kg body weight; maximum dose: 15 mL). The recommended dose of IGIV is 400 mL/kg. Data suggest that measles vaccine, if given within 72 hr of measles exposure, will provide protection in some cases. Measles vaccine and immunoglobulin should not be administered at the same time.

Two methods are available for **postexposure prophylaxis** against **hepatitis A** depending on the patient's age: hepatitis A immunization or

immunoglobulin. In those 12 mo-40 yr of age, hepatitis A immunization is preferred over immunoglobulin for postexposure prophylaxis and for protection of people traveling to areas where hepatitis A is endemic. Children 6-11 mo old should receive a dose of hepatitis A vaccine before international travel. However, the dose of hepatitis A vaccine received before 12 mo should not be counted in determining compliance with the recommended 2-dose schedule. In adults >40 yr, immunoglobulin may be administered for prophylaxis and for postexposure prophylaxis to people traveling internationally to hepatitis A–endemic areas (0.06 mL/kg). Immunoglobulin is preferred over hepatitis A immunization if there is an underlying immunodeficiency or chronic liver disease.

The most common adverse reactions to immunoglobulin are pain and discomfort at the injection site and, less commonly, flushing, headache, chills, and nausea. Serious adverse events are rare and include chest pain, dyspnea, anaphylaxis, and systemic collapse. Immunoglobulin should *not* be administered to people with selective IgA deficiency, who can produce antibodies against the trace amounts of IgA in immunoglobulin preparations and can develop reactions after repeat doses. These reactions can include fever, chills, and a shock-like syndrome. Because these reactions are rare, testing for selective IgA deficiencies is not recommended.

Intravenous Immunoglobulin

IGIV is a highly purified preparation of immunoglobulin antibodies prepared from adult plasma donors using alcohol fractionation and is modified to allow intravenous (IV) use. IGIV is more than 95% IgG and is tested to ensure minimum antibody titers to *Corynebacterium diphtheriae*, hepatitis B virus, measles virus, and poliovirus. Antibody concentrations against other pathogens vary widely among products and even among lots from the same manufacturer. Liquid and lyophilized powder preparations are available. IGIV does not contain thimerosal.

Not all IGIV products are approved by the U.S. Food and Drug Administration (FDA) for all indications. The major recommended FDA-approved indications for IGIV are:

◆ Replacement therapy for primary immunodeficiency disorders
◆ Kawasaki disease to prevent coronary artery abnormalities and shorten the clinical course
◆ Replacement therapy for prevention of serious bacterial infections in children infected with HIV
◆ Prevention of serious bacterial infections in people with hypogammaglobulinemia in chronic B-lymphocyte leukemia
◆ Immune-mediated thrombocytopenia to increase platelet count

IGIV may be helpful for patients with severe toxic shock syndrome, Guillain-Barré syndrome, and anemia caused by parvovirus B19. IGIV is also used for many other conditions based on clinical experience. IGIV may be used for varicella after exposure when varicella-zoster immune globulin is not available.

Reactions to IGIV may occur in up to 25% of patients. Some of these reactions appear to be related to the rate of infusion and can be mitigated by decreasing the rate. Such reactions include fever, headache, myalgia, chills, nausea, and vomiting. More serious reactions, including anaphylactoid events, thromboembolic disorders, aseptic meningitis, and renal insufficiency, have rarely been reported. Renal failure occurs mainly in patients with preexisting renal dysfunction.

Specific or hyperimmune immunoglobulin preparations are derived from donors with high titers of antibodies to specific agents and are designed to provide protection against those agents (see Table 197.2).

Subcutaneous Immunoglobulin

Subcutaneous administration of immunoglobulin (IGSC) is safe and effective in children and adults with primary immune deficiency disorders. Smaller doses administered weekly result in less fluctuation of serum IgG concentrations over time. Systemic reactions are less frequent than with IGIV, and the most common adverse effects of IGSC are injection-site reactions. There are no data on administration of IGIM by the subcutaneous route.

Hyperimmune Animal Antisera Preparations

Animal antisera preparations are derived from horses. The immunoglobulin fraction is concentrated using ammonium sulfate, and some products are further treated with enzymes to decrease reactions to foreign proteins. The following 2 equine antisera preparations are available for humans (as of 2018):

* **Diphtheria antitoxin**, which can be obtained from the U.S. Centers for Disease Control and Prevention (http://www.cdc.gov/diphtheria/dat.html) and is used to treat diphtheria.
* **Heptavalent botulinum antitoxin**, available from the CDC for use in adults with botulism. To request it, one can call the CDC's 24 hr line at 770-488-7100. This product contains antitoxin against all 7 (A-G) botulinum toxin types.

Great care must be exercised before administering animal-derived antisera because of the potential for severe allergic reactions. Due caution includes testing for sensitivity before administration, desensitization if necessary, and treating potential reactions, including febrile events, serum sickness, and anaphylaxis. *For infant botulism, IVIG (BabyBIG), a human-derived antitoxin, is licensed and should be used.*

Monoclonal Antibodies

Monoclonal antibodies (mAbs) are antibody preparations produced against a single antigen. They are mass-produced from a hybridoma, a hybrid cell used as the basis for production of large amounts of antibodies. A hybridoma is created by fusing an antibody-producing B lymphocyte with a fast-growing immortal cell such as a cancer cell. **Palivizumab** is used for prevention of severe disease from respiratory syncytial virus (RSV) among children ≤24 mo old with bronchopulmonary dysplasia (BPD, a form of chronic lung disease), a history of premature birth, or congenital heart lesions or neuromuscular diseases. The American Academy of Pediatrics (AAP) has developed specific recommendations for use of palivizumab (see Chapter 287). Monoclonal antibodies also are used to prevent transplant rejection and to treat some types of cancer, autoimmune diseases, and asthma. Use of mAbs against interleukin (IL)-2 and tumor necrosis factor (TNF)-α are being used as part of the therapeutic approach to patients with a variety of malignant and autoimmune diseases.

Serious adverse events associated with palivizumab are rare, primarily including cases of anaphylaxis and hypersensitivity reactions. Adverse reactions to mAbs directed at modifying the immune response, such as antibodies against IL-2 or TNF-α, can be more serious and include cytokine release syndrome, fever, chills, tremors, chest pain, immunosuppression, and infection with various organisms, including mycobacteria.

ACTIVE IMMUNIZATION

Vaccines are defined as whole or parts of microorganisms administered to prevent an infectious disease. Vaccines can consist of whole inactivated microorganisms (e.g., polio, hepatitis A), parts of the organism (e.g., acellular pertussis, HPV, hepatitis B), polysaccharide capsules (e.g., pneumococcal and meningococcal polysaccharide vaccines), polysaccharide capsules conjugated to protein carriers (e.g., Hib, pneumococcal, and meningococcal conjugate vaccines), live-attenuated microorganisms (e.g., measles, mumps, rubella, varicella, rotavirus, and live-attenuated influenza vaccines), and toxoids (e.g., tetanus, diphtheria) (Table 197.3). A **toxoid** is a bacterial toxin modified to be nontoxic but still capable of inducing an active immune response against the toxin.

Vaccines can contain a variety of other constituents besides the immunizing antigen. *Suspending fluids* may be sterile water or saline but can be a complex fluid containing small amounts of proteins or other constituents used to grow the immunobiologic culture. *Preservatives, stabilizers,* and *antimicrobial agents* are used to inhibit bacterial growth and prevent degradation of the antigen. Such components can include gelatin, 2-phenoxyethanol, and specific antimicrobial agents. Preservatives are added to multidose vials of vaccines, primarily to prevent bacterial contamination on repeated entry of the vial. In the past, many vaccines for children contained **thimerosal**, a preservative containing ethyl mercury. Removal of thimerosal as a preservative from vaccines for children began as a precautionary measure in 1999 in the absence of any data on harm from the preservative. This objective was accomplished by switching to single-dose packaging. Of the vaccines recommended for young children, only some preparations of influenza vaccine contain thimerosal as a preservative.*

Adjuvants are used in some vaccines to enhance the immune response. In the United States, the only adjuvants currently licensed by the FDA to be part of vaccines are **aluminum salts**; AsO_4, composed of 3-O-desacyl-4′-monophosphoryl 301 lipid A (MPL) adsorbed on to aluminum (as hydroxide salt); and MF59 and 1018 adjuvant. AsO_4 is found in 1 type of HPV vaccine, no longer available in the United States, but used in Europe. **MF59** is an oil-in-water emulsion found in 1 type of influenza vaccine approved for people ≥65 yr old. 1018 is an immunostimulatory sequence adjuvant used in HepB-CpG, a hepatitis B vaccine approved for persons > 18 yr. HepB-CpG contains yeast-derived recombinant HBsAg and is prepared by combining purified HBsAg with small synthetic immunostimulatory cytidine-phosphate-guanosine oligodeoxynucleotide motifs. The 1018 adjuvant binds to Toll-like receptor 9 to simulate a directed immune response to HBsAg. Vaccines with adjuvants should be injected deeply into muscle masses to avoid local irritation, granuloma formation, and necrosis associated with SC or intracutaneous administration.

Vaccines can induce immunity by stimulating antibody formation, cellular immunity, or both. Protection induced by most vaccines is thought to be mediated primarily by B lymphocytes, which produce antibodies. Such antibodies can inactivate toxins, neutralize viruses, and prevent their attachment to cellular receptors, facilitate phagocytosis and killing of bacteria, interact with complement to lyse bacteria, and prevent adhesion to mucosal surfaces by interacting with the bacterial cell surface.

Most B-lymphocyte responses require the assistance of CD4 helper T lymphocytes. These T-lymphocyte–dependent responses tend to induce high levels of functional antibody with high avidity. The T-dependent responses mature over time from primarily an IgM response to a persistent, long-term IgG response and induce immunologic memory that leads to enhanced responses on boosting. **T-lymphocyte–dependent vaccines**, which include protein moieties, induce good immune responses even in young infants. In contrast, polysaccharide antigens induce B-lymphocyte responses in the absence of T-lymphocyte help. These **T-lymphocyte–independent vaccines** are associated with poor immune responses in children <2 yr old and with short-term immunity and absence of an enhanced or booster response on repeat exposure to the antigen. With some polysaccharide vaccines, repeat doses actually are associated with reduced responses, as measured by antibody concentrations, compared to 1st doses (i.e., *hyporesponsive*). To overcome problems with plain polysaccharide vaccines, polysaccharides have been **conjugated**, or covalently linked, to protein carriers, converting the vaccine to a T-lymphocyte–dependent vaccine. In contrast to plain polysaccharide vaccines, conjugate vaccines induce higher-avidity antibody, immunologic memory leading to booster responses on repeat exposure to the antigen, long-term immunity, and community protection by decreasing carriage of the organism (Table 197.4). As of 2018 in the United States, licensed conjugate vaccines are available to prevent Hib, pneumococcal, and meningococcal diseases.

Serum antibodies may be detected as soon as 7-10 days after initial injection of antigen. Early antibodies are usually of the IgM class that can fix complement. IgM antibodies tend to decline as IgG antibodies increase. The IgG antibodies tend to peak approximately 1 mo after vaccination and with most vaccines persist for some time after a primary vaccine course. Secondary or booster responses occur more rapidly and result from rapid proliferation of memory B and T lymphocytes.

Assessment of the immune response to most vaccines is performed by measuring serum antibodies. Although detection of serum antibody at levels considered protective after vaccination can indicate immunity, loss of detectable antibody over time does not necessarily mean susceptibility to disease. Some vaccines induce immunologic memory, leading to a booster or anamnestic response on exposure to the microorganism, with resultant protection from disease. In some cases, cellular immune response is used to evaluate the status of the immune system.

---

*The thimerosal content in U.S.-licensed vaccines currently being manufactured is listed at http://www.fda.gov/BiologicsBloodVaccines/SafetyAvailability/VaccineSafety/ucm096228.htm#pres.

Table 197.3	Currently Available* Vaccines in the United States by Type		
PRODUCT	**TYPE**	**PRODUCT**	**TYPE**
Adenovirus	Live, oral vaccine indicated for active immunization for the prevention of febrile acute respiratory disease caused by adenovirus types 4 and 7, for use in military populations 17-50 yr of age	Japanese encephalitis vaccine	Purified, inactivated whole virus
Anthrax vaccine adsorbed	Cell-free filtrate of components including protective antigen	Measles, mumps, rubella (MMR) vaccine	Live-attenuated viruses
		Measles, mumps, rubella, varicella (MMRV) vaccine	Live-attenuated viruses
Bacille Calmette-Guérin (BCG) vaccine	Live-attenuated mycobacterial strain used to prevent tuberculosis in very limited circumstances	Meningococcal conjugate vaccine against serogroups A, C, W135, and Y (MCV4)	Polysaccharide from each serogroup conjugated to diphtheria toxoid CRM$_{197}$ protein
Cholera vaccine	Oral vaccine containing live-attenuated *Vibrio cholerae* CVD 103-HgR strain for protection against serogroup O1 in adults age 18-64 traveling to cholera-affected areas	Meningococcal polysaccharide vaccine against serogroups A, C, W135, and Y (MPSV4)	Polysaccharides from each of the serogroups conjugated to diphtheria toxoid protein
		Meningococcal B (MenB)	Recombinant proteins from serogroup B developed in *Escherichia coli*
Diphtheria and tetanus toxoids adsorbed	Toxoids of diphtheria and tetanus	Pneumococcal conjugate vaccine (13 valent) (PCV13)	Pneumococcal polysaccharides conjugated to diphtheria toxin CRM$_{197}$, contains 13 serotypes that accounted for >80% of invasive disease in young children prior to vaccine licensure
Diphtheria and tetanus toxoids and acellular pertussis (DTaP) vaccine	Toxoids of diphtheria and tetanus and purified and detoxified components from *Bordetella pertussis*		
DTaP–hepatitis B–inactivated polio vaccine (DTaP-HepB-IPV)	DTaP with hepatitis B surface antigen (HBsAg) produced through recombinant techniques in yeast with inactivated whole polioviruses	Pneumococcal polysaccharide vaccine (23 valent) (PPSV23)	Pneumococcal polysaccharides of 23 serotypes responsible for 85–90% of bacteremic disease in the United States
DTaP with IPV and *Haemophilus influenzae* type b (Hib) (DTaP-IPV/Hib)	DTaP with inactivated whole polioviruses and Hib polysaccharide conjugated to tetanus toxoid	Poliomyelitis (inactivated, enhanced potency) (IPV)	Inactivated whole virus highly purified from monkey kidney cells, trivalent types 1, 2, and 3
DTaP and inactivated polio vaccine (DTaP-IPV)	DTaP with inactivated whole polioviruses	Rabies vaccines (human diploid and purified chicken fibroblasts)	Inactivated whole virus
Hib conjugate vaccine (Hib)	Polysaccharide conjugated to either tetanus toxoid or meningococcal group B outer membrane protein	Rotavirus vaccines (RV5 and RV1)	Bovine rotavirus pentavalent vaccine (RV5) live reassortment attenuated virus, and human live-attenuated virus (RV1)
Hepatitis A vaccine (HepA)	Inactivated whole virus		
Hepatitis A–hepatitis B vaccine (HepA-HepB)	Combined hepatitis A and B vaccine	Smallpox vaccine	Vaccinia virus, an attenuated poxvirus that provides cross-protection against smallpox (variola)
Hepatitis B vaccine (HepB)	HBsAg produced through recombinant techniques in yeast	Tetanus and diphtheria toxoids, adsorbed (Td, adult use)	Tetanus toxoid plus a reduced quantity of diphtheria toxoid compared to diphtheria toxoid used for children <7 yr of age
Human papillomavirus vaccine 9-valent (9vHPV)	The L1 capsid proteins of HPV types 6 and 11 to prevent genital warts and types 16 18, 31, 33, 45, 52, and 58 to prevent cervical cancer (9vHPV).	Tetanus and diphtheria toxoids adsorbed plus acellular pertussis (Tdap) vaccine	Tetanus toxoid plus a reduced quantity of diphtheria toxoid plus acellular pertussis vaccine to be used in adolescents and adults and in children 7 through 10 yr of age who have not been appropriately immunized with DTaP
Influenza virus vaccine inactivated (IIV[†])	Available either as trivalent (A/H$_3$N$_2$, A/H$_1$N$_1$, and B) split and purified inactivated vaccines containing the hemagglutinin (H) and neuraminidase (N) of each type or as quadrivalent preparations (which include representative strains from 2 B strains in addition to the 2 influenza A strains in trivalent inactivated influenza vaccine)		
		Typhoid vaccine (polysaccharide)	Vi capsular polysaccharide of *Salmonella typhi* Ty2 strain
		Typhoid vaccine (oral)	Live-attenuated Ty21a strain of *S. typhi*
		Varicella vaccine	Live-attenuated Oka/Merck strain
		Yellow fever vaccine	Live-attenuated 17D-204 strain
Influenza virus vaccine live-attenuated, intranasal (LAIV)	Live-attenuated, temperature-sensitive, cold-adapted quadrivalent vaccine containing the H and N genes from the wild strains reassorted to have the 6 other genes from the cold-adapted parent	Herpes zoster (shingles) vaccine	Live-attenuated Oka/Merck strain for use in adults ≥60 yr old (Zostavax) Recombinant zoster vaccine, adjuvanted (Shingrix) for use in adults ≥50 years

*As of November 2018.

[†]There are various types of inactivated flu vaccines—IIV3, IIV4, RIV4, ccIIV4, aIIV3.

Data from US Food and Drug Administration: Vaccines licensed for use in the United States. http://www.fda.gov/BiologicsBloodVaccines/Vaccines/ApprovedProducts/ucm093833.htm.

Table 197.4	Characteristics of Polysaccharide and Conjugate Vaccines	
CHARACTERISTIC	**CONJUGATE**	**POLYSACCHARIDE**
T-lymphocyte–dependent immune response	Yes	No
Immune memory	Yes	No
Persistence of protection	Yes	No
Booster effect	Yes	No
Reduction of carriage	Yes	No
Community protection	Yes	No
Lack of hyporesponsiveness	Yes	No

Certain vaccines (e.g., acellular pertussis) do not have an accepted serologic correlate of protection.

Live-attenuated vaccines routinely recommended for children and adolescents include measles, mumps, and rubella (**MMR**); MMR and varicella (**MMRV**); rotavirus; and varicella. In addition, a cold-adapted, live-attenuated quadrivalent influenza vaccine (**LAIV**) is available in the past for persons 2-49 yr old who do not have conditions that place them at high risk for complications from influenza. Notably lower vaccine effectiveness during the 2013–2016 influenza seasons has resulted in LAIV not being recommended in the United States for the 2016–2017 and 2017–2018 seasons; LAIV is recommended for the 2018–1019 season. **Live-attenuated vaccines** tend to induce long-term immune responses. They replicate, often similarly to natural infections, until an immune response inhibits reproduction. Most live vaccines are administered in 1-dose or 2-dose schedules. The purpose of repeat doses, such as a 2nd dose of the MMR or MMRV vaccine, is to induce an initial immune response in those who failed to respond to the 1st dose. Because influenza viruses tend to mutate to evade preexisting immunity to prior strains, at least 1 of the strains in influenza vaccines each year is often different than in the previous year. Thus, influenza vaccines are recommended to be administered yearly.

The remaining vaccines in the recommended schedule for children and adolescents are inactivated vaccines. **Inactivated vaccines** tend to require multiple doses to induce an adequate immune response and are more likely than live-attenuated vaccines to need booster doses to maintain that immunity. However, some inactivated vaccines appear to induce long-term or perhaps lifelong immunity, after a primary series, including hepatitis B vaccine and inactivated polio vaccine.

VACCINATION SYSTEM IN THE UNITED STATES
Vaccine Production
Vaccine production is primarily a responsibility of private industry. Many of the vaccines recommended routinely for children are produced by only one vaccine manufacturer. Vaccines with multiple manufacturers include Hib, hepatitis B, rotavirus, **MCV4** (meningococcal conjugate vaccine against serogroups A, C, W135, and Y), diphtheria and tetanus toxoids and acellular pertussis (**DTaP**), and tetanus and diphtheria toxoids and acellular pertussis (Tdap) vaccines for adolescents and adults. Inactivated polio vaccine (**IPV**) as an IPV-only vaccine has only one manufacturer, but IPV is also available in combination products (DTaP–hepatitis B–IPV, DTaP-IPV/Hib, and DTaP-IPV) from different manufacturers. Influenza vaccine for children 6-35 mo of age is produced by fewer manufacturers (see http://www.cdc.gov/flu/protect/vaccine/vaccines.htm for available influenza vaccines). MMR, MMRV, varicella, pneumococcal conjugate vaccine (13 valent, **PCV13**), and tetanus and diphtheria (**Td**) vaccines also are produced by single manufacturers.

Vaccine Policy
Two major committees make vaccine policy recommendations for children: the Committee on Infectious Diseases (COID) of the AAP (the *Red Book* Committee) and the Advisory Committee on Immunization Practices (ACIP) of the CDC. Annually, the AAP, ACIP, American

Academy of Family Physicians (AAFP), and American College of Obstetricians and Gynecologists (ACOG) issue a harmonized childhood and adolescent immunization schedule (http://www.cdc.gov/vaccines/schedules/index.html). The ACIP recommendations (http://www.cdc.gov/vaccines/acip/recs/index.html) are official only after adoption by the CDC director, which leads to publication in the *Morbidity and Mortality Weekly Report (MMWR Morb Mortal Wkly Rep)*. The AAP recommendations are published in *Pediatrics* and the *Red Book*, which includes its continuously updated online version (aapredbook.org).

Vaccine Financing
Approximately 50% of vaccines routinely administered to children and adolescents <19 yr of age are purchased through a contract negotiated by the federal government with licensed vaccine manufacturers. Three major sources of funds are available to purchase vaccines through this contract. The greatest portion comes from the **Vaccines for Children** (**VFC**) program (http://www.cdc.gov/vaccines/programs/vfc/index.html), a federal entitlement program established in 1993. The VFC program covers children receiving Medicaid, children without insurance (uninsured), and Native Americans and Alaska Natives. In addition, underinsured children whose insurance does not cover immunization can be covered through VFC, but only if they go to a federally qualified health center (http://www.cms.gov/center/fqhc.asp). In contrast to other public funding sources that require approval of discretionary funding by legislative bodies, VFC funds are immediately available for new recommendations. These funds are only available if the ACIP votes the vaccine and the recommendation for its use into the VFC program, the federal government negotiates a contract, and the Office of Management and Budget (OMB) apportions funds. The VFC program can provide free vaccines to participating private providers for administration to children eligible for coverage under the program. The 2nd major federal funding source is the Section 317 **Discretionary Federal Grant Program** to states and selected localities. These funds must be appropriated annually by Congress, and in contrast to VFC, they do not have eligibility requirements for use. The 3rd major public source of funds is **state appropriations**.

The VFC program itself does not cover vaccine administration costs. Medicaid covers the administration fees for children enrolled in the program. Parents of other children eligible for VFC must pay administration fees out of pocket, although the law stipulates that no one eligible for the program can be denied vaccines because of inability to pay the administration fee. The Affordable Care Act (ACA) states that all vaccines recommended by ACIP and those included in the harmonized annual immunization schedules must be provided by qualified insurance programs with no copay and no deductible.

Vaccine Safety Monitoring
Monitoring vaccine safety is the responsibility of the FDA, CDC, and vaccine manufacturers. A critical part of that monitoring depends on reports provided to the **Vaccine Adverse Event Reporting System** (**VAERS**). Adverse events following immunization can be reported by completing a VAERS form, which can be obtained from http://www.vaers.hhs.gov or by calling 1-800-822-7967. Individual VAERS case reports may be helpful in generating hypotheses about whether vaccines are causing certain clinical syndromes. In general, however, the reports are not helpful in evaluating the causal role of vaccines in the adverse event, because most clinical syndromes that follow vaccination are similar to syndromes that occur in the absence of vaccination, which constitute background rates. For causality assessment, epidemiologic studies are often necessary, comparing the incidence rate of the adverse event after vaccination with the rate in unvaccinated individuals. A statistically significant higher rate in vaccinated individuals would be consistent with causation.

The **Vaccine Safety Datalink** consists of inpatient and outpatient records of some of the largest managed-care organizations in the United States and facilitates causality evaluation. In addition, the **Clinical Immunization Safety Assessment** (**CISA**) network has been established to advise primary care physicians on evaluation and management of adverse events (http://www.cdc.gov/vaccinesafety/Activities/CISA.html).

CISA facilitates CDC's collaboration with vaccine safety experts at leading academic medical centers and strengthens national capacity for vaccine safety monitoring. (For more information, refer to: https://www.cdc.gov/ vaccinesafety/ensuringsafety/monitoring/cisa/index.html.)

The Health and Medicine Division (HMD) of the National Academies of Sciences, Engineering and Medicine, previously the Institute of Medicine (IOM), has independently reviewed a variety of vaccine safety concerns and published reports summarizing its findings.* From 2001 through 2004, the IOM released 8 reports, concluding that the body of epidemiologic evidence did not show an association between vaccines and **autism**. In 2012 the IOM (HMD) report *Adverse Effects of Vaccines: Evidence and Causality*** reviewed a list of reported adverse effects associated with 8 vaccines to evaluate the scientific evidence, if any, of an event-vaccine relationship. The IOM committee had developed 158 causality conclusions and assigned each relationship between a vaccine and an adverse health problem to 1 of 4 causation categories. The committee concluded that available evidence convincingly supported a causal relationship between **anaphylaxis** and MMR, varicella-zoster, influenza, hepatitis B, meningococcal, and tetanus-containing vaccines. Additionally, the evidence favored rejection of 5 vaccine–adverse event relationships, including MMR vaccine and autism, inactivated influenza vaccines and asthma episodes and Bell palsy, and MMR and DTaP and type 1 diabetes mellitus. For the majority of cases (135 vaccine–adverse event pairs), the evidence was inadequate to accept or reject a causal relationship because of the rarity of the events. Overall, the committee concluded that few health problems are caused by or clearly associated with vaccines.

In 2013, the HMD released the report *Childhood Immunization Schedule and Safety: Stakeholder Concerns, Scientific Evidence, and Future Studies.*[†] The HMD uncovered no evidence of major safety concerns associated with adherence to the recommended childhood immunization schedule. The HMD specifically found no links between the immunization schedule and autoimmune diseases, asthma, hypersensitivity, seizures, child developmental disorders, learning or developmental disorders, or attention-deficit or disruptive disorders. Additionally, use of nonstandard schedules is harmful, because it increases the period of risk of acquiring vaccine-preventable diseases and increases the risk of incomplete immunization.[‡] In addition, the Agency for Healthcare Research and Quality (AHRQ) contracted with the Rand Corporation for an independent systematic review of the immunization schedule. That review concluded that while some vaccines are associated with serious adverse events, these events are extremely rare and must be weighed against the protective benefits that vaccines provide. AAP has summarized the information on a variety of safety issues and different vaccines.[§]

The National Vaccine Injury Compensation Program (VICP), established in 1988, is designed to compensate people injured by vaccines in the childhood and adolescent immunization schedule. The program is funded through an excise tax of $0.75 on vaccines recommended by the CDC per disease prevented per dose (e.g., the trivalent influenza vaccine is taxed $0.75 because it prevents one disease; the measles-mumps-rubella vaccine is taxed $2.25 because it prevents three diseases). As of 2018, this program covers all the routinely recommended vaccines that protect children against 16 diseases. The VICP was established to provide a no-fault system, with a table of related injuries and timeframes. In April 2018 the table was modified to reflect changes in the 21st Century Cures Act, requiring that the VICP cover vaccines recommended for routine administration in pregnant women. All people alleging injury from covered vaccines must first file with the program. If the injury meets the requirements of the table, compensation is automatic. If not, the claimant has the responsibility to prove causality. If compensation is accepted, the claimant cannot sue the manufacturer or physician administering the

vaccine. If the claimant rejects the judgment of the compensation system, the claimant can enter the tort system, which is uncommon. Information on the VICP is available at http://www.hrsa.gov/vaccinecompensation, or by calling 1-800-338-2382. All physicians administering a vaccine covered by the program are required by law to give the approved **Vaccine Information Statement (VIS)** to the child's parent or guardian at each visit before administering vaccines. Information on the VIS can be obtained from http://www.cdc.gov/vaccines/hcp/vis/index.html.

Vaccine Delivery

To ensure potency, vaccines should be stored at recommended temperatures before and after reconstitution. A comprehensive resource for providers on vaccine storage and handling recommendations and best practice strategies is available (https://www.cdc.gov/vaccines/hcp/ admin/storage/index.html). Expiration dates should be noted and expired vaccines discarded. Lyophilized vaccines often have long shelf lives. However, the shelf life of reconstituted vaccines generally is short, ranging from 30 min for varicella vaccine to 8 hr for MMR vaccine.

All vaccines have a preferred route of administration, which is specified in package inserts and in AAP and ACIP recommendations. Most inactivated vaccines, including DTaP, hepatitis A, hepatitis B, Hib, inactivated influenza vaccine (**IIV**), HPV, PCV13, MCV4, and Tdap, are administered IM. In contrast, MPSV4 and the more commonly used live-attenuated vaccines (MMR, MMRV, and varicella) should be dispensed by the SC route. Rotavirus vaccine is administered orally. IPV and **PPS23** (pneumococcal polysaccharide vaccine) can be given IM or SC. One influenza vaccine, LAIV, when recommended, is administered intranasally, and another influenza vaccine is administered by the intradermal route. For IM injections, the anterolateral thigh muscle is the preferred site for infants and young children. The recommended needle length varies depending on age and size: $\frac{5}{8}$ inch for newborn infants, 1 inch for infants 2-12 mo old, and 1-$1\frac{1}{4}$ inches for older children. For adolescents and adults, the deltoid muscle of the arm is the preferred site for IM administration with needle lengths of 1-$1\frac{1}{4}$ inches depending on patient size. Most IM injections can be made with 23-25 gauge needles. For SC injections, needle lengths generally range from $\frac{5}{8}$-$\frac{3}{4}$ inch with 23-25 gauge needles.

Additional aspects of immunization important for pediatricians and other healthcare providers are detailed on the websites listed in Table 197.5.

RECOMMENDED IMMUNIZATION SCHEDULE

All children in the United States should be vaccinated against 16 diseases (Figs. 197.1 and 197.2) (annually updated schedule available at http:// www.cdc.gov/vaccines/schedules/index.html).

Hepatitis B vaccine (**HepB**) is recommended in a 3-dose schedule starting at birth. The birth dose, as well as hepatitis B immunoglobulin, is critical for infants born to mothers who are hepatitis B surface antigen (HBsAg)–positive or whose hepatitis B immune status is unknown. The recommendation is to administer the 1st hepatitis B vaccine to all newborns within 24 hr of birth, the 2nd dose at 1-2 mo, with a minimal interval between the 1st and 2nd dose of 4 wk, and the 3rd dose from 6-18 mo of age ensuring that 8 wk has passed between the 2nd and 3rd dose. If the DTaP-HepB-IPV combination vaccine is used, a 4-dose schedule is permissible, which includes the stand-alone hepatitis B vaccine at birth and the combination vaccine for the next 3 doses.

The **DTaP** series consists of 5 doses administered at 2, 4, 6, and 15 through 18 mo of age, and 4 through 6 yr of age. The 4th dose of DTaP may be administered as early as 12 mo of age, provided at least 6 mo has elapsed since the 3rd dose. The 5th (booster) dose of DTaP vaccine is not necessary if the 4th dose was administered at 4 yr or older. One dose of an adult preparation of Tdap is recommended for all adolescents 11 through 12 yr of age, even if a dose of Tdap or DTaP was administered inadvertently or as part of the catch-up series at 7-10 yr of age. Adolescents 13 through 18 yr who missed the 11 through 12 yr Tdap booster dose should receive a single dose of Tdap if they have completed the diphtheria, tetanus, and pertussis (DTP)/DTaP series. Tdap may be given at any interval following the last Td. Table 197.6 lists preparations in which DTaP is combined with other vaccines. One dose of Tdap

---

*http://nationalacademies.org/hmd/Reports.aspx?filters=inmeta:activity=Immunization +Safety+Review.
**https://www.nap.edu/catalog/13164/adverse-effects-of-vaccines-evidence-and-causality.
[†]https://www.nap.edu/catalog/13563/the-childhood-immunization-schedule-and-safety -stakeholder-concerns-scientific-evidence.
[‡]For more information on the reports, see http://nationalacademies.org/hmd/Reports.aspx.
[§]https://www.healthychildren.org/English/safety-prevention/immunizations/Pages/Vaccine-Studies-Examine-the-Evidence.aspx.

Table 197.5	Vaccine Websites and Resources
ORGANIZATION	**WEBSITE**
HEALTH PROFESSIONAL ASSOCIATIONS	
American Academy of Family Physicians (AAFP)	http://www.familydoctor.org/online/famdocen/home.html
American Academy of Pediatrics (AAP)	http://www.aap.org/
AAP Childhood Immunization Support Program	http://www.aap.org/immunization/
American Association of Occupational Health Nurses (AAOHN)	http://www.aaohn.org/
American College Health Association (ACHA)	http://www.acha.org/
American College of Obstetricians and Gynecologists (ACOG)–Immunization for Women	http://www.immunizationforwomen.org/
American Medical Association (AMA)	http://www.ama-assn.org/
American Nurses Association (ANA)	http://www.nursingworld.org/
American Pharmacists Association (APhA)	http://www.pharmacist.com/
American School Health Association (ASHA)	http://www.ashaweb.org/
American Travel Health Nurses Association (ATHNA)	http://www.athna.org/
Association for Professionals in Infection Control and Epidemiology (APIC)	http://www.apic.org/
Association of State and Territorial Health Officials (ASTHO)	http://www.astho.org/
Association of Teachers of Preventive Medicine (ATPM)	http://www.atpm.org/
National Medical Association (NMA)	http://www.nmanet.org/
Society of Teachers of Family Medicine—Group on Immunization Education	http://www.immunizationed.org/
NONPROFIT GROUPS AND UNIVERSITIES	
Albert B. Sabin Vaccine Institute	http://www.sabin.org/
Brighton Collaboration	https://brightoncollaboration.org/public
Center for Vaccine Awareness and Research—Texas Children's Center	http://www.texaschildrens.org/departments/immunization-project
Children's Vaccine Program	http://www.path.org/vaccineresources/
Every Child by Two (ECBT)	http://www.ecbt.org/
Families Fighting Flu	http://www.familiesfightingflu.org/
GAVI, the Vaccine Alliance	http://www.gavialliance.org/
Health on the Net Foundation (HON)	http://www.hon.ch/
Immunization Action Coalition (IAC)	http://www.immunize.org/
Infectious Diseases Society of America (IDSA)	http://www.idsociety.org/Index.aspx
Institute for Vaccine Safety (IVS), Johns Hopkins Bloomberg School of Public Health	http://www.vaccinesafety.edu/
National Academies: Health and Medicine Division	http://www.nationalacademies.org/hmd/
National Alliance for Hispanic Health	http://www.hispanichealth.org/
National Foundation for Infectious Diseases (NFID)	http://www.nfid.org
National Foundation for Infectious Diseases (NFID)—Childhood Influenza Immunization Coalition (CIIC)	http://www.preventchildhoodinfluenza.com/
National Network for Immunization Information (NNii)	http://www.immunizationinfo.net/
Parents of Kids with Infectious Diseases (PKIDS)	http://www.pkids.org/
PATH Vaccine Resource Library	http://www.path.org/vaccineresources/
Vaccine Education Center at the Children's Hospital of Philadelphia	http://www.chop.edu/service/vaccine-education-center/home.html
Vaccinate Your Baby	http://www.vaccinateyourbaby.org/
GOVERNMENT ORGANIZATIONS	
Centers for Disease Control and Prevention (CDC)	
Advisory Committee on Immunization Practices (ACIP)	http://www.cdc.gov/vaccines/acip/index.html
ACIP Vaccine Recommendations	http://www.cdc.gov/vaccines/hcp/acip-recs/index.html
Current Vaccine Delays and Shortages	http://www.cdc.gov/vaccines/vac-gen/shortages/
Epidemiology and Prevention of Vaccine-Preventable Diseases (also known as the *Pink Book*)	https://www.cdc.gov/vaccines/pubs/pinkbook/index.html
Manual for the Surveillance of Vaccine-Preventable Diseases	www.cdc.gov/vaccines/pubs/surv-manual/index.html
Public Health Image Library	https://phil.cdc.gov/phil/home.asp
Travelers' Health	http://www.cdc.gov/travel/
CDC Health Information for International Travel (also known as the *Yellow Book*)	https://wwwnc.cdc.gov/travel/yellowbook/2016/table-of-contents
Vaccine Adverse Events Reporting System (VAERS)	http://www.cdc.gov/vaccinesafety/Activities/vaers.html
Vaccine Administration: Recommendations and Guidelines	http://www.cdc.gov/vaccines/recs/vac-admin/default.htm
Vaccines and Immunizations	http://www.cdc.gov/vaccines/
Vaccines for Children Program	http://www.cdc.gov/vaccines/programs/vfc/index.html
Vaccines for Children—Vaccine Price List	http://www.cdc.gov/vaccines/programs/vfc/awardees/vaccine-management/price-list/index.html
Vaccine Information Statements	www.cdc.gov/vaccines/hcp/vis/index.html
Vaccine Safety	http://www.cdc.gov/vaccinesafety/index.html
Vaccine Storage and Handling	http://www.cdc.gov/vaccines/recs/storage/default.htm
Department of Health and Human Services (HHS)	
National Vaccine Program Office (NVPO)	http://www.hhs.gov/nvpo/
Health Resources and Services Administration	
National Vaccine Injury Compensation Program	http://www.hrsa.gov/vaccinecompensation/
National Institute of Allergy and Infectious Diseases (NIAID)	
Vaccines	https://www.niaid.nih.gov/about/vrc
World Health Organization (WHO)	
Immunization, Vaccines, and Biologicals	http://www.who.int/immunization/en/

Recommended Child and Adolescent Immunization Schedule for ages 18 years or younger
United States, 2019

These recommendations must be read with the Notes that follow. For those who fall behind or start late, provide catch-up vaccination at the earliest opportunity as indicated by the green bars. To determine minimum intervals between doses, see the catch-up schedule (Fig.197.2). School entry and adolescent vaccine age groups are shaded in gray.

Vaccine	Birth	1 mo	2 mos	4 mos	6 mos	9 mos	12 mos	15 mos	18 mos	19-23 mos	2-3 yrs	4-6 yrs	7-10 yrs	11-12 yrs	13-15 yrs	16 yrs	17-18 yrs
Hepatitis B (HepB)	1st dose	2nd dose			←-------- 3rd dose --------→												
Rotavirus (RV) RV1 (2-dose series); RV5 (3-dose series)			1st dose	2nd dose	See Notes												
Diphtheria, tetanus, & acellular pertussis (DTaP: <7 yrs)			1st dose	2nd dose	3rd dose		←---- 4th dose ----→					5th dose					
Haemophilus influenzae type b (Hib)			1st dose	2nd dose	See Notes		3rd or 4th dose, See Notes										
Pneumococcal conjugate (PCV13)			1st dose	2nd dose	3rd dose		←---- 4th dose ----→										
Inactivated poliovirus (IPV: <18 yrs)			1st dose	2nd dose	←-------- 3rd dose --------→							4th dose					
Influenza (IIV) **or** Influenza (LAIV)					Annual vaccination 1 or 2 doses						Annual vaccination 1 or 2 doses			**or** Annual vaccination 1 dose only			Annual vaccination 1 dose only
Measles, mumps, rubella (MMR)						See Notes	←-- 1st dose --→					2nd dose					
Varicella (VAR)							←-- 1st dose --→					2nd dose					
Hepatitis A (HepA)						See Notes	2-dose series, See Notes										
Meningococcal (MenACWY-D ≥9 mos; MenACWY-CRM ≥2 mos)							See Notes							1st dose		2nd dose	
Tetanus, diphtheria, & acellular pertussis (Tdap: ≥7 yrs)														Tdap			
Human papillomavirus (HPV)														See Notes			
Meningococcal B															See Notes		
Pneumococcal polysaccharide (PPSV23)													See Notes				

■ Range of recommended ages for all children ■ Range of recommended ages for catch-up immunization ■ Range of recommended ages for certain high-risk groups ■ Range of recommended ages for non-high-risk groups that may receive vaccine, subject to individual clinical decision-making ■ No recommendation

Notes — Recommended Child and Adolescent Immunization Schedule for ages 18 years or younger, United States, 2019

For vaccine recommendations for persons 19 years of age and older, see the Recommended Adult Immunization Schedule.

Additional information
- Consult relevant ACIP statements for detailed recommendations at www.cdc.gov/vaccines/hcp/acip-recs/index.html.
- For information on contraindications and precautions for the use of a vaccine, consult the General Best Practice Guidelines for Immunization and relevant ACIP statements at www.cdc.gov/vaccines/hcp/acip-recs/index.html.
- For calculating intervals between doses, 4 weeks = 28 days. Intervals of ≥4 months are determined by calendar months.
- Within a number range (e.g., 12–18), a dash (–) should be read as "through."
- Vaccine doses administered ≤4 days before the minimum age or interval are considered valid. Doses of any vaccine administered ≥5 days earlier than the minimum age or minimum interval should not be counted as valid and should be repeated as age-appropriate. The repeat dose should be spaced after the invalid dose by the recommended minimum interval. For further details, see Table 3-1, Recommended and minimum ages and intervals between vaccine doses, in General Best Practice Guidelines for Immunization at www.cdc.gov/vaccines/hcp/acip-recs/general-recs/timing.html.
- Information on travel vaccine requirements and recommendations is available at wwwnc.cdc.gov/travel/.
- For vaccination of persons with immunodeficiencies, see Table 8-1, Vaccination of persons with primary and secondary immunodeficiencies, in General Best Practice Guidelines for Immunization at www.cdc.gov/vaccines/hcp/acip-recs/general-recs/immunocompetence.html, and Immunization in Special Clinical Circumstances (In: Kimberlin DW, Brady MT, Jackson MA, Long SS, eds. Red Book: 2018 Report of the Committee on Infectious Diseases. 31st ed. Itasca, IL: American Academy of Pediatrics; 2018:67–111).
- For information regarding vaccination in the setting of a vaccine-preventable disease outbreak, contact your state or local health department.
- The National Vaccine Injury Compensation Program (VICP) is a no-fault alternative to the traditional legal system for resolving vaccine injury claims. All routine child and adolescent vaccines are covered by VICP except for pneumococcal polysaccharide vaccine (PPSV23). For more information, see www.hrsa.gov/vaccinecompensation/index.html.

Diphtheria, tetanus, and pertussis (DTaP) vaccination (minimum age: 6 weeks [4 years for Kinrix or Quadracel])

Routine vaccination
- 5-dose series at 2, 4, 6, 15–18 months, 4–6 years
  - **Prospectively:** Dose 4 may be given as early as age 12 months if at least 6 months have elapsed since dose 3.
  - **Retrospectively:** A 4th dose that was inadvertently given as early as 12 months may be counted if at least 4 months have elapsed since dose 3.

Catch-up vaccination
- Dose 5 is not necessary if dose 4 was administered at age 4 years or older.
- For other catch-up guidance, see Fig. 197. 2.

Haemophilus influenzae type b vaccination (minimum age: 6 weeks)

Routine vaccination
- **ActHIB, Hiberix, or Pentacel:** 4-dose series at 2, 4, 6, 12–15 months
- **PedvaxHIB:** 3-dose series at 2, 4, 12–15 months

Catch-up vaccination
- **Dose 1 at 7–11 months:** Administer dose 2 at least 4 weeks later and dose 3 (final dose) at 12–15 months or 8 weeks after dose 2 (whichever is later).
- **Dose 1 at 12–14 months:** Administer dose 2 (final dose) at least 8 weeks after dose 1.
- **Dose 1 before 12 months and dose 2 before 15 months:** Administer dose 3 (final dose) 8 weeks after dose 2.
- **2 doses of PedvaxHIB before 12 months:** Administer dose 3 (final dose) at 12–59 months and at least 8 weeks after dose 2.
- **Unvaccinated at 15–59 months:** 1 dose
- For other catch-up guidance, see Fig. 197. 2.

Special situations
- **Chemotherapy or radiation treatment:**
  12–59 months
  - Unvaccinated or only 1 dose before age 12 months: 2 doses, 8 weeks apart
  - 2 or more doses before age 12 months: 1 dose at least 8 weeks after previous dose
  Doses administered within 14 days of starting therapy or during therapy should be repeated at least 3 months after therapy completion.
- **Hematopoietic stem cell transplant (HSCT):**
  - 3-dose series 4 weeks apart starting 6 to 12 months after successful transplant regardless of Hib vaccination history

- **Anatomic or functional asplenia (including sickle cell disease):**
  12–59 months
  - Unvaccinated or only 1 dose before 12 months: 2 doses, 8 weeks apart
  - 2 or more doses before 12 months:1 dose at least 8 weeks after previous dose
  Unvaccinated persons age 5 years or older*
  - 1 dose
- **Elective splenectomy:**
  Unvaccinated persons age 15 months or older*
  - 1 dose (preferably at least 14 days before procedure)
- **HIV infection:**
  12–59 months
  - Unvaccinated or only 1 dose before age 12 months: 2 doses, 8 weeks apart
  - 2 or more doses before age 12 months: 1 dose at least 8 weeks after previous dose
  Unvaccinated persons age 5–18 years*
  - 1 dose
- **Immunoglobulin deficiency, early component complement deficiency:**
  12–59 months
  - Unvaccinated or only 1 dose before age 12 months: 2 doses, 8 weeks apart
  - 2 or more doses before age 12 months: 1 dose at least 8 weeks after previous dose

Unvaccinated = Less than routine series (through 14 months) OR no doses (14 months or older)

Hepatitis A vaccination (minimum age: 12 months for routine vaccination)

Routine vaccination
- 2-dose series (**Havrix** 6–12 months apart or **Vaqta** 6–18 months apart, minimum interval 6 months); a series begun before the 2nd birthday should be completed even if the child turns 2 before the second dose is administered.

Catch-up vaccination
- Anyone 2 years of age or older may receive HepA vaccine if desired. Minimum interval between doses: 6 months
- Adolescents 18 years and older may receive the combined HepA and HepB vaccine, **Twinrix**, as a 3-dose series (0, 1, and 6 months) or 4-dose series (0, 7, and 21–30 days, followed by a dose at 12 months).

Fig. 197.1 Recommended immunization schedule for children and adolescents age 18 yr or younger—United States, 2019. (*Courtesy of US Centers for Disease Control and Prevention, Atlanta, 2019.* https://www.cdc.gov/vaccines/schedules/hcp/imz/child-adolescent.html.) *Continued*

International travel

- Persons traveling to or working in countries with high or intermediate endemic hepatitis A (wwwnc.cdc.gov/travel/):
  - **Infants age 6–11 months:** 1 dose before departure; revaccinate with 2 doses, separated by 6–18 months, between 12 to 23 months of age.
  - **Unvaccinated age 12 months and older:** 1st dose as soon as travel considered

Special situations

At risk for hepatitis A infection: 2-dose series as above
- **Chronic liver disease**
- **Clotting factor disorders**
- **Men who have sex with men**
- **Injection or non-injection drug use**
- **Homelessness**
- **Work with hepatitis A virus** in research laboratory or nonhuman primates with hepatitis A infection
- **Travel** in countries with high or intermediate endemic hepatitis A
- **Close, personal contact with international adoptee** (e.g., household or regular babysitting) in first 60 days after arrival from country with high or intermediate endemic hepatitis A (administer dose 1 as soon as adoption is planned, at least 2 weeks before adoptee's arrival)

Hepatitis B vaccination
(minimum age: birth)

Birth dose (monovalent HepB vaccine only)

- **Mother is HBsAg-negative:** 1 dose within 24 hours of birth for **all** medically stable infants ≥2,000 grams. Infants <2,000 grams: administer 1 dose at chronological age 1 month or hospital discharge.
- **Mother is HBsAg-positive:**
  - Administer **HepB vaccine** and **0.5 mL of hepatitis B immune globulin (HBIG)** (at separate anatomic sites) within 12 hours of birth, regardless of birth weight. For infants <2,000 grams, administer 3 additional doses of vaccine (total of 4 doses) beginning at age 1 month.
  - Test for HBsAg and anti-HBs at age 9–12 months. If HepB series is delayed, test 1–2 months after final dose.
- **Mother's HBsAg status is unknown:**
  - Administer **HepB vaccine** within 12 hours of birth, regardless of birth weight.
  - For infants <2,000 grams, administer **0.5 mL of HBIG** in addition to HepB vaccine within 12 hours of birth. Administer 3 additional doses of vaccine (total of 4 doses) beginning at age 1 month.
  - Determine mother's HBsAg status as soon as possible. If mother is HBsAg-positive, administer **0.5 mL of HBIG** to infants ≥2,000 grams as soon as possible, but no later than 7 days of age.

Routine series

- 3-dose series at 0, 1, 2, 6–18 months (use monovalent HepB vaccine for doses administered before age 6 weeks)
- Infants who did not receive a birth dose should begin the series as soon as feasible (see Fig. 197. 2).
- Administration of **4 doses** is permitted when a combination vaccine containing HepB is used after the birth dose.
- **Minimum age** for the final (3rd or 4th) dose: 24 weeks
- **Minimum intervals:** dose 1 to dose 2: 4 weeks / dose 2 to dose 3: 8 weeks / dose 1 to dose 3: 16 weeks (when 4 doses are administered, substitute "dose 4" for "dose 3" in these calculations)

Catch-up vaccination

- Unvaccinated persons should complete a 3-dose series at 0, 1–2, 6 months.
- Adolescents age 11–15 years may use an alternative 2-dose schedule with at least 4 months between doses (adult formulation **Recombivax HB** only).
- Adolescents 18 years and older may receive a 2-dose series of HepB (**Heplisav-B**) at least 4 weeks apart.
- Adolescents 18 years and older may receive the combined HepA and HepB vaccine, **Twinrix**, as a 3-dose series (0, 1, and 6 months) or 4-dose series (0, 7, and 21–30 days, followed by a dose at 12 months).
- For other catch-up guidance, see Fig. 197. 2.

Human papillomavirus vaccination
(minimum age: 9 years)

Routine and catch-up vaccination

- HPV vaccination routinely recommended for all adolescents **age 11–12 years** (can start at age 9 years) and through age 18 years if not previously adequately vaccinated
- 2- or 3-dose series depending on age at initial vaccination:
  - **Age 9 through 14 years at initial vaccination:** 2-dose series at 0, 6–12 months (minimum interval: 5 months; repeat dose if administered too soon)
  - **Age 15 years or older at initial vaccination:** 3-dose series at 0, 1–2 months, 6 months (minimum intervals: dose 1 to dose 2: 4 weeks / dose 2 to dose 3: 12 weeks / dose 1 to dose 3: 5 months; repeat dose if administered too soon)
- If completed valid vaccination series with any HPV vaccine, no additional doses needed

Special situations

- **Immunocompromising conditions, including HIV infection:** 3-dose series as above
- **History of sexual abuse or assault:** Start at age 9 years
- **Pregnancy:** HPV vaccination not recommended until after pregnancy; no intervention needed if vaccinated while pregnant; pregnancy testing not needed before vaccination

Inactivated poliovirus vaccination
(minimum age: 6 weeks)

Routine vaccination

- 4-dose series at ages 2, 4, 6–18 months, 4–6 years; administer the final dose on or after the 4th birthday and at least 6 months after the previous dose.
- 4 or more doses of IPV can be administered before the 4th birthday when a combination vaccine containing IPV is used. However, a dose is still recommended after the 4th birthday and at least 6 months after the previous dose.

Catch-up vaccination

- In the first 6 months of life, use minimum ages and intervals only for travel to a polio-endemic region or during an outbreak.
- IPV is not routinely recommended for U.S. residents 18 years and older.

Series containing oral polio vaccine (OPV), either mixed OPV-IPV or OPV-only series:
- Total number of doses needed to complete the series is the same as that recommended for the U.S. IPV schedule. See www.cdc.gov/mmwr/volumes/66/wr/mm6601a6.htm?s_cid=mm6601a6_w.
- Only trivalent OPV (tOPV) counts toward the U.S. vaccination requirements. For guidance to assess doses documented as "OPV," see www.cdc.gov/mmwr/volumes/66/wr/mm6606a7.htm?s_cid=mm6606a7_w.
- For other catch-up guidance, see Fig. 197. 2.

Influenza vaccination
(minimum age: 6 months [IIV], 2 years [LAIV], 18 years [RIV])

Routine vaccination

- 1 dose any influenza vaccine appropriate for age and health status annually (2 doses separated by at least 4 weeks for **children 6 months–8 years** who did not receive at least 2 doses of influenza vaccine before July 1, 2018)

Special situations

- **Egg allergy, hives only:** Any influenza vaccine appropriate for age and health status annually
- **Egg allergy more severe than hives** (e.g., angioedema, respiratory distress): Any influenza vaccine appropriate for age and health status annually in medical setting under supervision of health care provider who can recognize and manage severe allergic conditions
- **LAIV should not be used for** those with a history of severe allergic reaction to any component of the vaccine (excluding egg) or to a previous dose of any influenza vaccine, children and adolescents receiving concomitant aspirin or salicylate-containing medications, children age 2 through 4 years with a history of asthma or wheezing, those who are immunocompromised due to any cause (including immunosuppression caused by medications and HIV infection), anatomic and functional asplenia, cochlear implants, cerebrospinal fluid-oropharyngeal communication, close contacts and caregivers of severely immunosuppressed persons who require a protected environment, pregnancy, and persons who have received influenza antiviral medications within the previous 48 hours.

Measles, mumps, and rubella vaccination
(minimum age: 12 months for routine vaccination)

Routine vaccination

- 2-dose series at 12–15 months, 4–6 years
- Dose 2 may be administered as early as 4 weeks after dose 1.

Catch-up vaccination

- Unvaccinated children and adolescents: 2 doses at least 4 weeks apart
- The maximum age for use of *MMRV* is 12 years.

Special situations

International travel
- **Infants age 6–11 months:** 1 dose before departure; revaccinate with 2 doses at 12–15 months (12 months for children in high-risk areas) and dose 2 as early as 4 weeks later.
- **Unvaccinated children age 12 months and older:** 2-dose series at least 4 weeks apart before departure

Meningococcal serogroup A,C,W,Y vaccination
(minimum age: 2 months [MenACWY-CRM, Menveo], 9 months [MenACWY-D, Menactra])

Routine vaccination

- 2-dose series: 11–12 years, 16 years

Catch-up vaccination

- Age 13–15 years: 1 dose now and booster at age 16–18 years (minimum interval: 8 weeks)
- Age 16–18 years: 1 dose

Special situations

Anatomic or functional asplenia (including sickle cell disease), HIV infection, persistent complement component deficiency, eculizumab use:
- **Menveo**
  - Dose 1 at age 8 weeks: 4-dose series at 2, 4, 6, 12 months
  - Dose 1 at age 7–23 months: 2-dose series (dose 2 at least 12 weeks after dose 1 and after the 1st birthday)
  - Dose 1 at age 24 months or older: 2-dose series at least 8 weeks apart

- **Menactra**
  - **Persistent complement component deficiency:**
    - Age 9–23 months: 2 doses at least 12 weeks apart
    - Age 24 months or older: 2 doses at least 8 weeks apart
  - **Anatomic or functional asplenia, sickle cell disease, or HIV infection:**
    - Age 9–23 months: Not recommended
    - 24 months or older: 2 doses at least 8 weeks apart
  - **Menactra** must be administered at least 4 weeks after completion of PCV13 series.

Travel in countries with hyperendemic or epidemic meningococcal disease, including countries in the African meningitis belt or during the Hajj (wwwnc.cdc.gov/travel/):
- Children age less than 24 months:
  - **Menveo (age 2–23 months):**
    - Dose 1 at 8 weeks: 4-dose series at 2, 4, 6, 12 months
    - Dose 1 at 7–23 months: 2-dose series (dose 2 at least 12 weeks after dose 1 and after the 1st birthday)
  - **Menactra (age 9–23 months):**
    - 2-dose series (dose 2 at least 12 weeks after dose 1; dose 2 may be administered as early as 8 weeks after dose 1 in travelers)
- Children age 2 years or older: 1 dose **Menveo** or **Menactra**

First-year college students who live in residential housing (if not previously vaccinated at age 16 years or older) or military recruits:
- 1 dose **Menveo** or **Menactra**

Note: **Menactra** should be administered either before or at the same time as DTaP. For MenACWY booster dose recommendations for groups listed under "Special situations" above and additional meningococcal vaccination information, see meningococcal *MMWR* publications at www.cdc.gov/vaccines/hcp/acip-recs/vacc-specific/mening.html.

Meningococcal serogroup B vaccination
(minimum age: 10 years [MenB-4C, Bexsero; MenB-FHbp, Trumenba])

Clinical discretion

- MenB vaccine may be administered based on individual clinical decision to **adolescents not at increased risk** age 16–23 years (preferred age 16–18 years):
- **Bexsero:** 2-dose series at least 1 month apart
- **Trumenba:** 2-dose series at least 6 months apart; if dose 2 is administered earlier than 6 months, administer a 3rd dose at least 4 months after dose 2.

Special situations

Anatomic or functional asplenia (including sickle cell disease), persistent complement component deficiency, eculizumab use:
- **Bexsero:** 2-dose series at least 1 month apart
- **Trumenba:** 3-dose series at 0, 1–2, 6 months

Bexsero and Trumenba are not interchangeable; the same product should be used for all doses in a series.
For additional meningococcal vaccination information, see meningococcal *MMWR* publications at www.cdc.gov/vaccines/hcp/acip-recs/vacc-specific/mening.html.

Pneumococcal vaccination
(minimum age: 6 weeks [PCV13], 2 years [PPSV23])

Routine vaccination with PCV13

- 4-dose series at 2, 4, 6, 12–15 months

Catch-up vaccination with PCV13

- 1 dose for healthy children age 24–59 months with any incomplete* PCV13 series
- For other catch-up guidance, see Fig. 197. 2.

Special situations

High-risk conditions below: When both PCV13 and PPSV23 are indicated, administer PCV13 first. PCV13 and PPSV23 should not be administered during same visit.

Chronic heart disease (particularly cyanotic congenital heart disease and cardiac failure); chronic lung disease (including asthma treated with high-dose, oral corticosteroids); diabetes mellitus:
Age 2–5 years
- Any incomplete* series with:
  - 3 PCV13 doses: 1 dose PCV13 (at least 8 weeks after any prior PCV13 dose)
  - Less than 3 PCV13 doses: 2 doses PCV13 (8 weeks after the most recent dose and administered 8 weeks apart)
- No history of PPSV23: 1 dose PPSV23 (at least 8 weeks after any prior PCV13 dose)
Age 6–18 years
- No history of PPSV23: 1 dose PPSV23 (at least 8 weeks after any prior PCV13 dose)

Cerebrospinal fluid leak, cochlear implant:
Age 2–5 years
- Any incomplete* series with:
  - 3 PCV13 doses: 1 dose PCV13 (at least 8 weeks after any prior PCV13 dose)
  - Less than 3 PCV13 doses: 2 doses PCV13, 8 weeks after the most recent dose and administered 8 weeks apart
- No history of PPSV23: 1 dose PPSV23 (at least 8 weeks after any prior PCV13 dose)
Age 6–18 years
- No history of either PCV13 or PPSV23: 1 dose PCV13, 1 dose PPSV23 at least 8 weeks later
- Any PCV13 but no PPSV23: 1 dose PPSV23 at least 8 weeks after the most recent dose of PCV13
- PPSV23 but no PCV13: 1 dose PCV13 at least 8 weeks after the most recent dose of PPSV23

Fig. 197.1, cont'd

Sickle cell disease and other hemoglobinopathies; anatomic or functional asplenia; congenital or acquired immunodeficiency; HIV infection; chronic renal failure; nephrotic syndrome; malignant neoplasms, leukemias, lymphomas, Hodgkin disease, and other diseases associated with treatment with immunosuppressive drugs or radiation therapy; solid organ transplantation; multiple myeloma:

Age 2–5 years
• Any incomplete* series with:
 - 3 PCV13 doses: 1 dose PCV13 (at least 8 weeks after any prior PCV13 dose)
 - Less than 3 PCV13 doses: 2 doses PCV13 (8 weeks after the most recent dose and administered 8 weeks apart)
• No history of PPSV23: 1 dose PPSV23 (at least 8 weeks after any prior PCV13 dose) and a 2nd dose of PPSV23 5 years later

Age 6–18 years
• No history of either PCV13 or PPSV23: 1 dose PCV13, 2 doses PPSV23 (dose 1 of PPSV23 administered 8 weeks after PCV13 and dose 2 of PPSV23 administered at least 5 years after dose 1 of PPSV23)
• Any PCV13 but no PPSV23: 2 doses PPSV23 (dose 1 of PPSV23 administered 8 weeks after the most recent dose of PCV13 and dose 2 of PPSV23 administered at least 5 years after dose 1 of PPSV23)
• PPSV23 but no PCV13: 1 dose PCV13 at least 8 weeks after the most recent PPSV23 dose and a 2nd dose of PPSV23 administered 5 years after dose 1 of PPSV23 and at least 8 weeks after a dose of PCV13

Chronic liver disease, alcoholism:
Age 6–18 years
• No history of PPSV23: 1 dose PPSV23 (at least 8 weeks after any prior PCV13 dose)

*An incomplete series is defined as not having received all doses in either the recommended series or an age-appropriate catch-up series. See Tables 8, 9, and 11 in the ACIP pneumococcal vaccine recommendations (www.cdc.gov/mmwr/pdf/rr/rr5911.pdf) for complete schedule details.

Rotavirus vaccination
(minimum age: 6 weeks)

Routine vaccination
• **Rotarix:** 2-dose series at 2 and 4 months.
• **RotaTeq:** 3-dose series at 2, 4, and 6 months.
If any dose in the series is either **RotaTeq** or unknown, default to 3-dose series.

Catch-up vaccination
• Do not start the series on or after age 15 weeks, 0 days.
• The maximum age for the final dose is 8 months, 0 days.
• For other catch-up guidance, see Figure 2.

Tetanus, diphtheria, and pertussis (Tdap) vaccination
(minimum age: 11 years for routine vaccination, 7 years for catch-up vaccination)

Routine vaccination
• **Adolescents age 11–12 years:** 1 dose Tdap
• **Pregnancy:** 1 dose Tdap during each pregnancy, preferably in early part of gestational weeks 27–36
• Tdap may be administered regardless of the interval since the last tetanus- and diphtheria-toxoid-containing vaccine.

Catch-up vaccination
• **Adolescents age 13–18 years who have not received Tdap:** 1 dose Tdap, then Td booster every 10 years
• **Persons age 7–18 years not fully immunized with DTaP:** 1 dose Tdap as part of the catch-up series (preferably the first dose); if additional doses are needed, use Td.
• **Children age 7–10 years** who receive Tdap inadvertently or as part of the catch-up series should receive the routine Tdap dose at 11–12 years.
• **DTaP inadvertently given after the 7th birthday:**
 - **Child age 7–10 years:** DTaP may count as part of catch-up series. Routine Tdap dose at 11–12 should be administered.
 - **Adolescent age 11–18 years:** Count dose of DTaP as the adolescent Tdap booster.

• For other catch-up guidance, see Fig. 197. 2.
• For information on use of Tdap or Td as tetanus prophylaxis in wound management, see www.cdc.gov/mmwr/volumes/67/rr/rr6702a1.htm.

Varicella vaccination
(minimum age: 12 months)

Routine vaccination
• 2-dose series: 12–15 months, 4–6 years
• Dose 2 may be administered as early as 3 months after dose 1 (a dose administered after a 4-week interval may be counted).

Catch-up vaccination
• Ensure persons age 7–18 years without evidence of immunity (see MMWR at www.cdc.gov/mmwr/pdf/rr/rr5604.pdf) have 2-dose series:
 - **Ages 7–12 years:** routine interval: 3 months (minimum interval: 4 weeks)
 - **Ages 13 years and older:** routine interval: 4–8 weeks (minimum interval: 4 weeks).
 - The maximum age for use of MMRV is 12 years.

Fig. 197.1, cont'd

Table 197.6	Combination Vaccines Licensed and Available in the United States

VACCINE PRODUCT (MANUFACTURER)*	TRADE NAME (YEAR LICENSED)	COMPONENTS	RECOMMENDED AGES	
			Primary Series	**Booster Dose**
DTaP-IPV/Hib (Sanofi Pasteur)	Pentacel (2008)	DTaP-IPV + PRP-T	2, 4, and 6 mo	15 through 18 mo
DTaP-HepB-IPV (GlaxoSmithKline)	Pediarix (2002)	DTaP + HepB + IPV	2, 4, and 6 mo	
DTaP-IPV (GlaxoSmithKline)	Kinrix (2008), Quadracel (2015)	DTaP + IPV		4 through 6 yr. Booster for 5th dose of DTaP. Booster for 4th dose of IPV
HepA-HepB (GlaxoSmithKline)	Twinrix (2001)	HepA + HepB	>18 yr of age; 0, 1, and 6 mo schedule	
MMRV (Merck & Co)	ProQuad (2005)	MMR + varicella	†	4 through 6 yr

*Dash (-) indicates that products are supplied in their final form by the manufacturer and do not require mixing or reconstitution by user; slash (/) indicates that products are mixed or reconstituted by user.

†Although ProQuad is available for the 1st dose (at 12 through 15 mo of age), the CDC recommends that MMR vaccine and varicella vaccine should be administered for the 1st dose in this age-group, unless the parent or caregiver expresses a preference for MMRV vaccine.

DTaP, Diphtheria and tetanus toxoids and acellular pertussis vaccine; HepA, hepatitis A vaccine; HepB, hepatitis B vaccine; IPV/Hib, trivalent inactivated polio vaccine and Haemophilus influenzae type b vaccine; MMRV, measles-mumps-rubella and varicella vaccine; PRP-T, H. influenzae type b capsular polysaccharide (polyribosyl-ribitol279 phosphate [PRP]) covalently bound to tetanus toxoid (PRP-T).

Adapted from Cohn AC, MacNeil JR, Clark TA, et al: Prevention and control of meningococcal disease: recommendations of the Advisory Committee on Immunization Practices, MMWR 62(2):1–28, 2013.

vaccine is recommended for pregnant adolescents with each pregnancy, preferably between 27 and 36 wk gestation, regardless of time since last Tdap or Td. Currently available data suggest that vaccinating earlier in the 27 through 36 wk period will maximize passive antibody transfer to the infant. This recommendation was made in response to data predicting lack of infant protection when maternal Tdap had been received before pregnancy.

There are 3 licensed preparations of single-antigen **Hib** vaccines. The vaccine conjugated to tetanus toxoid (PRP-T) is given in a 4-dose series at 2, 4, 6, and 12 through 15 mo of age, and the Hib vaccine conjugated to meningococcal outer membrane protein (PRP-OMP) is recommended in a 3-dose series at 2, 4, and 12 through 15 mo of age. The 3rd Hib vaccine is licensed as a booster for children 15 mo through 4 yr of age. There are several vaccines in which Hib is a component, in addition to single-antigen Hib conjugate vaccines (see Tables 197.6 and 197.7).

Influenza vaccine is recommended for all children beginning at 6 mo old, with a minimum age of 6 mo for IIVs and 24 mo for LAIV. Various influenza vaccine preparations are FDA-licensed for different age-groups.* Children 6 mo through 8 yr of age being vaccinated for the first time should receive 2 doses at least 4 wk apart. If such children only received a single dose of IIV the prior season, they need 2 doses the following season. For additional guidelines, follow dosing instructions in the influenza statement, which is updated annually by both the CDC (https://www.cdc.gov/flu/professionals/acip/index.htm) and AAP (aapredbook.org). Influenza vaccine usually is given in October or November, although there are benefits even when administered as late as February or March because influenza seasons most frequently peak in February. People ≥9 yr old should receive 1 dose of influenza vaccine annually. For the 2016–2017 flu season, the ACIP voted that LAIV should not be used at all because of low vaccine effectiveness during the previous 3 influenza seasons.

*See http://www.cdc.gov/flu/protect/vaccine/vaccines.htm and http://aapredbook.aappublications.org/site/news/vaccstatus.xhtml#flu.

Catch-up immunization schedule for persons aged 4 months—18 years who start late or who are more than 1 month behind, United States, 2019

The figure below provides catch-up schedules and minimum intervals between doses for children whose vaccinations have been delayed. A vaccine series does not need to be restarted, regardless of the time that has elapsed between doses. Use the section appropriate for the child's age. Always use this table in conjunction with Fig. 197.1 and the notes that follow.

Vaccine	Minimum Age for Dose 1	Minimum Interval Between Doses			
		Dose 1 to Dose 2	Dose 2 to Dose 3	Dose 3 to Dose 4	Dose 4 to Dose 5
Children age 4 months through 6 years					
Hepatitis B	Birth	4 weeks	8 weeks *and* at least 16 weeks after first dose. Minimum age for the final dose is 24 weeks.		
Rotavirus	6 weeks Maximum age for first dose is 14 weeks, 6 days	4 weeks	4 weeks Maximum age for final dose is 8 months, 0 days.		
Diphtheria, tetanus, and acellular pertussis	6 weeks	4 weeks	4 weeks	6 months	6 months
Haemophilus influenzae type b	6 weeks	No further doses needed if first dose was administered at age 15 months or older. 4 weeks if first dose was administered before the 1st birthday. 8 weeks (as final dose) if first dose was administered at age 12 through 14 months.	No further doses needed if previous dose was administered at age 15 months or older. 4 weeks if current age is younger than 12 months *and* first dose was administered at younger than age 7 months, *and* at least 1 previous dose was PRP-T (ActHib, Pentacel, Hiberix) or unknown. 8 weeks *and* age 12 through 59 months (as final dose) if current age is younger than 12 months *and* first dose was administered at age 7 through 11 months; OR if current age is 12 through 59 months *and* first dose was administered before the 1st birthday, *and* second dose administered at younger than 15 months; OR if both doses were PRP-OMP (PedvaxHIB; Comvax) *and* were administered before the 1st birthday.	8 weeks (as final dose) This dose only necessary for children age 12 through 59 months who received 3 doses before the 1st birthday.	
Pneumococcal conjugate	6 weeks	No further doses needed for healthy children if first dose was administered at age 24 months or older. 4 weeks if first dose administered before the 1st birthday. 8 weeks (as final dose for healthy children) if first dose was administered at the 1st birthday or after.	No further doses needed for healthy children if previous dose administered at age 24 months or older. 4 weeks if current age is younger than 12 months and previous dose given at <7 months old. 8 weeks (as final dose for healthy children) if previous dose given between 7-11 months (wait until at least 12 months old); OR if current age is 12 months or older and at least 1 dose was given before age 12 months.	8 weeks (as final dose) This dose only necessary for children age 12 through 59 months who received 3 doses before age 12 months or for children at high risk who received 3 doses at any age.	
Inactivated poliovirus	6 weeks	4 weeks	4 weeks if current age is < 4 years. 6 months (as final dose) if current age is 4 years or older.	6 months (minimum age 4 years for final dose).	
Measles, mumps, rubella	12 months	4 weeks			
Varicella	12 months	3 months			
Hepatitis A	12 months	6 months			
Meningococcal	2 months MenACWY-CRM 9 months MenACWY-D	8 weeks	See Notes	See Notes	
Children and adolescents age 7 through 18 years					
Meningococcal	Not Applicable (N/A)	8 weeks			
Tetanus, diphtheria; tetanus, diphtheria, and acellular pertussis	7 years	4 weeks	4 weeks if first dose of DTaP/DT was administered before the 1st birthday. 6 months (as final dose) if first dose of DTaP/DT or Tdap/Td was administered at or after the 1st birthday.	6 months if first dose of DTaP/DT was administered before the 1st birthday.	
Human papillomavirus	9 years	Routine dosing intervals are recommended.			
Hepatitis A	N/A	6 months			
Hepatitis B	N/A	4 weeks	8 weeks *and* at least 16 weeks after first dose.		
Inactivated poliovirus	N/A	4 weeks	6 months A fourth dose is not necessary if the third dose was administered at age 4 years or older and at least 6 months after the previous dose.	A fourth dose of IPV is indicated if all previous doses were administered at <4 years or if the third dose was administered <6 months after the second dose.	
Measles, mumps, rubella	N/A	4 weeks			
Varicella	N/A	3 months if younger than age 13 years. 4 weeks if age 13 years or older.			

Fig. 197.2 Catch-up immunization schedule for persons age 4 mo-18 yr who start late or who are more than 1 mo behind—United States, 2019. *(Courtesy of US Centers for Disease Control and Prevention, Atlanta, 2019.* https://www.cdc.gov/vaccines/schedules/hcp/imz/child-adolescent.html.)

IPV should be administered at 2, 4, and 6 through 18 mo of age with a booster dose at 4 through 6 yr. The final dose in the series should be administered on or after 4 yr of age and at least 6 mo after the previous dose. The final dose in the IPV series should be administered at 4 yr or older regardless of the number of previous doses, and the minimal interval from dose 3 to dose 4 is 6 mo. For series that contain oral polio vaccine (OPV), the total number of doses needed to complete the series is the same as that recommended for the U.S. IPV schedule. Only documentation specifying receipt of trivalent OPV constitutes proof of vaccination according to the U.S. polio vaccination recommendations. This is important because since April 2016, trivalent OPV (tOPV) is no longer available with the type 2 serotype removed. Thus, children vaccinated since that time only received the type 1 and 3 components and are not immune to type 2. In contrast, IPV contains all 3 polio serotypes. For catch-up vaccine recommendations, see the recommended childhood immunization schedule at http://www.cdc.gov/vaccines/schedules/hcp/imz/catchup.html.

MMR should be administered at 12 through 15 mo of age followed by a 2nd dose at 4 through 6 yr. Before all international travel, infants 6 through 11 mo of age should receive 1 dose of MMR vaccine. These children should be revaccinated with the routinely recommended 2 doses of MMR vaccine beginning at 12 mo of age. For children 12 mo or older, administer 2 doses before international travel; the 2nd dose should be administered at least 4 wk after the 1st dose.

Two doses of **varicella** vaccine should be given, the 1st at 12 through 15 mo of age and the 2nd at 4 through 6 yr. The 2nd dose may be administered before 4 yr of age provided at least 3 mo have elapsed since the 1st dose. MMR and MMRV preparations are available. The **quadrivalent MMRV** vaccine is preferred in place of separate MMR

and varicella vaccines at the 4-6 yr old visit. Because of the slight increase in febrile seizures associated with combined MMRV vaccine compared to simultaneous administration of the separate products, use of MMRV is not preferred over use of separate MMR and varicella vaccines for the initial dose at 12-15 mo of age.

Protection against pneumococcal and meningococcal disease can be provided by either conjugated or polysaccharide vaccines. Conjugated vaccines offer several benefits over polysaccharide vaccines (see Table 197.4). **PCV13** is recommended as a 4-dose series at 2, 4, 6, and 12 through 15 mo of age. In the latest immunization schedule, PCV13 is the only pneumococcal vaccine that appears; references to the previously available 7-valent pneumococcal conjugate vaccine (PCV7) have been removed. All healthy children who may have received PCV7 as part of a primary series have now aged out of the recommendation for pneumococcal vaccine. PPSV23 is recommended for select children with conditions that place them at risk for pneumococcal disease.

A 2-dose series of MCV4 includes a recommended dose for all adolescents at 11 through 12 yr of age and a booster dose at 16 yr. If the 1st dose is administered at 13 through 15 yr of age, a booster dose should be administered at 16 through 18 yr. No booster dose is needed if the 1st dose is administered at 16 yr. In addition, MCV4 should be administered to people 2 mo through 55 yr of age with underlying conditions that place them at high risk of meningococcal disease. In addition, 2-3 doses of the **meningococcal B (MenB)** vaccine are recommended for persons ≥10 yr old at increased risk of meningococcal disease.

Hepatitis A vaccine, licensed for administration to children ≥12 mo old, is recommended for universal administration to all children at 12 through 23 mo of age and for certain high-risk groups. The 2 doses in

Table 197.7	Vaccines Recommended for Children and Adolescents With Underlying Conditions or at High Risk
VACCINES	**SPECIAL SITUATIONS**
PCV13 (and PPSV23 in certain conditions)	Chronic heart disease (particularly cyanotic congenital heart disease and cardiac failure), chronic lung disease (including asthma if treated with high-dose oral corticosteroid therapy), chronic liver disease, chronic renal failure Diabetes mellitus Cerebrospinal fluid leak Cochlear implant Sickle cell disease and other hemoglobinopathies Anatomic or functional asplenia HIV infection Nephrotic syndrome Diseases associated with treatment with immunosuppressive drugs or radiation therapy, including malignant neoplasms, leukemias, lymphomas, and Hodgkin disease Generalized malignancy Solid organ transplantation Congenital or acquired immunodeficiencies Multiple myeloma
Hep A	Chronic liver disease Clotting factor disorders Men who have sex with men Injection or non-injection drug use Homelessness Work with hepatitis A virus Travel in countries with high or intermediate endemic hepatitis A Close, personal contact with international adoptee (e.g.,household or regular babysitting)
Flu	Egg allergy more severe than hives
MCV4	Anatomic or functional asplenia (including sickle cell disease) Persistent complement component deficiency Residents of or travelers to countries in African meningitis belt or pilgrims on the Hajj During outbreaks caused by a vaccine serogroup HIV infection
MenB	Anatomic or functional asplenia (including sickle cell disease) Children with persistent complement component deficiency During serogroup B outbreaks
Hib	Persons at increased risk for Hib disease, including chemotherapy recipients and those with anatomic or functional asplenia (including sickle cell disease), human immunodeficiency virus (HIV) infection, immunoglobulin deficiency, or early component complement deficiency Recipients of hematopoietic stem cell transplant (HSCT) Elective splenectomy
Hep B	Infants born to HBsAg-positive mothers or mothers whose HBsAg status is unknown (administer vaccine within 12 hr of birth)
HPV	Immunocompromising conditions, including HIV infection History of sexual abuse or assault

From Centers for Disease Control and Prevention: Child and adolescent schedule. https://www.cdc.gov/vaccines/schedules/hcp/imz/child-adolescent.html

the series should be separated by at least 6 mo. Children who have received 1 dose of hepatitis A vaccine before 24 mo of age should receive a 2nd dose 6-18 mo after the 1st dose. For anyone 2 yr or older who has not yet received the 2-dose hepatitis A vaccine series, 2 doses of vaccine separated by 6-18 mo may be administered if immunity against hepatitis A infection is desired. This is particularly important in people with chronic liver disease, clotting factor disorders, men who have sex with men, injection or non-injection drug use, homelessness, people exposed to hepatitis A virus at work, travel, and people in close contact with international adoptees. Before all international travel, infants 6 through 11 mo of age should receive 1 dose of hepatitis A vaccine. These children should be revaccinated with the routinely recommended 2 doses of hepatitis A vaccine beginning at 12 mo of age. For unvaccinated children 12 mo or older, 2 doses should be administered before international travel to countries with high or intermediate endemic hepatitis A; the 2nd dose should be administered at least 6 mo after the 1st dose.

The **9vHPV** vaccine is recommended at age 11 or 12 yr but can be started as early as 9 yr for males and females. For those who initiate the series before their 15th birthday, the recommended schedule is 2 doses of 9vHPV vaccine. The minimum interval is 5 mo between the 1st and 2nd dose. If the 2nd dose is given at a shorter interval, a 3rd dose

should be administered a minimum of 12 wk after the 2nd dose and a minimum of 5 mo after the 1st dose. For those initiating the series on or after their 15th birthday, the recommended schedule is 3 doses of 9vHPV vaccine. The minimum intervals are 4 wk between the 1st and 2nd dose, 12 wk between the 2nd and 3rd dose, and 5 mo between the 1st and 3rd dose. For children with a history of sexual abuse or assault, ACIP recommends routine HPV vaccination beginning at age 9 yr. In males and females with primary or secondary immunocompromising conditions such as B-lymphocyte deficiencies, T-lymphocyte complete or partial defects, HIV, malignancy, transplantation, autoimmune disease, or immunosuppressive therapy, ACIP recommends vaccination with 3 doses of 9vHPV (0, 1-2, and 6 mo) because immune response to vaccination might be attenuated. 9vHPV may be used to continue or complete a vaccination series in patients who started with 4vHPV or 2vHPV.

Two **rotavirus** vaccines are available, RotaTeq (RV5) and Rotarix (RV1). With both vaccines, the 1st dose can be administered as early as 6 wk of age and must be administered by 14 wk 6 days. The final dose in the series must be administered no later than 8 mo of age. The RV5 vaccine is administered in 3 doses at least 4 wk apart. The RV1 vaccine is administered in 2 doses at least 4 wk apart. Immunization should not be initiated for infants ≥15 wk old, as stated in the immunization schedule.

The present schedule, excluding influenza vaccine, can require as many as 34 doses, including 31 that must be administered by injection. Of the doses, 25 are recommended before 2 yr of age, including 22 injections. Influenza vaccination, starting at age 6 mo, can add an additional 20 injections through 18 yr. To reduce the injection burdens, several combination vaccines are available (see Table 197.6).

The recommended childhood and adolescent immunization schedule establishes a routine adolescent visit at 11 through 12 yr of age. MCV4, a Tdap booster, and 9vHPV vaccine should be administered during this visit. Influenza vaccine should be administered annually. In addition, the 11-12 yr old visit is an opportune time to review all the immunizations the adolescent has received previously, to provide any doses that were missed, and to review other age-appropriate preventive services. The 11-12 yr visit establishes an important platform for incorporating other vaccines. Information on the current status of new vaccine licensure and recommendations for use is available.*

For children who are at least 1 mo behind in their immunizations, catch-up immunization schedules are available for children 4 mo through 18 yr of age (http://www.cdc.gov/vaccines/schedules/hcp/imz/catchup .html). Also, interactive immunization schedules are available for children <6 yr of age at https://www.vacscheduler.org. Only written/electronic, dated, authentic records should be accepted as evidence of immunization. In general, when in doubt, a person with unknown or uncertain immunization status should be considered "disease susceptible," and recommended immunizations should be initiated without delay on a schedule commensurate with the person's current age. No evidence suggests that administration of vaccines to already-immune recipients is harmful.

VACCINES RECOMMENDED IN SPECIAL SITUATIONS

There are 8 vaccines—PCV13, PPSV23, MCV4, MenB, Flu, Hib, HepA, and HepB—recommended for children and adolescents at increased risk for complications from vaccine-preventable diseases or children who have an increased risk for exposure to these diseases, who are outside the age-groups for which these vaccines are normally recommended (PPSV23 and MenB are not routinely recommended for any age-group of children and are only used for children with high-risk conditions; see Table 197.7). Specific recommendations for use of these vaccines in children with underlying conditions can be found in the recommended immunization schedule.

PCV13 is recommended for children 24 mo through 5 yr of age with certain medical conditions that place them at high risk for pneumococcal disease. This recommendation includes children with sickle cell disease and other hemoglobinopathies, including hemoglobin SS, hemoglobin S-C, or hemoglobin S–β-thalassemia, or children who are functionally or anatomically asplenic; children with HIV infection; and children who have chronic disease (Table 197.7). (For further recommendations on pneumococcal vaccine recommendations, see https://www.cdc.gov/ vaccines/vpd/pneumo/hcp/who-when-to-vaccinate.html.)

Children at high risk for pneumococcal disease also should receive **PPSV23** to provide immunity to serotypes not contained in the 13-valent conjugate vaccine. PPSV23 should be administered on or after the 2nd birthday and should follow completion of the PCV13 series by at least 6-8 wk. Two doses of PPSV23 are recommended, with an interval of 5 yr between doses. Immunization of children >5 yr old with high-risk conditions can be performed with PCV13 and/or PPSV23, depending on the condition and vaccination history. When both PCV13 and PPSV23 are indicated, PCV13 should be administered first. The 2 vaccines should not be administered during the same visit.

MCV4 is recommended for HIV-infected persons ≥2 mo old, children with anatomic or functional asplenia (including sickle cell disease), and children with persistent complement component deficiency (includes persons with inherited or chronic deficiencies in C3, C5–9, properdin, factor D or factor H or taking eculizumab).

Meningococcal B (**MenB**) vaccine is recommended for persons ≥10 yr old at increased risk of meningococcal disease. This includes people with complement deficiencies or anatomic or functional asplenia, people at increased risk due to serogroup B meningococcal disease outbreaks, and microbiologists who routinely are exposed to isolates of *Neisseria meningitidis*. Young adults age 16-23 (preferred range: 16-18 yr) who are not at increased risk for meningococcal disease may be vaccinated with either of the 2 MenB vaccines, which are not interchangeable, to provide short-term protection against most strains of serogroup B meningococcal disease.

Hib vaccine and HepA vaccine are recommended for children with certain high-risk conditions. **HepB** is recommended for infants born to HBsAg-positive mothers or mothers whose HBsAg status is unknown (administer vaccine within 12 hr of birth) (see Table 197.7).

In addition to vaccines in the recommended childhood and adolescent schedule, a variety of vaccines are available for children who will be **traveling** to areas of the world where certain infectious diseases are common (Table 197.8). Vaccines for travelers include typhoid fever, hepatitis A, hepatitis B, Japanese encephalitis, MCV4 or MPS4, cholera, rabies, and yellow fever, depending on the location and circumstances of travel. **Measles** is endemic in many parts of the world. Children 6-11 mo old should receive a dose of MMR and hepatitis A vaccines before international travel. However, doses of MMR and hepatitis A vaccines received before 12 mo should not be counted in determining compliance with the recommended 2-dose MMR schedule. For unvaccinated children ≥12 mo old, administer 2 doses before international travel following the recommended schedule. (Additional information on vaccines for international travel can be found at http://wwwnc.cdc.gov/ travel/.)

Vaccine recommendations for children with **immunocompromising conditions**, either primary (inherited) or secondary (acquired), vary according to the underlying condition, the degree of immune deficit, the risk for exposure to disease, and the vaccine (Table 197.9 and Fig. 197.3). Immunization of children who are immunocompromised poses the following potential concerns: the incidence or severity of some vaccine-preventable diseases is higher, and therefore certain vaccines are recommended specifically for certain conditions; vaccines may be less effective during the period of altered immunocompetence and may need to be repeated when immune competence is restored; and because of altered immunocompetence, some children and adolescents may be at increased risk for an adverse event following receipt of a live-virus vaccine. Live-attenuated vaccines generally are contraindicated in immunocompromised persons. The exceptions include **MMR**, which may be given to a child with HIV infection provided the child is asymptomatic or symptomatic without evidence of severe immunosuppression, and **varicella** vaccine, which may be given to HIV-infected children if the CD4+ lymphocyte count is at least 15%. MMRV is not recommended in these situations.

Altered immunocompetence is considered a precaution for rotavirus; however, the vaccine is contraindicated in children with severe combined immunodeficiency disease. Inactivated vaccines may be administered to immunocompromised children, although their effectiveness might not be optimal depending on the immune deficit. Children with complement deficiency disorders may receive all vaccines, including live-attenuated vaccines. In contrast, children with phagocytic disorders may receive both inactivated and live-attenuated viral vaccines but not live-attenuated bacterial vaccines.*

Corticosteroids can suppress the immune system. Children receiving corticosteroids (≥2 mg/kg/day or ≥20 mg/day of prednisone or equivalent) for ≥14 days should not receive live vaccines until therapy has been discontinued for at least 1 mo. Children on the same dose levels but for <2 wk may receive live-virus vaccines as soon as therapy is discontinued, although some experts recommend waiting 2 wk after therapy has been discontinued. Children receiving lower doses of corticosteroids may be vaccinated while receiving therapy.

Children and adolescents with malignancy, and those who have undergone solid organ or hematopoietic stem cell transplantation and

---

*http://aapredbook.aappublications.org/site/news/vaccstatus.xhtml and http://www.fda.gov/ BiologicsBloodVaccines/Vaccines/ApprovedProducts/UCM093833

*https://www.cdc.gov/vaccines/pubs/pinkbook/downloads/appendices/a/immuno-table.pdf

Table 197.8	Recommended Immunizations for International Travel*

| IMMUNIZATIONS | LENGTH OF STAY | |
	Brief, <1 mo	Long-Term/Residential, >1 mo
Review and complete age-appropriate childhood and adolescent schedule (see text for details) • DTaP, poliovirus, pneumococcal, and *Haemophilus influenzae* type b (Hib) vaccines may be given at 4 wk intervals if necessary to complete recommended schedule before departure. • Influenza • MMR: 2 additional doses given if <12 mo old at 1st dose • Meningococcal disease (MenACWY)[†] • Rotavirus • Varicella • Human papillomavirus (HPV) • Hepatitis A: 2 additional doses given if <12 mo old at 1st dose[†§] • Hepatitis B[§] • Tdap	+	+
Yellow fever[‖]	+	+
Typhoid fever[¶]	±	+
Rabies**	±	±
Japanese encephalitis[††]	±	+
Cholera[‡‡]	±	±

*See disease-specific chapters in the Centers for Disease Control and Prevention's *Yellow Book* for details. For further sources of information, see text.

[†]Recommended for regions of Africa with endemic infection and during local epidemics, and required for travel to Saudi Arabia for the Hajj.

[‡]For infants age 6-11 mo, 1st dose is recommended before departure for all international travel. For unvaccinated children 12 mo and older, this vaccine is indicated for travelers to areas with intermediate or high endemic rates of hepatitis A virus infection.

[§]If there is insufficient time to complete 6 mo primary series, accelerated series can be given.

[‖]For regions with endemic infection, see Health Information for International Travel (http://www.cdc.gov/travel). Because of the risk of serious adverse events after yellow fever vaccination, clinicians should only vaccinate people who (1) are at risk of exposure to yellow fever virus (YFV) or (2) require proof of vaccination to enter a country.

[¶]Indicated for travelers who will consume food and liquids in areas of poor sanitation.

**Indicated for people with high risk for animal exposure (especially to dogs) and for travelers to countries with endemic infection.

[††]For regions with endemic infection (see Health Information for International Travel). For high-risk activities in areas experiencing outbreaks, vaccine is recommended, even for brief travel.

[‡‡]Cholera vaccine (CVD 103-HgR, Vaxchora) is recommended for adult (18-64 yr old) travelers to an area of active toxigenic *V. cholerae* O1 transmission.

+, Recommended; ±, consider; DTaP, diphtheria and tetanus toxoids and acellular pertussis.

Data from Centers for Disease Control and Prevention: Travelers' health. https://wwwnc.cdc.gov/travel.

immunosuppressive or radiation therapy, should not receive live-virus and live-bacteria vaccines depending on their immune status. Children who have undergone chemotherapy for leukemia may need to be reimmunized with age-appropriate single doses of previously administered vaccines. Preterm infants generally can be vaccinated at the same chronological age as full-term infants according to the recommended childhood immunization schedule. An exception is the birth dose of HepB. Infants weighing ≥2 kg and who are stable should receive a birth dose within the 1st 24 hr of life. However, HepB should be deferred in infants weighing <2 kg at birth until chronological age 1 mo or hospital discharge, if born to an HBsAg-negative mother. All preterm, low-birthweight infants born to HBsAg-positive mothers should receive hepatitis B immunoglobulin (HBIG) and HepB vaccine (at separate anatomic sites) within 12 hr of birth. However, such infants should receive an additional 3 doses of vaccine starting at 30 days of age (see Fig. 197.2). Infants born to HBsAg-positive mothers should be tested for HBsAg and antibody at 9-12 mo, or 1-2 mo after completion of the HepB series if the series is delayed. If the test is negative for antibody against the surface antigen (anti-HBs), an additional dose of HepB is recommended with testing 1-2 mo after the dose. If the child is still antibody negative, an additional 2 doses of vaccine should be administered.

If the mother's HBsAg status is unknown within 12 hr of birth, administer HepB vaccine regardless of birthweight. For infants weighing <2,000 g, administer HBIG in addition to HepB within 12 hr of birth. Determine the mother's HBsAg status as soon as possible and, if the mother is HBsAg-positive, also administer HBIG to infants weighing ≥2,000 g as soon as possible, but no later than 7 days of age.

Varicella-zoster immunoglobulin (**VariZIG**) is recommended for patients without evidence of immunity to varicella who are at high risk for severe varicella and complications, who have been exposed to varicella or herpes zoster, and for whom varicella vaccine is contraindicated. This includes immunocompromised patients without evidence of immunity, newborn infants whose mothers have signs and symptoms of varicella around the time of delivery (i.e., 5 days before to 2 days after), hospitalized premature infants born at ≥28 wk gestation whose mothers do not have evidence of immunity to varicella, hospitalized premature infants born at <28 wk gestation or who weigh ≤1,000 g at birth, regardless of their mother's evidence of immunity to varicella, and pregnant women without evidence of immunity.

Some children have situations that are not addressed directly in current immunization schedules. Physicians can use general rules to guide immunization decisions in some of these instances. In general, vaccines may be given simultaneously on the same day, whether inactivated or live. Different inactivated vaccines can be administered at any interval between doses. However, because of theoretical concerns about viral interference, different live-attenuated vaccines (MMR, varicella), if not administered on the same day, should be given at least 1 mo apart. An inactivated and a live vaccine may be spaced at any interval from each other.

Immunoglobulin does not interfere with inactivated vaccines. However, immunoglobulin can interfere with the immune response to measles vaccine and by inference to varicella vaccine. In general, immunoglobulin, if needed, should be administered at least 2 wk after the measles vaccine. Depending on the dose of immunoglobulin received, MMR should be deferred for as long as 3-11 mo. Immunoglobulin is not expected to interfere with the immune response to LAIV or rotavirus vaccines.

Certain adult (including pregnancy) immunizations are recommended to decrease the risk of infection in their children; these include influenza virus and pertussis (Tdap).

Table 197.9	Vaccination of Persons With Primary and Secondary Immune Deficiencies

PRIMARY

CATEGORY	SPECIFIC IMMUNODEFICIENCY	CONTRAINDICATED VACCINES*	RISK-SPECIFIC RECOMMENDED VACCINES*	EFFECTIVENESS AND COMMENTS
B lymphocyte (humoral)	Severe antibody deficiencies (e.g., X-linked agammaglobulinemia and common variable immunodeficiency)	OPV[a] Smallpox[b] LAIV BCG Yellow fever virus (YFV) and live-bacteria vaccines[e] No data for rotavirus vaccines	Annual IIV is the only vaccine given to patients receiving IG therapy; routine inactivated vaccines can be given if not receiving IGIV.	The effectiveness of any vaccine will be uncertain if it depends only on the humoral response (e.g., PPSV23). IG therapy interferes with the immune response to live vaccines MMR and VAR.
	Less severe antibody deficiencies (e.g., selective IgA deficiency and IgG subclass deficiency)	OPV[a] BCG YFV vaccine Other live vaccines[d] appear to be safe.	Vaccines should be given as on the annual immunization schedule for immunocompetent people.[e] PPSV23 should be given at 2 yr of age.[f]	All vaccines are probably effective. Immune response may be attenuated.
T lymphocyte (cell-mediated and humoral)	Complete defects (e.g., SCID, complete DiGeorge syndrome)	All live vaccines[c,d,g]	The only vaccine that should be given if the patient is receiving IG is annual IIV if there is some residual antibody protection.	All inactivated vaccines are probably ineffective.
	Partial defects (e.g., most patients with DiGeorge syndrome, hyper-IgM syndrome, Wiskott-Aldrich syndrome, ataxia-telangiectasia)	All live vaccines[c,d,g]	Routine inactivated vaccines should be given.[e] PPSV23 should be given beginning at 2 yr of age.[f]	Effectiveness of any vaccine depends on degree of immune suppression.
	Interferon (IFN)-γ–interleukin (IL)-12 axis deficiencies	All live vaccines for IL-12/IL-12R deficiencies, IFN-γ, IFN-α, or STAT1 deficiencies	None	None
Complement	Persistent complement, properdin, MBL, or factor B deficiency; secondary deficiency because taking eculizumab (Solaris)	None	PPSV23 should be given beginning at 2 yr of age.[f] MCV series beginning in infancy.[h] MenB series beginning at 10 yr of age	All routine vaccines are probably effective.
Phagocytic function	Chronic granulomatous disease	Live-bacteria vaccines[c]	None	All inactivated vaccines are safe and probably effective. Live-virus vaccines are probably safe and effective.
	Phagocytic deficiencies that are undefined or accompanied by defect in T-cell and NK-cell dysfunction (e.g., Chédiak-Higashi syndrome, leukocyte adhesion defects, myeloperoxidase deficiency)	MMR, MMRV, OPV,[a] smallpox, LAIV, YF, all bacteria vaccines	PPSV23 should be given beginning at 2 yr of age.[f] MCV series beginning in infancy.[h]	All inactivated vaccines are safe and probably effective.

SECONDARY

SPECIFIC IMMUNODEFICIENCY	CONTRAINDICATED VACCINES*	RISK-SPECIFIC RECOMMENDED VACCINES*	EFFECTIVENESS AND COMMENTS
HIV/AIDS	OPV[a] Smallpox BCG Combined MMRV LAIV Withhold MMR, varicella, and zoster in severely immunocompromised persons. YF vaccine may have a contraindication or precaution depending on the indicators of immune function.[j]	PPSV23 should be given beginning at 2 yr of age.[f] MCV series beginning in infancy.[h] Consider Hib (if not administered in infancy).[i]	Rotavirus vaccine is recommended on standard schedule. MMR and VAR are recommended for HIV-infected children who are asymptomatic or only low-level immunocompromised.[k] All inactivated vaccines may be effective.

Continued

Table 197.9	Vaccination of Persons With Primary and Secondary Immune Deficiencies—cont'd

SECONDARY

SPECIFIC IMMUNODEFICIENCY	CONTRAINDICATED VACCINES*	RISK-SPECIFIC RECOMMENDED VACCINES*	EFFECTIVENESS AND COMMENTS
Generalized malignant neoplasm, transplantation, autoimmune disease, immunosuppressive or radiation therapy	Live-virus and live-bacteria vaccines, depending on immune status.[c,d,m]	PPSV23 should be given beginning at 2 yr of age.[f] Annual IIV (unless receiving intensive chemotherapy or anti-B cell antibodies). Hib vaccine may be indicated.[n]	Effectiveness of any vaccine depends on degree of immune suppression; inactivated standard vaccines are indicated if not highly immunosuppressed, but doses should be repeated after chemotherapy ends.
Asplenia (functional, congenital anatomic, surgical)	LAIV	PPSV23 should be given beginning at 2 yr of age.[f] MCV series beginning in infancy.[h] MenB series beginning at 10 yr of age. Hib (if not administered in infancy)[o]	All routine vaccines are probably effective.
Chronic renal disease	LAIV	PPSV23 should given beginning at 2 yr of age.[f] HepB is indicated if not previously immunized.	All routine vaccines are probably effective.
CNS anatomic barrier defect (cochlear implant, congenital dysplasia of the inner ear, persistent CSF communication with naso-/oropharynx)	None	PPSV23 should be given beginning at 2 yr of age.[f]	All standard vaccines are indicated.

*Other vaccines that are universally or routinely recommended should be given if not contraindicated.

[a]OPV is no longer available in the United States.

[b]This table refers to contraindications for nonemergency vaccination (i.e., ACIP recommendations)

[c]Live-bacteria vaccines: BCG and oral Ty21a *Salmonella typhi* vaccine.

[d]Live-virus vaccines: MMR, MMRV, VAR, OPV, LAIV, YF, zoster, rotavirus, and vaccinia (smallpox). Smallpox vaccine is not recommended for children or the general public.

[e]Children who are delayed or underimmunized should be immunized with routinely recommended vaccines, according to age and catch-up schedule.

[f]PPSV23 is begun at 2 yr or older. If PCV13 is required, PCV13 doses should be administered first, followed by PPSV23 at least 8 wk later; a 2nd dose of PPSV23 is given 5 yr after the 1st.

[g]Regarding T-lymphocyte immunodeficiency as a contraindication for rotavirus vaccine, data exist only for SCID.

[h]Age and schedule of doses depend on the product; repeated doses are required.

[i]Pneumococcal vaccine is not indicated for children with chronic granulomatous disease beyond age-based universal recommendations for PCV13. Children with chronic granulomatous disease are not at increased risk for pneumococcal disease.

[j]YF vaccine is contraindicated in HIV-infected children <6 yr old who are highly immunosuppressed. There is precaution for use of YF vaccine in asymptomatic HIV-infected children <6 yr with total lymphocyte percentage of 15–24%, and >6 yr old with $CD4^+$ T-lymphocyte counts of 200-499 cells/mm^3. (Data from Centers for Disease Control and Prevention: Yellow fever vaccine: recommendations of the Advisory Committee on Immunization Practices, *MMWR Recomm Rep* 59[RR-07]; 1–27, 2010.)

[k]HIV-infected children should receive immune globulin after exposure to measles and may receive varicella vaccine if $CD4^+$ T-lymphocyte percentage is ≥15% for those <6 yr old, or $CD4^+$ T-lymphocyte count ≥200 cells/mm^3 for those ≥6 yr old. People with perinatal HIV infection who were vaccinated with measles, rubella, or mumps–containing vaccine before the establishment of combination antiretroviral therapy (cART) should be considered unvaccinated and should receive 2 appropriately spaced doses of MMR vaccine once effective cART has been established (at least 6 mo with $CD4^+$ T-lymphocytes ≥15% for children <6 yr old, or $CD4^+$ T-lymphocyte count ≥200 cells/mm^3 for children ≥6 yr old).

[l]For patients 5-18 yr old who have not received a Hib primary series and a booster dose or at least 1 Hib dose after age 14 mo.

[m]Withholding inactivated vaccines also is recommended with some forms of immunosuppressive therapy, such as anti-CD20 antibodies, induction or consolidation chemotherapy, or patients with major antibody deficiencies receiving immune globulins. Inactivated influenza vaccine is an exception, but consideration should be given to repeating doses of any inactivated vaccine administered during these therapies.

[n]For persons <60 mo old undergoing chemotherapy or radiation therapy who have not received a Hib primary series plus a booster dose or at least 1 Hib dose after age 14 mo.

[o]For persons >59 mo old who are asplenic and persons ≥15 mo who are undergoing elective splenectomy and who have not received a Hib primary series and a booster dose or at least 1 Hib dose after age 14 mo.

BCG, Bacille Calmette-Guérin vaccine; CNS, central nervous system; Hib, *Haemophilus influenzae* type b vaccine; HIV/AIDS, human immunodeficiency virus/acquired immunodeficiency syndrome; IG, immune globulin; IIV, inactivated influenza vaccine; LAIV, live-attenuated influenza vaccine; MMR, measles, mumps, rubella vaccine; MMRV, measles-mumps-rubella-varicella; MCV, quadrivalent meningococcal polysaccharide vaccine; MenB, serogroup B meningococcal vaccine; OPV, oral poliovirus vaccine; PPSV23, pneumococcal polysaccharide vaccine; SCID, severe combined immunodeficiency disease; VAR, varicella; YF, yellow fever.

Adapted from Immunization in special circumstances. In Kimberlin DW, Brady MT, Jackson MA, Long SS, editors: *Red Book 2018: Report of the Committee on Infectious Diseases*, ed 31, Elk Grove Village, IL, 2018, American Academy of Pediatrics.

PRECAUTIONS AND CONTRAINDICATIONS

Observation of valid precautions and contraindications is critical to ensure that vaccines are used in the safest manner possible and to obtain optimal immunogenicity. When a child presents for immunization with a clinical condition considered a **precaution**, the physician must weigh benefits and risks to that individual child. If benefits are judged to outweigh risks, the vaccine or vaccines in question may be administered. A **contraindication** means the vaccine should not be administered under any circumstances.

A general contraindication for all vaccines is **anaphylactic reaction to a prior dose**. Anaphylactic hypersensitivity to vaccine constituents is also a contraindication. However, if a vaccine is essential, there are desensitizing protocols for some vaccines. The major constituents of concern are *egg proteins* for vaccines grown in eggs; *gelatin*, a stabilizer in many vaccines; and antimicrobial agents. The recommendations for persons with egg allergy were modified as follows: Persons with a history of egg allergy who have experienced only hives after exposure to egg should receive a flu vaccine. Persons who had reactions such

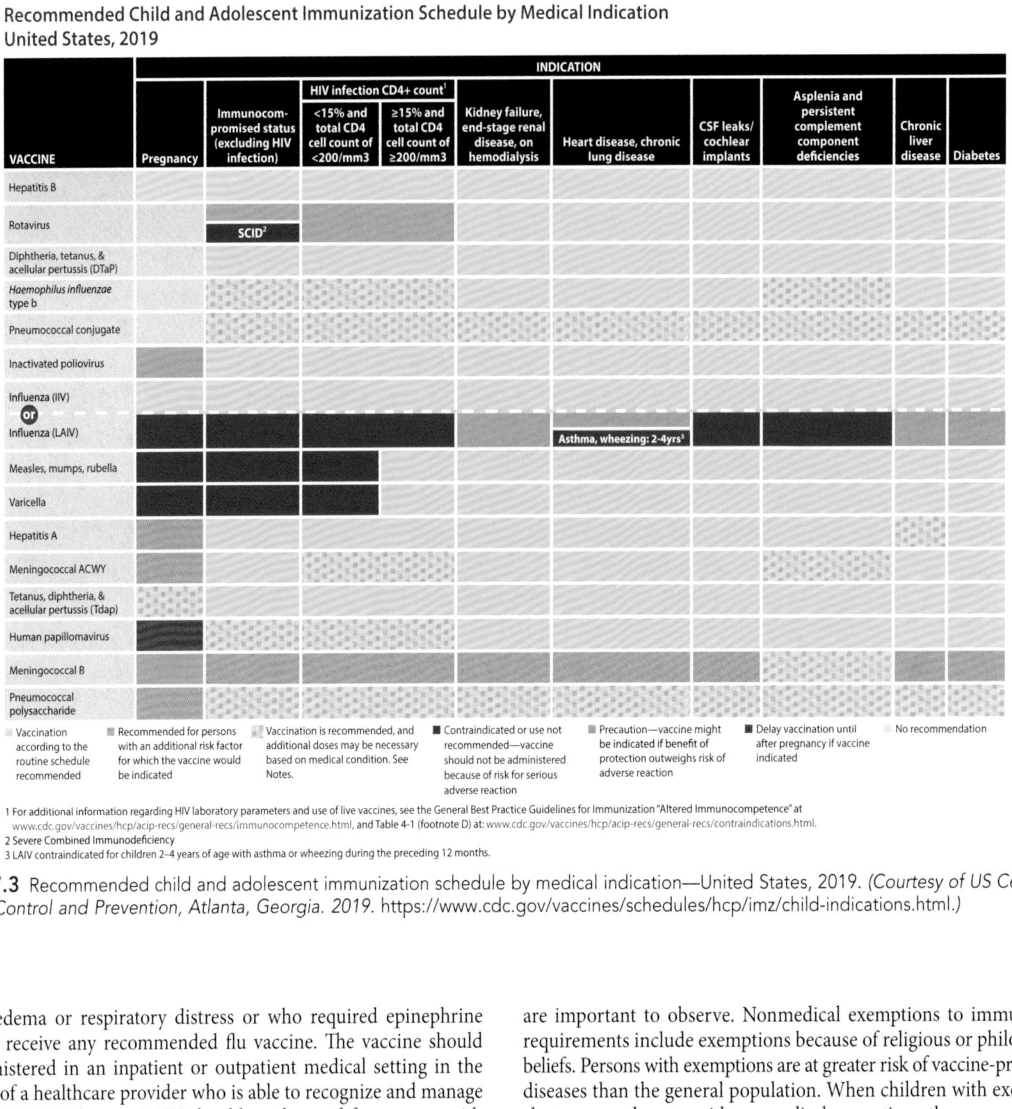

Recommended Child and Adolescent Immunization Schedule by Medical Indication
United States, 2019

VACCINE	Pregnancy	Immunocom-promised status (excluding HIV infection)	HIV infection CD4+ count[1]		Kidney failure, end-stage renal disease, on hemodialysis	Heart disease, chronic lung disease	CSF leaks/ cochlear implants	Asplenia and persistent complement component deficiencies	Chronic liver disease	Diabetes
			<15% and total CD4 cell count of <200/mm3	≥15% and total CD4 cell count of ≥200/mm3						
Hepatitis B										
Rotavirus		SCID[2]								
Diphtheria, tetanus, & acellular pertussis (DTaP)										
Haemophilus influenzae type b										
Pneumococcal conjugate										
Inactivated poliovirus										
Influenza (IIV) **or** Influenza (LAIV)						Asthma, wheezing: 2-4yrs[3]				
Measles, mumps, rubella										
Varicella										
Hepatitis A										
Meningococcal ACWY										
Tetanus, diphtheria, & acellular pertussis (Tdap)										
Human papillomavirus										
Meningococcal B										
Pneumococcal polysaccharide										

◾ Vaccination according to the routine schedule recommended   ◾ Recommended for persons with an additional risk factor for which the vaccine would be indicated   ◾ Vaccination is recommended, and additional doses may be necessary based on medical condition. See Notes.   ◾ Contraindicated or use not recommended—vaccine should not be administered because of risk for serious adverse reaction   ◾ Precaution—vaccine might be indicated if benefit of protection outweighs risk of adverse reaction   ◾ Delay vaccination until after pregnancy if vaccine indicated   No recommendation

1 For additional information regarding HIV laboratory parameters and use of live vaccines, see the General Best Practice Guidelines for Immunization "Altered Immunocompetence" at www.cdc.gov/vaccines/hcp/acip-recs/general-recs/immunocompetence.html, and Table 4-1 (footnote D) at: www.cdc.gov/vaccines/hcp/acip-recs/general-recs/contraindications.html.
2 Severe Combined Immunodeficiency
3 LAIV contraindicated for children 2–4 years of age with asthma or wheezing during the preceding 12 months.

Fig. 197.3 Recommended child and adolescent immunization schedule by medical indication—United States, 2019. *(Courtesy of US Centers for Disease Control and Prevention, Atlanta, Georgia. 2019.* https://www.cdc.gov/vaccines/schedules/hcp/imz/child-indications.html.*)*

as angioedema or respiratory distress or who required epinephrine also may receive any recommended flu vaccine. The vaccine should be administered in an inpatient or outpatient medical setting in the presence of a healthcare provider who is able to recognize and manage severe allergic conditions. LAIV should not be used for persons with a history of severe allergic reaction to any component of the vaccine (excluding egg) or to a previous dose of any influenza vaccine. The measles and mumps components of MMR are grown in chick embryo fibroblast tissue culture. However, the amount of egg protein in MMR is so small that there are no special procedures for administering the vaccine to someone with a history of anaphylaxis following egg ingestion.

Vaccines should usually be deferred in children with moderate to severe acute illnesses, regardless of the presence of fever, until the child recovers. *However, children with mild illnesses may be vaccinated.* Studies of undervaccinated children have documented opportunities that were missed because mild illness was used as an invalid contraindication. Complete tables of contraindications and contraindication misperceptions can be found at http://www.cdc.gov/vaccines/recs/vac-admin/contraindications.html.

MEDICAL EXEMPTIONS

All 50 states, the District of Columbia, and Puerto Rico have regulations requiring verification of immunization for child care and school attendance. This provides direct protection to the immunized population and indirect protection to those unable to be immunized. It also functions to improve timely immunization of children. Regulations also allow for medical exemption from immunization requirements in all 50 states, and the majority of states also have varied regulations that allow for nonmedical exemptions. Rare, medically recognized contraindications

are important to observe. Nonmedical exemptions to immunization requirements include exemptions because of religious or philosophical beliefs. Persons with exemptions are at greater risk of vaccine-preventable diseases than the general population. When children with exemptions cluster, as can happen with nonmedical exemptions, the community may be at risk for outbreaks, leading to exposure of children who cannot be protected by vaccination to vaccine-preventable diseases, such as children too young for vaccination and those with medical contraindications. (For more information, see: http://pediatrics.aappublications.org/content/early/2016/08/25/peds.2016-2145.)

IMPROVING IMMUNIZATION COVERAGE

Standards for child and adolescent immunization practices have been developed to support achievement of high levels of immunization coverage while providing vaccines in a safe and effective manner and educating parents about risks and benefits of vaccines (Table 197.10).

Despite benefits that vaccines have to offer, many children are underimmunized as a result of not receiving recommended vaccines or not receiving them at the recommended ages. Much of the underimmunization problem can be solved through physician actions. Most children have a regular source of healthcare. However, missed opportunities to provide immunizations at healthcare visits include but are not limited to failure to provide all recommended vaccines that could be administered at a single visit during that visit, failure to provide immunizations to children outside of well-child care encounters when contraindications are not present, and referral of children to public health clinics because of inability to pay for vaccines. Simultaneous administration of multiple vaccines is generally safe and effective. When the benefits of simultaneous vaccination are explained, many parents prefer such immunization to making an extra visit. Providing all needed vaccines simultaneously should be the standard of practice.

Only valid contraindications and precautions to vaccine administration should be observed. Ideally, immunizations should be provided during well-child visits; however, if no contraindications exist, it is important to administer vaccines at other visits, particularly if the child is behind in the schedule. There is no good evidence that providing immunizations outside of well-child care ultimately decreases the number of well-child visits.

Financial barriers to immunization should be minimized. Participation in the **Vaccines for Children (VFC)** program allows physicians to receive vaccines at no cost for their eligible patients, which helps such patients get immunized in their medical home.

Several interventions have been shown to help physicians increase immunization coverage in their practices. Reminder systems for children before an appointment or recall systems for children who fail to keep appointments have repeatedly been demonstrated to improve coverage. Assessment and feedback is also an important intervention. Many physicians overestimate the immunization coverage among patients they serve and thus are not motivated to make any changes in their practices to improve performance. Assessing the immunization

coverage of patients served by an individual physician with feedback of results can be a major motivator for improvement. Often, public health departments can be contacted to provide the assessments and feedback. Alternatively, physicians can perform self-assessment. Review of approximately 60 consecutive charts of 2 yr old children may provide a reasonable estimate of practice coverage. Another approach is to have a staff member review the chart of every patient coming in for a visit and placing immunization needs reminders on the chart for the physician. Electronic medical records can be designed to accomplish this goal.

VACCINE HESITANCY

The WHO characterized *vaccine hesitancy* as a delay in acceptance or refusal of vaccines despite availability of vaccination services. Factors implicated in vaccine hesitancy include complacency, convenience, and confidence. In a national telephone survey of parents of 6-23 mo olds, approximately 3% of parents refused all vaccines, and 20% refused or delayed at least 1 vaccine in the recommended schedule. Concerns about vaccine safety and questions about the necessity of vaccines are often cited as reasons for refusal. Vaccine-hesitant individuals are a heterogeneous group, and their individual concerns should be respected

Table 197.10	Standards for Child and Adolescent Immunization Practices

AVAILABILITY OF VACCINES

Vaccination services are readily available.

Vaccinations are coordinated with other healthcare services and provided in a medical home when possible.

Barriers to vaccination are identified and minimized.

Patient costs are minimized.

ASSESSMENT OF VACCINATION STATUS

Healthcare professionals review the vaccination and health status of patients at every encounter to determine which vaccines are indicated.

Healthcare professionals assess for and follow only medically accepted contraindications.

EFFECTIVE COMMUNICATION ABOUT VACCINE BENEFITS AND RISKS

Parents or guardians and patients are educated about the benefits and risks of vaccination in a culturally appropriate manner and in easy-to-understand language.*

Healthcare professionals offer strong and consistent recommendations for all universally recommended vaccines according to the current immunization schedule. They use presumptive language (e.g., these vaccines are routine) and deliver this recommendation in the same manner for all vaccines.

Healthcare professionals answer parents' or guardians' and patients' questions thoroughly and emphasize an unwavering commitment to the recommendation. If parents or guardians and patients are hesitant or refuse, healthcare professionals persevere and offer the vaccine again at the next most appropriate time.

PROPER STORAGE AND ADMINISTRATION OF VACCINES AND DOCUMENTATION OF VACCINATIONS

Healthcare professionals follow appropriate procedures for vaccine storage and handling.

Up-to-date, written vaccination protocols are accessible at all locations where vaccines are administered.

Persons who administer vaccines and staff who manage or support vaccine administration are knowledgeable and receive ongoing education.

Healthcare professionals simultaneously administer as many indicated vaccine doses as possible.

Vaccination records for patients are accurate, complete, and easily accessible.

Healthcare professionals report adverse events following vaccination promptly and accurately to the Vaccine Adverse Event Reporting System (VAERS) and are aware of a separate program, the National Vaccine Injury Compensation Program (VICP).

Healthcare professionals and personnel review the immunization timeline with parents or guardians and patients and schedule follow-up immunization visits before the family leaves the care setting.

All personnel who have contact with patients are appropriately vaccinated and communicate consistent messages about vaccines.

IMPLEMENTATION OF STRATEGIES TO IMPROVE VACCINATION COVERAGE

Systems are used to remind parents or guardians, patients, and healthcare professionals when vaccinations are due and to recall those who are overdue.

Office- or clinic-based patient record reviews and vaccination coverage assessments are performed annually.

Healthcare professionals practice community-based approaches.

Healthcare professionals understand cultural needs and disparities of different populations and use the most effective strategies for these populations.

Most healthcare visits (including acute care or sick visits) are viewed as opportunities to review immunization records, provide vaccines that are due, and catch up on missed vaccinations.

*Additional resources to help improve immunization rates include the following:
- Provider Resources for Vaccine Conversations with Parents from CDC, AAP, and American Academy of Family Physicians (www.cdc.gov/vaccines/hcp/conversations/index.html)
- American Academy of Pediatrics (AAP) Training Guide (https://shar.es/1JRNmJ)
- Centers for Disease Control and Prevention (CDC): *Pink Book*, Chapter 6: Vaccine administration (https://www.cdc.gov/vaccines/pubs/pinkbook/vac-admin.html); and quality improvement projects and educational materials (https://www.cdc.gov/vaccines/ed/index.html)
- Immunization Action Coalition: *Suggestions to improve your immunization services* (http://www.immunize.org/catg.d/p2045.pdf)

Adapted from National Vaccine Advisory Committee: Standards for child and adolescent immunization practices, *Pediatrics* 112:958–963, 2003; and Bernstein HH, Bocchini JA; AAP Committee on Infectious Diseases: The need to optimize adolescent immunization, *Pediatrics* 139(3):e20164186, 2017, and Practical approaches to optimize adolescent immunization, *Pediatrics* 139(3):e20164187, 2017.

and addressed. Multiple studies have shown that the most important factor in persuading parents to accept vaccines remains the *one-on-one contact* with an informed, caring, and concerned pediatrician. Parents should be reassured that vaccines are tested thoroughly before licensure, that ongoing mechanisms of monitoring safety exist after licensure, and that the current vaccine schedule is the only recommended schedule. It is important to stress that serious disease can occur if a child and family are not immunized, because unvaccinated children put medically exempt children who live in that same area at risk, as well as some children who have been vaccinated (while most vaccines are highly effective, no vaccine is 100% effective). Parental education can be provided through reputable sources for vaccine information (see Table 197.6). (For more information, see http://pediatrics.aappublications.org/content/early/2016/08/25/peds.2016-2146.) Provider resources for vaccine conversations with parents are available at http://www.cdc.gov/vaccines/hcp/patient-ed/conversations/index.html.

Physician concerns about liability should be addressed by appropriate documentation of discussions in the chart. The Committee on Bioethics of the AAP has published guidelines for dealing with parents' refusal of immunization. Physicians also might want to consider having parents sign a **refusal waiver**. A sample refusal-to-vaccinate waiver can be found at http://www2.aap.org/immunization/pediatricians/pdf/refusaltovaccinate.pdf.

Bibliography is available at Expert Consult.

197.1 International Immunization Practices

Jean-Marie Okwo-Bele, Tracey S. Goodman, and John David Clemens

Vaccines are used to prevent infectious diseases around the world. However, the types of vaccines in use, the indications and contraindications, and the immunization schedules vary substantially. Most developing countries follow the immunization schedules promulgated by the World Health Organization's Immunization Programme; the latest update is available at http://www.who.int/immunization/policy/Immunization_routine_table2.pdf.

According to this schedule, all children should be vaccinated at birth against tuberculosis with bacille Calmette-Guérin (BCG) vaccine. Many children also receive a dose of the live-attenuated oral polio vaccine (OPV) at this time. Immunization visits are scheduled for 6, 10, and 14 wk of age when DTP-containing vaccine and OPV are administered. At least 1 dose of injectable inactivated polio vaccine (IPV) is recommended at 14 wk of age or later for all countries using OPV. Two doses of measles vaccines are recommended, with the 1st dose given at 9-12 mo of age and the 2nd dose at 15-18 mo. Almost all developing countries have implemented hepatitis B vaccination. Two schedule options may be used, depending on epidemiologic and programmatic considerations. Hepatitis B vaccine can be given at the same time as DTP-containing vaccine doses at 6, 10, and 14 wk of age, often in combination vaccines. To prevent perinatal transmission, a birth dose of HepB should be administered as soon as possible after birth (<24 hr) and followed by 2 or 3 subsequent doses. Yellow fever and Japanese encephalitis vaccines are recommended for infants 9 mo of age living in endemic areas. Substantial efforts have been made to incorporate *Haemophilus influenzae* type b (Hib) vaccines into all but one country worldwide, in general within a DTP-containing combination vaccine.

In the past few years, the support from GAVI, the **Vaccine Alliance**, has facilitated the introduction of rotavirus and pneumococcal conjugate vaccines into developing-country immunization programs. The increased coverage with these additional vaccines will considerably reduce the global childhood morbidity and mortality caused by pneumonia, meningitis, and diarrheal diseases.

In 1988 the World Health Assembly endorsed the goal of eradicating polio from the world by the end of 2000. Although that goal has not yet been reached, endemic polio transmission was contained to 3 countries worldwide (Afghanistan, Nigeria, and Pakistan) by the end of 2016. The principal strategy is use of OPV both for routine immunization and mass campaigns in low-coverage areas, targeting all children <5 yr old for immunization, regardless of prior immunization status. Once interruption of wild poliovirus transmission is achieved, the goal is to stop the use of OPV, which in rare cases can cause vaccine-associated polio and can mutate and take on the phenotypic characteristics of the wild viruses.

Latin American countries have maintained the elimination of indigenous circulation of measles since 2002. The strategy called for attainment of high routine immunization coverage of infants with a dose at age 9 mo, a one-time mass campaign targeting all persons age 9 mo-15 yr regardless of prior immunization status, and follow-up campaigns of children born since the prior campaign, generally every 3-5 yr. Although global measles mortality has decreased by 79% worldwide in recent years, from 651,600 deaths in 2000 to 134,200 in 2015—measles is still common in many developing countries, particularly in parts of Africa and Asia. Latin American countries achieved the elimination of indigenous rubella and congenital rubella syndrome with strategies consisting of both routine immunization and mass campaigns.

Immunization schedules in the industrialized world are substantially more variable than in the developing world. Immunization recommendations for **Canada** are developed by the Canadian National Advisory Committee on Immunization but are implemented somewhat differently by each province. The Canadian schedule is similar to the U.S. immunization schedule, with a few exceptions.[*] A birth dose of hepatitis B vaccine is not specifically recommended as it is in the United States, although some northern Canadian provinces do provide a birth dose. Conjugate meningococcal C vaccine is recommended in a 1- or 2-dose series, depending on the age at the time of administration (1 dose if ≥12 mo). In contrast to the U.S. situation, hepatitis A vaccine is not recommended in Canada as a routine pediatric immunization.

There is tremendous variation in vaccines used and the immunization schedules recommended in Europe.[†] As an example, the **United Kingdom** developed an immunization schedule during the late 1980s that includes visits at 2, 3, and 4 mo of age, when a combination DTaP-Hib-IPV vaccine is administered. Following evidence that a 3-dose series of Hib vaccine at these ages was insufficient to ensure long-term, high-grade protection, a booster dose was added at 12 mo of age. MMR is recommended in a 2-dose schedule at 12 mo and 40 mo of age. During the 2nd MMR visit, a booster of DTaP and IPV is provided. A Td/IPV booster is recommended at age 14 yr. PCV13 is recommended at 2, 4, and 12 mon of age. The UK was the first country to use conjugate meningococcal C vaccine (**MCV-C**) during a massive catch-up campaign for children, adolescents, and young adults. The effectiveness of the vaccine in the 1st year was ≥88%, and herd immunity was induced with an approximate two-thirds reduction in the incidence among unvaccinated children. Given the success of this strategy, MenC vaccination at age 3 wk was discontinued as of July 2016. Now MenC is given in combination with the 4th dose of Hib at 12 mo. MenB is given at 2, 4, and 12 mo of age. In September 2008, HPV vaccine was recommended for girls 12-13 yr old. As of April 2013, the UK schedule did not include hepatitis B vaccine, varicella vaccine, or influenza vaccine for universal childhood immunization, although annual influenza vaccination is recommended for persons ≥65 yr old (see http://www.nhs.uk/conditions/vaccinations/pages/vaccination-schedule-age-checklist.aspx).

The **Japanese** immunization schedule in 2016 is substantially different from the Y.S. schedule.[‡] The Japanese do not use MMR, instead offering the choice of MR (preferred in principle) or single-antigen measles and rubella vaccination. Mumps vaccine is available on a voluntary basis. Japanese children are vaccinated routinely; against diphtheria, tetanus, pertussis, and polio with DTaP in combination with IPV; against Japanese encephalitis; and against tuberculosis with BCG. Hib, PCV, HepB, varicella, and HPV vaccines are also included in the routine vaccination

---

[*]https://www.canada.ca/en/public-health/services/provincial-territorial-immunization-information/provincial-territorial-routine-vaccination-programs-infants-children.html.
[†]http://apps.who.int/immunization_monitoring/globalsummary.
[‡]https://www.niid.go.jp/niid/images/vaccine/schedule/2016/EN20161001.pdf.

schedule and made available free of charge under the **Preventive Vaccinations Act**. Adults ≥65 yr old receive annual influenza vaccinations. Rotavirus, HepA (from age 1 yr and above), meningococcus (ACWY) (from age 2 yr and above), and yellow fever vaccines are available on a voluntary basis.

Some children come to the United States having started or completed international immunization schedules with vaccines produced outside the United States. In general, doses administered in other countries should be considered valid if administered at the same ages as recommended in the United States. For missing doses, age-inappropriate doses, lost immunization records, or other concerns, pediatricians have 2 options: administer or repeat missing or inappropriate doses, or perform serologic tests, and if they are negative, administer vaccines.

Bibliography is available at Expert Consult.

Chapter **198**
Infection Prevention and Control

Michael J. Chusid and Joan P. Moran

第一百九十八章
感染预防和控制

中文导读

　　本章主要介绍了手卫生、标准防护、隔离、其他措施、外科预防、雇员健康。在标准防护中详细阐述了接触传播和接触隔离、液滴传播和液滴隔离、空气传播和空气隔离，以及对患者进行分类管理等。在外科预防中详细介绍了清洁伤口、清洁污染伤口、污染伤口、脏的感染伤口的定义及预防措施。在雇员健康部分着重强调了预防接种疫苗的重要性。

Infection prevention and control (**IPC**) programs have an important role in pediatric medicine. To be fully effective, IPC programs require a functional infrastructure that addresses collaboration with the public health system, widespread immunizations, and use of appropriate techniques to prevent transmission of infection within the general population and within healthcare institutions. The national focus on preventing **healthcare-associated infection (HAI)** is exemplified by The Joint Commission's 2017 National Patient Safety Goals, with 5 of the 16 elements related to reduction and prevention of HAI. Governmental agencies and insurance providers have reduced or eliminated payment to institutions for expenses associated with certain HAIs, and a host of national organizations have been established to monitor and report rates of HAI at healthcare facilities.

HAIs or **nosocomial infections** refer to infections acquired during hospitalization or acquired in other healthcare settings, such as nursing homes or ambulatory surgical care centers. An estimated 3–5% of children admitted to hospitals acquire an HAI. Rates are highest in patients undergoing invasive procedures. Infections can also be acquired in emergency departments, physicians' offices, daycare, and long-term care settings. **Medical device–associated infections** occur in both the home and the hospital. Adequate education of home health providers as well as of families is essential to prevent or minimize device-associated infections, since increasing numbers of children are sent home from the hospital with intravenous (IV) catheters and other medical devices in place.

Susceptibility to HAI includes host factors, recent invasive procedures, presence of catheters or other devices, prolonged use of antibiotics, contaminated physical environment, and exposure to other patients, visitors, or healthcare providers with active contagious infections or colonized with invasive microorganisms. Host factors increasing the risk for HAI include anatomic abnormalities (dermal sinuses, cleft palate, obstructive uropathy), abnormal skin, organ dysfunction, malnutrition, and underlying diseases or comorbidities. Invasive procedures can introduce potential pathogens by breaching normal anatomic host barriers. IV and other catheters provide direct access to sterile anatomic sites for usually minimally pathogenic organisms, as well as adherent surfaces for microbial binding, and can disrupt patterns of normally protective flow of mucus (e.g., nasotracheal tubes and sinus ostia). Antibiotic use can alter the composition of bowel flora and encourage the multiplication and emergence of toxigenic or invasive organisms already present in small numbers in the gut, such as *Clostridium difficile* and *Salmonella* spp.

Transmission of infectious agents occurs by various routes, but by far the most common and important route is the **hands**. Medical equipment, toys, and hospital and office furnishings can become microbially contaminated and thus have a role in transmission of potential pathogens. Pagers, phones, computer keyboards, and even neckties become easily contaminated. These inanimate objects serve as **fomites** for bacteria. There is increasing recognition of the importance of the healthcare environment in the acquisition of organisms such as methicillin-resistant *Staphylococcus aureus* (MRSA), vancomycin-resistant enterococci (VRE), multidrug-resistant gram-negative bacilli (MDR-GNB), *C. difficile,* and respiratory syncytial virus (RSV). Thermometers and other equipment that come in contact with mucous membranes pose special risks. Some agents are easily disseminated by airborne transmission, such as varicella virus, measles virus, and *Mycobacterium tuberculosis.* Food can be contaminated and has been involved in hospital outbreaks of nosocomial infection. The hospital physical environment can also serve as a risk factor for infection, particularly for immunocompromised patients. Rainwater or plumbing leaks have been associated with bacterial and fungal infections, new construction or renovation with airborne fungal infection, and contamination of an institution's potable water supply with bacterial, fungal, and atypical mycobacterial nosocomial infections. Widespread outbreaks of infection have been associated with mycobacterial contamination of equipment during the manufacturing process.

Common causes of HAI in children are seasonal viruses such as rotavirus and respiratory viral agents, staphylococci, and gram-negative bacilli. Fungi and multidrug-resistant organisms are common causes of infection in immunocompromised children as well as those requiring intensive care and prolonged hospitalization. Common sites of infection are the respiratory tract, gastrointestinal (GI) tract, bloodstream, skin, and urinary tract.

Liberalization of visitation policies and in-hospital animal visitation has increased the likelihood of HAI acquisition. The use of contaminated pharmaceutical products such as injectable depot corticosteroids has led to outbreaks of fatal fungal HAIs.

HAIs cause considerable morbidity and occasional mortality of hospitalized children. Infections prolong hospital stays and increase healthcare costs. **Surveillance**, the initial step in identifying such infections and suggesting methods for prevention, is the responsibility of **infection preventionists**. Within hospitals, oversight of such surveillance is usually the responsibility of the **infection prevention and control committee**, a multidisciplinary group that collects and reviews surveillance data, establishes institutional policies, and investigates intrainstitutional infection outbreaks. The chair of the committee is often an infectious disease specialist. Surveillance in outpatient settings and during home care is often less well defined. Local, state, and federal health departments play important roles in identifying and controlling outbreaks and in establishing public health policy.

HAND HYGIENE

The most important tool in any IPC program is good hand hygiene. Although much attention is directed at the type of cleansing agent employed, the most important aspect of handwashing is *placing the hands under water and using friction with or without soap.* Studies show that a 15-second scrub removes the majority of transient, surface flora but does not alter deeper resident flora. A variety of hand gels and rubs can be used in place of handwashing. **Waterless hand hygiene** products increase hand hygiene compliance and save time; these agents are the preferred agents for routine hand hygiene when hands are not visibly soiled. These products are effective in killing most microbes but do not remove dirt or debris. However, they are ineffective against nonenveloped agents such as norovirus and *C. difficile* spores, requiring the use of other cleansing products during hospital *C. difficile* outbreaks. Hands should be cleaned before and after every patient encounter. In hospital handwashing compliance studies, physicians are usually the least compliant group studied, and compliance programs must pay special attention to this group of caregivers.

STANDARD PRECAUTIONS

Standard precautions, formerly known as u*niversal precautions*, are intended to protect healthcare workers from pathogens and should be used whenever there is direct contact with patients. Infected patients are often contagious before symptoms of disease develop. Asymptomatic infected patients are quite capable of transmitting infectious agents. Standard precautions involve the use of barriers—gloves, gowns, masks, goggles, and face shields—as needed, to prevent transmission of microbes associated with contact with blood and body fluids (Table 198.1).

ISOLATION

Isolation of patients infected with transmissible pathogens decreases the risk of nosocomial transmission of organisms to staff and other patients. The specific type of isolation depends on the infecting agent and potential route of transmission. **Transmission by contact** is the most common mode of pathogen transmission and involves direct contact with the patient or contact with a contaminated intermediate object. **Contact isolation** requires the use of gown and gloves when in contact with the patient or immediate surroundings. **Transmission by droplets** involves the propulsion of infectious large particles over a short distance (<3 ft), with deposition on another's mucous membranes or skin. **Droplet isolation** requires the use of gloves and gowns, as well as masks and eye guards when closer than 3 ft to the patient. **Airborne transmission** occurs by dissemination of evaporated droplet nuclei (≤5 μm) or dust particles carrying an infectious agent. **Airborne infection isolation** (**AII**) requires the use of masks and negative pressure air-handling systems to prevent spread of the infectious agent. In the case of active pulmonary tuberculosis in older children and adults, severe acute respiratory syndrome (SARS), or avian influenza, the use of special high-density masks (N-95) or self-contained breathing systems such as powered air-purifying respirators (**PAPRs**) or controlled air-purifying respirators (**CAPRs**) are recommended. Positive pressure HEPA-filtered air-handling systems are used in some institutions for housing seriously immunocompromised patients and negative pressure systems for the care of patients with highly contagious respiratory infections such as Ebola virus.

Standard precautions are indicated for all patients and are appropriate for use in the clinic as well as the hospital. Additionally, for hospitalized patients, further **transmission-based precautions** are indicated for certain infections (Table 198.2). For contact and droplet isolation, single rooms are preferred but not required. Cohorting children infected with the same pathogen is acceptable, but the etiologic diagnosis should be confirmed by laboratory methods before exposing infected children to one another. Transmission-based isolation precautions should be continued for as long as a patient is considered contagious.

The use of isolation techniques in outpatient settings has not been well studied. Professional offices should establish procedures to ensure that proper cleaning, disinfection, and sterilization methods are employed. Many practices and clinics provide separate waiting areas for sick and well children. **Triage** of patients is essential to ensure that contagious children or adults are not present in waiting areas. Outbreaks of measles and varicella in patients within the waiting area have been reported where the air exhaust from examination rooms enters the waiting area. Cleaning the clinic environment is important, especially in high-touch areas. Toys and items that are shared among patients should be cleaned between uses; if feasible, disposable toys should be used. Toys contaminated with blood or body fluids should be autoclaved or discarded.

ADDITIONAL MEASURES

Other preventive measures include aseptic technique, catheter care, prudent use of antibiotics through use of an effective **antibiotic stewardship program**, isolation of contagious patients, periodic cleansing of the environment, disinfection and sterilization of medical equipment, reporting of infections, safe handling of needles and other sharp instruments, and establishment of employee health services. Sterile technique must be used for all invasive procedures, including catheter placement and manipulation. The use of barrier techniques at the time of IV catheter placement has reduced the rate of catheter-related bloodstream infections

Table 198.1	Recommendations for Application of Standard Precautions for Care of All Patients in All Healthcare Settings
COMPONENT	**RECOMMENDATIONS**
Hand hygiene	Before and after each patient contact, regardless of whether gloves are used.
	After contact with blood, body fluids, secretions, excretions, or contaminated items; immediately after removing gloves; before and after entering patient rooms.
	Alcohol-containing antiseptic hand rubs preferred except when hands are visibly soiled with blood or other proteinaceous material or if exposure to spores (e.g., *Clostridium difficile, Bacillus anthracis*) or nonenveloped viruses (norovirus) is likely to have occurred; in these cases, soap and water is required.
PERSONAL PROTECTIVE EQUIPMENT (PPE)	
Gloves	For touching blood, body fluids, secretions, excretions, or contaminated items; for touching mucous membranes and nonintact skin.
	Employ hand hygiene before and after glove use.
Gown	During procedures and patient-care activities when contact of clothing or exposed skin with blood, body fluids, secretions, or excretions is anticipated.
Mask, eye protection (goggles), face shield	During procedures and patient-care activities likely to generate splashes or sprays of blood, body fluids, or secretions, such as suctioning and endotracheal intubation, to protect healthcare personnel.
	For patient protection, use of a mask by the person inserting an epidural anesthesia needle or performing myelograms when prolonged exposure of the puncture site is likely to occur.
Soiled patient-care equipment	Handle in a manner that prevents transfer of microorganisms to others and to the environment.
	Wear gloves if equipment is visibly contaminated.
	Perform hand hygiene.
ENVIRONMENT	
Environmental control	Develop procedures for routine care, cleaning, and disinfection of environmental surfaces, especially frequently touched surfaces in patient-care areas.
Textiles (linens) and laundry	Handle in a manner that prevents transfer of microorganisms to others and the environment.
PATIENT CARE	
Injection practices (use of needles and other sharps)	Do not recap, bend, break, or manipulate used needles; if recapping is required, use a one-handed scoop technique only.
	Use needle-free safety devices when available, placing used sharps in puncture-resistant container.
	Use a sterile, single-use, disposable needle and syringe for each injection.
	Single-dose medication vials preferred when medications may be administered to more than one patient.
Patient resuscitation	Use mouthpiece, resuscitation bag, or other ventilation devices to prevent contact with mouth and oral secretions.
Patient placement	Prioritize for single-patient room if patient is at increased risk for transmission, is likely to contaminate the environment, is unable to maintain appropriate hygiene, or is at increased risk for acquiring infection or developing adverse outcome following infection.
Respiratory hygiene/cough etiquette (source containment of infectious respiratory secretions in symptomatic patients) beginning at initial point of encounter, such as triage or reception areas in emergency department or physician office	Instruct symptomatic persons to cover nose/mouth when sneezing or coughing; use tissues with disposal in no-touch receptacles.
	Employ hand hygiene after soiling of hands with respiratory secretions.
	Wear surgical mask if tolerated or maintain spatial separation (>3 ft if possible).

Adapted from Kimberlin DW, Brady MT, Jackson MA, et al, editors: *Red Book 2018–2021: Report of the Committee on Infectious Diseases*, ed 31, Elk Grove Village, IL, 2018, American Academy of Pediatrics, pp 148–150.

by half. Appropriate catheter use also includes limiting the duration and number of catheters employed, scrubbing catheter hubs with every access, and removing catheters as soon as they become unnecessary.

SURGICAL PROPHYLAXIS

Surgical antibiotic prophylaxis should be employed when there is a high risk of postoperative infection or when the consequences of such infection would be catastrophic. The choice of prophylactic antibiotic depends on the surgical site and type of surgery. A useful classification of surgical procedures based on infectious risk recognizes 4 preoperative wound categories: clean wounds, clean-contaminated wounds, contaminated wounds, and dirty and infected wounds (Table 198.3). The American College of Surgeons, Surgical Infection Society, and American Academy of Pediatrics have made clinical recommendations regarding antibiotic prophylaxis.

Clean wounds are uninfected operative wounds where no inflammation is noted at the operative site and respiratory, alimentary, and genitourinary tracts and the oropharynx are not entered. Such wounds are often the result of nonemergent procedures with primary closure or drained by a closed system. Operative incisional wounds after nonpenetrating trauma are included in this category. For clean wounds, prophylactic antimicrobial therapy is *not* recommended except in patients at high risk for infection and in circumstances where the consequences of infection would be potentially life threatening, as with implantation of a foreign body such as a prosthetic heart valve or cerebrospinal fluid shunt, open heart surgery for repair of structural defects, and surgery in immunocompromised patients or small infants.

Clean-contaminated wounds are operative wounds in which the respiratory, alimentary, or genitourinary tract is entered under controlled conditions and that do not have unusual bacterial contamination

Table 198.2	Clinical Syndromes and Conditions Warranting Empirical Transmission-Based Precautions in Addition to Standard Precautions Pending Confirmation of Diagnosis*

CLINICAL SYNDROME OR CONDITION†	POTENTIAL PATHOGENS‡	EMPIRICAL PRECAUTIONS (ALWAYS INCLUDES STANDARD PRECAUTIONS)
DIARRHEA		
Acute diarrhea with a likely infectious cause in an incontinent or diapered patient	Enteric pathogens§	Contact precautions (pediatrics and adult)
Meningitis	*Neisseria meningitidis*	Droplet precautions for 1st 24 hr of antimicrobial therapy; mask and face protection for intubation
	Enteroviruses	Contact precautions for infants and children
	Mycobacterium tuberculosis	Airborne precautions if pulmonary infiltrate
		Airborne precautions plus contact precautions if potentially infectious draining body fluid present
RASH OR EXANTHEMS, GENERALIZED, ETIOLOGY UNKNOWN		
Petechial/ecchymotic with fever (general)	*N. meningitidis*	Droplet precautions for 1st 24 hr of antimicrobial therapy
If positive history of travel to an area with an ongoing outbreak of VHF in the 10 days before onset of fever	Ebola, Lassa, and Marburg viruses	Droplet precautions plus contact precautions, with face/eye protection, emphasizing safety sharps and barrier precautions when blood exposure likely Use N95 or higher respiratory protection when aerosol-generating procedure performed.
Vesicular	Varicella-zoster, herpes simplex, variola (smallpox), and vaccinia viruses	Airborne precautions plus contact precautions
	Vaccinia virus	Contact precautions only if herpes simplex, localized zoster in an immunocompetent host, or vaccinia viruses likely
Maculopapular with cough, coryza, and fever	Rubeola (measles) virus	Airborne precautions
RESPIRATORY INFECTIONS		
Cough/fever/upper lobe pulmonary infiltrate in HIV-negative patient or patient at low risk for HIV infection	*M. tuberculosis*, respiratory viruses, *Streptococcus pneumoniae*, *Staphylococcus aureus* (MSSA or MRSA)	Airborne precautions plus contact precautions
Cough/fever/pulmonary infiltrate in any lung location in HIV-infected patient or patient at high risk for HIV infection	*M. tuberculosis*, respiratory viruses, *S. pneumoniae*, *S. aureus* (MSSA or MRSA)	Airborne precautions plus contact precautions Use eye/face protection if aerosol-generating procedure performed or contact with respiratory secretions anticipated. If tuberculosis is unlikely and there are no AIIRs or respirators available, use droplet precautions instead of airborne precautions. Tuberculosis is more likely in HIV-infected than in HIV-negative patients.
Cough/fever/pulmonary infiltrate in any lung location in patient with history of recent travel (10-21 days) to countries with active outbreaks of SARS, avian influenza	*M. tuberculosis*, severe acute respiratory syndrome virus (SARS-CoV), avian influenza	Airborne precautions plus contact precautions plus eye protection If SARS and tuberculosis unlikely, use droplet precautions instead of airborne precautions.
Respiratory infections, particularly bronchiolitis and pneumonia, in infants and young children	Respiratory syncytial virus, parainfluenza virus, adenovirus, influenza virus, human metapneumovirus	Contact plus droplet precautions Droplet precautions may be discontinued when adenovirus and influenza have been ruled out.
SKIN OR WOUND INFECTION		
Abscess or draining wound that cannot be covered	*S. aureus* (MSSA or MRSA), group A streptococcus	Contact precautions Add droplet precautions for 1st 24 hr of appropriate antimicrobial therapy if invasive group A streptococcal disease is suspected.

*Infection control professionals should modify or adapt this table according to local conditions. To ensure that appropriate empirical precautions are always implemented, hospitals must have systems in place to evaluate patients routinely according to these criteria as part of their preadmission and admission care.

†Patients with the syndromes or conditions listed may present with atypical signs or symptoms (e.g., neonates and adults with pertussis may not have paroxysmal or severe cough). The clinician's index of suspicion should be guided by the prevalence of specific conditions in the community as well as clinical judgment.

‡The organisms listed are not intended to represent the complete, or even most likely, diagnoses, but rather possible etiologic agents that require additional precautions beyond standard precautions, until they can be ruled out.

§These pathogens include enterohemorrhagic *Escherichia coli* O157:H7, *Shigella* spp., hepatitis A virus, norovirus, rotavirus, *Clostridium difficile*.

AIIRs, Airborne infection isolation rooms; HIV, human immunodeficiency virus; MRSA, methicillin-resistant *S. aureus*; MSSA, methicillin-susceptible *S. aureus*; VHF, viral hemorrhagic fever.

Adapted from Centers for Disease Control and Preventionwebsite,http://www.cdc.gov/hicpac/2007ip/2007ip_table2.html.

preoperatively. These wounds occur in operations that involve the biliary tract, appendix, vagina, and oropharynx where no evidence of infection or major break in technique is encountered, as well as in urgent or emergency surgery in an otherwise clean procedure. In procedures involving clean-contaminated wounds, the risk for bacterial contamination and infection is variable. Recommendations for pediatric patients derived from adult data suggest that antibiotic prophylaxis be provided for procedures in children with obstructive jaundice, certain alimentary tract procedures, and urinary tract surgery or instrumentation in the presence of bacteriuria or obstructive uropathy.

Table 198.3	Common Surgical Procedures for Which Perioperative Prophylactic Antibiotics Are Recommended		
SURGICAL PROCEDURE	**LIKELY PATHOGENS**	**RECOMMENDED DRUGS**	**NON β-LACTAM ALTERNATIVE**
CLEAN WOUNDS			
Cardiac surgery (e.g., open heart surgery) Vascular surgery Neurosurgery Orthopedic surgery (e.g., joint replacement)	Skin flora, enteric gram-negative bacilli	Cefazolin or cefuroxime	Clindamycin or vancomycin
CLEAN-CONTAMINATED WOUNDS			
Head and neck surgery involving oral cavity or pharynx	Skin flora, oral anaerobes, oral streptococci	Cefazolin + metronidazole, ampicillin-sulbactam	Clindamycin
Gastrointestinal and genitourinary surgery	Enteric gram-negative bacilli, anaerobes, gram-positive cocci	Cefazolin + metronidazole, cefotetan or piperacillin-sulbactam If colon is involved, consider bacterial reduction with oral neomycin and erythromycin.	Clindamycin
CONTAMINATED WOUNDS			
Traumatic wounds (e.g., compound fracture)	Skin flora	Cefazolin	Clindamycin or vancomycin
DIRTY WOUNDS			
Appendectomy, penetrating abdominal wounds, colorectal surgery	Enteric gram-negative bacilli, anaerobes, gram-positive cocci	Cefazolin + metronidazole, cefoxitin, cefotetan or ampicillin-sulbactam	Clindamycin + aminoglycoside

Adapted from Bratzler DW, Dellinger PD, Olsen KM, et al: Clinical practice guidelines from antimicrobial prophylaxis in surgery, *Am J Health Syst Pharm* 70:195–283, 2013.

Contaminated wounds include open, fresh, and accidental wounds; major breaks in otherwise sterile operative technique; gross spillage from the GI tract; penetrating trauma occurring <4 hr earlier; and incisions where acute nonpurulent inflammation is encountered.

Dirty and infected wounds include penetrating traumatic wounds >4 hr before surgery, wounds with retained devitalized tissue, and those in which clinical infection is apparent or the viscera have been perforated. In contaminated and dirty or infected wound procedures, antimicrobial therapy is indicated and may need to be continued for several days. In these patients, antibiotic therapy is considered therapeutic rather than truly prophylactic.

Prophylactic antibiotics should be administered, preferably intravenously, within 1 hr before skin incision, with the intent of having peak serum concentrations of the drug present in blood and tissues at the time of incision. Adequate plasma and tissue concentration of the antibiotic should be maintained until the incision is closed. Intraoperative antibiotic dosing may be necessary if surgery is prolonged or the antibiotic being employed has a short intravascular half-life. Continuation of prophylactic therapy after the procedure is not recommended. In cases of contaminated surgical sites, antibiotics are continued as therapy for infection at the site. For patients undergoing colonic procedures, additional oral antibiotics may be employed and should also be given the day before surgery.

The selection of antibiotic regimen for prophylaxis is based on the procedure, the likely contaminating organisms, and antibiotic. Because of the variety of antibiotics available, many regimens are acceptable (see Table 198.3).

EMPLOYEE HEALTH

Employee health is important in hospital-based infection control because employees are at risk for acquiring infection from patients, and infected employees pose a potential risk to patients. This risk is minimized by use of standard precautions and hand hygiene before and after all patient contacts. Within hospitals, employee health services or departments of occupational safety and health manage employee health issues. New employees should be screened for the presence of infectious diseases. Their immunization history should be noted and necessary immunizations offered.

All healthcare workers (medical and nonmedical, paid or volunteer, full-time or part-time, student or nonstudent, with or without patient care responsibilities) who work within facilities providing healthcare, inpatient or outpatient, should be immune to **measles, rubella, and varicella**. All workers who are at risk of exposure to blood or body fluids should be immunized against **hepatitis B**. In pediatric institutions, employees with patient contact should be urged to receive the **pertussis booster** vaccine. Annual **influenza** immunization is strongly recommended for all healthcare workers, and institutions are being ranked publically regarding employee immunization rates as a measure of quality of care. Many healthcare facilities have now made annual influenza vaccination mandatory for employees unless there are legitimate medical reasons for nonimmunization. Such a program reduces staff illness and absenteeism and decreases HAI. Immunizations should be encouraged and provided free of charge whenever possible to enhance compliance. All healthcare workers with duties involving face-to-face contact with patients with suspected or confirmed **tuberculosis** (including transport staff) should be included in a tuberculosis screening program at the time of hiring and may require periodic retesting if the workplace is determined to be a high-prevalence environment for tuberculosis.

Each medical office and hospital must comply with the rules developed by the U.S. Occupational Safety and Health Administration (OSHA). Each office and hospital should have written policies about exclusion of infected and ill staff from direct patient care. Staff should be encouraged not to report for work if they are ill. Regular educational sessions should be performed to ensure that staff are aware of IPC methods and that they adhere to such policies.

Bibliography is available at Expert Consult.

Chapter 199

Childcare and Communicable Diseases

Ana M. Vaughan and Susan E. Coffin

第一百九十九章

儿童保育和传染病

中文导读

　　本章首先介绍了儿童保育过程中传染病的流行病学特点，随后详细介绍了呼吸道感染、胃肠道感染、皮肤病的常见病原菌及好发人群。另外，详细描述了在保育院的儿童比家庭看护的儿童更常见的侵入微生物、疱疹病毒、血液传播的病原体和耐药菌的感染现状。此外，针对预防措施及预防准则进行了详细阐述。其中，在预防措施中尤其强调了手卫生的重要性。

More than 20 million children <5 yr old attend a childcare facility. These facilities can include part-day or full-day programs at nursery schools or preschools and full-day programs based in either a licensed childcare center or another person's home. Regardless of the age at entry, children entering daycare are more prone to infections, largely from the exposure to greater numbers of children.

Childcare facilities can be classified on the basis of number of children enrolled, ages of attendees, health status of the children enrolled, and type of setting. As defined in the United States, **childcare facilities** consist of childcare centers, small and large family childcare homes, and facilities for ill children or for children with special needs. Centers are licensed and regulated by state governments and care for a larger number of children than are typically cared for in family homes. In contrast, **family childcare homes** are designated as small (1-6 children) or large (7-12 children), may be full-day or part-day and may be designed for either daily or sporadic attendance. Family childcare homes generally are not licensed or registered, depending on state requirements.

Although the majority of children who attend childcare facilities are cared for in family childcare homes, most studies of infectious diseases in infants and toddlers have been conducted in childcare centers. Almost any organism has the potential to be spread and to cause disease in a childcare setting. Epidemiologic studies have established that children in childcare facilities are 2-18 times more likely to acquire a variety of infectious diseases than children not enrolled in childcare (Table 199.1). Children who attend childcare facilities are more likely to receive more courses of antimicrobial agents for longer periods and to acquire antibiotic-resistant organisms. Transmission of infectious agents in group care depends on the age and immune status of the children, season, hygiene practices, crowding, and environmental characteristics of the facilities. The pathogen characteristics, including infectivity, survivability in the environment, and virulence, also influence transmission in childcare settings. Rates of infection, duration of illness, and risk for hospitalization tend to decrease among children in childcare facilities after the 1st 6 mo of attendance and decline to levels observed among homebound children after 3 yr of age. Adult caregivers are also at increased risk for acquiring and transmitting infectious diseases, particularly in the 1st yr of working in these settings.

EPIDEMIOLOGY

Respiratory tract infections and **gastroenteritis** are the most common diseases associated with childcare. These infections occur in children and their household contacts, as well as childcare workers, and can spread into the community. The severity of illness caused by a given respiratory and enteric pathogen depends on the person's underlying health status, the inoculum, and prior exposures to the pathogen, either by infection or immunization. Hepatitis B virus (HBV) transmission has been reported rarely in a childcare setting. Transmission of hepatitis C virus (HCV), hepatitis D virus (HDV), and HIV has not been reported in a childcare setting. Some organisms, such as hepatitis A virus (HAV), can cause subclinical disease in young children and produce overt and sometimes serious disease in older children and adults. Other diseases, such as otitis media and varicella, usually affect children rather than adults. Several agents, such as cytomegalovirus and parvovirus B19, can have serious consequences for the fetuses of pregnant women or for immunocompromised persons. Because many childcare workers are women of childbearing age, they should be encouraged to discuss possible risks with their physician if they become pregnant. Both

Table 199.1	Infectious Diseases in the Childcare Setting

DISEASE	INCREASED INCIDENCE WITH CHILDCARE
RESPIRATORY TRACT INFECTIONS	
Otitis media	Yes
Sinusitis	Probably
Pharyngitis	Probably
Pneumonia	Yes
GASTROINTESTINAL TRACT INFECTIONS	
Diarrhea (rotavirus, calicivirus, astrovirus, enteric adenovirus, *Giardia lamblia*, *Cryptosporidium*, *Shigella*, *Escherichia coli* O157:H7, and *Clostridium difficile*)	Yes
Hepatitis A	Yes
SKIN DISEASES	
Impetigo	Probably
Scabies	Probably
Pediculosis	Probably
Tinea (ringworm)	Probably
INVASIVE BACTERIA INFECTIONS	
Haemophilus influenzae type b	No*
Neisseria meningitidis	Probably
Streptococcus pneumoniae	Yes
ASEPTIC MENINGITIS	
Enteroviruses	Probably
HERPESVIRUS INFECTIONS	
Cytomegalovirus	Yes
Varicella-zoster virus	Yes
Herpes simplex virus	Probably
BLOODBORNE INFECTIONS	
Hepatitis B	Few case reports
HIV	No cases reported
Hepatitis C	No cases reported
VACCINE-PREVENTABLE DISEASES	
Measles, mumps, rubella, diphtheria, pertussis, tetanus	Not established
Polio	No
H. influenzae type b	No*
Varicella	Yes
Rotavirus	Yes

*Not in the post–vaccine era; yes in the pre–vaccine era.

infections and infestations of the skin and hair may be acquired through contact with contaminated linens or through close personal contact, which is inevitable in childcare settings.

RESPIRATORY TRACT INFECTIONS

Respiratory tract infections account for the majority of childcare-related illnesses. Children <2 yr old who attend childcare centers have more upper and lower respiratory tract infections than do age-matched children not in childcare. The organisms responsible for these illnesses are similar to those that circulate in the community and include respiratory syncytial virus (RSV), parainfluenza viruses, influenza viruses, human metapneumoviruses, adenoviruses, rhinoviruses, coronaviruses, parvovirus B19, and *Streptococcus pneumoniae*.

Upper respiratory tract infections, including **otitis media**, are among the most common manifestation of these infections. The risk for developing otitis media is 2-3 times greater among children who attend childcare centers than among children cared for at home. Most prescriptions for antibiotics for children <3 yr old in childcare are to treat otitis media. These children also are at increased risk for recurrent otitis media, further increasing use of antimicrobial agents in this population.

Studies have demonstrated reductions in both otitis media and antibiotic use subsequent to pneumococcal vaccination implementation. Pharyngeal carriage of group A streptococcus occurs earlier among children in childcare, although outbreaks of clinical infections with this organism are uncommon. **Influenza** vaccination of younger infants reduces influenza infection and secondary sequelae in both the children and the adults who care for them, in their home and in childcare settings. Following adoption of the acellular pertussis vaccine, increases in clusters and outbreaks of infection caused by *Bordetella pertussis* have led to the recognition of less durable immunity, with older children and adults serving as reservoirs of infection.

Transmission of these organisms typically occurs through either direct or indirect contact with the respiratory droplets of an infected child. In childcare settings, contamination of surfaces occurs frequently as children mouth toys, drool, and cough or sneeze. Additionally, some respiratory pathogens are spread through large droplets that typically can travel 3-6 ft. However, intimate contact between children is a routine part of the play and care of young children, thus facilitating transmission. The most common surfaces from which airborne droplets can be spread are the hands, so the most efficient form of infection control in the childcare setting is good handwashing.

GASTROINTESTINAL TRACT INFECTIONS

Acute infectious **diarrhea** is 2-3 times more common among children in childcare than among children cared for in their homes. Outbreaks of diarrhea, which occur frequently in childcare centers, are usually caused by enteric viruses such as caliciviruses, enteric adenoviruses, and astroviruses, or by enteric parasites such as *Giardia lamblia* or *Cryptosporidium*. A dramatic and sustained decline in the burden of rotavirus infection has been demonstrated since introduction of the rotavirus vaccination program in 2006, and this trend is likely reflected in the daycare population as well. Bacterial **enteropathogens** such as *Shigella* and *Escherichia coli* O157:H7, and less often *Campylobacter*, *Clostridium difficile*, and *Bacillus cereus*, also have caused outbreaks of diarrhea in childcare settings. *Salmonella* rarely is associated with outbreaks of diarrhea in childcare settings, because person-to-person spread of this organism is uncommon.

Outbreaks of **hepatitis A** in children enrolled in childcare facilities have resulted in community-wide outbreaks. Hepatitis A is typically mild or asymptomatic in young children and often is identified only after symptomatic illness becomes apparent among either older children or adult contacts of children in childcare. Enteropathogens and HAV are transmitted in childcare facilities by the fecal-oral route and can also be transmitted through contaminated food or water. Children in diapers constitute a high risk for the spread of gastrointestinal infections through the fecal-oral route. As such, enteric illness and HAV infection are more common in centers that care for children who are not toilet-trained and where proper hygienic practices are not followed. The most common enteropathogens, such as norovirus and *G. lamblia*, are characterized by low infective doses and high rates of asymptomatic excretion among children in childcare, characteristics that facilitate transmission and outbreaks.

SKIN DISEASES

The most commonly recognized skin infections or infestations in children in childcare are impetigo caused by *S. aureus* or group A streptococcus, pediculosis, scabies, tinea capitis and tinea corporis, and molluscum. Many of these diseases are spread by contact with infected linens, clothing, hairbrushes, and hats and through direct personal contact; they more often affect children >2 yr old. The magnitude of these infections and infestations in children in childcare is not known.

Parvovirus B19, which causes fifth disease (erythema infectiosum), is spread through the respiratory route and has been associated with outbreaks in childcare centers. The rash of fifth disease is a systemic manifestation of parvovirus B19 infection; the child is no longer contagious once the rash is present (see Chapter 278). The greatest health hazard is for pregnant women and immunocompromised hosts, because of their respective risks for fetal loss and aplastic crisis.

INVASIVE ORGANISMS

Prior to universal immunization, *Haemophilus influenzae* type b invasive disease was more common among children in childcare than children in homecare. Although the largest burden of invasive *H. influenza* infection in the pediatric population still occurs in children <5 yr old, infection is now caused primarily by nontypeable *H. influenzae*; there have been no reported outbreaks of nontypeable or type b *H. influenzae* in >5 yr in the United States.

Data suggest that the risk for primary disease caused by *Neisseria meningitidis* is higher among children in childcare than among children in homecare. Childcare attendance is also associated with nasopharyngeal carriage of penicillin-resistant *S. pneumoniae* and invasive pneumococcal disease, especially among children with a history of recurrent otitis media and use of antibiotics. Secondary spread of *S. pneumoniae* and *N. meningitidis* has been reported, indicating the potential for outbreaks to occur in this setting. Routine use of pneumococcal conjugate vaccine has decreased the incidence of invasive disease and reduced carriage of serotypes of *S. pneumoniae* contained in the vaccine both in the vaccinated child and in younger siblings. The universal use of conjugate meningococcal vaccine in children <2 yr old is anticipated in the near future and will alter the epidemiology of meningococcal disease in this age-group. Outbreaks of aseptic meningitis have been reported among children in childcare centers, as well as among their parents and their teachers.

HERPESVIRUSES

As many as 70% of diapered children who become infected with **cytomegalovirus** (CMV) shed virus in urine and saliva for prolonged periods. CMV-infected children often transmit the virus to other children with whom they have contact, as well as to their care providers and their mothers, at a rate of 8–20%/yr. Transmission occurs as a result of contact with either saliva or urine. The overwhelming majority of primary infections with and reactivation of CMV in otherwise healthy children result in asymptomatic shedding of CMV; nonetheless, this shedding can pose a health risk for previously uninfected pregnant childcare providers or immunocompromised persons. A licensed CMV vaccine is not yet available, but research is ongoing, with recent trials demonstrating tolerability and immunogenicity of candidate CMV vaccines (see Chapter 282).

Varicella often is transmitted in childcare centers, but routine use of varicella vaccine has reduced this risk. Vaccinated children who become infected with varicella often have mild, atypical symptoms and signs of disease that can result in delayed recognition and spread of infection to susceptible contacts. The role of childcare facilities in the spread of **herpes simplex virus**, especially during episodes of gingivostomatitis, requires further clarification.

BLOODBORNE PATHOGENS

Because it is impossible to identify every child who might have a bloodborne infection such as hepatitis B, C, or D or HIV, it is critical that standard precautions be observed routinely to reduce the risk for transmitting these viruses and other pathogens. Transmission of hepatitis B among children in childcare has been documented in a few instances but is rare, influenced in part by implementation of universal immunization of infants with hepatitis B vaccine. Transmission of hepatitis C or D in childcare settings has not been reported.

In the past, concerns have been raised about the risk of HIV transmission in childcare settings and the acquisition of opportunistic infections by HIV-infected children who attend childcare. It is important to note that no cases of HIV transmission in out-of-home childcare have been reported. Children with HIV infection enrolled in childcare facilities should be kept up-to-date on their vaccines and monitored for exposure to infectious diseases.

Transmission of bloodborne pathogens can theoretically occur when there is contact between blood or body fluids and a mucous membrane or an open wound. Although a common concern, bloodborne pathogens are unlikely to spread by toddler **biting** in a group setting. Most bites do not break the skin, and if a bite does break the skin, the mouth of the biter does not stay on the victim long enough for blood to transfer from the victim to the biter. If there are concerns about transmission of HBV, HCV, or HIV infection, it is recommended to check the status of the biter rather than the bite victim as part of the initial evaluation process.

ANTIBIOTIC USE AND BACTERIAL RESISTANCE

Antibiotic resistance has become a major global problem and threatens the health of children who attend childcare facilities, because the incidence of infection by organisms resistant to frequently used antimicrobial agents has increased dramatically. It is estimated that children in childcare are 2-4 times more likely to receive an antibiotic, and that they receive longer courses of antibiotics, compared to age-matched children in homecare. This frequency of antibiotic use combined with the propensity for person-to-person transmission of pathogens in a crowded environment has resulted in an increased prevalence of antibiotic-resistant bacteria in the respiratory and intestinal tracts, including *S. pneumoniae*, *H. influenzae*, *Moraxella catarrhalis*, *E. coli* O157:H7, and *Shigella* spp.

Historically found primarily in the healthcare setting, methicillin-resistant *Staphylococcus aureus* (**MRSA**) is now prevalent in the community setting. Daycare attendance is cited as a risk factor for colonization with MRSA, and carriage is associated with increased risk of infection and transmission. Population-based surveillance has demonstrated a rise in both invasive and noninvasive MRSA infections in community settings over the past 2 decades. Currently, large-scale studies investigating the epidemiology of *S. aureus* in the childcare setting are limited.

PREVENTION

Written policies designed to prevent or to control the spread of infectious agents in a childcare center should be available and should be reviewed regularly. All programs should use a health consultant to help with development and implementation of infection prevention and control (IPC) policies (see Chapter 198). Standards for environmental and personal hygiene should include maintenance of current immunization records for both children and staff; appropriate policies for exclusion of ill children and caretakers; targeting of potentially contaminated areas for frequent cleaning; adherence to appropriate procedures for changing diapers; appropriate handling of food; management of pets; and surveillance for and reporting of communicable diseases. Staff whose primary function is preparing food should not change diapers. Appropriate and thorough **hand hygiene** is the most important factor for reducing infectious diseases in the childcare setting. Strategies for improving adherence to these standards should be implemented. Children at risk for introducing an infectious disease should not attend childcare until they are no longer contagious (Tables 199.2 and 199.3).

Routine vaccination has had a proven significant beneficial effect on the health of children in childcare settings. In the United States, there are 16 diseases and organisms for which all children should be immunized unless there are contraindications: diphtheria, pertussis, tetanus, measles, mumps, rubella, polio, hepatitides A and B, varicella, *H. influenzae* type b, *S. pneumoniae*, rotavirus, *N. meningitidis,* influenza, and human papillomavirus (see Chapter 197). Rates of immunization among children in licensed childcare facilities are high, in part because of laws in almost all states that require age-appropriate immunizations of children who attend licensed childcare programs. Vaccines against influenza, *H. influenzae* type b, hepatitis B, rotavirus, varicella, *S. pneumoniae,* and hepatitis A are of particular benefit to children in childcare centers.

Childcare providers should receive all immunizations that are recommended routinely for adults, including Tdap (tetanus and diphtheria toxoids and acellular pertussis) booster, and have a preemployment health evaluation, with a tuberculin skin test or interferon-γ release blood assay. Local public health authorities should be notified of cases of reportable communicable disease that occur in children or providers in childcare settings.

STANDARDS

Every state has specific standards for licensing and reviewing childcare centers and family childcare homes. The American Academy of Pediatrics, American Public Health Association, and National Resource

Center jointly publish comprehensive health and safety performance standards that can be used by pediatricians and other healthcare professionals to guide decisions about management of infectious diseases in childcare facilities (available at http://nrckids.org/CFOC). Additionally, the **National Association for the Education of Young Children (NAEYC)**, a professional organization supporting early childhood education efforts and volunteer accreditation, is gaining recognition as a resource for health and safety standards for childcare facilities (http://www.naeyc.org/). Specific standards set by all states can be reviewed at the U.S. Department of Health and Human Services' **National Center on Early Childhood Quality Assurance** website (https://childcareta.acf.hhs.gov/licensing).

Bibliography is available at Expert Consult.

Table 199.2	Disease- or Condition-Specific Recommendations for Exclusion of Children in Out-of-Home Childcare	
CONDITION	**MANAGEMENT OF CASE**	**MANAGEMENT OF CONTACTS**
Clostridium difficile	Exclusion until stools are contained in the diaper or child is continent and stool frequency is no more than 2 stools above that child's normal frequency for the time the child is in the program. Stool consistency does not need to return to normal to be able to return to childcare. Neither test of cure nor repeat testing should be performed for asymptomatic children in whom *C. difficile* was diagnosed previously.	Symptomatic contacts should be excluded until stools are contained in the diaper or child is continent and stool frequency is no more than 2 stools above that child's normal frequency for the time the child is in the program. Testing is not required for asymptomatic contacts.
Hepatitis A virus (HAV) infection	Serologic testing to confirm HAV infection in suspected cases. Exclusion until 1 wk after onset of illness.	In facilities with diapered children, if 1 or more cases confirmed in child or staff attendees or 2 or more cases in households of staff or attendees, hepatitis A vaccine (HepA) or immune globulin intramuscular (IGIM) should be administered within 14 days of exposure to all unimmunized staff and attendees. In centers without diapered children, HepA or IGIM should be administered to unimmunized classroom contacts of index case. Asymptomatic IGIM recipients may return after receipt of IGIM.
Impetigo	No exclusion if treatment has been initiated and as long as lesions on exposed skin are covered.	No intervention unless additional lesions develop.
Measles	Exclusion until 4 days after beginning of rash and when the child is able to participate.	Immunize exposed children without evidence of immunity within 72 hr of exposure. Children who do not receive vaccine within 72 hr or who remain unimmunized after exposure should be excluded until at least 2 wk after onset of rash in the last case of measles.
Mumps	Exclusion until 5 days after onset of parotid gland swelling.	In outbreak setting, people without documentation of immunity should be immunized or excluded. Immediate readmission may occur following immunization. Unimmunized people should be excluded for 26 or more days following onset of parotitis in last case. A 2nd dose of MMR vaccine (or MMRV, if age appropriate) should be offered to all students (including those in postsecondary school) and to all healthcare personnel born in or after 1957 who have only received 1 dose of MMR vaccine. A 2nd dose of MMR also may be considered during outbreaks for preschool-age children who have received 1 MMR dose. People previously vaccinated with 2 doses of a mumps-containing vaccine who are identified by public health as at increased risk for mumps because of an outbreak should receive a 3rd dose of a mumps-containing vaccine to improve protection against mumps disease and related complications.
Pediculosis capitis (head lice) infestation	Treatment at end of program day and readmission on completion of 1st treatment. Children should not be excluded or sent home early from school because of head lice, because this infestation has low contagion within classrooms.	Household and close contacts should be examined and treated if infested. No exclusion necessary.
Pertussis	Exclusion until completion of 5 days of the recommended course of antimicrobial therapy if pertussis is suspected. Children and providers who refuse treatment should be excluded until 21 days have elapsed from cough onset.	Immunization and chemoprophylaxis should be administered as recommended for household contacts. Symptomatic children and staff should be excluded until completion of 5 days of antimicrobial therapy. Untreated adults should be excluded until 21 days after onset of cough.

Continued

Table 199.2	Disease- or Condition-Specific Recommendations for Exclusion of Children in Out-of-Home Childcare—cont'd

CONDITION	MANAGEMENT OF CASE	MANAGEMENT OF CONTACTS
Rubella	Exclusion for 7 days after onset of rash for postnatal infection.	During an outbreak, children without evidence of immunity should be immunized or excluded for 21 days after onset of rash of the last case in the outbreak. Pregnant contacts should be evaluated.
Infection with *Salmonella* serotypes Typhi or Paratyphi	Exclusion until 3 consecutive stool cultures obtained at least 48 hr after cessation of antimicrobial therapy are negative, stools are contained in the diaper or child is continent, and stool frequency is no more than 2 stools above that child's normal frequency for the time the child is in the program.	When *Salmonella* serotype Typhi infection is identified in a child care staff member, local or state health departments may be consulted regarding regulations for length of exclusion and testing, which may vary by jurisdiction.
Infection with nontyphoidal *Salmonella* spp., *Salmonella* of unknown serotype	Exclusion until stools are contained in the diaper or child is continent and stool frequency is no more than 2 stools above that child's normal frequency for the time the child is in the program. Stool consistency does not need to return to normal to be able to return to childcare. Negative stool culture results *not* required for nonserotype Typhi or Paratyphi *Salmonella* spp.	Symptomatic contacts should be excluded until stools are contained in the diaper or child is continent and stool frequency is no more than 2 stools above that child's normal frequency for the time the child is in the program. Stool cultures are not required for asymptomatic contacts.
Scabies	Exclusion until after treatment given.	Close contacts with prolonged skin-to-skin contact should receive prophylactic therapy. Bedding and clothing in contact with skin of infected people should be laundered.
Infection with Shiga toxin–producing *Escherichia coli* (STEC), including *E. coli* O157:H7	Exclusion until 2 stool cultures (obtained at least 48 hr after any antimicrobial therapy, if administered, has been discontinued) are negative, and stools are contained in the diaper or child is continent, and stool frequency is no more than 2 stools above that child's normal frequency. Some state health departments have less stringent exclusion policies for children who have recovered from less virulent STEC infection.	Meticulous hand hygiene; stool cultures should be performed for any symptomatic contacts. In outbreak situations involving virulent STEC strains, stool cultures of asymptomatic contacts may aid controlling spread. Center(s) with cases should be closed to new admissions during STEC outbreak.
Shigellosis	Exclusion until treatment complete and one or more posttreatment stool cultures are negative for *Shigella* spp., and stools are contained in the diaper or child is continent, and stool frequency is no more than 2 stools above that child's normal frequency for the time the child is in the program. Some states may require more than 1 negative stool culture.	Meticulous hand hygiene; stool cultures should be performed for any symptomatic contacts.
Staphylococcus aureus skin infections	Exclusion only if skin lesions are draining and cannot be covered with a watertight dressing.	Meticulous hand hygiene; cultures of contacts are not recommended.
Streptococcal pharyngitis	Exclusion until at least 12 hr after treatment has been initiated.	Symptomatic contacts of documented cases of group A streptococcal infection should be tested and treated if test results are positive.
Tuberculosis	Most children younger than 10 yr are not considered contagious. For those with active disease, exclusion until determined to be noninfectious by physician or health department authority. No exclusion for latent tuberculosis infection (LTBI).	Local health department personnel should be informed for contact investigation.
Varicella	Exclusion until all lesions have crusted or, in immunized people without crusts, until no new lesions appear within 24 hr period.	For people without evidence of immunity, varicella vaccine should be administered, ideally within 3 days, but up to 5 days after exposure, or when indicated, varicella-zoster immune globulin (VariZIG) should be administered up to 10 days after exposure; if VariZIG is not available, immune globulin intravenous (IGIV) should be considered as an alternative. If vaccine cannot be administered and VariZIG/IGIV is not indicated, preemptive oral acyclovir or valacyclovir can be considered.

From Kimberlin DW, Brady MT, Jackson MA, Long SS, editors: *Red Book 2018–2021: Report of the Committee on Infectious Diseases*, ed 31, Elk Grove Village, IL, 2018, American Academy of Pediatrics (Table 2.3, pp 130–135).

Table 199.3	General Recommendations for Exclusion of Children in Out-of-Home Childcare
SYMPTOM(S)	**MANAGEMENT**
Illness preventing participation in activities, as determined by childcare staff.	Exclusion until illness resolves and able to participate in activities.
Illness that requires more care than staff can provide without compromising health and safety of others.	Exclusion or placement in care environment where appropriate care can be provided without compromising care of others.
Severe illness suggested by fever with behavior changes, lethargy, irritability, persistent crying, difficulty breathing, or progressive rash.	Medical evaluation and exclusion until symptoms have resolved.
Persistent abdominal pain (≥2 hr) or intermittent abdominal pain associated with fever, dehydration, or other systemic signs and symptoms.	Medical evaluation and exclusion until symptoms have resolved.
Vomiting ≥2 times in preceding 24 hr.	Exclusion until symptoms have resolved, unless vomiting is determined to be caused by a noncommunicable condition and child is able to remain hydrated and participate in activities.
Diarrhea if stool not contained in diaper or if fecal accidents occur in a child who is normally continent; if stool frequency ≥2 above normal for child or stools contain blood or mucus.	Medical evaluation for stools with blood or mucus; exclusion until stools are contained in the diaper or when toilet-trained children no longer have accidents using the toilet and when stool frequency becomes <2 stools above child's normal frequency/24 hr.
Oral lesions	Exclusion if unable to contain drool, or if unable to participate because of other symptoms, or until child or staff member is considered to be noninfectious (lesions smaller or resolved).
Skin lesions	Exclusion if lesions are weeping and cannot be covered with a waterproof dressing.

From Kimberlin DW, Brady MT, Jackson MA, Long SS, editors: *Red Book 2018–2021: Report of the Committee on Infectious Diseases*, ed 31, Elk Grove Village, IL, 2018, American Academy of Pediatrics (Table 2.2, p 129).

Chapter **200**
Health Advice for Children Traveling Internationally
John C. Christenson and Chandy C. John

第二百章
国际旅行儿童保健建议

中文导读

　　本章主要介绍了儿科旅行医学咨询、安全和预防咨询、儿童旅行所需常规疫苗接种、特殊的儿科旅行疫苗、旅行者腹泻、虫媒传染病、疟疾化学预防、返回旅行者，以及青少年旅行者。具体描述了儿童旅行所需常规疫苗接种中的白喉－破伤风－百日咳疫苗、B型流感嗜血杆菌疫苗、甲肝疫苗、乙肝疫苗、流感及禽流感疫苗、麻疹腮腺炎风疹疫苗、肺炎球菌疫苗、脊髓灰质炎疫苗和水痘疫苗。还详细描述了特殊的儿科旅行疫苗，包括霍乱、甲型肝炎疫苗接种和暴露前免疫球蛋白、乙型脑炎、脑膜炎球菌疫苗及狂犬病、结核、伤寒和黄热病疫苗。

Children are traveling internationally with increasing frequency and to more exotic destinations that pose unique injury and disease risks. Compared to adults, children are *less* likely to receive pretravel advice and *more* likely to be seen by a medical provider or be hospitalized on return for a travel-related illness. Primary care providers are confronted with the challenge of trying to ensure safe, healthy travel for their patient, whether travel is occurring for purposes of tourism, study abroad, visiting friends and relatives, or volunteerism. Whenever possible, health professionals are encouraged to consult with **travel medicine specialists**, especially when uncertain about pretravel advice, unique travel medicine vaccines (e.g., yellow fever, Japanese encephalitis, typhoid, rabies), and recommendations for malaria medications.

Travel medicine is a unique specialty, and experienced travel medicine practitioners provide specialized guidance on the infectious and noninfectious risks based on age, itinerary, duration, season, purpose of travel, and underlying traveler characteristics (health and vaccination status). A **pretravel consultation** includes the essential elements of (1) safety and preventive counseling against injuries and diseases; (2) routine, recommended, and required vaccinations, based on individual risk assessment; (3) counseling and medications for self-treatment of traveler's diarrhea; and (4) when indicated by itinerary, malaria chemoprophylaxis.

In the United States, recommendations and vaccine requirements for travel to different countries are provided by the Centers for Disease Control and Prevention (CDC) and are available online at https://wwwnc.cdc.gov/travel/page/yellowbook-home. Some travel vaccines and medications may not be recommended based on specifics of travel itinerary, trip duration, or patient characteristics. Alternatively, some vaccinations are not approved for younger children because of lack of data or limited immunologic response but may still confer potential benefit to the young traveler with off-label vaccine administration. In both scenarios, consultation or referral to a knowledgeable travel medicine practitioner is encouraged, especially if uncertainty exists regarding pretravel recommendations.

THE PEDIATRIC TRAVEL MEDICINE CONSULTATION

Parents of traveling children should seek medical consultation at least one month before departure to review the travel itinerary, obtain safety and preventive counseling, ensure adequate vaccinations (routine, recommended, and required), receive necessary medications for chronic health conditions, and obtain important medications for self-treatment of traveler's diarrhea and, when indicated, malaria chemoprophylaxis with counseling. Preparing a child to travel internationally should begin with an emphasis on the positive aspects of the upcoming trip rather than solely focusing on travel risks and diseases. Subsequent advice, vaccinations, and medications should be emphasized as important measures, with the provider goal of keeping the child healthy during travel rather than to discourage traveling.

Pediatric Travelers Visiting Friends and Relatives

Compared to most children traveling internationally, the **pediatric visiting-friends-and-relatives (VFR) traveler** is the most vulnerable population uniquely at risk for travel-related illnesses. VFR travelers may include immigrants, refugees, migrants, students, or displaced persons who are traveling back to their country of origin for purposes of visiting friends and relatives. Pediatric VFR travelers are typically children accompanying their parents or family members back to their ancestral country, where relational, social, and cultural connections remain. Compared to tourist travelers, VFR travelers are more likely to travel for longer durations, visit more remote destinations, travel by higher-risk local transportation modes, experience closer contact with the local population, and utilize fewer insect, food, and water precautions. Adult and pediatric VFR travelers are also less likely to perceive a risk of travel-related illnesses, seek pretravel advice, receive travel immunizations, or use effective malaria prophylaxis on arrival in the destination country. VFR travel comprises 50–84% of imported malaria in U.S. children (i.e., malaria acquired outside the United States), and pediatric VFR travelers are reported to be 4 times more likely than tourist travelers

to acquire malaria. Among all travelers, unvaccinated pediatric VFR travelers remain at higher risk for contracting hepatitis A and having symptomatic illness. Several studies suggest that VFR travelers are at disproportionate risk of acquiring typhoid fever and possibly tuberculosis. Providers should inquire if their foreign-born patients will be traveling internationally and seek opportunities to encourage pretravel consultation for VFR travelers.

SAFETY AND PREVENTIVE COUNSELING TOPICS

Health and Evacuation Insurance, Underlying Health Conditions, and Medications

Parents should be made aware that their medical insurance policy might not provide coverage for hospitalizations or medical emergencies in foreign countries and is unlikely to cover the high cost of an emergency medical evacuation. Supplemental **travel medical insurance** and **evacuation insurance** may be purchased and are especially recommended for prolonged travel itineraries, for remote destinations, and for children with higher-risk preexistent health conditions going to countries where inpatient care at a level comparable to the traveler's home country may not be available. A list of medical and evacuation insurance providers can be found at the U.S. Department of State International Travel advisory website (https://travel.state.gov/content/travel/en/international-travel/emergencies.html).

Parents of children with medical conditions should take with them a brief medical summary and a sufficient supply of prescription medications for their children, with bottles that are clearly identified by prescription labels. For children requiring care by specialists, an international directory for that specialty can be consulted. A directory of physicians worldwide who speak English and who have met certain qualifications is available from the **International Association for Medical Assistance to Travelers** (https://www.iamat.org/). If medical care is needed urgently when abroad, sources of information include the U.S. embassy or consulate, hotel managers, travel agents catering to foreign tourists, and missionary hospitals.

A travel health kit consisting of prescription medications and nonprescription items, such as acetaminophen, an antihistamine, oral rehydration solution packets, antibiotic ointment, bandages, insect repellent (DEET or picaridin), and sunscreen, is highly recommended for all children. Children with persistent asthma should have bronchodilators and oral corticosteroids prescribed for treatment of any acute asthma exacerbations encountered during overseas travel. Children with a history of angioedema, anaphylaxis, or severe allergies to food or insects should have an epinephrine autoinjector (EpiPen) and antihistamines available for use during travel.

Parents and family members should be aware of the prevalence of counterfeit medication and lack of quality control of medications in many areas of the world, particularly in low- and middle-income countries. Critical medications, including insulin and newly prescribed antimalarials, should be purchased prior to international travel and packed in original prescription containers.

Safety and Injury Prevention

Motor vehicle accidents are a leading cause of traumatic injuries to, hospitalizations of, and deaths of pediatric and adult travelers. Differences in traffic patterns should be emphasized to children, and the use of safety belts should be reinforced. When possible, child safety seats should be taken on the trip. Parents should also be aware of additional risks for small children that may exist overseas, such as open balconies, windows without screens or bars, exposed wires and electrical outlets, paint chips, pest and rodent poison, and stray animals. **Water-related activities** also are associated with significant injuries in pediatric travelers, and pools and oceanfronts are often unsupervised and without lifeguards at overseas destinations.

Animal Contact

Among travelers, attacks from domestic or stray animals are much more likely to occur than attacks from wild animals. Wounds from animal bites present a risk for bacterial infections, tetanus, and rabies. **Dogs** are responsible for >95% of all **rabies** transmission in Asia, Africa, and Latin America. Globally, the World Health Organization (WHO) estimates that approximately 55,000 human deaths result from rabies each year, with the vast majority of cases occurring in South Asia, Southeast Asia, and Africa. Rabies transmission is reported less frequently after bites from cats and other carnivores, monkeys, and bats. Macaque monkeys native to Asia and North Africa can be found in urban centers and tourist sites and pose a risk for rabies and herpes B virus infections following bites and scratches.

Young children are more likely to be bitten and experience more severe facial wounds because of their short stature. As such, they are at higher risk for rabies exposure from dogs and other animals during travel and require greater supervision. Parents should always encourage their children to report bite injuries and to avoid petting, feeding, or handling dogs, monkeys, and stray animals. Before travel, **tetanus** vaccinations need to be current for all travelers. Children, long-term travelers, expatriates, and all individuals likely to come into contact with animals in a rabies-endemic region (primarily Africa and South and Southeast Asia) should consider **preexposure vaccination** for rabies before international travel (see Rabies later). Bite or scratch wounds should be washed thoroughly and for a prolonged time (15 min) with copious water and soap. Local wound care will substantially reduce the risk of canine and other mammalian rabies transmission. Rabies **postexposure vaccination** and rabies immunoglobulin should be considered. Antibiotics (amoxicillin-clavulanate) may need to be administered to a child to prevent secondary infections, especially for animal bites involving the hands and head/neck areas.

ROUTINE CHILDHOOD VACCINATIONS REQUIRED FOR PEDIATRIC TRAVEL

Parents should allow at least 4 wk before departure for optimal administration of vaccines to their children. All children who travel should be immunized according to the routine childhood immunization schedule with all vaccines appropriate for their age. The immunization schedule can be accelerated to maximize protection for traveling children, especially for unvaccinated or incompletely vaccinated children (see Fig. 197.2 in Chapter 197). Routine and catch-up childhood vaccine schedules for healthcare professionals can be found at the CDC website (https://www.cdc.gov/vaccines/schedules/).

Live-attenuated viral vaccines should be administered concurrently or ≥4 wk apart to minimize immunologic interference. Intramuscular immunoglobulin interferes with the immune response to measles immunization and possibly to varicella immunization. If a child requires measles or varicella immunization, the vaccines should be given either 2 wk before or 3 mo after immunoglobulin administration (longer with higher doses of intravenous immunoglobulin). Immunoglobulin does not interfere with the immune response to oral typhoid, poliovirus, or yellow fever vaccines.

Vaccine products produced in eggs (yellow fever, influenza) may be associated with hypersensitivity responses, including anaphylaxis in persons with known severe **egg sensitivity**. Screening by inquiring about adverse effects when eating eggs is a reasonable way to identify those at risk for anaphylaxis from receiving influenza or yellow fever vaccines. Although measles and mumps vaccines are produced in chick embryo cell cultures, children with egg allergy are at very low risk for anaphylaxis with these vaccines.

Diphtheria-Tetanus-Pertussis

Children traveling internationally should be fully vaccinated with diphtheria and tetanus toxoids and acellular pertussis (DTaP), having completed the 4th or 5th booster dose by 4-6 yr of age. A single dose of an adolescent/adult preparation of tetanus and diphtheria toxoids and acellular pertussis (Tdap) vaccine is recommended at 11-12 yr of age for those who have completed the recommended primary DTaP (or DTP) series.

Adolescents and adults should receive a single Tdap booster if >5 yr have elapsed since the last dose, since a tetanus-containing booster (Td or Tdap) may not be readily available for tetanus-prone wounds during international travel or in remote settings (adventure travel, wilderness).

Haemophilus influenzae Type b

Haemophilus influenzae type b (Hib) remains a leading cause of meningitis in children 6 mo to 3 yr of age in many low- and middle-income countries. Before they travel, all unimmunized children <5 yr old should be vaccinated (see Chapter 197). A single dose of Hib vaccine should also be administered to unvaccinated or partially vaccinated children ≥5 yr old if they have anatomic or functional asplenia, sickle cell disease, HIV infection, leukemia, malignancy, or other immunocompromising condition. Unvaccinated children >5 yr old do not need vaccination unless they have a high-risk condition.

Hepatitis A

Hepatitis A is a routine childhood vaccine in the United States but requires special considerations in the traveling pediatric patient, and protection from hepatitis A in specific children may also involve the provision of immunoglobulin. For this reason, hepatitis A vaccination is covered later in Specialized Pediatric Travel Vaccinations.

Hepatitis B

Hepatitis B is a travel-associated infection. Hepatitis B is highly prevalent throughout much of the world, including areas of South America, sub-Saharan Africa, eastern and southeastern Asia, and most of the Pacific basin. In certain parts of the world, 8–15% of the population may be chronically infected. Disease can be transmitted by blood transfusions not screened for hepatitis B surface antigen, exposure to unsterilized needles, close contact with local children who have open skin lesions, and sexual exposure. Exposure to hepatitis B is more likely for travelers residing for prolonged periods in endemic areas. Partial protection may be provided by 1 or 2 doses, but ideally 3 doses should be given before travel. For unvaccinated adolescents, the 1st 2 doses are 4 wk apart and are followed by a 3rd dose 8 wk later (at least 16 wk after 1st dose).

All unvaccinated children and adolescents should receive the accelerated hepatitis B vaccine series prior to travel. Because 1 or 2 doses provide some protection, hepatitis B vaccination should be initiated even if the full series cannot be completed before travel.

Influenza and Avian Influenza

Influenza remains the most common vaccine-preventable disease occurring among pediatric and adult travelers. The risk for exposure to influenza during international travel varies depending on the time of year, destination, and intermingling of persons from different parts of the world where influenza may be circulating. In tropical areas, influenza can occur throughout the year, whereas in the temperate regions of the Southern hemisphere, most activity occurs from April through September. In the Northern hemisphere, influenza generally occurs from November through March. Seasonal influenza vaccination is strongly recommended for all pediatric and adolescent travelers who do not have a contraindication or severe egg allergy.

Currently, there are no available vaccines effective against avian influenza strains such as influenza A H5N1 and H7N9, which have become a great concern worldwide. Because these strains of influenza virus are spread through contact with infected birds, these precautions include avoiding direct contact with birds or surfaces with bird droppings, avoiding poultry farms or bird markets, eating only well-cooked bird meat or products, and washing hands frequently. **Oseltamivir** is the antiviral of choice to treat infections caused by these viruses.

Measles-Mumps-Rubella

Measles is still endemic in many low- and middle-income countries and in some industrialized nations. It remains a leading cause of vaccine-preventable death in much of the world. Vaccine status for measles is important for all traveling children, particularly if they are traveling to low- and middle-income countries or areas with measles outbreaks. Measles vaccine, preferably in combination with mumps and rubella vaccines (MMR), should be given to all children at 12-15 mo and at 4-6 yr of age, unless there is a contraindication (see Chapter 197.2). In children traveling internationally, the 2nd vaccination can be given as soon as 4 wk after the 1st, to induce immunity among those children who did not respond to the 1st MMR vaccine.

Children 6-12 mo old traveling to low- and middle-income countries should be vaccinated. The monovalent measles vaccine is not available in the United States. Early vaccination (i.e., 6-12 mo of age) will provide some immunity to measles, but antibody response may not be durable or lasting. Any MMR vaccine before 12 mo of age does not count toward the routine vaccination schedule; children vaccinated early for purposes of international travel must be revaccinated on or after their 1st birthday with 2 doses, separated by at least 4 wk. Infants <6 mo old are generally protected by maternal antibodies and would not need early MMR vaccination before travel.

Pneumococcal Vaccines

Streptococcus pneumoniae is the leading cause of childhood **bacterial pneumonia** and is among the leading causes of bacteremia and bacterial meningitis in children in low- and middle-income and industrialized nations. Preparing a child to travel internationally includes routine or catch-up vaccination with 13-valent pneumococcal conjugate vaccine (PCV13) and, for children with certain high-risk conditions, use of 23-valent pneumococcal polysaccharide vaccine (PPSV23). A single dose of PCV13 should be administered to previously unvaccinated children 6-18 yr old with underlying high-risk medical conditions: anatomic or functional asplenia (including sickle cell disease), HIV infection, a congenital immunodeficiency or immunocompromising condition, chronic heart or lung disease, chronic renal failure or nephrotic syndrome, diabetes mellitus, cerebrospinal fluid leak, or cochlear implant. The Advisory Committee on Immunization Practices (ACIP) also recommends that high-risk children ≥2 yr old receive the PPSV23 vaccine ≥8 wk after their last PCV13 dose. ACIP recommendations on prevention of pneumococcal disease among infants and children using PCV13 and PPSV23 can be found at http://www.cdc.gov/vaccines/hcp/acip-recs/vacc-specific/pneumo.html.

Polio Vaccine

Poliomyelitis was eradicated from the Western hemisphere in 1991. Polio remains endemic in 3 countries—Afghanistan, Nigeria, and Pakistan—with additional surrounding countries at risk for importation of polio. The poliovirus vaccination schedule in the United States is now a 4-dose, all-inactivated poliovirus (IPV) regimen (see Chapter 197). Traveling infants should begin IPV series as early as 6 wk of age (for an accelerated dosing schedule for children, see Fig. 197.2). Length of immunity conferred by IPV immunization is not known; a single booster dose of IPV is therefore recommended for previously vaccinated adolescents and adults traveling to polio-endemic areas if approximately 10 yr has elapsed since they completed their primary series. Oral poliovirus vaccine is no longer available in the United States.

Varicella

All children ≥12 mo old who have no history of varicella vaccination or chickenpox should be vaccinated unless there is a contraindication to vaccination (see Chapter 197). Infants <6 mo old are generally protected by maternal antibodies. All children now require 2 doses, the 1st at 12 mo of age and the 2nd at 4-6 yr. The 2nd dose can be given as soon as 3 mo after the 1st dose. For unvaccinated children ≥13 yr old, the 1st and 2nd doses can be separated by 4 wk.

SPECIALIZED PEDIATRIC TRAVEL VACCINATIONS

Table 200.1 summarizes the dosages and age restrictions of vaccines specifically given to children traveling internationally.

Cholera

Cholera is present in many low- and middle-income countries, but the risk for infection among travelers to these countries is extremely low. At present, no cholera vaccine is available for travelers in the United States, although an effective vaccine is available in other countries. Travelers entering countries reporting cholera outbreaks are at minimal risk of acquiring cholera if they take adequate safe

food and water precautions and practice frequent handwashing. No country or territory currently requires cholera vaccination as a condition for entry.

Hepatitis A Vaccination and Preexposure Immunoglobulin

Hepatitis A virus (HAV) is endemic in most of the world, and travelers are at risk, even if their travel is restricted to the usual tourist routes. HAV infection can result from eating shellfish harvested from sewage-contaminated waters, eating unwashed vegetables or fruits, or eating food prepared by an asymptomatic HAV carrier. Young children infected with hepatitis A are often asymptomatic but can transmit infection to unvaccinated older children and adults, who are more likely to develop clinical hepatitis. Few areas carry no risk of HAV infection, and therefore immunization is recommended for all travelers. Hepatitis A vaccine (HepA) is recommended in the United States for universal immunization of all children ≥12 mo old, administered as 2 doses 6 mo apart. A single dose of HepA given to travelers will provide adequate protection. Protective immunity develops within 2 wk after the initial vaccine dose. A combined 3-dose HepA and hepatitis B vaccine (Twinrix, GlaxoSmith-Kline) is available in the United States but is licensed for use only in individuals >18 yr old. Pediatric combination hepatitis A–hepatitis B vaccine (HepA-HepB) (Twinrix-Junior, GlaxoSmithKline) is licensed for use in children 1-18 yr old in Canada and Europe.

Children <1 yr old are at lower risk of clinical HAV infection, especially if they are breastfed or residing in areas with safe water for formula reconstitution. Some experts recommend use of preexposure intramuscular immunoglobulin for children <6 mo who are traveling internationally to higher-risk destinations, particularly low-income destinations or regions where hygienic or sanitary conditions are limited. However, administration of immunoglobulin diminishes the immunogenicity of live-virus vaccines, in particular measles vaccine, that may be needed for infant travelers. Vaccination against measles should occur ≥2 wk before any immunoglobulin administration, and a 3 mo interval is suggested between immunoglobulin administration and subsequent measles immunization.

Because measles-endemic countries frequently overlap with higher-risk travel destinations for HAV infection hepatitis A vaccine is recommended for infant travelers 6-11 mo of age. Several studies demonstrate that infants as young as 6 mo will develop antibodies following HepA, especially if there are no interfering maternal antibodies from prior maternal vaccination or disease. There is potential for a more durable immune response to the hepatitis A vaccination especially in later infancy, when potential interfering maternal antibody concentrations are lower. If early hepatitis A vaccination is given rather than immunoglobulin to infant travelers (age 6-11 mo), it should not count toward the routine 2-dose vaccine series. Similar to MMR vaccination, an informed decision should be made, with the parents balancing the risk of travel-associated disease and vaccine adverse events with the potential protective benefit to the traveling infant.

Japanese Encephalitis

Japanese encephalitis is a disease transmitted by mosquitoes in many areas of Asia, especially in rural farming areas. Although it is a leading cause of vaccine-preventable encephalitis in children in many Asian countries and parts of western Pacific countries, the risk of disease to nonimmune travelers is low. A map showing where Japanese encephalitis transmission occurs can be found at https://wwwnc.cdc.gov/travel/yellowbook/2018/infectious-diseases-related-to-travel/japanese-encephalitis.

Most human infections with **Japanese encephalitis virus (JEV)** are asymptomatic, and <1% of individuals develop clinical disease. With symptomatic disease, the fatality rate is 20–30% and the incidence of neurologic or psychiatric sequelae in survivors is 30–50%. The risk of JEV disease for pediatric travelers is unknown, but among all travelers, it is estimated to be less than 1 case per 1 million travelers to Asia. However, if residing in a rural area with active JEV transmission in the raining season, the risk may increase to 5-50 cases per 100,000 population per year. Risk of Japanese encephalitis neurologic disease following

Table 200.1	Travel Vaccinations for Children

VACCINE	FORMULATION	ROUTE AND DOSE	SCHEDULE	INDICATIONS	COMMENTS
Hepatitis A	Pediatric: Havrix (GlaxoSmithKline); 720 EU VAQTA (Merck); 25 U	IM; 0.5 mL	Primary series: 2 doses, 6-18 mo apart Booster: currently not recommended	Children >6 months of age	Inactivated vaccine Lifelong protection is likely.
	Adult: Havrix (GlaxoSmithKline); 1440 EU VAQTA (Merck); 50 U	IM; 1.0 mL	Primary series: 2 doses, 6-18 mo apart Booster: currently not recommended	Adults ≥19 yr old	Inactivated vaccine Lifelong protection is likely.
Hepatitis A and B	Twinrix (GlaxoSmithKline)	IM; 1.0 mL	Primary series: 3 doses at 0, 1, and 6 mo Accelerated schedule: 0, 7, and 21 days; 4th dose 12 mo later Boosters: not needed	Adults ≥18 yr old	Inactivated vaccine Lifelong protection is likely. Accelerated schedule is as effective.
Immunoglobulin, human	Injectable	IM	Travel up to 1 mo duration: 0.1 mL/kg Travel up to 2 mo duration: 0.2 mL/kg Travel 2 mo or more: 0.2 mL/kg (repeat every 2 mo)	Infants <1 yr old	Passive immunizations against hepatitis A. Its use would require delay of measles and varicella vaccinations (at least 3 mo).
Japanese encephalitis virus (JEV)	Inactivated: Ixiaro (Intercell USA)	IM 2 mo to <3 yr old: 0.25 mL ≥3 yr old: 0.5 mL	Primary series: 2 doses at days 0 and 28 Booster: 1 dose 1 yr later if exposure to JEV expected	Travel to high-risk areas; prolonged stays	Booster recommendation is extrapolated from recommendation for individuals ≥17 yr old.
Meningococcal, polysaccharide	Quadrivalent: A, C, Y, W135	SC; 0.5 mL	Primary series: single dose Booster: 5 yr in persons ≥4 yr old; 2–3 yr in children 2–4 yr old	≥2 yr old	Required for entry to Saudi Arabia during the Hajj. Recommended for travelers visiting "meningitis belt" in sub-Saharan Africa during dry months. This vaccine is rarely used in U.S. since conjugate vaccines are more immunogenic.
Meningococcal, conjugate	Quadrivalent: ACWY-D: Menactra (Sanofi Pasteur)	IM: 0.5 mL	Children 9-23 mo old: 2 doses, 3 mo apart 2-55 yr old: 1 dose	Routine vaccination in U.S. at ≥11-12 yr old with recommended booster 5 yr later	Required for entry to Saudi Arabia during the Hajj. Recommended for travelers visiting "meningitis belt" in sub-Saharan Africa during dry months. This vaccine should not be used in infants <9 mo old since it may interfere with antibody production by pneumococcal conjugate vaccine.
	Quadrivalent: ACWY-CRM: Menveo (Novartis)	IM; 0.5 mL	Children initiating vaccination at 2 mo: doses at 2, 4, 6, and 12 mo old Children starting vaccination at 7-23 mo old: 2 doses, with 2nd dose after 2 yr old and at least 3 mo after 1st dose	Routine vaccination in U.S. at ≥11-12 yr old with recommended booster 5 yr later	Required for entry to Saudi Arabia during the Hajj. Recommended for travelers visiting "meningitis belt" in sub-Saharan Africa during dry months.
Rabies	Inactivated	IM; 1.0 mL	Preexposure series: 3 doses at days 0, 7, and 21 or 28 Booster: depends on risk category and serologic testing. Postexposure: rabies immune globulin; day 0; vaccines at days 0, 3, 7, and 14; 5th dose at day 28 is recommended if host is immunocompromised.		Consider for young travelers planning prolonged stays; especially away from large urban centers with adequate medical care systems and airport.

Continued

Table 200.1	Travel Vaccinations for Children—cont'd				
VACCINE	**FORMULATION**	**ROUTE AND DOSE**	**SCHEDULE**	**INDICATIONS**	**COMMENTS**
Typhoid fever	Live-attenuated Ty21a1	Oral	1 capsule every other day for 4 doses Boosters: every 5 yr	Persons ≥6 yr old	If series sequence not completed, all 4 doses need to be repeated. Contraindicated in immunocompromised hosts. Cannot be taken with hot beverage. Person must not be taking antibiotics.
	Injectable Polysaccharide Vi antigen	IM; 0.5 mL	Primary series: 1 dose Booster: every 2 yr	Persons ≥2 yr old	
Yellow fever	Live injectable	SC; 0.5 mL	Primary series: 1 dose Dose must be given at least 10 days before arrival to risk area. Booster: no longer required by WHO. U.S. travelers: recommended every 10 yr for high-risk travelers.	≥9 mo old	Contraindicated in immunocompromised hosts. Avoid in pregnancy and in breastfeeding mothers, unless high-risk travel cannot be avoided. Contraindicated in infants <4 mo old. Avoid in persons with thymus disorders. Infants 6-8 mo old: consider vaccination with caution if risk or travel cannot be avoided; consult travel medicine specialist. Caution in persons ≥60 yr old (high risk for vaccine-related infection). Requires official certificate of vaccination.

IM, Intramuscular; SC, subcutaneous; WHO, World Health Organization.

mosquito-bite transmission is thought to be higher in children than adults. The disease occurs primarily from June to September in temperate zones and throughout the entire year in tropical zones. Vaccination is recommended for travelers planning visits >1 mo to rural areas of Asia, where the disease is endemic, especially areas of rice or pig farming. Vaccination is recommended for shorter visits to such areas if the traveler will often be outdoors (e.g., camping or hiking). Risk for infection can be greatly reduced by following the standard precautions to avoid mosquito bites.

The inactivated Vero cell culture–derived Japanese encephalitis vaccine (Ixiaro) has replaced the older inactivated mouse brain–derived vaccine (JE-VAX), which is no longer manufactured. Japanese encephalitis vaccine efficacy is >95% in adults who receive 2 doses administered 28 days apart. The licensed range for Japanese encephalitis vaccine has been extended to include children as young as 2 mo, with a dose administered on days 0 and 28.

Meningococcal Vaccines

Currently, 3 forms of meningococcal vaccine are available in the United States: a quadrivalent polysaccharide A/C/Y/W-135 vaccine (Menomune); 2 quadrivalent conjugate A/C/Y/W-135 vaccines, MenACWY-CRM (Menveo) and MenACWY-D (Menactra); and 2 meningococcal B vaccines (Bexcero, Trumenba).

Children traveling to those equatorial countries in sub-Saharan Africa where the incidence of meningococcal disease (especially group A) is highest should receive a *Neisseria meningitidis* quadrivalent vaccine, especially if travel is prolonged or occurs during the dry season of December to June. Risk is greatest in the meningitis belt of sub-Saharan

Africa,* with rates of meningococcal disease in endemic regions reaching up to 1,000 cases per 100,000 population per year. Ongoing vaccination programs for resident populations with a monovalent group A vaccine in highly endemic areas has resulted in a decrease in cases of invasive disease. Children 9-23 mo old traveling to these equatorial African countries where meningococcal disease is hyperendemic or epidemic should receive a 2-dose series of MenACWY-D, 8-12 wk apart. Infants as young as 2 mo can receive the MenACWY-CRM vaccine, with doses administered at 2, 4, 6, and 12 mo of age. If the child is between 7 and 23 mo old, 2 doses of the vaccine are administered 8 wk apart. Conjugate vaccines are preferred in children over the less effective polysaccharide vaccine. Booster doses of conjugate A/C/Y/W-135 should occur every 3-5 yr for travelers returning to endemic areas, depending on the age of the pediatric traveler. Providers may also want to consider meningococcal vaccination for other pediatric travelers, especially if there is remote or rural travel to low-income countries with limited healthcare access, since meningococcal outbreaks can occur anywhere in the world. Proof of receipt of quadrivalent meningococcal vaccination is also necessary for individuals traveling to Saudi Arabia for the annual Hajj or Umrah pilgrimage.

Serogroups A and C are most often associated with epidemics of meningitis in sub-Saharan Africa, especially in the meningitis belt of equatorial Africa during the dry season months (December to June). Serogroups Y and W-135 have also been found in meningococcal outbreaks. Serogroup B is associated with more sporadic cases of invasive

---

*See the map at http://wwwnc.cdc.gov/travel/yellowbook/2016/chapter-3-infectious-diseases-related-to-travel/meningococcal-disease.

meningococcal disease in industrialized countries, including the United States. Routine vaccination of travelers with meningococcal B vaccine is currently not recommended. Additional vaccine information on meningococcal vaccination regimens and booster intervals can be found at the CDC website (https://www.cdc.gov/vaccines/vpd-vac/mening/default.html).

Rabies

Rabies is endemic in many countries in Africa, Asia, and Central and South America. Children are at particular risk because they are less likely to report bites and because facial bites are more common in children. Rabies has the potential for an extended latency period (months) and is uniformly fatal once the clinical symptoms emerge. **Preexposure prophylaxis** is recommended for ambulatory children with extended travel to high-risk regions, especially expatriate children and younger children traveling to or living in rural areas where enzootic dog rabies is endemic. Rabies preexposure vaccination should also be considered for adventure travelers (hikers, bikers), individuals likely to come into contact with rabies vectors (e.g., students working with animal or bat conservation), or travelers with itineraries to rabies-endemic regions where timely, effective **postexposure prophylaxis** might not be available following an animal bite. Most animal bites in a rabies-endemic area should be considered a medical emergency, especially bites from stray dogs, other carnivores, and bats. Immediate wound care washing should be followed by prompt administration of appropriate postexposure rabies prophylaxis at a medical facility. Postexposure prophylaxis is required even for persons who received preexposure vaccination. Algorithms for pre- and postexposure vaccination are the same regardless of patient age.

Numerous rabies vaccine formulations exist around the world. In the United States, 2 rabies vaccines are available: human diploid cell vaccine (HDCV; Imovax, Sanofi Pasteur, SA) and purified chick embryo cell (PCEC; RabAvert, Novartis) vaccine. Preexposure prophylaxis is given intramuscularly (HDCV or PCEC) as 3 doses (1 mL) on days 0, 7, and 21 or 28.

Postexposure prophylaxis is given as 4 doses (1 mL) of HDCV or PCEC vaccine intramuscularly on days 0, 3, 7, and 14. A 5th dose is recommended at day 28 for immunocompromised individuals. Two doses (1 mL) intramuscularly on days 0 and 3 are recommended for previously vaccinated individuals. Previously unvaccinated persons should also receive **rabies immunoglobulin** (**RIG**, 20 IU/kg), with as much of the dose as possible infiltrated around the wound site at the time of initial postexposure prophylaxis. Previously vaccinated persons do not require RIG. Unpurified or purified equine RIG preparations are still used in some low- and middle-income countries and are associated with a higher risk for severe reactions, including serum sickness and anaphylaxis. Purified cell culture–derived vaccines also are not always available abroad; travelers should be aware that any rabies vaccines derived from neural tissue carry an increased risk for adverse reactions, often with neurologic sequelae. If rabies prophylaxis is initiated abroad, neutralizing titers should be checked on return and immunization completed with a cell culture–derived vaccine. If rabies prophylaxis cannot be provided abroad, children with high-risk bites (e.g., stray dog) should be emergently transported to a site where they can receive prophylaxis, because the vaccinations should be started as soon as possible after the bite and ideally within 24 hr. Infants and young children respond well to rabies vaccine, and both pre- and postexposure vaccinations can be given at any age, using the same dose and schedule as adults. Individual travelers simultaneously receiving **mefloquine** or **chloroquine** may have limited immune reactions to intradermal (ID) rabies vaccine and should be vaccinated intramuscularly. The ID administration route is not currently recommended in the United States.

Tuberculosis

The risk for tuberculosis in the typical traveler is low. Pre- and posttravel testing for tuberculosis is controversial and should be done on an individualized basis depending on the itinerary, duration, and activities (e.g., working in a hospital setting). Immunization with bacille Calmette-Guérin (BCG) is even more controversial. BCG vaccine has variable efficacy in reducing severe tuberculosis disease in infants and young children, is not available in the United States, and is generally not recommended for pediatric travelers. Infection with *Mycobacterium bovis* can be prevented through avoiding consumption of unpasteurized dairy products.

Typhoid

Salmonella typhi infection, or **typhoid fever**, is common in many low- and middle-income countries in Asia, Africa, and Latin America (see Chapter 225). Typhoid vaccination is recommended for most children ≥2 yr old who are traveling to the Indian subcontinent, because the incidence of typhoid is 10-100 times higher for travelers to the Indian subcontinent than all other travel destinations. Vaccination should be strongly considered for other travelers to low- and middle-income countries, particularly if they are VFR travelers, lack access to reliable clean water and food, are traveling for a prolonged duration, or are adventurous eaters.

Two typhoid vaccines, the intramuscular (IM) Vi-polysaccharide vaccine and the oral Ty21a strain live-attenuated vaccine, are recommended for use in children in the United States. Both produce a protective response in 50–80% of recipients. The Ty21a vaccine may offer partial protection against *Salmonella paratyphi*, another cause of enteric fever. Travelers who have had prior diagnoses of typhoid fever should still receive vaccination, because past infection does not confer long-term immunity.

The IM Vi-polysaccharide vaccine is licensed for use in children ≥2 yr old. It can be given any time before departure, but it should ideally be administered 2 wk before travel, with a booster needed 2-3 yr later. The oral Ty21a vaccine can only be used in children ≥6 yr old and is given in 4 doses over 1 wk. Enteric-coated capsules are to be swallowed with a cool or room-temperature drink, at least 1 hr before a meal, every other day until the 4 doses are completed. Oral typhoid capsules must remain refrigerated (not frozen). Capsules should never be broken open, because vaccine efficacy depends on capsules being swallowed whole in order to pass through the acidic stomach contents. The oral vaccine is associated with an immune response lasting 5-7 yr (depending on national labeling). Antibiotics inhibit the immune response to the oral Ty21a vaccine; the vaccine should not be given within 72 hr of antibiotic treatment, and antibiotics should be avoided until 7 days after completing the vaccine series. Studies demonstrate that mefloquine, chloroquine, and atovaquone-proguanil can be given concurrently with the oral Ty21a vaccine without affecting the immunogenicity of the vaccine. Oral Ty21a vaccine should not be given to immunocompromised children; these children should receive the IM Vi-polysaccharide vaccine.

Yellow Fever

Yellow fever (see Chapter 296) is a mosquito-borne viral illness resembling other viral hemorrhagic fevers (Chapter 297) but with more prominent hepatic involvement. Yellow fever is present in tropical areas of South America and Africa.

Yellow fever vaccination is indicated in children >9 mo old traveling to an endemic area. Many countries require yellow fever vaccination by law for travelers arriving from endemic areas, and some African countries require evidence of vaccination from all entering travelers. Current recommendations can be obtained by contacting state or local health departments or the Division of Vector-Borne Infectious Diseases of the CDC (800-232-4636; http://wwwnc.cdc.gov/travel/yellowbook/2016/chapter-3-infectious-diseases-related-to-travel/yellow-fever). Most countries accept a medical waiver for children who are too young to be vaccinated (<6 mo) and for persons with a contraindication to vaccination. Children with asymptomatic HIV infection may be vaccinated if exposure to yellow fever virus (YFV) cannot be avoided.

Yellow fever vaccine (0.5 mL subcutaneously), a live-attenuated vaccine (17D strain) developed in chick embryos, is safe and highly effective in children >9 mo old, but in young infants is associated with a greatly increased risk for vaccine-associated encephalitis (0.5-4/1,000) and other severe reactions. Yellow fever vaccine should *never* be given to infants <6 mo old; infants 6-8 mo old should be vaccinated only in consultation with the CDC or a travel medicine expert to assess the current epidemiology, travel itinerary and duration, and whether the YFV exposure is greater than vaccine risks. In children >9 mo old, adverse effects are rare, although vaccine-associated neurotropic and viscerotropic disease associated with the vaccine have been reported. The risk of these reactions is higher in those with thymus disease, altered immune status, age >60 yr, or multiple sclerosis and in infants <9 mo old (neurotropic disease). Yellow fever vaccination is generally contraindicated in pregnancy and for nursing mothers, unless extended travel to a yellow fever–endemic area is unavoidable.

Children with immunodeficiency or an immunosuppressed state, a thymic disorder or dysfunction (e.g., DiGeorge syndrome), or a history of anaphylactic reactions to eggs should not receive yellow fever vaccine. Long-lived immunity develops with this vaccine, perhaps even lasting for a lifetime. Effective July 2016, WHO and countries following international health regulations no longer require revaccination every 10 yr. However, individuals traveling to high-risk areas with active yellow fever transmission and who anticipate frequent or prolonged stays should be reimmunized every 10 yr.

TRAVELER'S DIARRHEA
Ingestion of contaminated food or water makes travel-associated diarrhea the most common health complaint among international travelers. Traveler's diarrhea, characterized by a 2-fold or greater increase in the frequency of unformed bowel movements, occurs in as many as 40% of all travelers overseas (see Chapter 366.1). Children, especially those <3 yr old, have a higher incidence of diarrhea, more severe symptoms, and more prolonged symptoms than adults, with a reported attack rate of 60% for those <3 yr old in one study.

An important risk factor for traveler's diarrhea is the country of destination. High-risk areas (attack rates of 25–50%) include low- and middle-income countries of Latin America, Africa, the Middle East, and Asia. Intermediate risk occurs in Mediterranean countries, China, and Israel. Low-risk areas include North America, Northern Europe, Australia, and New Zealand. Fecal-oral diarrheal pathogens that children acquire during travel are similar to those acquired by adults and include enterotoxigenic and enteroaggregative *Escherichia coli, Campylobacter, Salmonella* (nontyphoidal serotypes predominate), and *Shigella* spp. Enteric protozoa are a much less common cause of traveler's diarrhea than bacterial pathogens; *Giardia lamblia* is the most likely protozoal cause of persistent diarrhea. Less common travel-associated protozoa include *Cryptosporidium* spp., *Entamoeba histolytica,* and *Cyclospora.* Viral infections, particularly rotavirus and norovirus infections, may also cause travel-associated diarrhea in children. Clinicians should be aware that not all diarrheal illness in children is food-borne or water-borne; febrile children with malaria may also present with vomiting and/or nonbloody diarrhea and may be misdiagnosed as having traveler's diarrhea.

Guidance on Prevention of Traveler's Diarrhea
Food and water hygiene remain important measures to reduce the incidence of traveler's diarrhea in children. However, creating long lists of foods to avoid or offering the popular, simple advice of "Boil it, peel it, cook it, or forget it!" is generally an ineffective method of reducing traveler's diarrhea. Most studies show that these types of dietary directives are difficult to keep and may have little impact on the incidence of traveler's diarrhea. In adult studies, the risk of developing traveler's diarrhea appears to be more associated with *where you eat rather than what you eat.* Eating in a relative's or friend's home is generally safer than eating in a restaurant, where restaurant kitchen hygiene and proper refrigeration may be lacking and employee handwashing may be sporadic.

In general, travel medicine providers can give some commonsense food and water advice to family travelers. Boiled or bottled water, hot beverages, and canned or bottled beverages are generally safe to consume. Ice should be avoided. In low- and middle-income countries, tap water is generally unsafe for drinking or brushing teeth. Boiling water for ≥1 min (or 3 min at altitudes >2,000 meters) remains a reliable method of disinfecting water. Food that is thoroughly cooked and served hot

is almost always safe to eat. Dry foods, such as pastry items, breads, and cookies, are generally safe to eat. Unpasteurized milk or other dairy products (cheese) should always be avoided. Breastfeeding should be encouraged for young children, especially infants <6 mo old, to reduce exposure to contaminated water or formula. All children should be reminded to wash their hands before eating and after playing around soil or animals. Chemoprophylactic agents for traveler's diarrhea are not recommended for children.

Management of Traveler's Diarrhea
Dehydration is the greatest threat presented by a diarrheal illness in a small child. Parents should be made aware of the symptoms and signs of dehydration and given instructions on how to administer rehydration solutions. Prepackaged WHO **oral rehydration solution** packets, which are available at stores or pharmacies in almost all low- and middle-income countries, should be part of a child's travel kit. Oral rehydration solution should be mixed as directed with bottled or boiled water and given slowly, as tolerated, to the child while symptoms persist.

Antimotility agents such as diphenoxylate (Lomotil) and loperamide (Imodium) should be avoided in infants and young children. The American Academy of Pediatrics (AAP) does not recommend their routine use in acute gastroenteritis. Use of antimotility agents may be beneficial in older children and adolescents with afebrile, nonbloody traveler's diarrhea. In general, antimotility agents should not distract parents from giving frequent oral rehydration solution, because ongoing intestinal fluid losses likely continue despite a decrease in stooling. Bismuth subsalicylate for acute gastroenteritis should be avoided because of concern for toxicity and Reye syndrome.

Presumptive Antibiotic Treatment
Oral rehydration is the mainstay of treatment for pediatric traveler's diarrhea. However, antibiotics should be prescribed for the pediatric traveler, with parental instructions to start presumptive treatment early in the diarrheal illness. Systemic antibiotics can shorten the duration and severity of diarrheal illness, especially if presumptive antibiotics are initiated immediately after onset of traveler's diarrhea. For children, the drug of choice is **azithromycin** (10 mg/kg once daily for up to 3 days, with maximum daily dose of 500 mg). **Ciprofloxacin** (10 mg/kg per dose twice daily for up to 3 days, maximum dose of 500 mg twice daily) is an alternative for children >1 yr old but should not be prescribed for travelers to the Indian subcontinent or Southeast Asia, where fluoroquinolone resistance is common. Shiga-toxin–producing *E. coli* such as *E. coli* O157:H7 is an extremely uncommon cause of pediatric traveler's diarrhea in nonindustrialized countries, and the benefit of presumptive antibiotic therapy in traveling children, even with bloody diarrhea, typically outweighs the low risk of developing hemolytic-uremic syndrome. Parents need to be aware that the use of antibiotics for the treatment of traveler's diarrhea has been associated with colonization with highly resistant organisms such as extended-spectrum β-lactamase–producing Enterobacteriaceae. These organisms could later cause infections once back home.

Azithromycin is highly effective against most bacterial pathogens that cause traveler's diarrhea and is the preferred antibiotic among many travel experts. Azithromycin can be prescribed in powder form that can be reconstituted with safe water into a liquid suspension when needed. Amoxicillin, trimethoprim-sulfamethoxazole (cotrimoxazole), and erythromycin should *not* be prescribed for self-treatment of traveler's diarrhea, because of widespread resistance among diarrheal pathogens. Traveler's diarrhea that results in bloody stools, persistently high fevers, systemic chills and rigors, severe or localizing abdominal pain, or continued fluid losses should prompt additional medical evaluation.

INSECT-BORNE INFECTIONS
Insect-borne infections for which traveling children are most at risk include malaria, dengue, chikungunya, yellow fever, Zika, and Japanese encephalitis, depending on the area of travel. **Malaria** is transmitted by nighttime biting *Anopheles* mosquitoes, whereas **dengue** occurs from mosquito species (*Culex, Aedes*) that are predominantly active during

the day. Families should be encouraged to protect children against daytime and nighttime biting mosquitoes, since many regions of the world where malaria is found also have diseases transmitted by daytime biting mosquitoes (dengue, Zika, chikungunya). Sexually active adolescents and young adults need to be advised on the risks of traveling to Zika-endemic regions in peak season. In addition to insect bite prevention using insect repellents, methods of contraception should be discussed with the traveler.

Exposure to insect bites can be reduced by wearing appropriate attire and using insect repellents containing *N,N*-diethyl-*m*-toluamide (**DEET**) or picaridin. The AAP recommends avoiding DEET-containing repellents in children <2 mo old. Rare cases of neurologic events have been reported in very young children with exposure to inappropriate, frequent applications of DEET-containing repellents (>10 times/day) or who licked off DEET. Concentrations of 25–30% DEET need be applied every 4-6 hr as needed, whereas 5–7% DEET provides only 1-2 hr of protection time. DEET concentrations >40–50% do not confer a substantially longer protection time for children and are not recommended.

Picaridin is fragrance-free, effective, and generally well tolerated on exposed skin and faces. It has similar efficacy to DEET but with less inhalational or dermal irritation. Picaridin at concentrations of 20% or higher provides adequate protection against *Anopheles* mosquitoes that have potential to transmit malaria. When applying sunscreen and insect repellent, sunscreen should be applied first, followed by DEET or picaridin.

Spraying or treating clothing with **permethrin**, a synthetic pyrethroid, is a safe and effective method of further reducing insect bites in children. Permethrin can be applied directly to clothing, bed nets, shoes, and hats and should be allowed to dry fully before use. As an insecticide, permethrin should never be applied to skin. Permethrin-treated garments retain both repellency and insecticidal activity, even with repeated laundering. Clothing will eventually need to be re-treated to maintain repellency, according to the product label. Bed nets, particularly permethrin-impregnated bed nets, also decrease the risk of insect bites, and their use is highly recommended in malarial areas.

MALARIA CHEMOPROPHYLAXIS

Malaria, a mosquito-borne infection, is the leading parasitic cause of death in children worldwide (see Chapter 314). Of the 5 *Plasmodium* species that infect humans, *Plasmodium falciparum* causes the greatest morbidity and mortality. Each year, >8 million U.S. citizens visit parts of the world where malaria is endemic (sub-Saharan Africa, Central and South America, India, Southeast Asia, Oceania). Children accounted for 15–20% of imported malaria cases in a WHO study in Europe. Given the major resurgence of malaria and increased travel among families with young children, physicians in industrialized countries are increasingly required to give advice on prevention, diagnosis, and treatment of malaria. **Risk factors** for severe malaria and death include inadequate adherence to chemoprophylaxis, delay in seeking medical care, delay in diagnosis, and nonimmune status, but the case fatality rate of imported malaria remains <1% in children from nonendemic countries. The CDC maintains updated information at http://www.cdc.gov/malaria/travelers/index.html, as well as a malaria hotline for physicians (770-488-7788). It is important to check this updated information, because recommendations for prophylaxis and treatment are often modified as a result of changes in the risk for developing malaria in different areas of the world, changing *Plasmodium* resistance patterns, and the availability of new antimalarial medications.

Avoidance of mosquitoes and **barrier protection** from mosquitoes are an important part of malaria prevention for travelers to endemic areas. The *Anopheles* mosquito feeds from dusk to dawn. Travelers should remain in well-screened areas, wear clothing that covers most of the body, sleep under a bed net (ideally impregnated with permethrin), and use insect repellents with DEET during these hours. Parents should be discouraged from taking a young child on a trip that will entail evening or nighttime exposure in areas endemic for *P. falciparum*.

Chemoprophylaxis is the cornerstone of malaria prevention for nonimmune children and adults who travel to malaria-endemic

areas, *but is not a replacement for other protective measures.* Travelers often do not take malaria prophylaxis as prescribed or at all. They are more likely to use prophylactic antimalarial drugs if their physicians provide appropriate recommendations and education before departure. However, in one survey, only 14% of persons who sought medical advice obtained correct information about malaria prevention and prophylaxis. Families with children visiting friends and relatives are particularly less likely to take malaria prophylaxis or seek pretravel medical advice.

Resistance of *P. falciparum* to the traditional chemoprophylactic agent, **chloroquine**, is widespread, and in most areas of the world other agents must be used (Table 200.2). Factors that must be considered in choosing appropriate chemoprophylaxis medications and dosing schedules include age of the child, travel itinerary (including whether the child will be traveling to areas of risk within a particular country and whether chloroquine-resistant *P. falciparum* is present in the country), vaccinations being given, allergies or other known adverse reactions to antimalarial agents, and the availability of medical care during travel.

Children traveling to areas with chloroquine-resistant *P. falciparum* can be given mefloquine, atovaquone-proguanil, or doxycycline (if >8 yr old) as malaria prophylaxis. For trips shorter than 4 wk, atovaquone-proguanil is the preferred medication, because it is given for only a short period before and after travel. Atovaquone-proguanil or doxycycline is also indicated for travel of any duration to western Cambodia and the Thailand-Cambodia and Thailand-Myanmar borders because of mefloquine resistance in these areas. For periods of travel >4 wk to all other areas with chloroquine-resistant *P. falciparum*, mefloquine is the preferred medication because it can be taken weekly.

Mefloquine is FDA-approved only for children weighing >15 kg, but the CDC recommends mefloquine prophylaxis for all children regardless of weight because the risk for acquiring severe malaria outweighs the risk for potential mefloquine toxicity. Adults taking mefloquine prophylaxis have a 10–25% incidence of sleep disturbance and dysphoria and, less frequently, more serious neuropsychiatric symptoms. These side effects appear to be less common in children. Other potential side effects of mefloquine therapy include nausea and vomiting.

The lack of a liquid or suspension formulations for all antimalarial agents can make administration difficult. For children who cannot take tablets, parents should take a chloroquine or mefloquine prescription to a compounding pharmacy, which can pulverize the tablets and place exact dosages into gel capsules. Parents can then open the gel capsules and sprinkle the powder into food. Disguising these medications, which have a bitter taste, is important; chocolate syrup has been used successfully as a vehicle for the medication. Persons with depression, neuropsychiatric disorders, seizure disorders, or cardiac conduction defects should not take mefloquine.

Atovaquone-proguanil fixed combination (Malarone) is an effective and safe chemoprophylaxis for travelers to chloroquine-resistant malaria-endemic areas. Adverse effects are infrequent and mild (abdominal pain, vomiting, and headache) and infrequently result in discontinuation of the medication. Atovaquone-proguanil prophylaxis must be taken every day with food, so it is better suited for prophylaxis during short periods of exposure. Recent data allow dosing down to 5 kg body weight, although the use of atovaquone-proguanil in children weighing 5-10 kg is considered off-label.

Daily **doxycycline** is an alternative chemoprophylaxis regimen for chloroquine-resistant *P. falciparum* malaria. Doxycycline has been used extensively and is highly effective, but it cannot be used in children <8 yr old because of the risk of permanent tooth staining. Adverse effects (nausea, vomiting, photosensitivity, vaginal candidiasis) are relatively uncommon. Persons given doxycycline prophylaxis should be warned to decrease exposure to direct sunlight to minimize the possibility of photosensitivity.

Primaquine has also been used successfully as chemoprophylaxis, especially in areas of high prevalence of *Plasmodium vivax* and *Plasmodium ovale*, but there are limited data about its use in nonimmune children. Primaquine prophylaxis for children should only be given in consultation with the CDC or a travel medicine specialist.

Chloroquine, chloroquine-proguanil, and azithromycin do not provide

Table 200.2	Antimalarial Chemoprophylaxis for Children					
AREA	**DRUG**	**ADULT DOSE**	**PEDIATRIC DOSE**	**ADVANTAGES**	**DISADVANTAGES**	**COMMENTS**
Chloroquine-resistant area	Mefloquine*†	250 mg salt (228 mg base) tablets One tablet weekly	Weight <10 kg: 5 mg salt (4.6 mg base)/kg/wk Weight 10-19 kg: ¼ tablet/wk Weight 20-30 kg: ½ tablet/wk Weight 31-45 kg: ¾ tablet/wk Weight >45 kg: 1 tablet/wk	Once-weekly dosing	Bitter taste No pediatric formulation Side effects of sleep disturbance, vivid dreams	Children going to malaria-endemic area for ≥4 wk Children unlikely to take daily medication
	Doxycycline‡	100 mg tablet One tablet daily	2 mg/kg daily (max: 100 mg)	Known safety profile Readily available in most pharmacies	Cannot give to children <8 yr old Daily dosing Must take with food or causes stomach upset Photosensitivity Yeast superinfections	Children ≥8 yr old going to area for <4 wk who cannot take or cannot obtain atovaquone-proguanil
	Atovaquone-proguanil§ (Malarone)	250/100 adult tablet One tablet daily	Pediatric tablet: 62.5 mg atovaquone/25 mg proguanil Weight 5-8 kg: ½ pediatric tablet once daily Weight >8-10 kg: ¾ pediatric tablet once daily Weight >10-20 kg: 1 pediatric tablet once daily Weight >20-30 kg: 2 pediatric tablets once daily Weight >30-40 kg: 3 pediatric tablets once daily Weight >40 kg: 1 adult tablet once daily	Pediatric tablet formulation available Generally well tolerated	Daily dosing Expensive Can cause stomach upset	Children going to malaria-endemic area for <4 wk
Chloroquine-susceptible area	Chloroquine phosphate	500 mg salt (300 mg base) One tablet weekly	8.3 mg/kg salt (5 mg/kg base) weekly	Once-weekly dosing Generally well tolerated Safe in pregnancy	Bitter taste No pediatric formulation	Best medication for children traveling to areas with *Plasmodium falciparum* or *P. vivax* that is chloroquine susceptible

Drugs used for chloroquine-resistant areas can also be used in chloroquine-susceptible areas.

*Chloroquine and mefloquine should be started 1-2 wk before departure and continued for 4 wk after last exposure.

†Mefloquine resistance exists in western Cambodia and along the Thailand–Cambodia and Thailand–Myanmar borders. Travelers to these areas should take doxycycline or atovaquone-proguanil. See text for precautions about mefloquine use.

‡Doxycycline should be started 1-2 days before departure and continued for 4 wk after last exposure. Do not use in children <8 yr old or in pregnant women.

§Atovaquone-proguanil (Malarone) should be started 1-2 days before departure and continued for 7 days after last exposure; should be taken with food or a milky drink. Not recommended in pregnant women, children who weigh <5 kg, and women breastfeeding infants who weigh <5 kg. Contraindicated in individuals with severe renal impairment (creatinine clearance <30 mL/min).

adequate protection for children traveling to a chloroquine-resistant malaria-endemic area.

In areas of the world where *P. falciparum* remains fully chloroquine-sensitive (Haiti, the Dominican Republic, Central America west of the Panama Canal, and some countries in the Middle East), weekly chloroquine is the drug of choice for malaria chemoprophylaxis. Updated information on chloroquine susceptibility and recommended malaria prophylaxis is available at http://wwwnc.cdc.gov/travel/yellowbook/2016/chapter-3-infectious-diseases-related-to-travel/malaria.

On leaving an area endemic for *P. vivax* or *P. ovale* after a prolonged visit (usually >3 mo), travelers should consider terminal prophylaxis with primaquine (0.5 mg/kg base) daily, up to a maximum dose of 30 mg base or 52.6 mg salt, for 14 days, to eliminate extraerythrocytic forms of *P. vivax* and *P. ovale* and prevent relapses. Screening for glucose-6-phosphate dehydrogenase deficiency is mandatory before primaquine treatment, since primaquine is contraindicated in G6PD-deficient persons because it can cause severe hemolysis.

Small amounts of antimalarial drugs are secreted into breast milk. The amounts of transferred drug are not considered to be either harmful or sufficient to provide adequate prophylaxis against malaria. Prolonged infant exposure to doxycycline through breast milk is not advisable.

Self-treatment of presumptive malaria during travel remains controversial. It should never be substituted for seeking appropriate medical care, but it can be considered in special circumstances such as travel to remote areas, intolerance of prophylaxis, or refusal of chemoprophylaxis by the traveler. Self-treatment medication should be different than the prescribed chemoprophylaxis. The CDC or a travel medicine specialist should be consulted if self-treatment medication is being considered for a traveler.

THE RETURNING TRAVELER

Posttravel evaluations are part of travel medicine and continuing care. Physicians unfamiliar with diseases that occur in low- and middle-income countries often misdiagnose the cause of illness in a child returning from travel abroad. Among returning patients identified from the GeoSentinel Surveillance Network sites who were ill, the common disorders included, in descending order of frequency, malaria, giardiasis,

Table 200.3	Common Causes of Fever by Geographic Area	
GEOGRAPHIC AREA	**COMMON TROPICAL DISEASE-CAUSING FEVER**	**OTHER INFECTIONS CAUSING OUTBREAKS OR CLUSTERS IN TRAVELERS**
Caribbean	Chikungunya, dengue, malaria (Haiti), Zika	Acute histoplasmosis, leptospirosis
Central America	Chikungunya, dengue, malaria (primarily *Plasmodium vivax*), Zika	Leptospirosis, histoplasmosis, coccidioidomycosis
South America	Chikungunya, dengue, malaria (primarily *P. vivax*), Zika	Bartonellosis, leptospirosis, enteric fever, histoplasmosis
South-Central Asia	Dengue, enteric fever, malaria (primarily non-falciparum)	Chikungunya
Southeast Asia	Dengue, malaria (primarily non-falciparum)	Chikungunya, leptospirosis
Sub-Saharan Africa	Malaria (primarily *P. falciparum*), tick-borne rickettsiae (main cause of fever in southern Africa), acute schistosomiasis, dengue	

From Wilson ME: Post-travel evaluation. In CDC *Yellow Book*, Chapter 5 (Table 5.2). https://wwwnc.cdc.gov/travel/yellowbook/2018/post-travel-evaluation/fever-in-returned-travelers.

Table 200.4	Common Infections by Incubation Period	
DISEASE	**USUAL INCUBATION PERIOD (RANGE)**	**DISTRIBUTION**
INCUBATION <14 DAYS		
Chikungunya	2-4 days (1-14 days)	Tropics, subtropics
Dengue	4-8 days (3-14 days)	Topics, subtropics
Encephalitis, arboviral (Japanese encephalitis, tick-borne encephalitis, West Nile virus, other)	3-14 days (1-20 days)	Specific agents vary by region
Enteric fever	7-18 days (3-60 days)	Especially in Indian subcontinent
Acute HIV	10-28 days (10 days to 6 wk)	Worldwide
Influenza	1-3 days	Worldwide, can also be acquired while traveling
Legionellosis	5-6 days (2-10 days)	Widespread
Leptospirosis	7-12 days (2-26 days)	Widespread, most common in tropical areas
Malaria, *Plasmodium falciparum*	6-30 days (98% onset within 3 mo of travel)	Tropics, subtropics
Malaria, *Plasmodium vivax*	8 days to 12 mo (almost half have onset >30 days after completion of travel)	Widespread in tropics and subtropics
Spotted-fever rickettsiae	Few days to 2-3 wk	Causative species vary by region
Zika virus infection	3-14 days	Widespread in Latin America, endemic through much of Africa, Southeast Asia, and Pacific Islands
INCUBATION 14 DAYS TO 6 WK		
Encephalitis, arboviral; enteric fever; acute HIV; leptospirosis; malaria	See above incubation periods for relevant diseases.	See above distribution for relevant diseases.
Amebic liver abscess	Weeks to months	Most common in resource-poor countries
Hepatitis A	28-30 days (15-50 days)	Most common in resource-poor countries
Hepatitis E	26-42 days (2-9 wk)	Widespread
Acute schistosomiasis (Katayama syndrome)	4-8 wk	Most common in sub-Saharan Africa
INCUBATION >6 WK		
Amebic liver abscess, hepatitis E, malaria, acute schistosomiasis	See above incubation periods for relevant diseases.	See above distribution for relevant diseases.
Hepatitis B	90 days (60-150 days)	Widespread
Leishmaniasis, visceral	2-10 mo (10 days to years)	Asia, Africa, Latin America, southern Europe, and the Middle East
Tuberculosis	Primary, weeks; reactivation, years	Global distribution, rates, and levels of resistance vary widely.

From Wilson ME: Post-travel evaluation. In CDC *Yellow Book*, Chapter 5 (Table 5.3). https://wwwnc.cdc.gov/travel/yellowbook/2018/post-travel-evaluation/fever-in-returned-travelers.

dengue fever, campylobacteriosis, cutaneous larva migrans, enteric fever, spotted fever (rickettsiosis), chikungunya fever, hepatitis A, and influenza. Returning pediatric travelers who are severely ill or with continued fevers should be seen in consultation with a pediatric travel medicine or infectious diseases specialist. The cause of fever may be suggested by the geographic area (Table 200.3) and incubation period (Table 200.4).

Among all persons returning from travel (children and adults), 3 major patterns of illness have been noted (Table 200.5). The etiology of each of these disease presentations in part depends on the country or geographic region visited (see Table 200.3). Table 200.6 provides suggestive clues to a diagnosis.

Fever is a particularly worrisome symptom. Children with a febrile/systemic illness following recent travel to a malarial destination should be promptly evaluated for malaria, especially if having traveled to sub-Saharan Africa and Papua New Guinea. *P. falciparum* malaria will generally present within 1-2 mo after return from travel to a malaria-endemic area, but can occur within the 1st yr after return. In contrast, symptoms of *P. vivax* or *P. ovale* malaria are typically later in onset following travel (i.e., several months), are milder in disease severity, and may occur in a relapsing pattern if undiagnosed or improperly untreated. Other symptoms of malaria can be nonspecific and include chills, malaise, headache, myalgias, vomiting, diarrhea, cough, and

Table 200.5	Patterns of Illness in Returning International Travelers

SYSTEMIC FEBRILE ILLNESS

Malaria
Dengue
Zika
Enteric fever (typhoid/paratyphoid)
Chikungunya virus
Spotted-fever rickettsiae
Hepatitis A
Acute HIV
Leptospirosis
Measles
Infectious mononucleosis
Respiratory causes (pneumonia, influenza)
Undetermined fever source

ACUTE DIARRHEA

Campylobacter
Shigella spp.
Salmonella spp.
Diarrheagenic *Escherichia coli* (enterotoxigenic *E. coli*, enteroadherent *E. coli*—not tested for by routine stool culture methods)

Giardiasis (acute, persistent, or recurrent)
Entamoeba histolytica
Cryptosporidium spp.
Cyclospora cayetanensis
Presumed viral enteritis

DERMATOLOGIC MANIFESTATIONS

Rash with fever (dengue)
Arthropod-related dermatitis (insect bites)
Cutaneous larva migrans (*Ancylostoma braziliense*)
Bacterial skin infections—pyoderma, impetigo, ecthyma, erysipelas
Myiasis (tumbu and botfly)
Scabies
Tungiasis
Superficial mycosis
Animal bites
Leishmaniasis
Rickettsial diseases
Marine envenomation/dermatitis
Photoallergic dermatitis and phytophotodermatitis

Table 200.6	Common Clinical Findings and Associated Infections

COMMON CLINICAL FINDINGS	INFECTIONS TO CONSIDER AFTER TROPICAL TRAVEL
Fever and rash	Dengue, chikungunya, Zika, rickettsial infections, enteric fever (skin lesions may be sparse or absent), acute HIV infection, measles
Fever and abdominal pain	Enteric fever, amebic liver abscess
Undifferentiated fever and normal or low white blood cell count	Dengue, malaria, rickettsial infection, enteric fever, chikungunya, Zika
Fever and hemorrhage	Viral hemorrhagic fevers (dengue and others), meningococcemia, leptospirosis, rickettsial infections
Fever and arthralgia or myalgia, sometimes persistent	Chikungunya, dengue, Zika
Fever and eosinophilia	Acute schistosomiasis, drug hypersensitivity reaction, fascioliasis and other parasitic infections (rare)
Fever and pulmonary infiltrates	Common bacterial and viral pathogens, legionellosis, acute schistosomiasis, Q fever, leptospirosis
Fever and altered mental status	Cerebral malaria, viral or bacterial meningoencephalitis, African trypanosomiasis, scrub typhus
Mononucleosis syndrome	Epstein-Barr virus (EBV) infection, cytomegalovirus (CMV) infection, toxoplasmosis, acute HIV infection
Fever persisting >2 wk	Malaria, enteric fever, EBV infection, CMV infection, toxoplasmosis, acute HIV infection, acute schistosomiasis, brucellosis, tuberculosis, Q fever, visceral leishmaniasis (rare)
Fever with onset >6 wk after travel	*Plasmodium vivax* or *P. ovale* malaria, acute hepatitis (B, C, or E), tuberculosis, amebic liver abscess

From Wilson ME: Post-travel evaluation. In CDC *Yellow Book*, Chapter 5 (Table 5.6). https://wwwnc.cdc.gov/travel/yellowbook/2018/post-travel-evaluation/fever-in-returned-travelers.

possible seizures. Children are more likely than adults to have higher fevers and also gastrointestinal symptoms, hepatomegaly, splenomegaly, and severe anemia. Thrombocytopenia (without increased bleeding) and fever in a child returning from an endemic area are highly suggestive of malaria.

Thick and thin blood smears need to be performed for diagnosis *if* malaria is clinically suspected. If results are negative initially, 2 or more additional smears should be done 12-24 hr after the initial smears. Rapid malaria antigen tests (BinaxNOW Malaria) are FDA-approved and sensitive for diagnosing falciparum malaria. Treatment should be initiated immediately once the diagnosis is confirmed or empirically if presentation is severe with suspected malaria. Treatment should be determined in consultation with a pediatric infectious disease specialist and/or the CDC for updated information on the drugs of choice, which are similar to those for adults (see Chapter 314). Great caution should be used with young children, nonimmune patients, and pregnant patients with falciparum malaria, and hospitalization of these patients should be strongly considered until reliable improvement is observed.

Enteric (typhoid) fever should be considered in children with persistent or recurrent fevers following return from the Indian subcontinent. Multiple blood cultures and a stool culture may both be necessary to diagnosis enteric fever. **Dengue** is another cause of fever and systemic illness in ill travelers, particularly when returning from Southeast Asia, the Caribbean, Central and South America, or the Indian subcontinent. Many bacterial and protozoal causes of acute traveler's diarrhea may also result in fever and systemic symptoms in children. Additional travel-associated febrile, diarrheal, and dermatologic illnesses exist, of which the most common etiologies can be found in Tables 200.5 and 200.6.

THE ADOLESCENT TRAVELER

The preparation of an adolescent interested in traveling abroad can pose a challenge for most clinicians. Study abroad, gap year, humanitarian volunteer work, adventure, and tourism are among many reasons for travel to countries with limited resources. While many travel-related problems discussed in this chapter are relevant to this group, other high-risk activities such as sexual intercourse, alcohol consumption, driving, use of illicit drugs, and adventure travel (mountain climbing, white water rafting, kayaking, biking) require special attention and discussion with the traveler and parents/guardians. Topics such as HIV exposure, sexually transmitted infections, sexual assault, and unplanned pregnancy may require specific preventive strategies such as condom use, contraception, and postexposure HIV prophylaxis.

Bibliography is available at Expert Consult.

Chapter **201**

Fever

Linda S. Nield and Deepak Kamat

第二百零一章
发热

中文导读

本章首先介绍了发热的定义，随后主要介绍了发热的发病机制、病因学、临床特征、评估和处理。在发热的病因中详细描述了发热病因的分类、不同病因的发热特点以及不同发热类型的常见疾病。其中，重点列举了感染性发热、非感染性发热和周期性发热综合征的常见疾病。在发热的评估中尤其强调了急性发热的评估内容及评估方法。在发热的处理中详细介绍了发热的处理原则、退热药的使用方法等内容。

Fever is defined as a rectal temperature ≥38°C (100.4°F), and a value >40°C (104°F) is called **hyperpyrexia**. Traditionally, body temperature fluctuates in a defined normal range (36.6-37.9°C [97.9-100.2°F] rectally), so that the highest point is reached in early evening and the lowest point is reached in the morning. Any abnormal rise in body temperature should be considered a symptom of an underlying condition. The range of normal temperature is broad, 35.5-37.7°C (96-100°F); if 37°C (98.6°F) is considered normal, many cluster around this temperature (36.1-37.5°C [97-99.5°F]).

PATHOGENESIS

Body temperature is regulated by thermosensitive neurons located in the preoptic or anterior hypothalamus that respond to changes in blood temperature, as well as by cold and warm receptors located in skin and muscles. Thermoregulatory responses include redirecting blood to or from cutaneous vascular beds, increased or decreased sweating, regulation of extracellular fluid (ECF) volume by arginine vasopressin, and behavioral responses, such as seeking a warmer or cooler environmental temperature.

Three different mechanisms can produce fever: pyrogens, heat production exceeding heat loss, and defective heat loss. The 1st mechanism involves endogenous and exogenous pyrogens that raise the hypothalamic temperature set point. **Endogenous pyrogens** include the cytokines interleukin (IL)-1 and IL-6, tumor necrosis factor (TNF)-α, and interferon (IFN)-β and IFN-γ. Stimulated leukocytes and other cells produce lipids that also serve as endogenous pyrogens. The best-studied lipid mediator is prostaglandin E_2, which attaches to the prostaglandin receptors in the hypothalamus to produce the new temperature set point. Along with infectious diseases and drugs, malignancy and inflammatory diseases can cause fever through the production of endogenous pyrogens. Some substances produced within the body are not pyrogens but are capable of stimulating endogenous pyrogens. Such substances include antigen-antibody complexes in the presence of complement, complement components, lymphocyte products, bile acids, and androgenic steroid metabolites. **Exogenous pyrogens** come from outside the body and consist of mainly infectious pathogens and drugs. Microbes, microbial toxins, or other products of microbes are the most common exogenous pyrogens, which stimulate macrophages and other cells to produce endogenous pyrogens. **Endotoxin** is one of the few substances that can directly affect thermoregulation in the hypothalamus as well as stimulate endogenous pyrogen release. Many drugs cause fever, and the mechanism for increasing body temperature varies with the class of drug. Drugs that are known to cause fever include vancomycin, amphotericin B, and allopurinol.

Heat production exceeding heat loss is the 2nd mechanism that leads to fever; examples include salicylate poisoning and malignant hyperthermia. **Defective heat loss**, the 3rd mechanism, may occur in children with ectodermal dysplasia or victims of severe heat exposure.

ETIOLOGY

The causes of fever can be organized into 4 main categories: *infectious, inflammatory, neoplastic,* and *miscellaneous.* Self-limited viral infections (common cold, influenza, gastroenteritis) and uncomplicated bacterial infections (otitis media, pharyngitis, sinusitis) are the most common causes of acute fever. The body temperature rarely rises above potentially lethal levels (42°C [107.6°F]) in the neurologically intact child unless extreme hyperthermic environmental conditions are present or other extenuating circumstances exist, such as underlying malignant hyperthermia or thyrotoxicosis.

The pattern of the fever can provide clues to the underlying etiology. Viral infections typically are associated with a slow decline of fever over 1 wk, whereas bacterial infections are often associated with a prompt resolution of fever after effective antimicrobial treatment. Although antimicrobials can result in rapid elimination of bacteria, if tissue injury has been extensive, the inflammatory response and fever can continue for days after all microbes have been eradicated.

Intermittent fever is an exaggerated circadian rhythm that includes a period of normal temperatures on most days; extremely wide fluctuations may be termed **septic** or **hectic fever**. **Sustained fever** is persistent and does not vary by >0.5°C (0.9°F)/day. **Remittent fever** is persistent and varies by >0.5°C/day. **Relapsing fever** is characterized by febrile periods separated by intervals of normal temperature; **tertian fever** occurs on the 1st and 3rd days (malaria caused by *Plasmodium vivax*), and **quartan fever** occurs on the 1st and 4th days (malaria caused by *Plasmodium malariae*). Diseases characterized by relapsing fevers should be distinguished from infectious diseases that have a tendency to relapse (Table 201.1). **Biphasic fever** indicates a single illness with 2 distinct periods (**camelback fever** pattern); poliomyelitis is the classic example. A biphasic course is also characteristic of other enteroviral infections, leptospirosis, dengue fever, yellow fever, Colorado tick fever, spirillary rat-bite fever *(Spirillum minus)*, and the African hemorrhagic fevers (Marburg, Ebola, and Lassa fevers). The term **periodic fever** is used narrowly to describe fever syndromes with a regular periodicity (cyclic neutropenia and periodic fever, aphthous stomatitis, pharyngitis, adenopathy) or more broadly to include disorders characterized by recurrent episodes of fever that do not follow a strictly periodic pattern (familial Mediterranean fever, TNF receptor–associated periodic syndrome [Hibernian fever], hyper-IgD syndrome, Muckle-Wells syndrome) (see Chapter 188). **Factitious fever**, or self-induced fever, may be caused by intentional manipulation of the thermometer or injection of pyrogenic material.

The **double quotidian fever** (or fever that peaks twice in 24 hr) is classically associated with inflammatory arthritis. In general, a single isolated fever spike is not associated with an infectious disease. Such a spike can be attributed to the infusion of blood products and some drugs, as well as some procedures, or to manipulation of a catheter on a colonized or infected body surface. Similarly, temperatures in excess of 41°C (105.8°F) are most often associated with a noninfectious cause. Causes for very high temperatures (>41°C [105.8°F]) include central fever (resulting from central nervous system dysfunction involving the hypothalamus or spinal cord injury), malignant hyperthermia, malignant neuroleptic syndrome, drug fever, or heat stroke. Temperatures that are lower than normal (<36°C [96.8°F]) can be associated with overwhelming sepsis but are more often related to cold exposure, hypothyroidism, or overuse of antipyretics.

CLINICAL FEATURES

The clinical features of fever can range from no symptoms to extreme malaise. Children might complain of feeling hot or cold, display facial flushing, and experience shivering. Fatigue and irritability may be evident. Parents often report that the child looks ill or pale and has a decreased appetite. The underlying etiology also produces accompanying symptoms. Although the underlying etiologies can manifest in varied ways clinically, there are some predictable features. For example, **fever with petechiae** in an ill-appearing patient indicates the high possibility of life-threatening conditions such as meningococcemia, Rocky Mountain spotted fever, or acute bacterial endocarditis.

Changes in heart rate, most frequently tachycardia, accompany fever. Normally heart rate rises by 10 beats/min per 1°C (1.8°F) rise in temperature for children >2 mo old. Relative tachycardia, when the pulse rate is elevated disproportionately to the temperature, is usually caused by noninfectious diseases or infectious diseases in which a toxin is responsible for the clinical manifestations. **Relative bradycardia** (temperature-pulse dissociation), when the pulse rate remains low in the presence of fever, can accompany typhoid fever, brucellosis, leptospirosis, or drug fever. Bradycardia in the presence of fever also may be a result of a conduction defect resulting from cardiac involvement with acute rheumatic fever, Lyme disease, viral myocarditis, or infective endocarditis.

EVALUATION

Most acute febrile episodes in a normal host can be diagnosed by a careful history and physical examination and require few, if any, laboratory tests. Because infection is the most likely etiology of the acute fever, the evaluation should initially be geared to discovering an underlying infectious cause (Table 201.2). The details of the history should include the onset and pattern of fever and any accompanying signs and symptoms. The patient often displays signs or symptoms that provide

---

Table 201.1	Fevers Prone to Relapse

INFECTIOUS CAUSES
Relapsing fever (*Borrelia recurrentis*)
Q fever (*Coxiella burnetii*)
Typhoid fever (*Salmonella typhi*)
Syphilis (*Treponema pallidum*)
Tuberculosis
Histoplasmosis
Coccidioidomycosis
Blastomycosis
Melioidosis (*Pseudomonas pseudomallei*)
Lymphocytic choriomeningitis (LCM) infection
Dengue fever
Yellow fever
Chronic meningococcemia
Colorado tick fever
Leptospirosis
Brucellosis
Oroya fever (*Bartonella bacilliformis*)
Acute rheumatic fever
Rat-bite fever (*Spirillum minus*)
Visceral leishmaniasis
Lyme disease (*Borrelia burgdorferi*)
Malaria
Babesiosis
Noninfluenza respiratory viral infection
Epstein-Barr virus infection

NONINFECTIOUS CAUSES
Behçet disease
Crohn disease
Weber-Christian disease (panniculitis)
Leukoclastic angiitis syndromes
Sweet syndrome
Systemic lupus erythematosus and other autoimmune disorders

PERIODIC FEVER SYNDROMES (see Chapter 188)
Familial Mediterranean fever
Cyclic neutropenia
Periodic fever, aphthous stomatitis, pharyngitis, and adenopathy (PFAPA)
Hyper–immunoglobulin D syndrome
Hibernian fever (tumor necrosis factor superfamily immunoglobulin A–associated syndrome [TRAPS])
Muckle-Wells syndrome
Others

Table 201.2	Evaluation of Acute Fever

Thorough history: onset, other symptoms, exposures (daycare, school, family, pets, playmates), travel, medications, other underlying disorders, immunizations
Physical examination: complete, with focus on localizing symptoms
Laboratory studies on a case-by-case basis:
• Rapid antigen testing
• Nasopharyngeal: respiratory viruses by polymerase chain reaction
• Throat: group A streptococcus
• Stool: NAAT for enteric pathogens, calprotectin
• Blood: complete blood count, blood culture, C-reactive protein, sedimentation rate, procalcitonin
• Urine: urinalysis, culture
• Cerebrospinal fluid: cell count, glucose, protein, Gram stain, culture
• Chest radiograph or other imaging studies on a case-by-case basis

NAAT, Nucleic acid amplification test.

clues to the cause of the fever. Exposures to other ill persons at home, daycare, and school should be noted, along with any recent travel or medications. The past medical history should include information about underlying immune deficiencies or other major illnesses and receipt of childhood vaccines.

Physical examination should begin with a complete evaluation of vital signs, which should include pulse oximetry because hypoxia may indicate lower respiratory infection. In the acutely febrile child, the physical examination should focus on any localized complaints, but a complete head-to-toe screen is recommended, because clues to the underlying diagnosis may be found. For example, palm and sole lesions may be discovered during a thorough skin examination and provide a clue for infection with **coxsackievirus**.

If a fever has an obvious cause, then laboratory evaluation may not be required, and management is tailored to the underlying cause with as-needed reevaluation. If the cause of the fever is not apparent, further diagnostic evaluation should be considered on a case-by-case basis. The history of presentation and abnormal physical examination findings guide the evaluation. The child with respiratory symptoms and hypoxia may require a chest radiograph or rapid antigen testing for **respiratory syncytial virus** or **influenza**. The child with pharyngitis can benefit from rapid antigen detection testing for **group A streptococcus** and a throat culture. Dysuria, back pain, or a history of vesicoureteral reflux should prompt a urinalysis and urine culture, and bloody diarrhea should prompt a stool culture. A complete blood count and blood culture should be considered in the ill-appearing child, along with cerebrospinal fluid studies if the child has neck stiffness or if the possibility of meningitis is considered. Well-defined high-risk groups require a more extensive evaluation on the basis of age, associated disease, or immunodeficiency status and might warrant prompt antimicrobial therapy before a pathogen is identified. Fever in neonates and young infants (0-3 mo old), fever in older children, and fever of unknown origin are discussed in Chapters 202, 203, and 204, respectively.

MANAGEMENT

Although fever is a common parental worry, no evidence supports the belief that high fever can result in brain damage or other bodily harm, except in rare instances of febrile status epilepticus and heat stroke. *Treating fever in self-limiting illnesses for the sole reason of bringing the body temperature back to normal is not necessary in the otherwise healthy child*. Most evidence suggests that fever is an adaptive response and should be treated only in select circumstances. In humans, increased temperatures are associated with decreased microbial replication and an increased inflammatory response. Although fever can have beneficial effects, it also increases oxygen consumption, carbon dioxide production,

and cardiac output and can exacerbate cardiac insufficiency in patients with heart disease or chronic anemia (e.g., sickle cell disease), pulmonary insufficiency in patients with chronic lung disease, and metabolic instability in patients with diabetes mellitus or inborn errors of metabolism. Children between 6 mo and 5 yr of age are at increased risk for simple febrile seizures. *The focus of the evaluation and treatment of febrile seizures is aimed at determining the underlying cause of the fever.* Children with idiopathic epilepsy also often have an increased frequency of seizures associated with a fever. High fever during pregnancy may be teratogenic.

Fever with temperatures <39°C (102.2°F) in healthy children generally does not require treatment. However, as temperatures become higher, patients tend to become more uncomfortable, and treatment of fever is then reasonable. If a child is included in one of the high-risk groups previously discussed or if the child's caregiver is concerned that the fever is adversely affecting the child's behavior and causing discomfort, treatment may be given to hasten the resolution of the fever. Other than providing symptomatic relief, antipyretic therapy does not change the course of infectious diseases. Encouraging good hydration is the 1st step to replace fluids that are lost related to the increased metabolic demands and insensible losses of fever. Antipyretic therapy is beneficial in high-risk patients and patients with discomfort. **Hyperpyrexia** (>41°C [105.8°F]) indicates high probability of hypothalamic disorders or central nervous system hemorrhage and should be treated with antipyretics. Some studies show that hyperpyrexia may be associated with a significantly increased risk of serious bacterial infection, but other studies have not substantiated this relationship. The most common antipyretics are acetaminophen, 10-15 mg/kg/dose every 4 hr, and ibuprofen in children >6 mo old at 5-10 mg/kg/dose every 8 hr. Antipyretics reduce fever by reducing production of prostaglandins. If used appropriately, antipyretics are safe; potential adverse effects include liver damage (acetaminophen) and gastrointestinal or kidney disturbances (ibuprofen). To reduce fever most safely, the caregiver should choose 1 type of medication and clearly record the dose and time of administration so that overdosage does not occur, especially if multiple caregivers are involved in the management. Physical measures such as tepid baths and cooling blankets are not considered effective to reduce fever. Evidence is also scarce for the use of complementary and alternative medicine interventions.

Fever caused by specific underlying etiologies resolves when the condition is properly treated. Examples include administration of intravenous immunoglobulin to treat Kawasaki disease or the administration of antibiotics to treat bacterial infections.

Bibliography is available at Expert Consult.

Chapter 202

Fever Without a Focus in the Neonate and Young Infant

Laura Brower and Samir S. Shah

第二百零二章

新生儿和婴儿无病灶发热

中文导读

本章主要介绍了新生儿和婴儿无病灶发热的病因学、流行病学、临床表现、诊断、实验室诊断、治疗和预后。在诊断部分详细介绍了病毒性呼吸道疾病、尿路感染和细菌性脑膜炎。在实验室诊断部分详细介绍了全血细胞计数、血培养、尿分析、脑脊液检查、单纯疱疹病毒检测、肠道病毒检测和其他诊断研究。在治疗部分详细介绍了抗生素的使用、出院标准等内容。

Fever is a common reason for neonates and young infants to undergo medical evaluation in the hospital or ambulatory setting. For this age-group (0-3 mo), **fever without a focus** refers to a rectal temperature of 38°C (100.4°F) or greater, without other presenting signs or symptoms. The evaluation of these patients can be challenging because of the difficulty distinguishing between a serious infection (bacterial or viral) and a self-limited viral illness. The etiology and evaluation of fever without a focus depend on the age of the child. Three age-groups are typically considered: neonates 0-28 days, young infants 29-90 days, and children 3-36 mo. This chapter focuses on neonates and young infants.

ETIOLOGY AND EPIDEMIOLOGY

Serious bacterial infection (SBI) occurs in 7% to 13% of neonates and young infants with fever. In this group, the most common SBIs are urinary tract infection (UTI; 5–13%), bacteremia (1–2%) and meningitis (0.2–0.5%). *Escherichia coli* is the most common organism causing SBI, followed by group B streptococcus (GBS). The decrease in GBS infections is related to increased screening of pregnant women and use of intrapartum antibiotic prophylaxis. Other, less common organisms include *Klebsiella* spp., *Enterococcus* spp., *Streptococcus pneumoniae*, *Neisseria meningitidis*, and *Staphylococcus aureus* (Table 202.1). *Listeria monocytogenes* is a rare cause of neonatal infections, potentially related to changes in public health education and improvements in food safety. Additional details about specific bacteria are available in the following chapters: *Escherichia coli* (Chapter 227), GBS (Chapter 211), *Streptococcus pneumoniae* (Chapter 209), *Neisseria meningitidis* (Chapter 218), *Staphylococcus aureus* (Chapter 208.1), and *Listeria monocytogenes* (Chapter 215). Specific bacterial infections that can present with fever in this age-group, although often with symptoms other than isolated fever, include pneumonia (Chapter 428), gastroenteritis (Chapter 366), osteomyelitis (Chapter 704), septic arthritis (Chapter 705), omphalitis (Chapter 125), cellulitis, and other skin and soft tissue infections (Chapter 685).

Herpes simplex virus (**HSV**) infections (Chapter 279) should also be considered in febrile neonates <28 days old, particularly given the high rate of mortality and significant morbidity among survivors.

Table 202.1	Bacterial Pathogens in Neonates and Young Infants With Urinary Tract Infection, Bacteremia, or Meningitis	
FREQUENCY	**URINARY TRACT INFECTION**	**BACTEREMIA AND MENINGITIS**
Common	*Escherichia coli*	*Escherichia coli* Group B streptococcus
Less common	*Klebsiella* spp. *Enterococcus* spp.	*Streptococcus pneumoniae* *Staphylococcus aureus* *Klebsiella* spp.
Rare	Group B 　streptococcus *Staphylococcus aureus* *Pseudomonas* 　*aeruginosa* *Enterobacter* spp. *Citrobacter* spp. *Proteus mirabilis*	*Listeria monocytogenes* *Neisseria meningitidis* *Salmonella* spp. *Enterobacter* spp. *Enterococcus* spp. *Cronobacter sakazakii*

Neonatal HSV is rare, with a prevalence of 0.2–0.3% among febrile neonates. Most of these infections are caused by HSV type 2, though HSV type 1 can also cause neonatal infection. Neonates with disseminated disease and skin, eye, and mouth (SEM) disease typically present at 5-12 days of life. Neonates with central nervous system (CNS) disease generally present at 16-19 days. Perinatally acquired HSV may occasionally manifests beyond 28 days of age, although some of these later-onset cases may represent postnatal acquisition.

In febrile infants who appear well, viral illnesses are much more common than bacterial or serious viral infections. The most common viruses include respiratory syncytial virus (**RSV**; Chapter 287), enteroviruses (Chapter 277), influenza viruses (Chapter 285), parainfluenza viruses (Chapter 286), human metapneumovirus (Chapter 288), adenovirus (Chapter 289), parechoviruses (Chapter 277), and rhinovirus (Chapter 290).

CLINICAL MANIFESTATIONS
In neonates and young infants, bacterial and viral infections can present with isolated fever or nonspecific symptoms, making diagnosis of serious illnesses challenging. Some neonates and young infants will have signs of systemic illness at presentation, including abnormal temperature (hypothermia <36°C [96.8°F], fever ≥38°C [100.4°F]), abnormal respiratory examination (tachypnea >60 breaths/min, respiratory distress, apnea), abnormal circulatory examination (tachycardia >180 beats/min, delayed capillary refill >3 sec, weak or bounding pulses), abnormal abdominal examination, abnormal neurologic examination (lethargy, irritability, alterations in tone), or abnormal skin examination (rash, petechiae, cyanosis). Infants with **septic arthritis** or **osteomyelitis** may appear well except for signs around the involved joint or bone or may only manifest with pseudoparalysis (disuse) and paradoxical irritability (pain when attempting to comfort the child).

DIAGNOSIS
No consensus exists on the diagnosis and empirical treatment of febrile neonates and young infants. Traditionally, all neonates <60 or <90 days of age were hospitalized; underwent laboratory evaluation of the blood, urine, and cerebrospinal fluid (CSF); and received empirical antibiotics. Additionally, some patients had stool cultures, chest radiographs, HSV evaluation, and/or received empirical antiviral agents. Under this approach, many infants without SBI or serious viral infection received evaluation, treatment, and hospitalization. Protocols were subsequently developed to identify infants at lower risk of SBI, who may be managed outside the hospital setting. The 3 most widely used are the Rochester, Philadelphia, and Boston criteria (Table 202.2). Clinical prediction rules are further discussed later in the Other Diagnostic Studies section. Despite these protocols, substantial variation continues to exist in the approach to and management of the febrile infant. *It must be emphasized that these criteria apply to the well-appearing child; those who appear*

Table 202.2	Protocols to Identify Febrile Infants at Low Risk of Serious Bacterial Infection (SBI)

BOSTON CRITERIA

Febrile infants 0-27 days
　1. Empirical antimicrobials
　2. Admit to hospital
Febrile infants 28-89 days: Non–low risk
　1. Empirical antimicrobials
　2. Admit to hospital
Febrile infants 28-89 days: Low risk
　1. One dose of IV Ceftriaxone
　2. Discharge to home with follow-up in 24 hr
　3. Risk of SBI 5.4%

Low Risk Criteria
1. Normal examination and well-appearing
2. Caregiver available by telephone
3. No antimicrobials, no DTaP vaccine in previous 48 hours
4. Meets all laboratory/radiographic criteria
　a. Peripheral blood: WBC count <20,000 per mm^3
　b. Urine
　　i. Urinalysis with <10 WBCs per hpf
　　ii. Dipstick negative for leukocyte esterase
　c. CSF: WBC count <10 per mm^3
　d. Chest radiograph: No infiltrate on chest radiograph (only obtained if signs of respiratory illness)

PHILADELPHIA CRITERIA

Febrile infants 0-28 days
　1. Empirical antimicrobials
　2. Admit to hospital
Febrile infants 29-56 days: Non–low risk
　1. Empirical antimicrobials
　2. Admit to hospital
Febrile infants 29-56 days: Low risk
　1. No antibiotics
　2. Discharge to home with follow-up in 24 hr
　3. Risk of SBI <1%

Low Risk Criteria
1. Normal examination and well-appearing
2. Caregiver available to be contacted
3. Meets all laboratory/ radiographic criteria
　a. Peripheral blood
　　i. WBC count <15,000 per mm^3
　　ii. Band-neutrophil ratio <0.2
　b. Urine
　　i. <10 WBCs per hpf
　　ii. No bacteria on Gram stain
　c. CSF
　　i. WBC count <8 per mm^3
　　ii. Negative Gram stain
　　iii. Non-bloody specimen
　d. Chest radiograph: No infiltrate
　e. Stool: (only obtained if loose, watery stool)
　　i. No blood
　　ii. Few or no WBC on smear

ROCHESTER CRITERIA

Febrile infants 0-60 days: Non–low risk
　1. Empirical antimicrobials
　2. Admit to hospital
Febrile infants 0-60 days: Low risk
　1. No antimicrobials
　2. Discharge to home with follow-up in 24 hr
　3. Risk of SBI 1%

Low Risk Criteria
1. Normal examination and well-appearing
2. Previously healthy, term gestation, no perinatal/recent antimicrobial therapy, no unexplained hyperbilirubinemia
3. Meets all laboratory/ radiographic criteria
　a. Peripheral blood
　　i. WBC count 5-15,000 per mm^3
　　ii. Absolute band count ≤1500 per mm^3
　b. Urine
　　i. ≤10 WBCs per hpf
　　ii. No bacteria on Gram stain
　c. CSF: Not included
　d. Chest radiograph: No infiltrate (only obtained if signs of respiratory illness)
　e. Stool (only obtained if loose, watery stool)
　　i. ≤5 WBC per hpf

DTaP, Diphtheria-tetanus-pertussis; WBC, white blood cell; CSF, cerebrospinal fluid; IV, intravenous; SBI, serious bacterial infection; hpf, high-power field *critically ill (septic) require prompt evaluation, resuscitation, and empirical antibiotic therapy (within 1 hr).*

Many experts advocate that all neonates ≤28 days old undergo a complete evaluation for serious infection, receive empirical antimicrobials, and be hospitalized. Of the 3 widely used criteria, only the Rochester criteria allow neonates ≤28 days to be designated as "low risk" and managed outside the hospital without antimicrobials. In one study, <1% of low-risk infants ≤28 days old had SBI; however, in another study applying the Boston and Philadelphia criteria to neonates, 3–4% of those classified as low risk had SBI.

Young febrile infants ≥29 days old who appear ill (with signs of systemic illness) require complete evaluation for SBI, including antimicrobials and hospitalization; however, well-appearing infants can be managed safely as outpatients using low-risk criteria as indicated in Table 202.2. In each of these approaches, infants must have a normal physical examination, must be able to reliably obtain close follow-up, and must meet certain laboratory and/or radiographic criteria. Based on these protocols, all infants following the Boston or Philadelphia criteria would undergo lumbar puncture (LP), whereas low-risk infants following the Rochester criteria would not. There is substantial variation in clinical practice in the performance of LPs in well-appearing infants >28 days. Clinicians should consider multiple factors, including the home situation and ability to contact the family, when deciding about LP in this age-group.

In addition, approximately 35% of infants with **bacterial meningitis** do not have a positive blood culture.

The protocols discussed in Table 202.2 were initially developed for use in the emergency department (ED). Infants evaluated in the office setting may warrant a different approach when a relationship between the physician and family already exists to facilitate clear communication and timely follow-up. In one large study of febrile infants <3 mo old who were initially evaluated for fever in the office setting, clinicians hospitalized only 36% of infants but initiated antibiotics in 61 of the 63 infants with bacteremia or bacterial meningitis. These findings suggest that, with very close follow-up (including multiple in person visits or frequent contacts by telephone), some febrile infants perceived to be at low risk for **invasive bacterial infection** (**IBI**; bacteremia and meningitis), on the basis of history, physical examination, and normal but limited laboratory testing, can be managed in an office-based setting. It is important to note that 3% of infants with SBI did not initially receive empirical antibiotics, necessitating careful consideration of risks and benefits of selective rather than universal testing and empirical antibiotic treatment of febrile infants evaluated in the office setting.

Viral Respiratory Illness
Several studies have demonstrated a decreased risk of SBI in infants with positive testing for influenza or RSV, although the risk of UTI remains significant. In one prospective study, the risk of SBI in neonates <28 days old was not altered by RSV status. Given these data, young febrile infants with bronchiolitis may not require LP, particularly if they can be closely observed or have close follow-up.

Urinary Tract Infection and Bacterial Meningitis
Traditionally, infants with abnormal findings on urinalysis (UA) would undergo complete evaluation for infection, including LP. In well-appearing infants >28 days old with an abnormal UA, some evidence suggests that the risk of bacterial meningitis is extremely low, <0.5%. For neonates 0-28 days, the risk of concomitant bacterial meningitis with UTI is 1–2%.

CSF pleocytosis in the absence of bacterial meningitis (i.e., **sterile pleocytosis**) has been reported in infants with UTI. The cause is uncertain, with some studies attributing this phenomenon to traumatic LPs or undetected viral infection rather than inflammation in the context of systemic illness.

LABORATORY DIAGNOSIS
Complete Blood Count
The peripheral complete blood cell count (CBC) and differential are frequently obtained by providers when evaluating febrile neonates and infants. The white blood cell (WBC) count alone cannot accurately predict SBI risk. In one series, isolated use of the WBC cutoffs in the Rochester criteria, outside 5-15,000 WBCs/mm³, would miss at least 33% of infants with bacteremia and 40% of those with meningitis. A prospective study found no increased risk of SBI in febrile, well-appearing infants with leukopenia (WBC count <5,000/mm³). The WBC count combined with other factors may help determine an infant's risk of SBI, but it should not be used in isolation to predict infection risk.

Blood Culture
The ability to identify pathogens in the blood depends on the volume of blood, the timing of the blood culture in relation to antimicrobial administration, and to a lesser degree, on the number of blood cultures obtained. A negative blood culture does not eliminate the risk of bacterial meningitis; in one study, 38% of infants with culture-proven bacterial meningitis had negative blood cultures. For additional information on the time to positivity of blood cultures in neonates and young infants, see "Discharge from the Hospital," later.

Urinalysis
Different methods can assist in making a presumptive diagnosis of UTI while awaiting results of a urine culture. *Traditional* UA consists of dipstick biochemical analysis of urine for nitrites or leukocyte esterase (LE) and microscopic examination of the urine for WBCs and bacteria. One study found that the traditional UA had a higher negative predictive value (NPV) than dipstick alone (99.2% vs 98.7%), but that dipstick alone had a higher positive predictive value (PPV, 66.8% for dipstick alone vs 51.2% for traditional UA). *Enhanced* UA includes hemocytometer cell count (to decrease variability of urine cell counts) and Gram stain on uncentrifuged urine. The enhanced UA has a higher sensitivity but comparable specificity to traditional UA. However, the enhanced UA has not been studied in the most common protocols for evaluation of the febrile infant, and many institutions/office practices do not perform this test.

Cerebrospinal Fluid
CSF evaluation consists of culture and Gram stain, cell count, glucose and protein. Polymerase chain reaction (PCR) testing may also be sent based on the clinical scenario, usually for enterovirus or HSV. Normal CSF parameters vary by age of the infant and should be interpreted in combination with other clinical and historical risk factors, given that some infants with normal CSF parameters may have CNS infections (Table 202.3). The CSF Gram stain can be a useful adjunct to other CSF parameters given the high specificity of the test (99.3–99.9%; i.e., relatively few false-positive results), although the range of reported sensitivity is much broader (67–94.1%).

The interpretation of CSF can be challenging in the setting of a traumatic LP, where the CSF is contaminated with peripheral blood. Some clinicians assume a ratio of WBCs to red blood cells (RBCs) of 1:500 in the CSF. Others advocate calculating the expected CSF WBCs based on the peripheral blood WBCs and RBCs and then using the observed-to-predicted ratio of CSF WBCs to aid in the identification of bacterial meningitis. This calculation assumes that the ratio of WBCs to RBCs in the peripheral blood remains constant after introduction into the CSF. The formula is:

$$\text{Predicted CSF WBCs} = \text{CSF RBCs} \times (\text{Peripheral blood WBCs}/ \text{Peripheral blood RBCs})$$

One retrospective cohort study concluded that an observed/predicted CSF WBC ratio of ≤0.01 was helpful in predicting the absence of bacterial meningitis; however, another retrospective cohort study and one case series of traumatic LPs concluded that adjustment of CSF WBC count does not improve the accuracy of diagnosis of meningitis in patients with traumatic LPs. Clinicians may consider hospitalization and empirical antimicrobials in patients with traumatic LPs (per the Philadelphia criteria) given the challenge of interpreting the CSF WBC count when there is blood contamination of the specimen.

Treatment with antibiotics prior to LP can complicate the interpretation of CSF parameters. CSF cultures are negative relatively rapidly

Table 202.3	Values of Cerebrospinal Fluid (CSF) Studies in Neonates and Infants by Age

CSF WHITE BLOOD CELL COUNTS	CELLS/mm³
Upper limit of normal by age*	
1-28 days	18
29-60 days	8.5
61-90 days	8.5
90th percentile by age[†]	
0-7 days	26
8-28 days	8–9
29-56 days	6–8
95th percentile by age[‡]	
0-28 days	19
29-56 days	9

CSF Protein	mg/dL
Upper limit of normal by age*	
1-28 days	131
29-60 days	105.5
61-90 days	71
90th percentile by age[†]	
0-7 days	153
8-28 days	84–106
29-56 days	84–105
95th percentile by age[§]	
0-14 days	132
15-28 days	100
29-42 days	89
43-56 days	83

CSF Glucose	mg/dL
Lower limit of normal by age*	
1-28 days	30
29-60 days	30.5
61-90 days	33.5
10th percentile for infants 0-56 days[†]	38–43

*Data from Byington CL, Kendrick J, Sheng X: Normative cerebrospinal fluid profiles in febrile infants, *J Pediatr* 158(1):130–134, 2011. All infants had nontraumatic lumbar puncture (LP) and no evidence of bacterial or viral infection.

[†]Data from Chadwick SL, Wilson JW, Levin JE, Martin JM: Cerebrospinal fluid characteristics of infants who present to the emergency department with fever: establishing normal values by week of age, *Pediatr Infect Dis J* 30(4):e63–e67, 2011. All infants were excluded if they had identified viral or bacterial meningitis, positive blood or urine cultures, a ventriculoperitoneal shunt, recent neurosurgery/antibiotics/seizure, or a traumatic LP.

[‡]Data from Kestenbaum LA, Ebberson J, Zorc JJ, et al: Defining cerebrospinal fluid white blood cell count reference values in neonates and young infants, *Pediatrics* 125(2):257–264, 2010. Infants were excluded for traumatic LP, serious bacterial infection, congenital infection, seizure, presence of ventricular shunt, or positive CSF testing for enterovirus.

[§]Data from Shah SS, Ebberson J, Kestenbaum LA, et al: Age-specific reference values for cerebrospinal fluid protein concentration in neonates and young infants, *J Hosp Med* 6(1):22–27, 2011. Infants were excluded for traumatic LP, serious bacterial infection, congenital infection, seizure, presence of a ventricular shunt, positive CSF testing for enterovirus, or elevated serum bilirubin.

after antibiotic administration, within 2 hr for *N. meningitidis* and 4-24 hr for *S. pneumoniae*. In patients with bacterial meningitis, CSF glucose increases to normal range, usually within 4-24 hr of antibiotic administration, while CSF protein concentrations, despite decreasing, remain abnormal for >24 hr after antibiotic administration. Changes in CSF WBC count and absolute neutrophil count (ANC) are minimal in the 1st 24 hr of antibiotic therapy. Therefore, CSF findings can provide relevant management information even in the setting of antibiotic administration before LP. Multiplex PCR testing for common bacterial pathogens should not be affected by prior antibiotic therapy.

Herpes Simplex Virus Testing

No consensus exists on which neonates should be tested and empirically treated for HSV infection. Historical and clinical features that should raise concern for HSV include exposure to individuals infected with HSV, particularly mothers with primary HSV infections or first-time genital infections, seizure or abnormal neurologic examination, vesicular rash, ill appearance, apnea, hypothermia, petechial rash/excessive bleeding, or a history of a scalp electrode. However, neonates with HSV can present without any high-risk clinical or historical features, particularly with early isolated CNS disease. Published approaches to neonatal HSV include (1) testing and empirical treatment of all neonates <21 days old who are evaluated for infection; (2) testing and empirical treatment of neonates with the presence of high-risk clinical features for HSV; and (3) testing and empirical treatment for all neonates with high-risk features plus testing the CSF of all neonates <21 days old while deferring empirical acyclovir in those without high-risk features, unless the CSF HSV PCR test is positive.

The American Academy of Pediatrics (AAP) Committee on Infectious Diseases recommends that neonates undergoing evaluation for HSV have the following laboratory studies performed: surface cultures of the mouth, conjunctiva, nasopharynx, rectum, and any vesicles; CSF PCR (sensitivity: 75–100%); whole blood PCR; and serum levels of alanine transaminase (ALT). HSV PCR testing of the mouth, conjunctiva, nasopharynx, rectum, and vesicles has been shown to be more sensitive than culture, with comparable specificity, although no direct comparisons have been performed in neonates.

Enterovirus Testing

Enterovirus is a common and typically benign cause of fever in febrile infants, although it can be difficult to distinguish from SBI on initial presentation. Enterovirus PCR testing of the CSF is a sensitive and rapid means to diagnose infection. One retrospective study of patients with CSF enterovirus testing found no cases of bacterial meningitis in patients with positive enterovirus PCR; this study did not include neonates ≤28 days old. Several studies have demonstrated shorter length of stay, fewer antibiotics, and lower cost among infants with positive CSF enterovirus test results. These results suggest that during local enterovirus seasons, and if PCR testing is available, testing for enterovirus may be of benefit in the evaluation of febrile infants and neonates. Some centers have implemented multiplex PCR panels, which permit testing for multiple viruses, including enterovirus and HSV (and bacteria), simultaneously.

Other Diagnostic Studies

Investigations have examined the utility of inflammatory markers such as C-reactive protein (CRP) and serum procalcitonin (PCT) in the diagnosis of SBI and, more specifically, IBI (bacteremia and meningitis). One meta-analysis reported that PCT is superior to WBC count and CRP for the detection of IBI in children <3 yr old, whereas another found that PCT was inferior to prediction rules in identifying SBI in young infants. A prospective multicenter cohort study of febrile infants 7-91 days old determined that the PCT was better at identifying patients with IBI than CRP, WBC count, or ANC. Building on these results, clinical prediction rules for febrile infants, such as the **Step-by-Step** approach, incorporate PCT (≥0.5 ng/mL) and CRP (>20 mg/L), along with age ≤21 days, ill appearance, ANC >10,000/mm³, and pyuria in a stepwise approach to determine which patients are high risk for IBI; only 0.7% of infants who met none of those criteria had IBI.

As previously described, older infants with positive RSV and influenza testing have a very low risk of SBI beyond UTI. One large case-based survey demonstrated decreased admission rates and antibiotic use for infants with positive respiratory viral tests, and another study demonstrated that implementation of a care algorithm incorporating viral testing led to shorter length of stay and antibiotic course.

Chest radiographs are unlikely to be clinically useful in the evaluation of the febrile infant without respiratory symptoms. Studies that have examined routine use of radiographs have found limited utility because in infants without respiratory symptoms, most results will be normal, and abnormal results can be difficult to interpret.

TREATMENT
Antimicrobials

Neonates and infants hospitalized for evaluation for SBI should receive antimicrobial therapy. Commonly used regimens include (1) a third-generation cephalosporin (typically cefepime), (2) a third-generation cephalosporin and ampicillin, or (3) an aminoglycoside and ampicillin.

Ampicillin is the preferred treatment of GBS and covers *L. monocytogenes* and many *Enterococcus* spp. For neonates 0-28 days, options 2 or 3 have been recommended, given the risk of *L. monocytogenes*. For young infants >28 days, option 1 (third-generation cephalosporin: ceftriaxone) can be a reasonable choice. For ill-appearing infants or those with positive CSF Gram stains, additional antibiotics may include **vancomycin** or broad-spectrum antibiotics such as carbapenems. Local epidemiology and resistance patterns may assist in these choices. Neonates with concern for HSV should be empirically treated with high-dose acyclovir (60 mg/kg/day).

Treatment duration and route of antimicrobial administration depend on the infection. Additional details based on specific infections and organisms are available in the following chapters: meningitis (Chapter 129), urinary tract infection (Chapter 553), *Escherichia coli* (Chapter 227), GBS (Chapter 211), and HSV (Chapter 279).

Discharge From the Hospital

Traditionally, infants remained in the hospital receiving antimicrobial therapy until bacterial cultures were negative for 48 hr or even longer. Multiple studies have suggested that shorter culture observation periods (i.e., 24 or 36 hr) may be reasonable since most pathogens in the blood grow within this time frame when automated blood culture monitoring systems are used. In one multicenter retrospective cross-sectional study, 91% of blood cultures were positive by 24 hr and 96% by 36 hr. Fewer studies have evaluated the **time to positivity** of CSF and urine cultures, but in one large study of febrile infants 28-90 days old, all positive CSF cultures grew within 24 hr (median time to positivity, 18 hr). For blood cultures, 1.3% grew after 24 hr (median time to positivity, 16 hr), and for urine cultures, 0.9% grew after 24 hr (median time to positivity, 16 hr). For neonates undergoing evaluation for HSV, it is reasonable to await results of HSV testing before discharge to home. For patients with identified bacterial infections or HSV infections, the duration of the hospital stay will be determined by the specific pathogen and site of infection.

PROGNOSIS

Most well-appearing neonates and young infants with fever recover completely and relatively quickly, depending on the etiology of the fever. Most infection-related mortality and long-term morbidity results from HSV infection and bacterial meningitis. For HSV, reported mortality rates for range from 27–31% for disseminated disease and 4–6% for CNS disease. Of those who survive, 83% of patients with disseminated disease and 31% of those with CNS disease will have normal development at 12 mo old. The mortality of bacterial meningitis varies by pathogen, but ranges from 4–15%. In one study of children who had meningitis as infants, 84% had normal development at age 5 yr.

Bibliography is available at Expert Consult.

Chapter **203**
Fever in the Older Child
Paul L. Aronson and Mark I. Neuman

第二百零三章
大年龄儿童发热

中文导读

本章主要介绍了大年龄儿童发热的诊断、发热评估的一般方法、评估和管理。在诊断部分详细介绍了病毒感染、细菌感染、隐匿性尿路感染、隐匿性菌血症；在评估发热原因的一般方法中详细介绍了一般方法及评估方法，具体包括整体外观和生命体征、症状、体格检查、实验室检测和影像学。在发热的管理中详细介绍了一般管理原则和其他方面等内容。

Fever is the most common reason for a child to seek medical care. While most infants and children have benign viral causes of fever, a small percentage will have more serious infections. Unlike the situation in infants <2 mo of age, in older children with fever, pediatricians can rely more readily on symptoms and physical examination findings to establish a diagnosis. Diagnostic testing, including laboratory testing and radiographic studies, is not routinely indicated unless diagnostic uncertainty exists after examination or the patient appears critically ill. Occult infections, such as urinary tract infection, may be present, and screening for such infections should be guided by patient age, patient gender, and degree of fever.

DIAGNOSIS

The many potential causes of fever in older infants and children can be broadly categorized into viral and bacterial infections, further organized by body region, as well as the less common inflammatory, oncologic, endocrine, and medication-induced causes (Table 203.1).

Viral Infections

Viral infections are the most common cause of fever, and the prevalence of specific viral infections varies by season. In the summer and early fall, enteroviruses (e.g., coxsackieviruses) predominate, usually presenting as hand-foot-and-mouth disease, herpangina, aseptic meningitis, or a

Table 203.1	Etiologies of Fever in Children >2 Mo of Age
INFECTIOUS *Central Nervous System* Bacterial meningitis Viral meningitis Viral encephalitis Epidural abscess Brain abscess *Ear, Nose, and Throat* Acute otitis media Mastoiditis Viral upper respiratory infection (i.e., common cold) Acute bacterial sinusitis Acute streptococcal pharyngitis Acute viral pharyngitis Retropharyngeal abscess Ludwig angina Peritonsillar abscess Herpangina Herpes simplex virus gingivostomatitis Acute bacterial lymphadenitis Viral laryngotracheobronchitis (i.e., croup) Bacterial tracheitis Epiglottitis Lemierre syndrome *Face and Ocular* Parotitis (viral and bacterial) Erysipelas Preseptal cellulitis Orbital cellulitis *Lower Respiratory Tract* Acute viral bronchiolitis Pneumonia (viral and bacterial) Complicated pneumonia (e.g., empyema, pleural effusion) Tuberculosis *Cardiac* Pericarditis Myocarditis Endocarditis *Gastrointestinal* Gastroenteritis (viral and bacterial) Mesenteric adenitis Acute appendicitis Hepatitis Pancreatitis Gallbladder disease (e.g., cholecystitis, cholangitis) Intraabdominal abscess *Genitourinary* Urinary tract infection/pyelonephritis Renal abscess Epididymitis Pelvic inflammatory disease Tuboovarian abscess	*Skin, Soft Tissue, and Muscle* Viral exanthemas (e.g., varicella, coxsackievirus, roseola, measles) Scarlet fever Syphilis Cellulitis Abscess Necrotizing fasciitis Myositis (viral and bacterial) *Bone and Joint* Osteomyelitis Septic arthritis Transient synovitis Discitis *Toxin Mediated* Toxic shock syndrome Staphylococcal scalded skin syndrome *Invasive Bacterial Infections* Occult bacteremia Bacterial sepsis Bacterial meningitis Disseminated gonococcal infection *Vector-Borne (Tick, Mosquito)* Lyme disease Rickettsiae (e.g., Rocky Mountain spotted fever, ehrlichiosis) Arboviruses (e.g., West Nile virus) Dengue fever **INFLAMMATORY** Kawasaki disease Acute rheumatic fever Systemic lupus erythematosus Inflammatory bowel disease Juvenile idiopathic arthritis Henoch-Schönlein purpura Other rheumatologic diseases (e.g., dermatomyositis) Periodic fever syndromes Serum-like sickness syndrome **ONCOLOGIC** Leukemia Lymphoma Solid tumors (e.g., neuroblastoma) **ENDOCRINE** Thyrotoxicosis/thyroid storm **MEDICATION INDUCED** Serotonin syndrome Anticholinergic toxidrome (e.g., antihistamines) Sympathomimetic toxidrome (e.g., cocaine) Salicylate toxicity **OTHER** Hemophagocytic lymphohistiocytosis Macrophage activation syndrome Ectodermal dysplasia Dysautonomia

variety of other manifestations. In the late fall and winter, viral upper and lower respiratory tract infections such as respiratory syncytial virus (RSV) and influenza and gastrointestinal (GI) viruses such as norovirus and rotavirus are common. Parainfluenza virus is a common cause of **laryngotracheobronchitis (croup)** and occurs primarily in the fall and spring, affecting mostly infants and toddlers. Varicella is a less common cause of fever than in the past because of childhood vaccination but still occurs, with the highest incidence in winter and early spring.

Bacterial Infections

Although viral infections are the most common cause of fever in older infants and children and are often diagnosed based on symptoms and physical examination findings, bacterial infections also occur. Common bacterial infections include acute **otitis media** and **streptococcal pharyngitis (strep throat)**. Acute otitis media is diagnosed by the presence of a bulging, erythematous, and nonmobile tympanic membrane upon insufflation. Strep throat occurs most frequently in the late fall and winter and is uncommon before age 3 yr. The presence of focal auscultatory findings, including crackles, is suggestive of a lower respiratory tract infection, such as bacterial pneumonia, but may also be present

among children with **bronchiolitis**. Atypical **pneumonia** caused by mycoplasma typically occurs in school-age children and is often associated with headache, malaise, and low-grade fever. The presence of neck pain or drooling may indicate a deep neck infection such as a **retropharyngeal abscess**, which occurs in infants and young children, or a **peritonsillar abscess**, which typically affects older children. Skin and soft tissue infections such as cellulitis and abscess may also present with fever, with the buttock a common area for abscesses in young children. Bone and joint infections such as **osteomyelitis** and **septic arthritis** may present with fever and refusal to bear weight or limp in the young child. Invasive bacterial infections, including **sepsis** and **bacterial meningitis**, must be considered in young children presenting with fever. While uncommon, these infections are potentially life-threatening and require prompt recognition and treatment. Ill appearance, lethargy, and tachycardia are typically present among children with severe sepsis, and petechiae may be an early finding among children with meningococcemia or other invasive bacterial diseases. Figs. 203.1 and 203.2 show age-related diagnoses and organisms producing bacterial sepsis in infants and children. Children with fever who are immunosuppressed, such as children receiving chemotherapy or those with sickle cell disease, are

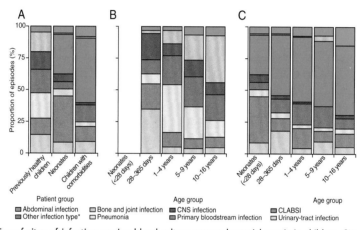

Fig. 203.1 Age distribution of sites of infection causing blood culture–proven bacterial sepsis in children. Sites of infection are shown for **A,** the 3 patient groups together, as well as separately for **B,** previously healthy children ≥28 days old, and **C,** neonates and children with comorbidities ≥28 days old. CLABSI, Central line–associated bloodstream infection; CNS, central nervous system. *Skin infection, wound infection, endocarditis, toxic shock syndrome; ear, nose, and throat infection; other, nonspecified focal infection. *(From Agyeman PKA, Schlapbach LJ, Giannoni E, et al: Epidemiology of blood culture-proven bacterial sepsis in children in Switzerland: a population-based cohort study, Lancet Child Adolesc 1:124–133, 2017, Fig 3.)*

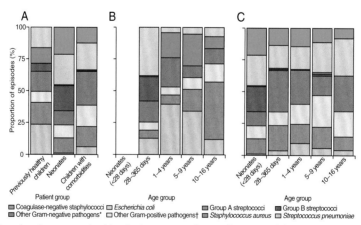

Fig. 203.2 Age distribution of pathogens causing blood culture–proven bacterial sepsis in children. Pathogens isolated in blood culture are shown for A, the 3 patient groups together, as well as separately for **B,** previously healthy children ≥28 days old, and **C,** neonates and children with comorbidities ≥28 days old. *Pseudomonas aeruginosa, Klebsiella spp., Neisseria meningitidis, Haemophilus influenzae, other gram-negative pathogens. †Enterococcus spp., viridans group streptococci, other gram-positive pathogens. *(From Agyeman PKA, Schlapbach LJ, Giannoni E, et al: Epidemiology of blood culture-proven bacterial sepsis in children in Switzerland: a population-based cohort study, Lancet Child Adolesc 1:124–133, 2017, Fig 4.)*

Table 203.2	Risk Factors for Urinary Tract Infection in Children 2-24 Mo of Age

FEMALE	MALE
White race	Uncircumcised boys at higher risk
Age <1 yr	Nonblack race
Temperature ≥39°C (102.2°F)	Temperature ≥39°C (102.2°F)
Fever duration ≥2 days	Fever duration >1 day
No obvious source of infection	No obvious source of infection

Adapted from Subcommittee on Urinary Tract Infection et al. Urinary tract infection: clinical practice guideline for the diagnosis and management of the initial UTI in febrile infants and children 2 to 24 months, *Pediatrics* 128(3):595–610, 2011.

at higher risk for invasive bacterial infection.

Infants and children age 2-24 mo merit special consideration because they have limited verbal skills, are at risk for occult bacterial infections, and may be otherwise asymptomatic except for fever (see Chapter 202).

Occult Urinary Tract Infection

Among children 2-24 mo old without symptoms or physical examination findings that identify another focal source of infection, the prevalence of urinary tract infection (UTI) may be as high as 5–10%. The highest risk of UTI occurs in females and uncircumcised males, with a very low rate of infection (<0.5%) in circumcised males. Table 203.2 lists risk factors for UTI.

Occult Bacteremia

Occult bacteremia is defined as a positive blood culture for a pathogen in a well-appearing child without an obvious source of infection. In the 1990s, before vaccination programs against *Haemophilus influenzae* type b (Hib) and *Streptococcus pneumoniae*, up to 5% of young children age 2 mo to 24 (up to 36) mo with fever ≥39°C (102.2°F) had occult bacteremia, most often caused by *S. pneumoniae*. Currently, the prevalence of occult bacteremia is <1% in febrile, well-appearing young children. The vast majority of pneumococcal occult bacteremia is transient, with a minority of these children developing new focal infections, sepsis, or other sequelae. Unimmunized and incompletely immunized young children remain at higher risk for occult bacteremia because of pneumococcus (see Chapter 209). Bacteremia caused by Hib or meningococcus should not be considered benign because subsequent serious invasive infection may rapidly follow the bacteremia.

GENERAL APPROACH

The general approach to fever in the older child begins with an assessment of the child's overall appearance and vital signs. A detailed history of the present illness and a thorough physical examination should be performed to identify the cause of the fever.

Overall Appearance and Vital Signs

Children who are ill or appear toxic or who have abnormal vital signs (e.g., tachycardia, tachypnea, hypotension) require rapid assessment, including a focused physical examination to evaluate for the presence of an invasive bacterial infection. A more detailed history and physical exam can be performed in the well-appearing child.

Symptoms

A thorough history should be obtained from the caregiver (and patient, when appropriate), including a characterization of the fever and any other associated symptoms. The degree and duration of the fever should be assessed, and the method of taking the temperature should be ascertained (e.g., rectal, oral, axillary). For children with prolonged fever, it is important to determine whether the fever has been episodic or persistent. Patients with prolonged fever may harbor occult infections, UTI, bone or soft tissue infections, or have an inflammatory or oncologic condition. Additionally, **Kawasaki disease** should be considered among

children with prolonged fever, and a careful evaluation for other stigmata associated with this condition is warranted (see Chapter 191).

Following characterization of the fever, it is important to ask systematically about the presence of symptoms that may indicate an etiology for the fever, including symptoms of common viral infections such as rhinorrhea, cough, vomiting, and diarrhea. Additionally, symptoms should be elicited for each body system: headache, ear pain, sore throat, neck pain or swelling, difficulty breathing, chest pain, abdominal pain, rash or changes in skin color, extremity pain or difficulty with ambulation (including refusal to bear weight in a young child), and overall activity level. In older children, the presence of dysuria, urinary frequency, or back pain may be indicative of UTI. Assessment of oral intake and urine output is also critical, because dehydration may accompany common childhood infections and is associated with higher rates of morbidity. Presence of weight loss or night sweats may indicate leukemia, lymphoma, or tuberculosis. Additionally, a thorough social history should be performed, inquiring about attendance at daycare, any travel, and any sick contacts at daycare, school, or in the household.

Physical Examination

Following an assessment of overall appearance, vital signs should be obtained, a thorough history of present illness should be elicited, and a complete physical examination should be performed, with particular attention given to body systems with associated symptoms (e.g., thorough exam of oropharynx for child with sore throat). A complete physical examination is particularly important in young children <24 mo old who have limited verbal skills to communicate localized pain. In older children the physical exam may proceed systematically from head to toe, but in younger children, who may be fearful of the exam, it is important to auscultate the heart and lungs first before proceeding to potentially painful aspects of the examination (e.g., inspection of ears or oropharynx). In addition to a careful evaluation of each body system, a complete examination should include an assessment of neck pain and mobility, which may be limited in children with **meningitis**. Additionally, the examiner should palpate carefully for the presence of **lymphadenopathy**, which may be present with infectious as well as oncologic causes of fever. Erythema and exudate of the tonsils with palatal petechiae suggest streptococcal pharyngitis. Erythema, bulging, and decreased mobility of the tympanic membrane are the cardinal signs of acute otitis media. Diffuse crackles and wheezes on auscultation of the lungs occur with acute viral bronchiolitis, while focal crackles or decreased breath sounds are more consistent with pneumonia. Focal tenderness in the right lower quadrant of the abdomen is suggestive of **appendicitis**, and suprapubic tenderness may indicate UTI (**cystitis**). Any focal bony tenderness may reflect a diagnosis of osteomyelitis, while erythema, swelling, and limitation of range of motion suggest a diagnosis of septic arthritis. Abnormal gait or pain with ambulation without focal findings may also reflect a bone or joint infection. A careful skin examination should also be performed. The presence of petechiae may suggest meningococcal or other invasive bacterial infection, whereas viral exanthems are typically associated with a blanching macular or maculopapular rash.

EVALUATION
Laboratory Testing

Laboratory testing is not routinely indicated in the well-appearing child without a focus of infection on examination. Urine testing should be considered based on the child's age and duration of fever. In general, the decision to perform laboratory testing should be guided by the overall appearance and vital signs of the child, the presence of specific symptoms or physical examination findings, and the child's age.

For children who are ill or appear toxic or who have vital sign abnormalities indicative of an invasive bacterial infection (tachycardia, hypotension), rapid laboratory evaluation should be performed. Testing should include a complete blood count (CBC) and blood culture and possibly urine and cerebrospinal fluid (CSF) cultures, depending on the age of the child and the presence or absence of physical exam findings indicative of UTI or bacterial meningitis. Children who are immunosuppressed or who have a central venous catheter should also undergo diagnostic testing and receive prompt antimicrobial therapy, given their higher risk of invasive bacterial infection.

For well-appearing children with symptoms or signs indicative of a viral upper respiratory or GI infection, routine viral testing is not generally indicated. **Influenza** testing may be indicated within 48 hr of symptom onset in certain higher-risk populations, with immunosuppression, chronic respiratory or cardiac disease, sickle cell disease, hospitalization, and age <2 yr influencing the decision to treat with an antiviral agent. Viral testing may also be useful with prolonged fever to identify a source of the fever and avoid extensive evaluation for inflammatory conditions such as Kawasaki disease.

Rapid strep testing of the oropharynx is indicated for children ≥3 yr old with signs of streptococcal pharyngitis on examination. Although strep throat is uncommon in children <3 yr old, this group should undergo rapid strep testing if they have signs of strep throat on exam and a household contact with streptococcal pharyngitis (see Chapter 210).

Febrile children 2-24 mo old with 2 or 3 of the risk factors for UTI listed in Table 203.2, particularly females and uncircumcised males, should undergo evaluation with urine dipstick, urine microscopy, and urine culture. Females and uncircumcised males 2-6 mo old with high fever or fever that lasts ≥2 days, may undergo urine testing even in the presence of respiratory tract infection, given the higher risk of UTI in this younger group (see Chapter 553).

Given the very low risk of occult bacteremia, routine performance of blood testing (e.g., CBC, blood culture) is not indicated in the vast majority of immunized children with fever. Unimmunized and underimmunized children <2 yr old remain at higher risk of occult pneumococcal bacteremia, and CBC and blood culture may be considered in this population in the absence of another source of infection.

Imaging

The presence of focal crackles or decreased breath sounds on auscultation in the febrile child is suggestive of **pneumonia**. Current guidelines recommend presumptive antibiotic treatment for pneumonia based on clinical grounds and reserve the use of chest radiography for children with hypoxemia or significant respiratory distress and for those who fail outpatient therapy. Chest radiography is indicated for hospitalized children to assess for complicated pneumonia, including **empyema**. The performance of other imaging should be dictated by physical exam findings. The presence of drooling and neck or throat pain in an infant or toddler may be suggestive of a retropharyngeal abscess, which is usually confirmed by imaging that may include a lateral radiograph of the soft tissue of the neck or computed tomography (CT) if clinical suspicion is high. Ultrasonography (US) may be performed to assess for **appendicitis** in children with fever and focal right lower quadrant pain or abdominal pain that is severe. However, definitive imaging, including CT or MRI, may be required if US is nondiagnostic or if clinical suspicion is high.

MANAGEMENT
General Management Principles

Management should be guided by the presence of specific symptoms by history or signs on physical examination. Based on the child's age and duration of fever, management may also be guided by focused diagnostic testing, such a urinalysis and selective urine culture testing among young febrile children (see Table 203.2 and Fig. 203.3). Supportive care, including the use of antipyretics and adequate hydration, should be reviewed with the patient and caregiver for all children with fever. Children with viral infections generally require supportive care only, except for children at higher risk of severe or complicated disease with **influenza virus** (see Chapter 285). Antibiotics should be reserved for children with evidence of bacterial infection on physical examination. A wait-and-see approach can be considered for children with acute **otitis media**, in whom a prescription for antibiotics can be provided to the family but instructions given to not fill the prescription unless severe or worsening symptoms develop (see Chapter 658). Oral antibiotics can be prescribed to young children >2 mo old with UTI, although

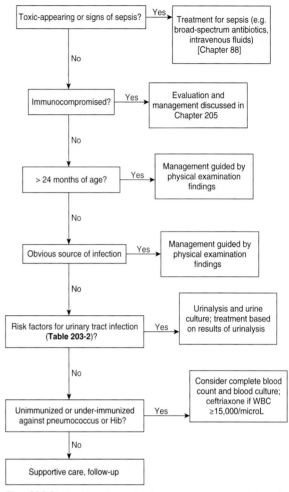

Fig. 203.3 Algorithm for evaluation and management of fever in infants and children >2 mo of age. Hib, *Haemophilus influenzae* type b; WBC, white blood cell count.

children who cannot tolerate oral intake, are vomiting or dehydrated, or appear toxic require parenteral antibiotics and hospitalization.

Blood tests, including CBC and blood culture, should be considered to evaluate for occult **bacteremia** in the unimmunized or ill-appearing child. One management strategy for these children is to administer a parenteral antibiotic (e.g., ceftriaxone) if leukocytosis is present (white blood cell count ≥15,000/μL) while awaiting results of blood culture. Children who appear toxic or who have signs of either sepsis or bacterial meningitis require emergent treatment with parenteral antibiotics as well as adjunct therapies to support the child's hemodynamics (see Chapter 88).

Importantly, anticipatory guidance should be provided to all families of children with fever, including the criteria to return to care and the importance of fever control and adequate hydration.

Other Considerations

Children who are unimmunized or underimmunized are at higher risk of invasive bacterial infection, as are children who are immunocompromised. Management of fever in these children is described further in Chapter 205. Additionally, the approach to fever in the returning traveler should be focused on identifying commonly encountered infections based on the region of travel (see Chapter 200).

Bibliography is available at Expert Consult.

Chapter **204**

Fever of Unknown Origin

Andrew P. Steenhoff

第二百零四章
不明原因发热

中 文 导 读

本章主要介绍了不明原因发热的病因学、诊断、管理和预后。首先介绍了不明原因发热的定义，随后具体介绍了四大分类，包括经典的不明原因发热、医疗相关的不明原因发热、免疫缺陷的不明原因发热和 HIV 相关发热。随后介绍了不明原因发热病因的诊断，包括感染性疾病、风湿免疫病、恶性肿瘤病、肉芽肿病、家族遗传病和其他类疾病。

Fever of unknown origin (**FUO**) is a diagnostic dilemma for pediatricians because it is often difficult to distinguish clinically between benign and potentially life-threatening causes. Pediatricians face the important challenge of not missing the diagnosis of a serious illness or an easily treatable condition that can result in increased morbidity. Fortunately, FUO usually an uncommon presentation of a common disease, with most of these common diseases being easily treatable.

The classification of FUO is best reserved for children with a temperature >38°C (100.4°F) documented by a healthcare provider and for which the cause could not be identified after at least 8 days of evaluation (Table 204.1). It is important to differentiate FUO from **fever without a source**; FWS is fever where the source has not yet been identified and is differentiated from FUO by the duration of the fever. FWS can progress to FUO if no cause is elicited after 7 days of evaluation.

ETIOLOGY

The many causes of FUO in children are infectious, rheumatologic (connective tissue or autoimmune), autoinflammatory, oncologic, neurologic, genetic, factitious, and iatrogenic processes (Table 204.2). Although oncologic disorders should be seriously considered, most children with malignancies do not have fever alone. The possibility of **drug fever** should be considered if the patient is receiving any drug. Drug fever is usually sustained and not associated with other symptoms. Discontinuation of the drug is associated with resolution of the fever, generally within 72 hr, although certain drugs, such as iodides, are excreted for a prolonged period, with fever that can persist for as long as 1 mo after drug withdrawal.

Most fevers of unknown origin result from atypical presentations of common diseases. In some cases, the presentation as an FUO is characteristic of the disease (e.g., JIA), but the definitive diagnosis can be established only after prolonged observation, because initially there are no associated or specific findings on physical examination, and all laboratory results are negative or normal.

In the United States the systemic infectious diseases most commonly implicated in children with FUO are salmonellosis, tuberculosis, rickettsial diseases, syphilis, Lyme disease, cat-scratch disease, atypical prolonged presentations of common viral diseases, Epstein-Barr virus (EBV) infection, cytomegalovirus (CMV) infection, viral hepatitis, coccidioidomycosis, histoplasmosis, malaria, and toxoplasmosis. Less common infectious causes of FUO include tularemia, brucellosis, leptospirosis, and rat-bite fever. Acquired immunodeficiency syndrome alone is not usually responsible for FUO, although febrile illnesses often occur in patients with AIDS as a result of opportunistic infections (see Table 204.1).

Juvenile idiopathic arthritis (JIA) and **systemic lupus erythematosus** (SLE) are the connective tissue diseases most often associated with FUO. **Inflammatory bowel disease** (IBD) and **Kawasaki disease** are also frequently reported as causes of FUO. If **factitious fever** (inoculation of pyogenic material or manipulation of the thermometer by the patient or parent) is suspected, the presence and pattern of fever should be documented in the hospital. Prolonged and continuous observation of the patient, which can include electronic or video surveillance, is imperative. FUO lasting >6 mo is uncommon in children and suggests granulomatous, autoinflammatory, or autoimmune disease. Repeat interval evaluation is required, including history, physical examination, laboratory evaluation, and imaging studies.

Historically, 90% of pediatric FUO cases in the United States had an identifiable cause: approximately 50% infectious, 10–20% collagen vascular, and 10% oncologic. Later studies from the 1990s had variable results: 20–44% infectious, 0–7% collagen vascular, 2–3% oncologic, and up to 67% undiagnosed. The reason for the paradoxical increase in undiagnosed cases of FUO ironically is likely caused by improved infectious and autoimmune diagnostic techniques. The advent of polymerase chain reaction (PCR), improved culture techniques, and better understanding of atypical viral and bacterial pathogenesis and autoimmune processes likely contribute to earlier diagnosis of these conditions and fewer children with these conditions advancing to the

| Table 204.1 | Summary of Definitions and Major Features of 4 Subtypes of Fever of Unknown Origin (FUO) |

FEATURE	CLASSIC FUO	HEALTHCARE-ASSOCIATED FUO	IMMUNE-DEFICIENT FUO	HIV-RELATED FUO
Definition	>38°C (100.4°F), >3 wk, >2 visits or 1 wk in hospital	≥38°C (100.4°F), >1 wk, not present or incubating on admission	≥38°C (100.4°F), >1 wk, negative cultures after 48 hr	≥38°C (100.4°F), >3 wk for outpatients, >1 wk for inpatients, HIV infection confirmed
Patient location	Community, clinic, or hospital	Acute care hospital	Hospital or clinic	Community, clinic, or hospital
Leading causes	Cancer, infections, inflammatory conditions, undiagnosed, habitual hyperthermia	Healthcare-associated infections, postoperative complications, drug fever	Majority caused by infections, but cause documented in only 40–60%	HIV itself, typical and atypical mycobacteria, CMV, lymphomas, toxoplasmosis, cryptococcosis, immune reconstitution inflammatory syndrome (IRIS)
History emphasis	Travel, contacts, animal and insect exposure, medications, immunizations, family history, cardiac valve disorder	Operations and procedures, devices, anatomic considerations, drug treatment	Stage of chemotherapy, drugs administered, underlying immunosuppressive disorder	Drugs, exposures, risk factors, travel, contacts, stage of HIV infection
Examination emphasis	Fundi, oropharynx, temporal artery, abdomen, lymph nodes, spleen, joints, skin, nails, genitalia, rectum or prostate, lower-limb deep veins	Wounds, drains, devices, sinuses, urine	Skin folds, IV sites, lungs, perianal area	Mouth, sinuses, skin, lymph nodes, eyes, lungs, perianal area
Investigation emphasis	Imaging, biopsies, sedimentation rate, skin tests	Imaging, bacterial cultures	CXR, bacterial cultures	Blood and lymphocyte count; serologic tests; CXR; stool examination; biopsies of lung, bone marrow, and liver for cultures and cytologic tests; brain imaging
Management	Observation, outpatient temperature chart, investigations, avoidance of empirical drug treatments	Depends on situation	Antimicrobial treatment protocols	Antiviral and antimicrobial protocols, vaccines, revision of treatment regimens, good nutrition
Time course of disease	Months	Weeks	Days	Weeks to months
Tempo of investigation	Weeks	Days	Hours	Days to weeks

CMV, Cytomegalovirus; CXR, chest radiograph; HIV, human immunodeficiency virus; IV, intravenous line.
Adapted from Mackowak PA, Durack DT: Fever of unknown origin. In Mandell GL, Bennett, JE, Dolin R, editors: *Mandell, Douglas, and Bennett's principles and practice of infectious diseases*, ed 7, Philadelphia, 2010, Elsevier (Table 51-1).

category of FUO. By contrast, causes of FUO remain primarily infectious in developing settings where there is a higher infectious disease burden, and advanced diagnostics techniques are more limited.

DIAGNOSIS

The evaluation of FUO requires a thorough history and physical examination supplemented by a few screening laboratory tests and additional laboratory and imaging evaluation informed by the history or abnormalities on examination or initial screening tests (see Table 204.2). Occasionally the **fever pattern** helps make a diagnosis (Fig. 204.1). Nonetheless, most diseases causing an FUO do not have a typical fever pattern.

History

A detailed fever history should be obtained, including onset, frequency, duration, response or nonresponse to therapy, recurrence, and associated symptoms. Repetitive chills and temperature spikes are common in children with **septicemia** (regardless of cause), particularly when associated with kidney disease, liver or biliary disease, infective endocarditis, malaria, brucellosis, rat-bite fever, or a loculated collection of pus.

The age of the patient is helpful in evaluating FUO. Children >6 yr old often have a respiratory or genitourinary tract infection, localized infection (abscess, osteomyelitis), JIA, or rarely, leukemia. Adolescent

patients are more likely to have IBD, autoimmune processes, lymphoma, or tuberculosis, in addition to the causes of FUO found in younger children.

A history of exposure to wild or domestic **animals** should be solicited. The incidence of **zoonotic infections** in the United States is increasing, and these infections are often acquired from pets that are not overtly ill. Immunization of dogs against specific disorders such as **leptospirosis** can prevent canine disease but does not always prevent the animal from carrying and shedding leptospires, which may be transmitted to household contacts. A history of ingestion of rabbit or squirrel meat might provide a clue to the diagnosis of oropharyngeal, glandular, or typhoidal **tularemia**. A history of tick bite or travel to tick- or parasite-infested areas should be obtained.

Any history of **pica** should be elicited. Ingestion of dirt is a particularly important clue to infection with *Toxocara canis* (visceral larva migrans) or *Toxoplasma gondii* (toxoplasmosis).

A history of unusual dietary habits or travel as early as the birth of the child should be sought. Tuberculosis, malaria, histoplasmosis, and coccidioidomycosis can reemerge years after visiting or living in an endemic area. It is important to identify prophylactic immunizations and precautions taken by the patient against ingestion of contaminated water or food during foreign travel. Rocks, dirt, and artifacts from

Table 204.2	Diagnostic Considerations for Fever of Unknown Origin in Children

ABSCESSES
Abdominal
Brain
Dental
Hepatic
Paraspinal
Pelvic
Perinephric
Rectal
Subphrenic
Psoas

BACTERIAL DISEASES
Actinomycosis
Bartonella henselae (cat-scratch disease)
Brucellosis
Campylobacter
Chlamydia
Francisella tularensis (tularemia)
Listeria monocytogenes (listeriosis)
Meningococcemia (chronic)
Mycoplasma pneumoniae
Rat-bite fever (*Streptobacillus moniliformis*; streptobacillary form of rat-bite fever)
Salmonella
Tuberculosis
Whipple disease
Yersiniosis

LOCALIZED INFECTIONS
Cholangitis
Infective endocarditis
Lymphogranuloma venereum
Mastoiditis
Osteomyelitis
Pneumonia
Pyelonephritis
Psittacosis
Sinusitis

SPIROCHETES
Borrelia burgdorferi (Lyme disease)
Relapsing fever (*Borrelia recurrentis*)
Leptospirosis
Rat-bite fever (*Spirillum minus*; spirillary form of rat-bite fever)
Syphilis

FUNGAL DISEASES
Blastomycosis (extrapulmonary)
Coccidioidomycosis (disseminated)
Histoplasmosis (disseminated)

RICKETTSIAE
African tick-bite fever
Ehrlichia canis
Q fever
Rocky Mountain spotted fever
Tick-borne typhus

VIRUSES
Cytomegalovirus
Hepatitis viruses
HIV
Epstein-Barr virus

PARASITIC DISEASES
Amebiasis
Babesiosis
Giardiasis
Malaria
Toxoplasmosis
Trichinosis
Trypanosomiasis
Visceral larva migrans (*Toxocara*)

RHEUMATOLOGIC DISEASES
Behçet disease
Juvenile dermatomyositis
Juvenile idiopathic arthritis
Rheumatic fever
Systemic lupus erythematosus

HYPERSENSITIVITY DISEASES
Drug fever
Hypersensitivity pneumonitis
Serum sickness
Weber-Christian disease

NEOPLASMS
Atrial myxoma
Cholesterol granuloma
Hodgkin disease
Inflammatory pseudotumor
Leukemia
Lymphoma
Pheochromocytoma
Neuroblastoma
Wilms tumor

GRANULOMATOUS DISEASES
Granulomatosis with polyangiitis
Crohn disease
Granulomatous hepatitis
Sarcoidosis

FAMILIAL AND HEREDITARY DISEASES
Anhidrotic ectodermal dysplasia
Autonomic neuropathies
Fabry disease
Familial dysautonomia
Familial Hibernian fever
Familial Mediterranean fever, many other autoinflammatory diseases (Chapter 188)
Hypertriglyceridemia
Ichthyosis
Sickle cell crisis
Spinal cord/brain injury

MISCELLANEOUS
Addison disease
Castleman disease
Chronic active hepatitis
Cyclic neutropenia
Diabetes insipidus (central and nephrogenic)
Drug fever
Factitious fever
Hemophagocytic syndromes
Hypothalamic-central fever
Infantile cortical hyperostosis
Inflammatory bowel disease
Kawasaki disease
Kikuchi-Fujimoto disease
Metal fume fever
Pancreatitis
Periodic fever syndromes
Poisoning
Pulmonary embolism
Thrombophlebitis
Thyrotoxicosis, thyroiditis

geographically distant regions that have been collected and brought into the home as souvenirs can serve as vectors of disease.

A **medication** history should be pursued rigorously. This history should elicit information about nonprescription preparations and topical agents, including eyedrops, that may be associated with atropine-induced fever.

The genetic background of a patient also is important. Descendants of the Ulster Scots may have FUO because they are afflicted with nephrogenic diabetes insipidus. **Familial dysautonomia** (Riley-Day syndrome), a disorder in which hyperthermia is recurrent, is more common among Jews than among other population groups. Ancestry from the Mediterranean region should suggest **familial Mediterranean fever**. Both familial Mediterranean fever and hyper-IgD syndrome are inherited as autosomal recessive disorders. Tumor necrosis factor receptor–associated periodic syndrome and Muckle-Wells syndrome are inherited as autosomal dominant traits.

Pseudo-FUO is defined as successive episodes of benign, self-limited infections with fever that the parents perceive as 1 prolonged fever episode. This needs to be carefully ruled out before undertaking an unnecessary evaluation. Usually, pseudo-FUO starts with a well-defined infection (frequently viral) that resolves but is followed by other febrile viral illnesses that may be less well defined. Diagnosis of pseudo-FUO usually requires a careful history, focusing on identifying afebrile periods between febrile episodes. If pseudo-FUO is suspected and the patient does not appear ill, keeping a *fever diary* can be helpful.

Physical Examination

A complete physical examination is essential to search for any clues to the underlying diagnosis, and often it is worthwhile to repeat a detailed examination on different days to detect signs that may have changed or been missed (Tables 204.3 and 204.4). The child's general appearance, including **sweating** during fever, should be noted. The continuing absence of sweat in the presence of an elevated or changing body temperature suggests dehydration caused by vomiting, diarrhea, or central or nephrogenic diabetes insipidus. It also should suggest anhidrotic ectodermal dysplasia, familial dysautonomia, or exposure to atropine. The general activity of the patient and the presence or absence of rashes should also be noted.

A careful ophthalmic examination is important. Red, weeping eyes may be a sign of connective tissue disease, particularly polyarteritis nodosa. Palpebral **conjunctivitis** in a febrile patient may be a clue to measles, coxsackievirus infection, tuberculosis, infectious mononucleosis, lymphogranuloma venereum, or cat-scratch disease. In contrast, bulbar conjunctivitis in a child with FUO suggests Kawasaki disease or leptospirosis. Petechial conjunctival **hemorrhages** suggest infective endocarditis. Uveitis suggests sarcoidosis, JIA, SLE, Kawasaki disease, Behçet

disease, and vasculitis. **Chorioretinitis** suggests CMV, toxoplasmosis, and syphilis. **Proptosis** suggests an orbital tumor, thyrotoxicosis, metastasis (neuroblastoma), orbital infection, Wegener granulomatosis (granulomatosis with polyangiitis), or pseudotumor.

The ophthalmoscope should also be used to examine nail-fold capillary abnormalities that are associated with connective tissue diseases such as juvenile dermatomyositis and systemic scleroderma. Immersion oil or lubricating jelly is placed on the skin adjacent to the nail bed, and the capillary pattern is observed with the ophthalmoscope set on +40.

FUO is sometimes caused by **hypothalamic dysfunction**. A clue to this disorder is failure of pupillary constriction because of absence of the sphincter constrictor muscle of the eye. This muscle develops embryologically when hypothalamic structure and function also are undergoing differentiation.

Fever resulting from familial dysautonomia may be suggested by lack of tears, an absent corneal reflex, or a smooth tongue with absence of fungiform papillae. Tenderness to tapping over the sinuses or the upper teeth suggests sinusitis. Recurrent oral candidiasis may be a clue to various disorders of the immune system, especially involving the T lymphocytes. Hyperactive deep tendon reflexes can suggest thyrotoxicosis as the cause of FUO.

Hyperemia of the pharynx, with or without exudate, suggests streptococcal infection, Epstein-Barr virus infection, CMV infection, toxoplasmosis, salmonellosis, tularemia, Kawasaki disease, gonococcal infection, or leptospirosis.

The muscles and bones should be palpated carefully. Point tenderness over a bone can suggest occult osteomyelitis or bone marrow invasion from neoplastic disease. Tenderness over the trapezius muscle may be a clue to subdiaphragmatic abscess. Generalized muscle tenderness suggests dermatomyositis, trichinosis, polyarteritis, Kawasaki disease, or mycoplasma or arboviral infection.

Rectal examination can reveal perirectal lymphadenopathy or tenderness, which suggests a deep pelvic abscess, iliac adenitis, or pelvic osteomyelitis. A guaiac test should be obtained; occult blood loss can suggest granulomatous colitis or ulcerative colitis as the cause of FUO.

Laboratory Evaluation

The laboratory evaluation of the child with FUO and whether inpatient or outpatient are determined on a case-by-case basis. Hospitalization may be required for laboratory or imaging studies that are unavailable or impractical in an ambulatory setting, for more-careful observation, or for temporary relief of parental anxiety. The **tempo** of diagnostic evaluation should be adjusted to the tempo of the illness; haste may be imperative in a critically ill patient, but if the illness is more chronic, the evaluation can proceed in a systematic manner and can be carried out in an outpatient setting. If there are no clues in the patient's history

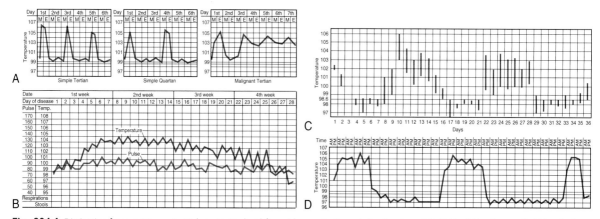

Fig. 204.1 Distinctive fever patterns. **A,** Malaria. **B,** Typhoid fever (demonstrating relative bradycardia). **C,** Hodgkin disease (Pel-Ebstein fever pattern). **D,** Borreliosis (relapsing fever pattern). *(From Woodward TE: The fever pattern as a clinical diagnostic aid. In Mackowiak PA, editor: Fever: basic mechanisms and management, ed 2, Philadelphia, 1997, Lippincott-Raven, pp 215–236.)*

or on physical examination that suggest a specific infection or area of suspicion, it is unlikely that diagnostic studies will be helpful. In this common scenario, continued surveillance and repeated reevaluations of the child should be employed to detect any new clinical findings.

Although ordering a large number of diagnostic tests in every child with FUO according to a predetermined list is discouraged, certain studies should be considered in the evaluation. A complete blood cell count (CBC) with a white blood cell (WBC) differential and a urinalysis should be part of the initial laboratory evaluation. An absolute neutrophil count (ANC) of <5,000/μL is evidence against indolent bacterial infection other than typhoid fever. Conversely, in patients with a polymorphonuclear leukocyte (PMN) count of >10,000/μL or a nonsegmented PMN count of >500/μL, a severe bacterial infection is highly likely. Direct examination of the blood smear with Giemsa or Wright stain can reveal organisms of malaria, trypanosomiasis, babesiosis, or relapsing fever.

An erythrocyte sedimentation rate (ESR) >30 mm/hr indicates inflammation and the need for further evaluation for infectious, autoimmune, autoinflammatory, or malignant diseases, tuberculosis, Kawasaki disease, or autoimmune disease. A low ESR does not eliminate the possibility of infection or JIA. C-reactive protein (CRP) is another acute-phase reactant that becomes elevated and returns to normal more rapidly than the ESR. Experts recommend checking either ESR or CRP, because there is no evidence that measuring both in the same patient with FUO is clinically useful.

Blood cultures should be obtained aerobically. Anaerobic blood cultures have an extremely low yield and should be obtained only if there are specific reasons to suspect anaerobic infection. Multiple or repeated blood cultures may be required to detect bacteremia associated with infective endocarditis, osteomyelitis, or deep-seated abscesses. Polymicrobial bacteremia suggests factitious or self-induced infection or GI pathology. The isolation of leptospires, *Francisella*, or *Yersinia* requires selective media or specific conditions not routinely used. Therefore, it is important to inform the laboratory what organisms are suspected in a particular case. Urine culture should be obtained in all cases.

Tuberculin skin testing (TST) should be performed with intradermal placement of 5 units of purified protein derivative that has been kept appropriately refrigerated. In children >2 yr old, it is reasonable to test for tuberculosis using an interferon-γ release assay (IGRA).

Imaging studies of the chest, sinuses, mastoids, or GI tract may be indicated by specific historical or physical findings. Radiographic evaluation of the GI tract for IBD may be helpful in evaluating selected children with FUO and no other localizing signs or symptoms.

Examination of the bone marrow can reveal leukemia; metastatic neoplasm; mycobacterial, fungal, or parasitic infections; histiocytosis; hemophagocytosis; or storage diseases. If a bone marrow aspirate is performed, cultures for bacteria, mycobacteria, and fungi should be obtained.

Serologic tests can aid in the diagnosis of EBV infection, CMV infection, toxoplasmosis, salmonellosis, tularemia, brucellosis, leptospirosis, cat-scratch disease, Lyme disease, rickettsial disease, and on some occasions JIA. The clinician should be aware that the reliability and the sensitivity and specificity of these tests vary; for example, serologic tests for Lyme disease outside of reference laboratories have been generally unreliable.

Radionuclide scans may be helpful in detecting abdominal abscesses as well as osteomyelitis, especially if the focus cannot be localized to a specific limb or multifocal disease is suspected. Gallium citrate localizes inflammatory tissues (leukocytes) associated with tumors or abscesses. Technetium-99m phosphate is useful for detecting osteomyelitis before plain radiographs demonstrate bone lesions. Granulocytes tagged with indium or iodinated IgG may be useful in detecting localized pyogenic processes. ^{18}F-fluorodeoxyglucose positron emission tomography (PET)

Table 204.3	Subtle Physical Findings with Special Significance in Patients with Fever of Unknown Origin	
BODY SITE	**PHYSICAL FINDING**	**DIAGNOSIS**
Head	Sinus tenderness	Sinusitis
Temporal artery	Nodules, reduced pulsations	Temporal arteritis
Oropharynx	Ulceration	Disseminated histoplasmosis, SLE, IBD, Behçet syndrome, periodic fever syndromes
	Tender tooth	Periapical abscess, sinus referred pain
Fundi or conjunctivae	Choroid tubercle	Disseminated granulomatosis*
	Petechiae, Roth spots	Endocarditis
Thyroid	Enlargement, tenderness	Thyroiditis
Heart	Murmur	Infective or marantic endocarditis
	Relative bradycardia	Typhoid fever, malaria, leptospirosis, psittacosis, central fever, drug fever
Abdomen	Enlarged iliac crest lymph nodes, splenomegaly	Lymphoma, endocarditis, disseminated granulomatosis*
	Audible abdominal aortic or renal artery bruit	Large vessel vasculitis such as Takayasu arteritis
	Costovertebral tenderness	Chronic pyelonephritis, perinephric abscess
Rectum	Perirectal fluctuance, tenderness	Abscess
	Prostatic tenderness, fluctuance	Abscess
Genitalia	Testicular nodule	Periarteritis nodosa, cancer
	Epididymal nodule	Disseminated granulomatosis
Spine	Spinal tenderness	Vertebral osteomyelitis
	Paraspinal tenderness	Paraspinal collection
Lower extremities	Deep venous tenderness	Thrombosis or thrombophlebitis
Upper or lower extremities	Pseudoparesis	Syphilitic bone disease
Skin and nails	Petechiae, splinter hemorrhages, subcutaneous nodules, clubbing	Vasculitis, endocarditis

*Includes tuberculosis, histoplasmosis, coccidioidomycosis, sarcoidosis, granulomatosis with polyangiitis, and syphilis.

Adapted from Mackowak PA, Durack DT: Fever of unknown origin. In Mandell GL, Bennett, JE, Dolin R, editors: *Mandell, Douglas, and Bennett's principles and practice of infectious diseases*, ed 7, Philadelphia, 2010, Elsevier (Table 51-8).

Table 204.4	Examples of Potential Diagnostic Clues to Infections Presenting as Fever of Unknown Origin	
ETIOLOGY	**HISTORICAL CLUES**	**PHYSICAL CLUES**
Anaplasmosis	Transmitted by bite of *Ixodes* tick in association with outdoor activity in northern-central and eastern United States	Fever, headache, arthralgia, myalgia, pneumonitis, thrombocytopenia, lymphopenia, elevated liver enzymes
Babesiosis	Transmitted by bite of *Ixodes* tick in association with outdoor activity in northeastern United States	Arthralgias, myalgias, relative bradycardia, hepatosplenomegaly, anemia, thrombocytopenia, elevated liver enzymes
Bartonellosis	Recent travel to Andes Mountains (Oroya fever; *Bartonella bacilliformis*), association with homelessness in urban settings (*Bartonella quintana*) or scratch of infected kitten or feral cat (*Bartonella henselae*)	Conjunctivitis, retroorbital pain, anterior tibial bone pain, macular rash, nodular plaque lesions, regional lymphadenopathy
Blastomycosis	Contact with soil adjacent to Mississippi and Ohio River valleys, Saint Lawrence River in New York and Canada, and North American Great Lakes or exposure to infected dogs	Arthritis, atypical pneumonia, pulmonary nodules, and/or fulminant adult respiratory distress syndrome; verrucous, nodular, or ulcerative skin lesions; prostatitis
Brucellosis	Associated with contact or consumption of products from infected goats, pigs, camels, yaks, buffalo, or cows and with abattoir work	Arthralgias, hepatosplenomegaly, suppurative musculoskeletal lesions, sacroiliitis, spondylitis, uveitis, hepatitis, pancytopenia
Coccidioidomycosis	Exposure to soil or dust in southwestern United States	Arthralgias, pneumonia, pulmonary cavities, pulmonary nodules, erythema multiforme, erythema nodosum
Ehrlichiosis	Transmitted by bite of *Amblyomma*, *Dermacentor*, or *Ixodes* tick in association with outdoor activity in midwestern and southeastern United States	Pneumonitis, hepatitis, thrombocytopenia, lymphopenia
Enteric fever (*Salmonella enterica* serovar *typhi*)	Recent travel to a low- or middle-income country (LMIC) with consumption of potentially contaminated food or water	Headache, arthritis, abdominal pain, relative bradycardia, hepatosplenomegaly, leukopenia
Histoplasmosis	Exposure to bat or blackbird excreta in roosts, chicken houses, or caves in region surrounding Ohio and Mississippi River valleys	Headache, pneumonia, pulmonary cavities, mucosal ulcers, adenopathy, erythema nodosum, erythema multiforme, hepatitis, anemia, leukopenia, thrombocytopenia
Leptospirosis	Occupational exposure among workers in sewers, rice and sugarcane fields, and abattoirs; recreational water sports and exposure to contaminated waters or infected dogs	Bitemporal and frontal headache, calf and lumbar muscle tenderness, conjunctival suffusion, hepatic and renal failure, hemorrhagic pneumonitis
Leishmaniasis (visceral disease)	Associated with recent travel to areas endemic for sand flies	Hepatosplenomegaly, lymphadenopathy, and hyperpigmentation of face, hand, foot, and abdominal skin (kala-azar)
Malaria	Recent travel to endemic areas in Asia, Africa, and Central/South America	Fever, headaches, nausea, emesis, diarrhea, hepatomegaly, splenomegaly, anemia
Psittacosis (*Chlamydia psittaci*)	Associated with contact with birds, especially psittacine birds	Fever, pharyngitis, hepatosplenomegaly, pneumonia, blanching maculopapular eruptions; erythema multiforme, marginatum, and nodosum
Q fever (*Coxiella burnetii*)	Associated with farm, veterinary, or abattoir work; consumption of unpasteurized milk; contact with infected sheep, goats, or cattle	Atypical pneumonia, hepatitis, hepatomegaly, relative bradycardia, splenomegaly
Rat-bite fever (*Streptobacillus moniliformis*)	Recent bite or scratch by rat, mouse, or squirrel; ingestion of food or water contaminated by rat excrement	Headaches, myalgias, polyarthritis, and maculopapular, morbilliform, petechial, vesicular, or pustular rash over the palms, soles, and extremities
Relapsing fever (*Borrelia recurrentis*)	Associated with poverty, crowding, and poor sanitation (louse-borne), or with camping (tick-borne), particularly in the Grand Canyon	High fever with rigors, headache, delirium, arthralgias, myalgias, and hepatosplenomegaly
Rocky Mountain spotted fever	Associated with outdoor activity in the South Atlantic or southeastern United States and exposure to *Dermacentor* tick bites	Headache, petechial rash involving the extremities, palms, and soles
Tuberculosis	Recent contact with tuberculosis; recent immigration from endemic country; work or residence in homeless shelters, correctional facilities, or healthcare facilities	Night sweats, weight loss, atypical pneumonia, cavitary pulmonary lesions
Tularemia	Associated with bites by *Amblyomma* or *Dermacentor* ticks, deer flies, and mosquitoes or direct contact with tissues of infected animals such as rabbits, squirrels, deer, raccoons, cattle, sheep, and swine	Ulcerated skin lesions at a bite site, pneumonia, relative bradycardia, lymphadenopathy, conjunctivitis
Whipple disease (*Tropheryma whipplei*)	Potential association with exposure to sewage	Chronic diarrhea, arthralgia, weight loss, malabsorption, malnutrition

Adapted from Wright WF, Mackowiak PA: Fever of unknown origin. In Bennett JF, Dolin R, Blaser MJ, editors: *Mandell, Douglas, and Bennett's principles and practice of infectious diseases*, ed 8, Philadelphia, 2015, Elsevier (Table 56-9).

is a helpful imaging modality in adults with an FUO and can contribute to an ultimate diagnosis in 30–60% of patients. Echocardiograms can demonstrate vegetation on the leaflets of heart valves, suggesting infective endocarditis. Ultrasonography (US) can identify intraabdominal abscesses of the liver, subphrenic space, pelvis, or spleen.

Total body CT or MRI (both with contrast) is usually the first imaging study of choice; both permit detection of neoplasms and collections of purulent material without the use of surgical exploration or radioisotopes. CT and MRI are helpful in identifying lesions of the head, neck, chest, retroperitoneal spaces, liver, spleen, intraabdominal and intrathoracic lymph nodes, kidneys, pelvis, and mediastinum. CT or US-guided aspiration or biopsy of suspicious lesions has reduced the need for exploratory laparotomy or thoracotomy. MRI is particularly useful for detecting osteomyelitis or myositis if there is concern about a specific limb. Diagnostic imaging can be very helpful in confirming or evaluating a suspected diagnosis. With CT scans, however, the child is exposed to large amounts of radiation. PET-CT or MRI may help localize an occult tumor.

Biopsy is occasionally helpful in establishing a diagnosis of FUO. Bronchoscopy, laparoscopy, mediastinoscopy, and GI endoscopy can provide direct visualization and biopsy material when organ-specific manifestations are present. When employing any of the more invasive testing procedures, the risk/benefit ratio for the patient must always be considered before proceeding further.

MANAGEMENT
The ultimate treatment of FUO is tailored to the underlying diagnosis. Fever and infection in children are not synonymous, and **antimicrobial agents** should only be used when there is evidence of infection, with avoidance of empirical trials of medication. An exception may be the use of antituberculous treatment in critically ill children with suspected disseminated tuberculosis. Empirical trials of other antimicrobial agents may be dangerous and can obscure the diagnosis of infective endocarditis, meningitis, parameningeal infection, or osteomyelitis. After a complete evaluation, **antipyretics** may be indicated to control fever associated with adverse symptoms.

PROGNOSIS
Children with FUO have a better prognosis than adults. The outcome in a child depends on the primary disease process. In many cases, no diagnosis can be established, and fever abates spontaneously. In as many as 25% of children in whom fever persists, the cause of the fever remains unclear, even after thorough evaluation.

In a series of 69 patients referred for "prolonged" unexplained fever, 10 were not actually having fever, and 11 had diagnoses that were readily apparent at the initial visit. The remaining 48 were classified as having FUO. The median duration of reported fever for these patients was 30 days. Fifteen received a diagnosis, and 10 (67%) had confirmed infections: acute EBV or CMV infection ($n = 5$; with 1 patient developing hemophagocytic lymphohistiocytosis); cat-scratch disease (3); and histoplasmosis (2). The other 5 patients had inflammatory conditions (systemic JIA, 2; IBD, 1; central fever (1), or malignancy (acute lymphoblastic leukemia, 1).

Bibliography is available at Expert Consult.

Chapter **205**
Infections in Immunocompromised Persons
Marian G. Michaels, Hey Jin Chong, and Michael Green
第二百零五章
免疫缺陷患者的感染

中文导读

本章主要介绍了原发免疫缺陷的感染、获得性免疫缺陷的感染和免疫缺陷患者感染的预防三大部分内容。在原发免疫缺陷的感染中详细介绍了吞噬系统的异常、脾功能缺陷、光化或补体活性、B细胞缺陷(体液免疫缺陷)、T细胞缺陷（细胞介导的免疫缺陷），以及B细胞和T细胞联合缺陷。在获得性免疫缺陷的感染中详细介绍了源自感染的获得性免疫缺陷、恶性肿瘤、发热和中性粒细胞减少、不伴有中性粒细胞减少的发热和移植。

Infection and disease develop when the host immune system fails to protect adequately against potential pathogens. In individuals with an intact immune system, infection occurs in the setting of naïveté to the microbe and absence of or inadequate preexisting microbe-specific immunity, or when protective barriers of the body such as the skin have been breached. Healthy children are able to meet the challenge of most infectious agents with an immunologic armamentarium capable of preventing significant disease. Once an infection begins to develop, an array of immune responses is set into action to control the disease and prevent it from reappearing. In contrast, immunocompromised children might not have this same capability. Depending on the level and type of immune defect, the affected child might not be able to contain the pathogen or develop an appropriate immune response to prevent recurrence.

General practitioners are likely to see children with an abnormal immune system in their practice because increasing numbers of children survive with primary immunodeficiencies or receive immunosuppressive therapy for treatment of malignancy, autoimmune disorders, or transplantation.

Primary immunodeficiencies are compromised states that result from genetic defects affecting one or more arms of the immune system. **Acquired**, or **secondary, immunodeficiencies** may result from infection (e.g., infection with HIV), from malignancy, or as an adverse effect of immunomodulating or immunosuppressing medications. The latter include medications that affect T cells (corticosteroids, calcineurin inhibitors, tumor necrosis factor [TNF] inhibitors, chemotherapy), neutrophils (myelosuppressive agents, idiosyncratic or immune-mediated neutropenia), specific immunoregulatory cells (TNF blockers, interleukin-2 inhibitors), or all immune cells (chemotherapy). Perturbations of the mucosal and skin barriers or the normal microbial flora can also be characterized as secondary immunodeficiencies, predisposing the host to infections, if only temporarily.

The major pathogens causing infections among immunocompetent hosts are also the main pathogens responsible for infections among children with immunodeficiencies. In addition, less virulent organisms, including normal skin flora, commensal bacteria of the oropharynx or gastrointestinal (GI) tract, environmental fungi, and common community viruses of low-level pathogenicity, can cause severe, life-threatening illnesses in immunocompromised patients (Table 205.1). For this reason, close communication with the diagnostic laboratory is critical to ensure that the laboratory does not disregard normal flora and organisms normally considered contaminants as being unimportant.

205.1 Infections Occurring With Primary Immunodeficiencies

Marian G. Michaels, Hey Jin Chong, and Michael Green

Currently, more than 300 genes involving inborn errors of immunity have been identified, accounting for a wide array of diseases presenting with susceptibility to infection, allergy, autoimmunity, and autoinflammation, as well as malignancy.

ABNORMALITIES OF THE PHAGOCYTIC SYSTEM

Children with abnormalities of the phagocytic and neutrophil system have problems with bacteria as well as environmental fungi. Disease manifests as recurrent infections of the skin, mucous membranes, lungs, liver, and bones. Dysfunction of this arm of the immune system can be a result of inadequate numbers, abnormal movement properties, or aberrant function of neutrophils (see Chapter 153).

Neutropenia is defined as an absolute neutrophil count (ANC) of <1,000 cells/mm³ and can be associated with significant risk for developing severe bacterial and fungal disease, particularly when the ANC is <500 cells/mm³. Although acquired neutropenia secondary to bone marrow suppression from a virus or medication is common, genetic causes of neutropenia also exist. Primary congenital neutropenia most

Table 205.1	Most Common Causes of Infections in Immunocompromised Children

BACTERIA, AEROBIC
Acinetobacter
Bacillus
Burkholderia cepacia
Citrobacter
Corynebacterium
Enterobacter spp.
Enterococcus faecalis
Enterococcus faecium
Escherichia coli
Klebsiella spp.
Listeria monocytogenes
Mycobacterium spp.
Neisseria meningitidis
Nocardia spp.
Pseudomonas aeruginosa
Staphylococcus aureus
Staphylococcus, coagulase-negative
Streptococcus pneumoniae
Streptococcus, viridans group

BACTERIA, ANAEROBIC
Bacillus
Clostridium
Fusobacterium
Peptococcus
Peptostreptococcus
Propionibacterium
Veillonella

FUNGI
Aspergillus
Candida albicans
Other *Candida* spp.
Cryptococcus neoformans
Fusarium spp.
Pneumocystis jiroveci
Zygomycoses (*Mucor, Rhizopus, Rhizomucor*)

VIRUSES
Adenoviruses
Cytomegalovirus
Epstein-Barr virus
Herpes simplex virus
Human herpesvirus 6
Polyomavirus (BK)
Respiratory and enteric community-acquired viruses
Varicella-zoster virus

PROTOZOA
Cryptosporidium parvum
Giardia lamblia
Toxoplasma gondii

often manifests during the 1st yr of life with cellulitis, perirectal abscesses, or stomatitis from *Staphylococcus aureus* or *Pseudomonas aeruginosa*. Episodes of severe disease, including bacteremia or meningitis, are also possible. Bone marrow evaluation shows a failure of maturation of myeloid precursors. Most forms of congenital neutropenia are autosomal dominant, but some, such as Kostmann syndrome (see Chapter 153) and Shwachman-Diamond syndrome, are caused by autosomal recessive mutations. Cyclic neutropenia can be associated with autosomal dominant inheritance or de novo sporadic mutations and manifests as fixed cycles of severe neutropenia between periods of normal granulocyte numbers. Often the ANC has normalized by the time the patient presents with symptoms, thus hampering the diagnosis. The cycles classically occur every 21 days (range: 14-36 days), with neutropenia lasting 3-6 days. Most often the disease is characterized by recurrent aphthous ulcers and stomatitis during the periods of neutropenia. However, life-threatening necrotizing myositis or cellulitis and systemic disease can occur, especially with *Clostridium septicum* or *Clostridium perfringens.* Many of the neutropenic syndromes respond to colony-stimulating factor.

Leukocyte adhesion defects are caused by defects in the β chain of integrin (CD18), which is required for the normal process of neutrophil aggregation and attachment to endothelial surfaces (see Chapter 153). In the most severe form there is a total absence of CD18. Children with this defect can have a history of delayed cord separation and recurrent infections of the skin, oral mucosa, and genital tract beginning early in life. Ecthyma gangrenosum also occurs. Because the defect involves leukocyte migration and adherence, the ANC in the peripheral blood is usually extremely elevated, but pus is not found at the site of infection. Survival is usually <10 yr in the absence of **hematopoietic stem cell transplantation (HSCT)**.

Chronic granulomatous disease (CGD) is an inherited neutrophil dysfunction syndrome, which can be either X-linked or autosomal recessive (see Chapter 156). In addition, CGD can develop in response to spontaneous mutations in the genes associated with heritable chronic granulomatous disease. Neutrophils and other myeloid cells have defects in their nicotinamide-adenine dinucleotide phosphate oxidase function, rendering them incapable of generating superoxide and thereby impairing intracellular killing. Accordingly, microbes that destroy their own hydrogen peroxide (*S. aureus, Serratia marcescens, Burkholderia cepacia, Nocardia* spp., *Aspergillus*) cause recurrent infections in these children. Less common but considered pathognomonic are *Granulibacter bethesdensis, Francisella philomiragia, Chromobacterium violaceum,* and *Paecilomyces* infections. Infections have a predilection to involve the lungs, liver, and bone. **Mulch pneumonitis** can be seen in patients with known CGD but also can be a unique presenting feature in adults with autosomal recessive CGD. Mulch pneumonitis can resemble hypersensitivity pneumonitis, and bronchoscopy may yield aspergillus but often may not identify a clear organism. Treatment with antifungals and corticosteroids for the inflammation is recommended. *S. aureus* abscesses can occur in the liver despite prophylaxis. In addition, these children can present with recurrent abscesses affecting the skin or perirectal region or lymph nodes. Sepsis can occur but is more common with certain gram-negative organisms such as *C. violaceum* and *F. philomiragia.*

Prophylaxis with trimethoprim-sulfamethoxazole (TMP-SMX), recombinant human interferon-γ, and oral antifungal agents with activity against *Aspergillus* spp., such as itraconazole or newer azoles, substantially reduces the incidence of severe infections. Patients with life-threatening infections are also reported to benefit from aggressive treatment with white blood cell transfusions in addition to antimicrobial agents directed against the specific pathogen. It is important to remember that patients with CGD do not make pus, and thus drain placement for liver abscesses may not be effective. In addition, HSCT can be curative, and gene therapy trials are also a consideration.

DEFECTIVE SPLENIC FUNCTION, OPSONIZATION, OR COMPLEMENT ACTIVITY

Children who have congenital asplenia or splenic dysfunction associated with polysplenia or hemoglobinopathies, such as sickle cell disease, as well as those who have undergone splenectomy, are at risk for serious infections from encapsulated bacteria and bloodborne protozoa such as *Plasmodium* and *Babesia.* Prophylaxis against bacterial infection with penicillin should be considered for these patients, particularly children <5 yr of age. The most common causative organisms include *S. pneumoniae, Haemophilus influenzae* type b (Hib), and *Salmonella,* which can cause sepsis, pneumonia, meningitis, and osteomyelitis. Defects in the early complement components, particularly C2 and C3, may also be associated with severe infection from these bacteria. **Terminal complement defects** (C5, C6, C7, C8, and C9) are associated with recurrent infections with *Neisseria.* Patients with complement deficiency also have an increased incidence of autoimmune disorders. Vaccines for *S. pneumoniae,* Hib, and *N. meningitidis* should be administered to all children with abnormalities in opsonization or complement pathways (see Chapters 159 and 160).

B CELL DEFECTS (HUMORAL IMMUNODEFICIENCIES)

Antibody deficiencies account for the majority of primary immunodeficiencies among humans (see Chapters 149 and 150). Patients with defects in the B cell arm of the immune system fail to develop appropriate antibody responses, with abnormalities that range from complete agammaglobulinemia to isolated failure to produce antibody against a specific antigen or organism. Antibody deficiencies found in children with diseases such as **X-linked agammaglobulinemia (XLA)** or common variable immunodeficiency predispose to infections with encapsulated organisms such as *S. pneumoniae* and *H. influenzae* type b. Other bacteria can also be problematic in these children (see Table 205.1). Patients with XLA can also have neutropenia, with one case series showing 12 of 13 patients with XLA having neutropenia as part of the initial presentation. Because of the neutropenia, patients with XLA can present with *Pseudomonas* septicemia. Viral infections can also occur, with rotavirus leading to chronic diarrhea. Enteroviruses can disseminate and cause a chronic meningoencephalitis syndrome in these patients. Paralytic polio has developed after immunization with live polio vaccine. Protozoan infections such as giardiasis can be severe and persistent. Children with B cell defects can develop bronchiectasis over time following chronic or recurrent pulmonary infections.

Children with antibody deficiencies are usually asymptomatic until 5-6 mo of age, when maternally derived antibody levels begin to wane. These children begin to develop recurrent episodes of otitis media, bronchitis, pneumonia, bacteremia, and meningitis. Many of these infections respond quickly to antibiotics, delaying the recognition of antibody deficiency.

Selective IgA deficiency leads to a lack of production of secretory antibody at the mucosal membranes (see Chapter 150). Even though most patients have no increased risk for infections, some have mild to moderate disease at sites of mucosal barriers. Accordingly, recurrent sinopulmonary infection and GI disease are the major clinical manifestations. These patients also have an increased incidence of allergies and autoimmune disorders compared with the normal population.

Hyper-IgM syndrome encompasses a group of genetic defects in immunoglobulin class switch recombination. The most common type is caused by a defect in the CD40 ligand on the T cell, leading to the inability of the B cell to class switch (see Chapter 150). Similar to other patients with humoral defects, these patients are at risk for bacterial sinopulmonary infections. However, unlike a true pure antibody defect, besides being important in T cell–B cell interactions, CD40 ligand is also important in the interaction between T cells and macrophages/monocytes, influencing opportunistic infections such as *Pneumocystis jiroveci* pneumonia (PCP) and *Cryptosporidium* intestinal infection.

T CELL DEFECTS (CELL-MEDIATED IMMUNODEFICIENCIES)

Children with primary cell-mediated immunodeficiencies, either isolated or more often in combination with B cell defects, present early in life and are susceptible to viral, fungal, and protozoan infections. Clinical manifestations include chronic diarrhea, mucocutaneous candidiasis, and recurrent pneumonia, rhinitis, and otitis media. In thymic hypoplasia (**DiGeorge syndrome**), hypoplasia or aplasia of the thymus and parathyroid glands occurs during fetal development in association with the presence of other congenital abnormalities. Hypocalcemia and cardiac anomalies are usually the presenting features of DiGeorge syndrome, which should prompt evaluation of the T cell system.

Chronic mucocutaneous candidiasis (CMC) is a group of immunodeficiencies leading to susceptibility to fungal infections of the skin, nails, oral cavity, and genitals. Most frequently caused by *Candida* spp., dermatophyte infections with *Microsporum, Epidermophyton,* and *Trichophyton* have also been described. Interestingly, patients with CMC do not have an increased risk for histoplasmosis, blastomycosis, or coccidioidomycosis. Despite chronic cutaneous and mucosal infection with *Candida* spp., these patients often lack a delayed hypersensitivity to skin tests for *Candida* antigen. Several gene defects make up this group of disorders, including *STAT1* gain-of-function mutations, *IL17R* defects, *CARD9* deficiency, and *ACT1* deficiency. Although patients with CMC generally do not develop invasive candidiasis, this differs depending on the gene defect. Endocrinopathies and autoimmunity can also be seen in affected people, especially in individuals with *STAT1* gain-of-function mutations.

COMBINED B CELL AND T CELL DEFECTS

Patients with defects in both the T cell and B cell components of the immune system have variable manifestations depending on the extent of the defect (see Chapters 149-152). Complete or almost complete immunodeficiency is found with **severe combined immunodeficiency disorder (SCID)**, whereas partial defects can be present in such states as ataxia-telangiectasia, Wiskott-Aldrich syndrome, hyper-IgE syndrome, and X-linked lymphoproliferative disorder. Rather than one disorder, it is now recognized that SCID represents a heterogeneous group of genetic defects that leave the infant globally immune deficient and present in the 1st 6 mo of life with recurrent and typically severe infections caused by a variety of bacteria, fungi, and viruses. Failure to thrive, chronic diarrhea, mucocutaneous or systemic candidiasis, PCP, or cytomegalovirus (CMV) infections are common early in life. Passive maternal antibody is relatively protective against the bacterial pathogens during the 1st few mo of life, but thereafter patients are susceptible to both gram-positive and gram-negative organisms. Exposure to live-virus vaccines can also lead to disseminated disease; accordingly, the use of live vaccines (including rotavirus vaccine) is contraindicated in patients with suspected or proven SCID. Without stem cell transplantation or gene therapy, most affected children succumb to opportunistic infections within the 1st yr of life.

Children with **ataxia-telangiectasia** develop late-onset recurrent sinopulmonary infections from both bacteria and respiratory viruses. In addition, these children experience an increased incidence of malignancies. **Wiskott-Aldrich syndrome** is an X-linked recessive disease associated with eczema, thrombocytopenia, reduced number of CD3 lymphocytes, moderately suppressed mitogen responses, and impaired antibody response to polysaccharide antigens. Accordingly, infections with *S. pneumoniae* or *H. influenzae* type b and PCP are common. Children with hyper-IgE syndrome have greatly elevated levels of IgE and present with recurrent episodes of *S. aureus* abscesses of the skin, lungs, and musculoskeletal system. Although the antibody abnormality is notable, these patients also have marked eosinophilia and poor cell-mediated responses to neoantigens and are at increased risk for fungal infections.

Bibliography is available at Expert Consult.

205.2 Infections Occurring With Acquired Immunodeficiencies

Marian G. Michaels, Hey Jin Chong, and Michael Green

Immunodeficiencies can be secondarily acquired as a result of infections or other underlying disorders, such as malignancy, cystic fibrosis, diabetes mellitus, sickle cell disease, or malnutrition. Immunosuppressive medications used to prevent rejection after organ transplantation, to prevent **graft-versus-host disease (GVHD)** after stem cell transplantation, or to treat malignancies may also leave the host vulnerable to infections. Similarly, medications used to control rheumatologic or other autoimmune diseases may be associated with an increased risk for developing infection. Surgical removal of the spleen likewise puts a person at increased risk for infections. Further, any process that disrupts the normal mucosal and skin barriers (e.g., burns, surgery, indwelling catheters) may lead to an increased risk for infection.

ACQUIRED IMMUNODEFICIENCY FROM INFECTIOUS AGENTS

Infection with HIV, the causative agent of AIDS, remains globally an important infectious cause of acquired immunodeficiency (see Chapter 302). Left untreated, HIV infection has profound effects on many parts of the immune system but in particular T cell–mediated immunity that leads to susceptibility to the same types of infections as with primary T cell immunodeficiencies.

Other organisms can also lead to temporary alterations of the immune system. Very rarely, transient neutropenia associated with community-acquired viruses can lead to significant disease with bacterial infections. Secondary infections can occur because of impaired immunity or disruption of normal mucosal immunity, as exemplified by the increased risk for pneumonia from *S. pneumoniae* or *S. aureus* following influenza infection and group A streptococcal cellulitis and fasciitis following varicella.

MALIGNANCIES

The immune systems of children with malignancies are compromised by the therapies used to treat the cancer and, at times, by direct effects of the cancer itself. The type, duration, and intensity of anticancer therapy remain the major risk factors for infections in these children and often affect multiple arms of the immune system. The presence of mucous membrane abnormalities, indwelling catheters, malnutrition, prolonged exposure to antibiotics, and frequent hospitalizations adds to the risk for infection in these children.

Even though several arms of the immune system can be affected, the major abnormality predisposing to infection in children with cancer is **neutropenia**. The depth and duration of neutropenia are the primary predictors of the risk of infection in children being treated for cancer. Patients are at particular risk for bacterial and fungal infections if the ANC decreases to <500 cells/mm^3, and the risk is highest in those with counts <100 cells/mm^3. Counts of >500 cells/mm^3 but <1,000 cells/mm^3 incur some increased risk for infection, but not nearly as great. The lack of neutrophils can lead to a diminution of inflammatory response, limiting the ability to localize sites of infection and potentially leaving fever as the only manifestation of infection. Accordingly, the absence of physical signs and symptoms does not reliably exclude the presence of infection, resulting in the need for empirical antibiotics (Fig. 205.1). Because patients with **fever and neutropenia** might only have subtle signs and symptoms of infection, the presence of fever warrants an intensive investigation, including a thorough physical examination with careful attention to the oropharynx, lungs, perineum and anus, skin, nail beds, and intravascular catheter insertion sites (Table 205.2).

A comprehensive laboratory evaluation, including a complete blood cell count, serum creatinine, blood urea nitrogen, and serum transaminases, should be obtained. Blood cultures should be taken from each port of any **central venous catheter** (CVC) and from a peripheral vein. Although the latter sampling is often omitted with continued fevers and neutropenia, it should be obtained before the initial antibiotic administration and reconsidered in children with 1 or more positive cultures from a CVC, facilitating localization of the source of the infection. Other microbiologic studies should be done if there are associated clinical symptoms, including a nasal aspirate for viruses in patients with upper respiratory findings; stool for viruses such as rotavirus or norovirus and for *Clostridium difficile* toxin in patients with diarrhea; urinalysis and culture in young children or in older patients with symptoms of urgency, frequency, dysuria, or hematuria; and biopsy and culture of cutaneous lesions. Chest radiographs should be obtained in any patient with lower respiratory tract symptoms, although pulmonary infiltrates may be absent in children with severe neutropenia. Sinus films should be obtained for children >2 yr of age if rhinorrhea is prolonged. Abdominal CT scans should also be considered in children with profound neutropenia and abdominal pain to evaluate for the presence of typhlitis. Chest CT scan and fungal biomarkers (e.g., galactomannan, β-D-glucan) testing should be considered for children not responding to broad-spectrum antibiotics who have continued fever and neutropenia for >96 hr. Biopsies for cytology, Gram stain, and culture should be considered if abnormalities are found during endoscopic procedures or if lung nodules are identified radiographically.

Classic studies by Pizzo and colleagues demonstrated that before the routine institution of empirical antimicrobial therapy for fever and

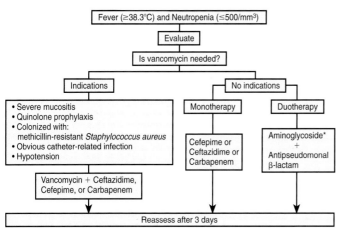

Fig. 205.1 Algorithm for the initial management of the febrile neutropenic patient. Monotherapy can be considered with cefepime, imipenem/cilastatin, meropenem, piperacillin-tazobactam, or ticarcillin–clavulanic acid. *Aminoglycoside antibiotics should be avoided if the patient is also receiving nephrotoxic, ototoxic, or neuromuscular blocking agents; has renal or severe electrolyte dysfunction; or is suspected of having meningitis (because of poor blood-brain perfusion). (Adapted from Freifeld AG, Bow EJ, Sepkowitz KA, et al: Clinical practice guideline for the use of antimicrobial agents in neutropenic patients with cancer: 2010 update by the Infectious Diseases Society of America, Clin Infect Dis 52: e56–e93, 2011.)

Table 205.2	Host Defense Defects and Common Pathogens by Time After Bone Marrow or Hematopoietic Stem Cell Transplantation		
TIME PERIOD	**HOST DEFENSE DEFECTS**	**CAUSES**	**COMMON PATHOGENS**
Pretransplant	Neutropenia Abnormal anatomic barriers	Underlying disease Prior chemotherapy	Aerobic gram-negative bacilli
Preengraftment	Neutropenia Abnormal anatomic barriers	Chemotherapy Radiation Indwelling catheters	Aerobic gram-positive cocci Aerobic gram-negative bacilli Candida Aspergillus Herpes simplex virus (in previously infected patients) Community-acquired viral pathogens
Postengraftment	Abnormal cell-mediated immunity Abnormal anatomic barriers	Chemotherapy Immunosuppressive medications Radiation Indwelling catheters Unrelated cord blood donor	Gram-positive cocci Aerobic gram-negative bacilli Cytomegalovirus Adenoviruses Community-acquired viral pathogens Pneumocystis jiroveci
Late posttransplant	Delayed recovery of immune function (cell-mediated, humoral, and abnormal anatomic barriers)	Time required to develop donor-related immune function Graft-versus-host disease	Varicella-zoster virus Streptococcus pneumoniae

neutropenia, 75% of children with fever and neutropenia were ultimately found to have a documented site of infection, suggesting that most children with fever and neutropenia will have an underlying infection (see Table 205.2). Currently, **gram-positive cocci** are the most common pathogens identified in these patients; however, gram-negative organisms such as *Pseudomonas aeruginosa, Escherichia coli,* and *Klebsiella* can cause life-threatening infection and must be considered in the empirical treatment regimen. Other multidrug-resistant Enterobacteriaceae are increasingly recovered in these children. Although coagulase-negative staphylococci often cause infections in these children in association with CVCs, these infections are typically indolent, and a short delay in treatment usually does not lead to a detrimental outcome. Other gram-positive bacteria, such as *S. aureus* and *S. pneumoniae,* can cause more fulminant disease and require prompt institution of therapy. Viridans streptococci are particularly important potential pathogens in patients with the oral mucositis that is often associated with use of cytarabine and in patients who experience selective pressure from treatment with certain antibiotics such as quinolones. Infection caused by this group of organisms can present as acute septic shock syndrome. Also, patients with prolonged neutropenia are at increased risk for opportunistic fungal

infections, with *Candida* and *Aspergillus* spp. being the most commonly identified fungi. Other fungi that can cause serious disease in these children include *Mucor* and *Fusarium* spp. and dematiaceous molds.

FEVER AND NEUTROPENIA

The use of empirical antimicrobial treatment as part of the management of fever and neutropenia decreases the risk of progression to sepsis, septic shock, acute respiratory distress syndrome, organ dysfunction, and death. In 2010 the Infectious Diseases Society of America (IDSA) updated a comprehensive guideline for the use of antimicrobial agents in neutropenic children and adults with cancer (see Fig. 205.1).

First-line antimicrobial therapy should take into consideration the types of microbes anticipated and the local resistance patterns encountered at each institution as well as the level of risk for severe infection associated with a given patient. In addition, antibiotic choices may be limited by specific circumstances, such as the presence of drug allergy and renal or hepatic dysfunction. The empirical use of oral antibiotics has been shown to be safe in some low-risk adults who have no evidence of bacterial focus or signs of significant illness (rigors, hypotension, mental status changes) and for whom a quick recovery of the bone marrow is anticipated. Guidelines for the management of fever and neutropenia in children with cancer and/or undergoing HSCT (2012) conclude that the use of oral antimicrobial therapy as either initial or stepdown therapy can be considered in low-risk children who can tolerate oral antibiotics and in whom careful monitoring can be ensured. However, the guideline emphasizes that oral medication use may present major challenges in children, including availability of liquid formulations of appropriate antibiotics, cooperation of young children, and presence of mucositis potentially interfering with absorption. Accordingly, decisions to implement this approach should be reserved for a select subset of these children presenting with fever and neutropenia.

The decision to initially use intravenous (IV) monotherapy vs an expanded regimen of antibiotics depends on the severity of illness of the patient, history of previous colonization with resistant organisms, and obvious presence of catheter-related infection. **Vancomycin** should be added to the initial empirical regimen if the patient has hypotension or other evidence of septic shock, an obvious catheter-related infection, or a history of colonization with methicillin-resistant *S. aureus*, or if the patient is at high risk for viridans streptococci (severe mucositis, acute myelogenous leukemia, or prior use of quinolone prophylaxis). Otherwise, use of monotherapy with an antibiotic such as cefepime or piperacillin-tazobactam can be considered. Ceftazidime should not be used as monotherapy if concern exists for gram-positive organisms or resistant gram-negative bacteria. Carbapenems such as imipenem/cilastin and meropenem should not be first line, aiming to prevent pressure on carbapenem-resistant Enterobacteriaceae. The addition of a 2nd anti–gram-negative bacterial agent (e.g., aminoglycoside) for empirical therapy can be considered in patients who are clinically unstable when multidrug-resistant organisms are suspected.

Regardless of the regimen chosen initially, it is critical to evaluate the patient carefully and continually for response to therapy, development of secondary infections, and adverse effects. Management recommendations for these children are evolving. Based on the 2012 guidelines, patients who have negative blood cultures at 48 hr, who have been afebrile for at least 24 hr, and who have evidence of bone marrow recovery (ANC >100 cells/mm³) can have antibiotics discontinued. However, if symptoms persist or evolve, IV antibiotics should be continued. Continuation of antibiotics in children whose fever has abated and who are clinically well but continue to have depression of neutrophils is more controversial. The 2012 pediatric guidelines advocate for discontinuing antibiotics in low-risk patients at 72 hr for children who have negative blood cultures and who have been afebrile for at least 24 hr regardless of bone marrow recovery, as long as careful follow-up is ensured. In contrast, others continue to advocate for continuing antibiotics in this circumstance to prevent recurrence of fever.

Patients without an identified etiology but with **persistent fever** should be reassessed daily. At day 3-5 of persistent fever and neutropenia, those remaining clinically well may continue on the same regimen, although consideration should be given to discontinuing vancomycin or double gram-negative bacterial coverage if they were included initially. Patients who remain febrile with clinical progression warrant the addition of vancomycin if it was not included initially and risk factors exist; clinicians should also consider changing the empirical antibacterial regimen to cover for potential antimicrobial resistance in these children. If fever persists for >96 hr, the addition of an **antifungal agent** with antimold activity should be considered, particularly for those at high risk for invasive fungal infection (those with acute myelogenous leukemia or relapsed acute lymphocytic leukemia or who are receiving highly myelosuppressive chemotherapies for other cancers or with allogeneic HSCT). Medications, including **liposomal amphotericin** products and **echinocandins**, have been studied in children; voriconazole itraconazole, and posaconazole have been successfully used in adults, with increasing experience in children. Studies comparing caspofungin to liposomal amphotericin for children with malignancies and fever and neutropenia showed caspofungin to be noninferior.

The use of **antiviral agents** in children with fever and neutropenia is not warranted without specific evidence of viral disease. Active herpes simplex or varicella-zoster lesions merit treatment to decrease the time of healing; even if these lesions are not the source of fever, they are potential portals of entry for bacteria and fungi. CMV is a rare cause of fever in children with cancer and neutropenia. If CMV infection is suspected, assays to evaluate viral load in the blood and organ-specific infection should be obtained. Ganciclovir, foscarnet, or cidofovir may be considered while evaluation is pending, although ganciclovir can cause bone marrow suppression and foscarnet and cidofovir can be nephrotoxic. If influenza is identified, specific treatment with an antiviral agent should be administered. Choice of treatment (oseltamivir, zanamivir) should be based on the anticipated susceptibility of the circulating influenza strains.

The use of **hematopoietic growth factors** shortens the duration of neutropenia but has not been proved to reduce morbidity or mortality. Accordingly, the 2010 IDSA recommendations do not endorse the routine use of hematopoietic growth factors in patients with established fever and neutropenia, although the recommendations do note that hematopoietic growth factors can be considered as prophylaxis in those with neutropenia at high risk for fever.

FEVER WITHOUT NEUTROPENIA

Infections occur in children with cancer in the absence of neutropenia. Most often these infections are viral in etiology. However, *Pneumocystis jiroveci* can cause pneumonia regardless of the neutrophil count. Administration of prophylaxis against *Pneumocystis* is an effective preventive strategy and should be provided to all children undergoing active treatment for malignancy. First-line therapy remains TMP-SMX, with second-line alternatives including pentamidine, atovaquone, dapsone, or dapsone-pyrimethamine. Environmental fungi such as *Cryptococcus, Histoplasma*, and *Coccidioides* can also cause disease. *Toxoplasma gondii* is an uncommon but occasional pathogen in children with cancer. Infections caused by pathogens encountered in healthy children (*S. pneumoniae*, group A streptococcus) can occur in children with cancer regardless of the granulocyte count.

TRANSPLANTATION

Transplantation of hematopoietic stem cells and solid organs (including heart, liver, kidney, lungs, pancreas, and intestines) is increasingly used as therapy for a variety of disorders. Children undergoing transplantation are at risk for infections caused by many of the same microbial agents that cause disease in children with primary immunodeficiencies. Although the types of infections after transplantation generally are similar among all recipients of these procedures, some differences exist between patients depending on the type of transplantation performed, the type and amount of immunosuppression given, and the child's preexisting immunity to specific pathogens.

Stem Cell Transplantation

Infections following HSCT can be classified as occurring during the **pretransplantation period, preengraftment period** (0-30 days after transplantation), **postengraftment period** (30-100 days), or **late posttransplantation period** (>100 days). Specific defects in host defenses predisposing to infection vary within each of these periods (Table 205.2). Neutropenia and abnormalities in cell-mediated and humoral immune function occur predictably during specific periods after transplantation. In contrast, breaches of anatomic barriers caused by indwelling catheters and mucositis secondary to radiation or chemotherapy create defects in host defenses that may be present any time after transplantation.

Pretransplantation Period

Children come to HSCT with a heterogeneous history of underlying diseases, chemotherapy exposure, degree of immunosuppression, and previous infections. Approximately 12% of all infections among adult HSCT recipients occur during the pretransplantation period. These infections are often caused by aerobic gram-negative bacilli and manifest as localized infections of the skin, soft tissue, and urinary tract. Importantly, the development of infection during this period does not delay or adversely affect the success of engraftment.

Preengraftment Period

Bacterial infections predominate in the preengraftment period (0-30 days). **Bacteremia** is the most common documented infection and occurs in as many as 50% of all HSCT recipients during the 1st 30 days after transplantation. Bacteremia is typically associated with the presence of either mucositis or an indwelling catheter but may also be seen with pneumonia. Similarly, >40% of children undergoing HSCT experienced 1 or more infections in the preengraftment period. Gram-positive cocci, gram-negative bacilli, yeast, and, less frequently, other fungi cause infection during this period. *Aspergillus* has been identified in 4–20% of HSCT recipients, most often after 3 wk of neutropenia. Infections caused by the emerging fungal pathogens *Fusarium* and *Pseudallescheria boydii* are associated with the prolonged neutropenia during the preengraftment period.

Viral infections also occur during the preengraftment period. Among adults, reactivation of herpes simplex virus (HSV) is the most common viral disease observed, but this is less common among children. A history of HSV infection or seropositivity indicates the need for prophylaxis. Nosocomial exposure to community-acquired viral pathogens, including respiratory syncytial virus (RSV), influenza virus, adenovirus, rotavirus, and norovirus, represents another important source of infection during this period. There is growing evidence that community-acquired viruses cause increased morbidity and mortality for HSCT recipients during this period. Adenovirus is a particularly important viral pathogen that can occur early, although it typically presents after engraftment.

Postengraftment Period

The predominant defect in host defenses in the postengraftment period is altered cell-mediated immunity. Accordingly, organisms historically categorized as "opportunistic pathogens" predominate during this period. The risk is especially accentuated 50-100 days after transplantation, when host immunity is lost and donor immunity is not yet established. *P. jiroveci* presents during this period if patients are not maintained on appropriate prophylaxis. Reactivation of *T. gondii*, a rare cause of disease among HSCT recipients, can also occur after engraftment. Hepatosplenic candidiasis often presents during the postengraftment period, although seeding likely occurs during the neutropenic phase.

Cytomegalovirus is an important cause of morbidity and mortality among HSCT recipients. Unlike patients undergoing solid-organ transplantation, where primary infection from the donor causes the greatest harm, CMV reactivation in an HSCT recipient whose donor is naïve to the virus can cause severe disease. Disease risk from CMV after HSCT is also increased in recipients of cord blood transplants or matched unrelated T cell–depleted transplants and those with GVHD. **Adenovirus**, another important viral pathogen, has been recovered from up to 5% of adult and pediatric HSCT recipients and causes invasive disease in approximately 20% of cases. Children receiving matched unrelated donor organs or unrelated cord blood cell transplants have an incidence of adenovirus infection as high as 14% during this early postengraftment period. **Polyomaviruses** such as BK virus have been increasingly recognized as a cause of renal dysfunction and hemorrhagic cystitis after bone marrow transplantation. Infections with other herpesviruses (Epstein-Barr virus [EBV] and human herpesvirus 6) as well as community-acquired pathogens are associated with excess morbidity and mortality during this period, similar to the preengraftment period.

Late Posttransplantation Period

Infection is unusual after 100 days in the absence of chronic GVHD. However, the presence of chronic GVHD significantly affects anatomic barriers and is associated with defects in humoral, splenic, and cell-mediated immune function. Viral infections, including primary infection with or reactivation of varicella-zoster virus (VZV), are responsible for >40% of infections during this period. This may decrease over time as the Oka varicella vaccine strain has a lower rate of reactivation than wild-type varicella. Bacterial infections, particularly of the upper and lower respiratory tract, account for approximately 30% of infections. These may be associated with deficiencies in immunoglobulin production, especially IgG2. Fungal infections account for <20% of confirmed infections during the late posttransplantation period.

Table 205.3	Risk Factors for Infections After Solid-Organ Transplantation in Children

PRETRANSPLANTATION FACTORS

Age of patient
Underlying disease, malnutrition
Specific organ transplanted
Previous exposures to infectious agents
Previous immunizations
Presence of infection in the donor

INTRAOPERATIVE FACTORS

Duration of transplant surgery
Exposure to blood products
Technical problems
Organisms transmitted with donor organ

POSTTRANSPLANTATION FACTORS

Immunosuppression
Induction immunosuppression type
Maintenance immunosuppression
Augmented treatment for rejection
Indwelling catheters
Nosocomial exposures
Community exposures

Solid-Organ Transplantation

Factors predisposing to infection after organ transplantation include those that either existed before transplantation or are secondary to intraoperative events or posttransplantation therapies (Table 205.3). Some of these additional risks cannot be prevented, and some risks acquired during or after the operation depend on decisions or actions of members of the transplant team. Organ recipients are at risk for infection from potential exposure to pathogens in the donor organ. Although some donor-derived infections can be anticipated through donor screening, many pathogens are not routinely screened for, and strategies defining when and how to screen for all but a small subset of potential pathogens have not been identified or implemented. Similar to other children who have undergone surgical procedures; surgical site infections are a frequent cause of infection early after transplantation. Beyond this, the need for immunosuppressive agents to prevent rejection is the major factor predisposing to infection following transplantation. Despite efforts to optimize immunosuppressive regimens to prevent or treat rejection with minimal impairment of immunity, all current regimens interfere with the ability of the immune system to prevent infection. The primary target of the majority of these immunosuppressive agents in organ recipients is the cell-mediated immune system, but regimens can and do impair many other aspects of the transplant recipient's immune system as well.

Timing

The timing of specific types of infections is generally predictable, regardless of which organ is transplanted. Infectious complications typically develop in 1 of 3 intervals: early (0-30 days after transplantation), intermediate (30-180 days), or late (>180 days); most infections present in the 1st 180 days after transplantation. Table 205.4 should be used as a general guideline to the types of infections encountered but may be modified with the introduction of newer immunosuppressive therapies and by the use of prophylaxis.

Early infections are usually the result of a complication of the transplant surgery itself, the unexpected acquisition of a bacterial or fungal pathogen from the donor, or the presence of an indwelling catheter. In contrast, infections during the intermediate period typically result from a complication of the immunosuppression, which tends to be at its greatest intensity during the 1st 6 mo after transplantation. This is the period of greatest risk for infections caused by opportunistic pathogens such as CMV, EBV, and *P. jiroveci*. Anatomic abnormalities, such as bronchial stenosis and biliary stenosis, that develop as a result of the transplant surgery can also predispose to recurrent infection in this period.

Table 205.4	Timing of Infectious Complications After Solid-Organ Transplantation

EARLY PERIOD (0-30 DAYS)
Bacterial Infections
Gram-negative enteric bacilli
• Small bowel, liver, neonatal heart
Pseudomonas, Burkholderia, Stenotrophomonas, Alcaligenes
• Cystic fibrosis lung
Gram-positive organisms
• All transplant types
Fungal Infections
• All transplant types
Viral Infections
Herpes simplex virus
• All transplant types
Nosocomial respiratory viruses
• All transplant types

MIDDLE PERIOD (1-6 MO)
Viral Infections
Cytomegalovirus
• All transplant types
• Seronegative recipient of seropositive donor
Epstein-Barr virus
• All transplant types (small bowel the highest-risk group)
• Seronegative recipient
Varicella-zoster virus
• All transplant types
• Opportunistic infections
Pneumocystis jiroveci
• All transplant types
Toxoplasma gondii
• Seronegative recipient of cardiac transplant from a seropositive donor
Bacterial Infections
Pseudomonas, Burkholderia, Stenotrophomonas, Alcaligenes
• Cystic fibrosis lung
Gram-negative enteric bacilli
• Small bowel

LATE PERIOD (>6 MO)
Viral Infections
Epstein-Barr virus
• All transplant types, but less risk than middle period
Varicella-zoster virus
• All transplant types
Community-acquired viral infections
• All transplant types
Bacterial Infections
Pseudomonas, Burkholderia, Stenotrophomonas, Alcaligenes
• Cystic fibrosis lung
• Lung transplants with chronic rejection
Gram-negative bacillary bacteremia
• Small bowel
Fungal Infections
Aspergillus
• Lung transplants with chronic rejection

Adapted from Green M, Michaels MG: Infections in solid organ transplant recipients. In Long SS, Prober C, Fisher M, editors: *Principles and practice of pediatric infectious disease*, ed 5, Philadelphia, 2018, Elsevier (Table 95-1).

Infections developing late after transplantation typically result from uncorrected anatomic abnormalities, chronic rejection, or exposure to community-acquired pathogens. Augmented immunosuppression as treatment for late, acute cellular rejection or chronic rejection can increase the risk for late presentations with CMV, EBV, and other potential opportunistic infections. Acquisition of infection from community-acquired pathogens such as RSV can result in severe infection secondary to the immunocompromised state of the transplant recipient during the early and intermediate periods. Compared with the earlier periods, community-acquired infections in the late period are usually benign, because immunosuppression is typically maintained at significantly lower levels. However, certain pathogens such as VZV and EBV may be associated with severe disease even at this late period.

Bacterial and Fungal Infections

Although there are important graft-specific considerations for bacterial and fungal infections following transplantation, some principles are generally applicable to all transplant recipients. Bacterial and fungal infections after organ transplantation are usually a direct consequence of the surgery, a breach in an anatomic barrier, a foreign body, or an abnormal anatomic narrowing or obstruction. With the exception of infections related to the use of indwelling catheters, sites of bacterial infection tend to occur at or near the transplanted organ. Infections following abdominal transplantation (liver, intestine, or renal) usually occur in the abdomen or at the surgical wound. The pathogens are typically enteric gram-negative bacteria, *Enterococcus,* and occasionally *Candida.* Infections after thoracic transplantation (heart, lung) usually occur in the lower respiratory tract or at the surgical wound. Pathogens associated with these infections include *S. aureus* and gram-negative bacteria. Patients undergoing lung transplantation for cystic fibrosis experience a particularly high rate of infectious complications, because they are often colonized with *P. aeruginosa* or *Aspergillus* before transplantation. Even though the infected lungs are removed, the sinuses and upper airways remain colonized with these pathogens, and subsequent reinfection of the transplanted lungs can occur. Children receiving organ transplants are often hospitalized for long periods and receive many antibiotics; thus recovery of bacteria with multiple antibiotic resistance patterns is common after all types of organ transplantation. Infections caused by *Aspergillus* are less common but occur after all types of organ transplantation and are associated with high rates of morbidity and mortality.

Viral Infections

Viral pathogens, especially herpesviruses, are a major source of morbidity and mortality following solid-organ transplantation. In addition, BK virus is a major cause of renal disease after kidney transplantation. The patterns of disease associated with individual viral pathogens are generally similar among all organ transplant recipients. However, the incidence, mode of presentation, and severity differ according to type of organ transplanted and, for many viral pathogens, pretransplant serologic status of the recipient.

Viral pathogens can be generally categorized as latent pathogens, which cause infection through reactivation in the host or acquisition from the donor (e.g., CMV, EBV) or as community-acquired viruses (e.g., RSV). For CMV and EBV, primary infection occurring after transplantation is associated with the greatest degree of morbidity and mortality. The highest risk is seen in a naïve host who receives an organ from a donor who previously was infected with one of these viruses. This mismatched state is frequently associated with severe disease. However, even if the donor is negative for CMV and EBV, primary infection can be acquired from a close contact or through blood products. Secondary infections (reactivation of a latent strain within the host or superinfection with a new strain) tend to result in milder illness unless the patient is highly immunosuppressed, which can occur in the setting of treatment of significant rejection.

CMV is one of the most commonly recognized transplant viral pathogens. Disease from CMV has decreased significantly with the use of preventive strategies, including antiviral prophylaxis as well as viral load monitoring to inform preemptive antiviral therapy. Some centers have implemented a hybrid approach where surveillance viral load monitoring follows a relatively short period (2-4 wk) of chemoprophylaxis. Clinical manifestations of CMV disease can range from a syndrome of fatigue and fever to tissue invasive disease that most often affects the liver, lungs, and GI tract.

Infection caused by EBV is another important complication of solid-organ transplantation. Clinical symptoms range from a mild mononucleosis syndrome to disseminated **posttransplant lymphoproliferative disorder**. Posttransplant lymphoproliferative disorder is more common among children than adults, because primary EBV infection in the immunosuppressed host is more likely to lead to uncontrolled proliferative disorders, including posttransplant lymphoma.

Other viruses, such as adenovirus, also have the capacity to be donor associated, but appear to be less common. The unexpected development of donor-associated viral pathogens, including hepatitis B virus, hepatitis C virus, and HIV, is rare today because of intensive donor screening. However, the changing epidemiology of some viruses (e.g., dengue, chikungunya, Zika) raises concerns for the donor-derived transmission of these emerging viral pathogens.

Community-acquired viruses, including those associated with respiratory tract infection (RSV, influenza virus, adenovirus, parainfluenza virus) and GI infection (enteroviruses, norovirus, and rotavirus), can cause important disease in children after organ transplantation. In general, risk factors for more severe infection include young age, acquisition of infection early after transplantation, and augmented immune suppression. Infection in the absence of these risk factors frequently results in a clinical illness that is comparable to that seen in immunocompetent children. However, some community-acquired viruses, such as adenovirus, can be associated with graft dysfunction even when acquired late after transplantation.

Opportunistic Pathogens

Children undergoing solid-organ transplantation are also at risk for symptomatic infections from pathogens that do not usually cause clinical disease in immunocompetent hosts. Although these typically present in the intermediate period, these infections can also occur late in patients, requiring prolonged and high levels of immunosuppression. *P. jiroveci* is a well-recognized cause of pneumonia after solid-organ transplantation, although routine prophylaxis has essentially eliminated this problem. *T. gondii* can complicate cardiac transplantations because of tropism of the organism for cardiac muscle and risk for donor transmission; less often it complicates other types of organ transplantation.

Bibliography is available at Expert Consult.

205.3 Prevention of Infection in Immunocompromised Persons

Marian G. Michaels, Hey Jin Chong, and Michael Green

Although infections cannot be completely prevented in children who have defects in one or more arms of their immune system, measures can be taken to decrease the risks for infection. Replacement immunoglobulin is a benefit to children with primary B cell deficiencies. Interferon (IFN)-γ, TMP-SMX, and oral antifungal agents have long been used to reduce the number of infections occurring in children with CGD, although the relative benefit of INF-γ has been questioned. Children who have depressed cellular immunity resulting from primary diseases, advanced HIV infection, or immunosuppressive medications benefit from prophylaxis against *P. jiroveci*. Immunizations prevent many infections and are particularly important for children with compromised immune systems who do not have a contraindication or inability to respond. For children rendered immunocompromised because of medication or splenectomy, immunizations should be administered before treatment. This timing allows for superior response to vaccine antigens, avoids the risk of live vaccines, which may be contraindicated depending on the immunosuppression, and importantly provides protection before the immune system is compromised.

Although immunodeficient children are a heterogeneous group, some principles of prevention are generally applicable. The use of inactivated vaccines does not lead to an increased risk for adverse effects, although their efficacy may be reduced because of an impaired immune response. In most cases, children with immunodeficiencies should receive all the recommended inactivated vaccines. Live-attenuated vaccinations can cause disease in some children with immunologic defects, and therefore alternative immunizations should be used whenever possible, such as inactivated influenza vaccine rather than live-attenuated influenza vaccine or inactivated typhoid vaccine rather than the oral live typhoid vaccine for travelers. In general, live-virus vaccines should not be used in children with primary T cell abnormalities; efforts should be made to ensure that close contacts are all immunized to decrease the risk of exposure. In some patients in whom wild-type viral infection can be severe, immunizations, even with live-virus vaccine, are warranted in the immunosuppressed child. For example, children with HIV infection and a CD4 level of >15% should receive vaccinations against measles and varicella. Some vaccines should be given to children with immunodeficiencies in addition to routine vaccinations. As an example, children with asplenia or splenic dysfunction should receive meningococcal vaccine and both the conjugate and the polysaccharide pneumococcal vaccines. Influenza vaccination is recommended for all individuals >6 mo old and should be emphasized for immunocompromised children as well as all household contacts, to minimize risk for transmission to the immunocompromised child.

Bibliography is available at Expert Consult.

Chapter 206
Infection Associated With Medical Devices
Joshua Wolf and Patricia M. Flynn

第二百零六章
与医疗器械相关的感染

中文导读

本章主要介绍了血管内置入装置、脑脊液分流、尿管、腹膜透析导管和矫形假肢。在血管内置入装置部分详细介绍了导管类型、导管相关皮肤和软组织感染、导管相关血流感染以及相关感染的预防。在脑脊液分流、尿管、腹膜透析导管和矫形假肢部分详细介绍了导管的种类、感染发生率、感染的类型、感染后的症状、诊断方法、常见病原、治疗措施、导管的移除以及感染预防等内容。

Use of implanted synthetic and prosthetic devices has revolutionized pediatric practice by providing long-term venous access, limb-salvage surgery, and successful treatment of hydrocephalus, urinary retention, and renal failure. However, infectious complications of these devices remain a major concern. These infections are related to the development of **biofilms**, organized communities of microorganisms on the device surface protected from the immune system and from antimicrobial therapy. A number of factors are important to the development of infection, including host susceptibility, device composition, duration of implantation, and exposure to colonizing organisms.

INTRAVASCULAR ACCESS DEVICES
Intravascular access devices range from short, stainless steel needles or plastic cannulae inserted for brief periods to multilumen implantable synthetic plastic catheters that are expected to remain in use for years. Infectious complications include local skin and soft tissue infections such as exit-site, tunnel-tract, and device-pocket infections, and **catheter-related bloodstream infections (CRBSIs)**. The use of central venous devices has improved the quality of life of high-risk patients but has also increased the risk of infection.

Catheter Types
Short-term peripheral cannulae are most often used in pediatric patients, and infectious complications occur infrequently. The rate of peripheral CRBSIs in children is <0.15%. Patient age <1 yr, duration of use >144 hr, and some infusates are associated with increased risk for catheter-related infection. Catheter-associated phlebitis is more common (1–6%) but is rarely infective and can be treated conservatively by cannula removal.

Central venous catheters (CVCs), which terminate in a central vein such as the superior or inferior vena cava, are widely used in both adult and pediatric patients and are responsible for the majority of catheter-related infections. These catheters are frequently used in critically ill patients, including neonates, who have many other risk factors for nosocomial infection. Patients in an intensive care unit (ICU) with a CVC in place have a 5-fold greater risk for developing a nosocomial bloodstream infection than those without.

The use of peripherally inserted central catheters, which are inserted into a peripheral vein and terminate in a central vein, has increased in pediatric patients. Infection rates seem to be similar to long-term tunneled CVCs (approximately 2 per 1,000 catheter-days), but other complications such as fracture, dislodgment, and occlusion are more common.

When prolonged intravenous (IV) access is required, a cuffed silicone rubber (Silastic) or polyurethane catheter may be inserted into the superior vena cava through the subclavian, cephalic, or jugular vein. The extravascular segment of the catheter passes through a subcutaneous (SC) tunnel before exiting the skin, usually on the superior aspect of the chest (e.g., Broviac or Hickman catheter). A cuff around the catheter near the exit site induces a fibrotic reaction to seal the tunnel. Totally implanted devices comprise a tunneled central catheter attached to an SC reservoir or port with a self-sealing silicone septum immediately under the skin that permits repeated percutaneous needle access.

The incidence of local (exit site, tunnel, and pocket) infection with long-term catheters is 0.2-2.8/1,000 catheter-days. The incidence of Broviac or Hickman CRBSI is 0.5-11.0/1,000 catheter-days. The incidence of CRBSI in implantable devices is much lower at 0.3-1.8/1,000 catheter-days; however, treatment with total parenteral nutrition (TPN) eliminates this risk reduction because of a much greater relative increase in infection rate in ports. The risk for CRBSI is increased among premature infants, young children, and TPN patients.

Catheter-Associated Skin and Soft Tissue Infection
A number of local infections can occur in the presence of a CVC. The clinical manifestations of local infection include erythema, tenderness, and purulent discharge at the exit site or along the SC tunnel tract of

the catheter. **Exit-site infection** denotes infection localized to the exit site, without significant tracking along the tunnel, often with purulent discharge. **Tunnel-tract infection** indicates infection in the SC tissues tracking along a tunneled catheter, which may also include serous or serosanguineous discharge from a draining sinus along the path. **Pocket infection** indicates suppurative infection of an SC pocket containing a totally implanted device. Bloodstream infection may coexist with local infection.

The diagnosis of local infection is established clinically, but a gram-stained smear and culture of any exit-site drainage should be performed to identify the microbiologic cause. The source is usually contamination by skin or gastrointestinal flora, and the most common organisms are *Staphylococcus aureus*, coagulase-negative staphylococci, *Pseudomonas aeruginosa*, *Candida* spp., and mycobacteria. Green discharge is strongly suggestive of mycobacterial infection, and appropriate stains and culture should be performed.

Treatment of local infection related to a short-term CVC should include device removal. Exit-site infection may resolve with device removal alone, but systemic symptoms should be managed with antimicrobial therapy as recommended next for treatment of CRBSI. In the case of long-term CVCs, exit-site infections usually respond to local care with topical or systemic antibiotics alone. However, tunnel or pocket infections require removal of the catheter and systemic antibiotic therapy in almost all cases. When a CVC is removed as a result of tunnel infection, the cuff should also be removed and sent for culture if possible. In cases of mycobacterial infection, wide surgical debridement of the tissues is usually required for cure.

Catheter-Related Bloodstream Infection

CRBSI occurs when microorganisms attached to the CVC are shed into the bloodstream, leading to bacteremia. The term **catheter-related bloodstream infection** is reserved for a bloodstream infection that is demonstrated by CVC tip culture or other techniques to have been caused by colonization of the device. In contrast, the more general term **central line–associated bloodstream infection (CLABSI)** is typically used for surveillance and can refer to any bloodstream infection that occurs in a patient with a CVC, unless there is an identified alternative source. On the device, the organisms are embedded in biofilms as organized communities. Colonization may be present even in the absence of symptoms or positive cultures.

Organisms may contaminate the external surface of the CVC during insertion or the intraluminal surface through handling of the catheter hub or contaminated infusate. Most cases of CRBSI appear to be caused by intraluminal colonization, but external colonization may play a greater role in infections related to recently inserted (<30 days) catheters. Gram-positive cocci predominate, with about half of infections caused by coagulase-negative staphylococci. Gram-negative enteric bacteria are isolated in approximately 20–30% of episodes, and fungi account for 5–10% of episodes.

Fever without an identifiable focus is the most common clinical presentation of CRBSI; local soft tissue symptoms and signs are usually absent. Onset of fever or rigors during or soon after flushing of a catheter is highly suggestive of CRBSI. Symptoms and signs of complicated infection, such as septic thrombophlebitis, endocarditis, or ecthyma gangrenosum, may also be present.

Blood cultures collected before beginning antibiotic therapy are generally positive from both the CVC and the peripheral blood. It is important not to collect cultures unless infection is suspected, as blood culture contamination may occur and can lead to inappropriate therapy. To help interpret positive cultures with common skin contaminants, blood cultures should be collected from at least 2 sites, preferably including all lumens of a CVC *and* the peripheral blood, before initiation of antibiotic therapy.

Tests to differentiate CRBSI from other sources of bacteremia in the presence of a CVC include culture of the catheter tip, quantitative blood cultures, or **differential time to positivity** of blood cultures drawn from different sites. Definitive diagnosis of CRBSI can be important to identify those patients who might benefit from catheter removal or adjunctive therapy. Although CVC tip culture can identify CRBSI, it

precludes salvage of the catheter. The most readily available technique to confirm CRBSI without catheter removal is calculation of differential time to positivity between blood cultures drawn through a catheter and from a peripheral vein or separate lumen. During CRBSI, blood obtained through the responsible lumen will usually indicate growth at least 2-3 hr before peripheral blood or uncolonized lumens because of a higher intraluminal microorganism burden. Identical volumes of blood must be collected simultaneously from each site, and a continuously monitored blood culture system is required. Specificity of this test is good (94–100%), and sensitivity is good when a peripheral blood culture is available (approximately 90%) but poorer when comparing 2 lumens of a CVC (64%). Where available, quantitative blood culture showing at least a 3-fold higher number of organisms from central compared with peripheral blood is similarly diagnostic.

Treatment of CRBSI related to **long-term vascular access devices** (Hickman, Broviac, totally implantable devices) with systemic antibiotics is successful for many bacterial infections without removal of the device. Antibiotic therapy should be directed to the isolated pathogen and given for a total of 10-14 days from the date of blood culture clearance. Until identification and susceptibility testing are available, empirical therapy, based on local antimicrobial susceptibility data and usually including **vancomycin** plus an antipseudomonal aminoglycoside (e.g., gentamicin), penicillin (e.g., piperacillin-tazobactam), or cephalosporin (e.g., ceftazidime or cefepime) is generally indicated. An echinocandin or azole antifungal should be initiated if fungemia is suspected. Patients who have a past history of CRBSI with a resistant organism treated without CVC removal should generally receive initial empirical therapy directed against that organism, since relapse is common.

Antibiotic lock or dwell therapy, with administration of solutions of high concentrations of antibiotics or ethanol that remain in the catheter for up to 24 hr, have been proposed to improve outcomes when used as an adjuvant to systemic therapy. Antibiotic locks are recommended in patients receiving dialysis who may not have antibiotics frequently delivered through the CVC, but evidence does not suggest that routine use of lock therapy is beneficial in other patient populations, and it may cause harm. Ethanol lock therapy increases the risk of CVC occlusion, and both can result in delays to necessary CVC removal.

If blood cultures remain positive after 72 hr of appropriate therapy, or if a patient deteriorates clinically, the device should be removed. Failure of CRBSI salvage therapy is common and can be serious in infections caused by *S. aureus* (approximately 50%), *Candida* spp. (>70%), and *Mycobacterium* spp. (>70%), although some case reports of cure with antimicrobial lock therapy are promising. Other indications for removing a long-term catheter include severe sepsis, suppurative thrombophlebitis, and endocarditis. Prolonged therapy (4-6 wk) is indicated for persistent bacteremia or fungemia despite catheter removal, since this may represent unrecognized infective endocarditis or thrombophlebitis. The decision to attempt catheter salvage should weigh the risk and clinical impact of persistent or relapsed infection against the risk of surgical intervention.

CRBSI may be complicated by other intravascular infections such as septic thrombophlebitis or endocarditis. Presence of these conditions may be suggested by preexisting risk factors (e.g., congenital heart disease), signs and symptoms, or persistent bacteremia or fungemia 72 hr after device removal and appropriate therapy. Screening for these complications in otherwise low-risk children, even those with *S. aureus* infection, is not recommended, because the overall frequency is low and the tests can be difficult to interpret and may lead to inappropriate therapy.

Prevention of Infection

Catheters should routinely be removed as soon as they are no longer needed. Although prevalence of infection increases with prolonged duration of catheter use, routine replacement of a required CVC, either at a new site or over a guidewire, results in significant morbidity and is not recommended. Optimal prevention of infections related to long-term vascular access devices includes "bundles" of interventions, including meticulous aseptic surgical insertion technique in an operating room–like environment, avoidance of bathing or swimming (except with totally implantable devices), and careful catheter care. Use of antibiotic, tau-rolidine, or ethanol lock solutions; heparin with preservatives; and alcohol-impregnated caps, as well as antimicrobial-impregnated/coated catheters, all reduce the risk of CRBSIs and may be appropriate in high-risk populations. There is no evidence that routine replacement of short-term peripheral catheters prevents phlebitis or other complications in children, so they should only be replaced when clinically indicated (e.g., phlebitis, dysfunction, dislodgment).

CEREBROSPINAL FLUID SHUNTS

Cerebrospinal fluid (CSF) shunting is required for the treatment of many children with **hydrocephalus**. The usual procedure uses a silicone rubber device with a proximal portion inserted into the ventricle, a unidirectional valve, and a distal segment that diverts the CSF from the ventricles to either the peritoneal cavity (**ventriculoperitoneal** [VP] shunt) or right atrium (**ventriculoatrial** [VA] shunt). The incidence of shunt infection ranges from 1–20% (average, 10%). The highest rates are reported in young infants, patients with prior shunt infections, and certain etiologies of hydrocephalus. Most infections result from intra-operative contamination of the surgical wound by skin flora. Accordingly, coagulase-negative staphylococci are isolated in more than half the cases. *S. aureus* is isolated in approximately 20% and gram-negative bacilli in 15% of cases.

Four distinct clinical syndromes have been described: colonization of the shunt, infection associated with wound infection, distal infection with peritonitis, and infection associated with meningitis. The most common type of infection is **colonization of the shunt**, with nonspecific symptoms that reflect shunt malfunction as opposed to frank infection. Symptoms associated with colonized VP shunts include lethargy, headache, vomiting, a full fontanel, and abdominal pain. Fever is common but may be <39°C (102.2°F). Symptoms usually occur within months of the surgical procedure. Colonization of a VA shunt results in more severe systemic symptoms, and specific symptoms of shunt malfunction are often absent. Septic pulmonary emboli, pulmonary hypertension, and infective endocarditis are frequently reported complications of VA shunt colonization. Chronic VA shunt colonization may cause hypo-complementemic glomerulonephritis from antigen-antibody complex deposition in the glomeruli, commonly called "shunt nephritis"; clinical findings include hypertension, microscopic hematuria, elevated blood urea nitrogen and serum creatinine levels, and anemia.

Diagnosis is by Gram stain, microscopy, biochemistry, and culture of CSF. CSF should be obtained by direct aspiration of the shunt before administration of antibiotics, because CSF obtained from either lumbar or ventricular puncture is often sterile. It is unusual to observe signs of ventriculitis, and CSF findings can be only minimally abnormal. Blood culture results are usually positive in VA shunt colonization but negative in cases of VP colonization.

Wound infection presents with obvious erythema, swelling, discharge, or dehiscence along the shunt tract and most often occurs within days to weeks of the surgical procedure. *S. aureus* is the most common isolate. In addition to the physical findings, fever is common, and signs of shunt malfunction eventually ensue in most cases.

Distal infection of VP shunts with **peritonitis** presents with abdominal symptoms, usually without evidence of shunt malfunction. The pathogenesis is likely related to perforation of bowel at VP shunt placement or translocation of bacteria across the bowel wall. Thus, gram-negative isolates predominate, and mixed infection is common. The infecting organisms are often isolated from only the distal portion of the shunt.

Common pathogens responsible for community-acquired **meningitis**, including *Streptococcus pneumoniae*, *Neisseria meningitidis*, and *Haemophilus influenzae* type b, can also rarely cause bacterial meningitis in patients with shunts. The clinical presentation is similar to that for acute bacterial meningitis in other children (see Chapter 621.1).

Treatment of shunt colonization includes removal of the shunt and systemic antibiotic therapy directed against the isolated organisms. Treatment without removal of the shunt is rarely successful and should not be routinely attempted. After collection of appropriate samples for culture, empirical therapy is usually with vancomycin plus an

antipseudomonal agent with relatively good CSF penetration, such as ceftazidime or meropenem. Definitive therapy should be directed toward the isolate and should account for poor penetration of most antibiotics into the CSF across noninflamed meninges. Accordingly, intraventricular antibiotics may be indicated but are usually reserved unless there is evidence of treatment failure. If the isolate is susceptible, a parenteral antistaphylococcal penicillin with or without intraventricular vancomycin is the treatment of choice. If the organism is resistant to penicillins, systemic vancomycin and possibly intraventricular vancomycin are recommended. In gram-negative infections, a third-generation cepha-losporin with or without intraventricular aminoglycoside is optimal. When using intraventricular antibiotics, monitoring CSF levels is neces-sary to avoid toxicity.

Removal of the colonized device is required for cure, and final replacement should be delayed until clearance of CSF cultures is documented. Many neurosurgeons immediately remove the shunt and place an external ventricular drain to relieve intracranial pressure (ICP), with a second-stage shunt replacement once CSF sterilization has been confirmed. Others opt initially to exteriorize the distal end of the shunt and replace the shunt in a single-stage procedure once CSF cultures remain sterile for 48-72 hr. Daily CSF cultures should be collected until clearance has been documented on 2-3 consecutive specimens, and antibiotics should be continued for at least 10 days after documented sterilization of the CSF. Gram-negative organisms may require a longer duration of therapy (up to 21 days). The CSF white cell count generally increases for the 1st 3-5 days of appropriate therapy and alone should not prompt concern for treatment failure. Distal shunt infection with peritonitis and wound infection are managed in a similar fashion.

Treatment of **bacterial meningitis** with typical community-acquired pathogens such as meningococcus or pneumococcus usually requires only systemic antibiotic therapy. Shunt replacement is not required in the absence of device malfunction, poor clinical response, persistent CSF culture positivity, or relapse of infection after antibiotic therapy.

Prevention of Infection

Prevention of shunt infection includes meticulous cutaneous prepara-tion and surgical technique. Systemic and intraventricular antibiotics, antibiotic-impregnated shunts, and soaking the shunt tubing in antibiotics are used to reduce the incidence of infection, with varying success. Systemic prophylactic antibiotics given before and during shunt insertion can reduce the risk for infection and should be used routinely but should not be continued for more than 24 hr postoperatively. Antibiotic-impregnated catheters also appear to reduce the risk of infection and may be used in high-risk patients where the devices are available.

URINARY CATHETERS

Urinary catheters are a frequent cause of nosocomial infection, with about 14 infections per 1,000 admissions. As with other devices, microorganisms adhere to the catheter surface and establish a biofilm that allows proliferation. The physical presence of the catheter reduces the normal host defenses by preventing complete emptying of the bladder, thus providing a medium for growth, distending the urethra, and blocking periurethral glands. Almost all patients catheterized >30 days develop bacteriuria. The organism burden in catheter-associated urinary tract infection (UTI) is typically ≥10,000 colony-forming units/mL. Lower thresholds may be used where there is a high index of suspicion, but these episodes may represent colonization rather than infection. Urine culture should only be performed in catheterized patients when infection is suspected, because asymptomatic colonization is ubiquitous and may lead to overtreatment and subsequent development of bacterial resistance. Gram-negative bacilli and *Enterococcus* spp. are the predominant organisms isolated in catheter-related UTI; coagulase-negative staphylococci are implicated in approximately 15% of cases. Symptomatic UTIs should be treated with antibiotics and catheter removal. Catheter colonization with *Candida* spp. is common but rarely leads to invasive infection, and treatment does not have a long-term impact on colonization. Treatment for asymptomatic candiduria or bacteriuria is not recom-mended, except in neonates, immunocompromised patients, and those with urinary tract obstruction.

Prevention of Infection

All urinary catheters introduce a risk for infection, and their casual use should be avoided. When in place, their duration of use should be minimized. Technologic advances have led to development of silver- or antibiotic-impregnated urinary catheters that are associated with lower rates of infection. Prophylactic antibiotics do not significantly reduce the infection rates for long-term catheters but clearly increase the risk for infection with antibiotic-resistant organisms.

PERITONEAL DIALYSIS CATHETERS

During the 1st yr of peritoneal dialysis for end-stage renal disease, 65% of children will have 1 or more episodes of peritonitis. Bacterial entry comes from luminal or periluminal contamination of the catheter or by translocation across the intestinal wall. Hematogenous infection is rare. Infections can be localized at the exit site or associated with peritonitis, or both. Organisms responsible for peritonitis include coagulase-negative staphylococci (30–40%), *Staphylococcus aureus* (10–20%), streptococci (10–15%), *Escherichia coli* (5-10%), *Pseudomonas* spp. (5–10%), other gram-negative bacteria (5–15%), *Enterococcus* spp. (3–6%), and fungi (2–10%). *S. aureus* is more common in localized exit-site or tunnel-tract infections (42%). Most infectious episodes are caused by a patient's own flora, and carriers of *S. aureus* have increased rates of infection compared with noncarriers.

The clinical manifestations of peritonitis may be subtle and include low-grade fever with mild abdominal pain or tenderness. Cloudy peritoneal dialysis fluid may be the first and predominant sign. With peritonitis, the peritoneal fluid cell count is usually >100 white blood cells/μL. When peritonitis is suspected, the effluent dialysate should be submitted for a cell count, Gram stain, and culture. The Gram stain is positive in up to 40% of cases of peritonitis.

Patients with cloudy fluid and clinical symptoms should receive empirical therapy, preferably guided by results of a Gram stain. If no organisms are visualized, vancomycin and either an aminoglycoside or a third- or fourth-generation cephalosporin with antipseudomonal activity should be given by the intraperitoneal route. Blood levels should be measured for glycopeptides and aminoglycosides. Patients without cloudy fluid and with minimal symptoms may have therapy withheld pending culture results. Once the cause is identified by culture, changes in the therapeutic regimen may be needed. Oral **rifampin** may be added as adjunctive therapy for *S. aureus* infections, but drug interactions must be considered. Candidal peritonitis should be treated with catheter removal and intraperitoneal or oral **fluconazole** or an intravenous **echinocandin** such as caspofungin or micafungin, depending on the *Candida* spp. Catheter retention has been associated with almost inevitable relapse and higher risk of mortality in adult studies. The duration of therapy is a minimum of 14 days, with longer treatment of 21-28 days for episodes of *S. aureus*, *Pseudomonas* spp., and resistant gram-negative bacteria and 28-42 days for fungi. Repeat episodes of peritonitis with the same organism within 4 wk of previous therapy should lead to consideration of catheter removal or attempt at salvage with administration of a fibrinolytic agent and a longer course of up to 6 wk of antibiotic therapy.

In all cases, if the infection fails to clear following appropriate therapy, or if a patient's condition is deteriorating, the catheter should be removed. Exit-site and tunnel-tract infections may occur independently of peritonitis or may precede it. Appropriate antibiotics should be administered on the basis of Gram stain and culture findings and are typically given systemically only, unless peritonitis is also present. Some experts recommend that the peritoneal catheter be removed if *Pseudomonas* spp. or fungal organisms are isolated.

Prevention of Infection

In addition to usual hygienic practices, regular application of **mupirocin** or **gentamicin** cream to the catheter exit site reduces exit-site infections and peritonitis. Some practitioners recommend against the use of gentamicin cream because of the risk of infection with gentamicin-resistant bacteria. Systemic antibiotic prophylaxis should be considered at catheter insertion, if there is accidental contamination, and at dental procedures. Antifungal prophylaxis with oral nystatin or fluconazole should be considered during antibiotic therapy to prevent fungal infection.

ORTHOPEDIC PROSTHESES

Orthopedic prostheses are used infrequently in children. Infection most often follows introduction of microorganisms at surgery through airborne contamination or direct inoculation, hematogenous spread, or contiguous spread from an adjacent infection. Early postoperative infection occurs within 2-4 wk of surgery, with manifestations typically including fever, pain, and local symptoms of wound infection. Rapid assessment, including isolation of the infecting organism by joint aspiration or intraoperative culture, operative debridement, and antimicrobial treatment, may allow salvage of the implant if the duration of symptoms is <1 mo, the prosthesis is stable, and the pathogen is susceptible to antibiotics. Chronic infection presents >1 mo after surgery and is often caused by organisms of low virulence that contaminated the implant at surgery or by failure of wound healing. Typical manifestations include pain and deterioration in function. Local symptoms such as erythema, swelling, or drainage may also occur. These infections respond poorly to antibiotic treatment and usually require removal of the implant using a 1- or 2-stage procedure. Surgical irrigation and debridement of the site with retention of the prosthesis and long-term suppressive antibiotic therapy may be considered, but eradication of infection appears uncommon. Acute hematogenous infections are most often observed ≥2 yr after surgery. Retention of the prosthesis is sometimes attempted, but inadequate long-term data exist to determine the success rate. If salvage therapy is attempted, prompt debridement and appropriate antibiotic therapy are recommended. As with other long-term implanted devices, the most common organisms are coagulase-negative staphylococci and *S. aureus*. With prior antibiotic therapy, the prosthesis culture may be negative; in these situations, molecular techniques to identify the organism are available, but sensitivity and specificity are poorly understood.

Systemic antibiotic prophylaxis, antibiotic-containing bone cement, and operating rooms fitted with laminar airflow have been proposed to reduce infection. To date, results from clinical studies are conflicting.

Bibliography is available at Expert Consult.

Section 3
Antibiotic Therapy

第三篇
抗生素治疗

Chapter **207**
Principles of Antibacterial Therapy

Mark R. Schleiss

第二百零七章
抗生素治疗原则

中文导读

本章主要介绍了与年龄相关的儿童应用抗生素的风险和儿科常用抗生素两部分。在关于与年龄相关的儿童应用抗生素的风险中具体描述了新生儿、年长儿、免疫受损与住院患者、与医疗装置相关的感染。在儿科常用抗生素中具体描述了青霉素类、头孢菌素类、碳青霉烯类、糖肽类、氨基糖苷类、四环素类、磺胺类、大环内酯类、林可酰胺类、喹诺酮类、链霉素类、噁唑烷酮类、达托霉素以及其他类常用抗生素。

Antibacterial therapy in infants and children presents many challenges. A daunting problem is the paucity of pediatric data regarding pharmacokinetics and optimal dosages; as a consequence, pediatric recommendations are frequently extrapolated from adult studies. A 2nd challenge is the need for the clinician to consider important differences among pediatric age-groups with respect to the pathogenic species most often responsible for bacterial infections. Age-appropriate antibiotic dosing and toxicities must be considered, taking into account the developmental status and physiology of infants and children. Finally, the style of how a pediatrician uses antibiotics in children, particularly young infants, has some important differences compared with how antibiotics are used adult patients.

Specific antibiotic therapy is optimally driven by a **microbiologic diagnosis**, predicated on isolation of the pathogenic organism from a sterile body site, and supported by antimicrobial susceptibility testing. However, given the inherent difficulties that can arise in collecting specimens from pediatric patients, and given the high risk of mortality and disability associated with serious bacterial infections in very young infants, much of pediatric infectious diseases practice is based on a clinical diagnosis with **empirical** use of antibacterial agents, administered before or even without eventual identification of the specific pathogen. Although there is increasing emphasis on the importance of using

empirical therapy sparingly (so as to not select for resistant organisms), there are some settings in which antimicrobials must be administered before the presence of a specific bacterial pathogen is proven. This is particularly relevant to the care of the febrile or ill-appearing neonate or young infant under 30 days of age.

Several key considerations influence decision-making regarding appropriate empirical use of antibacterial agents in infants and children. It is important to know the age-appropriate differential diagnosis with respect to likely pathogens. This information affects the choice of antimicrobial agent and also the dose, dosing interval, and route of administration (oral vs parenteral). A complete history and physical examination, combined with appropriate laboratory and radiographic studies, are necessary to identify specific diagnoses, information that in turn affects the choice, dosing, and degree of urgency of administration of antimicrobial agents. The vaccination history may confer reduced risk for some invasive infections (i.e., *Haemophilus influenzae* type b, *Streptococcus pneumoniae*, *Neisseria meningitidis*), but not necessarily elimination of risk. The risk of serious bacterial infection in pediatric practice is also affected by the child's immunologic status, which may be compromised by immaturity (neonates), underlying disease, and associated treatments (see Chapter 205). Infections in immunocompromised children may result from bacteria that are not considered pathogenic in immunocompetent children. The presence of foreign bodies (medical devices) also increases the risk of bacterial infections (see Chapter 206). The likelihood of central nervous system (CNS) involvement must be considered in all pediatric patients with serious bacterial infections, because many cases of bacteremia in childhood carry a significant risk for hematogenous spread to the CNS.

The patterns of **antimicrobial resistance** in the community and for the potential causative pathogen being empirically covered must also be considered. Resistance to penicillin and cephalosporins is commonplace among strains of *S. pneumoniae*, often necessitating the use of other classes of antibiotics. Similarly, the striking emergence of community-acquired methicillin-resistant *Staphylococcus aureus* (**MRSA**) infections has complicated antibiotic choices for this pathogen. Extended-spectrum β-lactamase (**ESBL**)–producing gram-negative bacteria (Enterobacteriaceae) have reduced the effectiveness of penicillins and cephalosporins. Furthermore, carbapenem-resistant Enterobacteriaceae are an increasing problem among hospitalized patients, particularly in children with an epidemiologic connection to regions of the world, such as India, where such strains are frequently encountered.

Antimicrobial resistance occurs through many modifications of the bacterial genome (Tables 207.1 and 207.2). Mechanisms include enzyme inactivation of the antibiotic, decreased cell membrane permeability to intracellularly active antibiotics, efflux of antibiotics out of the bacteria, protection or alteration of the antibiotic target site, excessive production of the target site, and bypassing the antimicrobial site of action.

Antimicrobial resistance has reached *crisis proportions*, driven by the emergence of new resistance mechanisms (e.g., carbapenemases, including *Klebsiella pneumoniae*–associated carbapenemases, or **KPCs**) and by overuse of antibiotics, both in healthcare and in other venues, such as agribusiness and animal husbandry. This increase in antibiotic resistance has rendered some bacterial infections encountered in clinical practice virtually untreatable. Accordingly, there is an urgent need to develop new antimicrobials, as well as rediscover some older antibiotics that have been out of use in recent decades but still retain activity against resistant organisms. It is vital that practitioners use antibiotics only as

necessary, with the narrowest feasible antimicrobial spectrum, to help thwart emergence of resistance. In addition, advocacy for **vaccines**, particularly conjugate pneumococcal vaccine, can also decrease the selective pressure that excessive antimicrobial use exerts on resistance.

Effective antibiotic action requires achieving therapeutic levels of the drug at the site of infection. Although measuring the level of antibiotic at the site of infection is not always possible, one may measure the serum level and use this level as a surrogate marker for achievement of the desired effect at the tissue level. Various target serum levels are appropriate for different antibiotic agents and are assessed by the peak and trough serum levels and the area under the therapeutic drug level curve (Fig. 207.1). These levels in turn are a reflection of the route of administration, drug absorption (IM, PO), volume of distribution, and drug elimination half-life, as well as of drug-drug interactions that might enhance or impede enzymatic inactivation of an antibiotic or result in antimicrobial synergism or antagonism (Fig. 207.2).

AGE- AND RISK-SPECIFIC USE OF ANTIBIOTICS IN CHILDREN
Neonates
The causative pathogens associated with neonatal infections are typically acquired around the time of delivery. Thus, empirical antibiotic selection must take into account the importance of these organisms (see Chapter 129). Among the causes of neonatal sepsis in infants, **group B streptococcus** (GBS) is the most common. Although intrapartum antibiotic prophylaxis administered to women at increased risk for transmission of GBS to the infant has greatly decreased the incidence of this infection in neonates, particularly with respect to early-onset disease, GBS infections are still frequently encountered in clinical practice (see Chapter 211). Gram-negative enteric organisms acquired from the maternal birth canal, in particular *Escherichia coli*, are also common causes of neonatal sepsis. Although less common, *Listeria monocytogenes* is an important pathogen to consider, insofar as the organism is intrinsically resistant to cephalosporin antibiotics, which are often used as empirical therapy for serious bacterial infections in young children. *Salmonella*

Table 207.1	Mechanisms of Resistance to β-Lactam Antibiotics

I. Alter target site (PBP)
  A. Decrease affinity of PBP for β-lactam antibiotic
    1. Modify existing PBP
      a. Create mosaic PBP
        (1) Insert nucleotides obtained from neighboring bacteria (e.g., penicillin-resistant *Streptococcus pneumoniae*)
        (2) Mutate structural gene of PBP(s) (e.g., ampicillin-resistant β-lactamase–negative *Haemophilus influenzae*)
    2. Import new PBP (e.g., mecA in methicillin-resistant *Staphylococcus aureus*)
II. Destroy β-lactam antibiotic
  A. Increase production of β-lactamases, carbapenemases
    1. Acquire more efficient promoter
      a. Mutate existing promoter
      b. Import new promoter
    2. Deregulate control of β-lactamase production
      a. Mutate regulator genes (e.g., ampD in "stably derepressed" *Enterobacter cloacae*)
  B. Modify structure of resident β-lactamase
    1. Mutate structural gene (e.g., ESBLs in *Klebsiella pneumoniae*)
  C. Import new β-lactamase(s) with different spectrum of activity
III. Decrease concentration of β-lactam antibiotic inside cell
  A. Restrict its entry (loss of porins)
  B. Pump it out (efflux mechanisms)

ESBLs, Extended-spectrum β-lactamases; PBP, Penicillin-binding protein.
Adapted from Opal SM, Pop-Vicas A: Molecular mechanisms of antibiotic resistance in bacteria. In Bennett JF, Dolin R, Blaser MJ, editors: *Mandell, Douglas, and Bennett's principles and practice of infectious diseases*, ed 8, Philadelphia, 2015, Elsevier (Table 18-4).

Table 207.2	Aminoglycoside-Modifying Enzymes*	
ENZYMES	**USUAL ANTIBIOTICS MODIFIED**	**COMMON GENERA**
PHOSPHORYLATION		
APH(2″)	K, T, G	SA, SR
APH(3′)-I	K	E, PS, SA, SR
APH(3′)-III	K ± A	E, PS, SA, SR
ACETYLATION		
AAC(2′)	G	PR
AAC(3)-I	±T, G	E, PS
AAC(3)-III, -IV, or -V	K, T, G	E, PS
AAC(6′)	K, T, A	E, PS, SA
ADENYLATION		
ANT(2″)	K, T, G	E, PS
ANT(4′)	K, T, A	SA
BIFUNCTIONAL ENZYMES		
AAC(6′)-APH(2″)	G, Ar	SA, Ent
AAC(6′)-Ibcr	G, K, T, FQ*	E

*Aminoglycoside-modifying enzymes confer antibiotic resistance through 3 general reactions: N-acetylation, O-nucleotidylation, and O-phosphorylation. For each of these general reactions, there are several different enzymes that attack a specific amino or hydroxyl group.

A, Amikacin; AAC, aminoglycoside acetyltransferase; ANT, aminoglycoside nucleotidyltransferase; APH, aminoglycoside phosphotransferase; cr, ciprofloxacin resistance; Ar, arbekacin, E, Enterobacteriaceae; Ent, enterococci, FQ, fluoroquinolone (acetylates the piperazine ring in some fluoroquinolones), G, gentamicin; K, kanamycin; PR, *Providencia-Proteus*; PS, pseudomonads; SA, staphylococci; SR, streptococci; T, tobramycin.
Adapted from Opal SM, Pop-Vicas A: Molecular mechanisms of antibiotic resistance in bacteria. In Bennett JF, Dolin R, Blaser MJ, editors: *Mandell, Douglas, and Bennett's principles and practice of infectious diseases*, ed 8, Philadelphia, 2015, Elsevier (Table 18-5).

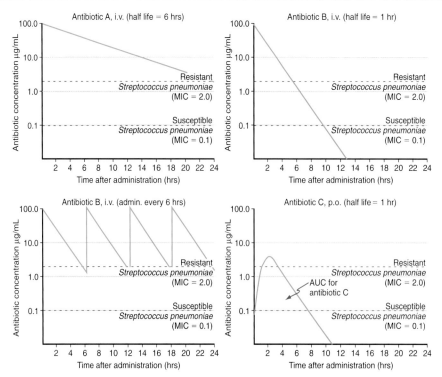

Fig. 207.1 Area under the curve (AUC; *shaded area*) for different antibiotics. The AUC provides a measure of antibiotic exposure to bacterial pathogens. The greatest exposure comes with antibiotics that have a long serum half-life and are administered parenterally (*upper left panel*, antibiotic A). The lowest exposure occurs with oral administration (*lower right panel*, antibiotic C). Dosing of antibiotic B once a day (*upper right panel*) provides far less exposure than dosing the same antibiotic every 6 hr (*lower left panel*). MIC, Minimal inhibitory concentration. (*From Pong AL, Bradley JS: Guidelines for the selection of antibacterial therapy in children, Pediatr Clin North Am 52:869–894, 2005.*)

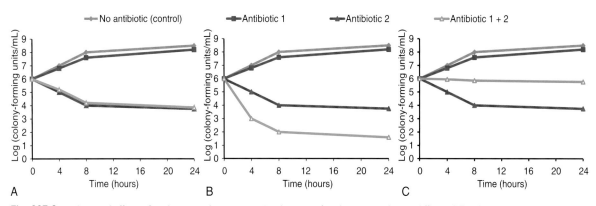

Fig. 207.2 Antibacterial effects of antibiotic combinations. **A,** Combination of antibiotics 1 and 2 is *indifferent*; killing by antibiotic 2 is unchanged when antibiotic 1 is added. **B,** Combination of antibiotics 1 and 2 results in *synergy*; killing by antibiotic 2 is significantly enhanced when antibiotic 1 is added at a subinhibitory concentration. **C,** Combination of antibiotics 1 and 2 is *antagonistic*; killing by antibiotic 2 is diminished in the presence of antibiotic 1. (*From Eliopoulos GM, Moellering RC Jr: Principles of anti-infective therapy. In Bennett JF, Dolin R, Blaser MJ, editors: Mandell, Douglas, and Bennett's principles and practice of infectious diseases, ed 8, Philadelphia, 2015, Elsevier, Fig 17-1.*)

bacteremia and **meningitis** on a global basis is a well-recognized infection in infants. All these organisms can be associated with meningitis in the neonate; therefore lumbar puncture should always be considered with bacteremic infections in this age-group, and if meningitis cannot be excluded, antibiotic management should include agents capable of crossing the blood-brain barrier.

Older Children

Antibiotic choices in toddlers and young children were once driven by the high risk of this age-group to invasive disease caused by *H. influenzae*

type b (**Hib**; see Chapter 221). With the advent of conjugate vaccines against Hib, invasive disease has declined dramatically. However, outbreaks still occur, and have been observed in the context of parental refusal of vaccines. Therefore, it is still important to use antimicrobials that are active against Hib in many clinical settings, particularly if meningitis is a consideration. Other important pathogens to consider in this age-group include *E. coli, S. pneumoniae, N. meningitidis,* and *S. aureus.* Strains of *S. pneumoniae* that are resistant to penicillin and cephalosporin antibiotics are frequently encountered in clinical practice. Similarly, MRSA is highly prevalent in children in the outpatient setting.

Resistance of *S. pneumoniae* as well as MRSA is a result of mutations that confer alterations in penicillin-binding proteins, the molecular targets of penicillin and cephalosporin activity (see Table 207.1).

Depending on the specific clinical diagnosis, other pathogens encountered among older children include *Moraxella catarrhalis*, nontypeable (nonencapsulated) strains of *H. influenzae*, and *Mycoplasma pneumoniae*, which cause upper respiratory tract infections and pneumonia; group A streptococcus, which causes pharyngitis, skin and soft tissue infections, osteomyelitis, septic arthritis, and rarely, bacteremia with toxic shock syndrome; *Kingella kingae*, which causes bone and joint infections; viridians group streptococci and *Enterococcus*, which cause endocarditis; and *Salmonella* spp., which cause enteritis, bacteremia, osteomyelitis, and septic arthritis. Vector-borne bacterial infections, including *Borrelia burgdorferi*, *Rickettsia rickettsii*, and *Anaplasma phagocytophilum*, are increasingly recognized in certain regions, with an evolving epidemiology triggered by climate change. These complexities underscore the importance of formulation of a complete differential diagnosis in children with suspected severe bacterial infections, including an assessment of the severity of the infection undertaken in parallel with consideration of local epidemiological disease trends, including knowledge of the antimicrobial susceptibility patterns in the community.

Immunocompromised and Hospitalized Patients

It is important to consider the risks associated with immunocompromising conditions (malignancy, solid-organ or hematopoietic stem cell transplantation) and the risks conferred by conditions leading to prolonged hospitalization (intensive care, trauma, burns). Serious viral infections, particularly influenza, can also predispose to invasive bacterial infections, especially those caused by *S. aureus*. Immunocompromised children are predisposed to develop a wide range of bacterial, viral, fungal, or parasitic infections. Prolonged hospitalization can lead to nosocomial infections, often associated with indwelling lines and catheters and caused by highly antibiotic-resistant gram-negative enteric organisms. In addition to bacterial pathogens already discussed, *Pseudomonas aeruginosa* and enteric organisms, including *E. coli*, *K. pneumoniae*, *Enterobacter*, and *Serratia*, are important opportunistic pathogens in these settings. Selection of appropriate antimicrobials is challenging because of the diverse causes and scope of antimicrobial resistance exhibited by these organisms. Many strains of enteric organisms have resistance because of ESBLs (see Table 207.1). Class B metallo-β-lactamases (also known as New Delhi metallo-β-lactamases) that hydrolyze all β-lactam antibiotics except aztreonam are increasingly being described, as well as KPCs that confer resistance to carbapenems. Reports of **carbapenemases** are increasingly being described for Enterobacteriaceae. Carbapenemase-producing Enterobacteriaceae are different from other multidrug-resistant microorganisms in that they are susceptible to few (if any) antibacterial agents.

Other modes of antimicrobial resistance are being increasingly recognized. *P. aeruginosa* encodes proteins that function as efflux pumps to eliminate multiple classes of antimicrobials from the cytoplasm or periplasmic space. In addition to these gram-negative pathogens, infections caused by *Enterococcus faecalis* and *E. faecium* are inherently difficult to treat. These organisms may cause urinary tract infection (UTI) or infective endocarditis in immunocompetent children and may be responsible for a variety of syndromes in immunocompromised patients, especially in the setting of prolonged intensive care. The emergence of infections caused by **vancomycin-resistant enterococcus (VRE)** has further complicated antimicrobial selection in high-risk patients and has necessitated the development of newer antimicrobials that target these highly resistant gram-positive bacteria.

Infections Associated With Medical Devices

A special situation affecting antibiotic use is the presence of an indwelling medical device, such as venous catheter, ventriculoperitoneal shunts, stents, or other catheters (see Chapter 206). In addition to *S. aureus*, coagulase-negative staphylococci are also a major consideration. Coagulase-negative staphylococci seldom cause serious disease in the absence of risk factors such as indwelling catheters. Empirical antibiotic regimens must take this risk into consideration. In addition to appropriate

antibiotic therapy, removal or replacement of the colonized prosthetic material is usually required for cure.

ANTIBIOTICS COMMONLY USED IN PEDIATRIC PRACTICE

Table 207.3 lists antibiotic medications and pediatric indications.

Penicillins

Although there has been ever-increasing emergence of resistance to penicillins, these agents remain valuable and are commonly used for management of many pediatric infectious diseases.

Penicillins remain the drugs of choice for pediatric infections caused by group A and group B streptococcus, *Treponema pallidum* (syphilis), *L. monocytogenes*, and *N. meningitidis*. The **semisynthetic penicillins** (nafcillin, cloxacillin, dicloxacillin) are useful for management of susceptible (non-MRSA) staphylococcal infections. The **aminopenicillins** (ampicillin, amoxicillin) were developed to provide broad-spectrum activity against gram-negative organisms, including *E. coli* and *H. influenzae*, but the emergence of resistance (typically mediated by a β-lactamase) has limited their utility in many clinical settings. The **carboxypenicillins** (ticarcillin) and **ureidopenicillins** (piperacillin, mezlocillin, azlocillin) also have bactericidal activity against most strains of *P. aeruginosa*.

Resistance to penicillin is mediated by a variety of mechanisms (see Table 207.1). The production of β-lactamase is a common mechanism exhibited by many organisms that may be overcome, with variable success, by including a β-lactamase inhibitor in the therapeutic formulation with the penicillin. Such combination products (ampicillin-sulbactam, amoxicillin-clavulanate, ticarcillin–clavulanic acid [no longer available in the U.S.], piperacillin-tazobactam) are potentially very useful for management of resistant isolates, but only if the resistance is β-lactamase mediated. Notably, MRSA and *S. pneumoniae* mediate resistance to penicillins through mechanisms other than β-lactamase production, rendering these combination agents of little value for the management of these infections.

Table 207.4 lists adverse reactions to penicillins.

Cephalosporins

Cephalosporins differ structurally from penicillins insofar as the β-lactam ring exists as a 6-member ring, compared to the 5-member ring structure of the penicillins. These agents are widely used in pediatric practice, both in oral and parenteral formulations (Table 207.5). The **first-generation cephalosporins** (e.g., cefazolin, a parenteral formulation, and cephalexin, an oral equivalent) are commonly used for management of skin and soft tissue infections caused by susceptible strains of *S. aureus* and group A streptococcus. The **second-generation cephalosporins** (e.g., cefuroxime, cefoxitin) have better activity against gram-negative bacterial infections than first-generation cephalosporins and are used to treat respiratory tract infections, UTIs, and skin and soft tissue infections. A variety of orally administered second-generation agents (cefaclor, cefprozil, loracarbef, cefpodoxime) are commonly used in the outpatient management of sinopulmonary infections and otitis media. The **third-generation cephalosporins** (cefotaxime [no longer available], ceftriaxone, and ceftazidime) are typically used for serious pediatric infections, including meningitis and sepsis. Ceftazidime is highly active against most strains of *P. aeruginosa*, making this a useful agent for febrile, neutropenic oncology patients. The U.S. Food and Drug Administration (FDA) approved the combination of ceftazidime and the novel β-lactamase inhibitor *avibactam* in 2015. Current indications include complicated intraabdominal infections and UTIs. The combination may also be useful for the treatment of infection caused by KPCs. Pediatric experience is limited. Ceftriaxone should not be mixed or reconstituted with a calcium-containing product, such as Ringer or Hartmann solution or parenteral nutrition containing calcium, because particulate formation can result. Cases of fatal reactions with ceftriaxone–calcium precipitates in lungs and kidneys in neonates have been reported. A **fourth-generation cephalosporin** called *cefepime* has activity against *P. aeruginosa* and retains good activity against methicillin-susceptible staphylococcal infections. A **fifth-generation cephalosporin**

Text continued on p. 1546

Table 207.3	Selected Antibacterial Medications (Antibiotics)*

DRUG (TRADE NAMES, FORMULATIONS)	INDICATIONS (MECHANISM OF ACTION) AND DOSING	COMMENTS
Amikacin sulfate Amikin Injection: 50 mg/mL, 250 mg/mL	Aminoglycoside antibiotic active against gram-negative bacilli, especially *Escherichia coli*, *Klebsiella*, *Proteus*, *Enterobacter*, *Serratia*, and *Pseudomonas* Neonates: Postnatal age ≤7 days, weight 1,200-2,000 g: 7.5 mg/kg q12-18h IV or IM; weight >2,000 g: 10 mg/kg q12h IV or IM; postnatal age >7 days, weight 1,200-2,000 g: 7.5 mg/kg q8-12h IV or IM; weight >2,000 g: 10 mg/kg q8h IV or IM Children: 15-25 mg/kg/24 hr divided q8-12h IV or IM Adults: 15 mg/kg/24 hr divided q8-12h IV or IM	*Cautions:* Anaerobes, *Streptococcus* (including *S. pneumoniae*) are resistant. May cause ototoxicity and nephrotoxicity. Monitor renal function. Drug eliminated renally. Administered IV over 30-60 min *Drug interactions:* May potentiate other ototoxic and nephrotoxic drugs *Target serum concentrations:* Peak 25-40 mg/L; trough <10 mg/L
Amoxicillin Amoxil, Polymox Capsule: 250, 500 mg Tablet: chewable: 125, 250 mg Suspension: 125 mg/5 mL, 250 mg/5 mL Drops: 50 mg/mL	Penicillinase-susceptible β-lactam: gram-positive pathogens except *Staphylococcus*; *Salmonella*, *Shigella*, *Neisseria*, *E. coli*, and *Proteus mirabilis* Children: 20-50 mg/kg/24 hr divided q8-12h PO. Higher dose of 80-90 mg/kg 24 hr PO for otitis media Adults: 250-500 mg q8-12h PO Uncomplicated gonorrhea: 3 g with 1 g probenecid PO	*Cautions:* Rash, diarrhea, abdominal cramping. Drug eliminated renally *Drug interaction:* Probenecid
Amoxicillin-clavulanate Augmentin Tablet: 250, 500, 875 mg Tablet, chewable: 125, 200, 250, 400 mg Suspension: 125 mg/5 mL, 200 mg/5 mL, 250 mg/5 mL, 400 mg/5 mL	β-Lactam (amoxicillin) combined with β-lactamase inhibitor (clavulanate) enhances amoxicillin activity against penicillinase-producing bacteria. *S. aureus* (not methicillin-resistant organism), *Streptococcus*, *Haemophilus influenzae*, *Moraxella catarrhalis*, *E. coli*, *Klebsiella*, *Bacteroides fragilis* Neonates: 30 mg/kg/24 hr divided q12h PO Children: 20-45 mg/kg 24 hr divided q8-12h PO. Higher dose 80-90 mg/kg/24 hr PO for otitis media	*Cautions:* Drug dosed on amoxicillin component. May cause diarrhea, rash. Drug eliminated renally *Drug interaction:* Probenecid *Comment:* Higher dose may be active against penicillin-tolerant/resistant *S. pneumoniae*
Ampicillin Polycillin, Omnipen Capsule: 250, 500 mg Suspension: 125 mg/5 mL, 250 mg/5 mL, 500 mg/5 mL Injection	β-Lactam with same spectrum of antibacterial activity as amoxicillin Neonates: Postnatal age ≤7 days weight ≤2,000 g: 50 mg/kg/24 hr IV or IM q12h (meningitis: 100 mg/kg/24 hr divided q12h IV or IM); weight >2,000 g: 75 mg/kg/24 hr divided q8h IV or IM (meningitis: 150 mg/kg/24 hr divided q8h IV or IM). Postnatal age >7 days weight <1,200 g: 50 mg/kg/24 hr IV or IM q12h (meningitis: 100 mg/kg/24 hr divided q12h IV or IM); weight 1,200-2,000 g: 75 mg/kg/24 hr divided q8h IV or IM (meningitis: 150 mg/kg/24 hr divided q8hr IV or IM); weight >2,000 g: 100 mg/kg/24 hr divided q6h IV or IM (meningitis: 200 mg/kg/24 hr divided q6h IV or IM) Children: 100-200 mg/kg/24 hr divided q6h IV or IM (meningitis: 200-400 mg/kg/24 hr divided q4-6h IV or IM) Adults: 250-500 mg q4-8h IV or IM	*Cautions:* Less bioavailable than amoxicillin, causing greater diarrhea *Drug interaction:* Probenecid
Ampicillin-sulbactam Unasyn Injection	β-Lactam (ampicillin) and β-lactamase inhibitor (sulbactam) enhances ampicillin activity against penicillinase-producing bacteria: *S. aureus*, *H. influenzae*, *M. catarrhalis*, *E. coli*, *Klebsiella*, *B. fragilis* Children: 100-200 mg/kg/24 hr divided q4-8h IV or IM Adults: 1-2 g q6-8h IV or IM (max daily dose: 8 g)	*Cautions:* Drug dosed on ampicillin component. May cause diarrhea, rash. Drug eliminated renally *Note:* Higher dose may be active against penicillin-tolerant/resistant *S. pneumoniae* *Drug interaction:* Probenecid
Azithromycin Zithromax Tablet: 250 mg Suspension: 100 mg/5 mL, 200 mg/5 mL	Azalide antibiotic with activity against *S. aureus*, *Streptococcus*, *H. influenzae*, *Mycoplasma*, *Legionella*, *Chlamydia trachomatis*, *Babesia microti* Children: 10 mg/kg PO on day 1 (max dose: 500 mg) followed by 5 mg/kg PO q24h for 4 days Group A streptococcus pharyngitis: 12 mg/kg/24 hr PO (max dose: 500 mg) for 5 days Adults: 500 mg PO day 1 followed by 250 mg for 4 days Uncomplicated *C. trachomatis* infection: single 1 g dose PO	*Note:* Very long half-life permitting once-daily dosing. No metabolic-based drug interactions (unlike erythromycin and clarithromycin), limited GI distress. Shorter-course regimens (e.g., 1-3 days) under investigation. 3 day, therapy (10 mg/kg/24 hr × 3 days) and single-dose therapy (30 mg/kg): use with increasing frequency (not for streptococcus pharyngitis)
Aztreonam Azactam Injection	β-Lactam (monobactam) antibiotic with activity against gram-negative aerobic bacteria, Enterobacteriaceae, and *Pseudomonas aeruginosa* Neonates: Postnatal age ≤7 days weight ≤2,000 g: 60 mg/kg/24 hr divided q12h IV or IM; weight >2,000 g: 90 mg/kg/24 hr divided q8h IV or IM; postnatal age >7 days weight <1,200 g: 60 mg/kg/24 hr divided q12h IV or IM; weight 1,200-2,000 g: 90 mg/kg/24 hr divided q8h IV or IM; weight >2,000 g: 120 mg/kg/24 hr divided q6-8h IV or IM Children: 90-120 mg/kg/24 hr divided q6-8h IV or IM. For cystic fibrosis, up to 200 mg/kg/24 hr IV Adults: 1-2 g IV or IM q8-12h (max dose: 8 g/24 hr)	*Cautions:* Rash, thrombophlebitis, eosinophilia. Renally eliminated *Drug interaction:* Probenecid

Continued

Table 207.3	Selected Antibacterial Medications (Antibiotics)—cont'd

DRUG (TRADE NAMES, FORMULATIONS)	INDICATIONS (MECHANISM OF ACTION) AND DOSING	COMMENTS
Cefadroxil Generic Capsule: 500 mg Tablet: 1,000 mg Suspension: 125 mg/5 mL, 250 mg/5 mL, 500 mg/5 mL	First-generation cephalosporin active against *S. aureus, Streptococcus, E. coli, Klebsiella,* and *Proteus* Children: 30 mg/kg/24 hr divided q12h PO (max dose: 2 g) Adults: 250-500 mg q8-12h PO	*Cautions:* β-Lactam safety profile (rash, eosinophilia). Renally eliminated. Long half-life permits q12-24h dosing *Drug interaction:* Probenecid
Cefazolin Ancef, Kefzol Injection	First-generation cephalosporin active against *S. aureus, Streptococcus, E. coli, Klebsiella,* and *Proteus* Neonates: Postnatal age ≤7 days 40 mg/kg/24 hr divided q12h IV or IM; >7 days 40-60 mg/kg/24 hr divided q8h IV or IM Children: 50-100 mg/kg/24 hr divided q8h IV or IM Adults: 0.5-2g q8h IV or IM (max dose: 12 g/24 hr)	*Caution:* β-Lactam safety profile (rash, eosinophilia). Renally eliminated. Does not adequately penetrate CNS *Drug interaction:* Probenecid
Cefdinir Omnicef Capsule: 300 mg Oral suspension: 125 mg/5 mL	Extended-spectrum, semisynthetic cephalosporin Children 6 mo-12 yr: 14 mg/kg/24 hr in 1 or 2 doses PO (max dose: 600 mg/24 hr) Adults: 600 mg q24h PO	*Cautions:* Reduce dosage in renal insufficiency (creatinine clearance <60 mL/min). Avoid taking concurrently with iron-containing products and antacids because absorption is markedly decreased; take at least 2 hr apart *Drug interaction:* Probenecid
Cefepime Maxipime Injection	Expanded-spectrum, fourth-generation cephalosporin active against many gram-positive and gram-negative pathogens, including *P. aeruginosa* and many multidrug-resistant pathogens Children: 100-150 mg/kg/24 hr q8-12h IV or IM Adults: 2-4 g/24 hr q12h IV or IM	*Adverse events:* Diarrhea, nausea, vaginal candidiasis *Cautions:* β-lactam safety profile (rash, eosinophilia). Renally eliminated *Drug interaction:* Probenecid
Cefixime Suprax Tablet: 200, 400 mg Suspension: 100 mg/5 mL	Third-generation cephalosporin active against streptococci, *H. influenzae, M. catarrhalis, Neisseria gonorrhoeae, Serratia marcescens,* and *Proteus vulgaris*. No antistaphylococcal or antipseudomonal activity Children: 8 mg/kg/24 hr divided q12-24h PO Adults: 400 mg/24 hr divided q12-24h PO	*Cautions:* β-Lactam safety profile (rash, eosinophilia). Renally eliminated. Does not adequately penetrate CNS *Drug interaction:* Probenecid
Cefoperazone sodium Cefobid Injection	Third-generation cephalosporin active against many gram-positive and gram-negative pathogens Neonates: 100 mg/kg/24 hr divided q12h IV or IM Children: 100-150 mg/kg/24 hr divided q8-12h IV or IM Adults: 2-4 g/24 hr divided q8-12h IV or IM (max dose: 12 g/24 hr)	*Cautions:* Highly protein-bound cephalosporin with limited potency reflected by weak antipseudomonal activity. Variable Gram-positive activity. Primarily hepatically eliminated in bile *Drug interaction:* Disulfiram-like reaction with alcohol
Cefotaxime sodium Claforan Injection	Third-generation cephalosporin active against Gram-positive and Gram-negative pathogens. No antipseudomonal activity Neonates: ≤7 days: 100 mg/kg/24 hr divided q12h IV or IM; >7 days: weight <1,200 g 100 mg/kg/24 hr divided q12h IV or IM; weight >1,200 g: 150 mg/kg/24 hr divided q8h IV or IM Children: 150 mg/kg/24 hr divided q6-8h IV or IM (meningitis: 200 mg/kg/24 hr divided q6-8h IV) Adults: 1-2 g q8-12h IV or IM (max dose: 12 g/24 hr)	*Cautions:* β-Lactam safety profile (rash, eosinophilia). Renally eliminated. Each gram of drug contains 2.2 mEq sodium. Active metabolite *Drug interaction:* Probenecid
Cefotetan disodium Cefotan Injection	Second-generation cephalosporin active against *S. aureus, Streptococcus, H. influenzae, E. coli, Klebsiella, Proteus,* and *Bacteroides*. Inactive against *Enterobacter* Children: 40-80 mg/kg/24 hr divided q12h IV or IM Adults: 2-4 g/24 hr divided q12h IV or IM (max dose: 6 g/24 hr)	*Cautions:* Highly protein-bound cephalosporin, poor CNS penetration; β-lactam safety profile (rash, eosinophilia), disulfiram-like reaction with alcohol. Renally eliminated (~20% in bile)
Cefoxitin sodium Mefoxin Injection	Second-generation cephalosporin active against *S. aureus, Streptococcus, H. influenzae, E. coli, Klebsiella, Proteus,* and *Bacteroides*. Inactive against *Enterobacter* Neonates: 70-100 mg/kg/24 hr divided q8-12h IV or IM Children: 80-160 mg/kg/24 hr divided q6-8h IV or IM Adults: 1-2 g q6-8h IV or IM (max dose: 12 g/24 hr)	*Cautions:* Poor CNS penetration; β-lactam safety profile (rash, eosinophilia). Renally eliminated. Painful given intramuscularly *Drug interaction:* Probenecid

Continued

Table 207.3	Selected Antibacterial Medications (Antibiotics)—cont'd

DRUG (TRADE NAMES, FORMULATIONS)	INDICATIONS (MECHANISM OF ACTION) AND DOSING	COMMENTS

Cefpodoxime proxetil
Vantin
Tablet: 100 mg, 200 mg
Suspension: 50 mg/5 mL,
  100 mg/5 mL
	Third-generation cephalosporin active against *S. aureus,*
	  Streptococcus, H. influenzae, M. catarrhalis,
	  N. gonorrhoeae, E. coli, Klebsiella, and *Proteus.*
	  No antipseudomonal activity
	Children: 10 mg/kg/24 hr divided q12h PO
	Adults: 200-800 mg/24 hr divided q12h PO (max dose:
	  800 mg/24 hr)
	Uncomplicated gonorrhea: 200 mg PO as single-dose therapy
		Cautions: β-Lactam safety profile (rash,
		  eosinophilia). Renally eliminated. Does not
		  adequately penetrate CNS. Increased
		  bioavailability when taken with food
		Drug interaction: Probenecid; antacids and H$_2$
		  receptor antagonists may decrease
		  absorption

Ceftaroline fosamil
Teflaro
Injection
	Fifth-generation cephalosporin active against *S. aureus*
	  (including MRSA when used for skin and soft tissue
	  infection), *Streptococcus pyogenes, Streptococcus
	  agalactiae, Escherichia coli, Klebsiella pneumoniae,
	  H. influenzae,* and *Klebsiella oxytoca*
	Children: skin/skin structure infections *or* community-acquired
	  pneumonia, 24 mg/kg/24 hr divided q8h IV (2-23 mo old)
	  ×5-14 days; 36 mg/kg/24 hr divided q8h IV (weight ≤33 kg)
	  ×5-14 days; 400 mg q8h IV (weight >33 kg)
	Adults: 600 mg q12h IV
		Caution: β-Lactam safety profile (rash,
		  eosinophilia)
		Drug interaction: Probenecid

Cefprozil
Cefzil
Tablet: 250, 500 mg
Suspension: 125 mg/5 mL,
  250 mg/5 mL
	Second-generation cephalosporin active against *S. aureus,*
	  Streptococcus, H. influenzae, E. coli, M. catarrhalis,
	  Klebsiella, and *Proteus* spp.
	Children: 30 mg/kg/24 hr divided q8-12h PO
	Adults: 500-1,000 mg/24 hr divided q12h PO (max dose:
	  1.5 g/24 hr)
		Cautions: β-Lactam safety profile (rash,
		  eosinophilia). Renally eliminated. Good
		  bioavailability; food does not affect
		  bioavailability
		Drug interaction: Probenecid

Ceftazidime
Fortaz, Ceptaz, Tazicef,
  Tazidime
Injection
	Third-generation cephalosporin active against gram-positive
	  and gram-negative pathogens, including *P. aeruginosa*
	Neonates: Postnatal age ≤7 days: 100 mg/kg/24 hr divided
	  q12h IV or IM; >7 days weight ≤1,200 g: 100 mg/kg/24 hr
	  divided q12h IV or IM; weight >1,200 g: 150 mg/kg/24 hr
	  divided q8h IV or IM
	Children: 150 mg/kg/24 hr divided q8h IV or IM (meningitis:
	  150 mg/kg/24 hr IV divided q8h)
	Adults: 1-2 g q8-12h IV or IM (max dose: 8-12 g/24 hr)
		Cautions: β-Lactam safety profile (rash,
		  eosinophilia). Renally eliminated. Increasing
		  pathogen resistance developing with
		  long-term, widespread use
		Drug interaction: Probenecid

Ceftizoxime
Cefizox
Injection
	Third-generation cephalosporin active against gram-positive
	  and gram-negative pathogens. No antipseudomonal
	  activity
	Children: 150 mg/kg/24 hr divided q6-8h IV or IM
	Adults: 1-2 g q6-8h IV or IM (max dose: 12 g/24 hr)
		Cautions: β-Lactam safety profile (rash,
		  eosinophilia). Renally eliminated
		Drug interaction: Probenecid

Ceftriaxone sodium
Rocephin
Injection
	Third-generation cephalosporin widely active against
	  gram-positive and gram-negative pathogens. No
	  antipseudomonal activity
	Neonates: 50-75 mg/kg q24h IV or IM
	Children: 50-75 mg/kg q24h IV or IM (meningitis: 75 mg/kg
	  dose once then 80-100 mg/kg/24 hr divided q12-24h
	  IV or IM)
	Adults: 1-2 g q24h IV or IM (max dose: 4 g/24 hr)
		Cautions: β-Lactam safety profile (rash,
		  eosinophilia). Eliminated via kidney (33–65%)
		  and bile; can cause sludging. Long half-life
		  and dose-dependent protein binding favors
		  q24h rather than q12h dosing. Can add 1%
		  lidocaine for IM injection
		Drug interaction: Probenecid. In neonates,
		  co-administration with calcium-containing
		  products can result in severe precipitation
		  and attendant embolic complications

**Cefuroxime (cefuroxime axetil
  for oral administration)**
Ceftin, Kefurox, Zinacef
Injection
Suspension: 125 mg/5 mL
Tablet: 125, 250, 500 mg
	Second-generation cephalosporin active against *S. aureus,*
	  Streptococcus, H. influenzae, E. coli, M. catarrhalis,
	  Klebsiella, and *Proteus*
	Neonates: 40-100 mg/kg/24 hr divided q12h IV or IM
	Children: 200-240 mg/kg/24 hr divided q8h IV or IM; PO
	  administration: 20-30 mg/kg/24 hr divided q8-12h PO
	Adults: 750-1,500 mg q8h IV or IM (max dose: 6 g/24 hr)
		Cautions: β-Lactam safety profile (rash,
		  eosinophilia). Renally eliminated. Food
		  increases PO bioavailability
		Drug interaction: Probenecid

Cephalexin
Keflex, Keftab
Capsule: 250, 500 mg
Tablet: 500 mg, 1 g
Suspension: 125 mg/5 mL,
  250 mg/5 mL, 100 mg/mL
  drops
	First-generation cephalosporin active against *S. aureus,*
	  Streptococcus, E. coli, Klebsiella, and *Proteus*
	Children: 25-100 mg/kg/24 hr divided q6-8h PO
	Adults: 250-500 mg q6h PO (max dose: 4 g/24 hr)
		Cautions: β-Lactam safety profile (rash,
		  eosinophilia). Renally eliminated
		Drug interaction: Probenecid

Cephradine
Velosef
Capsule: 250, 500 mg
Suspension: 125 mg/5 mL,
  250 mg/5 mL
	First-generation cephalosporin active against *S. aureus,*
	  Streptococcus, E. coli, Klebsiella, and *Proteus*
	Children: 50-100 mg/kg/24 hr divided q6-12h PO
	Adults: 250-500 mg q6-12h PO (max dose: 4 g/24 hr)
		Cautions: β-Lactam safety profile (rash,
		  eosinophilia). Renally eliminated
		Drug interaction: Probenecid

Continued

Table 207.3 | Selected Antibacterial Medications (Antibiotics)—cont'd

DRUG (TRADE NAMES, FORMULATIONS)	INDICATIONS (MECHANISM OF ACTION) AND DOSING	COMMENTS
Ciprofloxacin Cipro Tablet: 100, 250, 500, 750 mg Injection Ophthalmic solution and ointment Otic suspension Oral suspension: 250 and 500 mg/5 mL	Quinolone antibiotic active against *P. aeruginosa, Serratia, Enterobacter, Shigella, Salmonella, Campylobacter, N. gonorrhoeae, H. influenzae, M. catarrhalis,* some *S. aureus,* and some *Streptococcus* Neonates: 10 mg/kg q 12 hr PO or IV Children: 15-30 mg/kg/24 hr divided q12h PO or IV; cystic fibrosis: 20-40 mg/kg/24 hr divided q8-12h PO or IV Adults: 250-750 mg q12h; 200-400 mg IV q12h PO (max dose: 1.5 g/24 hr)	*Cautions:* Concerns of joint destruction in juvenile animals not seen in humans; tendonitis, superinfection, dizziness, confusion, crystalluria, some photosensitivity *Drug interactions:* Theophylline; magnesium-, aluminum-, or calcium-containing antacids; sucralfate; probenecid; warfarin; cyclosporine
Clarithromycin Biaxin Tablet: 250, 500 mg Suspension: 125 mg/5 mL, 250 mg/5 mL	Macrolide antibiotic with activity against *S. aureus, Streptococcus, H. influenzae, Legionella, Mycoplasma,* and *C. trachomatis* Children: 15 mg/kg/24 hr divided q12h PO Adults: 250-500 mg q12h PO (max dose: 1 g/24 hr)	*Cautions:* Adverse events less than erythromycin; GI upset, dyspepsia, nausea, cramping *Drug interactions:* Same as erythromycin: astemizole carbamazepine, terfenadine, cyclosporine, theophylline, digoxin, tacrolimus
Clindamycin Cleocin Capsule: 75, 150, 300 mg Suspension: 75 mg/5 mL Injection Topical solution, lotion, and gel Vaginal cream	Protein synthesis inhibitor active against most gram-positive aerobic and anaerobic cocci except *Enterococcus* Neonates: Postnatal age ≤7 days weight <2,000 g; 10 mg/kg/24 hr divided q12h IV or IM; weight >2,000 g: 15 mg/kg/24 hr divided q8h IV or IM; >7 days weight <1,200 g: 10 mg/kg/24 hr IV or IM divided q12h; weight 1,200-2,000 g: 15 mg/kg/24 hr divided q8h IV or IM; weight >2,000 g: 20 mg/kg/24 hr divided q8h IV or IM Children: 10-40 mg/kg/24 hr divided q6-8h IV, IM, or PO Adults: 150-600 mg q6-8h IV, IM, or PO (max dose: 5 g/24 hr IV or IM or 2 g/24 hr PO)	*Cautions:* Diarrhea, nausea, *Clostridium difficile*–associated colitis, rash. Administer slow IV over 30-60 min. Topically active as an acne treatment
Cloxacillin sodium Tegopen Capsule: 250, 500 mg Suspension: 125 mg/5 mL	Penicillinase-resistant penicillin active against *S. aureus* and other gram-positive cocci except *Enterococcus* and coagulase-negative staphylococci Children: 50-100 mg/kg/24 hr divided q6h PO Adults: 250-500 mg q6h PO (max dose: 4 g/24 hr)	*Cautions:* β-Lactam safety profile (rash, eosinophilia). Primarily hepatically eliminated; requires dose reduction in renal disease. Food decreases bioavailability *Drug interaction:* Probenecid
Colistin (Colistimethate sodium; polymyxin E) Injection Inhalation	Treatment of multidrug resistant gram-negative organisms (*Enterobacteriaceae* including extended-spectrum beta lactamase and carbapenemase-producing strains) Children: 2.5-5 mg/kg/day divided in 2-4 divided doses IV Adults: 300 mg/day in 2-4 divided doses IV	*Cautions:* Nephrotoxicity (~3% in young children; higher rates in adolescents and adults); adjust dose for renal insufficiency; neurotoxicity (headaches, paresthesia, ataxia) *Drug interactions:* Should not be administered concomitantly with polymyxins or aminoglycosides
Co-trimoxazole (trimethoprim-sulfamethoxazole; TMP-SMX) Bactrim, Cotrim, Septra, Sulfatrim Tablet: SMX 400 mg and TMP 80 mg Tablet DS: SMX 800 mg and TMP 160 mg Suspension: SMX 200 mg and TMP 40 mg/5 mL Injection	Antibiotic combination with sequential antagonism of bacterial folate synthesis with broad antibacterial activity: *Shigella, Legionella, Nocardia, Chlamydia, Pneumocystis jiroveci.* Dosage based on TMP component Children: 6-20 mg TMP/kg/24 hr or IV divided q12h PO *Pneumocystis carinii* pneumonia: 15-20 mg TMP/kg/24 hr divided q12h PO or IV *P. carinii* prophylaxis: 5 mg TMP/kg/24 hr or 3 times/wk PO Adults: 160 mg TMP q12h PO	*Cautions:* Drug dosed on TMP (trimethoprim) component. Sulfonamide skin reactions: rash, erythema multiforme, Stevens-Johnson syndrome, nausea, leukopenia. Renal and hepatic elimination; reduce dose in renal failure *Drug interactions:* Protein displacement with warfarin, possibly phenytoin, cyclosporine
Daptomycin Cubicin	Disrupts bacterial cell membrane function, causing depolarization leading to inhibition of protein, DNA and RNA synthesis, which results in bacterial cell death. Active against enterococci (including glycopeptide-resistant strains), staphylococci (including MRSA), streptococci, and corynebacteria. Approved for skin and soft tissue infections. Acceptable for bacteremia and right-sided endocarditis with susceptible strains Adults: In skin and soft tissue infections, 4 mg/kg daptomycin IV once daily. For *S. aureus* bacteremia or right-sided endocarditis, 6 mg/kg IV once daily Children: For skin/skin structure infections, 12-23 mo, 10 mg/kg IV q24h; 2-6 yr, 9 mg/kg IV q24h; 7-11 yr, 7 mg/kg q24h; 12-17 yr, 5 mg/kg q24h, all for up to 14 days. For staphylococcal bacteremia, 1-6 yr, 12 mg/kg q24h; 7-11 yr, 9 mg/kg q24h; 12-17 yr, 7 mg/kg q24h; all for up to 42 days. For staphylococcal endocarditis, 1-5 yr, 10 mg/kg IV q24h for at least 6 wk; ≥6 yr, 6 mg/kg IV q24h for at least 6 wk	*Cautions:* Should not be used for pneumonia because drug inactivated by surfactants. Associated with rash, renal failure, anemia, and headache. Is reported to cause myopathy, rhabdomyolysis, and eosinophilic pneumonia *Drug interactions:* Should not be administered with statins

Continued

Table 207.3	Selected Antibacterial Medications (Antibiotics)—cont'd

DRUG (TRADE NAMES, FORMULATIONS)	INDICATIONS (MECHANISM OF ACTION) AND DOSING	COMMENTS
Demeclocycline Declomycin Tablet: 150, 300 mg Capsule: 150 mg	Tetracycline active against most gram-positive cocci except *Enterococcus*, many gram-negative bacilli, anaerobes, *Borrelia burgdorferi* (Lyme disease), *Mycoplasma*, and *Chlamydia* Children: 8-12 mg/kg/24 hr divided q6-12h PO Adults: 150 mg PO q6-8h Syndrome of inappropriate antidiuretic hormone secretion: 900-1,200 mg/24 hr or 13-15 mg/kg/24 hr divided q6-8h PO with dose reduction based on response to 600-900 mg/24 hr	*Cautions:* Teeth staining, possibly permanent (if administered <8 yr old) with prolonged use; photosensitivity, diabetes insipidus, nausea, vomiting, diarrhea, superinfections *Drug interactions:* Aluminum-, calcium-, magnesium-, zinc- and iron-containing food, milk, dairy products may decrease absorption
Dicloxacillin Dynapen, Pathocil Capsule: 125, 250, 500 mg Suspension: 62.5 mg/5 mL	Penicillinase-resistant penicillin active against *S. aureus* and other gram-positive cocci except *Enterococcus* and coagulase-negative staphylococci Children: 12.5-100 mg/kg/24 hr divided q6h PO Adults: 125-500 mg q6h PO	*Cautions:* β-Lactam safety profile (rash, eosinophilia). Primarily renally (65%) and bile (30%) elimination. Food may decrease bioavailability *Drug interaction:* Probenecid
Doripenem Doribax Injection	Carbapenem antibiotic with broad-spectrum activity against gram-positive cocci and gram-negative bacilli, including *P. aeruginosa* and anaerobes Children: dose unknown. Adults: 500 mg q8h IV	*Cautions:* β-Lactam safety profile; does not undergo hepatic metabolism. Renal elimination (70–75%); dose adjustment for renal failure *Drug interactions:* Valproic acid, probenecid
Doxycycline Vibramycin, Doxy Injection Capsule: 50, 100 mg Tablet: 50, 100 mg Suspension: 25 mg/5 mL Syrup: 50 mg/5 mL	Tetracycline antibiotic active against most gram-positive cocci except *Enterococcus*, many gram-negative bacilli, anaerobes, *B. burgdorferi* (Lyme disease), *Mycoplasma*, and *Chlamydia* Children: 2-5 mg/kg/24 hr divided q12-24h PO or IV (max dose: 200 mg/24 hr) Adults: 100-200 mg/24 hr divided q12-24h PO or IV	*Cautions:* Teeth staining, possibly permanent (<8 yr old) with prolonged use; photosensitivity, nausea, vomiting, diarrhea, superinfections *Drug interactions:* Aluminum-, calcium-, magnesium-, zinc-, iron-, kaolin-, and pectin-containing products, food, milk, dairy products may decrease absorption. Carbamazepine, rifampin, and barbiturates may decrease half-life
Erythromycin E-Mycin, Ery-Tab, Eryc, Ilosone Estolate 125, 500 mg Tablet EES: 200 mg Tablet base: 250, 333, 500 mg Suspension: estolate 125 mg/5 mL, 250 mg/5 mL, EES 200 mg/5 mL, 400 mg/5 mL Estolate drops: 100 mg/mL. EES drops: 100 mg/2.5 mL. Available in combination with sulfisoxazole (Pediazole), dosed on erythromycin content	Bacteriostatic macrolide antibiotic most active against gram-positive organisms, *Corynebacterium diphtheriae*, and *Mycoplasma pneumoniae* Neonates: Postnatal age ≤7 days: 20 mg/kg/24 hr divided q12h PO; >7 days weight <1,200 g: 20 mg/kg/24 hr divided q12h PO; weight >1,200 g: 30 mg/kg/24 hr divided q8h PO (give as 5 mg/kg/dose q6h to improve feeding intolerance) Children: Usual max dose: 2 g/24 hr Base: 30-50 mg/kg/24 hr divided q6-8h PO Estolate: 30-50 mg/kg/24 hr divided q8-12h PO Stearate: 20-40 mg/kg/24 hr divided q6h PO Lactobionate: 20-40 mg/kg/24 hr divided q6-8h IV Gluceptate: 20-50 mg/kg/24 hr divided q6h IV; usual max dose: 4 g/24 hr IV Adults: Base: 333 mg PO q8h; estolate/stearate/base: 250-500 mg q6h PO	*Cautions:* Motilin agonist leading to marked abdominal cramping, nausea, vomiting, and diarrhea. Associated with hypertrophic pyloric stenosis in young infants. Many different salts with questionable tempering of GI adverse events. Rare cardiac toxicity with IV use. Dose of salts differ. Topical formulation for treatment of acne *Drug interactions:* Antagonizes hepatic CYP 3A4 activity: astemizole, carbamazepine, terfenadine, cyclosporine, theophylline, digoxin, tacrolimus, carbamazepine
Gentamicin Garamycin Injection Ophthalmic solution, ointment, topical cream	Aminoglycoside antibiotic active against gram-negative bacilli, especially *E. coli, Klebsiella, Proteus, Enterobacter, Serratia,* and *Pseudomonas* Neonates: Postnatal age ≤7 days weight 1,200-2,000 g: 2.5 mg/kg q12-18h IV or IM; weight <2,000 g: 2.5 mg/kg q12h IV or IM; postnatal age >7 days weight 1,200-2,000 g: 2.5 mg/kg q8-12h IV or IM; weight >2,000 g: 2.5 mg/kg q8h IV or IM Children: 2.5 mg/kg/24 hr divided q8-12h IV or IM. Alternatively, may administer 5-7.5 mg/kg/24 hr IV once daily Intrathecal: Preservative-free preparation for intraventricular or intrathecal use: neonate: 1 mg/24 hr; children: 1-2 mg/24 hr intrathecal; adults: 4-8 mg/24 hr Adults: 3-6 mg/kg/24 hr divided q8h IV or IM	*Cautions:* Anaerobes, *S. pneumoniae*, and other *Streptococcus* are resistant. May cause ototoxicity and nephrotoxicity. Monitor renal function. Drug eliminated renally. Administered IV over 30-60 min *Drug interactions:* May potentiate other ototoxic and nephrotoxic drugs *Target serum concentrations:* Peak 6-12 mg/L; trough >2 mg/L with intermittent daily dose regimens only

Continued

| Table 207.3 | Selected Antibacterial Medications (Antibiotics)—cont'd |

DRUG (TRADE NAMES, FORMULATIONS)	INDICATIONS (MECHANISM OF ACTION) AND DOSING	COMMENTS
Imipenem-cilastatin Primaxin Injection	Carbapenem antibiotic with broad-spectrum activity against gram-positive cocci and gram-negative bacilli, including *P. aeruginosa* and anaerobes. No activity against *Stenotrophomonas maltophilia* Neonates: Postnatal age ≤7 days weight <1,200 g: 20 mg/kg q18-24h IV or IM; weight >1,200 g: 40 mg/kg divided q12h IV or IM; postnatal age >7 days weight 1,200-2,000 g: 40 mg/kg q12h IV or IM; weight >2,000 g: 60 mg/kg q8h IV or IM Children: 60-100 mg/kg/24 hr divided q6-8h IV or IM Adults: 2-4 g/24 hr divided q6-8h IV or IM (max dose: 4 g/24 hr)	*Cautions:* β-Lactam safety profile (rash, eosinophilia), nausea, seizures. Cilastatin possesses no antibacterial activity; reduces renal imipenem metabolism. Primarily renally eliminated *Drug interaction:* Possibly ganciclovir
Linezolid Zyvox Tablet: 400, 600 mg Oral suspension: 100 mg/5 mL Injection: 100 mg/5 mL	Oxazolidinone antibiotic active against gram-positive cocci (especially drug-resistant organisms), including *Staphylococcus, Streptococcus, E. faecium,* and *Enterococcus faecalis*. Interferes with protein synthesis by binding to 50S ribosome subunit Children: 10 mg/kg q12h IV or PO Adults: Pneumonia: 600 mg q12h IV or PO; skin infections: 400 mg q12h IV or PO	*Adverse events:* Myelosuppression, pseudomembranous colitis, nausea, diarrhea, headache *Drug interaction:* Probenecid
Loracarbef Generic Capsule: 200 mg Suspension: 100 mg/5 mL, 200 mg/5 mL	Carbacephem very closely related to cefaclor (second-generation cephalosporin) active against *S. aureus, Streptococcus, H. influenzae, M. catarrhalis, E. coli, Klebsiella,* and *Proteus* Children: 30 mg/kg/24 hr divided q12h PO (max dose: 2 g) Adults: 200-400 mg q12h PO (max dose: 800 mg/24 hr)	*Cautions:* β-Lactam safety profile (rash, eosinophilia). Renally eliminated *Drug interaction:* Probenecid
Meropenem Merrem Injection	Carbapenem antibiotic with broad-spectrum activity against gram-positive cocci and gram-negative bacilli, including *P. aeruginosa* and anaerobes. No activity against *S. maltophilia* Children: 60 mg/kg/24 hr divided q8h IV meningitis: 120 mg/kg/24 hr (max dose: 6 g/24 hr) q8h IV Adults: 1.5-3 g q8h IV	*Cautions:* β-Lactam safety profile; appears to possess less CNS excitation than imipenem. 80% renal elimination *Drug interaction:* Probenecid
Metronidazole Flagyl, Metro I.V., Topical gel, vaginal gel Injection Tablet: 250, 500 mg	Highly effective in the treatment of infections caused by anaerobes. Oral therapy of *C. difficile* colitis Neonates: weight <1,200 g: 7.5 mg/kg/48 hr PO or IV; postnatal age ≤7 days weight 1,200-2,000 g: 7.5 mg/kg/24 hr q24h PO or IV; weight 2,000 g: 15 mg/kg/24 hr divided q12h PO or IV; postnatal age <7 days weight 1,200-2,000 g: 15 mg/kg/24 hr divided q12h PO or IV; weight >2,000 g: 30 mg/kg/24 hr divided q12 h PO or IV Children: 30 mg/kg/24 hr divided q6-8h PO or IV Adults: 30 mg/kg/24 hr divided q6h PO or IV (max dose: 4 g/24 hr)	*Cautions:* Dizziness, seizures, metallic taste, nausea, disulfiram-like reaction with alcohol. Administer IV slow over 30-60 min. Adjust dose with hepatic impairment *Drug interactions:* Carbamazepine, rifampin, phenobarbital may enhance metabolism; may increase levels of warfarin, phenytoin, lithium
Mezlocillin sodium Mezlin Infection	Extended-spectrum penicillin active against *E. coli, Enterobacter, Serratia,* and *Bacteroides*; limited antipseudomonal activity Neonates: Postnatal age ≤7 days: 150 mg/kg/24 hr divided q12h IV; >7 days: 225 mg/kg divided q8h IV Children: 200-300 mg/kg/24 hr divided q4-6h IV; cystic fibrosis 300-450 mg/kg/24 hr IV Adults: 2-4 g/dose q4-6h IV (max dose: 12 g/24 hr)	*Cautions:* β-Lactam safety profile (rash, eosinophilia); painful given intramuscularly; each gram contains 1.8 mEq sodium. Interferes with platelet aggregation with high doses; increases noted in liver function test results. Renally eliminated. Inactivated by β-lactamase enzyme *Drug interaction:* Probenecid
Mupirocin Bactroban Ointment	Topical antibiotic active against *Staphylococcus* and *Streptococcus* Topical application: Nasal (eliminate nasal carriage) and to the skin 2-4 times daily	*Caution:* Minimal systemic absorption because drug metabolized within the skin
Nafcillin sodium Nafcil, Unipen Injection Capsule: 250 mg Tablet: 500 mg	Penicillinase-resistant penicillin active against *S. aureus* and other gram-positive cocci, except *Enterococcus* and coagulase-negative staphylococci Neonates: Postnatal age ≤7 days weight 1,200-2,000 g: 50 mg/kg/24 hr divided q12h IV or IM; weight >2,000 g: 75 mg/kg/24 hr divided q8h IV or IM; postnatal age >7 days weight 1,200-2,000 g: 75 mg/kg/24 hr divided q8h; weight >2,000 g: 100 mg/kg/24 hr divided q6-8h IV (meningitis: 200 mg/kg/24 hr divided q6h IV) Children: 100-200 mg/kg/24 hr divided q4-6h IV Adults: 4-12 g/24 hr divided q4-6h IV (max dose: 12 g/24 hr)	*Cautions:* β-Lactam safety profile (rash, eosinophilia), phlebitis; painful given intramuscularly; oral absorption highly variable and erratic (not recommended) *Adverse effect:* Neutropenia

Continued

Table 207.3	Selected Antibacterial Medications (Antibiotics)—cont'd

DRUG (TRADE NAMES, FORMULATIONS)	INDICATIONS (MECHANISM OF ACTION) AND DOSING	COMMENTS
Nalidixic acid NegGram Tablet: 250, 500, 1,000 mg Suspension: 250 mg/5 mL	First-generation quinolone effective for short-term treatment of lower UTIs caused by *E. coli, Enterobacter, Klebsiella,* and *Proteus* Children: 50-55 mg/kg/24 hr divided q6h PO; suppressive therapy: 25-33 mg/kg/24 hr divided q6-8h PO Adults: 1 g q6h PO; suppressive therapy: 500 mg q6h PO	*Cautions:* Vertigo, dizziness, rash. Not for use in systemic infections *Drug interactions:* Liquid antacids
Neomycin sulfate Mycifradin Tablet: 500 mg Topical cream, ointment Solution: 125 mg/5 mL	Aminoglycoside antibiotic used for topical application or orally before surgery to decrease GI flora (nonabsorbable) and hyperammonemia Infants: 50 mg/kg/24 hr divided q6h PO Children: 50-100 mg/kg/24 hr divided q6-8h PO Adults: 500-2,000 mg/dose q6-8h PO	*Cautions:* In patients with renal dysfunction because small amount absorbed may accumulate *Adverse events:* Primarily related to topical application, abdominal cramps, diarrhea, rash Aminoglycoside ototoxicity and nephrotoxicity if absorbed
Nitrofurantoin Furadantin, Furan, Macrodantin Capsule: 50, 100 mg Extended-release capsule: 100 mg Macrocrystal: 50, 100 mg Suspension: 25 mg/5 mL	Effective in treatment of lower UTIs caused by gram-positive and gram-negative pathogens Children: 5-7 mg/kg/24 hr divided q6h PO (max dose: 400 mg/24 hr); suppressive therapy 1-2.5 mg/kg/24 hr divided q12-24h PO (max dose: 100 mg/24 hr) Adults: 50-100 mg/24 hr divided q6h PO	*Cautions:* Vertigo, dizziness, rash, jaundice, interstitial pneumonitis. Do not use with moderate to severe renal dysfunction *Drug interactions:* Liquid antacids
Ofloxacin Ocuflox 0.3% ophthalmic solution: 1, 5, 10 mL Floxin 0.3% otic solution: 5, 10 mL	Quinolone antibiotic for treatment of conjunctivitis or corneal ulcers (ophthalmic solution) and otitis externa or chronic suppurative otitis media (otic solution) caused by susceptible gram-positive, gram-negative, anaerobic bacteria, or *C. trachomatis* *Child >1-12 yr:* Conjunctivitis: 1-2 drops in affected eye(s) q2-4h for 2 days, then 1-2 drops qid for 5 days Corneal ulcers: 1-2 drops q 30 min while awake and at 4 hr intervals at night for 2 days, then 1-2 drops hourly for 5 days while awake, then 1-2 drops q6h for 2 days Otitis externa (otic solution): 5 drops into affected ear bid for 10 days Chronic suppurative otitis media: treat for 14 days *Child >12 yr and adults:* Ophthalmic solution doses same as for younger children. Otitis externa (otic solution): Use 10 drops bid for 10 or 14 days as for younger children	*Adverse events:* Burning, stinging, eye redness (ophthalmic solution), dizziness with otic solution if not warmed
Oxacillin sodium Prostaphlin Injection Capsule: 250, 500 mg Suspension: 250 mg/5 mL	Penicillinase-resistant penicillin active against *S. aureus* and other gram-positive cocci, except *Enterococcus* and coagulase-negative staphylococci Neonates: Postnatal age ≤7 days weight 1,200-2,000 g: 50 mg/kg/24 hr divided q12h IV; weight >2,000 g: 75 mg/kg/24 hr IV divided q8h IV; postnatal age >7 days weight <1,200 g: 50 mg/kg/24 hr IV divided q12h IV; weight 1,200-2,000 g: 75 mg/kg/24 hr divided q8h IV; weight >2,000 g: 100 mg/kg/24 hr divided q6h IV Infants: 100-200 mg/kg/24 hr divided q4-6h IV Children: PO 50-100 mg/kg/24 hr divided q4-6h IV Adults: 2-12 g/24 hr divided q4-6h IV (max dose: 12 g/24 hr)	*Cautions:* β-Lactam safety profile (rash, eosinophilia) Moderate oral bioavailability (35–65%) Primarily renally eliminated *Drug interaction:* Probenecid *Adverse effect:* Neutropenia
Penicillin G Injection Tablets	Penicillin active against most gram-positive cocci; *S. pneumoniae* (resistance is increasing), group A streptococcus, and some gram-negative bacteria (e.g., *N. gonorrhoeae, N. meningitidis*) Neonates: Postnatal age ≤7 days weight 1,200-2,000 g: 50,000 units/kg/24 hr divided q12h IV or IM (meningitis: 100,000 U/kg/24 hr divided q12h IV or IM); weight >2,000 g: 75,000 U/kg/24 hr divided q8h IV or IM (meningitis: 150,000 U/kg/24 hr divided q8h IV or IM); postnatal age >7 days weight ≤1,200 g: 50,000 U/kg/24 hr divided q12h IV (meningitis: 100,000 U/kg/24 hr divided q12h IV); weight 1,200-2,000 g: 75,000 U/kg/24 hr q8h IV (meningitis: 225,000 U/kg/24 hr divided q8h IV); weight >2,000 g: 100,000 U/kg/24 hr divided q6h IV (meningitis: 200,000 U/kg/24 hr divided q6h IV) Children: 100,000-250,000 units/kg/24 hr divided q4-6h IV or IM (max dose: 400,000 U/kg/24 hr) Adults: 2-24 million units/24 hr divided q4-6h IV or IM	*Cautions:* β-Lactam safety profile (rash, eosinophilia), allergy, seizures with excessive doses particularly in patients with marked renal disease. Substantial pathogen resistance. Primarily renally eliminated *Drug interaction:* Probenecid

Table 207.3 | Selected Antibacterial Medications (Antibiotics)—cont'd

DRUG (TRADE NAMES, FORMULATIONS)	INDICATIONS (MECHANISM OF ACTION) AND DOSING	COMMENTS
Penicillin G, benzathine Bicillin Injection	Long-acting repository form of penicillin effective in treatment of infections responsive to persistent, low penicillin concentrations (1-4 wk), e.g., group A streptococcus pharyngitis, rheumatic fever prophylaxis Neonates weight >1,200 g: 50,000 units/kg IM once Children: 300,000-1.2 million units/kg q 3-4 wk IM (max dose: 1.2-2.4 million units/dose) Adults: 1.2 million units IM q 3-4 wk	*Cautions:* β-Lactam safety profile (rash, eosinophilia), allergy. Administer by IM injection only. Substantial pathogen resistance. Primarily renally eliminated *Drug interaction:* Probenecid
Penicillin G, procaine Crysticillin Injection	Repository form of penicillin providing low penicillin concentrations for 12 hr Neonates weight >1,200 g: 50,000 units/kg/24 hr IM Children: 25,000-50,000 units/kg/24 hr IM for 10 days (max dose: 4.8 million units/dose) Gonorrhea: 100,000 units/kg (max dose: 4.8 million units/24 hr) IM once with probenecid 25 mg/kg (max dose: 1 g) Adults: 0.6-4.8 million units q12-24h IM	*Cautions:* β-Lactam safety profile (rash, eosinophilia) allergy. Administer by IM injection only. Substantial pathogen resistance. Primarily renally eliminated *Drug interaction:* Probenecid
Penicillin V Pen VK, V-Cillin K Tablet: 125, 250, 500 mg Suspension: 125 mg/5 mL, 250 mg/5 mL	Preferred oral dosing form of penicillin, active against most gram-positive cocci; *S. pneumoniae* (resistance is increasing), other streptococci, and some gram-negative bacteria (e.g., *N. gonorrhoeae, N. meningitidis*) Children: 25-50 mg/kg/24 hr divided q4-8h PO Adults: 125-500 mg q6-8h PO (max dose: 3 g/24 hr)	*Cautions:* β-Lactam safety profile (rash, eosinophilia), allergy, seizures with excessive doses particularly in patients with renal disease. Substantial pathogen resistance. Primarily renally eliminated. Inactivated by penicillinase *Drug interaction:* Probenecid
Piperacillin Pipracil Injection	Extended-spectrum penicillin active against *E. coli, Enterobacter, Serratia, P. aeruginosa,* and *Bacteroides* Neonates: Postnatal age ≤7 days 150 mg/kg/24 hr divided q8-12h IV; >7 days; 200 mg/kg/24 hr divided q6-8h IV Children: 200-300 mg/kg/24 hr divided q4-6h IV; cystic fibrosis: 350-500 mg/kg/24 hr IV Adults: 2-4 g/dose q4-6h (max dose: 24 g/24 hr) IV	*Cautions:* β-Lactam safety profile (rash, eosinophilia); painful given intramuscularly; each gram contains 1.9 mEq sodium. Interferes with platelet aggregation/serum sickness–like reaction with high doses; increases in liver function test results. Renally eliminated. Inactivated by penicillinase *Drug interaction:* Probenecid
Piperacillin-tazobactam Zosyn Injection	Extended-spectrum penicillin (piperacillin) combined with a β-lactamase inhibitor (tazobactam) active against *S. aureus, H. influenzae, E. coli, Enterobacter, Serratia, Acinetobacter, P. aeruginosa,* and *Bacteroides* Children: 300-400 mg/kg/24 hr divided q6-8h IV or IM Adults: 3.375 g q6-8h IV or IM	*Cautions:* β-Lactam safety profile (rash, eosinophilia); painful given intramuscularly; each gram contains 1.9 mEq sodium Interferes with platelet aggregation, serum sickness–like reaction with high doses, increases in liver function test results. Renally eliminated *Drug interaction:* Probenecid
Quinupristin/dalfopristin Synercid IV injection: powder for reconstitution, 10 mL contains 150 mg quinupristin, 350 mg dalfopristin	Streptogramin antibiotic (quinupristin) active against vancomycin-resistant *E. faecium* (VRE) and methicillin-resistant *S. aureus* (MRSA). Not active against *E. faecalis* Children and adults: VRE: 7.5 mg/kg q8h IV for VRE; skin infections: 7.5 mg/kg q12h IV	*Adverse events:* Pain, edema, or phlebitis at injection site, nausea, diarrhea *Drug interactions:* Synercid is a potent inhibitor of CYP 3A4
Sulfadiazine Tablet: 500 mg	Sulfonamide antibiotic primarily indicated for treatment of lower UTIs caused by *E. coli, P. mirabilis,* and *Klebsiella* Toxoplasmosis: Neonates: 100 mg/kg/24 hr divided q12h PO with pyrimethamine 1 mg/kg/24 hr PO (with folinic acid) Children: 120-200 mg/kg/24 hr divided q6h PO with pyrimethamine 2 mg/kg/24 hr divided q12h PO ≥3 days, then 1 mg/kg/24 hr (max dose: 25 mg/24 hr) with folinic acid Rheumatic fever prophylaxis: weight ≤30 kg: 500 mg/24 hr q24h PO; weight >30 kg: 1 g/24 hr q24h PO	*Cautions:* Rash, Stevens-Johnson syndrome, nausea, leukopenia, crystalluria. Renal and hepatic elimination; avoid use with renal disease. Half-life: ~10 hr *Drug interactions:* Protein displacement with warfarin, phenytoin, methotrexate
Sulfamethoxazole Gantanol Tablet: 500 mg Suspension: 500 mg/5 mL	Sulfonamide antibiotic used for treatment of otitis media, chronic bronchitis, and lower UTIs caused by susceptible bacteria Children: 50-60 mg/kg/24 hr divided q12h PO Adults: 1 g/dose q12h PO (max dose: 3 g/24 hr)	*Cautions:* Rash, Stevens-Johnson syndrome, nausea, leukopenia, crystalluria. Renal and hepatic elimination; avoid use with renal disease. Half-life: ~12 hr. Initial dose often a loading dose (doubled) *Drug interactions:* Protein displacement with warfarin, phenytoin, methotrexate

Continued

Table 207.3 | Selected Antibacterial Medications (Antibiotics)—cont'd

DRUG (TRADE NAMES, FORMULATIONS)	INDICATIONS (MECHANISM OF ACTION) AND DOSING	COMMENTS
Sulfisoxazole Gantrisin Tablet: 500 mg Suspension: 500 mg/5 mL Ophthalmic solution, ointment	Sulfonamide antibiotic used for treatment of otitis media, chronic bronchitis, and lower UTIs caused by susceptible bacteria Children: 120-150 mg/kg/24 hr divided q4-6h PO (max dose: 6 g/24 hr) Adults: 4-8 g/24 hr divided q4-6h PO	*Cautions:* Rash, Stevens-Johnson syndrome, nausea, leukopenia, crystalluria. Renal and hepatic elimination; avoid use with renal disease. Half-life: ~7-12 hr. Initial dose often a loading dose (doubled) *Drug interactions:* Protein displacement with warfarin, phenytoin, methotrexate
Tigecycline Tygacil Injection	Tetracycline-class antibiotic (glycylcycline) active against **Enterobacteriaceae, including extended spectrum β-lactamase producers; streptococci (including VRE); staphylococci (including MRSA); and anaerobes** Children: unknown Adults: 100 mg loading dose followed by 50 mg q12h IV	*Cautions:* Pregnancy; children <8 yr old; photosensitivity; hypersensitivity to tetracyclines; hepatic impairment (~60% hepatic clearance) *Drug interaction:* Warfarin; mycophenolate mofetil
Tobramycin Nebcin, Tobrex Injection Ophthalmic solution, ointment	Aminoglycoside antibiotic active against **gram-negative bacilli, especially *E. coli, Klebsiella, Enterobacter, Serratia, Proteus,* and *Pseudomonas*** Neonates: Postnatal age ≤7 days, weight 1,200-2,000 g: 2.5 mg/kg q12-18h IV or IM; weight >2,000 g: 2.5 mg/kg q12h IV or IM; postnatal age >7 days, weight 1,200-2,000 g: 2.5 mg/kg q8-12h IV or IM; weight >2,000 g: 2.5 mg/kg q8h IV or IM Children: 2.5 mg/kg/24 hr divided q8-12h IV or IM. Alternatively, may administer 5-7.5 mg/kg/24 hr IV. Preservative-free preparation for intraventricular or intrathecal use: neonate, 1 mg/24 hr; children, 1-2 mg/24 hr; adults, 4-8 mg/24 hr Adults: 3-6 mg/kg/24 hr divided q8h IV or IM	*Cautions: S. pneumoniae,* other *Streptococcus,* and anaerobes are resistant. May cause ototoxicity and nephrotoxicity. Monitor renal function. Drug eliminated renally. Administered IV over 30-60 min *Drug interactions:* May potentiate other ototoxic and nephrotoxic drugs *Target serum concentrations:* Peak 6-12 mg/L; trough <2 mg/L
Trimethoprim Proloprim, Trimpex Tablet: 100, 200 mg	Folic acid antagonist effective in prophylaxis and treatment of *E. coli, Klebsiella, P. mirabilis,* and *Enterobacter* UTIs; *P. carinii* pneumonia Children: For UTI: 4-6 mg/kg/24 hr divided q12h PO Children >12 yr and adults: 100-200 mg q12h PO. *P. carinii* pneumonia (with dapsone): 15-20 mg/kg/24 hr divided q6h for 21 days PO	*Cautions:* Megaloblastic anemia, bone marrow suppression, nausea, epigastric distress, rash *Drug interactions:* Possible interactions with phenytoin, cyclosporine, rifampin, warfarin
Vancomycin Vancocin, Lyphocin Injection Capsule: 125 mg, 250 mg Suspension	Glycopeptide antibiotic active against most **gram-positive pathogens including staphylococci (including MRSA and coagulase-negative staphylococci), *S. pneumoniae* including penicillin-resistant strains, *Enterococcus* (resistance is increasing), and *C. difficile*–associated colitis** Neonates: Postnatal age ≤7 days, weight <1,200 g: 15 mg/kg/24 hr divided q24h IV; weight 1,200-2,000 g: 15 mg/kg/24 hr divided q12-18h IV; weight >2,000 g: 30 mg/kg/24 hr divided q12h IV; postnatal age >7 days, weight <1,200 g: 15 mg/kg/24 hr divided q24h IV; weight 1,200-2,000 g: 15 mg/kg/24 hr divided q8-12h IV; weight >2,000 g: 45 mg/kg/24 hr divided q8h IV Children: 45-60 mg/kg/24 hr divided q8-12h IV; *C. difficile*–associated colitis: 40-50 mg/kg/24 hr divided q6-8h PO	*Cautions:* Ototoxicity and nephrotoxicity particularly when co-administered with other ototoxic and nephrotoxic drugs Infuse IV over 45-60 min. Flushing (red man syndrome) associated with rapid IV infusions, fever, chills, phlebitis (central line is preferred). Renally eliminated. *Target serum concentrations:* Peak (1 hr after 1 hr infusion) 30-40 mg/L; trough 5-10 mg/L

*In the Drug column, the generic drug name is in **bold**. In the Indications column, **bold** indicates major organisms targeted and mechanisms of action.

CNS, Central nervous system; GI, gastrointestinal; IM, intramuscular/ly; IV, intravenous/ly; PO, oral/ly; q12-24h, every 12 to 24 hours; bid, twice daily; qid, 4 times daily; UTIs, urinary tract infections.

called *ceftaroline* has been licensed. Ceftaroline is the active metabolite of the prodrug ceftaroline fosamil (which is the agent administered to the patient). Ceftaroline is a broad-spectrum cephalosporin with bactericidal activity against resistant gram-positive organisms, including MRSA, and common gram-negative pathogens. It has FDA approval and is licensed for use in children. Ceftaroline is indicated for MRSA in the treatment of skin and soft tissue infections. It is also licensed for treatment of community-acquired pneumonia but is not indicated for MRSA pneumonia. Ceftaroline's activity is attributed to its ability to bind to penicillin-binding protein 2a with higher affinity than other β-lactams. Another fifth-generation cephalosporin with a similar spectrum of activity, *ceftobiprole*, has been approved for use in Canada and the European Union.

Another fifth-generation cephalosporin, *ceftolozane*, is a derivative of ceftazidime with improved activity against *Pseudomonas* spp. It is not stable against most ESBLs or carbapenemases. It is marketed in combination with the β-lactam inhibitor tazobactam, to improve its activity against β-lactamase–producing Enterobacteriaceae. Experience with children is limited.

Table 207.6 lists adverse reactions to cephalosporins.

Carbapenems

The carbapenems include imipenem (formulated in combination with cilastatin), meropenem, ertapenem, and doripenem. The basic structure of these agents is similar to that of β-lactam antibiotics, and these drugs have a similar mechanism of action. The carbapenems provide the

Table 207.4	Adverse Reactions to Penicillins

TYPE OF REACTION	FREQUENCY (%)	OCCURS MOST FREQUENTLY WITH
ALLERGIC		
Immunoglobulin E antibody	0.04-0.015	Penicillin G
Anaphylaxis*		
Early urticaria* (<72 hr)		
Cytotoxic antibody	Rare	Penicillin G
Hemolytic anemia*		
Antigen-antibody complex disease	Rare	Penicillin G
Serum sickness*		
Delayed hypersensitivity	2-5	Ampicillin, amoxicillin
Contact dermatitis*		
IDIOPATHIC	2-5	Ampicillin
Skin rash		
Fever		
Late-onset urticaria		
GASTROINTESTINAL		
Diarrhea	3-11	Ampicillin
C. difficile–associated colitis	Rare	Ampicillin
HEMATOLOGIC		
Hemolytic anemia	Rare	Penicillin G
Neutropenia	10-17	Penicillin G, nafcillin, oxacillin[†]
Platelet dysfunction	43-73	Piperacillin
HEPATIC		
Elevated serum aspartate transaminase	0.01-22	Flucloxacillin, oxacillin
ELECTROLYTE DISTURBANCE		
Hypokalemia	Rare	Nafcillin, oxacillin
Hyperkalemia, acute	Rare	Penicillin G
NEUROLOGIC		
Seizures	Rare	Penicillin G
Bizarre sensations	Rare	Procaine penicillin
RENAL		
Interstitial nephritis*	Variable	Any penicillin

*Reaction can occur with any of the penicillins.
[†]With prolonged therapy.
Adapted from Doi Y, Chambers HF: Penicillins and β-lactamase inhibitors. In Bennett JF, Dolin R, Blaser MJ, editors: *Mandell, Douglas, and Bennett's principles and practice of infectious diseases*, ed 8, Philadelphia, 2015, Elsevier (Table 20-7).

broadest spectrum of antibacterial activity of any licensed class of antibiotics and are active against gram-positive, gram-negative, and anaerobic organisms. Among the carbapenems, **meropenem** is the only agent licensed for treatment of pediatric meningitis. At this time, ertapenem and doripenem are not approved for pediatric use. Importantly, MRSA and *E. faecium* are *not* susceptible to carbapenems. Carbapenems also tend to be poorly active against *Stenotrophomonas maltophilia*, rendering their use for cystic fibrosis patients who are infected with this organism problematic. Ertapenem is poorly active against *P. aeruginosa* and *Acinetobacter* species and should be avoided when these pathogens are encountered. Although imipenem-cilastatin is the first carbapenem approved for clinical use and the carbapenem with the greatest clinical experience, this antibiotic unfortunately has a propensity to cause seizures in children, particularly in the setting of intercurrent meningitis. Accordingly, meropenem is typically more suitable for pediatric use, where meningitis is commonly a consideration. A new agent called **meropenem-vaborbactam** was licensed. The addition of the β-lactamase inhibitor vaborbactam extends the spectrum of activity of meropenem to include some ESBL- and carbapenemase-producing bacteria. No dosage recommendations exist as yet for pediatric use.

Other carbapenems in various stages of clinical trials include panipenem, biapenem, razupenem, tomopenem, and tebipenem/pivoxil (the

first oral carbapenem). Panipenem and biapenem are licensed in Japan, but there is minimal experience with pediatric dosing.

Glycopeptides

Glycopeptide antibiotics include **vancomycin** and **teicoplanin**, the less commonly available analog. These agents are bactericidal and act by inhibition of cell wall biosynthesis. The antimicrobial activity of the glycopeptides is limited to gram-positive organisms, including *S. aureus*, coagulase-negative staphylococci, pneumococcus, enterococci, *Bacillus*, and *Corynebacterium*. Vancomycin is frequently employed in pediatric practice and is of particular value for serious infections, including meningitis, caused by MRSA and penicillin- and cephalosporin-resistant *S. pneumoniae*. Vancomycin is also commonly used for infections in the setting of fever and neutropenia in oncology patients, in combination with other antibiotics (see Chapter 205), and for infections associated with indwelling medical devices (Chapter 206). Oral formulations of vancomycin are occasionally used to treat pseudomembranous colitis caused by *Clostridium difficile* infections; intrathecal therapy may also be used for selected CNS infections. Vancomycin must be administered with care because of its propensity to produce **red man syndrome**, which is a reversible adverse effect that is rare in young children and can typically be readily managed by slowing the rate of drug infusion.

Newer FDA-approved glycopeptide antibiotics include televancin, dalbavancin, and oritavancin; pediatric experience is limited. **Televancin** is indicated for skin and skin structure infections caused by *S. aureus* (including MRSA), group A streptococcus, and *E. faecalis* (vancomycin-susceptible isolates only). It is also approved for hospital-acquired (including ventilator-associated) pneumonia caused by *S. aureus*. The recommended adult dose is 10 mg/kg intravenously (IV) every 24 hr for 7-21 days. Televancin appears to be more nephrotoxic than vancomycin and has been associated with prolongation of the QT interval. **Dalbavancin**'s unique characteristic is its long half-life, 150-250 hr. In adults with normal renal function, the dose is 1000 mg IV, followed 1 wk later by 500 mg IV. This agent can be considered when MRSA is confirmed or strongly suggested. Dalbavancin is not active against vancomycin-resistant *S. aureus*. It is FDA-approved for bacterial skin and soft tissue infections. **Oritavancin** is a vancomycin derivative with indications similar to those of dalbavancin. It has a half-life of approximately 250 hr. The dosage for adults is a single 1200 mg dose, administered IV over 3 hr. The FDA has approved dalbavancin and oritavancin for treatment of acute bacterial skin and skin structure infections caused by gram-positive bacteria, including MRSA.

Aminoglycosides

Aminoglycoside antibiotics include streptomycin, kanamycin, gentamicin, tobramycin, netilmicin, and amikacin. The most commonly used aminoglycosides in pediatric practice are **gentamicin** and **tobramycin**. They exert their mechanism of action by inhibition of bacterial protein synthesis. Although they are most often used to treat gram-negative infections, the aminoglycosides are broad-spectrum agents, with activity against *S. aureus* and synergistic activity against GBS, *L. monocytogenes*, viridans streptococci, corynebacteria JK, *Pseudomonas*, *Staphylococcus epidermidis*, and *Enterococcus* when co-administered with a β-lactam agent. Aminoglycoside use has decreased with the development of alternatives, but they still play a key role in pediatric practice in the management of neonatal sepsis, UTIs, gram-negative bacterial sepsis, and complicated intraabdominal infections; infections in cystic fibrosis patients (including both parenteral and aerosolized forms of therapy); and in oncology patients with fever and neutropenia. Aminoglycosides, in particular streptomycin, are also important in the management of *Francisella tularensis*, *Mycobacterium tuberculosis*, and atypical mycobacterial infections.

Toxicities of aminoglycoside therapy include nephrotoxicity and ototoxicity (cochlear and/or vestibular), and serum levels as well as renal function and hearing should be monitored in patients on long-term therapy. Toxicities of aminoglycosides may be reduced by the use of once-daily dosing regimens with appropriate monitoring of serum levels. Hypokalemia, volume depletion, hypomagnesemia, and other nephrotoxic drugs may increase the renal toxicity of aminoglycosides. A rare

| Table 207.5 | Classification of Parenteral and Oral Cephalosporins |

CEPHALOSPORINS	FIRST GENERATION	SECOND GENERATION	CEPHAMYCINS	THIRD GENERATION	FOURTH GENERATION	FIFTH GENERATION	MRSA-ACTIVE
Parenteral	Cefazolin (Ancef, Kefzol) Cephalothin (Keflin, Seffin)* Cephapirin (Cefadyl)* Cephradine (Velosef)*	Cefamandole (Mandol)* Cefonicid (Monocid)* Cefuroxime (Kefurox, Zinacef)	Cefmetazole (Zefazone)* Cefotetan (Cefotan) Cefoxitin (Mefoxin)	Cefoperazone (Cefobid)* Cefotaxime* (Claforan) Ceftazidime (Fortaz) Ceftizoxime (Cefizox)* Ceftriaxone (Rocephin) Moxalactam*	Cefepime (Maxipime) Cefpirome (Cefrom)* Ceftolozane (combined with tazobactam; CXA-101)	Ceftaroline (Teflaro) Ceftobiprole (Zevtera)*	Ceftaroline (Teflaro) Ceftobiprole (Zevtera)*
Oral	Cefadroxil (Duricef, Ultracef) Cephalexin (Keflex, Biocef, Keftab) Cephradine (Velosef)*	Cefaclor (Ceclor)* Cefprozil (Cefzil) Cefuroxime axetil (Ceftin) Loracarbef (Lorabid)*		Cefdinir (Omnicef) Cefditoren (Spectracef) Cefixime (Suprax) Cefpodoxime (Vantin) Ceftibuten (Cedax)			

*Not currently available in the United States.
Adapted from Craig WA, Andes DR: Cephalosporins. IN Bennett JF, Dolin R, Blaser MJ, editors: *Mandell, Douglas, and Bennett's principles and practice of infectious diseases*, ed 8, Philadelphia, 2015, Elsevier (Table 21-1).

| Table 207.6 | Potential Adverse Effects of Cephalosporins |

TYPE	SPECIFIC	FREQUENCY
Hypersensitivity	Rash	1–3%
	Urticaria	<1%
	Serum sickness	<1%
	Anaphylaxis	0.01%
Gastrointestinal	Diarrhea	1–19%
	Nausea, vomiting	1–6%
	Transient transaminase elevation	1–7%
	Biliary sludge	20–46%*
Hematologic	Eosinophilia	1–10%
	Neutropenia	<1%
	Thrombocytopenia	<1-3%
	Hypoprothrombinemia	<1%
	Impaired platelet aggregation	<1%
	Hemolytic anemia	<1%
Renal	Interstitial nephritis	<1%
Central nervous system	Seizures	<1%
	Encephalopathy	<1%
False-positive laboratory	Coombs positive	3%
	Glucosuria	Rare
	Serum creatinine	Rare
Other	Drug fever	Rare
	Disulfiram-like reaction[†]	Rare
	Superinfection	Rare
	Phlebitis	Rare
	Calcium-antibiotic precipitation*	Unknown; can be associated with embolic events

*Ceftriaxone.
[†]Cephalosporins with thiomethyl tetrazole ring (MTT) side chain.
Adapted from Craig WA, Andes DR: Cephalosporins. In Bennett JF, Dolin R, Blaser MJ, editors: *Mandell, Douglas, and Bennett's principles and practice of infectious diseases*, ed 8, Philadelphia, 2015, Elsevier (Table 21-6).

complication of aminoglycosides is **neuromuscular blockade**, which may occur in the presence of other neuromuscular blocking agents and in the setting of infant botulism.

Tetracyclines

The tetracyclines (tetracycline hydrochloride, doxycycline, demeclocycline, and minocycline) are bacteriostatic antibiotics that exhibit their antimicrobial effect by binding to the bacterial 30S ribosomal subunit, inhibiting protein translation. These agents have a broad spectrum of antimicrobial activity against gram-positive and gram-negative bacteria, rickettsia, and some parasites. The oral bioavailability of these agents facilitates oral dosing for many infections, including Rocky Mountain spotted fever, anaplasmosis, ehrlichiosis, Lyme disease, and malaria. Tetracyclines must be prescribed judiciously to children <9 yr old, because they can cause staining of teeth, hypoplasia of dental enamel, and abnormal bone growth in this age-group.

Tigecycline, a semisynthetic derivative of minocycline, is a parenteral agent of a new antibiotic class (**glycylcyclines**) and is licensed in the United States. It has a broader spectrum of activity (bacteriostatic) than traditional tetracyclines but retains the side effect profile of tetracyclines. Tigecycline is active against tetracycline-resistant gram-positive and gram-negative pathogens, including MRSA and possibly VRE, but not *Pseudomonas*. A novel tetracycline derivative, **eravacycline** (a fluorocycline), has completed phase 3 studies but is not yet licensed for use.

Complications of tetracyclines include eosinophilia, leukopenia and thrombocytopenia (tetracycline), pseudotumor cerebri, anorexia, emesis and nausea, candidal superinfection, hepatitis, photosensitivity, and a hypersensitivity reaction (urticaria, asthma exacerbation, facial edema, dermatitis) as well as a systemic lupus erythematosus–like syndrome (minocycline). The FDA issued a "black box" warning regarding tigecycline in 2013 based on a meta-analysis of 10 studies that showed increased mortality among patients receiving this drug.

A salutary side effect of **demeclocycline** has been identified; it is occasionally used as an off-label treatment of hyponatremia resulting from the syndrome of inappropriate antidiuretic hormone.

Sulfonamides

Trimethoprim and the sulfonamides are bacteriostatic agents that inhibit the bacterial folate synthesis pathway, in the process impairing both nucleic acid and protein synthesis. Sulfonamides interfere with the synthesis of dihydropteroic acid from paraaminobenzoic acid, whereas trimethoprim acts at a site further downstream, interfering with synthesis of tetrahydrofolic acid from dihydrofolic acid. The sulfonamides are available in both parenteral and oral formulations. Although there have historically been a large number of sulfonamide antibiotics developed for clinical use, relatively few remain available for pediatric practice. The most important agent is the combination of **trimethoprim-sulfamethoxazole** (TMP-SMX), used for treatment of UTIs. TMP-SMX has also emerged as a commonly prescribed agent for staphylococcal skin and soft tissue infections, since this antibiotic retains activity against MRSA. TMP-SMX also plays a unique role in immunocompromised patients, as a prophylactic and therapeutic agent for *Pneumocystis jiroveci* infection. Other common sulfonamides include **sulfisoxazole**, which is useful in the management of UTIs, and **sulfadiazine**, which is a drug of choice in the treatment of toxoplasmosis.

Macrolides

The macrolide antibiotics most often used in pediatric practice include **erythromycin**, **clarithromycin**, and **azithromycin**. This class of antimicrobials exerts its antibiotic effect through binding to the 50S subunit of the bacterial ribosome, producing a block in elongation of bacterial polypeptides. Clarithromycin is metabolized to 14-hydroxy clarithromycin, and interestingly this active metabolite also has potent antimicrobial activity. The spectrum of antibiotic activity includes many gram-positive bacteria. Unfortunately, resistance to these agents among *S. aureus* and group A streptococcus is fairly widespread, limiting the usefulness of macrolides for many skin and soft-tissue infections and for streptococcal pharyngitis. Azithromycin and clarithromycin have demonstrated efficacy for otitis media. All macrolide members have an important role in the management of pediatric respiratory infections, including atypical pneumonia caused by *M. pneumoniae, Chlamydophila pneumoniae,* and *Legionella pneumophila,* as well as infections caused by *Bordetella pertussis.*

Telithromycin, a ketolide antibiotic derived from erythromycin, was initially FDA-approved for the treatment in adults of mild to moderate community-acquired pneumonia, acute exacerbations of chronic bronchitis, and acute sinusitis, having good activity against the agents causing these infections (*S. pneumoniae, M. pneumoniae, C. pneumoniae,* and *L. pneumophila* for community-acquired pneumonia; *M. catarrhalis* and *H. influenzae* for sinusitis). Reports of liver failure and myasthenia gravis from telithromycin in particular prompted the withdrawal of drug from the market. **Solithromycin** is a related, next-generation oral and intravenous fluoroketolide in phase 3 clinical development for the treatment of community-acquired pneumonia.

Drug interactions are common with erythromycin and to a lesser extent with clarithromycin. These agents can inhibit the CYP 3A4 enzyme system, resulting in increased levels of certain drugs, such as astemizole, cisapride, statins, pimozide, and theophylline. Itraconazole may increase macrolide levels, whereas rifampin, carbamazepine, and phenytoin may decrease macrolide levels. There are few reported adverse drug interactions with azithromycin. Cross-resistance may develop between a macrolide and the subsequent use of clindamycin.

Lincosamides

The prototype of the lincosamide class of antibiotics is **clindamycin**, which acts at the ribosomal level to exert its antimicrobial effect. The 50S subunit of the bacterial ribosome is the molecular target of this agent. Its spectrum of activity includes gram-positive aerobes and anaerobes. Clindamycin has no significant activity against gram-negative organisms. An important role for clindamycin has emerged in the management of MRSA infections. Because of its outstanding penetration into body fluids (excluding the CNS) and tissues and bone, clindamycin can be used for therapy of serious infections caused by MRSA. Clindamycin is also useful in the management of invasive group A streptococcus infections and in the management of many anaerobic infections, often in combination with a β-lactam. A form of **inducible clindamycin resistance** is exhibited by some strains of MRSA; therefore consultation with the clinical microbiology laboratory is necessary before treating

a serious MRSA infection with clindamycin. Pseudomembranous colitis, a common complication of clindamycin therapy in adults, is seldom observed in pediatric patients. Clindamycin also plays an important role in the treatment of malaria and babesiosis (when co-administered with quinine), *P. jiroveci* pneumonia (when co-administered with primaquine), and toxoplasmosis.

Quinolones

The **fluoroquinolones** (ciprofloxacin, levofloxacin, moxifloxacin, gemifloxacin, besifloxacin [ophthalmic suspension], and delafloxacin) are antimicrobials that inhibit bacterial DNA replication by binding to the topoisomerases of the target pathogen, inhibiting the bacterial enzyme DNA gyrase. This class has broad-spectrum activity against both gram-positive and gram-negative organisms. Some fluoroquinolones exhibit activity against penicillin-resistant *S. pneumoniae* as well as MRSA. These agents uniformly show excellent activity against gram-negative pathogens, including the Enterobacteriaceae and respiratory tract pathogens such as *M. catarrhalis* and *H. influenzae.* Quinolones are also very active against pathogens associated with atypical pneumonia, particularly *M. pneumoniae* and *L. pneumophila.*

Although these agents are not approved for use in children, there is a reasonable body of evidence that the fluoroquinolones are generally safe, well tolerated, and effective against a variety of bacterial infections frequently encountered in pediatric practice. Parenteral quinolones are appropriate for critically ill patients with gram-negative infections. The use of oral quinolones in stable outpatients may also be reasonable for treatment of infections that would otherwise require parenteral antibiotics (e.g., *P. aeruginosa* soft tissue infections such as osteochondritis) or selected genitourinary tract infections. However, these agents should be reserved for situations where no other oral antibiotic alternative is feasible. In 2013 the FDA changed the warning labels for the fluoroquinolones to better describe the associated risk of permanent peripheral neuropathy. Additional risks include tendonitis, arrhythmias, and retinal detachment. Moreover, in situations of overuse (e.g., typhoid fever, gonococcal infection), organisms have been demonstrated to rapidly develop resistance. The FDA has advised against the use of quinolones for uncomplicated infections such as sinusitis and bronchitis. Thus, use of fluoroquinolones in pediatric practice should still be approached with continued caution, and consultation with an expert is recommended.

Streptogramins and Oxazolidinones

The emergence of highly resistant gram-positive organisms, in particular VRE, has necessitated development of new classes of antibiotics. One such class especially useful for resistant gram-positive infections is the streptogramins. The currently licensed agent in this category is **dalfopristin-quinupristin,** which is available in a parenteral formulation. It is appropriate for treatment of MRSA, coagulase-negative staphylococci, penicillin-susceptible and penicillin-resistant *S. pneumoniae,* and vancomycin-resistant *E. faecium* but not *E. faecalis.*

Another licensed class of antibiotics for highly resistant gram-positive infections is the oxazolidinone class. The prototype in this group is **linezolid**, available in both oral and parenteral formulations and approved for use in pediatric patients. Its mechanism of action involves inhibition of ribosomal protein synthesis. It is indicated for MRSA, VRE, coagulase-negative staphylococci, and penicillin-resistant *S. pneumoniae.* A related drug, **tedizolid phosphate,** is also FDA-approved for acute bacterial skin and skin structure infections. It is more potent in vitro than linezolid against MRSA and may be associated with less myelosuppression. It is available in both intravenous and oral formulations.

There is little information on streptogramins and oxazolidinones in treatment of CNS infections, and neither class is approved for pediatric meningitis. Linezolid can cause significant anemia and thrombocytopenia and is a monoamine oxidase inhibitor.

Daptomycin

Daptomycin is a novel member of the cyclic lipopeptide class of antibiotics. Its spectrum of activity includes virtually all gram-positive organisms, including *E. faecalis* and *E. faecium* (including VRE) and *S. aureus* (including MRSA). The structure of daptomycin is a 13-member amino acid peptide linked to a 10-carbon lipophilic tail, which results in a novel mechanism of action of disruption of the bacterial membrane through the formation of transmembrane channels. These channels cause leakage of intracellular ions, leading to depolarization of the cellular membrane and inhibition of macromolecular synthesis. A theoretical advantage of daptomycin for serious infections is its bactericidal activity against MRSA and enterococci. It is administered intravenously; experience in children is limited. Myopathy and elevations in creatine phosphokinase have been described. An FDA warning has been issued linking some cases of eosinophilic pneumonitis to the use of daptomycin. Daptomycin is inactivated by surfactant and should not be used to treat pneumonia.

Miscellaneous Agents

Metronidazole, which functions by disruption of DNA synthesis, has a unique role as an antianaerobic agent and also possesses antiparasitic and anthelmintic activity. In 2017 a related drug, **benznidazole**, was approved through the FDA's orphan drug Accelerated Approval Pathway. This antiprotozoal agent inhibits the synthesis of DNA, RNA, and proteins within *Trypanosoma cruzi* and is approved for adult and pediatric use for Chagas disease. **Rifampin** is a rifamycin antibiotic that inhibits bacterial RNA polymerase and has a major role in the management of tuberculosis. It is also of value in the management of other bacterial infections in pediatric patients, usually used as a 2nd (synergistic) agent

in the treatment of *S. aureus* infections or to eliminate nasopharyngeal colonization of *H. influenzae* type b or *N. meningitidis*. **Rifabutin** is a related drug that has an off-label indication for treatment of tuberculosis, an orphan drug indication for Crohn disease, and an indication for prevention or treatment of disseminated *Mycobacterium avium* complex disease in patients with HIV or immune deficiency. **Rifaximin** is a *nonabsorbed rifamycin* that has been used as an adjunct agent to treat patients with multiple recurrences of *C. difficile* infection. **Fidaxomicin** is a first-in-class member of a new category of narrow-spectrum macrocyclic antibiotic drugs. It is an RNA polymerase inhibitor with activity against *C. difficile* infection.

The emerging crisis in antimicrobial resistance has also necessitated the rediscovery of antimicrobial agents seldom used in clinical practice in recent decades, such as **colistin** (colistimethate sodium), a member of the polymyxin family of antibiotics (polymyxin E). Polymyxins' general structure consists of a cyclic peptide with hydrophobic tails. After binding to lipopolysaccharide in the outer membrane of gram-negative bacteria, polymyxins disrupt both outer and inner membranes, leading to cell death. Colistin is broadly active against the Enterobacteriaceae family, including *P. aeruginosa*. It is also active against ESBL- and carbapenemase-producing strains. Toxicities are chiefly renal and neurologic.

Bibliography is available at Expert Consult.

Section 4
Gram-Positive Bacterial Infections
第四篇
革兰阳性菌感染

Chapter 208
Staphylococcus
James T. Gaensbauer and James K. Todd
第二百零八章
葡萄球菌

中文导读

　　本章主要介绍了关于金黄色葡萄球菌感染、中毒性休克综合征和凝固酶阴性葡萄球菌感染的病因、流行病学、发病机制、临床表现、诊断、治疗、预后、预防等内容。在关于金黄色葡萄球菌的临床表现中具体描述了新生儿、皮肤、呼吸道、脓毒症、肌肉、骨及关节、中枢神经系统、心脏、肾脏、中毒性休克综合征和胃肠道的临床表现。在关于凝固酶阴性葡萄球菌的临床表现中具体描述了菌血症、心内膜炎、中心静脉导管感染、脑脊液分流和泌尿道感染的表现。

Staphylococci are hardy, aerobic, gram-positive bacteria that grow in pairs and clusters and are ubiquitous as normal flora of humans and present on fomites and in dust. They are resistant to heat and drying and may be recovered from nonbiologic environments weeks to months after contamination. Strains are classified as *Staphylococcus aureus* if they are coagulase positive or as one of the many species of **coagulase-negative staphylococci** (e.g., *Staphylococcus epidermidis, Staphylococcus saprophyticus, Staphylococcus haemolyticus*). *S. aureus* has many virulence factors that mediate various serious diseases, whereas coagulase-negative staphylococci tend to be less pathogenic unless an indwelling foreign body (e.g., intravascular catheter) is present. *S. aureus* strains resistant to β-lactam antibiotics, typically referred to as **methicillin-resistant Staphylococcus aureus (MRSA)**, have become a significant problem in both community and hospital settings.

208.1 *Staphylococcus aureus*

James T. Gaensbauer and James K. Todd

Staphylococcus aureus is the most common cause of pyogenic infection of the skin and soft tissues. **Bacteremia** (primary and secondary) is common and can be associated with or can result in osteomyelitis, suppurative arthritis, pyomyositis, deep abscesses, pneumonia, empyema, endocarditis, pericarditis, and rarely meningitis. **Toxin-mediated diseases,** including food poisoning, staphylococcal scarlet fever, scalded skin syndrome, and toxic shock syndrome (TSS), are caused by certain *S. aureus* strains.

ETIOLOGY

Strains of *S. aureus* can be identified and characterized by the virulence factors they produce. These factors tend to play 1 or more of 4 pathogenic roles in human disease: *S. aureus* protecting the organism from host defenses, localizing infection, causing local tissue damage, and affecting noninfected sites through toxin elaboration.

Most strains of *S. aureus* possess factors that protect the organism from host defenses. Many staphylococci produce a loose polysaccharide capsule, or **biofilm,** which may interfere with opsonophagocytosis. Production of clumping factor and coagulase differentiates *S. aureus* from coagulase-negative staphylococci. **Clumping factor** interacts with fibrinogen to create large clumps of organisms, interfering with effective phagocytosis. **Coagulase** causes plasma to clot by interacting with fibrinogen and may have an important role in abscess formation. **Protein A** is located on the outermost coat of the cell wall and can absorb serum immunoglobulins, preventing antibacterial antibodies from acting as opsonins and thus inhibiting phagocytosis. The staphylococcal enzyme **catalase** inactivates hydrogen peroxide, promoting intracellular survival.

Many strains of *S. aureus* produce substances that cause local tissue destruction. A number of immunologically distinct **hemolysins** that act on cell membranes and cause tissue necrosis have been identified (α-toxin, β-hemolysin, δ-hemolysin). Much attention has been given to the **Panton-Valentine leukocidin,** a protein that *S. aureus* combines with phospholipid in the leukocytic cell membrane, producing increased permeability and eventual death of the cell. Strains of *S. aureus* that produce Panton-Valentine leukocidin are associated with more-severe and invasive skin disease, pneumonia, and osteomyelitis. Many strains of *S. aureus* release 1 or more exotoxins. **Exfoliatins A and B** are serologically distinct proteins that produce localized (bullous impetigo) or generalized (scalded skin syndrome, staphylococcal scarlet fever) dermatologic manifestations (see Chapter 685).

S. aureus can produce >20 distinct enterotoxins (types A-V). Ingestion of preformed enterotoxin, particularly types A or B, can result in **food poisoning,** resulting in vomiting and diarrhea and, in some cases, profound hypotension.

Toxic shock syndrome toxin-1 (TSST-1) is associated with **toxic shock syndrome (TSS),** related to menstruation and focal staphylococcal infection (see Chapter 208.2). TSST-1 is a superantigen that induces production of interleukin (IL)-1 and tumor necrosis factor (TNF), resulting in hypotension, fever, and multisystem involvement. Focal infections associated with enterotoxins A or B also may be associated with nonmenstrual TSS.

S. aureus also possesses intrinsic factors that can contribute to pathogenesis, including proteins that promote adhesion to fibrinogen, fibronectin, collagen, and other human proteins. Expression of proteins that mediate antibiotic resistance is also of critical importance. Although historically sensitive to penicillin, *S. aureus* isolates now almost universally produce **penicillinase** or **β-lactamase,** which inactivates many β-lactamases at the molecular level and represents the major resistance mechanism against many penicillin and cephalosporin antibiotics. Thus, treatment of *S. aureus* with β-lactam antibiotics requires either a penicillinase resistant β-lactam ring or combination with a β-lactamase inhibitor. Production of altered **penicillin-binding proteins (PBPs)** in the bacterial cell wall mediates resistance to penicillinase resistant antibiotics: an **altered PBP-2A,** encoded by the gene *MECA*, is responsible for the methicillin and cephalosporin resistance of MRSA isolates.

EPIDEMIOLOGY

Approximately 20–40% of normal individuals carry at least 1 strain of *S. aureus* in the anterior nares at any given time, with intermittent carriage occurring in up to 70% of individuals. The organisms may be transmitted from the nose to the skin, where colonization is more transient. Persistent umbilical, vaginal, and perianal carriage may also occur. Many neonates are colonized within the 1st week of life, usually by a maternal strain. Rates of colonization with MRSA in the general pediatric population are typically <2% but may be higher in some locales and in children with significant healthcare exposure and chronic medical conditions.

Exposure to *S. aureus* generally occurs by autoinoculation or direct contact with the hands of other colonized individuals. Heavily colonized nasal carriers (often aggravated by a viral upper respiratory tract infection) are particularly effective disseminators. Spread by fomites is rare, although an outbreak occurring in a high school football team was attributed to sharing towels. Infection control policies in healthcare facilities, particularly those emphasizing good hand hygiene, have been shown to decrease rates of nosocomial staphylococcal infection.

Outside the hospital setting, outbreaks of staphylococcal disease, in particular disease caused by methicillin-resistant strains, have been reported among athletes, military personnel, young children, veterinarians, injection drug users, and inmates in correctional facilities. Increased disease frequency is noted among household contacts of a MRSA-colonized or infected individual. Skin infections caused by *S. aureus* are considerably more prevalent among persons living in low socio-economic circumstances and particularly among those in tropical climates.

The burden of staphylococcal disease is significant. Most important is the role of *S. aureus*, including MRSA, in **hospital-acquired infections,** including infections of the bloodstream, infection of surgical sites, and ventilator-associated pneumonia. *S. aureus* is a significant cause of morbidity and mortality in neonatal intensive care units (NICUs). Community-acquired staphylococcal infections are estimated to result in 14 million annual outpatient healthcare visits. In 2005 an estimated 478,000 hospitalizations were associated with *S. aureus* infection in the United States, more than half of which were caused by MRSA. Recent evidence shows a decline in rates of invasive MRSA infection in adults, but an opposite trend in U.S. pediatric patients was noted in 2013.

PATHOGENESIS

Except in the case of food poisoning resulting from ingestion of preformed enterotoxins, disease associated with *S. aureus* typically begins with colonization as previously described. Subsequent disease manifestations in susceptible individuals result either directly from tissue invasion or from injury caused by various toxins and enzymes produced by the organism (Fig. 208.1).

The most significant risk factor for the development of infection is **disruption of intact skin,** including breaches from wounds, skin disease such as eczema, epidermolysis bullosa or burns, ventriculoperitoneal shunts, and indwelling intravascular or intrathecal catheters. Additional risk factors include corticosteroid treatment, malnutrition, and azotemia.

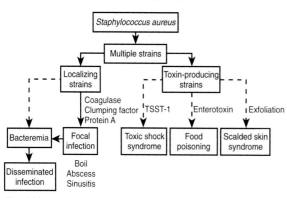

Fig. 208.1 Relationship of virulence factors and diseases associated with *Staphylococcus aureus*. TSST-1, toxic shock syndrome toxin-1.

Antibiotic therapy with a drug to which *S. aureus* is resistant favors colonization and the development of infection. Viral infections of the respiratory tract, especially influenza virus, may predispose to secondary bacterial infection with staphylococci in certain individuals.

Congenital defects in chemotaxis (e.g., Job, Chédiak-Higashi, and Wiskott-Aldrich syndromes) and defective phagocytosis and killing (e.g., neutropenia, chronic granulomatous disease) increase the risk for staphylococcal infections. Patients with HIV infection have neutrophils that are defective in their ability to kill *S. aureus* in vitro. Patients with recurrent staphylococcal infection should be evaluated for immune defects, especially those involving neutrophil dysfunction. Poor mucous clearance in children with cystic fibrosis frequently leads to chronic staphylococcal colonization and persistent inflammation in these patients.

Infants may acquire type-specific humoral immunity to staphylococci transplacentally. Older children and adults develop antibodies to staphylococci as a result of colonization or minor infections. Antibody to the various *S. aureus* toxins appears to protect against those specific toxin-mediated diseases, but humoral immunity does not necessarily protect against focal or disseminated *S. aureus* infection with the same organisms.

CLINICAL MANIFESTATIONS
Signs and symptoms vary with the location of the infection, which is usually the skin but may be any tissue. Disease states of various degrees of severity are generally a result of local suppuration, systemic dissemination with metastatic infection, or systemic effects of toxin production.

Newborn
S. aureus is an important cause of neonatal infections (see Chapter 129).

Skin
S. aureus is an important cause of **pyogenic** skin infections, including impetigo contagiosa, ecthyma, bullous impetigo, folliculitis, hydradenitis, furuncles (boils), carbuncles (multiple coalesced boils), and paronychia. **Toxigenic** infection with skin manifestations include staphylococcal scalded skin syndrome and staphylococcal scarlet fever. *S. aureus* is a frequent cause of superinfection of underlying dermatologic conditions, such as eczema or bug bites. Recurrent skin and soft tissue infections often are noted with community-associated MRSA and affect the lower extremities and buttocks. *S. aureus* is also an important cause of traumatic and surgical wound infections and can cause deep soft tissue involvement, including cellulitis and rarely, necrotizing fasciitis.

Respiratory Tract
Infections of the upper respiratory tract (otitis media, sinusitis) caused by *S. aureus* are rare, in particular considering the frequency with which the anterior nares are colonized. *S. aureus* sinusitis is relatively common in children with cystic fibrosis or defects in leukocyte function and

may be the only focus of infection in some children with TSS. Suppurative **parotitis** is a rare infection, but *S. aureus* is a common cause. A membranous **tracheitis** that complicates viral croup may result from infection with *S. aureus,* although other organisms may also be responsible. Patients typically have high fever, leukocytosis, and evidence of severe upper airway obstruction. Direct laryngoscopy or bronchoscopy shows a normal epiglottis with subglottic narrowing and thick, purulent secretions within the trachea. Treatment requires careful airway management and appropriate antibiotic therapy.

Pneumonia caused by *S. aureus* may be primary or secondary after a viral infection such as influenza (see Chapter 428). Hematogenous pneumonia may be secondary to septic emboli from right-sided endocarditis or septic thrombophlebitis, with or without intravascular devices. Inhalation pneumonia is caused by alteration of mucociliary clearance, leukocyte dysfunction, or bacterial adherence initiated by a viral infection. Common symptoms and signs include high fever, abdominal pain, tachypnea, dyspnea, and localized or diffuse bronchopneumonia or lobar disease. *S. aureus* often causes a **necrotizing pneumonitis** that may be associated with early development of empyema, pneumatoceles, pyopneumothorax, and bronchopleural fistulas. Chronic pulmonary infection with *S. aureus* contributes to progressive pulmonary dysfunction in children with cystic fibrosis (see Chapter 432).

Sepsis
S. aureus bacteremia and sepsis may be primary or associated with any localized infection. The onset may be acute and marked by nausea, vomiting, myalgia, fever, and chills. Organisms may localize subsequently at any site (usually a single deep focus) but are found especially in the heart valves, lungs, joints, bones, muscles, and deep tissue abscesses.

In some instances, especially in young adolescent males, disseminated *S. aureus* disease occurs, characterized by fever, persistent bacteremia despite antibiotics, and focal involvement of 2 or more separate tissue sites (skin, bone, joint, kidney, lung, liver, heart). These patients often have an endovascular nidus of infection, such as an infected venous thrombosis.

Muscle
Localized staphylococcal abscesses in muscle sometimes without septicemia have been called **pyomyositis**. This disorder is reported most frequently from tropical areas and is termed *tropical pyomyositis,* but also occurs in the United States in otherwise healthy children. Multiple abscesses occur in 30–40% of cases. History may include prior trauma at the site of the abscess. Surgical drainage and appropriate antibiotic therapy are essential.

Bones and Joints
S. aureus is the most common cause of osteomyelitis and suppurative arthritis in children (see Chapters 704 and 705).

Central Nervous System
Meningitis caused by *S. aureus* is uncommon; it is associated with penetrating cranial trauma and neurosurgical procedures (craniotomy, cerebrospinal fluid [CSF] shunt placement), and less frequently with endocarditis, parameningeal foci (epidural or brain abscess), complicated sinusitis, diabetes mellitus, or malignancy. The CSF profile of *S. aureus* meningitis is indistinguishable from that in other forms of bacterial meningitis (see Chapter 621.1).

Heart
S. aureus is a common cause of acute endocarditis on native valves and results in high rates of morbidity and mortality. Perforation of heart valves, myocardial abscesses, heart failure, conduction disturbances, acute hemopericardium, purulent pericarditis, and sudden death may ensue (see Chapter 464).

Kidney
S. aureus is a common cause of renal and perinephric abscess, usually of hematogenous origin. Pyelonephritis and cystitis caused by *S. aureus* are unusual (see Chapter 553).

Toxic Shock Syndrome

S. aureus is the principal cause of TSS, which should be suspected in anyone with fever, shock, and/or a scarlet fever–like rash (see Chapter 208.2).

Intestinal Tract

Staphylococcal enterocolitis may rarely follow overgrowth of normal bowel flora by *S. aureus*, which can result from broad-spectrum oral antibiotic therapy. Diarrhea is associated with blood and mucus. Peritonitis associated with *S. aureus* in patients receiving long-term ambulatory peritoneal dialysis usually involves the catheter tunnel.

Food poisoning may be caused by ingestion of *preformed* enterotoxins produced by staphylococci in contaminated foods (see Chapter 366). The source of contamination is often colonized or infected food workers. Approximately 2-7 hr after ingestion of the toxin, sudden, severe vomiting begins. Watery diarrhea may develop, but fever is absent or low. Symptoms rarely persist >12-24 hr. Rarely, shock and death may occur.

DIAGNOSIS

The diagnosis of *S. aureus* infection depends on isolation of the organism in culture from nonpermissive sites, such as cellulitis aspirates, abscess cavities, blood, bone, or joint aspirates, or other sites of infection. Swab cultures of surfaces are not as useful, because they may reflect surface contamination rather than the true cause of infection. Tissue samples or fluid aspirates in a syringe provide the best culture material. Cellulitic lesions may be cultured using a needle aspirate from the most inflamed area after thorough skin cleansing, inoculated directly into a blood culture bottle; use of injected saline and targeting the leading edge are less effective. Isolation from the nose or skin does not necessarily imply causation because these sites may be normally colonized sites. Because of the high prevalence of MRSA, the increasing severity of *S. aureus* infections, and the fact that bacteremia is not universally present even in severe *S. aureus* infections, it is important to obtain a culture of any potential focus of infection as well as a blood culture before starting antibiotic treatment. The organism can be grown readily in liquid and on solid media. After isolation, identification is made on the basis of Gram stain and coagulase, clumping factor, and protein A reactivity. Increasingly, molecular techniques such as polymerase chain reaction are used to supplement traditional culture methods. Automated PCR systems may allow rapid species identification from positive blood cultures and simultaneously identify genetic patterns associated with methicillin resistance, such as expression of the *MECA* gene produced by MRSA. PCR-based determination of MRSA nasal colonization on admission to hospitals or ICUs aids infection control procedures and identify patients at higher risk of infection.

Diagnosis of *S. aureus* food poisoning is usually made on the basis of epidemiologic and clinical findings. Food suspected of contamination may be cultured and can be tested for enterotoxin.

Differential Diagnosis

Many of the clinical entities previously discussed can also be caused by other bacterial pathogens, and consideration of the differential is particularly important when making empirical antibiotic choices before definitive identification of the offending pathogen. Skin lesions caused by *S. aureus* may be indistinguishable from those caused by group A streptococci, although the former usually expand slowly, while the latter are prone to spread more rapidly and can be very aggressive. Fluctuant skin and soft tissue lesions also can be caused by other organisms, including *Mycobacterium tuberculosis,* atypical mycobacteria, *Bartonella henselae* (cat-scratch disease), *Francisella tularensis,* and various fungi. *S. aureus* pneumonia is often suspected in very ill-appearing children or after failure to improve with standard treatment that does not cover *Staphylococcus,* or on the basis of chest radiographs that reveal pneumatoceles, pyopneumothorax, or lung abscess (Fig. 208.2). Other etiologies of cavitary pneumonias include *Klebsiella pneumoniae* and *M. tuberculosis.* In bone and joint infections, culture is the only reliable way to differentiate *S. aureus* from other, less common etiologies, including group A streptococci and in young children, *Kingella kingae.*

TREATMENT

Antibiotic therapy alone is rarely effective in individuals with undrained abscesses or with infected foreign bodies. Loculated collections of purulent material should be relieved by incision and drainage. Foreign bodies should be removed, if possible. Therapy always should be initiated with an antibiotic consistent with the local staphylococcal susceptibility patterns as well as the severity of infection. For most patients with serious *S. aureus* infection, intravenous (IV) treatment is recommended until the patient has become afebrile and other signs of infection have improved. Oral therapy is often continued for a time, especially in patients with chronic infection or underlying host defense problems. Serious *S. aureus* infections, with or without abscesses, tend to persist and recur, necessitating prolonged therapy.

Treatment of *S. aureus* osteomyelitis (Chapter 704), meningitis (Chapter 621.1), and endocarditis (Chapter 464) is discussed in the respective chapters on these diagnoses.

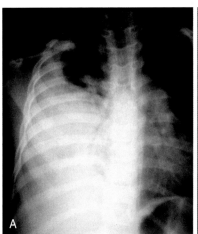 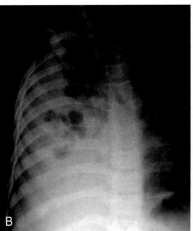 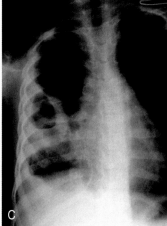

Fig. 208.2 Pneumatocele formation. A, *Staphylococcus aureus* pneumonia in 5 yr old child initially demonstrated consolidation of the right middle and lower zones. **B,** Seven days later, multiple lucent areas are noted as pneumatoceles develop. **C,** Two weeks later, significant resolution is evident, with a rather thick-walled pneumatocele persisting in the right midzone associated with significant residual pleural thickening. *(From Kuhn JP, Slovis TL, Haller JO: Caffey's pediatric diagnostic imaging, ed 10, Philadelphia, 2004, Mosby, pp 1003–1004.)*

Initial treatment for serious infections thought to be caused by **methicillin-susceptible S. aureus (MSSA)** should include semisynthetic penicillin (e.g., nafcillin) or a first-generation cephalosporin (e.g., cefazolin). Penicillin and ampicillin are not appropriate, because >90% of all staphylococci isolated, regardless of source, are resistant to these agents. Addition of a β-lactamase inhibitor (clavulanic acid, sulbactam, tazobactam) to a penicillin-based drug also confers antistaphylococcal activity but has no effect on MRSA. The spectrum of these agents (which includes gram-negative bacteria) can be an advantage when broad empirical coverage is needed, but narrower coverage should be selected once *S. aureus* is identified. *Antistaphylococcal penicillins and most cephalosporins do not provide activity against MRSA.*

For initial treatment for penicillin-allergic individuals and those with suspected serious infections caused by MRSA, **vancomycin** is the preferred therapy. Serum levels of vancomycin should be monitored, with serum trough concentrations of 10-20 μg/mL, depending on the location and severity of infection. Rare vancomycin intermediate and vancomycin-resistant strains of *S. aureus* have also been reported, mostly in patients being treated with vancomycin. For critically ill patients with suspected *S. aureus*, empirical therapy with both vancomycin and nafcillin should be considered until cultures results are available. *Initial treatment with IV **clindamycin**, followed by a transition to oral clindamycin, has been effective in bone, joint, and soft tissue infection; however, not all strains of MSSA or MRSA are susceptible to clindamycin.* Inducible clindamycin resistance in isolates initially reported as susceptible must be ruled out by D-test or molecular methods. Clindamycin is bacteriostatic and should not be used to treat endocarditis, persistent bacteremia, or CNS infections caused by *S. aureus*. Given that the mechanism of action of clindamycin involves inhibition or protein synthesis, many experts use clindamycin to treat *S. aureus* toxin–mediated illnesses (e.g., TSS) to inhibit toxin production.

Although the very-broad- spectrum carbapenems (meropenem, ertapenem, and imipenem) have activity against MSSA, they have no activity against MRSA. As a result, carbapenems are rarely used for empirical therapy of possible staphylococcal infection and are too broad in most cases for use in identified MSSA infections. Quinolone antibiotics have unpredictable activity against MSSA and no activity against MRSA. **Linezolid** and **daptomycin** are useful for serious *S. aureus* infections, particularly those caused by MRSA, when treatment with vancomycin is ineffective or not tolerated.(Table 208.1). A number of novel antistaphylococcal antibiotics have emerged for use in resistant or refractory MSSA and MRSA infection in adults that may be required for pediatric therapy in select patients under the guidance of a pediatric infectious disease specialist. These include **ceftaroline**, a broad-spectrum antistaphylococcal cephalosporin, and **oritavancin** and **dalbavancin**, lipoglycopeptides structurally related to vancomycin with very long half-lives and broad activity against gram-positive organisms. **Rifampin** or **gentamicin** may be added to a β-lactam or vancomycin for synergy in serious infections such as endocarditis, particularly when prosthetic valve material is involved.

In many infections, oral antimicrobials may be substituted to complete the course of treatment, after an initial period of parenteral therapy and determination of antimicrobial susceptibilities, or can be used as initial treatment in less severe infections. **Dicloxacillin** (50-100 mg/kg/24 hr divided 4 times daily PO) and **cephalexin** (25-100 mg/kg/24 hr divided 3-4 times daily PO) are absorbed well orally (PO) and are effective against MSSA. **Amoxicillin-clavulanate** (40-80 mg amoxicillin/kg/24 hr divided 3 times daily PO) is also effective when a broader spectrum of coverage is required. Clindamycin (30-40 mg/kg/24 hr divided 3-4 times daily PO) is highly absorbed from the intestinal tract and is frequently used for empirical coverage when both MRSA and MSSA are possible, as well as for suspectible MRSA infections or for MSSA in penicillin/cephalosporin-allergic patients. Compliance with oral clindamycin may be limited in small children because of poor palatability of oral formulations. **Trimethoprim-sulfamethoxazole** (TMP-SMX) may be an effective oral antibiotic for many strains of both MSSA and MRSA. Oral linezolid is an option for severe MRSA infections that have improved but require ongoing therapy when more common

Table 208.1	Parenteral Antimicrobial Agent(s) for Treatment of Serious *Staphylococcus aureus* Infections

SUSCEPTIBILITY	ANTIMICROBIALS	COMMENTS
I. INITIAL EMPIRICAL THERAPY (ORGANISM OF UNKNOWN SUSCEPTIBILITY)		
Drugs of choice:	Vancomycin + nafcillin or oxacillin	For life-threatening infections (e.g., septicemia, endocarditis, CNS infection); linezolid could be substituted if the patient has received several recent courses of vancomycin
	Vancomycin	For non–life-threatening infection without signs of severe sepsis (e.g., skin infection, cellulitis, osteomyelitis, pyarthrosis) when rates of MRSA colonization and infection in the community are substantial
	Cefazolin or nafcillin	For non–life-threatening infection when low likelihood of MRSA is suspected
	Clindamycin	For non–life-threatening infection without signs of severe sepsis when rates of MRSA colonization and infection in the community are substantial and prevalence of clindamycin resistance is low
II. METHICILLIN-SUSCEPTIBLE, PENICILLIN-RESISTANT *S. aureus*		
Drugs of choice:	Nafcillin*	
Alternatives (depending on susceptibility results):	Cefazolin	
	Clindamycin	Only for patients with a serious penicillin allergy and clindamycin-susceptible strain
	Vancomycin	Only for penicillin- and cephalosporin-allergic patients
	Ampicillin + sulbactam	When broader coverage, including gram-negative organisms is required
III. METHICILLIN-RESISTANT *S. aureus* (MRSA)		
Drugs of choice:	Vancomycin*	
Alternatives: susceptibility testing results available before alternative drugs are used	Clindamycin (if susceptible)	
	Daptomycin†	
	Linezolid†	
	Trimethoprim-sulfamethoxazole	

*One of the adjunctive agents, gentamicin or rifampin, should be added to the therapeutic regimen for life-threatening infections such as endocarditis or central nervous system (CNS) infection. Consultation with an infectious diseases specialist should be considered to determine which agent to use and duration of use.

†Linezolid and daptomycin are agents with activity in vitro and efficacy with multidrug-resistant, gram-positive organisms, including *S. aureus*. Because experience with these agents in children is limited, consultation with an infectious diseases specialist should be considered before use. Daptomycin is ineffective for treatment of pneumonia.

options are not tolerated or are ineffective due to resistance patterns. Despite in vitro susceptibility of *S. aureus* to ciprofloxacin and other quinolone antibiotics, these agents should *not* be used in serious staphylococcal infections, because their use is associated with rapid development of resistance.

The **duration** of oral therapy depends on the response, as determined by the clinical response and in some cases, radiologic and laboratory findings.

PROGNOSIS

Untreated *S. aureus* septicemia is associated with a high fatality rate, which has been reduced significantly by appropriate antibiotic treatment. *S. aureus* pneumonia can be fatal at any age but is more likely to be associated with high morbidity and mortality in young infants or in patients whose therapy has been delayed. Prognosis also may be influenced by numerous host factors, including nutrition, immunologic competence, and the presence or absence of other debilitating diseases. In most cases with abscess formation, surgical drainage is necessary.

PREVENTION

S. aureus infection is transmitted primarily by direct contact. Strict attention to **hand hygiene** is the most effective measure for preventing the spread of staphylococci from between individuals (see Chapter 198). Use of a hand wash containing chlorhexidine or alcohol is recommended. In hospitals or other institutional settings, all persons with acute *S. aureus* infections should be isolated until they have been treated adequately. There should be constant surveillance for nosocomial *S. aureus* infections within hospitals. When MRSA is recovered, strict isolation of affected patients has been shown to be the most effective method for preventing nosocomial spread of infection. When hospital-acquired infections do occur, clusters of nosocomial cases may be defined by molecular typing, and if associated with a singular molecular strain, it may also be necessary to identify colonized hospital personnel and attempt to eradicate carriage in affected individuals.

A number of protocols are aimed at **decolonization** in patients with recurrent *S. aureus* skin infection, particularly in individuals colonized with MRSA. These often involve various combinations of decontaminating baths (hypochlorite, 1 tsp common bleach solution per gallon of water, or chlorhexidine 4% soap used weekly), an appropriate oral antibiotic, nasal mupirocin twice daily for 1 wk, and cleaning of household linens in hot water. Although success is not universal, recurrent infections may be reduced, particularly when eradication is done in both the patient and frequent or household contacts. Most cases of mild, recurrent disease will resolve in time without these measures.

Because of the potential severity of infections with *S. aureus* and concerns about emerging resistance, much work has focused on developing a staphylococcal vaccine for use in high-risk patients, but to date, clinical trials have been disappointing. Because *S. aureus* is frequently a co-infection in severe influenza infections, an indirect preventive impact against staphylococcal pneumonia and tracheitis may be achieved though annual influenza vaccination.

Food poisoning may be prevented by excluding individuals with *S. aureus* infections of the skin from the preparation and handling of food. Prepared foods should be eaten immediately or refrigerated appropriately to prevent multiplication of *S. aureus* that may have contaminated the food (see Chapter 366).

Bibliography is available at Expert Consult.

208.2 Toxic Shock Syndrome

James T. Gaensbauer and James K. Todd

Toxic shock syndrome (TSS) is an acute and potentially severe illness characterized by fever, hypotension, erythematous rash with subsequent desquamation on the hands and feet, and multisystem involvement, including vomiting, diarrhea, myalgias, nonfocal neurologic abnormalities, conjunctival hyperemia, and strawberry tongue.

ETIOLOGY

TSS is caused by TSST-1–producing and some enterotoxin-producing strains of *S. aureus,* which may colonize the vagina or cause focal sites of staphylococcal infection.

EPIDEMIOLOGY

TSS continues to occur in the United States in men, women, and children, with highest rates in menstruating women 15-25 yr of age. **Nonmenstrual TSS** is associated with *S. aureus* infected nasal packing and wounds, sinusitis, tracheitis, pneumonia, empyema, abscesses, burns, osteomyelitis, and primary bacteremia. Most strains of *S. aureus* associated with TSS are methicillin susceptible because USA300, the predominant isolate of community-acquired MRSA in the United States, does not contain genes expressing the most common TSS superantigens.

PATHOGENESIS

The primary toxin associated with TSS is TSST-1, although a significant proportion of nonmenstrual TSS is caused by one or more staphylococcal enterotoxins. These toxins act as a **superantigens,** which trigger cytokine release causing massive loss of fluid from the intravascular space and end-organ cellular injury. Epidemiologic and in vitro studies suggest that these toxins are selectively produced in a clinical environment consisting of a neutral pH, a high P_{CO_2}, and an aerobic P_{O_2}, which are the conditions found in abscesses and the vagina with tampon use during menstruation. The risk factors for symptomatic disease include a nonimmune host colonized with a toxin-producing organism, which is exposed to focal growth conditions (menstruation plus tampon use or abscess) that induce toxin production. Some hosts may have a varied cytokine response to exposure to TSST-1, helping to explain a spectrum of severity of TSS that may include staphylococcal scarlet fever. The overall mortality rate of treated patients is 3–5% with early treatment.

Approximately 90% of adults have antibody to TSST-1 without a history of clinical TSS, suggesting that most individuals are colonized at some point with a toxin-producing organism at a site (anterior nares) where low-grade or inactive toxin exposure results in an immune response without disease.

CLINICAL MANIFESTATIONS

The diagnosis of TSS is based on clinical manifestations (Table 208.2). Milder cases and those with incomplete clinical characteristics may be common, particularly if the nidus of infection is addressed quickly (e.g., removal of a tampon). The onset of classic TSS is abrupt, with high fever, vomiting, and diarrhea, and is accompanied by sore throat, headache, and myalgias. A diffuse erythematous macular rash (sunburn-like or scarlatiniform) appears within 24 hr and may be associated with hyperemia of pharyngeal, conjunctival, and vaginal mucous membranes. A strawberry tongue is common. Symptoms may include alterations in the level of consciousness, oliguria, and hypotension, which in severe cases may progress to shock and disseminated intravascular coagulation. Complications, including acute respiratory distress syndrome (ARDS), myocardial dysfunction, and renal failure, are commensurate with the degree of shock. Recovery occurs within 7-10 days and is associated with desquamation, particularly of palms and soles; hair and nail loss have also been observed after 1-2 mo. Immunity to the toxins is slow to develop, so recurrences can occur, especially if there is inadequate antibiotic treatment and/or recurrent tampon use. Many cases of apparent scarlet fever without shock may be caused by TSST-1–producing *S. aureus* strains.

DIAGNOSIS

There is no specific laboratory test, and diagnosis depends on meeting certain clinical and laboratory criteria in the absence of an alternate diagnosis (see Fig. 208.2). Appropriate tests reveal involvement of multiple organ systems, including the hepatic, renal, muscular, gastrointestinal, cardiopulmonary, and central nervous systems. Bacterial cultures of the associated focus (vagina, abscess) before administration of antibiotics usually yield *S. aureus,* although this is not a required element of the definition.

Table 208.2	Diagnostic Criteria of Staphylococcal Toxic Shock Syndrome

MAJOR CRITERIA (ALL REQUIRED)

Acute fever; temperature >38.8°C (101.8°F)

Hypotension (orthostatic, shock; blood pressure below age-appropriate norms)

Rash (erythroderma with convalescent desquamation)

MINOR CRITERIA (ANY 3 OR MORE)

Mucous membrane inflammation (vaginal, oropharyngeal or conjunctival hyperemia, strawberry tongue)

Vomiting, diarrhea

Liver abnormalities (bilirubin or transaminase greater than twice the upper limit of normal)

Renal abnormalities (blood urea nitrogen or creatinine greater than twice the upper limit of normal, or greater than 5 white blood cells per high-power field)

Muscle abnormalities (myalgia or creatinine phosphokinase greater than twice the upper limit of normal)

Central nervous system abnormalities (alteration in consciousness without focal neurologic signs)

Thrombocytopenia ($\leq$100,000/mm^3)

EXCLUSIONARY CRITERIA

Absence of another explanation

Negative blood cultures (except occasionally for *Staphylococcus aureus*)

Data from Kimberlin DW, Brady MT, Jackson MA, Long SS, editors: *Red book: 2015 report of the Committee on Infectious Diseases*, ed 30, Elk Grove Village, IL, 2015, American Academy of Pediatrics.

Differential Diagnosis

Group A streptococci can cause a similar TSS-like illness, termed **streptococcal TSS** (see Chapter 210), which is often associated with severe streptococcal sepsis or a focal streptococcal infection such as cellulitis, necrotizing fasciitis, or pneumonia.

Kawasaki disease closely resembles TSS clinically but is usually not as severe or rapidly progressive. Both conditions are associated with fever unresponsive to antibiotics, hyperemia of mucous membranes, and an erythematous rash with subsequent desquamation. However, many of the clinical features of TSS are rare in Kawasaki disease, including diffuse myalgia, vomiting, abdominal pain, diarrhea, azotemia, hypotension, ARDS, and shock (see Chapter 191). Kawasaki disease typically occurs in children <5 yr old. Scarlet fever, Rocky Mountain spotted fever, leptospirosis, toxic epidermal necrolysis, sepsis, and measles must also be considered in the differential diagnosis.

TREATMENT

Identification and drainage/removal of any focal source of infection (e.g., abscess, tampon, nasal packing), when present, is essential. Recommended antibiotic therapy for TSS should include the combination of a β-lactamase–resistant antistaphylococcal antibiotic (nafcillin, oxacillin, or cefazolin) plus clindamycin to reduce toxin production. Although TSS is most often caused by MSSA, clinicians should consider use of vancomycin in place of the β-lactam in areas where MRSA rates are very high, when hospital acquired MRSA is suspected, and when the clinical picture overlaps with staphylococcal sepsis.

TSS often requires intensive supportive care, including aggressive **fluid replacement** to prevent or treat hypotension, renal failure, and cardiovascular collapse. Inotropic agents may be needed to treat shock; corticosteroids and intravenous immunoglobulin may be helpful in severe cases.

PREVENTION

The risk for acquiring menstrual TSS is low (1-2 cases/100,000 menstruating women). Changing tampons at least every 8 hr is recommended. If a fever, rash, or dizziness develops during menstruation, any tampon should be removed immediately and medical attention sought. Antistaphylococcal therapy and avoidance of tampon use with subsequent menstrual cycles may also reduce the risk for recurrent menstrual TSS.

Bibliography is available at Expert Consult.

208.3 Coagulase-Negative Staphylococci
James T. Gaensbauer and James K. Todd

At present, there are approximately 30 species of coagulase-negative staphylococci (**CoNS**) affecting or colonizing humans. *Staphylococcus epidermidis* and, less often, *Staphylococcus hominis, S. haemolyticus,* and others, are widely distributed on the skin and are significant causes of nosocomial infection, particularly in the bloodstream of neonatal and immunocompromised hosts, in surgical patients, and in those with indwelling catheters and other medical devices. *Staphylococcus saprophyticus* is a common cause of urinary tract infection (UTI). *Staphylococcus lugdunensis* has been increasingly recognized as a cause of potentially severe infection.

EPIDEMIOLOGY

In the United States, CoNS may be the most common cause of hospital-acquired infection, particularly in NICUs. In many instances, growth of CoNS from clinical specimens represents contamination from skin rather than a cause of true disease, posing significant challenges for clinicians and infection control specialists. CoNS are normal inhabitants of the human skin, throat, mouth, vagina, and urethra. *S. epidermidis* is the most common and persistent species, representing 65–90% of staphylococci present on the skin and mucous membranes. Colonization, sometimes with strains acquired from hospital staff, precedes infection. Alternatively, direct inoculation during surgery may initiate infection of CSF shunts, prosthetic valves, or indwelling vascular lines. For epidemiologic purposes, CoNS can be identified on the basis of molecular DNA methods.

PATHOGENESIS

CoNS produce an exopolysaccharide protective biofilm, particularly on indwelling medical devices, that surrounds the organism and may enhance adhesion to foreign surfaces, resist phagocytosis, and impair penetration of antibiotics. However, the low virulence of CoNS usually requires the presence of another factor for development of clinical disease. Of these, the most significant is the presence of an indwelling catheter or other medical device, including central venous catheters (CVCs), hemodialysis shunts and grafts, CSF shunts (meningitis), peritoneal dialysis catheters (peritonitis), pacemaker wires and electrodes (local infection), prosthetic cardiac valves (endocarditis), and prosthetic joints (arthritis). Other risk factors for the development of infection include immature or compromised immunity and significant exposure to antibiotics.

CLINICAL MANIFESTATIONS
Bacteremia

CoNS, specifically *S. epidermidis,* are the most common cause of nosocomial bacteremia, usually in association with central vascular catheters. In neonates, CoNS bacteremia, with or without a CVC, may be manifested as apnea, bradycardia, temperature instability, abdominal distention, hematochezia, meningitis in the absence of CSF pleocytosis, and cutaneous abscesses. Persistence of positive blood cultures despite adequate antimicrobial therapy is common, particularly when catheters are not removed. In older children, CoNS bacteremia is indolent and is not usually associated with overwhelming septic shock.

Endocarditis

Infection of native heart valves or the right atrial wall secondary to an infected thrombosis at the end of a central line may produce endocarditis. *S. epidermidis* and other CoNS may rarely produce native valve subacute endocarditis in previously normal patients without a CVC. CoNS is a common cause of prosthetic valve endocarditis, presumably a result of inoculation at surgery. Infection of the valve sewing ring, with abscess formation and dissection, produces valve dysfunction, dehiscence, arrhythmias, or valve obstruction (see Chapter 464). *S. lugdunensis* has been increasingly associated with severe endocardial infection in adults, but its role as a significant pediatric pathogen is unclear.

Central Venous Catheter Infection

CVCs become infected through the exit site and subcutaneous tunnel, which provide a direct path to the bloodstream. *S. epidermidis* is the most frequent pathogen, in part because of its high rate of cutaneous colonization. Line sepsis is usually manifested as fever and leukocytosis; tenderness and erythema may be present at the exit site or along the subcutaneous tunnel. Catheter thrombosis may complicate line sepsis. Disease severity with CoNS is often less severe than other etiologies of line infection.

Cerebrospinal Fluid Shunts

CoNS, introduced at surgery, is the most common pathogen associated with CSF shunt meningitis. Most infections (70–80%) occur within 2 mo of the operation and manifest as signs of meningeal irritation, fever, increased intracranial pressure (headache), or peritonitis from the intraabdominal position of the distal end of the shunt tubing.

Urinary Tract Infection

S. saprophyticus is a common cause of primary UTIs in sexually active females. Manifestations are similar to those characteristics of UTI caused by *Escherichia coli* (see Chapter 553). CoNS also cause asymptomatic UTI in hospitalized patients with urinary catheters and after urinary tract surgery or transplantation.

DIAGNOSIS

Because *S. epidermidis* is a common skin inhabitant and may contaminate poorly collected blood cultures, differentiating bacteremia from contamination is often difficult. True bacteremia should be suspected if blood cultures grow rapidly (within 24 hr), >1 blood culture is positive with the same CoNS strain, cultures from both line and peripheral sites are positive, and clinical and laboratory signs and symptoms compatible with CoNS sepsis are present and subsequently resolve with appropriate therapy. No blood culture that is positive for CoNS in a neonate or patient with an intravascular catheter should be considered contaminated without careful assessment of the foregoing criteria and examination of the patient. Before initiating presumptive antimicrobial therapy in such patients, it is always prudent to draw 2 separate blood cultures to facilitate subsequent interpretation if CoNS is grown. Increasingly, PCR techniques can allow rapid identification of CoNS in positive blood cultures; use of such methods may prevent unnecessary antibiotic exposure.

TREATMENT

Because most CoNS strains are resistant to methicillin, **vancomycin** is the initial drug of choice. The addition of rifampin to vancomycin may increase antimicrobial efficacy due to good penetration of this antibiotic into biofilms on indwelling medical devices. Other antibiotics with good in vitro activity against CoNS may be considered in certain circumstances. These include linezolid, quinupristin-dalfopristin, and daptomycin. Antibiotics with potential activity include teicoplanin, clindamycin, levofloxacin, and TMP-SMX. Removal of an infected catheter is ideal. However, this is not always possible because of the therapeutic requirements of the underlying disease (e.g., nutrition for short bowel syndrome, chemotherapy for malignancy). A trial of IV vancomycin (potentially with addition of rifampin) is indicated to attempt to preserve the use of the central line, as long as systemic manifestations of infection are not severe. Antibiotic therapy given through an infected CVC (alternating lumens if multiple) and the use of antibiotic locks in conjunction with systemic therapy may increase the likelihood of curing CoNS line sepsis without line removal. Prosthetic heart valves and CSF shunts usually need to be removed to treat the infection adequately.

Peritonitis caused by *S. epidermidis* in patients on continuous ambulatory peritoneal dialysis is an infection that may be treated with IV or intraperitoneal antibiotics without removing the dialysis catheter. If the organism is resistant to methicillin, vancomycin adjusted for renal function is appropriate therapy. Unlike most CoNS, *S. saprophyticus* is usually methicillin susceptible, and UTI can typically be treated with a first-generation cephalosporin (cephalexin), amoxicillin–clavulanic acid, or TMP-SMX.

PROGNOSIS

Most episodes of CoNS bacteremia respond successfully to antibiotics and removal of any foreign body that is present. Poor prognosis is associated with malignancy, neutropenia, and infected prosthetic or native heart valves. CoNS increases morbidity, duration of hospitalization, and mortality among patients with underlying complicated illnesses.

PREVENTION

Iatrogenic morbidity and resource utilization caused by contaminated blood cultures can be reduced by using gloves, good skin preparatory techniques, and trained, dedicated personnel to draw blood cultures. Prevention of CoNS infection of indwelling lines includes basic techniques such as central line care "bundles," which incorporate good hand hygiene, decontamination of hubs and ports before access, minimizing frequency of access, and frequent replacement of external connections and infusion materials. In a recent large randomized controlled trial in children, antibiotic-impregnated catheters significantly reduced rates of central line–associated bloodstream infections.

Bibliography is available at Expert Consult.

Chapter 209
Streptococcus pneumoniae (Pneumococcus)
Kacy A. Ramirez and Timothy R. Peters

第二百零九章
肺炎链球菌（肺炎球菌）

中文导读

　　本章首先阐述了肺炎链球菌（肺炎球菌）是儿童群体一种非常重要的病原体，可引起严重的甚至危及生命的疾病。肺炎链球菌多糖-蛋白质结合疫苗（PCV）的应用仍然是控制这一威胁的最佳方法。随后分别介绍了关于肺炎链球菌感染的病因、流行病学、发病机制、临床表现、诊断、治疗、预后和预防等内容。其中，着重介绍了易患侵袭性肺炎链球菌感染的高危儿童、肺炎链球菌结合疫苗推荐接种方案。

Streptococcus pneumoniae (pneumococcus) is an important pathogen that kills more than 1 million children each year. Childhood pneumococcal disease is prevalent and typically severe, causes numerous clinical syndromes, and is a major cause of life-threatening pneumonia, bacteremia, and meningitis. Antimicrobial resistance in pneumococcus is a major public health problem, with 15–30% of isolates worldwide classified as **multidrug resistant** (**MDR**; resistant to ≥3 classes of antibiotics). Pneumococcal polysaccharide-protein conjugate vaccines (**PCVs**) developed for infants have been highly successful in the control of disease caused by virulent vaccine-specific serotypes. Epidemiologic surveillance reveals a dynamic pneumococcal ecology with emergence of highly virulent, MDR serotypes. Ongoing vaccine development and distribution efforts remain the best approach to control this threat to childhood health.

ETIOLOGY

Streptococcus pneumoniae is a gram-positive, lancet-shaped, polysaccharide encapsulated diplococcus, occurring occasionally as individual cocci or in chains; >90 serotypes have been identified by type-specific capsular polysaccharides. Antisera to some pneumococcal polysaccharides cross-react with other pneumococcal types, defining serogroups (e.g., 6A and 6B). Encapsulated strains cause most serious disease in humans. Capsular polysaccharides impede phagocytosis. Virulence is related in part to capsular size, but pneumococcal types with capsules of the same size can vary widely in virulence.

On solid media, *S. pneumoniae* forms unpigmented, umbilicated colonies surrounded by a zone of incomplete (α) hemolysis. *S. pneumoniae* is bile soluble (i.e., 10% deoxycholate) and optochin sensitive. *S. pneumoniae* is closely related to the viridans groups of *Streptococcus mitis*, which typically overlap phenotypically with pneumococci. The conventional laboratory definition of pneumococci continues to rely on bile and optochin sensitivity, although considerable confusion occurs in distinguishing pneumococci and other α-hemolytic streptococci. Pneumococcal capsules can be microscopically visualized and typed by exposing organisms to type-specific antisera that combine with their unique capsular polysaccharide, rendering the capsule refractile (Quellung reaction). Specific antibodies to capsular polysaccharides confer protection on the host, promoting opsonization and phagocytosis. Additionally, CD4⁺ T cells have a direct role in antibody-independent immunity to pneumococcal nasopharyngeal colonization. Conjugated PCVs promote T-cell immunity and protect against pneumococcal colonization, in contrast to the pneumococcal polysaccharide vaccine (PPSV23) that is used in adults and certain high-risk pediatric populations and that does not affect nasopharyngeal colonization.

EPIDEMIOLOGY

Most healthy individuals carry various *S. pneumoniae* serotypes in their upper respiratory tract; >90% of children between 6 mo and 5 yr of age harbor *S. pneumoniae* in the nasopharynx at some time. A single serotype usually is carried by a given individual for an extended period (45 days to 6 mo). Carriage does not consistently induce local or systemic immunity sufficient to prevent later reacquisition of the same serotype. Rates of pneumococcal carriage peak during the 1st and 2nd yr of life and decline gradually thereafter. Carriage rates are highest in institutional setting and during the winter, and rates are lowest in summer. Nasopharyngeal carriage of pneumococci is common among young children attending out-of-home care, with rates of 21–59% in point prevalence studies.

Before the introduction of heptavalent pneumococcal conjugate vaccine (**PCV7**) in 2000, serotypes 4, 6B, 9V, 14, 18C, 19F, and 23F caused most invasive childhood pneumococcal infections in the United States. The introduction of PCVs resulted in a marked decrease in **invasive pneumococcal infections (IPIs)** in children. By 2005, however, IPIs began to increase slightly because of an increase in non-PCV7 serotypes, particularly serotype 19A. Serotype replacement can result from expansion of existing nonvaccine serotypes, as well as from vaccine-type pneumococci acquiring the polysaccharide capsule of a nonvaccine serotype (**serotype switching**). Since the introduction of PCV13 in 2010 in the United States, there has been a decline in IPIs caused by new vaccine serotypes, including 19A. Nonetheless, 19A remains an important cause of meningitis. Indirect protection of unvaccinated persons has occurred since PCV introduction, and this *herd protection* is likely a result of decreases in nasopharyngeal carriage of virulent pneumococcal vaccine serotypes.

S. pneumoniae is the most frequent cause of bacteremia, bacterial pneumonia, otitis media, and bacterial meningitis in children. The decreased ability in children <2 yr old to produce antibody against the T-cell–independent polysaccharide antigens and the high prevalence of colonization may explain an increased susceptibility to pneumococcal infection and the decreased effectiveness of polysaccharide vaccines. Children at increased risk of pneumococcal infections include those with sickle cell disease, asplenia, deficiencies in humoral (B-cell) and complement-mediated immunity, HIV infection, certain malignancies (e.g., leukemia, lymphoma), chronic heart, lung, or renal disease (particularly nephrotic syndrome), cerebrospinal fluid (CSF) leak, and cochlear implants. Table 209.1 lists other high-risk groups. Some American Indian, Alaska Native, and African American children may also be at increased risk. Children <5 yr old in out-of-home daycare are at increased risk (approximately 2-fold higher) of experiencing IPIs than other children. Males are more frequently affected than females. Because immunocompetent vaccinated children have had fever episodes

of IPI, the proportion of infected children with immunologic risk factors has increased (estimated at 20%).

Pneumococcal disease usually occurs sporadically but can be spread from person to person by respiratory droplet transmission. *S. pneumoniae* is an important cause of secondary bacterial pneumonia in patients with influenza. During influenza epidemics and pandemics, most deaths result from bacterial pneumonia, and pneumococcus is the predominant bacterial pathogen isolated in this setting. Pneumococcal copathogenicity may be important in disease caused by other respiratory viruses as well.

PATHOGENESIS

Invasion of the host is affected by a number of factors. Nonspecific defense mechanisms, including the presence of other bacteria in the nasopharynx, may limit multiplication of pneumococci. Aspiration of secretions containing pneumococci is hindered by the epiglottic reflex and by respiratory epithelial cell cilia, which move infected mucus toward the pharynx. Similarly, normal ciliary flow of fluid from the middle ear through the eustachian tube and sinuses to the nasopharynx usually prevents infection with nasopharyngeal flora, including pneumococci. Interference with these normal clearance mechanisms by allergy, viral infection, or irritants (e.g., smoke) may allow colonization and subsequent infection with these organisms in otherwise normally sterile sites.

Virulent pneumococci are intrinsically resistant to phagocytosis by alveolar macrophages. Pneumococcal disease frequently is facilitated by viral respiratory tract infection, which may produce mucosal injury, diminish epithelial cell ciliary activity, and depress the function of alveolar macrophages and neutrophils. Phagocytosis may be impeded by respiratory secretions and alveolar exudate. In the lungs and other tissues, the spread of infection is facilitated by the antiphagocytic properties of the pneumococcal capsule. Surface fluids of the respiratory tract contain only small amounts of immunoglobulin G and are deficient in complement. During inflammation, there is limited influx of IgG, complement, and neutrophils. Phagocytosis of bacteria by neutrophils may occur, but normal human serum may not opsonize pneumococci and facilitate phagocytosis by alveolar macrophages. In tissues, pneumococci multiply and spread through the lymphatics or bloodstream or, less often, by direct extension from a local site of infection (e.g., sinuses). In bacteremia the severity of disease is related to the number of organisms in the bloodstream and to the integrity of specific host defenses. A poor prognosis correlates with very large numbers of pneumococci and high concentrations of capsular polysaccharide in the blood and CSF.

Invasive pneumococcal disease is 30- to 100-fold more prevalent in children with sickle cell disease and other hemoglobinopathies and in children with congenital or surgical asplenia than in the general population. This risk is greatest in infants <2 yr old, the age when antibody production to most serotypes is poor. The increased frequency of pneumococcal disease in asplenic persons is related to both deficient opsonization of pneumococci and absence of clearance by the spleen of circulating bacteria. Children with sickle cell disease also have deficits in the antibody-independent properdin (alternative) pathway of complement activation, in addition to functional asplenia. Both complement pathways contribute to antibody-independent and antibody-dependent **opsonophagocytosis** of pneumococci. With advancing age (e.g., >5 yr), children with sickle cell disease produce anticapsular antibody, augmenting antibody-dependent opsonophagocytosis and greatly reducing, but not eliminating, the risk of severe pneumococcal disease. Deficiency of many of the complement components (e.g., C2 and C3) is associated with recurrent pyogenic infection, including *S. pneumoniae* infection. The efficacy of phagocytosis also is diminished in patients with B- and T-cell immunodeficiency syndromes (e.g., agammaglobulinemia, severe combined immunodeficiency) or loss of immunoglobulin (e.g., nephrotic syndrome) and is largely caused by a deficiency of opsonic anticapsular antibody. These observations suggest that opsonization of pneumococci depends on the alternative complement pathway in antibody-deficient persons, and that recovery from pneumococcal disease depends on the development of anticapsular antibodies that act as opsonins, enhancing phagocytosis and killing of pneumococci. Children with HIV infection also have high rates of IPI similar to or greater than rates in children with sickle cell disease, although rates of invasive pneumococcal disease

Table 209.1	Children at Increased Risk of Invasive Pneumococcal Infection
RISK GROUP	**CONDITION**
Immunocompetent children	Chronic heart disease* Chronic lung disease† Diabetes mellitus Cerebrospinal fluid leaks Cochlear implant
Children with functional or anatomic asplenia	Sickle cell disease and other hemoglobinopathies Congenital or acquired asplenia, or splenic dysfunction
Children with immunocompromising conditions	HIV infection Chronic renal failure and nephrotic syndrome Diseases associated with treatment with immunosuppressive drugs or radiation therapy, including malignant neoplasm, leukemia, lymphoma, and Hodgkin disease; or stem cell and solid-organ transplantation Congenital immunodeficiency‡ Toll-like receptor signaling defects (IRAK-4, IKBKG, MyD88) *NEMO* gene defects

*Particularly cyanotic congenital heart disease and cardiac failure.
†Including asthma if treated with high-dose oral corticosteroid therapy.
‡Includes B-(humoral) or T-lymphocyte deficiency; complement deficiencies, particularly C1,C2,C3, and C4 deficiency; and phagocytic disorders, excluding chronic granulomatous disease.
Adapted from Centers for Disease Control and Prevention: Licensure of a 13-valent pneumococcal conjugate vaccine (PCV13) and recommendations for use among children: Advisory Committee on Immunization Practices, *MMWR* 59(RR-11):1–18, 2010 (Table 2).

decreased after the introduction of highly active antiretroviral therapy (HAART).

CLINICAL MANIFESTATIONS

The signs and symptoms of pneumococcal infection are related to the anatomic site of disease. Common clinical syndromes include otitis media (Chapter 658), sinusitis (see Chapter 408), pneumonia (Fig. 209.1) (Chapter 428), and sepsis (Chapter 88). Before routine use of PCVs, pneumococci caused >80% of bacteremia episodes in infants 3-36 mo old with fever without an identifiable source (i.e., occult bacteremia). Bacteremia may be followed by meningitis (Chapter 621), osteomyelitis (Chapter 704), suppurative (septic) arthritis (Chapter 705), endocarditis (Chapter 464), and rarely, brain abscess (Chapter 622). Primary peritonitis (Chapter 398.1) may occur in children with peritoneal effusions caused by nephrotic syndrome and other ascites-producing conditions. Local complications of infection may occur, causing empyema, pericarditis, mastoiditis, epidural abscess, periorbital cellulitis, or meningitis. Hemolytic-uremic syndrome (Chapter 511.04) and disseminated intravascular coagulation also occur as rare complications of pneumococcal infections. Epidemic conjunctivitis caused by nonencapsulated or encapsulated pneumococci occurs as well.

DIAGNOSIS

The diagnosis of pneumococcal infection is established by recovery of *S. pneumoniae* from the site of infection or the blood/sterile body fluid. Although pneumococci may be found in the nose or throat of patients with otitis media, pneumonia, septicemia, or meningitis, cultures of these locations are generally not helpful for diagnosis, since they are not indicative of causation. Blood cultures should be obtained in children with pneumonia, meningitis, arthritis, osteomyelitis, peritonitis, pericarditis, or gangrenous skin lesions. Because of the implementation of universal vaccination with PCVs, there has been a substantial decrease in the incidence of occult bacteremia, but blood cultures should still be considered in febrile patients with clinical toxicity or significant leukocytosis. Leukocytosis often is pronounced, with total white blood cell counts frequently >15,000/μL. In severe cases of pneumococcal disease, WBC count may be low.

Pneumococci can be identified in body fluids as gram-positive, lancet-shaped diplococci. Early in the course of pneumococcal meningitis, many bacteria may be seen in relatively acellular CSF. With current methods of continuously monitored blood culture systems, the average time to isolation of pneumococcal organisms is 14-15 hr. Pneumococcal latex agglutination tests for urine or other body fluids suffer from poor sensitivity and add little to gram-stained fluids and standard cultures. Multiplex real-time polymerase chain reaction (PCR) assays are specific and more sensitive than culture of pleural fluid, CSF, and blood, particularly in patients who have recently received antimicrobial therapy. Additional investigational assays, including serotype-specific urinary antigen detection, have not been validated.

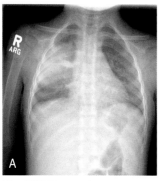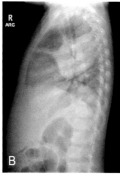

Fig. 209.1 Bacterial pneumonia. "Round" pneumonia caused by *Streptococcus pneumoniae* in 2 yr old girl with a 2-day history of cough, high fever, leukocytosis, and back pain.

TREATMENT

Antimicrobial resistance among *S. pneumoniae* continues to be a serious healthcare concern, especially for the widely used β-lactams, macrolides, and fluoroquinolones. Serotypes 6A, 6B, 9V, 14, 19A, 19F, and 23F are the most common serotypes associated with resistance to penicillin. Consequently, the introduction of the 7- and 13-valent pneumococcal conjugate vaccines (**PCV7** and **PCV13**) has altered antimicrobial resistance patterns.

Resistance in pneumococcal organisms to penicillin and the extended-spectrum cephalosporins cefotaxime and ceftriaxone is defined by the minimum inhibitory concentration (MIC), as well as clinical syndrome. Pneumococci are considered *susceptible, intermediate,* or *resistant* to various antibacterial agents based on specific MIC breakpoints. For patients with pneumococcal meningitis, penicillin-susceptible strains have MIC ≤0.06 μg/mL, and penicillin-resistant strains have MIC ≥0.12 μg/mL. For patients with nonmeningeal pneumococcal infections, breakpoints are higher; in particular, penicillin-susceptible strains have MIC ≤2 μg/mL, and penicillin resistant strains have MIC ≥8 μg/mL. For patients with meningitis, cefotaxime- and ceftriaxone-susceptible strains have MIC ≤0.5 μg/mL, and resistant strains have MIC ≥2.0 μg/mL. For patients with nonmeningeal pneumococcal disease, breakpoints are higher, and cefotaxime- and ceftriaxone-susceptible strains have MIC ≤1 μg/mL, and resistant strains have MIC ≥4 μg/mL. In cases when the pneumococcus is resistant to erythromycin but sensitive to clindamycin, *a D-test should be performed* to determine whether clindamycin resistance can be induced; if the D-test is positive, clindamycin should not be used to complete treatment of the patient. More than 30% of pneumococcal isolates are resistant to trimethoprim-sulfamethoxazole (TMP-SMX); levofloxacin resistance is low but has also been reported. All isolates from children with severe infections should be tested for antibiotic susceptibility, given widespread pneumococcal MDR strains. Resistance to vancomycin has not been seen at this time, but vancomycin-tolerant pneumococci that are killed at a slower rate have been reported, and these tolerant pneumococci may be associated with a worse clinical outcome. Linezolid is an oxazolidinone antibacterial with activity against MDR gram-positive organisms, including pneumococcus, and has been used in the treatment of MDR pneumococcal pneumonia, meningitis, and severe otitis. Despite early favorable studies, use of this drug is limited by myelosuppression and high cost, and linezolid resistance in pneumococcus is reported.

Children ≥1 mo old with suspected pneumococcal meningitis should be treated with combination therapy using **vancomycin** (60 mg/kg/24 hr divided every 6 hr IV), and high-dose **cefotaxime** (300 mg/kg/24 hr divided every 8 hr IV) or **ceftriaxone** (100 mg/kg/24 hr divided every 12 hr IV). Proven pneumococcal meningitis can be treated with penicillin alone, or cefotaxime or ceftriaxone alone, if the isolate is penicillin susceptible. If the organism is nonsusceptible (i.e., intermediate or full resistance) to penicillin but susceptible to cefotaxime and ceftriaxone, pneumococcal meningitis can be treated with cefotaxime or ceftriaxone alone. However, if the organism is nonsusceptible to penicillin and to cefotaxime or ceftriaxone, pneumococcal meningitis should be treated with combination vancomycin plus cefotaxime or ceftriaxone, not with vancomycin alone, and consideration should be given to the addition of **rifampin**. Some experts recommend use of corticosteroids in pneumococcal meningitis early in the course of disease, but data demonstrating clear benefit in children are lacking.

The 2011 Infectious Diseases Society of America guidelines recommend **amoxicillin** as first-line therapy for previously healthy, appropriately immunized infants and preschool children with mild to moderate, uncomplicated community-acquired pneumonia. **Ampicillin** or **penicillin G** may be administered to the fully immunized infant or school-age child admitted to a hospital ward with uncomplicated community-acquired pneumonia, when local epidemiologic data document lack of substantial high-level penicillin resistance for invasive *S. pneumoniae*. Empirical therapy with a parenteral **third-generation cephalosporin** (ceftriaxone or cefotaxime) should be prescribed for hospitalized infants and children who are not fully immunized, in regions where local epidemiology of invasive pneumococcal strains documents widespread penicillin resistance, or for infants and children with life-threatening

Table 209.2	Comparison of Pneumococcal Vaccines Licensed in United States*	
CARRIER PROTEIN	**PNEUMOCOCCAL CAPSULAR POLYSACCHARIDES**	**MANUFACTURER**
Diphtheria CRM₁₉₇ protein	**4, 6B, 9V, 14, 18C, 19F, 23F**	Wyeth Lederle (PCV7, Prevnar)
Diphtheria CRM₁₉₇ protein	1, 3, **4**, 5, 6A, **6B**, 7F, **9V, 14, 18C**, 19A, **19F, 23F**	Wyeth Lederle (PCV13, Prevnar 13)
None	1, 2, 3, **4**, 5, **6B**, 7F, 8, 9N, **9V**, 10A, 11A, 12F, **14**, 15B, 17F, **18C,** 19A, **19F**, 20, 22F, **23F**, 33F	Sanofi Pasteur MSD (PPSV23, Pneumovax II)

*PCV7 serotypes in **bold**.

infection, including those with empyema. Non–β-lactam agents, such as vancomycin, have not been shown to be more effective than third-generation cephalosporins in the treatment of pneumococcal pneumonia, given the degree of drug resistance currently seen in the United States.

Higher doses of amoxicillin (80-100 mg/kg/24 hr) have been successful in the treatment of otitis media caused by penicillin-nonsusceptible strains. If the patient has failed initial antibiotic therapy, alternative agents should be active against penicillin-nonsusceptible pneumococcus as well as β-lactamase–producing *Haemophilus influenzae* and *Moraxella catarrhalis*. These include high-dose oral amoxicillin-clavulanate (in the 14:1 formulation to reduce risk of diarrhea), oral cefdinir, cefpodoxime, or cefuroxime; or a 3-day course of intramuscular (IM) ceftriaxone if patients fail oral therapy. Empirical treatment of pneumococcal disease should be based on knowledge of susceptibility patterns in specific communities.

For individuals with a non–type I allergic reaction to penicillin, cephalosporins (standard dosing) can be used. For type I allergic reactions (immediate, anaphylactic) to β-lactam antibiotics, clindamycin and levofloxacin are preferred alternatives depending on the site of infection (e.g., clindamycin may be effective for pneumococcal infections other than meningitis). TMP-SMX may also be considered for susceptible strains, but erythromycin (or related macrolides; e.g., azithromycin, clarithromycin) should be avoided given high rates of resistance.

PROGNOSIS

Prognosis depends on the integrity of host defenses, virulence and numbers of the infecting organism, age of the host, site and extent of the infection, and adequacy of treatment. The mortality rate for pneumococcal meningitis is approximately 10% in most studies. Pneumococcal meningitis results in sensorineural hearing loss in 20–30% of patients and can cause other serious neurologic sequelae, including paralysis, epilepsy, blindness, and intellectual deficits.

PREVENTION

The highly successful PCVs have resulted in a marked decrease in IPIs in children. PCVs provoke protective antibody responses in 90% of infants given these vaccines at 2, 4, and 6 mo of age, and greatly enhanced responses (e.g., immunologic memory) are apparent after vaccine doses given at 12-15 mo of age (Table 209.2). In a large clinical trial, PCV7 was shown to reduce invasive disease caused by vaccine serotypes by up to 97% and to reduce invasive disease caused by all serotypes, including serotypes not in the vaccine, by 89%. Children who received PCV7 had 7% fewer episodes of acute otitis media and underwent 20% fewer tympanostomy tube placements than unvaccinated children. Following PCV13, a 64% reduction in IPIs caused by vaccine serotypes has been seen, particularly in children <5 yr old. The number of pneumococcal isolates and percentage of isolates with high-level penicillin resistance from cultures taken from children with otitis media or mastoiditis for clinical indications have decreased, largely related to decreases in serotype 19A. Rates of hospitalization for pneumococcal pneumonia among U.S. children decreased after PCV13 introduction. The number of cases of pneumococcal meningitis in children remain unchanged, but the proportion of PCV13 serotypes have decreased significantly. In addition, pneumococcal conjugate vaccines significantly reduce nasopharyngeal carriage of vaccine serotypes. PCVs have significantly decreased rates of invasive pneumococcal disease in children with sickle cell disease,

Table 209.3	Recommended Routine Vaccination Schedule for 13-Valent Pneumococcal Conjugate Vaccine (PCV13) Among Infants and Children Who Have Not Received Previous Doses of 7-Valent Vaccine (PCV7) or PCV13, by Age at 1st Dose—United States, 2010

AGE AT 1ST DOSE (mo)	PRIMARY PCV13 SERIES*	PCV13 BOOSTER DOSE†
2-6	3 doses	1 dose at age 12-15 mo
7-11	2 doses	1 dose at age 12-15 mo
12-23	2 doses	—
24-59 (healthy children)	1 dose	—
24-71 (children with certain chronic diseases or immunocompromising conditions‡)	2 doses	—

*Minimum interval between doses is 8 wk except for children vaccinated at age <12 mo, for whom minimum interval between doses is 4 wk. Minimum age for administration of 1st dose is 6 wk.
†Given at least 8 wk after the previous dose.
‡See Table 209.1.
From Centers for Disease Control and Prevention. Licensure of a 13-valent pneumococcal conjugate vaccine (PCV13) and recommendations for use among children: Advisory Committee on Immunization Practices, *MMWR* 59(RR-11):1–18 (Table 8); 59:258–261, 2010 (Table 3).

and studies suggest substantial protection for HIV-infected children and splenectomized adults. Adverse events after the administration of PCV have included local swelling and redness and slightly increased rates of fever, when used in conjunction with other childhood vaccines.

Immunologic responsiveness and efficacy after administration of pneumococcal polysaccharide vaccines (PPSV23) is unpredictable in children <2 yr old. PPSV23 contains purified polysaccharide of 23 pneumococcal serotypes responsible for >95% of invasive disease. The clinical efficacy of PPSV23 is controversial, and studies have yielded conflicting results.

Immunization with PCV13 is recommended for all infants on a schedule for primary immunization, in previously unvaccinated infants, and for transition for those partially vaccinated with PCV7 (Table 209.3). High-risk children ≥2 yr old, such as those with asplenia, sickle cell disease, some types of immune deficiency (e.g., antibody deficiencies), HIV infection, cochlear implant, CSF leak, diabetes mellitus, and chronic lung, heart, or kidney disease (including nephrotic syndrome), may benefit also from PPSV23 administered after 2 yr of age following priming with the scheduled doses of PCV13. Thus, it is recommended that children 2 yr of age and older with these underlying conditions receive supplemental vaccination with PPSV23. A 2nd dose of PPSV23 is recommended 5 yr after the 1st dose of PPSV23 for persons ≥2 yr old who are immunocompromised, have sickle cell disease, or functional or

		PCV13 RECOMMENDED	PPSV23 RECOMMENDED	REVACCINATION 5 YR AFTER 1ST DOSE
Table 209.4	Medical Conditions or Other Indications for Administration of PCV13,* and Indications for PPSV23[†] Administration, and Revaccination for Children Age 6–18 Yr[‡]			
RISK GROUP	**UNDERLYING MEDICAL CONDITION**			
Immunocompetent persons	Chronic heart disease[§]		✓	
	Chronic lung disease[ǁ]		✓	
	Diabetes mellitus		✓	
	Cerebrospinal fluid leaks	✓	✓	
	Cochlear implants	✓	✓	
	Alcoholism		✓	
	Chronic liver disease		✓	
	Cigarette smoking		✓	
Persons with functional or anatomic asplenia	Sickle cell disease, other hemoglobinopathies	✓	✓	✓
	Congenital or acquired asplenia	✓	✓	✓
Immunocompromised persons	Congenital or acquired immunodeficiencies[¶]	✓	✓	✓
	HIV infection	✓	✓	✓
	Chronic renal failure	✓	✓	✓
	Nephrotic syndrome	✓	✓	✓
	Leukemia	✓	✓	✓
	Lymphoma	✓	✓	✓
	Hodgkin disease	✓	✓	✓
	Generalized malignancy	✓	✓	✓
	Iatrogenic immunosuppression**	✓	✓	✓
	Solid-organ transplant	✓	✓	✓
	Multiple myeloma	✓	✓	✓

*13-valent pneumococcal conjugate vaccine.

[†]23-valent pneumococcal polysaccharide vaccine.

[‡]Children age 2-5 yr with chronic conditions (e.g., heart disease, diabetes), immunocompromising conditions (e.g., HIV), functional or anatomic asplenia (including sickle cell disease), cerebrospinal fluid leaks, or cochlear implants, and who have not previously received PCV13, have been recommended to receive PCV13 since 2010.

[§]Including congestive heart failure and cardiomyopathies.

[ǁ]Including chronic obstructive pulmonary disease, emphysema, and asthma.

[¶]Includes B- (humoral) or T-lymphocyte deficiency, complement deficiencies (particularly C1, C2, C3, and C4 deficiencies), and phagocytic disorders (excluding chronic granulomatous disease).

**Diseases requiring treatment with immunosuppressive drugs, including long-term systemic corticosteroids and radiation therapy.

From Centers for Disease Control and Prevention: Use of 13-valent pneumococcal conjugate vaccine and 23-valent pneumococcal polysaccharide vaccine among children aged 6-18 years with immunocompromising conditions: recommendations of the Advisory Committee on Immunization Practices, *MMWR* 62:521–524, 2013.

anatomic asplenia. Additional recommendations have been made for at-risk children 6-18 yr old (Table 209.4).

Immunization with pneumococcal vaccines also may prevent pneumococcal disease caused by nonvaccine serotypes that are serotypically related to a vaccine strain. However, because current vaccines do not eliminate all pneumococcal invasive infections, penicillin prophylaxis is recommended for children at high risk of invasive pneumococcal disease, including children with asplenia or sickle cell disease. Oral penicillin V potassium (125 mg twice daily for children <3 yr old; 250 mg twice daily for children ≥3 yr old) decreases the incidence of pneumococcal sepsis in children with sickle cell disease. Once-monthly IM benzathine penicillin G (600,000 units every 3-4 wk for children weighing <60 lb;

1,200,000 units every 3-4 wk for children weighing ≥60 lb) may also provide prophylaxis. Erythromycin may be used in children with penicillin allergy, but its efficacy is unproven. Prophylaxis in sickle cell disease has been safely discontinued after the 5th birthday in children who have received all recommended pneumococcal vaccine doses and who had not experienced invasive pneumococcal disease. Prophylaxis is often administered for at least 2 yr after splenectomy or up to 5 yr of age. Efficacy in children >5 yr old and adolescents is unproved. If oral antibiotic prophylaxis is used, strict compliance must be encouraged.

Given the rapid emergence of penicillin-resistant pneumococci, especially in children receiving long-term, low-dose therapy, prophylaxis cannot be relied on to prevent disease. High-risk children with fever should be promptly evaluated and treated regardless of vaccination or penicillin prophylaxis history.

Bibliography is available at Expert Consult.

Chapter **210**
Group A Streptococcus
*Stanford T. Shulman and
Caroline H. Reuter*

第二百一十章
A组链球菌

中文导读

本章主要介绍了关于A组链球菌感染的病因、流行病学、发病机制、临床表现、诊断、治疗、并发症、预后和预防等内容。在A组链球菌感染后的临床表现部分详细介绍了呼吸道感染、猩红热、脓疱病、丹毒、肛周皮炎、阴道炎和严重侵袭性疾病。另外，重点介绍了风湿热的病因、流行病学、发病机制、临床表现、诊断、治疗、并发症、预后和预防等内容。

Group A streptococcus (**GAS**), also known as *Streptococcus pyogenes*, is a common cause of infections of the upper respiratory tract (pharyngitis) and the skin (impetigo, pyoderma) in children. Less frequently, GAS causes perianal cellulitis, vaginitis, septicemia, pneumonia, endocarditis, pericarditis, osteomyelitis, suppurative arthritis, myositis, cellulitis, omphalitis, and other infections. This organism also causes distinct clinical entities (scarlet fever and erysipelas), as well as streptococcal toxic shock syndrome and monomicrobial necrotizing fasciitis. GAS is also the cause of 2 potentially serious nonsuppurative complications: rheumatic fever (Chapters 210.1 and 465) and acute glomerulonephritis (Chapter 537.4).

ETIOLOGY

Group A streptococci are gram-positive, coccoid-shaped bacteria that tend to grow in chains. They are broadly classified by their hemolytic activity on mammalian (typically sheep) red blood cells. The zone of complete hemolysis that surrounds colonies grown on blood agar distinguishes β-hemolytic (complete hemolysis) from α-hemolytic (green or partial hemolysis) and γ (nonhemolytic) species. The β-hemolytic streptococci can be divided into groups by a group-specific polysaccharide (**Lancefield C carbohydrate**) located in the bacterial cell wall. More than 20 serologic groups are identified, designated by the letters A through V. Serologic grouping by the Lancefield method is precise, but group A organisms can be identified more readily by any of a number of latex agglutination, coagglutination, molecular assays or enzyme immunoassays. Group A strains can also be distinguished from other groups by differences in sensitivity to bacitracin. A disk containing 0.04 unit of bacitracin inhibits the growth of most group A strains, whereas other groups are generally resistant to this antibiotic. This method is approximately 95% accurate. GAS can be subdivided into >220 serotypes on the basis of the **M protein** antigen, which is located on the cell surface and in fimbriae that project from the outer surface of the cell.

Currently, a molecular approach to M-typing GAS isolates using the polymerase chain reaction (PCR) is based on sequencing the terminal portion of the *emm* gene of GAS that encodes the M protein. More than 220 distinct M types have been identified using *emm* typing, with excellent correlation between known serotypes and *emm* types. The *emm* types can be grouped into *emm* clusters that share structural and binding properties. Immunity is largely based on type-specific opsonic anti-M antibody.

M/*emm* typing is valuable for epidemiologic studies; specific GAS diseases tend to be associated with certain M types. Types 1, 12, 28, 4, 3, and 2 (in that order) are the most common causes of uncomplicated streptococcal pharyngitis in the United States. M types usually associated with pharyngitis rarely cause skin infections, and the M types associated with skin infections rarely cause pharyngitis. A few **pharyngeal** strains (e.g., M type 12) are associated with glomerulonephritis, but many more **skin** strains (e.g., M types 49, 55, 57, and 60) are considered nephritogenic. Several pharyngeal serotypes (e.g., M types 1, 3, 5, 6, 18, and 29), but no skin strains, are associated with **acute rheumatic fever** in North America. Rheumatogenic potential is not solely dependent on serotype but is likely a characteristic of specific strains within several serotypes.

EPIDEMIOLOGY

Humans are the natural reservoir for GAS. These bacteria are highly communicable and can cause disease in normal individuals of all ages who do not have type-specific immunity against the particular serotype involved. Disease in neonates is uncommon in developed countries, probably because of maternally acquired antibody. The incidence of pharyngeal infections is highest in children 5-15 yr of age, especially in young school-age children. These infections are most common in the northern regions of the United States, especially during winter and early spring. Children with untreated acute pharyngitis spread GAS by airborne salivary droplets and nasal discharge. Transmission is favored by close proximity; therefore schools, military barracks, and homes are important environments for spread. The incubation period for pharyngitis is usually 2-5 days. GAS has the potential to be an important upper respiratory tract pathogen and to produce outbreaks of disease in the daycare setting. Foods contaminated by GAS occasionally cause explosive outbreaks of pharyngotonsillitis. Children are usually no longer infectious within 24 hr of starting appropriate antibiotic therapy. Chronic pharyngeal carriers of GAS rarely transmit this organism to others.

Streptococcal pyoderma (impetigo, pyoderma) occurs most frequently during the summer in temperate climates, or year-round in warmer climates, when the skin is exposed and abrasions and insect bites are more likely to occur (see Chapter 685). Colonization of healthy skin by GAS usually precedes the development of impetigo. Because GAS cannot penetrate intact skin, impetigo and other skin infections usually occur at the site of open lesions (insect bites, traumatic wounds, burns). Although impetigo serotypes may colonize the throat, spread is usually from skin to skin, not via the respiratory tract. Fingernails and the perianal region can harbor GAS and play a role in disseminating impetigo. Multiple cases of impetigo in the same family are common. Both impetigo and pharyngitis are more likely to occur among children living in crowded homes and in poor hygienic circumstances.

The incidence of **severe invasive** GAS infections, including bacteremia, streptococcal toxic shock syndrome, and necrotizing fasciitis, has increased in recent decades. The incidence appears to be highest in very young and elderly persons. Before the routine use of varicella vaccine, varicella was the most commonly identified risk factor for invasive GAS infection in children. Other risk factors include diabetes mellitus, HIV infection, intravenous drug use, and chronic pulmonary or chronic cardiac disease. The portal of entry is unknown in almost 50% of cases of severe invasive GAS infection; in most cases it is believed to be skin or less often mucous membranes. Severe invasive disease rarely follows clinically apparent GAS pharyngitis.

PATHOGENESIS

Virulence of GAS depends primarily on the M protein, and strains rich in M protein resist phagocytosis in fresh human blood, whereas M-negative strains do not. M protein stimulates the production of protective opsonophagocytic antibodies that are type specific, protecting against infection with a homologous M type but much less so against other M types. Therefore, multiple GAS infections attributable to various M types are common during childhood and adolescence. By adult life, individuals are probably immune to many of the common M types in the environment.

GAS produces a large variety of extracellular enzymes and toxins, including erythrogenic toxins, known as **streptococcal pyrogenic exotoxins**. Streptococcal pyrogenic exotoxins A, C, and SSA, alone or in combination, are responsible for the **rash of scarlet fever** and are elaborated by streptococci that contain a particular bacteriophage. These exotoxins stimulate the formation of specific antitoxin antibodies that provide immunity against the scarlatiniform rash but not against other streptococcal infections. GAS can produce up to 12 different pyrogenic exotoxins, and repeat attacks of scarlet fever are possible. Mutations in genes that are promoters of several virulence genes, including pyrogenic exotoxins, as well as several newly discovered exotoxins, appear to be involved in the pathogenesis of invasive GAS disease, including the streptococcal toxic shock syndrome.

The importance of other streptococcal toxins and enzymes in human disease is not yet established. Many of these extracellular substances are antigenic and stimulate antibody production after an infection. However, these antibodies do not confer immunity. Their measurement is useful for establishing evidence of a recent streptococcal infection to aid in the diagnosis of postinfectious illnesses. Tests for antibodies against streptolysin O (anti–streptolysin O) and DNase B (anti–DNase B) are the most frequently used antibody determinations. Because the immune response to extracellular antigens varies among individuals as well as with the site of infection, it is sometimes necessary to measure other streptococcal antibodies.

CLINICAL MANIFESTATIONS

The most common infections caused by GAS involve the respiratory tract and the skin and soft tissues.

Respiratory Tract Infections

GAS is an important cause of acute **pharyngitis** (Chapter 409) and pneumonia (Chapter 428).

Scarlet Fever

Scarlet fever is GAS pharyngitis associated with a characteristic rash, which is caused by an infection with **pyrogenic exotoxin** (erythrogenic toxin)–producing GAS in individuals who do not have antitoxin antibodies. It is now encountered less often and is less virulent than in the past, but the incidence is cyclic, depending on the prevalence of toxin-producing strains and the immune status of the population. The modes of transmission, age distribution, and other epidemiologic features are otherwise similar to those for GAS pharyngitis.

The rash appears within 24-48 hr after onset of symptoms, although it may appear with the first signs of illness (Fig. 210.1A). It often begins around the neck and spreads over the trunk and extremities. The rash is a diffuse, finely papular, erythematous eruption producing bright-red discoloration of the skin, which blanches on pressure. It is often accentuated in the creases of the elbows, axillae, and groin (Pastia lines). The skin has a goose-pimple appearance and feels rough. The cheeks are often erythematous with pallor around the mouth. After 3-4 days, the rash begins to fade and is followed by **desquamation**, initially on the face, progressing downward, and often resembling a mild sunburn. Occasionally, sheetlike desquamation may occur around the free margins of the fingernails, the palms, and the soles. Examination of the pharynx of a patient with scarlet fever reveals essentially the same findings as with GAS pharyngitis. In addition, the tongue is usually coated and the papillae are swollen (Fig. 210.1B). After desquamation, the reddened papillae are prominent, giving the tongue a strawberry appearance (Fig. 210.1C).

Typical scarlet fever is not difficult to diagnose; the milder form with equivocal pharyngeal findings can be confused with viral exanthems, Kawasaki disease, and drug eruptions. Staphylococcal infections are occasionally associated with a scarlatiniform rash. A history of recent exposure to a GAS infection is helpful. Identification of GAS in the pharynx confirms the diagnosis.

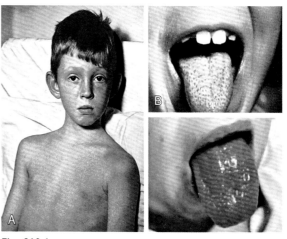

Fig. 210.1 Scarlet fever. **A,** Punctate, erythematous rash (2nd day). **B,** White strawberry tongue (1st day). **C,** Red strawberry tongue (3rd day). *(Courtesy of Dr. Franklin H. Top, Professor and Head of the Department of Hygiene and Preventive Medicine, State University of Iowa, College of Medicine, Iowa City, IA; and Parke, Davis & Company's Therapeutic Notes. From Gershon AA, Hotez PJ, Katz SL: Krugman's infectious diseases of children, ed 11, Philadelphia, 2004, Mosby, Plate 53.)*

Impetigo

Impetigo (or pyoderma) has traditionally been classified into 2 clinical forms: bullous and nonbullous (see Chapter 685). **Nonbullous impetigo** is the more common form and is a superficial infection of the skin that appears first as a discrete papulovesicular lesion surrounded by a localized area of redness. The vesicles rapidly become purulent and covered with a thick, confluent, amber-colored crust that gives the appearance of having been stuck onto the skin. The lesions may occur anywhere but are most common on the face and extremities. If untreated, nonbullous impetigo is a mild but chronic illness, often spreading to other parts of the body, but occasionally self-limited. Regional **lymphadenitis** is common. Nonbullous impetigo is generally not accompanied by fever or other systemic signs or symptoms. Impetiginized excoriations around the nares are seen with active GAS infections of the nasopharynx, particularly in young children. However, impetigo is rarely associated with overt streptococcal infection of the upper respiratory tract.

Bullous impetigo is less common and occurs most often in neonates and young infants. It is characterized by flaccid, transparent bullae usually <3 cm in diameter on previously untraumatized skin. The usual distribution involves the face, buttocks, trunk, and perineum.

Although *Staphylococcus aureus* has traditionally been accepted as the sole pathogen responsible for bullous impetigo, there has been confusion about the organisms responsible for nonbullous impetigo. In most episodes of nonbullous impetigo, either GAS or *S. aureus* (or both) is isolated. Earlier investigations suggested that GAS was the causative agent in most cases of nonbullous impetigo and that *S. aureus* was only a secondary invader. However, *S. aureus* has emerged as the causative agent in most cases of nonbullous impetigo. Culture of the lesions is the only way to distinguish nonbullous impetigo caused by *S. aureus* from that caused by GAS.

Erysipelas

Erysipelas is a now relatively rare acute GAS infection involving the deeper layers of the skin and the underlying connective tissue. The skin in the affected area is swollen, red, and very tender. Superficial blebs may be present. The most characteristic finding is a sharply defined, slightly elevated border. At times, reddish streaks of lymphangitis project out from the margins of the lesion. The onset is abrupt, and signs and symptoms of a systemic infection, such as high fever, are often present. Cultures obtained by needle aspirate of the advancing margin of the inflamed area often reveal the causative agent.

Perianal Dermatitis

Perianal dermatitis, also called perianal cellulitis or **perianal streptococcal disease,** is a distinct clinical entity characterized by well-demarcated, perianal erythema associated with anal pruritus, painful defecation, and occasionally blood-streaked stools. Most children are 2-7 yr old (range: 18 days to 12 yr). Physical examination reveals flat, pink to beefy-red perianal erythema with sharp margins extending as far as 2 cm from the anus. Erythema may involve the vulva and vagina. Lesions may be very tender and, particularly when chronic, may fissure and bleed. Systemic symptoms and fever are unusual. Culture or a rapid strep test of a perianal swab will yield group A streptococci or detect antigen.

Vaginitis

GAS is a common cause of vaginitis in prepubertal girls (see Chapter 564). Patients usually have a serous discharge with marked erythema and irritation of the vulvar area, accompanied by discomfort in walking and in urination.

Severe Invasive Disease

Invasive GAS infection is defined by isolation of GAS from a normally sterile body site and includes 3 overlapping clinical syndromes. **GAS toxic shock syndrome (TSS)** is differentiated from other types of invasive GAS infections by the presence of shock and multiorgan system failure early in the course of the infection (Table 210.1). The 2nd syndrome is **GAS necrotizing fasciitis**, characterized by extensive local necrosis of subcutaneous soft tissues and skin. The 3rd syndrome is the group of

Table 210.1	Definition of Streptococcal Toxic Shock Syndrome

CLINICAL CRITERIA

Hypotension *plus* 2 or more of the following:
  Renal impairment
  Coagulopathy
  Hepatic involvement
  Adult respiratory distress syndrome
  Generalized erythematous macular rash
    Soft tissue necrosis

DEFINITE CASE

Clinical criteria *plus* group A streptococcus from a normally sterile site

PROBABLE CASE

Clinical criteria *plus* group A streptococcus from a nonsterile site

---

focal and systemic infections that do not meet the criteria for TSS or necrotizing fasciitis and includes bacteremia with no identified focus, meningitis, pneumonia, peritonitis, puerperal sepsis, osteomyelitis, suppurative arthritis, myositis, and surgical wound infections. GAS TSS, necrotizing fasciitis, and focal and systemic infections can be present in any combination.

The pathogenic mechanisms responsible for severe, invasive GAS infections, including streptococcal TSS and necrotizing fasciitis, have yet to be defined completely, but an association with streptococcal pyrogenic exotoxins is strongly suspected. At least 2 of the 3 original streptococcal pyrogenic exotoxins (A and C), the newly discovered streptococcal pyrogenic exotoxins, and potentially other as yet unidentified toxins produced by GAS act as **superantigens**, which stimulate intense activation and proliferation of T lymphocytes and macrophages, resulting in the production of large quantities of proinflammatory cytokines. These cytokines are capable of inducing shock and tissue injury and appear to mediate many of the clinical manifestations of severe, invasive GAS infections.

DIAGNOSIS

When deciding whether to perform a diagnostic test on a patient presenting with acute pharyngitis, the clinical and epidemiologic findings should be considered. A history of close contact with a well-documented case of GAS pharyngitis is helpful, as is an awareness of a high prevalence of GAS infections in the community. The signs and symptoms of streptococcal and nonstreptococcal pharyngitis overlap too broadly to allow the requisite diagnostic precision on clinical grounds alone. The clinical diagnosis of GAS pharyngitis cannot be made with reasonable accuracy even by the most experienced physicians, and laboratory confirmation is required, except for patients with overt viral signs and symptoms (e.g., rhinorrhea, cough, mouth ulcers, hoarseness), who generally do not need a diagnostic test performed.

Culture of a throat swab on a sheep blood agar plate is effective for documenting the presence of GAS and for confirming the clinical diagnosis of acute GAS pharyngitis. When performed correctly, a single throat swab has a sensitivity of 90–95% for detecting the presence of GAS in the pharynx.

The significant disadvantage of culturing a throat swab on a blood agar plate is the delay (overnight or longer) in obtaining the culture result. **Streptococcal rapid antigen detection** tests are available for the identification of GAS directly from throat swabs. Their advantage over culture is the speed in providing results, often <10-15 min. Rapid identification and treatment of patients with streptococcal pharyngitis can reduce the risk for spread of GAS, allowing the patient to return to school or work sooner, and can reduce the acute morbidity of this illness.

Almost all currently available rapid antigen detection tests have excellent specificity of >95% compared with blood agar plate cultures. False-positive test results are quite unusual, and therefore therapeutic decisions can be made with confidence on the basis of a positive test result. Unfortunately, the sensitivity of most of these tests is 80–90%, sometimes lower, when compared with blood agar plate culture. Therefore, a negative rapid test does not completely exclude the presence of GAS, and a confirmatory throat culture should be performed in children and adolescents, but not necessarily in adults, who are at exceptionally low risk for developing acute rheumatic fever. Definitive studies are not available to determine whether some rapid antigen detection tests are significantly more sensitive than others, or whether any of these tests is sensitive enough to be used routinely in children and adolescents without throat culture confirmation of negative test results. Some experts believe that physicians who use a rapid antigen detection test without culture backup should compare the results with that specific test to those of throat cultures to confirm adequate sensitivity in their practice.

Some microbiology laboratories have replaced culture methods with rapid and very sensitive and specific GAS molecular assays. These molecular assays include PCR methods and nucleic acid amplification tests using isothermal loop amplification. The **isothermal loop amplification** methods have been reported to have sensitivity up to 100% and specificity >96% compared to culture or PCR. This very high sensitivity may lead to higher numbers of positive results, which in turn may contribute to identification of more patients with asymptomatic GAS colonization and unnecessary antibiotic therapy. However, the benefit of faster results, sometimes <10 min, ensures more expedited initiation of appropriate antibiotic therapy for patients with GAS pharyngitis.

GAS infection can also be diagnosed retrospectively on the basis of an elevated or increasing streptococcal antibody titer. The **anti–streptolysin O** assay is the streptococcal antibody test most often used. Because streptolysin O is also produced by groups C G streptococci, the test is not specific for group A infection. The anti–streptolysin O response can be feeble after streptococcal skin infection. In contrast, the anti–DNase B responses are generally present after either skin or throat infections. A significant antibody increase is usually defined as an increase in titer of 2 or more dilution increments (≥4-fold rise) between the acute-phase and convalescent-phase specimens, regardless of the actual height of the antibody titer. Physicians frequently misinterpret streptococcal antibody titers because of a failure to appreciate that the normal levels of these antibodies are substantially higher among school-age children than adults. Both the traditional anti–streptolysin O and the anti–DNase B tests are neutralization assays. Newer tests use **latex agglutination** or nephelometric assays. Unfortunately, these newer tests often have not been well standardized against the traditional neutralization assays. Physicians should be aware of these potential problems when interpreting the results of streptococcal serologic testing.

A commercially available **slide agglutination test** for the detection of antibodies to several streptococcal antigens is the Streptozyme test (Wampole Laboratories, Stamford, CT). This test is much less well standardized and less reproducible than other antibody tests, and it should not be used as a test for evidence of a preceding GAS infection.

Differential Diagnosis

Viruses are the most common cause of acute pharyngitis in children. Respiratory viruses such as influenza virus, parainfluenza virus, rhinovirus, coronavirus, adenovirus, and respiratory syncytial virus are frequent causes of acute pharyngitis. Other viral causes of acute pharyngitis include enteroviruses and herpes simplex virus. Epstein-Barr virus is a frequent cause of acute pharyngitis that is often accompanied by other clinical findings of infectious mononucleosis (e.g., splenomegaly, generalized lymphadenopathy). Systemic infections with other viral agents, including cytomegalovirus, rubella virus, measles virus, and HIV, may be associated with acute pharyngitis.

GAS is by far the most common cause of bacterial pharyngitis, accounting for 15–30% of cases of acute pharyngitis in children and a lower proportion in adults. Groups C and G β-hemolytic streptococcus also cause acute pharyngitis, typically in teens and young adults (see Chapter 212). *Arcanobacterium haemolyticum* and *Fusobacterium necrophorum* are additional, less common causes. *Neisseria gonorrhoeae*

can occasionally cause acute pharyngitis in sexually active adolescents. Other bacteria, such as *Francisella tularensis* and *Yersinia enterocolitica*, as well as mixed infections with anaerobic bacteria (Vincent angina), are rare causes of acute pharyngitis. *Chlamydia pneumoniae* and *Mycoplasma pneumoniae* have been implicated as causes of acute pharyngitis, particularly in adults. *Corynebacterium diphtheriae* is a serious cause of pharyngitis but is rare because of universal immunization (see Chapter 214). Although other bacteria (e.g., *S. aureus, Haemophilus influenzae, Streptococcus pneumoniae*) are frequently cultured from the throats of children with acute pharyngitis, their etiologic role in pharyngitis has not been established, because they are often isolated in healthy children.

GAS pharyngitis is the only common cause of acute pharyngitis for which antibiotic therapy is definitely indicated. Therefore, when confronted with a patient with acute pharyngitis, the clinical decision that usually needs to be made is whether or not the pharyngitis is attributable to GAS.

TREATMENT

Antibiotic therapy for patients with GAS pharyngitis can prevent **acute rheumatic fever** (RF), shorten the clinical course of the illness, reduce transmission of the infection to others, and prevent suppurative complications. *For the patient with classic scarlet fever, antibiotic therapy should be started immediately, but for the majority of patients, who present with much less distinctive findings, treatment should be withheld until there is laboratory confirmation, by throat culture, molecular assay, or rapid antigen detection test.* Rapid antigen detection tests, because of their high degree of specificity, allow initiation of antibiotic therapy immediately for the patient with a positive test result.

GAS is exquisitely sensitive to **penicillin** and **cephalosporins**, and resistant strains have never been encountered. Penicillin or amoxicillin is therefore the drug of choice (except in patients who are allergic to penicillins) for pharyngeal infections as well as for suppurative complications. Oral penicillin V (250 mg/dose 2 or 3 times daily [bid-tid] for children weighing ≤60 lb and 500 mg/dose bid-tid for children >60 lb) is recommended but must be taken for a full **10 days**, even though there is symptomatic improvement within 3-4 days. Penicillin V (phenoxymethylpenicillin) is preferred over penicillin G, because it may be given without regard to mealtime. The major concern with all forms of oral therapy is the risk that the drug will be discontinued before the 10-day course has been completed. Therefore, when oral treatment is prescribed, the necessity of completing a full course of therapy must be emphasized. If the parents seem unlikely to comply with oral therapy because of family disorganization, difficulties in comprehension, or other reasons, parenteral therapy with a single intramuscular (IM) injection of benzathine penicillin G (600,000 IU for children weighing ≤60 lb and 1.2 million IU for children >60 lb) is the most efficacious and often the most practical method of treatment. Disadvantages include soreness around the site of injection, which may last for several days, and potential for injection into nerves or blood vessels if not administered correctly. The local reaction is diminished when benzathine penicillin G is combined in a single injection with procaine penicillin G, although it is necessary to ensure that an adequate dose of benzathine penicillin G is administered.

In several comparative clinical trials, once-daily amoxicillin (50 mg/kg, maximum: 1,000 mg) for 10 days has been demonstrated to be effective in treating GAS pharyngitis. This somewhat broader-spectrum agent has the advantage of once-daily dosing, which may enhance adherence. In addition, amoxicillin is relatively inexpensive and is considerably more palatable than penicillin V suspension.

A 10-day course of a narrow-spectrum oral cephalosporin is recommended for most **penicillin-allergic** individuals. It has been suggested that a 10-day course with an oral cephalosporin is superior to 10 days of oral penicillin in eradicating GAS from the pharynx. Analysis of these data suggests that the difference in eradication is mainly the result of a higher rate of eradication of carriers included unintentionally in these clinical trials. Some penicillin-allergic persons (up to 10%) are also allergic to cephalosporins, and these agents should be avoided in patients with immediate (anaphylactic-type) hypersensitivity to penicillin.

Most oral broad-spectrum cephalosporins are considerably more expensive than penicillin or amoxicillin and are more likely to select for antibiotic-resistant flora.

Oral clindamycin is an appropriate agent for treating penicillin-allergic patients, and resistance to clindamycin among GAS isolates in the United States is currently only approximately 1%. An oral **macrolide** (erythromycin or clarithromycin) or **azalide** (azithromycin) is also an appropriate agent for patients allergic to penicillins. Ten days of therapy is indicated except for azithromycin, which is given at 12 mg/kg once daily for 5 days. Erythromycin is associated with substantially higher rates of gastrointestinal side effects than the other agents. In recent years, macrolide resistance rates among pharyngeal isolates of GAS in most areas of the United States have been approximately 5–8%. Sulfonamides and the tetracyclines are not recommended for treatment of GAS pharyngitis. However, studies showed that trimethoprim-sulfamethoxazole (TMP-SMX) is highly active in vitro against GAS and was comparable to IM penicillin for impetigo from GAS in clinical trials.

Most oral antibiotics must be administered for the conventional 10 days to achieve maximal pharyngeal eradication rates of GAS and prevention of RF, but certain newer agents are reported to achieve comparable bacteriologic and clinical cure rates when given for ≤5 days. However, definitive results from comprehensive studies are not available to allow full evaluation of these proposed shorter courses of oral antibiotic therapy, which therefore cannot be recommended at this time. In addition, these antibiotics have a much broader spectrum than penicillin and are generally more expensive, even when administered for short courses.

The majority of patients with GAS pharyngitis respond clinically to antimicrobial therapy, and GAS is eradicated from the pharynx. Post-treatment throat cultures are indicated only in the relatively few patients who remain symptomatic, whose symptoms recur, or who have had RF or rheumatic heart disease and are therefore at unusually high risk for recurrence.

Antibiotic therapy for a patient with nonbullous impetigo can prevent local extension of the lesions, spread to distant infectious foci, and transmission of the infection to others. However, the ability of antibiotic therapy to prevent poststreptococcal glomerulonephritis has not been definitively demonstrated. Patients with a few superficial, isolated lesions and no systemic signs can be treated with topical antibiotics. **Mupirocin** is a safe and effective agent that has become the topical treatment of choice. If there are widespread lesions or systemic signs, oral therapy with coverage for both GAS and *S. aureus* is needed. With the rapid emergence of methicillin-resistant *S. aureus* in many communities, one should consider using clindamycin alone or a combination of TMP-SMX and amoxicillin as first-line therapy. Oral cefuroxime is an effective treatment of perianal streptococcal disease.

Theoretical considerations and experimental data suggest that intravenous **clindamycin** is a more effective agent for the treatment of severe, invasive GAS infections than IV penicillin. However, because approximately 1% of GAS isolates in the United States are resistant to clindamycin, clindamycin initially should be used in combination with penicillin for these infections until susceptibility to clindamycin has been established. If **necrotizing fasciitis** is suspected, immediate surgical exploration or biopsy is required to identify a deep soft-tissue infection that should be debrided immediately. Patients with **streptococcal TSS** require rapid and aggressive fluid replacement, management of respiratory or cardiac failure, if present, and anticipatory management of multiorgan system failure. Limited data suggest that intravenous immune globulin (IVIG) is effective as adjunctive therapy in the management of streptococcal TSS.

COMPLICATIONS

Suppurative complications from the spread of GAS to adjacent structures were extremely common in the preantibiotic era. Cervical lymphadenitis, peritonsillar abscess, retropharyngeal abscess, otitis media, mastoiditis, and sinusitis still occur in children in whom the primary illness has gone unnoticed or in whom treatment of the pharyngitis has been inadequate. GAS pneumonia can also occur.

Acute rheumatic fever (Chapter 210.1) and acute poststreptococcal **glomerulonephritis** (Chapter 537.4) are both nonsuppurative sequelae of infections with GAS that occur after an asymptomatic latent period. They are both characterized by disease remote from the site of the primary GAS infection. Acute RF and acute glomerulonephritis differ in their clinical manifestations, epidemiology, and potential morbidity. In addition, acute glomerulonephritis follows a GAS infection of either the upper respiratory tract or the skin, but acute RF only follows an infection of the upper respiratory tract.

Poststreptococcal Reactive Arthritis

Poststreptococcal reactive arthritis (**PSRA**) describes a syndrome characterized by the onset of acute arthritis following an episode of GAS pharyngitis in a patient whose illness does not fulfill the Jones Criteria for diagnosis of acute RF. It is still unclear whether this entity represents a distinct syndrome or is a variant of acute RF. Although PSRA usually involves the large joints similar to the arthritis of acute RF, it may also involve small peripheral joints, as well as the axial skeleton, and is typically nonmigratory, characteristics distinct from the arthritis of acute RF. The latent period between the antecedent episode of GAS pharyngitis and PSRA may be considerably shorter (usually <10 days) than that typically seen with acute RF (usually 14-21 days). In contrast to the arthritis of acute RF, PSRA does not respond dramatically to therapy with aspirin or other nonsteroidal antiinflammatory drugs (NSAIDs). In addition, fewer patients with PSRA than with acute RF have temperature >38°C (100.4°F). Even though no more than half of PSRA patients with throat culture have GAS isolated, all have serologic evidence of a recent GAS infection. Because a very small proportion of patients with PSRA have been reported to develop valvular heart disease subsequently, these patients should be carefully observed for several months for clinical evidence of **carditis**. Some recommend that these patients receive secondary antistreptococcal prophylaxis for up to 1 yr. If clinical evidence of carditis is not observed, the prophylaxis can be discontinued. If valvular disease is detected, the patient should be classified as having had acute RF and should continue to receive secondary prophylaxis appropriate for RF patients.

Pediatric Autoimmune Neuropsychiatric Disorders Associated with *Streptococcus pyogenes*

Pediatric autoimmune neuropsychiatric disorders associated with *Streptococcus pyogenes* (**PANDAS**) is a term proposed for a group of neuropsychiatric disorders (originally obsessive-compulsive disorder (OCD), tic disorder, and Tourette syndrome, or only OCD or feeding abnormality) for which a possible relationship with GAS infections has been hypothesized (see Chapter 37). *This relationship has not been proved.* It has been proposed that this subset of patients with OCDs may produce autoimmune antibodies in response to a GAS infection that cross-react with brain tissue similar to the autoimmune response believed to be responsible for the manifestations of **Sydenham chorea**. It has also been suggested that secondary prophylaxis that prevents recurrences of rheumatic fever, including Sydenham chorea, might also be effective in preventing exacerbations of OCDs in these patients, but clinical trials have not confirmed this. It has also been proposed that these patients may benefit from immunoregulatory therapy such as plasma exchange or IVIG, but these unproven modalities should only be used in a clinical research trial. That PANDAS may represent an extension of the spectrum of acute RF is intriguing, but it should be considered only as a yet-unproven hypothesis. Until carefully designed and well-controlled studies have established a causal relationship between neurobehavioral abnormalities and GAS infections, routine diagnostic laboratory testing for GAS and antistreptococcal antibodies, long-term antistreptococcal prophylaxis, or immunoregulatory therapy (e.g., IVIG, plasma exchange) to treat exacerbations of this disorder clearly are not recommended (see Chapter 37). It has also been suggested that a broad spectrum of infectious agents may have the ability to trigger exacerbations in children with these neurobehavioral disorders.

PROGNOSIS

The prognosis for appropriately treated GAS pharyngitis is excellent, and complete recovery is the rule. When therapy is instituted within 9 days of the onset of symptoms and continued for the full course, acute RF is almost always prevented. There is no comparable evidence that acute poststreptococcal glomerulonephritis can be prevented once pharyngitis or pyoderma with a nephritogenic strain of GAS has occurred. In rare instances, particularly in neonates or in children whose response to infection is compromised, fulminant pneumonia, septicemia, and death may occur despite usually adequate therapy.

PREVENTION

The only specific indication for long-term use of an antibiotic to prevent GAS infections is for patients with a history of acute RF and/or rheumatic heart disease. Mass prophylaxis is generally not feasible except to reduce the number of infections during epidemics of impetigo and to control epidemics of pharyngitis in military populations and in schools. Because the ability of antimicrobial agents to prevent GAS infections is limited, a group A streptococcal vaccine offers the possibility of a more effective approach.

Several candidate vaccines are in development, including a 30-valent M protein–based recombinant vaccine, another recombinant vaccine that includes several conserved non–M protein epitopes that induce protective antibody, and an M-protein vaccine that includes an epitope in a very conserved region of M protein to provide broad immunity. All these vaccines are in relatively early stages of development.

Bibliography is available at Expert Consult.

210.1 Rheumatic Fever

Stanford T. Shulman and Caroline H. Reuter

ETIOLOGY

Considerable evidence supports the link between antecedent GAS pharyngitis and **acute rheumatic fever** (RF) and **rheumatic heart disease**. As many as two thirds of patients with an acute episode of RF have history of an upper respiratory tract infection several weeks before, and the peak age and seasonal incidence of acute RF closely parallel that of GAS pharyngitis. Patients with acute RF almost always have serologic evidence of a recent GAS infection. Their antibody titers are usually *considerably higher* than those seen in patients with uncomplicated GAS infections. Outbreaks of GAS pharyngitis in closed communities, such as boarding schools or military bases, may be followed by outbreaks of acute RF. Antimicrobial therapy that eliminates GAS from the pharynx also prevents initial episodes of acute RF, and long-term, continuous antibiotic prophylaxis that prevents GAS pharyngitis also prevents recurrences of acute RF.

Not all serotypes of GAS can cause rheumatic fever. When some GAS strains (e.g., M type 4) caused acute pharyngitis in a very susceptible rheumatic population, there were no recurrences of RF. In contrast, episodes of pharyngitis caused by other serotypes in the same population led to frequent recurrences of acute RF, suggesting that the latter organisms were rheumatogenic. The concept of *rheumatogenicity* is further supported by the observation that although serotypes of GAS frequently associated with skin infection can be isolated also from the upper respiratory tract, they rarely cause recurrences of RF in individuals with a previous history of RF or first episodes of RF. In addition, certain serotypes of GAS (M types 1, 3, 5, 6, 18, 29) are more frequently isolated from patients with acute RF than are other serotypes.

EPIDEMIOLOGY

The annual incidence of acute rheumatic fever in some developing countries exceeds 50 per 100,000 children, and very high rates are also seen in ethnic minority populations within Australia and New Zealand. Worldwide, **rheumatic heart disease** remains the most common form of acquired heart disease in all age-groups, accounting for up to 50% of all cardiovascular disease and 50% of all cardiac admissions in many developing countries. Striking differences in the incidence of acute RF and rheumatic heart disease among different ethnic groups are often evident within the same country; these differences are partially related to differences in socioeconomic status, and there is a genetic basis for increased susceptibility.

In the United States at the beginning of the 20th century, acute RF was a leading cause of death among children and adolescents, with annual incidence rates of 100-200 per 100,000 population. In addition, rheumatic heart disease was a leading cause of heart disease among adults <40 yr old. At that time, as many as 25% of pediatric hospital beds in the United States were occupied by patients with acute RF or its complications. By the 1940s, the annual incidence of acute RF had decreased to 50 per 100,000 population, and over the next 4 decades, the decline in incidence accelerated rapidly. By the early 1980s, the annual incidence in some areas of the United States was as low as 0.5 per 100,000 population. This sharp decline in the incidence of acute RF has been observed in other industrialized countries as well.

The explanation for this dramatic decline in the incidence of acute RF and rheumatic heart disease in the United States and other industrialized countries is not clear but is likely related in large part to a *decline in circulating rheumatogenic strains causing acute pharyngitis*. Historically, acute RF was associated with poverty and overcrowding, particularly in urban areas. Much of the decline in the incidence of acute RF in industrialized countries during the preantibiotic era was probably the result of improved living conditions. Of the various manifestations of poverty, **crowding**, which facilitates spread of GAS infections, is most closely associated with the incidence of acute RF. The decline in incidence of acute RF in industrialized countries over the past 4 decades is also attributable to the greater availability of medical care and to the widespread use of antibiotics. Antibiotic therapy of GAS pharyngitis is important in preventing initial attacks and, particularly, recurrences of the disease. In addition, the decline in the United States is attributed to a shift in the prevalent strains of GAS causing pharyngitis from mostly rheumatogenic to nonrheumatogenic.

A dramatic outbreak of acute RF in the Salt Lake City, UT, area began in early 1985, and 198 cases were reported by the end of 1989. Other outbreaks were reported between 1984 and 1988 in Columbus and Akron, OH; Pittsburgh, PA; Nashville and Memphis, TN; New York, NY; Kansas City, MO; Dallas, TX; and among Navy recruits in California and Army recruits in Missouri. In virtually all areas of the United States, rates have declined substantially.

Certain rheumatogenic serotypes (types 1, 3, 5, 6, and 18) that were isolated less often during the 1970s and early 1980s dramatically reappeared during rheumatic fever outbreaks, and their appearance in selected communities was probably a major factor. GAS that are associated with rheumatogenicity often form highly mucoid colonies on throat culture plates.

In addition to the specific characteristics of the infecting strain of GAS, the risk of developing acute RF also depends on various host factors. The incidence of both initial attacks and recurrences of acute RF peaks in children 5-15 yr old, the age of greatest risk for GAS pharyngitis. Patients who have had an attack of acute RF tend to have recurrences, and the clinical features of the recurrences tend to mimic those of the initial attack. In addition, there appears to be a genetic predisposition to acute RF. Studies in twins show a higher concordance rate of acute RF in monozygotic than in dizygotic twin pairs.

PATHOGENESIS

The **cytotoxicity theory** suggests that a GAS toxin is involved in the pathogenesis of acute rheumatic fever and rheumatic heart disease. GAS produces a number of enzymes that are cytotoxic for mammalian cardiac cells, such as streptolysin O, which has a direct cytotoxic effect on mammalian cells in tissue culture. Most proponents of the cytotoxicity theory have focused on this enzyme. However, a major problem with the cytotoxicity hypothesis is its inability to explain the substantial latent period (usually 10-21 days) between GAS pharyngitis and onset of acute RF.

An **immune-mediated pathogenesis** for acute RF and rheumatic heart disease has been suggested by its clinical similarity to other illnesses with an immunopathogenesis and by the latent period between the GAS infection and acute RF. The antigenicity of several GAS cellular and extracellular epitopes and their immunologic cross-reactivity with cardiac antigenic epitopes also lends support to the hypothesis of molecular mimicry. Common epitopes are shared between certain GAS components (e.g., M protein, cell membrane, group A cell wall carbohydrate, capsular hyaluronate) and specific mammalian tissues (e.g., heart valve, sarcolemma, brain, joint). For example, certain rheumatogenic M proteins (M1, M5, M6, and M19) share epitopes with human myocardial proteins such as tropomyosin and myosin. Additionally, the involvement of GAS superantigens such as pyrogenic exotoxins in the pathogenesis of acute RF has been proposed.

Another proposed pathogenetic hypothesis is that the binding of an M-protein N-terminal domain to a region of collagen type IV leads to an **antibody response to the collagen**, resulting in ground substance inflammation, especially in subendothelial areas such as cardiac valves and myocardium.

CLINICAL MANIFESTATIONS AND DIAGNOSIS

Because no clinical or laboratory finding is pathognomonic for acute rheumatic fever, T. Duckett Jones proposed guidelines in 1944 to aid in diagnosis and to limit overdiagnosis. The **Jones Criteria,** as revised in 2015 by the American Heart Association (AHA), are intended for diagnosis of the initial attack of acute RF and recurrent attacks (Table 210.2). There are **5 major and 4 minor criteria** and a requirement of evidence of recent GAS infection. The 2015 revision includes separate criteria for **Low-Risk populations** (defined as those with incidence ≤2 per 100,000 school-age children per year or all-age rheumatic heart disease prevalence of ≤1 per 1,000 population) and **Moderate/High-Risk populations** (defined as those with higher incidence or prevalence rates). Virtually all of the United States, Canada, and Western Europe are Low-Risk, whereas Moderate/High-Risk populations include Maoris in New Zealand, aborigines in Australia, Pacific Islanders, and most developing countries. Diagnosis of a first attack or recurrent attack of acute RF can be established when a patient fulfills 2 major or 1 major and 2 minor criteria and has evidence of preceding GAS infection. Diagnosis of recurrent acute RF can also be made only in the Moderate/High-Risk population by presence of 3 minor criteria with evidence of preceding GAS infection. In the 2015 Jones Criteria revision, a major change from previous versions expands the definition of the major criterion **carditis** to include *subclinical evidence* (e.g., in the absence of a murmur, echocardiographic evidence of mitral regurgitation [MR] meeting specific criteria to distinguish physiologic from pathologic MR) (see Table 465.1). Areas in which the Jones Criteria differ in Low-Risk from Moderate/High-Risk populations relate to the major criterion of **arthritis** and the minor criteria of arthralgia, definition of fever, and of elevated inflammatory markers (see Table 210.2 and text below). These changes are designed to make it easier to fulfill the Jones Criteria in patients from Moderate/High-Risk populations. Even with strict application of the criteria, overdiagnosis as well as underdiagnosis of acute RF may occur. The diagnosis of acute RF can be made without strict adherence to the Jones Criteria in 3 circumstances: (1) when chorea occurs as the only major manifestation of acute RF, (2) when indolent carditis is the only manifestation in patients who first come to medical attention only months after the apparent onset of acute RF, and (3) in a limited number of patients with recurrence of acute RF in particularly high-risk populations.

The 5 Major Criteria
Migratory Polyarthritis

Arthritis occurs in approximately 75% of patients with acute rheumatic fever and typically involves larger joints, particularly the knees, ankles, wrists, and elbows. Involvement of the spine, small joints of the hands and feet, or hips is uncommon. Rheumatic joints are classically hot, red, swollen, and exquisitely tender, with even the friction of bedclothes being uncomfortable. The pain can precede and can appear to be disproportionate to the objective findings. The joint involvement is characteristically migratory in nature; that is, a severely inflamed joint can become normal within 1-3 days without treatment, even as 1 or more other large joints become involved. Severe arthritis can persist for several weeks in untreated patients. Monoarticular arthritis is unusual unless antiinflammatory therapy is initiated prematurely, aborting the progression of the migratory polyarthritis. If a child with fever and arthritis is suspected to have acute RF, it is frequently useful to withhold salicylates and observe for migratory progression. A dramatic response to even low doses of salicylates is another characteristic feature of the arthritis, and the absence of such a response should suggest an alternative diagnosis.

Rheumatic arthritis is almost never deforming. Synovial fluid in acute RF usually has 10,000-100,000 white blood cells/μL with a predominance of neutrophils, protein level of approximately 4 g/dL, normal glucose level, and forms a good mucin clot. Frequently, arthritis is the earliest manifestation of acute RF and may correlate temporally with peak antistreptococcal antibody titers. There is often an inverse relationship between the severity of arthritis and the severity of cardiac involvement. In Moderate/High-Risk populations only, monoarthritis in the absence of prior inflammatory therapies, or even polyarthralgia without frank objective signs of arthritis, can fulfill this major criterion. Before **polyarthralgia** should be considered a major criterion in the Moderate/High-Risk population, other potential causes should be excluded.

Table 210.2	Guidelines for the Diagnosis of Initial or Recurrent Attack of Rheumatic Fever (Jones Criteria, Updated 2015)[1-5]

MAJOR MANIFESTATIONS	MINOR MANIFESTATIONS	SUPPORTING EVIDENCE OF ANTECEDENT GROUP A STREPTOCOCCAL INFECTION
Carditis	Clinical features:	Positive throat culture or rapid streptococcal antigen test
Polyarthritis	Arthralgia	Elevated or increasing streptococcal antibody titer
Erythema marginatum	Fever	
Subcutaneous nodules	Laboratory features:	
Chorea	Elevated acute-phase reactants:	
	Erythrocyte sedimentation rate	
	C-reactive protein	
	Prolonged P-R interval	

1. **Initial attack:** 2 major manifestations, or 1 major and 2 minor manifestations, plus evidence of recent GAS infection. **Recurrent attack:** 2 major, or 1 major and 2 minor, or 3 minor manifestations (the latter only in the Moderate/High-Risk population), plus evidence of recent GAS infection (see text).

2. **Low-Risk population** is defined as acute rheumatic fever (ARF) incidence <2 per 100,000 school-age children per year, or all-age rheumatic heart disease (RHD) prevalence of <1 per 1,000 population. **Moderate/High-Risk population** is defined as ARF incidence >2 per 100,000 school-age children per year, or all-age RHD prevalence of >1 per 1,000 population.

3. Carditis is now defined as clinical and/or subclinical (echocardiographic valvulitis). See Table 210.3.

4. Arthritis (major) refers only to polyarthritis in Low-Risk populations, but also to monoarthritis or polyarthralgia in Moderate/High-Risk populations.

5. Minor criteria for Moderate/High-Risk populations only include monoarthralgia (polyarthralgia for Low-Risk populations), fever of >38°C (>38.5°C in Low-Risk populations), ESR >30 mm/hr (>60 mm/hr in Low-Risk populations).

From Gewitz MH, Baltimore RS, Tani LY, et al: Revision of the Jones Criteria for the diagnosis of acute rheumatic fever in the era of Doppler echocardiography: a scientific statement from the American Heart Association, *Circulation* 131(20):1806–1818, 2015.

Carditis

A major change in the 2015 revision of the Jones Criteria is the acceptance of **subclinical carditis** (defined as without a murmur of valvulitis but with echocardiographic evidence of valvulitis) or **clinical carditis** (with a valvulitis murmur) as fulfilling the major criterion of carditis in all populations. The echocardiographic features of subclinical carditis must meet those included in Table 465.1, to distinguish pathologic from physiologic degrees of valve regurgitation. Subclinical (i.e. only echocardiographic) evidence of pathologic mitral regurgitation requires that a jet is seen in at least two views, the jet length is ≥2 cm in at least 1 view, peak jet velocity is >3 meters/second, and the peak systolic jet is in at least 1 envelope. Subclinical pathologic evidence of aortic regurgitation is similar except that the jet length is ≥1 cm in at least 1 view.

Carditis and resultant chronic rheumatic heart disease are the most serious manifestations of acute RF and account for essentially all the associated morbidity and mortality. Rheumatic carditis is characterized by **pancarditis**, with active inflammation of myocardium, pericardium, and endocardium (see Chapter 465). Cardiac involvement during acute RF varies in severity from fulminant, potentially fatal exudative pancarditis to mild, transient cardiac involvement. **Endocarditis** (valvulitis) is a universal finding in rheumatic carditis, whereas the presence of pericarditis or myocarditis is variable. Myocarditis and/or pericarditis without clinical evidence of endocarditis almost never is rheumatic carditis; alternate etiologies (especially viral) need to be sought. Most rheumatic heart disease is isolated mitral valvular disease or combined aortic and mitral valvular disease. Isolated aortic or right-sided valvular involvement is quite uncommon. Serious and long-term illness is related entirely to the severity of valvular heart disease as a consequence of a single attack or recurrent attacks of acute RF. Valvular insufficiency is characteristic of both acute and convalescent stages of acute RF, whereas mitral and/or aortic valvular stenosis usually appears years or even decades after the acute illness. However, in developing countries, where acute RF often occurs at a younger age, mitral stenosis and aortic stenosis may develop sooner after acute RF than in developed countries and can occur in young children.

Acute rheumatic carditis usually presents as tachycardia and cardiac murmurs, with or without evidence of myocardial or pericardial involvement. Moderate to severe rheumatic carditis can result in cardiomegaly and heart failure with hepatomegaly and peripheral and pulmonary edema. Echocardiographic findings include pericardial effusion, decreased ventricular contractility, and aortic and/or mitral regurgitation. **Mitral regurgitation** is characterized typically by a high-pitched apical holosystolic murmur radiating to the axilla. In patients with significant MR, this may be associated with an apical mid-diastolic murmur of relative mitral stenosis. Aortic insufficiency is characterized by a high-pitched decrescendo diastolic murmur at the left sternal border.

Carditis occurs in approximately 50–60% of all cases of acute RF. Recurrent attacks of acute RF in patients who had carditis with their initial attack are associated with high rates of carditis with increasing severity of cardiac disease. The major consequence of acute rheumatic carditis is chronic, progressive valvular disease, particularly valvular stenosis, which can require valve replacement.

Chorea

Sydenham chorea occurs in approximately 10–15% of patients with acute RF and usually presents as an isolated, frequently subtle, movement disorder. Emotional lability, incoordination, poor school performance, uncontrollable movements, and facial grimacing are characteristic, all exacerbated by stress and disappearing with sleep. Chorea occasionally is unilateral (hemichorea). The latent period from acute GAS infection to chorea is usually substantially longer than for arthritis or carditis and can be months. Onset can be insidious, with symptoms being present for several months before recognition. Clinical maneuvers to elicit features of chorea include (1) demonstration of *milkmaid's grip* (irregular contractions and relaxations of the muscles of the fingers while squeezing the examiner's fingers), (2) spooning and pronation of the hands when the patient's arms are extended, (3) wormian darting movements of the tongue on protrusion, and (4) examination of handwriting to evaluate fine motor movements. Diagnosis is based on clinical findings with supportive evidence of GAS antibodies. However, in the usual patient with a long latent period from the inciting streptococcal infection to onset of chorea, antibody levels have often declined to normal. Although the acute illness is distressing, chorea rarely if ever leads to permanent neurologic sequelae.

Erythema Marginatum

Erythema marginatum is a rare (approximately 1% of patients with acute RF) but characteristic rash of acute RF. It consists of erythematous, serpiginous, macular lesions with pale centers that are not pruritic (Fig. 210.2). It occurs primarily on the trunk and extremities, but not on the face, and it can be accentuated by warming the skin.

Subcutaneous Nodules

Subcutaneous nodules are a rare (≤1% of patients with acute RF) finding and consist of firm nodules approximately 0.5-1 cm in diameter along the extensor surfaces of tendons near bony prominences. There is a correlation between the presence of these nodules and significant rheumatic heart disease.

Minor Criteria

These are more *nonspecific* than major criteria, and the 2015 revised Jones Criteria have included some changes from previous criteria. The 1st of the 2 clinical minor criteria involve joint manifestations (only if arthritis is not used as a major criterion) and is defined as *polyarthralgia* in Low-Risk populations and *monoarthralgia* in Moderate/High-Risk populations. The 2nd clinical minor manifestation is fever, defined as *at least 38.5°C* in Low-Risk populations and *at least 38.0°C* in Moderate/High-Risk populations. The 2 laboratory minor criteria are (1) elevated acute-phase reactants, defined as erythrocyte sedimentation rate (ESR) at least 60 mm/hr and/or C-reactive protein (CRP) at least 3.0 mg/dL (30 mg/L) in Low-Risk populations, and ESR at least 30 mm/hr and/or CRP at least 3.0 mg/dL (30 mg/L) in Moderate/High-Risk populations, and (2) prolonged P-R interval on ECG (unless carditis is a major criterion). However, a prolonged P-R interval alone does not constitute evidence of carditis or predict long-term cardiac sequelae.

Recent Group A Streptococcus Infection

An absolute requirement for the diagnosis of acute RF is supporting evidence of a recent GAS infection. Acute RF typically develops 10-21 days after an acute episode of GAS pharyngitis at a time when clinical findings of pharyngitis are no longer present and when only 10–20% of patients still harbor GAS in the throat. One third of patients with acute RF have no history of an antecedent pharyngitis. Therefore, evidence of an antecedent GAS infection is usually based on elevated or rising serum antistreptococcal antibody titers. A slide agglutination test

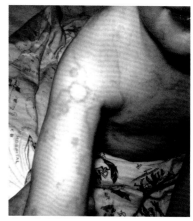

Fig. 210.2 Polycyclic red borders of erythema marginatum in a febrile child with acute rheumatic fever. *(From Schachner LA, Hansen RC, editors: Pediatric dermatology, ed 3, Philadelphia, 2003, Mosby, p 808.)*

(Streptozyme) purports to detect antibodies against 5 different GAS antigens. Although this test is rapid, relatively simple to perform, and widely available, it is less standardized and less reproducible than other tests and is not recommended as a diagnostic test for evidence of an antecedent GAS infection. If only a single antibody is measured (usually anti–streptolysin O), only 80–85% of patients with acute RF have an elevated titer; however, 95–100% have an elevation if 3 different antibodies (anti–streptolysin O, anti–DNase B, antihyaluronidase) are measured. Therefore, when acute RF is suspected clinically, multiple antibody tests should be performed. Except for chorea, the clinical findings of acute RF generally coincide with peak antistreptococcal antibody responses. Most patients with chorea have elevation of antibodies to at least 1 GAS antigen. However, in patients with a long latent period from the inciting GAS infection, antibody levels may have declined to within the normal range. The diagnosis of acute RF should *not* be made in those patients with elevated or increasing streptococcal antibody titers who do not fulfill the Jones Criteria.

Differential Diagnosis

The differential diagnosis of rheumatic fever includes many infectious as well as noninfectious illnesses (Table 210.3). When children present with arthritis, a collagen vascular disease must be considered. **Juvenile idiopathic arthritis** (JIA) must be distinguished from acute RF. Children with JIA tend to be younger and usually have less joint pain relative to their other clinical findings than those with acute RF. Spiking fevers, nonmigratory arthritis, lymphadenopathy, and splenomegaly are more suggestive of JIA than acute RF. The response to salicylate therapy is also much less dramatic with JIA than with acute RF. **Systemic lupus erythematosus** (SLE) can usually be distinguished from acute RF by antinuclear antibodies in SLE. Other causes of arthritis such as pyogenic arthritis, malignancies, serum sickness, Lyme disease, sickle cell disease, and reactive arthritis related to gastrointestinal infections (e.g., *Shigella*, *Salmonella*, *Yersinia*) should also be considered. Poststreptococcal reactive arthritis is discussed earlier (see Chapter 210).

When **carditis** is the sole major manifestation of suspected acute RF, viral myocarditis, viral pericarditis, Kawasaki disease, and infective endocarditis should also be considered. Patients with infective endocarditis may present with both joint and cardiac manifestations. These patients can usually be distinguished from patients with acute RF by blood cultures and the presence of extracardiac findings (e.g., hematuria, splenomegaly, splinter hemorrhages). When **chorea** is the sole major manifestation of suspected acute RF, Huntington chorea, Wilson disease, SLE, and various encephalitides should also be considered.

Table 210.3	Differential Diagnosis of Acute Rheumatic Fever	
ARTHRITIS	**CARDITIS**	**CHOREA**
Juvenile idiopathic arthritis	Viral myocarditis	Huntington chorea
Reactive arthritis (e.g., *Shigella*, *Salmonella*, *Yersinia*)	Viral pericarditis	Wilson disease
Serum sickness	Infective endocarditis	Systemic lupus erythematosus
Sickle cell disease	Kawasaki disease	Tic disorder
Malignancy	Congenital heart disease	Hyperactivity
Systemic lupus erythematosus	Mitral valve prolapse	Encephalitis
Lyme disease (*Borrelia burgdorferi*)	Innocent murmurs	
Pyogenic arthritis		
Poststreptococcal reactive arthritis		

TREATMENT

All patients with acute rheumatic fever should be placed on bed rest and monitored closely for evidence of carditis. They can be allowed to ambulate when the signs of acute inflammation have improved. However, patients with carditis require longer periods of bed rest.

Antibiotic Therapy

Once the diagnosis of acute RF has been established and regardless of the throat culture results, the patient should receive 10 days of orally administered penicillin or amoxicillin or a single intramuscular injection of benzathine penicillin to ensure eradication of GAS from the upper respiratory tract. If penicillin allergic, 10 days of erythromycin, 5 days of azithromycin, or 10 days of clindamycin is indicated. After this initial course of antibiotic therapy, long-term antibiotic prophylaxis for secondary prevention should be instituted (see later).

Antiinflammatory Therapy

Antiinflammatory agents (e.g., salicylates, corticosteroids) should be withheld if arthralgia or atypical arthritis is the only clinical manifestation of presumed acute RF. Premature treatment with one of these agents may interfere with the development of the characteristic migratory polyarthritis and thus obscure the diagnosis of acute RF. Acetaminophen can be used to control pain and fever while the patient is being observed for more definite signs of acute RF or for evidence of another disease.

Patients with typical migratory polyarthritis and those with carditis without cardiomegaly or congestive heart failure should be treated with oral salicylates. The usual dose of aspirin is 50-70 mg/kg/day in 4 divided doses orally (PO) for 3-5 days, followed by 50 mg/kg/day in 4 divided doses PO for 2-3 wk and half that dose for another 2-4 wk. Determination of the serum salicylate level is not necessary unless the arthritis does not respond or signs of salicylate toxicity (tinnitus, hyperventilation) develop. There is no evidence that NSAIDs are more effective than salicylates.

Patients with carditis and more than minimal cardiomegaly and/or congestive heart failure should receive **corticosteroids**. The usual dose of prednisone is 2 mg/kg/day in 4 divided doses for 2-3 wk, followed by half the dose for 2-3 wk and then tapering of the dose by 5 mg/24 hr every 2-3 days. When prednisone is being tapered, aspirin should be started at 50 mg/kg/day in 4 divided doses for 6 wk to prevent rebound of inflammation. Supportive therapies for patients with moderate to severe carditis include digoxin, fluid and salt restriction, diuretics, and oxygen. The cardiac toxicity of digoxin is enhanced with myocarditis.

Termination of the antiinflammatory therapy may be followed by the reappearance of clinical manifestations or of elevation in ESR and CRP (rebound). It may be prudent to increase salicylates or corticosteroids until near-normalization of inflammatory markers is achieved.

Sydenham Chorea

Because chorea often occurs as an isolated manifestation after the resolution of the acute phase of the disease, antiinflammatory agents are usually not indicated. Sedatives may be helpful early in the course of chorea; **phenobarbital** (16-32 mg every 6-8 hr PO) is the drug of choice. If phenobarbital is ineffective, **haloperidol** (0.01-0.03 mg/kg/24 hr divided twice daily PO) or **chlorpromazine** (0.5 mg/kg every 4-6 hr PO) should be initiated. Some patients may benefit from a few-week course of corticosteroids.

COMPLICATIONS

The arthritis and chorea of acute RF resolve completely without sequelae. Therefore, the long-term sequelae of RF are essentially limited to the heart (see Chapter 465).

The AHA has published updated recommendations regarding the use of prophylactic antibiotics to prevent infective endocarditis (see Chapter 464). The AHA recommendations no longer suggest routine endocarditis prophylaxis for patients with rheumatic heart disease who are undergoing dental or other procedures. However, the maintenance of optimal oral healthcare remains an important component of an overall healthcare program. For the relatively few patients with rheumatic heart disease in whom infective endocarditis prophylaxis remains recommended, such as those with a prosthetic valve or prosthetic material used in valve repair, the current AHA recommendations should be followed (see Chapter 464). These recommendations advise using an agent other than a penicillin to prevent infective endocarditis in those receiving penicillin prophylaxis for RF because oral α-hemolytic streptococci are likely to have developed resistance to penicillin.

PROGNOSIS

The prognosis for patients with acute rheumatic fever depends on the clinical manifestations present at the initial episode, the severity of the initial episode, and the presence of recurrences. Approximately 50–70% of patients with carditis during the initial episode of acute RF recover with no residual heart disease; the more severe the initial cardiac involvement, the greater the risk for residual heart disease. Patients without carditis during the initial episode are less likely to have carditis with recurrent attacks, but there is a stepwise increase in cardiac involvement as the number of episodes increases. In contrast, patients with carditis during the initial episode are very likely to have carditis with recurrences, and the risk for permanent heart damage increases with each recurrence. Patients who have had acute RF are susceptible to recurrent attacks following reinfection of the upper respiratory tract with GAS, with approximately 50% risk with each GAS pharyngitis. Therefore, these

Table 210.4	Chemoprophylaxis for Recurrences of Acute Rheumatic Fever (Secondary Prophylaxis)	
DRUG	**DOSE**	**ROUTE**
Penicillin G benzathine	600,000 IU for children weighing ≤60 lb and 1.2 million IU for children >60 lb, every 4 wk*	Intramuscular
or		
Penicillin V	250 mg, twice daily	Oral
or		
Sulfadiazine or sulfisoxazole	0.5 g, once daily for patients weighing ≤60 lb 1.0 g, once daily for patients weighing >60 lb	Oral
For People Who Are Allergic to Penicillin and Sulfonamide Drugs		
Macrolide or azalide	Variable	Oral

*In high-risk situations, administration every 3 wk is recommended.
Adapted from Gerber MA, Baltimore RS, Eaton CB, et al: Prevention of rheumatic fever and diagnosis and treatment of acute streptococcal pharyngitis: a scientific statement from the American Heart Association Rheumatic Fever, Endocarditis, and Kawasaki Disease Committee of the Council on Cardiovascular Disease in the Young, *Circulation* 119:1541–1551, 2009.

Table 210.5	Duration of Prophylaxis for People Who Have Had Acute Rheumatic Fever: AHA Recommendations
CATEGORY	**DURATION**
Rheumatic fever without carditis	5 yr or until 21 yr of age, whichever is longer
Rheumatic fever with carditis but without residual heart disease (no valvular disease*)	10 yr or until 21 yr of age, whichever is longer
Rheumatic fever with carditis and residual heart disease (persistent valvular disease*)	10 yr or until 40 yr of age, whichever is longer; sometimes lifelong prophylaxis

*Clinical or echocardiographic evidence.
Adapted from Gerber MA, Baltimore RS, Eaton CB, et al: Prevention of rheumatic fever and diagnosis and treatment of acute streptococcal pharyngitis: a scientific statement from the American Heart Association (AHA) Rheumatic Fever, Endocarditis, and Kawasaki Disease Committee of the Council on Cardiovascular Disease in the Young, *Circulation* 119:1541–1551, 2009.

patients require long-term continuous chemoprophylaxis.

Before antibiotic prophylaxis was available, 75% of patients who had an initial episode of acute RF had 1 or more recurrences in their lifetime. These recurrences were a major source of morbidity and mortality. The risk of recurrence is highest in the 1st 5 yr after the initial episode and decreases with time.

Approximately 20% of patients who present with "pure" chorea who are not given secondary prophylaxis develop rheumatic heart disease within 20 yr. Therefore, patients with chorea, even in the absence of other manifestations of RF, require long-term antibiotic prophylaxis (see Table 210.4).

PREVENTION

Prevention of both initial and recurrent episodes of acute rheumatic fever depends on controlling GAS infections of the upper respiratory tract. Prevention of initial attacks (primary prevention) depends on identification and eradication of GAS causing acute pharyngitis. A New Zealand study in a population with very high rates of acute RF showed that a school-based GAS pharyngitis screening and management program using oral amoxicillin substantially decreased pharyngeal GAS prevalence and rates of acute RF. Individuals who have already suffered an attack of acute RF are particularly susceptible to recurrences of RF with any subsequent GAS upper respiratory tract infection, whether or not they are symptomatic. Therefore, these patients should receive continuous antibiotic prophylaxis to prevent recurrences (secondary prevention).

Primary Prevention

Appropriate antibiotic therapy instituted before the 9th day of symptoms of acute GAS pharyngitis is highly effective in preventing first attacks of acute RF. However, approximately 30% of patients with acute RF do not recall a preceding episode of pharyngitis and did not seek therapy.

Secondary Prevention

Secondary prevention is directed at preventing acute GAS pharyngitis in patients at substantial risk of recurrent acute RF. Secondary prevention requires continuous antibiotic prophylaxis, which should begin as soon as the diagnosis of acute RF has been made and immediately after a full course of antibiotic therapy has been completed. Because patients who have had carditis with their initial episode of acute RF are at higher risk for having carditis with recurrences and for sustaining additional cardiac damage, they should receive long-term antibiotic prophylaxis well into adulthood and perhaps for life (Tables 210.4 and 210.5).

Patients who did not have carditis with their initial episode of acute RF have a relatively low risk for carditis with recurrences. Antibiotic prophylaxis should continue in these patients until the patient reaches 21 yr of age or until 5 yr have elapsed since the last rheumatic fever attack, whichever is longer. The decision to discontinue prophylactic antibiotics should be made only after careful consideration of potential risks and benefits and of epidemiologic factors such as the risk for exposure to GAS infections.

The regimen of choice for secondary prevention is a single intramuscular injection of benzathine penicillin G (600,000 IU for children weighing ≤60 lb and 1.2 million IU for those >60 lb) every 4 wk (Table 210.4). In certain high-risk patients, and in certain areas of the world where the incidence of rheumatic fever is particularly high, use of benzathine penicillin G every 3 wk may be necessary because serum concentrations of penicillin may decrease to marginally effective levels after 3 wk. In the United States, administration of benzathine penicillin G every 3 wk is recommended only for those who have recurrent acute RF despite adherence to a 4 wk regimen. In compliant patients, continuous oral antimicrobial prophylaxis can be used. Penicillin V (250 mg twice daily) and sulfadiazine or sulfisoxazole (500 mg for those weighing ≤60 lb or 1,000 mg for those >60 lb, once daily) are equally effective when used in such patients. For the exceptional patient who is allergic to both penicillin and sulfonamides, a macrolide (erythromycin or clarithromycin) or azalide (azithromycin) may be used. Table 210.5 notes the duration of secondary prophylaxis.

Bibliography is available at Expert Consult.

Chapter 211
Group B Streptococcus

Catherine S. Lachenauer
and Michael R. Wessels

第二百一十一章
B组链球菌

中文导读

本章首先阐述了B组链球菌或无乳链球菌是新生儿细菌性脓毒症的主要原因，进而介绍了关于B组链球菌的病因、流行病学、发病机制、临床表现、诊断、实验室检查、治疗、预后和预防等内容。在B组链球菌感染的临床表现部分详细介绍了早发型和晚发型B组链球菌疾病的临床特点及区别。在B组链球菌感染的预防部分详细介绍了化学预防和母体免疫。

Group B streptococcus (**GBS**), or *Streptococcus agalactiae,* is a major cause of **neonatal bacterial sepsis** in the United States. Although advances in prevention strategies have led to a decline in the incidence of neonatal disease, GBS remains a major pathogen for neonates, pregnant women, and nonpregnant adults.

ETIOLOGY

Group B streptococci are facultative anaerobic gram-positive cocci that form chains or diplococci in broth and small, gray-white colonies on solid medium. GBS is definitively identified by demonstration of the Lancefield group B carbohydrate antigen, such as with latex agglutination techniques widely used in clinical laboratories. Presumptive identification can be established on the basis of a narrow zone of β-hemolysis on blood agar, resistance to bacitracin and trimethoprim-sulfamethoxazole (TMP-SMX), lack of hydrolysis of bile esculin, and elaboration of CAMP factor (named for the discoverers, Christie, Atkins, and Munch-Petersen), an extracellular protein that, in the presence of the β toxin of *Staphylococcus aureus,* produces a zone of enhanced hemolysis on sheep blood agar. Individual GBS strains are serologically classified according to the presence of 1 of the structurally distinct capsular polysaccharides, which are important virulence factors and stimulators of antibody-associated immunity. Ten GBS capsular types have been identified: types Ia, Ib, II, III, IV, V, VI, VII, VIII, and IX.

EPIDEMIOLOGY

GBS emerged as a prominent neonatal pathogen in the late 1960s. For the next 2 decades, the incidence of neonatal GBS disease remained fairly constant, affecting 1.0-5.4 per 1,000 liveborn infants in the United States. Two patterns of disease were seen: **early-onset disease**, which presents at <7 days of age, and **late-onset disease**, which presents at ≥7 days of age. Since the early 1990s, widespread implementation of **maternal intrapartum chemoprophylaxis** has led to a striking decrease

in the incidence of early-onset neonatal GBS disease in the United States, from 1.7 to 0.25 per 1,000 live births in recent years. This strategy has *not* had a significant effect on the incidence of late-onset disease, which has remained stable at approximately 0.3-0.4 per 1,000 live births (Fig. 211.1). The incidence of neonatal GBS disease is higher in premature and low-birthweight infants, although most cases occur in full-term infants.

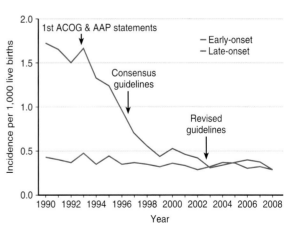

Fig. 211.1 Incidence of early- and late-onset, invasive group B streptococcal (GBS) disease–active bacterial core surveillance areas, 1990–2008, and activities for prevention of GBS disease. AAP, American Academy of Pediatrics; ACOG, American College of Obstetricians and Gynecologists. *(Adapted from Jordan HT, Farley MM, Craig A, et al: Revisiting the need for vaccine prevention of late-onset neonatal group B streptococcal disease, Pediatr Infect Dis J 27:1057–1064, 2008.)*

Rates of both early- and late-onset disease are higher in black infants.

Colonization by GBS in healthy adults is common. Vaginal or rectal colonization occurs in up to approximately 30% of pregnant women and is the usual source for GBS transmission to newborn infants. In the absence of maternal chemoprophylaxis, approximately 50% of infants born to colonized women acquire GBS colonization, and 1–2% of infants born to colonized mothers develop early-onset disease. Heavy maternal colonization increases the risk for infant colonization and development of early-onset disease. Additional risk factors for early-onset disease include prolonged rupture of membranes, intrapartum fever, prematurity, maternal bacteriuria during pregnancy, or previous delivery of an infant who developed GBS disease. Risk factors for late-onset disease are less well defined. Whereas late-onset disease may follow vertical transmission, horizontal acquisition from nursery or other community sources (family, healthcare providers, placental capsules) has also been described.

GBS is also an important cause of invasive disease in adults. GBS may cause urinary tract infections, bacteremia, endometritis, chorioamnionitis, and wound infection in pregnant and parturient women. In nonpregnant adults, especially those with underlying medical conditions such as diabetes mellitus, cirrhosis, or malignancy, GBS may cause serious infections such as bacteremia, skin and soft tissue infections, bone and joint infections, endocarditis, pneumonia, and meningitis. In the era of maternal chemoprophylaxis, most invasive GBS infections occur in nonpregnant adults. Unlike neonatal disease, the incidence of invasive GBS disease in adults has increased substantially, doubling between 1990 and 2007.

The serotypes most frequently associated with neonatal GBS disease are types Ia, III, and V; Ib and II are less common. Strains of serotype III are isolated in >50% of cases of late-onset disease and of meningitis associated with early- or late-onset disease. The serotype distribution of colonizing and invasive isolates from pregnant women is similar to that from infected newborns. In Japan, serotypes VI and VIII have been reported as common maternal colonizing serotypes, and case reports indicate that type VIII strains may cause neonatal disease indistinguishable from that caused by other serotypes.

PATHOGENESIS

A major risk factor for the development of early-onset neonatal GBS infection is maternal vaginal or rectal colonization by GBS. Infants acquire GBS by ascending infection or during passage through the birth canal. Fetal aspiration of infected amniotic fluid may occur. The incidence of early-onset GBS infection increases with the duration of rupture of membranes. Infection may also occur through seemingly intact membranes. In cases of late-onset infection, GBS may be vertically transmitted or acquired later from maternal or nonmaternal sources.

Several bacterial factors are implicated in the pathophysiology of invasive GBS disease, primarily the type-specific **capsular polysaccharide**. Strains that are associated with invasive disease in humans elaborate more capsular polysaccharide than do colonizing isolates. All GBS capsular polysaccharides are high-molecular-weight polymers composed of repeating oligosaccharide subunits that include a short side chain terminating in *N*-acetylneuraminic acid (**sialic acid**). Studies in type III GBS show that the sialic acid component of the capsular polysaccharide prevents activation of the alternative complement pathway in the absence of type-specific antibody. Sialylated capsular polysaccharide on the GBS surface also interacts with sialic acid–binding lectins or siglecs on human leukocytes to dampen inflammatory gene activation. Thus, the capsular polysaccharide appears to exert a virulence effect by protecting the organism from opsonophagocytosis in the nonimmune host and by downregulating leukocyte activation. In addition, type-specific virulence attributes are suggested by the fact that type III strains are implicated in most cases of late-onset neonatal GBS disease and meningitis. Type III strains are taken up by brain endothelial cells more efficiently in vitro than are strains of other serotypes, although studies using acapsular mutant strains demonstrate that it is not the capsule itself that facilitates cellular invasion. A single clone of type III GBS is highly associated with late-onset disease and meningitis. This clonal group, ST-17, produces a surface-anchored protein called hypervirulent GBS adhesin (**HvgA**) that is not present in other GBS isolates. HvgA contributes to GBS

adherence to intestinal and endothelial cells and mediates invasion into the central nervous system (CNS) in an experimental infection model in mice. Other putative GBS virulence factors include GBS surface proteins, which may play a role in adhesion to host cells; C5a peptidase, which is postulated to inhibit the recruitment of polymorphonuclear cells into sites of infection; β-hemolysin, which has been associated with cell injury in vitro; and hyaluronidase, which has been postulated to act as a spreading factor in host tissues.

In a classic study of pregnant women colonized with type III GBS, those who gave birth to healthy infants had higher levels of capsular polysaccharide–specific antibody than those who gave birth to infants who developed invasive disease. In addition, there is a high correlation of antibody titer to GBS type III in mother–infant paired sera. These observations indicate that transplacental transfer of maternal antibody is critically involved in neonatal immunity to GBS. Optimal immunity to GBS also requires an intact complement system. The classical complement pathway is an important component of GBS immunity in the absence of specific antibody; in addition, antibody-mediated opsonophagocytosis may proceed by the alternative complement pathway. These and other results indicate that anticapsular antibody can overcome the prevention of C3 deposition on the bacterial surface by the sialic acid component of the type III capsule.

The precise steps between GBS colonization and invasive disease remain unclear. In vitro studies showing GBS entry into alveolar epithelial cells and pulmonary vasculature endothelial cells suggest that GBS may gain access to the bloodstream by invasion from the alveolar space, perhaps following intrapartum aspiration of infected fluid. β-Hemolysin/cytolysin may facilitate GBS entry into the bloodstream following inoculation into the lungs. However, highly encapsulated GBS strains, which enter eukaryotic cells poorly in vitro compared with capsule-deficient organisms, are associated with virulence clinically and in experimental infection models.

GBS induces the release of proinflammatory cytokines. The group B antigen and the peptidoglycan component of the GBS cell wall are potent inducers of tumor necrosis factor-α release in vitro, whereas purified type III capsular polysaccharide is not. Even though the capsule plays a central role in virulence through avoidance of immune clearance, the capsule does not directly contribute to cytokine release and resultant inflammatory response.

The complete genome sequences of hundreds of GBS strains have been reported, emphasizing a genomic approach to better understanding GBS. Analysis of these sequences shows that GBS is closely related to *Streptococcus pyogenes* and *Streptococcus pneumoniae*. Many known and putative GBS virulence genes are clustered in pathogenicity islands that also contain mobile genetic elements, suggesting that interspecies acquisition of genetic material plays an important role in genetic diversity.

CLINICAL MANIFESTATIONS

Two syndromes of neonatal GBS disease are distinguishable on the basis of age at presentation, epidemiologic characteristics, and clinical features (Table 211.1). **Early-onset neonatal GBS disease** presents within the 1st 6 days of life and is often associated with maternal obstetric complications, including chorioamnionitis, prolonged rupture of membranes, and premature labor. Infants may appear ill at the time of delivery, and most infants become ill within 24 hr of birth. In utero infection may result in septic abortion or immediate distress after birth. More than 80% of early-onset GBS disease presents as sepsis; pneumonia and meningitis are other common manifestations. Asymptomatic bacteremia is uncommon but can occur. In symptomatic patients, nonspecific signs such as hypothermia or fever, irritability, lethargy, apnea, and bradycardia may be present. Respiratory signs are prominent regardless of the presence of pneumonia and include cyanosis, apnea, tachypnea, grunting, flaring, and retractions. A fulminant course with hemodynamic abnormalities, including tachycardia, acidosis, and shock, may ensue. Persistent fetal circulation may develop. Clinically and radiographically, pneumonia associated with early-onset GBS disease is difficult to distinguish from **respiratory distress syndrome**. Patients with meningitis often present with nonspecific findings, as described for sepsis or pneumonia, with more specific signs of CNS involvement initially absent.

Table 211.1	Characteristics of Early- and Late-Onset Group B Streptococcus Disease	
	EARLY-ONSET DISEASE	**LATE-ONSET DISEASE**
Age at onset	0-6 days	7-90 days
Increased risk after obstetric complications	Yes	No
Common clinical manifestations	Sepsis, pneumonia, meningitis	Bacteremia, meningitis, osteomyelitis, other focal infections
Common serotypes	Ia, Ib, II, III, V	III predominates
Case fatality rate	4.7%	2.8%

Adapted from Schrag SJ, Zywicki S, Farley MM, et al: Group B streptococcal disease in the era of intrapartum antibiotic prophylaxis, *N Engl J Med* 342:15–20, 2000.

Late-onset neonatal GBS disease presents at ≥7 days of life (may be seen in 1st 2-3 mo) and usually manifests as bacteremia (45–65%) and meningitis (25–35%). Focal infections involving bone and joints, skin and soft tissue, the urinary tract, or lungs may also be seen. Cellulitis and adenitis are often localized to the submandibular or parotid regions. In contrast to early-onset disease, maternal obstetric complications are not risk factors for the development of late-onset GBS disease. Infants with late-onset disease are often less severely ill on presentation than infants with early-onset disease, and the disease is often less fulminant.

Invasive GBS disease in children beyond early infancy is uncommon. Bacteremia without a focus is the most common syndrome associated with childhood GBS disease beyond early infancy. Focal infections may include meningitis, pneumonia, endocarditis, and bone and joint infections.

DIAGNOSIS

A major challenge is distinguishing between respiratory distress syndrome and invasive neonatal GBS infection in preterm infants because the 2 illnesses share clinical and radiographic features. Severe apnea, early onset of shock, abnormalities in the peripheral leukocyte count, and greater lung compliance may be more likely in infants with GBS disease. Other neonatal pathogens, including *Escherichia coli* and *Listeria monocytogenes*, may cause illness that is clinically indistinguishable from that caused by GBS.

The diagnosis of invasive GBS disease is established by isolation and identification of the organism from a normally sterile site, such as blood, urine, or cerebrospinal fluid (CSF). Isolation of GBS from gastric or tracheal aspirates or from skin or mucous membranes indicates colonization and is not diagnostic of invasive disease. CSF should be examined in all neonates suspected of having sepsis, because specific CNS signs are often absent in the presence of meningitis, especially in early-onset disease. Antigen detection methods that use group B polysaccharide–specific antiserum, such as latex particle agglutination, are available for testing of urine, blood, and CSF, but these tests are less sensitive than culture. Moreover, antigen is often detected in urine samples collected by bag from otherwise healthy neonates who are colonized with GBS on the perineum or rectum.

LABORATORY FINDINGS

Frequently present are abnormalities in the peripheral white blood cell count, including an increased or decreased absolute neutrophil count, elevated band count, increased ratio of bands to total neutrophils, or leukopenia. Elevated C-reactive protein level has been investigated as a potential early marker of GBS sepsis but is unreliable. Findings on chest radiograph are often indistinguishable from those of respiratory distress syndrome and may include reticulogranular patterns, patchy infiltrates, generalized opacification, pleural effusions, or increased interstitial markings.

TREATMENT

Penicillin G is the treatment of choice of confirmed GBS infection. Empirical therapy of neonatal sepsis that could be caused by GBS generally includes ampicillin and an aminoglycoside, both for the need for broad coverage pending organism identification and for synergistic

Table 211.2	Recommended Duration of Therapy for Manifestations of Group B Streptococcus Disease
TREATMENT	**DURATION**
Bacteremia without a focus	10 days
Uncomplicated meningitis	14 days
Ventriculitis	At least 4 wk
Septic arthritis or osteomyelitis	3-4 wk

Data from the American Academy of Pediatrics: Group B streptococcal infections. In Kimberlin DW, Brady MT, Jackson MA, Long SS, editors: *Red book: 2015 report of the Committee on Infectious Diseases*, ed 30. Elk Grove Village, IL, 2015, American Academy of Pediatrics, pp 746–747.

bactericidal activity. Once GBS has been definitively identified and a good clinical response has occurred, therapy may be completed with penicillin alone. Especially in patients with meningitis, high doses of penicillin (450,000-500,000 units/kg/day) or ampicillin (300 mg/kg/day) are recommended because of the relatively high mean inhibitory concentration (MIC) of penicillin for GBS as well as the potential for a high initial CSF inoculum. The duration of therapy varies according to the site of infection and should be guided by clinical circumstances (Table 211.2). Extremely ill near-term patients with respiratory failure have been successfully treated with extracorporeal membrane oxygenation.

In patients with GBS meningitis, some experts recommend that additional CSF be sampled at 24-48 hr to determine whether sterility has been achieved. Persistent GBS growth may indicate an unsuspected intracranial focus or an insufficient antibiotic dose.

For **recurrent neonatal GBS disease**, standard intravenous antibiotic therapy followed by attempted eradication of GBS mucosal colonization has been suggested. This suggestion is based on the findings in several studies that invasive isolates from recurrent episodes are usually identical to each other and to colonizing isolates from the affected infant. Rifampin has most frequently been used for this purpose, but one report demonstrates that eradication of GBS colonization in infants is not reliably achieved by rifampin therapy. Optimal management of this uncommon situation remains unclear.

PROGNOSIS

Studies from the 1970s and 1980s showed that up to 30% of infants surviving GBS meningitis had major long-term neurologic sequelae, including developmental delay, spastic quadriplegia, microcephaly, seizure disorder, cortical blindness, or deafness; less severe neurologic complications may be present in other survivors. A study of infants who survived GBS meningitis diagnosed from 1998 through 2006 found that 19% had severe **neurologic impairment** and 25% had mild to moderate impairment at long-term follow-up. Periventricular leukomalacia and severe developmental delay may result from GBS disease and accompanying shock in premature infants, even in the absence of meningitis. The outcome of focal GBS infections outside the CNS, such as bone or soft tissue infections, is generally favorable.

In the 1990s, the case fatality rates associated with early- and late-onset neonatal GBS disease were 4.7% and 2.8%, respectively. Mortality is higher in premature infants; one study reported a case fatality rate of 30% in infants at gestational age <33 wk and 2% in those ≥37 wk. The case fatality rate in children age 3 mo to 14 yr was 9%, and in nonpregnant adults, 11.5%.

PREVENTION

Persistent morbidity and mortality from perinatal GBS disease despite advances in neonatal care have spurred intense investigation into modes of prevention. Two basic approaches to GBS prevention have been investigated: elimination of colonization from the mother or infant (chemoprophylaxis) and induction of protective immunity (immunoprophylaxis).

Chemoprophylaxis

Administration of antibiotics to pregnant women *before* the onset of labor does not reliably eradicate maternal GBS colonization and is not an effective means of preventing neonatal GBS disease. Interruption of neonatal colonization is achievable through administration of antibiotics to the mother **during labor**. Infants born to GBS-colonized women with premature labor or prolonged rupture of membranes who were given **intrapartum chemoprophylaxis** had a substantially lower rate of GBS colonization (9% vs 51%) and early-onset disease (0% vs 6%) than did the infants born to women who were not treated. Maternal postpartum febrile illness was also decreased in the treatment group.

In the mid-1990s, guidelines for chemoprophylaxis were issued that specified administration of intrapartum antibiotics to women identified as *high risk* by either culture-based or risk factor–based criteria. These guidelines were revised in 2002 after epidemiologic data indicated the superior protective effect of the **culture-based** approach in the prevention of neonatal GBS disease, and further revised guidelines were issued in 2010. According to current recommendations, vaginorectal GBS screening cultures should be performed for all pregnant women at 35–37 wk gestation, except for those with GBS bacteriuria during the current pregnancy or a previous infant with invasive GBS disease. Any woman with a positive prenatal screening culture, GBS bacteriuria during pregnancy, or a previous infant with invasive GBS disease should receive intrapartum antibiotics. Women whose culture status is unknown (culture not done, incomplete, or results unknown) and who deliver prematurely (<37 wk gestation), experience prolonged rupture of membranes (≥18 hr), experience intrapartum fever (≥38°C [100.4°F]), or have a positive nucleic acid amplification test for GBS should also receive intrapartum chemoprophylaxis (Figs. 211.2 and 211.3). Routine intrapartum prophylaxis is not recommended for women with GBS colonization undergoing planned cesarean delivery who have not begun labor or had rupture of membranes.

Penicillin remains the preferred agent for **maternal chemoprophylaxis** because of its narrow spectrum and the universal penicillin susceptibility of GBS isolates associated with human infection. Ampicillin is an acceptable alternative. If amnionitis is suspected, broad-spectrum antibiotic therapy that includes an agent active against GBS should replace GBS prophylaxis. Occasional GBS isolates have demonstrated reduced in vitro susceptibility to penicillin and other β-lactam antibiotics in association with mutations in penicillin-binding proteins. However, the clinical significance of these higher MIC values is unclear. Because of frequent resistance of GBS to clindamycin (up to 38%), cefazolin should be used in most cases of intrapartum chemoprophylaxis for penicillin-intolerant women. For penicillin-allergic women at high risk for anaphylaxis, clindamycin should be used, if isolates are demonstrated to be susceptible. Vancomycin should be used if isolates are resistant to, or demonstrate inducible resistance to, clindamycin or if clindamycin susceptibility is unknown.

The U.S. Centers for Disease Control and Prevention (CDC) guidelines also provide recommendations for secondary prevention of early-onset GBS disease in newborns (Fig. 211.4). Extent of newborn evaluation and decision to institute empirical antibiotics are guided by clinical evaluation of the infant as well as gestational age, maternal risk factors, and receipt of intrapartum prophylaxis. In the era of maternal

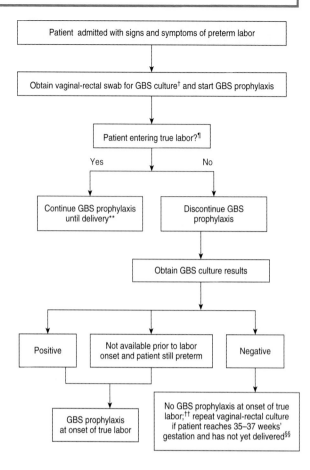

* At <37 weeks and 0 days' gestation.
† If patient has undergone vaginal-rectal GBS culture within the preceding 5 weeks, the results of that culture should guide management. GBS-colonized women should receive intrapartum antibiotic prophylaxis. No antibiotics are indicated for GBS prophylaxis if a vaginal-rectal screen within 5 weeks was negative.
¶ Patient should be regularly assessed for progression to true labor; if the patient is considered not to be in true labor, discontinue GBS prophylaxis.
** If GBS culture results become available prior to delivery and are negative, then discontinue GBS prophylaxis.
†† Unless subsequent GBS culture prior to delivery is positive.
§§ A negative GBS screen is considered valid for 5 weeks. If a patient with a history of PTL is re-admitted with signs and symptoms of PTL and had a negative GBS screen >5 weeks prior, she should be rescreened and managed according to this algorithm at that time.

Fig. 211.2 Algorithm for GBS intrapartum prophylaxis for women with preterm labor (PTL). *(From Verani JR, McGee L, Schrag SJ, Division of Bacterial Diseases, National Center for Immunization and Respiratory Diseases, Centers for Disease Control and Prevention (CDC): Prevention of perinatal group B streptococcal disease—revised guidelines from CDC 2010, MMWR Recomm Rep 59[RR-10]:22, 2010.)*

chemoprophylaxis, most cases of early-onset disease are seen in infants born to women with negative prenatal screening cultures. Data from a large epidemiologic study indicate that the administration of maternal intrapartum antibiotics does not change the clinical spectrum or delay the onset of clinical signs in infants who developed GBS disease despite maternal prophylaxis.

A significant concern with maternal intrapartum chemoprophylaxis has been that large-scale antibiotic use among parturient women might lead to increased rates of antimicrobial resistance or infection in infants with organisms other than GBS, but this has not been borne out. In a population-based study of early-onset neonatal infection from 2005–2014,

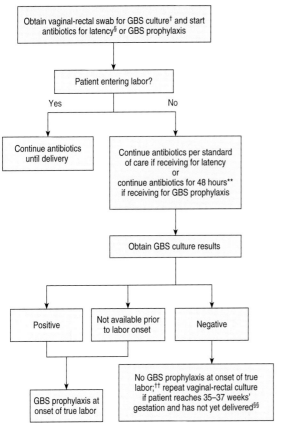

Fig. 211.3 Algorithm for screening for group B streptococcal (GBS) colonization and use of intrapartum prophylaxis for women with preterm premature rupture of membranes (pPROM). *(From Verani JR, McGee L, Schrag SJ, Division of Bacterial Diseases, National Center for Immunization and Respiratory Diseases, Centers for Disease Control and Prevention: Prevention of perinatal group B streptococcal disease—revised guidelines from CDC 2010. MMWR Recomm Rep 59[RR-10]:22, 2010.)*

* At <37 weeks and 0 days' gestation.

† If patient has undergone vaginal-rectal GBS culture within the preceding 5 weeks, the results of that culture should guide management. GBS-colonized women should receive intrapartum antibiotic prophylaxis. No antibiotics are indicated for GBS prophylaxis if a vaginal-rectal screen within 5 weeks was negative.

§ Antibiotics given for latency in the setting of pPROM that include ampicillin 2 g intravenously (IV) once, followed by 1 g IV every 6 hours for at least 48 hours are adequate for GBS prophylaxis. If other regimens are used, GBS prophylaxis should be initiated in addition.

** GBS prophylaxis should be discontinued at 48 hours for women with pPROM who are not in labor. If results from a GBS screen performed on admission become available during the 48-hour period and are negative, GBS prophylaxis should be discontinued at that time.

†† Unless subsequent GBS culture prior to delivery is positive.

§§ A negative GBS screen is considered valid for 5 weeks. If a patient with pPROM is entering labor and had a negative GBS screen >5 weeks prior, she should be rescreened and managed according to this algorithm at that time.

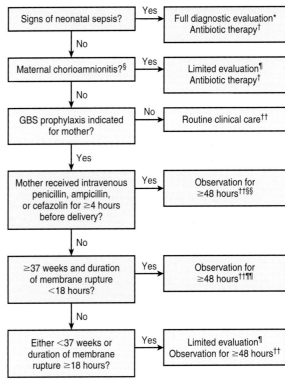

Fig. 211.4 Algorithm for secondary prevention of early-onset group B streptococcal disease among newborns. *(From Verani JR, McGee L, Schrag SJ, Division of Bacterial Diseases, National Center for Immunization and Respiratory Diseases, Centers for Disease Control and Prevention: Prevention of perinatal group B streptococcal disease—revised guidelines from CDC 2010, MMWR Recomm Rep 59[RR-10]:22, 2010.)*

* Full diagnostic evaluation includes a blood culture, a complete blood count (CBC) including white blood cell differential and platelet counts, chest radiograph (if respiratory abnormalities are present), and lumbar puncture (if patient is stable enough to tolerate procedure and sepsis is suspected).

† Antibiotic therapy should be directed toward the most common causes of neonatal sepsis, including intravenous ampicillin for GBS and coverage for other organisms (including *Escherichia coli* and other gram-negative pathogens) and should take into account local antibiotic resistance patterns.

§ Consultation with obstetric providers is important to determine the level of clinical suspicion for chorioamnionitis. Chorioamnionitis is diagnosed clinically and some of the signs are nonspecific.

¶ Limited evaluation includes blood culture (at birth) and CBC with differential and platelets (at birth and/or at 6–12 hours of life).

†† If signs of sepsis develop, a full diagnostic evaluation should be conducted and antibiotic therapy initiated.

§§ If ≥37 weeks' gestation, observation may occur at home after 24 hours if other discharge criteria have been met, access to medical care is readily available, and a person who is able to comply fully with instructions for home observation will be present. If any of these conditions is not met, the infant should be observed in the hospital for at least 48 hours and until discharge criteria are achieved.

¶¶ Some experts recommend a CBC with differential and platelets at age 6–12 hours.

the incidence of early-onset sepsis both overall and caused by *E. coli* remained stable. At present, the substantial decline in early-onset neonatal GBS disease favors continued broad-scale intrapartum chemoprophylaxis, but continued surveillance is required.

A limitation of the maternal chemoprophylaxis strategy is that intrapartum antibiotic use is unlikely to have an impact on late-onset neonatal disease, miscarriages, or stillbirths attributed to GBS, or adult GBS disease. In addition, with wider implementation of maternal chemoprophylaxis, an increasing percentage of early-onset neonatal disease has been in patients born to women with negative cultures, that is, false-negative screens.

Maternal Immunization

Human studies demonstrate that transplacental transfer of naturally acquired maternal antibody to the GBS capsular polysaccharide protects newborns from invasive GBS infection, and that efficient transplacental passage of vaccine-induced GBS antibodies occurs. Conjugate vaccines composed of the GBS capsular polysaccharides coupled to carrier proteins have been produced for human use. In early clinical trials, conjugate GBS vaccines were well tolerated and induced levels of functional antibodies well above the range believed to be protective in >90% of recipients. A vaccine containing type III polysaccharide coupled to tetanus toxoid was safely administered to pregnant women and elicited functionally active type-specific antibody that was efficiently transported to the fetus. Vaccines containing GBS surface proteins have been considered as a means to provide protection against strains of multiple serotypes, and availability of whole genome sequencing has enabled identification of vaccine protein candidates.

A successful GBS maternal vaccine administered before or during pregnancy should lead to transplacental passage of vaccine-induced antibody that protects the fetus and newborn against infection by several GBS serotypes. Such a vaccine would eliminate the need for cumbersome cultures during pregnancy, circumvent the various risks

associated with large-scale antibiotic prophylaxis, likely have an impact on both early- and late-onset disease, and provide a prevention strategy in middle and low income countries, where maternal chemoprophylaxis may not be feasible. Intrapartum chemoprophylaxis will likely remain an important aspect of prevention, particularly for women in whom opportunities for GBS immunization are missed and for infants born so early that levels of transplacentally acquired antibodies may not be high enough to be protective.

Bibliography is available at Expert Consult.

Chapter 212

Non–Group A or B Streptococci

David B. Haslam

第二百一十二章
非A组或B组链球菌

中文导读

本章首先阐述了链球菌菌属的多样性及主要分类，包括主要的人类病原体化脓性链球菌(A组链球菌)、无乳链球菌(B组链球菌)、肺炎链球菌和其他重要的病原体包括具有兰斯菲尔德型抗原的C组链球菌和G组链球菌。随后，重点介绍了C组链球菌和G组链球菌感染的病因、发病机制、临床表现、并发症、诊断、危险因素、治疗等内容。在治疗部分详细描述了β-内酰胺类、利奈唑胺、大环内酯类、喹诺酮类药物等。

The genus *Streptococcus* is exceptionally diverse and includes the major human pathogens *Streptococcus pyogenes* (group A streptococcus), *Streptococcus agalactiae* (group B streptococcus), and *Streptococcus pneumoniae*. Other important pathogens include large-colony species–bearing Lancefield groups C and G antigens and numerous small-colony variants that may or may not express Lancefield carbohydrate antigen among the viridians streptococci (Table 212.1). This chapter focuses on **Streptococcus dysgalactiae subspecies *equisimilis*,** commonly known as "group C and G streptococci"; Chapter 209 discusses *S. pneumoniae*, and Chapter 213 discusses enterococci.

All members of the genus *Streptococcus* are gram-positive, catalase-negative organisms. Lancefield carbohydrate antigen, hemolytic activity, and colony morphology have classically been used to further distinguish and classify streptococci. These features provide a useful framework for the clinician and are still the most commonly used classification schema. However, grouping based on these phenotypic features does not precisely correlate with genetic relatedness, and it is becoming clear that disease propensity is better correlated with sequence homology than with Lancefield grouping or hemolytic activity.

In this chapter, groups C and G streptococci refer exclusively to the large colony-forming organisms, often called "*S. pyogenes*–like," because their microbiologic and clinical features tend to mimic those of group A streptococcus. Despite their different Lancefield antigens, the group C and G streptococci are almost identical genetically and are placed within the *S. dysgalactiae* subsp. *equisimilis* (**SDSE**) group. Their genome sequences are approximately equidistant between *S. pyogenes* and animal pathogens that bear the group C antigen, which are classified as *S. dysgalactiae* subsp. *dysgalactiae*. These 2 subspecies of *S. dysgalactiae* likely will be split into distinct species in the future, when their sequence-based grouping will reflect their propensity to cause human (represented by subsp. *equisimilis*) and animal (represented by subsp. *dysgalactiae*) infections.

The groups C and G streptococci share a number of virulence factors with *S. pyogenes*, including the production of streptolysin O, M protein, streptococcal pyrogenic exotoxin B, and hyaluronidase. The M protein is similar to that of *S. pyogenes* and may account for postinfectious **glomerulonephritis** that is occasionally seen after infection with these organisms. A toxic shock–like syndrome associated with groups C and

| Table 212.1 | Relationship of Streptococci Identified by Hemolysis and Lancefield Grouping to Sites of Colonization and Disease |

	GROUP A STREPTOCOCCUS (*S. pyogenes*)	GROUP B STREPTOCOCCUS (*S. agalactiae*)	OTHER β-HEMOLYTIC STREPTOCOCCI	VIRIDANS STREPTOCOCCI
Hemolysis	β	β	β	α
Lancefield group	A	B	C-H, K-V Especially C and G	
Species or strains	M types (>180)	Serotypes (Ia, Ib, II, III, IV, V, VI, VII, and VIII)		*Streptococcus bovis* *Streptococcus mitis* *Streptococcus mutans* *Streptococcus sanguis* Many others
Normal flora	Pharynx, skin, anus	Gastrointestinal and genitourinary tract	Pharynx, skin, gastrointestinal and genitourinary tracts	Pharynx, nose, skin, genitourinary tract
Common human diseases	Pharyngitis, tonsillitis, erysipelas, impetigo, septicemia, wound infections, necrotizing fasciitis, cellulitis, meningitis, pneumonia, scarlet fever, toxic shock–like syndrome, rheumatic fever, acute glomerulonephritis	Puerperal sepsis chorioamnionitis, endocarditis, neonatal sepsis, meningitis, osteomyelitis, pneumonia	Wound infections, puerperal sepsis, cellulitis, sinusitis, endocarditis, brain abscess, sepsis, nosocomial infections, opportunistic infections	Endocarditis, human bite infections

α, Partial hemolysis; β, complete hemolysis; γ, no hemolysis (nonhemolytic).

G streptococcal infection has been related to M protein type and production of a pyrogenic exotoxin by SDSE.

SDSE organisms are common habitants of the pharynx, detected in up to 5% of asymptomatic children. Other potential sites of colonization include the skin and gastrointestinal tract. Colonization of the vagina is reported and may be the source of occasional SDSE isolated from the umbilicus of healthy neonates.

Clinical manifestations of disease caused by SDSE overlap those of disease caused by *S. pyogenes*. In children, these organisms are implicated most often in **pharyngitis**. The true role of these organisms as a cause of pharyngitis is difficult to determine because asymptomatic colonization is common. Nevertheless, several epidemics of SDSE pharyngitis have been reported, including food-borne outbreaks. A large study in Japan reported the detection of *S. pyogenes* in 15% and SDSE in 2% of children with pharyngitis. The clinical presentation of SDSE is indistinguishable from *S. pyogenes*–associated pharyngitis. Isolated case reports have described SDSE **pneumonia** in children, which is commonly complicated by abscess formation, empyema, and bacteremia. Additional respiratory infections include rare reports of epiglottitis and sinusitis.

SDSE are a significant cause of skin and soft tissue infections. As with *S. pyogenes*, **lymphangitis** can complicate superficial infections caused by SDSE. Musculoskeletal infections, particularly pyogenic arthritis, occasionally are caused by SDSE. Pediatric cases are uncommon but may be increasing in incidence.

Reactive arthritis has been described after SDSE infection; however, unlike the situation with *S. pyogenes*, the association between SDSE infection and acute rheumatic fever has not clearly been defined, and antibiotic prophylaxis is not recommended following reactive arthritis caused by SDSE.

Endocarditis, bacteremia, brain abscess, and toxic shock syndrome caused by SDSE have all been described but are uncommon in children. These infections generally occur in children with immune deficits or in adolescents after delayed recognition of sinusitis.

These organisms can cause neonatal **septicemia** similar to early-onset group B streptococcal disease. Risk factors include prematurity and prolonged rupture of membranes. Respiratory distress, hypotension, apnea, bradycardia, and disseminated intravascular coagulation may be seen, and associated maternal infection is common. Neonatal toxic shock syndrome associated with SDSE has also been described.

Treatment of SDSE infections is similar to that of *S. pyogenes*. These organisms retain susceptibility to penicillin and other β-lactams. Other agents with reliable activity include linezolid, quinupristin-dalfopristin, and vancomycin, although occasional isolates demonstrate tolerance to vancomycin. Clindamycin and macrolides have poor bactericidal activity against these organisms and are associated with significant resistance rates. Resistance to quinolones is reported, and up to 70% of SDSE cases are resistant to tetracycline.

Bibliography is available at Expert Consult.

Chapter 213
Enterococcus
David B. Haslam

第二百一十三章
肠球菌

中文导读

　　本章主要介绍了关于肠球菌感染的病因、流行病学、发病机制、临床表现、治疗、预防等内容。在关于肠球菌发病机制中具体描述了肠球菌抗生素耐药的内部机制以及获得性耐药的机制。在关于肠球菌的临床表现中具体描述了新生儿感染和大龄儿童感染的临床特点。在关于肠球菌的治疗中着重阐述了万古霉素耐药肠球菌的治疗，包括利奈唑胺、达托霉素、奎奴普丁-达福普汀、替吉环素和头孢洛林等药物治疗。

Enterococcus has long been recognized as a pathogen in select populations and has become a common and particularly troublesome cause of hospital-acquired infection over the past 2 decades. Formerly classified with *Streptococcus bovis* and *Streptococcus equinus* as Lancefield group D streptococci, enterococci are placed in a separate genus and are notorious for causing hospital-acquired infection and resisting antibiotics.

ETIOLOGY
Enterococci are gram-positive, catalase-negative facultative anaerobes that grow in pairs or short chains. Most are nonhemolytic (also called γ-hemolytic) on sheep blood agar, although some isolates have α- or β-hemolytic activity. Enterococci are distinguished from most Lancefield-groupable streptococci by their ability to grow in bile and hydrolyze esculin. They are able to grow in 6.5% NaCl and hydrolyze L-pyrrolidinyl-β-naphthylamide, features used by clinical laboratories to distinguish them from group D streptococcus. Identification at the species level is achieved by differing patterns of carbohydrate fermentation.

EPIDEMIOLOGY
Enterococci are normal inhabitants of the gastrointestinal (GI) tract of humans and organisms throughout the animal kingdom, suggesting they are highly evolved to occupy this niche. Oral secretions and dental plaque, the upper respiratory tract, skin, and vagina may also be colonized by *Enterococcus*. *Enterococcus faecalis* is the predominant organism, with colonization usually occurring in the 1st wk of life. By the time of adulthood, *E. faecalis* colonization is nearly ubiquitous but accounts for a minor fraction of the intestinal microbiota in the normal host. *Enterococcus faecium* colonization is less consistent, although approximately 25% of adults harbor this organism, generally at very low abundance. Disruption of the normal intestinal microbiota by antibiotic exposure or hematopoietic stem cell transplantation greatly enriches for fecal enterococcal abundance and dramatically increases the risk of subsequent bloodstream infection.

E. faecalis accounts for approximately 80% of enterococcal infections, with almost all the remaining infections caused by *E. faecium*. Only rarely are other species, such as *Enterococcus gallinarum* and *Enterococcus casseliflavus*, associated with invasive infection, but these organisms are notable for their intrinsic low-level vancomycin resistance. Whole genome sequencing suggests that the patient's indigenous flora is the source of enterococcal infection in most cases. However, direct spread from person to person or from contaminated medical devices may occur, particularly within newborn nurseries and intensive care units (NICUs), where nosocomial spread has resulted in hospital outbreaks.

PATHOGENESIS
Enterococci are not aggressively invasive organisms, usually causing disease only in children with damaged mucosal surfaces or impaired immune response. Their dramatic emergence as a cause of nosocomial infection is predominantly a result of their resistance to antibiotics commonly used in the hospital setting. **Hospital-associated enterococci** generally lack CRISPR (clustered regularly interspaced short palindromic repeat) elements. Their diverse antimicrobial resistance repertoire is likely related to deficient CRISPR-mediated defense against phage-mediated horizontal gene transfer. Secreted and cell surface molecules are implicated in pathogenesis. Adhesion-promoting factors such as the surface protein Eps likely account for the propensity of these organisms to cause endocarditis and urinary tract infections (UTIs). The ability to form biofilms likely facilitates the colonization of urinary and vascular catheters. Other proposed virulence factors include cytolysin, aggregation substance, gelatinase, and extracellular superoxide.

Antimicrobial Resistance
Enterococci are *highly resistant* to cephalosporins and semisynthetic penicillins such as nafcillin, oxacillin, and methicillin. They are moderately resistant to extended-spectrum penicillins such as ticarcillin and carbenicillin. Ampicillin, imipenem, and penicillin are the most

active β-lactams against these organisms. Some strains of *E. faecalis* and *E. faecium* demonstrate decreased resistance to β-lactam antibiotics because of mutations in penicillin-binding protein 5. In addition, occasional strains of *E. faecalis* produce a plasmid-encoded β-lactamase similar to that found in *Staphylococcus.* These isolates are completely resistant to penicillins, necessitating the combination of a penicillin plus a β-lactamase inhibitor or the use of imipenem or vancomycin. Any active drug may be insufficient if used alone for serious infections where high bactericidal activity is desired (Tables 213.1 and 213.2).

All enterococci have intrinsic *low-level resistance* to aminoglycosides because these antibiotics are poorly transported across the *Enterococcus* cell wall. Concomitant use of a cell wall active agent, such as a β-lactam or glycopeptide antibiotic, improves the permeability of the cell wall for the aminoglycosides, resulting in synergistic killing. However, some isolates demonstrate high-level resistance, defined as mean inhibitory concentration (MIC) >2,000 μg/mL, a result of modification or inactivation of aminoglycoside agents. Strains demonstrating high-level resistance and even some moderately resistant isolates are not affected synergistically by aminoglycosides and cell wall–active antibiotics.

Resistance to almost all other antibiotic classes, including tetracyclines, macrolides, and chloramphenicol, has been described among the enterococci, necessitating individual susceptibility testing for these antibiotics when their use is considered. Despite apparent susceptibility in vitro, trimethoprim-sulfamethoxazole (TMP-SMX) has poor activity in vivo and should not be used as the primary agent against *Enterococcus* infections.

Whereas ampicillin and vancomycin continue to have reliable activity against *E. faecalis*, resistance to both antibiotics is prevalent among *E. faecium.* Resistance to vancomycin, defined as MIC >32 μg/mL, and other glycopeptides, including teicoplanin, occurs in >30% of invasive *E. faecium* infections. Rates of vancomycin-resistant *Enterococcus* (**VRE**) have increased >2-fold since 2000 and have become a major challenge in the care of hospitalized patients. Mortality in patients with VRE bloodstream infections is considerable, and treatment is complicated

by frequent resistance of VRE to most other antibiotic classes. Both high- and moderate-level resistance are described in *E. faecalis* and *E. faecium.* High-level resistance (MIC ≥64 μg/mL) can be transferred by way of conjugation and usually results from plasmid-mediated transfer of the *vanA* gene. High-level resistance is most common among *E. faecium* but is increasingly seen among *E. faecalis* isolates. Moderate-level resistance (MIC 8-256 μg/mL) results from a chromosomal homolog of *vanA,* known as *vanB.* Isolates that harbor the *vanB* gene are only moderately resistant to vancomycin and initially demonstrate susceptibility to teicoplanin, although resistance can emerge during therapy. Resistance to newer agents, including linezolid and daptomycin, is rare thus far. **Linezolid** resistance is a result of mutations in the 26S ribosomal subunit, whereas **daptomycin** resistance is associated with mutations in genes required for membrane synthesis and repair.

CLINICAL MANIFESTATIONS

Enterococcus infections traditionally occurred predominantly in newborn infants; however, infection in older children is increasingly common. Most *Enterococcus* infections occur in patients with breakdown of normal physical barriers such as the GI tract, skin, or urinary tract. Other risk factors for *Enterococcus* infection include cancer chemotherapy, prolonged hospitalization, indwelling vascular catheters, prior use of antibiotics, and compromised immunity.

Neonatal Infections

Enterococcus accounts for up to 15% of all neonatal bacteremia and septicemia. As with group B streptococcus infections, *Enterococcus* infections are seen in 2 distinct settings in neonatal patients. Early-onset infection (<7 days of age) may mimic early-onset group B streptococcus septicemia but tends to be milder. Early-onset *Enterococcus* sepsis most often occurs in full-term infants who are otherwise healthy. Late-onset infection (≥7 days old) is associated with risk factors such as extreme prematurity, presence of an intravascular catheter, or **necrotizing enterocolitis** (NEC), or it follows an intraabdominal surgical procedure. Symptoms in late-onset disease are more severe than those in early-onset disease and include apnea, bradycardia, and deteriorating respiratory function. Associated focal infections include scalp abscess and catheter infection. Mortality rates range from 6% in early-onset septicemia to 15% in late-onset infections associated with NEC.

Enterococci are an occasional cause of **meningitis.** In neonates in particular, meningitis usually occurs as a complication of septicemia. Alternatively, the organism may gain access to the central nervous system by way of contiguous spread, such as through a neural tube defect or in association with an intraventricular shunt. *Enterococcus* meningitis can be associated with minimal abnormality of cerebrospinal fluid.

Infections in Older Children

Enterococcus rarely causes UTIs in healthy children but accounts for approximately 15% of cases of nosocomially acquired UTIs in both children and adults. Presence of an indwelling urinary catheter is the major risk factor for nosocomial UTIs. *Enterococcus* is frequently isolated in intraabdominal infections following intestinal perforation or surgery. The significance of enterococci in polymicrobial infections has been questioned, although reported mortality rates are higher when intraabdominal infections include enterococci. *Enterococcus* is increasingly common as a cause of nosocomial bacteremia, including catheter-associated bloodstream infections (**CLABSIs**); these organisms accounted for approximately 10% of CLABSIs in children, ranking 3rd after coagulase-negative staphylococci and *Staphylococcus aureus.* Predisposing factors for enterococcal bacteremia and endocarditis include an indwelling central venous catheter, GI surgery, immunodeficiency, and cardiovascular abnormalities. Risk factors for VRE bacteremia include residence on hematology/oncology unit, prolonged mechanical ventilation, immunosuppression, and recent broad-spectrum antibiotic exposure.

TREATMENT

Treatment of invasive *Enterococcus* infections must recognize that these organisms are resistant to antimicrobial agents frequently used as empirical therapy. In particular, **cephalosporins** should not be

Table 213.1	Intrinsic Resistance Mechanisms Among Enterococci
ANTIMICROBIAL	**MECHANISM**
Ampicillin, penicillin	Altered binding protein
Aminoglycoside (low level)	Decreased permeability, altered ribosomal binding
Clindamycin	Altered ribosomal binding
Erythromycin	Altered ribosomal binding
Tetracyclines	Efflux pump
Trimethoprim-sulfamethoxazole	Utilize exogenous folate

Table 213.2	Acquired Resistance Mechanisms Among Enterococci
ANTIMICROBIAL	**MECHANISM**
Ampicillin, penicillin (high level)	Mutation of PBP5
Aminoglycoside (high level)	Enzyme modification
Quinolones	DNA gyrase mutation
Chloramphenicol	Efflux pump
Glycopeptide	Altered cell wall binding
Quinupristin-dalfopristin	Ribosomal modification, efflux pump
Linezolid	Point mutation
Daptomycin	Unknown

relied on in situations where *Enterococcus* is known or suspected to be involved. In general, in the immunocompetent host, minor localized infections caused by susceptible *Enterococcus* can be treated with ampicillin alone. Antibiotics containing β-lactamase inhibitors (clavulanate or sulbactam) provide advantage only for the few organisms whose resistance results from production of β-lactamase. In uncomplicated UTIs, nitrofurantoin is efficacious when the organism is known to be sensitive to this antibiotic.

Invasive infections, such as sepsis, meningitis, and endocarditis, are usually treated with penicillin or ampicillin if the organism is susceptible. Addition of an aminoglycoside has traditionally been suggested but is associated with nephrotoxicity and may not be routinely indicated in uncomplicated enterococcal bloodstream infection. Vancomycin can be substituted for the penicillins in allergic patients but should be used with an aminoglycoside because vancomycin alone is not bactericidal. Endocarditis from strains possessing high-level aminoglycoside resistance may relapse even after prolonged therapy. High-dose or continuous infusion penicillin has been proposed for treatment of these infections in adults, yet ultimately valve replacement may be necessary. In patients with catheter-associated enterococcal bacteremia, the catheter should be removed promptly in most cases, although infected lines have been salvaged with the combined use of ampicillin or vancomycin and an aminoglycoside.

Vancomycin-Resistant Enterococci

The treatment of serious infections caused by multiresistant, vancomycin-resistant strains is particularly challenging. **Linezolid**, an oxazolidinone antibiotic that inhibits protein synthesis, is bacteriostatic against most *E. faecium* and *E. faecalis* isolates, including VRE isolates. Response rates are generally >90%, including cases of bacteremia and sepsis, and this antibiotic has become the preferred agent in treatment of VRE infections in many institutions. Anecdotal reports reveal the success of linezolid in treating meningitis caused by VRE. Unfortunately, as seen with other antibiotics, linezolid resistance is documented, and nosocomial spread of these organisms can occur. Linezolid frequently causes reversible bone marrow suppression after prolonged use and is associated with rare occurrences of lactic acidosis and irreversible peripheral neuropathy. **Serotonin syndrome** may be seen in patients taking concomitant selective serotonin reuptake inhibitor antidepressants. Oxazolidinones in development include **tedizolid**, which has better in vitro activity against enterococci and appears to have favorable pharmacokinetic and toxicity profiles compared to linezolid.

Daptomycin is a cyclic lipopeptide that is rapidly bactericidal against a broad range of gram-positive organisms. This antibiotic inserts into the bacterial cell wall, causing membrane depolarization and cell death. It has been approved for the treatment of adults with serious skin and soft tissue infections, right-sided endocarditis, and bacteremia caused by susceptible organisms. Most strains of VRE (both *E. faecium* and *E. faecalis*) are susceptible to daptomycin in vitro, and its efficacy in adult patients with VRE appears to be similar to that of linezolid. Experience with daptomycin in children is limited, particularly in the setting of *Enterococcus* infections. However, based on the experience with adult patients, daptomycin may be an alternative to linezolid when resistance or side effects limit utility of that antibiotic. Daptomycin dosages may need to be higher in children than adults because of more rapid renal clearance. The antibiotic has unreliable activity in the lung and therefore should not be used as a sole agent to treat pneumonia. Resistance of both *Staphylococcus aureus* and *Enterococcus* to daptomycin has rarely been described, sometimes arising during therapy.

Quinupristin-dalfopristin is a combined streptogramin antibiotic that inhibits bacterial protein synthesis at 2 different stages. It has activity against most *E. faecium* strains, including those with high-level vancomycin resistance. Approximately 90% of *E. faecium* strains are susceptible to quinupristin-dalfopristin in vitro. Notably, it is inactive against *E. faecalis* and therefore should not be used as the sole agent against gram-positive organisms until culture results exclude the presence of *E. faecalis*. Studies in children suggest that this antibiotic is effective and generally well tolerated, although episodes of arthralgia and myalgia during therapy are reported. Emergence of resistance to quinupristin-dalfopristin is rare but has been demonstrated.

Tigecycline is the first clinically available glycylcycline antibiotic, an expended-spectrum derivative of the tetracycline family. The agent inhibits protein synthesis by binding to the 30S ribosome and is bacteriostatic against susceptible organisms. Tigecycline has broad activity against gram-positive, gram-negative, and anaerobic organisms, including methicillin-resistant *Staphylococcus aureus* (MRSA) and VRE, and is approved for the treatment of adults with skin and soft tissue infections and intraabdominal infections caused by susceptible organisms. Its efficacy in VRE infections has not yet been demonstrated in clinical trials, and there is little published experience with the use of tigecycline in children thus far. As with other tetracycline antibiotics, tigecycline use may cause discoloration of the teeth, and its use in children <8 yr old should generally be avoided. GI side effects are common and may be intolerable.

Ceftaroline, a fifth-generation cephalosporin with activity against MRSA, has activity against many *E. faecalis* strains and may be highly synergistic with daptomycin against daptomycin-nonsusceptible strains. Ceftaroline has poor activity against *E. faecium* and should not be relied on as the sole agent to treat infections caused by this organism.

PREVENTION

Strategies for preventing enterococcal infections include timely removal of urinary and intravenous catheters and debridement of necrotic tissue. Infection control strategies, including surveillance cultures, patient and staff cohorting, and strict gown and glove isolation, are effective at decreasing colonization rates with VRE. Unfortunately, these organisms may persist on inanimate objects such as stethoscopes, complicating efforts to limit their nosocomial spread. To prevent the emergence and spread of vancomycin-resistant organisms, the U.S. Centers for Disease Control and Prevention (CDC) has developed a series of guidelines for prudent vancomycin use. Antibiotics with broad activity against anaerobic organisms are also thought to contribute to colonization with VRE, suggesting that prudent use of such antibiotics may also help limit spread of VRE. Decolonization strategies have been attempted but are generally ineffective in eradicating skin or GI carriage of VRE. In particular, antimicrobial therapy is not indicated for this purpose. The role of probiotic agents in eliminating VRE colonization is currently unclear but may be a useful adjunct to prudent antimicrobial usage and other infection control interventions in limiting nosocomial spread of VRE.

Bibliography is available at Expert Consult.

Chapter **214**
Diphtheria (*Corynebacterium diphtheriae*)

Amruta Padhye and Stephanie A. Fritz

第二百一十四章
白喉棒状杆菌（白喉杆菌）

中文导读

本章主要介绍了关于白喉棒状杆菌（白喉杆菌）感染的病因、流行病学、发病机制、临床表现、诊断、并发症、治疗、支持治疗、预后、预防等内容。在白喉棒状杆菌感染的临床表现部分详细介绍了呼吸道白喉、皮肤白喉和其他部位感染。在白喉棒状杆菌感染的并发症部分详细介绍了中毒性心肌病和中毒性神经病。在白喉棒状杆菌感染的预防部分详细介绍了无症状病例接触、无症状携带和疫苗。

Diphtheria is an acute toxic infection caused by *Corynebacterium* species, typically *Corynebacterium diphtheriae* and, less often, toxigenic strains of *Corynebacterium ulcerans*. Although diphtheria was reduced from a major cause of childhood death to a medical rarity in the Western hemisphere in the early 20th century, recurring reminders of the fragility of this success, particularly in conflict areas, emphasize the need to continue vigorous promotion of those same control principles across the global community.

ETIOLOGY

Corynebacteria are aerobic, nonencapsulated, non–spore-forming, mostly nonmotile, pleomorphic, gram-positive bacilli. *C. diphtheriae* is by far the most frequently isolated agent of diphtheria. *C. ulcerans* is more often isolated from animal sources and can cause human disease similar to *C. diphtheriae*. Selective medium (e.g., cystine-tellurite blood agar or Tinsdale agar) that inhibits growth of competing organisms is required for isolation and, when reduced by *C. diphtheriae*, renders colonies gray-black. Differentiation of *C. diphtheriae* from *C. ulcerans* is based on urease activity; *C. ulcerans* is urease-positive. Four *C. diphtheriae* biotypes (*mitis, intermedius, belfanti, gravis*) are capable of causing diphtheria and are differentiated by colony morphology, hemolysis, and fermentation reactions. The ability to produce diphtheritic toxin results from acquisition of a lysogenic corynebacteriophage by either *C. diphtheriae* or *C. ulcerans*, which encodes the diphtheritic toxin gene and confers diphtheria-producing potential on these strains. Thus, indigenous nontoxigenic *C. diphtheriae* can be rendered toxigenic and disease-producing after importation of a toxigenic *C. diphtheriae*. Demonstration of diphtheritic toxin production by the modified Elek test, an agar immunoprecipitin technique, alone or in conjunction with polymerase chain reaction (PCR) testing for carriage of the toxin gene, is necessary to confirm disease. Toxigenic and nontoxigenic strains are indistinguishable by colony type, microscopic features, or biochemical test results.

EPIDEMIOLOGY

Unlike other diphtheroids (coryneform bacteria), which are ubiquitous in nature, *C. diphtheriae* is an exclusive inhabitant of human mucous membranes and skin. Spread is primarily by airborne respiratory droplets, direct contact with respiratory secretions of symptomatic individuals, or exudate from infected skin lesions. Asymptomatic respiratory tract carriage is important in transmission. In areas where diphtheria is endemic, 3–5% of healthy individuals can carry toxigenic organisms, but carriage is exceedingly rare when diphtheria is rare. Skin infection and skin carriage are silent reservoirs of *C. diphtheriae*, and organisms can remain viable in dust or on fomites for up to 6 mo. Transmission through contaminated milk and through an infected food handler has been proved or suspected.

In the 1920s, >125,000 diphtheria cases, with 10,000 deaths, were reported annually in the United States, with the highest fatality rates among very young and elderly persons. The incidence then began to decrease and, with widespread use of diphtheria toxoid in the United States after World War II, declined steadily through the late 1970s. Since then, ≤5 cases have occurred annually in the United States, with no epidemics of respiratory tract diphtheria. Similar decreases occurred in Europe. Despite the worldwide decrease in disease incidence, diphtheria remains endemic in many developing countries with poor immunization rates against diphtheria.

When diphtheria was endemic, it primarily affected children <15 yr old. Since the introduction of toxoid immunization, the disease has shifted to adults who lack natural exposure to toxigenic *C. diphtheriae* in the vaccine era and have low rates of booster immunization. In the 27 sporadic cases of respiratory tract diphtheria reported in the United States in the 1980s, 70% occurred among persons >25 yr old. The largest outbreak of diphtheria in the developed world since the 1960s occurred from 1990–1996 in the newly independent countries of the former Soviet Union, involving >150,000 cases in 14 countries. Of these, >60% of cases occurred in individuals >14 yr old. Case fatality rates ranged from 3–23% by country. Factors contributing to the epidemic included a large population of underimmunized adults, decreased childhood immunization rates, population migration, crowding, and failure to respond aggressively during early phases of the epidemic. Cases of diphtheria among travelers from these endemic areas were transported to many countries in Europe.

Most proven cases of respiratory tract diphtheria in the United States in the 1990s were associated with **importation** of toxigenic *C. diphtheriae,* although clonally related toxigenic *C. diphtheriae* has persisted in this country and Canada for at least 25 yr. World Health Organization (WHO) surveillance reports indicate that most cases of diphtheria worldwide occur in the Southeast Asia and Africa regions. In Europe, increasing reports of respiratory and systemic infections have been attributed to *C ulcerans*; animal contact is the predominant risk factor.

Cutaneous diphtheria, a curiosity when diphtheria was common, accounted for more than 50% of reported *C. diphtheriae* isolates in the United States by 1975. This indolent local infection, compared with mucosal infection, is associated with more prolonged bacterial shedding, greater contamination of the environment, and increased transmission to the pharynx and skin of close contacts. Outbreaks are associated with homelessness, crowding, poverty, alcoholism, poor hygiene, contaminated fomites, underlying dermatosis, and introduction of new strains from exogenous sources. It is no longer a tropical or subtropical disease; 1,100 *C. diphtheriae* infections were documented in a neighborhood in Seattle (site of the last major U.S. outbreak), from 1971–1982; 86% were cutaneous, and 40% involved toxigenic strains. Cutaneous diphtheria is an important source for toxigenic *C. diphtheriae* in the United States, and its importation is frequently the source for subsequent sporadic cases of respiratory tract diphtheria. Cutaneous diphtheria caused by *C. ulcerans* from travel to tropical countries or animal contact has been increasingly reported.

PATHOGENESIS
Both toxigenic and nontoxigenic *C. diphtheriae* cause skin and mucosal infection and can rarely cause focal infection after bacteremia. The organism usually remains in the superficial layers of skin lesions or respiratory tract mucosa, inducing local inflammatory reaction. The major virulence of the organism lies in its ability to produce a potent polypeptide exotoxin, which inhibits protein synthesis and causes local tissue necrosis and resultant local inflammatory response. Within the first few days of respiratory tract infection (usually in the pharynx), a dense necrotic coagulum of organisms, epithelial cells, fibrin, leukocytes, and erythrocytes forms, initially white and advancing to become a gray-brown, leather-like adherent **pseudomembrane** (*diphtheria* is Greek for leather). Removal is difficult and reveals a bleeding edematous submucosa. Paralysis of the palate and hypopharynx is an early local effect of diphtheria toxin. Toxin absorption can lead to systemic manifestations: kidney tubule necrosis, thrombocytopenia, cardiomyopathy, and demyelination of nerves. Because the latter 2 complications can occur 2-10 wk after mucocutaneous infection, the pathophysiology in some cases is suspected to be immunologically mediated.

CLINICAL MANIFESTATIONS
The manifestations of *C. diphtheriae* infection are influenced by the anatomic site of infection, the immune status of the host, and the production and systemic distribution of toxin.

Respiratory Tract Diphtheria
In a classic description of 1,400 cases of diphtheria in California (1954), the primary focus of infection was the tonsils or pharynx (94%), with the nose and larynx the next 2 most common sites. After an average incubation period of 2-4 days (range 1-10 days), local signs and symptoms of inflammation develop. Infection of the anterior nares is more common among infants and causes serosanguineous, purulent, erosive rhinitis with membrane formation. Shallow ulceration of the external nares and upper lip is characteristic. In tonsillar and **pharyngeal diphtheria**, sore throat is the universal early symptom. Only half of patients have fever, and fewer have dysphagia, hoarseness, malaise, or headache. Mild pharyngeal injection is followed by unilateral or bilateral tonsillar membrane formation, which can extend to involve the uvula (which may cause toxin-mediated paralysis), soft palate, posterior oropharynx, hypopharynx, or glottic areas (Fig. 214.1). Underlying soft tissue edema and enlarged lymph nodes can cause a bull-neck appearance. The degree of local extension correlates directly with profound prostration, bull-neck appearance, and fatality due to airway compromise or toxin-mediated complications (Fig. 214.2).

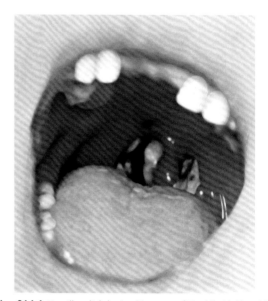

Fig. 214.1 Tonsillar diphtheria. *(Courtesy of Franklin H. Top, MD, Professor and Head of the Department of Hygiene and Preventive Medicine, State University of Iowa, College of Medicine, Iowa City, IA; and Parke, Davis & Company's Therapeutic Notes.)*

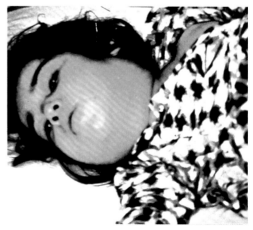

Fig. 214.2 Diphtheria. Bull-neck appearance of diphtheritic cervical lymphadenopathy. *(Courtesy of the Centers for Disease Control and Prevention.)*

The characteristic adherent membrane, extension beyond the faucial area, dysphagia, and relative lack of fever help differentiate diphtheria from **exudative pharyngitis** caused by *Streptococcus pyogenes* or Epstein-Barr virus. Vincent angina, infective phlebitis with thrombosis of the jugular veins (Lemierre syndrome), and mucositis in patients undergoing cancer chemotherapy are usually differentiated by the clinical setting. Infection of the larynx, trachea, and bronchi can be primary or a secondary extension from the pharyngeal infection. Hoarseness, stridor, dyspnea, and croupy cough are clues. Differentiation from bacterial epiglottitis, severe viral laryngotracheobronchitis, and staphylococcal or streptococcal tracheitis hinges partially on the relative paucity of other signs and symptoms in patients with diphtheria and primarily on visualization of the adherent pseudomembrane at laryngoscopy and intubation.

Patients with laryngeal diphtheria are at significant risk for suffocation because of local soft tissue edema and airway obstruction by the diphtheria membrane, a dense cast of respiratory epithelium, and necrotic coagulum. Establishment of an artificial airway and resection of the pseudomembrane can be lifesaving, but further obstructive complications are common, and systemic toxic complications are inevitable.

Cutaneous Diphtheria

Classic cutaneous diphtheria is an indolent, nonprogressive infection characterized by a superficial, ecthyma-like, nonhealing ulcer with a gray-brown membrane. Diphtheria skin infections cannot always be differentiated from streptococcal or staphylococcal impetigo, and these conditions frequently coexist. In most cases, a primary process, such as dermatosis, laceration, burn, bite, or impetigo, becomes secondarily infected with *C. diphtheriae*. Extremities are more often affected than the trunk or head. Pain, tenderness, erythema, and exudate are typical. Local hyperesthesia or hypesthesia is unusual. Respiratory tract colonization or symptomatic infection with toxic complications occurs in the minority of patients with cutaneous diphtheria. Among infected adults in the Seattle outbreak, 3% with cutaneous infections and 21% with symptomatic nasopharyngeal infection, with or without skin involvement, demonstrated toxic myocarditis, neuropathy, or obstructive respiratory tract complications. All had received at least 20,000 units of equine antitoxin at the time of hospitalization.

Infection at Other Sites

C. diphtheriae occasionally causes mucocutaneous infections at other sites, such as the ear (otitis externa), the eye (purulent and ulcerative conjunctivitis), and the genital tract (purulent and ulcerative vulvovaginitis). The clinical setting, ulceration, membrane formation, and submucosal bleeding help differentiate diphtheria from other bacterial and viral causes. Rare cases of septicemia are described and are universally fatal. Sporadic cases of endocarditis occur, and clusters among intravenous drug users have been reported in several countries; skin was the probable portal of entry, and almost all strains were nontoxigenic. Sporadic cases of pyogenic arthritis, mainly from nontoxigenic strains, have been reported in adults and children. Diphtheroids isolated from sterile body sites should not be routinely dismissed as contaminants without careful consideration of the clinical setting.

DIAGNOSIS

Specimens for culture should be obtained from the nose and throat and any other mucocutaneous lesion. A portion of membrane should be removed and submitted for culture along with underlying exudate. The laboratory must be notified to use selective medium. *C. diphtheriae* survives drying. If obtained in a remote area, a dry swab specimen can be placed in a silica gel pack and sent to the laboratory. Evaluation of a direct smear using Gram stain or specific fluorescent antibody is unreliable. Culture isolates of coryneform organisms should be identified to the species level, and toxigenicity and antimicrobial susceptibility tests should be performed for *C. diphtheriae* isolates. It is recommended that all isolates be sent to a reference laboratory. In the United States, the Centers for Disease Control and Prevention (CDC) Pertussis and Diphtheria Laboratory provides support to local and state health departments needing assistance with isolation, identification, and subtyping

of *C. diphtheriae* and *C. ulcerans*.

COMPLICATIONS

Respiratory tract obstruction by pseudomembranes may require bronchoscopy or intubation and mechanical ventilation. Two other tissues usually remote from sites of *C. diphtheriae* infection can be significantly affected by **diphtheritic toxin**: the heart and the nervous system.

Toxic Cardiomyopathy

Toxic cardiomyopathy occurs in 10–25% of patients with respiratory diphtheria and is responsible for 50–60% of deaths. Subtle signs of myocarditis can be detected in most patients, especially the elderly, but the risk for significant complications correlates directly with the extent and severity of exudative local oropharyngeal disease, as well as delay in administration of antitoxin. The first evidence of cardiac toxicity characteristically occurs during the 2nd and 3rd wk of illness as the pharyngeal disease improves, but can appear acutely as early as the 1st wk of illness, a poor prognostic sign, or insidiously as late as the 6th wk. Tachycardia disproportionate to fever is common and may be evidence of cardiac toxicity or autonomic nervous system dysfunction. A prolonged P-R interval and changes in the ST-T wave on an electrocardiographic tracing are relatively frequent findings; dilated and hypertrophic cardiomyopathy detected by echocardiogram has been described. Single or progressive cardiac **dysrhythmias** can occur, including first-, second-, and third-degree heart block. Temporary transvenous pacing may improve outcomes. Atrioventricular dissociation and ventricular tachycardia are also described, the latter having a high associated mortality. Heart failure may appear insidiously or acutely. Elevation of the serum aspartate transaminase concentration closely parallels the severity of myonecrosis. Severe dysrhythmia portends death. Histologic postmortem findings are variable: little or diffuse myonecrosis with acute inflammatory response. Recovery from toxic myocardiopathy is usually complete, although survivors of more severe dysrhythmias can have permanent conduction defects.

Toxic Neuropathy

Neurologic complications parallel the severity of primary infection and are multiphasic in onset. Acutely or 2-3 wk after onset of oropharyngeal inflammation, hypesthesia and local **paralysis** of the soft palate typically occur. Weakness of the posterior pharyngeal, laryngeal, and facial nerves may follow, causing a nasal quality in the voice, difficulty in swallowing, and risk for aspiration. **Cranial neuropathies** characteristically occur in the 5th wk, leading to oculomotor and ciliary paralysis, which can cause strabismus, blurred vision, or difficulty with accommodation. Symmetric demyelinating **polyneuropathy** has onset 10 days to 3 mo after oropharyngeal infection and causes principally motor deficits with diminished deep tendon reflexes. Nerve conduction velocity studies and cerebrospinal fluid findings in diphtheritic polyneuropathy are indistinguishable from those of Guillain-Barré syndrome. Paralysis of the diaphragm may ensue. Complete neurologic recovery is likely, but rarely vasomotor center dysfunction 2-3 wk after onset of illness can cause hypotension or cardiac failure.

Recovery from myocarditis and neuritis is often slow but usually complete. Corticosteroids do not diminish these complications and are not recommended.

TREATMENT

Specific **antitoxin** is the mainstay of therapy and should be administered on the basis of clinical diagnosis. Because it neutralizes only free toxin, antitoxin efficacy diminishes with elapsed time after the onset of mucocutaneous symptoms. Equine diphtheria antitoxin is available in the United States only from the CDC. Physicians treating a case of suspected diphtheria should contact the CDC Emergency Operations Center (770-488-7100 at all times). Antitoxin is administered as a single empirical dose of 20,000-100,000 units based on the degree of toxicity, site and size of the membrane, and duration of illness. Skin testing must be performed before administration of antitoxin. Patients with positive sensitivity testing or with a history of hypersensitivity reaction to horse equine protein should be desensitized. Antitoxin is probably of no value for local manifestations of cutaneous diphtheria, but its use is prudent because toxic sequelae can occur. Commercially available intravenous immunoglobulin preparations contain low titers of antibodies to diphtheria toxin; their use for therapy of diphtheria is not proved or approved. Antitoxin is not recommended for asymptomatic carriers.

The role of **antimicrobial therapy** is to halt toxin production, treat localized infection, and prevent transmission of the organism to contacts. *C. diphtheriae* is usually susceptible to various agents in vitro, including penicillins, erythromycin, clindamycin, rifampin, and tetracycline. Resistance to erythromycin is common in populations if the drug has been used broadly, and resistance to penicillin has also been reported. Only erythromycin or penicillin is recommended; erythromycin is marginally superior to penicillin for eradication of nasopharyngeal carriage. Appropriate therapy is **erythromycin** (40-50 mg/kg/day divided every 6 hr by mouth [PO] or intravenously [IV]; maximum 2 g/day), **aqueous crystalline penicillin G** (100,000-150,000 units/kg/day divided every 6 hr IV or intramuscularly [IM]), or **procaine penicillin** (300,000 units every 12 hr IM for those ≤10 kg in weight; 600,000 units every 12 hr IM for those >10 kg in weight) for 14 days. Once oral medications are tolerated, oral penicillin V (250 mg four times daily) may be used. *Antibiotic therapy is not a substitute for antitoxin therapy.* Some patients with cutaneous diphtheria have been treated for 7-10 days. Elimination of the organism should be documented by negative results of at least 2 successive cultures of specimens from the nose and throat (or skin) obtained 24 hr apart after completion of therapy. Treatment with erythromycin is repeated if either culture yields *C. diphtheriae.*

SUPPORTIVE CARE

Droplet precautions are instituted for patients with pharyngeal diphtheria; for patients with cutaneous diphtheria, **contact precautions** are observed until the results of cultures of specimens taken after cessation of therapy are negative. Cutaneous wounds are cleaned thoroughly with soap and water. Bed rest is essential during the acute phase of disease, usually for ≥2 wk until the risk for symptomatic cardiac damage has passed, with return to physical activity guided by the degree of toxicity and cardiac involvement.

PROGNOSIS

The prognosis for patients with diphtheria depends on the virulence of the organism (subspecies *gravis* has the highest fatality rate), patient age, immunization status, site of infection, and speed of administration of the antitoxin. Mechanical obstruction from laryngeal diphtheria or bull-neck diphtheria and the complications of myocarditis account for most diphtheria-related deaths. The case fatality rate of almost 10% for respiratory tract diphtheria has not changed in 50 yr; the rate was 8% in a Vietnamese series described in 2004. At recovery, administration of diphtheria toxoid is indicated to complete the primary series or booster doses of immunization, because not all patients develop antibodies to diphtheria toxin after infection.

PREVENTION

Protection against serious disease caused by imported or indigenously acquired *C. diphtheriae* depends on immunization. In the absence of a precisely determined minimum protective level for diphtheria antitoxin, the presumed minimum is 0.01-0.10 IU/mL. In outbreaks, 90% of individuals with clinical disease have had antibody values <0.01 IU/mL, and 92% of asymptomatic carriers have had values >0.1 IU/mL. In serosurveys in the United States and Western Europe, where almost universal immunization during childhood has been achieved, 25% to >60% of adults lack protective antitoxin levels, with typically very low levels in elderly persons.

All suspected diphtheria cases should be reported to local and state health departments. Investigation is aimed at preventing secondary cases in exposed individuals and at determining the source and carriers to halt spread to unexposed individuals. Reported rates of carriage in household contacts of case patients are 0–25%. The risk for development of diphtheria after household exposure to a case is approximately 2%, and the risk after similar exposure to a carrier is 0.3%.

Asymptomatic Case Contacts

All household contacts and people who have had intimate respiratory or habitual physical contact with a patient are closely monitored for illness for 7 days. Cultures of the nose, throat, and any cutaneous lesions are performed. Antimicrobial prophylaxis is presumed effective and is administered regardless of immunization status, using a single injection of benzathine penicillin G (600,000 units IM for patients <6 yr old, or 1,200,000 units IM for patients >6 yr old) or erythromycin (40-50 mg/kg/day divided qid PO for 10 days; max 2 g/day). Diphtheria toxoid vaccine, in age-appropriate form, is given to immunized individuals who have not received a booster dose within 5 yr. Children who have not received their 4th dose should be vaccinated. Those who have received fewer than 3 doses of diphtheria toxoid or who have uncertain immunization status should be immunized with an age-appropriate preparation on a primary schedule.

Asymptomatic Carriers

When an asymptomatic carrier is identified, antimicrobial prophylaxis is given for 10-14 days and an age-appropriate preparation of diphtheria toxoid is administered immediately if a booster has not been given within 1 yr. Droplet precautions (respiratory tract colonization) or contact precautions (cutaneous colonization only) are observed until at least 2 subsequent cultures obtained 24 hr apart after cessation of therapy have negative results.

Repeat cultures are performed about 2 wk after completion of therapy for cases and carriers; if results are positive, an additional 10-day course of oral erythromycin should be given and follow-up cultures performed. Susceptibility testing of isolates should be performed, as erythromycin resistance is reported. Neither antimicrobial agent eradicates carriage in 100% of individuals. In one report, a single course of therapy failed in 21% of carriers. Transmission of diphtheria in modern hospitals is rare. Only those who have an unusual contact with respiratory or oral secretions should be managed as contacts. Investigation of the casual contacts of patients and carriers or persons in the community without known exposure has yielded extremely low carriage rates and is not routinely recommended.

Vaccine

Universal immunization with diphtheria toxoid throughout life, to provide constant protective antitoxin levels and to reduce severity of *C. diphtheriae* disease, is the only effective control measure. Although immunization does not preclude subsequent respiratory or cutaneous carriage of toxigenic *C. diphtheriae,* it decreases local tissue spread, prevents toxic complications, diminishes transmission of the organism, and provides herd immunity when at least 70–80% of a population is immunized.

Diphtheria toxoid is prepared by formaldehyde treatment of toxin, standardized for potency, and adsorbed to aluminum salts, enhancing immunogenicity. Two preparations of diphtheria toxoids are formulated according to the *limit of flocculation* (Lf) content, a measure of the quantity of toxoid. The pediatric (6 mo to 6 yr) preparations (i.e., **DTaP** [diphtheria and tetanus toxoids with acellular pertussis vaccine], **DT** [diphtheria and tetanus toxoids vaccine]) contain 6.7-25.0 Lf units of diphtheria toxoid per 0.5 mL dose; the adult preparation (Td; 10% of pediatric diphtheria toxoid dose, Tdap [diphtheria and tetanus toxoids with acellular pertussis vaccine]) contain no more than 2-2.5 Lf units of toxoid per 0.5 mL dose. The *higher-potency* (D) formulation of toxoid is used for primary series and booster doses for children through 6 yr of age because of superior immunogenicity and minimal reactogenicity. For individuals ≥7 yr old, Td is recommended for the primary series and booster doses because the lower concentration of diphtheria toxoid is adequately immunogenic and increasing the content of diphtheria toxoid heightens reactogenicity with increasing age.

For children 6 wk to 6 yr of age, five 0.5 mL doses of diphtheria-containing (D) vaccine (DTaP preferred) are given in the primary series, including doses at 2, 4, and 6 mo of age, and a 4th dose, an integral part of the primary series, at 15-18 mo. A booster dose is given at 4-6 yr of age (unless the 4th primary dose was administered at ≥4 yr). For persons ≥7 yr old not previously immunized for diphtheria, three

0.5 mL doses of *lower-level* diphtheria-containing (d) vaccine are given in a primary series of 2 doses at least 4 wk apart and a 3rd dose 6 mo after the 2nd dose. The 1st dose should be Tdap, and subsequent doses should be Td. The only contraindication to tetanus and diphtheria toxoid is a history of neurologic or severe hypersensitivity reaction after a prior dose. For children <7 yr old in whom pertussis immunization is contraindicated, DT is used. Those whose immunization is begun with DTaP or DT before 1 yr of age should have a total of five 0.5 mL doses of diphtheria-containing (D) vaccines by 6 yr of age. For those whose immunization is begun at around 1 yr old, the primary series is three 0.5 mL doses of diphtheria-containing (D) vaccine, with a booster given at 4-6 yr, unless the 3rd dose was given after the 4th birthday.

A booster dose, consisting of the adult preparation of Tdap, is recommended at 11-12 yr of age. Adolescents 13-18 yr old who missed the Td or Tdap booster dose at 11-12 yr or in whom it has been ≥5 yr since the Td booster dose also should receive a single dose of Tdap if they have completed the DTP/DTaP series.

There is no association of DT or Td with convulsions. Local adverse effects alone do not preclude continued use. The rare patient who experiences an Arthus-type hypersensitivity reaction or a temperature >39.4°C (103°F) after a dose of Td usually has high serum tetanus antitoxin levels and should not be given Td more frequently than every 10 yr, even if the patient sustains a significant tetanus-prone injury. The DT or Td preparation can be given concurrently with other vaccines. *Haemophilus influenzae* type b (Hib), meningococcal, and pneumococcal conjugate vaccines containing diphtheria toxoid (PRP-D) or the variant of diphtheria toxin, CRM197 protein, are not substitutes for diphtheria toxoid immunization and do not affect reactogenicity.

Bibliography is available at Expert Consult.

Chapter **215**
Listeria monocytogenes
Thomas S. Murray and Robert S. Baltimore
第二百一十五章
单核细胞增多性李斯特菌

中文导读

　　本章主要介绍了关于单核细胞增多性李斯特菌感染的病因、流行病学、病理、发病机制、临床表现、诊断、治疗、预后、预防等内容。在关于单核细胞增多性李斯特菌感染的临床表现部分详细介绍了妊娠李斯特菌病、新生儿李斯特菌病（早发型和晚发型）和新生儿后感染。在关于单核细胞增多性李斯特菌感染的鉴别诊断部分详细描述了中枢神经系统感染的特点。

Listeriosis in humans is caused principally by *Listeria monocytogenes*, 1 of 6 species of the genus *Listeria* that are widely distributed in the environment and throughout the food chain. Human infections can usually be traced to an animal reservoir. Infection usually occurs at the extremes of age. In the pediatric population, perinatal infections predominate and usually occur secondary to maternal infection or colonization. Outside the newborn period, disease is most often encountered in *immunosuppressed* (usually T-cell deficiencies) children and adults and in elderly persons. For most people the major risk for infection with *Listeria* is **food-borne transmission**. In the United States, food-borne outbreaks are caused by improperly processed dairy products and contaminated vegetables and principally affect the same individuals at risk for sporadic disease.

ETIOLOGY

Members of the genus *Listeria* are facultatively anaerobic, non–spore-forming, motile, gram-positive bacilli that are catalase positive. In the laboratory, *Listeria* can be distinguished from other gram-positive bacilli by their characteristic tumbling motility and growth at cold temperature (4-10°C [39.2-50°F]). The 6 *Listeria* spp. are divided into 2 genomically distinct groups on the basis of DNA-DNA hybridization studies. One group contains the species *Listeria grayi*, considered nonpathogenic. The 2nd group contains 5 species: the nonhemolytic species *Listeria innocua* and *L. welshimeri* and the hemolytic species *Listeria monocytogenes*, *L. seeligeri*, and *L. ivanovii*. *Listeria ivanovii* is pathogenic primarily in animals, and the vast majority of both human and animal disease is caused by *L. monocytogenes*.

Subtyping of *L. monocytogenes* isolates for epidemiologic purposes has been attempted with the use of heat-stable somatic O and heat-labile flagellar H antigens, phage typing, pulsed-field gel electrophoresis, ribotyping, and multilocus enzyme electrophoresis. Electrophoretic typing demonstrates the clonal structure of populations of *L. monocytogenes* as well as the sharing of populations between human and animal sources. **Subtyping** is an important component of determining whether cases are connected or sporadic but usually requires collaboration with a specialized laboratory.

Selected biochemical tests, together with the demonstration of *tumbling motility*, umbrella-type formation below the surface in semisolid medium, hemolysis, and a typical cyclic adenosine monophosphate test, are usually sufficient to establish a presumptive identification of *L. monocytogenes*.

EPIDEMIOLOGY

Listeria monocytogenes is widespread in nature, has been isolated throughout the environment, and is associated with epizootic disease and asymptomatic carriage in >42 species of wild and domestic animals and 22 avian species. Epizootic disease in large animals (e.g., sheep, cattle) is associated with abortion and "circling disease," a form of basilar meningitis. *L. monocytogenes* is isolated from sewage, silage, and soil, where it survives for >295 days. Human-to-human transmission rarely occurs except in maternal-fetal transmission. The annual incidence of listeriosis decreased by 36% between 1996 and 2004 and has remained level since then. However, **food-borne outbreaks** continue to occur. In 2011, 84 cases and 15 deaths in 19 states were traced to cantaloupes from a single source. The cases were connected by use of pulsed-field gel electrophoresis, which showed that 4 different strains traced to the same source. The rate of *Listeria* infections varies among states. Epidemic human listeriosis has been associated with food-borne transmission in several large outbreaks, especially in association with aged soft cheeses; improperly pasteurized milk and milk products; contaminated raw and ready-to-eat beef, pork, and poultry, and packaged meats and salads; and vegetables both fresh and frozen harvested from farms where the ground is contaminated with the feces of colonized animals. Food-borne outbreaks in 2016 included raw milk, packaged salads, and frozen vegetables. The ability of *L. monocytogenes* to grow at temperatures as low as 4°C (39.2°F) increases the risk for transmission from aged soft cheeses and stored contaminated food. Listeriosis is an uncommon but important recognized etiology of neonatal sepsis and meningitis. Small clusters of nosocomial person-to-person transmission have occurred in hospital nurseries and obstetric suites. Sporadic endemic listeriosis is less well characterized. Likely routes include food-borne infection and zoonotic spread. **Zoonotic transmission** with cutaneous infections occurs in veterinarians and farmers who handle sick animals.

Reported cases of listeriosis are clustered at the extremes of age. Some studies show higher rates in males and a seasonal predominance in the late summer and fall in the Northern hemisphere. Outside the newborn period and during pregnancy, disease is usually reported in patients with underlying immunosuppression, with a 100-300 times increased risk in HIV-infected persons and in the elderly population (Table 215.1). In a recent surveillance study from England, malignancies accounted for one third of cases, with special risk associated with cancer in elderly persons.

The incubation period, which is defined only for common-source food-borne disease, is 21-30 days but in some cases may be longer. Asymptomatic carriage and fecal excretion are reported in 1–5% of healthy persons and 5% of abattoir workers, but duration of excretion, when studied, is short (<1 mo.).

PATHOLOGY

One of the major concepts of *Listeria* pathology and pathogenesis is its ability to survive as an intracellular pathogen. *Listeria* incites a mononuclear response and elaboration of cytokines, producing multisystem disease, particularly pyogenic meningitis. Granulomatous reactions and microabscess formation develop in many organs, including liver, lungs, adrenals, kidneys, central nervous system (CNS), and notably

Table 215.1	Types of *Listeria monocytogenes* Infections

Listeriosis in pregnancy
Neonatal listeriosis
  Early onset
  Late onset
Food-borne outbreaks/febrile gastroenteritis
Listeriosis in normal children and adults (rare)
Focal *Listeria* infections (e.g., meningitis, endocarditis, pneumonia, liver abscess, osteomyelitis, septic arthritis)
Listeriosis in immunocompromised persons
  Lymphohematogenous malignancies
  Collagen vascular diseases
  Diabetes mellitus
  HIV infection
  Transplantation
  Renal failure with peritoneal dialysis
Listeriosis in elderly persons

the placenta. Animal models demonstrate *translocation*, the transfer of intraluminal organisms across intact intestinal mucosa. Histologic examination of tissues, including the placenta, shows granulomatous inflammation and microabscess formation. Intracellular organisms can often be demonstrated with special stains.

PATHOGENESIS

Listeria organisms usually enter the host through the gastrointestinal (GI) tract. Gastric acidity provides some protection, and drugs that raise gastric pH may promote infection. Studies of intracellular and intercellular spread of *L. monocytogenes* have revealed a complex pathogenesis. Four pathogenic steps are described: internalization by phagocytosis, escape from the phagocytic vacuole, nucleation of actin filaments, and cell-to-cell spread. **Listeriolysin**, a hemolysin and the best-characterized virulence factor, probably mediates lysis of vacuoles and is responsible for the zone of hemolysis around colonies on blood-containing solid media. In cell-to-cell spread, locomotion proceeds via cytochalasin-sensitive polymerization of actin filaments, which extrude the bacteria in pseudopods, which in turn are phagocytosed by adjacent cells, necessitating escape from a double-membrane vacuole. This mechanism protects intracellular bacteria from the humoral arm of immunity and is responsible for the well-known requirement of T-cell–mediated activation of monocytes by lymphokines for clearance of infection and establishment of immunity. It appears that secretion of cyclic di-adenosine monophosphate by the bacteria induces the host to produce interferon, which activates the immune system to fight the organism. The significant risk for listeriosis in patients with depressed T-cell immunity speaks for the role of this arm of the immune system. The role of opsonizing antibody in protecting against infection is unclear. In addition, siderophores scavenge iron from the host, enhancing growth of the organism and likely explaining the relatively high risk of listeriosis in iron overload syndromes.

CLINICAL MANIFESTATIONS

The clinical presentation of listeriosis depends greatly on the age of the patient and the circumstances of the infection.

Listeriosis in Pregnancy

Pregnant women have increased susceptibility to *Listeria* infectious (approximately 20 times higher than nonpregnant women), probably because of a relative impairment in cell-mediated immunity. *L. monocytogenes* has been grown from placental and fetal cultures of pregnancies ending in spontaneous abortion. The usual presentation in the 2nd and 3rd trimesters is a flulike illness that may result in seeding of the uterine contents by bacteremia. Rarely is maternal listeriosis severe, but meningitis in pregnancy has been reported. Recognition and treatment at this stage are associated with normal pregnancy outcomes, but the fetus may not be infected even if listeriosis in the mother is not treated. In other instances, placental listeriosis develops with infection of the fetus that may be associated with stillbirth or premature delivery. Delivery of an infected premature fetus is associated with very high infant mortality. Disseminated disease is apparent at birth, often with a diffuse pustular rash. Infection in the mother usually resolves without specific therapy after delivery, but postpartum fever and infected lochia may occur.

Neonatal Listeriosis

Two clinical presentations are recognized for neonatal listeriosis: early-onset neonatal disease (<5 days, usually within 1-2 days of birth), which is a predominantly **septicemic** form, and late onset neonatal disease (>5 days, mean 14 days of life), which is a predominantly **meningitic** form (Table 215.2). The principal characteristics of the 2 presentations resemble the clinical syndromes described for group B streptococcus (see Chapter 211).

Early-onset disease occurs with milder transplacental or ascending infections from the female genital tract. There is a strong association with recovery of *L. monocytogenes* from the maternal genital tract, obstetric complications, prematurity, and neonatal sepsis with multiorgan involvement, including rash, but without CNS localization (Fig. 215.1). The mortality rate is approximately 20–30%.

The epidemiology of **late-onset disease** is poorly understood. Onset is usually after 5 days but before 30 days of age. Affected infants frequently are full-term, and the mothers are culture negative and asymptomatic. The presenting syndrome is usually purulent meningitis with parenchymal brain involvement, which, if adequately treated, has a mortality rate of <20%.

Table 215.2	Characteristic Features of Early- and Late-Onset Neonatal Listeriosis
EARLY ONSET (<5 DAYS)	**LATE ONSET (≥5 DAYS)**
Positive result of maternal *Listeria* culture	Negative results of maternal *Listeria* culture
Obstetric complications	Uncomplicated pregnancy
Premature delivery	Term delivery
Low birthweight	Normal birthweight
Neonatal sepsis	Neonatal meningitis
Mean age at onset 1.5 days	Mean age at onset 14.2 days
Mortality rate >30%	Mortality rate <10% Nosocomial outbreaks

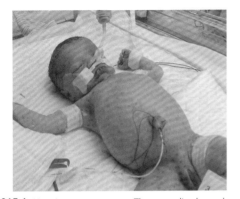

Fig. 215.1 *Listeria monocytogenes.* The generalized maculopapular rash present at birth disappeared within a few hours of life. *(From Benitez-Segura I, Fiol-Jaume M, Balliu PR, Tejedor M: Listeria monocytogenes: generalized maculopapular rash may be the clue, Arch Dis Child Fetal Neonatal Ed 98(1):F64, 2013, Fig 1.)*

Postneonatal Infections

Listeriosis beyond the newborn period may rarely occur in otherwise healthy children but is most often encountered in association with underlying malignancies (especially lymphomas) or immunosuppression. When associated with food-borne outbreaks, disease may cause GI symptoms or any of the *Listeria* syndromes. The clinical presentation is usually meningitis, less commonly sepsis, and rarely other CNS involvement, such as cerebritis, meningoencephalitis, brain abscess, spinal cord abscess, or a focus outside the CNS, such as suppurative arthritis, osteomyelitis, endocarditis, peritonitis (associated with peritoneal dialysis), or liver abscess. It is not known whether the frequent GI signs and symptoms result from enteric infection, because the mode of acquisition is often unknown.

DIAGNOSIS

Listeriosis should be included in the differential diagnosis of infections in pregnancy, of neonatal sepsis and meningitis, and of sepsis or meningitis in older children who have underlying malignancies (lymphomas), are receiving immunosuppressive therapy, or have undergone transplantation. The diagnosis is established by culture of *L. monocytogenes* from blood or cerebrospinal fluid (CSF). Cultures from the maternal cervix, vagina, lochia, and placenta, if possible, should be obtained when intrauterine infections lead to premature delivery or early-onset neonatal sepsis. Cultures from closed-space infections may also be useful. It is helpful to alert the laboratory to suspected cases so that *Listeria* isolates are not discarded as contaminating diphtheroids.

Histologic examination of the placenta is also useful. Molecular assays are now commercially available to detect *L. monocytogenes* from CNS samples. Serodiagnostic tests have not proved useful.

Differential Diagnosis

Listeriosis is indistinguishable clinically from neonatal sepsis and meningitis caused by other organisms. The presence of increased peripheral blood monocytes suggests listeriosis. Monocytosis or lymphocytosis may be modest or striking. Beyond the neonatal period, *L. monocytogenes* CNS infection is associated with fever, headache, seizures, and signs of meningeal irritation. The brainstem may be characteristically affected. The white blood cell concentration may vary from normal to slightly elevated, and the CSF laboratory findings are variable and less striking than in the more common causes of bacterial meningitis. Polymorphonuclear leukocytes or mononuclear cells may predominate, with shifts from polymorphonuclear to mononuclear cells in sequential lumbar puncture specimens. The CSF glucose concentration may be normal, but a low level mirrors the severity of disease. The CSF protein concentration is moderately elevated. *L. monocytogenes* is isolated from the blood in 40–75% of cases of meningitis caused by the organism. Deep focal infections from *L. monocytogenes,* such as endocarditis, osteomyelitis, and liver abscess, are also indistinguishable clinically from such infections from more common organisms. Cutaneous infections should be suspected in patients with a history of contact with animals, especially products of conception.

TREATMENT

The emergence of multiantibiotic resistance mandates routine susceptibility testing of all isolates. The recommended therapy is **ampicillin** (100-200 mg/kg/day divided every 6 hr intravenously [IV]; 200-400 mg/kg/day divided every 6 hr IV if meningitis is present) alone or in combination with an **aminoglycoside** (5.0-7.5 mg/kg/day divided every 8 hr IV). The aminoglycoside enhances the bactericidal activity and is generally recommended in cases of endocarditis and meningitis. The adult dose is ampicillin, 4-6 g/day divided every 6 hr, plus an aminoglycoside. The ampicillin dose is doubled if meningitis is present. Special attention to dosing is required for neonates, who require longer dosing intervals because of the longer half-lives of the antibiotics in their bodies. *L. monocytogenes* is not susceptible to the cephalosporins, including third-generation cephalosporins. If these agents are used for empirical therapy for neonatal sepsis or meningitis in a newborn, ampicillin must be added for possible *L. monocytogenes* infection.

Vancomycin, vancomycin plus an aminoglycoside, trimethoprim-sulfamethoxazole, and erythromycin are alternatives to ampicillin. The duration of therapy is usually 2-3 wk, with 3 wk recommended for immunocompromised persons and patients with meningitis. A longer course is needed for endocarditis, brain abscess, and osteomyelitis. Antibiotic treatment is unnecessary for gastroenteritis without invasive disease.

PROGNOSIS

Early gestational listeriosis may be associated with abortion or stillbirth, although maternal infection with sparing of the fetus has been reported. There is no convincing evidence that *L. monocytogenes* is associated with repeated spontaneous abortions in humans. The mortality rate is >50% for premature infants infected in utero, 30% for early-onset neonatal sepsis, 15% for late-onset neonatal meningitis, and <10% in older children with prompt institution of appropriate antimicrobial therapy. Mental retardation, hydrocephalus, and other CNS sequelae are reported in survivors of *Listeria* meningitis.

PREVENTION

Listeriosis can be prevented by pasteurization and thorough cooking of foods. Irradiation of meat products may also be beneficial. Consumption of unpasteurized or improperly processed dairy products should be avoided, especially aged soft cheeses, uncooked and precooked meat products that have been stored at 4°C (39.2°F) for extended periods, and unwashed vegetables (Table 215.3). This avoidance is particularly

Table 215.3	Prevention of Food-Borne Listeriosis

GENERAL RECOMMENDATIONS TO PREVENT *LISTERIA* INFECTION

FDA recommendations for washing and handling food:
- Rinse raw produce, such as fruits and vegetables, thoroughly under running tap water before eating, cutting, or cooking. Even if the produce will be peeled, it should still be washed first.
- Scrub firm produce, such as melons and cucumbers, with a clean produce brush.
- Dry the produce with a clean cloth or paper towel.
- Separate uncooked meats and poultry from vegetables, cooked foods, and ready-to-eat foods.

Keep your kitchen and environment cleaner and safer.
- Wash hands, knives, countertops, and cutting boards after handling and preparing uncooked foods.
- Be aware that *Listeria monocytogenes* can grow in foods in the refrigerator. Use an appliance thermometer, such as a refrigerator thermometer, to check the temperature inside your refrigerator. The refrigerator should be 4.5°C (40°F) or lower and the freezer −17.8°C (0°F) or lower.
- Clean up all spills in your refrigerator promptly, especially juices from hot dog and lunch meat packages, raw meat, and raw poultry.
- Clean the inside walls and shelves of your refrigerator with hot water and liquid soap, then rinse.

Cook meat and poultry thoroughly.
- Thoroughly cook raw food from animal sources, such as beef, pork, or poultry to a safe internal temperature. For a list of recommended temperatures for meat and poultry, visit the safe minimum cooking temperatures chart at http://www.FoodSafety.gov.

Store foods safely.
- Use precooked or ready-to-eat food as soon as you can. Do not store the product in the refrigerator beyond the use-by date; follow USDA refrigerator storage time guidelines:
  - Hot dogs: store opened package no longer than 1 wk and unopened package no longer than 2 wk in the refrigerator.
  - Luncheon and deli meat: store factory-sealed, unopened package no longer than 2 wk. Store opened packages and meat sliced at a local deli no longer than 3-5 days in the refrigerator.
- Divide leftovers into shallow containers to promote rapid, even cooling. Cover with airtight lids or enclose in plastic wrap or aluminum foil. Use leftovers within 3-4 days.

Choose safer foods.
- Do not drink raw (unpasteurized) milk, and do not eat foods that have unpasteurized milk in them.

RECOMMENDATIONS FOR PERSONS AT HIGHER RISK*

In addition to the recommendations listed above, include:

Meats
- Do not eat hot dogs, luncheon meats, cold cuts, other deli meats (e.g., bologna), or fermented or dry sausages unless they are heated to an internal temperature of 73.9°C (165°F) or until steaming hot just before serving.
- Avoid getting fluid from hot dog and lunch meat packages on other foods, utensils, and food preparation surfaces, and wash hands after handling hot dogs, luncheon meats, and deli meats.
- Pay attention to labels. Do not eat refrigerated pâté or meat spreads from a deli or meat counter or from the refrigerated section of a store. Foods that do not need refrigeration, such as canned or shelf-stable pâté and meat spreads, are safe to eat. Refrigerate after opening.

Cheeses
- Do not eat soft cheese such as feta, queso blanco, queso fresco, brie, Camembert, blue-veined, or panela (queso panela) unless it is labeled as made with pasteurized milk. Make sure the label says "MADE WITH PASTEURIZED MILK."

Seafood
- Do not eat refrigerated smoked seafood, unless it is contained in a cooked dish, such as a casserole, or unless it is a canned or shelf-stable product.
- Refrigerated smoked seafood, such as salmon, trout, whitefish, cod, tuna, and mackerel, is most often labeled as "nova-style," "lox," "kippered," "smoked," or "jerky."
  - These fish are typically found in the refrigerator section or sold at seafood and deli counters of grocery stores and delicatessens.
- Canned and shelf stable tuna, salmon, and other fish products are safe to eat.

Follow this general FDA advice for melon safety:
- Consumers and food preparers should wash their hands with warm water and soap for at least 20 sec before and after handling any whole melon, such as cantaloupe, watermelon, or honeydew.
- Scrub the surface of melons, such as cantaloupes, with a clean produce brush under running water and dry them with a clean cloth or paper towel before cutting. Be sure that your scrub brush is sanitized after each use, to avoid transferring bacteria between melons.
- Promptly consume cut melon or refrigerate promptly. Keep your cut melon refrigerated ≤4.5°C (40°F) (0-1.1°C [32-34°F] is best), for no more than 7 days.
- Discard cut melons left at room temperature for >4 hr.

*Including pregnant women, persons with weakened immune system, and older adults.
FDA, Food and Drug Administration; USDA, U.S. Department of Agriculture.
Adapted from Centers for Disease Control and Prevention: *Listeria* (listeriosis): prevention. http://www.cdc.gov/listeria/prevention.html.

important during pregnancy and for immunocompromised persons. Infected domestic animals should be avoided when possible. Education regarding risk reduction is aimed particularly at pregnant women and people being treated for cancer.

Careful handwashing is essential to prevent nosocomial spread within obstetric and neonatal units. Immunocompromised patients given prophylaxis with trimethoprim-sulfamethoxazole are protected from *Listeria* infections. Cases and especially outbreaks should be reported immediately to public health authorities so that timely investigation can be initiated in order to interrupt transmission from the contaminated source.

Bibliography is available at Expert Consult.

Chapter 216

Actinomyces

Brian T. Fisher

第二百一十六章

放线菌

中文导读

　　本章首先描述了放线菌是厌氧或微需氧、无孢子、无运动能力的革兰阳性菌，放线菌属可能是人类口咽、胃肠道或泌尿生殖道的内源性菌群的一部分，感染部位包括皮肤、子宫颈、腹部、骨盆、胸部、中枢神经系统（CNS）等。随后，进一步介绍了关于放线菌感染的病因、流行病学、发病机制、诊断、临床表现、鉴别诊断、治疗、预后等内容。在关于放线菌感染的临床表现部分详细介绍了颈面部放线菌病、腹部和盆腔放线菌病、胸部放线菌病、脑和其他形式的放线菌病。

Actinomyces species are anaerobic or microaerophilic, nonsporulating, nonmotile gram-positive bacteria that have a filamentous and branching structure. Infection caused by these bacteria is termed **actinomycosis**, which often presents as an indolent granulomatous, suppurative process with potential for direct extension to contiguous tissue across natural anatomic barriers and formation of draining fistulas and sinus tracts. Organisms from the genus *Actinomyces* can be part of the endogenous flora of the oropharynx, gastrointestinal (GI) tract, or urogenital tract of humans, and thus the site of infection usually is a local process involving the skin or the cervicofacial, abdominal, pelvic, or thoracic regions. However, the infection can disseminate to other locations, including the central nervous system (CNS).

ETIOLOGY AND EPIDEMIOLOGY

Almost 50 species of *Actinomyces* have been identified using 16S ribosomal RNA sequencing, with more than half these species associated with human infection. *Actinomyces israelii* is the predominant species causing human actinomycosis. Other species associated with infection include, but are not limited to, *Actinomyces odontolyticus*, *A. meyeri*, *A. naeslundii*, *A. gerencseriae*, and *A. viscosus*.

Although actinomycosis occurs worldwide, it is a rare infection. Accordingly, knowledge regarding the epidemiology of actinomycosis is limited to case reports and case series. Based on these reports, this infection appears to affect people of all ages, with no predilection for a particular race, season, or occupation. The infection rate may be higher among males, possibly related to increased trauma or poorer dental hygiene. In a review of 85 cases of actinomycosis, 27% were in persons <20 yr old, and 7% were among children <10 yr old. The youngest patient in this series was 28 days old. Risk factors in children include trauma, dental caries, debilitation, and poorly controlled diabetes mellitus. Although actinomycosis is not a common opportunistic infection, disease has been associated with corticosteroid use, leukemia, renal failure, congenital immunodeficiency diseases, and HIV infection.

PATHOGENESIS

The 3 most common sites of *Actinomyces* infection are, in order of frequency, cervicofacial, abdominal and pelvic, and thoracic regions, although infection may involve any organ in the body. Actinomycosis typically follows a breach in the local cutaneous or mucosal barrier, such as after a traumatic injury or surgery. Other medical interventions can result in mucosal barrier injuries and predispose to infection, such as the association between intrauterine devices and pelvic actinomycosis. Involvement of the thoracic region has been postulated to present after an aspiration event in patients with poor dentition or a recent dental procedure or after aspiration of a foreign body. Notably, more than one third of patients do not have an identifiable antecedent event that would explain the onset of actinomycosis.

The hallmark of actinomycosis is contiguous spread that fails to respect tissue or fascial planes. Sites of infection show dense cellular infiltrates and suppuration that form many interconnecting abscesses and sinus tracts. These abscesses and sinus tracts may be followed by cicatricial healing from which the organism spreads by burrowing along fascial planes, causing deep, communicating, scarred sinus tracts.

DIAGNOSIS

The presence of **sulfur granules** on macroscopic or microscopic evaluation of involved tissue is highly suggestive of a diagnosis of actinomycosis. On macroscopic appearance, the sulfur granules are typically yellow, accounting for their name, but may be white, gray, or brown. These granules microscopically can appear on hematoxylin-eosin or Gomori methenamine silver stains as a mass of gram-positive branching filamentous rods surrounded by the host immune response inclusive of polymorphonuclear neutrophils and a milieu of eosinophilic staining inert material often referred to as the **Splendore-Hoeppli phenomenon**. Notably, one species, *A. meyeri*, is nonbranching. *Nocardia* is indistinguishable from *Actinomyces* on Gram stain, but *Nocardia* stains with the modified acid-fast stain, contrasting with *Actinomyces*.

Although highly suggestive of actinomycosis, sulfur granules often are not present, and thus additional testing is necessary to make the diagnosis. Patients with actinomycosis in the absence of sulfur granules are typically diagnosed by culturing the organism from tissue procured from the involved site. Cultures on brain-heart infusion agar incubated at 37°C (98.6°F) anaerobically (95% nitrogen and 5% carbon dioxide) and a separate set incubated aerobically reveal organisms within the lines of streak at 24-48 hr. *A. israelii* colonies appear as loose masses of delicate, branching filaments with a characteristic spider-like growth. Colonies of other species, such as *A. naeslundii* and *A. viscosus* may have similar growth characteristics. Unfortunately, even under these conditions, it can be challenging to grow *Actinomyces,* and the yield of different culturing techniques can vary by species. Additionally, conventional biochemical testing for speciation is complex and may result in misclassification of an organism. The evolution of diagnostic tools such as 16S rRNA sequence analysis and matrix-assisted laser desorption/ionization (MALDI) time of flight (TOF) mass spectrometry has improved the accuracy of speciation of cultured organisms and highlighted the potential for detection of *Actinomyces* directly from the involved tissue without culture.

Importantly, actinomycosis is usually, if not always, **polymicrobial** in nature. In a large study of >650 cases, infection with *Actinomyces* was identified in pure culture in only 1 case and was usually identified with other endogenous flora, most notably members of the **HACEK group,** which includes *Aggregatibacter* (formerly *Haemophilus*) *aphrophilus, Aggregatibacter* (formerly *Actinobacillus*) *actinomycetemcomitans, Cardiobacterium hominis, Eikenella corrodens,* and *Kingella kingae. A. actinomycetemcomitans* is a fastidious, gram-negative bacillus that is part of the oral flora and has been implicated as a pathogen in periodontal disease. Other bacterial species frequently isolated concomitantly in human actinomycosis include *Fusobacterium, Bacteroides, Capnocytophaga,* and aerobic and anaerobic streptococci.

CT or MRI of the involved area is often employed in the initial patient evaluation. No pathognomonic radiographic findings exist for actinomycosis, but the identification of a process that invades across tissue planes and ignores anatomic boundaries can be highly suggestive of actinomycosis. Furthermore, radiographic imaging can be helpful to establish the extent of the infectious process, guide subsequent diagnostic and therapeutic interventions, and monitor for resolution of infection.

CLINICAL MANIFESTATIONS
Cervicofacial Actinomycosis

Cervicofacial actinomycosis in a pediatric patient often manifests as a mass in the neck or submandibular region that persists for weeks to months. Less than half of patients will have associated pain, and fewer than one third of patients will have fever. A minority of patients will

report dysphagia or have a draining sinus (Fig. 216.1). Less frequently, cervicofacial actinomycosis manifests clinically as an acute pyogenic infection with a tender, fluctuant mass with trismus, firm swelling, and fistulas with drainage containing the characteristic sulfur granules. Bone is not involved early in the disease, but periostitis, mandibular osteomyelitis, or perimandibular abscess may develop. Infection may spread through sinus tracts to the cranial bones, possibly giving rise to meningitis. The ability of *Actinomyces* to burrow through tissue planes, including the periosteum, is a key difference between actinomycosis and nocardiosis. While predisposing factors for cervicofacial actinomycosis are not well defined for children, adult cases are often preceded by a history of oral trauma, oral surgery, dental procedures, or caries, facilitating entry of organisms into cervicofacial tissues.

Abdominal and Pelvic Actinomycosis

Of all the forms of actinomycosis, delayed diagnosis is most typical for abdominal and pelvic infection. A disruption of the mucosa of the GI tract (e.g., acute GI perforation, abdominal trauma) is often postulated as the inciting event for adult-onset abdominopelvic actinomycosis. In pediatric patients, however, medical history frequently fails to identify prior evidence of mucosal barrier injury. In a contemporary pediatric case series of abdominal and pelvic actinomycosis, prior abdominal surgery (all appendectomies) was reported in only 21% of patients and dental caries in 11%. Most often, a child presents with abdominal pain and a palpable lump or mass on abdominal examination. Fever accompanies the abdominal pain in more than half of cases, with weight loss in almost one third. As with other forms of actinomycosis, abdominopelvic infection can spread across tissue planes by contiguous extension involving any tissue or organ, including muscle, solid abdominopelvic viscera, and walls of the intestinal tract. Likely because of delays in diagnosis, more than one third of pediatric cases present with a draining sinus fistula.

Thoracic Actinomycosis

Thoracic actinomycosis may manifest as an endobronchial infection, a tumor-like lesion, diffuse pneumonia, or a pleural effusion. In a retrospective review of reported pediatric cases of thoracic infection, almost half presented with a chest wall mass. Additional symptoms such as cough, fever, chest pain, and weight loss were reported in <40% of patients. Importantly, thoracic actinomycosis can be found incidentally on radiographs ordered for noninfectious concerns. The variation in presentation and indolent nature of thoracic actinomycosis often delay the diagnosis. Left untreated, the infectious process can dissect along tissue planes and extend through the chest wall or diaphragm, characteristically producing numerous sinus tracts that contain small abscesses and purulent drainage. Other complications include bony destruction of adjacent ribs, sternum, and vertebral bodies. Multiple lobe involvement of the lungs is occasionally found.

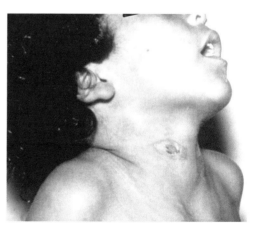

Fig. 216.1 A 2 yr old boy with HIV infection who has cervicofacial actinomycosis and a draining fistula.

Cerebral and Other Forms of Actinomycosis

CNS involvement of *Actinomyces* is often the result of hematogenous spread to the brain parenchyma from a distant site but can also result from contiguous spread from a cervicofacial lesion. The former often results in multiple brain abscesses. **Laryngeal** actinomycosis rarely has been reported in older teenagers. Oropharyngeal colonization with *Actinomyces* may be involved in the development of obstructive tonsillar hypertrophy. Severe forms of **periodontitis,** particularly localized juvenile periodontitis, are associated with *Actinomyces,* especially in children 10-19 yr old. *Actinomyces* has a propensity for infecting heart valves, a process that results in an insidious presentation of endocarditis, with fever present in less than half of cases.

DIFFERENTIAL DIAGNOSIS

Actinomycosis has been referred to as a "great imitator" with presentations that mimic appendicitis, pseudoappendicitis caused by *Yersinia enterocolitica,* amebiasis, malignancy, and inflammatory bowel disease. Actinomycosis must be differentiated from other chronic inflammatory infections, including tuberculosis, nocardiosis, polymicrobial bacterial infections, and fungal infections.

TREATMENT

As with any infection, prompt initiation of antibiotics is important to resolve the infection. Routine susceptibility testing is not typically performed, but most *Actinomyces* spp. are susceptible to penicillin G, which is considered the drug of choice. Because actinomycosis is often found to be polymicrobial in nature, broadening to an agent with a β-lactamase inhibitor, such as ampicillin-sulbactam or amoxicillin-clavulanate, may be warranted, especially if there is an initial poor response. In particular, *A. actinomycetemcomitans* is a **co-pathogen** in at least 30% of actinomycosis infections. Failure to recognize this organism and treat it adequately has resulted in clinical relapse and deterioration in patients with actinomycosis. *A. actinomycetemcomitans* is susceptible to penicillin and ampicillin in vitro, but sensitivity testing does not always correlate with clinical outcome. Transitioning to a cephalosporin, ampicillin-sulbactam, or amoxicillin-clavulanate may be necessary in these patients. Treating actinomycosis in a patient with a penicillin allergy can be challenging, because there is variation in susceptibility by *Actinomyces* spp. to other antibiotic classes. Notably, despite being an anaerobe, a large percentage of *Actinomyces* are not susceptible to metronidazole. It is recommended that an infectious diseases specialist be consulted to help guide antibiotic choices in patients with penicillin allergy or in patients with deep-seated infections such as brain abscesses, endocarditis, or osteomyelitis. Commercially available sensitivity testing methods are available and can be employed in patients with severe disease or poor response to initial therapy.

No definitive comparative effectiveness data exist to guide the optimal route and duration of therapy. Most experts would recommend initial parenteral administration of antibiotics with the opportunity to transition to enteral therapy on clinical improvement. The exception would be for endocarditis or CNS disease, for which parenteral administration should be continued for the entirety of therapy. Given concerns for relapsing infection, antibiotics are often continued for 3-12 mo. The ultimate duration is often dictated by the location of the infection and follow-up clinical exams and imaging. Courses of antibiotic therapy <3 mo have been used in cases of local disease with successful surgical resection.

Traditionally, an adjunctive surgical intervention was thought to be necessary for successful outcome. However, in some case series a subset of patients have responded well to medical management alone. In the setting of significant abscesses and/or sinus tracts, a surgical approach to establish source control and, if possible, completely resect involved issue can hasten clinical improvement. However, the morbidity of the surgical procedure needs to be weighed against the potential benefits for each patient.

PROGNOSIS

The prognosis is excellent with early diagnosis, prompt initiation of antibiotic therapy, and if necessary, adequate surgical debridement. Actinomycosis often presents in children without a known underlying immunodeficient state. However, disseminated or recalcitrant actinomycosis should raise suspicion for immunodeficiency.

Bibliography is available at Expert Consult.

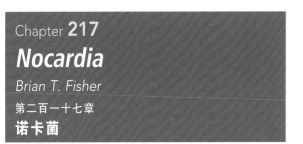

Chapter **217**
Nocardia
Brian T. Fisher

第二百一十七章
诺卡菌

中文导读

　　本章首先阐述了诺卡菌主要是免疫功能低下人群的机会感染病原体。诺卡菌病包括急性、亚急性或具有缓解和恶化趋势的慢性化脓性感染。随后，进一步介绍了关于诺卡菌感染的病因、流行病学、发病机制、临床表现、影像学表现、诊断、治疗、预后等内容。在关于诺卡菌感染治疗部分详细介绍了复方磺胺甲噁唑、利奈唑胺、外科引流等治疗措施。

A number of *Nocardia* species have been identified as the source of both local and disseminated disease in children and adults. These organisms are primarily opportunistic pathogens infecting immunocompromised persons. Infection caused by these bacteria is termed **nocardiosis**, which consists of acute, subacute, or chronic suppurative infections with a tendency for remissions and exacerbations.

ETIOLOGY

Nocardia spp. are obligate aerobes and will grow on a variety of culture media, including simple blood agar, brain-heart infusion agar, and Lowenstein-Jensen media. Colonies can appear as early as 48 hr, but typically growth of *Nocardia* is slower than in other bacteria and may take 1-2 wk. Growth appears as waxy, folded, or heaped colonies at the edges, and yield is best achieved in conditions that include a temperature of 37°C (98.6°F) with 10% carbon dioxide. However, many isolates of *Nocardia* are thermophilic and will grow at temperatures up to 50°C (122°F). Microscopically, *Nocardia* spp. are weakly gram-positive rod-shaped filamentous bacteria. For some isolates, there may be alternating areas of gram-positive and gram-negative staining, giving a beaded appearance often described with *Nocardia*. These organisms are also weakly acid fast, and the modified Kinyoun acid-fast staining technique can be helpful to identify organisms from clinical specimens such as a tissue biopsy or bronchoalveolar lavage (BAL).

Approximately 100 distinct *Nocardia* spp. have been identified, almost 20 of which have been associated with human infection. The distribution of *Nocardia* spp. causing disease varies across observational studies, partly because of variation in taxonomic classification over time. Currently, the predominant species to cause disease are *Nocardia farcinica*, *N. cyriacigeorgica*, *N. abscessus*, and *N. nova*. Species identification can be critical for optimal clinical outcomes because of variability in virulence strategies and antibiotic resistance profiles (see Treatment later). Traditional approaches to speciation require biochemical processing that can be laborious and inefficient. Techniques such as 16S rDNA polymerase chain reaction (PCR) or matrix-assisted laser desorption/ionization (MALDI) time of flight (TOF) mass spectrometry can more efficiently speciate *Nocardia*. Of these, MALDI-TOF technology is likely to become more available in clinical microbiology laboratories in the near future.

EPIDEMIOLOGY

Once thought to be a rare human disease, nocardiosis is being recognized more frequently and has been diagnosed in persons of all ages. Pediatric patients with compromised cellular immunity are at particular risk, including children receiving immune suppression after solid-organ or stem cell transplantation, chemotherapy for malignancy, prolonged corticosteroid therapy, children with poorly controlled HIV infection, or those with a primary immunodeficiency, especially **chronic granulomatous disease** (see Chapter 156). Notably, nocardiosis has been described in patients without an identified immune defect, although in these clinical scenarios, other predisposing factors such as bronchiectasis are often present.

Multiple contemporary retrospective studies have been performed in Australia, France, and Spain to better define the epidemiology of nocardiosis in children and adults. The incidence of nocardiosis has been estimated to be 6 cases per 100,000 hospital admissions. This rate is much higher in susceptible hosts, such as in solid-organ transplant recipients, in whom the rate is as high as 20 per 1000 transplants.

PATHOGENESIS

Nocardia organisms are environmental saprophytes that are ubiquitous in soil and decaying vegetable matter and have been isolated from soil worldwide. Infection does not result from human to human but typically by inhalation of the organism, presumably from aerosolized dust. Infection can also be acquired by direct cutaneous inoculation, including after arthropod and cat bites. From 70–80% of *Nocardia* infections originate in the pulmonary parenchyma, with 10–25% being primary cutaneous disease.

Nocardia can disseminate from the primary site of infection to any organ or any musculoskeletal location. Dissemination after primary lung infection is common, occurring in 15–50% of patients; those with an underlying immunocompromised condition are more likely to have disseminated disease. The central nervous system (CNS) is the most concerning and most common secondary site of infection, complicating as much as 25% of pulmonary disease. Although rare, isolated CNS disease has been described. Whereas most cases are the result of an environmental exposure, a description of *N. farcinica* sternal wound infections among patients undergoing open heart surgery highlights the possibility of a nosocomial source.

CLINICAL AND RADIOGRAPHIC MANIFESTATIONS

The clinical presentation can be nonspecific, with fever reported in approximately 60% of patients, cough in 30%, and dyspnea in 25%. Extrapulmonary signs and symptoms can correspond to the site of infection. In particular, neurologic deficit has been reported in up to 25% of all cases and in more than half of patients with CNS involvement. Neurologic complaints can include headache, confusion or altered mental status, weakness, and speech impairment. Renal nocardiosis can cause dysuria, hematuria, or pyuria, and gastrointestinal (GI) involvement may be associated with nausea, vomiting, diarrhea, abdominal distention, or melena. Skin infection manifests as **sporotrichoid nocardiosis** or superficial ulcers (Fig. 217.1). **Mycetoma** is a chronic, progressive infection developing days to months after inoculation, usually on a distal location on the limbs.

Given the nonspecific symptoms and signs of nocardiosis (with the exception of cutaneous lesions), radiographic imaging is often necessary to define the location and extent of disease. Pulmonary infection can appear as a consolidation consistent with typical bacterial pneumonia or even as a necrotizing pneumonia with or without a pleural effusion. Single or multiple nodules and cavitary lesions have also been described. Cavitary lesions are more common in patients with an underlying immunocompromising condition. CNS disease can take the form of meningitis or focal lesions. Meningitis presents as neutrophil- or lymphocyte-predominant pleocytosis, elevated cerebrospinal fluid protein, and hypoglycorrhachia. For focal lesions, CT or MRI of the brain often reveals single- or multiple-ring enhancing lesions. Similar to the brain, when other organs or soft tissues are involved, CT or MRI also typically reveals single- or multiple-ring enhancing lesions, suggestive of an abscess or abscesses.

DIAGNOSIS

Microbiologic evidence is necessary to confirm the diagnosis of nocardiosis. An estimated 25% of patients with nocardiosis will be diagnosed by routine blood culture. In the remaining patients, an invasive procedure such as bronchoscopy, tissue biopsy, or abscess aspiration is necessary to procure specimens for diagnostic testing. Histopathologic staining of such material can reveal beaded, weakly gram-positive or modified acid-fast filamentous bacteria. Histopathology can also show delicately

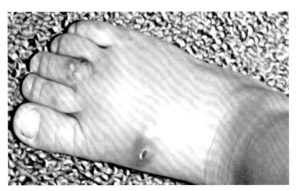

Fig. 217.1 A 2 yr old girl with multiple pustules on the dorsum of the right foot caused by *Nocardia brasiliensis*. (*Courtesy of Jaime E. Fergie, MD.*)

branching bacteria with proclivity to fragment. Speciation of *Nocardia* is becoming increasingly reliant on 16S rDNA PCR or MALDI-TOF technologies. Given that *Nocardia* spp. can colonize the respiratory airway, a sputum or BAL culture that yields a *Nocardia* species is not itself confirmatory of nocardiosis. However, a positive microbiologic test for a *Nocardia* species from one of these specimens in conjunction with the clinical and radiographic findings is strongly supportive of nocardiosis.

When a diagnosis of nocardiosis is made, strong consideration should be given to evaluation for disseminated disease, even in the absence of signs or symptoms, especially in the immunocompromised host. Although data are limited, most experts agree that at the minimum, MRI of the brain should be performed in the immunocompromised host with nocardiosis.

TREATMENT

The choice, dose, and duration of antimicrobial treatment depend on the site and extent of infection, immune status of the patient, initial clinical response, and species and susceptibility testing of the *Nocardia* isolate. A number of therapeutic options exist for the treatment of nocardiosis; however, there are no comparative effectiveness studies to inform the optimal therapeutic regimen. **Trimethoprim-sulfamethoxazole** (TMP-SMX) is the sulfonamide formulation that is recommended, although sulfadiazine and sulfisoxazole have been used. Increasing recognition of resistance to TMP-SMX across and within *Nocardia* spp. highlights the importance of speciation of *Nocardia* isolates and of performing sensitivity testing in a certified microbiology laboratory. TMP-SMX resistance rates range from 3–10%, with higher rates for specific species. In particular, some reports have identified resistance rates approximating 20% for the commonly identified species of *N. cyriacigeorgica* and *N. farcinica*. Interestingly, administration of TMP-SMX as prophylaxis against *Pneumocystis jiroveci* pneumonia is not always protective against nocardiosis, and thus clinicians should not exclude this diagnosis from the differential in patients receiving TMP-SMX prophylaxis.

Other antibacterial agents with in vitro activity against *Nocardia* spp. include but are not limited to amikacin, amoxicillin-clavulanate, ceftriaxone, ciprofloxacin, clarithromycin, imipenem, linezolid, and minocycline. Large studies reporting on the in vitro resistance of clinical isolates suggest that **linezolid** has the least amount of resistance across all species. Therefore, while awaiting sensitivity testing in patients with *Nocardia* isolated from a clinical specimen, it may be reasonable to administer linezolid empirically. Subsequent therapeutic decisions should be guided by final sensitivity results as well as consideration of the site of infection and pharmacokinetics of the available agents. It is not clear whether parenteral administration is superior to enteral formulations. However, most experts support the use of parenteral therapy for more severe disease, including endocarditis or CNS disease.

In vitro and in vivo animal models have suggested the benefit of combination regimens for the treatment of nocardiosis. There are no clinical data to confirm the need for combination therapy; however, based on the preclinical data, there is expert support for using combination therapy in disseminated disease and in children with an underlying immunocompromising condition. A variety of combination therapies have been suggested in case reports such as amikacin plus ceftriaxone or amikacin plus imipenem. Since data on combination therapy are limited, antibiotic choices should primarily be guided by sensitivity testing of the clinical *Nocardia* isolate.

Surgical drainage of abscesses can be helpful in hastening resolution of nocardiosis. However, no comparative data have documented improvement in overall outcomes with adjunctive surgical intervention, and success has been reported with medical management alone in resolving deep-seated abscesses, even in the CNS. Therefore, the decision to intervene surgically needs to be balanced with the potential consequences of a surgical procedure to drain an abscess.

The necessary duration of therapy for nocardiosis varies by the clinical presentation and the status of the patient. Generally, superficial cutaneous infection requires at least 6-12 wk, pulmonary or systemic nocardiosis is treated for 6-12 mo, and CNS infection for at least 12 mo. These intervals should only be considered as a guide for expected therapeutic durations. The ultimate duration should be dictated by clinical and radiographic resolution of disease.

PROGNOSIS

Historically, nocardiosis has been associated with significant mortality. Fortunately, more recent reports have documented an improved rate of complete cure to approximately 80%. Predictably, attributable case fatality rates vary by disease entity. There is no attributable case fatality associated with cutaneous disease, but 10–20% attributable case fatality has been assigned to disseminated and visceral disease. CNS disease has the highest attributable case fatality rates, reaching 25%. Importantly, much of the data on case fatality rates are informed by predominantly adult cohorts, and thus there may be fewer fatal outcomes in children. Nonetheless, early diagnosis and intervention are important to reduce the morbidity and mortality of nocardiosis, especially in immunocompromised patients at increased risk for disseminated disease.

Bibliography is available at Expert Consult.

Section 5
Gram-Negative Bacterial Infections

第五篇
革兰阴性菌感染

Chapter **218**
Neisseria meningitidis (Meningococcus)

Andrew J. Pollard and Manish Sadarangani

第二百一十八章
脑膜炎奈瑟菌

中文导读

本章主要介绍了脑膜炎奈瑟菌感染的病因、流行病学、发病机制、病理生理学、临床表现、诊断、治疗、并发症、预后、预防等内容。在脑膜炎奈瑟菌感染的发病机制和病理生理学部分详细介绍了免疫和宿主因素。在脑膜炎奈瑟菌感染的治疗部分详细介绍了抗生素治疗和支持治疗。在脑膜炎奈瑟菌感染的预防部分详细介绍了二级预防和预防接种。

Neisseria meningitidis (the meningococcus) is a commensal of the human nasopharynx in approximately 10% of the population and rarely enters the bloodstream to cause devastating invasive disease such as meningitis and meningococcal septicemia (meningococcemia). Although a rare endemic disease in most countries, the epidemiology of meningococcal disease varies widely over time and in different geographic regions, with both hyperendemic and epidemic disease patterns occurring. Onset of disease in susceptible individuals may be very rapid, within hours, and the case fatality rate is high, especially among those presenting with septic shock, despite access to modern critical care. Individual susceptibility is known to involve a complex relationship among environmental, host, and bacterial factors, and prevention of meningococcal disease through behavior modification (e.g., avoiding tobacco smoke) and vaccination offers the best prospect for control.

ETIOLOGY

Neisseria meningitidis is a gram-negative, fastidious, encapsulated, oxidase-positive, aerobic diplococcus. Differences in the chemistry of the polysaccharide capsule allow definition of 12 (previously thought to be 13) serologically distinct meningococcal capsular groups, of which 6, designated A, B, C, W (previously designated W135), X, and Y, are responsible for almost all cases of disease. Meningococcal strains may be subclassified on the basis of antigenic variation in 2 porin proteins found in the outer membrane, **PorB** (serotype) and **PorA** (serosubtype), and **lipopolysaccharide** (immunotype), using serology. Serologic typing is being replaced by molecular typing methods, which target genes under immune selection to provide **antigen sequence typing** (based on amino acid variation in various surface proteins, including PorA and FetA). Sequencing of antigen genes (e.g., *PorA, fHbp, NadA, NHBA*) is set to be an important means of monitoring pressure on meningococcal populations by protein-based vaccines. Because meningococci readily exchange genetic material, typing based on a few antigens cannot provide an accurate picture of relatedness of strains, an important goal in monitoring epidemiology. **Multilocus sequence typing**, which types meningococci using variation in 7 housekeeping genes, has been widely used to map the distribution of genetic lineages of meningococci (http://pubmlst.org/neisseria/) and provides a clearer picture of the genetic and epidemiologic relatedness of strains. To provide still better definition of genetic variation, in some countries, including the United Kingdom, **whole genome sequencing** is used to type meningococci and appears set to replace both antigen and multilocus sequence typing, as costs continue to fall. The application of molecular approaches to epidemiology has established that (1) endemic meningococcal disease is caused by genetically heterogeneous strains, although only a small number of genetic lineages are associated with the majority of cases of invasive disease; and (2) outbreaks are usually clonal, caused by single strains.

EPIDEMIOLOGY

Meningococci are transmitted during close contact through aerosol droplets or exposure to respiratory secretions, as by kissing. The organism does not survive for long periods in the environment. Enhanced rates of mucosal colonization and increased disease risk are associated with activities that increase the likelihood of exposure to a new strain or increase proximity to a carrier, thus facilitating transmission, including kissing, bar patronage, binge drinking, attendance at nightclubs, men having sex with men, and living in freshman college dormitories. Factors that damage the nasopharyngeal mucosa, such as smoking and respiratory viral infection (notably influenza), are also associated with increased rates of carriage and disease, perhaps by driving upregulation of host adhesion molecules that are receptors for meningococci. Carriage is unusual in early childhood and peaks during adolescence and young adulthood.

Meningococcal disease is a global problem, but disease rates vary by a factor of 10-100–fold in different geographic locations at one point in time and in the same location at different times. Most cases of meningococcal disease are sporadic, but small outbreaks (usually in schools or colleges, representing <3% of U.S. cases), **hyperendemic** disease (increased rates of disease persisting for a decade or more as a result of a single clone), and epidemic disease are all recognized patterns. However, over the last decade, rates of meningococcal disease have declined in most industrialized countries, partly through introduction of immunization programs, possibly aided by widespread legislation against smoking in public places. The arrival of hyperinvasive lineages and their eventual decline through development of natural immunity is recognized as a major driver of changes in disease rates over time. The U.S. disease rate was 1.1 cases per 100,000 population in 1999 but had fallen to 0.14 per 100,000 by 2014 (Fig. 218.1). By contrast, the rate

of disease in Ireland in 1999 was >12 per 100,000, and rates of 1,000 per 100,000 have been described during epidemic disease in sub-Saharan Africa. Disease caused by dominant hyperendemic clones has been recognized in the last decade in Oregon, United States; Quebec, Canada; Normandy, France; and across New Zealand. Laboratory data underreport meningococcal disease incidence rates, because up to 50% of cases are not culture confirmed, particularly where prehospital antibiotics are recommended for suspected cases. In the United Kingdom, polymerase chain reaction (PCR) methods are used routinely for diagnosis of suspected cases, doubling the number of confirmed cases.

The highest rate of meningococcal disease occurs in infants <1 yr old, probably as a result of *immunologic inexperience* (antibody that recognizes meningococcal antigens is naturally acquired during later childhood), immaturity of the alternative and lectin complement pathways, and perhaps the poor responses made by infants to bacterial polysaccharides. In the absence of immunization, incidence rates decline through childhood, except for a peak of disease among adolescence and young adults, which may be related to increased opportunity for exposure from social activities.

In the United States, most cases of disease in the 1st yr of life are caused by capsular **group B** strains. After age 1 yr, 85% of disease cases are about equally distributed among capsular groups B and C strains, with the remainder caused by **group Y** strains. In most other industrialized countries, capsular group B strains predominate at all ages, in part because of introduction of routine capsular **group C** meningococcal conjugate vaccine among infants and/or toddlers. For reasons not understood, disease in children caused by group Y strains was uncommon in the United States before the 1990s and then began to increase. Rates of disease caused by this capsular group have also increased in several other countries but are declining in the United States. Disease caused by capsular **group W** strains has increased in the United Kingdom as a result of a hyperinvasive clone, which appears to have originated in Latin America.

Large outbreaks of capsular **group A** meningococcal disease occurred during and immediately after the First World War and the Second World War in both Europe and the United States, but since the 1990s, almost all cases caused by capsular group A strains have occurred in Eastern Europe, Russia, and developing countries. The highest incidence of capsular group A disease has occurred in a band across sub-Saharan Africa, the *meningitis belt*, with annual endemic rates of 10-25 per 100,000 population. For more than a century, this region has experienced large capsular group A epidemics every 7-10 yr, with annual rates as high as 1,000 per 100,000 population. The onset of cases in the sub Saharan region typically begins during the dry season, possibly related to drying and damage to the nasopharyngeal mucosa; subsides with the rainy season; and may reemerge the following dry season. Rates of capsular group A meningococcal disease are currently falling across this region as a result of a mass vaccine implementation targeting strains bearing the A polysaccharide. However, both endemic and epidemic meningococcal disease in this region is also caused by capsular groups C, W, and X strains. Capsular group A and **group X** are infrequent causes of disease in other areas of the world, although both A and W strains have been associated with outbreaks among pilgrims returning from the Hajj.

PATHOGENESIS AND PATHOPHYSIOLOGY

Colonization of the nasopharynx by *N. meningitidis* is the first step in either carriage or invasive disease. Disease usually occurs 1-14 days after acquisition of the pathogen. Initial contact of meningococci with host epithelial cells is mediated by pili, which may interact with the host CD46 molecule or an integrin. Close adhesion is then mediated by Opa and Opc binding to carcinoembryonic antigen (CEA) cell adhesion molecule receptors and integrins, respectively. Subsequent internalization of meningococci by epithelial cells is followed by transcytosis through to the basolateral tissues and dissemination into the bloodstream. Immunoglobulin A$_1$ protease secreted by invasive bacteria degrades secretory IgA on the mucosal surface, circumventing this first-line host defense mechanism.

Once in the bloodstream, meningococci multiply rapidly to high levels to cause septicemia (**meningococcemia**). Patients with a higher

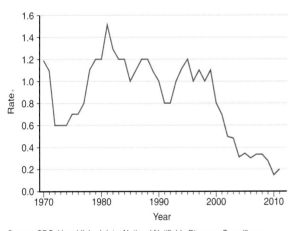

Fig. 218.1 Rate of meningococcal disease, by year—united states, 1970–2011. *(From Cohn AC, MacNeil JR, Clark TA, et al; Centers for Disease Control and Prevention: Prevention and control of meningococcal disease: recommendations of the Advisory Committee on Immunization Practices, MMWR Recomm Rep 62(RR-2):1–28, 2013.)*

Source: CDC, Unpublished data, National Notifiable Diseases Surveillance System (NNDSS) for 1970–1996 and Active Bacterial Core surveillance (ABCs) system for 1997–2011.

* Per 100,000 population.

† ABCs cases from 1997–2011 estimated to the U.S. population. In 2010, estimated case counts from ABCs were lower than cases reported to NNDSS and might not be representative.

bacterial load have a more rapid clinical deterioration and longer period of hospitalization, as well as a higher risk of death and permanent sequelae. Resistance to complement-mediated lysis and phagocytosis is largely mediated by the polysaccharide capsule and **lipopolysaccharide (LPS)**. Outer membrane vesicles released from the surface of the organism contain LPS, outer membrane proteins, periplasmic proteins, and phospholipid, and play a major role in the inflammatory cascade that leads to severe disease.

Much of the tissue damage is caused by host immune mechanisms activated by meningococcal components, in particular LPS. During invasive disease LPS is bound to a circulating plasma protein, known as LPS-binding protein. The host receptor complex for LPS consists of Toll-like receptor (TLR)-4, CD14, and myeloid differentiation protein 2. Binding of LPS to TLR-4, which is upregulated on circulating leukocytes during septicemia, results in activation of a number of different cell types. An intense inflammatory reaction results from secretion of proinflammatory cytokines such as tumor necrosis factor (TNF)-α, interleukin (IL)-1β, IL-6, IL-8, and granulocyte-macrophage colony-stimulating factor, levels of which are closely associated with plasma levels of LPS. The major antiinflammatory cytokines IL-1Rα, IL-2, IL-4, and IL-12 and transforming growth factor-β are present at very low levels. Both high and low levels have been observed for IL-10 and interferon-γ.

The pathophysiologic events that occur during meningococcal septicemia are largely related to microvascular injury. This leads to increased vascular permeability and the capillary leak syndrome, pathologic vasoconstriction and vasodilation, disseminated intravascular coagulation (DIC), and profound myocardial dysfunction. Increased vascular permeability can lead to dramatic fluid loss and severe hypovolemia. **Capillary leak syndrome** with or without aggressive fluid resuscitation (which is essential in severe cases) leads to pulmonary edema and respiratory failure. Initial vasoconstriction is a compensatory mechanism in response to hypovolemia and results in the clinical features of pallor and cold extremities. Following resuscitation, some patients experience **warm shock**, that is, intense vasodilation with bounding pulses and warm extremities, despite persistent hypotension and metabolic acidosis. Virtually all antithrombotic mechanisms appear to be dysfunctional during meningococcal sepsis, leading to a procoagulant state and DIC. All these factors contribute to depressed myocardial function, but there is also a direct negative cytokine effect on myocardial contractility, thought to be largely mediated by IL-6. Hypoxia, acidosis, hypoglycemia, hypokalemia, hypocalcemia, and hypophosphatemia are all common features in severe septicemia and further depress cardiac function. Some patients become unresponsive to the positive inotropic effects of catecholamines and require high levels of inotropic support during intensive care management. These processes result in impairment of microvascular blood flow throughout the body and ultimately lead to **multiorgan failure**, which is responsible for much of the mortality.

Following invasion of the circulation, meningococci may also penetrate the blood-brain barrier and enter the cerebrospinal fluid (CSF), facilitated by pili and possibly Opc. Once there, bacteria continue to proliferate and LPS and other outer membrane products can stimulate a proinflammatory cascade similar to that observed in the blood. This leads to upregulation of specific adhesion molecules and recruitment of leukocytes into the CSF. Central nervous system damage occurs directly by meningeal inflammation and indirectly by circulatory collapse and causes a high rate of neurologic sequelae in affected patients. Death can occur from cerebral edema, which leads to **increased intracranial pressure (ICP)** and cerebral or cerebellar herniation.

Immunity

There is an inverse correlation between the incidence of disease and the prevalence of complement-dependent **serum bactericidal antibody (SBA)**. The level of SBA is highest at birth and among adults and lowest in children between 6 mo and 2 yr of age, when the highest incidence of disease occurs. Such antibodies are naturally elicited by asymptomatic carriage of pathogenic and nonpathogenic *Neisseria*, such as *Neisseria lactamica*, and other antigenically related gram-negative bacteria. A similar relationship was described for capsular groups A, B, and C. Vaccine trials support these earlier findings. For the meningococcal

capsular group C conjugate vaccine, an SBA titer ≥1:8 correlated strongly with postlicensure vaccine effectiveness. For capsular group B disease the data are less certain, but the proportions of capsular group B vaccine recipients with ≥4-fold rises in SBA after vaccination or SBA titers ≥1:4 have been correlated with clinical effectiveness in studies of outer membrane vesicle vaccines. These cutoffs are therefore currently used for regulatory approval of new meningococcal vaccines. The strong association between disease risk and genetic variation in human complement factor H further supports the importance of complement-mediated protection against disease.

There is evidence that mechanisms other than complement-dependent bactericidal antibodies may be important in determining protection against meningococcal disease. Disease in individuals with complement deficiency has a different age distribution, has less severe clinical features, and often involves unusual capsular groups. In particular, complement deficiency does not appear strongly related to an increased risk of capsular group B disease. Alternative surrogate markers of protection include the opsonophagocytic assay and antibody avidity, but no studies have attempted to link these laboratory tests with vaccine efficacy or even population protection, as has been found with SBA.

Host Factors

Host susceptibility is strongly related to age, as previously described, indicating that immunologic responsiveness and/or naïveté in infancy and early childhood are key determinants of risk. **Complement** is a key factor in protection against meningococcal disease. Individuals with inherited deficiencies of properdin, factor D, or terminal complement components have up to a 1,000-fold higher risk for development of meningococcal disease than complement-sufficient people. The risk of meningococcal disease is also increased in patients with acquired complement deficiencies associated with diseases such as nephrotic syndrome, systemic lupus erythematosus (SLE), and hepatic failure and in patients treated with eculizumab, a monoclonal antibody against complement protein C5.

Among those with complement deficiencies, meningococcal disease is more prevalent during late childhood and adolescence, when carriage rates are higher than in children <10 yr old; meningococcal infections in these patients may be recurrent. Although meningococcal disease can occasionally be overwhelming in patients with late complement component deficiency, cases are more typically described as being less severe than in complement-sufficient persons (properdin deficiency being the exception), perhaps reflecting that these cases are often caused by unusual capsular groups. In one study, one third of individuals with meningococcal disease caused by capsular groups X, Y, and W had a complement deficiency. Although protective against early infection, extensive complement activation and bacteriolysis may contribute to the pathogenesis of severe disease once bacterial invasion has occurred.

The sibling risk ratio for meningococcal disease is similar to that for other diseases where susceptibility shows polygenic inheritance, and a number of host genetic factors have now been identified to affect either susceptibility to meningococcal disease or severity of disease. The molecules implicated include proteins on epithelial surfaces, the complement cascade, pattern recognition receptors, clotting factors, and inflammatory mediators. Deficiencies in the complement pathways are consistently associated with an increased risk of meningococcal disease, with specific polymorphisms in mannose-binding lectin and factor H found to be associated with disease susceptibility. A genome-wide association study of 7,522 individuals in Europe identified single nucleotide polymorphisms (SNPs) within genes encoding complement factor H (*CFH*) and CFH-related protein 3 (*CFHR3*), which were associated with host susceptibility to meningococcal disease. Complement-mediated bacteriolysis is known to be extremely important in protection against meningococcal disease, giving these associations biologic plausibility. In particular, factor H attaches to various binding proteins expressed on the bacterial surface, downregulating complement activation and allowing the organism to evade host responses.

In terms of disease severity, a meta-analysis of data from smaller studies found that SNPs in genes encoding plasminogen activator inhibitor 1 (*SERPINE1*), IL-1 receptor antagonist (*IL1RN*), and IL-1β

(*IL1B*) are associated with increased mortality from meningococcal disease, as reflected in pathophysiologic changes that occur during invasive disease.

CLINICAL MANIFESTATIONS

The most common form of meningococcal infection is asymptomatic carriage of the organism in the nasopharynx. In the rare cases where invasive disease occurs, the clinical spectrum of meningococcal disease varies widely, but the highest proportion of cases present with meningococcal meningitis (30–50%). Other recognized presentations include bacteremia without sepsis, meningococcal septicemia with or without meningitis, pneumonia, chronic meningococcemia, and occult bacteremia. Focal infections in various sites (e.g., myocardium, joints, pericardium, bone, eye, peritoneum, sinuses, middle ear) are well recognized, and all may progress to disseminated disease. Urethritis, cervicitis, vulvovaginitis, orchitis, and proctitis may also occur.

Acute meningococcal septicemia cannot be distinguished from other viral or bacterial infections early after onset of symptoms (Table 218.1). Typical nonspecific early symptoms include fever, irritability, lethargy, respiratory symptoms, refusal to drink, and vomiting. Less frequently, diarrhea, sore throat, and chills/shivering are reported. A maculopapular rash, which is indistinguishable from rashes seen after viral infections, is evident in approximately 10% of cases early in the course of infection (Fig. 218.2). Limb pain, myalgia, or refusal to walk may occur as the primary complaint in 7% of otherwise clinically unsuspected cases. As disease progresses, cold hands or feet and abnormal skin color may be important signs, capillary refill time becomes prolonged, and a nonblanching or petechial rash will develop in >80% of cases. In fulminant meningococcal septicemia, the disease progresses rapidly over several hours from fever with nonspecific signs to septic shock characterized by prominent petechiae and purpura (**purpura fulminans**) with poor peripheral perfusion, tachycardia (to compensate for reduced blood volume resulting from capillary leak), increased respiratory rate (to compensate for pulmonary edema), hypotension (a late sign of shock in young children), confusion, and coma (resulting from decreased cerebral perfusion). Coagulopathy, electrolyte disturbance (especially hypokalemia), acidosis, adrenal hemorrhage, renal failure, and myocardial failure may all develop (Fig. 218.3). Meningitis may be present.

Meningococcal meningitis is indistinguishable from meningitis caused by other bacteria. Nonspecific symptoms and signs (see Table 218.1), including fever and headache, predominate, especially in the young and early in the illness. Children <5 yr old rarely report headache. More specific symptoms of photophobia, nuchal rigidity, bulging of the fontanel, and clinical signs of meningeal irritation may develop but are unusual in infants. Seizures and focal neurologic signs occur less frequently than in patients with meningitis caused by *Streptococcus*

pneumoniae or *Haemophilus influenzae* type b. A meningoencephalitis-like picture can occur, associated with rapidly progressive cerebral edema and death from increased ICP, which may be more common with capsular group A infection.

Occult meningococcal bacteremia manifests as fever with or without associated symptoms that suggest a minor viral infection. Resolution of bacteremia may occur without antibiotics, but sustained bacteremia leads to meningitis in approximately 60% of cases and to distant infection of other tissues.

Chronic meningococcemia, which occurs rarely, is characterized by fever, nontoxic appearance, arthralgia, headache, splenomegaly, and a maculopapular or petechial rash (Fig. 218.4). Symptoms are intermittent, with a mean duration of illness of 6-8 wk. Blood culture results are usually positive, but cultures may initially be sterile. Chronic meningococcemia may spontaneously resolve, but meningitis may develop in untreated cases. Some cases have been associated with complement deficiency and others with sulfonamide therapy. One report indicates that up to 47% of isolates from patients with chronic meningococcemia (vs <10% in acute cases) have a mutation in the *lpxl1* gene, leading to a reduced inflammatory response and the milder course of infection.

DIAGNOSIS

The initial diagnosis of meningococcal disease should be made on clinical assessment to avoid delay in implementation of appropriate therapy.

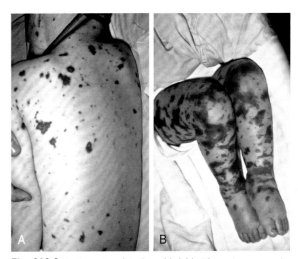

Fig. 218.3 A, Purpuric rash in 3 yr old child with meningococcemia. **B,** Purpura fulminans in 11 mo old child with meningococcemia. *(From Thompson ED, Herzog KD: Fever and rash. In Zaoutis L, Chiang V, editors: Comprehensive pediatric hospital medicine, Philadelphia, 2007, Mosby, Figs 62-6 and 62-7.)*

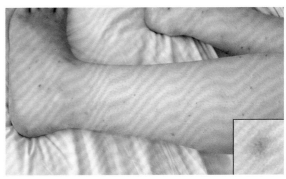

Fig. 218.4 Rash of chronic meningococcemia. *(From Persa OD, Jazmati N, Robinson N, et al: A pregnant woman with chronic meningococcaemia from Neisseria meningitidis with lpxL1-mutations, Lancet 384:1900, 2014.).*

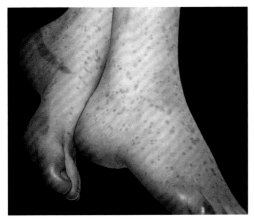

Fig. 218.2 Meningococcemia. A maculopapular, nonhemorrhagic rash that subsequently became petechial. *(From Habif TP: Clinical dermatology, ed 6, Philadelphia, 2016, Elsevier, Fig 9-59.)*

| **Table 218.1** | Prevalence of Symptoms and Signs in Children and Young People With Meningococcal Septicemia, Meningococcal Disease, and Bacterial Meningitis |

SYMPTOM OR SIGN	PREVALENCE RANGE (NUMBER OF STUDIES)		
	Bacterial Meningitis	**Meningococcal Disease**	**Meningococcal Septicemia**
Fever	66-97% (10)	58-97% (7)	98% (1)
Vomiting or nausea	18-70% (10)	44-76% (6)	
Rash	9-62% (6)	59-100% (9)	70% (1)
Headache	3-59% (7)	16-49% (5)	40% (1)
Lethargy	13-87% (6)	36-65% (3)	59% (1)
Coughing	N/A (0)	15-27% (2)	33% (1)
Irritable or unsettled	21-79% (8)	36-67% (3)	32% (1)
Runny nose	N/A (0)	24% (1)	31% (1)
Muscle ache or joint pain	23% (1)	7-65% (3)	30% (1)
Refusing food or drink	26-76% (4)	13-60% (3)	27% (1)
Altered mental state*	26-93% (6)	45-81% (3)	N/A (0)
Stiff neck	13-74% (13)	5-71% (6)	N/A (0)
Impaired consciousness	60-87% (4)	10-72% (2)	N/A (0)
Unconsciousness	4-18% (4)	N/A (0)	N/A (0)
Chills or shivering	N/A (0)	39% (1)	N/A (0)
Photophobia	5-16% (2)	2-31% (5)	N/A (0)
Respiratory symptoms	25-49% (4)	16-23% (2)	N/A (0)
Breathing difficulty	13-34% (4)	11% (1)	N/A (0)
Cold hands or feet	N/A (0)	43% (1)	N/A (0)
Shock	8-16% (2)	27-29% (2)	N/A (0)
Seizures	14-38% (12)	7-17% (3)	N/A (0)
Diarrhea	21-29% (2)	7-9% (2)	N/A (0)
Abdominal pain or distention	17% (1)	4% (1)	N/A (0)
Leg pain	N/A (0)	11-37% (2)	N/A (0)
Thirst	N/A (0)	8% (1)	N/A (0)
Sore throat, coryza or throat infection	18% (1)	24% (1)	N/A (0)
Ill appearance	N/A (0)	79% (1)	N/A (0)
Capillary refill time >2 sec	N/A (0)	83% (1)	N/A (0)
Hypotension	N/A (0)	28% (1)	N/A (0)
Abnormal skin color	N/A (0)	19% (1)	N/A (0)
Bulging fontanel[†]	13-45% (4)	N/A (0)	N/A (0)
Ear infection or ear, nose, and throat infections[‡]	18-49% (5)	N/A (0)	N/A (0)
Chest infection	14% (1)	N/A (0)	N/A (0)
Brudzinski sign	11-66% (2)	N/A (0)	N/A (0)
Kernig sign	10-53% (3)	N/A (0)	N/A (0)
Abnormal pupils	10% (1)	N/A (0)	N/A (0)
Cranial nerve pair involvement	4% (1)	N/A (0)	N/A (0)
Toxic or moribund state	3-49% (2)	N/A (0)	N/A (0)
Back rigidity	46% (1)	N/A (0)	N/A (0)
Paresis	6% (1)	N/A (0)	N/A (0)
Focal neurologic deficit	6-47% (3)	N/A (0)	N/A (0)

Classification of conditions presented in the table reflects the terminology used in the evidence.
*This includes confusion, delirium, and drowsiness.
[†]The age ranges in the 4 studies are 0-14 yr, 0-2 yr, 0-12 mo, and 0-13 wk.
[‡]One study reported the number of children and young people with ear, nose, and throat infections; the 4 other studies reported the number of ear infections only.
N/A, Not applicable.
Adapted from National Collaborating Center for Women's and Children's Health (UK): Bacterial meningitis and meningococcal septicaemia: management of bacterial meningitis and meningococcal septicaemia in children and young people younger than 16 years in primary and secondary care, *NICE clinical guidelines, No 102*, London, 2010, RCOG Press.

Laboratory findings are variable but may include leukocytopenia or leukocytosis, often with increased percentages of neutrophils and band forms, and anemia, thrombocytopenia, proteinuria, and hematuria. Elevations of erythrocyte sedimentation rate (ESR) and C-reactive protein (CRP) may occur, but in patients with rapid onset of disease, these values may be within normal limits at presentation. Increased CRP in the presence of fever and petechiae makes the diagnosis likely. Hypoalbuminemia, hypocalcemia, hypokalemia, hypomagnesemia, hypophosphatemia, hypoglycemia, and metabolic acidosis, often with increased lactate levels, are common in patients with meningococcal septicemia. Patients with coagulopathy have decreased serum concentrations of prothrombin and fibrinogen and prolonged coagulation times.

A confirmed diagnosis of meningococcal disease is established by isolation of *N. meningitidis* from a normally sterile body fluid such as blood, CSF, or synovial fluid. Meningococci may be identified in a Gram stain preparation and/or culture of petechial or purpuric skin lesions, although this procedure is rarely undertaken, and occasionally are seen on Gram stain of the buffy coat layer of a centrifuged blood sample. Although blood culture may be positive in more than two thirds of cases before antibiotic use, culture results often are negative if the patient has been treated with antibiotics prior to collection of the culture specimen; data suggest that <50% are culture positive. Isolation of the organism from the nasopharynx is not diagnostic of invasive disease because the organism is a common commensal.

PCR using primers specific for meningococcal genes (e.g., *ctrA*) has high sensitivity and specificity for detection of meningococci using whole blood samples and has increased confirmation of suspected cases by >40% in the United Kingdom.

Lumbar puncture should be undertaken to establish a diagnosis of meningococcal meningitis in patients without contraindications, including presence of septic shock, coagulopathy, thrombocytopenia, respiratory distress, seizures, increased ICP, or local infection. In patients with meningococcal meningitis, the cellular and chemical characteristics of the CSF are those of acute bacterial meningitis, showing gram-negative diplococci in up to 75% of cases. CSF culture results may be positive in patients with meningococcemia in the absence of CSF pleocytosis or clinical evidence of meningitis; conversely, positive CSF specimens that are gram positive are sometimes culture negative. Overdecolorized pneumococci in Gram stain preparations can be mistaken for meningococci, and therefore empirical therapy should not be narrowed to *N. meningitidis* infection on the basis of Gram stain findings alone.

Detection of capsular polysaccharide antigens using rapid latex agglutination tests on CSF can support the diagnosis in cases clinically consistent with meningococcal disease, but the tests have not performed adequately in clinical practice (poor sensitivity and cross-reactivity of capsular group B test with *Escherichia coli* K1 antigen) and have been replaced by molecular diagnostic methods. Urine antigen testing is insensitive and should not be used. PCR-based assays for detection of meningococci in blood and CSF have been developed, and multiplex PCR assays that detect several bacterial species associated with meningitis, including the meningococcus, are used in some laboratories.

Differential Diagnosis

Meningococcal disease can appear similar to sepsis or meningitis caused by many other gram-negative bacteria, *S. pneumoniae, Staphylococcus aureus,* or group A streptococcus; to Rocky Mountain spotted fever, ehrlichiosis, or epidemic typhus; and to bacterial endocarditis. Viral and other infectious etiologies of meningoencephalitis should be considered in some cases.

Petechial **rashes** are common in viral infections (enteroviruses, influenza and other respiratory viruses, measles virus, Epstein-Barr virus, cytomegalovirus, parvovirus) and may be confused with meningococcal disease. Petechial or purpuric rashes are also associated with protein C or S deficiency, platelet disorders (including idiopathic thrombocytopenic purpura), Henoch-Schönlein purpura, connective tissue disorders, drug eruptions, and trauma, including nonaccidental injury. The nonpetechial, blanching maculopapular rash observed in some cases of meningococcal disease, especially early in the course, may initially be confused with a viral exanthem.

TREATMENT
Antibiotics

Empirical antimicrobial therapy should be initiated immediately after the diagnosis of invasive meningococcal infection is suspected and cultures are obtained, using a **third-generation cephalosporin** to cover the most likely bacterial pathogens until the diagnosis is confirmed. In regions with a high rate of β-lactam–resistant *S. pneumoniae*, empirical *addition* of intravenous (IV) **vancomycin** is recommended (see Chapter 621.1) while awaiting the outcome of bacterial identification and sensitivity, but this is unnecessary in other settings where cephalosporin resistance of pneumococci is very rare (in these settings a risk assessment of each case should be made). Once the diagnosis of β-lactam–sensitive meningococcal disease is confirmed in the laboratory, some authorities recommend a switch to penicillin. Even with no evidence that survival outcomes are different, however, limited evidence from one study indicates that, in meningococcal purpura, necrotic skin lesions are less common among children treated with ceftriaxone than with penicillin. Furthermore, it may be cost-effective by using a once-daily dose of ceftriaxone for therapy in younger children, and this is the recommended practice in the United Kingdom (Table 218.2). No adequate studies have investigated the optimal duration of therapy for children, but the course is generally continued for 5-7 days.

Early treatment of meningococcal infections may prevent serious sequelae, but timely early diagnosis is often difficult in the absence of

Table 218.2	Treatment of *Neisseria Meningitidis* Invasive Infections				
DRUG	**ROUTE**	**DOSE**	**DOSING INTERVAL (hr)**	**MAXIMUM DAILY DOSE**	**NOTES**
Penicillin G	IM or IV	300,000 units/kg/day	4-6	12-24 million units	Does not clear carriage, and "prophylaxis" is required at the end of treatment.
Ampicillin	IM or IV	200-400 mg/kg/day	6	6-12 g	Does not clear carriage, and "prophylaxis" is required at the end of treatment.
Cefotaxime	IM or IV	200-300 mg/kg/day	6-8	8-12 g	Recommended in the neonate
Ceftriaxone	IM or IV	100 mg/kg/day	12-24	2-4 g	Preferred treatment as only once or twice daily, and may reduce skin complications.
ALTERNATIVE THERAPY IN THE FACE OF LIFE-THREATENING β-LACTAM ALLERGY					
Chloramphenicol*	IV	50-100 mg/kg/day	6	2-4 g	
Meropenem†	IV	60-120 mg/kg/day	8	1.5-6 g	

*Monitor blood levels to avoid toxicity.
†Rate of crossreactivity in penicillin-allergic adults is 2–3%.
IM, Intramuscular; IV, intravenous.

petechial or purpuric skin findings. Among children presenting with petechial rashes, 1–10% may have underlying meningococcal disease, and protocols have been established to ensure that these patients are identified without exposing the >90% of cases without meningococcal disease to unnecessary parenteral antibiotic therapy (Fig. 218.5).

Isolates of *N. meningitidis* with decreased susceptibility to penicillin (minimal inhibitory concentration of penicillin of 0.1-1.0 mg/mL) have been reported from Europe, Africa, Canada, and the United States (4% of isolates in 2006). Decreased susceptibility is caused at least in part by altered penicillin-binding protein 2 and does not appear to adversely affect the response to therapy. Isolates with reduced susceptibility to third-generation cephalosporins have been described in France, but the level of reduced susceptibility is not likely to affect therapeutic outcomes where these agents are used for treatment.

Supportive Care

Most children with meningococcal disease can be managed with antibiotics and simple supportive care and will improve rapidly. However, with an overall 5–10% case fatality rate, the priority in initiating management of children presenting with meningococcal disease is identification of the life-threatening features of the disease: shock and increased ICP. Delayed initiation of supportive therapy is associated with poor outcome, and protocols have therefore been established to aid clinicians in a step-by-step approach (http://www.meningitis.org). In all children presenting with meningococcal disease, assessment of the airway should be performed, since the airway could be compromised as a result of a depressed level of consciousness (elevated ICP in meningitis or poor cerebral perfusion in shock). In patients with meningococcal septicemia, supplementary oxygen should be used to treat hypoxia, which is caused

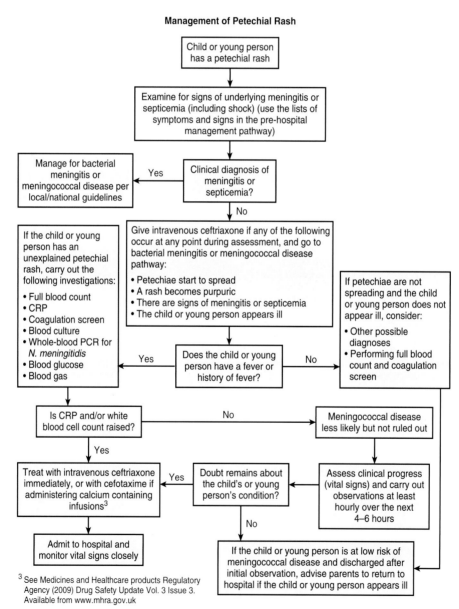

Management of Petechial Rash

Fig. 218.5 Treatment algorithm for petechial rash. CRP, C-reactive protein; PCR, polymerase chain reaction. *(From National Collaborating Center for Women's and Children's Health (UK): Bacterial meningitis and meningococcal septicaemia: management of bacterial meningitis and meningococcal septicaemia in children and young people younger than 16 years in primary and secondary care, NICE clinical guidelines, No 102, London, 2010, RCOG Press.)*

by pulmonary edema (from capillary leak), and some patients will require endotracheal intubation. Hypovolemia requires both volume replacement and inotropic support to maintain cardiac output. Because ongoing fluid resuscitation may lead to pulmonary edema, endotracheal intubation and ventilation should be initiated in a patient who remains in compensated shock after 40 mL/kg of fluid resuscitation to improve oxygenation and reduce work of breathing. Biochemical and hematologic abnormalities are common in meningococcal septicemia, and protocols recommend anticipation, assessment, and correction of glucose, potassium, calcium, magnesium, phosphate, clotting factors, and anemia.

Children with meningococcal meningitis should be cautiously managed with maintenance fluids (fluid restriction is not recommended and may be harmful), and those with increased ICP should be managed with close attention to maneuvers to maintain normal cerebral perfusion. If there is shock in the presence of elevated ICP, the shock should be carefully corrected to ensure that cerebral perfusion pressure is maintained.

Many adjunctive therapies have been attempted in patients with severe meningococcal septicemia, but few have been subjected to randomized controlled trials (RCTs). Data are insufficient to recommend use of anticoagulant or fibrinolytic agents, extracorporeal membrane oxygenation, plasmapheresis, or hyperbaric oxygen. In well-designed clinical trials, an antibody directed against endotoxin (HA1A) did not confer any benefit in children with meningococcal disease, and although initially promising in adult sepsis, activated protein C was not useful in pediatric sepsis and was associated with an increased risk of bleeding. Recombinant bactericidal permeability increasing protein was studied in an underpowered (survival end-point) trial and showed some potentially beneficial effects against secondary end-points (amputations, transfusions, functional outcome) and requires further investigation.

Although the benefits of **corticosteroids** for adjunctive therapy in pediatric *bacterial* meningitis caused by *H. influenzae* type b (Hib) are accepted, no pediatric data specifically demonstrate benefit in *meningococcal* meningitis. However, some authorities extrapolate from animal data, from experience with Hib, and from compelling data from adult meningitis and recommend corticosteroids as adjunctive therapy in pediatric meningococcal meningitis, given with or soon after the 1st dose of antibiotics. Therapeutic doses of corticosteroids should not be used routinely in meningococcal septicemia. Some intensivists recommend replacement doses of corticosteroids in patients with treatment-refractory septic shock, since severe sepsis caused by meningococcus is associated with adrenal insufficiency resulting from adrenal necrosis or hemorrhage (Waterhouse-Friderichsen syndrome).

COMPLICATIONS

Adrenal hemorrhage, endophthalmitis, arthritis, endocarditis, pericarditis, myocarditis, pneumonia, lung abscess, peritonitis, and renal infarcts can occur during acute infection. Renal insufficiency requiring dialysis may result from prerenal failure. Reactivation of latent herpes simplex virus infections is common during meningococcal infection.

A self-limiting immune complex vasculitis may occur, usually in the 1st 10 days after onset of the disease, resulting in various manifestations, including fever, rash, arthritis, and rarely iritis, pericarditis, or carditis. The arthritis is monoarticular or oligoarticular, involves large joints, and is associated with sterile effusions that respond to nonsteroidal antiinflammatory drugs. Because most patients with meningococcal meningitis become afebrile by the 7th hospital day, persistence or recrudescence of fever after 5 days of antibiotics warrants evaluation for immune complex–mediated complications.

The most common complication of acute severe meningococcal septicemia is focal skin infarction, which typically affects the lower limbs and can lead to substantial scarring and require skin grafting. Distal tissue necrosis in purpura fulminans may require amputation (which should be delayed to allow demarcation) in approximately 2% of survivors. Avascular necrosis of epiphyses and epiphyseal-metaphyseal defects can result from the generalized DIC and may lead to growth disturbance and late skeletal deformities.

Deafness is the most frequent neurologic sequela of meningitis, occurring in 5–10% of children. Cerebral arterial or venous thrombosis with resultant cerebral infarction can occur in severe cases. Meningococcal

meningitis is rarely complicated by subdural effusion or empyema or by brain abscess. Other rare neurologic sequelae include ataxia, seizures, blindness, cranial nerve palsies, hemiparesis or quadriparesis, and obstructive hydrocephalus (manifests 3-4 wk after onset of illness). Behavioral and psychosocial complications of the disease are frequently reported.

PROGNOSIS

The case fatality rate for invasive meningococcal disease is 5–10%, with clear differences related to age of the patient and meningococcal genotype. Most deaths occur within 48 hr of hospitalization in children with meningococcemia. Poor prognostic factors on presentation include hypothermia or extreme hyperpyrexia, hypotension or shock, purpura fulminans, seizures, leukopenia, thrombocytopenia (including DIC), acidosis, and high circulating levels of endotoxin and TNF-α. The presence of petechiae for <12 hr before admission, absence of meningitis, and low or normal ESR indicate rapid, fulminant progression and poorer prognosis.

Because complement deficiency is rare following capsular group B infection, screening is unlikely to be useful in detecting cases caused by this group, but some authorities recommend routine screening in these cases. However, with one third or more of cases of disease caused by groups X, Y, and W apparently associated with complement deficiency, it is clearly appropriate to screen after infection with non-B capsular groups.

PREVENTION
Secondary Prevention

Close contacts of patients with meningococcal disease are at increased risk of infection because such individuals are likely to be colonized with the index case's (hyperinvasive) strain. Antibiotic prophylaxis should be offered as soon as possible to individuals who have been exposed directly to a patient's oral secretions, for whom risk may be 1,000 times the background rate in the population. This includes household, kissing, and close family contacts of cases, as well as childcare and recent preschool contacts in the United States. Up to 30% of cases occur in the 1st wk, but risk persists for up to 1 yr after presentation of the index case. Although prophylaxis is effective in preventing secondary cases, co primary cases may occur in the days after presentation of the index case, and contacts should be carefully evaluated if they develop symptoms. Advice on management of nonclose contacts, such as those in daycare, nursery settings, or school and other institutions, varies in different countries because the risk of a secondary case in this situation is low and opinion on risk assessment varies. **Ceftriaxone** and **ciprofloxacin** are the most effective agents for prophylaxis, with ciprofloxacin the drug of choice in some countries. **Rifampin** is most widely used but fails to eradicate colonization in 15% of cases (Table 218.3). Prophylaxis is not routinely recommended for medical personnel except those with exposure to aerosols of respiratory secretions, such as through mouth-to-mouth resuscitation, intubation, or suctioning before or in the 24 hr after antibiotic therapy is initiated in the index case.

Neither penicillin nor ampicillin treatment eradicates nasopharyngeal carriage and should not be routinely used for prophylaxis. Patients with meningococcal infection treated solely with penicillin or ampicillin are therefore at risk of relapse or transmission to a close contact and should receive antimicrobial prophylaxis with one of the agents listed in Table 218.3 before hospital discharge. The preference is to use ceftriaxone for *treatment* of the index case, in which case further prophylaxis is not required. Droplet infection control precautions should be observed for hospitalized patients for 24 hr. after initiation of effective therapy. All confirmed or probable cases of meningococcal infection must be reported to the local public health department according to national or regional regulations.

Close contacts of cases could also be immunized to further reduce the risk of secondary infection, as described later.

Vaccination

Meningococcal plain *polysaccharide vaccines* containing capsular polysaccharides from capsular groups A + C or capsular groups A, C, W, Y have been available since the 1960s and used in the control of

Table 218.3	Antibiotic Prophylaxis to Prevent *Neisseria Meningitidis* Infection*		
AGE-GROUP	**DOSE**	**DURATION**	**EFFICACY**
Rifampin[†]			
Infants <1 mo	5 mg/kg PO every 12 hr	2 days (4 doses)	
Children ≥1 mo	10 mg/kg PO every 12 hr (max 600 mg)	2 days (4 doses)	90-95%
Adults	600 mg PO every 12 hr	2 days (4 doses)	90-95%
Ceftriaxone			
Children <15 yr	125 mg IM	1 dose	90-95%
Children ≥15 yr	250 mg IM	1 dose	90-95%
Ciprofloxacin			
Children ≥1 mo[†‡]	20 mg/kg (max 500 mg) PO	1 dose	90-95%
Azithromycin (Not Recommended Routinely)			
All ages	10 mg/kg (max 500 g) PO	1 dose	90%

*Recommended for household and kissing contacts. In the United States, chemoprophylaxis is recommended for:
- Household contact, especially children <2 yr old
- Childcare or preschool contact at any time during 7 days before onset of illness
- Direct exposure to index patient's secretions through kissing, sharing toothbrushes or eating utensils at any time during 7 days before onset of illness
- Mouth-to-mouth resuscitation, unprotected contact during endotracheal intubation during 7 days before onset of illness
- Frequently slept in same dwelling as index patient during 7 days before onset of illness
- Passengers seated directly next to the index case during airline flights lasting >8 hr

[†]Not recommended for pregnant women (ceftriaxone is agent of choice in this setting).
[‡]Not recommended routinely for young people <18 yr old; use only if fluoroquinolone-resistant strains of *N. meningitidis* have not been identified in the community.

IM, Intramuscularly; PO, orally (by mouth).

outbreaks and epidemics and for high-risk groups. However, polysaccharide vaccines are poorly immunogenic in infants, do not induce immunologic memory, and are associated with *immunologic hyporesponsiveness* (reduced response to future doses of polysaccharide). Plain polysaccharide vaccines have been superseded by meningococcal protein-polysaccharide *conjugate vaccines*, which are generally more immunogenic than plain polysaccharides, are immunogenic from early infancy, induce immunologic memory, and are not associated with hyporesponsiveness. The conjugate vaccines contain meningococcal polysaccharides that are chemically conjugated to a carrier protein. Three carrier proteins are used in various meningococcal conjugate vaccines: tetanus toxoid, diphtheria toxoid, and the mutant diphtheria toxin, CRM197. However, although plain polysaccharide vaccines should be considered redundant in most industrialized countries where the new-generation conjugates are available, they may still have a role in some regions where conjugates are not yet available.

The first meningococcal conjugate vaccine used was a monovalent capsular group C meningococcal conjugate vaccine (**MenC**), introduced in the United Kingdom in 1999 and administered to all children and young people <19 yr old in a mass catch-up campaign before establishment in the routine infant immunization schedule. The MenC vaccine has proved highly (>95%) effective in controlling disease through both direct protection of the vaccinated population and induction of herd immunity, protecting the wider population. *Herd immunity* is induced through the impact of conjugate vaccines on colonization, reducing carriage and blocking transmission of meningococci among adolescents and young adults. Monovalent MenC vaccines are used widely in the industrialized countries of Western Europe, Canada, and Australia, where disease

caused by capsular group C meningococci has virtually disappeared. However, serologic surveys show that antibody levels wane, especially after infant immunization, and booster doses are now recommended during adolescence to sustain individual and population immunity.

Quadrivalent meningococcal A, C, Y, W conjugate vaccines (**MenACWY**) have been available since 2005 and are routinely used for U.S. adolescents and as a single adolescent booster dose in some countries that had established MenC infant programs more than a decade ago. MenACWY was initially introduced as a single dose at 11 yr of age in the United States, but concerns about waning immunity led to the adoption of a 2nd dose. The initial reports on effectiveness (>80%) of MenACWY in the U.S. program indicates that these vaccines are likely to provide control of disease caused by capsular groups C, W, and Y (capsular group A being unimportant currently), although the program has taken some time to become fully established. As the population of immunized adolescents and young adults in the United States grows, the effects of these vaccines on carriage of meningococci likely will reduce disease among other segments of the population through herd immunity, assuming the transmission dynamics of Y and W meningococci are the same as for capsular group C. Although MenACWY vaccines are not currently recommended in the United States for routine use in younger age-groups in view of the low rate of disease caused by these capsular groups in infancy, they may provide broader protection in countries that are already using MenC vaccines in infant programs. Other combination vaccines containing various conjugates, including Hib-MenC (used in the United Kingdom as 12 mo booster) and Hib-MenCY, may have a role in broadening protection beyond MenC, in early life. Table 218.4 outlines the current U.S. programmatic recommendations.

Individuals at high risk of meningococcal disease, such as those with complement deficiency and travelers to regions where there is a risk of epidemic meningococcal disease caused by A or W, should receive MenACWY (see Table 218.4). The risk of disease among close contacts of cases of disease caused by vaccine capsular groups may be further reduced if they are offered MenACWY in addition to antimicrobial prophylaxis. A possible association between MenACWY-diphtheria and Guillain-Barré syndrome, which caused concern early after the vaccine was first used in the United States, has not been substantiated.

A capsular group A meningococcal conjugate vaccine (**MenA**) has been developed for use in the sub-Saharan African meningitis belt, and implementation in 2010 through mass vaccination appears already to have interrupted disease caused by this capsular group. More than 235 million people have been vaccinated since the introduction.

The majority of disease in infants and in most industrialized countries is caused by capsular *group B polysaccharide-bearing meningococci*. This polysaccharide capsule has chemical identity with glycosylated protein antigens in the human fetus and, as a "self" antigen, is therefore not immunogenic in humans and leads to the theoretical risk of induction of autoimmunity. Vaccine development has therefore focused on subcapsular protein antigens. Several countries (e.g., Cuba, Norway, New Zealand) successfully controlled capsular group B epidemics by immunizing with tailor-made outer membrane vesicle vaccines prepared from blebs of outer membrane harvested from the respective epidemic strains. The principal limitation of outer membrane vesicle vaccines is that the bactericidal antibody responses induced by immunization are limited to the vaccine strain, because the response is largely directed against the homologous PorA (serosubtype) protein, and they are therefore not considered for use in endemic settings, including the United States or most other industrialized countries.

Promising approaches for prevention of capsular group B disease have been developed over the past decade. One vaccine that was developed for adolescent immunization was licensed in the United States in 2014 and contains 2 variants of factor H–binding protein (**2fHbp**; Pfizer vaccines); it appears highly immunogenic in the target population, inducing bactericidal antibodies directed against a panel of strains bearing variants of fHbp. It is currently recommended for use in high-risk groups and during outbreaks (see Table 218.4). Factor H–binding protein appears to be an important virulence determinant, aiding survival of meningococci in blood, and is expressed by virtually all strains.

Table 218.4	Recommendations for Meningococcal Vaccination (United States, 2017)

GENERAL POPULATION

<2 YR	2-10 YR	11-18 YR	19-55 YR
Not recommended	Not recommended	A single dose of MenACWY-D or MenACWY-CRM at age 11-12 yr with a booster dose at age 16 yr	Not recommended

SPECIAL POPULATIONS AT INCREASED RISK OF MENINGOCOCCAL DISEASE

RISK FACTOR	2-18 MONTHS	7-23 MONTHS	2-55 YR
Persistent complement deficiencies, functional or anatomic asplenia	4 doses of MenACWY-CRM at 2, 4, 6, and 12-15 mo*	2 doses of MenACWY-CRM, with 2nd dose administered at age ≥12 mo and ≥3 mo after 1st dose, or 2 doses of MenACWY-D (not indicated for functional or anatomic asplenia†) at age 9 and 12 mo*†	2 doses of MenACWY-CRM or MenACWY-D 8-12 wk apart*§ and MenB vaccine (2 doses of 4CMenB or 3 doses of 2fHbp)†
At risk during a community outbreak with a vaccine capsular group covered by the relevant vaccine	4 doses of MenACWY-CRM at 2, 4, 6, and 12-15 mo	2 doses of MenACWY-CRM, with 2nd dose administered at age ≥12 mo and ≥3 mo after 1st dose, or 2 doses of MenACWY-D at age 9 and 12 mo†	1 dose of MenACWY-CRM or MenACWY-D MenB vaccine (2 doses of 4CMenB or 3 doses of 2fHbp) depending on capsular group associated with the outbreak†
Travel to or resident of countries where meningococcal disease is hyperendemic or epidemic‖	4 doses of MenACWY-CRM at 2, 4, 6, and 12-15 mo*	2 doses of MenACWY-CRM, with 2nd dose administered at age ≥12 mo and ≥3 mo after 1st dose, or 2 doses of MenACWY-D at 9 and age 12 mo (could be reduced to 8 wk if required for travel)*†	1 dose of MenACWY-CRM or MenACWY-D*†
Have HIV	4 doses of MenACWY-CRM at 2, 4, 6, and 12-15 mo*	2 doses of MenACWY-CRM or 2 doses of MenACWY-D at age 9-23 mo, 12 wk apart*†	2 doses of MenACWY-CRM or MenACWY-D 8-12 wk apart*†‖
Other risk factors	—	—	1 dose MenACWY

*Booster every 5 yr if ongoing risk (after 3 yr if <7 yr old).
†Assuming not previously vaccinated.
‡Because of high risk for invasive pneumococcal disease, children with functional or anatomic asplenia should not be immunized with MenACWY-D before age 2 yr, to avoid interference with the immune response to the pneumococcal conjugate vaccine (PCV).
§If MenACWY-D is used, it should be administered at least 4 wk. after completion of all PCV doses.
‖For example, visitors to the "meningitis belt" of sub-Saharan Africa. Vaccination also is required by the government of Saudi Arabia for all travelers to Mecca during the annual Hajj.
Adapted from https://www.cdc.gov/vaccines/hcp/acip-recs/vacc-specific/mening.html.

A 4-component meningococcal vaccine, **4CMenB** (Bexsero, GSK vaccines), is licensed in Europe and North America and available in various other regions. This vaccine contains an outer membrane vesicle (derived from the New Zealand outbreak strain) and 3 recombinant proteins: a single variant of factor H–binding protein, neisserial adhesin A, and neisserial heparin-binding antigen. 4CMenB vaccine induced bactericidal antibodies against strains containing the vaccine antigens in infants, toddlers, and adolescents in clinical trials. The vaccine appears to have a generally favorable safety profile, although induction of fever in infants and pain at the injection site in other age-groups are common. This vaccine has been used to control university outbreaks of capsular group B meningococcal disease in the United States and Canada and hyperendemic disease in Quebec, Canada. Current recommendations for use in the United States are outlined in Table 218.4. It was recommended for routine use in the infant immunization program in the United Kingdom in 2014 and deployed from September 2015. Early data indicate a vaccine effectiveness of 82.9% against all capsular group B meningococcal disease following 2 doses at age 2 and 4 mo, but vaccine effectiveness is anticipated to be higher against strains targeted by the vaccine antigens.

Bibliography is available at Expert Consult.

Chapter **219**
Neisseria gonorrhoeae (Gonococcus)

Katherine Hsu, Sanjay Ram, and Toni Darville

第二百一十九章
淋病奈瑟菌（淋病双球菌）

中文导读

本章主要介绍了淋病奈瑟菌（淋病双球菌）感染的病因、流行病学、发病机制、临床表现、诊断、治疗、并发症、预防等内容。在淋病奈瑟菌感染的临床表现部分详细介绍了无症状淋病、单纯局部淋病和播散性淋球菌感染。在淋病奈瑟菌感染的诊断部分详细介绍了革兰氏染色与培养和核酸扩增检测。在淋病奈瑟菌感染的治疗部分详细介绍了推荐治疗方案。

Neisseria gonorrhoeae is the causative agent of **gonorrhea**, an infection of the genitourinary tract mucous membranes and of the mucosa of the rectum, oropharynx, and conjunctiva. Gonorrhea transmitted by sexual contact or perinatally is second only to chlamydial infections in the number of cases reported to the U.S. Centers for Disease Control and Prevention (CDC). This high prevalence and the development of antibiotic-resistant strains have led to significant morbidity.

ETIOLOGY

Neisseria gonorrhoeae is a nonmotile, aerobic, non–spore-forming, gram-negative diplococcus with flattened adjacent surfaces. Optimal growth occurs at 35-37°C (95-98.6°F) and at pH 7.2-7.6 in an atmosphere of 3–5% carbon dioxide. The specimen should be inoculated immediately onto fresh, moist, modified Thayer-Martin or specialized transport media, because gonococci do not tolerate drying. Thayer-Martin medium contains antimicrobial agents that inhibit hardier normal flora present in clinical specimens from mucosal sites that may otherwise overgrow gonococci. Presumptive identification may be based on colony appearance, Gram stain appearance, and production of cytochrome oxidase. Gonococci are differentiated from other *Neisseria* spp. by the fermentation of glucose but not maltose, sucrose, or lactose. Gram-negative diplococci are seen in infected material, often within polymorphonuclear leukocytes (PMNs).

As with all gram-negative bacteria, *N. gonorrhoeae* possesses a cell envelope composed of an inner cytoplasmic membrane, a middle layer of peptidoglycan, and an outer membrane. The outer membrane contains **lipooligosaccharide** (**LOS**; also called **endotoxin**), phospholipid, and a variety of proteins that contribute to cell adherence, tissue invasion, and resistance to host defenses. Systems previously used to characterize gonococcal strains included auxotyping and serotyping. **Auxotyping** is based on genetically stable requirements of strains for specific nutrients or cofactors as defined by an isolate's ability to grow on chemically defined media. **Serotyping** systems were based on specific monoclonal antibodies directed against a porin protein called **PorB** (formerly Protein I or PorI), a trimeric outer membrane protein that makes up a substantial part of the gonococcal envelope structure. Changes in PorB proteins present in a community are believed to result, at least in part, from selective immune pressure. DNA-based typing methods have now supplanted auxo- and serotyping. Older gel-based DNA-based typing methods that included restriction fragment length polymorphism (RFLP) analysis of genomic DNA or rRNA (ribotyping), or typing of genes encoding opacity protein (*opa*) were labor intensive and sometimes lacked the ability to accurately discriminate among strains. Methods currently used include the *Neisseria gonorrhoeae* multiantigen sequence typing (**NG-MAST**), which examines the sequences of the variable internal fragments of 2 highly polymorphic *N. gonorrhoeae* genes (*porB* encoding PorB and *tbpB* encoding subunit B of transferrin-binding protein), and multilocus sequence typing (**MLST**), which analyzes the sequences of 7 chromosomal housekeeping genes.

EPIDEMIOLOGY

Since gonorrhea became a nationally notifiable disease in 1944, U.S. rates have ranged between a historic high of 467.7 cases per 100,000 population in 1975 and a historic low of 98.1 per 100,000 in 2009. However, rates have increased almost every year since 2009, with a total of 555,608 cases and a rate of 171.9/100,000 reported in 2017. Rates of reported gonorrhea are also highest in the South (194.0/100,000); among young adults age 20-24 (684.8 cases per 100,000 females age 20-24; 705.2 cases per 100,000 males age 20-24); among males (169.7/100,000 males vs 120.4/100,000 females); and among blacks (548.1/100,000 vs

66.4/100,000 among whites). During 2013–2017, the rate among males increased 86.3% and the rate among females increased 39.4%, suggesting either increased transmission or increased case ascertainment (e.g., through increased extragenital screening) among gay, bisexual, and other men who have sex with men (MSM).

Molecular typing methods (e.g., NG-MAST, MLST) are used to analyze the spread of individual strains of *N. gonorrhoeae* within a community. Maintenance and subsequent spread of gonococcal infections in a community are sustained through continued transmission by asymptomatically infected people and also by a **hyperendemic, high-risk** core group such as commercial sex workers, MSM, or adolescents with multiple sexual partners. This latter observation reflects that most persons who have gonorrhea cease sexual activity and seek care, unless economic need or other factors (e.g., drug addiction) drive persistent sexual activity. Thus, many core transmitters belong to a subset of infected persons who lack or ignore symptoms and continue to be sexually active, underscoring the importance of seeking out and treating the sexual contacts of infected persons who present for treatment. **Oral sex** has a role in sustaining gonorrhea in MSM by providing a pool of untreated asymptomatic pharyngeal infections and may account for as much as one third of symptomatic gonococcal urethritis in MSM.

Gonococcal infection of neonates usually results from peripartum exposure to infected exudate from the cervix of the mother. An acute infection begins 2-5 days after birth. The incidence of neonatal infection depends on the prevalence of gonococcal infection among pregnant women, prenatal screening for gonorrhea, and neonatal ophthalmic prophylaxis.

PATHOGENESIS AND PATHOLOGY

N. gonorrhoeae infects primarily columnar epithelium, because stratified squamous epithelium is relatively resistant to invasion. Mucosal invasion by gonococci results in a local inflammatory response that produces a purulent exudate consisting of PMNs, serum, and desquamated epithelium. The gonococcal LOS (endotoxin) exhibits direct cytotoxicity, causing ciliostasis and sloughing of ciliated epithelial cells. Tumor necrosis factor (TNF) and other cytokines are thought to mediate the cytotoxicity of gonococcal infections. LOS activates complement, which also contributes to the acute inflammatory response.

Gonococci may ascend the urogenital tract, causing urethritis or epididymitis in postpubertal males and acute endometritis, salpingitis, and peritonitis (collectively termed **acute pelvic inflammatory disease** or **PID**) in postpubertal females. Dissemination from the fallopian tubes through the peritoneum to the liver capsule results in **perihepatitis** (Fitz-Hugh–Curtis syndrome). Gonococci that invade the lymphatics and blood vessels may cause inguinal lymphadenopathy; perineal, perianal, ischiorectal, and periprostatic abscesses; and **disseminated gonococcal infection** (DGI).

A number of gonococcal virulence and host immune factors are involved in the penetration of the mucosal barrier and subsequent manifestations of local and systemic infection. Selective pressure from different mucosal environments probably leads to changes in the outer membrane of the organism, including expression of variants of pili, opacity or Opa proteins (formerly protein II), and LOS. These changes may enhance gonococcal attachment, invasion, replication, and evasion of the host's immune response.

For infection to occur, the gonococcus must first attach to host cells. Gonococci adhere to the microvilli of nonciliated epithelial cells by hairlike protein structures (pili) that extend from the cell wall. Pili undergo high-frequency antigenic variation that may aid in the organism's escape from the host immune response and may provide specific ligands for different cell receptors. Opacity proteins, most of which confer an opaque appearance to colonies, function as ligands for members of the carcinoembryonic antigen–related cell adhesion molecule (**CEACAM**) family of proteins or heparin sulfate proteoglycans (HSPGs) to facilitate binding to human cells. Interactions between complement receptor 3 (CR3) on cervical epithelial cells and iC3b, pili, and PorB on the gonococcal surface facilitates cellular entry of gonococci in women. In contrast, the interaction between LOS and asialoglycoprotein receptor (ASGP-R) permits gonococcal entry into male urethral epithelial cells.

Gonococci that express certain Opa proteins adhere to CEACAM3 and are phagocytosed by human neutrophils in the absence of serum. The interaction of Opa with CEACAM1 on CD4⁺ T lymphocytes may suppress their activation and proliferation and contribute to the immunosuppression associated with gonorrhea. A gonococcal IgA protease inactivates IgA_1 by cleaving the molecule in the hinge region and could contribute to colonization or invasion of host mucosal surfaces.

Other phenotypic changes that occur in response to environmental stresses allow gonococci to establish infection. Examples include iron-repressible proteins for binding transferrin or lactoferrin, anaerobically expressed proteins, and proteins that are synthesized in response to contact with epithelial cells. Gonococci may grow in vivo under anaerobic conditions or in an environment with a relative lack of iron.

Approximately 24 hr after attachment, the epithelial cell surface invaginates and surrounds the gonococcus in a phagocytic vacuole. This phenomenon is thought to be mediated by the insertion of the gonococcal outer membrane PorB into the host cell, causing alterations in membrane permeability. Subsequently, phagocytic vacuoles begin releasing gonococci into the subepithelial space by means of exocytosis. Viable organisms may then cause local disease (i.e., salpingitis) or disseminate through the bloodstream or lymphatics.

Serum IgG and IgM directed against gonococcal proteins and LOS activate complement on gonococci. Gonococci have evolved several mechanisms to dampen complement activation. Scavenging cytidine monophospho-*N*-acetyl neuraminic acid (CMP-Neu5Ac, the donor molecule for sialic acid) to sialylate its LOS is one such example, which reduces binding of bactericidal antibodies and simultaneously enhances binding of a complement inhibitor called **factor H** (FH). This property is often lost on subculturing gonococci on media that lacks CMP-Neu5Ac and is thus termed "unstable serum resistance." In contrast, "stable serum resistance"(complement resistance independent of LOS sialylation) is often seen in gonococci that express particular porin proteins (most PorB.1As and select PorB.1Bs),which enables them to bind to complement inhibitors such as FH and C4b-binding protein (C4BP). Such strains are often associated with disseminated disease. *N. gonorrhoeae* differentially subverts the effectiveness of complement and alters the inflammatory responses elicited in human infection. Isolates from cases of DGI typically are "stably" serum resistant, show less C3b deposition on their surface, inactivate C3b more rapidly, generate less C5a, and result in less inflammation at local sites. PID isolates are serum sensitive, deposit more C3b on their surface, inactivate C3b relatively slowly, generate more C5a, and result in more inflammation at local sites. IgG antibody directed against gonococcal reduction-modifiable protein (**Rmp**) blocks complement-mediated killing of *N. gonorrhoeae*. Anti-Rmp blocking antibodies may harbor specificity for outer membrane protein (e.g., OmpA) sequences shared with other *Neisseria* spp. or Enterobacteriaceae, may be directed against a unique Rmp sequence upstream of the OmpA-shared region that includes a cysteine loop, or both. Preexisting antibodies directed against Rmp facilitate transmission of gonococcal infection to exposed women; Rmp is highly conserved in *N. gonorrhoeae*, and the blocking of mucosal defenses may be one of its functions. Gonococcal adaptation also appears to be important in the evasion of killing by neutrophils. Examples include sialylation of LOS, increases in catalase production, and changes in the expression of surface proteins.

Host factors may influence the incidence and manifestations of gonococcal infection. Prepubertal girls are susceptible to vulvovaginitis and rarely experience salpingitis. *N. gonorrhoeae* infects noncornified epithelium, and the thin noncornified vaginal epithelium and alkaline pH of the vaginal mucin predispose this age group to infection of the lower genital tract. Estrogen-induced cornification of the vaginal epithelium in neonates and mature females resists infection. Postpubertal females are more susceptible to salpingitis, especially during menses, when diminished bactericidal activity of the cervical mucus and reflux of blood from the uterine cavity into the fallopian tubes facilitate passage of gonococci into the upper reproductive tract.

Populations at risk for DGI include asymptomatic carriers; neonates; menstruating, pregnant, and postpartum women; MSM; and individuals with defects in complement. The asymptomatic carrier state implies failure of the host immune system to recognize the gonococcus as a pathogen, the capacity of the gonococcus to avoid being killed, or both. **Pharyngeal colonization** has been proposed as a risk factor for DGI. The high rate of asymptomatic infection in pharyngeal gonorrhea may account for this phenomenon. Women are at greater risk for development of DGI during menstruation, pregnancy, and the postpartum period, presumably because of the maximal endocervical shedding and decreased peroxidase bactericidal activity of the cervical mucus during these periods. A lack of neonatal bactericidal IgM antibody is thought to account for the increased susceptibility of neonates to DGI. Persons with terminal complement component deficiencies (C5-C9) are at considerable risk for development of recurrent episodes of DGI.

CLINICAL MANIFESTATIONS
Gonorrhea is manifested by a spectrum of clinical presentations from asymptomatic carriage, to the characteristic localized mucosal infections, to disseminated systemic infection (see Chapter 146).

Asymptomatic Gonorrhea
The incidence of asymptomatic gonorrhea in children has not been ascertained. Gonococci have been isolated from the oropharynx of young children who have been abused sexually by male contacts; oropharyngeal symptoms are usually absent. Most genital tract infections produce symptoms in children. However, as many as 80% of sexually mature females with urogenital gonorrhea infections are asymptomatic in settings in which most infections are detected through screening or other case-finding efforts. This situation is in contrast to that in men, who are asymptomatic only 10% of the time. Asymptomatic rectal carriage of *N. gonorrhoeae* has been documented in 26–68% of females with urogenital infection. Most persons with positive rectal culture results are asymptomatic. Most pharyngeal gonococcal infections are asymptomatic, although rarely **acute tonsillopharyngitis** or **cervical lymphadenopathy** can occur. Pharyngeal gonorrhea is easily acquired through fellatio and may account for a significant proportion of urethral gonorrhea in MSM. Pharyngeal gonorrhea is increasingly prevalent, particularly among adolescents and young adults, and associated with overall increasing prevalence of oral sex behaviors.

Uncomplicated, Localized Gonorrhea
Genital gonorrhea has an incubation period of 2-5 days in men and 5-10 days in women. Primary infection develops in the urethra of males, the vulva and vagina of prepubertal females, and the cervix of postpubertal females. Neonatal ophthalmitis (ophthalmia neonatorum) occurs in both sexes.

Urethritis is usually characterized by a purulent discharge and by dysuria without urgency or frequency. Untreated urethritis in males resolves spontaneously in several weeks or may be complicated by epididymitis, penile edema, lymphangitis, prostatitis, or seminal vesiculitis. Gram-negative intracellular diplococci are found in the discharge. In MSM, the rectal mucosa can become infected after receptive anal intercourse. Symptoms range from painless mucopurulent discharge and scant rectal bleeding to overt proctitis with associated rectal pain and tenesmus.

In prepubertal females, **vulvovaginitis** is usually characterized by a purulent vaginal discharge with a swollen, erythematous, tender, and excoriated vulva. Dysuria may occur. Gonococcal infection should be considered in any girl with vaginal discharge, even when sexual abuse is not suspected; sexual abuse must be considered strongly when gonococcal infection is diagnosed in prepubertal children beyond the neonatal period. In postpubertal females, symptomatic gonococcal **cervicitis** and urethritis are characterized by purulent discharge, suprapubic pain, dysuria, intermenstrual bleeding, and dyspareunia. The cervix may be inflamed and tender. In urogenital gonorrhea limited to the lower genital tract, pain is not enhanced by moving the cervix, and the adnexa are not tender to palpation. Purulent material may be expressed from the urethra or ducts of the Bartholin gland. Rectal gonorrhea is often asymptomatic but may cause proctitis with symptoms of anal discharge, pruritus, bleeding, pain, tenesmus, and constipation. Asymptomatic rectal gonorrhea may not be from anal intercourse but may represent

translocation of infected secretions from cervicovaginal infection.

Gonococcal **ophthalmitis** may be unilateral or bilateral and may occur in any age group after inoculation of the eye with infected secretions. **Ophthalmia neonatorum** caused by *N. gonorrhoeae* usually appears from 1-4 days after birth (see Chapter 652). Ocular infection in older patients results from inoculation or autoinoculation from a genital site. The infection begins with mild inflammation and a serosanguineous discharge. Within 24 hr, the discharge becomes thick and purulent, and tense edema of the eyelids with marked chemosis occurs. If the disease is not treated promptly, corneal ulceration, rupture, and blindness may follow.

Disseminated Gonococcal Infection
Hematogenous dissemination occurs in 1–3% of all gonococcal infections, more frequently after asymptomatic primary infections than symptomatic infections. Women previously accounted for the majority of cases, with symptoms beginning 7-30 days after infection and within 7 days of menstruation in about one half of cases, but more recent case series describe more male than female cases. The most common manifestations are asymmetric arthralgia, petechial or pustular acral skin lesions, tenosynovitis, suppurative arthritis, and rarely carditis, meningitis, and osteomyelitis. The most common initial symptom is acute onset of **polyarthralgia with fever**. Only 25% of patients complain of skin lesions. Most deny genitourinary symptoms; however, primary mucosal infection is documented by genitourinary cultures. Results of approximately 80–90% of cervical cultures are positive in women with DGI. In males, urethral culture results are positive in 50–60%, pharyngeal culture results are positive in 10–20%, and rectal culture results are positive in 15% of cases.

DGI is classified into 2 clinical syndromes that have some overlapping features. The more common **tenosynovitis-dermatitis syndrome** is characterized by fever, chills, skin lesions, and polyarthralgia predominantly involving the wrists, hands, and fingers. Blood culture results are positive in approximately 30–40% of cases, and results of synovial fluid cultures are almost uniformly negative. In the **suppurative arthritis syndrome**, systemic symptoms and signs are less prominent, and monoarticular arthritis is more common, often involving the knee. A polyarthralgia phase may precede the monoarticular infection. In cases of monoarticular involvement, synovial fluid culture results are positive in approximately 45–55%, and synovial fluid findings are consistent with septic arthritis. Blood culture results are usually negative. DGI in neonates usually occurs as a polyarticular suppurative arthritis.

Dermatologic lesions usually begin as painful, discrete, 1-20 mm, pink or red macules that progress to maculopapular, vesicular, bullous, pustular, or petechial lesions. The typical necrotic pustule on an erythematous base is distributed unevenly over the extremities, including the palmar and plantar surfaces, usually sparing the face and scalp. The lesions number between 5 and 40, and 20–30% may contain gonococci. Although immune complexes may be present in DGI, complement levels are normal, and the role of the immune complexes in pathogenesis is uncertain.

Acute endocarditis is an uncommon (1–3%) but often fatal manifestation of DGI that usually leads to rapid destruction of the aortic valve. **Acute pericarditis** is a rarely described entity in patients with disseminated gonorrhea. **Meningitis** with *N. gonorrhoeae* has been documented, and signs and symptoms are similar to those of any acute bacterial meningitis.

DIAGNOSIS
Laboratory confirmation of gonococcal infection is essential, given the legal implications of potential sexual abuse in children and the need to refer sex partners of adolescents and adults for treatment. Given the advent of highly sensitive and specific nucleic acid amplification tests (NAATs), the use of less sensitive, nonamplified test technologies is no longer justified, such as nucleic acid hybridization/probe tests, nucleic acid genetic transformation tests, or enzyme immunoassays. Culture and susceptibility testing capability still need to be maintained, both because data are insufficient to recommend nonculture tests in cases of sexual assault in prepubescent boys and extragenital anatomic site exposure in prepubescent girls, and because culture is necessary to evaluate suspected cases of gonorrhea treatment failure and to monitor

developing resistance to current treatment regimens.

Gram Stain and Culture

Gram stains can be useful in the initial evaluation of patients with suspected gonococcal infection. In males with symptomatic urethritis, a presumptive diagnosis of gonorrhea can be made by identification of gram-negative intracellular diplococci (within leukocytes) in the urethral discharge. A similar finding in females is not sufficient because *Mima polymorpha* and *Moraxella*, which are normal vaginal flora, have a similar appearance. The sensitivity of the Gram stain for diagnosing gonococcal cervicitis and asymptomatic infections is also low. The presence of commensal *Neisseria* spp. in the oropharynx prevents the use of the Gram stain for diagnosis of pharyngeal gonorrhea.

Culture can be performed of any site, including nongenital sites. Advantages of culture include the availability of an isolate for further studies, including antibiotic susceptibility testing. Disadvantages of culture include more stringent transport and growth requirements, lower sensitivity than NAATs, and a delay in availability of results. Material for cervical cultures is obtained as follows. After the exocervix is wiped, a swab is placed in the cervical os and rotated gently for several seconds. Male urethral specimens are obtained by placement of a small swab 2-3 cm into the urethra. Rectal swabs are best obtained by passing of a swab 2-4 cm into the anal canal; specimens that are heavily contaminated by feces should be discarded. For optimal culture results, specimens should be obtained with noncotton swabs (e.g., a urethrogenital calcium alginate–tipped swab [Calgiswab, Puritan Medical Products, Guilford, ME]), inoculated directly onto culture plates, and incubated immediately. The choice of anatomic sites to culture depends on the sites exposed and the clinical manifestations. If symptoms are present, samples from the urethra and rectum can be cultured for men, and samples from the endocervix and rectum can be cultured for all females, regardless of a history of anal intercourse. A pharyngeal culture specimen should be obtained from both men and women if symptoms of pharyngitis are present with a history of recent oral exposure, or oral exposure to a person known to have genital gonorrhea. In a suspected case of **child sexual abuse**, culture remains the recommended method of detection for *N. gonorrhoeae* in urethral specimens from boys and for extragenital sites (conjunctiva, pharynx, and rectum) from all children because NAATs have not yet been sufficiently evaluated for these populations and sample sites. Culture of the endocervix should not be attempted until after puberty.

Specimens from sites that are normally colonized by other organisms (e.g., cervix, rectum, pharynx) should be inoculated on a selective culture medium, such as modified Thayer-Martin medium (fortified with vancomycin, colistin, nystatin, and trimethoprim to inhibit growth of indigenous flora). Specimens from sites that are normally sterile or minimally contaminated (i.e., synovial fluid, blood, cerebrospinal fluid) should be inoculated on a nonselective chocolate agar medium. If DGI is suspected, blood, pharynx, rectum, urethra, cervix, and synovial fluid (if involved) should be cultured. Cultured specimens should be incubated promptly at 35-37°C (95-98.6°F) in 3–5% carbon dioxide. When specimens must be transported to a central laboratory for culture plating, a reduced, nonnutrient holding medium (i.e., Amies-modified Stuart medium) preserves specimens with minimal loss of viability for up to 6 hr. When transport may delay culture plating by >6 hr, it is preferable to inoculate the sample directly onto a culture medium and transport it at an ambient temperature in CO_2-enriched atmosphere. The Transgrow and JEMBEC (John E. Martin Biological Environmental Chamber) systems of modified Thayer-Martin medium are alternative transport systems.

Nucleic Acid Amplification Tests

The U.S. Food and Drug Administration (FDA) has approved NAATs for use with endocervical swabs, vaginal swabs, male urethral swabs, and female and male first-catch urine. Advantages of using NAATs include less stringent transport conditions, more rapid turnaround time, flexibility in sampling source (providing additional feasibility of testing in settings where physical exam is not done), and patient preference for less invasive sampling. However, NAATs cannot provide antimicrobial susceptibility results, so in cases of persistent gonococcal infection after treatment,

clinicians should perform both culture and antimicrobial susceptibility testing. Although urine specimens are acceptable for women, the sensitivity for screening appears to be lower than with vaginal or endocervical swab samples. In contrast, the sensitivity and specificity of urine and urethral swab specimens from men are similar, so first-catch urine is the recommended sample type for urethral screening in men. Product inserts for each NAAT vendor must be carefully examined to assess current indications and allowable specimens. NAATs are not FDA cleared for use with specimens from the rectum, pharynx, conjunctiva, joint fluid, blood, or cerebrospinal fluid. However, most commercial and public health laboratories have established performance specifications to satisfy Centers for Medicare and Medicaid Services (CMMS) regulations for FDA Clinical Laboratory Improvement Amendments (CLIA) compliance in testing and reporting results for rectal and pharyngeal swab specimens, facilitating their use for clinical management (gonorrhea screening of rectal and pharyngeal sites with NAATs is recommended at least annually in MSM reporting rectal or pharyngeal receptive intercourse).

Data on use of NAATs are limited in children. In a multicenter study of NAATs using strand displacement amplification or transcription-mediated amplification in children being evaluated for sexual abuse, urine from prepubertal girls was a reliable alternative to vaginal culture for detection of *N. gonorrhoeae*. However, culture still remains the recommended method for testing for all other sample sites among prepubertal children. Because of the legal implications of a diagnosis of *N. gonorrhoeae* infection in a child, all positive specimens should be retained for additional confirmatory testing.

TREATMENT

All patients who are presumed or proven to have gonorrhea should be evaluated for concurrent syphilis, HIV, and *C. trachomatis* infection. The incidence of *Chlamydia* co-infection is 15–25% among males and 35–50% among females. Patients beyond the neonatal period should be treated presumptively for *Chlamydia trachomatis* infection unless a negative chlamydial NAAT result is documented at the time treatment is initiated for gonorrhea. However, if chlamydial test results are not available, or if a non-NAAT result is negative for *Chlamydia*, patients should be treated for both gonorrhea and *Chlamydia* infection (see Chapter 253.2). Persons who receive a diagnosis of gonorrhea should be instructed to abstain from sexual activity for 7 days after treatment and until all sex partners are adequately treated (7 days after receiving treatment and resolution of symptoms, if present). Sexual partners exposed in the preceding 60 days should be examined, specimens collected, and presumptive treatment started.

N. gonorrhoeae has progressively developed resistance to the antibiotics used to treat it over the years. Antimicrobial resistance in *N. gonorrhoeae* occurs as plasmid-mediated resistance to penicillin and tetracycline and chromosomally mediated resistance to penicillins, tetracyclines, spectinomycin, fluoroquinolones, cephalosporins, and azithromycin. Emergence of cephalosporin resistance worldwide has prompted designation of *N. gonorrhoeae* as antibiotic resistance threat level "Urgent" by the CDC. Surveillance data from the CDC Gonococcal Isolate Surveillance Project reveal concerning fluctuations in minimum inhibitory concentration (MIC) for the oral cephalosporin **cefixime** and the injectable third-generation cephalosporin **ceftriaxone**, leading the CDC to revise its U.S. gonorrhea treatment guidelines in 2012 to dual therapy in an attempt to preserve the last commercially available effective treatment. A theoretical basis exists for using 2 antimicrobials with different molecular targets to improve treatment efficacy and potentially delay emergence and spread of resistance to cephalosporins.

Table 219.1 summarizes first-line treatment regimens for neonate, child (weight ≤45 kg), adolescent, and adult gonococcal regimens. Mucosal, localized infections are treatable with single doses; disseminated infections are treated for a minimum of 1 wk. Although dual therapy is not recommended for neonatal and childhood infections, it is recommended for all adult and adolescent infections (inclusive of children >45 kg). The use of **azithromycin** as the 2nd antimicrobial is preferred to doxycycline because of the convenience and compliance advantages of single-dose therapy and the higher prevalence of gonococcal resistance to tetracycline compared to azithromycin among gonococcal surveillance isolates, particularly in strains with elevated MIC to cefixime.

Alternative regimens exist for adolescents and adults but are extremely limited. For patients with cephalosporin allergy, the combination of gentamicin (240 mg intramuscularly [IM]) plus azithromycin (2 g orally [PO]) cured 100% of uncomplicated urogenital cases in a trial of U.S. patients age 15-60 yr; the combination of gemifloxacin (320 mg PO) (not licensed for use in those <18 yr old) plus azithromycin (2 g PO) cured >99% of uncomplicated urogenital cases in the same trial but was limited by 8% of patients vomiting within 1 hr of dual–oral drug administration. For patients with azithromycin allergy, doxycycline (100 mg PO twice daily for 7 days) can be used in place of azithromycin as an alternative 2nd antimicrobial. If ceftriaxone is not available, alternative cephalosporins to be used in combination with azithromycin or doxycycline for uncomplicated anorectal and urogenital infection include oral cefixime (400 mg PO), which does not provide as high, or as sustained, bactericidal blood levels as a 250 mg IM dose of ceftriaxone

and has limited efficacy for pharyngeal gonorrhea, and other single-dose injectable cephalosporin regimens, such as ceftizoxime (500 mg IM), cefoxitin (2 g IM) with probenecid (1 g PO), or cefotaxime (500 mg IM), none of which offers any advantage over ceftriaxone for urogenital infection, and their efficacy against pharyngeal infection is less certain.

Pregnant women with gonococcal infection should be treated with standard adult dual therapy. If allergy precludes standard treatment, consultation with an infectious disease specialist is recommended. HIV–co-infected patients with gonococcal infection are treated the same as HIV-negative patients.

Follow-up test-of-cure is not recommended for persons diagnosed with uncomplicated urogenital or rectal gonorrhea receiving recommended or alternative regimens. However, any person with pharyngeal gonorrhea who is treated with an alternative regimen should return 14 days after treatment for a test-of cure using culture, NAAT, or both, because pharyngeal gonorrhea is more difficult to eradicate. Symptoms

Table 219.1	Recommended Treatment of Gonococcal Infections		
	INFECTION	**TREATMENT REGIMEN**	**LENGTH OF THERAPY**
Neonates	Ophthalmia neonatorum	Ceftriaxone,* 25-50 mg/kg IV or IM (max 250 mg), plus lavage infected eye frequently until discharge eliminated	Once
	Disseminated infection Scalp abscess Septic arthritis	Ceftriaxone,* 25-50 mg/kg IV or IM qd *or* Cefotaxime, 25-50 mg/kg IV or IM q8–12h[†]	7 days
	Meningitis	Ceftriaxone,* 25-50 mg/kg IV or IM qd *or* Cefotaxime, 25-50 mg/kg IV or IM q8-12h[†]	10-14 days
	Endocarditis	Ceftriaxone,* 25-50 mg/kg IV or IM qd *or* Cefotaxime, 25-50 mg/kg IV or IM q8-12h[†]	Minimum 28 days
Children ≤45 kg	Pharyngeal infection Anorectal infection Urogenital infection	Ceftriaxone, 25-50 mg/kg IV or IM (max 250 mg)	Once
	Conjunctivitis	Ceftriaxone, 50 mg/kg IM (max 1 g)[‡]	Once
	Disseminated infection Septic arthritis	Ceftriaxone, 50 mg/kg IV or IM qd (max 1 g daily)	7 days
	Meningitis	Ceftriaxone, 50 mg/kg IV or IM q12-24h (max 4 g daily)	10-14 days
	Endocarditis	Ceftriaxone, 50 mg/kg IV or IM q12-24h (max 4 g daily)	Minimum 28 days
Adults, adolescents, and children >45 kg	Pharyngeal infection Anorectal infection Urogenital infection	Ceftriaxone, 250 mg IM *plus* Azithromycin, 1 g PO	Once
	Conjunctivitis	Ceftriaxone, 1 g IM *plus* Azithromycin, 1 g PO[‡]	Once
	Disseminated infection Septic arthritis	Ceftriaxone, 1 g IV or IM qd[§] *plus* Azithromycin, 1 g PO	7 days Once
	Meningitis	Ceftriaxone, 1-2 g IV q12-24h *plus* Azithromycin, 1 g PO	10-14 days Once
	Endocarditis	Ceftriaxone, 1-2 g IV q12-24h *plus* Azithromycin, 1 g PO	Minimum 28 days Once

*When available, cefotaxime should be substituted for ceftriaxone in neonates with hyperbilirubinemia (particularly those who are premature) and in those <28 days old if receiving calcium-containing intravenous fluids. Consult neonatal dosing references.
[†]Dose and/or dosing frequency change after postnatal age >7 days. Consult neonatal dosing references.
[‡]Plus lavage of the infected eye with saline solution (once).
[§]Ceftriaxone should be continued for 24-48 hr after clinical improvement begins, at which time the switch may be made to an oral agent (e.g., cefixime or a quinolone) if antimicrobial susceptibility is documented by culture. If no organism is isolated and the diagnosis is secure, treatment with ceftriaxone should be continued for at least 7 days.
IM, Intramuscularly; IV, intravenously; PO, orally (by mouth); qd, every day; q8-12h, every 8 to 12 hours.
From Hsu KK, Wangu Z: *Neisseria gonorrhoeae.* In Long SS, Prober CG, Fischer M, editors: *Principles and practice of pediatric infectious diseases,* ed 5, Philadelphia, 2018, Elsevier, Table 126.1.

persisting after treatment should be evaluated by culture for *N. gonorrhoeae* (with or without simultaneous NAAT), and any gonococci isolated should be tested for antimicrobial susceptibility. **Treatment failure** should be considered in (1) persons whose symptoms do not resolve within 3–5 days after appropriate treatment and who report no sexual contact during posttreatment follow-up and (2) persons with a positive test-of-cure (i.e., positive culture >72 hr or positive NAAT ≥7 days after receiving recommended treatment) who report no sexual contact during posttreatment follow-up.

COMPLICATIONS

Prompt diagnosis and correct therapy ensure complete recovery from uncomplicated gonococcal disease. Complications of gonorrhea result from the spread of gonococci from a local site of invasion. Complications and permanent sequelae may be associated with delayed treatment, recurrent infection, metastatic sites of infection (meninges, aortic valve), and delayed or topical therapy of gonococcal ophthalmia.

The interval between primary infection and development of a complication is usually days to weeks. In postpubertal females, endometritis may occur, especially during menses, and may progress to salpingitis, tuboovarian abscess, and peritonitis (PID). Manifestations of PID include signs of lower genital tract infection (e.g., vaginal discharge, suprapubic pain, cervical tenderness) and upper genital tract infection (e.g., fever, leukocytosis, elevated erythrocyte sedimentation rate, and adnexal tenderness or mass). The differential diagnosis includes gynecologic diseases (ovarian cyst, ovarian tumor, ectopic pregnancy) and intraabdominal disorders (appendicitis, urinary tract infection, inflammatory bowel disease). Although *N. gonorrhoeae* and *C. trachomatis* are implicated in many cases of PID, this syndrome encompasses a spectrum of infectious diseases of the upper genital tract caused by *N. gonorrhoeae*, *C. trachomatis,* and endogenous flora (streptococci, anaerobes, gram-negative bacilli). Treatment must therefore be broad. For women with more severe symptoms (inability to exclude surgical emergency, presence of tuboovarian abscess, severe illness, nausea, vomiting or high fever), pregnancy, or lack of response to outpatient therapy within 72 hr, parenteral therapy should be initiated in the hospital. The decision to hospitalize adolescents with acute PID should be based on the same criteria used for older women, because the clinical response to outpatient treatment is similar among younger and older women.

Recommended parenteral regimens are cefotetan (2 g intravenously [IV] every 12 hr [q12h]) or cefoxitin (2 g IV q6h) plus doxycycline (100 mg PO or IV q12h), or clindamycin (900 mg IV q8h) plus a loading dose of gentamicin (2 mg/kg IV or IM) followed by maintenance gentamicin (1.5 mg/kg q8h). An alternative parenteral regimen is ampicillin-sulbactam (3 g IV q6h) plus doxycycline (100 mg PO or IV q12h). Clinical experience should guide transition to oral therapy, which usually can be initiated within 24 hr of improvement. Thereafter, oral clindamycin (450 mg PO 4 times daily [qid]) or doxycycline (100 mg PO twice daily [bid]) is given to complete 14 days of total therapy, unless tuboovarian abscess is present, in which case clindamycin (450 mg PO qid) or metronidazole (500 mg PO bid) should be added to doxycycline to complete 14 days of therapy with more effective anaerobic coverage. Parenteral therapy and intramuscular/oral therapy appear to be similar in clinical efficacy for younger and older women with PID of mild to moderate severity. Recommended regimens are as follows: a single dose of ceftriaxone (250 mg IM) plus doxycycline (100 mg PO bid) with or without metronidazole (500 mg PO bid) for 14 days; and single doses of cefoxitin (2 g IM) and probenecid (1 g PO) plus doxycycline (100 mg PO bid) with or without metronidazole (500 mg PO bid) for 14 days.

Once inside the peritoneum, gonococci may seed the liver capsule, causing a perihepatitis with right upper quadrant pain (**Fitz-Hugh–Curtis syndrome**), with or without signs of salpingitis. Perihepatitis may also be caused by *C. trachomatis*. Progression to PID occurs in approximately 20% of cases of gonococcal cervicitis, and *N. gonorrhoeae* is isolated in approximately 40% of cases of PID in the United States. Untreated cases may lead to hydrosalpinx, pyosalpinx, tuboovarian abscess, and eventual sterility. Even with adequate treatment of PID, the risk for sterility from

bilateral tubal occlusion approaches 20% after 1 episode of salpingitis and exceeds 60% after 3 or more episodes. The risk for ectopic pregnancy is increased approximately 7-fold after 1 or more episodes of salpingitis. Additional sequelae of PID include chronic pain, dyspareunia, and increased risk for recurrent PID.

Urogenital gonococcal infection acquired during the first trimester of pregnancy carries a high risk for septic abortion. After 16 wk of pregnancy, infection leads to **chorioamnionitis**, a major cause of premature rupture of the membranes and premature delivery.

In males, without treatment, gonococcal urethritis usually resolves spontaneously over several weeks to months. Epididymitis and acute or chronic prostatitis are uncommon complications; most men with gonococcal epididymitis also have overt urethritis. Even more unusual complications include penile edema associated with penile dorsal lymphangitis or thrombophlebitis, periurethral abscess or fistulas, seminal vesiculitis, and balanitis in uncircumcised men.

PREVENTION

Efforts to develop gonococcal vaccines that confer broad cross-protection have been unsuccessful thus far. A pilus vaccine elicited an antibody response and conferred protection against challenge with the homologous strain but did not protect against disease in a trial involving 3,250 volunteers. The high degree of interstrain and intrastrain antigenic variability of pili poses a formidable barrier to the development of a single effective pilus vaccine. An outer membrane vaccine that was enriched in PorB also elicited an antibody response but failed to protect male volunteers against challenge with the homologous strain, likely because small amounts of Rmp present in the vaccine preparation elicited subversive antibodies. A formalin-killed whole cell vaccine trial in 62 volunteers in an Inuvik population in Canada also failed to provide any protection. Gonococcal surface structures, such as the porin protein (isolated without contaminating Rmp), proteins expressed under various stress conditions that may be encountered in vivo and have been identified by proteomic and transcriptomic approaches, and lipooligosaccharides, may prove more promising as vaccine candidates.

In the absence of a vaccine, prevention of gonorrhea in adolescents and adults can be achieved through **education**, use of **barrier protection** (especially condoms), **screening** of high-risk populations as recommended by the U.S. Preventive Services Task Force (PSTF) and CDC (e.g., sexually active women ≤24 yr old, MSM, individuals previously infected with gonorrhea), and **early identification and treatment** of contacts—all sex partners within the 60 days preceding symptom onset or gonorrhea diagnosis, or, if none, the most recent sex partner, should be examined and treated presumptively. For heterosexual patients, expedited partner therapy (EPT) with cefixime (400 mg) and azithromycin (1 g) can be delivered to partners by the patient, a disease investigation specialist, or a collaborating pharmacy, as permitted by law (https://www.cdc.gov/std/ept/legal/). EPT has been shown to be safe and effective in prevention of reinfection with gonorrhea and is endorsed by the American Academy of Pediatrics, American Academy of Family Physicians, and Society of Adolescent Health and Medicine, as well as other clinical organizations, for use when in-person evaluation and treatment of the partner is impractical or unsuccessful. (Because of the high risk for coexisting undiagnosed sexually transmitted infections such as HIV, EPT is not considered a routine partner management strategy for MSM.)

An infant born to a woman with cervical gonococcal infection has an approximately 30% risk of acquiring ophthalmic infection, compared to a <5% risk if ocular prophylaxis is given. **Gonococcal ophthalmia neonatorum** can be prevented by instilling erythromycin (0.5%) ophthalmic ointment into the conjunctival sac (see Chapter 652). If erythromycin ointment is unavailable, infants at risk for *N. gonorrhoeae* (especially those born to a mother with untreated gonococcal infection or with no prenatal care) can be administered ceftriaxone 25-50 mg/kg IV or IM, not to exceed 250 mg, in a single dose.

Bibliography is available at Expert Consult.

Chapter **220**
Kingella kingae
Pablo Yagupsky

第二百二十章
金格杆菌

中文导读

本章主要介绍了金格杆菌感染的病因、流行病学、发病机制、临床疾病、诊断、治疗、预防等内容。在金格杆菌感染所致的临床疾病中首先介绍了感染所致的疾病谱和各个病种的发病率，随后详细介绍了化脓性关节炎、骨髓炎、脊椎病、隐匿菌血症和心内膜炎。在金格杆菌感染治疗中详细描述了头孢素、万古霉素、克林霉素等药物的用法及治疗疗程。

Kingella kingae is being increasingly recognized as the most common etiology of septic arthritis, osteomyelitis, and spondylodiscitis in young children.

ETIOLOGY
Kingella kingae is a fastidious, facultative anaerobic, β-hemolytic member of the Neisseriaceae family that appears as pairs or short chains of gram-negative coccobacilli with tapered ends (Fig. 220.1).

EPIDEMIOLOGY
K. kingae is asymptomatically carried in the posterior pharynx. **Colonization** usually starts after age 6 mo, reaches a prevalence of 10% between

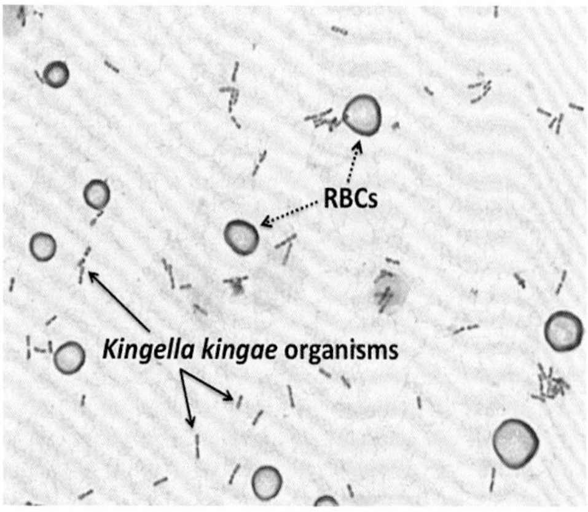

Fig. 220.1 Typical Gram stain of a positive blood culture vial from a child with *K. kingae* bacteremia showing pairs and short chains of plump gram-negative coccobacilli. RBCs, Red blood cells.

12 and 24 mo, and decreases in older children. Pharyngeal colonization plays a crucial role in the **transmission** of the organism through intimate contact between siblings and playmates. Daycare attendance increases the risk for colonization and transmission, and clusters of invasive infection have been reported in childcare facilities.

The species elaborates 4 different polysaccharide capsules (a-d),which appear to represent important virulence factors. Colonizing *K. kingae* strains differ in their invasive potential. Whereas certain clones are commonly found as respiratory colonizers but are seldom isolated from sites of disease, other clones, usually expressing polysaccharide capsule a or b, readily penetrate into the bloodstream and disseminate to the skeletal system or the endocardium, sites for which the organism has a particular tropism.

Invasive *K. kingae* disease is most frequently diagnosed in otherwise healthy children between ages 6 mo and 3 yr, coinciding with the peak prevalence of **pharyngeal carriage** (Fig. 220.2). In contrast, older children and adults with *K. kingae* infections often have underlying chronic diseases, immunosuppressing conditions, malignancy, or cardiac valve pathology. An annual incidence of 9.4 per 100,000 culture-proven invasive infections among Israeli children <5 yr old has been estimated, but because of the suboptimal culture recovery of *K. kingae* organisms, this figure can be considered only a minimal estimate.

PATHOGENESIS
The pathogenesis of *K. kingae* disease begins with adherence of the organism to the pharyngeal epithelium, mediated by pili and a nonpilus adhesin. *K. kingae* secretes a potent Repeats-in-Toxin (RTX) toxin that exhibits deleterious activity to respiratory epithelial cells, macrophages, and synoviocytes, suggesting that it may play a role in disrupting the respiratory mucosa, promoting survival of the bacterium in the bloodstream, and facilitating invasion of skeletal system tissues. Children with *K. kingae* disease frequently present with symptoms of an upper respiratory infection, hand-foot-and-mouth disease, herpetic stomatitis,

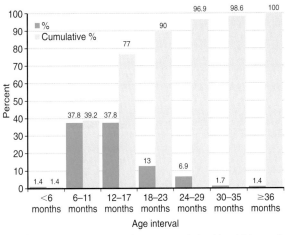

Fig. 220.2 Age distribution of 291 previously healthy children with invasive *K. kingae* infection. *(Data from Dubnov-Raz G, Ephros M, Garty BZ, et al: Invasive pediatric Kingella kingae infections: a nationwide collaborative study, Pediatr Infect Dis J 29:639–643, 2010.)*

Table 220.1	Clinical Spectrum and Relative Frequency of *Kingella kingae* Infections
CLINICAL DISEASE	**FREQUENCY**
SKELETAL SYSTEM	+++
Septic arthritis	+++
Osteomyelitis	++
Spondylodiscitis	+
Tenosynovitis	±
Dactylitis	±
Bursitis	±
Bacteremia with no focus	+++
CARDIAC	+
Endocarditis	+
Pericarditis	±
Meningitis	±
Peritonitis	±
Cellulitis	±
Soft tissue abscesses	±
LOWER RESPIRATORY TRACT	±
Laryngotracheobronchitis	±
Pneumonia	±
Pleural empyema	±
OCULAR	±
Keratitis	±
Corneal abscess	±
Endophthalmitis	±
Eyelid abscess	±

+++, Very common; ++, common; +, infrequent; ±, exceptional.

or buccal aphthous ulcers, suggesting that viral-induced damage to the colonized mucosal surface facilitates invasion of the bloodstream.

CLINICAL DISEASE

Septic arthritis is the most common invasive *K. kingae* infection in children, followed by bacteremia, osteomyelitis, and endocarditis (Table 220.1). The organism is the most frequent etiology of skeletal system infections in children 6 mo to 3 yr old in at least some countries. With the exception of patients with endocarditis, the presentation of invasive *K. kingae* infections is frequently mild, and a body temperature <38°C (100.4°F), a normal C-reactive protein (CRP) level, and a normal white blood cell (WBC) count are common, requiring a high index of clinical suspicion.

Septic Arthritis

Although *K. kingae*–driven arthritis especially affects the large, weight-bearing joints, involvement of the small metacarpophalangeal, sternoclavicular, and tarsal joints is not unusual (see Chapter 704). The disease has an acute presentation, and children are brought to medical attention after a median of 3 days. The leukocyte count in the synovial fluid shows <50,000 WBCs/μL in almost 25% of the patients, and the Gram stain of synovial fluid is positive in only a small percentage of cases. Involvement of the hip joint resembles toxic synovitis, and the possibility of a *K. kingae* infection should be always suspected in children <4 yr old presenting with hip pain or a limp.

Osteomyelitis

K. kingae osteomyelitis usually involves the long bones of the extremities (see Chapter 704). The calcaneus, talus, sternum, and clavicle are also frequently affected (and are rarely infected by other bacterial pathogens). Onset of *K. kingae* osteomyelitis is insidious, and the disease is diagnosed after ≥1 wk in 70% of patients. MRI shows mild bone and soft tissue changes. Involvement of the epiphyseal cartilage appears to be specifically associated with the organism. Despite the frequent diagnostic delay, chronic osteomyelitis and functional orthopedic disabilities are unusual.

SPONDYLODISCITIS

K. kingae is currently the 2nd most common bacterium isolated in children <4 yr old with spondylodiscitis. The organism presumably penetrates the rich network of blood vessels that traverse the cartilaginous vertebral endplates and enters the annulus in young children during a bacteremic episode. *K. kingae* spondylodiscitis usually involves the lumbar intervertebral spaces and, with decreasing frequency, the thoracolumbar, thoracic, lumbosacral, and cervical disks. Involvement of

multiple disks is uncommon. Patients present with limping, lumbar pain, back stiffness, refusal to sit or walk, neurologic symptoms, or abdominal complaints. Radiography or MRI studies demonstrate narrowing of the intervertebral space. Patients respond well to appropriate antibiotic treatment and recover without complications, although residual narrowing of the intervertebral space may occur.

Occult Bacteremia

Patients with *K. kingae* bacteremia and no focal infection (occult bacteremia) usually present with mild to moderate fever, symptoms suggestive of a viral upper respiratory infection, a mean CRP level of 2.2 mg/dL, and a mean WBC count of 12,700/μL. Children with *K. kingae* bacteremia respond favorably to a short course of antibiotics.

Endocarditis

In contrast to other *K. kingae* infections, endocarditis is also diagnosed in school-age children, adolescents, and adult patients. The disease may affect native as well as prosthetic valves. Predisposing factors include congenital cardiac malformations or rheumatic valvular disease, but some patients have previously normal hearts. Typically, the left side of the heart is involved, usually the mitral valve. Fever and acute-phase reactants are elevated more in patients with endocarditis than in those with uncomplicated bacteremia; no particular cutoff value accurately distinguishes between the 2 conditions. Despite the exquisite susceptibility of *K. kingae* to antibiotics, cardiac failure, septic shock, cerebrovascular accident (stroke), and other life-threatening complications are common, and the mortality rate is high (>10%). Because of the potential severity of *K. kingae* endocarditis, routine echocardiographic evaluation of children with isolated bacteremia is indicated.

DIAGNOSIS

The diagnosis of *K. kingae* disease is established by isolation of the bacterium or by a positive nucleic acid amplification test (NAAT; polymerase chain reaction) from a normally sterile site such as blood, synovial fluid, or bone tissue. Although *K. kingae* grows on routine bacteriologic media, its recovery from exudates is frequently unsuccessful. Detection is enhanced by inoculating synovial fluid specimens into blood culture vials, suggesting that diluting purulent samples in a large volume of nutrient broth reduces the concentration of detrimental factors, improving the isolation of this fastidious bacterium.

Testing bone and joint specimens by NAAT that targets specific *K. kingae* genes, such as *cpn* or those encoding the RTX toxin, results in a 4-fold improvement in the detection of the organism and reduces the fraction of *culture-negative septic arthritis* in young children.

TREATMENT

K. kingae is usually highly susceptible to penicillin and cephalosporins but exhibits decreased susceptibility to oxacillin. Although β-lactamase production is frequently detected in colonizing *K. kingae* strains, its prevalence among invasive organisms is low and shows wide geographic variation. Testing for β-lactamase production should be routinely performed in all isolates derived from normally sterile body sites.

Because of the lack of specific guidelines for treating *K. kingae* disease, patients have been administered a variety of antibiotic regimens according to protocols developed for infections caused by traditional bacterial pathogens. The first-line therapy for skeletal infections in young children usually consists of intravenous (IV) administration of a second- or third-generation **cephalosporin**, pending culture results. *K. kingae* is always *resistant* to glycopeptide antibiotics, and the majority of isolates are also *resistant* to clindamycin, a serious concern in areas where skeletal infections caused by community-associated methicillin-resistant *S. aureus* are common, and **vancomycin** or **clindamycin** are initially administered to children with presumptive septic arthritis or osteomyelitis. The initial antibiotic regimen is frequently changed to a cephalosporin (e.g., ceftriaxone) once *K. kingae* is identified or to ampicillin after β-lactamase production is excluded. A favorable clinical response and decreasing CRP levels to ≤20 μg/mL are used to guide switching to oral antibiotics and defining duration of therapy. Antibiotic treatment has ranged from 2-3 wk for *K. kingae* arthritis, from 3-6 wk for *K. kingae* osteomyelitis, and from 3-12 wk for *K. kingae* spondylodiscitis. Although

some children with septic arthritis have been managed with repeat joint aspirations and lavage, most patients respond promptly to conservative treatment with appropriate antibiotics and do not require invasive surgical procedures.

Children with *K. kingae* bacteremia without focal infection are initially treated with an intravenous β-lactam antibiotic and are subsequently switched to an oral drug once the clinical condition has improved. In most cases, duration of therapy is 1-2 wk.

Patients with *K. kingae* endocarditis are usually treated with an IV β-lactam antibiotic alone or in combination with an aminoglycoside for 4-7 wk. Early surgical intervention is necessary for life-threatening complications unresponsive to medical therapy.

PREVENTION

Because the risk of asymptomatic pharyngeal carriers for developing an invasive *K. kingae* infection is low (<1% per year), in the absence of clinical disease, there is no indication to eradicate the organism from the colonized mucosal surfaces. Nonetheless, in the reported outbreaks of *K. kingae* infections in child daycare centers, 31 of 199 (15.6%) classmates developed a proven or presumptive infection, including fatal endocarditis, within 1 mo, indicating that the causative strains combined unusual transmissibility and virulence. Under these circumstances, prophylactic antibiotic therapy to eradicate colonization in contacts and prevent further cases of disease has been employed, consisting of either rifampin alone, 10 mg/kg or 20 mg/kg twice daily for 2 days, or rifampin in combination with amoxicillin (80 mg/kg/day) for 2 days or 4 days. The effectiveness of these regimens has ranged between 47% and 80%, indicating that eradication of *K. kingae* from colonized mucosae is difficult to achieve. However, after antibiotic prophylaxis administration, no further cases of disease have been detected, suggesting that reduction of the bacterial density by antibiotics and/or induction of an effective immune response by prolonged carriage is enough to decrease transmissibility and prevent additional cases.

Bibliography is available at Expert Consult.

Chapter **221**
Haemophilus influenzae
Robert S. Daum

第二百二十一章
流感嗜血杆菌

中文导读

　　本章主要介绍了流感嗜血杆菌感染的病因、流行病学、发病机制、诊断、临床表现、治疗和预防等内容。在流感嗜血杆菌感染的发病机制中介绍了抗生素耐药和免疫。在流感嗜血杆菌感染的临床表现及治疗部分详细介绍了临床疾病、蜂窝织炎、声门上喉炎或急性会厌炎、肺炎、化脓性关节炎、心包炎、无相关病灶的菌血症、其他感染、新生儿的侵袭性疾病、中耳炎、结膜炎和鼻窦炎。

Effective vaccines to prevent **Haemophilus influenzae type b (Hib)** disease, introduced in the United States and most other countries, have resulted in a dramatic decrease in the incidence of infections caused by this organism. However, mortality and morbidity from Hib infection remain a problem worldwide, primarily in developing countries. Occasional cases of invasive disease caused by non–type b organisms continue to occur but are infrequent. Nontypeable members of the species are an important cause of otitis media, sinusitis, and chronic bronchitis.

ETIOLOGY

Haemophilus influenzae is a fastidious, gram-negative, pleomorphic coccobacillus that requires factor X (hematin) and factor V (phosphopyridine nucleotide) for growth. Some *H. influenzae* isolates are surrounded by a polysaccharide capsule and can be serotyped into 1 of 6 antigenically and biochemically distinct types designated a, b, c, d, e, and f.

EPIDEMIOLOGY

Before the advent of an effective Hib conjugate vaccine in 1988, *H. influenzae* type b was a major cause of serious disease among children. There was a striking age distribution of cases, with >90% in children <5 yr old and the majority in children <2 yr old. The annual attack rate of invasive disease was 64-129 cases per 100,000 children <5 yr old. Invasive disease caused by other capsular serotypes has been much less frequent but continues to occur. The incidence of invasive disease caused by type b and non–type b serotypes has been estimated at approximately 0.08 and 1.02 cases, respectively, per 100,000 children <5 yr old per year in the United States. Nonencapsulated (nontypeable) *H. influenzae* strains also occasionally cause invasive disease, especially in neonates, immunocompromised children, and children in developing countries. The estimated rate of invasive disease caused by nontypeable *H. influenzae* in the United States is 1.88 per 100,000 children <5 yr old per year. Nontypeable isolates are common etiologic agents in otitis media, sinusitis, and chronic bronchitis.

Humans are the only natural hosts for *H. influenzae,* which is part of the normal respiratory flora in 60–90% of healthy children. Most isolates are nontypeable. Before the advent of conjugate vaccine immunization, *H. influenzae* type b could be isolated from the pharynx of 2–5% of healthy preschool and school-age children, with lower rates among infants and adults. Asymptomatic colonization with Hib occurs at a much lower rate in immunized populations.

The continued circulation of the type b organism despite current vaccine coverage levels suggests that elimination of Hib disease may be a formidable task. The few cases of Hib invasive disease in the United States now occur in both unvaccinated and fully vaccinated children. Approximately 50% of cases occur in young infants who are too young to have received a complete primary vaccine series. Among the cases in patients who are old enough to have received a complete vaccine series, the majority are underimmunized. To highlight this point, during a shortage of Hib vaccine, invasive disease developed in 5 children in Minnesota, all of whom were incompletely immunized. Continued efforts are necessary to provide currently available Hib conjugate vaccines to children in developing countries, where affordability remains an important issue.

In the prevaccine era, certain groups and individuals had an increased incidence of invasive Hib disease, including Alaskan Natives, American Indians (Apache, Navajo), and African Americans. Persons with certain chronic medical conditions were also known to be at increased risk for invasive disease, including those with sickle cell disease, asplenia, congenital and acquired immunodeficiencies, and malignancies. Unvaccinated infants with invasive Hib infection are also at increased risk for recurrence, reflecting that they typically do not develop a protective immune response to *H. influenzae.*

Socioeconomic risk factors for invasive Hib disease include childcare outside the home, the presence of siblings of elementary school age or younger, short duration of breastfeeding, and parental smoking. A history of otitis media is associated with an increased risk for invasive disease. Much less is known about the epidemiology of invasive disease caused

by non–type b strains, and it is not clear whether the epidemiologic features of Hib disease apply to disease caused by non-Hib isolates.

Among age-susceptible household contacts who have been exposed to a case of invasive Hib disease, there is increased risk for secondary cases of invasive disease in the 1st 30 days, especially in susceptible children <24 mo old. Whether a similar increased risk occurs for contacts of individuals with non-Hib disease is unknown.

The mode of transmission is usually direct contact or inhalation of respiratory tract droplets containing *H. influenzae.* The incubation period for invasive disease is variable, and the exact period of communicability is unknown. Most children with invasive Hib disease are colonized in the nasopharynx before initiation of antimicrobial therapy; 25–40% may remain colonized during the 1st 24 hr of therapy.

With the decline of disease caused by type b organisms, disease caused by other serotypes (a, c-f) and nontypeable organisms has been recognized more clearly. There is no evidence that these non–type b infections have increased in frequency. However, clusters of type a and, less often, type f and type e infections have occurred. Data from Israel suggest that nontypeable *H. influenzae* is the most common case of invasive *H. influenzae* disease in that country.

PATHOGENESIS

The pathogenesis of Hib disease begins with adherence to respiratory epithelium and colonization of the nasopharynx, which is mediated by pilus and nonpilus adherence factors. The mechanism of entry into the intravascular compartment is unclear but appears to be influenced by cytotoxic factors. Once in the bloodstream, *H. influenzae* type b, and perhaps other encapsulated strains, resist intravascular clearance mechanisms at least in part because of a polysaccharide capsule. In the case of Hib, the magnitude and duration of bacteremia influence the likelihood of dissemination of bacteria to sites such as the meninges and joints.

Noninvasive *H. influenzae* infections such as otitis media, sinusitis, and bronchitis are usually caused by nontypeable strains. These organisms gain access to sites such as the middle ear and sinus cavities by direct extension from the nasopharynx. Factors facilitating spread from the pharynx include eustachian tube dysfunction and antecedent viral infections of the upper respiratory tract.

Antibiotic Resistance

Most *H. influenzae* isolates are susceptible to ampicillin or amoxicillin, but about one-third produce a β-lactamase and are therefore resistant to these antibiotics. β-Lactamase–negative ampicillin-resistant isolates have been identified and manifest resistance by production of a β-lactam–insensitive cell wall synthesis enzyme called PBP3.

Amoxicillin-clavulanate is uniformly active against *H. influenzae* clinical isolates except for the rare β-lactamase–negative ampicillin-resistant isolates. Among macrolides, azithromycin has in vitro activity against a high percentage of *H. influenzae* isolates; in contrast, the activity of erythromycin and clarithromycin against *H. influenzae* clinical isolates is poor. *H. influenzae* resistance to third-generation cephalosporins has not been documented. Resistance to trimethoprim-sulfamethoxazole (TMP-SMX) is infrequent (approximately 10%), and resistance to quinolones is believed to be rare.

Immunity

In the prevaccine era, the most important known element of host defense was antibody directed against the type b capsular polysaccharide polyribosylribitol phosphate (**PRP**). Anti-PRP antibody is acquired in an age-related fashion and facilitates clearance of *H. influenzae* type b from blood, in part related to opsonic activity. Antibodies directed against antigens such as outer membrane proteins or lipopolysaccharide (LPS) may also have a role in opsonization. Both the classical and alternative complement pathways are important in defense against Hib.

Before the introduction of vaccination, protection from Hib infection was presumed to correlate with the concentration of circulating anti-PRP antibody at the time of exposure. A serum antibody concentration of 0.15-1.0 μg/mL was considered protective against invasive infection. Unimmunized infants >6 mo old and young children usually lacked an anti-PRP antibody concentration of this magnitude and were susceptible to disease after encountering Hib. This lack of antibody in infants and young children may have reflected a maturational delay in the immunologic response to thymus-independent type 2 antigens such as unconjugated PRP, presumably explaining the high incidence of type b infections in infants and young children in the prevaccine era.

The conjugate vaccines act as thymus-dependent antigens and elicit serum antibody responses in infants and young children (Table 221.1). These vaccines are believed to prime memory antibody responses on subsequent encounters with PRP. The concentration of circulating anti-PRP antibody in a child primed by a conjugate vaccine may not correlate precisely with protection, presumably because a memory response may occur rapidly on exposure to PRP and provide protection.

Much less is known about immunity to other *H. influenzae* serotypes or to nontypeable isolates. For nontypeable isolates, evidence suggests that antibodies directed against 1 or more outer membrane proteins are bactericidal and protect against experimental challenge. A variety of antigens have been evaluated in an attempt to identify vaccine candidates for nontypeable *H. influenzae*, including outer membrane proteins (P1, P2, P4, P5, P6, D15, and Tbp A/B), LPS, various adhesins, and lipoprotein D.

DIAGNOSIS

Presumptive identification of *H. influenzae* is established by direct examination of the collected specimen after staining with Gram reagents. Because of its small size, pleomorphism, and occasional poor uptake of stain, as well as the tendency for proteinaceous fluids to have a red background, *H. influenzae* is sometimes difficult to visualize. Furthermore, given that identification of microorganisms on smear by either technique requires at least 10^5 bacteria/mL, failure to visualize them does not preclude their presence.

Culture of *H. influenzae* requires prompt transport and processing of specimens because the organism is fastidious. Specimens should not be exposed to drying or temperature extremes. Primary isolation of *H. influenzae* can be accomplished on chocolate agar or on blood agar plates using the staphylococcus streak technique.

Serotyping of *H. influenzae* is accomplished by slide agglutination with type-specific antisera. Accurate serotyping is essential to monitor progress toward elimination of type b invasive disease. Timely reporting of cases to public health authorities should be ensured.

CLINICAL MANIFESTATIONS AND TREATMENT

The initial antibiotic therapy of invasive infections possibly caused by *H. influenzae* should be a parenterally administered antimicrobial agent effective in sterilizing all foci of infection and effective against ampicillin-resistant strains, usually an **extended-spectrum cephalosporin** such as ceftriaxone. These antibiotics have achieved popularity because of their relative lack of serious adverse effects and ease of administration. After the antimicrobial susceptibility of the isolate has been determined, an appropriate agent can be selected to complete the therapy. **Ampicillin** remains the drug of choice for the therapy of infections caused by susceptible isolates. If the isolate is resistant to ampicillin, ceftriaxone can be administered once daily in selected circumstances for outpatient therapy.

Oral antimicrobial agents are sometimes used to complete a course of therapy initiated by the parenteral route and are typically initial therapy for noninvasive infections such as otitis media and sinusitis. If the organism is susceptible, amoxicillin is the drug of choice. An oral second- or third-generation cephalosporin or amoxicillin-clavulanate may be used when the isolate is resistant to ampicillin.

Meningitis

In the prevaccine era, meningitis accounted for more than half of all cases of invasive *H. influenzae* disease. Clinically, meningitis caused by *H. influenzae* type b cannot be differentiated from meningitis caused by *Neisseria meningitidis* or *Streptococcus pneumoniae* (see Chapter 621.1). It may be complicated by other foci of infection such as the lungs, joints, bones, and pericardium.

Antimicrobial therapy should be administered intravenously for 7-14 days for uncomplicated cases. Ceftriaxone, and ampicillin cross the blood-brain barrier during acute inflammation in concentrations adequate to treat *H. influenzae* meningitis. Intramuscular therapy with ceftriaxone may be an alternative in patients with normal organ perfusion.

The prognosis of Hib meningitis depends on the age at presentation, duration of illness before appropriate antimicrobial therapy, cerebrospinal fluid (CSF) capsular polysaccharide concentration, and rapidity with which organisms are cleared from CSF, blood, and urine. Clinically manifested inappropriate secretion of antidiuretic hormone and evidence of focal neurologic deficits at presentation are poor prognostic features. Approximately 6% of patients with Hib meningitis are left with some hearing impairment, probably because of inflammation of the cochlea and the labyrinth. **Dexamethasone** (0.6 mg/kg/day divided every 6 hr for 2 days), particularly when given shortly before or concurrent with the initiation of antimicrobial therapy, decreases the incidence of hearing loss. Major neurologic sequelae of Hib meningitis include behavior problems, language disorders, impaired vision, mental retardation, motor abnormalities, ataxia, seizures, and hydrocephalus.

Cellulitis

Children with Hib cellulitis often have an antecedent upper respiratory tract infection. They usually have no prior history of trauma, and the infection is thought to represent seeding of the organism to the involved soft tissues during bacteremia. The head and neck, particularly the cheek and preseptal region of the eye, are the most common sites of involvement. The involved region generally has indistinct margins and is tender and indurated. **Buccal cellulitis** is classically erythematous with a violaceous hue, although this sign may be absent. *H. influenzae* may often be recovered directly from an aspirate of the leading edge, although this procedure is seldom performed. The blood culture may also reveal the causative organism. Other foci of infection may be present concomitantly, particularly in children <18 mo old. A diagnostic lumbar puncture should be considered at diagnosis in these children.

Parenteral antimicrobial therapy is indicated until patients become afebrile, after which an appropriate oral antimicrobial agent may be substituted. A 7-10 day course is customary.

Preseptal Cellulitis

Infection involving the superficial tissue layers anterior to the orbital septum is termed preseptal cellulitis, which may be caused by *H. influenzae*. Uncomplicated preseptal cellulitis does not imply a risk for

Table 221.1	*Haemophilus influenzae* Type b (Hib) Conjugate Vaccines Available in the United States		
VACCINE	**TRADE NAME**	**COMPONENTS**	**MANUFACTURER**
PRP-T	ActHib	PRP conjugated to tetanus toxoid	Sanofi
PRP-T	Hibrix	PRP conjugated to tetanus toxoid	GlaxoSmithKline Biologicals
PRP-OMP	PedvaxHIB	PRP conjugated to OMP	Merck
PRP-T/DTaP-IPV	Pentacel	PRP-T + DTaP-IPV vaccines	Sanofi Pasteur

DTaP, Diphtheria and tetanus toxoids and acellular pertussis vaccine; HepB, hepatitis B vaccine; IPV, trivalent inactivated polio vaccine; OMP, outer membrane protein complex from *Neisseria meningitidis*; PRP, polyribosylribitol phosphate.

visual impairment or direct central nervous system (CNS) extension. However, concurrent bacteremia may be associated with the development of meningitis. *H. influenzae* preseptal cellulitis is characterized by fever, edema, tenderness, warmth of the lid, and, occasionally, purple discoloration. Evidence of interruption of the integument is usually absent. Conjunctival drainage may be associated. *S. pneumoniae, Staphylococcus aureus,* and group A streptococcus cause clinically indistinguishable preseptal cellulitis. The latter 2 pathogens are more likely when fever is absent and the integument is interrupted (e.g., insect bite, trauma).

Children with preseptal cellulitis in whom *H. influenzae* and *S. pneumoniae* are etiologic considerations (young age, high fever, intact integument) should undergo blood culture, and a diagnostic lumbar puncture should be considered.

Parenteral antibiotics are indicated for preseptal cellulitis. Because methicillin-susceptible and methicillin-resistant *S. aureus, S. pneumoniae,* and group A β-hemolytic streptococci are other causes, empirical therapy should include agents active against these pathogens. Patients with preseptal cellulitis without concurrent meningitis should receive parenteral therapy for about 5 days, until fever and erythema have abated. In uncomplicated cases, antimicrobial therapy should be given for 10 days.

Orbital Cellulitis

Infections of the orbit are infrequent and usually develop as complications of acute ethmoid or sphenoid sinusitis. Orbital cellulitis may manifest as lid edema but is distinguished by the presence of proptosis, chemosis, impaired vision, limitation of the extraocular movements, decreased mobility of the globe, or pain on movement of the globe. The distinction between preseptal and orbital cellulitis may be difficult and is best delineated by CT.

Orbital infections are treated with parenteral therapy for at least 14 days. Underlying sinusitis or orbital abscess may require surgical drainage and more prolonged antimicrobial therapy.

Supraglottitis or Acute Epiglottitis

Supraglottitis is a cellulitis of the tissues comprising the laryngeal inlet (see Chapter 412). It has become exceedingly rare since the introduction of conjugate Hib vaccines. Direct bacterial invasion of the involved tissues is probably the initiating pathophysiologic event. This dramatic, potentially lethal condition can occur at any age. Because of the risk of sudden, unpredictable airway obstruction, supraglottitis is a medical emergency. Other foci of infection, such as meningitis, are rare. Antimicrobial therapy directed against *H. influenzae* and other etiologic agents should be administered parenterally, but only after the airway is secured, and therapy should be continued until patients are able to take fluids by mouth. The duration of antimicrobial therapy is typically 7 days.

Pneumonia

The true incidence of *H. influenzae* pneumonia in children is unknown because invasive procedures required to obtain culture specimens are seldom performed (see Chapter 428). In the prevaccine era, type b bacteria were believed to be the usual cause. The signs and symptoms of pneumonia caused by *H. influenzae* cannot be differentiated from those of pneumonia caused by many other microorganisms. Other foci of infection may be present concomitantly.

Children <12 mo old in whom *H. influenzae* pneumonia is suspected should receive parenteral antimicrobial therapy initially because of their increased risk for bacteremia and its complications. Older children who do not appear severely ill may be managed with an oral antimicrobial. Therapy is continued for 7-10 days. Uncomplicated pleural effusion associated with *H. influenzae* pneumonia requires no special intervention. However, if empyema develops, surgical drainage is indicated.

Suppurative Arthritis

Large joints, such as the knee, hip, ankle, and elbow, are affected most often (see Chapter 705). Other foci of infection may be present concomitantly. Although single-joint involvement is the rule, multijoint

involvement occurs in approximately 6% of cases. The signs and symptoms of septic arthritis caused by *H. influenzae* are indistinguishable from those of arthritis caused by other bacteria.

Uncomplicated septic arthritis should be treated with an appropriate parenteral antimicrobial for at least 5-7 days. If the clinical response is satisfactory, the remainder of the course of antimicrobial treatment may be given orally. Therapy is typically given for 3 wk for uncomplicated septic arthritis, but it may be continued beyond 3 wk, until the C-reactive protein concentration is normal.

Pericarditis

H. influenzae is a rare cause of pericarditis (see Chapter 467). Affected children often have had an antecedent upper respiratory tract infection. Fever, respiratory distress, and tachycardia are consistent findings. Other foci of infection may be present concomitantly.

The diagnosis may be established by recovery of the organism from blood or pericardial fluid. Gram stain or detection of PRP in pericardial fluid, blood, or urine (when type b organisms are the cause) may aid the diagnosis. Antimicrobials should be provided parenterally in a regimen similar to that used for meningitis (see Chapter 621.1). Pericardiectomy is useful for draining the purulent material effectively and preventing tamponade and constrictive pericarditis.

Bacteremia Without an Associated Focus

Bacteremia caused by *H. influenzae* may be associated with fever without any apparent focus of infection (see Chapter 202). In this situation, risk factors for occult bacteremia include the magnitude of fever (≥39°C [102.2°F]) and the presence of leukocytosis (≥15,000 cells/μL). In the prevaccine era, meningitis developed in approximately 25% of children with occult Hib bacteremia if left untreated. In the vaccine era, this *H. influenzae* infection has become exceedingly rare. When it does occur, the child should be reevaluated for a focus of infection and a 2nd blood culture performed. The child should be hospitalized and given parenteral antimicrobial therapy after a diagnostic lumbar puncture and chest radiograph are obtained.

Miscellaneous Infections

Rarely, *H. influenzae* causes urinary tract infection, epididymoorchitis, cervical adenitis, acute glossitis, infected thyroglossal duct cysts, uvulitis, endocarditis, endophthalmitis, primary peritonitis, osteomyelitis, and periappendiceal abscess.

Invasive Disease in Neonates

Neonates rarely have invasive *H. influenzae* infection. In the infant with illness within the 1st 24 hr of life, especially in association with maternal chorioamnionitis or prolonged rupture of membranes, transmission of the organism to the infant is likely to have occurred through the maternal genital tract, which may be (<1%) colonized with nontypeable *H. influenzae*. Manifestations of neonatal invasive infection include bacteremia with sepsis, pneumonia, respiratory distress syndrome with shock, conjunctivitis, scalp abscess or cellulitis, and meningitis. Less frequently, mastoiditis, septic arthritis, and congenital vesicular eruption may occur.

Otitis Media

Acute otitis media is one of the most common infectious diseases of childhood (see Chapter 658). It results from the spread of bacteria from the nasopharynx through the eustachian tube into the middle ear cavity. Usually, because of a preceding viral upper respiratory tract infection, the mucosa in the area becomes hyperemic and swollen, resulting in obstruction and an opportunity for bacterial multiplication in the middle ear.

The most common bacterial pathogens are *H. influenzae, S. pneumoniae,* and *Moraxella catarrhalis.* Most *H. influenzae* isolates causing otitis media are nontypeable. Ipsilateral conjunctivitis may also be present. Amoxicillin (80-90 mg/kg/day) is a suitable first-line oral antimicrobial agent, because the probability that the causative isolate is resistant to amoxicillin and the risk for invasive potential are sufficiently low to justify this approach. Alternatively, in certain cases, a single dose of ceftriaxone constitutes adequate therapy.

In the case of treatment failure or if a β-lactamase–producing isolate is obtained by tympanocentesis or from drainage fluid, amoxicillin-clavulanate (Augmentin) is a suitable alternative.

Conjunctivitis

Acute infection of the conjunctivae is common in childhood (see Chapter 644). In neonates, *H. influenzae* is an infrequent cause. However, it is an important pathogen in older children. Most *H. influenzae* isolates associated with conjunctivitis are nontypeable, although type b isolates and other serotypes are occasionally found. Empirical treatment of conjunctivitis beyond the neonatal period usually consists of topical antimicrobial therapy with sulfacetamide. Topical fluoroquinolone therapy is to be avoided because of its broad spectrum, high cost, and high rate of emerging resistance among many bacterial species. Ipsilateral otitis media caused by the same organism may be present and requires oral antibiotic therapy.

Sinusitis

H. influenzae is an important cause of acute sinusitis in children, 2nd in frequency only to *S. pneumoniae* (see Chapter 408). Chronic sinusitis lasting >1 yr or severe sinusitis requiring hospitalization is often caused by *S. aureus* or anaerobes such as *Peptococcus, Peptostreptococcus,* and *Bacteroides.* Nontypeable *H. influenzae* and viridans group streptococci are also frequently recovered.

For uncomplicated sinusitis, amoxicillin is acceptable initial therapy. However, if clinical improvement does not occur, a broader-spectrum agent, such as amoxicillin-clavulanate, may be appropriate. A 10-day course is sufficient for uncomplicated sinusitis. Hospitalization for parenteral therapy is rarely required; the usual reason is suspicion of progression to orbital cellulitis.

PREVENTION

Immunization with Hib conjugate vaccine is recommended for all infants. Prophylaxis is indicated if close contacts of an index patient with type b disease are unvaccinated. The contagiousness of non-Hib infections is not known, and prophylaxis is not recommended.

Vaccine

Several Hib conjugate vaccines are currently marketed in the United States, containing either PRP–outer membrane protein (**PRP-OMP**) or PRP–tetanus toxoid (**PRP-T**), which differ in the carrier protein used and the method of conjugating the polysaccharide to the protein (see Table 221.1 and Chapter 197). One of the combination vaccines consists of PRP-OMP combined with hepatitis B vaccine (Comvax, Merck, Whitehouse Station, NJ) and can be used for doses recommended at 2, 4, and 12-15 mo of age. Another consists of PRP-T combined with DTaP vaccine (diphtheria and tetanus toxoids and acellular pertussis) and IPV vaccine (trivalent, inactivated polio vaccine) (Pentacel, Sanofi Pasteur, Swiftwater, PA) and can be used for doses recommended at 2, 4, 6, and 12-15 mo of age. A third consists of PRP-T combined with *N. meningitidis* serogroups C and Y (GlaxoSmithKline Biologicals) and can be used for doses recommended at 2, 4, 6, and 12-15 mo of age for children at increased risk for *N. meningitidis* disease. PRP-T by itself is licensed for doses scheduled for children ≥15 mo old.

The Hib conjugate vaccines stimulate circulating anticapsular antibody and provide long-term immunity through B-cell memory.

Prophylaxis

Unvaccinated children <48 mo old who are in close contact with an index case of invasive Hib infection are at increased risk for invasive infection. The risk for secondary disease for children >3 mo old is inversely related to age. About half the secondary cases among susceptible household contacts occur in the 1st wk after hospitalization of the index case. Because many children are now protected against *H. influenzae* type b by prior immunization, the need for prophylaxis has greatly decreased. When prophylaxis is used, **rifampin** is indicated for all members of the household or close-contact group, including the index patient, if the group includes 1 or more children <48 mo old who are not fully immunized.

Parents of children hospitalized for invasive Hib disease should be informed of the increased risk for secondary infection in other young children in the same household if they are not fully immunized. Parents of children exposed to a single case of invasive Hib disease in a child-care center or nursery school should be similarly informed, although there is disagreement about the need for rifampin prophylaxis for these children.

For prophylaxis, children should be given rifampin orally (0-1 mo old, 10 mg/kg/dose; >1 mo old, 20 mg/kg/dose, not to exceed 600 mg/dose) once daily for 4 consecutive days. The adult dose is 600 mg once daily. Rifampin prophylaxis is not recommended for pregnant women.

Bibliography is available at Expert Consult.

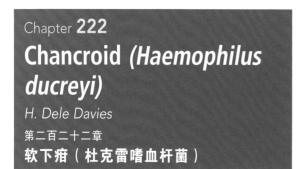

Chapter **222**

Chancroid *(Haemophilus ducreyi)*

H. Dele Davies

第二百二十二章

软下疳（杜克雷嗜血杆菌）

中文导读

本章首先阐述了软下疳（杜克雷嗜血杆菌）是　　一种性传播疾病，其特征为疼痛的生殖器溃疡和腹股沟淋巴结肿大，进一步介绍了软下疳的病因、流行病 学、临床表现、诊断、治疗和并发症等内容。在关于 软下疳治疗部分详细描述了软下疳对青霉素和氨苄青

霉素耐药情况，并就阿奇霉素、头孢曲松、红霉素、 环丙沙星及相关评估内容等进行了详细介绍。

Chancroid is a sexually transmitted disease characterized by painful genital ulceration and inguinal lymphadenopathy.

ETIOLOGY AND EPIDEMIOLOGY

Chancroid is caused by *Haemophilus ducreyi,* a fastidious gram-negative bacillus. It is prevalent in many developing countries but occurs sporadically in the developed world. Most Western cases occur in returning travelers (90% are male) from endemic areas or occasionally in localized urban outbreaks associated with commercial sex workers. Chancroid is a risk factor for transmission of HIV. Diagnosis of chancroid in infants and children is strong evidence of sexual abuse. Male circumcision lowers the risk for chancroid. The incidence of chancroid has declined significantly since 1981 and remains low in the United States.

CLINICAL MANIFESTATIONS

The incubation period is 4-7 days, with a small, inflammatory papule on the preputial orifice or frenulum in men and on the labia, fourchette, or perineal region in women. The lesion becomes pustular, eroded, and ulcerative within 2-3 days. The ulcer edge is classically ragged and undermined. Without treatment, the ulcers may persist for weeks to months. Painful, tender inguinal lymphadenitis occurs in >50% of cases, more often among men. The lymphadenopathy can become fluctuant to form **buboes,** which can spontaneously rupture.

DIAGNOSIS

Diagnosis is usually established by the clinical presentation and the exclusion of both syphilis (*Treponema pallidum*) and herpes simplex virus infections. Gram stain of ulcer secretions may show gram-negative coccobacilli in parallel clusters ("school of fish"). Culture requires expensive, special media and has a sensitivity of only 80%. Polymerase chain reaction (PCR) and indirect immunofluorescence using monoclonal antibodies are available as research tools and are performed by some clinical laboratories using their own in-house Clinical Laboratory Improvement Amendments (CLIA)–verified kits. There are currently no U.S. Food and Drug Administration (FDA)–approved PCR tests for *H. ducreyi.* The ulcer of chancroid is accompanied by concurrent **lymphadenopathy** that is usually unilateral, unlike lymphogranuloma venereum (see Chapter 253.4). Genital herpes is characterized by vesicular lesions with a history of recurrence (see Chapter 279).

TREATMENT

Most *H. ducreyi* organisms are resistant to penicillin and ampicillin because of plasmid-mediated β-lactamase production. Spread of plasmid-mediated resistance among *H. ducreyi* has resulted in lack of efficacy of previously useful drugs such as sulfonamides and tetracyclines. Chancroid is easy to treat if recognized early. The current treatment recommendation is for **azithromycin** (1 g as a single dose orally [PO]) or **ceftriaxone** (250 mg as a single dose intramuscularly). Alternative regimens include **erythromycin** (500 mg 3 times daily PO for 7 days), which is most often used in developing countries, and ciprofloxacin (500 mg twice daily PO for 3 days, for persons ≥18 yr old). Fluctuant nodes may require drainage. Symptoms usually resolve within 3-7 days. Relapses can usually be treated successfully with the original treatment regimen. Patients with HIV infection may require longer duration of treatment. Persistence of the ulcer and the organism following therapy should raise suspicion of resistance to the prescribed antibiotic.

Patients with chancroid should be evaluated for other sexually transmitted infections, including syphilis, hepatitis B virus, HIV, chlamydia, and gonorrhea; an estimated 10% have concomitant syphilis or genital herpes. If initial HIV or syphilis testing is negative, patients should be tested for again in 3 mo because of the high rates of co-infections. In developing countries, patients with a compatible genital ulcer are treated for both chancroid and syphilis. All sexual contacts of patients with chancroid should be evaluated and treated.

COMPLICATIONS

Complications include **phimosis** in men and secondary bacterial infection. Bubo formation may occur in untreated cases. Genital ulceration as a syndrome increases the risk for transmission of HIV.

Bibliography is available at Expert Consult.

Chapter 223
Moraxella catarrhalis
Timothy F. Murphy

第二百二十三章
卡他莫拉菌

中文导读

    本章首先阐述了卡他莫拉菌是革兰阴性双球菌，是一种在婴儿期就开始定植于呼吸道的人类特异性病原体，随后详细介绍了卡他莫拉菌感染的病因、流行病学、发病机制、临床表现、诊断、治疗和预防等内容。在卡他莫拉菌感染的临床表现部分详细描述了急性中耳炎、复发性中耳炎和渗出性中耳炎、鼻窦炎和菌血症。在卡他莫拉菌感染的治疗部分详细描述了治疗指南、相关抗生素的耐药情况等内容。

Moraxella catarrhalis is an unencapsulated gram-negative diplococcus and is a **human-specific pathogen** that colonizes the respiratory tract beginning in infancy. Patterns of colonization and infection with *M. catarrhalis* are changing in countries where pneumococcal conjugate vaccines are used widely. The most important clinical manifestation of *M. catarrhalis* infection in children is **otitis media**.

ETIOLOGY

Moraxella catarrhalis has long been considered to be an upper respiratory tract commensal. Substantial genetic heterogeneity exists among strains of *M. catarrhalis*. Several outer membrane proteins demonstrate sequence differences among strains, particularly in regions of the proteins that are exposed on the bacterial surface. *M. catarrhalis* endotoxin lacks repeating polysaccharide side chains and is thus a lipooligosaccharide (LOS). In contrast to other gram-negative respiratory pathogens, such as *Haemophilus influenzae* and *Neisseria meningitidis*, the LOS of *M. catarrhalis* is relatively conserved among strains; only 3 serotypes (A, B, and C) based on oligosaccharide structure have been identified. Genetic and antigenic differences among strains account for the observation that resolving an infection by one strain does not induce protective immunity to other strains. *M. catarrhalis* causes recurrent infections, which generally represent reinfection by new strains.

EPIDEMIOLOGY

The ecologic niche of *M. catarrhalis* is the human respiratory tract. The bacterium has not been recovered from animals or environmental sources. **Age** is the most important determinant of the prevalence of upper respiratory tract colonization. Common throughout infancy, nasopharyngeal colonization is a dynamic process with active turnover as a result of acquisition and clearance of strains of *M. catarrhalis*. Some geographic variation in rates of colonization is observed. On the basis of monthly or bimonthly cultures, colonization during the 1st yr of life may range from 33–100%. Several factors likely account

for this variability among studies, including living conditions, daycare attendance, hygiene, environmental factors (e.g., household smoking), and genetics of the population. The prevalence of colonization steadily decreases with age. Understanding nasopharyngeal colonization patterns is important, because the pathogenesis of otitis media involves migration of the bacterium from the nasopharynx to the middle ear via the eustachian tube.

The widespread use of pneumococcal polysaccharide vaccines in many countries has resulted in alteration of patterns of nasopharyngeal colonization in the population. A relative increase in colonization by nonvaccine pneumococcal serotypes, nontypeable *H. influenzae*, and *M. catarrhalis* has occurred. Whether changes in colonization patterns will result in a true increase in new episodes of otitis media and sinusitis caused by nontypeable *H. influenzae* and *M. catarrhalis* requires continuous surveillance.

PATHOGENESIS OF INFECTION

Strains of *M. catarrhalis* differ in their virulence properties. The species is composed of complement-resistant and complement-sensitive genetic lineages, the **complement-resistant** strains being more strongly associated with virulence. Strains that cause infection in children differ in several phenotypic characteristics from strains that cause infection in adults, in whom the most common clinical manifestation is lower respiratory tract infection in the setting of chronic obstructive pulmonary disease.

The presence of several **adhesin** molecules with differing specificities for various host cell receptors reflects the importance of adherence to the human respiratory epithelial surface in the pathogenesis of infection. *M. catarrhalis* has long been viewed as an exclusively extracellular pathogen. However, the bacterium is now known to invade multiple cell types, including bronchial epithelial cells, small airway cells, and type 2 alveolar cells. In addition, *M. catarrhalis* resides intracellularly in lymphoid tissue, providing a reservoir for persistence in the human respiratory tract. As with many gram-negative bacteria, *M. catarrhalis* sheds vesicles from its surface during growth. These vesicles are internalized by respiratory epithelial cells and mediate several virulence mechanisms, including B-cell activation, induction of inflammation, and delivery of β-lactamases. Analysis of genomes reveals modest genetic heterogeneity among strains.

M. catarrhalis forms biofilms in vitro and in the middle ears of children with chronic and recurrent otitis media. **Biofilms** are communities of bacteria encased in a matrix attached to a surface. Bacteria in biofilms are more resistant to antibiotics and to host immune responses than bacteria growing individually in planktonic form.

CLINICAL MANIFESTATIONS

M. catarrhalis causes predominantly mucosal infections in children. The mechanism of infection is **migration** of the infecting strains from the nasopharynx to the middle ear in the case of otitis media or to the sinuses in the case of sinusitis. The inciting event for both otitis media and sinusitis is often a preceding viral infection.

Acute Otitis Media

Approximately 80% of children have 1 or more episodes of otitis media by age 3 yr. Otitis media is the most common reason that children receive antibiotics. On the basis of culture of middle ear fluid obtained by tympanocentesis, the predominant causes of acute otitis media are *Streptococcus pneumoniae, H. influenzae,* and *M. catarrhalis. M. catarrhalis* is cultured from the middle ear fluid in 15–20% of patients with acute otitis media. When more sensitive methods (e.g., PCR) are used, the number of middle ear fluid samples from children with otitis media in which *M. catarrhalis* is detected is substantially greater than by culture alone. The distribution of the causative agents of otitis media is changing as a result of widespread administration of pneumococcal conjugate vaccines, with a relative increase in *H. influenzae* and *M. catarrhalis.*

Acute otitis media caused by *M. catarrhalis* is clinically milder than otitis media caused by *H. influenzae* or *S. pneumoniae,* with less fever and lower prevalence of a red, bulging tympanic membrane. However, substantial overlap in symptoms is seen, making it impossible to predict etiology in an individual child on the basis of clinical features. Tympanocentesis is required to make an etiologic diagnosis but is not performed routinely, and thus, treatment of otitis media is generally empirical.

Recurrent Otitis Media and Otitis Media With Effusion

Otitis media with effusion refers to the presence of fluid in the middle ear in the absence of signs and symptoms of acute infection. Children who experience 4 or more episodes of acute otitis media in a year or who have at least 8 mo of middle ear effusion in a year are defined as **otitis prone.** These children have conductive hearing loss, which may lead to delays in speech and language development. Analysis of middle ear fluid from children with otitis media with effusion using sensitive molecular techniques (e.g., PCR) indicates that bacterial DNA is present in up to 80% of samples from such children. Indeed, *M. catarrhalis* DNA is present, both alone and as a co-pathogen, in a larger proportion of cases of otitis media with effusion than of acute otitis media. Biofilms may account for these observations, although definitive evidence is lacking.

Sinusitis

A small proportion of viral upper respiratory tract infections are complicated by bacterial sinusitis. According to findings of studies that use sinus puncture, *M. catarrhalis* accounts for approximately 20% of cases of acute bacterial sinusitis in children and a smaller proportion in adults. Sinusitis caused by *M. catarrhalis* is clinically indistinguishable from that caused by *S. pneumoniae* or *H. influenzae.*

Bacteremia

M. catarrhalis rarely causes bacteremia or invasive infections in children. When bacteremia occurs, the usual source is the respiratory tract. Some children have underlying immunocompromising conditions, but no particular immunodeficiency is associated with invasive *M. catarrhalis* infections.

DIAGNOSIS

The clinical diagnosis of otitis media is made by demonstration of fluid in the middle ear by pneumatic otoscopy. A tympanocentesis is required to establish an etiologic diagnosis, but this procedure is not performed routinely. Thus, the choice of antibiotic for otitis media is empirical and generally based on guidelines. Management of bacterial sinusitis is also empirical, because determining the etiology of sinusitis requires a **sinus puncture**, also a procedure that is not performed routinely.

The key to making a microbiologic diagnosis is distinguishing *M. catarrhalis* from commensal *Neisseria* organisms that are part of the normal upper respiratory tract flora. Indeed, the difficulty in distinguishing colonies of *M. catarrhalis* from *Neisseria* spp. explains in part why *M. catarrhalis* has been overlooked in the past as a respiratory tract pathogen. *M. catarrhalis* produces round, opaque colonies that can be slid across the agar surface without disruption, the "hockey puck sign." In addition, after 48 hr, *M. catarrhalis* colonies tend to be larger than *Neisseria* and take on a pink color. A variety of biochemical tests distinguish *M. catarrhalis* from *Neisseria* spp., and commercially available kits based on these tests are available.

Sensitive tests that employ polymerase chain reaction (PCR) to detect respiratory tract bacterial pathogens in human respiratory tract secretions are in development. Their application will likely contribute new information about the epidemiology and disease patterns of *M. catarrhalis.*

TREATMENT

A proportion of cases of *M. catarrhalis* otitis media resolve spontaneously. Treatment of otitis media is empirical, and clinicians are advised to follow guidelines of the American Academy of Pediatrics (see Chapter 658).

Strains of *M. catarrhalis* rapidly acquired β-lactamase worldwide in the 1970s and 1980s, rendering essentially all strains resistant to amoxicillin. When *M. catarrhalis* is present as a co-pathogen in otitis media, its β-lactamase reduces susceptibility of nontypeable *H. influenzae* and *S. pneumoniae* to amoxicillin. Antimicrobial susceptibility patterns have remained relatively stable for decades. However, strains of *M. catarrhalis* that are resistant to macrolides and fluoroquinolones have been isolated in several centers in Asia. Careful surveillance will be important to track the potential emergence of resistant strains more widely. Most strains of *M. catarrhalis* are susceptible to amoxicillin/clavulanic acid, extended-spectrum cephalosporins, macrolides (azithromycin, clarithromycin), trimethoprim-sulfamethoxazole, and fluoroquinolones.

PREVENTION

Vaccines to prevent otitis media and other infections caused by *M. catarrhalis* are under development, but none is yet available.

Bibliography is available at Expert Consult.

Chapter **224**
Pertussis (*Bordetella pertussis* and *Bordetella parapertussis*)

Emily Souder and Sarah S. Long

第二百二十四章
百日咳鲍特菌（百日咳杆菌）

中文导读

本章主要介绍了百日咳鲍特菌感染的病因、流行病学、发病机制、临床表现、诊断、治疗、并发症和预防。在百日咳鲍特菌感染的治疗部分详细介绍了抗生素、辅助治疗、隔离、家庭照护和其他的密切联系等内容。其中，详细描述了百日咳暴露后预防的抗生素推荐治疗方案。在百日咳鲍特菌感染的预防部分详细介绍了白喉–破伤风–百日咳三联疫苗和白喉–百日咳–破伤风三联疫苗。

Pertussis is an acute respiratory tract infection; the term *pertussis* means "intense cough" and is preferable to *whooping cough,* because most infected individuals do not "whoop."

ETIOLOGY

Bordetella pertussis is the cause of epidemic pertussis and the usual cause of sporadic pertussis. *Bordetella parapertussis* is an occasional cause of sporadic pertussis that contributes significantly to total cases of pertussis in Eastern and Western Europe, but increasingly has been detected during regional pertussis outbreaks in the United States. *B. pertussis* and *B. parapertussis* are exclusive pathogens of humans and some primates. *Bordetella holmesii*, first identified as a cause of bacteremia in immunocompromised hosts without cough illness, also is reported to cause pertussis-like cough illness in small outbreaks in healthy persons. *Bordetella bronchiseptica* is a common animal pathogen. Occasional reports in humans describe a variety of body sites involved, and cases typically occur in immunocompromised persons or young children with intense exposure to animals. Protracted coughing (which in some cases is paroxysmal) is attributable sporadically to *Mycoplasma,* parainfluenza viruses, influenza viruses, enteroviruses, respiratory syncytial virus (RSV), or adenoviruses.

EPIDEMIOLOGY

The World Health Organization (WHO) estimated that in 2008, 16 million cases of pertussis and 195,000 childhood deaths occurred worldwide, 95% of which were in developing countries. The WHO also estimated that 82% of infants worldwide received 3 doses of pertussis vaccine and that global vaccination against pertussis averted 687,000 deaths in 2008. Before vaccination was available, pertussis was the leading cause of death from communicable disease among U.S. children <14 yr old, with 10,000 deaths annually. Widespread use of whole cell pertussis vaccine (DTP) led to a >99% decline in cases. After the low U.S. number of 1,010 cases reported in 1976, there was an increase in annual pertussis incidence to 1.2 cases per 100,000 population from 1980 through 1989, with epidemic pertussis in many states in 1989–1990, 1993, and 1996. Since then, pertussis has become increasingly endemic, with shifting burden of disease to young infants, adolescents, and adults. By 2004, the incidence of reported pertussis in the United States was 8.9 cases per 100,000 in the general population and approximately 150 per 100,000 in infants <2 mo old, with 25,827 total cases reported, the highest since 1959. A total of 40 pertussis-related deaths were reported in 2005, and 16 were reported in 2006; >90% of these cases occurred in infants.

Prospective and serologic studies suggested that pertussis is *underrecognized*, especially among adolescents and adults, in whom the actual number of U.S. cases is estimated to be 600,000 annually. A number of studies documented pertussis in 13–32% of adolescents and adults with cough illness for >7 days. Responding to these changes in epidemiology, tetanus toxoid, reduced-content diphtheria toxoid, and acellular pertussis antigens (**Tdap**) was recommended in 2006 for 11-12 yr olds and was aimed to enhance control. With >70% uptake of Tdap in adolescents, the burden of disease in young adolescents fell commensurately, but without evidence of protection of the community (herd) of young infants, older adolescents, and adults. An epidemiologic shift has occurred due to substantial and rapid waning of protection following both DTaP and Tdap in the aging cohort of children and adolescents who were not primed with DTP (whole cell) vaccine, which was no longer used in the United States after 1997. The >42,000 cases of pertussis and 20 deaths reported in 2012 were the highest numbers in >50 yr. A shift in disease burden was observed among 7-10 yr olds in 2010, 13-14 yr olds in 2012, and 14-16 yr olds in 2014, as the cohort of solely DTaP-vaccinated cohort aged.

Neither natural disease nor vaccination provides complete or lifelong immunity against pertussis reinfection or disease. Subclinical reinfection undoubtedly contributed significantly to immunity against disease ascribed previously to both vaccine and prior infection. The resurgence of pertussis can be attributed to a variety of factors, including partial control of pertussis leading to less continuous exposure as well as increased awareness and improved diagnostics. Rapidly waning vaccine-induced immunity and pathogen adaptation are most important currently. Although the DTaP series is protective short-term, vaccine effectiveness wanes rapidly, with estimates of only 10% protection 8.5 yr after the 5th dose. Tdap protection also is short-lived, with efficacy falling from >70% initially to 34% within 2-4 yr. Divergence of circulating strains from vaccine strains began with the introduction of DTP, but with the exclusive use of acellular pertussis vaccines, **pertactin-deficient strains** emerged and have become dominant in countries where these vaccines are used. Pertactin-deficient *B. pertussis* was first reported in the United States from a Philadelphia infant case collection from 2008 to 2011. The Centers for Disease Control and Prevention (CDC) subsequently reported the earliest U.S. isolate from 1994 and rapid dominance of pertactin-deficient strains in the United States since 2010. Despite the role of pertactin as a bacterial virulence factor, illness severity in infants with pertactin-deficient *B. pertussis* is similar to that of pertactin-producing strains. Until development of new pertussis vaccine(s), pertussis will continue to be endemic, with cycling epidemics.

PATHOGENESIS

Bordetella organisms are small, fastidious, gram-negative coccobacilli that colonize only ciliated epithelium. The exact mechanism of disease symptomatology remains unknown. *Bordetella* species share a high degree of DNA homology among virulence genes. Only *B. pertussis* expresses **pertussis toxin** (PT), the major virulence protein. PT has numerous proven biologic activities (e.g., histamine sensitivity, insulin secretion, leukocyte dysfunction). Injection of PT in experimental animals causes lymphocytosis immediately by rerouting lymphocytes to remain in the circulating blood pool but does not cause cough. PT appears to have a central, but not a singular, role in pathogenesis. *B. pertussis* produces an array of other biologically active substances, many of which are postulated to have a role in disease and immunity. After aerosol acquisition, filamentous **hemagglutinin**, some **agglutinogens** (especially fimbriae [Fim] types 2 and 3), and the 69-kDa **pertactin** (Prn) protein are important for attachment to ciliated respiratory epithelial cells. **Tracheal cytotoxin**, adenylate cyclase, and PT appear to inhibit clearance of organisms. Tracheal cytotoxin, dermonecrotic factor, and adenylate cyclase are postulated to be predominantly responsible for the local epithelial damage that produces respiratory symptoms and facilitates absorption of PT. Both antibody and cellular immune responses follow infection and immunization. Antibody to PT neutralizes toxin, and antibody to Prn enhances opsonophagocytosis. Disease as well as DTP appear to drive a mixed cellular and antibody (Th1) immunologic response, while DTaP and Tdap drive a narrow antibody-dominant (Th2) response.

Pertussis is *extremely contagious*, with attack rates as high as 100% in susceptible individuals exposed to aerosol droplets at close range. High airborne transmission rates were shown in a baboon model of pertussis despite vaccination with the acellular vaccine. *B. pertussis* does not survive for prolonged periods in the environment. Chronic carriage by humans is not documented. After intense exposure as in households, the rate of subclinical infection is as high as 80% in fully immunized or previously infected individuals. When carefully sought, a symptomatic source case can be found for most patients; usually a sibling or related adult.

CLINICAL MANIFESTATIONS

Classically, pertussis is a prolonged disease, divided into catarrhal, paroxysmal, and convalescent stages. The **catarrhal stage** (1-2 wk) begins insidiously after an incubation period ranging from 3-12 days with nondistinctive symptoms of congestion and rhinorrhea variably accompanied by low-grade fever, sneezing, lacrimation, and conjunctival suffusion. As initial symptoms wane, coughing marks the onset of the **paroxysmal stage** (2-6 wk). The cough begins as a dry, intermittent, irritative hack and evolves into the inexorable paroxysms that are the hallmark of pertussis. A well-appearing, playful toddler with insignificant provocation suddenly expresses an anxious aura and may clutch a parent or comforting adult before beginning a machine-gun burst of uninterrupted cough on a single exhalation, chin and chest held forward, tongue protruding maximally, eyes bulging and watering, face purple, until coughing ceases and a loud whoop follows as inspired air traverses the still partially closed airway. **Posttussive emesis** is common, and exhaustion is universal. The number and severity of paroxysms escalate over days to a week and remain at that plateau for days to weeks. At the peak of the paroxysmal stage, patients may have >1 episode hourly. As the paroxysmal stage fades into the **convalescent stage** (≥2 wk), the number, severity, and duration of episodes diminish.

Infants <3 mo old do not display the classic stages. The catarrhal phase lasts only a few days or is unnoticed, and then, after the most insignificant startle from a draft, light, sound, sucking, or stretching, a well-appearing young infant begins to choke, gasp, gag, and flail the extremities, with face reddened. Cough may not be prominent, especially in the early phase, and whoop is infrequent. Apnea and cyanosis can follow a coughing paroxysm, or apnea can occur as the only symptom (without cough). Both are more common with pertussis than with neonatal viral infections. The paroxysmal and convalescent stages in young infants are lengthy. Paradoxically, in infants, cough and whooping may become louder and more classic in convalescence. "Exacerbations" of paroxysmal coughing can occur throughout the 1st yr. of life with subsequent respiratory illnesses; these are not a result of recurrent infection or reactivation of *B. pertussis*.

Adolescents and previously immunized children have foreshortening of all stages of pertussis. Adults have no distinct stages. Classically, adolescents and adults describe a sudden feeling of strangulation followed by uninterrupted coughs, feeling of suffocation, bursting headache, diminished awareness, and then a gasping breath, usually without a whoop. Posttussive emesis and intermittency of paroxysms separated by hours of well-being are specific clues to the diagnosis. At least 30% of adolescents and adults with pertussis have nonspecific cough illness, distinguished only by duration, which usually is >21 days.

Findings on physical examination generally are uninformative. Signs of lower respiratory tract disease are not expected unless complicating secondary bacterial pneumonia is present. Conjunctival hemorrhages and petechiae on the upper body are common.

DIAGNOSIS

Pertussis should be suspected in any individual who has a pure or predominant complaint of cough, especially if the following features *are absent*: fever, malaise or myalgia, exanthem or enanthem, sore throat, hoarseness, tachypnea, wheezes, and rales. For sporadic cases, a clinical case definition of cough of ≥14 days' duration with at least 1 associated symptom of paroxysms, whoop, or posttussive vomiting has sensitivity of 81% and specificity of 58% for confirmation of pertussis. Pertussis should be suspected in older children whose cough illness is *escalating* at 7-10 days and whose coughing *is not* continuous, but rather comes in bursts. Pertussis should be suspected in infants <3 mo old with gagging, gasping, apnea, cyanosis, or an apparent life-threatening event. Sudden infant death occasionally is caused by *B. pertussis*.

Adenoviral infections usually are distinguishable by associated features, such as fever, sore throat, and conjunctivitis. *Mycoplasma* causes protracted episodic coughing, but patients usually have a history of fever, headache, and systemic symptoms at the onset of disease as well as more continuous cough and frequent finding of rales on auscultation of the chest. Epidemics of *Mycoplasma* and *B. pertussis* in young adults can be difficult to distinguish on clinical grounds. Although pertussis often is included in the differential diagnosis of young infants with afebrile pneumonia, *B. pertussis* is not associated with staccato cough (breath with every cough), purulent conjunctivitis, tachypnea, rales or wheezes that typify infection by *Chlamydia trachomatis,* or predominant lower respiratory tract signs that typify infection by RSV. Unless an infant with pertussis has secondary pneumonia (and then appears ill), the findings on examination between paroxysms, including respiratory rate, are entirely normal. Foreign body aspiration should be considered in the differential diagnosis.

Leukocytosis (15,000-100,000 cells/μL) caused by *absolute lymphocytosis* is characteristic in the catarrhal stage. Lymphocytes are normal small cells, rather than the large, atypical lymphocytes seen with viral infections. Adults, partially immune children, and occasionally infants may have less impressive lymphocytosis. Absolute increase in neutrophils suggests a different diagnosis or secondary bacterial infection. Eosinophilia is not a manifestation of pertussis. A severe course and death are correlated with rapid-rise and extreme leukocytosis (median peak white blood cell count in fatal vs nonfatal cases, 94,000 vs 18,000/μL, respectively) and thrombocytosis (median peak platelet count in fatal vs nonfatal cases, 782,000 vs 556,000/μL, respectively). Chest radiographic findings are only mildly abnormal in the majority of hospitalized infants, showing perihilar infiltrate or edema (sometimes with a butterfly appearance) and variable atelectasis. Parenchymal consolidation suggests secondary bacterial infection. Pneumothorax, pneumomediastinum, and subcutaneous emphysema can be seen occasionally.

Methods for confirmation of infection by *B. pertussis* (culture, PCR, serology) have limitations in sensitivity, specificity, or practicality, and tests' relative values depend on the setting, phase of disease, and purpose of use (e.g., as clinical diagnostic vs epidemiologic tools). Polymerase chain reaction (PCR) testing on nasopharyngeal wash specimens is the laboratory test of choice for *B. pertussis* identification. Both stand-alone and multiplex assays are U.S. Food and Drug Administration (FDA) cleared and available commercially. PCR assays using only single primers (IS481) cannot differentiate between some *Bordetella* spp. Multiplex assays using multiple targets can distinguish species. All assays detect pertactin-deficient strains. For **culture**, a specimen is obtained by deep nasopharyngeal aspiration or with the use of a flexible swab (Dacron or calcium alginate–tipped), held in the posterior nasopharynx for 15-30 sec (or until cough occurs). A 1% casamino acid liquid is acceptable for holding a specimen up to 2 hr; Stainer-Scholte broth or Regan-Lowe semisolid transport medium is used for longer transport periods, up to 4 days. The preferred isolation media are Regan-Lowe charcoal agar with 10% horse blood and 5-40 μg/mL cephalexin, and Stainer-Scholte media with cyclodextrin resins. Cultures are incubated at 35-37°C in a humid environment and examined daily for 7 days for slow-growing, tiny, glistening colonies. Direct fluorescent antibody testing of potential isolates using specific antibody for *B. pertussis* and *B. parapertussis* maximizes recovery rates.

Results of culture and PCR are expected to be positive in unimmunized, untreated children during the catarrhal and early paroxysmal stages of disease. *However, fewer than 20% of culture or PCR tests have positive results in partially or remotely immunized individuals tested in the paroxysmal stage.* Serologic tests for detection of change in antibodies to *B. pertussis* antigens between acute and convalescent samples are the most sensitive tests in immunized individuals and are useful epidemiologically. A single serum sample showing IgG antibody to PT >90 IU/mL (>2 SD above the mean of the immunized population) indicates recent symptomatic infection and usually is positive in the mid-paroxysmal phase. Tests for IgA and IgM pertussis antibody, or antibody to antigens other than PT, are not reliable methods for serologic diagnosis of pertussis.

TREATMENT

Infants <3 mo old with suspected pertussis usually are hospitalized, as are many 3-6 mo old, unless witnessed paroxysms are not severe, as well as patients of any age if significant complications occur. Prematurely born young infants have a high risk for severe, potentially fatal disease, and children with underlying cardiac, pulmonary, muscular, or

neurologic disorders have increased risk of poor outcome beyond infancy. Table 224.1 lists caveats in assessment and care of infants with pertussis. The specific, limited goals of hospitalization are to (1) assess progression of disease and likelihood of life-threatening events at peak of disease; (2) maximize nutrition; (3) prevent or treat complications; and (4) educate parents in the natural history of the disease and in care that will be given at home. Heart rate, respiratory rate, and pulse oximetry are monitored continuously with alarm settings so that paroxysms can be witnessed and recorded by healthcare personnel. Detailed cough records and documentation of feeding, vomiting, and weight change provide data to assess severity. Typical paroxysms that are not life threatening have the following features: duration <45 sec; red but not blue color change; tachycardia, bradycardia (not <60 beats/min in infants), or oxygen desaturation that spontaneously resolves at the end of the paroxysm; whooping or strength for brisk self-rescue at the end of the paroxysm; self-expectorated mucus plug; and posttussive exhaustion but not unresponsiveness. Assessing the need to provide oxygen, stimulation, or suctioning requires skilled personnel who can watchfully observe an infant's ability for self-rescue but who will intervene rapidly and expertly when necessary. The benefit of a quiet, dimly lighted, undisturbed, comforting environment cannot be overestimated or forfeited in a desire to monitor and intervene. Feeding children with pertussis is challenging. The risk of precipitating cough by nipple feeding does not warrant nasogastric, nasojejunal, or parenteral alimentation in most infants. The composition or thickness of formula does not affect the quality of secretions, cough, or retention. Large-volume feedings are avoided.

Within 48-72 hr, the direction and severity of disease are obvious from analysis of recorded information. Hospital discharge is appropriate if, over 48 hr, disease severity is unchanged or diminished, intervention is not required during paroxysms, nutrition is adequate, no complication has occurred, and parents are adequately prepared for care at home. Apnea and seizures occur in the incremental phase of illness and in patients with complicated disease. Portable oxygen, monitoring, or suction apparatus should not be needed at home.

Infants who have apnea, paroxysms that lead to life-threatening events, or respiratory failure require escalating respiratory support and frequently require intubation and pharmaceutically induced paralysis.

Antibiotics

An antimicrobial agent always is given when pertussis is suspected or confirmed to decrease contagiousness and to afford possible clinical benefit. *Azithromycin is the drug of choice in all age-groups, for treatment or postexposure prophylaxis* (Table 224.2). Macrolide resistance has been reported rarely, and recent isolates have retained susceptibility despite genetic strain adaptations. **Infantile hypertrophic pyloric stenosis (IHPS)** is associated with macrolide use in young infants, especially in those <14 days old, with highest risk in those receiving erythromycin vs azithromycin. Benefits of postexposure prophylaxis or treatment of

Table 224.1	Caveats in Assessment and Care of Infants With Pertussis

- Infants with potentially fatal pertussis may appear well between episodes.
- A paroxysm must be witnessed before a decision is made between hospital and home care.
- Only analysis of carefully compiled cough record permits assessment of severity and progression of illness.
- Suctioning of nose, oropharynx, or trachea should not be performed on a "preventive" schedule.
- Feeding in the period following a paroxysm may be more successful than after napping.
- Family support begins at the time of hospitalization with empathy for the child's and family's experience to date, transfer of the burden of responsibility for the child's safety to the healthcare team, and delineation of assessments and treatments to be performed.
- Family education, recruitment as part of the team, and continued support after discharge are essential.

Table 224.2	Recommended Antimicrobial Treatment and Postexposure Prophylaxis for Pertussis			
	PRIMARY AGENTS		**ALTERNATE AGENT***	
AGE-GROUP	**Azithromycin**	**Erythromycin**	**Clarithromycin**	**TMP-SMX**
<1 mo	Recommended agent 10 mg/kg/day in a single dose for 5 days	Not preferred Erythromycin is substantially associated with infantile hypertrophic pyloric stenosis. Use if azithromycin is unavailable; 40-50 mg/kg/day in 4 divided doses for 14 days.	Not recommended (safety data unavailable)	Contraindicated for infants <2 mo of age (risk for kernicterus)
1-5 mo	10 mg/kg/day in a single dose for 5 days	40-50 mg/kg/day in 4 divided doses for 14 days	15 mg/kg/day in 2 divided doses for 7 days	Contraindicated at age <2 mo For infants age ≥2 mo: TMP 8 mg/kg/day plus SMX 40 mg/kg/day in 2 divided doses for 14 days
Infants age ≥6 mo and children	10 mg/kg in a single dose on day 1 (max 500 mg), then 5 mg/kg/day (max 250 mg) on days 2-5	40-50 mg/kg/day (max 2 g/day) in 4 divided doses for 14 days	15 mg/kg/day in 2 divided doses (max 1 g/day) for 7 days	TMP 8 mg/kg/day plus SMX 40 mg/kg/day in 2 divided doses (max TMP: 320 mg/day) for 14 days
Adults	500 mg in a single dose on day 1, then 250 mg/day on days 2-5	2 g/day in 4 divided doses for 14 days	1 g/day in 2 divided doses for 7 days	TMP 320 mg/day–SMX 1600 mg/day in 2 divided doses for 14 days

*Trimethoprim-sulfamethoxazole (TMP-SMX) can be used as an alternative agent to macrolides in patients ≥2 mo old who are allergic to macrolides, who cannot tolerate macrolides, or who are infected with a rare macrolide-resistant strain of *Bordetella pertussis.*

Adapted from Centers for Disease Control and Prevention (CDC): Recommended antimicrobial agents for treatment and postexposure prophylaxis of pertussis: 2005 CDC guidelines, *MMWR* 54:1–16, 2005.

infants far outweigh risk of IHPS. Young infants should be managed expectantly if projectile vomiting occurs. The FDA also warns of risk of fatal heart rhythms with use of azithromycin in patients already at risk for cardiovascular events, especially those with prolongation of the QT interval. Trimethoprim-sulfamethoxazole (TMP-SMX) is an alternative to azithromycin for infants >2 mo old and children unable to receive azithromycin. Because of limited effectiveness, treatment of *B. parapertussis* is based on clinical judgment and is considered in high-risk populations. Agents are the same as for *B. pertussis.* Treatment of infections caused by other *Bordetella* spp. should be undertaken with consultation of a subspecialist.

Adjunct Therapies

No rigorous clinical trial has demonstrated a beneficial effect of β_2-adrenergic stimulants such as salbutamol and albuterol. Fussing associated with aerosol treatment triggers paroxysms. No randomized, blinded clinical trial of sufficient size has been performed to evaluate the usefulness of corticosteroids in the management of pertussis; their clinical use is not warranted. A randomized, double-blind, placebo-controlled trial of pertussis immunoglobulin intravenous (IGIV) was halted prematurely because of expiration/lack of additional supply of study product; there was no indication of clinical benefit. Standard immunoglobulin has not been studied and should not be used for treatment or prophylaxis.

Isolation

Patients with suspected pertussis are placed in isolation with **droplet precautions** to reduce close respiratory or mucous membrane contact with respiratory secretions. All healthcare personnel should wear a mask on entering the room. Screening for cough should be performed on entrance of patients to emergency departments, offices, and clinics to begin isolation immediately and until 5 days after initiation of azithromycin therapy. Children and staff with pertussis in childcare facilities or schools should be excluded until therapy has been taken for 5 days.

Care of Household and Other Close Contacts

Azithromycin should be given promptly to all household contacts and other close contacts, such as those in daycare, regardless of age, history of immunization, or symptoms (see Table 224.2). The same drugs and age-related doses used for treatment are used for prophylaxis. Visitation and movement of coughing family members in the hospital must be assiduously controlled until therapy has been taken for 5 days. In close contacts <7 yr old who have received <4 doses of DTaP, DTaP should be given to complete the recommended series. Children <7 yr old who received a 3rd DTaP dose >6 mo before exposure, or a 4th dose ≥3 yr before exposure, should be given a booster dose. Individuals ≥9 yr old should be given Tdap. Unmasked healthcare personnel exposed to untreated cases should be evaluated for postexposure prophylaxis and follow-up. Coughing healthcare personnel with or without known exposure to pertussis should be evaluated promptly for pertussis.

COMPLICATIONS

Infants <6 mo old have excessive mortality and morbidity; infants <2 mo old have the highest reported rates of pertussis-associated hospitalization (82%), pneumonia (25%), seizures (4%), encephalopathy (1%), and death (1%). Infants <4 mo old account for 90% of cases of fatal pertussis. Preterm birth and young maternal age are significantly associated with fatal pertussis. Neonates with pertussis have substantially longer hospitalizations, greater need for oxygen, and greater need for mechanical ventilation than neonates with viral respiratory tract infection.

The principal complications of pertussis are **apnea**, **secondary infections** (e.g., otitis media, pneumonia), and **physical sequelae** of forceful coughing. Fever, tachypnea or respiratory distress between paroxysms and absolute neutrophilia are clues to pneumonia. Expected pathogens include *Staphylococcus aureus, Streptococcus pneumoniae,* and bacteria of oropharyngeal flora. Increased intrathoracic and intraabdominal pressure during coughing can result in conjunctival and scleral hemorrhage, petechiae on the upper body, epistaxis, pneumothorax and subcutaneous emphysema, umbilical or inguinal hernia, and rarely hemorrhage in the central nervous system or retina. Laceration of the lingual frenulum occurs occasionally.

The need for intensive care and mechanical ventilation usually is limited to infants <3 mo old and children with underlying conditions. Respiratory failure from apnea may mandate intubation and ventilation through the days when disease peaks; prognosis is good. Progressive **pulmonary hypertension** in very young infants and secondary **bacterial pneumonia** are severe complications of pertussis and are the usual causes of death. Pulmonary hypertension and cardiogenic shock with fatal outcome are associated with extreme elevation of lymphocyte and platelet counts. Autopsies in fatal cases show luminal aggregates of leukocytes in the pulmonary vasculature. Extracorporeal membrane oxygenation of infants with pertussis in whom mechanical ventilation failed has been associated with >80% fatality (questioning the advisability of this procedure). Exchange transfusion or leukapheresis is associated with marked reduction in lymphocyte and platelet counts. Although recovery has been reported in several cases, benefit is unproven. Echocardiography should be performed in critically ill infants with pertussis to detect presence of pulmonary hypertension and to intervene expeditiously.

Acute neurologic events during pertussis almost always are the result of **hypoxemia** or **hemorrhage** associated with coughing or apnea in young infants. Apnea or bradycardia or both may result from apparent laryngospasm or vagal stimulation just before a coughing episode, from obstruction during an episode, or from hypoxemia following an episode. Seizures usually are a result of hypoxemia, but hyponatremia from excessive secretion of antidiuretic hormone during pneumonia can occur. The only neuropathology documented in pertussis is parenchymal hemorrhage and ischemic necrosis.

Bronchiectasis has been reported rarely after pertussis. Children who have pertussis before age 2 yr may have abnormal pulmonary function into adulthood.

PREVENTION

Universal immunization of children with pertussis vaccine, beginning in infancy with reinforcing dose(s) through adolescence and adulthood, is central to the *control* of pertussis. *Prevention* of pertussis mortality in young infants depends on universal maternal immunization during each pregnancy and focused full immunization of contacts, both children and adults of all ages.

DTaP Vaccines

Several diphtheria and tetanus toxoids combined with acellular pertussis vaccines (**DTaP**) or combination products currently are licensed in the United States for children <7 yr old. Acellular pertussis vaccines all contain inactivated PT and 2 or more additional antigens (filamentous hemagglutinin, Prn, and Fim 2 and 3). Clinical effectiveness immediately at completion of the 5-dose series is approximately 80% for illness defined as "paroxysmal cough" for >21 days. Mild local and systemic adverse events are not uncommon, but more serious events (persistent crying for ≥3 hr, hypotonic hyporesponsive episodes, seizures) are rare. DTaP-containing vaccines can be administered simultaneously with any other vaccines used in the standard schedule for children.

Four doses of DTaP should be administered during the 1st 2 yr of life, generally at ages 2, 4, 6, and 15-18 mo. In high-risk settings, infants may be given DTaP as early as 6 wk of age, with monthly doses through the 3rd dose. The 4th dose may be administered as early as 12 mo of age, provided that 6 mo have elapsed since the 3rd dose. When feasible, the same DTaP product is recommended for all doses of the primary vaccination series. The 5th dose of DTaP is recommended for children at 4-6 yr of age; a 5th dose is not necessary if the 4th dose in the series is administered on or after the 4th birthday.

Local reactions increase modestly in rate and severity with successive doses of DTaP. Swelling of the entire thigh or upper arm, sometimes accompanied by pain, erythema, and fever, has been reported in 2–3% of vaccinees after the 4th or 5th dose of a variety of DTaP products. Limitation of activity is less than might be expected. Swelling subsides spontaneously without sequelae. The pathogenesis is unknown. Extensive limb swelling after the 4th dose of DTaP usually is not associated with a similar reaction to the 5th dose and is not a contraindication to subsequent dose(s) of pertussis vaccines.

Exempting children from pertussis immunization should be considered only within the narrow limits as recommended. Exemptors have significantly increased risk for pertussis and play a role in outbreaks of pertussis among immunized populations. Although well-documented pertussis confers short-term protection, the duration of protection is unknown; immunization should be completed on schedule in children diagnosed with pertussis.

Tdap Vaccines

Two tetanus toxoid, reduced-diphtheria toxoid and acellular pertussis antigen vaccine (Tdap) products were licensed in 2005 and recommended universally in 2006 for adolescents. The preferred age for Tdap vaccination is 11-12 yr. All adolescents and adults of any age (including ≥65 yr) who have not received Tdap should receive a single dose of Tdap promptly, regardless of interval since Td, or at least in place of one Td booster at the 10 yr interval, or when indicated during wound management.

Pregnant women should be given Tdap during every pregnancy to provide passive antibody protection to the infant until administration of DTaP. Although Tdap can be given at any time during pregnancy, optimal administration is early in the period between 27 and 36 wk of gestation to maximize antibody concentration at birth. Safety of Tdap during pregnancy and effectiveness in reducing fatal pertussis in infants are proven. Special effort should be made to ensure that contacts of infants have received DTaP or Tdap as recommended. There is no recommendation for Tdap revaccination of persons other than pregnant women. Although no safety issues are associated with Tdap revaccination, rapidly waning protection following receipt of currently available vaccines does not support cost-effectiveness of universal revaccination.

There is no contraindication to concurrent administration of any other indicated vaccine. When Td is indicated and only Tdap is available, a previously Tdap-immunized person can be given Tdap. A single dose of Tdap is recommended for children 7-10 yr old who had incomplete DTaP vaccination before age 7 yr. Another dose of Tdap can be given in adolescence.

Bibliography is available at Expert Consult.

Chapter **225**
Salmonella
Jeffrey S. McKinney
第二百二十五章
沙门菌

中文导读

　　本章主要介绍了非伤寒沙门菌感染的病因、流行病学、发病机制、临床表现、并发症、诊断、治疗、预后和预防，以及肠热（伤寒）的病因、流行病学、发病机制、临床表现、并发症、诊断、鉴别诊断、治疗、预后和预防等内容。其中，在非伤寒沙门菌感染的临床表现部分详细介绍了急性肠炎、菌血症、肠外局灶性感染和慢性沙门菌携带。在菌血症部分详细描述了非洲新兴疾病非伤寒沙门菌菌血症和其他地区的非伤寒沙门菌菌血症。

Salmonellosis is a common and widely distributed food-borne disease that is a global major public health problem affecting millions of individuals and resulting in significant mortality. **Salmonellae** live in the intestinal tracts of warm- and cold-blooded animals. Some species are ubiquitous, whereas others are specifically adapted to a particular host.

The sequencing of the *Salmonella enterica* serovar Typhi (previously called *Salmonella typhi*) and *Salmonella typhimurium* genomes indicates an almost 95% genetic homology between the organisms. However, the clinical diseases caused by the 2 organisms differ considerably. Orally ingested salmonellae survive at the low pH of the stomach and evade the multiple defenses of the small intestine so as to gain access to the epithelium. Salmonellae preferentially enter M cells, which transport them to the lymphoid cells (T and B) in the underlying Peyer patches. Once across the epithelium, *Salmonella* serotypes that are associated with systemic illness enter intestinal macrophages and disseminate throughout the reticuloendothelial system (RES). By contrast, most **nontyphoidal *Salmonella* (NTS)** serovars induce an early local inflammatory response, which results in the infiltration of polymorphonuclear leukocytes (PMNs) into the intestinal lumen and diarrhea. These NTS serovars cause a gastroenteritis of rapid onset and brief duration, in contrast to **typhoid fever**, which has a considerably longer incubation period and duration of illness and in which systemic illness predominates and only a small proportion of children have diarrhea.

These differences in the manifestations of infection by the 2 groups of pathogens, one predominantly causing intestinal inflammation and the other leading to systemic disease, may be related to specific genetic pathogenicity islands in the organisms. Most NTS serovars seem unable to overcome defense mechanisms that limit bacterial dissemination from the intestine to systemic circulation in immunocompetent individuals and produce a self-limiting **gastroenteritis**. In contrast, *S. typhi* and *S. paratyphi* (i.e., typhoidal strains of *Salmonella*) may possess unique virulence traits that allow them to overcome mucosal barrier functions in immunocompetent hosts, and cause severe systemic illness. Interestingly, the frequencies of typhoid fever in immunocompetent and immunocompromised individuals do not differ. Intriguingly, some invasive NTS strains have been noted in Africa, particularly among HIV-positive adults and among children with HIV, malaria, or malnutrition (see Chapter 225.1). The presentation may resemble typhoid fever more than gastroenteritis.

From a taxonomic, Linnaean, perspective, the genus *Salmonella* belongs to the family Enterobacteriaceae. Two *Salmonella* spp. exist: *Salmonella enterica* and *Salmonella bongori*. The medically relevant species is *Salmonella enterica*, which is further divided into serotypes and often named based on presumed syndromes they cause or where they were discovered geographically.

From a medical perspective, among the salmonellae causing human disease, serotypes are also clinically grouped as either being **typhoidal** or **nontyphoidal**. There are only a few typhoidal *Salmonella* serotypes, including *Salmonella enterica* var. Typhi, also known as *S.* Typhi, and *Salmonella enterica* var. Paratyphi A. By contrast, there are 1000s of nontyphoidal *Salmonella* serotypes, collectively called **NTS serotypes**. NTS serotypes have a broad host range, whereas *S.* Typhi and *S.* Paratyphi A are restricted to human hosts.

225.1 Nontyphoidal Salmonellosis
Jeffrey S. McKinney

ETIOLOGY
Salmonellae are motile, nonsporulating, nonencapsulated, gram-negative rods that grow aerobically and are capable of facultative anaerobic growth. They are resistant to many physical agents but can be killed by heating to 54.4°C (130°F) for 1 hr or 60°C (140°F) for 15 min. They remain

viable at ambient or reduced temperatures for days and may survive for weeks in sewage, dried foodstuffs, pharmaceutical agents, and fecal material. As with other members of the family Enterobacteriaceae, *Salmonella* possesses somatic O antigens and flagellar H antigens.

With the exception of a few serotypes that affect only one or a few animal species, such as *Salmonella dublin* in cattle and *S. choleraesuis* in pigs, most serotypes have a broad host spectrum. Typically, such strains cause gastroenteritis that is often uncomplicated and does not need treatment but can be severe in the young, the elderly, and patients with weakened immunity. The causes are typically **Salmonella** **Enteritidis** (*Salmonella enterica* var. Enteritidis) and **Salmonella Typhimurium** (*S. enterica* var. Typhimurium), the 2 most important serotypes for salmonellosis transmitted from animals to humans. Nontyphoidal salmonellae have emerged as a major cause of **bacteremia** in Africa, especially among populations with a high incidence of HIV infection.

EPIDEMIOLOGY

Salmonellosis constitutes a major public health burden and represents a significant cost to society in many countries. Typhoid fever caused by this organism is a global problem, with >27 million cases worldwide each year, culminating in an estimated 217,000 deaths. Although there is little information on the epidemiology and the burden of *Salmonella* gastroenteritis in developing countries, *Salmonella* infections are recognized as major causes of childhood diarrheal illness. With the burden of HIV infections and malnutrition in Africa, NTS bacteremic infections have emerged as a major cause of morbidity and mortality among children and adults.

NTS infections have a worldwide distribution, with an incidence proportional to the standards of hygiene, sanitation, availability of safe water, and food preparation practices. In the developed world, the incidence of *Salmonella* infections and outbreaks has increased several-fold over the past few decades, which may be related to modern practices of mass food production that increase the potential for epidemics. Infections with NTS serovars such as S. Typhimurium and S. Enteritidis cause a significant disease burden, with an estimated 93.8 million cases worldwide and 155,000 deaths each year. Traditionally, *Salmonella* gastroenteritis accounts for more than half of all episodes of bacterial diarrhea in the United States, with incidence peaks at the extremes of ages, among young infants and elderly persons. Most human infections have been caused by S. Enteritidis; with S. Typhimurium incidence overtaking it in some countries. Recently, however, a surveillance program testing human stool specimens from 10 U.S. sites showed a relative decline in the incidence of S. Typhimurium vs other salmonellae, perhaps related to the use of a live-attenuated S. Typhimurium vaccine in poultry and more stringent performance standards for *Salmonella* contamination of poultry carcasses.

Salmonella infections in many parts of the world may also be related to intensive **animal husbandry practices**, which selectively promote the rise of certain strains, especially drug-resistant varieties that emerge in response to the use of antimicrobials in food animals. Poultry products were traditionally regarded as a common source of salmonellosis, but consumption of a range of foods is now also associated with outbreaks, including fruits and vegetables, and factory-processed foods such as peanut butter or cookies. It appears that some **multidrug-resistant** (MDR) strains of *Salmonella* are also more virulent than susceptible strains, and that poorer outcome does not simply relate to the delay in treatment response because of empirical choice of an ineffective antibiotic. Strains of MDR *Salmonella*, such as S. Typhimurium phage type DT104, harbor a genomic island that contains many of the drug-resistance genes. These *integrons* also contain genes that encode virulence factors.

Several risk factors are associated with outbreaks of *Salmonella* infections. Animals constitute the principal source of human NTS disease, with cases occurring in individuals who have had contact with infected animals, including domestic animals such as cats, dogs, reptiles, pet rodents, and amphibians; **high-risk pets** include turtles, iguanas, bearded dragons, lizards, various snakes, salamanders, and geckos. Specific serotypes may be associated with particular animal hosts; children with *S. enterica* var. Marina typically have exposure to pet lizards. NTS serovars usually cause self-limiting diarrhea, with secondary bacteremia occurring

in <10% of patients. The NTS serovars have a broad host range, including poultry and cattle, and NTS infection is usually from food poisoning in developed countries.

Domestic animals probably acquire the infection in the same way that humans do, through oral ingestion. Animal feeds contaminated with *Salmonella* are an important source of infection for animals. Moreover, subtherapeutic concentrations of antibiotics are often added to animal feed to promote growth. Such practices promote the emergence of **antibiotic-resistant bacteria**, including *Salmonella*, in the gut flora of the animals, with subsequent contamination of their meat. There is strong evidence to link resistance of S. Typhimurium to fluoroquinolones with the use of this group of antimicrobials in animal feeds. Animal-to-animal transmission can occur, with most infected animals being asymptomatic.

Although almost 80% of *Salmonella* infections are discrete, outbreaks can pose an inordinate burden on public health systems. During 1998–2008, a total of 1,491 outbreaks of *Salmonella* infections were reported to the Foodborne Disease Outbreak Surveillance System, and 80% of these were caused by a single serotype. Of the single-serotype outbreaks, 50% had an implicated food, and 34% could be assigned to a single food commodity. Of the 47 serotypes reported, the 4 most common, causing more than two thirds of the outbreaks, were Enteritidis, Typhimurium, Newport, and Heidelberg. Overall, eggs were the most frequently implicated food, followed by chicken, pork, beef, fruit, and turkey. *Salmonella* infections in chickens increase the risk for contamination of eggs, and both poultry and eggs are regarded as a dominant cause of common-source outbreaks. However, a growing proportion of *Salmonella* outbreaks are also associated with other food sources. The food sources include many fruits and vegetables, such as tomatoes, sprouts, watermelon, cantaloupe, lettuce, and mangoes. Geographically distributed infections are increasingly possible from foods (e.g., peanut butter) processed at a "point source" and then broadly distributed. Contemporary surveillance and reporting networks (e.g., ProMED, FoodNet) may help alert physicians and microbiologists to such events.

In addition to the effect of antibiotic use in animal feeds, the relationship of *Salmonella* infections to prior antibiotic use among children in the previous month is well recognized. This increased risk for infection in people who have received antibiotics for an unrelated reason may be related to alterations in gut microbial ecology, which predispose them to colonization and infection with antibiotic-resistant *Salmonella* isolates. These resistant strains of *Salmonella* can also be more virulent. The Centers for Disease Control and Prevention (CDC) reports resistance to **ceftriaxone** in approximately 3% of NTS tested and some level of resistance to **ciprofloxacin** in 3% of isolates. Approximately 5% of NTS tested by the CDC are resistant to 5 or more types of drugs. Consequently, costs are also expected to be higher for resistant than for susceptible infections because of the severity of the former. These patients are more likely to be hospitalized, and treatment is rendered less effective. The CDC is seeing some level of resistance to ciprofloxacin in two thirds of S. Typhi tested. Resistance to ceftriaxone or **azithromycin** has been seen in other parts of the world. *Variation in resistance among different strains makes* Salmonella *microbiologic culture and antibacterial susceptibility testing very important.*

Given the ubiquitous nature of the organism, nosocomial infections with NTS strains can also occur through contaminated equipment and diagnostic or pharmacologic preparations, particularly those of animal origin (pancreatic extracts, pituitary extracts, bile salts, rattlesnake tail). Hospitalized children are at increased risk for severe and complicated *Salmonella* infections, especially with drug-resistant organisms.

PATHOGENESIS

The estimated number of bacteria that must be ingested to cause symptomatic disease in healthy adults is 10^6-10^8 *Salmonella* organisms. The gastric acidity inhibits multiplication of salmonellae, and most organisms are rapidly killed at gastric pH ≤2.0. Achlorhydria, buffering medications, rapid gastric emptying after gastrectomy or gastroenterostomy, and a large inoculum enable viable organisms to reach the small intestine. Neonates and young infants have hypochlorhydria and rapid gastric emptying, which contribute to their increased vulnerability

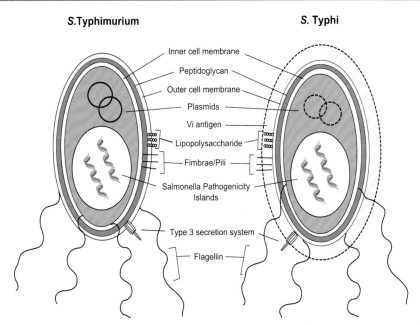

Fig. 225.1 Overlapping and distinct virulence systems in *Salmonella typhi* and nontyphoidal *Salmonella*. *(From de Jong HK, Parry CM, van der Poll T, Wiersinga WJ. Host-pathogen interaction in invasive Salmonellosis. PLoSPathog 2012;8(10):e1002933.)*

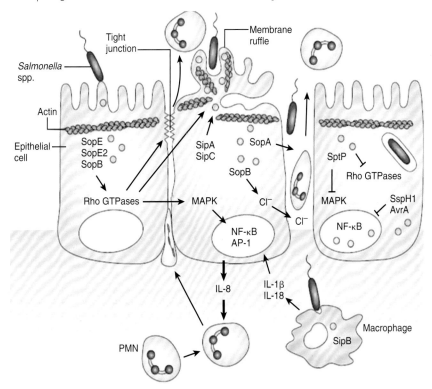

Fig. 225.2 On contact with the epithelial cell, salmonellae assemble the *Salmonella* pathogenicity island 1–encoded type III secretion system (TTSS-1) and translocate effectors (*yellow spheres*) into the eukaryotic cytoplasm. Effectors such as SopE, SopE2, and SopB then activate host Rho guanosine triphosphatase (GTPase), resulting in the rearrangement of the actin cytoskeleton into membrane ruffles, induction of mitogen-activated protein kinase (MAPK) pathways, and destabilization of tight junctions. Changes in the actin cytoskeleton, which are further modulated by the actin-binding proteins SipA and SipC, lead to bacterial uptake. MAPK signaling activates the transcription factors activator protein-1 (AP-1) and nuclear factor-κB (NF-κB), which turn on production of the proinflammatory polymorphonuclear leukocyte (PMN) chemokine interleukin (IL)-8. SipB induces caspase-1 activation in macrophages, with the release of IL-1β and IL-18, augmenting the inflammatory response. In addition, SopB stimulates Cl⁻ secretion by its inositol phosphatase activity. The destabilization of tight junctions allows the transmigration of PMNs from the basolateral to the apical surface, paracellular fluid leakage, and access of bacteria to the basolateral surface. However, the transmigration of PMNs also occurs in the absence of tight-junction disruption and is further promoted by SopA. The actin cytoskeleton is restored, and MAPK signaling is turned off by the enzymatic activities of SptP. This also results in the downmodulation of inflammatory responses, to which SspH1 and AvrA also contribute by inhibiting activation of NF-κB. *(From Haraga A, Ohlson MB, Miller SI: Salmonellae interplay with host cells, Nat Rev Microbiol 6:53–66, 2008.)*

to symptomatic salmonellosis. In infants who typically take fluids, the inoculum size required to produce disease is also comparatively smaller because of faster transit through the stomach.

Once they reach the small and large intestines, the ability of *Salmonella* organisms to multiply and cause infection depends on both the infecting dose and competition with normal flora. Prior antibiotic therapy may alter this relationship, as might factors such as co-administration of antimotility agents. The typical intestinal mucosal response to NTS infection is an **enterocolitis** with diffuse mucosal inflammation and edema, sometimes with erosions and microabscesses. *Salmonella* organisms are capable of penetrating the intestinal mucosa, although destruction of epithelial cells and ulcers are usually not found. Intestinal inflammation with PMNs and macrophages usually involves the lamina propria. Underlying intestinal lymphoid tissue and mesenteric lymph nodes enlarge and may demonstrate small areas of necrosis. Such lymphoid hypertrophy may cause interference with the blood supply to the gut mucosa. Hyperplasia of the RES is also found within the liver and spleen. If bacteremia develops, it may lead to localized infection and suppuration in almost any organ.

Both *S.* Typhi and NTS possess overlapping and distinct virulence systems (Fig. 225.1). Although *S.* Typhimurium can cause systemic disease in humans, intestinal infection usually results in a localized enteritis that is associated with a secretory response in the intestinal epithelium. Intestinal infection also induces secretion of interleukin (IL)-8 from the basolateral surface and other chemoattractants from the apical surface, directing recruitment and transmigration of neutrophils into the gut lumen and thus preventing the systemic spread of the bacteria (Fig. 225.2).

Central to *S.* Typhimurium pathogenesis are 2 **type III secretion** systems encoded within the pathogenicity islands **SPI-1** and **SPI-2**, which are responsible for the secretion and translocation of a set of bacterial proteins termed **effectors** into host cells; effectors are able to alter host cell physiology to facilitate bacterial entry and survival. Once delivered by the type III secretion systems, the secreted effectors play critical roles in manipulating the host cell to allow bacterial invasion, induction of inflammatory responses, and assembly of an intracellular protective niche conducive to bacterial survival and replication. The type III secretion system encoded on SPI-1 mediates invasion of the intestinal epithelium, whereas the type III secretion system encoded on SPI-2 is required for survival within macrophages. In addition, the expression of strong agonists of innate pattern recognition receptors (lipopolysaccharide and flagellin) is important for triggering a Toll-like receptor (TLR)–mediated inflammatory response.

Salmonella spp. invade epithelial cells in vitro by a process of bacteria-mediated endocytosis involving cytoskeletal rearrangement, disruption of the epithelial cell brush-border, and subsequent formation of membrane ruffles (Fig. 225.3). An adherent and invasive phenotype of *S.* Enterica is activated under conditions similar to those found in the human small intestine (high osmolarity, low oxygen). The invasive phenotype is mediated in part by SPI-1, a 40-kb region that encodes regulator proteins such as HilA and a variety of other products.

Shortly following invasion of the gut epithelium, invasive *Salmonella* organisms encounter macrophages within the gut-associated lymphoid tissue (GALT). The interaction between *Salmonella* and macrophages results in alteration in the expression of a number of host genes, including those encoding proinflammatory mediators (inducible nitric

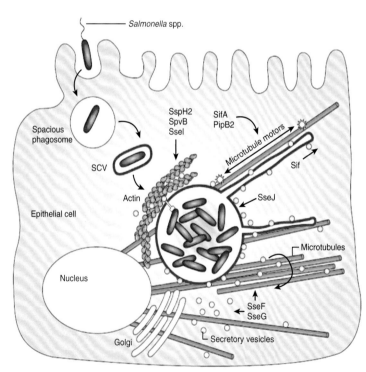

Fig. 225.3 Formation of the *Salmonella*-containing vacuole (SCV) and induction of the *Salmonella* pathogenicity island 2 (SPI-2) type III secretion system (TTSS) within the host cell. Shortly after internalization by macropinocytosis, salmonellae are enclosed in a spacious phagosome that is formed by membrane ruffles. Later, the phagosome fuses with lysosomes, acidifies, and shrinks to become adherent around the bacterium, and is called the SCV. It contains the endocytic marker lysosomal-associated membrane protein 1 (LAMP-1; *purple*). The *Salmonella* SPI-2 is induced within the SCV and translocates effector proteins *(yellow spheres)* across the phagosomal membrane several hours after phagocytosis. The SPI-2 effectors SifA and PipB2 contribute to formation of *Salmonella*-induced filament along microtubules *(green)* and regulate microtubule motor *(yellow star shape)* accumulation on the Sif and the SCV. SseJ is a deacylase that is active on the phagosome membrane. SseF and SseG cause microtubule bundling adjacent to the SCV and direct Golgi-derived vesicle traffic toward the SCV. Actin accumulates around the SCV in an SPI-2–dependent manner, in which SspH2, SpvB, and SseI are thought to have a role. *(From Haraga A, Ohlson MB, Miller SI: Salmonellae interplay with host cells, Nat Rev Microbiol 6:53–66, 2008.)*

oxide synthase, chemokines, IL-1β), receptors or adhesion molecules (tumor necrosis factor [TNF]-α receptor, CD40, intercellular adhesion molecule 1), and antiinflammatory mediators (transforming growth factor-β1, TGF-β2). Other upregulated genes include those involved in cell death or apoptosis (intestinal epithelial cell protease, TNF-R1, Fas) and transcription factors (early growth response 1, interferon [IFN] regulatory factor 1). *S.* Typhimurium can induce rapid macrophage death in vitro, which depends on the host cell protein caspase-1 and is mediated by the effector protein **SipB** (*Salmonella* invasion protein B). Intracellular *S.* Typhimurium is found within specialized vacuoles that have diverged from the normal endocytic pathway. This ability to survive within monocytes/macrophages is essential for *S.* Typhimurium to establish a systemic infection in the mouse. The mucosal proinflammatory response to *S.* Typhimurium infection and the subsequent recruitment of phagocytic cells to the site may also facilitate systemic spread of the bacteria.

Some virulence traits are shared by all salmonellae, but others are serotype restricted. These virulence traits have been defined in tissue culture and murine models, and it is likely that clinical features of human *Salmonella* infection will eventually be related to specific DNA sequences. With most diarrhea-associated nontyphoidal salmonelloses, the infection does not extend beyond the lamina propria and the local lymphatics. Specific virulence genes are related to the ability to cause bacteremia. These genes are found significantly more often in strains of *S.* Typhimurium isolated from the blood than in strains recovered from stool. Although both *S. dublin* and *S. choleraesuis* have a greater propensity to rapidly invade the bloodstream with little or no intestinal involvement, the development of disease after infection with *Salmonella* depends on the number of infecting organisms, their virulence traits, and several host defense factors. Various host factors may also affect the development of specific complications or clinical syndromes (Table 225.1); of these factors, HIV infections are assuming greater importance in Africa in all age-groups.

Bacteremia is possible with any *Salmonella* serotype, especially in individuals with reduced host defenses and especially in those with altered reticuloendothelial or cellular immune function. Thus, children with HIV infection, chronic granulomatous disease, and leukemia are more likely to develop bacteremia after *Salmonella* infection, although the majority of children with *Salmonella* bacteremia are HIV-negative. Children with *Schistosoma mansoni* infection and hepatosplenic involvement, as well as chronic malarial anemia, are also at a greater risk for development of chronic salmonellosis. Children with sickle cell disease are at increased risk for *Salmonella* septicemia and osteomyelitis. This risk may be related to the presence of numerous infarcted areas in the gastrointestinal (GI) tract, bones, and RES, as well as reduced phagocytic and opsonizing capacity of patients.

CLINICAL MANIFESTATIONS
Acute Enteritis
The most common clinical presentation of salmonellosis is acute enteritis. After an incubation period of 6-72 hr (mean: 24 hr), there is an abrupt onset of nausea, vomiting, and crampy abdominal pain, located primarily in the periumbilical area and right lower quadrant, followed by mild to severe watery diarrhea and sometimes by diarrhea containing blood and mucus. A large proportion of children with acute enteritis are febrile, although younger infants may exhibit a normal or subnormal temperature. Symptoms usually subside within 2-7 days in healthy children, and fatalities are rare. However, some children experience severe disease with a septicemia-like picture (high fever, headache, drowsiness, confusion, meningismus, seizures, abdominal distention). The stool typically contains a moderate number of PMNs and occult blood. Mild leukocytosis may be detected.

Bacteremia
Although the precise incidence of bacteremia following *Salmonella* gastroenteritis is unclear, transient bacteremia can occur in 1–5% of children with *Salmonella* diarrhea. Bacteremia can occur with minimal associated symptoms in newborns and very young infants, but in older infants it typically follows gastroenteritis and can be associated with fever, chills, and septic shock. In patients with AIDS, recurrent septicemia appears despite antibiotic therapy, often with a negative stool culture result for *Salmonella* and sometimes with no identifiable focus of infection. NTS GI infections typically cause bacteremia in developing countries.

Nontyphoidal *Salmonella* Bacteremia as Emerging Disease in Africa
In Africa, particularly sub-Saharan, NTS has been increasingly appreciated as among the most common causes of *all* bacteremia cases in febrile adults and children. Bacteremia from NTS in Africa has had an accompanying case fatality rate of 20–25%. Notably, children age 6-36 mo and adults age 30-50 yr are at greatest risk.

Clinical features among children with invasive NTS infections can be confusing, in that diarrhea is often *not* a prominent feature. Furthermore, 60% of children have an apparent lower respiratory tract infection focus (perhaps from co-infection or comorbidity). Fever is present in 95% of cases but may have no apparent focus. Fig. 225.4 summarizes other clinical features. Importantly, the lack of specificity of these clinical features severely compromises the ability of current clinical algorithms to identify invasive NTS infections. Accordingly, blood culture and clinical microbiology systems for bacterial growth, isolation, speciation, and antibacterial drug sensitivity testing are required for diagnosis and well-informed treatment decision-making. Among

Table 225.1	Host Factors and Conditions Predisposing to Development of Systemic Disease with Nontyphoidal *Salmonella* (NTS) Strains

Neonates and young infants (≤3 mo old)
HIV/AIDS
Other immunodeficiencies and chronic granulomatous disease
Defects in interferon γ production or action
Immunosuppressive and corticosteroid therapies
Malignancies, especially leukemia and lymphoma
Hemolytic anemia, including sickle cell disease, malaria, and
 bartonellosis
Collagen vascular disease
Inflammatory bowel disease
Achlorhydria or use of antacid medications
Impaired intestinal motility
Schistosomiasis, malaria
Malnutrition

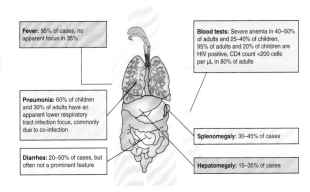

Fig. 225.4 Clinical features of invasive nontyphoidal *Salmonella* (NTS) disease in adults and children in Africa. (*From Feasey NA, Dougan G, Kingsley RA, et al: Invasive non-typhoidal* Salmonella *disease: an emerging and neglected tropical disease in Africa, Lancet 379: 2489–2499, 2012.*)

NTS isolates causing invasive systemic disease, the serotypes *S.* Typhimurium and *S.* Enteritidis have been frequently reported, but several other serotypes can cause invasive disease as well.

It remains unclear exactly why invasive infections by NTS seem so much more frequent in Africa, compared with the dominance of typhoidal *Salmonellae* in Asia. HIV infection is one identified host risk factor for NTS infection. Indeed, recurrent NTS infection was part of early CDC case definitions for the AIDS. However, only 20% of African children with NTS disease are HIV positive. Other risks for pediatric NTS may include recent or severe malaria infections, sickle cell anemia, active schistosomiasis, and malnutrition.

The epidemiologic patterns thus far appreciated for invasive infections by NTS in Africa suggest epidemics may occur over several years, peaking in the rainy season. However, it remains unclear as to the extent that invasive NTS infections are related to human diarrheal disease or GI carriage. Likewise, obvious food or animal sources of invasive NTS in humans have not been conclusively identified, and the relative role(s) of zoonotic and/or anthroponotic transmission is uncertain. Thus, optimal strategies for interrupting transmission of invasive NTS infections remain unclear. This is particularly problematic, given the emergence of antibacterial drug resistance that has also been noted among NTS organisms, including the multidrug-resistant strain referred to as (DNA multilocus "sequence type") ST313.

For invasive NTS infections in Africa, resistance to ampicillin, chloramphenicol, and co-trimoxazole may force increasing reliance on more expensive treatment options. Depending on local resistance patterns, drug availability, and patient state, empirical treatments may require third-generation cephalosporins (e.g., ceftriaxone), fluoroquinolones (e.g., ciprofloxacin), or macrolide/azalides (e.g., azithromycin). Of note, while *Salmonella* strains may be killed in culture in vitro by aminoglycosides, this drug class is not appropriate for treatment of invasive salmonellae, because aminoglycosides are not able to penetrate the intracellular niches in hosts that salmonellae so effectively exploit as part of their life cycle.

Nontyphoidal *Salmonella* Bacteremia in Other Geographic Regions

The emergence of invasive, high-mortality NTS infections in sub-Saharan Africa suggests that historical clinical divisions of *Salmonella* infections into typhoidal and nontyphoidal may become problematic oversimplification. Currently, however, in settings outside sub-Saharan Africa, NTS infections still tend to be self-limiting and noninvasive and are low-mortality events for most children who are immunocompetent. Risk factors for systemic spread of NTS include HIV infection, diabetes, sickle cell disease, systemic corticosteroid use, malignancy, chronic liver or kidney disease, chronic granulomatous disease, B-cell deficiencies, and dysfunction of proinflammatory cytokine pathways. Neonates and infants are also at particular risk for disseminated infection and thus warrant more aggressive evaluation and treatment.

Extraintestinal Focal Infections

Following bacteremia, salmonellae have the propensity to seed and cause focal suppurative infection of many organs. The most common focal infections involve the skeletal system, meninges, intravascular sites, and sites of preexisting abnormalities. The peak incidence of *Salmonella* meningitis is in infancy, and the infection may be associated with a florid clinical course, high mortality, and neurologic sequelae in survivors.

Chronic *Salmonella* Carriage

While traditionally viewed primarily as a complication of *Salmonella* infection among adults, *Salmonella* chronic carriage has important medical and epidemiologic implications, and may occur in children. Colonization of the gallbladder by *Salmonella typhi* has long been appreciated, but reports suggest that some nontyphoidal *Salmonella* (e.g., invasive NTS currently in Africa) can also establish long-term asymptomatic carriage states.

Antibacterial treatments of *Salmonella* infections are paradoxical, in that the prospect of becoming a chronic carrier is believed to be increased by exposure to antibacterial agents. Yet, clearance of established chronic carrier status requires prolonged medical treatment using antibacterial agents to which the relevant *Salmonella* strain is susceptible and sometimes requires gallstone or gallbladder removal. Chronic carriers of *Salmonella* may only have intermittently positive stool cultures and are often asymptomatic, which makes approaches to diagnosis and treatment especially complex.

COMPLICATIONS

Salmonella gastroenteritis can be associated with acute dehydration and complications that result from delayed presentation and inadequate treatment. Bacteremia in younger infants and immunocompromised individuals can have serious consequences and potentially fatal outcomes. *Salmonella* organisms can seed many organ systems, including causing osteomyelitis in children, particularly among children with sickle cell disease. Reactive arthritis may follow *Salmonella* gastroenteritis, especially in adolescents with the HLA-B27 antigen.

In certain high-risk groups, especially those with impaired immunity, the course of *Salmonella* gastroenteritis may be more complicated. Neonates, infants <6 mo old, and children with primary or secondary immunodeficiency may have symptoms that persist for several weeks. The course of illness and complications may also be affected by coexisting pathologies. In children with AIDS, *Salmonella* infection frequently becomes widespread and overwhelming, causing multisystem involvement, septic shock, and death. In patients with inflammatory bowel disease, especially active ulcerative colitis, *Salmonella* gastroenteritis may lead to rapid development of toxic megacolon, bacterial translocation, and sepsis. In children with schistosomiasis, the *Salmonella* may persist and multiply within schistosomes, leading to chronic infection unless the schistosomiasis is effectively treated. Prolonged or intermittent bacteremia is associated with low-grade fever, anorexia, weight loss, diaphoresis, and myalgias and may occur in children with RES dysfunction, which can be associated with underlying problems such as hemolytic anemia or malaria.

DIAGNOSIS

Few clinical features are specific to *Salmonella* gastroenteritis to allow differentiation from other bacterial causes of diarrhea. Definitive diagnosis of *Salmonella* infection is based on clinical correlation of the presentation and culture of and subsequent identification of *Salmonella* organisms from feces or other body fluids. In children with gastroenteritis, stool cultures have higher yields than rectal swabs. In children with NTS gastroenteritis, prolonged fever lasting ≥5 days and young age should be recognized as associated with development of bacteremia. In patients with sites of local suppuration, aspirated specimens should be Gram-stained and cultured. *Salmonella* organisms grow well on nonselective or enriched media, such as blood agar, chocolate agar, and nutrient broth, but stool specimens containing mixed bacterial flora require a selective medium, such as MacConkey, xylose-lysine-deoxycholate, bismuth sulfite, or *Salmonella-Shigella* (SS) agar for isolation of *Salmonella*.

Culture-independent diagnostic tests have some utility for screening or epidemiologic studies, but *without susceptibility results,* these tests do not show which drugs will be effective for any given patient.

TREATMENT

Appropriate therapy relates to the specific clinical presentation of *Salmonella* infection. In children with gastroenteritis, rapid clinical assessment, correction of dehydration and electrolyte disturbances, and supportive care are key. Antibiotics are not generally recommended for the treatment of isolated uncomplicated *Salmonella* gastroenteritis, because they may disrupt normal intestinal flora and prolong the excretion of *Salmonella* and increase the risk for creating a chronic carrier state. However, given the risk for bacteremia in young infants (<3 mo old) and the risk of disseminated infection in high-risk groups with immune compromise (HIV, malignancies, immunosuppressive therapy, sickle cell anemia, immunodeficiency states), these children must receive an appropriate empirically chosen antibiotic until culture results are available (Table 225.2). The *S.* Typhimurium phage type

Table 225.2	Treatment of *Salmonella* Gastroenteritis

ORGANISM AND INDICATION

Salmonella infections in infants <3 mo old or in
immunocompromised persons (in addition to appropriate
treatment for underlying disorder)

DOSE AND DURATION OF TREATMENT

Cefotaxime,[†] 100-200 mg/kg/day every 6-8 hr for 5-14 days*
or
Ceftriaxone, 75 mg/kg/day once daily for 7 days*
or
Ampicillin, 100 mg/kg/day every 6-8 hr for 7 days*
or
Cefixime, 15 mg/kg/day for 7-10 days*

*A blood culture should be obtained prior to antibiotic therapy. In a well
appearing immunocompetent child without evidence of disseminated disease,
a single dose of ceftriaxone may be given followed by oral azithromycin;
ampicillin, trimethoprim-sulfamethoxazole, or a fluoroquinolone may be
substituted once sensitivities are known.

    [†]If available.

DT104 strain is usually resistant to the following 5 drugs: ampicillin,
chloramphenicol, streptomycin, sulfonamides, and tetracycline. An
increasing proportion of *S.* Typhimurium phage type DT104 isolates
also have reduced susceptibility to fluoroquinolones. *Given the higher
mortality associated with multidrug-resistant* Salmonella i*nfections, it is
necessary to perform susceptibility tests on all human isolates. Infections
with suspected drug-resistant* Salmonella *should be closely monitored and
treated with appropriate antimicrobial therapy.*

PROGNOSIS

Most healthy children with *Salmonella* gastroenteritis recover fully.
However, malnourished children and children who do not receive optimal
supportive treatment are at risk for development of prolonged diarrhea
and complications. Young infants and immunocompromised patients
often have systemic involvement, a prolonged course, and extraintestinal
foci. In particular, children with HIV infection and *Salmonella* infections
can have a florid course.

After infection, NTS are excreted in feces for a median of 5 wk. A
prolonged carrier state after nontyphoidal salmonellosis is rare but may
be seen in children, particularly those with biliary tract disease and
cholelithiasis after chronic hemolysis. During the period of *Salmonella*
excretion, the individual may infect others, directly by the fecal-oral
route or indirectly by contaminating foods.

PREVENTION

Control of the transmission of *Salmonella* infections to humans requires
control of the infection in the animal reservoir, judicious use of antibiotics in dairy and livestock farming, prevention of contamination of
foodstuffs prepared from animals, and use of appropriate standards
in food processing in commercial and private kitchens. Because large
outbreaks are often related to mass food production, it should be recognized that contamination of just one piece of machinery used in food
processing may cause an outbreak; meticulous cleaning of equipment
is essential. Clean water supply and education in handwashing and
food preparation and storage are critical to reducing person-to-person
transmission. *Salmonella* may remain viable when cooking practices
prevent food from reaching a temperature >65.5°C (150°F) for >12 min.
Parents should be advised of the risk of various pets(classically including
reptiles and amphibians but also rodents) and be given recommendations for preventing transmission from these frequently infected hosts
(Table 225.3).

In contrast to the situation in developed countries, relatively little is
known about the transmission of NTS infections in developing countries,
and person-to-person transmission may be relatively more important
in some settings. Although some vaccines have been used in animals,
no human vaccine against NTS infections is currently available. Infections
should be reported to public health authorities so that outbreaks can

Table 225.3	Recommendations for Preventing Transmission of *Salmonella* from Reptiles and Amphibians to Humans

Pet store owners, healthcare providers, and veterinarians should
   provide information to owners and potential purchasers of reptiles
   and amphibians about the risks for and prevention of
   salmonellosis from these pets.
Persons at increased risk for infection or serious complications from
   salmonellosis (e.g., children <5 yr old, immunocompromised
   persons) should avoid contact with reptiles and amphibians and
   any items that have been in contact with reptiles and amphibians.
Reptiles and amphibians should be kept out of households that
   include children <5 yr old or immunocompromised persons.
   A family expecting a child should remove any pet reptile or
   amphibian from the home before the infant arrives.
Reptiles and amphibians should not be allowed in childcare
   centers.
Persons should always wash their hands thoroughly with soap and
   water after handling reptiles and amphibians or their cages.
Reptiles and amphibians should not be allowed to roam freely
   throughout a home or living area.
Pet reptiles and amphibians should be kept out of kitchens and
   other food preparation areas. Kitchen sinks should not be used to
   bathe reptiles and amphibians or to wash their dishes, cages, or
   aquariums. If bathtubs are used for these purposes, they should
   be cleaned thoroughly and disinfected with bleach.
Reptiles and amphibians in public settings (e.g., zoos, exhibits)
   should be kept from direct or indirect contact with patrons except
   in designated "animal contact" areas equipped with adequate
   handwashing facilities. Food and drink should not be allowed in
   animal contact areas.

From Centers for Disease Control and Prevention: Reptile-associated
salmonellosis—selected states, 1998–2002, *MMWR* 52:1206–1210, 2003.

be recognized and investigated. Given the rapid rise of antimicrobial
resistance among *Salmonella* isolates, it is imperative that there is rigorous
regulation of the use of antimicrobials in animal feeds.

Bibliography is available at Expert Consult.

225.2 Enteric Fever (Typhoid Fever)
Jeffrey S. McKinney

Enteric fever (more commonly termed *typhoid fever*) remains endemic
in many developing countries. Given the ease of modern travel, cases
are regularly reported from most developed countries, usually from
returning travelers.

ETIOLOGY

Typhoid fever is caused by *S. enterica* serovar Typhi (*S.* Typhi), a gram-
negative bacterium. A very similar but often less severe disease is caused
by *Salmonella* Paratyphi A and rarely by *S.* Paratyphi B (Schotmulleri)
and *S.* Paratyphi C (Hirschfeldii). The ratio of disease caused by *S.*
Typhi to that caused by *S.* Paratyphi is approximately 10:1, although
the proportion of *S.* Paratyphi A infections is increasing in some parts
of the world, for reasons that are unclear. Although *S.* Typhi shares
many genes with *Escherichia coli* and at least 95% of genes with *S.*
Typhimurium, several unique gene clusters known as *pathogenicity
islands* and other genes have been acquired during evolution. The
inactivation of single genes as well as the acquisition or loss of single
genes or large islands of DNA may have contributed to host adaptation
and restriction of *S.* Typhi.

EPIDEMIOLOGY

It is estimated that >26.9 million typhoid fever cases occur annually,
of which 1% result in death. The vast majority of this disease burden

is witnessed in Asia. Additionally, an estimated 5.4 million cases caused by paratyphoid occur each year. In 2010, 13.5 million cases of typhoid fever were recorded, and both typhoid and paratyphoid fevers together accounted for >12 million disability-adjusted life-years. The mortality caused by typhoid fever in the same year was found to be 7.2 per 100,000 population for sub-Saharan Africa. Given the paucity of microbiologic facilities in developing countries, these figures may be more representative of the clinical syndrome rather than of culture-proven disease. In most developed countries, the incidence of typhoid fever is <15 cases per 100,000 population, with most cases occurring in travelers. In contrast, the incidence may vary considerably in the developing world, with estimated rates ranging from 100-1,000 cases per 100,000 population. There are significant differences in the age distribution and population at risk. Population-based studies from South Asia also indicate that the age-specific incidence of typhoid fever may be highest in children <5 yr old, in association with comparatively higher rates of complications and hospitalization.

Typhoid fever is notable for the emergence of drug resistance. Following sporadic outbreaks of chloramphenicol-resistant *S.* Typhi infections, many strains of *S.* Typhi have developed plasmid-mediated multidrug resistance to all 3 of the primary antimicrobials: ampicillin, chloramphenicol, and trimethoprim-sulfamethoxazole. There is also a considerable increase in nalidixic acid–resistant and even ceftriaxone-resistant isolates of *S.* Typhi, as well as the emergence of fluoroquinolone-resistant isolates. Nalidixic acid–resistant isolates first emerged in Southeast Asia and India and now account for the majority of travel-associated cases of typhoid fever in the United States. Given the ongoing global movement of resistant *S.* Typhi, an international awareness of resistance patterns is needed for effective patient care.

S. Typhi is highly adapted to infection of humans to the point that it has lost the ability to cause transmissible disease in other animals. The discovery of the large number of pseudogenes in *S.* Typhi suggests that the genome of this pathogen has undergone degeneration to facilitate a specialized association with the human host. Thus, direct or indirect contact with an infected person (sick or chronic carrier) is a prerequisite for infection. Ingestion of foods or water contaminated with *S.* Typhi from human feces is the most common mode of transmission, although water-borne outbreaks as a consequence of poor sanitation or contamination have been described in developing countries. In other parts of the world, oysters and other shellfish cultivated in water contaminated by sewage and the use of night soil as fertilizer may also cause infection.

PATHOGENESIS

Enteric fever occurs through the ingestion of the organism, and a variety of sources of fecal contamination have been reported, including street foods and contamination of water reservoirs.

Human volunteer experiments established an infecting dose of about 10^5-10^9 organisms, with an incubation period ranging from 4-14 days, depending on the inoculating dose of viable bacteria. After ingestion, *S.* Typhi organisms are thought to invade the body through the gut mucosa in the terminal ileum, possibly through specialized antigen-sampling cells known as *M cells* that overlie GALT, through enterocytes, or via a paracellular route. *S.* Typhi crosses the intestinal mucosal barrier after attachment to the microvilli by an intricate mechanism involving membrane ruffling, actin rearrangement, and internalization in an intracellular vacuole. In contrast to NTS, *S.* Typhi expresses virulence factors that allow it to downregulate the pathogen recognition receptor–mediated host inflammatory response. Within the Peyer patches in the terminal ileum, *S.* Typhi can traverse the intestinal barrier through several mechanisms, including the M cells in the follicle-associated epithelium, epithelial cells, and dendritic cells. At the villi, *Salmonella* can enter through the M cells or by passage through or between compromised epithelial cells.

On contact with the epithelial cell, *S.* Typhi assembles type III secretion system encoded on SPI-1 and translocates effectors into the cytoplasm. These effectors activate host Rho guanosine triphosphatases, resulting in the rearrangement of the actin cytoskeleton into membrane ruffles, induction of mitogen-activated protein kinase (MAPK) pathways, and

destabilization of tight junctions. Changes in the actin cytoskeleton are further modulated by the actin-binding proteins SipA and SipC and lead to bacterial uptake. MAPK signaling activates the transcription factors activator protein (AP)-1 and nuclear factor (NF)-κB, which turn on production of IL-8. The destabilization of tight junctions allows the transmigration of PMNs from the basolateral surface to the apical surface, paracellular fluid leakage, and access of bacteria to the basolateral surface. Shortly after internalization of *S.* Typhi by macropinocytosis, salmonellae are enclosed in a spacious phagosome formed by membrane ruffles. Later, the phagosome fuses with lysosomes, acidifies, and shrinks to become adherent around the bacterium, forming the *Salmonella*-containing vacuole. A 2nd type III secretion system encoded on SPI-2 is induced within the *Salmonella*-containing vacuole and translocates effector proteins SifA and PipB2, which contribute to *Salmonella*-induced filament formation along microtubules.

After passing through the intestinal mucosa, *S.* Typhi organisms enter the mesenteric lymphoid system and then pass into the bloodstream via the lymphatics. This primary bacteremia is usually asymptomatic, and blood culture results are frequently negative at this stage of the disease. The bloodborne bacteria are disseminated throughout the body and are thought to colonize the organs of the RES, where they may replicate within macrophages. After a period of bacterial replication, *S.* Typhi organisms are shed back into the blood, causing a secondary bacteremia that coincides with the onset of clinical symptoms and marks the end of the incubation period (Fig. 225.5).

In vitro studies with human cell lines have shown qualitative and quantitative differences in the epithelial cell response to *S.* Typhi and *S.* Typhimurium with regard to cytokine and chemokine secretion. Thus, perhaps by avoiding the triggering of an early inflammatory response in the gut, *S.* Typhi can instead colonize deeper tissues and organ systems. Infection with *S.* Typhi produces an inflammatory response in the deeper mucosal layers and underlying lymphoid tissue, with hyperplasia of Peyer patches and subsequent necrosis and sloughing of overlying epithelium. The resulting ulcers can bleed but usually heal without scarring or stricture formation. The inflammatory lesion may occasionally penetrate the muscularis and serosa of the intestine and produce perforation. The mesenteric lymph nodes, liver, and spleen are hyperemic and generally have areas of focal necrosis as well. A mononuclear response may be seen in the bone marrow in association with areas of focal necrosis. The morphologic changes of *S.* Typhi infection are less prominent in infants than in older children and adults.

Several virulence factors, including the type III secretion system encoded on SPI-2, may be necessary for the virulence properties and ability to cause systemic infection. The surface Vi (virulence) polysaccharide capsular antigen found in *S.* Typhi interferes with phagocytosis by preventing the binding of C3 to the surface of the bacterium. The ability of organisms to survive within macrophages after phagocytosis is an important virulence trait encoded by the PhoP regulon and may be related to metabolic effects on host cells. The occasional occurrence of diarrhea may be explained by the presence of a toxin related to cholera toxin and *E. coli* heat-labile enterotoxin. *The clinical syndrome of fever and systemic symptoms is produced by a release of proinflammatory cytokines (IL-6, IL-1β, and TNF-α) from the infected cells.*

Characterization of a toxin, referred to as the **typhoid toxin**, represents a major advance in understanding *Salmonella* biology; with implications for longstanding observations about typhoidal vs nontyphoidal disease features, and the human host restriction of typhoidal infections. Although the exact role of typhoid toxin in disease pathophysiology is still being elucidated, the enzymatically active subunits of typhoid toxin are CdtB and PltA, which are, respectively, a cytothelial distending toxin (a DNase that causes double-stranded breaks in host cell DNA) and a pertussis-like toxin (with ADP-ribosyltransferase activity). These 2 active "A" subunits form a unique A_2B_5 architecture with a heptomeric set of PltB "B" subunits. The trafficking of the A_2B_5 typhoid toxin uses an elegant autocrine/paracrine delivery mechanism, which passes through the *Salmonella*-containing vesicle environment, where it is dependent on effectors released by the *Salmonella* pathogenicity island 2–encoded type III secretion system. After assembly in this host intracellular niche so characteristic of *Salmonella* biology, the typhoid exotoxin is exported

Pathogenesis of typhoid fever

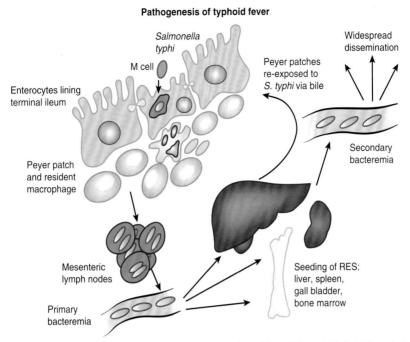

Fig. 225.5 Pathogenesis of typhoid fever. *RES*, Reticuloendothelial system. *(Adapted from Richens J: Typhoid fever. In Cohen J, Powderly WG, Opal SM, editors: Infectious diseases, ed 2, London, 2004, Mosby, pp 1561–1566.)*

into the *extracellular* space. Typhoid toxin binds a range of different glycans but has a preference for those with terminal sialic acids, notably sialoglycans terminated in Neu5Ac. Intriguingly, humans have a dominance of these glycans compared with other species. Accordingly, typhoid toxin binding preferences may help explain the human restriction of typhoidal infections and pathophysiology at a molecular level.

Importantly, S. Typhi and S. Paratyphi both express typhoid toxin, whereas "nontyphoidal" *Salmonella* spp. do not. Not only does this offer the prospect that typhoid toxin may help explain important clinical distinctions between typhoidal and nontyphoidal *Salmonella* infections, it raises hopes for new approaches to disease treatment and diagnostics. For example, antitoxin-based vaccines, therapeutics, or diagnostic tests might finally address the full microbiologic range of typhoid fever(s), because the typhoid toxin is conserved among not only S. Typhi but also S. Paratyphi isolates.

In addition to the virulence of the infecting organisms, host factors and immunity may also play an important role in predisposition to infection. Patients who are infected with HIV are at significantly higher risk for clinical infection with S. Typhi and S. Paratyphi. Similarly, patients with *Helicobacter pylori* infection have an increased risk of acquiring typhoid fever.

CLINICAL MANIFESTATIONS

The incubation period of typhoid fever is usually 7-14 days but depends on the infecting dose and ranges between 3 and 30 days. The clinical presentation varies from a mild illness with low-grade fever, malaise, and slight, dry cough to a severe clinical picture with abdominal discomfort and multiple complications.

Many factors influence the severity and overall clinical outcome of the infection. They include the duration of illness before the initiation of appropriate therapy, choice of antimicrobial treatment, age, previous exposure or vaccination history, virulence of the bacterial strain, quantity of inoculum ingested, and several host factors affecting immune status.

The presentation of typhoid fever may also differ according to age. Although data from South America and parts of Africa suggest that typhoid may manifest as a mild illness in young children, presentation may vary in different parts of the world. There is emerging evidence from South Asia that the presentation of typhoid may be more dramatic

in children <5 yr old, with comparatively higher rates of complications and hospitalization. Diarrhea, toxicity, and complications such as disseminated intravascular coagulation (DIC) are also more common in infancy, resulting in higher case fatality rates. However, some of the other features and complications of typhoid fever seen in adults, such as neurologic manifestations and GI bleeding, are rare in children.

Typhoid fever usually manifests as high-grade fever with a wide variety of associated features, such as generalized myalgia, abdominal pain, hepatosplenomegaly, and anorexia (Table 225.4). In children, diarrhea may occur in the earlier stages of the illness and may be followed by constipation. In the absence of localizing signs, the early stage of the disease may be difficult to differentiate from other endemic diseases, such as malaria and dengue fever. In approximately 25% of cases, a macular or maculopapular rash ("rose spots") may be visible around the 7th-10th day of the illness, and lesions may appear in crops of 10-15 on the lower chest and abdomen and last 2-3 days (Fig. 225.6). These lesions may be difficult to see in dark-skinned children. Patients managed as outpatients present with fever (99%) but have less emesis, diarrhea, hepatomegaly, splenomegaly, and myalgias than patients who require hospital admission.

The presentation of typhoid fever may be modified by coexisting morbidities and early diagnosis and administration of antibiotics. In malaria-endemic areas and in parts of the world where schistosomiasis is common, the presentation of typhoid may also be atypical. *It is also recognized that multidrug-resistant (MDR) S. Typhi infection is a more severe clinical illness with higher rates of toxicity, complications, and case fatality rates, which may be related to the greater virulence as well as higher numbers of circulating bacteria.* The emergence of typhoid infections resistant to nalidixic acid and fluoroquinolones is associated with higher rates of morbidity and treatment failure. These findings may have implications for treatment algorithms, especially in endemic areas with high rates of MDR and nalidixic acid– or fluoroquinolone-resistant typhoid.

If no complications occur, the symptoms and physical findings gradually resolve within 2-4 wk; however, the illness may be associated with malnutrition in a number of affected children. Although enteric fever caused by S. Paratyphi organisms has been classically regarded as a milder illness, there have been several outbreaks of infection with

Table 225.4	Common Clinical Features of Typhoid Fever in Children*	
FEATURE		**RATE (%)**
High-grade fever		95
Coated tongue		76
Anorexia		70
Vomiting		39
Hepatomegaly		37
Diarrhea		36
Toxicity		29
Abdominal pain		21
Pallor		20
Splenomegaly		17
Constipation		7
Headache		4
Jaundice		2
Obtundation		2
Ileus		1
Intestinal perforation		0.5

*Data collected in Karachi, Pakistan, from 2,000 children.

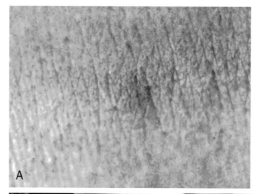
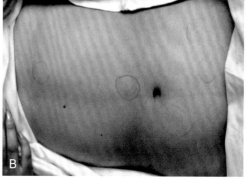

Fig. 225.6 A, "Rose spot" in volunteer with experimental typhoid fever. **B,** Small cluster of rose spots is usually located on the abdomen. These lesions may be difficult to identify, especially in dark-skinned people. *(From Huang DB, DuPont HL: Problem pathogens: extra-intestinal complications of* Salmonella enterica *serotype* Typhi *infection,* Lancet Infect Dis 5:341–348, 2005.)

drug-resistant *S.* Paratyphi A, suggesting that paratyphoid fever may also be severe, with significant morbidity and complications.

COMPLICATIONS

Although altered liver function is found in many patients with enteric fever, clinically significant hepatitis, jaundice, and cholecystitis are relatively rare and may be associated with higher rates of adverse outcome. Intestinal hemorrhage (<1%) and perforation (0.5–1%) are infrequent among children. Intestinal perforation may be preceded by a marked increase in abdominal pain (usually in the right lower quadrant), tenderness, vomiting, and features of peritonitis. Intestinal perforation and peritonitis may be accompanied by a sudden rise in pulse rate, hypotension, marked abdominal tenderness and guarding, and subsequent abdominal rigidity. A rising white blood cell count with a left shift and free air on abdominal radiographs may be seen in such cases.

Rare complications include toxic myocarditis, which may manifest as arrhythmias, sinoatrial block, or cardiogenic shock (Table 225.5). Neurologic complications are also relatively uncommon among children; they include delirium, psychosis, increased intracranial pressure, acute cerebellar ataxia, chorea, deafness, and Guillain-Barré syndrome. Although case fatality rates may be higher with neurologic manifestations, recovery usually occurs with no sequelae. Other reported complications include fatal bone marrow necrosis, DIC, hemolytic-uremic syndrome, pyelonephritis, nephrotic syndrome, meningitis, endocarditis, parotitis, orchitis, and suppurative lymphadenitis.

The propensity to become a carrier follows the epidemiology of gallbladder disease, increasing with patient age and the antibiotic resistance of the prevalent strains. Although limited data are available, rates of chronic carriage are generally lower in children than adults.

DIAGNOSIS

The mainstay of the diagnosis of typhoid fever is a positive result of culture from the blood or another anatomic site. Results of blood cultures are positive in 40–60% of the patients seen early in the course of the disease, and serial blood cultures may be required to identify *Salmonella* bacteremia. Stool and urine culture results may become positive after the 1st wk. The stool culture result is also occasionally positive during the incubation period. The sensitivity of blood cultures in diagnosing typhoid fever in many parts of the developing world is limited. Widespread liberal antibiotic use may render bacteriologic confirmation even more difficult. Bone marrow cultures may increase the likelihood of bacteriologic confirmation of typhoid and may provide a diagnosis for patients with classic fever of unknown origin caused by *Salmonella*. Still, collection of bone marrow specimens is difficult and relatively invasive.

Results of other laboratory investigations are nonspecific. Although blood leukocyte counts are frequently low in relation to the fever and toxicity, there is a wide range in counts; in younger children leukocytosis is common and may reach 20,000-25,000 cells/µL. Thrombocytopenia may be a marker of severe illness and may accompany DIC. Liver function test results may be deranged, but significant hepatic dysfunction is rare.

The classic **Widal test** measures antibodies against O and H antigens of *S.* Typhi but lacks sensitivity and specificity in endemic areas. Because many false-positive and false-negative results occur, diagnosis of typhoid fever by Widal test alone is prone to error. Other relatively newer diagnostic tests using monoclonal antibodies have been developed that directly detect *S.* Typhi–specific antigens in the serum or *S.* Typhi Vi antigen in the urine. However, few have proved sufficiently robust in large-scale evaluations. A nested polymerase chain reaction (PCR) analysis using *H1-d* primers has been used to amplify specific genes of *S.* Typhi in the blood of patients; it is a promising means of making a rapid diagnosis, especially given the low level of bacteremia in enteric fever. Despite these innovations, the mainstay of diagnosis of typhoid remains clinical in much of the developing world, and several diagnostic algorithms have been evaluated in endemic areas.

Table 225.5	Extraintestinal Infectious Complications of Typhoid Fever Caused by *Salmonella enterica* Serotype Typhi		
ORGAN SYSTEM	**PREVALENCE (%)**	**RISK FACTORS**	**COMPLICATIONS**
Central nervous system	3-35	Residence in endemic region, malignancy, endocarditis, congenital heart disease, paranasal sinus infections, pulmonary infections, meningitis, trauma, surgery, osteomyelitis of skull	Encephalopathy, cerebral edema, subdural empyema, cerebral abscess, meningitis, ventriculitis, transient Parkinsonism, motor neuron disorders, ataxia, seizures, Guillain-Barré syndrome, psychosis
Cardiovascular system	1-5	Cardiac abnormalities—e.g., existing valvular abnormalities, rheumatic heart disease, congenital heart defects	Endocarditis, myocarditis, pericarditis, arteritis, congestive heart failure
Pulmonary system	1-6	Residence in endemic region, past pulmonary infection, sickle cell anemia, alcohol abuse, diabetes, HIV infection	Pneumonia, empyema, bronchopleural fistula
Bone and joint	<1	Sickle cell anemia, diabetes, systemic lupus erythematosus, lymphoma, liver disease, previous surgery or trauma, extremes of age, corticosteroid use	Osteomyelitis, septic arthritis
Hepatobiliary system	1-26	Residence in endemic region, pyogenic infections, intravenous drug use, splenic trauma, HIV, hemoglobinopathy	Cholecystitis, hepatitis, hepatic abscesses, splenic abscess, peritonitis, paralytic ileus
Genitourinary system	<1	Urinary tract abnormalities, pelvic pathology, systemic abnormalities	Urinary tract infection, renal abscess, pelvic infections, testicular abscess, prostatitis, epididymitis
Soft tissue infections	At least 17 cases reported in English-language literature	Diabetes	Psoas abscess, gluteal abscess, cutaneous vasculitis
Hematologic	At least 5 cases reported in English-language literature		Hemophagocytosis syndrome

From Huang DB, DuPont HL: Problem pathogens: extra-intestinal complications of *Salmonella enterica* serotype Typhi infection, *Lancet Infect Dis* 5:341–348, 2005.

DIFFERENTIAL DIAGNOSIS

In endemic areas, typhoid fever may mimic many common febrile illnesses without localizing signs. In children with multisystem features and no localizing signs, the early stages of enteric fever may be confused with alternative conditions, such as acute gastroenteritis, bronchitis, and bronchopneumonia. Subsequently, the differential diagnosis includes malaria; sepsis with other bacterial pathogens; infections caused by intracellular microorganisms, such as tuberculosis, brucellosis, tularemia, leptospirosis, and rickettsial diseases; and viral infections such as Dengue fever, acute hepatitis, and infectious mononucleosis.

Infection by *Salmonella* in general, and typhoid or paratyphoid fever in particular, should be thoroughly considered in the differential diagnosis and workup for fever in a returned traveler.

TREATMENT

An early diagnosis of typhoid fever and institution of appropriate treatment are essential. The vast majority of children with typhoid fever can be managed at home with oral antibiotics and close medical follow-up for complications or failure of response to therapy. Patients with persistent vomiting, severe diarrhea, and abdominal distention may require hospitalization and parenteral antibiotic therapy.

There are general principles of typhoid fever management. Adequate rest, hydration, and attention are important to correct fluid and electrolyte imbalance. Antipyretic therapy (acetaminophen 10-15 mg/kg every 4-6 hr PO) should be provided as required. A soft, easily digestible diet should be continued unless the patient has abdominal distention or ileus. Antibiotic therapy is critical to minimize complications (Table 225.6). It has been suggested that traditional therapy with either chloramphenicol or amoxicillin is associated with relapse rates of 5–15% and 4–8%, respectively, whereas use of the azithromycin, quinolones and third-generation cephalosporins is associated with higher cure rates. The antibiotic treatment of typhoid fever in children is also influenced by the prevalence of antimicrobial resistance. Over the past 2 decades, emergence of MDR strains of S. Typhi (i.e., isolates fully resistant to amoxicillin, trimethoprim-sulfamethoxazole, and chloramphenicol) has necessitated treatment with **fluoroquinolones**, which are the antimicrobial drug of choice for treatment of salmonellosis in adults, with cephalosporins as an alternative. Some regions are also reporting S. Typhi that produce extended-spectrum β-lactamases. shows known worldwide distribution patterns of antimicrobial resistance among S. Typhi isolates.

Given the global movement of humans, foods, and bacteria, contemporary resistance tracking is a highly dynamic and international endeavor. Accordingly, pediatricians should seek to use important updates from reporting networks such as the World Health Organization's **Global Foodborne Infections Network** (WHO-GFN, formerly WHO Salmonella Surveillance Network), PulseNet, and ProMED.

Yet again, a strong microbiology laboratory infrastructure is important for optimal medical decision-making, because *Salmonella* susceptibilities and viable treatment options are often highly dependent on local, and changing, conditions. *Salmonella* strains that are highly resistant to the drugs listed for treatment in Table 225.6 still may have in vitro susceptibility to (notably expensive) newer therapeutics, such as carbapenem class drugs and tigecycline. In some locales, a reemergence of susceptibility to conventional drugs has been noted among some clinical isolates of S. Typhi.

Although some investigators suggest that children with typhoid fever should be treated with fluoroquinolones like adults, others question this approach because of the potential development of further resistance to fluoroquinolones and because quinolones are still not approved for widespread use in children. A Cochrane review of the treatment of typhoid fever also indicates that there is little evidence to support the protocolized administration of fluoroquinolones in all cases of typhoid fever. *Azithromycin may be an alternative antibiotic for children with uncomplicated typhoid fever.* The European Committee on Antibiotic Susceptibility Testing has characterized azithromycin

Table 225.6	Treatment of Typhoid Fever in Children						
	OPTIMAL THERAPY			**ALTERNATIVE EFFECTIVE DRUGS**			
SUSCEPTIBILITY	**Antibiotic**	**Daily Dose (mg/kg/day)**	**Days**	**Antibiotic**	**Daily Dose (mg/kg/day)**	**Days**	
UNCOMPLICATED TYPHOID FEVER							
Fully sensitive	Chloramphenicol	50-75	14-21	Fluoroquinolone, e.g., ofloxacin or ciprofloxacin	15	5-7*	
	Amoxicillin	75-100	14				
Multidrug resistant	Fluoroquinolone	15	5-7	Azithromycin	8-10	7	
	or						
	Cefixime	15-20	7-14	Cefixime	15-20	7-14	
Quinolone resistant†	Azithromycin	8-10	7	Cefixime	20	7-14	
	or						
	Ceftriaxone	75	10-14				
SEVERE TYPHOID FEVER							
Fully sensitive	Fluoroquinolone (e.g., ofloxacin)	15	10-14	Chloramphenicol	100	14-21	
				Amoxicillin	100		
Multidrug resistant	Fluoroquinolone	15	10-14	Ceftriaxone	60	10-14	
				or			
				Cefotaxime‡	80	10-14	
Quinolone resistant	Ceftriaxone	60	10-14	Azithromycin	10-20	7	
	Cefotaxime‡	80	10-14	Fluoroquinolone	20	7-14	

*A 3-day course is also effective, particularly for epidemic containment.

†The optimum treatment for quinolone-resistant typhoid fever has not been determined. Azithromycin, third-generation cephalosporins, or high-dose fluoroquinolones for 10-14 days is effective.

‡If available.

Adapted from World Health Organization: Treatment of typhoid fever. In *Background document: the diagnosis, prevention and treatment of typhoid fever. Communicable disease surveillance and response: vaccines and biologicals*, Geneva, 2003, WHO, pp 19–23. http://whqlibdoc.who.int/hq/2003/WHO_V&B_03.07.pdf.

susceptible *S. typhi* isolates as those with minimal inhibitory concentration of ≤16 mg/L.

In addition to antibiotics, the importance of supportive treatment and maintenance of appropriate fluid and electrolyte balance must be underscored. Although additional treatment with dexamethasone (3 mg/kg for the initial dose, followed by 1 mg/kg every 6 hr for 48 hr) is recommended for severely ill patients with shock, obtundation, stupor, or coma, corticosteroids should be administered only under strict controlled conditions and supervision, because their use may mask signs of abdominal complications.

PROGNOSIS

The prognosis for a patient with enteric fever depends on the rapidity of diagnosis and institution of appropriate antibiotic therapy. Other factors are the patient/s, age, general state of health, and nutrition; the causative *Salmonella* serotype; and the appearance of complications. Infants and children with underlying malnutrition and patients infected with MDR isolates are at higher risk for adverse outcomes.

Despite appropriate therapy, 2–4% of infected children may experience relapse after initial clinical response to treatment. Individuals who excrete *S. Typhi* for ≥3 mo after infection are regarded as chronic carriers. The risk for becoming a carrier is low in most children (<2% for all infected children) and increases with age. A chronic urinary carrier state can develop in children with schistosomiasis.

PREVENTION

Of the major risk factors for outbreaks of typhoid fever, **contamination of water supplies** with sewage is the most important. Other risk factors for development of typhoid fever are congestion, contact with another acutely infected individual or a chronic carrier, and lack of water and sanitation services. During outbreaks, central chlorination as well as domestic water purification is important. In endemic situations, consumption of street foods, especially ice cream and cut fruit, is recognized as an important risk factor. The human-to-human spread by chronic carriers is also important, and attempts should be made to target food handlers and high-risk groups for *S. Typhi* carriage screening. Once identified,

chronic carriers must be counseled as to the risk for disease transmission and the importance of handwashing.

A variety of vaccines targeting typhoid fever exist, but this remains a disease for which our vaccination protection for children lags, despite that disease risk factors, transmission patterns, and antibacterial drug resistance among salmonellae should make effective immunization an important element of effective control.

The classic heat-inactivated whole cell vaccine for typhoid is associated with an unacceptably high rate of side effects and has been largely withdrawn from public health use.

An oral, live-attenuated preparation of the **Ty21a strain** of *S.* Typhi has efficacy in endemic regions of 67–82% for up to 5 yr. Significant adverse effects are rare, but as a live-attenuated vaccine, Ty21a should not be used by immunocompromised persons. Proguanil, mefloquine, and antibiotics should be stopped from 3 days before until 3 days after the administration of Ty21a. The duration of protection following Ty21a immunization may vary with vaccine dose, and probably with subsequent "booster-like" exposures to *S. typhi*. Indeed, the recommended vaccination schedules for Ty21a vary in different countries.

The Vi capsular polysaccharide can be used in persons ≥2 yr old. It is given as a single intramuscular dose, with a booster every 2 yr, and has a protective efficacy of 70–80%. The vaccines are currently recommended for anyone traveling into endemic areas, but a few countries have introduced large-scale vaccination strategies. Several large-scale projects using the Vi polysaccharide vaccine in Asia have demonstrated protective efficacy against typhoid fever across all age-groups, but the data on protection among young children (<5 yr old) showed intriguing differences between studies.

Protein-conjugated Vi polysaccharide vaccines have been shown to have high efficacy in young children and thus may offer protection in parts of the world where a large proportion of preschool children are at risk for typhoid fever. These conjugated vaccines have been licensed in some countries but are not currently licensed or available in the United States.

Bibliography is available at Expert Consult.

Chapter **226**
Shigella
Patrick C. Seed

第二百二十六章
志贺菌

中文导读

本章主要介绍了志贺菌感染的病因、流行病学、发病机制、免疫、临床表现、鉴别诊断、诊断、治疗和预防等内容。在志贺菌感染的临床表现部分详细描述了5岁以下儿童急性感染的临床特征，以及感染后的诸多并发症。在志贺菌感染的治疗部分详细介绍了志贺菌病的治疗指南及治疗流程，并强调了营养、补液等对症支持治疗的重要性。

Shigellosis, infection by *Shigella* species, is acute invasive enteric infection clinically manifested by diarrhea that is often bloody. The term **dysentery** describes a syndrome of bloody diarrhea with fever, abdominal cramps, rectal pain, and mucoid stools. **Bacillary dysentery** is a term often used to distinguish dysentery caused by *Shigella* from amebic dysentery caused by *Entamoeba histolytica*.

ETIOLOGY
Four species of *Shigella* are responsible for shigellosis: *Shigella dysenteriae* (group A), *Shigella flexneri* (group B), *Shigella boydii* (group C), and *Shigella sonnei* (group D). Serotypes are used to distinguish members of each group: 15, 19, 19, and 1 in groups A-D, respectively. Species/group distributions vary geographically and have important therapeutic implications because of variations in species antimicrobial susceptibility.

EPIDEMIOLOGY
The World Health Organization (WHO) estimates 80-165 million cases of shigellosis each year worldwide and 600,000 deaths annually. *Shigella* spp. are endemic to temperate and tropical climates. Most of these cases and deaths occur in developing countries where public health sanitation and hygiene are inadequate. In the U.S. Foodborne Disease Active Surveillance Network (**FoodNet**), *Shigella* remains the 3rd most important pathogen. In 2016 the top 3 pathogens, *Salmonella*, *Campylobacter*, and *Shigella*, had laboratory-confirmed incidence rates (cases per 100,000 population) of 15.74, 12.82, and 5.39, respectively. Although infection can occur at any age, children <10 yr old have the highest incidence rates, with males having an approximately 1.3-fold higher incidence than females. Approximately 70% of all episodes and 60% of all *Shigella*-related deaths involve children <5 yr old. Infection in the 1st 6 mo of life is rare for reasons that are not clear. Breast milk from women living in endemic areas contains antibodies to both virulence plasmid-coded antigens and lipopolysaccharides, and breastfeeding might partially explain the age-related incidence.

Asymptomatic infection of children and adults occurs frequently in endemic areas. In cases of *Shigella* dysentery, up to 75% of family member contacts may have asymptomatic infection. Infection with *Shigella* occurs most often during the warm months in temperate climates and during the rainy season in tropical climates. In industrialized societies, up to 50% of locally diagnosed cases are associated with international travel; the highest-risk travel designation is Africa, followed by Central America, South America, and parts of Asia. In recent years in the United States, travel to Haiti, the Dominican Republic, and India, in particular, have been associated with antibiotic-resistant (fluoroquinolone) *S. sonnei* infections. Additional risk factors include men who have sex with men (MSM), including recent U.S. outbreaks of azithromycin-resistant *S. sonnei* infections among affected individuals in the Midwest.

In developed countries, *S. sonnei* is the most common cause and *S. flexneri* is the 2nd most common cause of bacillary dysentery; in preindustrial societies, *S. flexneri* is most common, and *S. sonnei* 2nd in frequency. *S. boydii* is found primarily in India. *S. dysenteriae* serotype 1 tends to occur in massive epidemics, but is also endemic in Asia and Africa, where it is associated with high mortality rates (5–15%). The epidemiologic transition has favored the emergence of *S. sonnei* as the dominant serogroup in some countries, although the reason for this epidemiologic shift is not clear.

Contaminated food (often a salad or other item requiring extensive handling of the ingredients) and water are important vectors. Exposure to both contaminated fresh water and contaminated salt water is a risk factor for infection. Rapid spread within families, custodial institutions, and childcare centers demonstrates the ability of *Shigella* to be transmitted from one individual to the next and the requirement for ingestion of very few organisms to cause illness. Human challenge studies have demonstrated the high infectivity and low infectious dose for *Shigella* spp. Ten bacteria of the species *S. sonnei* and *S. dysenteriae* can cause dysentery. In contrast, ingestion of 10^8-10^{10} *Vibrio cholerae* is necessary to cause cholera.

PATHOGENESIS

Shigella has specialized mechanisms to survive the low gastric pH. *Shigella* survives the acid environment in the stomach and moves through the gut to the colon, its target organ. The basic virulence trait shared by all shigellae is the ability to invade colonic epithelial cells by turning on a series of temperature-regulated and host-dependent proteins. This invasion mechanism is encoded on a large (220 kb) plasmid that at body temperature results in synthesis of a group of polypeptides involved in cell invasion and killing. Shigellae that lose the virulence plasmid are no longer pathogenic. **Enteroinvasive** *Escherichia coli* (EIEC) that harbor a closely related plasmid containing these invasion genes behave clinically similar to shigellae (see Chapter 227). The virulence plasmid encodes a type III secretion system required to trigger entry into epithelial cells and apoptosis in macrophages. This secretion system translocates effector molecules from the bacterial cytoplasm to the membrane and cytoplasm of target host cells through a needle-like appendage. The **type III secretion system** is composed of approximately 50 proteins, including the Mxi and Spa proteins involved in assembly and regulation of the type III secretion system, chaperones (IpgA, IpgC, IpgE, and Spa15), transcription activators (VirF, VirB, and MxiE), translocators (IpaB, IpaC, and IpaD), and approximately 30 effector proteins. In addition to the major plasmid-encoded virulence traits, chromosomally encoded factors are also required for full virulence.

The pathologic changes of shigellosis take place primarily in the colon. The changes are most intense in the distal colon, although pancolitis can occur. Shigellae cross the colonic epithelium through M cells in the follicle-associated epithelium overlying the Peyer patches. Grossly, localized or diffuse mucosal edema, ulcerations, friable mucosa, bleeding, and exudate may be seen. Microscopically, ulcerations, pseudomembranes, epithelial cell death, infiltration extending from the mucosa to the muscularis mucosae by PMNs and mononuclear cells, and submucosal edema occur.

After *Shigella* transcytosis through M cells, it encounters resident macrophages and subverts macrophage killing by activating the inflammasome and inducing pyroptosis, apoptosis, and proinflammatory signaling. Free bacteria invade the epithelial cells from the basolateral side, move into the cytoplasm by actin polymerization, and spread to adjacent cells. Proinflammatory signaling by macrophages and epithelial cells further activates the innate immune response involving natural killer cells and attracts polymorphonuclear leukocytes (PMNs). The influx of PMNs disintegrates the epithelial cell lining, which initially exacerbates the infection and tissue destruction by facilitating the invasion of more bacteria. Ultimately, PMNs phagocytose and kill *Shigella*, thus contributing to the resolution of the infection.

Some shigellae make toxins, including Shiga toxin and enterotoxins. **Shiga toxin** is a potent exotoxin that inhibits protein synthesis. It is produced in significant amounts by *S. dysenteriae* serotype 1, by a subset of *E. coli*, which are known as **enterohemorrhagic** *E. coli* (EHEC), or Shiga toxin–producing *E. coli*, and occasionally by other *Shigella* spp. Shiga toxin inhibits protein synthesis to injure vascular endothelial cells and trigger the severe complication of hemolytic-uremic syndrome (see Chapter 227). Targeted deletion of the genes for other enterotoxins (*ShET1* and *ShET2*) decreases the incidence of fever and dysentery in human challenge studies. Lipopolysaccharides are virulence factors for all shigellae; other traits are important for only a few serotypes (e.g., Shiga toxin synthesis by *S. dysenteriae* serotype 1 and *ShET1* by *S. flexneri* 2a).

IMMUNITY

In symptomatic infection, *Shigella* activates an intense innate immune response through triggering extra- and intracellular pathogen recognition systems. The induction of acute inflammation with a massive recruitment of PMNs produces intensive local tissue destruction. In rectal biopsies of infected patients, acute-phase proinflammatory cytokines are induced, including interleukin (IL)-1β, IL-6, IL-8, tumor necrosis factor-α, and TNF-β. Concurrently, antiinflammatory genes encoding IL-10 and transforming growth factor-β are also upregulated to mitigate uncontrolled inflammation. Furthermore, interferon-γ expression is induced during human infection and is required to limit *Shigella* invasion in intestinal epithelial cells and macrophages. *Shigella*-specific immunity elicited upon natural infection is characterized by the induction of a humoral response. Local secretory immunoglobulin A (IgA) and serum IgG are produced against lipopolysaccharide and some protein effectors (Ipas). Protection is thought to be serotype specific. Natural protective immunity arises only after several episodes of infection, is of short duration, and seems to be effective in limiting reinfection, particularly in young children. However, children have delayed and reduced antigen-specific antibody-secreting cells with late and reduced mucosa IgA production against *Shigella*. Less effective adaptive immunity may put children at more risk for increased disease severity, mortality, and recurrences.

CLINICAL MANIFESTATIONS AND COMPLICATIONS

Shigellae produce intra- and extraintestinal symptoms. *Bacillary dysentery is clinically similar regardless of infecting serotype.* However, different species produce illnesses with different severity and risk for mortality, with *S. dysenteriae* type 1 most likely to produce any single manifestation and with greater severity. Ingestion of shigellae is followed by an incubation period of 12 hr to several days before symptoms ensue. Severe abdominal pain, emesis, anorexia, generalized toxicity, urgency, and painful defecation characteristically occur (Table 226.1). The typically high **fever** with shigellosis distinguishes it from EHEC. The **diarrhea** may be watery and of large volume initially, evolving into frequent, small-volume, bloody mucoid stools. Most children never progress to the stage of bloody diarrhea, but some have bloody stools from the outset. Significant dehydration is related to the fluid and electrolyte losses in feces and emesis. Untreated diarrhea can last 7-10 days; only approximately 10% of patients have diarrhea persisting for >10 days. Persistent diarrhea occurs in malnourished infants, children with AIDS, and occasionally previously normal children. Even nondysenteric disease can be complicated by persistent illness.

Physical examination initially shows abdominal distention and tenderness, hyperactive bowel sounds, and a tender rectum on digital examination. **Rectal prolapse** may be present, particularly in malnourished children. Neurologic findings are among the most common extraintestinal manifestations of bacillary dysentery, occurring in as many as 40% of hospitalized children. EIEC can cause similar neurologic toxicity. Convulsions, headache, lethargy, confusion, nuchal rigidity, or hallucinations may be present before or after the onset of diarrhea. The cause of these neurologic findings is not understood. Infections with Shiga toxin positive and negative strains can lead to neurologic features. **Seizures** sometimes occur when little fever is present, suggesting that simple febrile convulsions do not explain their appearance. Hypocalcemia or hyponatremia may be associated with seizures in a small number of patients. Although symptoms often suggest central nervous system infection, and cerebrospinal fluid pleocytosis with minimally elevated protein levels can occur, meningitis caused by shigellae is rare. Based on animal studies, it has been suggested that proinflammatory mediators, including TNF-α and IL-1β, nitric oxide, and corticotropin-releasing

Table 226.1	Acute Clinical Manifestations of Shigellosis in Children <5 Yr Old	
MANIFESTATION	**DYSENTERY** (*n* = 757)	**WATERY DIARRHEA** (*n* = 288)
Fever	607 (80%)	207 (72%)
Abdominal cramps	616 (81%)	137 (48%)
Vomiting	136 (18%)	89 (31%)
WHO-defined dehydration	95 (13%)	134 (47%)
Tenesmus	511 (68%)	32 (11%)
Rectal prolapse	19 (3%)	4 (1%)

From Kotloff KL, Riddle MS, Platts-Mills JA, et al: Shigellosis, *Lancet* 391:801–810, 2018.

hormone, all play a role in the enhanced susceptibility to *Shigella*-mediated seizures and encephalopathy.

The most common complication of shigellosis is **dehydration** (Table 226.2). Inappropriate secretion of antidiuretic hormone with profound hyponatremia can complicate dysentery, particularly when *S. dysenteriae* is the etiologic agent. Hypoglycemia and protein-losing enteropathy are common and are decreased by early appropriate antibiotic therapy. Severe protein-losing enteropathy is associated with prolonged illness and linear growth shortfalls. **Bacteremia** is uncommon except in girls or women infected with HIV, malnourished children, young infants, and children with *S. dysenteriae* serotype 1 infection. When bacteremia occurs with dysentery (<5%), it is as likely to be caused by other enteric bacteria as by *Shigella* itself. The presence of *E. coli, Klebsiella*, and other enteric bacteria in blood cultures of children with shigellosis may reflect the loss of the barrier function during severe colitis. The mortality rate is high (approximately 20%) when sepsis occurs, with a greater likelihood of occurrence in HIV-infected persons. Other major complications include **disseminated intravascular coagulation** (DIC), particularly in very young, malnourished children. Despite the extent to which the intestinal epithelial barrier is lost, bacteremia and DIC are uncommon.

Neonatal shigellosis is rare, particularly among the exclusively breastfed. Neonates may have only low-grade fever with mild, nonbloody diarrhea. However, complications occur more often in neonates than in older children and include septicemia, meningitis, dehydration, colonic perforation, and toxic megacolon.

S. dysenteriae serotype 1 infection is frequently complicated by hemolysis, anemia, and **hemolytic-uremic syndrome**. HUS is caused by Shiga toxin–mediated vascular endothelial injury. Shiga-toxin–producing non-*dysenteriae Shigella* and *E. coli* that produce Shiga toxins (e.g., *E. coli* O157:H7, *E. coli* O111:NM, *E. coli* O26:H11, and less often, many other serotypes) also cause HUS (see Chapter 538.5).

Rectal prolapse, toxic megacolon or pseudomembranous colitis (usually associated with *S. dysenteriae*), cholestatic hepatitis, conjunctivitis, iritis,

corneal ulcers, pneumonia, arthritis (usually 2-5 wk after enteritis), reactive arthritis, cystitis, myocarditis, and vaginitis (typically with blood-tinged discharge associated with *S. flexneri*) are uncommon events. Although rare, surgical complications of shigellosis can be severe; the most common are intestinal obstruction and appendicitis with and without perforation.

On average, the severity of illness and risk of death are least with disease caused by *S. sonnei* and greatest with infection by *S. dysenteriae* type 1. Risk groups for severe illness and poor outcomes include infants; children who are not breastfed; children with HIV; children recovering from measles; malnourished children and adults; adults >50 yr old; and patients with dehydration, unconsciousness, hypo- or hyperthermia, hyponatremia, or lesser stool frequency who have a history of convulsion when first seen. Death is a rare outcome in well-nourished older children. Multiple factors contribute to death in malnourished children with shigellosis, including illness in the 1st yr of life, altered consciousness, dehydration, hypothermia, thrombocytopenia, anemia, hyponatremia, renal failure, hyperkalemia hypoglycemia, bronchopneumonia, and bacteremia.

The rare syndrome of severe toxicity, convulsions, extreme hyperpyrexia, and headache, followed by brain edema and a rapidly fatal outcome without sepsis or significant dehydration (Ekiri syndrome or "lethal toxic encephalopathy"), is not well understood.

DIFFERENTIAL DIAGNOSIS
Although clinical features suggest shigellosis, they are insufficiently specific to allow confident diagnosis. Infection by *Campylobacter jejuni, Salmonella* spp., EIEC, Shiga toxin–producing *E. coli* (e.g., *E. coli* O157:H7), *Yersinia enterocolitica, Clostridium difficile*, and *Entamoeba histolytica*, as well as inflammatory bowel disease, produce overlapping features and may challenge the clinician.

DIAGNOSIS
Presumptive data supporting a diagnosis of bacillary dysentery include the finding of fecal leukocytes (usually >50 or 100 PMNs per high-power field, confirming the presence of colitis), fecal blood, and demonstration in peripheral blood of leukocytosis with a dramatic left shift (often with more bands than segmented neutrophils). The total peripheral white blood cell count is usually 5,000-15,000 cells/µL, although leukopenia and leukemoid reactions occur.

Culture of both stool and rectal swab specimens optimizes the chance of diagnosing *Shigella* infection. Culture media should include MacConkey agar as well as selective media such as xylose-lysine-deoxycholate and *Salmonella-Shigella* agar. Transport media should be used if specimens cannot be cultured promptly. Appropriate media should be used to exclude *Campylobacter* and *Salmonella* spp. and other agents. Studies of outbreaks and illness in volunteers show that the laboratory is often not able to confirm the clinical suspicion of shigellosis even when the pathogen is present. Multiple fecal cultures improve the yield of *Shigella*.

Culture-based diagnosis of *Shigella* infection, as with other enteric infections, is being displaced by molecular methods, often multiplexed, allowing testing for a panel of potential agents in a single assay. Studies using molecular methods such as polymerase chain reaction (PCR) suggest that culture significantly underestimates the true frequency of infection. Quantitative PCR improves ascertainment of *Shigella* burden in children with moderate to severe diarrhea in low-income countries. The generally **high negative predictive value** (NPV) of many molecular tests for *Shigella* (generally >95–97%) make the tests useful for decisions regarding antibiotic discontinuation and the necessity to test for addition etiologies of diarrhea. The diagnostic inadequacy of cultures makes it incumbent on the clinician to use judgment in the management of clinical syndromes consistent with shigellosis. In children who appear toxic, blood cultures should be obtained, especially in very young or malnourished infants, because of their increased risk of bacteremia.

TREATMENT
As with gastroenteritis from other causes, the first concern in a child with suspected shigellosis should be for fluid and electrolyte correction and maintenance (see Chapter 366). Drugs that impair intestinal motility

---

Table 226.2 | Clinical Complications of Shigellosis

INTESTINAL COMPLICATIONS
Rectal prolapse*
Toxic megacolon
Intestinal perforation
Intestinal obstruction
Appendicitis
Persistent diarrhea

EXTRAINTESTINAL COMPLICATIONS
Dehydration
Severe hyponatremia (serum sodium <126 mmol/L)*
Hypoglycemia
Focal infections (e.g., meningitis, osteomyelitis, arthritis, splenic
   abscesses, vaginitis)
Sepsis, usually in malnourished or immunocompromised persons
Seizure or encephalopathy
Leukemoid reaction (peripheral leukocytes >40000/µL)*

POSTINFECTIOUS MANIFESTATIONS
Hemolytic-uremic syndrome (HUS)*
Reactive arthritis[†]
Irritable bowel syndrome (IBS)[‡]
Malnutrition

*Significantly more common in episodes with *Shigella dysenteriae* type 1 than with all other *Shigella* spp. among Bangladeshi children younger than 15 yr during the 1990s (rectal prolapse [52% vs 15%], severe hyponatremia [58% vs 26%], leukemoid reaction [22% vs 2%], and HUS [8% vs 1%]).

[†]Typical acute symptoms include asymmetric oligoarthritis (usually lower limb), enthesitis, dactylitis, and back pain. Extraarticular manifestations include conjunctivitis and uveitis; urethritis and other genitourinary tract manifestations; oral, skin, and nail lesions; and rarely, cardiac abnormalities.

[‡]IBS follows approximately 4% of *Shigella* episodes in studies from high-resource settings.

Adapted from Kotloff KL, Riddle MS, Platts-Mills JA, et al: Shigellosis, *Lancet* 391:801–810, 2018.

(e.g., diphenoxylate hydrochloride with atropine [Lomotil] or loperamide [Imodium]) should not be used because of the risk of prolonging the illness.

Nutrition is a key concern in areas where malnutrition is common. A high-protein and high-caloric diet during convalescence enhances growth in 6 mo after infection. Controlled studies show that cooked green bananas, a food rich in amylase-resistant starches, significantly improves outcome in severe disease. A single large dose of **vitamin A** (200,000 IU) lessens the severity of shigellosis in settings where vitamin A deficiency is common. **Zinc** supplementation (20 mg elemental zinc for 14 days) significantly decreases the duration of diarrhea, improves weight gain during recovery, enhances adaptive immunity to the *Shigella*, and decreases diarrheal disease in malnourished children.

The decision to use **antibiotics** remains challenging (Fig. 226.1). Many experts recommend withholding antibacterial therapy because of the self-limited nature of the infection, the cost of drugs, the risk of emergence of resistant organisms, the risk of prolonging carriage (if *Salmonella* is present), or increasing the risk for HUS (EHEC). However, a counter argument of empirical treatment for all children with suspected shigellosis has validity. Untreated illness can cause a child to have prolonged illness; chronic or recurrent diarrhea can ensue. Malnutrition can develop or worsen during prolonged illness, particularly in children in developing countries. The risk of continued excretion and subsequent infection of family contacts further argues against the strategy of withholding antibiotics.

Shigella antimicrobial susceptibility varies by species and geography. In the United States, strains are frequently resistant to ampicillin (74%) and trimethoprim-sulfamethoxazole (TMP-SMX) (36%). In general, the proportion of antibiotic-resistant isolates is lower in North America and Europe than in Asia or Africa. Previously, *Shigella* was widely regarded as susceptible in vitro to azithromycin, ceftriaxone, cefotaxime, cefixime, nalidixic acid, and quinolones. However, the CDC reports that 87% of *S. sonnei*–related U.S. cases are ciprofloxacin nonsusceptible, of which only approximately half followed international travel. Among MSM, clusters of shigellosis caused by *S. sonnei* and to a lesser extent *S. flexnerii* were reported with up to 87% azithromycin resistance. International travel increases the risk for antibiotic-resistant infection. For example, Chinese isolates of *S. sonnei* are often resistant to TMP-SMX (94.5%), ampicillin (40.3%), piperacillin (36.5%), and ceftriaxone (12.8%).

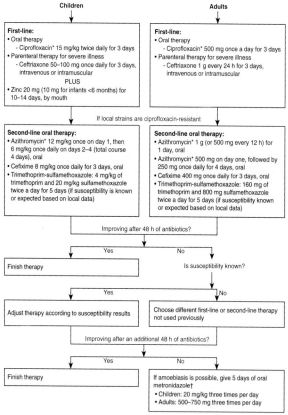

Fig. 226.1 Management algorithm: guidelines for treatment of shigellosis. Empirical therapy should be directed by hospital, clinical laboratory, or public health antibiograms whenever possible. Minimal inhibitory concentrations of 0·12-1·0 µg/mL for ciprofloxacin might be considered susceptible by laboratory standards but could harbor resistance genes known to confer decreased susceptibility. *Azithromycin and fluoroquinolones should be used with caution in patients taking the antimalarial artemether, because these drugs can prolong the QT interval on the electrocardiogram and trigger arrhythmias. †Per WHO recommendations. Another acceptable regimen is a 7-10 day course of metronidazole followed by a luminal agent such as paromomycin or diiodohydroxyquinoline. (*From World Health Organization: The selection and use of essential medicines, March, 2017.* http://www.who.int/medicines/publications/essentialmedicines/en/.)

Currently, in most developed and developing countries, *Shigella* strains are often resistant to ampicillin and TMP-SMX. Therefore, these drugs should not be used for empirical treatment of suspected shigellosis; they should be instituted only if the strain is known to be susceptible (e.g., in an outbreak caused by a defined strain). Empirical therapy in children with dysentery should be given based on considerations of regional infection cluster data and international travel history. Therapy may include azithromycin, a third-generation cephalosporin, or ciprofloxacin. **Ceftriaxone** (50-100 mg/kg/24 hr as a single daily dose intravenously or intramuscularly) can be used for empirical therapy, especially for small infants. The oral third-generation cephalosporin **cefixime** (8 mg/kg/24 hr divided every 12-24 hr) can also be used; however, oral first- and second-generation cephalosporins are inadequate as alternative drugs despite in vitro susceptibility. **Azithromycin** (12 mg/kg/24 hr orally for the 1st day, followed by 6 mg/kg/24 hr for the next 4 days) has proved to be an effective alternative drug for shigellosis. **Ciprofloxacin** (20-30 mg/kg/24 hr divided into 2 doses) is the drug of choice recommended by WHO for all patients with bloody diarrhea, regardless of age. Concurrent zinc supplementation is recommended with antibiotic therapy.

Although **quinolones** are reported to cause arthropathy in immature animals and are associated with neuropathy, these risks are low in children and are outweighed by the value of these drugs for the treatment of this potentially life-threatening disease. However, some experts recommend that the quinolones be reserved for seriously ill children with bacillary dysentery caused by an organism suspected or known to be resistant to other agents, because overuse of quinolones promotes the development of resistance to these drugs.

Treatment of patients in whom *Shigella* infection is suspected on clinical grounds should be initiated when these patients are first evaluated. Molecular stool testing or culture is obtained to exclude other pathogens and, in the case of culture, to assist in antibiotic changes should a child fail to respond to empirical therapy. A child who has typical dysentery and who responds to initial empirical antibiotic treatment should be continued on that drug for a full 5-day course even if the stool culture is negative, due to the method's low NPV. The logic of this recommendation is based on the proven difficulty of culturing *Shigella* from stools of ill patients during adult volunteer infection studies. In a child who fails to respond to therapy of a dysenteric syndrome in the presence of initially negative stool culture results, additional cultures should be obtained, or molecular testing, where available and cost permissive, should be performed, and the child should be reevaluated for other possible diagnoses. In the child with negative molecular stool testing for shigellae, the high NPV makes the diagnosis less likely, and alternative diagnoses should be considered.

PREVENTION

Numerous measures have been recommended to decrease the risk of *Shigella* transmission to children. Mothers should be encouraged to *prolong breastfeeding* of infants. Families and daycare personnel should be educated in *proper handwashing* techniques and encouraged to wash hands after using the toilet, changing diapers, or engaging in preparation of foods. They should be taught how to manage potentially contaminated materials such as raw vegetables, soiled diapers, and diaper-changing areas. Children with diarrhea should be excluded from childcare facilities. Children should be supervised when handwashing after they use the toilet. Caretakers should be informed of the risk of transmission if they prepare food when they are ill with diarrhea. Families should be educated regarding danger of swallowing contaminated water from ponds, lakes, or untreated pools. In developing countries, a safe water supply and appropriate sanitation systems are important measures for reducing the risk for shigellosis. **Measles immunization** can substantially reduce the incidence and severity of diarrheal diseases, including shigellosis. There is not yet a vaccine that is effective for preventing infection by *Shigella*. Every infant should be immunized against measles at the recommended age.

Bibliography is available at Expert Consult.

Chapter **227**
Escherichia coli
Patrick C. Seed

第二百二十七章
大肠埃希菌

中文导读

　　本章主要介绍了肠道产毒素性大肠埃希菌、肠道侵袭性大肠埃希菌、肠道致病性大肠埃希菌、产志贺样毒素大肠埃希菌、肠集聚性大肠埃希菌、弥散黏附性大肠埃希菌、肠溶性出血性大肠埃希菌的病因、流行病学、发病机制、临床表现等内容。其中，就大肠埃希菌腹泻的临床特征、发病机制和诊断进行了详细描述。随后系统地介绍了大肠埃希菌的诊断、治疗、预防等内容。

Escherichia coli is an important cause of intraintestinal and extraintestinal infections. **Intraintestinal infections** present as different diarrheal illnesses. **Extraintestinal infections** include disease of the urinary tract (see Chapter 553) and bloodstream (Chapters 129, 202, and 203). Intraintestinal **pathogenic** *E. coli*, also called **enteric** *E. coli*, produce diarrheal diseases. *E. coli* causing extra- and intraintestinal infections are highly specialized with unique genetic attributes that encode different sets of virulence factors and genetic programs. Extraintestinal pathogenic *E. coli* increasingly harbor multidrug resistances, including transferrable plasmids resulting in extended-spectrum β-lactamase (ESBL) production. This results in resistance to penicillins, cephalosporins, and aztreonam. Carbapenemase-bearing *E. coli* have also emerged, often in combination with multi–antibiotic class resistance, resulting in highly drug-resistant strains.

Escherichia coli species are members of the Enterobacteriaceae family. They are facultative anaerobic, gram-negative bacilli that usually ferment lactose. Most fecal *E. coli* organisms are commensal, are ubiquitous among humans starting in the 1st mo of life, and do not cause diarrhea. Six major groups of **diarrheagenic** *E. coli* pathotypes have been characterized on the basis of clinical, biochemical, and molecular-genetic criteria: enterotoxigenic *E. coli* (ETEC); enteroinvasive *E. coli* (EIEC); enteropathogenic *E. coli* (EPEC); *Shiga* toxin–producing *E. coli* (STEC), also known as enterohemorrhagic *E. coli* (EHEC) or verotoxin-producing *E. coli* (VTEC); enteroaggregative *E. coli* (EAEC or EggEC); and diffusely adherent *E. coli* (DAEC).

E. coli strains can also be categorized by their serogroup, where *O* refers to the lipopolysaccharide (LPS) O-antigen or serotype and *H* refers to the flagellar antigen, for example, *E. coli* O157:H7. However, because each pathotype contains many serotypes (e.g., 117 ETEC serotypes have been identified), and some serotypes can belong to more than 1 pathotype (e.g., O26:H11 can be either EPEC or EHEC, depending on which specific virulence genes are present), serotyping frequently does not provide definitive identification of pathotypes.

Because *E. coli* are normal fecal flora, pathogenicity is defined by demonstration of virulence characteristics and association of those traits with illness (Table 227.1). The mechanism by which *E. coli* produces **diarrhea** typically involves adherence of organisms to a glycoprotein or glycolipid receptor on a target intestinal cell, followed by production of a factor that injures or disturbs the function of intestinal cells. The genes for virulence properties and antibiotic resistance are often carried on transferable plasmids, pathogenicity islands, or bacteriophages. In the developing world, the various diarrheagenic *E. coli* strains cause frequent infections in the 1st years of life; diarrheagenic *E. coli* as a group are responsible for 30-40% of all diarrhea cases in children worldwide. They occur with increased frequency during the warm months in temperate climates and during rainy season months in tropical climates. Most diarrheagenic *E. coli* strains (except STEC) require a large inoculum of organisms to induce disease, thus necessitating exposure to grossly contaminated ingestible materials. Infection is most likely when food-handling or sewage-disposal practices are suboptimal. The diarrheagenic *E. coli* pathotypes are also important in North America and Europe, although their epidemiology is less well defined in these areas than in the developing world. In North America, the various diarrheagenic *E. coli* strains may cause as much as 30% of infectious diarrhea in children <5 yr old.

Many studies have found diarrheagenic *E. coli* pathotypes in a significant proportion of asymptomatic healthy children living in developing countries. **Fecal contamination** (human and animal), which is common in the low-resource environments where many young children live, facilitates the transmission of pathogens. Also, with modern, highly sensitive microbiologic methods, small numbers of bacteria can be detected in stool samples. Therefore, it is important to assess the prevalence of various enteropathogens in children with and without diarrhea to interpret results. Excretion of enteropathogens by children without diarrhea may be explained by characteristics of the pathogens (virulence heterogeneity), the host (host susceptibility, age, nutritional status,

Table 227.1	Clinical Characteristics, Pathogenesis, and Diagnosis of Diarrheagenic *E. coli*

PATHOGEN	POPULATIONS AT RISK	CHARACTERISTICS OF DIARRHEA			MAIN VIRULENCE FACTORS		DIAGNOSIS
		Watery	Bloody	Duration	Adherence Factors	Toxins	
ETEC	>1 yr old and travelers	+++	—	Acute	Colonization factor antigens (CFs or CFAs); ECP	Heat-labile enterotoxin (LT) Heat-stable enterotoxin (ST)	Detection of enterotoxins (LT and ST) by enzyme immunoassays or PCR (*lt, st*)
EIEC	>1 yr old	+	++	Acute	Invasion plasmid antigen (IpaABCD)		Detection of invasion plasmid antigen of *Shigella* (*ipaH*) by PCR
EPEC	<2 yr old	+++	+	Acute, prolonged or persistent	A/E lesion, intimin/Tir, EspABD, Bfp	EspF, Map, EAST1, SPATEs (*EspC*)	Detection of intimin gene (*eae*) ± bundle-forming pili (*bfpA*) by PCR, and absence of *Shiga* toxins; HEp-2 cells adherence assay (LA, LLA)
STEC (EHEC/ VTEC)	6 mo-10 yr and elderly persons	+	+++	Acute	A/E lesion, intimin/Tir, EspABD	*Shiga* toxins (Stx1, Stx2, and variants of Stx2)	Detection of *Shiga* toxins by enzyme immunoassays or PCR (*Stx1, Stx2*); stool culture on MacConkey-sorbitol media to detect *E. coli* O157. Simultaneous culture for O157 and nonculture assays to detect *Shiga* toxins
EAEC	<2 yr old, HIV-infected patients, and travelers	+++	+	Acute, prolonged, or persistent	Aggregative adherence fimbriae (AAF)	SPATEs (Pic, Pet), ShET1, EAST1	Detection of *AggR*, AA plasmid, and other virulence genes: *aap, aatA, astA, set1A* by PCR; HEp-2 cells adherence assay (AA)
DAEC	>1 yr old and travelers	++	—	Acute	Afa/Dr, AIDA-I	SPATEs (Sat)	Detection of Dr adhesins (daaC or daaD) and Dr-associated genes by PCR; HEp-2 cells adherence assay (DA)

—, Not present; +, present; ++, common; +++, very common; A/E lesion, attaching and effacing lesion; AA, aggregative adherence; Bfp, bundle-forming pili; DA, diffuse adherence; DAEC, diffusely adherent *E. coli*; EAEC, enteroaggregative *E. coli*; EAST1, enteroaggregative heat-stable toxin; ECP, *E. coli* common pilus; EHEC, enterohemorrhagic *E. coli*; EIEC, enteroinvasive *E. coli*; FPEC, enteropathogenic *E. coli*; EspABD, *E. coli*–secreted proteins A, B, and D; ETEC, enterotoxigenic *E. coli*; LA, localized adherence; LLA, localized-like adherence; PCR, polymerase chain reaction; ShET1, *Shigella* enterotoxin 1; SPATEs, serine-protease autotransporter of Enterobacteriaceae; STEC, *Shiga* toxin–producing *E. coli*; Tir, translocated intimin receptor; VTEC, verotoxin-producing *E. coli*.

breastfeeding, immunity), and environmental factors (inoculum size).

ENTEROTOXIGENIC *ESCHERICHIA COLI*

ETEC accounts for a sizable fraction of dehydrating infantile diarrhea in the developing world (10–30%) and of **traveler's diarrhea** (20–60% of cases); ETEC is the most common cause of traveler's diarrhea. In the Global Enteric Multicenter Study (GEMS) conducted across Asia and Africa, *heat-stable* enterotoxin (ST)–expressing ETEC (with or without coexpression of *heat-labile* enterotoxin [LT]) was among the most important causes of diarrhea in young children in developing countries and was associated with increased risk of death. The typical signs and symptoms include explosive watery, nonmucoid, nonbloody diarrhea; abdominal pain; nausea; vomiting; and little or no fever. The illness is usually self-limited and resolves in 3-5 days but occasionally lasts >1 wk.

ETEC causes few or no structural alterations in the gut mucosa. Diarrhea follows colonization of the small intestine and elaboration of enterotoxins. ETEC strains secrete an LT and/or an ST. LT, a large molecule consisting of 5 receptor-binding subunits and 1 enzymatically active subunit, is structurally, functionally, and neutralizing antibody cross-reactive with cholera toxin produced by *Vibrio cholerae*. LT stimulates adenylate cyclase, resulting in increased cyclic adenosine monophosphate. ST is a small molecule not related to cholera toxin. ST stimulates guanylate cyclase, resulting in increased cyclic guanosine monophosphate. Each toxin induces ion and water secretion into the intestinal lumen, resulting in profuse watery diarrhea. The genes for these toxins are encoded on plasmids.

Colonization of the intestine requires fimbrial **colonization factor antigens (CFAs)**, which promote adhesion to the intestinal epithelium. Over 25 CFA types exist and can be expressed alone or in combinations. Prevalent colonization factors include CFA/I, CS1-CS7, CS14, and CS17. However, CFAs have not been detected on all ETEC strains. Although 30–50% of ETEC isolates have no characterized CFA by phenotypic screening, novel CFAs continue to be identified. CFAs are highly immunogenic. However, the multiple CFAs and their allelic variants have made the definition of immunity and development of useful vaccines difficult. A large proportion of strains produce a type IV pilus called *longus*, which functions as a colonization factor and is found among several other gram-negative bacterial pathogens. ETEC strains also have the common pilus, produced by commensal and pathogenic *E. coli* strains. Among the nonfimbrial adhesions, TibA is a potent bacterial adhesin that mediates bacterial attachment and invasion of cells. For many years, the O serogroup was used to distinguish pathogenic from commensal *E. coli*. Because the pathogenic *E. coli* are now defined and classified by using probes or primers for specific virulence genes, determining the O serogroup has become less important. Of the >180 *E. coli* serogroups, only a relatively small number typically are ETEC. The most common O groups are O6, O8, O128, and O153, and based on some large retrospective studies, these serogroups account for only half the ETEC strains.

ENTEROINVASIVE *ESCHERICHIA COLI*

Clinically, EIEC infections present either with watery diarrhea or a dysentery syndrome with blood, mucus, and leukocytes in the stools, as well as fever, systemic toxicity, crampy abdominal pain, tenesmus, and urgency. The illness resembles **bacillary dysentery** because EIEC shares virulence genes with *Shigella* spp. Sequencing of multiple housekeeping genes indicates that EIEC is more related to *Shigella* than to noninvasive *E. coli*. EIEC diarrhea occurs mostly in outbreaks; however, endemic disease occurs in developing countries. In some areas of the developing world as many as 5% of sporadic diarrhea episodes and 20% of bloody diarrhea cases are caused by EIEC (see Chapter 226).

EIEC disease resembles **shigellosis**. EIEC cause colonic lesions with ulcerations, hemorrhage, mucosal and submucosal edema, and infiltration by polymorphonuclear leukocytes (PMNs). EIEC strains behave like *Shigella* in their capacity to invade gut epithelium and produce a dysentery-like illness. The invasive process involves initial entry into cells, intracellular multiplication, intracellular and intercellular spread, and host cell death. All bacterial genes necessary for entry into the host cell are clustered within a 30-kb region of a large virulence plasmid; these genes are closely related to those found on the invasion plasmid of *Shigella* spp. This region carries genes encoding the entry-mediating proteins, including proteins that form a needle-like injection apparatus called type III secretion, required for secreting the invasins (IpaA-D and IpgD). The Ipas are the primary effector proteins of epithelial cell invasion. The type III secretion apparatus is a system triggered by contact with host cells; bacteria use it to transport proteins into the host cell plasma membrane and inject toxins into the host cell cytoplasm.

EIEC encompasses a small number of serogroups (O28ac, O29, O112ac, O124, O136, O143, O144, O152, O159, O164, O167, and some untypeable strains). These serogroups have LPS antigens related to *Shigella* LPS, and as with shigellae, are nonmotile (they lack H or flagellar antigens) and are usually non–lactose fermenting.

ENTEROPATHOGENIC *ESCHERICHIA COLI*
EPEC causes acute, prolonged, and persistent diarrhea, primarily in children <2 yr old in developing countries, where the organism may account for 20% of infant diarrhea. In developed countries, EPEC cause occasional daycare center and pediatric ward outbreaks. Profuse watery, nonbloody diarrhea with mucus, vomiting, and low-grade fever are common symptoms. Prolonged diarrhea (>7 days) and persistent diarrhea (>14 days) can lead to **malnutrition**, a potentially mortality-associated outcome of EPEC infection in infants in the developing world. Studies show that breastfeeding is protective against diarrhea caused by EPEC.

EPEC colonization causes blunting of intestinal villi, local inflammatory changes, and sloughing of superficial mucosal cells; EPEC-induced lesions extend from the duodenum through the colon. EPEC induces a characteristic attaching and effacing histopathologic lesion, which is defined by the intimate attachment of bacteria to the epithelial surface and effacement of host cell microvilli. Factors responsible for the attaching and effacing lesion formation are encoded by the *locus of enterocyte effacement* (LEE), a pathogenicity island with genes for a type III secretion system, the translocated intimin receptor (Tir) and intimin, and multiple effector proteins such as the *E. coli*–secreted proteins (EspA-B-D). Some strains adhere to the host intestinal epithelium in a pattern known as *localized adherence*, a trait that is mediated in part by the type IV bundle-forming pilus (Bfp) encoded by a plasmid (the EAF plasmid). After initial contact, proteins are translocated through filamentous appendages forming a physical bridge between the bacteria and the host cell; bacterial effectors (EspB, EspD, Tir) are translocated through these conduits. Tir moves to the surface of host cells, where it is bound by a bacterial outer membrane protein intimin (encoded by the *eae* gene). Intimin-Tir binding triggers polymerization of actin and other cytoskeletal components at the site of attachment. These cytoskeletal changes result in intimate bacterial attachment to the host cell, enterocyte effacement, and pedestal formation.

Other LEE-encoded effectors include Map, EspF, EspG, EspH, and SepZ. Various other effector proteins are encoded outside the LEE and secreted by the type III secretion system (the non–LEE-encoded proteins, or Nle). The contribution of these putative effectors (NleA/EspI, NleB, NleC, NleD, etc.) to virulence is still under investigation. The presence and expression of virulence genes vary among EPEC strains.

The *eae* (intimin) and *bfp*A genes are useful for identifying EPEC

and for subdividing this group of bacteria into typical and atypical strains. *E. coli* strains that are *eae+/bfp*A+ are classified as "typical" EPEC; most of these strains belong to common O:H serotypes. *E. coli* strains that are *eae+/bfp*A− are classified as "atypical" EPEC. Typical EPEC has been considered for many years to be a leading cause of infantile diarrhea in developing countries and was considered rare in industrialized countries. However, current data suggest that atypical EPEC are more prevalent than typical EPEC in both developed and developing countries, even in persistent diarrhea cases. Determining which of these heterogeneous strains are true pathogens remains a work in progress. In the GEMS, typical EPEC was the main pathogen associated with increased risk of mortality, particularly in infants in Africa.

The classic EPEC serogroups include strains of 12 O serogroups: O26, O55, O86, O111, O114, O119, O125, O126, O127, O128, O142, and O158. However, various *E. coli* strains defined as EPEC based on the presence of the intimin gene belong to nonclassic EPEC serogroups, especially the atypical strains.

SHIGA TOXIN–PRODUCING *ESCHERICHIA COLI*
STEC causes a broad spectrum of diseases. STEC infections may be asymptomatic. Patients who develop intestinal symptoms can have mild diarrhea or severe hemorrhagic colitis. Abdominal pain with initially watery diarrhea that may become bloody over several days characterizes STEC illness. Infrequent fever differentiates STEC disease from the otherwise similar appearance of shigellosis or EIEC disease. Most persons with STEC recover from the infection without further complication. However, 5–10% of children with STEC hemorrhagic colitis go on within a few days to develop systemic complications such as **hemolytic-uremic syndrome** (HUS), characterized by acute kidney failure, thrombocytopenia, and microangiopathic hemolytic anemia (see Chapter 538). Severe illness occurs most often among children 6 mo to 10 yr old. Young children with STEC-associated bloody diarrhea and neutrophilic leukocytosis in the early course of their diarrhea are at risk for HUS progression. Older individuals can also develop HUS or thrombotic thrombocytopenic purpura.

STEC is transmitted person to person (e.g., in families and daycare centers) as well as by food and water; ingestion of a small number of organisms is sufficient to cause disease with some strains. Poorly cooked hamburger is a common cause of food-borne outbreaks, although many other foods (apple cider, lettuce, spinach, mayonnaise, salami, dry fermented sausage, and unpasteurized dairy products) have also been incriminated in STEC transmission.

STEC affects the colon most severely. These organisms adhere to intestinal cells, and most strains that affect humans produce attaching-effacing lesions such as those seen with EPEC and contain related genes (e.g., *intimin, Tir, EspA-D*). Unlike EPEC, STEC produces **Shiga toxins** (Stx; previously called verotoxins and Shiga-like) as key virulence factors. There are 2 major Shiga toxin families, Stx1 and Stx2, with multiple subtypes identified by letters (e.g., Stx2a, Stx2c). Some STEC produce only Stx1, and others produce only 1 of the variants of Stx2; many STEC have genes for several toxins. **Stx1** is essentially identical to Shiga toxin, the protein synthesis–inhibiting exotoxin of *Shigella dysenteriae* serotype 1. **Stx2** and variants of Stx2 are more distantly related to Shiga toxin, although they share conserved sequences.

These ETEC Shiga toxins are composed of a single A subunit noncovalently associated with a pentamer composed of identical B subunits. The B subunits bind to globotriaosylceramide (Gb_3), a glycosphingolipid receptor on host cells. The A subunit is taken up by endocytosis. The toxin target is the 28S rRNA, which is depurated by the toxin at a specific adenine residue, causing protein synthesis to cease and affected cells to die. These toxins are carried on bacteriophages that are normally inactive (lysogenic) in the bacterial chromosome; when the phages are induced to replicate (e.g., by the stress induced by many antibiotics), they cause lysis of the bacteria and release of large amounts of toxin. Toxin translocation across the intestinal epithelium into the systemic circulation can lead to damage of vascular endothelial cells, resulting in activation of the coagulation cascade, formation of microthrombi, intravascular hemolysis, and ischemia.

The clinical outcome of an STEC infection depends on a strain-specific combination of epithelial attachment and the toxin factors. The Stx2 family of toxins is associated with a higher risk of causing HUS. Strains that make only Stx1 often cause only watery diarrhea and are infrequently associated with HUS.

The most common STEC serotypes are *E. coli* O157:H7, *E. coli* O111:NM, and *E. coli* O26:H11, although several hundred other STEC serotypes have also been described. *E. coli* **O157:H7** is the most virulent serotype and the serotype most frequently associated with HUS; however, other non-O157 serotypes also cause this illness.

ENTEROAGGREGATIVE *ESCHERICHIA COLI*

EAEC is associated with (1) acute, prolonged and persistent pediatric diarrhea in developing countries, most prominently in children <2 yr old and in malnourished children; (2) acute and persistent diarrhea in HIV-infected adults and children; and (3) acute traveler's diarrhea; EAEC is the 2nd most common cause of traveler's diarrhea after ETEC. Typical EAEC illness is manifested by watery, mucoid, secretory diarrhea with low-grade fever and little or no vomiting. The watery diarrhea can persist for ≥14 days. In some studies, many patients have grossly bloody stools, indicating that EAEC cannot be excluded on stool characteristics. EAEC strains are associated with growth retardation and malnutrition in infants in the developing world.

EAEC organisms form a characteristic biofilm on the intestinal mucosa and induce shortening of the villi, hemorrhagic necrosis, and inflammatory responses. The proposed model of pathogenesis of EAEC infection involves 3 phases: adherence to the intestinal mucosa by way of the aggregative adherence fimbriae or related adhesins; enhanced production of mucus; and production of toxins and inflammation that results in damage to the mucosa and intestinal secretion. Diarrhea caused by EAEC is predominantly secretory. The intestinal inflammatory response (elevated fecal lactoferrin, interleukin [IL]-8 and IL-1β) may be related to growth impairment and malnutrition.

EAEC strains are recognized by adherence to HEp-2 cells in an aggregative, stacked-brick pattern, called *aggregative adherence* (AA). EAEC virulence factors include the AA fimbriae (AAF-I, -II, and -III) that confer the AA phenotype. Some strains produce toxins, including the plasmid-encoded enterotoxin EAST1 (encoded by *ast*A), a homolog of the ETEC ST; an autotransporter toxin called Pet; other STATE toxins; and the chromosomally encoded enterotoxin ShET1 (encoded by *set*A and *set*B). Other virulence factors include outer membrane and secreted proteins, such as dispersin (*aap*), and the dispersin transport complex (aatPABCD). EAEC is a heterogeneous group of *E. coli*. The original diagnostic criteria (HEp-2 cell adherence pattern) identified many strains that are probably not true pathogens; genetic criteria appear to more reliably identify true pathogens. A transcriptional activator called **AggR** controls the expression of plasmid-borne and chromosomal virulence factors. Identification of AggR appears to reliably identify illness-associated pathogenic EAEC strains ("typical" EAEC). EAEC *aggR*-positive strains carrying 1-3 of the genes *aap*, *ast*A, and *set1A* are significantly associated with diarrhea compared with EAEC isolates lacking these genes. Other than the factors AAF and AggR, EAEC strains are genetically diverse and thus display variable virulence. EAEC strains belong to multiple serogroups, including O3, O7, O15, O44, O77, O86, O126, and O127.

DIFFUSELY ADHERENT *ESCHERICHIA COLI*

Although the status of DAEC strains as true pathogens has been in doubt, multiple studies in both developed and developing countries have associated these organisms with diarrhea, particularly in children after the 1st 1-2 yr of life. DAEC strains isolated from children and adults seem to represent 2 different bacterial populations. **Age-dependent susceptibility** may explain discrepancies among epidemiologic studies to diarrhea or by the use of inappropriate detection methods. Data suggest that these organisms also cause traveler's diarrhea in adults. DAEC produces acute watery diarrhea that is usually not dysenteric but is often prolonged.

DAEC strains produce diffuse adherence in cultured epithelial cells. They express surface fimbriae (designated F1845) that are responsible for the **diffuse adherence** phenotype in a prototype strain. These fimbriae

are homologous with members of the Afa/Dr family of adhesins, which are identified by hybridization with a specific probe, *daaC*, common to operons encoding Afa/Dr adhesions. A 2nd putative adhesin associated with the diffuse adherence pattern phenotype is an outer membrane protein, designated AIDA-I. The contribution of other putative effectors (*icuA, fimH, afa, agg-3A, pap, astA, shET1*) to virulence is still under investigation. The only documented secreted factor associated with DAEC infection is the serine-protease autotransporters of Enterobacteriaceae (SPATE) cytotoxin Sat. Bacteria expressing Afa/Dr adhesins interact with membrane-bound receptors, including decay-accelerating factor (DAF). The structural and functional lesions induced by DAEC include loss of microvilli and a decrease in the expression and enzyme activities of functional brush-border–associated proteins. Afa/Dr DAEC isolates produce a secreted autotransporter toxin that induces marked fluid accumulation in the intestine. DAEC strains typically induce IL-8 production in vitro. Serogroups of DAEC strains are less well defined than those of other diarrheagenic *E. coli*.

ENTEROAGGREGATIVE HEMORRHAGIC *ESCHERICHIA COLI*

In 2011, a massive outbreak of an unusual O104:H4 strain of diarrheagenic *E. coli* began in Germany. Eventually, >4,000 individuals were sickened with hemorrhagic colitis; the outbreak involved primarily adults (<100 children were reported affected). More than 800 people developed HUS, and >50 of these individuals died. Genomic analysis suggested the outbreak strain was most closely related to EAEC and had acquired a lambdoid bacteriophage with genes for Shiga toxin Stx2a. It was thus a **hybrid** pathogen with colonization mechanisms similar to a typical EAEC strain and toxin production typical of an STEC strain. This outbreak strain carries Pic on the chromosome and a pAA-like plasmid encoding AAF, AggR, Pet, ShET1, and dispersin. A 2nd virulence plasmid encodes multiple antibiotic resistances. The high morbidity and mortality associated with this strain may reflect the stronger adherence of EAEC compared with STEC, delivering more Stx to target cells. Alternative terminology for this strain includes **enteroaggregative hemorrhagic *E. coli*** and **Shiga toxin–producing EAEC**. Whether Shiga toxin production in an EAEC background merits separate classification is unclear. Organisms with Shiga toxin genes in an atypical EPEC background were designated as a separate group (referred to as **STEC, EHEC,** or **verotoxin-producing *E. coli***) before the relative importance of the various genes was clear. EPEC strains are a heterogeneous group themselves. The important issue is not the nomenclature but rather the concept that virulence genes can move between *E. coli*, resulting in new variants.

DIAGNOSIS

The features of illness are seldom distinctive enough to allow confident diagnosis strictly on clinical observations, and routine laboratory studies such as blood counts rarely prove effective in the diagnosis. Practical, non–DNA-dependent methods for routine diagnosis of diarrheagenic *E. coli* have been developed primarily for STEC. Serotype O157:H7 is suggested by isolation of an *E. coli* that fails to ferment sorbitol on MacConkey sorbitol medium; latex agglutination confirms that the organism contains O157 LPS. Other STEC strains can be detected in routine hospital laboratories using commercially available enzyme immunoassay or latex agglutination assays to detect Shiga toxins, although the variable sensitivity of commercial immunoassays has limited their value.

Although some STEC (O157:H7 strains) can be detected in routine microbiology laboratories using selective media and appropriate antisera, the diagnosis of other diarrheagenic *E. coli* infection is traditionally made based on tissue culture assays (e.g., HEp-2-cells assay for EPEC, EAEC, DAEC) or identification of specific virulence factors of the bacteria by phenotype (e.g., toxins) or genotype. Multiplex, real-time, or conventional polymerase chain reaction (PCR) can be used for presumptive diagnosis of isolated *E. coli* colonies. The genes commonly used for diagnostic PCR are *lt* and *st* for ETEC; *IpaH* or *iaL* for EIEC; *eae* and *bfp*A for EPEC; *eae, Stx1,* and *Stx2* for STEC; *AggR* or the AA plasmid for EAEC; and *daaC* or *daaD* for DAEC. Commercial assays such as the FilmArray Gastrointestinal Panel and Eurofins Diatherix Panel now detect genetic markers for EPEC, EAEC, ETEC, STEC, and EIEC, among other pathogen genes, directly from a fecal sample in several hours.

Serotyping does not provide definitive identification of pathotypes (except for selected cases such as O157:H7) because each pathotype contains many serotypes and some serotypes can belong to >1 pathotype. Consequently, serotyping should not be used routinely for diarrheagenic *E. coli* identification in clinical laboratories (e.g., to diagnose EPEC in infantile diarrhea), except during an outbreak investigation.

Other laboratory data are at best *nonspecific* indicators of etiology. Fecal leukocyte examination of the stool is often positive with EIEC or occasionally positive with other diarrheagenic *E. coli*. With EIEC and STEC there may be an elevated peripheral blood PMN count with a left shift. Determination of *Stx2* blood levels in the early, postbloody diarrhea period may be useful to identify children at risk of HUS; however, this method requires further evaluation. Fecal lactoferrin, IL-8, and IL-1β can be used as inflammatory markers. Electrolyte changes are nonspecific, reflecting only fluid loss.

TREATMENT

The cornerstone of management is appropriate fluid and electrolyte therapy. In general, this therapy should include oral replacement and maintenance with rehydration solutions such as those specified by the World Health Organization. Pedialyte and other readily available oral rehydration solutions are acceptable alternatives. After refeeding, continued supplementation with oral rehydration fluids is appropriate to prevent recurrence of dehydration. Early refeeding (within 6-8 hr of initiating rehydration) with breast milk or infant formula or solid foods should be encouraged. Prolonged withholding of feeding can lead to chronic diarrhea and malnutrition. If the child is malnourished, oral zinc should be given to speed recovery and decrease the risk of future diarrheal episodes.

Specific antimicrobial therapy of diarrheagenic *E. coli* is improving with accurate, rapid molecular diagnostic panels using direct fecal samples. However, the unpredictability of antibiotic susceptibilities remains problematic. Treatment is complicated by these organisms often being multiply resistant to antibiotics because of their previous exposure to inappropriate antibiotic therapy. Multiple studies in developing countries have found that diarrheagenic *E. coli* strains typically are resistant to antibiotics such as trimethoprim-sulfamethoxazole (TMP-SMX) and ampicillin (60–70%). Most data come from case series or clinical trials in adults with traveler's diarrhea. ETEC responds to antimicrobial agents such as TMP-SMX when the *E. coli* strains are susceptible. ETEC cases from traveler's diarrhea trials respond to ciprofloxacin, azithromycin, and rifaximin. However, other than for a child recently returning from travel in the developing world, empirical treatment of severe *watery diarrhea* with antibiotics is seldom appropriate.

In resource-poor settings where rapid molecular panel tests are not available, EIEC infections may be treated before culture results are finalized because the clinician suspects shigellosis and has begun empirical therapy. If the organisms prove to be susceptible, TMP-SMX is an appropriate choice. Although treatment of EPEC infection with TMP-SMX intravenously or orally for 5 days may be effective in speeding resolution, the lack of a rapid diagnostic test in the resource-poor setting makes treatment decisions difficult. Ciprofloxacin or rifaximin is useful for EAEC traveler's diarrhea, but pediatric data are sparse. Specific therapy for DAEC has not been defined.

The STEC strains represent a particularly difficult therapeutic dilemma; many antibiotics can induce bacterial stress, toxin production, and phage-mediated bacterial lysis with toxin release. Antibiotics should not be given for STEC infection because they can increase the risk of HUS (see Chapter 538). In settings with rapid molecular diagnostics, a delay in providing antibiotics is rarely consequential and can allow the clinician to more confidently recommend or exclude antibiotics from the therapeutic plan.

PREVENTION OF ILLNESS

In the developing world, prevention of disease caused by pediatric diarrheagenic *E. coli* is probably best done by maintaining prolonged breastfeeding, paying careful attention to personal hygiene, and following proper food- and water-handling procedures. People traveling to these places can be best protected by handwashing, consuming only processed water, bottled beverages, breads, fruit juices, fruits that can be peeled, or foods that are served steaming hot.

Prophylactic antibiotic therapy is effective in adult travelers but has not been studied in children and is not recommended. Public health measures, including sewage disposal and food-handling practices, have made pathogens that require large inocula to produce illness relatively uncommon in industrialized countries. Food-borne outbreaks of STEC are a problem for which no adequate solution has been found. During the occasional hospital outbreak of EPEC disease, attention to enteric isolation precautions and cohorting may be critical.

Protective immunity against diarrheagenic *E. coli* remains an active area of research, and no vaccines are available for clinical use in children. Multiple vaccine candidates based on bacterial toxins and colonization factors have shown promise for prevention of ETEC in adult travelers, but long-term protection with these vaccines has not been optimal, particularly in children.

Bibliography is available at Expert Consult.

Chapter **228**
Cholera
Anna Lena Lopez

第二百二十八章
霍乱

中文导读

　　本章主要介绍了霍乱的病因、流行病学、发病机制、临床表现、实验室检查、诊断与鉴别诊断、并发症、治疗和预防。其中，在发病机制部分就霍乱发病机制与霍乱毒素进行了详细描述。在治疗部分首先介绍了补液的重要性，随后详细介绍了推荐用于治疗霍乱的抗感染药以及补锌等内容。在预防部分详细描述了霍乱疫苗的应用现状和用法。

Cholera is a dehydrating diarrheal disease that rapidly leads to death in the absence of immediate initiation of appropriate treatment. Worldwide, 1.3 billion people are at risk for cholera, resulting in an estimated 1 to 4 million cases and 95,000 deaths annually. Cholera is highly prone to producing outbreaks, and the ongoing outbreaks in Yemen and Haiti emphasize how cholera and potentially other infectious diseases can easily reemerge in areas that have long been considered free of the disease after a natural disaster or war-related conflicts.

ETIOLOGY

Cholera is caused by *Vibrio cholerae*, a gram-negative, comma-shaped bacillus, subdivided into serogroups by its somatic O antigen. Of the >200 serogroups, only serogroups O1 and O139 have been associated with epidemics, although some non-O1, non-O139 *V. cholerae* strains (e.g., O75, O141) are pathogenic and can cause small outbreaks. A flagellar H antigen is present but is not used for species identification. The O1 serogroup is further divided into classical and the El Tor biotypes based on its biochemical characteristics. Since the turn of the 21st century, only **O1 El Tor** has been reported; hybrids and variants of *V. cholerae* O1 El Tor possessing classical genes have been reported worldwide. These hybrid and variant strains have been associated with more severe disease.

Each biotype of *V. cholerae* can be further subdivided into Inaba, Ogawa, and Hikojima serotypes based on the antigenic determinants on the O antigen. **Inaba** strains have A and C antigenic determinants, whereas **Ogawa** strains have A and B antigenic determinants. **Hikojima** strains produce all 3 antigenic determinants but are unstable and rare. Recent studies reveal that serotype switching results from a selection process as yet unidentified.

EPIDEMIOLOGY

The 1st 6 cholera pandemics originated in the Indian subcontinent and were caused by classical O1 *V. cholerae*. The 7th pandemic is the most extensive of all and is caused by *V. cholerae* O1 El Tor. This pandemic began in 1961 in Sulawesi, Indonesia, and has spread to the Indian subcontinent, Southeast Asia, Africa, Oceania, Southern Europe, and the Americas. In 1991, *V. cholerae* O1 El Tor first appeared in Peru before rapidly spreading in the Americas. Cholera becomes **endemic** in areas following outbreaks when a large segment of the population develops immunity to the disease after recurrent exposure. The disease is now endemic in parts of Africa and Asia and in Haiti.

In 1992 the first non-O1 *V. cholerae* that resulted in epidemics was identified in India and Bangladesh and was designated *V. cholerae* **O139**. From 1992–1994, this organism replaced O1 as the predominant cause of cholera in South Asia but has since been an uncommon etiologic agent.

The hybrid El Tor strains were first identified sporadically in Bangladesh. In 2004, during routine surveillance in Mozambique, isolates of *V. cholerae* O1 El Tor carrying classical genes were identified. Since then, hybrid and variant El Tor strains have been reported in other parts of Asia and Africa and have caused outbreaks in India and Vietnam. Although the classical biotype has virtually disappeared, its genes remain within the El Tor biotype. The current circulating strain in Haiti is closely related to the South Asian strain.

Humans are the only known hosts for *V. cholerae*, but free-living and plankton-associated *V. cholerae* exist in the marine environment. The organism thrives best in moderately salty water but can survive in rivers and fresh water if nutrient levels are high, as occurs when there is organic pollution such as human feces. The formation of a biofilm on abiotic surfaces and the ability to enter a viable but nonculturable state have been hypothesized as factors that allow *V. cholerae* to persist in the environment. Surface sea temperature, pH, chlorophyll content, the presence of iron compounds and chitin, and climatic conditions such as amount of rainfall and sea level rise are all important environmental factors that influence the survival of *V. cholerae* in the environment and the expression of cholera toxin, an important virulence determinant.

Consumption of **contaminated water** and ingestion of **undercooked**

shellfish are the main modes of transmission, with the latter more often seen in developed countries. In cholera-endemic areas, the incidence is highest among children <2 yr old; however, in epidemics, all age-groups are usually affected. Persons with blood group O, decreased gastric acidity, malnutrition, immunocompromised state, and absence of local intestinal immunity (prior exposure by infection or vaccination) are at increased risk for developing severe disease. Household contacts of cholera-infected patients are at high risk for the disease, because the stools of infected patients contain high concentrations of *V. cholerae*. Moreover, as *V. cholerae* organisms are shed, they enter into a hyperinfective state, requiring an infectious dose that is reduced by one-tenth to one-hundredth compared to organisms that were not shed by humans.

PATHOGENESIS

Large inocula of bacteria (>10^8 colony-forming units) are required for severe cholera to occur; however, for persons whose gastric barrier is disrupted, a much lower dose (10^5 CFUs) is required. After ingestion of *V. cholerae* from the environment, several changes occur in the vibrios as they traverse the human intestine: increased expression of genes required for nutrient acquisition, downregulation of chemotactic response, and expression of motility factors. Together these changes allow the vibrios to reach a hyperinfectious state, leading to lower infectious doses required to secondarily infect other persons. This hyperinfectivity may remain for 5-24 hr after excretion and is believed to be the predominant pathway for person-to-person transmission during epidemics.

If the vibrios survive gastric acidity, they colonize the small intestine through various factors such as toxin–co-regulated pili and motility, leading to efficient delivery of cholera toxin (Fig. 228.1). The cholera toxin consists of 5 binding B subunits and 1 active A subunit. The B subunits are responsible for binding to the GM_1 ganglioside receptors located in the small intestinal epithelial cells. After binding, the A subunit is released into the cell, where it stimulates adenylate cyclase and initiates a cascade of events. An increase in cyclic adenosine monophosphate leads to an increase in chloride secretion by the crypt cells, which in turn leads to inhibition of absorption of sodium and chloride by the microvilli. These events eventually lead to massive purging of electrolyte rich isotonic fluid in the small intestine that exceeds the absorptive capacity of the colon, resulting in rapid dehydration and depletion of electrolytes, including sodium, chloride, bicarbonate, and potassium. Metabolic acidosis and hypokalemia then ensue.

CLINICAL MANIFESTATIONS

Most cases of cholera are mild or inapparent. Among symptomatic individuals, approximately 20% develop severe **dehydration** that can rapidly lead to death. Following an incubation period of 1-3 days (range: several hours to 5 days), acute watery **diarrhea** and **vomiting** ensue. The onset may be sudden, with profuse watery diarrhea, but some patients have a prodrome of anorexia and abdominal discomfort and the stool may initially be brown. Diarrhea can progress to painless purging of profuse *rice-water stools* (suspended flecks of mucus) with a fishy smell, which is the hallmark of the disease (Figs. 228.2 and 228.3). Vomiting with clear watery fluid is usually present at the onset of the disease.

Cholera gravis, the most severe form of the disease, results when purging rates of 500-1,000 mL/hr occur. This purging leads to dehydration manifested by decreased urine output, a sunken fontanel (in infants), sunken eyes, absence of tears, dry oral mucosa, shriveled hands and feet ("washerwoman's hands"), poor skin turgor, thready pulse, tachycardia, hypotension, and vascular collapse (Fig. 228.3). Patients with metabolic acidosis can present with typical Kussmaul breathing. Although patients may be initially thirsty and awake, they rapidly progress to obtundation and coma. If fluid losses are not rapidly corrected, death can occur within hours.

LABORATORY FINDINGS

Findings associated with dehydration such as elevated urine specific gravity and hemoconcentration are evident. **Hypoglycemia** is a common finding that is caused by decreased food intake during the acute illness. Serum potassium may be initially normal or even high in the presence of metabolic acidosis; however, as the acidosis is corrected, hypokalemia may become evident. Metabolic acidosis due to bicarbonate loss is a prominent finding in severe cholera. Serum sodium and chloride levels may be normal or decreased, depending on the severity of the disease.

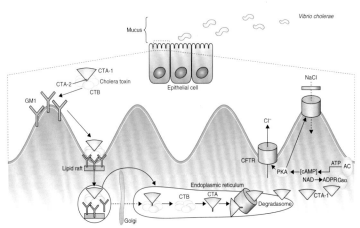

Fig. 228.1 Cholera pathogenesis and cholera toxin action. After ingestion, *Vibrio cholerae* colonize the small intestine and secrete cholera toxin, which has a doughnut-like structure with a central enzymatic toxic-active A (CTA-1 + CTA-2) subunit associated with a pentameric B subunit (CTB). After binding to GM_1 ganglioside receptors on small intestinal epithelial cells, which are mainly localized in lipid rafts on the cell surface, the cholera toxin is endocytosed and transported to the degradosome via the endoplasmic reticulum (ER) by a retrograde pathway, which, dependent on cell type, may or may not involve passage through the Golgi apparatus. In the ER, CTA dissociates from CTB, allowing CTA-1 to reach the cytosol by being translocated through the degradosome pathway. In the cytosol, CTA-1 subunits rapidly refold and bind to the Gsα subunit of adenylate cyclase (AC) in the cell membrane; on binding, CTA-1 adenosine diphosphate (ADP)-ribosylates the Gsα subunit, which stimulates AC activity, leading to an increase in intracellular concentration of cyclic adenosine monophosphate (cAMP), activation of protein kinase A (PKA), phosphorylation of the cystic fibrosis transmembrane conductance regulator (CFTR), a major chloride channel, and extracellular secretion of chloride ions (Cl⁻) and water. Cholera toxin–induced Cl⁻ (and bicarbonate ion) secretion is particularly pronounced in intestinal crypt cells, whereas the increased intracellular cAMP concentrations in villus cells mainly inhibit the uptake of sodium chloride (NaCl) and water. *(Adapted from Clemens J, Shin S, Sur D, et al: New-generation vaccines against cholera, Nat Rev Gastroenterol Hepatol 8:701–710, 2011; by permission of Nature Publishing Group.)*

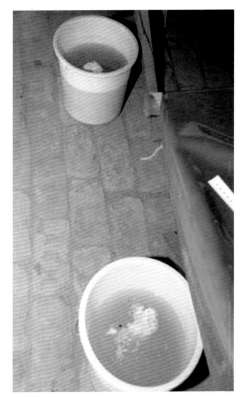

Fig. 228.2 Rice-water stool in a patient with cholera. *(Modified from Harris JB, LaRocque RC, Qadri F: Cholera, Lancet 379:2466–2474, 2012.)*

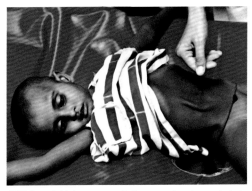

Fig. 228.3 A child, lying on a cholera cot, showing typical signs of severe dehydration from cholera. The patient has sunken eyes, lethargic appearance, and poor skin turgor, but within 2 hr was sitting up, alert, and eating normally. *(From Sack DA, Sack RB, Nair GB, et al: Cholera, Lancet 363:223–233, 2004.)*

DIAGNOSIS AND DIFFERENTIAL DIAGNOSIS

In children who have acute watery diarrhea with severe dehydration residing in a cholera-endemic area or who have recently traveled to an area known to have cholera, the disease may be suspected pending laboratory confirmation. Cholera differs from other diarrheal diseases in that it often occurs in *large outbreaks affecting both adults and children.* Treatment of dehydration should begin as soon as possible. Diarrhea caused by other etiologic causes (e.g., enterotoxigenic *Escherichia coli* or rotavirus) may be difficult to distinguish from cholera clinically. Microbiologic isolation of *V. cholerae* remains the gold standard for diagnosis. Although definitive diagnosis is not required for treatment

to be initiated, laboratory confirmation is necessary for epidemiologic surveillance. *V. cholerae* may be isolated from stools, vomitus, or rectal swabs. Specimens may be transported on Cary-Blair media if they cannot be processed immediately. Selective media such as thiosulfate-citrate–bile salts sucrose agar that inhibit normal flora should be used. Because most laboratories in industrialized countries do not routinely culture for *V. cholerae*, clinicians should request appropriate cultures for clinically suspected cases.

Stool examination reveals few fecal leukocytes and erythrocytes because cholera does not cause inflammation. Dark-field microscopy may be used for rapid identification of typical *darting motility* in wet mounts of rice-water stools, a finding that disappears once specific antibodies against *V. cholerae* O1 or O139 are added. Rapid diagnostic tests are currently available and may be especially useful in areas with limited laboratory capacity, allowing early identification of cases at the onset of an outbreak and facilitating a timely response. Molecular identification with the use of polymerase chain reaction and DNA probes is available but often not used in areas where cholera exists.

COMPLICATIONS

Delayed initiation of rehydration therapy or inadequate rehydration often leads to complications. Renal failure from prolonged hypotension can occur. Unless potassium supplementation is provided, **hypokalemia** can lead to nephropathy and focal myocardial necrosis. Hypoglycemia is common among children and can lead to seizures unless it is appropriately corrected.

TREATMENT

Rehydration is the mainstay of therapy (see Chapter 69). Effective and timely case management decreases mortality considerably. Children with mild or moderate dehydration may be treated with oral rehydration solution (ORS) unless the patient is in shock, is obtunded, or has intestinal ileus. Vomiting is not a contraindication to ORS. Severely dehydrated patients require intravenous fluid, ideally with lactated Ringer solution. When available, rice-based ORS should be used during rehydration, because this fluid has been shown to be superior to standard ORS in children and adults with cholera. Close monitoring is necessary, especially during the 1st 24 hr of illness, when large amounts of stool may be passed. After rehydration, patients should be reassessed every 1-2 hr, or more frequently if profuse diarrhea is ongoing. Feeding should not be withheld during diarrhea. Frequent, small feedings are better tolerated than less frequent, large feedings.

Antibiotics should only be given in patients with moderately severe to severe dehydration (Table 228.1). As soon as vomiting stops (usually within 4-6 hr after initiation of rehydration therapy), an antibiotic to which local *V. cholerae* strains are sensitive must be administered. Antibiotics shorten the duration of illness, decrease fecal excretion of vibrios, decrease the volume of diarrhea, and reduce the fluid requirement during rehydration. Single-dose antibiotics increase compliance; doxycycline, ciprofloxacin, and azithromycin are effective against cholera. There are increasing reports of resistance to tetracyclines, trimethoprim-sulfamethoxazole, and other drugs. Because of these multidrug-resistant strains, antibiotic treatment must be tailored based on available susceptibility results from the area. The 2013 WHO guidelines recommend cotrimoxazole (4 mg trimethoprim/kg and 20 mg/kg sulfamethoxazole/kg twice daily) and chloramphenicol (20 mg/kg IM every 6 hr for 3 days) as possible alternative antibiotics for treatment. A recent systematic review, however, recommended the use of single-dose azithromycin (20 mg/kg) due to widespread antimicrobial resistance. Cephalosporins and aminoglycosides are not clinically effective against cholera and therefore should not be used, even if in vitro tests show strains to be sensitive.

Zinc should be given as soon as vomiting stops. Zinc deficiency is common among children in many developing countries. Zinc supplementation in children <5 yr old shortens the duration of diarrhea and reduces subsequent diarrhea episodes when given daily for 14 days at the time of the illness. Children <6 mo old should receive 10 mg of oral zinc daily for 2 wk, and children >6 mo should receive 20 mg of oral zinc daily for 2 wk.

Table 228.1	Recommended Antimicrobials for Cholera*	
RECOMMENDING BODY	**ANTIBIOTIC OF CHOICE**	**ALTERNATIVE**
WHO[†] (antibiotics recommended for cases with severe dehydration)	**Adults** Doxycycline, 300 mg given as a single dose orally (PO) or Tetracycline, 500 mg 4 times a day × 3 days PO **Children** Tetracycline, 12.5 mg/kg/dose 4 times a day × 3 days (up to 500 mg/dose × 3 days) PO	**Adults** Erythromycin, 250 mg 4 times a day × 3 days PO **Children** Erythromycin, 12.5 mg/kg/dose 4 times a day × 3 days (up to 250 mg 4 times a day × 3 days) PO
PAHO[‡] (antibiotics recommended for cases with moderate to severe dehydration)	**Adults** Doxycycline, 300 mg PO given as a single dose **Children** Erythromycin, 12.5 mg/kg/dose 4 times a day × 3 days (up to 500 mg/dose × 3 days) or Azithromycin, 20 mg/kg as a single dose (up to 1 g)	**Adults** Ciprofloxacin, 1 g PO single dose or Azithromycin, 1 g PO single dose (first line for pregnant women) **Children** Ciprofloxacin, 20 mg/kg PO as a single dose or Doxycycline, 2-4 mg/kg PO as a single dose

*Antibiotic selection must be based on sensitivity patterns of strains of *Vibrio cholerae* O1 or O139 in the area.
[†]Adapted from World Health Organization: *The treatment of diarrhea: a manual for physicians and other senior health workers*, 4th revision, Geneva, 2005, WHO.
[‡]Adapted from Pan American Health Organization: *Recommendations for clinical management of cholera*, Washington, DC, 2010. http://new.paho.org/hq/index.php?option=com_docman&task=doc_download&gid=10813&Itemid=.

Table 228.2	Available Oral Cholera Vaccines*	
VACCINE TRADE NAME	**CONTENTS**	**DOSING SCHEDULE**

Dukoral (Crucell)	1 mg of recombinant B subunit of cholera toxin plus 2.5×10^{10} colony-forming units of the following strains of *V. cholerae*:
	  Formalin-killed El Tor Inaba (Phil 6973)
	  Heat-killed classical Inaba (Cairo 48)
	  Heat-killed classical Ogawa (Cairo 50)
	  Formalin-killed classical Ogawa (Cairo 50)
		Children 2-6 yr old: 3 doses, 1-6 wk apart
		Adults and children >6 yr old: 2 doses, 1-6 wk apart

Shanchol (Shantha Biotech)
Euvichol (Eubiologics)
	V. cholerae O1:
	  600 EU Formalin-killed El Tor Inaba (Phil 6973)
	  300 EU Heat-killed classical Inaba (Cairo 48)
	  300 EU Heat-killed classical Ogawa (Cairo 50)
	  300 EU Formalin-killed classical Ogawa (Cairo 50)
	V. cholerae O139-600 EU of Formalin-killed strain 4260B
		Adults and children ≥1 yr old: 2 doses, 2 wk apart

*WHO-prequalified vaccines.

PREVENTION

Improved personal hygiene, access to clean water, and sanitation are the mainstays of cholera control. Appropriate case management substantially decreases case fatalities to <1%. Travelers from developed countries often have no prior exposure to cholera and are therefore at risk of developing the disease. Children traveling to cholera-affected areas should avoid drinking potentially contaminated water and eating high-risk foods such as raw or undercooked fish and shellfish. No country or territory requires vaccination against cholera as a condition for entry.

In 2016, a live oral cholera vaccine, CVD 103 Hg-R (Vaxchora, PaxVax), was licensed in the United States for use in adults age 18-64 yr traveling to cholera-affected areas.

Alarmed by the increasing prevalence of cholera, in 2011 the World Health Assembly recommended the use of oral cholera vaccines to complement existing water, sanitation, and hygiene initiatives for cholera control. Older-generation parenteral cholera vaccines have not been recommended by World Health Organization (WHO) because of the limited protection they confer and their high reactogenicity. Oral cholera vaccines are safe, are protective for approximately 2-5 yr duration, and confer moderate herd protection. Three oral cholera vaccines are currently available internationally and recognized by WHO (Table 228.2). An internationally licensed killed whole cell oral cholera vaccine with recombinant B subunit (Dukoral, Crucell) has been available in >60 countries, including the European Union, and provides protection against cholera in endemic areas as well as cross-protection against certain strains of enterotoxigenic *E. coli*. The 2 other vaccines (Shanchol, Shantha Biotech; and Euvichol, Eubiologics) are variants of the 1st vaccine and contain the *V. cholerae* O1 and O139 antigens but do not contain the B subunit. Without the B subunit, these vaccines do not require buffer for administration, thereby reducing administration costs and resources, making them easier to deploy.

Oral cholera vaccines have been available for >2 decades, and with the WHO declaration, countries are now using oral cholera vaccines in mass vaccination campaigns where cholera remains a substantial problem. A cholera vaccine stockpile, established by WHO, is now available and can be accessed by countries at risk for cholera, supplementing efforts to lessen the impact of this ongoing cholera scourge.

Bibliography is available at Expert Consult.

Chapter **229**
Campylobacter
Ericka V. Hayes

第二百二十九章
弯曲菌

中文导读

　　本章主要介绍了弯曲菌感染的病因、流行病学、发病机制、临床表现、诊断、并发症、治疗、预后和预防。在弯曲菌感染的病因部分详细描述了与人类疾病相关的弯曲杆菌菌种。在弯曲菌感染的临床表现部分详细介绍了急性胃肠炎、菌血症、局灶性肠外感染和围产期感染。在弯曲菌感染的并发症部分详细介绍了反应性关节炎、吉兰-巴雷综合征和其他并发症。

Campylobacter, typically *Campylobacter jejuni* and *Campylobacter coli*, are found globally and are among the most common causes of human intestinal infections. Clinical presentation varies by age and underlying conditions.

ETIOLOGY

Twenty-six species and 9 subspecies of *Campylobacter* are recognized (as of December 2014). Most of these have been isolated from humans, and many are considered pathogenic. The most significant of these are *C. jejuni* and *C. coli,* which are believed to cause the majority of human enteritis. More than 100 serotypes of *C. jejuni* have been identified. *C. jejuni* has been subspeciated into *C. jejuni* subsp. *jejuni* and *C. jejuni* subsp. *doylei*. Although *C. jejuni* subsp. *doylei* has been isolated from humans, it is much less common, less hardy, and more difficult to isolate. Other species, including *Campylobacter fetus, Campylobacter lari,* and *Campylobacter upsaliensis,* have been isolated from patients with diarrhea, although much less frequently (Table 229.1). Emerging *Campylobacter* spp. have been implicated in acute gastroenteritis, inflammatory bowel disease, and peritonitis, including *C. concisus,* and *C. ureolyticus*. Additional *Campylobacter* spp. have been isolated from clinical specimens, but their roles as pathogens have not been established.

Campylobacter organisms are gram-negative, curved, thin (0.2-0.8 μm wide), non–spore-forming rods (0.5-5 μm long) that usually have tapered ends. They are smaller than most other enteric bacterial pathogens and have variable morphology, including short, comma-shaped or **S**-shaped organisms and long, multispiraled, filamentous, seagull-shaped organisms. Individual organisms are usually motile with a flagellum at one or both poles depending on the species. Such morphology enables these bacteria to colonize the mucosal surfaces of both the gastrointestinal (GI) and respiratory tracts and move through them in a spiraling motion. Most *Campylobacter* organisms are microaerophilic, occasionally partially anaerobic, and oxidase positive. Most can transform into coccoid forms under adverse conditions, especially oxidation.

EPIDEMIOLOGY

Worldwide, *Campylobacter* enteritis is a leading cause of acute diarrhea. Efforts to reduce *Campylobacter* contamination and use of safe handling practices have led to decreased incidence. *Campylobacter* infections can be both food-borne and water-borne and most frequently result from ingestion of contaminated **poultry** (chicken, turkey) or **raw milk**. Less often, the bacteria come from drinking water, household pets (cats, dogs, hamsters), and farm animals. Infections are more common in resource-limited settings, are prevalent year-round in tropical areas, and can exhibit seasonal peaks in temperate regions (late spring with a peak midsummer in most of the United States, with a smaller secondary peak in late fall). In industrialized countries, *Campylobacter* infections peak in early childhood and again in young adulthood (15-44 yr). This 2nd peak is not seen with *Salmonella* and *Shigella* infections. In developing countries, repeated infections are common in childhood, leading to increased immunity and rare disease in adulthood. Each year in the United States, there are an estimated 2.5 million cases of *Campylobacter* infection. Of these, death is rare, with 50-150 reports annually. In The Netherlands, medical record review shows that on average each resident acquires asymptomatic *Campylobacter* colonization every 2 yr, progressing to symptomatic infection in approximately 1% of colonized people.

Food-borne infection is most common and can be seen with the consumption of raw or undercooked meat, as well as by cross-contamination of other foods. Although **chickens** are the classic source of *Campylobacter,* many animal sources of human food can also harbor *Campylobacter,* including seafood. *C. coli* has been linked to swine. Poultry is more likely to be heavily contaminated, whereas red meats often have fewer organisms. Unpasteurized milk products are also a documented source. Additionally, many pets can carry *Campylobacter,* and flies inhabiting contaminated environments can acquire the organism. Shedding from animals can contaminate water sources. Humans can acquire infection from water, although much less frequently than from contaminated food. **Airborne** (droplet) **transmission** of *Campylobacter*

Table 229.1	*Campylobacter* Species Associated With Human Disease	
SPECIES	**DISEASES IN HUMANS**	**COMMON SOURCES**
C. jejuni	Gastroenteritis, bacteremia, Guillain-Barré syndrome	Poultry, raw milk, cats, dogs, cattle, swine, monkeys, water
C. coli	Gastroenteritis, bacteremia	Poultry, raw milk, cats, dogs, cattle, swine, monkeys, oysters, water
C. fetus	Bacteremia, meningitis, endocarditis, mycotic aneurysm, diarrhea	Sheep, cattle, birds, dogs
C. hyointestinalis	Diarrhea, bacteremia, proctitis	Swine, cattle, deer, hamsters, raw milk, oysters
C. lari	Diarrhea, colitis, appendicitis, bacteremia, UTI	Seagulls, water, poultry, cattle, dogs, cats, monkeys, oysters, mussels
C. upsaliensis	Diarrhea, bacteremia, abscesses, enteritis, colitis, hemolytic-uremic syndrome	Cats, dogs, other domestic pets
C. concisus	Diarrhea, gastritis, enteritis, periodontitis	Human oral cavity, dogs
C. sputorum	Diarrhea, bedsores, abscesses, periodontitis	Human oral cavity, cattle, swine, dogs
C. rectus	Periodontitis	
C. mucosalis	Enteritis	Swine, dogs
C. jejuni subsp. *doylei*	Diarrhea, colitis, appendicitis, bacteremia, UTI	Swine
C. curvus	Gingivitis, alveolar abscess	Poultry, raw milk, cats, dogs, cattle, swine, monkeys, water, human oral cavity
C. gracilis	Head and neck abscesses, abdominal abscesses, empyema	Dogs
C. cryaerophila	Diarrhea	Swine

UTI, Urinary tract infection.

has occurred in poultry workers. Use of antimicrobials in animal foods may increase the prevalence of antibiotic-resistant *Campylobacter* isolated from humans.

Human infection can result from exposure to as few as 500 bacteria, although a higher dose (>9,000 bacteria) is often needed to cause illness reproducibly. Inoculum effectiveness is dependent on host factors, including immune status and stomach acidification. *C. jejuni* and *C. coli* spread person to person, perinatally, and at childcare centers where diapered toddlers are present. People infected with *C. jejuni* usually shed the organism for weeks, but some can shed for months, with children tending toward longer shedding. **Handwashing** is critical to preventing spread in these environments.

PATHOGENESIS

Most *Campylobacter* isolates are acid sensitive and should, in theory, be eradicated in the stomach. Therefore, models for the pathogenesis of *C. jejuni* enteritis include mechanisms to transit the stomach, adhere to intestinal mucosal cells, and initiate intestinal lumen fluid accumulation. Host conditions associated with reduced gastric acidity, such as proton pump inhibitor use, and foods capable of shielding organisms in transit through the stomach may help allow *Campylobacter* to reach the intestine. Once there, *Campylobacter* is able to adhere to and invade intestinal mucosal cells through motility, including use of flagellae, as well as by the use of surface proteins (e.g., PEB1, CadF), large plasmids (e.g., pVir), surface adhesins (e.g., JlpA), and chemotactic factors. Lumen fluid accumulation is associated with direct damage to mucosal cells resulting from bacterial invasion and potentially from an enterotoxin and other cytotoxins. Additionally, *C. jejuni* has mechanisms that enable transit away from the mucosal surface. The factors used depend on the species involved.

Campylobacter spp. differ from other enteric bacterial pathogens in that they have both *N*- and *O*-linked glycosylation capacities. *N*-linked glycosylation is associated with molecules expressed on the bacterial surface, and *O*-linked glycosylation appears limited to flagellae. Slipped-strand mispairing in glycosylation loci results in modified, antigenically distinct surface structures. It is hypothesized that antigenic variation provides a mechanism for immune evasion.

C. fetus possesses a high-molecular-weight S-layer protein that mediates high-level resistance to serum-mediated killing and phagocytosis and is therefore thought to be responsible for the propensity to produce bacteremia. *C. jejuni* and *C. coli* are generally sensitive to serum-mediated killing, but serum-resistant variants exist. Some suggest these serum-resistant variants may be more capable of systemic dissemination.

Campylobacter infections can be followed by **Guillain-Barré syndrome**, **reactive arthritis**, and **erythema nodosum**. Such complications are thought to be from molecular mimicry between nerve, joint, and dermal tissue and *Campylobacter* surface antigens. Most *Campylobacter* infections are not followed by immunoreactive complications, indicating that host conditions as well as other factors, in addition to molecular mimicry, are required for these complications. It is proposed that low-grade inflammation caused by *Campylobacter*, below the threshold that can be detected by endoscopy, results in crosstalk with gut nerves, leading to symptoms.

CLINICAL MANIFESTATIONS

There are a variety of clinical presentations of *Campylobacter* infections, depending on host factors such as age, immunocompetence, and underlying conditions. Infection presents most often as gastroenteritis, but also as bacteremia, neonatal infections, and, less often, extraintestinal infections.

Acute Gastroenteritis

Acute gastroenteritis with diarrhea is usually caused by *C. jejuni* (90–95%) or *C. coli*, and rarely by *C. lari*, *C. hyointestinalis*, or *C. upsaliensis*. Infections with *C. jejuni* and *C. coli* are indistinguishable by clinical presentation. The average incubation period is 3 days (range: 1-7 days). One third of symptomatic patients can have a prodrome with fever, headache, dizziness, and myalgias; 1-3 days later, they develop cramping abdominal pain and loose, watery stools, or, less frequently, mucus-containing bloody stools. In severe cases (approximately 15%), blood appears in the stools 2-4 days after the onset of symptoms. In younger children, >50% may develop blood in their stools. Some patients do not develop diarrhea at all, most often children who are 6-15 yr old.

Fever may be the only manifestation initially and is most pronounced in patients >1 yr old. From 60–90% of older children also complain of abdominal pain. The abdominal pain is most frequently periumbilical and sometimes persists after the stools return to normal. The abdominal pain can mimic appendicitis, colitis, or intussusception. Nausea is common, with up to 25% of adults developing vomiting. Vomiting tends to be more common the younger the patient and is most frequent in infants. Infection with species other than *C. jejuni* and *C. coli* may have milder symptoms.

Diarrhea lasts approximately 7 days and will resolve spontaneously. More mild disease can last 1-2 days; 20–30% of patients will have symptoms for 2 wk, and 5–10% are symptomatic for >2 wk. Relapse can occur in 5–10% of patients. Persistent or recurrent *Campylobacter* gastroenteritis has been reported in immunocompetent patients, in patients with hypogammaglobulinemia (both congenital and acquired), and in patients with AIDS. Persistent infection can mimic chronic **inflammatory bowel disease** (IBD); therefore *Campylobacter* infection should also be considered when evaluating for IBD. Some evidence supports that *Campylobacter* infection may also be the trigger for development of IBD. Fecal shedding of the organisms in untreated patients usually lasts for 2-3 wk, with a range from a few days to several months. Shedding tends to occur longer in young children. Acute appendicitis, mesenteric lymphadenitis, and ileocolitis have been reported in patients who have had appendectomy during *C. jejuni* infection.

Bacteremia
Transient bacteremia has been shown in early acute infection in 0.1–1% of patients. With the exception of bacteremia caused by *C. fetus*, bacteremia with *Campylobacter* occurs most often among patients with chronic illnesses or immunodeficiency (e.g., HIV), severe malnutrition, and in extremes of age. However, bacteremia is also well described in patients without underlying disease. The majority of cases of bacteremia are asymptomatic. *C. fetus* causes bacteremia in adults with or without identifiable focal infection, usually in the setting of underlying conditions such as malignancy, immunodeficiency, or diabetes mellitus. When symptomatic, *C. jejuni* bacteremia is associated with fever, headache, malaise, and abdominal pain. Relapsing or intermittent fever is associated with night sweats, chills, and weight loss when the illness is prolonged. Lethargy and confusion can occur, but focal neurologic signs are unusual without cerebrovascular disease or meningitis. Moderate leukocytosis with left shift may be found. Variable presentations have been described, including transient asymptomatic bacteremia, rapidly fatal septicemia, and prolonged bacteremia of 8-13 wk.

Focal Extraintestinal Infections
Focal infections caused by *C. jejuni* are rare and occur mainly among neonates and immunocompromised patients. Multiple sites have been reported, including meningitis, pneumonia, thrombophlebitis, pancreatitis, cholecystitis, ileocecitis, urinary tract infection, arthritis, peritonitis, ileocecitis, pericarditis, and endocarditis. *C. fetus* shows a predilection for vascular endothelium, leading to endocarditis, pericarditis, thrombophlebitis, and mycotic aneurysms. *C. hyointestinalis* has been associated with proctitis, *C. upsaliensis* with breast abscesses, and *C. rectus* with periodontitis.

Perinatal Infections
Perinatal infections are most often acquired at birth from a mother infected with or shedding *Campylobacter*. Maternal *C. fetus* and *C. jejuni* infections may be asymptomatic and can result in abortion, stillbirth, premature delivery, or neonatal infection with sepsis and meningitis. Severe perinatal infections are uncommon and are caused most often by *C. fetus* and rarely by *C. jejuni*. Neonatal infection with *C. jejuni* is associated with diarrhea that may be bloody. Nosocomial infections in nurseries have also been described.

DIAGNOSIS
The clinical presentation of *Campylobacter* enteritis can be similar to that of enteritis caused by other bacterial pathogens. The differential diagnosis includes *Shigella*, *Salmonella*, *Escherichia coli*, *Yersinia enterocolitica*,

Aeromonas, *Vibrio parahaemolyticus*, and amebiasis. Fecal leukocytes are found in as many as 75% of cases, and fecal blood is present in 50% of cases (higher in pediatric patients). *Campylobacter* should be considered in patients with bloody stools, fever, and abdominal pain.

The diagnosis of *Campylobacter* enteritis is usually confirmed by identification of the organism in cultures of stool or rectal swabs. Isolation is most likely from selective media such as CAMPY-agar grown in microaerophilic conditions (5–10% oxygen), 1–10% carbon dioxide, with some hydrogen. Some *C. jejuni* grow best at 42°C (107.6°F). Growth on solid media results in small (0.5-1.0 mm), slightly raised, smooth colonies. Organisms can be identified from stool microscopically in approximately 50% of known *Campylobacter* cases. Gram stain is even less sensitive. Stool culture is >90% sensitive and is the standard method of diagnosis. Visible growth on stool culture is most often present in 1-2 days. Visible growth in blood cultures is often not apparent until 5-14 days after inoculation.

Routine culture may be adequate for isolation of *C. jejuni* because of the large numbers of bacteria that are often present. However, because *Campylobacter* organisms grow more slowly under routine conditions than do other enteric bacteria, routine culture can result in failure because of overgrowth of other enteric bacteria. *Campylobacter* culture can be enhanced, when necessary, with selective media. However, selective culture media developed to enhance isolation of *C. jejuni* may inhibit the growth of other *Campylobacter* spp. Filtration methods are available and can preferentially enrich for *Campylobacter* by selecting for their small size. These methods allow subsequent culture of the enriched sample on antibiotic-free media, enhancing rates of isolation of *Campylobacter* organisms inhibited by the antibiotics included in standard selective media. Isolation of *Campylobacter* from normally sterile sites does not require enhancement procedures. Clinically, it is not necessary to speciate *Campylobacter*, because clinical disease is the same. Speciation can be done, when needed, and specialized laboratories can perform strain typing when required for epidemiologic purposes.

For rapid diagnosis of *Campylobacter* enteritis, direct carbolfuchsin stain of fecal smear, indirect fluorescence antibody test, dark-field microscopy, or latex agglutination were used historically. Polymerase chain reaction testing is more specific and sensitive and is becoming more widely available for rapid testing, often grouped with testing for other bacterial, viral, and parasitic stool pathogens in a multiplex assay. At this time, the recommendation remains to confirm all positive rapid tests with culture, which also allows for susceptibility testing and epidemiologic investigations. Serologic diagnosis is also possible and is most helpful in patients with late-onset reactive arthritis or Guillain-Barré syndrome, since these patients may have negative stool cultures by the time of presentation with these late complications.

COMPLICATIONS
Severe, prolonged *C. jejuni* infection can occur in patients with immunodeficiencies, including hypogammaglobulinemia, malnutrition, and acquired immunodeficiency syndrome (AIDS). In patients with AIDS, increased frequency and severity of *C. jejuni* infection occurs; severity correlates inversely with CD4 count. Complications can include acute complications, as described earlier, and late-onset complications that may present after the acute infection has resolved. The most common late-onset complications include reactive arthritis and Guillain-Barré syndrome.

Reactive Arthritis
Reactive arthritis can accompany *Campylobacter* enteritis in adolescents and adults, especially in patients who are positive for HLA-B27 (see Chapter 182). Reactive arthritis occurs in up to 3% of patients, although up to 13% may have joint symptoms. This manifestation usually appears 1-2 wk after the onset of diarrhea but has been seen 5-40 days later. It involves mainly large joints and resolves without sequelae. The arthritis is typically migratory and occurs without fever. Synovial fluid lacks bacteria. The arthritis responds well to nonsteroidal antiinflammatory drugs and typically resolves after 1 wk to several months. Reactive arthritis with conjunctivitis, urethritis, and rash (including erythema nodosum) also occurs but is less common.

Guillain-Barré Syndrome

Guillain-Barré syndrome (GBS) is an acute demyelinating disease of the peripheral nervous system characterized clinically by acute flaccid paralysis and is the most common cause of neuromuscular paralysis worldwide (see Chapter 634). GBS carries a mortality rate of approximately 2%, and approximately 20% of patients develop major neurologic sequelae. *C. jejuni* has been identified as the trigger in up to 40% of patients with GBS and is most closely linked to the serotypes Penner O19 and O41. It has been reported 1-12 wk after *C. jejuni* gastroenteritis in 1 of every 1,000 *C. jejuni* infections. Stool cultures obtained from patients with GBS at the onset of neurologic symptoms have yielded *C. jejuni* in >25% of the cases. Serologic studies suggest that 20–45% of patients with GBS have evidence of recent *C. jejuni* infection. Molecular mimicry between nerve tissue GM_1 ganglioside and *Campylobacter* surface antigens may be the triggering factor in *Campylobacter*-associated GBS. The Miller-Fisher variant, which more often affects cranial nerves, is characterized by ataxia, areflexia, and ophthalmoplegia and is linked to cross-reacting antibodies to the GQ1b ganglioside found in cranial nerve myelin; the most common serotype for this variant is Penner O2. When associated with *Campylobacter,* GBS is more likely to be the axonal form and has a worse prognosis with slower recovery and more neurologic disability. The management of GBS includes supportive care, intravenous immunoglobulin, and plasma exchange.

Other Complications

Immunoglobulin A nephropathy and immune complex glomerulonephritis with *C. jejuni* antigens in the kidneys have been reported. *Campylobacter* infection has also been associated with hemolytic anemia and hemolytic-uremic syndrome.

Treatment

Fluid replacement, correction of electrolyte imbalance, and supportive care are the mainstays of treatment of children with *Campylobacter* gastroenteritis. Antimotility agents are contraindicated because they can cause prolonged or fatal disease. The need for antibiotic therapy in healthy patients with uncomplicated gastroenteritis is controversial. Data suggest a shortened duration of symptoms (by an average of 1.3 days) and intestinal shedding of organisms if antibiotics are initiated early in the disease. Antibiotics are recommended for patients with bloody stools, high fever, or a severe course, as well as for children who are immunosuppressed or have underlying diseases, and individuals at high risk of developing severe disease (e.g., pregnancy). Extraintestinal infections (e.g., bacteremia) should also be treated with antibiotics.

Most *Campylobacter* isolates are susceptible to macrolides, fluoroquinolones, aminoglycosides, chloramphenicol, tetracyclines, and clindamycin (though there is no clinical efficacy data for these last three agents, only in vitro data) and are resistant to cephalosporins, penicillins, and trimethoprim. Resistance to tetracyclines, macrolides, and more often fluoroquinolones has been described. **Antibiotic resistance** among *C. jejuni* has become a serious worldwide problem. Macrolide resistance is increased in areas such as Thailand and Ireland, whereas fluoroquinolone resistance has been reported in Spain, Hungary, and multiple developing countries in >50% of cultured *Campylobacter*. Fluoroquinolone resistance continues to increase in the United States and is related to the use of quinolones in veterinary medicine and food products, as well as acquisition from travelers. Erythromycin-resistant *Campylobacter* isolates are uncommon in the United States; therefore, **azithromycin** is the drug of choice if therapy is required, particularly in pediatric patients. Drug sensitivities should be determined for patients who do not respond to therapy or any patient with invasive or extraintestinal infection. Sepsis is treated with parenteral antibiotics such as meropenem or imipenem, with or without an aminoglycoside. For extraintestinal infection caused by *C. fetus*, prolonged therapy is advised. *C. fetus* isolates resistant to erythromycin and fluoroquinolones have been reported; therefore empirical therapy for serious *C. fetus* infection should avoid these agents pending susceptibilities.

PROGNOSIS

Although *Campylobacter* gastroenteritis is usually self-limited, immunosuppressed children (including children with AIDS) can experience a protracted or severe course. Septicemia in newborns and immunocompromised hosts has a poor prognosis, with an estimated mortality rate of 30–40%. Additional prognosis is based on the secondary sequelae that may develop.

PREVENTION

Most human *Campylobacter* infections are sporadic and are acquired from infected animals or contaminated foods or water. Interventions to minimize transmission include cooking meats thoroughly, preventing recontamination after cooking by not using the same surfaces, utensils, or containers for both uncooked and cooked food, and avoiding unpasteurized dairy products. Also, it is important to ensure that water sources are not contaminated and that water is kept in clean containers. Contact with infected animals should be avoided. No specific isolation is required; **standard precautions** are sufficient, although in a hospital or clinic setting with an incontinent child, **contact precautions** are indicated. However, children in diapers should be kept out of daycare until the diarrhea resolves. Breastfeeding appears to decrease symptomatic *Campylobacter* disease but does not reduce colonization.

Several approaches at immunization have been studied, including the use of live-attenuated organisms, subunit vaccines, and killed–whole cell vaccines. No vaccine is currently available.

Bibliography is available at Expert Consult.

Chapter **230**
Yersinia
Ericka V. Hayes

第二百三十章
耶尔森菌

中 文 导 读

本章首先阐述了耶尔森菌属包括14个菌种，其中对人有致病性的有3种：小肠结肠炎耶尔森菌、假结核耶尔森菌和鼠疫耶尔森菌。随后，详细介绍了小肠结肠炎耶尔森菌感染的病因、流行病学、发病机制、临床表现、诊断、鉴别诊断、治疗、并发症和预防，

假结核耶尔森菌感染的病因、流行病学、发病机制、临床表现、诊断、鉴别诊断、治疗、并发症和预防，以及瘟疫（鼠疫耶尔森菌）的病因、流行病学、发病机制、临床表现、诊断、鉴别诊断、治疗和预防。

The genus *Yersinia* is a member of the family Enterobacteriaceae and comprises more than 14 named species, 3 of which are established as human pathogens. *Yersinia enterocolitica* is by far the most common *Yersinia* species causing human disease and produces fever, abdominal pain that can mimic appendicitis, and diarrhea. *Yersinia pseudotuberculosis* is most often associated with mesenteric lymphadenitis. *Yersinia pestis* is the agent of **plague** and typically causes an acute febrile lymphadenitis (bubonic plague) and less often occurs as septicemic, pneumonic, pharyngeal, or meningeal plague. Other *Yersinia* species are uncommon causes of infections of humans, and their identification is often an indicator of immunodeficiency.

Yersinia is enzootic and can colonize pets. Infections in humans are incidental and most often result from contact with infected animals or their tissues; ingestion of contaminated water, milk, or meat; or for *Y. pestis,* the bite of infected fleas or inhalation of respiratory droplets (human, dog, cat). Association with human disease is less clear for *Yersinia frederiksenii, Yersinia intermedia, Yersinia kristensenii, Yersinia aldovae, Yersinia bercovieri, Yersinia mollaretii, Yersinia rohdei,* and *Yersinia ruckeri.* Some *Yersinia* isolates replicate at low temperatures (1-4°C [33.8-39.2°F]) or survive at high temperatures (50-60°C [122-140°F]). Thus, common food preparation and storage and common pasteurization methods might not limit the number of bacteria. Most are sensitive to oxidizing agents.

230.1 *Yersinia enterocolitica*
Ericka V. Hayes

ETIOLOGY
Yersinia enterocolitica is a large, gram-negative coccobacillus that exhibits little or no bipolarity when stained with methylene blue and carbolfuchsin.

It ferments glucose and sucrose but not lactose, is oxidase negative, and reduces nitrate to nitrite. These facultative anaerobes grow well on common culture media and are motile at 22°C (71.6°F) but not 37°C (98.6°F). Optimal growth temperature is 25-28°C (77-82.4°F); however, the organism can grow at refrigerator temperature. *Y. enterocolitica* includes pathogenic and nonpathogenic members. It has 6 different biotypes (1A, 1B, and 2-5). *Y. enterocolitica* relies on other bacteria for iron uptake, and conditions associated with **iron overload** increase risk of infection.

EPIDEMIOLOGY
Y. enterocolitica is transmitted to humans through food, water, animal contact, and contaminated blood products. Transmission can occur from mother to newborn. *Y. enterocolitica* appears to have a global distribution but is seldom a cause of tropical diarrhea. In 2014, incidence of culture-confirmed *Y. enterocolitica* infection in the United States was 0.28 per 100,000 population (52% decrease from incidence in 1996–1998). Infection may be more common in Northern Europe. Most infections occur among children <5 yr old (incidence: 1.6-1.9 per 100,000 population), with the majority among children <1 yr old. It is estimated that *Y. enterocolitica* accounts for 5% of illnesses secondary to major bacterial enteric pathogens in children <5 yr old in the United States. Cases are more common in colder months and among males.

Natural reservoirs of *Y. enterocolitica* include pigs, rodents, rabbits, sheep, cattle, horses, dogs, and cats, with **pigs** being the major animal reservoir. Direct or indirect contact with animals, including pets, other domesticated animals, and wild animals, may be responsible for <1% of cases of enteric illnesses caused by *Y. enterocolitica*. Culture and molecular techniques have found the organism in a variety of foods and beverages, including vegetable juice, pasteurized milk, carrots, and water. Consumption of contaminated water or food, particularly undercooked pork, is the most common form of transmission to humans. A source of sporadic *Y. enterocolitica* infections is **chitterlings** (pig intestines, "chitlins"), a traditional dish in the southeastern United States as well as Latin America, often in celebration of winter holidays. The infection is often seen in young infants in the household due to contamination of bottle and food preparation when chitterlings are prepared. In one study, 71% of human isolates were indistinguishable from the strains isolated from pigs. *Y. enterocolitica* is an occupational threat to butchers.

In part because of its capacity to multiply at refrigerator temperatures, *Y. enterocolitica* can be transmitted by intravenous injection of contaminated fluids, including blood products.

Patients with conditions leading to iron overload are at higher risk of developing *Yersinia* infections.

PATHOGENESIS

The *Yersinia* organisms most often enter by the alimentary tract and cause mucosal ulcerations in the ileum. Necrotic lesions of Peyer patches and **mesenteric lymphadenitis** occur. If septicemia develops, suppurative lesions can be found in infected organs. Infection can trigger **reactive arthritis** and **erythema nodosum**, particularly in HLA-B27–positive individuals.

Virulence traits of pathogenic biotypes(1B and 2-5) are encoded by chromosomal genes and a highly conserved 70 kb virulence plasmid (pYV/pCD). The chromosomal genes control the production of heat-stable enterotoxins, and the plasmid allows penetration through the intestinal wall. Adherence, invasion, and toxin production are the essential mechanisms of pathogenesis. The bacteria mainly invade the intestinal epithelium in the Peyer patches of the ileum. After invasion, plasmid-encoded type III secretion of 3 antiphagocytic proteins protects *Yersinia* against the immunologic response of local macrophages. From Peyer patches, bacteria can disseminate to cause local or systemic disease. Motility appears to be required for *Y. enterocolitica* pathogenesis. Serogroups that predominate in human illness are O:3, O:8, O:9, and O:5,27. *Yersinia* does not produce siderophores and uses analogous siderophores from other bacteria or host-chelated iron stores to thrive, placing patients with iron overload, as in hemochromatosis, thalassemia, and sickle cell disease, at higher risk for infection.

CLINICAL MANIFESTATIONS

Disease occurs most often as enterocolitis with diarrhea, fever, and abdominal pain. Acute enteritis is more common among younger children, and mesenteric lymphadenitis that can mimic appendicitis may be found in older children and adolescents. Incubation period is usually 4-6 days after exposure (range 1-14 days). Stools may be watery or contain leukocytes, less often, frank blood and mucus. Duration of diarrhea is often longer for *Y. enterocolitica* than for other causes of acute gastroenteritis, ranging from 12-22 days in several studies. Fever is common. Notably, prominent pharyngitis may be seen in 20% of patients at presentation, which may help distinguish it from other causes of gastroenteritis. *Y. enterocolitica* is excreted in stool for 1-4 wk. Family contacts of a patient are often found to be asymptomatically colonized with *Y. enterocolitica*. *Y. enterocolitica* septicemia is less common and is most often found in very young children (<3 mo old) and immunocompromised persons. Systemic infection can be associated with splenic and hepatic abscesses, osteomyelitis, septic arthritis, meningitis, endocarditis, and mycotic aneurysms. Exudative pharyngitis, pneumonia, empyema, lung abscess, and acute respiratory distress syndrome occur infrequently.

Reactive complications include erythema nodosum, reactive arthritis, and rarely uveitis. These manifestations may be more common in select populations (northern Europeans), in association with HLA-B27, and in females.

DIAGNOSIS

Diagnosis is made typically through isolation of the organism, usually from the stool. *Y. enterocolitica* is easily cultured from normally sterile sites but requires special procedures for isolation from stool, where other bacteria can outgrow it. *Yersinia* should be cultured on selective agar (CIN, cefsulodin-irgasan-novobiocin) at 25-28°C to increase yield. If O:3 serogroup is suspected, MacConkey agar should be used at 25-28°C. Multiplex polymerase chain reaction (PCR) testing is also available. Many laboratories do not routinely perform the tests required to detect *Y. enterocolitica*; procedures targeted to this organism must be specifically requested. A history indicating contact with environmental sources of *Yersinia* and detection of fecal leukocytes are helpful indicators of a need to test for *Y. enterocolitica*. The isolation of a *Yersinia* from stool should be followed by tests to confirm that the isolate is a pathogen. Serodiagnosis is not readily available, and utility is limited by cross-reactivity.

Differential Diagnosis

The clinical presentation is similar to other forms of bacterial enterocolitis. The most common considerations include *Shigella*, *Salmonella*, *Campylobacter*, *Clostridium difficile*, enteroinvasive *Escherichia coli*, *Y. pseudotuberculosis*, and occasionally *Vibrio*-related diarrheal disease. Amebiasis, appendicitis, Crohn disease, ulcerative colitis, diverticulitis, and pseudomembranous colitis should also be considered.

TREATMENT

Enterocolitis in an immunocompetent patient is a self-limiting disease, and no benefit from antibiotic therapy is established. Patients with systemic infection and very young children (in whom septicemia is common) should be treated. *Yersinia* organisms are typically susceptible to trimethoprim-sulfamethoxazole (TMP-SMX), aminoglycosides, third-generation cephalosporins, and quinolones, although strains resistant to quinolones have been reported. *Y. enterocolitica* produces β-lactamases, which are responsible for resistance to penicillins and first-generation cephalosporins. TMP-SMX is the recommended empirical treatment in children for **enterocolitis** (generally a 5-day course), because it has activity against most strains and is well tolerated. In **severe infections** such as bacteremia, third-generation cephalosporins, with or without aminoglycosides, are effective, and usually a 3 wk course of therapy is administered, with possible transition to oral therapy. Patients on deferoxamine should discontinue iron chelation therapy during treatment for *Y. enterocolitica*, especially if they have complicated gastrointestinal (GI) infection or extraintestinal infection.

COMPLICATIONS

Reactive arthritis, erythema nodosum, erythema multiforme, hemolytic anemia, thrombocytopenia, and systemic dissemination of bacteria have been reported in association with *Y. enterocolitica* infection. Septicemia is more common in younger children, and reactive arthritis is more common in older patients. Arthritis appears to be mediated by immune complexes, which form as a result of antigenic mimicry, and viable organisms are not present in involved joints.

PREVENTION

Prevention centers on reducing contact with environmental sources of *Yersinia*. Families should be warned of the high risk of chitterling preparation, especially with young infants and children in the household. Breaking or sterilization of the chain from animal reservoirs to humans holds the greatest potential to reduce infections, and the techniques applied must be tailored to the reservoirs in each geographic area. There is no licensed vaccine.

Bibliography is available at Expert Consult.

230.2 *Yersinia pseudotuberculosis*
Ericka V. Hayes

Yersinia pseudotuberculosis has a worldwide distribution; *Y. pseudotuberculosis* disease is less common than *Y. enterocolitica* disease. The most common form of disease is a **mesenteric lymphadenitis** that produces an appendicitis-like syndrome. *Y. pseudotuberculosis* is associated with a Kawasaki syndrome–like illness in approximately 8% of cases.

ETIOLOGY

Y. pseudotuberculosis is a small, gram-negative, aerobic and facultative anaerobic coccobacillus. As with *Y. enterocolitica,* it ferments glucose and does not ferment lactose, is oxidase negative, catalase producing, urea splitting, and shares a number of morphologic and culture characteristics. It is differentiated biochemically from *Y. enterocolitica* on the basis of ornithine decarboxylase activity, fermentation of sucrose, sorbitol, and cellobiose, and other tests, although some overlap between species occurs. Antisera to somatic O antigens and sensitivity to *Yersinia* phages can also be used to differentiate the 2 species. Subspecies-specific DNA sequences that allow direct probe- and primer-specific differentiation of *Y. pestis, Y. pseudotuberculosis,* and *Y. enterocolitica* have been described. *Y. pseudotuberculosis* is more closely related phylogenetically to *Y. pestis* than to *Y. enterocolitica.*

EPIDEMIOLOGY

Y. pseudotuberculosis is zoonotic, with reservoirs in wild rodents, rabbits, deer, farm animals, various birds, and domestic animals, including cats and canaries. Transmission to humans is by consumption of or contact with contaminated animals or contact with an environmental source contaminated by animals (often water). Direct evidence of transmission of *Y. pseudotuberculosis* to humans by consumption of lettuce and raw carrots has been reported. The organism has a worldwide distribution; however, infections are more commonly reported in Europe, in boys, and in the winter. During 1996–2014, FoodNet reported 224 cases of infections secondary to *Y. pseudotuberculosis* in the United States, with an annual average incidence of 0.03 per 100,000 persons. Compared with *Y. enterocolitica* infections, those caused by *Y. pseudotuberculosis* are more likely to be invasive and occur in adolescents and adults. Iron-overloading conditions, AIDS, other immunodeficiencies, and other debilitating diseases (including liver cirrhosis) may predispose to invasive *Y. pseudotuberculosis* infection.

PATHOGENESIS

Ileal and colonic mucosal ulceration and mesenteric lymphadenitis are hallmarks of the infection. Necrotizing epithelioid granulomas may be seen in the mesenteric lymph nodes, but the appendix is often grossly and microscopically normal. The mesenteric nodes are often the only source of isolation of the organism. *Y. pseudotuberculosis* antigens bind directly to human leukocyte antigen (HLA) class II molecules and can function as **superantigens,** which might account for the clinical illness resembling **Kawasaki syndrome.**

CLINICAL MANIFESTATIONS

Pseudoappendicitis and mesenteric lymphadenitis with abdominal pain, right lower quadrant tenderness, fever, and leukocytosis constitute the most common clinical presentation. Enterocolitis and extraintestinal spread are uncommon. Iron overload, diabetes mellitus, and chronic liver disease are often found concomitantly with extraintestinal *Y. pseudotuberculosis* infection. Renal involvement with tubulointerstitial nephritis, azotemia, pyuria, and glucosuria can occur. *Y. pseudotuberculosis* can present as a Kawasaki syndrome–like illness with fever of 1-6 days' duration, strawberry tongue, pharyngeal erythema, scarlatiniform rash, cracked red swollen lips, conjunctivitis, sterile pyuria, periungual desquamation, and thrombocytosis. Some of these children have had coronary changes. Other uncommon manifestations include septic arthritis, massive lower GI bleeding, postaneurysmal prosthetic vascular infection, and acute encephalopathy.

DIAGNOSIS

PCR of involved tissue can be used to identify *Y. pseudotuberculosis;* isolation by culture can require an extended interval. Involved mesenteric lymph nodes removed at appendectomy can yield the organism by culture. Abdominal CT scan or ultrasound examination of children

with unexplained fever and abdominal pain can reveal a characteristic picture of enlarged mesenteric lymph nodes and thickening of the terminal ileum with or without peritoneal findings including appendiceal inflammation and periappendiceal fluid. *Y. pseudotuberculosis* is rarely recovered from stool. Serologic testing is available in specialized labs.

Differential Diagnosis

Appendicitis (most common), inflammatory bowel disease, and other intraabdominal infections should be considered. Kawasaki syndrome, staphylococcal or streptococcal disease, leptospirosis, Stevens-Johnson syndrome, and collagen vascular diseases, including acute-onset juvenile idiopathic arthritis, can mimic the syndrome with prolonged fever and rash. *C. difficile* colitis, meningitis, encephalitis, enteropathic arthropathies, acute pancreatitis, sarcoidosis, toxic shock syndrome, typhoid fever, and ulcerative colitis may also be considered.

TREATMENT

Uncomplicated mesenteric lymphadenitis caused by *Y. pseudotuberculosis* is a self-limited disease, and antimicrobial therapy is not required. Few data exist on optimal treatment and duration of therapy. Infections with *Y. pseudotuberculosis* can generally be managed the same as those caused by *Y. enterocolitica.* Culture-confirmed bacteremia should be treated with a third-generation cephalosporin with or without an aminoglycoside, TMP-SMX, fluoroquinolones, or chloramphenicol.

COMPLICATIONS

Erythema nodosum and reactive arthritis can follow infection. Coronary aneurysm formation has been described with disease presenting as Kawasaki syndrome–like illness. Rare local complications of GI disease include perforation, obstruction, and intussusception.

PREVENTION

Avoiding exposure to potentially infected animals and good food-handling practices can prevent infection. The sporadic nature of the disease makes application of targeted prevention measures difficult.

Bibliography is available at Expert Consult.

230.3 Plague *(Yersinia pestis)*
Ericka V. Hayes

ETIOLOGY

Yersinia pestis is a gram-negative, facultative anaerobe that is a pleomorphic nonmotile, non–spore-forming coccobacillus and a potential agent of bioterrorism. It evolved from *Y. pseudotuberculosis* through acquisition of chromosomal changes and plasmid-associated factors that are essential to its virulence and survival in mammalian hosts and fleas. *Y. pestis* shares bipolar staining appearance with *Y. pseudotuberculosis* and can be differentiated by biochemical reactions, serology, phage sensitivity, and molecular techniques. *Y. pestis* exists in 3 biovars: Antigua (Africa), Medievalis (central Asia), and Orientalis (widespread).

EPIDEMIOLOGY

Plague is endemic in at least 24 countries. Approximately 3,000 cases are reported worldwide per year, with 100-200 deaths. Plague is uncommon in the United States (0-40 reported cases/yr); most of these cases occur west of a line from east Texas to east Montana, with 80% of cases in California, New Mexico, Arizona, and Colorado. In 2015, there was a cluster of 11 cases (with 3 deaths) in 4 mo related to exposure at Yosemite National Park in California's Sierra Nevada Mountains. The epidemic form of disease killed approximately 25% of the population of Europe in the Middle Ages in one of several epidemics and pandemics. The epidemiology of **epidemic** plague involves extension of infection from the zoonotic reservoirs to urban rats, *Rattus rattus* and *Rattus norvegicus,* and from fleas of urban rats to humans. Epidemics are no longer seen. Selective pressure exerted by plague pandemics in medieval Europe is hypothesized for enrichment of a deletion mutation in the gene encoding CCR5 (CCR5-Δ32). The enhanced frequency of this mutation in European populations endows approximately 10% of European descendants with relative resistance to acquiring HIV-1.

The most common mode of transmission of *Y. pestis* to humans is through **flea bites**. Historically, most human infections are thought to have resulted from bites of fleas that acquired infection from feeding on infected urban rats. Less frequently, infection is caused by contact with infectious body fluids or tissues or inhalation of respiratory secretions of infected animals. Currently, most cases of plague secondary to direct animal contact or inhalation of animal secretions are related to domestic **cats** or **dogs**. Direct transmission from human to human through droplet inhalation is possible but extremely rare. Laboratory transmission of *Y. pestis* has been described as well. **Sylvatic plague** can exist as a stable enzootic infection or as an epizootic disease with high host mortality. Ground squirrels, rock squirrels, prairie dogs, rats, mice, bobcats, cats, rabbits, and chipmunks may be infected. Transmission among animals is usually by flea bite or by ingestion of contaminated tissue. *Xenopsylla cheopis* is the flea usually associated with transmission to humans, but >30 species of fleas have been demonstrated as vector competent, and *Pulex irritans,* the human flea, can transmit plague and might have been an important vector in some historical epidemics. Both sexes are similarly affected by plague, and transmission is more common in colder regions and seasons, possibly because of temperature effects on *Y. pestis* infections in vector fleas.

PATHOGENESIS

In the most common form of plague, infected fleas regurgitate organisms into a patient's skin during feeding. The bacteria translocate via lymphatics to regional lymph nodes, where *Y. pestis* replicates, resulting in bubonic plague. In the absence of rapidly implemented specific therapy, bacteremia can occur, resulting in purulent, necrotic, and hemorrhagic lesions in many organs. Both plasmid and chromosomal genes are required for full virulence. Pneumonic plague can be secondary to bacteremia or primary when infected material is inhaled. The organism is highly transmissible from persons with pneumonic plague and from domestic cats with pneumonic infection. This high transmissibility and high morbidity and mortality have provided an impetus for attempts to use *Y. pestis* as a biologic weapon.

CLINICAL MANIFESTATIONS

Y. pestis infection can manifest as several clinical syndromes; infection can also be subclinical. The 3 principal clinical presentations of plague are bubonic, septicemic, and pneumonic. **Bubonic plague** is the most common form and accounts for 80–90% of cases in the United States. From 2-8 days after a flea bite, lymphadenitis develops in lymph nodes closest to the inoculation site, including the inguinal (most common), axillary, or cervical region. These buboes are remarkable for tenderness. Fever, chills, weakness, prostration, headache, and the development of septicemia are common. The skin might show insect bites or scratch marks. Purpura and gangrene of the extremities can develop as a result of disseminated intravascular coagulation (DIC). These lesions may be the origin of the name Black Death. Untreated plague results in death in >50% of symptomatic patients. Death can occur within 2-4 days after onset of symptoms.

Occasionally, *Y. pestis* establishes systemic infection and induces the systemic symptoms seen with bubonic plague without causing a bubo (**primary septicemic plague**). Because of the delay in diagnosis linked to the lack of the bubo, septicemic plague carries an even higher case fatality rate than bubonic plague. In some regions, bubo-free septicemic plague accounts for 25% of cases.

Pneumonic plague is the least common but most dangerous and lethal form of the disease. Pneumonic plague can result from hematogenous dissemination, or, rarely, as primary pneumonic plague after inhalation of the organism from a human or animal with plague pneumonia or potentially from a biologic attack. Signs of pneumonic plague include severe pneumonia with high fever, dyspnea, and hemoptysis.

Meningitis, tonsillitis, or gastroenteritis can occur. Meningitis tends to be a late complication following inadequate treatment. Tonsillitis and gastroenteritis can occur with or without apparent bubo formation or lymphadenopathy.

DIAGNOSIS

Plague should be suspected in patients with fever and history of exposure to small animals in endemic areas. Thus, bubonic plague is suspected in a patient with a painful swollen lymph node, fever, and prostration who has been potentially exposed to fleas or rodents in the western United States. A history of camping or the presence of flea bites increases the index of suspicion.

Y. pestis is readily transmitted to humans by some routine laboratory manipulations. Thus, it is imperative to clearly notify a laboratory when submitting a sample suspected of containing *Y. pestis***.** Laboratory diagnosis is based on bacteriologic culture or direct visualization using Gram, Giemsa, or Wayson stain of lymph node aspirates, blood, sputum, or exudates. Fluorescent antibody staining can also be done on specimens. *Y. pestis* grows slowly under routine culture conditions and best at temperatures that differ from those used for routine cultures in many clinical laboratories. Note some automated blood culture identification systems may misidentify *Y. pestis*. A rapid antigen test detecting *Y. pestis* F1 antigen in sputum and serum samples exists. Suspected isolates of *Y. pestis* should be forwarded to a reference laboratory for confirmation. Special containment shipping precautions are required. Cases of plague should be reported to local and state health departments and the Centers for Disease Control and Prevention (CDC). Serologic testing is also available.

Differential Diagnosis

The Gram stain of *Y. pestis* may be confused with *Enterobacter agglomerans.* Mild and subacute forms of bubonic plague may be confused with other disorders causing localized lymphadenitis and lymphadenopathy, including tularemia and cat-scratch adenitis. Septicemic plague may be indistinguishable from other forms of overwhelming bacterial sepsis.

Pulmonary manifestations of plague are similar to those of anthrax, Q fever, and tularemia, all agents with **bioterrorism** and **biologic warfare** potential. Thus, the presentation of a suspected case, and especially any cluster of cases, requires immediate reporting. Additional information on this aspect of plague and procedures can be found at http://www.bt.cdc.gov/agent/plague/.

TREATMENT

Patients with suspected plague should be placed on **droplet isolation** until pneumonia is ruled out, sputum cultures are negative, and antibiotic treatment has been administered for 48 hr. The treatment of choice for bubonic plague historically has been **streptomycin** (30 mg/kg/day, maximum 2 g/day, divided every 12 hr intramuscularly [IM] for 10 days). Intramuscular streptomycin is inappropriate for septicemia because absorption may be erratic when perfusion is poor. The poor central nervous system penetration of streptomycin also makes this an inappropriate drug for meningitis. Furthermore, streptomycin might not be widely and immediately available. **Gentamicin** (children, 7.5 mg/kg IM or intravenously [IV] divided every 8 hr; adults, 5 mg/kg IM or IV once daily) has been shown to be as efficacious as streptomycin; in patients with abscesses, an additional agent may be needed in addition to an aminoglycoside because of poor abscess penetration. Alternative treatments include **doxycycline** (in children who weigh <45 kg: 4.4 mg/kg/day divided every 12 hr IV, maximum 200 mg/day; not recommended for children <8 yr of age; in children who weigh ≥45 kg, 100 mg every 12 hr orally [PO]), c**iprofloxacin** (30 mg/kg/day divided every 12 hr, maximum 400 mg every 12 hr IV), and **chloramphenicol** (100 mg/kg/day IV divided every 6 hr, for children >2 yr; maximum dose 4 g/day; not widely available in the United States). Meningitis is usually treated with chloramphenicol or a fluoroquinolone. Resistance to these agents and relapses are rare. *Y. pestis* is susceptible in vitro to **fluoroquinolones**, which are effective in treating experimental plague in animals. *Y. pestis* is susceptible in vitro to penicillin, but penicillin is ineffective in treatment of human disease. Mild disease may be treated with oral chloramphenicol or tetracycline in children >8 yr old. Clinical improvement is noted within 48 hr of initiating treatment. Typical duration of therapy is 10-14 days, with a switch to oral therapy 2 days after defervescence and clinical improvement. Drainage of suppurative buboes may be needed; material is infectious, and appropriate precautions should be taken intraoperatively.

Postexposure prophylaxis should be given to close contacts of patients with pneumonic plague. Antimicrobial prophylaxis is recommended within 7 days of exposure for persons with direct, close contact with patient with pneumonic plague or those exposed to an accidental or terrorist-induced aerosol. Recommended regimens for children >8 yr old include doxycycline or ciprofloxacin; for children <8 yr old, doxycycline, chloramphenicol and ciprofloxacin are options for a 7-day course at the treatment doses above. Contacts of cases of uncomplicated bubonic plague do not require prophylaxis. *Y. pestis* is a potential agent of bioterrorism that can require mass casualty prophylaxis.

PREVENTION

Avoidance of exposure to infected animals and fleas is the best method of prevention of infection. In the United States, special care is required in environments inhabited by rodent reservoirs of *Y. pestis* and their ectoparasites. Patients with plague should be isolated if they have pulmonary symptoms, and infected materials should be handled with extreme care. There is currently no available licensed vaccine for *Y. pestis* in the United States. Several vaccine development trials are underway, and recombinant subunit vaccines based on rF1 and rV antigens seem to be the most promising. Using baits containing live vaccines for oral immunization of wild animals may be a helpful alternative for control of epidemics.

Bibliography is available at Expert Consult.

Chapter **231**

Aeromonas and *Plesiomonas*

Ameneh Khatami and Adam J. Ratner

第二百三十一章
气单胞菌和邻单胞菌

中文导读

本章主要介绍了气单胞菌感染的病因、流行病学、发病机制、临床表现、诊断、治疗和预防，以及邻单胞菌感染的病因、流行病学、发病机制、临床表现、诊断和治疗。在气单胞菌感染的临床表现部分详细介绍了肠炎、皮肤和软组织感染、败血症和其他感染。在邻单胞菌感染的治疗部分详细描述了补液的重要性，以及应用抗生素的指征和用药的选择等内容。

Aeromonas and *Plesiomonas* are gram-negative bacilli that include species capable of causing enteritis and, less frequently, skin and soft tissue infections and invasive disease. They are common in fresh water and brackish water and colonize animals and plants in these environments.

231.1 *Aeromonas*

Ameneh Khatami and Adam J. Ratner

ETIOLOGY

Aeromonas is a member of the Aeromonadaceae family and includes 2 major groups of isolates: the nonmotile *psychrophilic* organisms that infect cold-blooded animals, most often fish, and the motile *mesophilic* organisms that infect humans and other warm-blooded animals. *Aeromonas* species are oxidase- and catalase-positive, facultatively anaerobic, gram-negative bacilli that ferment glucose. *Aeromonas* is a diverse genus with difficult taxonomy and species differentiation because of high nucleotide variability and has undergone multiple reclassifications of species and taxa in recent years. Eleven species are recognized as clinically significant human pathogens, with *Aeromonas hydrophila*, *Aeromonas veronii* biotype sobria, and *Aeromonas caviae* most frequently associated with human infection. *Aeromonas dhakensis*, which was first isolated from children with diarrhea in Dhaka, Bangladesh and initially classified as a subspecies of *A. hydrophila*, has been recognized as a distinct species and an important cause of human infection.

EPIDEMIOLOGY

Aeromonas organisms are found in fresh and brackish aquatic sources, including rivers and streams, well water, both treated and bottled drinking water, and sewage. These organisms are most often detected in aquatic sources during warm-weather months, when they reach greater population densities. Rates of human infection may also exhibit seasonality depending on local conditions. For example, *Aeromonas* is isolated with increased frequency from May to October in the Northern hemisphere. Some species resist chlorination of water and exhibit tolerance to high salt concentrations. *Aeromonas* has been isolated from meats, milk, seafood, seaweed, and vegetables consumed by humans. Asymptomatic colonization occurs in humans and is more common in inhabitants of tropical regions. Most human infections with *Aeromonas* are associated with exposure to contaminated water but may also be contracted via other routes, including ingestion of contaminated food. A systematic review of cases of traveler's diarrhea worldwide implicated *Aeromonas* in 0.8–3.3% of infections, with highest frequencies in travelers to Southeast Asia and Africa. A study in Bangladesh of >56,000 stool samples from patients with diarrhea found that approximately 25% had a bacterial etiology detected, 13% of which were *Aeromonas*. *Aeromonas* infections have also been acquired at various sites of natural disasters. For example, following the 2004 Thailand tsunami, *Aeromonas* was the leading cause of skin and soft tissue infection among survivors.

PATHOGENESIS

Clinical and epidemiologic data seem to support that *Aeromonas* organisms are **enteric** pathogens, although this point is not universally accepted. Reasons for uncertainty include a lack of outbreaks with clonally distinct isolates, infrequent person-to-person transmission, absence of a robust animal model, and overlapping prevalence in symptomatic and asymptomatic individuals. In addition, there are conflicting data when comparing the human challenge model with characteristics of suspected outbreaks of *Aeromonas* enteritis, further complicating interpretation.

Aeromonas isolates possess a variety of potential virulence factors, including constitutive *polar* and inducible *lateral* flagella, fimbriae, outer membrane proteins, endotoxin (lipopolysaccharide), capsules, extracellular hydrolytic enzymes, enterotoxins, hemolysins, and multiple secretion systems. The mechanistic role of many of these factors in human pathogenicity remains unclear. Polar flagella provide motility in liquid media, and lateral flagella may act as adhesins. There are numerous hemolysins and heat-labile and heat-stable enterotoxins. *Aeromonas* cytotoxic enterotoxin (**Act/aerolysin**) is secreted by a type II secretion system and is able to lyse erythrocytes, inhibit phagocytosis, and induce cytotoxicity in eukaryotic cells. *Aeromonas* also has a type III secretion system with an effector protein that causes actin reorganization and eventual apoptosis in vitro. A type VI secretion system has been described and functions analogously to a phage tail, with antimicrobial activity.

Aeromonas sobria is the most enterotoxic among clinical isolates, and cytotoxic activity with cytopathic and intracellular effects is found in 89% of isolates. A few strains produce Shiga toxin. Some clinically important species have also been shown to harbor a cholera-like toxin (**Asao toxin**). *Aeromonas* has serine proteases that can cause a cascade of inflammatory mediators, leading to vascular leakage, and in vitro studies show induction of apoptosis in murine macrophages by human isolates of *Aeromonas*. There are limited data on *quorum-sensing* molecules, which coordinate gene expression according to local density and may be involved in biofilm production or population control.

CLINICAL MANIFESTATIONS

Aeromonas may colonize humans asymptomatically or cause illness, including enteritis, focal invasive infections, and septicemia. Although apparently immunologically normal individuals may present with any of these manifestations, invasive disease is more common among immunocompromised persons.

Enteritis

The most common clinical manifestation of infection with *Aeromonas* is enteritis, which occurs primarily among children <3 yr old. *Aeromonas* is the 3rd or 4th most common cause of childhood **bacterial diarrhea** and has been isolated from 2–10% of patients with diarrhea and 1–5% of asymptomatic controls. One study demonstrated isolation from hospitalized neonates with diarrhea at rates of 0–19% depending on the season. Isolation from human feces also varies geographically based on food habits, level of sanitation, population demographics, aquaculture and farming practices, and laboratory isolation methods used. *Aeromonas* diarrhea is often watery and self-limited, although a dysentery-like syndrome with blood and mucus in the stool has also been described. Fever, abdominal pain, and vomiting are common in children. Enteritis caused by *A. hydrophila* and *A. sobria* tends to be acute and self-limited, whereas 30% of the patients with *A. caviae* enteritis have chronic or intermittent diarrhea that may last 4-6 wk. *A. sobria* and *A. caviae* are most frequently associated with traveler's diarrhea. Complications of *Aeromonas* enteritis include intussusception, failure to thrive, hemolytic-uremic syndrome, bacteremia, and postinfectious chronic colitis. *Aeromonas* infection may also present as acute segmental colitis, mimicking inflammatory bowel disease or ischemic colitis.

Skin and Soft Tissue Infections

Skin and soft tissue infections are the 2nd most common presentation of *Aeromonas*. Predisposing factors include local trauma and exposure to contaminated fresh water. *Aeromonas* soft tissue infections have been reported following bites from a number of animal species, including alligators, tigers, bears, and snakes, as well as from tick bites. These infections have also been reported after sports injuries and medicinal leech therapy. Antibiotic prophylaxis is generally used in conjunction with leech therapy because of the presence of *A. hydrophila* in the gastrointestinal (GI) tract of leeches, where they aid in the breakdown of ingested red blood cells. The spectrum of skin and soft tissue infections is broad, ranging from a localized skin nodule to life-threatening necrotizing fasciitis, myonecrosis, and gas gangrene. Soft tissue infections are most frequently found on the extremities, are often polymicrobial, and are 3 times more likely in men than in women. *Aeromonas* **cellulitis**, the most common skin manifestation, clinically presents similar to other forms of bacterial cellulitis but should be suspected in wounds after contact with a water source, especially during the summer.

Septicemia

Aeromonas septicemia is the 3rd most common presentation of infection and is associated with a mortality rate of 27–73%, with higher incidence during summer months or during the wet season in the tropics. Patients often present with fever and GI symptoms, including abdominal pain, nausea, vomiting, and diarrhea. From 2–4% of patients may present with ecthyma gangrenosum–like lesions. *Aeromonas* may be the only organism isolated or may be part of a polymicrobial bacteremic illness. Most cases (approximately 80%) occur in immunocompromised adults or those with hepatobiliary disease and in young children in whom the source of infection is probably *Aeromonas* in the GI tract. Less frequently, bacteremia can be secondary to trauma-related myonecrosis or infected burns. In such patients, mortality is often higher than in those with primary bacteremia, because of the underlying trauma. Rarely, *Aeromonas* bacteremia occurs in otherwise healthy adults exposed to fresh water.

Other Infections

Aeromonas is a rare cause of GI infections such as necrotizing gastroenteritis, peritonitis, cholecystitis, appendicitis, and liver and pancreas abscess formation; cardiovascular infections, including endocarditis and septic embolism; and pulmonary infections, including tracheobronchitis, pneumonia, empyema, and lung abscess formation. *Aeromonas* is also associated with musculoskeletal infections, including osteomyelitis, pyogenic arthritis, pyomyositis, and necrotizing fasciitis, as well as ear, nose, and throat infections, including endophthalmitis, keratitis, orbital cellulitis, otitis media, and epiglottitis. Other rare infections include meningitis, urinary tract infection, pelvic inflammatory disease, lymphadenitis, hot tub folliculitis, and surgical wound infections. *Aeromonas* is associated with tracheobronchitis and aspiration pneumonia after near-drowning.

DIAGNOSIS

Diagnosis is established by isolation of *Aeromonas* in culture. The organism is generally grown on standard media when the source material is normally sterile. Isolation and identification of the organism from nonsterile sites are more difficult. Often, *Aeromonas* is not identified by typical laboratory protocols for examining stool specimens. If *Aeromonas* is suspected, the yield may increase if the laboratory is notified before testing, because overnight enrichment in alkaline peptone water and culture on selective agars may be useful. Most strains (approximately 90%) produce β-hemolysis on blood agar. Lactose-fermenting strains of *Aeromonas* may not be identified if the clinical laboratory does not routinely perform oxidase tests on lactose fermenters isolated on MacConkey agar. Aeromonads are resistant to vibriostatic agent O129; however, differentiation of *Aeromonas* from *Vibrio* spp. and identification of *Aeromonas* spp. and subspp. is not reliable using biochemical testing, particularly when commercial identification systems are used. Similarly, classification of *Aeromonas* strains at the species and subspecies level is difficult to achieve by sequencing regions of the 16S rRNA gene. Sequencing of housekeeping genes, such as *gyrB* and *rpoD*, and multilocus sequence typing are accurate for species identification but are time-, cost- and labor-intensive. Increasingly, laboratories use matrix-assisted laser desorption/ionization time-of-flight (MALDI-TOF) mass spectrometry to rapidly identify organisms, because this method is accurate for *Aeromonas* as a genus and for many of the clinically important species.

TREATMENT

Aeromonas **enteritis** is usually self-limited, and antimicrobial therapy may not be indicated, although some studies suggest that antimicrobial therapy may shorten the course of the illness. Antimicrobial therapy is reasonable to consider in patients with protracted diarrhea, dysentery-like illness, or underlying conditions such as hepatobiliary disease or an immunocompromised state. Antibiotic sensitivity varies among species and also by geography; therefore it is important to perform susceptibility testing. Chromosomally mediated class B, C, and D β-lactamases are found in most species and can be difficult to identify because many are inducible. These include metallo- and AmpC β-lactamases, which can lead to clinical failure if carbapenems or third-generation cephalosporins are used as monotherapy in high-organism-load infections. There is near-uniform resistance to penicillins. **Septicemia** can be treated with a fourth-generation cephalosporin (e.g., cefepime) or ciprofloxacin, with or without an aminoglycoside, although specific therapy should be guided by susceptibility data. Another option for less severe infections includes trimethoprim-sulfamethoxazole (TMP-SMX). Evidence-based recommendations for duration of treatment are lacking, and thus treatment is typically guided by clinical response. In general, diarrhea is treated for 3 days, wound infections for 7-10 days, and bacteremia for 14-21 days, depending on clinical response and host characteristics.

PREVENTION

Reducing contact with contaminated environmental fresh and brackish water and contaminated foods should reduce the risk for *Aeromonas* infections. Some *Aeromonas* outer membrane proteins are immunogenic and are candidate antigens for preclinical vaccine development.

Bibliography is available at Expert Consult.

231.2 *Plesiomonas shigelloides*
Ameneh Khatami and Adam J. Ratner

ETIOLOGY

Plesiomonas shigelloides is a facultatively anaerobic, gram-negative, non–spore-forming bacillus that ferments glucose. It is a catalase-, oxidase-, and indole-positive motile organism with polar flagella. A high level of genetic diversity has been recognized among *P. shigelloides* strains, reflecting frequent homologous recombination.

EPIDEMIOLOGY

P. shigelloides is ubiquitous in fresh water and, because it can tolerate salinity of up to 4%, can be found in estuarine or brackish water, as well as in animal inhabitants of these ecosystems, including fish, shellfish, crustaceans, water mammals, amphibians, reptiles, and other vertebrates. *P. shigelloides* has been recovered from healthy (colonized) and diseased animals, including cats. It can cause both sporadic infections and outbreaks in a range of animals. As a mesophile with optimal growth temperature of 35-39°C (95-102.2°F), *P. shigelloides* has been found most often in tropical waters or during warmer months, although there are increasing reports of isolation from surface water in colder climates. Similarly, most cases of infection occur during the warmer months of the year. *P. shigelloides* is not a usual commensal organism in the human GI tract, and infection of humans is thought to be the result of consumption of contaminated water or raw seafood or possibly through contact with colonized animals. The frequency of isolation of *P. shigelloides* from diarrheal stools in these circumstances has been reported to range from 2% to >10%. Mixed infection with *Salmonella*, *Aeromonas*, rotavirus, or other enteric pathogens may occur in almost one third of patients. The majority of symptomatic patients in North America have a known exposure to potentially contaminated water or seafood (notably oysters) or have traveled abroad. *Plesiomonas* has been reported to be associated with 1.3–5.4% of episodes of traveler's diarrhea, with the highest rates associated with travel to South and Southeast Asia. Other risk factors include immune compromise (in particular HIV infection), blood dyscrasias (including sickle cell disease), and young age. The highest rates of *Plesiomonas* enteritis occur in children <2 yr old. Although *P. shigelloides* has a worldwide distribution, there is unexplained geographic variability in the incidence of enteritis that may be related to water temperatures as well as lack of hygiene and sanitation.

PATHOGENESIS

Epidemiologic and microbiologic evidence in the form of a series of food-borne outbreaks attributable to *P. shigelloides* indicates that this organism is an **enteropathogen**. However, the pathogenic capacity of *P. shigelloides* has not been confirmed through oral challenge studies, and these organisms have been isolated from the stools of healthy individuals at a low rate. The mechanism of enteritis is not known, but putative virulence factors have been described, including cholera-like toxin, heat-labile and heat-stable enterotoxins, and lipopolysaccharide. Most strains of *P. shigelloides* also secrete a β-hemolysin, which is thought to be a major virulence factor. In vitro studies show that isolates of *P. shigelloides* can invade and induce apoptosis in cells of enteric origin, as well as exhibiting evidence of modulation of host defenses through inhibition of cathepsins involved in antigen processing and presentation.

CLINICAL MANIFESTATIONS

Clinical disease in humans generally begins 24-48 hr after exposure to the organism, although incubation periods in excess of 4 days have been reported. Diarrhea can occur in all age-groups, including neonates, is typically secretory, and less often presents as invasive dysentery. Secretory enteritis usually presents as a mild self-limiting disease with watery diarrhea and abdominal pain, but in 13% of cases diarrhea can persist for >2 wk. Dehydration, hypokalemia, and peritonitis are uncommon complications; however, there have been several reports of a cholera-like presentation with severe secretory diarrhea. The frequency of secretory vs dysenteric presentation seems to cluster by individual outbreak, suggesting that either the human populations or the bacterial populations involved are associated with each particular presentation. **Dysentery** presents with macroscopic blood and/or mucus in the stool, significant abdominal pain, and vomiting, with more severe cases also associated with fever. Fatal outcomes have been reported with severe cases of *Plesiomonas* dysentery, although in most of these cases the exact role of *P. shigelloides* is unclear.

Extraintestinal infections, usually bacteremia, are rare and usually occur in patients with underlying immunodeficiency. About 90% of these cases are monomicrobial, and in almost half, *P. shigelloides* is also isolated from a site other than blood. Rarely, bacteremia accompanying enteritis has been documented in apparently otherwise normal children. Septicemia also appears to result from ingestion of contaminated water or seafood and has a high mortality rate in adults. Other extraintestinal diseases include pneumonia, meningitis, osteomyelitis, septic arthritis, reactive arthritis, abscesses, and focal infections of the GI or reproductive tracts. Almost one third of all bacteremias occur in neonates who present with early-onset sepsis and meningitis, and although rare, these make up most of the reported cases of *P. shigelloides* meningitis and have a very high mortality rate (80%). In several cases of neonatal disease, *Plesiomonas* has also been isolated from maternal feces, suggesting intrapartum vertical transmission. Compared to *Aeromonas* and *Vibrio* spp., traumatic wounds sustained in aquatic environments less often contain *P. shigelloides*.

DIAGNOSIS

P. shigelloides is a non–lactose-fermenting organism and grows well on traditional enteric media with optimal growth at 30°C (86°F), although selective techniques may be required to isolate the organism from mixed cultures and to differentiate *P. shigelloides* from *Shigella* spp. If enrichment is necessary, alkaline peptone water or bile peptone broth may be used. Colonies are nonhemolytic on 5% blood agar. Many strains cross-react with *Shigella* on serologic testing but can be differentiated easily as oxidase-positive organisms. *P. shigelloides* has a unique biochemical profile and can generally be identified using commercial kits. Rapid identification systems, including MALDI-TOF, can also be used to identify *P. shigelloides*. *P. shigelloides* is included in at least one U.S. Food and Drug Administration (FDA)–approved commercial panel that detects a range of enteropathogens directly from diarrheal stools (culture independent) by polymerase chain reaction.

TREATMENT

Enteritis caused by *P. shigelloides* is usually mild and self-limited. In cases associated with dehydration or with a cholera-like disease, patients usually respond favorably to **oral rehydration solution**. Consideration of **antimicrobial therapy** is reserved for patients with prolonged or bloody diarrhea, those who are immunocompromised, the elderly, and the very young. Data from uncontrolled studies suggest that antimicrobial therapy may decrease the duration of symptoms, although no difference was found in an exclusively pediatric study.

P. shigelloides produces a chromosomally encoded, noninducible β-lactamase, which generally renders strains resistant to the penicillins, including broad-spectrum penicillins. *P. shigelloides* is also usually resistant to aminoglycosides and tetracyclines. Most strains of *P. shigelloides* are susceptible to β-lactam/β-lactamase inhibitor combinations as well as to TMP-SMX, some cephalosporins, carbapenems, and fluoroquinolones; however, therapy should be guided by antimicrobial susceptibility testing, since resistance to TMP-SMX, fluoroquinolones, and other agents has been reported.

Severe cases of *P. shigelloides* dysentery should be treated similarly to shigellosis (with empirical azithromycin or a third-generation cephalosporin for children and ciprofloxacin or azithromycin for adults). Antibiotics are essential for therapy of extraintestinal disease. Empirical therapy with a third-generation cephalosporin is often first-line management, because most isolates are susceptible in vitro. Alternatives include imipenem, aztreonam, β-lactam/β-lactamase inhibitor combinations, and quinolones. Definitive therapy should be guided by the susceptibility of the individual isolate. Duration of therapy ranges from 1-2 wk but may be extended depending on underlying chronic conditions and clinical response.

Bibliography is available at Expert Consult.

Chapter 232

Pseudomonas, Burkholderia, and *Stenotrophomonas*

第二百三十二章

铜绿假单胞菌、洋葱伯克霍尔德菌复合体和窄食单胞菌

中文导读

本章主要介绍了铜绿假单胞菌、洋葱伯克霍尔德   菌复合体和窄食单胞菌。在铜绿假单胞菌部分详细介

绍了铜绿假单胞菌感染的病因、流行病学、病理、发病机制、临床表现、诊断、治疗、支持治疗、预后和预防。其中在关于铜绿假单胞菌感染的治疗部分，详细描述了烧伤和伤口感染、囊性纤维化、免疫缺陷患者、医院肺炎和婴儿。在洋葱伯克霍尔德菌复合体部分详细介绍了鼻疽伯克霍尔德菌(鼻疽病)和假单胞菌(类鼻疽)。在窄食单胞菌部分详细介绍了病因、发病机制、治疗等内容。

232.1 *Pseudomonas aeruginosa*

Thomas S. Murray and Robert S. Baltimore

ETIOLOGY

Pseudomonas aeruginosa is a gram-negative rod and is a strict aerobe. It can multiply in a great variety of environments that contain minimal amounts of organic compounds. Strains from clinical specimens do not ferment lactose, are oxidase positive, and may produce β-hemolysis on blood agar. Many strains produce pigments, including pyocyanin, pyoverdine, and pyorubin, that diffuse into and color the surrounding medium. Strains of *P. aeruginosa* are differentiated for epidemiologic purposes by a variety of genotyping methods, including restriction fragment length polymorphisms using pulsed-field gel electrophoresis, multilocus sequence typing, and more recently, whole genome sequencing.

EPIDEMIOLOGY

P. aeruginosa is a classic "opportunist." It rarely causes disease in people who do not have a predisposing risk factor. Compromised host defense mechanisms resulting from trauma, neutropenia, mucositis, immunosuppression, or impaired mucociliary transport explain the predominant role of this organism in producing opportunistic infections. In pediatric settings, it is most frequently seen in the respiratory secretions of children with **cystic fibrosis** (CF). *P. aeruginosa* was found in 1% of neonates with fever and bacteremia in a review of 6 U.S. centers. One series of neonatal intensive care unit (NICU) infections reported that 3.8%episodes of neonatal bacteremia from 1989–2003 were caused by *P. aeruginosa*. Another children's hospital reported 232 episodes of *P. aeruginosa* bacteremia over a 10 yr period, with half the infected children diagnosed with an underlying malignancy.

P. aeruginosa and other pseudomonads frequently enter the hospital environment on the clothes, skin, or shoes of patients or hospital personnel, with plants or vegetables brought into the hospital, and in the gastrointestinal (GI) tract of patients. Colonization of any moist or liquid substance may ensue; the organisms may be found growing in any water reservoir, including distilled water, and in hospital kitchen sinks and laundries, some antiseptic solutions, and equipment used for respiratory therapy and urinary procedures. Colonization of skin, throat, stool, and nasal mucosa of patients is low at admission to the hospital but increases to as high as 50–70% with prolonged hospitalization and with the use of broad-spectrum antibiotics, chemotherapy, mechanical ventilation, and urinary catheters. Patients' intestinal microbial flora may be altered by the broad-spectrum antibiotics, reducing resistance to colonization and permitting *P. aeruginosa* in the environment to populate the GI tract. Intestinal mucosal breakdown associated with medications, especially cytotoxic agents, and nosocomial enteritis may provide a pathway by which *P. aeruginosa* spreads to the lymphatics or bloodstream.

PATHOLOGY

The pathologic manifestations of *P. aeruginosa* infections depend on the site and type of infection. Because of its elaboration of toxins and invasive factors, the organism can often be seen invading blood vessels and causing vascular necrosis. In some infections there is spread through tissues with necrosis and microabscess formation. In patients with CF, focal and diffuse bronchitis/bronchiolitis leading to bronchiolitis obliterans has been reported.

Pathogenesis

Invasiveness of *P. aeruginosa* is mediated by a host of virulence factors. Bacterial attachment is facilitated by pili that adhere to epithelium damaged by prior injury or infection. Extracellular proteins, proteases, elastases, and cytotoxins disrupt cell membranes, and in response, host-produced cytokines cause capillary vascular permeability and induce an inflammatory response. Dissemination and bloodstream invasion follow extension of local tissue damage and are facilitated by the antiphagocytic properties of endotoxin, the exopolysaccharide, and protease cleavage of immunoglobulin G. *P. aeruginosa* also produces numerous exotoxins, including exotoxin A, which causes local necrosis and facilitates systemic bacterial invasion. *P. aeruginosa* possesses a type III secretion system composed of a needle structure that inserts into host cell membranes and allows secretion of exotoxins directly into host cells. *P. aeruginosa* strains with the gene encoding the type III secretion system–dependent phospholipase ExoU are associated with increased mortality compared with ExoU-negative strains, in retrospective studies of patients with *P. aeruginosa* **ventilator-associated pneumonia**. The host responds to infection with a robust inflammatory response, recruiting neutrophils to the infection site and producing antibodies to *P. aeruginosa* proteins such as exotoxin A and endotoxin. There is a lack of convincing data that these antibodies are protective against the establishment of infection.

In addition to acute infection, *P. aeruginosa* is also capable of chronic persistence thought to be partly a result of the formation of **biofilms**, organized communities of bacteria encased in an extracellular matrix that protects the organisms from the host immune response and the effects of antibiotics. Biofilm formation requires pilus-mediated attachment to a surface, proliferation of the organism, and production of exopolysaccharide as the main bacterial component of the extracellular matrix. A mature biofilm can persist despite an intense host immune response, is resistant to many antimicrobials, and is difficult to eradicate with current therapies.

CLINICAL MANIFESTATIONS

Most clinical patterns are related to opportunistic infections in immunocompromised hosts (see Chapter 205) or are associated with shunts and indwelling catheters (Chapter 206). *P. aeruginosa* may be introduced into a minor wound of a healthy person as a secondary invader, and cellulitis and a localized abscess that exudes green or blue pus may follow. The characteristic skin lesions of *P. aeruginosa*, **ecthyma gangrenosum**, whether caused by direct inoculation or a metastatic focus secondary to septicemia, begin as pink macules and progress to hemorrhagic nodules and eventually to ulcers with ecchymotic and gangrenous centers with eschar formation, surrounded by an intense red areola (Table 232.1 and Fig. 232.1).

Outbreaks of dermatitis and urinary tract infections (UTIs) caused by *P. aeruginosa* have been reported in healthy persons after use of pools or hot tubs. Skin lesions of folliculitis develop several hours to 2 days after contact with these water sources. Skin lesions may be erythematous, macular, papular, or pustular. Illness may vary from a few scattered lesions to extensive truncal involvement. In some children, malaise, fever, vomiting, sore throat, conjunctivitis, rhinitis, and swollen breasts may be associated with dermal lesions. UTIs caused by *P. aeruginosa* are most often nosocomial and are often associated with the presence of an indwelling urinary catheter, urinary tract malformations, and previous antibiotic use. UTIs may be minimized or prevented

Table 232.1	*Pseudomonas aeruginosa* Infections
INFECTION	**COMMON CLINICAL CHARACTERISTICS**
Endocarditis	Native right-sided (tricuspid) valve disease with intravenous drug abuse
Pneumonia	Compromised local (lung) or systemic host defense mechanisms; nosocomial (respiratory), bacteremic (malignancy), or abnormal mucociliary clearance (cystic fibrosis) may be pathogenetic; cystic fibrosis is associated with mucoid *P. aeruginosa* organisms producing capsular slime
Central nervous system infection	Meningitis, brain abscess; contiguous spread (mastoiditis, dermal sinus tracts, sinusitis); bacteremia or direct inoculation (trauma, surgery)
External otitis	Swimmer's ear; humid warm climates, swimming pool contamination
Malignant otitis externa	Invasive, indolent, febrile toxic, destructive necrotizing lesion in young infants, immunosuppressed neutropenic patients, or diabetic patients; associated with 7th nerve palsy and mastoiditis
Chronic mastoiditis	Ear drainage, swelling, erythema; perforated tympanic membrane
Keratitis	Corneal ulceration; contact lens keratitis
Endophthalmitis	Penetrating trauma, surgery, penetrating corneal ulceration; fulminant progression
Osteomyelitis/septic arthritis	Puncture wounds of foot and osteochondritis; intravenous drug abuse; fibrocartilaginous joints, sternum, vertebrae, pelvis; open fracture osteomyelitis; indolent pyelonephritis and vertebral osteomyelitis
Urinary tract infection	Iatrogenic, nosocomial; recurrent UTIs in children, instrumented patients, and those with obstruction or stones
Intestinal tract infection	Immunocompromised, neutropenia, typhlitis, rectal abscess, ulceration, rarely diarrhea; peritonitis in peritoneal dialysis
Ecthyma gangrenosum	Metastatic dissemination; hemorrhage, necrosis, erythema, eschar, discrete lesions with bacterial invasion of blood vessels; also subcutaneous nodules, cellulitis, pustules, deep abscesses
Primary and secondary skin infections	Local infection; burns, trauma, decubitus ulcers, toe web infection, green nail (paronychia); whirlpool dermatitis; diffuse, pruritic folliculitis; vesiculopustular or maculopapular, erythematous lesions

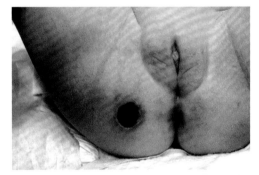

Fig. 232.1 Round, nontender skin lesion on 2 yr old female's buttock. Note the black ulcerated center of the lesion and its red margin. *(From Ghanaiem H, Engelhard D: A healthy 2-year-old child with a round black skin lesion, J Pediatr 163:1225, 2013.)*

by prompt removal of the catheter and by early identification and corrective surgery of obstructive lesions when present.

Burns and Wound Infection
The surfaces of burns or wounds are frequently populated by *P. aeruginosa* and other gram-negative organisms; this initial colonization with a low number of adherent organisms is a prerequisite to invasive disease. *P. aeruginosa* colonization of a burn site may develop into **burn wound sepsis**, which has a high mortality rate when the density of organisms reaches a critical concentration. Administration of antibiotics may diminish the susceptible microbiologic flora, permitting strains of relatively resistant *P. aeruginosa* to flourish. Multiplication of organisms in devitalized tissues or associated with prolonged use of intravenous or urinary catheters increases the risk for septicemia with *P. aeruginosa*, a major problem in burned patients (see Chapter 92).

Cystic Fibrosis
P. aeruginosa is common in children with CF, with a prevalence that increases with increasing age and severity of pulmonary disease (see Chapter 432). Initial infection is caused by **nonmucoid environmental strains** of *P. aeruginosa*, but after a variable period, **mucoid strains** of *P. aeruginosa* that produce the antiphagocytic exopolysaccharide alginate, which is rarely encountered in other conditions, predominate. Repeated isolation of mucoid *P. aeruginosa* from the sputum is associated with increased morbidity and mortality. The infection begins insidiously or even asymptomatically, and the progression has a highly variable pace. In children with CF, antibody does not eradicate the organism, and antibiotics are only partially effective; thus, after infection becomes chronic, it cannot be completely eradicated. Repeated courses of antibiotics select for *P. aeruginosa* strains that are resistant to multiple antibiotics.

Immunocompromised Persons
Children with leukemia or other malignancies, particularly those who are receiving immunosuppressive therapy and who are neutropenic, typically with intravascular catheters, are extremely susceptible to septicemia caused by invasion of the bloodstream by *P. aeruginosa* that is colonizing the respiratory or GI tract. Signs of sepsis are often accompanied by a generalized vasculitis, and hemorrhagic necrotic lesions may be found in all organs, including the skin (ecthyma gangrenosum) (see Fig. 232.1). Hemorrhagic or gangrenous perirectal cellulitis or abscesses may occur, associated with ileus and profound hypotension.

Nosocomial Pneumonia
Although not a frequent cause of community-acquired pneumonia in children, *P. aeruginosa* does cause nosocomial pneumonia, especially ventilator-associated pneumonia, in patients of all ages. *P. aeruginosa* has historically been found to contaminate ventilators, tubing, and humidifiers. Such contamination is uncommon now because of disinfection practices and routine changing of equipment. Nevertheless, colonization of the upper respiratory tract and the GI tract may be followed by

aspiration of *P. aeruginosa*–contaminated secretions, resulting in severe pneumonia. Prior use of broad-spectrum antibiotics is a risk factor for colonization with antibiotic-resistant strains of *P. aeruginosa*. One of the most challenging situations is distinguishing between colonization and pneumonia in intubated patients. This distinction can often only be resolved by using invasive culture techniques such as quantitative bronchoalveolar lavage.

Infants

P. aeruginosa is an occasional cause of **nosocomial bacteremia** in newborns and accounts for 2–5% of positive blood culture results in NICUs. A frequent focus preceding bacteremia is **conjunctivitis**. Older infants rarely present with community-acquired sepsis caused by *P. aeruginosa*. In the few reports describing community-acquired sepsis, preceding conditions included ecthyma-like skin lesions, virus-associated transient neutropenia, and prolonged contact with contaminated bath water or a hot tub.

DIAGNOSIS

P. aeruginosa infection is rarely clinically distinctive. Diagnosis depends on recovery of the organism from the blood, cerebrospinal fluid (CSF), urine, or needle aspirate of the lung, or from purulent material obtained by aspiration of subcutaneous abscesses or areas of cellulitis. In the appropriate clinical setting, recovery of *P. aeruginosa* from a coughed or suctioned sputum may represent infection; but it also may only represent colonization, and clinical judgment is required. Rarely, skin lesions that resemble *P. aeruginosa* infection may follow septicemia caused by *Aeromonas hydrophila,* other gram-negative bacilli, and *Aspergillus.* When *P. aeruginosa* is recovered from nonsterile sites such as skin, mucous membranes, or voided urine, quantitative cultures may be useful to differentiate colonization from invasive infection. In general, ≥100,000 colony-forming units/mL of fluid or gram of tissue is evidence suggestive of invasive infection. Quantitative cultures of tissue and skin are not routine and require consultation with the clinical microbiology laboratory.

TREATMENT

Systemic infections with *P. aeruginosa* should be treated promptly with an antibiotic to which the organism is susceptible in vitro. Response to treatment may be limited, and prolonged treatment may be necessary for systemic infection in immunocompromised hosts.

Septicemia and other aggressive infections should be treated with either 1 or 2 bactericidal agents. Although the number of agents required is controversial, the evidence continues to suggest that the benefit of adding a 2nd agent is questionable, even when studies have included immunosuppressed patients. Whether the use of 2 agents delays the development of resistance is also controversial, with evidence both for and against. Appropriate antibiotics for single-agent therapy include ceftazidime, cefepime, ticarcillin-clavulanate, and piperacillin-tazobactam. Gentamicin or another aminoglycoside may be used concomitantly for synergistic effect.

Ceftazidime has proved to be extremely effective in patients with CF, at 150-250 mg/kg/day divided every 6-8 hr intravenously (IV) to a maximum of 6 g/day. Piperacillin or piperacillin-tazobactam, 300-450 mg/kg/day divided every 6-8 hr IV to a maximum of 12 g/day, also has proved to be effective therapy for susceptible strains of *P. aeruginosa* when combined with an aminoglycoside. Studies of acute *Pseudomonas* infection in ICUs show that continuous infusions of piperacillin-tazobactam are more effective than the same daily dose given as pulse infusions.

Additional effective antibiotics include imipenem-cilastatin, meropenem, and aztreonam. Ciprofloxacin is an effective outpatient therapy, and while commonly used in children with CF, it is not approved in the United States for persons <18 yr old, except for oral treatment of UTIs or when there are no other agents to which the organism is susceptible. Inhaled therapy with either tobramycin or aztreonam is also used for chronic pulmonary infection, with inhaled colistin reserved for the treatment of resistant pseudomonads. It is important to base continued treatment on the results of susceptibility tests because

antibiotic resistance of *P. aeruginosa* to 1 or more antibiotics is increasing. Macrolide therapy decreases pulmonary exacerbations in patients with chronic lung disease and *P. aeruginosa* infection. The mechanism likely relates to altering the virulence properties of *P. aeruginosa* rather than direct bacterial killing.

P. aeruginosa displays intrinsic and acquired resistance to antibiotics. It has many mechanisms for resistance to multiple classes of antibiotics, including but not limited to genetic mutation, production of β-lactamases, and drug efflux pumps. Throughout the United States there has been an alarming increase in multidrug-resistant (MDR) *P. aeruginosa* isolates recovered from children, with resistance to at least 3 classes of antibiotics. The rate of MDR *P. aeruginosa* increased to 26% in 2012 from 15.9% in 1999. Also, the rate of carbapenem-resistant *P. aeruginosa* increased from 12% to 20% during the same period. A newer agent with efficacy against many MDR *P. aeruginosa* isolates is ceftazidime/avibactam, a drug that combines ceftazidime with a β-lactamase inhibitor.

Meningitis can occur by spread from a contiguous focus, as a secondary focus when there is bacteremia, or after invasive procedures. *P. aeruginosa* meningitis is best treated with ceftazidime in combination with an aminoglycoside such as gentamicin, both given IV. Concomitant intraventricular or intrathecal treatment with gentamicin may be required when IV therapy fails but is not recommended for routine use.

SUPPORTIVE CARE

P. aeruginosa infections vary in severity from *superficial* to *intense* septic presentations. With severe infections there is often multisystem involvement and a systemic inflammatory response. Supportive care is similar to care for severe sepsis caused by other gram-negative bacilli and requires support of blood pressure, oxygenation, and appropriate fluid management.

PROGNOSIS

The prognosis is dependent primarily on the nature of the underlying factors that predisposed the patient to *P. aeruginosa* infection. In severely immunocompromised patients, the prognosis for patients with *P. aeruginosa* sepsis is poor unless susceptibility factors such as neutropenia or hypogammaglobulinemia can be reversed. The overall mortality rate was 12.3% in one series of 232 children with *P. aeruginosa* bacteremia, with 3% dying within 48 hr of admission. Resistance of the organism to first-line antibiotics also decreases the chance of survival. The outcome may be improved when there is a urinary tract portal of entry, absence of neutropenia or recovery from neutropenia, and drainage of local sites of infection.

P. aeruginosa is recovered from the lungs of most children who die of CF and adds to the slow deterioration of these patients. The prognosis for normal development is poor in the few infants who survive *P. aeruginosa* meningitis.

PREVENTION

Prevention of infections is dependent on limiting contamination of the healthcare environment and preventing transmission to patients. Effective hospital infection control programs are necessary to identify and eradicate sources of the organism as quickly as possible. In hospitals, infection can be transmitted to children by the hands of personnel, from washbasin surfaces, from catheters and other hospital equipment, and from solutions used to rinse suction catheters.

Strict attention to hand hygiene before and between contacts with patients may prevent or interdict epidemic disease. Meticulous care and sterile procedures in suctioning of endotracheal tubes, insertion and maintenance of indwelling catheters, and removal of catheters as soon as medically reasonable greatly reduce the hazard of extrinsic contamination by *P. aeruginosa* and other gram-negative organisms. Prevention of follicular dermatitis caused by *P. aeruginosa* contamination of whirlpools or hot tubs is possible by maintaining pool water at a pH of 7.2-7.8. Antimicrobial stewardship programs that promote the appropriate use of antibiotics in the hospital setting are critical for reducing the rates of MDR *P. aeruginosa* by limiting unnecessary antibiotic use.

Infections in burned patients may be minimized by protective isolation, debridement of devitalized tissue, and topical applications of bactericidal cream. Administration of intravenous immunoglobulin may be used. Approaches under investigation to prevent infection include development of a *P. aeruginosa* vaccine. No vaccine is currently licensed in the United States.

Bibliography is available at Expert Consult.

232.2 *Burkholderia cepacia* Complex
Thomas S. Murray and Robert S. Baltimore

Burkholderia cepacia is a filamentous gram-negative rod now recognized to be a group of related species or **genomovars** (*B. cepacia, B. cenocepacia, B. multivorans*). It is ubiquitous in the environment but may be difficult to isolate from respiratory specimens in the laboratory, requiring an enriched, selective media oxidation-fermentation base supplemented with polymyxin B–bacitracin-lactose agar (OFPBL) and as long as 3 days of incubation.

B. cepacia is a classic opportunist that rarely infects normal tissue but can be a pathogen for individuals with preexisting damage to respiratory epithelium, especially persons with CF or with immune dysfunction such as chronic granulomatous disease. *B. cepacia* has multiple virulence factors, including lipopolysaccharide, flagella, and a type III secretion system that promotes invasion of respiratory epithelial cells. Resistance to many antibiotics and disinfectants appears to be a factor in the emergence of *B. cepacia* as a nosocomial pathogen. In critical care units it may colonize the tubing used to ventilate patients with respiratory failure. In some patients this colonization may lead to invasive pneumonia and septic shock. Although *B. cepacia* is found throughout the environment, human-to-human spread among CF patients occurs either directly by inhalation of aerosols or indirectly from contaminated equipment or surfaces, accounting for the strict infection control measures for children with CF who are colonized with *B. cepacia*. For example, CF patients colonized with *B. cepacia* are asked not to attend events where other persons with CF will be present. *B. cepacia* infections in persons with CF may represent chronic infection in some patients, but others, especially those with *Burkholderia cenocepacia*, genomovar III, can develop an acute respiratory syndrome of fever, leukocytosis, and progressive respiratory failure, with more rapid decline in pulmonary function and lower survival rate.

Treatment in hospitals should include standard precautions and avoidance of placing colonized and uncolonized patients in the same room. The use of antibiotics is guided by susceptibility studies of a patient's isolates, because the susceptibility pattern of this species is quite variable, and multiply resistant strains are common. Trimethoprim-sulfamethoxazole (TMP-SMX) and doxycycline or minocycline are potential oral therapies for *B. cepacia* complex. For IV therapy, meropenem with a 2nd agent such as TMP-SMX, doxycycline, minocycline, ceftazidime, or amikacin are potential options. Even though there is primary resistance to aminoglycosides, these agents may be useful in combination with other antibiotics. Treatment with 2 or more agents may be necessary to control the infection and avoid the development of resistance. No vaccine is currently available.

BURKHOLDERIA MALLEI (GLANDERS)

Glanders is a severe infectious disease of horses and other domestic and farm animals that is caused by *Burkholderia mallei*, a nonmotile gram-negative bacillus that is occasionally transmitted to humans. It is acquired by inoculation into the skin, usually at the site of a previous abrasion, or by inhalation of aerosols. Laboratory workers may acquire it from clinical specimens. The disease is relatively common in Asia, Africa, and the Middle East. The clinical manifestations include septicemia, acute or chronic pneumonitis, and hemorrhagic necrotic lesions of the skin, nasal mucous membranes, and lymph nodes. The diagnosis is usually made by recovery of the organism in cultures of affected tissue. Glanders is treated with sulfadiazine, tetracyclines, or chloramphenicol and streptomycin over many months. The disease has been eliminated from the United States, but interest in this organism has

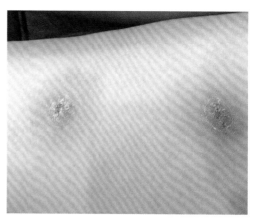

Fig. 232.2 Thigh abscesses at the sites of mosquito bites in 15 yr old Pennsylvania resident who had recently returned from Thailand, July 2016. Photo was taken 7 wk after onset. *(From Mitchell PK, Campbell C, Montgomery MP, et al: Notes from the field: travel–associated melioidosis and resulting laboratory exposures—United States, 2016, MMWR 66(37):1001–1002, 2017.)*

increased because of the possibility of its use as a bioterrorism agent (see Chapter 741). Although standard precautions are appropriate when caring for hospitalized infected patients, biosafety level 3 precautions are required for laboratory staff working with *B. mallei*. No vaccine is available.

BURKHOLDERIA PSEUDOMALLEI (MELIOIDOSIS)

Melioidosis is an important disease of Southeast Asia and northern Australia and occurs in the United States mainly in persons returning from endemic areas. The causative agent is *Burkholderia pseudomallei*, an inhabitant of soil and water in the tropics. It is ubiquitous in endemic areas, and infection follows inhalation of dust, ingestion, or direct contamination of abrasions or wounds. Human-to-human transmission has only rarely been reported. Serologic surveys demonstrate that asymptomatic infection occurs in endemic areas. The disease may remain latent and appear when host resistance is reduced, sometimes years after the initial exposure. Diabetes mellitus is a risk factor for severe melioidosis.

Melioidosis may present as a **primary skin lesion** (vesicle, bulla, or urticaria) (Fig. 232.2). Pulmonary infection may be subacute and mimic tuberculosis or may present as an acute necrotizing pneumonia. Occasionally, septicemia occurs and numerous abscesses are noted in various organs of the body. Myocarditis, pericarditis, endocarditis, intestinal abscess, cholecystitis, acute gastroenteritis, UTIs, septic arthritis, paraspinal abscess, osteomyelitis, mycotic aneurysm, and generalized lymphadenopathy all have been observed. Melioidosis may also present as an encephalitic illness with fever and seizures. It is also an agent of severe wound infections after contact with contaminated water following a tsunami. Diagnosis is based on visualization of characteristic small, gram-negative rods in exudates or growth on laboratory media such as eosin–methylene blue or MacConkey agar. Serologic tests are available, and diagnosis can be established by a 4-fold or greater increase in antibody titer in an individual with an appropriate syndrome. It has been recognized as a possible agent of bioterrorism (see Chapter 741).

B. pseudomallei is susceptible to many antimicrobial agents, and the U.S. Centers for Disease Control and Prevention (CDC) recommends meropenem or ceftazidime as IV therapies and TMP-SMX or doxycycline as oral therapy. Other choices include aminoglycosides, tetracycline, chloramphenicol, and amoxicillin-clavulanate. Therapy should be guided by antimicrobial susceptibility tests; 2 or 3 agents such as ceftazidime or meropenem plus either TMP-SMX, sulfisoxazole, or an aminoglycoside are usually chosen for severe or septicemic disease. For severe disease, prolonged treatment for 2-6 mo is recommended to prevent relapses. Appropriate antibiotic therapy generally results in recovery.

Bibliography is available at Expert Consult.

232.3 *Stenotrophomonas*
Thomas S. Murray and Robert S. Baltimore

Stenotrophomonas maltophilia (formerly *Xanthomonas maltophilia* or *Pseudomonas maltophilia*) is a short to medium-sized, straight gram-negative bacillus. It is ubiquitous in nature and can be found in the hospital environment, especially in tap water or standing water, and may contaminate sinks and hospital equipment such as nebulizers. Strains isolated in the laboratory may be contaminants, may be a commensal from the colonized surface of a patient, or may represent an invasive pathogen. The species is an opportunist and is often recovered from immunosuppressed patients and patients with CF after multiple courses of antimicrobial therapy. Serious infections usually occur among those requiring intensive care, including neonatal intensive care, typically patients with ventilator-associated pneumonia or catheter-associated infections. Prolonged antibiotic exposure appears to be a frequent factor in nosocomial *S. maltophilia* infections, probably because of its endogenous antibiotic resistance pattern. Common types of infection include pneumonia following airway colonization and aspiration, bacteremia, soft tissue infections, endocarditis, and osteomyelitis. *S. maltophilia* bacteremia is a **nosocomial infection** associated with the presence of a central venous catheter.

Strains vary as to antibiotic susceptibility, and the treatment of *S. maltophilia* can be difficult because of inherent antimicrobial resistance. Data are lacking on whether there is clinical benefit to treat *S. maltophilia* recovered from the respiratory tract of a patient with CF. For invasive infections, **TMP-SMX** is the treatment of choice and is the only antimicrobial for which susceptibility is routinely reported. **Minocycline** monotherapy has recently been shown to be a viable alternative to TMP-SMX with fewer adverse effects and similar clinical outcomes. Mean inhibitory concentration testing is available for other antibiotics, such as ticarcillin-clavulanate, and reserved for TMP-SMX–resistant isolates. For resistant organisms or for patients who cannot tolerate sulfa drugs, other options based on clinical outcome include ciprofloxacin, as well as ceftazidime alone, or in combination with other agents such as aminoglycosides. **Tigecycline** is a newer agent reported to have efficacy for treating a highly resistant isolate.

Bibliography is available at Expert Consult.

Chapter **233**
Tularemia *(Francisella tularensis)*
Kevin J. Downes
第二百三十三章
兔热病（土拉菌病）

中文导读

　　本章主要介绍了兔热病（土拉菌病）的病因、流行病学、发病机制、临床表现、诊断、鉴别诊断、治疗、预后和预防。在关于兔热病的流行病学部分详细介绍了该病好发区域、儿童发病年龄和性别分布等内容。在关于兔热病的临床表现部分详细介绍了该病各种临床症状和体征的发生率以及主要的6大临床综合征。在关于兔热病的治疗部分详细介绍了推荐治疗方案，以及暴露后的预防治疗方案。

Tularemia is a **zoonosis** caused by the gram-negative bacterium *Francisella tularensis*. Tularemia is primarily a disease of wild animals; human disease is incidental and usually results from tick or deer fly bites or contact with infected live or dead wild animals. The illness caused by *F. tularensis* is manifest by multiple clinical syndromes, the most common consisting of an ulcerative lesion at the site of inoculation with regional lymphadenopathy or lymphadenitis. *F. tularensis* is also a potential agent of bioterrorism (see Chapter 741).

ETIOLOGY

Francisella tularensis is a small, nonmotile, pleomorphic, catalase-positive gram-negative coccobacillus. It can be classified into 4 main subspecies: *Francisella tularensis* subsp. *tularensis* (type A), *F. tularensis* subsp. *holarctica* (type B), *F. tularensis* subsp. *mediasiatica*, and *F. tularensis* subsp. *novicida*. Type A can be further subdivided into 4 distinct genotypes designated A1a, A1b, A2a, and A2b, with **A1b** appearing to produce more serious disease in humans. Although all subspecies of *F. tularensis* can cause human infections, types A and B are most common and type A is the most virulent. *F. tularensis* is an intracellular organism than can infect a number of host cell types, including macrophages, hepatocytes, and epithelial cells. It is one of the most virulent bacterial pathogens known, with as few as 10 microorganisms causing infections in humans and animals.

EPIDEMIOLOGY

Tularemia is primarily found in the Northern hemisphere. Type A is found predominantly in North America, whereas type B is found throughout the Northern hemisphere, including North America, Europe, and Asia. Human infections with type B are usually milder and have lower mortality rates compared to infections with type A. *F. tularensis* subsp. *mediasiatica* appears to be restricted to central Asia, whereas *F. tularensis* subsp. *novicida* has been isolated in North America, Australia, and Southeast Asia.

According to the Centers for Disease Control and Prevention (CDC), the number of annual reported cases of tularemia in the United States from 2005 to 2015 ranged from 93 to 315 per year. In 2015 the number of cases reported in the United States was the highest it had been over the past 50 years. Tularemia occurs all over the Unites States, with the majority of cases reported from central states (Fig. 233.1). The overall U.S. incidence of tularemia in 2015 was 0.10 per 100,000 residents; Wyoming (3.58/100,000), South Dakota (2.91/100,000), Nebraska (1.32/100,000), Kansas (1.17/100,000), and Colorado (0.95/100,000) were states with the highest incidence.

Although cases of tularemia occur all year, most cases and outbreaks occur in warm, summer months (May-August). Tularemia is more common in males, and there is a bimodal distribution based on age, with peaks in childhood (5-9 yr) and later adulthood (65-69 yr), potentially because of greater opportunities for environmental and animal exposures at these ages. Fig. 233.2 shows the distribution of tularemia by age and gender from 2001 to 2010 in the United States.

PATHOGENESIS

Of all the zoonotic diseases, tularemia is unusual because of the different modes of transmission of disease. A large number of animals serve as a reservoir for this organism. In the United States, **rabbits** and **ticks** are the principal reservoirs. Dogs may be an intermediate vector. In the United States, *Amblyomma americanum* (lone star tick), *Dermacentor variabilis* (dog tick), and *Dermacentor andersoni* (wood tick) are the most common tick vectors. These ticks usually feed on infected small rodents and later feed on humans. **Deer flies** (*Chrysops* spp.) can also transmit tularemia and are present in the western United States. *F. tularensis* subsp. *tularensis* is carried by rabbits, ticks, and tabanid flies (e.g., deer flies), whereas subsp. *holarctica* is associated with aquatic habitats and transmitted primarily by mosquitoes, but also aquatic rodents (beavers, muskrats), hares, voles, ticks, tabanid flies, and ingestion of contaminated water (e.g., ponds, rivers).

The organism can penetrate both intact skin and mucous membranes (eyes, mouth, gastrointestinal [GI] tract, or lungs). Transmission can occur through the bite of infected ticks or other biting insects, by contact with infected animals or their carcasses, by consumption of contaminated foods or water, or through inhalation, as might occur in a laboratory setting or if a machine (e.g., lawn mower) runs over infected animal carcasses. However, this organism is not transmitted from person to person. The most common portal of entry for human infection is through the skin or mucous membrane. Hunting or skinning infected wild rodents, such as rabbits or prairie dogs, has been the source of infection in numerous reports. Domesticated animals such as cats and hamsters can also transmit tularemia.

Usually >10^8 organisms are required to produce infection if *F. tularensis* bacteria are ingested, but as few as 10 organisms may cause disease if they are inhaled or injected into the skin (i.e., insect bite). Infection with *F. tularensis* stimulates the host to produce antibodies, which have

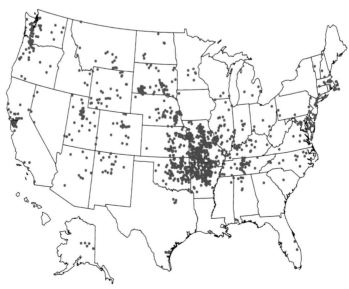

* One dot is placed randomly within county of residence for each reported case.

Fig. 233.1 Reported cases of tularemia—United States, 2001–2010. *(From Centers for Disease Control and Prevention: Tularemia—United States, 2001–2010. MMWR 62:963–966, 2013).*

only recently been recognized as important in the immune response to this organism. The *F. tularensis* envelope is largely responsible for virulence and plays major roles in the ability of the organism to evade the immune system, attach to and invade cells, and cause severe disease. The body is most dependent on cell-mediated immunity to contain and eradicate *F. tularensis*. Tularemia is usually followed by specific protection; thus chronic infection or reinfection is unlikely.

CLINICAL MANIFESTATIONS

Symptoms of tularemia vary based on the mode of transmission. The average incubation period from infection until clinical symptoms is 3 days (range: 1-21 days). Early symptoms of infection are generally nonspecific: fever, chills, myalgias, arthralgias, headache, and fatigue. Bacteremia may be common in the early stages of infection. A sudden onset of fever is common, and a pulse-temperature dissociation may be present. Findings on physical examination may include lymphadenopathy, hepatosplenomegaly, or skin lesions. Table 233.1 shows the frequency of various symptoms and examination findings.

The clinical manifestations of tularemia have been divided into 6 major clinical syndromes (Table 233.2). **Ulceroglandular** and **glandular** disease are the 2 most common forms of tularemia diagnosed in children. Infections following the bites of ticks or deer flies take these forms. Mortality with these forms of tularemia is rare, especially with implementation of effective treatment. Glandular disease, which is associated with lymphadenopathy without skin ulceration, may also result from minor skin abrasions. Within 48-72 hr after inoculation of the skin, an

erythematous, tender, or pruritic papule may appear at the portal of entry. This papule may enlarge and form an ulcer with a black base. Ulcers are generally erythematous and painful with raised borders and may last several weeks, especially if untreated. Various other skin lesions have been described, including erythema multiforme and erythema nodosum. Approximately 20% of patients may develop a generalized maculopapular rash that occasionally becomes pustular.

The unifying manifestation of glandular and ulceroglandular forms of tularemia is painful regional **lymphadenopathy**. Adenopathy may develop before, concurrent with, or after skin ulceration in ulceroglandular disease. Cervical or posterior auricular nodes are involved following bites on the head or neck, whereas enlarged axillary or epitrochlear nodes signal exposure on the arms. Nodes may vary in size from 0.5-10 cm (⅕-4 inches) and appear singly or in clusters. These affected nodes may become fluctuant and drain spontaneously and are often associated with overlying skin changes. Late suppuration of the involved nodes has been described in 25–30% of patients despite effective therapy. Examination of this material from such lymph nodes usually reveals sterile necrotic material.

Oropharyngeal tularemia results from consumption of poorly cooked meats or contaminated water. This syndrome is characterized by acute pharyngitis, with or without tonsillitis, and cervical lymphadenitis. Infected tonsils may become large and develop a yellowish white membrane that may resemble the membranes associated with diphtheria. GI disease may also occur and usually presents with mild, unexplained diarrhea or emesis but may progress to rapidly fulminant and fatal disease. GI bleeding can develop in more severe forms associated with intestinal ulcers.

Oculoglandular tularemia is uncommon, but when it does occur, the portal of entry is the conjunctiva. Contact with contaminated fingers or debris from crushed insects is the most common mechanism of this form of tularemia. Disease is generally unilateral, and the conjunctiva is painful and inflamed with yellowish nodules and pinpoint ulcerations. Purulent conjunctivitis with ipsilateral preauricular or submandibular

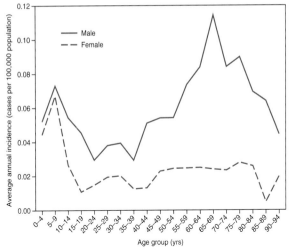

Fig. 233.2 Incidence of tularemia, by age and gender—United States, 2001–2010. (*From Centers for Disease Control and Prevention (CDC): Tularemia—United States, 2001–2010, MMWR 62:963–966, 2013*).

Table 233.1	Common Clinical Manifestations of Tularemia in Children
SIGN OR SYMPTOM	**FREQUENCY**
Lymphadenopathy	96%
Fever (>38.3°C [100.9°F])	87%
Ulcer/eschar/papule	45%
Pharyngitis	43%
Myalgias/arthralgias	39%
Nausea/vomiting	35%
Hepatosplenomegaly	35%

Table 233.2	Clinical Syndromes of Tularemia in Children	
CLINICAL SYNDROME	**CHARACTERISTICS OF SYNDROME**	**FREQUENCY**
Ulceroglandular	Skin ulcer/eschar, painful regional adenopathy	45%
Glandular	Regional adenopathy without detectable skin ulceration	25%
Pneumonia	Nonproductive cough, dyspnea, pleuritic chest pain; multilobar/diffuse infiltrates > lobar infiltrates on chest radiography	14%
Oropharyngeal	Pharyngitis, mucosal ulcers, cervical adenopathy	4%
Oculoglandular	Unilateral, painful, and often purulent conjunctivitis; chemosis; conjunctival ulcers; preauricular adenopathy	2%
Typhoidal	Severe systemic disease (sepsis-like syndrome): high fever, headaches, myalgias, arthralgias, neurologic symptoms	2%

lymphadenopathy can develop and is referred to as *Parinaud oculo-glandular syndrome*. Corneal ulceration and perforation are uncommon but serious complications of this form of disease.

Typhoidal tularemia is usually associated with a large inoculum of organisms and is a term used to describe severe, bacteremic disease regardless of the mode of transmission or portal of entry. Patients are critically ill, and symptoms mimic those with other forms of sepsis: high fevers, confusion, rigors, myalgias, vomiting, and diarrhea. Clinicians practicing in tularemia-endemic regions must always consider this diagnosis in critically ill children. Complications of bacteremia with *F. tularensis* can include the development of meningitis, pericarditis, hepatitis, peritonitis, endocarditis, skin/soft tissue abscesses, and osteomyelitis. Because of its increased virulence, *F. tularensis* subsp. *tularensis* (type A disease) is more often associated with typhoidal tularemia. Patients with tularemia meningitis usually develop a marked cerebrospinal fluid (CSF) with a monocytic predominance. As with other causes of bacterial meningitis, CSF glucose is low and protein is high.

Pneumonia caused by *F. tularensis* (**pneumonic tularemia**) can develop following inhalation (primary pulmonary infection) or secondary to hematogenous spread in other forms of tularemia, particularly the typhoidal form. Inhalation-related infection has been described in laboratory workers who are working with the organism and results in a relatively high mortality rate. Aerosols from farming activities involving rodent contamination (haying, threshing) or animal carcass destruction with lawn mowers have been reported to cause pneumonia as well. Patients generally complain of a nonproductive cough, dyspnea, or pleuritic chest pain. Chest radiographs of patients with pneumonic tularemia typically reveal diffuse, patchy infiltrates rather than focal areas of consolidation. Pleural effusions may also be present. In pulmonary infections, hilar or mediastinal adenopathy can develop, and in severe forms, necrotizing or hemorrhagic pneumonitis. Mortality with pneumonic tularemia is high if untreated.

DIAGNOSIS

The diagnosis can be delayed since symptoms are often similar to other, more common infections. The history and physical examination of the patient may suggest the diagnosis, especially if the patient has a history of animal or tick exposure. Routine hematologic blood tests are non-diagnostic. Definitive diagnosis is made by growth of *F. tularensis* in culture. *F. tularensis* can be isolated in culture of lymph node biopsies or aspirates, blood, wounds, pharyngeal swabs, pleural fluid, or sputum specimens, although cultures are positive in only approximately 10% of cases. *F. tularensis* can be cultured in the microbiology laboratory on cysteine-glucose–blood agar, but care should be taken to alert the personnel in the laboratory if this is attempted so that they can take the proper precautions to protect themselves from acquiring infection; biosafety level 3 containment is necessary to avoid occupational exposure. Histopathologic findings of involved lymph nodes demonstrate granulomas with central necrosis (early) and caseation (late). Unfortunately, these findings cannot distinguish tularemia from other causes of granulomatous lymphadenitis, such as tuberculosis, cat-scratch disease (*Bartonella henselae* infection), or sarcoidosis. Polymerase chain reaction of tissue specimens may be more sensitive than culture but is currently only used to make a presumptive diagnosis.

The diagnosis of tularemia is usually established through the use of a standard and highly reliable serum agglutination test. In the standard tube agglutination test, a single titer of ≥1:160 in a patient with a compatible history and physical findings can establish the diagnosis. A microagglutination test is also available, and ≥1:128 is considered positive. A 4-fold increase in titer from paired serum samples collected >2 wk apart (acute to convalescent phase) can also be considered diagnostic. False-negative serologic responses can be obtained early in the infection or if paired sera are collected too close together. Once infected, patients may have a positive agglutination test result (1:20 to 1:80) that persists for life. Other testing techniques available include enzyme-linked immunosorbent assay, analysis of urine for tularemia antigen, direct fluorescent antibody, and immunohistochemical staining; these studies have limited roles in establishing the diagnosis of tularemia.

Differential Diagnosis

The differential diagnosis of **ulceroglandular** or **glandular** tularemia is broad and includes infestation with pathogens that cause acute or subacute lymphadenitis: cat-scratch disease *(B. henselae)*, infectious mononucleosis, typical bacterial pathogens (*Staphylococcus aureus*, group A streptococcus), *Mycobacterium tuberculosis*, nontuberculous mycobacteria, *Toxoplasma gondii*, *Sporothrix schenckii*, plague (*Yersinia pestis*), anthrax (*Bacillus anthracis*), melioidosis (*Burkholderia pseudomallei*), and rat-bite fever (*Streptobacillus moniliformis*, *Spirillum minus*). Noninfectious processes such as sarcoidosis and Kawasaki disease can also present similarly. **Oculoglandular** disease may also occur with other infectious agents, such as *B. henselae*, *Treponema pallidum*, *Coccidioides immitis*, herpes simplex virus (HSV), adenoviruses, and the bacterial agents responsible for purulent conjunctivitis. **Oropharyngeal** tularemia must be differentiated from the same diseases that cause ulceroglandular/glandular disease and from cytomegalovirus, HSV, adenovirus, and other viral or bacterial etiologies. **Pneumonic** tularemia must be differentiated from the other non–β-lactam–responsive organisms that cause community-acquired pneumonia, such as *Mycoplasma* and *Chlamydophila*, as well as mycobacteria, fungi, and rickettsiae. Inhalation plague, anthrax, and Q fever could present similarly. **Typhoidal** tularemia must be differentiated from other forms of sepsis as well as from enteric fever (typhoid and paratyphoid fever) and brucellosis.

TREATMENT

Aminoglycosides are the mainstay of treatment of tularemia: gentamicin is the drug of choice for the treatment of tularemia in children and streptomycin is the drug of choice in adults. Table 233.3 displays therapeutic options for treatment of tularemia as well for postexposure prophylaxis. Chloramphenicol and tetracyclines have been used, but the high relapse rate has limited their use in children. They are often used as adjunctive therapy for treatment of tularemia meningitis. Fluoroquinolones (ciprofloxacin) have been successful in mild-moderate cases of illness, especially those caused by subsp. *holarctica*. β-Lactam agents demonstrate poor activity against *F. tularensis* and should not be used.

Therapy with aminoglycosides is typically continued for 7-10 days, but a longer course is needed in more severe disease. In mild cases, 5-7 days may be sufficient. Treatment with chloramphenicol or doxycycline should be continued for 14-21 days because of an increased risk of relapse, likely because of their bacteriostatic nature. Postexposure prophylaxis is generally recommended for 14 days.

Table 233.3	Recommended Treatment for Patients With Tularemia
INDICATION	**DRUG AND DOSAGE**
Moderate-severe disease	Gentamicin, 5 mg/kg/day IV or IM divided every 8-12 hr, *or* Streptomycin, 15 mg/kg/dose IM every 12 hr (max 1 g/dose)
Mild disease	Gentamicin, 5 mg/kg/day IV or IM divided every 8-12 hr, *or* Ciprofloxacin, 15 mg/kg/dose every 12 hr (max 500 mg/dose)
Meningitis	Streptomycin or gentamicin, in doses given for moderate-severe disease, *plus* chloramphenicol, 50-100 mg/kg/day IV divided every 6 hr (max 1000 mg/dose), *or* doxycycline, 2.2 mg/kg/dose IV every 12 hr (max 100 mg/dose)
Postexposure prophylaxis	Doxycycline, 2.2 mg/kg/dose every 12 hr (max 100 mg/dose), *or* Ciprofloxacin, 15 mg/kg/dose every 12 hr (max 500 mg/dose)

IM, Intramuscularly; IV, intravenously.

PROGNOSIS

Poor outcomes are associated with a delay in appropriate treatment, but with rapid recognition and treatment, fatalities are exceedingly rare. The mortality rate for severe untreated disease (e.g., pneumonia, typhoidal disease) can be as high as 30% in these situations, but in general the overall mortality rate is <1%. Subspecies *tularensis* is associated with more aggressive disease and worse outcomes than subsp. *holarctica*.

Relapses are uncommon if gentamicin or streptomycin is used. Patients typically defervesce within 24-48 hr after starting therapy, although lymphadenopathy can take several weeks to resolve fully. Late suppuration of involved lymph nodes may occur despite adequate therapy. Patients who have not started on appropriate therapy early may respond more slowly to antimicrobial therapy.

PREVENTION

Prevention of tularemia is based on *avoiding exposure*. Children living in tick-endemic regions should be taught to avoid tick-infested areas. Families should have a tick control plan for their immediate environment and for their pets. Protective clothing should be worn when entering a tick-infested area. Insect repellents can be used safely in infants and children. Children should undergo frequent tick checks during and after their time in tick-infested areas. If ticks are found on the child, **forceps** should be used to pull the tick straight out. The skin should be cleansed before and after this procedure.

Children should also be taught to avoid sick and dead animals. Dogs and cats are most likely to bring these animals to a child's attention. Children should be encouraged to wear gloves, masks, and eye protection while cleaning wild game. Families should cook wild game thoroughly before eating.

Prophylactic antimicrobial agents are not effective in preventing tularemia and should not be used after exposure. No tularemia vaccine is currently available for the general public. **Standard precautions** are adequate for hospitalized children with tularemia, since no cases of person-to-person transmission have been identified.

Bibliography is available at Expert Consult.

Chapter **234**
Brucella
Kevin J. Downes
第二百三十四章
布鲁氏菌

中文导读

本章主要介绍了布鲁氏菌感染的病因、流行病学、发病机制、临床表现、诊断、鉴别诊断、治疗、预后和预防等内容。在关于布鲁氏菌病的诊断部分详细介绍了病原培养、血清凝集试验、酶联免疫法等内容。在关于布鲁氏菌病的治疗部分首先强调了选用具有良好的细胞内杀菌作用药物的重要性，进而详细介绍了布鲁氏菌病的推荐治疗方案，包括适应证、药物种类、具体剂量、使用方法和治疗疗程等内容。

Human **brucellosis** is caused by organisms of the genus *Brucella* and continues to be a major public health problem worldwide. Humans are accidental hosts and acquire this zoonosis from direct contact with an infected animal (cattle, sheep, camels, goats, and pigs) or consumption of products of an infected animal. Although brucellosis is widely recognized as an occupational risk among adults working with livestock, much of the brucellosis in children is food-borne and is associated with consumption of unpasteurized dairy products. *Brucella* spp. are also potential agents of bioterrorism (see Chapter 741).

ETIOLOGY

Brucella abortus (cattle), *Brucella melitensis* (goats and sheep), *Brucella suis* (swine), and *Brucella canis* (dogs) are the most common organisms responsible for human disease. These organisms are small, aerobic, non–spore-forming, nonmotile, gram-negative coccobacillary bacteria. *Brucella* spp. are fastidious in their growth but can be grown on various laboratory media, including blood and chocolate agars.

EPIDEMIOLOGY

Brucellosis is endemic in many parts of the world and is especially prevalent in the Mediterranean basin, Persian Gulf, Indian subcontinent, and parts of Mexico and Central and South America. There are approximately 500,000 new cases annually worldwide, although accurate estimates of the prevalence of disease are lacking because of underreporting and underdiagnosis. Childhood brucellosis accounts for 10–30% of cases. *B. melitensis* is the most prevalent species causing human brucellosis and is most often carried by sheep, goats, camels, and buffalo. Because of improved sanitation and animal vaccination, brucellosis has become rare in industrialized countries where recreational or occupational exposure to infected animals is a major risk factor for the development of disease. A history of travel to endemic regions or consumption of exotic food or unpasteurized dairy products may be an important clue to the diagnosis of human brucellosis. In the United States, >50% of cases occur in California, Florida, and Texas; hunting **feral swine** in these states is a recently recognized risk factor. All age-groups can be infected by *Brucella,* and infections are more common in males, likely because of more frequent occupational and environmental exposures.

PATHOGENESIS

Modes of transmission for these organisms include *inoculation* through cuts or abrasions in the skin, inoculation of the conjunctiva, *inhalation* of infectious aerosols, or *ingestion* of contaminated meat or dairy products. **Infected livestock** are the most common source of human infection. In children the primary means of infection is through eating or drinking unpasteurized or raw dairy products. Individuals in endemic areas with occupational exposures to animals, such as farmers and veterinarians, are at highest risk. Laboratory workers are more often exposed to infected aerosols. The risk for infection depends on the nutritional and immune status of the host, the route of inoculum, and the species of *Brucella.* For reasons that remain unclear, it has been suggested that *B. melitensis* and *B. suis* are more virulent than *B. abortus* or *B. canis.*

The major virulence factor for *Brucella* appears to be its cell wall **lipopolysaccharide** (LPS). Strains containing smooth LPS have been demonstrated to have greater virulence and are more resistant to killing by polymorphonuclear leukocytes. These organisms are facultative intracellular pathogens that can survive and replicate within the mononuclear phagocytic cells (monocytes, macrophages) of the reticuloendothelial system. Even though *Brucella* spp. are chemotactic for entry of leukocytes into the body, the leukocytes are less efficient at killing these organisms than other bacteria despite the assistance of serum factors such as complement. *Brucella* spp. possess multiple strategies to evade immune responses and establish and maintain chronic infection. Specifically, during chronic stages of infection, organisms persist within the liver, spleen, lymph nodes, and bone marrow and result in granuloma formation.

Antibodies are produced against the LPS and other cell wall antigens, providing a means of diagnosis and probably playing a role in long-term immunity. The major factor in recovery from infection appears to be development of a cell-mediated response, resulting in macrophage activation and enhanced intracellular killing. Specifically, sensitized T lymphocytes release cytokines (e.g., interferon-γ, tumor necrosis factor-α), which activate the macrophages and enhance their intracellular killing capacity.

CLINICAL MANIFESTATIONS

Brucellosis is a systemic illness that can be very difficult to diagnose in children. Symptoms can be acute or insidious in nature and are usually nonspecific. The incubation period is generally 2-4 wk but may be shorter with *B. melitensis.* Fever is present in >75% of cases, and the fever pattern can vary widely. The most common physical complaints are arthralgia, myalgia, and back pain. Systemic symptoms, such as fatigue, sweats, chills, anorexia, headache, weight loss, and malaise, are reported in the majority of adult cases but are less frequent in children. Other associated symptoms include abdominal pain, diarrhea, rash, vomiting, cough, and pharyngitis.

The most common physical manifestation of brucellosis is hepatic and splenic enlargement, which is present in approximately half of cases. Whereas arthralgia is common, arthritis occurs in a minority of cases. Arthritis is typically monoarticular and most often involves the knee or hip in children and the sacroiliac joint in adolescents and adults. A number of skin lesions have been described with brucellosis, but there is no typical rash for this infection. Epididymo-orchitis is more common in adolescents and adults.

In endemic countries, *Brucella* spp. are an important cause of occult bacteremia in young children. Because of the organism's ability to establish chronic infection, hepatic and splenic abscesses may develop. Serious manifestations of brucellosis include endocarditis, meningitis, osteomyelitis, and spondylitis. Although headache, mental inattention, and depression may be demonstrated in patients with uncomplicated brucellosis, invasion of the nervous system occurs in only 1–4% of cases. Neonatal and congenital infections with these organisms have also been described, resulting from transplacental transmission, breast milk, and blood transfusions. The signs and symptoms associated with congenital/neonatal brucellosis are nonspecific.

Hematologic abnormalities are common with brucellosis; thrombocytopenia, leukopenia, anemia, or pancytopenia may occur. Hemolytic complications can include microangiopathic hemolytic anemia, thrombotic microangiopathy, and autoimmune hemolytic anemia. Elevations of liver enzymes occur in approximately half of cases.

DIAGNOSIS

A definitive diagnosis of brucellosis is established by recovering the organisms from the blood, bone marrow, or other tissues. Unfortunately, cultures are insensitive and positive only in a minority of cases. Isolation of the organism may require as long as 4 wk from a blood culture sample unless the laboratory is using an automated culture system such as the lysis-centrifugation method, where the organism can be recovered in 5-7 days. Therefore, it is prudent to alert the clinical microbiology laboratory that brucellosis is suspected so that cultures can be held longer. Bone marrow cultures may be superior to blood cultures when evaluating patients who have received previous antimicrobial therapy.

Because of the low yield of cultures, various serologic tests have been applied to the diagnosis of brucellosis. The serum agglutination test is the most widely used and detects antibodies against *B. abortus, B. melitensis,* and *B. suis.* This method does not detect antibodies against *B. canis* because this species lacks the smooth LPS; *B. canis*–specific antigen is required to diagnose this species. No single titer is ever diagnostic, but most patients with acute infections have titers of ≥1:160. Antibodies can generally be detected within 2-4 wk after infection. Low titers may be found early in the course of the illness, requiring the use of acute and convalescent sera testing to confirm the diagnosis: 4-fold increase in titers drawn ≥2 wk apart. Because patients with active infection have both an immunoglobulin M (IgM) and an IgG response and the serum agglutination test measures the total quantity of agglutinating antibodies, the total quantity of IgG is measured by treatment of the serum with 2-mercaptoethanol. This fractionation is important in determining the significance of the antibody titer, because low levels of IgM can remain in the serum for weeks to months after the infection has been treated. IgG titers decrease with effective therapy, and a negative 2-mercaptoethanol test after treatment indicates a favorable response.

It is important to remember that all serologic results must be interpreted in light of a patient's history and physical examination. False-positive results from cross-reacting antibodies to other gram-negative organisms, such as *Yersinia enterocolitica, Francisella tularensis,* and *Vibrio cholerae,* can occur. In addition, the prozone effect can give false-negative results in the presence of high titers of antibody. To avoid this issue, serum that is being tested should be diluted to ≥1:320.

The enzyme immunoassay should only be used for suspected cases with negative serum agglutination tests or for the evaluation of patients in the following situations: (1) complicated cases, (2) suspected chronic brucellosis, or (3) reinfection. Polymerase chain reaction assays have been developed but are not available in most clinical laboratories.

Differential Diagnosis

Brucellosis should be considered in the differential diagnosis of fever of unknown origin in endemic areas. It may present similar to other infections such as tularemia, cat-scratch disease, malaria, typhoid fever, histoplasmosis, blastomycosis, and coccidioidomycosis. Infections caused by *Mycobacterium tuberculosis*, atypical mycobacteria, rickettsiae, and *Yersinia* can also present similar to brucellosis.

TREATMENT

Many antimicrobial agents are active in vitro against *Brucella* spp., but the clinical effectiveness does not always correlate with these results. Agents that provide good intracellular killing are required for elimination of *Brucella* infections. Because of the risk of relapse with monotherapy, combination therapy is generally recommended. In children, **doxycycline** or trimethoprim-sulfamethoxazole (TMP-SMX) in combination with **rifampin** are most often used for uncomplicated (e.g., nonfocal) infections (Table 234.1). While data support that the combination of doxycycline plus an aminoglycoside (streptomycin, gentamicin) is superior to the above oral combination therapies, with fewer treatment failures and relapses, the inconvenience of parenteral therapy may limit this approach in uncomplicated cases, particularly in resource-limited settings. Fluoroquinolones may be a viable alternative to doxycycline or TMP-SMX but have not been studied in children. For uncomplicated infections, a 6 wk course of therapy is recommended.

In more serious infections (e.g., endocarditis, meningitis, osteoarticular), 3-drug therapy is advised. An aminoglycoside (streptomycin, gentamicin) should be administered for the 1st 7-14 days along with doxycycline or TMP-SMX plus rifampin, which are then continued for 4-6 mo. Treatment may need to be continued for up to 1 yr in severe cases of central nervous system (CNS) disease.

Although **relapse** occurs in approximately 5–15% of cases, antimicrobial resistance is rare. Relapse is confirmed by isolation of *Brucella* within weeks to months after therapy has ended. Prolonged treatment is the key to preventing disease relapse, and steps should be taken to assure compliance with the long courses of therapy needed to achieve eradication.

PROGNOSIS

The primary indication of clinical response is resolution of symptoms, which may be slow; the average time to defervescence is 4-5 days. The prognosis after therapy is excellent if patients are compliant with the prolonged therapy. Patients should be followed clinically and serologically for 1-2 yr. Before the use of antimicrobial agents, the course of brucellosis was often prolonged and associated with death. Since the institution of specific therapy, most deaths are a result of specific organ system involvement (e.g., endocarditis) in complicated cases. Initiation of antimicrobial therapy may precipitate a Jarisch-Herxheimer–like reaction, presumably because of a large antigen load, but these reactions are rarely associated with serious complications.

PREVENTION

Prevention of brucellosis depends on effective eradication of the organism from livestock. **Pasteurization** of milk and dairy products for human consumption remains an important aspect of prevention. It should be noted that certification of raw milk does not eliminate the risk of brucellosis acquisition. No vaccine currently exists for use in children, and therefore education of the public continues to have a prominent role in prevention of brucellosis.

Bibliography is available at Expert Consult.

Table 234.1 | Recommended Therapy for Treatment of Brucellosis

AGE/CONDITIONS	ANTIMICROBIAL AGENT	DOSE	ROUTE*	DURATION†
≥8 yr	Doxycycline	4.4 mg/kg/day divided twice daily; max 200 mg/day	PO	≥6 wk
	plus			
	Rifampin	15-20 mg/kg/day in 1 or 2 divided doses; max 600-900 mg/day	PO	≥6 wk
	Alternative:			
	Doxycycline	4.4 mg/kg/day divided twice daily; max 200 mg/day	PO	≥6 wk
	plus			
	Streptomycin	20-40 mg/kg/day in 2-4 divided doses; max 1 g/day	IM	2-3 wk
	or			
	Gentamicin	6-7.5 mg/kg/day in 3 divided doses	IM/IV	1-2 wk
<8 yr	Trimethoprim-sulfamethoxazole (TMP-SMX)	TMP (10 mg/kg/day; max 480 mg/day) and SMX (50 mg/kg/day; max 2.4 g/day)	PO	≥6 wk
	plus			
	Rifampin	15-20 mg/kg/day in 1 or 2 divided doses; max 600-900 mg/day	PO	≥6 wk
Meningitis, osteomyelitis/ spondylitis endocarditis	Doxycycline	4.4 mg/kg/day divided twice daily; max 200 mg/day	PO	≥4-6 mo
	plus			
	Gentamicin	6-7.5 mg/kg/day in 3 divided doses	IV	1-2 wk
	plus			
	Rifampin	15-20 mg/kg/day in 1 or 2 divided doses; max 600-900 mg/day	PO	≥4-6 mo

*PO, Oral (by mouth): IM, intramuscular; IV, intravenous.
†Longer courses of therapy may be needed for more severe or complicated cases.

Chapter **235**
Legionella
Jeffrey S. Gerber

第二百三十五章
军团菌

中文导读

本章主要介绍了军团菌感染的病因、流行病学、发病机制、临床表现、诊断、鉴别诊断、治疗和预后等内容。在关于军团菌病的流行病学部分详细介绍了军团菌生存环境、传播方式、院内感染机制、发病率、流行季节等内容。在关于军团菌病的临床表现部分详细介绍了该病的症状、体征、影像学特点、患病的危险因素、庞蒂亚克热。在关于军团菌病的治疗部分详细介绍了该病推荐的治疗方案以及当前研究现状。

Legionellosis comprises **legionnaires disease** (*Legionella* pneumonia), other invasive extrapulmonary *Legionella* infections, and an acute flulike illness known as **Pontiac fever.** In contrast to the syndromes associated with invasive disease, Pontiac fever is a self-limited illness that develops after aerosol exposure and may represent a toxic or hypersensitivity response to *Legionella*.

ETIOLOGY

Legionellaceae are aerobic, non–spore-forming, nonencapsulated, gram-negative bacilli that stain poorly with Gram stain when performed on smears from clinical specimens. Stained smears of *Legionella pneumophila* taken from colonial growth resemble *Pseudomonas*. Unlike other *Legionella* species, *Legionella micdadei* stains acid fast. Although 58 species of the genus have now been identified, the majority (90%) of clinical infections are caused by *L. pneumophila*, and most of the remainder are caused by *L. micdadei, Legionella bozemanii, Legionella dumoffii,* and *Legionella longbeachae.*

The organisms are fastidious and require L-cysteine, ferric ion, and α-keto acids for growth. Colonies develop within 3-5 days on buffered charcoal yeast extract agar, which may contain selected antibiotics to inhibit overgrowth by other microorganisms; *Legionella* rarely grows on routine laboratory media.

EPIDEMIOLOGY

The environmental reservoir of *Legionella* in nature is fresh water (lakes, streams, thermally polluted waters, potable water), and invasive pneumonia (legionnaires disease) is related to exposure to potable water or to aerosols containing the bacteria. Growth of *Legionella* occurs more readily in warm water, and exposure to warm-water sources is an important risk factor for disease. *Legionella* organisms are facultative intracellular parasites that grow inside protozoa present in biofilms, consisting of organic and inorganic material found in plumbing and water storage tanks and various other bacterial species. Epidemic and sporadic cases of community-acquired legionnaires disease can be attributed to potable water in the local environment of the patient. Risk factors for acquisition of sporadic community-acquired pneumonia include exposure to cooling towers, nonmunicipal water supply, residential plumbing repairs, and lower water heater temperatures, which facilitate growth of bacteria or lead to release of a bolus of biofilm containing *Legionella* into potable water. The mode of transmission may be by inhalation of aerosols or by microaspiration. Outbreaks of legionnaires disease have been associated with protozoa in the implicated water source; replication within these eukaryotic cells presumably amplifies and maintains *Legionella* within the potable-water distribution system or in cooling towers. Outbreaks of community-acquired pneumonia and some nosocomial outbreaks have been linked to common sources, including potable hot-water heaters, evaporative condensers, cooling towers, whirlpool baths, water births, humidifiers, and nebulizers. Travel-associated legionnaires disease and Pontiac fever are increasingly recognized in major outbreaks. Although person-to-person transmission has been reported, if it does occur, it is extremely rare.

Hospital-acquired infections are most often linked to potable water. Exposure may occur through 3 general mechanisms: (1) inhalation of contaminated water vapor through artificial ventilation; (2) aspiration of ingested microorganisms, including those in gastric feedings that are mixed with contaminated tap water; and (3) inhalation of aerosols from showers, sinks, and fountains. Extrapulmonary legionellosis may occur through topical application of contaminated tap water into surgical or traumatic wounds. In contrast to legionnaires disease, Pontiac fever outbreaks have occurred through exposure to aerosols from whirlpool baths and ventilation systems.

The incidence of legionellosis in the United States increased from 1,100 cases in 2000 to >6000 cases in 2015, for a national incidence rate of 1.9 per 100,000 population based on reporting to the Centers for Disease Control and Prevention (CDC) through the National Notifiable Disease Surveillance System. Because this is a passive reporting system, these are likely underestimates of the incidence of disease. An active laboratory-based and population-based surveillance system for tracking *Legionella* infections was recently launched by CDC, which will help to better assess its true incidence and epidemiology. (For up-to-date information, see https://www.cdc.gov/legionella/.)

Legionellosis demonstrates geographic differences, and the vast majority of cases are classified as legionnaires disease (99.5%), with a small fraction as Pontiac fever (0.5%). *Legionella* infections are reported most frequently in fall and summer, and recent studies show an association with total monthly rainfall and humidity. Approximately 0.5–5.0% of those exposed to a common source develop pneumonia, whereas the attack rate in Pontiac fever outbreaks is very high (85–100%). Although *Legionella* is associated with 0.5–10% of pneumonia cases in adults, it is a rare cause of pneumonia in children, accounting for <1% of cases; however, infrequent testing for *Legionella* might underestimate its prevalence. Acquisition of antibodies to *L. pneumophila* in healthy children occurs progressively over time, although these antibodies presumably reflect subclinical infection or mild respiratory disease or antibodies that cross-react with other bacterial species. Community-acquired legionnaires disease in children is increasingly reported (1.7% of reported cases), and most cases occur in children 15-19 yr old, followed by infants. The incidence in infants is reported to be 0.11 per 100,000. Legionnaires disease is particularly severe in neonates. The epidemiology of hospital-acquired legionnaires disease in children is derived almost exclusively from case reports, so the true incidence of this entity is unknown.

PATHOGENESIS

Although *Legionella* can be grown on artificial media, the intracellular environment of eukaryotic cells provides the definitive site of growth. *Legionella* organisms are facultative intracellular parasites of eukaryotic cells. In nature, *Legionella* replicate within protozoa found in fresh water. In humans the main target cell for *Legionella* is the alveolar macrophage, although other cell types may also be invaded. After entry, virulent strains of *L. pneumophila* stimulate the formation of a special phagosome that permits bacterial replication to proceed. The phagosome consists of components of the endoplasmic reticulum and escapes the degradative lysosomal pathway. Growth in macrophages occurs to the point of cell death, followed by reinfection of new cells, until these cells are activated and can subsequently kill intracellular microorganisms. Acute, severe infection of the lung provokes an acute inflammatory response and necrosis. Early on, more bacteria are found in extracellular spaces as a result of intracellular replication, lysis, and release of bacteria. Subsequently, macrophage activation and other immune responses produce intense infiltration of tissue by macrophages that contain intracellular bacteria, ultimately leading to control of bacterial replication and killing.

Corticosteroid therapy poses a high risk for infection by interfering with T-cell and macrophage function. Although community-acquired legionnaires disease may occur in healthy, immunocompetent patients without other comorbid conditions, those who have defects in cellular-mediated immunity are at higher risk for infection. As in other diseases caused by facultative intracellular microorganisms, the outcome is critically dependent on the specific and nonspecific immune responses of the host, particularly macrophage and T-cell responses.

CLINICAL MANIFESTATIONS

Legionnaires disease was originally believed to cause atypical pneumonia associated with extrapulmonary signs and symptoms, including diarrhea, confusion, hyponatremia, hypophosphatemia, abnormal liver function test results, and renal dysfunction. Although a subset of patients may exhibit these classic manifestations, *Legionella* infection typically causes pneumonia that is indistinguishable from pneumonia produced by other infectious agents. Fever, cough, and chest pain are common presenting symptoms; the cough may be productive of purulent sputum or may be nonproductive. Although the classic chest radiographic appearance demonstrates rapidly progressive alveolar filling infiltrates, the chest radiographic appearance is widely variable, with tumor-like shadows, evidence of nodular infiltrates, unilateral or bilateral infiltrates, or cavitation, although cavitation is rarely seen in immunocompetent patients. This picture overlaps substantially with disease caused by *Streptococcus pneumoniae*. Although pleural effusion is less often associated with

legionnaires disease, its frequency varies so widely that neither the presence nor absence of effusion is helpful in the differential diagnosis.

Most reports of nosocomial *Legionella* pneumonia in children demonstrate the following clinical features: rapid onset, temperature >38.5°C (101.3°F), cough, pleuritic chest pain, tachypnea, and dyspnea. Abdominal pain, headache, and diarrhea are also common. Chest radiographs reveal lobar consolidations or diffuse bilateral infiltrates, and pleural effusions may be noted. Usually there is no clinical response to broad-spectrum β-lactam (penicillins and cephalosporins) or aminoglycoside antibiotics. Concomitant infection with other pathogens, including *M. pneumoniae* and *C. pneumoniae*, occurs in 5–10% of cases of legionnaires disease; therefore detection of another potential pulmonary pathogen does not preclude the diagnosis of legionellosis.

Risk factors for legionnaires disease in adults include chronic diseases of the lung (smoking, bronchitis), older age, diabetes and renal failure, immunosuppression associated with organ transplantation, corticosteroid therapy, and episodes of aspiration. In surveys of community-acquired infection, a significant number of adults have no identified risk factors. The number of reported cases of community-acquired legionnaires disease in children is small. Among these, immunocompromised status, especially corticosteroid treatment, coupled with exposure to contaminated potable water, is the major risk factor. Infection in a few children with chronic pulmonary disease without immune deficiency has also been reported, but infection in children lacking any risk factors is uncommon. The modes of transmission of community-acquired disease in children include exposure to mists, fresh water, water coolers, and other aerosol-generating apparatuses. Nosocomial *Legionella* infection has been reported more frequently than community-acquired disease in children and usually occurs in those who are immunocompromised (e.g., stem cell transplants, solid organ transplants), those with structural lung disease, or neonates receiving mechanical ventilation. The modes of acquisition include **microaspiration**, frequently associated with nasogastric tubes, and **aerosol inhalation**. Bronchopulmonary *Legionella* infections are reported in patients with cystic fibrosis and have been associated with aerosol therapy or mist tents. Legionnaires disease is also reported in children with asthma and tracheal stenosis. Chronic corticosteroid therapy for asthma is a reported risk factor for *Legionella* infections in children. Molecular fingerprinting of strains has demonstrated that potable water serves as the major reservoir and source of nosocomial infection.

Pontiac Fever

Pontiac fever in adults and children is characterized by high fever, myalgia, headache, and extreme debilitation, lasting for 3-5 days. Cough, breathlessness, diarrhea, confusion, and chest pain may occur, but there is no evidence for invasive infection. The disease is self-limited without sequelae. Virtually all exposed individuals seroconvert to *Legionella* antigens. A very large outbreak in Scotland that affected 35 children was attributed to *L. micdadei*, which was isolated from a whirlpool spa. The onset of illness was 1-7 days (median: 3 days), and all exposed children developed significant titers of specific antibodies to *L. micdadei*. The pathogenesis of Pontiac fever is not known. In the absence of evidence of true infection, the most likely hypothesis is that this syndrome is caused by a toxic or hypersensitivity reaction to microbial, or protozoan, antigens.

DIAGNOSIS

Culture of *Legionella* from sputum, other respiratory tract specimens, blood, or tissue is the gold standard against which indirect methods of detection should be compared. If present, pleural fluid should be obtained for culture. Specimens obtained from the respiratory tract that are contaminated with oral flora must be treated and processed to reduce contaminants and plated onto selective media. Because these are costly and time-consuming methods, many laboratories do not process specimens for culture.

The urinary antigen assay that detects *L. pneumophila* serogroup I has revolutionized the diagnosis of *Legionella* infection and has 80% sensitivity and 99% specificity. The assay is a useful method in the prompt diagnosis of legionnaires disease caused by this serogroup, which accounts for the majority of symptomatic infections. In the United States, this test is frequently used because it is widely available in reference laboratories. Where available, polymerase chain reaction is used to identify *L. pneumophila* from bronchoscopic lavage and other clinical specimens to the exclusion of other respiratory pathogens. Other methods, including direct immunofluorescence, have low sensitivity and are generally not employed. Retrospective diagnosis can be made serologically using an enzyme immunoassay to detect specific antibody production. Seroconversion may not occur for several weeks after onset of infection, and the available serologic assays do not detect all strains of *L. pneumophila* or all species.

In view of the low sensitivity of direct detection and the slow growth of the microorganism in culture, the diagnosis of legionellosis should be pursued actively when there is suggestive clinical evidence, including the lack of response to usual antibiotics, even when results of other laboratory studies are negative.

TREATMENT

In community-acquired pneumonia in adults who are hospitalized, guidelines recommend empirical treatment with a broad-spectrum cephalosporin plus a macrolide or quinolone for treatment of atypical microorganisms *(Legionella, Chlamydophila pneumoniae, Mycoplasma pneumoniae)*. Evidence-based guidelines for management of community-acquired pneumonia in children do not yet include *Legionella* in the differential diagnosis or empirical treatment recommendations. Effective treatment of legionnaires disease is based in part on the intracellular concentration of antibiotics. **Azithromycin**, **clarithromycin**, or the **quinolones** (ciprofloxacin and levofloxacin) have generally replaced erythromycin as therapy for patients with diagnosed *Legionella* infection. **Doxycycline** is an acceptable alternative. In serious infections or in high-risk patients, parenteral therapy is recommended initially, although

oral conversion if favored when tolerated, particularly due to the generally high bioavailability of oral macrolides, quinolones, and tetracyclines. The duration of antibiotic therapy for legionnaires disease in adults is typically for a minimum of 5 days, although therapy may be continued for 10-14 days in more seriously ill or immunocompromised patients. Treatment of extrapulmonary infections, including prosthetic valve endocarditis and sternal wound infections, may require prolonged therapy. In vitro data and case reports suggest that trimethoprim-sulfamethoxazole (15 mg TMP/kg/day and 75 mg SMX/kg/day) may also be effective. A large, retrospective study of hospitalized adults with *Legionella* pneumonia found no difference in mortality between those treated with azithromycin and with quinolones. The role of combination therapy is unknown.

PROGNOSIS

The mortality rate for community-acquired legionnaires disease in adults who are hospitalized is approximately 15% but may exceed 50% in immunocompromised patients, although reporting bias might inflate these estimates. The prognosis depends on underlying host factors and possibly on the duration of illness before initiation of appropriate therapy. Despite appropriate antibiotic therapy, patients may succumb to respiratory complications, such as acute respiratory distress syndrome. A high mortality rate is noted in case reports of premature infants and children, virtually all of whom have been immunocompromised. Delay in diagnosis is also associated with increased mortality. Consequently, *Legionella* should be considered in the differential diagnosis of both community-acquired and nosocomial pneumonia in children, especially in those refractory to empirical therapy or with epidemiologic risk factors for legionellosis.

Bibliography is available at Expert Consult.

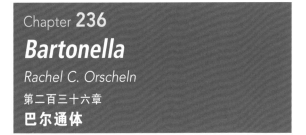

Chapter **236**

Bartonella

Rachel C. Orscheln

第二百三十六章
巴尔通体

中文导读

　　本章主要介绍了汉塞巴尔通体（猫抓病）、杆菌状巴尔通体（巴尔通体病）、五日热巴尔通体（战壕热）及杆菌性血管瘤病和杆菌性肝紫癜(汉塞巴尔通体和五日热巴尔通体)。关于猫抓病详细介绍了其病因、流行病学、发病机制、临床表现、诊断、鉴别诊断、治疗、并发症、预后和预防。关于巴尔通体病详细介绍了其病因、流行病学、发病机制、临床表现、诊断、治疗和预防。关于战壕热详细介绍了其病因、流行病学、临床表现、诊断和治疗。关于杆菌性血管瘤病和杆菌性肝紫癜详细介绍了杆菌性血管瘤病、杆菌性紫癜、菌血症和心内膜炎、诊断、治疗和预防。

The spectrum of disease resulting from human infection with *Bartonella* species includes the association of **bacillary angiomatosis** and **cat-scratch disease** with *Bartonella henselae*. There are more than 30 validated species of *Bartonella*, but 6 major species are responsible for most human disease: *B. henselae, B.quintana, B. bacilliformis, B. elizabethae, B. vinsonii,* and *B. clarridgeiae* (Table 236.1). The remaining *Bartonella* spp. have been found primarily in animals, particularly rodents and moles. However, zoonotic infections from animal-associated strains of *Bartonella* spp. have been reported. In 2013 a novel *Bartonella* agent with the proposed name *Candidatus* Bartonella ancashi *(Bartonella ancashensis)* was described as a cause of **verruga peruana**.

Members of the genus *Bartonella* are gram-negative, oxidase-negative, fastidious aerobic rods that ferment no carbohydrates. *B. bacilliformis* is the only species that is motile, achieving motility by means of polar flagella. Optimal growth is obtained on fresh media containing ≥5% sheep or horse blood in the presence of 5% carbon dioxide. The use of lysis centrifugation for specimens from blood on chocolate agar for extended periods (2-6 wk) enhances recovery.

Bibliography is available at Expert Consult.

236.1 Cat-Scratch Disease (*Bartonella henselae*)

Rachel C. Orscheln

The most common presentation of *Bartonella* infection is cat-scratch disease **(CSD)**, which is a subacute, regional lymphadenitis caused most frequently by *B. henselae*. It is the most common cause of chronic lymphadenitis that persists for >3 wk.

ETIOLOGY

Bartonella henselae can be cultured from the blood of healthy cats. *B. henselae* organisms are the small pleomorphic gram-negative bacilli visualized with Warthin-Starry stain in affected lymph nodes from patients with CSD. Development of serologic tests that showed prevalence of antibodies in 84–100% of cases of CSD, culturing of *B. henselae* from CSD nodes, and detection of *B. henselae* by polymerase chain reaction (PCR) in the majority of lymph node samples and pus from patients with CSD, confirmed the organism as the cause of CSD. Occasional cases of CSD may be caused by other organisms, including *Bartonella clarridgeiae, B. grahamii, B. alsatica,* and *B. quintana*.

EPIDEMIOLOGY

CSD is common, with >24,000 estimated cases per year in the United States. It is transmitted most frequently by cutaneous inoculation through the bite or scratch of a cat. However, transmission may occur through other routes, such as flea bites. Most patients (87–99%) have had contact with cats, many of which are kittens <6 mo old, and >50% of patients have a definite history of a cat scratch or bite. Cats have high-level *Bartonella* bacteremia for months without any clinical symptoms; kittens are more frequently bacteremic than adult cats. Transmission between cats occurs through the cat flea, *Ctenocephalides felis*. In temperate zones, most cases occur between September and March, perhaps in relation to the seasonal breeding of domestic cats or to the close proximity of family pets in the fall and winter. In tropical zones, there is no seasonal prevalence. Distribution is worldwide, and infection occurs in all races.

Cat scratches appear to be more common among children, and males are affected more often than females. CSD is a sporadic illness; usually only 1 family member is affected, even though many siblings play with the same kitten. However, clusters do occur, with family cases within weeks of one another. Anecdotal reports have implicated other sources, such as dog scratches, wood splinters, fishhooks, cactus spines, and porcupine quills.

PATHOGENESIS

The pathologic findings in the primary inoculation **papule** and affected lymph nodes are similar. Both show a central avascular necrotic area with surrounding lymphocytes, giant cells, and histiocytes. Three stages of involvement occur in affected nodes, sometimes simultaneously in the same node. The 1st stage consists of generalized enlargement with thickening of the cortex and hypertrophy of the germinal center and with a predominance of lymphocytes. Epithelioid granulomas with Langerhans giant cells are scattered throughout the node. The 2nd stage is characterized by granulomas that increase in density, fuse, and become infiltrated with polymorphonuclear leukocytes, with beginning central necrosis. In the 3rd stage, necrosis progresses with formation of large, pus-filled sinuses. This purulent material may rupture into surrounding tissue. Similar granulomas have been found in the liver, spleen, and osteolytic lesions of bone when those organs are involved.

CLINICAL MANIFESTATIONS

After an incubation period of 7-12 days (range: 3-30 days), 1 or more 3-5 mm red papules develop at the site of cutaneous inoculation, often reflecting a linear cat scratch. These lesions are often overlooked because of their small size but are found in at least 65% of patients when careful examination is performed (Fig. 236.1). Lymphadenopathy is generally evident within 1-4 wk (Fig. 236.2). **Chronic regional lymphadenitis** is the hallmark, affecting the1st or 2nd set of nodes draining the entry site. Affected lymph nodes in order of frequency include the axillary, cervical, submandibular, preauricular, epitrochlear, femoral, and inguinal nodes. Involvement of >1 group of nodes occurs in 10–20% of patients, although at a given site, half the cases involve several nodes.

Nodes involved are usually tender and have overlying erythema but without cellulitis. They usually range between 1 and 5 cm in size, although they can become much larger. From 10–40% eventually suppurate. The

Table 236.1	*Bartonella* Species Causing Majority of Human Disease		
DISEASE	**ORGANISM**	**VECTOR**	**PRIMARY RISK FACTOR**
Bartonellosis (Carrión disease)	*B. bacilliformis*	Sandfly (*Lutzomyia verrucarum*)	Living in endemic areas (Andes Mountains)
Cat-scratch disease	*B. henselae* *B. clarridgeiae*	Cat	Cat scratch or bite
Trench fever	*B. quintana*	Human body louse	Body louse infestation during outbreak
Bacteremia, endocarditis	*B. henselae* *B. elizabethae* *B. vinsonii* *B. quintana*	Cat for *B. henselae* Rat for *B. elizabethae* Vole for *B. vinsonii* Human body louse for *B. quintana*	Severe immunosuppression
Bacillary angiomatosis	*B. henselae* *B. quintana*	Cat for *B. henselae* Human body louse for *B. quintana*	Severe immunosuppression
Peliosis hepatis	*B. henselae* *B. quintana*	Cat for *B. henselae* Human body louse for *B. quintana*	Severe immunosuppression

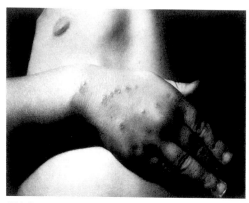

Fig. 236.1 A child with typical cat-scratch disease demonstrating the original scratch injuries and the primary papule that soon thereafter developed proximal to the middle finger. *(Courtesy of Dr. V.H. San Joaquin, University of Oklahoma Health Sciences Center, Oklahoma City.)*

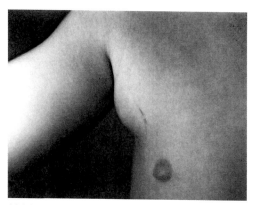

Fig. 236.2 Right axillary lymphadenopathy followed the scratches and development of a primary papule in this child with typical cat-scratch disease. *(From Mandell GL, Bennett JE, Dolin R, editors: Principles and practice of infectious diseases, ed 6, Philadelphia, 2006, Elsevier, p 2737.)*

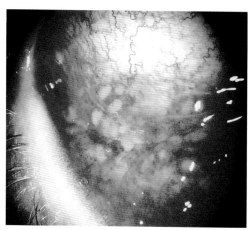

Fig. 236.3 The granulomatous conjunctivitis of Parinaud oculoglandular syndrome is associated with ipsilateral local lymphadenopathy, usually preauricular and less often submandibular. *(From Mandell GL, Bennett JE, Dolin R, editors: Principles and practice of infectious diseases, ed 6, Philadelphia, 2006, Elsevier, p 2739.)*

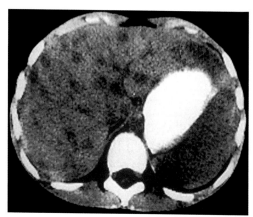

Fig. 236.4 In this CT scan of a patient with hepatic involvement of cat-scratch disease, the absence of enhancement of the multiple lesions after contrast infusion is consistent with the granulomatous inflammation of this entity. Treated empirically with various antibiotics without improvement before establishment of this diagnosis, the patient subsequently recovered fully with no further antimicrobial therapy. *(Courtesy of Dr. V.H. San Joaquin, University of Oklahoma Health Sciences Center, Oklahoma City.)*

duration of enlargement is usually 1-2 mo, with persistence up to 1 yr in rare cases. Fever occurs in approximately 30% of patients, usually 38-39°C (100.4-102.2°F). Other nonspecific symptoms, including malaise, anorexia, fatigue, and headache, affect less than one third of patients. Transient rashes, which may occur in approximately 5% of patients, are mainly truncal maculopapular rashes. Erythema nodosum, erythema multiforme, and erythema annulare are also reported.

CSD is usually a self-limited infection that spontaneous resolves within a few weeks to months. The most common ocular presentation of CSD is **Parinaud oculoglandular syndrome,** which is unilateral conjunctivitis followed by preauricular lymphadenopathy and occurs in 5% of patients with CSD (Fig. 236.3). Direct eye inoculation as a result of rubbing with the hands after cat contact is the presumed mode of spread. A conjunctival granuloma may be found at the inoculation site. The involved eye is usually not painful and has little or no discharge but may be quite red and swollen. Submandibular or cervical lymphadenopathy may also occur.

More severe, disseminated illness occurs up to 14% of patients and is characterized by presentation with high fever, often persisting for several weeks. Other prominent symptoms include significant abdominal pain and weight loss. **Hepatosplenomegaly** may occur, although hepatic dysfunction is rare (Fig. 236.4). Granulomatous changes may be seen in the liver and spleen. Another common site of dissemination is bone, with the development of multifocal **granulomatous osteolytic lesions,** associated with localized pain but without erythema, tenderness, or swelling. Other, uncommon manifestations are neuroretinitis with papilledema and stellate macular exudates, encephalitis, endocarditis, and atypical pneumonia.

DIAGNOSIS

In most cases the diagnosis can be strongly suspected on clinical grounds in a patient with history of exposure to a cat. Serologic testing can be used to confirm the diagnosis. Most patients have elevated IgG antibody titers at presentation. However, the IgM response to *B. henselae* has frequently resolved by the time testing is considered. There is cross-reactivity among *Bartonella* spp., particularly *B. henselae* and *B. quintana.*

If tissue specimens are obtained, bacilli may be visualized with Warthin-Starry and Brown-Hopps tissue stains. *Bartonella* DNA can be identified through PCR analysis of tissue specimens. Culturing of the organism is not generally practical for clinical diagnosis.

Differential Diagnosis

The differential diagnosis of CSD includes virtually all causes of lymphadenopathy (see Chapter 517). The more common entities include pyogenic (suppurative) lymphadenitis, primarily from staphylococcal or streptococcal infections, atypical mycobacterial infections, and malignancy. Less common entities are tularemia, brucellosis, and sporotrichosis. Epstein-Barr virus, cytomegalovirus, and *Toxoplasma gondii* infections usually cause more generalized lymphadenopathy.

LABORATORY FINDINGS

Routine laboratory tests are not helpful. The erythrocyte sedimentation rate is often elevated. The white blood cell count may be normal or mildly elevated. Hepatic transaminases are often normal but may be elevated in systemic disease. Ultrasonography or CT may reveal many granulomatous nodules in the liver and spleen; the nodules appear as hypodense, round, irregular lesions and are usually multiple. However, CSD presenting as a solitary splenic lesion has been reported.

TREATMENT

Antibiotic treatment of CSD is not always needed and is not clearly beneficial. For most patients, treatment consists of conservative symptomatic care and observation. Studies show a significant discordance between in vitro activity of antibiotics and clinical effectiveness. For many patients, diagnosis is considered in the context of failure to respond to β-lactam antibiotic treatment of presumed staphylococcal lymphadenitis.

A small prospective study of oral azithromycin (500 mg on day 1, then 250 mg on days 2-5; for smaller children, 10 mg/kg/24 hr on day 1 and 5 mg/kg/24 hr on days 2-5) showed a decrease in initial lymph node volume in 50% of patients during the 1st 30 days, but after 30 days there was no difference in lymph node volume. No other clinical benefit was found. For the majority of patients, CSD is self-limited, and resolution occurs over weeks to months without antibiotic treatment. Azithromycin, clarithromycin, trimethoprim-sulfamethoxazole (TMP-SMX), rifampin, ciprofloxacin, and gentamicin appear to be the best agents if treatment is considered.

Suppurative lymph nodes that become tense and extremely painful should be drained by **needle aspiration**, which may need to be repeated. Incision and drainage of nonsuppurative nodes should be avoided because chronic draining sinuses may result. Surgical excision of the node is rarely necessary.

Children with hepatosplenic CSD appear to respond well to rifampin at a dose of 20 mg/kg for 14 days, either alone or in combination with a 2nd agent such as azithromycin, gentamicin, or TMP-SMX.

COMPLICATIONS

Encephalopathy can occur in as many as 5% of patients with CSD and typically manifests 1-3 wk after the onset of lymphadenitis as the sudden onset of neurologic symptoms, which often include seizures, combative or bizarre behavior, and altered level of consciousness. Imaging studies are generally normal. The cerebrospinal fluid is normal or shows minimal pleocytosis and protein elevation. Recovery occurs without sequelae in almost all patients but may take place slowly over many months.

Other neurologic manifestations include peripheral facial nerve paralysis, myelitis, radiculitis, compression neuropathy, and cerebellar ataxia. One patient has been reported to have encephalopathy with persistent cognitive impairment and memory loss.

Stellate macular retinopathy is associated with several infections, including CSD. Children and young adults present with unilateral or rarely bilateral loss of vision with central scotoma, optic disc swelling, and macular star formation from exudates radiating out from the macula. The findings usually resolve completely, with recovery of vision, generally within 2-3 mo. The optimal treatment for the neuroretinitis is unknown, although treatment of adults with doxycycline and rifampin for 4-6 wk has had good results.

Hematologic manifestations include hemolytic anemia, thrombocytopenic purpura, nonthrombocytopenic purpura, and eosinophilia. **Leukocytoclastic vasculitis,** similar to Henoch-Schönlein purpura, has been reported in association with CSD in one child. A systemic presentation of CSD with pleurisy, arthralgia or arthritis, mediastinal masses,

enlarged nodes at the head of the pancreas, and atypical pneumonia also has been reported.

PROGNOSIS

The prognosis for CSD in a normal host is generally excellent, with resolution of clinical findings over weeks to months. Recovery is occasionally slower and may take as long as 1 yr.

PREVENTION

Person-to-person spread of *Bartonella* infections is not known. Isolation of the affected patient is not necessary. Prevention would require elimination of cats from households, which is not practical or necessarily desirable. Awareness of the risk of cat (and particularly kitten) scratches should be emphasized to parents. Cat scratches or bites should be washed immediately. Cat flea control is helpful.

Bibliography is available at Expert Consult.

236.2 Bartonellosis *(Bartonella bacilliformis)*

Rachel C. Orscheln

The first human *Bartonella* infection described was **bartonellosis**, a geographically distinct disease caused by *B. bacilliformis*. There are 2 predominant forms of illness caused by *B. bacilliformis*: **Oroya fever**, a severe, febrile hemolytic anemia, and **verruca peruana** (verruga peruana), an eruption of hemangioma-like lesions. *B. bacilliformis* also causes asymptomatic infection. Bartonellosis is also called **Carrión disease**.

ETIOLOGY

Bartonella bacilliformis is a small, motile, gram-negative organism with a brush of ≥10 unipolar flagella, which appear to be important components for invasiveness. An obligate aerobe, it grows best at 28°C (82.4°F) in semisolid nutrient agar containing rabbit serum and hemoglobin.

EPIDEMIOLOGY

Bartonellosis is a zoonosis found only in mountain valleys of the Andes Mountains in Peru, Ecuador, Colombia, Chile, and Bolivia at altitudes and environmental conditions favorable for the vector, which is the **sandfly,** *Lutzomyia verrucarum*.

PATHOGENESIS

After the sandfly bite, *Bartonella* organisms enter the endothelial cells of blood vessels, where they proliferate. Found throughout the reticuloendothelial system, they then reenter the bloodstream and parasitize erythrocytes. They bind on the cells, deform the membranes, and then enter intracellular vacuoles. The resultant hemolytic anemia may involve as many as 90% of circulating erythrocytes. Patients who survive this acute phase may or may not experience the cutaneous manifestations, which are nodular hemangiomatous lesions or verrucae ranging in size from a few millimeters to several centimeters.

CLINICAL MANIFESTATIONS

The incubation period is 2-14 wk. Patients may be totally asymptomatic or may have nonspecific symptoms such as headache and malaise without anemia.

Oroya fever is characterized by fever with rapid development of anemia. Clouding of the sensorium and delirium are common symptoms and may progress to overt psychosis. Physical examination demonstrates signs of severe hemolytic anemia, including icterus and pallor, sometimes in association with generalized lymphadenopathy.

In the preeruptive stage of **verruca peruana** (Fig. 236.5), patients may complain of arthralgias, myalgias, and paresthesias. Inflammatory reactions such as phlebitis, pleuritis, erythema nodosum, and encephalitis may develop. The appearance of verrucae is pathognomonic of the eruptive phase. Lesions vary greatly in size and number.

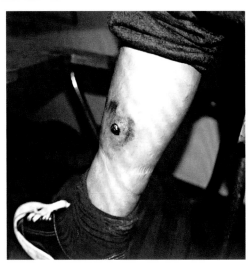

Fig. 236.5 A single, large lesion of verruca peruana on the leg of an inhabitant of the Peruvian Andes. Such lesions are prone to superficial ulceration, and their vascular nature may lead to copious bleeding. Ecchymosis of the skin surrounding the lesion is also evident. *(Courtesy of Dr. J.M. Crutcher, Oklahoma State Department of Health, Oklahoma City.)*

DIAGNOSIS

The diagnosis of bartonellosis is established on clinical grounds in conjunction with a blood smear demonstrating organisms or with blood culture. The anemia is macrocytic and hypochromic, with reticulocyte counts as high as 50%. *B. bacilliformis* may be seen on Giemsa stain preparation as red-violet rods in the erythrocytes. In the recovery phase, organisms change to a more coccoid form and disappear from the blood. In the absence of anemia, the diagnosis depends on blood cultures. In the eruptive phase, the typical verruca confirms the diagnosis. Antibody testing has been used to document infection.

TREATMENT

B. bacilliformis is sensitive to many antibiotics, including rifampin, tetracycline, and chloramphenicol. Treatment is very effective in rapidly diminishing fever and eradicating the organism from the blood. **Chloramphenicol** (50-75 mg/kg/day) is considered the drug of choice, because it is also useful in the treatment of concomitant infections such as *Salmonella*. Fluoroquinolones are used successfully as well. Blood transfusions and supportive care are critical in patients with severe anemia. Antimicrobial treatment for verruca peruana is considered when there are >10 cutaneous lesions, if the lesions are erythematous or violaceous, or if the onset of the lesions was <1 mo before presentation. Oral rifampin is effective in the healing of lesions. Surgical excision may be needed for lesions that are large and disfiguring or that interfere with function.

PREVENTION

Prevention depends on avoidance of the vector, particularly at night, by the use of protective clothing and insect repellents (see Chapter 200)

Bibliography is available at Expert Consult.

236.3 Trench Fever (*Bartonella quintana*)
Rachel C. Orscheln

ETIOLOGY

The causative agent of trench fever was first designated *Rickettsia quintana,* was then assigned to the genus *Rochalimaea,* and now has been reassigned as *Bartonella quintana.*

EPIDEMIOLOGY

Trench fever was first recognized as a distinct clinical entity during World War I, when more than a million troops in the trenches were infected. Infection with *B. quintana* is currently rare in the United states and primarily occurs in the setting of conditions favorable to body lice infestations, such as homelessness, crowding, and poor sanitation. When pooled samples of head and body lice have been collected from homeless populations, up to 33% of individuals have lice pools that test positive for *B. quintana.*

Humans are the only known reservoir. No other animal is naturally infected, and usual laboratory animals are not susceptible. The **human body louse**, *Pediculus humanus* var. *corporis,* is the vector and is capable of transmission to a new host 5-6 days after feeding on an infected person. Lice excrete the organism for life; transovarian passage does not occur. Humans may have prolonged asymptomatic bacteremia for years.

CLINICAL MANIFESTATIONS

The incubation period for trench fever averages about 22 days (range: 4-35 days). The clinical presentation is highly variable. Symptoms can be very mild and brief. About half of infected persons have a single febrile illness with abrupt onset lasting 3-6 days. In other patients, prolonged, sustained fever may occur. More commonly, patients have periodic febrile illness with 3-8 episodes lasting 4-5 days each, sometimes occurring over 1 yr or more. This form is reminiscent of malaria or **relapsing fever** *(Borrelia recurrentis).* Afebrile bacteremia can occur.

Clinical findings usually consist of fever (typically with a temperature of 38.5-40°C [101.3-104°F]), malaise, chills, sweats, anorexia, and severe headache. Common findings include marked conjunctival injection, tachycardia, myalgias, arthralgias, and severe pain in the neck, back, and legs. Crops of erythematous macules or papules may occur on the trunk on as many as 80% of patients. Splenomegaly and mild liver enlargement may be noted.

DIAGNOSIS

In nonepidemic situations, it is impossible to establish a diagnosis of trench fever on clinical grounds, because the findings are not distinctive. A history of body louse infection or having been in an area of epidemic disease should heighten suspicions. *B. quintana* can be cultured from the blood with modification to include culture on epithelial cells. Serologic tests for *B. quintana* are available, but there is cross-reaction with *B. henselae.*

TREATMENT

There are no controlled trials of treatment, but bacteremia with *Bartonella* treated with a combination of gentamicin and doxycycline increases the rate of cure compared to other regimens, such as doxycycline or β-lactam antibiotics alone.

Bibliography is available at Expert Consult.

236.4 Bacillary Angiomatosis and Bacillary Peliosis Hepatis (*Bartonella henselae* and *Bartonella quintana*)
Rachel C. Orscheln

Both *B. henselae* and *B. quintana* cause vascular proliferative disease called bacillary angiomatosis and bacillary peliosis in severely immunocompromised persons, primarily adult patients with acquired immunodeficiency syndrome (AIDS) or cancer and organ transplant recipients. Subcutaneous and lytic bone lesions are strongly associated with *B. quintana,* whereas peliosis hepatis is associated exclusively with *B. henselae.*

BACILLARY ANGIOMATOSIS

Lesions of cutaneous bacillary angiomatosis, also known as **epithelioid**

angiomatosis, are the most easily identified and recognized form of *Bartonella* infection in immunocompromised hosts. They are found primarily in patients with AIDS who have very low CD4 counts. The clinical appearance can be quite diverse. The vasoproliferative lesions of bacillary angiomatosis may be cutaneous or subcutaneous and may resemble the vascular lesions (verruca peruana) of *B. bacilliformis* in immunocompetent persons, characterized by erythematous papules on an erythematous base with a collarette of scale. They may enlarge to form large, pedunculated lesions and may ulcerate. Trauma may result in profuse bleeding.

Bacillary angiomatosis may be clinically indistinguishable from Kaposi sarcoma. Other considerations in the differential diagnosis are pyogenic granuloma and verruca peruana *(B. bacilliformis)*. Deep, soft tissue masses caused by bacillary angiomatosis may mimic a malignancy.

Osseous bacillary angiomatosis lesions typically involve the long bones. These lytic lesions are very painful and highly vascular and are occasionally associated with an overlying erythematous plaque. The high degree of vascularity produces a very positive result on a technetium-99m methylene diphosphonate bone scan, resembling that of a malignant lesion.

Lesions can be found in virtually any organ, producing similar vascular proliferative lesions. They may appear raised, nodular, or ulcerative when seen on endoscopy or bronchoscopy. They may be associated with enlarged lymph nodes with or without an obvious local cutaneous lesion. Brain parenchymal lesions have been described.

BACILLARY PELIOSIS

Bacillary peliosis affects the reticuloendothelial system, primarily the liver (**peliosis hepatis**) and less frequently the spleen and lymph nodes. It is a vasoproliferative disorder characterized by random proliferation of venous lakes surrounded by fibromyxoid stroma harboring numerous bacillary organisms. Clinical findings include fever and abdominal pain in association with abnormal liver function test results, particularly a greatly increased alkaline phosphatase level. Cutaneous bacillary angiomatosis with splenomegaly may be associated with thrombocytopenia or pancytopenia. The vascular proliferative lesions in the liver and spleen appear on CT scan as hypodense lesions scattered throughout the parenchyma. The differential diagnosis includes hepatic Kaposi sarcoma, lymphoma, and disseminated infection with *Pneumocystis jirovecii* or *Mycobacterium avium* complex.

BACTEREMIA AND ENDOCARDITIS

Bartonella henselae, B. quintana, B. vinsonii, and *B. elizabethae* all are reported to cause bacteremia or endocarditis. They are associated with symptoms such as prolonged fevers, night sweats, and profound weight loss. A cluster of cases in Seattle in 1993 occurred in a homeless population with chronic alcoholism. These patients with high fever or hypothermia were thought to represent *urban trench fever,* but no body louse infestation was associated. Some cases of culture-negative endocarditis may represent *Bartonella* endocarditis. One report described central nervous system involvement with *B. quintana* infection in 2 children.

DIAGNOSIS

Diagnosis of bacillary angiomatosis is made initially by biopsy. The characteristic small-vessel proliferation with mixed inflammatory response and the staining of bacilli by Warthin-Starry silver distinguish bacillary angiomatosis from pyogenic granuloma or Kaposi sarcoma (see Chapter 284). Travel history can usually preclude verruca peruana.

Culture is impractical for CSD but is the diagnostic procedure for suspected bacteremia or endocarditis. Lysis centrifugation technique or fresh chocolate or heart infusion agar with 5% rabbit blood and prolonged incubation may increase the yield of culture. PCR on tissue can also be a useful tool, and positive serologic testing can provide support for the diagnosis.

TREATMENT

Bartonella infections in immunocompromised hosts caused by both *B. henselae* and *B. quintana* have been treated successfully with antimicrobial agents. Bacillary angiomatosis responds rapidly to erythromycin, azithromycin, and clarithromycin, which are the drugs of choice. Alternative choices are doxycycline or tetracycline. Severely ill patients with peliosis hepatis or patients with osteomyelitis may be treated initially with a macrolide or doxycycline and the addition of rifampin or gentamicin. The use of doxycycline for 6 wk with the addition of an aminoglycoside for a minimum of 2 wk is associated with improved prognosis in endocarditis. A Jarisch-Herxheimer reaction may occur. Relapses may follow, and prolonged treatment for several months may be necessary.

PREVENTION

Immunocompromised persons should consider the potential risks of cat ownership because of the risks for *Bartonella* infections as well as toxoplasmosis and enteric infections. Those who elect to obtain a cat should adopt or purchase a cat >1 yr old and in good health. Prompt washing of any wounds from cat bites or scratches is essential.

Bibliography is available at Expert Consult.

Anaerobic Bacterial Infections

第六篇

厌氧菌感染

Chapter **237**

Botulism (Clostridium botulinum)

Laura E. Norton and Mark R. Schleiss

第二百三十七章

肉毒中毒（肉毒杆菌）

中文导读

　　本章主要介绍了肉毒中毒的病原学、流行病学、发病机制、临床表现、诊断及鉴别诊断、治疗、支持治疗、并发症、预后和防治。其中流行病学、发病机制、临床表现分别从婴儿肉毒中毒、食源性肉毒中毒和创伤性肉毒中毒三种疾病类别做了详细介绍。诊断部分包括特征性的临床表现和实验室诊断，其中实验室诊断方法主要有病原学、血清学检测、肌电图等。在鉴别诊断中主要描述了与多发性神经根神经病、重症肌无力以及中枢神经系统疾病的鉴别要点。治疗部分主要介绍了免疫球蛋白、肉毒素抗毒素以及抗生素在治疗中的作用。

There are 3 naturally occurring forms of human botulism, characterized by mode of acquisition: **infant botulism** (intestinal toxemia), **foodborne botulism**, and **wound botulism**. Infant botulism is the most common form in the United States. Under rare circumstances of altered intestinal anatomy, physiology, and microflora, older children and adults may contract infant-type botulism (**adult intestinal toxemia**). Two other forms, both human-made, also occur: **inhalational botulism**, from inhaling accidentally aerosolized toxin, and **iatrogenic botulism**, from overdosage of botulinum toxin used for therapeutic or cosmetic purposes.

ETIOLOGY

Botulism is the acute, flaccid paralysis caused by the neurotoxin produced by *Clostridium botulinum* or, infrequently, an equivalent neurotoxin produced by rare strains of *Clostridium butyricum* and *Clostridium baratii*. *C. botulinum* is a gram-positive, spore-forming, obligate anaerobe whose natural habitat worldwide is soil, dust, and marine sediments.

The organism is found in a wide variety of fresh and cooked agricultural products. Spores of some *C. botulinum* strains endure boiling for several hours, enabling the organism to survive efforts at food preservation. In contrast, botulinum toxin is heat labile and easily destroyed by heating at ≥85°C (185°F) for 5 min. **Neurotoxigenic *C. butyricum*** has been isolated from soils near Lake Weishan in China, the site of foodborne botulism outbreaks associated with this organism, as well as from vegetables, soured milk, and cheeses. Although first recognized in China, cases of infant botulism due to *C. butyricum* have now been identified in Japan, Europe, and the United States. Little is known about the ecology of neurotoxigenic *C. baratii*.

Botulinum toxin is synthesized as a 150-kDa precursor protein that enters the circulation and is transported to the neuromuscular junction. The toxin is only released by actively replicating (vegetative) bacteria and not the spore form. At the neuromuscular junction, toxin binds to the neuronal membrane on the presynaptic side of the neural synapse.

It undergoes autoproteolysis to a 100-kDa heavy chain and a 50-kDa light chain. These chains are joined via disulfide bond formation. The heavy chain contains the neuronal attachment sites that mediate binding to presynaptic nerve terminals. It also mediates translocation of the light chain into the cell cytoplasm after binding. The light chain, a key component of the toxin, is a member of the zinc metalloprotease family and mediates cleavage of the fusogenic SNARE protein family member, SNAP-25. Cleavage of this protein precludes release of acetylcholine from axon at the presynaptic terminal, abrogating nerve signaling and producing paralysis. Botulinum toxin is among the most potent poisons known to humankind; indeed, the parenteral human lethal dose is estimated to be on the order of 10^{-6} mg/kg. The toxin blocks neuromuscular transmission and causes death through airway and respiratory muscle paralysis. At least 7 antigenic toxin types, designated by letters A-G, are distinguished serologically, by demonstration of the inability of neutralizing antibody against one toxin type to protect against a different type. Toxin types are further differentiated into subtypes by differences in the nucleotide sequences of their toxin genes. As with the gene for tetanus toxin, the gene for botulinum toxin for some toxin types and subtypes resides on a plasmid.

The toxin types serve as convenient clinical and epidemiologic markers. Toxin types A, B, E, and F are well-established causes of human botulism, whereas types C and D cause illness in other animals. Toxin types A and B cause the majority of cases of infant botulism in the United States. Neurotoxigenic *C. butyricum* strains produce a type E toxin, whereas neurotoxigenic *C. baratii* strains produce a type F toxin. Type G toxin has not been established as a cause of either human or animal disease.

EPIDEMIOLOGY

Infant botulism has been reported from all inhabited continents except Africa. Notably, the infant is the only family member who is ill. The most striking epidemiologic feature of infant botulism is its age distribution, with 95% of cases involving infants 3 wk to 6 mo old, with a broad peak from 2-4 mo old. Cases have been recognized in infants as young as 1.5 days or as old as 382 days at onset. The male/female ratio of hospitalized cases is approximately 1:1, and cases occur in all racial and ethnic groups. Identified risk factors for the illness include breastfeeding, the ingestion of honey, a slow intestinal transit time (<1 stool/day), and ingestion of untreated well water. Although breastfeeding appears to provide protection against fulminant sudden death from infant botulism, cases can occur in breastfed infants at the time of introduction of nonhuman milk for feeding.

Although infant botulism is an uncommon and often unrecognized illness, it is the most common form of human botulism in the United States, with approximately 80-140 hospitalized cases diagnosed annually. The Council of State and Territorial Epidemiologists (CSTE) maintains a **National Botulism Surveillance System** for intensive surveillance for cases of botulism in the United States (https://www.cdc.gov/botulism/surveillance.html). In 2015, 141 confirmed cases of infant botulism were reported to the Centers for Disease Control and Prevention (CDC). There were no deaths. Approximately 56% of infant botulism cases were caused by type B, 43% by type A, and the remainder by other types. Cases were identified in 33 states and the District of Columbia, with California reporting the highest number of cases. Consistent with the known asymmetric soil distribution of *C. botulinum* toxin types, most cases west of the Mississippi River have been caused by type A strains, whereas most cases east of the Mississippi River have been caused by type B strains.

Foodborne botulism results from the ingestion of a food in which *C. botulinum* has multiplied and produced toxin. Although the traditional view of foodborne botulism has been thought of as resulting chiefly from ingestion of home-canned foods, in fact, outbreaks in North America have recently been more often associated with restaurant-prepared foods, including potatoes, sautéed onions, and chopped garlic. Other outbreaks in the United States have occurred from commercial foods sealed in plastic pouches that relied solely on refrigeration to prevent outgrowth of *C. botulinum* spores. Uncanned foods responsible for foodborne botulism cases include peyote tea, hazelnut flavoring added to yogurt, sweet cream cheese, sautéed onions in patty melt sandwiches, potato salad, and fresh and dried fish.

Many types of preserved foods have been implicated in foodborne botulism, but common foods implicated with exposure include low-acid (pH ≥6.0) home-canned foods such as jalapeño peppers, carrots, potatoes, asparagus, olives, and beans. The potential for foodborne botulism exists throughout the world, but outbreaks typically occur in the temperate zones rather than the tropics, where preservation of fruits, vegetables, and other foods is less commonly undertaken.

Approximately 5-10 outbreaks and 15-25 cases of foodborne botulism occur annually in the United States. There were 39 cases of confirmed foodborne botulism reported in the United States in 2015, including a large outbreak of 27 cases associated with a potluck meal in Ohio. Most of the continental U.S. outbreaks resulted from proteolytic type A or type B strains, which produce a strongly putrefactive odor in the food that some people find necessary to verify by tasting, exposing themselves to toxin in the process. In contrast, in Alaska and Canada, most foodborne outbreaks have resulted from nonproteolytic type E strains in Native American foods, such as fermented salmon eggs and seal flippers, which do not exhibit signs of spoilage. A further hazard of type E strains is their ability to grow at the temperatures maintained by household refrigerators (5°C [41°F]).

Wound botulism is an exceptionally rare disease, with <400 cases reported worldwide, but it is important to pediatrics because adolescents and children may be affected. Although many cases have occurred in young, physically active males who are at the greatest risk for traumatic injury, wound botulism also occurs with crush injuries in which no break in the skin is evident. In the past 15 yr, wound botulism from injection has become increasingly common in adult heroin abusers in the western United States and in Europe, not always with evident abscess formation or cellulitis.

A single outbreak of **inhalational botulism** was reported in 1962 in which 3 laboratory workers in Germany were exposed unintentionally to aerosolized botulinum toxin. Some patients in the United States have been hospitalized by accidental overdose of therapeutic or cosmetic botulinum toxin.

PATHOGENESIS

All forms of botulism produce disease through a final common pathway. Botulinum toxin is carried by the bloodstream to peripheral cholinergic synapses, where it binds irreversibly, blocking acetylcholine release and causing impaired neuromuscular and autonomic transmission. **Infant botulism** is an infectious disease that results from ingesting the spores of botulinum toxin–producing strains, with subsequent spore germination, multiplication, and production of botulinum toxin in the large intestine. This sequence is distinct from **foodborne botulism**, which is an intoxication that results when preformed botulinum toxin contained in an improperly preserved or inadequately cooked food is swallowed. **Wound botulism** results from spore germination and colonization of traumatized tissue by *C. botulinum;* the pathogenesis of this form of botulism is similar in this respect to that of tetanus. **Inhalational botulism** occurs when aerosolized botulinum toxin is inhaled. A bioterrorist attack could result in large or small outbreaks of inhalational or foodborne botulism (see Chapter 741).

Since botulinum toxin is not a *cytotoxin,* it does not cause overt macroscopic or microscopic pathology. Pathologic changes (pneumonia, petechiae on intrathoracic organs) may be found at autopsy, but these are secondary changes and not primarily attributable to botulinum toxin. No diagnostic technique is available to identify botulinum toxin binding at the neuromuscular junction. Nerve conduction velocity studies are typically normal. Electromyography (EMG) findings are often nonspecific and nondiagnostic (see later). The healing process in botulism consists of sprouting of new terminal unmyelinated motor neurons. Movement resumes when these new nerve terminals locate noncontracting muscle fibers and reinnervate them by inducing formation of a new motor end plate. In experimental animals, this process takes about 4 wk.

CLINICAL MANIFESTATIONS

The full clinical spectrum of infant botulism ranges from mild to fulminant sudden death. Botulinum toxin is distributed hematogenously.

Because relative blood flow and density of innervation are greatest in the bulbar musculature, all forms of botulism manifest neurologically as a symmetric, descending, flaccid paralysis beginning with the cranial nerve musculature and progressing over hours to days. **Bulbar palsies** may manifest with symptoms as poor feeding, weak suck, feeble cry, drooling, and even obstructive apnea. These clinical clues unfortunately may not be recognized as bulbar in origin (Fig. 237.1). Patients with evolving illness may already have generalized weakness and hypotonia in addition to bulbar palsies when first examined. The brain itself is spared in infant botulism, since botulinum toxin does not cross the blood-brain barrier.

In contrast to botulism caused by *C. botulinum*, a majority of the rare cases caused by intestinal colonization with *C. butyricum* are associated with a Meckel diverticulum accompanying abdominal distention, often leading to misdiagnosis as an acute abdomen. The also rare *C. baratii* type F infant botulism cases have been characterized by very young age at onset, rapidity of onset, and greater severity but shorter duration of paralysis.

In older children with **foodborne** or **wound botulism**, the onset of neurologic symptoms follows a characteristic pattern of diplopia, ptosis, dry mouth, dysphagia, dysphonia, and dysarthria, with decreased gag and corneal reflexes. Importantly, because the toxin acts only on motor nerves, paresthesias are not seen in botulism, except when a patient hyperventilates from anxiety. The sensorium remains clear, but this fact may be difficult to ascertain because of the slurred speech.

Foodborne botulism begins with gastrointestinal (GI) symptoms of nausea, vomiting, or diarrhea in approximately 30% of cases. These symptoms are thought to result from metabolic by-products of growth of *C. botulinum* or from the presence of other toxic contaminants in the food, because GI distress is rarely observed in wound botulism. Constipation may occur in foodborne botulism once flaccid paralysis becomes evident. Illness usually begins 12-36 hr after ingestion of the contaminated food but can range from as short as 2 hr to as long as 8 days. The incubation period in **wound botulism** is 4-14 days. Fever may be present in wound botulism but is absent in foodborne botulism unless a secondary infection (often pneumonia) is present. All forms of botulism display a wide spectrum of clinical severity, from the very mild, with minimal ptosis, flattened facial expression, minor dysphagia, and dysphonia, to the fulminant, with rapid onset of extensive paralysis, frank apnea, and fixed, dilated pupils. *Fatigability with repetitive muscle activity* is the clinical hallmark of botulism.

Infant botulism differs in apparent initial symptoms of illness only because the infant cannot verbalize them. Clinical progression can be more rapid and more severe in very young infants. The incubation period in infant botulism is estimated to be 3-30 days. Usually, the first indication of illness is a decreased frequency or even absence of defecation, and indeed constipation may be the chief complaint (although this sign is also frequently overlooked). Parents typically notice inability to feed, lethargy, weak cry, and diminished spontaneous movement. Dysphagia may be evident, and an increase in secretions drooling from the mouth may be noted. Gag, suck, and corneal reflexes all diminish as the paralysis advances. Oculomotor palsies may be evident. Paradoxically, the pupillary light reflex may be unaffected until the child is severely paralyzed, or it may be initially sluggish. Loss of head control is typically a prominent sign. Opisthotonos may be observed. Respiratory arrest may occur suddenly from airway occlusion by unswallowed secretions or from obstructive flaccid pharyngeal musculature. Death from botulism results either from airway obstruction or paralysis of the respiratory muscles. Occasionally, the diagnosis of infant botulism is suggested by a respiratory arrest that occurs after the infant is curled into position for lumbar puncture, or following the administration of an aminoglycoside antibiotic administered for suspected sepsis (see later).

In mild cases or in the early stages of illness, the physical signs of infant botulism may be subtle and easily missed. Eliciting cranial nerve palsies and fatigability of muscular function requires careful examination. Ptosis may not be seen unless the head of the child is kept erect.

DIAGNOSIS

Definitive diagnosis of botulism is made by specialized laboratory testing that requires hours to days to complete. Therefore, clinical diagnosis is the foundation for early recognition of and response to all forms of botulism. Routine laboratory studies, including those of the cerebrospinal fluid (CSF), are normal in botulism unless dehydration, undernourishment (metabolic acidosis and ketosis), or secondary infection is present.

The **classic triad** of botulism is the acute onset of a symmetric flaccid descending paralysis with clear sensorium, no fever, and no paresthesias. Suspected botulism represents a medical and public health emergency that is immediately reportable by telephone in most U.S. health jurisdictions. State health departments (first call) and the CDC (770-488-7100

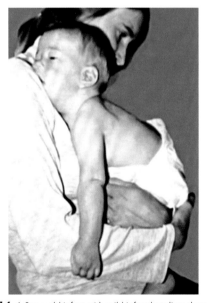

Fig. 237.1 A 3 mo old infant with mild infant botulism showing signs of ptosis, an expressionless face, and hypotonia of the neck, trunk, and limbs. The additional bulbar palsies—ophthalmoplegia, weak cry, weak sucking, and dysphagia (drooling)—are not apparent in the photograph. *(From Arnon SS, Schechter R, Maslanka SE, et al: Human botulism immune globulin for the treatment of infant botulism, N Engl J Med 354:462–471, 2006.)*

Table 237.1	Diagnoses Considered in Subsequently Laboratory-Confirmed Cases of Infant Botulism
ADMISSION DIAGNOSIS	**SUBSEQUENTLY CONSIDERED DIAGNOSES**
Suspected sepsis, meningitis	Guillain-Barré syndrome
Pneumonia	Myasthenia gravis
Dehydration	Disorders of amino acid metabolism
Viral syndrome	Hypothyroidism
Hypotonia of unknown etiology	Drug ingestion Organophosphate poisoning
Constipation	Brainstem encephalitis
Failure to thrive	Heavy metal poisoning (Pb, Mg, As)
Spinal muscular atrophy type 1 (Werdnig-Hoffmann disease)	Poliomyelitis Viral polyneuritis Hirschsprung disease Metabolic encephalopathy Medium-chain acetyl–coenzyme A dehydrogenase deficiency

at any time) can arrange for diagnostic testing, epidemiologic investigation, and provision of equine antitoxin.

The diagnosis of botulism is unequivocally established by demonstration of the presence of botulinum toxin in serum or of *C. botulinum* toxin or organisms in wound material, enema fluid, or feces. *C. botulinum* is not part of the normal resident intestinal flora of humans, and its presence in the setting of acute flaccid paralysis is diagnostic. An epidemiologic diagnosis of foodborne botulism can be established when *C. botulinum* organisms and toxin are found in food eaten by patients.

Electromyography can sometimes distinguish between causes of acute flaccid paralysis, although results may be variable, including normal, in patients with botulism. The distinctive EMG finding in botulism is facilitation (potentiation) of the evoked muscle action potential at high-frequency (50 Hz) stimulation. In infant botulism, a characteristic pattern known as **BSAP** (brief, small, abundant motor unit action potentials), is present only in clinically weak muscles. Nerve conduction velocity and sensory nerve function are normal in botulism.

Infant botulism requires a high index of suspicion for early diagnosis (Table 237.1). Rule out sepsis remains the most common admission diagnosis. If a previously healthy infant (usually 2-4 mo old) demonstrates weakness with difficulty in sucking, swallowing, crying, or breathing, infant botulism should be considered a likely diagnosis. A careful cranial nerve examination is then very helpful. Rare instances of co-infection with *C. difficile*, respiratory syncytial virus, or influenza virus have occurred.

Differential Diagnosis

Botulism is frequently misdiagnosed, most often as a **polyradiculo-neuropathy** (Guillain-Barré or Miller Fisher syndrome), myasthenia gravis, or a central nervous system (CNS) disease (Table 237.2). In the United States, botulism is more likely than **Guillain-Barré syndrome**, intoxication, or poliomyelitis to cause a cluster of cases of acute flaccid paralysis. Botulism differs from other flaccid paralyses in its initial and prominent cranial nerve palsies that are disproportionate to milder weakness and hypotonia below the neck; in its symmetry; and in its absence of sensory nerve damage. Spinal muscular atrophy may closely mimic infant botulism at presentation.

Additional diagnostic procedures may be useful in rapidly excluding botulism as the cause of paralysis. The CSF is unchanged in botulism but is abnormal in many CNS diseases. Although the CSF protein concentration is eventually elevated in Guillain-Barré syndrome, it may be normal early in illness. Imaging of the brain, spine, and chest may reveal hemorrhage, inflammation, or neoplasm. A test dose of edrophonium chloride briefly reverses paralytic symptoms in many patients with myasthenia gravis and, reportedly, in some with botulism, although this is rarely performed in infants. A close inspection of the skin, especially the scalp, may reveal an attached tick that is causing paralysis. Possible organophosphate intoxication should be pursued aggressively, because specific antidotes (oximes) are available and because the patient may be part of a commonly exposed group, some of whom have yet to demonstrate illness. Other tests that require days for results include stool culture for *Campylobacter jejuni* as a precipitant of Guillain-Barré syndrome, spinal muscular atrophy and other genetic (including mitochondrial) disorders, and assays for the autoantibodies that cause myasthenia gravis, Lambert-Eaton syndrome, and Guillain-Barré syndrome.

TREATMENT

Human botulism immune globulin, given intravenously (BIG-IV, also referred to as BabyBIG), is licensed for the treatment of infant botulism caused by type A or B botulinum toxin. Treatment with BIG-IV consists of a single intravenous infusion of 50-100 mg/kg (see package insert) that should be given as soon as possible after infant botulism is suspected so as to immediately end the toxemia that is the cause of the illness and arrest progression of paralysis. *When the diagnosis of infant botulism is suspected, treatment should not be delayed for laboratory confirmation.* In the United States, BIG-IV may be obtained from the California Department of Public Health (24 hr telephone: 510-231-7600; http://www.infantbotulism.org). The use of BIG-IV shortens mean hospital stay from approximately 6 wk to approximately 2 wk. Most of the decrease in hospital stay results from shorter duration of mechanical ventilation and reduced days in intensive care. Hospital costs are reduced by >$100,000 per case (in 2012 U.S. dollars).

Older patients with suspected food, wound, or inhalational botulism may be treated with 1 vial of licensed equine heptavalent (A-G) botulinum antitoxin (HBAT; https://www.cdc.gov/mmwr/preview/mmwrhtml/mm5910a4.htm), available in the United States through the CDC by way of state and local health departments.

Antibiotic therapy is not part of the treatment of uncomplicated infant or foodborne botulism, because the toxin is primarily an intracellular molecule that is released into the intestinal lumen with vegetative bacterial cell death and lysis. Indeed, there is theoretical concern that antibiotics with clostridiocidal activity may increase the amount of free toxin in the large bowel and actually worsen an infant's clinical status. Antibiotic use in infant botulism patients is indicated only for the treatment of secondary infections. In these patients, aminoglycosides should be avoided, since this class of antibiotics can potentiate the action of botulinum toxin at the neuromuscular junction. Wound botulism requires aggressive treatment with antibiotics and antitoxin in a manner analogous to that for tetanus (see Chapter 238) and may require wound debridement to remove the source of the toxin.

SUPPORTIVE CARE

Management of botulism rests on the following 3 principles: (1) fatigability with repetitive muscle activity is the clinical hallmark of the disease; (2) complications are best avoided by anticipating them; and (3) meticulous supportive care is a necessity. The 1st principle applies mainly to feeding and breathing. Correct positioning is imperative to protect the airway and improve respiratory mechanics. The patient should be positioned face-up on a rigid-bottomed crib (or bed), the head of which is tilted at 30 degrees. A small cloth roll is placed under the cervical vertebrae to tilt the head back so that secretions drain to the posterior pharynx and away from the airway. In this tilted position, the abdominal viscera pull the diaphragm down, thereby improving respiratory mechanics. The patient's head and torso should not be elevated by bending the middle of the bed; in such a position, the hypotonic thorax would slump into the abdomen, and breathing would be compromised.

About half of patients with infant botulism require endotracheal intubation, which is best done prophylactically. The indications include diminished gag and cough reflexes and progressive airway obstruction by secretions.

Feeding should be done by a nasogastric or nasojejunal tube until sufficient oropharyngeal strength and coordination enable allow oral

Table 237.2	Conditions Considered in Differential Diagnosis of Foodborne Botulism and Wound Botulism

Acute gastroenteritis
Myasthenia gravis
Guillain-Barré syndrome
Organophosphate poisoning
Meningitis
Encephalitis
Psychiatric illness
Cerebrovascular accident
Poliomyelitis
Hypothyroidism
Aminoglycoside-associated paralysis
Tick paralysis
Hypocalcemia
Hypermagnesemia
Carbon monoxide poisoning
Hyperemesis gravidarum
Laryngeal trauma
Diabetic complications
Inflammatory myopathy
Overexertion

feeding by breast or bottle. Expressed breast milk is the most desirable food for infants, in part because of its immunologic components (e.g., secretory IgA, lactoferrin, leukocytes). Tube feeding also assists in the restoration of peristalsis, a nonspecific but probably essential part of eliminating *C. botulinum* from the intestinal flora. Intravenous feeding (hyperalimentation) is discouraged because of the potential for infection and the advantages of tube feeding.

Because sensation and cognitive function remain fully intact, providing auditory, tactile, and visual stimuli is beneficial. Maintaining strong central respiratory drive is essential, so sedatives and CNS depressants should be avoided. Full hydration and stool softeners such as lactulose may mitigate the protracted constipation. Cathartics are not recommended. Patients with foodborne and infant botulism excrete *C. botulinum* toxin and organisms in their feces, often for many weeks, and care should be taken in handling their excreta, with full engagement of hospital infection control staff. When bladder palsy occurs in severe cases, gentle suprapubic pressure with the patient in the sitting position with the head supported may help attain complete voiding and reduce the risk for urinary tract infection (UTI). Families of affected patients may require emotional and financial support, especially when the paralysis of botulism is prolonged.

COMPLICATIONS

Almost all the complications of botulism are *nosocomial*, and a few are iatrogenic (Table 237.3). Some critically ill, toxin-paralyzed patients who must spend weeks or months on ventilators in intensive care units inevitably experience some of these complications. Suspected "relapses" of infant botulism usually reflect premature hospital discharge or an inapparent underlying complication such as pneumonia, UTI, or otitis media.

PROGNOSIS

When the regenerating nerve endings have induced formation of a new motor end plate, neuromuscular transmission is restored. In the absence of complications, particularly those related to hypoxia, the prognosis in infant botulism is for full and complete recovery. Hospital stay in untreated infant botulism averages 5.7 wk but differs significantly by toxin type, with patients with untreated type B disease being hospitalized a mean of 4.2 wk and those with untreated type A disease being hospitalized a mean of 6.7 wk.

In the United States, the case fatality ratio for hospitalized cases of infant botulism is <1%. After recovery, patients with untreated infant botulism appear to have an increased incidence of strabismus that requires timely screening and treatment.

Table 237.3	Complications of Infant Botulism

Acute respiratory distress syndrome
Aspiration
Clostridium difficile enterocolitis
Hypotension
Inappropriate antidiuretic hormone secretion
Long bone fractures
Misplaced or plugged endotracheal tube
Nosocomial anemia
Otitis media
Pneumonia
Pneumothorax
Recurrent atelectasis
Seizures secondary to hyponatremia
Sepsis
Subglottic stenosis
Tracheal granuloma
Tracheitis
Transfusion reaction
Urinary tract infection

The case fatality ratio in foodborne and wound botulism varies by age, with younger patients having the best prognosis. Some adults with botulism have reported chronic weakness and fatigue for >1 yr as sequelae.

PREVENTION

Foodborne botulism is best prevented by adherence to safe methods of home canning (pressure cooker and acidification), by avoiding suspicious foods, and by heating all home-canned foods to 85°C (185°F) for ≥5 min. Wound botulism is best prevented by not using illicit drugs and by treatment of contaminated wounds with thorough cleansing, surgical debridement, and provision of appropriate antibiotics.

Many patients with infant botulism are presumed to have inhaled and then swallowed airborne clostridial spores; these cases cannot be prevented. However, a clearly identified and avoidable source of botulinum spores for infants is **honey**. *Honey is an unsafe food for any child <1 yr old.* Corn syrups were once thought to be a possible source of botulinum spores, but evidence indicates otherwise. Breastfeeding appears to slow the onset of infant botulism and to diminish the risk for sudden death in infants in whom the disease develops.

Bibliography is available at Expert Consult.

Chapter **238**
Tetanus *(Clostridium tetani)*
Mark R. Schleiss
第二百三十八章
破伤风（破伤风梭菌）

中文导读

　　本章主要介绍了破伤风的病原学、流行病学、发病机制、临床表现、诊断及鉴别诊断、治疗、支持治疗、并发症、预后和防治。该病是由破伤风梭菌感染导致，破伤风毒素为主要致病因子，对毒素产生的过程和作用机制作了详细阐述。在临床表现部分对全身性破伤风、局限性破伤风、头部破伤风、婴儿型破伤风的作了详细介绍。同时对如何预防破伤风作了详细介绍。

ETIOLOGY

Tetanus is an acute, spastic paralytic illness caused by a neurotoxin produced by *Clostridium tetani*. Thus, tetanus can be considered more as a toxin-mediated process than an acute infectious process, since there are few, if any, symptoms elicited by the presence of replicating microorganisms or host inflammatory response. Unlike other pathogenic clostridia species, *C. tetani* is not a tissue-invasive organism and instead causes illness through the toxin, **tetanospasmin**, more commonly referred to as **tetanus toxin**. Tetanospasmin is the 2nd most poisonous substance known, surpassed in potency only by botulinum toxin. The human lethal dose of tetanus toxin is estimated to be 10^{-5} mg/kg.

Clostridium tetani is a motile, gram-positive, spore-forming obligate anaerobe. The organism's natural habitat worldwide is soil, dust, and the alimentary tracts of various animals. *C. tetani* forms spores terminally, with a classic morphologic appearance resembling a drumstick or tennis racket microscopically. The formation of spores is a critical aspect of the organism's persistence in the environment. Spores can survive boiling but not autoclaving, whereas the vegetative cells are killed by antibiotics, heat, and standard disinfectants.

EPIDEMIOLOGY

Tetanus occurs worldwide and is endemic in many developing countries, although its incidence varies considerably. Public health efforts in recent years have had an impressive impact on tetanus-associated mortality, although many challenges remain. Approximately 57,000 deaths were caused by tetanus globally in 2015. Of these, approximately 20,000 deaths occurred in neonates and 37,000 in older children and adults. Most mortality from **neonatal (or umbilical) tetanus** occurs in South Asia and Sub-Saharan Africa. Mortality in adults is largely caused by **maternal tetanus,** which results from postpartum, postabortal, or postsurgical wound infection with *C. tetani*. Reported tetanus cases in the United States have declined >95% since 1947, and deaths from tetanus have declined by >99% in that same period. From 2009 through 2015, a total of 197 cases and 16 deaths from tetanus were reported in the United States. The majority of U.S. childhood cases of tetanus have occurred in unimmunized children whose parents objected to vaccination.

Most non-neonatal cases of tetanus are associated with a traumatic injury, often a penetrating wound inflicted by a dirty object such as a nail, splinter, fragment of glass, or unsterile injection. Tetanus may also occur in the setting of illicit drug injection. The disease has been associated with the use of contaminated suture material and after intramuscular injection of medicines, most notably quinine for chloroquine-resistant falciparum malaria. The disease may also occur in association with animal bites, abscesses (including dental abscesses), ear and other body piercing, chronic skin ulceration, burns, compound fractures, frostbite, gangrene, intestinal surgery, ritual scarification, infected insect bites, and female circumcision. Rarely, cases may present to clinical attention without an antecedent history of trauma.

PATHOGENESIS

Tetanus typically occurs after spores (introduced by traumatic injury) germinate, multiply, and produce tetanus toxin. A plasmid carries the toxin gene. Toxin is produced only by the vegetative cell, not the spore. It is released after the vegetative phase of replication, with replication occurring under anaerobic conditions. The low oxidation-reduction potential of an infected injury site therefore provides an ideal environment for transition from the spore to the vegetative stage of growth. Following bacterial cell death and lysis, tetanospasmin is produced. The toxin has no known function for clostridia in the soil environment where they normally reside. Tetanus toxin is a 150 kDa simple protein consisting of a heavy (100 kDa) and a light (50 kDa) chain joined by a single disulfide bond. Tetanus toxin binds at the neuromuscular junction and enters the motor nerve by endocytosis, after which it undergoes retrograde axonal transport, facilitated by dyneins, to the cytoplasm of the α-motoneuron. In the sciatic nerve, the transport rate was found to be 3.4 mm/hr. The toxin exits the motoneuron in the spinal cord and next enters adjacent spinal inhibitory interneurons, where it prevents release of the neurotransmitters glycine and γ-aminobutyric acid (GABA). Tetanus toxin thus blocks the normal inhibition of antagonistic muscles on which voluntary coordinated movement depends; as a consequence, affected muscles sustain maximal contraction and cannot relax. This aspect of pathogenesis led to the term **lockjaw**, classically applied to the clinical manifestations of tetanus in the affected individual. The autonomic nervous system is also rendered unstable in tetanus.

The phenomenal potency of tetanus toxin is enzymatic. The 50 kDa light chain (A-chain) of tetanus toxin is a zinc-containing endoprotease whose substrate is synaptobrevin, a constituent protein of the docking complex that enables the synaptic vesicle to fuse with the terminal neuronal cell membrane. The cleavage of synaptobrevin is the final target of tetanus toxin, and even in low doses the neurotoxin will inhibit neurotransmitter exocytosis in the inhibitory interneurons. The blockage of GABA and glycine causes the physiologic effects of tetanus toxin. The 100 kDa heavy chain (B-chain) of the toxin contains its binding and internalization domains. It binds to disialogangliosides (GD2 and GD1b) on the neuronal membrane. The translocation domain aids the movement of the protein across that membrane and into the neuron.

Because *C. tetani* is not an invasive organism, its toxin-producing vegetative cells remain where introduced into the wound, which may display local inflammatory changes and a mixed bacterial flora.

CLINICAL MANIFESTATIONS

Tetanus is most often generalized but may also be localized. The incubation period typically is 2-14 days but may be as long as months after the injury. In **generalized tetanus** the presenting symptom in about half of cases is **trismus** (masseter muscle spasm, or lockjaw). Headache, restlessness, and irritability are early symptoms, often followed by stiffness, difficulty chewing, dysphagia, and neck muscle spasm. The so-called sardonic smile of tetanus (**risus sardonicus**) results from intractable spasms of facial and buccal muscles. When the paralysis extends to abdominal, lumbar, hip, and thigh muscles, the patient may assume an arched posture of extreme hyperextension of the body, or **opisthotonos**, with the head and the heels bent backward and the body bowed forward. In severe cases, only the back of the head and the heels of the patient are noted to be touching the supporting surface. Opisthotonos is an equilibrium position that results from unrelenting total contraction of opposing muscles, all of which display the typical boardlike rigidity of tetanus. Laryngeal and respiratory muscle spasm can lead to airway obstruction and asphyxiation. Because tetanus toxin does not affect sensory nerves or cortical function, the patient unfortunately remains conscious, in extreme pain, and in fearful anticipation of the next tetanic seizure. The seizures are characterized by sudden, severe tonic contractions of the muscles, with fist clenching, flexion, and adduction of the arms and hyperextension of the legs. Without treatment, the duration of these seizures may range from a few seconds to a few minutes in length with intervening respite periods. As the illness progresses, the spasms become sustained and exhausting. The smallest disturbance by sight, sound, or touch may trigger a tetanic spasm. Dysuria and urinary retention result from bladder sphincter spasm; forced defecation may occur. Fever, occasionally as high as 40°C (104°F), is common and is caused by the substantial metabolic energy consumed by spastic muscles. Notable autonomic effects include tachycardia, dysrhythmias, labile hypertension, diaphoresis, and cutaneous vasoconstriction. The tetanic paralysis usually becomes more severe in the 1st wk after onset, stabilizes in the 2nd wk, and ameliorates gradually over the ensuing 1-4 wk.

Neonatal tetanus, the infantile form of generalized tetanus, typically manifests within 3-12 days of birth. It presents as progressive difficulty in feeding (sucking and swallowing), associated hunger, and crying. Paralysis or diminished movement, stiffness and rigidity to the touch, and spasms, with or without opisthotonos, are characteristic. The umbilical stump, which is typically the portal of entry for the microorganism, may retain remnants of dirt, dung, clotted blood, or serum, or it may appear relatively benign.

Localized tetanus results in painful spasms of the muscles adjacent to the wound site and may precede generalized tetanus. **Cephalic tetanus** is a rare form of localized tetanus involving the bulbar musculature that occurs with wounds or foreign bodies in the head, nostrils, or face. It also occurs in association with chronic otitis media. Cephalic tetanus is characterized by retracted eyelids, deviated gaze, trismus, risus sardonicus, and spastic paralysis of the tongue and pharyngeal musculature.

DIAGNOSIS

The picture of tetanus is one of the most dramatic in medicine, and the diagnosis may be established clinically. The typical setting is an unimmunized patient (and/or mother) who was injured or born within the preceding 2 wk, who presents with trismus, dysphagia, generalized muscle rigidity and spasm, and a clear sensorium.

Results of routine laboratory studies are usually normal. A peripheral leukocytosis may result from a secondary bacterial infection of the wound or may be stress-induced from the sustained tetanic spasms. The cerebrospinal fluid analysis is normal, although the intense muscle contractions may raise intracranial pressure. Serum muscle enzymes (creatine kinase, aldolase) may be elevated. Neither the electroencephalogram nor the electromyogram shows a characteristic pattern, although EMG may show continuous discharge of motor subunits and shortening, or absence of the silent interval normally observed after an action potential. An assay for antitoxin levels is not readily available, although a serum antitoxin level of ≥0.01 IU/mL is generally considered protective and makes the diagnosis of tetanus less likely. *C. tetani* is not always visible on Gram stain of wound material and is isolated by culture in only approximately 30% of cases. The **spatula test** is a simple diagnostic bedside test that involves touching the oropharynx with a spatula or tongue blade. Normally this maneuver will elicit a gag reflex, as the patient tries to expel the spatula (negative test). If tetanus is present, patients develop a reflex spasm of the masseter muscles and bite the spatula (positive test). This bedside diagnostic maneuver is said to have a high sensitivity and specificity.

Differential Diagnosis

Florid and generalized tetanus is typically not mistaken for any other disease. However, trismus may result from parapharyngeal, retropharyngeal, or dental abscesses or rarely from acute encephalitis involving the brainstem. Either rabies or tetanus may follow an animal bite, and rabies may manifest as trismus with seizures. **Rabies** may be distinguished from tetanus by hydrophobia, marked dysphagia, predominantly clonic seizures, and pleocytosis (see Chapter 300). Although **strychnine poisoning** may result in tonic muscle spasms and generalized seizure activity, it seldom produces trismus, and unlike in tetanus, general relaxation usually occurs between spasms. Hypocalcemia may produce tetany that is characterized by laryngeal and carpopedal spasms, but trismus is absent. Occasionally, epileptic seizures, narcotic withdrawal, or other drug reactions may suggest tetanus.

TREATMENT

Management of tetanus requires eradication of *C. tetani*, correction of wound environment conditions conducive to its anaerobic replication, neutralization of all accessible tetanus toxin, control of seizures and respiration, palliation, provision of meticulous supportive care, and prevention of recurrences.

Surgical wound excision and debridement are often needed to remove the foreign body or devitalized tissue that created the anaerobic growth conditions necessary for vegetative replication. Surgery should be performed promptly after administration of **human tetanus immuno-globulin** (TIG) and antibiotics. Excision of the umbilical stump in the neonate with tetanus is no longer recommended.

Tetanus toxin cannot be neutralized by TIG after it has begun its axonal ascent to the spinal cord. However, TIG should be given as soon as possible, toward the goal of neutralizing toxin that diffuses from the wound into the circulation before the toxin can bind at distant muscle groups. The optimal dose of TIG has not been determined. Some experts recommend a single intramuscular injection of 500 units of TIG to neutralize systemic tetanus toxin, but total doses as high as 3,000-6,000 U are also recommended. Infiltration of part of the dose of TIG into the wound is recommended by the Red Book Committee of the American Academy of Pediatrics, although the efficacy of this approach has not been proved. If TIG is unavailable, use of human intravenous immu-noglobulin may be necessary. IVIG contains 4-90 U/mL of TIG; the optimal dosage of IVIG for treating tetanus is not known, and its use is not approved for this indication. In parts of the world where it is available, another alternative may be equine-derived tetanus antitoxin (TAT). This product is no longer available in the United States. A dose of 1,500-3,000 U is recommended and should be administered after appropriate testing for sensitivity and desensitization, since up to 15% of patients given the usual dose of TAT will experience serum sickness. The human-derived immunoglobulins are much preferred because of their longer half-life (30 days) and the virtual absence of allergic and serum sickness adverse effects. Results of studies examining the potential benefit of intrathecal administration of TIG are conflicting. The TIG preparation available for use in the United States is neither licensed nor formulated for intrathecal or intravenous use.

Oral (or intravenous) **metronidazole** (30 mg/kg/day, given at 6 hr intervals; maximum dose, 4 g/day) decreases the number of vegetative forms of *C. tetani* and is currently considered the antibiotic of choice. Parenteral penicillin G (100,000 U/kg/day, administered at 4-6 hr intervals, with a daily maximum 12 million U) is an alternative treatment. Antimicrobial therapy for a total duration of 7-10 days is recommended.

Supportive care and pharmacologic interventions targeted at control of tetanic spasms are of critical importance in the management of tetanus. Toward this goal, all patients with generalized tetanus should receive **muscle relaxants**. Diazepam provides both relaxation and seizure control. The initial dose of 0.1-0.2 mg/kg every 3-6 hr intravenously is subsequently titrated to control the tetanic spasms, after which the effective dose is sustained for 2-6 wk before a tapered withdrawal. Magnesium sulfate, other benzodiazepines (midazolam), chlorpromazine, dantrolene, and baclofen are also used. Intrathecal baclofen produces such complete muscle relaxation that apnea often ensues; as with most other agents listed, baclofen should be used only in an intensive care unit setting. Favorable survival rates in generalized tetanus have been described with the use of neuromuscular blocking agents such as vecuronium and pancuronium, which produce a general flaccid paralysis that is then managed by mechanical ventilation. Autonomic instability is regulated with standard α- or β-adrenergic (or both) blocking agents; morphine has also proved useful.

SUPPORTIVE CARE

Meticulous supportive care in a quiet, dark, secluded setting is most desirable. Because tetanic spasms may be triggered by minor stimuli, the patient should be sedated and protected from all unnecessary sounds, sights, and touch, and all therapeutic and other manipulations must be carefully scheduled and coordinated. Endotracheal intubation may not be required, but it should be done to prevent aspiration of secretions before laryngospasm develops. A tracheostomy kit should be immediately at hand for unintubated patients. Endotracheal intubation and suctioning easily provoke reflex tetanic seizures and spasms, so early tracheostomy should be considered in severe cases not managed by pharmacologically induced flaccid paralysis. Therapeutic botulinum toxin has been used to overcome trismus.

Cardiorespiratory monitoring, frequent suctioning, and maintenance of the patient's substantial fluid, electrolyte, and caloric needs are fundamental. Careful nursing attention to mouth, skin, bladder, and bowel function is needed to avoid ulceration, infection, and obstipation. Prophylactic subcutaneous heparin may be of value, but it must be balanced with the risk of hemorrhage. Enoxaparin would be an alternative for the patient for whom deep vein thrombosis prophylaxis is warranted.

COMPLICATIONS

The seizures and the severe, sustained rigid paralysis of tetanus predispose the patient to many complications. Aspiration of secretions with attendant pneumonia is an important complication to consider and may be present at initial diagnosis. Maintaining airway patency often mandates endotracheal intubation and mechanical ventilation with their attendant hazards, including pneumothorax and mediastinal emphysema. The seizures may result in lacerations of the mouth or tongue, in intramuscular hematomas or **rhabdomyolysis** with myoglobinuria and renal failure, or in long-bone or spinal fractures. Venous thrombosis, pulmonary embolism, gastric ulceration with or without hemorrhage, paralytic ileus, and decubitus ulceration are described as complications. Excessive use of muscle relaxants, which are an integral part of care, may produce iatrogenic apnea. Cardiac arrhythmias, including asystole, unstable blood pressure, and labile temperature regulation reflect disordered autonomic nervous system control that may be aggravated by inattention to maintenance of intravascular volume needs.

PROGNOSIS

Recovery in tetanus occurs through regeneration of synapses within the spinal cord that results in restoration of muscle relaxation. Interestingly, an episode of tetanus does not result in the production of toxin-neutralizing antibodies, presumably because the infinitesimally small amounts of toxin required to cause disease are not sufficient to elicit an immune response. Therefore, active immunization with tetanus toxoid during convalescence and/or at discharge, with provision for completion of the primary vaccine series, is mandatory.

The most important factor that influences outcome is the quality of supportive care. Mortality is highest in very young and very old patients. A favorable prognosis is associated with a long incubation period, absence of fever, and localized disease. An unfavorable prognosis is associated with onset of trismus <7 days after injury and onset of generalized tetanic spasms <3 days after onset of trismus. Sequelae of hypoxic brain injury, especially in infants, include cerebral palsy, diminished mental abilities, and behavioral difficulties. Most fatalities occur within the 1st wk of illness. Reported case fatality rates for generalized tetanus are 5–35%, and for neonatal tetanus they extend from <10% with intensive care treatment to >75% without it. Cephalic tetanus has an especially poor prognosis because of breathing and feeding difficulties.

PREVENTION

Tetanus is an entirely and easily preventable disease. A serum antibody titer of ≥0.01 U/mL is considered protective. Active immunization should begin in early infancy with combined diphtheria toxoid–tetanus toxoid–acellular pertussis (DTaP) vaccine at 2, 4, 6, and 15-18 mo of age, with boosters at 4-6 yr (DTaP) and 11-12 yr (Tdap) of age, and at 10 yr intervals thereafter throughout adult life with tetanus and reduced diphtheria toxoid (Td). Immunization of women with tetanus toxoid prevents neonatal tetanus, and pregnant women should receive 1 dose of reduced diphtheria and pertussis toxoids (Tdap) during each pregnancy, preferably at 27-36 wk of gestation. Recommended immunization schedules are regularly updated (http://www.cdc.gov/vaccines/schedules).

Arthus reactions (type III hypersensitivity reactions), a localized vasculitis associated with deposition of immune complexes and activation of complement, are reported rarely after tetanus vaccination. Mass immunization campaigns in developing countries have occasionally provoked a widespread hysterical reaction.

Wound Management

Tetanus prevention measures after trauma consist of inducing active immunity to tetanus toxin and of passively providing antitoxic antibody (Table 238.1). Tetanus prophylaxis is an essential part of all wound management, but specific measures depend on the nature of the injury and the immunization status of the patient. Prevention of tetanus must be included in planning for the consequences of bombings, natural disasters, and other possible civilian mass-casualty events.

Tetanus toxoid should always be given after a dog or other animal bite, even though *C. tetani* is infrequently found in canine mouth flora. Non-minor wounds require human TIG except those in a fully immunized patient (i.e., ≥3 doses of adsorbed tetanus toxoid). In any other circumstances (e.g., patients with an unknown or incomplete immunization history; crush, puncture, or projectile wounds; wounds contaminated with saliva, soil, or feces; avulsion injuries; compound fractures; or frostbite), TIG 250 units should be administered intramuscularly, regardless of the patient's age or weight. If TIG is unavailable, use of human IVIG may be considered. If neither of these products is available, 3,000-5,000 units of equine-derived TAT (in regions of the world where it is available) may be given intramuscularly after testing for hypersensitivity. Serum sickness may occur with this agent.

The wound should undergo immediate, thorough surgical cleansing and debridement to remove foreign bodies and any necrotic tissue in which anaerobic conditions might develop. Tetanus toxoid should be given to stimulate active immunity and may be administered concurrently with TIG (or TAT) if given in separate syringes at widely separated sites. A tetanus toxoid booster (preferably Tdap) is administered to all persons with any wound if the tetanus immunization status is unknown or incomplete. A booster is administered to injured persons who have completed the primary immunization series if (1) the wound is clean and minor but ≥10 yr have passed since the last booster or (2) the wound is more serious and ≥5 yr have passed since the last booster (Table 238.1). Persons who experienced an Arthus reaction after a dose of tetanus toxoid–containing vaccine should not receive Td more frequently than every 10 yr, even for tetanus prophylaxis as part of wound management. In a situation of delayed wound care, active immunization should be started at once.

Bibliography is available at Expert Consult.

Table 238.1	Tetanus Vaccination and Immune Globulin Use in Wound Management				
HISTORY OF ABSORBED TETANUS TOXOID	**CLEAN, MINOR WOUNDS**		**ALL OTHER WOUNDS***		
	DTaP, Tdap, *or* Td[†]	TIG[‡]	DTaP, Tdap, *or* TD[†]	TIG[‡]	
Uncertain or <3 doses	Yes	No	Yes	Yes	
≥3 doses	No if <10 yr since last dose of tetanus-containing vaccine	No	No if <5 yr since last tetanus-containing vaccine[§]	No	
	Yes if ≥10 yr since last dose of tetanus-containing vaccine	No	Yes if ≥5 yr since last tetanus-containing vaccine dose	No	

*Such as, but not limited to, wounds contaminated with dirt, feces, and saliva; puncture wounds; avulsions; and wounds resulting from missiles, crushing, burns, and frostbite.
[†]DTaP is used for children <7 yr old. Tdap is preferred over Td for underimmunized children ≥7 yr old who have not received Tdap previously.
[‡]Intravenous immune globulin should be used when TIG is unavailable.
[§]More frequent boosters are not needed and can accentuate adverse events.
DT, Diphtheria and tetanus toxoid vaccine; DTaP, combined diphtheria toxoid–tetanus toxoid–acellular pertussis vaccine; Td, tetanus toxoid and reduced diphtheria toxoid vaccine; Tdap, tetanus toxoid, reduced diphtheria toxoid, and acellular pertussis vaccine; TIG, tetanus immune globulin.
Data from Tetanus (lockjaw). In Kimberlin DW, Brady MT, Jackson MA, Long SS, editors: *Red book: 2015 report of the Committee on Infectious Diseases,* ed 30, Elk Grove Village, IL, 2015, American Academy of Pediatrics.

Chapter **239**
Clostridium difficile Infection

Osman Z. Ahmad and Mitchell B. Cohen

第二百三十九章
艰难梭菌感染

中文导读

　　本章主要介绍了艰难梭菌感染的病原学、流行病学、传播途径、发病机制、临床表现、诊断、治疗、预后和预防。艰难梭菌感染多表现为抗生素相关腹泻的常见原因。该菌产生毒素A和毒素B，毒素在体内引起炎症反应和细胞死亡导致症状。临床表现以消化道症状为主，可发生假膜性结肠炎，部分患儿存在反应性关节炎，诊断方法主要介绍了酶联免疫试验和PCR检测。治疗部分主要介绍轻中度感染口服甲硝唑，重度感染予以万古霉素治疗。本病易复发，在预后部分详细介绍了改善预后的方法，粪便移植可用于解决肠道菌群的破坏。

Clostridium difficile infection (**CDI**), also known as pseudomembranous colitis or *C. difficile*–associated diarrhea, refers to gastrointestinal (GI) colonization with *C. difficile* resulting in a diarrheal illness. It is a common cause of **antibiotic-associated diarrhea** and the most common cause of healthcare-associated infections in the United States, accounting for 12% of these infections. An increase in inpatient and outpatient acquisition of CDI has been observed, and new risk factors have been identified, fueling the development of new therapeutic options.

ETIOLOGY

Clostridium difficile (which has been renamed *Clostridioides difficile*) is a gram-positive, spore-forming, anaerobic bacillus that is resistant to killing by alcohol. It is acquired from the environment or by the fecal-oral route. Organisms causing symptomatic intestinal disease produce 1 or both of the following: **toxin A** and **toxin B**. These toxins affect intracellular signaling pathways, resulting in inflammation and cell death. The cytotoxic **binary toxin**, an AB toxin, is not present in the majority of strains but has been detected in epidemic strains.

EPIDEMIOLOGY

Once thought to be an infrequent infection of chronically ill and hospitalized patients, the incidence of CDI is increasing in pediatric patients, and the setting of acquisition is changing. The incidence in pediatric patients increased 48%, from 2.5 to 3.7 cases per 1,000 admissions between 2001 and 2006. A population-based cohort study over a similar period found that 75% of cases were community acquired and 16% had no preceding hospitalization or antibiotic exposure. Similar 2011 CDC national data estimate3 cases of community-acquired CDI in children

for every healthcare-acquired case. In addition to an overall increase in all strains, a *hypervirulent strain*, denoted **NAP1/BI/027** (also called **BI**), has emerged and is estimated to cause 10–20% of pediatric infections. This strain produces binary toxin and exhibits 16- and 23-fold increases in the production of toxins A and B, respectively. The specific role of this hypervirulent strain in the changing epidemiology of CDI is not completely understood.

Asymptomatic carriage occurs with potentially pathogenic strains and is common in neonates and infants ≤1 yr old. A carrier frequency rate of 50% may occur in children <1 yr old, but the rate declines by age 3 yr. Carriers can infect other susceptible individuals.

Risk factors for CDI include the use of broad-spectrum antibiotics, hospitalization (particularly if the prior room occupant was infected), GI surgery, inflammatory bowel disease (IBD), chemotherapy, enteral tube feeding, proton pump inhibitor (PPI) or H_2-receptor antagonist use, and chronic illness.

PATHOGENESIS

Disease is caused by GI infection with a toxin-producing strain. Any process that disrupts normal flora, impairs the acid barrier defense, alters the normal GI immune response (e.g., IBD), or inhibits intestinal motility may lead to infection. Normal bowel flora appears to be protective, conferring colonization resistance.

By affecting intracellular signaling pathways and cytoskeletal organization, toxins induce an inflammatory response and cell death, leading to diarrhea and pseudomembrane formation. Antibodies against toxin A have been shown to confer protection against symptomatic disease, and failure of antibody production occurs in patients with recurrent disease.

CLINICAL MANIFESTATIONS

Infection with toxin-producing strains of *C. difficile* leads to a spectrum of disease ranging from mild, self-limited diarrhea to explosive, watery diarrhea with occult blood or mucus, to pseudomembranous colitis, and even death. **Pseudomembranous colitis** describes a bloody diarrhea with accompanying fever, abdominal pain/cramps, nausea, and vomiting. Rarely, small-gut involvement, toxic megacolon, bacteremia, abscess formation, intestinal perforation, and even death can occur.

Symptoms of CDI generally begin <1 wk after colonization and may develop during or weeks after antibiotic exposure. They are generally more severe in certain populations, including patients receiving chemotherapy, patients with chronic GI disease (e.g., IBD), and some patients with cystic fibrosis (CF). CDI-associated **reactive arthritis** is an occasional complication, occurring in approximately 1.4% of children with CDI. Reactive arthritis may begin a median of 10.5 days after initial GI symptoms, often accompanied by fever or rash. Joint involvement may be migratory or polyarticular and may resemble septic arthritis.

DIAGNOSIS

Evaluation for CDI should be reserved for children with **diarrhea**, defined as the passage of at least 3 loose stools within a 24 hr period or bloody diarrhea (Fig. 239.1). CDI is diagnosed by the detection of a *C. difficile* **toxin** in the stool of a symptomatic patient. Most patients present with a history of recent antibiotic use, but the absence of antibiotic exposure should not dissuade the astute clinician from considering this diagnosis and ordering the appropriate test. Conversely, high carriage rates without illness among infants should prompt careful consideration when testing and treating children <3 yr old.

The cell culture cytotoxicity assay was replaced as the standard test for toxin detection by **enzyme immunoassay** (EIA), a same-day test for toxin A and/or toxin B with sufficient specificity (94–100%) but less-than-ideal sensitivity (88–93%). Many laboratories use **nucleic acid amplification tests** (NAATs) to supplement or supplant EIA with the goal of improving sensitivity. The sensitivities of the real-time polymerase chain reaction (PCR) assay for toxin A/B were superior compared with EIA for toxin A/B (95% vs 35%, respectively), and the specificity was equal (100%). However, some have questioned the clinical significance of low copy number–positive tests. For example, positive *C. difficile* PCR results occur with similar frequency in patients with IBD with and without an IBD exacerbation. A positive result in a highly sensitive PCR assay that detects low copy numbers of a toxin gene in *C. difficile* may reflect colonization in a subset of patients with IBD, confounding clinical decision-making in managing disease exacerbations. To address this, NAAT-positive tests may be "confirmed" by toxin assays. In addition, eliminating certain high carrier populations from testing (e.g., children under 1 yr of age) will increase the positive predictive value of laboratory testing. Culture for organism isolation is a sensitive test but is labor intensive, taking several days. Culture alone is not specific because it does not differentiate between toxin-producing and non–toxin-producing strains.

Pseudomembranous nodules and characteristic plaques may be seen on colonoscopy or sigmoidoscopy.

TREATMENT

Initial treatment of CDI involves discontinuation of any nonvital antibiotic therapy and administration of fluid and electrolyte replacement. For mild cases, this treatment may be curative. Persistent symptoms or moderate to severe disease warrant antimicrobial therapy directed against *C. difficile*.

Oral **metronidazole** remains the first-line therapy for mild to moderate CDI in children (Table 239.1). For more severe infection, oral **vancomycin** is approved by the U.S. Food and Drug Administration (FDA) for CDI. Vancomycin exhibits ideal pharmacologic properties for treatment of this enteric pathogen, since it is not absorbed in the gut. Vancomycin is suggested as a first-line agent for severe disease, as manifested by hypotension, peripheral leukocytosis, or severe pseudomembranous colitis. Concerns about cost and the emergence of vancomycin-resistant enterococci limit its use as first-line therapy in mild to moderate disease. **Fidaxomicin**, a second-line agent not yet approved for pediatric use, is a narrow-spectrum macrolide antibiotic with noninferior efficacy to vancomycin but superior recurrence prevention. The cost of a course of fidaxomicin can be twice that of vancomycin and 125-fold higher than metronidazole. Reports have demonstrated high treatment efficacy for donor (unaffected) fecal therapy (transplant).

Treatment of adults is different (Table 239.2). Because treatment of CDI continues to evolve, adult-based protocols may be relevant to older children and adolescents.

PROGNOSIS

The response rate to initial treatment of CDI is >95%; however, both the treatment failure rate and the recurrence rate have increased since the late 1990s. Additionally, the risk of subsequent reappearance increases with each recurrence.

Initial recurrence rates are 5–20%, are diagnosed clinically, and generally occur within 4 wk of treatment. Some recurrences result from incomplete eradication of the original strain, and others are caused by reinfection with a different strain. Treatment for the initial recurrence involves retreatment with the original antibiotic course.

Recurrences of CDI may be caused by a suboptimal immune response, failure to kill organisms that have sporulated, or failure of delivery of antibiotic to the site of infection, in the case of ileus or toxic megacolon. Subsequent treatment with pulsed or tapered vancomycin decreases recurrence rates. In addition to this approach, other antibiotics (rifaximin or nitazoxanide), toxin-binding polymers (Tolevamer), and probiotics (*Saccharomyces boulardii* or *Lactobacillus* GG) have been used as adjunctive therapy. Although not well studied in children, *S. boulardii* significantly decreases recurrence rates when used as an adjunct to vancomycin therapy in adults. Because failure to manifest an adequate antitoxin immune response is associated with a higher frequency of recurrent CDI, intravenous immune globulin has been used to treat recurrent disease. In the case of ileus or toxic megacolon, an enema of vancomycin may be used to place the antibiotic directly at the site of infection, although most often intravenous therapy is first attempted in this circumstance.

Fecal microbiota transplantation (FMT) has been used to address the disruption in normal gut flora thought to allow colonization with *C.*

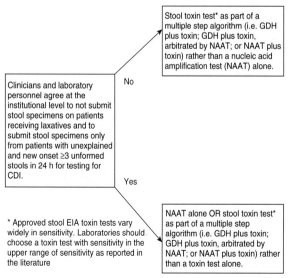

Fig. 239.1 *Clostridium difficile* infection (CDI) laboratory test recommendations based on pre-agreed institutional criteria for patient stool submission. EIA, Enzyme immunoassay; GDH, glutamate dehydrogenase. (*From McDonald LC, Gerding DN, Johnson S, et al: Clinical practice guidelines for* Clostridium difficile *infection in adults and children: 2017 update by the Infectious Diseases Society of America [IDSA] and Society for Healthcare Epidemiology of America [SHEA],* Clin Infect Dis 66(7):e1–e48, 2018, Fig 2.)

difficile (see Table 239.2). FMT involves the instillation of fecal material from a healthy donor into the patient's GI tract by nasoenteric tube, enema, capsules, or colonoscopy. Published FMT results in children with recurrent CDI are limited to case reports and small case series. There are few data to guide clinicians on the indications, route, efficacy, and safety of FMT in children, but investigation is ongoing. Initial reports indicate an overall success rate of approximately 90% in patients with recurrent CDI. Current approaches to FMT are not specific and involve complete reconstitution of the gut microbiome. The gut microbiota has been shown to influence susceptibility to genetic and environmentally acquired conditions. Transplantation of healthy donor fecal material to patients with CDI may reestablish the "normal" composition of the gut microbiota but has the theoretical concern of adding new, microbiome-based susceptibilities derived from the donor microbiome.

It is important to recognize that postinfectious diarrhea may result from other causes, such as postinfectious irritable bowel syndrome, microscopic colitis, and IBD. A test-of-cure is not recommended in the asymptomatic patient, and a positive test for recurrence is not useful until at least 4 wk after the initial test.

PREVENTION

Currently, the strategies for prevention of CDI include recognition of common sites of acquisition (hospitals, childcare settings, extended-care facilities); effective environmental cleaning (i.e., use of chlorinated cleaning solutions); appropriate antibiotic and PPI prescription practices; cohorting of infected patients; **contact precautions**; and proper handwashing with soap and water. Moderate evidence shows that probiotics may reduce the incidence of *C. difficile*–associated diarrhea.

Lastly, with the increasing incidence, morbidity, mortality, and rising healthcare costs from CDI, **immunization** to prevent the disease itself could become an effective paradigm. Although a strong immune response against toxins A and B may prevent the development of CDI, it does not prevent colonization of the host by the bacterium. Therefore, surface proteins involved in adherence have been studied as potential vaccine candidates in animals. Vaccines targeting nontoxin antigens will likely be needed to prevent colonization, reduce spore production, and interrupt disease transmission, especially in high-risk populations.

Bibliography is available at Expert Consult.

Table 239.1	Recommendations for the Treatment of *Clostridium difficile* Infection in Children			
CLINICAL DEFINITION	**RECOMMENDED TREATMENT**	**PEDIATRIC DOSE**	**MAXIMUM DOSE**	**STRENGTH OF RECOMMENDATION/ QUALITY OF EVIDENCE**
Initial episode, nonsevere	Metronidazole × 10 days PO *or*	7.5 mg/kg/dose tid or qid	500 mg tid or qid	Weak/Low
	Vancomycin × 10 days PO	10 mg/kg/dose qid	125 mg qid	Weak/Low
Initial episode, severe/fulminant	Vancomycin × 10 days PO or PR *with or without*	10 mg/kg/dose qid	500 mg qid	Strong/Moderate
	Metronidazole × 10 days IV*	10 mg/kg/dose tid	500 mg tid	Weak/Low
First recurrence, nonsevere	Metronidazole × 10 days PO *or*	7.5 mg/kg/dose tid or qid	500 mg tid or qid	Weak/Low
	Vancomycin × 10 days PO	10 mg/kg/dose qid	125 mg qid	Weak/Low
Second or subsequent recurrence	Vancomycin in a tapered and pulsed regimen† *or*	10 mg/kg/dose qid	125 mg qid	Weak/Low
	Vancomycin × 10 days, followed by rifaximin‡ × 20 days *or*	Vancomycin, 10 mg/kg/dose qid; rifaximin: no pediatric dosing	Vancomycin, 500 mg qid; rifaximin, 400 mg tid	Weak/Low
	Fecal microbiota transplantation			Weak/Very low

*In cases of severe or fulminant *Clostridium difficile* infection associated with critical illness, consider addition of intravenous metronidazole to oral vancomycin.
†Tapered and pulsed regimen: vancomycin, 10 mg/kg with max of 125 mg 4 times daily for 10-14 days, then 10 mg/kg with max of 125 mg twice daily for 1 wk, then 10 mg/kg with max of 125 mg once daily for 1 wk, and then 10 mg/kg with max of 125 mg every 2 or 3 days for 2-8 wk.
‡No pediatric dosing for rifaximin; not approved by the U.S. Food and Drug Administration for use in children <12 yr old.
IV, Intravenously; PO, orally; PR, rectally; tid, 3 times daily; qid, 4 times daily.
Adapted from McDonald LC, Gerding DN, Johnson S, et al: Clinical practice guidelines for *Clostridium difficile* infection in adults and children: 2017 update by the Infectious Diseases Society of America (IDSA) and Society for Healthcare Epidemiology of America (SHEA), *Clin Infect Dis* 66(7):e1–e48, 2018 (Table 2).

Table 239.2	Recommendations for the Treatment of *Clostridium difficile* Infection in Adults		
CLINICAL DEFINITION	**SUPPORTIVE CLINICAL DATA**	**RECOMMENDED TREATMENT***	**STRENGTH OF RECOMMENDATION/ QUALITY OF EVIDENCE**
Initial episode, nonsevere	Leukocytosis with white blood cell count of ≤15,000 cells/mL and serum creatinine level <1.5 mg/dL	VAN, 125 mg qid × 10 days *or*	Strong/High
		FDX, 200 mg bid × 10 days	Strong/High
		Alternate if above agents are unavailable: metronidazole, 500 mg tid PO × 10 days	Weak/High
Initial episode, severe†	Leukocytosis with a white blood cell count of ≥15,000 cells/mL or a serum creatinine level >1.5 mg/dL	VAN, 125 mg qid PO × 10 days *or*	Strong/High
		FDX, 200 mg bid × 10 days	Strong/High

Continued

Table 239.2 | Recommendations for the Treatment of *Clostridium difficile* Infection in Adults

CLINICAL DEFINITION	SUPPORTIVE CLINICAL DATA	RECOMMENDED TREATMENT*	STRENGTH OF RECOMMENDATION/ QUALITY OF EVIDENCE
Initial episode, fulminant	Hypotension or shock, ileus, megacolon	VAN, 500 mg qid PO or by nasogastric tube. If ileus, consider adding rectal instillation of VAN. Intravenous metronidazole (500 mg every 8 hr) should be administered with oral or rectal VAN, particularly if ileus is present.	Strong/Moderate (oral VAN) Weak/Low (rectal VAN) Strong/Moderate (intravenous metronidazole)
First recurrence		VAN, 125 mg qid × 10 days, if metronidazole was used for the initial episode *or*	Weak/Low
		Use prolonged tapered and pulsed VAN regimen if standard regimen was used for initial episode (e.g., 125 mg qid for 10-14 days, bid for 1 wk, qd for 1 wk, and then every 2 or 3 days for 2-8 wk) *or*	Weak/Low
		FDX, 200 mg bid ×for 10 days if VAN was used for the initial episode	Weak/Moderate
Second or subsequent recurrence		VAN in a tapered and pulsed regimen *or*	Weak/Low
		VAN, 125 mg qid PO × 10 days, followed by rifaximin, 400 mg tid × 20 days *or*	Weak/Low
		FDX, 200 mg bid × 10 days *or*	Weak/Low
		Fecal microbiota transplantation‡	Strong/Moderate

*All randomized trials have compared 10-day treatment courses, but some patients (particularly those treated with metronidazole) may have delayed response to treatment, and clinicians should consider extending treatment duration to 14 days in those circumstances.

†The criteria proposed for defining severe or fulminant *Clostridium difficile* infection (CDI) are based on expert opinion. These may need to be reviewed in the future on publication of prospectively validated severity scores for patients with CDI.

‡The opinion of the panel is that appropriate antibiotic treatments for at least 2 recurrences (i.e., 3 CDI episodes) should be tried before offering fecal microbiota transplantation.

FDX, Fidaxomicin; VAN, vancomycin; PO, orally (by mouth); qd, once daily; bid, twice daily; tid, 3 times daily; qid, 4 times daily.

Adapted from McDonald LC, Gerding DN, Johnson S, et al: Clinical practice guidelines for *Clostridium difficile* infection in adults and children: 2017 update by the Infectious Diseases Society of America (IDSA) and Society for Healthcare Epidemiology of America (SHEA), *Clin Infect Dis* 66(7):e1–e48, 2018 (Table 1).

Chapter 240
Other Anaerobic Infections
Sindhu Mohandas and Michael J. Chusid

第二百四十章
其他厌氧菌感染

中文导读

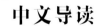

　　本章集中讨论与专性厌氧细菌感染有关的情况。厌氧菌感染通常是由内源菌群引起的，多发生于黏膜，常与需氧菌混合感染，可发生血行播散，影响于身体各个系统。在临床表现部分详解介绍了菌血症、中枢神经系统、上呼吸道、下呼吸道、腹腔、生殖系统、皮肤和软组织等各部分感染的临床表现，培养和

核酸检测为病原菌诊断的主要方法，厌氧菌感染的治疗通常需要充分的引流和适当的抗感染治疗，抗感染药的选择需根据病原体确定。常见的厌氧菌有梭状芽孢杆菌、拟杆菌和普氏菌属、梭杆菌、韦荣氏球菌、厌氧球菌，并对各类病原体的感染部位、感染的临床表现等作了详细介绍。

Anaerobic bacteria are among the most numerous organisms colonizing humans. Anaerobes are present in soil and are normal inhabitants of all living animals, but infections caused by anaerobes are relatively uncommon. **Obligate anaerobes** are markedly or entirely intolerant of exposure to oxygen. **Facultative anaerobes** can survive in the presence of environmental oxygen but grow better in settings of reduced oxygen tension. This chapter concentrates on conditions associated with obligate anaerobic bacterial infection.

Infections with anaerobes frequently occur adjacent to mucosal surfaces, often as **mixed infections** with aerobes. Conditions of reduced oxygen tension provide the optimal conditions for proliferation of anaerobes. Traumatized areas, devascularized areas, and areas of crush injury are all ideal sites for anaerobic infection. Frequently, both aerobic and anaerobic organisms invade devitalized areas, with local extension and bacteremia most often caused by the more virulent aerobes. Abscess formation evolves over days to weeks and generally involves both aerobes and anaerobes. Examples of such infections include appendicitis and periappendiceal, pelvic, perirectal, peritonsillar, retropharyngeal, parapharyngeal, pulmonary, and dental abscesses. **Septic thrombophlebitis,** as a consequence of appendicitis, chronic sinusitis, pharyngitis, and otitis media, provides a route for hematogenous spread of anaerobic infection to parenchymal organs such as the liver, brain, and lungs.

Anaerobic infection is usually caused by endogenous flora. Combinations of impaired physical barriers to infection, compromised tissue viability, ecologic alterations in normal flora, impaired host immunity, and anaerobic bacterial virulence factors contribute to infection with normal anaerobic inhabitants of mucous membranes. Bacterial virulence factors include capsules, toxins, enzymes, and fatty acids.

CLINICAL MANIFESTATIONS

Anaerobic infections occur in a variety of sites throughout the body (Table 240.1). Anaerobes often coexist synergistically with aerobes. Infections with anaerobes are usually polymicrobial, including an aerobic component.

Bacteremia

Anaerobes account for approximately 5% of bloodstream bacterial isolates in adults, but this rate is lower in children. The most common blood isolates of anaerobic bacteria in children are *Bacteroides fragilis* group, *Peptostreptococcus, Clostridium,* and *Fusobacterium* spp.

Isolation of anaerobes from the blood is often an indication of a serious primary anaerobic infection. The lower gastrointestinal (GI) tract and wound infections are the 2 most common sources for bacteremia. Risk factors for anaerobic bacteremia include malignancy, hematologic disorders, solid-organ transplant, recent surgery (GI, obstetric, gynecologic), intestinal obstruction, decubiti, dental extraction, early infancy, sickle cell disease, diabetes mellitus, splenectomy, and chemotherapy or other immunosuppressive drug use.

As with certain aerobes, the cell wall of gram-negative anaerobes may contain **endotoxins,** which can be associated with the development of hypotension and shock when present in the circulatory system. Clostridia produce **hemolysins,** and the presence of these organisms in the blood can result in massive hemolysis and cardiovascular collapse.

Central Nervous System

Anaerobic **meningitis** is rare but can occur in neonates as a complication of ear or neck infections or from anatomic defects of meninges (dural sinus tracts). Anaerobic cerebrospinal fluid (CSF) shunt infections may occur when the distal end of the ventriculoperitoneal shunt perforates the intestinal tract.

Brain abscess and subdural empyema are usually polymicrobial, with anaerobes typically involved (see Chapter 622). Brain abscess usually occurs because of spread from infected sinuses, middle ear, or lung and rarely from endocarditis. *Clostridium perfringens* can cause brain abscess and meningitis after head injuries or after intracranial surgery. Brain abscesses may require surgical drainage combined with a prolonged course of antibiotic therapy.

Upper Respiratory Tract

The respiratory tract is colonized by both aerobes and anaerobes. Anaerobic bacteria are involved in chronic sinusitis, chronic otitis media, peritonsillar infections, parapharyngeal and retropharyngeal abscesses, and periodontal infections. The predominant organisms involved are *Prevotella, Porphyromonas, Bacteroides, Fusobacterium,* and *Peptostreptococcus* spp.

Anaerobic periodontal disease is most common in patients with poor dental hygiene or who are receiving drugs that induce gingival hypertrophy. **Vincent angina,** also known as **acute necrotizing ulcerative gingivitis** or **trench mouth,** is an acute, fulminating, mixed anaerobic bacterial-spirochetal infection of the gingival margin and floor of the mouth. It is characterized by gingival pain, foul breath, and pseudomembrane formation. **Ludwig angina** is an acute, life-threatening cellulitis of dental origin of the sublingual and submandibular spaces. Infection spreads rapidly in the neck and may cause sudden airway obstruction.

Lemierre syndrome, or **postanginal sepsis,** is a suppurative infection of the lateral pharyngeal space, of increasing prevalence, that often begins as pharyngitis (see Chapter 409). It may complicate Epstein-Barr virus or other viral and bacterial infections of the pharynx. It usually manifests as a unilateral septic thrombophlebitis of the jugular venous system with septic pulmonary embolization. Patients present with prolonged pharyngitis, neck pain and fever. Clinical signs include unilateral painful cervical swelling, trismus, and dysphagia, culminating with signs of sepsis and respiratory distress. *Fusobacterium necrophorum* is the most commonly isolated organism, although polymicrobial infection may occur. Metastatic infections involving muscles, bones, internal organs (often lungs), and the brain can occur as a complication of Lemierre syndrome.

Lower Respiratory Tract

Anaerobic lung abscess, empyema, and anaerobic pneumonia are most often encountered in children who have disordered swallowing or seizures or in whom an inhaled foreign body is occluding a bronchus. Infections are usually polymicrobial. Children and adults can aspirate oral or gastric contents during sleep, seizure, or periods of unconsciousness. In most cases, lung cilia and phagocytes clear particulate matter and microbes. If the aspiration is of increased volume or frequency or a foreign body blocks normal ciliary clearance, normal pulmonary clearance mechanisms are overcome and infection ensues. Appropriate cultures need to avoid specimen contamination with oral flora through use of bronchoalveolar lavage, lung biopsy, or thoracentesis.

In unusual cases, particularly in patients with poor dental hygiene, aspirated mouth contents may contain the anaerobe *Actinomyces israelii,* resulting in pulmonary actinomycosis (see Chapter 216). Anaerobic pneumonitis associated with this microorganism is remarkable for the ability of the infection to traverse tissue planes. Affected patients often develop fistulas on their chest walls overlying areas of intrathoracic

Table 240.1	Infections Associated With Anaerobic Bacteria	
SITE AND INFECTION	**MAJOR RISK FACTORS**	**ANAEROBIC BACTERIA***
CENTRAL NERVOUS SYSTEM		
Cerebral abscess	Cyanotic heart disease Cystic fibrosis Penetrating trauma	Polymicrobial *Prevotella* *Porphyromonas* *Bacteroides* *Fusobacterium* *Peptostreptococcus*
Epidural and subdural empyemas, meningitis	Direct extension from contiguous sinusitis, otitis media, mastoiditis, or anatomic defect involving the dura	*Bacteroides fragilis*[†] *Fusobacterium* *Peptostreptococcus* *Veillonella*
UPPER RESPIRATORY TRACT		
Dental abscess	Poor periodontal hygiene	*Peptostreptococcus*
Ludwig angina (cellulitis of sublingual-submandibular space)	Drugs producing gingival hypertrophy	*Fusobacterium*
Necrotizing gingivitis (Vincent stomatitis)		*Prevotella melaninogenica* *Fusobacterium*
Chronic otitis-mastoiditis-sinusitis	Tympanic perforation Tympanostomy tubes	*Prevotella* *Bacteroides* *Fusobacterium* *Peptostreptococcus*
Peritonsillar abscess	Streptococcal pharyngitis	*Fusobacterium*
Retropharyngeal abscess	Penetrating injury	*Prevotella* *Porphyromonas*
Lemierre syndrome	Preexisting viral or bacterial pharyngitis	*Fusobacterium*
LOWER RESPIRATORY TRACT		
Aspiration pneumonia	Periodontal disease	Polymicrobial *Prevotella* *Porphyromonas* *Fusobacterium* *Peptostreptococcus*
Necrotizing pneumonitis	Bronchial obstruction	*P. melaninogenica*
Lung abscess	Altered gag or consciousness Aspirated foreign body Sequestered lobe Vascular anomaly	*Bacteroides intermedius* *Fusobacterium* *Peptostreptococcus* *Eubacterium* *B. fragilis* *Veillonella*
Septic pulmonary emboli		*Fusobacterium*
INTRAABDOMINAL		
Abscess	Appendicitis	Polymicrobial *B. fragilis* *Bilophila wadsworthia* *Peptostreptococcus* *Clostridium* spp.
Secondary peritonitis	Penetrating trauma (especially of the colon)	*Bacteroides* *Clostridium* *Peptostreptococcus* *Eubacterium* *Fusobacterium*
FEMALE GENITAL TRACT		
Bartholin abscess	Vaginosis	*B. fragilis*
Tuboovarian abscess	Intrauterine device	*Bacteroides bivius*
Endometritis		*Peptostreptococcus*
Pelvic thrombophlebitis		*Clostridium*
Salpingitis		*Mobiluncus*
Chorioamnionitis		*Actinomyces*
Septic abortion		*Clostridium*
SKIN AND SOFT TISSUE		
Cellulitis	Decubitus ulcers	Varies with site and contamination with oral or enteric flora
Perirectal cellulitis	Abdominal wounds	*Clostridium perfringens* (myonecrosis)
Myonecrosis (gas gangrene)	Pilonidal sinus	*Bacteroides* *Clostridium*
Necrotizing fasciitis and synergistic gangrene	Trauma Human and animal bites Immunosuppressed or neutropenic patients Varicella	*Fusobacterium* *Clostridium tertium* *Clostridium septicum* Anaerobic streptococci

Continued

Table 240.1	Infections Associated With Anaerobic Bacteria——cont'd	
SITE AND INFECTION	**MAJOR RISK FACTORS**	**ANAEROBIC BACTERIA***
BLOOD Bacteremia	Intraabdominal infection, abscesses, myonecrosis, necrotizing fasciitis	B. fragilis Clostridium Peptostreptococcus Fusobacterium

*Infections may also be from or may involve aerobic bacteria as the sole agent or as part of a mixed infection; brain abscess may contain microaerophilic streptococci; intraabdominal infections may contain gram-negative enteric organisms and enterococci; and salpingitis may contain *Neisseria gonorrhoeae* and *Chlamydia trachomatis*.
†*Bacteroides fragilis* is usually isolated from infections below the diaphragm except for brain abscesses.

infection. These may extrude distinctive, pathognomonic particles composed of bacterial colonies, called "sulfur granules."

Intraabdominal Infection
The entire digestive tract is heavily colonized with anaerobes. The density of organisms is highest in the colon, where anaerobes outnumber aerobes 1,000 : 1. Perforation of the gut leads to leakage of intestinal flora into the peritoneum, resulting in peritonitis involving both aerobes and anaerobes. Secondary sepsis caused by aerobes often occurs early. As the peritoneal infection is walled off, an abscess containing both aerobes and anaerobes often evolves. The predominant aerobic organisms are *Escherichia coli* and *Streptococcus* spp. (including *Enterococcus* spp.), and the anaerobes are the *B. fragilis* group, *Peptostreptococcus*, *Clostridium*, and *Fusobacterium* spp.

Secondary hepatic abscesses may then develop as complications of appendicitis, intestinal perforation, inflammatory bowel disease, or biliary tract disease. In children with malignancy receiving chemotherapy, the intestinal mucosa is often damaged, leading to translocation of bacteria and focal invasion of bowel wall. **Typhlitis** is a mixed infection of the gut wall in neutropenic patients, usually located in the ileocecum and characterized by abdominal pain, diarrhea, fever, and abdominal distention. Similarly, a mixed aerobic-anaerobic infection of the intestinal wall and peritoneum may develop in a small infant as a complication of **necrotizing enterocolitis**, believed to be a result of the relative vascular insufficiency of the gut and hypoxia (see Chapter 123.2).

Genital Tract
Pelvic inflammatory disease and tuboovarian abscesses are frequently caused by mixed aerobic-anaerobic infection. Vaginitis can be caused by overgrowth of anaerobic flora. Anaerobes frequently contribute to chorioamnionitis and premature labor and may result in anaerobic bacteremia of the newborn. Although these bacteremias are often transient, anaerobes occasionally cause invasive disease in the newborn, including central nervous system (CNS) infection.

Skin and Soft Tissue
Anaerobic skin infections occur in the setting of bites, foreign bodies, and skin and tissue ulceration because of pressure necrosis or lack of adequate blood supply. Animal bites and human bites inoculate oral and skin flora into damaged and hypoxic cutaneous tissue. The extent of the infection depends on the depth of the bite and the associated crush injury to the tissues. In immunocompromised patients, unusual oral anaerobes such as *Capnocytophaga canimorsus* can cause life-threatening infection.

Clostridial myonecrosis, or **gas gangrene**, is a rapidly progressive infection of deep soft tissues, primarily muscles, associated with *Clostridium perfringens*. **Necrotizing fasciitis** is a more superficial, polymicrobial infection of the subcutaneous space with acute onset and rapid progression that has significant morbidity and mortality (see Chapter 685.2). Group A streptococcus, known in the lay press as the "flesh-eating bacteria," and *Staphylococcus aureus* are occasionally the causative pathogens. Typically, necrotizing fasciitis is produced by combined infection of *S. aureus* or gram-negative bacilli and anaerobic streptococci, termed **synergistic gangrene**. This infection is often seen as a complication of varicella following secondary infection of a cutaneous vesicle. Diabetic patients may develop a particularly aggressive and destructive synergistic gangrene of the inguinal area and adjacent scrotum or vulva known as **Fournier gangrene**. Early recognition with aggressive surgical debridement and antimicrobial therapy is necessary to limit disfiguring morbidity and mortality.

Other Sites
Occasionally, the bone adjacent to an anaerobic infection becomes infected by direct extension from a contiguous infection in cranial and facial bones or by direct inoculation associated with trauma to tubular bones. Anaerobic septic arthritis is rare, and risk factors include trauma and prosthetic joints. Most infections are monomicrobial, and the organism isolated is related to the route of infection. *Peptostreptococcus* and *P. acnes* are isolated in prosthetic joint infections, *B. fragilis* and fusobacteria in hematogenous infections, and clostridia following trauma.

Anaerobic infections of the kidneys (renal and perirenal abscesses) and heart (pericarditis) are rare. **Enteritis necroticans** ("pigbel") is a rare but often fatal GI infection that can follow ingestion of a large meal in a chronically starved child or adult. It is associated with the consumption of pork and is believed to be caused by *Clostridium welchii* type C (an organism not usually present in the human intestine), the organism being transmitted by contaminated pig meat. Anaerobic **osteomyelitis**, particularly of fingers and toes, can complicate any process capable of producing hypoxic necrosis, including diabetes, neuropathies, vasculopathies, and coagulopathies.

DIAGNOSIS
The diagnosis of anaerobic infection requires a high index of suspicion and the collection of appropriate and adequate specimens for anaerobic culture (Table 240.2). Culture specimens should be obtained in a manner that protects them from contamination with mucosal bacteria and from exposure to ambient oxygen. Swab samples from mucosal surfaces, nasal secretions, respiratory specimens, and stool should *not* be sent for anaerobic culture because these sites normally harbor anaerobic flora. Aspirates of infected sites, abscess material, and biopsy specimens are appropriate for anaerobic culturing. Specimens should be protected from atmospheric oxygen and transported to the laboratory immediately. Anaerobic transport medium is used to increase the likelihood of recovery of obligate anaerobes. Gram staining of abscess fluid from suspected anaerobic infections is useful because even if the organisms do not grow in culture, they can be seen on the smear.

Antimicrobial resistance among anaerobes has consistently increased over time, and the susceptibility of anaerobic agents to antimicrobial agents has become less predictable. A rapid and simple screening test for antibiotic susceptibility can be used to detect β-lactamase production and presumptive penicillin resistance. More detailed susceptibility testing, available at reference laboratories, is recommended for isolates recovered from sterile body sites or those that are clinically important and are known to have variable or unique susceptibilities.

Recent advances in direct detection of anaerobes from clinical samples include 16S ribosomal RNA (16S rRNA) gene-based methods, DNA hybridization, matrix-assisted laser desorption/ionization time-of-flight

Table 240.2	Clues to Presumptive Diagnosis of Anaerobic Infections*

Infection contiguous to or near a mucosal surface colonized with anaerobic bacteria (oropharynx, intestinal-genitourinary tract)

Putrid odor

Severe tissue necrosis, abscesses, gangrene, or fasciitis

Gas formation in tissues (crepitus on exam or visible on plain radiograph)

Failure to recover organisms using conventional aerobic microbiologic methods, despite the presence of mixed pleomorphic organisms on smears

Failure of organisms to grow after pretreatment with antibiotics effective against anaerobes

Failure of clinical response to antibiotic therapy poorly effective against anaerobic bacteria (e.g., aminoglycosides)

"Sulfur granules" in discharges caused by actinomycosis

Toxin-mediated syndromes: botulism, tetanus, gas gangrene, food poisoning, pseudomembranous colitis

Infections associated with anaerobic bacteria (see Table 240.1)

Septic thrombophlebitis

Septicemic syndrome with jaundice or intravascular hemolysis

Typical appearance on Gram stain:
  Bacteroides spp.—small, delicate, pleomorphic, pale, gram-negative bacilli
  Fusobacterium nucleatum—thin, gram-negative bacilli with fusiform shape, pointed ends
  Fusobacterium necrophorum—pleomorphic gram-negative bacilli with rounded ends
  Peptostreptococcus—chained, gram-positive cocci similar to aerobic cocci
  Clostridium perfringens—large, short, fat (boxcar-shaped) gram-positive bacilli

*Suspicion of anaerobic infection is critical before specimens are sampled for culture, to ensure optimal microbiologic techniques and prompt, appropriate therapy.

mass spectrometry (MALDI-TOF MS), multiplex PCR, and oligonucleotide array technologies. MALDI-TOF MS has been used as a rapid method to identify infectious agents, including many anaerobes. 16S rRNA gene sequencing can be used for isolates whose identification by MS is unreliable.

TREATMENT

Treatment of anaerobic infections usually requires adequate drainage and appropriate antimicrobial therapy. Antibiotic therapy varies depending on the suspected or proven anaerobe involved. Many oral anaerobic bacterial species are susceptible to penicillins, although some strains may produce a β-lactamase. Drugs that are active against such strains include metronidazole, penicillins combined with β-lactamase inhibitors (ampicillin-sulbactam, ticarcillin-clavulanate, piperacillin-tazobactam), carbapenems (imipenem, meropenem, doripenem, ertapenem), clindamycin, tigecycline, linezolid, and cefoxitin. Penicillin and vancomycin are active against the gram-positive anaerobes.

Increasing resistance to antimicrobials has been noted among anaerobes, particularly with *Bacteroides* spp. Clindamycin is no longer recommended in the empirical treatment of abdominal infections due to increasing resistance among *Bacteroides*. Aerobes are usually present with the anaerobes, necessitating broad-spectrum antibiotic combinations for empirical therapy. Specific therapy is based on culture results and clinical course.

For **soft tissue infections**, providing adequate perfusion to the area is critical. At times, a muscle flap or skin flap procedure is needed to ensure that nutrients and antimicrobial agents are brought to the affected area and adequate oxygen tension is maintained. Drainage of infected areas is often necessary for cure. Bacteria may survive in abscesses because of high bacterial inoculum, lack of bactericidal activity, and local conditions that facilitate bacterial proliferation. Aspiration is sometimes effective for small collections, whereas incision and drainage may be required for larger abscesses. Extensive debridement and resection

of all devitalized tissue are needed to control fasciitis and myonecrosis. Adjunctive **hyperbaric oxygen** (HBO) therapy has been found to be beneficial in a few uncontrolled studies. However, it should be recognized that surgical treatment is critical and should never be delayed for the provision of HBO therapy.

Uncomplicated infections caused by anaerobic organisms are generally treated for 2-4 wk. Some infections, including osteomyelitis and brain abscess, may need longer treatment of 6-8 wk.

COMMON ANAEROBIC PATHOGENS
Clostridium
Strains of *Clostridium* cause disease by proliferation and often by production of toxins. Of the >60 species that have been identified, only a few cause infections in humans. The most frequently implicated *Clostridium* spp. are *C. difficile* (Chapter 239), *C. perfringens*, *C. botulinum* (Chapter 237), *C. tetani* (Chapter 238), *C. butyricum*, *C. septicum*, *C. sordellii*, *C. tertium*, and *C. histolyticum*.

Clostridia can cause unique histotoxic syndromes produced by specific toxins (e.g., gas gangrene, food poisoning) as well as nonsyndromic infections (e.g., abscess, local infections, sepsis).Based on the clinical syndrome produced, clostridial species are categorized into 3 groups: **histotoxic** (*C. perfringens*, *C. ramosum*, *C. novyi*, *C. septicum*, *C. bifermentans*, and *C. sordellii*), **enterotoxigenic** (*C. perfringens* and *C. difficile*), and **neurotoxic** (*C. tetani* and *C. botulinum*).

C. perfringens produces a variety of toxins and virulence factors. Strains of *C. perfringens* are designated A through E. **Alpha toxin** is a phospholipase that hydrolyzes sphingomyelin and lecithin and is produced by all strains. This toxin causes hemolysis, platelet lysis, increased capillary permeability, and hepatotoxicity. **Beta toxin**, produced by strains B and C, causes hemorrhagic necrosis of the small bowel. **Epsilon toxin** is produced by B and D strains and injures vascular endothelial cells, leading to increased vascular permeability, edema, and organ dysfunction. **Iota toxin,** produced by E strains, causes dermal edema. An enterotoxin is produced by type A and some type C and D strains. Hemolysins and a variety of enzymes are produced by many *C. perfringens* strains.

Clostridia can be involved in various other polymicrobial pediatric infections: arthritis, osteomyelitis, skin and soft tissue infections (often after trauma or foreign body penetration), intraabdominal, pulmonary, intracranial, and pelvic infections; abscesses; and panophthalmitis.

Clostridial species invade the bloodstream shortly before, during, or just after death, leading to contamination of tissues that may be donated for transplantation. A large outbreak of *Clostridium* infections in tissue graft recipients was reported in 14 patients who received musculoskeletal grafts processed at a single tissue bank. Because of this outbreak, recommendations for tissue processing now include a processing method that kills bacterial spores.

Myonecrosis (Gas Gangrene)
Clostridium perfringens is the major etiologic cause of myonecrosis, a rapidly progressive anaerobic soft tissue infection. Gas gangrene usually affects muscles compromised by surgery, trauma, or vascular insufficiency that become contaminated with *C. perfringens* spores, usually from foreign material or a medical device. Wounds can be contaminated by *C. perfringens* spores from the skin, dirt, soil, and clothing, especially wounds in the lower trunk.

In immunocompromised persons, especially patients receiving cancer chemotherapy, *C. septicum* is a classic cause of rapidly fatal gas gangrene. A clue to the diagnosis of gas gangrene is pain out of proportion to the clinical appearance of the wound. Infection progresses rapidly with edema, swelling, myonecrosis, and sometimes crepitation of soft tissues. Hypotension, mental confusion, shock, and renal failure are common. A characteristic sweet odor is present in the serosanguineous discharge. The exudate reveals gram-positive bacilli but few leukocytes. Early and complete debridement with excision of necrotic tissue is key to controlling the infection. Repeated, frequent assessment of tissue viability in the operating room is required. High-dose penicillin (250,000 units/kg/day divided every 4-6 hr [q4-6h] intravenously [IV]) or clindamycin (25-40 mg/kg/day divided q6-8h IV) can be employed in pure clostridial infections. If, as is often the case, a mixed bacterial infection is suspected, broader antibiotic coverage is warranted, with an agent such as piperacillin-tazobactam (300 mg/kg/day divided q6hr IV) or meropenem (60 mg/kg/day divided q8h IV). Addition of clindamycin or vancomycin is warranted if staphylococcal or streptococcal co-infection is suspected.

Aggressive supportive care is essential, and amputation of affected limbs is often required. HBO therapy can reduce tissue loss and thus the extent of debridement and has been beneficial in a few studies. However, HBO should only be used as an adjunct to surgical treatment, which is primary.

The prognosis for patients with myonecrosis is poor, even with early, aggressive therapy.

Food Poisoning

Clostridium perfringens type A produces an enterotoxin that causes food poisoning. This intoxication results in the acute onset of watery diarrhea and crampy abdominal pain. The usual foods containing toxin are improperly prepared or stored meats and gravies. A specific etiologic diagnosis is rarely made in children with food poisoning. Therapy consists of rehydration and electrolyte replacement if necessary. The illness resolves spontaneously within 24 hr of onset. Prevention requires the maintenance of hot food at a temperature ≥74°C (165.2°F).

Bacteroides and Prevotella

Bacteroides fragilis is one of the more virulent anaerobic pathogens and is most frequently recovered from blood cultures and cultures of tissue or pus. The most common *B. fragilis* infection in children occurs as a complication of **appendicitis**. The organism is part of normal colonic flora but is not common in the mouth or respiratory tract. *B. fragilis* is usually found as part of polymicrobial appendiceal and other intraabdominal abscesses and is often involved in genital tract infections such as pelvic inflammatory disease and tuboovarian abscess. *Prevotella* organisms are normal oral flora, and *Prevotella* infection typically involves gums, teeth, tonsils, and parapharyngeal spaces. Both *B. fragilis* and *Prevotella* may be involved in aspiration pneumonitis and lung abscess.

Strains of *B. fragilis* and *Prevotella melaninogenica* produce β-lactamase and are resistant to penicillins. Recommended treatment is with ticarcillin-clavulanate, piperacillin-tazobactam, cefoxitin, metronidazole, clindamycin, imipenem, or meropenem. Increasing rates of antimicrobial resistance has been seen in *Bacteroides* spp. over the last few decades. *B. fragilis* resistance to clindamycin is increasing worldwide and has reached 40% in some locales. Therefore, clindamycin is no longer recommended as empirical therapy for intraabdominal infections.

Because infections involving *B. fragilis* and *P. melaninogenica* are usually polymicrobial, therapy should include antimicrobial agents active against likely concomitant aerobic pathogens. Drainage of abscesses and debridement of necrotic tissue are often required for control of these infections.

Fusobacterium

Fusobacterium organisms inhabit the intestine, respiratory tract, and female genital tracts. These organisms, which are more virulent than most of the normal anaerobic flora, cause bacteremia and a variety of rapidly progressive infections. **Lemierre syndrome**, bone and joint infections, and abdominal and genital tract infections are most common. Some strains produce a β-lactamase and are resistant to penicillins, requiring therapy with drugs such as ampicillin-sulbactam and clindamycin.

Veillonella

Veillonella spp. are normal flora of the mouth, upper respiratory tract, intestine, and vagina. These anaerobes rarely cause infection. Strains are recovered as part of the polymicrobial flora causing abscess, chronic sinusitis, empyema, peritonitis, and wound infection. *Veillonella* spp. are susceptible to penicillins, cephalosporins, clindamycin, metronidazole, and carbapenems.

Anaerobic Cocci

Peptostreptococcus spp. are normal flora of the skin, respiratory tract, and gut. These organisms are often present in brain abscesses, chronic sinusitis, chronic otitis, and lung abscesses. Such infections are often polymicrobial, and therapy is aimed at the accompanying aerobes as well as the anaerobes. Most of the gram-positive cocci are susceptible to penicillin, cephalosporins, carbapenems, and vancomycin.

Bibliography is available at Expert Consult.

Section **7**

Mycobacterial Infections

第七篇
分枝杆菌感染

Chapter **241**

Principles of Antimycobacterial Therapy

Stacene R. Maroushek

第二百四十一章
抗分枝杆菌治疗原则

中文导读

本章主要介绍了结核分枝杆菌、麻风分枝杆菌、非结核分枝杆菌的治疗原则。对于结核分枝杆菌的治疗主要分为一线药物和二线药物两大板块，对作用机制、用药剂量以及药物的副作用进行了详细介绍，并详细介绍了不同类型的结核病的治疗方案。详细介绍了治疗麻风分枝杆菌的药物（氨苯砜、氯法齐明）的药理、药量及副作用。在非结核分支杆菌部分详细介绍了各个药物的药理、用量及副作用，并针对不同的非结核分枝杆菌给出了针对性的治疗方案。

The treatment of mycobacterial infection and disease can be challenging. Patients require therapy with multiple agents, the offending pathogens commonly exhibit complex drug resistance patterns, and patients often have underlying conditions that affect drug choice and monitoring. Several of the drugs have not been well studied in children, and current recommendations are extrapolated from the experience in adults.

Single-drug therapy of *Mycobacterium tuberculosis* and nontuberculous mycobacteria is not recommended because of the high likelihood of developing antimicrobial resistance. Susceptibility testing of mycobacterial isolates often can aid in therapeutic decision-making.

AGENTS USED AGAINST *MYCOBACTERIUM TUBERCULOSIS*
Commonly Used Agents
Isoniazid
Isoniazid (**INH**) is a hydrazide form of isonicotinic acid and is bactericidal for rapidly growing *M. tuberculosis*. The primary target of INH involves the *INHA* gene, which encodes the enoyl ACP (acyl carrier protein) reductase needed for the last step of the mycolic acid biosynthesis pathway of cell wall production. Resistance to INH occurs following mutations in the *INHA* gene or in other genes encoding enzymes that activate INH, such as *katG*.

INH is indicated for the treatment of *M. tuberculosis*, *M. kansasii*, and *M. bovis*. The pediatric dosage is 10-15 mg/kg/day orally (PO) in a single dose, not to exceed 300 mg/day. The adult dosage is 5 mg/kg/day PO in a single dose, not to exceed 300 mg/day. Alternative pediatric dosing is 20-30 mg/kg PO in a single dose, not to exceed 900 mg/dose, given twice weekly under **directly observed therapy (DOT)**, in which patients are observed to ingest each dose of antituberculosis medication to maximize the likelihood of completing therapy. The duration of treatment depends on the disease being treated (Table 241.1). INH needs to be taken 1 hr before or 2 hr after meals because food decreases absorption. It is available in liquid, tablet, intravenous (IV; not approved

Table 241.1	Recommended Usual Treatment Regimens for Drug-Susceptible Tuberculosis in Infants, Children, and Adolescents

INFECTION/DISEASE CATEGORY	REGIMEN	COMMENTS
LATENT *MYCOBACTERIUM TUBERCULOSIS* INFECTION[a]		
Isoniazid susceptible	12 weeks of isoniazid plus rifapentine, once a week *or* 4 mo of rifampin, once a day *or* 9 mo of isoniazid, once a day	Continuous daily therapy is required. Intermittent therapy even by DOT is not recommended. If daily therapy is not possible, DOT twice a week can be used for 9 mo.
Isoniazid resistant	4 mo of rifampin, once a day	Continuous daily therapy is required. Intermittent therapy even by DOT is not recommended.
Isoniazid-rifampin resistant	Consult a tuberculosis specialist.	Moxifloxacin or levofloxacin with or without ethambutol or pyrazinamide.
PULMONARY AND EXTRAPULMONARY INFECTION		
Except meningitis[b]	2 mo of isoniazid, rifampin, pyrazinamide, and ethambutol daily or twice weekly, followed by 4 mo of isoniazid and rifampin[c] by DOT[d] for drug-susceptible *M. tuberculosis*	Some experts recommend a 3-drug initial regimen (isoniazid, rifampin, and pyrazinamide) if the risk of drug resistance is low. DOT is highly desirable. If hilar adenopathy only and the risk of drug resistance is low, 6 mo course of isoniazid and rifampin is sufficient. Drugs can be given 2 or 3 times/wk under DOT.
Meningitis	9-12 mo of isoniazid and rifampin for drug-susceptible *Mycobacterium bovis* 2 mo of isoniazid, rifampin, pyrazinamide, and an aminoglycoside[e] or ethionamide, once daily, followed by 7-10 mo of isoniazid and rifampin, once daily or twice weekly (9-12 mo total) for drug-susceptible *M. tuberculosis* At least 12 mo of therapy without pyrazinamide for drug-susceptible *M. bovis*	For patients who may have acquired tuberculosis in geographic areas where resistance to streptomycin is common, kanamycin, amikacin, or capreomycin can be used instead of streptomycin.

[a]Positive TST or IGRA result, no disease. See text for comments and additional acceptable/alternative regimens.

[b]Duration of therapy may be longer for human immunodeficiency virus (HIV)-infected people, and additional drugs and dosing intervals may be indicated

[c]Medications should be administered daily for the 1st 2 wk to 2 mo of treatment and then can be administered 2-3 times/wk by DOT. (Twice-weekly therapy is not recommended for HIV-infected people.)

[d]If initial chest radiograph shows pulmonary cavities, and sputum culture after 2 mo of therapy remains positive, the continuation phase is extended to 7 mo, for a total treatment duration of 9 mo.

[e]Streptomycin, kanamycin, amikacin, or capreomycin.

DOT, Directly observed therapy; IGRA, interferon-γ release assay; TST, tuberculin skin test.

Adapted from American Academy of Pediatrics: *Red book: 2018–2021 report of the Committee on Infectious Diseases*, ed 31, Elk Grove Village, IL, 2018, AAP (Table 3.85).

by the FDA), and intramuscular (IM) preparations.

Major **adverse effects** include hepatotoxicity in 1% of children and approximately 3% of adults (increasing with age) and dose-related peripheral neuropathy. Pyridoxine can prevent the peripheral neuropathy and is indicated for breastfeeding infants and their mothers, children and youth on milk- or meat-deficient diets, pregnant adolescents, and symptomatic HIV-infected children. Minor adverse events include rash, worsening of acne, epigastric pain with occasional nausea and vomiting, decreased vitamin D levels, and dizziness. The liquid formulation of INH contains sorbitol, which often causes diarrhea and stomach upset.

INH is accompanied by significant drug-drug interactions (Table 241.2). The metabolism of INH is by acetylation. Acetylation rates have minimal effect on efficacy, but **slow acetylators** have an increased risk for hepatotoxicity, especially when used in combination with rifampin. Routine baseline liver function testing or monthly monitoring is only indicated for persons with underlying hepatic disease or receiving concomitant hepatotoxic drugs, including other antimycobacterial agents, acetaminophen, or alcohol. Monthly clinic visits while taking INH alone are encouraged to monitor adherence, adverse effects, and worsening of infection.

Rifamycins

The rifamycins (rifampin, rifabutin, rifapentine) are a class of macrolide antibiotics developed from *Streptomyces mediterranei*. Rifampin is a synthetic derivative of rifamycin B, and rifabutin is a derivative of rifamycin S. Rifapentine is a cyclopentyl derivative. The rifamycins inhibit the DNA-dependent RNA polymerase of mycobacteria, resulting

Table 241.2	Isoniazid Drug-Drug Interactions

DRUG USED WITH ISONIAZID	EFFECTS
Acetaminophen, alcohol, rifampin	Increased hepatotoxicity of isoniazid or listed drugs
Aluminum salts (antacids)	Decreased absorption of isoniazid
Carbamazepine, phenytoin, theophylline, diazepam, warfarin	Increased level, effect, or toxicity of listed drugs due to decreased metabolism
Itraconazole, ketoconazole, oral hypoglycemic agents	Decreased level or effect of listed drugs due to increased metabolism
Cycloserine, ethionamide	Increased central nervous system adverse effects of cycloserine and ethionamide
Prednisolone	Increased isoniazid metabolism

in decreased RNA synthesis. These agents are generally bactericidal at treatment doses, but they may be bacteriostatic at lower doses. Resistance is from a mutation in the DNA-dependent RNA polymerase gene (*rpoB*) that is often induced by previous incomplete therapy. Cross-resistance between rifampin and rifabutin has been demonstrated.

Rifampin is active against *M. tuberculosis, M. leprae, M. kansasii,* and *M. avium* complex. Rifampin is an integral drug in standard combination treatment of active *M. tuberculosis* disease and can be used as an alternative to INH in the treatment of latent tuberculosis infection in children who cannot tolerate INH. **Rifabutin** has a similar spectrum, with increased activity against *M. avium* complex. **Rifapentine** is undergoing pediatric clinical trials and appears to have activity similar to the activity of rifampin. The pediatric dosage of rifampin is 10-15 mg/kg/day PO in a single dose, not to exceed 600 mg/day. The adult dosage of rifampin is 5-10 mg/kg/day PO in a single dose, not to exceed 600 mg/day. Commonly used rifampin preparations include 150 and 300 mg capsules and a suspension that is usually formulated at a concentration of 10 mg/mL. The shelf life of rifampin suspension is short (approximately 4 wk), so it should not be compounded with other antimycobacterial agents. An IV form of rifampin is also available for initial treatment of patients who cannot take oral preparations. Dosage adjustment is needed for patients with liver failure. Other rifamycins (rifabutin and rifapentine) have been poorly studied in children and are not recommended for pediatric use.

Rifampin can be associated with **adverse effects** such as transient elevations of liver enzymes; gastrointestinal (GI) upset with cramps, nausea, vomiting, and anorexia; headache; dizziness; and immunologically mediated fever and flulike symptoms. Thrombocytopenia and hemolytic anemias can also occur. Rifabutin has a similar spectrum of toxicities, except for an increased incidence of rash (4%) and neutropenia (2%). Rifapentine has fewer adverse effects but is associated with hyperuricemia and cytopenias, especially lymphopenia and neutropenia. All rifamycins can turn urine and other secretions (tears, saliva, stool, sputum) *orange*, which can stain contact lenses. Patients and families should be warned about this common but otherwise innocuous adverse effect.

Rifamycins induce the hepatic cytochrome P450 (CYP) isoenzyme system and are associated with the increased metabolism and decreased level of several drugs when administered concomitantly. These drugs include digoxin, corticosteroids such as prednisone and dexamethasone, dapsone, fluconazole, phenytoin, oral contraceptives, warfarin, and many antiretroviral agents, especially protease inhibitors and nonnucleoside reverse transcriptase inhibitors. Rifabutin has less of an effect on lowering protease inhibitor levels.

The use of pyrazinamide in combination with rifampin for short-course latent tuberculosis therapy has been associated with serious liver dysfunction and death. This combination has never been well studied or recommended for pediatric patients and should not be used.

No routine laboratory monitoring for rifamycins is indicated unless the patient is symptomatic. In patients with signs of toxicity, complete blood count (CBC) and kidney and liver function tests are indicated.

Pyrazinamide

Pyrazinamide (**PZA**) is a synthetic pyrazide analog of nicotinamide that is bactericidal against intracellular *M. tuberculosis* organisms in acidic environments, such as within macrophages or inflammatory lesions. A bacteria-specific enzyme (pyrazinamidase) converts PZA to pyrazinoic acid, which leads to low pH levels not tolerated by *M. tuberculosis*. Resistance is poorly understood but can arise from bacterial pyrazinamidase alterations.

PZA is indicated for the initial treatment phase of active tuberculosis in combination with other antimycobacterial agents. The pediatric dosage is 15-30 mg/kg/day PO in a single dose, not to exceed 2,000 mg/day. Twice-weekly dosing with directly observed therapy only is with 50 mg/kg/day PO in a single dose, not to exceed 4,000 mg/day. It is available in a 500 mg tablet and can be made into a suspension of 100 mg/mL.

Adverse effects include GI upset (e.g., nausea, vomiting, poor appetite) in approximately 4% of children, dosage-dependent hepatotoxicity, and elevated serum uric acid levels that can precipitate gout in susceptible adults. Approximately 10% of pediatric patients have elevated uric acid levels but with no associated clinical sequelae. Minor reactions include arthralgias, fatigue, and, rarely, fever.

Use of PZA in combination with rifampin for short-course treatment of latent tuberculosis is associated with serious liver dysfunction and death, and this combination should be avoided.

No routine laboratory monitoring for PZA is required, but monthly visits to reinforce the importance of therapy are desirable.

Ethambutol

Ethambutol is a synthetic form of ethylenedi-imino-di-1-butanol dihydrochloride that inhibits RNA synthesis needed for cell wall formation. At standard dosages ethambutol is bacteriostatic, but at dosages >25 mg/kg it has bactericidal activity. The mechanism of resistance to ethambutol is unknown, but resistance develops rapidly when ethambutol is used as a single agent against *M. tuberculosis*.

Ethambutol is indicated for the treatment of infections caused by *M. tuberculosis, M. kansasii, M. bovis,* and *M. avium* complex. Ethambutol should only be used as part of a combination treatment regimen for *M. tuberculosis*. Daily dosing is 15-20 mg/kg PO in a single dose, not to exceed 2,500 mg/day. Twice-weekly dosing is with 50 mg/kg PO in a single dose, not to exceed 2,500 mg/day. Dosage adjustment is needed in renal insufficiency. Ethambutol is available in 100 and 400 mg tablets.

The major adverse effect with ethambutol is **optic neuritis**, and thus ethambutol should generally be reserved for children old enough to have visual acuity and color discrimination reliably monitored. Visual changes are usually dosage dependent and reversible. Other adverse events include headache, dizziness, confusion, hyperuricemia, GI upset, peripheral neuropathy, hepatotoxicity, and cytopenias, especially neutropenia and thrombocytopenia.

Routine laboratory monitoring includes baseline and periodic visual acuity and color discrimination testing, CBC, serum uric acid levels, and kidney and liver function tests.

Less Commonly Used Agents
Aminoglycosides

The aminoglycosides used for mycobacterial infections include streptomycin, amikacin, kanamycin, and capreomycin. **Streptomycin** is isolated from *Streptomyces griseus* and was the first drug used to treat *M. tuberculosis*. **Capreomycin**, a cyclic polypeptide from *Streptomyces capreolus*, and **amikacin**, a semisynthetic derivative of kanamycin, are newer agents that are recommended when streptomycin is unavailable. Aminoglycosides act by binding irreversibly to the 30S subunit of ribosomes and inhibiting subsequent protein synthesis. Streptomycin exhibits concentration-dependent bactericidal activity, and capreomycin is bacteriostatic. Resistance results from mutation in the binding site of the 30S ribosome, by decreased transport into cells, or by inactivation by bacterial enzymes. Cross-resistance between aminoglycosides has been demonstrated.

The aminoglycosides are indicated for the treatment of *M. tuberculosis* and *M. avium* complex. All are considered second-line drugs in the treatment of *M. tuberculosis* and should be used only when resistance patterns are known. Aminoglycosides are poorly absorbed orally and are administered by IM injection. Pediatric dosing ranges for streptomycin are 20 mg/kg/day if given daily and 20-40 mg/kg/day if given twice weekly; dosing is IM in a single daily dose. Capreomycin, amikacin, and kanamycin dosages are 15-30 mg/kg/day IM in a single dose, not to exceed 1 g/day. Dosage adjustment is necessary in renal insufficiency.

Aminoglycosides have **adverse effects** on proximal renal tubules, the cochlea, and the vestibular apparatus of the ear. Nephrotoxicity and ototoxicity account for most of the significant adverse events. Rarely, patients exhibit fever or rash with administration of aminoglycosides. Concomitant use of other nephrotoxic or ototoxic agents should be avoided, because adverse effects may be additive. An infrequent but serious, synergistic, dosage-dependent aminoglycoside effect with nondepolarizing neuromuscular blockade agents can result in respiratory depression or paralysis.

Hearing and kidney function should be monitored at baseline and periodically. Early signs of ototoxicity include tinnitus, vertigo, and hearing loss. Ototoxicity appears to be irreversible, but early kidney damage may be reversible. As with other aminoglycosides, peak and trough drug levels are helpful in dosing and managing early toxicities.

Cycloserine

Cycloserine, derived from *Streptomyces orchidaceus* or *Streptomyces garyphalus,* is a synthetic analog of the amino acid D-alanine that interferes with bacterial cell wall synthesis through competitive inhibition of D-alanine components to be incorporated into the cell wall. It is bacteriostatic, and the mechanism of resistance is unknown.

Cycloserine is used to treat *M. tuberculosis* and *M. bovis.* The dosage is 10-20 mg/kg/day PO divided into 2 doses, not to exceed 1 g/day. It is available in a 250 mg capsule.

The major adverse effect is **neurotoxicity** with significant psychologic disturbance, including seizures, acute psychosis, headache, confusion, depression, and personality changes. The neurotoxic effects are additive with ethionamide and INH. Cycloserine has also been associated with megaloblastic anemia. It must be dosage-adjusted in patients with kidney impairment and should be used with caution in patients with underlying psychiatric illness.

Routine laboratory monitoring includes kidney and hepatic function, CBC, and cycloserine levels. Psychiatric symptoms are less common at blood levels <30 μg/mL.

Ethionamide

Ethionamide is structurally related to INH and is an ethyl derivative of thioisonicotinamide that inhibits peptide synthesis by an unclear mechanism thought to involve nicotinamide adenine dinucleotide and NAD phosphate dehydrogenase disruptions. Ethionamide is bacteriostatic at most therapeutic levels. Resistance develops quickly if ethionamide used as a single-agent therapy, although the mechanism is unknown.

Ethionamide is used as an alternative to streptomycin or ethambutol in the treatment of *M. tuberculosis* and has some activity against *M. kansasii* and *M. avium* complex. A metabolite, ethionamide sulfoxide, is bactericidal against *M. leprae.* Ethionamide has been shown to have good central nervous system (CNS) penetration and has been used as a 4th drug in combination with rifampin, INH, and PZA. The pediatric dosing is 15-20 mg/kg/day PO in 2 divided doses, not to exceed 1 g/day. It is available as a 250 mg tablet.

Gastrointestinal upset is common, and other **adverse effects** include neurologic disturbances (anxiety, dizziness, peripheral neuropathy, seizures, acute psychosis), hepatic enzyme elevations, hypothyroidism, hypoglycemia, and hypersensitivity reaction with rash and fever. Ethionamide should be used with caution in patients with underlying psychiatric or thyroid disease. The psychiatric adverse effects can be potentiated with concomitant use of cycloserine.

In addition to close assessment of mood, routine monitoring includes thyroid and liver function tests. In diabetic patients taking ethionamide, blood glucose levels should be monitored.

Fluoroquinolones

The fluoroquinolones are fluorinated derivatives of the quinolone class of antibiotics. Ciprofloxacin is a first-generation fluoroquinolone, and levofloxacin is the more active l-isomer of ofloxacin. **Moxifloxacin** and **gatifloxacin** are agents with emerging use in pediatric mycobacterial disease. Fluoroquinolones are not indicated for use in children <18 yr old, but studies of their use in pediatric patients continue to indicate that they may be used in special circumstances. Fluoroquinolones are bactericidal and exert their effect by inhibition of DNA gyrase. The alterations in DNA gyrase result in relaxation of supercoiled DNA and breaks in double-stranded DNA. The mechanism of resistance is not well defined but likely involves mutations in the DNA gyrase.

Levofloxacin is an important second-line drug in the treatment of multidrug-resistant (MDR) *M. tuberculosis.* **Ciprofloxacin** has activity against *Mycobacterium fortuitum* complex and against *M. tuberculosis.* The pediatric dosage of ciprofloxacin is 20-30 mg/kg/day PO or intravenously (IV), not to exceed 1.5 mg/day PO or 800 mg/day IV. The adult dosage of ciprofloxacin is 500-750 mg/dose PO in 2 divided doses or 200-400 mg/dose IV every 12 hr. Ciprofloxacin is available in 100, 250, 500, and 750 mg tablets and can be made in 5% (50 mg/mL) or 10% (100 mg/mL) suspensions. The dosage of levofloxacin for children is 5-10 mg/kg/day given once daily either PO or IV, not to exceed 1,000 mg/day, and for adults, 500-1,000 mg/day PO or IV, not to exceed 1,000 mg/day. Levofloxacin is available in 250, 500, and 750 mg tablets, and a 50 mg/mL suspension can be extemporaneously compounded.

The suspension has a shelf life of only 8 wk.

The most common adverse effect of fluoroquinolones is **GI upset**, with nausea, vomiting, abdominal pain, and diarrhea, including pseudomembranous colitis. Other, less common adverse effects include bone marrow depression, CNS effects (e.g., lowered seizure threshold, confusion, tremor, dizziness, headache), elevated liver transaminases, photosensitivity, and arthropathies. The potential for arthropathies (e.g., tendon ruptures, arthralgias, tendinitis) is the predominant reason that fluoroquinolones are not recommended for pediatric use. The mechanism of injury appears to involve the disruption of extracellular matrix of cartilage and depletion of collagen, a particular concern related to the bone and joint development of children.

Fluoroquinolones induce the CYP isoenzymes that can increase the concentrations of dually administered theophylline and warfarin. Nonsteroidal antiinflammatory drugs (NSAIDs) can potentiate the CNS effects of fluoroquinolones and should be avoided while taking a fluoroquinolone. Both ciprofloxacin and levofloxacin should be dosage-adjusted in patients with significant renal dysfunction.

While taking fluoroquinolones, patients should be monitored for hepatic and renal dysfunction, arthropathies, and hematologic abnormalities.

Linezolid

Linezolid is a synthetic oxazolidinone derivative. This drug is not currently approved for use against mycobacterial infection in pediatric or adult patients but has activity against some mycobacterial species. Studies on efficacy of treatment of mycobacterial infections are under way. Linezolid inhibits translation by binding to the 23S ribosomal component of the 50S ribosome subunit, preventing coupling with the 70S subunit. Resistance is thought to be from a point mutation at the binding site but is poorly studied because only a few cases of resistance have been reported.

The approved indications for linezolid are for bacterial infections other than mycobacteria, but studies reveal in vitro activity against rapidly growing mycobacteria (*M. fortuitum* complex, *M. chelonae, M. abscessus*), *M. tuberculosis,* and *M. avium* complex. The dosage for 0-11 yr old children is 10 mg/kg/day PO or IV in divided doses every 8-12 hr. For persons >12 yr old, the dosage is 600 mg PO or IV every 12 hr. Linezolid is available in 400 and 600 mg tablets and as a 20 mg/mL suspension.

Adverse effects of linezolid include GI upset (e.g., nausea, vomiting, diarrhea), CNS disturbances (e.g., dizziness, headache, insomnia, peripheral neuropathy), lactic acidosis, fever, myelosuppression, and pseudomembranous colitis. Linezolid is a weak inhibitor of monoamine oxidase A, and patients are advised to avoid foods with high tyramine content. Linezolid should be used cautiously in patients with preexisting myelosuppression.

In addition to monitoring for GI upset and CNS perturbations, routine laboratory monitoring includes CBC at least weekly.

Paraaminosalicylic Acid

Paraaminosalicylic acid (**PAS**) is a structural analog of paraaminobenzoic acid (PABA). It is bacteriostatic and acts by competitively inhibiting the synthesis of folic acid, similar to the action of sulfonamides. Resistance mechanisms are poorly understood.

PAS acts against *M. tuberculosis.* The dosage is 150 mg/kg/day PO in 2 or 3 divided doses. PAS is dispensed in 4 g packets, and the granules should be mixed with liquid and swallowed whole.

Common **adverse effects** include GI upset, and less common events include hypokalemia, hematuria, albuminuria, crystalluria, and elevations of hepatic transaminases. PAS can decrease the absorption of rifampin, and co-administration with ethionamide potentiates the adverse effects of PAS.

In addition to monitoring for weight loss, routine laboratory monitoring includes liver and kidney function tests.

Bedaquiline Fumarate

This oral diarylquinoline has been recommended for the treatment of MDR tuberculosis. Bedaquiline fumarate should be used as part of combination therapy and administered by direct observation. Although approved for patients ≥18 yr old, bedaquiline may be considered for children on a case-by-case basis.

Serious **adverse effects** include hepatotoxicity and a prolonged QT interval.

Delamanid

Delamanid is a dihydro-nitroimidazooxazole derivative recently approved for use in the treatment of MDR tuberculosis. It acts by inhibiting the synthesis of mycobacterial cell wall compounds such as methoxymycolic acid and ketomycolic acid. Limited studies are available in the pediatric population, and delamanid should be used only in conjunction with a tuberculosis specialist.

Adverse effects include nausea, vomiting, dizziness, anxiety, shaking, and QT prolongation.

AGENTS USED AGAINST *MYCOBACTERIUM LEPRAE*
Dapsone

Dapsone is a sulfone antibiotic with characteristics similar to sulfon-amides. Similar to other sulfonamides, dapsone acts as a competitive antagonist of PABA, which is needed for the bacterial synthesis of folic acid. Dapsone is bacteriostatic against *M. leprae.* Resistance is not well understood but is thought to occur after alterations at the PABA-binding site.

Dapsone is used in the treatment of *M. leprae* in combination with other antileprosy agents (rifampin, clofazimine, ethionamide). The pediatric dosage is 1-2 mg/kg/day PO as a single dose, not to exceed 100 mg/day, for a duration of 3-10 yr. The adult dosage is 100 mg/day PO as a single dose. Dapsone is available in 25 and 100 mg scored tablets and as an oral suspension of 2 mg/mL. The dosage should be adjusted in renal insufficiency.

Dapsone has many reported **adverse effects**, including dosage-related hemolytic anemia, especially in patients with glucose-6-phosphate dehydrogenase (G6PD) deficiency, pancreatitis, renal complications (acute tubular necrosis, acute renal failure, albuminuria), increased liver enzymes, psychosis, tinnitus, peripheral neuropathy, photosensitivity, and a hypersensitivity syndrome with fever, rash, hepatic damage, and malaise. Treatment may produce a *lepra reaction,* which is a nontoxic, paradoxical worsening of lepromatous leprosy with the initiation of therapy. This hypersensitivity reaction is not an indication to discontinue therapy. Dapsone should be used with caution in patients with G6PD deficiency or taking other folic acid antagonists. Dapsone levels can decrease with concomitant rifampin and can increase with concomitant clotrimazole.

Routine laboratory monitoring includes CBC weekly during the 1st mo of therapy, weekly through 6 mo of therapy, and then every 6 mo thereafter. Other periodic assessments include kidney function with creatine levels, urinalysis, and liver function tests.

Clofazimine

Clofazimine is a synthetic phendimetrazine tartrate derivative that acts by binding to the mycobacterial DNA at guanine sites. It has a slow bactericidal activity against *M. leprae.* Mechanisms of resistance are not well studied. No cross-resistance between clofazimine and dapsone or rifampin has been shown.

Clofazimine is indicated as part of a combination therapy for the treatment of *M. leprae.* It appears there may be some activity against other mycobacteria such as *M. avium* complex, although treatment failures are common. Safety and efficacy of clofazimine are poorly studied in children. The pediatric dosage is 1 mg/kg/day PO as a single dose, not to exceed 100 mg/day, in combination with dapsone and rifampin, for 2 yr and then additionally as a single agent for >1 yr. The adult dosage is 100 mg/day PO. Clofazimine should be taken with food to increase absorption.

The most common adverse effect is a dosage-related, reversible, pink to tan-brown discoloration of the skin and conjunctiva. Other **adverse effects** include a dry, itchy skin rash, headache, dizziness, abdominal pain, diarrhea, vomiting, peripheral neuropathy, and elevated hepatic transaminases.

Routine laboratory monitoring includes periodic liver function tests.

AGENTS USED AGAINST NONTUBERCULOUS MYCOBACTERIA
Cefoxitin

Cefoxitin, a cephamycin derivative, is a second-generation cephalosporin that, like other cephalosporins, inhibits cell wall synthesis by linking with penicillin-binding proteins to create an unstable bacterial cell wall. Resistance develops by alterations in penicillin-binding proteins.

Cefoxitin is often used in combination therapy for mycobacterial disease (Table 241.3). Pediatric dosing is based on disease severity, with a range of 80-160 mg/kg/day divided every 4-8 hr, not to exceed 12 g/day. Adult dosages are 1-2 g/day, not to exceed 12 g/day. Cefoxitin is available in IV and IM formulations. Increased dosing intervals are needed with renal insufficiency.

Adverse effects are primarily hematologic (eosinophilia, granulocytopenia, thrombocytopenia, hemolytic anemia), GI (nausea, vomiting, diarrhea with possible pseudomembranous colitis), and CNS related (dizziness, vertigo). Potential additive adverse effects can occur when cefoxitin is used with aminoglycosides.

Routine laboratory monitoring with long-term use includes CBC and liver and renal function tests.

Doxycycline

Doxycycline is in the tetracycline family of antibiotics and has limited use in pediatrics. As with other tetracyclines, doxycycline acts to decrease protein synthesis by binding to the 30S ribosome and to transfer RNA. It can also cause alterations to the cytoplasmic membrane of susceptible bacteria.

Doxycycline is used to treat *M. fortuitum* (see Table 241.3). Although it can be used to treat *Mycobacterium marinum,* adult treatment failures have occurred. Pediatric dosing is based on age and weight. For children >8 yr old who weigh <45 kg, the dosage is 4.4 mg/kg/day divided twice daily. Dosing for larger children and adults is 100 mg twice daily. Doxycycline is available as 50 and 100 mg capsules or tablets and in 25 mg/5 mL and 50 mg/5 mL suspensions.

Doxycycline use in children is limited by a **permanent tooth discoloration**, which becomes worse with long-term use. Other **adverse effects** include photosensitivity, liver and kidney dysfunction, and esophagitis, which can be minimized by dosing with large volumes of liquid. Doxycycline can decrease the effectiveness of oral contraceptives. Rifampin, carbamazepine, and phenytoin can decrease the concentration of doxycycline.

Routine laboratory monitoring with long-term use includes kidney and liver function tests as well as CBC.

Macrolides

Clarithromycin and azithromycin belong to the macrolide family of antibiotics. Clarithromycin is a methoxy derivative of erythromycin. Macrolides act by binding the 50S subunit of ribosomes, subsequently inhibiting protein synthesis. Resistance mechanisms for mycobacteria are not well understood but might involve binding site alterations. Clarithromycin appears to have synergistic antimycobacterial activity when combined with rifamycins, ethambutol, or clofazimine.

Clarithromycin is widely used for the prophylaxis and treatment of *M. avium* complex disease and also has activity against *Mycobacterium abscessus, M. fortuitum,* and *M. marinum.* Azithromycin has significantly different pharmacokinetics compared with other macrolide agents and has not been studied and is not indicated for mycobacterial infections. The pediatric dosage of clarithromycin for primary prophylaxis of *M. avium* complex infections is 7.5 mg/kg/dose PO given twice daily, not to exceed 500 mg/day. This dosage is used for recurrent *M. avium* complex disease in combination with ethambutol and rifampin. The adult dosage is 500 mg PO twice daily to be used as a single agent for primary prophylaxis or as part of combination therapy with ethambutol and rifampin. Dosage adjustment is needed for renal insufficiency but not liver failure. Clarithromycin is available in 250 and 500 mg tablets and suspensions of 125 mg/5 mL and 250 mg/5 mL.

Table 241.3	Treatment of Nontuberculous Mycobacteria Infections in Children

ORGANISM	DISEASE	INITIAL TREATMENT
SLOWLY GROWING SPECIES		
Mycobacterium avium complex (MAC); *Mycobacterium haemophilum; Mycobacterium lentiflavum*	Lymphadenitis	Complete excision of lymph nodes; if excision incomplete or disease recurs, clarithromycin or azithromycin plus ethambutol and/or rifampin (or rifabutin).
	Pulmonary infection	Clarithromycin or azithromycin plus ethambutol with rifampin or rifabutin (pulmonary resection in some patients who fail to respond to drug therapy). For severe disease, an initial course of amikacin or streptomycin often is included. Clinical data in adults with mild to moderate disease support that 3-times-weekly therapy is as effective as daily therapy, with less toxicity. For patients with advanced or cavitary disease, drugs should be given daily.
Mycobacterium chimaera	Prosthetic valve endocarditis	Valve removal, prolonged antimicrobial therapy based on susceptibility testing.
	Disseminated	See text.
Mycobacterium kansasii	Pulmonary infection	Rifampin plus ethambutol with isoniazid daily. If rifampin resistance is detected, a 3-drug regimen based on drug susceptibility testing should be used.
	Osteomyelitis	Surgical debridement and prolonged antimicrobial therapy using rifampin plus ethambutol with isoniazid.
Mycobacterium marinum	Cutaneous infection	None, if minor; rifampin, TMP-SMX, clarithromycin, or doxycycline* for moderate disease; extensive lesions may require surgical debridement. Susceptibility testing not routinely required.
Mycobacterium ulcerans	Cutaneous and bone infections	Daily intramuscular streptomycin and oral rifampin for 8 wk; excision to remove necrotic tissue, if present; potential response to thermotherapy.
RAPIDLY GROWING SPECIES		
Mycobacterium fortuitum group	Cutaneous infection	Initial therapy for serious disease is amikacin plus meropenem IV, followed by clarithromycin, doxycycline,* TMP-SMX, or ciprofloxacin PO, on the basis of in vitro susceptibility testing; may require surgical excision. Up to 50% of isolates are resistant to cefoxitin.
	Catheter infection	Catheter removal and amikacin plus meropenem IV; clarithromycin, TMP-SMX, or ciprofloxacin, orally, on the basis of in vitro susceptibility testing.
Mycobacterium abscessus	Otitis media; cutaneous infection	There is no reliable antimicrobial regimen because of variability in drug susceptibility. Clarithromycin plus initial course of amikacin plus cefoxitin or imipenem/meropenem; may require surgical debridement on the basis of in vitro susceptibility testing (50% are amikacin resistant).
	Pulmonary infection (in cystic fibrosis)	Serious disease, clarithromycin, amikacin, and cefoxitin or imipenem/ meropenem on the basis of susceptibility testing; most isolates have very low MIC to tigecycline; may require surgical resection.
Mycobacterium chelonae	Catheter infection, prosthetic valve endocarditis	Catheter removal; debridement, removal of foreign material; valve replacement; and tobramycin (initially) plus clarithromycin, meropenem, and linezolid.
	Disseminated cutaneous infection	Tobramycin and meropenem or linezolid (initially) plus clarithromycin.

*Doxycycline can be used for short durations (i.e., ≤21 days) without regard to patient age, but for longer treatment durations is not recommended for children <8 yr old. Only 50% of isolates of *M. marinum* are susceptible to doxycycline.

IV, Intravenously; MIC, minimum inhibitory concentration; PO, orally (by mouth); TMP-SMX, trimethoprim-sulfamethoxazole.

From American Academy of Pediatrics: *Red book: 2018–2021 report of the Committee on Infectious Diseases*, ed 31, Elk Grove Village, IL, 2018, AAP (Table 3.90).

The primary adverse effect of clarithromycin is **GI upset**, including vomiting (6%), diarrhea (6%), and abdominal pain (3%). Other **adverse effects** include taste disturbances, headache, and QT prolongation if used with inhaled anesthetics, clotrimazole, antiarrhythmic agents, or azoles. Clarithromycin should be used cautiously in patients with renal insufficiency or liver failure.

Routine laboratory monitoring with prolonged use of clarithromycin includes periodic liver enzyme tests. Diarrhea is an early sign of pseudomembranous colitis.

Trimethoprim-Sulfamethoxazole

Trimethoprim-sulfamethoxazole (TMP-SMX) is formulated in a fixed ratio of 1 part TMP to 5 parts SMX. SMX is a sulfonamide that inhibits synthesis of dihydrofolic acid by competitively inhibiting PABA, similar to dapsone. TMP blocks production of tetrahydrofolic acid and downstream biosynthesis of nucleic acids and protein by reversibly binding to dihydrofolate reductase. The combination of the 2 agents is synergistic and often bactericidal.

TMP-SMX is often used in combination therapy for mycobacterial disease (see Table 241.3). Oral or IV pediatric dosage for serious infections is TMP 15-20 mg/kg/day divided every 6-8 hr, and for mild infections, TMP 6-12 mg/kg/day divided every 12 hr. The adult dosage is 160 mg TMP and 800 mg SMX every 12 hr. Dosage reduction may be needed in renal insufficiency. TMP-SMX is available in single-strength tablets (80/400 mg TMP/SMX) and double-strength tablets (160/800 mg TMP/ SMX) and in a suspension of 40 mg TMP and 200 mg SMX per 5 mL.

The most common adverse effect with TMP-SMX is **myelosuppression**. It must be used with caution in patients with G6PD deficiency. Other **adverse effects** include renal abnormalities, rash, aseptic meningitis, GI disturbances (e.g., pancreatitis, diarrhea), and prolonged QT interval if co-administered with inhaled anesthetics, azoles, or macrolides.

Routine laboratory monitoring includes monthly CBC and periodic electrolytes and creatinine to monitor renal function.

Bibliography is available at Expert Consult.

Chapter **242**
Tuberculosis (*Mycobacterium tuberculosis*)

Lindsay Hatzenbuehler Cameron and Jeffrey R. Starke

第二百四十二章
结核病（结核分枝杆菌）

中文导读

　　本章节主要介绍了结核病的病因、流行病学、传播途径、发病机制、临床表现、诊断方法、治疗以及预防接种。具体描述了其临床分期、免疫学机制。详细描述了原发性肺结核、进展性肺结核、再活化结核病、胸腔积液、心包结核、血行播散性结核、上呼吸道结核、淋巴结核、中枢神经系统结核、皮肤结核、骨和关节结核、腹腔和消化道结核、泌尿系结核、孕

期结核病、围产期结核病、新生儿结核病，以及感染艾滋病毒儿童结核病的临床表现。详细描述了结核菌素皮肤试验、γ–干扰素释放试验、细菌培养、核酸检测等诊断方法。具体介绍了耐药结核病的治疗，糖皮质激素的使用以及随访观察。同时对BCG疫苗的接种以及围产期结核病的预防作了详细介绍。

Tuberculosis has caused human disease for more than 4,000 yr and is one of the most important infectious diseases worldwide.

ETIOLOGY

There are 5 closely related mycobacteria in the *Mycobacterium tuberculosis* complex: *M. tuberculosis, M. bovis, M. africanum, M. microti,* and *M. canetti. M. tuberculosis* is the most important cause of tuberculosis (TB) disease in humans. The tubercle bacilli are non–spore-forming, nonmotile, pleomorphic, weakly gram-positive curved rods 1-5 μm long, typically slender and slightly bent. They can appear beaded or clumped under microscopy. They are obligate aerobes that grow in synthetic media containing glycerol as the carbon source and ammonium salts as the nitrogen source (Löwenstein-Jensen culture media). These mycobacteria grow best at 37-41°C (98.6-105.8°F), produce niacin, and lack pigmentation. A lipid-rich cell wall accounts for resistance to the bactericidal actions of antibody and complement. A hallmark of all mycobacteria is **acid fastness**—the capacity to form stable mycolate complexes with arylmethane dyes (crystal violet, carbolfuchsin, auramine, and rhodamine). They resist decoloration with ethanol and hydrochloric or other acids.

Mycobacteria grow slowly, with a generation time of 12-24 hr. Isolation from clinical specimens on solid synthetic media usually takes 3-6 wk, and drug susceptibility testing requires an additional 2-4 wk. Growth can be detected in 1-3 wk in selective liquid medium using radiolabeled

nutrients (e.g., BACTEC radiometric system), and drug susceptibilities can be determined in an additional 3-5 days. Once mycobacterial growth is detected, the species of mycobacteria present can be determined within hours using high-pressure liquid chromatography analysis (identifying the mycolic acid fingerprint of each species) or DNA probes. Restriction fragment length polymorphism profiling of mycobacteria is a helpful tool to study the epidemiology of tuberculosis strain relatedness in both outbreaks and routine epidemiology of tuberculosis in a community.

Clinical Stages

There are 3 major clinical stages of tuberculosis: exposure, infection, and disease. **Exposure** means a child has had significant contact (shared the air) with an adult or adolescent with infectious tuberculosis but lacks proof of infection. In this stage, the **tuberculin skin test (TST)** or **interferon-γ release assay (IGRA)** result is negative, the chest radiograph is normal, the physical examination is normal, and the child lacks signs or symptoms of disease. However, the child may be infected and develop TB disease rapidly, since there may not have been enough time for the TST or IGRA to turn positive. **Tuberculosis infection (TBI)** occurs when the individual inhales droplet nuclei containing *M. tuberculosis*, which survive intracellularly within the lung and associated lymphoid tissue. The hallmark of TBI is a positive TST or IGRA result. In this stage the child has no signs or symptoms, a normal physical

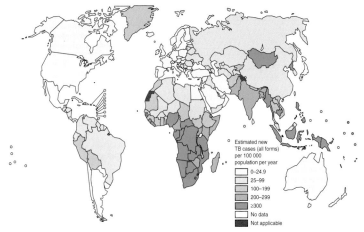

Fig. 242.1 Estimated 2015 tuberculosis (TB) incidence rates. (From the World Health Organization: Global tuberculosis report 2016, Geneva, 2016, WHO.)

examination, and the chest radiograph is either normal or reveals only granuloma or calcifications in the lung parenchyma. **Disease** occurs when signs or symptoms or radiographic manifestations caused by *M. tuberculosis* become apparent. Not all infected individuals have the same risk of developing disease. An immunocompetent adult with untreated TBI has approximately a 5–10% lifetime risk of developing disease. In contrast, an infected child <1 yr old has a 40% chance of developing TB disease within 9 mo.

EPIDEMIOLOGY

The World Health Organization (WHO) estimates that since 2015, tuberculosis has surpassed human immunodeficiency virus infection and acquired immunodeficiency syndrome (HIV/AIDS) as the leading cause of death from an infectious disease worldwide, and that almost one third of the world's population (2.5 billion people) is infected with *M. tuberculosis*. Approximately 95% of TB cases occur in the developing world. The highest numbers of cases are in Asia, Africa, and the eastern Mediterranean region. An estimated 10.4 million incident cases and 1.8 million TB-associated deaths occurred worldwide in 2015 (Fig. 242.1). The WHO 2016 Global Tuberculosis Report estimates that in 2015 there were 1 million childhood incident cases, 170,000 TB-associated deaths among non–HIV-infected children, and 40,000 TB-associated deaths among HIV-infected children. The global burden of tuberculosis is influenced by several factors, including: the HIV pandemic; the development of **multidrug-resistant (MDR) tuberculosis**; and the disproportionately low access of populations in low-resource settings worldwide to both diagnostic tests and effective medical therapy.

In the United States, TB case rates decreased steadily during the 1st half of the 20th century, long before the advent of antituberculosis drugs, as a result of improved living conditions and likely, genetic selection favoring persons resistant to developing disease. A resurgence of tuberculosis in the late 1980s was associated primarily with the HIV epidemic, transmission of the organism in congregate settings including healthcare institutions, disease occurring in recent immigrants, and poor conduct of community TB control. Since 1992, the number of reported TB cases decreased each year until 2015, when it increased by 1.6% from 2014, to 9,557 cases (Fig. 242.2). Despite the increase in the number of reported cases in 2015, TB incidence in the United States has remained stable at 3 cases per 100,000 persons. Of the cases in 2015, 439 (4.6%) occurred in children <15 yr old (rate: 1.5/100,000 population), 55% of whom were ≤5 yr old. Racial and ethnic minorities and foreign-born persons, including children in these groups, are disproportionately affected by tuberculosis in the United States. In 2015 the Centers for Disease Control and Prevention (CDC) reported that 87% of all TB cases were among ethnic minority populations. The TB case rate among Asian, non-Hispanic black, and Hispanic children was

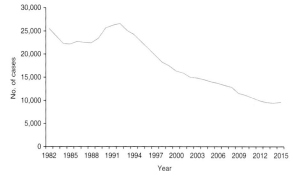

Fig. 242.2 Reported tuberculosis cases in the United States for 1982–2015 (as of June 9, 2016). (From Centers for Disease Control and Prevention: Reported tuberculosis in the United States, 2015, Atlanta, 2015, US Department of Health and Human Services.)

27, 13, and 12 times as high, respectively, as among non-Hispanic white children (Fig. 242.3). The TB rate among foreign-born persons in the United States was 13 times higher than among U.S.-born persons and accounted for 66% of all TB cases in 2015 (Fig. 242.4). Foreign-born children accounted for 22% of the total number of childhood TB cases in 2015. Of U.S.-born children with tuberculosis, 66% have at least 1 foreign-born parent, and 75% of all pediatric patients have some international connection through a family member or previous travel or residence in a TB-endemic country.

Most children are infected with *M. tuberculosis* in their home by someone close to them, but outbreaks of childhood tuberculosis also have occurred in elementary and high schools, nursery schools, daycare centers and homes, churches, school buses, and sports teams. HIV-infected adults with tuberculosis can transmit *M. tuberculosis* to children, and children with HIV infection are at increased risk for developing tuberculosis after infection. Specific groups are at high risk for acquiring TBI and progressing to tuberculosis (Table 242.1).

The incidence of **drug-resistant tuberculosis** has increased dramatically throughout the world. **MDR-TB** is defined as resistance to at least isoniazid and rifampin; **extensively drug-resistant tuberculosis** includes MDR-TB plus resistance to any fluoroquinolone and at least 1 of 3 injectable drugs (kanamycin, capreomycin, amikacin). In 2015 the estimate for MDR-TB was 3.9% of incident cases, but rates as high as 32% have been reported in countries formerly part of the Soviet Union. In 2015 in the United States, a total of 89 patients with MDR-TB were reported, 70.8% of whom were foreign-born (Fig. 242.5). The CDC

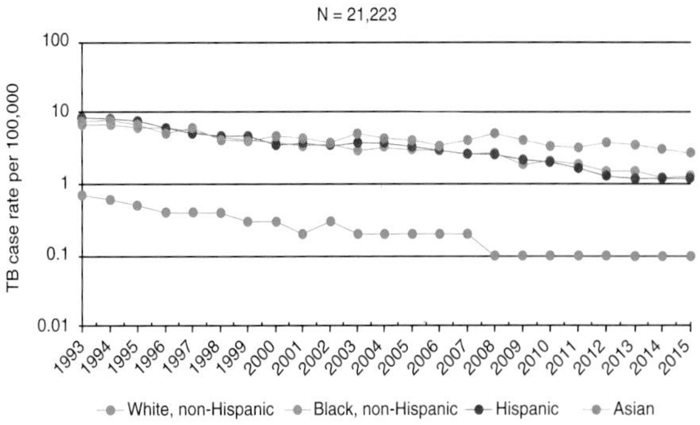

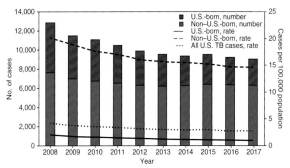

Note: Rates presented in a logarithmic scale

*Rates are per 100,000 persons

Multiple race/ethnicity, American Indian/Alaska Native and Native Hawaiian and other Pacific Islander rate not show because of small denominators

Fig. 242.3 Reported pediatric tuberculosis (TB) cases in the United States by race/ethnicity for the years 1993-2015. *(From Centers for Disease Control and Prevention, National Center for HIV/AIDS, Viral Hepatitis, STD and TB Prevention: Epidemiology of Pediatric Tuberculosis in United States, 1993-2015. Atlanta, 2015, U.S. Department of Health and Human Services.)*

Fig. 242.4 Number of tuberculosis (TB) cases and rate, by national origin—United States, 2008–2017. *(From Stewart RJ, Tsang CA, Pratt RH, et al: Tuberculosis—United States, 2017, MMWR 67(11):317–322, 2018.)*

Table 242.1	Groups at High Risk for Acquiring Tuberculosis Infection and Developing Disease in Countries With Low Incidence

RISK FACTORS FOR TUBERCULOSIS INFECTION

Children exposed to high-risk adults
Foreign-born persons from high-prevalence countries
Homeless persons
Persons who inject drugs
Present and former residents or employees of correctional institutions, homeless shelters, and nursing homes
Healthcare workers caring for high-risk patients (if infection control is not adequate)

RISK FACTORS FOR PROGRESSION OF TUBERCULOSIS INFECTION TO TUBERCULOSIS DISEASE

Infants and children ≤4 yr old, especially those <2 yr old
Adolescents and young adults
Persons co-infected with human immunodeficiency virus
Persons with skin test conversion in the past 1-2 yr
Persons who are immunocompromised, especially in cases of malignancy and solid-organ transplantation, immunosuppressive medical treatments including anti–tumor necrosis factor therapies, diabetes mellitus, chronic renal failure, silicosis, and malnutrition

RISK FACTORS FOR DRUG-RESISTANT TUBERCULOSIS

Personal or contact history of treatment for tuberculosis
Contacts of patients with drug-resistant tuberculosis
Birth or residence in a country with a high rate of drug resistance
Poor response to standard therapy
Positive sputum smears (acid-fast bacilli) or culture ≥2 mo after initiating appropriate therapy

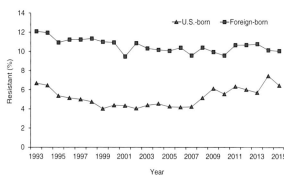

Fig. 242.5 Primary isoniazid resistance in U.S.-born vs foreign-born persons in the United States, 1993–2015 (as of June 9, 2016). Based on initial isolates from persons with no prior history of tuberculosis. *(From Centers for Disease Control and Prevention: Reported tuberculosis in the United States, 2015, Atlanta, 2015, US Department of Health and Human Services.)*

reported that among children with culture-confirmed tuberculosis in the United States in 2014, 17.4% had resistance to at least 1 first-line drug, and 0.9% had MDR-TB.

TRANSMISSION

Transmission of *M. tuberculosis* is usually by inhalation of airborne mucus droplet nuclei, particles 1-5 μm in diameter that contain *M. tuberculosis*. Transmission rarely occurs by direct contact with an infected discharge or a contaminated fomite. The chance of transmission increases when the patient has a positive acid-fast smear of sputum, an extensive upper lobe infiltrate or cavity, copious production of thin sputum, and severe and forceful cough. Environmental factors such as poor air circulation enhance transmission. Most adults no longer transmit the organism within several days to 2 wk after beginning adequate chemotherapy, but some patients remain infectious for many weeks. Young children with tuberculosis rarely infect other children or adults. Tubercle bacilli are sparse in the endobronchial secretions of children with pulmonary tuberculosis, and cough is often absent or lacks the tussive force required to suspend infectious particles of the correct size. Children and adolescents with adult-type cavitary or endobronchial pulmonary tuberculosis can transmit the organism.

Airborne transmission of *M. bovis* and *M. africanum* also occurs. *M. bovis* can penetrate the gastrointestinal (GI) mucosa or invade the lymphatic tissue of the oropharynx when large numbers of the organism are ingested. Human infection with *M. bovis* is rare in developed countries as a result of the pasteurization of milk and effective TB control programs for cattle. Approximately 46% of culture-proven childhood TB cases from the San Diego, California, region since 1994 were caused by *M. bovis*, likely acquired by children when visiting Mexico or another country, or consuming dairy products from countries with suboptimal veterinary TB control programs.

Zoonotic transmission is an uncommon source of *M. tuberculosis* that has been reported in adults exposed to elephants and potentially cattle.

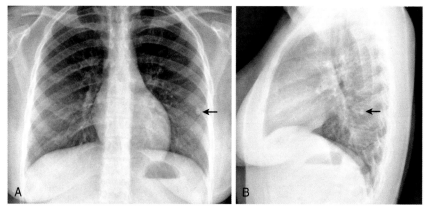

Fig. 242.6 Posteroanterior (**A**) and lateral (**B**) chest radiograph images of an adolescent showing a 7 mm calcified granuloma in the left lower lobe (arrows). *(From Lighter J, Rigaud M: Diagnosing childhood tuberculosis: traditional and innovative modalities, Curr Probl Pediatr Adolesc Health Care 39:55–88, 2009.)*

PATHOGENESIS

The **primary complex** (or Ghon complex) of tuberculosis includes local infection at the portal of entry and the regional lymph nodes that drain the area. The lung is the portal of entry in >98% of cases. The tubercle bacilli multiply initially within alveoli and alveolar ducts. Most of the bacilli are killed, but some survive within nonactivated macrophages, which carry them through lymphatic vessels to the regional lymph nodes. When the primary infection is in the lung, the hilar lymph nodes usually are involved, although an upper lobe focus can drain into paratracheal nodes. The tissue reaction in the lung parenchyma and lymph nodes intensifies over the next 2-12 wk as the organisms grow in number and **tissue hypersensitivity** develops. The parenchymal portion of the primary complex often heals completely by fibrosis or calcification after undergoing caseous necrosis and encapsulation (Fig. 242.6). Occasionally, this portion continues to enlarge, resulting in focal pneumonitis and pleuritis. If caseation is intense, the center of the lesion liquefies and empties into the associated bronchus, leaving a residual cavity.

The foci of infection in the regional lymph nodes develop some fibrosis and encapsulation, but healing is usually less complete than in the parenchymal lesion. Viable *M. tuberculosis* can persist for decades within these foci. In most cases of initial TBI, the lymph nodes remain normal in size. However, hilar and paratracheal lymph nodes that enlarge significantly as part of the host inflammatory reaction can encroach on a regional bronchus (Figs. 242.7 and 242.8). Partial obstruction of the bronchus caused by external compression can cause hyperinflation in the distal lung segment. Complete obstruction results in atelectasis. Inflamed caseous nodes can attach to the bronchial wall and erode through it, causing endobronchial tuberculosis or a fistula tract. The caseum causes complete obstruction of the bronchus. The resulting lesion is a combination of pneumonitis and atelectasis and has been called a **collapse-consolidation lesion** or **segmental lesion** (Fig. 242.9).

During the development of the primary complex, tubercle bacilli are carried to most tissues of the body through the blood and lymphatic vessels. Although seeding of the organs of the reticuloendothelial system is common, bacterial replication is more likely to occur in organs with conditions that favor their growth, such as the lung apices, brain, kidneys, and bones. **Disseminated tuberculosis** occurs if the number of circulating bacilli is large and the host's cellular immune response is inadequate. More often, the number of bacilli is small, leading to clinically inapparent metastatic foci in many organs. These remote foci usually become encapsulated, but they may be the origin of both **extrapulmonary tuberculosis** and **reactivation pulmonary tuberculosis**.

The time between initial infection and clinically apparent TB disease is variable. Disseminated and meningeal tuberculosis are early manifestations, often occurring within 2-6 mo of acquisition. Significant lymph node or endobronchial tuberculosis usually appears within 3-9 mo.

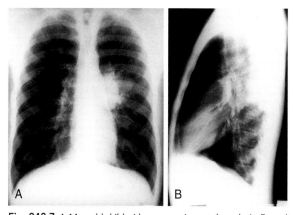

Fig. 242.7 A 14 yr old child with proven primary tuberculosis. Frontal (**A**) and lateral (**B**) views of the chest show hyperinflation, prominent left hilar lymphadenopathy, and alveolar consolidation involving the posterior segment of the left upper lobe as well as the superior segment of the left lower lobe. *(From Hilton SVW, Edwards DK, editors: Practical pediatric radiology, ed 3, Philadelphia, 2003, Saunders, p 334.)*

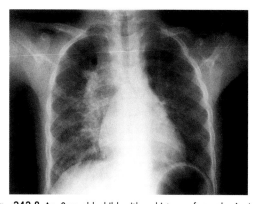

Fig. 242.8 An 8 yr old child with a history of cough. A single frontal view of the chest shows marked right hilar and paratracheal lymphadenopathy with alveolar disease involving the right middle and lower lung fields. This was also a case of primary tuberculosis. *(From Hilton SVW, Edwards DK, editors: Practical pediatric radiology, ed 3, Philadelphia, 2003, Saunders, p. 335.)*

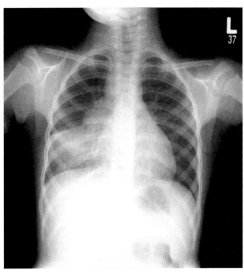

Fig. 242.9 Right-sided hilar lymphadenopathy and collapse-consolidation lesions of primary tuberculosis in a 4 yr old child.

Lesions of the bones and joints take several years to develop, whereas renal lesions become evident decades after infection. Extrapulmonary manifestations are more common in children than adults and develop in 25–35% of children with tuberculosis, vs approximately 10% of immunocompetent adults.

Pulmonary tuberculosis that occurs >1 yr after the primary infection is usually caused by endogenous regrowth of bacilli persisting in partially encapsulated lesions. This reactivation tuberculosis is rare in children but is common among adolescents and young adults. The most common form is an infiltrate or cavity in the apex of the upper lobes, where oxygen tension and blood flow are highest.

The risk for dissemination of *M. tuberculosis* is very high in HIV-infected persons. Reinfection also can occur in persons with advanced HIV or AIDS. In immunocompetent persons the response to the initial infection with *M. tuberculosis* usually provides protection against reinfection when a new exposure occurs. However, exogenous reinfection has been reported to occur in adults and children without immune compromise in highly endemic areas.

Immunity
Conditions that adversely affect cell-mediated immunity predispose to progression from TBI to disease. Rare specific genetic defects associated with deficient cell-mediated immunity in response to mycobacteria include interleukin (IL)-12 receptor B1 deficiency and complete and partial interferon (IFN)-γ receptor 1 chain deficiencies. TBI is associated with a humoral antibody response, which plays little known role in host defense. Shortly after infection, tubercle bacilli replicate in both free alveolar spaces and inactivated alveolar macrophages. Sulfatides in the mycobacterial cell wall inhibit fusion of the macrophage phagosome and lysosomes, allowing the organisms to escape destruction by intracellular enzymes. **Cell-mediated immunity** develops 2-12 wk after infection, along with tissue hypersensitivity (Fig. 242.10). After bacilli enter macrophages, lymphocytes that recognize mycobacterial antigens proliferate and secrete lymphokines and other mediators that attract other lymphocytes and macrophages to the area. Certain lymphokines activate macrophages, causing them to develop high concentrations of lytic enzymes that enhance their mycobactericidal capacity. A discrete subset of regulator helper and suppressor lymphocytes modulates the immune response. Development of specific cellular immunity prevents progression of the initial infection in most persons.

The pathologic events in the initial TBI seem to depend on the balance among the mycobacterial antigen load; cell-mediated immunity, which enhances intracellular killing; and tissue hypersensitivity, which promotes

extracellular killing. When the antigen load is small and the degree of tissue sensitivity is high, granuloma formation results from the organization of lymphocytes, macrophages, and fibroblasts. When both antigen load and degree of sensitivity are high, granuloma formation is less organized. Tissue necrosis is incomplete, resulting in formation of caseous material. When the degree of tissue sensitivity is low, as often occurs in infants or immunocompromised persons, the reaction is diffuse and the infection is not well contained, leading to dissemination and local tissue destruction. Tumor necrosis factor (TNF) and other cytokines released by specific lymphocytes promote cellular destruction and tissue damage in susceptible persons.

CLINICAL MANIFESTATIONS
Primary Pulmonary Disease
The **primary complex** includes the parenchymal pulmonary focus and the regional lymph nodes. Approximately 70% of lung foci are subpleural, and localized pleurisy is common. The initial parenchymal inflammation usually is not visible on chest radiograph, but a localized, nonspecific infiltrate may be seen before the development of tissue hypersensitivity. All lobar segments of the lung are at equal risk for initial infection. Two or more primary foci are present in 25% of cases. The hallmark of primary tuberculosis in the lung is the relatively large size of the regional lymphadenitis compared with the relatively small size of the initial lung focus (see Figs. 242.7 and 242.8). As delayed-type hypersensitivity develops, the hilar lymph nodes continue to enlarge in some children, especially infants, compressing the regional bronchus and causing obstruction. The usual sequence is *hilar lymphadenopathy, focal hyperinflation,* and then *atelectasis.* The resulting radiographic shadows have been called *collapse-consolidation* or *segmental* tuberculosis (see Fig. 242.9). Rarely, inflamed caseous nodes attach to the endobronchial wall and erode through it, causing endobronchial tuberculosis or a fistula tract. The caseum causes complete obstruction of the bronchus, resulting in extensive infiltrate and collapse. Enlargement of the subcarinal lymph nodes can cause compression of the esophagus and rarely a bronchoesophageal fistula.

Most cases of tuberculous bronchial obstruction in children resolve fully with appropriate treatment. Occasionally, there is residual calcification of the primary focus or regional lymph nodes. The appearance of calcification implies that the lesion has been present for at least 6-12 mo. Healing of the segment can be complicated by scarring or contraction associated with cylindrical bronchiectasis, but this is rare.

Children can have lobar pneumonia without impressive hilar lymphadenopathy. If the primary infection is progressively destructive, liquefaction of the lung parenchyma can lead to formation of a thin-walled primary TB cavity. Rarely, bullous tuberculous lesions occur in the lungs and lead to pneumothorax if they rupture. Erosion of a parenchymal focus of tuberculosis into a blood or lymphatic vessel can result in dissemination of the bacilli and a **miliary** pattern, with small nodules evenly distributed on the chest radiograph (Fig. 242.11).

The symptoms and physical signs of primary pulmonary tuberculosis in children are surprisingly meager considering the degree of radiographic changes often present. When active case finding is performed, up to 50% of infants and children with radiographically moderate to severe pulmonary tuberculosis have no physical findings. Infants are more likely to experience signs and symptoms. Nonproductive cough and mild dyspnea are the most common symptoms. Systemic complaints such as fever, night sweats, anorexia, and decreased activity occur less often. Some infants have difficulty gaining weight or develop a true failure-to-thrive syndrome that often does not improve significantly until several months of effective treatment have been taken. Pulmonary signs are even less common. Some infants and young children with bronchial obstruction have localized wheezing or decreased breath sounds that may be accompanied by tachypnea or, rarely, respiratory distress. These pulmonary symptoms and signs are occasionally alleviated by antibiotics, suggesting bacterial superinfection.

Progressive Primary Pulmonary Disease
A rare but serious complication of tuberculosis in a child occurs when the primary focus enlarges steadily and develops a large caseous center.

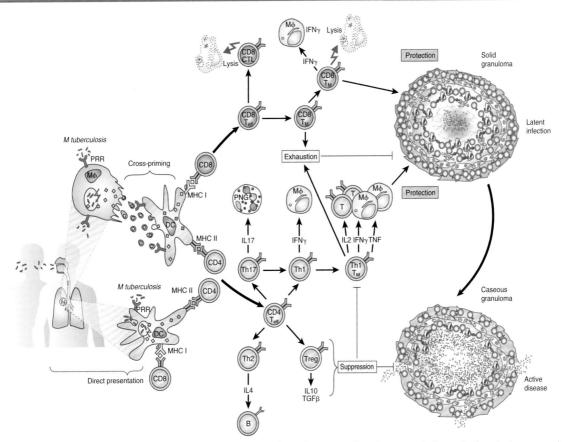

Fig. 242.10 Overview of the immune response in tuberculosis. Control of *Mycobacterium tuberculosis* is mainly the result of productive teamwork between T-cell populations and macrophages (Mø). *M. tuberculosis* survives within macrophages and dendritic cells (DCs) inside the phagosomal compartment. Gene products of major histocompatibility complex (MHC) class II are loaded with mycobacterial peptides that are presented to CD4 T cells. CD8 T-cell stimulation requires loading of MHC I molecules by mycobacterial peptides in the cytosol, either by egression of mycobacterial antigens into the cytosol or cross-priming, by which macrophages release apoptotic bodies carrying mycobacterial peptides. These vesicles are taken up by DCs and peptides presented. The CD4 T-helper (Th) cells polarize into different subsets. DCs and macrophages express pattern recognition receptors (PRRs), which sense molecular patterns on pathogens. Th1 cells produce interleukin (IL)-2 for T-cell activation, interferon-γ (IFN-γ), or tumor necrosis factor (TNF) for macrophage activation. Th17 cells, which activate polymorphonuclear granulocytes (PNGs), contribute to the early formation of protective immunity in the lung after vaccination. Th2 cells and regulatory T cells (Treg) counterregulate Th1-mediated protection via IL-4, transforming growth factor β (TGF-β), or IL-10. CD8 T cells produce IFN-γ and TNF, which activate macrophages. They also act as cytolytic T lymphocytes (CTL) by secreting perforin and granulysin, which lyse host cells and directly attack *M. tuberculosis*. These effector T cells (Teff) are succeeded by memory T cells (T_M). T_M cells produce multiple cytokines, notably IL2, IFN-γ, and TNF. During active containment in solid granuloma, *M. tuberculosis* recesses into a dormant stage and is immune to attack. Exhaustion of T cells is mediated by interactions between T cells and DCs through members of the programmed death 1 system. Treg cells secrete IL-10 and TGF-β, which suppress Th1. This process allows resuscitation of *M. tuberculosis*, which leads to granuloma caseation and active disease. B, B cell. (*From Kaufman SHE, Hussey G, Lambert PH: New vaccines for tuberculosis. Lancet 375:2110–2118, 2010.*)

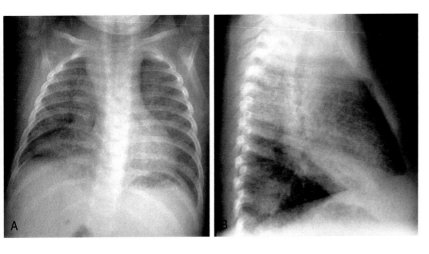

Fig. 242.11 Posteroanterior **(A)** and lateral **(B)** chest radiographs of an infant with miliary tuberculosis. The child's mother had failed to complete treatment for pulmonary tuberculosis twice within 3 yr of this child's birth.

Liquefaction can cause formation of a primary cavity associated with large numbers of tubercle bacilli. The enlarging focus can slough necrotic debris into the adjacent bronchus, leading to further intrapulmonary dissemination. Significant signs or symptoms are common in locally progressive disease in children. High fever, severe cough with sputum production, weight loss, and night sweats are common. Physical signs include diminished breath sounds, rales, and dullness or egophony over the cavity. The prognosis for full recovery is excellent with appropriate therapy.

Reactivation Tuberculosis

Pulmonary tuberculosis in adults usually represents endogenous reactivation of a site of TBI established previously in the body. This form of tuberculosis is rare in childhood but can occur in adolescence. Children with a healed TBI acquired when they were <2 yr old rarely develop chronic reactivation pulmonary disease, which is more common in those who acquire the initial infection when they are >7 yr old. The most common pulmonary sites are the original parenchymal focus, lymph nodes, or the apical seedings (**Simon foci**) established during the hematogenous phase of the early infection. This form of TB disease usually remains localized in the lungs, because the established immune response prevents further extrapulmonary spread. The most common radiographic findings are extensive infiltrates and thick-walled cavities in the upper lobes.

Older children and adolescents with reactivation tuberculosis are more likely to experience fever, anorexia, malaise, weight loss, night sweats, productive cough, hemoptysis, and chest pain than children with primary pulmonary tuberculosis. However, physical examination findings usually are minor or absent, even when cavities or large infiltrates are present. Most signs and symptoms improve within several weeks of starting effective treatment, although the cough can last for several months. This form of tuberculosis may be highly contagious if there is significant sputum production and cough. The prognosis for full recovery is excellent with appropriate therapy.

Pleural Effusion

Tuberculous pleural effusions, which can be local or general, originate in the discharge of bacilli into the pleural space from a subpleural pulmonary focus or caseated lymph node. Asymptomatic local pleural effusion is so common in primary tuberculosis that it is considered as part of the primary complex. Larger and clinically significant effusions occur months to years after the primary infection. Tuberculous pleural effusion is uncommon in children <6 yr old and rare in children <2 yr old. Effusions are usually unilateral but can be bilateral. They are rarely associated with a segmental pulmonary lesion and are uncommon in disseminated tuberculosis. Often the radiographic abnormality is more extensive than would be suggested by physical findings or symptoms (Fig. 242.12).

Clinical onset of tuberculous pleurisy is often sudden, characterized by low to high fever, shortness of breath, chest pain on deep inspiration, and diminished breath sounds. The fever and other symptoms can last for several weeks after the start of antituberculosis chemotherapy. The TST is positive in only 70–80% of cases. The prognosis is excellent, but radiographic resolution often takes months. Scoliosis is a rare complication from a long-standing effusion.

Examination of pleural fluid and the pleural membrane is important to establish the diagnosis of tuberculous **pleurisy**. The pleural fluid is usually yellow and only occasionally tinged with blood. The specific gravity is usually 1.012-1.025, the protein level is usually 2-4 g/dL, and the glucose concentration may be low, although it is usually in the low-normal range (20-40 mg/dL). Typically there are several hundred to several thousand white blood cells per microliter (WBCs/μL), with an early predominance of polymorphonuclear leukocytes (PMNs) followed by a high percentage of lymphocytes. Acid-fast smears of the pleural fluid are rarely positive. Cultures of the fluid are positive in <30% of cases. Measurement of adenosine deaminase (ADA) levels may enhance the diagnosis of pleural tuberculosis. Biopsy of the pleural membrane is more likely to yield a positive acid-fast stain or culture, and granuloma formation can be demonstrated.

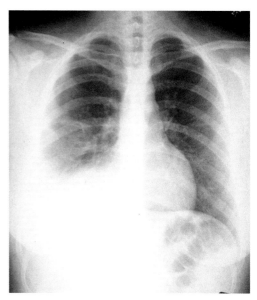

Fig. 242.12 Pleural tuberculosis in 16 yr old girl.

Pericardial Disease

The most common form of cardiac tuberculosis is **pericarditis**. It is rare, occurring in 0.5–4% of TB cases in children. Pericarditis usually arises from direct invasion or lymphatic drainage from subcarinal lymph nodes. The presenting symptoms are nonspecific, including low-grade fever, malaise, and weight loss. Chest pain is unusual in children. A pericardial friction rub or distant heart sounds with pulsus paradoxus may be present. The pericardial fluid is typically serofibrinous or hemorrhagic. Acid-fast smear of the fluid rarely reveals the organism, but cultures are positive in 30–70% of cases. ADA levels are elevated in TB pericarditis. The culture yield from pericardial biopsy may be higher, and the presence of granulomas often suggests the diagnosis. Partial or complete pericardiectomy may be required when constrictive pericarditis develops.

Lymphohematogenous (Disseminated) Disease

Tubercle bacilli are disseminated to distant sites, including liver, spleen, skin, and lung apices, in all cases of TBI. Lymphohematogenous spread is usually asymptomatic. Rare patients experience protracted hematogenous tuberculosis caused by the intermittent release of tubercle bacilli as a caseous focus erodes through the wall of a blood vessel in the lung. The clinical picture subsequent to lymphohematogenous dissemination depends on the burden of organisms released from the primary focus to distant sites and the adequacy of the host's immune response. Although the clinical picture may be acute, more often it is indolent and prolonged, with spiking fever accompanying the release of organisms into the bloodstream. Multiple organ involvement is common, leading to hepatomegaly, splenomegaly, lymphadenitis in superficial or deep nodes, and papulonecrotic tuberculids appearing on the skin. Bones and joints or kidneys also can become involved. Meningitis occurs only late in the course of the disease. Early pulmonary involvement is surprisingly mild, but diffuse involvement becomes apparent with prolonged infection.

The most clinically significant form of disseminated tuberculosis is miliary disease, which occurs when massive numbers of tubercle bacilli are released into the bloodstream, causing disease in 2 or more organs. **Miliary tuberculosis** usually complicates the primary infection, occurring within 2-6 mo of the initial infection. Although this form of disease is most common in infants and young children, it is also found in adolescents and older adults, resulting from the breakdown of a previously healed primary pulmonary lesion. The clinical manifestations of miliary tuberculosis are protean, depending on the number of organisms that disseminate and where they lodge. Lesions are often larger and more numerous in the lungs, spleen, liver, and bone marrow than other tissues. Because this form of tuberculosis is most common in infants and malnourished or immunosuppressed patients, the host's immune incompetence likely plays a role in pathogenesis.

Rarely, the onset of miliary tuberculosis is explosive, and the patient can become gravely ill in several days. More often, the onset is insidious, with early systemic signs, including anorexia, weight loss, and low-grade fever. At this time, abnormal physical signs are usually absent. Generalized lymphadenopathy and hepatosplenomegaly develop within several weeks in approximately 50% of cases. The fever can then become higher and more sustained, although the chest radiograph usually is normal and respiratory symptoms are minor or absent. Within several more weeks, the lungs can become filled with tubercles, and dyspnea, cough, rales, or wheezing occur. The lesions of miliary tuberculosis are usually <2-3 mm in diameter when first visible on chest radiograph (see Fig. 242.11). The smaller lesions coalesce to form larger lesions and sometimes extensive infiltrates. As the pulmonary disease progresses, an alveolar air block syndrome can result in frank respiratory distress, hypoxia, and pneumothorax, or pneumomediastinum. Signs or symptoms of meningitis or peritonitis are found in 20–40% of patients with advanced disease. Chronic or recurrent headache in a patient with miliary tuberculosis usually indicates the presence of meningitis, whereas the onset of abdominal pain or tenderness is a sign of tuberculous peritonitis. **Cutaneous lesions** include papulonecrotic tuberculids, nodules, or purpura. Choroid tubercles occur in 13–87% of patients and are highly specific for the diagnosis of miliary tuberculosis. Unfortunately, the TST is nonreactive in up to 40% of patients with disseminated tuberculosis.

Diagnosis of disseminated tuberculosis can be difficult, and a high index of suspicion by the clinician is required. Often the patient presents with fever of unknown origin. Early sputum or gastric aspirate cultures have a low sensitivity. Biopsy of the liver or bone marrow with appropriate bacteriologic and histologic examinations more often yields an early diagnosis. The most important clue is usually history of recent exposure to an adult with infectious tuberculosis.

The resolution of miliary tuberculosis is slow, even with proper therapy. Fever usually declines within 2-3 wk of starting chemotherapy, but the chest radiographic abnormalities might not resolve for many months. Occasionally, corticosteroids hasten symptomatic relief, especially when air block, peritonitis, or meningitis is present. The prognosis is excellent with early diagnosis and adequate chemotherapy.

Upper Respiratory Tract Disease

Tuberculosis of the upper respiratory tract is rare in developed countries but is still observed in developing countries. Children with laryngeal tuberculosis have a croup-like cough, sore throat, hoarseness, and dysphagia. Most children with laryngeal tuberculosis have extensive upper lobe pulmonary disease, but occasional patients have primary laryngeal disease with a normal chest radiograph. Tuberculosis of the middle ear results from aspiration of infected pulmonary secretions into the middle ear or from hematogenous dissemination in older children. The most common signs and symptoms are painless unilateral otorrhea, tinnitus, decreased hearing, facial paralysis, and a perforated tympanic membrane. Enlargement of lymph nodes in the preauricular or anterior cervical chains can accompany this infection. Diagnosis is difficult, because stains and cultures of ear fluid are often negative, and histology of the affected tissue often shows a nonspecific acute and chronic inflammation without granuloma formation.

Lymph Node Disease

Tuberculosis of the superficial lymph nodes, often referred to as **scrofula,** is the most common form of extrapulmonary tuberculosis in children (Figs. 242.13 to 242.15). Historically, scrofula was usually caused by drinking unpasteurized cow's milk laden with *M. bovis.* Most current cases occur within 6-9 mo of initial infection by *M. tuberculosis,* although some cases appear years later. The tonsillar, anterior cervical, submandibular, and supraclavicular nodes become involved secondary to

extension of a primary lesion of the upper lung fields or abdomen. Infected nodes in the inguinal, epitrochlear, or axillary regions result from regional lymphadenitis associated with tuberculosis of the skin or skeletal system. The nodes usually enlarge gradually in the early stages of lymph node disease. They are discrete, nontender, and firm but not hard. The nodes often feel fixed to underlying or overlying tissue. Disease is most often **unilateral**, but bilateral involvement can occur because of the crossover drainage patterns of lymphatic vessels in the chest and lower neck. As infection progresses, multiple nodes are infected, resulting in a mass of matted nodes. Systemic signs and symptoms other than a low-grade fever are usually absent. The TST is usually reactive, but the chest radiograph is normal in 70% of cases. The onset of illness is occasionally more acute, with rapid enlargement, tenderness, and fluctuance of lymph nodes and with high fever. The

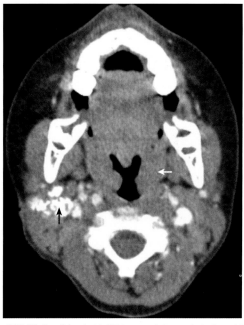

Fig. 242.13 Scrofula. Axial CT image of the neck in 8 yr old boy shows calcified right cervical lymphadenopathy *(black arrow)* with tonsillar swelling *(white arrow)*. (From Lighter J, Rigaud M: Diagnosing childhood tuberculosis: traditional and innovative modalities, Curr Probl Pediatr Adolesc Health Care 39:55–88, 2009.)

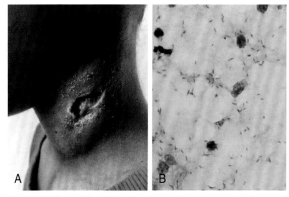

Fig. 242.14 Scrofula. **A,** Ulcerative lesion 3.2 × 2.1 cm with undermined edges and necrotic base with surrounding induration. **B,** Acid-fast bacilli. (From Sharawat IK: Scrofula, J Pediatr 189:236, 2017).

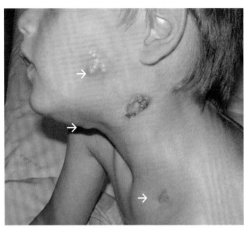

Fig. 242.15 Scrofula. Tuberculous lymphadenitis with fistula in 4 yr old boy associated with scrofuloderma *(arrows). (From Pereira C, Cascais M, Felix M, Salgado M: Scrofula in a child, J Pediatr 189:235, 2017).*

initial presentation is rarely a fluctuant mass with overlying cellulitis or skin discoloration.

Lymph node tuberculosis can resolve if left untreated but more often progresses to caseation and necrosis. The capsule of the node breaks down, resulting in the spread of infection to adjacent nodes. Rupture of the node usually results in a draining sinus tract that can require surgical removal. **Tuberculous lymphadenitis** can usually be diagnosed by fine-needle aspiration (FNA) of the node and responds well to antituberculosis therapy, although the lymph nodes do not return to normal size for months or even years. Surgical removal is not usually necessary and must be combined with antituberculosis medication, because the lymph node disease is only 1 part of a systemic infection.

A definitive diagnosis of tuberculous adenitis usually requires histologic or bacteriologic confirmation, which is best accomplished by FNA for culture, stain, and histology. If FNA is not successful in establishing a diagnosis, excisional biopsy of the involved node is indicated. Culture of lymph node tissue yields the organism in only approximately 50% of cases. Many other conditions can be confused with tuberculous adenitis, including infection caused by **nontuberculous mycobacteria (NTM)**, cat-scratch disease *(Bartonella henselae)*, tularemia, brucellosis, toxoplasmosis, pyogenic infection, or noninfectious causes, including tumor, branchial cleft cyst, and cystic hygroma. The most common problem is distinguishing infection caused by *M. tuberculosis* from lymphadenitis caused by NTM in geographic areas where NTM is common. Both conditions are usually associated with a normal chest radiograph and a reactive TST. An important clue to the diagnosis of tuberculous adenitis is an epidemiologic link to an adult with infectious tuberculosis. In areas where both diseases are common, culture of the involved tissue may be necessary to establish the exact cause of the disease.

Central Nervous System Disease

Tuberculosis of the central nervous system (CNS) is the most serious complication in children and is fatal without prompt and appropriate treatment. **Tuberculous meningitis** usually arises from the formation of a metastatic caseous lesion in the cerebral cortex or meninges that develops during the lymphohematogenous dissemination of the primary infection. This initial lesion increases in size and discharges small numbers of tubercle bacilli into the subarachnoid space. The resulting gelatinous exudate infiltrates the corticomeningeal blood vessels, producing inflammation, obstruction, and subsequent infarction of cerebral cortex. The brainstem is often the site of greatest involvement, which accounts for the commonly associated dysfunction of cranial nerves III, VI, and VII. The exudate also interferes with the normal flow of cerebrospinal fluid (CSF) in and out of the ventricular system at the level of the basilar cisterns, leading to a communicating hydrocephalus. The combination

of vasculitis, infarction, cerebral edema, and hydrocephalus results in the severe damage that can occur gradually or rapidly. Profound abnormalities in electrolyte metabolism from salt wasting or the syndrome of inappropriate antidiuretic hormone secretion (SIADH) also contribute to the pathophysiology of tuberculous meningitis.

Tuberculous meningitis complicates approximately 0.3% of untreated TBIs in children. It is most common in children 6 mo to 4 yr old. Occasionally, tuberculous meningitis occurs many years after the infection, when rupture of 1 or more of the subependymal tubercles discharges tubercle bacilli into the subarachnoid space. The clinical progression of tuberculous meningitis may be rapid or gradual. Rapid progression tends to occur more often in infants and young children, who can experience symptoms for only several days before the onset of acute hydrocephalus, seizures, and cerebral edema. More often, the signs and symptoms progress slowly over weeks and are divided into 3 stages.

The **1st stage** typically lasts 1-2 wk and is characterized by nonspecific symptoms such as fever, headache, irritability, drowsiness, and malaise. Focal neurologic signs are absent, but infants can experience a stagnation or loss of developmental milestones. The **2nd stage** usually begins more abruptly. The most common features are lethargy, nuchal rigidity, seizures, positive Kernig and Brudzinski signs, hypertonia, vomiting, cranial nerve palsies, and other focal neurologic signs. The accelerating clinical illness usually correlates with the development of hydrocephalus, increased intracranial pressure, and vasculitis. Some children have no evidence of meningeal irritation but can have signs of encephalitis, such as disorientation, movement disorders, or speech impairment. The **3rd stage** is marked by coma, hemi- or paraplegia, hypertension, decerebrate posturing, deterioration of vital signs, and eventually death.

The prognosis of tuberculous meningitis correlates most closely with the clinical stage of illness at the time treatment is initiated. The majority of patients in the 1st stage have an excellent outcome, whereas most patients in the 3rd stage who survive have permanent disabilities, including blindness, deafness, paraplegia, diabetes insipidus, or mental retardation. The prognosis for young infants is generally worse than for older children. *It is imperative that antituberculosis treatment be considered for any child who develops basilar meningitis and hydrocephalus, cranial nerve palsy, or stroke with no other apparent etiology.* Often the key to the correct diagnosis is identifying an adult who has infectious tuberculosis and is in contact with the child. Because of the short incubation period of tuberculous meningitis, the illness has not yet been diagnosed in the adult in many cases.

The diagnosis of tuberculous meningitis can be difficult early in its course, requiring a high degree of suspicion on the part of the clinician. The TST is nonreactive in up to 50% of cases, and 20–50% of children have a normal chest radiograph. The most important laboratory test for the diagnosis of tuberculous meningitis is examination and culture of the lumbar CSF. The CSF leukocyte count usually ranges from 10-500 cells/µL. PMNs may be present initially, but lymphocytes predominate in the majority of cases. The CSF glucose is typically <40 mg/dL but rarely <20 mg/dL. The protein level is elevated and may be extremely high (400-5,000 mg/dL) secondary to hydrocephalus and spinal block. Although the lumbar CSF is grossly abnormal, ventricular CSF can have normal chemistries and cell counts because this fluid is obtained from a site proximal to the inflammation and obstruction. During early stage 1, the CSF can resemble that of viral aseptic meningitis, only to progress to the more severe CSF profile over several weeks. The success of the microscopic examination of acid-fast–stained CSF and mycobacterial culture is related directly to the volume of the CSF sample. Examinations or culture of small amounts of CSF are unlikely to demonstrate *M. tuberculosis*. When 5-10 mL of lumbar CSF can be obtained, the acid-fast stain of the CSF sediment is positive in up to 30% of cases and the culture is positive in 50–70% of cases. Polymerase chain reaction (PCR) testing of the CSF and ADA levels can improve diagnosis. Cultures of other body fluids can help confirm the diagnosis.

Radiographic studies can aid in the diagnosis of tuberculous meningitis. CT or MRI of the brain of patients with tuberculous meningitis may be normal during early stages of the disease. As disease progresses, basilar enhancement and communicating hydrocephalus with signs of cerebral edema or early focal ischemia are the most common findings

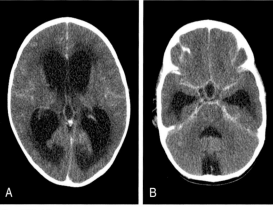

Fig. 242.16 Tuberculous meningitis in a child. **A** and **B,** Postcontrast CT images demonstrate intense enhancement in the suprasellar cistern, sylvian cistern, and prepontine cistern. Dilation of the ventricular system is seen, consistent with associated hydrocephalus. *(From Lerner A, Rajamohan A, Shiroishi MS, et al: Cerebral infections and inflammation. In Haaga JR, Boll DT, editors: CT and MRI of the whole body, ed 6, Philadelphia, 2017, Elsevier, Fig 10-20.)*

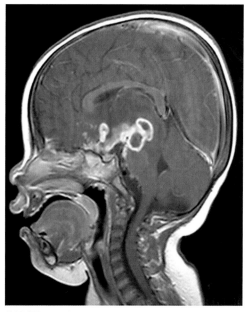

Fig. 242.17 MRI of brain of 3 yr old child showing multiple pontine tuberculomas.

(Fig. 242.16). Some small children with tuberculous meningitis have one or several clinically silent tuberculomas, occurring most often in the cerebral cortex or thalamic regions.

Another manifestation of CNS tuberculosis is the **tuberculoma,** a tumor-like mass resulting from aggregation of caseous tubercles that usually manifests clinically as a brain tumor. Tuberculomas account for up to 30% of brain tumors in some areas of the world but are rare in North America. In adults, tuberculomas are most often supratentorial, but in children they are often infratentorial, located at the base of the brain near the cerebellum (Fig. 242.17). Lesions are most often singular but may be multiple. The most common symptoms are headache, fever, focal neurologic findings, and convulsions. The TST is usually reactive, but the chest radiograph is usually normal. Surgical excision is sometimes necessary to distinguish tuberculoma from other causes of brain tumor. However, surgical removal is not necessary because most tuberculomas resolve with medical management. Corticosteroids are usually administered during the 1st few wk of treatment or in the immediate postoperative period to decrease cerebral edema. On CT or MRI of the brain, tuberculomas usually appear as discrete lesions with a significant amount of surrounding edema. Contrast medium enhancement is often impressive and can result in a ringlike lesion. Since the advent of CT, the paradoxical development of tuberculomas in patients with tuberculous meningitis who are receiving ultimately effective chemotherapy has been recognized. The cause and nature of these tuberculomas are poorly understood, but they do not represent failure of antimicrobial treatment. This phenomenon should be considered whenever a child with tuberculous meningitis deteriorates or develops focal neurologic findings during treatment. Corticosteroids can alleviate the occasionally severe clinical signs and symptoms that occur. These lesions can persist for months or years.

Cutaneous Disease
Cutaneous tuberculosis is rare in the United States but occurs worldwide and accounts for 1–2% of tuberculosis (see Chapter 685).

Bone and Joint Disease
Bone and joint infection complicating tuberculosis is most likely to involve the vertebrae. The classic manifestation of **tuberculous spondylitis** is progression to **Pott disease,** in which destruction of the vertebral bodies leads to gibbus deformity and kyphosis (Fig. 242.18) (see Chapter 699.4). **Skeletal tuberculosis** is a late complication of tuberculosis and has become a rare entity since the availability of antituberculosis therapy, but is more likely to occur in children than in adults. Tuberculous bone lesions can resemble pyogenic and fungal infections or bone tumors.

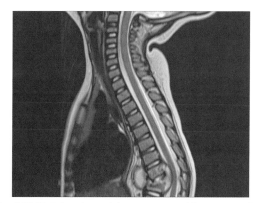

Fig. 242.18 Tuberculosis of the spine in a toddler. *(From Feder Jr HM, Rigos L, Teti K: Pott's disease in a Connecticut toddler, Lancet 388:504–505, 2016).*

Multifocal bone involvement can occur. A bone biopsy is essential to confirm the diagnosis. Surgical intervention is generally not necessary for cure, and prognosis is excellent with adequate medical treatment. A sterile polyarticular (large joints) arthritis may also be noted in patients with active tuberculosis at another site.

Abdominal and Gastrointestinal Disease
Tuberculosis of the oral cavity or pharynx is quite unusual. The most common lesion is a painless ulcer on the mucosa, palate, or tonsil with enlargement of the regional lymph nodes. Tuberculosis of the parotid gland has been reported rarely in endemic countries. Tuberculosis of the esophagus is rare in children but may be associated with a tracheo-esophageal fistula in infants. These forms of tuberculosis are usually associated with extensive pulmonary disease and swallowing of infectious respiratory secretions. They can occur in the absence of pulmonary disease, by spread from mediastinal or peritoneal lymph nodes.

Tuberculous peritonitis occurs most often in young men and is uncommon in adolescents and rare in children. Generalized peritonitis can arise from subclinical or miliary hematogenous dissemination.

Localized peritonitis is caused by direct extension from an abdominal lymph node, intestinal focus, or genitourinary tuberculosis. Rarely, the lymph nodes, omentum, and peritoneum become matted and can be palpated as a doughy, irregular, nontender mass. Abdominal pain or tenderness, ascites, anorexia, and low-grade fever are typical manifestations. The TST is usually reactive. The diagnosis can be confirmed by paracentesis with appropriate stains and cultures, but this procedure must be performed carefully to avoid entering a bowel that is adherent to the omentum.

Tuberculous enteritis is caused by hematogenous dissemination or by swallowing tubercle bacilli discharged from the patient's own lungs. The jejunum and ileum near Peyer patches and the appendix are the most common sites of involvement. The typical findings are shallow ulcers that cause pain, diarrhea or constipation, weight loss, and low-grade fever. Mesenteric adenitis usually complicates the infection. The enlarged nodes can cause intestinal obstruction or erode through the omentum to cause generalized peritonitis. The clinical presentation of tuberculous enteritis is nonspecific, mimicking other infections and conditions that cause diarrhea. The disease should be suspected in any child with chronic GI complaints and a reactive TST or positive IGRA. Biopsy, acid-fast stain, and culture of the lesions are usually necessary to confirm the diagnosis.

Genitourinary Disease
Renal tuberculosis is rare in children, because the incubation period is several years or longer. Tubercle bacilli usually reach the kidney during lymphohematogenous dissemination. The organisms often can be recovered from the urine in cases of miliary tuberculosis and in some patients with pulmonary tuberculosis in the absence of renal parenchymal disease. In true renal tuberculosis, small caseous foci develop in the renal parenchyma and release *M. tuberculosis* into the tubules. A large mass develops near the renal cortex that discharges bacteria through a fistula into the renal pelvis. Infection then spreads locally to the ureters, prostate, or epididymis. Renal tuberculosis is often clinically silent in its early stages, marked only by sterile pyuria and microscopic hematuria. Dysuria, flank or abdominal pain, and gross hematuria develop as the disease progresses. Superinfection by other bacteria is common and can delay recognition of the underlying tuberculosis. Hydronephrosis or ureteral strictures can complicate the disease. Urine cultures for *M. tuberculosis* are positive in 80–90% of cases, and acid-fast stains of large volumes of urine sediment are positive in 50–70% of cases. The TST is nonreactive in up to 20% of patients. A pyelogram or CT scan often reveals mass lesions, dilation of the proximal ureters, multiple small filling defects, and hydronephrosis if ureteral stricture is present. Disease is most often unilateral.

Genital tract tuberculosis is uncommon in prepubescent boys and girls. This condition usually originates from lymphohematogenous spread, although it can be caused by direct spread from the intestinal tract or bone. Adolescent girls can develop genital tract tuberculosis during the primary infection. The fallopian tubes are most often involved (90–100% of cases), followed by the endometrium (50%), ovaries (25%), and cervix (5%). The most common symptoms are lower abdominal pain and dysmenorrhea or amenorrhea. Systemic manifestations are usually absent, and the chest radiograph is normal in the majority of cases. The TST is usually reactive. Genital tuberculosis in adolescent boys causes epididymitis or orchitis. The condition usually manifests as a painless, unilateral nodular swelling of the scrotum. Involvement of the glans penis is extremely rare. Genital abnormalities and a positive TST in an adolescent boy or girl suggest genital tract tuberculosis.

Pregnancy and the Newborn
Pulmonary and particularly extrapulmonary tuberculosis other than lymphadenitis in a pregnant woman is associated with increased risk for prematurity, fetal growth retardation, low birthweight, and perinatal mortality. **Congenital tuberculosis** is rare because the most common result of female genital tract tuberculosis is infertility. Primary infection in the mother just before or during pregnancy is more likely to cause congenital infection than is reactivation of a previous infection. Congenital transmission usually occurs from a lesion in the placenta through the umbilical vein, when tubercle bacilli infect the fetal liver, where a primary focus with periportal lymph node involvement can occur. Organisms pass through the liver into the main fetal circulation and infect many organs. The bacilli in the lung usually remain dormant until after birth, when oxygenation and pulmonary circulation increase significantly. Congenital tuberculosis can also be caused by aspiration or ingestion of infected amniotic fluid. However, the most common route of infection for the neonate is postnatal airborne transmission from an adult with infectious pulmonary tuberculosis.

Perinatal Disease
Symptoms of congenital tuberculosis may be present at birth but usually begin by the 2nd or 3rd wk of life. The most common signs and symptoms are respiratory distress, fever, hepatic or splenic enlargement, poor feeding, lethargy or irritability, lymphadenopathy, abdominal distention, failure to thrive, ear drainage, and skin lesions. The clinical manifestations vary in relation to the site and size of the caseous lesions. Many infants have an abnormal chest radiograph, most often with a miliary pattern. Some infants with no pulmonary findings early in the course of the disease later develop profound radiographic and clinical abnormalities. Hilar and mediastinal lymphadenopathy and lung infiltrates are common. Generalized lymphadenopathy and meningitis occur in 30–50% of patients.

The clinical presentation of tuberculosis in newborns is similar to that caused by bacterial sepsis and other congenital infections, such as syphilis, toxoplasmosis, and cytomegalovirus. The diagnosis should be suspected in an infant with signs and symptoms of bacterial or congenital infection whose response to antibiotic and supportive therapy is poor and in whom evaluation for other infections is unrevealing. The most important clue for rapid diagnosis of congenital tuberculosis is a maternal or family **history** of tuberculosis. Often, the mother's disease is discovered only after the neonate's diagnosis is suspected. The infant's TST is negative initially but can become positive in 1-3 mo. A positive acid-fast stain of an early-morning gastric aspirate from a newborn usually indicates tuberculosis. Direct acid-fast stains on middle ear discharge, bone marrow, tracheal aspirate, or tissue biopsy (especially liver) can be useful. The CSF should be examined, cultured, and sent for PCR testing. The mortality rate of congenital tuberculosis remains very high because of delayed diagnosis. Many children have a complete recovery if the diagnosis is made promptly and adequate chemotherapy is started.

Disease in HIV-Infected Children
Most cases of tuberculosis in HIV-infected children are seen in developing countries. However, the rate of TB disease in untreated HIV-infected children is 30 times higher than in non–HIV-infected children in the United States. Establishing the diagnosis of tuberculosis in an HIV-infected child may be difficult, because TST reactivity can be absent (also with a negative IGRA), culture confirmation is difficult, and the clinical features of tuberculosis are similar to many other HIV-related infections and conditions. Tuberculosis in HIV-infected children is often more severe, progressive, and likely to occur in extrapulmonary sites. Radiographic findings are similar to those in children with normal immune systems, but lobar disease and lung cavitation are more common. Nonspecific respiratory symptoms, fever, and weight loss are the most common complaints. Rates of drug-resistant tuberculosis tend to be higher in HIV-infected adults and probably are also higher in HIV-infected children. Recurrent disease and relapse occur more frequently in HIV-infected children. The prognosis generally is good if TB disease is not far advanced at diagnosis and appropriate antituberculosis drugs are available.

The mortality rate of HIV-infected children with tuberculosis is high, especially as the CD4 lymphocyte numbers decrease. In adults the host immune response to TBI appears to enhance HIV replication and accelerate the immune suppression caused by HIV. Increased mortality rates are attributed to progressive HIV infection rather than tuberculosis. Therefore, HIV-infected children with potential exposures and/or recent infection should be promptly evaluated and treated for tuberculosis. Conversely, all children with TB disease should be tested for HIV infection.

Children with HIV infection who are given highly active antiretroviral therapy (HAART) are at high risk of developing **immune reconstitution inflammatory syndrome**. IRIS should be suspected in patients who experience a worsening of TB symptoms during antituberculosis therapy (*paradoxical* IRIS) or who develop new-onset TB symptoms and radiographic findings after initiation of HAART (*unmasking* IRIS). Factors suggesting IRIS are temporal association (within 3 mo of starting HAART), unusual clinical manifestations, unexpected clinical course, exclusion of alternative explanations, evidence of preceding immune restoration (rise in CD4 lymphocyte count), and decrease in HIV viral load. The most common clinical manifestations of IRIS in children are fever, cough, new skin lesions, enlarging lymph nodes in the thorax or neck, and appearance or enlargement of tuberculomas in the brain, with or without accompanying meningitis. The treatment of IRIS in HIV-positive children with tuberculosis should be undertaken by a clinician with specific expertise in TB treatment.

DIAGNOSTIC TOOLS
Tuberculin Skin Testing (TST)
The development of delayed-type hypersensitivity in most persons infected with the *M. tuberculosis* complex organisms makes the TST a useful diagnostic tool. The **Mantoux TST** is the intradermal injection of 0.1 mL purified protein derivative stabilized with Tween 80. T cells sensitized by prior infection are recruited to the skin, where they release lymphokines that induce induration through local vasodilation, edema, fibrin deposition, and recruitment of other inflammatory cells to the area. The amount of induration in response to the test should be measured by a trained person 48-72 hr after administration. In some patients, the onset of induration is >72 hr after placement; this is also a positive result. Immediate hypersensitivity reactions to tuberculin or other constituents of the preparation are short-lived (<24 hr) and not considered a positive result. Tuberculin sensitivity develops 3 wk to 3 mo (most often in 4-8 wk) after inhalation of organisms.

Host-related factors, including very young age, malnutrition, immunosuppression by disease or drugs, viral infections (measles, mumps, varicella, influenza), vaccination with live-virus vaccines, and overwhelming tuberculosis, can depress the skin test reaction in a child infected with *M. tuberculosis*. Corticosteroid therapy can decrease the reaction to tuberculin, but the effect is variable; TST done at the time of initiating corticosteroid therapy is usually reliable. Approximately 10% of immunocompetent children with TB disease (up to 50% of those with meningitis or disseminated disease) do not react initially to purified protein derivative; most become reactive after several months of antituberculosis therapy. False-positive reactions to tuberculin can be caused by cross-sensitization to antigens of NTM, which generally are more prevalent in the environment as one approaches the equator. These cross-reactions are usually transient over months to years and produce <10-12 mm of induration, but larger areas of induration can occur. Previous vaccination with bacille Calmette-Guérin (BCG) also can cause a reaction to a TST, especially if a person has received 2 or more BCG vaccinations. Approximately 50% of the infants who receive a BCG vaccine never develop a reactive TST, and the reactivity usually wanes in 2-3 yr in those with initially positive skin test results. Older children and adults who receive a BCG vaccine are more likely to develop tuberculin reactivity, but most lose the reactivity by 5-10 yr after vaccination. However, some individuals maintain tuberculin reactivity from BCG vaccine for many years. When present, skin test reactivity usually causes <10 mm of induration, although larger reactions occur in some persons.

The appropriate size of induration indicating a positive Mantoux TST result varies with related epidemiologic and risk factors. In children with no TB risk factors, skin test reactions are usually false-positive results. The American Academy of Pediatrics (AAP) and CDC discourage routine testing of all children and recommend targeted tuberculin testing of children at risk identified through periodic screening questionnaires (Table 242.2). Possible exposure to an adult with or at high risk for infectious pulmonary tuberculosis is the most crucial risk factor for children. Reaction size limits for determining a positive TST result vary with the person's risk for infection (Table 242.3). In those at

Table 242.2	Tuberculin Skin Test (TST) or Interferon-γ Release Assay (IGRA): Recommendations for Infants, Children, and Adolescents*

CHILDREN FOR WHOM IMMEDIATE TST OR IGRA IS INDICATED[†]

Contacts of people with confirmed or suspected contagious tuberculosis (contact investigation)

Children with radiographic or clinical findings suggesting tuberculosis disease

Children immigrating from countries with endemic infection (e.g., Asia, Middle East, Africa, Latin America, countries from former Soviet Union), including international adoptees

Children with travel histories to countries with endemic infection and substantial contact with indigenous people from such countries[‡]

Children who should have annual TST or IGRA:
- Children infected with human immunodeficiency virus

CHILDREN AT INCREASED RISK FOR PROGRESSION OF TUBERCULOSIS INFECTION TO TUBERCULOSIS DISEASE

Children with other medical conditions, including diabetes mellitus, chronic renal failure, malnutrition, and congenital or acquired immunodeficiencies and children receiving tumor necrosis factor (TNF) antagonists deserve special consideration. Without recent exposure, these children are not at increased risk of acquiring tuberculosis infection. Underlying immune deficiencies associated with these conditions theoretically would enhance the possibility for progression to severe disease. Initial histories of potential exposure to tuberculosis should be included for all of these patients. If these histories or local epidemiologic factors suggest a possibility of exposure, immediate and periodic TST or IGRA should be considered. **An initial TST or IGRA should be performed before initiation of immunosuppressive therapy, including prolonged corticosteroid administration, organ transplantation, or use of TNF-α antagonists or blockers, or immunosuppressive therapy in any child requiring these treatments.**

*Bacille Calmette-Guérin immunization is not a contraindication to a TST.
[†]Beginning as early as 3 mo of age.
[‡]If the child is well and has no history of exposure, the TST or IGRA should be delayed up to 10 wk after return.

From American Academy of Pediatrics: *Red book: 2018 report of the Committee on Infectious Diseases,* ed 30, Elk Grove Village, IL, 2015, AAP, p 831.

highest risk of progression to TB disease, TST sensitivity is most important, whereas specificity is more important for persons at low risk of progression.

Interferon-γ Release Assay (IGRA)
Two blood tests—T-SPOT.*TB* (Oxford Immunotec; Marlborough, MA) and QuantiFERON-TB (QFT, Qiagen; Germantown, MD) detect IFN-γ generation by the patient's T cells in response to specific *M. tuberculosis* antigens (ESAT-6, CFP-10, and TB7.7). The QFT test measures whole blood concentrations of IFN-γ, and the T-SPOT.*TB* test measures the number of lymphocytes/monocytes producing IFN-γ. The test antigens are not present on *M. bovis*–BCG and *Mycobacterium avium* complex, the major group of environmental mycobacteria, so one would expect higher specificity compared with the TST and fewer false-positive results. Both IGRAs have internal positive and negative controls. Internal positive controls allows for detection of an anergic test response, which is useful in children who are young and immunocompromised. Indeterminate (QFT)/invalid (T-SPOT.*TB*) responses occur when the test sample is negative but the positive control has insufficient activity or if the negative control has high background activity. Indeterminate/invalid results are also caused by technical factors (e.g., insufficient shaking of QFT tubes, delayed processing time). Most studies report indeterminate or invalid rates in children of 0–10%, which is influenced by a child's age and immune status. In children <2 yr old, indeterminate rates can be as high as 8.1%, vs 2.7% in older children, although more recent studies generally report much lower rates. *An indeterminate or invalid*

Table 242.3	Definitions of Positive Tuberculin Skin Test (TST) Results in Infants, Children, and Adolescents*

INDURATION ≥5 mm

Children in close contact with known or suspected contagious people with tuberculosis disease
Children suspected to have tuberculosis disease:
- Findings on chest radiograph consistent with active or previously tuberculosis disease
- Clinical evidence of tuberculosis disease[†]

Children receiving immunosuppressive therapy[‡] or with immunosuppressive conditions, including HIV infection

INDURATION ≥10 mm

Children at increased risk of disseminated tuberculosis disease:
- Children <4 yr old
- Children with other medical conditions, including Hodgkin disease, lymphoma, diabetes mellitus, chronic renal failure, or malnutrition (see Table 242.2)

Children with increased exposure to tuberculosis disease:
- Children born in high-prevalence regions of the world
- Children often exposed to adults with HIV infection, homeless, users of illicit drugs, residents of nursing homes, incarcerated or institutionalized, or migrant farm workers
- Children who travel to high-prevalence regions of the world

INDURATION ≥15 mm

Children ≥4 yr old without any risk factors

*These definitions apply regardless of previous BCG immunization; erythema at TST site does not indicate a positive test result. Tests should be read at 48-72 hr after placement.
[†]Evidence by physical examination or laboratory assessment that would include tuberculosis in the working differential diagnosis (e.g., meningitis).
[‡]Including immunosuppressive doses of corticosteroids or tumor necrosis factor-α antagonists.
BCG, Bacille Calmette-Guérin; HIV, human immunodeficiency virus.
From American Academy of Pediatrics: *Red book: 2015 report of the Committee on Infectious Diseases*, ed 30, Elk Grove Village, IL, 2018, American Academy of Pediatrics, p 830.

Table 242.4	Recommendations for Use of Tuberculin Skin Test (TST) and Interferon-γ Release Assay (IGRA) in Children

TST preferred, IGRA acceptable
- Children <2 yr of age*

IGRA preferred, TST acceptable
- Children >2 yr of age who have received BCG vaccine
- Children >2 yr of age who are unlikely to return for TST reading

TST *and* IGRA should be considered when:
The initial and repeat IGRAs are indeterminate or invalid.
The initial test (TST or IGRA) is *negative,* and:
- Clinical suspicion for TB disease is moderate to high.[†]
- The child has TB risk factor and is at high risk of progression and poor outcome (especially therapy with immunomodulating biologic agent, e.g., TNF-α antagonist).[†]

The initial TST is *positive* and:
- >2 yr old and history of BCG vaccination.
- Additional evidence needed to increase adherence with therapy.

*Some experts do not use an IGRA for children younger than 2 yr because of a relative lack of data for this age-group and the high risk of progression to disease.
[†]Positive result of either test is considered significant in these groups.
BCG, Bacille Calmette-Guérin; TB, tuberculosis; TNF, tumor necrosis factor.
Adapted from Starke JR, AAP Committee of Infectious Diseases: Interferon-γ release assays for diagnosis of tuberculosis infection and disease in children, *Pediatrics* 134(6):e1771, 2014.

IGRA result is neither negative nor positive and cannot be used to guide treatment decisions.

As with the TST, IGRAs cannot differentiate between TBI and TB disease. Two clear advantages of the IGRAs are the need for only one patient encounter (vs two with TST) and the lack of cross-reaction with BCG vaccination and most other mycobacteria, thereby increasing test specificity for TBI. Studies comparing IGRA and TST performance in children have shown comparable sensitivity (85% in culture-confirmed children) between the 2 tests, and superior IGRA specificity (95% vs 49%) in BCG-immunized, low-risk children.

Neither the TST nor the IGRAs perform well in infants and young children who are malnourished, severely immunocompromised, or have disseminated TB disease. Studies have evaluated the use of IGRAs in young children and support their use in children 2-5 yr old. Among immunocompetent children 0-5 yr old with culture-confirmed TB disease, 60% of those <2 yr old had a positive QFT compared to 100% of children 2-5 yr old, rates comparable to the TST.

Additional studies among healthy, exposed children <5 yr old have demonstrated that IGRA and TST agreement reaches 89%, and that IGRA test performance was confirmed to be adequate in children 2-5 yr old. Therefore, most experts support the use of IGRAs for the evaluation of TBI in young children at low risk of infection, especially in those who have received a BCG vaccine. IGRAs are also preferred in children who are unlikely to return for TST. *The use of both TST and IGRA should be considered in children whose initial TST or IGRA testing is negative and who are highly suspect for TB disease or risk of progression from infection to disease,* as well as in those with an indeterminate initial and repeat IGRA testing; those ≥2 yr old who have a positive TST and have received the BCG vaccine; those whose family is reluctant to treat infection based on a TST result alone; and those in whom nontuberculous mycobacterial

disease is suspected (Table 242.4). Most studies have shown no consistent, significant difference between the 2 commercially available IGRAs, and the CDC recommends no preference. Because of cost constraints, WHO does not indorse IGRA use in low- and middle-income countries, even in those with a high prevalence of tuberculosis.

MYCOBACTERIAL SAMPLING, SUSCEPTIBILITY AND CULTURE

The most specific confirmation of pulmonary tuberculosis is isolation of *M. tuberculosis* from a clinical sample. Sputum specimens for culture should be collected from adolescents and older children who are able to expectorate. Induced sputum with a jet nebulizer, inhaled saline, and chest percussion followed by nasopharyngeal suctioning is effective in children as young as 1 yr. Sputum induction provides samples for both culture and acid-fast bacilli staining. The traditional culture specimen in young children is the early-morning gastric acid obtained before the child has arisen and peristalsis has emptied the stomach of the pooled respiratory secretions that have been swallowed overnight. However, even under optimal conditions, 3 consecutive morning gastric aspirates yield the organisms in <50% of cases. The culture yield from bronchoscopy is even lower, but this procedure can demonstrate the presence of endobronchial disease or a fistula. *Negative cultures never exclude the diagnosis of tuberculosis in a child.* The presence of a positive TST or IGRA, an abnormal chest radiograph consistent with tuberculosis, and history of recent exposure to an adult with infectious tuberculosis is highly suggestive of the clinical diagnosis of TB disease. If a likely adult source case has been identified, drug susceptibility test results of the isolate from the adult source usually can be used to determine the best therapeutic regimen for the child, except in very high incidence areas, where the apparent source case might not be the actual one. Cultures should be always obtained from the child whenever the source case is unknown, there are multiple possible source cases, or the source case has possible or confirmed drug-resistant tuberculosis.

Confirmation of extrapulmonary tuberculosis is best achieved with a positive culture. However, for many forms of tuberculosis, the culture yield is only 25–50%, and probable diagnosis is by a combination of clinical signs and symptoms, analysis of body fluids when possible, radiographic or histopathologic evidence of tuberculosis, and elimination of other possible diagnoses.

Nucleic Acid Amplification Tests

The main nucleic acid amplification test (NAAT) studied in children with tuberculosis is PCR, which uses specific DNA sequences as markers for microorganisms. Compared with a clinical diagnosis of pulmonary tuberculosis in children, the sensitivity of PCR has varied from 25–83%, and specificity has varied from 80–100%. A negative PCR result never eliminates the diagnosis of tuberculosis, and the diagnosis is not confirmed by a positive PCR result.

Gene Xpert MTB/RIF (Xpert; Cepheid, Sunnyvale, CA) is a real-time PCR assay for *M. tuberculosis* that simultaneously detects **rifampin resistance**, which is often used as a proxy for MDR tuberculosis. This assay uses a self-contained cartridge system, which yields results from direct specimens in 2 hr and is less operator dependent than traditional PCR detection methods. Sensitivity and specificity of Xpert have averaged 72–77% and 99% in acid-fast bacilli (AFB) sputum smear–negative adults and 98–99% and 99–100% in AFB sputum smear–positive adults, respectively. Pediatric studies reveal that, compared with culture, the sensitivity and specificity of Xpert is 62% and 98% on induced or expectorated sputa and 66% and 98% on gastric aspirates, respectively. Compared with smear microscopy, Xpert improved the sensitivity of detecting pediatric TB cases by 36–44%. Xpert's sensitivity and specificity to detect rifampin resistance in sputum samples from adults with tuberculosis was 86% and 98%, respectively. Although cartridges for the Xpert system are expensive, it offers advantages in rapid detection of MDR-TB and is especially useful in settings lacking laboratory infrastructure. In low-resource settings, Xpert may replace smear microscopy; however, it should never replace mycobacterial cultures and drug susceptibility studies.

TREATMENT

The basic principles of management of TB disease in children and adolescents are the same as in adults. Several drugs are used to affect a relatively rapid cure and prevent the emergence of secondary drug resistance during therapy (Tables 242.5 and 242.6). The choice of regimen depends on the extent of TB disease, the host, and the likelihood of drug resistance (see Chapter 241, Table 241.1). As recommended by WHO and AAP, *the standard therapy of intrathoracic tuberculosis (pulmonary disease and/or hilar lymphadenopathy) in children is a 6 mo regimen of isoniazid and rifampin supplemented in the 1st 2 mo of treatment by pyrazinamide and ethambutol.* Several clinical trials have shown that this regimen yields a success rate approaching 100%, with an

incidence of clinically significant adverse reactions of <2%. Nine-month regimens of only isoniazid and rifampin are also effective for drug-susceptible tuberculosis, but the necessary length of treatment, the need for good adherence by the patient, and the relative lack of protection against possible initial drug resistance have led to the favoring of treatment regimens with additional drugs for a short period. Most experts recommend that all drug administration be directly observed, meaning that a healthcare worker watches when the medications are administered to the patients. When **directly observed therapy (DOT)** is used, intermittent (twice or thrice weekly) administration of drugs after an initial period as short as 2 wk of daily therapy is as effective for drug-susceptible tuberculosis in children as daily therapy for the entire course.

Extrapulmonary tuberculosis is usually caused by small numbers of mycobacteria. In general, the treatment for most forms of extrapulmonary tuberculosis in children, including cervical lymphadenopathy, is the same as for pulmonary tuberculosis. *Exceptions are bone and joint, disseminated, and CNS tuberculosis, for which there are inadequate data to recommend 6 mo of therapy; these conditions are treated for 9-12 mo.* Surgical debridement in bone and joint disease and ventriculoperitoneal shunting in CNS disease may be necessary adjuncts to medical therapy.

The optimal treatment of tuberculosis in HIV-infected children has not been established. HIV-seropositive adults with tuberculosis can be treated successfully with standard regimens that include isoniazid, rifampin, pyrazinamide, and ethambutol. The total duration of therapy should be 6-9 mo, or 6 mo after culture of sputum becomes sterile, whichever is longer. Data for children are limited to relatively small series. *Most experts believe that HIV-infected children with drug-susceptible tuberculosis should receive the standard 4-drug regimen for the 1st 2 mo followed by isoniazid and rifampin, for a total duration of at least 9 mo. However, all treatment should be daily, not intermittent.* Children with HIV infection appear to have more frequent adverse reactions to antituberculosis drugs and must be monitored closely during therapy. Co-administration of rifampin and some antiretroviral agents results in subtherapeutic blood levels of protease inhibitors and nonnucleoside reverse transcriptase inhibitors and toxic levels of rifampin. Concomitant administration of these drugs is not recommended. Treatment of HIV-infected children is often empirically based on epidemiologic and radiographic information, because the radiographic appearance of other pulmonary complications of HIV in children, such as lymphoid interstitial pneumonitis and bacterial pneumonia, may be similar to that of tuberculosis. Therapy should be

Table 242.5	Commonly Used Drugs for Treatment of Tuberculosis in Infants, Children, and Adolescents				
DRUG	**DOSAGE FORMS**	**DAILY DOSAGE (mg/kg)**	**TWICE-WEEKLY DOSAGE (mg/kg/dose)**	**MAXIMUM DOSE**	**ADVERSE REACTIONS**
Ethambutol	Tablets: 100 mg 400 mg	20	50	2.5 g	Optic neuritis (usually reversible), decreased red-green color discrimination, gastrointestinal tract disturbances, hypersensitivity
Isoniazid*	Scored tablets: 100 mg 300 mg Syrup: 10 mg/mL	10-15[†]	20-30	Daily: 300 mg Twice weekly: 900 mg	Mild hepatic enzyme elevation, hepatitis,[†] peripheral neuritis, hypersensitivity
Pyrazinamide*	Scored tablets: 500 mg	30-40	50	2 g	Hepatotoxic effects, hyperuricemia, arthralgias, gastrointestinal tract upset
Rifampin*	Capsules: 150 mg 300 mg Syrup formulated from capsules	15-20	15-20	600 mg	Orange discoloration of secretions or urine, staining of contact lenses, vomiting, hepatitis, influenza-like reaction, thrombocytopenia, pruritus Oral contraceptives may be ineffective.

*Rifamate is a capsule containing 150 mg of isoniazid and 300 mg of rifampin. Two capsules provide the usual adult (i.e., person weighing >50 kg) daily doses of each drug. Rifater, in the United States, is a capsule containing 50 mg of isoniazid, 120 mg of rifampin, and 300 mg of pyrazinamide. Isoniazid and rifampin also are available for parenteral administration. Many experts recommend using a daily rifampin dose of 20–30 mg/kg/day for infants and toddlers and for serious forms of tuberculosis such as meningitis and disseminated disease.
[†]When isoniazid in a dosage exceeding 10 mg/kg/day is used in combination with rifampin, the incidence of hepatotoxic effects may be increased.
From American Academy of Pediatrics: *Red book: 2018 report of the Committee on Infectious Diseases*, ed 30, Elk Grove Village, IL, 2015, AAP, p 842.

Table 242.6	Less Commonly Used Drugs for Treating Drug-Resistant Tuberculosis in Infants, Children, and Adolescents*			
DRUGS	**DOSAGE, FORMS**	**DAILY DOSAGE (mg/kg)**	**MAXIMUM DOSE**	**ADVERSE REACTIONS**
Amikacin†	Vials: 500 mg, 1 g	15-30 (IV or IM administration)	1 g	Auditory and vestibular toxic effects, nephrotoxic effects
Bedaquiline	Tablets: 100 mg	Adults and children ≥12 yr, >33 kg: 400 mg for 14 days, then 200 mg 3 times weekly for 22 wk		QTc prolongation, reduced levels with efavirenz co-administration
Capreomycin†	Vials: 1 g	15-30 (IM administration)	1 g	Auditory and vestibular toxicity and nephrotoxic effects
Clofazimine	Gelcaps: 50 mg 100 mg	2-3 mg/kg per day	100 mg	QTc prolongation, reversible skin pigmentation
Cycloserine	Capsules: 250 mg	10-20, given in 2 divided doses	1 g	Psychosis, personality changes, seizures, rash
Delamanid	Tablets: 50 mg 100 mg	Adults and children ≥13 yr, ≥35 kg: 100 mg twice daily Children 6-12 yr, 20-34 kg: 50 mg twice daily		QTc prolongation, adverse events with hypoalbuminemia, avoid if metronidazole allergic
Ethionamide	Tablets: 250 mg	15-20, given in 2-3 divided doses	1 g	GI tract disturbances, hepatotoxic effects, hypersensitivity reactions, hypothyroidism
Kanamycin	Vials: 75 mg/2 mL 500 mg/2 mL 1 g/3 mL	15-30 (IM or IV administration)	1 g	Auditory and vestibular toxic effects, nephrotoxic effects
Levofloxacin	Tablets: 250 mg 500 mg 750 mg Oral solution: 25/mL Vials: 25 mg/mL	Adults: 750-1000 mg (daily) Children: 15-20 mg/kg daily	1 g	Theoretic effect on growing cartilage, joint pain, GI tract disturbances, rash, headache, restlessness, confusion
Linezolid	Tablets: 400 mg 600 mg Syrup: 20 mg/mL	Children ≥12 yr: 10 mg/kg daily Children <12 yr: 10 mg/kg twice daily	600 mg	Bone marrow suppression, peripheral neuropathy, lactic acidosis, potential overlapping toxicity with nucleoside reverse transcriptase inhibitors
Ofloxacin	Tablets: 200 mg 300 mg 400 mg Vials: 20 mg/mL 40 mg/mL	Adults/adolescents: 800 mg Children 15-20 mg/kg daily	800 mg	Arthropathy, arthritis
Moxifloxacin	Tablets: 400 mg IV solution: 400 mg/250 mL in 0.8% saline	Adults/adolescents: 400 mg Children: 7.5-10 mg/kg daily	400 mg	Arthropathy, arthritis
Paraaminosalicylic acid (PAS)	Packets: 3 g	200-300 (2-4 times a day)	10 g	GI tract disturbances, hypersensitivity, hepatotoxic effects
Streptomycin†	Vials: 1 g 4 g	20-40 (IM administration)	1 g	Auditory and vestibular toxic effects, nephrotoxic effects, rash

*These drugs should be used in consultation with a specialist in tuberculosis.
†Dose adjustment in renal insufficiency.
GI, Gastrointestinal; IM, intramuscular; IV, intravenous.
From American Academy of Pediatrics: *Red book: 2018 Report of the Committee on Infectious Diseases*, ed 30. Elk Grove Village, IL, 2015, AAP, p 843–844; and Harausz EP, Garcia-Prats AJ, Seddon JA, et al: New/repurposed drugs for pediatric multidrug-resistant tuberculosis: practice-based recommendations, *Am J Respir Crit Care Med* 195(10):1300-1310, 2017.

considered when tuberculosis cannot be excluded.

Drug-Resistant Tuberculosis

The incidence of drug-resistant tuberculosis is increasing in many areas of the world, including North America. There are 2 major types of drug resistance. **Primary resistance** occurs when a person is infected with *M. tuberculosis* that is already resistant to a particular drug. **Secondary resistance** occurs when drug-resistant organisms emerge as the dominant population during treatment. The major causes of secondary drug resistance are poor adherence to the medication by the patient or inadequate treatment regimens prescribed by the physician. Nonadherence to one drug is more likely to lead to secondary resistance than is failure to take all drugs. Secondary resistance is rare in children because of the small size of their mycobacterial population. Consequently, most drug resistance in children is primary, and patterns of drug resistance among children tend to mirror those found among adults in the same population. The main predictors of drug-resistant tuberculosis among adults are history of previous antituberculosis treatment, co-infection with HIV, and exposure to another adult with infectious drug-resistant tuberculosis.

Treatment of drug-resistant tuberculosis is successful only when at least 2 bactericidal drugs are given to which the infecting strain of M. tuberculosis *is susceptible.* When a child has possible drug-resistant tuberculosis, usually at least 4 or 5 drugs should be administered initially until the susceptibility pattern is determined and a more-specific regimen can be designed. The specific treatment plan must be individualized for each patient according to the results of susceptibility testing on the isolates from the child or the adult source case. *Treatment duration of 9 mo with rifampin, pyrazinamide, and ethambutol is usually adequate for isoniazid-resistant tuberculosis in children. When resistance to isoniazid and rifampin is present, the total duration of therapy often must be extended to 12-24 mo, and intermittent regimens should not be used.* In 2016, WHO endorsed 9-12 mo shorter treatment regimen for adults and children with MDR-TB who were not previously treated with second-line drugs, or in whom resistance to second-line fluoroquinolones or injectable agents is unlikely. This recommendation was based the results of adult observational studies and extrapolated for use in children based on biologic plausibility.

As second-line treatment options for MDR-TB in children, there is increasing use of new antituberculosis medications (bedaquiline and delamanid) and repurposed drugs (linezolid and clofazimine). **Delamanid** is endorsed for use in children ≥6 years and ≥20 kg in whom a 4-drug regimen plus pyrazinamide cannot be used because of drug resistance, in those who experience significant drug intolerance, or those at high risk of treatment failure. There is less evidence to support the use of **bedaquiline** in children. It is considered acceptable in children ≥12 yr old and >33 kg, with the same indications specified for delamanid. A baseline electrocardiogram and QTc monitoring is recommended in patients receiving bedaquiline or delamanid. Both **linezolid** and **clofazimine** are now included as core second-line agents in treatment regimens for children with MDR-TB. Both drugs require close monitoring for adverse effects and toxicity. The prognosis of single-drug–resistant or MDR tuberculosis in children is usually good if the drug resistance is identified early in the treatment, if appropriate drugs are administered under DOT, if adverse reactions from the drugs are minor, and if the child and family are in a supportive environment. The treatment of drug-resistant tuberculosis in children always should be undertaken by a clinician with specific expertise in TB treatment.

Corticosteroids

Corticosteroids are useful in treating some children with TB disease. They are most beneficial when the host inflammatory reaction contributes significantly to tissue damage or impairment of organ function. There is convincing evidence that corticosteroids decrease mortality rates and long-term neurologic sequelae in some patients with **tuberculous meningitis** by reducing vasculitis, inflammation, and ultimately intracranial pressure. Lowering the intracranial pressure limits tissue damage and favors circulation of antituberculosis drugs through the brain and meninges. Short courses of corticosteroids also may be effective for children with **endobronchial tuberculosis** that causes respiratory distress, localized emphysema, or segmental pulmonary lesions. Several randomized clinical trials have shown that corticosteroids can help relieve symptoms and constriction associated with acute tuberculous **pericardial effusion.** Corticosteroids can cause dramatic improvement in symptoms in some patients with tuberculous pleural effusion and shift of the mediastinum. However, the long-term course of disease is probably unaffected. Some children with severe **miliary tuberculosis** have dramatic improvement with corticosteroid therapy if the inflammatory reaction is so severe that alveolocapillary block is present. There is no convincing evidence to support a specific corticosteroid preparation. The most common regimen is **prednisone**, 1-2 mg/kg/day in 1-2 divided doses orally for 4-6 wk, followed by a taper.

Supportive Care

Children receiving treatment should be followed carefully to promote **adherence** to therapy, to monitor for toxic reactions to medications, and to ensure that the tuberculosis is being adequately treated. Adequate **nutrition** is important. Patients should be seen at monthly intervals and should be given just enough medication to last until the next visit. **Anticipatory guidance** with regard to the administration of medications to children is crucial. The physician should foresee difficulties that the family might have in introducing several new medications in inconvenient dosage forms to a young child. The clinician must report all cases of suspected tuberculosis in a child to the local health department to be sure that the child and family receive appropriate care and evaluation.

Nonadherence to treatment is the major problem in TB therapy. The patient and family must know what is expected of them through verbal and written instructions in their primary language. Approximately 30–50% of patients taking long-term treatment are significantly nonadherent with self-administered medications, and clinicians are usually not able to determine in advance which patients will be nonadherent. Preferably, DOT should be instituted by the local health department.

Mycobacterium tuberculosis Infection

The following aspects of the natural history and treatment of TBI, often referred to as *latent tuberculosis infection,* in children must be considered in the formulation of recommendations about therapy: (1) infants and children <5 yr old with TBI have been infected recently; (2) the risk for progression to disease is high; (3) untreated infants with TBI have up to a 40% chance of development of TB disease; (4) the risk for progression decreases gradually through childhood, until adolescence when the risk increases; (5) infants and young children are more likely to have life-threatening forms of tuberculosis, including meningitis and disseminated disease; and (6) children with TBI have more years at risk for development of disease than adults. Because of these factors, and the excellent safety profile of isoniazid, rifampin, and rifapentine in children, there is a tendency to err on the side of overtreatment in infants, young children, and adolescents.

The main TBI treatment regimens used in children include 6-9 mo of **isoniazid** (daily, or twice weekly by DOT), 3 mo of daily **rifampin** and isoniazid, 4-6 mo of daily rifampin, and once-weekly isoniazid and **rifapentine**, for 12 total doses. Isoniazid therapy for TBI appears to be more effective for children than adults, with several large clinical trials demonstrating risk reduction of 70–90%. The risk of isoniazid-related hepatitis is minimal in infants, children, and adolescents, who tolerate the drug better than adults.

Analysis of data from several studies demonstrates that the efficacy decreased significantly if isoniazid was taken for <9 mo. However, the international standard is 6 mo of treatment with isoniazid because of resource considerations. Isoniazid given twice weekly has been used extensively to treat TBI in children, especially schoolchildren and close contacts of case patients. DOT should be considered when it is unlikely that the child and family will adhere to daily self-administration, or if the child is at increased risk for rapid development of disease (newborns and infants, recent contacts, immunocompromised children). For healthy children taking isoniazid but no other potentially hepatotoxic drugs, routine biochemical monitoring and supplementation with pyridoxine are not necessary. A 3 mo daily regimen of rifampin and isoniazid has been used in Europe, with programmatic data suggesting that the regimen is effective, but this regimen is not recommended in the United States. Rifampin alone for 4-6 mo is now frequently used for the treatment of TBI in infants, children, and adolescents. This regimen is most often used when a shorter, self-administered treatment regimen is preferred, when isoniazid cannot be tolerated, or the child has had contact with a source case infected with an isoniazid-resistant but rifamycin-susceptible organism. Rifapentine is a rifamycin with a very long half-life, allowing for weekly administration in conjunction with isoniazid. Studies have demonstrated that 12 doses of once-weekly isoniazid and rifapentine are as effective for treating TBI and as safe as 9 mo of daily isoniazid in children as young as 2 yr. This is becoming the preferred regimen for the treatment of TBI in age-eligible children who are exposed to a contact with presumed pan-susceptible TB. Given the risk of selecting for drug-resistant isolates by missing intermittent doses of rifamycins, this treatment regimen currently is recommended only with DOT under the supervision of local health departments. Studies have revealed that the shorter treatment regimens for TBI in children are equally efficacious as 9 mo of isoniazid and are associated with superior treatment completion rates.

For children with MDR-TB, the regimen will depend on the drug-susceptibility profile of the contract case's organism; an expert in tuberculosis should be consulted.

Few controlled studies have been published regarding the efficacy of any form of treatment for TBI in HIV-infected children. A 9 mo course of daily isoniazid is recommended. Most experts recommend that routine monitoring of serum hepatic enzyme concentrations be performed and pyridoxine be given when HIV-infected children are treated with isoniazid. The optimal duration of rifampin therapy in HIV-infected children with TBI is not known, but many experts recommend at least a 6 mo course.

Isoniazid should be given to children <5 yr old who have a negative TST or IGRA result but who have a known recent exposure to an adult with potentially contagious TB disease. This practice is often referred to as **window prophylaxis**. By the time delayed hypersensitivity develops (2-3 mo), an untreated child already may have developed severe tuberculosis. For these children, tuberculin skin or IGRA testing is repeated 8-10 wk after contact with the source case for tuberculosis has been broken (*broken contact* is defined as physical separation or adequate initial treatment of the source case). If the 2nd test result is positive, the child should complete a treatment course for TBI (either 9 mo of INH or one of the shorter treatment options). If a new TBI treatment course is started (either 4 mo of rifampin or 12 weekly doses of isoniazid and rifapentine), the treatment start date is day one of the new regimen. If the 2nd test result is negative, TBI treatment can be stopped.

PREVENTION

The highest priority of any TB control program should be case finding and treatment, which interrupts transmission of infection between close contacts. All children and adults with symptoms suggestive of TB disease and those in close contact with an adult with suspected infectious pulmonary tuberculosis should be tested for TBI (by TST or IGRA) and examined as soon as possible. On average, 30–50% of household contacts to infectious cases are infected, and 1% of contacts already have overt disease. This scheme relies on effective and adequate public health response and resources. Children, particularly young infants, should receive high priority during contact investigations, because their risk for infection is high, and they are more likely to rapidly develop severe forms of tuberculosis.

Mass testing of large groups of children for TBI is an inefficient process. When large groups of children at low risk for tuberculosis are tested, the vast majority of TST reactions are actually false-positive reactions because of biologic variability or cross-sensitization with NTM. However, testing of high-risk groups of adults or children should be encouraged, because most of these persons with positive TST or IGRA results have TBI. Testing should take place only if effective mechanisms are in place to ensure adequate evaluation and treatment of the persons who test positive.

Bacille Calmette-Guérin Vaccination

The only available vaccine against tuberculosis is the BCG vaccine. The original vaccine organism was a strain of *M. bovis* attenuated by subculture every 3 wk for 13 yr. This strain was distributed to dozens of laboratories that continued to subculture the organism on different media under various conditions. The result has been production of many BCG vaccines that differ widely in morphology, growth characteristics, sensitizing potency, and animal virulence.

The administration route and dosing schedule for the BCG vaccines are important variables for efficacy. The preferred route of administration is intradermal injection with a syringe and needle, because it is the only method that permits accurate measurement of an individual dose.

The BCG vaccines are extremely safe in immunocompetent hosts. Local ulceration and regional suppurative adenitis occur in 0.1–1%

of vaccine recipients. Local lesions do not suggest underlying host immune defects and do not affect the level of protection afforded by the vaccine. Most reactions are mild and usually resolve spontaneously, but chemotherapy is needed occasionally. Surgical excision of a suppurative draining node is rarely necessary and should be avoided if possible. **Osteitis** is a rare complication of BCG vaccination that appears to be related to certain strains of the vaccine that are no longer in wide use. Systemic complaints such as fever, convulsions, loss of appetite, and irritability are extraordinarily rare after BCG vaccination. Profoundly immunocompromised patients can develop disseminated BCG infection after vaccination. Children with HIV infection appear to have rates of local adverse reactions to BCG vaccines that are comparable with rates in immunocompetent children. However, the incidence in these children of disseminated infection months to years after vaccination is currently unknown.

Recommended vaccine schedules vary widely among countries. The official WHO recommendation is a single dose administered during infancy, in populations where the risk for tuberculosis is high. However, *infants with known or suspected HIV infection should not receive a BCG vaccination.* In some countries, repeat vaccination is universal, although no clinical trials support this practice. In others, it is based on either TST or the absence of a typical scar. The optimal age for administration and dosing schedule are unknown because adequate comparative trials have not been performed.

Although dozens of BCG trials have been reported in various human populations, the most useful data have come from several controlled trials. The results of these studies have been disparate. Some demonstrated substantial protection from BCG vaccines, but others showed no efficacy at all. A meta-analysis of published BCG vaccination trials suggested that BCG is 50% effective in preventing pulmonary tuberculosis in adults and children. The protective effect for disseminated and meningeal tuberculosis appears to be slightly higher, with BCG preventing 50–80% of cases. A variety of explanations for the varied responses to BCG vaccines have been proposed, including methodologic and statistical variations within the trials, interaction with NTM that either enhances or decreases the protection afforded by BCG, different potencies among the various BCG vaccines, and genetic factors for BCG response within the study populations. BCG vaccination administered during infancy has little effect on the ultimate incidence of tuberculosis in adults, suggesting waning protection with time.

BCG vaccination has worked well in some situations but poorly in others. Clearly, BCG vaccination has had little effect on the ultimate control of tuberculosis throughout the world, because >5 billion doses have been administered but tuberculosis remains epidemic in most regions. BCG vaccination does not substantially influence the chain of transmission, because cases of contagious pulmonary tuberculosis in adults that can be prevented by BCG vaccination constitute a small fraction of the sources of infection in a population. The best use of BCG vaccination is to prevent life-threatening forms of tuberculosis in infants and young children.

BCG vaccination has never been adopted as part of the strategy for TB control in the United States. Widespread use of the vaccine would render subsequent TSTs less useful. However, BCG vaccination can contribute to TB control in select population groups. BCG is recommended for TST-negative, HIV-negative infants and children who are at high risk for intimate and prolonged exposure to persistently untreated or ineffectively treated adults with infectious pulmonary tuberculosis and who cannot be removed from the source of infection or placed on long-term preventive therapy. It also is recommended for those who are continuously exposed to persons with tuberculosis who have bacilli that are resistant to isoniazid and rifampin. Any child receiving BCG vaccination should have a documented negative TST before receiving the vaccine. After receiving the vaccine, the child should be separated from the possible sources of infection until it can be demonstrated that the child has had a vaccine response, demonstrated by tuberculin reactivity, which usually develops within 1-3 mo.

Active research to develop new TB vaccines has led to the creation and preliminary testing of several vaccine candidates based on attenuated strains of mycobacteria, subunit proteins (H4:IC31), or DNA. The genome of *M. tuberculosis* has been sequenced, allowing researchers to further study and better understand the pathogenesis and host immune responses to tuberculosis.

Prevention of Perinatal Tuberculosis

The most effective way of preventing TB infection and disease in the neonate or young infant is through appropriate testing and treatment of the mother and other family members. High-risk pregnant women should be tested with a TST or IGRA, and those with a positive test result should receive a chest radiograph with appropriate abdominal shielding. If the mother has a negative chest radiograph and is clinically well, no separation of the infant and mother is needed after delivery. The child needs no special evaluation or treatment if the child remains asymptomatic. Other household members should undergo testing for TBI and further evaluation as indicated.

If the mother has suspected tuberculosis at the time of delivery, the newborn should be separated from the mother until the chest radiograph is obtained. If the mother's chest radiograph is abnormal, separation should be maintained until the mother has been evaluated thoroughly, including examination of the sputum. If the mother's chest radiograph is abnormal but the history, physical examination, sputum examination, and evaluation of the radiograph show no evidence of current active tuberculosis, it is reasonable to assume that the infant is at low risk for infection. The mother should receive appropriate treatment, and she and her infant should receive careful follow-up care.

If the mother's chest radiograph or AFB sputum smear shows evidence of current TB disease, additional steps are necessary to protect the infant. Isoniazid therapy for newborns has been so effective that separation of the mother and infant is no longer considered mandatory. Separation should occur only if the mother is ill enough to require hospitalization, has been or is expected to become nonadherent to treatment, or has suspected drug-resistant tuberculosis. Isoniazid treatment for the infant should be continued until the mother is sputum culture negative for ≥3 mo. At that time, a Mantoux TST should be placed on the child. If the test is positive, isoniazid is continued for a total duration of 9-12 mo; if the test is negative, isoniazid can be discontinued. Once the mother and child are taking adequate therapy, it is usually safe for the mother to breastfeed, because the medications, although found in milk, are present in low concentrations. If isoniazid resistance is suspected or the mother's adherence to medication is in question, continued separation of the infant from the mother should be considered. The duration of separation must be at least as long as is necessary to render the mother noninfectious. A TB expert should be consulted if the young infant has potential exposure to the mother or another adult with TB disease caused by an isoniazid-resistant strain of *M. tuberculosis*.

Although isoniazid is not thought to be teratogenic, the treatment of pregnant women who have asymptomatic TBI is often deferred until after delivery. However, symptomatic pregnant women or those with radiographic evidence of TB disease should be appropriately evaluated. Because pulmonary tuberculosis is harmful to both the mother and the fetus and represents a great danger to the infant after delivery, tuberculosis in pregnant women always should be treated. The most common regimen for drug-susceptible tuberculosis is isoniazid, rifampin, and ethambutol. The aminoglycosides and ethionamide should be avoided because of their teratogenic effect. The safety of pyrazinamide in pregnancy has not been established.

Bibliography is available at Expert Consult.

Chapter **243**

Hansen Disease (*Mycobacterium leprae*)

Cristina Garcia-Mauriño and Asuncion Mejias

第二百四十三章

汉森病（麻风分枝杆菌）

中文导读

本章主要介绍了汉森病的病原学、流行病学、传播途径、发病机制、临床表现、诊断方法、治疗以及预防接种。该病是由麻风分枝杆菌引起的表现多样、可治愈的疾病。具有地方性及遗传易感性特点，主要通过呼吸道传播，因为宿主对麻风分枝杆菌发生免疫反应而发病。主要依据Ridley-Jopling scale和WHO分类两种方法进行临床分期。临床表现主要累及皮肤、周围神经系统，也可累及其他器官。急性加重期可发生严重免疫反应。诊断主要依赖于临床表现，全层皮肤活检及PCR检测是重要的实验室诊断手段。治疗主要包括多药物联合抗感染治疗和控制麻风反应。易发生永久性神经损害，早期治疗可以减少远期并发症。应加强该病预防保护，接种卡介苗具有一定的保护作用。

Leprosy (Hansen disease) is a heterogeneous, curable infection caused by *Mycobacterium leprae* that primarily affects the upper airway, skin, and peripheral nerves. Disease manifestations are mainly determined by the host's immunologic response to infection, resulting in a wide clinical spectrum. The majority of exposed individuals never develop clinical disease. Hansen disease (**HD**) is currently the accepted designation of leprosy, and contrary to popular folklore, HD is *not* highly transmissible and *is* treatable. In addition, the associated morbidity and disability can be prevented with early diagnosis and appropriate treatment.

MICROBIOLOGY

Mycobacterium leprae is an obligate intracellular acid-fast gram-positive bacillus of the family Mycobacteriaceae measuring 1-8 μm in length. It grows optimally at 27-33°C (80.6-91.4°F) yet cannot be cultured in vitro. The bacillus multiplies slowly, with a doubling time of 11-13 days. It is the only bacterium known to infect **Schwann cells** of peripheral nerves. Identification of acid-fast bacilli in peripheral nerves is pathognomonic of leprosy.

EPIDEMIOLOGY

The prevalence of leprosy is variable, with the majority of cases being identified in tropical and subtropical areas. The World Health Organization (WHO) goal to eliminate leprosy as a public health problem, defined as a reduction in its prevalence to less than 1 case per 10,000 population, was achieved at the global level in 2000. Despite an overall decline in reported prevalence, HD continues to afflict more than 2 million people worldwide. Approximately 213,899 new cases were reported globally in 2014, with >94% of cases occurring in Southeast Asia (mostly India), Africa, and South America (mostly Brazil). A total of 8.8% of these cases occurred in children. In 2016, WHO released *Global Leprosy Strategy 2016–2020: Accelerating Towards a Leprosy-Free World*.

Since 1984, HD has been a *notifiable disease* in the United States, with 13,950 registered cases by the end of 2015. Of the 178 new U.S. cases reported in 2015, 72% were identified in Texas, Louisiana, Hawaii, California, Florida, New York, and Arkansas. Of the U.S. cases, 57% were identified in immigrants, mainly Asian or South Pacific Islanders; however, over one third of U.S. cases are **autochthonous** and do not report contact with foreign countries or people with leprosy. Less than 3% of U.S. cases in 2015 occurred in children <16 yr old. Younger patients predominate in areas with high endemicity.

The likelihood of developing HD is determined by several variables: age (with 2 incidence peaks: 10-14 yr and 30 yr), gender (male/female ratio 2:1, with no differences observed in children), genetics, immune status, type of leprosy (with higher risk in those exposed to patients with multibacillary disease), and possibly through exposure to **armadillos**. Whole genome sequencing has allowed identification of genes and polymorphisms associated with increased susceptibility to leprosy (approximately 5% of people are genetically susceptible to *M. leprae* infection). HD in immunocompromised hosts has been reported in solid-organ and bone marrow transplant recipients and patients receiving tumor necrosis factor (TNF)–blocking monoclonal antibodies. Patients with HIV infection do not appear to be at increased risk of acquiring leprosy, increased disease severity, or poor response to treatment. However, clinicians should be aware that concomitant HIV infection and leprosy can result in worsening of symptoms of leprosy during HIV treatment as a result of an immune reconstitution inflammatory syndrome.

The exact mechanism of transmission is not fully understood but is thought to occur primarily by the respiratory route. Natural infection occurs in humans and armadillos, which are the only recognized nonhuman reservoir. The risk of transmission from armadillos to humans seems low, and again the mechanism is not fully understood. The incubation period between natural infection and overt clinical disease in humans ranges from 3 mo to 20 yr, with a mean of 4 yr for **tuberculoid** leprosy and 10 yr for **lepromatous** leprosy. Up to 10^7 viable bacilli per day can be shed in the respiratory secretions of patients with **multibacillary** leprosy. The relative risk for developing disease in household contacts is 8-10 fold for lepromatous disease and 2-4–fold for the tuberculoid form. Transmissions by breast milk, the transplacental route, and through broken skin have been reported. Environmental factors and subclinically infected humans may also play a role in disease transmission. The infectivity of patients with HD becomes negligible within 24 hr of the first administration of effective therapy.

PATHOGENESIS

In the skin, *M. leprae* shows affinity for keratinocytes, macrophages, and histiocytes, and in peripheral nerves the organism can be found in the Schwann cells. The mechanism of mycobacterial dissemination from the respiratory tract to the skin and nerves is thought to occur hematogenously but has not been completely elucidated. *M. leprae* induces demyelination and binds to the laminin-2 glycoprotein present in the basal lamina of Schwann cells in peripheral nerves, where it replicates slowly over several years. Infection stimulates the dedifferentiation of Schwann cells to immature cells through the activation of the Erk1/2 pathway. This reprogramming of Schwann cells seems to be linked to disease dissemination. In addition to the direct nerve invasion, the immune response to infection also contributes to nerve damage. Schwann cells express human leukocyte antigen (HLA) class II molecules and present mycobacterial peptides to the HLA class II–restricted CD4$^+$ T cells, which initiate an inflammatory response. These events explain the nerve damage seen in paucibacillary disease and in reversal reactions. Swelling within the perineurium leads to ischemia, further nerve damage, and eventually fibrosis and axonal death.

DISEASE CLASSIFICATION

Disease classification is important to determine potentially infectious cases and prognosis. Based on the cellular immune response and disease dissemination, 2 classification schemes for leprosy are frequently used: the Ridley-Jopling scale and the WHO classification:

A. The **Ridley-Jopling scale** is used in the United States and describes the 5 types of leprosy, according to clinical spectrum of disease, bacillary load, and findings on histopathology.

1. *Tuberculoid form*: Patients usually have a vigorous and specific cellular immune response to *M. leprae* antigens and have a small number of skin lesions, generally, 1-3 well-demarcated macules or plaques with elevated borders (Fig. 243.1) and reduced or absent sensation. The lesions are infiltrated by T-helper 1 (Th1) cells producing abundant interferon (IFN)-γ and TNF-α, forming well-demarcated granulomas, with few, if any bacilli found within the lesions.

2. *Borderline tuberculoid form*

3. *Borderline form*

4. *Borderline lepromatous*

5. *Lepromatous form*: Patients have an absence of specific cellular immunity to *M. leprae* (but intact immunity to *Mycobacterium tuberculosis*) and present the most severe form of disease. They manifest clinically apparent infiltration of peripheral nerves and skin lesions (usually many lesions and not all hypoesthetic or

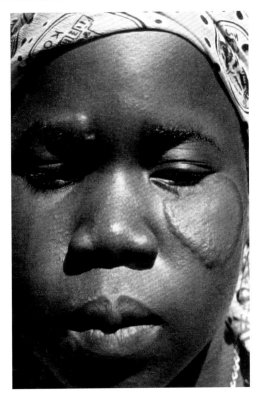

Fig. 243.1 Tuberculous leprosy in a patient who has a single skin lesion with a raised border and flattened center.

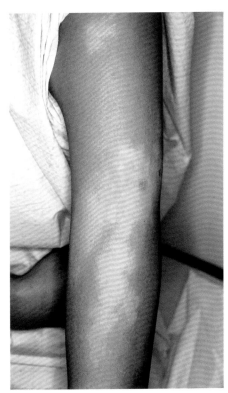

Fig. 243.2 Borderline leprosy in a patient who has numerous, hypopigmented lesions with poorly defined borders.

anesthetic), with a high load of bacilli in the absence of an effective cell-mediated immune response. Skin biopsies reveal extensive infiltration of the skin and nerves, containing messenger RNA for Th2 cytokines such as interleukin (IL)-4 and IL-10, poorly formed granulomas, and uncontrolled proliferation of bacilli within foamy macrophages. A large amount of circulating antibody to *M. leprae* is present but does not confer protective immunity. Over time, patients with the lepromatous form develop a systemic disease with symmetric peripheral nerve involvement and a diffuse infiltrative dermopathy that includes thickening of the facial skin and hair loss of the eyelashes and eyebrows (madarosis), leading to the classic presentation of the *leonine facies*. They also have involvement of the nasal mucosa causing nasal congestion and epistaxis.

The majority of patients will present with a borderline form. From borderline tuberculoid to borderline lepromatous forms, there is a progressive reduction in cellular immune responses, an increase in bacillary load, more frequent hypopigmented skin lesions and nerve involvement, and higher antibody titers (Fig. 243.2). Patients with the extreme forms of the disease (tuberculoid and lepromatous) are considered to have stable cell-mediated immunity, because their disease manifestations do not change much over time. In contrast, patients with borderline disease have unstable cell-mediated immunity and demonstrate changes in their clinical manifestations over time toward the polar forms (downgrade) or present sudden reversal reactions (upgrade). *Indeterminate leprosy* is the earliest form of the disease and is seen most frequently in young children. Patients usually have a single hypopigmented macule with poorly defined borders, without erythema or induration. Anesthesia is minimal or absent, especially if the lesion is on the face. The diagnosis is usually one of exclusion in the setting of a contact investigation. Tissue biopsies show diagnostic evidence of leprosy but do not meet sufficient criteria for classification. Up to 50–75%

of these lesions will heal spontaneously, and the rest will progress to another form of leprosy.
B. The **WHO classification** can be used when histologic evaluation and confirmatory diagnosis is unavailable, a common scenario in the field. This simplified scheme is based on the number of skin lesions:
1. Paucibacillary (1-5 patches)
2. Multibacillary (>5 patches)

CLINICAL MANIFESTATIONS

The host immune response determines the clinical spectrum of leprosy. Skin and serologic studies suggest that up to 90% of infected people develop immunity after exposure, without manifesting clinical disease. In genetically susceptible individuals with sufficient exposure to become infected, the cellular host's immunologic response to infection and unique tropism for peripheral nerves determines the wide spectrum of clinical (and histologic) manifestations. Regardless of the disease subtype, HD affects the skin and peripheral nerves. Leprosy lesions usually do not itch or hurt.

Skin Involvement

The most common skin lesions are **macules** or **plaques** with unclear outer limits, with or without neurologic symptoms. Diffuse infiltrative lesions and subcutaneous nodules are less common. Initial lesions are insidious hypopigmented macules, although they may appear erythematous on pale skin. Lesions may involve any area of the body, are more pronounced in cooler areas (e.g., earlobes, nose), and occur less frequently in the scalp, axillae, or perineum. Approximately 70% of skin lesions have reduced sensation; the degree of hypoesthesia depends on the location and size of the lesion and the degree of Th1 immune response. Examination of the skin should ideally be performed in natural sunlight and be tested for hypoesthesia to light touch, pinprick, temperature, and anhidrosis.

Studies in endemic areas in children <15 yr old have shown predominance of **paucibacillary** forms, with predominance of single lesions.

Nerve Involvement

Peripheral nerves are most frequently affected early in the disease and should be palpated for thickness and tenderness (Fig. 243.3), as well as evaluated for both motor and sensory function, particularly temperature and light touch. The posterior tibial nerve (medial malleolus) is the most common nerve affected, followed by the ulnar (elbow), median (wrist), lateral popliteal (fibular neck), and facial nerves. The skin lesions overlying a nerve trunk distribution predict the involvement of nerves in the vicinity. There is a pure **neuritic** form of leprosy, usually occurring in India and Nepal, in which patients present with asymmetric neuropathy, but lack skin lesions.

Other Organ Involvement

Ocular involvement leading to vision loss results from both direct bacillary invasion of the eye and optic nerve damage. **Lagophthalmos** occurs when there is destruction of the facial nerve (cranial nerve VII), and trigeminal nerve (cranial nerve V) destruction causes anesthesia of the cornea and conjunctiva, leading to abrasions. Facial skin lesions are associated with a 10-fold higher risk of facial nerve damage. Systemic involvement of other organs is seen mainly in patients with lepromatous leprosy where a high bacillary burden leads to infiltration of the nasal mucosa, bones, and testes. Renal involvement and amyloidosis are rare findings.

Immunologic Reactions

Leprosy reactions are acute clinical exacerbations reflecting disturbances of the immunologic balance to *M. leprae* infection and occurring in 30–50% of all leprosy patients. These sudden changes occur in patients with borderline and lepromatous leprosy, typically during the initial years after infection (sometimes as the initial presentation), but can occur before, during, or after completion of treatment. There are 2 main types of leprosy reactions, which require immediate treatment so as to prevent long-term complications. In children <15 yr old, leprosy reactions range from 1–30% and are mainly type 1 reactions.

Type 1 reactions (also known as **reversal reactions**) occur in one third of patients with borderline disease. These reactions are characterized by acute edema and increased erythema, warmth, and painful inflammation of preexisting cutaneous plaques or nodules, with acute swelling and tenderness of peripheral nerves that can quickly progress to cause nerve abscesses and necrosis. There may be a peripheral lymphocytosis and an increased cytokine response, but systemic symptoms are uncommon and appear to be associated with an increase in Th1-mediated reactivity to mycobacterial antigens. Increased serum concentrations of CXCL10 have been found in type 1 reactions. Rapid and sustained reversal of the inflammatory process using corticosteroids is essential to prevent continued nerve damage.

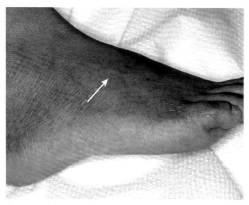

Fig. 243.3 Thickened, superficial peroneal nerve of leprosy.

Type 2 reactions, or **erythema nodosum leprosum (ENL)**, occur in borderline lepromatous and lepromatous forms, as these patients have the highest levels of *M. leprae* antigens and antibodies, most often in the 1st 2 yr after starting therapy. ENL is distinguished from reversal reactions by the development of new painful, erythematous subcutaneous nodules with an accompanying systemic inflammatory response. ENL is accompanied by high circulating concentrations of TNF-α. Patients develop high fever and signs of systemic toxicity, and in severe cases, ENL can be life threatening, presenting with features similar to septic shock. Deposition of extravascular immune complexes leads to neutrophil infiltration and activation of complement in the skin and other organs. Tender, erythematous dermal papules or nodules (resembling erythema nodosum) occur in clusters, typically on extensor surfaces of the lower extremities and face. Immune complex deposition also contributes to migrating polyarthralgias, painful swelling of lymph nodes and spleen, iridocyclitis, vasculitis, orchitis, and, rarely, nephritis. Patients may present with either a single acute episode, a relapsing form comprised of multiple acute episodes, or a chronic continuous form. Management of type two reactions is usually more complicated because of recurrence and systemic involvement.

Lucio phenomenon (erythema necroticans) is an uncommon, but potentially fatal reaction distinct from type 1 or 2 reactions and occurs in patients with untreated lepromatous leprosy, in patients whose ancestry is from Mexico. It is a necrotizing vasculitis caused by *M. leprae* directly invading the endothelium. Clinically, patients develop violaceous or hemorrhagic plaques, followed by ulcerations in the absence of systemic complaints. Secondary bacterial infections are common.

DIAGNOSIS

The diagnosis of HD requires high clinical suspicion and should be considered in any patient with a hypoesthetic or anesthetic skin lesion that does not respond to standard treatment, especially if there is a history of travel or residence in an endemic region or a history of contact with leprosy patients or armadillos. There are no reliable tests to diagnose subclinical leprosy. Full-thickness skin biopsy and PCR are the main laboratory tests to aid in the diagnosis. Patients are considered to have HD if they have 1 or more of the 3 cardinal signs: loss of sensation in a localized skin lesion, thickened peripheral nerve with loss of sensation or weakness of muscles enervated by that nerve, or the presence of acid-fast bacilli (AFB) on biopsy. The positive predictive value for the diagnosis of leprosy in patients meeting all 3 criteria is 98%.

To confirm the diagnosis and determine the extent of nerve involvement and the type of infiltrate, a full-thickness skin biopsy from the most active lesion should be performed. *M. leprae* is best identified in tissue using the *Fite stain*. Lesions from patients with the lepromatous form reveal numerous AFB in clumps (globi), whereas patients with the tuberculoid form rarely have mycobacteria identified, but the diagnosis can be made by demonstration of well-formed noncaseating granulomas and nerve involvement. The presence of **neural inflammation** differentiates leprosy from other granulomatous disorders. Mycobacterial culture of lesions should be performed to exclude *M. tuberculosis* and nontuberculous cutaneous infections. If no resources are available, slit-skin (skin smear) biopsies represent an alternative. Slit-skin smears have high specificity but low sensitivity; only 30% of adults and 10–30% of children <15 yr old are smear positive (usually patients with the lepromatous form). The bacterial index can range from 0 (no bacilli in 100 oil-immersion fields), as generally seen in paucibacillary disease, to 6+ (>1,000 bacilli/field), as can be seen in multibacillary disease.

Diagnostic and histopathologic consultation in the United States is available through the **National Hansen's Disease Program** (**NHDP**; http://www.hrsa.gov/hansens or 800-642-2477). Specimens (formalin or paraffin embedded) can be sent to the NHDP for pathologic analysis free of charge. A polymerase chain reaction (PCR) test for *M. leprae* is not readily available in clinical practice but may be performed at the NHDP. In nonendemic areas, PCR may be useful for diagnosis when AFB are discernible in tissue, but clinical and histopathologic features are not typical. *M. leprae* DNA is detectable by PCR in 95% of lepromatous disease (sensitivity >90%) and 55% of tuberculoid lepra (sensitivity of 34–80%). PCR has also allowed detection of the organism in nasal secretions from asymptomatic people. Molecular testing for mutations causing drug resistance is also available through the NHDP and is usually used in the setting of relapse.

Antibodies to *M. leprae* are present in 90% of patients with untreated lepromatous disease, 40–50% of patients with paucibacillary disease, and 1–5% of healthy controls. However, serologic testing is insensitive and is not used for diagnosis.

TREATMENT

The primary goal of treatment is early antimicrobial therapy to prevent permanent neuropathy. Leprosy is curable. Effective treatment requires multidrug therapy (MDT) with **dapsone**, **clofazimine**, and **rifampin**. Combination therapy is employed to prevent antimicrobial resistance. In the United States, clinical providers considering a diagnosis and treatment of a patient with HD should obtain consultation from the NHDP. The recommended combination MDT can be obtained free of charge from the NHDP (Table 243.1) and in other countries through WHO (Table 243.2). Compared to WHO, the NHDP advocates for a longer duration of treatment and daily rather than monthly administration of rifampin, because shorter antimicrobial regimens have been associated with greater risk of relapse. The recommended duration by the WHO for tuberculoid disease is 6 mo and for lepromatous disease, 12 mo.

Before starting combination MDT, patients should be tested for glucose-6-phosphate dehydrogenase deficiency, have a baseline complete blood cell count and liver function testing, and be evaluated for evidence of active tuberculosis, in which monotherapy with rifampin should be avoided. Response to therapy is seen clinically as flattening or disappearance of skin lesions and improvement in nerve function, usually

within 1-2 mo after initiating MDT. Complete resolution or improvement may take 6-12 mo, depending on the severity of infection. Most skin lesions heal without scarring.

Alternative agents to treat HD include minocycline, clarithromycin, and some fluoroquinolones (levofloxacin, ofloxacin, moxifloxacin). Given limited data, these alternative antimicrobials are used in selected cases of intolerance to the routine combination MDT regimen or for documented resistance. It is important to note that some patients who have been adequately treated for HD may later show evidence of chronic reversal reactions and late neuropathies, but these are bacillus negative and thus should not be considered relapses. Neuritis must be treated promptly to minimize nerve injury and disability. Treatment with corticosteroids appears to improve nerve function in two third of patients.

Bone marrow suppression and hepatotoxicity have been reported and should be monitored every 3 mo during therapy. A screening urinalysis should be performed annually. Other reactions, such as methemoglobinemia and hypersensitivity reactions to dapsone, are rare. An ophthalmologic evaluation should routinely be performed in all patients with HD because ocular complications can occur. Given the proclivity for testicular invasion in multibacillary leprosy with resultant testicular dysfunction and infertility, males should be screened for elevated follicle-stimulating hormone or luteinizing hormone concentrations and decreased testosterone levels.

After completion of MDT, annual follow-up for ≥5 yr for paucibacillary and ≥10 yr for multibacillary disease is warranted. Relapse of the disease after completion of MDT is rare (0.01–4.0%) and must be distinguished from the more common leprosy immunologic reactions. Patients who have a bacillary index of ≥4 pre-MDT or ≥3 at the completion of MDT

Table 243.1	NHDP-Recommended Multidrug Therapy Regimens for Hansen Disease in the United States		
TYPE OF LEPROSY	**PATIENT POPULATION**	**ANTIMICROBIAL THERAPY**	**DURATION OF THERAPY**
Multibacillary (LL, BL, BB)	Adult	Dapsone, 100 mg/day, *and* Rifampin, 600 mg/day, *and* Clofazimine, 50 mg/day	24 mo
	Pediatric*	Dapsone, 1 mg/kg/day, *and* Rifampin, 10-20 mg/kg/day, *and* Clofazimine, 1 mg/kg/day[†]	
Paucibacillary (TT, BT)	Adult	Dapsone, 100 mg/day, *and* Rifampin, 600 mg/day	12 mo
	Pediatric*	Dapsone, 1 mg/kg/day, *and* Rifampin, 10-20 mg/kg/day	

NHDP multidrug therapy is daily and of longer duration than WHO-recommended regimen. All drugs are administered orally.
*Daily pediatric mg/kg dose should not exceed adult daily maximum.
[†]Clofazimine is only available through NHDP Investigational New Drug (IND) program; minimum formulation is 50 mg, and capsules should not be cut. Alternative dosing includes clofazimine, 2 mg/kg every other day, *or* clarithromycin, 7.5 mg/kg/day.
NHDP, National Hansen's Disease Program; BB, Borderline; BL, borderline lepromatous; BT, borderline tuberculoid; LL, lepromatous; TT, tuberculoid.

Table 243.2	WHO-Recommended Multidrug Therapy (MDT) Regimens for Hansen Disease		
TYPE OF LEPROSY	**PATIENT POPULATION**	**ANTIMICROBIAL THERAPY**	**DURATION OF THERAPY**
Multibacillary (LL, BL, BB)	Adult	Rifampicin, 600 mg once monthly, *and* Dapsone, 100 mg/day, *and* Clofazimine, 300 mg once monthly and 50 mg/day	12 mo
	Pediatric*	Rifampicin, 450 mg once monthly, *and* Dapsone, 50 mg/day, *and* Clofazimine, 150 mg once monthly and 50 mg every other day	
Paucibacillary (TT, BT)	Adult	Rifampicin, 600 mg once monthly, *and* Dapsone, 100 mg/day	6 mo
	Pediatric*	Rifampicin, 450 mg once monthly, *and* Dapsone, 50 mg/day	

*In children <10 yr old, MDT dosages should be in mg/kg, not to exceed the adult daily maximum: rifampicin, 10 mg/kg once monthly; dapsone, 2 mg/kg/day; and clofazimine, 1 mg/kg on alternate days.
WHO, World Health Organization; BB, Borderline; BL, borderline lepromatous; BT, borderline tuberculoid; LL, lepromatous; TT, tuberculoid.

have the highest risk of relapse (approximately 20%). When relapse occurs, it is usually within 5-10 yr of MDT completion and a result of reactivation of drug-susceptible mycobacteria. Thus, patients who are expected to relapse are generally treated with the same MDT regimen. Resistance to dapsone and rifampicin has been documented, although it rarely occurs with combination therapy.

Leprosy Reactions

Immunologic reactions can occur before, during, and years after treatment and should be treated aggressively to prevent peripheral nerve damage. In general, antimycobacterial drugs should be continued. Fatigue, malaise, or fever can be present, and the inflammation associated with these reactions can cause severe nerve injury. Prompt therapy with corticosteroids with or without other antiinflammatory agents, adequate analgesia, and physical support are essential for patients with active neuritis to prevent nerve damage. If corticosteroids are indicated for a prolonged time, the frequency of rifampicin administration should be decreased from daily to monthly administration (to avoid drug interaction).

For **type 1 reactions**, prednisone is recommended, 1 mg/kg/day orally (40-60 mg) with a slow taper (decreasing by 5 mg every 2-4 wk after evidence of improvement over 3-6 mo), in addition to standard MDT. If there is evidence of peripheral nerve deterioration, higher doses and longer tapers may be needed. Nerve function improves after corticosteroid treatment in 30–80% of patients who did not have preexisting neuritis. In patients not responding to corticosteroids, cyclosporine may be used as a second-line agent.

For **type 2 reactions**, prednisone is routinely used at 1 mg/kg/day for 12 wk. However, given the recurrence and chronicity of ENL, corticosteroid-sparing agents should be considered to avoid complications associated with their prolonged use. **Thalidomide** (100-400 mg/daily for 48-72 hr, tapering over 2 wk to 100 mg/daily) is effective in treating these types of reactions. Given the teratogenicity of thalidomide (contraindicated for children <12 yr old and woman of childbearing age), the drug is only available through a restrictive distribution program approved by the U.S. Food and Drug Administration (FDA). Low dose **clofazimine** (50-100 mg 3 times weekly) alone or in combination with corticosteroids (300 mg/day, tapering to <100 mg/day, for 12 mo) has also been useful in managing patients with chronic ENL and is generally used until all signs of the reaction have abated. Other immunosuppressive drugs have been used to treat type-2 reactions with inconsistent results, including cyclosporine, mycophenolate, and methotrexate. Lucio phenomenon is managed with corticosteroids and treatment of underlying infections.

LONG-TERM COMPLICATIONS

Leprosy is a leading cause of permanent physical disability among communicable diseases worldwide. The major chronic complications and deformities of leprosy are caused by **nerve injury**. Nerve impairment may be purely sensory, motor, or autonomic, or may be a combination. The prognosis for arresting progression of tissue and nerve damage is good if therapy is started early, but recovery of lost sensory and motor function is variable and frequently incomplete. Nerve function impairment can occur before diagnosis, during MDT, or after MDT and can develop without overt signs of skin or nerve inflammation (silent neuropathy). Patients at highest risk of nerve impairment are those with multibacillary leprosy and preexisting nerve damage. These patients should undergo regular monthly surveillance during therapy and for at least 2 yr from the time of diagnosis. In children, deformities can occur in 3–10% of cases and mainly in those with nerve enlargement. Other factors contributing to risk of deformities include increasing age in children, delay in accessing medical care, multiple skin lesions, multibacillary disease, smear positivity, multiple nerve involvement, and leprosy reaction at presentation.

PREVENTION

In addition to treating active leprosy cases, control measures for HD include the management of **contacts** of index patients. In endemic countries, close monitoring of household contacts of HD patients, particularly HD patients with multibacillary disease, is warranted to ensure that early treatment can be implemented if evidence of early HD develops. These household contacts should be examined at baseline and then yearly for 5 yr. In nonendemic areas, disease presenting in the contacts of patients with HD is rare. A single dose of bacille Calmette-Guérin (BCG) vaccine has variable protective efficacy against leprosy, ranging from 10–80%; an additional dose results in increased protection. Any suspected or newly diagnosed case of leprosy in the United States should be reported to local and state public health departments, the Centers for Disease Control and Prevention (CDC), and NHDP. There are no leprosy vaccines available or recommended for use in the United States. In the hospital setting, **standard precautions** should be implemented. Hand hygiene is recommended for all people in contact with a patient with lepromatous leprosy.

Bibliography is available at Expert Consult.

Chapter **244**
Nontuberculous Mycobacteria

Ericka V. Hayes

第二百四十四章
非结核分枝杆菌

中文导读

本章主要介绍了非结核分枝杆菌病的病原学、流行病学、发病机制、临床表现、诊断和治疗。非结核分枝杆菌是一组高度多样化的细菌群，在环境中广泛存在。典型的病理损害为干酪样肉芽肿。儿童以淋巴结炎为主要表现，也可发生皮肤、耳部、肺部感染，以及罕见的弥散性疾病。其中鸟分枝杆菌复合群常与播散性感染相关。本病诊断困难，依赖于临床表现、组织病理、影像学及微生物的联合诊断。本病治疗时间长，治疗困难，往往需要辅助手术干预，抗感染治疗需根据细菌药物敏感实验选择药物。

Nontuberculous mycobacteria (**NTM**), also referred to as **atypical mycobacteria** and **mycobacteria other than tuberculosis** (MOTT), are all members of the genus *Mycobacterium* and include species other than *Mycobacterium tuberculosis* complex and *Mycobacterium leprae*. The NTM constitute a highly diverse group of bacteria that differ from *M. tuberculosis* complex bacteria in their pathogenicity, interhuman transmissibility, nutritional requirements, ability to produce pigments, enzymatic activity, and drug susceptibility. In contrast to the *M. tuberculosis* complex, NTM are acquired from environmental sources and not by person-to-person spread, although the latter is under debate, especially in patients with cystic fibrosis. Their omnipresence in the environment means that the clinical relevance of NTM isolation from clinical specimens is sometimes unclear; a positive culture might reflect occasional presence or contamination rather than true NTM disease. NTM are associated with pediatric lymphadenitis, otomastoiditis, serious lung infections, and, rarely, disseminated disease. Treatment is long-term and cumbersome and often requires adjunctive surgical intervention. Comprehensive guidelines on diagnosis and treatment are provided by the American Thoracic Society (ATS) and British Thoracic Society (BTS).

ETIOLOGY

NTM are ubiquitous in the environment all over the world, existing as saprophytes in soil and water (including municipal water supplies, tap water, hot tubs, and shower heads), environmental niches that are the supposed sources of human infections. With the introduction of molecular identification tools such as 16S recombinant DNA gene sequencing, the number of identified NTM species has grown to more than 150; the *clinical relevance* (i.e., percentage of isolates that are causative agents of true NTM disease, rather than occasional contaminants) differs significantly by species.

Mycobacterium avium complex (**MAC**; i.e., *M. avium*, *Mycobacterium intracellulare*, and several closely related but rarer species) and *Mycobacterium kansasii* are most often isolated from clinical samples, yet the isolation frequency of these species differs significantly by geographic area. MAC bacteria have been frequently isolated from natural and synthetic environments, and cases of MAC disease have been successfully linked to home exposure to shower and tap water. Although the designation *M. avium* suggests that human infections are acquired from birds (Latin *avium*), molecular typing has established that *M. avium* strains that cause pediatric lymphadenitis and adult pulmonary disease represent the *M. avium hominis suis* subgrouping, mainly found in humans and pigs and not in birds.

Some NTM have well-defined ecologic niches that help explain infection patterns. The natural reservoir for *Mycobacterium marinum* is fish and other cold-blooded animals, and the **fish tank granuloma**, a localized skin infection caused by *M. marinum*, follows skin injury in an aquatic environment. *Mycobacterium fortuitum* complex bacteria and *Mycobacterium chelonae* are ubiquitous in water and have caused clusters of nosocomial surgical wound and venous catheter–related infections. *Mycobacterium ulcerans* is associated with severe, chronic skin infections (**Buruli ulcer disease**) and is endemic mainly in West Africa and Australia, although other foci exist. Its incidence is highest in children <15 yr old. *M. ulcerans* had been detected in environmental samples by polymerase chain reaction (PCR) but was only recently recovered by culture from a water strider (an insect of the *Gerris* genus) from Benin.

EPIDEMIOLOGY

Humans are exposed to NTM on a daily basis. In rural U.S. counties, where *M. avium* is common in swamps, the prevalence of asymptomatic infections with *M. avium* complex, as measured by skin test sensitization, approaches 70% by adulthood. Still, the incidence and prevalence of the various NTM disease types remain largely unknown, especially for pediatric NTM disease. In Australian children the overall incidence of NTM infection is 0.84 per 100,000, with lymphadenitis accounting for two thirds of cases. The incidence of pediatric NTM disease in the Netherlands is estimated at 0.77 infections per 100,000 children per year, with lymphadenitis making up 92% of all infections.

In comparison, estimations of the prevalence of NTM from respiratory samples in adults are 5-15 per 100,000 persons per year, with important differences between countries or regions. Because pulmonary NTM disease progresses slowly, over years rather than months, and usually takes several years to cure, the prevalence of pulmonary NTM disease is much higher than incidence rates would suggest.

The paradigm that NTM disease is a rare entity limited to developed countries is changing. In recent studies in African countries with a high prevalence of HIV infection, it has been found that NTM might play a much larger role as a cause of tuberculosis-like disease of children and adults than previously assumed and thus confuse the diagnosis of tuberculosis.

Although it is generally believed that NTM infections are contracted from environmental sources, recent whole genome sequence analysis of *Mycobacterium abscessus* strains of patients in a cystic fibrosis (CF) clinic in the United Kingdom has raised the possibility of nosocomial transmission among CF patients.

PATHOGENESIS

The histologic appearances of lesions caused by *M. tuberculosis* and NTM are often indistinguishable. The classic pathologic lesion consists of caseating granulomas. Compared to *M. tuberculosis* infections, NTM infections are more likely to result in *granulomas that are noncaseating*, poorly defined (nonpalisading), irregular or serpiginous or even absent, with only chronic inflammatory changes observed. The histology likely reflects the immune status of the patient.

In patients with AIDS and disseminated NTM infection, the inflammatory reaction is usually scant, and tissues are filled with large numbers of histiocytes packed with acid-fast bacilli (AFB). These disseminated NTM infections typically occur only after the number of CD4 T lymphocytes has fallen below 50/μL, suggesting that specific T-cell products or activities are required for immunity to mycobacteria.

The pivotal roles of interferon (IFN)-γ, interleukin (IL)-12, and tumor necrosis factor (TNF)-α in disease pathogenesis are demonstrated by the high incidence of mostly disseminated NTM disease in children with IFN-γ and IL-12 pathway deficiencies and in persons treated with agents that neutralize TNF-α.

Observed differences in pathogenicity, clinical relevance, and spectrum of clinical disease associated with the various NTM species emphasize the importance of bacterial factors in the pathogenesis of NTM disease, although exact virulence factors remain largely unknown.

CLINICAL MANIFESTATIONS

Lymphadenitis of the superior anterior cervical or submandibular lymph nodes is the most common manifestation of NTM infection in children (Table 244.1). Preauricular, posterior cervical, axillary, and inguinal nodes are involved occasionally. Lymphadenitis is most common in children 1-5 yr of age and has been related to soil exposure (e.g., playing in sandboxes) and teething, although exact predisposing conditions have not been found. Given the constant environmental exposure to NTM, the occurrence of these infections might also reflect an atypical immune response of a subset of the infected children during or after their first contact with NTM. However, in healthy children with isolated NTM lymphadenitis, immunodeficiency is very rare.

Affected children usually lack constitutional symptoms and present with a unilateral subacute and slowly enlarging lymph node or group of closely approximated nodes >1.5 cm in diameter that are firm, painless, freely movable, and not erythematous (Fig. 244.1). The involved nodes occasionally resolve without treatment, but most undergo rapid suppuration after several weeks (Fig. 244.2). The center of the node becomes fluctuant, and the overlying skin thins and becomes erythematous and often even violaceous. Eventually, the nodes rupture and can form cutaneous sinus tracts that can drain persistently, reminiscent of scrofula from tuberculosis (Fig. 244.3).

In the United States and Western Europe, *M. avium* complex accounts for approximately 80% of NTM lymphadenitis in children. *M. kansasii* accounts for most other cases of lymphadenitis in the United States. *Mycobacterium malmoense* and *Mycobacterium haemophilum* have also been described as causative agents of lymphadenitis. *M. malmoense* is only common in Northwestern Europe. For *M. haemophilum*, underestimation of its importance is likely because the bacteria require specific culture conditions (hemin-enriched media, low incubation temperatures). On the basis of PCR analysis of lymph node samples from lymphadenitis cases in The Netherlands, *M. haemophilum* is the 2nd most common cause of this infection, after *M. avium* complex. One study suggests that children with *M. avium* complex lymphadenitis are significantly younger than those infected by *M. haemophilum*, possibly related to age-specific environmental exposures. *Mycobacterium lentiflavum* is also an emerging NTM associated with lymphadenitis.

Cutaneous disease caused by NTM is rare in children (see Table 244.1). Infection usually follows percutaneous inoculation with fresh or salt water contaminated by *M. marinum*. Within 2-6 wk after exposure, an erythematous papule develops at the site of minor abrasions on the elbows, knees, or feet (**swimming pool granuloma**) and on the hands and fingers of fish tank owners, mostly inflicted during tank cleaning (**fish tank granuloma**). These lesions are usually nontender and enlarge over 3-5 wk to form violaceous plaques. Nodules or pustules can develop and occasionally will ulcerate, resulting in a serosanguineous discharge. The lesions sometimes resemble sporotrichosis, with satellite lesions near the site of entry, extending along the superficial lymphatics. Lymphadenopathy is usually absent. Although most infections remain localized to the skin, penetrating *M. marinum* infections can result in tenosynovitis, bursitis, osteomyelitis, or arthritis.

M. ulcerans infection is the 3rd most common mycobacterial infection in immunocompetent patients, after *M. tuberculosis* and *M. leprae* infection, and causes cutaneous disease in children living in tropical regions of Africa, South America, Asia, and parts of Australia. In some communities in West Africa, up to 16% of people have been affected. Children <15 yr old are particularly affected in rural tropical counties, accounting for 48% of infected individuals in Africa. Infection follows percutaneous inoculation from minor trauma, such as pricks and cuts from plants or insect bites. After an incubation period of approximately 3 mo, lesions appear as an erythematous nodule, usually on legs or arms. The lesion undergoes central necrosis and ulceration. The lesion, often called a **Buruli ulcer** after the region in Uganda where a large case series was reported, has a characteristic undermined edge, expands over several weeks, and can result in extensive, deep soft tissue destruction or bone involvement. Lesions are typically painless, and constitutional symptoms are unusual. Lesions might heal slowly over 6-9 mo or might continue to spread, leading to deformities, contractures, and disability.

Skin and soft tissue infections caused by **rapidly growing mycobacteria**, such as *M. fortuitum*, *M. chelonae*, or *M. abscessus*, are rare in children and usually follow percutaneous inoculation from puncture or surgical wounds, minor abrasions, or tattooing. There has been a large outbreak of *M. fortuitum* furunculosis related to nail salon footbaths. Clinical disease usually arises after a 4-6 wk incubation period and manifests as localized cellulitis, painful nodules, or a draining abscess. *M. haemophilum* can cause painful subcutaneous nodules, which often ulcerate and suppurate in immunocompromised patients, particularly after kidney transplantation.

NTM are an uncommon cause of **catheter-associated infections** but are becoming increasingly recognized in this respect. Infections caused by *M. fortuitum*, *M. chelonae*, or *M. abscessus* can manifest as bacteremia or localized catheter tunnel infections.

Otomastoiditis, or chronic otitis media, is a rare extrapulmonary

Table 244.1	Major Clinical Syndromes Associated with Nontuberculous Mycobacterial Infection	
SYNDROME	**MOST COMMON CAUSES**	**LESS FREQUENT CAUSES***
Chronic nodular disease (adults with bronchiectasis; cystic fibrosis)	MAC (*M. intracellulare, M. avium*), *M. kansasii, M. abscessus*	*M. xenopi, M. malmoense, M. szulgai, M. smegmatis, M. celatum, M. simiae, M. goodii, M. asiaticum, M. heckeshornense, M. branderi, M. lentiflavum, M. triplex, M. fortuitum, M. arupense, M. abscessus* subsp. *bolletii, M. phocaicum, M. aubagnense, M. florentinum, M. abscessus* subsp. *massiliense, M. nebraskense, M. saskatchewanense, M. seoulense, M. senuense, M. paraseoulense, M. europaeum, M. sherrisii, M. kyorinense, M. noviomagense, M. mantenii, M. shinjukuense, M. koreense, M. heraklionense, M. parascrofulaceum, M. arosiense*
Cervical or other lymphadenitis (especially children)	MAC	*M. scrofulaceum, M. malmoense* (northern Europe)*, M. abscessus, M. fortuitum, M. lentiflavum, M. tusciae, M. palustre, M. interjectum, M. elephantis, M. heidelbergense, M. parmense, M. bohemicum, M. haemophilum, M. europaeum, M. florentinum, M. triplex, M. asiaticum, M. kansasii, M. heckeshornense*
Skin and soft tissue disease	*M. fortuitum* group*, M. chelonae, M. abscessus, M. marinum, M. ulcerans* (Australia, tropical countries only)	*M. kansasii, M. haemophilum, M. porcinum, M. smegmatis, M. genavense, M. lacus, M. novocastrense, M. houstonense, M. goodii, M. immunogenum, M. mageritense, M. abscessus* subsp. *massiliense, M. arupense, M. monacense, M. bohemicum, M. branderi, M. shigaense, M. szulgai, M. asiaticum, M. xenopi, M. kumamotense, M. setense, M. montefiorense* (eels)*, M. pseudoshottsii* (fish)*, M. shottsii* (fish)
Skeletal (bone, joint, tendon) infection	*M. marinum*, MAC*, M. kansasii, M. fortuitum* group*, M. abscessus, M. chelonae*	*M. haemophilum, M. scrofulaceum, M. heckeshornense, M. smegmatis, M. terrae/chromogenicum* complex*, M. wolinskyi, M. goodii, M. arupense, M. xenopi, M. triplex, M. lacus, M. arosiense*
Disseminated infection		*M. genavense, M. haemophilum, M. xenopi*
HIV-seropositive host	*M. avium, M. kansasii*	*M. marinum, M. simiae, M. intracellulare, M. scrofulaceum, M. fortuitum, M. conspicuum, M. celatum, M. lentiflavum, M. triplex, M. colombiense, M. sherrisii, M. heckeshornense*
HIV-seronegative host	*M. abscessus, M. chelonae*	*M. marinum, M. kansasii, M. haemophilum, M. chimaera, M. conspicuum, M. shottsii* (fish)*, M. pseudoshottsii* (fish)
Catheter-related infections	*M. fortuitum, M. abscessus, M. chelonae*	*M. mucogenicum, M. immunogenum, M. mageritense, M. septicum, M. porcinum, M. bacteremicum, M. brumae*
Hypersensitivity pneumonitis	Metal workers; hot tub	*M. immunogenum M. avium*

*The available information is sparse for selected pathogens such as *M. xenopi, M. malmoense, M. szulgai, M. celatum,* and *M. asiaticum* and the newly described species.
HIV, Human immunodeficiency virus; MAC, *Mycobacterium avium* complex.
From Brown-Elliott BA, Wallace Jr. RJ: Infections caused by nontuberculous mycobacteria other than *Mycobacterium avium* complex. In Bennett JF, Dolin R, Blaser MJ, editors: *Mandell, Douglas, and Bennett's principles and practice of infectious diseases,* ed 8, Philadelphia, 2015, Elsevier (Table 254-1).

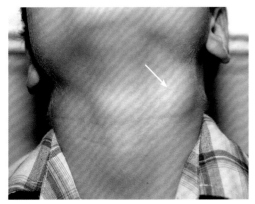

Fig. 244.1 Enlarging cervical lymph node infected with *Mycobacterium avium* complex infection. The node is firm, painless, freely movable, and not erythematous.

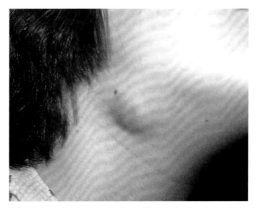

Fig. 244.2 Suppurating cervical lymph node infected with *Mycobacterium avium* complex.

NTM disease type that specifically affects children with tympanostomy tubes and a history of topical antibiotic or steroid use. *M. abscessus* is the most common causative agent, followed by *M. avium* complex (see Table 244.1). Patients present with painless, chronic otorrhea resistant to antibiotic therapy. CT can reveal destruction of the mastoid bone with mucosal swelling (Fig. 244.4).

Delayed or unsuccessful treatment can result in permanent hearing loss. In unusual circumstances, NTM causes other bone and joint infections that are indistinguishable from those produced by *M. tuberculosis* or other bacterial agents. Such infections usually result from operative incision or accidental puncture wounds. *M. fortuitum* infections from puncture wounds of the foot resemble infections caused by *Pseudomonas aeruginosa* and

Staphylococcus aureus.

Pulmonary infections are the most common form of NTM illness in adults but are rare in children. *M. avium* complex bacteria, the most commonly identified organisms (see Table 244.1), are capable of causing acute pneumonitis, chronic cough, or wheezing associated with paratracheal or peribronchial lymphadenitis and airway compression in normal children. Associated constitutional symptoms such as fever, anorexia, and weight loss occur in 60% of these children. Chest radiographic findings are very similar to those for primary tuberculosis, with unilateral infiltrates and hilar lymphadenopathy (Fig. 244.5). Pleural effusion is uncommon. Rare cases of progression to endobronchial granulation tissue have been reported.

Pulmonary infections usually occur in adults with underlying chronic lung disease. The onset is insidious and consists of cough and fatigue, progressing to weight loss, night sweats, low-grade fever, and generalized malaise in severe cases. Thin-walled cavities with minimal surrounding parenchymal infiltrates are characteristic, but radiographic findings can resemble those of tuberculosis. A separate disease manifestation occurs in postmenopausal women and is radiologically characterized by bronchiectasis and nodular lesions, often affecting the middle lobe and lingula.

Chronic pulmonary infections specifically affect children with CF and are generally caused by *M. abscessus* and *M. avium* complex. *M. abscessus* primarily affects children, and *M. avium* complex is most common among adults. The percentage of CF patients with at least 1 sputum culture positive for NTM is 6–8.1% overall and increases with age; in CF patients <12 yr old, a prevalence of 3.9% has been reported. The strong representation of *M. abscessus* in these patients is remarkable, because this bacterium is an uncommon isolate in other categories of patients. There are indications that NTM infections in CF patients further accelerate the decline in lung function; antimycobacterial therapy can result in weight gain and improved lung function in affected patients.

Disseminated disease is usually associated with *M. avium* complex infection and occurs in immunocompromised children. The 1st category of patients with disseminated disease includes persons with mutations in genes coding for the interferon-γ receptor (IFNGR) or the IL-12 receptor, or for IL-12 production. Patients with complete **IFNGR deficiency** have severe, difficult-to-treat disease. Those with partial IFNGR deficiency or IL-12 pathway mutations have milder disease that can respond to IFN-γ and antimycobacterial therapy. **Multifocal osteomyelitis** is particularly prevalent in persons with the IFNGR1 818del4 mutation. Recurrences, even years after a course of treatment, and multiple infections are well documented. The 2nd category of patients affected by disseminated disease is patients with acquired immunodeficiency syndrome (**AIDS**). Disseminated NTM disease in patients with AIDS usually appears when CD4 cell counts are <50 cells/μL; in younger children, especially those <2 yr old, these infections occur at higher CD4 cell counts. The most recent estimate of the incidence of disseminated NTM disease is 0.14-0.2 episodes per 100 person-years, a 10-fold decrease from its incidence before highly active antiretroviral therapy (HAART) was available.

Colonization of the respiratory or gastrointestinal (GI) tract probably precedes disseminated *M. avium* complex infections, but screening studies of respiratory secretions or stool samples are not useful to predict dissemination. Continuous high-grade bacteremia is common, and multiple organs are infected, typically including lymph nodes, liver, spleen, bone marrow, and GI tract. Thyroid, pancreas, adrenal gland, kidney, muscle, and brain can also be involved. The most common signs and symptoms of disseminated *M. avium* complex infections in patients with AIDS are fever, night sweats, chills, anorexia, marked weight loss, wasting, weakness, generalized lymphadenopathy, and hepatosplenomegaly. Jaundice, elevated alkaline phosphatase or lactate dehydrogenase levels, anemia, and neutropenia can occur. Imaging studies usually demonstrate massive lymphadenopathy of hilar, mediastinal, mesenteric, or retroperitoneal nodes. The survival in children with AIDS has improved considerably with the availability of HAART.

Disseminated disease in children without any apparent immunodeficiency is exceedingly rare.

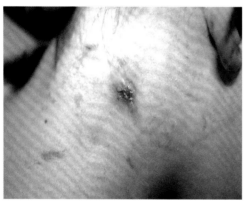

Fig. 244.3 Ruptured cervical lymph node infected with *Mycobacterium avium* complex, which resembles the classic scrofula of tuberculosis.

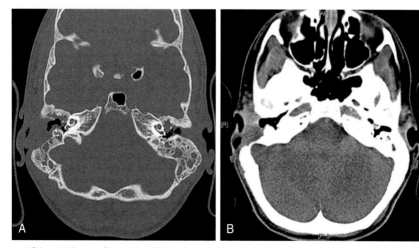

Fig. 244.4 CT images of the middle ear of 6 yr old child infected with *Mycobacterium abscessus*, demonstrating extensive bone destruction in the right mastoid and associated right-sided mucosal swelling. **A,** Bone tissue window setting. **B,** Soft tissue window setting.

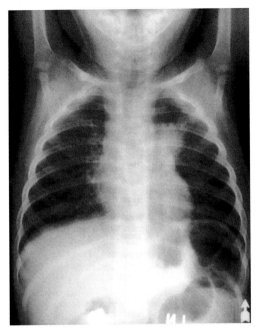

Fig. 244.5 Chest radiograph of 2 yr old child infected with *Mycobacterium avium* complex, demonstrating a left upper lobe infiltrate and left hilar lymphadenopathy.

Table 244.2	American Thoracic Society Diagnostic Criteria for Nontuberculous Mycobacteria (NTM) Lung Disease

The **minimum evaluation** of a patient for NTM lung disease should include:
1. Chest radiograph or, when no cavitation is present, HRCT
2. At least 3 sputum or respiratory samples for AFB culture
3. Exclusion of other disease, such as tuberculosis

Clinical diagnosis of NTM is based on pulmonary symptoms, presence of nodules or cavities, as seen on chest radiograph or an HRCT scan, with multifocal bronchiectasis with multiple small nodules, and exclusion of other diagnoses.

Microbiologic diagnosis of NTM:
At least 2 expectorated sputa (or at least 1 bronchial wash or lavage) with positive cultures for NTM, or transbronchial or other lung biopsy showing the presence of granulomatous inflammation or AFB, with 1 or more sputum or bronchial washings that are culture positive for NTM.

AFB, Acid-fast bacilli; HRCT, high-resolution computed tomography.
Data from Griffith DE, Aksamit T, Brown-Elliott BA, et al: An official ATS/IDSA statement: diagnosis, treatment and prevention of nontuberculous mycobacterial diseases, *Am J Respir Crit Care Med* 175:367–416, 2007.
From Brown-Elliott BA, Wallace Jr. RJ: Infections caused by nontuberculous mycobacteria other than *Mycobacterium avium* complex. In Bennett JF, Dolin R, Blaser MJ, editors: *Mandell, Douglas, and Bennett's principles and practice of infectious diseases*, ed 8, Philadelphia, 2015, Elsevier (Table 254-3).

days of inoculation in almost all patients by automated blood culture systems. In adults, some studies have shown that liver biopsy cultures and stains are more sensitive than blood culture or bone marrow biopsy workup. Commercially available DNA probes differentiate NTM from *M. tuberculosis*. If DNA probes cannot identify the causative mycobacteria, DNA sequencing of bacterial housekeeping genes will always yield a clue to the identity of these NTM. Identification of histiocytes containing numerous AFB from bone marrow and other biopsy tissues provides a rapid presumptive diagnosis of disseminated mycobacterial infection.

TREATMENT

Therapy for NTM infections is long-term and cumbersome; expert consultation is advised. Therapy involves medical, surgical, or combined treatment (see Chapter 241, Table 241.3). Isolation of the infecting strain followed by drug-susceptibility testing is ideal, because it provides a baseline for drug susceptibility. Important discrepancies exist between in vitro drug susceptibility and in vivo response to treatment, explained in part by synergism, mainly among first-line antituberculosis drugs. In vitro, **slow growers** (*M. kansasii, M. marinum, Mycobacterium xenopi, M. ulcerans, M. malmoense*) are usually susceptible to the first-line antituberculosis drugs **rifampicin** and **ethambutol**; *M. avium* complex bacteria are often resistant to these drugs alone but susceptible to the combination and have variable susceptibility to other antibiotics, most importantly the macrolides. **Rapid growers** (*M. fortuitum, M. chelonae, M. abscessus*) are highly resistant to antituberculosis drugs and often have inducible macrolide-resistance mechanisms. Susceptibility to macrolides, aminoglycosides, carbapenems, tetracyclines, and glycylcyclines are most relevant for therapy guidance. In all NTM infections, multidrug therapy (MDT) is essential to avoid development of resistance.

The preferred treatment of NTM lymphadenitis is complete surgical excision. Clinical trials revealed that surgery is more effective than antibiotic treatment (see Table 241.3). Nodes should be removed while still firm and encapsulated. Excision is more difficult if extensive caseation with extension to surrounding tissue has occurred, and complications of facial nerve damage or recurrent infection are more likely in such cases. Incomplete surgical excision is not advised, because chronic drainage can develop. If there are concerns or risk factors for possible *M. tuberculosis* infection, therapy with isoniazid, rifampin, ethambutol, and pyrazinamide should be administered until cultures confirm the cause to be NTM (see Chapter 242). If surgery of NTM lymphadenitis

DIAGNOSIS

For infections of lymph nodes, skin, bone, and soft tissues, isolation of the causative NTM bacteria by *Mycobacterium* culture, preferably with histologic confirmation of granulomatous inflammation, normally suffices for diagnosis (Table 244.2). The differential diagnosis of NTM lymphadenitis includes acute bacterial lymphadenitis, tuberculosis, cat-scratch disease (*Bartonella henselae*), mononucleosis, toxoplasmosis, brucellosis, tularemia, and malignancies, especially lymphomas. Differentiation between NTM and *M. tuberculosis* may be difficult, but children with NTM lymphadenitis usually have a Mantoux tuberculin skin test reaction of <15 mm induration, unilateral anterior cervical node involvement, a normal chest radiograph, and no history of exposure to adult tuberculosis. Definitive diagnosis requires excision of the involved nodes for culture and histology. Fine-needle aspiration for PCR and culture can enable earlier diagnosis, before excisional biopsy.

The diagnosis of pulmonary NTM infection in children is difficult because many species of NTM, including *M. avium* complex, are omnipresent in our environment and can contaminate clinical samples or be present but not causative of disease. As a result, isolation of these bacteria from nonsterile specimens (respiratory and digestive tract) does not necessarily reflect true disease. To determine the clinical relevance of isolation of NTM, the ATS/BTS diagnostic criteria are an important support. These criteria take into consideration clinical features and radiologic, pathologic, and microbiologic findings. Their hallmark is the need for multiple positive cultures yielding the same NTM species to make a definitive diagnosis of pulmonary NTM disease. In children, definitive diagnosis often requires invasive procedures such as bronchoscopy and pulmonary or endobronchial biopsy; in CF patients, more aggressive sample pretreatment is necessary to prevent overgrowth by other species, especially *Pseudomonas*. The chance of NTM isolation being clinically relevant differs significantly by species; some species are more likely causative agents of true pulmonary disease (*M. avium, M. kansasii, M. abscessus, M. malmoense*), whereas others are more likely contaminants (*Mycobacterium gordonae, M. fortuitum, M. chelonae*).

Blood cultures are 90–95% sensitive in AIDS patients with disseminated infection. *M. avium* complex may be detected within 7-10 cannot be performed for some reason, or removal of infected tissue is incomplete, or recurrence or chronic drainage develops, a 3 mo trial of chemotherapy is warranted. **Clarithromycin** or **azithromycin** combined with rifabutin or ethambutol are the most common therapy regimens reported (see Table 241.3). Suppuration may still occur on antibiotic therapy. In select patients, a wait-and-see approach can be chosen because the disease can resolve spontaneously, although resolution can take several months.

Posttraumatic cutaneous NTM lesions in immunocompetent patients usually heal spontaneously after incision and drainage without other therapy (see Table 241.3). *M. marinum* is susceptible to rifampin, amikacin, ethambutol, sulfonamides, trimethoprim-sulfamethoxazole, and tetracycline. Therapy with a combination of these drugs, particularly clarithromycin and ethambutol, may be given until 1 mo after the lesion has disappeared. Corticosteroid injections should not be used. Superficial infections with *M. fortuitum* or *M. chelonae* usually resolve after surgical incision and open drainage, but deep-seated or catheter-related infections require removal of infected central lines and therapy with parenteral amikacin plus cefoxitin, ciprofloxacin, or clarithromycin.

Some localized forms of *M. ulcerans* skin disease (Buruli ulcer) can heal spontaneously; for most forms, excisional surgery with primary closure or skin grafting is recommended. Provisional guidelines by the World Health Organization recommend treatment with rifampin and streptomycin, with or without surgery. Currently, all-oral regimens of rifampicin and fluoroquinolones or macrolides are being tested in clinical trials. In clinical experience, a drug treatment duration of 8 wk generally leads to low recurrence levels. **Physiotherapy** after surgery is essential to prevent contractures and functional disabilities.

Pulmonary infections should be treated initially with isoniazid, rifampin, ethambutol, and pyrazinamide pending culture identification and drug-susceptibility testing particularly if their is high suspicion for tuberculosis. For slow-growing NTM, a combination of rifampin or rifabutin, ethambutol, and clarithromycin (or azithromycin) is recommended; exceptions are *M. kansasii*, for which a regimen of isoniazid, rifampicin, and ethambutol is advised, and *M. simiae*, for which no effective regimen is known, and regimens are usually designed on the basis of in vitro drug susceptibilities. After culture conversion, treatment should be continued for at least 1 yr. For pulmonary disease caused by rapidly growing NTM, a combination of macrolides, fluoroquinolones, aminoglycosides, cefoxitin, and carbapenems is the optimal therapy; 3- or 4-drug regimens are selected on drug-susceptibility testing results. In patients with CF, inhaled antibiotics may have a role.

Patients with disseminated *M. avium* complex and IL-12 pathway defects or IFNGR deficiency should be treated for at least 12 mo with clarithromycin or azithromycin combined with rifampin or rifabutin and ethambutol. In vitro susceptibility testing for clarithromycin is important to guide therapy. Once the clinical illness has resolved, lifelong daily prophylaxis with azithromycin or clarithromycin is advisable to prevent recurrent disease. The use of interferon adjunctive therapy is determined by the specific genetic defect.

In children with AIDS, prophylaxis with azithromycin or clarithromycin is indicated to prevent infection with *M. avium* complex. Although few pediatric studies exist, the U.S. Public Health Service recommends either **azithromycin** (20 mg/kg once weekly PO, maximum 1,200 mg/dose; *or* 5 mg/kg once daily PO, maximum 250 mg/dose in patients intolerant of larger dose) or **clarithromycin** (7.5 mg/kg/dose twice daily PO; maximum 500 mg/dose) for HIV-infected children with significant immune deficiency, as defined by the CD4 count (children ≥6 yr old, CD4 count <50 cells/μL; 2-6 yr old, <75/μL; 1-2 yr old, <500/μL; <1 yr old, <750/μL). Primary prophylaxis may be safely discontinued in children >2 yr old receiving stable HAART for >6 mo and experiencing sustained (>3 mo) CD4 cell recovery well above the age-specific target for initiation of prophylaxis: >100 cells/μL for children ≥6 yr old and >200/μL for children 2-5 yr old. For children <2 yr old, no specific recommendations for discontinuing MAC prophylaxis exist.

Bibliography is available at Expert Consult.

Section **8**

Spirochetal Infections

第八篇

螺旋体感染

Chapter **245**

Syphilis *(Treponema pallidum)*

Maria Jevitz Patterson and H. Dele Davies

第二百四十五章

梅毒（梅毒螺旋体）

中文导读

本章主要介绍了梅毒的病原学、流行病学、临床表现及实验室检查、诊断、治疗和预防。本病由苍白密螺旋体导致，主要通过胎盘和性接触传播，近几年有上升趋势，根据出现的时间临床表现分为三期。先天性梅毒分为早期表现和晚期表现。诊断需结合病史、临床表现和实验室诊断。实验室诊断包括暗视野显微镜或PCR检测找到密螺旋体，非梅毒螺旋体抗原血清试验和密螺旋体抗体实验。详细介绍了先天性梅毒的诊断方法，指出需注意母体疾病史。治疗首选青霉素，对获得性梅毒、孕期梅毒、先天性梅毒的治疗作了详细介绍。该病是可预防的，加强感染母亲的产前管理是预防先天性梅毒的关键。

Syphilis is a chronic systemic sexually or vertically (mother to child) transmitted infection that can be easily treated if detected early but manifests with protean clinical symptoms and significant morbidity if left unchecked.

ETIOLOGY

Syphilis is caused by *Treponema pallidum,* a delicate, tightly spiraled, motile spirochete with finely tapered ends belonging to the family Spirochaetaceae. The pathogenic members of this genus include *T. pallidum* subspecies *pallidum* (venereal syphilis), *T. pallidum* subspecies *pertenue* (yaws), *T. pallidum* subspecies *endemicum* (bejel or endemic syphilis), and *T. pallidum* subspecies *carateum* (pinta). Because these microorganisms stain poorly and are below the detection limits of conventional light microscopy, detection in clinical specimens requires dark-field, phase contrast microscopy or direct immunofluorescent or silver staining. *T. pallidum* cannot be cultured in vitro. In recent years, advanced detection using nucleic acid amplification testing by polymerase chain reaction (PCR) has been increasingly used by specialized laboratories.

EPIDEMIOLOGY

In addition to presentation at sexually transmitted disease clinics, patients with syphilis are increasingly seen by primary care providers in private practice settings. Two forms of syphilis occur in children and adolescents.

Acquired syphilis is transmitted almost exclusively by sexual contact, including vaginal, anal, and oral exposure. Less-common modes of transmission include transfusion of contaminated blood or direct contact with infected tissues. After an epidemic resurgence of primary and secondary syphilis in the United States that peaked in 1989, the annual rate declined 90% to the lowest ever rate by 2000. The total number of cases of primary and secondary syphilis has subsequently rebounded since 2000, particularly among men who have sex with men and men and women with HIV. Despite a decrease among women for almost a decade, their rates increased every year from 2004 to 2008. Cases of congenital syphilis reached an historic low in 2005 but have subsequently increased, reflecting the rates among women. Since 2012 the rates of congenital syphilis have increased to the highest since 2001 (Fig. 245.1). The increase occurs across every region and all races and ethnicities.

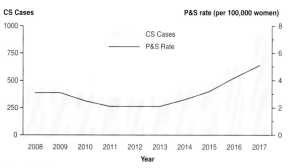

Fig. 245.1 Congenital syphilis—reported cases by year of birth and rates of reported cases of primary and secondary syphilis among women aged 15-44 yr, United States, 2008-2017. *CS,* congenital syphilis; *P&S,* primary and secondary syphilis. *(From Centers for Disease Control and Prevention (CDC): Sexually transmitted disease surveillance 2017, Atlanta, 2018. US Department of Health and Human Services. Fig. 49. Available at: https://www.cdc.gov/std/stats17/2017-STD-Surveillance-Report_CDC -clearance-9.10.18.pdf.)*

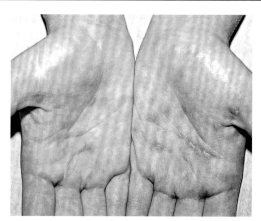

Fig. 245.2 Secondary syphilis. Ham-colored palmar macules on an adolescent with secondary syphilis. *(From Weston WL, Lane AT, Morelli JG: Color textbook of pediatric dermatology, ed 3, St. Louis, 2002, Mosby.)*

Congenital syphilis results from transplacental transmission of spirochetes or occasionally by intrapartum contact with infectious lesions. Women with primary and secondary syphilis and spirochetemia are more likely to transmit infection to the fetus than are women with latent infection. Transmission can occur at any stage of pregnancy, resulting in early fetal loss, preterm or low birthweight infants, stillbirths, neonatal deaths, or infants born with congenital disease. The incidence of congenital infection in offspring of untreated or inadequately treated infected women remains highest during the first 4 yr after acquisition of primary infection, secondary infection, and early latent disease. Maternal factors associated with congenital syphilis include limited access to healthcare, late or no prenatal care, drug use, multiple sex partners, unprotected sexual contact, incarceration, work in the sex trade, and inadequate treatment of syphilis during pregnancy. Congenital syphilis may be seen in the context of untreated, inadequately treated, or undocumented treatment prior to or during pregnancy. In addition, the mother may have been treated appropriately but did not have an adequate serologic response to therapy and the infant was inadequately evaluated or the infant had documented congenital syphilis. Confirmed cases of both acquired and congenital syphilis must be reported to the local health department.

CLINICAL MANIFESTATIONS AND LABORATORY FINDINGS

Many persons infected with syphilis are *asymptomatic for years* or do not recognize the early signs of disease or seek treatment. The Centers for Disease Control and Prevention (CDC) recommends testing all pregnant women and selective testing of adolescents, based on lesions or risk factors (those with other sexually transmitted diseases including HIV, men who have sex with men, incarcerated individuals, or persons who exchange sex for money or drugs). Periods of active clinical disease alternate with periods of latency. **Primary syphilis** is characterized by a chancre and regional lymphadenitis. A **painless papule** (which may be overlooked) appears at the site of entry (usually the genitalia) 2-6 wk after inoculation and develops into a clean, painless, but highly contagious ulcer with raised borders (**chancre**) containing abundant *T. pallidum.* Extragenital chancres can occur at other sites of primary entry and pose a diagnostic challenge. Oral lesions can be mistaken for aphthous ulcers or herpes. Lesions on the nipple can be confused with cellulitis or eczema. Adjacent lymph nodes are generally enlarged and nontender. The chancre heals spontaneously within 4-6 wk, leaving a thin scar.

Untreated patients develop manifestations of **secondary syphilis** related to spirochetemia 2-10 wk after the chancre heals. Manifestations of secondary syphilis include a generalized nonpruritic maculopapular rash, notably involving the palms and soles (Fig. 245.2). Pustular lesions can also develop. **Condylomata lata,** gray-white to erythematous wart-like plaques, can occur in moist areas around the anus, scrotum, or vagina, and white plaques (**mucous patches**) may be found in mucous membranes. Secondary syphilis should be considered in the differential diagnosis of virtually any rash of unknown etiology. A **flu-like illness** with low-grade fever, headache, malaise, anorexia, weight loss, sore throat, myalgias, arthralgias, and generalized lymphadenopathy is often present. Renal, hepatic, or ocular manifestations may be present. Meningitis occurs in 30% of patients with secondary syphilis and is characterized by cerebrospinal fluid (CSF) pleocytosis and elevated protein level. Patients with meningitis might not show neurologic symptoms. Even without treatment, secondary infection becomes **latent** within 1-2 mo after onset of rash. Relapses with secondary manifestations can occur during the 1st yr of latency (the **early latent period**). **Late syphilis** follows and may be either asymptomatic (**late latent**) or symptomatic (**tertiary**). Tertiary disease follows in about one-third of untreated cases and is marked by neurologic, cardiovascular, and **gummatous lesions** (nonsuppurative granulomas of the skin, bone, and liver, resulting from the host cytotoxic T-cell response). In the preantibiotic era, neurologic manifestations of tertiary syphilis (**tabes dorsalis** and **paresis**) were very common. The clinical course of syphilis and its tissue manifestations reflect the immunopathobiology of the host humoral and delayed-type hypersensitivity responses. A robust timeline of progression through the overlapping stages occurs in immunocompromised HIV patients

Congenital Infection

Untreated syphilis during pregnancy results in a vertical transmission rate approaching 100%, with profound effects on pregnancy outcome, reflecting obliterating endarteritis. Fetal or perinatal death occurs in 40% of affected infants. Premature delivery can also occur. Neonates can also be infected at delivery by contact with an active genital lesion. Most infected infants are asymptomatic at birth, including up to 40% with CSF seeding, and are identified only by routine prenatal screening. In the absence of treatment, symptoms develop within weeks or months. Among infants symptomatic at birth or in the first few months of life, manifestations have traditionally been divided into early and late stages. All stages of congenital syphilis are characterized by a vasculitis, with progression to necrosis and fibrosis. The **early signs** appear during the first 2 yr of life, and the **late signs** appear gradually during the first 2 decades. Early manifestations vary and involve multiple organ systems, resulting from transplacental spirochetemia and are analogous to the secondary stage of acquired syphilis. Hepato-splenomegaly, jaundice, and elevated liver enzymes are common. Histologically, liver involvement includes bile stasis, fibrosis, and extramedullary hematopoiesis. Lymphadenopathy tends to be diffuse and resolve spontaneously, although shotty nodes can persist.

Coombs-negative hemolytic anemia is characteristic. Thrombocytopenia is often associated with platelet trapping in an enlarged spleen. Characteristic **osteochondritis and periostitis** (Fig. 245.3) and a mucocutaneous rash (Fig. 245.4A and B) manifesting with erythematous maculopapular or vesiculobullous lesions followed by desquamation involving hands and feet (see Fig. 245.4C) are common. Mucous patches, persistent rhinitis (**snuffles**), and condylomatous lesions (Fig. 245.5) are highly characteristic features of mucous membrane involvement containing abundant spirochetes. Blood and moist open lesions from infants with congenital syphilis and children with acquired primary or secondary syphilis are infectious until 24 hr of appropriate treatment.

Bone involvement is common. Roentgenographic abnormalities include **Wimberger lines** (demineralization of the medial proximal tibial metaphysis), multiple sites of osteochondritis at the wrists, elbows, ankles, and knees, and periostitis of the long bones and rarely the skull. The osteochondritis is painful, often resulting in irritability and refusal to move the involved extremity (**pseudoparalysis of Parrot**).

Congenital neurosyphilis is often asymptomatic in the neonatal period, although CSF abnormalities can occur even in asymptomatic infants. Failure to thrive, chorioretinitis, nephritis, and nephrotic syndrome can also be seen. Manifestations of renal involvement include hypertension, hematuria, proteinuria, hypoproteinemia, hypercholesterolemia, and hypocomplementemia, probably related to glomerular deposition of circulating immune complexes. Less-common clinical manifestations of early congenital syphilis include gastroenteritis, peritonitis, pancreatitis, pneumonia, eye involvement (glaucoma and chorioretinitis), nonimmune hydrops, and testicular masses.

Late manifestations (children > 2 yr of age) are rarely seen in developed countries. These result primarily from chronic granulomatous inflammation of bone, teeth, and central nervous system and are summarized in Table 245.1. Skeletal changes are caused by persistent or recurrent periostitis and associated thickening of the involved bone. Dental abnormalities, such as **Hutchinson teeth** (Fig. 245.6), are common. Defects in enamel formation lead to repeated caries and eventual tooth destruction. **Saddle nose** (Fig. 245.7) is a depression of the nasal root and may be associated with a perforated nasal septum.

Other late manifestations of congenital syphilis can manifest as hypersensitivity phenomena. These include unilateral or bilateral interstitial keratitis and the **Clutton joint** (see Table 245.1). Other common ocular manifestations include choroiditis, retinitis, vascular occlusion, and optic atrophy. Soft-tissue gummas (identical to those of acquired disease) and paroxysmal cold hemoglobinuria are rare hypersensitivity phenomena.

DIAGNOSIS

Fundamental limitations of the currently available tests for syphilis are vexing, but results must always be interpreted in the context of patient history and physical examination. Physicians should remain aware of their local prevalence rates and treat presumptively when syphilis is suspected by clinical and epidemiologic data. Diagnosis of primary syphilis is confirmed when *T. pallidum* is demonstrated by darkfield microscopy or direct fluorescent antibody testing on specimens from skin lesions, placenta, or umbilical cord. Nucleic acid–based amplification assays, such as PCR, are also used in some specialized laboratories, but are not commercially available. Despite the absence of a true gold standard serologic assay, serologic testing for syphilis remains the principal means for diagnosis and traditionally involves a 2-step screening process with a nontreponemal test followed by a confirmatory treponemal test (Fig. 245.8A).

The **Venereal Disease Research Laboratory** (VDRL) and **rapid plasma reagin** (RPR) tests are sensitive *nontreponemal tests* that detect antibodies against phospholipid antigens on the treponeme surface that cross react with cardiolipin-lecithin-cholesterol antigens of damaged host cells. The quantitative results of these tests are helpful both in screening and in monitoring therapy. Titers increase with active disease, including treatment failure or reinfection, and decline with adequate treatment (Fig. 245.9). Nontreponemal tests usually become nonreactive within 1 yr of adequate therapy for primary syphilis and within 2 yr of

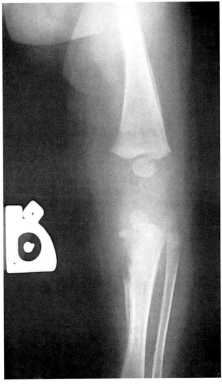

Fig. 245.3 Osteochondritis and periostitis in a newborn with congenital syphilis.

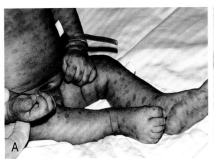
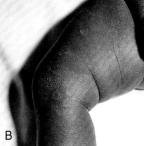
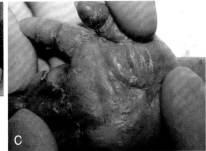

Fig. 245.4 A and **B,** Papulosquamous plaques in 2 infants with syphilis. **C,** Desquamation on the palm of a newborn's hand. (*A and B from Eichenfeld LF, Frieden IJ, Esterly NB, editors: Textbook of neonatal dermatology, Philadelphia, 2001, WB Saunders, p. 196; C, courtesy Dr. Patricia Treadwell.*)

adequate treatment for secondary disease. 15–20% of patients become **serofast** (nontreponemal titers persisting at low levels for long periods). In congenital infection, these tests become nonreactive within a few months after adequate treatment. Certain conditions such as infectious mononucleosis and other viral infections, autoimmune diseases, and pregnancy can give false-positive VDRL results. False-positive results are less common with the use of purified cardiolipin-lecithin-cholesterol antigen. All pregnant women should be screened early in pregnancy and at delivery. All positive maternal serologic tests for syphilis, regardless of titer, necessitate thorough investigation. Antibody excess can give a false-negative reading unless the serum is diluted (**prozone effect**). False-negative results can also occur in early primary syphilis, in latent syphilis of long duration, and in late congenital syphilis.

Treponemal tests traditionally are used to confirm diagnosis and measure specific *T. pallidum* antibodies (immunoglobulin [Ig] G, IgM, and IgA), which appear earlier than nontreponemal antibodies. These treponemal tests include the *T. pallidum* particle agglutination test, the *T. pallidum* hemagglutination assay, and the fluorescent treponemal antibody absorption test. Treponemal antibody titers become positive soon after initial infection and usually remain positive for life, even with adequate therapy (see Fig. 245.9). These antibody titers do not correlate with disease activity. Traditionally they are useful for diagnosis of a first episode of syphilis and for distinguishing false-positive results of nontreponemal antibody tests but cannot accurately identify length of time of infection, response to therapy, or reinfection.

There is limited cross reactivity of treponemal antibody tests with other spirochetes, including the causative organisms of Lyme disease *(Borrelia burgdorferi)*, yaws, endemic syphilis, and pinta. Only venereal syphilis and Lyme disease are found in the United States. *Nontreponemal tests (VDRL, RPR)* are uniformly nonreactive in Lyme disease.

Various enzyme-linked, chemiluminescence, and multiplex flow immunoassays to detect treponemal IgG and IgM have been developed. These assays have increased sensitivity and are amenable to automation and high-volume use. Rapid point-of-care tests are available to allow

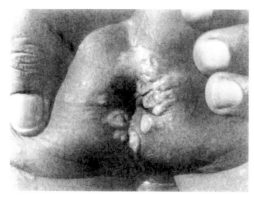

Fig. 245.5 Perianal condylomata lata. *(From Karthikeyan K, Thappa DM: Early congenital syphilis in the new millennium, Pediatr Dermatol 19:275–276, 2002.)*

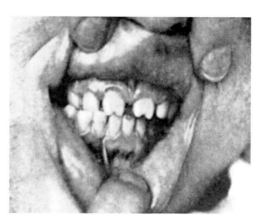

Fig. 245.6 Hutchinson teeth as a late manifestation of congenital syphilis.

Table 245.1	Late Manifestations of Congenital Syphilis
SYMPTOM/SIGN	**DESCRIPTION/COMMENTS**
Olympian brow	Bony prominence of the forehead caused by persistent or recurrent periostitis
Clavicular or Higoumenaki's sign	Unilateral or bilateral thickening of the sternoclavicular third of the clavicle
Saber shins	Anterior bowing of the midportion of the tibia
Scaphoid scapula	Convexity along the medial border of the scapula
Hutchinson teeth	Peg-shaped upper central incisors; they erupt during 6th yr of life with abnormal enamel, resulting in a notch along the biting surface
Mulberry molars	Abnormal 1st lower (6 yr) molars characterized by small biting surface and excessive number of cusps
Saddle nose*	Depression of the nasal root, a result of syphilitic rhinitis destroying adjacent bone and cartilage
Rhagades	Linear scars that extend in a spoke-like pattern from previous mucocutaneous fissures of the mouth, anus, and genitalia
Juvenile paresis	Latent meningovascular infection; it is rare and typically occurs during adolescence with behavioral changes, focal seizures, or loss of intellectual function
Juvenile tabes	Rare spinal cord involvement and cardiovascular involvement with aortitis
Hutchinson triad	Hutchinson teeth, interstitial keratitis, and 8th nerve deafness
Clutton joint	Unilateral or bilateral painless joint swelling (usually involving knees) from synovitis with sterile synovial fluid; spontaneous remission usually occurs after several weeks
Interstitial keratitis	Manifests with intense photophobia and lacrimation, followed within weeks or months by corneal opacification and complete blindness
8th nerve deafness	May be unilateral or bilateral, appears at any age, manifests initially as vertigo and high-tone hearing loss, and progresses to permanent deafness

*A perforated nasal septum may be an associated abnormality.

quality screening programs in resource-limited settings where the World Health Organization otherwise relies on syndromic management of sexually transmitted infections and patients are treated for all likely causes of their constellation of signs and symptoms. In the United States, use of immunoassays has confounded screening because it switches the traditional algorithm: the treponemal-specific testing is done before

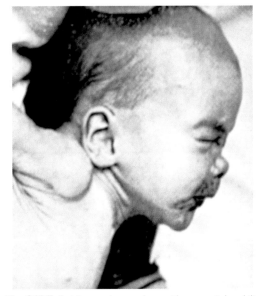

Fig. 245.7 Saddle nose in a newborn with congenital syphilis.

the nontreponemal testing. Because the former remain positive for life, clinical and epidemiologic data are required to provide guidelines to distinguish cured disease, early syphilis, untreated late latent disease, and true false-positive tests. Benefits of reverse screening are increased detection of transmissible early syphilis and of late latent disease to afford monitoring for tertiary disease. Although the CDC continues to recommend the traditional screen (see Fig. 245.8A), they have provided guidelines for interpretation of the reverse screening algorithm (see Fig. 245.8B). Interpretation of nontreponemal and treponemal serologic tests in the newborn can be confounded by maternal IgG antibodies transferred to the fetus. Passively acquired antibody is suggested by a neonatal titer at least 4-fold (i.e., a 2 tube dilution) less than the maternal titer. This conclusion can be verified by gradual decline in antibody in the infant, usually becoming undetectable by 3-6 mo of age.

Neurologic involvement can occur at any stage of syphilis. The diagnosis of neurosyphilis remains difficult but is often established by demonstrating pleocytosis and increased protein in the CSF and a positive CSF VDRL test along with neurologic symptoms. The CSF VDRL test is specific but relatively insensitive (22–69%) for neurosyphilis. CSF PCR and IgM immunoblot tests are under development to assist in diagnosis of neurosyphilis.

Darkfield or direct fluorescent antibody microscopy of scrapings from primary lesions or congenital or secondary lesions can reveal *T. pallidum*, often before serology becomes positive, but these modalities are usually not available in clinical practice. Since 2015 different methods of PCR, including routine PCR, nested PCR, reverse-transcriptase PCR, and quantitative PCR targeting different DNA gene sequences have been used by many laboratories as methods to detect *T. pallidum* in primary disease. However, there are currently no commercially available test kits, and each test must be validated for use in each laboratory. Furthermore, these tests are not useful for asymptomatic patients and interpretation may be complicated by the fact that they amplify both

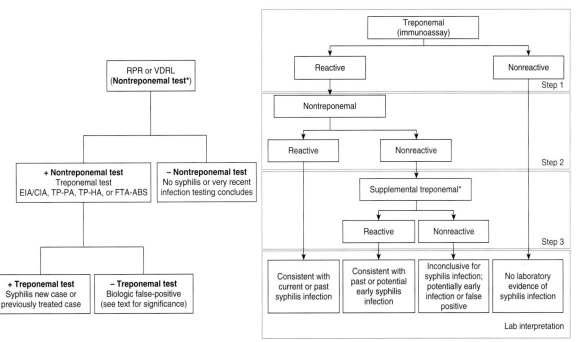

The supplemental treponemal test should use a unique platform and/or antigen, different from the first treponemal test.

B

Fig. 245.8 A, Traditional laboratory testing algorithm for syphilis. **B,** Suggested alternate testing algorithm. *EIA/CIA,* enzyme immunoassay/chemiluminescence immunoassay; *FTA-ABS,* fluorescent treponemal antibody absorption; *RPR,* rapid plasma reagin; *TP-HA, Treponema pallidum* hemagglutination; *TP-PA, Treponema pallidum* particle agglutination; *VDRL,* Venereal Disease Research Laboratory. *If nontreponemal test is positive qualitatively, a titer is then quantitated. (**A,** Based on data from Workowski KA, Berman S; Centers for Diseases Control and Prevention [CDC]: Sexually transmitted diseases treatment guidelines, 2010. MMWR Recomm Rep 59[RR-12]:1–110, 26–29, 2010.)*

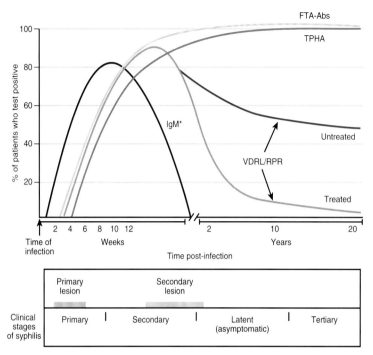

Fig. 245.9 Common patterns of serologic reactivity in syphilis patients. *FTA-Abs*, fluorescent treponemal antibody absorption (test); *RPR*, rapid plasma reagin (test); *TPHA*, *Treponema pallidum* hemagglutination assay; *VDRL*, Venereal Disease Research Laboratory (test). IgM by immunoassay. *(From Peeling R, Ye H: Diagnostic tools for preventing and managing maternal and congenital syphilis: an overview. Bull World Health Organ 82(6):439–446, 2004.)*

dead and living organisms. Placental examination by gross and microscopic techniques can be useful in the diagnosis of congenital syphilis. The disproportionately large placentas are characterized histologically by focal proliferative villitis, endovascular and perivascular arteritis, and focal or diffuse immaturity of placental villi.

Congenital Syphilis
Diagnosis of congenital syphilis requires thorough review of maternal history of syphilis treatment preconception and testing, treatment, and the dynamics of response during the current pregnancy. Regardless of maternal treatment and the presence/absence of symptoms in the infant, proactive evaluation and treatment of exposed neonates is critical (Fig. 245.10 and Table 245.2). Symptomatic infants should be thoroughly evaluated and treated. Fig. 245.10 describes the guidelines for evaluating and managing asymptomatic infants who are considered at risk for congenital syphilis because the maternal nontreponemal and treponemal serology is positive. Internationally adopted, refugee, and immigrant children should also be screened, regardless of history or report of treatment.

Diagnosis of neurosyphilis in the newborn with syphilitic infection is confounded by poor sensitivity of the CSF VDRL test in this age group and lack of CSF abnormalities. A positive CSF VDRL test in a newborn warrants treatment for neurosyphilis, even though it might reflect passive transfer of antibodies from serum to CSF. It is now accepted that all infants with a presumptive diagnosis of congenital syphilis should be treated with regimens effective for neurosyphilis because central nervous system involvement cannot be reliably excluded. Diagnosis of syphilis beyond early infancy should lead to consideration of possible child abuse.

For infants with proven or highly probable disease or abnormal physical findings, complete evaluation, including serologic tests (RPR or VDRL), complete blood count with differential and platelet count, liver function tests, long-bone radiographs, ophthalmology examination, auditory brainstem response, and other tests as indicated, should be performed. For infants with a positive VDRL or RPR test result and normal physical examination whose mothers were inadequately treated, further evaluation is not necessary if 10 days of parenteral therapy are administered.

TREATMENT
The goals of early detection and treatment include treatment of current infection and prevention of both late stage disease and sexual or vertical transmission. *T. pallidum* remains extremely sensitive to penicillin, with no evidence of emerging penicillin resistance, and thus penicillin remains the treatment drug of choice (Table 245.3 and http://www.cdc.gov/std/treatment). Parenteral penicillin G is the only documented effective treatment for congenital syphilis, syphilis during pregnancy, and neurosyphilis. Aqueous crystalline penicillin G is preferred over procaine penicillin, because it better achieves and sustains the minimum concentration of 0.018 µg/mL (0.03 units/mL) needed for 7-10 days to achieve the prolonged treponemicidal levels required for the long dividing time of *T. pallidum*. Although nonpenicillin regimens are available to the penicillin-allergic patient, desensitization followed by standard penicillin therapy is the most reliable strategy. Success of treatment also depends upon the integrity of the host immune response. A transient acute systemic febrile reaction called the **Jarisch-Herxheimer reaction** (caused by massive release of endotoxin-like antigens during bacterial lysis) occurs in 15–20% of patients with acquired or congenital syphilis treated with penicillin. It is not an indication for discontinuing penicillin therapy.

Acquired Syphilis
Primary, secondary, and early latent disease is treated with a single dose of benzathine penicillin G (50,000 units/kg IM, maximum 2.4 million units). Persons with late latent or tertiary disease require 3 doses at 1 wk intervals. Nonpregnant penicillin-allergic patients without neurosyphilis may be treated with either doxycycline (100 mg PO twice daily for 2 wk) or tetracycline (500 mg PO 4 times daily for 2 wk). Emerging *azalide* and *macrolide resistance* has been documented throughout the U.S. (a 23S rRNA point mutation at position 2058) and more recently worldwide (a 23S rRNA point mutation at position 2059), compromising the effective use of these antibiotics. Careful serologic follow-up is always necessary. Documentation of serologic cure is an essential part of syphilis treatment. Less than a 4-fold decline in titer reflects treatment failure.

The CDC recommends that all persons with syphilis be tested for HIV. Patients coinfected with HIV are at increased risk for neurologic complications and higher rates of treatment failure. CDC guidelines

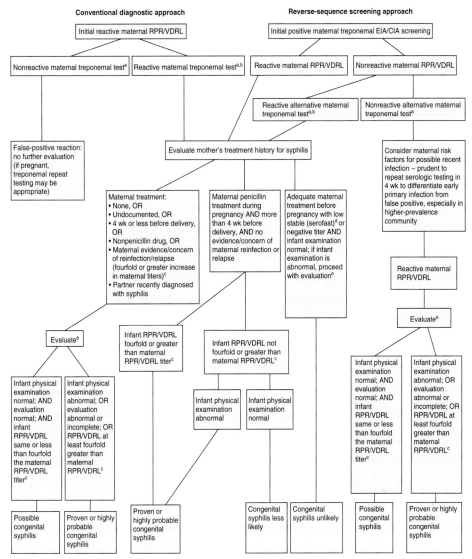

Conventional diagnostic approach

Initial reactive maternal RPR/VDRL

Nonreactive maternal treponemal test[a] | Reactive maternal treponemal test[a,b]

Reverse-sequence screening approach

Initial positive maternal treponemal EIA/CIA screening

Reactive maternal RPR/VDRL | Nonreactive maternal RPR/VDRL

Reactive alternative maternal treponemal test[a,b] | Nonreactive alternative maternal treponemal test[a]

False-positive reaction: no further evaluation (if pregnant, treponemal repeat testing may be appropriate)

Evaluate mother's treatment history for syphilis

Consider maternal risk factors for possible recent infection – prudent to repeat serologic testing in 4 wk to differentiate early primary infection from false positive, especially in higher-prevalence community

Maternal treatment:
• None, OR
• Undocumented, OR
• 4 wk or less before delivery, OR
• Nonpenicillin drug, OR
• Maternal evidence/concern of reinfection/relapse (fourfold or greater increase in maternal titers)[c]
• Partner recently diagnosed with syphilis

Maternal penicillin treatment during pregnancy AND more than 4 wk before delivery, AND no evidence/concern of maternal reinfection or relapse

Adequate maternal treatment before pregnancy with low stable (serofast)[d] or negative titer AND infant examination normal; if infant examination is abnormal, proceed with evaluation[e]

Reactive maternal RPR/VDRL

Evaluate[e]

Infant RPR/VDRL fourfold or greater than maternal RPR/VDRL titer[c]

Infant RPR/VDRL not fourfold or greater than maternal RPR/VDRL[c]

Infant physical examination normal; AND evaluation normal; AND infant RPR/VDRL same or less than fourfold the maternal RPR/VDRL titer[c]

Infant physical examination abnormal; OR evaluation abnormal or incomplete; OR RPR/VDRL at least fourfold greater than maternal RPR/VDRL[c]

Infant physical examination abnormal

Infant physical examination normal

Infant physical examination normal; AND evaluation normal; AND infant RPR/VDRL same or less than fourfold the maternal RPR/VDRL titer[c]

Infant physical examination abnormal; OR evaluation abnormal or incomplete; OR RPR/VDRL at least fourfold greater than maternal RPR/VDRL[c]

Possible congenital syphilis

Proven or highly probable congenital syphilis

Proven or highly probable congenital syphilis

Congenital syphilis less likely

Congenital syphilis unlikely

Possible congenital syphilis

Proven or highly probable congenital syphilis

RPR indicates rapid plasma reagin; VDRL, Venereal Disease Research Laboratory.

[a] *Treponema pallidum* particle agglutination (TP-PA) (which is the preferred treponemal test), fluorescent treponemal antibody absorption (FTA-ABS), or microhemagglutination test for antibodies to *T pallidum* (MHA-TP).

[b] Test for human immunodeficiency virus (HIV) antibody. Infants of HIV-infected mothers do not require different evaluation or treatment for syphilis.

[c] A fourfold change in titer is the same as a change of 2 dilutions. For example, a titer of 1:64 is fourfold greater than a titer of 1:16, and a titer of 1:4 is fourfold lower than a titer of 1:16. When comparing titers, the same type of nontreponemal test should be used (eg, if the initial test was an RPR, the follow-up test should also be an RPR).

[d] Stable VDRL titers 1:2 or less or RPR 1:4 or less beyond 1 year after successful treatment are considered low serofast.

[e] Complete blood cell (CBC) and platelet count; cerebrospinal fluid (CSF) examination for cell count, protein, and quantitative VDRL; other tests as clinically indicated (eg, chest radiographs, long-bone radiographs, eye examination, liver function tests, neuroimaging, and auditory brainstem response).

Fig. 245.10 Algorithm for evaluation and treatment of infants born to mothers with reactive serologic tests for syphilis. *(From American Academy of Pediatrics: Red book: 2018-2021 report of the committee on infectious diseases, ed 31, Elk Grove Village, IL, 2018, American Academy of Pediatrics, Fig. 3.10, p. 779).*

recommend the same treatment of primary and secondary syphilis as for patients who are not infected with HIV, but some experts recommend 3 weekly doses of benzathine penicillin G. HIV-infected patients with late latent syphilis or latent syphilis of unknown duration should have a CSF evaluation for neurosyphilis before treatment.

Sex partners of infected persons of any stage should be evaluated and treated. Persons exposed for 90 days or less preceding diagnosis in a sex partner should be treated presumptively even if seronegative. Persons exposed for more than 90 days before the diagnosis in a sex partner should be treated if seropositive or if serologic tests are not available. Follow-up serology should be performed on treated patients

to establish adequacy of therapy, and all patients should be tested for other sexually transmitted diseases, including HIV.

Syphilis in Pregnancy

When clinical or serologic findings suggest active infection or when diagnosis of active syphilis cannot be excluded with certainty, treatment is indicated. The goals of treatment of the pregnant woman include eradication of maternal disease, prevention of mother to child transmission, and treatment of fetal infection. Patients should be treated immediately with the penicillin regimen appropriate for the woman's stage of syphilis. Women who have been adequately treated in the past do not require

Table 245.2	Clues That Suggest a Diagnosis of Congenital Syphilis

EPIDEMIOLOGIC BACKGROUND	CLINICAL FINDINGS
Untreated early syphilis in the mother	Osteochondritis, periostitis
Untreated latent syphilis in the mother	Snuffles, hemorrhagic rhinitis
An untreated mother who has contact with a known syphilitic during pregnancy	Condylomata lata
	Bullous lesions, palmar or plantar rash
Mother treated less than 30 days prior to delivery	Mucous patches
Mother treated for syphilis during pregnancy with a drug other than penicillin	Hepatomegaly, splenomegaly
	Jaundice
Mother treated for syphilis during pregnancy without follow-up to demonstrate 4-fold decrease in titer	Nonimmune hydrops fetalis
	Generalized lymphadenopathy
Mother coinfected with HIV	Central nervous system signs; elevated cell count or protein in cerebrospinal fluid
	Hemolytic anemia, diffuse intravascular coagulation, thrombocytopenia
	Pneumonitis
	Nephrotic syndrome
	Placental villitis or vasculitis (unexplained enlarged placenta)
	Intrauterine growth restriction

Arranged in decreasing order of confidence of diagnosis.

Modified from Remington JS, Klein JO, Wilson CB, et al., editors: *Infectious diseases of the fetus and newborn infant*, ed 6, Philadelphia, 2006, WB Saunders, p. 556.

Table 245.3	Recommended Treatment for Syphilis in People Older Than 1 Mo

STATUS	CHILDREN	ADULTS
Congenital syphilis	Aqueous crystalline penicillin G, 200,000-300,000 U/kg/day, IV, administered as 50,000 U/kg, every 4-6 hr for 10 days*	
Primary, secondary, and early latent syphilis[†]	Penicillin G benzathine,[‡] 50,000 U/kg, IM, up to the adult dose of 2.4 million U in a single dose	Penicillin G benzathine, 2.4 million U, IM, in a single dose OR *If allergic to penicillin and not pregnant,* Doxycycline, 100 mg, orally, twice a day for 14 days OR Tetracycline, 500 mg, orally, 4 times/day for 14 days
Late latent syphilis[§]	Penicillin G benzathine, 50,000 U/kg, IM, up to the adult dose of 2.4 million U, administered as 3 single doses at 1-wk intervals (total 150,000 U/kg, up to the adult dose of 7.2 million U)	Penicillin G benzathine, 7.2 million U total, administered as 3 doses of 2.4 million U, IM, each at 1-wk intervals OR *If allergic to penicillin and not pregnant,* Doxycycline, 100 mg, orally, twice a day for 4 wk OR Tetracycline, 500 mg, orally, 4 times/day for 4 wk
Tertiary		Penicillin G benzathine 7.2 million U total, administered as 3 doses of 2.4 million U, IM, at 1-wk intervals *If allergic to penicillin and not pregnant, consult an infectious diseases expert*
Neurosyphilis[‖]	Aqueous crystalline penicillin G, 200,000-300,000 U/kg/day, IV, every 4-6 hr for 10-14 days, in doses not to exceed the adult dose	Aqueous crystalline penicillin G, 18-24 million U per day, administered as 3-4 million U, IV, every 4 hr for 10-14 days[¶] OR Penicillin G procaine,[‡] 2.4 million U, IM, once daily PLUS probenecid, 500 mg, orally, 4 times/day, both for 10-14 days[¶]

*If the patient has no clinical manifestations of disease, the cerebrospinal fluid *(CSF)* examination is normal, and the CSF Venereal Disease Research Laboratory *(VDRL)* test result is negative, some experts would treat with up to 3 weekly doses of penicillin G benzathine, 50,000 U/kg, IM. Some experts also suggest giving these patients a single dose of penicillin G benzathine, 50,000 U/kg, IM, after the 10-day course of intravenous aqueous penicillin.

[†]Early latent syphilis is defined as being acquired within the preceding year.

[‡]Penicillin G benzathine and penicillin G procaine are approved for intramuscular administration only.

[§]Late latent syphilis is defined as syphilis beyond 1 yr duration.

[‖]Patients who are allergic to penicillin should be desensitized.

[¶]Some experts administer penicillin G benzathine, 2.4 million U, IM, once per week for up to 3 wk after completion of these neurosyphilis treatment regimens.

IV, intravenously; *IM,* intramuscularly.

From American Academy of Pediatrics: *Red book: 2015 report of the committee on infectious diseases*, ed 30, Elk Grove Village, IL, 2015, American Academy of Pediatrics, Table 3.74.

additional therapy unless quantitative serology suggests evidence of reinfection (**4-fold elevation in titer**). Doxycycline and tetracycline *should not be* administered during pregnancy, and macrolides do not effectively prevent fetal infection. Pregnant patients who are allergic to penicillin should be desensitized and treated with penicillin.

Congenital Syphilis

Adequate maternal treatment at least 30 days prior to delivery is likely to prevent congenital syphilis. All infants born to mothers with syphilis should be followed until nontreponemal serology is negative. The infant should be treated if there is any uncertainty about the adequacy of maternal treatment. The goal of infant treatment is prevention of organ damage, skeletal deformity, and developmental delay. Any infant at risk of congenital syphilis should be evaluated for HIV.

Congenital syphilis is treated with aqueous penicillin G (100,000-150,000 units/kg/24 hr divided every 12 hr IV for the 1st wk of life, and every 8 hr thereafter) or procaine penicillin G (50,000 units/kg IM once daily) given for 10 days. Both penicillin regimens are recognized as adequate therapy for congenital syphilis, but higher concentrations of penicillin are achieved in the CSF of infants treated with intravenous aqueous penicillin G than in those treated with intramuscular procaine penicillin. Treated infants should be followed every 2-3 mo to confirm at least a 4-fold decrease in nontreponemal titers. Treated infants with congenital neurosyphilis should undergo clinical and CSF evaluation at 6-mo intervals until CSF is normal. At age 2 these infants should receive a full developmental assessment. In a very-low-risk neonate who is asymptomatic and whose mother was treated appropriately, without evidence of relapse or reinfection, but with a low and stable VDRL titer (serofast), no evaluation is necessary. Some specialists would treat such an infant with a single dose of benzathine penicillin G 50,000 units/kg IM.

PREVENTION

Syphilis, including congenital syphilis, is a reportable disease in all 50 states and the District of Columbia. Testing is indicated at any time for persons with suspicious lesions, a history of recent sexual exposure to a person with syphilis, or diagnosis of another sexually transmitted infection, including HIV infection. The resurgence of syphilis compels clinicians to remain cognizant of its protean manifestations to avoid missed or late diagnosis. Timely treatment lessens risk of community spread. Despite the genome sequencing of *T. pallidum* in 1998, vaccine prevention remains elusive, confounded by the treponeme's ability to evade the immune system.

Congenital Syphilis

Congenital syphilis is a preventable disease, a sentinel event indicating multiple missed opportunities. Primary prevention is tied to prevention of syphilis in women of childbearing age and secondary prevention with early diagnosis and prompt treatment of women and their partners. Access to and use of comprehensive prenatal care is key, with careful history taking (including interim sexual partners) at each visit. Routine prenatal screening for syphilis remains the most important factor in identifying infants at risk for developing congenital syphilis. Screening all women at the beginning of prenatal care is an evidence-based standard of care and legally required in all states. In pregnant women without optimal prenatal care, serologic screening for syphilis should be performed at the time pregnancy is diagnosed. Any woman who is delivered of a stillborn infant at 20 wk or fewer of gestation should be tested for syphilis. In communities and populations with a high prevalence of syphilis and in patients at high risk (women with a history of incarceration, drug use, or multiple or concurrent partners), testing should be performed at least 2 additional times: at the beginning of the 3rd trimester (28 wk) and at delivery. Some states mandate repeat testing at delivery for all women, underscoring the importance of preventive screening. Women at high risk for syphilis should be screened even more frequently, either monthly or pragmatically in the case of inconsistent prenatal care, at every medical encounter because they can have repeat infections during pregnancy or reinfection late in pregnancy. Follow-up serologic testing of all treated women should be done after treatment to document titer decline, relapse, or reinfection.

No newborn should leave the hospital without the mother's syphilis status having been determined at least once during pregnancy or at delivery. In states conducting newborn screening for syphilis, both the mother's and infant's serologic results should be known before discharge. In addition, all previously uninvestigated infants of an infected mother should be screened. Strong linkages between clinicians and public health practitioners remain essential for comprehensive prevention of acquired and congenital syphilis.

Bibliography is available at Expert Consult.

Chapter **246**
Nonvenereal Treponemal Infections
Stephen K. Obaro and H. Dele Davies
第二百四十六章
非性病性密螺旋体感染

中文导读

　　本章主要介绍了雅司病、非性病性梅毒、品他病3种非性病性螺旋体病，主要通过接触传播。雅司病最常见，儿童对该病相对易感，病变主要累及皮肤和骨骼，病程迁延，诊断需结合流行病史、典型的临床表现和实验室检查，需注意与其他相似皮肤疾病和镰状细胞病导致的指炎相鉴别，治疗主要采用苄星青霉素G，过敏者可用红霉素或四环素，口服单剂阿奇霉素疗效与青霉素疗效相同。此外还大致介绍了非性病性梅毒和品他病的流行病学、临床表现、诊断和治疗。

Nonvenereal treponemal infections—yaws, bejel (endemic syphilis), and pinta—are caused by different subspecies of *Treponema pallidum* and occur in tropical and subtropical areas. The causative agents of nonvenereal treponematoses—*T. pallidum pertenue*, *T. pallidum* subspecies *endemicum*, and *Treponema carateum*—cannot be distinguished from *T. pallidum* subspecies *pallidum* by morphologic or serologic tests.

In general, nonvenereal treponematoses have prominent cutaneous manifestations and relapsing courses, as in venereal syphilis, but they are not found in urban centers, they are not sexually transmitted, and they are not congenitally acquired. Transmission is primarily through body contact, poor hygiene, crowded conditions, and poor access to healthcare. Children also serve as the primary reservoirs for these organisms, spreading infection via skin-to-skin and skin-to-mucous membrane contact, and possibly via fomites as well.

Penicillin remains the treatment of choice for syphilis and nonvenereal treponemal infections.

Bibliography is available at Expert Consult.

246.1 Yaws *(Treponema pertenue)*
Stephen K. Obaro and H. Dele Davies

Yaws is the most prevalent nonvenereal treponematosis. The causative agent, *Treponema pertenue*, bears very close genomic resemblance to *T. pallidum* subspecies *pallidum*. The overall sequence identity between the genomes of *T. pallidum pertenue* and *T. pallidum* subspecies *pallidum* is 99.8%. Yaws is a contagious, chronic, relapsing infection involving the skin and bony structures caused by the spirochete *T. pertenue*, which is identical to *T. pallidum* microscopically and serologically. It occurs in tropical regions with heavy rainfall and annual temperatures ≥27°C (80°F). Almost all cases occur in children in tropical and subtropical countries. It is also referred to as "framboesia," "pian," "parangi," and "bouba." A high percentage of the population is infected in endemic areas.

T. pertenue is transmitted by direct contact from an infected lesion through a skin abrasion or laceration. Transmission is facilitated by overcrowding and poor personal hygiene in the rain forest areas of the world. Yaws predominantly affects children, with approximately 75% of cases being reported in children younger than 15 yr of age. This population also constitutes the reservoir for disease transmission. The initial papular lesion, which constitutes **primary yaws**, also described as the **mother yaw**, occurs 2-8 wk after inoculation. This lesion typically involves the buttocks or lower extremities. The papule develops into a raised, raspberry-like papilloma and is often accompanied by regional lymphadenopathy. The skin pathology is very similar to that of venereal syphilis, consisting of epidermal hyperplasia and papillomatosis (Fig. 246.1). Healing of the mother yaw leaves a hypopigmented scar. The **secondary stage** lesions can erupt anywhere on the body before or after the healing of the mother yaw and may be accompanied by lymphadenopathy, anorexia, and malaise. Multiple cutaneous lesions (daughter yaws, pianomas, or frambesias) appear, spread diffusely, ulcerate, and are covered by exudates containing treponemes. Secondary lesions heal without scarring. Recurrent lesions are common within 5 yr after the primary lesion.

The lesions are often associated with bone pain resulting from underlying periostitis or osteomyelitis, especially of the fingers, nose, and tibia. The initial period of clinical activity is followed by a 5-10 yr period of latency. The appearance of tertiary stage lesions develops in approximately 10% of infected patients, with onset typically at puberty with solitary and destructive lesions. These lesions occur as painful papillomas on the hands and feet, gummatous skin ulcerations, or osteitis. Bony destruction and deformity, juxta-articular nodules, depigmentation, and painful hyperkeratosis (**dry crab yaws**) of the palms and soles are common. Approximately 10% of patients may progress and develop tertiary stage lesions after 5 yr or more of untreated infection, although this outcome is now rare.

The diagnosis is based on the characteristic clinical manifestations of the disease in an endemic area. Darkfield examination of cutaneous lesions for treponemes and both treponemal and nontreponemal

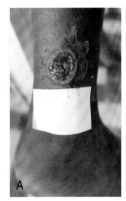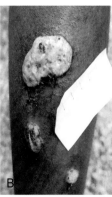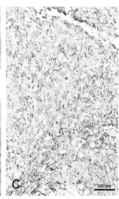

Fig. 246.1 Yaws lesions in a patient with treatment failure associated with macrolide-resistant *T p pertenue*. **A,** Primary lesion (*red*, moist 2.5 cm ulcer) on the left leg of an 11 yr old patient with yaws observed at the 30-mo survey. Lesional swab PCR was positive for *T p pertenue* with wild-type 23S rRNA. **B,** Secondary yaws papillomas (multiple nodules with yellow color granular surface) seen at 36-mo survey. These lesions were PCR positive for *T p pertenue* with A2059G mutation in 23S rRNA. **C,** Photomicrograph of skin biopsy of the larger papilloma lesion in panel **B** with abundant spirochete organisms stained bright red by the *Treponema pallidum* immunohistochemical stain (×400 magnification). *T p pertenue, Treponema pallidum* subspecies *pertenue*. (*From Mitja O, Godornes C, Houinei W, et al: Re-emergence of yaws after single mass azithromycin treatment followed by targeted treatment: a longitudinal study, Lancet 391:1599–1606, 2018. Fig. 2*).

serologic tests for syphilis, which are positive because of cross reactivity, are used to confirm the diagnosis. The nontreponemal agglutination tests such as the rapid plasma reagin and Venereal Diseases Research Laboratory tests are positive in untreated cases, and these tests can be used for test of cure, because they revert to negative following treatment. However, the treponemal tests (*T. pallidum* hemagglutination assay, *T. pallidum* particle agglutination assay, and fluorescent treponemal antibody absorption) are more specific and remain positive for life. New immunochromatographic test strips that can be applied for testing both whole blood and serum are simple, cheap, and easy to use and do not require refrigeration. However, they have lower sensitivity compared to the antibody assays and appear to work best in persons with more active disease.

Differential diagnosis includes other conditions with similar cutaneous manifestations such as eczema, psoriasis, excoriated chronic scabies, tungiasis, leishmaniasis, tropical ulcer cutaneous mycoses, and verrucae. Involvement of the bone may mimic dactylitis that is commonly associated with sickle cell disease

Treatment of yaws consists of a single dose of the long-acting benzathine penicillin G (1.2 million units IM for adults and 0.6 million units for children < 10 yr) for index patients and all contacts. Patients allergic to penicillin may be treated with erythromycin, doxycycline, or tetracycline at appropriate doses for venereal syphilis (see Chapter 245). One oral dose of azithromycin (30 mg/kg; maximum: 2 g) is as effective as benzathine penicillin. Treatment cures the lesions of active yaws, renders them noninfectious, and prevents relapse. Family members, contacts, and patients with latent infection should receive the same dose as those with active disease. Eradication of yaws from some endemic areas has been accomplished by treating the entire population (mass treatment) with azithromycin, although reemergence has been reported in those who did not receive mass treatment.

Bibliography is available at Expert Consult.

246.2 Bejel (Endemic Syphilis; *Treponema pallidum* endemicum)
Stephen K. Obaro and H. Dele Davies

Bejel, or endemic syphilis, affects children in remote rural communities living in poor hygienic conditions. Unlike yaws, bejel can occur in temperate as well as dry, hot climates. Infection with *T. pallidum* subspecies *endemicum* follows penetration of the spirochete through traumatized skin or mucous membranes. In experimental infections, a primary papule forms at the inoculation site after an incubation period of 3 wk. A primary lesion is almost never visualized in human infections; however, primary ulcers have been described surrounding the nipples of nursing mothers with infected children.

The clinical manifestations of the **secondary stage** typically occur 3-6 mo after inoculation and are confined to the skin and mucous membranes. They consist of highly infectious mucous patches on the oral mucosa and condyloma-like lesions on the moist areas of the body, especially the axilla and anus. These mucocutaneous lesions resolve spontaneously over a period of several months, but recurrences are common. The secondary stage is followed by a variable latency period before the onset of late or tertiary bejel. The tertiary stage can occur as

early as 6 mo or as late as several years after resolution of initial symptoms. The lesions in the tertiary stage are identical to those of yaws and include gumma formation in skin, subcutaneous tissue, and bone, resulting in painful destructive ulcerations, swelling, and deformity.

The diagnosis is based on the characteristic clinical manifestations of the disease in an endemic area. Dark-field examination of cutaneous lesions for treponemes and both treponemal and nontreponemal serologic tests for syphilis, which are positive because of cross reactivity, are used to confirm the diagnosis.

Differentiation from venereal syphilis is extremely difficult in an endemic area. Bejel is distinguished by the absence of a primary chancre and lack of involvement of the central nervous system and cardiovascular system during the late stage.

Treatment of early infection consists of a single dose of benzathine penicillin G (1.2 million units IM for adults and 0.6 million units for children < 10 yr). Late infection is treated with 3 injections of the same dosage at intervals of 7 days. Patients allergic to penicillin may be treated with erythromycin or tetracycline.

Bibliography is available at Expert Consult.

246.3 Pinta *(Treponema carateum)*
Stephen K. Obaro and H. Dele Davies

Pinta is a chronic, nonvenereally transmitted infection caused by *T. pallidum* subsp. *carateum*, a spirochete morphologically and serologically indistinguishable from other human treponemes. This is perhaps the mildest of the nonvenereal treponematoses. The disease is endemic in Mexico, Central America, South America, and parts of the West Indies and largely affects children younger than 15 yr of age.

Infection follows direct inoculation of the treponeme through abraded skin. After a variable incubation period of days, the **primary** lesion appears at the inoculation site as a small asymptomatic erythematous papule resembling localized psoriasis or eczema. The regional lymph nodes are often enlarged. Spirochetes can be visualized on darkfield examination of skin scrapings or from biopsy of the involved lymph nodes. After a period of enlargement, the primary lesion disappears. Unlike primary yaws, the lesion does not ulcerate but can expand with central depigmented resolution. **Secondary** lesions follow within 6-8 mo and consist of small macules and papules on the face, scalp, and other sun-exposed portions of the body. These pigmented, highly infectious lesions are scaly and nonpruritic and can coalesce to form large plaque-like elevations resembling psoriasis. In the late or **tertiary** stage, atrophic and depigmented lesions develop on the hands, wrists, ankles, feet, face, and scalp. Hyperkeratosis of palms and soles is uncommon.

The diagnosis is based on the characteristic clinical manifestations of the disease in an endemic area. Darkfield examination of cutaneous lesions for treponemes and both treponemal and nontreponemal serologic tests for syphilis, which are positive because of cross reactivity, are used to confirm the diagnosis.

Treatment consists of a single dose of benzathine penicillin G (1.2 million units IM for adults and 0.6 million units for children < 10 yr). Tetracycline and erythromycin are alternatives for patients allergic to penicillin. Treatment campaigns and improvement of standards of living are necessary for reduction and elimination of disease.

Chapter 247
Leptospira
H. Dele Davies and Kari A. Simonsen

第二百四十七章
钩端螺旋体病

中文导读

本章主要介绍了钩端螺旋体病的病原学、流行病学、病理学和发病机制、临床表现、诊断、治疗和预防。该病是由致病性的钩端螺旋体导致的，为常见的人畜共患病。病原体经皮肤黏膜进入人体，形成菌血症，产生全身小血管损害。从无症状到重症表现多样，根据临床表现可分为无黄疸型和有黄疸型。诊断需注意流行病学和接触史，实验室诊断常用血清学检查，金标准为显微凝集试验，也可通过PCR检测病原体进行诊断。早期治疗可缩短病程，建议首选青霉素，对青霉素过敏者可用强力霉素。预防包括控制传染源，切断传播途径，保护易感人群，暂无儿童预防治疗的数据。

Leptospirosis is a common and widespread zoonosis caused by aerobic, motile spirochetes of the genus *Leptospira*.

ETIOLOGY

Leptospira spp. are thin, helix-shaped members of the phylum Spirochaetes. There are 22 species identified within the genus *Leptospira*, and these are further divided into over 300 serovars. There are at least 10 pathogenic *Leptospira* species, with serovars demonstrating preferential host specificity.

EPIDEMIOLOGY

Leptospirosis has a worldwide distribution, but most human cases occur in tropical and subtropical countries with disease burden disproportionately affecting resource-poor populations. Leptospires survive for days to weeks in warm and damp environmental conditions, including water and moist soil. In the United States, the CDC estimates 100-200 annual cases. Hawaii reports about 50% of US cases, with Pacific coastal and Southern states having higher incidence than the remainder of the country. Leptospires infect many species of animals, including rats, mice, and moles; livestock such as cattle, goats, sheep, horses, and pigs; wild mammals like raccoons or opossums; and domestic dogs. Infected animals excrete spirochetes in their urine for prolonged periods. Globally, most human cases result from exposure to water or soil contaminated with rat urine; however, the major animal reservoir in the United States is the dog. Groups at high risk for leptospirosis include persons exposed occupationally or recreationally to contaminated soil, water, or infected animals. High-risk occupations include agricultural workers, veterinarians, abattoir workers, meat inspectors, rodent control workers, laboratory workers, sewer workers, and military personnel. Exposure to contaminated floodwaters is also a documented source of infection. Transmission via animal bites and directly from person to person has been rarely reported.

PATHOLOGY AND PATHOGENESIS

Leptospires enter human hosts through mucous membranes (primarily eyes, nose, and mouth), transdermally through abraded skin, or by ingestion of contaminated water. After penetration, they circulate in the bloodstream, causing endothelial damage of small blood vessels with secondary ischemic damage to end organs.

CLINICAL MANIFESTATIONS

The spectrum of human leptospirosis ranges from asymptomatic infection to severe disease (5–10% of infections) with multiorgan dysfunction and death. The onset is usually abrupt, and the illness may follow a monophasic or the classically described biphasic course (Fig. 247.1). The incubation period ranges from 2 to 30 days, following which there is an **initial** or **septicemic phase** lasting 2-7 days, during which leptospires can be isolated from the blood, cerebrospinal fluid (CSF), and other tissues. This phase may be followed by a brief period of well-being before onset of a second symptomatic **immune** or **leptospiruric phase**. This phase is associated with the appearance of circulating IgM antibody, disappearance of organisms from the blood and CSF, and appearance of signs and symptoms associated with localization of leptospires in the tissues. Despite the presence of circulating antibody, leptospires can persist in the kidney, urine, and aqueous humor. The immune phase can last for several weeks. Symptomatic infection may be anicteric or icteric.

Anicteric Leptospirosis

The **septicemic phase** of anicteric leptospirosis has an abrupt onset with flulike signs of fever, shaking chills, lethargy, severe headache, malaise, nausea, vomiting, and severe debilitating myalgia most prominent in the lower extremities, lumbosacral spine, and abdomen. Bradycardia and hypotension can occur, but circulatory collapse is uncommon. Conjunctival suffusion with photophobia and orbital pain (in the absence of chemosis and purulent exudate), generalized lymphadenopathy, and hepatosplenomegaly may also be present. A transient (<24 hr) erythematous maculopapular, urticarial, petechial, purpuric, or desquamating rash occurs in 10% of cases. Rarer manifestations include pharyngitis, pneumonitis, arthritis, carditis, cholecystitis, and orchitis. The **second** or **immune phase** can follow a brief asymptomatic interlude and is characterized by recurrence of fever and aseptic meningitis. Although 80% of infected children have abnormal CSF profiles, only 50% have clinical meningeal manifestations. CSF abnormalities include a modest elevation in pressure, pleocytosis with early polymorphonuclear leukocytosis followed by mononuclear predominance rarely exceeding 500 cells/mm³, normal or slightly elevated protein levels, and normal glucose values. Encephalitis, cranial and peripheral neuropathies, papilledema, and paralysis are uncommon. A self-limited unilateral or bilateral uveitis can occur during this phase, rarely resulting in permanent visual impairment. Central nervous system symptoms usually resolve spontaneously within 1 wk, with almost no mortality.

Icteric Leptospirosis (Weil Syndrome)

Weil syndrome is a severe form of leptospirosis seen more commonly in adults (>30 yr) than in children. The initial manifestations are similar to those described for anicteric leptospirosis. The immune phase, however, is characterized by jaundice, acute renal dysfunction, thrombocytopenia, and, in fulminant cases, pulmonary hemorrhage and cardiovascular collapse. Hepatic involvement leads to right upper quadrant pain, hepatomegaly, direct and indirect hyperbilirubinemia, and modestly elevated serum levels of hepatic enzymes. Liver function usually returns to normal after recovery. Patients have abnormal findings on urinalysis (hematuria, proteinuria, and casts), and azotemia is common, often associated with oliguria or anuria. Acute kidney failure occurs in 16–40% of cases. Abnormal electrocardiograms are present in 90% of cases, but congestive heart failure is uncommon. Transient thrombocytopenia occurs in >50% of cases. Rarely, hemorrhagic manifestations occur, including epistaxis, hemoptysis, and pulmonary, gastrointestinal, and adrenal hemorrhage. Patients with pulmonary hemorrhage syndrome may have >50% mortality rate, although the overall mortality rate for severe disease is lower, about 5–15%.

DIAGNOSIS

Leptospirosis should be considered in the differential diagnosis of acute flulike febrile illnesses with a history of direct contact with animals or with soil or water contaminated with animal urine. The disease may be difficult to distinguish clinically from dengue or malaria in endemic areas.

The diagnosis is most often confirmed by serologic testing and less often confirmed by isolation of the infecting organism from clinical specimens. The gold standard diagnostic method is the microscopic agglutination test, a serogroup-specific assay using live antigen suspension of leptospiral serovars and dark-field microscopy for agglutination. A 4-fold or greater increase in titer in paired sera confirms the diagnosis. Agglutinins usually appear by the 12th day of illness and reach a maximum titer by the 3rd wk. Low titers can persist for years. Approximately 10% of infected persons do not have detectable agglutinins, presumably because available antisera do not identify all *Leptospira* serotypes. Additionally, enzyme-linked immunosorbent assay (ELISA) methods, latex agglutination, and immunochromatography are commercially available, and DNA PCR diagnostics have been developed. Phase-contrast and dark-field microscopy are insensitive for spirochete detection, but organisms may be identified using Warthin-Starry silver stain or fluorescent antibody staining of tissue or body fluids. Unlike other pathogenic spirochetes, leptospires can be recovered from the blood or CSF during the first 10 days of illness and from urine after the 2nd wk by repeated culture of small inoculum (i.e., one drop of blood or CSF in 5 mL of medium) on commercially available selective media. However, the inoculum in clinical specimens is small, and growth can take up to 16 wk.

TREATMENT

Leptospira spp. demonstrate in vitro susceptibility to penicillin and tetracyclines, but in vivo effectiveness of these antibiotics in treating human leptospirosis is unclear due to the naturally high spontaneous recovery rates. Some studies suggest that initiation of treatment before the 7th day shortens the clinical course and decreases the severity of the infection; thus treatment with penicillin G, cefotaxime, ceftriaxone, or doxycycline (in children ≥8 yr of age) should be instituted early when the diagnosis is suspected. There is evidence that a short (<2 wk) course of doxycycline may be safely used in children >2 yr of age. Parenteral penicillin G (6-8 million U/m²/day divided every 4 hr IV for 7 days) is recommended, with doxycycline 2 mg/kg/day divided in 2 doses with maximum of 100 mg twice daily as an alternative for patients allergic to penicillin. Cefotaxime, ceftriaxone, and azithromycin have been evaluated in clinical trials and have demonstrated equivalent effectiveness with doxycycline. These antibiotics can be used as alternatives in patients for whom doxycycline is contraindicated. In mild illness, oral doxycycline, amoxicillin, and ampicillin have been used successfully. In severe illness, supportive care with specific attention given to cardiopulmonary status, renal function, coagulopathy, and fluid and electrolyte balance is warranted.

PREVENTION

Prevention of human leptospirosis infection is facilitated through rodent control measures and avoidance of contaminated water and soil. Immunization of livestock and domestic dogs is recommended as a

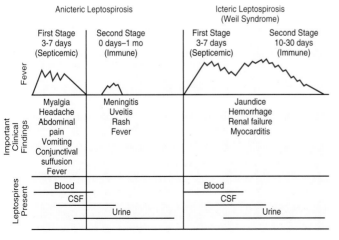

Fig. 247.1 Stages of anicteric and icteric leptospirosis. Correlation between clinical findings and presence of leptospires in body fluids, *CSF*, cerebrospinal fluid. *(Reprinted with permission from Feigin RD, Anderson DC: Human leptospirosis, CRC Crit Rev Clin Lab Sci 5:413–467, 1975. Copyright CRC Press, Inc., Boca Raton, FL.)*

means of reducing animal reservoirs. Human vaccine development has been challenging due to the diversity of *Leptospira* serovars and their variable geographic distribution. Protective clothing (i.e., boots, gloves, and goggles) should be worn by persons at risk for occupational exposure. In hospital settings, in addition to standard precautions, contact precautions are recommended for potential exposures to infected urine. Leptospirosis was successfully prevented in American soldiers stationed

in the tropics by administering prophylactic doxycycline (200 mg PO once a week). This approach may be similarly effective for travelers to highly endemic areas for short periods; however, there are no specific pediatric data to support any prophylaxis regimen.

Bibliography is available at Expert Consult.

Chapter **248**
Relapsing Fever *(Borrelia)*
H. Dele Davies and Stephen K. Obaro

第二百四十八章
回归热（疏螺旋体）

中文导读

本章主要介绍了回归热的病原学、流行病学、病理学和发病机制、临床表现、诊断、治疗、预后和预防。该病是由疏螺旋体导致的，包括虱传（流行性）回归热和蜱传（地方性）回归热。病原体经皮肤或黏膜入血，发热期大量在体内繁殖循环。临床表现以反复发热和流感样症状为主要表现，可发生中枢神经系统和周围神经受损表现，严重者可有心肌炎、肝衰竭和弥散性血管内凝血病。诊断依赖于找到病原体，常用外周血涂片，也可用特异性的PCR检测。首选四环素或强力霉素。目前还没有疫苗，疾病控制需要避免或消除节肢动物病媒介。

Relapsing fever is characterized by recurring fevers and flu-like symptoms such as headaches, myalgia, arthralgia, and rigors.

ETIOLOGY
Relapsing fever is an arthropod (lice or ticks)-transmitted infection caused by spirochetes of the genus *Borrelia*.

Louse-borne (epidemic) relapsing fever is caused by *Borrelia recurrentis* and is transmitted from person to person by *Pediculus humanus*, the human body louse. Human infection occurs as a result of crushing lice during scratching, facilitating entry of infected hemolymph through abraded or normal skin or mucous membranes.

Tick-borne (endemic) relapsing fever is caused by several species of *Borrelia* and is transmitted to humans by *Ornithodoros* ticks. *Borrelia hermsii* and *Borrelia turicatae* are the common species in the western United States, while *Borrelia dugesii* is the major cause of disease in Mexico and Central America. Human infection occurs when saliva, coxal fluid, or excrement is released by the tick during feeding, thereby permitting spirochetes to penetrate the skin and mucous membranes.

EPIDEMIOLOGY
Louse-borne relapsing fever tends to occur in epidemics associated with war, poverty, famine, and poor personal hygiene, often in association

with typhus. This form of relapsing fever is no longer seen in the United States but is endemic in parts of East Africa. Using 16S rRNA polymerase chain reaction assays for molecular detection, up to 20.5% of all unexplained fever in the horn of Africa, including northwestern Morocco where the population traditionally lives in mud huts, is caused by tickborne relapsing fever, making this the most common cause of bacterial infections.

Ornithodoros ticks, which transmit endemic relapsing fever and are distributed worldwide, including in the western United States, prefer warm, humid environments and high altitudes and are found in rodent burrows, caves, and other nesting sites (Fig. 248.1). Rodents (e.g., squirrels and chipmunks) are the principal reservoirs. Infected ticks gain access to human dwellings on the rodent host. Human contact is often unnoticed because these soft ticks have a painless bite and detach immediately after a short blood meal.

PATHOLOGY AND PATHOGENESIS
Relapsing fever is cyclical because the *Borrelia* organisms undergo antigenic (phase) variation. Multiple variants evolve simultaneously during the first relapse, with one type becoming predominant. Spirochetes isolated during the primary febrile episode differ antigenically from those recovered during a subsequent relapse. During febrile episodes,

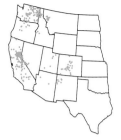 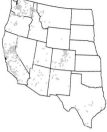

● Each dot, placed randomly within the county of exposure (where known), represents one case.

● Each dot, placed randomly within the county of residence, represents one case.

Fig. 248.1 Cases of tickborne relapsing fever–United States, 1990-2011. During the years 1990-2011, 483 cases of tickborne relapsing fever were reported in the western United States, with infections being transmitted most frequently in California, Washington, and Colorado. *(From Centers for Disease Control and Prevention [CDC]: Tick-borne relapsing fever: distribution. Available at: http://www.cdc.gov/relapsing-fever/distribution).*

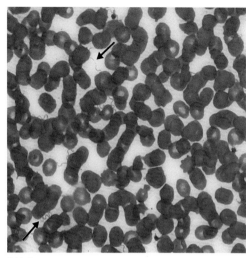

Fig. 248.2 Stained thin smear of a newborn's peripheral blood, showing the presence of numerous spirochetes (indicated by *black arrows*) at ×63 magnification—Colorado, 2011. *(From Centers for Disease Control and Prevention [CDC]: Tickborne relapsing fever in a mother and newborn child–Colorado, 2011. MMWR Morb Mortal Wkly Rep 61:174–176, 2012.)*

spirochetes enter the bloodstream, induce the development of specific immunoglobulin M and G antibodies, and undergo agglutination, immobilization, lysis, and phagocytosis. During remission, *Borrelia* spirochetes may remain in the bloodstream, but spirochetemia is insufficient to produce symptoms. The number of relapses in untreated patients depends on the number of antigenic variants of the infecting strain.

CLINICAL MANIFESTATIONS

Relapsing fever is characterized by febrile episodes lasting 2-9 days, separated by afebrile intervals of 2-7 days. Louse-borne disease has an incubation period of 2-14 days, longer periods of pyrexia, fewer relapses, and longer remission periods than tickborne disease. The incubation period of tickborne disease is usually 7 days (range: 2-9 days). Each form of relapsing fever is characterized by sudden onset of high fever, lethargy, headache, photophobia, nausea, vomiting, myalgia, and arthralgia. Additional symptoms may appear later and include abdominal pain, a productive cough, mild respiratory distress, and bleeding manifestations, including epistaxis, hemoptysis, hematuria, and hematemesis. During the end of the primary febrile episode, a diffuse, erythematous, macular, or petechial rash lasting up to 2 days may develop over the trunk and shoulders. There may also be lymphadenopathy, pneumonia, and splenomegaly. Hepatic tenderness associated with hepatomegaly is a common sign, with jaundice in half of affected children. Central nervous system manifestations include lethargy, stupor, meningismus, convulsions, peripheral neuritis, focal neurologic deficits, and cranial nerve paralysis and may be the principal feature of late relapses in tickborne disease. Severe manifestations include myocarditis, hepatic failure, and disseminated intravascular coagulopathy.

The initial symptomatic period characteristically ends with a crisis in 2-9 days, marked by abrupt diaphoresis, hypothermia, hypotension, bradycardia, profound muscle weakness, and prostration. In untreated patients, the 1st relapse occurs within 1 wk, followed by usually 3 but up to 10 relapses, with symptoms during each relapse becoming milder and shorter as the afebrile remission period lengthens.

DIAGNOSIS

Diagnosis depends on demonstration of spirochetes by darkfield microscopy or in thin or thick blood smears stained with Giemsa or Wright stain and by blood culture (Fig. 248.2). During afebrile remissions, spirochetes are not found in the blood. Serologic tests have not been standardized, are generally not available, and produce cross reactions with other spirochetes, including *Borrelia burgdorferi*, the agent of Lyme disease. Molecular methods, including nested polymerase chain reaction or 16S rRNA polymerase chain reaction assays, have been used for detection of tickborne and louse-borne recurrent fever and have been found to have improved sensitivity and specificity compared to blood smears. However, these assays are not yet routinely available for commercial use.

TREATMENT

Oral or parenteral tetracycline or doxycycline is the drug of choice for louse-borne and tickborne relapsing fever. For children older than 8 yr of age and young adults, tetracycline 500 mg PO every 6 hr or doxycycline 100 mg PO every 12 hr for 10 days is effective. Single-dose treatment with tetracycline (500 mg PO) or erythromycin is efficacious in adults, but experience in children is limited. In children younger than 8 yr of age, erythromycin (50 mg/kg/day divided every 6 hr PO) for a total of 10 days is recommended, although there is evidence that doxycycline given for durations of less than 2 wk is safe in children > 2 yr of age. Penicillin and chloramphenicol are also effective.

Resolution of each febrile episode either by natural crisis or as a result of antimicrobial treatment is often accompanied by the Jarisch-Herxheimer reaction, which is caused by massive antigen release. Corticosteroid or antipyretic pretreatment do not prevent the reaction.

PROGNOSIS

With adequate therapy, the mortality rate for relapsing fever is <5%. A majority of patients recover from their illness with or without treatment after the appearance of anti-*Borrelia* antibodies, which agglutinate, kill, or opsonize the spirochete. However, pregnant women and their neonates are at increased risk for tickborne recurrent fever-associated complications, including adult respiratory distress syndrome, Jarisch-Herxheimer reaction, and precipitous or premature delivery. Neonates have up to a 33% case-fatality rate.

PREVENTION

No vaccine is available. Disease control requires avoidance or elimination of the arthropod vectors. In epidemics of louse-borne disease, good personal hygiene and delousing of persons, dwellings, and clothing with commercially available insecticides can prevent dissemination. The risk for tickborne disease can be minimized in endemic areas by maintaining rodent-free dwellings. Giving prophylactic doxycycline for 4 days after a tick bite may prevent tickborne relapsing fever caused by *Borrelia persica.*

Bibliography is available at Expert Consult.

Chapter 249

Lyme Disease *(Borrelia burgdorferi)*

Stephen C. Eppes and Neal D. Goldstein

第二百四十九章

莱姆病（伯氏疏螺旋体）

中文导读

　　本章主要介绍了莱姆病的病原学、流行病学、传播途径、病理学和发病机制、临床表现、实验室检查、诊断、治疗、预后和预防。该病是由伯氏疏螺旋体引起的人畜共患病，主要传播媒介为蜱，在流行地区居住是儿童最重要的风险因素。病原体经皮肤进入人体，发生血液播散，机体体液、细胞免疫与病原体相互作用发生炎症。临床表现缺乏特异性，分为先天性莱姆病、早期表现和晚期表现。早期表现进一步分为早期局限性或早期播散性疾病。常规实验室检查缺乏特异性，常用血清学检测协助诊断，病原培养和检测困难。治疗方面主要介绍了抗感染药的选择，存在关节症状时可使用非甾体抗炎药缓解症状。本病治疗困难，慢性症状和复发常见。预防主要是避免蜱虫咬伤。

Lyme disease is the most common vector-borne disease in the United States and is an important public health problem.

ETIOLOGY

Lyme disease is caused by the spirochete *Borrelia burgdorferi* sensu lato (broad sense). In North America, *B. burgdorferi* sensu stricto (strict sense) causes almost all cases; a recently discovered species in the upper Midwestern United States, *Borrelia mayonii* (belonging to the group *B. burgdorferi* sensu lato), also causes Lyme disease, but the illness is slightly different, with more diffuse rashes and gastrointestinal symptoms. In Europe, the species *Borrelia afzelii* and *Borrelia garinii* also cause disease. The 3 major outer-surface proteins, called OspA, OspB, and OspC (which are highly charged basic proteins of molecular weights of about 31, 34, and 23 kDa, respectively), and the 41 kDa flagellar protein are important targets for the immune response. Differences in the molecular structure of the different species are associated with differences in the clinical manifestations of Lyme borreliosis in Europe and the United States. These differences include the greater incidence of radiculoneuritis in Europe.

EPIDEMIOLOGY

Lyme disease has been reported from more than 50 countries, predominately distributed in forested areas of Asia; northwestern, central, and eastern Europe; and in the northeastern and midwestern United States. In Europe, most cases occur in the Scandinavian countries and in central Europe, especially Germany, Austria, and Switzerland, while in the United States, 95% of cases occurred in 16 states in 2017: Connecticut, Delaware, Maine, Maryland, Massachusetts, Minnesota, New Hampshire, New Jersey, New York, North Carolina, Pennsylvania, Rhode Island, Vermont, Virginia, West Virginia, and Wisconsin (Fig. 249.1).

In the United States, in excess of 20,000 confirmed cases have been reported annually to the Centers for Disease Control and Prevention (CDC) over the last decade, and reported cases have trended upward since 1995, with an approximate 9% increase of reported cases in 2017 compared to 2016. In 2017, the most recent year national data are available, more than 29,000 confirmed cases and more than 13,000 probable cases were reported. The 3-yr averaged national incidence is estimated at 8.5 cases per 100,000 population, and for the last decade the national incidence has ranged from a low of 7.0 cases per 100,000 (2012) to a high of 9.8 cases per 100,000 (2009). In endemic areas, the reported annual incidence ranges from 20 to 100 cases per 100,000 population, although this figure may be as high as 600 cases per 100,000 population in hyperendemic areas. The reported incidence of disease is bimodal. There is an initial peak among children 5-14 yr of age followed by a second peak among adults 55-69 yr of age. In the United States, Lyme disease is diagnosed in boys slightly more often than in girls, and 94% of patients are of European descent. Early Lyme disease usually occurs from spring to early fall, corresponding to deer tick activity. Late disease (chiefly arthritis) occurs year round. Among adults, outdoor occupation and leisure activities are risk factors; for children, location of residence in an endemic area is the most important risk for infection.

Lyme disease is designated a nationally notifiable disease by the CDC

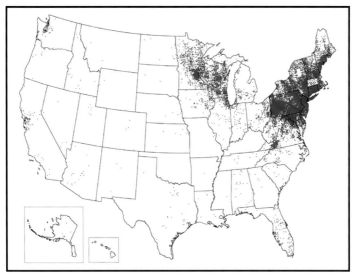

Fig. 249.1 The geographic distribution of Lyme disease cases in the United States. *(From the Centers for Disease Control and Prevention [CDC]: Reported cases of Lyme disease—United States, 2017. Available at: https://www.cdc.gov/lyme/datasurveillance/maps-recent.html.)*

and Council for State and Territorial Epidemiologists. Healthcare providers, hospitals, laboratories, and other parties are required by law to notify local health departments when a confirmed or probable case of Lyme disease occurs. The local health departments in turn report cases to the state and territorial health departments; it is voluntary in turn for these authorities to report data to the CDC, and therefore the actual number of Lyme disease cases as well as incidence is likely underreported and underestimated. Lyme disease was the 6th most common notifiable disease reported to the CDC in 2017.

TRANSMISSION

Lyme disease is a zoonosis caused by the transmission of *B. burgdorferi* to humans through the bite of an infected tick of the *Ixodes* genus. In the eastern and midwestern United States, the vector is ***Ixodes scapularis***, the black-legged tick that is commonly known as the **deer tick**, which is responsible for most cases of Lyme disease in the United States. The vector on the Pacific Coast is *Ixodes pacificus,* the western black-legged tick. *Ixodes* ticks have a 2-yr, 3-stage life cycle. The larvae hatch in the early summer and are usually uninfected with *B. burgdorferi*. The tick can become infected at any stage of its life cycle by feeding on a host, usually a small mammal such as the white-footed mouse *(Peromyscus leucopus)*, which is a natural reservoir for *B. burgdorferi*. The larvae overwinter and emerge the following spring in the nymphal stage, which is the stage of the tick most likely to transmit the infection. The nymphs molt to adults in the fall, and then adults spend the 2nd winter attached to white-tailed deer *(Odocoileus virginianus)*. The females lay their eggs the following spring before they die, and the 2-yr life cycle begins again.

Several factors are associated with increased risk for transmission of *B. burgdorferi* from ticks to humans. The proportion of infected ticks varies by geographic area and by stage of the tick's life cycle. In endemic areas in the northeastern and midwestern United States, 15–25% of nymphal ticks and 35–50% of adult ticks are infected with *B. burgdorferi*. By contrast, *I. pacificus* often feeds on lizards, which are not a competent reservoir for *B. burgdorferi,* reducing the chance that these ticks will be infected. The risk for transmission of *B. burgdorferi* from infected *Ixodes* ticks is related to the duration of feeding. Experiments in animals show that infected nymphal ticks must feed for 36-48 hr, and infected adults must feed for 48-72 hr, before the risk for transmission of *B. burgdorferi* becomes substantial. If the tick is recognized and removed promptly, transmission of *B. burgdorferi* will not occur. Most patients with Lyme disease do not remember the tick bite that transmitted the infection.

The tick species that carry *B. burgdorferi* may be geographically expanding in the U.S. *I. scapularis* also transmits other microorganisms, namely *Anaplasma phagocytophilum* and *Babesia microti,* as well as a recently described species, *Borrelia miyamotoi.* Simultaneous transmission can result in coinfections with these organisms and *B. burgdorferi.*

PATHOLOGY AND PATHOGENESIS

Similar to other spirochetal infections, untreated Lyme disease is characterized by asymptomatic infection, clinical disease that can occur in stages, and a propensity for cutaneous and neurologic manifestations.

The skin is the initial site of infection by *B. burgdorferi*. Inflammation induced by *B. burgdorferi* leads to the development of the characteristic rash, **erythema migrans**. Early disseminated Lyme disease results from the spread of spirochetes through the bloodstream to tissues throughout the body. The spirochete adheres to the surfaces of a wide variety of different types of cells, but the principal target organs are skin, central and peripheral nervous system, joints, heart, and eyes. Because the organism can persist in tissues for prolonged periods, symptoms can appear very late after initial infection.

The symptoms of early disseminated and late Lyme disease are a result of inflammation mediated by interleukin-1 and other lymphokines in response to the presence of the organism. It is likely that relatively few organisms actually invade the host, but cytokines serve to amplify the inflammatory response and lead to much of the tissue damage. Lyme disease is characterized by inflammatory lesions that contain both T and B lymphocytes, macrophages, plasma cells, and mast cells. The refractory symptoms of late Lyme disease can have an immunogenetic basis. Persons with certain HLA-DR allotypes may be genetically predisposed to develop chronic Lyme arthritis. An autoinflammatory response in the synovium can result in clinical symptoms long after the bacteria have been killed by antibiotics.

CLINICAL MANIFESTATIONS

The clinical manifestations of Lyme disease are divided into early and late stages (Table 249.1). Early Lyme disease is further classified as early localized or early disseminated disease. Untreated patients can progressively develop clinical symptoms of each stage of the disease, or they can present with early disseminated or with late disease without apparently having had any symptoms of the earlier stages of Lyme disease.

Early Localized Disease

The first clinical manifestation of Lyme disease in most patients is erythema migrans (Fig. 249.2). Although it usually occurs 7-14 days after the bite, the onset of the rash has been reported from 3 to 30 days later. The initial lesion occurs at the site of the bite. The rash is generally either uniformly erythematous or a target lesion with central clearing; rarely, there are vesicular or necrotic areas in the center of the rash. Occasionally the rash is itchy or painful, although usually it is asymptomatic. The lesion can occur anywhere on the body, although the most common locations are the axilla, periumbilical area, thigh, and groin. It is not unusual for the rash to occur on the neck or face, especially in young children. Without treatment, the rash gradually expands (hence the name *migrans*) to an average diameter of 15 cm and typically remains present for 1-2 wk. Erythema migrans may be associated with systemic features, including fever, myalgia, headache, or malaise. Coinfection with *B. microti* or *A. phagocytophilum* during early infection with *B. burgdorferi* is associated with more severe systemic symptoms. **Coinfections** should be suspected with unusual features of Lyme disease, poor response to treatment, and prolonged fever, anemia, leukopenia, elevated liver enzymes, or thrombocytopenia.

Early Disseminated Disease

In the United States, approximately 20% of patients with acute *B. burgdorferi* infection develop secondary (multiple) erythema migrans lesions, a common manifestation of early disseminated Lyme disease, caused by hematogenous spread of the organisms to multiple skin sites

Table 249.1	Clinical Stages of Lyme Disease	
DISEASE STAGE	**TIMING AFTER TICK BITE**	**TYPICAL CLINICAL MANIFESTATIONS**
Early localized	3-30 days	Erythema migrans (single), variable constitutional symptoms (headache, fever, myalgia, arthralgia, fatigue)
Early disseminated	3-12 wk	Erythema migrans (single or multiple), worse constitutional symptoms, cranial neuritis, meningitis, carditis, ocular disease
Late	>2 mo	Arthritis

(Fig. 249.3). The secondary lesions, which can develop several days or weeks after the first lesion, are usually smaller than the primary lesion and are often accompanied by more-severe constitutional symptoms. The most common early neurologic manifestations are **peripheral facial nerve palsy** and **meningitis**. Lyme meningitis usually has an indolent onset with days to weeks of symptoms that can include headache, neck pain and stiffness, and fatigue. Fever is variably present.

The clinical findings of papilledema, cranial neuropathy (especially cranial nerve VII), and erythema migrans, which are present individually or together in 90% of cases, help differentiate Lyme meningitis from viral meningitis, in which these findings are rarely present. The aseptic meningitis due to Lyme disease can be accompanied by significant elevations of intracranial pressure, which can sometimes last weeks or even months. All of the cranial nerves except the olfactory have been reported to be involved with Lyme disease, but the most common are VI and especially VII. In endemic areas, Lyme disease is the leading cause of peripheral facial nerve palsy. It is often the initial or the only manifestation of Lyme disease and is sometimes bilateral. Cerebrospinal fluid (CSF) findings indicating meningitis are present in more than half of the cases of peripheral facial nerve palsy. The facial paralysis usually lasts 2-8 wk and resolves completely in most cases. Radiculoneuritis and other peripheral neuropathies can occur but are more common in Europe.

Cardiac involvement occurs in 5–15% of early disseminated Lyme disease and usually takes the form of heart block, which can be 1st, 2nd, or 3rd degree, and the rhythm can fluctuate rapidly. Rarely, myocardial (myocarditis) dysfunction can occur. Patients presenting with suspected or proven early disseminated Lyme disease should have a careful cardiac examination, and electrocardiography should be strongly considered. Lyme carditis is a treatable condition and is the only manifestation of Lyme disease that has been fatal.

Of the ocular conditions reported in Lyme disease, papilledema and uveitis are most common.

Late Disease

Arthritis is the usual manifestation of late Lyme disease and begins weeks to months after the initial infection. Arthritis typically involves the large joints, especially the knee, which is affected in 90% of cases; involvement is usually monoarticular or oligoarticular; occasionally it may be migratory. The hallmark of Lyme arthritis is joint swelling, which is a result of synovial effusion and sometimes synovial hypertrophy. The swollen joint may be only mildly symptomatic or it may be painful and tender, although patients usually do not experience the severe pain and systemic toxicity that are common in pyogenic arthritis. If untreated, the arthritis can last several weeks, resolve, and then be followed by recurrent attacks in the same or other joints.

Late manifestations of Lyme disease involving the central nervous system, sometimes termed *late neuroborreliosis*, are rarely reported in

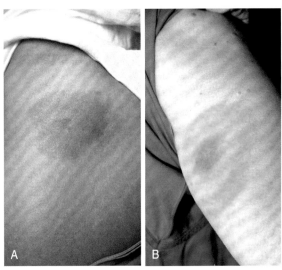

Fig. 249.2 Skin manifestations of Lyme borreliosis. **A,** Erythema migrans on the upper leg, showing central clearing. **B,** Erythema migrans of the arm showing "bulls-eye" appearance. (**A,** *from Stanek G, Strle F: Lyme borreliosis,* Lancet 362:1639–1647, 2003).

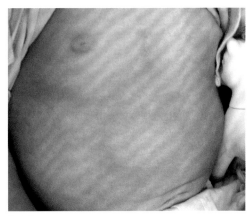

Fig. 249.3 Multiple erythema migrans in a boy with early disseminated Lyme disease.

children. In adults, chronic encephalitis and polyneuritis have been attributed to Lyme disease. The term *Lyme encephalopathy* has been used to describe chronic encephalitis (demonstrable by objective measures), but other literature has also used this term in reference to memory loss and other cognitive sequelae after Lyme disease has been treated. At times, the vague and mistaken term *chronic Lyme disease* has been used to describe symptomatology in persons who might have never had well-documented infection with *B. burgdorferi* at all, have serologic evidence of prior infection but current symptoms not consistent with Lyme disease, or have persistent symptoms after having received appropriate antibiotic therapy. Prolonged treatment does not treat the chronic neuropsychiatric symptoms and at times has harmed the patient.

Congenital Lyme Disease

In endemic areas, infection can occur during pregnancy, although congenital infection appears to be a rare event. *B. burgdorferi* has been identified from several abortuses and from a few liveborn children with congenital anomalies; however, the tissues in which the spirochete has been identified usually have not shown histologic evidence of inflammation. Severe skin and cardiac manifestations have been described in a few cases, but no consistent pattern of fetal damage has been identified to suggest a clinical syndrome of congenital infection. Furthermore, studies conducted in endemic areas have indicated that there is no difference in the prevalence of congenital malformations among the offspring of women with serum antibodies against *B. burgdorferi* and the offspring of those without such antibodies.

LABORATORY FINDINGS

Standard laboratory tests rarely are helpful in diagnosing Lyme disease because any associated laboratory abnormalities usually are nonspecific. The peripheral white blood cell count may be either normal or elevated. The erythrocyte sedimentation rate (ESR) may be mildly elevated. Liver transaminases are occasionally mildly elevated. In Lyme arthritis, the white blood cell count in joint fluid can range from 25,000 to 100,000/mL, often with a preponderance of polymorphonuclear cells. A lower ESR and C-reactive protein and a peripheral blood absolute neutrophil count of less than 10,000 may help to differentiate Lyme from septic arthritis. When meningitis is present, there usually is a low-grade pleocytosis with a lymphocytic and monocytic predominance. The CSF protein level may be elevated, but the glucose concentration usually is normal. Gram stain and routine bacterial cultures are negative. Imaging of the central nervous system (e.g., MRI and single-photon emission computed tomography) occasionally reveals abnormalities, but there is no definitive pattern in Lyme disease. The main role of imaging is to exclude other diagnoses.

DIAGNOSIS

In the appropriate epidemiologic setting (endemic area, season) typical erythema migrans is pathognomonic. Occasionally, the diagnosis of erythema migrans may be difficult because the rash initially can be confused with nummular eczema, tinea corporis, granuloma annulare, an insect bite, southern tick-associated rash illness, or cellulitis. The relatively rapid expansion of erythema migrans helps distinguish it from these other skin lesions. The other clinical manifestations of Lyme disease are less specific and may be confused with other conditions; the monoarticular or pauciarticular arthritis sometimes is confused with a septic joint or other causes of arthritis in children, such as juvenile idiopathic arthritis or rheumatic fever; the facial nerve palsy caused by Lyme disease is clinically indistinguishable from idiopathic Bell palsy, although bilateral involvement is much more common with Lyme disease; Lyme meningitis generally occurs in the warmer months, the same period that enteroviral meningitis is prevalent. Therefore, for all disease manifestations other than erythema migrans, it is recommended to have laboratory confirmation of infection with *B. burgdorferi*.

Although *B. burgdorferi* has been isolated from blood, skin, CSF, myocardium, and the synovium of patients with Lyme disease, the organism is difficult to isolate in culture (cultivation is largely relegated to research laboratories). Infection is usually identified by the detection of antibody in serum. Although some laboratories offer polymerase chain reaction as a diagnostic test for Lyme disease, its sensitivity may be poor because of the low concentrations of bacteria in many sites, especially CSF. Other antigen-based tests, including a test for *B. burgdorferi* antigens in urine, are unreliable. Clinicians should be aware that some laboratories use alternative diagnostic tests and/or alternative interpretive criteria that are not evidence based, leading to a false diagnosis of Lyme disease. The CDC and the Food and Drug Administration recommend against using these tests.

Serology

Following the transmission of *B. burgdorferi* from a tick bite, specific immunoglobulin (Ig) M antibodies appear first, usually within 2 wk, peak at 6-8 wk, and subsequently decline. Sometimes a prolonged or recurrent elevation of IgM antibodies occurs despite effective antimicrobial treatment. Elevated IgM levels after 6-8 wk are often false positives. Specific IgG antibodies usually appear between 2 and 6 wk, peak after 4-6 mo, and can remain elevated for years, particularly in patients with arthritis. The antibody response to *B. burgdorferi* may be blunted in patients with early Lyme disease who are treated promptly with an effective antimicrobial agent. *Serodiagnosis during the first 4 wk of infection is not sensitive and may need to be repeated.*

By far the most common method used to detect IgG and IgM antibodies is the enzyme-linked immunosorbent assay (ELISA). *This method is sensitive but not optimally specific.* The ELISA sometimes produces false-positive results because of antibodies that cross react with other spirochetal infections (e.g., *B. miyamotoi*, syphilis, leptospirosis, or relapsing fever), or certain viral infections (e.g., Epstein-Barr virus), or that occur in certain autoimmune diseases (e.g., systemic lupus erythematosus). The positive predictive value of the ELISA result depends primarily on the plausibility that the patient has Lyme disease based on the clinical and epidemiologic history and the physical examination (**the pretest probability**). For patients who have been in endemic areas with opportunities for *Ixodes* tick exposure and who have typical clinical manifestations of Lyme disease, the pretest probability is high and positive ELISA results are usually true positives. For patients who are from nonendemic areas and/or who have little risk for *Ixodes* tick exposures and/or have nonspecific symptoms (low pretest probability), rates of false-positive results are high. Infection with *B. miyamotoi* may cause false-positive ELISA tests for Lyme disease. This syndrome of relapsing fever, headache, myalgia, but no rash with neutropenia or thrombocytopenia are uncommon in Lyme disease.

Western immunoblotting is well standardized, and there are accepted criteria for interpretation. Five of 10 IgG bands and 2 of 3 IgM bands are considered reactive. The Western blot is not as sensitive as ELISA, especially in early infection, but is highly specific. Any positive or equivocal ELISA must be confirmed with Western blotting. The CDC recommends using IgM and IgG Western blot confirmation when symptoms have been present ≤30 days and IgG only when symptoms have been present longer than 30 days. This 2-tier testing is the recommended laboratory evaluation of most cases of Lyme disease and is associated with a high degree of sensitivity and specificity when used appropriately. There are discussions to eliminate the second-tier Western blot assay and substitute it with a second-tier ELISA that is easier to perform and interpret.

Clinicians should be aware that Lyme disease might not be the cause of a patient's symptoms despite the presence of antibodies to *B. burgdorferi*. The test result may be falsely positive (as described for ELISA), or the patient might have been infected previously. Antibodies to *B. burgdorferi* that develop with infection can persist for many years despite adequate treatment and clinical cure of the disease. In addition, because some people who become infected with *B. burgdorferi* are asymptomatic, the background rate of seropositivity among patients who have never had clinically apparent Lyme disease may be substantial in endemic areas. Finally, because antibodies against *B. burgdorferi* persist after successful treatment, there is no reason to obtain follow-up serologic tests.

TREATMENT

Table 249.2 provides treatment recommendations. Most patients can be treated with an oral regimen of antibiotic therapy. Young children are generally treated with amoxicillin. Doxycycline has the advantages of good central nervous system penetration and activity against *A. phagocytophilum*, which may be transmitted at the same time as *B. burgdorferi* in certain geographic areas. In general, children younger than 8 yr of age should not be treated with doxycycline because of the risk of permanent staining of the teeth (although courses of ≤2 wk are usually safe in this regard). Patients who are treated with doxycycline should be alerted to the risk for developing photosensitivity in sun-exposed areas while taking the medication; long sleeves, long pants, and hat are recommended for activities in direct sunlight. The only oral cephalosporin proved to be effective for the treatment of Lyme disease is cefuroxime axetil, which is an alternative for persons who cannot take doxycycline or who are allergic to penicillin. Macrolide antibiotics, including azithromycin, appear to have limited activity.

Parenteral therapy is usually recommended for patients with higher degrees of heart block or central nervous system involvement, though oral therapy for meningitis is now considered acceptable for ambulatory patients. Patients with arthritis that fails to resolve after an initial course of oral therapy can be retreated with an oral regimen or can receive intravenous antibiotic therapy. Ceftriaxone is favored because of its excellent anti-*Borrelia* activity, tolerability, and once-daily dosing regimen, which can usually be done on an outpatient basis.

Peripheral facial nerve palsy can be treated using an oral antibiotic. However, these patients may have concomitant meningitis; patients with meningitis may need to receive a parenteral antibiotic. Experts are divided on whether every patient with Lyme-associated facial palsy needs a CSF analysis, but clinicians should consider lumbar puncture for patients with significant headache, neck pain or stiffness, or papilledema.

Patients with symptomatic cardiac disease, 2nd- or 3rd-degree heart block, or significantly prolonged PR interval should be hospitalized and monitored closely. These patients should receive a parenteral antibiotic. Patients with mild 1st-degree heart block can be treated with an oral antibiotic.

Some patients develop a Jarisch-Herxheimer reaction soon after treatment is initiated; this results from lysis of the *Borrelia*. The manifestations of this reaction are low-grade fever and achiness. These symptoms resolve spontaneously within 24-48 hr, although administration of nonsteroidal antiinflammatory drugs often is beneficial. Nonsteroidal antiinflammatory drugs also may be useful in treating symptoms of early Lyme disease and of Lyme arthritis. Coinfections with other pathogens transmitted by *Ixodes* ticks should be treated according to standard recommendations.

Criteria for the post–Lyme disease syndrome have been proposed by the Infectious Disease Society of America. There is no clear evidence that this condition is related to persistence of the organism. Studies in adults show little benefit associated with prolonged or repeated treatment with oral or parenteral antibiotics.

PROGNOSIS

There is a widespread misconception that Lyme disease is difficult to cure and that chronic symptoms and clinical recurrences are common. The most likely reason for apparent treatment failure is an incorrect diagnosis of Lyme disease.

The prognosis for children treated for Lyme disease is excellent. Children treated for erythema migrans rarely progress to late Lyme disease. The long-term prognosis for patients who are treated beginning in the later stages of Lyme disease also is excellent. Although chronic and recurrent arthritis may occur, especially among patients with certain human leukocyte antigen allotypes (an autoimmune process), most children who are treated for Lyme arthritis are cured and have no sequelae. Although there are rare reports of adults who have developed late neuroborreliosis, usually among persons with Lyme disease in whom treatment was delayed for months or years, similar cases in children are rare.

PREVENTION

The best way to avoid Lyme disease is to avoid tick-infested areas. Children should be examined for deer ticks after known or potential exposure (although many people are not able to identify the species or the stage of the tick). If a tick attachment is noted, the tick should be grasped at the mouthparts with a forceps or tweezers; if these are not available, the tick should be covered with a tissue. The recommended method of tick removal is to pull directly outward without twisting. Infection is usually preventable if the tick is removed before 36 hr of attachment; at this time the ticks are flat and non-engorged. The overall risk for acquiring Lyme disease after a tick bite is low (1–3%) in most endemic areas. If the tick is engorged and present for >72 hr (high-risk tick bite), the risk of infection may increase to 25% in hyperendemic areas. Patients and families can be advised to watch the area for development of erythema migrans and to seek medical attention if the rash or constitutional symptoms occur. If infection develops, early treatment of the infection is highly effective. Prophylaxis after a high-risk tick bite with a single dose of doxycycline in adults (200 mg PO) or 4.4 mg/kg in children is effective in reducing the risk of Lyme disease. The routine testing of ticks that have been removed from humans for evidence of *B. burgdorferi* is not recommended, because the value of a positive test result for predicting infection in the human host is unknown.

Personal protective measures that may be effective in reducing the chance of tick bites include wearing protective clothing (long pants tucked into socks, long-sleeved shirts) when entering tick-infested areas, checking for and promptly removing ticks, and using tick repellent such as *N,N*-diethyl-3-methylbenzamide (DEET). This chemical can safely be used on pants, socks, and shoes; care must be used with heavy or repeated application on skin, particularly in infants, because of the risk of systemic absorption and toxicity. Permethrin treatment of clothing is also an effective prevention strategy.

Bibliography is available at Expert Consult.

Table 249.2	Recommended Treatment of Lyme Disease
DRUG	**PEDIATRIC DOSING**
Amoxicillin	50 mg/kg/day in 3 divided doses (max: 1,500 mg/day)
Doxycycline	4.4 mg/kg/day in 2 divided doses (max: 200 mg/day) (see text regarding doxycycline use in children)
Cefuroxime axetil	30 mg/kg/day in 2 divided doses (max: 1,000 mg/day)
Ceftriaxone (IV)*,†	50-75 mg/kg/day once daily (max: 2,000 mg/day)
Azithromycin‡	10 mg/kg/day once daily ×7 days
RECOMMENDED THERAPY BASED ON CLINICAL MANIFESTATION	
Erythema migrans	Doxycycline ×10 days Amoxicillin ×14 days
Meningitis	Doxycycline ×14 days or Ceftriaxone ×14 days (14-21 for hospitalized patients)
Cranial nerve palsy§	Doxycycline ×14 days
Cardiac disease	Oral regimen or ceftriaxone, 14-21 days (see text for specifics)
Arthritis	Oral regimen, 28 days
Persistent arthritis after initial treatment	Oral regimen ×28 days or Ceftriaxone, 14-28 days

*Penicillin G is an alternative parenteral agent but requires more frequent dosing.
†Doses of 100 mg/kg/day should be used for meningitis.
‡For those unable to take amoxicillin or doxycycline.
§Treatment is to prevent late disease not to treat the cranial palsy; avoid corticosteroids.

Section **9**

Mycoplasmal Infections

第九篇

支原体感染

Chapter **250**

Mycoplasma pneumoniae

Asuncion Mejias and Octavio Ramilo

第二百五十章

肺炎支原体

中文导读

本章主要介绍了肺炎支原体病的病原学、流行病学、发病机制、临床表现、诊断、治疗和预防。肺炎支原体是常见学龄期儿童和青少年呼吸道感染病原。主要通过呼吸道传播，多发生于夏季或初秋。主要因病原体细胞外附着和宿主免疫反应致病。临床表现主要描述了呼吸道症状和肺外表现。气管支气管炎和非典型肺炎是主要呼吸道表现，病原体定植于呼吸道可引起儿童哮喘。肺外表现可累及中枢神经系统、皮肤黏膜、血液系统、骨骼肌肉等。诊断方法主要描述了支原体培养、血清学试验、冷凝集素试验和PCR检测。治疗主要包括抗感染药治疗和辅助治疗。8岁以下儿童首选大环内脂类药物，重点讲述了大环内酯类药物耐药支原体的治疗。严重病例可加用类固醇激素治疗。

Among the 7 *Mycoplasma* species isolated from the human respiratory tract, *Mycoplasma pneumoniae* remains the most common species causing respiratory infections in school-age children and young adults.

THE ORGANISM

Mycoplasmas are the smallest self-replicating prokaryotes known to cause disease in humans. Their size of 150-250 nm is more on the order of viruses than bacteria. *Mycoplasma pneumoniae* is a fastidious double-stranded DNA bacterium that is distinguished by a small genome (~800,000 base pairs) and a long doubling time, which makes culturing it a slow process (5-20 days) compared to other bacteria. *M. pneumoniae* isolates can be classified in 2 major genetic groups (subtype 1 and 2) based on the P1 adhesion protein. Distinguishing these 2 subtypes is important for epidemiologic and clinical purposes. Like other mycoplasmas, *M. pneumoniae* is distinguished by the complete absence of a cell wall that results in (1) their dependence to host cells for obtaining essential nutrients, (2) the intrinsic resistance to β-lactam agents, and (3) their pleomorphic shape and lack of visibility on Gram staining.

EPIDEMIOLOGY

M. pneumoniae infections occur worldwide and throughout the year. This organism is a frequent cause of community-acquired pneumonia (CAP) in children and adults, accounting for ~20% of all CAP in middle and high school children and up to 50% of CAP in college students and military recruits. The proportion of cases increases according to age, as recently shown in a population-based study of CAP conducted in the United States (5% in < 5 yr; 16% in 5-9 yr; and 23% in 10-17 yr).

In contrast to the acute, short-lived epidemics associated with some respiratory viruses, *M. pneumoniae* infection occurs endemically worldwide. Infections tend to occur most commonly during summer or early fall, although mycoplasma infections have been described all year long. Epidemic outbreaks of variable intensity occur every few years and they are likely related to the alternative circulation of the two *M. pneumoniae* subtypes. Transmission occurs through the respiratory route by large droplet spread during close contact with a symptomatic person. Community outbreaks have been described in closed settings (colleges, boarding schools, military bases) and can spread largely through school contacts. Attack rates within families are high, with transmission rates of 40 to > 80% for household adult and children contacts, respectively. In contrast to many other respiratory infections, the incubation period is 2-3 wk; hence, the course of infection in a specific population (family) may last several weeks.

The occurrence of mycoplasma illnesses is related, in part, to age and preexposure immunity. Overt illness is less common before 3 yr of age but can occur. Children younger than 5 yr of age appear to have milder illnesses associated with upper respiratory tract involvement, vomiting, and diarrhea. Immunity after infection is not long lasting, as evidenced by the frequency of reinfections over time. The 2 mycoplasma subtypes are immunologically different, and infection with 1 subtype does not appear to confer immunity against the other. *Asymptomatic carriage* after infection can last up to 4 mo despite antibiotic therapy and may contribute to prolonged outbreaks. Children are often the reservoir from whom mycoplasma spreads. In the clinical setting, there are no available tools yet to differentiate carriage vs. infection.

PATHOGENESIS

The pathogenicity of *M. pneumoniae* is dependent upon its extracellular attachment and the initiation of the host cell immune response. Cells of the ciliated respiratory epithelium are the target cells of *M. pneumoniae* infection. The organism is an elongated snake-like structure with a one-end organelle, which mediates the attachment to sialic acid receptors in the cilia through a complex set of adhesion proteins (P1, P30, proteins B and C, P116, and HMW1-3). *M. pneumoniae* rarely invades beyond the respiratory tract basement membrane. Virulent organisms attach to ciliated respiratory epithelial cell surfaces located in the bronchi, bronchioles, alveoli, and possibly upper respiratory tract and burrow down between cells, resulting in ciliostasis and eventual sloughing of the cells. *M. pneumoniae* also causes cytolytic injury to the host cells in part by the production of hydrogen peroxide and possibly through the adenosine diphosphate–ribosylating and vacuolating toxin termed CARDS (community-acquired respiratory distress syndrome). This exotoxin is associated with more severe or even fatal disease. This bacterium facilitates the formation of biofilms, with strain-specific phenotypic differences, which hinder antibiotic penetration and recognition by the immune system.

Once *M. pneumoniae* reaches the lower respiratory tract, it promotes the polyclonal activation of B lymphocytes and CD4+ T cells, and amplifies the immune response with the production of various proinflammatory and antiinflammatory cytokines and chemokines, such as tumor necrosis factor-α, interleukin (IL)-8, IL-1β, Il-6, and IL-10.

Although it is well documented that specific cell-mediated immunity and antibody titers against *M. pneumoniae* increase with age (and therefore probably follow repeated infections), the immune mechanisms that protect against or clear the infection are not well defined. In humans, nasal IgA antibodies correlated with protection after experimental challenge. A distinct aspect of *M. pneumoniae* is its ability to induce the production of cold agglutinins (IgM antibodies) directed against the I antigen expressed in the surface of erythrocytes. Even though antibody responses do not confer complete protection against reinfections, the importance of a robust humoral response is apparent, since patients with congenital antibody deficiencies, such as those with hypogammaglobulinemia, can develop severe and prolonged disease and have a higher risk of extrapulmonary manifestations. In children with sickle cell disease or sickle-related hemoglobinopathies, *M. pneumoniae* is a common infectious trigger of acute chest syndrome. These children and also children with Down syndrome can develop more severe forms of *Mycoplasma* pneumonia. On the other hand, *M. pneumoniae* does not seem to be a common opportunistic agent in patients with AIDS.

M. pneumoniae has been detected by polymerase chain reaction (PCR) in many nonrespiratory sites, including blood, pleural fluid, cerebrospinal fluid (CSF), and synovial fluid. The mechanisms of extrapulmonary disease associated with *M. pneumoniae* are unclear and appear to be different according to the duration of symptoms at the time of presentation: direct invasion vs. immune-mediated.

CLINICAL MANIFESTATIONS

Most of the *M. pneumoniae* infections are symptomatic and most of them occur in children and adolescents.

Respiratory Tract Disease

Tracheobronchitis and atypical pneumonia are the most commonly recognized clinical syndromes associated with *M. pneumoniae*. This agent is responsible for up to 20% of all cases of CAP. Although the onset of illness may be abrupt, it is usually characterized by gradual development of headache, malaise, fever, and sore throat, followed by progression of lower respiratory symptoms, including hoarseness and nonproductive cough. The gradual onset in children with atypical pneumonia is in contrast to the sudden onset of lobar pneumonia. Coryza and gastrointestinal complaints are unusual and usually suggest a viral etiology. Although the clinical course in untreated patients is variable, cough, the clinical hallmark of *M. pneumoniae* infection, usually worsens during the 1st wk of illness, and symptoms generally resolve within 2 wk. Cough can last up to 4 wk and may be accompanied by wheezing. Patients generally recover without complications, although some individuals can develop prolonged wheezing.

Chest examination may be unrevealing, even in patients with severe cough. There may be no auscultative or percussive findings or only minimum dry rales. Clinical findings are often less severe than suggested by the patient chest radiograph, explaining why the term walking pneumonia is often used to describe CAP caused by *M. pneumoniae*. Radiographic findings are variable and nonspecific, not allowing differentiation from viral or bacterial pathogens. Pneumonia is usually described as interstitial or bronchopneumonic, and involvement is most common in the lower lobes. Bilateral diffuse infiltrates, lobar pneumonia, or hilar lymphadenopathy can occur in up to 30% of patients. Although unusual, large pleural effusions associated with lobar infiltrates and necrotizing pneumonia have been described in patients with sickle cell disease, immunodeficiencies, Down syndrome, and chronic cardiopulmonary disease. Bronchiolitis obliterans has also been described as a complication of *M. pneumoniae* in otherwise healthy children. The white blood cell and differential counts are usually normal, whereas the erythrocyte sedimentation rate and C-reactive protein are often elevated. Appropriate antibiotics shorten the duration of illness but do not reliably eradicate the bacteria from the respiratory tract.

Other respiratory illnesses caused occasionally by *M. pneumoniae* include undifferentiated upper respiratory tract infections, intractable, nonproductive cough, pharyngitis (usually without marked cervical lymphadenopathy), sinusitis, croup, and bronchiolitis. *M. pneumoniae* is a common trigger of wheezing in asthmatic children and can cause chronic colonization in the airways, resulting in lung dysfunction in adolescents and adult asthmatic patients. Otitis media and bullous myringitis, which also occur with other viral and bacterial infections, have been described but are rare, and their absence should not exclude the diagnosis of *M. pneumoniae*.

Extrapulmonary Disease

Despite the reportedly rare isolation of *M. pneumoniae* from nonrespiratory sites, the improved sensitivity of PCR for *M. pneumoniae* DNA detection has led to increasing identification of this bacterium in nonrespiratory sites, particularly the central nervous system (CNS). Patients with or without respiratory symptoms can have involvement of the skin, CNS, blood, heart, gastrointestinal tract, and joints. Nonrespiratory manifestations of *M. pneumoniae* include:

1. *CNS disease:* occurs in 0.1% of all patients with *M. pneumoniae* infection and in 7–16% of those requiring hospitalization. Manifestations include encephalitis, acute disseminated encephalomyelitis (ADEM), transverse myelitis, cerebellar ataxia, aseptic meningitis, Guillain-Barré syndrome, Bell palsy, and peripheral neuropathy. CNS disease manifestations occur 3-23 days (mean: 10 days) after onset of respiratory illness but may not be preceded by any signs of respiratory infection in up to 20% of cases. Studies in children suggest that there are two pathogenic mechanisms for *M. pneumoniae*-associated

neurologic disease: the first pattern is characterized by almost absent or no prodromal respiratory symptoms (<7 days) and non-reactive IgM responses. On the other hand, the second pattern is characterized by the presence of respiratory symptoms (most commonly cough) for ≥7 days and reactive IgM in acute serum. In the first group *M. pneumoniae* is usually identified in cerebrospinal fluid by PCR but not in the respiratory tract, while in children presenting with ≥7 days of respiratory symptoms the opposite is true. These studies suggest that encephalitis occurring more than 7 days after onset of prodromal symptoms is more likely to be caused by an autoimmune response to *M. pneumonia*, while its occurrence early in the course of the disease may be associated with direct bacterial invasion of the CNS. Involvement of the brainstem can result in severe dystonia and movement disorders. The CSF may be normal or have mild mononuclear pleocytosis and/or increase CSF protein concentrations. Diagnosis is confirmed with positive CSF PCR, positive PCR from a throat swab, or demonstration of seroconversion. Findings on MRI include focal ischemic changes, ventriculomegaly, diffuse edema, or multifocal white matter inflammatory lesions consistent with postinfectious ADEM. Long-term sequelae have been reported in 23–64% of cases.

2. ***Dermatologic disease:*** a variety of exanthems have been associated with *M. pneumoniae*, most notably maculopapular rash, urticaria and the mycoplasma associated rash and mucositis syndrome previously called erythema multiforme or Stevens-Johnson syndrome (SJS). Gianotti-Crosti syndrome and erythema nodosum are also associated with *M. pneumoniae* infections. Approximately 10% of children with *M. pneumoniae* CAP will exhibit a maculopapular rash. Mycoplasma-associated rash and mucositis usually develops 3-21 days after initial respiratory symptoms, lasts less than 14 days, and is rarely associated with severe complications (Figs. 250.1 and 250.2). *M. pneumoniae* may also produce an isolated oral mucositis in absence of rash.

3. ***Hematologic abnormalities:*** include mild degrees of hemolysis with a positive Coombs test and minor reticulocytosis 2-3 wk after the onset of illness. Severe hemolysis is associated with high titers of cold hemagglutinins (≥1:512) and occurs rarely. Thrombocytopenia, aplastic anemia, and coagulation defects occur occasionally.

4. ***Musculoskeletal:*** arthritis appears to be less common in children than in adults, but monoarthritis, polyarthritis, and migratory arthritis have been described. Rhabdomyolysis has also been documented, often associated with other organ system manifestations.

5. ***Other conditions,*** such as mild hepatitis, pancreatitis, acute glomerulonephritis, iritis or uveitis, and cardiac complications (pericarditis, myocarditis, and rheumatic fever-like syndrome, most commonly seen in adults) are also described. Fatal *M. pneumoniae* infections are rare.

DIAGNOSIS

No specific clinical, epidemiologic, or laboratory parameters allow for a definite diagnosis of *M. pneumoniae* infection. Nevertheless, pneumonia in school-age children and young adults with a gradual onset and cough as a prominent finding suggests *M. pneumoniae* infection. The best method for diagnosis is a combination of PCR from respiratory samples and serology (acute and convalescent).

Cultures on special media (SP4 agar media) of the throat or sputum might demonstrate the classic *M. pneumoniae* "mulberry" colonies, but growth generally requires incubation for 2-3 wk, and few laboratories maintain the capability of culturing *M. pneumoniae*. The fastidious nutritional requirements of *Mycoplasma* make cultures slow and impractical.

Serologic tests (immunofluorescence tests, enzyme-linked immune assays [EIAs], or complement fixation) to detect serum immunoglobulin (Ig) M and IgG antibodies against *M. pneumoniae* are commercially available. IgM antibodies have a high rate of false-positive and false-negative results. In most cases, IgM antibodies are not detected within the 1st wk after onset of symptoms or in children with recurrent infections and may be positive for up to 6-12 mo after infection. A 4-fold or greater increase in IgG antibody titers against *M. pneumoniae* between acute and convalescent sera obtained 2-4 wk apart is diagnostic.

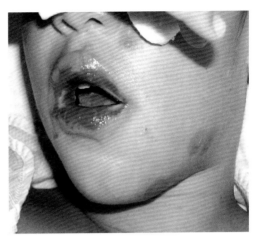

Fig. 250.1 Lip changes found in *Mycoplasma pneumoniae*–associated mucositis.

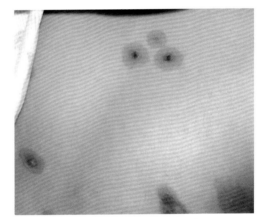

Fig. 250.2 Classic skin lesions found in *Mycoplasma pneumoniae*–associated rash.

Cold hemagglutinins (cold-reacting antibodies [IgM] against red blood cells) can be detected in approximately 50% of patients with *M. pneumoniae* pneumonia. These antibodies are nonspecific, especially at titers <1:64, as modest increases in cold hemagglutinins can be observed in other viral infections. Cold agglutinin antibodies should not be used for the diagnosis of *M. pneumoniae* infections if other methods are available.

PCR-based tests for *M. pneumoniae* have replaced other diagnostic tests. PCR of a nasopharyngeal or throat swab (the combination of both increases sensitivity) for *M. pneumoniae* genomic DNA carries a sensitivity and a specificity of 80 to >97%. In adults, sputum samples are more likely than nasopharyngeal or throat swabs to yield positive results. Different primers have been used to identify gene sequences of the P1 cytoadhesion protein or the ribosomal (r) 16S RNA. PCR allows a more rapid diagnosis in acutely ill patients and can be positive earlier in the course of infection than serologic tests. Mycoplasma PCR from respiratory samples may be positive in asymptomatic subjects. Nonetheless, identification of *M. pneumoniae* by PCR (or culture) from a patient with compatible clinical manifestations suggests causation.

Other diagnostic methods: The matrix-assisted laser desorption ionization-time of flight mass spectrometry (MALDI-TOF MS) could represent an accurate tool for identification and subtyping of *M. pneumoniae*. However, the need for culture to subsequently be able to perform MALDI-TOF MS limits its applicability in the clinical setting.

Silver nanorod array-surface enhanced Raman spectroscopy (NA-SERS) is an investigational system that does not require growth of the bacterium. It appears a promising and sensitive tool for mycoplasma detection and strain characterization.

The diagnosis of extrapulmonary disease associated with *M. pneumoniae* is challenging. Although *M. pneumoniae* has been identified by PCR in the CSF of children with encephalitis, there are currently no reliable tests for the diagnosis of CNS or other nonrespiratory sites associated with *M. pneumoniae*. Since the extrapulmonary manifestations of *M. pneumoniae* may have an immunologic base, measuring acute and convalescent IgM and IgG antibody levels is advisable.

TREATMENT

M. pneumoniae illness is usually mild, and most cases of pneumonia can be managed without the need for hospitalization. Because mycoplasmas lack a cell wall, they inherently are resistant to β-lactam agents that act by inhibiting the cell wall synthesis. In addition, other drug classes, such as trimethoprim, rifampin, or linezolid are inactive against *M. pneumoniae*. Studies regarding the effectiveness of antimicrobial therapy for *M. pneumoniae* infections in children are contradictory. Nevertheless, empiric treatment is often initiated based on clinical suspicion due to the difficulty of a definitive diagnosis.

Antimicrobial Therapy

M. pneumoniae is typically sensitive to macrolides (erythromycin, clarithromycin, azithromycin), tetracyclines, and quinolones in vitro. Treatment of mycoplasma does not assure eradication. Data from observational studies showed that macrolide treatment of children with *M. pneumoniae* CAP markedly shortened the course of illness. Treatment may be more effective when started within 3-4 days of illness onset. Although macrolides do not have bactericidal activity, they are preferred in children younger than 8 yr of age. Two multicenter studies of pediatric CAP demonstrated comparable clinical and bacteriologic success rates between erythromycin and clarithromycin or azithromycin. However, the newer macrolides were better tolerated. The recommended treatment is clarithromycin (15 mg/kg/day divided into 2 doses PO for 10 days) or azithromycin (10 mg/kg once PO on day 1 and 5 mg/kg once daily PO on days 2-5). In addition to the antibacterial effect, macrolides may have immunomodulatory properties, but the relevance of the antiinflammatory properties of macrolides for the treatment of *M. pneumoniae* CAP is not known. Tetracyclines (doxycycline 100 mg twice a day for 7-14 days) are also effective and may be used for children older than 8 yr of age. Fluoroquinolones such as levofloxacin (750 mg once a day for 7-14 days) are effective and bactericidal but have higher minimum inhibitory concentrations (MIC) compared with macrolides and currently are not recommended as a first-line therapy in children.

Macrolide-resistant strains, mostly associated with mutations in the 23S rRNA, have been increasingly reported in Asia (>90% in Japan and China) and are also present in Europe with great variability from country to country (0% in the Netherlands vs. 26% in Italy). In the United States and Canada, the rates of resistance varied from 3.5 to 13% of cases. Although not routinely performed at clinical laboratories, identification of macrolide-resistant strains can be performed by sequencing and identification of specific mutations in the 23S rRNA gene. The clinical significance of macrolide-resistant infections has not been completely elucidated, however, studies in children indicated that the clinical efficacy of macrolide-susceptible *M. pneumoniae* infections is >4-fold higher compared with infections caused by resistant strains (91% vs. 22% respectively). Thus, for patients with severe infections not responding to macrolide therapy within the first 48 hr of treatment, the possibility of macrolide-resistant *M. pneumoniae* should be considered and switching to a non-macrolide antimicrobial regimen might be prudent. Doxycycline (2-4 mg/kg in one or two divided doses for 10 days; max 200 mg or 100 mg q12h) for children >8 yr, or levofloxacin (10 mg/kg per dose every 12 hr in children <5 yr or once a day in older children) after assessment of risk and benefits of using quinolones in children, are potential alternatives for macrolide-resistant *M. pneumoniae* infections. Other quinolones such as tosufloxacin or garenoxacin are used in Japan. There are new ketolides in development that appear promising.

Adjunctive Therapy

There is no evidence that treatment of upper respiratory tract or nonrespiratory tract disease with antimicrobial agents alters the course of illness. However, patients with severe manifestations of extrapulmonary disease may benefit from antimicrobial treatment, since direct involvement of the bacterium cannot be excluded. Oftentimes antibiotics are administered in combination with immunomodulatory therapy. In this regard, corticosteroids with or without intravenous immunoglobulin are the most commonly used agents for managing severe *M. pneumoniae* extrapulmonary manifestations, particularly for patients with CNS involvement or rash and mucositis. Although definitive data are lacking, case studies suggest the associated clinical benefit of steroids in the management of severe lung disease, SJS, and hemolytic anemia.

PREVENTION

Trials with inactivated and live attenuated vaccines for *M. pneumoniae* have been conducted with disappointing results. In hospitalized patients standard and droplet precautions are recommended for the duration of symptoms. It is important to emphasize that mycoplasma infection remains contagious as long as cough persists and despite successful antibiotic therapy. Prophylaxis with tetracyclines or azithromycin substantially reduces the secondary attack rates in institutional outbreaks and family close contacts. Antimicrobial prophylaxis is not recommended routinely; however, it can be considered in patients at high risk for severe disease, such as children with sickle cell disease.

Bibliography is available at Expert Consult.

Chapter 251

Genital Mycoplasmas (*Mycoplasma hominis, Mycoplasma genitalium,* and *Ureaplasma urealyticum*)

Rosa Rodríguez-Fernández and Asuncion Mejias

第二百五十一章
生殖器支原体（人型支原体、生殖支原体、解脲支原体）

中文导读

　　本章主要介绍了人型支原体、生殖支原体和解脲支原体3种生殖道支原体的病原学、流行病学、传播途径、发病机制、临床表现、诊断和治疗。该类病原体多定植在女性生殖道，可通过性接触和母婴垂直传播。可引起泌尿生殖道和羊膜的慢性炎症。临床表现主要介绍了宫内和新生儿感染、泌尿生殖系统感染和非生殖器感染3部分。宫内和新生儿感染主要表现为绒毛膜羊膜炎、支气管肺发育异常、中枢神经系统感染。PCR检测为诊断的首选方法，并介绍了生殖道感染和新生儿感染的实验室检测。在治疗部分主要对新生儿、青少年和成人介绍了不同的治疗方案。

ETIOLOGY

Mycoplasma species are small pleomorphic bacteria that typically lack a cell wall and are bound by a cell membrane. Many of the biologic properties of mycoplasmas are in fact due to the absence of a rigid cell wall, including resistance to β-lactam antibiotics. These ubiquitous organisms are difficult to cultivate and belong to the family Mycoplasmataceae in the class Mollicutes and represent the smallest self-replicating organisms known to date. The entire genome of many of the *Mycoplasma* species is among the smallest of prokaryotic genomes. The family Mycoplasmataceae is composed of two genera responsible for human infection: *Mycoplasma* and *Ureaplasma*. Of those, *Mycoplasma hominis, Mycoplasma genitalium,* and *Ureaplasma* spp., which include *Ureaplasma urealyticum* (biovar 2) and *Ureaplasma parvum* (biovar 1), are considered human urogenital pathogens and are reviewed in this chapter.

Genital mycoplasmas are often associated with sexually transmitted infections such as cervicitis and nongonococcal urethritis (NGU) or with puerperal infections such as endometritis. *M. hominis* and *Ureaplasma* spp. commonly colonize the female genital tract and can cause chorioamnionitis, colonization of neonates, and perinatal infections. Two other genital *Mycoplasma* species, *Mycoplasma fermentans* and *Mycoplasma penetrans,* have been identified in respiratory or genitourinary secretions primarily in HIV-infected patients.

EPIDEMIOLOGY

M. hominis and *Ureaplasma* spp. are commensal organisms in the lower genital and urinary tract of postpubertal women and men. The prevalence of colonization with these bacteria has been directly associated with low socioeconomic status, hormonal changes, and ethnicity and increases proportionally according to sexual activity, being highest among individuals with multiple sexual partners. Female colonization is greatest in the vagina and lower in the endocervix, urethra, and endometrium, with rates varying from 40% to 80% for *Ureaplasma* spp. and 21–50% for *M. hominis* among sexually active asymptomatic women. *Ureaplasma* is isolated less often from urine than from the cervix, but *M. hominis* is present in the urine and in the cervix with approximately the same frequency. Male colonization is less common and occurs primarily in the urethra. Among prepubertal children and sexually inactive adults, colonization rates are <10%. *M. genitalium* is implicated in approximately 15–20% of NGU cases in men and plays a role in cervicitis and pelvic inflammatory disease in women. Studies using polymerase chain reaction (PCR) show that colonization of the female lower urogenital tract with *M. genitalium* is less common than with *M. hominis* or *Ureaplasma* spp.

TRANSMISSION

Genital mycoplasmas are transmitted by sexual contact or by vertical transmission from mother to infant. As with other perinatal infections, vertical transmission can occur through ascending intrauterine infection, hematogenous spread from placental infection, or through a colonized birth canal at the time of delivery. Transmission rates among neonates born to women colonized with *Ureaplasma* spp. range from 18 to 88%. Neonatal colonization rates are higher among infants who weigh <1,000 g, are born in the presence of chorioamnionitis, or are born to mothers of lower socioeconomic status. Neonatal colonization is transient and decreases proportionally with age. Organisms may be recovered from the newborn's throat, vagina, rectum, and, occasionally, conjunctiva for as long as 3 mo after birth.

PATHOGENESIS

Genital mycoplasmas can cause chronic inflammation of the genitourinary tract and amniotic membranes. These bacteria usually live in a state of adherence to the respiratory or urogenital tract, but can disseminate to other organs when there is a disruption of the mucosa or a weakened or immature immune system, such as in premature infants. *Ureaplasma* spp. can infect the amniotic sac early in gestation without rupturing the amniotic membranes, resulting in a clinically silent, chronic chorioamnionitis characterized by an intense inflammatory response. Attachment to fetal human tracheal epithelium can cause ciliary disarray, clumping, and loss of epithelial cells. *In vitro* studies show that *Ureaplasma* spp. stimulates macrophage production of interleukin (IL)-6 and tumor necrosis factor-α. In addition, high concentrations of proinflammatory cytokines possibly associated with development of bronchopulmonary dysplasia (BPD) of prematurity, such as monocyte chemoattractant protein-1 and IL-8, have been found in tracheal secretions from very-low-birthweight infants colonized with *Ureaplasma* spp. Immunity appears to require serotype-specific antibody. Thus, lack of maternal antibodies might account for a higher disease risk in premature newborns.

CLINICAL MANIFESTATIONS

The main syndromes associated with *Ureaplasma* spp., *M. genitalium*, and *M. hominis* are displayed in Table 251.1.

Intrauterine and Neonatal Infections
Chorioamnionitis and Early Onset Infections

Genital mycoplasmas are associated with a variety of fetal and neonatal infections. *Ureaplasma* spp. can cause clinically inapparent chorioamnionitis, resulting in spontaneous abortion, increased fetal death, or premature delivery. The role of *Ureaplasma* in clinical chorioamnionitis is still unclear. The association between preterm birth and ureaplasmas remains uncertain. Studies have shown that women with *Ureaplasma* spp. detected by PCR in amniotic fluid between 12 to 20 wk of gestation have an increased risk of preterm labor and delivery. *Ureaplasma* spp. can also be recovered from tracheal, blood, cerebrospinal fluid (CSF), or lung biopsy specimens in up to 50% of sick infants younger than 34 wk gestation. In a study of 351 mother/infant dyads, isolation of *Ureaplasma* spp. or *M. hominis* from cord blood was documented in 23% of infants born between 23 and 32 wk gestation, and correlated with the development of systemic inflammatory response syndrome.

Bronchopulmonary Dysplasia

The role of these organisms in causing severe respiratory insufficiency, the need for mechanical ventilation, the development of BPD, or death remains controversial. Nevertheless, meta-analyses of published studies have identified respiratory colonization with *Ureaplasma* spp. as an independent risk factor for the development of BPD. However, trials

Table 251.1	Clinical Syndromes and Antibiotic Therapy for Ureaplasmas and Mycoplasmas Infection		
	UREAPLASMA SPP.	**M. HOMINIS**	**M. GENITALIUM**
INTRAUTERINE AND NEONATAL INFECTIONS			
Chorioamnionitis	++	++	–
Preterm delivery	++	++	++
Postpartum fever	++	+++	UK
BPD	+++	+	UK
CNS infections	+	+	UK
NEC	+	UK	UK
GENITOURINARY INFECTIONS			
NGU (acute/chronic)	++*	–	+++
Cervicitis	–	–	+++
PID	+	++	+++
NON-NEONATAL/NON-GENITOURINARY INFECTIONS			
CNS disease[†]	+	++	–
Bacteremia	+	++	–
Surgical wound infections	++	++	–
Arthritis	+	++	–
TREATMENT			
Macrolides	++	–	++
Quinolones[‡]	+	++	+
Clindamycin	–	++	+
Tetracyclines (doxycycline)	++	+	+

BPD: bronchopulmonary dysplasia; *CNS*: central nervous system; *NEC*: necrotizing enterocolitis; *NGU*: nongonococcal urethritis; *PID*: pelvic inflammatory disease; *UK*: unknown.
*Only *Ureaplasma urealyticum* (not *parvum*).
[†]CNS disease includes: meningitis, brain abscess, subdural empyema, and nonfunctioning CNS shunts.
[‡]The most commonly used quinolones are ciprofloxacin and moxifloxacin.

using erythromycin therapy in high-risk preterm infants with tracheobronchial colonization of *U. urealyticum* have failed to show any difference in the development of BPD in treated vs. nontreated infants. To date there is not enough evidence to support the use of antibiotic therapy in preterm infants at-risk or with confirmed *Ureaplasma* spp. infection to prevent the development of BPD.

Central Nervous System Infections

M. hominis and *Ureaplasma* spp. have been isolated from the CSF of premature infants and, less commonly, full-term infants. However, the clinical significance of recovering these bacteria from the CSF is uncertain, simultaneous isolation of other pathogens is unusual, and most infants have no overt signs of CNS disease. These bacteria may represent true pathogens and may be associated with CNS disease based on the host susceptibility/gestational age and bacteria pathogenicity. Overall, CSF pleocytosis is not consistent, and spontaneous clearance of mycoplasmas has been documented without specific therapy. *Ureaplasma* spp. meningitis has been associated with intraventricular hemorrhage and hydrocephalus. Limited data suggest that meningitis caused by *M. hominis* can be associated with significant morbidity and mortality. In a review of 29 reported neonatal cases with *M. hominis* meningitis, 8 (28%) neonates died and 8 (28%) developed neurologic sequelae. The age of onset of meningitis ranges from 1 to 196 days of life, and organisms can persist in the CSF without therapy for days to weeks. Pachymeningitis may be evident on MRI.

Other: *M. hominis* and *Ureaplasma* spp. have also been associated with neonatal conjunctivitis, abscesses (mainly at the scalp electrode site and associated with *M. hominis*), bacteremia, and necrotizing enterocolitis (NEC).

Genitourinary Infections

In sexually active adolescents and adults, genital mycoplasmas are associated with sexually transmitted diseases and are rarely associated with focal infections outside the genital tract. *U. urealyticum* (not *U. parvum*) and *M. genitalium* are recognized etiologic agents of NGU, mainly in men. Approximately 20% of NGU may be caused by these organisms either alone or associated with *Chlamydia trachomatis*. Rare complications of NGU include epididymitis and prostatitis. Salpingitis, cervicitis, pelvic inflammatory disease, and endometritis have been described in women associated with *M. genitalium* and to a lesser extent with *M. hominis*.

Nongenital Infections

Ureaplasma spp. and *M. hominis* infections are rarely described outside the neonatal period. These infections have been reported in both immunocompetent and immunocompromised children, including patients with hypogammaglobulinemia, lymphoma, or solid organ transplant recipients, who appear to be at higher risk of infection.

Cases of *Ureaplasma* spp. pneumonia, osteomyelitis, arthritis, meningitis, mediastinitis, bacteremia, infection of aortic grafts, and post-cesarean wound infections have been reported. Recent data suggest that *Ureaplasma* spp. is associated with post-transplant hyperammonemia syndrome, a rare but potentially fatal complication.

M. hominis is most commonly reported in systemic infections and has been associated with CNS disease (including meningitis, brain abscesses, subdural empyema, and nonfunctioning shunts), surgical wound infections, arthritis (associated in up to 50% of cases with prior manipulation of the GU tract), prosthetic and naïve endocarditis, osteomyelitis, and pneumonia. There are reports of life-threatening mediastinitis, sternal wound infections, pleuritis, peritonitis, and pericarditis, with high mortality rates in patients following organ transplantation. These infections should be suspected in culture-negative systemic or local infections, when samples have been properly collected and before initiation of antibiotic therapy.

DIAGNOSIS

All Mollicutes lack a cell wall and are therefore not visible on Gram stain. *M. hominis* and *Ureaplasma* spp. can grow in cell-free media and require sterols for growth, producing characteristic colonies on agar. Colonies of *M. hominis* are 200-300 μm in diameter with a fried-egg appearance, while colonies of *Ureaplasma* spp. are smaller (16-60 μm in diameter). *M. genitalium* is a fastidious organism and can be isolated with difficulty in cell culture systems. Most hospital diagnostic microbiology laboratories are not prepared to culture these pathogens, and nucleic acid-based tests are the preferred method for diagnosis. PCR-based assays have greater sensitivity and provide a more practical method for detection. Serologic assays have limited value in the clinical setting and are not commercially available for diagnostic purposes.

Genital Tract Infection

Confirmation of genital tract infection is challenging because of the high colonization rates in the vagina and urethra. NGU is typically defined as new-onset urethral discharge or dysuria with Gram stain of urethral discharge showing ≥ 5 polymorphonuclear leukocytes per oil-immersion field in the absence of gram-negative diplococci (i.e., *Neisseria gonorrhoeae*). The lack of cell wall prevents the identification of these bacteria by routine Gram stain. Detection of *Ureaplasma* spp. or *M. hominis* by PCR is available for a variety of specimens, including urine, amniotic fluid, placental tissue, respiratory specimens, synovial fluid, and swabs of the cervix, urethra, and vagina. *M. genitalium* is often identified by nucleic acid amplification test (NAAT) testing of first-void urine specimens in men and vaginal swabs in women.

Neonates

Ureaplasma spp. and *M. hominis* have been isolated from urine, blood, CSF, tracheal aspirates, pleural fluid, abscesses, and lung tissue. Premature neonates who are clinically ill with pneumonitis, focal abscesses, or CNS disease (particularly progressive hydrocephalus with or without pleocytosis) for whom bacterial cultures are negative or in whom there is no improvement with standard antibiotic therapy warrant further work-up to rule out genital mycoplasmas. Isolation requires special media using urea for ureaplasmas and arginine for *M. hominis*, and clinical specimens must be cultured immediately or frozen at −70°C (−94°F) to prevent loss of organisms. When inoculated into broth containing arginine (for *M. hominis*) or urea (for *Ureaplasma* spp.), growth is indicated by an alkaline pH. Identification of *Ureaplasma* spp. on agar requires 1-2 days of growth and visualization with the dissecting microscope, whereas *M. hominis* is apparent to the eye but can require 2-7 days to grow. PCR-based assays are available and will shed light to the causality of these pathogens when sterile sites are tested (CSF, joint fluid, etc.).

TREATMENT

These organisms lack a cell wall, and thus β-lactam agents are not effective. These bacteria are also resistant to sulfonamides and trimethoprim because they do not produce folic acid. Rifamycins do not have activity against Mollicutes (see Table 251.1).

Unlike other mycoplasmas and ureaplasmas, *M. hominis* is resistant to macrolides but generally susceptible to clindamycin and quinolones. Most *Ureaplasma* spp. are susceptible to macrolides and advanced generation quinolones, such as moxifloxacin, but are often resistant to ciprofloxacin and clindamycin. Susceptibility to tetracyclines is variable for both organisms, with increasing resistance being reported. *M. genitalium* is typically susceptible to macrolides and moxifloxacin, with variable resistance to tetracyclines and clindamycin.

Adolescents and Adults

Recommended treatment for NGU should include antibiotics with activity against *C. trachomatis* with either doxycycline (100 mg PO twice daily for 7 days) or azithromycin (1 g PO as a single dose). Recurrent NGU after completion of treatment suggests the presence of doxycycline or azithromycin-resistant *M. genitalium*. If the initial empiric regimen did not include macrolides, retreatment with azithromycin may be indicated. Azithromycin is also preferred in children younger than 8 yr, and in those with allergy to tetracyclines. On the other hand if patients received azithromycin initially, retreatment with moxifloxacin may be most effective. Before the introduction of azithromycin up to 60% of patients with *M. genitalium* NGU developed recurrent or chronic urethritis despite 1-2 wk of treatment with doxycycline.

Sexual partners should also be treated to avoid recurrent disease in the index case. Nongenital mycoplasmal infections may require surgical drainage and prolonged antibiotic therapy.

Neonates

Treatment of these infections in neonates is challenging. Doxycycline and quinolones are generally avoided at this age due to their associated toxicities. In addition, attributing causality may be difficult. In general, therapy for neonates with genital mycoplasma infections is indicated if infections are associated with pure growth of the organism or if the organism is detected by PCR from a normally sterile site in conjunction with compatible disease manifestations to assure the treatment of an infectious process rather than merely colonization.

Treatment is usually based on predictable antimicrobial sensitivities, because susceptibility testing is not readily available for individual isolates (see Table 251.1). For infants with symptomatic CNS infection, cures have been described with chloramphenicol, doxycycline, and moxifloxacin. The long-term consequences of asymptomatic CNS infection associated with genital mycoplasmas, especially in the absence of pleocytosis, are unknown. Because mycoplasmas can spontaneously clear from the CSF, therapy should involve minimal risks.

Bibliography is available at Expert Consult.

Section **10**

Chlamydial Infections

第十篇
衣原体感染

Chapter **252**
Chlamydia pneumoniae

Stephan A. Kohlhoff and
Margaret R. Hammerschlag

第二百五十二章
肺炎衣原体

中文导读

　　本章主要介绍了肺炎衣原体的病原学、流行病学、发病机制、临床表现、诊断、治疗和预后。该病原体是引起下呼吸道感染的常见病原体，主要通过呼吸道飞沫传播，发病较为隐匿，无明显的临床症状。主要引起呼吸道感染症状，严重者可表现为胸腔积液和脓胸，可诱发哮喘，大多数情况与其他细菌合并感染。组织培养衣原体是特异性诊断，可以采用PCR检测进行诊断，常用的血清学方法为微量免疫荧光法。主要采用大环内酯类药物治疗，治疗后可能会存在长期咳嗽。

Chlamydia pneumoniae is a common cause of lower respiratory tract diseases, including pneumonia in children and bronchitis and pneumonia in adults.

ETIOLOGY

Chlamydiae are obligate intracellular pathogens that have established a unique niche in host cells. Chlamydiae cause a variety of diseases in animal species at virtually all phylogenic levels. The most significant human pathogens are *C. pneumoniae* and *Chlamydia trachomatis* (see Chapter 253). *Chlamydia psittaci* is the cause of psittacosis, an important zoonosis (see Chapter 254). There are now 9 recognized chlamydial species.

Chlamydiae have a gram-negative envelope without detectable peptidoglycan, although recent genomic analysis has revealed that both *C. pneumoniae* and *C. trachomatis* encode proteins forming a nearly complete pathway for synthesis of peptidoglycan, including penicillin-binding proteins. Chlamydiae also share a group-specific lipopolysaccharide antigen and use host adenosine triphosphate for the synthesis of chlamydial proteins. Although chlamydiae are auxotrophic for 3 of 4 nucleoside triphosphates, they encode functional glucose-catabolizing enzymes that can be used to generate adenosine triphosphate. As with peptidoglycan synthesis, for some reason these genes are turned off.

All chlamydiae also encode an abundant surface-exposed protein called the *major outer membrane protein*. The major outer membrane protein is the major determinant of the serologic classification of *C. trachomatis* and *C. psittaci* isolates.

EPIDEMIOLOGY

C. pneumoniae is primarily a human respiratory pathogen. The organism has also been isolated from nonhuman species, including horses, koalas, reptiles, and amphibians, where it also causes respiratory infection, although the role that these infections might play in transmission to humans is unknown. *C. pneumoniae* appears to affect individuals of all ages. The proportion of community-acquired pneumonias associated with *C. pneumoniae* infection is 2–19%, varying with geographic location, the age group examined, and the diagnostic methods used. Several studies of the role of *C. pneumoniae* in lower respiratory tract infection in pediatric populations have found evidence of infection in 0–18% of patients based on serology or culture for diagnosis. In 1 study, almost 20% of the children with *C. pneumoniae* infection were coinfected with *Mycoplasma pneumoniae*. *C. pneumoniae* may also be responsible for 10–20% of episodes of acute chest syndrome in children with sickle cell disease, up to 10% of asthma exacerbations, 10% of episodes of bronchitis, and 5–10% of episodes of pharyngitis in children.

Asymptomatic infection appears to be common based on epidemiologic studies.

Transmission probably occurs from person to person through respiratory droplets. Spread of the infection appears to be enhanced by close proximity, as is evident from localized outbreaks in enclosed populations, such as military recruits and in nursing homes.

PATHOGENESIS

Chlamydiae are characterized by a unique developmental cycle (Fig. 252.1) with morphologically distinct infectious and reproductive forms: the elementary body (EB) and reticulate body (RB). Following infection, the infectious EBs, which are 200-400 μm in diameter, attach to the host cell by a process of electrostatic binding and are taken into the cell by endocytosis that does not depend on the microtubule system. Within the host cell, the EB remains within a membrane-lined phagosome. The phagosome does not fuse with the host cell lysosome. The inclusion membrane is devoid of host cell markers, but lipid markers traffic to the inclusion, which suggests a functional interaction with the Golgi apparatus. The EBs then differentiate into RBs that undergo binary fission. After approximately 36 hr, the RBs differentiate into EBs. At approximately 48 hr, release can occur by cytolysis or by a process of exocytosis or extrusion of the whole inclusion, leaving the host cell intact. Chlamydiae can also enter a persistent state after treatment with certain cytokines such as interferon-γ, treatment with antibiotics, or restriction of certain nutrients. While chlamydiae are in the persistent state, metabolic activity is reduced. The ability to cause prolonged, often subclinical, infection is one of the major characteristics of chlamydiae.

CLINICAL MANIFESTATIONS

Infections caused by *C. pneumoniae* cannot be readily differentiated from those caused by other respiratory pathogens, especially *M. pneumoniae*. The pneumonia usually occurs as a classic atypical (or nonbacterial) pneumonia characterized by mild to moderate constitutional symptoms, including fever, malaise, headache, cough, and often pharyngitis. Severe pneumonia with pleural effusions and empyema has been described. Milder respiratory infections have been described, manifesting as a pertussis-like illness.

C. pneumoniae can serve as an infectious trigger for asthma, can cause pulmonary exacerbations in patients with cystic fibrosis, and can produce acute chest syndrome in patients with sickle cell anemia. *C. pneumoniae* has been isolated from middle ear aspirates of children with acute otitis media, most of the time as co-infection with other bacteria. Asymptomatic respiratory infection has been documented in 2–5% of adults and children and can persist for 1 yr or longer.

DIAGNOSIS

It is not possible to differentiate *C. pneumoniae* from other causes of atypical pneumonia on the basis of clinical findings. Auscultation reveals the presence of rales and often wheezing. The chest radiograph often appears worse than the patient's clinical status would indicate and can show mild, diffuse involvement or lobar infiltrates with small pleural effusions. The complete blood count may be elevated with a left shift but is usually unremarkable.

Specific diagnosis of *C. pneumoniae* infection has been based on isolation of the organism in tissue culture. *C. pneumoniae* grows best in cycloheximide-treated HEp-2 and HL cells. The optimum site for culture is the posterior nasopharynx; the specimen is collected with wire-shafted swabs in the same manner as that used for *C. trachomatis*. The organism can be isolated from sputum, throat cultures, bronchoalveolar lavage fluid, but few laboratories perform such cultures because of technical difficulties. A multiplexed nucleic acid amplification testing assay (Film Array, Biofire Diagnostics, Salt Lake City, UT) received FDA clearance in 2012 for the detection of 17 viruses and *C. pneumoniae*, *M. pneumoniae*, and *Bordetella pertussis*. The Film Array system combines nucleic acid extraction, nested polymerase chain reaction, detection, and data analysis.

Serologic diagnosis can be accomplished using the microimmunofluorescence (MIF) or the complement fixation tests. The complement fixation test is genus specific and is also used for diagnosis of lymphogranuloma venereum (see Chapter 253.4) and psittacosis (see Chapter 254). Its sensitivity in hospitalized patients with *C. pneumoniae* infection and children is variable. The Centers for Disease Control and Prevention (CDC) has proposed modifications in the serologic criteria for diagnosis. Although the MIF test was considered to be the only currently acceptable serologic test, the criteria were made significantly more stringent. Acute infection, using the MIF test, was defined by a 4-fold increase in immunoglobulin (Ig) G titer or an IgM titer of ≥16; use of a single elevated IgG titer was discouraged. An IgG titer of ≥16 was thought to indicate past exposure, but neither elevated IgA titers nor any other serologic marker was thought to be a valid indicator of persistent or chronic infection. Because diagnosis would require paired sera, this would be a retrospective diagnosis. The CDC did not recommend the use of any enzyme-linked immune assay for detection of antibody to *C. pneumoniae* because of concern about the inconsistent correlation of these results with culture results. Studies of *C. pneumoniae* infection in children with pneumonia and asthma show that more than 50% of children with culture-documented infection have no detectable MIF antibody.

TREATMENT

The optimum dose and duration of antimicrobial therapy for *C. pneumoniae* infections remain uncertain. Most treatment studies have used only serology for diagnosis, and thus microbiologic efficacy cannot be assessed. Prolonged therapy for 2 wk or longer is required for some patients, because recrudescent symptoms and persistent positive cultures have been described following 2 wk of erythromycin and 30 days of tetracycline or doxycycline.

Tetracyclines, macrolides (erythromycin, azithromycin, and clarithromycin), and quinolones show *in vitro* activity. Like *C. psittaci*, *C. pneumoniae* is resistant to sulfonamides. The results of treatment studies have shown that erythromycin (40 mg/kg/day PO divided twice a day for 10 days), clarithromycin (15 mg/kg/day PO divided twice a day for 10 days), and azithromycin (10 mg/kg PO on day 1, and then 5 mg/kg/day PO on days 2-5) are effective for eradication of *C. pneumoniae* from the nasopharynx of children with pneumonia in approximately 80% of cases.

PROGNOSIS

Clinical response to antibiotic therapy varies. Coughing often persists for several weeks even after therapy.

Bibliography is available at Expert Consult.

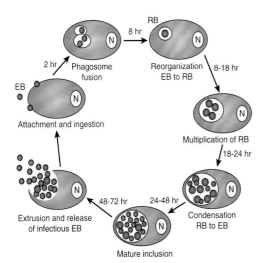

Fig. 252.1 Life cycle of chlamydiae in epithelial cells. *EB*, elementary body; *RB*, reticulate body. (*From Hammerschlag MR: Infections due to* Chlamydia trachomatis *and* Chlamydia pneumoniae *in children and adolescents.* Pediatr Rev 25:43–50, 2004.)

Chapter **253**
Chlamydia trachomatis
Margaret R. Hammerschlag
第二百五十三章
沙眼衣原体

中文导读

本章主要介绍了沙眼衣原体感染导致的疾病，主要为沙眼、生殖道感染、新生儿结膜炎和肺炎、性病淋巴节肉芽肿四部分介绍。简要讲述了沙眼的病原体血清型、临床表现、诊断方法和治疗。生殖道感染主要是通过性接触传播，部分患者可无症状，主要通过分子检测确诊，阿奇霉素和强力霉素为一线治疗药物，易发生并发症，对性活跃人群筛查和治疗可有效控制传播。新生儿结膜炎和肺炎主要是通过分娩垂直传播，可有结膜、鼻咽、直肠和阴道多部位感染，分子检测为主要诊断方法，治疗主要采用红霉素或阿奇霉素，孕妇的围产期筛查和治疗可有效控制该病。性病淋巴节肉芽肿是由性病淋巴节肉芽肿变种的L1、L2和L3血清型引起的全身性传播疾病，详细介绍了该病的临床表现、诊断方法和治疗。

Chlamydia trachomatis is subdivided into 2 biovars: lymphogranuloma venereum (LGV) and trachoma, which is the agent of human oculogenital diseases other than LGV. Although the strains of both biovars have almost complete DNA homology, they differ in growth characteristics and virulence in tissue culture and animals. In developed countries, *C. trachomatis* is the most prevalent sexually transmitted disease, causing urethritis in men, cervicitis and salpingitis in women, and conjunctivitis and pneumonia in infants.

253.1 Trachoma
Margaret R. Hammerschlag

Trachoma is the most important preventable cause of blindness in the world. It is caused primarily by the A, B, Ba, and C serotypes of *C. trachomatis*. It is endemic in the Middle East and Southeast Asia and among Navajo Indians in the southwestern United States. In areas that are endemic for trachoma, such as Egypt, genital chlamydial infection is caused by the serotypes responsible for oculogenital disease: D, E, F, G, H, I, J, and K. The disease is spread from eye to eye. Flies are a common vector.

Trachoma begins as a **follicular conjunctivitis,** usually in early childhood. The follicles heal, leading to conjunctival scarring that can result in an entropion, with the eyelid turning inward so that the lashes abrade the cornea. It is the corneal ulceration secondary to the constant trauma that leads to scarring and blindness. Bacterial superinfection can also contribute to scarring. Blindness occurs years after the active disease.

Trachoma can be diagnosed clinically. The World Health Organization suggests that at least 2 of 4 criteria must be present for a diagnosis of trachoma: lymphoid follicles on the upper tarsal conjunctivae, typical conjunctival scarring, vascular pannus, and limbal follicles. The diagnosis is confirmed by culture or staining tests for *C. trachomatis* performed during the active stage of disease. Serologic tests are not helpful clinically because of the long duration of the disease and the high seroprevalence in endemic populations.

Poverty and lack of sanitation are important factors in the spread of trachoma. As socioeconomic conditions improve, the incidence of the disease decreases substantially. Endemic trachoma is managed by mass drug administration (MDA) with azithromycin in affected communities. Endemic communities should receive MDA until clinical signs of active disease in children, 1-9 yr of age, falls below 5%. MDA with a single dose of azithromycin to all the residents of a village dramatically reduced the prevalence and intensity of infection. This effect continued for 2 yr after treatment, probably by interrupting the transmission of ocular *C. trachomatis* infection.

Bibliography is available at Expert Consult.

253.2 Genital Tract Infections
Margaret R. Hammerschlag

EPIDEMIOLOGY
There are an estimated 3 million new cases of chlamydial sexually transmitted infections each year in the United States. *C. trachomatis* is

a major cause of epididymitis and is the cause of 23–55% of all cases of nongonococcal urethritis, although the proportion of chlamydial nongonococcal urethritis has been gradually declining. As many as 50% of men with gonorrhea may be coinfected with *C. trachomatis*. The prevalence of chlamydial cervicitis among sexually active women is 2–35%. Rates of infection among girls 15-19 yr of age exceed 20% in many urban populations but can be as high as 15% in suburban populations as well.

Children who have been sexually abused can acquire anogenital *C. trachomatis* infection, which is usually asymptomatic. However, because perinatally acquired rectal and vaginal *C. trachomatis* infections can persist for 3 yr or longer, the detection of *C. trachomatis* in the vagina or rectum of a young child is not absolute evidence of sexual abuse.

CLINICAL MANIFESTATIONS

The trachoma biovar of *C. trachomatis* causes a spectrum of disease in sexually active adolescents and adults. Up to 75% of women with *C. trachomatis* have no symptoms of infection. *C. trachomatis* can cause urethritis (acute urethral syndrome), epididymitis, cervicitis, salpingitis, proctitis, and pelvic inflammatory disease. The symptoms of chlamydial genital tract infections are less acute than those of gonorrhea, consisting of a discharge that is usually mucoid rather than purulent. Asymptomatic urethral infection is common in sexually active men. Autoinoculation from the genital tract to the eyes can lead to concomitant inclusion conjunctivitis.

DIAGNOSIS

Diagnosis of genital chlamydial infection is now accomplished by nucleic acid amplification tests (NAATs). These tests have high sensitivity, perhaps even detecting 10–20% greater than culture, while retaining high specificity. 6 FDA-approved NAATs are commercially available for detecting *C. trachomatis*, including polymerase chain reaction (PCR; Amplicor Chlamydia test, Roche Molecular Diagnostics, Nutley, NJ), strand displacement amplification (ProbeTec, BD Diagnostic Systems, Sparks, MD), transcription-mediated amplification (Amp CT, Hologic, San Diego, CA), and GeneXpert CT/NG assay (Cepheid, Sunnyvale, CA). PCR and strand displacement amplification are DNA amplification tests that use primers that target gene sequences on the cryptogenic *C. trachomatis* plasmid that is present at approximately 10 copies in each infected cell. Transcription-mediated amplification is a ribosomal RNA amplification assay. GeneXpert is an on-demand qualitative real-time PCR. All these assays are also available as coamplification tests for simultaneously detecting *C. trachomatis* and *Neisseria gonorrhoeae*.

The available commercial NAATs are FDA approved for cervical and vaginal swabs from adolescent girls and women, urethral swabs from adolescent boys and men, and urine from adolescents and adults. Use of urine avoids the necessity for a clinical pelvic examination and can greatly facilitate screening in certain populations, especially adolescents, although several studies have now demonstrated that endocervical specimens and vaginal swabs are superior to urine for NAAT. Self-collected vaginal specimens appear to be as reliable as specimens obtained by a healthcare professional.

Data on use of NAATs for vaginal specimens or urine from children are very limited and insufficient to allow making a recommendation for their use. The CDC recommends that NAATs be used as an alternative to culture only if confirmation is available. Confirmation tests should consist of a second FDA-approved NAAT that targets a different gene sequence from the initial test.

The etiology of most cases of nonchlamydial nongonococcal urethritis is unknown, although *Ureaplasma urealyticum* and possibly *Mycoplasma genitalium* are implicated in up to one-third of cases (see Chapter 251). Proctocolitis may develop in individuals who have a rectal infection with an LGV strain (see Chapter 253.4).

TREATMENT

The first-line treatment regimens recommended by the CDC for uncomplicated *C. trachomatis* genital infection in men and nonpregnant women include azithromycin (1 g PO as a single dose) and doxycycline (100 mg PO twice a day for 7 days). Alternative regimens are erythromycin base (500 mg PO 4 times a day for 7 days), erythromycin ethylsuccinate (800 mg PO 4 times a day for 7 days), ofloxacin (300 mg PO twice a day for 7 days), and levofloxacin (500 mg PO once daily for 7 days). The high erythromycin dosages might not be well tolerated. Doxycycline and quinolones are contraindicated in pregnant women, and quinolones are contraindicated in persons younger than 18 yr. For pregnant women, the recommended treatment regimen is azithromycin (1 g PO as a single dose) or amoxicillin (500 mg PO 3 times a day for 7 days). Alternative regimens for pregnant women are erythromycin base (250 mg PO 4 times a day for 14 days) and erythromycin ethylsuc-cinate (800 mg PO 4 times a day for 7 days or 400 mg PO 4 times a day for 14 days).

Empirical treatment without microbiologic diagnosis is recommended only for patients at high risk for infection who are unlikely to return for follow-up evaluation, including adolescents with multiple sex partners. These patients should be treated empirically for both *C. trachomatis* and gonorrhea.

Sex partners of patients with nongonococcal urethritis should be treated if they have had sexual contact with the patient during the 60 days preceding the onset of symptoms. The most recent sexual partner should be treated even if the last sexual contact was more than 60 days from onset of symptoms.

COMPLICATIONS

Complications of genital chlamydial infections in women include perihepatitis (Fitz-Hugh-Curtis syndrome) and salpingitis. Of women with untreated chlamydial infection who develop pelvic inflammatory disease, up to 40% will have significant sequelae; approximately 17% will suffer from chronic pelvic pain, approximately 17% will become infertile, and approximately 9% will have an ectopic (tubal) pregnancy. Adolescent girls may be at higher risk for developing complications, especially salpingitis, than older women. Salpingitis in adolescent girls is also more likely to lead to tubal scarring, subsequent obstruction with secondary infertility, and increased risk for ectopic pregnancy. Approximately 50% of neonates born to pregnant women with untreated chlamydial infection will acquire *C. trachomatis* infection (see Chapter 253.3). Women with *C. trachomatis* infection have a 3-5–fold increased risk for acquiring HIV infection.

PREVENTION

Timely treatment of sex partners is essential for decreasing risk for reinfection. Sex partners should be evaluated and treated if they had sexual contact during the 60 days preceding onset of symptoms in the patient. The most recent sex partner should be treated even if the last sexual contact was > 60 days. Patients and their sex partners should abstain from sexual intercourse until 7 days after a single-dose regimen or after completion of a 7-day regimen.

Annual routine screening for *C. trachomatis* is recommended for all sexually active female adolescents, for all women 20-25 yr of age, and for older women with risk factors such as new or multiple partners or inconsistent use of barrier contraceptives. Sexual risk assessment might indicate more frequent screening of some women.

Bibliography is available at Expert Consult.

253.3 Conjunctivitis and Pneumonia in Newborns

Margaret R. Hammerschlag

EPIDEMIOLOGY

Chlamydial genital infection is reported in 5–30% of pregnant women, with a risk for vertical transmission at parturition to newborn infants of approximately 50%. The infant may become infected at 1 or more sites, including the conjunctivae, nasopharynx, rectum, and vagina. Transmission is rare following cesarean section with intact membranes. The introduction of systematic prenatal screening for *C. trachomatis* infection and treatment of pregnant women has resulted in a dramatic decrease in the incidence of neonatal chlamydial infection in the United States. However, in countries where prenatal screening is not done, such as the Netherlands, *C. trachomatis* remains an important cause of neonatal infection, accounting for >60% of neonatal conjunctivitis.

Inclusion Conjunctivitis

Approximately 30–50% of infants born to mothers with active, untreated chlamydial infection develop clinical conjunctivitis. Symptoms usually develop 5-14 days after delivery, or earlier in infants born after prolonged rupture of membranes. The presentation is extremely variable and ranges from mild conjunctival injection with scant mucoid discharge to severe conjunctivitis with copious purulent discharge, chemosis, and pseudomembrane formation. The conjunctiva may be very friable and might bleed when stroked with a swab. Chlamydial conjunctivitis must be differentiated from gonococcal ophthalmia, which is sight threatening. At least 50% of infants with chlamydial conjunctivitis also have nasopharyngeal infection.

Pneumonia

Pneumonia caused by *C. trachomatis* can develop in 10–20% of infants born to women with active, untreated chlamydial infection. Only approximately 25% of infants with nasopharyngeal chlamydial infection develop pneumonia. *C. trachomatis* pneumonia of infancy has a very characteristic presentation. Onset usually occurs between 1 and 3 mo of age and is often insidious, with persistent cough, tachypnea, and absence of fever. Auscultation reveals rales; wheezing is uncommon. The absence of fever and wheezing helps to distinguish *C. trachomatis* pneumonia from respiratory syncytial virus pneumonia. A distinctive laboratory finding is the presence of peripheral eosinophilia (>400 cells/μL). The most consistent finding on chest radiograph is hyperinflation accompanied by minimal interstitial or alveolar infiltrates.

Infections at Other Sites

Infants born to mothers with *C. trachomatis* can develop infection in the rectum or vagina. Although infection in these sites appears to be totally asymptomatic, it can cause confusion if it is identified at a later date. Perinatally acquired rectal, vaginal, and nasopharyngeal infections can persist for 3 yr or longer.

DIAGNOSIS

Definitive diagnosis is achieved by isolation of *C. trachomatis* in cultures of specimens obtained from the conjunctiva or nasopharynx. Data on use of NAATs for diagnosis of *C. trachomatis* in children are limited. Limited data suggest that PCR may be equivalent to culture for detecting *C. trachomatis* in the conjunctiva of infants with conjunctivitis. However, NAATs are not currently FDA-cleared for use with conjunctival or nasopharyngeal specimens from infants. Laboratories can do internal validation delineated in the CDC 2014 *C. trachomatis* and *N. gonorrhoeae* laboratory guidelines.

TREATMENT

The recommended treatment regimens for *C. trachomatis* conjunctivitis or pneumonia in infants are erythromycin (base or ethylsuccinate, 50 mg/kg/day divided 4 times a day PO for 14 days) and azithromycin suspension (20 mg/kg/day once daily PO for 3 days). The rationale for using oral therapy for conjunctivitis is that 50% or more of these infants have concomitant nasopharyngeal infection or disease at other sites, and studies demonstrate that topical therapy with sulfonamide drops and erythromycin ointment is not effective. The failure rate with oral erythromycin remains 10–20%, and some infants require a second course of treatment. Mothers (and their sexual contacts) of infants with *C. trachomatis* infections should be empirically treated for genital infection. An association between treatment with both oral erythromycin and azithromycin and infantile hypertrophic pyloric stenosis has been reported in infants younger than 6 wk of age.

PREVENTION

Neonatal gonococcal prophylaxis with topical erythromycin ointment does not prevent chlamydial ophthalmia or nasopharyngeal colonization with *C. trachomatis* or chlamydial pneumonia. The most effective method of controlling perinatal chlamydial infection is screening and treatment of pregnant women. In 2015, the Canadian Pediatric Society recommended that neonatal ocular prophylaxis be discontinued in Canada and recommended enhanced prenatal screening for chlamydia. The program was implemented in 2016. In the United States, implementation of prenatal screening and treatment of pregnant women has resulted in a dramatic decrease in perinatal chlamydial infections. For treatment of *C. trachomatis* infection in pregnant women, the CDC currently recommends either azithromycin (1 g PO as a single dose) or amoxicillin (500 mg PO 3 times a day for 7 days) as first-line regimens. Erythromycin base (250 mg PO 4 times a day for 14 days) and erythromycin ethylsuccinate (800 mg 4 times a day for 7 days, or 400 mg PO 4 times a day for 14 days) are listed as alternative regimens. Reasons for failure of maternal treatment to prevent infantile chlamydial infection include poor compliance and reinfection from an untreated sexual partner.

Bibliography is available at Expert Consult.

253.4 Lymphogranuloma Venereum

Margaret R. Hammerschlag

LGV is a systemic sexually transmitted disease caused by the L_1, L_2, and L_3 serotypes of the LGV biovar of *C. trachomatis*. Unlike strains of the trachoma biovar, LGV strains have a predilection for lymphoid tissue. Less than 1,000 cases are reported in adults in the United States annually. There has been a resurgence of LGV infections among men who have sex with men in Europe and the United States. Many of the men were HIV infected and used illicit drugs, specifically methamphetamines. The only pediatric case that has been reported since the emergence of the new clusters of HIV-associated cases in 2003 was a 16 yr old boy who presented with LGV proctocolitis after having receptive unprotected anal intercourse with a 30 yr old man he met on the Internet. This history was obtained after the boy was found to be HIV-positive. The diagnosis of LGV, particularly when it presents with proctocolitis, relies on a high index of suspicion that would lead to emphasizing certain aspects of the history and ordering the pertinent diagnostic tests. Many pediatricians and pediatric gastroenterologists might not be very familiar with the entity and might not entertain it as a diagnostic consideration in the pediatric patients. The diagnosis can be further suggested by *C. trachomatis* testing: commonly by NAATs or culturing the organism if culture is available. Currently available NAATs will not differentiate LGV from other *C. trachomatis* serovars. NAATs for *C. trachomatis* are also not FDA-cleared for testing rectal specimens, but laboratories can do an internal validation as recommended in the CDC 2014 *C. trachomatis* and *N. gonorrhoeae* laboratory guidelines. NAATs have been found in several clinical studies to perform well with rectal specimens. Typing of the *C. trachomatis* specimen can be done by sequencing from the NAAT specimen by many state laboratories. Trying to ascertain the *C. trachomatis* serovar for confirmation of LGV has therapeutic implications, as LGV needs to be treated with a 3 wk course of doxycycline; a single-dose of azithromycin will not eradicate the infection.

CLINICAL MANIFESTATIONS

The **first stage of LGV** is characterized by the appearance of the primary lesion, a painless, usually transient papule on the genitals. The **second stage** is characterized by usually unilateral femoral or inguinal lymphadenitis with enlarging, painful buboes. The nodes may break down and drain, especially in men. In women, the vulvar lymph drains to the retroperitoneal nodes. Fever, myalgia, and headache are common. The **third stage** is a genitoanorectal syndrome with rectovaginal fistulas, rectal strictures, and urethral destruction. Among men who have sex with men, rectal infection with LGV can produce a severe, acute proctocolitis, which can be confused with inflammatory bowel disease or malignancy.

DIAGNOSIS

LGV can be diagnosed by serologic testing or by culture of *C. trachomatis* or molecular testing for *C. trachomatis* from a specimen aspirated from a bubo. Most patients with LGV have complement-fixing antibody titers of >1:16. Chancroid and herpes simplex virus can be distinguished clinically from LGV by the concurrent presence of painful genital ulcers. Syphilis can be differentiated by serologic tests. However, co-infections can occur.

TREATMENT

Doxycycline (100 mg PO bid for 21 days) is the recommended treatment. The alternative regimen is erythromycin base (500 mg PO 4 times a day for 21 days). Azithromycin (1 g PO once weekly for 3 wk) may also be effective, but clinical data are lacking. Sex partners of patients with LGV should be treated if they have had sexual contact with the patient during the 30 days preceding the onset of symptoms.

Bibliography is available at Expert Consult.

Chapter 254

Psittacosis (*Chlamydia psittaci*)

Stephan A. Kohlhoff and Margaret R. Hammerschlag

第二百五十四章
鹦鹉热衣原体

中文导读

本章主要介绍了鹦鹉热衣原体感染的病原学、流行病学、临床表现、诊断、治疗、预后和预防。该病原体主要存在禽类体内，在人类较少感染，接触禽类为感染高危因素。临床表现多样，可累及肺部及多器官。主要诊断方法包括病原体分离、PCR检测和免疫学方法。详细介绍了治疗方案，强力霉素和四环素为首选治疗药物，儿童和孕妇可选用红霉素和阿奇霉素替代治疗。合理治疗可明显降低死亡率。感染禽类隔离和危险人群防护可有效预防。

Chlamydia psittaci, the agent of psittacosis (also known as **parrot fever** and **ornithosis**), is primarily an animal pathogen and rarely causes human disease. In birds, *C. psittaci* infection is known as *avian chlamydiosis*.

ETIOLOGY

C. psittaci affects both psittacine birds (e.g., parrots, parakeets, macaws) and nonpsittacine birds (ducks, turkeys); the known host range includes 130 avian species. The life cycle of *C. psittaci* is the same as for *C. pneumoniae* (see Chapter 252). Strains of *C. psittaci* have been analyzed by patterns of pathogenicity, inclusion morphology in tissue culture, DNA restriction endonuclease analysis, and monoclonal antibodies, which indicate that there are 7 avian serovars. The organism has also been found in non-avian domestic animals, including cattle, sheep, pigs, goats, and cats. Non-avian *C. psittaci* has rarely caused disease in humans. Two of the avian serovars, psittacine and turkey, are of major importance in the avian population of the United States. Each is associated with important host preferences and disease characteristics.

EPIDEMIOLOGY

From 2005 to 2009 there were 66 reported cases of psittacosis in the United States. Of these, 85% of these cases were associated with exposure to birds, including 70% following exposure to caged pet birds, which were usually psittacine birds, including cockatiels, parakeets, parrots, and macaws. Chlamydiosis among caged nonpsittacine birds occurs most often in pigeons, doves, and mynah birds. Persons at highest risk for acquiring psittacosis include bird fanciers and owners of pet birds (43% of cases) and pet shop employees (10% of cases). Reported cases most likely underestimate the number of actual infections owing to a lack of awareness.

Inhalation of aerosols from feces, fecal dust, and nasal secretions of animals infected with *C. psittaci* is the primary route of infection. *Source birds are either asymptomatic or have anorexia, ruffled feathers, lethargy, and watery green droppings.* Psittacosis is uncommon in children, in part because children may be less likely to have close contact with infected birds. One high-risk activity is cleaning the cage. Several major outbreaks of psittacosis have occurred in turkey-processing plants; workers exposed to turkey viscera are at the highest risk for infection.

CLINICAL MANIFESTATIONS

Infection with *C. psittaci* in humans ranges from clinically inapparent to severe disease, including pneumonia and multiorgan involvement. The mean incubation period is 15 days after exposure, with a range of 5-21 days. *Onset of disease is usually abrupt, with fever, cough, headache, myalgia, and malaise.* The fever is high and is often associated with rigors and sweats. The headache can be so severe that meningitis is considered. The cough is usually nonproductive. Gastrointestinal symptoms are occasionally reported. Crackles may be heard on auscultation. Chest radiographs are usually abnormal and are characterized by the presence of variable infiltrates, sometimes accompanied by pleural effusions. The white blood cell count is usually normal but is sometimes mildly elevated. Elevated levels of aspartate aminotransferase, alkaline phosphatase, and bilirubin are common. Nonpulmonary complications include pericarditis, endocarditis, and myocarditis. Mortality occurs in 5% of cases.

DIAGNOSIS

Psittacosis can be difficult to diagnose because of the varying clinical presentations. A history of exposure to birds or association with an active case can be important clues, but as many as 20% of patients with psittacosis have no known contact. Person-to-person spread has been suggested but not proved. Other infections that cause pneumonia with high fever, unusually severe headache, and myalgia include routine bacterial and viral respiratory infections as well as *Coxiella burnetii* infection (Q fever), *Mycoplasma pneumoniae* infection, *C. pneumoniae* infection, tularemia, tuberculosis, fungal infections, and Legionnaires disease.

A patient is considered to have a confirmed case of psittacosis if clinical illness is compatible with psittacosis and the case is laboratory confirmed by either isolation of *C. psittaci* from respiratory specimens (e.g., sputum, pleural fluid, or tissue) or blood, or 4-fold or greater increase in antibody (immunoglobulin G) against *C. psittaci* by complement fixation or microimmunofluorescence between paired acute- and convalescent-phase serum specimens obtained at least 2-4 wk apart. A patient is considered to have a probable case of psittacosis if the clinical illness is compatible with psittacosis and 1 of the 2 following laboratory results is present: supportive serology (e.g., *C. psittaci* antibody titer [Immunoglobulin M] ≥ 32 in at least 1 serum specimen obtained after onset of symptoms), or detection of *C. psittaci* DNA in a respiratory specimen (e.g., sputum, pleural fluid, or tissue) via amplification of a specific target by polymerase chain reaction assay.

Although microimmunofluorescence has greater specificity to *C. psittaci* than complement fixation, cross reactions with other *Chlamydia* species can occur. Therefore acute- and convalescent-phase serum specimens should be analyzed at the same time in the same laboratory. False-negative microimmunofluorescence results can occur in acutely ill patients. Early treatment of psittacosis with tetracycline can abrogate the antibody response.

Although *C. psittaci* will grow in the same culture systems used for isolation of *Chlamydia trachomatis* and *C. pneumoniae*, very few laboratories culture for *C. psittaci*, mainly because of the potential biohazard. Real-time polymerase chain reaction assays have been developed for use in the detection of *C. psittaci* in respiratory specimens. These assays can distinguish *C. psittaci* from other chlamydial species and identify different *C. psittaci* genotypes. However, polymerase chain reaction–based tests have not been cleared by the FDA for use as diagnostic tests in human samples.

TREATMENT

Recommended treatment regimens for psittacosis are doxycycline (100 mg PO twice daily) or tetracycline (500 mg PO 4 times a day) for at least 10-14 days after the fever abates. The initial treatment of severely ill patients is doxycycline hyclate (4.4 mg/kg/day divided every 12 hr IV; maximum: 100 mg/dose). Erythromycin (500 mg PO 4 times a day) and azithromycin (10 mg/kg PO day 1, not to exceed 500 mg, followed by 5 mg/kg PO on days 2-5, not to exceed 250 mg) are alternative drugs if tetracyclines are contraindicated (e.g., children < 8 yr of age and pregnant women) but may be less effective. Remission is usually evident within 48-72 hr. Initial infection does not appear to be followed by long-term immunity. Reinfection and clinical disease can develop within 2 mo of treatment.

PROGNOSIS

The mortality rate of psittacosis is 15–20% with no treatment but is <1% with appropriate treatment. Severe illness leading to respiratory failure and fetal death has been reported among pregnant women.

PREVENTION

Several control measures are recommended to prevent transmission of *C. psittaci* from birds. Bird fanciers should be cognizant of the potential risk. *C. psittaci* is susceptible to heat and to most disinfectants and detergents but is resistant to acid and alkali. Accurate records of all bird-related transactions aid in identifying sources of infected birds and potentially exposed persons. Newly acquired birds, including birds that have been to shows, exhibitions, fairs, or other events, should be isolated for 30-45 days or tested or treated prophylactically before adding them to a group of birds. Care should be taken to prevent transfer of fecal material, feathers, food, or other materials between birdcages. Birds with signs of avian chlamydiosis (e.g., ocular or nasal discharge, watery green droppings, or low body weight) should be isolated and should not be sold or purchased. Their handlers should wear protective clothing and a disposable surgical cap and use a respirator with an N95 or higher efficiency rating (not a surgical mask) when handling them or cleaning their cages. Infected birds should be isolated until fully treated, which is generally 45 days.

Bibliography is available at Expert Consult.

Section **11**
Rickettsial Infections
第十一篇
立克次体感染

Chapter **255**
Spotted Fever Group Rickettsioses
J. Stephen Dumler and Megan E. Reller
第二百五十五章
斑疹热组立克次体感染

中文导读

本章主要介绍了斑疹热组立克次体引起的疾病，分为落矶山立克次体病、地中海斑疹热或南欧斑疹热、立克次体痘和蚤传播的斑疹热三大部分。落矶山立克次体病是由立氏立克次体感染所致，在美国是最常见和最严重的立克次体病，详细介绍了本病的流行病学、传播途径、致病机制，典型的临床症状有发热、头痛和皮疹，可有中枢神经系统表现及其他系统损伤表现，早期诊断困难，诊断方法有PCR检测、免疫学试验等，还详细介绍了本病的鉴别诊断、治疗、预后和预防。地中海斑疹热或南欧斑疹热是由康氏立克次体感染导致的，详细介绍了本病的病原、流行病学、发病机制、临床表现和实验室检测、诊断和鉴别诊断、治疗、并发症和预防。还简要介绍了立克次体痘和蚤传播的斑疹热。

Rickettsia species were classically divided into *spotted fever* and *typhus* groups based on serologic reactions and the presence or absence of the outer membrane protein A *(ompA)* gene. Sequencing of at least 45 complete genomes has refined distinctions. However, there is controversy regarding phylogeny, and some data suggest that diversity and pathogenicity are the result of gene loss and lateral gene transfer from other prokaryotes or even eukaryotes, which further obscures accurate taxonomic classification. One proposal is to divide existing species into spotted fever and *transitional* groups based on genetic relatedness; both include pathogenic species and species not now known to cause human disease (Table 255.1). Although increasingly more is understood about the molecular basis by which these bacteria cause human illness, an alternative classification system based on pathogenetic mechanisms has not been defined. The list of pathogens and potential pathogens in the spotted fever group has expanded dramatically in recent years. Among them are the tickborne agents *Rickettsia rickettsii,* the cause of Rocky Mountain or Brazilian spotted fever (RMSF); *R. conorii,* the cause of

Mediterranean spotted fever (MSF) or boutonneuse fever; *R. sibirica,* the cause of North Asian tick typhus; *R. japonica,* the cause of Oriental spotted fever; *R. honei,* the cause of Flinders Island spotted fever or Thai tick typhus; *R. africae,* the cause of African tick bite fever; *R. akari,* the cause of mite-transmitted rickettsialpox; *R. felis,* the cause of cat flea–transmitted typhus; and *R. australis,* the cause of tick-transmitted Queensland tick typhus. One proposal creates subspecies of *R. conorii,* including subsp. *conorii* (classical MSF), subsp. *indica* (Indian tick typhus), subsp. *caspia* (Astrakhan fever), and subsp. *israelensis* (Israeli spotted fever). The recognition that *R. parkeri* and "*R. philippi*" (*Rickettsia* 364D) both cause mild spotted fever in North America and the association of high seroprevalence for spotted fever group *Rickettsia* infections in humans where *Amblyomma* ticks frequently contain *R. amblyommatis* suggest that the full range of agents that can cause spotted fever is still to be discerned.

Infections with other members of the spotted fever and transitional groups are clinically similar to MSF, with fever, maculopapular rash,

Table 255.1 | Summary of Rickettsial Diseases of Humans, Including *Rickettsia*, *Orientia*, *Ehrlichia*, *Anaplasma*, *Neorickettsia*, and *Coxiella*

GROUP OR DISEASE	AGENT	ARTHROPOD VECTOR, TRANSMISSION HOSTS		GEOGRAPHIC DISTRIBUTION	PRESENTING CLINICAL FEATURES*	COMMON LAB ABNORMALITIES*	DIAGNOSTIC TESTS	TREATMENT†
SPOTTED FEVER GROUP								
Rocky Mountain spotted fever	*Rickettsia rickettsii*	Tick bite: *Dermacentor* species (wood tick, dog tick) *Rhipicephalus sanguineus* (brown dog tick)	Dogs Rodents	Western hemisphere	Fever, headache, rash,* emesis, diarrhea, myalgias	AST, ALT ↓Na (mild) ↓Platelets ±Leukopenia Left shift	Early: IH, DFA, PCR After 1st wk: IFA	**Doxycycline** Tetracycline Chloramphenicol
Mediterranean spotted fever (boutonneuse fever)	*Rickettsia conorii*	Tick bite: *R. sanguineus* (brown dog tick)	Dogs Rodents	Africa, Mediterranean, India, Middle East	Painless eschar (tache noir) with regional lymphadenopathy, fever, headache, rash,* myalgias	AST, ALT ↓Na (mild) ↓Platelets ±Leukopenia Left shift	Early: IH, DFA, PCR After 1st wk: IFA	**Doxycycline** Tetracycline Chloramphenicol Azithromycin Clarithromycin Fluoroquinolones
African tick-bite fever	*Rickettsia africae*	Tick bite	Cattle Goats?	Sub-Saharan Africa, Caribbean	Fever, single or multiple eschars, regional lymphadenopathy, rash* (can be vesicular)	AST, ALT ↓Platelets	Early: IH, DFA After 1st wk: IFA	**Doxycycline**
Tickborne lymphadenopathy (TIBOLA); Dermacentor-borne necrosis and lymphadenopathy (DEBONEL)	*Rickettsia slovaca, Rickettsia raoultii, Rickettsia sibirica mongolotimonae*	Tick bite: *Dermacentor*	?	Europe	Eschar (scalp), painful lymphadenopathy	?	PCR	Doxycycline
Rickettsia sp, 364D genotype	"*Rickettsia philippi*"	*Dermacentor occidentalis* (Pacific coast tick)		California	Eschar, fever, headache, lymphadenopathy, malaise	Unremarkable	PCR	Doxycycline
Flea-borne spotted fever	*Rickettsia felis*	Flea bite	Opossums Cats Dogs	Western hemisphere, Europe	Fever, rash,* headache	?	Early: PCR After 1st wk: IFA	Doxycycline
TRANSITIONAL GROUP								
Rickettsialpox	*Rickettsia akari*	Mite bite	Mice	North America, Russia, Ukraine, Adriatic, Korea, South Africa	Painless eschar, ulcer or papule; tender regional lymphadenopathy, fever, headache, rash* (can be vesicular)	↓WBC	Early: IH, DFA After 1st wk: IFA	**Doxycycline** Chloramphenicol
Queensland tick typhus	*Rickettsia australis*	*Ixodes holocyclus, I. tasmani*	Bandicoots and Rodents	Australia, Tasmania	Fever, eschar, headache, myalgia, lymphadenopathy	↓WBC, ↓platelets	Early: PCR on eschar or eschar swab; After 1st wk: IFA	**Doxycycline**
TYPHUS GROUP								
Murine typhus	*Rickettsia typhi*	Flea feces	Rats Opossums	Worldwide	Fever, headache, rash,* myalgias, emesis, lymphadenopathy, hepatosplenomegaly	AST, ALT ↓Na (mild) ↓WBC ↓ Platelets	Early: DFA After 1st wk: IFA	**Doxycycline** Chloramphenicol

Disease	Organism	Reservoir	Transmission	Geographic Distribution	Clinical Features	Laboratory Findings	Diagnosis	Treatment†
Epidemic (louse-borne) typhus (recrudescent form: Brill-Zinsser disease)	*Rickettsia prowazekii*	Humans	Louse feces	South America, Central America, Mexico, Africa, Asia, Eastern Europe	Fever, headache, abdominal pain, rash,* CNS involvement	AST, ALT ↓Platelets	Early: none; After 1st wk: IgG/IgM, IFA	**Doxycycline** Tetracycline Chloramphenicol
Flying squirrel (sylvatic) typhus	*Rickettsia prowazekii*	Flying squirrels	Louse feces? Flea feces or bite?	Eastern United States	Same as above (often milder)	AST, ALT ↓Platelets	Early: none; After 1st wk: IFA	**Doxycycline** Tetracycline Chloramphenicol
SCRUB TYPHUS Scrub typhus	*Orientia tsutsugamushi*	Rodents?	Chigger bite: *Leptotrombidium*	South Asia, Japan, Indonesia, Korea, China, Russia, Australia	Fever, rash,* headache, painless eschar, hepatosplenomegaly, gastrointestinal symptoms	↓Platelets AST, ALT	Early: none; After 1st wk: IFA	**Doxycycline** Tetracycline Chloramphenicol *If doxycycline resistant:* **rifampicin** Azithromycin
EHRLICHIOSIS AND ANAPLASMOSIS Human monocytic ehrlichiosis	*Ehrlichia chaffeensis*	Deer Dogs	Tick bite: *Amblyomma americanum* (lone star tick)	United States Europe? Africa? Asia?	Fever, headache, malaise, myalgias, rash*‡ hepatosplenomegaly,‡ swollen hands/feet‡	AST, ALT ↓WBC ↓Platelets ↓Na (mild)	Early: PCR; After 1st wk: IFA	**Doxycycline** Tetracycline
Human granulocytic anaplasmosis	*Anaplasma phagocytophilum*	Rodents Deer Ruminants	Tick bite: *Ixodes* species *Haemaphysalis longicornis*	United States, Europe, Asia	Fever, headache, malaise, myalgias	AST, ALT ↓WBC, ↓ANC ↓Platelets	Early: PCR, blood smear; After 1st wk: IFA	**Doxycycline** Tetracycline Rifampin
Ewingii ehrlichiosis	*Ehrlichia ewingii*	Dogs Deer	Tick bite: *Amblyomma americanum* (lone star tick)	United States (south-central, southeast)	Fever, headache, malaise, myalgias	AST, ALT, ↓WBC ↓Platelets	Early: PCR serology not available	**Doxycycline** Tetracycline
Ehrlichia muris euclairensis infection	*Ehrlichia muris euclairensis*	?	*Ixodes scapularis*	Minnesota, Wisconsin	Fever, headache, malaise, myalgias	AST, ALT ↓WBC, ↓Platelets	Early: PCR specific serology not available	**Doxycycline**
Sennetsu neorickettsiosis	*Neorickettsia sennetsu*	fish, trematodes	Ingestion of fish helminth?, ingestion of fermented fish	Japan, Malaysia, Laos	Fever, "mononucleosis" symptoms, postauricular and posterior cervical lymphadenopathy	Atypical lymphocytosis	Early: none; After 1st wk: IFA	**Doxycycline** Tetracycline
Q FEVER Q Fever: acute (for chronic, see text)	*Coxiella burnetii*	Cattle Sheep Goats Cats Rabbits	Inhalation of infected aerosols: contact with parturient animals, abattoir, contaminated cheese and milk, ?ticks	Worldwide	Fever, headache, arthralgias, myalgias, gastrointestinal symptoms, cough, pneumonia, rash (children)	AST, ALT WBC ↓ Platelets Interstitial infiltrate	Early: PCR; After 1st wk: IFA	**Doxycycline** Tetracycline Fluoroquinolones Trimethoprim-sulfamethoxazole

*Rash is infrequently present at initial presentation but appears during the 1st wk of illness.
†Preferred treatment is in **bold**.
‡Often present in children but not adults.

ALT, alanine aminotransferase; ANC, absolute neutrophil count; AST, aspartate aminotransferase; CNS, central nervous system; DFA, direct fluorescent antibody; IFA, indirect fluorescent antibody; IgG, immunoglobulin G; IgM, immunoglobulin M; IH, immunohistochemistry; PCR, polymerase chain reaction; WBC, white blood cell count.

and eschar at the site of the tick bite. Israeli spotted fever is generally associated with a more severe course, including death, in children. African tick bite fever is relatively mild, can include a vesicular rash, and often manifests with multiple eschars. New potentially pathogenic rickettsial species have been identified, including *R. slovaca*, the cause of tickborne lymphadenopathy or *Dermacentor*-borne necrosis and lymphadenopathy. *R. aeschlimannii*, *R. heilongjiangensis*, *R. helvetica*, *R. massiliae*, and *R. raoultii* are all reported to cause mild to moderate illnesses in humans, although few cases have been described. Fortunately, the vast majority of infections respond well to doxycycline treatment if instituted early in illness; however, this is a significant challenge.

Bibliography is available at Expert Consult.

255.1 Rocky Mountain Spotted Fever (*Rickettsia rickettsii*)

Megan E. Reller and J. Stephen Dumler

RMSF is the most frequently identified and most severe rickettsial disease in the United States. It is also the most common vector-borne disease in the United States after Lyme disease. Although considered uncommon, RMSF is believed to be greatly underdiagnosed and underreported. RMSF should be considered in the differential diagnosis of fever, headache, and rash in the summer months, especially after tick exposure. Because fulminant disease and death are associated with delays in treatment, patients in whom the illness is clinically suspected should be treated promptly.

ETIOLOGY

RMSF results from systemic infection of endothelial cells by the obligate intracellular bacterium *Rickettsia rickettsii*.

EPIDEMIOLOGY

The term **Rocky Mountain spotted fever** is historical, because the agent was discovered in the Bitterroot Range of the Rocky Mountains of Montana. Few cases are reported from this region. Cases have been reported throughout the continental United States (except Vermont

and Maine), southwestern Canada, Mexico, Central America, and South America, but not from outside of the Western Hemisphere. In 2010, the Centers for Disease Control and Prevention (CDC) reporting criteria for Rocky Mountain spotted fever changed to **spotted fever group rickettsiosis,** because serology often does not distinguish *R. rickettsii* from infection by other spotted fever group *Rickettsia*. Additionally, cases detected by enzyme immunoassay were classified as probable. Thus, in 2012, 2,802 confirmed and probable cases of spotted fever rickettsiosis were reported in Morbidity and Mortality Weekly Reports Summary of Notifiable Diseases. Unlike in prior years, most cases were reported from the west south-central states, especially from Arkansas, Oklahoma, and Missouri; high numbers of cases were also reported from North Carolina, Tennessee, Virginia, New Jersey, Georgia, Alabama, and Arizona (Fig. 255.1). The incidence of RMSF cycles over 25-35 yr intervals but has generally increased over the past decades. The mean number of cases reported each year to the CDC has steadily increased (515 during 1993–1998, 946 during 1999–2004, 2,068 during 2005–2010, and 3,692 during 2011–2016), of which approximately 14% occur in those younger than 19 yr. Habitats favored by ticks, including wooded areas or coastal grassland and salt marshes, and, in the southwestern United States and Mexico, shaded areas where dogs congregate and acquire infected ticks are those that place children at increased risk for infection. Foci of intense risk for infection are found both in rural and urban areas, most recently in Mexico. Clustering of cases within families likely reflects shared environmental exposures. In the United States, 90% of cases occur between April and September, months in which humans spend the most time outdoors. The highest age-specific incidence of RMSF among children is seen in those older than 10 yr of age, with males outnumbering females; however, the highest case fatality rate for RMSF is observed in those less than 10 yr of age.

TRANSMISSION

Ticks are the natural hosts, reservoirs, and vectors of *R. rickettsii* and maintain the infection in nature by transovarial transmission (passage of the organism from infected ticks to their progeny). Ticks harboring rickettsiae are substantially less fecund than uninfected ticks; thus, horizontal transmission (acquisition of rickettsiae by taking a blood meal from transiently rickettsemic hosts such as small mammals or dogs) contributes to maintenance of rickettsial infections in ticks.

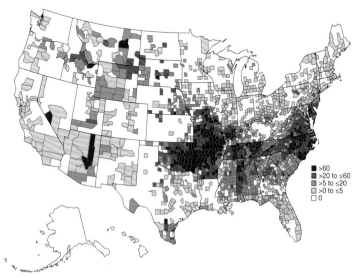

Fig. 255.1 Reported incidence rate* of spotted fever rickettsiosis,† by county—United States, 2000–2013. *As reported through national surveillance, per 1,000,000 persons per year. Cases are reported by county of residence, which is not always where the infection was acquired. †Includes Rocky Mountain spotted fever (RMSF) and other spotted fever group rickettsioses. In 2010, the name of the reporting category changed from RMSF to spotted fever rickettsiosis. *(From Biggs HM, Behravesh CB, Bradley KK, et al: Diagnosis and management of tickborne rickettsial diseases: Rocky Mountain spotted fever and other spotted fever group rickettsioses, ehrlichioses, and anaplasmosis—United States, MMWR Recomm Rep 65:1–44, 2016, Fig. 1.)*

Uninfected ticks that simultaneously feed (cofeed) with infected transmitting ticks easily become infected, even if feeding on an immune host and are also likely to be major contributors to natural transmission and maintenance. Ticks transmit the infectious agent to mammalian hosts (including humans) via infected saliva during feeding. The pathogen *R. rickettsii* in ticks becomes virulent after exposure to blood or increased temperature; thus, the longer the tick is attached, the greater the risk of transmission. The principal tick hosts of *R. rickettsii* are *Dermacentor variabilis* (the American dog tick) in the eastern United States and Canada, *Dermacentor andersoni* (the wood tick) in the western United States and Canada, *Rhipicephalus sanguineus* (the common brown dog tick) in the southwestern United States and in Mexico, and *Amblyomma cajennense* and *Amblyomma aureolatum* in Central and South America (Fig. 255.2).

Dogs can serve as reservoir hosts for *R. rickettsii*, can develop RMSF themselves, and can bring infected ticks into contact with humans. Serologic studies suggest that many patients with RMSF likely acquired the illness from ticks carried by the family dog.

Humans can also become infected when trying to remove an attached tick, because *R. rickettsii*–containing tick fluids or feces can be rubbed into the open wound at the bite site or into the conjunctivae by contaminated fingers. Inhalation of aerosolized rickettsiae has caused severe infections and deaths in laboratory workers, highlighting another mechanism of infection.

PATHOLOGY AND PATHOGENESIS

Systemic infection is most obvious on the skin (rash), but nearly all organs and tissues are affected. Following inoculation of tick saliva into the dermis, rickettsial outer surface proteins bind to the vascular endothelial cell surface proteins, which signals focal cytoskeletal changes and endocytosis. Thereafter, rickettsia phospholipase-mediated dissolution of the endosomal membranes allows escape into the cytosol. Members of the spotted fever group actively nucleate actin polymerization on 1 pole to achieve directional movement, allowing some rickettsiae to propel into neighboring cells despite minimal initial damage to its host cell. The rickettsiae proliferate and damage the host cells by oxidative membrane alterations, protease activation, or continued phospholipase activity. It is likely that some aspects of intracellular infection are mediated by rickettsial protein effectors delivered into the host cell by bacterial secretion systems.

The histologic correlate of the initial macular or maculopapular rash is perivascular infiltration of lymphoid and histiocytic cells with edema but without significant endothelial damage. Proliferation of rickettsiae within the cytoplasm of infected endothelial cells leads to endothelial injury and **lymphohistiocytic or leukocytoclastic vasculitis** of small venules and capillaries, which allows extravasation of intravascular erythrocytes into the dermis and manifests as a petechial rash (Fig. 255.3). This process is systemic and ultimately results in widespread microvascular leakage, tissue hypoperfusion, and possibly end-organ ischemic injury. Infrequently, inflammation leads to nonocclusive thrombi. Very rarely, small and large vessels become completely obliterated by thrombi, leading to tissue infarction or hemorrhagic necrosis. Interstitial pneumonitis and vascular leakage in the lungs can lead to non-cardiogenic pulmonary edema, and meningoencephalitis can cause significant cerebral edema and herniation.

The presence of the infectious agent initiates an inflammatory cascade, including release of cytokines and chemokines such as tumor necrosis factor-α, interleukin-1β, interferon-γ, and regulated upon activation, normal T-cell expressed and secreted (RANTES). Infection of endothelial cells by *R. rickettsii* induces surface E-selectin expression and procoagulant activity followed by chemokine recruitment of lymphocytes, macrophages, and, occasionally, neutrophils. Local inflammatory and immune responses are suspected to contribute to the vascular injury; however, the benefits of effective inflammation and immunity are greater. Blockade of tumor necrosis factor-α and interferon-γ action in animal models diminishes survival and increases morbidity; reactive oxygen intermediates, nitric oxide expression, and sequestration of tryptophan from rickettsiae are mechanisms by which rickettsiae are killed within cells. Direct contact of infected endothelial cells with perforin-producing CD8 T lymphocytes and interferon-γ–producing natural killer cells, accompanied by rickettsia antibody, helps control the infection. The timing and balance between rickettsia-mediated increases in vascular permeability and the benefits of induction of innate and adaptive immunity are likely the major determinants of severity and outcome.

CLINICAL MANIFESTATIONS

The incubation period of RMSF in children varies from 2 to 14 days (median: 7 days). In 49% of cases, patients or their parents report a history of removing an attached tick, although the site of the tick bite is usually inapparent. Epidemiologic clues include living in or visiting an endemic area, playing or hiking in the woods, typical season, similar illness in family members, and close contact with a dog. In patients

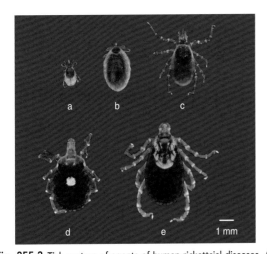

Fig. 255.2 Tick vectors of agents of human rickettsial diseases. An unengaged nymph **(A)**, engorged nymph **(B)**, and adult female **(C)** of *Ixodes scapularis* (deer tick), the vector of *Anaplasma phagocytophilum* and *Ehrlichia muris*–like agent (EMLA), the causes of human granulocytic anaplasmosis and EMLA ehrlichiosis, respectively. An adult female **(D)** of *Amblyomma americanum* (lone star tick), the vector of *Ehrlichia chaffeensis* and *Ehrlichia ewingii*, the causes of human monocytic ehrlichiosis and ewingii ehrlichiosis, respectively. An adult female **(E)** of *Dermacentor variabilis* (American dog tick), the vector of *Rickettsia rickettsii*, the cause of Rocky Mountain spotted fever.

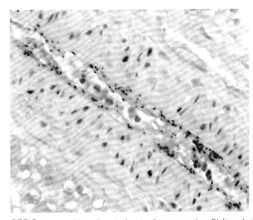

Fig. 255.3 Immunohistochemical stain demonstrating *Rickettsia* (red) in infection of blood vessel endothelial cells. (*From Biggs HM, Behravesh CB, Bradley KK, et al: Diagnosis and management of tickborne rickettsial diseases: Rocky Mountain spotted fever and other spotted fever group rickettsioses, ehrlichioses, and anaplasmosis—United States, MMWR Recomm Rep 65:1–44, 2016, Fig. 20.)*

presenting for care, the illness is initially nonspecific, and most patients are not diagnosed during their first visit with a healthcare practitioner. Manifestations often (>50%) include fever, rash (frequently involving the palms or soles), nausea and vomiting, and headache, and less often (<50%) myalgias, abdominal pain, diarrhea, conjunctival injection, altered mental status, lymphadenopathy, and peripheral edema. Pain and tenderness of calf muscles are particularly common in children.

The typical **clinical triad of fever, headache, and rash** is observed in 58% of pediatric patients overall, and rash involving soles and palms first appearing after day 3 is associated with significantly higher risk of death among Mexican children. Fever and headache persist if the illness is untreated. Fever can exceed 40°C (104°F) and can remain persistently elevated or can fluctuate dramatically. Headache is severe, unremitting, and unresponsive to analgesics.

Rash usually appears after only 1-2 days of illness, and an estimated 3–5% of children never develop a rash that is recognized. Initially, discrete, pale, rose-red blanching macules or maculopapules appear; characteristically this initial rash is observed on the extremities, including the wrists, ankles, or lower legs (Fig. 255.4). In 65% of patients, the initial rash spreads rapidly to involve the entire body, including the soles and palms. The rash can become petechial or even hemorrhagic, sometimes with palpable purpura.

In severe disease, the petechiae can enlarge into ecchymoses, which can become necrotic (Fig. 255.5). Severe vascular obstruction secondary to the rickettsial vasculitis and thrombosis is uncommon but can result in gangrene of the digits, earlobes, scrotum, nose, or an entire limb. **Central nervous system** infection usually manifests as changes in mental status (33%) or as photophobia (18%), seizure (17%), or meningismus (16%). Patients can also manifest ataxia, coma, or auditory deficits. Cerebrospinal fluid parameters are usually normal, but one-third have pleocytosis (<10-300 cells/μL), either mononuclear or less often neutrophil-dominated. Some (20%) have elevated protein (<200 mg/dL) in the cerebrospinal fluid; hypoglycorrhachia is rare. Neuroimaging studies often reveal only subtle abnormalities. However, with advanced disease and neurologic signs, a unique but nonspecific "starry sky" appearance may be observed on brain MRI that reflects the same systemic vasculitis observed with skin lesions.

Other

Pulmonary disease occurs more often in adults than in children. However, 33% of children examined have a chest radiograph interpreted as an infiltrate or pneumonia. The clinical presentation in these cases can manifest as rales, infiltrates, and noncardiogenic pulmonary edema.

Other findings can include conjunctival suffusion, periorbital edema, dorsal hand and foot edema, and hepatosplenomegaly. Severe disease can include myocarditis, acute renal failure, and vascular collapse.

Persons with glucose-6-phosphate dehydrogenase deficiency are at increased risk for fulminant RMSF, defined as death from *R. rickettsii* infection within 5 days. The clinical course of fulminant RMSF is characterized by profound coagulopathy and extensive thrombosis leading to kidney, liver, and respiratory failure. Features associated with increased risk of death include altered mental status, admission to an intensive care unit, need for inotropic support, coma, and need for rapidly administered intravenous fluid.

Occasionally, clinical signs and symptoms suggest a localized process such as appendicitis or cholecystitis. Thorough evaluation usually reveals evidence of a systemic process, and unnecessary surgical interventions are avoided.

LABORATORY FINDINGS

Laboratory abnormalities are common but nonspecific. Thrombocytopenia occurs in 60%, and the total white blood cell count is most often normal, with leukocytosis in 24% and leukopenia in 9%. Other characteristic abnormalities include a left-shifted leukocyte differential, anemia (33%), hyponatremia (<135 mEq/mL in 52%), and elevated serum aminotransferase levels (50%).

DIAGNOSIS

Delays in diagnosis and treatment are associated with severe disease and death. Because no reliable diagnostic test is readily available to confirm RMSF during acute illness, the decision to treat must be based on compatible epidemiologic, clinical, and laboratory features. RMSF should be considered in patients presenting spring through fall with an acute febrile illness accompanied by headache and myalgia (particularly if they report exposure to ticks or contact with a dog or have been in forested or tick-infested rural areas). A history of tick exposure, a rash (especially if on the palms or soles), a normal or low leukocyte count with a marked left shift, a relatively low or decreasing platelet count, and a low serum sodium concentration are all clues that can support a diagnosis of RMSF. In patients without a rash or in dark-skinned patients in whom a rash can be difficult to appreciate, the diagnosis can be exceptionally elusive and delayed. One half of pediatric deaths occur within 9 days of onset of symptoms. Thus, treatment should not be withheld pending definitive laboratory results for a patient with clinically suspected illness. Further, prompt response to early treatment is diagnostically helpful.

If a rash is present, a vasculotropic rickettsial infection can be diagnosed as early as day 1 or 2 of illness with biopsy of a petechial

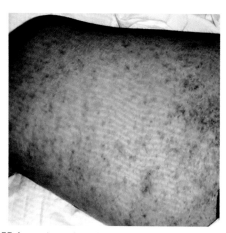

Fig. 255.4 Maculopapular rash with central petechiae associated with Rocky Mountain spotted fever. *(From Biggs HM, Behravesh CB, Bradley KK, et al: Diagnosis and management of tickborne rickettsial diseases: Rocky Mountain spotted fever and other spotted fever group rickettsioses, ehrlichioses, and anaplasmosis—United States, MMWR Recomm Rep 65:1–44, 2016, Fig. 21.)*

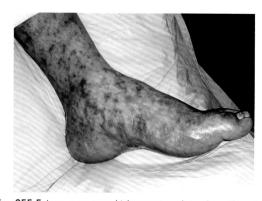

Fig. 255.5 Late-stage petechial purpuric rash involving the sole of the foot in a patient with Rocky Mountain spotted fever. *(From Biggs HM, Behravesh CB, Bradley KK, et al: Diagnosis and management of tickborne rickettsial diseases: Rocky Mountain spotted fever and other spotted fever group rickettsioses, ehrlichioses, and anaplasmosis—United States, MMWR Recomm Rep 65:1–44, 2016, Fig. 22.)*

lesion and immunohistochemical or immunofluorescent demonstration of specific rickettsial antigen in the endothelium. Although very specific, the sensitivity of this method is probably 70% at most. Furthermore, it can be adversely influenced by prior antimicrobial therapy, suboptimal selection of skin lesions for biopsy, and examination of insufficient tissue because of the focal nature of the infection. Tissue or blood can also be evaluated for *R. rickettsii* nucleic acids by polymerase chain reaction (PCR) at the CDC and selected public health or reference laboratories; PCR on blood is less sensitive than PCR on tissue and of similar sensitivity to tissue immunohistology, probably because the level of rickettsemia is generally very low (<6 rickettsiae/mL). Since eschars are rare with RMSF, scab scrapings or skin swabs are not useful specimens for the detection of rickettsemia by PCR.

Definitive diagnosis is most often accomplished by serology, which is retrospective, because a rise in titer is not seen until after the 1st wk of illness. The gold standard for the diagnosis of RMSF is a 4-fold increase in immunoglobulin G antibody titer by indirect fluorescent antibody assay between paired acute and convalescent (at 2-4 wk) sera or demonstration of seroconversion with a minimum convalescent titer higher than the positive cutoff (e.g., 128). A single titer is neither sensitive (patients can die before seroconversion) nor specific (an elevated titer can represent prior infection). Despite the historic role of IgM testing, its role in early diagnosis has recently become controversial and cannot be advocated. With current serologic methods, RMSF cannot be reliably distinguished from other spotted fever group rickettsiae infections. Cross reactions with typhus group rickettsiae also occur, but titers may be lower for the typhus group. Cross reactions are not seen with *Ehrlichia* or *Anaplasma* infections. Currently, ELISA serologic methods can only provide "probable" rather than confirmed evidence of infection. Weil-Felix antibody testing should not be performed, because it lacks both sensitivity and specificity. RMSF and other spotted fever group rickettsioses are reportable diseases in the United States.

DIFFERENTIAL DIAGNOSIS

Other rickettsial infections are easily confused with RMSF, especially all forms of human ehrlichiosis and murine typhus and novel spotted fever group rickettsioses that result from *R. parkeri* or "*R. philipii* str. 364D" infections. RMSF can also mimic a variety of other diseases, such as meningococcemia and enteroviral infections. Negative blood cultures can exclude meningococcemia. PCR can differentiate enterovirus from *R. rickettsii* in patients with aseptic meningitis and cerebrospinal fluid pleocytosis. Other diseases in the differential diagnosis are typhoid fever, secondary syphilis, Lyme disease, leptospirosis, rat-bite fever, scarlet fever, toxic shock syndrome, rheumatic fever, rubella, parvovirus infection, Kawasaki disease, idiopathic thrombocytopenic purpura, thrombotic thrombocytopenic purpura, Henoch-Schönlein purpura, hemolytic uremic syndrome, aseptic meningitis, acute gastrointestinal illness, acute abdomen, hepatitis, infectious mononucleosis, hemophagocytic and macrophage activation syndromes, dengue fever, and drug reactions.

TREATMENT

The time-proven effective therapies for RMSF are tetracyclines and chloramphenicol. The treatment of choice for suspected RMSF in patients of all ages, including children under 8 years of age, is doxycycline (4 mg/kg/day divided every 12 hr PO or IV; maximum: 200 mg/day). Tetracycline (25-50 mg/kg/day divided every 6 hr PO; maximum: 2 g/day) is an alternative. Chloramphenicol (50-100 mg/kg/day divided every 6 hr IV; maximum: 4 g/day) should be reserved for patients with doxycycline allergy and for pregnant women, because chloramphenicol is an independent risk factor for increased mortality vs tetracyclines. If used, chloramphenicol should be monitored to maintain serum concentrations of 10-30 μg/mL. Chloramphenicol is preferred for pregnant women because of potential adverse effects of doxycycline on fetal teeth and bone and maternal liver function. RMSF is a life-threatening illness for which prompt therapy is imperative, and multiple recent studies demonstrate a negligible risk for tooth discoloration in children younger than 8 yr of age with the use of doxycycline. Chloramphenicol is rarely associated with aplastic anemia and is no longer available as an oral preparation in the United States. An additional benefit of doxycycline over chloramphenicol is its effectiveness against potential concomitant *Ehrlichia* or *Anaplasma* infection. Sulfonamides should not be used, because they are associated with greater morbidity and mortality with all rickettsial infections. Other antibiotics, including penicillins, cephalosporins, and aminoglycosides, are not effective. The use of alternative antimicrobial agents, such as fluoroquinolones and the macrolides (azithromycin and clarithromycin), has not been evaluated.

Therapy should be continued for a minimum of 5-7 days and until the patient has been afebrile for at least 3 days. Treated patients usually defervesce within 48 hr, so the duration of therapy is usually <10 days.

SUPPORTIVE CARE

Most infections resolve rapidly with appropriate antimicrobial therapy and do not require hospitalization or other supportive care. Among those hospitalized, 36% require intensive care. Particular attention to hemodynamic status is mandatory in severely ill children, because iatrogenic pulmonary or cerebral edema could be easily precipitated owing to diffuse microvascular injury of the lungs, meninges, and brain. Judicious use of corticosteroids for meningoencephalitis has been advocated by some, but no controlled trials have been conducted.

COMPLICATIONS

Complications of RMSF include noncardiogenic pulmonary edema from pulmonary microvascular leakage, cerebral edema from meningoencephalitis, and multiorgan damage (hepatitis, pancreatitis, cholecystitis, epidermal necrosis, and gangrene) mediated by rickettsial vasculitis and/or the accumulated effects of hypoperfusion and ischemia (acute renal failure). Long-term neurologic sequelae can occur in any child with RMSF but are more likely to occur in those hospitalized for ≥2 wk. Examples of neurologic sequelae include speech or swallowing disorders; global encephalopathy; cerebellar, vestibular, and motor dysfunction; hearing loss; and cortical blindness. Learning disabilities and behavioral problems are the most common neurologic sequelae among children who have survived severe disease.

PROGNOSIS

Delays in diagnosis and therapy are significant factors associated with severe illness or death. Before the advent of effective antimicrobial therapy for RMSF, the case fatality rate was 10% for children and 30% for adults. The overall case fatality rate decreased to an historic low (0.3–0.4%) from 2003 to 2012; however, many experts attribute this decrease to detection and reporting of other less virulent emerging forms of spotted fever group rickettsioses that cannot be readily differentiated from RMSF using current serologic tests. The overall case fatality rate of children 5-9 yr of age was 2.4%, and rates as high as 8.5% and 11.8% were documented in Texas (1986–1996) and in Arizona (1999–2007), respectively, and rates as high as 30–40% are now reported from outbreaks in Mexico. Diagnosis based on serology alone underestimates the true mortality of RMSF, because death often occurs within 14 days (before developing a serologic response). Deaths occur despite the availability of effective therapeutic agents, indicating the need for clinical vigilance and a low threshold for early empiric therapy. Even with administration of appropriate antimicrobials, delayed therapy can lead to irreversible vascular or end-organ damage and long-term sequelae or death. Early therapy in uncomplicated cases usually leads to rapid defervescence within 1-3 days and recovery within 7-10 days. A slower response may be seen if therapy is delayed. In those who survive despite no treatment, fever subsides in 2-3 wks.

PREVENTION

No vaccines are available. Prevention of RMSF is best accomplished by preventing or treating tick infestation in dogs, avoiding areas where ticks reside, using insect repellents containing N, N-diethyl-3-methylbenzamide (DEET) or new alternatives (https://www.epa.gov/insect-repellents/find-repellent-right-you), wearing protective clothing, and carefully inspecting children after play in areas where they are potentially exposed to ticks. Recovery from infection yields lifelong immunity.

Prompt and complete removal of attached ticks helps reduce the risk for transmission because rickettsiae in the ticks need to be reactivated to become virulent, and this requires at least several hours to days of exposure to body heat or blood. Contrary to popular belief, the application of petroleum jelly, 70% isopropyl alcohol, fingernail polish, or a hot match are not effective in removing ticks. A tick can be safely removed by grasping the mouth parts with a pair of forceps at the site of attachment to the skin and applying gentle and steady pressure to achieve retraction without twisting, thereby removing the entire tick and its mouth parts. The site of attachment should then be disinfected. Ticks should not be squeezed or crushed, because their fluids may be infectious. The removed tick should be soaked in alcohol or flushed down the toilet, and hands should be washed to avoid accidental inoculation into conjunctivae, mucous membranes, or breaks in skin. Typically, prophylactic antimicrobial therapy is not recommended because tetracyclines and chloramphenicol are only rickettsiastatic; however, the evidence to support this position is meager.

Bibliography is available at Expert Consult.

255.2 Mediterranean Spotted Fever or Boutonneuse Fever (*Rickettsia conorii*)

Megan E. Reller and J. Stephen Dumler

MSF or boutonneuse fever is caused by *R. conorii* and its related subspecies; it is also called by other names, such as Kenya tick typhus, Indian tick typhus, Israeli spotted fever, and Astrakhan fever. It is a moderately severe vasculotropic rickettsiosis in adults but comparatively milder in children, with more frequent lymphadenopathy; often, MSF is initially associated with an eschar at the site of the tick bite. Minor differences in clinical presentation could be associated with genetic diversity of the rickettsial subspecies.

ETIOLOGY

MSF is caused by systemic endothelial cell infection by the obligate intracellular bacterium *R. conorii*. Similar species are distributed globally, such as *R. sibirica*, *R. heilongjiangensis*, and *R. mongolotimonae* in Russia, China, Mongolia, and Pakistan; *R. australis* and *R. honei* in Australia; *R. japonica* in Japan; *R. africae* in South Africa; and *R. parkeri* and "*R. philippi* str. 364D" in the Americas (see Table 255.1). Analysis of antigens and related DNA sequences show that all are closely related within a broad genetic clade that includes spotted fever group *Rickettsia* species such as *R. rickettsii*, the cause of RMSF.

EPIDEMIOLOGY

R. conorii is distributed over a large geographic region, including India, Pakistan, Russia, Ukraine, Georgia, Israel, Morocco, southern Europe, Ethiopia, Kenya, and South Africa. Reported cases of MSF in southern Europe have steadily increased since 1980, and the seroprevalence is 11–26% in some areas. The peak in reported cases occurs during July and August in the Mediterranean basin; in other regions it occurs during warm months when ticks are active.

TRANSMISSION

Transmission occurs after the bite of the brown dog tick, *R. sanguineus*, or for other *Rickettsia* spp. tick genera such as *Dermacentor*, *Haemaphysalis*, *Amblyomma*, *Hyalomma*, and *Ixodes*. Clustering of human cases of boutonneuse fever, infected ticks, and infected dogs implicate the household dog as a potential vehicle for transmission.

PATHOLOGY AND PATHOGENESIS

The underlying pathology seen with MSF is nearly identical to that of RMSF, except that eschars are often present at the site of tick bite where inoculation of rickettsiae occurs. The histopathology of the resultant lesion includes necrosis of dermal and epidermal tissues with a superficial crust; a dermis densely infiltrated by lymphocytes, histiocytes, and

scattered neutrophils; and damaged capillaries and venules in the dermis. Immunohistochemical stains and nucleic acid amplification tests confirm that the lesions contain rickettsia-infected endothelial cells, and potentially other cells such as macrophages. The necrosis results from both direct rickettsia-mediated vasculitis and resultant extensive local inflammation. Thus, rickettsiae have ready access to lymphatics and venous blood and disseminate to cause systemic disease.

CLINICAL MANIFESTATIONS AND LABORATORY FINDINGS

Typical findings in children include fever (37–100%), a maculopapular rash that appears 3–5 days after onset of fever (94–100%), hepatosplenomegaly (20–83%), myalgias and arthralgias (10–42%), headache (8–63%), nausea, vomiting, or diarrhea (5–28%), and lymphadenopathy (52–54%). In 60–90% of patients, a **painless eschar** or **tache noire** appears at the site of the tick bite, often on the scalp, with accompanying regional lymphadenopathy (50–60%) (Fig. 255.6). The infection can be severe, mimicking RMSF, although morbidity and fatalities in children are less frequent than in adults. Findings can include seizures, purpuric skin lesions, meningitis and neurologic deficits, respiratory and/or acute renal failure, and severe thrombocytopenia. Even though the case fatality rate can be as high as 10% in adults and severe infections occur in approximately 9% of children, pediatric deaths are rare. As with RMSF, a particularly severe form occurs in patients with glucose-6-phosphate dehydrogenase deficiency and in patients with underlying conditions such as alcoholic liver disease or diabetes mellitus.

DIAGNOSIS

Laboratory diagnosis of MSF and related spotted fever group rickettsioses is the same as that for RMSF. Cases can be confirmed by immunohistologic or immunofluorescent or demonstration of or amplification of nucleic acids from rickettsiae in skin biopsies, in vitro cultivation via centrifugation-assisted shell vial tissue culture, or demonstration of seroconversion or accompanied by a 4-fold rise in serum antibody titer to spotted fever group rickettsiae between acute and convalescent sera. Antibodies to spotted fever group antigens cross react, so RMSF or other spotted fever group rickettsiosis in the United States or MSF in Europe, Africa, and Asia cannot be distinguished by these methods. When eschars are present, biopsy of the eschar with submission of tissue or a swab of the base for PCR provides considerably higher sensitivity than PCR on blood and is advocated, if available. Treatment should not be withheld while waiting for diagnostic test results.

DIFFERENTIAL DIAGNOSIS

The differential diagnosis includes conditions also associated with single eschars, such as anthrax, bacterial ecthyma, brown recluse spider bite, rat-bite fever (caused by *Spirillum minus*), and other rickettsioses (such as rickettsialpox, African tick-bite fever, *R. parkeri* or *R. philipii* str. 364D rickettsiosis, and scrub typhus). The spotted fever group rickettsia *R. africae* causes African tick-bite fever, a milder illness than MSF that is often associated with multiple eschars and occasionally a vesicular

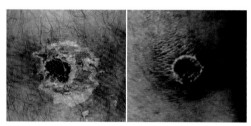

Fig. 255.6 Various appearances of eschars associated with *Rickettsia parkeri* rickettsiosis. (*From Biggs HM, Behravesh CB, Bradley KK, et al: Diagnosis and management of tickborne rickettsial diseases: Rocky Mountain spotted fever and other spotted fever group rickettsioses, ehrlichioses, and anaplasmosis—United States, MMWR Recomm Rep 65:1–44, 2016, Fig. 24.*)

rash. African tick-bite fever can be contracted in North Africa, where MSF also occurs and is a common infection of travelers to sub-Saharan Africa who encounter bush or high grasslands on safari. *R. parkeri* and *R. philipii* str. 364D rickettsiosis are emerging infections in North and South America and in the U.S. western states, respectively. Both often present with an eschar and milder clinical manifestations similar to those observed with African tick-bite fever.

TREATMENT AND SUPPORTIVE CARE

In adults, MSF is effectively treated with tetracycline, doxycycline, chloramphenicol, ciprofloxacin, ofloxacin, levofloxacin, azithromycin, or clarithromycin. For children, the treatment of choice is doxycycline (4 mg/kg/day divided every 12 hr PO or IV; maximum: 200 mg/day). Tetracycline and chloramphenicol are alternatives, as for RMSF. Azithromycin (10 mg/kg/day once daily PO for 3 days), azithromycin (10 mg/kg/day once daily) and clarithromycin (15 mg/kg/day divided twice daily PO for 7 days) are also used. Specific fluoroquinolones regimens effective for children have not been established, although recent reports suggest the use of fluoroquinolones is associated with increased disease severity as compared with doxycycline. Intensive care may be required.

COMPLICATIONS

The complications of MSF are similar to those of RMSF. Overall, the case fatality rate is less than 2%, but fatalities are rare in children. Particularly severe infections have been noted in patients with underlying medical conditions, including glucose-6-phosphate dehydrogenase deficiency and diabetes mellitus.

PREVENTION

MSF is transmitted by tick bites, and prevention is the same as recommended for RMSF. No vaccine is currently available.

Bibliography is available at Expert Consult.

255.3 Rickettsialpox (Rickettsia akari) and Flea-Borne Spotted Fever

Megan E. Reller and J. Stephen Dumler

Rickettsialpox is caused by *R. akari*, a transitional group *Rickettsia* species

that is transmitted by the mouse mite, *Allodermanyssus sanguineus.* The mouse host for this mite is widely distributed in cities in the United States, Europe, and Asia. Seroepidemiologic studies suggest a high prevalence of this infection in urban settings. The disease is uncommon and is usually mild. Unlike the situation with most forms of rickettsiosis, the macrophage is an important target cell for *R. akari.*

Rickettsialpox is best known because of its association with a varicelliform rash. In fact, this rash is a modified form of an antecedent typical macular or maculopapular rash like those seen in other vasculotropic rickettsioses and is occasionally seen with other rickettsioses such as African tick-bite fever. Clinical descriptions in children are infrequent. At presentation, most patients have fever, headache, and chills. In up to 90% of cases, there is a painless papular, ulcerative lesion, or eschar, at the initial site of inoculation, which can be associated with tender regional lymphadenopathy. In some patients, the maculopapular rash becomes vesicular, involving the trunk, head, and extremities. The infection generally resolves spontaneously and does not require therapy. However, a short course of doxycycline hastens resolution and is sometimes used in patients older than 8 yr of age and in young children with relatively severe illness. Complications and fatalities are rare; however, clear examples of severe disease in children like that observed with RMSF are described.

Flea-borne spotted fever, caused by *Rickettsia felis*, is often considered within the typhus group because of flea transmission; however, phylogenetic studies place it close to the *Rickettsia* genus spotted fever or within the "transitional" group. Similarly, a related cat flea-associated agent, *R. asembonensis*, was isolated from cat fleas and has been identified in environmental samples over broad geographic regions. Since the discovery of *R. felis* in a febrile patient from Texas by use of molecular amplification methods, and its subsequent isolation from infected cat fleas, molecular and cross-reactive serologic tests have purported to identify human infections globally, some at high rates of prevalence. Clinical isolates have yet to be made from infected humans, and many patients identified by molecular methods lack serologic responses or even clinical signs. Its identification within mosquitoes and in conjunction with malaria further confound its role as a human pathogen. Until many of the discrepant findings observed with *R. felis* are resolved, its role as an important infectious agent in humans remains to be resolved.

Bibliography is available at Expert Consult.

Chapter 256
Scrub Typhus *(Orientia tsutsugamushi)*

Megan E. Reller and J. Stephen Dumler

第二百五十六章
恙虫病（恙虫病东方体）

中文导读

　　本章主要介绍了恙虫病的病原学、流行病学、传播途径、病理和发病机制、临床表现和实验室检查、诊断和鉴别诊断、治疗和维持治疗、并发症和预防。该病是由恙虫病东方体感染传播导致，经恙螨叮咬传播。发病机制主要是感染引起免疫炎症导致弥漫性血管炎及血管周围炎症。临床表现可涉及多个器官，可有发热、皮疹、肝脾大、消化道症状、血液系统异常等。诊断主要依靠血清学检测，病原学检测敏感度低，需与不明原因发热、伤寒、登革出血热、其他立克次氏体病等多种疾病鉴别。治疗首选强力霉素，并介绍了其他替代治疗。可发生肺炎、脑膜炎等严重并发症。切断传播途径为主要预防方法。

Scrub typhus is an important cause of acute febrile illness in South and East Asia and the Pacific and could be emerging in the Middle East and South America. The causative agent is distinct from, but related to, *Rickettsia* species. The infection is transmitted via chigger (larval mite) bites and involves many antigenically diverse strains of *Orientia tsutsugamushi*, hampering vaccine development.

ETIOLOGY

The causative agent of scrub typhus, or tsutsugamushi fever, is *O. tsutsugamushi,* which is distinct from other spotted fever and typhus group rickettsiae (see Table 255.1 in Chapter 255). *O. tsutsugamushi* lacks both lipopolysaccharide and peptidoglycan in its cell wall. Like other vasculotropic rickettsiae, *O. tsutsugamushi* infects endothelial cells and causes vasculitis, the predominant clinicopathologic feature of the disease. However, the organism also infects macrophages and cardiac myocytes. A new *Candidatus* species, *Orientia chuto*, was isolated from a patient in the Middle East, and definitive evidence of infection based on serology and/or PCR amplification of *O. tsutsugamushi* genes from acute phase blood suggests a wider range for scrub typhus and related infections.

EPIDEMIOLOGY

More than 1 million infections occur each year, and it is estimated that more than 1 billion people are at risk. Scrub typhus occurs mostly in Asia, including areas delimited by Korea, Pakistan, and northern Australia. Outside these tropical and subtropical regions, the disease occurs in Japan, the Primorsky of far eastern Russia, Tajikistan, Nepal, and nontropical China, including Tibet. Cases imported to the United States and other parts of the world are reported. Endemic scrub typhus has historically been confined to Asia and Oceania and the tsutsugamushi triangle; however, *Orientia* may be distributed more broadly, with confirmed cases in South America and possible cases in Africa. Most infections in children are acquired in rural areas. In Thailand and Sri Lanka, scrub typhus is the cause of 1–8% of acute fevers of unknown origin. Infections are most common during rainy months, usually June through November. Reported cases in boys are higher than in girls.

TRANSMISSION

O. tsutsugamushi is transmitted via the bite of the larval stage (chigger) of a trombiculid mite *(Leptotrombidium),* which serves as both vector and reservoir. Vertical transovarial transmission (passage of the organism from infected mites to their progeny) is the major mechanism for maintenance in nature. Because only the larval stage takes blood meals, a role for horizontal transmission from infected rodent hosts to uninfected mites has not been proved, but transmission among co-feeding larval mites is a possibility. Multiple serotypes of *O. tsutsugamushi* are recognized, and some share antigenic cross reactivity; however, they do not stimulate protective cross-immunity.

PATHOLOGY AND PATHOGENESIS

The pathogenesis of scrub typhus is uncertain. The process may be stimulated by widespread infection of vascular endothelial cells, which corresponds to the distribution of disseminated vasculitic and perivascular inflammatory lesions observed in histopathologic examinations. In autopsy series, the major result of the vascular injury appears to be hemorrhage. However, data support the concept that vascular injury nitiated by the infection is sustained by immune-mediated inflammation that together cause significant vascular leakage. The net result is significant vascular compromise and ensuing end-organ injury, most often manifested in the brain and lungs, as with other vasculotropic rickettsioses.

CLINICAL MANIFESTATIONS AND LABORATORY FINDINGS

Scrub typhus can be mild or severe in children and can affect almost every organ system. Most patients present with fever for 9-11 days (range: 1-30 days) before seeking medical care. Regional or generalized lymphadenopathy is reported in 23–93% of patients, hepatomegaly in about two-thirds, and splenomegaly in about one-third of children with scrub typhus. Gastrointestinal symptoms, including abdominal pain, vomiting, and diarrhea, occur in up to 40% of children at presentation. A **single painless eschar** with an erythematous rim at the site of the chigger bite is seen in 7–68% of cases, and a maculopapular rash is present in less than half; both can be absent. Hemophagocytic lymphohistiocytosis has been described. Leukocyte and platelet counts are most commonly within normal ranges, although thrombocytopenia occurs in one-quarter to one-third of children, and leukocytosis is observed in approximately 40% of children. Clinical manifestations often respond dramatically to appropriate treatment. Adverse outcomes in fetuses and newborn infants of infected mothers have been described, resulting from vertical transmission.

DIAGNOSIS AND DIFFERENTIAL DIAGNOSIS

Owing to the potential for severe complications, diagnosis and decision to initiate treatment should be based on clinical suspicion and confirmed by *O. tsutsugamushi* serologic tests such as indirect fluorescent antibody. The indirect fluorescent antibody assay is >90% sensitive with 11 days or more of fever, but interpretations vary with prevalence of infection in endemic regions. Although the rickettsiae can be cultivated using tissue culture methods, polymerase chain reaction tests are not highly sensitive, and these diagnostic methods are not widely available. The differential diagnosis includes fever of unknown origin, enteric fever, typhoid fever, dengue hemorrhagic fever, other rickettsioses, tularemia, anthrax, dengue, leptospirosis, malaria, and infectious mononucleosis.

TREATMENT AND SUPPORTIVE CARE

The recommended treatment regimen for scrub typhus is doxycycline 4 mg/kg/day PO or IV divided every 12 hr; maximum: 200 mg/day).

Alternative regimens include tetracycline (25-50 mg/kg/day PO divided every 6 hr; maximum: 2 g/day) or chloramphenicol (50-100 mg/kg/day divided every 6 hr IV; maximum: 4 g/24 hr). If used, chloramphenicol should be monitored to maintain serum concentrations of 10-30 µg/mL. Alternatives, now supported by data from randomized trials, include azithromycin (10 mg/kg PO on day 1, then 5 mg/kg PO; maximum: 500 mg/day) or clarithromycin (15-30 mg/kg/day PO divided every 12 hr; maximum: 1 g/day). Therapy should be continued for a minimum of 5 days and until the patient has been afebrile for at least 3 days to avoid relapse. However, a single dose of oral doxycycline was reported effective for all 38 children treated with this regimen in a large series of children with scrub typhus from Thailand. Most children respond rapidly to doxycycline or chloramphenicol within 1-2 days (range: 1-5 days). Strains of *O. tsutsugamushi* with modestly higher doxycycline minimal inhibitory concentrations are reported in some regions of Thailand. Clinical trials showed that azithromycin could be as effective, and that rifampicin is superior to doxycycline in such cases and could have a role as an alternative therapy, especially for pregnant women. The use of ciprofloxacin in pregnant women resulted in an adverse outcome in 5 of 5 pregnancies among Indian women. Intensive care may be required for hemodynamic management of severely affected patients.

COMPLICATIONS

Serious complications include pneumonitis in 20–35% and meningoencephalitis in approximately 10–25% of children. Acute renal failure, myocarditis, and a septic shock–like syndrome occur much less often. Cerebrospinal fluid examination shows a mild mononuclear pleocytosis with normal glucose levels. Chest radiographs reveal transient perihilar or peribronchial interstitial infiltrates in most children who are examined. Among 883 patients <20 yr of age in 18 published studies, the case fatality rate was 11%; the median for the studies was 1.6–1.8% and ranged as high as 33%.

PREVENTION

Prevention is based on avoidance of the chiggers that transmit *O. tsutsugamushi*. Protective clothing is the next most useful mode of prevention. Infection provides immunity to reinfection by homologous but not heterologous strains; however, because natural strains are highly heterogeneous, infection does not always provide complete protection against reinfection. No vaccines are currently available.

Bibliography is available at Expert Consult.

Chapter **257**

Typhus Group Rickettsioses

Megan E. Reller and J. Stephen Dumler

第二百五十七章
斑疹伤寒群立克次体

中文导读

　　本章主要介绍了地方性斑疹伤寒和流行性斑疹伤寒两种疾病。地方性斑疹伤寒是指由斑疹伤寒立克次体经鼠蚤为媒介而引起的急性传染病，主要表现为病原体感染引起的全身血管炎症状，部分患儿为自限性，详细介绍了本病的临床表现，诊断部分指出比较

急性期和恢复期抗体滴度为常用诊断方法。流行性斑疹伤寒是普氏立克次体通过体虱传播的急性传染病。临床表现多样，中枢神经系统症状明显。在治疗部分均指出首选强力霉素，替代疗法包括四环素或氯霉素，切断传播媒介可有效控制该病传播。

Members of the typhus group of rickettsiae (see Table 255.1 in Chapter 255) include *Rickettsia typhi,* the cause of murine typhus, and *Rickettsia prowazekii,* the cause of louse-borne or epidemic typhus. *R. typhi* is transmitted to humans by fleas, and *R. prowazekii* is transmitted in the feces of body lice. Louse-borne or epidemic typhus is widely considered to be the most virulent of the rickettsial diseases, with a high case fatality rate even with treatment. Murine typhus is moderately severe and likely underreported worldwide. The genomes of both *R. typhi* and *R. prowazekii* are similar.

Bibliography is available at Expert Consult.

257.1 Murine (Endemic or Flea-Borne) Typhus *(Rickettsia typhi)*

Megan E. Reller and J. Stephen Dumler

ETIOLOGY

Murine typhus is caused by *R. typhi,* a rickettsia transmitted from infected fleas to rats, other rodents, or opossums and back to fleas. Transovarial transmission (passage of the organism from infected fleas to their progeny) in fleas is inefficient. Transmission depends on infection from the flea to uninfected mammals that then sustain transient rickettsemia and serve as sources of the bacterium for uninfected fleas that bite during the period of rickettsemia.

EPIDEMIOLOGY

Murine typhus has a worldwide distribution and occurs especially in warm coastal ports, where it is maintained in a cycle involving rat fleas (*Xenopsylla cheopis*) and rats (*Rattus* species). Peak incidence occurs when rat populations are highest during spring, summer, and fall. Sentinel surveillance studies suggest that travel-acquired murine typhus occurs most often in those visiting Southeast Asia and Africa. In the United States, the disease is recognized most often in south Texas and Southern California. However, seroprevalence studies among children indicate that murine typhus is acquired across the southeast and south-central United States, thus expanding the endemic areas in which pediatricians must be alert for this infection. In the coastal areas of south Texas and in Southern California, the disease is seen predominantly from March through June and is associated with a *sylvatic cycle* involving opossums and cat fleas (*Ctenocephalides felis*).

TRANSMISSION

R. typhi normally cycles between rodents or midsize animals such as opossums and their fleas. Human acquisition of murine typhus occurs when rickettsiae-infected flea feces contaminate flea bite wounds. Direct inoculation via flea bite is possible, but inefficient.

PATHOLOGY AND PATHOGENESIS

R. typhi is a vasculotropic rickettsia that causes disease in a manner similar to *Rickettsia rickettsii* (see Chapter 255.1). *R. typhi* organisms in flea feces deposited on the skin as part of the flea feeding reflex are inoculated into the pruritic flea bite wound. After an interval for local proliferation, the rickettsiae spread systemically via lymphatics to the blood, after which they infect the endothelium in many tissues. As with spotted fever group rickettsiae, typhus group rickettsiae infect endothelial cells, but unlike the spotted fever group rickettsiae, they polymerize intracellular actin poorly, have limited intracellular mobility, and probably cause cellular injury by either enzymatic membrane or mechanical lysis after accumulating in large numbers within the endothelial cell cytoplasm. Intracellular infection leads to endothelial cell damage, recruitment of inflammatory cells, and vasculitis. The inflammatory cell infiltrates bring in a number of effector cells, including macrophages that produce proinflammatory cytokines, and CD4, CD8, and natural killer lymphocytes, which can produce immune cytokines such as interferon-γ or participate in cell-mediated cytotoxic responses. Intracellular rickettsial proliferation of typhus group rickettsiae is inhibited by cytokine-mediated mechanisms and nitric oxide–dependent and –independent mechanisms.

Pathologic findings include systemic vasculitis in response to rickettsiae within endothelial cells. This vasculitis manifests as interstitial pneumonitis, meningoencephalitis, interstitial nephritis, myocarditis, and mild hepatitis with periportal lymphohistiocytic infiltrates. As vasculitis and inflammatory damage accumulate, multiorgan damage can ensue.

CLINICAL MANIFESTATIONS

In children, murine typhus is a generally a self-limited infection, but can be severe, similar to other vasculotropic rickettsioses. The incubation period varies from 1 to 2 wk. The initial presentation is often nonspecific and mimics typhoid fever; fever of undetermined origin is the most common presentation. Pediatric patients with murine typhus exhibit symptoms classically attributed to other vasculotropic rickettsioses, such as rash (48–80%), myalgias (29–57%), vomiting (29–45%), cough (15–40%), headache (19–77%), and diarrhea or abdominal pain (10–40%). A petechial rash is observed in <15% of children, and the usual appearance is that of macules or maculopapules distributed on the trunk and extremities. The rash can involve both the soles and palms. Among common clinical features, only abdominal pain, diarrhea, and sore throat are more common in children than in adults, underscoring the mild nature of most cases in children. Murine-typhus associated hemophagocytic syndrome was recently described. Although neurologic involvement is a common finding in adults with murine typhus, photophobia, confusion, stupor, coma, seizures, meningismus, and ataxia are seen in <20% of hospitalized children and <6% of infected children treated as outpatients. Poor neonatal outcomes are reported with infection during pregnancy; however, both the frequency and clinical spectrum are not well documented.

LABORATORY FINDINGS

Although nonspecific, laboratory findings are less severe than in adults. Helpful findings include mild leukopenia (28–40%) with a moderate left shift, mild to marked thrombocytopenia (30–60%), hyponatremia (20–66%), hypoalbuminemia (30–87%), and elevated aspartate aminotransferase (82%) and alanine aminotransferase (38%). Elevations in serum urea nitrogen are usually a result of prerenal mechanisms.

DIAGNOSIS AND DIFFERENTIAL DIAGNOSIS

Delays in diagnosis and therapy are associated with increased morbidity and mortality; thus, diagnosis must be based on clinical suspicion. Occasionally, patients present with findings suggesting pharyngitis, bronchitis, hepatitis, gastroenteritis, or sepsis; thus, the differential diagnosis may be extensive.

Confirmation of the diagnosis is usually accomplished by comparing acute and convalescent-phase antibody titers obtained with the indirect fluorescent antibody assay to demonstrate a 4-fold rise in titer. Current objective studies of the diagnostic yield of *R. typhi* nucleic acid amplification from acute-phase whole blood show disappointingly low sensitivity, and rickettsial culture is not readily available. Thus, paired (acute and convalescent) serology to demonstrate a 4-fold rise in IgG antibody titer by IFA remains the standard for confirming acute infection. Use of IgM serologic tests is discouraged for diagnosis of rickettsial infections, because of both limited sensitivity and specificity.

TREATMENT

A meta-analysis of murine typhus in children reviewed treatment in 261 children, including 54 who received no antimicrobial therapy. Although 15% had complications, there we no deaths. The standard therapy for murine typhus in children was similar to that for adults and focused on use of tetracyclines or chloramphenicol. No controlled trials of other antimicrobial agents have been performed. Quinolones have been used in children, and limited clinical studies show that ciprofloxacin is as effective as doxycycline and chloramphenicol to treat murine typhus; however, treatment failures are reported. In vitro experiments suggest that minimal inhibitory concentrations of azithromycin and clarithromycin for *R. typhi* should be easily achieved.

Therefore, the time-honored recommended treatment for murine typhus remains doxycycline (4 mg/kg/day divided every 12 hr PO or IV; maximum: 200 mg/day). Alternative regimens include tetracycline (25-50 mg/kg/day divided every 6 hr PO; maximum: 2 g/day) or chloramphenicol (50-100 mg/kg/day divided every 6 hr IV; maximum: 4 g/day). Therapy should be for a minimum of 5 days continued until the patient has been afebrile for at least 3 days.

SUPPORTIVE CARE

Although disease is usually mild, 15% of children have complications and 2–7% require intensive care for management of meningoencephalitis, a disseminated intravascular coagulation–like condition, or other conditions. As for other rickettsial infections with significant systemic vascular injury, careful hemodynamic management is mandatory to avoid pulmonary or cerebral edema.

COMPLICATIONS

Complications of murine typhus in pediatric patients are uncommon; however, relapse, stupor, facial edema, dehydration, splenic rupture, and meningoencephalitis are reported. Predominance of abdominal pain has led to surgical exploration to exclude a perforated viscus.

PREVENTION

Control of murine typhus was dependent on elimination of the flea reservoir and control of flea hosts, and this approach remains important. However, with the recognition of cat fleas as potentially significant reservoirs and vectors, the presence of these flea vectors and their mammalian hosts in suburban areas where close human exposures occur poses increasingly difficult control problems. It is not known with certainty if infection confers protective immunity; reinfection appears to be rare.

Bibliography is available at Expert Consult.

257.2 Epidemic (Louse-Borne) Typhus (*Rickettsia prowazekii*)

Megan E. Reller and J. Stephen Dumler

ETIOLOGY

Humans are considered the principal reservoir of *R. prowazekii,* the causative agent of epidemic or louse-borne typhus and its recrudescent form, Brill-Zinsser disease. Another reservoir exists in flying squirrels, their ectoparasites, and potentially ticks, in a sylvatic cycle with small rodents. *R. prowazekii* is the most pathogenic member of the genus *Rickettsia* and multiplies to very large intracellular quantities before rupture of infected endothelial cells.

EPIDEMIOLOGY

The infection is characteristically seen in winter or spring and especially during times of poor hygienic practices associated with crowding, war, famine, extreme poverty, and civil strife. As observed in a recent outbreak among youths at a rehabilitation center in Rwanda, infections in children under these conditions can lead to severe adverse outcomes. *R. prowazekii* has also been associated with sporadic cases of a mild, typhus-like illness in the United States; such cases are associated with exposure to flying squirrels harboring infected lice or fleas. *R. prowazekii* organisms isolated from these squirrels appear to be genetically similar to isolates obtained during typical outbreaks.

Most cases of louse-borne typhus in the developed world are sporadic, but outbreaks have been identified in Africa (Ethiopia, Nigeria, Rwanda, and Burundi), Mexico, Central America, South America, Eastern Europe, Afghanistan, Russia, northern India, and China within the past 25 yr. Following the Burundi Civil War in 1993, 35,000-100,000 cases of epidemic typhus were diagnosed in displaced refugees, resulting in an estimated 6,000 deaths.

TRANSMISSION

Human body lice (Pediculus humanus corporis) become infected by feeding on persons who have rickettsiae circulating in their blood owing to endothelial infection. The ingested rickettsiae infect the midgut epithelial cells of the lice and are passed into the feces, which, in turn, are introduced into a susceptible human host through abrasions or perforations in the skin, through the conjunctivae, or rarely through inhalation as fomites in clothing, bedding, or furniture.

CLINICAL MANIFESTATIONS

Louse-borne typhus can be mild or severe in children. The incubation period is usually <14 days. The typical clinical manifestations include fever, severe headache, abdominal tenderness, and rash in most patients, as well as chills (82%), myalgias (70%), arthralgias (70%), anorexia (48%), nonproductive cough (38%), dizziness (35%), photophobia (33%), nausea (32%), abdominal pain (30%), tinnitus (23%), constipation (23%), meningismus (17%), visual disturbances (15%), vomiting (10%), and diarrhea (7%). However, investigation of recent African outbreaks has shown a lower incidence of rash (25%) and a high incidence of delirium (81%) and cough associated with pneumonitis (70%). The rash is initially pink or erythematous and blanches. In one-third of patients, red, nonblanching macules and petechiae appear predominantly on the trunk. Infections identified during the preantibiotic era typically produced a variety of central nervous system findings, including delirium (48%), coma (6%), and seizures (1%). Estimates of case fatality rates range between 3.5% and 20% in outbreaks.

Brill-Zinsser disease is a form of typhus that becomes recrudescent months to years after the primary infection, thus rarely affecting children. When bacteremic with rickettsiae, these infected patients can transmit the agent to lice, potentially providing the initial event that triggers an outbreak if hygienic conditions permit.

TREATMENT

Recommended treatment regimens for louse-borne or sylvatic typhus are identical to those used for murine typhus. The treatment of choice is doxycycline (4 mg/kg/day divided every 12 hr PO or IV; maximum: 200 mg/day). Alternative treatments include tetracycline (25-50 mg/kg/day divided every 6 hr PO; maximum: 2 g/day) or chloramphenicol (50-100 mg/kg/day divided every 6 hr IV; maximum: 4 g/day). Therapy should be continued for a minimum of 5 days and until the patient is afebrile for at least 3 days. Evidence exists that doxycycline as a single 200 mg oral dose (4.4 mg/kg if < 45 kg) is also efficacious.

PREVENTION

Immediate destruction of vectors with an insecticide is important in the control of an epidemic. Lice live in clothing rather than on the skin; thus, searches for ectoparasites should include examination of clothing. For epidemic typhus, antibiotic therapy and delousing measures interrupt transmission, reduce the prevalence of infection in the human reservoir, and diminish the impact of an outbreak. Dust containing excreta from infected lice is stable and capable of transmitting typhus, and care must be taken to prevent its inhalation. Infection confers solid protective immunity. However, recrudescence can occur years later with Brill-Zinsser disease, implying that immunity is not complete.

Bibliography is available at Expert Consult.

Chapter 258

Ehrlichiosis and Anaplasmosis

J. Stephen Dumler and Megan E. Reller

第二百五十八章
埃立克体病和无形体病

中文导读

　　本章主要介绍了埃立克体病和无形体病。人埃立克体病是指菲埃立克体感染引起的人单核细胞埃立克体病，人无形体病主要指嗜吞噬细胞无形体感染所致的人粒细胞无形体病。详细讲述了两种疾病病原的发现与分类，病原的传播媒介及途径，介绍了疾病的病理和发病机制，两种疾病均与病原体导致的血管炎症和免疫损伤相关。详细介绍了两种疾病的临床表现及实验室检查，诊断学方法，因临床表现缺乏特异性，需与其他因节肢动物传播的感染、皮疹和弥散性血管内凝血为主要表现的疾病相鉴别，详细介绍了治疗方法，指出四环素类药物为首选治疗。患者可发生机会性感染、呼吸窘迫综合征、弥散性血管内凝血等严重并发症，避免蜱虫叮咬为主要预防手段。

ETIOLOGY

Ehrlichiosis in humans was 1st described in 1987, when clusters of bacteria confined within cytoplasmic vacuoles of circulating leukocytes (morulae), particularly **mononuclear** leukocytes, were detected in the peripheral blood of a patient with suspected Rocky Mountain spotted fever (RMSF). The etiologic agent, *Ehrlichia chaffeensis,* was cultivated from blood of an infected patient in 1990 and identified as the predominant cause of human ehrlichiosis. Investigations showed that infection by *E. chaffeensis* is transmitted by *Amblyomma americanum* ticks and occurs more often than RMSF in some geographic areas. By 1994, other cases in which morulae were found only in **neutrophils** and lacked serologic evidence for *E. chaffeensis* infection led to the recognition of the species classified as *Anaplasma phagocytophilum,* which encompasses several previously described veterinary pathogens on at least 2 different continents and causing **anaplasmosis**.

Since these 1st discoveries in humans, additional species in the *Anaplasmataceae* family were identified as human pathogens, including (1) *Ehrlichia ewingii* in 1996, a veterinary pathogen of canine neutrophils transmitted by *A. americanum* ticks; (2) the *Ixodes scapularis*–transmitted *Ehrlichia muris* subsp. *euclairensis* in 2009, only present so far in patients from Minnesota and Wisconsin in the United States; (3) infections by *Candidatus* Neoehrlichia mikurensis, presumably *Ixodes* spp. or *Haemaphysalis concinna* tick-transmitted, recognized in 2010 as a cause of sepsis-like infections of immune compromised patients in Europe, and later as a cause of mild febrile illness in healthy individuals in China; (4) Panola Mountain *Ehrlichia,* a bacterium rarely associated with infections in human but present in *A. americanum* ticks in the United States and with genetic features of the ruminant pathogen *Ehrlichia ruminantium*; (5) *Ehrlichia canis,* the established canine pathogen that has infected humans in Venezuela; and (6) *Anaplasma capra,* the cause of mild fever after *Ixodes persulcatus* tick bites, so far only identified in China. The latter 5 have not yet been established as causes of infection in children.

Although the infections caused by these various genera have been called ehrlichiosis, further study has identified substantial differences in biology and diagnostic approaches such that the CDC now generally separates these into ehrlichiosis, anaplasmosis, or undetermined ehrlichiosis/anaplasmosis. **Human monocytic ehrlichiosis (HME)** describes disease characterized by infection of predominantly monocytes and is caused by *E. chaffeensis,* **human granulocytic anaplasmosis (HGA)** describes disease related to infection of circulating neutrophils by *Anaplasma phagocytophilum,* and **ewingii ehrlichiosis** is caused by infection of granulocytes by *E. ewingii* (see Table 255.1 in Chapter 255).

All of these organisms are tick-transmitted and are small, obligate intracellular bacteria with gram-negative-type cell walls. *Neorickettsia sennetsu* is another related bacterium that is rarely recognized as a cause of human disease and is not transmitted by ticks. *E. chaffeensis* alters host signaling and transcription once inside the cell. It survives in an endosome that enters a receptor recycling pathway to avoid phagosome-lysosome fusion and growth into a **morula,** an intravacuolar aggregate of bacteria. *A. phagocytophilum* survives in a unique vacuole that becomes decorated by microbial proteins that prevent endosomal trafficking and lysosome fusion. Little is known about the vacuoles in which *E. ewingii* and *E. muris* subsp. *euclairensis* grow. These bacteria are pathogens of phagocytic cells in mammals, and characteristically each species has a specific host cell affinity: *E. chaffeensis* infects mononuclear phagocytes, and *A. phagocytophilum* and *E. ewingii* infect neutrophils. Infection leads to direct modifications in function, in part the result of changes in intracellular signal transduction or modulation of transcription of the host cell that diminishes host defenses toward the bacterium. Yet, host immune and inflammatory reactions are still activated and in part account for many of the clinical manifestations in ehrlichiosis, such as overlaps with macrophage activation or hemophagocytic lymphohistiocytosis syndromes.

EPIDEMIOLOGY

Infections with *E. chaffeensis* occur across the southeastern, south central, and mid-Atlantic states of the United States in a distribution that parallels that of RMSF; cases have also been reported in northern California. Suspected cases with appropriate serologic and occasionally molecular evidence have been reported in Europe, Africa, South America, and the Far East, including China and Korea. Human infections with *E. ewingii* have only been identified in the United States in areas where *E. chaffeensis* also exists, perhaps owing to the shared tick vector. Canine infections are documented in both sub-Saharan Africa and in South America.

Although the median age of patients with HME and HGA is generally older (>51 yr), many infected children have been identified, and for HME the case fatality rate is 4% in those <5 yr of age. Little is known about the epidemiology of *E. ewingii* infections; although infections in children occur, they are recognized at a rate 100-fold less than for *E. chaffeensis.* All infections are strongly associated with tick exposure and tick bites and are identified predominantly during May through September. Although both nymphal and adult ticks can transmit infection, nymphs are more likely to transmit disease, because they are most active during the summer.

TRANSMISSION

The predominant tick species that harbors *E. chaffeensis* and *E. ewingii* is *A. americanum,* the Lone Star tick (see Fig. 255.1D in Chapter 255). The tick vectors of *A. phagocytophilum* are *Ixodes* spp., including *I. scapularis* (black-legged or deer tick) in the eastern United States (see Fig. 255.1 in Chapter 255), *Ixodes pacificus* (western black-legged tick) in the western United States, *Ixodes ricinus* (sheep tick) in Europe, *Ixodes persulcatus* in Eurasia, and *Haemaphysalis concinna* in China. The *Ixodes* spp. ticks also transmit *Borrelia burgdorferi, Borrelia miyamotoi, Babesia microti,* and tick-borne encephalitis-associated flaviviruses in Europe, Powassan viruses, and *E. muris* subsp. *euclairensis* in North America. Co-infections with these agents and *A. phagocytophilum* are documented in children and adults.

Ehrlichia and *Anaplasma* species are maintained in nature predominantly by horizontal transmission (tick to mammal to tick), because the organisms are not transmitted to the progeny of infected adult female ticks (transovarial transmission). The major reservoir for *E. chaffeensis* is the white-tailed deer (*Odocoileus virginianus*), which is found abundantly in many parts of the United States. A reservoir for *A. phagocytophilum* in the eastern United States appears to be the white-footed mouse, *Peromyscus leucopus.* Deer or domestic ruminants can sustain persistent asymptomatic infections, but the genetic variants in these reservoirs might not be infectious for humans. Efficient transmission requires persistent infections of mammals. Although *E. chaffeensis* and *A. phagocytophilum* can cause persistent infections in animals, the documentation of chronic infections in humans is exceedingly rare. Transmission of *Ehrlichia* can occur within hours of tick attachment, in contrast to the 1-2 days of attachment required for transmission of *B. burgdorferi* to occur. Transmission of *A. phagocytophilum* is via the bite of the small nymphal stage of *Ixodes* spp., including *I. scapularis* (see Fig. 255.1A in Chapter 255), which is very active during late spring and early summer in the eastern United States.

PATHOLOGY AND PATHOGENESIS

Although HME and anaplasmosis often clinically mimic RMSF or typhus, vasculitis is rare. Pathologic findings include mild, diffuse perivascular lymphohistiocytic infiltrates; Kupffer cell hyperplasia and mild lobular hepatitis with infrequent apoptotic hepatocytes and less frequently centrilobular necrosis, cholestasis, and steatosis; infiltrates of mononuclear phagocytes in the spleen, lymph nodes, and bone marrow with occasional hemophagocytosis; granulomas of the liver and bone marrow in patients with *E. chaffeensis* infections; and hyperplasia of 1 or more bone marrow hematopoietic lineages.

The exact pathogenetic mechanisms are poorly understood, but histopathologic examinations suggest diffuse macrophage activation and poorly regulated host immune and inflammatory reactions. This activation results in moderate to profound leukopenia and thrombocytopenia despite a hypercellular bone marrow, and deaths often are related to severe hemorrhage or secondary opportunistic infections. Hepatic and other organ-specific injury occurs by a mechanism that appears to be triggered by the bacterium but more closely related to induction of innate and adaptive immune effectors. Meningoencephalitis with a mononuclear cell pleocytosis in the cerebrospinal fluid (CSF) occurs with HME but is rare with HGA.

CLINICAL MANIFESTATIONS

The clinical manifestations of HME, HGA, and ewingii ehrlichiosis are similar. Many well-characterized infections of HME and HGA of variable severity have been reported in children, including deaths. Children with ehrlichiosis are often ill for 4-12 days, shorter than in adults. In series of children with HME, most required hospitalization and many (25%) required intensive care; these statistics might represent preferential reporting of severe cases. However, review of case reports and electronic surveillance of HGA to the Centers for Disease Control and Prevention identified that 42% of patients 5-9 yr of age required hospitalization and the case fatality rate is 4% among children <5 yr of age. Population-based studies document that seroconversion often occurs in children who are well or who have only a mild illness. Many fewer pediatric cases of *E. ewingii* infection are reported, so the clinical manifestations related to this infection are less well characterized. The incubation period (time from last tick bite or exposure) appears to range from 2 days to 3 wk. Nearly 25% of patients do not report a tick bite.

Clinically, ehrlichioses are undifferentiated febrile illnesses. In HME, fever (~100%), headache (77%), and myalgia (77%) are most common, but many patients also report abdominal pain, nausea, and vomiting. Altered mental status accompanied by other signs of central nervous system involvement is present in 36%. Rash is a common feature (~60%) in children. The rash is usually macular or maculopapular, but petechial lesions can occur. Photophobia, conjunctivitis, pharyngitis, arthralgias, and lymphadenopathy can occur but are less consistently present. Lymphadenopathy, hepatomegaly, and splenomegaly are detected in nearly 50% of children with ehrlichiosis. Edema of the face, hands, and feet occurs more commonly in children than in adults, but arthritis is uncommon in both groups.

Similar but less severe manifestations occur with HGA in children, including fever (93%), headache (73%), myalgia (73%), rigors (60%); nausea, vomiting, abdominal pain, and anorexia occur in 30% or less. Cough is present in 20%; rash is very infrequent and most often is erythema migrans that results from concurrent Lyme disease.

Meningoencephalitis with a lymphocyte-predominant CSF pleocytosis is an uncommon but potentially severe complication of HME that appears to be rare with HGA. CSF protein may be elevated, and glucose may be mildly depressed in adults with HME meningoencephalitis, but CSF protein and glucose in affected children are typically normal. In 1 series, 19% of adult patients with central nervous system symptoms and abnormal CSF died despite normal CTs of the brain.

Chronic or persistent disease with low or absent fever is very unlikely to be any form of ehrlichiosis.

LABORATORY FINDINGS

Characteristically, most children with HME and HGA present with leukopenia (57–80%) and thrombocytopenia (38–93%); cytopenias reach a nadir several days into the illness. Lymphopenia is common in both HME and HGA, and neutropenia is reported in adults with HGA. Leukocytosis can also occur, but usually after the 1st wk of illness or with effective antimicrobial treatment. Adults with pancytopenia often have a cellular or reactive bone marrow examination, and in nearly 75% of bone marrow specimens from adults with HME, granulomas and granulomatous inflammation are present; this finding is not a feature of adults with HGA. Mild to severely elevated serum hepatic transaminase levels are frequent in both HME (85–92%) and HGA (40–50%). Hyponatremia (<135 mEq/L) is present in most cases. A clinical picture similar to disseminated intravascular coagulopathy has also been reported.

DIAGNOSIS

Any delays in diagnosis or treatment are major contributors to increased morbidity or mortality in adults, where those not started on doxycycline at hospital admission are much more likely to require intensive care and a significantly longer course of illness and hospitalization. Thus treatment must begin as early as possible based on clinical suspicion. Because both HME and anaplasmosis can be fatal, therapy should not be withheld while waiting for the results of confirmatory testing. In fact, prompt response to therapy supports the diagnosis.

While several reports document pediatric patients with *E. chaffeensis* infection diagnosed based on typical *Ehrlichia* morulae in peripheral blood leukocytes (Fig. 258.1A), this finding is too infrequent to be considered a useful diagnostic approach. In contrast, HGA in adults presents with a small but significant percentage (1–40%) of circulating neutrophils (Fig. 258.1B) containing typical morulae in 20–60% of patients.

E. chaffeensis and *A. phagocytophilum* infections can be confirmed by demonstrating a 4-fold change in immunoglobulin G titer by indirect immunofluorescence assay between paired sera. Serologic tests during the acute phase of infection are often negative; consequently, confirmation of acute infection requires demonstration a 4-fold rise in IgG titer in paired samples. Infection can also be established by specific polymerase chain reaction, demonstration of specific antigen in a tissue sample by immunohistochemistry, or isolation of the organism in cell culture. A single specific titer of ≥128 or identification of morulae in monocytes or macrophages for *E. chaffeensis* or in neutrophils or eosinophils for *A. phagocytophilum* by microscopy is suggestive. *E. ewingii* infection can only be confirmed by polymerase chain reaction, because it has not been cultured and serologic antigens are not available. *E. ewingii* antibodies cross react with *E. chaffeensis* in routine serologic tests. Up to 15% of patients with HGA have serologic cross-reactions with *E. chaffeensis*; thus serodiagnosis depends on testing with both *E. chaffeensis* and *A. phagocytophilum* antigens and demonstrating a 4-fold or higher difference between titers. During the acute phase of illness when antibodies are often not detected, polymerase chain reaction amplification of *E. chaffeensis* or *A. phagocytophilum* DNA is sensitive in >86% of cases. Although *E. chaffeensis* and *A. phagocytophilum* can be cultivated in tissue culture, this method is not timely or widely available.

DIFFERENTIAL DIAGNOSIS

Because of the nonspecific presentation, ehrlichiosis mimics other arthropod-borne infections such as RMSF, tularemia, babesiosis, Lyme disease, murine typhus, relapsing fever, and Colorado tick fever. Other potential diagnoses often considered include otitis media, streptococcal pharyngitis, infectious mononucleosis, Kawasaki disease, endocarditis, respiratory or gastrointestinal viral syndromes, hepatitis, leptospirosis, Q fever, collagen–vascular diseases, hemophagocytic syndromes, and leukemia. If rash and disseminated intravascular coagulopathy predominate, meningococcemia, bacterial sepsis, and toxic shock syndrome are also suspected. Meningoencephalitis might suggest aseptic meningitis caused by enterovirus or herpes simplex virus, bacterial meningitis, or RMSF. Severe respiratory disease may be confused with bacterial, viral, and fungal causes of pneumonia. Mounting evidence suggests that ehrlichiosis or anaplasmosis may be precipitating factors for hemophagocytic lymphohistiocytosis.

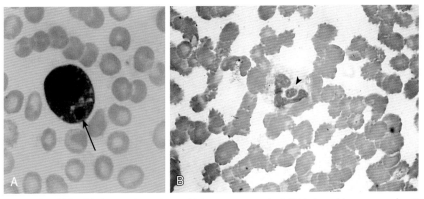

Fig. 258.1 Morulae in peripheral blood leukocytes in patients with human monocytic ehrlichiosis and human granulocytic anaplasmosis. **A,** A morula *(arrow)* containing *Ehrlichia chaffeensis* in a monocyte. **B,** A morula *(arrowhead)* containing *Anaplasma phagocytophilum* in a neutrophil. Wright stains, original magnifications ×1,200. *E. chaffeensis* and *A. phagocytophilum* have similar morphologies but are serologically and genetically distinct.

TREATMENT

Both HME and HGA are effectively treated with tetracyclines, especially doxycycline, and the majority of patients improve within 48 hr. In vitro tests document that both *E. chaffeensis* and *A. phagocytophilum* have minimal inhibitory concentrations to chloramphenicol above blood levels that can be safely achieved. Therefore, a short course of doxycycline is the recommended regimen. Doxycycline is used safely in children younger than 8 yr of age because tooth discoloration is dose dependent and the need for multiple courses is unlikely; experience has demonstrated that adverse consequences of doxycycline use in children <8 yr of age are extremely rare. Few data exist to recommend alternative therapies; however, both *E. chaffeensis* and *A. phagocytophilum* are susceptible in vitro to rifampin, which has been used successfully to treat HGA in pregnant women and children.

The recommended regimen for patients of all ages with severe or complicated HME and HGA is doxycycline (for those who weigh <45 kg, 4 mg/kg/day PO or IV divided every 12 hr; maximum dose: 100 mg/dose). An alternative regimen is tetracycline (25-50 mg/kg/day divided every 6 hr PO; maximum 2 g/day). For children who weigh more than 45 kg, the adult dose, 100 mg twice daily by oral or intravenous route, can be used. Therapy should be continued for ≥5 days and until the patient has been afebrile for ≥2-4 days.

Other broad-spectrum antibiotics, including penicillins, cephalosporins, aminoglycosides, and macrolides, are not effective. In vitro studies suggest that fluoroquinolones are active against *A. phagocytophilum*, although at least 1 patient relapsed when levofloxacin was discontinued. *E. chaffeensis* is naturally resistant to fluoroquinolones owing to a single nucleotide change in *gyrA*, which suggests that *A. phagocytophilum* could also become resistant to fluoroquinolones rapidly.

COMPLICATIONS AND PROGNOSIS

Fatal HME is reported in several pediatric patients, where the findings included pulmonary involvement and respiratory failure in patients with or without immune compromise. The pattern of severe pulmonary involvement culminating in diffuse alveolar damage and acute respiratory distress syndrome and secondary nosocomial or opportunistic infections is now well-documented with HME and HGA in adults. One child with HGA died after 3 wk of fever, thrombocytopenia, and lymphadenopathy suspected to be a hematologic malignancy. Patients who are immuno-compromised (e.g., HIV infection, high-dose corticosteroid therapy, cancer chemotherapy, immunosuppression for organ transplantation) are at high risk for fulminant *E. chaffeensis* infection, for *E. ewingii* infection, and for severe HGA.

PREVENTION

HME, HGA, and ewingii ehrlichiosis are tick-borne diseases, and any activity that increases exposure to ticks increases risk. Avoiding tick-infested areas, wearing appropriate light-colored clothing, spraying tick repellents on clothing, carefully inspecting for ticks after exposure, and promptly removing any attached ticks diminish the risk. The interval between tick attachment and transmission of the agents may be as short as 4 hr; thus attached ticks should be removed promptly. A role of prophylactic therapy for ehrlichiosis and anaplasmosis after tick bites has not been investigated. It is not known if infection confers protective immunity; however, reinfection appears to be exceedingly rare.

Bibliography is available at Expert Consult.

Chapter 259
Q Fever (*Coxiella burnetii*)
Megan E. Reller and J. Stephen Dumler

第二百五十九章
Q热（贝纳柯克斯体）

中文导读

本章主要介绍了Q热的病原学、流行病学、传播途径、病理和发病机制、临床表现和并发症、实验室检查、诊断和鉴别诊断、治疗、并发症和预后，以及预防。Q热是由贝纳柯克斯体所致的急性传染病，家畜为主要传染源，蜱为传播媒介，主要通过呼吸道、接触、消化道传播。在临床表现部分详细介绍了原发性Q热和局部持续性Q热的不同表现。主要介绍了血清学诊断和PCR检测方法，需根据临床表现做出相应鉴别诊断，在治疗部分详细介绍了不同临床类型的治疗方案，预防需有效识别患病家畜并采取一定的消毒措施。

Q fever (for query fever, the name given following an outbreak of febrile illness in an abattoir in Queensland, Australia) is rarely reported in children but is probably underdiagnosed. Symptomatic patients can have acute or chronic disease.

ETIOLOGY

Although previously classified within the order Rickettsiales, *Coxiella burnetii* (the causative agent of Q fever) is genetically distinct from the genera *Rickettsia, Orientia, Ehrlichia,* and *Anaplasma*. Hence, based on small genome analysis, it best aligns within the order Legionellales, family Coxiellaceae. *C. burnetii* is highly infectious for both humans and animals; even a single organism can cause infection. The agent has been nationally notifiable since 1999 and is listed as a Category B agent of bioterrorism by the Centers for Disease Control and Prevention (CDC). Unlike *Rickettsia,* the organism can enter a sporogenic differentiation cycle, which renders it highly resistant to chemical and physical treatments.

C. burnetii resides intracellularly within macrophages. In vitro, the organism undergoes a lipopolysaccharide phase variation similar to that described for smooth and rough strains of Enterobacteriaceae. Unlike *Ehrlichia, Anaplasma,* and *Chlamydia, C. burnetii* survives and proliferates within acidified phagosomes to form aggregates of >100 bacteria.

EPIDEMIOLOGY

The disease is reported worldwide, except in New Zealand. Although seroepidemiologic studies suggest that infection occurs just as often in children as in adults, children less often present with clinical disease than adults. During the large outbreak of Q fever in the Netherlands in 2007–2009, only 3.5% of those diagnosed with Q fever were age 19 yr or younger. Although infections are recognized more often in men than in women, reported cases in boys and girls are equal. Approximately 60% of infections are asymptomatic, and only 5% of symptomatic patients require hospitalization. Seroprevalence surveys show that 6–70% of children in endemic European and African communities have evidence of past infection. In France, the overall incidence of Q fever is estimated to be 50 cases per 100,000 persons. A similar estimate is not available for Africa, where cases are likely misdiagnosed as malaria. The seroprevalence of Q fever in the United States is estimated to be 3.1%. Reported cases of Q fever in the United States have been received from every state, but 35% are reported from 4 states (California, Texas, Colorado, and Illinois). In the United States, reported Q fever cases increased by greater than 9-fold from 17 cases in 2000 to 167 cases in 2008, reflecting an increase in incidence, increased reporting after September 11, 2001, improved diagnostic tools, or a combination of factors. Cases decreased significantly in 2008–2013 relative to 2007 but returned to previous high levels in 2014 (173 cases, including 147 acute and 39 chronic). Beginning in 2008, reported cases in the United States have been classified as acute or chronic. Between 2002 and 2014, more than 50% of recognized cases in the United States required hospitalization. Reported cases in Asia and Australia have also increased. Most infections in children are identified during the lamb birthing season in Europe (January through June), following farm visits, or after exposure to placentas of dogs, cats, and rabbits. The largest (~4,000 human cases) community outbreak ever described occurred in the Netherlands in 2007–2012 and was associated with intensive farming of dairy goats and dairy sheep. In 2011, the 1st multistate outbreak of Q fever in humans was linked to interstate sale of infected goats; an outbreak of unknown source was also reported. From 2000 to 2010, 60% of cases reported to CDC occurred in individuals without reported exposure to livestock.

More than 20% of cases of clinically recognized acute or chronic Q fever occur in immunosuppressed hosts or in persons with prosthetic valves or damaged native valves or vessels. These findings highlight the need for considering Q fever in those with clinically compatible illness, especially but not exclusively in those with likely exposures and in vulnerable hosts. Epidemiologic investigations and control efforts require a One Health approach, with consideration of the interactions between humans, animals, environment, and public health.

TRANSMISSION

In contrast to other rickettsial infections, humans usually acquire *C. burnetii* by inhaling infectious aerosols (e.g., contaminated barnyard dust) or ingesting (and likely aspirating) contaminated foods. Ticks are rarely implicated. Cattle, sheep, and goats are the primary reservoirs, but infection in other livestock and domestic pets is also described. Organisms are excreted in milk, urine, and feces of infected animals, but especially in amniotic fluids and the placenta. An increase in incidence is associated with the seasonal mistral winds in France that coincide with lamb birthing season and with consumption of cheese among children in Greece. In Nova Scotia and Maine, exposure to newborn animals, especially kittens, has been associated with small outbreaks of Q fever in families. Exposure to domestic ruminants is the major risk in Europe and Australia, although many urban dwellers in France also acquire Q fever without such an exposure. Person-to-person transmission is possible but rare. Clinical Q fever during pregnancy can result from primary infection or reactivation of latent infection and is associated with miscarriage, intrauterine growth retardation, and premature births. Obstetricians and other related healthcare workers are at risk for acquiring infection because of the quantity of *C. burnetii* sequestered in the placenta. Sexual transmission and cases attributable to blood transfusion or bone marrow transplantation are also reported. Transmission following *live cell therapy* (injected live animal cells) has also been reported.

PATHOLOGY AND PATHOGENESIS

The pathology of Q fever depends on the mode of transmission, route of dissemination, specific tissues involved, and course of the infection. When acquired via inhalation, a mild interstitial lymphocytic pneumonitis and macrophage- and organism-rich intraalveolar exudates are often seen. When the liver is involved, a mild to moderate lymphocytic lobular hepatitis can be seen. Inflammatory pseudotumors can develop in the pulmonary parenchyma or other tissues. Classic fibrin-ring ("doughnut") granulomas, generally associated with acute, self-limited infections, are occasionally identified in liver, bone marrow, meninges, and other organs. Typically, infected tissues are also infiltrated by lymphocytes and histiocytes.

Recovery from symptomatic or asymptomatic acute infection can result in persistent subclinical infection, possibly maintained by dysregulated cytokine responses. The persistence of *C. burnetii* in tissue macrophages at sites of preexisting tissue damage elicits low-grade chronic inflammation and, depending on the site of involvement, can result in irreversible cardiac valve damage, persistent vascular injury, or osteomyelitis. Endocarditis of native or prosthetic valves is characterized by infiltrates of macrophages and lymphocytes in necrotic fibrinous valvular vegetations and an absence of granulomas.

CLINICAL MANIFESTATIONS AND COMPLICATIONS

Children are less likely to develop symptoms compared with adults. Only approximately 40–50% of people infected with *C. burnetii* develop symptoms. Historically, 2 forms of symptomatic disease have been thought to occur. **Acute Q fever**, now better characterized as **primary Q fever,** is more common and usually manifests as self-limited undifferentiated fever or an influenza-like illness with interstitial pneumonitis. Persistent localized infection with *C. burnetii* can cause what has historically been referred to as **chronic Q fever**. In adults, persistent localized infection usually involves the cardiovascular system—native heart valves, especially those with preexisting valvulopathy, prosthetic valves, or other endovascular prostheses. Q fever osteomyelitis is less common

but proportionally more common in children. Less common persistent localized *C. burnetii* infections include lymphadenitis, genital infection, and pericarditis.

Primary (Acute) Q Fever

Acute Q fever develops approximately 3 wk (range: 14-39 days) after exposure to the causative agent. The severity of illness in children ranges from subclinical infection to a systemic illness of sudden onset characterized by high fever, severe frontal headache, nonproductive cough, chest pain, vomiting, diarrhea, abdominal pain, arthralgias, and myalgias. Approximately 40% of children with acute Q fever present with fever, 25% with pneumonia or an influenza-like illness, >10% with meningoencephalitis, and >10% with myocarditis. Other manifestations include pericarditis, hepatitis, hemophagocytosis, rhabdomyolysis, and a hemolytic uremic–like syndrome. Rash, ranging from maculopapular to purpuric lesions, is an unusual finding in adults with Q fever but is observed in approximately 50% of pediatric patients. Rigors and night sweats are common in adults with Q fever and occur less often in children. Prominent clinical findings that can create diagnostic confusion include fatigue, vomiting, abdominal pain, and meningismus. Hepatomegaly and splenomegaly may be detected in some patients.

Routine laboratory investigations in pediatric acute Q fever are usually normal but can reveal mild leukocytosis and thrombocytopenia. Up to 85% of children have modestly elevated serum hepatic transaminase levels that usually normalize within 10 days. Hyperbilirubinemia is uncommon in the absence of complications. C-reactive protein is uniformly elevated in pediatric Q fever. Chest radiographs are abnormal in 27% of all patients; in children, the most common findings include single or multiple bilateral infiltrates with reticular markings in the lower lobes.

Primary Q fever in children is usually a self-limited illness, with fever persisting for only 7-10 days compared with 2-3 wk in adults. However, severe manifestations of acute illness, such as myocarditis requiring cardiac transplantation, meningoencephalitis, pericarditis, hemophagocytosis, thrombosis with antiphospholipid antibody syndrome, as well as a relapsing febrile illness lasting for several months, have been reported.

Persistent Localized Q Fever Infection

The risk for developing persistent localized Q fever infection, historically called *chronic Q fever,* is strongly correlated with advancing age and underlying conditions such as cardiac valve damage or immunosuppression; persistent localized Q fever infection is rarely diagnosed in children. A review identified only 5 cases of Q fever endocarditis and 6 cases of osteomyelitis among children, none of whom had known predisposing immune deficiencies. Four of the 5 cases of endocarditis occurred in children with underlying congenital heart abnormalities and involved the aortic, pulmonary, and tricuspid valves. Four of the 6 children with Q fever osteomyelitis had a prior diagnosis or clinical course consistent with idiopathic chronic recurrent multifocal osteomyelitis. A long interval before diagnosis and lack of high fever are common in pediatric cases of persistent localized Q fever infection—historically chronic Q fever.

Although Q fever endocarditis often results in death (23–65% of cases) in adults, mortality has not been reported for children. Endocarditis associated with persistent or chronic Q fever can occur months to years after acute infection and can occur in the absence of recognized acute Q fever and in the absence of clinically recognized valvulopathy. Chronic hepatitis has also been reported.

LABORATORY FINDINGS

Laboratory features in children with chronic Q fever are poorly documented; adult patients often have an erythrocyte sedimentation rate of >20 mm/hr (80% of cases), hypergammaglobulinemia (54%), and hyperfibrinogenemia (67%). In children, the presence of rheumatoid factor in >50% of cases, and circulating immune complexes in nearly 90% suggests an autoimmune process. The presence of antiplatelet antibodies, anti–smooth muscle antibodies, antimitochondrial antibodies, circulating anticoagulants, positive direct Coombs tests, and antiphospholipid antibodies also suggest this possibility.

DIAGNOSIS AND DIFFERENTIAL DIAGNOSIS

Although uncommonly diagnosed, Q fever in children most often mimics other childhood respiratory infections. It should be considered in children who have an influenza-like illness, lower or upper respiratory tract infection, fever of unknown origin, myocarditis, meningoencephalitis, culture-negative endocarditis, or recurrent osteomyelitis, and who live in rural areas or who are in close contact with domestic livestock, cats, or animal products.

The diagnosis of primary (acute) Q fever is most easily and commonly confirmed by testing acute and convalescent sera (3-6 wk apart), which show a 4-fold increase in indirect fluorescent immunoglobulin G antibody titers to phase II *C. burnetii* antigens. The phase II antibody response to *C. burnetii* appears 1st and is higher than the phase I antibody response. Phase II immunoglobulin G antibodies can remain elevated for months to years, regardless of initial symptoms or lack thereof. In contrast, persistent localized (chronic) Q fever is characterized by a phase I immunoglobulin G antibody titer greater than 800 that is sustained for 6 mo or more, such as occurs with Q fever endocarditis in patients with valvular heart disease. Cross-reactions with antibodies to *Legionella* and *Bartonella* can occur.

Although culture has been considered the gold standard, sensitivity (compared with a composite standard including serology and polymerase chain reaction) is low. *C. burnetii* has been cultivated in tissue culture cells, which can become positive within 48 hr, but isolation and antimicrobial susceptibility testing of *C. burnetii* should be attempted only in specialized biohazard facilities. Testing by polymerase chain reaction can be performed on blood, serum, and tissue samples and is available only in some public health, reference, or research laboratories. Polymerase chain reaction (PCR) has been helpful in patients with equivocal titers, as occurs with early infection. PCR usually remains positive for 7-10 days after acute infection. Sensitivity has been improved by real-time methods and the use of repeated sequences as targets. Immunohistochemical staining has also been used, but is not readily available. PCR should be performed either before or shortly after initiation of treatment. PCR can also confirm a serologic diagnosis of endocarditis in untreated patients. Genotyping has aided epidemiologic investigations to confirm source of infection. The differential diagnosis depends on the clinical presentation. In patients with respiratory disease, *Mycoplasma pneumoniae*, *Chlamydophila pneumoniae*, legionellosis, psittacosis, and Epstein-Barr virus infection should be considered. In patients with granulomatous hepatitis, tuberculous and nontuberculous mycobacterial infections, salmonellosis, visceral leishmaniasis, toxoplasmosis, Hodgkin disease, monocytic ehrlichiosis, granulocytic anaplasmosis, brucellosis, cat scratch disease (*Bartonella henselae*), or autoimmune disorders such as sarcoidosis should be considered. **Culture-negative endocarditis** suggests infection with *Brucella*, *Bartonella*, HACEK organisms *(Haemophilus, Aggregatibacter, Cardiobacterium hominis, Eikenella corrodens, Kingella)*, partially treated bacterial endocarditis, nonbacterial endocarditis, or potentially noninfectious inflammatory conditions, including chronic recurrent multifocal osteomyelitis and antiphospholipid syndrome.

TREATMENT

Selection of an appropriate antimicrobial regimen for children is difficult owing to the lack of rigorous studies, the limited therapeutic window for drugs that are known to be efficacious, and the potential length of therapy required to preclude relapse.

Most pediatric patients with Q fever have a self-limited illness that is identified only on retrospective serologic evaluation. However, to prevent potential complications, treatment should be considered for patients who present with acute Q fever within 3 days of onset of symptoms, because therapy started more than 3 days after onset of illness has little effect on the course of acute Q fever. Because confirmatory testing in early acute infection is not possible, and because tetracycline and doxycycline can be associated with tooth discoloration in children younger than 9 yr of age, empirical therapy is warranted in those with clinically suspected Q fever who are 8 yr of age or older or at high risk for severe illness. Doxycycline (4 mg/kg/day PO or IV divided every 12 hr; maximum: 200 mg/day) is the drug of choice; the usual course is 2 wk. Children at high risk include those hospitalized or with severe illness, those diagnosed after prolonged (>2 wk) unremitting symptoms, and those with preexisting valvular heart disease or who are immunocompromised. Because tooth discoloration is both dose and duration dependent and few children require multiple courses, younger children with mild Q fever could be treated with 5 days of doxycycline followed by 14 days of trimethoprim-sulfamethoxazole if symptoms persist. During pregnancy, Q fever is best treated with trimethoprim-sulfamethoxazole. The fluoroquinolones are also effective, and success with a combination of a fluoroquinolone and rifampin is also achieved with prolonged therapy (16-21 days). Macrolides, including erythromycin and clarithromycin, are less-effective alternatives.

For persistent focal Q fever, especially endocarditis and mostly in adults, therapy for 18-36 mo is mandatory. The current recommended regimen for Q fever endocarditis is a combination of doxycycline and hydroxychloroquine for 18 mo or longer. For patients with heart failure, valve replacement could be necessary. Interferon-γ therapy has been used as adjunct therapy for intractable Q fever.

PREVENTION

Recognition of the disease in livestock or other domestic animals should alert communities to the risk for human infection by aerosol exposures within 15 km. Milk from infected herds must be pasteurized at temperatures sufficient to destroy *C. burnetii*. *C. burnetii* is resistant to significant environmental conditions but can be inactivated with a solution of 1% Lysol, 1% formaldehyde, or 5% hydrogen peroxide. Special isolation measures are not required because person-to-person transmission is rare, except when others are exposed to the placenta of an infected patient. A vaccine is available and provides protection against Q fever for at least 5 yr in abattoir workers. Because the vaccine is strongly reactogenic and no trials in children have been conducted, it should only be used when extreme risk is judged to exist. Clusters of cases resulting from intense natural exposures, such as in slaughterhouses or on farms, are well documented. Clusters of cases that occur in the absence of such an exposure should be investigated as potential sentinel events for bioterrorism.

Bibliography is available at Expert Consult.

Section 12
Fungal Infections
第十二篇
真菌感染

Chapter **260**
Principles of Antifungal Therapy

William J. Steinbach,
Michael Cohen-Wolkowiez,
and Daniel K. Benjamin Jr.

第二百六十章
抗真菌治疗原则

中 文 导 读

　　本章主要介绍了多烯类、嘧啶类似物、唑类和棘白菌素类抗真菌药的临床使用。其中多烯类药物着重介绍两性霉素B，嘧啶类似物着重介绍氟胞嘧啶，唑类药物中分别介绍氟康唑、伊曲康唑、伏立康唑、泊沙康唑和艾沙康唑，棘白霉素类药物分别介绍卡泊芬净、米卡芬净和阿尼芬净。本章结合临床研究，对上述药物的作用机制、药物代谢动力学特征、用药剂量、副作用等进行详细阐述，同时对常见病原真菌给予治疗建议。

Invasive fungal infections are a major cause of morbidity and mortality in the growing number of immunocompromised children. Fortunately, the therapeutic armamentarium for invasive fungal infections has markedly increased since the turn of the century (Tables 260.1 and 260.2).

POLYENES
Amphotericin B
The prototype of the oldest antifungal class, the polyene macrolides, is amphotericin B deoxycholate. Amphotericin B was once the preferred treatment for most invasive fungal infections as well as the standard of comparison for all newer antifungal agents. Amphotericin B is so named because it is amphoteric, forming soluble salts in both acidic and basic environments. However, because of its insolubility in water, amphotericin B for clinical use is actually amphotericin B mixed with the detergent deoxycholate. Amphotericin B binds to ergosterol, the major sterol found in fungal cytoplasmic membranes, and acts by creating transmembrane channels. The fungicidal activity is due to a damaged barrier and subsequent cell death through leakage of essential nutrients from the fungal cell.

Amphotericin B is released from its carrier and distributes very efficiently with lipoproteins and is then taken up preferentially by organs of the reticuloendothelial system. Following an initial 24-48 hr distributional half-life there is very slow release and a subsequent terminal elimination half-life of up to 15 days. In addition to conventional amphotericin B deoxycholate, 3 fundamentally different lipid-associated formulations have been developed that offer the advantage of an increased daily dosage of the parent drug, better delivery to the primary reticuloendothelial organs (lungs, liver, spleen), and reduced toxicity. Amphotericin B lipid complex (ABLC) is a tightly packed ribbon-like structure of a bilayered membrane, amphotericin B colloidal dispersion (ABCD) is composed of disk-like structures of cholesteryl sulfate complexed with amphotericin B, and liposomal amphotericin B (L-amphotericin B) consists of small uniformly sized vesicles of a lipid bilayer of amphotericin B. Lipid formulations of amphotericin B generally have a slower onset of action, presumably owing to the required disassociation of free amphotericin B from the lipid vehicle. The ability to safely administer higher daily doses of the parent drugs improves their efficacy, comparing favorably with amphotericin B deoxycholate but with less toxicity. Lipid formulations

Table 260.1	Suggested Dosing of Antifungal Agents in Children and Neonates		
DRUG	**FORMULATIONS**	**SUGGESTED PEDIATRIC DOSAGE**	**COMMENTS**
Amphotericin B deoxycholate	IV	1 mg/kg/day	Generally less toxicity in children than adults; do not start with smaller test doses
Lipid amphotericin B formulations	IV	5 mg/kg/day	Generally, all lipid formulations are dosed the same; there is no clear indication of one formulation over another for clinical efficacy
Fluconazole	IV, PO	12 mg/kg/day	Loading dose (25 mg/kg) is recommended in neonates based on pharmacokinetic simulations and likely suggested in children, but insufficiently studied
Itraconazole	PO	2.5 mg/kg/dose bid	Divide dosage twice daily in children; follow trough levels
Voriconazole	IV, PO	8 mg/kg/dose bid IV maintenance; 9 mg/kg/dose bid oral maintenance	Linear pharmacokinetics in children requires higher dosing than in adults; 9 mg/kg/dose bid IV loading, followed by maintenance dosing; follow trough levels
Posaconazole	IV, PO	Suspected to be 12-24 mg/kg/day divided tid (oral suspension)	Dosage unclear in children at present. In adults, max dosage for oral suspension is 800 mg/day, and optimally divide this into 2 or 3 doses; follow trough levels. Adult dosing for IV and extended-release tablet is 300 mg twice on 1st day, then 300 mg once daily.
Isavuconazole	PO, IV	No dosing in children	Adult dosing for IV and tablet is 200 mg 3 times on 1st day, then 200 mg once daily.
Micafungin	IV	2-10 mg/kg/day	Highest dosages in neonates (10 mg/kg/day), and lower dosages in children; >8 yr of age, use adult dosage
Anidulafungin	IV	1.5 mg/kg/day	Loading dose of 3 mg/kg/day
Caspofungin	IV	50 mg/m^2/day	Load with 70 mg/m^2/day, then 50/mg/m^2/day as maintenance dosage

have the added benefit of increased tissue concentrations compared to conventional amphotericin B, specifically in the liver, lungs, and spleen. However, it is not entirely clear if these higher concentrations in tissue are truly available to the microfoci of infection.

Tolerance to amphotericin B deoxycholate is limited by its acute and chronic toxicities. In addition to interacting with fungal ergosterol, the drug also interacts with cholesterol in human cell membranes, likely accounting for its toxicity. Up to 80% of patients receiving amphotericin B develop either infusion-related toxicity or nephrotoxicity, especially with concomitant therapy with nephrotoxic drugs such as aminoglycosides, vancomycin, cyclosporine, or tacrolimus. Renal function usually returns to normal after cessation of amphotericin B, although permanent renal impairment can occur after larger doses. Amphotericin B nephrotoxicity is generally less severe in infants and children than in adults, likely due to the more rapid clearance of the drug in children. Lipid formulations appear to stabilize amphotericin B in a self-associated state so that it is not available to interact with the cholesterol of human cellular membranes.

Unlike older approaches, there is no total dosage of amphotericin B recommended, and the key to success is to give high dosages in the initial phase of therapy and to reduce the frequency of administration (not necessarily the daily dose) if toxicity develops. There are no data or consensus opinions among authorities indicating improved efficacy of any new amphotericin B lipid formulation over conventional amphotericin B deoxycholate. One exception is that L-amphotericin B has shown fewer infusion-related adverse events than the other lipid formulations or conventional amphotericin B.

PYRIMIDINE ANALOGS
5-Fluorocytosine
5-Fluorocytosine (5-FC) is a fluorinated analog of cytosine and has antifungal activity results from the rapid conversion into 5-fluorouracil (5-FU) within susceptible fungal cells. Clinical and microbiologic antifungal resistance develops quickly to 5-FC monotherapy, so clinicians have reserved it for combination approaches to augment other more potent antifungals. Fungistatic 5-FC is thought to enhance the antifungal

activity of amphotericin B, especially in anatomic sites where amphotericin B penetration is often suboptimal, such as cerebrospinal fluid (CSF), heart valves, and the vitreal body. 5-FC penetrates well into most body sites because it is small, highly water-soluble, and not bound by serum proteins to any great extent. One explanation for the synergy detected with the combination of amphotericin B plus 5-FC is that the membrane-permeabilizing effects of low concentrations of amphotericin B facilitate penetration of 5-FC to the cell interior. 5-FC is only available as an oral formulation in the United States, and the dosage is 150 mg/kg/day in 4 divided doses.

5-FC can exacerbate myelosuppression in patients with neutropenia, and toxic levels can develop when used in combination with amphotericin B, owing to nephrotoxicity of the amphotericin B and decreased renal clearance of 5-FC. Routine serum 5-FC level monitoring is warranted in high-risk patients, and levels should be obtained after 3-5 days of therapy, with a goal to achieve a 2-hr post-dose peak <100 µg/mL (and ideally 30-80 µg/mL). Levels >100 µg/mL are associated with bone marrow aplasia. Toxicities can include azotemia, renal tubular acidosis, leukopenia, thrombocytopenia, and others and appear in approximately 50% of patients in the 1st 2 wk of therapy.

Nearly all clinical studies involving 5-FC are combination antifungal protocols for cryptococcal meningitis, owing to the inherently rather weak antifungal activity of 5-FC monotherapy. The use of 5-FC for *Candida* meningitis in premature neonates is discouraged. A study evaluating risk factors and mortality rates of neonatal candidiasis among extremely premature infants showed that infants with *Candida* meningitis who received amphotericin B in combination with 5-FC had a prolonged time to sterilization of the CSF compared to infants receiving amphotericin B monotherapy.

AZOLES
The azole antifungals inhibit the fungal cytochrome P450$_{14DM}$ (also known as lanosterol 14α-demethylase), which catalyzes a late step in fungal cell membrane ergosterol biosynthesis. Of the older 1st-generation, itraconazole has activity against *Aspergillus* but fluconazole is ineffective against *Aspergillus* and other molds. Second-generation

Table 260.2 Suggested Antifungals for Specific More Common Fungal Pathogens

FUNGAL SPECIES	AMPHOTERICIN B FORMULATIONS	FLUCONAZOLE	ITRACONAZOLE	VORICONAZOLE	POSACONAZOLE	ISAVUCONAZOLE	FLUCYTOSINE	CASPOFUNGIN, MICAFUNGIN, OR ANIDULAFUNGIN
Aspergillus calidoustus	++	-	-	-	-	-	-	++
Aspergillus fumigatus	+	-	+/-	++	+	++	-	+
Aspergillus terreus	-	-	+	++	+	++	-	+
Blastomyces dermatitidis	++	+	++	+	+	+	-	-
Candida albicans	+	++	+	+	+	+	+	++
Candida glabrata	+	-	+/-	+/-	+/-	+/-	+	+/-
Candida krusei	+	-	-	+	+	+	+	++
Candida lusitaniae	-	++	+	+	+	+	+	+
Candida parapsilosis	++	++	+	+	+	+	+	+/-
Coccidioides immitis	++	+	++	+	++	+	-	-
Cryptococcus spp.	++	+	+	++	+	+	++	-
Fusarium spp.	+/-	-	-	++	+	+	-	-
Histoplasma capsulatum	++	+	++	+	+	+	-	-
Mucor spp.	++	-	+/-	-	+	+	-	-
Scedosporium apiospermum	-	-	+/-	+	+	+	-	+/-
Scedosporium prolificans	-	-	+/-	+/-	+/-	+/-	-	+/-

++, preferred therapy(ies); +, usually active; +/–, variably active; –, usually not active.

triazoles (voriconazole, posaconazole, and isavuconazole) have an expanded antifungal spectrum of activity, including activity against molds, and generally greater *in vitro* antifungal activity.

Fluconazole

Fluconazole is fungistatic, and this activity is not influenced by concentration once the maximal fungistatic concentration is surpassed (concentration independent), in contrast to the concentration-dependent fungicidal activity of amphotericin B. Fluconazole is available as either an oral or intravenous form, and oral administration has a bioavailability of approximately 90% relative to intravenous administration. Fluconazole passes into tissues and fluids very rapidly, probably due to its relatively low lipophilicity and limited degree of binding to plasma proteins. Concentrations of fluconazole are 10-20–fold higher in the urine than blood, making it an ideal agent for treating fungal urinary tract infections. Concentrations in the CSF and vitreous humor of the eye are approximately 80% of those found simultaneously in blood.

Simple conversion of the corresponding adult dosage of fluconazole on a weight basis is inappropriate for pediatric patients. Fluconazole clearance is generally more rapid in children than adults, with a mean plasma half-life of approximately 20 hr in children and approximately 30 hr in adult patients. Therefore, to achieve comparable exposure in pediatric patients, the daily fluconazole dosage needs to be essentially doubled. Correct pediatric fluconazole dosages should be proportionately higher than adult dosages, generally 12 mg/kg/day. In neonates the volume of distribution is significantly greater and more variable than in infants and children, and doubling the dosage for neonatal patients is necessary to achieve comparable plasma concentrations. The increased volume of distribution is thought to be due to the larger amount of body water found in the total body volume of neonates. A pharmacokinetic study in premature infants suggests that maintenance fluconazole dosages of 12 mg/kg/day are necessary to achieve exposures similar to those in older children and adults. In addition, a loading dose of 25 mg/kg in neonates has achieved steady-state concentrations sooner. While this fluconazole loading dose has been studied in adult and neonatal patients, this approach has never been formally studied in children. Side effects of fluconazole are uncommon but generally include gastrointestinal upset (vomiting, diarrhea, nausea) and skin rash.

Fluconazole plays an important role in the treatment of invasive candidiasis. Consensus guidelines suggest that use of the fungistatic fluconazole for invasive candidiasis is an acceptable alternative to an echinocandin as initial therapy in selected patients, including those who are not critically ill and who are considered unlikely to have a fluconazole-resistant *Candida* species. Although most isolates of *Candida albicans* remain susceptible to fluconazole, for certain *Candida* species fluconazole is not an ideal agent: *C. krusei* is generally resistant and *C. glabrata* is often resistant. In treating infection caused by these *Candida* species, it is critical to treat with an echinocandin or amphotericin B rather than fluconazole. There is no confirmed role for combination antifungal therapy with fluconazole and another antifungal against invasive candidiasis.

Prophylaxis with fluconazole to prevent neonatal candidiasis remains a controversial topic. In the 1st prospective, randomized double-blind trial of 100 infants with birthweights <1,000 g, infants who received fluconazole for 6 wk had a decrease in fungal colonization and a decrease in the development of invasive fungal infection (0% vs. 20%) compared to placebo. Other studies have yielded similarly encouraging results and have demonstrated that use of fluconazole prophylaxis for 4-6 wk in high-risk infants does not increase the incidence of fungal colonization and infections caused by natively fluconazole-resistant *Candida* species. A more recent large trial studied fluconazole prophylaxis in extremely low birthweight infants in nurseries with a lower incidence of candidiasis and found that fluconazole prophylaxis led to a decreased incidence of candidiasis but had no effect on mortality. The universal implementation of such a strategy across nurseries is discouraged, because the rate of *Candida* infections varies greatly among centers. Consensus guidelines now recommend fluconazole prophylaxis only in centers with high rates (>10%) of neonatal candidiasis.

Itraconazole

Compared to fluconazole, itraconazole has the benefit of antifungal activity against *Aspergillus* species but comes with several practical constraints, such as erratic oral absorption in high-risk patients and significant drug interactions. These pharmacokinetic concerns have been addressed with both an intravenous formulation (now no longer available) and a better-absorbed oral solution to replace the unpredictable capsules used earlier. Itraconazole has a high volume of distribution and accumulates in tissues, and tissue-bound levels are probably more clinically relevant to infection treatment than serum levels. Dissolution and absorption of itraconazole are affected by gastric pH. Patients with achlorhydria or taking H_2-receptor antagonists might demonstrate impaired absorption, and co-administration of the capsule with acidic beverages such as colas or cranberry juice can enhance absorption. Administration with food significantly increases the absorption of the capsule formulation, but the oral suspension with a cyclodextrin base is better absorbed on an empty stomach.

Side effects are relatively few and include nausea and vomiting (10%), elevated transaminases (5%), and peripheral edema. There have been reports in adults of development of cardiomyopathy. Because of important drug interactions, prior or concurrent use of rifampin, phenytoin, carbamazepine, and phenobarbital should be avoided.

Itraconazole has a role in treating less-serious infections with endemic mycoses (histoplasmosis, coccidioidomycosis, and blastomycosis), as well as use in prophylaxis against invasive fungal infections in high-risk patients. The plethora of drug interactions make itraconazole a concern in complex patients receiving other medications. As with most azole antifungals, monitoring itraconazole serum levels is a key principle in management (generally itraconazole trough levels should be >0.5-1 μg/mL; trough levels >5 μg/mL may be associated with increased toxicity). Concentrations should be checked after 1-2 wk of therapy to ensure adequate drug exposure. When measured by high-pressure liquid chromatography, both itraconazole and its bioactive hydroxy-itraconazole metabolite are reported, the sum of which should be considered in assessing drug levels. Itraconazole is no longer recommended for primary therapy of invasive aspergillosis.

Voriconazole

Voriconazole is a 2nd-generation triazole and a synthetic derivative of fluconazole. Voriconazole generally has the spectrum of activity of itraconazole and the high bioavailability of fluconazole. Importantly, it is fungicidal against *Aspergillus* and fungistatic against *Candida*. It is extensively metabolized by the liver and has approximately 90% oral bioavailability. The cytochrome P-450 2C19 (CYP2C19) enzyme appears to play a major role in the metabolism of voriconazole, and polymorphisms in CYP2C19 are associated with slow voriconazole metabolism. As many as 20% of non-Indian Asians have low CYP2C19 activity and develop voriconazole levels as much as 4-fold higher than those in homozygous subjects, leading to potentially increased toxicity.

Voriconazole is available as an oral tablet, an oral suspension, and an intravenous solution. In adults, voriconazole exhibits nonlinear pharmacokinetics, has a variable half-life of approximately 6 hr with large interpatient variation in blood levels, and achieves good CSF penetration. In contrast to the situation in adults, elimination of voriconazole is linear in children. A multicenter safety, population pharmacokinetic study of intravenous voriconazole dosages in immunocompromised pediatric patients showed that body weight was more influential than age in accounting for the observed variability in voriconazole pharmacokinetics, and voriconazole needs to be dosed higher in pediatric patients than adult patients. Adult patients load with 6 mg/kg/dose and then transition to a maintenance dosage of 4 mg/kg/dose, but children should begin and continue with 9 mg/kg/dose intravenously (see Table 260.1) and continue maintenance dosing at 8 mg/kg/dose. This need for an increased dosage in treating children is crucial to understand and is mandated by the fundamentally different pharmacokinetics of this drug in pediatric patients. Obtaining voriconazole serum levels (to achieve ≥1-2 μg/mL) is critical for therapeutic success. Oral voriconazole is best absorbed on an empty stomach. Generally a trough level greater than the minimum inhibitory concentration (MIC) of the infecting organism is preferred, and very high voriconazole levels have been associated with toxicity (generally >6 μg/mL). However, many studies have shown an inconsistent relationship between dosing and levels, highlighting the need for close monitoring after the initial dosing scheme and then dose adjustment as needed in the individual patient. The main side effects of voriconazole include reversible dosage-dependent visual disturbances (increased brightness, blurred vision) in as many as one-third of treated patients, elevated hepatic transaminases with increasing dosages, and occasional skin reactions likely caused by photosensitization. In some rare long-term (mean of 3 yr of therapy) cases, this voriconazole phototoxicity has developed into cutaneous squamous cell carcinoma. Discontinuing voriconazole is recommended in patients experiencing chronic phototoxicity.

The largest prospective clinical trial of voriconazole as primary therapy for invasive aspergillosis compared initial randomized therapy with voriconazole versus amphotericin B and demonstrated improved response and survival with voriconazole over amphotericin B. *Voriconazole is guideline-recommended as the preferred primary therapy against invasive aspergillosis.* Voriconazole also has a role in treating candidiasis, but its fungistatic nature makes it often less than ideal for treating critically ill or neutropenic patients where the fungicidal echinocandin antifungals are preferred.

Posaconazole

Posaconazole is a 2nd-generation triazole that is a derivative of itraconazole and is currently available as an oral suspension, an intravenous formulation, and an extended release tablet. The antimicrobial spectrum of posaconazole is similar to that of voriconazole; however, the former is active against *Zygomycetes* such as mucormycosis, and voriconazole is not active against these particular mold infections.

Effective absorption of the oral suspension strongly requires taking the medication with food, ideally a high-fat meal; taking posaconazole on an empty stomach will result in approximately one-fourth of the absorption as in the fed state, emphasizing the importance of diet to increase serum levels of oral suspension posaconazole (the opposite of voriconazole). Posaconazole exposure is maximized with acidic beverages, administration in divided doses, and the absence of proton pump inhibitors. The tablet formulation has better absorption due to its delayed release in the small intestine, but absorption will still be slightly increased with food. If the patient can take the large tablets, the extended-release tablet is the preferred form due to the ability to easily obtain higher and more consistent drug levels. Due to the low pH (<5) of IV posaconazole, a central venous catheter is required for administration. The IV formulation contains only slightly lower amounts of the cyclodextrin vehicle than voriconazole, so similar theoretical renal accumulation concerns exist. Posaconazole causes transient hepatic reactions, including mild to moderate elevations in liver transaminases, alkaline phosphatase, and total bilirubin.

The correct pediatric dosage of posaconazole is not known, because initial studies are still ongoing. In adult patients, dosages >800 mg/day do not result in increased serum levels, and division of daily dosing into 3 or 4 doses/day results in greater serum levels than a once- or twice-daily dosing scheme when using the oral suspension. Similar to itraconazole and voriconazole, posaconazole should be monitored with trough levels (to achieve ≥0.7 μg/mL).

In an international randomized, single-blinded study of posaconazole versus fluconazole or itraconazole in neutropenic patients undergoing chemotherapy for acute myelogenous leukemia or myelodysplastic syndromes, posaconazole was superior in preventing invasive fungal infections. Fewer patients in the posaconazole group had invasive aspergillosis, and survival was significantly longer among recipients of posaconazole than among recipients of fluconazole or itraconazole. Another multisite international randomized, double-blinded study in patients with allogeneic hematopoietic stem-cell transplantation and graft versus host disease showed that posaconazole was not inferior to fluconazole in the prevention of invasive fungal infections. *Posaconazole is approved for prophylaxis against invasive fungal infections but has shown great efficacy in clinical experience with recalcitrant mold infections.*

In patients with chronic granulomatous disease (CGD) and proven invasive fungal infection refractory to standard therapy, posaconazole was proved to be well tolerated and quite effective. This agent might prove to be very useful in this patient population where long-term therapy with an oral agent is required.

Isavuconazole

Isavuconazole is triazole that was FDA approved in March 2015 for treatment of invasive aspergillosis and invasive mucormycosis with oral (capsules only) and IV formulations. Isavuconazole has a similar antifungal spectrum as voriconazole and some activity against *Zygomycetes* (yet potentially not as potent against *Zygomycetes* as posaconazole). A phase 3 clinical trial in adult patients demonstrated non-inferiority versus voriconazole against invasive aspergillosis and other mold infections, while another study showed good clinical activity against mucormycosis. Isavuconazole is dispensed as the prodrug isavuconazonium sulfate. Dosing in adult patients is loading with isavuconazole 200 mg (equivalent to 372-mg isavuconazonium sulfate) every 8 hr for 2 days (6 doses), followed by 200 mg once daily for maintenance dosing. The half-life is long (>5 days), there is 98% bioavailability in adults, and there is no reported food effect with oral isavuconazole. Unlike voriconazole, the IV formulation does not contain the vehicle cyclodextrin, possibly making it more attractive in patients with renal failure. Early experience suggests a much lower rate of photosensitivity and skin disorders as well as visual disturbances compared with voriconazole. No specific pediatric dosing data exist for isavuconazole, yet pediatric pharmacokinetic trials are beginning.

ECHINOCANDINS

The echinocandins are a class of antifungals that interfere with cell wall biosynthesis by noncompetitive inhibition of 1,3-β-D-glucan synthase, an enzyme present in fungi but absent in mammalian cells. 1,3-β-glucan is an essential cell wall polysaccharide and provides structural integrity for the fungal cell wall. Echinocandins are generally fungicidal in vitro against *Candida* species, although not as rapidly as amphotericin B, and are fungistatic against *Aspergillus*. As a class these agents are not metabolized through the CYP enzyme system, lessening some of the drug interactions and side effects seen with the azole class. The echinocandins appear to have a prolonged and dosage-dependent fungicidal antifungal effect on *C. albicans,* compared to the fungistatic fluconazole. Three compounds in this class (caspofungin, micafungin, and anidulafungin) are FDA approved for use. Owing to the large size of the molecules, the current echinocandins are only available in an intravenous formulation. Because 1,3-β-glucan is a selective target present only in fungal cell walls and not in mammalian cells, drug-related toxicity is minimal, with no apparent myelotoxicity or nephrotoxicity with the agents. *The echinocandins are the preferred primary therapy for invasive candidiasis.*

Caspofungin

At present there is no known maximum tolerated dosage and no toxicity-determined maximum length of therapy for caspofungin. The usual course is to begin with a loading dose followed by a lesser daily maintenance dosage, which is 70 mg followed by 50 mg daily in adult patients. Much of the dosage accumulation is achieved in the 1st wk of dosing, and renal insufficiency has little effect on the pharmacokinetics of caspofungin. Caspofungin has been evaluated at double the recommended dosage (100 mg/day in adults) with no adverse effects, and it is unclear if higher dosage of this relatively safe agent results in greater clinical efficacy.

Pharmacokinetics are slightly different in children, with caspofungin levels lower in smaller children and with a reduced half-life. A study evaluated the pharmacokinetics of caspofungin in children with neutropenia and showed that in patients receiving 50 mg/m^2/day (maximum, 70 mg/day), the levels were similar to those in adults receiving 50 mg/day and were consistent across age ranges. In this study, weight-based dosing (1 mg/kg/day) was suboptimal when compared to body surface area regimens, so caspofungin should be appropriately dosed in children as a loading dose of 70 mg/m^2/day, followed by daily maintenance dosing of 50 mg/m^2/day.

Caspofungin was approved for refractory aspergillosis or intolerance to other therapies and for candidemia and various other sites of invasive

Candida infections. In the pivotal clinical study, patients with acute invasive aspergillosis underwent salvage therapy after failing primary therapy, and recipients had a 41% favorable response with caspofungin. In a multicenter trial of patients with invasive candidiasis, 73% of patients who received caspofungin had a favorable response at the end of therapy, compared to 62% in the amphotericin B group. Importantly, caspofungin treatment performed equally well to amphotericin B treatment for all the major *Candida* species, but other studies have shown that some infections with *C. parapsilosis* do not potentially clear as effectively with an echinocandin. Caspofungin was also evaluated against L-amphotericin B in the empirical treatment of patients with persistent fever and neutropenia and was not inferior to liposomal amphotericin B in >1,000 patients.

Caspofungin in children has been reported to be safe. Caspofungin pharmacokinetics were evaluated in older infants and toddlers at 50 mg/m^2/day and found to be similar to adults receiving the standard 50 mg daily dose. Caspofungin in newborns has been used as single or adjuvant therapy for refractory cases of disseminated candidiasis. Neonates with invasive candidiasis are at high risk for central nervous system involvement; it is not known if the dosages of caspofungin studied provide sufficient exposure to penetrate the central nervous system at levels necessary to cure infection. Therefore, caspofungin is not recommended as monotherapy in neonatal candidiasis.

Micafungin

The pharmacokinetics of micafungin have been evaluated in children and young infants. An inverse relation between age and clearance was observed, where mean systemic clearance was significantly greater and mean half-life was significantly shorter in patients 2-8 yr of age compared to patients 9-17 yr of age. Therefore, dosing of micafungin in children is age-related and needs to be higher in children <8 yr old. To achieve micafungin exposures equivalent to exposures in adults receiving 100, 150, and 200 mg daily, as evidenced by simulation profiles, children require dosages >3 mg/kg.

Several pharmacokinetic studies of micafungin in term and preterm infants have shown that micafungin in infants has a shorter half-life and a more rapid rate of clearance compared with published data in older children and adults. These results suggest that young infants should receive 10 mg/kg daily of micafungin if used to treat invasive candidiasis.

The safety profile of micafungin is optimal when compared to other antifungal agents. Clinical trials including those of micafungin used for treatment of localized and invasive candidiasis as well as prophylaxis studies in patients following stem cell transplantation have demonstrated fewer adverse events compared to liposomal amphotericin B and fluconazole. The most common adverse events experienced by these patients are related to the gastrointestinal tract (nausea, diarrhea). Hypersensitivity reactions associated with micafungin have been reported, and liver enzymes are elevated in 5% of patients receiving this agent. Hyperbilirubinemia, renal impairment, and hemolytic anemia related to micafungin use have also been identified in postmarketing surveillance of the drug.

An open-label, noncomparative, multinational study in adult and pediatric patients with a variety of diagnoses evaluated the use of micafungin monotherapy and combination therapy in 225 patients with invasive aspergillosis. Of those only treated with micafungin, favorable responses were seen in 50% of the primary and 41% of the salvage therapy group.

Micafungin at dosages of 100 and 150 mg daily was also noninferior to caspofungin in an international, randomized, double-blinded study of adults with candidemia or invasive candidiasis and was found to be superior to fluconazole in the prevention of invasive fungal infections in a randomized study of adults undergoing hematopoietic stem cell transplantation.

Of the 3 drugs within the echinocandin class, micafungin has been the one most extensively studied in children, including several pharmacokinetic studies in neonates. A pediatric substudy as part of a double-blind, randomized, multinational trial comparing micafungin (2 mg/kg/day) with liposomal amphotericin B (3 mg/kg/day) as 1st-line treatment for invasive candidiasis showed similar success for micafungin and liposomal amphotericin B. In general, micafungin was better tolerated than liposomal amphotericin B as evidenced by fewer adverse events leading to discontinuation of therapy.

Anidulafungin

Anidulafungin has the longest half-life of all the echinocandins (approximately 18 hr). In a study of 25 neutropenic children receiving anidulafungin as empirical therapy, 4 patients in the group receiving 0.75 mg/kg/day experienced adverse events such as facial erythema and rash, elevation in serum blood urea nitrogen, and fever and hypotension. In a pharmacokinetic study in neonates and young infants, anidulafungin exposures comparable to adults were achieved with doses of 1.5 mg/kg/day (3 mg/kg loading dose). One infant in this cohort supported by extracorporeal membrane oxygenation achieved the lowest exposure, which suggests that dose adjustments are required in this population.

A randomized, double-blind study in adult patients without neutropenia with invasive candidiasis showed that anidulafungin was not inferior to fluconazole in the treatment of invasive candidiasis. In this study, the incidence and types of adverse events were similar in the 2 groups, and all-cause mortality was 31% in the fluconazole group and 23% in the anidulafungin group. No clinical studies of anidulafungin in pediatric patients are currently available.

Bibliography is available at Expert Consult.

Chapter **261**
Candida
Jessica E. Ericson and
Daniel K. Benjamin Jr.

第二百六十一章
念珠菌属

中文导读

本章主要介绍了念珠菌属在新生儿、免疫功能正常的儿童和青少年以及免疫缺陷儿童和青少年人群中的感染情况。详细阐述了新生儿念珠菌属感染的流行病学、发病机制、临床表现、诊断、预防、治疗和预后。阐述了在免疫功能正常的儿童和青少年中口腔念珠菌病、尿布性皮炎、甲周感染和外阴阴道炎的治疗。介绍了免疫缺陷儿童和青少年对念珠菌属感染的病因、临床表现、诊断和治疗，在临床表现中对HIV感染、肿瘤和移植以及导管相关感染三类人群的不同特点进行了描述。同时也对原发性免疫缺陷病中的慢性皮肤黏膜念珠菌病进行了简单介绍。

Candidiasis encompasses many clinical syndromes that may be caused by several species of *Candida*. Invasive candidiasis (*Candida* infections of the blood and other sterile body fluids) is a leading cause of infection-related mortality in hospitalized immunocompromised patients.

Candida exists in 3 morphologic forms: oval to round **blastospores or yeast cells** (3-6 mm in diameter); double-walled **chlamydospores** (7-17 mm in diameter), which are usually at the terminal end of a pseudohypha; and **pseudomycelium,** which is a mass of pseudohyphae and represents the tissue phase of *Candida*. **Pseudohyphae** are filamentous processes that elongate from the yeast cell without the cytoplasmic connection of a true hypha. *Candida* grows aerobically on routine laboratory media but can require several days of incubation for visible growth.

Candida albicans accounts for most human infections, but *Candida parapsilosis, Candida tropicalis, Candida krusei, Candida lusitaniae, Candida glabrata,* and several other species are commonly isolated from hospitalized children. Species identification and susceptibility testing are important owing to increasing frequency of fluconazole resistance and increasing prevalence of non-albicans *Candida* species. *Candida auris* is an emerging multi-resistant invasive pathogen that has a global presence and affects immunocompromised patients; nosocomial spread has been reported.

Treatment of invasive *Candida* infections is complicated by the emergence of non-*albicans* strains. Amphotericin B deoxycholate is inactive against approximately 20% of strains of *C. lusitaniae*. Fluconazole is useful for many *Candida* infections but is inactive against all strains of *C. krusei* and 5–25% of strains of *C. glabrata*. Susceptibility testing of these clinical isolates is recommended.

261.1 Neonatal Infections
Jessica E. Ericson and Daniel K. Benjamin Jr.

Candida is a common cause of oral mucous membrane infections (**thrush**) and perineal skin infections (***Candida* diaper dermatitis**) in young infants. Rare presentations include **congenital cutaneous candidiasis,** caused by an ascending infection into the uterus during gestation, and **invasive fungal dermatitis,** a postnatal skin infection resulting in positive blood cultures. Invasive candidiasis is a common infectious complication in the neonatal intensive care unit (NICU) because of improved survival of extremely preterm infants.

EPIDEMIOLOGY

Candida species are the third most common cause of bloodstream infection in premature infants. The cumulative incidence is <0.3% among infants >2,500 g birthweight admitted to the NICU. The cumulative incidence increases to 8% for infants <750 g birthweight. In addition, the incidence varies greatly by individual NICU. Among centers in the National Institutes of Health-sponsored Neonatal Research Network, the cumulative incidence of candidiasis among infants <1,000 g birthweight ranges from 2% to 28%. Colonization is associated with a significantly increased risk of future invasive *Candida* infection. Up to 10% of full-term infants are colonized as the result of vertical transmission from the mother at birth, with slightly higher rates of colonization in premature infants. Colonization rates increase to >50% among infants admitted to the NICU by 1 mo of age. Histamine-2 blockers, corticosteroids, and broad-spectrum antibiotics facilitate *Candida* colonization and overgrowth.

Significant risk factors for neonatal invasive candidiasis include prematurity, low birthweight, exposure to broad-spectrum antibiotics, abdominal surgery, endotracheal intubation, and presence of a central venous catheter.

PATHOGENESIS

Immunologic immaturity along with an underdeveloped layer of skin, need for invasive measures (endotracheal tubes, central venous catheters), and exposure to broad-spectrum antibiotics places preterm infants at great risk for invasive candidiasis. Premature infants are also at high risk for spontaneous intestinal perforations and necrotizing enterocolitis. Both conditions require abdominal surgery, prolonged exposure to broad-spectrum antibiotics, and total parenteral nutrition administration requiring placement of central venous catheters. Each of these factors increases the risk of invasive candidiasis by decreasing the physiologic barriers that protect against invasive infection.

CLINICAL MANIFESTATIONS

The manifestations of neonatal candidiasis vary in severity from oral thrush and *Candida* diaper dermatitis (see Chapter 261.2) to invasive candidiasis that can manifest with overwhelming sepsis (see Chapter 261.3). Signs of invasive candidiasis among premature infants are often nonspecific and include temperature instability, lethargy, apnea, hypotension, respiratory distress, abdominal distention, and thrombocytopenia.

Central nervous system involvement is common and is most accurately described as meningoencephalitis. *Candida* infections involving the central nervous system often result in abscesses, leading to unremarkable cerebrospinal fluid parameters (white blood cell count, glucose, protein) even though central nervous system infection is present. Endophthalmitis is an uncommon complication affecting <5% of infants with invasive candidiasis. In addition, candidemia is associated with an increased risk of severe retinopathy of prematurity. Renal involvement commonly complicates neonatal invasive candidiasis. Renal involvement may be limited to candiduria or can manifest with diffuse infiltration of *Candida* throughout the renal parenchyma or the presence of *Candida* and debris within the collecting system. Due to the poor sensitivity of blood cultures for *Candida*, candiduria should be considered a surrogate marker of candidemia in premature infants. Other affected organs include the heart, bones, joints, liver, and spleen.

DIAGNOSIS

Mucocutaneous infections are most often diagnosed by direct clinical exam. Scrapings of skin lesions may be examined with a microscope after Gram staining or suspension in KOH. Definitive diagnosis of invasive disease requires histologic demonstration of the fungus in tissue specimens or recovery of the fungus from normally sterile body fluids. Hematologic parameters are sensitive but not specific. Thrombocytopenia occurs in more than 80% of premature infants with invasive candidiasis, but also occurs in 75% of premature infants with Gram-negative bacterial sepsis and nearly 50% of infants with Gram-positive bacterial sepsis. Blood cultures have very low sensitivity for invasive candidiasis. In a study of autopsy-proven candidiasis in adult patients, the sensitivity of multiple blood cultures for detecting single-organ disease was 28%. Blood culture volumes in infants are often only 0.5-1 mL, making the sensitivity in this population almost certainly lower. Blood culture volume should be maximized as much as possible to increase sensitivity. Fungal-specific media can improve sensitivity when *Candida* is present as a coinfection with bacteria and can also decrease the time to positivity, leading to more rapid diagnosis.

Further assessment of infants in the presence of documented candidemia should include ultrasound or computerized tomography of the head to evaluate for abscesses; ultrasound of the liver, kidney, and spleen; cardiac echocardiography; ophthalmologic exam; lumbar puncture; and urine culture. These tests are necessary to determine if more than 1 body system is infected, which is commonly the case.

PROPHYLAXIS

NICUs with a high incidence of invasive candidiasis should consider prophylaxis with fluconazole in infants <1,000 g birthweight as a cost-effective method of reducing invasive candidiasis. Twice-weekly fluconazole at 3 or 6 mg/kg/dose decreases rates of both colonization with *Candida* species and invasive fungal infections. Use of this dosing strategy has not been shown to increase the frequency of infections caused by fluconazole-resistant strains, but use of an alternative antifungal class for cases of breakthrough infection is suggested.

TREATMENT

In the absence of systemic manifestations, topical antifungal therapy is the treatment of choice for congenital cutaneous candidiasis in full-term infants. Congenital cutaneous candidiasis in preterm infants can progress to systemic disease, and therefore systemic therapy is warranted.

Every attempt should be made to remove or replace central venous catheters once the diagnosis of candidemia is confirmed. Delayed removal has been consistently associated with increased mortality and morbidity, including poor neurodevelopmental outcomes.

Although no well-powered randomized, controlled trials exist to guide length and type of therapy, 21 days of systemic antifungal therapy from the last positive *Candida* culture is recommended in infants. Antifungal therapy should be targeted based on susceptibility testing. Amphotericin B deoxycholate has been the mainstay of therapy for systemic candidiasis and is active against both yeast and mycelial forms. Nephrotoxicity, hypokalemia, and hypomagnesemia are common, but amphotericin B deoxycholate is better tolerated in infants than in adult patients. *C. lusitaniae*, an uncommon pathogen in infants, is often resistant to amphotericin B deoxycholate. Liposomal amphotericin is associated with worse outcomes in infants and should be used only when urinary tract involvement can reliably be excluded. Fluconazole is often used instead of amphotericin B deoxycholate for treatment of invasive neonatal *Candida* infections because of its effectiveness and low incidence of side effects. It is particularly useful for urinary tract infections, obtaining high concentrations in the urine. A loading dose should be given to obtain therapeutic serum concentrations in a timely manner. Fluconazole is inactive against all strains of *C. krusei* and some isolates of *C. glabrata*. Additionally, in centers where fluconazole prophylaxis is used, another agent, such as amphotericin B deoxycholate, should be used for treatment. The echinocandins have excellent activity against most *Candida* species and have been used successfully in patients with resistant organisms or in whom other therapies have failed. Several studies have described the pharmacokinetics of antifungals in infants (Table 261.1).

PROGNOSIS

Mortality following invasive candidiasis in premature infants has been consistently reported to be around 20% in large studies but can be as high as 50% in infants <1,500 g birthweight. Candidiasis is also associated with poor neurodevelopmental outcomes, chronic lung disease, and severe retinopathy of prematurity.

Bibliography is available at Expert Consult.

261.2 Infections in Immunocompetent Children and Adolescents

Jessica E. Ericson and Daniel K. Benjamin Jr.

ORAL CANDIDIASIS

Oral thrush is a superficial mucous membrane infection that affects approximately 2–5% of normal neonates. *C. albicans* is the most commonly isolated species. Oral thrush can develop as early as 7-10 days of age. The use of antibiotics, especially in the 1st yr of life, can lead to recurrent or persistent thrush. It is characterized by pearly white, curdish material visible on the tongue, palate, and buccal mucosa. Oral thrush may be asymptomatic or can cause pain, fussiness, and decreased feeding,

Table 261.1	Dosing of Antifungal Agents in Infants* and Number of Infants Younger Than 1 Yr of Age Studied With Reported Pharmacokinetic Parameters

DRUG	INFANTS STUDIED	SUGGESTED DOSE
Amphotericin B deoxycholate	27	1 mg/kg/day
Amphotericin B lipid complex	28	5 mg/kg/day
Liposomal amphotericin B	17	5 mg/kg/day
Amphotericin B colloidal dispersion	0	5 mg/kg/day
Fluconazole[†]	65	12 mg/kg/day
Micafungin[‡]	138	10 mg/kg/day
Caspofungin[§]	22	50 mg/m²/day
Anidulafungin[‡]	15	1.5 mg/kg/day

*Voriconazole dosing has not been investigated in the nursery.
[†]A loading dose of 25 mg/kg of fluconazole is necessary to achieve therapeutic serum concentrations in the early days of therapy.
[‡]Micafungin has been studied in infants <120 days of life at this dosage.
[§]Caspofungin and anidulafungin should generally be avoided because dosing sufficient to penetrate brain tissue has not been studied.

leading to inadequate nutritional intake and dehydration. It is uncommon after 1 yr of age but can occur in older children treated with antibiotics. Persistent or recurrent thrush with no obvious predisposing reason, such as recent antibiotic treatment, warrants investigation of an underlying immunodeficiency, especially vertically transmitted HIV infection or a primary congenital immune defect.

Treatment of mild cases might not be necessary. When treatment is warranted, the most commonly prescribed antifungal agent is topical nystatin. For recalcitrant or recurrent infections, a single dose of fluconazole may be useful. In breastfed infants, simultaneous treatment of infant and mother with topical nystatin or oral fluconazole may be indicated.

DIAPER DERMATITIS

Diaper dermatitis is the most common infection caused by *Candida* (see Chapter 686) and is characterized by a confluent erythematous rash with satellite pustules. *Candida* diaper dermatitis often complicates other noninfectious diaper dermatitides and often occurs following a course of oral antibiotics.

A common practice is to presumptively treat any diaper rash that has been present for longer than 3 days with topical antifungal therapy such as nystatin, clotrimazole, or miconazole. If significant inflammation is present, the addition of hydrocortisone 1% may be useful for the 1st 1-2 days, but topical corticosteroids should be used cautiously in infants because the relatively potent topical corticosteroid can lead to adverse effects. Frequent diaper changes and short periods without diapers are important adjunctive treatments.

UNGUAL AND PERIUNGUAL INFECTIONS

Paronychia and onychomycosis may be caused by *Candida*, although *Trichophyton* and *Epidermophyton* are more common causes (see Chapter 686). *Candida* onychomycosis differs from tinea infections by its propensity to involve the fingernails and not the toenails, and by the associated paronychia. *Candida* paronychia often responds to treatment consisting of keeping the hands dry and using a topical antifungal agent. Psoriasis and immune dysfunction, including HIV and primary immunodeficiencies, predispose to *Candida* ungual infections. Ungual infections often require systemic antifungal therapy. Once-weekly fluconazole for 4-12 mo is an effective treatment strategy with fairly low toxicity.

VULVOVAGINITIS

Vulvovaginitis is a common *Candida* infection of pubertal and post-pubertal female patients (see Chapter 564). Predisposing factors include pregnancy, use of oral contraceptives, and use of oral antibiotics.

Prepubertal girls with *Candida* vulvovaginitis usually have a predisposing factor such as diabetes mellitus or prolonged antibiotic treatment. Clinical manifestations can include pain or itching, dysuria, vulvar or vaginal erythema, and an opaque white or cheesy exudate. More than 80% of cases are caused by *C. albicans*.

Candida vulvovaginitis can be effectively treated with either vaginal creams or troches of nystatin, clotrimazole, or miconazole. Oral therapy with a single dose of fluconazole is also effective.

Bibliography is available at Expert Consult.

261.3 Infections in Immunocompromised Children and Adolescents

Jessica E. Ericson and Daniel K. Benjamin Jr.

ETIOLOGY

Candida albicans is the most common cause of invasive candidiasis among immunocompromised pediatric patients and is associated with higher rates of mortality and end-organ involvement than are non-*albicans* species.

CLINICAL MANIFESTATIONS
HIV-Infected Children

Oral thrush and diaper dermatitis are the most common *Candida* infections in HIV-infected children. Besides oral thrush, 3 other types of oral *Candida* infections can occur in HIV-infected children: atrophic candidiasis, which manifests as a fiery erythema of the mucosa or loss of papillae of the tongue; chronic hyperplastic candidiasis, which presents with oral symmetric white plaques; and angular cheilitis, in which there is erythema and fissuring of the angles of the mouth. Topical antifungal therapy may be effective, but systemic treatment with fluconazole or itraconazole is usually necessary. Symptoms of dysphagia or poor oral intake can indicate progression to *Candida* esophagitis, requiring systemic antifungal therapy. In HIV patients, esophagitis can also be caused by cytomegalovirus, herpes simplex virus, reflux, or lymphoma; *Candida* is the most common cause, and *Candida* esophagitis can occur in the absence of thrush.

Candida dermatitis and onychomycosis are more common in HIV-infected children. These infections are generally more severe than they are in immunocompetent children and can require systemic antifungal therapy.

Cancer and Transplant Patients

Fungal infections, especially *Candida* and *Aspergillus* infections, are a significant problem in oncology patients with chemotherapy-associated neutropenia (see Chapter 205). Greater than 5 days of fever during a neutropenic episode is associated with presence of an invasive fungal infection. Accordingly, empirical antifungal therapy should be started if fever and neutropenia persist for 5 or more days. An echinocandin should be used until sensitivity testing results are available. High-risk oncology patients warrant prophylaxis against invasive *Candida* infection. Both fluconazole and echinocandins are used for this indication, typically at lower doses than those used for treatment. If an echinocandin is used for prophylaxis, liposomal amphotericin B should be used if empirical treatment becomes warranted.

Bone marrow transplant recipients have a much higher risk of fungal infections because of the dramatically prolonged duration of neutropenia. Voriconazole prophylaxis decreases the incidence of candidemia in bone marrow transplant recipients with the additional benefit over fluconazole of mold prophylaxis. The use of granulocyte colony-stimulating factor reduces the duration of neutropenia after chemotherapy and is associated with decreased risk for candidemia. When *Candida* infection occurs in this population, the lung, spleen, kidney, and liver are involved in more than 50% of cases.

Solid-organ transplant recipients are also at increased risk for superficial and invasive *Candida* infections. Studies in liver transplant recipients demonstrate the utility of antifungal prophylaxis with amphotericin B deoxycholate, fluconazole, voriconazole, or caspofungin in high-risk patients (those with prolonged surgical time, comorbidities, recent antibiotic exposure, or bile leak).

Catheter-Associated Infections

Central venous catheter infections occur most often in oncology patients but can affect any patient with a central catheter (see Chapter 206). Neutropenia, use of broad-spectrum antibiotics, and parenteral alimentation are associated with increased risk for *Candida* central catheter infection. Treatment typically requires removing or replacing the catheter followed by a 2-3-wk course of systemic antifungal therapy. Removal of the central catheter in place at time of positive blood culture and use of a peripheral IV or enteral support for at least 48 hr prior to obtaining central access is advocated. Removal of the original catheter followed by immediate replacement with a new central catheter in a different anatomic location is acceptable if an interval without central access is not feasible. Delays in catheter removal are associated with increased risks of metastatic complications and death.

DIAGNOSIS

The diagnosis is often presumptive in neutropenic patients with prolonged fever because positive blood cultures for *Candida* occur only in a minority of patients who are later found to have disseminated infection. If isolated, *Candida* grows readily on routine blood culture media, with ≥90% of positive cultures identified within 72 hr. CT may demonstrate findings consistent with invasive fungal infection but also is limited by nonspecific findings and false negatives. The role of screening by CT scan has not been well defined. In high-risk patients, serial serum assays for (1,3)-β-D-glucan, a polysaccharide component of the fungal cell wall, may contribute to the diagnosis of invasive Candida infection. However, this test is not sensitive or specific enough to be used without a careful assessment of the limitations of the assay.

TREATMENT

Echinocandins are favored as empirical therapy for moderately or severely ill children and for those with neutropenia; fluconazole is acceptable for those who are infected with a susceptible organism and are less critically ill; amphotericin B products are also acceptable. Definitive antifungal selection should be made based on susceptibility testing results. Fluconazole is not effective against *C. krusei* and some isolates of *C. glabrata*. *C. parapsilosis* has occasional resistance to the echinocandins, but the overall rate is still low. Amphotericin B deoxycholate is inactive against approximately 20% of the strains of *C. lusitaniae,* and therefore susceptibility testing should be performed for all strains (Table 261.2). *C. auris,* a species first identified in 2009 that has caused nosocomial infections worldwide, is resistant to most antifungals. An echinocandin should be used until sensitivity results are available.

Table 261.2	Dosing of Antifungal Agents in Children Older Than 1 Yr of Age for Treatment of Invasive Disease
DRUG	**SUGGESTED DOSAGE**
Amphotericin B deoxycholate	1 mg/kg/day
Amphotericin B lipid complex	5 mg/kg/day
Liposomal amphotericin B	5 mg/kg/day
Amphotericin B colloidal dispersion	5 mg/kg/day
Fluconazole[†]	12 mg/kg/day
Voriconazole[*,‡]	8 mg/kg every 12 hr
Micafungin	2-4 mg/kg/day
Caspofungin	50 mg/m²/day
Anidulafungin	1.5 mg/kg/day

*Use adult dosages in children older than 12 yr of age for voriconazole and older than 8 yr of age for micafungin.
[†]Loading doses should be used for fluconazole (25 mg/kg), voriconazole (9 mg/kg q 12 × 24 hr), caspofungin (70 mg/m²), and anidulafungin (3 mg/kg).
[‡]Dosing should be adjusted based on the results of therapeutic drug monitoring.

PRIMARY IMMUNE DEFECTS

Chronic mucocutaneous candidiasis involves *Candida* infections of the oral cavity, esophagus, and/or genital mucosa, as well as involvement of skin and nails, that is recurrent or persistent and difficult to treat. There is a broad spectrum of genetic immune defects associated with chronic mucocutaneous candidiasis mostly related to severe T-cell defects or disorders of interleukin-17 production (see Chapter 151). Genes or disorders associated with chronic mucocutaneous candidiasis include severe combined immunodeficiency syndrome, NEMO or IKBG deficiency, DOCK8 deficiency, STAT3 deficiency (autosomal dominant hyperimmunoglobulin E syndrome), autoimmune polyendocrinopathy type 1, CARD9 deficiency, *STAT1* gain-of-function mutations, and *IL17RA* mutations.

Primary immunodeficiencies associated with an increased risk of invasive *Candida* infections include severe congenital neutropenia, CARD 9 deficiency, chronic granulomatous disease, and leukocyte adhesion deficiency type 1.

Bibliography is available at Expert Consult.

Chapter **262**
Cryptococcus neoformans and *Cryptococcus gattii*
David L. Goldman

第二百六十二章
新生隐球菌和格特隐球菌

中文导读

本章主要介绍了隐球菌感染的情况，因在众多分类中新生隐球菌和格特隐球菌是主要病原，故着重介绍上述两种菌。详细阐述了新生隐球菌和格特隐球菌感染的流行病学、发病机制、临床表现、诊断、治疗和预防。在临床表现中根据感染部位不同，分别介绍了与新生隐球菌和格特隐球菌感染相关的脑膜炎、肺炎、皮肤感染、骨骼感染和脓毒症的特征。

ETIOLOGY

While more than 30 cryptococcal species have been described, 2 species (*Cryptococcus neoformans* and *C. gattii*) are responsible for the vast majority of disease. These species can be further classified by serologic and molecular typing techniques. Both *C. neoformans* and *C. gattii* are encapsulated, facultative intracellular pathogens. There is significant overlap in the disease caused by these pathogens; however, important differences in epidemiology and clinical presentation exist. Cryptococcal disease may rarely also be caused by other species (e.g., *C. laurentii* and *C. albidus*), especially in immunocompromised individuals (including neonates).

EPIDEMIOLOGY

C. neoformans is distributed in temperate climates predominantly in soil contaminated with droppings from certain avian species, including pigeons, canaries, and cockatoos. It may also be found on rotting wood, fruits, and vegetables and may be carried by cockroaches. Disease secondary to *C. neoformans* primarily occurs in immunocompromised individuals and especially in those with defects in cellular immunity, though apparently normal individuals can also be affected. A large increase in the incidence of cryptococcosis was noted in association with the AIDS epidemic, with disease generally occurring with severe immunosuppression (CD4$^+$T cells < 100/μL). However, since the development of highly active anti-retroviral therapy (HAART), the incidence of AIDS-associated cryptococcosis has decreased dramatically, except in resource-limited areas of the world such as sub-Saharan Africa, where HAART is not readily available.

Other risk factors for cryptococcal infection include immunosuppression associated with organ transplantation, diabetes mellitus, renal failure, cirrhosis, corticosteroids, rheumatologic conditions, chemotherapeutics, and immune modulating monoclonal antibodies (e.g., etanercept, infliximab, and alemtuzumab). In patients who have undergone organ transplantation, cryptococcosis is the third most common fungal infection after candidiasis and aspergillosis. Children with certain primary immunodeficiency diseases may also be at increased risk for cryptococcosis, including those with hyper-IgM syndrome, severe combined immunodeficiency, idiopathic CD4$^+$ lymphopenia, autoantibodies to granulocyte-macrophage colony-stimulating factor or interferon-γ, CD40 ligand deficiency, and monoMAC syndrome (monocytopenia, B and natural killer cell lymphopenia).

C. gattii was initially recognized for its tendency to cause disease in tropical regions, especially among the native peoples of Australasia, where the organism can be found in association with Eucalyptus trees. In these regions, affected individuals are typically immunocompetent. More recently, *C. gattii* disease has been observed outside these tropical regions. An outbreak of *C. gattii* disease involving British Columbia and extending into the Pacific Northwest region of the United States was first recognized in 1999. Affected individuals were typically adults, with disease occurring in both immunocompetent and immunocompromised individuals. Comorbid conditions were often present, with examples including chronic lung and heart disease. A disproportionate fraction of patients (relative to those infected with *C. neoformans*) presented with pulmonary disease. An incubation period ranging from 2 to 12 mo is typical. In the appropriate clinical context, cryptococcosis should be considered in the differential diagnosis of residents of the Pacific Northwest as well as returning travelers.

Overall, cryptococcosis is significantly less common in children than in adults. The basis for this discrepancy is poorly understood but could be related to differences in exposure or immune response. Serologic studies suggest that subclinical infection is common among children living in urban areas after age 2 yr. During the early AIDS epidemic, the incidence of cryptococcosis in the United States was reported to be on the order of 10% in adults and 1% in children. The largest series of pediatric cryptococcosis comes from South Africa and describes 361 cases, accounting for 2% of the cryptococcosis cases over a 2-yr period. More recent series of pediatric cases, including those from Asia, the United States, and Colombia, highlight the potential for Cryptococcus (including *C. neoformans*) to cause disease in immunosuppressed and non-immunosuppressed children.

PATHOGENESIS

Like many fungi, *C. neoformans* and *C. gattii* survive as saprophytes in the environment. Their virulence characteristics appear to have evolved as an adaptive response to environmental stressors. Several key factors have been identified, including the ability to grow at 37°C, encapsulation, and melanin production. The polysaccharide capsule exhibits a variety of biologic activities that are important in the pathogenesis of disease, including interference with opsonization, inhibition of chemotaxis, and enhancement of non-protective TH2 inflammation. Capsular material is shed by the organism into body tissues and fluids during infection and has been implicated in the development of increased intracranial pressure (ICP), a hallmark of cryptococcal meningoencephalitis. Detection of shed capsular antigen in the serum and CSF are key to the diagnosis of cryptococcal disease. The organism also has the ability to undergo phenotypic variation in response to environmental changes through a variety of mechanisms and can form large giant cells (on the order 20 times its normal size), which are resistant to phagocytosis.

In most cases, infection is acquired by inhalation of desiccated forms of the organism, which upon deposition within the lungs are engulfed by alveolar macrophages. An additional portal of entry can be seen with organ transplantation of infected tissue. Furthermore, direct inoculation can lead to cutaneous or ophthalmic infection. After entry into the respiratory tract, infection can be latent and later progress in the context of immunodeficiency. Alternatively, infection can progress and disseminate to produce symptomatic disease. Cell-mediated immunity that leads to macrophage activation is the most important host defense for producing granulomatous inflammation and containing cryptococcal infection. Entry of the organism into the CNS may occur via several mechanisms, including infected macrophages, through infected endothelial cells, and between the tight junctions of endothelial cells.

CLINICAL MANIFESTATIONS

The manifestations of cryptococcal infection reflect the route of inoculation, the infecting strain, and immune status of the host. Sites of infection include lung, CNS, blood, skin, bone, eyes, and lymph nodes.

Meningitis

CNS disease is the most commonly recognized manifestation of cryptococcosis. The disease is characteristically subacute or chronic, and affected patients may develop intracerebral masses, known as cryptococcomas and increased ICP. Importantly meningeal signs and fever (typical of other pediatric meningitides) may be lacking. In a review of pediatric cryptococcosis from Colombia, the most common symptoms were headache (78%), fever (69%), nausea and vomiting (66%), confusion (50%), and meningismus (38%).

Despite antifungal therapy, the mortality rate for cryptococcosis remains high, ranging from 15% to 40%. Most deaths occur within several weeks of diagnosis. Factors associated with a poor prognosis reflect a high fungal burden and poor host response, including altered mentation, high CSF fungal burden, low CSF WBC number (<10 cells/mm³), and failure to rapidly sterilize the CSF. Increased ICP is a key factor in the morbidity and mortality of cryptococcal meningitis and is especially problematic for patients with *C. gattii* disease. Appropriate management of increased ICP is therefore essential to the appropriate management of cryptococcal meningitis (see below). Post-infectious sequelae are common and include hydrocephalus, decreased visual acuity, deafness, cranial nerve palsies, seizures, and ataxia.

Pneumonia

After CNS disease, pneumonia is the most commonly recognized form of cryptococcosis. As with meningitis, pneumonia occurs in both immunocompetent and immunocompromised individuals. Pulmonary disease can present in isolation or in the context of disseminated disease, meningitis, which is typical among immunocompromised individuals. Along these lines, among adults with AIDS-associated cryptococcal pneumonia, over 90% had concomitant CNS infection. Clinicians should have a high suspicion for cryptococcal meningitis/disseminated disease in patients with cryptococcal pneumonia, especially among immuno-compromised individuals.

Cryptococcal pneumonia is often asymptomatic and may be detected because of radiographs performed for other reasons. In this regard, the detection of asymptomatic pulmonary nodules secondary to *C. neoformans* has been described in children with sarcomas, who are being evaluated for metastatic disease. Among symptomatic patients, a wide array of symptoms has been reported, including fever, cough, pleuritic chest pain, and constitutional symptoms like weight loss. In a review of 24 patients with pulmonary cryptococcosis, cough was the most common symptom. Severe disease may result in respiratory failure. The findings of chest radiographs are variable and may demonstrate a poorly localized bronchopneumonia, nodules, masses, or lobar consolidations. However, cavities and pleural effusions are rare. Immunocompromised patients can have alveolar and interstitial infiltrates that mimic *Pneumocystis* pneumonia and usually represent disseminated disease.

Cutaneous Infection

Cutaneous disease most commonly follows disseminated cryptococcosis and rarely local inoculation. Early lesions are erythematous, may be single or multiple, and are variably indurated and tender. Lesions often become ulcerated with central necrosis and raised borders. Cutaneous cryptococcosis in immunocompromised patients can resemble molluscum contagiosum.

Skeletal Infection

Skeletal infection occurs in approximately 5% of patients with disseminated infection but rarely in HIV-infected patients. The onset of symptoms is insidious and chronic. Bone involvement is typified by soft tissue swelling and tenderness, and arthritis is characterized by effusion, erythema, and pain on motion. Skeletal disease is unifocal in approximately 75% of cases. The vertebrae are the most common sites of infection, followed by the tibia, ileum, rib, femur, and humerus. Concomitant bone and joint disease results from contiguous spread.

Sepsis Syndrome

Sepsis syndrome is a rare manifestation of cryptococcosis and occurs almost exclusively among HIV-infected patients. Fever is followed by respiratory distress and multiorgan system disease that is often fatal.

Cryptococcal-associated immune reconstitution inflammatory syndrome (C-IRIS) occurs in the setting of AIDS. Improvement of immune function due to the administration of HAART in AIDS patients (or the reduction of immunosuppression in transplant recipients) may enhance inflammation to the organism, resulting in exacerbation of symptoms. This situation is similar to IRIS seen with other opportunistic pathogens. IRIS may present as a worsening of symptoms in someone with a known diagnosis of cryptococcosis or in someone in whom the diagnosis of cryptococcosis is sub-clinical (unmasking-IRIS). IRIS is particularly problematic in CNS cryptococcosis and may result in worsening of increased ICP. The extent of C-IRIS in pediatric cryptococcosis is not well characterized.

DIAGNOSIS

Recovery of the fungus by culture or demonstration of the fungus in histologic sections of infected tissue or body fluids by India ink staining is definitive. Cryptococci can grow easily on standard fungal and bacterial culture media. Colonies can be seen within 48-72 hr when grown aerobically at standard temperatures. The CSF profile in patients with cryptococcal meningitis may reveal a mild lymphocytosis and elevated protein but is often normal. A latex agglutination test, which detects cryptococcal antigen in serum and CSF, is the most useful diagnostic test. Titers of >1:4 in bodily fluid strongly suggest infection, and titers of >1:1,024 reflect high burden of yeast, poor host immune response, and greater likelihood of therapeutic failure. Serial monitoring of cryptococcal antigen levels is not useful in guiding therapy, as the polysaccharide antigen is actively shed into the tissue and may persist for prolonged periods. Patients with localized pneumonia typically do not have elevated serum antigen levels (though occasionally low levels of antigen, <1:4 may be detected). Higher serum antigen levels in patients with pulmonary disease are indicative of dissemination outside the lungs. A point of care lateral flow assay based on polysaccharide antigen detection has been developed for use in resource limited areas.

TREATMENT

The choice of treatment depends on the sites of involvement and the host immune status. Treatment regimens have not been rigorously studied in children and generally represent extrapolations from studies done in adults. The immunocompetent patient with asymptomatic or mild disease limited to the lungs should be treated with oral fluconazole (pediatric dose 6-12 mg/kg/day and adult dose 400 mg/day) for 6-12 mo to prevent dissemination of disease. Alternative treatments include itraconazole (pediatric dose 5-10 mg/kg/day divided every 12 hr and adult dose 400 mg/day), voriconazole, and posaconazole. Fluconazole therapy can also be used for immunocompromised individuals with isolated mild-moderate pulmonary disease in the absence of dissemination or CNS disease, as evidenced by unremarkable CSF studies. Longer maintenance therapy with fluconazole to prevent recurrence should be considered in this cohort, especially among AIDS patients if CD4+ T cells remain less than 100/μL. Adjunctive surgical management of pulmonary lesions that are not responsive to surgical management should be considered.

For more severe forms of disease including meningitis and any form of disseminated disease, an initial induction regimen to promote rapid decline in fungal burden is indicated. Induction therapy should consist of amphotericin B (1 mg/kg/day) plus flucytosine (100-150 mg/kg/day divided every 6 hr assuming normal kidney function) for a minimum of 2 wk, keeping serum flucytosine concentrations between 40 and 60 μg/mL. Longer periods of induction (4-6 wk) should be considered in the following scenarios: (1) Immunocompetent patients with cryptococcal meningitis; (2) Meningitis secondary to *C. gattii*; (3) Neurological complications (including cryptococcomas); and (4) Absence of flucytosine in the induction regimen. Lipid-complex amphotericin B (3-6 mg/kg/day) can be used in place of amphotericin B for patients with underlying renal injury or those receiving nephrotoxic drugs. Following induction, consolidation therapy with oral fluconazole (pediatric dose 10-12 mg/

kg/day, adult dose 400-800 mg/day) should be given for 8 wk. In patients with ongoing immunosuppression, maintenance fluconazole should be used to prevent recurrence. In organ transplant recipients, current recommendations are for 6-12 mo of maintenance therapy with fluconazole (pediatric dose 6 mg/kg/day, adult dose 200-400 mg/day). In patients with AIDS, prolonged maintenance therapy should be given. Studies in adults suggest that maintenance therapy can be discontinued once the patient has achieved immune reconstitution (as indicated by CD4+ T cells >100/μL and undetectable or very low HIV RNA level that is sustained for greater than 3 mo). A minimum of 12 mo of antifungal therapy is indicated. Use of adjuvant interferon gamma for patients with refractory cryptococcal meningitis has been described in adults, but not in pediatric patients.

Increased ICP. Increased ICP contributes greatly to the morbidity and mortality of cryptococcal meningitis, and aggressive management of this phenomenon is indicated. Current guidelines indicate that in patients with increased ICP (>25 cm H$_2$O), CSF should be removed to establish a pressure ≤ 20 cm H$_2$O or by 50% if ICP is extremely high. Ventriculoperitoneal shunts may be required for patients with persistently elevated increased ICP. Corticosteroids, mannitol, and acetazolamide are generally not indicated in the treatment of increased ICP, though anecdotal reports describe use in association with cryptococcoma and C-IRIS.

C-IRIS. To prevent the development of C-IRIS, most experts recommend delaying the institution of HAART for 4-10 wk after the initiation of antifungal therapy. Recurrence of disease and emergence of antifungal resistance should be excluded in the context of a diagnosis of C-IRIS. Treatment strategies have not been well studied but generally consist of antifungal therapy along with antiinflammatory agents (e.g., NSAIDs and corticosteroids). Reduction of increased ICP through therapeutic lumbar puncture may be necessary.

PREVENTION

Persons at high risk should avoid exposures such as bird droppings. Effective HAART for persons with HIV infection reduces the risk of cryptococcal disease. Fluconazole prophylaxis is effective for preventing cryptococcosis in patients with AIDS and CD4+ lymphocyte counts <100/μL. An alternative approach involves serial monitoring of serum cryptococcal antigen with pre-emptive antifungal therapy.

Bibliography is available at Expert Consult.

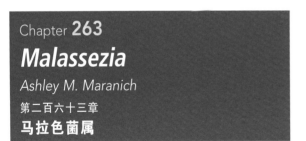

Chapter **263**

Malassezia

Ashley M. Maranich

第二百六十三章

马拉色菌属

中文导读

　　本章主要介绍了马拉色菌属的命名、生物学特性、致病性、易感人群、临床表现和治疗。马拉色菌属为亲脂性酵母菌，感染好发于皮脂腺丰富部位。临床表现以皮肤和头皮病变为主，包括花斑癣、新生儿

痤疮、脂溢性皮炎和头皮屑、头皮银屑病、毛囊炎、头颈部特应性皮炎等。治疗分为局部涂抹和口服用药

两种方式。治疗成功后可维持数月，易出现复发。

Members of the genus *Malassezia* include the causative agents of **tinea versicolor** (also **pityriasis versicolor**) (Fig. 263.1) and are associated with other dermatologic conditions and with fungemia in patients with indwelling catheters. *Malassezia* species are commensal lipophilic yeasts with a predilection for the sebum-rich areas of the skin. They are considered a part of the normal skin flora, with presence established by 3-6 mo of age.

The history of *Malassezia* nomenclature is complex and can be confusing. Because the yeast forms may be oval or round, these organisms were formally designated *Pityrosporum ovale* and *Pityrosporum orbiculare*. Newer technologies have allowed an improved classification system, with 13 recognized species. Only *Malassezia pachydermatis*, a zoophilic yeast that causes dermatitis in dogs, is not lipophilic.

Transformation of the yeast form to a hyphal form facilitates invasive disease. The clusters of thick-walled blastospores together with the hyphae produce the characteristic spaghetti-and-meatballs appearance of *Malassezia* species.

M. globosa, *M. sympodialis*, *M. restricta*, and *M. furfur* are the major causes of tinea versicolor (see Chapter 686). *Malassezia* organisms are also increasingly associated with other dermatologic conditions. *M. sympodialis* and *M. globosa* are implicated in neonatal acne, and *M. globosa* and *M. restricta* are most closely associated with seborrheic dermatitis and dandruff. *Malassezia* are also causally associated with scalp psoriasis, *Pityrosporum* folliculitis, and head and neck atopic

dermatitis. *Malassezia* may be isolated from sebum-rich areas of asymptomatic persons, emphasizing that demonstration of the fungus does not equate with infection.

The traditional primary therapy for tinea versicolor is topical selenium sulfide 2.5% applied daily for at least 10 min for a week, followed by weekly to monthly applications for several months to prevent relapse. Additional topical agents that have efficacy include terbinafine, clotrimazole, topical azoles, and tacrolimus. *Malassezia*-associated skin diseases limited to the head and neck can be managed with either 1% ciclopirox, ketoconazole, or zinc pyrithione shampoos.

Oral therapy for tinea versicolor with fluconazole or itraconazole is easier to administer but is more expensive, has higher side effect risks, and may be less effective than topical therapy. Various dosing regimens have been used with success, including fluconazole 300 mg weekly for 2-4 wk, fluconazole as a single 400 mg dose, and itraconazole 200 mg daily for 5-7 days or 100 mg daily for 2 wk. Regardless of the regimen chosen, patients should be encouraged to exercise while taking these medications so as to increase the skin concentration of the drug through sweating.

Despite successful treatment, repigmentation might not occur for several months. Relapses are common and can require repeat or alternative therapies.

M. furfur is the species most commonly causing fungemia, and *M. pachydermatis* has been implicated in several outbreaks in neonatal intensive care units. The use of lipid emulsions containing medium-chain triglycerides inhibits the growth of *Malassezia* and can prevent infection. Infection is most common in premature infants, although immunocompromised patients, especially those with malignancies, can also be infected. Symptoms of catheter-associated fungemia are indistinguishable from other causes of catheter-associated infections but should be suspected in patients, especially neonates, receiving intravenous lipid infusions. Compared with other causes of fungal sepsis, it is unusual for catheter-related *Malassezia* fungemia to be associated with secondary focal infection.

Malassezia species do not grow readily on standard fungal media, and successful culture requires overlaying the agar with olive oil. Recovery of *Malassezia* from blood culture is optimized by supplementing the medium with olive oil or palmitic acid.

Fungemia caused by *M. furfur* or other species can be successfully treated in most cases by immediately discontinuing the lipid infusion and removing the involved catheter. For persistent or invasive infections, amphotericin B (deoxycholate or lipid-complex formulations), fluconazole, and itraconazole are effective. Flucytosine has no activity against *Malassezia*.

Bibliography is available at Expert Consult.

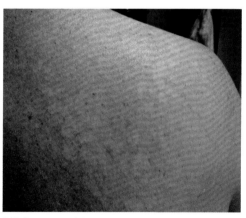

Fig. 263.1 A young adult with tinea versicolor. Notice the characteristic hypopigmented scaling macules. The asymmetric pattern seen in this patient is not characteristic of all patients with this infection. *(Courtesy Ashley M Maranich, MD.)*

Chapter **264**
Aspergillus
William J. Steinbach

第二百六十四章
曲霉属

中文导读

　　本章主要介绍了曲霉属感染相关疾病。过敏性疾病（超敏反应综合征）中包括哮喘、外源性肺泡炎、过敏性支气管肺曲霉病、变应性曲霉性鼻窦炎；非侵袭性综合征包括肺曲霉球、慢性肺曲霉病、鼻窦炎、耳部曲霉病；侵袭性疾病包括侵袭性肺曲霉病、皮肤曲霉病、侵袭性鼻窦炎以及中枢神经系统、眼、心脏等不同器官受累导致的疾病。侵袭性肺曲霉病在临床中最常见，详细阐述了其临床表现、诊断、经验性治疗和易感人群。

The aspergilli are ubiquitous fungi whose normal ecological niche is that of a soil saprophyte that recycles carbon and nitrogen. The genus *Aspergillus* contains approximately 250 species, but most human disease is caused by *Aspergillus fumigatus, A. flavus, A. niger, A. terreus,* and *A. nidulans.* Invasive disease is most commonly caused by *A. fumigatus. Aspergillus* reproduces asexually via production of spores (conidia). Most cases of *Aspergillus* disease (**aspergillosis**) are due to inhalation of airborne conidia that subsequently germinate into fungal hyphae and invade host tissue. People are likely exposed to conidia on a daily basis. When inhaled by an immunocompetent person, conidia are rarely deleterious, presumably because they are efficiently cleared by phagocytic cells. Macrophage- and neutrophil-mediated host defenses are required for resistance to invasive disease.

Aspergillus is a relatively unusual pathogen in that it can create very different disease states depending on the host characteristics, including allergic (hypersensitivity), saprophytic (noninvasive), chronic, or invasive disease. Immunodeficient hosts are at risk for invasive disease, whereas immunocompetent atopic hosts tend to develop allergic disease. Disease manifestations include primary allergic reactions; colonization of the lungs or sinuses; localized infection of the lung or skin; chronic infection of the lung; invasive pulmonary disease; or widely disseminated disease of the lungs, brain, skin, eye, bone, heart, and other organs. Clinically, these syndromes often manifest with mild, nonspecific, and late-onset symptoms, particularly in the immunosuppressed host, complicating accurate diagnosis and timely treatment.

264.1 Allergic Disease (Hypersensitivity Syndromes)
William J. Steinbach

ASTHMA
Attacks of atopic asthma can be triggered by inhalation of *Aspergillus* conidia, producing allergic responses and subsequent bronchospasm. Exposure to fungi, especially *Aspergillus,* needs to be considered as a trigger in a patient with an asthma flare, especially in those patients with severe or recalcitrant asthma.

EXTRINSIC ALVEOLAR ALVEOLITIS
Extrinsic alveolar alveolitis is a hypersensitivity pneumonitis that occurs due to repetitive inhalational exposure to inciting materials, including *Aspergillus* conidia. Symptoms typically occur shortly after exposure and include fever, cough, and dyspnea. Neither blood nor sputum eosinophilia is present. Chronic exposure to the triggering material can lead to pulmonary fibrosis.

ALLERGIC BRONCHOPULMONARY ASPERGILLOSIS
Allergic bronchopulmonary aspergillosis (ABPA) is a hyper-sensitivity disease resulting from immunologic sensitization to *Aspergillus* antigens. It is primarily seen in patients with asthma or cystic fibrosis. Inhalation of conidia produces non-invasive colonization of the bronchial airways, resulting in persistent inflammation and development of hypersensitivity inflammatory responses. Disease manifestations are due to abnormal immunologic responses to *A. fumigatus* antigens and include wheezing, pulmonary infiltrates, bronchiectasis, and even fibrosis.

There are 8 primary diagnostic criteria for ABPA: episodic bronchial obstruction, peripheral eosinophilia, immediate cutaneous reactivity to **Aspergillus** antigens, precipitating IgE antibodies to **Aspergillus** antigen, elevated total IgE, serum precipitin (specific IgG) antibodies to *A. fumigatus,* pulmonary infiltrates, and central bronchiectasis. Secondary diagnostic criteria include repeated detection of **Aspergillus** from sputum by identification of morphologically consistent fungal elements or direct culture, coughing brown plugs or specks. Radiologically, bronchial wall thickening, pulmonary infiltrates, and central bronchiectasis can be seen.

Treatment depends on relieving inflammation via an extended course of systemic corticosteroids. Addition of oral antifungal agents, such as itraconazole or voriconazole, is used to decrease the fungal burden and diminish the inciting stimulus for inflammation. Because disease activity is correlated with serum IgE levels, these levels are used as one marker to define duration of therapy. An area of research interest is the utility of anti-IgE antibody therapy in the management of ABPA.

ALLERGIC *ASPERGILLUS* SINUSITIS

Allergic *Aspergillus* sinusitis is thought to be similar in etiology to ABPA. It has been primarily described in young adult patients with asthma and may or may not be seen in combination with ABPA. Patients often present with symptoms of chronic sinusitis or recurrent acute sinusitis, such as congestion, headaches, and rhinitis, and are found to have nasal polyps and opacification of multiple sinuses on imaging. Laboratory findings can include elevated IgE levels, precipitating antibodies to *Aspergillus* antigen, and immediate cutaneous reactivity to *Aspergillus* antigens. Sinus tissue specimens might contain eosinophils, Charcot-Leyden crystals, and fungal elements consistent with *Aspergillus* species. Surgical drainage is an important aspect of treatment, often accompanied by courses of either systemic or inhaled steroids. Use of an antifungal agent may also be considered.

Bibliography is available at Expert Consult.

264.2 Saprophytic (Noninvasive) Syndromes
William J. Steinbach

PULMONARY ASPERGILLOMA

Aspergillomas are masses of fungal hyphae, cellular debris, and inflammatory cells that proliferate without vascular invasion, generally in the setting of preexisting cavitary lesions or ectatic bronchi. These cavitary lesions can occur as a result of infections such as tuberculosis, histoplasmosis, or resolved abscesses, or secondary to congenital or acquired defects such as pulmonary cysts or bullous emphysema. Patients may be asymptomatic, with diagnosis made through imaging for other reasons, or they might present with hemoptysis, cough, or fever. On imaging, initially there may be thickening of the walls of a cavity, and later on there is a solid round mass separated from the cavity wall, as the fungal ball develops. Detection of *Aspergillus* antibody in the serum suggests this diagnosis. Treatment is indicated for control of complications, such as hemoptysis. Surgical resection is the definitive treatment but has been associated with significant risks. Systemic antifungal treatment with azole-class agents may be indicated in certain patients.

CHRONIC PULMONARY ASPERGILLOSIS

Chronic aspergillosis can occur in patients with normal immune systems or mild degrees of immunosuppression, including intermittent corticosteroids. Three major categories, each with overlapping clinical features, have been proposed to describe different manifestations of chronic aspergillosis. The first is chronic cavitary pulmonary aspergillosis (CCPA), which is similar to aspergilloma, except that multiple cavities form and expand with occupying fungal balls. The second is chronic fibrosing pulmonary aspergillosis, where the multiple individual lesions progress to significant pulmonary fibrosis. The final is subacute invasive aspergillosis (IA), which was previously called chronic necrotizing pulmonary aspergillosis, a slowly progressive subset found in patients with mild to moderate immune impairment.

Treatment based on new consensus guidelines can sometimes involve surgical resection, although long-term antifungal therapy is often indicated. Management of semi-IA is similar to that of invasive pulmonary aspergillosis; however, the disease is more indolent, and thus there is a greater emphasis on oral therapy. Direct instillation of antifungals into the lesion cavity has been employed with some success.

SINUSITIS

Sinus aspergillosis typically manifests with chronic sinus symptoms that are refractory to antibacterial treatment. Imaging can demonstrate mucosal thickening in the case of *Aspergillus* sinusitis or a single mass within the maxillary or ethmoid sinus in the case of sinus aspergilloma. If untreated, sinusitis can progress and extend into the ethmoid sinuses and orbits. Therapy of sinusitis depends on surgical debridement and drainage, including surgical removal of the fungal mass in cases of sinus aspergilloma. Treatment of invasive sinus aspergillosis is identical to treatment of invasive pulmonary aspergillosis.

OTOMYCOSIS

Aspergillus can colonize the external auditory canal, with possible extension to the middle ear and mastoid air spaces if the tympanic membrane is disrupted by concurrent bacterial infection. Symptoms include pain, itching, decreased unilateral hearing, or otorrhea. Otomycosis is more often seen in patients with impaired mucosal immunity, such as patients with hypogammaglobulinemia, diabetes mellitus, chronic eczema, or HIV and those using chronic steroids. Treatments have not been well studied, but topical treatment with acetic or boric acid instillations or azole creams as well as oral azoles such as voriconazole, itraconazole, and posaconazole have been described.

Bibliography is available at Expert Consult.

264.3 Invasive Disease
William J. Steinbach

IA occurs after conidia enter the body, escape immunologic control mechanisms, and germinate into fungal hyphae that subsequently invade tissue parenchyma and vasculature. The invasion of the vasculature can result in thrombosis and localized necrosis and facilitates hematogenous dissemination. The incidence of IA increased over the last several decades, likely due to more use of severely immunosuppressive therapies for a widening array of underlying diseases and better management of other infections found in the at-risk populations. The most common site of primary infection is the lung, but primary invasive infection is also seen in the sinuses and skin and rarely elsewhere. Secondary infection can be seen after hematogenous spread, often to the skin, central nervous system (CNS), eye, bone, and heart.

IA is primarily a disease of immunocompromised hosts, and common risk factors in adults include cancer or chemotherapy-induced neutropenia, particularly if severe and/or prolonged; hematopoietic stem cell transplantation, especially during the initial pre-engraftment phase or if complicated by graft vs. host disease; neutrophil or macrophage dysfunction, as occurs in severe combined immunodeficiency (SCID) or chronic granulomatous disease (CGD); prolonged high-dose steroid use; solid organ transplantation; and rarely HIV. Adults with severe influenza virus pneumonia may also be at risk for IA. Studies in the pediatric age group have identified similar risk factors for IA, but a well-defined incidence of IA among pediatric patients has not been determined to date.

INVASIVE PULMONARY ASPERGILLOSIS

Invasive pulmonary aspergillosis is the most common form of aspergillosis. It plays a significant role in morbidity and mortality in the patient populations mentioned at increased risk for IA. Presenting symptoms can include fever despite initiation of empirical broad-spectrum antibacterial therapy, cough, chest pain, hemoptysis, and pulmonary infiltrates. Patients on high-dose steroids are less likely to present with fever. Symptoms in these immunocompromised patients can be very vague, and thus maintaining a high index of suspicion when confronted with a high-risk patient is essential.

Diagnosis

Imaging can be helpful, although no finding is pathognomonic for invasive pulmonary aspergillosis. Characteristically, multiple, ill-defined nodules can be seen, though lobar or diffuse consolidation is not uncommon and normal chest X-rays do not rule out disease. Classic radiologic signs on CT during neutropenia include the **halo sign,** when angioinvasion produces a hemorrhagic nodule surrounded by ischemia (Fig. 264.1). Early on there is a rim of ground-glass opacification surrounding a nodule. Over time, these lesions evolve into cavitary lesions or lesions with an **air crescent sign** when the lung necroses around the fungal mass, often seen during recovery from neutropenia. Unfortunately, these findings are not specific to invasive pulmonary aspergillosis and can also be seen in other pulmonary fungal infections, as well as pulmonary hemorrhage and organizing pneumonia. In addition, several reviews of imaging results of pediatric aspergillosis cases suggest that cavitation and air crescent formation are less common among these patients than among adult patients. On MRI, the typical finding for pulmonary disease is the **target sign,** a nodule with lower central signal compared to the rim-enhancing periphery.

Diagnosis of IA can be complicated for a number of reasons. Conclusive diagnosis requires culture of *Aspergillus* from a normally sterile site and histologic identification of tissue invasion by fungal hyphae consistent with *Aspergillus* morphology. However, obtaining tissue specimens is often impractical in critically ill, often thrombocytopenic, patients. In addition, depending on the specimen type, a positive result from culture can represent colonization rather than infection; however, this should be interpreted conservatively in high-risk patients. Isolation of *Aspergillus* from blood cultures is uncommon, likely because fungemia is low-level and intermittent.

Serology can be useful in the diagnosis of allergic *Aspergillus* syndromes as well as aspergilloma but is low yield for invasive disease, likely because of deficient immune responses in the high-risk immunocompromised population. Bronchoalveolar lavage (BAL) can be useful, but negative culture results cannot be used to rule out disease, owing to inadequate sensitivity. Addition of molecular biologic assays such as antigen detection and polymerase chain reaction (PCR) can greatly improve the diagnostic yield of BAL for aspergillosis. An enzyme-linked immunosorbent assay (ELISA)-based test for galactomannan, one of the components of the *Aspergillus* cell wall, is the molecular biomarker of choice for the diagnosis of IA in serum, BAL fluid, and CSF. This assay is best used in serial monitoring for development of infection and has been shown to be the most sensitive in detecting disease in cancer patients or hematopoietic stem cell transplant recipients, with less utility in solid organ transplant recipients. Earlier reports of increased false-positive reactions in children versus adults have been refuted, and the galactomannan assay is effective in diagnosing IA in children. This test does possess high rates of false negativity in patients with congenital immunodeficiency (e.g., CGD) and invasive *Aspergillus* infections. Another molecular assay, the beta-glucan assay, is a nonspecific fungal assay that detects the major component of the fungal cell wall and has been used to diagnose IA.

Unlike the galactomannan assay, which is specific for *Aspergillus*, despite some cross-reactivity with other fungi, the beta-glucan assay will not discriminate which fungal infection is infecting the patient. PCR-based assays are in development for the diagnosis of aspergillosis but are still being optimized and are not yet commercially available.

Treatment

Successful treatment of IA hinges on the ability to reconstitute normal immune function and use of effective antifungal agents until immune recovery can be achieved. Therefore, lowering overall immunosuppression, specifically via cessation of corticosteroid use, is vital to improve the ultimate outcome. In 2016, updated treatment guidelines for *Aspergillus* infections were published by the Infectious Diseases Society of America, continuing the shift in management to voriconazole from previous recommendations for amphotericin B. Primary therapy for all forms of IA is the azole-class antifungal voriconazole, based on multiple studies showing both improved response rates and survival in patients receiving voriconazole when compared to amphotericin B. In addition, voriconazole is better tolerated than amphotericin B and can be given orally as well as intravenously. Guideline-recommended alternative therapies include liposomal amphotericin B, isavuconazole, or other lipid formulations of amphotericin B.

Azoles are metabolized through the cytochrome P-450 system, and thus medication interactions can be a significant complication, especially with some chemotherapeutic agents (e.g., vincristine). Other triazole antifungals are also available, including posaconazole, which is approved for antifungal prophylaxis and may be an alternative agent for first-line treatment of IA. Although the dosing of itraconazole and voriconazole has been established for pediatric patients, the pharmacokinetic studies for posaconazole have not yet been completed. Importantly, the dose of voriconazole used in children is higher than that used in adults (see Chapter 260).

The echinocandin class of antifungals may also a play a role in treatment of IA, but to date, these agents are generally employed as second-line medications, particularly for salvage therapy. Combination antifungal therapy has revealed disparate results. Combination primary antifungal therapy with voriconazole plus an echinocandin may be considered in select patients with documented IA but is not recommended. However, it is possible that combination therapy may be beneficial to certain specific patient groups. Importantly, primary therapy with an echinocandin is not recommended, but an echinocandin can be used in the settings in which azole or polyene antifungal are contraindicated. Unfortunately, even with newer antifungals, complete or partial response rates for treatment of IA are only approximately 50%. To augment antifungal therapies, patients have been treated with growth factors to increase neutrophil counts, granulocyte transfusions, interferon-γ, and surgery.

Special Populations

Patients with CGD represent a pediatric population at particular risk for pulmonary aspergillosis. Invasive pulmonary aspergillosis can be the first serious infection identified in these patients, and the lifetime risk of development is estimated to be 33%. Unlike classical IA in cancer patients, the onset of symptoms is often gradual, with slow development of fever, fatigue, pneumonia, and elevated sedimentation rate. The neutrophils of patients with CGD surround the collections of fungal elements but cannot kill them, thereby permitting local invasion with extension of disease to the pleura, ribs, and vertebrae, though angioinvasion is not seen. Imaging in these patients is much less likely to reveal the halo sign, infarcts, or cavitary lesions and instead generally shows areas of tissue destruction due to the ongoing inflammatory processes.

CUTANEOUS ASPERGILLOSIS

Cutaneous aspergillosis can occur as a primary disease or as a consequence of hematogenous dissemination or spread from underlying structures. Primary cutaneous disease classically occurs at sites of skin disruption, such as intravenous access device locations, adhesive dressings, or sites of injury or surgery. Premature infants are at particular risk, given their immature skin and need for multiple access devices. Cutaneous disease in transplant recipients tends to reflect hematogenous distribution from

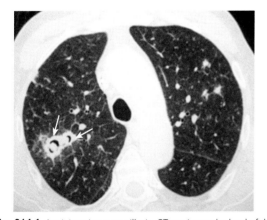

Fig. 264.1 Angioinvasive aspergillosis. CT section at the level of the lower trachea shows a consolidation with an eccentric cavitation and air crescent sign *(arrows).* This finding in this neutropenic patient is highly diagnostic of angioinvasive aspergillosis. *(From Franquet T: Nonneoplastic parenchymal lung disease. In Haaga JR, Boll DT, editors: CT and MRI of the Whole Body, ed 6, Philadelphia, 2017, Elsevier, Fig. 36.14.)*

a primary site of infection, often the lungs. Lesions are erythematous indurated papules that progress to painful, ulcerated, necrotic lesions. Treatment depends on the combination of surgical debridement and antifungal therapy, with systemic voriconazole recommended as primary therapy.

INVASIVE SINONASAL DISEASE

Invasive *Aspergillus* sinusitis represents a difficult diagnosis, because the clinical presentation tends to be highly variable. Patients can present with congestion, rhinorrhea, epistaxis, headache, facial pain or swelling, orbital swelling, fever, or abnormal appearance of the nasal turbinates. Because noninvasive imaging can be normal, diagnosis rests on direct visualization via endoscopy and biopsy. Sinus mucosa may be pale, discolored, granulating, or necrotic, depending on the stage and extent of disease. The infection can invade adjacent structures, including the eye and brain. This syndrome is difficult to distinguish clinically from other types of invasive fungal disease of the sinuses such as zygomycosis, rendering obtaining specimens for culture and histology extremely important. If the diagnosis is confirmed, treatment should be with voriconazole similar to invasive pulmonary disease. Because voriconazole is not active against mucormycosis, amphotericin B formulations should be considered in invasive fungal sinusitis pending definitive identification.

CENTRAL NERVOUS SYSTEM

The primary site of *Aspergillus* infection tends to be the lungs, but as the hyphae invade into the vasculature, fungal elements can dislodge and travel through the bloodstream, permitting establishment of secondary infection sites. One of the sites commonly involved in disseminated disease is the CNS. Cerebral aspergillosis can also arise secondary to local extension of sinus disease. The presentation of cerebral aspergillosis is highly variable but can include changes in mental status, seizures, paralysis, coma, and ophthalmoplegia. As the hyphae invade the CNS vasculature, hemorrhagic infarcts develop that convert to abscesses. Biopsy is required for definitive diagnosis, but patients are often too ill to tolerate surgery. Imaging can be helpful for diagnosis, and MRI is preferred. Lesions tend to be multiple, to be located in the basal ganglia, to have intermediate intensity with no enhancement, and to have no mass effect. CT shows hypodense, well-demarcated lesions, sometimes with ring enhancement and edema. Diagnosis often depends on characteristic imaging findings in a patient with known aspergillosis at other sites. Galactomannan assay testing of CSF has been studied and may become a future methodology to confirm the diagnosis. In general, the prognosis for CNS aspergillosis is extremely poor, likely owing to the late onset at presentation. Reversal of immunosuppression is extremely important. Surgical resection of lesions may be useful. Voriconazole, usually at high doses, is the best therapy, and itraconazole, posaconazole, and liposomal formulations of amphotericin B are alternative options.

EYE

Fungal endophthalmitis and keratitis may be seen in patients with disseminated *Aspergillus* infection. Pain, photophobia, and decreased visual acuity may be present, though many patients are asymptomatic. Emergent ophthalmologic evaluation is important when these entities are suspected. Endophthalmitis is treated with intravitreal injection of either amphotericin B or voriconazole along with surgical intervention and systemic antifungal therapy with voriconazole. Keratitis requires topical and systemic antifungal therapy.

BONE

Aspergillus osteomyelitis can occur, most commonly in the vertebrae. Rib involvement occurs owing to extension of disease in patients with CGD and is most often caused by *A. nidulans*. Treatment depends on the combination of surgical debridement and systemic antifungals. Arthritis can develop owing to hematogenous dissemination or local extension, and treatment depends on joint drainage combined with antifungal therapy. Amphotericin B has been the most commonly employed agent in the past, although voriconazole is the preferred first-line therapy.

HEART

Cardiac infection can occur as a result of surgical contamination, secondary to disseminated infection, or as a result of direct extension from a contiguous focus of infection and includes endocarditis, myocarditis, and pericarditis. Treatment requires surgical intervention in the case of endocarditis and pericarditis, along with systemic antifungals, sometimes lifelong due to the possibility of recurrent infection.

EMPIRICAL ANTIFUNGAL THERAPY

Because the diagnosis of invasive *Aspergillus* infections is often complicated and delayed, empirical initiation of antifungal therapy is often considered in high-risk patients. At present, antifungal coverage with amphotericin B (conventional or liposomal), voriconazole, itraconazole, or the echinocandin caspofungin should be considered in patients at risk for prolonged neutropenia or with findings suggesting invasive fungal infections. At this time, our ability to diagnose and treat infections due to *Aspergillus* remains suboptimal. Additional study of antigen detection assays based on galactomannan and other *Aspergillus* cell wall components as well as standardization of PCR-based assays will facilitate diagnosis. The optimal treatment remains another challenging question, because current therapeutic regimens tend to produce complete or partial response only approximately half of the time. Novel antifungals currently under development offer a future with hopefully improved survival, but immune reconstitution remains of paramount importance.

Bibliography is available at Expert Consult.

Chapter **265**
Histoplasmosis (*Histoplasma capsulatum*)

Matthew C. Washam and
Lara A. Danziger-Isakov

第二百六十五章
组织胞浆菌病（荚膜组织包浆菌）

中文导读

　　本章主要介绍了组织胞浆菌病的病因学、流行病学、发病机制、临床表现、诊断和治疗。本病由荚膜组织包浆菌感染导致。分别阐述了急性肺组织包浆菌病、肺组织包浆菌病并发症、慢性肺组织包浆菌病的临床表现。诊断性检测方法包括抗原检测、抗体检测、组织或体液培养、组织学检查、PCR等。分别介绍了急性肺组织包浆菌病和进行性播散性组织包浆菌病的治疗方案。

ETIOLOGY

Histoplasmosis is caused by *Histoplasma capsulatum*, a dimorphic fungus found in the environment as a saprobe in the mycelial (mold) form and in tissues in the parasitic form as yeast.

EPIDEMIOLOGY

Two varieties of *Histoplasma* cause human histoplasmosis. The most common variety, *H. capsulatum* var. *capsulatum*, is found in soil as the saprotrophic form throughout the midwestern United States, primarily along the Ohio and Mississippi rivers. In parts of Kentucky and Tennessee, almost 90% of the population older than 20 yr of age have positive skin test results for histoplasmin. Sporadic cases have also been reported in nonendemic states in patients without a travel history. Worldwide, *H. capsulatum* var. *capsulatum* is endemic to parts of Central and South America, the Caribbean, China, India, Southeast Asia, and the Mediterranean. The less common variety, *H. capsulatum* var. *duboisii*, is endemic to certain areas of western and central sub-Saharan Africa.

　　H. capsulatum thrives in soil rich in nitrates such as areas that are heavily contaminated with bird or bat droppings or decayed wood. Fungal spores are often carried on the wings of birds. Focal outbreaks of histoplasmosis have been reported after aerosolization of microconidia resulting from construction in areas previously occupied by starling roosts or chicken coops or by chopping decayed wood or burning bamboo exposed to a blackbird roost. Unlike birds, bats are actively infected with *Histoplasma*. Focal outbreaks of histoplasmosis have also been reported after intense exposure to bat guano in caves and along bridges frequented by bats. Horizontal person-to-person transmission does not occur, although transplacental transmission of *H. capsulatum* has been reported in immunocompromised mothers.

PATHOGENESIS

Inhalation of microconidia (fungal spores) is the initial stage of human infection. The conidia reach the alveoli, germinate, and proliferate as yeast. Alternatively, spores can remain as mold with the potential for activation. Most infections are asymptomatic or self-limited. When disseminated disease occurs, any organ system can be involved. The initial infection is a bronchopneumonia. As the initial pulmonary lesion ages, giant cells form, followed by formation of caseating or noncaseating granulomas and central necrosis. Granulomas contain viable yeast, and disease can relapse. At the time of spore germination, yeast cells are phagocytosed by alveolar macrophages, where they replicate and gain access to the reticuloendothelial system via the pulmonary lymphatic system and hilar lymph nodes. Dissemination with splenic involvement typically follows the primary pulmonary infection. In normal hosts, specific cell-mediated immunity follows in approximately 2 wk, enabling sensitized T cells to activate macrophages and kill the organism. The initial pulmonary lesion resolves within 2-4 mo but may undergo calcification resembling the Ghon complex of tuberculosis. Alternatively, buckshot calcifications involving the lung and spleen may be seen. Unlike tuberculosis, reinfection with *H. capsulatum* may occur and can lead to exaggerated host responses in some cases.

　　Children with immune deficiencies, specifically deficiencies involving cell-mediated immunity, are at increased risk for disseminated histoplasmosis. Primary immunodeficiencies involving mutations in the IL-12/IFN-γ pathway have been reported in children with disseminated histoplasmosis, including IL-12Rβ1 deficiency and IFN-γ R1 deficiency. Other primary immunodeficiencies identified in children with disseminated disease include *STAT1* gain-of-function mutations, idiopathic CD4 lymphopenia, AR-DOCK8 deficiency, AD-GATA2 deficiency, and

X-linked CD40L deficiency. Children with certain secondary immunodeficiencies (cancer patients, solid organ transplant recipients, children with HIV infection, and children receiving immunomodulatory therapy with TNF-α inhibitors) are also at increased risk for disseminated disease.

CLINICAL MANIFESTATIONS

Exposure to *Histoplasma* is common in endemic areas, although the large majority of infections are subclinical. Less than 1% of those infected display the following clinical manifestations:

Acute pulmonary histoplasmosis follows initial or recurrent respiratory exposure to microconidia. Symptomatic disease occurs more often in young children; in older patients, symptoms follow exposure to large inocula in closed spaces (e.g., chicken coops or caves) or prolonged exposure (e.g., camping on contaminated soil, chopping decayed wood). The median incubation time is 14 days. The prodrome is not specific and usually consists of flu-like symptoms, including headache, fever, chest pain, cough, and myalgias. Hepatosplenomegaly occurs more often in infants and young children. Symptomatic infections may be associated with significant respiratory distress and hypoxia and can require intubation, mechanical ventilation, and steroid therapy. Acute pulmonary disease can also manifest with a prolonged illness (10 days to 3 wk) consisting of weight loss, dyspnea, high fever, asthenia, and fatigue. Children with symptomatic disease typically have a patchy bronchopneumonia; hilar lymphadenopathy is variably present (Fig. 265.1). In young children, the pneumonia can coalesce. Focal or buckshot calcifications are convalescent findings in patients with acute pulmonary infection.

Complications of pulmonary histoplasmosis occur secondary to exaggerated host responses to fungal antigens within the lung parenchyma or hilar lymph nodes. **Histoplasmomas** are of parenchymal origin and are usually asymptomatic. These fibroma-like lesions are often concentrically calcified and single. Rarely, these lesions produce broncholithiasis associated with "stone spitting," wheezing, and hemoptysis. In endemic regions, these lesions can mimic parenchymal tumors and are occasionally diagnosed at lung biopsy. **Mediastinal granulomas** form when reactive hilar lymph nodes coalesce and mat together. Although these lesions are usually asymptomatic, huge granulomas can compress the mediastinal structures, producing symptoms of esophageal, bronchial, or vena caval obstruction. Local extension and necrosis can produce pericarditis or pleural effusions. **Mediastinal fibrosis** is a rare complication of mediastinal granulomas and represents an uncontrolled fibrotic reaction arising from the hilar nodes. Structures within the mediastinum become encased within a fibrotic mass, producing obstructive symptomatology. Superior vena cava syndrome, pulmonary venous obstruction with a mitral stenosis-like syndrome, and pulmonary artery obstruction with congestive heart failure have been described. Dysphagia accompanies esophageal entrapment, and a syndrome of cough, wheeze, hemoptysis, and dyspnea accompanies bronchial obstruction. Rarely, children develop a sarcoid-like disease with arthritis or arthralgia, erythema nodosum, keratoconjunctivitis, iridocyclitis, and pericarditis. **Pericarditis**, with effusions both pericardial and pleural, is a self-limited benign condition that develops as a result of an inflammatory reaction to adjacent mediastinal disease. The effusions are exudative, and the organism is rarely culturable from fluid. **Progressive disseminated histoplasmosis** can occur in infants as well as children with deficient cell-mediated immunity. Disseminated disease may occur either during the initial acute infection in children with primary or secondary immunodeficiencies affecting T-cell function (see Pathogenesis above), in infants, or as a reactivation of a latent focus of infection within the reticuloendothelial system in children who acquire an immunosuppressive condition years following primary infection. Disseminated histoplasmosis in an HIV-infected patient is an AIDS-defining illness. Fever is the most common finding and can persist for weeks to months before the condition is diagnosed. The majority of patients have hepatosplenomegaly, lymphadenopathy, and interstitial pulmonary disease. Extrapulmonary infection is a characteristic of disseminated disease and can include destructive bony lesions, Addison disease, meningitis, multifocal chorioretinitis, and endocarditis. Some patients develop mucous membrane ulcerations and skin findings such as nodules, ulcers, or molluscum-like papules. A sepsis-like syndrome has been identified in a small number of HIV-infected patients with disseminated histoplasmosis and is characterized by the rapid onset of shock, multiorgan failure, and coagulopathy. Reactive hemophagocytic syndrome has been described in immunocompromised patients with severe disseminated histoplasmosis. Many children with disseminated disease experience transient hyperglobulinemia. Elevated acute-phase reactants and hypercalcemia are typically seen but are nonspecific. Anemia, thrombocytopenia, and pancytopenia are variably present; elevated liver function tests and high serum concentrations of angiotensin-converting enzyme may be observed. Chest radiographs are normal in more than half of children with disseminated disease.

Chronic pulmonary histoplasmosis is an opportunistic infection in adult patients with centrilobular emphysema. **Chronic progressive disseminated histoplasmosis** is a slowly progressive infection due to *Histoplasma* that occurs in older adults without obvious immunosuppression that is uniformly fatal if untreated. These entities are rare in children.

DIAGNOSIS

Optimal diagnosis of suspected histoplasmosis depends on the clinical presentation and underlying immune status of the patient. Utilizing serum and urine antigen tests along with serum antibody tests via complement fixation and immunodiffusion yields a diagnostic sensitivity >90% for acute pulmonary and disseminated forms of histoplasmosis. Diagnostic testing options include:

Antigen detection is the most widely available diagnostic study for patients with suspected pulmonary histoplasmosis or progressive disseminated histoplasmosis. Enzyme immunoassay has replaced radioimmunoassay in many laboratories as the method to detect *H. capsulatum* polysaccharide antigen in urine, blood, bronchoalveolar lavage fluid, and cerebrospinal fluid. In patients at risk for disseminated disease, antigen can be demonstrated in the urine, blood, or bronchoalveolar lavage fluid in more than 90% of cases. Antigenuria has been shown to correlate with severity of disseminated histoplasmosis. Serum, urine, and bronchoalveolar lavage fluid from patients with acute or chronic pulmonary infections are variably antigen positive. In 1 study, antigenuria was present in 83% of patients with acute pulmonary disease and 30% of patients with subacute pulmonary disease. False-positive results on urinary antigen testing can occur in patients with *Blastomyces dermatitidis, Coccidioides immitis, Coccidioides posadasii, Paracoccidioides*

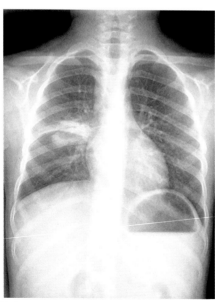

Fig. 265.1 Radiograph of a 5 yr old child with acute pulmonary histoplasmosis showing right perihilar lymphadenopathy.

brasiliensis, and *Penicillium marneffei.* Testing both urine and serum samples for histoplasma antigen increases the sensitivity compared with testing only the urine or serum alone. Sequential measurement of urinary antigen in patients with disseminated disease is useful for monitoring response to therapy; however, persistent low-level antigenuria may occur in some patients who have completed therapy and have no evidence of active infection.

Antibody tests continue to be useful for the diagnosis of acute pulmonary histoplasmosis, its complications, and chronic pulmonary disease. Serum antibody to yeast and mycelium-associated antigens is classically measured by complement fixation. Although titers of >1:8 are found in more than 80% of patients with histoplasmosis, titers of ≥1:32 are most significant for the diagnosis of recent infection. Complement-fixation antibody titers are often not significant early in the infection and do not become positive until 4-6 wk after exposure. A 4-fold increase in either yeast or mycelial-phase titers or a single titer of ≥1:32 is presumptive evidence of active infection. Complement-fixation titers may be falsely positive in patients with other systemic mycoses such as *B. dermatitidis* and *C. immitis* and may be falsely negative in immunocompromised patients. Antibody detection by immunodiffusion is less sensitive but more specific than complement fixation and is used to confirm questionably positive complement-fixation titers. The highest sensitivity for antibody testing can be achieved by combining complement fixation and immunodiffusion testing.

Culture sensitivity of tissue or body fluid samples is generally highest for children with progressive disseminated histoplasmosis or acute pulmonary histoplasmosis due to a large inoculum of organisms. *Histoplasma* typically grows within 6 wk on Sabouraud agar at 25°C (77°F). Identification of tuberculate macroconidia allows for only a presumptive diagnosis, because *Sepedonium* species form similar structures. A confirmatory test using a chemiluminescent DNA probe for *H. capsulatum* is necessary to establish a definitive identification. The yeast can be recovered from blood or bone marrow in >90% of patients with progressive disseminated histoplasmosis. Sputum cultures are rarely obtained and are variably positive in normal hosts with acute pulmonary histoplasmosis; cultures of bronchoalveolar lavage fluid appear to have a slightly higher yield than sputum cultures. Blood cultures are sterile in patients with acute pulmonary histoplasmosis, and cultures from any source are typically sterile in patients with the sarcoid form of the disease.

Histological examination can identify yeast forms in tissue from patients with complicated forms of acute pulmonary disease (histoplasmoma and mediastinal granuloma). Tissue should be stained with methenamine silver or periodic acid-Schiff stains, and yeast can be found within or outside of macrophages. In children with disseminated disease, organisms can be identified from bone marrow, liver, and mucocutaneous lesions. In those who are severely ill, Wright stain of peripheral blood can demonstrate fungal elements within leukocytes. Examination of fibrotic tissue from children with mediastinal fibrosis usually demonstrates no organisms.

Real-time polymerase chain reaction has been used on formalin-fixed, paraffin-embedded biopsy tissue and has an analytical sensitivity of at least 6 pg/μL from tissue-extracted DNA and a clinical sensitivity and specificity of 88.9% and 100%, respectively. Although not widely available, molecular methods may ultimately provide a more timely and accurate diagnosis.

Skin testing is useful only for epidemiologic studies, as cutaneous reactivity is lifelong and intradermal injection can elicit an immune response in otherwise seronegative persons. Reagents are no longer commercially available.

TREATMENT

Acute pulmonary histoplasmosis does not require antifungal therapy for asymptomatic or mildly symptomatic children. Oral itraconazole (4-10 mg/kg/day in 2 divided doses, not to exceed 400 mg daily) for 6-12 wk should be considered in patients with acute pulmonary infections who fail to improve clinically within 1 mo. Although it appears to be less effective, fluconazole may be considered as an alternative therapy in children intolerant to itraconazole. Clinical experience in treating histoplasmosis with the newer azoles (voriconazole and posaconazole) is increasing, although these medications are not currently recommended at this time. *Patients with pulmonary histoplasmosis who become hypoxemic or require ventilatory support* should receive amphotericin B deoxycholate (0.7-1.0 mg/kg/day) or amphotericin B lipid complex (3-5 mg/kg/day) until improved; continued therapy with oral itraconazole for a minimum of 12 wk is also recommended. The lipid preparations of amphotericin are not preferentially recommended in children with pulmonary histoplasmosis, as the classic preparation is generally well tolerated in this patient population. Patients with severe obstructive symptoms caused by granulomatous mediastinal disease may be treated sequentially with amphotericin B followed by itraconazole for 6-12 mo. Patients with milder mediastinal disease may be treated with oral itraconazole alone. Some experts recommend that surgery be reserved for patients who fail to improve after 1 mo of intensive amphotericin B therapy. Sarcoid-like disease with or without pericarditis may be treated with nonsteroidal antiinflammatory agents for 2-12 wk.

Progressive disseminated histoplasmosis usually requires amphotericin B deoxycholate (1 mg/kg/day for 4-6 wk) as the cornerstone of therapy. Lipid preparations of amphotericin may be substituted in patients intolerant to the classic drug preparation. Alternatively, amphotericin B may be given for 2-4 wk followed by oral itraconazole (4-10 mg/kg/day in 2 divided doses) as maintenance therapy for 3 mo, depending on *Histoplasma* antigen status. Longer therapy may be needed in patients with severe disease, immunosuppression, or primary immunodeficiency syndromes. It is recommended to monitor blood levels of itraconazole during treatment, aiming for a concentration of ≥1 μg/mL but <10 μg/mL to avoid potential drug toxicity. It is also recommended to monitor urine antigen levels during therapy and for 12 mo after therapy has ended to ensure cure. Relapses in immunocompromised patients with progressive disseminated histoplasmosis are relatively common. Lifelong suppressive therapy with daily itraconazole (5 mg/kg/day up to adult dose of 200 mg/day) may be required if immunosuppression cannot be reversed. For severely immunocompromised HIV-infected children living in endemic regions, itraconazole (2-5 mg/kg every 12-24 hr) may be used prophylactically. Care must be taken to avoid interactions between antifungal azoles and protease inhibitors.

Bibliography is available at Expert Consult.

Chapter 266
Blastomycosis (*Blastomyces dermatitidis* and *Blastomyces gilchristii*)

Gregory M. Gauthier and Bruce S. Klein

第二百六十六章

芽生菌病（皮肤芽生菌和吉尔克里斯蒂芽生菌）

中文导读

本章主要介绍了芽生菌病的病因学、流行病学、发病机制、临床表现、诊断和治疗。本病由皮肤芽生菌和吉尔克里斯蒂芽生菌感染导致。最常见的临床表现是肺炎，肺外芽生菌病以皮肤或骨受累多见，中枢神经系统芽生菌病好发于合并获得性免疫缺陷综合征（AIDS）的儿童。芽生菌病易误诊，诊断需依靠组织或体液培养，其他方法包括真菌涂片、血清学检测、抗原或抗体检测。根据患病人群及疾病严重程度不同，给予相应的治疗建议。

ETIOLOGY

Blastomyces dermatitidis and *Blastomyces gilchristii* belong to a group of fungi that exhibit thermal dimorphism. In the soil (22-25°C [71.6-77°F]), these fungi grow as mold and produce spores, which are the infectious particles. Following soil disruption, aerosolized mycelial fragments and spores inhaled into the lungs (37°C [98.6°F]) convert into pathogenic yeast and cause infection. In addition to *B. dermatitidis* and *B. gilchristii*, 4 additional species have been recently identified including *B. percursus, B. helicus, B. parvus,* and *B. silverae*.

EPIDEMIOLOGY

B. dermatitidis and *B. gilchristii* cause disease in immunocompetent and immunocompromised children. Only 2–13% of blastomycosis cases occur in the pediatric population (average age: 9.1-11.5 yr; range: 19 days to 18 yr). Blastomycosis of newborns and infants is rare. In North America, the geographic distribution of blastomycosis cases is restricted to the Midwest, south-central, and southeastern United States and parts of Canada bordering the Great Lakes and Saint Lawrence River Valley. In these geographic regions, several areas are hyperendemic for blastomycosis (e.g., Marathon and Vilas Counties, Wisconsin; Washington Parish, Louisiana; central and south-central Mississippi; Kenora, Ontario). Outside of North America, autochthonous infections have been reported from Africa (≈100 cases) and India (<12 cases). *B. dermatitidis* is not considered endemic to the Middle East, Central America, South America, Europe Asia, or Australia. In North America, *Blastomyces* grows in an ecologic niche characterized by forested, sandy soils with an acidic pH that have decaying vegetation and are near water. Most *Blastomyces* infection are sporadic; however, more than 17 outbreaks have been reported, and most of these outbreaks have involved pediatric patients. Outbreaks are associated with construction or outdoor activities (camping, hiking fishing, rafting on a river, using a community compost pile); however some outbreaks have no identifiable risk factors other than geography. The severity of infection is influenced by the size of the inhaled inoculum and the integrity of the patient's immune system. Those immunosuppressed by solid organ transplantation, AIDS, and tumor necrosis factor-α inhibitors are at risk for developing severe or disseminated infection.

PATHOGENESIS

The ability of mycelial fragments and spores to convert to yeast in the lung is a crucial event in the pathogenesis of infection with *Blastomyces* and other dimorphic fungi. This temperature-dependent morphologic shift, which is known as the phase transition, enables *Blastomyces* to evade the host immune system and establish infection. In the yeast form, the essential virulence factor BAD1 (*Blastomyces* adhesin-1 formerly WI-1) is secreted into the extracellular milieu and binds back to chitin on the fungal cell wall. BAD1 is a multifunctional protein that promotes binding of yeast to alveolar macrophages (via CR3 and CD14 receptors) and lung tissue (via heparan sulfate), blocks the deposition of complement on the yeast surface, binds calcium, suppresses the host's ability to produce cytokines (tumor necrosis factor-α, interleukin-17, interferon-gamma), and inhibits activation of CD4$^+$ T lymphocytes. Deletion of *BAD1* abolishes virulence of *Blastomyces* yeast in a murine model of pulmonary infection.

The phase transition between mold and yeast forms is a complex event that involves alteration in cell wall composition, metabolism, intracellular signaling, and gene expression. The morphologic shift to yeast is regulated in part by a histidine kinase known as DRK1 (*dimorphism regulating kinase-1*). This sensor kinase controls not only the conversion of mold to yeast but also spore production, cell wall composition, and *BAD1* expression; the loss of *DRK1* gene expression through gene disruption renders *B. dermatitidis* avirulent in a murine model of pulmonary blastomycosis. The function of DRK1 is conserved in other thermally dimorphic fungi, including *Histoplasma capsulatum* and *Talaromyces marneffei* (formerly *Penicillium marneffei*).

The phase transition is reversible, and following a drop in temperature from 37°C (98.6°F) to 22°C (71.6°F), yeast convert to sporulating mold. Growth as mold promotes survival in the soil, allows for sexual reproduction to enhance genetic diversity, and facilitates transmission to new hosts (via spores and mycelial fragments). The transition from yeast to mold is influenced by SREB (siderophore biosynthesis repressor in *Blastomyces*) and *N*-acetylglucosamine transporters (NGT1, NGT2). Deletion of *SREB*, which encodes a GATA transcription factor, results in the failure of *B. dermatitidis* yeast to complete the conversion to mold at 22°C. *N*-Acetylglucosamine, which polymerizes to form chitin, accelerates the transition to hyphae via NGT1 and NGT2 transporters.

Innate and adaptive immune systems are required to effectively control infection; humoral immunity is dispensable. Macrophages and neutrophils are capable of ingesting and killing *Blastomyces* conidia. In contrast, yeast are poorly killed by nonactivated macrophages, are resistant to reactive oxygen species, and suppress nitric oxide production. Adaptive immunity is mediated by T lymphocytes (Th1 and Th17), which activate macrophages and neutrophils to facilitate clearance of infection. Following infection, cell-mediated immunity against *Blastomyces* can last for at least 2 yr.

CLINICAL MANIFESTATIONS

The clinical manifestations of blastomycosis are diverse and include subclinical infection, symptomatic pneumonia, and disseminated disease. Clinical disease develops 3 wk-3 mo following inhalation of spores or mycelial fragments. Asymptomatic or subclinical infections are estimated to occur in 50% of patients.

The most common clinical manifestation of blastomycosis is **pneumonia**, which can range from acute to chronic. Acute symptoms resemble community-acquired pneumonia and include fever, dyspnea, cough, chest pain, and malaise (Fig. 266.1). Respiratory failure, including acute respiratory distress syndrome (ARDS), can occur in patients with an overwhelming burden of infection. Chest imaging typically demonstrates air space consolidation, which can involve the upper or lower lobes. Other radiographic features include nodular, reticulonodular, and miliary patterns. Hilar adenopathy and pleural effusions are uncommon. Because the clinical and radiographic features can mimic bacterial pneumonia, patients can be mistakenly treated with antibiotics, resulting in disease progression, which can result in disseminated disease or respiratory failure, including ARDS. Patients with subacute or chronic pneumonia experience fevers, chills, night sweats, cough, weight loss, hemoptysis, dyspnea, and chest pain. Mass lesions and cavitary disease on chest roentgenography can mimic malignancy and tuberculosis, respectively.

Extrapulmonary blastomycosis most often affects the skin or bone but can involve almost any organ. The incidence of **extrapulmonary blastomycosis** in children ranges from 38% to 50%, similar to rates in adult patients (25–40%). The skin is the most common site for

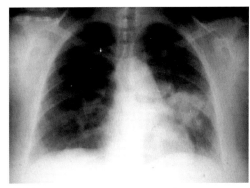

Fig. 266.1 Left lung infection in a patient with symptoms resembling acute bacterial pneumonia. Organisms of *Blastomyces dermatitidis* in sputum seen with potassium hydroxide preparation, and subsequent culture confirmed the diagnosis. *(From Bradsher Jr RW: Blastomycoses. In Bennett JF, Dolin R, Blaser MJ, editors: Mandell, Douglas, and Bennett's Principles and Practice of Infectious Diseases, ed 8. Philadelphia, 2015, Elsevier, Fig. 266-5.)*

extrapulmonary blastomycosis, which is usually the result of hematogenous dissemination. Direct inoculation of *B. dermatitidis* into the skin from trauma or a laboratory accident can result in primary cutaneous blastomycosis. Skin manifestations include plaques, papules, ulcers, nodules, and verrucous lesions. Erythema nodosum is rare in blastomycosis. Dissemination of *B. dermatitidis* to the bone results in lytic destruction, pain, soft tissue swelling, sinus tract formation, and ulceration. The ribs, skull, spine, and long bones are most commonly affected. Patients with osteomyelitis often have pulmonary or cutaneous involvement. Vertebral osteomyelitis can be complicated by paraspinal abscess, psoas abscess, and vertebral body collapse. Extension of long bone osteomyelitis can result in pathologic fracture or septic arthritis. Genitourinary blastomycosis occurs in <10% of adults but is rare in children.

Central nervous system (CNS) blastomycosis (brain abscess, meningitis) occurs in <10% of immunocompetent patients but in up to 40% of persons with AIDS. The majority of patients with CNS blastomycosis have clinically apparent infection at non-CNS sites (e.g., lung, skin). Symptoms of CNS infection include headache, altered mental status, memory loss, seizure, cranial nerve deficits, and focal neurologic deficits. Complications include hydrocephalus, cerebral herniation, infarction, panhypopituitarism, residual weakness, and poor functioning in school. Lumbar puncture demonstrates leukocytosis with a neutrophil or lymphocyte predominance, elevated protein, and low glucose. Growth of *Blastomyces* in culture from cerebral spinal fluid occurs in less than 50% of affected patients.

Blastomycosis can complicate pregnancy, and clinical information is limited to case reports. Disseminated infection involving the lungs, skin, and bone is common. Spread of infection to the placenta has been documented by histopathology; however, the frequency of placental blastomycosis remains unknown. Transmission of *Blastomyces* to the fetus is uncommon and is postulated to occur through transplacental transmission or aspiration of infected vaginal secretions. Although clinical data are limited, blastomycosis during pregnancy does not appear to increase the risk for congenital malformations.

DIAGNOSIS

The diagnosis of blastomycosis requires a high index of suspicion because the clinical and radiographic manifestations can mimic other diseases, including community-acquired pneumonia, tuberculosis, and malignancy. The misdiagnosis of blastomycosis, most often as community-acquired pneumonia, results in delay of therapy and progression of disease including dissemination and respiratory failure. Blastomycosis should be included in the differential diagnosis for patients with pneumonia who (1) live in or visit areas in which this pathogen is endemic; (2) fail to respond to a treatment course of antibiotics; or (3) have concomitant skin lesions or osteomyelitis. A detailed medical history regarding exposure risks (e.g., canoeing, rafting, hiking, fishing, playing in outdoor forts, beaver dam exploration, home remodeling, nearby road or building construction, woodpile for a wood burning stove, and use of a community compost pile) should be obtained. In addition, the health of family pets such as dogs should also be ascertained, as canine disease may be a harbinger of human infection. The incidence of blastomycosis in dogs is 10-fold higher than in humans, and canine infection suggests a common source of environmental *Blastomyces* exposure.

Growth of *Blastomyces* in culture from sputum, skin, bone, or other clinical specimens provides a definitive diagnosis. Sputum specimens should be stained with 10% potassium hydroxide or calcofluor white. Histopathology shows neutrophilic infiltration with noncaseating granulomas (pyogranulomas). *Blastomyces* yeast in tissue samples can be visualized using Gomori methenamine silver or periodic acid–Schiff stains. Yeasts are 8-20 μm in size, have a double refractile cell wall, and are characterized by broad-based budding between mother and daughter cells.

Nonculture diagnostic techniques should be used in conjunction with fungal smears and cultures to facilitate the diagnosis of blastomycosis. The development of a *Blastomyces* antigen test has supplanted insensitive serologic methods such as complement fixation and immunodiffusion. Urine, serum, cerebrospinal fluid, and bronchoalveolar fluid specimens can be collected for the *Blastomyces* antigen test. Sensitivity of the urine antigen test ranges from 76.3% to 92.9% and is influenced by the burden of infection. The antigen test can cross-react with other dimorphic fungi, including *Histoplasma capsulatum, Paracoccidioides brasiliensis,* and *Penicillium marneffei,* decreasing the specificity to 76.9–79%. An antibody test against the BAD1 protein has been developed and has a sensitivity of 87.8% and a specificity of 94–99%; however, this test is not yet commercially available. Combination antigen and BAD1 antibody testing can increase diagnostic sensitivity to 97.6%.

TREATMENT

Antifungal therapy is influenced by the severity of the infection, involvement of the central nervous system, the integrity of the host's immune system, and pregnancy. All persons diagnosed with blastomycosis should receive antifungal therapy. **Newborns** with blastomycosis should be treated with amphotericin B deoxycholate 1 mg/kg/day. **Children with mild to moderately severe infection** can be treated with itraconazole 10 mg/kg/day (maximum: 400 mg/day) for 6-12 mo. **Children with severe disease, immunodeficiency, or immunosuppression** should be treated with amphotericin B deoxycholate 0.7-1.0 mg/kg/day or lipid amphotericin B 3-5 mg/kg/day until there is clinical improvement, generally 7-14 days, and then itraconazole 10 mg/kg/day (maximum: 400 mg/day) for a total of 12 mo. **Central nervous system blastomycosis** requires therapy with lipid amphotericin B 5 mg/kg/day for 4-6 wk, followed by itraconazole, fluconazole, or voriconazole for ≥12 mo.

All pediatric patients of childbearing age should undergo pregnancy testing prior to initiation of azole antifungals. Itraconazole can increase the risk for spontaneous abortion, and fluconazole can cause craniofacial defects resembling Antley-Bixler syndrome. Voriconazole and posaconazole cause skeletal abnormalities in animal models. Treatment of blastomycosis in **pregnant patients** consists of lipid amphotericin B 3-5 mg/kg/day.

For patients receiving itraconazole, the oral antifungal of choice, *therapeutic drug monitoring* should be performed 14 days into therapy (goal total itraconazole level 1-5 μg/mL), and liver function tests should be monitored periodically. Due to the long half-life of itraconazole, serum drug levels can be obtained at any time of the day, irrespective of when the drug was administered. Total itraconazole level is determined by adding itraconazole and hydroxyitraconazole concentrations; hydroxyitraconazole is a metabolite that possesses antifungal activity. Voriconazole, posaconazole, and isavuconazonium sulfate have activity against *B. dermatitidis.* Clinical experience with these drugs appears promising but remains limited. Therapeutic drug monitoring is needed for voriconazole and posaconazole (goal trough levels 1-5 μg/mL). The echinocandins (caspofungin, micafungin, and anidulafungin) *should not be used* to treat blastomycosis. Serial measurement of urine antigen levels to assess response to therapy can be helpful adjunct in monitoring response to antifungal therapy.

Bibliography is available at Expert Consult.

Chapter **267**
Coccidioidomycosis (*Coccidioides* Species)
Rebecca C. Brady
第二百六十七章
球孢子菌病（球孢子菌属）

中文导读

　　本章主要介绍了球孢子菌病的病因学、流行病学、发病机制、临床表现、诊断、治疗和预防。临床表现分为原发性球孢子菌病、并发肺部感染、残留的肺部球孢子菌病和播散性（肺外）感染。实验室诊断方法包括培养、组织病理学检查、抗原检测、血清学检测和影像学。治疗以抗真菌药为主，若空腔位于外周、反复出血或胸膜浸润，需考虑行外科切除。

ETIOLOGY

Coccidioidomycosis (valley fever, San Joaquin fever, desert rheumatism, coccidioidal granuloma) is caused by *Coccidioides* spp., a soil-dwelling dimorphic fungus. *Coccidioides* spp. grow in the environment as spore-bearing (arthroconidia-bearing) mycelial forms. In their parasitic form, they appear as unique, endosporulating spherules in infected tissue. The 2 recognized species, *C. immitis* and *C. posadasii,* cause similar illnesses.

EPIDEMIOLOGY

Coccidioides spp. inhabit soil in arid regions. *C. immitis* is primarily found in California's San Joaquin Valley. *C. posadasii* is endemic to southern regions of Arizona, Utah, Nevada, New Mexico, western Texas, and regions of Mexico and Central and South America.

Population migrations into endemic areas and increasing numbers of immunosuppressed persons have caused coccidioidomycosis to become an important health problem. From 2000 to 2012, there were 3,453 incidents of pediatric coccidioidomycosis cases reported in California, about 9.6% of the total coccidioidomycosis cases. During the same time period, there were 1,301 hospitalizations and 11 deaths associated with coccidioidomycosis in the California pediatric population. Case and hospitalization rates per 100,000 population increased from 0.7 to 3.9 and from 0.2 to 1.2, respectively. These case and hospitalization rates were highest in males, those in the 12-17 age group, and residents of the California endemic region.

Infection results from inhalation of aerosolized spores. Incidence increases during windy, dry periods that follow rainy seasons. Seismic events, archaeologic excavations, and other activities that disturb contaminated sites have caused outbreaks. Person-to-person transmission does not occur. Rarely, infections result from spores that contaminate fomites or grow beneath casts or wound dressings of infected patients. Infection has also resulted from transplantation of organs from infected donors and from mother to fetus or newborn. Visitors to endemic areas can acquire infections, and diagnosis may be delayed when they are evaluated in nonendemic areas. Spores are highly virulent, and *Coccidioides* spp. are potential agents of bioterrorism (see Chapter 741).

PATHOGENESIS

Inhaled spores reach terminal bronchioles, where they transform into septated spherules that resist phagocytosis and within which many endospores develop. Released endospores transform into new spherules, and the process results in an acute focus of infection. Endospores can also disseminate lymphohematogenously. Eventually, a granulomatous reaction predominates. Both recovery and protection upon reexposure depend on effective cellular immunity.

Children with **congenital primary immunodeficiency** disorders may be at increased risk for infection; these disorders include interleukin-12Rβ1 deficiency, interferon-γR1 deficiency, and *STAT1* gain-of-function mutations.

CLINICAL MANIFESTATIONS

The clinical spectrum (Fig. 267.1) encompasses pulmonary and extrapulmonary disease. Pulmonary infection occurs in 95% of cases and can be divided into primary, complicated, and residual infections. Approximately 60% of infections are asymptomatic. Symptoms in children are often milder than those in adults. The incidence of extrapulmonary dissemination in children approaches that of adults.

Primary Coccidioidomycosis

The incubation period is 1-4 wk, with an average of 10-16 days. Early symptoms include malaise, chills, fever, and night sweats. Chest discomfort occurs in 50–70% of patients and varies from mild tightness to severe pain. Headache and/or backache are sometimes reported. An

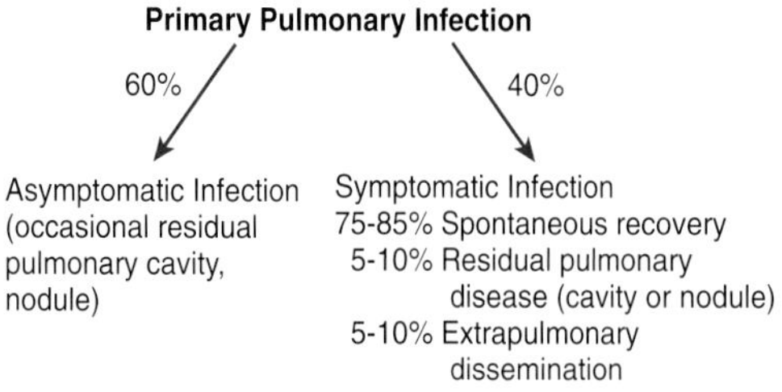

Primary Pulmonary Infection

60% / 40%

Asymptomatic Infection (occasional residual pulmonary cavity, nodule)

Symptomatic Infection
75-85% Spontaneous recovery
5-10% Residual pulmonary
    disease (cavity or nodule)
5-10% Extrapulmonary
    dissemination

Fig. 267.1 Natural history of coccidioidomycosis.

Table 267.1	Risk Factors for Poor Outcome in Patients With Active Coccidioidomycosis

PRIMARY INFECTIONS

Severe, prolonged (≥6 wk), or progressive infection

RISK FACTORS FOR EXTRAPULMONARY DISSEMINATION

Primary or acquired cellular immune dysfunction (including patients receiving tumor necrosis factor inhibitors)
Neonates, infants, the elderly
Male sex (adult)
Filipino, African, Native American, or Latin American ethnicity
Late-stage pregnancy and early postpartum period
Standardized complement fixation antibody titer >1:16 or increasing titer with persisting symptoms
Blood group B
Human leukocyte antigen class II allele-DRBI*1301

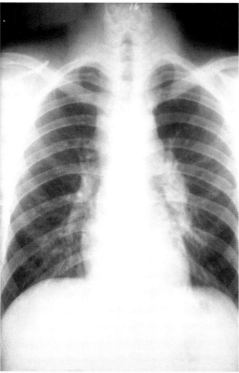

Fig. 267.2 Chest radiograph of a 19 yr old man with acute primary coccidioidomycosis. There is prominent hilar lymphadenopathy and mediastinal widening.

evanescent, generalized, fine macular erythematous or urticarial eruption may be seen within the first few days of infection. Erythema nodosum can occur (more often in women) and is sometimes accompanied by an erythema multiforme rash, usually 3-21 days after the onset of symptoms. The clinical constellation of erythema nodosum, fever, chest pain, and arthralgias (especially knees and ankles) has been termed *desert rheumatism* and *valley fever*. The chest examination is often normal even if radiographic findings are present. Dullness to percussion, friction rub, or fine rales may be present. Pleural effusions can occur and can become large enough to compromise respiratory status. Hilar and mediastinal lymphadenopathy are common (Fig. 267.2).

Complicated Pulmonary Infection

Complicated infections include severe and persistent pneumonia, progressive primary coccidioidomycosis, progressive fibrocavitary disease, transient cavities that develop in areas of pulmonary consolidation, and empyema that follows rupture of a cavity into the pleural space. Some cavities persist, are thin walled and peripheral, and cause no symptoms; occasionally there is mild hemoptysis, and rarely there is serious hemorrhage. Rarely, acute respiratory insufficiency occurs following intense exposure; this condition is associated with high mortality rates.

Residual Pulmonary Coccidioidomycosis

Residual pulmonary coccidioidomycosis includes fibrosis as well as persisting pulmonary nodules. Nodules are present in 5–7% of infections and sometimes require differentiation from malignancy in adults.

Disseminated (Extrapulmonary) Infection

Clinically apparent dissemination occurs in 0.5% of patients. Its incidence is increased in infants; men; persons of Filipino, African, and Latin American ancestry; and persons from other Asian backgrounds. Primary or acquired disorders of cellular immunity (Table 267.1) markedly increase the risk of dissemination.

Symptoms usually occur within 6 mo of primary infection. Prolonged fever, toxicity, skin lesions, subcutaneous and/or osseous cold abscesses, and laryngeal lesions can herald the onset. Organism-specific skin lesions have a predilection for the nasolabial area and appear initially as papules, which evolve to form pustules, plaques, abscesses, and verrucous plaques. Biopsy of these lesions demonstrates spherules. **Basilar meningitis** is the most common manifestation and may be accompanied by ventriculitis, ependymitis, cerebral vasculitis, abscess, and syringomyelia. Headache, vomiting, meningismus, and cranial nerve dysfunction are often present. Untreated meningitis is almost invariably fatal. Bone infections account for 20–50% of extrapulmonary manifestations, are often multifocal, and can affect adjacent structures. Miliary dissemination and peritonitis can mimic tuberculosis.

DIAGNOSIS

Nonspecific tests have limited usefulness. The complete blood count might show an elevated eosinophil count, and marked eosinophilia can accompany dissemination.

Culture, Histopathologic Findings, and Antigen Detection

Although diagnostic, culture is positive in only 8.3% of respiratory tract specimens and in only 3.2% of all other sites. *Coccidioides* is isolated from clinical specimens as the spore-bearing mold form, and thus the laboratory should be informed and use special precautions when the diagnosis is suspected. The observation of endosporulating spherules in histopathologic specimens is also diagnostic.

A quantitative enzyme immunoassay (EIA) (MiraVista Diagnostics) that detects coccidioidal galactomannan in urine, serum, plasma, cerebrospinal fluid, or bronchoalveolar lavage fluid has excellent specificity and is positive in 70% of patients with severe infections. Although the EIA can cross-react with other endemic mycoses, interpretation is often straightforward because there is negligible geographic overlap with areas endemic for other mycoses. In addition, a real-time polymerase chain reaction assay has been developed to directly detect the fungus in tissue samples and is undergoing validation but is not yet commercially available.

Cerebrospinal fluid (CSF) analysis should be performed in patients with suspected dissemination. The findings in meningitis are similar to those seen with tuberculous meningitis (see Chapter 242). Eosinophilic pleocytosis may be present. Fungal stains and culture are usually negative. Volumes of 10 mL in adults have improved the yield of culture.

Serology

Serologic tests provide valuable diagnostic information but may be falsely negative early in self-limited infections and in immunocompromised patients. Three major methods are used, including EIA, complement fixation (CF), and immunodiffusion. EIA and CF tests are best done in experienced reference laboratories.

Immunoglobulin (Ig) M–specific antibody becomes measurable in 50% of infected patients 1 wk after onset and in 90% of infected patients by 3 wk. EIA is sensitive and can detect IgM and IgG antibody; it is less specific than other methods, and confirmation with immunodiffusion or CF may be needed. IgG antibodies measured by CF appear between the 2nd and 3rd wk but can take several months; follow-up testing is needed if tests are negative and clinical suspicion persists. In the presence of CF titers of 1:2 or 1:4, a positive immunodiffusion test can help corroborate significance. IgG-specific antibody can persist for months, with titers elevated in proportion to the severity of illness. CF titers >1:16 are suggestive of dissemination. Direct comparison of the results of CF (IgG) antibody tests measured by different methodologies should be interpreted with caution. IgG antibody titers used to monitor disease activity should be tested concurrently with serum samples taken earlier in the illness using the same methodology.

C. immitis antibody is present in CSF in 95% of patients with meningitis and is usually diagnostic. Rarely, "spillover" in patients without meningitis but with high IgG titers in serum can be present in CSF. Isolation of *Coccidioides* from CSF culture of patients with meningitis is uncommon, although culture of large volumes of CSF may improve sensitivity.

Imaging Procedures

During primary infection, chest radiography may be normal or demonstrate consolidation, single or multiple circumscribed lesions, or soft pulmonary densities. Hilar and subcarinal lymphadenopathy is often present (see Fig. 267.2). Cavities tend to be thin walled (Fig. 267.3). Pleural effusions vary in size. The presence of miliary or reticulonodular lesions is prognostically unfavorable. Isolated or multiple osseous lesions are usually lytic and often affect cancellous bone. Lesions can affect adjacent structures, and vertebral lesions can impact the spinal cord.

TREATMENT

Based on the few rigorous clinical trials performed in adults and the opinions of experts in the management of coccidioidomycosis, consensus treatment guidelines have been developed (Table 267.2). Consultation with experts in an area of endemicity should be considered when formulating a plan of management.

Patients should be followed closely because late relapse can occur, especially in patients who are immunosuppressed or have severe manifestations. Treatment is recommended for all HIV-infected patients with active coccidioidomycosis and CD4 counts <250/μL. Following successful treatment, antifungals may be stopped if the CD4 count exceeds 250/μL. Treatment should be continued if the CD4 count remains less than 250/μL and should be given indefinitely in all HIV-infected patients with coccidioidal meningitis.

First-line agents include oral and intravenous preparations of fluconazole (12 mg/kg/day IV or PO) and itraconazole (10 mg/kg/day). Serum levels of itraconazole should be monitored.

Amphotericin B is preferred for initial treatment of severe infections. Amphotericin B deoxycholate is less costly than lipid formulations and is often well tolerated in children. Once a daily dose of amphotericin B deoxycholate of 1-1.5 mg/kg/day is achieved, the frequency of administration can be reduced to 3 times weekly. The recommended total dosage ranges from 15 to 45 mg/kg and is determined by the clinical response. Lipid formulations of amphotericin are recommended for patients with impaired renal function, for patients receiving other nephrotoxic agents, or if amphotericin B deoxycholate is not tolerated. Some experts prefer liposomal amphotericin to treat central nervous system infections because it achieves higher levels in brain parenchyma.

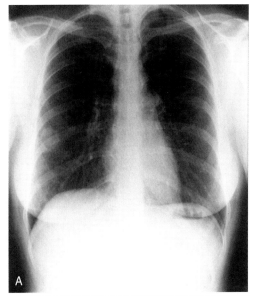
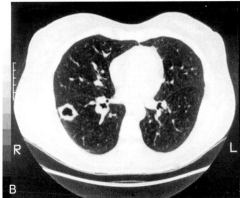

Fig. 267.3 A, Chest radiograph revealing a chronic cavitary lesion in the right lung of a woman with coccidioidomycosis. **B,** CT showing the same cavity in the right lung.

Amphotericin B preparations do not cross the blood-brain barrier to effectively treat *Coccidioides* spp., but they can mask the signs of meningitis. Infections during pregnancy should be treated with amphotericin B, because the azoles are potentially teratogenic. Voriconazole and posaconazole have been used successfully as salvage therapy in infections failing the standard agents.

Primary Pulmonary Infection

Primary pulmonary coccidioidomycosis resolves in 95% of patients without risk factors for dissemination; antifungal therapy does not lessen the frequency of dissemination or pulmonary residua. When it is elected to defer antifungal therapy, visits are recommended at 1-3 mo intervals for 2 yr and as needed.

Patients with significant or prolonged symptoms are more likely to incur benefit from antifungal agents, but there are no established criteria upon which to base the decision. Table 267.2 summarizes commonly used indicators in adults. A treatment trial in adults with primary respiratory infections examined outcomes of antifungal therapy prescribed on the basis of severity and compared them to an untreated group with less-severe symptoms; complications occurred only in patients in the treatment group and only in those in whom treatment was stopped. If treatment is elected, a 3-6 mo course of fluconazole (12 mg/kg/day) or itraconazole (10 mg/kg/day) is recommended.

Table 267.2	Indications for Treatment of Coccidioidomycosis in Adults
INDICATION	**TREATMENT**
Acute pneumonia, mild	Observe without antifungal treatment at 1-3 mo intervals for 2 yr; some experts recommend antifungal treatment
Weight loss >10%; night sweats >3 wk; infiltrates at least half of 1 lung or parts of both lungs; prominent or persistent hilar lymphadenopathy; complement fixation titers >1:16; inability to work, symptoms >2 mo	Treat with an azole daily for 3-6 mo, with follow-up at 1-3 mo intervals for 2 yr
Uncomplicated acute pneumonia, special circumstances: immunosuppression, late pregnancy, Filipino or African ancestry, age >55 yr, other chronic diseases (diabetes, cardiopulmonary disease), symptoms >2 mo	Treat with an azole daily for 3-6 mo, with follow-up at 1-3 mo intervals for 2 yr Treat with amphotericin B if in late pregnancy
Diffuse pneumonia: reticulonodular or miliary infiltrates suggest underlying immunodeficiency and possible fungemia, pain	Treat initially with amphotericin B if significant hypoxia or rapid deterioration, followed by an azole for ≥1 yr In mild cases, an azole for ≥1 yr
Chronic pneumonia	Treat with an azole for ≥1 yr
Disseminated disease, nonmeningeal	Treat with an azole for ≥1 yr except in severe or rapidly worsening cases, for which amphotericin B is recommended
Disseminated disease, meningeal	Treat with fluconazole (some add intrathecal amphotericin B) and treat indefinitely

Diffuse Pneumonia

Diffuse reticulonodular densities or miliary infiltrates, sometimes accompanied by severe illness, can occur in dissemination or follow exposure to a large fungal inoculum. In this setting, amphotericin B is recommended for initial treatment, followed thereafter by extended treatment with high-dose fluconazole (see Table 267.2).

Disseminated (Extrapulmonary) Infection

For nonmeningeal infection (see Table 267.2), oral fluconazole and itraconazole are effective for treating disseminated coccidioidomycosis that is not extensive, is not progressing rapidly, and has not affected the central nervous system. Some experts recommend higher doses for adults than were used in clinical trials. A subgroup analysis showed a tendency for improved response of skeletal infections that were treated with itraconazole. Amphotericin B deoxycholate is used as an alternative, especially if there is rapid worsening and lesions are in critical locations. Voriconazole has been used successfully as salvage therapy. The optimal duration of therapy with the azoles has not been clearly defined. Late relapses have occurred after lengthy treatment and favorable clinical response.

Meningitis

Therapy with oral or IV fluconazole is currently preferred for coccidioidal meningitis. In adults, a dosage of 400-1,200 mg/day is recommended. For children, the dose is 12 mg/kg/day. Some experts use intrathecal, intraventricular, or intracisternally administered amphotericin B in addition to an azole, believing that the clinical response may be faster.

Patients who respond to the azole should continue treatment indefinitely. Hydrocephalus is a common occurrence and is not necessarily a marker of treatment failure. In the event of treatment failure with azoles, intrathecal therapy with amphotericin B deoxycholate is indicated, with or without the azole treatment. Cerebral vasculitis can occur and can predispose to cerebral ischemia, infarction, or hemorrhage. The efficacy of steroids in high dosage is unresolved. Salvage therapy with voriconazole has been found to be effective.

Surgical Management

If a cavity is located peripherally or there is recurrent bleeding or pleural extension, excision may be needed. Infrequently, bronchopleural fistula or recurrent cavitation occurs as a surgical complication; rarely, dissemination can result. Perioperative intravenous therapy with amphotericin B may be considered. Drainage of cold abscesses, synovectomy, and curettage or excision of osseous lesions is sometimes needed. Local and systemic administration of amphotericin B can be used to treat coccidioidal articular disease.

PREVENTION

Prevention relies on education about ways to reduce exposure. Physicians practicing in nonendemic regions should incorporate careful travel histories when evaluating patients with symptoms compatible with coccidioidomycosis.

Bibliography is available at Expert Consult.

Chapter **268**
Paracoccidioides brasiliensis
Andrew P. Steenhoff
第二百六十八章
副球孢子菌病（巴西副球孢子菌）

中文导读

　　本章主要介绍了巴西副球孢子菌感染引起副球孢子菌病的病因学、流行病学、发病机制、临床表现、诊断和治疗。临床表现形式分为急性和慢性，其中急性罕见，几乎只发生在儿童和免疫功能受损人群，表现为发热、消瘦、腹腔淋巴结肿大、肝脾大等。成年人发病为慢性进行性病程。治疗药物以唑类为主，首选伊曲康唑口服，其他药物包括两性霉素B、磺胺类药物、泼尼松等。

ETIOLOGY

Paracoccidioidomycosis (South American or Brazilian blastomycosis, Lutz-Splendore-Almeida disease) is the most common systemic mycosis in Latin America. It is a fungal infection that is endemic in South America, with cases reported in Central America and Mexico. Brazil accounts for more than 80% of all reported cases. The etiologic agent, *Paracoccidioides brasiliensis*, is a thermally dimorphic fungus found in the environment in the mycelial (mold) form and in tissues as yeast.

EPIDEMIOLOGY

P. brasiliensis is a soil-inhabiting microorganism and is ecologically unique to Central and South America. Endemic outbreaks occur mainly in the tropical rain forests of Brazil, with cases scattered in Argentina, Colombia, and Venezuela. There is an increased incidence in areas with moderately high altitude, with high humidity and rainfall, and where coffee and tobacco are grown. Armadillos appear to be a natural reservoir for *P. brasiliensis*. The most common route of infection is by inhalation of conidia. The disease is not usually thought to be contagious, and person-to-person transmission has not been confirmed. Paracoccidioidomycosis is more common among boys after puberty because of the role of estrogen in preventing the transition of conidia to the yeast form. Children account for <10% of the total number of cases.

PATHOGENESIS

Invasion of *P. brasiliensis* into the human body is based on a myriad of fungal components and strategies to bypass host defense mechanisms. With the emergence of CRISPR technology and full access to diverse databanks (such as genomes, transcriptomes, proteomes, metabolomes, lipidomes), investigators are poised to better understand the virulence processes of *P. brasiliensis*, hopefully allowing translation into benefits for patients.

The entry route into the body is via the respiratory tract, and the lungs are the site of primary infection, although not all patients have respiratory symptoms. Once the conidia or hyphal fragments reach the alveoli, yeast transformation takes place. The infection then spreads to the mucous membranes of the nose, mouth, and gastrointestinal tract. Cell-mediated immunity, mainly through lymphocytes and the production of Th-1 cytokines, is crucial to containing the infection. Tumor necrosis factor-α and interferon-γ activated macrophages are responsible for intracellular killing of *P. brasiliensis*. If the initial immune response is not successful, the response may shift toward a Th-2 pattern, which is unable to contain the infection, resulting in clinical progression. The yeast can disseminate by the lymphohematogenous route to skin, lymph nodes, and other organs and remain dormant in lymph nodes, producing a latent infection with reactivation occurring later on in life. There are cases of patients who developed disease 30 or more years after leaving an endemic region.

Histopathologically, the yeast-like cells are round, with the parent cell being quite large and surrounded by small buds, giving it the appearance of a ship's wheel. A mixed suppurative and granulomatous inflammatory reaction with areas of necrosis is seen in pulmonary infections. In chronic infections fibrosis and calcification may be seen. Mucocutaneous infections are typified by ulceration and pseudoepitheliomatous hyperplasia.

CLINICAL MANIFESTATIONS

There are 2 clinical forms of disease. The **acute** form (juvenile paracoccidioidomycosis) is rare, occurs almost exclusively in children and persons with impaired immunity, and targets the reticuloendothelial system. Pulmonary symptoms may be absent, although chest radiographs often show patchy, confluent, or nodular densities. Patients typically present acutely with fever, malaise, wasting, lymphadenopathy, and abdominal enlargement from intraabdominal lymphadenopathy. Hepatomegaly and splenomegaly are nearly constant. Localized bony lesions have been reported in children and can progress to systemic disease. Multifocal osteomyelitis, arthritis, and pericardial effusions can also occur. Nonspecific laboratory findings include anemia, eosinophilia, and hypergammaglobulinemia. Acute paracoccidioidomycosis has a 25% mortality rate. Hepatic involvement associated with jaundice may confer a worse prognosis.

Adults develop a **chronic,** progressive illness that manifests initially with flu-like symptoms, fever, and weight loss (adult paracoccidioidomycosis). Pulmonary infection develops with dyspnea, cough, chest pain, and hemoptysis. Findings on physical examination are scant, although chest radiographs can show infiltrates that are disproportionate with mild clinical findings. Mucositis involving the mouth and its structures as well as the nose can manifest as localized pain, change in voice, or dysphagia. Lesions can extend beyond the oral cavity onto the skin. Generalized lymphadenopathy, hepatosplenomegaly, and adrenal involvement (seen in 15–50% of cases) can lead to Addison disease. Meningoencephalitis and central nervous system granulomas can occur as presenting or secondary symptoms. Adults with extensive exposure to soil, such as farmers, are most likely to develop the chronic form of the disease.

DIAGNOSIS

Demonstration of the fungus by direct wet mount (potassium hydroxide) preparation of sputum, exudate, or pus supports the diagnosis in many cases. Histopathologic examination of biopsy specimens using special fungal staining techniques is also diagnostic. Immunohistochemistry using monoclonal antibodies to specific glycoproteins can also be done on tissue sections. Culture of the fungus on Sabouraud-dextrose or yeast extract agar confirms the diagnosis. Antibodies to *P. brasiliensis* can be demonstrated in most patients. Serial antibody titers and lymphocyte proliferative responses to fungal antigens are useful for monitoring the response to therapy. The 43 kDa glycoprotein (gp43) is present in sera of more than 90% of patients with paracoccidioidomycosis by immunodiffusion (the most commonly used diagnostic test) and in 100% by immunoblotting. A latex particle agglutination test using pooled crude fungal exoantigens is being developed for the detection of anti–*P. brasiliensis* antibodies and has shown 92% agreement with the double immunodiffusion test. Newer diagnostic methods that might prove to be very useful in the future include polymerase chain reaction, detection of gp43, and capture enzyme-linked immunosorbent assay to detect specific immunoglobulin E in patient sera. Skin testing with paracoccidioidin is not reliable, because 30–50% of patients with active disease are nonreactive initially and a positive test indicates previous exposure but not necessarily active disease.

TREATMENT

Itraconazole (5-10 mg/kg/day with maximum dose of 200 mg/day) orally for 6 mo is the treatment of choice for paracoccidioidomycosis. Fluconazole has also been used, but high doses ($\geq$600 mg/day) and longer treatment periods are required. A small number of patients have been treated with other azoles, including voriconazole, posaconazole, and isavuconazole. These drugs are potential substitutes for itraconazole but are more costly and can have interactions with other drugs. Terbinafine is an allylamine that has potent in vitro activity against *P. brasiliensis* and has been used for successful treatment of paracoccidioidomycosis. Amphotericin B is recommended for disseminated disease and if other therapies fail. Therapy with sulfonamide compounds, including sulfadiazine, TMP-SMX (trimethoprim 8-10 mg/kg/day to maximum of 160 mg, sulfamethoxazole 40-50 mg/kg/day to maximum of 800 mg), and dapsone, have been used historically and are generally less expensive than the newer azoles and allylamines. The primary disadvantage is that the treatment course is very long, lasting months to years, depending on the agent selected. Relapse can occur following any form of therapy, including with amphotericin B. In selected patients with intense inflammation in sites such as the central nervous system or with lung lesions causing respiratory insufficiency, there is some evidence that use of prednisone for 1-2 wk concomitantly with antifungal therapy reduces inflammation more effectively and may be of benefit. Occasionally children develop paradoxical clinical worsening during treatment, including new lymph node enlargement, fistula formation, fever, and weight loss. In this circumstance, steroids are also recommended.

Two therapies currently under investigation include the use of curcumin, an antioxidant found in the Indian spice turmeric, and the calcineurin inhibitor cyclosporine. Curcumin was found to have more antifungal activity than fluconazole against *P. brasiliensis* when studied in vitro using human buccal epithelial cells. Cyclosporine blocks the thermodimorphism of *P. brasiliensis*. Animal models demonstrate that fungal whole cells, purified antigens, peptides, and DNA vaccines have great potential toward the development of a vaccine for use in humans.

Bibliography is available at Expert Consult.

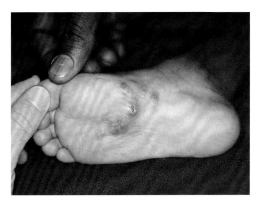

Chapter **269**
Sporotrichosis (Sporothrix schenckii)

Andrew P. Steenhoff

第二百六十九章
孢子丝菌病（申克孢子丝菌）

中文导读

　　本章主要介绍了孢子丝菌病的病因学、流行病学、发病机制、临床表现、诊断和治疗。临床表现中以皮肤孢子丝菌病最常见，分为皮肤淋巴管型或皮肤固定型。皮肤以外病变在儿童中少见，为骨和关节的感染；肺孢子丝菌病可表现为慢性肺炎。伊曲康唑是治疗中枢神经系统感染以外的首选药物，其他治疗药物包括饱和碘化钾溶液、两性霉素B等。

ETIOLOGY

Sporotrichosis is a rare fungal infection that occurs worldwide both sporadically and in outbreaks. The etiologic agent, *Sporothrix schenckii,* exhibits temperature dimorphism, existing as a mold at environmental temperatures (25-30°C [77-86°F]) and as a yeast in vivo (37°C [98.6°F]).

EPIDEMIOLOGY

S. schenckii is found throughout the world, but most cases of sporotrichosis are reported from North America, South America, and Japan. In the United States, the majority of cases have occurred in the Midwest, particularly in areas along the Mississippi and Missouri rivers. The fungus is found in decaying vegetation and has been isolated most commonly from sphagnum moss, rosebushes, barberry, straw, and some types of hay. Sporotrichosis can occur as an occupational disease among farmers, gardeners, veterinarians, and laboratory workers. Transmission from bites and scratches of animals, most commonly cats and armadillos, has occurred. Reports of human-to-human transmission are rare. Sporotrichosis has rarely been reported in infants. The mechanism of transmission in children may be zoonotic but usually is unclear. In 1 endemic area of Peru, the incidence of infection is greater in children than in adults; risk factors for infection in these children are playing in crop fields, living in houses with dirt floors, and owning a cat.

PATHOGENESIS

Disease in humans usually follows cutaneous inoculation of the fungus into a minor wound. Pulmonary infection can result from the inhalation of large numbers of spores. Disseminated infection is unusual but can occur in immunocompromised patients following ingestion or inhalation of spores. The cellular immune response to *S. schenckii* infection is both neutrophilic and monocytic. Histologically, the coexistence of noncaseating granulomas and microabscess formation is characteristic.

T-cell–mediated immunity appears to be important in limiting infection, and antibody does not protect against infection. As a result of the paucity of organisms, it is usually difficult to demonstrate the fungi in biopsy specimens.

CLINICAL MANIFESTATIONS

Cutaneous sporotrichosis is the most common form of disease in all age groups. Cutaneous disease may either be lymphocutaneous or fixed cutaneous, the former being much more common (Fig. 269.1). Lymphocutaneous sporotrichosis accounts for more than 75% of reported

Fig. 269.1 Sporotrichosis. Erythematous papules and nodules on the plantar surface with early lymphangitic (sporotrichoid) spread. *(From Paller AS, Mancini AJ: Hurwitz clinical pediatric dermatology, ed 5, Philadelphia, 2016, Elsevier, Fig. 17.48.)*

cases in children and occurs after traumatic subcutaneous inoculation. After a variable and often prolonged incubation period (1-12 wk), an isolated, painless erythematous papule develops at the inoculation site. The initial lesion is usually on an extremity in adults but is often on the face in children. The original papule enlarges and ulcerates. Although the infection might remain limited to the inoculation site (fixed cutaneous form), satellite lesions follow lymphangitic spread and appear as multiple tender subcutaneous nodules tracking along the lymphatic channels that drain the lesion. These secondary nodules are subcutaneous granulomas that adhere to the overlying skin and subsequently ulcerate. Sporotrichosis does not heal spontaneously, and these ulcerative lesions can persist for years if untreated. Systemic signs and symptoms are uncommon.

Extracutaneous sporotrichosis is rare in children, and most cases are reported in adults with underlying medical conditions, including AIDS and other immunosuppressing diseases. The most common form of extracutaneous sporotrichosis involves infection of the bones and joints. Pulmonary sporotrichosis usually manifests as a chronic pneumonitis similar to the presentation of pulmonary tuberculosis.

DIAGNOSIS

Cutaneous and lymphocutaneous sporotrichosis must be differentiated from other causes of nodular lymphangitis, including atypical mycobacterial infection, nocardiosis, leishmaniasis, tularemia, melioidosis, cutaneous anthrax, and other systemic mycoses, including coccidioidomycosis. Definitive diagnosis requires isolation of the fungus from the site of infection by culture. Special histologic staining such as periodic acid–Schiff and methenamine silver is required to identify yeast forms in tissues, which are typically oval or cigar-shaped. In spite of special staining techniques, diagnostic yield from biopsy specimens is low because of the small number of organisms present in the tissues. In cases of disseminated disease, demonstration of serum antibody against *S. schenckii*–related antigens can be diagnostically useful. Serologic testing is not commercially available but is offered by specialized laboratories, including the Centers for Disease Control and Prevention in the United States.

TREATMENT

Although comparative trials and extensive experience in children are not available, itraconazole is the recommended treatment of choice for infections outside the central nervous system. The recommended dosage for children is 5-10 mg/kg/day orally, with an initial maximum dose of 200 mg daily, which may be increased up to 400 mg daily if there is no initial response. Alternatively, younger children with cutaneous disease only may be treated with a saturated solution of potassium iodide (1 drop, 3 times daily, increasing as tolerated to a maximum of 1 drop/kg of body weight or 40 to 50 drops, 3 times daily, whichever is lowest). Adverse reactions, usually in the form of nausea and vomiting, should be managed with temporary cessation of therapy and reinstitution at a lower dosage. Therapy is continued 2 to 4 wk after cutaneous lesions have resolved, which usually takes at least 6-12 wk. Terbinafine, an allylamine, has been used successfully to treat cutaneous sporotrichosis but is reported to have lower cure rates and higher relapse rates than itraconazole. Further clinical efficacy data are needed to routinely recommend its use. Amphotericin B is the treatment of choice for pulmonary infections, disseminated infections, central nervous system disease, and infections in immunocompromised persons. Oral fluconazole 12 mg/kg daily (maximum dose, 400-800 mg daily) can be used if other agents are not tolerated. Posaconazole shows promise, but further data are needed.

Therapy with azoles or a saturated solution of potassium iodide should not be used in pregnant women. Amphotericin B can be used safely for cases of pulmonary or disseminated disease in pregnancy. Pregnant patients with cutaneous disease can be treated with local hyperthermia or can have therapy delayed until the pregnancy is completed. Hyperthermia involves heating the affected area to 42-45°C (107.6-113°F) using water baths or heating pads and works by inhibiting growth of the fungus. Dissemination to the fetus does not occur, and the disease is not worsened by pregnancy. Surgical debridement has a role in the treatment of some cases of sporotrichosis, particularly in osteoarticular disease.

Bibliography is available at Expert Consult.

Chapter 270

Mucormycosis

Rachel L. Wattier and William J. Steinbach

第二百七十章

毛霉病

中文导读

　　本章主要介绍了毛霉病的病因学、流行病学、发病机制、临床表现、诊断和治疗。本病是毛霉目真菌引起的机会性感染，临床表现包括鼻窦和鼻脑型感染、肺毛霉病、胃肠毛霉病、播散性毛霉病和皮肤软组织毛霉病。诊断依靠培养或组织的真菌形态学鉴定。大多数毛霉病为侵袭性，治疗困难，死亡率高，治疗药物包括两性霉素B、泊沙康唑、伊沙康唑等。

ETIOLOGY

Mucormycosis refers to a group of opportunistic fungal infections caused by fungi of the order Mucorales, which are primitive, fast-growing fungi that are largely saprophytic and ubiquitous. These organisms are found commonly in soil, in decaying plant and animal matter, and on moldy cheese, fruit, and bread. Mucormycosis was previously called zygomycosis, and the causative organisms were referred to as Zygomycetes, but this terminology has been abandoned due to re-classification of organisms from the former phylum Zygomycota using molecular phylogenetic analysis.

The most common disease-causing genera of Mucorales are *Rhizopus, Mucor,* and *Lichtheimia* (formerly *Absidia*). Infections caused by organisms of the genera *Actinomucor, Apophysomyces, Cokeromyces, Cunninghamella, Rhizomucor, Saksenaea,* and *Syncephalastrum* are seen less often. Mucormycosis in humans is characterized by a rapidly evolving course, tissue necrosis, and blood vessel invasion.

EPIDEMIOLOGY

Mucormycosis is primarily a disease of persons with underlying conditions that impair host immunity. Predisposing factors include diabetes, hematologic malignancies, stem cell or organ transplantation, persistent acidosis, corticosteroid or deferoxamine therapy, prematurity, and, less commonly, AIDS. Mucormycosis is the 2nd most common invasive mold infection in immunocompromised hosts, after aspergillosis.

PATHOGENESIS

The primary route of infection is inhalation of spores from the environment. In immunocompromised persons, if spores are not cleared by macrophages, they germinate into hyphae, resulting in local invasion and tissue destruction. Cutaneous or percutaneous routes of infection can lead to cutaneous and subcutaneous mucormycosis. Ingestion of contaminated food or supplements has been linked to gastrointestinal disease. Typically these infections are characterized by extensive angioinvasion, resulting in thrombosis, infarction, and tissue necrosis, which can limit the delivery of antifungal agents and leukocytes to the site of infection and contribute to dissemination of the infection to other organs.

Macrophages and neutrophils are the main host defense against the Mucorales and other filamentous fungi and provide almost complete immunity against mucormycosis by phagocytosis and oxidative killing of spores, perhaps explaining the predilection for mucormycosis in patients with neutropenia or neutrophil dysfunction. Many of the Mucorales have virulence mechanisms that scavenge iron, an element essential for cell growth, from the host. The iron chelator deferoxamine paradoxically increases iron availability and uptake by members of the Mucorales. Acidosis diminishes the phagocytic and chemotactic ability of neutrophils while increasing the availability of unbound iron, likely explaining the susceptibility to mucormycosis among individuals with uncontrolled acidosis.

CLINICAL MANIFESTATIONS

There are no unique signs or symptoms of mucormycosis. It can occur as any of several clinical syndromes, including sinus/rhinocerebral, pulmonary, gastrointestinal, disseminated, or cutaneous or subcutaneous disease.

Sinus and rhinocerebral infection have historically been the most common forms of mucormycosis and occur primarily in persons with diabetes mellitus or who are immunocompromised. Infection typically originates in the paranasal sinuses. Initial symptoms are consistent with sinusitis and include headache, retroorbital pain, fever, and nasal discharge. Infection can evolve rapidly or be slowly progressive. Orbital involvement manifesting as periorbital edema, proptosis, ptosis, and ophthalmoplegia can occur early in the disease. The nasal discharge is often dark and bloody; involved tissues become red, then violaceous, and then black as vessel thrombosis and tissue necrosis occur. Extension beyond the nasal cavity into the mouth is common. Direct bony involvement is common as a result of contiguous pressure effects or because of direct invasion and infarction. Destructive paranasal sinusitis with intracranial extension can be demonstrated by computed tomography (CT) or magnetic resonance imaging (MRI) (Fig. 270.1). Cases complicated by cavernous sinus thrombosis or thrombosis of the internal carotid artery have been reported. Brain abscesses can occur in patients with rhinocerebral infection that extends directly from the nasal cavity and sinuses, usually to the frontal or frontotemporal lobes. In patients with hematogenous disseminated disease, abscesses can involve the occipital lobe or brainstem.

Pulmonary mucormycosis usually occurs in severely neutropenic patients and has become more common in recent epidemiologic series. It is characterized by fever, tachypnea, and productive cough with pleuritic chest pain and hemoptysis. A wide range of pulmonary radiographic findings, including solitary pulmonary nodule, segmental or lobar consolidation, and cavitary and bronchopneumonic changes, are recognized (see Fig. 270.1). Although the radiographic findings overlap with other pulmonary invasive fungal infections, the presence of multiple nodules (≥10), pleural effusions, or the reversed halo sign are more suggestive of mucormycosis.

Gastrointestinal mucormycosis is uncommon. Often the diagnosis is delayed; only 25% of cases are diagnosed antemortem, and the subsequent mortality is as high as 85%. It can occur as a complication of disseminated disease or as an isolated intestinal infection in individuals with diabetes, immunosuppressed or malnourished children, or preterm infants. Any part of the gastrointestinal tract can be involved, with the

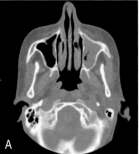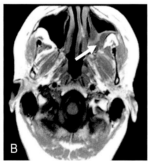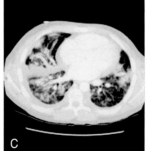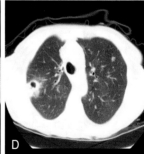

Fig. 270.1 Radiographic findings in sinopulmonary mucormycosis. **A,** Left maxillary sinus air-fluid level is evident in this computed tomography (CT) scan that is indistinguishable from bacterial sinusitis. **B,** Magnetic resonance image reveals T2 signal hyperintensity in the left pterygoid musculature *(arrow)* in conjunction with a left maxillary sinus air-fluid level. **C,** Multiple heterogeneous nodular and consolidative lesions with a large pulmonary vessel infarct *(wedge)* and modest pleural effusions are shown in a cancer patient with cancer and pulmonary mucormycosis. **D,** Contrast-enhanced CT scan demonstrates a cavity within a dense infiltrate in a patient with acute myelogenous leukemia and pulmonary mucormycosis. *(From Konotoyiannis DP, Lewis RE: Agents of mucormycosis and entomophthoramycosis. In Bennett JF, Dolin R, Blaser MJ, editors: Mandell, Douglas, and Bennett's principles and practice of infectious diseases, ed 8, Philadelphia, 2015, Elsevier, Fig. 260-5; courtesy Dr. Edith Marom, University of Texas, MD Anderson Cancer Center, Houston, Texas.)*

stomach followed by colon and ileum being the most commonly affected. Abdominal pain and distention with hematemesis, hematochezia, or melena can occur. Stomach or bowel wall perforation is not uncommon.

Disseminated mucormycosis is associated with a very high mortality rate, especially among immunocompromised persons. Disseminated infection can originate from any of the primary sites of infection but often originates from pulmonary infection. Clinical presentation varies based on the involved sites.

Cutaneous and soft tissue mucormycosis can complicate burns and surgical or traumatic wounds. Primary cutaneous disease may be invasive locally, progressing through all tissue layers, including muscle, fascia, and bone (Fig. 270.2). Necrotizing fasciitis may occur. Infection manifests as an erythematous papule that ulcerates, leaving a black necrotic center. The skin lesions are painful, and affected patients may be febrile. In contrast, secondary cutaneous lesions from hematogenous seeding tend to be nodular, with minimal destruction of the epidermis.

DIAGNOSIS

The diagnosis relies on direct morphologic identification of mycotic elements from culture or tissue biopsy specimens obtained at the site of disease. Mucorales appear as broad (5-25 μm in diameter), infrequently septate, thin-walled hyphae, branching irregularly at right angles when stained with Gomori methenamine silver (GMS) or hematoxylin and eosin. Secondary to their thin-walled structure and lack of regular septation, they often appear twisted, collapsed, or folded. Organisms may be challenging to identify reliably by morphology from tissue specimens; immunohistochemistry or PCR can provide more reliable identification when the morphology is not characteristic. Angioinvasion within tissue is a hallmark of mucormycosis.

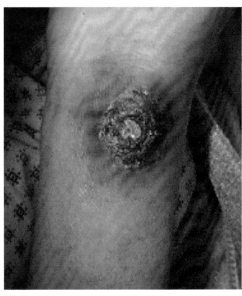

Fig. 270.2 Cutaneous presentation of mucormycosis. Chronic, nonhealing ulcer with necrosis following traumatic inoculation. *(From Konotoyiannis DP, Lewis RE: Agents of mucormycosis and entomophthoramycosis. In Bennett JF, Dolin R, Blaser MJ, editors: Mandell, Douglas, and Bennett's principles and practice of infectious diseases, ed 8, Philadelphia, 2015, Elsevier, Fig. 260-6A.)*

Mucorales can be cultured on standard laboratory media from sputum, bronchoalveolar lavage fluid, skin lesions, or biopsy material. Cultures from non-tissue specimens, such as bronchoalveolar lavage fluid, have poor sensitivity. Polymerase chain reaction (PCR)-based methods may improve detection over culture but have not been evaluated on a wide scale. Though Mucorales can be culture contaminants, isolation in a susceptible host should prompt consideration of clinical disease. Noninvasive fungal biomarkers, such as galactomannan, or 1,3-β-D-glucan, do not detect the causative agents of mucormycosis.

TREATMENT

Most forms of mucormycosis can be aggressive and difficult to treat, with high mortality rates, except for localized cutaneous disease, which has relatively favorable outcomes. The optimal therapy for mucormycosis in children requires early diagnosis and prompt institution of medical therapy combined with extensive surgical debridement of all devitalized tissue. Correction of predisposing factors, such as neutropenia, hyperglycemia, and/or acidosis, if possible, is an essential component of management.

Lipid formulations of amphotericin B, either liposomal amphotericin, or amphotericin B lipid complex, are the mainstay of antifungal therapy for mucormycosis. Doses of at least 5 mg/kg/day and up to 10 mg/kg/day are recommended, though the benefit of increasing up to 10 mg/kg/day is not well defined. The duration of therapy is individualized, depending on clinical response and immune reconstitution.

Other antifungals with activity against the Mucorales include posaconazole and isavuconazole. Importantly, voriconazole is not active against agents of mucormycosis and in some studies has been identified as a predisposing factor for mucormycosis. This association is not completely understood; some studies suggest that it may be a marker for higher-risk patients rather than actually influencing susceptibility. Posaconazole is active against many of the Mucorales and has shown promise when used as salvage therapy, though it has not been evaluated for primary therapy of mucormycosis. Concerns have been raised about its activity against *Rhizopus oryzae* and *Mucor circinelloides*, 2 of the most common causative agents of mucormycosis. Posaconazole is presently not recommended for primary therapy but may be used for salvage therapy or step down from an amphotericin B-based regimen. Isavuconazole was recently licensed for primary therapy of mucormycosis based on a single arm study in which it showed favorable outcomes compared to contemporary response rates with amphotericin B-based therapy. However, there are currently no pediatric dosing data for isavuconazole.

Although the echinocandins lack significant activity against the Mucorales, animal models have demonstrated potential synergy when they are used with amphotericin B in treatment of experimental mucormycosis. Caspofungin has been shown to uncover β-glucan in the cell wall of *Rhizopus*, resulting in an increase in neutrophil activity. However, clinical studies evaluating combination therapy with addition of either an echinocandin or posaconazole to an amphotericin B-based regimen have shown conflicting results. Currently combination therapy is not recommended as primary therapy but may be considered as salvage therapy for refractory disease. Hyperbaric oxygen has been used anecdotally as an adjunctive therapy. Iron chelation with deferasirox has been tried as salvage therapy in refractory mucormycosis but is currently not recommended due to adverse outcomes in a small clinical trial.

Bibliography is available at Expert Consult.

Chapter **271**
Pneumocystis jirovecii
Francis Gigliotti and Terry W. Wright

第二百七十一章
耶氏肺孢子菌肺炎

中文导读

　　本章主要介绍了耶氏肺孢子菌肺炎的病因、流行病学、发病机制、病理学、临床表现、实验室检查、诊断、治疗、并发症、预后和预防。本病在免疫缺陷人群中为致命性感染，根据感染人群不同，至少有三种不同的临床表现类型。诊断需有感染的临床症状、体征，并证实肺中存在耶氏肺孢子虫。推荐治疗药物为甲氧苄啶磺胺甲噁唑。重症联合免疫缺陷患者、接受免疫抑制治疗、器官移植等人群需予药物预防。

Pneumocystis jirovecii pneumonia (interstitial plasma cell pneumonitis) in an immunocompromised person is a life-threatening infection. Primary infection in the immunocompetent person is usually subclinical and goes unrecognized. The disease most likely results from new or repeat acquisition of the organism rather than reactivation of latent organisms. Even in the most severe cases, with rare exceptions, the organisms remain localized to the lungs.

ETIOLOGY

P. jirovecii is a common extracellular parasite found worldwide in the lungs of mammals. The taxonomic placement of this organism has not been unequivocally established, but nucleic acid homologies place it closest to fungi despite sharing morphologic features and drug susceptibility with protozoa. Detailed studies of the basic biology of the organism are not possible because of the inability to maintain *P. jirovecii* in culture. Phenotypic and genotypic analyses demonstrate that each mammalian species is infected by a unique strain (or possibly species) of *Pneumocystis*. A biologic correlate of these differences is evidenced by animal experiments that have shown organisms are not transmissible from one mammalian species to another. These observations have led to the suggestion that organisms be renamed, with those infecting humans renamed *P. jirovecii*.

EPIDEMIOLOGY

Serologic surveys show that most humans are infected with *P. jirovecii* before 4 yr. of age. In the immunocompetent child, these infections are usually asymptomatic. *P. jirovecii* DNA can occasionally be detected in nasopharyngeal aspirates of normal infants. Pneumonia caused by *P. jirovecii* occurs almost exclusively in severely immunocompromised hosts, including those with congenital or acquired immunodeficiency disorders, malignancies, or transplanted organs. Patients with primary immunodeficiency diseases at risk for infection include severe combined immunodeficiency disease, X-linked CD40 ligand deficiency, major histocompatibility complex class II deficiency, nuclear factor kappa B essential modulator deficiency, dedicator of cytokinesis 8 deficiency, Wiskott-Aldrich syndrome, and caspase recruitment domain 11 deficiency. Small numbers of *P. jirovecii* can be found in the lungs of infants who have died with the diagnosis of sudden infant death syndrome. This observation could indicate a cause-and-effect relationship or simply that there is overlap in the timing of the primary infection with *P. jirovecii* and sudden infant death syndrome.

Without chemoprophylaxis, approximately 40% of infants and children with AIDS, 70% of adults with AIDS, 12% of children with leukemia, and 10% of patients with organ transplants experience *P. jirovecii* pneumonia. Epidemics that occurred among debilitated infants in Europe during and after World War II are attributed to malnutrition. The use of new biologic immunosuppressive agents has expanded at-risk populations. The addition of tumor necrosis factor-α inhibitors to the management of patients with inflammatory bowel disease has resulted in a demonstrable increase in *P. jirovecii* pneumonia in this patient population, as has the use of rituximab in patients with hematologic malignancies.

The natural habitat and mode of transmission to humans are unknown, but animal studies clearly demonstrate airborne transmission. Animal-to-human transmission is unlikely because of the host specificity of *P. jirovecii*. Thus person-to-person transmission is likely but has not been conclusively demonstrated.

PATHOGENESIS

Two forms of *P. jirovecii* are found in the alveolar spaces: cysts, which are 5-8 μm in diameter and contain up to 8 pleomorphic intracystic sporozoites (or intracystic bodies), and extracystic trophozoites (or trophic forms), which are 2-5 μm cells derived from excysted sporozoites. The terminology of sporozoite and trophozoite is based on the morphologic similarities to protozoa, because there are no exact correlates for these forms of the organism among the fungi. *P. jirovecii* attaches to type I alveolar epithelial cells, possibly by adhesive proteins such as fibronectin or mannose-dependent ligands.

Control of infection depends on intact cell-mediated immunity. Studies in patients with AIDS show an increased incidence of *P. jirovecii* pneumonia with markedly decreased CD4+ T-lymphocyte counts. The CD4+ cell count provides a useful indicator in both older children and adults of the need for prophylaxis for *P. jirovecii* pneumonia. Although normally functioning CD4+ T cells are central to controlling infection by *P. jirovecii*, the final effector pathway for destruction of *P. jirovecii* is poorly understood but likely depends on alveolar macrophages. A role for CD4+ T cells could be to provide help for the production of specific antibody that is then involved in the clearance of organisms through interaction with complement, phagocytes, or T cells or through direct activation of alveolar macrophages.

In the absence of an adaptive immune response, as can be modeled in severe combined immunodeficient mice, infection with *P. murina* produces little alteration in lung histology or function until late in the course of the disease. If functional lymphocytes are given to severe combined immunodeficient mice infected with *P. murina,* there is rapid onset of an inflammatory response that results in an intense cellular infiltrate, markedly reduced lung compliance, and significant hypoxia, mimicking the characteristic changes of *P. jirovecii* pneumonia in humans. These inflammatory changes are also associated with marked disruption of surfactant function. T-cell subset analysis has shown that CD4+ T cells produce an inflammatory response that clears the organisms but also results in lung injury. CD8+ T cells are ineffective in the eradication of *P. jirovecii.* CD8+ T cells do help to modulate the inflammation produced by CD4+ T cells, but in the absence of CD4+ T cells the ineffectual inflammatory response of CD8+ T cells contributes significantly to lung injury. These various T-cell effects are likely responsible for the variations in presentation and outcome of *P. jirovecii* pneumonia observed in different patient populations.

PATHOLOGY

The histopathologic features of *P. jirovecii* pneumonia are of 2 types. The 1st type is infantile interstitial plasma cell pneumonitis, which was seen in epidemic outbreaks in debilitated infants 3-6 mo of age. Extensive infiltration with thickening of the alveolar septum occurs, and plasma cells are prominent. The 2nd type is a diffuse desquamative alveolar pneumonitis found in immunocompromised children and adults. The alveoli contain large numbers of *P. jirovecii* in a foamy exudate with alveolar macrophages active in the phagocytosis of organisms. The alveolar septum is not infiltrated to the extent it is in the infantile type, and plasma cells are usually absent.

CLINICAL MANIFESTATIONS

There are at least three distinct clinical presentations of *P. jirovecii* pneumonia. In patients with profound congenital immunodeficiency or in AIDS patients with very few CD4+ T cells, the onset of hypoxia and symptoms is subtle, with tachypnea progressing to nasal flaring, often without fever; intercostal, suprasternal, and infrasternal retractions; and cyanosis in severe cases. In cases of *P. jirovecii* pneumonia occurring in children and adults with immunodeficiency resulting from immunosuppressive medications, the onset of hypoxia and symptoms is often more abrupt, with fever, tachypnea, dyspnea, and cough, progressing to severe respiratory compromise. This type accounts for the majority of cases, although the severity of clinical expression can vary. *Rales are usually not detected on physical examination.* The 3rd pattern of disease is seen in severely immunocompromised patients with *P. jirovecii* pneumonia who appear to be responding to therapy but then have an acute and seemingly paradoxical deterioration thought to be associated with return of immune function. This condition is referred to as *immune reconstitution inflammatory syndrome* and is most commonly seen in patients with newly diagnosed AIDS who present with *P. jirovecii* pneumonia and who have a rapid response to antiretroviral therapy that is instituted at the same time as anti-*Pneumocystis* therapy. It can also occur in stem cell transplant recipients who engraft while infected with *P. jirovecii.*

LABORATORY FINDINGS

The chest radiograph reveals bilateral diffuse interstitial or alveolar ground glass infiltrates (Fig. 271.1). The earliest densities are perihilar, and progression proceeds peripherally, sparing the apical areas until last. The arterial oxygen tension (PaO_2) is invariably decreased. The major role of the laboratory in establishing a diagnosis of *P. jirovecii* pneumonia is in identifying organisms in lung specimens by a variety of methods. Once obtained, the specimens are typically stained with 1 of 4 commonly used stains: Grocott-Gomori silver stain and toluidine blue stain for the cyst form, polychrome stains such as Giemsa stain for the trophozoites and sporozoites, and the fluorescein-labeled monoclonal antibody stains for both trophozoites and cysts. Polymerase chain reaction analysis of respiratory specimens offers promise as a rapid diagnostic method, but a standardized system for clinical use has not been established. Serum lactate dehydrogenase levels are often elevated but are not specific.

DIAGNOSIS

Definitive diagnosis requires demonstration of *P. jirovecii* in the lung in the presence of clinical signs and symptoms of the infection. Organisms can be detected in specimens collected by bronchoalveolar lavage (BAL), tracheal aspirate, transbronchial lung biopsy, bronchial brushings, percutaneous transthoracic needle aspiration, and open lung biopsy. Hypertonic saline–induced sputum samples are helpful if *P. jirovecii* is found, but the absence of the organisms in induced sputum does not exclude the infection and BAL should be performed. Open lung biopsy is the most reliable method, although BAL is more practical in most cases. Estimates of the diagnostic yield of the various specimens are 20–40% for induced sputum, 50–60% for tracheal aspirate, 75–95% for BAL, 75–85% for transbronchial biopsy, and 90–100% for open lung biopsy.

TREATMENT

The recommended therapy for *P. jirovecii* pneumonia is trimethoprim-sulfamethoxazole (TMP-SMX) (15-20 mg TMP and 75-100 mg SMX/kg/day in 4 divided doses) administered intravenously, or orally if there is mild disease and no malabsorption or diarrhea. The duration of treatment is 3 wk for patients with AIDS and 2 wk for other patients. Unfortunately, adverse reactions often occur with TMP-SMX, especially rash and neutropenia in patients with AIDS. For patients who cannot tolerate or who fail to respond to TMP-SMX after 5-7 days, pentamidine isethionate (4 mg/kg/day as a single dose IV) may be used. Adverse

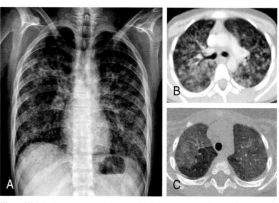

Fig. 271.1 *Pneumocystis jiroveci* infection in a 17 yr old boy with acute lymphoblastic leukemia and immunodeficiency, who presented with dyspnea, fever, nonproductive cough, and decreased white blood cell counts. **A,** The radiograph shows diffuse bilateral interstitial opacity throughout the lungs. **B,** Contrast-enhanced computed tomography *(CT)* confirms the bilateral patchy and ground-glass opacities in both lungs. The diagnosis was confirmed by a positive polymerase chain reaction test from bronchial lavage fluid. **C,** CT in a different patient demonstrates a typical "crazy paving" pattern in both upper lobes. *(From Westra SJ, Yikilmaz A, Lee EY: Pulmonary infection. In Coley BD, editor:* Caffey's pediatric diagnostic imaging, *ed 13, Philadelphia, 2019, Elsevier, Fig. 54-30.)*

reactions are frequent and include renal and hepatic dysfunction, hyperglycemia or hypoglycemia, rash, and thrombocytopenia. Atovaquone (750 mg twice daily with food, for patients >13 yr of age) is an alternative treatment that has been used primarily in adults with mild to moderate disease. Limited experience is available for younger children. Pharmacokinetic studies of atovaquone show that a dose of 30 mg/kg/day PO in 2 divided doses for children 0-3 mo of age and older than 2 yr of age is adequate and safe; a dose of 45 mg/kg/day PO in 2 divided doses is needed for children between 4 mo and 2 yr of age. Other effective therapies include trimetrexate glucuronate or combinations of trimethoprim plus dapsone or clindamycin plus primaquine.

Some studies in adults suggest that administration of corticosteroids as adjunctive therapy to suppress the inflammatory response increases the chances for survival in moderate and severe cases of *P. jirovecii* pneumonia. The recommended regimen of corticosteroids for adolescents older than 13 yr of age and for adults is oral prednisone, 80 mg/day PO in 2 divided doses on days 1-5, 40 mg/day PO once daily on days 6-10, and 20 mg/day PO once daily on days 11-21. A reasonable regimen for children is oral prednisone, 2 mg/kg/day for the 1st 7-10 days, followed by a tapering regimen for the next 10-14 days.

SUPPORTIVE CARE

Basic supportive care is dictated by the condition of the patient, with careful attention to maintain appropriate hydration and oxygenation. Only 5-10% of AIDS patients require mechanical ventilation compared with 50-60% of patients without AIDS, consistent with the hypothesis that the patient's ability to mount an inflammatory response correlates with severity and outcome. There are anecdotal reports of giving surfactant to children with severe *P. jirovecii* pneumonia, although the use of surfactant to treat adult-type respiratory distress syndrome is controversial.

COMPLICATIONS

Most complications occur as adverse events associated with the drugs used or the mechanical ventilation used for treatment. The most severe pulmonary complication of *P. jirovecii* pneumonia is adult-type respiratory distress syndrome. Rarely, *P. jirovecii* infection affects extrapulmonary sites (e.g., retina, spleen, and bone marrow), but such infections are usually not symptomatic and also respond to treatment.

PROGNOSIS

Without treatment, *P. jirovecii* pneumonitis is fatal in almost all immunocompromised hosts within 3-4 wk of onset. The mortality rate varies with patient population and is related to inflammatory response rather than organism burden. AIDS patients have a mortality rate of 5–10%, and patients with other diseases such as malignancies have mortality rates as high as 20–25%. Patients who require mechanical ventilation have mortality rates of 60–90%. Patients remain at risk for *P. jirovecii* pneumonia as long as they are immunocompromised. Continuous prophylaxis should be initiated or reinstituted at the end of therapy for patients with AIDS (see Chapter 302).

PREVENTION

Patients at high risk for *P. jirovecii* pneumonia should be placed on chemoprophylaxis. Prophylaxis in infants born to HIV-infected mothers and for HIV-infected infants and children is based on age and CD4 cell counts (see Chapter 302). Because CD4 counts fluctuate rapidly during the first year of life, infants born to HIV-infected mothers should be placed on prophylaxis during the 1st year of life until HIV infection is ruled out. Patients with severe combined immunodeficiency syndrome, patients receiving intensive immunosuppressive therapy for cancer or other diseases, and organ transplant recipients are also candidates for prophylaxis. TMP-SMX (5 mg/kg TMP and 25 mg SMX/kg PO once daily or divided into 2 doses daily) is the drug of choice and may be given for 3 consecutive days each wk, or, alternatively, each day. Alternatives for prophylaxis include dapsone (2 mg/kg/day PO, maximum: 100 mg/dose; or 4 mg/kg PO once weekly, maximum: 200 mg/dose), atovaquone (30 mg/kg/day PO for infants 1-3 mo. and ≥24 mo of age; 45 mg/kg/day for infants and toddlers 4-23 mo of age), and aerosolized pentamidine (300 mg monthly by Respirgard II nebulizer), but all of these agents are inferior to TMP-SMX. Finally, limited clinical experience suggests that pentamidine can be given intravenously once monthly to prevent *P. jirovecii* pneumonia. Prophylaxis must be continued as long as the patient remains immunocompromised. Some AIDS patients who reconstitute adequate immune response during highly active antiretroviral therapy may have prophylaxis withdrawn.

Bibliography is available at Expert Consult.

Section **13**

Viral Infections

第十三篇

病毒感染

Chapter **272**

Principles of Antiviral Therapy

Mark R. Schleiss

第二百七十二章

抗病毒治疗原则

中文导读

　　本章主要介绍了抗病毒治疗原则，包括针对不同感染类型的抗病毒药和抗病毒免疫球蛋白的使用。用于疱疹病毒感染的药物大部分为核苷类似物，包括阿昔洛韦、更昔洛韦和缬更昔洛韦等；用于呼吸道病毒感染的药物包括利巴韦林、金刚烷胺和金刚乙胺、奥司他韦、扎那米韦和帕拉米韦等；用于肝炎的抗病毒药可分为干扰素和核苷或核苷酸类似物，包括拉米夫定、恩替卡韦等。

Antiviral chemotherapy typically requires a delicate balance between targeting critical steps in viral replication without interfering with host cellular function. Because viruses require cellular functions to complete replication, many antiviral agents exert significant host cellular toxicity, a limitation that has hindered antiviral drug development. In spite of this limitation, a number of agents are licensed for use against viruses, particularly herpesviruses, respiratory viruses, and hepatitis viruses (Table 272.1).

In making the decision to commence antiviral drugs, it is important for the clinician to obtain appropriate diagnostic specimens, which can help clarify the antiviral of choice. The choice of a specific antiviral is based on the recommended agent of choice for a particular clinical condition, pharmacokinetics, toxicities, cost, and the potential for development of resistance (Table 272.2). Intercurrent conditions in the patient, such as renal insufficiency, should also be considered. Clinicians must monitor antiviral therapy closely for adverse events or toxicities, both anticipated and unanticipated.

In vitro sensitivity testing of virus isolates to antiviral compounds usually involves a complex tissue culture system. The potency of an antiviral is determined by the **50% inhibitory dose (ID$_{50}$),** which is the antiviral concentration required to inhibit the growth in cell culture of a standardized viral inoculum by 50%. Because of the complexity of these assays, the results vary widely, and the actual relationship between antiviral sensitivity testing and antiviral therapy outcomes is sometimes unclear. Because these assays are often not readily available and take considerable time to complete, **genotypic analysis** for antiviral susceptibility is increasingly being offered. Such assays may be useful for patients on long-term antiviral therapy.

Clinical context is essential in making decisions about antiviral treatment, along with knowledge of a patient's immune status. For example, antiviral treatment is rarely if ever indicated in an immunocompetent child shedding cytomegalovirus (CMV) but may be lifesaving when administered to an immunocompromised solid organ transplant (SOT) or hematopoietic stem cell transplant (HSCT) patient. Antivirals can be used with a variety of clinical goals in mind. Antivirals can be used for **treatment** of active end-organ disease, as **prophylaxis** to prevent viral infection or disease, or as **preemptive therapy** aimed at reducing risk of progression to disease (i.e., a positive signal indicating viral replication but in the absence of clinical evidence of end-organ disease). In preemptive therapy, a patient will usually have a positive signal for polymerase chain reaction–based identification of viral nucleic acids in a clinical sample (blood or body fluid) but have no symptoms. However, SOT and HSCT patients are at high risk of developing disease in this setting (particularly due to CMV infection), a scenario that warrants preemptive

Table 272.1	Currently Licensed Antiviral Drugs	
ANTIVIRAL	**TRADE NAME**	**MECHANISM OF ACTION**
Acyclovir	Zovirax	Inhibits viral DNA polymerase
Adefovir	Hepsera	Nucleotide reverse transcriptase inhibitor
Amantadine*	Symmetrel	Blocks M2 protein ion channel
Baloxavir	Xofluza	Inhibits polymerase acidic endonuclease, blocking viral replication
Beclabuvir	BMS-791325	Inhibitor of HCV NS5B
Boceprevir†	Victrelis	Inhibitor of HCV NS3 serine protease
		Active against HCV genotype 1
Cidofovir	Vistide	Inhibits viral DNA polymerase
Daclatasvir	Daklinza	Inhibitor of HCV NS5A
		Used in varying combinations with sofosbuvir, ribavirin, and interferon
Dasabuvir	Exviera	Inhibitor of HCV NS5B
		Used together with the combination medication ombitasvir/paritaprevir/ ritonavir (Vikiera Pak)
		Activity limited to HCV genotype 1
Elbasvir	(Zepatier)	Inhibitor of HCV NS5A
		Used in combination with the NS3/4A protease inhibitor grazoprevir under the trade name Zepatier, either with or without ribavirin
Entecavir	Baraclude	Nucleoside reverse transcriptase inhibitor
		Active against HBV
Famciclovir	Generic	Inhibits viral DNA polymerase
Fomivirsen†	Vitravene	Phosphorothioate oligonucleotide inhibits viral replication via antisense mechanism
Foscarnet	Foscavir	Inhibits viral DNA polymerase and reverse transcriptase at pyrophosphate-binding site
Ganciclovir	Cytovene	Inhibits viral DNA polymerase
Grazoprevir	(Zepatier)	Inhibitor of HCV NS3-4A serine protease Used in combination with elbasvir under the trade name Zepatier, either with or without ribavirin
Idoxuridine	Herplex	Inhibits viral DNA polymerase
Interferon-α	Intro-A (interferon-α2b) Roferon-A (interferon-α2a) Infergen (interferon alfacon-1)	Produces multiple effector proteins that exert antiviral effects; also directly interacts with immune system components
Interferon-α2b plus ribavirin	Rebetron	Not established
Lamivudine (3TC)	Epivir	Inhibits viral DNA polymerase and reverse transcriptase; active against HBV
Ledipasvir	(with Sofosbuvir: Harvoni)	Inhibitor of HCV NS5A
Ombitasvir	(Viekira Pak)	Inhibitor of HCV NS5A
		Used in combination with paritaprevir, ritonavir and dasabuvir in Viekira Pak
		Active against HCV genotype 1
Oseltamivir	Tamiflu	Neuraminidase inhibitor; interference with deaggregation and release of viral progeny
Paritaprevir	(Viekira Pak) (Technivie/Viekirax)	Inhibitor of HCV NS3-4A serine protease Used in combination with ombitasvir, ritonavir and dasabuvir (Viekira Pak), or in combination with ombitasvir and ritonavir (Technivie/Viekirax)
Pegylated interferon	PEG-Intron (α2b), Pegasys (α2a)	Same as interferon
Penciclovir	Denavir	Inhibits viral DNA polymerase
Peramivir	Rapivab	Neuraminidase inhibitor
Ribavirin	Virazole, Rebetol, Copegus	Interference with viral messenger RNA
Rimantadine*	Flumadine	Blocks M2 protein ion channel
Simeprevir	Olysio	Inhibitor of HCV NS3-4A serine protease Active against genotype 1 ± genotype 4
		Used with include sofosbuvir or ribavirin and pegylated interferon-alfa
Sofosbuvir	(Harvoni)	Inhibitor of HCV NS5B
		Used in combination with Ledipasvir (Harvoni)
Telaprevir	Incivek Incivio	Inhibitor of HCV NS3-4A serine protease
		Active against HCV genotype 1
Telbivudine	Tyzeka	Interferes with HBV DNA replication
Tenofovir	Viread	Nucleoside reverse transcriptase inhibitor
		Active against HBV
Trifluridine	Viroptic	Inhibits viral DNA polymerase
Valacyclovir	Valtrex	Same as acyclovir
Valganciclovir	Valcyte	Same as ganciclovir
Velpatasvir	(Epclusa, Sofosvel, Velpanat)	Inhibitor of HCV NS5A
		Used in combination with sofosbuvir (Epclusa, Sofosvel, Velpanat)
		Active against all 6 HCV genotypes
Vidarabine	ara-A	Inhibits viral DNA polymerase (and to lesser extent, cellular DNA polymerase)
Zanamivir	Relenza	Neuraminidase inhibitor; interference with deaggregation and release of viral progeny

Continued

Table 272.1	Currently Licensed Antiviral Drugs—cont'd	
ANTIVIRAL	**TRADE NAME**	**MECHANISM OF ACTION**
FDA-APPROVED COMBINATION THERAPIES		
Interferon-α2b + ribavirin	Rebetron (Intron-A plus Rebetol)	
Interferon-α2a + ribavirin	Roferon-A + ribavirin	
Pegylated interferon-α2b + ribavirin (3 yr and older)	PEG-Intron + Rebetol	
Pegylated interferon-α2a + ribavirin (5 yr and older)	Pegasys + Copegus	

*No longer recommended by Centers for Disease Control and Prevention for treatment of influenza.
†No longer marketed in United States.
‡No longer available.

Table 272.2	Antiviral Therapies for Non-HIV Clinical Conditions*		
VIRUS	**CLINICAL SYNDROME**	**ANTIVIRAL AGENT OF CHOICE**	**ALTERNATIVE ANTIVIRAL AGENTS**
Influenza A and B	Treatment	Oseltamivir (>2 wk old)	Zanamivir (>7 yr old) Peramivir (>2 yr old)
	Prophylaxis	Oseltamivir (>3 mo old)	Zanamivir (>5 yr old)
Respiratory syncytial virus	Bronchiolitis or pneumonia in high-risk host	Ribavirin aerosol	
Adenovirus	In immunocompromised patients: Pneumonia Viremia Nephritis Hemorrhagic cystitis	Cidofovir	
CMV	Congenital CMV infection	Ganciclovir (IV)	Valganciclovir (if oral therapy appropriate; long-term oral valganciclovir investigational but may improve developmental and hearing outcomes)
	Retinitis in AIDS patients	Valganciclovir	Ganciclovir Cidofovir Foscarnet Ganciclovir ocular insert
	Pneumonitis, colitis; esophagitis in immunocompromised patients	Ganciclovir (IV)	Foscarnet Cidofovir Valganciclovir
HSV	Neonatal herpes	Acyclovir (IV)	
	Suppressive therapy following neonatal herpes with central nervous system involvement	Acyclovir (PO)	
	HSV encephalitis	Acyclovir (IV)	
	HSV gingivostomatitis	Acyclovir (PO)	Acyclovir (IV)
	First episode genital infection	Acyclovir (PO)	Valacyclovir Famciclovir Acyclovir (IV) (severe disease)
	Recurrent genital herpes	Acyclovir (PO)	Valacyclovir Famciclovir
	Suppression of genital herpes	Acyclovir (PO)	Valacyclovir Famciclovir
	Cutaneous HSV (whitlow, herpes gladiatorum)	Acyclovir (PO)	Penciclovir (topical)
	Eczema herpeticum	Acyclovir (PO)	Acyclovir (IV) (severe disease)
	Mucocutaneous infection in immunocompromised host (mild)	Acyclovir (IV)	Acyclovir (PO) (if outpatient therapy acceptable)
	Mucocutaneous infection in immunocompromised host (moderate to severe)	Acyclovir (IV)	
	Prophylaxis in bone marrow transplant recipients	Acyclovir (IV)	Valacyclovir
	Acyclovir-resistant HSV	Foscarnet	Cidofovir
	Keratitis or keratoconjunctivitis	Trifluridine	Vidarabine
Varicella-zoster virus	Chickenpox, healthy child	Supportive care	Acyclovir (PO)
	Chickenpox, immunocompromised child	Acyclovir (IV)	
	Zoster (not ophthalmic branch of trigeminal nerve), healthy child	Supportive care	Acyclovir (PO)
	Zoster (ophthalmic branch of trigeminal nerve), healthy child	Acyclovir (IV)	
	Zoster, immunocompromised child	Acyclovir (IV)	Valacyclovir

*For antiviral agents for hepatitis B and hepatitis C, see Table 272.1.
CMV, cytomegalovirus; HSV, herpes simplex virus.

treatment with an antiviral agent. In contrast, prophylaxis is administered to seropositive patients who are at risk to reactivate latent viral infection but do not yet have evidence of active viral replication or shedding.

A fundamental concept important in the understanding of the mechanism of action of most antivirals is that viruses must use host cell components to replicate. Thus mechanisms of action for antiviral compounds must be selective to virus-specific functions whenever possible, and antiviral agents may have significant toxicities to the host if these compounds impact cellular physiology. Some of the more commonly targeted sites of action for antiviral agents include viral entry, absorption, penetration, and uncoating (amantadine, rimantadine); transcription or replication of the viral genome (acyclovir, valacyclovir, cidofovir, famciclovir, penciclovir, foscarnet, ganciclovir, valganciclovir, ribavirin, trifluridine); viral protein synthesis (interferons) or protein modification (protease inhibitors); and viral assembly, release, or deaggregation (oseltamivir, zanamivir, interferons).

An understudied and underappreciated issue in antiviral therapy is emergence of resistance, particularly in the setting of high viral load, high intrinsic viral mutation rate, and prolonged or repeated courses of antiviral therapy. Resistant viruses are more likely to develop or be selected for in immunocompromised patients because these patients are more likely to have multiple or long-term exposures to an antiviral agent.

ANTIVIRALS USED FOR HERPESVIRUSES

The herpesviruses are important pediatric pathogens, particularly in newborns and immunocompromised children. Most of the licensed antivirals are nucleoside analogs that inhibit viral DNA polymerase, inducing premature chain termination during viral DNA synthesis in infected cells.

Acyclovir

Acyclovir is a safe and effective therapy for herpes simplex virus (HSV) infections. The favorable safety profile of acyclovir derives from its requirement for activation to its active form via phosphorylation by a viral enzyme, thymidine kinase (TK). Thus acyclovir can be activated only in cells already infected with HSV that express the viral TK enzyme, a strategy that maximizes selectivity and reduces the potential for cellular toxicity in uninfected cells. Acyclovir is most active against HSV and is also active against varicella-zoster virus (VZV); therapy is indicated for infections with these viruses in a variety of clinical settings. Activity of acyclovir against CMV is less pronounced, and activity against Epstein-Barr virus is minimal, both in vitro and clinically. Therefore, under most circumstances, acyclovir should not be used to treat CMV or Epstein-Barr virus infections.

The biggest impact of acyclovir in clinical practice is in the treatment of primary and recurrent genital HSV infections. Oral nucleoside therapy plays an important role in the management of acute primary genital herpes, treatment of episodic symptomatic reactivations, and prophylaxis against reactivation. Acyclovir is also indicated in the management of suspected or proven HSV encephalitis in patients of all ages and for treatment of neonatal HSV infection, with or without central nervous system (CNS) involvement. With respect to neonatal HSV infection, the routine empirical use of acyclovir as empiric therapy against presumptive or possible HSV infection in infants admitted with fever and no focus in the 1st 4 wk of life is controversial. Acyclovir should be used routinely in infants born to women with risk factors for primary genital herpes or infants presenting with any combination of vesicular lesions, seizures, meningoencephalitis, hepatitis, pneumonia, or disseminated intravascular coagulation. Some advocate initiation of acyclovir in all febrile neonates. Other experts have argued that a selective approach based on the history and physical exam is more appropriate when making decisions about the use of acyclovir in febrile infants. Given the safety of the drug, prudence would dictate the use of acyclovir in such patients if HSV infection cannot be excluded.

Acyclovir is indicated for the treatment of primary HSV gingivostomatitis and for primary genital HSV infection. Long-term suppressive therapy for genital HSV and for recurrent oropharyngeal infections (herpes labialis) is also effective. Acyclovir is also recommended for less commonly encountered HSV infections, including herpetic whitlow, eczema herpeticum, and herpes gladiatorum. In addition, acyclovir is commonly used for prophylaxis against HSV reactivation in SOT and HSCT patients. Severe end-organ HSV disease, including disseminated infection, is occasionally encountered in immunocompromised or pregnant patients, representing another clinical scenario where acyclovir therapy is warranted.

Acyclovir modifies the course of primary VZV infection, although the effect is modest. Acyclovir or another nucleoside analog should always be used in localized or disseminated VZV infections, such as pneumonia, particularly in immunocompromised patients. Primary VZV infection in pregnancy is another setting where acyclovir is indicated; this is a high-risk scenario and can be associated with a substantial risk of maternal mortality, particularly if pneumonia is present.

Acyclovir is available in topical (5% ointment), parenteral, and oral formulations, including an oral suspension formulation for pediatric use. Topical therapy has little role in pediatric practice and should be avoided in favor of alternative modes of delivery, particularly in infants with vesicular lesions compatible with herpetic infection, where topical therapy should never be used. The bioavailability of oral formulations is modest, with only 15–30% of the oral dose being absorbed. There is widespread tissue distribution following systemic administration, and high concentrations of drug are achieved in the kidneys, lungs, liver, myocardium, and skin vesicles. Cerebrospinal fluid concentrations are approximately 50% of plasma concentrations. Acyclovir crosses the placenta, and breast milk concentrations are approximately 3 times plasma concentrations, although there are no data on efficacy of in utero therapy or impact of acyclovir therapy on nursing infants. Acyclovir therapy in a nursing mother is not a contraindication to breastfeeding. The main route of elimination is renal, and dosage adjustments are necessary for renal insufficiency. Hemodialysis also eliminates acyclovir.

Acyclovir has an exceptional safety profile. Toxicity is observed typically only in exceptional circumstances: for example, if administered by rapid infusion to a dehydrated patient or a patient with underlying renal insufficiency, acyclovir can crystallize in renal tubules and produce a reversible obstructive uropathy. High doses of acyclovir are associated with neurotoxicity, and prolonged use can cause neutropenia. The favorable safety profile of acyclovir is underscored by recent studies of its safe use during pregnancy, and suppressive therapy in pregnant women with histories of recurrent genital HSV infection, typically with valacyclovir (see later), has become standard of care among many obstetricians. One uncommon but important complication of long-term use of acyclovir is the selection for acyclovir-resistant HSV strains, which usually occurs from mutations in the HSV TK gene. Resistance is rarely observed in pediatric practice but should be considered in any patient who has been on long-term antiviral therapy and who has an HSV or VZV infection that fails to clinically respond to acyclovir therapy.

Valacyclovir

Valacyclovir is the L-valyl ester of acyclovir and is rapidly converted to acyclovir following oral administration. This agent has a safety and activity profile similar to that of acyclovir but has a bioavailability of >50%, 3-5-fold greater than that of acyclovir. Plasma concentrations approach those observed with intravenous acyclovir. Valacyclovir is available only for oral administration. A suspension formulation is not commercially available, but an oral suspension (25 mg/mL or 50 mg/mL) may be prepared extemporaneously from 500-mg caplets for use in pediatric patients for whom a solid dosage form is not appropriate. Suppressive therapy with valacyclovir is commonly prescribed in the 2nd and 3rd trimesters of pregnancy in women who have a clinical history of recurrent genital herpes. *It is important to be aware that perinatal transmission of HSV can occur, leading to symptomatic disease in spite of maternal antenatal antiviral prophylaxis.* In such settings, the possibility of emergence of acyclovir-resistant virus should be considered.

Penciclovir and Famciclovir

Penciclovir is an acyclic nucleoside analog that, like acyclovir, inhibits the viral DNA polymerase following phosphorylation to its active form. Compared with acyclovir, penciclovir has a substantially longer intracellular half-life, which in theory can confer superior antiviral activity at the intracellular level; however, there is no evidence that this effect confers clinical superiority. Penciclovir is licensed only as a topical formulation (1% penciclovir cream), and this formulation is indicated for therapy of cutaneous HSV infections. Topical therapy for primary or recurrent herpes labialis or cutaneous HSV infection is an appropriate use of penciclovir in children older than 2 yr of age.

Famciclovir is the prodrug formulation (diacetyl ester) of penciclovir. In contrast to penciclovir, famciclovir may be administered orally and has bioavailability of approximately 70%. Following oral administration, famciclovir is deacetylated to the parent drug, penciclovir. The efficacy of famciclovir for HSV and VZV infections appears equivalent to that of acyclovir, although the pharmacokinetic profile is more favorable. Famciclovir is indicated for oral therapy of HSV and VZV infections. There is currently no liquid or suspension formulation available, and experience with pediatric use is very limited. The toxicity profile is identical to that of acyclovir. In a clinical trial, valacyclovir was found to be superior to famciclovir in prevention of reactivation and reduction of viral shedding in the setting of recurrent genital HSV infection.

Ganciclovir and Valganciclovir

Ganciclovir is a nucleoside analog with structural similarity to acyclovir. Like acyclovir, ganciclovir must be phosphorylated for antiviral activity, which is targeted against the viral polymerase. The gene responsible for ganciclovir phosphorylation is not TK but rather the virally encoded UL97 phosphotransferase gene. Antiviral resistance in CMV can be observed with prolonged use of nucleoside antivirals, and resistance should be considered in patients on long-term therapy who appear to fail to respond clinically and virologically. Ganciclovir is broadly active against many herpesviruses, including HSV and VZV, but is most valuable for its activity against CMV. Ganciclovir was the first antiviral agent licensed specifically to treat and prevent CMV infection. It is indicated for prophylaxis against and therapy of CMV infections in high-risk patients, including HIV-infected patients and SOT or HSCT recipients. Of particular importance is the use of ganciclovir in the management of CMV retinitis, a sight-threatening complication of HIV infection. Ganciclovir is also of benefit for newborns with symptomatic congenital CMV infection and may be of value in partially ameliorating the sensorineural hearing loss and developmental disabilities that are common complications of congenital CMV infection.

Ganciclovir is supplied as parenteral and oral formulations. Ganciclovir ocular implants are also available for the management of CMV retinitis. The bioavailability of oral ganciclovir is poor, <10%, and hence oral ganciclovir therapy has been supplanted by the oral prodrug, valganciclovir, which is well absorbed from the gastrointestinal tract and quickly converted to ganciclovir by intestinal or hepatic metabolism. Bioavailability of ganciclovir (from valganciclovir) is approximately 60% from tablet and solution formulations. Significant concentrations are found in aqueous humor, subretinal fluid, cerebrospinal fluid, and brain tissue (enough to inhibit susceptible strains of CMV). Subretinal concentrations are comparable with plasma concentrations, but intravitreal concentrations are lower. Drug concentrations in the CNS range from 24% to 70% of plasma concentrations. The main route of elimination is renal, and dosage adjustments are necessary for renal insufficiency. Dose reduction is proportional to the creatinine clearance. Hemodialysis efficiently eliminates ganciclovir, so administration of additional doses after dialysis is necessary.

Ganciclovir has several important toxicities. Reversible myelosuppression is the most important toxicity associated with ganciclovir therapy and commonly requires either discontinuation of therapy or the intercurrent administration of granulocyte colony–stimulating factor. There are also the theoretical risks for carcinogenicity and gonadal toxicity; although these effects have been observed in some animal models, they have never been observed in patients. The decision to administer ganciclovir to a pediatric patient is complex and should be made in consultation with a pediatric infectious disease specialist.

Foscarnet

Foscarnet has a unique profile, insofar as it is not a nucleoside analog but rather a pyrophosphate analog. The drug has broad activity against most herpesviruses. Like the nucleoside analogs, foscarnet inhibits viral DNA polymerase. On the other hand, foscarnet does not require phosphorylation to exert its antiviral activity, thus differing from the nucleoside analogs. It binds to a different site on the viral DNA polymerase to exert its antiviral effect and therefore retains activity against strains of HSV and CMV that are resistant to nucleoside analogs. Its clinical utility is as a second-line agent for management of CMV infections in high-risk patients who cannot tolerate ganciclovir and as an alternative for patients with persistent or refractory HSV, CMV, or VZV disease with suspected or documented antiviral drug resistance.

Foscarnet is available only as a parenteral formulation and is a toxic agent that must be administered cautiously. Nephrotoxicity is common, and reversible renal insufficiency is often observed, as evidenced by an increase in serum creatinine. Abnormalities in calcium and phosphorus homeostasis are common, and electrolytes and renal function must be monitored carefully during treatment.

Cidofovir

Cidofovir is an acyclic nucleotide analog that requires phosphorylation to its active form, cidofovir diphosphate, to exert its antiviral effect. Analogous to penciclovir, it has an extended intracellular half-life that contributes to its prolonged antiviral activity. Cidofovir is active against HSV, VZV, and CMV. In contrast to most of the other agents with activity against herpesviruses, cidofovir also exhibits broad-spectrum activity against other DNA viruses, most notably the poxviruses. Cidofovir has activity against the BK virus, a polyomavirus, and therapy may be warranted in some settings of BK reactivation post HSCT and post SOT. Cidofovir is useful in the management of adenovirus infections in the immunocompromised host. Cidofovir is also useful in the management of CMV disease caused by strains with documented ganciclovir resistance.

Cidofovir is administered intravenously and is cleared renally by tubular secretion. Extensive prehydration and co-administration of probenecid are recommended. Nephrotoxicity is commonly encountered, even with appropriate prehydration; cidofovir must be co-administered with care with other nephrotoxic medications. Other potential toxicities include reproductive toxicity and carcinogenesis.

Trifluridine

Trifluridine is a pyrimidine nucleoside analog with activity against HSV, CMV, and adenovirus. It is formulated as a 1% ophthalmic solution and approved for topical use in the treatment of HSV keratitis and keratoconjunctivitis. Trifluridine is the treatment of choice for HSV keratitis, a disease that should always be managed in consultation with an ophthalmologist.

Vidarabine

Vidarabine is a nucleoside analog that has activity against HSV. It was the first parenteral antiviral agent for HSV infection, although it is no longer available for intravenous administration. A topical preparation remains available to treat HSV keratitis and is considered a second-line agent for this indication.

Fomivirsen

Fomivirsen is an anti-CMV compound that was used as a second-line agent for CMV retinitis by direct injection into the vitreous space. It is an antisense 21-mer DNA oligonucleotide that binds directly to complementary messenger RNA. This agent is of interest because it was the first antisense antiviral agent approved by the US Food and Drug Administration (FDA). The drug is no longer marketed.

New Agents

There is a major need for development of new, nontoxic antivirals for HSV infection. Two new agents are approaching licensure and will be very useful in the management of HSCT and SOT patients. The oral lipid conjugate prodrug of cidofovir, CMX001, has improved activity against herpesviruses compared with parenterally administered cidofovir and a markedly reduced risk of nephrotoxicity. Another novel agent, letermovir (AIC246), is highly orally bioavailable and has a novel mechanism of action, exerting its antiviral effect by interfering with the viral terminase complex. This agent demonstrates substantial promise as an alternative to more toxic antivirals in patients at high risk for

CMV disease, particularly in the transplantation setting. It is also active against BK virus and poxviruses.

ANTIVIRALS USED FOR RESPIRATORY VIRAL INFECTIONS

Antiviral therapies are available for many respiratory pathogens, including respiratory syncytial virus (RSV), influenza A, and influenza B. Antiviral therapy for respiratory viral infections is of particular value for infants, children with chronic lung disease, and immunocompromised children.

Ribavirin

Ribavirin is a guanosine analog that has broad-spectrum activity against a variety of viruses, particularly RNA viruses. Its precise mechanism of action is incompletely understood but is probably related to interference with viral messenger RNA processing and translation. Ribavirin is available in oral, parenteral, and aerosolized formulations. Although intravenous ribavirin is highly effective in the management of Lassa fever and other hemorrhagic fevers, this formulation is not licensed for use in the United States. The only licensed formulations in the United States are an aqueous formulation for aerosol administration (indicated for RSV infection) and an oral formulation that is combined with interferon-α for the treatment of hepatitis C. (For more information about antivirals for hepatitis, see Chapter 385.) Administration of ribavirin by aerosol should be considered for serious RSV lower respiratory tract disease in immunocompromised children, young infants with serious RSV-associated illness, and high-risk infants and children (children with chronic lung disease or cyanotic congenital heart disease). In vitro testing and uncontrolled clinical studies also suggest efficacy of aerosolized ribavirin for parainfluenza, influenza, and measles infections.

Ribavirin is generally nontoxic, particularly when administered by aerosol. Oral ribavirin is used in combination with other agents for therapy of hepatitis C (discussed later). There is no role for the use of oral ribavirin in the treatment of community-acquired viral respiratory tract infections. Ribavirin and its metabolites concentrate in red blood cells and can persist for several weeks and, in rare instances, may be associated with anemia. Conjunctivitis and bronchospasm have been reported following exposure to aerosolized drug. Care must be taken when using aerosolized ribavirin in children undergoing mechanical ventilation to avoid precipitation of particles in ventilator tubing; the drug is not formally approved for use in the mechanically ventilated patient, although there is published experience with this approach, which can be considered for mechanically ventilated patients, particularly in a "high-dose, short-duration" regimen (6 g/100 mL water given for a period of 2 hr 3 times a day). Concerns regarding potential teratogenicity from animal studies have not been borne out in clinical practice, although care should be taken to prevent inadvertent exposure to aerosolized drug in pregnant healthcare providers.

Amantadine and Rimantadine

Amantadine and rimantadine are tricyclic amines (adamantanes) that share structural similarity. Both were indicated for prophylaxis and therapy of influenza A. The mechanism of action of the tricyclic amines against influenza A virus was unclear, but they appeared to exert their antiviral effect at the level of uncoating of the virus. Both agents are extremely well absorbed after oral administration and are eliminated via the kidneys (90% of the dose is unchanged), necessitating dosage adjustments for renal insufficiency. The toxicities of the tricyclic amines are modest and include CNS adverse effects such as anxiety, difficulty concentrating, and lightheadedness and gastrointestinal adverse effects such as nausea and loss of appetite.

Although these agents are still manufactured and available, the Centers for Disease Control and Prevention (CDC) no longer recommends the use of the adamantane agents in treatment or prophylaxis against influenza, due to emergence of widespread resistance.

Oseltamivir, Zanamivir, and Peramivir

Oseltamivir and zanamivir are active against both influenza A and B, although the importance of this broader spectrum of antiinfluenza activity in disease control is modest because influenza B infection is typically a much milder illness. Emerging strains of influenza, including H5N1 and the 2009-2010 pandemic strain, H1N1 (swine flu), are susceptible to oseltamivir and zanamivir but resistant to amantadine. Therefore these agents are emerging as the antivirals of choice for influenza infection. Neither agent has appreciable activity against other respiratory viruses. The mechanism of antiviral activity of these agents is via inhibition of the influenza neuraminidase.

Zanamivir has poor oral bioavailability and is licensed only for inhalational administration. With inhaled administration, >75% of the dose is deposited in the oropharynx and much of it is swallowed. The actual amount distributed to the airways and lungs depends on factors such as the patient's inspiratory flow. Approximately 13% of the dose appears to be distributed to the airways and lungs, with approximately 10% of the inhaled dose distributed systemically. Local respiratory mucosal drug concentrations greatly exceed the drug concentration needed to inhibit influenza A and B viruses. Elimination is via the kidneys, and no dosage adjustment is necessary with renal insufficiency, because the amount that is systemically absorbed is low.

Oseltamivir is administered as an esterified prodrug that has high oral bioavailability. It is eliminated by tubular secretion, and dosage adjustment is required for patients with renal insufficiency. Gastrointestinal adverse effects, including nausea and vomiting, are occasionally observed. The drug is indicated for both treatment and prophylaxis. The usual adult dosage for treatment of influenza is 75 mg twice daily for 5 days. Treatment should be initiated within 2 days of the appearance of symptoms. Recommended treatment dosages for children vary by age and weight. The recommended dose for children younger than 1 yr of age is 3 mg/kg/dose twice a day. For children older than 1 yr of age, doses are 30 mg twice a day for children weighing ≤15 kg, 45 mg twice a day for children weighing 15-23 kg, 60 mg twice a day for those weighing 23-40 kg, and 75 mg twice a day for children weighing ≥40 kg. Dosages for chemoprophylaxis are the same for each weight group in children older than 1 yr of age, but the drug should be administered only once daily rather than twice daily. Oseltamivir is FDA approved for therapy of influenza A and B treatment in children 2 wk of age and older, whereas zanamivir is recommended for treatment of children 7 yr of age and older. Current treatment and dosage recommendations for treatment of influenza in children and for chemoprophylaxis are available at: https://www.cdc.gov/flu/professionals/antivirals/summary-clinicians.htm. Oseltamivir has been described to produce neuropsychiatric (narcolepsy) and psychologic (suicidal events) side effects in some patient populations; the drug should be discontinued if behavioral or psychiatric side effects are observed. In late 2014 the FDA approved another neuraminidase inhibitor, peramivir, for treatment of influenza. It is available as a single-dose, intravenous option. The drug is currently approved for use in children >2 yr of age. The dose is 12 mg/kg dose, up to 600 mg maximum, via intravenous infusion for a minimum of 15 min in children from 2 to 12 yr of age. Children 13 and older should receive the adult dose (600 mg IV in a single, 1-time dose).

Baloxavir

Oral baloxavir marboxil (Xofluza) is approved by the FDA for treatment of acute uncomplicated influenza within 2 days of illness onset in people ≥12 yr. The safety and efficacy of baloxavir for the treatment of influenza have been established in pediatric patients ≥12 yr and older weighing at least 40 kg. Safety and efficacy in patients <12 yr or weighing less than 40 kg have not been established. Baloxavir efficacy is based on clinical trials in outpatients 12 to 64 yr of age; people with underlying medical conditions and adults >65 yr were not included in the initial published clinical trials. There are no available data for baloxavir treatment of hospitalized patients with influenza.

ANTIVIRALS USED FOR HEPATITIS

Seven antiviral agents have been approved by the FDA for treatment of adults with chronic hepatitis B in the United States. These agents are categorized as either interferons (IFN-α2b and peginterferon-α2a) or nucleoside or nucleotide analogs (lamivudine, adefovir, entecavir, tenofovir, telbivudine). Lamivudine is currently considered the first-line therapy in adult patients, but experience in children is limited. In 2012 tenofovir was FDA approved for children with chronic hepatitis B aged 12 yr or older weighing >35 kg. Entecavir was approved in the United States for use in children 2 yr and older with chronic HBV and evidence of active viral replication and disease activity and, with IFN-α, is emerging as a first-line antiviral regimen for children with hepatitis B who are candidates for antiviral therapy.

Adefovir demonstrates a favorable safety profile and is less likely to select for resistance than lamivudine, but virologic response was limited to adolescent patients and was lower than that of lamivudine. Most experts recommend watchful waiting of children with chronic hepatitis B infection, because current therapies are only modestly effective at best and evidence of long-term benefit is scant. Young children are often believed to be immune tolerant of hepatitis B infection (i.e., they have viral DNA present in serum but normal transaminase levels and no evidence of active hepatitis). These children should have transaminases and viral load monitored but are not typically considered to be candidates for antiviral therapy.

Only various combinations of interferons and ribavirin were approved by the FDA to treat adults and children with chronic hepatitis C (see Tables 272.1 and 272.2). The development of novel and highly effective antivirals for HCV has revolutionized the care of hepatitis C patients. These drugs are not yet licensed for pediatric use. Novel drugs include ledipasvir, sofosbuvir, daclatasvir, elbasvir, beclabuvir, grazoprevir, paritaprevir, ombitasvir, velpatasvir, and dasabuvir. Ledipasvir, ombitasvir, daclatasvir, elbasvir, and velpatasvir inhibit the virally encoded phosphoprotein, NS5A, which is involved in viral replication, assembly, and secretion, whereas sofosbuvir is metabolized to a uridine triphosphate mimic, which functions as an RNA chain terminator when incorporated into the nascent RNA by the NS5B polymerase enzyme. Dasabuvir and beclabuvir are also NS5B inhibitors. Paritaprevir and grazoprevir inhibit the nonstructural protein 3 (NS3/4) serine protease, a viral nonstructural protein that is the 70-kDa cleavage product of the hepatitis C virus polyprotein.

Past efforts to treat HCV prior to the advent of these new direct therapies had yielded mixed results. Although only 10–25% of adults treated with interferon had a sustained remission of disease, treatment with a combination of interferon and ribavirin achieves remission in close to half of treated adults. Randomized controlled trials indicated that patients treated with pegylated interferons (so called because they are formulated and stabilized with polyethylene glycol), both as dual therapy with ribavirin and as monotherapy, experienced higher sustained viral response rates than did those treated with nonpegylated interferons. The advent of new, direct therapies has led to permanent remission of HCV disease in adult patients. Data on the use of these agents in infants and children are limited. In early 2017 the combination of sofosbuvir with ribavirin and the fixed-dose combination of sofosbuvir/ledipasvir was approved by the FDA for treatment of children with chronic HCV infection 12 yr of age and older. The only drugs currently approved for children younger than 12 yr remain pegylated interferon and ribavirin. The use of IFN-α2b in combination with ribavirin has been approved by the FDA for chronic hepatitis C in this age group.

There are significant genotype-dependent differences in responsiveness to antiviral therapy; patients with genotype 1 had the lowest levels of sustained virologic response, and patients with genotype 2 or 3 had the highest response. The use of IFN-ααb in combination with ribavirin provides a much more favorable sustained virologic response in children with HCV genotype 2/3 than in those with HCV genotype 1. For genotype 1 hepatitis C treated with pegylated interferons combined with ribavirin, it has been shown that genetic polymorphisms near the human *IL28B* gene, encoding interferon lambda 3, are associated with significant differences in response to the treatment.

ANTIVIRAL IMMUNE GLOBULINS

Immune globulins are useful adjuncts in the management of viral disease. However, they are most valuable when administered as prophylaxis against infection and disease in high-risk patients; their value as therapeutic agents in the setting of established infection is less clear. **Varicella-zoster immune globulin (human)** is valuable for prophylaxis against VZV in high-risk children, particularly newborns and immunocompromised children (see Chapter 280). **Cytomegalovirus immune globulin** is warranted for children at high risk for CMV disease, particularly SOT and HSCT patients, and can play a role in preventing injury to the infected fetus when administered to the pregnant patient (see Chapter 282). **Palivizumab,** a monoclonal antibody with anti-RSV activity, is effective for preventing severe RSV lower respiratory tract disease in high-risk premature infants and has replaced **RSV immune globulin** (see Chapter 287). **Hepatitis B immune globulin** is indicated in infants born to hepatitis B surface antigen-positive mothers (see Chapter 385).

Bibliography is available at Expert Consult.

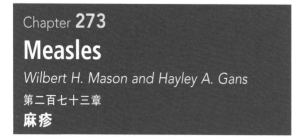

Chapter **273**

Measles

Wilbert H. Mason and Hayley A. Gans

第二百七十三章

麻疹

<hr/>

中文导读

本章主要介绍了麻疹的病因学、流行病学、传播途径、病理学、发病机制、临床表现、实验室检查、诊断、鉴别诊断、并发症、治疗、预后和预防。本病为麻疹病毒感染所致，病程分为潜伏期、前驱期、出疹期和恢复期。临床表现包括发热、咳嗽、黏膜疹、结膜炎等，需与风疹、EB病毒、肠道病毒等感染相鉴别。并发症包括肺炎、急性喉炎、麻疹脑炎、心肌炎等，其中亚急性硬化性全脑炎为慢性并发症。麻疹治疗以支持为主，同时建议补充维生素A。预防措施包括接种疫苗和暴露后预防。

Measles is highly contagious, but endemic transmission has been interrupted in the United States as a result of widespread vaccination; indigenous or imported cases have occasionally resulted in epidemics in the United States in unimmunized or partially immunized American or foreign-born children (adopted children, refugees, returning tourists). In some areas of the world, measles remains a serious threat to children (Fig. 273.1).

ETIOLOGY

Measles virus is a single-stranded, lipid-enveloped RNA virus in the family Paramyxoviridae and genus *Morbillivirus*. Other members of the genus *Morbillivirus* affect a variety of mammals, such as rinderpest virus in cattle and distemper virus in dogs, but humans are the only host of measles virus. Of the 6 major structural proteins of measles virus, the 2 most important in terms of induction of immunity are the hemagglutinin (H) protein and the fusion (F) protein. The neutralizing antibodies are directed against the H protein, and antibodies to the F protein limit proliferation of the virus during infection. Small variations in genetic composition have also been identified that result in no effect on protective immunity but provide molecular markers that can distinguish between viral types. Related genotypes have been grouped by clades, and the World Health Organization recognizes 8 clades, A-H, and 23 genotypes. These markers have been useful in the evaluation of endemic and epidemic spread of measles.

EPIDEMIOLOGY

The measles vaccine has changed the epidemiology of measles dramatically. Once worldwide in distribution, endemic transmission of measles has been interrupted in many countries where there is widespread vaccine coverage. Historically, measles caused universal infection in childhood in the United States, with 90% of children acquiring the infection before 15 yr of age. Morbidity and mortality associated with measles decreased prior to the introduction of the vaccine as a result of improvements in healthcare and nutrition. However, the incidence declined dramatically following the introduction of the measles vaccine in 1963. The attack rate fell from 313 cases per 100,000 population in 1956–1960 to 1.3 cases per 100,000 in 1982–1988.

A nationwide indigenous measles outbreak occurred in the United States in 1989–1991, resulting in more than 55,000 cases, 11,000 hospitalizations, and 123 deaths, demonstrating that the infection had not yet been controlled. This resurgence was attributed to vaccine failure in a small number of school-age children, low coverage of preschool-age children, and more rapid waning of maternal antibodies in infants born to mothers who had never experienced wild-type measles infection. Implementation of the 2-dose vaccine policy and more intensive immunization strategies resulted in interruption of endemic transmission and in 2,000 measles was declared eliminated from the United States. The current rate is <1 case per 1,000,000 population.

Measles continues to be imported into the United States from abroad; therefore continued maintenance of >90% immunity through vaccination is necessary to prevent widespread outbreaks from occurring (see Fig. 273.1).

In 2014 the United States encountered a record number of cases since elimination in 2000, with 667 cases of measles reported to the U.S. Centers for Disease Control and Prevention (CDC). There were 23 outbreaks reported compared with a median of 4 outbreaks reported annually during 2001–2010. The majority of cases were associated with importations from other countries (returning tourists, adoptees, refugees), particularly from the Philippines, with prior year epidemics associated with epidemics in the World Health Organization European Region. Measles cases are largely restricted to unvaccinated individuals. Since 2014, cases continue to result from importations causing multistate outbreaks, but due to increased awareness and vaccination efforts, cases remain <200/annually, with 86 reported in 2016 and 120 to date in 2017.

High levels of measles immunity in a population of ~95% are required to interrupt the endemic spread of measles. In the United States this can be achieved through the current 2-dose immunization strategies when coverage rates are high (>90% 1-dose coverage at 12-15 mo and >95% 2-dose coverage in school-age children). Although measles-mumps-rubella coverage remains high (90–91.5% in children 19-35 mo for 2000–2015), pockets of lower coverage rates exist because of reluctance of parents to vaccinate their children. This variability in vaccination has contributed to outbreaks among school-age children in recent years.

TRANSMISSION

The portal of entry of measles virus is through the respiratory tract or conjunctivae following contact with large droplets or small-droplet aerosols in which the virus is suspended. Patients are infectious from 3 days before to up to 4-6 days after the onset of rash. Approximately 90% of exposed susceptible individuals experience measles. Face-to-face contact is not necessary, because viable virus may be suspended in air for as long as 1 hr after the patient with the source case leaves a room. Secondary cases from spread of aerosolized virus have been reported in airplanes, physicians' offices, and hospitals.

PATHOLOGY

Measles infection causes necrosis of the respiratory tract epithelium and an accompanying lymphocytic infiltrate. Measles produces a small-vessel vasculitis on the skin and on the oral mucous membranes. Histology of the rash and exanthem reveals intracellular edema and dyskeratosis associated with formation of epidermal syncytial giant cells with up to 26 nuclei. Viral particles have been identified within these giant cells. In lymphoreticular tissue, lymphoid hyperplasia is prominent. Fusion of infected cells results in multinucleated giant cells, the **Warthin-Finkeldey giant cells** that are pathognomonic for measles, with up to 100 nuclei and intracytoplasmic and intranuclear inclusions.

PATHOGENESIS

Measles infection consists of 4 phases: incubation period, prodromal illness, exanthematous phase, and recovery. During incubation, measles virus migrates to regional lymph nodes. A primary viremia ensues that disseminates the virus to the reticuloendothelial system. A secondary viremia spreads virus to body surfaces. The prodromal illness begins after the secondary viremia and is associated with epithelial necrosis and giant cell formation in body tissues. Cells are killed by cell-to-cell plasma membrane fusion associated with viral replication that occurs in many body tissues, including cells of the central nervous system. Virus shedding begins in the prodromal phase. With onset of the rash, antibody production begins, and viral replication and symptoms begin to subside. Measles virus also infects $CD4^+$ T cells, resulting in suppression of the Th1 immune response and a multitude of other immunosuppressive effects.

Measles virus attaches to specific cell receptors to infect host cells. Studies in primates show that the initial targets for measles virus are alveolar macrophages, dendritic cells, and lymphocytes. The cell receptor used appears to be the signaling lymphocyte activating molecule or more properly CD150. Subsequently, respiratory epithelial cells become infected but do not express CD150. The mechanism of infection of

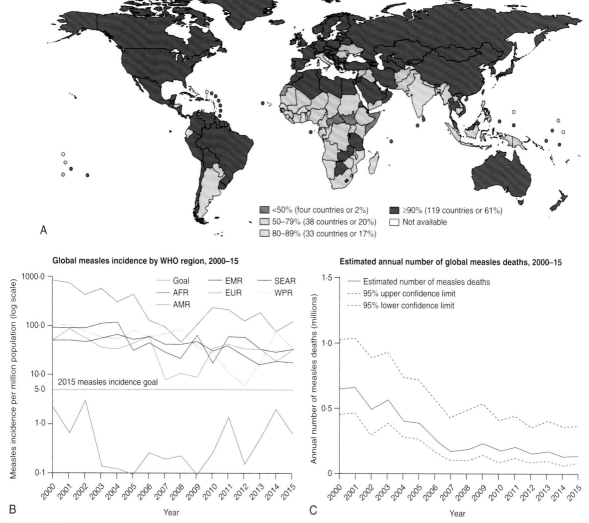

Fig. 273.1 Progress toward achieving global measles milestones for measles vaccine coverage (**A**), measles incidence (**B**), and measles mortality (**C**). **A,** Milestone 1: increase routine coverage with the 1st dose of measles-containing vaccine (MCV1) for children aged 1 yr to ≥90% nationally and ≥80% in every district. Progress: The number of countries with ≥90% MCV1 coverage increased from 84 (44%) in 2000 to 119 (61%) in 2015. Among countries with ≥90% MCV1 coverage nationally, the percentage with ≥80% coverage in every district was only 39% of 119 countries in 2015. **B,** Milestone 2: reduce global measles incidence to less than 5 cases per 1 million population. Progress: reported global annual measles incidence decreased 75% from 2000 to 2015, but only the Region of the Americas achieved the milestone of less than 5 cases per 1 million population. **C,** Milestone 3: reduce global measles mortality by 95% from the 2000 estimate. Progress: the number of estimated global annual measles deaths decreased 79% from 2000 to 2015. AFR, African Region; AMR, Region of the Americas; EMR, Eastern Mediterranean Region; EUR, European Region; SEAR, South-East Asia Region; WPR, Western Pacific Region. *(From Moss WJ: Measles,* Lancet *390:2490–2502, 2017, Fig. 2, with data from Patel MK, Gacic-Dobo M, Strebel PM, et al: Progress toward regional measles elimination—worldwide, 2000–2015. MMWR Morb Mortal Wkly Rep 65:1228–1233, 2016.)*

respiratory tissues is attachment to the PVRL4 receptor (Nectin4) that is expressed on cells in the trachea, oral mucosa, nasopharynx, and lungs. These 2 receptors, CD150 and PVRL4, account for the lymphotropic and epitheliotropic nature of natural measles virus infection and, along with the prolonged immunosuppressive effects of measles, suggest that it is more characteristic of human immunodeficiency virus infection than a respiratory illness.

CLINICAL MANIFESTATIONS

Measles is a serious infection characterized by high fever, an enanthem, cough, coryza, conjunctivitis, and a prominent exanthem (Fig. 273.2). After an incubation period of 8-12 days, the prodromal phase begins with a mild fever followed by the onset of conjunctivitis with photophobia,

coryza, a prominent cough, and increasing fever. **Koplik spots** represent the enanthem and are the pathognomonic sign of measles, appearing 1-4 days prior to the onset of the rash (Fig. 273.3). They first appear as discrete red lesions with bluish white spots in the center on the inner aspects of the cheeks at the level of the premolars. They may spread to involve the lips, hard palate, and gingiva. They also may occur in conjunctival folds and in the vaginal mucosa. Koplik spots have been reported in 50–70% of measles cases but probably occur in the great majority.

Symptoms increase in intensity for 2-4 days until the 1st day of the rash. The rash begins on the forehead (around the hairline), behind the ears, and on the upper neck as a red maculopapular eruption. It then spreads downward to the torso and extremities, reaching the palms and

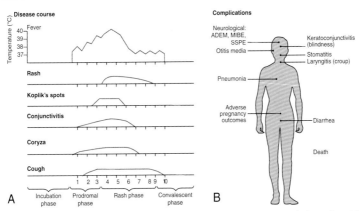

Fig. 273.2 Measles disease course **(A)** and complications **(B)**. ADEM, acute demyelinating encephalomyelitis; MIBE, measles inclusion body encephalitis; SSPE, subacute sclerosing panencephalitis. *(Modified from Moss WJ: Measles, Lancet 390:2490–2502, 2017, Fig. 4.)*

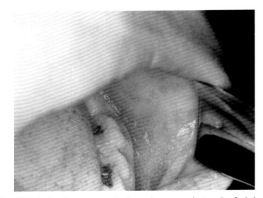

Fig. 273.3 Koplik spots on the buccal mucosa during the 3rd day of rash. *(From Centers for Disease Control and Prevention (CDC): Public health image library, image #4500. Available at: http://phil.cdc.gov/phil/details.asp.)*

soles in up to 50% of cases. The exanthem frequently becomes confluent on the face and upper trunk (Fig. 273.4).

With the onset of the rash, symptoms begin to subside. The rash fades over about 7 days in the same progression as it evolved, often leaving a fine desquamation of skin in its wake. Of the major symptoms of measles, the cough lasts the longest, often up to 10 days. In more severe cases, generalized lymphadenopathy may be present, with cervical and occipital lymph nodes especially prominent.

MODIFIED MEASLES INFECTION
In individuals with passively acquired antibody, such as infants and recipients of blood products, a subclinical form of measles may occur. The rash may be indistinct, brief, or, rarely, entirely absent. Likewise, some individuals who have received a vaccine, when exposed to measles, may have a rash but few other symptoms. Persons with modified measles are not considered highly contagious.

LABORATORY FINDINGS
The diagnosis of measles is almost always based on clinical and epidemiologic findings. Laboratory findings in the acute phase include reduction in the total white blood cell count, with lymphocytes decreased more than neutrophils. However, absolute neutropenia has been known to occur. In measles not complicated by bacterial infection, the erythrocyte sedimentation rate and C-reactive protein level are usually normal.

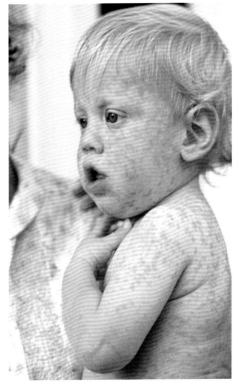

Fig. 273.4 A child with measles displaying the characteristic red blotchy pattern on his face and body. *(From Kremer JR, Muller CP: Measles in Europe—there is room for improvement, Lancet 373:356–358, 2009.)*

DIAGNOSIS
In the absence of a recognized measles outbreak, confirmation of the clinical diagnosis is often recommended. Serologic confirmation is most conveniently made by identification of immunoglobulin (Ig) M antibody in serum. IgM antibody appears 1-2 days after the onset of the rash and remains detectable for about 1 mo. If a serum specimen is collected <72 hr after onset of rash and is negative for measles antibody, a 2nd specimen should be obtained. Serologic confirmation may also be made by demonstration of a 4-fold rise in IgG antibodies in acute and convalescent specimens collected 2-4 wk apart. Viral isolation from blood, urine, or respiratory secretions can be accomplished by culture at the CDC or local or state laboratories. Molecular detection by polymerase

chain reaction is available through some state and local health departments and through the CDC.

DIFFERENTIAL DIAGNOSIS

Typical measles is unlikely to be confused with other illnesses, especially if Koplik spots are observed. Measles in the later stages or modified or atypical infections may be confused with a number of other exanthematous immune-mediated illnesses and infections, including rubella, adenovirus infection, enterovirus infection, and Epstein-Barr virus infection. Exanthem subitum (in infants) and erythema infectiosum (in older children) may also be confused with measles. *Mycoplasma pneumoniae* and group A streptococcus may also produce rashes similar to that of measles. Kawasaki syndrome can cause many of the same findings as measles but lacks discrete intraoral lesions (Koplik spots) and a severe prodromal cough and typically leads to elevations of neutrophils and acute-phase reactants. In addition, the characteristic thrombocytosis of Kawasaki syndrome is absent in measles (see Chapter 191). Drug eruptions may occasionally be mistaken for measles.

COMPLICATIONS

Complications of measles are largely attributable to the pathogenic effects of the virus on the respiratory tract and immune system (Table 273.1, Fig. 273.2). Several factors make complications more likely. Morbidity and mortality from measles are greatest in individuals younger than 5 yr of age (especially <1 yr of age) and older than 20 yr of age. In developing countries, higher case fatality rates have been associated with crowding, possibly attributable to larger inoculum doses after household exposure. Severe malnutrition in children results in a suboptimal immune response and higher morbidity and mortality with measles infection. Low serum retinol levels in children with measles are associated with higher measles morbidity and mortality in developing countries and in the United States. Measles infection lowers serum retinol concentrations, so subclinical cases of hyporetinolemia may be made symptomatic during measles. Measles infection in immunocompromised persons is associated with increased morbidity and mortality. Among patients with malignancy in whom measles develops, pneumonitis occurs in 58% and encephalitis occurs in 20%.

Pneumonia is the most common cause of death in measles. It may manifest as **giant cell pneumonia** caused directly by the viral infection or as superimposed bacterial infection. The most common bacterial pathogens are *Streptococcus pneumoniae, Haemophilus influenzae,* and *Staphylococcus aureus.* Following severe measles pneumonia, the final common pathway to a fatal outcome is often the development of bronchiolitis obliterans.

Croup, tracheitis, and bronchiolitis are common complications in infants and toddlers with measles. The clinical severity of these complications frequently requires intubation and ventilatory support until the infection resolves.

Acute otitis media is the most common complication of measles and was of particularly high incidence during the epidemic of the late 1980s and early 1990s because of the relatively young age of affected children. Sinusitis and mastoiditis also occur as complications. Viral and/or bacterial tracheitis is seen and can be life-threatening. Retropharyngeal abscess has also been reported.

Measles infection is known to suppress skin test responsiveness to purified tuberculin antigen. There may be a higher rate of activation of pulmonary tuberculosis in populations of individuals infected with *Mycobacterium tuberculosis* who are then exposed to measles.

Diarrhea and vomiting are common symptoms associated with acute measles, and diffuse giant cell formation is found in the epithelium in the gastrointestinal tract. Dehydration is a common consequence, especially in young infants and children. Appendicitis or abdominal pain may occur from obstruction of the appendiceal lumen by lymphoid hyperplasia.

Febrile seizures occur in <3% of children with measles. Encephalitis following measles is a long-associated complication, often with an unfavorable outcome. Rates of 1-3 per 1,000 cases of measles have been reported, with greater numbers occurring in adolescents and adults than in preschool- or school-age children. Encephalitis is a postinfectious, immunologically mediated process and is not the result of a direct effect by the virus. Clinical onset begins during the exanthem and manifests as seizures (56%), lethargy (46%), coma (28%), and irritability (26%). Findings in cerebrospinal fluid include lymphocytic pleocytosis in 85% of cases and elevated protein concentrations. Approximately 15% of patients with measles encephalitis die. Another 20–40% of patients suffer long-term sequelae, including cognitive impairment, motor disabilities, and deafness.

Measles encephalitis in immunocompromised patients results from direct damage to the brain by the virus. Subacute measles encephalitis manifests 1-10 mo after measles in immunocompromised patients, particularly those with AIDS, lymphoreticular malignancies, and immunosuppression. Signs and symptoms include seizures, myoclonus, stupor, and coma. In addition to intracellular inclusions, abundant viral nucleocapsids and viral antigen are seen in brain tissue. Progressive disease and death almost always occur.

A severe form of measles rarely seen nowadays is **hemorrhagic measles** or **black measles.** It manifested as a hemorrhagic skin eruption and was often fatal. Keratitis, appearing as multiple punctate epithelial foci, resolved with recovery from the infection. Thrombocytopenia sometimes occurred following measles.

Myocarditis is a rare complication of measles. Miscellaneous bacterial infections have been reported, including bacteremia, cellulitis, and toxic shock syndrome. Measles during pregnancy is associated with high rates of maternal morbidity, fetal wastage, and stillbirths, with congenital malformations in 3% of liveborn infants.

Subacute Sclerosing Panencephalitis

Subacute sclerosing panencephalitis (SSPE) is a chronic complication of measles with a delayed onset and an outcome that is nearly always fatal. It appears to result from a persistent infection with an altered

| Table 273.1 | Complications by Age for Reported Measles Cases, United States, 1987–2000 |

COMPLICATION	OVERALL (67,032 CASES WITH AGE INFORMATION)	NO. (%) OF PERSONS WITH COMPLICATION BY AGE GROUP				
		<5 yr (N = 28,730)	5-9 yr (N = 6,492)	10-19 yr (N = 18,580)	20-29 yr (N = 9,161)	<30 yr (N = 4,069)
Any	19,480 (29.1)	11,883 (41.4)	1,173 (18.1)	2,369 (12.8)	2,656 (29.0)	1,399 (34.4)
Death	177 (0.3)	97 (0.3)	9 (0.1)	18 (0.1)	26 (0.3)	27 (0.7)
Diarrhea	5,482 (8.2)	3,294 (11.5)	408 (6.3)	627 (3.4)	767 (8.4)	386 (9.5)
Encephalitis	97 (0.1)	43 (0.2)	9 (0.1)	13 (0.1)	21 (0.2)	11 (0.3)
Hospitalization	12,876 (19.2)	7,470 (26.0)	612 (9.4)	1,612 (8.7)	2,075 (22.7)	1,107 (27.2)
Otitis media	4,879 (7.3)	4,009 (14.0)	305 (4.7)	338 (1.8)	157 (1.7)	70 (1.7)
Pneumonia	3,959 (5.9)	2,480 (8.6)	183 (2.8)	363 (2.0)	554 (6.1)	379 (9.3)

From Perry RT, Halsey NA: The clinical significance of measles: a review, *Clin Infect Dis* 189(Suppl. 1):S4–S16, 2004.

measles virus that is harbored intracellularly in the central nervous system for several yr. After 7-10 yr the virus apparently regains virulence and attacks the cells in the central nervous system that offered the virus protection. This "slow virus infection" results in inflammation and cell death, leading to an inexorable neurodegenerative process.

SSPE is a rare disease and generally follows the prevalence of measles in a population. The incidence in the United States in 1960 was 0.61 cases per million persons younger than age 20 yr. By 1980 the rate had fallen to 0.06 cases per million. Between 1956 and 1982 a total of 634 cases of SSPE had been reported to the national SSPE registry. After 1982 approximately 5 cases/yr were reported annually in the United States, and only 2-3 cases/yr were reported in the early 1990s. However, between 1995 and 2000, reported cases in the United States increased and 13 cases were reported in 2000. Nine of the 13 cases occurred in foreign-born individuals. This "resurgence" may be the result of an increased incidence of measles between 1989 and 1991. Although the age of onset ranges from <1 yr to <30 yr, the illness is primarily one of children and adolescents. Measles at an early age favors the development of SSPE: 50% of patients with SSPE had primary measles before 2 yr of age, and 75% had measles before 4 yr of age. Males are affected twice as often as females, and there appear to be more cases reported from rural than urban populations. Recent observations from the registry indicate a higher prevalence among children of Hispanic origin.

The pathogenesis of SSPE remains enigmatic. Factors that seem to be involved include defective measles virus and interaction with a defective or immature immune system. The virus isolated from brain tissue of patients with SSPE is missing 1 of the 6 structural proteins, the matrix or M protein. This protein is responsible for assembly, orientation, and alignment of the virus in preparation for budding during viral replication. Immature virus may be able to reside, and possibly propagate, within neuronal cells for long periods. The fact that most patients with SSPE were exposed at a young age suggests that immune immaturity is involved in pathogenesis.

Clinical manifestations of SSPE begin insidiously 7-13 yr after primary measles infection. Subtle changes in behavior or school performance appear, including irritability, reduced attention span, and temper outbursts. This initial phase (**stage I**) may at times be missed because of brevity or mildness of the symptoms. Fever, headache, and other signs of encephalitis are absent. The hallmark of the **2nd stage** is massive myoclonus, which coincides with extension of the inflammatory process site to deeper structures in the brain, including the basal ganglia. Involuntary movements and repetitive myoclonic jerks begin in single muscle groups but give way to massive spasms and jerks involving both axial and appendicular muscles. Consciousness is maintained. In the **3rd stage**, involuntary movements disappear and are replaced by choreoathetosis, immobility, dystonia, and lead pipe rigidity that result from destruction of deeper centers in the basal ganglia. The sensorium deteriorates into dementia, stupor, and then coma. The **4th stage** is characterized by loss of critical centers that support breathing, heart rate, and blood pressure. Death soon ensues. Progression through the clinical stages may follow courses characterized as acute, subacute, or chronic progressive.

The diagnosis of SSPE can be established through documentation of a compatible clinical course and at least 1 of the following supporting findings: (1) measles antibody detected in cerebrospinal fluid, (2) characteristic electroencephalographic findings, and (3) typical histologic findings in and/or isolation of virus or viral antigen from brain tissue obtained by biopsy or postmortem examination.

Cerebrospinal fluid analysis reveals normal cells but elevated IgG and IgM antibody titers in dilutions >1 : 8. Electroencephalographic patterns are normal in stage I, but in the myoclonic phase, suppression-burst episodes are seen that are characteristic of, but not pathognomonic for, SSPE. Brain biopsy is no longer routinely indicated for diagnosis of SSPE.

Management of SSPE is primarily supportive and similar to care provided to patients with other neurodegenerative diseases. Clinical trials using isoprinosine with or without interferon suggest significant benefit (30–34% remission rate) compared with patients without treatment (5–10% with spontaneous remissions).

It is recognized that carbamazepine is of significant benefit in the control of myoclonic jerks in the early stages of the illness.

Virtually all patients eventually succumb to SSPE. Most die within 1-3 yr of onset from infection or loss of autonomic control mechanisms. Prevention of SSPE depends on prevention of primary measles infection through vaccination. SSPE has been described in patients who have no history of measles infection and exposure only to the vaccine virus. However, wild-type virus, not vaccine virus, has been found in brain tissue of at least some of these patients, suggesting that they had had subclinical measles previously.

TREATMENT

Management of measles is supportive because there is no specific antiviral therapy approved for treatment of measles. Maintenance of hydration, oxygenation, and comfort are goals of therapy. Antipyretics for comfort and fever control are useful. For patients with respiratory tract involvement, airway humidification and supplemental oxygen may be of benefit. Respiratory failure from croup or pneumonia may require ventilatory support. Oral rehydration is effective in most cases, but severe dehydration may require intravenous therapy. Prophylactic antimicrobial therapy to prevent bacterial infection is not indicated.

Measles infection in immunocompromised patients is highly lethal. Ribavirin is active in vitro against measles virus. Anecdotal reports of ribavirin therapy with or without intravenous gamma globulin suggest some benefit in individual patients. However, no controlled trials have been performed, and ribavirin is not licensed in the United States for treatment of measles.

Vitamin A

Vitamin A deficiency in children in developing countries has long been known to be associated with increased mortality from a variety of infectious diseases, including measles. In the United States, studies in the early 1990s documented that 22–72% of children with measles had low retinol levels. In addition, 1 study demonstrated an inverse correlation between the level of retinol and severity of illness. Several randomized controlled trials of vitamin A therapy in the developing world and the United States have demonstrated reduced morbidity and mortality from measles. Vitamin A therapy is indicated for all patients with measles. Vitamin A should be administered once daily for 2 days at doses of 200,000 IU for children 12 mo of age or older; 100,000 IU for infants 6 mo through 11 mo of age; and 50,000 IU for infants younger than 6 mo of age.

In children with signs and symptoms of vitamin A deficiency, a 3rd age-appropriate dose is recommended 2-4 wk after the 2nd dose.

PROGNOSIS

In the early 20th century, deaths from measles in the United States varied between 2,000 and 10,000 per year, or about 10 deaths per 1,000 cases of measles. With improvements in healthcare and antimicrobial therapy, better nutrition, and decreased crowding, the death:case ratio fell to 1 per 1,000 cases. Between 1982 and 2002, the CDC estimated that there were 259 deaths caused by measles in the United States, with a death:case ratio of 2.5-2.8 per 1,000 cases of measles. Pneumonia and encephalitis were complications in most of the fatal cases, and immunodeficiency conditions were identified in 14–16% of deaths. In 2011, of the 222 cases reported in the United States, 70 (32%) were hospitalized, including 17 (24%) with diarrhea, 15 (21%) with dehydration, and 12 (17%) with pneumonia. No cases of encephalitis or deaths were reported. In the 1st half of 2015, of 159 reported cases 22 (14%) were hospitalized, with 5 pneumonia cases and no deaths.

PREVENTION

Patients shed measles virus from 7 days after exposure to 4-6 days after the onset of rash. Exposure of susceptible individuals to patients with measles should be avoided during this period. In hospitals, standard and airborne precautions should be observed for this period. Immunocompromised patients with measles will shed virus for the duration of the illness, so isolation should be maintained throughout the disease.

Vaccine

Vaccination against measles is the most effective and safe prevention strategy. Measles vaccine in the United States is available as a combined vaccine with measles-mumps-rubella vaccine, the last of which is the recommended form in most circumstances (Table 273.2). Following the measles resurgence of 1989-1991, a 2nd dose of measles vaccine was added to the schedule. The current recommendations include a 1st dose at 12-15 mo of age, followed by a 2nd dose at 4-6 yr of age. However, the 2nd dose can be given any time after 30 days following the 1st dose, and the current schedule is a convenience schedule. Seroconversion is slightly lower in children who receive the 1st dose before or at 12 mo of age (87% at 9 mo, 95% at 12 mo, and 98% at 15 mo) because of persisting maternal antibody; however, this is an evolving situation, with children currently as young as 6 mo unprotected from maternal antibodies and susceptible to measles infection. For children who have not received 2 doses by 11-12 yr of age, a 2nd dose should be provided. Infants who receive a dose before 12 mo of age should be given 2 additional doses at 12-15 mo and 4-6 yr of age. Children who are traveling should be offered either primary measles immunization even as young as 6 mo or a 2nd dose even if <4 yr.

Adverse events from the measles-mumps-rubella vaccine include fever (usually 6-12 days following vaccination), rash in approximately 5% of vaccinated persons, and, rarely, transient thrombocytopenia. Children prone to febrile seizures may experience an event following vaccination, so the risks and benefits of vaccination should be discussed with parents. Encephalopathy and autism have not been shown to be causally associated with the measles-mumps-rubella vaccine or vaccine constituents.

A review of the effect of measles vaccination on the epidemiology of SSPE has demonstrated that measles vaccination protects against SSPE and does not accelerate the course of SSPE or trigger the disease in those already infected with wild measles virus.

Passively administered immune globulin may inhibit the immune response to live measles vaccine, and administration should be delayed for variable amounts of time based on the dose of Ig (Table 273.3).

Live vaccines should not be administered to pregnant women or to immunodeficient or immunosuppressed patients. However, patients with HIV who are not severely immunocompromised should be immunized. Because measles virus may suppress the cutaneous response to tuberculosis antigen, skin testing for tuberculosis should be performed before or at the same time as administration of the vaccine. Individuals infected with *M. tuberculosis* should be receiving appropriate treatment at the time of administration of measles vaccine.

Postexposure Prophylaxis

Susceptible individuals exposed to measles may be protected from infection by either vaccine administration or with Ig. The vaccine is effective in prevention or modification of measles if given within 72 hr of exposure. Ig may be given up to 6 days after exposure to prevent or modify infection. Immunocompetent children should receive 0.5 mL/kg (maximum dose in both cases is 15 mL/kg) intramuscularly (IM). For severely immunocompromised children and pregnant woman without

Table 273.2	Recommendations for Measles Immunization	
CATEGORY	**RECOMMENDATIONS**
Unimmunized, no history of measles (12-15 mo of age)	MMR or MMRV vaccine is recommended at 12-15 mo of age; a 2nd dose is recommended at least 28 days after the 1st dose (or 90 days for MMRV) and usually is administered at 4 through 6 yr of age
Children 6-11 mo of age in epidemic situations or before international travel	Immunize with MMR vaccine, but this dose is not considered valid, and 2 valid doses administered on or after the 1st birthday are required. The 1st valid dose should be administered at 12-15 mo of age; the 2nd valid dose is recommended at least 28 days later and usually is administered at 4 through 6 yr of age. MMRV should not be administered to children <12 mo of age.
Students in kindergarten, elementary, middle, and high school who have received 1 dose of measles vaccine at 12 mo of age or older	Administer the 2nd dose
Students in college and other postsecondary institutions who have received 1 dose of measles vaccine at 12 mo of age or older	Administer the 2nd dose
History of immunization before the 1st birthday	Dose not considered valid; immunize (2 doses)
History of receipt of inactivated measles vaccine or unknown type of vaccine, 1963–1967	Dose not considered valid; immunize (2 doses)
Further attenuated or unknown vaccine administered with IG	Dose not considered valid; immunize (2 doses)
Allergy to eggs	Immunize; no reactions likely
Neomycin allergy, nonanaphylactic	Immunize; no reactions likely
Severe hypersensitivity (anaphylaxis) to neomycin or gelatin	Avoid immunization
Tuberculosis	Immunize; if patient has untreated tuberculosis disease, start antituberculosis therapy before immunizing
Measles exposure	Immunize or give IG, depending on circumstances
HIV infected	Immunize (2 doses) unless severely immunocompromised; administration of IG if exposed to measles is based on degree of immunosuppression and measles vaccine history
Personal or family history of seizures	Immunize; advise parents of slightly increased risk of seizures
Immunoglobulin or blood recipient	Immunize at the appropriate interval

MMR, measles-mumps-rubella vaccine; MMRV, measles-mumps-rubella-varicella vaccine.
From American Academy of Pediatrics: Measles. In Kimberlin DW, Brady MT, Jackson MA, Long SS, editors: *Red book 2018 report of the committee on infectious diseases*, ed 31, Itasca, IL, 2018, American Academy of Pediatrics, Table 3.39, p. 543.

Table 273.3 | Suggested Intervals Between Immunoglobulin Administration and Measles Immunization*

INDICATION FOR IMMUNOGLOBULIN	Route	Units (U) or Milliliters (mL)	mg IgG/kg	Interval (mo)[†]
Tetanus (as tetanus Ig)	IM	250 U	10	3
Hepatitis A prophylaxis (as Ig):				
Contact prophylaxis	IM	0.02 mL/kg	3.3	3
International travel	IM	0.06 mL/kg	10	3
Hepatitis B prophylaxis (as hepatitis B Ig)	IM	0.06 mL/kg	10	3
Rabies prophylaxis (as rabies Ig)	IM	20 IU/kg	22	4
Varicella prophylaxis (as VariZIG)	IM	125 U/10 kg (maximum 625 U)	20-40	5
Measles prophylaxis (as Ig):				
Standard	IM	0.50 mL/kg	80	6
Immunocompromised host	IV		400 mg/kg	8
Respiratory syncytial virus prophylaxis (palivizumab monoclonal antibody)[‡]	IM	—	15 mg/kg (monoclonal)	None
Cytomegalovirus immune globulin	IV	3 mL/kg	150	6
Blood transfusion:				
Washed RBCs	IV	10 mL/kg	Negligible	0
RBCs, adenine-saline added	IV	10 mL/kg	10	3
Packed RBCs	IV	10 mL/kg	20-60	6
Whole blood	IV	10 mL/kg	80-100	6
Plasma or platelet products	IV	10 mL/kg	160	7
Replacement (or therapy) of immune deficiencies (as IVIG)	IV	—	300-400	8
ITP (as IVIG)	IV	—	400	8
ITP	IV	—	1,000	10
ITP or Kawasaki disease	IV	—	1,600-2,000	11

*Immunization in the form of measles-mumps-rubella (MMR), measles-mumps-rubella-varicella (MMRV), or monovalent measles vaccine.

[†]These intervals should provide sufficient time for decreases in passive antibodies in all children to allow for an adequate response to measles vaccine. Physicians should not assume that children are fully protected against measles during these intervals. Additional doses of Ig or measles vaccine may be indicated after exposure to measles.

[‡]Monoclonal antibodies, such as palivizumab, do not interfere with the immune response to vaccines.

Ig, immunoglobulin; IgG, immunoglobulin G; ITP, immune (formerly termed "idiopathic") thrombocytopenic purpura; IVIG, intravenous Ig; RBCs, red blood cells.

From American Academy of Pediatrics: *Red book: 2015 report of the Committee on Infectious Diseases*, ed 30, Elk Grove Village, IL, 2015, American Academy of Pediatrics, Table 1.10, p. 39.

evidence of measles immunity, Ig intravenously is the recommended IG at 400 mg/kg. Ig is indicated for susceptible household contacts of measles patients, especially infants younger than 6 mo of age, pregnant women, and immunocompromised persons.

Bibliography is available at Expert Consult.

Chapter **274**

Rubella

Wilbert H. Mason and Hayley A. Gans

第二百七十四章
风疹

中文导读

　　本章主要介绍了风疹的病因学、流行病学、病理学、发病机制、临床表现、实验室检查、诊断、鉴别诊断、并发症、治疗、预后、预防和疫苗。临床表现包括低热、咽痛、淋巴结病变等前驱症状，儿童中首要表现为皮疹。最常见的诊断检测方法为风疹IgM。并发症包括血小板减少、关节炎、脑炎、进行性风疹性全脑炎等，其中先天性风疹综合征可导致多系统病变。本病无特异性治疗，以支持治疗为主。

Rubella (**German measles** or **3-day measles**) is a mild, often exanthematous disease of infants and children that is typically more severe and associated with more complications in adults. Its major clinical significance is transplacental infection and fetal damage as part of the **congenital rubella syndrome (CRS)**.

ETIOLOGY

Rubella virus is a member of the family Togaviridae and is the only species of the genus *Rubivirus*. It is a single-stranded RNA virus with a lipid envelope and 3 structural proteins, including a nucleocapsid protein that is associated with the nucleus and 2 glycoproteins, E1 and E2, that are associated with the envelope. The virus is sensitive to heat, ultraviolet light, and extremes of pH but is relatively stable at cold temperatures. Humans are the only known host.

EPIDEMIOLOGY

In the prevaccine era, rubella appeared to occur in major epidemics every 6-9 yr, with smaller peaks interspersed every 3-4 yr, and was most common in preschool-age and school-age children. During the rubella epidemic of 1964-1965 there were an estimated 12.5 million cases of rubella associated with 2,000 cases of encephalitis, more than 13,000 abortions or perinatal deaths, and 20,000 cases of CRS. Following introduction of the rubella vaccine in 1969, the incidence of rubella fell 78% and CRS cases fell 69% by 1976 (Fig. 274.1). Further decline in rubella and CRS cases occurred when certain at-risk populations were added to those for whom rubella immunization is indicated, including adolescents and college students. After years of decline, a resurgence of rubella and CRS cases occurred during 1989-1991 in association with the epidemic of measles during that period (see Fig. 274.1). Subsequently, a 2-dose recommendation for rubella vaccine was implemented and resulted in a decrease in incidence of rubella from 0.45 per 100,000 population in 1990 to 0.1 per 100,000 population in 1999 and a corresponding decrease of CRS, with an average of 6 infants with CRS reported annually from 1992 to 2004. Mothers of these infants tended to be young, Hispanic, or foreign born. The number of reported cases of rubella continued to decline through the 1990s and the 1st decade of this century.

The endemic spread of rubella was declared eliminated in the United States in 2004 and eliminated in the Americas in 2015. However, cases of rubella continue to be imported into the United States from countries where it remains endemic, with more than 100,000 cases of CRS annually worldwide. From 2004 to 2016 there were 101 cases of rubella and 11 cases of CRS reported in the United States, all of which were imported cases of unknown source. Three of the CRS cases were acquired in

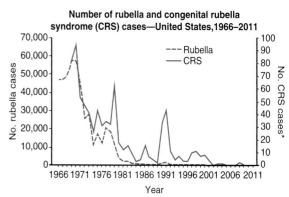

Number of rubella and congenital rubella syndrome (CRS) cases—United States, 1966-2011

*By year of birth.

Fig. 274.1 Number of rubella and congenital rubella syndrome cases—United States, 1966-2011. Rubella and CRS data provided were reported voluntarily to Centers for Disease Control and Prevention from state health departments. *(From McLean HQ, Fiebelkorn AP, Temte JL, et al: Prevention of measles, rubella, congenital rubella syndrome, and mumps, 2013, MMWR Recomm Rep 62[RR-04]:1–34, 2013.)*

Africa. Worldwide in 2016, 22,106 cases of rubella and 358 cases of CRS were reported, demonstrating that the elimination of rubella internationally has not been achieved and highlighting that continued vigilance and maintenance of high levels of immunity in the United States are necessary.

PATHOLOGY

Little information is available on the pathologic findings in rubella occurring postnatally. The few reported studies of biopsy or autopsy material from cases of rubella revealed only nonspecific findings of lymphoreticular inflammation and mononuclear perivascular and meningeal infiltration. The pathologic findings for CRS are often severe and may involve nearly every organ system (Table 274.1).

PATHOGENESIS

The viral mechanisms for cell injury and death in postnatal or congenital rubella are not well understood. Following infection, the virus replicates in the respiratory epithelium and then spreads to regional lymph nodes (Fig. 274.2). Viremia ensues and is most intense from 10 to 17 days after infection. Viral shedding from the nasopharynx begins approximately 10 days after infection and may be detected up to 2 wk following onset of the rash. The period of highest communicability is from 5 days before to 6 days after the appearance of the rash.

Congenital infection occurs during maternal viremia. After infecting the placenta, the virus spreads through the vascular system of the developing fetus and may infect any fetal organ. The most important risk factor for severe congenital defects is the stage of gestation at the time of infection. Maternal infection during the first 8 wk of gestation results in the most severe and widespread defects. The risk for congenital defects has been estimated at 90% for maternal infection before 11 wk of gestation, 33% at 11-12 wk, 11% at 13-14 wk, and 24% at 15-16 wk. Defects occurring after 16 wk of gestation are uncommon, even if fetal infection occurs.

Causes of cellular and tissue damage in the infected fetus may include tissue necrosis due to vascular insufficiency, reduced cellular multiplication time, chromosomal breaks, and production of a protein inhibitor causing mitotic arrests in certain cell types. The most distinctive feature of congenital rubella is chronicity. Once the fetus is infected early in gestation, the virus persists in fetal tissue until well beyond delivery. Persistence suggests the possibility of ongoing tissue damage and reactivation, most notably in the brain.

CLINICAL MANIFESTATIONS

Postnatal infection with rubella is a mild disease not easily discernible from other viral infections, especially in children. Following an incubation period of 14-21 days, a prodrome consisting of low-grade fever, sore throat, red eyes with or without eye pain, headache, malaise, anorexia, and lymphadenopathy begins. Suboccipital, postauricular, and anterior cervical lymph nodes are most prominent. In children, the 1st manifestation of rubella is usually the rash, which is variable and not distinctive. It begins on the face and neck as small, irregular pink macules that coalesce, and it spreads centrifugally to involve the torso and extremities, where it tends to occur as discrete macules (Fig. 274.3). About the time

Table 274.1	Pathologic Findings in Congenital Rubella Syndrome
SYSTEM	**PATHOLOGIC FINDINGS**
Cardiovascular	Patent ductus arteriosus Pulmonary artery stenosis Ventriculoseptal defect Myocarditis
Central nervous system	Chronic meningitis Parenchymal necrosis Vasculitis with calcification
Eye	Microphthalmia Cataract Iridocyclitis Ciliary body necrosis Glaucoma Retinopathy
Ear	Cochlear hemorrhage Endothelial necrosis
Lung	Chronic mononuclear interstitial pneumonitis
Liver	Hepatic giant cell transformation Fibrosis Lobular disarray Bile stasis
Kidney	Interstitial nephritis
Adrenal gland	Cortical cytomegaly
Bone	Malformed osteoid Poor mineralization of osteoid Thinning cartilage
Spleen, lymph node	Extramedullary hematopoiesis
Thymus	Histiocytic reaction Absence of germinal centers
Skin	Erythropoiesis in dermis

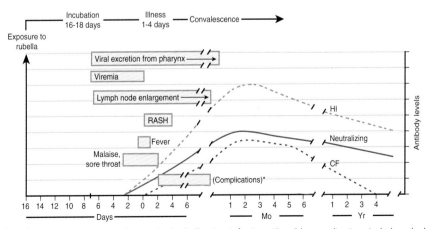

Fig. 274.2 Pathophysiologic events in postnatally acquired rubella virus infection. *Possible complications include arthralgia and/or arthritis, thrombocytopenic purpura, and encephalitis. CF, complement fixation titer; HI, hemagglutination-inhibition titer. *(From Lamprecht CL: Rubella virus. In Beshe RB, editor: Textbook of human virology, ed 2, Littleton, MA, 1990, PSG Publishing, p. 685.)*

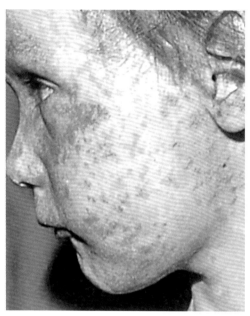

Fig. 274.3 Rash of rubella.

of onset of the rash, examination of the oropharynx may reveal tiny, rose-colored lesions (**Forchheimer spots**) or petechial hemorrhages on the soft palate. The rash fades from the face as it extends to the rest of the body so that the whole body may not be involved at any one time. The duration of the rash is generally 3 days, and it usually resolves without desquamation. Subclinical infections are common, and 25–40% of children may not have a rash. Teenagers and adults tend to be more symptomatic and have systemic manifestations, with up to 70% of females demonstrating arthralgias and arthritis.

LABORATORY FINDINGS
Leukopenia, neutropenia, and mild thrombocytopenia have been described during postnatal rubella.

DIAGNOSES
A specific diagnosis of rubella is important for epidemiologic reasons, for diagnosis of infection in pregnant women, and for confirmation of the diagnosis of congenital rubella. The most common diagnostic test is rubella immunoglobulin (Ig) M enzyme immunosorbent assay, which is typically present about 4 days after the appearance of the rash. As with any serologic test, the positive predictive value of testing decreases in populations with low prevalence of disease and in immunized individuals. Tests should be performed in the context of a supportive history of exposure or consistent clinical findings. The relative sensitivity and specificity of commercial kits used in most laboratories range from 96% to 99% and 86% to 97%, respectively. A caveat for testing of congenitally infected infants early in infancy is that false-negative results may occur owing to competing IgG antibodies circulating in these patients. In such patients, an IgM capture assay, reverse transcriptase polymerase chain reaction (PCR) test, or viral culture should be performed for confirmation. Viral isolation by culture of nasopharyngeal secretions, urine in the newborn, or cord blood or placenta can be used to diagnose congenital infection. PCR testing of amniotic fluid during pregnancy is also an appropriate approach to diagnose congenital infection.

DIFFERENTIAL DIAGNOSES
Rubella may manifest as distinctive features suggesting the diagnosis. It is frequently confused with other infections because it is uncommon, is similar to other viral exanthematous diseases, and demonstrates variability in the presence of typical findings. In severe cases, it may resemble measles. The absence of Koplik spots and a severe prodrome,

as well as a shorter course, allow for differentiation from measles. Other diseases frequently confused with rubella include infections caused by adenoviruses, parvovirus B19 (erythema infectiosum), Epstein-Barr virus, enteroviruses, roseola, and *Mycoplasma pneumoniae*.

COMPLICATIONS
Complications following postnatal infection with rubella are infrequent and generally not life threatening.

Postinfectious **thrombocytopenia** occurs in approximately 1 in 3,000 cases of rubella and occurs more frequently among children and in girls. It manifests about 2 wk following the onset of the rash as petechiae, epistaxis, gastrointestinal bleeding, and hematuria. It is usually self-limited.

Arthritis following rubella occurs more commonly among adults, especially women. It begins within 1 wk of onset of the exanthem and classically involves the small joints of the hands. It is self-limited and resolves within weeks without sequelae. There are anecdotal reports and some serologic evidence linking rubella with rheumatoid arthritis, but a true causal association remains speculative.

Encephalitis is the most serious complication of postnatal rubella. It occurs in 2 forms: a postinfectious syndrome following acute rubella and a rare progressive panencephalitis manifesting as a neurodegenerative disorder years following rubella.

Postinfectious encephalitis is uncommon, occurring in 1 in 5,000 cases of rubella. It appears within 7 days after onset of the rash, consisting of headache, seizures, confusion, coma, focal neurologic signs, and ataxia. Fever may recrudesce with the onset of neurologic symptoms. Cerebrospinal fluid may be normal or have a mild mononuclear pleocytosis and/or elevated protein concentration. Virus is rarely, if ever, isolated from cerebrospinal fluid or brain, suggesting a noninfectious pathogenesis. Most patients recover completely, but mortality rates of 20% and long-term neurologic sequelae have been reported.

Progressive rubella panencephalitis (PRP) is an extremely rare complication of either acquired rubella or CRS. It has an onset and course similar to those of the subacute sclerosing panencephalitis associated with measles (see Chapter 273). However, unlike in the postinfectious form of rubella encephalitis, rubella virus may be isolated from brain tissue of the patient with PRP, suggesting an infectious pathogenesis, albeit a slow one. The clinical findings and course are undistinguishable from those of subacute sclerosing panencephalitis and transmissible spongiform encephalopathies (see Chapter 304). Death occurs 2-5 yr after onset.

Other neurologic syndromes rarely reported with rubella include Guillain-Barré syndrome and peripheral neuritis. Myocarditis is a rare complication.

Congenital Rubella Syndrome
In 1941 an ophthalmologist first described a syndrome of cataracts and congenital heart disease that he correctly associated with rubella infections in the mothers during early pregnancy (Table 274.2). Shortly after the first description, hearing loss was recognized as a common finding often associated with microcephaly. In 1964-1965 a pandemic of rubella occurred, with 20,000 cases reported in the United States, leading to more than 11,000 spontaneous or therapeutic abortions and 2,100 neonatal deaths. From this experience emerged the expanded definition of CRS that includes numerous other transient or permanent abnormalities.

Nerve deafness is the single most common finding among infants with CRS. Most infants have some degree of intrauterine growth restriction. Retinal findings described as **salt-and-pepper retinopathy** are the most common ocular abnormality but have little early effect on vision. Unilateral or bilateral cataracts are the most serious eye finding, occurring in about a third of infants (Fig. 274.4). Cardiac abnormalities occur in half of the children infected during the first 8 wk of gestation. Patent ductus arteriosus is the most frequently reported cardiac defect, followed by lesions of the pulmonary arteries and valvular disease. Interstitial pneumonitis leading to death in some cases has been reported. Neurologic abnormalities are common and may progress following birth. Meningoencephalitis is present in 10–20% of infants with CRS and may persist for up to 12 mo. Longitudinal follow-up through 9-12 yr of

Table 274.2	Clinical Manifestations of Congenital Rubella Syndrome in 376 Children Following Maternal Rubella*	
MANIFESTATION		**RATE (%)**
Deafness		67
Ocular		71
Cataracts		29
Retinopathy		39
Heart disease[†]		48
Patent ductus arteriosus		78
Right pulmonary artery stenosis		70
Left pulmonary artery stenosis		56
Valvular pulmonic stenosis		40
Low birthweight		60
Psychomotor retardation		45
Neonatal purpura		23
Death		35

*Other findings: hepatitis, linear streaking of bone, hazy cornea, congenital glaucoma, delayed growth.
[†]Findings in 87 patients with congenital rubella syndrome and heart disease who underwent cardiac angiography.
From Cooper LZ, Ziring PR, Ockerse AB, et al: Rubella: clinical manifestations and management, *Am J Dis Child* 118:18–29, 1969.

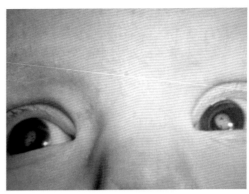

Fig. 274.4 Bilateral cataracts in infant with congenital rubella syndrome.

infants without initial retardation revealed progressive development of additional sensory, motor, and behavioral abnormalities, including hearing loss and autism. PRP has also been recognized rarely after CRS. Subsequent postnatal growth retardation and ultimate short stature have been reported in a minority of cases. Rare reports of immunologic deficiency syndromes have also been described.

A variety of late-onset manifestations of CRS have been recognized. In addition to PRP, they include diabetes mellitus (20%), thyroid dysfunction (5%), and glaucoma and visual abnormalities associated with retinopathy, which had previously been considered benign.

TREATMENT
There is no specific treatment available for either acquired rubella or CRS.

SUPPORTIVE CARE
Postnatal rubella is generally a mild illness that requires no care beyond antipyretics and analgesics. Intravenous immunoglobulin or corticosteroids can be considered for severe, nonremitting thrombocytopenia.

Management of children with CRS is more complex and requires pediatric, cardiac, audiologic, ophthalmologic, and neurologic evaluation and follow-up because many manifestations may not be readily apparent initially or may worsen with time. Hearing screening is of special importance because early intervention may improve outcomes in children with hearing problems caused by CRS.

PROGNOSIS
Postnatal infection with rubella has an excellent prognosis. Long-term outcomes of CRS are less favorable and somewhat variable. In an Australian cohort evaluated 50 yr after infection, many had chronic conditions but most were married and had made good social adjustments. A cohort from New York from the mid-1960s epidemic had less-favorable outcomes, with 30% leading normal lives, 30% in dependent situations but functional, and 30% requiring institutionalization and continuous care.

Reinfection with wild virus occurs postnatally in both individuals who were previously infected with wild-virus rubella and vaccinated individuals. Reinfection is defined serologically as a significant increase in IgG antibody level and/or an IgM response in an individual who has a documented preexisting rubella-specific IgG above an accepted cutoff. Reinfection may result in an anamnestic IgG response, an IgM and IgG response, or clinical rubella. There are 29 reports in the literature of CRS following maternal reinfection. Reinfection with serious adverse outcomes to adults or children is rare and of unknown significance.

PREVENTION
Patients with postnatal infection should be isolated from susceptible individuals for 7 days after onset of the rash. Standard plus droplet precautions are recommended for hospitalized patients. Children with CRS may excrete the virus in respiratory secretions up to 1 yr of age, so contact precautions should be maintained for them until 1 yr of age, unless repeated cultures of urine and pharyngeal secretions are negative. Similar precautions apply to patients with CRS with regard to attendance in school and out-of-home childcare.

Exposure of susceptible pregnant women poses a potential risk to the fetus. For pregnant women exposed to rubella, a blood specimen should be obtained as soon as possible for rubella IgG-specific antibody testing; a frozen aliquot also should be saved for later testing. If the rubella antibody test result is positive, the mother is likely immune. If the rubella antibody test is negative, a 2nd specimen should be obtained 2-3 wk later and tested concurrently with the saved specimen. If both of these samples test negative, a 3rd specimen should be obtained 6 wk after exposure and tested concurrently with the saved specimen. If both the 2nd and 3rd specimens test negative, infection has not occurred. A negative first specimen and a positive test result in either the 2nd and 3rd specimen indicate that seroconversion has occurred in the mother, suggesting recent infection. Counseling should be provided about the risks and benefits of termination of pregnancy. The routine use of immunoglobulin for susceptible pregnant women exposed to rubella is not recommended and is considered only if termination of pregnancy is not an option because of maternal preferences. In such circumstances, immunoglobulin 0.55 mL/kg IM may be given with the understanding that prophylaxis may reduce the risk for clinically apparent infection but does not guarantee prevention of fetal infection.

VACCINATION
Rubella vaccine in the United States consists of the attenuated Wistar RA 27/3 strain that is usually administered in combination with measles and mumps (MMR) or also with varicella (MMRV) in a 2-dose regimen at 12-15 mo and 4-6 yr of age. It theoretically may be effective as postexposure prophylaxis if administered within 3 days of exposure. Vaccine should not be administered to severely immunocompromised patients (e.g., transplant recipients). Patients with HIV infection who are not severely immunocompromised may benefit from vaccination. Fever is not a contraindication, but if a more serious illness is suspected, immunization should be delayed. Immunoglobulin preparations may inhibit the serologic response to the vaccine (see Chapter 197). Vaccine should not be administered during pregnancy. If pregnancy occurs within 28 days of immunization, the patient should be counseled on the theoretical risks to the fetus. Studies of more than 200 women who had been inadvertently immunized with rubella vaccine during pregnancy

showed that none of their offspring developed CRS. Therefore interruption of pregnancy is probably not warranted.

Following a single dose of rubella RA 27/3 vaccine, 95% of persons 12 mo of age and older develop serologic immunity, and after 2 doses 99% have detectable antibody. Rubella RA 27/3 vaccine is highly protective, because 97% of those vaccinated are protected from clinical disease after 1 dose. Detectable antibodies remain for 15 yr in most individuals vaccinated following 1 dose, and 91–100% had antibodies after 12-15 yr after 2 doses. Although antibody levels may wane, especially after 1 dose of vaccine, increased susceptibility to rubella disease does not occur.

Adverse reactions to rubella vaccination are uncommon in children. MMR administration is associated with fever in 5–15% of vaccinees and with rash in approximately 5% of vaccinees. Arthralgia and arthritis are more common following rubella vaccination in adults. Approximately 25% of postpubertal women experience arthralgia, and 10% of postpubertal women experience arthritis. Peripheral neuropathies and transient thrombocytopenia may also occur.

As part of the worldwide effort to eliminate endemic rubella virus transmission and occurrence of CRS, maintaining high population immunity through vaccination coverage and high-quality integrated measles-rubella surveillance have been emphasized as being vital to its success.

Bibliography is available at Expert Consult.

Chapter 275
Mumps
Wilbert H. Mason and Hayley A. Gans

第二百七十五章
腮腺炎

中文导读

本章主要介绍了腮腺炎的病因学、流行病学、病理学、发病机制、临床表现、诊断、鉴别诊断、并发症、治疗、预后和预防。本病为腮腺炎病毒感染所致，临床表现包括发热、头痛等前驱症状，继之出现单侧或双侧腮腺炎。并发症包括脑膜炎和脑膜脑炎、睾丸炎和卵巢炎、胰腺炎、心脏受累、关节炎和甲状腺炎。治疗以缓解症状为主，目前尚无特异性抗病毒药。

Mumps is an acute self-limited infection that was once commonplace but is now uncommon in developed countries because of widespread use of vaccination. It is characterized by fever, bilateral or unilateral parotid swelling and tenderness, and the frequent occurrence of meningoencephalitis and orchitis. Although infrequent in countries with extensive vaccination programs, mumps remains endemic in the rest of the world, warranting continued vaccine protection. Nonetheless, outbreaks of mumps have been reported in highly vaccinated populations in the United States, particularly among students.

ETIOLOGY
Mumps virus is in the family Paramyxoviridae and the genus *Rubulavirus*. It is a single-stranded pleomorphic RNA virus encapsulated in a lipoprotein envelope possessing 7 structural proteins. Surface glycoproteins called HN (hemagglutinin-neuraminidase) and F (fusion) mediate absorption of the virus to host cells and penetration of the virus into cells, respectively. Both proteins stimulate production of protective antibodies. Mumps virus exists as a single serotype with up to 12 known genotypes, and humans are the only natural host.

EPIDEMIOLOGY
In the prevaccine era, mumps occurred primarily in young children between the ages of 5 and 9 yr and in epidemics about every 4 yr. Mumps infection occurred more often in the winter and spring months. In 1968, just after the introduction of the mumps vaccine, 185,691 cases were reported in the United States. Following the recommendation for routine use of mumps vaccine in 1977, the incidence of mumps fell dramatically in young children (Fig. 275.1) and shifted instead to older children, adolescents, and young adults. Outbreaks continued to occur *even in highly vaccinated* populations as a result of primary vaccine failure with 1 dose of vaccine and because of undervaccination of susceptible persons. After implementation of the 2-dose recommendation for the measles-mumps-rubella (MMR) vaccine for measles control in 1989, the number of mumps cases declined further. During 2001-2003, fewer than 300 mumps cases were reported each year. In 2006 the largest mumps epidemic in the past 20 yr occurred in the United States. A

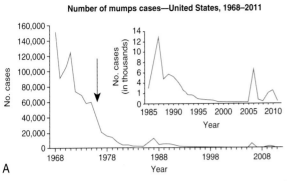

Number of mumps cases—United States, 1968–2011

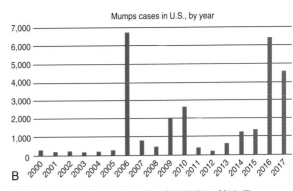

Mumps cases in U.S., by year

Fig. 275.1 **A,** Mumps cases in the United States from 1968, right after the live mumps vaccine was introduced in 1967, to 2011. There was a steady decline following introduction of the vaccine and recommendation for routine vaccination in 1977 *(arrow)*. Note national increases in activity in 1986-1987, 2006. Mumps data provided were reported voluntarily to Centers for Disease Control and Prevention from state health departments. **B,** Mumps cases in the United States from 2000 to 2017 showing the increased activity in 2006, 2009, 2010, and 2014-2017. Mumps data provided were reported voluntarily to Centers for Disease Control and Prevention from state health departments. *(**A,** From McLean HQ, Fiebelkorn AP, Temte JL, et al: Prevention of measles, rubella, congenital rubella syndrome and mumps, MMWR Recomm Rep 62[RR-04]:1–34, 2013; **B,** From Morbidity and Mortality Weekly Report (MMWR): Notifiable Diseases and Mortality Tables. https://www.cdc.gov/mumps/outbreaks.html.)*

total of 6,584 cases occurred, 85% of them in 8 midwestern states. Twenty-nine percent of the cases occurred in patients 18-24 yr old, most of whom were attending college. An analysis of 4,039 patients with mumps seen in the 1st 7 mo of the epidemic indicated that 63% had received more than 2 doses of the MMR vaccine. Subsequently, several outbreaks of mumps have been documented in highly vaccinated populations in the United States, several in school settings including Universities and in Guam. This phenomenon is reported globally as well. The majority of cases in vaccinated persons represent close contact thought to provide intense exposure that may overcome vaccine immunity and perhaps genotype mismatch between circulating mumps genotypes and those in the vaccine.

Mumps is spread from person to person by respiratory droplets. Virus appears in the saliva from up to 7 days before to as long as 7 days after onset of parotid swelling. The period of maximum infectiousness is 1-2 days before to 5 days after onset of parotid swelling. Viral shedding before onset of symptoms and in asymptomatic infected individuals impairs efforts to contain the infection in susceptible populations. The U.S. Centers for Disease Control and Prevention, the American Academy of Pediatrics, and the Health Infection Control Practices Advisory Committee recommend an isolation period of 5 days after onset of parotitis for patients with mumps in both community and healthcare settings.

PATHOLOGY AND PATHOGENESIS

Mumps virus targets the salivary glands, central nervous system (CNS), pancreas, testes, and, to a lesser extent, thyroid, ovaries, heart, kidneys, liver, and joint synovia.

Following infection, initial viral replication occurs in the epithelium of the upper respiratory tract. Infection spreads to the adjacent lymph nodes by the lymphatic drainage, and viremia ensues, spreading the virus to targeted tissues. Mumps virus causes necrosis of infected cells and is associated with a lymphocytic inflammatory infiltrate. Salivary gland ducts are lined with necrotic epithelium, and the interstitium is infiltrated with lymphocytes. Swelling of tissue within the testes may result in focal ischemic infarcts. The cerebrospinal fluid (CSF) frequently contains a mononuclear pleocytosis, even in individuals without clinical signs of meningitis.

CLINICAL MANIFESTATIONS

The incubation period for mumps ranges from 12 to 25 days but is usually 16-18 days. Mumps virus infection may result in clinical presentation ranging from asymptomatic (in the prevaccine era 15–24% of infections were asymptomatic, accurate estimates in the postvaccination era are difficult to measure) or nonspecific symptoms to the typical illness associated with parotitis with or without complications involving

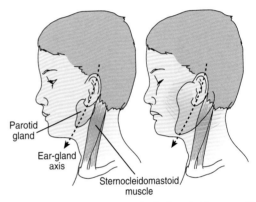

Fig. 275.2 Schematic of a parotid gland infected with mumps *(right)* compared with a normal gland *(left)*. An imaginary line bisecting the long axis of the ear divides the parotid gland into 2 equal parts. These anatomic relationships are not altered in the enlarged gland. An enlarged cervical lymph node is usually posterior to the imaginary line. *(From Mumps [epidemic parotitis]. In Krugman S, Ward R, Katz SL, editors: Infectious diseases in children, ed 6, St. Louis, 1977, Mosby, p. 182.)*

several body systems. The typical patient presents with a prodrome lasting 1-2 days consisting of fever, headache, vomiting, and achiness. Parotitis follows and may be unilateral initially but becomes bilateral in approximately 70% of cases (Fig. 275.2). The parotid gland is tender, and parotitis may be preceded or accompanied by ear pain on the ipsilateral side. Ingestion of sour or acidic foods or liquids may enhance pain in the parotid area. As swelling progresses, the angle of the jaw is obscured and the ear lobe may be lifted upward and outward (see Figs. 275.2 and 275.3). The opening of the Stensen duct may be red and edematous. The parotid swelling peaks in approximately 3 days and then gradually subsides over 7 days. Fever and the other systemic symptoms resolve in 3-5 days. A morbilliform rash is rarely seen. Submandibular salivary glands may also be involved or may be enlarged without parotid swelling. Edema over the sternum as a result of lymphatic obstruction may also occur. Symptoms in immunized individuals are the same but tend to be less severe, and parotitis may be absent.

DIAGNOSIS

When mumps was highly prevalent, the diagnosis could be made on the basis of a history of exposure to mumps infection, an appropriate incubation period, and development of typical clinical findings. Confirmation of the presence of parotitis could be made with demonstration of

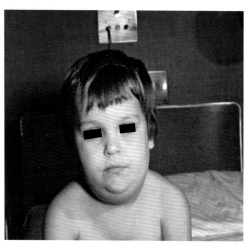

Fig. 275.3 A child with mumps showing parotid swelling. *(From the Centers for Disease Control and Prevention [CDC]: Public health image library [PHIL], image #4491. Available at: http://phil.cdc.gov/phil/home .asp.)*

an elevated serum amylase value. Leukopenia with a relative lymphocytosis was a common finding. Currently, in highly immunized populations patients with parotitis lasting longer than 2 days and of unknown cause, a specific diagnosis of mumps should be confirmed or ruled out by virologic or serologic means. This step may be accomplished by isolation of the virus in cell culture, detection of viral antigen by direct immunofluorescence, or identification of nucleic acid by reverse transcriptase polymerase chain reaction (PCR). Virus can be isolated from upper respiratory tract secretions (buccal and oropharyngeal [OP] mucosa), CSF, or urine during the acute illness; however, PCR from the OP becomes negative quickly especially in immunized individuals and thus should be run within 3 days of parotid swelling. Serologic testing is usually a more convenient and available mode of diagnosis. A significant increase in serum mumps immunoglobulin G antibody between acute and convalescent serum specimens as detected by complement fixation, neutralization hemagglutination, or enzyme immunoassay tests establishes the diagnosis. Mumps immunoglobulin G antibodies may cross react with antibodies to parainfluenza virus in serologic testing. More commonly, an enzyme immunoassay for mumps immunoglobulin M antibody is used to identify recent infection. All serologic tests are difficult to interpret in immunized individuals, and negative test results do not rule out mumps infection. Skin testing for mumps is neither sensitive nor specific and should not be used.

DIFFERENTIAL DIAGNOSIS

Parotid swelling may be caused by many other infectious and noninfectious conditions, especially in sporadic cases. Viruses that cause parotitis include parainfluenza 1 and parainfluenza 3 viruses, influenza A virus, cytomegalovirus, Epstein-Barr virus, enteroviruses, lymphocytic choriomeningitis virus, and HIV. Purulent parotitis, usually caused by *Staphylococcus aureus,* is unilateral, is extremely tender, is associated with an elevated white blood cell count and may involve purulent drainage from the Stensen duct. Submandibular or anterior cervical adenitis from a variety of pathogens may also be confused with parotitis. Other noninfectious causes of parotid swelling include obstruction of the Stensen duct, collagen vascular diseases such as Sjögren syndrome, systemic lupus erythematosus, immunologic diseases, tumor, and drugs.

COMPLICATIONS

The most common complications of mumps are meningitis, with or without encephalitis, and gonadal (orchitis, oophoritis) involvement. Uncommon complications include conjunctivitis, optic neuritis,

pneumonia, nephritis, pancreatitis, mastitis, and thrombocytopenia. Complications can occur in the absence of parotitis especially in immunized individuals, and overall complications rates in immunized individuals are lower than in unimmunized and are shifted towards the adult populations.

Maternal infection with mumps during the first trimester of pregnancy results in increased fetal wastage. No fetal malformations have been associated with intrauterine mumps infection. However, perinatal mumps disease has been reported in infants born to mothers who acquired mumps late in gestation.

Meningitis and Meningoencephalitis

Mumps virus is neurotropic and is thought to enter the CNS via the choroid plexus and infect the choroidal epithelium and ependymal cells, both of which can be found in CSF along with mononuclear leukocytes. Symptomatic CNS involvement occurs in 10–30% of infected individuals, but CSF pleocytosis has been found in 40–60% of patients with mumps parotitis. The meningoencephalitis may occur before, along with, or following the parotitis. It most commonly manifests 5 days after the parotitis. Clinical findings vary with age. Infants and young children have fever, malaise, and lethargy, whereas older children, adolescents, and adults complain of headache and demonstrate meningeal signs. In 1 series of children with mumps and meningeal involvement, findings were fever in 94%, vomiting in 84%, headache in 47%, parotitis in 47%, neck stiffness in 71%, lethargy in 69%, and seizures in 18%. In typical cases, symptoms resolve in 7-10 days. CSF in mumps meningitis has a white blood cell pleocytosis of 200-600 µL with a predominance of lymphocytes. The CSF glucose content is normal in most patients, but a moderate hypoglycorrhachia (glucose content 20-40 mg/dL) may be seen in 10–20% of patients. The CSF protein content is normal or mildly elevated.

Less-common CNS complications of mumps include transverse myelitis, acute disseminated encephalomyelitis (**ADEM**), aqueductal stenosis, and facial palsy. Sensorineural hearing loss is rare and has been estimated to occur in 0.5-5.0 in 100,000 cases of mumps. The hearing loss can be transient, with permanent unilateral hearing loss in 1 in 20,000 and bilateral loss occurring rarely. There is some evidence that this sequela is more likely in patients with meningoencephalitis.

Orchitis and Oophoritis

In adolescent and adult males, orchitis is 2nd only to parotitis as a common finding in mumps. Involvement in prepubescent boys is extremely rare, but after puberty, orchitis occurs in 30–40% of males. It begins within days following onset of parotitis in most cases and is associated with moderate to high fever, chills, and exquisite pain and swelling of the testes. In 30% or less of cases, the orchitis is bilateral. Atrophy of the testes may occur, but sterility is rare even with bilateral involvement.

Oophoritis is uncommon in postpubertal females but may cause severe pain and may be confused with appendicitis when located on the right side.

Pancreatitis

Pancreatitis may occur in mumps with or without parotid involvement. Severe disease is rare, but fever, epigastric pain, and vomiting are suggestive. Epidemiologic studies have suggested that mumps may be associated with the subsequent development of diabetes mellitus, but a causal link has not been established.

Cardiac Involvement

Myocarditis has been reported in mumps, and molecular studies have identified mumps virus in heart tissue taken from patients with endocardial fibroelastosis.

Arthritis

Arthralgia, monoarthritis, and migratory polyarthritis have been reported in mumps. Arthritis is seen with or without parotitis and usually occurs within 3 wk of onset of parotid swelling. It is generally mild and self-limited.

Thyroiditis

Thyroiditis is rare following mumps. It has not been reported without parotitis and may occur weeks after the acute infection. Most cases resolve, but some become relapsing and result in hypothyroidism.

TREATMENT

No specific antiviral therapy is available for mumps. Management should be aimed at reducing the pain associated with meningitis or orchitis and maintaining adequate hydration. Antipyretics may be given for fever.

PROGNOSIS

The outcome of mumps is nearly always excellent, even when the disease is complicated by encephalitis, although fatal cases from CNS involvement or myocarditis have been reported. No mumps deaths have occurred in the recent outbreaks in the United States.

PREVENTION

Immunization with the live mumps vaccine is the primary mode of prevention used in the United States. It is given as part of the MMR 2-dose vaccine schedule, at 12-15 mo of age for the 1st dose and 4-6 yr of age for the 2nd dose. If not given at 4-6 yr, the 2nd dose should be given before children enter puberty. In those traveling, 2 doses are recommended in individuals older than 12 mo administered at least 28 days apart. Antibody develops in 94% (range: 89–97%) of vaccines after 1 dose. Antibody levels achieved following vaccination are lower than following natural infection.

The median vaccine effectiveness of mumps vaccine after 1 dose of vaccine is 78% (range: 49–92%) and after 2 doses is 88% (range: 66–95%). Duration of effectiveness is ≥10 yr after 1 dose and ≥15 yr after 2 doses.

During outbreaks, *a 3rd MMR dose* administered to the at-risk population was associated with improved outbreak control with significantly fewer cases in those receiving the 3rd dose compared with those not receiving it. Despite these results, modeling supports the current 2-dose schedule without a routine 3rd booster dose because the current regimen significantly controls size of outbreaks, severity of disease, and number of hospitalizations, whereas the 3rd dose appears to be a possible strategy during an outbreak.

As a live-virus vaccine, MMR should not be administered to pregnant women or to severely immunodeficient or immunosuppressed individuals. HIV-infected patients who are not severely immunocompromised may receive the vaccine, because the risk for severe infection with mumps outweighs the risk for serious reaction to the vaccine. Individuals with anaphylactoid reactions to egg or neomycin may be at risk for immediate-type hypersensitivity reactions to the vaccine. Persons with other types of reactions to egg or reactions to other components of the vaccine are not restricted from receiving the vaccine.

In 2006, in response to the multistate outbreak in the United States, evidence of immunity to mumps through vaccination was redefined. Acceptable presumptive evidence of immunity to mumps now consists of 1 of the following: (1) documentation of adequate vaccination at age 12 mo or older, (2) laboratory evidence of immunity, (3) birth before 1957, and (4) documentation of physician-diagnosed mumps. Evidence of immunity through documentation of adequate vaccination is defined as 1 dose of a live mumps virus vaccine for preschool-age children and adults not at high risk and 2 doses for school-age children (i.e., grades K-12) and for adults at high risk (e.g., healthcare workers, international travelers, and students at post–high school educational institutions).

All persons who work in healthcare facilities should be immune to mumps. Adequate mumps vaccination for healthcare workers born during or after 1957 consists of 2 doses of a live mumps virus vaccine. Healthcare workers with no history of mumps vaccination and no other evidence of immunity should receive 2 doses, with >28 days between doses. Healthcare workers who have received only 1 dose previously should receive a 2nd dose. Because birth before 1957 is only presumptive evidence of immunity, healthcare facilities should consider recommending 1 dose of a live mumps virus vaccine for unvaccinated workers born before 1957 who do not have a history of physician-diagnosed mumps or laboratory evidence of mumps immunity. During an outbreak, healthcare facilities should strongly consider recommending 2 doses of a live mumps virus vaccine to unvaccinated workers born before 1957 who do not have evidence of mumps immunity.

Adverse reactions to mumps virus vaccine are rare. Parotitis and orchitis have been reported rarely. There is inadequate information to make a causal relationship to other reactions, such as febrile seizures, deafness, rash, purpura, encephalitis, and meningitis with the strain of mumps vaccine virus used for immunization in the United States. Higher rates of aseptic meningitis following vaccination for mumps are associated with vaccine strains used elsewhere in the world, including the Leningrad 3 and Urabe Am 9 strains. Transient suppression of reactivity to tuberculin skin testing has been reported after mumps vaccination.

In 2005 the quadrivalent measles, mumps, rubella, and varicella (MMRV) vaccine was made available. However, in 2010, studies showed a greater risk of febrile seizures in children 12-23 mo of age 5-12 days following administration of the vaccine. No increased risk of seizures was seen in children receiving the 1st dose of the MMRV at older than 48 mo of age. As a result, the American Academy of Pediatrics currently recommends either the MMR vaccine and separate varicella vaccine or the MMRV vaccine in children 12-47 mo of age. After 48 mo of age, the MMRV is generally preferred.

Bibliography is available at Expert Consult.

Chapter 276

Polioviruses

Eric A.F. Simões

第二百七十六章

脊髓灰质炎病毒

中文导读

　　本章主要介绍了脊髓灰质炎病毒感染的病因学、流行病学、传播、发病机制、临床表现、诊断、鉴别诊断、治疗、并发症、预后和预防。临床表现包括无症状性感染、顿挫型脊髓灰质炎、非瘫痪型脊髓灰质炎和瘫痪型脊髓灰质炎。在瘫痪型脊髓灰质炎中根据累及部位不同详细阐述了脊髓型、延髓型和脑型的临床特点。实验室诊断包括从粪便中进行病毒分离和鉴定，血清学检测等。详细阐述了不同临床类型的治疗方案。

ETIOLOGY

The polioviruses are nonenveloped, positive-stranded RNA viruses belonging to the Picornaviridae family, in the genus *Enterovirus,* species Enterovirus C and consist of 3 antigenically distinct serotypes (types 1, 2, and 3). Polioviruses spread from the intestinal tract to the central nervous system (CNS), where they cause aseptic meningitis and poliomyelitis, or polio. The polioviruses are extremely hardy and can retain infectivity for several days at room temperature.

EPIDEMIOLOGY

The most devastating result of poliovirus infection is paralysis, although 90–95% of infections are inapparent. Despite the absence of symptoms, clinically inapparent infections induce protective immunity. Clinically apparent but nonparalytic illness occurs in approximately 5% of all infections, with paralytic polio occurring in approximately 1 in 1,000 infections among infants to approximately 1 in 100 infections among adolescents. In industrialized countries prior to universal vaccination, epidemics of paralytic poliomyelitis occurred primarily in adolescents. Conversely, in developing countries with poor sanitation, infection early in life results in infantile paralysis. Improved sanitation explains the virtual eradication of polio from the United States in the early 1960s, when only approximately 65% of the population was immunized with the Salk vaccine, which contributed to the disappearance of circulating wild-type poliovirus in the United States and Europe.

TRANSMISSION

Humans are the only known reservoir for the polioviruses, which are spread by the fecal-oral route. Poliovirus has been isolated from feces for longer than 2 wk before paralysis to several wk after the onset of symptoms.

PATHOGENESIS

Polioviruses infect cells by adsorbing to the genetically determined **poliovirus receptor (CD155).** The virus penetrates the cell, is uncoated,

and releases viral RNA. The RNA is translated to produce proteins responsible for replication of the RNA, shutoff of host cell protein synthesis, and synthesis of structural elements that compose the capsid. Mature virus particles are produced in 6-8 hr and are released into the environment by disruption of the cell.

In the contact host, wild-type and vaccine strains of polioviruses gain host entry via the gastrointestinal tract. Recent studies in nonhuman primates demonstrate that the primary sites of replication are in the CD155+ epithelial cells lining the mucosa of the tonsil follicle and small intestine, as well as see the macrophages/dendritic cells in the tonsil follicle and Peyer patches. Regional lymph nodes are infected, and primary viremia occurs after 2-3 days. The virus seeds multiple sites, including the reticuloendothelial system, brown fat deposits, and skeletal muscle. Wild-type poliovirus probably accesses the CNS along peripheral nerves. Vaccine strains of polioviruses do not replicate in the CNS, a feature that accounts for the safety of the live-attenuated vaccine. Occasional **revertants** (by nucleotide substitution) of these vaccine strains develop a neurovirulent phenotype and cause **vaccine-associated paralytic poliomyelitis (VAPP).** Reversion occurs in the small intestine and probably accesses the CNS via the peripheral nerves. Poliovirus has almost never been cultured from the cerebrospinal fluid (CSF) of patients with paralytic disease, and patients with aseptic meningitis caused by poliovirus never have paralytic disease. With the 1st appearance of non-CNS symptoms, a secondary viremia probably occurs as a result of enormous viral replication in the reticuloendothelial system.

The exact mechanism of entry into the CNS is not known. However, once entry is gained, the virus may traverse neural pathways and multiple sites within the CNS are often affected. The effect on motor and vegetative neurons is most striking and correlates with the clinical manifestations. Perineuronal inflammation, a mixed inflammatory reaction with both polymorphonuclear leukocytes and lymphocytes, is associated with extensive neuronal destruction. Petechial hemorrhages and considerable inflammatory edema also occur in areas of poliovirus infection. The poliovirus primarily infects motor neuron cells in the spinal cord (**the** anterior horn cells) and the medulla oblongata (the cranial nerve nuclei). Because of the overlap in muscle innervation by 2-3 adjacent segments of the spinal cord, clinical signs of weakness in the limbs develop when more than 50% of motor neurons are destroyed. In the medulla, less-extensive lesions cause paralysis, and involvement of the reticular formation that contains the vital centers controlling respiration and circulation may have a catastrophic outcome. Involvement of the intermediate and dorsal areas of the horn and the dorsal root ganglia in the spinal cord results in hyperesthesia and myalgias that are typical of acute poliomyelitis. Other neurons affected are the nuclei in the roof and vermis of the cerebellum, the substantia nigra, and, occasionally, the red nucleus in the pons; there may be variable involvement of thalamic, hypothalamic, and pallidal nuclei and the motor cortex.

Apart from the histopathology of the CNS, inflammatory changes occur generally in the reticuloendothelial system. Inflammatory edema and sparse lymphocytic infiltration are prominently associated with hyperplastic lymphocytic follicles.

Infants acquire immunity transplacentally from their mothers. Transplacental immunity disappears at a variable rate during the 1st 4-6 mo of life. Active immunity after natural infection is probably lifelong but protects against the infecting serotype only; infections with other serotypes are possible. Poliovirus-neutralizing antibodies develop within several days after exposure as a result of replication of the virus in the tonsils and in the intestinal tract and deep lymphatic tissues. This early production of circulating immunoglobulin (Ig) G antibodies protects against CNS invasion. Local (mucosal) immunity, conferred mainly by secretory IgA, is an important defense against subsequent reinfection of the gastrointestinal tract.

CLINICAL MANIFESTATIONS

The incubation period of poliovirus from contact to initial clinical symptoms is usually considered to be 8-12 days, with a range of 5-35 days. Poliovirus infections with wild-type virus may follow 1 of several courses: **inapparent infection,** which occurs in 90–95% of cases and causes no disease and no sequelae; abortive poliomyelitis; nonparalytic poliomyelitis; or paralytic poliomyelitis. Paralysis, if it occurs, appears 3-8 days after the initial symptoms. The clinical manifestations of paralytic polio caused by wild or vaccine strains are comparable, although the incidence of abortive and nonparalytic paralysis with vaccine-associated poliomyelitis is unknown.

Abortive Poliomyelitis

In approximately 5% of patients, a nonspecific influenza-like syndrome occurs 1-2 wk after infection, which is termed *abortive poliomyelitis*. Fever, malaise, anorexia, and headache are prominent features, and there may be sore throat and abdominal or muscular pain. Vomiting occurs irregularly. The illness is short lived, lasting up to 2-3 days. The physical examination may be normal or may reveal nonspecific pharyngitis, abdominal or muscular tenderness, and weakness. Recovery is complete, and no neurologic signs or sequelae develop.

Nonparalytic Poliomyelitis

In approximately 1% of patients infected with wild-type poliovirus, signs of abortive poliomyelitis are present, as are more intense headache, nausea, and vomiting, as well as soreness and stiffness of the posterior muscles of the neck, trunk, and limbs. Fleeting paralysis of the bladder and constipation are frequent. Approximately two thirds of these children have a short symptom-free interlude between the 1st phase (**minor illness**) and the 2nd phase (CNS disease or **major illness**). Nuchal rigidity and spinal rigidity are the basis for the diagnosis of nonparalytic poliomyelitis during the 2nd phase.

Physical examination reveals nuchal-spinal signs and changes in superficial and deep reflexes. Gentle forward flexion of the occiput and neck elicits nuchal rigidity. The examiner can demonstrate head drop by placing the hands under the patient's shoulders and raising the patient's trunk. Although normally the head follows the plane of the trunk, in poliomyelitis it often falls backward limply, but this response is not attributable to true paresis of the neck flexors. In struggling infants, it may be difficult to distinguish voluntary resistance from clinically important true

nuchal rigidity. The examiner may place the infant's shoulders flush with the edge of the table, support the weight of the occiput in the hand, and then flex the head anteriorly. True nuchal rigidity persists during this maneuver. When open, the anterior fontanel may be tense or bulging.

In the early stages the reflexes are normally active and remain so unless paralysis supervenes. Changes in reflexes, either increased or decreased, may precede weakness by 12-24 hr. The superficial reflexes, the cremasteric and abdominal reflexes, and the reflexes of the spinal and gluteal muscles are usually the first to diminish. The spinal and gluteal reflexes may disappear before the abdominal and cremasteric reflexes. Changes in the deep tendon reflexes generally occur 8-24 hr after the superficial reflexes are depressed and indicate impending paresis of the extremities. Tendon reflexes are absent with paralysis. Sensory defects do not occur in poliomyelitis.

Paralytic Poliomyelitis

Paralytic poliomyelitis develops in approximately 0.1% of persons infected with poliovirus, causing 3 clinically recognizable syndromes that represent a continuum of infection differentiated only by the portions of the CNS most severely affected. These are (1) spinal paralytic poliomyelitis, (2) bulbar poliomyelitis, and (3) polioencephalitis.

Spinal paralytic poliomyelitis may occur as the 2nd phase of a biphasic illness, the 1st phase of which corresponds to abortive poliomyelitis. The patient then appears to recover and feels better for 2-5 days, after which severe headache and fever occur with exacerbation of the previous systemic symptoms. Severe muscle pain is present, and sensory and motor phenomena (e.g., paresthesia, hyperesthesia, fasciculations, and spasms) may develop. On physical examination the distribution of paralysis is characteristically spotty. Single muscles, multiple muscles, or groups of muscles may be involved in any pattern. Within 1-2 days, *asymmetric flaccid paralysis or paresis occurs*. Involvement of 1 leg is most common, followed by involvement of 1 arm. The proximal areas of the extremities tend to be involved to a greater extent than the distal areas. To detect mild muscular weakness, it is often necessary to apply gentle resistance in opposition to the muscle group being tested. Examination at this point may reveal nuchal stiffness or rigidity, muscle tenderness, initially hyperactive deep tendon reflexes (for a short period) followed by absence or diminution of reflexes, and paresis or flaccid paralysis. In the spinal form, there is weakness of some of the muscles of the neck, abdomen, trunk, diaphragm, thorax, or extremities. *Sensation is intact; sensory disturbances, if present, suggest a disease other than poliomyelitis.*

The paralytic phase of poliomyelitis is extremely variable; some patients progress during observation from paresis to paralysis, whereas others recover, either slowly or rapidly. The extent of paresis or paralysis is directly related to the extent of neuronal involvement; paralysis occurs if >50% of the neurons supplying the muscles are destroyed. The extent of involvement is usually obvious within 2-3 days; only rarely does progression occur beyond this interval. Bowel and bladder dysfunction ranging from transient incontinence to paralysis with constipation and urinary retention often accompany paralysis of the lower limbs.

The onset and course of paralysis are variable in developing countries. The biphasic course is rare; typically the disease manifests in a single phase in which prodromal symptoms and paralysis occur in a continuous fashion. In developing countries, where a history of intramuscular injections precedes paralytic poliomyelitis in approximately 50–60% of patients, patients may present initially with fever and paralysis (**provocation paralysis**). The degree and duration of muscle pain are also variable, ranging from a few days usually to a wk. Occasionally, spasm and increased muscle tone with a transient increase in deep tendon reflexes occur in some patients, whereas in most patients, flaccid paralysis occurs abruptly. Once the temperature returns to normal, progression of paralytic manifestations stops. Little recovery from paralysis is noted in the 1st days or wk, but, if it is to occur, it is usually evident within 6 mo. The return of strength and reflexes is slow and may continue to improve for as long as 18 mo after the acute disease. Lack of improvement from paralysis within the 1st several wk or mo after onset is usually evidence of permanent paralysis. Atrophy of the limb, failure of growth, and deformity are common and are especially evident in the growing child.

Bulbar poliomyelitis may occur as a clinical entity without apparent involvement of the spinal cord. Infection is a continuum, and designation of the disease as bulbar implies only dominance of the clinical manifestations by dysfunctions of the cranial nerves and medullary centers. The clinical findings seen with bulbar poliomyelitis with respiratory difficulty (other than paralysis of extraocular, facial, and masticatory muscles) include (1) nasal twang to the voice or cry caused by palatal and pharyngeal weakness (hard-consonant words such as cookie and candy bring this feature out best); (2) inability to swallow smoothly, resulting in accumulation of saliva in the pharynx, indicating partial immobility (holding the larynx lightly and asking the patient to swallow will confirm such immobility); (3) accumulated pharyngeal secretions, which may cause irregular respirations that appear interrupted and abnormal even to the point of falsely simulating intercostal or diaphragmatic weakness; (4) absence of effective coughing, shown by constant fatiguing efforts to clear the throat; (5) nasal regurgitation of saliva and fluids as a result of palatal paralysis, with inability to separate the oropharynx from the nasopharynx during swallowing; (6) deviation of the palate, uvula, or tongue; (7) involvement of vital centers in the medulla, which manifest as irregularities in rate, depth, and rhythm of respiration; as cardiovascular alterations, including blood pressure changes (especially increased blood pressure), alternate flushing and mottling of the skin, and cardiac arrhythmias; and as rapid changes in body temperature; (8) paralysis of 1 or both vocal cords, causing hoarseness, aphonia, and, ultimately, asphyxia unless the problem is recognized on laryngoscopy and managed by immediate tracheostomy; and (9) the **rope sign,** an acute angulation between the chin and larynx caused by weakness of the hyoid muscles (the hyoid bone is pulled posteriorly, narrowing the hypopharyngeal inlet).

Uncommonly, bulbar disease may culminate in an ascending paralysis (Landry type), in which there is progression cephalad from initial involvement of the lower extremities. Hypertension and other autonomic disturbances are common in bulbar involvement and may persist for a week or more or may be transient. Occasionally, hypertension is followed by hypotension and shock and is associated with irregular or failed respiratory effort, delirium, or coma. This kind of bulbar disease may be rapidly fatal.

The course of bulbar disease is variable; some patients die as a result of extensive, severe involvement of the various centers in the medulla; others recover partially but require ongoing respiratory support, and others recover completely. Cranial nerve involvement is seldom permanent. Atrophy of muscles may be evident, patients immobilized for long periods may experience pneumonia, and renal stones may form as a result of hypercalcemia and hypercalciuria secondary to bone resorption.

Polioencephalitis is a rare form of the disease in which higher centers of the brain are severely involved. Seizures, coma, and spastic paralysis with increased reflexes may be observed. Irritability, disorientation, drowsiness, and coarse tremors are often present with peripheral or cranial nerve paralysis that coexists or ensues. Hypoxia and hypercapnia caused by inadequate ventilation due to respiratory insufficiency may produce disorientation without true encephalitis. The manifestations are common to encephalitis of any cause and can be attributed to polioviruses only with specific viral diagnosis or if accompanied by flaccid paralysis.

Paralytic poliomyelitis with ventilatory insufficiency results from several components acting together to produce ventilatory insufficiency resulting in hypoxia and hypercapnia. It may have profound effects on many other systems. Because respiratory insufficiency may develop rapidly, close continued clinical evaluation is essential. Despite weakness of the respiratory muscles, the patient may respond with so much respiratory effort associated with anxiety and fear that overventilation may occur at the outset, resulting in respiratory alkalosis. Such effort is fatiguing and contributes to respiratory failure.

There are certain characteristic patterns of disease. Pure spinal poliomyelitis with respiratory insufficiency involves tightness, weakness, or paralysis of the respiratory muscles (chiefly the diaphragm and intercostals) without discernible clinical involvement of the cranial nerves or vital centers that control respiration, circulation, and body temperature. The cervical and thoracic spinal cord segments are chiefly

affected. Pure bulbar poliomyelitis involves paralysis of the motor cranial nerve nuclei with or without involvement of the vital centers. Involvement of the 9th, 10th, and 12th cranial nerves results in paralysis of the pharynx, tongue, and larynx with consequent airway obstruction. Bulbospinal poliomyelitis with respiratory insufficiency affects the respiratory muscles and results in coexisting bulbar paralysis.

The clinical findings associated with involvement of the respiratory muscles include (1) anxious expression; (2) inability to speak without frequent pauses, resulting in short, jerky, breathless sentences; (3) increased respiratory rate; (4) movement of the ala nasi and of the accessory muscles of respiration; (5) inability to cough or sniff with full depth; (6) paradoxical abdominal movements caused by diaphragmatic immobility caused by spasm or weakness of 1 or both leaves; and (7) relative immobility of the intercostal spaces, which may be segmental, unilateral, or bilateral. When the arms are weak, and especially when deltoid paralysis occurs, there may be impending respiratory paralysis because the phrenic nerve nuclei are in adjacent areas of the spinal cord. Observation of the patient's capacity for thoracic breathing while the abdominal muscles are splinted manually indicates minor degrees of paresis. Light manual splinting of the thoracic cage helps to assess the effectiveness of diaphragmatic movement.

DIAGNOSIS

Poliomyelitis should be considered in any unimmunized or incompletely immunized child with paralytic disease. Although this guideline is most applicable in poliomyelitis endemic countries (Afghanistan, Pakistan, and Nigeria), the spread of polio in 2013 from endemic countries to many nonendemic countries (Niger, Chad, Cameroon, Ethiopia, Kenya, Somalia, and Syria) and the isolation of wild poliovirus type 1 in Israel in 2014 and circulating type 1 vaccine-associated paralytic polio in Ukraine in 2015 suggest that the diagnosis of polio should be entertained in all countries. VAPP should be considered in any child with paralytic disease occurring 7-14 days after receiving the orally administered polio vaccine (OPV). VAPP can occur at later times after administration and should be considered in any child with paralytic disease in countries or regions where wild-type poliovirus has been eradicated and the OPV has been administered to the child or a contact. The combination of fever, headache, neck and back pain, asymmetric flaccid paralysis without sensory loss, and pleocytosis does not regularly occur in any other illness.

The World Health Organization (WHO) recommends that the laboratory diagnosis of poliomyelitis be confirmed by isolation and identification of poliovirus in the stool, with specific identification of wild-type and vaccine-type strains. In suspected cases of acute flaccid paralysis, 2 stool specimens should be collected 24-48 hr apart as soon as possible after the diagnosis of poliomyelitis is suspected. Poliovirus concentrations are high in the stool in the 1st wk after the onset of paralysis, which is the optimal time for collection of stool specimens. Polioviruses may be isolated from 80–90% of specimens from acutely ill patients, whereas <20% of specimens from such patients may yield virus within 3-4 wk after onset of paralysis. Because most children with spinal or bulbospinal poliomyelitis have constipation, rectal straws may be used to obtain specimens; ideally a minimum of 8-10 g of stool should be collected. In laboratories that can isolate poliovirus, isolates should be sent to either the U.S. Centers for Disease Control and Prevention or to 1 of the WHO-certified poliomyelitis laboratories where DNA sequence analysis can be performed to distinguish between wild poliovirus and neurovirulent, revertant OPV strains. With the current WHO plan for global eradication of poliomyelitis, most regions of the world (the Americas, Europe, and Australia) have been certified wild-poliovirus free; in these areas, poliomyelitis is most often caused by vaccine strains. Hence it is critical to differentiate between wild-type and revertant vaccine-type strains.

The CSF is often normal during the minor illness and typically contains a pleocytosis with 20-300 cells/μL with CNS involvement. The cells in the CSF may be polymorphonuclear early during the course of the disease but shift to mononuclear cells soon afterward. By the 2nd wk of major illness, the CSF cell count falls to near-normal values. In contrast, the CSF protein content is normal or only slightly elevated at the outset of CNS disease but usually rises to 50-100 mg/dL by the 2nd wk of illness. In polioencephalitis, the CSF may remain normal or show minor changes. Serologic testing demonstrates seroconversion or a 4-fold or greater increase in antibody titers from the acute phase of illness to 3-6 wk later.

DIFFERENTIAL DIAGNOSIS

Poliomyelitis should be considered in the differential diagnosis of any case of paralysis and is only 1 of many causes of acute flaccid paralysis in children and adults. There are numerous other causes of acute flaccid paralysis (Table 276.1). In most conditions, the clinical features are sufficient to differentiate between these various causes, but in some cases nerve conduction studies and electromyograms, in addition to muscle biopsies, may be required.

The possibility of polio should be considered in any case of acute flaccid paralysis, even in countries where polio has been eradicated. The diagnoses most often confused with polio are VAPP, West Nile virus infection, and infections caused by other enteroviruses (including EV-A71 and EV-D68), as well as Guillain-Barré syndrome, transverse myelitis, and traumatic paralysis. In **Guillain-Barré syndrome**, which is the most difficult to distinguish from poliomyelitis, the paralysis is characteristically symmetric, and sensory changes and pyramidal tract signs are common, contrasting with poliomyelitis. Fever, headache, and meningeal signs are less notable, and the CSF has few cells but an elevated protein content. **Transverse myelitis** progresses rapidly over hr to days, causing an acute symmetric paralysis of the lower limbs with concomitant anesthesia and diminished sensory perception. Autonomic signs of hypothermia in the affected limbs are common, and there is bladder dysfunction. The CSF is usually normal. **Traumatic neuritis** occurs from a few hr to a few days after the traumatic event, is asymmetric, is acute, and affects only 1 limb. Muscle tone and deep tendon reflexes are reduced or absent in the affected limb with pain in the gluteus. The CSF is normal.

Conditions causing pseudoparalysis do not present with nuchal-spinal rigidity or pleocytosis. These causes include unrecognized trauma, transient (toxic) synovitis, acute osteomyelitis, acute rheumatic fever, scurvy, and congenital syphilis (pseudoparalysis of Parrot).

TREATMENT

There is no specific antiviral treatment for poliomyelitis. The management is supportive and aimed at limiting progression of disease, preventing ensuing skeletal deformities, and preparing the child and family for the prolonged treatment required and for permanent disability if this seems likely. Patients with the nonparalytic and mildly paralytic forms of poliomyelitis may be treated at home. All intramuscular injections and surgical procedures are contraindicated during the acute phase of the illness, especially in the 1st wk of illness, because they might result in progression of disease.

Abortive Poliomyelitis

Supportive treatment with analgesics, sedatives, an attractive diet, and bed rest until the child's temperature is normal for several days is usually sufficient. Avoidance of exertion for the ensuing 2 wk is desirable, and careful neurologic and musculoskeletal examinations should be performed 2 mo later to detect any minor involvement.

Nonparalytic Poliomyelitis

Treatment for the nonparalytic form is similar to that for the abortive form; in particular, relief is indicated for the discomfort of muscle tightness and spasm of the neck, trunk, and extremities. Analgesics are more effective when they are combined with the application of hot packs for 15-30 min every 2-4 hr. Hot tub baths are sometimes useful. A firm bed is desirable and can be improvised at home by placing table leaves or a sheet of plywood beneath the mattress. A footboard or splint should be used to keep the feet at a right angle to the legs. Because muscular discomfort and spasm may continue for some wk, even in the nonparalytic form, hot packs and gentle physical therapy may be necessary. Patients with nonparalytic poliomyelitis should also be carefully examined 2 mo after apparent recovery to detect minor residual effects that might cause postural problems in later yr.

Paralytic Poliomyelitis

Most patients with the paralytic form of poliomyelitis require hospitalization with complete physical rest in a calm atmosphere for the 1st 2-3 wk. **Suitable body alignment** is necessary for comfort and to avoid excessive skeletal deformity. A neutral position with the feet at right angles to the legs, the knees slightly flexed, and the hips and spine straight is achieved by use of boards, sandbags, and, occasionally, light splint shells. The position should be changed every 3-6 hr. **Active and passive movements** are indicated as soon as the pain has disappeared. Moist hot packs may relieve muscle pain and spasm. Opiates and sedatives are permissible only if no impairment of ventilation is present or impending. Constipation is common, and fecal impaction should be prevented. When bladder paralysis occurs, a parasympathetic stimulant such as bethanechol may induce voiding in 15-30 min; some patients show no response to this agent, and others respond with nausea, vomiting, and palpitations. Bladder paresis rarely lasts more than a few days. If bethanechol fails, manual compression of the bladder and the psychologic effect of running water should be tried. If catheterization must be performed, care must be taken to prevent urinary tract infections. An appealing diet and a relatively high fluid intake should be started at once unless the patient is vomiting. Additional salt should be provided if the environmental temperature is high or if the application of hot packs induces sweating. Anorexia is common initially. Adequate dietary and fluid intake can be maintained by placement of a central venous catheter. An orthopedist and a physiatrist should see patients as early in the course of the illness as possible and should assume responsibility for their care before fixed deformities develop.

The management of pure bulbar poliomyelitis consists of maintaining the airway and avoiding all risk of inhalation of saliva, food, and vomitus. Gravity drainage of accumulated secretions is favored by using the head-low (foot of bed elevated 20-25 degrees) prone position with the face to 1 side. Patients with weakness of the muscles of respiration or swallowing should be nursed in a lateral or semiprone position. Aspirators with rigid or semirigid tips are preferred for direct oral and pharyngeal aspiration, and soft, flexible catheters may be used for nasopharyngeal aspiration. Fluid and electrolyte equilibrium is best maintained by intravenous infusion because tube or oral feeding in the 1st few days may incite vomiting. In addition to close observation for respiratory insufficiency, the blood pressure should be measured at least twice daily because hypertension is not uncommon and occasionally leads to hypertensive encephalopathy. Patients with pure bulbar poliomyelitis may require tracheostomy because of vocal cord paralysis or constriction of the hypopharynx; most patients who recover have little residual impairment, although some exhibit mild dysphagia and occasional vocal fatigue with slurring of speech.

Impaired ventilation must be recognized early; mounting anxiety, restlessness, and fatigue are early indications for preemptive intervention. Tracheostomy is indicated for some patients with pure bulbar poliomyelitis, spinal respiratory muscle paralysis, or bulbospinal paralysis because such patients are generally unable to cough, sometimes for many months. Mechanical respirators are often needed.

COMPLICATIONS

Paralytic poliomyelitis may be associated with numerous complications. Acute gastric dilation may occur abruptly during the acute or convalescent stage, causing further respiratory embarrassment; immediate gastric aspiration and external application of ice bags are indicated. Melena severe enough to require transfusion may result from single or multiple superficial intestinal erosions; perforation is rare. Mild hypertension for days or weeks is common in the acute stage and probably related to lesions of the vasoregulatory centers in the medulla and especially to underventilation. In the later stages, because of immobilization, hypertension may occur along with hypercalcemia, nephrocalcinosis, and vascular lesions. Dimness of vision, headache, and a lightheaded feeling associated with hypertension should be regarded as premonitory of a frank convulsion. Cardiac irregularities are uncommon, but electrocardiographic abnormalities suggesting myocarditis occur with some frequency. Acute pulmonary edema occurs occasionally, particularly in patients with arterial hypertension. Hypercalcemia occurs because

Table 276.1 Differential Diagnosis of Acute Flaccid Paralysis

SITE, CONDITION, FACTOR, OR AGENT	CLINICAL FINDINGS	ONSET OF PARALYSIS	PROGRESSION OF PARALYSIS	SENSORY SIGNS AND SYMPTOMS	REDUCTION OR ABSENCE OF DEEP TENDON REFLEXES	RESIDUAL PARALYSIS	PLEOCYTOSIS
ANTERIOR HORN CELLS OF SPINAL CORD							
Poliomyelitis (wild and vaccine-associated paralytic poliomyelitis)	Paralysis	Incubation period 7-14 days (range: 4-35 days)	24-48 hr to onset of full paralysis; proximal → distal, asymmetric	No	Yes	Yes	Aseptic meningitis (moderate polymorphonuclear leukocytes at 2-3 days)
Nonpolio enteroviruses (including EV-A71, EV D68)	Hand-foot-and-mouth disease, aseptic meningitis, acute hemorrhagic conjunctivitis, possibly idiopathic epidemic flaccid paralysis	As in poliomyelitis	As in poliomyelitis	No	Yes	Yes	As in poliomyelitis
West Nile virus	Meningitis encephalitis	As in poliomyelitis	As in poliomyelitis	No	Yes	Yes	Yes
OTHER NEUROTROPIC VIRUSES							
Rabies virus		Mo–Yr	Acute, symmetric, ascending	Yes	Yes	No	±
Varicella-zoster virus	Exanthematous vesicular eruptions	Incubation period 10-21 days	Acute, symmetric, ascending	Yes	±	±	Yes
Japanese encephalitis virus		Incubation period 5-15 days	Acute, proximal, asymmetric	±	±	±	Yes
GUILLAIN-BARRÉ SYNDROME							
Acute inflammatory polyradiculo-neuropathy	Preceding infection, bilateral facial weakness	Hr to 10 days	Acute, symmetric, ascending (days to 4 wk)	Yes	Yes	±	No
Acute motor axonal neuropathy	Fulminant, widespread paralysis, bilateral facial weakness, tongue involvement	Hr to 10 days	1-6 days	No	Yes	±	No

Disease	Signs and symptoms	Progression of paralysis				
ACUTE TRAUMATIC SCIATIC NERITIS						
Intramuscular gluteal injection		Acute, asymmetric; Hr to 4 days; Complete, affected limb	Yes	Yes	±	No
Acute transverse myelitis	Preceding Mycoplasma pneumoniae, Schistosoma, other parasitic or viral infection	Acute, symmetric hypotonia of lower limbs; Hr to days	Yes, early	Yes	Yes	Yes
Epidural abscess	Headache, back pain, local spinal tenderness, meningismus	Complete; Hr to days	Yes	Yes	±	Yes
Spinal cord compression; trauma		Complete; Hr to days	Yes	Yes	±	±
NEUROPATHIES						
Exotoxin of Corynebacterium diphtheriae	In severe cases, palatal paralysis, blurred vision	Incubation period 1-8 wk (paralysis 8-12 wk after onset of illness)	Yes	Yes		±
Toxin of Clostridium botulinum	Abdominal pain, diplopia, loss of accommodation, mydriasis	Rapid, descending, symmetric; Incubation period 18-36 hr	No	±		No
Tick bite paralysis	Ocular symptoms	Acute, symmetric, ascending; Latency period 5-10 days	Yes	No		No
DISEASES OF THE NEUROMUSCULAR JUNCTION						
Myasthenia gravis	Weakness, fatigability, diplopia, ptosis, dysarthria	Multifocal	No	No	No	No
DISORDERS OF MUSCLE						
Polymyositis	Neoplasm, autoimmune disease	Subacute, proximal → distal; Wk to mo	Yes	No		No
Viral myositis		Pseudoparalysis; Hr to days	No	No		No
METABOLIC DISORDERS						
Hypokalemic periodic paralysis	Proximal limb, respiratory muscles	Sudden postprandial	Yes	No	±	No
INTENSIVE CARE UNIT WEAKNESS						
Critical illness polyneuropathy	Flaccid limbs and respiratory weakness	Acute, following systemic inflammatory response syndrome/sepsis; Hr to days	Yes	±	±	No

Modified from Marx A, Glass JD, Sutter RW: Differential diagnosis of acute flaccid paralysis and its role in poliomyelitis surveillance, *Epidemiol Rev* 22:298–316, 2000.

of skeletal decalcification that begins soon after immobilization and results in hypercalciuria, which in turn predisposes the patient to urinary calculi, especially when urinary stasis and infection are present. High fluid intake is the only effective prophylactic measure.

PROGNOSIS

The outcome of inapparent, abortive poliomyelitis and aseptic meningitis syndromes is uniformly good, with death being exceedingly rare and with no long-term sequelae. The outcome of paralytic disease is determined primarily by degree and severity of CNS involvement. In severe bulbar poliomyelitis, the mortality rate may be as high as 60%, whereas in less-severe bulbar involvement and/or spinal poliomyelitis, the mortality rate varies from 5% to 10%, death generally occurring from causes other than the poliovirus infection.

Maximum paralysis usually occurs 2-3 days after the onset of the paralytic phase of the illness, with stabilization followed by gradual return of muscle function. The recovery phase lasts usually about 6 mo, beyond which persisting paralysis is permanent. In general, paralysis is more likely to develop in male children and female adults. Mortality and the degree of disability are greater after the age of puberty. Pregnancy is associated with an increased risk for paralytic disease. Tonsillectomy and intramuscular injections may enhance the risk for acquisition of bulbar and localized disease, respectively. Increased physical activity, exercise, and fatigue during the early phase of illness have been cited as factors leading to a higher risk for paralytic disease. Finally, it has been clearly demonstrated that type 1 poliovirus has the greatest propensity for natural poliomyelitis and type 3 poliovirus has a predilection for producing VAPP.

Postpolio Syndrome

After an interval of 30-40 yr, as many as 30–40% of persons who survived paralytic poliomyelitis in childhood may experience muscle pain and exacerbation of existing weakness or development of new weakness or paralysis. This entity, referred to as postpolio syndrome, has been reported only in persons who were infected in the era of wild-type poliovirus circulation. Risk factors for postpolio syndrome include increasing length of time since acute poliovirus infection, presence of permanent residual impairment after recovery from acute illness, and female sex.

PREVENTION

Vaccination is the only effective method of preventing poliomyelitis. Hygienic measures help to limit the spread of the infection among young children, but immunization is necessary to control transmission among all age groups. Both the inactivated polio vaccine (IPV), which is currently produced using better methods than those for the original vaccine and is sometimes referred to as enhanced IPV, and the live-attenuated OPV have established efficacy in preventing poliovirus infection and paralytic poliomyelitis. Both vaccines induce production of antibodies against the 3 strains of poliovirus. IPV elicits higher serum IgG antibody titers, but the OPV also induces significantly greater mucosal IgA immunity in the oropharynx and gastrointestinal tract, which limits replication of the wild poliovirus at these sites. Transmission of wild poliovirus by fecal spread is limited in OPV recipients. The immunogenicity of IPV is not affected by the presence of maternal antibodies, and IPV has no adverse effects. Live vaccine may undergo reversion to neurovirulence as it multiplies in the human intestinal tract and may cause VAPP in vaccinees or in their contacts. The overall risk for recipients varies from 1 case per 750,000 immunized infants in the United States to 1 in 143,000 immunized infants in India. The risk for paralysis in the B-cell–immunodeficient recipient may be as much as 6,800 times that in normal subjects. HIV infection has not been found to result in long-term excretion of virus. *As of January 2000, the IPV-only schedule is recommended for routine polio vaccination in the United States.* All children should receive 4 doses of IPV, at 2 mo, 4 mo, 6-18 mo, and 4-6 yr of age.

In 1988 the World Health Assembly resolved to eradicate poliomyelitis globally by 2000, and remarkable progress had been made toward reaching this target. To achieve this goal, the WHO used 4 basic strategies: routine immunization, National Immunization Days, acute flaccid paralysis surveillance, and mop-up immunization. This strategy has resulted in a >99% decline in poliomyelitis cases; in early 2002, there were only 10 countries in the world endemic for poliomyelitis. In 2012 there were the fewest cases of poliomyelitis ever, and the virus was endemic in only 3 countries (Afghanistan, Pakistan, and Nigeria). India has not had a child paralyzed with wild poliovirus type 2 since February 2011. The last case of wild poliovirus type 3 infection occurred in Nigeria in November 2012, and the last case of wild poliovirus type 2 infection occurred in India in October 1999. This progress prompted the WHO assembly, in May 2013, to recommend the development of a *Polio Eradication and Endgame Strategic Plan 2013-2018*. This plan included the withdrawal of trivalent OPV (tOPV) with bivalent OPV (bOPV) in all countries by 2016 and the introduction of initially 1 dose of IPV followed by the replacement of bOPV with IPV in all countries of the world by 2019. As long as the OPV is being used, there is the potential that vaccine-derived poliovirus (VDPV) will acquire the neurovirulent phenotype and transmission characteristics of the wild-type polioviruses. VDPV emerges from the OPV because of continuous replication in immunodeficient persons (iVDPV) or by circulation in populations with low vaccine coverage (cVDPVs). The risk was highest with the type 2 strain. Between 2000 and 2012, 90% of the 750 paralytic cases of cVDPV and 40% of VAPP were caused by type 2 strains. Between 17 April and 1 May 2016, 155 countries and territories in the world switched from the use of tOPV to bOPV. tOPV is no longer used globally in any routine or supplemental immunization activities.

Several countries are global priorities because they face challenges in eradication of the disease. Polioviruses remain endemic in Pakistan, Afghanistan, and Nigeria. For these 3 countries, there are several reasons for the failure to eradicate polio. The rejection of poliovirus vaccine initiatives and campaign quality in security-compromised areas in parts of these countries are still the main difficulties faced in 2019. Following an emergency committee meeting in November 2018 that reviewed data on WPV1 and cVDPV, new recommendations for international travelers to certain countries were made by the WHO and endorsed by the CDC. There has been an increase in WPV1 (21 cases each in Afghanistan and Nigeria and 12 in Pakistan in 2018). In addition, outbreaks of cVDPV2 in Syria, Somalia, Kenya, DR Congo, Niger, and Mozambique, cVDPV1 in Papua New Guinea, and cVDPV3 in Somalia, with spread of cVDPV2 between Somalia and Kenya and between Nigeria and Niger, highlight that routine immunization coverage remains very poor in many areas of these countries. Continuing spread due to poor herd immunity and now international spread pose a significant threat to the eradication effort. The committee recommended that for countries with WPV1, cVDPV1, or cVDPV3 with potential risk of international spread, all residents and long-term visitors (i.e., >4 weeks) of all ages receive a dose of bOPV or IPV between 4 wk and 12 mo before travel to these countries (currently Afghanistan, Pakistan, Nigeria, Papua New Guinea, and Somalia). Such travelers should be provided with an International Certificate of Vaccination of Prophylaxis to record their polio vaccination and service proof of vaccination. These countries have been advised to restrict at the point of departure the international travel of any resident lacking documentation of full vaccination, whether by air, sea, or land. For countries infected with cVDPV2 with potential risk of international spread (DR Congo, Kenya, Nigeria, Niger, and Somalia as of January 2019), visitors should be encouraged to follow these recommendations (not mandated).

In October 2016, cVDPV2 was isolated from the sewage in different parts of India, most probably due to the use of tOPV, which was still being used in private dispensaries and was not destroyed as was mandated. This illustrates the dangers of purely using bOPV. The WHO has mandated that infants in all countries still using bOPV should receive a dose of IPV, to offer protection against polio virus type 2. All countries have complied with this requirement; see Fig. 276.1 for the status as of November 2016. In this regard, recent studies from India have shown that following a course of OPV, IPV boosts serologic and mucosal immunity that lasts for at least 11 mo. It is estimated that between 12 and 24 mo after withdrawal of Sabin poliovirus type 2 vaccine, the world would have eradicated type 2 poliovirus circulation in humans. The switch from bOPV to IPV worldwide is slated to occur soon thereafter. These efforts

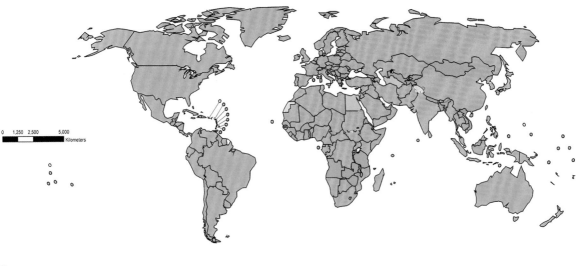

Introduced to date* *(173 countries or 89%)*
Gavi countries with formal commitment to introduce in
  2017 *(18 countries or 9%)*
Non Gavi countries with formal commitment to introduce in
  2017 *(3 countries or 2%)*
Not available
Not applicable
Including partial introduction in india

Fig. 276.1 Countries identified by the World Health Organization as using IPV vaccine to date and introductions planned according to Gavi eligibility status. WHO/IVB Database as of 7 November 2016. World Health Organization 2016. *(Courtesy World Health Organization.* http://www.who.int/immunization/diseases/poliomyelitis/endgame_objective2/en/. *Accessed June 6, 2017.)*

may be stymied because of the global inability to produce IPV in a large enough volume to cover all the 128 million babies born annually in the world. This problem was a crisis during the global synchronized introduction of bOPV, when several countries (e.g., India) had to use 2 fractional doses of IPV (⅕ dose) administered intradermally. To enhance scale up of IPV production in countries such as India, Brazil, and China, IPV using Sabin strains of poliovirus have been developed in Japan and China. These mitigate the stringent requirements for wild-type poliovirus culture that are normally required for IPV production. Other strategies include developing adjuvants for IPV that could potentially lower the antigen quantities needed for each dose.

In countries where bOPV is included in routine immunization, it is best if it follows at least 1 dose of IPV or 2 doses of fractional intradermal IPV. This follows the experience in the United States and Hungary that reported no VAPP following a sequential use of IPV followed by OPV. Global synchronous cessation of OPV will need to be coordinated by the WHO, but the recent experiences in the horn of Africa and Israel/West Bank suggest that stopping transmission of wild poliovirus type 1 in the 3 endemic countries is of the utmost urgency, if we are to stop using OPV.

Bibliography is available at Expert Consult.

Chapter **277**
Nonpolio Enteroviruses
Kevin Messacar and Mark J. Abzug

第二百七十七章
非脊髓灰质炎肠道病毒

中文导读

　　本章主要介绍了除脊髓灰质炎外的肠道病毒感染的病因学、发病机制、临床表现、诊断、鉴别诊断、治疗、并发症和预后。详细阐述了感染后导致病毒血症、中枢神经系统感染、脑炎、心肌炎、新生儿感染的发病机制。临床表现包括非特异性发热、手足口病、疱疹性咽峡炎、心肌炎和心包炎、各系统表现、肌炎和关节炎、新生儿感染等。实验室诊断包括病毒培养、核酸检测和血清学检测。本病尚无特异性抗病毒药，以支持治疗为主。

The genus *Enterovirus* contains a large number of viruses spread via the gastrointestinal and respiratory routes that produce a broad range of illnesses in patients of all ages. Many of the manifestations predominantly affect infants and young children.

ETIOLOGY

Enteroviruses are nonenveloped, single-stranded, positive-sense viruses in the Picornaviridae ("small RNA virus") family, which also includes the rhinoviruses, hepatitis A virus, and parechoviruses. The original human enterovirus subgroups—polioviruses (see Chapter 276), coxsackieviruses, and echoviruses—were differentiated by their replication patterns in tissue culture and animals (Table 277.1). Enteroviruses have been reclassified on the basis of genetic similarity into 4 species, human enteroviruses A-D. Specific enterovirus types are distinguished by antigenic and genetic sequence differences, with enteroviruses discovered after 1970 classified by species and number (e.g., enterovirus D68 and A71). Although more than 100 types have been described, 10-15 account for the majority of disease. No disease is uniquely associated with any specific serotype, although certain manifestations are preferentially associated with specific serotypes. *The closely related human parechoviruses can cause clinical presentations similar to those associated with enteroviruses.*

Epidemiology

Enterovirus infections are common, with a worldwide distribution. In temperate climates, annual epidemic peaks occur in summer/fall, although some transmission occurs year-round. Enteroviruses are responsible for 33–65% of acute febrile illnesses and 55–65% of hospitalizations for suspected sepsis in infants during the summer and fall in the United States. In tropical and semitropical areas, enteroviruses typically circulate year-round. In general, only a few serotypes circulate simultaneously. Infections by different serotypes can occur within the same season.

Factors associated with increased incidence and/or severity include young age, male sex, exposure to children, poor hygiene, overcrowding, and low socioeconomic status. More than 25% of symptomatic infections occur in children younger than 1 yr of age. Breastfeeding reduces the risk for infection, likely via enterovirus-specific antibodies.

Humans are the only known natural reservoir for human enteroviruses. Virus is primarily spread person to person, by the fecal-oral and respiratory routes, although types causing acute hemorrhagic conjunctivitis may be spread via airborne transmission. Virus can be transmitted vertically prenatally or in the peripartum period, or, possibly, via breastfeeding. Enteroviruses can survive on environmental surfaces, permitting transmission via fomites. Enteroviruses also can frequently be isolated from water sources, sewage, and wet soil. Although contamination of drinking water, swimming pools and ponds, and hospital water reservoirs may occasionally be responsible for transmission, such contamination is often considered the result rather than the cause of human infection. Transmission is common within families (≥50% risk of spread to nonimmune household contacts), daycare centers, playgrounds, summer camps, orphanages, and hospital nurseries; severe secondary infections may occur in nursery outbreaks. Transmission risk is increased by diaper changing and decreased by handwashing. Tickborne transmission has been suggested.

Large enterovirus outbreaks have included meningitis epidemics (echoviruses 4, 6, 9, 13, and 30 commonly); epidemics of hand-foot-and-mouth disease with severe central nervous system (CNS) and/or cardiopulmonary disease caused by enterovirus A71 in Asia and Australia; outbreaks of atypical, severe hand-foot-and-mouth disease caused by coxsackievirus A6 in the United States and United Kingdom; outbreaks of human enterovirus D68 respiratory illness associated with acute flaccid myelitis in the United States and Europe; outbreaks of acute hemorrhagic conjunctivitis caused by enterovirus D70, coxsackievirus A24, and coxsackievirus A24 variant in tropical and temperate regions;

Table 277.1	Classification of Human Enteroviruses
Family	Picornaviridae
Genus	*Enterovirus*
Subgroups*	Poliovirus serotypes 1-3
	Coxsackie A virus serotypes 1-22, 24 (23 reclassified as echovirus 9)
	Coxsackie B virus serotypes 1-6
	Echovirus serotypes 1-9, 11-27, 29-33 (echoviruses 10 and 28 reclassified as non-enteroviruses; echovirus 34 reclassified as a variant of coxsackie A virus 24; echoviruses 22 and 23 reclassified within the genus *Parechovirus*)
	Numbered enterovirus serotypes (enterovirus 72 reclassified as hepatitis A virus)

*The human enteroviruses have been alternatively classified on the basis of nucleotide and amino acid sequences into 4 species (human enteroviruses A-D).

and community outbreaks of uveitis. Reverse transcription polymerase chain reaction (RT-PCR) and genomic sequencing help identify outbreaks and demonstrate, depending on the outbreak, commonality of outbreak strains, differences among epidemic strains and older prototype strains, changes in circulating viral subgroups over time, cocirculation of multiple genetic lineages, coinfections with different enterovirus serotypes, and associations between specific genogroups and/or genetic substitutions and epidemiologic and clinical characteristics. Genetic analyses have demonstrated recombination and genetic drift that lead to evolutionary changes in genomic sequence and antigenicity and extensive genetic diversity. For example, emergence of new subgenotypes and genetic lineages of enterovirus A71 may contribute to sequential outbreaks and increases in circulation.

The incubation period is typically 3-6 days, except for a 1-3 day incubation period for acute hemorrhagic conjunctivitis. Infected children, both symptomatic and asymptomatic, frequently shed cultivable enteroviruses from the respiratory tract for <1-3 wk, whereas fecal shedding continues for as long as 7-11 wk. Enterovirus RNA can be shed from mucosal sites for comparable, and, possibly, longer periods.

PATHOGENESIS

Cell surface macromolecules, including poliovirus receptor, integrin very-late-activation antigen (VLA)-2, decay-accelerating factor/complement regulatory protein (DAF/CD55), intercellular adhesion molecule-1 (ICAM-1), ICAM-5, and coxsackievirus-adenovirus receptor, serve as viral receptors. In addition, respiratory epithelial cell sialic acids serve as receptors for enterovirus D68, enterovirus D70, and coxsackievirus A24 variants, and human scavenger receptor class B2 (SCARB2), human P-selectin glycoprotein ligand-1, and DC-SIGN are receptors for enterovirus A71. After virus attaches to a cell surface receptor, a conformational change in surface capsid proteins expels a hydrophobic pocket factor, facilitating penetration and uncoating with release of viral RNA in the cytoplasm. Translation of the positive-sense RNA produces a polyprotein that undergoes cleavage by proteases encoded in the polyprotein. Several proteins produced guide synthesis of negative-sense RNA that serves as a template for replication of new positive-sense RNA. The genome is approximately 7,500 nucleotides long and includes a highly conserved 5′ noncoding region important for replication efficiency and a highly conserved 3′ polyA region; these flank a continuous region encoding viral proteins. The 5′ end is covalently linked to a small viral protein (VPg) necessary for initiation of RNA synthesis. There is significant variation within genomic regions encoding the structural proteins, leading to variability in antigenicity. Replication is followed by further cleavage of proteins and assembly into 30 nm icosahedral virions. Of the 4 structural proteins (VP1-VP4) in the capsid, VP1 is the most important determinant of serotype specificity. Additional regulatory proteins such as an RNA-dependent RNA polymerase and proteases are also present in the virion. Approximately 10^4-10^5 virions are released from an infected cell by lysis within 5-10 hr of infection.

Following oral or respiratory acquisition, initial replication for most enteroviruses occurs in the pharynx and intestine, possibly within mucosal M cells. The acid stability of most enteroviruses favors survival in the gastrointestinal tract. Two or more enteroviruses may invade and replicate in the gastrointestinal tract simultaneously, but interference

due to replication of 1 type often hinders growth of the heterologous type. Initial replication of most enteroviruses in the pharynx and intestine is followed within days by multiplication in lymphoid tissue such as tonsils, Peyer patches, and regional lymph nodes. A primary, transient viremia (**minor viremia**) results in spread to distant parts of the reticuloendothelial system, including the liver, spleen, bone marrow, and distant lymph nodes. Host immune responses may limit replication and progression beyond the reticuloendothelial system, resulting in subclinical infection. Clinical infection occurs if replication proceeds in the reticuloendothelial system and virus spreads via a secondary, sustained viremia (**major viremia**) to target organs such as the CNS, heart, and skin. *Tropism to target organs is determined in part by the infecting serotype.* Some enteroviruses, such as enterovirus D68, can be acid-labile and bind sialic acid receptors on respiratory epithelial cells in the upper and lower respiratory tract and primarily produce respiratory illness. Cytokine responses may contribute to development of respiratory disease by these viruses. Transient early viremia following respiratory enterovirus D68 infection has also been demonstrated.

Enteroviruses can damage a wide variety of organs and systems, including the CNS, heart, liver, lungs, pancreas, kidneys, muscle, and skin. Damage is mediated by necrosis and the inflammatory response. **CNS infections** are often associated with pleocytosis of the cerebrospinal fluid (CSF), composed of macrophages and activated T lymphocytes, and a mixed meningeal inflammatory response. Parenchymal involvement may affect the cerebral white and gray matter, cerebellum, basal ganglia, brainstem, and spinal cord with perivascular and parenchymal mixed or lymphocytic inflammation, gliosis, cellular degeneration, and neuronophagocytosis. **Encephalitis** during enterovirus A71 epidemics has been characterized by severe involvement of the brainstem, spinal cord gray matter, hypothalamus, and subthalamic and dentate nuclei, and can be complicated by pulmonary edema, pulmonary hemorrhage, and/or interstitial pneumonitis, presumed secondary to brainstem damage, sympathetic hyperactivity, myoclonus, ataxia, autonomic dysfunction, and CNS and systemic inflammatory responses (including cytokine and chemokine overexpression). Immunologic cross-reactivity with brain tissue has been postulated as 1 mechanism responsible for neurologic damage and sequelae following enterovirus A71 infection.

Enterovirus **myocarditis** is characterized by perivascular and interstitial mixed inflammatory infiltrates and myocyte damage, possibly mediated by viral cytolytic (e.g., cleavage of dystrophin or serum response factor) and innate and adaptive immune-mediated mechanisms. Chronic inflammation may persist after viral clearance.

The potential for enteroviruses to cause persistent infection is controversial. Persistent infection in dilated cardiomyopathy and in myocardial infarction has been suggested, but enterovirus RNA sequences and/or antigens have been demonstrated in cardiac tissues in some, but not other, series. Infections with enteroviruses such as coxsackievirus B4, during gestation or subsequently, have been implicated as a trigger for development of β-cell autoantibodies and/or type 1 diabetes in genetically susceptible hosts. Persistent infection in the pancreas, intestine, or peripheral blood mononuclear cells, with downstream immunomodulatory effects, has been suggested, but data are inconsistent. Similarly, persistent infection has been implicated in a variety of conditions, including amyotrophic lateral sclerosis, Sjögren syndrome, chronic fatigue syndrome, and gastrointestinal tumors. Early enterovirus infection was associated with reduced risk of developing lymphocytic and myeloid leukemia in 1 large retrospective Taiwanese cohort study.

Severe **neonatal infections** can produce hepatic necrosis, hemorrhage, inflammation, endotheliitis, and venoocclusive disease; myocardial mixed inflammatory infiltrates, edema, and necrosis; meningeal and brain inflammation, hemorrhage, gliosis, necrosis, and white matter damage; inflammation, hemorrhage, thrombosis, and necrosis in the lungs, pancreas, and adrenal glands; and disseminated intravascular coagulation. In utero infections are characterized by placentitis and infection of multiple fetal organs such as heart, lung, and brain.

Development of type-specific neutralizing antibodies appears to be the most important immune defense, mediating prevention against and recovery from infection. Immunoglobulin (Ig) M antibodies, followed by long-lasting IgA and IgG antibodies, and secretory IgA, mediating mucosal immunity, are produced. Although local reinfection of the gastrointestinal tract can occur, replication is usually limited and not associated with disease. In vitro and animal experiments suggest that heterotypic antibody may enhance disease caused by a different serotype. Evidence also suggests that subneutralizing concentrations of serotype-specific antibody may lead to antibody-dependent enhancement of enterovirus A71 infection. Innate and cellular defenses (macrophages and cytotoxic T lymphocytes) may play important roles in recovery from infection. Altered cellular responses to enterovirus A71, including T lymphocyte and natural killer cell depletion, were associated with severe meningoencephalitis and pulmonary edema.

Hypogammaglobulinemia and *agammaglobulinemia predispose to severe, often chronic enterovirus infections.* Similarly, perinatally infected neonates lacking maternal type-specific antibody to the infecting virus are at risk for severe disease. Enterovirus A71 disease increases after 6 mo of age, when maternal serotype-specific antibody levels have declined. Other risk factors for significant illness include young age, immune suppression (posttransplantation and lymphoid malignancy), and, according to animal models and/or epidemiologic observations, exercise, cold exposure, malnutrition, and pregnancy. Specific human leukocyte antigen genes, immune response gene (e.g., interleukin-10 and interferon-γ) polymorphisms, and low vitamin A levels have been linked to enterovirus A71 susceptibility and severe disease.

CLINICAL MANIFESTATIONS

Manifestations are protean, ranging from asymptomatic infection to undifferentiated febrile or respiratory illnesses in the majority, to, less frequently, severe diseases such as meningoencephalitis, myocarditis, and neonatal sepsis. A majority of individuals are asymptomatic or have very mild illness, yet may serve as important sources for spread of infection. Symptomatic disease is generally more common in young children.

Nonspecific Febrile Illness

Nonspecific febrile illnesses are the most common symptomatic manifestations, especially in infants and young children. These are difficult to clinically differentiate from serious infections such as urinary tract infection, bacteremia, and bacterial meningitis, often necessitating hospitalization with diagnostic testing and presumptive antibiotic therapy for suspected bacterial infection in young infants.

Illness usually begins abruptly with fever of 38.5-40°C (101-104°F), malaise, and irritability. Associated symptoms may include lethargy, anorexia, diarrhea, nausea, vomiting, abdominal discomfort, rash, sore throat, and respiratory symptoms. Older children may have headaches and myalgias. Findings are generally nonspecific and may include mild conjunctivitis, pharyngeal injection, and cervical lymphadenopathy. Meningitis may be present, but specific clinical features such as meningeal findings or bulging anterior fontanelle distinguishing those with meningitis are often lacking in infants. Fever lasts a mean of 3 days and occasionally is biphasic. Duration of illness is usually 4-7 days but can range from 1 day to >1 wk. White blood cell (WBC) count and results of routine laboratory tests are generally normal, although transient neutropenia can be seen. Concomitant enterovirus and bacterial infection is rare but has been observed in a small number of infants.

Enterovirus illnesses may be associated with a wide variety of skin manifestations, including macular, maculopapular, urticarial, vesicular, and petechial eruptions. Rare cases of idiopathic thrombocytopenic purpura have been reported. Enteroviruses have also been implicated in cases of pityriasis rosea. In general, the frequency of cutaneous manifestations is inversely related to age. Serotypes commonly associated with rashes are echoviruses 9, 11, 16, and 25; coxsackie A viruses 2, 4, 6, 9, and 16; coxsackie B viruses 3-5; and enterovirus A71. Virus can occasionally be recovered from vesicular skin lesions.

Hand-Foot-and-Mouth Disease

Hand-foot-and-mouth disease, one of the more distinctive rash syndromes, is most frequently caused by coxsackievirus A16, sometimes in large outbreaks, and can also be caused by enterovirus A71; coxsackie A viruses 5, 6, 7, 9, and 10; coxsackie B viruses 2 and 5; and some echoviruses. It is usually a mild illness, with or without low-grade fever. When the mouth is involved, the oropharynx is inflamed and often contains scattered, painful vesicles on the tongue, buccal mucosa, posterior pharynx, palate, gingiva, and/or lips (Fig. 277.1). These may ulcerate, leaving 4-8 mm shallow lesions with surrounding erythema. Maculopapular, vesicular, and/or pustular lesions may occur on the hands and fingers, feet, and buttocks and groin (see Figs. 277.1 and 277.2). Skin lesions occur more commonly on the hands than feet and are more common on dorsal surfaces, but frequently also affect palms and soles. Hand and feet lesions are usually tender, 3-7 mm vesicles that resolve in about 1 wk. Buttock lesions do not usually progress to vesiculation. Disseminated vesicular

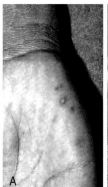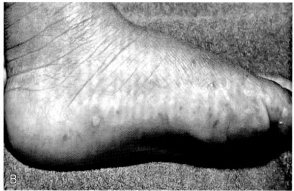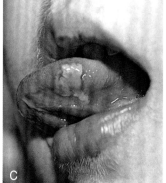

Fig. 277.1 A, Oval blisters of the palms in a child with hand-foot-and-mouth disease (coxsackievirus A16 infection). **B,** Oval blisters on the feet of a child with hand-foot-and-mouth disease. **C,** Erosion of the tongue in a child with hand-foot-and-mouth disease. *(From Weston WL, Lane AT, Morelli JG: Color textbook of pediatric dermatology, ed 3, St. Louis, 2002, Mosby, p. 109.)*

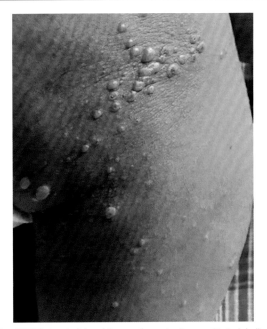

Fig. 277.2 Atypical hand-foot-and-mouth disease. Vesiculobullous rash on the right buttock and posterior thigh. *(From Waldman A, Thomas L, Thacker S, et al: Vesiculobullous eruption as an atypical hand, foot, and mouth presentation. J Pediatr 179:273, 2016, Fig. B.)*

rashes described as **eczema coxsackium** may complicate preexisting eczema. Coxsackievirus A6, in particular, is responsible for relatively severe, atypical hand-foot-and-mouth disease (and herpangina) affecting adults and children that is characterized by fever, generalized rash (face, proximal extremities, and trunk, in addition to hands, feet, and buttocks), pain, dehydration, and desquamation of palms and soles (Fig. 277.2). **Onychomadesis** (nail shedding) has been observed following coxsackievirus A6 and other coxsackievirus infections. Hand-foot-and-mouth disease caused by enterovirus A71 can be associated with neurologic and cardiopulmonary involvement, especially in young children (see Neurologic Manifestations below). Hand-foot-and-mouth disease caused by coxsackievirus A16 also can occasionally be associated with complications such as encephalitis, acute flaccid paralysis, myocarditis, pericarditis, and shock.

Herpangina

Herpangina is characterized by sudden onset of fever, sore throat, dysphagia, and painful lesions in the posterior pharynx. Temperatures range from normal to 41°C (106°F); fever tends to be higher in younger patients. Headache and backache may occur in older children, and vomiting and abdominal pain occur in 25% of cases. Characteristic lesions, present on the anterior tonsillar pillars, soft palate, uvula, tonsils, posterior pharyngeal wall, and, occasionally, the posterior buccal surfaces, are discrete 1-2 mm vesicles and ulcers that enlarge over 2-3 days to 3-4 mm and are surrounded by erythematous rings that vary in size up to 10 mm. The number of lesions can range from 1 to >15, but is most commonly around 5. The remainder of the pharynx appears normal or minimally erythematous. Most cases are mild and have no complications. However, dehydration due to decreased oral intake may occur and some cases are associated with meningitis or more severe illness. Fever generally lasts 1-4 days, and resolution of symptoms occurs in 3-7 days. A variety of enteroviruses cause herpangina, including enterovirus A71, but coxsackie A viruses are implicated most often.

Respiratory Manifestations

Symptoms such as sore throat and coryza frequently accompany and sometimes dominate enterovirus illnesses. Other respiratory findings may include wheezing, exacerbation of asthma, apnea, respiratory distress,

pneumonia, otitis media, bronchiolitis, croup, parotitis, and pharyngotonsillitis, which may occasionally be exudative. Lower respiratory tract infection may be significant in immunocompromised patients. Clusters and outbreaks of cases of severe respiratory disease, including pneumonia and wheezing (both in children with a history of asthma and those unaffected by asthma), have been increasingly recognized in association with multiple lineages of enterovirus D68.

Pleurodynia (Bornholm disease), caused most frequently by coxsackie B viruses 3, 5, 1, and 2 and echoviruses 1 and 6, is an epidemic or sporadic illness characterized by paroxysmal thoracic pain, due to myositis involving chest and abdominal wall muscles and, possibly, pleural inflammation. In epidemics, which occur every 10-20 yr, children and adults are affected, but most cases occur in persons younger than age 30 yr. Malaise, myalgias, and headache are followed by sudden onset of fever and spasmodic, pleuritic pain in the chest or upper abdomen aggravated by coughing, sneezing, deep breathing, or other movement. During spasms, which last from a few minutes to several hours, pain may be severe and respirations are usually rapid, shallow, and grunting, suggesting pneumonia or pleural inflammation. A pleural friction rub is noted during pain episodes in <10% of patients. Chest radiographs are generally normal but can demonstrate pulmonary infiltrates or pleural effusions. Pain localized to the abdomen may suggest colic, intestinal obstruction, appendicitis, or peritonitis. Pain usually subsides within 3-6 days but can persist for up to weeks. Symptoms may occur in a biphasic or, rarely, recurrent pattern, with less prominent fever during recurrences. Pleurodynia may be associated with meningitis, orchitis, myocarditis, or pericarditis.

Life-threatening noncardiogenic pulmonary edema, hemorrhage, and/or interstitial pneumonitis may occur in patients with enterovirus A71 brainstem encephalitis.

Ocular Manifestations

Epidemics of **acute hemorrhagic conjunctivitis,** primarily caused by enterovirus D70 and coxsackievirus A24/A24 variant, are explosive and marked by high contagiousness, with spread mainly via eye-hand-fomite-eye transmission. School-age children, teenagers, and adults 20-50 yr of age have the highest attack rates. Sudden onset of severe eye pain is associated with photophobia, blurred vision, lacrimation, conjunctival erythema and congestion, lid edema, preauricular lymphadenopathy, and, in some cases, subconjunctival hemorrhages and superficial punctate keratitis. Subconjunctival hemorrhage is the hallmark of enterovirus D70 cases (>70%) but is more rare with coxsackievirus infections. Eye discharge is initially serous but becomes mucopurulent with secondary bacterial infection. Systemic symptoms including fever and headache occur in up to 20% of cases; manifestations suggestive of pharyngoconjunctival fever occasionally occur. Recovery is usually complete within 1-2 wk. Polyradiculoneuropathy or acute flaccid paralysis following enterovirus D70 infection occurs occasionally. Other enteroviruses have occasionally been implicated as causes of keratoconjunctivitis.

Epidemic and sporadic uveitis in infants caused by subtypes of enteroviruses 11 and 19 can be associated with severe complications, including destruction of the iris, cataracts, and glaucoma. Enteroviruses have been implicated in cases of chorioretinitis, uveoretinitis, optic neuritis, and unilateral acute idiopathic maculopathy.

Myocarditis and Pericarditis

Enteroviruses account for approximately 25–35% of cases of myocarditis and pericarditis of proven etiology (see Chapters 466 and 467). Coxsackie B viruses are most commonly implicated, although coxsackie A viruses and echoviruses also may be causative. Adolescents and young adults (especially physically active males) are disproportionately affected. Myopericarditis may be the dominant feature or it may be 1 manifestation of disseminated disease, as in neonates. Disease ranges from relatively mild to severe. Upper respiratory symptoms frequently precede fatigue, dyspnea, chest pain, congestive heart failure, and dysrhythmias. Presentations may mimic myocardial infarction; sudden death may also occur (including apparent sudden infant death syndrome). A pericardial friction rub indicates pericardial involvement. Chest radiography often demonstrates cardiac enlargement and echocardiography may confirm ventricular dilation, reduced contractility, and/or pericardial effusion. Electrocardiography frequently reveals ST segment, T wave, and/or rhythm abnormalities, and serum myocardial enzyme concentrations are often elevated. The acute mortality of enterovirus myocarditis is 0–4%. Recovery is complete without residual disability in the majority of patients. Occasionally, chronic cardiomyopathy, inflammatory ventricular microaneurysms, or constrictive pericarditis may result. The role of persistent infection in chronic dilated cardiomyopathy is controversial. Enteroviruses have also been implicated in late adverse cardiac events following heart transplantation and in acute coronary events, including myocardial infarction, endocarditis, and peripartum cardiomyopathy. Cardiopulmonary dysfunction observed in enterovirus A71 epidemics most commonly occurs without evidence of myocarditis and may be of neurogenic origin; however, true myocarditis has also been described.

Gastrointestinal and Genitourinary Manifestations

Gastrointestinal symptoms such as emesis (especially with meningitis), diarrhea (rarely severe), and abdominal pain are frequent but generally not dominant. Diarrhea, hematochezia, pneumatosis intestinalis, and necrotizing enterocolitis have occurred in premature infants during nursery outbreaks. Enterovirus infection has been implicated in acute and chronic gastritis, intussusception, chronic intestinal inflammation in hypogammaglobulinemic patients, sporadic hepatitis in normal children, severe hepatitis in neonates, and pancreatitis, which may result in transient exocrine pancreatic insufficiency.

Coxsackie B viruses are second only to mumps as causes of orchitis, most commonly presenting in adolescents. The illness is frequently biphasic; fever and pleurodynia or meningitis are followed approximately 2 wk later by orchitis, often with epididymitis. Enteroviruses have also been implicated in cases of nephritis and IgA nephropathy.

Neurologic Manifestations

Enteroviruses are the most common cause of viral **meningitis** in mumps-immunized populations, accounting for up to 90% or more of cases in which a cause is identified. Meningitis is particularly common in infants, especially in those younger than 3 mo of age, often during community epidemics. Frequently implicated serotypes include coxsackie B viruses 2-5; echoviruses 4, 6, 7, 9, 11, 13, 16, and 30; and enteroviruses D70 and A71. Most cases in infants and young children are mild and lack specific meningeal signs, whereas nuchal rigidity is apparent in more than half of children older than 1-2 yr of age. Fever is present in 50–100% and may be accompanied by irritability, malaise, headache, photophobia, nausea, emesis, anorexia, lethargy, hypotonia, rash, cough, rhinorrhea, pharyngitis, diarrhea, and/or myalgia. Some cases are biphasic, with fever and nonspecific symptoms lasting a few days and followed by return of fever with meningeal signs several days later. Fever usually resolves in 3-5 days, and other symptoms in infants and young children usually resolve within 1 wk. In adults, symptoms tend to be more severe and of longer duration. CSF findings include pleocytosis (generally <500 but occasionally as high as 1,000-8,000 WBCs/µL; often predominantly polymorphonuclear cells in the first 48 hr before becoming mostly mononuclear); normal or slightly low glucose content (10% <40 mg/dL); and normal or mildly increased protein content (generally <100 mg/dL). *CSF parameters are normal in up to half of young infants despite detection of enterovirus in CSF and may also be normal in older children early after illness onset.* Acute complications occur in approximately 10% of young children, including simple and complex seizures, obtundation, increased intracranial pressure, syndrome of inappropriate antidiuretic hormone secretion, ventriculitis, transient cerebral arteriopathy, and coma. The long-term prognosis for most children, even in those with acute complications, is good.

Enteroviruses are also responsible for ≥10–20% of cases of **encephalitis** with an identified cause. Frequently implicated serotypes include echoviruses 3, 4, 6, 9, and 11; coxsackie B viruses 2, 4, and 5; coxsackie A virus 9; and enterovirus A71. After initial nonspecific symptoms, there is progression to encephalopathy characterized by confusion, weakness, lethargy, and/or irritability. Symptoms are most commonly generalized, although focal findings, including focal motor seizures,

hemichorea, acute cerebellar ataxia, aphasia, extrapyramidal symptoms, and/or focal imaging abnormalities, may occur. Meningeal signs and CSF indices similar to enteroviral meningitis are commonly present, leading to characterization of most cases as **meningoencephalitis**. Severity ranges from mild alteration in mental status to coma and decerebrate status. Long-term sequelae, including epilepsy, weakness, cranial nerve palsy, spasticity, psychomotor retardation, and hearing loss, or death may follow severe disease. Persistent or recurrent cases have been observed rarely.

Neurologic manifestations have been prominent in epidemics in Asia and Australia of enterovirus A71 and, to a lesser extent, coxsackievirus A16 disease. Many affected children have had hand-foot-and-mouth disease, some have had herpangina, and others have had no mucocutaneous manifestations. Neurologic syndromes in a fraction of children have included meningitis, meningoencephalomyelitis, **acute flaccid paralysis**, Guillain-Barré syndrome, transverse myelitis, acute disseminated encephalomyelitis, cerebellar ataxia, opsoclonus-myoclonus syndrome, benign intracranial hypertension, and **brainstem encephalitis** (**rhombencephalitis** involving the midbrain, pons, and medulla). Enterovirus A71 rhombencephalitis is characterized by altered consciousness, myoclonus, vomiting, ataxia, nystagmus, tremor, cranial nerve abnormalities, autonomic dysfunction, and MRI demonstrating lesions in the brainstem, thalamus, and cerebellum. Although the disease has been mild and reversible in some children, others have had rapid progression to noncardiogenic (presumed neurogenic) pulmonary edema and hemorrhage, cardiopulmonary failure, shock, and coma. High mortality rates have been reported in children younger than 5 yr of age, especially in those younger than 1 yr of age. Deficits such as central hypoventilation, bulbar dysfunction, neurodevelopmental delay, cerebellar defects, attention deficit/hyperactivity–related symptoms, persistent limb weakness, and muscle atrophy have been observed among survivors, especially those who experienced cardiopulmonary failure or acute flaccid paralysis during their acute illness. Although the most severe cases have been associated with enterovirus A71, similar clinical pictures have been produced by other enterovirus serotypes (e.g., coxsackieviruses A16 and B5, echovirus 7).

Patients with **antibody or combined immunodeficiencies** (including human immunodeficiency virus infection, acute lymphocytic leukemia, and transplantation) and patients receiving anti-CD20 antibody therapy are at risk for acute or, more commonly, **chronic enterovirus meningoencephalitis**. The latter is characterized by persistent CSF abnormalities, viral detection in CSF or brain tissue for years, and recurrent encephalitis and/or progressive neurologic deterioration, including insidious intellectual or personality deterioration, altered mental status, seizures, motor weakness, and increased intracranial pressure. Although disease may wax and wane, deficits generally become progressive and ultimately are frequently fatal or lead to long-term sequelae. A **dermatomyositis-like syndrome,** hepatitis, arthritis, myocarditis, or disseminated infection may also occur. Chronic enterovirus meningoencephalitis has become less common with prophylactic high-dose intravenous immunoglobulin replacement in agammaglobulinemic patients.

A variety of nonpoliovirus enteroviruses, including enteroviruses D68, D70, A71, coxsackie A viruses 7 and 24, coxsackie B viruses, and several echoviruses, have been associated with acute flaccid paralysis with motor weakness due to spinal cord anterior horn cell involvement. **Acute flaccid myelitis** is used to designate the clinical syndrome of acute flaccid limb weakness with longitudinal magnetic resonance imaging abnormalities in the spinal cord gray matter. Neurologic abnormalities are commonly preceded by a febrile respiratory or gastrointestinal prodromal illness around 1 wk prior to onset. Limb involvement tends to be asymmetric and varies from 1 to all 4 limbs, with severity ranging from mild weakness to complete paralysis. Cranial nerve dysfunction, including bulbar paralysis, and respiratory failure requiring ventilator support, similar to poliovirus poliomyelitis, have been described in acute flaccid myelitis cases associated with enterovirus D68. Sensory involvement, encephalopathy, seizures, and supratentorial imaging changes are uncommon. Functional improvements can be seen over time, but muscle atrophy with limb weakness and some degree of disability frequently persist.

Other neurologic syndromes include cerebellar ataxia; transverse myelitis; Guillain-Barré syndrome (including Miller-Fisher variant) and axonal polyneuropathy; acute disseminated encephalomyelitis; peripheral neuritis; optic neuritis; sudden hearing loss, tinnitus, and inner ear disorders such as vestibular neuritis; and other cranial neuropathies.

Myositis and Arthritis

Although myalgia is common, direct evidence of muscle involvement, including rhabdomyolysis, muscle swelling, focal myositis, and polymyositis, has uncommonly been reported. A dermatomyositis-like syndrome and arthritis can be seen in enterovirus-infected hypogammaglobulinemic patients. Enteroviruses are a rare cause of arthritis in normal hosts.

Neonatal Infections

Neonatal infections are relatively common, with a disease incidence comparable to or greater than that of symptomatic neonatal herpes simplex virus, cytomegalovirus, and group B streptococcus infections. Infection frequently is caused by coxsackie B viruses 2-5 and echoviruses 6, 9, 11, and 19, although many serotypes have been implicated, including coxsackie B virus 1 and echovirus 30 in more recent years. Enteroviruses may be acquired vertically before, during, or after delivery, including possibly via breast milk; horizontally from family members; or by sporadic or epidemic transmission in nurseries. In utero infection can lead to fetal demise, nonimmune hydrops fetalis, or neonatal illness. Additionally, maternal and intrauterine infections have been speculatively linked to congenital anomalies; prematurity, low birthweight, and intrauterine growth restriction; neurodevelopmental sequelae; unexplained neonatal illness and death; and increased risk of type 1 diabetes and schizophrenia.

The majority of neonatal infections are asymptomatic, and symptomatic presentations range from benign febrile illness to severe multisystem disease. Most affected newborns are full term and previously well. Maternal history often reveals a recent viral illness preceding or immediately following delivery, which may include fever and abdominal pain. Neonatal symptoms may occur as early as day 1 of life, with onset of severe disease generally within the first 2 wk of life. Frequent findings include fever or hypothermia, irritability, lethargy, anorexia, rash (usually maculopapular, occasionally petechial or papulovesicular), jaundice, respiratory symptoms, apnea, hepatomegaly, abdominal distention, emesis, diarrhea, and decreased perfusion. Most patients have benign courses, with resolution of fever in an average of 3 days and of other symptoms in about 1 wk. A biphasic course may occur occasionally. A minority have severe disease dominated by any combination of sepsis, meningoencephalitis, myocarditis, hepatitis, coagulopathy, and/or pneumonitis. Meningoencephalitis may be manifested by focal or complex seizures, bulging fontanelle, nuchal rigidity, and/or reduced level of consciousness. Myocarditis, most often associated with coxsackie B virus infection, may be suggested by tachycardia, dyspnea, cyanosis, and cardiomegaly. Hepatitis and pneumonitis are most often associated with echovirus infection, although they may also occur with coxsackie B viruses. Gastrointestinal manifestations may be prominent in premature neonates. Laboratory and radiographic evaluation may reveal leukocytosis, thrombocytopenia, CSF pleocytosis, CNS white matter damage, elevations of serum transaminases and bilirubin, coagulopathy, pulmonary infiltrates, and electrocardiographic changes.

Complications of severe neonatal disease include CNS necrosis and generalized or focal neurologic compromise; arrhythmias, congestive heart failure, myocardial infarction, and pericarditis; hepatic necrosis and failure; coagulopathy with intracranial or other bleeding; adrenal necrosis and hemorrhage; and rapidly progressive pneumonitis and pulmonary hypertension. Myositis, arthritis, necrotizing enterocolitis, inappropriate antidiuretic hormone secretion, hemophagocytic lymphohistiocytosis-like presentation, bone marrow failure, and sudden death are rare events. Mortality with severe disease is significant and is most often associated with hepatitis and bleeding complications, myocarditis, and/or pneumonitis.

Survivors of severe neonatal disease may have gradual resolution of hepatic and cardiac dysfunction, although persistent hepatic dysfunction and residual cardiac impairment, chronic calcific myocarditis, and

ventricular aneurysm can occur. Meningoencephalitis may be associated with speech and language impairment; cognitive deficits; spasticity, hypotonicity, or weakness; seizure disorders; microcephaly or hydrocephaly; and ocular abnormalities. However, many survivors appear to have no long-term sequelae. Risk factors for severe disease include illness onset in the first few days of life; maternal illness just prior to or after delivery; prematurity; male sex; infection by echovirus 11 or a coxsackie B virus; positive serum viral culture; absence of neutralizing antibody to the infecting virus; and evidence of severe hepatitis, myocarditis, and/or multisystem disease.

Transplant Recipients and Patients With Malignancies

Enterovirus infections in stem cell and solid organ transplant recipients may be severe and/or prolonged, causing progressive pneumonia, severe diarrhea, pericarditis, heart failure, meningoencephalitis, and disseminated disease. Enterovirus-associated hemophagocytic lymphohistiocytosis, meningitis, encephalitis, and myocarditis have been reported in children with malignancies and patients treated with anti-CD20 monoclonal antibody. Infections in these groups are associated with high fatality rates.

DIAGNOSIS

Clues to enterovirus infection include characteristic findings such as hand-foot-and-mouth disease or herpangina lesions, consistent seasonality, known community outbreak, and exposure to enterovirus-compatible disease. In the neonate, history of maternal fever, malaise, and/or abdominal pain near delivery during enterovirus season is suggestive.

Traditionally, enterovirus infection has been confirmed with viral culture using a combination of cell lines. Sensitivity of culture ranges from 50% to 75% and can be increased by sampling of multiple sites (e.g., CSF plus oropharynx and rectum in children with meningitis). In neonates, yields of 30–70% are achieved when blood, urine, CSF, and mucosal swabs are cultured. A major limitation is the inability of most coxsackie A viruses to grow in culture. Yield may also be limited by neutralizing antibody in patient specimens, improper specimen handling, or insensitivity of the cell lines used. Culture is relatively slow, with 3-8 days usually required to detect growth. Although cultivation of an enterovirus from any site can generally be considered evidence of recent infection, isolation from the rectum or stool can reflect more remote shedding. Similarly, recovery from a mucosal site may suggest an association with an illness, whereas recovery from a normally sterile site (e.g., CSF, blood, or tissue) is more conclusive evidence of causation. Serotype identification by type-specific antibody staining or neutralization of a viral isolate is generally required only for investigation of an outbreak or an unusual disease manifestation, surveillance, or to distinguish nonpoliovirus enteroviruses from vaccine or wild-type polioviruses.

Direct testing for nucleic acid has replaced culture due to increased sensitivity and more rapid turnaround. RT-PCR detection of highly conserved areas of the enterovirus genome can detect the majority of enteroviruses in CSF; serum; urine; conjunctival, nasopharyngeal, oropharyngeal, tracheal, rectal, and stool specimens; dried blood spots; and tissues such as myocardium, liver, and brain. However, the closely related parechoviruses are not detected by most enterovirus RT-PCR primers. Sensitivity and specificity of RT-PCR are high, with results available in as short as 1 hr. Real-time, quantitative PCR assays and nested PCR assays with enhanced sensitivity have been developed, as have enterovirus-containing multiplex PCR assays, nucleic acid sequence–based amplification assays, reverse transcription-loop-mediated isothermal amplification, culture-enhanced PCR assays, and PCR-based microarray assays. PCR testing of CSF from children with meningitis and from hypogammaglobulinemic patients with chronic meningoencephalitis is frequently positive despite negative cultures. Routine PCR testing of CSF in infants and young children with suspected meningitis during enterovirus season decreases the number of diagnostic tests, duration of hospital stay, antibiotic use, and overall costs. PCR testing of tracheal aspirates of children with myocarditis has good concordance with testing of myocardial specimens. In ill neonates and young infants, PCR testing of serum and urine has higher yields than culture. Viral load in blood of neonates is correlated with disease severity; viral nucleic acid may persist in blood of severely ill newborns for up to 2 mo.

Sequence analysis of amplified nucleic acid can be used for serotype identification and phylogenetic analysis and to establish a transmission link among cases. Serotype-specific (e.g., enterovirus A71, enterovirus D68, and coxsackievirus A16) PCR assays have been developed. For enterovirus A71, the yield of specimens other than CSF and blood (oropharyngeal, nasopharyngeal, rectal, vesicle swabs, and CNS tissue) is greater than the yield of CSF and blood, which are infrequently positive. Enterovirus D68 is more readily detected in respiratory specimens (i.e., nasal wash or nasopharyngeal swab) compared to stool/rectal or CSF specimens. Of note, commercially available multiplex respiratory PCR assays generally are unable to distinguish enteroviruses (including enterovirus D68) from rhinoviruses. Antigen detection assays that target specific serotypes such as enterovirus A71 with monoclonal antibodies have also been developed.

Enterovirus infections can be detected serologically by a rise in serum or CSF of neutralizing, complement fixation, enzyme-linked immunosorbent assay, or other type-specific antibody or by detection of serotype-specific IgM antibody. However, serologic testing requires presumptive knowledge of the infecting serotype or an assay with sufficiently broad cross-reactivity. Sensitivity and specificity may be limiting, and cross-reactivity among serotypes may occur. Except for epidemiologic studies or cases characteristic of specific serotypes (e.g., enterovirus A71), serology is generally less useful than culture or nucleic acid detection.

DIFFERENTIAL DIAGNOSIS

The differential diagnosis of enterovirus infections varies with the clinical presentation (Table 277.2).

Human parechoviruses, members of the Picornaviridae family, produce many manifestations similar to the nonpolio enteroviruses. They are small RNA viruses that were originally classified as echoviruses. Nineteen parechoviruses have been identified that infect humans; serotypes 1 and 3 are the most common causes of symptomatic infection. Parechovirus epidemics occur in the same season as enterovirus infections, with a biennial pattern of circulation noted in Europe. Outbreaks have been described in the nursery setting. In young infants, parechoviruses can cause a sepsis-like illness similar to enterovirus illness and are a common, underrecognized cause of viral meningoencephalitis. More frequently than with enteroviruses, infants with parechovirus CNS infection often have no CSF pleocytosis. There is also a higher incidence of white matter MRI abnormalities and long-term neurodevelopmental deficits with parechovirus encephalitis compared with enterovirus encephalitis. Rarely, parechoviruses have been identified in cases of hepatitis or myocarditis. Infections in older children are often unrecognized or cause acute, benign febrile, respiratory, or gastrointestinal illnesses with few specific findings.

Infants suspected of having an enterovirus infection should also be considered as possibly having a parechovirus infection, because the 2 may be indistinguishable. A distinctive rash involving the extremities with palm and sole erythema or peripheral leukopenia in the setting of high fever during the summer-fall season are clinical findings that should also prompt consideration of parechovirus infection. The diagnosis of parechovirus infection is confirmed by human parechovirus-specific PCR on CSF, blood, stool, and oropharyngeal or nasopharyngeal specimens.

TREATMENT

In the absence of a proven antiviral agent for enterovirus infections, supportive care is the mainstay of treatment. Newborns and young infants with nonspecific febrile illnesses and children with meningitis frequently require diagnostic evaluation and hospitalization for presumptive treatment of bacterial and herpes simplex virus infection. Neonates with severe disease and infants and children with concerning disease manifestations (e.g., myocarditis, enterovirus A71 neurologic and cardiopulmonary disease, enterovirus D68 respiratory failure, and acute flaccid myelitis) may require intensive cardiorespiratory support. Milrinone has been suggested as a useful agent in severe enterovirus A71 cardiopulmonary disease. Liver and cardiac transplantation have been performed for neonates with progressive end-organ failure.

Immunoglobulin has been utilized to treat enterovirus infections based on the importance of the humoral immune response to enterovirus infection and the observation that absence of neutralizing antibody is a risk factor for symptomatic infection. Immunoglobulin products contain neutralizing antibodies to many commonly circulating serotypes, although titers vary with serotype and among products and lots. Anecdotal and retrospective, uncontrolled use of intravenous immunoglobulin or infusion of maternal convalescent plasma to treat newborns with severe disease has been associated with varying outcomes. The 1 randomized, controlled trial was too small to demonstrate significant clinical benefits, although neonates who received immunoglobulin containing high neutralizing titers to their own isolates had shorter periods of viremia and viruria. Immunoglobulin has been administered intravenously and intraventricularly to treat hypogammaglobulinemic patients with chronic enterovirus meningoencephalitis and intravenously in transplant and oncology patients with severe infections, with variable success. Intravenous immunoglobulin and corticosteroids have been used for patients with neurologic disease caused by enterovirus A71, enterovirus D68, and other enteroviruses. Modulation of cytokine profiles after administration of intravenous immunoglobulin for enterovirus A71–associated brainstem encephalitis has been demonstrated. High-titer enterovirus A71 immunoglobulin appeared promising in animal models.

Table 277.2	Differential Diagnosis of Enterovirus Infections	
CLINICAL MANIFESTATION	**BACTERIAL PATHOGENS**	**VIRAL PATHOGENS**
Nonspecific febrile illness	*Streptococcus pneumoniae, Haemophilus influenzae* type b, *Neisseria meningitidis*	Influenza viruses, human herpesviruses 6 and 7, human parechoviruses
Exanthems/enanthems	Group A streptococcus, *Staphylococcus aureus, N. meningitidis*	Herpes simplex virus, adenoviruses, varicella-zoster virus, Epstein-Barr virus, measles virus, rubella virus, human herpesviruses 6 and 7, human parechoviruses
Respiratory illness/conjunctivitis	*S. pneumoniae, H. influenzae* (nontypeable and type b), *N. meningitidis, Mycoplasma pneumoniae, Chlamydia pneumoniae*	Adenoviruses, influenza viruses, respiratory syncytial virus, parainfluenza viruses, rhinoviruses, human metapneumovirus, coronaviruses
Myocarditis/pericarditis	*S. aureus, H. influenzae* type b, *M. pneumoniae*	Adenoviruses, influenza virus, parvovirus, cytomegalovirus
Meningitis/encephalitis	*S. pneumoniae, H. influenzae* type b, *N. meningitidis, Mycobacterium tuberculosis, Borrelia burgdorferi, M. pneumoniae, Bartonella henselae, Listeria monocytogenes*	Herpes simplex virus, West Nile virus, influenza viruses, adenoviruses, Epstein-Barr virus, mumps virus, lymphocytic choriomeningitis virus, arboviruses, human parechoviruses
Neonatal infections	Group B streptococcus, Gram-negative enteric bacilli, *L. monocytogenes, Enterococcus*	Herpes simplex virus, adenoviruses, cytomegalovirus, rubella virus, human parechoviruses

and clinical trials in regions with epidemic enterovirus A71 disease are ongoing. Anti–enterovirus A71 monoclonal antibodies have also been generated and evaluated in vitro and in animal models. A retrospective study suggested that treatment of presumed viral myocarditis with immunoglobulin was associated with improved outcome; however, virologic diagnoses were not made. Evaluation of corticosteroids and cyclosporine and other immunosuppressive therapy for myocarditis has been inconclusive. Successful treatment of enterovirus myocarditis with interferon-α has been reported anecdotally, and interferon-β treatment was associated with viral clearance, improved cardiac function, and survival in chronic cardiomyopathy associated with persistence of enterovirus (or adenovirus) genome. Activity of interferon-α against enterovirus 71 has been demonstrated in in vitro and animal models, but potency varies with interferon-α type.

Antiviral agents that act at various steps in the enterovirus life cycle—attachment, penetration, uncoating, translation, polyprotein processing, protease activity, replication, and assembly—are being evaluated. Candidates include pharmacologically active chemical compounds, small interfering RNAs and DNA-like antisense agents, purine nucleoside analogs, synthetic peptides, enzyme inhibitors of signal transduction pathways, interferon-inducers, and herbal compounds. Pleconaril, an inhibitor of attachment and uncoating, was associated with benefit in some controlled studies of enterovirus meningitis and picornavirus upper respiratory tract infections, and uncontrolled experience suggested possible benefits in high-risk infections. A randomized, controlled trial of pleconaril in neonates with severe hepatitis, coagulopathy, and/or myocarditis suggested possible virologic and clinical benefits of treatment. Pocapavir, an agent with a similar mechanism of action that is in development for treatment of poliovirus infections, has been used in a small number of cases of severe neonatal enterovirus sepsis. Vapendavir is another attachment inhibitor that is in clinical trials for rhinovirus infections and has in vitro activity against enteroviruses (including enterovirus A71) but has not entered clinical trials for enterovirus infections. Pleconaril, pocapavir, and vapendavir are not currently available for clinical use.

Design and evaluation of candidate agents active against enterovirus A71 and enterovirus D68 are high priorities. Challenges for therapies of enterovirus A71 include limited cross-genotypic activity of candidate compounds and high viral mutagenicity that favors emergence of resistance. Lactoferrin and ribavirin have demonstrated activity in in vitro and/or animal models. The investigational agents rupintrivir and V-7404, which inhibit the 3C-protease conserved among many enteroviruses and essential for infectivity, have broad activity in vitro, including against both enterovirus A71 and enterovirus D68. DAS181 is an investigational, inhaled drug with sialidase activity that has in vitro activity against recently circulating strains of enterovirus D68. The antidepressant fluoxetine interacts with the enterovirus 2C protein and has in vitro activity against group B and D enteroviruses; it has been used anecdotally for chronic enterovirus encephalitis associated with agammaglobulinemia and enterovirus D68-associated acute flaccid myelitis. A retrospective study did not demonstrate a signal of efficacy in the latter condition.

COMPLICATIONS AND PROGNOSIS

The prognosis in the majority of enterovirus infections is excellent. Morbidity and mortality are associated primarily with myocarditis, neurologic disease, severe neonatal infections, and infections in immune compromised hosts.

Prevention

The first line of defense is prevention of transmission through good hygiene, such as handwashing, avoidance of sharing utensils and drinking containers and other potential fomites, disinfection of contaminated surfaces, and avoiding community settings where exposures are likely to occur. Chlorination of drinking water and swimming pools may be important. Contact precautions should be used for all patients with enterovirus infections in the hospital setting; droplet precautions should also be included for patients with respiratory syndromes and, possibly, enterovirus A71 infection. Infection control techniques such as cohorting have proven effective in limiting nursery outbreaks. Prophylactic administration of immunoglobulin or convalescent plasma has been used in nursery epidemics; simultaneous use of infection control interventions makes it difficult to determine efficacy.

Pregnant women near term should avoid contact with individuals ill with possible enterovirus infections. If a pregnant woman experiences a suggestive illness, it is advisable not to proceed with emergency delivery unless there is concern for fetal compromise or obstetric emergencies cannot be excluded. Rather, it may be advantageous to extend pregnancy, allowing the fetus to passively acquire protective antibodies. A strategy of prophylactically administering immunoglobulin (or maternal convalescent plasma) to neonates born to mothers with enterovirus infections is untested.

Maintenance antibody replacement with high-dose intravenous immunoglobulin for patients with hypogammaglobulinemia has reduced the incidence of chronic enterovirus meningoencephalitis, although breakthrough infections occur. Inactivated vaccines to prevent enterovirus A71 infections have been demonstrated to be safe and effective (>90% against enterovirus A71 hand-foot-and-mouth disease and >80% against enterovirus A71 serious disease) in phase 3 clinical trials. Inactivated enterovirus A71 vaccines have been approved for prevention of severe hand-foot-and-mouth disease in China and are being studied in other Asian countries. Other vaccine strategies for enterovirus A71, including VP1 capsid protein-based subunit, DNA, and vector vaccines; combined peptide vaccines; live-attenuated vaccines; virus-like particles; breast milk enriched with VP1 capsid protein or lactoferrin; and interferon-γ–expressing recombinant viral vectors, are also under investigation. Circulation of multiple enterovirus A71 types, antigenic drift, viral recombination, and potential immunologic cross-reactivity with brain tissue may pose challenges to development of enterovirus A71 vaccines.

Bibliography is available at Expert Consult.

Chapter **278**

Parvoviruses

William C. Koch

第二百七十八章

细小病毒

中文导读

本章主要介绍了细小病毒感染的病因学、流行病学、发病机制、临床表现、诊断、鉴别诊断、治疗、并发症和预防，其中重点介绍了细小病毒B19和人博卡病毒。细小病毒B19感染的临床表现包括传染性红斑（第五病）、关节病变、再生障碍性危象、心肌炎、胎儿感染、免疫功能低下者感染，其他皮肤表现包括丘疹-紫癜性手套袜子综合征。人博卡病毒感染临床表现包括上呼吸道感染、肺炎、病毒血症等。实验室诊断包括血清学和DNA检测。本病尚无特异性抗病毒药，治疗可给予免疫球蛋白。

The parvoviruses are small, single-stranded DNA viruses. They are common infectious agents of a variety of animal species, including mammals, birds, and insects. Parvoviruses as a group include a number of important animal pathogens. There are 5 different types of parvoviruses known to infect humans: the dependoviruses, also called adeno-associated viruses (AAV), parvovirus B19 (B19V), human bocaviruses (HBoV), parvovirus 4 (PARV4), and human bufavirus (HBuV). B19V and HBoV are the only 2 parvoviruses known to be pathogenic in humans. B19V is the most well studied and clinically important of the human parvoviruses and the cause of **erythema infectiosum** or **fifth disease**. *The more recently described human bocavirus is an emerging human pathogen.*

ETIOLOGY

The 5 human parvoviruses are distinct enough from each other to represent 5 different genera within the Parvoviridae family. B19V is a member of the genus *Erythroparvovirus*. The virus is composed of an icosahedral protein capsid without an envelope and contains a single-stranded DNA genome of approximately 5.5 kb. It is relatively heat and solvent resistant. It is antigenically distinct from other mammalian parvoviruses and has only 1 known serotype, with 3 distinct genotypes described. The relatively short parvovirus genome does not encode a DNA polymerase, so all parvoviruses require either host cell factors present in late S phase or coinfection with another virus to replicate their DNA. B19V can be propagated effectively in vitro only in CD36+ erythroid progenitor cells derived from human bone marrow, umbilical cord blood, or peripheral blood.

HBoV is a member of the genus *Bocaparvovirus*. HBoV was first isolated from nasopharyngeal specimens from children with respiratory tract infection in 2005. It was identified using random polymerase chain reaction (PCR) amplification and sequencing methods specifically designed to detect previously unknown viral sequences. Analysis of the gene sequences showed similarities to both bovine and canine parvoviruses, and thus the virus was named human bocavirus. Later, 3 other HBoVs were identified in stool samples and named HBoV types 2, 3, and 4, with the initial respiratory isolate called HBoV1. The HBoV capsid structure and genome size are similar to those of B19V, but the genomic organization and replication are different (though not fully characterized to date). HBoVs cannot be propagated in conventional cell culture but have been grown in a pseudostratified human airway epithelial cell culture system.

The AAVs are members of the genus *Dependoparvovirus* and were the first parvoviruses to be found in humans. They were originally identified as contaminants in adenovirus preparations, resulting in the designation AAV. They were later isolated directly from human tissue samples, and now several AAV serotypes are known to commonly infect humans. AAVs have a unique life cycle that can take 1 of 2 paths: (1) a lytic infection with replication of viral DNA and production of new virus, or (2) viral integration into the host cell DNA. In the presence of a "helper" virus, usually an adenovirus or a herpesvirus, AAV can replicate its DNA, produce capsids, and release new virions by cell lysis. In the absence of a helper virus infection, the AAV genome becomes integrated into the host cell DNA. This feature has drawn interest in AAVs as potential vectors for gene therapy. Although human infection with AAVs is common, there is no known disease association and no evidence of pathogenicity, so this virus will not be discussed further in this chapter.

PARV4 was initially identified in 2005 from the blood of an adult patient with acute viral syndrome, who was also an intravenous drug user co-infected with hepatitis C. Subsequently, this virus has been found in blood donors and donated plasma pools in many different countries. It appears to be present in approximately 3% of blood donors in the United States and 4% of plasma pools. There is currently no known disease association or clinical symptomology associated with infection. Likewise, BuV is a parvovirus that has recently been found to infect humans but its role as a pathogen is undetermined. It was first identified in 2012 in the feces from children <5 yr of age with acute diarrhea. BuV is a member of the genus *Protoparvovirus*, and PARV4 has been assigned to a new parvovirus genus, *Tetraparvovirus*. The full epidemiology and clinical relevance of both of these viruses await further study.

EPIDEMIOLOGY
Parvovirus B19

Infections with B19V are common and occur worldwide. Clinically apparent infections, such as the rash illness of erythema infectiosum and transient aplastic crisis, are most prevalent in school-age children (70% of cases occur in patients between 5 and 15 yr of age). Seasonal peaks occur in the late winter and spring, with sporadic infections throughout the year. Seroprevalence increases with age, with 40–60% of adults having evidence of prior infection.

Transmission of B19V is by the respiratory route, presumably via large-droplet spread from nasopharyngeal viral shedding. The transmission rate is 15–30% among susceptible household contacts, and mothers are more commonly infected than fathers. In outbreaks of erythema infectiosum in elementary schools, the secondary attack rates range from 10% to 60%. Nosocomial outbreaks also occur, with secondary attack rates of 30% among susceptible healthcare workers.

Although respiratory spread is the primary mode of transmission, B19V is also transmissible in blood and blood products, as documented among children with hemophilia receiving pooled-donor clotting factor. Given the resistance of the virus to solvents, fomite transmission could be important in childcare centers and other group settings, but this mode of transmission has not been established.

Human Bocaviruses

The majority of published studies have used molecular methods to detect HBoV DNA in respiratory secretions, fecal samples, blood, and other tissues. HBoV DNA (HBoV1) can be found commonly in respiratory secretions from children hospitalized with acute lower respiratory tract infections (LRTIs). It is more prevalent in children younger than 2 yr of age and seems to be associated with wheezing respiratory illness. However, it can be isolated from respiratory secretions from asymptomatic children and can often be found as a coinfection with other common respiratory pathogens of children this age, including respiratory syncytial virus, human metapneumovirus, and rhinoviruses. This has caused some confusion as to the pathogenic role of HBoV in acute LRTI, including whether it can persist in secretions long after a subclinical infection or requires a helper virus. A limited number of seroepidemiologic studies have been performed, and these suggest that infection is common in children younger than 5 yr of age. The most recent studies provide evidence that the virus is in fact pathogenic, especially in children younger than 2 yr with wheezing and LRTI, as HBoV1 is more likely to be the only virus isolated in these patients and more likely to have an acute antibody response when coupled with antibody testing. When quantitative PCR is used, the virus is found to be much higher in titer in these symptomatic cases.

HBoV DNA (HBoV2, HBoV3, and HBoV4) has also been found in fecal samples in studies from various countries, but its role as a cause of viral gastroenteritis is still undetermined.

PATHOGENESIS
Parvovirus B19

The primary target of B19 infection is the erythroid cell line, specifically erythroid precursors near the pronormoblast stage. Viral infection produces cell lysis, leading to a progressive depletion of erythroid precursors and a transient arrest of erythropoiesis. The virus has no apparent effect on the myeloid cell line. The tropism for erythroid cells is related to the erythrocyte P blood group antigen, which is the primary cell receptor for the virus and is also found on endothelial cells, placental cells, and fetal myocardial cells. Thrombocytopenia and neutropenia are often observed clinically, but the pathogenesis of these abnormalities is unexplained.

Experimental infection of normal volunteers with B19V revealed a biphasic illness. From 7 to 11 days after inoculation, subjects had viremia and nasopharyngeal viral shedding with fever, malaise, and rhinorrhea. Reticulocyte counts dropped to undetectable levels but resulted in only a mild, clinically insignificant fall in serum hemoglobin. With the appearance of specific antibodies, symptoms resolved and serum hemoglobin returned to normal. Several subjects experienced a rash associated with arthralgia 17-18 days after inoculation. Some manifestations of B19 infection, such as transient aplastic crisis, appear to be a direct result of viral infection, whereas others, including the exanthem and arthritis, appear to be **postinfectious phenomena** related to the immune response. Skin biopsy of patients with erythema infectiosum reveals edema in the epidermis and a perivascular mononuclear infiltrate compatible with an immune-mediated process.

Individuals with **chronic hemolytic anemia** and increased red blood cell (RBC) turnover are very sensitive to minor perturbations in erythropoiesis. Infection with B19V leads to a transient arrest in RBC production and a precipitous fall in serum hemoglobin, often requiring transfusion. The reticulocyte count drops to undetectable levels, reflecting the lysis of infected erythroid precursors. Humoral immunity is crucial in controlling infection. Specific immunoglobulin (Ig) M appears within 1-2 days of infection and is followed by anti-B19 IgG, which leads to control of the infection, restoration of reticulocytosis, and a rise in serum hemoglobin.

Individuals with **impaired humoral immunity** are at increased risk for more serious or persistent infection with B19V, which usually manifests as chronic RBC aplasia, although neutropenia, thrombocytopenia, and marrow failure are also described. Children undergoing chemotherapy for leukemia or other forms of cancer, transplant recipients, and patients with congenital or acquired immunodeficiency states (including AIDS) are at risk for chronic B19V infections.

Infections in the **fetus** and **neonate** are somewhat analogous to infections in immunocompromised persons. B19V is associated with nonimmune fetal hydrops and stillbirth in women experiencing a primary infection but does not appear to be teratogenic. Like most mammalian parvoviruses, B19V can cross the placenta and cause fetal infection during primary maternal infection. Parvovirus cytopathic effects are seen primarily in erythroblasts of the bone marrow and sites of extramedullary hematopoiesis in the liver and spleen. Fetal infection can presumably occur as early as 6 wk of gestation, when erythroblasts are first found in the fetal liver; after the 4th mo of gestation, hematopoiesis switches to the bone marrow. In some cases, fetal infection leads to profound fetal anemia and subsequent high-output cardiac failure (see Chapter 124). **Fetal hydrops** ensues and is often associated with fetal death. There may also be a direct effect of the virus on myocardial tissue that contributes to the cardiac failure. However, most infections during pregnancy result in normal deliveries at term. Some of the asymptomatic infants from these deliveries have been reported to have chronic postnatal infection with B19V that is of unknown significance.

Human Bocaviruses

Mechanisms of HBoV replication and pathogenesis are poorly characterized to date. Growth of HBoV1 in tissue culture is difficult, though the virus has been cultured in primary respiratory epithelial cells as noted above. The primary site of viral replication appears to be the respiratory tract, as the virus has been detected most frequently and in highest copy numbers here. HBoV1 has also been found occasionally in the serum, suggesting the potential for systemic spread. HBoV1 has also been detected in stool, but copy numbers are very low. In contrast, HBoV types 2-4 are found predominantly in the stool, but host cell types are not known.

CLINICAL MANIFESTATIONS
Parvovirus B19

Many infections are clinically inapparent. Infected children characteristically demonstrate the rash illness of erythema infectiosum. Adults, especially women, frequently experience acute polyarthropathy with or without a rash.

Erythema Infectiosum (Fifth Disease)

The most common manifestation of B19V is erythema infectiosum, also known as *fifth disease*, which is a benign, self-limited exanthematous illness of childhood.

The incubation period for erythema infectiosum is 4-28 days (average: 16-17 days). The prodromal phase is mild and consists of low-grade fever in 15–30% of cases, headache, and symptoms of mild upper respiratory tract infection. The hallmark of erythema infectiosum is the characteristic rash, which occurs in 3 stages that are not always distinguishable. The initial stage is an erythematous facial flushing, often described as a **slapped-cheek appearance** (Fig. 278.1). The rash spreads rapidly or concurrently to the trunk and proximal extremities as a diffuse macular erythema in the second stage. Central clearing of macular lesions occurs promptly, giving the rash a **lacy, reticulated appearance** (Fig. 278.2). The rash tends to be more prominent on extensor surfaces, sparing the palms and soles. Affected children are afebrile and do not appear ill. Some have petechiae. Older children and adults often complain of mild pruritus. The rash resolves spontaneously without desquamation, but tends to wax and wane over 1-3 wk. It can recur with exposure to sunlight, heat, exercise, and stress. Lymphadenopathy and atypical papular, purpuric, vesicular rashes are also described.

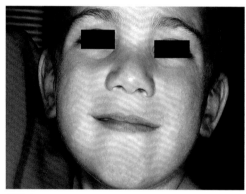

Fig. 278.1 Erythema infectiosum. Erythema of the bilateral cheeks, which has been likened to a "slapped-cheek" appearance. (*From Paller AS, Macini AJ: Hurwitz clinical pediatric dermatology, ed 3, Philadelphia, 2006, WB Saunders, p. 431.*)

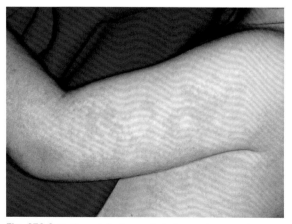

Fig. 278.2 Erythema infectiosum. Reticulate erythema on the upper arm of a patient with erythema infectiosum. (*From Paller AS, Macini AJ: Hurwitz clinical pediatric dermatology, ed 3, Philadelphia, 2006, WB Saunders, p. 431.*)

Arthropathy

Arthritis and arthralgia may occur in isolation or with other symptoms. Joint symptoms are much more common among adults and older adolescents with B19V infection. Females are affected more frequently than males. In 1 large outbreak of fifth disease, 60% of adults and 80% of adult women reported joint symptoms. Joint symptoms range from diffuse polyarthralgia with morning stiffness to frank arthritis. The joints most often affected are the hands, wrists, knees, and ankles, but practically any joint may be affected. The joint symptoms are self-limited and, in the majority of patients, resolve within 2-4 wk. Some patients may have a prolonged course of many months, suggesting rheumatoid arthritis. Transient rheumatoid factor positivity is reported in some of these patients but with no joint destruction.

Transient Aplastic Crisis

The transient arrest of erythropoiesis and absolute reticulocytopenia induced by B19V infection leads to a sudden fall in serum hemoglobin in individuals with chronic hemolytic conditions. This B19V-induced RBC aplasia or transient aplastic crisis occurs in patients with all types of chronic hemolysis and/or rapid RBC turnover, including sickle cell disease, thalassemia, hereditary spherocytosis, and pyruvate kinase deficiency. In contrast to children with erythema infectiosum only, patients with aplastic crisis are ill with fever, malaise, and lethargy and have signs and symptoms of profound anemia, including pallor, tachycardia, and tachypnea. Rash is rarely present. The incubation period for transient aplastic crisis is shorter than that for erythema infectiosum because the crisis occurs coincident with the viremia. Children with sickle cell hemoglobinopathies may also have a concurrent vasoocclusive pain crisis, further confusing the clinical presentation.

Immunocompromised Persons

Persons with impaired humoral immunity are at risk for chronic B19V infection. Chronic anemia is the most common manifestation, sometimes accompanied by neutropenia, thrombocytopenia, or complete marrow suppression. Chronic infections occur in persons receiving cancer chemotherapy or immunosuppressive therapy for transplantation and persons with congenital immunodeficiencies, AIDS, and functional defects in IgG production who are thereby unable to generate neutralizing antibodies.

Fetal Infection

Primary maternal infection is associated with nonimmune fetal hydrops and intrauterine fetal demise, with the risk for fetal loss after infection estimated at 2–5%. The mechanism of fetal disease appears to be a viral-induced RBC aplasia at a time when the fetal erythroid fraction is rapidly expanding, leading to profound anemia, high-output cardiac failure, and fetal hydrops. Viral DNA has been detected in infected abortuses. The second trimester seems to be the most sensitive period, but fetal losses are reported at every stage of gestation. If maternal B19V infection is suspected, fetal ultrasonography and measurement of the peak systolic flow velocity of the middle cerebral artery are sensitive, noninvasive procedures to diagnose fetal anemia and hydrops. Most infants infected in utero are born normally at term, including some who have had ultrasonographic evidence of hydrops. A small subset of infants infected in utero may acquire a chronic or persistent postnatal infection with B19V that is of unknown significance. Congenital anemia associated with intrauterine B19V infection has been reported in a few cases, sometimes following intrauterine hydrops. This process may mimic other forms of congenital hypoplastic anemia (e.g., Diamond-Blackfan syndrome). Fetal infection with B19V has been associated with bone lesions but has not been associated with other birth defects. B19V is only 1 of many causes of hydrops fetalis (see Chapter 124.2).

Myocarditis

B19V infection has been associated with myocarditis in fetuses, infants, children, and a few adults. Diagnosis has often been based on serologic findings suggestive of a concurrent B19V infection, but in many cases B19V DNA has been demonstrated in cardiac tissue. B19-related myocarditis is plausible because fetal myocardial cells are known to express P antigen, the cell receptor for the virus. In the few cases in which histology is reported, a predominantly lymphocytic infiltrate is described. Outcomes have varied from complete recovery to chronic cardiomyopathy to fatal cardiac arrest. Although B19-associated myocarditis seems to be a rare occurrence, there appears to be enough evidence to consider B19V as a potential cause of lymphocytic myocarditis, especially in infants and immunocompromised persons.

Other Cutaneous Manifestations

A variety of atypical skin eruptions have been reported with B19V infection. Most of these are petechial or purpuric in nature, often with evidence of vasculitis on biopsy. Among these rashes, the **papular-purpuric gloves-and-socks syndrome (PPGSS)** is well established in the dermatologic literature as distinctly associated with B19V infection (Fig. 278.3). PPGSS is characterized by fever, pruritus, and painful edema and erythema localized to the distal extremities in a distinct gloves-and-socks distribution, followed by acral petechiae and oral lesions. The syndrome is self-limited and resolves within a few weeks. Although PPGSS was initially described in young adults, a number of reports of the disease in children have since been published. In those cases linked to B19V infection, the eruption is accompanied by serologic evidence of acute infection. Generalized petechiae have also been reported.

Human Bocaviruses

Many studies have reported an association between respiratory tract infection and HBoV1 infection as detected by PCR of respiratory secretions, primarily nasopharyngeal secretions. Clinical manifestations in these studies have ranged from mild upper respiratory symptoms to pneumonia. However, the role of HBoV1 as a pathogen has been challenged by the detection of the virus in asymptomatic children and by the frequent detection of other respiratory viruses in the same samples. Nonetheless, studies that have included some combination of quantitative PCR, serum PCR, and serology have been more convincing about HBoV1 as a human pathogen. The use of a quantitative PCR method also seems to differentiate between HBoV1 infection (and wheezing) and prolonged viral shedding, as patients with higher viral titers were more likely to be symptomatic, to be viremic, and to have HBoV1 isolated without other viruses.

HBoV type 2 DNA has been found in the stool of 3–25% of children with gastroenteritis, but often with another enteric virus. DNA of HBoV types 2, 3, and 4 has also been found in the stool of healthy, asymptomatic individuals. At present, there are few data linking HBoV2, HBoV3, or HBoV4 to gastroenteritis or any clinical illness. Further studies are required to determine if any of the HBoVs are associated with some cases of childhood gastroenteritis.

DIAGNOSIS
Parvovirus B19 Infection

The diagnosis of erythema infectiosum is usually based on clinical presentation of the typical rash and rarely requires virologic confirmation. Similarly, the diagnosis of a typical transient aplastic crisis in a child with sickle cell disease is generally made on clinical grounds without specific virologic testing.

Serologic tests for the diagnosis of B19V infection are available. B19-specific IgM develops rapidly after infection and persists for 6-8 wk. Anti-B19 IgG serves as a marker of past infection or immunity. Determination of anti-B19 IgM is the best marker of recent/acute infection on a single serum sample; seroconversion of anti-B19 IgG antibodies in paired sera can also be used to confirm recent infection. Demonstration of anti-B19 IgG in the absence of IgM, even in high titer, is not diagnostic of recent infection.

Serologic diagnosis is unreliable in immunocompromised persons; diagnosis in these patients requires methods to detect viral DNA. Because the virus cannot be isolated by standard cell culture, methods to detect viral particles or viral DNA, such as PCR and nucleic acid hybridization, are necessary to establish the diagnosis. These tests are not widely available outside of research centers or reference laboratories. Prenatal diagnosis of B19V-induced fetal hydrops can be accomplished by detection of viral DNA in fetal blood or amniotic fluid by these methods.

Human Bocavirus Infections

HBoV1 infections cannot be differentiated from other viral respiratory infections on clinical grounds. HBoV DNA can be readily detected by PCR methods and is now included in several commercially available multiplex respiratory virus PCR assays. Quantitative PCR is useful to differentiate acute infection from persistent viral shedding, as higher viral copy numbers ($>10^4$ HBoV1 genomes/mL) correlate with acute illness, but this test is not widely available. Likewise, serologic methods to detect specific IgM and IgG antibodies have been developed, but these too are not routinely available and there are problems with cross-reactivity among antibodies to the various HBoV types. The most reliable method to diagnose HBoV1 infection would include detection of viral DNA in serum by PCR and in respiratory tract samples by quantitative PCR, with concurrent detection of IgM or a diagnostic IgG response in paired samples.

DIFFERENTIAL DIAGNOSIS
Parvovirus B19

The rash of erythema infectiosum must be differentiated from rubella, measles, enteroviral infections, and drug reactions. Rash and arthritis in older children should prompt consideration of juvenile rheumatoid arthritis, systemic lupus erythematosus, serum sickness, and other connective tissue disorders.

Human Bocavirus

Respiratory illness and wheezing caused by HBoV1 cannot be differentiated clinically from other common viral respiratory infections, especially respiratory syncytial virus, human metapneumovirus, rhinoviruses, enterovirus D68, and parainfluenza viruses. HBoV1 infection in young children seems to most closely resemble that of respiratory syncytial virus and human metapneumovirus, as the clinical symptoms and age ranges will overlap.

TREATMENT
Parvovirus B19

There is no specific antiviral therapy for B19V infection. Commercial lots of intravenous immunoglobulin (IVIG) have been used with some success to treat B19V-related episodes of anemia and bone marrow failure in immunocompromised children. Specific antibody may facilitate clearance of the virus but is not always necessary, because cessation of cytotoxic chemotherapy with subsequent restoration of immune function often

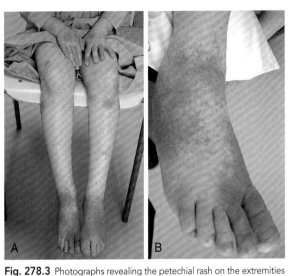

Fig. 278.3 Photographs revealing the petechial rash on the extremities **(A)** that was sharply demarcated on the ankles **(B)** in a 6 yr old child. *(From Parez N, Dehee A, Michel Y, et al: Papular-purpuric gloves and socks syndrome associated with B19V infection in a 6-yr-old child. J Clin Virol 44:167–169, 2009, Fig. 1.)*

suffices. In patients whose immune status is not likely to improve, such as patients with AIDS, administration of IVIG may give only a temporary remission, and periodic reinfusions may be required. In patients with AIDS, clearance of B19V infection has been reported after initiation of highly active antiretroviral therapy (HAART) without the use of IVIG.

No controlled studies have been published regarding dosing of IVIG for B19V-induced RBC aplasia. Multiple case reports and limited clinical series have reported successful treatment of severe anemia secondary to chronic B19V infection utilizing several different IVIG dosing regimens. A starting dose of 400 mg/kg/day for 5 days is usually recommended. The dose and duration of IVIG may be adjusted based on the response to therapy.

B19V-infected fetuses with anemia and hydrops have been managed successfully with intrauterine RBC transfusions, but this procedure has significant attendant risks. Once fetal hydrops is diagnosed, regardless of the suspected cause, the mother should be referred to a fetal therapy center for further evaluation because of the high risk for serious complications (see Chapter 124.2).

Human Bocavirus

There is no specific antiviral therapy available. Appropriate supportive treatment for viral LRTI and pneumonia is recommended, as directed by clinical severity. For children with wheezing illness specifically caused by HBoV1 infection, there are no data examining their response to bronchodilator therapy.

COMPLICATIONS
Parvovirus B19

Erythema infectiosum is often accompanied by arthralgias or arthritis in adolescents and adults that may persist after resolution of the rash. B19V may rarely cause thrombocytopenic purpura. Neurologic conditions, including aseptic meningitis, encephalitis, and peripheral neuropathy, have been reported in both immunocompromised and healthy individuals in association with B19V infection. The incidence of stroke may be increased in children with sickle cell disease following B19V-induced transient aplastic crisis. B19V is also a cause of infection-associated hemophagocytic syndrome, usually in immunocompromised persons.

Human Bocavirus

There are no studies reporting on complications of HBoV1 infection. Complications of wheezing and viral pneumonia would be possible, including hypoxemia and secondary bacterial infection, among others.

PREVENTION
Parvovirus B19

Children with erythema infectiosum are not likely to be infectious at presentation because the rash and arthropathy represent immune-mediated, postinfectious phenomena. Isolation and exclusion from school or child care are unnecessary and ineffective after diagnosis.

Children with B19V-induced RBC aplasia, including the transient aplastic crisis, are infectious upon presentation and demonstrate a more intense viremia. Most of these children require transfusions and supportive care until their hematologic status stabilizes. They should be isolated in the hospital to prevent spread to susceptible patients and staff. Isolation should continue for at least 1 wk and until fever has resolved. Pregnant caregivers should not be assigned to these patients. Exclusion of pregnant women from workplaces where children with erythema infectiosum may be present (e.g., primary and secondary schools) is not recommended as a general policy because it is unlikely to reduce their risk. There are no data to support the use of IVIG for postexposure prophylaxis in pregnant caregivers or immunocompromised children. No vaccine is currently available, though this is a topic of ongoing research.

Human Bocavirus

There are no studies that have addressed the prevention of transmission of this infection. In the hospital setting, standard precautions should be observed to limit spread of the virus. Since HBoV1 causes respiratory infection and can be detected in respiratory secretions sometimes in very high titer, measures to limit contact with respiratory secretions should be considered, including contact and droplet isolation for severely symptomatic young children. No vaccine is available, and no other preventive measures have been reported.

Bibliography is available at Expert Consult.

Chapter **279**

Herpes Simplex Virus

Lawrence R. Stanberry

第二百七十九章
单纯疱疹病毒

中文导读

　　本章主要介绍了单纯疱疹病毒感染的病因学、流行病学、发病机制、临床表现、诊断、实验室检查、治疗、预后和预防。临床表现包括急性口咽部感染、唇疱疹、皮肤感染、生殖器疱疹、眼感染、中枢神经

系统感染、免疫功能低下者感染和围产期感染。实验
室诊断包括病毒培养、DNA测定、血清学和抗原检

测。治疗药物有阿昔洛韦、伐昔洛韦和泛昔洛韦，详
细阐述了不同临床表现的治疗方案。

The 2 closely related herpes simplex viruses (HSVs), HSV type 1 (HSV-1) and HSV type 2 (HSV-2), cause a variety of illnesses, depending on the anatomic site where the infection is initiated, the immune state of the host, and whether the symptoms reflect primary or recurrent infection. Common infections involve the skin, eye, oral cavity, and genital tract. Infections tend to be mild and self-limiting, except in the immunocompromised patient and newborn infant, in whom they may be severe and life-threatening.

Primary infection occurs in individuals who have not been infected previously with either HSV-1 or HSV-2. Because these individuals are HSV seronegative and have no preexisting immunity to HSV, primary infections can be severe. **Nonprimary first infection** occurs in individuals previously infected with 1 type of HSV (e.g., HSV-1) who have become infected for the first time with the other type of HSV (in this case, HSV-2). Because immunity to 1 HSV type provides some cross-protection against disease caused by the other HSV type, nonprimary first infections tend to be less severe than true primary infections. During primary and nonprimary initial infections, HSV establishes latent infection in regional sensory ganglion neurons. Virus is maintained in this latent state for the life of the host but periodically can reactivate and cause **recurrent infection.** Symptomatic recurrent infections tend to be less severe and of shorter duration than 1st infections. Asymptomatic recurrent infections are extremely common and cause no physical distress, although patients with these infections are contagious and can transmit the virus to susceptible individuals. Reinfection with a new strain of either HSV-1 or HSV-2 at a previously infected anatomic site (e.g., the genital tract) can occur but is relatively uncommon, suggesting that host immunity, perhaps site-specific local immunity, resulting from the initial infection affords protection against exogenous reinfection.

ETIOLOGY

HSVs contain a double-stranded DNA genome of approximately 152 kb that encodes at least 84 proteins. The DNA is contained within an icosadeltahedral capsid, which is surrounded by an outer envelope composed of a lipid bilayer containing at least 12 viral glycoproteins. These glycoproteins are the major targets for humoral immunity, whereas other nonstructural proteins are important targets for cellular immunity. Two encoded proteins, viral DNA polymerase and thymidine kinase, are targets for antiviral drugs. HSV-1 and HSV-2 have a similar genetic composition with extensive DNA and protein homology. One important difference in the 2 viruses is their glycoprotein G genes, which have been exploited to develop a new generation of commercially available, accurate, type-specific serologic tests that can be used to discriminate whether a patient has been infected with HSV-1 or HSV-2 or both.

EPIDEMIOLOGY

HSV infections are ubiquitous, and there are no seasonal variations in risk for infection. The only natural host is humans, and the mode of transmission is direct contact between mucocutaneous surfaces. There are no documented incidental transmissions from inanimate objects such as toilet seats.

All infected individuals harbor latent infection and experience recurrent infections, which may be symptomatic or may go unrecognized and thus are periodically contagious. This information helps explain the widespread prevalence of HSV.

HSV-1 and HSV-2 are equally capable of causing initial infection at any anatomic site but differ in their capacity to cause recurrent infections. HSV-1 has a greater propensity to cause recurrent oral infections, whereas HSV-2 has a greater proclivity to cause recurrent genital infections. For this reason, HSV-1 infection typically results from contact with contaminated oral secretions, whereas HSV-2 infection most commonly results from anogenital contact.

HSV seroprevalence rates are highest in developing countries and among lower socioeconomic groups, although high rates of HSV-1 and HSV-2 infections are found in developed nations and among persons of the highest socioeconomic strata. Incident HSV-1 infections are more common during childhood and adolescence but are also found throughout later life. Data from the U.S. population–based National Health and Nutrition Examination Survey conducted between 1999 and 2004 showed a consistent increase of HSV-1 prevalence with age, which rose from 39% in adolescents 14-19 yr of age to 65% among those 40-49 yr of age. HSV-1 seroprevalence was not influenced by gender, but rates were highest in Mexican-Americans (80.8%), intermediate in non-Hispanic blacks (68.3%), and lowest in non-Hispanic whites (50.1%). The National Health and Nutrition Examination Survey study conducted between 2007 and 2010 found an overall HSV-2 prevalence of 15.5%, with a steady increase with age from 1.5% in the 14-19 yr old age group to 25.6% in the 40-49 yr old group. The rate was higher among females than males (20.3% and 10.6%, respectively) and varied by race and ethnic group, with an overall seroprevalence of 41.8% in non-Hispanic blacks, 11.3% in Mexican-Americans, and 11.3% in whites. Modifiable factors that predict HSV-2 seropositivity include less education, poverty, cocaine use, and a greater lifetime number of sexual partners. Studies show that only approximately 10–20% of HSV-2–seropositive subjects report a history of genital herpes, emphasizing the asymptomatic nature of most HSV infections.

A 3 yr longitudinal study of Midwestern adolescent females 12-15 yr of age found that 44% were seropositive for HSV-1 and 7% for HSV-2 at enrollment. At the end of the study, 49% were seropositive for HSV-1 and 14% for HSV-2. The attack rates, based on the number of cases per 100 person-years, were 3.2 for HSV-1 infection among all females and 4.4 for HSV-2 infection among girls who reported being sexually experienced. Findings of this study indicate that sexually active young women have a high attack rate for genital herpes and suggest that genital herpes should be considered in the differential diagnosis of any young woman who reports recurrent genitourinary complaints. In this study, participants with preexisting HSV-1 antibodies had a significantly lower attack rate for HSV-2 infection, and those who became infected were less likely to have symptomatic disease than females who were HSV seronegative when they entered the study. Prior HSV-1 infection appears to afford adolescent females some protection against becoming infected with HSV-2; in adolescent females infected with HSV-2, the preexisting HSV-1 immunity appears to protect against development of symptomatic genital herpes.

Neonatal herpes is an uncommon but potentially fatal infection of the fetus or more likely the newborn. It is not a reportable disease in most states, and therefore there are no solid epidemiologic data regarding its frequency in the general population. In King County, Washington, the estimated incidence of neonatal herpes was 2.6 cases per 100,000 live births in the late 1960s, 11.9 cases per 100,000 live births from 1978 to 1981, and 31 cases per 100,000 live births from 1982 to 1999. This increase in neonatal herpes cases parallels the increase in cases of genital herpes. The estimated rate of neonatal herpes is 1 per 3,000-5,000 live births, which is higher than reported for the reportable perinatally acquired sexually transmitted infections such as congenital syphilis and gonococcal ophthalmia neonatorum. More than 90% of the cases are the result of maternal-child transmission. The risk for transmission is greatest during a primary or nonprimary first infection (30–50%) and much lower when the exposure is during a recurrent infection (<2%). HSV viral suppression therapy in mothers does not consistently eliminate the possibility of neonatal infection. Infants born to mothers dually infected with HIV and HSV-2 are also at higher risk for acquiring HIV than infants born to HIV-positive mothers who are not HSV-2 infected. It is estimated that approximately 25% of pregnant women are HSV-2 infected and that approximately 2% of pregnant women acquire HSV-2 infection during pregnancy.

HSV is a leading cause of sporadic, fatal encephalitis in children and adults. In the United States the annual hospitalization rate for HSV encephalitis has been calculated to be 10.3 ± 2.2 cases/million in neonates, 2.4 ± 0.3 cases/million in children, and 6.4 ± 0.4 cases/million in adults.

PATHOGENESIS

In the immunocompetent host the pathogenesis of HSV infection involves viral replication in skin and mucous membranes followed by replication and spread in neural tissue. Viral infection typically begins at a cutaneous portal of entry such as the oral cavity, genital mucosa, ocular conjunctiva, or breaks in keratinized epithelia. Virus replicates locally, resulting in the death of the cell, and sometimes produces clinically apparent inflammatory responses that facilitate the development of characteristic herpetic vesicles and ulcers. Virus also enters nerve endings and spreads beyond the portal of entry to sensory ganglia by intraneuronal transport. Virus replicates in some sensory neurons, and the progeny virions are sent via intraneuronal transport mechanisms back to the periphery, where they are released from nerve endings and replicate further in skin or mucosal surfaces. It is virus moving through this neural arc that is primarily responsible for the development of characteristic herpetic lesions, although most HSV infections do not reach a threshold necessary to cause clinically recognizable disease. Although many sensory neurons become productively infected during the initial infection, some infected neurons do not initially support viral replication. It is in these neurons that the virus establishes a latent infection, a condition in which the viral genome persists within the neuronal nucleus in a largely metabolically inactive state. Intermittently throughout the life of the host, undefined changes can occur in latently infected neurons that trigger the virus to begin to replicate. This replication occurs despite the host's having established a variety of humoral and cellular immune responses that successfully controlled the initial infection. With reactivation of the latent neuron, progeny virions are produced and transported within nerve fibers back to cutaneous sites somewhere in the vicinity of the initial infection, where further replication occurs and causes recurrent infections. Recurrent infections may be symptomatic (with typical or atypical herpetic lesions) or asymptomatic. In either case, virus is shed at the site where cutaneous replication occurs and can be transmitted to susceptible individuals who come in contact with the site or with contaminated secretions. Latency and reactivation are the mechanisms by which the virus is successfully maintained in the human population.

Viremia, or hematogenous spread of the virus, does not appear to play an important role in HSV infections in the immunocompetent host but can occur in neonates, individuals with eczema, and severely malnourished children. It is also seen in patients with depressed or defective cell-mediated immunity, as occurs with HIV infection or some immunosuppressive therapies. Viremia can result in dissemination of the virus to visceral organs, including the liver and adrenals. Hematogenous dissemination of virus to the central nervous system appears to only occur in neonates.

The pathogenesis of HSV infection in newborns is complicated by their relative immunologic immaturity. The source of virus in neonatal infections is typically but not exclusively the mother. Transmission generally occurs during delivery, although it is well documented to occur even with cesarean delivery with intact fetal membranes. The most common portals of entry are the conjunctiva, mucosal epithelium of the nose and mouth, and breaks or abrasions in the skin that occur with scalp electrode use or forceps delivery. With prompt antiviral therapy, virus replication may be restricted to the site of inoculation (the skin, eye, or mouth). However, virus may also extend from the nose to the respiratory tract to cause pneumonia, move via intraneuronal transport to the central nervous system to cause encephalitis, or spread by hematogenous dissemination to visceral organs and the brain. Factors that may influence neonatal HSV infection include the virus type, portal of entry, inoculum of virus to which the infant is exposed, gestational age of the infant, and presence of maternally derived antibodies specific to the virus causing infection. Latent infection is established during neonatal infection, and survivors may experience recurrent cutaneous and neural infections. Persistent central nervous system infection may impact the neurodevelopment of the infant.

CLINICAL MANIFESTATIONS

The hallmarks of common HSV infections are skin vesicles and shallow ulcers. Classic infections manifest as small, 2-4 mm vesicles that may be surrounded by an erythematous base. These may persist for a few days before evolving into shallow, minimally erythematous ulcers. The vesicular phase tends to persist longer when keratinized epithelia is involved and is generally brief and sometimes just fleeting when moist mucous membranes are the site of infection. Because HSV infections are common and their natural history is influenced by many factors, including portal of entry, immune status of the host, and whether it is an initial or recurrent infection, the typical manifestations are seldom classic. Most infections are asymptomatic or unrecognized, and nonclassic presentations, such as small skin fissures and small erythematous nonvesicular lesions, are common.

Acute Oropharyngeal Infections

Herpes gingivostomatitis most often affects children 6 mo to 5 yr of age but is seen across the age spectrum. It is an extremely painful condition with sudden onset, pain in the mouth, drooling, refusal to eat or drink, and fever of up to 40.0-40.6°C (104-105.1°F). The gums become markedly swollen, and vesicles may develop throughout the oral cavity, including the gums, lips, tongue, palate, tonsils, pharynx and perioral skin (Fig. 279.1). The vesicles may be more extensively distributed than typically seen with enteroviral herpangina. During the initial phase of the illness there may be tonsillar exudates suggestive of bacterial pharyngitis. The vesicles are generally present only a few days before progressing to form shallow indurated ulcers that may be covered with a yellow-gray membrane. Tender submandibular, submaxillary, and cervical lymphadenopathy is common. The breath may be foul as a result of overgrowth of anaerobic oral bacteria. Untreated, the illness resolves in 7-14 days, although the lymphadenopathy may persist for several weeks.

In older children, adolescents, and college students, the initial HSV oral infection may manifest as pharyngitis and tonsillitis rather than gingivostomatitis. The vesicular phase is often over by the time the patient presents to a healthcare provider, and signs and symptoms may be indistinguishable from those of streptococcal pharyngitis, consisting of fever, malaise, headache, sore throat, and white plaques on the tonsils. The course of illness is typically longer than for untreated streptococcal pharyngitis.

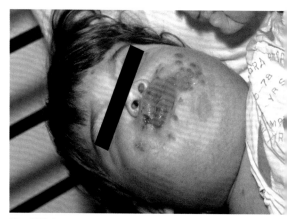

Fig. 279.1 Clustered perioral vesicles and erosions in an infant with primary herpetic gingivostomatitis. *(From Schachner LA, Hansen RC, editors: Pediatric dermatology, ed 3, Philadelphia, 1988, Mosby, p. 1078.)*

Herpes Labialis

Fever blisters (cold sores) are the most common manifestation of *recurrent* HSV-1 infections. The most common site of herpes labialis is the vermilion border of the lip, although lesions sometimes occur on the nose, chin, cheek, or oral mucosa. Older patients report experiencing burning, tingling, itching, or pain 3-6 hr (rarely as long as 24-48 hr) before the development of the herpes lesion. The lesion generally begins as a small grouping of erythematous papules that over a few hours progress to create a small, thin-walled vesicle. The vesicles may form shallow ulcers or become pustular. The short-lived ulcer dries and develops a crusted scab. Complete healing without scarring occurs with reepithelialization of the ulcerated skin, usually within 6-10 days. Some patients experience local lymphadenopathy but no constitutional symptoms.

Cutaneous Infections

In the healthy child or adolescent, cutaneous HSV infections are generally the result of skin trauma with macro or micro abrasions and exposure to infectious secretions. This situation most often occurs in play or contact sports such as wrestling (**herpes gladiatorum**) and rugby (**scrum pox**). An initial cutaneous infection establishes a latent infection that can subsequently result in recurrent infections at or near the site of the initial infection. Pain, burning, itching, or tingling often precedes the herpetic eruption by a few hours to a few days. Like herpes labialis, lesions begin as grouped, erythematous papules that progress to vesicles, pustules, ulcers, and crusts and then heal without scarring in 6-10 days. Although herpes labialis typically results in a single lesion, a cutaneous HSV infection results in multiple discrete lesions and involves a larger surface area. Regional lymphadenopathy may occur but systemic symptoms are uncommon. Recurrences are sometimes associated with local edema and lymphangitis or local neuralgia.

Herpes whitlow is a term generally applied to HSV infection of fingers or toes, although strictly speaking it refers to HSV infection of the paronychia. Among children, this condition is most commonly seen in infants and toddlers who suck the thumb or fingers and who are experiencing either a symptomatic or a subclinical oral HSV-1 infection (Fig. 279.2). An HSV-2 herpes whitlow occasionally develops in an adolescent as a result of exposure to infectious genital secretions. The onset of the infection is heralded by itching, pain, and erythema 2-7 days after exposure. The cuticle becomes erythematous and tender and may appear to contain pus, although if it is incised, little fluid is present. Incising the lesion is discouraged, as this maneuver typically prolongs recovery and increases the risk for secondary bacterial infection. Lesions and associated pain typically persist for about 10 days, followed by rapid improvement and complete recovery in 18-20 days. Regional lymphadenopathy is common, and lymphangitis and neuralgia may occur. Unlike other recurrent herpes infections, recurrent herpetic whitlows are often as painful as the primary infection but are generally shorter in duration.

Cutaneous HSV infections can be severe or life-threatening in patients with disorders of the skin such as eczema (eczema herpeticum), pemphigus, burns, and Darier disease and following laser skin resurfacing. The lesions are frequently ulcerative and nonspecific in appearance, although typical vesicles may be seen in adjacent normal skin (Fig. 279.3). If untreated, these lesions can progress to disseminated infection and death. Recurrent infections are common but generally less severe than the initial infection.

Genital Herpes

Genital HSV infection is common in sexually experienced adolescents and young adults, but up to 90% of infected individuals are *unaware* they are infected. Infection may result from genital-genital transmission (usually HSV-2) or oral-genital transmission (usually HSV-1). Symptomatic and asymptomatic individuals periodically shed virus from anogenital sites and hence can transmit the infection to sexual partners or, in the case of pregnant women, to their newborns. Classic primary genital herpes may be preceded by a short period of local burning and tenderness before vesicles develop on genital mucosal surfaces or keratinized skin and sometimes around the anus or on the buttocks

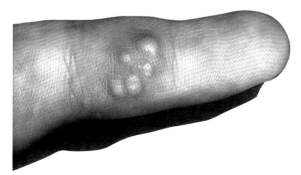

Fig. 279.2 Herpes simplex infection of finger (whitlow). *(From Schachner LA, Hansen RC, editors:* Pediatric dermatology, *ed 3, Philadelphia, 1988, Mosby, p. 1079.)*

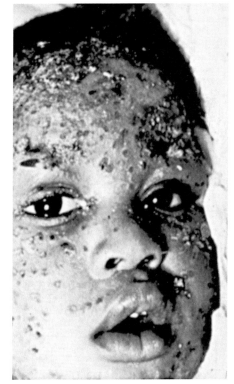

Fig. 279.3 Widespread cutaneous herpes infection in a child with underlying eczema (eczema herpeticum).

and thighs. Vesicles on mucosal surfaces are short lived and rupture to produce shallow, tender ulcers covered with a yellowish gray exudate and surrounded by an erythematous border. Vesicles on keratinized epithelium persist for a few days before progressing to the pustular stage and then crusting.

Patients may experience urethritis and dysuria severe enough to cause urinary retention and bilateral, tender inguinal and pelvic lymphadenopathy. Women may experience a watery vaginal discharge, and men may have a clear mucoid urethral discharge. Significant local pain and systemic symptoms such as fever, headache, and myalgia are common. Aseptic meningitis develops in an estimated 15% of cases. The course of classic primary genital herpes from onset to complete healing is 2-3 wk.

Most patients with symptomatic primary genital herpes experience at least 1 recurrent infection in the following year. Recurrent genital herpes is usually less severe and of shorter duration than the primary infection. Some patients experience a sensory prodrome with pain, burning, and tingling at the site where vesicles subsequently develop. Asymptomatic recurrent anogenital HSV infections are common, and all HSV-2–seropositive individuals appear to periodically shed virus from anogenital sites. *Most sexual transmissions and maternal-neonatal transmissions of virus result from asymptomatic shedding episodes.*

Genital infections caused by HSV-1 and HSV-2 are indistinguishable, but HSV-1 causes significantly fewer subsequent episodes of recurrent infection; hence, knowing which virus is causing the infection has important prognostic value. Genital HSV infection increases the risk for acquiring HIV infection.

Rarely, genital HSV infections are identified in young children and preadolescents. Although genital disease in children should raise concerns about possible sexual abuse, there are documented cases of autoinoculation, in which a child has inadvertently transmitted virus from contaminated oral secretions to his or her own genitalia.

Ocular Infections

HSV ocular infections may involve the conjunctiva, cornea, or retina and may be primary or recurrent. Conjunctivitis or keratoconjunctivitis is usually unilateral and is often associated with blepharitis and tender preauricular lymphadenopathy. The conjunctiva appears edematous but there is rarely purulent discharge. Vesicular lesions may be seen on the lid margins and periorbital skin. Patients typically have fever. Untreated infection generally resolves in 2-3 wk. Obvious corneal involvement is rare, but when it occurs it can produce ulcers that are described as appearing dendritic or geographic. Extension to the stroma is uncommon although more likely to occur in patients inadvertently treated with corticosteroids. When it occurs, it may be associated with corneal edema, scarring, and corneal perforation. Recurrent infections tend to involve the underlying stroma and can cause progressive corneal scarring and injury that can lead to blindness.

Retinal infections are rare and are more likely among infants with neonatal herpes and immunocompromised persons with disseminated HSV infections.

Central Nervous System Infections

HSV encephalitis is the leading cause of sporadic, nonepidemic encephalitis in children and adults in the United States. It is an acute necrotizing infection generally involving the frontal and/or temporal cortex and the limbic system and, beyond the neonatal period, is almost always caused by HSV-1. The infection may manifest as nonspecific findings, including fever, headache, nuchal rigidity, nausea, vomiting, generalized seizures, and alteration of consciousness. Injury to the frontal or temporal cortex or limbic system may produce findings more indicative of HSV encephalitis, including anosmia, memory loss, peculiar behavior, expressive aphasia and other changes in speech, hallucinations, and focal seizures. The untreated infection progresses to coma and death in 75% of cases. Examination of the cerebrospinal fluid (CSF) typically shows a moderate number of mononuclear cells and polymorphonuclear leukocytes, a mildly elevated protein concentration, a normal or slightly decreased glucose concentration, and often a moderate number of erythrocytes. HSV has also been associated with autoimmune encephalitis (see Chapter 616.4).

HSV is also a cause of aseptic meningitis and is the most common cause of recurrent aseptic meningitis (**Mollaret meningitis**).

Infections in Immunocompromised Persons

Severe, life-threatening HSV infections can occur in patients with compromised immune functions, including neonates, the severely malnourished, those with primary or secondary immunodeficiency diseases (including AIDS), and those receiving some immunosuppressive regimens, particularly for cancer and organ transplantation. Mucocutaneous infections, including mucositis and esophagitis, are most common, although their presentations may be atypical and can result in lesions that slowly enlarge, ulcerate, become necrotic, and extend to deeper tissues. Other HSV infections include tracheobronchitis, pneumonitis, and anogenital infections. Disseminated infection can result in a sepsis-like presentation, with liver and adrenal involvement, disseminated intravascular coagulopathy, and shock.

Perinatal Infections

HSV infection may be acquired in utero, during the birth process, or during the neonatal period. Intrauterine and postpartum infections are well described but occur infrequently. Postpartum transmission may be from the mother or another adult with a nongenital (typically HSV-1) infection such as herpes labialis. Most cases of neonatal herpes result from maternal infection and transmission, usually during passage through an infected birth canal of a mother with asymptomatic genital herpes. Transmission is well documented in infants delivered by cesarean section. Fewer than 30% of mothers of an infant with neonatal herpes have a history of genital herpes. The risk for infection is higher in infants born to mothers with primary genital infection (>30%) than with recurrent genital infection (<2%). Use of scalp electrodes may also increase risk. There also have been rare cases of neonatal herpes associated with Jewish ritual circumcisions, but only with ritual oral contact with the circumcision site.

Neonatal HSV infection is thought to never be asymptomatic. Its clinical presentation reflects timing of infection, portal of entry, and extent of spread. Infants with **intrauterine infection** typically have skin vesicles or scarring, eye findings including chorioretinitis and keratoconjunctivitis, and microcephaly or hydranencephaly that are present at delivery. Few infants survive without therapy, and those who do generally have severe sequelae. Infants infected during delivery or the postpartum period present with 1 of the following 3 patterns of disease: (1) disease localized to the skin, eyes, or mouth; (2) encephalitis with or without skin, eye, and mouth disease; and (3) disseminated infection involving multiple organs, including the brain, lungs, liver, heart, adrenals, and skin (Fig. 279.4). Approximately 20% present between 5 and 9 wk of age.

Infants with **skin, eye, and mouth disease** generally present at 5-11 days of life and typically demonstrate a few small vesicles, particularly on the presenting part or at sites of trauma such as sites of scalp electrode placement. If untreated, skin, eye, and mouth disease in infants may progress to encephalitis or disseminated disease.

Infants with encephalitis typically present at 8-17 days of life with clinical findings suggestive of bacterial meningitis, including irritability, lethargy, poor feeding, poor tone, and seizures. Fever is relatively uncommon, and skin vesicles occur in only approximately 60% of cases (Fig. 279.5). If untreated, 50% of infants with HSV encephalitis die and most survivors have severe neurologic sequelae.

Infants with disseminated HSV infections generally become ill at 5-11 days of life. Their clinical picture is similar to that of infants with

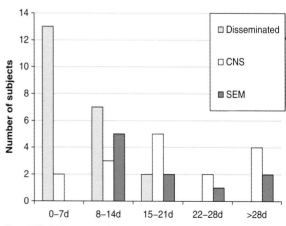

Fig. 279.4 Herpes simplex virus (HSV). Age at presentation by HSV disease type. (*From Curfman AL, Glissmeyer EW, Ahmad FA, et al: Initial presentation of neonatal herpes simplex virus infection, J Pediatr 172:121–126, 2016, p. 124*).

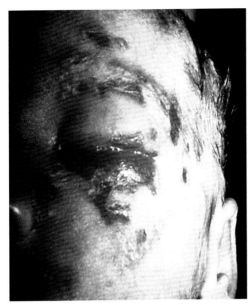

Fig. 279.5 Vesicular-pustular lesions on the face of a neonate with herpes simplex virus infection. *(From Kohl S: Neonatal herpes simplex virus infection, Clin Perinatol 24:129–150, 1997.)*

bacterial sepsis, consisting of hyperthermia or hypothermia, irritability, poor feeding, and vomiting. They may also exhibit respiratory distress, cyanosis, apneic spells, jaundice, purpuric rash, and evidence of central nervous system infection; seizures are common. Skin vesicles are seen in approximately 75% of cases. If untreated, the infection causes shock and disseminated intravascular coagulation; approximately 90% of these infants die, and most survivors have severe neurologic sequelae.

Infants with neonatal herpes whose mothers received antiherpes antiviral drugs in the weeks prior to delivery may present later than their untreated counterparts; whether the natural history of the infection in these infants is different is an unanswered question.

DIAGNOSIS

The clinical diagnosis of HSV infections, particularly life-threatening infections and genital herpes, should be confirmed by laboratory test, preferably isolation of virus or detection of viral DNA by polymerase chain reaction (PCR). Histologic findings or imaging studies may support the diagnosis but should not substitute for virus-specific tests. HSV immunoglobulin M tests are notoriously unreliable, and the demonstration of a 4-fold or greater rise in HSV-specific immunoglobulin G titers between acute and convalescent serum samples is useful only in retrospect.

The highest yield for virus cultures comes from rupturing a suspected herpetic vesicle and vigorously rubbing the base of the lesion to collect fluid and cells. Culturing dried, crusted lesions is generally of low yield. Although not as sensitive as viral culture, direct detection of HSV antigens can be done rapidly and has very good specificity. The use of DNA amplification methods such as PCR for detection of HSV DNA is highly sensitive and specific and in some instances can be performed rapidly. It is the test of choice in examining CSF in cases of suspected HSV encephalitis.

Evaluation of the neonate with suspected HSV infection should include cultures of suspicious lesions as well as eye and mouth swabs and PCR of both CSF and blood. In neonates testing for elevation of liver enzymes may provide indirect evidence of HSV dissemination to visceral organs. Culture or antigen detection should be used in evaluating lesions associated with suspected acute genital herpes. HSV-2 type-specific antibody tests are useful for evaluating sexually experienced adolescents or young adults who have a history of unexplained recurrent nonspecific urogenital signs and symptoms, but these tests are less useful for general screening in populations in which HSV-2 infections are of low prevalence.

Because most HSV diagnostic tests take at least a few days to complete, treatment should not be withheld but rather initiated promptly so as to ensure the maximum therapeutic benefit.

LABORATORY FINDINGS

Most self-limited HSV infections cause few changes in routine laboratory parameters. Mucocutaneous infections may cause a moderate polymorphonuclear leukocytosis. In HSV meningoencephalitis there can be an increase in mononuclear cells and protein in CSF, the glucose content may be normal or reduced, and red blood cells may be present. The electroencephalogram and MRI of the brain may show temporal lobe abnormalities in HSV encephalitis beyond the neonatal period. Encephalitis in the neonatal period tends to be more global and not limited to the temporal lobe (Fig. 279.6). Disseminated infection may cause elevated liver enzymes, thrombocytopenia, and abnormal coagulation.

TREATMENT

See Chapter 272 for more information about principles of antiviral therapy.

Three antiviral drugs are available in the United States for the management of HSV infections, namely acyclovir, valacyclovir, and famciclovir. All 3 are available in oral form, but only acyclovir is available in a suspension form. Acyclovir has the poorest bioavailability and hence requires more frequent dosing. Valacyclovir, a prodrug of acyclovir, and famciclovir, a prodrug of penciclovir, both have very good oral bioavailability and are dosed once or twice daily. Acyclovir and penciclovir are also available in a topical form, but these preparations provide limited or no benefit to patients with recurrent mucocutaneous HSV infections. Only acyclovir has an intravenous formulation. Early initiation of therapy results in the maximal therapeutic benefit. All 3 drugs have exceptional safety profiles and are safe to use in pediatric patients. *Doses should be modified in patients with renal impairment.*

Resistance to acyclovir and penciclovir is rare in immunocompetent persons but does occur in immunocompromised persons. Virus isolates from immunocompromised persons whose HSV infection is not responding or is worsening with acyclovir therapy should be tested for drug sensitivities. Foscarnet and cidofovir have been used in the treatment of HSV infections caused by acyclovir-resistant mutants.

Topical trifluridine and topical ganciclovir are used in the treatment of herpes keratitis.

Patients with genital herpes also require counseling to address psychosocial issues, including possible stigma, and to help them understand the natural history and management of this chronic infection.

Acute Mucocutaneous Infections

For gingivostomatitis, oral acyclovir (15 mg/kg/dose 5 times a day PO for 7 days; maximum: 1 g/day) started within 72 hr of onset reduces the severity and duration of the illness. Pain associated with swallowing may limit oral intake of infants and children, putting them at risk for dehydration. Intake should be encouraged through the use of cold beverages, ice cream, and yogurt.

For **herpes labialis**, oral treatment is superior to topical antiviral therapy. For treatment of a recurrence in adolescents, oral valacyclovir (2,000 mg bid PO for 1 day), acyclovir (200-400 mg 5 times daily PO for 5 days), or famciclovir (1,500 mg once daily PO for 1 day) shortens the duration of the episode. Long-term daily use of oral acyclovir (400 mg bid PO) or valacyclovir (500 mg once daily PO) has been used to prevent recurrences in individuals with frequent or severe recurrences.

Anecdotal reports suggest that treatment of adolescents with **herpes gladiatorum** with oral acyclovir (200 mg 5 times daily PO for 7-10 days) or valacyclovir (500 mg bid PO for 7-10 days) at the first signs of the outbreak can shorten the course of the recurrence. For patients with a history of recurrent herpes gladiatorum, chronic daily prophylaxis with valacyclovir (500-1,000 mg daily) has been reported to prevent recurrences.

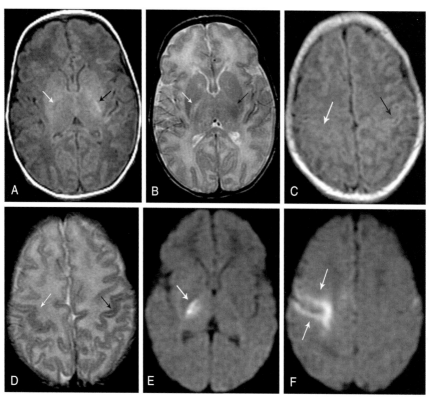

Fig. 279.6 Involvement of corticospinal tract and thalamus in a 2 wk old infant. **A,** MRI with axial T1-weighted image demonstrating subtle loss of T1 hyperintensity corresponding to myelination in the posterior limb of the right internal capsule *(white arrow)*. T1 hyperintensity in the left posterior limb of the internal capsule is maintained *(black arrow)*. **B,** T2-weighted image showing findings similar to those seen on T1-weighted imaging. **C,** Axial T1- and **(D)** T2-weighted images through the vertex demonstrating subtle indistinct margins of the cortex around the right central sulcus *(white arrow)* compared with the normal appearance on the left side *(black arrow)*. **E** and **F,** Diffusion-weighted images with more extensive diffusion restriction in the posterior limb of the right internal capsule and lateral thalamus *(arrows)*, and in the right pre- and postcentral gyrus *(arrows)*. *(From Bajaj M, Mody S, Natarajan G: Clinical and neuroimaging findings in neonatal herpes simplex virus infection, J Pediatr 165:404–407, 2014, Fig. 1.)*

There are no clinical trials assessing the benefit of antiviral treatment for **herpetic whitlow.** High-dose oral acyclovir (1,600-2,000 mg/day divided in 2-3 doses PO for 10 days) started at the first signs of illness has been reported to abort some recurrences and reduce the duration of others in adults.

A clinical trial in adults has established the effectiveness of oral acyclovir (200 mg 5 times a day PO for 5 days) in the treatment of **eczema herpeticum;** however, serious infections should be treated with intravenous acyclovir. Oral-facial HSV infections can reactivate after cosmetic facial laser resurfacing, causing extensive disease and scarring. Treatment of adults beginning the day before the procedure with either valacyclovir (500 mg twice daily PO for 10-14 days) or famciclovir (250-500 mg bid PO for 10 days) has been reported to be effective in preventing the infections. HSV infections in **burn patients** can be severe or life-threatening and have been treated with intravenous acyclovir (10-20 mg/kg/day divided every 8 hr IV).

Antiviral drugs are not effective in the treatment of HSV-associated **erythema multiforme,** but their daily use as for herpes labialis prophylaxis prevents *reoccurrences* of erythema multiforme.

Genital Herpes

Pediatric patients, usually adolescents or young adults, with suspected first-episode genital herpes should be treated with antiviral therapy. Treatment of the initial infection reduces the severity and duration of the illness but has no effect on the frequency of subsequent recurrent infections. Treatment options for adolescents include acyclovir (400 mg tid PO for 7-10 days), famciclovir (250 mg tid PO for 7-10 days), or valacyclovir (1,000 mg bid PO for 7-10 days). The twice-daily valacyclovir

option avoids treatment during school hours. For smaller children, acyclovir suspension can be used at a dose of 10-20 mg/kg/dose 4 times daily not to exceed the adult dose. The 1st episode of genital herpes can be extremely painful, and use of analgesics is generally indicated. All patients with genital herpes should be offered counseling to help them deal with psychosocial issues and understand the chronic nature of the illness.

There are 3 strategic options regarding the management of recurrent infections. The choice should be guided by several factors, including the frequency and severity of the recurrent infections, the psychologic impact of the illness on the patient, and concerns regarding transmission to a susceptible sexual partner. Option 1 is no therapy; option 2 is episodic therapy; and option 3 is long-term suppressive therapy. For **episodic therapy,** treatment should be initiated at the first signs of an outbreak. Recommended choices for episodic therapy in adolescents include famciclovir (1,000 mg bid PO for 1 day), acyclovir (800 mg tid PO for 2 days), or valacyclovir (500 mg bid PO for 3 days or 1,000 mg once daily for 5 days). Long-term suppressive therapy offers the advantage that it prevents most outbreaks, improves patient quality of life in terms of the psychosocial impact of genital herpes, and, with daily valacyclovir therapy, also reduces (but does not eliminate) the risk for sexual transmission to a susceptible sexual partner. Options for **long-term suppressive therapy** are acyclovir (400 mg bid PO), famciclovir (250 mg bid PO), and valacyclovir (500 or 1,000 mg qd PO).

Ocular Infections

HSV ocular infections can result in blindness. Management should involve consultation with an ophthalmologist.

Central Nervous System Infections

Patients older than neonates who have herpes encephalitis should be promptly treated with intravenous acyclovir (10 mg/kg every 8 hr given as a 1 hr infusion for 14-21 days). Treatment for increased intracranial pressure, management of seizures, and respiratory compromise may be required.

Infections in Immunocompromised Persons

Severe mucocutaneous and disseminated HSV infections in immunocompromised patients should be treated with intravenous acyclovir (30 mg/kg per day, in 3 divided doses for 7-14 days) until there is evidence of resolution of the infection. Oral antiviral therapy with acyclovir, famciclovir, or valacyclovir has been used for treatment of less-severe HSV infections and for suppression of recurrences during periods of significant immunosuppression. Drug resistance does occur occasionally in immunocompromised patients, and in individuals whose HSV infection does not respond to antiviral drug therapy, viral isolates should be tested to determine sensitivity. Acyclovir-resistant viruses are often also resistant to famciclovir but may be sensitive to foscarnet or cidofovir.

Perinatal Infections

All infants with proven or suspected neonatal HSV infection should be treated immediately with high-dose intravenous acyclovir (60 mg/kg/day divided every 8 hr IV). Treatment may be discontinued in infants shown by laboratory testing not to be infected. Infants with HSV disease limited to skin, eyes, and mouth should be treated for 14 days, whereas those with disseminated or central nervous system disease should receive 21 days of therapy. Patients receiving high-dose therapy should be monitored for neutropenia.

Suppressive oral acyclovir therapy for 6 mo after completion of the intravenous therapy has been shown to improve the neurodevelopment of infants with central nervous system infection and to prevent cutaneous recurrences in infants regardless of disease pattern. Infants should receive 300 mg/m^2 per dose 3 times daily for 6 mo. The absolute neutrophil count should be measured at weeks 2 and 4 after initiation of treatment and then monthly.

PROGNOSIS

Most HSV infections are self-limiting, last from a few days (for recurrent infections) to 2-3 wk (for primary infections), and heal without scarring. Recurrent oral-facial herpes in a patient who has undergone dermabrasion or laser resurfacing can be severe and lead to scarring. Because genital herpes is a sexually transmitted infection, it can be stigmatizing, and its psychologic consequences may be much greater than its physiologic effects. Some HSV infections can be severe and may have grave consequences without prompt antiviral therapy. Life-threatening conditions include neonatal herpes, herpes encephalitis, and HSV infections in immunocompromised patients, burn patients, and severely malnourished infants and children. Recurrent ocular herpes can lead to corneal scarring and blindness.

PREVENTION

Transmission of infection occurs through exposure to virus either as the result of skin-to-skin contact or from contact with contaminated secretions. Good handwashing and, when appropriate, the use of gloves provide healthcare workers with excellent protection against HSV infection in the workplace. Healthcare workers with active oral-facial herpes or herpetic whitlow should take precautions, particularly when caring for high-risk patients such as newborns, immunocompromised individuals, and patients with chronic skin conditions. Patients and parents should be advised about good hygienic practices, including handwashing and avoiding contact with lesions and secretions, during active herpes outbreaks. Schools and daycare centers should clean shared toys and athletic equipment such as wrestling mats at least daily after use. Athletes with active herpes infections who participate in contact sports such as wrestling and rugby should be excluded from practice or games until the lesions are completely healed. Genital herpes can be prevented by avoiding genital-genital and oral-genital contact. The risk for acquiring genital herpes can be reduced but not eliminated through the correct and consistent use of condoms. Male circumcision is associated with a reduced risk of acquiring genital HSV infection. The risk for transmitting genital HSV-2 infection to a susceptible sexual partner can be reduced but not eliminated by the daily use of oral valacyclovir by the infected partner.

For **pregnant women** with **active genital herpes** at the time of delivery, the risk for mother-to-child transmission can be reduced but not eliminated by delivering the baby via a cesarean section. The risk for recurrent genital herpes, and therefore the need for cesarean delivery, can be reduced but not eliminated in pregnant women with a history of genital herpes by the daily use of oral acyclovir, valacyclovir, or famciclovir during the last 4 wk of gestation, which is recommended by the American College of Obstetrics and Gynecology. There are documented cases of neonatal herpes occurring in infants delivered by cesarean section, as well as in infants born to mothers who have been appropriately treated with antiherpes antiviral drugs for the last month of gestation. Hence a history of cesarean delivery or antiviral treatment at term does not rule out consideration of neonatal herpes.

Infants delivered vaginally to women with *first-episode* genital herpes are at *very high risk* for acquiring HSV infection. The nasopharynx, mouth, conjunctivae, rectum, and umbilicus should be cultured (some add PCR surface testing) at delivery and 12 to 24 hr after birth. Some also recommend HSV-PCR on blood. Some authorities recommend that these infants receive anticipatory acyclovir therapy for at least 2 wk, and others treat such infants if signs develop or if surface cultures beyond 12-24 hr of life are positive. Infants delivered to women with a history of *recurrent genital herpes* are at low risk for development of neonatal herpes. In this setting, parents should be educated about the signs and symptoms of neonatal HSV infection and should be instructed to seek care without delay at the first suggestion of infection. When the situation is in doubt, infants should be evaluated and tested with surface culture (and PCR) for neonatal herpes as well as with PCR on blood *and* CSF; intravenous acyclovir is begun until culture and PCR results are negative or until another explanation can be found for the signs and symptoms.

Recurrent genital HSV infections can be prevented by the daily use of oral acyclovir, valacyclovir, or famciclovir, and these drugs have been used to prevent recurrences of oral-facial (labialis) and cutaneous (gladiatorum) herpes. Oral and intravenous acyclovir has also been used to prevent recurrent HSV infections in immunocompromised patients. Use of sun blockers is reported to be effective in preventing recurrent oral-facial herpes in patients with a history of sun-induced recurrent disease.

Bibliography is available at Expert Consult.

Chapter **280**

Varicella-Zoster Virus*

Philip S. LaRussa, Mona Marin, and Anne A. Gershon

第二百八十章

水痘–带状疱疹病毒

中文导读

本章主要介绍了水痘–带状疱疹病毒感染的病因学、流行病学、发病机制、临床表现、并发症、诊断、治疗、预后和预防。临床表现涵盖未接种疫苗的水痘患者、接种疫苗者的水痘样皮疹、新生儿水痘、先天性水痘综合征。阐述了感染后的并发症，包括细菌感染、脑炎与小脑共济失调、肺炎、进行性水痘、带状疱疹等。详细介绍了水痘和带状疱疹的治疗方案。预防中包括疫苗、与疫苗相关不良反应和暴露后预防。

Varicella-zoster virus (VZV) causes primary, latent, and reactivation infections. The primary infection is manifested as varicella (chickenpox) and results in establishment of a lifelong latent infection of sensory ganglionic neurons. Reactivation of the latent infection causes herpes zoster (shingles). Although often a mild illness of childhood, varicella can cause substantial morbidity and mortality in otherwise healthy children. Morbidity and mortality are higher in immunocompetent infants, adolescents, and adults as well as in immunocompromised persons. Varicella predisposes to severe group A streptococcus and staphylococcus aureus infections. A clinically modified disease can occur among vaccinated persons (breakthrough varicella), usually with milder presentation. Varicella and herpes zoster can be treated with antiviral drugs. Primary clinical disease can be prevented by immunization with live-attenuated varicella vaccine. Two herpes zoster vaccines are available for persons 50 yr of age and older to boost their immunity to VZV and prevent herpes zoster and its major complication, painful postherpetic neuralgia. One is a recombinant subunit (non-live) adjuvanted vaccine, and the other is a live vaccine that contains the same VZV strain used in the varicella vaccine but with a higher potency.

ETIOLOGY

VZV is a neurotropic human herpesvirus with similarities to herpes simplex virus. VZV enveloped viruses contain double-stranded DNA genomes that encode 71 proteins, including proteins that are targets of cellular and humoral immunity.

EPIDEMIOLOGY

Before the introduction of varicella vaccine in 1995, varicella was an almost universal communicable infection of childhood in the United States. Most children were infected by 10 yr of age, with fewer than 5% of adults remaining susceptible. This pattern of infection at younger ages remains characteristic in all countries in temperate climates. In contrast, in tropical areas, children acquire varicella at older ages and a higher proportion of young adults remain susceptible, leading to a higher proportion of cases occurring among adults. In the United States, prior to introduction of varicella vaccination, annual varicella epidemics occurred in winter and spring, and there were about 4 million cases of varicella, 11,000-15,000 hospitalizations, and 100-150 deaths every year. Varicella is a more serious disease in young infants, adults, and immunocompromised persons, in whom there are higher rates of complications and deaths than in healthy children. Within households, transmission of VZV to susceptible individuals occurs at a rate of 65–86%; more casual contact, such as occurs in a school classroom, is associated with lower attack rates among susceptible children. Persons with varicella may be contagious 24-48 hr before the rash is evident and until vesicles are crusted, usually 3-7 days after onset of rash, consistent with evidence that VZV is spread by aerosolization of virus in cutaneous lesions; spread from oropharyngeal secretions may occur but to a much lesser extent. Susceptible persons may also acquire varicella after close, direct contact with adults or children who have herpes zoster, again via aerosolization of virus in skin lesions.

Since implementation of the varicella vaccination program in 1996, there have been substantial declines in varicella morbidity and mortality in the United States. By 2006, prior to implementation of the 2-dose program, 1-dose vaccination coverage had reached 90% and varicella incidence had declined 90–91% since 1995 in sites where active surveillance was being conducted; varicella-related hospitalizations had declined 84% from prevaccine years. Varicella-related deaths decreased by 88% from 1990-1994 to 2005-2007; in persons younger than 20 yr of age there was a 97% decline in deaths. Declines in morbidity and mortality were seen in all age groups, including infants younger than 12 mo of age who were not eligible for vaccination, indicating protection from

---

*The findings and conclusions in this report are those of the authors and do not necessarily represent the official position of the Centers for Disease Control and Prevention, US Department of Health and Human Services.

exposure by indirect vaccination effects. Although the age-specific incidence has declined in all age groups, the median age at infection has increased, and cases occur predominantly in children in upper elementary school rather than in the preschool years. This change in varicella epidemiology highlights the importance of offering vaccine to every susceptible child, adolescent, and adult. The continued occurrence of breakthrough infections and of outbreaks in settings with high 1-dose varicella vaccine coverage, together with the evidence that 1 dose is only approximately 85% effective against all varicella, prompted adoption in 2006 of a routine 2-dose childhood varicella vaccination program with catch-up vaccination of all individuals without evidence of immunity. Between 2006 and 2014, varicella incidence declined further by approximately 85% and fewer outbreaks were reported; varicella-related hospitalizations too declined 38% during the 2-dose period (through 2012). Overall, from prevaccine years varicella incidence declined by 97% and hospitalizations by 93% through 2014 and 2012, respectively.

Herpes zoster is caused by the reactivation of latent VZV. It is not common in childhood and shows no seasonal variation in incidence. Zoster is not caused by exposure to a patient with varicella; in fact, exposures to varicella boost the cell-mediated immune response to VZV in individuals with prior infection, decreasing the likelihood of reactivation of latent virus. The lifetime risk for herpes zoster for individuals with a history of varicella is at least 30%, with 75% of cases occurring after 45 yr of age. Herpes zoster is unusual in healthy children younger than 10 yr of age, with the exception of those infected with VZV in utero or in the 1st yr of life, who have an increased risk for development of zoster in the 1st few yr of life. Herpes zoster in otherwise healthy children tends to be milder than herpes zoster in adults, is less frequently associated with acute pain, and is generally not associated with postherpetic neuralgia. In children receiving immunosuppressive therapy for malignancy or other diseases and in those who have HIV infection, herpes zoster occurs more frequently, occasionally multiple times, and may be severe. The attenuated VZV in the varicella vaccine can establish latent infection and reactivate as herpes zoster. However, the risk for development of subsequent herpes zoster is lower after vaccination than after natural VZV infection among both healthy and immunocompromised children. Although the Oka vaccine type VZV is attenuated, the severity of zoster caused by the Oka strain seems to be similar to that caused by the natural or wild type VZV; some reports indicated milder clinical features among vaccine recipients but without being statistically significant. Vaccinated children who do develop zoster may have disease resulting from either vaccine or wild-type VZV, due to breakthrough varicella or subclinical infection of some vaccinees with wild-type VZV occurring at some point after immunization.

PATHOGENESIS

Primary infection (varicella) results from inoculation of the virus onto the mucosa of the upper respiratory tract and tonsillar lymphoid tissue. During the early part of the 10-21 day incubation period, virus replicates in the local lymphoid tissue and spreads to T lymphocytes, causing a viremia that delivers the virus to skin where innate immunity controls VZV replication for some days. After innate immunity is overcome in skin, widespread cutaneous lesions develop as the incubation period ends. Adaptive host immune responses, especially cellular immunity, limit viral replication and lead to recovery from infection. In the immunocompromised child, the failure of adaptive immunity, especially cellular immune responses, results in continued viral replication that may lead to prolonged and/or disseminated infection with resultant complications of infection in the lungs, liver, brain, and other organs.

Latent infection develops during the incubation period or the disease itself. VZV is transported in a retrograde manner through sensory axons to the dorsal root ganglia throughout the spinal cord and to cranial nerve ganglia. Latency may also develop from viremia, infecting spinal and cranial nerve ganglia as well autonomic ganglia which do not project to the skin, including the enteric nervous system of the intestine. Latency of VZV occurs only in ganglionic neurons. Subsequent **reactivation** of latent VZV causes **herpes zoster,** usually manifested by a vesicular rash that is unilateral and dermatomal in distribution.

Reactivation of VZV may also occur without a rash; examples are unilateral dermatomal pain without rash (**zoster sine herpete**), aseptic meningitis, and gastrointestinal illness (enteric zoster). During herpes zoster, necrotic changes may be produced in the neurons and surrounding satellite cells in associated ganglia. The skin lesions of varicella and herpes zoster have identical histopathology, and infectious VZV is present in both. Varicella elicits humoral and cell-mediated immunity that is highly protective against symptomatic reinfection. Suppression of cell-mediated immunity to VZV correlates with an increased risk for VZV reactivation as herpes zoster.

CLINICAL MANIFESTATIONS

Varicella is an acute febrile rash illness that was common in children in the United States before the universal childhood vaccination program. It has variable severity but is usually self-limited. It may be associated with severe complications, including bacterial superinfection, especially with staphylococci and group A streptococci, pneumonia, encephalitis, bleeding disorders, congenital infection, and life-threatening perinatal infection. Herpes zoster is not common in children and typically causes localized cutaneous symptoms, but may disseminate in immunocompromised patients.

Varicella in Unvaccinated Individuals

The illness usually begins 14-16 days after exposure, although the incubation period can range from 10 to 21 days. Subclinical varicella is rare; almost all exposed, susceptible persons experience a rash, albeit so mild in some cases that it may go unnoticed. Prodromal symptoms may be present, particularly in older children and adults. Fever, malaise, anorexia, headache, and occasionally mild abdominal pain may occur 24-48 hr before the rash appears. Temperature elevation is usually 37.8-38.9°C (100-102°F) but may be as high as 41.1°C (106°F); fever and other systemic symptoms usually resolve within 2-4 days after the onset of the rash.

Varicella lesions often appear first on the scalp, face, or trunk. The initial exanthem consists of intensely pruritic erythematous macules that evolve through the papular stage to form clear, fluid-filled vesicles. Clouding and umbilication of the lesions begin in 24-48 hr. While the initial lesions are crusting, new crops form on the trunk and then the extremities; the simultaneous presence of lesions in various stages of evolution is characteristic of varicella (Fig. 280.1). The distribution of the rash is predominantly central or centripetal, with the greatest concentration on the trunk and proximally on the extremities. Ulcerative lesions involving the mucosa of the oropharynx and vagina are also common; many children have vesicular lesions on the eyelids and conjunctivae, but corneal involvement and serious ocular disease are rare. The average number of varicella lesions is about 300, but healthy children may have fewer than 10 to more than 1,500 lesions. In cases resulting from secondary household spread and in older children, more lesions usually occur, and new crops of lesions may continue to develop

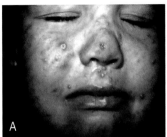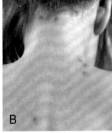

Fig. 280.1 A, Varicella lesions in unvaccinated persons display the characteristic "cropping" distribution, or manifest themselves in clusters; the simultaneous presence of lesions in various stages of evolution is characteristic. **B,** Breakthrough varicella lesions are predominantly maculopapular, and vesicles are less common; the illness is most commonly mild with <50 lesions. (*A, Courtesy Centers for Disease Control and Prevention [CDC]; B, courtesy CDC and Dr. John Noble, Jr.*)

for more than 7 days. The exanthem may be much more extensive in children with skin disorders, such as eczema or recent sunburn. Hypopigmentation or hyperpigmentation of lesion sites persists for days to weeks in some children, but severe scarring is unusual unless the lesions were secondarily infected.

The differential diagnosis of varicella includes vesicular rashes caused by other infectious agents, such as herpes simplex virus, enterovirus, monkey pox, rickettsial pox, and *S. aureus;* drug reactions; disseminated herpes zoster; contact dermatitis; and insect bites (especially for breakthrough varicella). Severe varicella was the most common illness confused with smallpox before the eradication of smallpox.

Varicelliform Rashes in Vaccinated Individuals

Varicelliform rashes that occur after vaccination could be a result of wild-type VZV, vaccine strain VZV, or other etiologies (e.g., insect bites, coxsackievirus). During days 0-42 after vaccination, the likelihood of rash from wild-type or vaccine strain VZV varies depending on the stage of a country's vaccination program. In the early stages of a vaccine program, rash within 1-2 wk is still most commonly caused by wild-type VZV, reflecting exposure to varicella before vaccination could provide protection. Rash occurring 14-42 days after vaccination is a result of either wild-type or vaccine strains, reflecting exposure and infection before protection from vaccination or an adverse event of vaccination (vaccine-associated rash), respectively. As wild-type varicella continues to decline as a consequence of the vaccination program, wild-type VZV circulation will also decline and rashes in the interval 0-42 days after vaccination will be less commonly caused by wild-type VZV. Spread of vaccine type VZV from a vaccinee with skin lesions has occurred, but is rare. The resulting illness in contacts is either asymptomatic or extremely mild with only a few vesicular lesions. Clinical reversion of the vaccine virus to virulence has not been described.

Breakthrough varicella is disease that occurs in a person vaccinated more than 42 days before rash onset and is caused by **wild-type** virus. One dose of varicella vaccine is 98% effective in preventing moderate and severe varicella and is 82% (95% confidence interval [CI]: 79–85%; range: 44–100%) effective in preventing all disease after exposure to wild-type VZV. This means that after close exposure to VZV, as may occur in a household or an outbreak setting in a school or daycare center, about 1 of every 5 children who received 1 dose of vaccine may experience breakthrough varicella. Exposure to VZV may also result in asymptomatic infection in the previously immunized child. The rash in breakthrough disease is frequently atypical and predominantly maculopapular, and vesicles are seen less commonly. The illness is most commonly mild with <50 lesions, shorter duration of rash, fewer complications, and little or no fever. However, approximately 25–30% of breakthrough cases in vaccines who received 1 dose are not mild, with clinical features more similar to those of wild-type infection. Breakthrough cases are overall **less contagious** than wild-type infections within household settings, but contagiousness varies proportionally with the number of lesions; typical breakthrough cases (<50 lesions) is about one-third as contagious as disease in unvaccinated cases, whereas breakthrough cases with ≥50 lesions are as contagious as wild-type cases. Consequently, children with breakthrough disease should be considered potentially infectious and excluded from school until lesions have crusted or, if there are no vesicles present, until no new lesions are occurring. Transmission has been documented to occur from breakthrough cases in household, childcare, and school settings.

Two doses of varicella vaccine provide better protection than a 1-dose schedule. One clinical trial estimated the 2-dose vaccine effectiveness for preventing all disease at 98%; the estimate is 92% (95% CI: 88–95%; range: 84–98%) in conditions of everyday clinical practice. Institution of 2 doses routinely in the United States substantially reduced the school outbreaks that were occurring among children who had received only 1 dose. Breakthrough cases have been reported among 2-dose vaccines; however, recipients of 2 doses of varicella vaccine are less likely to have breakthrough disease than those who received 1 dose. Additionally, data suggest that breakthrough varicella may be further attenuated among 2-dose vaccine recipients.

Neonatal Varicella

Mortality is particularly high in neonates born to susceptible mothers who contract varicella around the time of delivery. Infants whose mothers demonstrate varicella in the period from 5 days prior to delivery to 2 days afterward are at high risk for severe varicella. These infants acquire the infection transplacentally as a result of maternal viremia, which may occur up to 48 hr prior to onset of maternal rash. The infant's rash usually occurs toward the end of the 1st wk to the early part of the 2nd wk of life (although it may be as soon as 2 days). Because the mother has not yet developed a significant antibody response, the infant receives a large dose of virus without the moderating effect of maternal anti-VZV antibody. If the mother demonstrates varicella more than 5 days prior to delivery, she still may pass virus to the soon-to-be-born child, but infection is attenuated because of transmission of maternal VZV-specific antibody across the placenta. This moderating effect of maternal antibody is present if delivery occurs after about 30 wk of gestation, when maternal immunoglobulin (Ig) G is able to cross the placenta in significant amounts. *The recommendations for use of human varicella-zoster immunoglobulin (VZIG) differ based on when the infant is exposed to varicella.* Newborns whose mothers develop varicella during the period of 5 days before to 2 days after delivery should receive VZIG as soon as possible after birth. Although neonatal varicella may occur in about half of these infants despite administration of VZIG, it is milder than in the absence of VZIG administration. All premature infants born < 28 wk of gestation to a mother with active varicella at delivery (even if the maternal rash has been present for >1 wk) should receive VZIG. If VZIG is not available, intravenous immunoglobulin (IVIG) may provide some protection, although varicella-specific antibody titers may vary from lot to lot. Because perinatally acquired varicella may be life threatening, the infant should usually be treated with acyclovir (10 mg/kg every 8 hr IV) when lesions develop. Neonatal varicella can also follow a postpartum exposure of an infant delivered to a mother who was susceptible to VZV, although the frequency of complications declines rapidly in the weeks after birth. Recommendations for VZIG administration for these infants are presented in the postexposure prophylaxis section. Neonates with community-acquired varicella who experience severe varicella, especially those who have a complication such as pneumonia, hepatitis, or encephalitis, should also receive treatment with intravenous acyclovir (10 mg/kg every 8 hr). Infants with neonatal varicella who receive prompt antiviral therapy have an excellent prognosis.

Congenital Varicella Syndrome

In utero transmission of VZV can occur; however, because most adults in temperate climates are immune, pregnancy complicated by varicella is unusual in these settings. When pregnant women do contract varicella early in pregnancy, experts estimate that as many as 25% of the fetuses may become infected. Fortunately, clinically apparent disease in the infant is uncommon: the congenital varicella syndrome occurs in approximately 0.4% of infants born to women who have varicella during pregnancy before 13 wk of gestation and in approximately 2% of infants born to women with varicella between 13 and 20 wk of gestation. Rarely, cases of congenital varicella syndrome have been reported in infants of women infected after 20 wk of pregnancy, the latest occurring at 28 wk of gestation. Before availability of varicella vaccine in the United States, 44 cases of congenital varicella syndrome were estimated to occur each year. The congenital varicella syndrome is characterized by cicatricial skin scarring in a zoster-like distribution; limb hypoplasia; and abnormalities of the neurologic system (e.g., microcephaly, cortical atrophy, seizures, and mental retardation), eye (e.g., chorioretinitis, microphthalmia, and cataracts), renal system (e.g., hydroureter and hydronephrosis), and autonomic nervous system (e.g., neurogenic bladder, swallowing dysfunction, and aspiration pneumonia). Low birthweight is common among infants with congenital varicella syndrome. Most of the stigmata can be attributed to virus-induced injury to the nervous system, although there is no obvious explanation why certain regions of the body are preferentially infected during fetal VZV infection. The characteristic cutaneous lesion has been called a cicatrix, a zigzag scarring, in a *dermatomal* distribution, often associated with atrophy of the affected limb (Fig. 280.2). Many infants with severe manifestations of congenital varicella syndrome (atrophy and scarring of a limb) have significant neurologic deficiencies. Alternatively, there may be neither skin nor limb abnormalities but the infant may show cataracts or even extensive aplasia of the entire brain.

There are rare case reports of fetal abnormalities following the development of herpes zoster in the mother; whether or not these cases truly represent the congenital varicella syndrome is unclear. If it does occur, the congenital syndrome acquired as a result of maternal herpes zoster is exceedingly rare. Maternal herpes zoster was associated with typical congenital varicella syndrome in one case, but the mother had disseminated herpes zoster (at 12 wk of gestation).

The diagnosis of VZV fetopathy is based mainly on the history of gestational varicella combined with the presence of characteristic abnormalities in the newborn infant. Virus cannot be cultured from the affected newborn, but viral DNA may be detected in tissue samples by polymerase chain reaction (PCR). Since many infants with congenital varicella syndrome develop zoster before a year of age, it may be possible to isolate VZV from that rash. Alternatively, use of PCR to identify VZV DNA in vesicular fluid or scabs from zoster lesions in such an infant may be diagnostic. VZV-specific IgM antibody is detectable in the cord blood sample in some infants, although the IgM titer drops quickly in the postpartum period and can be nonspecifically positive. Chorionic villus sampling and fetal blood collection for the detection of viral DNA, virus, or antibody have been used in an attempt to diagnose fetal infection and embryopathy. The usefulness of these tests for patient management and counseling has not been defined. Because these tests may not distinguish between infection and disease, their utility may primarily be that of reassurance when the result is negative. Ultrasound may be useful to try to identify limb atrophy, which is common in congenital varicella syndrome. A persistently positive VZV IgG antibody titer at 12-18 mo of age is a reliable indicator of prenatal infection in the asymptomatic child, as is the development of zoster in the 1st yr of life without evidence of postnatal infection.

VZIG has often been administered to the susceptible mother exposed to varicella to modify maternal disease severity; it is uncertain whether this step modifies infection in the fetus, although some evidence suggests that it may be beneficial for the fetus too. Similarly, acyclovir treatment

may be given to the mother with severe varicella. A prospective registry of acyclovir use in the 1st trimester demonstrated that the occurrence of birth defects approximates that found in the general population. Acyclovir is a class B drug for pregnancy and should be considered when the benefit to the mother outweighs the potential risk to the fetus. The efficacy of acyclovir treatment of the pregnant woman in preventing or modifying the severity of congenital varicella is not known, but its use should be considered to protect the mother from severe disease. Because the damage caused by fetal VZV infection does not progress in the postpartum period, antiviral treatment of infants with congenital VZV syndrome is not indicated.

COMPLICATIONS

The complications of VZV infection (varicella or zoster) occur more commonly in immunocompromised patients. In the otherwise healthy child, asymptomatic transient varicella hepatitis is relatively common. Mild thrombocytopenia occurs in 1–2% of children with varicella and may be associated with petechiae. Purpura, hemorrhagic vesicles, hematuria, and gastrointestinal bleeding are rare complications that may have serious consequences. Other complications of varicella, some of them rare, include acute cerebellar ataxia, encephalitis, pneumonia, nephritis, nephrotic syndrome, hemolytic-uremic syndrome, arthritis, myocarditis, pericarditis, pancreatitis, orchitis, and acute retinal necrosis. A reduction in the number and rates of varicella-related complications is seen in vaccinated populations. Reports of serious varicella-related complications in vaccinated persons (breakthrough) are rare (meningitis, pneumonia, acute transverse myelitis, encephalitis [1 fatal case in an apparently immunocompetent child], and sepsis). Severe breakthrough varicella can occur among healthy persons, but cases appear to be more common among immunocompromised persons who are usually not recommended to receive varicella vaccine.

Declines in varicella-related hospitalizations and deaths in the United States since implementation of the varicella vaccination program provide supporting evidence that varicella vaccine reduces severe complications from varicella. Approximately 105 deaths (with varicella listed as the underlying cause of death) occurred in the United States annually before the introduction of the varicella vaccine; during 2008-2011 the annual average number of varicella deaths was 17. In both the pre- and postvaccine era, the majority of deaths (>80%) have been among persons without high-risk preexisting conditions.

Bacterial Infections

Secondary bacterial infections of the skin, usually caused by group A streptococcus or *S. aureus,* may occur in children with varicella. These range from impetigo to cellulitis, lymphadenitis, and subcutaneous abscesses. An early manifestation of secondary bacterial infection is erythema of the base of a new vesicle. Recrudescence of fever 3-4 days after the initial exanthem may also herald a secondary bacterial infection. Varicella is a well-described risk factor for serious invasive infections caused by group A streptococcus, which can have a fatal outcome. The more invasive infections, such as varicella gangrenosa, bacterial sepsis, pneumonia, arthritis, osteomyelitis, cellulitis, and necrotizing fasciitis, account for much of the morbidity and mortality of varicella in otherwise healthy children. Bacterial toxin–mediated diseases (e.g., toxic shock syndrome) also may complicate varicella. A substantial decline in varicella-related invasive bacterial infections is associated with the use of the varicella vaccine.

Encephalitis and Cerebellar Ataxia

Encephalitis (1 per 50,000 cases of varicella in unvaccinated children) and acute cerebellar ataxia (1 per 4,000 cases of varicella in unvaccinated children) are well-described neurologic complications of varicella; morbidity from central nervous system complications is highest among patients younger than 5 yr and older than 20 yr. Nuchal rigidity, altered consciousness, and seizures characterize meningoencephalitis. Patients with cerebellar ataxia have a gradual onset of gait disturbance, nystagmus, and slurred speech. Neurologic symptoms usually begin 2-6 days after the onset of the rash but may occur during the incubation period or after resolution of the rash. Clinical recovery is typically rapid, occurring

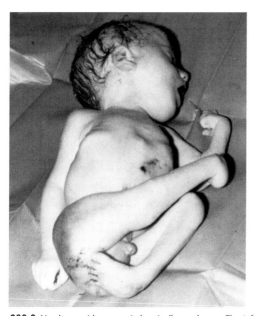

Fig. 280.2 Newborn with congenital varicella syndrome. The infant had severe malformations of both lower extremities and cicatricial scarring over his left abdomen.

within 24-72 hr, and is usually complete. Although severe hemorrhagic encephalitis, analogous to that caused by herpes simplex virus, is very rare in children with varicella, the consequences are similar to those of herpes simplex virus encephalitis. Reye syndrome (hepatic dysfunction with hypoglycemia and encephalopathy) associated with varicella and other viral illnesses such as influenza is rare now that salicylates are no longer used as antipyretics in these situations (see Chapter 384).

Pneumonia

Varicella pneumonia is a severe complication that accounts for most of the increased morbidity and mortality from varicella in adults and other high-risk populations, but pneumonia may also complicate varicella in young children. Respiratory symptoms, which may include cough, dyspnea, cyanosis, pleuritic chest pain, and hemoptysis, usually begin within 1-6 days after the onset of the rash. Smoking has been described as a risk factor for severe pneumonia complicating varicella. The frequency of varicella pneumonia may be greater in the parturient.

Progressive Varicella

Progressive varicella, with visceral organ involvement, coagulopathy, severe hemorrhage, and continued vesicular lesion development after 7 days, is a severe complication of primary VZV infection. Severe abdominal pain, which may reflect involvement of mesenteric lymph nodes or the liver, or the appearance of hemorrhagic vesicles in otherwise healthy adolescents and adults, immunocompromised children, pregnant women, and newborns, may herald severe, and potentially fatal, disease. Although rare in healthy children, the risk for progressive varicella is highest in children with congenital cellular immune deficiency disorders and those with malignancy, particularly if chemotherapy, and especially corticosteroids, had been given during the incubation period and the absolute lymphocyte count is <500 cells/μL. The mortality rate for children who acquired varicella while undergoing treatment for malignancy and who were not treated with antiviral therapy approached 7%; varicella-related deaths usually occurred within 3 days after the diagnosis of varicella pneumonia. Children who acquire varicella after organ transplantation are also at risk for progressive VZV infection. Children undergoing long-term, low-dose systemic or inhaled corticosteroid therapy are not considered to be at higher risk for severe varicella, but progressive varicella does occur in patients receiving high-dose corticosteroids. There are case reports in patients receiving inhaled corticosteroids as well as in asthmatic patients receiving multiple short courses of systemic corticosteroid therapy. Unusual clinical findings of varicella, including lesions that develop a hyperkeratotic appearance and continued new lesion formation for weeks or months, have been described in children with untreated, late-stage HIV infection. Immunization of HIV-infected children who have a CD4+ T-lymphocyte percent ≥15%, as well as children with leukemia and solid organ tumors who are in remission and whose chemotherapy can be interrupted for 2 wk around the time of immunization or has been terminated, have reduced frequency of severe disease. Moreover, since the advent of the universal immunization program in the United States, many children who would become immunocompromised later in life because of disease or treatment are protected before the immunosuppression occurs; also, as a result of reductions in varicella incidence, immunocompromised children are less likely to be exposed to varicella.

Herpes Zoster

Herpes zoster manifests as vesicular lesions clustered within 1 or, less commonly, 2 adjacent dermatomes (Fig. 280.3). In the elderly, herpes zoster typically begins with burning pain or itching followed by clusters of skin lesions in a dermatomal pattern. Almost half of the elderly with herpes zoster experience complications; the most frequent complication is postherpetic neuralgia, a painful condition that affects the nerves despite resolution of the skin lesions. Approximately 4% of patients suffer a 2nd episode of herpes zoster; 3 or more episodes are rare. Unlike herpes zoster in adults, zoster in children is infrequently associated with localized pain, hyperesthesia, pruritus, low-grade fever, or complications. In children, the rash is mild, with new lesions appearing for a few days (Fig. 280.4); symptoms of acute neuritis are minimal; and

complete resolution usually occurs within 1-2 wk. Unlike in adults, postherpetic neuralgia is unusual in children. An increased risk for herpes zoster early in childhood has been described in children who acquire infection with VZV in utero or in the 1st yr of life.

Immunocompromised children may have more severe herpes zoster, similar to the situation in adults, including postherpetic neuralgia. Immunocompromised patients may also experience disseminated cutaneous disease that mimics varicella, with or without initial dermatomal rash, as well as visceral dissemination with pneumonia, hepatitis, encephalitis, and disseminated intravascular coagulopathy. Severely immunocompromised children, particularly those with advanced HIV infection, may have unusual, chronic, or relapsing cutaneous disease, retinitis, or central nervous system disease without rash. The finding of a lower risk for herpes zoster among vaccinated children with leukemia than in those who have had varicella suggested that the vaccine virus reactivates less commonly than wild-type VZV. A study of HIV-infected vaccinated children found no cases of zoster 4.4 yr after immunization, which was significantly different than the rate in children who had experienced varicella. Studies to date indicate that the risk for herpes zoster in healthy children who have received 1 dose of vaccine is lower than in children who had wild-type varicella. Many more years of follow-up are needed to determine whether this lower risk is maintained among older persons who are at greatest risk for herpes zoster. The risk for herpes zoster in healthy children following 2 doses of varicella vaccine has not been evaluated.

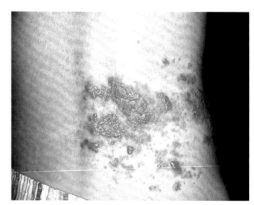

Fig. 280.3 Herpes zoster involving the lumbar dermatome. (*From Mandell GL, Bennett JE, Dolin R, editors: Principles and practice of infectious diseases, ed 6, Philadelphia, 2005, Elsevier, p. 1783.*)

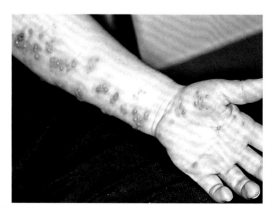

Fig. 280.4 Many groups of blisters occurring over the arm in a child with herpes zoster. (*From Weston WL, Lane AT, Morelli JG: Color textbook of pediatric dermatology, ed 3, Philadelphia, 2002, Mosby, Fig. 8-28.*)

DIAGNOSIS

Varicella and herpes zoster are usually diagnosed primarily by their clinical appearance. Laboratory evaluation has not been considered necessary for diagnosis or management. However, as varicella disease has declined to low levels, laboratory confirmation has become increasingly useful. The atypical nature of breakthrough varicella, with a higher proportion of papular rather than vesicular rashes, poses both clinical and laboratory diagnostic challenges.

Leukopenia is typical during the first 72 hr after onset of rash; it is followed by a relative and absolute lymphocytosis. Results of liver function tests are also usually (75%) mildly elevated. Patients with neurologic complications of varicella or uncomplicated herpes zoster have a mild lymphocytic pleocytosis and a slight to moderate increase in protein content of the cerebrospinal fluid; the cerebrospinal fluid glucose concentration is usually normal.

Rapid laboratory diagnosis of VZV is often important in high-risk patients and can be important for infection control, especially for breakthrough cases that have mild or atypical presentations. Confirmation of VZV infections can be accomplished by many referral hospital laboratories and all state health laboratories. VZV can be identified quickly by direct fluorescence assay of cells from cutaneous lesions (vesicular fluid) in 15-20 min; by PCR amplification testing (vesicular fluid, crusts) in hours to days, depending on availability; and by rapid culture with specific immunofluorescence staining (shell vial technique) in 48-72 hr. In the absence of vesicles or scabs, scrapings of maculopapular lesions can be collected for PCR or direct fluorescence assay testing. Infectious virus may be recovered by means of tissue culture methods; such methods require specific expertise, and virus may take days to weeks to grow. Of available tests, PCR is the most sensitive and allows for differentiation of wild-type and vaccine strains. Direct fluorescence assay is specific and less sensitive than PCR but when available allows for rapid diagnosis. Although multinucleated giant cells can be detected with nonspecific stains (Tzanck smear), they have poor sensitivity and do not differentiate VZV from herpes simplex virus infections. Strain identification (genotyping) can distinguish wild-type VZV from the vaccine strain in a vaccinated child; however, genotyping is available only at specialized reference laboratories. Laboratory tests of lesions cannot be used to distinguish between varicella and disseminated herpes zoster. VZV IgG antibodies can be detected by several methods, and a 4-fold or greater rise in IgG antibodies is confirmatory of acute infection (although this requires a 2-3 wk delay to collect a convalescent specimen); in vaccinated persons, commercially available tests are not sufficiently sensitive to always detect antibody following vaccination and a 4-fold rise in IgG antibody may not occur. VZV IgG antibody tests can also be valuable to determine the immune status of individuals whose clinical history of varicella is unknown or equivocal. However, caution must be taken in interpreting tests for immunity to VZV, especially in immunocompromised patients after a close exposure to VZV. Due to the possibility of false-positive results, it is preferable to rely on clinical rather than laboratory information, and if doubt, assume the individual is susceptible to varicella and proceed accordingly. Testing for VZV IgM antibodies is not useful for routine confirmation or ruling out of varicella because commercially available methods are unreliable and the kinetics of the IgM response have not been well defined. Reliable VZV-specific IgM assays are available in certain reference laboratories, including a capture-IgM assay available at the national VZV laboratory at the Centers for Disease Control and Prevention. Serologic tests are not useful for the initial diagnosis of herpes zoster, but a large rise in IgG titer in convalescent titer in the presence of an atypical zoster rash is confirmatory. As with any laboratory test, a negative varicella test should be considered in the context of the clinical presentation. Clinicians should use clinical judgment to decide on the best course of therapy.

TREATMENT

Antiviral treatment modifies the course of both varicella and herpes zoster. Antiviral drug resistance is rare for VZV but has occurred, primarily in children with HIV infection and other immunocompromising conditions where frequent relapse of VZV infections has resulted in multiple courses of antiviral therapy. Foscarnet and cidofovir may be useful for the treatment of acyclovir-resistant VZV infections, but consultation of an infectious disease specialist is recommended.

Varicella

The only antiviral drug available in liquid formulation that is licensed for treatment of varicella for pediatric use is acyclovir. Given the safety profile of acyclovir and its demonstrated efficacy in the treatment of varicella, treatment of all children, adolescents, and adults with varicella is acceptable. However, acyclovir therapy is not recommended routinely by the American Academy of Pediatrics for treatment of uncomplicated varicella in the otherwise healthy child because of the marginal benefit, the cost of the drug, and the low risk for complications of varicella. Oral therapy with acyclovir (20 mg/kg/dose; maximum: 800 mg/dose) given as 4 doses/day for 5 days can be used to treat uncomplicated varicella in individuals at increased risk for moderate to severe varicella: nonpregnant individuals older than 12 yr of age and individuals older than 12 mo of age with chronic cutaneous or pulmonary disorders; individuals receiving short-term, intermittent, or aerosolized corticosteroid therapy; individuals receiving long-term salicylate therapy; and possibly secondary cases among household contacts. To be most effective, treatment should be initiated as early as possible, preferably within 24 hr of the onset of the exanthem. There is less clinical benefit if treatment is initiated more than 72 hr after onset of the exanthem. Acyclovir therapy does not interfere with the induction of VZV immunity. Acyclovir has been successfully used to treat varicella in pregnant women. Some experts recommend the use of famciclovir or valacyclovir in older children who can swallow tablets. These drugs are highly active against VZV by the same mechanism as acyclovir and are better absorbed by the oral route than acyclovir. Valacyclovir (20 mg/kg/dose; maximum: 1,000 mg/dose, administered 3 times daily for 5 days) is licensed for treatment of varicella in children 2 to <18 yr of age, and both valacyclovir and famciclovir are approved for treatment of herpes zoster in adults. The oral adult dose of valacyclovir is 1 g TID. Patients receiving these antivirals should be well hydrated, and for prolonged use, renal function and white blood cell counts (especially neutrophils) should be monitored frequently. Common adverse symptoms during valacyclovir treatment are neurologic (headache, agitation, dizziness) and gastrointestinal (nausea, abdominal pain).

Intravenous therapy is indicated for severe disease and for varicella in immunocompromised patients (even if begun more than 72 hr after onset of rash). Any patient who has signs of disseminated VZV, including pneumonia, severe hepatitis, thrombocytopenia, or encephalitis, should receive immediate treatment. IV acyclovir therapy (500 mg/m^2 every 8 hr) initiated within 72 hr of development of initial symptoms decreases the likelihood of progressive varicella and visceral dissemination in high-risk patients. Treatment is continued for 7-10 days or until no new lesions have appeared for 48 hr. Delaying antiviral treatment in high-risk individuals until it is obvious that prolonged new lesion formation is occurring is not recommended because visceral dissemination occurs during the same period.

Acyclovir-resistant VZV has been identified primarily in children infected with HIV. These children may be treated with intravenous foscarnet (120 mg/kg/day divided every 8 hr for up to 3 wk). The dose should be modified in the presence of renal insufficiency. Resistance to foscarnet has been reported with prolonged use. Cidofovir is also useful in this situation. Because of the increased toxicity profile of foscarnet and cidofovir, these 2 drugs should be initiated in collaboration with an infectious disease specialist.

Herpes Zoster

Antiviral drugs are effective for treatment of herpes zoster. In healthy adults, acyclovir (800 mg 5 times a day PO for 5-7 days), famciclovir (500 mg tid PO for 7 days), and valacyclovir (1,000 mg tid PO for 7 days) reduce the duration of the illness but do not prevent development of postherpetic neuralgia. In otherwise healthy children, herpes zoster is a less-severe disease, and postherpetic neuralgia usually does not occur. Therefore, treatment of uncomplicated herpes zoster in the child with an antiviral agent may not always be necessary, although some experts would treat with oral acyclovir (20 mg/kg/dose; maximum: 800 mg/dose) to shorten the duration of the illness. It is important to start antiviral therapy as soon as possible. Delay beyond 72 hr from onset of rash limits its effectiveness.

In contrast, herpes zoster in immunocompromised children can be severe, and disseminated disease may be life-threatening. Patients at high risk for disseminated disease should receive IV acyclovir (500 mg/m^2 or 10 mg/kg every 8 hr). Oral acyclovir, famciclovir, and valacyclovir are options for immunocompromised patients with uncomplicated herpes zoster, who are considered at low risk for visceral dissemination. Neuritis with herpes zoster should be managed with appropriate analgesics.

Use of corticosteroids in the treatment of herpes zoster in children is not recommended.

PROGNOSIS

Primary varicella has a mortality rate of 2-3 per 100,000 cases, with the lowest case fatality rates among children 1-9 yr of age (~1 death per 100,000 cases). Compared with these age groups, infants have a 4 times greater risk of dying and adults have a 25 times greater risk of dying. The most common complications among people who died from varicella were pneumonia, central nervous system complications, secondary infections, and hemorrhagic conditions. The mortality rate of untreated primary infection was 7% in immunocompromised children in the 1960s. In the era of antiviral therapy and improved supportive care, the prognosis has improved with treatment administered early in the course of illness, but deaths have continued to occur.

Herpes zoster among healthy children has an excellent prognosis and is usually self-limited. Severe presentation with complications and sometimes fatalities can occur in immunocompromised children.

PREVENTION

VZV transmission is difficult to prevent, especially from persons with varicella, because a person with varicella may be contagious for 24-48 hr before the rash is apparent. Herpes zoster is less infectious than varicella; nonetheless, transmission has been reported even in the absence of direct contact with the patient. Infection control practices, including caring for patients with varicella in isolation rooms with filtered air systems, are essential. All healthcare workers should have evidence of varicella immunity (Table 280.1). Unvaccinated healthcare workers without other evidence of immunity who have had a close exposure to VZV should be furloughed for days 8-21 after exposure because they are potentially infectious during this period.

Vaccine

Varicella is a vaccine-preventable disease. Varicella vaccine contains live, attenuated VZV (Oka strain) and is indicated for subcutaneous administration. In the United States, varicella vaccine is recommended for routine administration as a 2-dose regimen to healthy children at ages 12-15 mo and 4-6 yr. Administration of the 2nd dose earlier than 4-6 yr of age is acceptable, but it must be at least 3 mo after the 1st dose. Catch-up vaccination with the 2nd dose is recommended for children and adolescents who received only 1 dose. Vaccination with 2 doses is recommended for all persons without evidence of immunity. The minimum interval between the 2 doses is 3 mo for persons 12 yr of age or younger and 4 wk for older children, adolescents, and adults. Administration of varicella vaccine within 4 wk of measles-mumps-rubella (MMR) vaccination is associated with a higher risk for breakthrough disease; therefore, it is recommended that the varicella and MMR vaccines either be administered simultaneously at different sites or be given at least 4 wk apart. Varicella vaccine can be administered as a monovalent vaccine (for all healthy persons ≥12 mo of age) or as the quadrivalent measles-mumps-rubella-varicella (MMRV) vaccine (for children age 12 mo through 12 yr only).

Varicella vaccine is contraindicated for persons who have a history of anaphylactic reaction to any component of the vaccine; pregnant women; persons with cell-mediated immune deficiencies, including those with leukemia, lymphoma, and other malignant neoplasms affecting the bone marrow or lymphatic systems; persons receiving

Table 280.1	Evidence of Immunity to Varicella

Evidence of immunity to varicella consists of any of the following:
- Documentation of age-appropriate vaccination with a varicella vaccine:
  - Preschool-age children (i.e., age ≥12 mo): 1 dose
  - School-age children, adolescents, and adults: 2 doses*
- Laboratory evidence of immunity[†] or laboratory confirmation of disease
- Birth in the United States before 1980[‡]
- Diagnosis or verification of a history of varicella disease by a healthcare provider[§]
- Diagnosis or verification of a history of herpes zoster by a healthcare provider

*For children who received their 1st dose at younger than age 13 yr and for whom the interval between the 2 doses was 28 or more days, the 2nd dose is considered valid.
[†]Commercial assays can be used to assess disease-induced immunity, but they lack sensitivity to always detect vaccine-induced immunity (i.e., they might yield false-negative results).
[‡]For healthcare personnel, pregnant women, and immunocompromised persons, birth before 1980 should not be considered evidence of immunity.
[§]Verification of history or diagnosis of typical disease can be provided by any healthcare provider (e.g., school or occupational clinic nurse, nurse practitioner, physician assistant, or physician). For persons reporting a history of, or reporting with, atypical or mild cases, assessment by a physician or his/her designee is recommended, and one of the following should be sought: (1) an epidemiologic link to a typical varicella case or to a laboratory-confirmed case or (2) evidence of laboratory confirmation if it was performed at the time of acute disease. When such documentation is lacking, persons should not be considered as having a valid history of disease, because other diseases might mimic mild atypical varicella.

immunosuppressive therapy; and persons who have a family history of congenital or hereditary immunodeficiency in 1st-degree relatives unless the immune competence of the potential vaccine recipient is demonstrated. Children with isolated humoral immunodeficiencies may receive varicella vaccine. The monovalent varicella vaccine has been studied in clinical trial settings in children with acute lymphocytic leukemia and certain solid tumors who are in remission but this practice is not recommended except in a research setting. Varicella vaccine can be administered to patients with leukemia, lymphoma, or other malignancies whose disease is in remission, who have restored immunocompetence, and whose chemotherapy has been terminated for at least 3 mo.

The vaccine should be considered for HIV-infected children with a CD4+ T-lymphocyte percentage ≥15%. These children should receive 2 doses of vaccine, 3 mo apart. Specific guidelines for immunizing these children should be reviewed before vaccination. Data indicate that varicella vaccine is highly effective in preventing herpes zoster among children infected with HIV. MMRV should not be administered as a substitute for the component vaccines in HIV-infected children.

Two zoster vaccines are licensed for use for prevention of herpes zoster and to decrease the frequency of postherpetic neuralgia among individuals 50 yr of age and older, with the recombinant vaccine being preferred over the live vaccine. Zoster vaccines are not indicated for the treatment of zoster or postherpetic neuralgia.

Vaccine-Associated Adverse Events

Varicella vaccine is safe and well tolerated. The incidence of injection site complaints observed ≤3 days after vaccination was slightly higher after dose 2 (25%) than after dose 1 (22%). A mild vaccine-associated varicelliform rash was reported in approximately 1–5% of healthy vaccinees, consisting of 6-10 papular-vesicular, erythematous lesions with peak occurrence 8-21 days after vaccination. Serious adverse reactions confirmed to be caused by the vaccine strain are rare and include pneumonia, hepatitis, meningitis, recurrent herpes zoster, severe rash, and four deaths. Transmission of vaccine virus to susceptible contacts is a very rare event from healthy vaccine recipients (11 instances from 9 vaccinees, all in the presence of a rash in the vaccinee). MMRV vaccine is associated with a greater risk for febrile seizures 5-12 days after the 1st dose among children 12-23 mo of age compared with simultaneous MMR and varicella vaccines (one extra febrile seizure for every 2,500 children vaccinated).

Postexposure Prophylaxis

Vaccine given to healthy children within 3-5 days after exposure (as soon as possible is preferred) is effective in preventing or modifying varicella. Varicella vaccine is now recommended for postexposure use and for outbreak control. Oral acyclovir administered late in the incubation period may modify subsequent varicella in the healthy child; however, its use in this manner is not recommended until it can be further evaluated.

High-titer anti-VZV immune globulin as postexposure prophylaxis is recommended for immunocompromised children, pregnant women, and newborns exposed to varicella. Since 2012 the product licensed for use in the United States is VariZIG. VariZIG is commercially available from a broad network of specialty distributors in the United States (list available at www.varizig.com). The recommended dose is 1 vial (125 units) for each 10 kg increment of body weight (maximum: 625 units), except for infants weighing ≤2 kg who should receive 0.5 vial. VariZIG should be given intramuscularly as soon as possible but may be efficacious up to 10 days after exposure.

Newborns whose mothers have varicella 5 days before to 2 days after delivery should receive VariZIG (0.5 vial for those weighing ≤2 kg and 1 vial for those weighing >2 kg). VariZIG is also indicated for pregnant women and immunocompromised persons without evidence of varicella immunity; hospitalized premature infants born at <28 wk of gestation (or weight <1,000 g) who were exposed to varicella, regardless of maternal varicella immunity; and hospitalized premature infants born at ≥28 wk of gestation who were exposed to varicella and whose mothers have no evidence of varicella immunity. Patients given VariZIG should be monitored closely and treated with acyclovir if necessary once lesions develop.

Close contact between a susceptible high-risk patient and a patient with herpes zoster is also an indication for VariZIG prophylaxis. Passive antibody administration or treatment does not reduce the risk for herpes zoster or alter the clinical course of varicella or herpes zoster when given after the onset of symptoms.

Although licensed pooled IVIG preparations contain anti-VZV antibodies, the titer varies from lot to lot. In situations in which administration of VariZIG is not possible, IVIG can be administered (400 mg/kg administered once within 10 days of exposure). Immunocompromised patients who have received high-dose IVIG (>400 mg/kg) for other indications within 2-3 wk before VZV exposure can be expected to have serum antibodies to VZV.

Bibliography is available at Expert Consult.

Chapter **281**

Epstein-Barr Virus

Jason B. Weinberg

第二百八十一章

EB病毒

中文导读

　　本章主要介绍了EB病毒感染的病因学、流行病学、发病机制、临床表现、诊断、并发症、致癌性、治疗、预后和预防。EB病毒感染导致的最常见疾病是传染性单核细胞增多症，临床表现包括发热、咽痛、腹痛、皮疹、眼睑水肿等，阳性体征有淋巴结肿大、肝脾大、扁桃体肿大。在诊断中介绍了鉴别诊断和实验室诊断。在实验室诊断中详细阐述了嗜异性抗体、EB病毒特异性抗体和病毒DNA的检测。并发症包括脾破裂、呼吸道阻塞、神经系统后遗症、血液系统受累等。描述了与EB病毒相关的淋巴恶性肿瘤。本病不推荐抗病毒药，以对症支持治疗为主。

Infectious mononucleosis is the best-known clinical syndrome caused by Epstein-Barr virus (EBV). It is characterized by systemic somatic complaints consisting primarily of fatigue, malaise, fever, sore throat, and generalized lymphadenopathy. Originally described as glandular fever, it derives its name from the mononuclear lymphocytosis with atypical-appearing lymphocytes that accompany the illness.

ETIOLOGY

EBV is a double-stranded DNA virus that is a member of the gammaherpesviruses and causes >90% of cases of infectious mononucleosis. Two distinct types of EBV, type 1 and type 2 (also called type A and type B), have been characterized and have 70–85% sequence homology. EBV-1 is more prevalent worldwide, although EBV-2 is more common in Africa than in the United States and Europe. Both types lead to persistent, lifelong, latent infection. Dual infections with both types have been documented among immunocompromised persons. EBV-1 induces in vitro growth transformation of B lymphocytes more efficiently than does EBV-2, but no type-specific disease manifestations or clinical differences have been identified.

As many as 5–10% of infectious mononucleosis–like illnesses are caused by other types of primary infections, particularly cytomegalovirus but also pathogens such as *Toxoplasma gondii,* adenovirus, hepatitis viruses and HIV. In the majority of EBV-negative cases of infectious mononucleosis, the exact cause remains unknown.

EPIDEMIOLOGY

EBV infects more than 95% of the world's population. It is transmitted primarily via oral secretions. Among children, transmission may occur by exchange of saliva from child to child, such as occurs between children in out-of-home childcare. EBV is shed in oral secretions consistently for more than 6 mo after acute infection and then intermittently for life. As many as 20–30% of healthy EBV-infected persons shed virus at any particular time. EBV is also found in male and female genital secretions, and some studies suggest the possibility of spread through sexual contact. Nonintimate contact, environmental sources, and fomites do not contribute to transmission of EBV.

Infection with EBV in developing countries and among socioeconomically disadvantaged populations in developed countries usually occurs during infancy and early childhood. In central Africa, almost all children are infected by 3 yr of age. Among more affluent populations in industrialized countries, half of the population is infected by 6-8 yr of age with approximately 30% of infections occurring during adolescence and young adulthood. In the United States, seroprevalence increases with age, from approximately 54% for 6-8 yr olds to 83% for 18-19 yr olds. Seroprevalence at each age is substantially higher for Mexican-Americans and non-Hispanic blacks than non-Hispanic whites. Large differences are seen by family income, with highest seroprevalence in children of families with lowest income.

The epidemiology of the disease manifestations of infectious mononucleosis is related to the age of acquisition of EBV infection. Primary infection with EBV during childhood is usually asymptomatic or mild and indistinguishable from other childhood infections. Primary EBV infection in adolescents and adults manifests in 30–50% of cases as the **classic triad of fatigue, pharyngitis, and generalized lymphadenopathy**, which constitute the major clinical manifestations of infectious mononucleosis. This syndrome may be seen at all ages but is rarely apparent in children younger than 4 yr of age, when most EBV infections are asymptomatic, or in adults older than 40 yr of age, when most individuals have already been infected by EBV. The true incidence of the syndrome of infectious mononucleosis is unknown but is estimated to occur in 20-70 per 100,000 person-years. In young adults, the incidence increases to approximately 100 per 100,000 person-years. The prevalence of serologic evidence of past EBV infection increases with age; almost all adults in the United States are seropositive.

PATHOGENESIS

After transmission by saliva to the oral cavity, EBV infects both oral epithelial cells and tonsillar B lymphocytes, although it is unclear which cells are the primary initial targets. Ongoing viral replication leads to viremia and dissemination of infected B lymphocytes into peripheral blood and the lymphoreticular system, including the liver and spleen. Clinical manifestations of infectious mononucleosis, which are due to the host immune response to EBV infection, occur after a 6-wk incubation period following acute infection. The atypical lymphocytes that are frequently detected in patients with infectious mononucleosis are primarily CD8 T lymphocytes. Polyclonal CD8 T lymphocyte activation occurs early during the incubation period following infection, while expansion of EBV-specific CD8 T lymphocytes is detected closer to the time of symptom onset. Natural killer (NK) cells also expand in frequency and number following infection, particularly a $CD56^{dim}$ $CD16^-$ NK cell subset that is more effective than other NK cell subsets at recognizing infected cells. The host immune response is effective in rapidly reducing the EBV viral load, although persistent shedding of high levels of virus can be detected in the oropharynx for up to 6 mo. Intermittent shedding from the oropharynx occurs for many years following primary infection.

EBV, like the other herpesviruses, establishes lifelong latent infection after the primary infection. Latent virus persists primarily in memory B lymphocytes. The EBV genome persists as an episome in the nucleus of an infected cell and replicates with cell division. Viral integration into the cell genome is not typical. Only a few viral proteins, including the EBV-determined nuclear antigens (EBNAs), are produced during latency. These proteins are important in maintaining the viral episome during the latent state. Reactivation and new viral replication occurs at a low rate in populations of latently infected cells and is responsible for intermittent viral shedding in oropharyngeal secretions of infected individuals. Reactivation is unlikely to be accompanied by distinctive clinical symptoms.

CLINICAL MANIFESTATIONS

The incubation period of infectious mononucleosis in adolescents is 30-50 days. In children, it may be shorter. The majority of cases of primary EBV infection in infants and young children are clinically silent. In older patients, the onset of illness is usually insidious and vague. Patients may complain of malaise, fatigue, acute or prolonged (>1 wk) fever, headache, sore throat, nausea, abdominal pain, and myalgia. This prodromal period may last 1-2 wk. The complaints of sore throat and fever gradually increase until patients seek medical care. Splenic enlargement may be rapid enough to cause left upper quadrant abdominal discomfort and tenderness, which may be the presenting complaint.

The **classic physical examination findings** are generalized lymphadenopathy (90% of cases), splenomegaly (50% of cases), and hepatomegaly (10% of cases). Lymphadenopathy occurs most commonly in the anterior and posterior cervical nodes and the submandibular lymph nodes and less commonly in the axillary and inguinal lymph nodes. Epitrochlear lymphadenopathy is particularly suggestive of infectious mononucleosis. Although liver enzymes are often elevated, symptomatic hepatitis or jaundice is uncommon. Splenomegaly to 2-3 cm below the costal margin is typical (15–65% of cases); massive enlargement is uncommon.

The sore throat is often accompanied by moderate to severe pharyngitis with marked tonsillar enlargement, occasionally with exudates (Fig. 281.1). Palatal petechiae at the junction of the hard and soft palate are frequently seen. The pharyngitis is similar to that caused by streptococcal infection. Other clinical findings may include rashes and edema of the eyelids. Rashes are usually maculopapular and have been reported in 3-15% of patients. Patients with infectious mononucleosis who are treated with ampicillin or amoxicillin may experience an **ampicillin rash,** which may also occur with other β-lactam antibiotics (Fig. 281.2). This morbilliform, vasculitic rash is probably immune mediated and resolves without specific treatment. EBV can also be associated with Gianotti-Crosti syndrome, a symmetric rash on the cheeks with multiple erythematous papules, which may coalesce into plaques and persist for 15-50 days. The rash has the appearance of atopic dermatitis and may appear on the extremities and buttocks.

DIAGNOSIS

A presumptive diagnosis of infectious mononucleosis may be made by the presence of classical clinical symptoms with atypical lymphocytosis

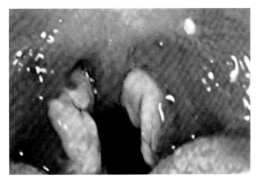

Fig. 281.1 Tonsillitis with membrane formation in infectious mononucleosis. *(Courtesy of Alex J. Steigman, MD.)*

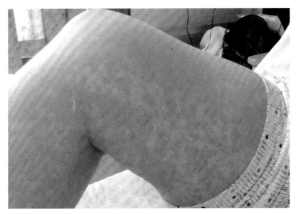

Fig. 281.2 Amoxicillin-induced rash in Epstein-Barr virus infection. Morbilliform maculopapular rash on the leg, which appeared shortly after starting amoxicillin. The rash is typical of that seen in the context of Epstein-Barr virus infection in patients treated with amoxicillin or ampicillin. *(From Norman SD, Murray IA, Shetty D, et al: Jaundice, abdominal pain, and fever in a young woman, Lancet 390:1713–1714, 2017, Fig. A, p. 1713.)*

in the peripheral blood. The diagnosis is usually confirmed by serologic testing, either for heterophile antibody or specific EBV antibodies.

Differential Diagnosis
EBV is the most common cause of infectious mononucleosis. Infectious mononucleosis–like illnesses may also be caused by primary infection with other pathogens, such as cytomegalovirus, *T. gondii*, adenovirus, and HIV. Streptococcal pharyngitis may cause sore throat and cervical lymphadenopathy indistinguishable from that of infectious mononucleosis, but it is not typically associated with hepatosplenomegaly. Approximately 5% of cases of EBV-associated infectious mononucleosis have positive throat cultures for group A streptococcus, representing pharyngeal streptococcal carriage. Failure of a patient with presumed streptococcal pharyngitis to improve within 48-72 hr should evoke suspicion of infectious mononucleosis. Hematologic malignancies should also be considered in a patient with an infectious mononucleosis–like illness, particularly when lymphadenopathy and hepatosplenomegaly are appreciated and the results of an initial laboratory evaluation are not consistent with an infectious etiology.

Laboratory Diagnosis
The majority of patients (>90%) have a leukocytosis of 10,000-20,000 cells/μL, of which at least two thirds are lymphocytes; atypical lymphocytes usually account for 20–40% of the total number. The atypical cells are mature T lymphocytes that have been antigenically activated. Compared with regular lymphocytes microscopically, **atypical lymphocytes** are

larger overall, with larger, eccentrically placed indented and folded nuclei with a lower nuclear-to-cytoplasm ratio. Although atypical lymphocytosis may be seen with many other infections associated with lymphocytosis, the highest degree of atypical lymphocytes is classically seen with EBV infection. Mild thrombocytopenia to 50,000-200,000 platelets/μL occurs in more than 50% of patients but only rarely is associated with purpura. Mild elevation of hepatic transaminases occurs in approximately 75% of uncomplicated cases, but it is usually asymptomatic and without jaundice.

Detection of Heterophile Antibodies
Heterophile antibodies are cross-reactive immunoglobulin M (IgM) antibodies that agglutinate mammalian erythrocytes but are not EBV-specific. Heterophile antibody tests, such as the **monospot** test, are positive in 90% of cases of EBV-associated infectious mononucleosis in adolescents and adults during the second week of illness, but in only up to 50% of cases in children younger than 4 yr of age. Test results can remain positive for up to 12 mo. The false-positive rate is low, generally <10%. A positive heterophile antibody test in a patient with classic clinical manifestations of mononucleosis strongly supports that diagnosis. However, because of the nonspecific nature of heterophile antibody testing, EBV-specific antibody testing should be performed when a precise diagnosis is necessary.

Detection of Epstein-Barr Virus–Specific Antibodies
If the heterophile test result is negative and an EBV infection is suspected, EBV-specific antibody testing is indicated. Measurement of antibodies to EBV proteins including viral capsid antigen (VCA), Epstein-Barr nuclear antigen (EBNA), and early antigen (EA) are used most frequently (Fig. 281.3 and Table 281.1). The acute phase of infectious mononucleosis is characterized by rapid IgM and IgG antibody responses to VCA in all cases and an IgG response to EA in most cases. The IgM response to VCA is transient but can be detected for at least 4 wk and occasionally up to 3 mo. The IgG response to VCA usually peaks late in the acute phase, declines slightly over the next several weeks to months, and then persists at a relatively stable level for life.

Anti-EA IgG antibodies are usually detectable for several months but may persist or be detected intermittently at low levels for many years. Antibodies to the diffuse-staining component of EA (EA-D) are found transiently in 80% of patients during the acute phase of infectious mononucleosis. Antibodies to the cytoplasmic-restricted component of EA (EA-R) emerge transiently in the convalescence from infectious mononucleosis. High levels of antibodies to EA-D or EA-R may be found also in immunocompromised patients with persistent EBV infections and active EBV replication.

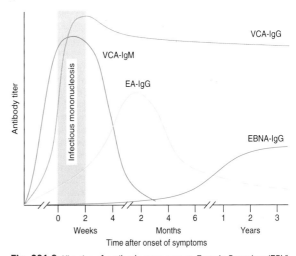

Fig. 281.3 Kinetics of antibody responses to Epstein-Barr virus (EBV) antigens in infectious mononucleosis. EA, early antigen; EBNA, EBV-determined nuclear antigens; IgG, immunoglobulin G; IgM, immunoglobulin M; VCA, viral capsid antigen.

Table 281.1	Correlation of Clinical Status and Antibody Responses to Epstein-Barr Virus Infection			
CLINICAL STATUS	VCA IgM	VCA IgG	EA IgG	EBNA IgG
Susceptible	–	–	–	–
Acute primary infection	+	+	+/–	–
Recent primary infection	+/–	+	+/–	+/–
Past infection	–	+	+/–	+

EA, early antigen (typically the diffuse staining component, or EA-D); EBNA, EBV-determined nuclear antigens; EBV, Epstein-Barr virus; IgG, immunoglobulin G; IgM, immunoglobulin M; VCA, viral capsid antigen.

Anti-EBNA IgG antibodies are the last to develop in infectious mononucleosis and gradually appear 3-4 mo after the onset of illness and remain at low levels for life. Absence of anti-EBNA when other antibodies are present implies recent infection, whereas the presence of anti-EBNA implies infection occurring more than 3-4 mo previously. The wide range of individual antibody responses and the various laboratory methods used can occasionally make interpretation of an antibody profile difficult. The detection of IgM antibody to VCA is the most valuable and specific serologic test for the diagnosis of acute EBV infection and is generally sufficient to confirm the diagnosis.

Detection of Viral DNA
EBV DNA can be detected and viral genome copy number quantified in whole blood, peripheral blood mononuclear cells (PBMC), and plasma using real-time polymerase chain reaction (PCR). EBV DNA can be detected in PBMC and plasma of patients with infectious mononucleosis for a brief period of time after the onset of symptoms and in PBMC for an extended period of time. However, detection of EBV DNA is usually not necessary to diagnose infectious mononucleosis in immunocompetent patients with typical manifestations of disease. In contrast, serial measurements of EBV genome copy number are often used following solid organ or hematopoietic stem cell transplantation as surveillance for posttransplant lymphoproliferative disease (PTLD). Very high or consistently increasing EBV genome copy number suggests an increased risk for PTLD, although definitive diagnosis is typically based on tissue biopsy. The frequency and duration of monitoring EBV genome copy number is determined by the time after transplant and risk factors such as the type of transplant and the degree of immunosuppression. Serial measurement of EBV genome copy number can be useful in monitoring response to therapy for PTLD. Measurement of EBV genome copy number can also be used for screening and to determine prognosis for some EBV-associated malignancies, such as nasopharyngeal carcinoma and Hodgkin lymphoma.

COMPLICATIONS
Severe complications are unusual in patients with infectious mononucleosis. Splenic rupture, either spontaneous or following mild trauma, may occur in approximately 0.1% of cases but is rarely fatal. Airway obstruction due to swelling of oropharyngeal lymphoid tissue occurs in <5% of cases. A variety of neurologic conditions have been associated with EBV infectious mononucleosis. Headache is a common symptom, but symptomatic meningitis or encephalitis is uncommon. More severe neurologic manifestations, such as seizures and ataxia, may occur in 1–5% of cases. Perceptual distortions of sizes, shapes, and spatial relationships, known as the **Alice in Wonderland syndrome (metamorphopsia)**, may be a presenting symptom. Some reports suggest an association between infectious mononucleosis and the possible development of multiple sclerosis. Hematologic abnormalities such as mild hemolytic anemia, thrombocytopenia and neutropenia are relatively common, but aplastic anemia, severe thrombocytopenia, and severe neutropenia are rare. Other rare complications include myocarditis, interstitial pneumonia, pancreatitis, parotitis, and orchitis.

Patients with dysregulated immune responses to primary infection, such as individuals with primary or secondary **hemophagocytic lymphohistiocytosis (HLH)**, can develop severe, life-threatening complications with primary EBV infection. Patients with other primary immunodeficiencies that result in failure to control EBV infection and/or abnormal inflammatory responses to infection are at risk for severe manifestations of EBV infection, often with fulminant infectious mononucleosis, chronic viremia, dysgammaglobulinemia, and lymphoproliferation. Immunodeficiencies most commonly linked to severe EBV infection tend to be those affecting aspects of NK cell, T lymphocyte, and NKT lymphocyte function. Examples include X-linked lymphoproliferative (XLP) syndrome, which is caused by mutations in genes encoding the signaling lymphocytic activation molecule (SLAM)-associated protein (SAP) or X-linked inhibitor of apoptosis (XIAP); X-linked immunodeficiency with magnesium defect, EBV infection, and neoplasia (XMEN), caused by mutations in *MAGT1*, which encodes a magnesium transporter protein; and deficiencies in IL-2-inducible T-cell kinase (ITK), CD27, or CD70.

ONCOGENESIS
Infection with EBV, the first human virus to be associated with malignancy, accounts for up to 2% of cancers worldwide. Manipulation of infected cells by EBV to establish and maintain latency can lead to transformation and oncogenesis. EBV is associated with lymphoid malignancies, such as Burkitt lymphoma, Hodgkin lymphoma, aggressive NK cell leukemia, T- and NK cell lymphoproliferative disorder, and epithelial cell malignancies such as nasopharyngeal carcinoma and gastric carcinoma.

Endemic Burkitt lymphoma is the most common childhood cancer in equatorial East Africa and New Guinea. These regions are holoendemic for *Plasmodium falciparum* malaria and have a high rate of EBV infection early in life. Constant exposure to malaria is thought to act as a B lymphocyte mitogen that contributes to the polyclonal B-lymphocyte proliferation with EBV infection, impairs T lymphocyte surveillance of EBV-infected B lymphocytes, and increases the risk for developing Burkitt lymphoma. Approximately 98% of cases of endemic Burkitt lymphoma contain the EBV genome compared with only 20% of nonendemic (sporadic) Burkitt lymphoma cases in other areas of the world.

The incidence of **Hodgkin lymphoma** peaks in childhood in developing countries and in young adulthood in developed countries. Infection with EBV increases the risk for Hodgkin lymphoma by a factor of 2-4, with the risk of developing Hodgkin lymphoma peaking at 2.4 yr following infectious mononucleosis. EBV is associated with more than half of cases of mixed cellularity Hodgkin lymphoma and approximately one quarter of cases of the nodular sclerosing subtype, but it is rarely associated with lymphocyte-predominant Hodgkin lymphoma. Immunohistochemical studies have localized EBV to the Reed-Sternberg cells and their variants, the pathognomonic malignant cells of Hodgkin lymphoma.

Numerous congenital and acquired immunodeficiency syndromes are associated with an increased incidence of EBV-associated B-lymphocyte lymphoma, especially central nervous system lymphoma and leiomyosarcoma. Congenital immunodeficiencies predisposing to EBV-associated lymphoproliferation include XLP syndrome, common-variable immunodeficiency, ataxia-telangiectasia, Wiskott-Aldrich syndrome, and Chédiak-Higashi syndrome. Individuals with acquired immunodeficiencies resulting from anticancer chemotherapy, immunosuppression after solid organ or hematopoietic cell transplantation, or HIV infection have a significantly increased risk for EBV-associated lymphoproliferation. The lymphomas may be focal or diffuse and are usually histologically polyclonal but may become monoclonal. EBV-associated PTLD can occur following solid organ transplantation and, less commonly, allogeneic hematopoietic cell transplantation. The most important risk factors for PTLD are the degree of T lymphocyte immunosuppression and recipient EBV serostatus.

TREATMENT
There is no specific treatment for infectious mononucleosis. The mainstays of management are rest, adequate fluid and nutrition intake, and

symptomatic treatment to manage fever, throat discomfort, and malaise. Bed rest is necessary only when the patient has debilitating fatigue. As soon as there is definite symptomatic improvement, the patient should be encouraged to resume normal activities. Because blunt abdominal trauma may predispose patients to splenic rupture, it is customary and prudent to advise against participation in contact sports and strenuous athletic activities during the first 2-3 wk of illness or while splenomegaly is present.

Antiviral therapy is not recommended. Although nucleoside analogs such as acyclovir inhibit viral replication in vitro and decrease the duration of oropharyngeal viral shedding in patients with infectious mononucleosis, they have not been shown to not provide consistent clinical benefit for patients with infectious mononucleosis or EBV-associated malignancies. Short courses of corticosteroids may be helpful for selected complications of infectious mononucleosis, such as airway obstruction, but there are insufficient data to support the use of corticosteroids to control typical symptoms in patients with infectious mononucleosis. Adoptive immunotherapy involving the infusion of EBV-specific cytotoxic T lymphocytes has shown some promise in early trials for transplant recipients with PTLD and for other patients with EBV-associated malignancies.

PROGNOSIS

The prognosis for complete recovery is excellent. The major symptoms typically last 2-4 wk, followed by gradual recovery within 2 mo of symptom onset. Cervical lymphadenopathy and fatigue may resolve more slowly. Prolonged and debilitating fatigue and malaise may wax and wane for several weeks to 6 mo and are common complaints even in otherwise unremarkable cases. Occasional persistence of fatigue for a few years after infectious mononucleosis is well recognized. There is no convincing evidence linking EBV infection or EBV reactivation to chronic fatigue syndrome.

PREVENTION

Vaccination against EBV would be appealing strategy to prevent acute disease (infectious mononucleosis) and complications such as EBV-associated malignancies. Early clinical trials using strategies targeting the EBV gp350 envelope glycoprotein demonstrated some protection against symptomatic infectious mononucleosis, although vaccination did not prevent EBV infection. No EBV vaccine is currently approved for clinical use.

Bibliography is available at Expert Consult.

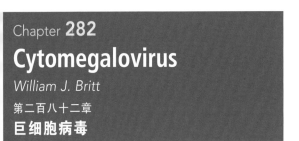

Chapter **282**
Cytomegalovirus
William J. Britt

第二百八十二章
巨细胞病毒

中文导读

本章主要介绍了巨细胞病毒与宿主的相互作用、流行病学、临床表现、诊断、治疗和预防。详细阐述了正常人群、免疫功能低下人群、先天性感染和围产期感染不同的临床表现。实验室诊断包括血清学和 DNA检测，分别介绍了先天性感染和非先天性感染的诊断。治疗中介绍了特异性抗病毒药和巨细胞免疫球蛋白。预防包括主动免疫、被动免疫和免疫咨询。

Human cytomegalovirus (CMV) is ubiquitous in the population, and individuals who become infected remain persistently infected for life, with intermittent shedding of infectious virus from mucosal surfaces. Although CMV rarely causes symptoms in normal individuals, it is an important cause of morbidity and sometimes death in immunocompromised hosts. CMV remains a well-recognized cause of disease in the newborn infant following intrauterine infection (congenital CMV) and the allograft recipients undergoing posttransplantation immunosuppression. CMV emerged as the most common opportunistic infection in HIV/AIDS patients prior to the advent of effective retroviral therapy. Invasive CMV infections can be observed in patients treated with immunosuppressive biologics such as anti-tumor necrosis factor (TNF) antibodies. In each of these clinical situations, the association of disease with CMV infection has been linked to high levels of virus replication and end organ disease, usually associated with virus dissemination. In contrast, there is likely another group of disease states associated with chronic effects of persistent CMV infection that reflects the robust inflammatory response induced by this virus. Such associations have included coronary artery disease, transplant vasculopathy and cardiac allograft loss, tubular sclerosis and renal allograft loss, exacerbations of inflammatory bowel disease, and possibly some cancers such as glioblastoma. In addition, there continues to be debate surrounding the role of CMV in immune senescence and the decrease in immune responsiveness observed in aging. Whether definitive evidence will eventually directly link CMV to these disease states is uncertain, but it is clear that understanding the complex biology of CMV infections, including the virus-mediated control of ensuing host responses to infection with this virus, will provide new insight into each of these diseases.

THE VIRUS AND ITS INTERACTION WITH THE HOST

CMV is the largest of the human herpesviruses, with an estimated size of 190 nm. The 230 kb double-stranded DNA genome is about 50% larger than the herpes simplex virus genome and encodes over 200 open reading frames, which include 100 unique virion proteins and an unknown number of nonstructural proteins. Viral DNA replication takes place in the nucleus of the infected cell followed by virus assembly in both the nucleus and cytoplasm. The structure of the virus is typical of herpesviruses and includes a complex envelope composed of host cell–derived membrane studded with virion glycoproteins, an amorphous area between the envelope and the capsid called the tegument layer, and an icosahedral capsid that contains the virion DNA. The tegument layer is highly immunogenic and induces strong adaptive immune responses, including CMV specific CD8+ cytotoxic T lymphocytes that are thought to play a pivotal role in controlling CMV replication in the infected host. Likewise, the protein components of the viral envelope are also immunogenic and believed to induce protective antibody responses that have been correlated with virus neutralization. In vivo, CMV appears to replicate in nearly all tissue and cell types whereas in vitro productive virus replication (production of infectious progeny) occurs in primary cells derived from epithelial tissue and the dermis. Literature from the 1990s suggested that each strain of CMV isolated from epidemiologically unrelated individuals was genetically unique, a finding suggesting that an infinite number of distinct viruses existed in the human population. This observation has been validated with next-generation sequencing technologies, which have provided evidence that CMV exists as genetically diverse forms within an individual. This finding has argued that during replication, CMV DNA synthesis is fraught with error rates that are much higher than previous studies would predict and/or potential recombination events if permissive cells are infected with genetically diverse populations of viruses. Thus repeated exposures to CMV over time could result in an individual acquiring a library of CMVs as reinfection of previously infected individuals with new strains of CMV appears commonplace. These observations have led many investigators to argue that CMV must express an armamentarium of immune evasion functions that allow it to remain hidden from protective host immunity. This relationship between host and virus is best illustrated by the finding that over years a persistently infected individual can maintain a stable virus load, unwavering antiviral antibody responses, and in some individuals, up to 15% of a total peripheral blood CD8+ CTL activity dedicated to recognition of CMV infected cells, suggesting that a détente has been established between virus replication and host innate and adaptive antiviral immunity. Thus CMV efficiently persists in an infected host for a lifetime while inducing chronic immune activation. This latter characteristic of the biology of CMV infection has supported a linkage between CMV and many of the chronic diseases that have been associated with this ubiquitous virus.

EPIDEMIOLOGY

CMV infections are acquired through several settings: (1) community exposure, (2) nosocomial transmission, and (3) intrauterine infection. **Community acquisition** occurs throughout life and is linked by exposure to CMV that is shed from mucosal surfaces such as saliva, genital secretions, and urine. Peaks in exposure occur during childhood and in adolescents and young adults, presumably in the latter cases secondary to sexual activity. Common routes of infection of the very young infant include perinatal exposure to infected genital secretions during birth and ingestion of CMV-containing breast milk. Breastfeeding is the most common route of CMV infection in early childhood. Ingestion of breast milk from seropositive women results in a rate of infection of about 60% in infants. Infection is most common during the first several months of breastfeeding, but the risk continues for the duration of breastfeeding. Infants infected through breast milk excrete virus in the saliva and urine for prolonged periods of time measured in months to years and thus serve as a reservoir of virus for spread to other infants, children, and adults. After this period of intense exposure to CMV during the first year of life, infection in the remainder of childhood and early teenage years depends on specific exposures such as enrollment in group childcare facilities and/or exposure to infected, similarly aged siblings. Up to 50% of young infants and children attending group care facilities can be excreting CMV, a source of virus that can result in infection of children enrolled in the facility and in some cases the adult workers in the facility. Furthermore, once infected at a group care facility, infants can then transmit virus to their parents and siblings, thus providing a mechanism for spread of CMV within the community. Throughout childhood and early adulthood, CMV is transmitted by exposure to saliva and urine. However, as noted above, in adolescence and early adulthood there is a spike in infection presumably associated with sexual exposure. CMV is considered a sexually transmitted infection, and a wealth of data has shown an increased rate of infection in the sexually active population as well as transmission in CMV-discordant couples. In summary, exposure to young children and sexual exposure represent the most consistent risk factors for acquisition of CMV infection.

Nosocomial infections with CMV are well described and are associated with exposure to blood products containing CMV and less commonly through allograft transplantation following transplantation of an organ from a CMV-infected donor. Prior to improvements in blood banking that limited the number of leukocytes in red cell transfusions and that more efficiently identified CMV infected donors, transmission of CMV by blood transfusion was not uncommon and closely related to the volume of blood that was transfused. Transfusion-acquired CMV infections often resulted in symptomatic illness, with laboratory findings including hepatitis and thrombocytopenia in children and adults. In newborn infants lacking antibodies to CMV secondary to being born to women without seroimmunity to CMV or in cases of extreme prematurity, severe and sometimes fatal infections could develop. Similarly, immunocompromised patients who received CMV-containing blood were also at risk for severe infection, regardless of their prior exposure to CMV. Methodologies that more efficiently deplete contaminating leukocytes and the use of blood products from CMV seronegative donors have greatly decreased the incidence of transfusion-associated CMV infections. Finally, CMV transmission through infected allografts is well described and infections arising from CMV transferred in the allograft are a major cause of morbidity in both the early and late period after transplantation. Severe infections and graft loss are more often associated with mismatches between the donor and recipient, as occurs if the donor has a history of CMV infection (donor, CMV positive) and the recipient has not been exposed to CMV (recipient, CMV negative; D+/R− mismatch). Even with effective antiviral therapy to modify CMV infections in the early posttransplant period, CMV infection remains linked to long-term graft dysfunction and graft loss, a particularly important problem in cardiac and lung transplant recipients.

Congenital CMV infection (present at birth) occurs following intrauterine transmission of CMV. Rates of congenital infection between 0.4% and 1.0% have been reported in the United States, with perhaps the best estimate being about 0.4% based on a large multicenter study. Rates as high 2% in some areas in Asia and Africa have also been described. Although the mechanism of transmission remains an active area of investigation, CMV is thought to be transferred to the developing fetus following hematogenous spread of CMV to the placenta, presumably followed by cell-free transfer of virus to the fetal blood system. The rate of transmission to the fetus is about 30% in women with primary infection during pregnancy; in utero infections also occur in previously immune women (nonprimary infection), albeit at a reduced rate that has been suggested to be on the order of 1–2%. This latter rate is an estimate because the number of previously immune women who experience active infection during pregnancy is not known. It is important to note that although the rate of transmission of CMV is more frequent following primary maternal infection, the absolute number of congenitally infected infants born to women with nonprimary infections in most populations outnumber those resulting from primary maternal infection by 3-4-fold. This is particularly true in Africa, South America, and Asia, where maternal seroimmunity to CMV often exceeds 95%. Interestingly, these populations also have the highest rates of congenital CMV infections. The source of nonprimary infection is also somewhat controversial. Older reports suggested that nonprimary infection followed reactivation (recurrence) of virus infection in seroimmune women, whereas more recent literature has demonstrated that reinfection by genetically distinct strains of CMV occurs in previously infected women and these newly acquired viruses can be transmitted to the developing fetus. In some studies, the reinfection rates are about 15–20%, with annualized rates as high as 25%. Thus immunity to CMV is far from protective, although it has been inferred from existing epidemiological data that it can modify the risk of transmission to the developing fetus.

Mechanisms of Disease Associated With Cytomegalovirus Infections

The mechanism(s) of disease associated with CMV infections remains undefined for most clinical syndromes that follow CMV infection. Several reasons have contributed to the overall lack of understanding of the pathogenesis of CMV infections and include: (1) the asymptomatic nature of infections in almost all immunocompetent individuals; (2) the complexity of the underlying disease processes in immunocompromised hosts that often confound the assignment of specific manifestations of CMV infection; (3) the species-specific tropism of human CMV; and perhaps most importantly, (4) limitations inherent in observational studies in humans. The strict species specificity of most CMVs has been a major limitation in the development of animal models that closely recapitulate human CMV infections. However, models have been developed in nonhuman primates, guinea pigs, and rodents to address specific aspects of the biology of CMVs. Although CMV replicates in a limited number of cells types in vitro, CMV inclusions, antigens, and nucleic acids can be demonstrated in almost all organ systems and cell types in individuals with severe, disseminated infections. The virus does not exhibit strict cellular or organ system tropism in vivo. Hematogenous dissemination has been argued to be associated primarily with cell-associated virus, and significant levels of plasma virus are usually detected only in severely immunocompromised hosts with high total-blood viral loads. Virus and viral DNA can be recovered from neutrophils, monocytes, and endothelial cells present in peripheral blood. High levels of virus replication can result in end-organ disease, secondary to direct virus-mediated cellular damage. These manifestations of CMV infections are thought to result from uncontrolled virus replication and dissemination, secondary to deficits in innate and adaptive immune responses to CMV. In some cases, clinical disease has been observed in patients without significant levels of virus replication, a finding suggesting indirect mechanisms of disease such as immunopathologic responses to CMV. Such a mechanism was clearly operative in patients with immune recovery vitritis, a pathological T-lymphocyte–mediated response to CMV in HIV/AIDS patients with CMV retinitis that closely followed the reconstitution of their virus-specific T lymphocyte responses following active retroviral therapy. Likewise, the level of virus replication has not been closely correlated with several chronic diseases thought to be linked to CMV, an observation that is consistent with indirect mechanisms of disease such as immunopathologic responses. These mechanisms are better described in animal models of human CMV disease.

From early observations in patients with invasive CMV infections in allograft recipients it was apparent that immunosuppressive therapies that resulted in altered T lymphocyte function predisposed these patients to severe infections. These observations that were first described in the 1970s were confirmed in multiple studies over the following decade. Definitive evidence consistent with this mechanism was provided by a clinical study that demonstrated that in vitro expanded, CMV-specific cytotoxic T lymphocytes could limit invasive infection in hematopoietic cell transplant recipients. Invasive infections such as retinitis and colitis in

HIV/AIDS patients with very low CD4+ T-lymphocyte counts also clearly demonstrated the importance of T lymphocyte responses and invasive CMV infections. Other studies in solid organ transplant (SOT) recipients have demonstrated that the passive transfer of immune globulins containing high titers of anti-CMV antibodies could provide some degree of protection from invasive disease, a finding that was consistent with the proposed role of antiviral antibodies in limiting CMV dissemination and disease in animal models of invasive CMV infections. The importance of innate immune responses such as natural killer (NK) cells and $\gamma\delta$ T lymphocytes in limiting invasive infections have been well documented in representative animal models but definitive evidence for a key role in resistance to CMV infections in humans is limited. Lastly, effector molecules such as γ-interferon appear to a play an important role in controlling local CMV infections in animal models, but evidence of a similar role in humans has not been shown experimentally.

The control of acute CMV infection is clearly dependent on an effective adaptive immune response; however, even a vigorous T lymphocyte response is not sufficient to eliminate CMV from the infected host, as CMV persists for the lifetime of the host either as a low level chronic infection or as a latent infection with limited transcription from specific regions of its genome. The inability of the host to completely clear CMV remains incompletely understood, but the large array of immune evasion functions encoded by this virus likely contributes to the blunted innate and adaptive immune response. These functions include: (1) inhibition of apoptotic and necroptotic functions of infected cells; (2) inhibition of interferon regulated responses; (3) inhibition of NK cell activation; (4) downregulation of class I MHC expression, inhibition of class II MHC function; and (5) mechanisms to limit antibody recognition of envelope proteins such as carbohydrate masking of antibody recognition sites and extensive variation in amino acid sequences in virion envelop proteins. Although each of these functions by itself could potentially have only limited effects on virus clearance secondary to the redundancy of antiviral activities of the host immune system, when acting in concert they likely provide the virus an advantage that leads to its persistence. The importance of these evasion functions has been shown in animal models, and specific immune evasion functions have been shown to facilitate virus dissemination and persistence, reinfection with genetically similar viruses, as well as reinfections with new strains of virus in animals with existing immunity to CMV.

CLINICAL MANIFESTATIONS

The clinical manifestations of CMV infection reflect the level of virus replication and the end-organ involvement. The manifestations of invasive CMV infections have been most commonly identified with syndromes that could be associated with a primary infection defined as an infection in an individual without existing immunity to the virus. Chronic CMV infections that have been associated with disease syndromes almost always have concurrent manifestations of the underlying causes of the primary disease, thus confounding the role of CMV in the primary disease process and its contribution to the clinical syndromes in these patients.

Normal Host

In the overwhelming majority of patients with acute CMV infections, there are no specific symptoms or clinical findings. In patients with symptomatic, acute CMV infection, clinical findings most commonly resemble a mononucleosis-like syndrome, with fatigue and occasionally cervical adenopathy. It has been reported that up to 20% of heterophile antibody negative mononucleosis could be attributed to CMV. Laboratory findings could include mild elevation of hepatic transaminases and decreased platelet counts.

Immunocompromised Host

The clinical presentation of CMV infection in immunocompromised hosts often reflects the magnitude of the immunodeficiency. Profoundly immunocompromised hosts such as hematopoietic stem cell transplantation (HSCT) recipients can present with disseminated infection and clinical manifestations reflecting disease in multiple organ systems, including liver, lung, gastrointestinal tract, and, less frequently, the CNS. Organ-threatening and life-threatening disease is not infrequent. In less immunocompromised patients such as most SOT recipients, CMV infection can present with fever, hematological abnormalities including leukopenia and thrombocytopenia, and mild hepatocellular dysfunction. In contrast to renal and liver SOT recipients, heart-lung and lung transplant recipients are at high risk for severe manifestations from CMV infection, presumably because the transplanted organ is a site of virus replication, disease, and life-threatening dysfunction. Prior to widespread use of antivirals for prophylaxis of allograft recipients, clinical disease usually developed between 30 and 60 day posttransplantation. More recently, prolonged antiviral prophylaxis has nearly eliminated CMV disease in the early posttransplant period in most SOTs, but late manifestations of CMV infection often become apparent after discontinuation of antiviral prophylaxis. These late manifestations are most worrisome in HSCT recipients, as they may signal deficits in graft function leading to invasive CMV infections. Finally, long-term graft function has been reported to be influenced by CMV infection. This has been most well studied in the renal allograft recipients and is thought by some investigators to represent a significant cause of chronic graft dysfunction and loss. Perhaps the most dramatic impact of CMV infection late in the posttransplant period can be seen in heart transplant recipients, where CMV is believed to play a major role in transplant vascular sclerosis, a vasculopathy of the coronary arteries in the allograft leading to loss of the transplanted heart.

Congenital Infection

Congenital infection with CMV can present with symptomatic infections (Table 282.1) in about 10% of infected newborns, whereas 90% of infected infants will have *no clinical manifestations* of infection in the newborn period and can be identified only by newborn screening programs. **Severe multiorgan disease** is infrequent and occurs in less than 5% of infants with congenital CMV infections. The clinical findings in infants with symptomatic congenital CMV infections can include hepatosplenomegaly, petechial rashes, jaundice, and microcephaly. These findings were utilized for decades in natural history studies to classify infants has having symptomatic or asymptomatic infections; however, more recently several authors have included intrauterine growth restriction as a finding of symptomatic congenital CMV infection. Laboratory findings are consistent with the clinical findings and include direct hyperbilirubinemia, elevation of hepatic transaminases, thrombocytopenia, and abnormal findings on cranial ultrasonography/computed tomography. If cerebrospinal fluid is obtained, there can be evidence of encephalitis, with elevation of mononuclear cell number and, in some cases, elevation of protein. A small number of symptomatically infected infants (<10%) will be found to have chorioretinitis. Finally, because hearing loss is the most common long-term sequelae associated with congenital CMV infection, the failure of an infant to pass a newborn hearing screening exam should alert caregivers to the possibility of congenital CMV infection. Hearing loss in the older infant and young child should also alert the clinician to the possibility of congenital CMV infection as about 50% of infants with hearing loss associated with congenital CMV infection will pass an initial hearing screening exam but develop hearing loss in later infancy and early childhood. Importantly, hearing loss can be progressive in infants with hearing loss secondary to congenital CMV infections. Lastly, the diagnosis of congenital CMV infection must be made within the first 2-3 wk of life, and congenital CMV infection cannot be assumed to be the cause of hearing loss in older infants without evidence of CMV infection in the newborn period.

An organized plan for follow-up is an important component of the clinical management of infants with congenital CMV infection. Because permanent sequelae are limited to disorders of the nervous system, long-term follow-up should include appropriate assessment of development and neuromuscular function in infected infants, with referral to specialized care if necessary. Hearing loss will develop in about 11% of infected infants, and in some infants hearing loss will progress during infancy. Thus audiologic testing and follow-up are mandatory in these patients. Other sequelae such as vision loss are infrequent, but vision testing and comprehensive eye examinations should be included in the care plan of infants with congenital CMV infection.

Perinatal Infection

Perinatal infections can be acquired during birth or following ingestion of CMV-containing breast milk. In almost all cases perinatal infections have not been associated with any clinical manifestations of infection and perhaps more importantly, have not been associated with any long-term sequelae. In rare cases such as is seen in breast milk transmission of CMV to extremely premature infants or infants born to nonimmune women, perinatal infection can result in severe, disseminated infections associated with end-organ disease and death. These more severe infections are thought to develop in infants that lack transplacentally acquired antiviral antibodies, either secondary to extreme prematurity, or as the product of a mother lacking anti-CMV antibodies. However, definitive evidence supporting this explanation is lacking.

DIAGNOSIS

In the nonimmunocompromised individual, diagnosis of CMV infection requires evidence of a primary infection. Serological reactivity for CMV is lifelong following primary infection; therefore the presence of immunoglobulin G (IgG) antibody to CMV does not provide evidence of acute infection. In addition, IgM reactivity for CMV can be detected for prolonged periods after acute infection and cannot be used to reliably estimate the duration of infection. Furthermore, recovery of virus from body fluids such as saliva or urine does not in itself permit diagnosis of CMV infection, because persistently infected individuals can intermittently shed virus. In the immunocompromised host, CMV can frequently be recovered from patients in the absence of evidence of invasive CMV infection. Thus assignment of CMV as a cause of disease in this patient population must be made carefully, and other potential causes of symptoms and clinical findings in these patients must also be considered. Serological assays are of limited value in the transplant recipient secondary to impact of immunosuppression on antibody responses in the allograft recipient. Moreover, IgM antibodies can be produced following a nonprimary infection in these patients. Sequential viral load measurements by polymer chain reaction (PCR) in relevant body fluids such as blood and measurements of CMV DNA in biopsy tissue can be of great value in establishing CMV as a cause of disease in allograft recipients. Histopathological detection of characteristic owl eye inclusion–bearing cells is insensitive but can point to a diagnosis of invasive CMV infection. The addition of immunohistochemistry for the detection of CMV-encoded proteins and/or in situ hybridization for the detection of CMV nucleic acids has greatly improved histologic detection of CMV in tissue specimens.

Table 282.1	Findings in Infants With Symptomatic Congenital Cytomegalovirus Infection

FINDINGS	% OF INFANTS
CLINICAL FINDINGS	
Prematurity (<37 wk)	24
Jaundice (direct bilirubin >2 mg/dL)	42
Petechiae	54
Hepatosplenomegaly	19
Purpura	3
Microcephaly	35
IUGR	28
1 clinical finding	41
2 clinical findings	59
LABORATORY FINDINGS	
Elevated ALT (>80 IU/mL)	71
Thrombocytopenia (<100,000 k/mm³)	43
Direct hyperbilirubinemia (>2 mg/dL)	54
Head CT abnormalities	42

Findings in 70 infants with symptomatic congenital CMV infection identified during newborn screening program for infants with congenital CMV infection at the University of Alabama Hospitals over an approximate 20 yr interval.
   CMV, cytomegalovirus; IUGR, in utero growth retardation; ALT, alanine aminotransferase.

Congenital Infections

The diagnosis of congenital CMV infections requires the recovery of replicating virus and/or viral nucleic acids within the first 2-3 wk of life. Sources of virus and viral nucleic acids include urine, saliva, and blood. Methods of detection include routine virus culture combined with immunofluorescence and PCR. Although quantification of virus in various specimens can suggest the likelihood of long-term sequelae such as hearing loss for a population of infected newborns, the predictive value for the individual patient remains limited. A considerable amount of effort has been devoted to identifying screening assays that would be suitable for populations of newborn infants. Initial interest centered on dried blood spots, because these samples are routinely collected as a component of newborn screening programs. Unfortunately, studies have indicated that the sensitivity of dried blood spots is too low to be considered useful for screening. In contrast, newborn screening using saliva has proven sensitive and specific and is now standard for newborn screening in some institutions. Identification of an infected infant by screening of saliva requires confirmation, preferably by assaying urine for the presence of CMV.

Early studies suggested that congenitally infected newborn infants could be identified by CMV-specific IgM reactivity and that elevated levels of CMV-specific IgM correlated with severity of disease. Subsequent studies have demonstrated that although this assay was of some value, the limited sensitivity of most assays employed to detect newborn IgM has also limited their clinical utility.

Noncongenital Infections

In nonimmunocompromised patients, demonstration of CMV-specific IgG seroconversion or the presence of CMV-specific IgM antibodies represents evidence of a newly acquired CMV infection. IgM anti-CMV antibody reactivity can persist for months depending on the sensitivity of the particular assay, thus limiting the use of IgM detection to precisely time the acquisition of CMV. The use of the IgG avidity assays in which CMV-specific binding antibodies are eluted with increasing concentrations of chaotropic agents such as urea can be used to estimate the duration of infection. This assay has been used almost exclusively in the management of CMV infections during pregnancy to aid in defining primary maternal infections. Detection of CMV in urine, saliva, blood, and tissue specimens obtained at biopsy can most reliably be accomplished by PCR-based methods, and because findings can be quantified, treatment responses can be monitored. However, conventional culture of CMV using human dermal fibroblasts often combined with immunofluorescence detection of CMV-encoded immediate early antigens also remains standard in many institutions. Routine histological stains allow detection of characteristic nuclear inclusions in tissue specimens (see above).

TREATMENT

Treatment of *immunocompromised hosts* with invasive CMV disease has been shown to limit both the morbidity and the mortality in the patient with disseminated CMV infections with end-organ disease. This has been shown in allograft transplant recipients and patients with HIV/AIDS. Similarly, antiviral prophylaxis can limit the development of clinically important CMV disease in allograft recipients and is the standard of care in most transplant centers. Several agents are currently licensed for CMV infections, including ganciclovir, foscarnet, and cidofovir, and all have appreciable toxicity. Newer agents such as letermovir have been licensed for use in adults and it is expected that indications for this agent will extend into pediatrics. In some transplant centers, high-titer CMV immunoglobulins have been included as a component of prophylaxis. Early on, when the treatment of CMV infections with antiviral agents was in its infancy, treatment with CMV immunoglobulins was shown to alter the natural history of CMV infection in renal and liver allograft recipients. The effectiveness of antiviral agents when used as prophylaxis in the immediate posttransplant period has resulted in less frequent use of these biologics.

Treatment of **congenitally infected infants** with ganciclovir has been studied in several clinical trials, and a significant number of infected infants have been treated off-label with this agent because of severe CMV infections. Two studies conducted by the Collaborative Antiviral Study Group (CASG) sponsored by the NIH have suggested that 6 wk of intravenously administered ganciclovir or 6 mo of an oral preparation of ganciclovir could limit hearing loss and possibly improve developmental outcome of infected infants. Long-term outcomes of treated infants are not known; thus it is difficult to definitively interpret these studies. In addition, infants with severe perinatal CMV infection following breast milk ingestion with documented end-organ disease have been successfully treated with ganciclovir. Currently, there are no recommendations for the treatment of infants with congenital CMV infection, although the results from a larger study that will determine the efficacy of treatment in infants with asymptomatic congenital CMV infections may provide sufficient data to firmly establish treatment guidelines.

PREVENTION

Passive Immunoprophylaxis

As was described in the preceding section, passive transfer of anti-CMV antibodies has been utilized to limit disease but not infection in allograft recipients. A similar approach has also been considered for prevention of intrauterine transmission of CMV and disease based on studies in animal models and limited observational data that suggested a role of antiviral antibodies in limiting disease following CMV infections in the perinatal period. An uncontrolled trial of human immune globulin reported in 2005 provided provocative evidence that passive transfer of anti-CMV antibodies to pregnant women undergoing primary CMV infection could limit transmission and disease. This study was seriously flawed in design, and findings from this trial were controversial. A second study utilizing the same immune globulin preparation failed to demonstrate that immune globulins provided protection from intrauterine transmission or disease. Thus it remains to be determined if passively transferred anti-CMV antibodies can modulate infection and disease following intrauterine exposure to CMV. A larger multicenter trial sponsored by the NIH (NICHD) has been terminated and results of this study should be available in the near future.

Active Immunoprophylaxis

Active immunization for the prevention of congenital CMV infection (and in transplant recipients) has been a goal of biomedical research for over 3 decades. A number of different vaccine platforms have been explored, including replicating attenuated CMV as vaccines, protein-based vaccines, heterologous virus-vectored CMV vaccines, and DNA vaccines. In all cases, some level of immunity has been induced in volunteers. Larger scale trials have been carried out using replication competent, attenuated CMV vaccines and adjuvanted recombinant protein vaccines. Current approaches are directed toward development of an adequately attenuated replicating CMV that retains sufficient immunogenicity to induce protective responses. In contrast to current status of candidate attenuated CMV vaccines, considerable progress has been made in the testing of adjuvanted recombinant viral proteins. An adjuvanted recombinant glycoprotein B, a major protein component of the envelope and target of neutralizing antibodies, has been shown to induce virus neutralizing antibodies and CD4+ T lymphocyte proliferative responses. Moreover, this vaccine reduced virus acquisition by about 50% in a trial carried out in young women. However, closer examination of this vaccine trial revealed that protection was very short-lived and that the effectiveness of the vaccine was not convincingly demonstrated because of the small numbers of subjects in the trial, despite the statistical significance. A follow-up trial in adolescent women using the same vaccine preparation failed to show any statistically significant difference between vaccine and placebo recipients. Finally, a major question that will face all vaccine programs is whether existing immunity in seropositive women can be augmented to a level to prevent damaging infection in their offspring. The maternal population with existing immunity to CMV prior to childbearing age is responsible for the greatest number of congenitally infected infants in almost all regions of the world; thus merely recapitulating naturally acquired adaptive immunity to CMV with a vaccine may not be sufficient to prevent congenital CMV infection and/or limit disease.

Counseling

Studies of the natural history of CMV have repeatedly demonstrated that transmission requires close, often direct contact with infected material such as secretions from the oral or genitourinary tract. Although limited data suggest that CMV can be transmitted on fomites, infectivity can persist for hours on surfaces such as toys. Limiting exposure to such secretions and attention to hygiene such as handwashing can drastically limit acquisition of CMV. Counseling has been shown to be very effective in the prevention of CMV infection in women of childbearing age. In fact, counseling programs have been shown to be more effective in limiting CMV infection during pregnancy than any vaccine that has been tested to date. Sexual transmission is an important route of infection, and CMV is considered to be a sexually transmitted infection. Limiting sexual transmission through education and counseling should be considered in sexually active individuals. Finally, the acquisition of CMV by hospital workers and other healthcare providers has been shown to be less than in age-matched individuals in the general public. Importantly, these studies were carried out prior to universal precautions that are in place in most hospitals today. Thus patient education with an emphasis on describing the sources of infectious virus in communities and attention to general hygiene could dramatically reduce CMV spread in the community, and particularly in women of childbearing age.

Bibliography is available at Expert Consult.

Chapter **283**

Roseola (Human Herpesviruses 6 and 7)

Brenda L. Tesini and Mary T. Caserta

第二百八十三章

玫瑰疹（人疱疹病毒6型和7型）

中文导读

本章主要介绍了人疱疹病毒6型和7型感染的病因学、流行病学、病理学和发病机制、临床表现、实验室检查、诊断、并发症、治疗、预后和预防。人疱疹病毒6B型感染是引起婴儿玫瑰疹的主要原因，临床表现主要为发热，热退后出现玫瑰色样皮疹。其他感染常见的表现包括发热、皮疹、易激惹、鼻塞流涕、消化道症状等。实验室诊断包括DNA和血清学检测。鉴别诊断包括麻疹、风疹、猩红热、肠道病毒感染和药物超敏反应。根据临床表现不同，治疗包括对症支持，更昔洛韦、膦甲酸钠和西多福韦等。

Human herpesvirus 6 (HHV-6A and HHV-6B) and human herpesvirus 7 (HHV-7) cause ubiquitous infection in infancy and early childhood. HHV-6B is responsible for the majority of cases of **roseola infantum** (**exanthem subitum** or **sixth disease**) and is associated with other diseases, including encephalitis, especially in immunocompromised hosts. A small percentage of children with roseola have primary infection with HHV-7.

ETIOLOGY

HHV-6A, HHV-6B, and HHV-7 are the sole members of the *Roseolovirus* genus in the Betaherpesvirinae subfamily of human herpesviruses. Human cytomegalovirus, the only other β-herpesvirus, shares limited sequence homology with HHV-6 and HHV-7. Morphologically all human herpesviruses are composed of an icosahedral nucleocapsid, protein-dense tegument, and lipid envelope. Within the nucleocapsid, HHV-6 and HHV-7 both contain large, linear, double-stranded DNA genomes that encode more than 80 unique proteins.

Initially, 2 strain groups of HHV-6 were recognized, HHV-6 variant A and HHV-6 variant B. Despite sharing highly conserved genomes with approximately 90% sequence identity, the 2 variants could be distinguished by restriction fragment length polymorphisms, reactivity with monoclonal antibodies, differential cell tropism, and epidemiology. Because of these differences, the two were reclassified as separate species in the genus *Roseolovirus* by the International Committee on the Taxonomy of Viruses in 2012.

HHV-6A detection is quite rare, and HHV-6B is the overwhelmingly predominant virus found in both normal and immunocompromised hosts by both culture and polymerase chain reaction (PCR). Previous reports of HHV-6A detection in children in Africa have not been substantiated in a recent large cohort using a more specific PCR target.

EPIDEMIOLOGY

Primary infection with HHV-6B is acquired rapidly by essentially all children following the loss of maternal antibodies in the 1st few mo of infancy, 95% of children being infected with HHV-6 by 2 yr of age. The peak age of primary HHV-6B infection is 6-9 mo of life, with infections occurring sporadically and without seasonal predilection or contact with other ill individuals. Infection with HHV-7 is also widespread but occurs later in childhood and at a slower rate; only 50% of children have evidence of prior infection with HHV-7 by 3 yr of age. Seroprevalence reaches 75% at 3-6 yr of age. In a small study of children with primary HHV-7 infection, the mean age of the patients was 26 mo, significantly older than that of children with primary HHV-6 infection.

Preliminary data suggest that the majority of children acquire primary infection with HHV-6 from the saliva or respiratory droplets of asymptomatic adults or older children. However, congenital infection with HHV-6 occurs in 1% of newborns. Two mechanisms of vertical transmission of HHV-6 have been identified, transplacental infection and chromosomal integration. HHV-6 is unique among the human herpesviruses in that it is integrated at the telomere end of human chromosomes at a frequency of 0.2–2.2% of the population and is passed from parent to child via the germline. Chromosomal integration of HHV-7 has only been suggested in a single case report thus far. Chromosomal integration has been identified as the major mechanism by which HHV-6 is vertically transmitted, accounting for 86% of congenital infections, with one third resulting from HHV-6A, a percentage much higher than in primary infection in the United States. The clinical consequences of chromosomal integration or transplacental infection with HHV-6 have yet to be determined. However, reactivation of chromosomally integrated HHV-6 virus has been demonstrated following hematopoietic stem cell transplantation (HSCT). In one series of infants identified with HHV-6 congenital infection, no evidence of disease was present in the early neonatal period. Primary infection with HHV-7 is presumed to be spread by the saliva of asymptomatic individuals. DNA of both HHV-6 and HHV-7 has been identified in the cervical secretions of pregnant women, suggesting an additional role for sexual or perinatal transmission of these viruses. Breast milk does not appear to play a role in transmission of either HHV-6 or HHV-7.

PATHOLOGY/PATHOGENESIS

Primary HHV-6B infection causes a viremia that can be demonstrated by co-culture of the patient's peripheral blood mononuclear cells with mitogen-stimulated cord blood mononuclear cells. HHV-6 has a recognizable cytopathic effect, consisting of the appearance of large refractile mononucleated or multinucleated cells with intracytoplasmic and/or intranuclear inclusions. Infected cells exhibit a slightly prolonged life span in culture; however, lytic infection predominates. HHV-6 infection also induces apoptosis of T cells. In vitro, HHV-6 can infect a broad range of cell types, including primary T cells, monocytes, natural killer cells, dendritic cells, and astrocytes. HHV-6 has also been documented to infect B-cell, megakaryocytic, endothelial, and epithelial cell lines. Human astrocytes, oligodendrocytes, and microglia have been infected with HHV-6 ex vivo. The broad tropism of HHV-6 is consistent with the recognition that CD46, present on the surface of all nucleated cells, is a cellular receptor for HHV-6, HHV-6A in particular. CD134, a member of the TNFR superfamily, is the main entry receptor for HHV-6B and may explain some of the differences in tissue tropism noted between HHV-6A and HHV-6B. The CD4 molecule has been identified as a receptor for HHV-7. HHV-7 has been demonstrated to reactivate HHV-6 from latency in vitro, but whether this phenomenon occurs in vivo is not clear.

Primary infection with HHV-6 and HHV-7 is followed by **lifelong latency** or persistence of virus at multiple sites. HHV-6 exists in a true state of viral latency in monocytes and macrophages. The detection of replicating HHV-6 in cultures of primary CD34+ hematopoietic stem cells has also been described, suggesting that cellular differentiation is a trigger for viral reactivation. This observation is clinically significant

because HHV-6 may cause either primary or reactivated infection during HSCT. Additionally, HHV-6 and HHV-7 infection may be persistent in salivary glands, and DNA of both HHV-6 and HHV-7 can be routinely detected in the saliva of both adults and children. HHV-7 can also be isolated in tissue culture from saliva, but HHV-6 cannot. HHV-6 DNA has been identified in the cerebrospinal fluid (CSF) of children, both during and subsequent to primary infection, as well as in brain tissue from immunocompetent adults at autopsy, implicating the central nervous system as an additional important site of either viral latency or persistence. HHV-7 DNA has also been found in adult brain tissue but at a significantly lower frequency.

CLINICAL MANIFESTATIONS

Roseola infantum (**exanthem subitum**, or **sixth disease**) is an acute, self-limited disease of infancy and early childhood. It is characterized by the abrupt onset of high fever, which may be accompanied by fussiness. The fever usually resolves acutely after 72 hr (crisis) but may gradually fade over a day (lysis) coincident with the appearance of a faint pink or rose-colored, nonpruritic, 2-3 mm morbilliform rash on the trunk (Fig. 283.1). The rash usually lasts 1-3 day but is often described as evanescent and may be visible only for hours, spreading from the trunk to the face and extremities. Because the rash is variable in appearance, location, and duration, it is not distinctive and may be missed. Associated signs are few but can include mild injection of the pharynx, palpebral conjunctivae, or tympanic membranes and enlarged suboccipital nodes. In Asian countries, ulcers at the uvulopalatoglossal junction (**Nagayama spots**) are commonly reported in infants with roseola.

High fever (mean: 39.7°C [103.5°F]) is the most consistent finding associated with primary HHV-6B infection. Rash detected either during the illness or following defervescence has been reported in approximately 20% of infected children in the United States. Additional symptoms and signs include irritability, inflamed tympanic membranes, rhinorrhea and congestion, gastrointestinal complaints, and encephalopathy. Symptoms of lower respiratory tract involvement such as cough are identified significantly less frequently in children with primary HHV-6B infection than in children with other febrile illnesses. The mean duration of illness caused by primary HHV-6B infection is 6 days, with 15% of children having fever for 6 or more days. Primary infection with HHV-6B accounts for a significant burden of illness on the healthcare system; one study found that 24% of visits to emergency departments by infants between 6 and 9 mo of age were because of primary HHV-6B infection. A population-based study of primary HHV-6B infection confirmed

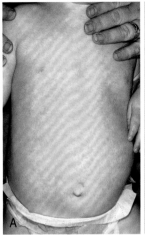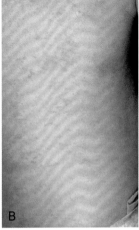

Fig. 283.1 Roseola infantum. Erythematous, blanching macules and papules **(A)** in an infant who had high fever for 3 days preceding development of the rash. On closer inspection **(B)**, some lesions reveal a subtle peripheral halo of vasoconstriction. (From Paller AS, Mancinin AJ, editors: Hurwitz clinical pediatric dermatology, ed 3, Philadelphia, 2006, Elsevier, p. 434.)

that 93% of infants had symptoms and were more likely to visit a physician than noninfected infants. Fever was less likely to be present with HHV-6B infection in children younger than 6 mo of age but was significantly more common in older infants and children.

Much less is known about the clinical manifestations of HHV-7 infection. Primary infection with HHV-7 has been identified in a small number of children with roseola in whom the illness is indistinguishable from that caused by HHV-6B. Secondary cases of roseola caused by infection with HHV-7 have also been reported. Additionally, primary infection with HHV-7 may be asymptomatic or may cause a nonspecific febrile illness lasting approximately 3 days.

LABORATORY FINDINGS

The most characteristic laboratory findings noted in children with primary HHV-6B infection are lower mean numbers of total white blood cells (8,900/μL), lymphocytes (3,400/μL), and neutrophils (4,500/μL) than in febrile children without primary HHV-6B infection. Similar hematologic findings have been reported during primary infection with HHV-7. Thrombocytopenia, elevated serum transaminase values, and atypical lymphocytes have also been noted sporadically in children with primary HHV-6B infection.

Results of CSF analyses reported in patients with encephalitis thought to be caused by HHV-6 have been normal or demonstrated only minimal CSF pleocytosis with mild elevations of protein, especially early in the course of the disease, which may progress with time. Areas of hyperintense signal on T2-weighted and fluid attenuation inversion recovery images of the hippocampus, uncus, and amygdala have been found on MRI, and increased metabolism within the hippocampus has been observed on positron emission tomography scanning.

DIAGNOSIS

Although roseola is generally a benign self-limited disease, its diagnosis can exclude other, more serious disorders that cause fever and rash. A history of 3 days of high fever in an otherwise nontoxic 10 mo old infant with a blanching maculopapular rash on the trunk suggests a diagnosis of roseola. Likewise, a specific diagnosis of HHV-6 is not usually necessary except in situations in which the manifestations of the infection are severe or unusual and might benefit from antiviral therapy.

The diagnosis of primary infection with either HHV-6 or HHV-7 is confirmed by demonstrating the presence of actively replicating virus in the patient's blood sample coupled with seroconversion. Viral culture is the gold standard method to document active viral replication. Unfortunately, culture is expensive, time consuming, and available only in research laboratories. Two other methods used to identify active HHV-6 replication are the detection of viral DNA by PCR on acellular fluids such as plasma or reverse transcriptase PCR on peripheral blood mononuclear cell samples designed to detect viral transcription and protein production. Quantitative PCR for HHV-6 genome copy numbers on various specimens is also frequently reported and is commercially available. However, the role of this methodology is not clear, as a specific value of DNA that can discriminate between patients with viremia and those who are culture negative has not been determined. Complicating the use of molecular assays for the detection of active replication of HHV-6 is the recognition that individuals with chromosomally integrated HHV-6 have persistent HHV-6 DNA in plasma, peripheral blood mononuclear cells, and CSF in the absence of disease and replicating virus.

Serologic methods such as indirect immunofluorescence assays, enzyme-linked immunosorbent assays, neutralization assays, and immunoblot have been described for the measurement of concentrations of antibodies to HHV-6 and HHV-7 in serum or plasma and are commercially available. Although immunoglobulin M antibody is produced early in infection with HHV-6, assays designed to measure this response have not proved useful in the diagnosis of primary or reactivated infection. The absence of immunoglobulin G antibody in an infant older than 6 mo of age combined with the presence of replicating virus is strong evidence of primary infection with either HHV-6 or HHV-7. Alternatively, the demonstration of seroconversion between acute and convalescent samples also confirms primary infection but is not clinically useful in the acute care setting. Unfortunately,

serologic assays have not been found reliable in the detection of HHV-6 reactivation and cannot be used to differentiate between infection with HHV-6A and infection with HHV-6B. Additionally, limited antibody cross-reactivity has been demonstrated between HHV-6 and HHV-7, complicating the interpretation of serologic assays, especially if low titers are reported.

Differential Diagnosis

Primary infection with either HHV-6B or HHV-7 usually causes an undifferentiated febrile illness that may be very difficult to distinguish from other common viral infections of childhood. This difficulty also applies to the early stages of roseola, before the development of rash. Once the rash is present, roseola may be confused with other exanthematous diseases of childhood, especially measles and rubella. Children with **rubella** often have a prodrome characterized by mild illness with low-grade fever, sore throat, arthralgia, and gastrointestinal complaints, unlike those with roseola. On physical examination, suboccipital and posterior auricular lymph nodes are prominent up to 1 wk before the rash of rubella is evident and persist during the exanthematous phase. Additionally, the rash of rubella usually begins on the face and spreads to the chest, like that in measles. The associated symptoms of **measles** virus infection include cough, coryza, and conjunctivitis, with high fever coincident with the development of rash, unlike in roseola. Roseola may also be confused with scarlet fever, though the latter is rare in children younger than 2 yr of age and causes a characteristic sandpaperlike rash concurrent with fever.

Roseola may be confused with illness caused by **enterovirus infections**, especially in the summer and fall months. Drug hypersensitivity reactions may also be difficult to distinguish from roseola. Antibiotics are frequently prescribed for children with fever from roseola before the appearance of rash. A child who then demonstrates rash after the resolution of fever may erroneously be labeled as being drug allergic.

COMPLICATIONS

Convulsions are the most common complication of roseola and are recognized in up to one third of patients. Seizures are also the most common complication of children with primary HHV-6B infection, occurring in approximately 15%, with a peak age of 12-15 mo. Children with primary HHV-6B infection are also reported to have a higher frequency of partial seizures, prolonged seizures, postictal paralysis, and repeated seizures than are children with febrile seizures not associated with HHV-6. In a study limited to children with primary HHV-6B infection and seizures, 30% of patients had prolonged seizures, 29% had focal seizures, and 38% had repeated seizures. A prospective study of children 2-35 mo of age with suspected encephalitis or severe febrile illness with convulsions found that 17% had primary infection with either HHV-6 or HHV-7, and status epilepticus was the most common presentation. Among children with febrile status epilepticus (FSE), primary or reactivated infection with HHV-6B or HHV-7 has been identified in approximately one third.

An association between recurrent seizures and reactivated or persistent infection of the central nervous system by HHV-6 has also been suggested. Studies evaluating brain tissue specimens implicate HHV-6 in as many as 35% of patients with temporal lobe epilepsy (TLE), high viral loads being found in the hippocampus or lateral temporal lobe regions. HHV-6 protein production has also been identified in a small number of resected tissue specimens. Primary astrocytes obtained from these samples had undetectable levels of a glutamate transporter, suggesting the loss of ability to control glutamate levels as a possible mechanism for the development of recurrent seizures. Additional evidence has demonstrated upregulation of genes related to monocyte chemotaxis in the amygdala of patients with TLE and HHV-6 DNA in specimens. Contrary to these findings, limited clinical data suggest that there may be a decreased risk of recurrent seizures after primary infection with HHV-6 and febrile seizures from other causes. Additionally, children with FSE associated with HHV-6B and HHV-7 had similar seizure characteristics and a similar proportion of electroencephalography and MRI hippocampal abnormalities as children with FSE not associated with HHV-6B or HHV-7, suggesting a shared pathogenesis to other etiologies of FSE.

Case reports and small-patient series have described additional complications in children with primary HHV-6B infection, including encephalitis, acute disseminated demyelination, autoimmune encephalitis, acute cerebellitis, hepatitis, and myocarditis. Late-developing long-term sequelae, including developmental disabilities and autistic-like features, are reported rarely in children who have central nervous system symptoms during primary HHV-6B infection.

Reactivation of HHV-6 has been reported in several different populations with and without disease with the use of various methods of detection. The best documentation of HHV-6 reactivation has been in immunocompromised hosts, especially those patients who have undergone HSCT. Such reactivation occurs in approximately 50% of patients, typically at 2-4 wk after transplantation. Many of the clinical complications seen following HSCT have been associated with HHV-6B reactivation, including fever, rash, delayed engraftment of platelets or monocytes, and graft-versus-host disease, with variable degrees of support in the literature for each. HHV-6 reactivation has been associated with worse overall survival compared to HSCT recipients who did not experience reactivation.

HHV-6B reactivation has also been reported as a cause of encephalitis in both normal and immunocompromised hosts. A distinct syndrome of **posttransplant acute limbic encephalitis (PALE)** has been described primarily in patients following HSCT, especially cord blood stem cell transplantation; it is characterized by short-term memory dysfunction, confusion, and insomnia with seizures noted either clinically or on prolonged electroencephalography monitoring. HHV-6B DNA has been identified in the CSF in the majority of these patients, with additional evidence of reactivation by detection of HHV-6B DNA in plasma. HHV-6 proteins were identified in the astrocytes of the hippocampus in one postmortem specimen, consistent with active HHV-6B infection at the time of death. The development of PALE is associated with increased mortality and long-term neurocognitive sequelae.

TREATMENT

Supportive care is usually all that is needed for infants with roseola. Parents should be advised to maintain hydration and may use antipyretics if the child is especially uncomfortable with the fever. Specific antiviral therapy is not recommended for routine cases of primary HHV-6B or HHV-7 infection. Unusual or severe manifestations of primary or presumed reactivated HHV-6B infection such as encephalitis/PALE, especially in immunocompromised patients, may benefit from treatment. Ganciclovir, foscarnet, and cidofovir all demonstrate inhibitory activity against HHV-6 in vitro, similar to their activity against cytomegalovirus. Case reports suggest that all 3 drugs, alone or in combination, can decrease HHV-6 viral replication, as evidenced by decreased viral loads in plasma and CSF. However, clinical data regarding efficacy are sparse and contradictory, with no randomized trials to guide use. Additionally, in vitro resistance of HHV-6 to all 3 drugs has been described. Despite these drawbacks, treatment with ganciclovir or foscarnet as first-line agents has been recommended for a minimum of 3 wk in patients with PALE. Foscarnet appears to be most likely to have activity against HHV-7 on the basis of in vitro testing, but no clinical data are available.

PROGNOSIS

Roseola is generally a self-limited illness associated with complete recovery. The majority of children with primary infections with HHV-6B and HHV-7 also recover uneventfully without sequelae. Although seizures are a common complication of primary infection with HHV-6B and HHV-7, the risk of recurrent seizures does not appear to be higher than that associated with other causes of simple febrile seizures.

PREVENTION

Primary infections with HHV-6 and HHV-7 are widespread throughout the human population with no current means of interrupting transmission.

Bibliography is available at Expert Consult.

Chapter **284**

Human Herpesvirus 8

Brenda L. Tesini and Mary T. Caserta

第二百八十四章
人疱疹病毒8型

中文导读

　　本章主要介绍了人疱疹病毒8型感染的病因学、流行病学、病理学和发病机制、临床表现、诊断和治疗。详细描述了感染在免疫功能低下人群中的临床表现，包括发热、肝脾大、全血细胞减少和淋巴组织增生。人疱疹病毒8型感染后可导致恶性疾病，分别介绍了卡波西肉瘤、原发性渗出性淋巴瘤和多中心卡斯特曼病。实验室诊断包括血清学检测及对组织样本进行分子学和免疫组织化学法检测。治疗原则为抗病毒和控制恶性增殖。

Human herpesvirus 8 (HHV-8) is an oncogenic virus identified in tissue specimens from patients with Kaposi sarcoma (KS). Because of this association, it is also known as **Kaposi sarcoma–associated herpesvirus**. HHV-8 is the etiologic agent of two additional lymphoproliferative disorders: **primary effusion–based lymphoma (PEL)** and **multicentric Castleman disease (MCD)**.

ETIOLOGY

HHV-8 is a γ_2-human herpesvirus similar to Epstein-Barr virus. The virus contains a large DNA genome encoding 85-95 unique proteins. Infection is followed by both lytic and latent viral states with different degrees of viral replication associated with distinct disease manifestations.

EPIDEMIOLOGY

The prevalence of infection with HHV-8 varies both geographically and by population and roughly matches the epidemiology of KS. HHV-8 infection is endemic in Africa and parts of South America, with infection rates of up to 30–60% by adolescence. Seroprevalence >20% has also been found in regions bordering the Mediterranean. In contrast, infection rates <5% are noted in North America, central Europe, and Asia. However, within geographic regions, the prevalence of infection varies with risk behaviors, rates of 30–75% being found among men who have sex with men in North America and Europe. HHV-8 DNA can be detected in saliva, blood, semen, and tissues. Based upon large-scale epidemiologic studies and the high prevalence of viral shedding in oral secretions, saliva is believed to be the major mode of transmission. Other less-common routes of HHV-8 transmission include blood transfusion, bone marrow transplantation, and solid organ transplantation. Vertical transmission and transmission via breast milk may occur in regions where HHV-8 is highly endemic, but the risk appears low.

PATHOLOGY AND PATHOGENESIS

HHV-8 contains multiple genes that impact cell-cycle regulation and the host immune response. Viral proteins interfere with the function of the tumor suppressor molecules, induce the expression of proangiogenesis factors, and lead to upregulation of the rapamycin pathway target, which is instrumental in the control of cell growth and metabolism. HHV-8 also encodes a homolog of human interleukin-6, which can bind and activate cytokine receptors and serve as a host cell autocrine growth factor. Additionally, viral proteins are associated with the constitutive expression of the transcription factor nuclear factor-κB. All of these proteins may be potential targets for therapeutic intervention.

CLINICAL MANIFESTATIONS

Although subclinical infection appears to be common, symptomatic primary HHV-8 infection has been described in immunocompetent children. Patients commonly have fever and a maculopapular rash or a mononucleosis-like syndrome, with full recovery the rule. In immunocompromised patients, primary infection has been associated with fever, rash, splenomegaly, pancytopenia, and lymphoid hyperplasia, and may be quite severe. Additionally, preliminary data suggest that transfusion-associated primary infection with HHV-8 is associated with an increased risk of mortality.

Even in regions with high rates of seroprevalence, the development of KS is uncommon. KS has several different clinical forms; each includes multifocal, angiogenic lesions arising from vascular endothelial cells infected with HHV-8. Classic KS is an indolent disorder seen in elderly men with limited involvement of the skin of the lower extremities. Endemic KS is more aggressive, occurring in children and young people, primarily in Africa, and can include visceral involvement as well as widespread cutaneous lesions (patches, plaques, or nodules). Post-transplantation KS and AIDS-related KS are the most severe forms, with disseminated lesions, often in the gastrointestinal tract and lungs, with or without cutaneous findings.

Primary effusion–based lymphoma is a rare disease caused by HHV-8 that is seen most commonly in HIV-infected individuals. It consists of lymphomatous invasion of the serosal surfaces of the pleura, pericardium, and peritoneum. Similarly, **multicentric Castleman disease** is an unusual lymphoproliferative disorder characterized by anemia, thrombocytopenia, generalized lymphadenopathy, and constitutional symptoms and frequently associated with HHV-8 infection and a high degree of viral replication.

DIAGNOSIS

Serologic assays, including immunofluorescence and enzyme-linked immunosorbent assays, are the primary methods of diagnosing infection with HHV-8. However, testing has limited sensitivity, specificity, and reproducibility and is primarily a research tool with no universally recognized standard assays. Additionally, the loss of antibodies over time, referred to as *seroreversion,* has been described, further complicating serodiagnosis. Immunohistochemistry and molecular methods are available for the detection of HHV-8 in tissue samples and are utilized in the diagnosis of KS, PEL, and MCD, alongside their disease-specific clinical manifestations.

TREATMENT

Treatment for KS, PEL, and MCD is multifaceted and includes attempts to control malignant proliferations with traditional chemotherapeutic regimens and biologic agents as well as agents aimed at specific cellular pathways targeted by HHV-8 proteins. Combined antiretroviral therapy (ART) is a mainstay of both prevention and therapy for HHV-8 related disease in HIV-infected patients. In HIV-associated KS, treatment with ART alone is often used for the control of mild (i.e., cutaneous) disease, while ART plus chemotherapy is utilized for more severe disease. In transplantation-associated KS, the first line of treatment includes decreasing immunosuppression, often in association with a switch from calcineurin inhibitors to sirolimus (rapamycin) to block the mammalian target of rapamycin pathway. Severe disease frequently requires the use of traditional chemotherapy as well. The role of specific antiherpesvirus antiviral treatment is unclear. Oral valganciclovir decreases the detection of HHV-8 in saliva, and ganciclovir treatment has been associated with decreased rates of development of KS in HIV-infected individuals. However, results of using antivirals in the treatment of established disease have been generally disappointing. The prognosis for PEL tends to be poor despite the use of traditional chemotherapy, while rituximab (anti-CD20)–based therapy has been highly successful for MCD treatment. However, relapse and the development of lymphoma following treatment can still occur. Rituximab treatment may also worsen concurrent KS without additional agents.

Bibliography is available at Expert Consult.

Chapter 285

Influenza Viruses*

Fiona P. Havers and Angela J.P. Campbell

第二百八十五章

流行性感冒病毒

中文导读

　　本章主要介绍了流行性感冒病毒感染的病因学、流行病学、发病机制、临床表现、并发症、实验室检查、诊断、鉴别诊断、治疗、预后和预防。流行病学中详细阐述了抗原变异和季节性流行性感冒（简称流感）。临床表现包括发热、头痛、厌食等全身症状，呼吸道症状及消化道症状。具体描述了并发症，包括中耳炎、肺炎、肺外表现、中枢神经系统并发症等。详细说明了流感的诊断依据及实验室检测方法。治疗药物包括神经氨酸酶抑制剂、巴洛沙韦和金刚烷胺，具体介绍了药物的适用人群、剂量和疗程。

Influenza viral infections cause a broad array of respiratory illnesses that are responsible for significant morbidity and mortality in children during **seasonal epidemics**. Influenza A viruses also have the potential to cause **global pandemics**, which can happen when a **new (novel) influenza A virus** emerges and transmits efficiently from person to person.

ETIOLOGY

Influenza viruses are large, single-stranded RNA viruses belonging to the family Orthomyxoviridae, which includes three genera (or types): A, B, and C. Influenza A and B viruses are the primary human pathogens causing seasonal epidemics, while influenza virus type C is a sporadic cause of predominantly mild upper respiratory tract illness. Influenza A viruses are further divided into subtypes based on two surface proteins that project as spikes from the lipid envelope, the hemagglutinin (HA) and neuraminidase (NA) proteins (Fig. 285.1). Strain variants are identified by antigenic differences in their HA and NA and are designated by the geographic area from which they were originally isolated, isolate number, and year of isolation—for example, influenza A/Victoria/361/2011(H3N2). The HA and NA antigens from influenza B and C viruses do not receive subtype designations, as there is less variation among influenza B and C antigens. However, influenza B viruses can be further broken down into lineages; currently circulating influenza B viruses belong to the B/Yamagata or B/Victoria lineage.

EPIDEMIOLOGY

Influenza has generally been thought to be transmitted primarily via respiratory droplets, but transmission through contact with secretions and small-particle aerosols may also occur. The typical incubation period ranges from 1 to 4 days, with an average of 2 days. Healthy adults are generally considered potentially infectious from a day before symptoms develop until 5-7 days after becoming ill. Children with primary influenza infection have higher influenza viral loads and more prolonged viral shedding than adults; therefore children may be able to infect others for a longer time. Influenza outbreaks occur commonly in schools and childcare settings. Healthcare-associated influenza infections can also occur in healthcare settings, and outbreaks in long-term care facilities and hospitals may cause significant morbidity.

In the United States, seasonal influenza viruses can be detected year round, but circulating viruses are most common during the fall and winter. Transmission through a community is rapid, with the highest incidence of illness occurring within 2-3 wk of introduction.

Antigenic Variation

Influenza A and B viruses contain a genome consisting of 8 single-stranded RNA segments. Minor changes within a subtype continually occur through point mutations during viral replication, particularly in the HA gene, and result in new influenza strains of the same HA type. This phenomenon, termed **antigenic drift**, occurs in both influenza A and B viruses. Variation in antigenic composition of influenza virus surface proteins occurs almost yearly, which confers a selective advantage to a new strain and contributes to annual epidemics. For this reason, the formulation of the influenza vaccine is reviewed each year and updated as needed.

Less frequent but more dramatic, major changes in virus subtype can occur, resulting in a new influenza A subtype to which most people have little to no immunity. This process is called antigenic shift and can occur through reassortment of viral gene segments when there is simultaneous infection by more than one strain of influenza in a single host, or by direct adaptation of an animal virus to a human host. Antigenic shift occurs in influenza A viruses, which have multiple avian and mammalian hosts acting as reservoirs for diverse strains.

Through the process of **reassortment**, potentially any of 18 HA and 11 NA proteins currently known to reside in influenza A viruses of nonhuman hosts could be introduced into humans, who may have little existing immunologic cross protection to emerging viruses. A global pandemic can result if an influenza A virus with a novel HA or NA

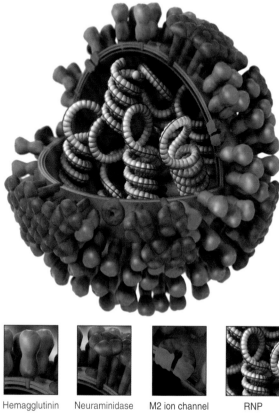

Hemagglutinin   Neuraminidase   M2 ion channel   RNP

Fig. 285.1 Graphical representation of influenza virus. The key at bottom identifies the surface protein constituents: the hemagglutinin, neuraminidase, matrix protein 2 (M2) ion channel, and ribonucleoprotein *(RNP). (From Centers for Disease Control and Prevention Public Health Image Library, Image ID#11822, Available at https://phil.cdc.gov/phil/details.asp; courtesy CDC/Douglas Jordan and Dan Higgins, 2009.)*

enters a nonimmune human population and acquires the capacity for sustained and efficient transmission between people. Four major **global pandemics** have occurred since 1900: in 1918 caused by an influenza A(H1N1) virus, 1957 caused by an influenza A(H2N2) virus, 1968 caused by an influenza A(H3N2) virus, and 2009 caused by an influenza A virus designated A(H1N1)pdm09. The most severe pandemic in recorded history occurred in 1918, when the virus was estimated to have killed at least 50 million people. The 1918 pandemic virus was likely the result of direct adaptation of an avian influenza virus to the human host, rather than from reassortment. The 2009 pandemic virus stemmed from reassortment of genes from swine, avian, and human viruses (Fig. 285.2). This resulted in the emergence of a novel influenza A(H1N1)pdm09 virus that spread quickly from North America across the globe and replaced the previously circulating seasonal H1N1 viruses.

Several novel influenza viruses, all originating in animals, have also caused outbreaks of human infections. Avian influenza A(H5N1), a virulent avian influenza virus that was first identified in 1997, has caused more than 800 documented cases in 16 countries, with a mortality rate over 50%. Another novel avian influenza, A(H7N9) virus, has caused more than 1,300 documented cases and also appears highly virulent. This virus first caused an outbreak of human infections in China during the spring of 2013, with annual epidemics in China occurring in subsequent years. During the first 4 yearly epidemics, infection was fatal in approximately 40% of documented cases.

In addition, novel influenza A variant viruses have caused human infections (Table 285.1). These include H3N2v viruses, which caused 372 confirmed human infections in the United States from 2011 to 2016 and were primarily transmitted through swine contact at agricultural fairs. Influenza viruses that normally circulate in swine are designated variant ("v") viruses when detected in humans, and H3N2v and other variant viruses, including H1N1v and H1N2v, have sporadically infected humans. In contrast to avian influenza A(H5N1) and A(H7N9) viruses, variant viruses generally cause mild illness and have been primarily detected in children. However, none of these viruses has exhibited sustained, efficient human-to-human transmission.

Seasonal Influenza

An estimated 11,000-45,000 children younger than 18 yr of age are hospitalized annually in the United States as a result of seasonal influenza-associated complications, with approximately 6,000-26,000 hospitalizations in children younger than 5 yr of age. Since 2004, the annual number of reported influenza-associated pediatric deaths in the United States has ranged from 37 to 171 during regular influenza seasons (358 were reported to have occurred during the 2009 H1N1 pandemic). Influenza disproportionately affects children with specific chronic conditions, such as underlying pulmonary, cardiac, or neurologic and neuromuscular disorders. Very young children, especially those younger than 2 yr of age, and children with chronic medical conditions are more likely to develop severe influenza-related complications, including viral and

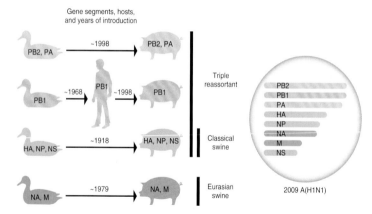

Fig. 285.2 Host and lineage origins for the gene segments of the 2009 A(H1N1) virus. PB2, polymerase basic 2; PB1, polymerase basic 1; PA, polymerase acidic; HA, hemagglutinin; NP, nucleoprotein; NA, neuraminidase; M, matrix gene; NS, nonstructural gene. Color of gene segment in circle indicates host. *(From Garten RJ, Davis CT, Russell CA, et al: Antigenic and genetic characteristics of swine-origin 2009 A(H1N1) influenza viruses circulating in humans, Science 325(5937):197–201, 2009.)*

Table 285.1	Subtypes of Novel Influenza A Viruses and Clinical Syndromes in Human Infections		
	LPAI VIRUSES	**HPAI VIRUSES**	**VARIANT VIRUSES***
Conjunctivitis	H7N2, H7N3, H7N7, H10N7	H7N3, H7N7	H1N1v, H3N2v
Upper respiratory tract illness	H6N1, H7N2, H7N3, H7N9, H9N2, H10N7	H5N1, H5N6, H7N7	H1N1v, H1N2v, H3N2v
Lower respiratory tract disease, pneumonia	H7N2, H7N9, H9N2, H10N8	H5N1, H5N6, H7N7, H7N9	H1N1v, H3N2v
Respiratory failure, acute respiratory distress syndrome	H7N9, H10N8	H5N1, H5N6, H7N7, H7N9	H1N1v, H3N2v
Multiorgan failure	H7N9, H10N8	H5N1, H5N6, H7N7, H7N9	—
Encephalopathy or encephalitis	H7N9	H5N1	—
Fatal outcomes†	H7N9, H9N2, H10N8	H5N1, H5N6, H7N7, H7N9	H1N1v, H3N2v

*Variant viruses of swine origin.
†High mortality in reported cases: about 40% for LPAI H7N9, about 50% for HPAI H5N1, and about 70% for HPAI H5N6.
LPAI, low-pathogenic avian influenza; HPAI, highly pathogenic avian influenza.
From Uyeki TM, Katz JM, Jernigan DB: Novel influenza A viruses and pandemic threats, *Lancet* 389:2172–2174, 2017.

bacterial pneumonia, hospitalization, respiratory failure, and death. However, while children with underlying medical conditions are at higher risk of complications, many healthy children are hospitalized with influenza, and nearly half of pediatric influenza-associated deaths are in children that have no known underlying medical condition.

Influenza also causes a substantial burden of disease in outpatient settings. It contributes to an estimated 600,000 to 2,500,000 outpatient medical visits annually in children younger than 5 yr of age, and has been identified in 10–25% of outpatient visits among all children with respiratory symptoms during influenza season. Influenza may also be underdiagnosed. Many who seek medical care for influenza do not have laboratory testing performed and do not receive a diagnosis of influenza. Every year, 3-4 influenza virus types or subtypes typically co-circulate, including influenza A(H3N2), influenza A(H1N1), and B viruses. Although 1 subtype usually predominates in any given season, it is difficult to predict which will be predominant. Thus, the influenza vaccine varies annually and contains 3 or 4 antigens representing the expected circulating types.

PATHOGENESIS
Influenza viruses infect the respiratory tract epithelium, primarily the ciliated columnar epithelial cells, by using the HA to attach to sialic acid residues. After viral entry into cells, virus replication occurs usually within 4-6 hr, and new virus particles are assembled and released to infect neighboring cells. With primary infection, virus replication continues for 10-14 days. Influenza virus causes a lytic infection of the respiratory epithelium with loss of ciliary function, decreased mucus production, and desquamation of the epithelial layer. These changes permit secondary bacterial invasion, either directly through the epithelium or, in the case of the middle ear space, through obstruction of the normal drainage through the eustachian tube.

The exact immune mechanisms involved in termination of primary infection and protection against reinfection are complex. Induction of cytokines that inhibit viral replication, such as interferon and tumor necrosis factor, as well as other host defenses, such as cell-mediated immune responses and local and humoral antibody defenses, all likely play a role. Secretory immunoglobulin A antibodies produced by the respiratory mucosa are thought to be an effective and immediate response generated during influenza infection. Serum antibody levels inhibiting HA activity can usually be detected by the second week after infection. These antibodies are also generated by vaccines, and high HA inhibition titers correlate with protection.

CLINICAL MANIFESTATIONS
The onset of influenza illness is *often abrupt,* with a predominance of systemic symptoms including fever, myalgias, chills, headache, malaise, and anorexia. Coryza, pharyngitis, and dry cough are also usually present at the onset of illness but may be less prominent than systemic symptoms. Respiratory manifestations can include isolated upper respiratory tract

illness, including croup, or progression to lower tract disease, such as bronchiolitis or pneumonia. More than other respiratory viruses, influenza virus typically causes systemic manifestations such as high temperature, myalgia, malaise, and headache. Less common clinical manifestations can include parotitis and rash.

Abdominal pain, vomiting, and diarrhea may also occur in children; in some studies, diarrhea was reported to be more often associated with influenza A(H1N1)pdm09 compared with influenza A(H3N2) or influenza B viruses. Influenza is a less distinct illness in younger children and infants. The infected young infant or child may be highly febrile and toxic in appearance, prompting a full diagnostic work-up. The typical duration of the febrile illness is 2-4 days. Cough may persist for longer periods, and evidence of small airway dysfunction is often found weeks later. Owing to the high transmissibility of influenza, other family members or close contacts of an infected person often experience a similar illness.

COMPLICATIONS
Otitis media and pneumonia are common complications of influenza in young children. Acute otitis media may be seen in up to 25% of cases of documented influenza. Pneumonia accompanying influenza may be a primary viral process or a secondary bacterial infection (such as with *Staphylococcus aureus*) facilitated through damaged respiratory epithelium. Influenza may cause acute myositis or rhabdomyolysis marked by muscle weakness and pain, particularly in the calf muscles, and myoglobinuria. Other extrapulmonary complications include acute renal failure, myocarditis, and sepsis. Central nervous system complications, such as encephalitis, myelitis, and Guillain-Barré syndrome, can occur and are seen more commonly in children than adults. Although it has essentially disappeared in the United States, Reye syndrome can result with the use of salicylates during influenza infection (see Chapter 388). Bacterial coinfection may also exacerbate respiratory complications of influenza and lead to sepsis, bacteremia, toxic shock syndrome, and other manifestations.

Influenza is particularly severe in some children, including those with underlying cardiopulmonary disease, including congenital and acquired valvular disease, cardiomyopathy, bronchopulmonary dysplasia, asthma, cystic fibrosis, and neurologic conditions. Pregnant women and adolescent females are at high risk for severe influenza. Children receiving cancer chemotherapy and children with immunodeficiency also have a higher risk of complications and may shed virus for longer periods than immunocompetent children.

LABORATORY FINDINGS
The clinical laboratory abnormalities associated with influenza are nonspecific. Chest radiographs may show evidence of atelectasis or infiltrate.

DIAGNOSIS AND DIFFERENTIAL DIAGNOSIS
The diagnosis of influenza depends on epidemiologic, clinical, and laboratory considerations. In the context of an epidemic, the clinical

Table 285.2	Influenza Virus Testing Methods		
METHOD	**ACCEPTABLE SPECIMENS**	**TEST TIME**	**COMMENTS**
Rapid Influenza Diagnostic Tests (antigen detection)	Nasopharyngeal (NP) swab, aspirate or wash, nasal swab, aspirate, or wash, throat swab	<15 min	Rapid turnaround; suboptimal sensitivity
Rapid Molecular Assay (influenza nucleic acid amplification)	NP swab, nasal swab	15-30 min	Rapid turnaround, high sensitivity
Immunofluorescence, Direct (DFA) or Indirect (IFA) Fluorescent Antibody Staining (antigen detection)	NP swab or wash, bronchial wash, nasal or endotracheal aspirate	1-4 hr	Relatively rapid turnaround; requires laboratory expertise and experience
RT-PCR (singleplex and multiplex; real-time and other RNA-based) and other molecular assays (influenza nucleic acid amplification)	NP swab, throat swab, NP or bronchial wash, nasal or endotracheal aspirate, sputum	Varies by assay (generally 1-8 hr)	Excellent sensitivity, relatively rapid turnaround compared with conventional methods
Rapid cell culture (shell vials, cell mixtures; yields live virus)	NP swab, throat swab, NP or bronchial wash, nasal or endotracheal aspirate, sputum	1-3 day	Culture isolates important for strain information and antiviral resistance monitoring
Viral tissue cell culture (conventional; yields live virus)	NP swab, throat swab, NP or bronchial wash, nasal or endotracheal aspirate, sputum	3-10 day	Not recommended for routine patient diagnosis
Serologic tests (antibody detection)	Paired (appropriately timed) acute and convalescent serum specimens	N/A (not performed during acute infection)	Not recommended for routine patient diagnosis, useful for research studies

N/A, not applicable; NP, nucleoprotein; RT-PCR, reverse transcription-polymerase chain reaction.
Modified from Centers for Disease Control and Prevention (CDC): *Influenza virus testing methods.* Available at https://www.cdc.gov/flu/professionals/diagnosis/table-testing-methods.htm in Information for Health Professionals (https://www.cdc.gov/flu/professionals/index.htm); and from 2018 IDSA Clinical Practice Guidelines.

diagnosis of influenza in a child who has fever, malaise, and respiratory symptoms may be made based on clinical discretion; however, clinical presentation is often indistinguishable from infection with other respiratory viruses, including respiratory syncytial virus, parainfluenza virus, human metapneumovirus, adenovirus, and even rhinovirus. Confirmation of influenza virus infection by diagnostic testing is not required for clinical decisions to prescribe antiviral medications, and prompt suspicion or diagnosis of influenza may allow for early antiviral therapy to be initiated and may reduce inappropriate use of antibiotics.

A number of diagnostic tests may be used for laboratory confirmation of influenza (Table 285.2). Although rapid influenza diagnostic tests are often employed because of their ease of use and fast results, they can have suboptimal sensitivity to detect influenza virus infection, particularly for novel influenza viruses. Sensitivities of rapid diagnostic tests are generally 50–70% compared to viral culture or reverse-transcription polymerase chain reaction. Specificities are higher, approximately 95–100%. Therefore false-negative results occur more often than false-positive results, particularly when the prevalence of influenza is high (i.e., during peak influenza activity in the community). The interpretation of negative results should take into account the clinical characteristics and the patient's risk for complications. If there is clinical suspicion for influenza in a patient at high risk for complications (Table 285.3), early empiric treatment should be given regardless of a negative rapid diagnostic test result, and another type of test (e.g., reverse-transcription polymerase chain reaction or direct fluorescent antibody testing) may be performed for confirmation.

TREATMENT

Antiviral medications are an important adjunct to influenza vaccination. Three classes of antiviral drugs are licensed for treatment of influenza in children. The neuraminidase inhibitors (NAIs), oral oseltamivir and inhaled zanamivir, may be used for treatment of children from birth and 7 yr, respectively (Table 285.4). In December 2012, the U.S. Food and Drug Administration (FDA) approved the use of oseltamivir for the treatment of influenza in infants as young as 2 wk of age, and the Centers for Disease Control and Prevention (CDC), American Academy of Pediatrics, and the Infectious Diseases Society of America recommend its use in infants of any age. A third NAI, peramivir, is given as an

Table 285.3	Children and Adolescents Who Are at Higher Risk for Influenza Complications for Whom Antiviral Treatment is Recommended*

Children younger than 2 yr of age[†]
Persons with chronic pulmonary (including asthma), cardiovascular (except hypertension alone), renal, hepatic, hematologic (including sickle cell disease), and metabolic disorders (including diabetes mellitus); or neurologic and neurodevelopmental conditions (including disorders of the brain, spinal cord, peripheral nerve, and muscle such as cerebral palsy, epilepsy [seizure disorders], stroke, intellectual disability, moderate to severe developmental delay, muscular dystrophy, or spinal cord injury)
Persons with immunosuppression, including that caused by medications or by HIV infection
Adolescents who are pregnant, or postpartum (within 2 wk after delivery)
Persons younger than 19 yr of age who are receiving long-term aspirin- or salicylate-containing medications therapy
American Indians/Alaska Natives
Persons who are extremely obese (body mass index ≥40)
Residents of long-term care facilities
Hospitalized patients at high risk for influenza complications

Current for 2018-2019 influenza season.
*Antiviral treatment is recommended for high-risk children with confirmed or suspected influenza; antivirals are also recommended for children who are hospitalized or have severe or progressive disease.
[†]Although all children younger than 5 yr of age are considered at higher risk for complications from influenza, the highest risk is for those younger than 2 yr of age, with the highest hospitalization and death rates among infants younger than 6 mo of age.
Adapted from Centers for Disease Control and Prevention (CDC): *Influenza antiviral medications: summary for clinicians.* Available at https://www.cdc.gov/flu/professionals/antivirals/summary-clinicians.htm. For current details, consult annually updated recommendations at https://www.cdc.gov/flu/professionals/index.htm.

Table 285.4	Recommended Dosage and Schedule of Influenza Antiviral Medications for Treatment and Chemoprophylaxis in Children for the 2018-2019 Influenza Season: United States

MEDICATION	TREATMENT DOSING**	CHEMOPROPHYLAXIS DOSING**
ORAL OSELTAMIVIR*		
Adults	75 mg twice daily	75 mg once daily
Children ≥12 mo		
Body wt		
≤15 kg (≤33 lb)	30 mg twice daily	30 mg once daily
>15-23 kg (33-51 lb)	45 mg twice daily	45 mg once daily
>23-40 kg (>51-88 lb)	60 mg twice daily	60 mg once daily
>40 kg (>88 lb)	75 mg twice daily	75 mg once daily
Infants 0-11 mo[†]	3 mg/kg per dose once daily	3 mg/kg per dose once daily
Term infants ages 0-8 mo[†]	3 mg/kg per dose twice daily	3 mg/kg per dose once daily for infants 3-8 mo old; not recommended for infants <3 mo old unless situation judged critical because of limited safety and efficacy data in this age group
Preterm infants	See details in footnote[‡]	Not recommended
INHALED ZANAMIVIR[§]		
Adults	10 mg (two 5 mg inhalations) twice daily	10 mg (two 5 mg inhalations) once daily
Children (≥7 yr old for treatment; ≥5 yr old for chemoprophylaxis)	10 mg (two 5 mg inhalations) twice daily	10 mg (two 5 mg inhalations) once daily
INTRAVENOUS PERAMIVIR		
Adults	600 mg intravenous infusion once given over 15-30 min	Not recommended
Children (2-12 yr old)	One 12 mg/kg dose, up to 600 mg maximum, via intravenous infusion for 15-30 min	Not recommended
Children (13-17 yr old)	One 600 mg dose via intravenous infusion for 15-30 min	Not recommended
ORAL BALOXAVIR[††]		
Adults		
40 to <80 kg	One 40 mg dose	Not recommended
>80 kg	One 80 mg dose	Not recommended
Children		
2-11 yr	Not recommended	Not recommended
12-17 yr, 40 to <80 kg	One 40 mg dose	Not recommended
12-17 yr, >80 kg	One 80 mg dose	Not recommended

*Oseltamivir is administered orally without regard to meals, although administration with meals may improve gastrointestinal tolerability. Oseltamivir is available as Tamiflu or as a generic formulation as capsules and as a powder for oral suspension that is reconstituted to provide a final concentration of 6 mg/mL.

[†]Approved by the FDA for children as young as 2 wk of age. Given preliminary pharmacokinetic data and limited safety data, oseltamivir can be used to treat influenza in both term and preterm infants from birth because benefits of therapy are likely to outweigh possible risks of treatment. CDC and US Food and Drug Administration (FDA)–approved dosing is 3 mg/kg per dose twice daily for children aged 9-11 mo; the American Academy of Pediatrics recommends 3.5 mg/kg per dose twice daily. The dose of 3 mg/kg provides oseltamivir exposure in children similar to that achieved by the approved dose of 75 mg orally twice daily for adults, as shown in two studies of oseltamivir pharmacokinetics in children. The AAP has recommended an oseltamivir treatment dose of 3.5 mg/kg orally twice daily for infants 9-11 mo, on the basis of data that indicated that a higher dose of 3.5 mg/kg was needed to achieve the protocol-defined targeted exposure for this cohort as defined in the CASG 114 study. It is unknown whether this higher dose will improve efficacy or prevent the development of antiviral resistance. However, there is no evidence that the 3.5 mg/kg dose is harmful or causes more adverse events to infants in this age group.

[‡]Oseltamivir dosing for preterm infants. The wt-based dosing recommendation for preterm infants is lower than for term infants. Preterm infants may have lower clearance of oseltamivir because of immature renal function, and doses recommended for term infants may lead to high drug concentrations in this age group. Limited data from the National Institute of Allergy and Infectious Diseases Collaborative Antiviral Study Group provide the basis for dosing preterm infants by using their postmenstrual age (gestational age plus chronological age): 1.0 mg/kg per dose orally twice daily for those <38 wk postmenstrual age; 1.5 mg/kg per dose orally twice daily for those 38-40 wk postmenstrual age; and 3.0 mg/kg per dose orally twice daily for those >40 wk postmenstrual age. For extremely preterm infants (<28 wk), please consult a pediatric infectious diseases physician.

[§]Zanamivir is administered by inhalation by using a proprietary Diskhaler device distributed together with the medication. Zanamivir is a dry powder, not an aerosol, and should not be administered by using nebulizers, ventilators, or other devices typically used for administering medications in aerosolized solutions. Zanamivir is not recommended for people with chronic respiratory diseases, such as asthma or chronic obstructive pulmonary disease, which increase the risk of bronchospasm.

**Antiviral treatment duration for uncomplicated influenza is 5 days for oral oseltamivir or inhaled zanamivir, and a single dose for intravenous peramivir or oral baloxavir. Recommended post-exposure chemoprophylaxis with oseltamivir or zanamivir in a non-outbreak setting is 7 days after last known exposure.

[††]Oral baloxavir marboxil is approved by the FDA for treatment of acute uncomplicated influenza within 2 days of illness onset in people 12 yr and older. The safety and efficacy of baloxavir for the treatment of influenza have been established in pediatric patients 12 yr and older weighing at least 40 kg. Safety and efficacy in patients <12 yr of age or weighing <40 kg have not been established. Baloxavir efficacy is based on clinical trials in outpatients 12 to 64 yr of age; people with underlying medical conditions and adults >65 yr were not included in the initial published clinical trials (Hayden F et al; Clin Infect Dis 2018). There are no available data for baloxavir treatment of hospitalized patients with influenza.

Adapted from Centers for Disease Control and Prevention (CDC): Influenza antiviral medications: summary for clinicians. Available at https://www.cdc.gov/flu/professionals/antivirals/summary-clinicians.htm. For current details, consult annually updated recommendations at https://www.cdc.gov/flu/professionals/index.htm; 2018 IDSA Clinical Practice Guidelines; and from Kimberlin DW, Acosta EP, Prichard MN, et al: National Institute of Allergy and Infectious Diseases Collaborative Antiviral Study Group. Oseltamivir pharmacokinetics, dosing, and resistance among children aged <2 yr with influenza, J Infect Dis 207(5):709–720, 2013. For current details, consult annually updated recommendations at https://www.cdc.gov/flu/professionals/index.htm.

intravenous infusion and is approved for treatment in persons 2 yr of age and older.

The second class of drugs is represented by a new influenza antiviral called baloxavir marboxil that was approved by the FDA in October 2018. Baloxavir is active against both influenza A and B viruses but has a different mechanism of action than neuraminidase inhibitors. Baloxavir

is a cap-dependent endonuclease inhibitor that interferes with viral RNA transcription and blocks virus replication. It is approved for treatment of acute uncomplicated influenza in people 12 yr and older.

The third class of drugs, adamantanes, includes oral amantadine and oral rimantadine, which are effective only against influenza A viruses. Genetic mutations have conferred widespread adamantane resistance

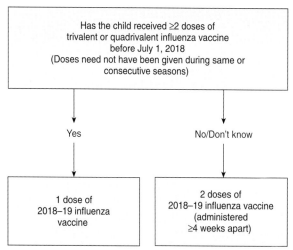

Fig. 285.3 Influenza vaccine dosing algorithm for children aged 6 mo through 8 yr—Advisory Committee on Immunization Practices, United States, 2018-2019 influenza season. (From Grohskopf LA, Sokolow LZ, Broder KR, Walter EB, Fry AM, Jernigan DB: Prevention and control of seasonal influenza with vaccines: recommendations of the advisory committee on immunization practices—United States, 2018-19 Influenza Season, MMWR Recomm Rep 67 (No. RR-3):1–20, 2018.)

among circulating influenza A viruses, including seasonal influenza viruses and many H5N1 and H7N9 avian influenza viruses; *therefore this class of antivirals is not currently recommended for use.*

When initiated early in the course of uncomplicated influenza illness, antiviral agents can reduce the duration of symptoms and the likelihood of complications. Among hospitalized patients, observational studies suggest that early treatment reduces disease severity and mortality. Although most data regarding potential benefit are for adults, a few studies support the use of antiviral agents in children. Antiviral treatment within 2 days of illness onset has been reported to reduce illness duration, the risk of otitis media, and the likelihood of hospitalization in children. Clinical benefit is greatest when antiviral treatment is administered early, especially within 48 hr of influenza illness onset.

CDC recommends treatment as early as possible for (1) hospitalized patients, (2) patients with complicated or progressive illness, and (3) patients at high risk for influenza complications (see Table 285.3). Decisions about starting antiviral treatment should not wait for laboratory confirmation of influenza. Although early treatment is desired, treatment even more than 48 hr from onset may be beneficial and is recommended for these 3 categories of patients.

The recommended treatment course for uncomplicated influenza is 1 dose of an oral oseltamivir or inhaled zanamivir given twice daily for 5 days; intravenous peramivir and oral baloxavir are both given as a single dose. Currently, for hospitalized patients and patients with severe or complicated illness, treatment with oral or enterically administered oseltamivir is recommended. The optimal duration and dose are uncertain for severe or complicated influenza and longer courses of treatment (e.g., 10 days of treatment) may be considered.

Clinical judgment, on the basis of the patient's disease severity, age, underlying medical conditions, likelihood of influenza, and time since onset of symptoms, is important when making antiviral treatment decisions for outpatients at high risk for complications. Antiviral treatment can also be considered for any previously healthy, symptomatic outpatient not at high risk with confirmed or suspected influenza on the basis of clinical judgment, if treatment can be initiated within 48 hr of illness onset.

It is possible that some influenza viruses may become resistant during antiviral treatment; this has been reported most often for oseltamivir resistance in influenza A(H1N1) viruses. Following treatment with baloxavir, emergence of viruses with molecular markers associated with reduced susceptibility to baloxavir has been observed in clinical trials.

Antiviral resistance and reduced susceptibility can also occasionally occur spontaneously with no known exposure to antiviral drugs. It is important to review annual recommendations and updates published by CDC before prescribing influenza antiviral medications (see https://www.cdc.gov/flu/professionals/antivirals/index.htm).

SUPPORTIVE CARE

Adequate fluid intake and rest are important in the management of influenza. Bacterial superinfections are relatively common and should be appropriately treated with antibiotic therapy. Bacterial superinfection should be suspected with recrudescence of fever, prolonged fever, or deterioration in clinical status. With uncomplicated influenza, people should usually start to feel better after the first 48-72 hr of symptoms.

PROGNOSIS

The prognosis for recovery from uncomplicated influenza is generally excellent, although full return to normal level of activity and freedom from cough may require weeks rather than days. Fatigue may also persist for weeks. However, severe influenza disease can be associated with hospitalizations and death, even among previously healthy children.

PREVENTION

Influenza vaccination is the best means of preventing influenza illness. In studies of children who are fully vaccinated, influenza vaccine is 40% to 60% effective in reducing the risk of laboratory-confirmed influenza illness. Vaccine effectiveness can vary from year to year and among different age and risk groups. Recommendations for use of the influenza vaccine have broadened as the impact of influenza is appreciated in such groups as pregnant women and young infants. Starting in the 2008-2009 influenza season, the United States Advisory Committee on Immunization Practices (ACIP) recommended that all children from 6 mo to 18 yr of age be vaccinated for influenza unless they have a specific contraindication to receiving the vaccine. Since the 2010-2011 season, annual flu vaccination is recommended for everyone 6 mo and older, with rare exception. In 2012, the Department of Health in the United Kingdom extended their influenza vaccination program to include all children between the ages of 2 and 17 yr. To protect infants younger than 6 mo who are too young to receive vaccine, household contacts and out-of-home caregivers are groups for whom additional vaccination efforts should be made. Chemoprophylaxis with antiviral medications is a secondary means of prevention and is not a substitute for vaccination.

Vaccines

There are 2 main categories of seasonal influenza vaccines available for children: inactivated influenza vaccine (IIV) and live-attenuated influenza vaccine (LAIV). Previously referred to as the trivalent inactivated vaccine, IIV is given intramuscularly; it uses killed virus components. The LAIV vaccine uses weakened influenza virus and is administered as an intranasal spray. Neither IIV nor LAIV can cause influenza. Although in 2014-2015 ACIP and CDC recommended the use of the LAIV nasal spray vaccine for healthy children 2 through 8 yr of age, this preferential recommendation was removed for the 2015-2016 season, and for the 2016-2017 and 2017-2018 seasons, ACIP and CDC made the interim recommendation that LAIV should not be used. This decision was based on concerns regarding low effectiveness against influenza A(H1N1)pdm09 in the United States noted during the 2013-2014 and 2015-2016 seasons. After review of additional data, LAIV containing an updated influenza A(H1N1)pdm09-like vaccine virus, was again recommended by CDC and ACIP as an option for vaccination for the 2018-2019 season. For the 2018-2019 season, ACIP and CDC made the interim recommendation that LAIV4 may be used.

Special vaccination instructions for children 6 mo to 8 yr of age should be followed: children in this age group who have not previously received a total of ≥2 previous doses of trivalent or quadrivalent vaccine require 2 doses (at least 4 weeks apart) of the current season's influenza vaccine to optimize immune response (Fig. 285.3). Influenza vaccines have an excellent safety profile, with the most common side effects being soreness, redness, tenderness, or swelling from the injection, and nasal congestion after the nasal spray.

Seasonal influenza vaccines become available in the late summer and early fall each year. The formulation reflects the strains of influenza viruses that are expected to circulate in the coming influenza season. Beginning in the 2013-2014 season, IIVs were available in both trivalent and quadrivalent formulations. The trivalent vaccine (IIV3) contains 2 influenza A strains and 1 influenza B strain; the quadrivalent vaccine (IIV4) contains a second influenza B strain of an antigenically distinct lineage. In addition to IIV and LAIV, a third vaccine category, recombinant hemagglutinin influenza vaccine, became available as a trivalent formulation in the 2013-2014 season but this is not licensed for children.

Ideally, vaccination should be given before the onset of influenza circulation in the community, so that there is time for antibodies to reach protective levels. Healthcare providers should offer vaccination by the end of October, if possible. The ACIP publishes guidelines for vaccine use each year when the vaccines are formulated and released; these should be referred to each season. These guidelines are widely publicized but appear initially in the *Morbidity and Mortality Weekly Report* published by CDC (https://www.cdc.gov/flu/index.htm).

Chemoprophylaxis

Routine use of antiviral medications for chemoprophylaxis is not recommended. Examples for which the use of chemoprophylaxis may be considered to prevent influenza after exposure to an infectious person include (1) unvaccinated persons at high risk of influenza complications, (2) persons for whom vaccine is contraindicated or expected to have low effectiveness, and (3) residents/patients in care facilities during institutional influenza outbreaks. Oral oseltamivir or inhaled zanamivir may be used for chemoprophylaxis of influenza; peramivir and baloxavir are not recommended for chemoprophylaxis because of a lack of data, and adamantanes are not currently recommended because of widespread adamantane resistance. Table 285.4 shows the recommendations for dosage and duration of treatment and chemoprophylaxis for the 2018-2019 influenza season, but updated recommendations from the ACIP and CDC should be consulted every season (https://www.cdc.gov/flu/professionals/antivirals/index.htm).

In general, if chemoprophylaxis can be started within 48 hr of exposure to an infectious person, postexposure chemoprophylaxis for persons at high risk of influenza complications (see Table 285.3) is recommended for 7 days after the last known exposure. An alternative to chemoprophylaxis for some persons after a suspected exposure is close monitoring and early initiation of antiviral treatment if symptoms develop. For control of influenza outbreaks among high-risk persons living in institutional settings, such as long-term care facilities, antiviral chemoprophylaxis is recommended for all vaccinated and unvaccinated residents and for unvaccinated healthcare providers. CDC and the Infectious Diseases Society of America recommend antiviral chemoprophylaxis for a minimum of 2 wk and up to 1 wk after the last known case is identified, whichever is longer.

Bibliography is available at Expert Consult.

Chapter **286**

Parainfluenza Viruses*

Holly M. Biggs and Angela J.P. Campbell

第二百八十六章

副流感病毒

中文导读

　　本章主要介绍了副流感病毒感染的病因学、流行病学、发病机制、临床表现、诊断和鉴别诊断、治疗、并发症、预后和预防。副流感病毒是婴幼儿急性呼吸道疾病的常见病因，引起呼吸道疾病，其他临床表现包括低热、流涕、消化道症状等。诊断基于临床和流行病学标准。本病尚无特异性抗病毒药，治疗包括雾化吸入、糖皮质激素、缓解呼吸道梗阻症状等。

Human parainfluenza viruses (HPIVs) are common causes of acute respiratory illness in infants and children and are important causes of lower respiratory tract disease in young children and immunocompromised persons. These viruses cause a spectrum of upper and lower respiratory tract illnesses but are particularly associated with **croup** (laryngotracheitis or laryngotracheobronchitis), **bronchiolitis**, and **pneumonia**.

ETIOLOGY

HPIVs are members of the Paramyxoviridae family. Four HPIVs cause illness in humans, classified as types 1-4, with diverse manifestations of infection. Type 4 is divided into two antigenic subtypes, 4a and 4b. HPIVs have a nonsegmented, single-stranded RNA genome with a lipid-containing envelope derived from budding through the host cell membrane. The major antigenic moieties are the hemagglutinin neuraminidase (HN) and fusion (F) surface glycoproteins.

EPIDEMIOLOGY

By 5 yr of age, most children have experienced primary infection with HPIV types 1, 2, and 3. HPIV-3 infections generally occur earliest, with half of infants infected by age 1 yr, and over 90% by age 5 yr. HPIV-1 and HPIV-2 are more common after infancy, with approximately 75% infected by age 5 yr. Although HPIV-4 is not recognized as often, about half of children have antibody by the age of 5 yr. In the United States and temperate climates, HPIV-1 has typically been reported to have biennial epidemics in the fall in odd-numbered years (Fig. 286.1). HPIV-2 has been reported to cause yearly outbreaks in the fall, but is less common than HPIV-1 or HPIV-3. HPIV-3 can be endemic throughout the year but typically peaks in late spring. In years with less HPIV-1 activity, the HPIV-3 season has been observed to extend longer or to have a second peak in the fall (see Fig. 286.1). The epidemiology of HPIV-4 is less well defined, because it is difficult to grow in tissue culture and was often excluded from previous studies, but a recent study suggests it may circulate throughout the year and peak in fall of odd-numbered years. National HPIV trends are created from weekly laboratory test result data that are reported on a voluntary basis, and are available at the Centers for Disease Control and Prevention (CDC) National Respiratory and Enteric Virus Surveillance System (NREVSS) website (https://www.cdc.gov/surveillance/nrevss).

HPIVs are spread primarily from the respiratory tract by inhalation of large respiratory droplets or contact with infected nasopharyngeal secretions. HPIVs are notable for causing outbreaks of respiratory illness in hospital wards, clinics, neonatal nurseries, and other institutional settings. The incubation period from exposure to symptom onset may range from 2 to 6 days. Children are likely to excrete virus from the oropharynx for 2-3 wk, but shedding can be more prolonged, especially in immunocompromised children, and may persist for months. Primary infection does not confer permanent immunity, and reinfections are common throughout life. Reinfections are usually mild and self-limited, but can cause serious lower respiratory tract illness, particularly in children with compromised immune systems.

PATHOGENESIS

HPIVs replicate in the respiratory epithelium. The propensity to cause illness in the upper large airways is presumably related to preferential replication in the larynx, trachea, and bronchi in comparison with other viruses. Some HPIVs induce cell-to-cell fusion. During the budding process, cell membrane integrity is lost, and viruses can induce cell death through the process of apoptosis. In children, the most severe illness generally coincides with the time of maximal viral shedding. However, disease severity is likely related to the host immune response to infection as much as to direct cytopathic effects of the virus. Virus-specific immunoglobulin A antibody levels and serum antibodies to the surface HN and F glycoproteins are able to neutralize HPIV, and both likely contribute to host immunity. Cell-mediated cytotoxicity is also important for controlling and terminating HPIV infection.

*Disclaimer: The findings and conclusions in this document are those of the authors and do not necessarily represent the official position of the Centers for Disease Control and Prevention.

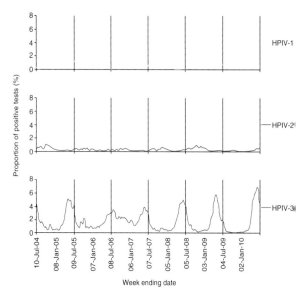

Fig. 286.1 Percentage of antigen tests positive for human parainfluenza virus-1–3 by 3-wk running average from July 2004 to June 2010 reported to the National Respiratory and Enteric Virus Surveillance System. *(Data from Abedi GR, Prill MM, Langley GE, et al: Estimates of parainfluenza virus-associated hospitalizations and cost among children aged less than 5 years in the United States, 1998-2010, J Pediatr Infect Dis Soc 5:7–13, 2016; Fig. 1.)*

CLINICAL MANIFESTATIONS

The most common type of illness caused by HPIV infection consists of some combination of low-grade fever, rhinorrhea, cough, pharyngitis, and hoarseness, and may be associated with vomiting or diarrhea. Rarely, HPIV infection is associated with parotitis. HPIVs have also been associated with a variety of skin manifestations, including typical maculopapular viral exanthems, erythema multiforme, and papular acrodermatitis, or Gianotti-Crosti syndrome (see Chapter 687). Although often mild, more serious HPIV illness may result in hospitalization, with common discharge diagnoses of bronchiolitis, fever/possible sepsis, and apnea among younger children, and croup, pneumonia, and asthma among older children (Fig. 286.2). HPIVs account for 50% of hospitalizations for croup and at least 15% of cases of bronchiolitis and pneumonia. HPIV-1, and to a lesser extent HPIV-2, cause more cases of croup, whereas HPIV-3 is more likely to infect the small air passages and cause pneumonia, bronchiolitis, or bronchitis. HPIV-4 causes a similar range of illness as the other types. Any HPIV can cause lower respiratory tract disease, particularly during primary infection or in patients with compromised immune systems. In children and adult patients with hematologic malignancies and undergoing hematopoietic stem cell transplantation, lymphopenia has repeatedly been shown to be an independent risk factor for progression from upper to lower respiratory tract disease.

DIAGNOSIS AND DIFFERENTIAL DIAGNOSIS

The diagnosis of HPIV infection in children is often based on only clinical and epidemiologic criteria. Croup is a clinical diagnosis and must be distinguished from other diagnoses, including foreign body aspiration, epiglottitis, retropharyngeal abscess, angioedema, and subglottic stenosis or hemangioma. Although the radiographic **steeple sign**, consisting of progressive narrowing of the subglottic region of the trachea, is characteristic of croup, differential considerations include acute epiglottitis, thermal injury, angioedema, and bacterial tracheitis. Manifestation of HPIV lower respiratory tract disease may be similar to that of a number of other respiratory viral infections; therefore identification of virus should be sought by the most sensitive diagnostic means available for certain severe illnesses, such as pneumonia in immunocompromised children.

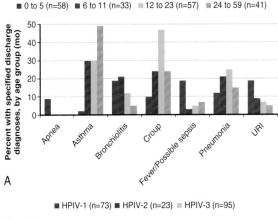

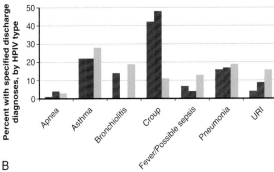

Fig. 286.2 Selected discharge diagnoses of hospitalized children with parainfluenza (HPIV) infection, by **(A)** age in months and **(B)** virus type. *(Data from Weinberg GA, Hall CB, Iwane MK, et al: Parainfluenza virus infection of young children: estimates of the population-based burden of hospitalization, J Pediatr 154:694–699, 2009, Table II.)*

Sensitive, specific, and rapid molecular assays such as multiplex polymerase chain reaction assays, have become more widely available and greatly increase sensitivity of HPIV detection. For immunocompromised patients, these highly sensitive platforms provide the critical ability to make a prompt diagnosis by detecting a wide range of viral pathogens, including HPIVs, thus allowing for early implementation of infection prevention measures and potential treatment. Conventional laboratory diagnosis is accomplished by HPIV isolation in tissue culture, although time to result can take up to a week or longer; this can be shortened to 1-3 days using a rapid shell viral culture system. Direct immunofluorescent staining is available in some laboratories for rapid identification of virus antigen in respiratory secretions.

TREATMENT

There are no specific antiviral medications approved for the treatment of HPIV infections. For croup, the possibility of rapid respiratory compromise should influence the level of care and treatment given (see Chapter 412). Humidified air has not been shown to be effective. Corticosteroids, including dexamethasone orally or by injection and less often budesonide via nebulizer, improve symptoms within 6 hr after treatment, lessen the need for other medications, and shorten hospital stays. In general, because of its safety, efficacy, and cost-effectiveness, a single dose of oral dexamethasone (0.6 mg/kg) is the primary treatment for croup in the office or emergency room setting. A single dose of intramuscular dexamethasone or budesonide (2 mg [2 mL solution] via nebulizer) may provide an alternative to dexamethasone for children with severe respiratory distress or vomiting. The dose may be repeated, but this should not be necessary on a routine basis, and there are no guidelines to compare outcomes of single- and multiple-dose treatment schedules. Moderate to severe symptoms that persist for more than a few days should prompt investigation for other causes of airway obstruction.

The severity assessment of croup generally incorporates a number of clinical features, which include the presence and degree of chest wall retractions, whether stridor is present at rest, and evaluation of the child's mental status (e.g., for agitation, anxiety, lethargy). For obstructive airway symptoms associated with moderate to severe croup, nebulized epinephrine (either racemic epinephrine 2.25% solution, 0.05 to 0.1 mL/kg/dose, maximum dose 0.5 mL, diluted, in 3 mL of normal saline; or L-epinephrine, 0.5 mL/kg/dose of 1 : 1,000 solution in normal saline, maximum dose 5 mL) is recommended and may also provide temporary symptomatic improvement. Children should be observed for at least 2 hr after receiving epinephrine treatment for return of obstructive symptoms. Repeated treatments may be provided, depending on the duration of symptoms. Oxygen should be administered for hypoxia, and supportive care with analgesics and antipyretics is reasonable for fever and discomfort associated with HPIV infections. The indications for antibiotics are limited to well-documented secondary bacterial infections of the middle ear(s) or lower respiratory tract.

Ribavirin has some antiviral activity against HPIVs in vitro and in animal models. Inhaled ribavirin has been given to severely immunocompromised children with HPIV pneumonia; however, the majority of data have not shown improved outcomes, and randomized, controlled studies are lacking. Some institutions use intravenous immunoglobulin for HPIV pneumonia in children with hematologic malignancies or who have undergone hematopoietic stem cell transplantation; the impact of this treatment strategy on clinical outcomes is also limited by lack of controlled studies. Use of investigational antiviral DAS181, a novel sialidase fusion protein inhibitor, has shown clinical potential when used for treatment of HPIV lower respiratory tract disease among solid-organ and hematopoietic stem cell transplant recipients, but further study is needed. Other potential strategies for drug development include hemagglutinin-neuraminidase inhibitors, transcription inhibitors, and synthetic small interfering RNAs.

COMPLICATIONS

Eustachian tube obstruction can lead to secondary bacterial invasion of the middle ear space and acute otitis media in 30–50% of HPIV infections. Similarly, obstruction of the paranasal sinuses can lead to sinusitis. The destruction of cells in the upper airways can lead to secondary bacterial invasion and resultant bacterial tracheitis, and antecedent HPIV infection of lower airways may predispose to bacterial pneumonia. Nonrespiratory complications of HPIV are rare but include aseptic meningitis, encephalitis, acute disseminated encephalomyelitis, rhabdomyolysis, myocarditis, and pericarditis.

PROGNOSIS

The prognosis for full recovery from HPIV infection in the immunocompetent child is excellent, with no long-term pulmonary sequelae. Deaths may rarely occur, particularly in immunocompromised children with lower respiratory tract infection.

PREVENTION

Vaccine development has focused largely on live-attenuated intranasal HPIV-3 vaccines. Candidates include a recombinant human HPIV-3 virus (rcp45) derived from complementary DNA, as well as a complementary DNA–derived chimeric bovine/human HPIV-3 virus; these candidates are well tolerated and immunogenic in infants and young children. Constructs using chimeric bovine/human HPIV-3 virus in addition to the F or both F and G proteins of respiratory syncytial virus are also under investigation. Although at a less advanced state in development, live attenuated candidate HPIV-1 and HPIV-2 vaccines have undergone phase 1 clinical studies (www.clinicaltrials.gov). The measure of protection afforded by vaccines will be difficult to assess, because symptomatic reinfection occurs and the frequency of serious infection in the general population is low. Nonetheless, it is clear that prevention of acute respiratory illness caused by HPIVs, particularly lower respiratory tract infections among infants and young children, is a worthwhile goal.

Bibliography is available at Expert Consult.

Chapter **287**

Respiratory Syncytial Virus

James E. Crowe Jr.

第二百八十七章

呼吸道合胞病毒

中文导读

本章主要介绍了呼吸道病毒感染的病因学、流行病学、发病机制、临床表现、诊断、治疗、预后和预防。在流行病学中详细介绍了呼吸道合胞病毒感染的流行季节、易感人群、易感因素及传播途径。临床表现包括流涕、咳嗽、低热、喘息；严重者表现为咳嗽、喘息加重、烦躁、发绀等。实验室诊断依靠呼吸道分泌物病毒培养和分子学检测方法。治疗中详述了呼吸支持、糖皮质激素和抗病毒药。

Respiratory syncytial virus (RSV) is the major cause of bronchiolitis (see Chapter 418) and viral pneumonia in children younger than 1 yr of age and is the most important respiratory tract pathogen of early childhood.

ETIOLOGY

RSV is an enveloped RNA virus with a single-stranded negative-sense genome that replicates entirely in the cytoplasm of infected cells and matures by budding from the apical surface of the cell membrane. Because this virus has a nonsegmented genome, it cannot undergo antigenic shift by reassortment like the influenza viruses do. The virus belongs to the family Pneumoviridae, which comprises large enveloped, negative-sense RNA viruses. This taxon was formerly a subfamily within the Paramyxoviridae but was reclassified in 2016 as a family with two genera, *Orthopneumovirus* (which includes RSV) and *Metapneumovirus* (which includes human metapneumovirus; see Chapter 288). There are two antigenic subgroups of RSV (subgroups A and B), distinguished based primarily on sequence and antigenic variation in one of the two surface proteins, the G glycoprotein that is responsible for attachment to host cells. This antigenic variation, which is caused by point mutations from infidelity of the viral RNA polymerase, may contribute to some degree to the frequency with which RSV reinfects children and adults. However, adult human challenge experiments have shown that the same RSV strain can reinfect in the upper respiratory tract repetitively, suggesting that mucosal immunity in that site is incomplete or short-lived.

RSV replicates in a wide variety of cell line monolayer cultures in the laboratory. In HeLa and HEp-2 cell monolayers, the virus causes cell-to-cell fusion that produces characteristic cytopathology called syncytia (multinucleate enlarged cells), from which the virus derives its name. Identification of syncytia in diagnostic cultures of respiratory secretions is helpful in identifying RSV, but it is not clear whether syncytium formation occurs to any significant degree in the airway epithelium in patients.

EPIDEMIOLOGY

RSV is distributed worldwide and appears in yearly epidemics. In temperate climates, these epidemics occur each winter over a 4- to 5-mo period. During the remainder of the year, infections are sporadic and much less common. In the Northern hemisphere, epidemics usually peak in January, February, or March, but peaks have been recognized as early as December and as late as June. Some areas in the United States, such as Florida, report a moderate incidence year-round. In the Southern hemisphere, outbreaks also occur during the winter months in that hemisphere. RSV outbreaks often overlap with outbreaks of influenza virus or human metapneumovirus but are generally more consistent from year to year and result in more disease overall, especially among infants younger than 6 mo of age. In the tropics, the epidemic pattern is less clear. The pattern of widespread annual outbreaks and the high incidence of infection during the first 3-4 mo of life are unique among human viruses.

Transplacentally acquired anti-RSV maternal immunoglobulin G (IgG) serum antibodies, if present in high concentration, appear to provide partial protection for the neonate. The age of peak incidence of severe lower respiratory tract disease and hospitalization is about 6 wk. Maternal IgGs may account for the lower severity and incidence of RSV infections during the first 4-6 wk of life, except among infants born prematurely, who receive less maternal immunoglobulin. Breastfeeding provides some protection against severe disease, an effect that may pertain only to female and not male infants. RSV is one of the most contagious viruses that affect humans. Infection is nearly universal among children by their second birthday. Reinfection occurs at a rate of at least 10–20% per epidemic throughout childhood, with a lower frequency among adults. In situations of high exposure, such as daycare centers, attack rates are nearly 100% among previously uninfected infants and 60–80% for second and subsequent infections.

Reinfection may occur as early as a few weeks after recovery but usually takes place during subsequent annual outbreaks. Antigenic variation is not required for reinfection, as shown by the fact that a proportion of adults inoculated repeatedly with the same experimental preparation of wild-type virus could be reinfected multiple times. The immune response of infants is poor in quality, magnitude, and durability. The severity of illness during reinfection in childhood is usually lower than that in first infection and appears to be a function of partial acquired immunity, more robust airway physiology, and increased age.

Asymptomatic RSV infection is unusual in young children. Most infants experience coryza and pharyngitis, often with fever and frequently with otitis media caused by virus in the middle ear or bacterial superinfection following eustachian tube dysfunction. The lower respiratory tract is involved to a varying degree, with bronchiolitis and bronchopneumonia in about a third of children. The hospitalization rate for RSV infection in otherwise healthy infants is typically 0.5–4%, depending on region, gender, socioeconomic status, exposure to cigarette smoke, gestational age, and family history of atopy. The admitting diagnosis is usually bronchiolitis with hypoxia, although this condition is often indistinguishable from RSV pneumonia in infants, and, indeed, the two processes frequently coexist. All RSV diseases of the lower respiratory tract (excluding croup) have their highest incidence at 6 wk to 7 mo of age and decrease in frequency thereafter. The syndrome of bronchiolitis is much less common after the 1st birthday. The terminology used for the diagnosis of virus-associated wheezing illnesses in toddlers can be confusing, because these illnesses are variably termed *wheezing-associated respiratory infection, wheezy bronchitis, exacerbation of reactive airways disease,* or *asthma attack.* Because many toddlers wheeze during RSV infection but do not go on to have lifelong asthma, it is best to use the diagnostic term *asthma* only later in life. Acute viral pneumonia is a recurring problem throughout childhood, although RSV becomes less prominent as the etiologic agent after the first year. RSV plays a causative role in an estimated 40–75% of cases of hospitalized bronchiolitis, 15–40% of cases of childhood pneumonia, and 6–15% of cases of croup.

Bronchiolitis and pneumonia resulting from RSV are more common in males than in females by a ratio of approximately 1.5 : 1. Other risk factors with a similar impact in the United States include one or more siblings in the home, white race, rural residence, maternal smoking, and maternal education < 12 yr. The medical factors in infants associated with the highest risk are chronic lung disease of prematurity, congenital heart disease, immunodeficiency, and prematurity. Still, most infants admitted to the hospital because of RSV infection do not have strong, easily identifiable risk factors. Therefore, any strategy for prophylaxis focused only on individuals with strong risk factors probably could prevent only approximately 10% of hospitalizations, even if the prophylaxis was 100% effective in treated high-risk individuals.

The incubation period from exposure to first symptoms is approximately 3–5 days. The virus is excreted for variable periods, probably depending on the severity of illness and immunologic status. Most infants with lower respiratory tract illness shed infectious viruses for 1–2 wk after hospital admission. Excretion for 3 wk and even longer has been documented. Spread of infection occurs when large, infected droplets, either airborne or conveyed on hands or other fomites, are inoculated in the nasopharynx of a susceptible subject. RSV is probably introduced into most families by young schoolchildren experiencing reinfection. Typically, in the space of a few days, 25–50% of older siblings and one or both parents acquire upper respiratory tract infections, but infants become more severely ill with fever, otitis media, or lower respiratory tract disease.

Nosocomial infection during RSV epidemics is an important concern. Virus is usually spread from child to child on the hands of caregivers or other fomites. Adults experiencing reinfection also have been implicated in the spread of the virus. Contact precautions are sufficient to prevent spread when compliance is meticulous, because the virus is not spread by small particle aerosol to an appreciable degree, and a distance of about 6 ft is likely sufficient to avoid aerosol transmission. However, in practice, adherence to isolation procedures by caregivers often is not complete.

PATHOGENESIS

Bronchiolitis is caused by obstruction and collapse of the small airways during expiration. Infants are particularly apt to experience small airway obstruction because of the small size of their normal bronchioles; airway resistance is proportional to $1/radius^4$. There has been relatively little pathologic examination of RSV disease in the lower airways of otherwise healthy subjects. Airway narrowing likely is caused by virus-induced necrosis of the bronchiolar epithelium, hypersecretion of mucus, and round-cell infiltration and edema of the surrounding submucosa. These changes result in the formation of mucus plugs obstructing bronchioles, with consequent hyperinflation or collapse of the distal lung tissue. In interstitial pneumonia, the infiltration is more generalized, and epithelial shedding may extend to both the bronchi and the alveoli. In older subjects, smooth muscle hyperreactivity may contribute to airway narrowing, but the airways of young infants typically do not exhibit a high degree of reversible smooth muscle hyperreactivity during RSV infection.

Several facts suggest that elements of the host response may cause inflammation and contribute to tissue damage. The immune response required to eliminate virus-infected cells (mostly containing cytolytic T cells) is a double-edged sword, reducing the cells producing virus but also causing host cell death in the process. A large number of soluble factors, such as cytokines, chemokines, and leukotrienes, are released in the process, and skewing of the patterns of these responses may predispose some individuals to more severe disease. There is also evidence that genetic factors may predispose to more severe bronchiolitis.

Children who received a formalin-inactivated, parenterally administered RSV vaccine in the 1960s experienced more severe and more frequent bronchiolitis upon subsequent natural exposure to wild-type RSV than did their age-matched controls. Several children died during naturally acquired RSV infections after FI-RSV vaccinations. This event greatly inhibited the progress in RSV vaccine development, because of both an incomplete understanding of the mechanism and a reluctance to test new experimental vaccines that might induce the same type of response.

Some studies have identified the presence of both RSV and human metapneumovirus viral RNA in airway secretions in a significant proportion of infants requiring assisted ventilation and intensive care. It may be that coinfection is associated with more severe disease. Positive results of polymerase chain reaction (PCR) analysis must be interpreted carefully because this positivity can remain for prolonged periods after infection, even when infectious virus can no longer be detected.

It is not clear how often superimposed bacterial infection plays a pathogenic role in RSV lower respiratory tract disease. RSV bronchiolitis in infants is probably exclusively a viral disease, although there is evidence that bacterial pneumonia can be triggered by respiratory viral infection, including with RSV. A large clinical study of pneumococcal vaccine showed that childhood vaccination reduced the incidence of viral pneumonia by approximately 30%, suggesting viral-bacterial interactions that we currently do not fully understand.

CLINICAL MANIFESTATIONS

Typically, the first sign of infection in infants with RSV is rhinorrhea. Cough may appear simultaneously but more often does so after an interval of 1–3 days, at which time there may also be sneezing and a low-grade fever. Soon after the cough develops, the child who experiences bronchiolitis begins to wheeze audibly. If the disease is mild, the symptoms may not progress beyond this stage. Auscultation often reveals diffuse fine inspiratory crackles and expiratory wheezes. Rhinorrhea usually persists throughout the illness, with intermittent fever. Chest radiograph findings at this stage are frequently normal.

If the illness progresses, cough and wheezing worsen and air hunger ensues, with an increased respiratory rate, intercostal and subcostal retractions, hyperexpansion of the chest, restlessness, and peripheral cyanosis. Signs of severe, life-threatening illness are central cyanosis, tachypnea of > 70 breaths/min, listlessness, and apneic spells. At this stage, the chest may be significantly hyperexpanded and almost silent to auscultation because of poor air movement.

Chest radiographs of infants hospitalized with RSV bronchiolitis have normal findings in approximately 30% of cases, with the other 70% showing hyperexpansion of the chest, peribronchial thickening, and interstitial infiltrates. Segmental or lobar consolidation is unusual, and pleural effusion is rare.

In some infants, the course of the illness may resemble that of pneumonia, the prodromal rhinorrhea and cough being followed by dyspnea, poor feeding, and listlessness. Although the clinical diagnosis is pneumonia, wheezing is often present intermittently, and the chest radiographs may show air trapping.

Fever is an inconsistent sign in RSV infection. In young infants, particularly those who were born prematurely, periodic breathing and apneic spells have been distressingly frequent signs, even with relatively mild bronchiolitis. Apnea is not necessarily caused by respiratory exhaustion but rather appears to be a consequence of alterations in the central control of breathing.

RSV infections in profoundly immunocompromised hosts may be severe at any age of life. The mortality rates associated with RSV pneumonia in the 1st few weeks after hematopoietic stem cell or solid-organ transplantation in both children and adults are high. RSV infection does not appear to be more severe in HIV-infected patients with reasonable control of HIV disease, although these patients may shed virus in respiratory secretions for prolonged periods.

DIAGNOSIS

Bronchiolitis is a clinical diagnosis. RSV can be suspected with varying degrees of certainty on the basis of the season of the year and the presence of the virus in the community. Other epidemiologic features that may be helpful are the presence of common colds in older household contacts and the age of the child. The other respiratory viruses that attack infants frequently during the first few months of life are human metapneumovirus, influenza viruses, parainfluenza virus type 3, rhinoviruses, enteroviruses, and coronaviruses.

Routine laboratory tests are of minimal diagnostic use in most cases of bronchiolitis or pneumonia caused by RSV. The white blood cell count is normal or elevated, and the differential cell count may be normal with either a neutrophilic or mononuclear predominance. Hypoxemia as measured by pulse oximetry or arterial blood gas analysis is frequent and tends to be more marked than anticipated from the clinical findings. A normal or elevated blood CO_2 value in a patient with a markedly elevated respiratory rate is a sign of respiratory failure.

The most important diagnostic concern is to differentiate viral infection from bacterial or chlamydial infection. When bronchiolitis is not accompanied by infiltrates on chest radiographs, there is little likelihood of a bacterial component. In infants 1-4 mo of age, interstitial pneumonitis may be caused by *Chlamydia trachomatis* (see Chapter 253). With *C. trachomatis* pneumonia, there may be a history of conjunctivitis, and the illness tends to be of subacute onset. Coughing and inspiratory crackles may be prominent; wheezing is not. Fever is usually absent.

Lobar consolidation without other signs or with pleural effusion should be considered of bacterial etiology until proved otherwise. Other signs suggesting bacterial pneumonia are neutrophilia, neutropenia in the presence of severe disease, ileus or other abdominal signs, high temperature, and circulatory collapse. In such instances, antibiotics should be initiated.

The definitive diagnosis of RSV infection is based on the detection in respiratory secretions of live virus by cell culture. Molecular diagnostic tests are more available, however. The presence of viral RNA (detected by a molecular diagnostic test using reverse transcription PCR) or viral antigens (detected by a rapid diagnostic test, usually a membrane blotting test incorporating antibody detection of viral proteins) is strongly supportive in the right clinical setting. The antigen test is less sensitive than virus culture, whereas reverse transcription PCR analysis is more sensitive than culture. An aspirate of mucus or a nasopharyngeal wash from the child's posterior nasal cavity is the optimal specimen. Nasopharyngeal or throat swabs are less preferable but are acceptable. A tracheal aspirate is unnecessary, but endotracheal tube lavage fluid from patients intubated for mechanical ventilation can be tested. The specimen should be placed on ice, taken directly to the laboratory, and processed immediately for culture, antigen detection, or PCR analysis. RSV is thermolabile, so it degrades over relatively short periods of time unless it is frozen at a low temperature such as −80°C (−112°F) in freezers used in research settings.

TREATMENT

The treatment of uncomplicated cases of bronchiolitis is symptomatic. Many infants are slightly to moderately dehydrated, and therefore fluids should be carefully administered in amounts somewhat greater than those for maintenance. Often, intravenous or tube feeding is helpful when sucking is difficult because of tachypnea. Humidified oxygen and suctioning usually are indicated for hospitalized infants who are hypoxic. High-flow nasal cannula therapy is used for respiratory distress, which is mostly useful for pressure support. Nasal continuous positive airway pressure is used in the intensive care unit for infants who have increased work of breathing, and mechanical ventilation is used for respiratory failure. Heliox (helium blended with oxygen) may improve ventilation in infants who have severe respiratory distress but who do not require large amounts of oxygen.

There is disagreement among experts regarding the usefulness of aerosolized saline or hypertonic saline, epinephrine, or β$_2$-agonists in RSV bronchiolitis. Most patients do not receive lasting benefit from prolonged therapy, which is associated with a relatively high frequency of side effects. Corticosteroid therapy is not indicated except in older children with an established diagnosis of asthma, because its use is associated with prolonged virus shedding and is of no proven clinical benefit. The 2014 American Academy of Pediatrics bronchiolitis clinical practice guideline suggests limitations on the use of α- and β-adrenergic agents and corticosteroids.

In nearly all instances of bronchiolitis, antibiotics are not useful, and their inappropriate use contributes to the development of antibiotic resistance. Interstitial pneumonia in infants 1-4 mo old may be caused by *C. trachomatis,* and macrolide therapy may be indicated for that infection.

Ribavirin is an antiviral agent delivered through an oxygen hood, face mask, or endotracheal tube with use of a small-particle aerosol generator most of the day for 3-5 days. Early small trials of its use suggested a modest beneficial effect on the course of RSV pneumonia, with some reduction in the duration of both mechanical ventilation and hospitalization. However, subsequent studies failed to document a clear beneficial effect of ribavirin, and therefore this drug is no longer used for routine therapy of RSV disease. The monoclonal antibody palivizumab is licensed for prophylaxis in high-risk infants during the RSV season and does prevent about half of the expected hospitalizations in that population. Small clinical trials using palivizumab as a therapy during established infection have not shown benefit to date. Next-generation monoclonal antibodies for RSV that are more potent and longer-lasting are in clinical trials.

PROGNOSIS

The mortality rate of hospitalized infants with RSV infection of the lower respiratory tract is very low in the developed world. Almost all deaths occur among young, premature infants or infants with underlying disease of the neuromuscular, pulmonary, cardiovascular, or immunologic system. However, it is estimated that more than 160,000 children worldwide in resource-poor settings die each year from RSV. In addition, thousands of elderly patients die of RSV infection each year in the United States.

There is recurrent wheezing in 30–50% of children who have severe RSV bronchiolitis in infancy, and many older children who are diagnosed with asthma have a history of severe bronchiolitis in infancy. The likelihood of the recurrence of wheezing is increased in the presence of an allergic diathesis (e.g., eczema, hay fever, or a family history of asthma). With a clinical presentation of bronchiolitis in a patient older than 1 yr of age, there is an increasing probability that, although the episode may be virus-induced, the event is likely the first of multiple wheezing attacks that will later be diagnosed as hyperreactive airways disease or asthma. Asthma is difficult to diagnose in the first year of life. It is not fully clear at this time whether early, severe RSV wheezing disease causes some cases of asthma or whether subjects destined to suffer asthma present with symptoms first when provoked by RSV infection during infancy. Results from a long-term follow-up study of infants who received palivizumab prophylaxis suggested that the prevention of severe RSV infection may reduce the incidence of reactive airways disease later in life.

PREVENTION

In the hospital, the most important preventive measures are aimed at blocking nosocomial spread. During RSV season, high-risk infants should be separated from all infants with respiratory symptoms. Gowns, gloves, and careful handwashing (contact isolation) should be used for the care of all infants with suspected or established RSV infection. A high level of compliance with contact isolation is essential. Viral laboratory tests are adequate for diagnosis in the setting of acute disease when levels of virus are high, but they are not designed to detect low levels of virus. Therefore, contact precaution isolation should be observed for most patients admitted for acute disease assigned for the duration of hospitalization. Rapid antigen tests should not be used to determine whether or not a patient still requires isolation, because low concentrations of virus may be present in respiratory secretions that are infectious for humans but below the lower limit of detection for such assays. Ideally, patients with RSV or metapneumovirus infections are housed separately, because coinfection with the two viruses may be associated with more severe disease.

Passive Immunoprophylaxis

Administration of palivizumab (15 mg/kg intramuscularly once a month), a neutralizing humanized murine monoclonal antibody against RSV, is recommended for protecting high-risk children against serious complications from RSV disease. Immunoprophylaxis reduces the frequency and total days of hospitalization for RSV infections in high-risk infants in about half of cases. Palivizumab is administered monthly from the beginning to the end of the RSV season. Palivizumab prophylaxis may be considered for the following infants and children:
Infants born before 29 wk of gestation in the first year of life
Infants born before 32 wk of gestation, who have chronic lung disease of prematurity (required > 21% FIO_2 [fraction of inspired oxygen] for ≥ 28 days after birth), in the first year of life
Infants younger than 1 yr of age with hemodynamically *significant* congenital heart disease following cardiac transplantation (children < 2 yr age)
Children 24 mo of age or younger with profound immunocompromising conditions during RSV season
Infants in the first year of life who have either congenital abnormalities of the airway or neuromuscular disease that compromises the handling of respiratory secretions

Administration in the second year of life is recommended for children who required 28 or more days of oxygen after birth and who have ongoing treatment for chronic pulmonary disease (oxygen, steroids, diuretics)

Recommendations for initiation and termination of prophylaxis reflect current descriptions from the Centers for Disease Control and Prevention of RSV seasonality in different geographic locations within the United States. Initiation in different areas of the United States may be recommended for different months, because of variation in the onset of the season in different regions, with special recommendations for Alaska and Florida. Regardless of the month in which the first dose is administered, the recommendation for a maximal number of five doses for all geographic locations is emphasized for high-risk infants. Categories of infants at increased risk of severe disease include those with hemodynamically significant congenital heart disease, chronic lung disease of prematurity, or birth before 32 wk, 0 days of gestation, congenital anatomic pulmonary abnormalities or neuromuscular disorder, and immunocompromised state; Down syndrome, cystic fibrosis, or Alaska Native infants are at increased risk, but passive immunization is not indicated unless another high-risk condition is present. A second season of palivizumab prophylaxis is recommended only for preterm infants < 32 weeks, 0 days gestation who required at least 28 days of oxygen after birth and who continue to require supplemental oxygen, chronic systemic corticosteroid therapy, or diuretic therapy within 6 mo of the start of the second RSV season.

Vaccine

There is no licensed vaccine against RSV. The challenge for the development of live virus vaccines has been to produce attenuated vaccine strains that infect infants in the nasopharynx after topical inoculation without producing unacceptable symptoms, that remain genetically stable during shedding, and that induce protection against severe disease following reinfection. The most promising live-attenuated virus candidates have been engineered in the laboratory from cold-passaged strains of RSV, according to a basic strategy that yielded the live poliovirus and influenza virus vaccine strains. A variety of nonreplicating experimental vaccines are being tested in early clinical trials. Subunit vaccine candidates are being tested in maternal immunization trials. The rationale of such studies is to test whether boosting the serum level of RSV-neutralizing antibodies in the mother can enhance immunity in neonates following transplacental transfer of those boosted levels of maternal antibodies to the infant.

Bibliography is available at Expert Consult.

Chapter **288**

Human Metapneumovirus

James E. Crowe Jr.

第二百八十八章

人偏肺病毒

中文导读

本章主要介绍了人偏肺病毒感染的病因学、流行病学、病理学、发病机制、临床表现、实验室检查、诊断和鉴别诊断、并发症、治疗、预后和预防。临床表现包括普通感冒、毛细支气管炎、肺炎等呼吸道疾病。实验室检测方法包括PCR、抗原和抗体检测。本病尚无特异性抗病毒药。大部分患者预后好，预防的唯一方法是减少暴露。

ETIOLOGY

Human metapneumovirus (HMPV) is a respiratory virus that has emerged as one of the most common causes of serious lower respiratory tract illness in children throughout the world.

ETIOLOGY

HMPV is an enveloped, single-stranded, nonsegmented, negative-sense RNA genome of the family Pneumoviridae, which comprises large enveloped negative-sense RNA viruses. This taxon was formerly a subfamily within the Paramyxoviridae, but was reclassified in 2016 as a family with two genera, *Metapneumovirus* (which includes HMPV) and *Orthopneumovirus* (which includes respiratory syncytial virus [RSV], see Chapter 287). HMPV and the avian pneumoviruses are highly related and are separated into the separate genus *Metapneumovirus* because the gene order in the nonsegmented genome is slightly altered and because avian pneumoviruses/HMPVs lack the genes for two nonstructural proteins, NS1 and NS2, which are encoded at the 3′ end of RSV genomes. These proteins are thought to counteract host type I interferons. The absence of NS1/NS2 in the metapneumoviruses (compared with RSV) may contribute to an overall slightly reduced pathogenicity relative to wild-type RSV strains.

The HMPV genome encodes nine proteins in the order 3′-N-P-M-F-M2-(orf1 and 2)-SH-G-L-5′. The genome also contains noncoding 3′ leader, 5′ trailer, and intergenic regions, consistent with the organization of most paramyxoviruses, with a viral promoter contained in the 3′ end of the genome. The F (fusion), G (glycosylated), and SH (short hydrophobic) proteins are integral membrane proteins on the surfaces of infected cells and virion particles. The F protein is a classic type I integral membrane viral fusion protein that contains two heptad repeats in the extracellular domain that facilitate membrane fusion. There is a predicted protein cleavage site near a hydrophobic fusion peptide that likely is cleaved by an extracellular protease, activating the F protein for fusion. The predicted attachment (G) protein of HMPV exhibits the

basic features of a glycosylated type II mucin-like protein. The HMPV G protein differs from the RSV G protein in that it lacks a cysteine noose structure. This protein may inhibit innate immune responses. The internal proteins of the virus appear similar in function to those of other paramyxoviruses.

EPIDEMIOLOGY

HMPV outbreaks occur in annual epidemics during late winter and early spring in temperate climates, often overlapping with the second half of the annual RSV epidemic (Fig. 288.1). Sporadic infections occur year round. The usual period of viral shedding is likely to be many days or even several weeks after primary infection in infants. The incubation period is approximately 3-5 days. Humans are the only source of virus; there is no known animal or environmental reservoir. Transmission occurs by close or direct contact with contaminated secretions involving large-particle aerosols, droplets, or contaminated surfaces. Nosocomial infections have been reported, and contact isolation with excellent handwashing for healthcare providers is critical in medical settings. This virus also affects the elderly, immunocompromised patients, and patients with reactive airways disease more severely than otherwise healthy individuals.

PATHOLOGY

Infection is usually limited to the superficial layer of airway epithelial cells and is associated with a local inflammatory infiltrate consisting of lymphocytes and macrophages. Immunocompromised individuals have evidence of both acute and organizing injuries during prolonged infection.

PATHOGENESIS

Infection occurs via inoculation of the upper respiratory tract. Infection can spread rapidly to the lower respiratory tract, but it is not clear whether the dissemination is mediated by cell-to-cell spread or by aspiration of infected materials from the upper tract. Severe lower respiratory tract

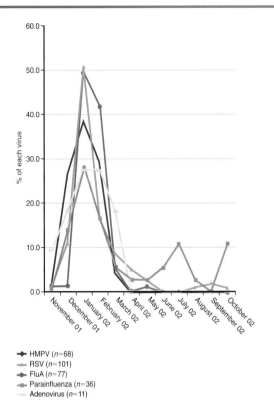

Fig. 288.1 Temporal distribution of respiratory viruses among children hospitalized with lower respiratory tract infections from November 2001 through October 2002. Data are displayed as the proportion of each virus detected monthly. FluA, influenza A; HMPV, human metapneumovirus; RSV, respiratory syncytial virus. *(From Wolf DG, Greenberg D, Kalkstein D, et al: Comparison of human metapneumovirus, respiratory syncytial virus and influenza A virus lower respiratory tract infections in hospitalized young children, Pediatr Infect Dis J 25:320–324, 2006.)*

Table 288.1	Clinical Manifestations of Human Metapneumovirus in Children

COMMON (>50%)
Fever > 38°C (100.4°F)
Cough
Rhinitis, coryza
Wheezing
Tachypnea, retractions
Hypoxia (O_2 saturation < 94%)
Chest radiograph demonstration of infiltrates or hyperinflation

LESS COMMON
Otitis media
Pharyngitis
Rales

RARE
Conjunctivitis
Hoarseness
Encephalitis
Fatal respiratory failure in immunocompromised children

illness, especially wheezing, occurs mainly during the first year of life, at a time when the airways are of a very small diameter and thus a high resistance. Maternal serum-neutralizing antibodies that cross the placenta may afford a relative protection against severe disease for several weeks or months after birth. Once infection is established, it is likely that cytotoxic T cells recognize and eliminate virus-infected cells, thus terminating the infection but also causing some cytopathology. The virus appears to have specific mechanisms for inhibiting T-cell responses during acute infection. Individuals with an underlying predisposition for reactive airways disease (including adults) are susceptible to severe wheezing during reinfection later in life, suggesting that HMPV may cause smooth muscle hyperactivity, inflammation, or increased mucus production in such individuals. Infection in otherwise healthy individuals resolves without apparent long-term consequences in most cases. HMPV infection is associated with exacerbations of asthma later in life.

CLINICAL MANIFESTATIONS

HMPV is associated with the common cold (complicated by otitis media in approximately 30% of cases) and with lower respiratory tract illnesses such as bronchiolitis, pneumonia, croup, and exacerbation of reactive airways disease. The profile of signs and symptoms caused by HMPV is very similar to that caused by RSV (Table 288.1). Approximately 5–10% of outpatient lower respiratory tract illnesses in otherwise healthy young children is associated with HMPV infection, which is second in incidence only to RSV. Children with RSV or HMPV infection require supplemental oxygen and medical intensive care at similar frequencies.

About half of the cases of HMPV lower respiratory tract illness in children occur in the first 6 mo of life, suggesting that young age is a major risk factor for severe disease. Both young adults and the elderly

can have HMPV infection that requires medical care including hospitalization, but severe disease occurs at much lower frequencies in adults than in young children. Severe disease in pediatric and older subjects is most common in immunocompromised patients or those with complications of preterm birth, congenital heart disease, and neuromuscular disease and can be fatal. A significant number of both adult and pediatric patients with asthma exacerbations have HMPV infection; it is not clear whether the virus causes long-term wheezing. RSV and HMPV coinfections have been reported; coinfections may be more severe than infection with a single virus, resulting in pediatric intensive care unit admissions. It is difficult to define true coinfections because these viral RNA genomes can be detected by a reverse transcriptase polymerase chain reaction (PCR) in respiratory secretions for at least several weeks after illness, even when virus shedding has terminated.

LABORATORY FINDINGS

The virus can be visualized only with electron microscopy. The virus grows in primary monkey kidney cells or LLC-MK2 cell or Vero cell–line monolayer cultures in reference or research laboratories, but efficient isolation of the virus requires an experienced laboratory technician. Conventional bright-field microscopy of infected cell monolayer cultures often reveals a cytopathic effect only after multiple passages in the cell culture. The characteristics of the cytopathic effect are not sufficiently distinct to allow identification of the virus on this basis alone, even by a trained observer. The most sensitive test for identification of HMPV in clinical samples is reverse transcriptase PCR, usually performed with primers directed to conserved viral genes. Detection by this modality is also available in some multiplex PCR tests for panels of respiratory viruses. Real-time reverse transcriptase PCR tests offer enhanced sensitivity and specificity, including assays designed to detect viruses from the four known genetic lineages. Direct antigen tests for identification of HMPV antigens in nasopharyngeal secretions are available but are less efficient than nucleic acid–based detection. Some laboratories have success with the use of immunofluorescence staining with monoclonal or polyclonal antibodies to detect HMPV in nasopharyngeal secretions and shell vial cultures or in monolayer cultures in which virus has been cultivated, with reported sensitivities varying from about 65% to 90%. A four-fold rise in serum antibody titer to HMPV from the acute to convalescent time point can be used in research settings to confirm infection.

DIAGNOSIS AND DIFFERENTIAL DIAGNOSIS

In temperate areas, the diagnosis should be suspected during the late winter in infants or young children with wheezing or pneumonia and a negative RSV diagnostic test result. The diseases caused by RSV and HMPV cannot be distinguished clinically. Many other common respiratory viruses, such as parainfluenza viruses, influenza viruses, adenoviruses, rhinoviruses, enteroviruses, and coronaviruses, can cause similar disease in young children. Some of these viruses can be identified by PCR genetic testing or conventional cell culture means. Chest radiographs are not very specific, mostly showing parahilar opacities, hyperinflation, atelectasis, and, occasionally, consolidation, but not pleural effusion or pneumothorax.

COMPLICATIONS

Bacterial superinfection of the lower airways is unusual but does occur. The local complication of otitis media is common, likely a result of eustachian tube dysfunction caused by the virus.

TREATMENT

There is no specific treatment at this time for HMPV infection. Management consists of supportive care similar to that used for RSV (see Chapter 287). The rate of bacterial lung infection or bacteremia associated with HMPV infection is not fully defined but is suspected to be low. Antibiotics are usually not indicated in the treatment of infants hospitalized for HMPV bronchiolitis or pneumonia.

Supportive Care

Treatment is supportive and includes careful attention to hydration; monitoring of respiratory status by physical examination and measurement of oxygen saturation; the use of supplemental oxygen, high-flow nasal cannula therapy, and nasal continuous positive airway pressure in an intensive care unit for increased work of breathing; and, if necessary in the case of respiratory failure, mechanical ventilation.

PROGNOSIS

Most infants and children recover from acute HMPV infection without apparent long-term consequences. Many experts believe an association exists between severe HMPV infections in infancy and the risk for recurrent wheezing or the development of asthma; however, it is not clear whether the virus causes these conditions or precipitates their first manifestations.

PREVENTION

The only method of prevention of HMPV infection is reduction of exposure. Contact precautions are recommended for the duration of HMPV-associated illness among hospitalized infants and young children. Patients known to have HMPV infection should be housed in single rooms or with a cohort of HMPV-infected patients. When feasible, it is wise to care for patients with RSV infection in a separate cohort from HMPV-infected patients, so as to prevent coinfection, which may be associated with more severe disease. Preventive measures include limiting exposure to contagious settings during annual epidemics (such as daycare centers) as much as possible and an emphasis on hand hygiene in all settings, including the home, especially during periods when the contacts of high-risk children have respiratory infections. However, providers should keep in mind that infection is universal in the first several years of life. Therefore, reduction of exposure makes the most sense during the first 6 mo of life, when infants are at the highest risk for severe disease.

Bibliography is available at Expert Consult.

Chapter **289**

Adenoviruses

Jason B. Weinberg and John V. Williams

第二百八十九章
腺病毒

中文导读

　　本章主要介绍了腺病毒感染的病因学、流行病学、发病机制、临床表现、诊断、并发症、治疗和预防。详细介绍了腺病毒的亚属、型别及对应的最常见感染部位。临床表现包括急性呼吸系统疾病、眼部感染、胃肠道感染、出血性膀胱炎以及心肌炎、肝炎和脑炎等少见并发症。详述了在免疫缺陷人群中感染的临床表现。支持治疗为腺病毒感染主要的治疗方式。

Human adenoviruses (HAdVs) are a common cause of human disease. Conjunctivitis is a familiar illness associated with the HAdVs, but these viruses also cause upper and lower respiratory disease, pharyngitis, gastroenteritis, and hemorrhagic cystitis. HAdVs can cause severe disease in immunocompromised hosts. Outbreaks of HAdV infection occur in communities and closed populations, notably the military. No currently approved antiviral drugs are highly effective against HAdVs. Vaccines are available for HAdV types 4 and 7 but are used only for military populations.

ETIOLOGY

Adenoviruses are nonenveloped viruses with an icosahedral protein capsid. The double-stranded DNA genome is contained within the particle complexed with several viral proteins. Antigenic variability in surface proteins of the virion and genomic sequencing define at least 70 serotypes grouped into seven species. Species differ in their tissue tropism and target organs, causing distinct clinical infections (Table 289.1). HAdVs can be shed from the gastrointestinal tract for prolonged periods and can establish persistent infection of the tonsils and adenoids.

EPIDEMIOLOGY

HAdVs circulate worldwide and cause endemic infections year-round in immunocompetent hosts. Asymptomatic infections are also common. Only about one third of all known HAdV types are associated with clinically apparent disease. The most prevalent types in recent surveillance studies are HAdV types 3, 2, 1, and 5. Epidemics of conjunctivitis (often severe), pharyngitis, and respiratory disease occur, especially in schools and military settings. Outbreaks of febrile respiratory illness caused by HAdV-4 and HAdV-7 are a major source of morbidity in military barracks, with attack rates ranging from 25% to > 90%. The spread of HAdV occurs by respiratory and fecal-oral routes. An important factor in HAdV transmission, especially in epidemics, is the ability of the nonenveloped particle to survive on inanimate objects in the environment. Nosocomial outbreaks have been reported.

PATHOGENESIS

HAdVs bind to cell surface receptors and trigger internalization by endocytosis. Acidification of the endosome induces conformational changes in the capsid, leading to eventual translocation of the genome to the cell nucleus. Viral messenger RNA transcription and genomic replication occur in the nucleus. Progeny virion particles assemble in the nucleus. Lysis of the cell releases new infectious particles and causes damage to epithelial mucosa, sloughing of cell debris, and inflammation. Host responses to HAdV infection include the recruitment of neutrophils, macrophages, and natural killer cells to the site of infection and the elaboration by those cells of a number of cytokines and chemokines. This host immune response is likely to contribute to the symptoms of HAdV infection, but specific mechanisms of pathogenesis are poorly understood. The strict species specificity of the adenoviruses has

Table 289.1	Adenovirus Types With Associated Infections	
SPECIES	**TYPE**	**PREFERRED SITE OF INFECTION**
A	12, 18, 31, 61	Gastrointestinal
B	3, 7, 11, 14, 16, 21, 34, 35, 50, 55, 66	Respiratory; renal/urinary tract epithelium
C	1, 2, 5, 6, 57	Respiratory
D	8-10, 13, 15, 17, 19, 20, 22-30, 32, 33, 36-39, 42-49, 51, 53, 54, 56, 58-60, 63-67	Ocular
E	4	Respiratory
F	40, 41	Gastrointestinal
G	52	Gastrointestinal

precluded the development of an animal model for HAdVs, although recent work with HAdV in a humanized mouse model shows promise. Mouse adenovirus has also been used to study adenovirus pathogenesis using a murine model.

CLINICAL MANIFESTATIONS

HAdVs cause a variety of common clinical syndromes in both immunocompetent and immunocompromised hosts. These syndromes are difficult to distinguish reliably from similar illnesses caused by other pathogens, such as respiratory syncytial virus, human metapneumovirus, human rhinovirus, rotavirus, group A streptococcus, and other common viral and bacterial pathogens.

Acute Respiratory Disease

Respiratory tract infections are common manifestations of HAdV infections in children and adults. HAdVs cause an estimated 5–10% of all childhood respiratory diseases. Primary infections in infants may manifest as bronchiolitis or pneumonia. HAdV pneumonia may present with features more typical of bacterial disease (lobar infiltrates, high fever, parapneumonic effusions). HAdV-14 has emerged as a significant cause of severe acute respiratory disease in military and civilian populations, in some cases leading to hospitalization and death. Pharyngitis caused by HAdV typically includes symptoms of coryza, sore throat, and fever. The virus can be identified in 15–20% of children with isolated pharyngitis, mostly in preschool children and infants.

Ocular Infections

The common follicular conjunctivitis caused by HAdV is self-limiting and requires no specific treatment. A more severe form called *epidemic keratoconjunctivitis* involves the cornea and conjunctiva. Pharyngoconjunctival fever is a distinct syndrome that includes a high temperature, pharyngitis, nonpurulent conjunctivitis, and preauricular and cervical lymphadenopathy.

Gastrointestinal Infections

HAdV can be detected in the stools of 5–10% of children with acute diarrhea. Most cases of acute diarrhea are self-limiting, although severe disease can occur. Enteric infection with HAdV is often asymptomatic, and shedding of virus after acute infection can be prolonged, so the causative role in these episodes is frequently uncertain. HAdV may also cause mesenteric adenitis.

Hemorrhagic Cystitis

Hemorrhage cystitis consists of a sudden onset of hematuria, dysuria, frequency, and urgency with negative urine bacterial culture results. Urinalysis may show sterile pyuria in addition to red blood cells. This illness occurs more frequently in young males and typically resolves on its own in 1-2 wk.

Other Complications

Less frequently, HAdVs are associated with myocarditis, hepatitis, or meningoencephalitis in immunocompetent individuals.

Adenoviruses in Immunocompromised Patients

Immunocompromised persons, particularly recipients of hematopoietic stem cell transplants (HSCTs) and solid-organ transplants, are at high risk for severe and fatal disease caused by HAdV. These patients may experience primary HAdV infection. Reactivation of persistent virus in a transplant recipient and transmission of virus from a donor organ may also occur. Organ failure as a consequence of pneumonia, hepatitis, gastroenteritis, and disseminated infection occurs primarily in these patients. HAdV infection in HSCT recipients commonly manifests as pulmonary or disseminated disease and is most likely to occur in the first 100 days after transplantation. Hemorrhagic cystitis caused by HAdV can be severe in HSCT recipients. Infections caused by HAdV in solid-organ transplant recipients usually involve the transplanted organ. Immunocompromised children are at greater risk than immunocompromised adults for complicated HAdV infection, presumably because of a lack of preexisting immunity. Additional risk factors include

T-cell–depleted grafts, high-level immunosuppression, and the presence of graft-versus-host disease. Some experts advocate a preemptive screening approach to detect and treat HAdV infection early in immunocompromised patients, with the intent to prevent dissemination and severe illness in this vulnerable population, though no highly effective antiviral therapy exists.

DIAGNOSIS

HAdV may be suspected as the etiology of an illness on the basis of epidemiologic or clinical features, but neither of these categories is specific enough to firmly establish the diagnosis. The frequency of asymptomatic shedding of HAdV makes assigning causality to this pathogen difficult at times. Most HAdV serotypes grow well in culture, although this method requires several days and thus is not helpful for early identification. Cells from respiratory or ocular specimens can be tested using immunofluorescent staining with antibodies to detect HAdV protein. Commercially available enzyme-linked immunoassays can be used to rapidly detect HAdV in patient specimens, usually in stool. Molecular techniques, such as polymerase chain reaction, offer a rapid, sensitive, and specific diagnosis of HAdV infections and are most useful clinically for the management of suspected HAdV infections in immunocompromised hosts. In these patients, measurement of the *HAdV genome copy number* using a quantitative real-time polymerase chain reaction can facilitate the diagnosis, and repeated measurements can aid in assessing a patient's response to treatment. Multiplex molecular assays capable of identifying HAdV in addition to other pathogens are increasingly available and useful for rapid diagnosis. Serology is generally useful only in epidemiologic investigations.

COMPLICATIONS

HAdV pneumonia can lead to respiratory failure requiring mechanical ventilation, especially in immunocompromised patients. Secondary bacterial pneumonia does not appear to be as common following HAdV infection as it is after influenza infection, but data that address this issue are limited. Severe HAdV pneumonia has been linked to chronic lung disease and bronchiolitis obliterans in a minority of cases. Epidemic keratoconjunctivitis is a vision-threatening form of HAdV infection. Nearly any form of HAdV infection can be fatal in an HSCT or solid-organ transplant recipient. Refractory severe anemia requiring repeated blood transfusions can develop in HSCT recipients with hemorrhagic cystitis. Mortality rates of up to 60–80% have been reported in transplant recipients with disseminated HAdV or HAdV pneumonia.

TREATMENT

Supportive care is the mainstay of HAdV treatment in most cases. Patients with severe HAdV conjunctivitis should be referred for ophthalmologic consultation. No specific antiviral therapy produces a definite clinical benefit against HAdV infection. The nucleoside analog cidofovir has in vitro activity against most HAdV serotypes. Cidofovir is used topically to treat epidemic keratoconjunctivitis, often in conjunction with topical steroids or other immunosuppressive agents to limit the inflammatory component. Cidofovir may be used intravenously for HAdV infections in immunocompromised patients. Cidofovir is highly nephrotoxic; however, prehydration, concomitant administration of probenecid, and weekly dosing may reduce renal toxicity. Clinical studies suggest some benefit from cidofovir, but there are no prospective, randomized controlled trials of cidofovir for HAdV infection. In addition, no formal guidelines or recommendations for treatment exist. The cidofovir derivative brincidofovir is better tolerated than cidofovir and shows promise as an approach to the prevention and treatment of HAdV disease in immunocompromised patients, but experience remains limited. There are anecdotal descriptions of benefit from intravenous immunoglobulin. Adoptive immunotherapy involving the infusion of HAdV-specific T cells may also provide some benefit for immunocompromised patients with life-threatening HAdV infections, but this intervention is not yet considered standard therapy.

PREVENTION

Environmental and fomite transmission of HAdV occurs readily; therefore, simple measures such as handwashing and cleaning are likely to reduce spread. HAdVs are highly immunogenic and have been used as gene therapy vectors and vaccine vectors for other pathogens, including malaria and HIV, but no HAdV-specific vaccines are available for routine use. Live-attenuated HAdV-4 and HAdV-7 vaccines were used effectively in the United States military from the 1970s until 1999. Cessation of their use led to widespread outbreaks in barracks, and those vaccines were subsequently reintroduced into military use.

Bibliography is available at Expert Consult.

Chapter **290**

Rhinoviruses

Santiago M.C. Lopez and John V. Williams

第二百九十章
鼻病毒

中文导读

　　本章主要介绍了鼻病毒感染的病因学、流行病学、发病机制、临床表现、诊断、并发症、治疗和预防。鼻病毒是引起成人和儿童感冒最常见的原因。许多人为无症状感染，也可出现鼻塞、流涕、咽痛、咳嗽、声嘶，发热少见，在儿童中临床症状重且持续时间长。目前尚无获批疫苗和特异性抗病毒药，支持治疗为鼻病毒感染主要的治疗方式。

Human rhinoviruses (HRVs) are the most frequent cause of the **common cold** in both adults and children. Although HRVs were once thought to cause only the common cold, it is now known that they are also associated with lower respiratory infections in adults and children. Many HRVs do not grow in culture. Recent studies using molecular diagnostic tools such as the polymerase chain reaction (PCR) have revealed that HRVs are leading causes of both mild and serious respiratory illnesses in children.

ETIOLOGY

HRVs are members of the Picornaviridae family ("pico" = small; "rna" = RNA genome). Traditional methods of virus typing using immune antiserum have identified approximately 100 serotypes, classified into HRVA, HRVB, and, recently, HRVC species on the basis of the genetic sequence similarity. HRVCs can be detected by reverse transcriptase PCR but have been cultured only using highly specialized methods. Virus gene sequence analysis demonstrates that HRVCs are a genetically distinct and diverse species. The increased proportions of HRV reported in recent PCR-based studies are likely the result of detection of these previously unknown HRVC viruses in addition to improved detection of known HRVA and HRVB strains.

EPIDEMIOLOGY

Rhinoviruses are distributed worldwide. There is no consistent correlation between serotypes and epidemiologic or clinical characteristics. Several studies suggest that HRVCs may be more strongly associated with lower respiratory infection and asthma than other HRVs, but the overall disease severity is not increased. Multiple types circulate in a community simultaneously, and particular HRV strains may be isolated during consecutive epidemic seasons, suggesting persistence in a community over an extended period. In temperate climates, the incidence of HRV infection peaks in the fall, with another peak in the spring, but HRV infections occur year-round. HRVC appears to circulate with seasonal variation, exchanging dominance with HRVA. HRVs are the major infectious trigger for asthma among young children, and numerous studies have described a sharp increase in asthmatic attacks in this age-group when school opens in the fall. The peak HRV incidence in the tropics occurs during the rainy season, from June to October.

HRVs are present in high concentrations in nasal secretions and can be detected in the lower airways. HRV particles are nonenveloped and quite hardy, persisting for hours to days in secretions on hands or other surfaces such as telephones, light switches, doorknobs, and stethoscopes. Sneezing and coughing are inefficient methods of transfer. Transmission occurs when infected secretions carried on contaminated fingers are rubbed onto the nasal or conjunctival mucosa. HRVs are present in aerosols produced by talking, coughing, and sneezing. Children are the most important reservoir of these viruses.

PATHOGENESIS

The majority of HRVs infect respiratory epithelial cells via intercellular adhesion molecule-1, but some HRV strains utilize the low-density lipoprotein receptor. The receptor for HRVC is cadherin-related family member 3 (CDHR3); however, distinct genetic alleles of this protein confer different susceptibility to HRVC infection. Infection begins in the nasopharynx and spreads to the nasal mucosa and, in some cases, to bronchial epithelial cells in the lower airway. There is no direct cellular damage from the virus, and it is thought that many of the pathogenic effects are produced by the host immune response. Infected epithelial cells release a number of cytokines and chemokines, which induce an influx of neutrophils to the upper airway. Both innate and adaptive immune mechanisms are important in HRV pathogenesis and clearance. HRV-specific nasal immunoglobulin (Ig) A can be detected on day 3 after infection, followed by the production of serum IgM and IgG after 7-8 days. Neutralizing IgG to HRVs may prevent or limit the severity of illness following reinfection. However, cross protection by antibodies to different HRV serotypes is limited in breadth and duration, allowing recurrent infection. Both allergen exposure and elevated IgE values predispose patients with asthma to more severe respiratory symptoms in response to HRV infection. Abnormalities in the host cellular response to HRV infection that result in impaired apoptosis, and increased viral replication, may be responsible for the severe and prolonged symptoms in individuals with asthma.

CLINICAL MANIFESTATIONS

Most HRV infections produce clinical symptoms, but many are asymptomatic; however, symptomatic HRV infection induces a much more robust host immune response in the blood than asymptomatic infection. Typical symptoms of sneezing, nasal congestion, rhinorrhea, and sore throat develop following an incubation period of 1-4 days. Cough and hoarseness are present in one third of cases. Fever is less common with HRV than with other common respiratory viruses, including influenza virus, respiratory syncytial virus, and human metapneumovirus. Symptoms are frequently more severe and last longer in children, with 70% of children compared with 20% of adults still reporting symptoms by day 10. Virus can be shed for as long as 3 wk.

HRVs are the most prevalent agents associated with acute wheezing, otitis media, and hospitalization for respiratory illness in children and are an important cause of severe pneumonia and exacerbation of asthma or chronic obstructive pulmonary disease in adults. HRV-associated hospitalizations are more frequent in young infants than in older children and in children with a history of wheezing or asthma. HRV infection in immunocompromised hosts may be life threatening. Certain strains or species of HRV, namely HRVC, may be more pathogenic than others.

DIAGNOSIS

Culturing HRVs is labor intensive and of relatively low yield; HRVC has only been cultivated in a polarized primary airway epithelial cell culture, a highly specialized method. Sensitive and specific diagnostic methods based on reverse transcriptase PCR are commercially available. However, because commercially available reverse transcriptase PCR tests do not identify the HRV types, it can be difficult to distinguish prolonged shedding from newly acquired infection. An important caveat of HRV detection is the fact that HRV infection can be asymptomatic, and thus the presence of the virus does not prove causality in all cases. Serology is impractical because of the great number of HRV serotypes. A presumptive clinical diagnosis based on symptoms and seasonality is not specific, because many other viruses cause similar clinical illnesses. Rapid detection techniques for HRV might lessen the use of unnecessary antibiotics or procedures.

COMPLICATIONS

Possible complications of HRV infection include sinusitis, otitis media, asthma exacerbation, bronchiolitis, pneumonia, and, rarely, death. HRV-associated wheezing during infancy is a significant risk factor for the development of childhood asthma. This effect appears to remain until adulthood, but the mechanisms have not been elucidated. One large study determined that genetic variants at the 17q21 locus were associated with asthma in children who had experienced HRV wheezing illnesses during infancy. A prospective study on a preterm cohort showed that a single nucleotide polymorphism on the gene coding for the vitamin

D receptor was associated with development of lower respiratory infection with HRV. Further studies are required to determine the likely multiple genetic and environmental factors that contribute to HRV-related asthma.

TREATMENT
Supportive care is the mainstay of HRV treatment. The symptoms of HRV infection are commonly treated with analgesics, decongestants, antihistamines, or antitussives. Data are limited on the effectiveness of such nonprescription cold medications for children. If bacterial superinfections are highly suspected or diagnosed, antibiotics may be appropriate. Antibiotics are not indicated for uncomplicated viral upper respiratory infection. Vaccines have not been successfully developed because of the numerous HRV serotypes and limited cross protection between serotypes.

PREVENTION
Good handwashing remains the mainstay of the prevention of HRV infection and should be reinforced frequently, especially in young children, the predominant "vectors" for disease. A polyvalent inactivated vaccine showed promise in a nonhuman primate model, but there are no licensed vaccines or antivirals.

Bibliography is available at Expert Consult.

Chapter **291**

Coronaviruses
Kevin W. Graepel and Mark R. Denison

第二百九十一章
冠状病毒

中文导读

本章主要介绍了冠状病毒感染的病因学、流行病学、SARS和MERS的发病机制、临床表现、诊断、治疗和预防。具体描述了在人类中造成流行的冠状病毒。临床表现包括呼吸道感染，胃肠道疾病、神经系统疾病等非呼吸道表现。详细阐述了严重急性呼吸道综合征相关冠状病毒和中东呼吸综合征冠状病毒感染的临床特点。实验室诊断方法包括病毒培养、血清学检测及PCR检测。目前无特异性抗病毒药。

Coronaviruses are increasingly recognized as important human pathogens. They cause up to 15% of common colds and have been implicated in more serious diseases, including croup, asthma exacerbations, bronchiolitis, and pneumonia. Evidence also suggests that coronaviruses may cause enteritis or colitis in neonates and infants and may be underappreciated as agents of meningitis or encephalitis. Four coronaviruses are endemic in humans: human coronaviruses (HCoVs) 229E, OC43, NL63, and HKU1. In addition, two epidemics of previously unknown coronaviruses caused significant respiratory distress and high mortality rates among infected individuals. The discoveries of **SARS-associated coronavirus (SARS-CoV)**, the cause of **severe acute respiratory syndrome (SARS),** and of **Middle East respiratory syndrome coronavirus (MERS-CoV)** support the potential for coronaviruses to emerge from animal hosts such as bats and camels and become important human pathogens.

ETIOLOGY
Coronaviruses are enveloped viruses of medium to large size (80-220 nm) that possess the largest known single-stranded positive-sense RNA genomes. These viruses encode the protein nsp14-ExoN, which is the first known RNA proofreading enzyme and is likely responsible for the evolution of the large and complex coronavirus genome. Coronaviruses derive their name from the characteristic surface projections of the spike protein, giving a corona or crown-like appearance on negative-stain electron microscopy. Coronaviruses are organized taxonomically by a lettering system based on genomic phylogenetic relationships. Alphacoronaviruses include HCoV-229E and HCoV-NL63. Betacoronaviruses include four human pathogens and are commonly divided into four lineages, without formal taxonomic recognition. HCoV-OC43 and HCoV-HKU1 are in lineage A, whereas SARS-CoV falls in lineage B. Lineages C and D were exclusively comprised of bat coronaviruses until the discovery of MERS-CoV, which aligns with lineage C. Gammacoronaviruses and deltacoronaviruses presently include exclusively nonhuman pathogens.

Coronaviruses received international attention during the SARS outbreak, which was responsible for more than 800 deaths in 30 countries. SARS-CoV, a novel coronavirus at the time of the epidemic, was found to be the causative agent of SARS. The detection of SARS-like coronaviruses in a live animal market in the Guangdong province in Southern China, along with serologic evidence of exposure in food handlers in the same market, suggest that these markets may have facilitated the spread of SARS-CoV to humans from an animal reservoir. Subsequent studies identified SARS-like coronaviruses in fecal specimens from asymptomatic Chinese horseshoe bats that are very closely related, but not direct precursors to, SARS-CoV and are capable of infecting human cells. Thus, although bats are a reservoir for SARS-CoV-like precursors, the precise antecedent to SARS-CoV remains to be identified.

Another novel coronavirus, **MERS-CoV,** was isolated from a man with acute pneumonia and renal failure in Saudi Arabia. As of March 1, 2017, the WHO had recorded nearly 2000 confirmed cases of MERS, with nearly 700 deaths worldwide (~35% mortality rate). MERS-CoV differs from SARS in that it seems to be less communicable, although human-to-human transmission has been documented. MERS-CoV uses dipeptidyl peptidase 4 and carcinoembryonic antigen–like cell-adhesion molecule 5 as its cellular and co-receptor, respectively; SARS-CoV utilizes ACE-2. With this receptor specificity, MERS-CoV can infect cells from several animal lineages, including human, pig, and bat, suggesting the possibility of movement between multiple species.

EPIDEMIOLOGY
Seroprevalence studies have demonstrated that antibodies against 229E and OC43 increase rapidly during early childhood, so that by adulthood 90–100% of persons are seropositive. Although less information is available for HKU1 and NL63, available studies demonstrate similar patterns of seroconversion to these viruses during early childhood. Although some degree of strain-specific protection may be afforded by recent infection, reinfections are common and occur despite the presence of strain-specific antibodies. Attack rates are similar in different age-groups. Although infections occur throughout the year, there is a peak during the winter and early spring for each of these HCoVs. In the United States, outbreaks of OC43 and 229E have occurred in 2- to 3-yr alternating cycles. Independent studies of viral etiologies of upper and lower respiratory infections during the same period, but from different countries, have confirmed that all known HCoVs have a worldwide distribution. Studies using both viral culture and polymerase chain reaction (PCR) multiplex assays demonstrate that coronaviruses often appear in coinfections with other respiratory viruses, including respiratory syncytial virus, adenovirus, rhinovirus, and human metapneumovirus. Volunteer studies demonstrated that OC43 and 229E are transmitted predominantly through the respiratory route. Droplet spread appears to be most important, although aerosol transmission may also occur.

There have been no identified natural or laboratory-acquired cases of SARS-CoV since 2004, but the mechanisms of introduction, spread, and disease remain important for potential animal-to-human transmission and disease. The primary mode of SARS-CoV transmission occurred through direct or indirect contact of mucous membranes with infectious droplets or fomites. Aerosol transmission was less common, occurring primarily in the setting of endotracheal intubation, bronchoscopy, or treatment with aerosolized medications. Fecal-oral transmission did not appear to be an efficient mode of transmission, but may have occurred because of the profuse diarrhea observed in some patients. The seasonality of SARS-CoV remains unknown. SARS-CoV is not highly infectious, with generally only two to four secondary cases resulting from a single infected adult. During the SARS epidemic, a small number of infected individuals, "superspreaders," transmitted infection to a much larger number of persons, but the mechanism for this high degree of spread remains unknown. In contrast, persons with mild disease, such as children younger than 12 yr of age, rarely transmitted the infection to others. Infectivity correlated with disease stage; transmission occurred almost exclusively during symptomatic disease. During the 2003 outbreak, most individuals with SARS-CoV infection were hospitalized within 3-4 days of symptom onset. Consequently, most subsequent infections occurred within hospitals and involved either healthcare workers or other hospitalized patients.

As of March 1, 2017, the WHO had recorded cases of MERS-CoV in 27 countries, all of which were linked to exposures in the Arabian peninsula (~80% in Saudi Arabia). Though the route of transmission between animals and humans is not fully understood, MERS-CoV is proposed to have repeatedly entered the human population through contact with respiratory secretions of dromedary camels and possibly with raw camel products (e.g., unpasteurized milk). Antibodies to MERS-CoV are found in dromedaries throughout the Middle East, and strains identical to human MERS-CoV isolates have been found in camels in Egypt, Oman, Qatar, and Saudi Arabia. These strains do not appear to be highly pathogenic or virulent in camels and have likely circulated within dromedaries for > 30 years. Despite well-documented zoonotic transmission, most reported cases occur through linked human-to-human transmission in healthcare settings, including outbreaks in Jordan, South Korea, and Saudi Arabia in 2015 and 2016. Risk factors for nosocomial MERS-CoV outbreaks include overcrowded emergency departments, delayed diagnosis or isolation, and poor infection control practices. Transmission most likely occurs through respiratory droplets and is thus a greater risk during aerosol-generating procedures. Outside of healthcare settings, human-to-human transmission has been infrequently documented and is primarily associated with close contact within households. No sustained human-to-human transmission has yet been reported.

PATHOGENESIS OF SARS AND MERS
Severe disease in SARS and MERS likely results from both direct virologic damage and subsequent immunopathology. Studies with SARS-CoV in human airway epithelial cell cultures indicate that ciliated cells are principal targets for infection, whereas MERS-CoV preferentially infects bronchial epithelial cells, type I and II pneumocytes, and vascular endothelial cells. Substantial viral loads can be detected in the lower respiratory tract and in blood for both viruses. However, late progression to severe disease appears independent of the quantity and timing of viremia. Thus, excessive host immune responses likely play an important role in the progression to lower respiratory disease and acute respiratory distress syndrome. CoV infections are associated with massive elaboration of inflammatory cytokines and recruitment of inflammatory cells. The roles for inflammatory cells are controversial, with cytotoxic T cells and macrophages implicated variously in immune protection and immunopathology. Recapitulation of human clinical features in animal models of MERS-CoV infection remains challenging, but promising new models are in development.

CLINICAL MANIFESTATIONS
Respiratory Infections
Even though up to 50% of respiratory tract infections with OC43 and 229E are asymptomatic, coronaviruses are still responsible for up to 15% of common colds and can cause fatal disease. Cold symptoms caused by HCoVs are indistinguishable from those caused by rhinoviruses and other respiratory viruses. The average incubation period is 2-4 days, with symptoms typically lasting 4-7 days. Rhinorrhea, cough, sore throat, malaise, and headache are the most common symptoms. Fever occurs in up to 60% of cases. Coronavirus NL63 is a cause of croup in children younger than 3 yr of age. Coronavirus infections are linked to episodes of wheezing in asthmatic children, albeit at a lower frequency and severity than observed with rhinovirus and respiratory syncytial virus infections. Lower respiratory tract infections, including bronchiolitis and pneumonia, are also reported in immunocompetent and immunocompromised children and adults. As with respiratory syncytial virus or rhinovirus, coronavirus detection in upper respiratory infections is frequently associated with acute otitis media and can be isolated from middle ear fluid.

Nonrespiratory Sequelae
There is some evidence to support a role for coronaviruses in human gastrointestinal disease, particularly in young children. Coronavirus-like particles have been detected by electron microscopy in the stools of infants with nonbacterial gastroenteritis. In addition, several outbreaks in neonatal intensive care units of gastrointestinal disease characterized by diarrhea, bloody stools, abdominal distention, bilious gastric aspirates, and classic necrotizing enterocolitis have also been associated with the presence of coronavirus-like particles in stools. In older children and

adults, coronavirus-like viruses have been observed with similar frequency in symptomatic and asymptomatic individuals, making it difficult to discern if they are pathogenic in the gastrointestinal tract. Coronaviruses are well-known causes of neurologic disease in animals, including demyelinating encephalitis, but their role in causing human neurologic disease remains unclear. They have been detected by culture, in situ hybridization, and reverse transcriptase PCR (RT-PCR) in brain tissue from a few patients with multiple sclerosis. HCoV-OC43 has been detected by RT-PCR in the spinal fluid, nasopharynx, or brain biopsy specimens of two children with acute encephalomyelitis. However, coronavirus RNA has also been recovered from the spinal fluid and brain tissue of adults without neurologic disease.

Severe Acute Respiratory Syndrome–Associated Coronavirus

SARS-CoV infections in teenagers and adults included a viral replication phase and an immunologic phase. During the viral replication phase, there was a progressive increase in viral load that reached its peak during the second week of illness. The appearance of specific antibodies coincided with peak viral replication. The clinical deterioration that typified the second and third week of illness was characterized by a decline in the viral load and evidence of tissue injury, likely from cytokine-mediated immunity. The explanation for milder clinical disease in children younger than 12 yr of age has not been determined. Seroepidemiologic studies suggest that asymptomatic SARS-CoV infections were uncommon. The incubation period ranged from 1-14 days, with a median of 4-6 days. The clinical manifestations were nonspecific, most commonly consisting of fever, cough, malaise, coryza, chills or rigors, headache, and myalgia. Coryza was more common in children younger than 12 yr of age, whereas systemic symptoms were seen more often in teenagers. Some young children had no respiratory symptoms. Gastrointestinal symptoms, including diarrhea and nausea or vomiting, occurred in up to one third of cases. The clinical course of SARS-CoV infection varied with age. Adults were most severely affected, with initial onset of fever, cough, chills, myalgia, malaise, and headache. Following an initial improvement at the end of the first week, fever recurred and respiratory distress developed, with dyspnea, hypoxemia, and diarrhea. These symptoms progressed in 20% of patients to acute respiratory distress syndrome and respiratory failure. Acute renal failure with histologic acute tubular necrosis was present in 6.9% of patients, likely a result of hypoxic kidney damage. Of SARS patients, 28.8% had abnormal urinalysis, with viral genome detectable by quantitative RT-PCR. In contrast, children younger than 12 yr of age had a relatively mild nonspecific illness, with only a minority experiencing significant lower respiratory tract disease and illness typically lasting less than 5 days. There were no deaths or cases of acute respiratory distress syndrome in children younger than 12 yr of age from SARS-CoV infection. Adolescents manifested increasing severity in direct correlation to increasing age; respiratory distress and hypoxia were observed in 10–20% of patients, one third of whom required ventilator support. The case fatality rate from SARS-CoV infection during the 2003 outbreak was 10–17%. No pediatric deaths were reported. The estimated case fatality rate according to age varied from < 1% for those younger than 20 yr of age to > 50% for those older than 65 yr of age.

Middle East Respiratory Syndrome Coronavirus

The incubation period of MERS-CoV is between 2-14 days. The syndrome usually presents with nonspecific clinical features typical of acute febrile respiratory illnesses, including low-grade fever, rhinorrhea, sore throat, and myalgia. In mildly symptomatic cases, radiographic findings are typically normal. Severe disease is characterized by the acute respiratory distress syndrome with multilobular airspace disease, ground-glass opacities, and occasional pleural effusions on radiography. The median time between hospitalization and ICU transfer for critical illness is 2 days. Risk factors for severe disease include age > 50 yr and comorbidities such as obesity, diabetes, COPD, end-stage renal disease, cancer, and immunosuppression. Specific host genetic risk factors have not been identified. Variation in clinical outcomes does not appear to be explained by viral strain-specific sequence variability. As with SARS, extrapul-

monary manifestations are common in severe MERS disease. Gastrointestinal symptoms such as nausea, vomiting, and diarrhea occur in one third of patients, and acute kidney injury has been documented in half of critically ill patients. Encephalitis-like neurologic manifestations have been observed in three cases. Laboratory analyses typically detect leukopenia and lymphopenia, with occasional thrombocytopenia, anemia, and aminotransferase elevations. The case fatality rate remains at 35%, though the true incidence of MERS-CoV infection is likely underestimated by existing data. Most patients have been adults, although children as young as 9 mo of age have been infected. It is not known whether children are less susceptible to MERS-CoV or present with a different clinical picture.

DIAGNOSIS

In the past, specific diagnostic tests for coronavirus infections were not available in most clinical settings. The use of conserved PCR primers for coronaviruses in multiplex RT-PCR viral diagnostic panels now allows widely available and sensitive detection of the viruses. Virus culture of primary clinical specimens remains a challenge for HCoVs HKU1, OC43, 229E, and NL63, even though both SARS-CoV and MERS-CoV can successfully be grown in culture from respiratory samples. Serodiagnosis with complement fixation, neutralization, hemagglutination inhibition, enzyme immunoassay, and Western blots have been used in the research setting. The diagnosis of SARS-CoV infection can be confirmed by serologic testing, detection of viral RNA using RT-PCR, or isolation of the virus in cell culture. Even though the serology for SARS-CoV has a sensitivity and specificity approaching 100%, antibodies are not detectable until 10 days after the onset of symptoms, and immunoglobulin G seroconversion may be delayed for up to 4 wk. In addition, the SARS epidemic resulted in the inclusion of coronavirus-conserved primers in many diagnostic PCR multiplex assays such that coronaviruses may be more readily detected.

The diagnosis of MERS-CoV should be guided by clinical features and an epidemiologic link. The mainstay for laboratory confirmation of MERS-CoV infection is real-time RT-PCR. Screening should target the region upstream of the envelope gene (upE), followed by confirmation with an assay targeting open reading frame 1a. The best diagnostic sensitivity is achieved from lower respiratory tract samples collected within the first week of infection, though MERS-CoV RNA can be detected in upper respiratory and blood samples. Alternatively, seroconversion can be documented by screening enzyme-linked immunosorbent assays followed by immunofluorescence microscopy. For all known endemic and emerging HCoVs, respiratory specimens (nasopharyngeal swabs or aspirates) are most likely to be positive, but in a setting of a possible novel coronavirus, serum or stool may be positive.

TREATMENT AND PREVENTION

Coronavirus infections of humans are acute and self-limited, although persistent infection and shedding occurs in multiple animal models in the setting of minimal or no symptoms. There are no available antiviral agents for clinical use against coronaviruses, although strategies targeting conserved coronavirus proteases and coronavirus polymerases have been shown to block replication of the viruses in vitro and are in the drug development pipeline. Thus, treatment of SARS-CoV and MERS-CoV infections is primarily supportive. The role of antiviral and immune-modulating agents remains inconclusive, though several clinical trials are ongoing. Ribavirin was extensively used during the 2003 SARS-CoV outbreak, but is of questionable benefit given its poor in vitro activity against SARS-CoV at clinically relevant concentrations. The identification of the proofreading nsp14-exonuclease in multiple coronaviruses suggests that this activity may be important in resistance to antiviral nucleosides and RNA mutagens such as ribavirin. Systemic corticosteroid therapy may be associated with increased mortality rates in SARS-CoV and MERS-CoV and is thus not recommended unless indicated for another clinical condition. Meta-analysis of observational studies suggests that human convalescent plasma may reduce SARS mortality rates; the use of blood products has not been well-studied in MERS. Several monoclonal antibody preparations have shown positive results against SARS-CoV and MERS-CoV in animal studies.

Challenges for the development of effective vaccines targeted against OC43, 229E, HKU1, and NL63 include the fact that infections are rarely life-threatening and reinfection is the rule, even in the presence of natural immunity from previous infections. The durability of immunity to SARS-CoV and MERS-CoV is poorly understood. Nevertheless, effective vaccines for SARS-CoV and MERS-CoV are highly desirable but not yet available. A potential vaccine target is the viral spike protein, which could be delivered as a recombinant protein or by viral or DNA vectors. This approach appears to be effective against closely related strains of SARS-CoV but not necessarily early animal or human variants. A SARS-CoV vaccine approach that recently has shown success in animal models used a live recombinant SARS-CoV mutant with inactivated ExoN, demonstrating attenuation and protection in aged, immunocompromised mice. Approaches for the rapid development of stably attenuated live viruses or broadly immunogenic and cross-protective protein immunogens continues to be a key area for future research. Although SARS-CoV demonstrated characteristics of symptomatic transmission that made it controllable by public health measures such as quarantine, these characteristics cannot be assumed for future novel HCoVs. The recent discovery of MERS-CoV serves as a reminder that coronavirus emergence is both likely and unpredictable, making it important to continue studies of the replication, emergence, and transmission of coronaviruses. Additionally, strategies for rapid recovery, testing, and development of vaccines and neutralizing human monoclonal antibodies may be essential to prevent the high morbidity and mortality rates associated with previous epidemics.

Bibliography is available at Expert Consult.

Chapter **292**

Rotaviruses, Caliciviruses, and Astroviruses

Dorsey M. Bass

第二百九十二章

轮状病毒、杯状病毒和星状病毒

中文导读

　　本章主要介绍了胃肠道感染病毒的病因学、流行病学、发病机制、临床表现、诊断、实验室检查、鉴别诊断、治疗、预后和预防。病因学和流行病学中具体描述了轮状病毒、杯状病毒、星状病毒和肠道腺病毒的特点。临床表现中主要介绍了轮状病毒感染的症状，简单提及了星状病毒、肠道腺病毒和诺瓦克病毒。治疗目标是防止和治疗脱水以及维持营养状况，具体阐述了支持治疗相关内容。详细介绍了轮状病毒疫苗。

Diarrhea is a leading cause of childhood death in the world, accounting for 5-10 million deaths per year. In early childhood, the single most important cause of severe dehydrating diarrhea is rotavirus infection. Rotavirus and other gastroenteric viruses are not only major causes of pediatric deaths but also lead to significant morbidity. Children in the United States, before vaccine was available, were estimated to have a risk of hospitalization for rotavirus diarrhea of 1:43, corresponding to 80,000 hospitalizations annually.

ETIOLOGY

Rotaviruses, astroviruses, caliciviruses such as the Norwalk agent, and enteric adenoviruses are the medically important pathogens of human viral gastroenteritis (see Chapter 366).

　　Rotaviruses are in the Reoviridae family and cause disease in virtually all mammals and birds. These viruses are wheel-like, triple-shelled icosahedrons containing 11 segments of double-stranded RNA. The diameter of the particles on electron microscopy is approximately 80 nm. Rotaviruses are classified by serogroup (A, B, C, D, E, F, and G) and subgroup (I or II). Rotavirus strains are species specific and do not cause disease in heterologous hosts. Group A includes the common human pathogens as well as a variety of animal viruses. Group B rotavirus is reported as a cause of severe disease in infants and adults in China only. Occasional human outbreaks of group C rotavirus are reported. The other serogroups infect only nonhumans.

　　Subgrouping of rotaviruses is determined by the antigenic structure of the inner capsid protein, VP6. Serotyping of rotaviruses, described for group A only, is determined by classic cross-neutralization testing and depends on the outer capsid glycoproteins, VP7 and VP4. The VP7 serotype is referred to as the *G type* (for glycoprotein). There are ten G serotypes, of which four cause most illness and vary in occurrence from year to year and region to region. The VP4 serotype is referred to as the P type. There are eleven P serotypes. Although both VP4 and VP7 elicit neutralizing immunoglobulin G antibodies, the relative role of these systemic antibodies compared with that of mucosal immunoglobulin A antibodies and cellular responses in protective immunity remains unclear.

Caliciviruses, which constitute the Caliciviridae family, are small, 27- to 35-nm viruses that are the most common cause of gastroenteritis outbreaks in older children and adults. Caliciviruses also cause a rotavirus-like illness in young infants. They are positive-sense, single-stranded RNA viruses with a single structural protein. Human caliciviruses are divided into two genera, the noroviruses and sapoviruses. Caliciviruses have been named for locations of initial outbreaks: Norwalk, Snow Mountain, Montgomery County, Sapporo, and others. Caliciviruses and astroviruses are sometimes referred to as **small, round viruses** on the basis of appearance on electron microscopy.

Astroviruses, which constitute the Astroviridae family, are important agents of viral gastroenteritis in young children, with a high incidence in both the developing and developed worlds. Astroviruses are positive-sense, single-stranded RNA viruses. They are small particles, approximately 30 nm in diameter, with a characteristic central five- or six-pointed star when viewed on electron microscopy. The capsid consists of three structural proteins. There are eight known human serotypes.

Enteric adenoviruses are a common cause of viral gastroenteritis in infants and children. Although many adenovirus serotypes exist and are found in human stool, especially during and after typical upper respiratory tract infections (see Chapter 289), only serotypes 40 and 41 cause gastroenteritis. These strains are very difficult to grow in tissue culture. The virus consists of an 80-nm–diameter icosahedral particle with a relatively complex double-stranded DNA genome.

Aichi virus is a picornavirus that is associated with gastroenteritis and was initially described in Asia. Several other viruses that may cause diarrheal disease in animals have been postulated but are not well established as human gastroenteritis viruses. These include coronaviruses, toroviruses, and pestiviruses. The **picobirnaviruses** are an unclassified group of small (30-nm), single-stranded RNA viruses that have been found in 10% of patients with HIV-associated diarrhea.

EPIDEMIOLOGY

Worldwide, rotavirus is estimated to cause more than 111 million cases of diarrhea annually in children younger than 5 yr of age. Of these, 18 million cases are considered at least moderately severe, with approximately 500,000 deaths per year. Rotavirus causes 3 million cases of diarrhea, 80,000 hospitalizations, and 20-40 deaths annually in the United States.

Rotavirus infection is most common in winter months in temperate climates. In the United States, the annual winter peak historically spread from west to east. Unlike the spread of other winter viruses, such as influenza, this wave of increased incidence was not caused by a single prevalent strain or serotype. Since widespread adoption of vaccine, this geographic phenomenon has vanished. Typically, several serotypes predominate in a given community for one or two seasons but nearby locations may harbor unrelated strains. Disease tends to be most severe in patients 3-24 mo of age, although 25% of the cases of severe disease occur in children older than 2 yr of age, with serologic evidence of infection developing in virtually all children by 4-5 yr of age. Infants younger than 3 mo are relatively protected by transplacental antibody and possibly breastfeeding. Infections in neonates and in adults in close contact with infected children are generally asymptomatic. Some rotavirus strains have stably colonized newborn nurseries for years, infecting virtually all newborns without causing any overt illness.

Rotavirus and the other gastrointestinal viruses spread efficiently via a fecal-oral route, and outbreaks are common in children's hospitals and childcare centers. The virus is shed in stool at a very high concentration before and for days after the clinical illness. Very few infectious virions are needed to cause disease in a susceptible host.

The epidemiology of **astroviruses** is not as thoroughly studied as that of rotavirus, but these viruses are a common cause of mild to moderate watery winter diarrhea in children and infants and an uncommon pathogen in adults. Hospital outbreaks are common. **Enteric adenovirus** gastroenteritis occurs year-round, mostly in children younger than 2 yr of age. Nosocomial outbreaks occur but are less common than with rotavirus and astrovirus. **Calicivirus** is best known for causing large, explosive outbreaks among older children and adults, particularly in settings such as schools, cruise ships, and hospitals. Often a single food, such as shellfish or water used in food preparation, is identified as a source. Like astrovirus and rotavirus, caliciviruses are also commonly found in winter infantile gastroenteritis.

PATHOGENESIS

Viruses that cause human diarrhea selectively infect and destroy villus tip cells in the small intestine. Biopsies of the small intestines show variable degrees of villus blunting and round cell infiltrate in the lamina propria. Pathologic changes may not correlate with the severity of clinical symptoms and usually resolve before the clinical resolution of diarrhea. The gastric mucosa is not affected despite the commonly used term *gastroenteritis,* although delayed gastric emptying has been documented during Norwalk virus infection.

In the small intestine, the upper villus enterocytes are differentiated cells, which have both digestive functions, such as hydrolysis of disaccharides, and absorptive functions, such as the transport of water and electrolytes via glucose and amino acid cotransporters. Crypt enterocytes are undifferentiated cells that lack the brush-border hydrolytic enzymes and are net secretors of water and electrolytes. Selective viral infection of intestinal villus tip cells thus leads to (1) decreased absorption of salt and water and an imbalance in the ratio of intestinal fluid absorption to secretion, and (2) diminished disaccharidase activity and malabsorption of complex carbohydrates, particularly lactose. Most evidence supports altered absorption as the more important factor in the genesis of viral diarrhea. It has been proposed that a rotavirus nonstructural protein (NSP4) functions as an enterotoxin.

Viremia may occur often in severe, primary infections, but symptomatic **extraintestinal infection** is extremely rare in immunocompetent persons—although immunocompromised patients may rarely experience central nervous system, hepatic, and renal involvement. The increased vulnerability of infants (compared with older children and adults) to severe morbidity and mortality from gastroenteritis viruses may relate to a number of factors, including decreased intestinal reserve function, lack of specific immunity, and decreased nonspecific host defense mechanisms such as gastric acid and mucus. Viral enteritis greatly enhances intestinal permeability to luminal macromolecules and has been postulated to increase the risk for food allergies.

CLINICAL MANIFESTATIONS

Rotavirus infection typically begins after an incubation period of < 48 hr (range: 1-7 days) with mild to moderate fever as well as vomiting, followed by the onset of frequent, watery stools. All three symptoms are present in about 50–60% of cases. Vomiting and fever typically abate during the second day of illness, but diarrhea often continues for 5-7 days. The stool is without gross blood or white blood cells. Dehydration may develop and progress rapidly, particularly in infants. The most severe disease typically occurs among children 4-36 mo of age. Malnourished children and children with underlying intestinal disease, such as short-bowel syndrome, are particularly likely to acquire severe rotavirus diarrhea. Rarely, immunodeficient children experience severe and prolonged illness. Rotavirus has rarely been associated with mild encephalopathy with reversible splenium lesions; this may progress to cerebellitis. Although most newborns infected with rotavirus are asymptomatic, some outbreaks of necrotizing enterocolitis have been associated with the appearance of a new rotavirus strain in the affected nurseries.

The clinical course of **astrovirus** infection appears to be similar to that of rotavirus gastroenteritis, with the notable exception that the disease tends to be milder, with less significant dehydration. **Adenovirus enteritis** tends to cause diarrhea of longer duration, often 10-14 days. The **Norwalk virus** has a short (12-hr) incubation period. Vomiting and nausea tend to predominate in an illness associated with the Norwalk virus, and the duration is brief, usually consisting of 1-3 days of symptoms. The clinical and epidemiologic picture of Norwalk virus often closely resembles so-called food poisoning from preformed toxins such as *Staphylococcus aureus* and *Bacillus cereus*.

DIAGNOSIS

In most cases, a satisfactory diagnosis of acute viral gastroenteritis can be made on the basis of the clinical and epidemiologic features. Many hospitals now offer multiplex PCR stool testing for multiple diarrheal pathogens, including a variety of bacterial and protozoan and all five common viral agents in one test. Enzyme-linked immunosorbent assays, which offer > 90% specificity and sensitivity, are available for the detection of group A rotaviruses, caliciviruses, and enteric adenoviruses in stool samples. Latex agglutination assays are also available for group A rotavirus and are less sensitive than the enzyme-linked immunosorbent assay. Research tools include electron microscopy of stools, RNA polymerase chain reaction analysis to identify G and P antigens, and culture. The diagnosis of viral gastroenteritis should always be questioned in patients with persistent or high fever, blood or white blood cells in the stool, or persistent severe or bilious vomiting, especially in the absence of diarrhea.

LABORATORY FINDINGS

Isotonic dehydration with acidosis is the most common finding in children with severe viral enteritis. The stools are free of blood and leukocytes. Although the white blood cell count may be moderately elevated secondary to stress, the marked left shift seen with invasive bacterial enteritis is absent.

DIFFERENTIAL DIAGNOSIS

The differential diagnosis includes other infectious causes of enteritis, such as bacteria and protozoa. Occasionally, surgical conditions such as appendicitis, bowel obstruction, and intussusception may initially mimic viral gastroenteritis.

TREATMENT

Avoiding and treating dehydration are the main goals in the treatment of viral enteritis. A secondary goal is maintenance of the nutritional status of the patient (see Chapters 69 and 366).

There is no routine role for antiviral drug treatment of viral gastroenteritis. Controlled studies show limited benefits for antidiarrheal drugs, and there is a significant risk for serious side effects with these types of agents. Antibiotics are similarly of no benefit. Antiemetics such as ondansetron may help alleviate vomiting in children older than 2 yr. Immunoglobulins have been administered orally to both normal and immunodeficient patients with severe rotavirus and norovirus gastroenteritis, but this treatment is currently considered experimental. Therapy with probiotic organisms such as *Lactobacillus* species has been shown to be helpful only in mild cases and not in dehydrating disease.

Supportive Treatment

Rehydration via the oral route can be accomplished in most patients with mild to moderate dehydration (see Chapters 69 and 366). Severe dehydration requires immediate intravenous therapy followed by oral rehydration. Modern oral rehydration solutions containing appropriate quantities of sodium and glucose promote the optimum absorption of fluid from the intestine. There is no evidence that a particular carbohydrate source (rice) or the addition of amino acids improves the efficacy of these solutions for children with viral enteritis. Other clear liquids, such as flat soda, fruit juice, and sports drinks, are inappropriate for the rehydration of young children with significant stool loss. Rehydration via the oral (or nasogastric) route should be done over 6-8 hr, and feedings should be initiated immediately thereafter. Providing the rehydration fluid at a slow, steady rate, typically 5 mL/min, reduces vomiting and improves the success of oral therapy. Rehydration solution should be continued as a supplement to make up for ongoing excessive stool loss. Initial intravenous fluids are required for the infant in shock or the occasional child with intractable vomiting.

After rehydration has been achieved, resumption of a normal diet for age has been shown to result in a more rapid recovery from viral gastroenteritis. Prolonged (>12 hr) administration of exclusive clear liquids or dilute formula is without clinical benefit and actually prolongs the duration of diarrhea. Breastfeeding should be continued even during rehydration. Selected infants may benefit from lactose-free feedings (such as soy formula and lactose-free cow's milk) for several days, although this step is not necessary for most children. Hypocaloric diets low in protein and fat such as BRAT (*b*ananas, *r*ice, cereal, *a*pplesauce, and *t*oast) have not been shown to be superior to a regular diet.

PROGNOSIS

Most fatalities occur in infants with poor access to medical care and are attributed to dehydration. Children may be infected with rotavirus each year during the first 5 yr of life, but each subsequent infection decreases in severity. Primary infection results in a predominantly serotype-specific immune response, whereas reinfection, which is usually with a different serotype, induces a broad immune response with cross-reactive heterotypic antibody. After the initial natural infection, children have limited protection against subsequent asymptomatic infection (38%) and greater protection against mild diarrhea (73%) and moderate to severe diarrhea (87%). After the second natural infection, protection increases against subsequent asymptomatic infection (62%) and mild diarrhea (75%) and is complete (100%) against moderate to severe diarrhea. After the third natural infection, there is even more protection against subsequent asymptomatic infection (74%) and near-complete protection against even mild diarrhea (99%).

PREVENTION

Good hygiene reduces the transmission of viral gastroenteritis, but even in the most hygienic societies, virtually all children become infected as a result of the efficiency of infection of the gastroenteritis viruses. Good handwashing and isolation procedures can help control nosocomial outbreaks. The role of breastfeeding in prevention or amelioration of rotavirus infection may be slight, given the variable protection observed in a number of studies. Vaccines offer the best hope for control of these ubiquitous infections.

Vaccines

A trivalent rotavirus vaccine was licensed in the United States in 1998 and was subsequently linked to an increased risk for intussusception, especially during the 3- to 14-day period after the first dose and the 3- to 7-day period after the second dose. The vaccine was withdrawn from the market in 1999. Subsequently, two new live, oral rotavirus vaccines have been approved in the United States after extensive safety and efficacy testing.

A live, oral, pentavalent rotavirus vaccine was approved in 2006 for use in the United States. The vaccine contains five reassortant rotaviruses isolated from human and bovine hosts. Four of the reassortant rotaviruses express one serotype of the outer protein VP7 (G1, G2, G3, or G4), and the fifth expresses the protein P1A (genotype P[8]) from the human rotavirus parent strain. The pentavalent vaccine protects against rotavirus gastroenteritis when administered as a three-dose series at 2, 4, and 6 mo of age. The first dose should be administered between 6 and 12 wk of age, with all three doses completed by 32 wk of age. The vaccine provides substantial protection against rotavirus gastroenteritis, with a primary efficacy of 98% against severe rotavirus gastroenteritis caused by G1-G4 serotypes and 74% efficacy against rotavirus gastroenteritis of any severity through the first rotavirus season after vaccination. It provides a 96% reduction in hospitalizations for rotavirus gastroenteritis through the first 2 yr after the third dose. In a study of more than 70,000 infants, the pentavalent vaccine did not increase the risk for intussusception, although other studies suggest a slight increased risk.

Another new monovalent rotavirus vaccine was licensed in the United States and also appears to be safe and effective. It is an attenuated monovalent human rotavirus and is administered as two oral doses at 2 and 4 mo of age. The vaccine has 85% efficacy against severe gastroenteritis and was found to reduce hospital admissions for all diarrhea by 42%. Despite being monovalent, the vaccine is effective in prevention of all four common serotypes of human rotavirus.

Preliminary surveillance data on the rotavirus incidence from the

U.S. Centers for Disease Control and Prevention suggest that rotavirus vaccination greatly reduced the disease burden in the United States during the 2007-2008 rotavirus season and thereafter. Given the incomplete vaccine coverage during this period, the results suggest a degree of "herd immunity" from rotavirus immunization. Studies from several developed countries show greater than 90% protection against severe rotavirus disease. Studies from developing countries show 50–60%

protection from severe disease. Vaccine-associated disease has been reported in vaccine recipients who have severe combined immunodeficiency disease (a contraindication). In addition, vaccine-derived virus may undergo reassortment and become more virulent, producing diarrhea in unvaccinated siblings.

Bibliography is available at Expert Consult.

Chapter 293
Human Papillomaviruses
Kristen A. Feemster
第二百九十三章
人乳头瘤病毒

中文导读

　　本章主要介绍了人乳头瘤病毒感染的病因学、流行病学、发病机制、临床表现、诊断、鉴别诊断、治疗、并发症、预后和预防。临床表现包括皮肤病灶、生殖器疣、鳞状上皮内病变和癌症、喉乳头瘤。诊断可依靠活检、细胞涂片、阴道镜检查。详细阐述了治疗方法，包括水杨酸制剂、冷冻治疗、激光治疗、药物涂抹等。细致地介绍了HPV疫苗。

See also Chapter 687.

Human papillomaviruses (HPVs) cause a variety of proliferative cutaneous and mucosal lesions, including common skin warts, benign and malignant anogenital tract lesions, oral pharyngeal cancers, and life-threatening respiratory papillomas. Most HPV-related infections in children and adolescents are benign (see also Chapter 687).

ETIOLOGY

The papillomaviruses are small (55 nm), DNA-containing viruses that are ubiquitous in nature, infecting most mammalian and many nonmammalian animal species. Strains are almost always species specific. Viral DNA is divided into an early region, which encodes proteins associated with viral replication and transcription, and a late region, which encodes capsid proteins necessary for virion assembly. These structural proteins are also the immunodominant antigens leading to type-specific immune responses. More than 100 different types of HPVs have been identified through the comparison of sequence homologies. The different HPV types typically cause disease in specific anatomic sites; more than 30 HPV types have been identified from genital tract specimens.

EPIDEMIOLOGY

HPV infections of the skin are common, and most individuals are probably infected with one or more HPV types at some times. There

are no animal reservoirs for HPV; all transmission is presumably from person to person. There is little evidence to suggest that HPV is transmitted by fomites. Common warts, including palmar and plantar warts, are frequently seen in children and adolescents and typically infect the hands and feet, common areas of frequent minor trauma.

Human papillomavirus is also the most prevalent viral sexually transmitted infection in the United States. Up to 80% of sexually active women will acquire HPV through sexual transmission; most have their first infection within 3 yr of beginning sexual intercourse. Thus, HPV disproportionately affects youth, with 75% of new infections occurring in 15- to 24-yr-olds. The greatest risk for HPV in sexually active adolescents is exposure to new sexual partners, but HPV can still be acquired even with a history of one partner, underscoring the ease of transmission of this virus through sexual contact. It is estimated that after 11 acts of sexual intercourse, 100% of all HPV types infecting an individual will be transmitted to the other sexual partner. Couple studies show that there is high concordance in the genital area as well as between the hand and the genital area in the other partner. Whether the DNA detected in the hand is capable of transmitting infectious particles is unknown. Unlike other sexually transmitted infections, female-to-male transmission appears greater than male-to-female transmission. This may be because males in general have superficial transient infections or deposition. In turn, males do not develop an adequate immune response, so reinfections are quite common. The prevalence of HPV in women decreases with time, suggesting immune protection, whereas in men, the prevalence of HPV remains high across all ages.

As with many other genital pathogens, perinatal transmission to newborns can occur. Transmission from caregiver to child during the early childhood years has also been documented. However, both perinatal and early childhood infections appear transient. It remains unclear whether these HPV DNA detections are simply a deposition of caregiver DNA or a true infection. Detection of HPV DNA in older preadolescent children is rare. HPV DNA detection in nonsexually active adolescents has been reported, but a history of sexual activity in adolescents is not always disclosed and is therefore difficult to confirm. While caregivers can spread HPV to young children, if lesions are detected in a child older than 3 yr of age, the possibility of sexual transmission should be raised.

In adolescents, HPV DNA is most commonly detected without evidence of any lesion. Some of these detections are thought to be the result of partner deposition and hence do not represent a true infection. In older women, detection of HPV DNA is more commonly associated with a lesion. This is because the HPV DNA detected in older women reflects those HPV infections that became established persistent infections. Persistence is now the known necessary prerequisite for the development of significant precancerous lesions and cervical cancer.

Approximately 15–20% of sexually active adolescents have detectable HPV at any given time and have normal cytologic findings. The most common clinically detected lesion in adolescent women is the cervical lesion termed **low-grade squamous intraepithelial lesion (LSIL)** (Table 293.1). LSILs can be found in 25–30% of adolescents infected with HPV. External genital warts are much less common, occurring in < 1% of adolescents, but approximately 10% of individuals will develop genital warts in their lifetime. LSIL is a cytologic and histologic term to reflect the benign changes caused by an active viral infection and is likely present in most, if not all, women with HPV infection. The majority of women, however, have very minute or subtle lesions not easily detected by cytology. As with HPV DNA detection, most LSILs regress spontaneously in young women and do not require any intervention or therapy. Less commonly, HPV can induce more severe cellular changes termed **high-grade squamous intraepithelial lesions (HSILs)** (see Chapter 568).

Although HSILs are considered precancerous lesions, they rarely progress to invasive cancer. HSILs occur in approximately 0.4–3% of sexually active women, whereas invasive cervical cancer occurs in 8 cases per 100,000 adult women. In true virginal populations, including children who are not sexually abused, rates of clinical disease are close to zero. In the United States, there are approximately 12,000 new cases and 3,700 deaths from cervical cancer each year. Worldwide, cervical cancer is the second most common cause of cancer deaths among women. HPV is also associated with a range of other anogenital cancers, including an estimated 4,600 cases of anal cancer and 11,100 cases of oropharyngeal cancers in men and women each year.

Some infants may acquire papillomaviruses during passage through an infected birth canal, leading to recurrent **juvenile laryngeal papillomatosis** (also referred to as *respiratory papillomatosis*). Cases also have been reported after cesarean section. The incubation period for emergence of clinically apparent lesions (genital warts or laryngeal papillomas) after perinatally acquired infection is unknown but is estimated to be around 3-6 mo (see Chapter 417.2). It may be that infections can also occur during hygienic care from an infected parent.

Genital warts may represent a sexually transmitted infection even in some very young children. As such, genital warts appearing in childhood should raise suspicion for possible sexual abuse with HPV transmission during the abusive contact. A child with genital warts should therefore be provided with a complete evaluation for evidence of possible abuse (see Chapter 16.1), including the presence of other sexually transmitted infections (see Chapter 146). However, the presence of genital warts in a child does not confirm sexual abuse, because perinatally transmitted genital warts may go undetected until the child is older. Typing for specific genital HPV types in children is not helpful in diagnosis or to confirm sexual abuse status, because the same genital types occur in both perinatal transmission and abuse.

PATHOGENESIS

Initial HPV infection of the cervix or other anogenital surfaces is thought to begin by viral invasion of the basal cells of the epithelium, a process that is enhanced by disruption of the epithelium caused by trauma or inflammation. It is thought that the virus initially remains relatively dormant because virus is present without any evidence of clinical disease. The life cycle of HPV depends on the differentiation program of keratinocytes. The pattern of HPV transcription varies throughout the epithelial layer as well as through different stages of disease (LSIL, HSIL, invasive cancer). Understanding of HPV transcription enhances understanding of its ability to behave as an oncovirus. Early region proteins, E6 and E7, function as transactivating factors that regulate cellular transformation. Complex interactions between E6- and E7-transcribed proteins and host proteins result in the perturbation of normal processes that regulate cellular DNA synthesis. The perturbations

Table 293.1	Terminology for Reporting Cervical Cytology and Histology	
DESCRIPTIVE DIAGNOSIS OF EPITHELIAL CELL ABNORMALITIES		**EQUIVALENT TERMINOLOGY**
SQUAMOUS CELL		
Atypical squamous cells of undetermined significance (ASC-US)		Squamous atypia
Atypical squamous cells, cannot exclude HSIL (ASC-H)		
Low-grade squamous intraepithelial lesion (LSIL)		Mild dysplasia, condylomatous atypia, HPV-related changes, koilocytic atypia, cervical intraepithelial neoplasia (CIN) 1
High-grade squamous intraepithelial lesion (HSIL)		Moderate dysplasia, CIN 2, severe dysplasia, CIN 3, carcinoma in situ
GLANDULAR CELL		
Endometrial cells, cytologically benign, in a postmenopausal woman		
Atypical		
Endocervical cells, NOS		
Endometrial cells, NOS		
Glandular cells, NOS		
Endocervical cells, favor neoplastic		
Glandular cells, favor neoplastic		
Endocervical adenocarcinoma in situ		
Adenocarcinoma		
Endocervical		
Endometrial		
Extrauterine		
NOS		

NOS, not otherwise specified.

caused by E6 and E7 are primarily disruption of the anti-oncoprotein p53 and retinoblastoma protein (Rb), respectively, contributing to the development of anogenital cancers. Disruption of these proteins results in continued cell proliferation, even under the circumstances of DNA damage, which leads to basal cell proliferation, chromosomal abnormalities, and aneuploidy, hallmarks of squamous intraepithelial lesion (SIL) development.

Evidence of productive viral infection occurs in benign lesions such as external genital warts and LSILs, with the abundant expression of viral capsid proteins in the superficial keratinocytes. The appearance of the HPV-associated koilocyte is a result of the expression of E4, a structural protein that causes collapse of the cytoskeleton. Low-level expression of E6 and E7 proteins results in cell proliferation seen in the basal cell layer of LSILs. LSILs are a manifestation of active viral replication and protein expression. In HSILs, expression of E6 and E7 predominates throughout the epithelium, with little expression of the structural proteins L1 and L2. This results in the chromosomal abnormalities and aneuploidy characteristic of the higher-grade lesions. The critical events that lead to cancer have not been verified; however, several mechanisms are thought to be critical, including viral integration into the host chromosome and activation of telomerase to lengthen chromosomes and avoid physiologic cell senescence. Over 150 HPV types have been documented and are classified by extent of their DNA homology into 5 genera, with the different types having different life-cycle and disease characteristics. The predominant group is α HPV types, which are associated with cutaneous and mucosal anogenital infections and cancers. β, γ, µ, and ν cause predominantly benign cutaneous lesions but can be difficult to manage in severely immunocompromised individuals. B types are commonly detected on the skin without any apparent lesions but are associated with the development of skin cancers in those with epidermodysplasia verruciformis or other forms of immunodeficiencies. Genital lesions caused by the α HPV types may be broadly grouped into those with little to no malignant potential (low risk) and those with greater malignant potential (high risk). Low-risk HPV types 6 and 11 are most commonly found in genital warts and are rarely found isolated in malignant lesions. High-risk HPV types are those types that are associated with anogenital cancers, specifically cervical cancer. HPV 16 and 18 are thought to be more oncogenic than other HPV types because they comprise 70% of cervical cancers, whereas each of the other 12 high-risk types (31, 33, 35, 39, 45, 51, 52, 56, 58, 59, 68, and 73) contributes less than 1–9%. HPV 16 appears to be even more important in anal and HPV-associated oropharyngeal cancers, comprising close to 90% of these cancers. HPV 16 is also commonly found in women without lesions or in those with LSILs, making the connection with cancer confusing. Genital warts and SIL are commonly associated with the detection of multiple HPV types, including a combination of low- and high-risk HPV types. Data show that it is likely that a single lesion arises from a single HPV type. Detection of multiple HPV types reflects the presence of cervical and anal coexisting lesions. Almost all (95%) incident low-risk and high-risk HPV DNA detections, with or without detectable SIL, will spontaneously resolve within 1-3 yr. Although HPV 16 has a slower rate of regression than some of the other high-risk types, the majority of incident HPV 16 detections also will resolve. Data suggest that clearance of an HPV type results in natural immune protection against reinfection with that same type. Redetections of the same type are not common and when found are often associated with a history of a new sexual partner, suggesting that these are not reactivated infections but are due to new exposures. These redetections rarely result in high-grade disease. Persistent high-risk–type infections are associated with increased risk for development of HSILs and invasive cancer. Progression of HSIL to invasive cancer is still rare, with only 5–15% showing progression. Approximately 50% of HPV 16–associated HSILs and 80% of non–HPV 16 HSILs will spontaneously regress in young women. Genital and common warts in general also resolve without therapy but may take years to do so. Genital warts in only extremely rare conditions can become malignant.

Most infants with recognized genital warts are infected with the low-risk types. In contrast, children with a history of sexual abuse have a clinical picture more like that of adult genital warts, consisting of mixed low- and high-risk types. There are rare reports of HPV-associated genital malignancies occurring in preadolescent children and adolescents. On the other hand, precancerous HSILs do occur in sexually active adolescents. There is a concern that younger age of sexual debut has contributed to the increase in invasive cervical cancers seen in women younger than 50 yr of age in the United States, specifically cervical adenocarcinomas. Persistent HPV infections are considered necessary but not sufficient for the development of invasive cancers. Other risk factors for which there is relatively strong suggestive evidence of association include smoking cigarettes, prolonged oral contraceptive use, greater parity, and *Chlamydia trachomatis* and herpes simplex virus infections.

CLINICAL MANIFESTATIONS

The clinical findings in HPV infection depend on the site of epithelial infection.

Skin Lesions

The typical HPV-induced lesions of the skin are proliferative, papular, and hyperkeratotic. Common warts are raised circinate lesions with a keratinized surface (Fig. 293.1). Plantar and palmar warts are practically flat. Multiple warts are common and may create a mosaic pattern. Flat warts appear as small (1- to 5-mm), flat, flesh-colored papules.

Genital Warts

Genital warts may be found throughout the perineum around the anus, vagina, and urethra, as well as in the cervical, intravaginal, and intraanal areas (Fig. 293.2). Intraanal warts occur predominantly in patients who have had receptive anal intercourse, in contrast with perianal warts, which may occur in men and women without a history of anal sex. Although rare, lesions caused by genital genotypes can also be found on other mucosal surfaces, such as the conjunctivae, tongue, gingivae, and nasal mucosa. They may be single or multiple lesions and are frequently found in multiple anatomic sites, including the cervix. External genital warts can be flat, dome shaped, keratotic, pedunculated, and cauliflower shaped and may occur singly, in clusters, or as plaques. On mucosal epithelium, the lesions are softer. Depending on the size and anatomic location, lesions may be pruritic and painful, may cause burning with urination, may be friable and bleed, or may become superinfected. Adolescents are frequently disturbed by the development of genital lesions. Other rarer lesions caused by HPV of the external genital area include Bowen disease, bowenoid papulosis, squamous cell carcinomas, Buschke-Löwenstein tumors, and vulvar intraepithelial neoplasias.

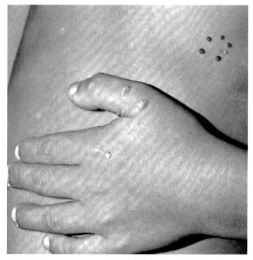

Fig. 293.1 Common warts of the left hand and the chest wall. *(From Meneghini CL, Bonifaz E: An Atlas of Pediatric Dermatology, Chicago, 1986, Year Book, p. 45.)*

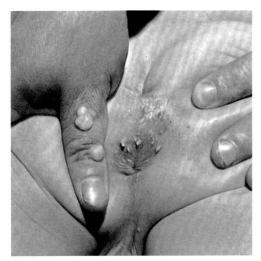

Fig. 293.2 Common warts of the hand in a mother and perianal condylomata acuminata in her son. *(From Meneghini CL, Bonifaz E: An Atlas of Pediatric Dermatology, Chicago, 1986, Year Book, p. 44.)*

Squamous Intraepithelial Lesions and Cancers
Squamous intraepithelial lesions detected with cytology are usually invisible to the naked eye and require the aid of colposcopic magnification and acetic acid. With aid, the lesions appear white and show evidence of neovascularity. SILs can occur on the cervix, vagina, vulva, penis, and intraanus. HPV-associated squamous cell lesions can also be found in the oropharynx. Invasive cancers tend to be more exophytic, with aberrant-appearing vasculature. These lesions are rarely found in non–sexually active individuals.

Laryngeal Papillomatosis
The median age at diagnosis of recurrent laryngeal papillomatosis is 3 yr. Children present with hoarseness, an altered cry, and sometimes stridor. Rapid growth of respiratory papillomas can occlude the upper airway, causing respiratory compromise. These lesions may recur within weeks of removal, requiring frequent surgery. The lesions do not become malignant unless treated with irradiation.

DIAGNOSIS
The diagnosis of external genital warts and common warts may be reliably determined by visual inspection of a lesion by an experienced observer and does not require additional tests for confirmation. A biopsy should be considered if the diagnosis is uncertain, the lesions do not respond to therapy, or the lesions worsen during therapy.

Screening for cervical cancer in young women begins with cytology, which is either performed by Papanicolaou smear or liquid-based cytology. Screening guidelines, which were updated in 2012 by the American Cancer Society and the U.S. Preventive Services Task Force, recommend starting screening at age 21 yr. Screening earlier is more likely to result in unnecessary referrals for colposcopy, because most lesions, including both LSILs and HSILs in this age-group, are likely to regress. Guidelines recommend screening with cytology every 3 yr. At 30 yr of age, screening can also include co-testing with HPV DNA at an interval of every 5 yr. This is not recommended earlier, because HPV infections are extremely common in young women, resulting in a very low positive-predictive value in this age-group.

The recommended terminology used for cytologic evaluation is based on the Bethesda system (see Table 293.1). Recent updates to the terminology used for histology uses similar terms. Many clinicians still prefer the World Health Organization terminology using cervical intraepithelial neoplasia (CIN) 1, 2, and 3 (see Table 293.1). Although the purpose of screening is to identify CIN 3+ lesions, the majority of CIN lesions are found in women who were referred for **atypical squamous cells of**

undetermined significance (**ASC-US**) or LSILs on cytology. On the other hand, few CIN 3 or cancers exist in women younger than 24 yr of age. Thus, for women 21-24 yr of age, ASC-US and LSILs are treated the same. The current preferred recommendation for young women with ASC-US or LSILs is to repeat cytology every 12 mo for up to 24 mo. For persistent ASC-US or LSILs at 2 yr of follow-up, referral for colposcopy is recommended. Women 21-24 yr of age with HSIL at any visit should be referred for colposcopy and biopsy. In adult women, HSIL can be treated without histologic confirmation. However, this approach should be avoided in those 21-24 yr of age, because HSIL is often misdiagnosed in this group or will resolve spontaneously.

In women older than 21 yr of age, high-risk HPV testing is acceptable to assist in ASC-US triage. This recommendation is based on the observations that adult women with ASC-US and a positive HPV test result for high-risk types are more likely to have CIN 2/3 than women with a negative HPV test result. However, in women with ASC-US and a positive HPV test for high-risk types, repeat cytology is recommended for confirmation. In women 21-24 yr of age referred for colposcopy and found to have no lesion or biopsy-confirmed LSIL after ASC-US or LSIL cytology, repeat cytology is recommended at 12 mo intervals. If ASC-US or LSIL has persisted after 2 yr or if HSIL is present at any time, referral for colposcopy is recommended. In women with biopsy-confirmed LSIL after atypical squamous cells of high grade (ASC-H) or HSIL, observation with cytology and colposcopy is recommended at 6 mo intervals for up to 2 yr. For persistent ASC-H or HSIL at 2 yr or progression at any time, treatment is recommended. Any young woman with histology-confirmed HSIL can be followed by colposcopy and cytology at 6 mo intervals if the patient is compliant. If HSIL continues to persist after 2 yr of follow-up, treatment is recommended. When CIN 3 is specified, treatment is recommended. These guidelines and updates can be found at http://www.asccp.org.

Very sensitive tests for the presence of HPV DNA, RNA, and proteins are becoming generally available, although they are not required for the diagnosis of external genital warts or related conditions. There are no indications for HPV DNA testing in women younger than 21 yr of age or children. HPV DNA testing is not recommended in women 21-30 yr of age but is acceptable for ASC-US triage.

Diagnosis of juvenile laryngeal papillomatosis (JRP) is made based on laryngeal examination.

There are no routine screening recommendations for noncervical or oropharyngeal lesions.

DIFFERENTIAL DIAGNOSIS
A number of other conditions should be considered in the differential diagnosis of genital warts, including condyloma latum, seborrheic keratoses, dysplastic and benign nevi, molluscum contagiosum, pearly penile papules, neoplasms, Bowen disease, bowenoid papulosis, Buschke-Löwenstein tumors, and vulvar intraepithelial neoplasias.

Condyloma latum is caused by secondary syphilis and can be diagnosed with darkfield microscopy and standard serologic tests for syphilis. Seborrheic keratoses are common, localized, hyperpigmented lesions that are rarely associated with malignancy. Molluscum contagiosum is caused by a poxvirus, is highly infectious, and is often umbilicated. Pearly penile papules occur at the penile corona and are normal variants that require no treatment.

TREATMENT
Most common (plantar, palmar, skin) warts eventually resolve spontaneously (see Chapter 687). Symptomatic lesions should be removed. Removal includes a variety of self-applied therapies, including salicylic acid preparations and provider-applied therapies (cryotherapy, laser therapy, electrosurgery). Genital warts are benign and usually remit, but only over an extended period. It is recommended that genital lesions be treated if the patient or the parent requests therapy. Treatments for genital warts are categorized into self-applied and provider-applied. No one therapy has been shown to be more efficacious than any other. Recommended patient-applied treatment regimens for external genital warts include topical podofilox, imiquimod, and sinecatechins. Podofilox 0.5% solution (using a cotton swab) or gel (using a finger) is applied

to visible warts in a cycle of applications twice a day for 3 days followed by 4 days of no therapy, repeated for up to a total of 4 cycles. Imiquimod 5% cream is applied at bedtime, 3 times a week, every other day, for up to 16 wk; the treated area should be washed with mild soap and water 6-10 hr after treatment. Sinecatechins (15% ointment) is a topical product from green tea extract used for external genital wart treatment that can be used 3 times daily for up to 16 wk. Provider-applied therapies include surgical treatments (electrosurgery, surgical excision, laser surgery) and office-based treatment (cryotherapy with liquid nitrogen or a cryoprobe, podophyllin resin 10–25%, and bichloroacetic or trichloroacetic acid). Office-based treatments are usually applied once a week for 3-6 wk. Podophyllin resins have lost favor to other methods because of the variability in preparations. Intralesional interferon is associated with significant adverse effects and is reserved for treatment of recalcitrant cases.

Many therapies are painful, and children should not undergo painful genital treatments unless adequate pain control is provided. Parents and patients should not be expected to apply painful therapies themselves. None of the patient-applied therapies are approved for use during pregnancy, and podophyllin resin is contraindicated in pregnancy. For any of the nonsurgical treatments, prescription is contraindicated in a patient with any history of hypersensitivity to any product constituents.

If HPV exposure as a result of sexual abuse is suspected or known, the clinician should ensure that the child's safety has been achieved and is maintained.

When indicated, the most common treatments for CIN 2/3 are ablative and excisional treatments, including cryotherapy, laser, and loop electrosurgical excisional procedures. Once confirmed by histology with CIN 1, LSILs can be observed indefinitely. The decision to treat a persistent CIN 1 rests between the provider and patient. Risks of treatment, including premature delivery in a future pregnancy, should be discussed prior to any treatment decision. Treatment in pregnancy is not recommended unless invasive cancer is present.

JRP is commonly treated with surgical removal of lesions, but laser and microdebriders are also used. There are also several reports describing the use of adjunctive treatments, including antivirals and the quadrivalent human papillomavirus vaccine. However, the effectiveness of adjunctive therapy is not consistent.

COMPLICATIONS

The presence of HPV lesions in the genital area may be a cause of profound embarrassment to a child or parent. Complications of therapy are uncommon; chronic pain (vulvodynia) or hypoesthesia may occur at the treatment site. Lesions may heal with hypopigmentation or hyperpigmentation and less commonly with depressed or hypertrophic scars. Surgical therapies can lead to infection and scarring. Premature delivery and low birthweight in future pregnancies are complications of excisional therapy for CIN.

It is estimated that 5–15% of untreated CIN 3 lesions will progress to cervical cancer. Most cancer is prevented by early detection and treatment of these lesions. Despite screening, cervical cancer develops rapidly in a few adolescents and young women. The reason for the rapid development of cancer in these rare cases remains unknown, but host genetic defects are likely underlying causes. Juvenile laryngeal papillomas rarely become malignant, unless they have been treated with irradiation. Vulvar condylomas rarely become cancerous. HPV-associated cancers of the vagina, vulva, anus, penis, and oral cavity are much rarer than cervical tumors, and therefore screening for them is not currently recommended. However, anal, vaginal, and vulvar cancers are more common in women with cervical cancer; hence, it is recommended to screen women with cervical cancer for other anogenital or oropharyngeal tumors with visual and/or digital inspection.

PROGNOSIS

With all forms of therapy, genital warts commonly recur, and approximately half of children and adolescents require a second or third treatment. Recurrence is also evident in patients with juvenile laryngeal papillomatosis. Patients and parents should be warned of this likelihood. Combination therapy for genital warts (imiquimod and podofilox) does

not improve response and may increase complications. Prognosis of cervical disease is better, with 85–90% cure rates after a single treatment with the loop electrosurgical excision procedure. Cryotherapy has a slightly lower cure rate. Recalcitrant disease should prompt an evaluation and is common in immunocompromised individuals, specifically men and women infected with HIV.

PREVENTION

The only means of preventing HPV infection is to avoid direct contact with lesions. Condoms may reduce the risk for HPV transmission; condoms also prevent other sexually transmitted infections, which are risk factors associated with SIL development. In addition, condoms appear to hasten the regression of LSILs in women. Avoiding smoking cigarettes is important in preventing cervical cancer. Prolonged oral contraceptive use and parity have been shown to be risks for cervical cancer. However, the mechanisms associated with these factors have not been identified, and consequently no change in counseling is recommended.

HPV vaccines show efficacy against type-specific persistence and development of type-specific disease, including the cervix, vagina, vulva, and anus. A quadrivalent HPV vaccine containing types 6, 11, 16, and 18 was licensed in the United States in 2006, and a bivalent HPV vaccine containing types 16 and 18 was licensed in the United States in 2009. A 9-valent vaccine containing types 6, 11, 16, 18, 31, 33, 45, 52, and 58 was approved in 2014. The types targeted by the nonavalent vaccine account for up to 85% of cervical cancer cases. The efficacy of these vaccines is mediated by the development of neutralizing antibodies. Prelicensure studies demonstrate 90–100% efficacy in the prevention of persistent HPV infection, CIN 2/3, adenocarcinoma in situ, anogenital warts, and precancerous vaginal and vulvar lesions. Since vaccine introduction, data from Sweden and Australia show a decrease in national rates of genital warts within 4 yr of implementing vaccination programs. Recent data from the United States show significant reductions in the prevalence of the HPV types contained in the quadrivalent vaccine among adolescent and young adult females in the years 2009-2012 (postvaccine) compared with 2003-2006 (prevaccine). Additionally, the HPV vaccine–type prevalence was 2.1% in vaccinated compared with 16.9% in unvaccinated 14- to 24-yr-old sexually active females. A systematic review of 20 studies conducted in nine high-income countries showed reductions of at least 68% in the prevalence of HPV 16 and 18 among 13- to 19-yr-olds in countries with HPV vaccination rates > 50%. Available effectiveness data suggest that HPV vaccination confers herd immunity in addition to individual protection.

Vaccination in the United States is recommended routinely for all adolescents at 11-12 yr of age and is administered intramuscularly in the deltoid region in a two-dose series at 0 and 6 -12 mo. A two-dose series was approved and recommended in 2016 for younger adolescents who initiate the HPV vaccine series prior to age 15 yr based upon immunogenicity data showing a comparable immune response among younger adolescents who receive a two-dose series compared with older adolescents who receive a three-dose series. Vaccination is also recommended for adults through age 45 yr if they have not been previously vaccinated.

It is important that vaccination take place in children before they become sexually active, because the rate of HPV acquisition is high shortly after the onset of sexual activity. Vaccine can be given to adolescents as young as 9 yr of age, and a catch-up vaccination is recommended in girls 13-26 yr and in boys 13-21 yr. For males who are gay, bisexual, or have sex with males, who are immunocompromised (including HIV infection), or who are transgender, catch-up vaccination can continue through age 45. For any adolescent who receives his or her first HPV vaccine dose at age 15 or older, a three-dose series at 0, 1-2, and 6 mo is recommended. The three-dose series is also recommended for adolescents and young adults 9-26 yr old who have an immunocompromising condition. Individuals who are already infected with one or more vaccine-related HPV types prior to vaccination are protected from clinical disease caused by the remaining vaccine HPV types. Therefore, a history of prior HPV infection is not a contraindication to vaccine receipt. However, HPV vaccines are not therapeutic.

Postlicensure vaccine safety surveillance has not identified any serious adverse events attributable to HPV vaccine receipt. Three large observational studies and safety monitoring through active and passive surveillance networks among more than 1 million individuals have not identified any association between HPV vaccination and outcomes such as autoimmune disorders, stroke, or venous thrombotic emboli. Vaccination can cause fever in approximately 1 in 60 and discomfort at the injection site for 1 in 30 vaccine recipients. Syncope has also been found to be correlated with vaccine administration in 0.1% of vaccine recipients. Therefore, it is advised that adolescents remain seated for 15 min following vaccination.

Despite an excellent safety and efficacy profile, HPV vaccine uptake has been slow. Immunization rates consistently lag behind rates for the other vaccines included in the adolescent immunization platform. In 2015, only 56.1% of 13- to 17-yr-olds received at least one HPV vaccine dose compared with 81.6% who received at least one dose of the quadrivalent meningococcal vaccine and 86.4% who received Tdap. Reasons for the slow uptake include inconsistent provider recommendation, lack of knowledge about HPV, parental belief that vaccination is not necessary for younger adolescents, and misconceptions about vaccine safety, among others. There is a growing body of literature evaluating interventions to improve HPV vaccine uptake. One important strategy is a strong, consistent recommendation in which HPV vaccines are presented in the same way as Tdap and meningococcal vaccines.

Bibliography is available at Expert Consult.

Chapter **294**
Arboviral Infections
Scott B. Halstead

第二百九十四章
虫媒病毒感染

中文导读

本章主要介绍了虫媒病毒感染的病因学、诊断和预防。感染后导致的疾病包括东方马脑炎、西方马脑炎、圣路易脑炎、西尼罗脑炎、波瓦生脑炎、拉克罗斯和加利福尼亚脑炎、科罗拉多蜱传热、基孔肯雅病、委内瑞拉马脑炎、日本脑炎、蜱传脑炎和寨卡病毒。其中详细阐述了寨卡病毒感染的流行病学、临床特点、治疗、实验室诊断、预后、鉴别诊断和预防。

The arthropod-borne viral infections are a group of mosquito- or tick-transmitted pathogens of several taxa manifested clinically mostly as neurologic infections, influenza-like illnesses, or acute viral exanthems. In temperate countries, arboviruses are transmitted during warmer weather; however, in tropical and subtropical countries, arboviruses may be transmitted year around either in an urban cycle (human to mosquito to human) or by arthropods that feed on other vertebrate species and then feed on humans.

ETIOLOGY

The principal arthropod-borne viral infections in North America are West Nile encephalitis (WNE), St. Louis encephalitis (StLE), Powassan (POW) encephalitis, a complex of California encephalitis group viruses, and, less frequently, western equine encephalitis (WEE), eastern equine encephalitis (EEE), and Colorado tick fever (Fig. 294.1). In 2013, chikungunya virus (CHIK) emerged from its original African zoonosis via Asia into the Western Hemisphere, exposing many residents of the United States who were traveling in the region. A few cases occurred domestically in southern states. In 2015, Zika virus (ZIKV), a flavivirus also maintained in Africa zoonoses, was introduced into the Americas, again from endemic areas in Asia. Limited transmission occurred within the continental United States. The major source of infection among Americans for each of these viruses has been travel to tropical and subtropical countries.

Throughout the world outside North America, there are many arboviruses that pose major health problems (Fig. 294.2). In descending order, these are the dengue viruses (DENV; Chapter 295), transmitted in all subtropical and tropical countries; Japanese encephalitis (JE), transmitted in northern, southern, and Southeast Asia; tick-borne encephalitis (TBE), transmitted across Europe and into northern and eastern Asia; yellow fever (YF; Chapter 296), transmitted from zoonotic cycles in Africa and South America; and Venezuelan equine encephalitis (VEE), transmitted in parts of South and Central America.

The etiologic agents belong to different viral taxa: *alphaviruses* of the family Togaviridae (CHIK, EEE, VEE, WEE), *flaviviruses* of the family Flaviviridae (DENV, JE, POW, STLE, TBE, WNE, YF, ZIKV), the

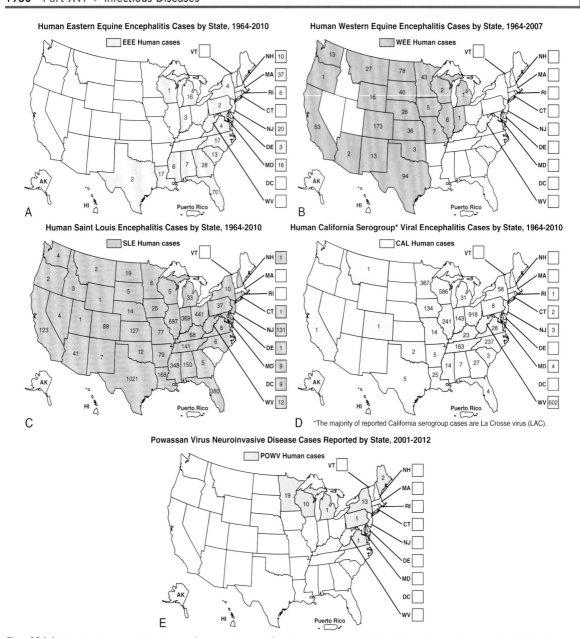

Fig. 294.1 The distribution and incidence of reported cases of eastern equine encephalitis **(A)**, western equine encephalitis **(B)**, St. Louis encephalitis **(C)**, California serogroup encephalitis **(D)**, and Powassan encephalitis; **(E)**, reported by state to the Centers for Disease Control and Prevention, 1964 to 2010. *(From Division of Vector-Borne Diseases, Centers for Disease Control and Prevention. Available at:* http://www.cdc.gov/ncidod/dvbid/arbor/arbocase/htm.)

California complex of the family Bunyaviridae (California encephalitis), and Reoviridae (Colorado tick fever virus). *Alphaviruses* are 69 nm, enveloped, positive-sense RNA viruses. Studies suggest that this group of viruses had a marine origin (specifically the southern ocean) and that they have subsequently spread to both the Old and New Worlds. VEE circulates in nature in six subtypes. Virus types I and III have multiple antigenic variants. Types IAB and IC have caused epizootics and human epidemics. *Flaviviruses* are 40- to 50-nm, enveloped, positive-sense RNA viruses that evolved from a common ancestor. They are mosquito-borne (WNE, STLE, JE, YF, DENV, ZIKV) and tick-borne (POW, TBE) agents, globally distributed, and responsible for many important human viral diseases. The California serogroup, 1 of 16 Bunyavirus groups, are 75- to 115-nm enveloped viruses possessing a three-segment, negative-sense RNA genome. Reoviruses are 60- to 80-nm double-stranded RNA viruses.

DIAGNOSIS

For arboviral infections not described separately, the etiologic diagnosis is established by testing either an acute-phase serum to detect the virus, viral antigen, or viral RNA (influenza-like illnesses or viral exanthems) or by recovery of virus from CNS tissue or CSF. More commonly, the diagnosis is established serologically. Serum obtained ≥ 5 days after the onset of illness is tested for the presence of virus-specific immunoglobulin (Ig) M antibodies using an enzyme-linked immunosorbent assay IgM capture test, an indirect immunofluorescence test, or a precipitin test. Alternatively, acute and convalescent sera can be tested for a four-fold

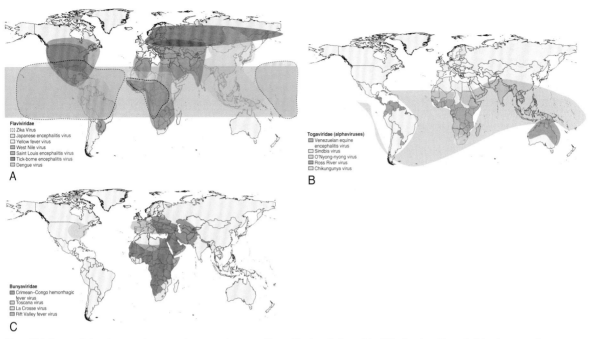

Fig. 294.2 World distribution of major arbovirus infections. *(From Charlier C, Beaudoin MC, Couderc T, et al: Arboviruses and pregnancy: maternal, fetal, and neonatal effects, Lancet Child Adolesc 1:134-146, 2017, Fig. 1.)*

or greater increase in enzyme-linked immunosorbent assay, hemagglutination inhibition, or neutralizing antibody titers. Commercial serologic diagnostic kits are marketed for DENV, CHIK, JE, TBE, WN, YF, or ZIKV viral infections. The serum and CSF should be tested for JE or WN virus–specific IgM. However, IgM may reflect past infection, because it may be present up to 12 mo after infection. For suspected flavivirus infections, including Zika virus, it may be possible to establish infection using a serologic test, calling upon the specificity of neutralizing antibodies. The most common of these is the plaque or focus-reduction neutralizing antibody test. Reference laboratories offer tests for all of the pathogenic flaviviruses. The diagnosis may also be established by the isolation of virus in cell cultures, by identification of viral RNA, or by detection of viral proteins (e.g., dengue NS1) from blood, brain tissue obtained by brain biopsy, or tissues obtained at autopsy.

PREVENTION

Several vaccines for Japanese encephalitis and tick-borne encephalitis are licensed in endemic and nonendemic countries. An experimental vaccine for VEE is available to protect laboratory workers. Travelers who plan to be in rural areas of Asia during the expected period of seasonal transmission should receive JE vaccine. Similarly, travelers who plan to travel, camp, or picnic in rural areas of Europe and East Asia should consult local health authorities concerning the need to be vaccinated against TBE. An inactivated vaccine manufactured in Japan by intracerebral injection of young mice and available throughout the world has been taken off the market owing to a high incidence of adverse events. In 2008-2009, tissue culture–based JE vaccine (Ixiaro) was licensed in Europe, Australia, and the United States. In the United States, this vaccine is licensed for use in children and adults and is distributed by Novartis (Basel). This vaccine is administered intramuscularly as two doses of 0.5 mL each, 28 days apart. The final dose should be completed at least 1 wk prior to the patient's expected arrival in a JE endemic area. This vaccine contains alum and protamine sulfate and has exhibited only mild adverse events. A highly efficacious live-attenuated single-dose JE vaccine developed in China for children is licensed and marketed in Asian countries. This vaccine can be coadministered with live-attenuated measles vaccine without altering the immune responses

to either vaccine. In humans, prior dengue virus infection provides partial protection from clinical JE.

No TBE vaccines are licensed or available in the United States. Two inactivated cell culture–derived TBE vaccines are available in Europe, in adult and pediatric formulations: FSME-IMMUN (Baxter, Austria) and Encepur (Novartis, Germany). The adult formulation of FSME-IMMUN is also licensed in Canada. Two other inactivated TBE vaccines are available in Russia: TBE-Moscow (Chumakov Institute, Russia) and EnceVir (Microgen, Russia). Immunogenicity studies suggest that the European and Russian vaccines should provide cross-protection against all three TBE virus subtypes. For both FSME-IMMUN and Encepur, the primary vaccination series consists of three doses. The specific recommended intervals between doses vary by country and vaccine. Because the routine primary vaccination series requires ≥ 6 mo for completion, most travelers to TBE-endemic areas will find avoiding tick bites to be more practical than vaccination.

For all viral diseases discussed in this chapter, personal measures should be taken to reduce exposure to mosquito or tick bites, especially for short-term residents in endemic areas. These measures include avoiding evening outdoor exposure, using insect repellents, covering the body with clothing, and using bed nets or house screening. Commercial pesticides, widely used by rice farmers, may be useful in reducing populations of vector mosquitoes or ticks. Fenthion, fenitrothion, and phenthoate are effectively adulticidal and larvicidal. Insecticides may be applied from portable sprayers or from helicopters or light aircraft.

Bibliography is available at Expert Consult.

294.1 Eastern Equine Encephalitis
Scott B. Halstead

In the United States, EEE is a disease with a very low incidence, with a median of eight cases occurring annually in the Atlantic and Gulf states from 1964 to 2007 (Fig. 294.1). Transmission occurs often in focal endemic areas of the coast of Massachusetts, the six southern counties of New Jersey, and northeastern Florida. In North America, the virus is maintained in freshwater swamps in a zoonotic cycle involving *Culiseta melanura* and birds. Various other mosquito species obtain viremic meals from birds and transmit the virus to horses and humans. Virus activity varies markedly from year to year in response to still unknown ecologic factors. Most infections in birds are silent, but infections in pheasants are often fatal, and epizootics in these species are used as sentinels for periods of increased viral activity. Cases have been recognized on Caribbean islands. The case:infection ratio is lowest in children (1 : 8) and somewhat higher in adults (1 : 29).

EEE virus infections result in fulminant encephalitis with a rapid progression to coma and death in one third of cases. In infants and children, abrupt onset of fever, irritability, and headache are followed by lethargy, confusion, seizures, and coma. High temperature, bulging fontanel, stiff neck, and generalized flaccid or spastic paralysis are observed. There may be a brief prodrome of fever, headache, and dizziness. Unlike most other viral encephalitides, the peripheral white blood cell count usually demonstrates a marked leukocytosis, and the cerebrospinal fluid (CSF) may show marked pleocytosis. Pathologic changes are found in the cortical and gray matter, with viral antigens localized to neurons. There is necrosis of neurons, neutrophilic infiltration, and perivascular cuffing by lymphocytes.

The prognosis in EEE is better for patients with a prolonged prodrome; the occurrence of convulsions conveys a poor prognosis. Patient fatality rates are 33–75% and are highest in the elderly. Residual neurologic defects are common, especially in children.

The diagnosis of encephalitis may be aided by CT or MRI and by electroencephalography. Focal seizures or focal findings on CT or MRI or electroencephalography should suggest the possibility of herpes simplex encephalitis, which should be treated with acyclovir (see Chapter 279).

294.2 Western Equine Encephalitis
Scott B. Halstead

WEE infections occur principally in the United States and Canada west of the Mississippi River (see Fig. 294.1), mainly in rural areas where water impoundments, irrigated farmland, and naturally flooded land provide breeding sites for *Culex tarsalis*. The virus is transmitted in a cycle involving mosquitoes, birds, and other vertebrate hosts. Humans and horses are susceptible to encephalitis. The case:infection ratio varies by age, having been estimated at 1 : 58 in children younger than 4 yr of age and 1 : 1,150 in adults. Infections are most severe at the extremes of life; one third of cases occur in children younger than 1 yr of age. Recurrent human epidemics have been reported from the Yakima Valley in Washington State and the Central Valley of California; the largest outbreak on record resulted in 3,400 cases and occurred in Minnesota, North and South Dakota, Nebraska, and Montana, as well as Alberta, Manitoba, and Saskatchewan, Canada. Epizootics in horses precede human epidemics by several weeks. For the past 20 yr, only three cases of WEE have been reported, presumably reflecting successful mosquito abatement.

In WEE, there may be a prodrome with symptoms of an upper respiratory tract infection. The onset is usually sudden with chills, fever, dizziness, drowsiness, increasing headache, malaise, nausea and vomiting, stiff neck, and disorientation. Infants typically present with the sudden cessation of feeding, fussiness, fever, and protracted vomiting. Convulsions and lethargy develop rapidly. On physical examination, patients are somnolent, exhibit meningeal signs, and have generalized motor weakness and reduced deep tendon reflexes. In infants, a bulging fontanel, spastic paralysis, and generalized convulsions may be observed. On pathologic examination, disseminated small focal abscesses, small focal hemorrhages, and patchy areas of demyelination are distinctive.

Patient fatality rates in WEE are 3–9% and are highest in the elderly. Major neurologic sequelae have been reported in up to 13% of cases and may be as high as 30% in infants. Parkinsonian syndrome has been reported as a residual in adult survivors.

294.3 St. Louis Encephalitis
Scott B. Halstead

Cases of STLE are reported from nearly all states; the highest attack rates occur in the gulf and central states (see Fig. 294.1). Epidemics frequently occur in urban and suburban areas; the largest, in 1975, involved 1,800 persons living in Houston, Chicago, Memphis, and Denver. Cases often cluster in areas where there are ground water or septic systems, which support mosquito breeding. The principal vectors are *Culex pipiens* and *Culex quinquefasciatus* in the central gulf states, *Culex nigripalpus* in Florida, and *C. tarsalis* in California. STLE virus is maintained in nature in a bird–mosquito cycle. Viral amplification occurs in bird species abundant in residential areas (e.g., sparrows, blue jays, and doves). Virus is transmitted in the late summer and early fall. The case:infection ratio may be as high as 1 : 300. Age-specific attack rates are lowest in children and highest in individuals older than age 60 yr. The most recent small outbreaks were in Florida in 1990 and Louisiana in 2001. For the past 15 yr, there have been a mean of 18 cases annually.

Clinical manifestations of STLE vary from a mild flulike illness to fatal encephalitis. There may be a prodrome of nonspecific symptoms with subtle changes in coordination or mentation of several days to 1 wk in duration. Early signs and symptoms include fever, photophobia, headache, malaise, nausea, vomiting, and neck stiffness. About half of patients exhibit an abrupt onset of weakness, incoordination, disturbed sensorium, restlessness, confusion, lethargy, and delirium or coma. The peripheral white blood cell count is modestly elevated, with 100-200 cells/μL found in the CSF. On autopsy, the brain shows scattered foci of neuronal damage and perivascular inflammation.

The principal risk factor for fatal outcome of STLE is advanced age, with patient fatality rates being as high as 80% in early outbreaks. In children, mortality rates are 2–5%. In adults, underlying hypertensive cardiovascular disease has been a risk factor for fatal outcome. Recovery from STLE is usually complete, but the rate of serious neurologic sequelae has been reported to be as high as 10% in children.

294.4 West Nile Encephalitis
Scott B. Halstead

West Nile (WN) virus was imported into the United States in 1999 and survives in a broad enzootic cycle across the United States and Canada. Every state in the continental United States plus nine provinces in Canada have reported mosquito, bird, mammalian, or human WN virus infection, most frequently during the summer or fall months. Through the end of 2015, 43,937 total cases had been reported in the United States, 40–50% of which were neuroinvasive, with 1,911 deaths (Fig. 294.3). WN virus transmission cycles appear to resemble those of Japanese encephalitis with large epizootics and human cases every 5-10 yr. WN virus has entered the blood supply through asymptomatic viremic potential blood donors. Since 2003, blood banks screen for WN virus RNA. During the major outbreak of 2012, 597 viremic potential blood donors were identified and the donation was rejected. WN virus has also been transmitted to humans via the placenta, breast milk, and organ transplantation. Throughout its range, the virus is maintained in nature by transmission between mosquitoes of the *Culex* genus and various species of birds. In the United States, human infections are largely acquired from *C. pipiens*. Horses are the nonavian vertebrates most likely to exhibit disease with WN virus infection. During the 2002 transmission season, 14,000 equine cases were reported, with a mortality rate of 30%. Disease occurs predominantly in individuals >50 yr of age. WN virus has been implicated as the cause of sporadic summertime cases of human encephalitis and meningitis in Israel, India, Pakistan, Romania, Russia, Canada, the United States, and parts of Central and South America. All American WN viruses are genetically similar and are related to a virus recovered from a goose

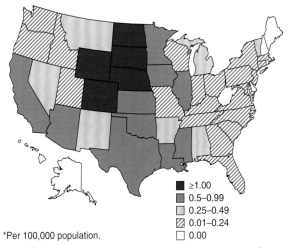

≥1.00
0.5–0.99
0.25–0.49
0.01–0.24
0.00

*Per 100,000 population.

Fig. 294.3 Rate (per 100,000 population) of reported cases of West Nile virus neuroinvasive disease, United States, 2016. *(From Burakoff A, Lehman J, Fischer M, et al: West Nile virus and other nationally notifiable arboviral diseases, United States, 2016, MMWR 67(1):13-17, 2018.)*

in Israel in 1998.

West Nile encephalitis (WNE) may be asymptomatic, but when clinical features appear, they include an abrupt onset of high fever, headache, myalgias, and nonspecific signs of emesis, rash, abdominal pain, or diarrhea. Most infections manifest as a flulike febrile illness, whereas a minority of patients demonstrate meningitis or encephalitis, or both. Rarely there may be cardiac dysrhythmias, myocarditis, rhabdomyolysis, optic neuritis, uveitis, retinitis, orchitis, pancreatitis, or hepatitis. WN virus disease in the United States has been accompanied by prolonged lymphopenia and an acute asymmetric polio-like paralytic illness with CSF pleocytosis involving the anterior horn cells of the spinal cord. A striking but uncommon feature has been parkinsonism and movement disorders (with tremor and myoclonus). WN virus infections have been shown to lead to chronic kidney disease in a small group of patients.

Cases of WNE and deaths due to the disease occur mainly in the elderly, although many serologic surveys show that persons of all ages are infected. In 2015, among a total of 2,175 human cases, 1,455 were neuroinvasive disease, which resulted in 146 deaths, a 10% mortality rate (see Fig. 294.2). Paralysis may result in permanent weakness.

Bibliography is available at Expert Consult.

294.5 Powassan Encephalitis
Scott B. Halstead

POW virus is transmitted by *Ixodes cookei* among small mammals in eastern Canada and the United States; it has been responsible for 39 deaths in the United States since 2008 (see Fig. 294.1). Other ticks may transmit the virus in a wider geographic area, and there is some concern that *Ixodes scapularis* (also called *Ixodes dammini*), a competent vector in the laboratory, may become involved as it becomes more prominent in the United States.

In a limited experience, POW encephalitis has occurred mainly in adults with vocational or recreational exposure and has a high fatality rate.

POW encephalitis has occurred mostly in adults living in enzootic areas with vocational or recreational exposure; it is associated with significant long-term morbidity and has a case-fatality rate of 10–15%.

Bibliography is available at Expert Consult.

294.6 La Crosse and California Encephalitis
Scott B. Halstead

La Crosse viral infections are endemic in the United States, occurring annually from July to September, principally in the north-central and central states (see Fig. 294.1). Infections occur in peridomestic environments as the result of bites from *Aedes triseriatus* mosquitoes, which often breed in tree holes. The virus is maintained vertically in nature by transovarial transmission and can be spread between mosquitoes by copulation and amplified in mosquito populations by viremic infections in various vertebrate hosts. Amplifying hosts include chipmunks, squirrels, foxes, and woodchucks. A case:infection ratio of 1 : 22-300 has been surmised. La Crosse encephalitis is principally a disease of children, who may account for up to 75% of cases. A mean of 100 cases has been reported annually for the past 10 yr.

The clinical spectrum includes a mild febrile illness, aseptic meningitis, and fatal encephalitis. Children typically present with a prodrome of 2-3 days of fever, headache, malaise, and vomiting. The disease evolves with clouding of the sensorium, lethargy, and, in severe cases, focal or generalized seizures. On physical examination, children are lethargic but not disoriented. Focal neurologic signs, including weakness, aphasia, and focal or generalized seizures, have been reported in 16–25% of cases. CSF shows low to moderate leukocyte counts. On autopsy, the brain shows focal areas of neuronal degeneration, inflammation, and perivascular cuffing.

Recovery from California encephalitis is usually complete. The case fatality rate is approximately 1%.

294.7 Colorado Tick Fever
Scott B. Halstead

Colorado tick fever virus is transmitted by the wood tick *Dermacentor andersoni,* which inhabits high-elevation areas of states extending from the central plains to the Pacific coast. The tick is infected with the virus at the larval stage and remains infected for life. Squirrels and chipmunks serve as primary reservoirs. Human infections typically occur in hikers and campers in indigenous areas during the spring and early summer.

Colorado tick fever begins with the abrupt onset of a flulike illness, including high temperature, malaise, arthralgia and myalgia, vomiting, headache, and decreased sensorium. Rash is uncommon. The symptoms rapidly disappear after 3 days of illness. However, in approximately half of patients, a second identical episode reoccurs 24-72 hr after the first one, producing the typical saddleback temperature curve of Colorado tick fever. Complications, including encephalitis, meningoencephalitis, and a bleeding diathesis, develop in 3–7% of infected persons and may be more common in children younger than 12 yr of age.

Recovery from Colorado tick fever is usually complete. Three deaths have been reported, all in persons with hemorrhagic signs.

294.8 Chikungunya Fever
Scott B. Halstead

Chikungunya virus is enzootic in several species of African subhuman primates but also is endemic in urban *Aedes aegypti* or *Aedes albopictus* transmission cycles in Africa and Asia. Chikungunya exited Africa historically producing Asian pandemics in 1790, 1824, 1872, 1924, 1963, and 2005. In 1827, chikungunya reached the Western Hemisphere, predominantly the Caribbean region, probably brought by the slave trade. In 2005, another Asian pandemic proceeded east from an initial outbreak on Reunion and then traveling to Asia across the Indian Ocean. In 2013, chikungunya virus from this epidemic was introduced into Latin America.

Clinical manifestations begin 3-7 days after a mosquito bite; the onset is abrupt, with high fever and often severe joint symptoms (hands, feet, ankles, wrists) that include symmetric bilateral polyarthralgia or arthritis.

Most pediatric patients are relatively asymptomatic, but all ages are vulnerable to classic disease. There may be headache, myalgias, conjunctivitis, weakness, lymphopenia, and a maculopapular rash. Mortality is rare; some individuals develop prolonged joint symptoms (tenosynovitis, arthritis) lasting over a year. The acute episode lasts 7-10 days. The differential diagnosis includes dengue, West Nile, enterovirus diseases, leptospirosis, rickettsial disease, measles, parvovirus disease, rheumatologic diseases, and other alphavirus diseases (e.g., Ross River virus) in endemic areas. Fig. 294.4 lists the diagnostic criteria.

The incidence of febrile convulsions is high in infants. The prognosis is generally good, although in large outbreaks in Africa and India, severe disease and deaths have been attributed to chikungunya infections, predominantly in adults.

Bibliography is available at Expert Consult.

294.9 Venezuelan Equine Encephalitis

Scott B. Halstead

VEE virus was isolated from an epizootic in Venezuelan horses in 1938. Human cases were first identified in 1943. Hundreds of thousands of equine and human cases have occurred over the past 70 yr. During 1971, epizootics moved through Central America and Mexico to southern Texas. After two decades of quiescence, epizootic disease emerged again in Venezuela and Colombia in 1995. Between December 1992 and January 1993, the Venezuelan state of Trujillo experienced an outbreak of this virus. Overall, 28 cases of the disease were reported, along with 12 deaths. June 1993 saw a bigger outbreak, in which 55 humans died, as well as 66 horses. A much larger outbreak in Venezuela and Colombia occurred in 1995. On May 23, 1995, equine encephalitis-like cases were reported in the northwest portion of the country. Eventually, the outbreak spread toward the north, as well as to the south. The outbreak caused about 11,390 febrile cases in humans, as well as 16 deaths. About 500 equine cases were reported with 475 deaths.

The incubation period is 2-5 days, followed by the abrupt onset of fever, chills, headache, sore throat, myalgia, malaise, prostration, photophobia, nausea, vomiting, and diarrhea. In 5–10% of cases, there is a biphasic illness; the second phase is heralded by seizures, projectile vomiting, ataxia, confusion, agitation, and mild disturbances in consciousness. There is cervical lymphadenopathy and conjunctival suffusion. Cases of meningoencephalitis may demonstrate cranial nerve palsy, motor weakness, paralysis, seizures, and coma. Microscopic examination of tissues reveals inflammatory infiltrates in lymph nodes, spleen, lung,

liver, and brain. Lymph nodes show cellular depletion, necrosis of germinal centers, and lymphophagocytosis. The liver shows patchy hepatocellular degeneration, the lungs demonstrate a diffuse interstitial pneumonia with intraalveolar hemorrhages, and the brain shows patchy cellular infiltrates.

There is no specific treatment for VEE. The treatment is intensive supportive care (see Chapter 85), including control of seizures (see Chapter 611).

In patients with VEE meningoencephalitis, the fatality rate ranges from 10% to 25%. Sequelae include nervousness, forgetfulness, recurrent headache, and easy fatigability.

Several veterinary vaccines are available to protect equines. VEE virus is highly infectious in laboratory settings, and biosafety level three containment should be used. An experimental vaccine is available for use in laboratory workers. Several vaccine constructs are in the pipeline for potential use in humans.

294.10 Japanese Encephalitis

Scott B. Halstead

JE is a mosquito-borne viral disease of humans, as well as horses, swine, and other domestic animals. The virus causes human infections and acute disease in a vast area of Asia, northern Japan, Korea, China, Taiwan, the Philippines, and the Indonesian archipelago and from Indochina through the Indian subcontinent. *Culex tritaeniorhynchus summarosus,* a night-biting mosquito that feeds preferentially on large domestic animals and birds but only infrequently on humans, is the principal vector of zoonotic and human JE in northern Asia. A more complex ecology prevails in southern Asia. From Taiwan to India, *C. tritaeniorhynchus* and members of the closely related *Culex vishnui* group are vectors. Before the introduction of JE vaccine, summer outbreaks of JE occurred regularly in Japan, Korea, China, Okinawa, and Taiwan. Over the past decade, there has been a pattern of steadily enlarging recurrent seasonal outbreaks in Vietnam, Thailand, Nepal, and India, with small outbreaks in the Philippines, Indonesia, and the northern tip of Queensland, Australia. Seasonal rains are accompanied by increases in mosquito populations and JE transmission. Pigs serve as an amplifying host.

The annual incidence in endemic areas ranges from 1-10 per 10,000 population. Children younger than 15 yr of age are principally affected, with nearly universal exposure by adulthood. The case:infection ratio for JE virus has been variously estimated at 1:25 to 1:1,000. Higher ratios have been estimated for populations indigenous to enzootic areas.

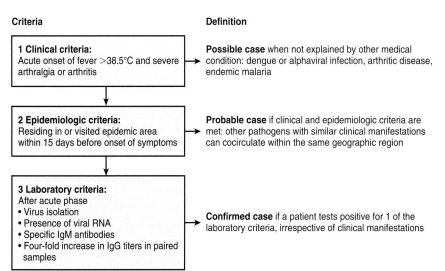

Criteria	Definition
1 Clinical criteria: Acute onset of fever >38.5°C and severe arthralgia or arthritis	**Possible case** when not explained by other medical condition: dengue or alphaviral infection, arthritic disease, endemic malaria
2 Epidemiologic criteria: Residing in or visited epidemic area within 15 days before onset of symptoms	**Probable case** if clinical and epidemiologic criteria are met: other pathogens with similar clinical manifestations can cocirculate within the same geographic region
3 Laboratory criteria: After acute phase • Virus isolation • Presence of viral RNA • Specific IgM antibodies • Four-fold increase in IgG titers in paired samples	**Confirmed case** if a patient tests positive for 1 of the laboratory criteria, irrespective of clinical manifestations

Fig. 294.4 Diagnostic criteria for chikungunya virus fever. *(From Burt FJ, Rolph MS, Rulli NE, et al: Chikungunya: a re-emerging virus, Lancet 379:662-668, 2012, Fig. 6.)*

JE occurs in travelers visiting Asia; therefore, a travel history in the diagnosis of encephalitis is critical.

After a 4- to 14-day incubation period, cases typically progress through the following four stages: prodromal illness (2-3 days), acute stage (3-4 days), subacute stage (7-10 days), and convalescence (4-7 wk). The onset may be characterized by an abrupt onset of fever, headache, respiratory symptoms, anorexia, nausea, abdominal pain, vomiting, and sensory changes, including psychotic episodes. Grand mal seizures are seen in 10–24% of children with JE; parkinsonian-like nonintention tremor and cogwheel rigidity are seen less frequently. Particularly characteristic are rapidly changing central nervous system signs (e.g., hyperreflexia followed by hyporeflexia or plantar responses that change). The sensory status of the patient may vary from confusion through disorientation and delirium to somnolence, progressing to coma. There is usually a mild pleocytosis (100-1,000 leukocytes/μL) in the cerebrospinal fluid, initially polymorphonuclear but in a few days predominantly lymphocytic. Albuminuria is common. Fatal cases usually progress rapidly to coma, and the patient dies within 10 days.

JE should be suspected in patients reporting exposure to night-biting mosquitoes in endemic areas during the transmission season. The etiologic diagnosis of JE is established by testing acute-phase serum collected early in the illness for the presence of virus-specific IgM antibodies or, alternatively, demonstrating a fourfold or greater increase in IgG antibody titers by testing paired acute and convalescent sera. The virus can also be identified by the polymerase chain reaction.

There is no specific treatment for JE. The treatment is intensive supportive care (see Chapter 85), including control of seizures (see Chapter 611).

Patient fatality rates for JE are 24–42% and are highest in children 5-9 yr of age and in adults older than 65 yr of age. The frequency of sequelae is 5–70% and is directly related to the age of the patient and severity of disease. Sequelae are most common in patients younger than 10 yr at the onset of disease. The more common sequelae are mental deterioration, severe emotional instability, personality changes, motor abnormalities, and speech disturbances.

Bibliography is available at Expert Consult.

294.11 Tick-Borne Encephalitis
Scott B. Halstead

TBE refers to neurotropic tick-transmitted flaviviral infections occurring across the Eurasian land mass. In the Far East, the disease is called *Russian spring-summer encephalitis*; the milder, often biphasic form in Europe is simply called TBE. TBE is found in all countries of Europe except Portugal and the Benelux countries. The incidence is particularly high in Austria, Poland, Hungary, Czech Republic, Slovakia, former Yugoslavia, and Russia. The incidence tends to be very focal. Seroprevalence is as high as 50% in farm and forestry workers. The majority of cases occur in adults, but even young children may be infected while playing in the woods or on picnics or camping trips. The seasonal distribution of cases is midsummer in southern Europe, with a longer season in Scandinavia and the Russian Far East. TBE can be excreted from the milk of goats, sheep, or cows. Before World War II, when unpasteurized milk was consumed, milk-borne cases of TBE were common.

Viruses are transmitted principally by hard ticks of *Ixodes ricinus* in Europe and *Ixodes persulcatus* in the Far East. Viral circulation is maintained by a combination of transmission from ticks to birds, rodents, and larger mammals and transstadial transmission from larval to nymphal and adult stages. In some parts of Europe and Russia, ticks feed actively during the spring and early fall, giving rise to the name *spring-summer encephalitis*.

After an incubation period of 7-14 days, the European form begins as an acute nonspecific febrile illness that is followed in 5–30% of cases by meningoencephalitis. The Far Eastern variety more often results in encephalitis with higher case fatality and sequelae rates. The first phase of illness is characterized by fever, headache, myalgia, malaise, nausea, and vomiting for 2-7 days. Fever disappears but after 2-8 days may

return, accompanied by vomiting, photophobia, and signs of meningeal irritation in children and more severe encephalitic signs in adults. This phase rarely lasts more than 1 wk.

There is no specific treatment for TBE. The treatment is intensive supportive care (see Chapter 85), including control of seizures (see Chapter 611).

The main risk for a fatal outcome is advanced age; the fatality rate in adults is approximately 1%, but sequelae in children are rare. Transient unilateral paralysis of an upper extremity is a common finding in adults. Common sequelae include chronic fatigue, headache, sleep disorders, and emotional disturbances.

Bibliography is available at Expert Consult.

294.12 Zika Virus
Scott B. Halstead

EPIDEMIOLOGY
Zika virus (ZIKV), a member of the *Flavivirus* genus, is maintained in complex African zoonotic cycles, spilling over from time to time into the *Aedes aegypti/Aedes albopictus* urban transmission cycles, possibly over a period of many years (Fig. 294.5). After the virus was discovered in Africa in 1947, human antibodies were found widely dispersed throughout tropical Asia. However, in all these locations, human ZIKV disease was mild and rare until 2007, when there was an outbreak of a mild febrile exanthem on the Yap Islands in the western Pacific. Soon thereafter, an outbreak on Tahiti in 2013-2014 was followed by 4 wk by a small outbreak of Guillain-Barré syndrome (GBS). In 2015, a massive epidemic in South America was accompanied by focal reports, particularly in Brazil, of ZIKV infections of pregnant women that produced infected and damaged fetuses or newborns. The epidemiology of ZIKV infections is essentially identical to that of the dengue and chikungunya viruses. Residents of urban areas, particularly those without adequate sources of piped water, are at highest risk. *Aedes aegypti*, the principal vector mosquito, is very abundant and widespread throughout South and Central America, Mexico, and the Caribbean region. During the American pandemic, ZIKV was found to infect the male reproductive tract, be secreted in urine and saliva, and be sexually transmitted. By 2017, the ZIKV epidemic in the American tropics appeared to wane. During 2015-2016, large numbers of imported Zika infections, some in pregnant women, were reported in the United States and other temperate-zone developed countries. Small outbreaks of endogenous human Zika infections were reported in South Florida during the summer of 2016.

From the pediatric perspective, the most important outcome of human ZIKV infection is termed the *congenital Zika syndrome (CZS)*, which consists of microcephaly, facial disproportion, hypertonia/spasticity, hyperreflexia, irritability, seizures, arthrogryposis, ocular abnormalities, and sensorineural hearing loss (Table 294.1). A comprehensive understanding of the precise antecedents to CZS is not known. It appears that the earlier during pregnancy that ZIKV infections occur, the greater the likelihood of and the more severe the CZS. Vertical transmission appears to follow viremia with ZIKV, transiting the uterus to infect the placenta and then the fetus. However, factors that affect the occurrence or severity of CZS, such as age, ethnicity, or prior immune status of the mother, are not known. In vitro studies have demonstrated that dengue antibodies can enhance ZIKV infection in vitro, in Fc-receptor–bearing cells, but, as yet, there is no evidence that a prior dengue infection alters the chance of ZIKV crossing the placenta or increases the risk of CZS. Maternal-fetal transmission of ZIKV can occur during labor and delivery. There are no reports of ZIKV infection acquired by an infant at the time of delivery leading to microcephaly. There are no data to contraindicate breastfeeding, although the virus has been identified in breast milk. Maternal and newborn laboratory testing is indicated during the first 2 wk of life if the mother had relevant epidemiologic exposure within 2 wk of delivery and had clinical manifestations of ZIKV infection (e.g., rash, conjunctivitis, arthralgia, or fever). Infants and children who acquire ZIKV infection postnatally appear to have a mild course, similar to that seen in adults.

CLINICAL FEATURES

Congenital Zika syndrome may be defined in a fetus with diagnostic evidence of ZIKV infection, including (1) severe microcephaly (>3 SD below the mean), partially collapsed skull, overlapping cranial sutures, prominent occipital bone, redundant scalp skin, and neurologic impairment; (2) brain anomalies, including cerebral cortex thinning, abnormal gyral patterns, increased fluid spaces, subcortical calcifications, corpus callosum anomalies, reduced white matter, and cerebellar vermis hypoplasia; (3) ocular findings, such as macular scarring, focal pigmentary retinal mottling, structural anomalies (microphthalmia, coloboma, cataracts, and posterior anomalies), chorioretinal atrophy, or optic nerve hypoplasia/atrophy; (4) congenital contractures, including unilateral or bilateral clubfoot and arthrogryposis multiplex congenita; and (5) neurologic impairment, such as pronounced early hypertonia/spasticity with extrapyramidal symptoms, motor disabilities, cognitive disabilities, hypotonia, irritability/excessive crying, tremors, swallowing dysfunction, vision impairment, hearing impairment, and epilepsy (see Table 294.1).

Acquired Zika virus infection may present with nonspecific viral syndrome–like features. Nonetheless, patients are at increased risk of myelitis and Guillain-Barré syndrome. In addition, the virus may remain present in the blood and body fluids for months after resolution of clinical symptoms.

MANAGEMENT

For infants with confirmed Zika virus infection, close follow-up is necessary. The appropriate follow-up evaluation depends upon whether or not the infant has clinical signs and symptoms of congenital Zika syndrome. All infants should have close monitoring of growth and development, repeat ophthalmologic examinations, and auditory brainstem response testing (see Table 294.1).

LABORATORY DIAGNOSIS

Laboratory testing for Zika virus infection in the neonate includes the following: serum and urine for Zika virus RNA via real-time reverse transcription polymerase chain reaction (rRT-PCR) and serum Zika virus immunoglobulin M (IgM) enzyme-linked immunosorbent assay (ELISA). If the IgM is positive, the plaque reduction neutralization test (PRNT) is used to confirm the specificity of the IgM antibodies against Zika virus and to exclude a false-positive IgM result. If CSF is available, it should be tested for Zika virus RNA (via rRT-PCR), as well as Zika virus IgM. CSF specimens need not be collected for the sole purpose of Zika virus testing but may be reasonable for the evaluation of infants with microcephaly or intracranial calcifications. A definitive diagnosis of congenital Zika virus infection is confirmed by the presence of Zika virus RNA in samples of serum, urine, or CSF collected within the first 2 days of life; IgM antibodies may be positive or negative. A negative rRT-PCR result with a positive Zika virus IgM test result indicates probable congenital Zika virus infection.

Fetuses or infants born to mothers who test positive for ZIKV infection should be studied sonographically or for clinical evidence of congenital Zika syndrome, a comprehensive evaluation (including ophthalmologic examination, laboratory tests, and specialist consultation) should be performed prior to hospital discharge.

PROGNOSIS

The prognosis of newborns with congenital Zika syndrome is unclear. Reported acute mortality rates among live-born infants range from 4% to 6%. The combination of Zika virus–related microcephaly and severe

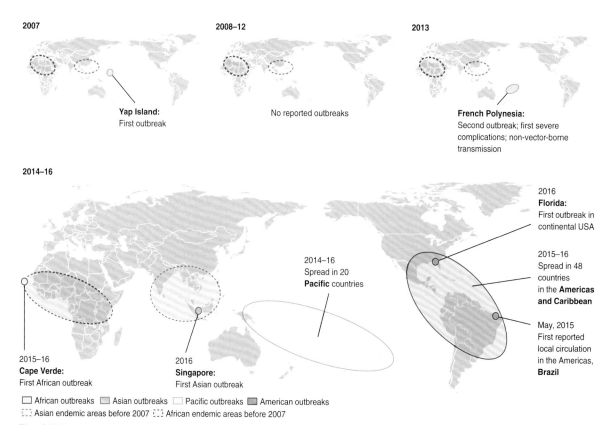

Fig. 294.5 Zika virus outbreaks from 2007 to 2016. *(From Baud D, Gubler DJ, Schaub B, et al: An update on Zika virus infection, Lancet 390:2099-2109, 2017, Fig. 2.)*

Table 294.1	Surveillance Case Classification: Children, Neonate to 2 Years of Age, Born to Mothers With Any Evidence of Zika Virus Infection During Pregnancy

ZIKA-ASSOCIATED BIRTH DEFECTS

Selected structural anomalies of the brain or eyes present at birth (congenital) and detected from birth to age 2 yr. Microcephaly at birth, with or without low birthweight, was included as a structural anomaly.

- **Selected congenital brain anomalies:** intracranial calcifications; cerebral atrophy; abnormal cortical formation (e.g., polymicrogyria, lissencephaly, pachygyria, schizencephaly, gray matter heterotopia); corpus callosum abnormalities; cerebellar abnormalities; porencephaly; hydranencephaly; ventriculomegaly/hydrocephaly.
- **Selected congenital eye anomalies:** microphthalmia or anophthalmia; coloboma; cataract; intraocular calcifications; chorioretinal anomalies involving the macula (e.g., chorioretinal atrophy and scarring, macular pallor, and gross pigmentary mottling), excluding retinopathy of prematurity; optic nerve atrophy, pallor, and other optic nerve abnormalities.
- **Microcephaly at birth:** birth head circumference < 3rd percentile for infant sex and gestational age based on INTERGROWTH-21st online percentile calculator (http://intergrowth21.ndog.ox.ac.uk/).

NEURODEVELOPMENTAL ABNORMALITIES POSSIBLY ASSOCIATED WITH CONGENITAL ZIKA VIRUS INFECTION

Consequences of neurologic dysfunction detected from birth (congenital) to age 2 yr. Postnatal-onset microcephaly was included as a neurodevelopmental abnormality.

- **Hearing abnormalities:** Hearing loss or deafness documented by testing, most frequently auditory brainstem response (ABR). Includes sensorineural hearing loss, mixed hearing loss, and hearing loss not otherwise specified. Failed newborn hearing screening is not sufficient for diagnosis.
- **Congenital contractures:** Multiple contractures (arthrogryposis) and isolated clubfoot documented at birth. Brain anomalies must be documented for isolated clubfoot but not for arthrogryposis.
- **Seizures:** Documented by electroencephalogram or physician report. Includes epilepsy or seizures not otherwise specified; excludes febrile seizures.
- **Body tone abnormalities:** Hypertonia or hypotonia documented at any age in conjunction with (1) a failed screen or assessment for gross motor function; (2) suspicion or diagnosis of cerebral palsy from age 1 to 2 yr; or (3) assessment by a physician or other medical professional, such as a physical therapist.
- **Movement abnormalities:** Dyskinesia or dystonia at any age; suspicion or diagnosis of cerebral palsy from age 1 to 2 yr.
- **Swallowing abnormalities:** Documented by instrumented or noninstrumented evaluation, presence of a gastrostomy tube, or physician report.
- **Possible developmental delay:** Abnormal result from most recent developmental screening (i.e., failed screen for gross motor domain or failed screen for two or more developmental domains at the same time point or age); developmental evaluation; or assessment review by developmental pediatrician. Results from developmental evaluation are considered the gold standard if available.
- **Possible visual impairment:** Includes strabismus (esotropia or exotropia), nystagmus, failure to fix and follow at age < 1 yr; diagnosis of visual impairment at age ≥ 1 yr.
- **Postnatal-onset microcephaly:** Two most recent head circumference measurements reported from follow-up care < 3rd percentile for child's sex and age based on World Health Organization child growth standards; downward trajectory of head circumference percentiles with most recent measurement < 3rd percentile. Age at measurement was adjusted for gestational age in infants born at < 40 wk of gestational age through age 24 mo chronologic age.

From Rice ME, Galang RR, Roth NM, et al: Vital signs: Zika-associated birth defects and neurodevelopmental abnormalities possibly associated with congenital Zika virus infection: US territories and freely associated states, 2018. MMWR 67(31):858-866, 2018.

cerebral abnormalities generally has a poor prognosis, but little is known about the prognosis for congenitally infected infants with less severe or no apparent abnormalities at birth.

DIFFERENTIAL DIAGNOSIS

The differential diagnosis for congenital Zika virus infection includes other congenital infections and other causes of microcephaly.

PREVENTION

The prevention of the congenital Zika syndrome includes avoidance, if possible, of travel to endemic regions; if travel to endemic regions cannot be avoided, careful contraception (male and female) is essential, especially with the knowledge that Zika virus can persist in semen for months after a primary infection (Table 294.2).

Bibliography is available at Expert Consult.

Table 294.2	CDC Recommendations for Preconception Counseling and Prevention of Sexual Transmission of Zika Virus Among Persons With Possible Zika Virus Exposure: United States, August 2018
EXPOSURE SCENARIO	**RECOMMENDATIONS (UPDATE STATUS)**
Only the male partner travels to an area with risk for Zika virus transmission and couple is planning to conceive	The couple should use condoms or abstain from sex for at least 3 mo after the male partner's symptom onset (if symptomatic) or last possible Zika virus exposure (if asymptomatic). **(Updated recommendation)**
Only the female partner travels to an area with risk for Zika virus transmission and couple is planning to conceive	The couple should use condoms or abstain from sex for at least 2 mo after the female partner's symptom onset (if symptomatic) or last possible Zika virus exposure (if asymptomatic). **(No change in recommendation)***
Both partners travel to an area with risk for Zika virus transmission and couple is planning to conceive	The couple should use condoms or abstain from sex for at least 3 mo from the male partner's symptom onset (if symptomatic) or last possible Zika virus exposure (if asymptomatic). **(Updated recommendation)**
One or both partners have ongoing exposure (i.e., live in or frequently travel to an area with risk for Zika virus transmission) and couple is planning to conceive	The couple should talk with their health care provider about their plans for pregnancy, their risk for Zika virus infection, the possible health effects of Zika virus infection on a baby, and ways to protect themselves from Zika. If either partner develops symptoms of Zika virus infection or tests positive for Zika virus infection, the couple should follow the suggested timeframes listed above before trying to conceive. **(No change in recommendation)***
Men with possible Zika virus exposure whose partner is pregnant	The couple should use condoms or abstain from sex for the duration of the pregnancy. **(No change in recommendation)***

*Petersen EE, Meaney-Delman D, Neblett-Fanfair R, et al: Update: interim guidance for preconception counseling and prevention of sexual transmission of Zika virus for persons with possible Zika virus exposure—United States, September 2016, MMWR Morb Mortal Wkly Rep 65:1077–1081, 2016.
From Polen KD, Gilboa SM, Hills S, et al: Update: interim guidance for preconception counseling and prevention of sexual transmission of Zika virus for men with possible Zika virus exposure: United States, August 2018, MMWR 67(31):868–870, 2018.

Chapter **295**

Dengue Fever, Dengue Hemorrhagic Fever, and Severe Dengue

Scott B. Halstead

第二百九十五章
登革热、登革热出血热和严重登革热

中文导读

　　本章主要介绍了登革病毒感染的病因学、流行病学、发病机制、临床表现、诊断、鉴别诊断、实验室检查、治疗、并发症、预后和预防。临床表现包括登革热、登革热出血热和登革热休克综合征、严重登革热。实验室检测包括分离病毒、抗原或基因检测以及血清学检测。非单纯性登革热以支持治疗为主，详述了登革热、登革热出血热和登革热休克综合征的治疗。

Dengue fever is a benign syndrome caused by several arthropod-borne viruses and is characterized by biphasic fever, myalgia or arthralgia, rash, leukopenia, and lymphadenopathy. **Dengue hemorrhagic fever** (Philippine, Thai, or Singapore hemorrhagic fever; hemorrhagic dengue; acute infectious thrombocytopenic purpura) is a severe, often fatal, febrile disease caused by one of four dengue viruses. It is characterized by capillary permeability, abnormalities of hemostasis, and, in severe cases, a protein-losing shock syndrome (**dengue shock syndrome**), which is thought to have an immunopathologic basis.

A revised case definition adopted by the World Health Organization (WHO) in 2009 includes as **severe dengue** those cases accompanied by fluid loss leading to shock, fluid loss with respiratory distress, liver damage evidenced by elevations of ALT or AST to > 1000 U/L, severe bleeding, and altered consciousness or significant heart abnormalities.

ETIOLOGY

There are at least four distinct antigenic types of dengue virus (dengue 1, 2, 3, and 4), members of the family Flaviviridae. In addition, three other arthropod-borne viruses (arboviruses) cause similar dengue fever syndromes with rash (Table 295.1; see also Chapter 294).

EPIDEMIOLOGY

Dengue viruses are transmitted by mosquitoes of the Stegomyia family. *Aedes aegypti,* a daytime biting mosquito, is the principal vector, and all four virus types have been recovered from it. Transmission occurs from viremic humans by bite of the vector mosquito where virus multiplies during an extrinsic incubation period and then by bite is passed on to a susceptible human in what is called the urban transmission cycle. In most tropical areas, *A. aegypti* is highly urbanized, breeding in water stored for drinking or bathing and in rainwater collected in any container. Dengue viruses have also been recovered from *Aedes albopictus,* as in the 2001 and 2015 Hawaiian epidemics, whereas outbreaks in the Pacific area have been attributed to several other *Aedes* species. These species breed in water trapped in vegetation. In Southeast Asia and West Africa, dengue virus may be maintained in a cycle involving canopy-feeding jungle monkeys and *Aedes* species, which feed on monkeys.

In the 19th and 20th centuries, epidemics were common in temperate areas of the Americas, Europe, Australia, and Asia. Dengue fever and dengue-like disease are now endemic in tropical Asia, the South Pacific Islands, northern Australia, tropical Africa, the Arabian Peninsula, the Caribbean, and Central and South America. Dengue fever occurs frequently among travelers to these areas. Locally acquired disease has been reported in Florida, Arizona, and Texas, and imported cases in the United States occur in travelers to endemic areas. More than 390 million dengue infections occur annually; approximately 96 million have clinical disease.

Dengue outbreaks in urban areas infested with *A. aegypti* may be explosive; in virgin soil epidemics, up to 70–80% of the population may be involved. Most overt disease occurs in older children and adults. Because *A. aegypti* has a limited flight range, spread of an epidemic occurs mainly through viremic human beings and follows the main lines of transportation. Sentinel cases may infect household mosquitoes; a large number of nearly simultaneous secondary infections give the appearance of a contagious disease. Where dengue is highly endemic, children and susceptible foreigners may be the only persons to acquire overt disease, because adults have become immune.

Dengue-Like Diseases

Dengue-like diseases may occur in epidemics. Epidemiologic features depend on the vectors and their geographic distribution (see Chapter 294). Chikungunya virus is enzootic in subhuman primates throughout much of West, Central, and South Africa. Periodic introductions of virus into the urban transmission cycle have led to pandemics, resulting in widespread endemicity in the most populous areas of Asia. In Asia, *A. aegypti* is the principal vector; in Africa, other Stegomyia species may be important vectors. In Southeast Asia, dengue and chikungunya outbreaks occur concurrently in the urban cycle. Outbreaks of o'nyong-nyong fever usually involve villages or small towns, in contrast to the urban outbreaks of dengue and chikungunya. West Nile virus is enzootic in Africa. Chikungunya is now endemic in urban cycles in tropical countries throughout the world. Intense transmission in Caribbean and Central and South American countries beginning in 2013 results in the emergence of limited chikungunya transmission in the United States.

Dengue Hemorrhagic Fever

Dengue hemorrhagic fever occurs where multiple types of dengue virus are simultaneously or sequentially transmitted. It is endemic in tropical America, Asia, the Pacific Islands, and parts of Africa, where warm temperatures and the practices of water storage in homes plus outdoor breeding sites result in large, permanent populations of *A. aegypti.* Under these conditions, infections with dengue viruses of all types are common. A first infection, referred to as a primary infection, may be followed by infection with a different dengue virus, referred to as a secondary infection. In areas of high endemicity, secondary infections are frequent.

Secondary dengue infections are relatively mild in the majority of instances, ranging from an inapparent infection through an undifferentiated upper respiratory tract or dengue-like disease, but may also progress to dengue hemorrhagic fever. Nonimmune foreigners, both adults and children, who are exposed to dengue virus during outbreaks of hemorrhagic fever have classic dengue fever or even milder disease. The differences in clinical manifestations of dengue infections between natives and foreigners in Southeast Asia are related to immunologic status. Dengue hemorrhagic fever can occur during primary dengue infections, most frequently in infants whose mothers are immune to dengue. Dengue hemorrhagic fever or severe dengue occurs rarely in individuals of African ancestry because of an as yet incompletely described resistance gene that is consistent with the low incidence of severe dengue throughout much of Africa and among African populations in the American tropics despite high rates of dengue infection.

PATHOGENESIS

The pathogenesis of dengue hemorrhagic fever is incompletely understood, but epidemiologic studies usually associate this syndrome with second heterotypic infections with dengue types 1-4 or in infants born to mothers who have had two or more lifetime dengue infections. Retrospective studies of sera from human mothers whose infants acquired dengue hemorrhagic fever and prospective studies in children acquiring sequential dengue infections have shown that the circulation of infection-enhancing antibodies at the time of infection is the strongest risk factor for development of severe disease. The absence of cross-reactive neutralizing antibodies and presence of enhancing antibodies from passive transfer or active production are the best correlates of risk for dengue hemorrhagic fever. Monkeys that are infected sequentially or are receiving small quantities of enhancing antibodies have enhanced viremias. In humans studied early during the course of secondary dengue infections, viremia levels directly predicted disease severity. When dengue virus immune complexes attach to monocyte/macrophage Fc receptors, a signal is sent that suppresses innate immunity, resulting in enhanced viral production. In the Americas, dengue hemorrhagic fever and dengue

VIRUS	GEOGRAPHIC GENUS AND DISEASE	VECTOR	DISTRIBUTION
Togavirus	Chikungunya	*Aedes aegypti* *Aedes africanus* *Aedes albopictus*	Africa, India, Southeast Asia, Latin America, United States
Togavirus	O'nyong-nyong	*Anopheles funestus*	East Africa
Flavivirus	West Nile fever	*Culex molestus* *Culex univittatus*	Europe, Africa, Middle East, India

Table 295.1 Vectors and Geographic Distribution of Dengue-Like Diseases

shock syndrome have been associated with dengue types 1-4 strains of recent Southeast Asian origin. Outbreaks of dengue hemorrhagic fever in all areas of the world are correlated with secondary dengue infections while recent outbreaks in India, Pakistan, and Bangladesh are related to imported dengue strains.

Early in the acute stage of secondary dengue infections, there is rapid activation of the complement system. Shortly before or during shock, blood levels of soluble tumor necrosis factor receptor, interferon-γ, and interleukin-2 are elevated. C1q, C3, C4, C5-C8, and C3 proactivators are depressed, and C3 catabolic rates are elevated. Circulating viral nonstructural protein 1 (NS1) is a viral toxin that activates myeloid cells to release cytokines by attaching to toll receptor 4. It also contributes to increased vascular permeability by activating complement, interacting with and damaging endothelial cells, and interacting with blood clotting factors and platelets. The mechanism of bleeding in dengue hemorrhagic fever is not known, but a mild degree of disseminated intravascular coagulopathy, liver damage, and thrombocytopenia may operate synergistically. Capillary damage allows fluid, electrolytes, small proteins, and, in some instances, red blood cells to leak into extravascular spaces. This internal redistribution of fluid, together with deficits caused by fasting, thirsting, and vomiting, results in hemoconcentration, hypovolemia, increased cardiac work, tissue hypoxia, metabolic acidosis, and hyponatremia.

Usually no pathologic lesions are found to account for death. In rare instances, death may be a result of gastrointestinal or intracranial hemorrhages. Minimal to moderate hemorrhages are seen in the upper gastrointestinal tract, and petechial hemorrhages are common in the interventricular septum of the heart, on the pericardium, and on the subserosal surfaces of major viscera. Focal hemorrhages are occasionally seen in the lungs, liver, adrenals, and subarachnoid space. The liver is usually enlarged, often with fatty changes. Yellow, watery, and at times blood-tinged effusions are present in serous cavities in approximately 75% of patients at autopsy.

Dengue virus is frequently absent in tissues at the time of death; viral antigens or RNA have been localized to hepatocytes and macrophages in the liver, spleen, lung, and lymphatic tissues.

CLINICAL MANIFESTATIONS
Dengue Fever
The incubation period is 1-7 days. The clinical manifestations are variable and are influenced by the age of the patient. In infants and young children, the disease may be undifferentiated or characterized by fever for 1-5 days, pharyngeal inflammation, rhinitis, and mild cough. A majority of infected older children and adults experience sudden onset of fever, with temperature rapidly increasing to 39.4-41.1°C (103-106°F), usually accompanied by frontal or retroorbital pain, particularly when pressure is applied to the eyes. Occasionally, severe back pain precedes the fever (back-break fever). A transient, macular, generalized rash that blanches under pressure may be seen during the first 24-48 hr of fever. The pulse rate may be slow relative to the degree of fever. Myalgia and arthralgia occur soon after the onset of fevers and increase in severity over time. From the second to sixth day of fever, nausea and vomiting are apt to occur, and generalized lymphadenopathy, cutaneous hyperesthesia or hyperalgesia, taste aberrations, and pronounced anorexia may develop.

Approximately 1-2 days after defervescence, a generalized, morbilliform, maculopapular rash appears that spares the palms and soles. It disappears in 1-5 days; desquamation may occur. Rarely there is edema of the palms and soles. About the time this second rash appears, the body temperature, which has previously decreased to normal, may become slightly elevated and demonstrate the characteristic biphasic temperature pattern.

Dengue Hemorrhagic Fever and Dengue Shock Syndrome (DHF/DSS)
The differentiation between dengue fever and dengue hemorrhagic fever is difficult early in the course of illness. A relatively mild first phase with abrupt onset of fever, malaise, vomiting, headache, anorexia, and cough may be followed after 2-5 days by rapid clinical deterioration and collapse. In this second phase, the patient usually has cold, clammy extremities, a warm trunk, flushed face, diaphoresis, restlessness, irritability, midepigastric pain, and decreased urinary output. Frequently, there are scattered petechiae on the forehead and extremities; spontaneous ecchymoses may appear, and easy bruising and bleeding at sites of venipuncture are common. A macular or maculopapular rash may appear, and there may be circumoral and peripheral cyanosis. Respirations are rapid and often labored. The pulse is weak, rapid, and thready, and the heart sounds are faint. The liver may enlarge to 4-6 cm below the costal margin and is usually firm and somewhat tender. Approximately 20–30% of cases of dengue hemorrhagic fever are complicated by shock (dengue shock syndrome). Dengue shock can be subtle, arising in patients who are fully alert, and is accompanied by increased peripheral vascular resistance and raised diastolic blood pressure. Shock is not from congestive heart failure but from venous pooling. With increasing cardiovascular compromise, the diastolic pressure rises toward the systolic level and the pulse pressure narrows. Fewer than 10% of patients have gross ecchymosis or gastrointestinal bleeding, usually after a period of uncorrected shock. After a 24- to 36-hr period of crisis, convalescence is fairly rapid in the children who recover. The temperature may return to normal before or during the stage of shock. Bradycardia and ventricular extrasystoles are common during convalescence.

Dengue With Warning Signs and Severe Dengue
In hyperendemic areas, among Asian children, the DHF/DSS continues to be the dominant life-threatening event, always challenging to an identifying physician using classical WHO diagnostic criteria. When the four dengue viruses spread to the American hemisphere and to South Asia, there were millions of primary and secondary dengue infections, many of them adults of all ages. Dengue disease in these areas presented a wider clinical spectrum resulting in a new diagnostic algorithm and case definitions (see below).

DIAGNOSIS
A clinical diagnosis of dengue fever derives from a high index of suspicion and knowledge of the geographic distribution and environmental cycles of causal viruses (for nondengue causes see Chapter 294). Because clinical findings vary and there are many possible causative agents, the term *dengue-like disease* should be used until a specific diagnosis is established. A case is confirmed by isolation of the virus, viral antigen, or genome by polymerase chain reaction analysis, the detection of IgM dengue antibodies as well as demonstration of a four-fold or greater increase in antibody titers. A probable case is a typical acute febrile illness with supportive serology and occurrence at a location where there are confirmed cases.

The WHO criteria for **dengue hemorrhagic fever** are fever (2-7 days in duration or biphasic), minor or major hemorrhagic manifestations including a positive tourniquet test, thrombocytopenia (≤100,000/μL), and objective evidence of increased capillary permeability (hematocrit increased by ≥ 20%), pleural effusion or ascites (by chest radiography or ultrasonography), or hypoalbuminemia. **Dengue shock syndrome** criteria include those for dengue hemorrhagic fever as well as hypotension, tachycardia, narrow pulse pressure (≤20 mm Hg), and signs of poor perfusion (cold extremities).

In 2009, the WHO promulgated guidelines for the diagnosis of probable dengue, dengue with warning signs, and a category called severe dengue (Fig. 295.1). The presence of warning signs in an individual with probable dengue alerts the physician to the possible need for hospitalization. Severe dengue is a mixture of syndromes associated with dengue infection, including classical DHF/DSS, but also rare instances of encephalitis or encephalopathy, liver damage, or myocardial damage. Severe dengue also includes respiratory distress, a harbinger of pulmonary edema caused by overhydration, an all too common outcome of inexpert treatment (see Treatment and Complications sections).

Virologic diagnosis can be established by serologic tests, by detection of viral proteins or viral RNA, or by the isolation of the virus from blood leukocytes or acute-phase serum. Following primary and secondary dengue infections, there is an appearance of antidengue (immunoglobulin [Ig] M) antibodies. These disappear after 6-12 wk, a feature that can be used to date a dengue infection. In secondary dengue infections, most dengue antibody is of the IgG class. Serologic diagnosis depends on a four-fold or greater increase in IgG antibody titer in paired sera by hemagglutination inhibition, complement fixation, enzyme immunoassay, or neutralization test. Carefully standardized IgM and IgG capture enzyme commercial immunoassays are now widely used to identify acute-phase antibodies from patients with primary or secondary dengue infections in single-serum samples. Usually such samples should be collected not earlier than 5 days and not later than 6 wk after onset. It may not be possible to distinguish the infecting virus by serologic methods alone, particularly when there has been prior infection with another member of the same arbovirus group. Virus can be recovered from acute-phase serum after inoculating tissue culture or living mosquitoes. Viral RNA can be detected in blood or tissues by specific complementary RNA probes or amplified first by polymerase chain reaction or by real-time polymerase chain reaction. A viral nonstructural protein, NS1, is released by infected cells into the circulation and can be detected in acute-stage blood samples using monoclonal or polyclonal antibodies. The detection of NS1 is the basis of commercial tests, including rapid lateral flow tests. These tests offer a reliable point-of-care diagnosis of acute dengue infection.

DIFFERENTIAL DIAGNOSIS

The differential diagnosis of dengue fever includes dengue-like diseases, viral respiratory and influenza-like diseases, the early stages of malaria, mild yellow fever, scrub typhus, viral hepatitis, and leptospirosis.

Four arboviral diseases have dengue-like courses but without rash: Colorado tick fever, sandfly fever, Rift Valley fever, and Ross River fever (see Chapter 294). Colorado tick fever occurs sporadically among campers and hunters in the western United States; sandfly fever in the Mediterranean region, the Middle East, southern Russia, and parts of the Indian subcontinent; and Rift Valley fever in North, East, Central, and South Africa. Ross River fever is endemic in much of eastern Australia, with epidemic extension to Fiji. In adults, Ross River fever often produces protracted and crippling arthralgia involving weight-bearing joints.

Because meningococcemia, yellow fever (see Chapter 296), other viral hemorrhagic fevers (see Chapter 297), many rickettsial diseases, and other severe illnesses caused by a variety of agents may produce a clinical picture similar to dengue hemorrhagic fever, the etiologic diagnosis should be made only when epidemiologic or serologic evidence suggests the possibility of a dengue infection.

LABORATORY FINDINGS

In dengue fever, pancytopenia may develop after the 3-4 days of illness. Neutropenia may persist or reappear during the latter stage of the disease and may continue into convalescence, with white blood cell counts < 2,000/μL. Platelet counts rarely fall below 100,000/μL. Venous clotting, bleeding and prothrombin times, and plasma fibrinogen values are within normal ranges. The tourniquet test result may be positive. Mild acidosis, hemoconcentration, increased transaminase values, and hypoproteinemia may occur during some primary dengue virus infections. The electrocardiogram may show sinus bradycardia, ectopic ventricular foci, flattened T waves, and prolongation of the P-R interval.

The most common hematologic abnormalities during dengue hemorrhagic fever and dengue shock syndrome are hemoconcentration with an increase of > 20% in the hematocrit, thrombocytopenia, a prolonged bleeding time, and a moderately decreased prothrombin level that is seldom < 40% of control. Fibrinogen levels may be subnormal, and fibrin split-product values are elevated. Other abnormalities include moderate elevations of serum transaminase levels, consumption of complement, mild metabolic acidosis with hyponatremia, occasionally hypochloremia, slight elevation of serum urea nitrogen, and hypoalbuminemia. Roentgenograms of the chest reveal pleural effusions (right > left) in nearly all patients with dengue shock syndrome. Ultrasonography can be used to detect serosal effusions of the thorax or abdomen. Thickening of the gallbladder wall and the presence of perivesicular fluid are characteristic signs of increased vascular permeability.

TREATMENT

Treatment of uncomplicated dengue fever is supportive. Bed rest is advised during the febrile period. Antipyretics should be used to keep the body temperature < 40°C (104°F). Analgesics or mild sedation may be required to control pain. Aspirin is contraindicated and should not be used because of its effects on hemostasis. Fluid and electrolyte replacement is required for deficits caused by sweating, fasting, thirsting, vomiting, and diarrhea.

Dengue Hemorrhagic Fever and Dengue Shock Syndrome

Dengue shock syndrome is a medical emergency that may occur in any child who lives in or has a recent travel history to a tropical

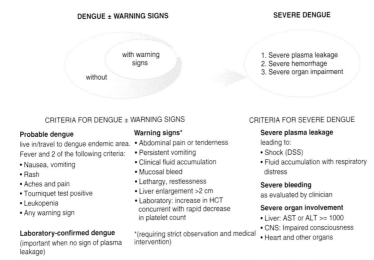

Fig. 295.1 Suggested dengue case classification and levels of severity. (*From World Health Organization (WHO) and Special Programme for Research and Training in Tropical Diseases (TDR): 2009 Dengue: guidelines for diagnosis, treatment, prevention and control, Fig. 1.4, http://apps. who.int/iris/bitstream/handle/10665/44188/9789241547871_eng.pdf?sequence=1.)*

destination. Management begins with diagnostic suspicion and the understanding that shock often accompanies defervescence. Detailed instructions for case management are available at the Geneva or New Delhi WHO websites: http://www.who.int/csr/don/archive/disease/dengue_fever/dengue.pdf. Management of dengue hemorrhagic fever and dengue shock syndrome includes immediate evaluation of vital signs and degrees of hemoconcentration, dehydration, and electrolyte imbalance. Close monitoring is essential for at least 48 hr because shock may occur or recur precipitously, usually several days after the onset of fever. Patients who are cyanotic or have labored breathing should be given oxygen. Rapid intravenous replacement of fluids and electrolytes can frequently sustain patients until spontaneous recovery occurs. Normal saline is more effective than the more expensive Ringer lactated saline in treating shock. When the pulse pressure is ≤10 mm Hg or when elevation of the hematocrit persists after the replacement of fluids, plasma or colloid preparations are indicated. Oral rehydration of children who are being monitored is useful. Prophylactic platelet transfusions have not been shown to reduce the risk of hemorrhaging or improve low platelet counts and may be associated with adverse effects.

Care must be taken to avoid overhydration, which may contribute to cardiac failure. Transfusions of fresh blood may be required to control bleeding but should not be given during hemoconcentration but only after evaluation of hemoglobin or hematocrit values. Salicylates are contraindicated because of their effect on blood clotting.

Sedation may be required for children who are markedly agitated. Use of vasopressors has not resulted in a significant reduction of mortality rates over that observed with simple supportive therapy. Disseminated intravascular coagulation may require treatment (see Chapter 510). Corticosteroids do not shorten the duration of disease or improve the prognosis in children receiving careful supportive therapy.

COMPLICATIONS

Hypervolemia during the fluid reabsorptive phase may be life-threatening and is heralded by a decrease in hematocrit with wide pulse pressure. Diuretics and digitalization may be necessary.

Primary infections with dengue fever and dengue-like diseases are usually self-limited and benign. Fluid and electrolyte losses, hyperpyrexia, and febrile convulsions are the most frequent complications in infants and young children. Epistaxis, petechiae, and purpuric lesions are uncommon but may occur at any stage. Blood from epistaxis that is swallowed, vomited, or passed by rectum may be erroneously interpreted as gastrointestinal bleeding. In adults and possibly in children, underlying conditions may lead to clinically significant bleeding. Convulsions may occur during a high temperature. Infrequently, after the febrile stage, prolonged asthenia, mental depression, bradycardia, and ventricular extrasystoles may occur in children.

In endemic areas, dengue hemorrhagic fever should be suspected in children with a febrile illness suggestive of dengue fever who experience hemoconcentration and thrombocytopenia.

PROGNOSIS
Dengue Fever
The prognosis for dengue fever is good. Care should be taken to avoid the use of drugs that suppress platelet activity.

Dengue Hemorrhagic Fever
The prognosis of dengue hemorrhagic fever is adversely affected by a late diagnosis and delayed or improper treatment. Death has occurred in 40–50% of patients with shock, but with adequate intensive care, deaths should occur in < 1% of cases. Infrequently, there is residual brain damage as a consequence of prolonged shock or occasionally of intracranial hemorrhage. Many fatalities are caused by overhydration.

PREVENTION
Dengue vaccines have been under development continuously since the 1970s. One such vaccine, Dengvaxia, developed by Sanofi Pasteur, is a mixture of four chimeras, DENV structural genes coupled with nonstructural genes of yellow fever 17D. In 2015, Dengvaxia completed phase III per protocol analyses on 32,568 children, vaccinated and controls, ages 2-16 yr. These studies revealed poor protection of seronegatives and good protection of seropositives with a reduction of hospitalization and severe disease in vaccinated children 9 yr old versus controls. Based on these data, this vaccine was endorsed by the WHO for targeted use in individuals 9 yr of age and older, living in countries that are highly endemic for dengue; it now is licensed for use in 14 countries. Other dengue type 1-4 vaccines are under development by the U.S. National Institutes of Health and Instituto Butantan in Sao Paulo, Brazil, and Takeda, Inc. Dengvaxia seronegative recipients who were incompletely protected were apparently sensitized to experience the enhanced disease of hospitalized dengue.

Prophylaxis in the absence of vaccine consists of avoiding daytime household-based mosquito bites through the use of insecticides, repellents, body covering with clothing, screening of houses, and destruction of *A. aegypti* breeding sites. If water storage is mandatory, a tight-fitting lid or a thin layer of oil may prevent egg laying or hatching. A larvicide, such as Abate (O,O′-[thiodi-*p*-phenylene] O,O,O′-tetramethyl phosphorothioate), available as a 1% sand-granule formation and effective at a concentration of 1 ppm, may be added safely to drinking water. Ultra-low-volume spray equipment effectively dispenses the adulticide malathion from trucks or airplanes for rapid intervention during an epidemic. Mosquito repellants and other personal antimosquito measures are effective in preventing mosquito bites in the field, forest, or jungle.

Bibliography is available at Expert Consult.

Chapter **296**
Yellow Fever
Scott B. Halstead

第二百九十六章
黄热病

中文导读

本章主要介绍了黄热病的病因学、流行病学、发病机制、临床表现、诊断、治疗、并发症和预防。本病由黄热病毒感染导致，通过蚊子叮咬传播。典型临床表现包括发热、头痛、肌痛、腰骶部疼痛、厌食、恶心和呕吐。实验室诊断方法包括抗原、抗体和基因检测。目前无特异性抗病毒药，以支持治疗为主。详细介绍了黄热病疫苗。

Yellow fever is an acute infection characterized in its most severe form by fever, jaundice, proteinuria, and hemorrhage. The virus is mosquito-borne and occurs in epidemic or endemic form in South America and Africa. Seasonal epidemics occurred in cities located in temperate areas of Europe and the Americas until 1900, and epidemics continue in West, Central, and East Africa.

ETIOLOGY

Yellow fever is the prototype of the *Flavivirus* genus of the family Flaviviridae, which are enveloped single-stranded RNA viruses 35-50 nm in diameter.

Yellow fever circulates zoonotically as five genotypes: type IA in West Central Africa, type IB in South America, type II in West Africa, type III in East Central Africa, and type IV in East Africa. Types IA and IB virus are capable of urban transmission between human beings by *Aedes aegypti*. Sometime in the 1600s, yellow fever virus was brought to the American tropics through the African slave trade. Subsequently, yellow fever caused enormous coastal and riverine epidemics in the Atlantic and Caribbean basins until the 20th century, when the virus and its urban and sylvan mosquito cycles were identified, mosquito control methods were perfected, and a vaccine was developed. The East and East/Central African genotypes have not fully entered the urban cycle and have not spread to the East Coast of Africa or to the countries of Asia.

EPIDEMIOLOGY

Human and nonhuman primate hosts acquire the yellow fever infection by the bite of infected mosquitoes. After an incubation period of 3-6 days, virus appears in the blood and may serve as a source of infection for other mosquitoes. The virus must replicate in the gut of the mosquito and pass to the salivary gland before the mosquito can transmit the virus. Yellow fever virus is transmitted in an urban cycle—human to *A. aegypti* to human—and a jungle cycle—monkey to jungle mosquitoes to monkey. Classic yellow fever epidemics in the United States, South America, the Caribbean, and parts of Europe were of the urban variety.

Since 2000, West Africa has experienced five urban epidemics, including in the capital cities of Abidjan (Cote d'Ivoire), Conakry (Guinea), and Dakar (Senegal). In 2012-2013, large outbreaks of East and East/Central yellow fever occurred across a large, predominantly rural area of war-ravaged Darfur in southwestern Sudan and in adjacent areas of northern Uganda. Beginning in 2015 and continuing to mid-2016, there were sharp outbreaks of yellow fever in and around Rwanda, Angola, and the bordering Democratic Republic of Congo, where there were 7,000 reported cases and 500 deaths. Eleven cases were imported into China by workers in Angola. In South America, all of the approximately 200 cases reported each year are jungle yellow fever. In late 2016 and continuing through 2018, a widespread zoonosis resulted in an estimated 2,000 yellow fever cases in Brazil. In colonial times, urban yellow fever attack rates in white adults were very high, suggesting that subclinical infections are uncommon in this age-group. Yellow fever may be less severe in children, with subclinical infection:clinical case ratios ≥ 2:1. In areas where outbreaks of urban yellow fever are common, most cases involve children because many adults are immune. Transmission in West Africa is highest during the rainy season, from July to November.

In tropical forests, yellow fever virus is maintained in a transmission cycle involving monkeys and tree hole–breeding mosquitoes (*Haemagogus* in Central and South America; the *Aedes africanus* complex in Africa). In the Americas, most cases involve tourists, campers, those who work in forested areas, and vacationers exposed to infected mosquitoes. In Africa, enzootic virus is prevalent in moist savanna and savanna transition areas, where other tree hole–breeding *Aedes* vectors transmit the virus between monkeys and humans and between humans.

PATHOGENESIS

Pathologic changes seen in the liver include (1) coagulative necrosis of hepatocytes in the midzone of the liver lobule, with sparing of cells around the portal areas and central veins; (2) eosinophilic degeneration of hepatocytes (**Councilman bodies**); (3) microvacuolar fatty change; and (4) minimal inflammation. The kidneys show acute tubular necrosis.

In the heart, myocardial fiber degeneration and fatty infiltration are seen. The brain may show edema and petechial hemorrhages. Direct viral injury to the liver results in impaired ability to perform functions of biosynthesis and detoxification; this is the central pathogenic event of yellow fever. Hemorrhage is postulated to result from decreased synthesis of vitamin K–dependent clotting factors and, in some cases, disseminated intravascular clotting. However, because the pathogenesis of shock in patients with yellow fever appears similar to that described for dengue shock syndrome and the other viral hemorrhagic fevers, viral damage to platelets and endothelial cells resulting in the release of prohemorrhagic factors may be the central mechanism of hemorrhage in yellow fever. Death and severe disease rates are lower in susceptible subSaharan African blacks than in other racial groups, suggesting existence of a resistance gene.

Renal dysfunction has been attributed to hemodynamic factors (prerenal failure progressing to acute tubular necrosis).

CLINICAL MANIFESTATIONS

In Africa, inapparent, abortive, or clinically mild infections are frequent; some studies suggest that children experience a milder disease than do adults. Abortive infections, characterized by fever and headache, may be unrecognized except during epidemics.

In its classic form, yellow fever begins with a sudden onset of fever, headache, myalgia, lumbosacral pain, anorexia, nausea, and vomiting. Physical findings during the early phase of illness, when virus is present in the blood, include prostration, conjunctival injection, flushing of the face and neck, reddening of the tongue at the tip and edges, and relative bradycardia. After 2-3 days, there may be a brief period of remission, followed in 6-24 hr by the reappearance of fever with vomiting, epigastric pain, jaundice, dehydration, gastrointestinal and other hemorrhages, albuminuria, hypotension, renal failure, delirium, convulsions, and coma. Death may occur after 7-10 days, with the fatality rate in severe cases approaching 50%. Some patients who survive the acute phase of illness later succumb to renal failure or myocardial damage. Laboratory abnormalities include leukopenia; prolonged clotting, prothrombin, and partial thromboplastin times; thrombocytopenia; hyperbilirubinemia; elevated serum transaminase values; albuminuria; and azotemia. Hypoglycemia may be present in severe cases. Electrocardiogram abnormalities such as bradycardia and ST-T changes are described.

DIAGNOSIS

Yellow fever should be suspected when fever, headache, vomiting, myalgia, and jaundice appear in residents of enzootic areas or in unimmunized visitors who have recently traveled (within 2 wk Before the onset of symptoms) to endemic areas. There are clinical similarities between yellow fever and dengue hemorrhagic fever. In contrast to the gradual onset of acute viral hepatitis resulting from hepatitis A, B, C, D, or E virus, jaundice in yellow fever appears after 3-5 days of high temperature and is often accompanied by severe prostration. Mild yellow fever is dengue-like and cannot be distinguished from a wide variety of other infections. Jaundice and fever may occur in any of several other tropical diseases, including malaria, viral hepatitis, louse-borne relapsing fever, leptospirosis, typhoid fever, rickettsial infections, certain systemic bacterial infections, sickle cell crisis, Rift Valley fever, Crimean-Congo hemorrhagic fever, and other viral hemorrhagic fevers. Outbreaks of yellow fever always include cases with severe gastrointestinal hemorrhage.

The specific diagnosis depends on the detection of the virus or viral antigen in acute-phase blood samples or antibody assays. The immunoglobulin M enzyme immunoassay is particularly useful. Sera obtained during the first 10 days after the onset of symptoms should be kept in an ultra-low-temperature freezer (−70°C [−94°F]) and shipped on dry ice for virus testing. Convalescent-phase samples for antibody tests are managed by conventional means. In handling acute-phase blood specimens, medical personnel must take care to avoid contaminating themselves or others on the evacuation trail (laboratory personnel and others). The postmortem diagnosis is based on virus isolation from liver or blood, identification of Councilman bodies in liver tissue, or detection of antigen or viral genome in liver tissue.

TREATMENT

It is customary to keep patients with yellow fever in a mosquito-free area, with use of mosquito nets if necessary. Patients are viremic during the febrile phase of the illness. Although there is no specific treatment for yellow fever, medical care is directed at maintaining the physiologic status with the following measures: (1) sponging and acetaminophen to reduce a high temperature, (2) vigorous fluid replacement of losses resulting from fasting, thirsting, vomiting, or plasma leakage, (3) correcting an acid-base imbalance, (4) maintaining nutritional intake to lessen the severity of hypoglycemia, and (5) avoiding drugs that are either metabolized by the liver or toxic to the liver, kidney, or central nervous system.

COMPLICATIONS

Complications of acute yellow fever include severe hemorrhage, liver failure, and acute renal failure. Bleeding should be managed by transfusion of fresh whole blood or fresh plasma with platelet concentrates if necessary. Renal failure may require peritoneal dialysis or hemodialysis.

PREVENTION

Yellow fever 17D is a live-attenuated vaccine with a long record of safety and efficacy. It is administered as a single 0.5-mL subcutaneous injection at least 10 days before arrival in a yellow fever–endemic area. YF-VAX, manufactured by Sanofi Pasteur, is licensed for use in the United States. With the exceptions noted later, individuals traveling to endemic areas in South America and Africa should be considered for vaccination, but the length of stay, exact locations to be visited, and environmental or occupational exposure may determine the specific risk and individual need for vaccination. Persons traveling from yellow fever–endemic to yellow fever–receptive countries may be required by national authorities to obtain a yellow fever vaccine (e.g., from South America or Africa to India). Usually, countries that require travelers to obtain a yellow fever immunization do not issue a visa without a valid immunization certificate. Vaccination is valid for 10 yr for international travel certification, although immunity lasts at least 40 yr and probably for life. Immunoglobulin M antibodies circulate for years after administration of yellow fever vaccine.

Since 1996, there have been a number of reports of *yellow fever vaccine–associated viscerotropic disease* with a higher risk in elderly vaccine recipients and a few cases in persons with previous thymectomies. Yellow fever vaccine should not be administered to persons who have symptomatic immunodeficiency diseases, are taking immunosuppressant drugs, have HIV, or have a history of thymectomy. A recent study has shown that individuals taking maintenance corticosteroids may be successfully vaccinated. Although the vaccine is not known to harm fetuses, its administration during pregnancy is not advised. The vaccine virus may be rarely transmitted through breastfeeding. In very young children, there is a small risk of encephalitis and death after yellow fever 17D vaccination. The 17D vaccine should not be administered to infants younger than 6 mo. Residence in or travel to areas of known or anticipated yellow fever activity (e.g., forested areas in the Amazon basin), which puts an individual at high risk, warrants immunization of infants 6-8 mo of age. Immunization of children 9 mo of age and older is routinely recommended before entry into endemic areas. Immunization of persons older than 60 yr of age should be weighed against their risk for sylvatic yellow fever in the American tropics and for urban or sylvatic yellow fever in Africa. Vaccination should be avoided in persons with a history of egg allergy. Alternatively, a skin test can be performed to determine whether a serious allergy exists that would preclude vaccination.

Bibliography is available at Expert Consult.

Chapter **297**

Ebola and Other Viral Hemorrhagic Fevers

Scott B. Halstead

第二百九十七章

埃博拉和其他病毒性出血热

中文导读

　　本章主要介绍了病毒性出血热的病因学、流行病学、临床表现、诊断、治疗和预防。详细阐述了克里米亚–刚果出血热、科萨努尔森林病、鄂木斯克出血热、裂谷热、阿根廷出血热、玻利维亚出血热、委内瑞拉出血热、拉萨热、马尔堡病、埃博拉出血热和肾综合征出血热的流行病学特点及临床特征。治疗方案包括利巴韦林、输血、肾脏替代治疗等。同时介绍了疫苗使用的现状。

Viral hemorrhagic fevers are a loosely defined group of clinical syndromes in which hemorrhagic manifestations are either common or especially notable in severe illness. Both the etiologic agents and clinical features of the syndromes differ, but coagulopathy may be a common pathogenetic feature.

ETIOLOGY

Six of the viral hemorrhagic fevers are caused by arthropod-borne viruses (arboviruses) (Table 297.1). Four are caused by togaviruses of the family **Flaviviridae:** Kyasanur Forest disease, Omsk hemorrhagic fever, dengue (see Chapter 295), and yellow fever (see Chapter 296) viruses. Three are caused by viruses of the family **Bunyaviridae:** Congo fever, Hantaan fever, and Rift Valley fever (RVF) viruses. Four are caused by viruses of the family **Arenaviridae:** Junin fever, Machupo fever, Guanarito fever, and Lassa fever. Two are caused by viruses in the family **Filoviridae:** Ebola virus and Marburg virus, enveloped, filamentous RNA viruses that are sometimes branched, unlike any other known virus.

EPIDEMIOLOGY

With some exceptions, the viruses causing viral hemorrhagic fevers are transmitted to humans via a nonhuman entity. The specific ecosystem required for viral survival determines the geographic distribution of disease. Although it is commonly thought that all viral hemorrhagic fevers are arthropod borne, seven may be contracted from environmental contamination caused by animals or animal cells or from infected humans (see Table 297.1). Laboratory and hospital infections have occurred with many of these agents. Lassa fever and Argentine and Bolivian hemorrhagic fevers are reportedly milder in children than in adults.

Crimean-Congo Hemorrhagic Fever

Sporadic human infection with Crimean-Congo hemorrhagic fever in Africa provided the original virus isolation. Natural foci are recognized in Bulgaria, western Crimea, and the Rostov-on-Don and Astrakhan regions; disease occurs in Central Asia from Kazakhstan to Pakistan. Index cases were followed by nosocomial transmission in Pakistan and Afghanistan in 1976, in the Arabian Peninsula in 1983, and in South Africa in 1984. In the Russian Federation, the vectors are ticks of the species *Hyalomma marginatum* and *Hyalomma anatolicum,* which, along with hares and birds, may serve as viral reservoirs. Disease occurs from June to September, largely among farmers and dairy workers.

Table 297.1	Viral Hemorrhagic Fevers	
MODE OF TRANSMISSION	**DISEASE**	**VIRUS**
Tick-borne	Crimean-Congo hemorrhagic fever (HF)*	Congo
	Kyasanur Forest disease	Kyasanur Forest disease
	Omsk HF	Omsk
Mosquito-borne[†]	Dengue HF	Dengue (4 types)
	Rift Valley fever	Rift Valley fever
	Yellow fever	Yellow fever
Infected animals or materials to humans	Argentine HF	Junin
	Bolivian HF	Machupo
	Lassa fever*	Lassa
	Marburg disease*	Marburg
	Ebola HF*	Ebola
	HF with renal syndrome	Hantaan

*Patients may be contagious; nosocomial infections are common.
[†]Chikungunya virus is associated infrequently with petechiae and epistaxis. Severe hemorrhagic manifestations have been reported in some cases.

Kyasanur Forest Disease

Human cases of Kyasanur Forest disease occur chiefly in adults in an area of Mysore State, India. The main vectors are two Ixodidae ticks, *Haemaphysalis turturis* and *Haemaphysalis spinigera.* Monkeys and forest rodents may be amplifying hosts. Laboratory infections are common.

Omsk Hemorrhagic Fever

Omsk hemorrhagic fever occurs throughout south-central Russia and northern Romania. Vectors may include *Dermacentor pictus* and *Dermacentor marginatus,* but direct transmission from moles and muskrats to humans seems well established. Human disease occurs in a spring–summer–autumn pattern, paralleling the activity of vectors. This infection occurs most frequently in persons with outdoor occupational exposure. Laboratory infections are common.

Rift Valley Fever

The virus causing RVF is responsible for epizootics involving sheep, cattle, buffalo, certain antelopes, and rodents in North, Central, East, and South Africa. The virus is transmitted to domestic animals by *Culex theileri* and several *Aedes* species. Mosquitoes may serve as reservoirs by transovarial transmission. An epizootic in Egypt in 1977-1978 was accompanied by thousands of human infections, principally among veterinarians, farmers, and farm laborers. Smaller outbreaks occurred in Senegal in 1987, Madagascar in 1990, and Saudi Arabia and Yemen in 2000-2001. Humans are most often infected during the slaughter or skinning of sick or dead animals. Laboratory infection is common.

Argentine Hemorrhagic Fever

Before the introduction of vaccine, hundreds to thousands of cases of Argentine hemorrhagic fever occurred annually from April through July in the maize-producing area northwest of Buenos Aires that reaches to the eastern margin of the Province of Cordoba. Junin virus has been isolated from the rodents *Mus musculus, Akodon arenicola,* and *Calomys laucha.* It infects migrant laborers who harvest the maize and who inhabit rodent-contaminated shelters.

Bolivian Hemorrhagic Fever

The recognized endemic area of Bolivian hemorrhagic fever consists of the sparsely populated province of Beni in Amazonian Bolivia. Sporadic cases occur in farm families who raise maize, rice, yucca, and beans. In the town of San Joaquin, a disturbance in the domestic rodent ecosystem may have led to an outbreak of household infection caused by Machupo virus transmitted by chronically infected *Calomys callosus,* ordinarily a field rodent. Mortality rates are high in young children.

Venezuelan Hemorrhagic Fever

In 1989, an outbreak of hemorrhagic illness occurred in the farming community of Guanarito, Venezuela, 200 miles south of Caracas. Subsequently, in 1990-1991, there were 104 cases reported with 26 deaths caused by Guanarito virus. Cotton rats *(Sigmodon alstoni)* and cane rats *(Zygodontomys brevicauda)* have been implicated as likely reservoirs of Venezuelan hemorrhagic fever.

Lassa Fever

Lassa virus has an unusual potential for human-to-human spread, which has resulted in many small epidemics in Nigeria, Sierra Leone, and Liberia. In 2012, an outbreak of more than 1,000 cases of Lassa fever occurred in east-central Nigeria. Medical workers in Africa and the United States have also contracted the disease. Patients with acute Lassa fever have been transported by international aircraft, necessitating extensive surveillance among passengers and crews. The virus is probably maintained in nature in a species of African peridomestic rodent, *Mastomys natalensis.* Rodent-to-rodent transmission and infection of humans probably operate via mechanisms established for other arenaviruses.

Marburg Disease

Previously, the world experience of human infections caused by Marburgvirus had been limited to 26 primary and 5 secondary cases in Germany and Yugoslavia in 1967 and to small outbreaks in Zimbabwe in 1975, Kenya in 1980 and 1988, and South Africa in 1983. However, in 1999 a large outbreak occurred in the Republic of Congo, and in 2005 a still larger outbreak occurred in Uige Province, Angola, with 252 cases and 227 deaths. In laboratory and clinical settings, transmission occurs by direct contact with tissues of the African green monkey or with infected human blood or semen. A reservoir in bats has been demonstrated. It appears that the virus is transmitted by close contact between fructivorous bats and from bats by aerosol to humans.

Ebola Hemorrhagic Fever

Ebola virus was isolated in 1976 from a devastating epidemic involving small villages in northern Zaire and southern Sudan; smaller outbreaks have occurred subsequently. Outbreaks have initially been nosocomial. Attack rates have been highest in children from birth to 1 yr of age and persons from 15 to 50 yr of age. The virus is in the *Filovirus* family and closely related to viruses of the genus Marburg virus. An Ebola virus epidemic occurred in Kikwit, Zaire, in 1995, followed by scattered outbreaks in Uganda and Central and West Africa. The virus has been recovered from chimpanzees, and antibodies have been found in other subhuman primates, which apparently acquire infection from a zoonotic reservoir in bats. The natural reservoir of Ebola is believed to be fruit bats. Reston virus, related to Ebola virus, has been recovered from Philippine monkeys and pigs and has caused subclinical infections in humans working in monkey colonies in the United States.

In 2014, West Africa experienced the largest outbreak of Ebola virus disease (EVD) in history and the first transmission in a large urban area (Fig. 297.1). Countries primarily affected were Liberia, Sierra Leone, and Guinea, with imported cases reported in Nigeria, Mali, and Senegal, as well as Europe and the United States. The outbreak was caused by the Zaire Ebola virus (species of Ebola virus include the Zaire, Sudan, Bundibugyo, Reston, and Tai Forest species), which has a mortality rate of approximately 55–65%. As of 8 May 2016, the World Health Organization (WHO) and respective governments reported a total of 28,616 suspected cases and 11,310 deaths (39.5%), though the WHO believes that this substantially understates the magnitude of the outbreak. The outbreak had largely subsided by the end of 2015. In 2018, an outbreak occurred in the Democratic Republic of the Congo, affecting more than 500 people (aged 8-80 yr), with a case fatality of approximately 50% (Fig. 297.2).

EVD may occur following exposure to fruit bats or bushmeat but most often occurs through exposure to body fluids of infected individuals (blood, sweat, saliva, vomitus, diarrhea, and less often human milk or semen) (Table 297.2). Persistent infection after recovery from acute EVD has been well documented, with virus particles present in body fluids such as semen for many months in apparently healthy survivors. Patients are infectious once they are symptomatic; the incubation period is 2-21 days (mean: 11 days). The age range in the West African epidemic was broad, but most patients were between 15 and 44 yr old.

Hemorrhagic Fever With Renal Syndrome

The endemic area of hemorrhagic fever with renal syndrome (HFRS), also known as *epidemic hemorrhagic fever* and *Korean hemorrhagic fever,* includes Japan, Korea, far eastern Siberia, north and central China, European and Asian Russia, Scandinavia, Czechoslovakia, Romania, Bulgaria, Yugoslavia, and Greece. Although the incidence and severity of hemorrhagic manifestations and the mortality rates are lower in Europe than in northeastern Asia, the renal lesions are the same. Disease in Scandinavia, **nephropathia epidemica,** is caused by a different although antigenically related virus, Puumala virus, associated with the bank vole, *Clethrionomys glareolus.* Cases occur predominantly in the spring and summer. There appears to be no age factor in susceptibility, but because of occupational hazards, young adult men are most frequently attacked. Rodent plagues and evidence of rodent infestation have accompanied endemic and epidemic occurrences. Hantaan virus has been detected in the lung tissue and excreta of *Apodemus agrarius coreae.* Antigenically related agents have been detected in laboratory rats and in urban rat populations around the world, including Prospect Hill

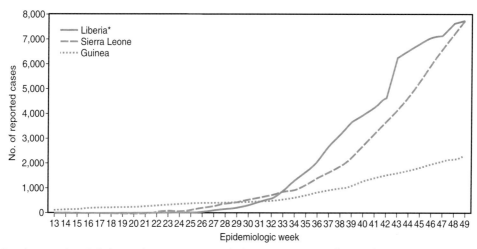

Fig. 297.1 Cumulative number of Ebola virus disease cases reported—three countries, West Africa, April 13, 2016. Reported from Sierra Leone (14,124 cases) and Liberia (10,678), followed by Guinea (3,814). *(Data from the number of cases and deaths in Guinea, Liberia, and Sierra Leone during the 2014-2016 West Africa Ebola Outbreak. Accessed at https://www.cdc.gov/vhf/ebola/outbreaks/2014-west-africa/case-counts.html.)*

virus in the wild rodent *Microtus pennsylvanicus* in North America and *sin nombre* virus in the deer mouse in the southern and southwestern United States; these viruses are causes of hantavirus pulmonary syndrome (see Chapter 299). Rodent-to-rodent and rodent-to-human transmission presumably occurs via the respiratory route.

CLINICAL MANIFESTATIONS

Dengue hemorrhagic fever (see Chapter 295) and yellow fever (see Chapter 296) cause similar syndromes in children in endemic areas.

Crimean-Congo Hemorrhagic Fever

The incubation period of 3-12 days is followed by a febrile period of 5-12 days and a prolonged convalescence. Illness begins suddenly with fever, severe headache, myalgia, abdominal pain, anorexia, nausea, and vomiting. After 1-2 days, the fever may subside until the patient experiences an erythematous facial or truncal flush and injected conjunctivae. A second febrile period of 2-6 days then develops, with a hemorrhagic enanthem on the soft palate and a fine petechial rash on the chest and abdomen. Less frequently, there are large areas of purpura and bleeding from the gums, nose, intestines, lungs, or uterus. Hematuria and proteinuria are relatively rare. During the hemorrhagic stage, there is usually tachycardia with diminished heart sounds and occasionally hypotension. The liver is usually enlarged, but there is no icterus. In protracted cases, central nervous system signs include delirium, somnolence, and progressive clouding of the consciousness. Early in the disease, leukopenia with relative lymphocytosis, progressively worsening thrombocytopenia, and gradually increasing anemia occur. In convalescence there may be hearing and memory loss. The mortality rate is 2–50%.

Kyasanur Forest Disease and Omsk Hemorrhagic Fever

After an incubation period of 3-8 days, both Kyasanur Forest disease and Omsk hemorrhagic fever begin with the sudden onset of fever and headache. Kyasanur Forest disease is characterized by severe myalgia, prostration, and bronchiolar involvement; it often manifests without hemorrhage but occasionally with severe gastrointestinal bleeding. In Omsk hemorrhagic fever, there is moderate epistaxis, hematemesis, and a hemorrhagic enanthem but no profuse hemorrhage; bronchopneumonia is common. In both diseases, severe leukopenia and thrombocytopenia, vascular dilation, increased vascular permeability, gastrointestinal hemorrhages, and subserosal and interstitial petechial hemorrhages occur. Kyasanur Forest disease may be complicated by acute degeneration of the renal tubules and focal liver damage. In many patients, recurrent febrile illness may follow an afebrile period of 7-15 days. This second phase takes the form of a meningoencephalitis.

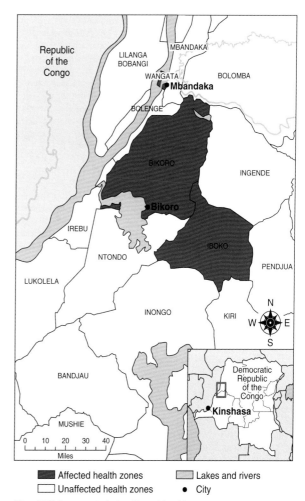

Fig. 297.2 Map of Ebola-affected health zones in the Democratic Republic of the Congo (DRC), 2018. *(Courtesy of the Centers for Disease Control and Prevention, 2018. Accessed at https://www.cdc.gov/vhf/ebola/outbreaks/drc/drc-map.html.)*

Table 297.2	Clinical Recommendations for Ebola Virus Infection	
RECOMMENDATION	**POPULATION**	**INTERVENTION**
1	Oral rehydration	Patients with suspected, probable, or confirmed Ebola virus disease
2	Parenteral administration of fluids	Patients with suspected, probable, or confirmed Ebola virus disease who are unable to drink or who have inadequate oral intake
3	Systematic monitoring and charting of vital signs and volume status	Patients with suspected, probable, or confirmed Ebola virus disease
4	Serum biochemistry	Patients with suspected, probable, or confirmed Ebola virus disease
5	Staffing ratio	Patients with suspected, probable, or confirmed Ebola virus disease
6	Communication with family and friends	Patients with suspected, probable, or confirmed Ebola virus disease
7	Analgesic therapy	Patients with suspected, probable, or confirmed Ebola virus disease who are in pain
8	Antibiotics	Patients with suspected, probable, or confirmed Ebola virus disease with high severity of illness

*Confidence is based on the quality of the evidence for the main outcome.
Modified from Lamontagne F, Fowler RA, Adhikari NK, et al: Evidence-based guidelines for supportive care of patients with Ebola virus disease, Lancet 391:700-708, 2018,Table 2.

Rift Valley Fever

Most RVF infections have occurred in adults with signs and symptoms resembling those of dengue fever (see Chapter 295). The onset is acute, with fever, headache, prostration, myalgia, anorexia, nausea, vomiting, conjunctivitis, and lymphadenopathy. The fever lasts 3-6 days and is often biphasic. The convalescence is often prolonged. In the 1977-1978 outbreak, many patients died after showing signs that included purpura, epistaxis, hematemesis, and melena. RVF affects the uvea and posterior chorioretina; macular scarring, vascular occlusion, and optic atrophy occur, resulting in permanent visual loss in a high proportion of patients with mild to severe RVF. At autopsy, extensive eosinophilic degeneration of the parenchymal cells of the liver has been observed.

Argentine, Venezuelan, and Bolivian Hemorrhagic Fevers and Lassa Fever

The incubation period in Argentine, Venezuelan, and Bolivian hemorrhagic fevers and Lassa fever is commonly 7-14 days; the acute illness lasts for 2-4 wk. Clinical illnesses range from undifferentiated fever to the characteristic severe illness. **Lassa fever** is most often clinically severe in white persons. The onset is usually gradual, with increasing fever, headache, diffuse myalgia, and anorexia (Table 297.3). During the first wk., signs frequently include a sore throat, dysphagia, cough, oropharyngeal ulcers, nausea, vomiting, diarrhea, and pains in the chest and abdomen. Pleuritic chest pain may persist for 2-3 wk. In Argentine and Bolivian hemorrhagic fevers and less frequently in Lassa fever, a petechial enanthem appears on the soft palate 3-5 days after onset and at about the same time on the trunk. The tourniquet test may be positive. The clinical course of Venezuelan hemorrhagic fever has not been well described.

In 35–50% of patients, these diseases may become severe, with persistent high temperature, increasing toxicity, swelling of the face or neck, microscopic hematuria, and frank hemorrhages from the stomach, intestines, nose, gums, and uterus. A syndrome of **hypovolemic shock** is accompanied by pleural effusion and renal failure. **Respiratory distress** resulting from airway obstruction, pleural effusion, or congestive heart failure may occur. A total of 10–20% of patients experience late neurologic involvement, characterized by intention tremor of the tongue and associated speech abnormalities. In severe cases, there may be intention tremors of the extremities, seizures, and delirium. The cerebrospinal fluid is normal. In Lassa fever, nerve deafness occurs in early convalescence in 25% of cases. Prolonged convalescence is accompanied by alopecia and, in Argentine and Bolivian hemorrhagic fevers, by signs of autonomic nervous system lability, such as postural hypotension, spontaneous flushing or blanching of the skin, and intermittent diaphoresis.

Laboratory studies reveal marked leukopenia, mild to moderate thrombocytopenia, proteinuria, and, in Argentine hemorrhagic fever,

Table 297.3	Clinical Stages of Lassa Fever
STAGE	**SYMPTOMS**
1 (days 1-3)	General weakness and malaise. High fever > 39°C (102.2°F), constant with peaks of 40-41°C (104-105.8°F)
2 (days 4-7)	Sore throat (with white exudative patches) very common; headache; back, chest, side, or abdominal pain; conjunctivitis; nausea and vomiting; diarrhea; productive cough; proteinuria; low blood pressure (systolic < 100 mm Hg); anemia
3 (after 7 days)	Facial edema; convulsions; mucosal bleeding (mouth, nose, eyes); internal bleeding; confusion or disorientation
4 (after 14 days)	Coma and death

From Richmond JK, Baglole DJ: Lassa fever: epidemiology, clinical features, and social consequences, BMJ 327:1271-1275, 2003.

moderate abnormalities in blood clotting, decreased fibrinogen, increased fibrinogen split products, and elevated serum transaminases. There is focal, often extensive eosinophilic necrosis of the liver parenchyma, focal interstitial pneumonitis, focal necrosis of the distal and collecting tubules, and partial replacement of splenic follicles by amorphous eosinophilic material. Usually bleeding occurs by diapedesis with little inflammatory reaction. The mortality rate is 10–40%.

Marburg Disease and Ebola Hemorrhagic Fever

After an incubation period of 4-7 days, the illness begins abruptly, with severe frontal headache, malaise, drowsiness, lumbar myalgia, vomiting, nausea, and diarrhea. A **maculopapular** eruption begins 5-7 days later on the trunk and upper arms. It becomes generalized and often hemorrhagic and exfoliates during convalescence. The exanthem is accompanied by a dark red enanthem on the hard palate, conjunctivitis, and scrotal or labial edema. Gastrointestinal hemorrhage occurs as the severity of illness increases. Late in the illness, the patient may become tearfully depressed, with marked hyperalgesia to tactile stimuli. In fatal cases, patients become hypotensive, restless, and confused and lapse into coma. Convalescent patients may experience alopecia and may have paresthesias of the back and trunk. There is a marked leukopenia with necrosis of granulocytes. Dysfunction in bleeding and clotting and thrombocytopenia are universal and correlated with the severity of disease; there are moderate abnormalities in concentrations of clotting proteins and elevations of serum transaminases and amylase. Pregnant women and young children are at high risk of severe disease with a fatal outcome. The mortality rate of Marburg disease is 25–85%, and the mortality rate of Ebola hemorrhagic fever 50–90%. High viral loads in acute-phase blood samples convey a poor prognosis. Viral RNA persists in tissues long after symptoms subside, and the virus has been excreted in semen more than 1 yr after recovery.

Manifestations of EVD may come in stages, but most EVD begins with the sudden onset of fever accompanied by fatigue, weakness, myalgias, headache, and sore throat. This is followed by gastrointestinal involvement, including anorexia, nausea, abdominal pain, vomiting, and diarrhea. Hemorrhage (defined by any evidence of bleeding) is seen in more than 50% and is a serious later phase, often accompanied by vascular leakage, multiorgan failure, and death. Those who survive improve on approximately days 6-11 of EVD. One late relapse, producing meningoencephalitis, has been reported.

Hemorrhagic Fever With Renal Syndrome
In most cases, HFRS is characterized by fever, petechiae, mild hemorrhagic phenomena, and mild proteinuria, followed by a relatively uneventful recovery. In 20% of recognized cases, the disease may progress through four distinct phases. The febrile phase is ushered in with fever, malaise, and facial and truncal flushing. It lasts 3-8 days and ends with thrombocytopenia, petechiae, and proteinuria. The hypotensive phase, of 1-3 days, follows defervescence. Loss of fluid from the intravascular compartment may result in marked hemoconcentration. Proteinuria and ecchymoses increase. The oliguric phase, usually 3-5 days in duration, is characterized by a low output of protein-rich urine, increasing nitrogen retention, nausea, vomiting, and dehydration. Confusion, extreme restlessness, and hypertension are common. The diuretic phase, which may last for days or weeks, usually initiates clinical improvement. The kidneys show little concentrating ability, and rapid loss of fluid may result in severe dehydration and shock. Potassium and sodium depletion may be severe. Fatal cases manifest as abundant protein-rich retroperitoneal edema and marked hemorrhagic necrosis of the renal medulla. The mortality rate is 5–10%.

DIAGNOSIS
The diagnosis of these viral hemorrhagic fevers depends on a high index of suspicion in endemic areas. In nonendemic areas, histories of recent travel, recent laboratory exposure, or exposure to an earlier case should evoke suspicion of a viral hemorrhagic fever.

In all viral hemorrhagic fevers, the viral agent circulates in the blood at least transiently during the early febrile stage. Togaviruses and bunyaviruses can be recovered from acute-phase serum samples by inoculation into a tissue culture or living mosquitoes. Argentine, Bolivian, and Venezuelan hemorrhagic fever viruses can be isolated from acute-phase blood or throat washings by intracerebral inoculation into guinea pigs, infant hamsters, or infant mice. Lassa virus may be isolated from acute-phase blood or throat washings by inoculation into tissue cultures. For Marburg disease and Ebola hemorrhagic fever, acute-phase throat washings, blood, and urine may be inoculated into a tissue culture, guinea pigs, or monkeys. The viruses are readily identified on electron microscopy, with a filamentous structure differentiating them from all other known agents. Specific complement-fixing and immunofluorescent antibodies appear during convalescence. The virus of HFRS is recovered from acute-phase serum or urine by inoculation into a tissue culture. A variety of antibody tests using viral subunits is becoming available. The serologic diagnosis depends on the demonstration of seroconversion or a four-fold or greater increase in immunoglobulin G antibody titer in acute and convalescent serum specimens collected 3-4 wk apart. Viral RNA may also be detected in blood or tissues with the use of reverse transcriptase polymerase chain reaction analysis.

The diagnosis of EVD is confirmed by enzyme-linked immunosorbent assay immunoglobulin M and polymerase chain reaction (which may need to be repeated if initially negative) testing. Criteria to aid in the diagnosis of EVD include temperature > 38.6°C (101.5°F) plus symptoms; contact with an affected patient, the patient's body fluids, or the funeral; residence in or travel to an endemic region; or a history of handling bats, rodents, or primates from an endemic area.

Handling blood and other biologic specimens is hazardous and must be performed by specially trained personnel. Blood and autopsy specimens should be placed in tightly sealed metal containers, wrapped in absorbent material inside a sealed plastic bag, and shipped on dry ice to laboratories with biocontainment safety level 4 facilities. Even routine hematologic and biochemical tests should be done with extreme caution.

Differential Diagnosis
Mild cases of hemorrhagic fever may be confused with almost any self-limited systemic bacterial or viral infection. More severe cases may suggest typhoid fever; epidemic, murine, or scrub typhus; leptospirosis; or a rickettsial spotted fever, for which effective chemotherapeutic agents are available. Many of these disorders may be acquired in geographic or ecologic locations endemic for a viral hemorrhagic fever.

The differential diagnosis of EVD includes malaria, typhoid, Lassa fever, influenza infection, and meningococcemia.

TREATMENT
Ribavirin administered intravenously is effective in reducing mortality rates in Lassa fever and HFRS. Further information and advice about the management, control measures, diagnosis, and collection of biohazardous specimens can be obtained from the Centers for Disease Control and Prevention, National Center for Infectious Diseases, Viral Special Pathogens Branch, Atlanta, Georgia 30333 (470-312-0094).

The therapeutic principle involved in all of these diseases, especially HFRS, is the reversal of dehydration, hemoconcentration, renal failure, and protein, electrolyte, or blood losses (see Table 297.2). The contribution of disseminated intravascular coagulopathy to the hemorrhagic manifestations is unknown, and the management of hemorrhage should be individualized. Transfusions of fresh blood and platelets are frequently given. Good results have been reported in a few patients after the administration of clotting factor concentrates. The efficacy of corticosteroids, ε-aminocaproic acid, pressor amines, and α-adrenergic blocking agents has not been established. Sedatives should be selected with regard to the possibility of kidney or liver damage. The successful management of HFRS may require renal dialysis.

Whole-blood transfusions from Ebola virus–immune donors and administration of Ebola monoclonal antibodies have been shown to be effective in lowering case fatality rates.

Patients suspected of having Lassa fever, Ebola fever, Marburg fever, or Congo-Crimean hemorrhagic fever should be placed in a private room on standard contact and droplet precautions. Caretakers should use barrier precautions to prevent skin or mucous membrane exposure. All persons entering the patient's room should wear gloves and gowns and face shields. Before exiting the patient's room, caretakers should safely remove and dispose of all protective gear and should clean and disinfect shoes. Protocols require two-person clinical care teams, one observer and one caregiver (see CDC website: www.cdc.gov/vhf/ebola).

Treatment of EVD often requires an intensive care unit and management of multiorgan system dysfunction, including correction of hypovolemia, hyponatremia, hypokalemia, hypoalbuminemia, hypocalcemia, and hypoxia, often with renal replacement therapy as well as ventilation support (Table 297.2). Convalescent serum and monoclonal antibodies have been employed on an experimental basis. Strict isolation and appropriate barrier protection of healthcare workers is mandatory. Several vaccines have been shown to be immunogenic, and one used late in the epidemic was protective. Epidemic control measures, isolation, and quarantine have been used to attempt to decrease the spread of the West African epidemic.

PREVENTION
A live-attenuated vaccine (Candid-I) for Argentine hemorrhagic fever (Junin virus) is highly efficacious. A form of inactivated mouse brain vaccine is reported to be effective in preventing Omsk hemorrhagic fever. Inactivated RVF vaccines are widely used to protect domestic animals and laboratory workers. HFRS inactivated vaccine is licensed in Korea, and killed and live-attenuated vaccines are widely used in

China. A vaccinia-vector glycoprotein vaccine provides protection against Lassa fever in monkeys. Single doses of recombinant vesicular stomatitis virus or adenovirus type 3 vaccines containing surface glycoproteins from Ebola and Marburg viruses have been shown to protect monkeys against Ebola virus and Marburg virus disease. The vesicular stomatitis-vectored Ebola vaccine was shown to be effective in preventing Ebola cases in a ring vaccination trial in Guinea and has been used widely in the 2018 Congo outbreak.

Prevention of mosquito-borne and tick-borne infections includes use of repellents, wearing of tight-fitting clothing that fully covers the extremities, and careful examination of the skin after exposure, with removal of any vectors found. Diseases transmitted from a rodent-infected environment can be prevented through methods of rodent control; elimination of refuse and breeding sites is particularly successful in urban and suburban areas.

Patients should be isolated until they are virus-free or for 3 wk after illness. Patient urine, sputum, blood, clothing, and bedding should be disinfected. Disposable syringes and needles should be used. Prompt and strict enforcement of barrier nursing may be lifesaving. The mortality rate among medical workers contracting these diseases is 50%. A few entirely asymptomatic Ebola infections result in strong antibody production.

Bibliography is available at Expert Consult.

Chapter 298
Lymphocytic Choriomeningitis Virus
Daniel J. Bonthius

第二百九十八章
淋巴细胞性脉络丛脑膜炎病毒

中文导读

　　本章主要介绍了淋巴细胞性脉络丛脑膜炎病毒感染的病因学、流行病学、发病机制、临床表现、实验室检查、诊断和鉴别诊断、并发症、治疗、预后和预防。临床表现包括获得性（产后）和先天性淋巴细胞性脉络丛脑膜炎病毒感染。其中获得性感染分为非特异性病毒综合征和无菌性脑膜炎两个临床阶段；先天性感染的临床特点为视力损害和脑功能障碍。目前无特异性抗病毒药，主要介绍了支持治疗。

Lymphocytic choriomeningitis virus (LCMV) is a prevalent human pathogen and an important cause of meningitis in children and adults. Capable of crossing the placenta and infecting the fetus, LCMV is also an important cause of neurologic birth defects and encephalopathy in the newborn.

ETIOLOGY
LCMV is a member of the family Arenaviridae, which are enveloped, negative-sense single-stranded RNA viruses. The name of the arenaviruses is derived from *arenosus,* the Latin word for "sandy," because of the fine granularities observed within the virion on ultrathin electron microscopic sections.

EPIDEMIOLOGY
Like all arenaviruses, LCMV utilizes rodents as its reservoir. The common house mouse, *Mus musculus,* is both the natural host and primary reservoir for the virus, which is transferred vertically from one generation of mice to the next via intrauterine infection. Hamsters and guinea pigs are also potential reservoirs. Although heavily infected with LCMV, rodents that acquire the virus transplacentally often remain asymptomatic because congenital infection provides rodents with immunologic tolerance for the virus. Infected rodents shed the virus in large quantities in nasal secretions, urine, feces, saliva, and milk throughout their lives.

Humans typically acquire LCMV by contacting fomites contaminated with infectious virus or by inhaling aerosolized virus. Most human infections occur during the fall and early winter, when mice move into human habitations. Humans can also acquire the virus via organ transplantation. Congenital LCMV infection occurs when a woman acquires a primary LCMV infection during pregnancy. The virus passes through the placenta to the fetus during maternal viremia. The fetus may also acquire the virus during passage through the birth canal from exposure to infected vaginal secretions. Outside of organ transplantation and vertical transmission during pregnancy, there have been no cases of human-to-human transmission of LCMV.

LCMV is prevalent in the environment, has a great geographic range, and infects large numbers of humans. The virus is found throughout the world's temperate regions and probably occurs wherever the genus *Mus* has been introduced (which is every continent but Antarctica). An epidemiologic study found that 9% of house mice are infected and that substantial clustering occurs, where the prevalence is higher. Serologic studies demonstrate that approximately 5% of adult humans possess antibodies to LCMV, indicating prior exposure and infection.

PATHOGENESIS

LCMV is not a cytolytic virus. Thus, unlike many other nervous system pathogens that directly damage the brain by killing host brain cells, LCMV pathogenesis involves other underlying mechanisms. Furthermore, the pathogenic mechanisms are different in postnatal (acquired) infection than in prenatal (congenital) infection. A critical difference in the pathogenesis of postnatal versus prenatal infection is that the virus infects brain parenchyma in the case of prenatal infection, but is restricted to the meninges and choroid plexus in postnatal cases.

In postnatal infections, LCMV replicates to high titers in the choroid plexus and meninges. Viral antigen within these tissues becomes the target of an acute mononuclear cell infiltration driven by CD8+ T lymphocytes. The presence of lymphocytes in large numbers within the meninges and cerebrospinal fluid leads to the symptoms of meningitis that mark acquired LCMV infection. As the lymphocytes clear the virus from the meninges and cerebrospinal fluid, the density of lymphocytes declines, and the symptoms of meningitis resolve. Thus, symptoms of acquired (postnatal) LCMV infection are immune mediated and are a result of the presence of large numbers of lymphocytes.

Prenatal infection likewise inflames the tissues surrounding the brain parenchyma, and this inflammation leads to some of the signs of congenital LCMV. In particular, within the ventricular system, congenital LCMV infection often leads to ependymal inflammation, which may block the egress of cerebrospinal fluid (CSF) at the cerebral aqueduct and lead to hydrocephalus. However, unlike postnatal cases, prenatal infection with LCMV includes infection of the substance of the brain rather than just the meninges or ependyma. This infection of brain parenchyma leads to the substantial neuropathologic changes typically accompanying congenital LCMV infection. In particular, LCMV infects the mitotically active neuroblasts, located at periventricular sites. Through an unknown mechanism, the presence of the virus kills these periventricular cells, leading to periventricular calcifications, a radiographic hallmark of this disorder. Within the fetal brain, LCMV infection of neurons and glial cells also disrupts neuronal migration, leading to abnormal gyral patterns, and interferes with neuronal mitosis, leading to microcephaly and cerebellar hypoplasia.

CLINICAL MANIFESTATIONS

The clinical manifestations of LCMV infection depend on whether the infection occurs prenatally or postnatally. Congenital infection with LCMV is unique, as it involves both the postnatal infection of a pregnant woman and the prenatal infection of a fetus.

Acquired (Postnatal) Lymphocytic Choriomeningitis Virus Infection

LCMV infection during postnatal life (during childhood or adulthood) typically consists of a brief febrile illness, from which the patient fully recovers. The illness classically consists of two clinical phases. In the first phase, the symptoms are those of a nonspecific viral syndrome and include fever, myalgia, malaise, nausea, anorexia, and vomiting. These symptoms usually resolve after several days but are followed by a second phase, consisting of central nervous system disease. The symptoms of this second phase are those of aseptic meningitis, including headache, fever, nuchal rigidity, photophobia, and vomiting. The entire course of the biphasic disease is typically 1-3 wk.

The clinical spectrum of LCMV infection is broad. One third of postnatal infections are asymptomatic. Other patients develop extraneural disease that extends beyond the usual symptoms and may include orchitis,

pneumonitis, myocarditis, parotitis, dermatitis, alopecia, and pharyngitis. In others, the neurologic disease may be considerably more severe than usual and may include transverse myelitis, Guillain-Barré syndrome, hydrocephalus, and encephalitis. Recovery from acquired LCMV infection is usually complete, but fatalities occasionally occur.

LCMV infections acquired via solid-organ transplantation always induce severe disease. Several weeks following the transplantation, recipients of infected organs develop fever, leukopenia, and lethargy. Following these nonspecific symptoms, the course of the disease rapidly progresses to multiorgan system failure and shock. These cases are almost always fatal.

Congenital Lymphocytic Choriomeningitis Virus Infection

LCMV infection during pregnancy can kill the fetus and induce spontaneous abortion. Among surviving fetuses, the two clinical hallmarks of congenital LCMV infection are vision impairment and brain dysfunction.

The vision impairment in congenital LCMV infection is a result of **chorioretinitis** and the formation of chorioretinal scars. The scarring is usually bilateral and most commonly located in the periphery of the fundus, but involvement of the macula also occurs.

Although the retinal injuries from congenital LCMV infection are often severe, it is the *brain* effects that cause the greatest disability. Prenatal infection with LCMV commonly induces either macrocephaly or microcephaly. **Macrocephaly** following LCMV infection is almost invariably caused by noncommunicating hydrocephalus, stemming from inflammation within the ventricular system. **Microcephaly** is a result of the virus-induced failure of brain growth. In addition to disturbances of head size, periventricular calcifications are also cardinal features of congenital LCMV infection.

Although hydrocephalus, microcephaly, and periventricular calcifications are by far the most commonly observed abnormalities of the brain in congenital LCMV, other forms of neuropathology, alone or in combination, can also occur. These include periventricular cysts, porencephalic cysts, encephalomalacia, intraparenchymal calcifications, cerebellar hypoplasia, and neuronal migration disturbances.

Infants with congenital LCMV infection typically present during the newborn period with evidence of brain dysfunction. The most common signs are lethargy, seizures, irritability, and jitteriness.

Within the fetus, LCMV has a specific tropism for the brain. Thus, unlike many other congenital infections, LCMV usually does not induce systemic manifestations. Birthweight is typically appropriate for gestational age. Skin rashes and thrombocytopenia, which are common in several other prominent congenital infections, are unusual in congenital LCMV infection. Hepatosplenomegaly is only rarely observed, and serum liver enzyme levels are usually normal. Auditory deficits are unusual.

LABORATORY FINDINGS

In acquired (postnatal) LCMV infection, the hallmark laboratory abnormality occurs during the second (central nervous system) phase of the disease and is CSF pleocytosis. The CSF typically contains hundreds to thousands of white blood cells, almost all of which are lymphocytes. However, CSF eosinophilia may also occur. Mild elevations of CSF protein and hypoglycorrhachia are common.

In congenital LCMV infection, laboratory findings in the newborn depend on whether the infant is still infected or not. If the infant still harbors the infection, then examination of the CSF may reveal a lymphocytic pleocytosis. Unlike many other congenital infections, LCMV does not typically induce elevations in liver enzymes, thrombocytopenia, or anemia. In many cases, the most reliably abnormal test is the head CT scan, which typically reveals a combination of microencephaly, hydrocephalus, and periventricular calcifications (Fig. 298.1).

DIAGNOSIS AND DIFFERENTIAL DIAGNOSIS

Acute LCMV infections can be diagnosed by isolating the virus from CSF. Polymerase chain reaction has also been used to detect LCMV RNA in patients with active infections. However, by the time of birth,

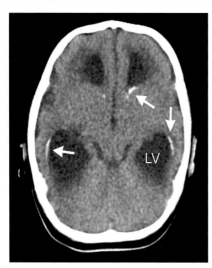

Fig. 298.1 Head CT scan from a 2 mo old microcephalic baby with congenital lymphocytic choriomeningitis virus infection. The scan reveals enlargement of the lateral ventricles *(LV)* and periventricular calcifications *(arrows)*.

a baby prenatally infected with LCMV may no longer harbor the virus. Thus, congenital LCMV infection is more commonly diagnosed by serologic testing. The immunofluorescent antibody test detects both immunoglobulin (Ig) M and IgG and has greater sensitivity than the more widely available complement fixation method. The immunofluorescent antibody test is commercially available, and its specificity and sensitivity make it an acceptable diagnostic tool. A more sensitive test for detecting congenital LCMV infection is the enzyme-linked immunosorbent assay, which measures titers of LCMV IgG and IgM and is performed at the Centers for Disease Control and Prevention.

For acquired (postnatal) LCMV infection, the principal items in the differential diagnosis are the other infectious agents that can induce meningitis. These include bacteria, fungi, viruses, and some other forms of pathogens. The most common viral causes of meningitis are the enteroviruses, including coxsackieviruses and echoviruses, and the arboviruses, including La Crosse encephalitis virus and equine encephalitis virus. Unlike LCMV, which is most common in winter, the enteroviruses and arboviruses are most commonly acquired in summer and early fall.

The principal items in the differential diagnosis of congenital LCMV infection are the other infectious pathogens that can cross the placenta and damage the developing fetus. These infectious agents are linked by the acronym TORCHS and include *Toxoplasma gondii,* rubella virus, cytomegalovirus, herpes simplex virus, and syphilis. Toxoplasmosis, Zika virus infection, and cytomegalovirus infection are particularly difficult to differentiate from LCMV, because all of these infectious agents can produce microcephaly, intracerebral calcifications, and chorioretinitis. Although clinical clues may aid in distinguishing one congenital infection from another, definitive identification of the causative infectious agent usually requires laboratory data, including cultures and serologic studies.

COMPLICATIONS

Complications in children with congenital LCMV infection are nonspecific and include the medical problems that commonly arise in scenarios, involving ventriculoperitoneal shunts, severe seizure disorders, and static encephalopathy. These complications include shunt failure or infection, aspiration pneumonia, injuries from falls, and joint contractures.

TREATMENT

There is no specific treatment for acquired or congenital LCMV infection. An effective antiviral therapy for LCMV infection has not yet been developed. Ribavirin is active against LCMV and other arenaviruses in vitro, but its utility in vivo is unproven. Immunosuppressive therapy, if present, should be reduced.

Supportive Care

Children with hydrocephalus from congenital LCMV infection often require placement of a ventriculoperitoneal shunt during infancy for treatment of hydrocephalus. Seizures often begin during early postnatal life, are often difficult to control, and require administration of multiple antiepileptic medications. The mental retardation induced by congenital LCMV infection is often profound. In most cases, affected children should be referred for educational intervention during early life. The spasticity accompanying congenital LCMV infection is often severe. Although physical therapy can help to maintain the range of motion and minimize painful spasms and contractures, implantation of a baclofen pump is often helpful.

PROGNOSIS

The great majority of patients with postnatally acquired LCMV infection have a full recovery with no permanent sequelae. Rarely, postnatal infections induce hydrocephalus and require shunting. Rarer yet, postnatal LCMV infection is fatal.

In contrast to the usual benign outcome of postnatal infections, prenatal infections typically lead to severe and permanent disability. In children with congenital LCMV infection, brain function is nearly always impaired and chorioretinitis is invariably present. Mental retardation, cerebral palsy, ataxia, epilepsy, and blindness are common neurologic sequelae. However, children with congenital LCMV infection have diverse outcomes. All children with the combination of microencephaly and periventricular calcifications are profoundly neurologically impaired. Blindness, medically refractory epilepsy, spastic quadriparesis, and mental retardation are typical of this group. However, other children with congenital LCMV infection who do not have the combination of microencephaly and periventricular calcifications often have a more favorable outcome, with less severe motor, mental, and vision impairments. Children with isolated cerebellar hypoplasia may be ataxic but have only mild or moderate mental retardation and vision loss.

PREVENTION

No vaccine exists to prevent LCMV infection. However, measures can be taken to reduce the risk of infection. Because rodents, especially house mice, are the principal reservoir of LCMV, people can reduce their risk of contracting LCMV by minimizing their exposure to the secretions and excretions of mice. This can be accomplished most effectively by eliminating cohabitation with mice. Congenital LCMV infection will not occur unless a woman contracts a primary infection with LCMV during pregnancy. Thus, women should be especially careful to avoid contact or cohabitation with mice during pregnancy. Pregnant women should also avoid contact with pet rodents, especially mice and hamsters. These facts should be stressed during prenatal visits.

Acquisition of LCMV from solid-organ transplantation represents a substantial risk to organ recipients. Prospective donors with LCMV meningitis or encephalitis pose a clear risk for transmitting a fatal infection to recipients. Healthcare providers, transplantation centers, and organ procurement organizations should be aware of the risks posed by LCMV and should consider LCMV in any potential donor with signs of aseptic meningitis but no identified infectious agent. The risks and benefits of offering and receiving organs from donors with possible LCMV infection should be carefully considered.

Bibliography is available at Expert Consult.

Chapter **299**
Hantavirus Pulmonary Syndrome
Scott B. Halstead
第二百九十九章
汉坦病毒肺综合征

中文导读

本章主要介绍了汉坦病毒肺综合征的病因学、流行病学、发病机制、临床表现、诊断、鉴别诊断、治疗、预后和预防。临床表现中具体介绍了前驱期和心肺期。前驱期中包括发热、肌痛、咳嗽或呼吸困难、胃肠道症状；心肺期中包括进行性咳嗽和呼吸急促，重症病例中出现急性肺水肿、缺氧和休克等。治疗需给予氧气以及对心脏功能密切的监测，多巴酚丁胺用于防止肺水肿加重。

The hantavirus pulmonary syndrome (HPS) is caused by multiple closely related hantaviruses that have been identified from the western United States, with sporadic cases reported from the eastern United States (Fig. 299.1) and Canada and important foci of disease in several countries in South America. HPS is characterized by a febrile prodrome followed by the rapid onset of noncardiogenic pulmonary edema and hypotension or shock. Sporadic cases in the United States caused by related viruses may manifest with renal involvement. Cases in Argentina and Chile sometimes include severe gastrointestinal hemorrhaging; nosocomial transmission has been documented in this geographic region only.

ETIOLOGY

Hantaviruses are a genus in the family Bunyaviridae, which are lipid-enveloped viruses with a negative-sense RNA genome composed of three unique segments. Several pathogenic viruses that have been recognized within the genus include Hantaan virus, which causes the most severe form of hemorrhagic fever with renal syndrome (HFRS) seen primarily in mainland Asia (see Chapter 297); Dobrava virus, which causes the most severe form of HFRS seen primarily in the Balkans; Puumala virus, which causes a milder form of HFRS with a high proportion of subclinical infections and is prevalent in northern Europe; and Seoul virus, which results in moderate HFRS and is transmitted predominantly in Asia by urban rats or worldwide by laboratory rats. Prospect Hill virus, a hantavirus that is widely disseminated in meadow voles in the United States, is not known to cause human disease. There are an increasing number of case reports of European hantaviruses causing HPS.

HPS is associated with *sin nombre* virus, isolated from deer mice, *Peromyscus maniculatus,* in New Mexico. Multiple HPS-like agents in the

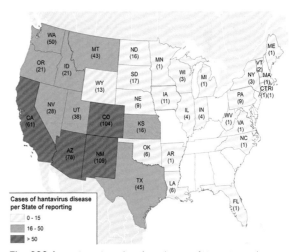

Fig. 299.1 Total number of confirmed cases of Hantavirus pulmonary syndrome, by state reporting, United States, 1993-2016. N = 728 as of January 2017. *(From Viral Special Pathogens Branch, Centers for Disease Control and Prevention. Available at: http://www.cdc.gov/hantavirus/surveillance/reporting-state.html).*

American hemisphere isolated to date belong to a single genetic group of hantaviruses and are associated with rodents of the family Muridae, subfamily Sigmodontinae. These rodent species are restricted to the Americas, suggesting that HPS may be a Western hemisphere disease.

EPIDEMIOLOGY

Persons acquiring HPS generally have a history of recent outdoor exposure or live in an area with large populations of deer mice. Clusters of cases have occurred among individuals who have cleaned houses that were rodent infested. *P. maniculatus* is one of the most common North American mammals and, where found, is frequently the dominant member of the rodent community. About half of the average of 30+ cases seen annually occurs between the months of May and July. Patients are almost exclusively 12-70 yr of age; 60% of patients are 20-39 yr of age. Rare cases are reported in children younger than 12 yr of age. Two thirds of patients are male, probably reflecting their greater outdoor activities. It is not known whether almost complete absence of disease in young children is a reflection of innate resistance or simply lack of exposure. Evidence of human-to-human transmission has been reported in Argentine outbreaks.

Hantaviruses do not cause apparent illness in their reservoir hosts, which remain asymptomatically infected for life. Infected rodents shed virus in saliva, urine, and feces for many weeks, but the duration of shedding and the period of maximum infectivity are unknown. The presence of infectious virus in saliva, the sensitivity of these animals to parenteral inoculation with hantaviruses, and field observations of infected rodents indicate that biting is important for rodent-to-rodent transmission. Aerosols from infective saliva or excreta of rodents are implicated in the transmission of hantaviruses to humans. Persons visiting animal care areas housing infected rodents have been infected after exposure for as little as 5 min. It is possible that hantaviruses are spread through contaminated food and breaks in skin or mucous membranes; transmission to humans has occurred by rodent bites. Person-to-person transmission is distinctly uncommon but has been documented in Argentina.

PATHOGENESIS

HPS is characterized by sudden and catastrophic pulmonary edema, resulting in anoxia and acute heart failure. The virus is detected in pulmonary capillaries, suggesting that pulmonary edema is the consequence of a T-cell attack on virus-infected capillaries. The disease severity is predicted by the level of acute-phase viremia titer. A useful hamster model of HPS is available.

CLINICAL MANIFESTATIONS

HPS is characterized by a prodrome and a cardiopulmonary phase. The mean duration after the onset of prodromal symptoms to hospitalization is 5.4 days. The mean duration of symptoms to death is 8 days (median: 7 days; range: 2-16 days). The most common **prodromal symptoms** are fever and myalgia (100%); cough or dyspnea (76%); gastrointestinal symptoms, including vomiting, diarrhea, and midabdominal pain (76%); and headache (71%). The **cardiopulmonary phase** is heralded by progressive cough and shortness of breath. The most common initial physical findings are tachypnea (100%), tachycardia (94%), and hypotension (50%). Rapidly progressive acute pulmonary edema, hypoxia, and shock develop in most severely ill patients. Pulmonary vascular permeability is complicated by cardiogenic shock associated with increased vascular resistance. The clinical course of the illness in patients who die is characterized by pulmonary edema accompanied by severe hypotension, frequently terminating in sinus bradycardia, electromechanical dissociation, ventricular tachycardia, or fibrillation. Hypotension may be progressive even with adequate oxygenation. HPS virus is excreted in the urine during the acute illness phase, and survivors may demonstrate evidence of chronic renal damage.

DIAGNOSIS

The diagnosis of HPS should be considered in a previously healthy patient presenting with a febrile prodrome, acute respiratory distress, and thrombocytopenia who has had outdoor exposure in the spring and summer months. A specific diagnosis of HPS is made by serologic tests that detect hantavirus immunoglobulin M antibodies. The early appearance of immunoglobulin G antibodies signals probable recovery. Hantavirus antigen can be detected in tissue by immunohistochemistry and amplification of hantavirus nucleotide sequences detected by reverse transcriptase polymerase chain reaction. The state health department or the Centers for Disease Control and Prevention should be consulted to assist in the diagnosis, epidemiologic investigations, and outbreak control.

Laboratory Findings

Laboratory findings include leukocytosis (median: 26,000 cells/μL), an elevated hematocrit resulting from hemoconcentration, thrombocytopenia (median: 64,000 cells/μL), prolonged prothrombin and partial thromboplastin times, elevated serum lactate dehydrogenase concentration, decreased serum protein concentrations, proteinuria, and microscopic hematuria. Patients who die often experience disseminated intravascular coagulopathy including frank hemorrhage and exceptionally high leukocyte counts.

DIFFERENTIAL DIAGNOSIS

The differential diagnosis includes adult respiratory distress syndrome, pneumonic plague, psittacosis, severe mycoplasmal pneumonia, influenza, leptospirosis, inhalation anthrax, rickettsial infections, pulmonary tularemia, atypical bacterial and viral pneumonial diseases, legionellosis, meningococcemia, and other sepsis syndromes. The key determinant in the diagnosis of HPS is thrombocytopenia.

TREATMENT

Management of patients with hantavirus infection requires maintenance of adequate oxygenation and careful monitoring and support of cardiovascular function. The pathophysiology of HPS somewhat resembles that of dengue shock syndrome (see Chapter 295). Pressor or inotropic agents, such as dobutamine, should be administered in combination with judicious volume replacement to treat symptomatic hypotension or shock while avoiding exacerbation of the pulmonary edema. Intravenous ribavirin, which is lifesaving if given early in the course of HFRS and is effective in preventing death in the hamster model, has not yet been demonstrated to be of value in HPS.

Further information and advice about management, control measures, diagnosis, and collection of biohazardous specimens can be obtained from the Centers for Disease Control and Prevention, National Center for Infectious Diseases, Viral Special Pathogens Branch, Atlanta, Georgia 30333 (470-312-0094).

PROGNOSIS

In some geographic areas, fatality rates for HPS have been 50%. Severe abnormalities in hematocrit, white blood cell count, lactate dehydrogenase value, and partial thromboplastin time, and a high viral load predict death with high specificity and sensitivity. The early appearance of immunoglobulin G antibodies may signal a hopeful prognosis.

PREVENTION

Avoiding contact with rodents is the only preventive strategy against HPS. Rodent control in and around the home is important. Barrier nursing is advised, and biosafety level 3 facilities and practices are recommended for laboratory handling of blood, body fluids, and tissues from suspect patients or rodents, because the virus may be aerosolized.

Bibliography is available at Expert Consult.

Chapter **300**
Rabies
Rodney E. Willoughby Jr.

第三百章
狂犬病

中文导读

本章主要介绍了狂犬病的流行病学、传播、发病机制、临床表现、鉴别诊断、诊断、治疗和预后、预防。本病几乎只通过患狂犬病的哺乳动物咬伤或抓伤传播，临床表现包括狂躁型狂犬病和麻痹型狂犬病。

实验室检测方法包括逆转录聚合酶链式反应、抗原及血清学检测和分离病毒。详细地阐述了预防方法，包括对宿主进行免疫及控制繁殖、暴露后预防和暴露前预防。

Rabies virus is a bullet-shaped, negative-sense, single-stranded, enveloped RNA virus from the family Rhabdoviridae, genus *Lyssavirus*. There currently are 14 species of *Lyssavirus*. The classic rabies virus (genotype 1) is distributed worldwide and naturally infects a large variety of animals. The other genotypes are more geographically confined, with none found in the Americas. Seven *Lyssavirus* genotypes are associated with rabies in humans, although genotype 1 accounts for the great majority of cases. Within genotype 1, a number of genetic variants have been defined. Each variant is specific to a particular animal reservoir, although cross-species transmission can occur.

EPIDEMIOLOGY

Rabies is present on all continents except Antarctica. Rabies predominantly afflicts underaged, poor, and geographically isolated populations. Approximately 59,000 cases of human rabies occur in Africa and Asia annually. Theoretically, rabies virus can infect any mammal (which then can transmit disease to humans), but true animal reservoirs that maintain the presence of rabies virus in the population are limited to terrestrial carnivores and bats. Worldwide, transmission from dogs accounts for > 90% of human cases. In Africa and Asia, other animals serve as prominent reservoirs, such as jackals, mongooses, and raccoon dogs. In industrialized nations, canine rabies has been largely controlled through the routine immunization of pets. In the United States, raccoons are the most commonly infected wild animal along the eastern seaboard. Three phylogenies of skunk rabies are endemic in the Midwest (north and south) and California, gray foxes harbor rabies in Arizona and Texas, red foxes and arctic foxes harbor rabies in Alaska, and mongooses carry rabies in Puerto Rico. Rabies occurs infrequently in livestock. Among American domestic pets, infected cats outnumber infected dogs, probably because cats frequently prowl unsupervised and are not uniformly subject to vaccine laws. Rabies is rare in small mammals, including mice, squirrels, and rabbits; to date, no animal-to-human transmission from these animals has been documented.

The epidemiology of human rabies in the United States is dominated by cryptogenic bat rabies. Bats are migratory in the spring and fall; rabid bats are identified in every state of the union except Hawaii. In one study, the largest proportion of cases of human rabies were infected with a bat variant, and in almost all cases of bat-associated human rabies there was no history of a bat bite. Among inhabitants of the Peruvian Amazon region who have exposure to rabies-infected vampire bats, there are some who have rabies virus–neutralizing antibodies and have survived. Antibody-positive patients remember bat bites but do not recall symptoms of rabies.

In the United States, 30,000 episodes of rabies postexposure prophylaxis (PEP) occur annually. Between one and three endemic human cases are diagnosed annually, half postmortem. There have been five outbreaks of rabies associated with solid-organ and corneal transplantations.

TRANSMISSION

Rabies virus is found in large quantities in the saliva of infected animals, and transmission occurs almost exclusively through inoculation of the infected saliva through a bite or scratch from a rabid mammal. Approximately 35–50% of people who are bitten by a known rabies-infected animal and receive no PEP actually contract rabies. The transmission rate is increased if the victim has suffered multiple bites and if the inoculation occurs in highly innervated parts of the body such as the face and the hands. Infection does not occur after exposure of intact skin to infected secretions, but virus may enter the body through intact mucous membranes. Claims that spelunkers may experience rabies after inhaling bat excreta have come under doubt, although inhalational exposure can occur during laboratory accidents.

No case of nosocomial transmission to a healthcare worker has been documented to date, but caregivers of a patient with rabies are advised to use full barrier precautions. The virus is rapidly inactivated in the environment, and contamination of fomites is not a mechanism of spread.

PATHOGENESIS

After inoculation, rabies virus replicates slowly and at low levels in muscle or skin. This slow initial step likely accounts for the disease's long incubation period. Virus then enters the peripheral motor nerve, utilizing the nicotinic acetylcholine receptor and possibly several other receptors for entry. Once in the nerve, the virus travels by fast axonal transport, crossing synapses roughly every 12 hr. Rapid dissemination occurs throughout the brain and spinal cord before symptoms appear. Infection of the dorsal root ganglia is apparently futile but causes characteristic radiculitis. Infection concentrates in the brainstem, accounting for autonomic dysfunction and relative sparing of cognition. Despite severe neurologic dysfunction with rabies, histopathology reveals limited damage, inflammation, or apoptosis. The pathologic hallmark of rabies, the Negri body, is composed of clumped viral nucleocapsids that create cytoplasmic inclusions on routine histology. Negri bodies can be absent in documented rabies virus infection. Rabies may be a metabolic disorder of neurotransmission; tetrahydrobiopterin deficiency in human rabies causes severe deficiencies in dopamine, norepinephrine, and serotonin metabolism.

After infection of the central nervous system, the virus travels anterograde through the peripheral nervous system to virtually all innervated organs, further exacerbating dysautonomia. It is through this route that the virus infects the salivary glands. Many victims of rabies die from uncontrolled cardiac dysrhythmia.

Deficiency of tetrahydrobiopterin, an essential cofactor for neuronal nitric oxide synthase, is predicted to lead to spasm of the basilar arteries. Onset of vasospasm has been confirmed in a few patients within 5-8 days of the first hospitalization, at about the time coma supervenes in the natural history. Increased intracranial pressure is regularly measured early in rabies in association with elevated N-acetylaspartate in cerebrospinal fluid (CSF), but is rarely radiologically apparent. Metabolites in CSF consistent with ketogenesis are associated with demise.

CLINICAL MANIFESTATIONS

The incubation period for rabies is 1-3 mo. In severe wounds to the head, symptoms may occur within 5 days after exposure, and occasionally the incubation period can extend to 8 yr. Rabies has two principal clinical forms. **Encephalitic** or **furious rabies** begins with nonspecific symptoms, including fever, sore throat, malaise, headache, nausea and vomiting, and weakness. These symptoms are often accompanied by paresthesia and pruritus at or near the site of the bite that then extend along the affected limb. Soon thereafter the patient begins to demonstrate symptoms of encephalitis, with agitation, sleep disturbance, or depressed mentation. Characteristically, patients with rabies encephalitis initially have periods of lucidity alternating with periods of profound encephalopathy. Hydrophobia and aerophobia are the cardinal signs of rabies; they are unique to humans and are not universal or specific. Phobic spasms are manifested by agitation and fear created by being offered a drink or fanning of air in the face, which in turn produce choking and aspiration through spasms of the pharynx, neck, and diaphragm. Seizures are rare and should point to an alternative diagnosis; orofacial dyskinesias and myoclonia may be confused with seizures. The illness is relentlessly progressive. There is a dissociation of electrophysiologic or encephalographic activity with findings of brainstem coma caused by anterograde denervation. Death almost always occurs within 1-2 days of hospitalization in developing countries and by 18 days of hospitalization with intensive care.

A second form of rabies known as **paralytic** or **dumb rabies** is seen much less frequently and is characterized principally by fevers and ascending motor weakness affecting both the limbs and the cranial nerves. Most patients with paralytic rabies also have some element of encephalopathy as the disease progresses subacutely.

Case reports suggest that milder forms of rabies encephalitis may exist, and 28 rabies survivors are known. Rabies should be considered earlier and more frequently than current practice to improve outcomes.

DIFFERENTIAL DIAGNOSIS

The differential diagnosis of rabies encephalitis includes all forms of severe cerebral infections, tetanus, and some intoxications and enven-omations. Rabies can be confused with autoimmune (anti–N-methyl-D-aspartate receptor, NMDAR) encephalitis, other infectious forms of encephalitis, psychiatric illness, drug abuse, and conversion disorders. Paralytic rabies is frequently confused with Guillain-Barré syndrome. The diagnosis of rabies is frequently delayed in Western countries because of the unfamiliarity of the medical staff with the infection. These considerations highlight the need to pursue a history of contact with an animal belonging to one of the known reservoirs for rabies or to establish a travel history to a rabies-endemic region.

DIAGNOSIS

The Centers for Disease Control and Prevention (CDC) require a number of tests to confirm a clinically suspected case of rabies. Reverse transcription polymerase chain reaction is the most sensitive available assay for the diagnosis of rabies when done iteratively. Rabies virus RNA has been detected in saliva, skin, and brain by the reverse transcription polymerase chain reaction. The virus can be grown both in cell culture and after animal injection, but identification of rabies by these methods is slow. Rabies antigen is detected through immunofluorescence of saliva or biopsies of hairy skin or brain. Corneal impressions are not recommended. Rabies-specific antibody can be detected in serum or CSF samples, but most patients die while seronegative. Antirabies antibodies are present in the sera of patients who have received an incomplete course of the rabies vaccine, precluding a meaningful interpretation in this setting. Recent treatment with intravenous immunoglobulin may result in a false-positive antibody test. Antibody in CSF is rarely detected after vaccination and is considered diagnostic of rabies regardless of immunization status. CSF abnormalities in cell count, glucose, and protein content are minimal and are not diagnostic. MRI findings in the brain are late.

TREATMENT AND PROGNOSIS

Rabies is generally fatal. Conventional critical care yielded 6 survivors from 79 attempts since 1990. Seventeen of 80 patients survived with use of the Milwaukee Protocol (MP) (http://www.mcw.edu/rabies); neurologic outcomes are poor in half of patients. Neither rabies immunoglobulin (RIG) nor rabies vaccine provides benefit once symptoms have appeared. Among 10 survivors of rabies after use of biologics, 7 had poor neurologic outcomes. Among 7 vaccine-naïve survivors, 2 had poor outcomes. Antiviral treatments have not been effective; favipiravir has been administered to 4 patients as compassionate use. Ribavirin and RIG delay the immune response and should be avoided. In contrast, appearance of the normal antibody response by 7 days is associated with clearance of salivary viral load and survival.

PREVENTION

Primary prevention of rabies infection includes vaccination of domestic animals and education to avoid wild animals, stray animals, and animals with unusual behavior.

Immunization and Fertility Control of Animal Reservoirs

The introduction of routine rabies immunization for domestic pets in the United States and Europe during the middle of the 20th century virtually eliminated infection in dogs. In the 1990s, control efforts in Europe and North America shifted to immunization of wildlife reservoirs of rabies, where rabies was newly emerging. These programs employed bait laced with either an attenuated rabies vaccine or a recombinant rabies surface glycoprotein inserted into vaccinia, distributed by air or hand into areas inhabited by rabid animals. Human contact with vaccine-laden bait has been infrequent. Adverse events after such contact have been rare, but the vaccinia vector poses a threat to the same population at risk for vaccinia itself, namely, pregnant women, immunocompromised patients, and people with atopic dermatitis. Mass culling of endemic reservoirs has never worked; vaccination and fertility control stop outbreaks. Bats are ubiquitous and very important for insect control. Less than 1% of free-flying bats but > 8% of downed bats and bats found in dwellings are rabid.

Postexposure Prophylaxis

The relevance of rabies for most pediatricians centers on evaluating whether an animal exposure warrants PEP (Table 300.1). No case of rabies has been documented in a person receiving the recommended schedule of PEP since introduction of modern cellular vaccines in the 1970s.

Given the incubation period for rabies, PEP is a medical urgency, not emergency. Algorithms have been devised to aid practitioners in deciding when to initiate rabies PEP (Fig. 300.1). The decision to proceed ultimately depends on the local epidemiology of animal rabies as determined by active surveillance programs, information that can be obtained from local and state health departments. *In general, bats, raccoons, skunks, coyotes, and foxes should be considered rabid unless proven otherwise through euthanasia and testing of brain tissue,* whereas bites from small herbivorous animals (squirrels, hamsters, gerbils, chipmunks, rats, mice, and rabbits) can be discounted. The response to bites from a pet, particularly a dog, cat, or ferret, depends on local surveillance statistics and on whether the animal is vaccinated and available for observation.

The approach to nonbite bat exposures is controversial. In response to the observation that most cases of rabies in the United States have been caused by bat variants and that the majority of affected patients had no recollection of a bat bite, the CDC has recommended that rabies PEP be considered after any physical contact with bats and when a bat is found in the same room as persons who may not be able to accurately report a bite, assuming that the animal is unavailable for testing. Such people include young children, the mentally disabled, and intoxicated individuals. Other nonbite contacts (e.g., handling a carcass, exposure to an animal playing with a carcass, or coming into contact with blood or excreta from a potentially rabid animal) usually do not require PEP.

In all instances of a legitimate exposure, effort should be made to recover the animal for quarantine and observation or brain examination after euthanasia. Testing obviates the need for PEP more than half the time. In most instances, PEP can be deferred until the results of observation or brain histology are known. In dogs, cats, and ferrets, symptoms of rabies always occur within several days of viral shedding; therefore, in these animals a 10-day observation period is sufficient to eliminate the possibility of rabies.

No duration of time between exposure and onset of symptoms should preclude rabies prophylaxis. Rabies PEP is most effective when applied expeditiously. Nevertheless, the series should be initiated in

Table 300.1	Rabies Postexposure Prophylaxis Guide	
ANIMAL TYPE	**EVALUATION AND DISPOSITION OF ANIMAL**	**POSTEXPOSURE PROPHYLAXIS RECOMMENDATIONS**
Dogs, cats, and ferrets	Healthy and available for 10 days of observation	Prophylaxis only if animal shows signs of rabies*
	Rabid or suspected of being rabid†	Immediate immunization and RIG
	Unknown (escaped)	Consult public health officials for advice
Bats, skunks, raccoons, foxes, and most other carnivores; woodchucks	Regarded as rabid unless geographic area is known to be free of rabies or until animal proven negative by laboratory tests†	Immediate immunization and RIG
Livestock, rodents, and lagomorphs (rabbits, hares, and pikas)	Consider individually	Consult public health officials. Bites of squirrels, hamsters, guinea pigs, gerbils, chipmunks, rats, mice and other rodents, rabbits, hares, and pikas almost never require antirabies treatment

*During the 10-day observation period, at the first sign of rabies in the biting dog, cat, or ferret, treatment of the exposed person with RIG (human) and vaccine should be initiated. The animal should be euthanized immediately and tested

†The animal should be euthanized and tested as soon as possible. Holding for observation is not recommended. Immunization is discontinued if the immunofluorescent test result for the animal is negative.

RIG, rabies immunoglobulin.

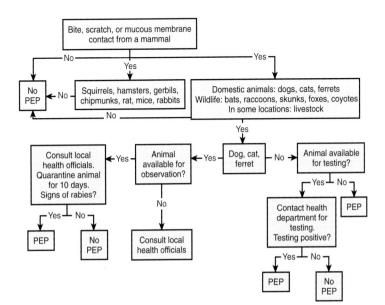

Fig. 300.1 Algorithm for evaluating a child for rabies postexposure prophylaxis. This and any other algorithm should be used in concert with local epidemiologic information regarding the incidence of animal rabies in any given location.

the asymptomatic person as soon as possible, regardless of the length of time since the bite. *The vaccine and RIG are contraindicated once symptoms develop.*

The first step in rabies PEP is to **cleanse the wound thoroughly.** Soapy water is sufficient to inactivate an enveloped virus, and its effectiveness is supported by broad experience. Other commonly used disinfectants, such as iodine-containing preparations, are virucidal and should be used in addition to soap when available. Probably the most important aspect of this component is that the wound is cleansed with copious volumes of disinfectant. **Primary closure is avoided;** wounds may be bacterially infected as well, so cosmetic repair should follow. Antibiotics and tetanus prophylaxis (see Chapter 238) should be applied with the use of usual wound care criteria.

The second component of rabies PEP consists of passive immunization with RIG. Most failures of PEP are attributed to not using RIG. Human RIG, the formulation used in industrialized countries, is administered at a dose of 20 IU/kg. **As much of the dose is infused around the wound as possible,** and the remainder is injected intramuscularly in a limb distant from the one injected with the killed vaccine. Like other immunoglobulin preparations, RIG interferes with the take of live viral vaccines for at least 4 mo after administration of the RIG dose. Human RIG is not available in many parts of the developing world. Equine RIG serves as a substitute for the human immunoglobulin preparation in some areas. Modern preparations of equine RIG are associated with fewer side effects than prior products composed of crude horse serum. Regrettably, for a large segment of the world's population, no passive immunization product is available at all. Monoclonal antibody products are in clinical trials and may alleviate this deficiency.

The third component of rabies PEP is immunization with inactivated vaccine. In most of the world, cell-based vaccines have replaced previous preparations. Two formulations currently are available in the United States, namely, RabAvert (Chiron Behring Vaccines, Maharashtra, India), a purified chick-embryo cell cultivated vaccine, and Imovax Rabies (Aventis Pasteur, Bridgewater, NJ), cultivated in human diploid cell cultures. In both children and adults, both vaccines are administered intramuscularly in a 1-mL volume in the deltoid or anterolateral thigh on days 0, 3, 7, and 14 after presentation. Injection into the gluteal area is associated with a blunted antibody response, so this area should not be used. The rabies vaccines can be safely administered during pregnancy. In most persons the vaccine is well tolerated; most adverse effects are related to booster doses. Pain and erythema at the injection site occur commonly, and local adenopathy, headache, and myalgias occur in 10–20% of patients. Approximately 5% of patients who receive the human diploid cell vaccine experience an immune complex–mediated allergic reaction, including rash, edema, and arthralgias, several days after a booster dose. The World Health Organization has approved schedules using smaller amounts of vaccine, administered intradermally, that are immunogenic and protective (http://www.who.int/rabies/human/post _exp_prophylaxis/en/), but none is approved for use in the United States. Other cell culture–derived rabies virus vaccines are available in the developing world. A few countries still produce nerve tissue–derived vaccines; these preparations are poorly immunogenic, and cross reactivity with human nervous tissue may occur with their use, producing severe neurologic symptoms even in the absence of rabies infection.

Preexposure Prophylaxis

The killed rabies vaccine can be given to prevent rabies in persons at high risk for exposure to wild-type virus, including laboratory personnel working with rabies virus, veterinarians, and others likely to be exposed to rabid animals as part of their occupation. Preexposure prophylaxis should be considered for persons traveling to a rabies-endemic region where there is a credible risk for a bite or scratch from a rabies-infected animal, particularly if there is likely to be a shortage of RIG or cell culture–based vaccine (see Chapter 200). Rabies vaccine as part of the routine vaccine series is under investigation in some countries. The schedule for preexposure prophylaxis consists of three intramuscular injections on days 0, 7, and 21 or 28. PEP in the patient who has received preexposure prophylaxis or a prior full schedule of PEP consists of two doses of vaccine (one each on days 0 and 3) and does not require RIG. Immunity from preexposure prophylaxis wanes after several years and requires boosting if the potential for exposure to rabid animals recurs.

Bibliography is available at Expert Consult.

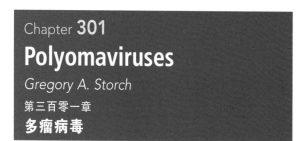

Chapter **301**

Polyomaviruses

Gregory A. Storch

第三百零一章

多瘤病毒

中文导读

　　本章主要介绍了多瘤病毒感染的病因、流行病学、发病机制、临床表现、诊断和治疗。多瘤病毒是双链DNA病毒，可能与人类肿瘤形成有关，JC病毒和BK病毒为人感染的常见病原体。临床表现可能与感染病毒类型相关，包括棘状毛发育不良、瘙痒性皮疹、进行性多灶性白质脑病、移植性肾病等。PCR法是检测BK和JC病毒的首选方法。目前尚无获批的特 异性抗病毒药。

The polyomaviruses are small (45 nm), nonenveloped, circular, double-stranded DNA viruses with genomes of approximately 5,000 bp. Because of the association of animal polyomaviruses with tumors in the animals they infect, there has been concern for a relationship to neoplasia in humans; however, there is strong evidence for an etiologic role in neoplasia only for Merkel cell polyomavirus (see below). Among the other polyomaviruses, the traditional human pathogens are JC virus and BK virus. The number of human polyomaviruses has expanded dramatically, with discovery of up to 12 additional viruses. Two polyomaviruses, designated KI virus and WU virus, can be detected in respiratory samples from children; however, a pathogenic role for these viruses has not been proven to date. Merkel cell polyomavirus is associated with Merkel cell carcinoma, an unusual neuroectodermal tumor of the skin that occurs primarily in elderly and immunocompromised individuals. Clonal integration of Merkel cell polyomavirus DNA is present in Merkel cell carcinoma cells, supporting an etiologic role for the virus in the development of the tumor. Another human polyomavirus has been isolated from patients with the dermatologic condition **trichodysplasia spinulosa** and has been named trichodysplasia spinulosa–associated polyomavirus. Trichodysplasia spinulosa is a condition of the skin that occurs in immunocompromised individuals and involves the development of follicular papules and keratin spines, usually involving the face. Two other viruses, designated human polyomaviruses 6 and 7, have also been found in human skin samples. They have been implicated in pruritic skin rashes in immunocompromised individuals. Human polyomavirus 9 was detected in serum from a renal transplant recipient. Other recently discovered viruses, named Malawi virus and St. Louis virus, were first detected in stool samples, but a role in gastrointestinal or other disease has not been established at this time.

JC and BK viruses are tropic for renal epithelium; JC virus also infects brain oligodendrocytes and is the etiologic agent of **progressive multifocal leukoencephalopathy (PML),** a rare and often fatal demyelinating disease of immunocompromised persons, especially those with AIDS. PML is known to occur in individuals receiving the immunomodulatory agents natalizumab (Tysabri), used to treat multiple sclerosis and Crohn disease, efalizumab (Raptiva), used to treat psoriasis, the anti-CD20 monoclonal antibody rituximab (Rituxan), and the anti-CD52 monoclonal antibody alemtuzumab (Campath), as well as multiple other immunomodulatory agents. BK virus is the cause of **transplant nephropathy** in renal transplant recipients and of hemorrhagic cystitis in hematopoietic stem cell and bone marrow transplant recipients. Several million persons in the United States were exposed to simian virus 40 (SV40), an oncogenic polyomavirus of Asian macaques, from contaminated poliovirus vaccines administered during the years 1955 to 1963. There were no recognized sequelae and no demonstrable increased risk for cancer.

Seroepidemiologic studies have shown that infection with all of the human polyomaviruses appears to be widespread, often occurring during childhood. Primary infection with these viruses is not recognized clinically. Approximately half of children in the United States are infected with BK virus by 3-4 yr of age and with JC virus by 10-14 yr of age, and approximately 60–80% of adults are seropositive for one or both viruses. Infection with polyomaviruses is thought to persist throughout life, with JC and BK viruses remaining latent in renal epithelium, oligodendrocytes, and peripheral blood mononuclear cells. The site of latency of the other human polyomaviruses is not currently known. Approximately 30–50% of healthy persons have detectable BK or JC virus in renal tissue at autopsy. Reactivation and viruria occur with increased frequency with advancing age and are more common in immunocompromised persons. On the basis of polymerase chain reaction results, BK and JC viruria occurs in 2.6% and 13.2%, respectively, of persons younger than 30 yr of age and in approximately 9% and 50%, respectively, of persons older than 60 yr of age.

Reactivation of BK and JC viruses with asymptomatic viruria occurs in 10–50% of hematopoietic stem cell and bone marrow transplant recipients and in 30% of renal transplant recipients. Of those renal transplant recipients who demonstrate BK viruria, approximately one third also have plasma viremia. Recipients with plasma viremia are at risk for development of nephropathy, which can clinically mimic allograft rejection and can result in failure of the allograft. Reduction of immunosuppression has been effective in preventing progression from viremia to nephropathy, and thus posttransplantation monitoring of either urine or plasma by polymerase chain reaction is important. It is particularly important to distinguish BK nephropathy from rejection because the treatments are different—increase in immunosuppression for rejection but decrease in immunosuppression for BK nephropathy.

Polymerase chain reaction is the preferred means for detecting the BK and JC viruses. The high seroprevalence in the general population and lack of clear relationship to clinical illness limit the usefulness of serologic testing, although recent studies suggest that high levels of anti-BK antibodies in renal transplant donors are associated with an increased risk of BK disease in the recipient. There are no proven antiviral treatments for BK or JC virus infection, although cidofovir may be effective in some cases of BK-related transplant nephropathy. Effective treatment of AIDS with antiretroviral therapy can prevent the progression of progressive multifocal leukoencephalopathy. Allogeneic BK virus–specific T cells are a potentially beneficial therapy for PML.

Bibliography is available at Expert Consult.

Chapter 302
Human Immunodeficiency Virus and Acquired Immunodeficiency Syndrome

Ericka V. Hayes

第三百零二章
人类免疫缺陷病毒和获得性免疫缺陷综合征

中文导读

本章主要介绍了人类免疫缺陷病毒感染的病因、流行病学、发病机制、临床表现、诊断、治疗、预后和预防。临床表现包括感染，中枢神经系统、呼吸道、心血管系统、胃肠和肝胆道受累，肾病，皮肤表现，血液系统与恶性病；感染中具体描述了机会性感染、非结核分枝杆菌、真菌、寄生虫和病毒感染，免疫重建炎症综合征；中枢神经系统疾病中具体描述了脑病、CNS淋巴瘤、CNS弓形虫病和进行性多灶性白质脑病。实验室检测包括血清学、DNA及RNA检测。具体阐述了HIV的治疗原则，详细介绍了不同种类药物名称、剂量和副作用。

Advances in research and major improvements in the treatment and management of HIV infection have brought about a substantial decrease in the incidence of new HIV infections and AIDS in children. Globally, from 2000 to 2015, there has been an estimated 70% decline in new infections in children aged 0-14 yr, largely the result of antiretroviral treatment (ART) of HIV-infected pregnant women for the prevention of mother-to-child transmission. Seventy percent of adults and children with HIV infection live in sub-Saharan Africa, where the disease continues to have a devastating impact (Fig. 302.1). Children experience more rapid disease progression than adults, with up to half of untreated children dying within the first 2 yr of life. This rapid progression is correlated with a higher viral burden and faster depletion of infected CD4 lymphocytes in infants and children than in adults. Accurate diagnostic tests and the early initiation of potent drugs to inhibit HIV replication have dramatically increased the ability to prevent and control this disease.

ETIOLOGY
HIV-1 and HIV-2 are members of the Retroviridae family and belong to the *Lentivirus* genus, which includes cytopathic viruses causing diverse diseases in several animal species. The HIV-1 genome contains two copies of single-stranded RNA that is 9.2 kb in size. At both ends of the genome there are identical regions, called **long terminal repeats,** which contain the regulation and expression genes of HIV. The remainder of the genome includes three major sections: the **GAG** region, which encodes the viral core proteins (p24 [capsid protein: CA], p17 [matrix protein: MA], p9, and p6, which are derived from the precursor p55); the **POL** region, which encodes the viral enzymes (i.e., reverse transcriptase [p51], protease [p10], and integrase [p32]); and the **ENV** region, which encodes the viral envelope proteins (gp120 and gp41, which are derived from the precursor gp160). Other regulatory proteins, such as transactivator of transcription (tat: p14), regulator of virion (rev: p19), negative regulatory factor (nef: p27), viral protein r (vpr: p15), viral infectivity factor (vif: p23), viral protein u (vpu in HIV-1: P16), and viral protein x (vpx in HIV-2: P15), are involved in transactivation, viral messenger RNA expression, viral replication, induction of cell cycle arrest, promotion of nuclear import of viral reverse transcription complexes, downregulation of the CD4 receptors and class I major histocompatibility complex, proviral DNA synthesis, and virus release and infectivity (Fig. 302.2).

The HIV tropism to the target cell is determined by its envelope glycoprotein (Env). Env consists of two components, namely, the surface, heavily glycosylated subunit, gp120 protein and the associated transmembrane subunit glycoprotein gp41. Both gp120 and gp41 are produced from the precursor protein gp160. The glycoprotein gp41 is very immunogenic and is used to detect HIV-1 antibodies in diagnostic

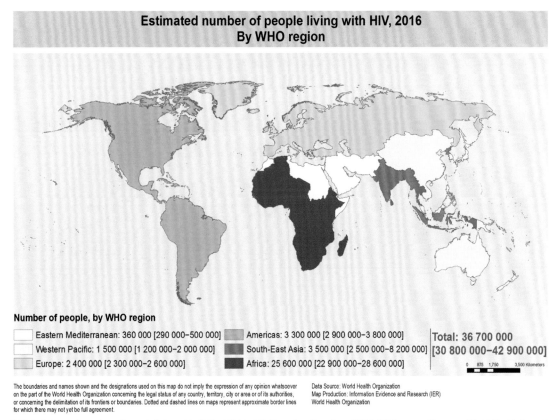

Fig. 302.1 Estimated number of people living with HIV in 2016 by WHO region. Data from WHO 2017 report. *(Courtesy World Health Organization, 2017. Global Health Observatory (GHO) data. http://www.who.int/gho/hiv/epidemic_status/cases_all/en/.)*

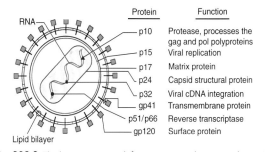

Protein	Function
p10	Protease, processes the gag and pol polyproteins
p15	Viral replication
p17	Matrix protein
p24	Capsid structural protein
p32	Viral cDNA integration
gp41	Transmembrane protein
p51/p66	Reverse transcriptase
gp120	Surface protein

Fig. 302.2 The human immunodeficiency virus and associated proteins and their functions.

assays; gp120 is a complex molecule that includes the highly variable **V3 loop.** This region is immunodominant for neutralizing antibodies. The heterogeneity of gp120 presents major obstacles in establishing an effective HIV vaccine. The gp120 glycoprotein also carries the binding site for the CD4 molecule, the most common host cell surface receptor of T lymphocytes. This tropism for $CD4^+$ T cells is beneficial to the virus because of the resulting reduction in the effectiveness of the host immune system. Other CD4-bearing cells include macrophages and microglial cells. The observations that $CD4^-$ cells are also infected by HIV and that some $CD4^+$ T cells are resistant to such infections suggests that other cellular attachment sites are needed for the interaction between HIV and human cells. Several chemokines serve as coreceptors for the envelope glycoproteins, permitting membrane fusion and entry into the cell. Most HIV strains have a specific tropism for one of the

chemokines, including the fusion-inducing molecule **CXCR-4,** which acts as a coreceptor for HIV attachment to lymphocytes, and **CCR-5,** a β chemokine receptor that facilitates HIV entry into macrophages. Several other chemokine receptors (CCR-3) have also been shown in vitro to serve as virus coreceptors. Other mechanisms of attachment of HIV to cells use nonneutralizing antiviral antibodies and complement receptors. The Fab portion of these antibodies attaches to the virus surface, and the Fc portion binds to cells that express Fc receptors (macrophages, fibroblasts), thus facilitating virus transfer into the cell. Other cell-surface receptors, such as the mannose-binding protein on macrophages or the DC-specific, C-type lectin (DC-SIGN) on dendritic cells, also bind to the HIV-1 envelope glycoprotein and increase the efficiency of viral infectivity. Cell-to-cell transfer of HIV without formation of fully formed particles is a more rapid mechanism of spreading the infection to new cells than is direct infection by the virus.

Following viral attachment, gp120 and the CD4 molecule undergo conformational changes, and gp41 interacts with the fusion receptor on the cell surface (Fig. 302.3). Viral fusion with the cell membrane allows entry of viral RNA into the cell cytoplasm. This process involves accessory viral proteins (nef, vif) and binding of cyclophilin A (a host cellular protein) to the capsid protein (p24). The p24 protein is involved in virus uncoating, recognition by restriction factors, and nuclear importation and integration of the newly created viral DNA. Viral DNA copies are then transcribed from the virion RNA through viral reverse transcriptase enzyme activity, which builds the first DNA strand from the viral RNA and then destroys the viral RNA and builds a second DNA strand to produce double-stranded circular DNA. The HIV-1 reverse transcriptase is error prone and lacks error-correcting mechanisms. Thus, many mutations arise, creating a wide genetic variation in HIV-1 isolates even within an individual patient. Many of the drugs used to fight HIV infection were designed to block the reverse

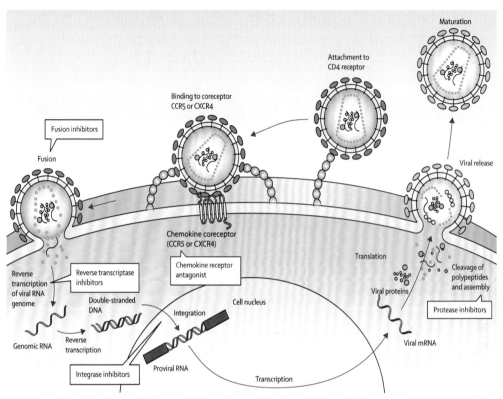

Fig. 302.3 HIV life cycle showing the sites of action and different classes of antiretroviral drugs. *(Adapted from Walker BN, Colledge NR, Ralston SH, Penman I, editors: Davidson's principles and practice of medicine, ed 22, London, 2014, Churchill Livingstone.)*

transcriptase action. The circular DNA is transported into the cell nucleus, using viral accessory proteins such as vpr, where it is integrated (with the help of the virus integrase) into the host chromosomal DNA and referred to as the *provirus.* The provirus has the advantage of latency, because it can remain dormant for extended periods, making it extremely difficult to eradicate. The infected CD4+ T cells that survive long enough to revert to resting memory state become the HIV latent reservoir where the virus persists indefinitely even in patients who respond favorably to potent antiretroviral therapy. The molecular mechanisms of this latency are complex and involve unique biologic properties of the latent provirus (e.g., absence of tat, epigenetic changes inhibiting HIV gene expression) and the nature of the cellular host (e.g., absence of transcription factors such as nuclear factor κB). Integration usually occurs near active genes, which allow a high level of viral production in response to various external factors such as an increase in inflammatory cytokines (by infection with other pathogens) and cellular activation. Anti-HIV drugs that block the integrase enzyme activity have been developed. Depending on the relative expression of the viral regulatory genes (tat, rev, nef), the proviral DNA may encode production of the viral RNA genome, which, in turn, leads to production of viral proteins necessary for viral assembly.

HIV-1 transcription is followed by translation. A capsid polyprotein is cleaved to produce the virus-specific protease (p10), among other products. This enzyme is critical for HIV-1 assembly because it cleaves the long polyproteins into the proper functional pieces. Several HIV-1 antiprotease drugs have been developed, targeting the increased sensitivity of the viral protease, which differs from the cellular proteases. The regulatory protein vif is active in virus assembly and Gag processing. The RNA genome is then incorporated into the newly formed viral capsid that requires zinc finger domains (p7) and the matrix protein (MA: p17). The matrix protein forms a coat on the inner surface of the viral membrane, which is essential for the budding of the new virus from the host cell's surface. As new virus is formed, it buds through

specialized membrane areas, known as *lipid rafts,* and is released. The virus release is facilitated by the viroporin vpu, which induces rapid degradation of newly synthesized CD4 molecules that impede viral budding. In addition, vpu counteracts host innate immunity (e.g., hampering natural killer T-cell activity).

Full-length sequencing of the HIV-1 genome demonstrated three different groups (M [main], O [outlier], and N [non-M, non-O]), probably occurring from multiple zoonotic infections from primates in different geographic regions. The same technique identified eight groups of HIV-2 isolates. Group M diversified to nine subtypes (or clades A to D, F to H, J, and K). In each region of the world, certain clades predominate, for example, clade A in Central Africa, clade B in the United States and South America, clade C in South Africa, clade E in Thailand, and clade F in Brazil. Although some subtypes were identified within group O, none was found in any of the HIV-2 groups. Clades are mixed in some patients as a result of HIV recombination, and some crossing between groups (i.e., M and O) has been reported.

HIV-2 has a similar life cycle to HIV-1 and is known to cause infection in several monkey species. Subtypes A and B are the major causes of infection in humans, but rarely cause infection in children. HIV-2 differs from HIV-1 in its accessory genes (e.g., it has no *vpu* gene but contains the *vpx* gene, which is not found in HIV-1). It is most prevalent in western Africa, but increasing numbers of cases are reported from Europe and southern Asia. The diagnosis of HIV-2 infection is more difficult because of major differences in the genetic sequences between HIV-1 and HIV-2. Thus, several of the standard confirmatory assays (immunoblot), which are HIV-1 specific, may give indeterminate results with HIV-2 infection. If HIV-2 infection is suspected, a combination screening test that detects antibody to HIV-1 and HIV-2 peptides should be used. In addition, the rapid HIV detection tests have been less reliable in patients suspected to be dually infected with HIV-1 and HIV-2, because of lower antibody concentrations against HIV-2. HIV-2 viral loads also have limited availability. Notably, HIV-2 infection demonstrates a longer asymptomatic stage of infection and slower declines of CD4+ T-cell counts than HIV-1, as well as is less efficiently transmitted from mother to child, likely related to lower levels of viremia with HIV-2.

EPIDEMIOLOGY

In 2015, the World Health Organization (WHO) estimated that 1.8 million children younger than 15 yr of age worldwide were living with HIV-1 infection; the 150,000 new infections annually in children was a 70% reduction since 2000. Approximately 80% of new infections in this age-group occur in sub-Saharan Africa. These trends reflect the slow but steady expansion of services to prevent perinatal transmission of HIV to infants. Notably, there are still 110,000 deaths worldwide of children < 15 yr of age with HIV. Unfortunately, through 2016, an estimated 16.5 million children have been orphaned by AIDS, defined as having one or both parents die from AIDS.

Globally, the vast majority of HIV infections in childhood are the result of **vertical transmission** from an HIV-infected mother. In the United States, approximately 11,700 children, adolescents, or young adults were reported to be living with perinatally acquired HIV infection in 2014. The number of U.S. children with AIDS diagnosed each year increased from 1984 to 1992 but then declined by more than 95% to < 100 cases annually by 2003, largely from the success of prenatal screening and perinatal antiretroviral treatment of HIV-infected mothers and infants. From 2009 to 2013, there were 497 infants born with perinatally acquired HIV in the United States and Puerto Rico. Children of racial and ethnic minority groups are disproportionately overrepresented, particularly non-Hispanic African-Americans and Hispanics. Race and ethnicity are not risk factors for HIV infection but more likely reflect other social factors that may be predictive of an increased risk for HIV infection, such as lack of educational and economic opportunities. As of 2014, New York, Florida, Texas, Georgia, Illinois, and California are the states with the highest numbers of perinatally acquired cases of HIV in the United States.

Adolescents (13-24 yr of age) constitute an important growing population of newly infected individuals; in 2015, 22% of all new HIV infections occurred in this age-group, with 81% of youth cases occurring in young males who have sex with males (MSM); 8% of cases of AIDS also occurred in this age-group. Targeted efforts have decreased new cases by 18% among youth MSM from 2008 to 2014. It is estimated than 50% of HIV-positive youth are unaware of their diagnosis, the highest of any age-group. Considering the long latency period between the time of infection and the development of clinical symptoms, reliance on AIDS case definition surveillance data significantly underrepresents the impact of the disease in adolescents. Based on a median incubation period of 8-12 yr, it is estimated that 15–20% of all AIDS cases were acquired between 13 and 19 yr of age.

Risk factors for HIV infection vary by gender in adolescents. For example, 91–93% of males between the ages of 13 and 24 yr with HIV acquire infection through sex with males. In contrast, 91–93% of adolescent females with HIV are infected through heterosexual contact. Adolescent racial and ethnic minority populations are overrepresented, especially among females.

Transmission

Transmission of HIV-1 occurs via sexual contact, parenteral exposure to blood, or vertical transmission from mother to child via exposure to vaginal secretions during birth or via breast milk. The primary route of infection in the pediatric population (<15 yr) is vertical transmission. Rates of transmission of HIV from mother to child have varied in high- and low-resource countries; the United States and Europe have documented transmission rates in untreated women of between 12% and 30%, whereas transmission rates in Africa and Haiti have been higher (25–52%), likely because of more advanced maternal disease and the presence of coinfections. *Perinatal treatment of HIV-infected pregnant women with antiretroviral drugs has dramatically decreased the rate to < 2%.*

Vertical transmission of HIV can occur before delivery (**intrauterine**), during delivery (**intrapartum**), or after delivery (**postpartum** through **breastfeeding**). Although intrauterine transmission has been suggested by identification of HIV by culture or polymerase chain reaction (PCR) in fetal tissue as early as 10 wk, statistical modeling data suggest that the majority of in utero transmissions likely occur in late gestation, when the vascular integrity of the placenta weakens and microtransfusions across the maternal–fetal circulation occur. It is generally accepted that 20–30% of infected newborns are infected in utero, because this percentage of infants has laboratory evidence of infection (positive viral culture or PCR) within the first week of life. Some studies have found that viral detection soon after birth is also correlated with an early onset of symptoms and rapid progression to AIDS, consistent with more long-standing infection during gestation.

A higher percentage of HIV-infected children acquire the virus intrapartum, evidenced by the fact that 70–80% of infected infants do not demonstrate detectable virus until after 1 wk of age. The mechanism of transmission appears to be mucosal exposure to infected blood and cervicovaginal secretions in the birth canal, and intrauterine contractions during active labor/delivery could also increase the risk of late micro-transfusions. Breastfeeding is the least-common route of vertical transmission in high resource nations, but is responsible for as much as 40% of perinatal infections in resource-limited countries. Both free and cell-associated viruses have been detected in breast milk from HIV-infected mothers. The risk for transmission through breastfeeding is approximately 9–16% in women with established infection, but is 29–53% in women who acquire HIV postnatally, suggesting that the viremia experienced by the mother during primary infection at least triples the risk for transmission. Where replacement feeding is readily available and safe, it seems reasonable for women to substitute infant formula for breast milk if they are known to be HIV infected or are at risk for ongoing sexual or parenteral exposure to HIV. However, the WHO recommends that in low-resource countries where other diseases (diarrhea, pneumonia, malnutrition) substantially contribute to a high infant mortality rate, the benefit of breastfeeding outweighs the risk for HIV transmission, and HIV-infected women in developing countries should exclusively breastfeed their infants for at least the first 6 mo of life (see Prevention later in this chapter).

Several risk factors influence the rate of vertical transmission: maternal viral load at delivery, preterm delivery (<34 wk gestation), and low maternal antenatal CD4 count. The most important variable appears to be the level of maternal viremia; the odds of transmission may be increased more than two-fold for every $\log_{10}$ increase in viral load at delivery. Elective cesarean delivery was shown to decrease transmission by 87% if used in conjunction with zidovudine therapy in the mother and infant. However, because these data predated the advent of **combined antiretroviral therapy** (**cART,** also called **HAART),** the additional benefit of cesarean section appears to be negligible if the mother's viral load is < 1,000 copies/mL. It should be noted that rarely (≤0.1%), transmission may occur with maternal viral loads < 50 copies/mL.

Transfusions of infected blood or blood products have accounted for 3–6% of all pediatric AIDS cases. The period of highest risk was between 1978 and 1985, before the availability of HIV antibody–screened blood products. Whereas the prevalence of HIV infection in individuals with hemophilia treated before 1985 was as high as 70%, heat treatment of factor VIII concentrate and HIV antibody screening of donors has virtually eliminated HIV transmission in this population. Donor screening has dramatically reduced, but not eliminated, the risk for blood transfusion–associated HIV infection: nucleic acid amplification testing of minipools (pools of 16-24 donations) performed on antibody-nonreactive blood donations (to identify donations made during the window period before seroconversion) reduced the residual risk of transfusion-transmitted HIV-1 to approximately 1 in 2 million blood units. However, in many resource-limited countries, screening of blood is not uniform, and the risk for transmitting HIV infection via transfusion remains in these settings.

Although HIV can be isolated rarely from saliva, it is in very low titers (<1 infectious particle/mL) and has not been implicated as a transmission vehicle. Studies of hundreds of household contacts of HIV-infected individuals have found that the risk for household HIV transmission is essentially nonexistent. Only a few cases have been reported in which urine or feces (possibly devoid of visible blood) have been proposed as a possible vehicle of HIV transmission, though these cases have not been fully verified.

In the pediatric population, sexual transmission is infrequent, but a small number of cases resulting from sexual abuse have been reported. Sexual contact is a major route of transmission in the adolescent population, accounting for most of the cases.

PATHOGENESIS

HIV infection affects most of the immune system and disrupts its homeostasis (see Fig. 302.3). In most cases, the initial infection is caused by low amounts of a single virus. Therefore, disease may be prevented by prophylactic drug(s) or vaccine. When the mucosa serves as the portal of entry for HIV, the first cells to be affected are the dendritic cells. These cells collect and process antigens introduced from the periphery and transport them to the lymphoid tissue. HIV does not infect the dendritic cell but binds to its DC-SIGN surface molecule, allowing the virus to survive until it reaches the lymphatic tissue. In the lymphatic tissue (e.g., lamina propria, lymph nodes), the virus selectively binds to cells expressing CD4 molecules on their surface, primarily helper T lymphocytes (CD4+ T cells) and cells of the monocyte-macrophage lineage. Other cells bearing CD4, such as microglia, astrocytes, oligodendroglia, and placental tissue containing villous Hofbauer cells, may also be infected by HIV. Additional factors (coreceptors) are necessary for HIV fusion and entry into cells. These factors include the chemokines CXCR4 (fusion) and CCR5. Other chemokines (CCR1, CCR3) may be necessary for the fusion of certain HIV strains. Several host genetic determinants affect the susceptibility to HIV infection, the progression of disease, and the response to treatment. These genetic variants vary in different populations. A deletion in the CCR5 gene that is protective against HIV infection (CCR5Δ32) is relatively common in whites but is rare in individuals of African descent. Several other genes that regulate chemokine receptors, ligands, the histocompatibility complex, and cytokines also influence the outcome of HIV infection. Usually, CD4+ lymphocytes migrate to the lymphatic tissue in response to viral antigens and then become activated and proliferate, making them highly susceptible to HIV infection. This antigen-driven migration and accumulation of CD4 cells within the lymphoid tissue may contribute to the generalized lymphadenopathy characteristic of the acute retroviral syndrome in adults and adolescents. HIV preferentially infects the very cells that respond to it (HIV-specific memory CD4 cells), accounting for the progressive loss of these cells and the subsequent loss of control of HIV replication. The continued destruction of memory CD4+ cells in the gastrointestinal tract (in the gut-associated lymphoid tissue or GALT) leads to reduced integrity of the gastrointestinal epithelium followed by leakage of bacterial particles into the blood and increased inflammatory response, which cause further CD4+ cell loss. When HIV replication reaches a threshold (usually within 3-6 wk from the time of infection), a burst of plasma viremia occurs. This intense viremia causes acute HIV infection, formerly known as **acute retroviral syndrome** which can present similar to the **flu or mononucleosis** (fever, rash, pharyngitis, lymphadenopathy, malaise, arthralgia, fatigue, elevated liver enzymes) in 50–70% of infected adults. With establishment of a cellular and humoral immune response within 2-4 mo, the viral load in the blood declines substantially, and patients enter a phase characterized by a lack of symptoms and a return of CD4 cells to only moderately decreased levels. Typically, adult patients who are not treated eventually progress to achieve a virologic set point (steady state), usually ranging from 10,000-100,000 during this clinical latency. This is in contrast to untreated infants with vertically acquired HIV who can achieve viral loads that are much higher, resulting in faster CD4 count declines and earlier onset of significant immunodeficiency. HIV rapidly responds to the immune system pressure by developing a genetically complex population (quasispecies) that successfully evades it. In addition, inappropriate use of antiretroviral treatment increases the ability of the virus to diverge even further by selecting for mutants with fitness or resistance advantages in the presence of subtherapeutic drug levels. Early HIV-1 replication in children has no apparent clinical manifestations. Whether tested by virus isolation or by PCR for viral nucleic acid sequences, fewer than 40% of HIV-1–infected infants demonstrate

evidence of the virus at birth. The viral load increases by 1-4 mo, and essentially all perinatally HIV-infected infants have detectable HIV-1 in peripheral blood by 4 mo of age, except for those who may acquire infection via ongoing breast feeding.

In adults, the long period of clinical latency (8-12 yr) is not indicative of viral latency. In fact, there is a very high turnover of virus and CD4 lymphocytes (more than a billion cells per day), gradually causing deterioration of the immune system, marked by depletion of CD4 cells. Several mechanisms for the depletion of CD4 cells in adults and children have been suggested, including HIV-mediated single cell killing, formation of multinucleated giant cells of infected and uninfected CD4 cells (**syncytia formation**), virus-specific immune responses (natural killer cells, antibody-dependent cellular cytotoxicity), superantigen-mediated activation of T cells (rendering them more susceptible to infection with HIV), autoimmunity, and programmed cell death (apoptosis). The viral burden is greater in the lymphoid organs than in the peripheral blood during the asymptomatic period. As HIV virions and their immune complexes migrate through the lymph nodes, they are trapped in the network of dendritic follicular cells. Because the ability of HIV to replicate in T cells depends on the state of activation of the cells, the immune activation that takes place within the microenvironment of the lymph nodes in HIV disease serves to promote infection of new CD4 cells, as well as subsequent viral replication within these cells. Monocytes and macrophages can be productively infected by HIV yet resist the cytopathic effect of the virus and, with their long lifespan, explain their role as reservoirs of HIV and as effectors of tissue damage in organs such as the brain. In addition, they reside in anatomic viral sanctuaries where current treatment agents are less effective.

The innate immune system responds almost immediately following HIV infection by recognizing the viral nucleic acids, once the virus fuses to the infected cell, by the toll-like receptor 7. This engagement leads to activation of proinflammatory cytokines and interferon (IFN-α), which blocks virus replication and spread. The virus uses its Nef protein to downregulate the expression of major histocompatibility complex (MHC) and non-MHC ligands to reduce the natural killer (NK) cell–mediated anti-HIV activity. It also modulates NK cell differentiation and maturation, dysregulates cytokine production, and increases apoptosis. Although the mechanism by which the innate system triggers the adaptive immune responses is not yet fully understood, cell-mediated and humoral responses occur early in the infection. CD8 T cells play an important role in containing the infection. These cells produce various ligands (macrophage inflammatory proteins 1α and 1β, RANTES), which suppress HIV replication by blocking the binding of the virus to the coreceptors (CCR5). HIV-specific cytotoxic T lymphocytes (CTLs) develop against both the structural (ENV, POL, GAG) and regulatory (tat) viral proteins. The CTLs appear at the end of the acute infection, as viral replication is controlled by killing HIV-infected cells before new viruses are produced and by secreting potent antiviral factors that compete with the virus for its receptors (CCR5). Neutralizing antibodies appear later in the infection and seem to help in the continued suppression of viral replication during clinical latency. There are at least two possible mechanisms that control the steady-state viral load level during the chronic clinical latency. One mechanism may be the limited availability of activated CD4 cells, which prevent a further increase in the viral load. The other mechanism is the development of an active immune response, which is influenced by the amount of viral antigen and limits viral replication at a steady state. There is no general consensus about which of these two mechanisms is more important. The CD4 cell limitation mechanism accounts for the effect of antiretroviral therapy, whereas the immune response mechanism emphasizes the importance of immune modulation treatment (cytokines, vaccines) to increase the efficiency of immune-mediated control. A group of cytokines that includes tumor necrosis factor TNF-α, TNF-β, interleukin IL-1, IL-2, IL-3, IL-6, IL-8, IL-12, IL-15, granulocyte-macrophage colony-stimulating factor, and macrophage colony-stimulating factor plays an integral role in upregulating HIV expression from a state of quiescent infection to active viral replication. Other cytokines such as IFN-γ, IFN-β, and IL-13 exert a suppressive effect on HIV replication. Certain cytokines (IL-4, IL-10, IFN-γ, transforming growth factor-β) reduce or enhance viral replication depending on the infected cell type. The interactions among these cytokines influence the concentration of viral particles in the tissues. Plasma concentrations of cytokines need not be elevated for them to exert their effect, because they are produced and act locally in the tissues. The activation of virtually all the cellular components of the immune system (i.e., T and B cells, NK cells, and monocytes) plays a significant role in the pathologic aspects of HIV infection. Further understanding of their interactions during the infection will expand our treatment options. Commonly, HIV isolated during the clinical latency period grows slowly in culture and produces low titers of reverse transcriptase. These isolates from earlier in clinical latency use CCR5 as their coreceptor. By the late stages of clinical latency, the isolated virus is phenotypically different. It grows rapidly and to high titers in culture and uses CXCR4 as its coreceptor. The switch from CCR5 receptor to CXCR4 receptor increases the capacity of the virus to replicate, to infect a broader range of target cells (CXCR4 is more widely expressed on resting and activated immune cells), and to kill T cells more rapidly and efficiently. As a result, the clinical latency phase is over and progression toward AIDS is noted. The **progression of disease** is related temporally to the gradual disruption of lymph node architecture and degeneration of the follicular dendritic cell network with loss of its ability to trap HIV particles. The virus is freed to recirculate, producing high levels of viremia and an increased disappearance of CD4 T cells during the later stages of disease.

The clinical course of HIV infection shows substantial heterogeneity. This variation is determined by both viral and host factors. HIV viruses that use coreceptor CXCR4 in the course of the infection are associated with an accelerated deterioration of the immune system and more rapid progression to AIDS. In addition, several known host genetic determinants (e.g., variants in the human leukocyte antigen region, polymorphisms in the CCR5 region such as CCR5Δ32) were already identified as affecting the disease course. There are likely additional host and viral factors yet to be identified that contribute to the variable course of HIV infection in individuals, as well. **Three distinct patterns of disease** are described in children. Approximately 15–25% of HIV-infected newborns in developed countries present with a **rapid progression** course, with onset of AIDS and symptoms during the first few months of life and a median survival time of 6-9 mo if untreated. In resource-limited countries, the majority of HIV-infected newborns will have this rapidly progressing disease course. It has been suggested that if intrauterine infection coincides with the period of rapid expansion of CD4 cells in the fetus, the virus could effectively infect the majority of the body's immunocompetent cells. The normal migration of these cells to the marrow, spleen, and thymus would result in efficient systemic delivery of HIV, unchecked by the immature immune system of the fetus. Thus, infection would be established before the normal ontogenic development of the immune system, causing more-severe impairment of immunity. Most children in this group have detectable virus in the plasma (median level: 11,000 copies/mL) in the first 48 hr of life. This early evidence of viral presence suggests that the newborn was infected in utero. The viral load rapidly increases, peaking by 2-3 mo of age (median: 750,000 copies/mL) and staying high for at least the first 2 yr of life.

Sixty percent to 80% of perinatally infected newborns in high resource countries present with a much **slower progression** of disease, with a median survival time of 6 yr representing the second pattern of disease. Many patients in this group have a negative PCR in the first week of life and are therefore considered to be infected intrapartum. In a typical patient, the viral load rapidly increases, peaking by 2-3 mo of age (median: 100,000 copies/mL) and then slowly declines over a period of 24 mo. The slow decline in viral load is in sharp contrast to the rapid decline after primary infection seen in adults. This observation can be explained only partially by the immaturity of the immune system in newborns and infants.

The third pattern of disease occurs in < 5% of perinatally infected children, referred to as **long-term survivors** or **long-term nonprogressors,** who have minimal or no progression of disease with relatively normal CD4 counts and very low viral loads for longer than 8 yr. Mechanisms for the delay in disease progression include effective humoral

immunity and/or CTL responses, host genetic factors (e.g., human leukocyte antigen profile), and infection with an attenuated (defective-gene) virus. A subgroup of the long-term survivors called elite survivors or elite suppressors has no detectable virus in the blood and may reflect different or greater mechanisms of protection from disease progression. Note that both groups warrant long-term close follow-up because later in their course they may begin to progress with their disease.

HIV-infected children have changes in the immune system that are similar to those in HIV-infected adults. Absolute CD4 cell depletion may be less dramatic because infants normally have a relative lymphocytosis. A value of 750 CD4 cells/μL in children younger than 1 yr of age is indicative of severe CD4 depletion and is comparable to < 200 CD4 cells/μL in adults. Lymphopenia is relatively rare in perinatally infected children and is usually only seen in older children or those with end-stage disease. Although cutaneous anergy is common during HIV infection, it is also frequent in healthy children younger than 1 yr of age, and thus its interpretation is difficult in infected infants. The depletion of CD4 cells also decreases the response to soluble antigens such as the in vitro mitogens phytohemagglutinin and concanavalin A.

Polyclonal activation of B cells occurs in most children early in the infection, as evidenced by elevation of immunoglobulins IgA, IgM, IgE, and, particularly, IgG (**hypergammaglobulinemia),** with high levels of anti–HIV-1 antibody. This response may reflect both dysregulation of the T-cell suppression of B-cell antibody synthesis and active CD4 enhancement of the B-lymphocyte humoral response. As a result, the antibody response to routine childhood vaccinations may be abnormal. The B-cell dysregulation precedes the CD4 depletion in many children and may serve as a surrogate marker of HIV infection in symptomatic children in whom specific diagnostic tests (PCR, culture) are not available or are too expensive. Despite the increased levels of immunoglobulins, some children lack specific antibodies or protective antibodies. Hypogammaglobulinemia is very rare (<1%).

Central nervous system (CNS) involvement is more common in pediatric patients than in adults. Macrophages and microglia play an important role in HIV neuropathogenesis, and data suggest that astrocytes may also be involved. Although the specific mechanisms for encephalopathy in children are not yet clear, the developing brain in young infants is affected by at least two mechanisms. The virus itself may directly infect various brain cells or cause indirect damage to the nervous system by the release of cytokines (IL-1α, IL-1β, TNF-α, IL-2) or reactive oxygen damage from HIV-infected lymphocytes or macrophages.

CLINICAL MANIFESTATIONS

The clinical manifestations of HIV infection vary widely among infants, children, and adolescents. In most infants, physical examination at birth is normal. Initial symptoms may be subtle, such as lymphadenopathy and hepatosplenomegaly, or nonspecific, such as failure to thrive, chronic or recurrent diarrhea, respiratory symptoms, or oral thrush and may be distinguishable only by their persistence. Whereas systemic and pulmonary findings are common in the United States and Europe, chronic diarrhea, pneumonia, wasting, and severe malnutrition predominate in Africa. Clinical manifestations found more commonly in children than adults with HIV infection include recurrent bacterial infections, chronic parotid swelling, lymphocytic interstitial pneumonitis (LIP), and early onset of progressive neurologic deterioration; note that chronic parotid swelling and LIP are associated with a slower progression of disease.

The CDC Surveillance Case Definition for HIV infection is based on the age-specific CD4+ T-lymphocyte count or the CD4+ T-lymphocyte percentage of total lymphocytes (Table 302.1), except when a stage 3–defining opportunistic illness (Table 302.2) supersedes the CD4 data. Age adjustment of the absolute CD4 count is necessary because counts that are relatively high in normal infants decline steadily until age 6 yr, when they reach adult norms. The CD4 count takes precedence over the CD4 T-lymphocyte percentage, and the percentage is considered only if the count is unavailable.

Infections

Approximately 20% of AIDS-defining illnesses in children are recurrent bacterial infections caused primarily by encapsulated organisms such

Table 302.1	HIV Infection Stage* Based on Age-Specific CD4+ T-Lymphocyte Count or CD4+ T-Lymphocyte Percentage of Total Lymphocytes

| | AGE ON DATE OF CD4+ T-LYMPHOCYTE TEST | | | | | |
| | <1 Yr | | 1-5 Yr | | ≥6 Yr | |
STAGE	CELLS/μL	%	CELLS/μL	%	CELLS/μL	%
1	≥1,500	≥34	≥1,000	≥30	≥500	≥26
2	750-1,499	26-33	500-999	22-29	200-499	14-25
3	<750	<26	<500	<22	<200	<14

*Stage is based primarily on the CD4+ T-lymphocyte count. The CD4+ T-lymphocyte count takes precedence over the CD4+ T-lymphocyte percentage, and the percentage is considered only if the count is missing.
From Centers for Disease Control and Prevention: Revised surveillance case definition for HIV infection—United States, 2014, MMWR 63(No RR-3):1-10, 2014.

Table 302.2	Stage 3–Defining Opportunistic Illnesses in HIV Infection

Bacterial infections, multiple or recurrent*
Candidiasis of bronchi, trachea, or lungs
Candidiasis of esophagus
Cervical cancer, invasive[†]
Coccidioidomycosis, disseminated or extrapulmonary
Cryptococcosis, extrapulmonary
Cryptosporidiosis, chronic intestinal (>1 mo duration)
Cytomegalovirus disease (other than liver, spleen, or nodes), onset at age > 1 mo
Cytomegalovirus retinitis (with loss of vision)
Encephalopathy attributed to HIV[‡]
Herpes simplex: chronic ulcers (>1 mo duration) or bronchitis, pneumonitis, or esophagitis (onset at age > 1 mo)
Histoplasmosis, disseminated or extrapulmonary
Isosporiasis, chronic intestinal (>1 mo duration)
Kaposi sarcoma
Lymphoma, Burkitt (or equivalent term)
Lymphoma, immunoblastic (or equivalent term)
Lymphoma, primary, of brain
Mycobacterium avium complex or *Mycobacterium kansasii*, disseminated or extrapulmonary
Mycobacterium tuberculosis of any site, pulmonary,[†] disseminated, or extrapulmonary
Mycobacterium, other species or unidentified species, disseminated or extrapulmonary
Pneumocystis jiroveci (previously known as *Pneumocystis carinii*) pneumonia
Pneumonia, recurrent[†]
Progressive multifocal leukoencephalopathy
Salmonella septicemia, recurrent
Toxoplasmosis of brain, onset at age > 1 mo
Wasting syndrome attributed to HIV[‡]

*Only among children aged < 6 yr.
[†]Only among adults, adolescents, and children aged ≥ 6 yr.
[‡]Suggested diagnostic criteria for these illnesses, which might be particularly important for HIV encephalopathy and HIV wasting syndrome, are described in the following references: Centers for Disease Control and Prevention: 1994 Revised classification system for human immunodeficiency virus infection in children less than 13 years of age, MMWR 43(No. RR-12), 1994; Centers for Disease Control and Prevention: 1993 Revised classification system for HIV infection and expanded surveillance case definition for AIDS among adolescents and adults, MMWR 41(No. RR-17), 1992.
From Centers for Disease Control and Prevention: Revised surveillance case definition for HIV infection—United States, 2014, MMWR 63(No RR-3):1-10, 2014.

as *Streptococcus pneumoniae* and *Salmonella* as a result of disturbances in humoral immunity. Other pathogens, including *Staphylococcus, Enterococcus, Pseudomonas aeruginosa,* and *Haemophilus influenzae,* and other Gram-positive and Gram-negative organisms may also be seen. The most common serious infections in HIV-infected children are bacteremia, sepsis, and bacterial pneumonia, accounting for more than 50% of infections in these patients. Meningitis, urinary tract infections, deep-seated abscesses, and bone/joint infections occur less frequently. Milder recurrent infections, such as otitis media, sinusitis, and skin and soft tissue infections, are very common and may be chronic with atypical presentations.

Opportunistic infections are generally seen in children with severe depression of the CD4 count. In adults, these infections often represent reactivation of a latent infection acquired early in life. In contrast, young children generally have primary infection and often have a more fulminant course of disease reflecting the lack of prior immunity. In addition, infants < 1 yr of age have a higher incidence of developing stage 3–defining opportunistic infections and mortality rates compared with older children and adults even at higher CD4 counts, reflecting that the CD4 count may overpredict the immune competence in young infants. This principle is best illustrated by *Pneumocystis jiroveci* (formerly *Pneumocystis carinii*) pneumonia, the most common opportunistic infection in the pediatric population (see Chapter 271). The peak incidence of *Pneumocystis* pneumonia occurs at age 3-6 mo in the setting of undiagnosed perinatally acquired disease, with the highest mortality rate in children younger than 1 yr of age. Aggressive approaches to treatment have improved the outcome substantially. Although the overall incidence of opportunistic infections has markedly declined since the era of combination antiretroviral therapy, opportunistic infections still occur in patients with severe immunodepletion as the result of unchecked viral replication, which often accompanies poor antiretroviral therapy adherence.

The classic clinical presentation of *Pneumocystis* pneumonia includes an acute onset of fever, tachypnea, dyspnea, and marked hypoxemia; in some children, more indolent development of hypoxemia may precede other clinical or x-ray manifestations. In some cases, fever may be absent or low grade, particularly in more indolent cases. Chest x-ray findings most commonly consist of interstitial infiltrates or diffuse alveolar disease, which rapidly progresses. Chest x-ray in some cases can have very subtle findings and can mimic the radiologic appearance of viral bronchiolitis. Nodular lesions, streaky or lobar infiltrates, or pleural effusions may occasionally be seen. The diagnosis is established by demonstration of *P. jiroveci* with appropriate staining of induced sputum or bronchoalveolar fluid lavage; rarely, an open lung biopsy is necessary. Bronchoalveolar lavage and open lung biopsy have significantly improved sensitivity (75–95%) for *Pneumocystis* testing than induced sputum (20–40%), such that if an induced sputum is negative it does not exclude the diagnosis. PCR testing on respiratory specimens is also available and is more sensitive than microscopy but also has less specificity; it is also not widely available.

The first-line therapy for *Pneumocystis* pneumonia is trimethoprim-sulfamethoxazole (TMP-SMX) (15-20 mg/kg/day of the TMP component divided every 6 hr intravenously) with adjunctive corticosteroids for moderate to severe disease, usually defined as if the PaO$_2$ is < 70 mm Hg while breathing room air. After improvement, therapy with oral TMP-SMX should continue for a total of 21 days while the corticosteroids are weaned. An alternative therapy for *Pneumocystis* pneumonia includes intravenous administration of pentamidine (4 mg/kg/day). Other regimens such as TMP plus dapsone, clindamycin plus primaquine, or atovaquone are used as alternatives in adults but have not been widely used in children to date.

Nontuberculous mycobacteria (NTM), with *Mycobacterium avium-intracellulare* complex (MAC) being most common, may cause disseminated disease in HIV-infected children who are severely immunosuppressed. The incidence of MAC infection in antiretroviral therapy–naïve children >6 yr with < 100 CD4 cells/μL is estimated to be as high as 10%, but effective cART that results in viral suppression makes MAC infections rare. Disseminated MAC infection is characterized by fever, malaise, weight loss, and night sweats; diarrhea, abdominal pain, and, rarely, intestinal perforation or jaundice (a result of biliary tract obstruction by lymphadenopathy) may also be present. Labs may be notable for significant anemia. The diagnosis is made by the isolation of MAC from blood, bone marrow, or tissue; the isolated presence of MAC in the stool does not confirm a diagnosis of disseminated MAC. Treatment can reduce symptoms and prolong life but is at best only capable of suppressing the infection if severe CD4 depletion persists. Therapy should include at least two drugs: clarithromycin or azithromycin and ethambutol. A third drug (rifabutin, rifampin, ciprofloxacin, levofloxacin, or amikacin) is generally added to decrease the emergence of drug-resistant isolates. Careful consideration of possible drug interactions with antiretroviral agents is necessary before initiation of disseminated MAC therapy. Drug susceptibilities should be ascertained, and the treatment regimen should be adjusted accordingly in the event of an inadequate clinical response to therapy. Because of the great potential for toxicity with most of these medications, surveillance for adverse effects should be ongoing. Less commonly, NTM infections can also be focal in these patients, including lymphadenitis, osteomyelitis, tenosynovitis, and pulmonary disease.

Oral candidiasis is the most common **fungal infection** seen in HIV-infected children. Oral nystatin suspension (2-5 mL qid) is often effective. Clotrimazole troches or fluconazole (3-6 mg/kg orally qd) are effective alternatives. Oral thrush progresses to involve the esophagus in as many as 20% of children with severe CD4 depletion, presenting with symptoms such as anorexia, dysphagia, vomiting, and fever. Treatment with oral fluconazole for 7-14 days generally results in rapid improvement in symptoms. Fungemia rarely occurs, usually in the setting of indwelling venous catheters, and up to 50% of cases may be caused by non-*albicans* species. Disseminated histoplasmosis, coccidioidomycosis, and cryptococcosis are rare in pediatric patients but may occur in endemic areas.

Parasitic infections such as intestinal cryptosporidiosis and microsporidiosis and rarely isosporiasis or giardiasis are other opportunistic infections that cause significant morbidity. Although these intestinal infections are usually self-limiting in healthy hosts, they cause severe chronic diarrhea in HIV-infected children with low CD4 counts, often leading to malnutrition. Nitazoxanide therapy is partially effective at improving cryptosporidia diarrhea, but immune reconstitution with cART is the most important factor for clearance of the infection. Albendazole has been reported to be effective against most microsporidia (excluding *Enterocytozoon bieneusi*), and TMP-SMX appears to be effective for isosporiasis.

Viral infections, especially with the herpesvirus group, pose significant problems for HIV-infected children. HSV causes recurrent gingivostomatitis, which may be complicated by local and distant cutaneous dissemination. Primary varicella-zoster virus infection (chickenpox) may be prolonged and complicated by bacterial superinfections or visceral dissemination, including pneumonitis. Recurrent, atypical, or chronic episodes of herpes zoster are often debilitating and require prolonged therapy with acyclovir; in rare instances, varicella-zoster virus has developed a resistance to acyclovir, requiring the use of foscarnet. Disseminated cytomegalovirus infection occurs in the setting of severe CD4 depletion (<50 CD4 cells/μL for >6 yr) and may involve single or multiple organs. Retinitis, pneumonitis, esophagitis, gastritis with pyloric obstruction, hepatitis, colitis, and encephalitis have been reported, but these complications are rarely seen if cART is given. Ganciclovir and foscarnet are the drugs of choice and are often given together in children with sight-threatening cytomegalovirus retinitis. Intraocular injections of foscarnet or intraocular ganciclovir implants plus oral valganciclovir have also been efficacious in adults and older children with cytomegalovirus retinitis. Measles may occur despite immunization and may present without the typical rash. It often disseminates to the lung or brain with a high mortality rate in these patients. HIV-infected children with low CD4 counts can also develop extensive cutaneous molluscum contagiosum infection. Respiratory viruses such as respiratory syncytial virus and adenovirus may present with prolonged symptoms and persistent viral shedding. In parallel with the increased prevalence of genital tract human papillomavirus infection, cervical intraepithelial neoplasia and anal intraepithelial neoplasia also occur with increased frequency among HIV-1–infected adult women compared with HIV-seronegative women. The relative risk for cervical intraepithelial neoplasia is 5-10 times higher for HIV-1 seropositive women. Multiple modalities are used to treat human papillomavirus infection (see Chapter 293), although none is uniformly effective and the recurrence rate is high among HIV-1–infected persons.

Appropriate therapy with antiretroviral agents may result in **immune reconstitution inflammatory syndrome (IRIS),** which is characterized by an increased inflammatory response from the recovered immune system to subclinical opportunistic infections (e.g., *Mycobacterium* infection, HSV infection, toxoplasmosis, CMV infection, *Pneumocystis* infection, cryptococcal infection). This condition is more commonly observed in patients with progressive disease and severe CD4+ T-lymphocyte depletion. Patients with IRIS develop fever and worsening of the clinical manifestations of the opportunistic infection or new manifestations (e.g., enlargement of lymph nodes, pulmonary infiltrates), typically within the first few weeks after initiation of antiretroviral therapy. Determining whether the symptoms represent IRIS, worsening of a current infection, a new opportunistic infection, or drug toxicity is often very difficult. If the syndrome does represent IRIS, adding nonsteroidal antiinflammatory agents or corticosteroids may alleviate the inflammatory reaction, although the use of corticosteroids is controversial. The inflammation may take weeks or months to subside. In most cases, continuation of cART while treating the opportunistic infection (with or without antiinflammatory agents) is sufficient. If opportunistic infection is suspected prior to the initiation of antiretroviral therapy, appropriate antimicrobial treatment should be started first.

Central Nervous System

The incidence of CNS involvement in perinatally infected children is as high as 50–90% in resource-limited countries but significantly lower in high income countries, with a median onset at 19 mo of age. Manifestations may range from subtle developmental delay to progressive encephalopathy with loss or plateau of developmental milestones, cognitive deterioration, impaired brain growth resulting in acquired microcephaly, and symmetric motor dysfunction. **Encephalopathy** may be the initial manifestation of the disease or may present much later when severe immune suppression occurs. With progression, marked apathy, spasticity, hyperreflexia, and gait disturbance may occur, as well as loss of language and oral, fine, and/or gross motor skills. The encephalopathy may progress intermittently, with periods of deterioration followed by transiently stable plateaus. Older children may exhibit behavioral problems and learning disabilities. Associated abnormalities identified by neuroimaging techniques include cerebral atrophy in up to 85% of children with neurologic symptoms, increased ventricular size, basal ganglia calcifications, and, less frequently, leukomalacia.

Fortunately, since the advent of cART, the incident rate of encephalopathy has dramatically declined to as low as 0.08% in 2006. However, as HIV-infected children progress through adolescence and young adulthood, other subtle manifestations of CNS disease are evident, such as cognitive deficits, attention problems, and psychiatric disorders. Living with a chronic, often stigmatizing, disease; parental loss; and the requirement for lifelong pristine medication adherence compounds these issues, making it challenging for these youth as they inherit responsibility for managing their disease as adults.

Focal neurologic signs and seizures are unusual and may imply a comorbid pathologic process such as a CNS tumor, opportunistic infection, or stroke. **CNS lymphoma** may present with new-onset focal neurologic findings, headache, seizures, and mental status changes. Characteristic findings on neuroimaging studies include a hyperdense or isodense mass with variable contrast enhancement or a diffusely infiltrating contrast-enhancing mass. **CNS toxoplasmosis** is exceedingly rare in young infants but may occur in vertically HIV-infected adolescents and is typically associated with serum antitoxoplasma IgG as a marker of infection. Other opportunistic infections of the CNS are rare and include infection with CMV, JC virus (**progressive multifocal leuko-encephalopathy**), HSV, *Cryptococcus neoformans,* and *Coccidioides immitis.* Although the true incidence of cerebrovascular disorders (both hemorrhagic and nonhemorrhagic strokes) is unclear, 6–10% of children from large clinical series have been affected.

Respiratory Tract

Recurrent upper respiratory tract infections such as otitis media and sinusitis are very common. Although the typical pathogens *(S. pneumoniae, H. influenzae, Moraxella catarrhalis)* are most common, unusual pathogens such as *P. aeruginosa,* yeast, and anaerobes may be present in chronic infections and result in complications such as invasive sinusitis and mastoiditis.

LIP (lymphocytic interstitial pneumonia) is the most common chronic lower respiratory tract abnormality reported to the Centers for Disease Control and Prevention (CDC) for HIV-infected children; historically this occurred in approximately 25% of HIV-infected children, although the incidence has declined in the cART era. LIP is a chronic process with nodular lymphoid hyperplasia in the bronchial and bronchiolar epithelium, often leading to progressive alveolar capillary block over months to years. It has a characteristic chronic diffuse reticulonodular pattern on chest radiography rarely accompanied by hilar lymphadenopathy, allowing a presumptive diagnosis to be made radiographically before the onset of symptoms. There is an insidious onset of tachypnea, cough, and mild to moderate hypoxemia with normal auscultatory findings or minimal rales. Progressive disease presents with symptomatic hypoxemia, which usually resolves with oral corticosteroid therapy, accompanied by digital clubbing. Several studies suggest that LIP is a lymphoproliferative response to a primary Epstein-Barr virus infection in the setting of HIV infection. It is also associated with a slower immunologic decline.

Most symptomatic HIV-infected children experience at least one episode of pneumonia during their disease. *S. pneumoniae* is the most common bacterial pathogen, but *P. aeruginosa* and other Gram-negative bacterial pneumonias may occur in end-stage disease and are often associated with acute respiratory failure and death. Rarely, severe recurrent bacterial pneumonia results in bronchiectasis. *Pneumocystis* pneumonia is the most common opportunistic infection, but other pathogens, including CMV, *Aspergillus, Histoplasma,* and *Cryptococcus* can cause pulmonary disease. Infection with common respiratory viruses, including respiratory syncytial virus, parainfluenza, influenza, and adenovirus, may occur simultaneously and have a protracted course and period of viral shedding from the respiratory tract. Pulmonary and extrapulmonary tuberculosis (TB) has been reported with increasing frequency in HIV-infected children in low-resource countries, although it is considerably more common in HIV-infected adults. Because of drug interactions between rifampin and ritonavir-based antiretroviral therapy and poor tolerability of the combination of multiple drugs required, treatment of TB/HIV coinfection is particularly challenging in children.

Cardiovascular System

Cardiac dysfunction, including left ventricular hypertrophy, left ventricular dilation, reduced left ventricular fractional shortening, and/or heart failure occurred in 18–39% of HIV-infected children in the pre-cART era; among those affected, a lower nadir CD4 percentage and a higher viral load were associated with lower cardiac function. However, a more current evaluation of HIV-infected children taking long-term cART found that echocardiographic findings were closer to normal and none had symptomatic heart disease, suggesting that cART has a cardioprotective effect. What is still unclear is whether an increased rate of premature cardiovascular disease that has been seen in adults will be seen in children who have disease- or treatment-related hyperlipidemia, and prospective studies will be needed to assess this risk. Because of this risk, regular monitoring of cholesterol and lipids, as well as education regarding a heart-healthy lifestyle, is an important part of pediatric HIV care.

Gastrointestinal and Hepatobiliary Tract

Oral manifestations of HIV disease include erythematous or pseudo-membranous candidiasis, periodontal disease (e.g., ulcerative gingivitis or periodontitis), salivary gland disease (i.e., swelling, xerostomia), and, rarely, ulcerations or oral hairy leukoplakia. Gastrointestinal tract involvement is common in HIV-infected children. A variety of pathogens can cause gastrointestinal disease, including bacteria (*Salmonella, Campylobacter, Shigella,* MAC), protozoa (*Giardia, Cryptosporidium, Isospora,* microsporidia), viruses (CMV, HSV, rotavirus), and fungi *(Candida).* MAC and the protozoal infections are most severe and protracted in patients with severe CD4 cell depletion. Infections may be localized or disseminated and affect any part of the gastrointestinal tract from the oropharynx to the rectum. Oral or esophageal ulcerations, either viral in origin or idiopathic, are painful and often interfere with eating. AIDS enteropathy, a syndrome of malabsorption with partial villous atrophy not associated with a specific pathogen, has been postulated to be a result of direct HIV infection of the gut. Disaccharide intolerance is common in HIV-infected children with chronic diarrhea.

The most common symptoms of gastrointestinal disease are chronic or recurrent diarrhea with malabsorption, abdominal pain, dysphagia, and failure to thrive. Prompt recognition of weight loss or poor growth velocity in the absence of diarrhea is critical. Linear growth impairment is often correlated with the level of HIV viremia. Supplemental enteral feedings should be instituted, either by mouth or with nighttime nasogastric tube feedings in cases associated with more severe chronic growth problems; placement of a gastrostomy tube for nutritional supplementation may be necessary in severe cases. The wasting syndrome, defined as a loss of > 10% of body weight, is not as common as failure to thrive in pediatric patients, but the resulting malnutrition is associated with a grave prognosis. Chronic liver inflammation evidenced by fluctuating serum levels of transaminases with or without cholestasis is relatively common, often without identification of an etiologic agent. Cryptosporidial cholecystitis is associated with abdominal pain, jaundice, and elevated γ-glutamyltransferase. In some patients, chronic hepatitis caused by CMV, hepatitis B, hepatitis C, or MAC may lead to portal hypertension and liver failure. Several of the antiretroviral drugs or other drugs such as didanosine, protease inhibitors, nevirapine, and dapsone may also cause reversible elevation of transaminases.

Pancreatitis with increased pancreatic enzymes with or without abdominal pain, vomiting, and fever may be the result of drug therapy (e.g., with pentamidine, didanosine, or stavudine) or, rarely, opportunistic infections such as MAC or CMV.

Renal Disease

Nephropathy is an unusual presenting symptom of HIV infection, more commonly occurring in older symptomatic children. A direct effect of HIV on renal epithelial cells has been suggested as the cause, but immune complexes, hyperviscosity of the blood (secondary to hyperglobulinemia), and nephrotoxic drugs are other possible factors. A wide range of histologic abnormalities has been reported, including focal glomerulosclerosis, mesangial hyperplasia, segmental necrotizing glomerulonephritis, and minimal change disease. Focal glomerulosclerosis generally progresses to renal failure within 6-12 mo, but other histologic abnormalities in children may remain stable without significant renal insufficiency for prolonged periods. **Nephrotic syndrome** is the most common manifestation of pediatric renal disease, with edema, hypoalbuminemia, proteinuria, and azotemia with normal blood pressure. Cases resistant to steroid therapy may benefit from cyclosporine therapy. Polyuria, oliguria, and hematuria have also been observed in some patients.

Skin Manifestations

Many cutaneous manifestations seen in HIV-infected children are inflammatory or infectious disorders that are not unique to HIV infection. These disorders tend to be more disseminated and respond less consistently to conventional therapy than in the uninfected child. Seborrheic dermatitis or eczema that is severe and unresponsive to treatment may be an early nonspecific sign of HIV infection. Recurrent or chronic episodes of HSV, herpes zoster, molluscum contagiosum, flat warts, anogenital warts, and candidal infections are common and may be difficult to control.

Allergic drug eruptions are also common, in particular related to nonnucleoside reverse transcription inhibitors; they generally respond to withdrawal of the drug but also may resolve spontaneously without drug interruption; rarely, progression to Stevens-Johnson syndrome has been reported. Epidermal hyperkeratosis with dry, scaling skin is frequently observed, and sparse hair or hair loss may be seen in the later stages of the disease.

Hematologic and Malignant Diseases

Anemia occurs in 20–70% of HIV-infected children, more commonly in children with AIDS. The anemia may be a result of chronic infection, poor nutrition, autoimmune factors, virus-associated conditions (hemophagocytic syndrome, parvovirus B19 red cell aplasia), or the adverse effect of drugs (zidovudine).

Leukopenia occurs in almost 30% of untreated HIV-infected children, and neutropenia often occurs. Multiple drugs used for treatment or prophylaxis for opportunistic infections, such as *Pneumocystis* pneumonia (TMP-SMX), MAC, and CMV (ganciclovir), or antiretroviral drugs (zidovudine) may also cause leukopenia and/or neutropenia. In cases in which therapy cannot be changed, treatment with subcutaneous granulocyte colony-stimulating factor may be necessary.

Thrombocytopenia has been reported in 10–20% of patients. The etiology may be immunologic (i.e., circulating immune complexes or anti-platelet antibodies) or, less commonly, from drug toxicity, or idiopathic. Antiretroviral therapy (cART) may also reverse thrombocytopenia in ART-naïve patients. In the event of sustained severe thrombocytopenia (<10,000 platelets/μL), treatment with intravenous immunoglobulin or anti-D immune globulin offers temporary improvement in most patients already taking cART. If ineffective, a course of steroids may be an alternative, but consultation with a hematologist should be sought. Deficiency of clotting factors (factors II, VII, IX) is not rare in children with advanced HIV disease and is often easy to correct with vitamin K. A novel disease of the thymus has been observed in a few HIV-infected children. These patients were found to have characteristic anterior medi-astinal multilocular thymic cysts without clinical symptoms. Histologic examination shows focal cystic changes, follicular hyperplasia, and diffuse plasmacytosis and multinucleated giant cells. Treatment with cART may result in resolution, or spontaneous involution occurs in some cases.

Malignant diseases have been reported infrequently in HIV-infected children, representing only 2% of AIDS-defining illnesses. Non-Hodgkin lymphoma (including Burkitt lymphoma), primary CNS lymphoma, and leiomyosarcoma are the most commonly reported neoplasms among HIV-infected children. Epstein-Barr virus is associated with most lymphomas and with all leiomyosarcomas (see Chapter 281). Kaposi sarcoma, which is caused by human herpesvirus 8, occurs frequently among HIV-infected adults but is exceedingly uncommon among HIV-infected children in resource-rich countries (see Chapter 284).

DIAGNOSIS

All infants born to HIV-infected mothers test antibody-positive at birth because of passive transfer of maternal HIV antibody across the placenta during gestation; therefore, antibody should not be used to establish the diagnosis of HIV in an infant. Most uninfected infants without ongoing exposure (i.e., who are not breastfed) lose maternal antibody between 6 and 18 mo of age and are known as **seroreverters**. Because a small proportion of uninfected infants continue to test HIV antibody-positive for up to 24 mo of age, positive IgG antibody tests, including the rapid tests, cannot be used to make a definitive diagnosis of HIV infection in infants younger than 24 mo of age. The presence of IgA or IgM anti-HIV in the infant's circulation can indicate HIV infection, because these immunoglobulin classes do not cross the placenta; however, IgA and IgM anti-HIV assays have been both insensitive and nonspecific and therefore are not valuable for clinical use. In any child older than 24 mo of age, demonstration of IgG antibody to HIV by a repeatedly reactive enzyme immunoassay and confirmatory HIV PCR establishes the diagnosis of HIV infection. Breastfed infants should have antibody testing performed 12 wk following cessation of breastfeeding to identify

those who became infected at the end of lactation by the HIV-infected mother. Certain diseases (e.g., syphilis, autoimmune diseases) may cause false-positive or indeterminate results. In such cases, specific viral diagnostic tests (see later) have to be done.

Several rapid HIV tests are currently available with sensitivity and specificity better than those of the standard enzyme immunoassay. Many of these tests require only a single step that allows test results to be reported within less than 30 min. Performing rapid HIV testing during delivery or immediately after birth is crucial for the care of HIV-exposed newborns whose mother's HIV status was unknown during pregnancy. A positive rapid test in the mother has to be confirmed by a second different rapid test (testing different HIV-associated antibodies) or by HIV RNA PCR (viral load). Given the earlier detection of fourth-generation HIV ELISA testing (p24 antigen + HIV-1, HIV-2 IgG and IgM antibodies), Western blots are not appropriate to confirm testing, because the fourth generation assays can be positive before the Western blot becomes positive (i.e., in acute infection). In infants who are at risk of exposure to HIV-2 infection (e.g., born to an HIV-infected woman from West Africa or who has an HIV+ partner from West Africa), a rapid test that can detect both HIV-1 and HIV-2 should be used. However, if the HIV testing is negative or the Western blot test reveals an unusual pattern, further diagnostic tests should be considered. In addition, they should be tested with an HIV-2–specific DNA PCR assay; this assay has very limited availability.

Viral diagnostic assays, such as HIV DNA or RNA PCR, are consider-ably more useful in young infants, allowing a definitive diagnosis in most infected infants by 1-4 mo of age (Table 302.3). By 4 mo of age, HIV PCR testing identifies all infected nonbreastfed infants. Historically, HIV DNA PCR testing was the preferred virologic assay over HIV RNA PCR testing in developed countries for young infants due to what was thought to be a modest advantage in detecting intrapartum acquired infection for DNA PCR in the first month of life. The perinatal use of ART prophylaxis (either single drug or combination) to prevent vertical transmission has not affected the predictive value of viral diagnostic testing. The FDA-approved HIV DNA PCR test is no longer commercially available in the United States, but other assays exist; however, the sensitivity and specificity of noncommercial HIV-1 DNA tests (using individual laboratory reagents) may differ from the sensitivity and specificity of the FDA-approved commercial test. HIV RNA PCR also has increased sensitivity for non-subtype B HIV (rare in the United States). Almost 40% of infected newborns have positive test results in the first 2 days of life, with > 90% testing positive by 2 wk of age. Plasma HIV RNA PCR assays, which detect viral replication, are as sensitive as the DNA PCR for early diagnosis. Either the DNA or RNA PCR is considered acceptable for infant testing. The commercially available HIV-1 assays are not designed for quantification of HIV-2 RNA and thus should not be used to monitor patients with this infection.

Viral diagnostic testing should be performed within the first 12-24 hr of life, particularly for high-risk infants (i.e., those of mothers without

Table 302.3	Laboratory Diagnosis of HIV Infection
TEST	**COMMENT**
HIV DNA PCR	Historically preferred test to diagnose HIV-1 subtype B infection in infants and children younger than 24 mo of age; highly sensitive and specific by 2 wk of age and available; performed on peripheral blood mononuclear cells. False negatives can theoretically occur in non-B subtype HIV-1 infections. Historically had been preferred for testing in young infants.
HIV RNA PCR	Preferred test to identify non–B subtype HIV-1 infections. Similar sensitivity and specificity to HIV DNA PCR in infants and children younger than 24 mo of age

PCR, polymerase chain reaction.
Data from American Academy of Pediatrics, Committee of Pediatric AIDS: Diagnosis of HIV-1 infection in children younger than 18 months in the United States, Pediatrics 120:e1547-e1562, 2007.

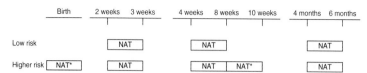

Fig. 302.4 Recommended virologic testing schedules for infants exposed to HIV by perinatal HIV transmission risk. Low Risk: Infants born to mothers who received standard ART during pregnancy with sustained viral suppression (usually defined as a confirmed HIV RNA level below the lower limits of detection of an ultrasensitive assay) and no concerns related to maternal adherence. Higher Risk: Infants born to mothers living with HIV who did not receive prenatal care, did not receive antepartum or intrapartum ARVs, received intrapartum ARV drugs only, initiated ART late in pregnancy (late second or third trimester), were diagnosed with acute HIV infection during pregnancy, or had detectable HIV viral loads close to the time of delivery, including those who received combination ARV drugs and did not have sustained viral suppression. *For higher-risk infants, additional virologic diagnostic testing should be considered at birth and 2-4 wk after cessation of ARV prophylaxis (i.e., at 8-10 wk of life). NAT, nucleic acid test. (*From Panel on Antiretroviral Therapy and Medical Management of Children Living with HIV. Guidelines for the Use of Antiretroviral Agents in Pediatric HIV Infection. Available at: http://aidsinfo.nih.gov/contentfiles/lvguidelines/pediatricguidelines.pdf. Accessed 1/13/18, Figure 1.*)

sustained virologic suppression, a late cART start, or a diagnosis with acute HIV during the pregnancy); the tests can identify almost 40% of HIV-infected children. It seems that many of these children have a more rapid progression of their disease and deserve more aggressive therapy. Data suggest that if cART treatment starts at this point, the outcome will be much better. In exposed children with negative virologic testing at 1-2 days of life, additional testing should be done at 2-3 wk of age, 4-8 wk of age, and 4-6 mo of age. For higher-risk infants, additional virologic diagnostic testing should be considered at 2 to 4 wk after cessation of ARV prophylaxis (i.e., at 8-10 wk of life) (Fig. 302.4). A positive virologic assay (i.e., detection of HIV by PCR) suggests HIV infection and should be confirmed by a repeat test on a second specimen as soon as possible because false-positive tests can occur. A confirmed diagnosis of HIV infection can be made with two positive virologic test results obtained from different blood samples. HIV infection can be presumptively excluded in nonbreastfed infants with two or more negative virologic tests (one at age ≥ 14 days and one at age ≥ 4 wk) or one negative virologic test (i.e., negative NAT [RNA or DNA]) at age ≥ 8 wk or one negative HIV antibody test at age ≥ 6 mo. Definitive exclusion of HIV infection in nonbreastfed infants is based on two or more negative virologic tests, with one obtained at age ≥ 1 mo and one at age ≥ 4 mo, or two negative HIV antibody tests from separate specimens obtained at age ≥ 6 mo. Some experts recommend documentation of seroreversion by testing for antibody at 12-18 mo of age; in low-risk infants with subtype B virus, this is likely not necessary, but antibody testing should be strongly considered in high-risk infants or infants infected with non–subtype B viruses.

TREATMENT

The currently available therapies do not eradicate the virus and cure the patient; instead they suppress the virus for extended periods of time and changes the course of the disease to a chronic process. Decisions about ART for pediatric HIV-infected patients are based on the magnitude of viral replication (viral load), CD4 lymphocyte count or percentage, and clinical condition. Because cART therapy changes as new drugs become available, decisions regarding therapy should be made in consultation with an expert in pediatric HIV infection. Plasma viral load monitoring and measurement of CD4 values have made it possible to implement rational treatment strategies for viral suppression, as well as to assess the efficacy of a particular drug combination. The following principles form the basis for cART:

1. Uninterrupted HIV replication causes destruction of the immune system and progression to AIDS.
2. The magnitude of the viral load predicts the rate of disease progression, and the CD4 cell count reflects the risk of opportunistic infections and HIV infection complications.
3. cART, which includes at least three drugs with at least two different mechanisms of action, should be the initial treatment. Potent combination therapy that suppresses HIV replication to an undetectable level restricts the selection of ART-resistant mutants; drug-resistant strains are the major factor limiting successful viral suppression and delay of disease progression.
4. The goal of sustainable suppression of HIV replication is best achieved by the simultaneous initiation of combinations of ART to which the

patient has not been exposed previously and that are not cross resistant to drugs with which the patient has been treated previously.
5. Drug-related interactions and toxicities should be minimal.
6. Adherence to the complex drug regimens is crucial for a successful outcome.

Increasing data have shown a benefit in adult studies to starting treatment earlier, which has led to recommendations to treat earlier in children, as well. There are strong data to support the treatment of all infants < 12 mo of age, regardless of the clinical symptoms, viral load, or CD4 count from the Children with HIV Early Antiretroviral (CHER) study. Urgent treatment is recommended for older children with stage 3 opportunistic infections or immunologic suppression. Treatment is recommended for all other children, as well. Rarely, treatment may need to be deferred on a case-by-case basis based on clinical or psychosocial factors that may affect adherence with the caregivers and child.

Combination Therapy

As of January 2019, 20 individual ART drugs, with 21 coformulated combination tablets as well as two pharmacokinetic boosters, were approved by the FDA for use in HIV-infected adults and adolescents. Of these, 19 were approved for at least some portion of the pediatric population (0-12 yr of age), with many but not all of them available as a liquid, powder, or small tablet/capsule (Table 302.4). ART drugs are categorized by their mechanism of action, such as preventing viral entrance into CD4+ T cells, inhibiting the HIV reverse transcriptase or protease enzymes, or inhibiting integration of the virus into the human DNA. Within the reverse transcriptase inhibitors, a further subdivision can be made: **nucleoside (or nucleotide) reverse transcriptase inhibitors (NRTIs)** and **nonnucleoside reverse transcriptase inhibitors (NNRTIs)** (see Fig. 302.3). The NRTIs have a structure similar to that of the building blocks of DNA (e.g., thymidine, cytosine). When incorporated into DNA, they act like chain terminators and block further incorporation of nucleosides, preventing viral DNA synthesis. Among the NRTIs, thymidine analogs (e.g., stavudine, zidovudine) are found in higher concentrations in activated or dividing cells, producing > 99% of the HIV virion population, and nonthymidine analogs (e.g., didanosine, lamivudine) have more activity in resting cells, which account for < 1% of the HIV virions but may serve as a reservoir for HIV. Suppression of replication in both populations is thought to be an important component of long-term viral control. NNRTIs (i.e., nevirapine, efavirenz, etravirine, rilpivirine) act differently than the NRTIs. They attach to the reverse transcriptase and cause a conformational change, reducing the activity of the enzyme. The **protease inhibitors (PIs)** are potent agents that act farther along the viral replicative cycle. They bind to the site where the viral long polypeptides are cut into individual, mature, and functional core proteins that produce the infectious virions before they leave the cell. The virus entry into the cell is a complex process that involves several cellular receptors and fusion. Several drugs have been developed to prevent this process. The **fusion inhibitor** enfuvirtide (T-20), which binds to viral gp41, causes conformational changes that prevent fusion of the virus with the CD4+ cell and entry into the cell.

Text continued on p. 1798

Table 302.4	Summary of Antiretroviral Therapies Available in 2019

DRUG (TRADE NAMES, FORMULATIONS)	DOSING	SIDE EFFECTS	COMMENTS
NUCLEOSIDE/NUCLEOTIDE REVERSE TRANSCRIPTASE INHIBITORS		Class adverse effects: Lactic acidosis with hepatic steatosis, particularly for older members of the class	
Abacavir (Ziagen, ABC): tablet: 300 mg; oral solution: 20 mg/mL Trizivir: combination of zidovudine (ZDV), lamivudine, ABC (300, 150, 300 mg) Epzicom: combination of lamivudine, ABC (300, 600 mg) Triumeq: combination of ABC, lamivudine, dolutegravir (600, 300, 50 mg)	Children: ≥3 mo to 13 yr: 8 mg/kg/ dose bid (maximum dose: 300 mg bid) >25 kg: 300 mg bid Children with stable CD4 counts and undetectable viral load > 6 mo while taking ABC can transition to 16 mg/kg once daily (max: 600 mg) Adolescents and adults: 600 mg once daily Trizivir (>40 kg): 1 tablet bid Epzicom (>25 kg): 1 tablet qd Triumeq: 1 tablet qd	Common: nausea, vomiting, anorexia, fever, headache, diarrhea, rash Less common: hypersensitivity, which can be fatal, Rare: lactic acidosis with hepatic steatosis, pancreatitis, elevated triglycerides, myocardial infarction	Can be given with food Genetic screening for HLAB*5701 must be done prior to initiation of ABC-containing treatment. If test is positive, avoid ABC. Do not restart ABC in patients who had hypersensitivity-like symptoms (e.g., flu-like symptoms)
Didanosine (Videx, ddI): powder for oral solution (prepared with solution containing antacid): 10 mg/mL	2 wk to < 3 mo: 50 mg/m²/dose bid 3-8 mo: 100 mg/m²/dose bid >8 mo: 120 mg/m²/dose (max: 200 mg/dose) bid Adolescents (>13 yr) and adults < 60 kg: 250 mg once daily >60 kg: 400 mg once daily (to increase adherence)	Common: diarrhea, abdominal pain, nausea, vomiting Less common: pancreatitis, peripheral neuropathy, electrolyte abnormalities, lactic acidosis with hepatic steatosis, hepatomegaly, retinal depigmentation	Food decreases bioavailability by up to 50%. Take 30 min before or 2 hr after meal. Tablets dissolved in water are stable for 1 hr (4 hr in buffered solution) Drug interactions: antacids/gastric acid antagonists may increase bioavailability; possible decreased absorption of fluoroquinolones, ganciclovir, ketoconazole, itraconazole, dapsone, and some protease inhibitors. Combination with d4T enhances toxicity; also common if combined with tenofovir. **Note: Due to increased side effects compared with other NRTIs, ddI is no longer recommended for treatment of HIV in children in the US.**
Enteric-coated didanosine (Videx EC): capsule, delayed release: 125, 200, 250, 400 mg; generic: 200, 250, 400 mg	20-25 kg: 200 mg once daily 25-60 kg: 250 mg once daily ≥60 kg: 400 mg once daily	Same as for ddI	Same as for ddI
Emtricitabine (Emtriva, FTC): capsule: 200 mg; oral solution: 10 mg/mL Truvada: combination of FTC, tenofovir disoproxil fumarate (TDF) (200, 300 mg) Truvada Low Strength: combinations of FTC/TDF (100, 150 mg); (133, 200 mg); (167, 250 mg) Atripla: combination of FTC, TDF, efavirenz (EFV) (200, 300, 600 mg) Descovy: combination of FTC, tenofovir disoproxil alafenamide (TAF) (200, 25 mg) Complera: combination of FTC, TDF, rilpivirine (RPV) (200, 300, 25 mg) Odefsey: combination of FTC, TAF, RPV (25, 200, 25 mg) Stribild: combination of FTC, TDF, elvitegravir (EVG), cobicistat (COBI) (200, 300, 150, 150 mg) Genvoya: combination of FTC, TAF, EVG, COBI (200, 10, 150, 150 mg) Biktarvy: combination of bictegravir (BIC), FTC, TAF (50, 200, 25 mg)	Infants: 0-3 mo: 3 mg/kg once daily Children ≥ 3 mo to 17 yr, oral solution: 6 mg/kg (max: 240 mg) once daily >33 kg, adolescents and adults: 200 mg capsule or 240 mg solution once daily Truvada, Descovy, Atripla, Complera, Descovy, Stribild, Genvoya or Biktarvy: adult dose: 1 tablet once daily	Common: headache, insomnia, diarrhea, nausea, skin discoloration Less common: lactic acidosis with hepatic steatosis, neutropenia	Patient should be tested for hepatitis B virus (HBV) because HBV exacerbation can occur when emtricitabine is discontinued. Can be given without regard to food. Oral solution should be refrigerated if temperature above 25°C (77°F) COBI is a pharmacokinetc enhancer (boosting agent) used to optimize drug levels; it is not interchangeable with ritonavir. It can alter renal tubular secretion of Cr, resulting in elevated Cr with normal GFR. Note oral solution is less bioavailable and has a max dose of 240 mg, while the max dose for capsules is 200 mg.

Continued

Table 302.4	Summary of Antiretroviral Therapies Available in 2019—cont'd

DRUG (TRADE NAMES, FORMULATIONS)	DOSING	SIDE EFFECTS	COMMENTS
Lamivudine (Epivir, Epivir HBV, 3TC): tablet: 150 (scored), 300 mg (Epivir, generic), 100 mg (Epivir HBV); Solution: 5 mg/mL (Epivir HBV), 10 mg/mL (Epivir) Combivir: combination of ZDV, lamivudine (300, 150 mg) Trizivir, Epzicom, and Triumeq combination (see abacavir) Symfi Lo combination of 3TC, TDF, EFV (300, 300, 400 mg)	Neonates (≥32 wk gestational age through 4 wk of age for term infants): 2 mg/kg/dose bid ≥4 wk to <3 mo: 4 mg/kg/dose bid ≥3 mo to <3 yr: 5 mg/kg/dose bid (max 150 mg) ≥3 yr: 5 mg/kg/dose bid (max 150 mg) or 10 mg/kg/dose qd (max 300 mg) For ≥14 kg with scored tablet (150 mg) 14 to <20 kg: 75 mg bid or 150 mg qd (if >3 yr) ≥20 to <25 kg: 75 mg qAM and 150 mg qPM or 225 mg qd (if >3 yr) ≥25 kg: 150 mg bid or 300 mg qd Children should be switched to once-daily dosing of lamivudine (oral solution or tablets) from twice-daily dosing at ≥3 yr if clinically stable for 36 wk with an undetectable viral load and stable CD4 T lymphocyte count Adolescents and adults: Combivir (>30 kg), Trizivir (>40 kg): 1 tablet bid Epzicom (>25 kg): 1 tablet qd Triumeq (>40 kg): 1 tablet qd Symfi Lo (>35 kg): 1 tablet qd	Common: headache, nausea Less common: pancreatitis, peripheral neuropathy, lactic acidosis with hepatic steatosis, lipodystrophy	No food restrictions Patient should be tested for hepatitis B virus (HBV) because HBV exacerbation can occur when lamivudine is discontinued. M184V mutation for this drug decreases viral fitness and can be advantageous to maintain including inducing AZT hypersusceptibility.
Stavudine (Zerit, d4T): capsule: 15, 20, 30, 40 mg; solution: 1 mg/mL	≥14 days and < 30 kg: 1 mg/kg/dose bid >30 kg: 30 mg bid	Common: headache, nausea, hyperlipidemia, fat maldistribution Less common: peripheral neuropathy, pancreatitis, lactic acidosis, hepatic steatosis	No food restrictions. Should not be administered with ZDV because of virologic antagonism. Higher incidence of lactic acidosis. Increased toxicity if combined with ddl. **Note: Due to increased side effects compared with other NRTIs, d4T is no longer recommended for treatment of HIV in children in the US.**
Tenofovir disoproxil fumarate (Viread, TDF): tablet: 150, 200, 250, 300 mg; powder: 40 mg/1 g powder Truvada: combination of FTC, TDF (200, 300 mg) Truvada Low Strength: combinations of FTC/TDF (100, 150 mg); (133, 200 mg); (167, 250 mg) Atripla: Combination of FTC, TDF, EFV (200, 300, 600 mg) Complera: combination of FTC, TDF, RPV (200, 300, 25 mg) Stribild: combination of FTC, TDF, EVG, COBI (200, 300, 150, 150 mg) Symfi Lo combination of 3TC, TDF, EFV (300, 300, 400 mg)	2 to <12 yr: 8 mg/kg/dose qd >12 yr and 35 kg, adolescents >12 yr and 35 kg and adults: 300 mg once daily Truvada, Atripla, Complera, Symfi Lo, and Stribild: 1 tablet qd Weight probands for ≥2 yr and ≥17 kg: 17 to <22 kg: 150 mg qd 22 to <28 kg: 200 mg qd 28 to <35 kg: 250 mg qd ≥35 kg: 300 mg qd	Common: nausea, vomiting, diarrhea Less common: lactic acidosis with hepatic steatosis, hepatomegaly, reduced bone density, renal toxicity	High-fat meal increases absorption; coadministration with ddl increased ddl toxicity, decreases atazanavir (ATV) levels (therefore, boosting ATV with ritonavir is required). ATV and lopinavir (LPV) increase TDF levels and potential toxicity. Screen for HBV before TDF is given, because exacerbation of hepatitis may occur when TDF is discontinued

Continued

Table 302.4	Summary of Antiretroviral Therapies Available in 2019—cont'd		
DRUG (TRADE NAMES, FORMULATIONS)	**DOSING**	**SIDE EFFECTS**	**COMMENTS**
Tenofovir alafenamide (Vemlidy, TAF) Descovy: combination of TAF, FTC (25, 200 mg) Genvoya: combination of TAF, FTC, EVG, COBI (10, 200, 150, 150 mg) Odefsey: combination of FTC, TAF, RPV (25, 200, 25 mg) Biktarvy: combination of BIC, FTC, TAF (50, 200, 25 mg)	Adolescents (≥13 yr, ≥35 kg): Descovy, Genvoya, or Odefsey: 1 tablet qd Biktarvy: ≥18 yr 1 tablet qd; >12 yr to 18 yr and >35 kg investigational dose 1 tablet qd based on limited data	Common: headache, diarrhea, nausea, increased serum lipids	Newer version of TDF that has less renal and bone toxicity. Screen for HBV before TAF is given, because exacerbation of hepatitis may occur when TAF is discontinued. Concentrates in cells more so than TDF, so is not approved for pregnant women given lack of data.
Zidovudine (Retrovir, AZT, ZDV): capsule: 100 mg; tablet: 300 mg; syrup: 10 mg/mL; intravenous injection: 10 mg/mL (all available generic) Combivir: combination of ZDV, lamivudine (300, 150 mg) Trizivir: Combination of ZDV, lamivudine, ABC (300, 150, 300 mg)	**Low Risk Prophylaxis:** <u>≥35 wk gestation at birth:</u> *Birth to age 4-6 wk:* 4 mg/kg/dose PO bid (or 3 mg/kg/dose IV q12h) <u>≥30 to <35 wk gestation at birth:</u> *Birth to age 2 wk:* 2 mg/kg/dose PO bid (or 1.5 mg/kg/dose IV q12h) THEN *Age 2 wk to 4-6 wk:* 3 mg/kg/dose PO bid (or 2.3 mg/kg/dose IV q12h) <u><30 wk gestation at birth</u> *Birth to age 4-6 wk:* 2 mg/kg/dose PO bid (or 1.5 mg/kg/dose IV q12h) **High Risk Prophylaxis and Treatment:** <u>≥35 wk gestation at birth:</u> Birth to age 4 wk: 4 mg/kg/dose PO bid THEN Age >4 wk: 12 mg/kg/dose PO bid <u>≥30 to <35 wk gestation at birth:</u> Birth to age 2 wk: 2 mg/kg/dose PO bid THEN Age 2 wk to 6-8 wk: 3 mg/kg/dose PO bid THEN Age >6-8 wk: 12 mg/kg/dose PO bid <u><30 wk gestation at birth:</u> Birth to age 4 wk: 2 mg/kg/dose PO bid THEN Age 4 wk to 8-10 wk: 3 mg/kg/dose PO bid THEN Age >8-10 wk: 12 mg/kg/dose PO bid <u>Infants >4 kg and ≥4 wk post delivery and children:</u> 4 kg to <9 kg: 12 mg/kg/dose PO bid 9 kg to <30 kg: 9 mg/kg/dose PO bid >30 kg, adolescents and adults: 300 mg bid Alternative body surface area dosing: 180-240 mg/m²/dose PO bid Combivir *or* Trizivir: 1 tablet bid	Common: bone marrow suppression (e.g., macrocytic anemia, neutropenia), headache, nausea, vomiting, anorexia Less common: liver toxicity, lactic acidosis with hepatic steatosis, myopathy, fat redistribution	No food restrictions Drug interactions: should not be given with d4T or doxorubicin. Rifampin may increase metabolism. Cimetidine, fluconazole, valproic acid may decrease metabolism. Ganciclovir, IFN-α, ribavirin increase ZDV toxicity. Only antiretroviral with an IV formulation currently.

Continued

Table 302.4	Summary of Antiretroviral Therapies Available in 2019—cont'd		
DRUG (TRADE NAMES, FORMULATIONS)	**DOSING**	**SIDE EFFECTS**	**COMMENTS**
NONNUCLEOSIDE REVERSE TRANSCRIPTASE INHIBITORS		Class adverse effects: Rash is mild to severe, usually within first 6 wk. Discontinue the drug if severe rash (with blistering, desquamation, muscle involvement, or fever)	
Efavirenz (Sustiva, EFV): capsule: 50, 200 mg; tablet: 600 mg Atripla: combination of EFV, FTC, TDF (600, 200, 300 mg) Symfi Lo combination of 3TC, TDF, EFV (300, 300, 400 mg)	Children < 3 yr: consult with expert Children ≥ 3 yr: 10 to < 15 kg: 200 mg qd 15 to < 20 kg: 250 mg qd 20 to < 25 kg: 300 mg qd 25 to < 32.5 kg: 350 mg qd 32.5 to < 40 kg: 400 mg qd ≥40 kg: 600 mg qd or 367 mg/m² body surface area Atripla (>40 kg, adult dose): 1 tablet qd Symfi Lo (>35 kg, adult dose): 1 tablet qd	Common: skin rashes, CNS abnormalities (e.g., vivid dreams, impaired concentration, insomnia, depression, hallucination) Less common: increased liver enzymes; potentially teratogenic, QTc prolongation (be careful with other QT-prolonging medications), false positives on some cannabinoid and benzodiazepine tests	Capsules can be opened for mixing in food. Administer at bedtime on empty stomach to minimize CNS side effects. Taking with food, especially fatty meal, can increase absorption and CNS side effects. Drug interactions: Efavirenz induces/inhibits CYP3A4 enzymes. Increase clearance of drugs metabolized by this pathway (e.g., antihistamines, sedatives and hypnotics, cisapride, ergot derivatives, warfarin, ethinyl estradiol) and several other ARVs (i.e., protease inhibitors). Drugs that induce CYP3A4 (e.g., phenobarbital, rifampin, rifabutin) decrease efavirenz levels. Clarithromycin levels decrease with EFV, and azithromycin should be considered. Use with caution in female adolescents with reproductive potential because of potential teratogenicity. Avoid using in individuals with a history of past or active psychiatric issues and use with caution in adolescents and young adults owing to possible affective side effects, including increased suicidality.
Etravirine (ETR, Intelence): tablet: 25, 100, 200 mg	Children <6 yr: consult with expert 16 to < 20 kg: 100 mg bid 20 to < 25 kg: 125 mg bid 25 to < 30 kg: 150 mg bid >30 kg, adolescents and adults: 200 mg bid	Common: nausea, rash, diarrhea Less common: hypersensitivity reactions	Always administer following a meal for absorption; taking on empty stomach decreases absorption by 50%. Tablets can be dispersed in water Inducer of CYP3A4 enzymes and inhibitor of CYP2C9 and CYP2C19, causing multiple interactions that should be checked before initiating ETR. Should not be given in combination with TPV, FPV, ATV, or other nonnucleoside reverse transcriptase inhibitors

Continued

Table 302.4	Summary of Antiretroviral Therapies Available in 2019—cont'd		
DRUG (TRADE NAMES, FORMULATIONS)	**DOSING**	**SIDE EFFECTS**	**COMMENTS**
Nevirapine (Viramune, NVP): tablet: 200 mg; extended-release (XR) tablet: 100, 400 mg; suspension: 10 mg/mL	**High risk Prophylaxis:** 3-dose series for high-risk infants >32 wk gestation at birth (including those born to mothers not taking HAART) NOTE: DOSES ARE A FLAT DOSE, NOT PER KG Dosing intervals: Within 48 hr of birth, 48 hr after first dose, 96 hr after second dose Birth weight 1.5-2 kg: 8 mg/dose PO Birth weight >2 kg: 12 mg/dose PO **Treatment (including higher risk prophylaxis with empiric therapy):** ≥37 wk gestation at birth: Birth to age 4 wk: 6 mg/kg/dose bid THEN Age >4 wk: 200 mg/m²/dose bid 34 to <37 wk gestation at birth: Birth to age 1 wk: 4 mg/kg/dose bid Age 1 to 4 wk: 6 mg/kg/dose bid Age >4 wk: 200 mg/m²/dose bid Note dose adjustment is optional at 4 wk for empiric HIV therapy for high risk infants with negative testing ≥1 mo to < 8 yr: 200 mg/m² once daily for 14 days; then same dose bid (max: 200 mg/dose) ≥8 yr: 120-150 mg/m² once daily for 14 days; then bid (max: 200 mg/dose) Adolescents and adults: 200 mg once daily for 14 days; then 200 mg bid or XR 400 mg qd (after 14 day lead in)	Common: skin rash, headache, fever, nausea, abnormal liver function tests Less common: hepatotoxicity (rarely life-threatening), hypersensitivity reactions	No food restrictions Drug interactions: induces hepatic CYP450A enzymes (including CYP3A and CYP2B6) activity and decreases protease inhibitor concentrations (e.g., IND, SQV, LPV). Should not be given with ATV. Reduces ketoconazole concentrations (fluconazole should be used as an alternative). Rifampin decreases nevirapine serum levels. Anticonvulsants and psychotropic drugs using same metabolic pathways as NVP should be monitored. Oral contraceptives may also be affected. XR formulation must be swallowed whole. For children ≤2 yr, some experts start with bid dosing without the 14 day lead-in of qd dosing. Lead-in dosing decreases occurrence of rash by allowing induction of cytochrome p450 metabolizing enzymes.
Rilpivirine (Edurant, RPV): tablet: 25 mg Complera: combination of RPV, FTC, TDF (25, 200, 300 mg) Odefsey: combination of FTC, TAF, RPV (25, 200, 25 mg) Juluca: combination of RPV, Dolutegravir (DTG) (25, 50 mg)	Pediatric patients: consult with expert Adolescents (>12 yr and 35 kg) and adults: 25 mg PO qd Complera or Odefsey: 1 tablet qd Juluca (>18 yr): 1 tablet qd; only for use in adults with ≥6 mo virologic suppression with no resistance to replace current regimen	Headache, insomnia, rash, depression, mood changes	Given with food only, 500 kcal meal. Do not use with proton pump inhibitors; antacids have to be spaced from dose by 2 h before or 4 h after. Should not be used if viral load > 100,000 copies/μL or drugs that induce CYP3A or with proton pump inhibitors

Continued

Table 302.4	Summary of Antiretroviral Therapies Available in 2019—cont'd		
DRUG (TRADE NAMES, FORMULATIONS)	**DOSING**	**SIDE EFFECTS**	**COMMENTS**
PROTEASE INHIBITORS		Class adverse effects: Gi side effects, hyperglycemia, hyperlipidemia (except atazanavir and darunavir), lipodystrophy, increased transaminases, increased bleeding disorders in hemophiliacs. Can induce metabolism of ethinyl estradiol; use alternate contraception (other than estrogen-containing oral contraceptives). All of these drugs undergo hepatic metabolism, mostly by CYP3A4, with many drug interactions. Treatment note: except in rare instances, always administer with boosting agent (ritonavir [RTV] or cobicistat [COBI]).	
Atazanavir (Reyataz, ATV): powder packet: 50 mg/packet; capsule: 150, 200, 300 mg (Note: capsules and packets are *not* interchangeable) Evotaz: combination of ATV, COBI (300, 150 mg)	Infants and children ≥ 3 mo and ≥ 5 kg: 5 to < 15 kg: ATV 200 mg (4 packets) + RTV 80 mg qd 15 to < 25 kg: ATV 250 mg (5 packets) + RTV 80 mg qd Note: Capsules are not approved for < 6 yr or < 15 kg Children ≥6 yr and ≥15 kg capsule dosing: 15 to <35 kg: 200 mg + RTV 100 mg ≥35 kg: 300 mg + RTV 100 mg Adolescents and adults: 300 mg + RTV 100 mg Adults (>18 yr): Evotaz: 1 tablet qd	Common: elevation of indirect bilirubin; headache, arthralgia, depression, insomnia, nausea, vomiting, diarrhea, paresthesias Less common: prolongation of PR interval on electrocardiogram (ECG); rash, rarely Stevens-Johnson syndrome, diabetes mellitus, nephrolithiasis	Administer with food to increase absorption. Review drug interactions before initiating because ATV inhibits CYP3A4, CYP1A2, CYP2C9, and UGT1A1 enzymes. Use with caution with cardiac conduction disease or liver impairment. Combination with EFV should not be used in treatment-experienced patients because it decreases ATV levels. TDF, antacids, H_2-receptor antagonists, and proton-pump inhibitors decrease ATV concentrations. Patients taking buffered ddI should take it at least 2 hr before ATV COBI is a pharmacokinetc enhancer (boosting agent) used to optimize drug levels; it is not interchangeable with ritonavir. It can alter renal tubular secretion of Cr, resulting in elevated Cr with normal GFR.
Darunavir (Prezista, DRV): tablets: 75, 150, 600, 800 mg; suspension: 100 mg/mL Prezcobix: combination DRV, COBI (800, 150 mg)	<3 yr or < 10 kg: do not use 3 to < 12 yr: 10 to < 11 kg: DRV 200 mg + RTV 32 mg bid 11 to < 12 kg: DRV 220 mg + RTV 32 mg bid 12 to < 13 kg: DRV 240 mg + RTV 40 mg bid 13 to < 14 kg: DRV 260 mg + RTV 40 mg bid 14 to < 15 kg: DRV 280 mg + RTV 48 mg bid 15 to < 30 kg: DRB 375 mg + RTV 48 mg bid 30 to < 40 kg: DRV 450 mg + RTV 100 mg bid ≥40 kg: DRV 600 mg + RTV 100 mg bid Adolescents ≥ 40 kg and adults with no DRV mutations: DRV 800 mg + RTV 100 mg qd Adults (>18 yr) with no DRV mutations: Prezcobix: 1 tablet qd Adolescents ≥ 40 kg and adults *with* DRV mutation(s): DRV 600 mg + RTV 100 mg bid	Common: diarrhea, nausea, vomiting, abdominal pain, fatigue, headache Less common: skin rashes (including Stevens-Johnson syndrome), lipid and liver enzyme elevations, hyperglycemia, fat maldistribution	DRV should be given with food. Contraindicated for concurrent therapy with cisapride, ergot alkaloids, benzodiazepines, pimozide, or any major CYP3A4 substrates. Use with caution in patients taking strong CYP3A4 inhibitors, or moderate/strong CYP3A4 inducers. Adjust dose with concurrent rifamycin therapy. Contains sulfa moiety: potential for cross-sensitivity with sulfonamide class

Continued

Table 302.4 | Summary of Antiretroviral Therapies Available in 2019—cont'd

DRUG (TRADE NAMES, FORMULATIONS)	DOSING	SIDE EFFECTS	COMMENTS
Fosamprenavir (Lexiva, FPV): tablet: 700 mg; suspension: 50 mg/mL	6 mo to 18 yr: <11 kg: FPV 45 mg/kg/dose + RTV 7 mg/kg/dose bid 11 to < 15 kg: FPV 30 mg/kg/dose + RTV 3 mg/kg/dose bid 15 to < 20 kg: FPV 23 mg/kg/dose + RTV 3 mg/kg/dose bid >20 kg: FPV 18 mg/kg/dose (max: 700 mg) + RTV 3 mg/kg/dose (max: 100 mg) bid Adolescents > 18 yr and adults: FPV 700 mg + RTV 100 mg bid *or* FPV 1,400 mg + RTV 200 mg qd For protease inhibitor (PI)–experienced, the once-daily dose is not recommended	Common: nausea, vomiting, perioral paresthesias, headache, rash, lipid abnormalities Less common: Stevens-Johnson syndrome, fat redistribution, neutropenia, elevated creatine kinase, hyperglycemia, diabetes mellitus, elevated liver enzymes, angioedema, nephrolithiasis	Should be given with food. FPV is an inhibitor of the CYP450 system and an inducer, inhibitor, and substrate of CYP3A4, which can cause multiple drug interactions. Use with caution in sulfa-allergic individuals.
Indinavir (Crixivan, IDV): capsule: 100, 200, 400 mg	Not approved for use in infants or children Adolescents and adults: IDV 800 mg IDV + RTV (100 mg to 200 mg) bid	Common: nausea, abdominal pain, hyperbilirubinemia, headache, dizziness, lipid abnormalities, nephrolithiasis, metallic taste Less common: fat redistribution, hyperglycemia, diabetes mellitus, hepatitis, acute hemolytic anemia	Reduce dose (600 mg IDV every 8 hr) with mild to moderate liver dysfunction. Adequate hydration (at least 48 oz fluid/day in adults) necessary to minimize risk of nephrolithiasis. IDV is cytochrome P450 3A4 inhibitor and substrate, which can cause multiple drug interactions: rifampin reduces levels; ketoconazole, ritonavir, and other protease inhibitors increase IDV levels. Do not coadminister with EFV, astemizole, cisapride, terfenadine
Lopinavir/Ritonavir (Kaletra, LPV/r): tablet: 100/25 mg, 200/50 mg; solution: 80/20 mg per/mL (contains 42% alcohol, 15% propylene glycol)	14 days to 18 yr: LPV 300 mg/m^2/dose + RTV 75 mg/m^2/dose bid In treatment naive children >1 yr a dose of 230 mg/m^2/dose bid can be used. Adolescents (>18 yr) and adults: LPV 400 mg + RTV 100 mg bid *or* 800 mg LPV + 200 mg RTV qd If taken with NVP, EFV, FPV, or NFV: LPV 600 mg + RTV 150 mg bid	Common: diarrhea, headache, nausea and vomiting, lipid elevation Less common: fat redistribution, hyperglycemia, diabetes mellitus, pancreatitis, hepatitis, PR interval prolongation	**Do not administer before postmenstrual age of 42 wk and postnatal age of 14 days owing to potential severe toxicities.** No food restrictions but has better GI tolerability when given with or after a meal. Pills must be swallowed whole. Oral solution should be given with high-fat meal to increase absorption. Poor palatability of oral solution is difficult to mask with flavorings or foods. Once-daily dosing is poorly tolerated in most children, and plasma concentration variability makes qd dosing contraindicated in children. Interacts with drugs using CYP3A4, which can cause multiple drug interactions
Nelfinavir (Viracept, NFV): tablet: 250, 625 mg	<2 yr: not recommended Children 2-13 yr: 45-55 mg/kg/dose bid (max: 1,250 mg/dose) Adolescents and adults: 1,250 mg bid	Common: diarrhea, asthenia, abdominal pain, skin rashes, lipid abnormalities Less common: exacerbation of liver disease, fat redistribution, hyperglycemia, diabetes mellitus, elevation of liver enzymes	Administer with a meal to optimize absorption; avoid acidic food or drink (e.g., orange juice). Tablet can be crushed or dissolved in water to administer as a solution. Nelfinavir inhibits CYP3A4 activity, which may cause multiple drug interactions. Rifampin, phenobarbital, and carbamazepine reduce levels. Ketoconazole, ritonavir, indinavir, and other protease inhibitors increase levels. Do not coadminister astemizole, cisapride, terfenadine. NFV is no longer recommended for treatment for HIV due to inferior potency compared to newer agents and unpredictable pharmacokinetics particularly in adolescents.

Continued

Table 302.4	Summary of Antiretroviral Therapies Available in 2019—cont'd

DRUG (TRADE NAMES, FORMULATIONS)	DOSING	SIDE EFFECTS	COMMENTS
Ritonavir (Norvir, RTV): capsule: 100 mg; tablet: 100 mg; solution: 80 mg/mL (contains 43% alcohol)	Only use is to enhance other PIs; dose varies (see information for specific PI)	Common: nausea, headache, vomiting, abdominal pain, diarrhea, taste aversion, lipid abnormalities, perioral paresthesias Less common: fat redistribution, hyperglycemia, diabetes mellitus, pancreatitis, hepatitis, PR interval prolongation, allergic reactions	Administration with food enhances bioavailability and reduces gastrointestinal symptoms. RTV solution should not be refrigerated (store at 20-25°C) RTV is potent inhibitor of CYP3A4 and CYP2D6 and inducer of CYP3A4 and CYP1A2 that leads to many drug interactions (e.g., protease inhibitors, antiarrhythmics, antidepressants, cisapride). Use cautiously with inhaled steroids (Cushing syndrome has been reported)
Saquinavir (Invirase, SQV): capsule: 200 mg; tablet: 500 mg	Infants and children < 16 yr: not approved for use Adolescents and adults: SQV 1,000 mg + RTV 100 mg bid	Common: diarrhea, abdominal pain, headache, nausea, skin rashes, lipid abnormalities Less common: exacerbation of chronic liver disease, diabetes mellitus, pancreatitis, elevated liver transaminases, fat maldistribution, increase in both QT and PR in ECG	Administer with a high-fat meal to enhance bioavailability. SQV is metabolized by CYP3A4, which may cause many drug interactions: rifampin, phenobarbital, and carbamazepine decrease serum levels. Saquinavir may decrease metabolism of calcium channel antagonists, azoles (e.g., ketoconazole), macrolides. Pretherapy EKG recommended and contraindicated in patients with prolonged QT interval.
Tipranavir (Aptivus, TPV): capsule: 250 mg; solution: 100 mg/mL (contains 116 IU vitamin E/mL)	<2 yr: not approved 2-18 yr (treatment-experienced only): TPV 375 mg/m^2/dose + RTV 150 mg/m^2 (max: TPV 500 mg + RTV 200 mg) bid or TPV 14 mg/kg/dose + RTV 6 mg/kg/dose (max: same) bid Adolescents (>18 yr) and adult: TPV 500 mg + RTV 200 mg bid	Common: diarrhea, nausea, vomiting, fatigue, headache, skin rashes, elevated liver enzymes, lipid abnormalities Less common: fat redistribution, hepatitis, hyperglycemia, diabetes mellitus, intracranial hemorrhage	No food restrictions. Better tolerated with meal. Can inhibit human platelet aggregation: use with caution in patients at risk for increased bleeding (trauma, surgery, etc.) or in patients receiving concurrent medications that may increase the risk of bleeding. TPV is metabolized by CYP3A4, which may cause many drug interactions. Contraindicated in patients with hepatic insufficiency or in those receiving concurrent therapy with amiodarone, cisapride, ergot alkaloids, benzodiazepines, pimozide. TPV contains sulfonamide moiety, and caution should be taken in patients with sulfonamide allergy
FUSION INHIBITORS			
Enfuvirtide (Fuzeon, ENF): injection: lyophilized powder of 108 mg reconstituted in 1.1 mL of sterile water delivers 90 mg/mL	<6 yr: not approved Children ≥6 yr to 16 yr: 2 mg/kg/dose SQ (max: 90 mg) bid Adolescents (>16 yr) and adults: 90 mg SQ bid	Common: Local injection site reactions in 98% (e.g., erythema, induration nodules, cysts, ecchymoses) Less common: increased incidence of bacterial pneumonia, hypersensitivity, fever, nausea, vomiting, chills, elevated liver enzymes, hypotension, immune-mediated reactions (e.g., glomerulonephritis, Guillain-Barré syndrome, respiratory distress)	Must be given subcutaneously. Severity of reactions increased if given intramuscularly. Apply ice after injection and massage the area to reduce local reactions. Injection sites should be rotated; recommended sites are upper arm, anterior thigh, or abdomen.

Continued

| Table 302.4 | Summary of Antiretroviral Therapies Available in 2019—cont'd | | |

DRUG (TRADE NAMES, FORMULATIONS)	DOSING	SIDE EFFECTS	COMMENTS
ENTRY INHIBITORS			
Maraviroc (Selzentry, MVC): oral solution: 20 mg/mL; tablet: 25, 75, 150, 300 mg	Neonates/infants: not approved ≥2 yr and ≥ 10 kg: Given with CYP3A inhibitors (EVG, RTV, PIs except TPV/r): 10 to < 20 kg: 50 mg bid 20 to < 30 kg: 75 mg bid 30 to < 40 kg: 100 mg bid >40 kg: 150 mg bid Given with NRTIs, T-20, TPV/r, NVP, RAL, or other drugs not affecting CYP3A: 10 to < 30 kg: not recommended 30 to < 40 kg: 300 mg bid >40 kg: 300 mg bid Given with EFV, ETR: not recommended Adolescents > 16 yr and adults: 150 mg bid if given with potent CYP3A inhibitor (e.g., protease inhibitor except TPV) 300 mg bid if given with not potent CYP3A4 inhibitors (e.g., NRTI, TPV, NVP, ENF, RAL) 600 mg bid if given with potent CYP3A4 inducer (e.g., EFV, ETR, rifampin, phenobarbital)	Common: fever, upper respiratory infection–like symptoms, rash, abdominal pain, musculoskeletal symptoms, dizziness Less common: cardiovascular abnormalities, cholestatic jaundice, rhabdomyolysis, myositis, osteonecrosis	Testing for CCR5-tropic virus required; virus must not have mixed tropism (i.e., CCR5/CXC4) to have efficacy. No food restrictions. MVC is a CYP3A4 and P-glycoprotein (Pgp) substrate, which may cause many drug interactions. Tropism assay to exclude the presence of CXCR4 HIV is required before using MVC. Caution should be used when given to patients with hepatic impairment or cardiac disease or receiving CYP3A4 or P-glycoprotein-modulating drugs.
INTEGRASE INHIBITORS (INSTI)			
Bictegravir (BIC) Only available as Biktarvy: combination of BIC, TAF, FTC (50, 25, 200 mg)	Biktarvy: ≥18 yr 1 tablet qd; >12 yr to 18 yr and >35 kg: investigational dose 1 tablet qd based on limited data	Diarrhea, nausea, headache	No food restrictions Metabolized by UGT1A1 and CYP450 (CYP) 3A
Dolutegravir (Tivicay, DTG): tablet: 10, 25, 50 mg Triumeq: combination of ABC, 3TC, DTG (600, 300, 50 mg) Juluca: combination of RPV, Dolutegravir (DTG) (25, 50 mg)	Neonates and infants: not approved ≥30 to < 40 kg: 35 mg qd (ARV-naïve or INSTI-naïve) >12 yr and ≥ 40 kg adolescents and adults: 50 mg qd (INSTI-naïve) If taken with EFV, FPV/RTV, TPV/RTV, or rifampin: 50 mg bid If INSTI-experienced with associated resistance or suspected resistance: 50 mg bid Triumeq: 1 tablet qd (INSTI-naïve, ≥ 40 kg) Juluca (>18 yr): 1 tablet qd; only for use in adults with ≥6 mo virologic suppression with no resistance to replace current regimen	Insomnia, headache, neuropsychiatric illness Rare: rash, hepatotoxicity, hypersensitivity reactions	No food restrictions. UGT1A1 and CYP450 (CYP) 3A substrate. Should be taken 2 hr before or 6 hr after taking laxatives, sucralfate, iron or calcium supplements, or buffered medications. DTG decreases tubular secretion of Cr and slightly increases measured Cr but does not affect GFR.
Elvitegravir (EVG): only found in 2 coformulated fixed-dose combination (FDC) tablets Stribild: combination of EVG, FTC, TDF, COBI (150, 200, 300, 150 mg) Genvoya: combination of FTC, TAF, EVG, COBI (200, 10, 150, 150 mg)	Genvoya: Not approved for <25 kg. Child and Adolescent (Weighing ≥25 kg; Any Sexual Maturity Rating [SMR]) and Adult Dose: 1 tablet qd Stribild: Not approved for <35 kg. Adolescent (Weighing ≥35 kg and SMR 4 or 5) and Adult Dose: 1 tablet qd	Nausea, diarrhea, headache	Administer with food. EVG is metabolized by CYP3A4 and modestly induces CYP2D6 that can cause multiple drug interactions. Cautiously use with nephrotoxic drugs. Do not use Stribild or Genvoya with ritonavir. COBI is a pharmacokinetc enhancer (boosting agent) used to optimize drug levels; it is not interchangeable with ritonavir. It can alter renal tubular secretion of Cr, resulting in elevated Cr with normal GFR.

Continued

Table 302.4	Summary of Antiretroviral Therapies Available in 2019—cont'd			

DRUG (TRADE NAMES, FORMULATIONS)	DOSING	SIDE EFFECTS	COMMENTS
Raltegravir (Isentress, RAL): film-coated tablet: 400 mg; HD tablet: 600 mg chewable tablet: 25, 100 mg (scored); granules for oral suspension: 100 mg suspended in 10 mL of water for final concentration of 10 mg/mL	**Treatment and high-risk prophylaxis (empiric therapy) for neonates:** >37 wk gestation at birth and >2 kg (oral suspension): Birth to Age 1 wk: approximately 1.5 mg/kg/dose qd 2 to <3 kg: 4 mg qd 3 to <4 kg: 5 mg qd 4 to <5 kg: 7 mg qd If mother on raltegravir in 2-24 h prior to delivery, delay first dose 24 to 48 hr after birth. Start other ART ASAP. Age 1-4 wk: approximately 3 mg/ kg/dose bid 2 to <3 kg: 8 mg bid 3 to <4 kg: 10 mg bid 4 to <5 kg: 15 mg bid THEN **Infant and Pediatrics dosing** (Oral suspension) Children aged ≥4 wk and ≥3 kg to <20 kg: approximately 6 mg/kg/dose bid 3 to <4 kg: 25 mg bid 4 to <6 kg: 30 mg bid 6 to <8 kg: 40 mg bid 8 to <11 kg: 60 mg bid 11 to <14 kg: 80 mg bid 14 to <20 kg: 100 mg bid Chewable tablet: 11 to <14 kg: 75 mg bid 14 to <20 kg: 100 mg bid 20 to <28 kg: 150 mg bid 28 to <40 kg: 200 mg bid ≥40 kg: 300 mg bid Child or adolescent ≥ 25 kg and adults: 400 mg film-coated tablet bid Child and Adolescent Weighing ≥50 kg (HD tablet): 1200 mg qd (2 tablets) For treatment-naive or virologically suppressed patients on an initial regimen of 400 mg twice daily (HD tablet): 1200 mg qd (2 tablets)	Common: nausea, headache, dizziness, diarrhea, fatigue Less common: itching, creatine phosphokinase elevation, myopathy, rhabdomyolysis, depression, hypersensitivity Rare: rash including Stevens-Johnson, TEN, hypersensitivity reaction	No food restrictions Oral suspension, film-coated tablet and chewable tablet are not interchangeable; chewable tablets and suspension have better oral bioavailability than film-coated tablet; hence, higher-dose film-coated tablet can be taken at 25 kg. RAL is metabolized by UGT1A1 glucuronidation, and inducers of this system (e.g., rifampin, TPV) will reduce RGV levels, whereas inhibitors of this system (e.g., ATV) will increase RGV levels. Do not administer rifampin with once daily raltegravir (HD). Aluminum and magnesium containing antacids should not be co-administered. UGT1A1 metabolism is low at birth and increases rapidly over first 4-6 wk of life. No data for preterm infants.

Antiretroviral drugs often have significant drug–drug interactions, with each other and with other classes of medicines, which should be reviewed before initiating any new medication.

The information in this table is not all-inclusive. Updated and additional information on dosages, drug–drug interactions, and toxicities is available on the AIDSinfo website at http://www.aidsinfo.nih.gov.

Modified from the Guidelines for use of antiretroviral agents in pediatric HIV infection. http://aidsinfo.nih.gov/contentfiles/pediatricguidelines.pdf.

Maraviroc is an example of a selective CCR5 coreceptor antagonist that blocks the attachment of the virus to this chemokine (an essential process in the viral binding and fusion to the CD4+ cells). **Integrase inhibitors (INSTIs)** (i.e., raltegravir, dolutegravir, elvitegravir, bictegravir) block the enzyme that catalyzes the incorporation of the viral genome into the host's DNA.

By targeting different points in the viral life cycle and stages of cell activation and by delivering drug to all tissue sites, maximal viral suppression is feasible. Combinations of three drugs consisting of a two-NRTI backbone of (1) a thymidine analog NRTI (abacavir or zidovudine) or tenofovir and (2) a nonthymidine analog NRTI (lamivudine or emtricitabine) to suppress replication in both active and resting cells added to (3) a ritonavir-boosted PI (lopinavir/ritonavir, atazanavir, or darunavir), an NNRTI (efavirenz or nevirapine), or an

INSTI (raltegravir or dolutegravir) can produce prolonged suppression of the virus. The use of three drugs from three different classes generally should be avoided but may be necessary in children with highly resistant viruses; the drugs in these regimens should only be chosen by an HIV specialist with pharmacist input. Combination treatment increases the rate of toxicities (see Table 302.4), and complex drug–drug interactions occur among many of the antiretroviral drugs. Many PIs are inducers or inhibitors of the cytochrome P450 system and are therefore likely to have serious interactions with multiple drug classes, including nonsedating antihistamines and psychotropic, vasoconstrictor, antimycobacterial, cardiovascular, anesthetic, analgesic, and gastrointestinal drugs (cisapride). Whenever new medications are added to an antiretroviral treatment regimen, especially a protease inhibitor or cobicistat containing regimen, a pharmacist and/or HIV specialist should be consulted to address possible drug interactions. The inhibitory effect of ritonavir (a PI) on the cytochrome P450 system has been exploited, and small doses of the drug are added to several other protease inhibitors (e.g., lopinavir, atazanavir, darunavir) to slow their metabolism by the P450 system and to improve their pharmacokinetic profile. This strategy provides more effective drug levels with less toxicity and less-frequent dosing. Recently, the development of cobicistat provides an alternative to ritonavir. Although cobicistat is a potent inhibitor of cytochrome P450 3A, it is a weak inhibitor of CYP2D6 and other CYP isoforms (e.g., CYP1A2), making pharmacologic interactions with many drugs more predictable than for ritonavir, which is also active against these isoforms. Preliminary studies with cobicistat suggest that it has a good tolerability profile and less effect on adipocytes (resulting in lesser accumulations of lipid and a milder response to insulin). The better solubility of cobicistat compared with ritonavir has helped the development of more single-tablet combination regimens with cobicistat. However, cobicistat is currently only approved for adolescents and adults; it is not approved for use in pregnancy.

Adherence

Adherence to the medication schedules and dosages is fundamental to cART success. Therefore, assessment of the likelihood of adherence to treatment is an important factor in deciding when to initiate therapy as well as choice of regimen. Numerous studies show that compliance of < 90% results in less-successful suppression of the viral load. In addition, several studies document that almost half of the pediatric patients surveyed were nonadherent to their regimen. Poor adherence to prescribed medication regimens results in subtherapeutic drug concentrations and enhances the development of resistant viruses. Several barriers to adherence are unique to children with HIV infection. Combination antiretroviral regimens are often unpalatable and require extreme dedication on the part of the caregiver and child; a reluctance to disclose the child's disease to others reduces social support; there may be a tendency to skip doses if the caregiver is not around or when the child is in school. Adolescents have other issues that reduce adherence. Denial and/or fear of their infection, an unstructured lifestyle, conduct or emotional disorders, wishing to be the same as their peers, depression, fatigue from taking a lifelong regimen, anxiety, and alcohol and substance abuse are just a few of the barriers to long-term adherence in this growing population. These and other barriers make participation of the family in the decision to initiate therapy essential. Intensive education on the relationship of drug adherence to viral suppression, training on drug administration, frequent follow-up visits, peer support, text messaging, and commitment of the caregiver and the patient (despite the inconvenience of adverse effects or the dosing schedule) are critical for successful antiviral treatment. Multiple methods such as the viral load response, self-reporting of missed doses during the last 3-7 days, and pharmacy/pill counting should be used to assess adherence. Assessing for emergence of resistant virus on sequencing (genotype) can also be a helpful tool.

Initiation of Therapy

The decision on when to initiate cART is evolving. When cART was first introduced, medication regimens had significant side effects. This led to decisions to delay therapy until it would be most beneficial, usually after advanced immunologic suppression had developed. In a large adult cohort, the Strategic Timing of Antiretroviral Treatment (START) trial demonstrated a strong benefit in starting therapy earlier in adults, even before CD4 counts fell into an immunosuppressed range; this became more feasible with the development of safer, better-tolerated medications. In adults, it has also been found that receiving suppressive cART eliminates the risk of the sexual transmission of HIV to others. Current adult guidelines recommend the initiation of cART in all adults with HIV. As with adult guidelines, the Panel on Antiretroviral Therapy and Medical Management of Children Living with HIV also recommends treatment for all children with HIV. However, the urgency of when to start treatment and the strength of the recommendations vary by age and pretreatment CD4 count. This is due to limited pediatric-specific data, as well as knowing that once pediatric patients are started on

medications, treatment will need to continue for life; this means that potential concerns about adherence and toxicities will go on for an extended period. For children < 1 yr of age, the CHER trial has clearly demonstrated the benefit of early immediate ART. Data in older children suggest that mortality rates are lower and growth is more normal in children < 10 yr of age who are started on immediate cART. More studies are needed for confirmation, however.

Children younger than 1 yr of age are at high risk for disease progression, and immunologic and virologic tests to identify those likely to develop rapidly progressive disease are less predictive than in older children. Therefore, HIV-infected infants younger than 1 yr of age should be treated with cART as soon as the diagnosis of HIV infection has been confirmed, regardless of their clinical or immunologic status or viral load. Data suggest that HIV-infected infants who are treated before the age of 3 mo control their HIV infection better than infants whose cART started later than 3 mo of age.

For children 1 yr to under 6 yr of age, urgent treatment is recommended if the children have stage 3–defining opportunistic infections or stage 3 immunodeficiency (CD4 < 500 cells/μL). For children with moderate HIV-related symptoms or CD4 counts of 500-999 cells/μL, treatment is strongly recommended. Treatment is also recommended for asymptomatic or mildly symptomatic children with CD4 counts ≥ 1,000 cells/μL.

For children ≥ 6 yr, urgent treatment is recommended if the children have stage 3–defining opportunistic infections or stage 3 immunodeficiency (CD4 < 200 cells/μL). For children with moderate HIV-related symptoms or CD4 counts of 200-499 cells/μL, treatment is again strongly recommended. Treatment is also recommended for asymptomatic or mildly symptomatic children with CD4 counts ≥ 500 cells/μL. *These guidelines are reviewed yearly, and care providers should check for revisions regularly at http://aidsinfo.nih.gov.*

Dosages

Children are usually treated with higher doses (per kg weight) than adults because of reduced absorption or increased drug metabolism. Data on ART drug dosages for neonates, especially premature infants, are often limited. Because of the immaturity of the neonatal liver, there must often be an increase in the dosing interval of drugs primarily cleared through hepatic glucuronidation.

Adolescents should have ART dosages prescribed on the basis of the Tanner staging of puberty rather than on the basis of age. Pediatric dosing ranges should be used during early puberty (Tanner stages I, II, and III), whereas adult dosing schedules should be followed in adolescents in late puberty (Tanner stages IV and V). Dolutegravir and Efavirenz should be avoided in females who may become pregnant and do not use effective contraception because of potential teratogenicity; however, if an HIV-positive female becomes pregnant while taking a dolutegravir or efavirenz-containing regimen, the regimen can be continued, assuming that virologic suppression is maintained, because by the time the pregnancy is typically determined, the period of teratogenesis has past, specifically for neural tube defects. Because some ART agents may alter the metabolism of some hormonal contraceptives and decrease their effectiveness, interactions should be considered when choosing contraceptive agents. A comprehensive table of interactions of HIV medications with hormonal contraceptives can be found here: https://aidsinfo.nih.gov/guidelines/htmltables/3/5803. Medroxyprogesterone (DMPA) is a reasonable choice outside of regimens containing cobicistat. Alternative contraception options, such as use of an intrauterine device, should also be considered.

Changing Antiretroviral Therapy

Therapy should be changed when the current regimen is judged ineffective as evidenced by an increase in viral load, deterioration of the CD4 cell count, or clinical progression. Development of toxicity or intolerance to drugs is another reason to consider a change in therapy. When a change is considered, the patient and family should be reassessed for adherence concerns. Because adherence is a major issue in this population, resistance testing (while the patient is taking antiretroviral medications) is important in identifying adherence issues (e.g., detectable virus sensitive to current drugs suggests a lack of adherence) or the development of resistance (e.g., evidence of resistance mutations to given drugs). In both situations, other contributing factors, such as poor absorption, an incorrect dose, or drug–drug interactions, should be carefully reviewed. While considering possible new drug choices, the potential for cross-resistance should be addressed. In starting a new regimen in a patient with virologic failure, the new regimen should include at least two, but preferably three, fully active antiretroviral medications, with assessment of the anticipated activity based on the treatment history and resistance testing (genotype or phenotype). The goal is to achieve and maintain virologic suppression. If virologic suppression cannot be achieved, the goals of therapy should focus on preserving the immunologic function and preventing further disease progression, as well as preventing the emergence of additional drug resistance (which could limit future treatment options).

Monitoring Antiretroviral Therapy

To ensure proper monitoring, the CD4 cell count, viral load, complete blood count, chemistries, urinalysis, and serum lipids should be obtained before an initiation of or change in cART to have a baseline for comparisons during treatment. At entry into care genotypic resistance testing should be done as well. Children need to be seen within 1-2 wk after initiation of new cART to reinforce and counsel regarding adherence and to screen for potential side effects. Virologic and immunologic surveillance (using the quantitative HIV RNA PCR and CD4 lymphocyte count), as well as clinical assessment, should be performed regularly while on cART. The initial virologic response (i.e., at least a five-fold [0.7 $\log_{10}$] reduction in viral load) should be achieved within 4-8 wk of initiating antiretroviral therapy. The maximum response to therapy usually occurs within 12-16 wk, but may be later (24 wk) in very young infants. Thus, HIV RNA levels should be measured at 4 wk and 3-4 mo after therapy initiation. Once an optimal response has occurred, the viral load should then be measured at least every 3-6 mo. If the response is unsatisfactory, another viral load should be determined as soon as possible to verify the results before a change in therapy is considered. Virologic failure is defined as a repeated plasma viral load ≥200 copies/mL after 6 mo of therapy. The CD4 cells respond more slowly to successful treatment particularly in patients with long standing infection and CD4 suppression. CD4 counts should be monitored every 3-4 mo and potentially can be done less frequently in adolescents and adults with documented virologic suppression. Potential toxicity should be monitored closely for the first 8-12 wk (including complete blood count, serum chemistries), and if no clinical or laboratory toxicity is documented, a follow-up visit every 3-4 mo is adequate. Monitoring for potential toxicity should be tailored to the drugs taken. These toxicities include but are not limited to hematologic complications (e.g., zidovudine); hypersensitivity rash (e.g., efavirenz); lipodystrophy (e.g., redistribution of body fat seen with NRTIs, protease inhibitors, which can take several years to emerge); hyperlipidemia (elevation of cholesterol and triglyceride concentrations); hyperglycemia, and insulin resistance (e.g., protease inhibitors); mitochondrial toxicity leading to severe lactic acidosis (e.g., stavudine, didanosine); electrocardiogram abnormalities (e.g., atazanavir, lopinavir); abnormal bone mineral metabolism (e.g., tenofovir disoproxil fumarate but not tenofovir alafenamide); and hepatic toxicity, including severe hepatomegaly with steatosis. After a patient is on a stable regimen, labs outside of CD4 count and viral load can be done every 6-12 mo. An important part of every visit is ongoing adherence counseling given the need for excellent adherence to cART to avoid the emergence of resistance. *Detailed current guidelines for monitoring HIV-infected children during therapy can be found at http://aidsinfo.nih.gov.*

Resistance to Antiretroviral Therapy

Young children usually are at greater risk than adults for developing resistance because they have higher viral loads than adults and are more limited by which ART options are available. The high mutation rate of HIV (mainly as a result of the absence of error-correcting mechanisms) results in the generation of viruses with multiple mutations everyday in the absence of cART. Failure to reduce the viral load to < 40 copies/mL on cART due to nonadherence resulting in subtherapeutic drug levels increases the risk for developing resistance by selecting those mutant viruses with a competitive advantage (i.e. drug resistance mutations). Even effectively treated patients do not completely suppress all viral replication, and persistence of HIV transcription and evolution of envelope sequences continues in the latent cellular reservoirs, though recent data show that this evolution does not appear to affect the emergence of resistance to cART in virologically suppressed patients. Accumulation of resistance mutations, particularly in nonadherent patients, progressively diminishes the potency of the cART and challenges the physician to find new regimens. For some drugs (e.g., nevirapine, lamivudine), a single mutation is associated with resistance, whereas for other drugs (e.g., zidovudine, lopinavir), several mutations are needed before significant resistance develops. Testing for drug resistance, especially when devising a new regimen, is the standard of care. Two types of tests are available; genotype is most commonly used but the phenotype may be helpful in select patients with complex viral resistance due to exposure to multiple cART regimens.

1. The **phenotype** measures the virus susceptibility in various concentrations of the drug. This allows calculation of the drug concentration that will inhibit the viral replication by 50% (IC_{50}). The ratio of the IC_{50} and a reference virus IC_{50} is reported as the fold resistance change. Note this test is usually combined with a genotype when used but is largely reserved for patients with extremely complex mutations.

2. The **genotype** predicts the virus susceptibility from mutations identified in the HIV genome isolated from the patient and is the more commonly used test. Several online sites (e.g., http://hivdb.stanford.edu) can assist in interpreting the test's results. Several studies show that the treatment success is higher in patients whose cART was guided by genotype or phenotype testing.

Neither method may detect drug resistance if the amount of the resistant virus is < 10% of the circulating population or if it is present only in the latent reservoir. Note that if a patient has not been taking cART for several weeks, the absence of selective drug pressure will make the dominant population of circulating viruses revert to the wild type, and resistance mutations can be missed.

It is recommended to test for drug resistance before initiating therapy and before changing treatment because of virologic failure. When changing therapy, the resistance test results should be considered in the context of previous resistance tests results, if done, and drugs used in previous regimens.

Supportive Care

Even before ART drugs were available, a significant impact on the quality of life and survival of HIV-infected children was achieved when supportive care was given. A multidisciplinary team approach is desirable for successful management. Following the initiation or change of cART, more frequent visits or contacts with the patient/caregivers for support and education will help in their acceptance and adjustment to the new regimen and will contribute to a better adherence. Close attention should be paid to the nutritional status, which is often delicately balanced and may require aggressive supplementation, especially in children with advanced disease. Painful oropharyngeal lesions and dental caries may interfere with eating, and thus routine dental evaluations and careful attention to oral hygiene should be encouraged. Paradoxically, an increasing number of adolescents with perinatally acquired or behavioral risk-acquired disease are obese. Some teens experience ART-related central lipoaccumulation (usually related to older agents), but others have poor dietary habits and inactivity as the cause of their obesity, just as others do who are obese in epidemic numbers in the United States. Their development should be evaluated regularly, with the provision of necessary physical, occupational, and/or speech therapy. Recognition of pain in the young child may be difficult, and effective nonpharmacologic and pharmacologic protocols for pain management should be instituted when indicated.

All HIV-exposed and HIV-infected children should receive standard pediatric immunizations. Live oral polio vaccine should not be given due to poor immunologic response in HIV+ children as well as concern for live vaccination in potentially immunocompromised children (Fig. 302.5). The risk and benefits of rotavirus vaccination should be considered in infants born to HIV-infected mothers. Because < 1% of these infants

Vaccine	Birth	1 mo	2 mo	4 mo	6 mo	12 mo	15 mo	18 mo	24 mo	4-6 yr	11-12 yr	14-16 yr
Hepatitis B	Hep B	Hep B			Hep B							
Measles, Mumps, Rubella*						MMR†	MMR†					
Influenza					Influenza‡							
Pneumococcal Conjugate and Hemophilus b			PCV Hib	PCV Hib	PCV Hib	PCV Hib					Pneumococcal§	
Diphtheria, Tetanus, Pertussis			DTap	DTap	DTap		DTap					
Polio (inactivated)			Polio	Polio	Polio							
Varicella						Varicella†						
Hepatitis A						Hep A[]						
Rotavirus*			RV¶	RV	RV							

* See text.
† Contraindicated in children with AIDS or CD4+ absolute count <500 for age 1-5 yr or <15%. Give 2 doses 1-3 mo apart. In immune reconstituted children on cART, CD4 count has to be sustained above threshold for at least 6 mo before live virus vaccination.
‡ Revaccination is recommended every year. Inactivated vaccine only should be used, not LAIV.
§ Revaccination with pneumococcal polysaccharide vaccine (PPV) every 5 yr.
[] Two doses at least 6 mo apart.
¶ First dose 6 through 14 wk of age and final dose no later than 8 mo 0 days of age. If using Rotarix, only 2 doses (2 and 4 mo) are needed.

Fig. 302.5 Routine childhood immunization schedule for HIV-infected children.

in resource-rich countries will develop HIV infection, the vaccine should be given. In other situations, the considerable attenuation of the vaccine's strains should be considered, and unless the infant has clinical symptoms of AIDS or a CD4 percentage of < 15%, vaccination is likely appropriate. Other live bacterial vaccines (e.g., bacillus Calmette-Guérin) should be avoided because of the high incidence of bacillus Calmette-Guérin–related disease in HIV-infected infants. Varicella and measles mumps–rubella vaccines are recommended for children who are not severely immunosuppressed (i.e., CD4 cell percentage ≥ 15%, absolute CD4 count > 500 cells/μL for ages 1-5 yr), but these vaccines should not be given to severely immunocompromised children (i.e., CD4 cell percentage < 15%, absolute CD4 count < 500 cells/μL for age 1-5 yr). Of note, prior immunizations do not always provide protection, as evidenced by outbreaks of measles and pertussis in immunized HIV-infected children. The durability of vaccine-induced titers is often short, especially if vaccines are administered when the child's CD4 cell count is low, and reimmunization when the CD4 count has increased may be indicated. It is recommended that children with HIV receive quadrivalent meningococcal conjugate vaccine at a younger age than the routine schedule. Adolescent vaccines are also important, including the Tdap booster and HPV vaccine. The current recommended annotated vaccine schedule for HIV-infected children is found here: https://www.cdc.gov/vaccines/schedules/hcp/child-adolescent.html.

Prophylactic regimens are integral for the care of HIV-infected children. All infants between 4-6 wk and 1 yr of age who are proven to be HIV-infected should receive prophylaxis to prevent *P. jiroveci* pneumonia regardless of the CD4 count or percentage (Tables 302.5 and 302.6). Infants exposed to HIV-infected mothers should receive the same prophylaxis until they are proven to be noninfected; however, prophylaxis does not have to be initiated if there is strong presumptive evidence of noninfection (i.e., non–breastfed infant with two negative HIV PCR tests at older than 14 days and 4 wk of age, respectively). When the HIV-infected child is older than 1 yr of age, prophylaxis should be given according to the CD4 lymphocyte count (see Table 302.5). The best prophylactic regimen is 150 mg/m²/day of TMP and 750 mg/m²/day of SMX (maximum: 320/1,600 mg) given as 1-2 daily doses 3 days (consecutively or every other day) per wk. For severe

adverse reactions to TMP-SMX, alternative therapies include dapsone, atovaquone, and aerosolized pentamidine.

Prophylaxis against MAC should be offered to HIV-infected children with advanced immunosuppression (i.e., CD4 lymphocyte count < 750 cells/μL in children younger than 1 yr of age, < 500 cells/μL in children 1-2 yr of age, < 75 cells/μL in children 2-5 yr of age, and < 50 cells/μL in children > 6 yr of age) (see Table 302.6). The drugs of choice are azithromycin (20 mg/kg [maximum: 1,200 mg] once a week orally or 5 mg/kg [maximum: 250 mg] once daily orally) or clarithromycin (7.5 mg/kg bid orally). In rare situations, rifabutin 300 mg qd can be an alternative for children older than 6 yr of age though efficacy data in children is very limited.

Based on adult data, primary prophylaxis against most opportunistic infections may be discontinued if patients have experienced sustained (>6 mo duration) immune reconstitution with cART, even if they had previous opportunistic infections such as *Pneumocystis* pneumonia or disseminated MAC. HIV-infected children are at higher risk for TB and thus should have tuberculin skin testing (5 tuberculin units purified protein derivation) or interferon gamma release assay (IGRA) testing for TB at least once per year; an induration of 5 mm or more should be considered positive for the PPD. If the child is living in close contact with a person with TB, the child should be tested more frequently. Of note, the sensitivity of purified protein derivation and IGRA is reduced in severely immunocompromised patients. The Guidelines for Prevention and Treatment of Opportunistic Infections Among HIV-Exposed and HIV-Infected Children (http://aidsinfo.nih.gov) should be consulted for these and other opportunistic infections that may occur in these populations. To reduce the incidence of opportunistic infections, parents should be counseled about (1) the importance of good hand washing, (2) avoiding raw or undercooked food *(Salmonella)*, (3) avoiding drinking or swimming in lake or river water or being in contact with young farm animals *(Cryptosporidium)*, and (4) the risk of playing with pets *(Toxoplasma* and *Bartonella* from cats, *Salmonella* from reptiles).

PROGNOSIS

The improved understanding of the pathogenesis of HIV infection in children and the availability of more effective antiretroviral drugs has

Table 302.5	Recommendations for PJP Prophylaxis and CD4 Monitoring for HIV-Exposed Infants and HIV-Infected Children, by Age and HIV Infection Status

AGE/HIV INFECTION STATUS	PJP PROPHYLAXIS	CD4 MONITORING
Birth to 4-6 wk, HIV-exposed	No prophylaxis	None
HIV infection reasonably excluded*	No prophylaxis	None
<1 yr, HIV-infected or HIV-indeterminate	Prophylaxis regardless of CD4 count or percentage	According to local practice for initiation or follow-up of cART
1-5 yr, HIV-infected	Prophylaxis if CD4 < 500 cells/μL or < 15%[†]	According to local practice for initiation or follow-up of cART
>6 yr, HIV-infected	Prophylaxis if CD4 < 200 cells/μL or < 15%[††]	According to local practice for initiation or follow-up of cART

The National Perinatal HIV Hotline (1-888-448-8765) provides consultation on all aspects of perinatal HIV care.

*See text.

[†]More frequent monitoring (e.g., monthly) is recommended for children whose CD4 counts or percentages are approaching the threshold at which prophylaxis is recommended.

[‡]Prophylaxis should be considered on a case-by-case basis for children who might otherwise be at risk for PJP, such as children with rapidly declining CD4 counts or percentages or children with category C conditions. Children who have had PJP should receive PJP prophylaxis until their CD4 count is ≥200 cells/mm³ for patients aged ≥6 yr, CD4 percentage is ≥15% or CD4 count is ≥500 cells/mm³ for patients aged 1 to <6 yr for >3 consecutive mo after receiving cART for ≥6 mo.

cART, combined antiretroviral therapy; PJP, *Pneumocystis jiroveci* pneumonia.

Table 302.6	Prophylaxis to Prevent First Episode of Opportunistic Infections Among HIV-Exposed and HIV-Infected Infants and Children, United States*

PATHOGEN	INDICATION	PREVENTIVE REGIMEN FIRST CHOICE	PREVENTIVE REGIMEN ALTERNATIVE
STRONGLY RECOMMENDED AS STANDARD OF CARE			
Pneumocystis pneumonia[†]	HIV-infected or HIV-indeterminate infants aged 1-12 mo; HIV-infected children aged 1-5 yr with CD4 count of < 500 cells/μL or CD4 percentage of < 15%; HIV-infected children aged 6-12 yr with CD4 count of < 200 cells/μL or CD4 percentage of < 15%; >13 yr with CD4 count <200 or <15%	TMP-SMX, 150/750 mg/m² body surface area per day or 5-10 mg/kg/day (TMP)/25-50 mg/kg/day (SMX) (max: 320/1,600 mg) orally qd or bid 3 times weekly on consecutive days *or* qd or bid orally 3 times weekly on alternate days	Dapsone: age ≥ 1 mo: 2 mg/kg (max: 100 mg) orally qd; or 4 mg/kg (max: 200 mg) orally once a week Atovaquone: age 1-3 mo and > 24 mo-12 yr: 30-40 mg/kg orally qd with food; age 4-24 mo: 45 mg/kg orally qd with food; ≥ 13 yr 1500 mg orally qd Aerosolized pentamidine: age ≥ 5 yr: 300 mg once a month by Respirgard II (Marquest, Englewood, CO) nebulizer
Malaria	Living or traveling to area in which malaria is endemic	Same for HIV-infected and HIV-uninfected children. Refer to http://www.cdc.gov/malaria/ for the most recent recommendations. Mefloquine, 5 mg/kg orally 1 time weekly (max: 250 mg) Atovaquone/proguanil (Malarone) qd 11-20 kg: 62.5 mg/25 mg (1 pediatric tablet) 21-30 kg: 2 pediatric tablets 31-40 kg: 3 pediatric tablets >40 kg: 1 adult tablet (250 mg/100 mg)	Doxycycline, 2.2 mg/kg body weight (maximum 100 mg) orally qd for children >8 yr Chloroquine, 5 mg/kg base (equal 7.5 mg/kg chloroquine phosphate) orally up to 300 mg weekly (only for regions where the parasite is sensitive)
Mycobacterium tuberculosis Isoniazid-sensitive	TST reaction ≥ 5 mm or Prior positive TST result without treatment or Close contact with any person who has contagious TB. TB disease must be excluded before start of treatment	Isoniazid, 10-15 mg/kg body weight (max: 300 mg) qd for 9 mo or 20-30 mg/kg body weight (max: 900 mg) orally 2 times weekly for 9 mo; DOT highly recommended	Rifampin, 10-20 mg/kg body weight (max: 600 mg) orally daily for 4-6 mo
Isoniazid-resistant	Same as previous pathogen; increased probability of exposure to isoniazid-resistant TB	Rifampin, 10-20 mg/kg body weight (max: 600 mg) orally daily for 4-6 mo	Consult TB expert

Continued

Table 302.6	Prophylaxis to Prevent First Episode of Opportunistic Infections Among HIV-Exposed and HIV-Infected Infants and Children, United States—cont'd		
		PREVENTIVE REGIMEN	
PATHOGEN	**INDICATION**	**FIRST CHOICE**	**ALTERNATIVE**
Multidrug-resistant (isoniazid and rifampin)	Same as previous pathogen; increased probability of exposure to multidrug-resistant TB	Choice of drugs requires consultation with public health authorities and depends on susceptibility of isolate from source patient	
Mycobacterium avium complex[‡]	For children age ≥ 6 yr with CD4 count of < 50 cells/μL; age 2-5 yr with CD4 count of < 75 cells/μL; age 1-2 yr with CD4 count of < 500 cells/μL; age < 1 yr with CD4 count of < 750 cells/μL	**Clarithromycin,** 7.5 mg/kg (max: 500 mg) orally bid *or* **Azithromycin,** 20 mg/kg (max: 1,200 mg) orally once a week	**Azithromycin,** 5 mg/kg body weight (max: 250 mg) orally qd *or* Children age ≥ 5 yr **Rifabutin,** 300 mg orally qd
Varicella-zoster virus[§]	Exposure to varicella or shingles with no history of varicella *or* Zoster or seronegative status for VZV *or* Lack of evidence for age-appropriate vaccination	Varicella-zoster immunoglobulin (VariZIG), 125 IU/10 kg (max: 625 IU) IM, administered ideally within 96 hr after exposure; potential benefit up to 10 days after exposure	If VariZIG is not available and < 96 hr from exposure, **acyclovir** 20 mg/kg (max: 800 mg) 4 times a day for 5-7 days *or* IVIG, 400 mg/kg, administered once
Vaccine-preventable pathogens	Standard recommendations for HIV-exposed and HIV-infected children	Routine vaccinations (see Fig. 302.5)	
USUALLY RECOMMENDED			
Toxoplasma gondii[¶]	Seropositive IgG to Toxoplasma and severe immunosuppression: age < 6 yr with CD4 percentage < 15%; age ≥ 6 yr with CD4 count < 100 cells/μL	TMP-SMX, 150/750 mg/m^2 orally qd or divided bid *or* Same dosage qd 3 times weekly on consecutive days *or* bid 3 times weekly on alternate days	**Dapsone,** age ≥ 1 mo: 2 mg/kg or 15 mg/m^2 (max: 25 mg) orally qd plus **Pyrimethamine,** 1 mg/kg (max: 25 mg) orally qd plus **Leucovorin,** 5 mg orally every 3d
Invasive bacterial infections	Hypogammaglobulinemia (i.e., IgG < 400 mg/dL)	IVIG 400 mg/kg body weight every 2-4 wk	
Cytomegalovirus	CMV antibody positivity and severe immunosuppression (CD4 count < 50 cells/μL for >6 yr; CD4 percentage <5% for ≤6 yr) For children aged 4 mo–16 yr, valganciclovir oral solution 50 mg/mL at dose in milligrams = 7 × BSA × CrCl (up to maximum CrCl of 150 mL/min/1.73 m^2) orally qd with food (maximum dose 900 mg/day)	**Valganciclovir,** 900 mg orally qd with food for older children who can receive adult dosing	

*Information in these guidelines might not represent FDA approval or FDA-approved labeling for products or indications. Specifically, the terms *safe* and *effective* might not be synonymous with the FDA-defined legal standards for product approval.

†Daily trimethoprim-sulfamethoxazole (TMP-SMX) reduces the frequency of certain bacterial infections. Compared with weekly dapsone, daily dapsone is associated with a lower incidence of PCP but higher hematologic toxicity and mortality rates. Patients receiving therapy for toxoplasmosis with sulfadiazine-pyrimethamine are protected against PCP and do not need TMP-SMX. TMP-SMX, dapsone-pyrimethamine, and possibly atovaquone (with or without pyrimethamine), protect against toxoplasmosis; however, data have not been prospectively collected.

‡Substantial drug interactions can occur between rifamycins (i.e., rifampin and rifabutin) and protease inhibitors and nonnucleoside reverse transcriptase inhibitors. A specialist should be consulted.

§Children routinely being administered intravenous immunoglobulin (IVIG) should receive VariZIG if the last dose of IVIG was administered more than 21 days before exposure.

¶Protection against toxoplasmosis is provided by the preferred anti-*Pneumocystis* regimens and possibly by atovaquone.

CMV, cytomegalovirus; FDA, U.S. Food and Drug Administration; HIV, human immunodeficiency virus; IgG, immunoglobulin G; IM, intramuscularly; IVIG, intravenous immunoglobulin; PCP, *Pneumocystis* pneumonia; TB, tuberculosis; TMP-SMX, trimethoprim-sulfamethoxazole; TST, tuberculin skin test; VZV, varicella-zoster virus.

From Centers for Disease Control and Prevention (CDC): Guidelines for the prevention and treatment of opportunistic infections among HIV-exposed and HIV-infected children, MMWR Recomm Rep 58(RR-11):127-128, 2009, Table 1.

changed the prognosis considerably for children with HIV infection. The earlier cART is started, the better the prognosis. In settings with ready access to early diagnosis and antiretroviral therapy, progression of the disease to AIDS has significantly diminished. Since the advent of cART in the mid-1990s, mortality rates in perinatally infected children have declined more than 90% and many children survive to adolescence and adulthood. Even with only partial reduction of the viral load, children may have both significant immunologic and clinical benefits. In general, the best prognostic indicators are the sustained suppression of the plasma viral load and the restoration of a normal CD4+ lymphocyte count. If determinations of the viral load and CD4 lymphocytes are available, the results can be used to evaluate the prognosis. It is unusual to see rapid progression in an infant with a viral load < 100,000 copies/mL. In contrast, a high viral load (>100,000 copies/mL) over time is associated with a greater risk for disease progression and death. CD4 count is also another prognostic indicator with mortality rate significantly higher in profoundly immunosuppressed individuals. To define the prognosis more accurately, the use of changes in both markers (CD4 lymphocyte percentage and plasma viral load) is recommended.

Even in resource-limited countries where cART and molecular diagnostic tests are less available, the use of cART has had a substantial benefit on the survival of HIV-infected children and has reduced the likelihood of mortality by > 75%. Children with opportunistic infections (e.g., *Pneumocystis* pneumonia, MAC), encephalopathy and regressing developmental milestones, or wasting syndrome, which are all AIDS defining conditions, have the worst prognosis, with 75% dying before 3 yr of age. A higher risk of death was documented in children who did not receive TMP-SMX preventive therapy. Persistent fever and/or oral thrush, serious bacterial infections (meningitis, pneumonia, sepsis), hepatitis, persistent anemia (<8 g/dL), and/or thrombocytopenia (<100,000/μL) also suggest a poor outcome, with > 30% of such children dying before 3 yr of age. In contrast, lymphadenopathy, splenomegaly, hepatomegaly, lymphoid interstitial pneumonitis, and parotitis are associated with a slower progression of disease and a better prognosis. With sustained virologic suppression and maintained immunologic function, life expectancy is quite good. For adults and adolescents acquiring HIV, effective cART can restore life expectancy to near normal.

PREVENTION

Use of antiretroviral therapy for interruption of perinatal transmission from mother to child has been one of the greatest achievements of HIV research. Maternal cART is documented to decrease the rate of perinatal HIV-1 transmission to < 2%, and to < 1% if the mother's viral RNA level is < 1,000 copies/mL at delivery. Therefore, it is recommended that **all pregnant women** be tested for HIV, and if they are positive, should be treated with a cART regimen, irrespective of the viral load or CD4 count during pregnancy. All infants born to HIV-infected mothers should receive zidovudine prophylaxis for 6 wk; prophylaxis for 4 wk can be done in low-risk infants. Additional ARV therapy should be considered if the risk of acquiring HIV by the newborn is high. High-risk scenarios include infants born to mothers who received neither antepartum nor intrapartum ARV drugs or only intrapartum ARV drugs, infants born to mothers with a significant detectable viral load (>1,000 copies/mL) near delivery despite cART (particularly if it was a vaginal delivery), infants born to mothers of unknown HIV status who test positive at delivery or postpartum, or infants who have a positive HIV antibody test on screening after delivery. In these scenarios, three regimen options can be considered: (1) the addition of three doses of nevirapine (at birth, 48 hr, and 144 hr of life); (2) an empirical HIV therapy regimen of zidovudine, lamivudine, and nevirapine at treatment doses or (3) an empirical HIV therapy regimen of zidovudine, lamivudine, and raltegravir at treatment doses (note treatment doses of raltegravir for neonates are different than for older children with an escalating dose over the 6 wk of therapy due to evolving liver metabolism in neonates). Enthusiasm and support for treatment regimens (particularly option 2) have been driven by a case of an apparent functional cure in an infant in 2013 who went 2 yr without cART with virologic suppression before rebound of the infection occurred (the so-called Mississippi baby), as well as a large cohort of high-risk, exposed infants in Canada. The most experience and data exist for zidovudine, which can cause transient anemia or neutropenia in exposed infants. There is also a strong pool of data supporting the safety of lamivudine. For the remaining drugs for treatment of high risk infants, nevirapine has the most experience of use but neither has robust data in premature infants. Dosing recommendations exist for nevirapine down to 32 wk but raltegravir can only be used in 37 wk and up. *In high-risk infants, consultation with an experienced HIV specialist is highly recommended. The National Perinatal HIV Hotline (888-448-8765) provides 24-7 support from experienced HIV specialists to help in managing high-risk infants. Guidelines and current recommended doses for prophylaxis in newborns are updated at least yearly and can be accessed at http://www.aidsinfo.nih.gov.* A complete blood count, differential leukocyte count, and platelet count should be performed at 4-8 wk of age to monitor zidovudine toxicity. This should be in conjunction with 4-6 wk of zidovudine prophylaxis for the infant. If the child is found to be HIV infected, baseline laboratory assessment (e.g., CD4 count, HIV RNA, complete blood count,

chemistries, lipids, genotype) should be done and cART should be started as soon as possible. The viral load and CD4 lymphocyte counts should be determined at 1 and 3 mo of age and should be repeated every 3 mo. Cesarean section (C-section) as a prevention strategy was examined in a multinational meta-analysis, which showed that the combination of elective C-section and maternal zidovudine treatment reduced transmission by 87%. However, these data were obtained prior to the advent of cART, and the additional benefit of elective C-section to the cART-treated mother whose viral load is < 1,000 copies/mL is negligible. Thus, elective C-section at 38 wk of gestation should be considered only for women whose viral load is > 1,000 copies/mL in late gestation, to further reduce the risk of vertical transmission.

The WHO recommends that all pregnant women receive a cART regimen appropriate for their own health, which should be continued for the remainder of their lives. This approach has the potential to reduce transmission during breastfeeding and future pregnancies, lowers the transmission risk to sexual partners, improves maternal survival, and promotes simplified universal treatment regimens. It is not currently recommended that HIV+ women breastfeed in resource rich countries and there has been a least one case of mother-to-child-transmission via breastfeeding in a virologically suppressed mother.

Although the most effective way to prevent postpartum transmission of HIV is to eliminate breastfeeding altogether and substitute replacement feeding, there is evidence that early weaning may not be safe in resource-limited settings because of the high risk of malnutrition and diarrhea in formula-fed infants without a consistent source of clean water. Furthermore, exclusive breastfeeding (no additional solids or fluids other than water) results in less transmission than mixed feeding. Guidelines have evolved to recommend that HIV-infected mothers living in resource-limited settings should breastfeed their infants until at least 12 mo of age, with exclusive breastfeeding for the first 6 mo, and cART should continue to be provided to the mother. In settings where there are safe alternatives to breastfeeding, formula feeding is recommended. *U.S. guidelines for prevention of mother-to-child transmission are regularly updated at http://aidsinfo.nih.gov/ and the international guidelines are regularly updated at the WHO website (http://www.who.int/hiv/topics/mtct/en/).*

Because perinatal transmission can be reduced dramatically by treating pregnant mothers, prenatal testing and identification of HIV-1 infection as early as possible in the mother is extremely important. The benefit of therapy both for the mother's health and to prevent transmission to the infant cannot be overemphasized. The recommended universal prenatal HIV-1 counseling and HIV-1 testing for all pregnant women has reduced the number of new infections dramatically in many areas of the United States and Europe. For women not tested during pregnancy, the use of rapid HIV antibody testing during labor or on the first day of the infant's life is a way to provide perinatal prophylaxis to an additional group of at-risk infants. Perinatal recommendations also now endorse the testing of pregnant women's partners to identify HIV+ partners who may transmit, leading to acute HIV infection which carries and extremely high risk of mother-to-child transmission.

Prevention of sexual transmission involves avoiding the exchange of bodily fluids. In sexually active adolescents, condoms should be an integral part of programs to reduce sexually transmitted diseases, including HIV-1. Unprotected sex with older partners or with multiple partners and the use of recreational drugs are often associated with acquisition of HIV-1 infection in adolescents and young adults. Educational efforts about avoidance of risk factors are essential for older school-age children and adolescents and should begin before the onset of sexual activity. In addition, promising research for sexually active adults may translate to increased prevention for adolescents. Three African trials demonstrated that male circumcision was associated with a 50–60% reduction in the risk of HIV acquisition in young men. For women, use of a 1% vaginal gel formulation of tenofovir during intercourse was found to reduce HIV acquisition by nearly 40% in one study, though subsequent trials have had variable efficacy; other topical microbicides are being investigated. A double-blind study of preexposure prophylaxis (PrEP) in MSM using once-daily dosing of coformulated tenofovir and emtricitabine resulted in a 44% reduction in the incidence of HIV. The incidence of HIV transmission was reduced by 73% when participants took the drug on 90% or more days. Studies of this regimen in other groups, including serodiscordant heterosexual couples, heterosexual individuals not in committed relationships, and intravenous drug users, showed excellent efficacy, as well (70–92%). All studies to date for PrEP have been in individuals 18 yr and up, however in adolescent patients with sufficiently high risk for acquisition, consideration should be given to using PrEP for HIV prevention. In addition, a large randomized multinational clinical trial of HIV serodiscordant adults demonstrated that effective ARV therapy in the HIV-infected partner reduced secondary transmission to an uninfected sexual partner by 96%. Further trials have confirmed that virologic suppression eliminates sexual transmission in heterosexual partners as well as men who have sex with men, spurning the catchphrase "U=U" or undetectable = untransmittable. The majority of these trials have been in adults, with limited participation by adolescents and young adults. Although much of the efficacy will likely be seen in young people, as well, further studies should be done on efficacy and acceptability in this age-group.

The course and prognosis of HIV infection has been radically improved by cART for all ages, particularly newer agents with less side effects. With good adherence, prolonged virologic suppression can be achieved and immune function can be preserved or reconstituted. However, lifelong adherence and side effects of medications are important challenges to recognize that can prevent patients from achieving good outcomes. Globally, great strides have been made in preventing mother-to-child transmission and increasing access to cART for children and adults, which is important for maintaining health as well as driving down sexual and vertical transmission with virologic suppression. However, there is still much work to be done in order to ensure the end of the global HIV epidemic, including continued advancement of our understanding of the immunology of HIV latency and reservoirs, HIV vaccines, and continued increasing of access to cART worldwide.

Bibliography is available at Expert Consult.

Chapter **303**
Human T-Lymphotropic Viruses (1 and 2)
Paul Spearman and Lee Ratner

第三百零三章
人T淋巴细胞病毒（1型和2型）

中文导读

本章主要介绍了人T淋巴细胞病毒1型和2型感染的病因、流行病学和传播方式、诊断、临床表现和预防。病毒可以在母婴间进行传播，通过生殖器分泌物、受污染的血液制品和静脉注射药物传播。临床表现中包括HLV-1相关关节炎、葡萄膜炎和皮炎，成人T细胞白血病/淋巴瘤，人嗜T淋巴细胞病毒1型相关性脊髓病，人类嗜T淋巴细胞病毒2型。

ETIOLOGY

Human T-lymphotropic viruses 1 (HTLV-1) and 2 (HTLV-2) are members of the *Deltaretrovirus* genus of the Retroviridae family and are single-stranded RNA viruses that encode reverse transcriptase, an RNA-dependent DNA polymerase that transcribes the single-stranded viral RNA into a double-stranded DNA copy. HTLV-1 was the first human retrovirus discovered, isolated in 1979 by the Gallo laboratory from a cutaneous T-cell lymphoma. The closely related virus HTLV-2 was subsequently identified in 1981. HTLV-1 is associated with adult T-cell leukemia/lymphoma (ATL) and HTLV-1–associated myelopathy/tropical spastic paraparesis (HAM/TSP), whereas HTLV-2 is less pathogenic and is rarely associated with leukemia or neurologic diseases.

HTLV-1 and -2 share a genome homology of approximately 65%. The genome contains *gag, pol,* and *env* genes and the pX region, which encodes nonstructural proteins. The nonstructural proteins include the Tax and Rex regulatory proteins, the novel proteins essential for virus spread (p30, p12, and p13), and the antisense-encoded HTLV-1 basic leucine zipper factor HBZ. HTLV-1 and -2 infect cells via the ubiquitous glucose transporter type or via Neuropilin-1, which serve as virus receptors. HTLV-1 and -2 can infect a variety of cells, with HTLV-1 most often found in CD4+ T cells and HTLV-2 showing a preference for CD8+ T cells. Following viral entry, reverse transcription produces a double-stranded DNA copy of the RNA genome that is transported into the nucleus and integrated into chromosomal DNA (the provirus), evading the typical mechanisms of immune surveillance and facilitating lifelong infection.

EPIDEMIOLOGY AND MODES OF TRANSMISSION

HTLV-1 infects 15-20 million persons globally. It is endemic in southwestern Japan (where > 10% of adults are seropositive), areas of the Caribbean, including Jamaica and Trinidad (≤6%), and in parts of sub-Saharan Africa (≤5%). Lower seroprevalence rates are found in South America (≤2%) and Taiwan (0.1–1%). There is microclustering with marked variability within geographic regions.

The seroprevalence of HTLV-1 and HTLV-2 in the United States in the general population is 0.01–0.03% for each virus, with higher rates with increasing age. The prevalence of HTLV-1 infection is highest in babies born in endemic areas or in persons who have had sexual contact with persons from endemic areas. The prevalence of HTLV-2 infection is highest in intravenous drug users, with a seroprevalence of 8.8–17.6% in this population.

HTLV-1 and -2 are transmitted as cell-associated viruses from mother to child and transmission through genital secretions, contaminated blood products, and intravenous drug use. **Mother-to-child transmission** during the intrauterine period or peripartum period is estimated to occur in less than 5% of cases but increases to approximately 20% with breastfeeding. A higher maternal HTLV-1 proviral load and prolonged breastfeeding are associated with a greater risk of mother-to-child transmission. In Japan, approximately 20–25% of children born to HTLV-1–infected mothers became infected prior to recommendations that seropositive mothers should avoid breastfeeding, with a marked reduction to 2.5% transmission following restriction of breastfeeding. HTLV-2 may also be transmitted via breastfeeding, but it has a slightly lower reported transmission rate via breast milk of approximately 14%.

DIAGNOSIS

HTLV-1 and HTLV-2 infections are diagnosed by screening using a second-generation enzyme immunoassay, with confirmation by immunoblot, indirect immunofluorescence, or line immunoassays. The polymerase chain reaction can also be used to distinguish HTLV-1 from HTLV-2 infection.

CLINICAL MANIFESTATIONS

The lifetime risk of disease associated with HTLV-1 infection is estimated at 5–10% and is highest following vertical transmission. HTLV-1 is associated with ATL and several nonmalignant conditions, including the neurodegenerative disorder HTLV-1–associated myelopathy (HAM), also known as tropical spastic paraparesis and sometimes termed HAM/tropical spastic paraparesis. The geographic epidemiologic characteristics of ATL and HAM are similar. **HTLV-1–associated arthropathy** mimics rheumatoid arthritis, including a positive rheumatoid factor. Treatment is with antiinflammatory agents. **HTLV-1–associated uveitis** may be unilateral or bilateral, is more common among females, and resolves spontaneously, although it often recurs within 1-3 yr. Topical corticosteroids hasten recovery. **HTLV-1–associated infective dermatitis** is a chronic and recurrent eczematous disease occurring during childhood and adolescence, which predisposes to staphylococcal infection. HTLV-1 infection predisposes to disseminated and recurrent *Strongyloides stercoralis* infection, an increased risk of developing tuberculosis disease following latent infection, and severe scabies.

ADULT T-CELL LEUKEMIA/LYMPHOMA

The age distribution of ATL peaks at approximately 50 yr, underscoring the long latent period of HTLV-1 infection. HTLV-1–infected persons remain at risk for ATL even if they move to an area of low HTLV-1

prevalence, with a lifetime risk for ATL of 2–4%. Most cases of ATL are associated with monoclonal integration of the HTLV-1 provirus into the cellular genome of CD4+ T lymphocytes, resulting in unchecked proliferation of CD4 T cells. There is a spectrum of disease that is categorized into different forms: acute, lymphomatous, chronic, primary cutaneous smoldering, and primary cutaneous tumoral. The acute form of ATL comprises 55–75% of all cases. Smoldering, subclinical lymphoproliferation may spontaneously resolve (the outcome in approximately half of cases) or progress to chronic leukemia or lymphomatous or even acute ATL. **Chronic, low-grade, HTLV-1–associated lymphoproliferation (pre-ATL)** may persist for years with abnormal lymphocytes with or without peripheral lymphadenopathy before progressing to the acute form. Acute ATL is characterized by hypercalcemia, lytic bone lesions, lymphadenopathy that spares the mediastinum, hepatomegaly, splenomegaly, cutaneous lymphomas, and opportunistic infections. Leukemia may develop with circulating polylobulated malignant lymphocytes, called flower cells, possessing mature T-cell markers. Antiviral therapy with zidovudine and interferon-α is the standard therapy for leukemic-type ATL in the United States and Europe. In lymphoma-type ATL, response rates may be improved using the anti-CCR4 monoclonal antibody mogamulizumab with chemotherapy. Allogeneic hematopoietic stem cell transplantation is sometimes employed.

HUMAN T-CELL LYMPHOTROPIC VIRUS-1–ASSOCIATED MYELOPATHY

HAM is more common in females than in males and has a relatively short incubation period of 1-4 yr after HTLV-1 infection, compared with 40-60 yr for ATL. HAM occurs in up to 4% of persons with HTLV-1 infection, usually developing during middle age. It is characterized by infiltration of mononuclear cells into the gray and white matter of the thoracic spinal cord, leading to severe white matter degeneration and fibrosis. HTLV-1 is found near but not directly within the lesions, suggesting that reactive inflammation is a major mechanism of disease. The cerebrospinal fluid typically shows a mildly elevated protein and a modest monocytic pleocytosis, along with anti–HTLV-1 antibodies. Neuroimaging studies are normal or show periventricular lesions in the white matter. Clinical manifestations include a gradual onset of slowly progressive, symmetric neurologic degeneration of the corticospinal tracts and, to a lesser extent, the sensory system that leads to lower-extremity spasticity or weakness, lower back pain, and hyperreflexia of the lower extremities with an extensor plantar response. The bladder and intestines may become dysfunctional, and men may become impotent. Some patients develop dysesthesias of the lower extremities with diminished sensation to vibration and pain. Upper-extremity function and sensation, cranial nerves, and cognitive function are usually preserved. Treatment regimens have been attempted with corticosteroids, danazol, interferon, plasmapheresis, high-dose vitamin C, and antivirals, all with minimal effects.

HUMAN T-CELL LYMPHOTROPIC VIRUS-2

HTLV-2 was originally identified in patients with hairy cell leukemia, although most patients with hairy cell leukemia are seronegative for HTLV-2 infection. HTLV-2 has been rarely isolated from patients with leukemias or with myelopathies resembling HAM, and there is limited evidence of disease specifically associated with HTLV-2 infection.

PREVENTION

Routine antibody testing of all blood products for HTLV-1 and -2 is performed in many developed countries and is effective in preventing blood transfusion–associated infections. Unfortunately, this routine testing is not always available in low and middle-income countries with higher endemicity. Prenatal screening and avoidance of breastfeeding by HTLV-1–infected mothers is an effective means of reducing mother-to-child transmission of HTLV-1. Safe sexual practices to avoid sexually transmitted infections, such as condom use and avoiding multiple sexual partners, may reduce transmission of both HTLV-I and HTLV-2. No vaccine is available.

Bibliography is available at Expert Consult.

Chapter **304**
Transmissible Spongiform Encephalopathies

David M. Asher

第三百零四章
传染性海绵状脑病

中文导读

　　本章主要介绍了传染性海绵状脑病的病因、流行病学、发病机制和病理学、临床表现、诊断、实验室检查、治疗、遗传咨询、预后和预防。详细介绍了疯牛病及其变异型、库鲁病、格斯特曼综合征和致命性家族性失眠症的临床特点、感染源、地理分布和流行、辅助检查。诊断依赖于临床表现、检查和活检。目前没有有效的治疗方法。

The transmissible spongiform encephalopathies (TSEs, prion diseases) are slow infections of the human nervous system, consisting of at least four diseases of humans (Table 304.1): kuru; Creutzfeldt-Jakob disease (CJD) with its variants—sporadic CJD (sCJD), familial CJD (fCJD), iatrogenic CJD (iCJD), and new-variant or variant CJD (vCJD); Gerstmann-Sträussler-Scheinker syndrome (GSS); and fatal familial insomnia (FFI), or the even more rare sporadic fatal insomnia syndrome. TSEs also affect animals; the most common and best-known TSEs of animals are scrapie in sheep, bovine spongiform encephalopathy (BSE or mad cow disease) in cattle, and a chronic wasting disease (CWD) of deer, elk, and moose found in parts of the United States, Canada, Norway, and Finland. All TSEs have similar clinical and histopathologic manifestations, and all are slow infections with very long asymptomatic incubation periods (often years), durations of several months or more, and overt disease affecting only the nervous system. TSEs are relentlessly progressive after illness begins and are invariably fatal. The most striking neuropathologic change that occurs in each TSE, to a greater or lesser extent, is spongy degeneration of the cerebral cortical gray matter.

ETIOLOGY

The TSEs are transmissible to susceptible animals by inoculation of tissues from affected subjects. Although the infectious agents replicate in some cell cultures, they do not achieve the high titers of infectivity found in brain tissues or cause recognizable cytopathic effects in cultures. Most previous studies of TSE agents have used in vivo assays, relying on the transmission of typical neurologic disease to animals as evidence that the agent was present and intact. Inoculation of susceptible recipient animals with small amounts of the infectious TSE agent results, months later, in the accumulation in tissues of large amounts of the agent with the same physical and biologic properties as the original agent. The TSE agents display a spectrum of extreme resistance to inactivation by a variety of chemical and physical treatments that is unknown among conventional pathogens. This characteristic, as well as their partial sensitivity to protein-disrupting treatments and their consistent association with abnormal isoforms of a normal host-encoded protein (prion protein or PrP), stimulated the hypothesis that the TSE agents are probably subviral in size, composed of protein, and devoid of nucleic acid.

The term **prion** (for proteinaceous infectious agent), coined by S.B. Prusiner, is now widely used for such agents. The prion hypothesis proposes that the molecular mechanism by which the pathogen-specific information of TSE agents is propagated involves a self-replicating change in the folding host-encoded PrP associated with a transition from an α-helix–rich structure in the native protease-sensitive conformation (cellular PrP or PrP^C) to a β-sheet–rich structure in the protease-resistant conformation associated with infectivity. The existence of a second host-encoded protein—termed protein X—that participates in the transformation was also postulated to explain certain otherwise puzzling findings but has never been identified.

The prion hypothesis is still not universally accepted; it relies on the postulated existence of a genome-like coding mechanism based on differences in protein folding that have not been satisfactorily explained at a molecular level. In addition, it has yet to account convincingly for the many biologic strains of TSE agent that have been observed, although strain-specific differences in the abnormal forms of the PrP have been found and proposed as providing a plausible molecular basis for the coding. It fails to explain why pure PrP uncontaminated with nucleic acid from an infected host has not transmitted a convincingly typical spongiform encephalopathy consistently associated with a serially self-propagating agent. A finding that was also troubling, in several experimental models and human illnesses, was that abnormal PrP and infectivity were not consistently associated. Particularly problematic is the finding that some illnesses associated with mutations in the *PRNP*

Table 304.1	Clinical and Epidemiologic Features of Human Transmissible Spongiform Encephalopathies (Prion Diseases)

DISEASE	CLINICAL FEATURES	SOURCE OF INFECTION	GEOGRAPHIC DISTRIBUTION AND PREVALENCE	USEFUL ANCILLARY TESTS	DURATION OF ILLNESS
sCJD	Dementia, myoclonus, ataxia	Unknown	Worldwide; ≈1/1 million/yr; 85–95% of all CJD cases in United States	EEG—PSWCs; CSF 14-3-3; MRI/DWI	1-24 mo (mean: 4-6 mo)
fCJD	Dementia, myoclonus, ataxia	Genetic association (*PRNP* mutations) ?? Possible exogenous source of infection	Worldwide—geographic clusters; >100 known families; 5–15% of CJD cases	Gene testing; EEG—PSWC rare; MRI/DWI (?)	Mean ≈15 mo
iCJD	Incoordination, dementia (late)	Cadaver dural grafts, human pituitary hormones, corneal transplantation, neurosurgical instruments, EEG depth electrodes	≈1% of CJD cases in toto (cadaver dural grafts), > 100 cases (human pituitary hormones), > 100 cases; corneal transplantation, 3 cases; neurosurgical instruments, 6 cases, including 2 from cortical depth electrodes; RBC transfusions, 4 cases of vCJD infection, 3 clinical, 1 preclinical (United Kingdom); human plasma–derived factor VIII, 1 preclinical case of vCJD (United Kingdom)		1 mo-10 yr
vCJD	Mood and behavioral abnormalities, paresthesias, dementia	Linked to BSE in cattle, transfusion plasma products	>230 clinical cases (see iatrogenic vCJD, above): none living, May 2017	Tonsil biopsy may show PrP^TSE MRI/FLAIR	8-36 mo (mean 14 mo)
Kuru	Incoordination, ataxia, tremors, dementia (late)	Linked to cannibalism	Fore people of Papua New Guinea (≈2,600 known cases)	EEG—no PSWCs; CSF 14-3-3 often negative; MRI (?)	3-24 mo
GSS	Incoordination, chronic progressive ataxia, corticospinal tract signs, dementia (late), myoclonus (rare)	90% genetic (*PRNP* mutations)	Worldwide; >50 families; ≈1-10/100 million/yr	*PRNP* gene sequencing	2-12 yr (mean ≈ 57 mo)
FFI	Disrupted sleep, intractable insomnia; autonomic hyperactivity; myoclonus, ataxia; corticospinal tract signs; dementia	*PRNP* gene mutation (D 178L); very rare sporadic cases	≈27 families in Europe, United Kingdom, United States, Finland, Australia, China, Japan	EEG—PSWCs only rarely positive; MRI—no DWI abnormalities; CSF 14-3-3 positive in ≈ 50%	8 mo to 6 yr (mean: *PRNP* 129 MM 12 ± 4 mo 129 MV 21 ± 15 mo)

BSE, bovine spongiform encephalopathy; CSF, cerebrospinal fluid; CJD, Creutzfeldt-Jakob disease; DWI, diffusion-weighted image; EEG, electroencephalography; fCJD, familial Creutzfeldt-Jakob disease; FFI, fatal familial insomnia; FLAIR, fluid attenuation inversion recovery MRI; GSS, Gerstmann-Sträussler-Scheinker syndrome; iCJD, iatrogenic Creutzfeldt-Jakob disease; *PRNP*, prion protein encoding gene; PrP^TSE, abnormal prion protein; PSWCs, periodic sharp wave complexes; RBC, red blood cell; sCJD, sporadic Creutzfeldt-Jakob disease; vCJD, variant Creutzfeldt-Jakob disease.

NOTE: PRNP 129 MM, homozygous, encoding the amino acid methionine at both codons 129 of the prion-protein-encoding (PRNP) gene on chromosome 20; 129 MV, heterozygous at PRNP codon 129, encoding methionine on one chromosome 20 and valine on the other.

Modified from Mandell GL, Bennett JE, Dolin R (eds): Principles and practice of infectious diseases, 6e, Philadelphia, 2005, Elsevier, p. 2222; and Love S, Louis DN, Ellison DW (eds): Greenfield's neuropathology, 8e, London, 2008, Hodder Arnold, p. 1239.

gene and accompanied by abnormal PrP failed to transmit infection to animals. If the TSE agents ultimately prove to consist of protein and only protein, without any obligatory nucleic acid component, then the term *prion* will indeed be appropriate and the early proponents of the prion hypothesis will prove to have been prescient. If the agents are ultimately found to contain small nucleic acid genomes, then they might better be considered atypical viruses, for which the term *virino* has been suggested. Until the actual molecular structure of the infectious TSE pathogens and the presence or absence of a nucleic acid genome are rigorously established, it seems less contentious to continue calling them TSE agents, although most authorities have accepted the term *prion* (sometimes referring to the agent of a TSE and sometimes to the abnormal protein, even when nontransmissible).

The earliest evidence that abnormal proteins are associated with the TSE was morphologic: Scrapie-associated fibrils were found in extracts of tissues from patients and animals with spongiform encephalopathies but not in normal tissues. Scrapie-associated fibrils resemble but are distinguishable from the amyloid fibrils that accumulate in the brains of patients with Alzheimer disease. A group of antigenically related

protease-resistant proteins (PrPs) proved to be components of scrapie-associated fibrils and to be present in the amyloid plaques found in the brains of patients and animals with TSEs. The abnormal forms of PrP are variously designated PrP^Sc (scrapie-type PrP), PrP-res (protease-resistant PrP), PrP^TSE (TSE-associated PrP), or PrP^D (disease-associated PrP) by different authorities.

It remains unclear whether abnormal PrP constitutes the complete infectious particle of spongiform encephalopathies, is a component of those particles, or is a pathologic host protein not usually separated from the actual infectious entity by currently used techniques. The demonstration that PrP is encoded by a normal host gene seemed to favor the last possibility. Several studies suggest that agent-specific pathogenic information can be transmitted and replicated by different conformations of a protein with the same primary amino acid sequence in the absence of agent-specific nucleic acids. Properties of two fungal proteins were found to be heritable without encoding in nucleic acid, although these properties have not been naturally transmitted to recipient fungi as infectious elements. Whatever its relationship to the actual infectious TSE particles, PrP clearly plays a central role in the susceptibility to infection, because the normal PrP must be expressed in mice and cattle if they are to acquire a TSE or to sustain replication of the infectious agents. Furthermore, inherited normal variations in the PrP phenotype are associated with increased susceptibility to vCJD and (to a lesser extent) to sCJD and with occurrence of familial TSEs (fCJD and GSS).

PrPs are glycoproteins; protease-resistant PrPs, when aggregated, have the physical properties of amyloid proteins. The PrPs of different species of animals are very similar in their amino acid sequences and antigenicity but are not identical in structure. The primary structure of PrP is encoded by the host and is not altered by the source of the infectious agent provoking its formation. The function of the ubiquitous protease-sensitive PrP precursor (designated PrP^C, for cellular PrP, or PrP-sen, for protease-sensitive PrP) in normal cells is unknown; it binds copper and may play some role in normal synaptic transmission, but it is not required for life or for relatively normal cerebral function in mice and cattle. As noted, animals must express PrP to develop scrapie disease and to support replication of the TSE agents. The degree of homology between amino acid sequences of PrPs in different animal species may correlate with the species barrier that affects the susceptibility of animals of one species to infection with a TSE agent adapted to grow in another species, although the degree of sequence homology does not always predict susceptibility to the same TSE agent.

Attempts to find particles resembling those of viruses or virus-like agents in brain tissues of humans or animals with spongiform encephalopathies have been unsuccessful. Peculiar tubulovesicular structures reminiscent of some viruses have been seen repeatedly in thin sections of TSE-infected brain tissues and cultured cells but not in normal cells. It has never been established that those structures are associated with infectivity.

EPIDEMIOLOGY

Kuru once affected many children of both sexes ≥ 4 yr of age, adolescents, and young adults (mainly females) living in one limited area of Papua New Guinea. The complete disappearance of kuru among people born after 1957 suggests that the practice of ritual cannibalism (thought to have ended that year) was probably the only mechanism by which the infection spread in Papua New Guinea.

CJD, the most common human spongiform encephalopathy, was formerly thought to occur only in older adults; however, iCJD and, much more rarely, sCJD (to date, seven reports in adolescents, one a 14 yr old female) have affected young people. A single case of sporadic fatal insomnia was recognized in a U.S. adolescent. GSS has not been diagnosed in children or adolescents. vCJD has a peculiar predilection for younger people. Of 174 cases of vCJD reported through 2010 in the United Kingdom, all except 23 were in people younger than 40 yr of age and 22 were in people younger than 20 yr of age; the youngest age at onset was 12 yr. sCJD has been recognized worldwide, at yearly rates of 0.25-2 cases/million population (not age-adjusted), with CJD foci of considerably higher incidence among Libyan Jews in Israel, in isolated villages of Slovakia, and in other limited areas. Sporadic CJD has not been convincingly linked to any common exposure, and the source of infection remains unknown. Proponents of the prion hypothesis are convinced that PrP can spontaneously misfold, becoming self-replicating and causing sCJD; skeptics favor infection with some ubiquitous TSE agent, which, fortunately, has a very low attack rate except in persons with certain mutations in the *PRNP* gene. Neither of those possible etiologies has been proven. Person-to-person spread has been confirmed only for iatrogenic cases. Spouses and household contacts of patients are not at risk of acquiring CJD, although two instances of conjugal CJD have been reported. However, medical personnel exposed to brains of patients with CJD may be at some increased risk; at least 20 healthcare workers have been recognized with the disease.

The striking resemblance of CJD to scrapie prompted a concern that infected sheep tissues might be a source of spongiform encephalopathy in humans. No reliable epidemiologic evidence suggests that exposure to potentially scrapie-contaminated animals, meat, meat products, or experimental preparations of the scrapie agent have transmitted a TSE to humans. The potential of the CWD agent to infect human beings has also not been demonstrated but remains under investigation; deer,

elk, and moose in 15 U.S. states and 2 Canadian provinces have been naturally infected; cases of CWD were recently detected in wild reindeer and moose (European elk) in Norway and Finland. Consumption of contaminated meat, including venison from animals infected with the CWD agent, has not been implicated as a risk factor for human TSE by epidemiologic studies; however, a recent unpublished study requiring several years yielded evidence that CWD was experimentally transmitted to monkeys fed venison from overtly healthy infected deer, prompting a health advisory from Canadian authorities. The outbreak of BSE among cattle (possibly infected by eating scrapie-agent–contaminated meat-and-bone meal added to feed) was first recognized in the United Kingdom in 1986 and later reported in cattle of 27 other countries, including Canada and the United States. More than 190,000 cases of BSE have been reported to the World Organization for Animal Health (OIE), almost 97% of those from the United Kingdom. Cases in the United Kingdom progressively declined after 1992 and later in other countries; in 2016 only 2 cases worldwide were reported to OIE (from France and Spain) and none from the United Kingdom. The finding of a new TSE in ungulate and feline animals in British zoos and later in domestic cats raised a fear that the BSE agent had acquired a range of susceptible hosts broader than that of scrapie, posing a potential danger for humans. That remains the most plausible explanation for the occurrence of vCJD, first described in adolescents in Britain in 1996 and, as of May 2017, eventually affecting at least 178 people in the United Kingdom. (not counting a disturbing number of people with evidence of possible asymptomatic or "preclinical" vCJD infection) and more than 50 in 11 other countries (total 231 cases worldwide): 27 in France, 5 in Spain, 4 in Ireland, 3 in the Netherlands, 2 each in Italy and Portugal, and single cases in Japan and Saudi Arabia. Variant CJD has also occurred in former U.K. residents (>6 mo) living in Ireland (two cases), France (one case), Canada (one case), Taiwan (one case), and the United States (two cases). Two cases of vCJD—one in the United States and one in Canada—have been reported in former long-time residents of Saudi Arabia, a country that has not recognized BSE but might have imported contaminated meat products from the United Kingdom. A third case of vCJD was previously confirmed in a Saudi citizen residing in Saudi Arabia. The most recent case of vCJD diagnosed in the United States occurred in an immigrant deemed by the CDC to have most likely been infected during early years spent in Kuwait.

No case of vCJD has been confirmed in anyone born in the United Kingdom after 1989. However, examination of resected appendixes in the United Kingdom for evidence of subclinical infection with prions suggested that about 1 in 2,000 people tested had a detectable accumulation of PrP^{TSE} in lymphoid follicles. It remains controversial whether those accumulations resulted from subclinical vCJD or another TSE; none of the subjects to date has presented to medical attention with overt TSE.

Iatrogenic transmissions of CJD have been recognized for more than 30 yr (Table 304.2). Such accidental transmissions of CJD have been attributed to use of contaminated neurosurgical instruments (no case reported since 1980) or operating facilities, use of cortical electrodes contaminated during epilepsy surgery, injections of human cadaveric pituitary growth hormone and gonadotropin (no longer marketed in the United States), and transplantation of contaminated corneas and allografts of human dura mater, still in limited use in the United States as a surgical patching material. Pharmaceuticals and tissue grafts derived from or contaminated with human neural tissues, particularly if obtained from unselected donors and large pools of donors, pose special risks.

Studies of animals experimentally infected with TSE agents first suggested that blood and blood components from humans with preclinical CJD infections might pose a risk of transmitting disease to recipients, and since the 1980s such blood components have been withdrawn as a precaution in the United States when a donor was later found to have CJD and blood products were still in-date. A surveillance program in the United Kingdom reported vCJD in three recipients of nonleukoreduced red blood cells from donors later diagnosed with vCJD; there was autopsy evidence of a preclinical vCJD infection in a fourth red cell recipient who died of another disease. (vCJD has not occurred in any recipient of leukoreduced red blood cells from a donor who later developed

Table 304.2	Iatrogenic Transmission of Creutzfeldt-Jakob Disease by Products of Human Origin		

| PRODUCT | NO. OF PATIENTS | INCUBATION TIME | |
		Mean	Range
Cornea	3	17 mo	16-18 mo
Dura mater allograft	>100	7.4 yr	1.3-16 yr
Pituitary extract			
Growth hormone	>100*	12 yr	5-38.5 yr
Gonadotropin	4	13 yr	12-16 yr
Red blood cells	4	? 6 yr	6.3-8.5 yr†
Plasma-derived coagulation factor VIII	1	? > 11 yr‡	

*There have been 28 cases reported among approximately 8,000 recipients of human cadaveric growth hormone in the United States; the remaining cases have been reported in other countries.

†The second transfusion-transmitted case of vCJD (Peden AH, Head MW, Ritchie DL, et al: Preclinical vCJD after blood transfusion in a *PRNP* codon 129 heterozygous patient, *Lancet* 364:527-529, 2004) died of unrelated causes about 5 yr after transfusion but was found to have accumulations of abnormal PrP in the spleen and cervical lymph node—a finding unique to vCJD and interpreted as probable preclinical infection.

‡The diagnosis of vCJD infection attributed to treatment with human plasma–derived coagulation factor VIII (UK Health Protection Agency: vCJD abnormal prion protein found in a patient with haemophilia at post mortem, Press release 17 February 2009, http://webarchive.nationalarchives.gov.uk/20140714084352/http://www.hpa.org.uk/webw/HPAweb&HPAwebStandard/HPAweb_C/1234859690542?p=1231252394302) was also supported by immunohistochemical testing for abnormal PrP in the spleen of a person who died of other causes. Both patients with "preclinical" infections are thought to have died during the asymptomatic incubation period of vCJD.

vCJD.) A study conducted over more than 20 yr by the American Red Cross and CDC found no recipient of blood components obtained from donors later diagnosed with sporadic CJD (and from one donor with familial CJD) developed a TSE.

Evidence of a preclinical vCJD infection was found at autopsy in a U.K. patient with hemophilia A treated with a human plasma–derived coagulation factor VIII to which at least one vCJD-infected donor contributed; the coagulation factor involved was never licensed in the United States. U.K. authorities have described two recipients of plasma-derived coagulation factors (both having a history of a transfusion with blood components, as well) who later developed sporadic CJD, concluding that the finding, while of concern, might be coincidental.

PATHOGENESIS AND PATHOLOGY

The probable portal of entry for the TSE agent in kuru is thought to have been either through the gastrointestinal tract or lesions in the mouth or integument incidentally exposed to the agent during cannibalism. Patients with vCJD (and animals with BSE and BSE-related TSEs) are thought to have been similarly infected with the BSE agent by consuming contaminated beef products. Except after direct introduction into the nervous system, the first site of replication of TSE agents appears to be in tissues of the reticuloendothelial system. TSE agents have been detected in low titers in the blood of experimentally infected animals (mice, monkeys, hamsters, and sheep and in the blood of persons with vCJD and perhaps sCJD); infectivity was mainly associated with nucleated cells, although the plasma contained a substantial portion of total infectivity in blood. Circulating lymphoid cells seem to be required to infect mice by peripheral routes. Limited evidence suggests that TSE agents also spread to the central nervous system by ascending peripheral nerves. Several research groups claimed to detect the CJD agent in human blood, although other attempts failed.

In human kuru, it seems probable that the only portal of exit of the agent from the body, at least in quantities sufficient to infect others, was through infected tissues exposed during cannibalism. In iatrogenically transmitted CJD, the brains and eyes of patients with CJD have been the probable sources of contamination. Experimental transmission of the agent to animals from the kidney, liver, lung, lymph node, and spleen showed that those tissues as well as the cerebrospinal fluid (CSF) sometimes contain the CJD agent; none of those sources has been implicated in accidental transmission of CJD to humans. At no time during the course of any TSE have antibodies or cell-mediated immunity to the infectious agents been convincingly demonstrated in either patients or animals. However, mice must be immunologically competent to be infected with the scrapie agent by peripheral routes of inoculation.

Typical changes in TSE include vacuolation and loss of neurons with hypertrophy and proliferation of glial cells, most pronounced in the cerebral cortex in patients with CJD and in the cerebellum in those with kuru. The central nervous system lesions are usually most severe in or even confined to gray matter, at least early in the disease. Loss of myelin appears to be secondary to the degeneration of neurons. There generally is no inflammation, but a marked increase in the number and size of astrocytes is usual. Spongiform changes are not a striking autopsy finding in patients with FFI, and neuronal degeneration and gliosis are largely restricted to thalamic nuclei.

Amyloid plaques are found in the brains of all patients with GSS and in at least 70% of those with kuru. These plaques are less common in patients with CJD. Amyloid plaques are most common in the cerebellum but occur elsewhere in the brain, as well. In brains of patients with vCJD, plaques surrounded by halos of vacuoles (described as flower-like or florid plaques) have been a consistent finding. TSE amyloid plaques react with antiserum prepared against PrP. Even in the absence of plaques, extracellular PrP can be detected in the brain parenchyma by immunostaining.

CLINICAL MANIFESTATIONS

Kuru, no longer seen, is a progressive degenerative disease of the cerebellum and brainstem with less obvious involvement of the cerebral cortex. The first sign of kuru was usually cerebellar ataxia followed by progressive incoordination. Coarse, shivering tremors were characteristic. Variable abnormalities in cranial nerve function appeared, frequently with impairment in conjugate gaze and swallowing. Patients died of inanition and pneumonia or of burns from cooking fires, usually within 1 yr after onset. Although changes in mentation were common, there was no frank dementia or progression to coma, as in CJD. There were no signs of acute encephalitis, such as fever, headaches, and convulsions.

CJD occurs throughout the world. Patients initially have either sensory disturbances (most often visual) or confusion and inappropriate behavior, progressing over weeks or months to frank dementia, akinetic mutism, and, ultimately, coma. Some patients have cerebellar ataxia early in the disease, and most patients experience myoclonic jerking movements. The mean survival time of patients with sCJD has been < 1 yr from the earliest signs of illness, although approximately 10% live for 2 yr. Variant CJD (Table 304.3) differs from the more common sCJD; patients with vCJD are much younger at onset (as young as 12 yr) and more often present with complaints of dysesthesia and subtle behavioral changes, often mistaken for psychiatric illness. Severe mental deterioration occurs later in the course of vCJD. Patients with vCJD have survived substantially longer than those with sCJD. Attempts have been made to subclassify cases of CJD based on the electrophoretic differences in PrP^TSE and variation in its sensitivity to digestion with the proteolytic enzyme proteinase (PK); the different variants are said to have somewhat different clinical features, including the duration of illness, though all are ultimately fatal.

GSS is a familial disease resembling CJD but with more prominent cerebellar ataxia and amyloid plaques. Dementia may appear only late in the course, and the average duration of illness is longer than typical sCJD. Progressively severe insomnia and dysautonomia, as well as ataxia, myoclonus, and other signs resembling those of CJD and GSS, characterize FFI and sporadic fatal insomnia. A case of sporadic **fatal insomnia** has been described in a young adolescent. GSS has not been diagnosed in children or adolescents.

A novel prion disease has been reported that is expressed in several

Table 304.3	**Clinical and Histopathologic Features of Patients With Variant and Typical Sporadic Creutzfeldt-Jakob Disease**	

FEATURE	VARIANT CJD (FIRST 10 PATIENTS)	SPORADIC CJD (185 PATIENTS)
Years of age at death* (range)	29 (19-74)	65
Duration of illness, mo (range)	12 (8-23)	4
Presenting signs	Abnormal behavior, dysesthesia	Dementia
Later signs	Dementia, ataxia, myoclonus	Ataxia, myoclonus
Periodic complexes on EEG	Rare	Most
PRNP 129 Met/Met	All tested (except one transfusion-transmitted case, one plasma-derivative transmitted case; one possible clinical case in United Kingdom where no tissue was available to confirm)	83%
Histopathologic changes	Vacuolation, neuronal loss, astrocytosis, plaques (100%)	Vacuolation, neuronal loss, astrocytosis, plaques (≤15%)
Florid PrP plaques[†]	100%	0
PrP^{TSE} glycosylation pattern	BSE-like[‡]	Not BSE-like

*Median age and duration for variant CJD; averages for typical sporadic CJD.
[†]Dense plaques with a pale periphery of surrounding vacuolated cells.
[‡]Characterized by an excess of high-molecular-mass band (diglycosylated) and 19-kDa nonglycosylated band glycoform of PrP-res (Collinge J, Sidle KC, Meads J, et al: Molecular analysis of prion strain variation and the aetiology of "new variant" CJD, Nature 383:685-690, 1996).
BSE, bovine spongiform encephalopathy; CJD, Creutzfeldt-Jakob disease; EEG, electroencephalogram; Met, codon 129 of one *PRNP* gene encoding for methionine; *PRNP*, prion protein–encoding gene; PrP, prion protein.
Modified from Will RG, Ironside JW, Zeidler M, et al: A new variant of Creutzfeldt-Jakob disease in the UK, Lancet 347:921-925, 1996.

generations with an autosomal dominant pattern associated with a unique mutation in the *PRNP* gene. The affected persons were middle-aged with a history of chronic diarrhea for years plus autonomic neuropathy and modest mental impairment but without full-blown dementia; PK-resistant PrP deposits with amyloid properties occurred in the brain, lymphoid tissues, kidney, spleen, and intestinal tract. The disease was not successfully transmitted to three lines of mice susceptible to several TSEs. It is not clear that such a syndrome—not a spongiform encephalopathy and apparently not associated with an infectious agent—should be lumped together with TSEs. It might well result from the abnormal *PRNP* gene product itself; if so, it would not pose the same potential threat to public health as do the TSEs.

DIAGNOSIS

The diagnosis of spongiform encephalopathies is most often determined on clinical grounds after excluding other diseases. The presence of 14-3-3 protein (see Laboratory Findings) in CSF may aid in distinguishing between CJD and Alzheimer disease—not a consideration in children. Elevations of 14-3-3 protein levels in the CSF are not specific to TSEs and are common in viral encephalitis and other conditions causing rapid necrosis of brain tissue. Brain biopsy may be diagnostic of CJD, but it can be recommended only if a potentially treatable disease remains to be excluded or if there is some other compelling reason to make an antemortem diagnosis. The definitive diagnosis usually requires the microscopic examination of brain tissue obtained at autopsy. The demonstration of protease-resistant PrP in brain extracts augments the histopathologic diagnosis. Accumulation of the abnormal PrP in lymphoid tissues, even before the onset of neurologic signs, is typical of vCJD. Tonsil biopsy may avoid the need for brain biopsy when antemortem diagnosis of vCJD is indicated. To date, no blood-based test has been validated for antemortem testing of either humans or animals. Transmission of disease to susceptible animals by inoculation of brain suspension, while sensitive, specific, and reliable, must be reserved for cases of special research interest.

LABORATORY FINDINGS

Virtually all patients with typical sporadic, iatrogenic, and familial forms of CJD have abnormal electroencephalograms (EEGs) as the disease progresses; the background becomes slow and irregular with diminished amplitude. A variety of paroxysmal discharges such as slow waves, sharp waves, and spike-and-wave complexes may also appear, and these may be unilateral or focal or bilaterally synchronous. Paroxysmal discharges may be precipitated by a loud noise. Many patients have typical periodic suppression-burst complexes of high-voltage slow activity on EEG at some time during the illness. Patients with vCJD have had only generalized slowing, without periodic bursts of high-voltage discharges on EEG. The CT or MRI may show cortical atrophy and large ventricles late in the course of CJD. Many patients with vCJD have an increase in density of the pulvinar on MRI. Reliable interpretation of the images is best left to experienced radiologists.

There may be a modest elevation of CSF protein content in patients with TSE. Unusual protein spots were observed in CSF specimens after two-dimensional separation in gels and silver staining; the spots were identified as 14-3-3 proteins, normal proteins (not related to PrP) abundant in neurons but not ordinarily detected in CSF. However, 14-3-3 protein has also been detected in CSF specimens from some patients with acute viral encephalitides and recent cerebral infarctions and is not specific to CJD. Finding the 14-3-3 protein in CSF is neither sensitive nor specific but has been of some help in confirming the diagnosis of vCJD, especially when accompanied by increases in other cellular proteins. The diagnosis usually rests on recognizing the typical constellation of clinical findings, clinical course, and testing (CSF examination, CT or MRI, EEG), confirmed by histopathology and detection of PrP^{TSE} in brain tissues at autopsy (or, less often, by tonsil or brain biopsy). Research techniques that amplify PrP^{TSE} in CSF, nasal brushings, and blood may eventually improve antemortem diagnosis but remain inadequately validated for routine use.

TREATMENT

No treatment has proven effective. Studies of cell cultures and rodents experimentally infected with TSE agents suggested that treatment with chlorpromazine, quinacrine, and tetracyclines might be of benefit, especially during the incubation period. Results of clinical trials based on those studies have been discouraging, and it seems unlikely that the severe brain damage found in late disease can be reversed by treatment. Infusions with pentosan polysulfate directly into the cerebral ventricles appear to have delayed the progression of vCJD in a least one patient but did not reverse earlier brain damage. Appropriate supportive care should be provided to all CJD patients as for other progressive fatal neurologic diseases. On the basis of experimental studies in animals, several prophylactic postexposure treatment regimens have been suggested, but none has been widely accepted.

GENETIC COUNSELING

TSEs sometimes occur in families in a pattern consistent with an autosomal dominant mode of inheritance. In patients with a family history of CJD, the clinical and histopathologic findings are similar to those seen in sporadic cases. In the United States, only approximately 10% of cases of CJD are familial. GSS and FFI are always familial. In some affected families, approximately 50% of siblings and children of a patient with a familial TSE eventually acquire the disease; in other families, the penetrance of illness may be less.

The gene coding for PrP is closely linked if not identical to that controlling the incubation periods of scrapie in sheep and both scrapie and CJD in mice. The gene encoding PrP in humans is designated the *PRNP* gene and is located on the short arm of chromosome 20. It has an open reading frame of 759 nucleotides (253 codons), in which more than 20 different point mutations and a variety of inserted sequences encoding extra tandem-repeated octapeptides are linked to the occurrence of spongiform encephalopathy in families with a pattern consistent with autosomal dominance of variable penetrance.

The same nucleotide substitution at codon 178 of the *PRNP* gene associated with CJD in some families has been found in all patients with FFI. Homozygosity for valine (V) and especially for methionine (M) at codon 129 seems to increase the susceptibility to iCJD and sCJD. Almost all patients with vCJD to be genotyped have been homozygous for methionine at codon 129 of the *PRNP* gene. A few probable preclinical vCJD infections and two clinically typical cases of vCJD (one confirmed and another not completely evaluated) occurred in persons with the 129 MV heterozygous genotype. It is of interest that when the *PRNP* genes from appendices containing accumulations of what appears to be PrP^{TSE} in the UK were sequenced, a surprising number were homozygous for V—the genotype of only approximately 10% of U.K. subjects and never found in a case of vCJD. The significance of this finding is not clear. U.K. authorities have adopted the precautionary assumption that some persons with PrP^{TSE} in lymphoid tissues may have latent infections. Whether the blood of such persons is infectious remains unknown.

Although the interpretation of these findings in regard to the prion hypothesis is in dispute, persons from families with CJD or GSS who have the associated mutations in the *PRNP* gene clearly have a high probability of eventually acquiring spongiform encephalopathy. Bearers of TSE-associated mutations have employed a preimplantation genetic diagnosis and in vitro selection of embryos to avoid passing the mutant gene to offspring. The significance of mutations in the *PRNP* genes of individuals from families with no history of spongiform encephalopathy is not known. It seems wise to avoid alarming those from unaffected families who have miscellaneous mutations in the *PRNP* gene, because the implications are not yet clear. In the United States, persons are deferred from donating blood if a blood relative has been diagnosed with a TSE unless the donor does not have a TSE-related mutation.

PROGNOSIS

The prognosis of all spongiform encephalopathies is uniformly poor. Approximately 10% of patients may survive for longer than 1 yr, but the quality of life is poor.

FAMILY SUPPORT

The CJD Foundation (http://www.cjdfoundation.org), organized and maintained by family members and friends of patients with CJD and related disorders, working closely with the Centers for Disease Control and Prevention (www.cdc.gov/prions/index.html) and with the National Prion Disease Pathology Surveillance Center, Case Western Reserve University, Cleveland (http://www.cjdsurveillance.com), is a support and educational group and a useful source of information regarding available resources for those dealing with the diseases.

PREVENTION

Exposure to the BSE agent in meat products clearly poses a special danger—now greatly reduced. Authorities in Canada, the United States, and other countries responded by implementing progressively more stringent agricultural and public health measures during the past 20 yr, with elimination of most bovine-derived materials from animal feeds probably the most effective measure. Three cases of BSE in native cattle were recognized in the United States from 2004 through 2012; a case was also found in a Canadian cow imported into the United States in 2003. Canada found 20 native cattle with BSE between 2003 and 2015 (and imported a case from the United Kingdom in 1993). In spite of encouraging epidemiologic studies that failed to implicate exposure to scrapie or CWD agents in human TSEs, it seems prudent to avoid exposing children to meat and other products likely to be contaminated with any TSE agent.

The safety of human blood, blood components, and plasma derivatives in the United States and Canada is protected by deferring those donors with histories suggesting an increased risk of TSEs: persons treated with cadaveric pituitary hormones (no longer used) or dura mater allografts, patients with a family history of CJD (unless sequencing shows that the TSE-affected blood relative or the donor has revealed no TSE-related mutation in either *PRNP* gene), and persons who spent substantial periods of time in specified countries during years when BSE was prevalent. Persons transfused with blood in the United Kingdom and France after 1980 should be deferred from donating blood (similar deferral policies are in place for donors of human cells and tissues). U.K. authorities have warned persons treated with U.K.-sourced pooled coagulation factor concentrates or antithrombin between 1989 and 2001 that they may be "at risk of vCJD for public health purposes" and that "special infection control precautions" apply to them.

In principle, it would be better to identify the few blood and tissue donors actually infected with a TSE rather than deferring all those at increased risk of exposure, because most of them are unlikely to have been infected. Antemortem screening tests that might eventually identify donors with preclinical TSE infections are currently under development though not clinically validated. It is unlikely that any test will be adopted to screen blood donors without simultaneously implementing a highly specific validated confirmatory test to avoid the serious adverse implications of inevitable false-positive screening results.

Standard precautions should be used to handle all human tissues, blood, and body fluids. Materials and surfaces contaminated with tissues or fluids from patients suspected of having CJD must be treated with great care. Whenever possible, discard contaminated instruments by careful packaging and incineration. Contaminated tissues and biologic products probably cannot be completely freed of infectivity without destroying their structural integrity and biologic activity; therefore, the medical and family histories of individual tissue donors should be carefully reviewed to exclude a diagnosis of TSE. Histopathologic examination of brain tissues of cadaveric donors and testing for abnormal PrP might be performed where feasible to provide an additional assurance of safety. Although no method of sterilization can be relied on to remove all infectivity from contaminated surfaces, exposures to moist heat, sodium hydroxide, chlorine bleach, concentrated formic acid, acidified detergent, and guanidine salts markedly reduced infectivity in experimental studies.

Bibliography is available at Expert Consult.

Section **14**

Antiparasitic Therapy
第十四篇
抗寄生虫治疗

Chapter **305**

Principles of Antiparasitic Therapy

Beth K. Thielen and Mark R. Schleiss

第三百零五章
抗寄生虫治疗的原则

中文导读

本章主要介绍了抗寄生虫治疗的原则，包括针对原生动物的抗寄生虫药、针对糯虫和外寄生虫的抗寄生虫药。针对原生动物的抗寄生虫药中，详细介绍了硝唑尼特、替硝唑、阿托伐醌、青蒿素衍生物及相关药物的联合治疗。针对糯虫和外寄生虫的抗寄生虫药中，详细介绍了阿苯达唑、伊维菌素、吡喹酮等药物。

Parasites are divided into three main groups taxonomically: **protozoans,** which are unicellular, and **helminths** and **ectoparasites,** which are multicellular. Chemotherapeutic agents appropriate for one group may not be appropriate for the others, and not all drugs are readily available (Table 305.1). Some drugs are not available in the United States, and some are available only from the manufacturer, specialized compounding pharmacies, or the Centers for Disease Control and Prevention (CDC). Information on the availability of drugs and expert guidance in management can be obtained by contacting the CDC Parasitic Diseases Branch (1-404-718-4745; e-mail parasites@cdc.gov (M-F, 8 AM-4 PM, Eastern time). For assistance in the management of malaria, healthcare providers should call the CDC Malaria Hotline: 1-770-488-7788 or 1-855-856-4713 toll-free (M-F, 9 AM-5 PM, Eastern time). For all emergency consultations after hours, clinicians can contact the CDC Emergency Operations Center at 1-770-488-7100 and request to speak with a CDC Malaria Branch clinician or on-call parasitic diseases physician. Some antiparasitic drugs are not licensed for use in the United States but can be obtained as investigational new drugs (INDs) from the CDC; providers should call the CDC Drug Service, Division of Scientific Resources and Division of Global Migration and Quarantine, at 1-404-639-3670.

SELECTED ANTIPARASITIC DRUGS FOR PROTOZOANS
Nitazoxanide (Alinia)
Nitazoxanide is a nitrothiazole benzamide, initially developed as a veterinary anthelmintic. Nitazoxanide inhibits pyruvate-ferredoxin oxidoreductase, which is an enzyme necessary for anaerobic energy metabolism. In humans, nitazoxanide is effective against many **protozoans** and **helminths.** Nitazoxanide is approved for the treatment of diarrhea caused by *Cryptosporidium parvum* and *Giardia intestinalis* in patients 1 yr of age and older.

Nitazoxanide is available as a tablet and an oral suspension (100 mg/5 mL), which has a pink color and strawberry flavor. The bioavailability of the suspension is ~ 70% compared with the tablet. The drug is well absorbed from the gastrointestinal tract but should be taken with food due to approximately two-fold higher absorption. One third is excreted in urine, and two thirds is excreted in feces as the active metabolite, tizoxanide. Although in vitro metabolism studies have not demonstrated cytochrome P450 enzyme effects, no pharmacokinetic studies have been performed yet in patients with compromised

Text continued on p. 2011

Table 305.1	Drugs for Parasitic Infections

Parasitic infections are found throughout the world. With increasing travel, immigration, use of immunosuppressive drugs, and the spread of HIV, physicians anywhere may see infections caused by previously unfamiliar parasites. The table below lists first-choice and alternative drugs for most parasitic infections.

INFECTION	DRUG	ADULT DOSAGE	PEDIATRIC DOSAGE
Acanthamoeba keratitis			
Drug of choice:	See footnote 1		
Amebiasis *(Entamoeba histolytica)*			
Asymptomatic infection			
Drug of choice:	Iodoquinol (Yodoxin)[2]	650 mg PO tid × 20 days	30-40 mg/kg/day (max 1950 mg) in 3 doses PO × 20 days
or	Paromomycin	25-35 mg/kg/day PO in 3 doses × 7 days	25-35 mg/kg/day PO in 3 doses × 7 days
Alternative:	Diloxanide furoate[3]	500 mg tid PO × 10 days	20 mg/kg/day PO in 3 doses × 10 days
Mild to moderate intestinal disease			
Drug of choice:	Metronidazole	500-750 mg tid PO × 7-10 days	35-50 mg/kg/day PO in 3 doses × 7-10 days
or	Tinidazole[4]	2 g PO once daily × 3 days	50 mg/kg/day PO (max 2 g) in 1 dose × 3 days
Either followed by:	Iodoquinol[2]	650 mg PO tid × 20 days	30-40 mg/kg/day PO in 3 doses × 20 days (max 2 g)
or	Paromomycin	25-35 mg/kg/day PO in 3 doses × 7 days	25-35 mg/kg/day PO in 3 doses × 7 days
Alternative:	Nitazoxanide[5]	500 mg bid × 3 days	1-3 yr: 100 mg bid × 3 days 4-11 yr: 100 mg bid × 3 days 12+ yr: use adult dosing
Severe intestinal and extraintestinal disease			
Drug of choice:	Metronidazole	750 mg PO tid × 7-10 days	35-50 mg/kg/day PO in 3 doses × 7-10 days
or	Tinidazole[4]	2 g PO once daily × 5 days	50 mg/kg/day PO (max 2 g) × 5 days
Either followed by:	Iodoquinol[2]	650 mg PO tid × 20 days	30-40 mg/kg/day PO in 3 doses × 20 days (max 2 g)
or	Paromomycin	25-35 mg/kg/day PO in 3 doses × 7 days	25-35 mg/kg/day PO in 3 doses × 7 days
Amebic meningoencephalitis, primary and granulomatous			
Naegleria fowleri			
Drug of choice:	Amphotericin B deoxycholate[6,7]	1.5 mg/kg/day IV in 2 divided doses × 3 days, then 1 mg/kg daily IV × 11 days	1.5 mg/kg/day IV in 2 divided doses × 3 days, then 1 mg/kg daily IV × 11 days
	plus Amphotericin B deoxycholate[6,7]	1.5 mg/kg intrathecally daily × 2 days, then 1 mg/kg intrathecally every other day × 8 days	1.5 mg/kg intrathecally daily × 2 days, then 1 mg/kg intrathecally every other day × 8 days
	plus Rifampin[7]	10 mg/kg (max 600 mg) IV or PO daily × 28 days	10 mg/kg (max 600 mg) IV or PO daily × 28 days
	plus Fluconazole[7]	10 mg/kg (max 600 mg) IV or PO daily × 28 days	10 mg/kg (max 600 mg) IV or PO daily × 28 days
	plus Azithromycin[7]	500 mg IV or PO daily × 28 days	10 mg/kg (max 500 mg) IV or PO daily × 28 days
	plus Miltefosine[6,7,8]	50 mg PO tid × 28 days	<45 kg: 50 mg bid (max 2.5 mg/kg) × 28 days ≥45 kg: use adult dosing
	plus Dexamethasone	0.6 mg/kg/day IV in 4 divided doses × 4 days	0.6 mg/kg/day IV in 4 divided doses × 4 days

[1]For treatment of keratitis caused by *Acanthamoeba*, 0.02% topical polyhexamethylene biguanide (PHMB) and 0.02% chlorhexidine have been successfully used individually and in combination in a large number of patients (Tabin G, et al: *Cornea* 20:757, 2001; Wysenbeek YS, et al: *Cornea* 19:464, 2000). The expected treatment course is 6-12 mo. PHMB is no longer available from Leiter's Park Avenue Pharmacy but is available from the O'Brien Pharmacy (1-800-627-4360; distributes in many states) and the Greenpark Pharmacy (1-713-432-9855; Texas only). Combinations with either 0.1% propamidine isethionate (Brolene) or hexamidine (Desmodine) have been used (Seal DV: *Eye* 17:893, 2003) successfully, but these are not available in the United States. Neomycin is no longer recommended due to high levels of resistance (*Acanthamoeba* keratitis: Treatment guidelines from The Medical Letter 143, 8/1/2013). In addition, the combination of chlorhexidine, natamycin (pimaricin), and debridement also has been successful (Kitagawa K, et al: *Jpn J Ophthalmol* 47:616, 2003).

[2]The drug is not available commercially but can be compounded by Expert Compounding Pharmacy, 6744 Balboa Blvd, Lake Balboa, CA 91406 (1-800-247-9767 or 1-818-988-7979 or info@expertpharmacy.org).

[3]The drug is not available commercially in the United States.

[4]A nitroimidazole similar to metronidazole, tinidazole was approved by the FDA in 2004 and appears to be as effective and better tolerated than metronidazole. It should be taken with food to minimize GI adverse effects. For children and patients unable to take tablets, a pharmacist may crush the tablets and mix them with cherry syrup (Humco, and others). The syrup suspension is good for 7 days at room temperature and must be shaken before use. Ornidazole, a similar drug, is also used outside the United States.

[5]Nitazoxanide is FDA approved as a pediatric oral suspension for treatment of *Cryptosporidium* in immunocompetent children ≥ 1 yr of age. It has also been used in some small studies for *Balantidium coli* infection. It may also be effective for mild to moderate amebiasis (Diaz E, et al: *Am J Trop Med Hyg* 68:384, 2003; Rossignol JF, et al: *Trans R Soc Trop Med Hyg* 101:1025, 2007). Nitazoxanide is available in 500 mg tablets and an oral suspension; it should be taken with food.

[6]*Naegleria* infection has been treated successfully with IV and intrathecal use of both amphotericin B and miconazole plus rifampin and with amphotericin B, rifampin, and ornidazole (Seidel J, et al: *N Engl J Med* 306:346, 1982; Jain R, et al: *Neurol India* 50:470, 2002). Other reports of successful therapy are less-well documented.

[7]An approved drug, but usage is considered off-label for this condition by the FDA.

[8]If you have a patient with suspected free-living amoeba infection, please contact the CDC Emergency Operations Center at 1-800-CDC-INFO to consult with a CDC expert regarding the use of this drug. Miltefosine has been reported to successfully treat primary amebic meningoencephalitis due to *Naegleria fowleri*, although controlled trials have not been conducted (Linam M, et al: *Pediatrics* 135:e744-e748, 2015).

Continued

Table 305.1	Drugs for Parasitic Infections—cont'd		
INFECTION	**DRUG**	**ADULT DOSAGE**	**PEDIATRIC DOSAGE**
Acanthamoeba			
Drug of choice:	See footnotes 7, 8		
Balamuthia mandrillaris			
Drug of choice:	See footnotes 7, 9a, 9b		
Sappinia diploidea			
Drug of choice:	See footnote 10		
Ancylostoma caninum (eosinophilic enterocolitis)			
Drug of choice:	Albendazole[7]	400 mg PO once	<10 kg/2 yr:[11] ≥2 yr: see adult dosing
or	Mebendazole	100 mg PO bid × 3 days	100 mg PO bid × 3 days[12]
or	Pyrantel pamoate (OTC)[7]	11 mg/kg PO (max 1 g) × 3 days	11 mg/kg PO (max 1 g) × 3 days
or	Endoscopic removal		
Ancylostoma duodenale, see Hookworm			
Angiostrongyliasis (*Angiostrongylus cantonensis, Angiostrongylus costaricensis*)			
Drug of choice:	See footnote 13		
Anisakiasis (*Anisakis* spp.)			
Treatment of choice:	Surgical or endoscopic removal		
Alternative:	Albendazole[7,14]	400 mg PO bid × 6-21 days	<10 kg/2 yr:[11] ≥2 yr: see adult dosing
Ascariasis (*Ascaris lumbricoides,* roundworm)			
Drug of choice:	Albendazole[7]	400 mg PO once	<10 kg/2 yr: see adult dosing[11] ≥2 yr: see adult dosing
or	Mebendazole	100 mg PO bid × 3 days or 500 mg PO once	100 mg PO bid × 3 days or 500 mg PO once[12]
or	Ivermectin[7]	150-200 µg/kg PO once	<15 kg: not indicated ≥15 kg: see adult dosing

[9a]Strains of *Acanthamoeba* isolated from fatal granulomatous amebic encephalitis are usually susceptible in vitro to pentamidine, ketoconazole, flucytosine, and (less so) amphotericin B. Chronic *Acanthamoeba* meningitis has been successfully treated in two children with a combination of oral trimethoprim-sulfamethoxazole, rifampin, and ketoconazole (Singhal T, et al: *Pediatr Infect Dis J* 20:623, 2001), and in an AIDS patient with fluconazole, sulfadiazine, and pyrimethamine combined with surgical resection of the CNS lesion (Seijo Martinez M, et al: *J Clin Microbiol* 38:3892, 2000). Disseminated cutaneous infection in an immunocompromised patient has been treated successfully with IV pentamidine isethionate, topical chlorhexidine, and 2% ketoconazole cream, followed by oral itraconazole (Slater CA, et al: *N Engl J Med* 331:85, 1994).

[9b]A free-living leptomyxid ameba that causes subacute to fatal granulomatous CNS disease. Several cases of *Balamuthia* encephalitis have been successfully treated with flucytosine, pentamidine, fluconazole, and sulfadiazine plus either azithromycin or clarithromycin (phenothiazines were also used) combined with surgical resection of the CNS lesion (Deetz TR, et al: *Clin Infect Dis* 37:1304, 2003; Jung S, et al: *Arch Pathol Lab Med* 128:466, 2004). Case reports and in vitro data suggest miltefosine may have some antiamebic activity (Aichelburg AC, et al: *Emerg Infect Dis* 14:1743, 2008; Martinez DY, et al: *Clin Infect Dis* 51:e7, 2010; Schuster FL, et al: *J Eukaryot Microbiol* 53:121, 2006). Miltefosine (Impavido) is now commercially available. Contact the Centers for Disease Control/Agency for Toxic Substances Disease Registry at 1-770-488-7100 or 1-800-232-4636 (main number) for guidance on treatment.

[10]A free-living ameba not previously known to be pathogenic to humans. It has been successfully treated with azithromycin, IV pentamidine, itraconazole, and flucytosine combined with surgical resection of the CNS lesion (Gelman BB, et al: *J Neuropathol Exp Neurol* 62:990, 2003).

[11]Limited data in children < 2 yr but has been used successfully for treatment of cutaneous larva migrans in children as young as 8 mo at a dose of 200 mg daily × 3 days (Black MD, et al: *Australas J Dermatol* 51:281-284, 2010). The WHO also recommends albendazole in children < 2 yr for treatment of taeniasis, strongyloidiasis, filariasis, hookworms, roundworms, pinworms, and threadworms.

[12]Limited safety data in children < 2 yr of age.

[13]Most patients have a self-limited course and recover completely. Analgesics, corticosteroids, and careful removal of CSF at frequent intervals can relieve symptoms from increased intracranial pressure (Lo Re V III, Gluckman SJ: *Am J Med* 114:217, 2003). No anthelmintic drug is proven to be effective, and some patients have worsened with therapy (Slom TJ, et al: *N Engl J Med* 346:668, 2002). Mebendazole or albendazole and a corticosteroid appeared to shorten the course of infection (Sawanyawisuth K, Sawanyawisuth K: *Trans R Soc Trop Med Hyg* 102:990, 2008; Chotmongkol V, et al: *Am J Trop Med Hyg* 81:443, 2009).

[14](Repiso Ortega A, et al: *Gastroenterol Hepatol* 26:341, 2003.) Successful treatment of a patient with anisakiasis with albendazole has been reported (Moore DA, et al: *Lancet* 360:54, 2002).

Continued

Table 305.1	Drugs for Parasitic Infections—cont'd

INFECTION	DRUG	ADULT DOSAGE	PEDIATRIC DOSAGE
Babesiosis *(Babesia microti)*			
Drugs of choice:[15]	Atovaquone[7] *plus* Azithromycin[7]	750 mg PO bid × 7-10 days 500-1000 mg once, then 250 mg daily × 7-10 days. Higher doses (600-1000 mg) and/or prolonged therapy (6 wk or longer) may be required for immunocompromised patients.	20 mg/kg (max 750 mg) PO bid × 7-10 days 10 mg/kg PO on day 1 (max 500 mg/dose), then 5 mg/kg/day (max 250 mg/dose) PO on days 2-10
or	Clindamycin[7]	300-600 mg IV qid or 600 mg tid PO × 7-10 days	20-40 mg/kg/day IV or PO in 3 or 4 doses × 7-10 days (max 600 mg/dose)
	plus Quinine[7]	648 mg tid PO × 7-10 days	10 mg/kg (max 648 mg) PO tid × 7-10 days
Balamuthia mandrillaris, see Amebic meningoencephalitis, primary			
Balantidiasis *(Balantidium coli)*			
Drug of choice:	Tetracycline[7,16]	500 mg PO qid × 10 days	<8 yr: not indicated ≥8 yr: 10 mg/kg (max 500 mg) PO qid × 10 days
Alternative:	Metronidazole[7]	750 mg PO tid × 5 days	35-50 mg/kg/day PO in 3 divided doses × 5 days
or	Iodoquinol[2,7]	650 mg PO tid × 20 days	30-40 mg/kg/day (max 2 g) PO in 3 divided doses × 20 days
or	Nitazoxanide[4,7]	500 mg PO bid × 3 days	1-3 yr: 100 mg PO bid × 3 days 4-11 yr: 200 mg PO bid × 3 days 12+ yr: see adult dosing
Baylisascariasis *(Baylisascaris procyonis)*			
Drug of choice:	Albendazole[7,17]	400 mg PO BID × 10-20 days	<10 kg/2 yr: 25-50 mg/kg/day PO in 1-2 divided doses × 10-20 days[11] ≥2 yr: 25-50 mg/kg/day PO in 1-2 divided doses × 10-20 days
Blastocystis hominis infection			
Drug of choice:	See footnote 18		
Capillariasis *(Capillaria philippinensis)*			
Drug of choice:	Mebendazole[7]	200 mg PO bid × 20 days	200 mg PO bid × 20 days[12]
Alternative:	Albendazole[7]	400 mg PO daily × 10 days	<10 kg/2 yr:[11] ≥2 yr: see adult dosing
Chagas disease, see Trypanosomiasis			
Clonorchis sinensis, see Fluke infection			
Cryptosporidiosis *(Cryptosporidium parvum)*			
Immunocompetent			
Drug of choice:	Nitazoxanide[4]	500 mg PO bid × 3 days	1-3 yr: 100 mg PO bid × 3 days 4-11 yr: 200 mg PO bid × 3 days 12+ yr: see adult dosing
HIV infected			
Drug of choice:	See footnote 19		

[15]Exchange transfusion has been used in severely ill patients and those with high (>10%) parasitemia (Hatcher JC, et al: *Clin Infect Dis* 32:1117, 2001). Clindamycin and quinine is the preferred therapy for severely ill patients. In patients who were not severely ill, combination therapy with atovaquone and azithromycin was as effective as clindamycin and quinine and may have been better tolerated (Krause PJ, et al: *N Engl J Med* 343:1454, 2000). Highly immunosuppressed patients should be treated for a minimum of 6 wk and at least 2 wk past the last positive smear (Krause PJ, et al: *Clin Infect Dis* 46:370, 2008). High doses of azithromycin (600-1,000 mg) have been used in combination with atovaquone for the treatment of immunocompromised patients (Weiss LM, et al: *N Engl J Med* 344:773, 2001). Resistance to atovaquone plus azithromycin has been reported in immunocompromised patients treated with a single subcurative course of this regimen (Wormser GP, et al: *Clin Infect Dis* 50:381, 2010). Most asymptomatic patients do not require treatment unless parasitemia persists > 3 mo (Wormser GP, et al: *Clin Infect Dis* 43:1089-1134, 2006).

[16]Use of tetracyclines is contraindicated in pregnancy and in children younger than 8 yr old.

[17]No drugs have been consistently demonstrated to be effective. The combination of albendazole 37 mg/kg/day PO and high-dose steroids has been used successfully (Peters JM, et al: *Pediatrics* 129:e806, 2012; Haider S: *Emerg Infect Dis* 18:347, 2012). Albendazole 25 mg/kg/day PO × 20 days started as soon as possible (up to 3 days after possible infection) might prevent clinical disease and is recommended for children with known exposure, as in the setting of ingestion of raccoon stool or contaminated soil (Murray WJ, Kazacos KR: *Clin Infect Dis* 39:1484, 2004). Mebendazole, levamisole, or ivermectin could be tried if albendazole is not available. Ocular baylisascariasis has been treated successfully using laser photocoagulation therapy to destroy the intraretinal larvae.

[18]Clinical significance of these organisms is controversial; metronidazole 750 mg tid × 10 days, iodoquinol 650 mg tid × 20 days, or trimethoprim-sulfamethoxazole 1 DS tablet bid × 7 days has been reported to be effective (Stenzel DJ, Borenam PFL: *Clin Microbiol Rev* 9:563, 1996; Ok UZ, et al: *Am J Gastroenterol* 94:3245, 1999). Metronidazole resistance may be common (Haresh K, et al: *Trop Med Int Health* 4:274, 1999). Nitazoxanide has been effective in children (Diaz E, et al: *Am J Trop Med Hyg* 68:384, 2003).

[19]Nitazoxanide has not consistently been shown to be superior to placebo in HIV-infected patients (Amadi B, et al: *Lancet* 360;1375, 2002). For HIV-infected patients, potent antiretroviral therapy (ART) is the mainstay of treatment. Nitazoxanide 500-1,000 mg for 14 days, paromomycin 500 mg 4 times daily × 14-21 days, or a combination of paromomycin and azithromycin may be tried to decrease diarrhea and recalcitrant malabsorption of antimicrobial drugs, which can occur with chronic cryptosporidiosis (Pantenburg B, et al: *Expert Rev Anti Infect Ther* 7:385, 2009).

Continued

Table 305.1	Drugs for Parasitic Infections—cont'd		
INFECTION	**DRUG**	**ADULT DOSAGE**	**PEDIATRIC DOSAGE**
Cutaneous larva migrans (*Ancylostoma braziliense, A. caninum,* dog and cat hookworm, creeping eruption)			
Drug of choice:	Albendazole[7,20]	400 mg PO daily × 3-7 days	<10 kg/2 yr: 200 mg PO daily × 3 days[11] ≥2 yr: see adult dosing
or	Ivermectin[7]	200 μg/kg PO daily × 1-2 days	<15 kg: not indicated ≥15 kg: see adult dosing
Alternative:	Thiabendazole	Apply topically tid × 7 days	Apply topically tid × 7 days
Cyclosporiasis (*Cyclospora cayetanensis*)			
Drug of choice:	Trimethoprim-sulfamethoxazole (TMP-SMX)[7,21]	TMP 160 mg/SMX 800 mg (1 DS tab) PO bid × 7-10 days	4-5 mg/kg TMP component (max 160 mg) PO bid × 7-10 days
Cysticercosis, see Tapeworm infection			
Cystoisosporiasis (*Cystoisospora belli,* formerly known as *Isospora*)			
Drug of choice:	Trimethoprim-sulfamethoxazole (TMP-SMX)[7]	TMP 160 mg/SMX 800 mg (1 DS tablet) PO bid × 10 days	4-5 mg/kg TMP component (max 160 mg) PO bid × 10 days
Alternative:	Pyrimethamine *plus* Leukovorin	50-75 mg PO divided bid × 10 days 10-25 mg PO daily × 10 days	— —
or	Ciprofloxacin[7]	500 mg PO bid × 7-10 days	—
Dientamoeba fragilis infection[22]			
	Paromomycin[7]	25-35 mg/kg/day PO in 3 doses × 7 days	25-35 mg/kg/day PO in 3 divided doses × 7 days
or	Iodoquinol[2]	650 mg PO tid × 20 days	30-40 mg/kg/day PO (max 2 g) in 3 divided doses × 20 days
or	Metronidazole[7]	500-750 mg tid × 10 days	35-50 mg/kg/day in 3 divided doses × 10 days
Diphyllobothrium latum, see Tapeworm infection			
Dracunculus medinensis (guinea worm) infection			
Treatment of choice:	Slow mechanical extraction of worm[23]		
Echinococcus, see Tapeworm infection			
Entamoeba histolytica, see Amebiasis			
Enterobius vermicularis (pinworm) infection[24]			
Drug of choice:	Albendazole[7]	400 mg PO once; repeat in 2 wk	<10 kg/2 yr: 200 mg PO once; repeat in 2 wk[11] ≥2 yr: see adult dosing
or	Mebendazole	100 mg PO once; repeat in 3 wk	100 mg PO once; repeat in 3 wk[12]
or	Pyrantel pamoate (OTC)	11 mg/kg base PO once (max 1 g); repeat in 2 wk	11 mg/kg base PO once (max 1 g); repeat in 2 wk
Fasciola hepatica, see Fluke infection			
Filariasis[25]			

[20]Albanese G, et al: *Int J Dermatol* 40:67, 2001.

  [21]HIV-infected patients may need a higher dosage and long-term maintenance (Kansouzidou A, et al: *J Trav Med* 11:61, 2004).

[22]Norberg A, et al: *Clin Microbiol Infect* 9:65, 2003.

[23]Treatment of choice is slow extraction of worm combined with wound care (*MMWR Morbid Mortal Wkly Rep* 60:1450, 2011). Instructions for this can be found at https://www.cdc.gov/parasites/guineaworm/treatment.html. Ten days of treatment with metronidazole 250 mg tid in adults and 25 mg/kg/day in 3 doses in children is not curative, but it decreases inflammation and facilitates removal of the worm. Mebendazole 400-800 mg/day × 6 days has been reported to kill the worm directly.

[24]Because all family members are usually infected, treatment of the entire household is recommended.

[25]Antihistamines or corticosteroids may be required to decrease allergic reactions due to disintegration of microfilariae from treatment of filarial infections, especially those caused by *Loa loa.* Endosymbiotic *Wolbachia* bacteria may have a role in filarial development and host response and may represent a new target for therapy. Treatment with doxycycline 100 or 200 mg/day × 4-6 wk in lymphatic filariasis and onchocerciasis has resulted in substantial loss of *Wolbachia* with subsequent blocking of microfilariae production and absence of microfilaria when followed for 24 mo after treatment (Hoerauf A, et al: *Med Microbiol Immunol* 192:211, 2003; Hoerauf A, et al: *BMJ* 326:207, 2003).

Continued

Table 305.1	Drugs for Parasitic Infections—cont'd		
INFECTION	**DRUG**	**ADULT DOSAGE**	**PEDIATRIC DOSAGE**
Lymphatic filariasis (*Wuchereria bancrofti, Brugia malayi, Brugia timori*)			
Drug of choice:[26]	Diethylcarbamazine[27,28]	6 mg/kg once or 6 mg/kg PO in 3 divided doses × 12 days[29]	<18 mo: no indication ≥18 mo: see adult dosing
Loa loa			
<8,000 microfilaria/mL[28]			
Drug of choice:	Diethylcarbamazine[27,28]	9 mg/kg PO in 3 doses × 14 days[29]	<18 mo: no indication ≥18 mo: see adult dosing
Alternative:	Albendazole[27]	200 mg PO bid × 21 days	<10 kg/2 yr:[11] ≥2 yr: see adult dosing
≥8,000 microfilaria/mL[28,30]			
Treatment of choice:	Apheresis		
or	Albendazole[27]	200 mg PO bid × 21 days	<10 kg/2 yr:[11] ≥2 yr: see adult dosing
Either followed by:	Diethylcarbamazine[27,28]	8-10 mg/kg PO in 3 doses × 21 days[29]	<18 mo: no indication ≥18 mo: see adult dosing
Mansonella ozzardi			
Drug of choice:	See footnote 31		
Mansonella perstans			
Drug of choice:	Doxycycline[7,16,32]	100 mg bid PO × 6 wk	4 mg/kg/day in 2 doses PO × 6 wk
Mansonella streptocerca[33]			
Drug of choice:	Diethylcarbamazine	6 mg/kg/day PO × 14 days	6 mg/kg/day PO × 14 days
or	Ivermectin[7]	150 µg/kg PO once	<15 kg: not indicated ≥15 kg: see adult dosing
Tropical pulmonary eosinophilia (TPE)[34]			
Drug of choice:	Diethylcarbamazine[27]	6 mg/kg once or 6 mg/kg PO in 3 divided doses × 14-21 days[26]	<18 mo: no indication ≥18 mo: see adult dosing
Onchocerca volvulus (river blindness)			
Drug of choice:	Ivermectin[35]	150 µg/kg PO once, repeated every 6-12 mo until asymptomatic	<15 kg: not indicated ≥15 kg: see adult dosing

[26]Most symptoms caused by adult worm. Single-dose combination of albendazole (400 mg) with either ivermectin (200 µg/kg) or diethylcarbamazine (6 mg/kg) is effective for reduction or suppression of *Wuchereria bancrofti* microfilaria but does not kill the adult forms (Addiss D, et al: *Cochrane Database Syst Rev* (1):CD003753, 2004).

[27]This drug is not FDA approved and not commercially available but is available under IND application through the CDC Drug Service (CDC Drug Service, Division of Scientific Resources, telephone at 1-404-639-3670.

[28]DEC is contraindicated in patients coinfected with *Oncocerca volvulus* due to risk of a life-threatening Mazzotti reaction and in patients with *Loa loa* infection and microfilaria levels ≥ 8,000 mm³ due to risk of encephalopathy and renal failure. Some experts use a cutoff of ≥ 2,500 mm³.

[29]For patients with microfilaria in the blood, *Medical Letter* consultants would start with a lower dosage and scale up: day 1, 50 mg; day 2, 50 mg tid; day 3, 100 mg tid; day 4-14, 6 mg/kg in 3 doses (for *Loa loa*, day 4-14, 9 mg/kg in 3 doses). Multidose regimens have been shown to provide more rapid reduction in microfilaria than single-dose diethylcarbamazine, but microfilaria levels are similar 6-12 mo after treatment (Andrade LD, et al: *Trans R Soc Trop Med Hyg* 89:319, 1995; Simonsen PE, et al: *Am J Trop Med Hyg* 53:267, 1995). A single dose of 6 mg/kg is used in endemic areas for mass treatment (Figueredo-Silva J, et al: *Trans R Soc Trop Med Hyg* 90:192, 1996; Noroes J, et al: *Trans R Soc Trop Med Hyg* 91:78, 1997).

[30]In heavy infections with *Loa loa*, rapid killing of microfilariae can provoke an encephalopathy. Apheresis has been reported to be effective in lowering microfilarial counts in patients heavily infected with *Loa loa* (Ottesen ES: *Infect Dis Clin North Am* 7:619, 1993). Albendazole or ivermectin has also been used to reduce microfilaremia; albendazole is preferred because of its slower onset of action and lower risk for encephalopathy (Klion AD, et al: *J Infect Dis* 168:202, 1993; Kombila M, et al: *Am J Trop Med Hyg* 58:458, 1998). Albendazole may be useful for treatment of loiasis when diethylcarbamazine is ineffective or cannot be used, but repeated courses may be necessary (Klion AD, et al: *Clin Infect Dis* 29:680, 1999). Diethylcarbamazine, 300 mg once/wk, has been recommended for prevention of loiasis (Nutman TB, et al: *N Engl J Med* 319:752, 1988).

[31]Diethylcarbamazine has no effect. Ivermectin 200 µg/kg once has been effective.

[32]Doxycycline is preferred for strains that carry *Wolbachia* bacteria. Combination therapy with diethylcarbamazine and mebendazole and monotherapy with mebendazole have been used successfully in strains that do not carry *Wolbachia*. Evidence is limited, and optimal therapy is uncertain. Ivermectin and albendazole appear to be ineffective.

[33]Diethylcarbamazine is potentially curative because of activity against both adult worms and microfilariae. Ivermectin is only active against microfilariae. (*The Medical Letter*: Drugs for parasitic infections, vol 11, 2013.)

[34]Relapse occurs and can be treated with diethylcarbamazine.

[35]Annual treatment with ivermectin, 150 µg/kg, can prevent blindness from ocular onchocerciasis (Mabey D, et al: *Ophthalmology* 103:1001, 1996). Ivermectin kills only the microfilaria but not the adult worms; emerging evidence suggests doxycycline is effective in killing adult worms and sterilizing females. The recommended regimen from the CDC is doxycycline 100-200 mg PO daily for 6 wk begun 1 wk after a dose of ivermectin is given to reduce the microfilaria burden. Diethylcarbamazine and suramin were formerly used for treatment of this disease but should no longer be used owing to the availability of less toxic therapies.

Continued

Table 305.1	Drugs for Parasitic Infections—cont'd		
INFECTION	**DRUG**	**ADULT DOSAGE**	**PEDIATRIC DOSAGE**

Fluke, hermaphroditic, infection

Clonorchis sinensis (Chinese liver fluke)

Drug of choice:	Praziquantel	25 mg/kg PO tid × 2 days	25 mg/kg PO tid × 2 days[36]
or	Albendazole[7]	10 mg/kg PO × 7 days	<10 kg/2 yr:[11] ≥2 yr: see adult dosing

Fasciola hepatica (sheep liver fluke)

Drug of choice:	Triclabendazole[7,37,38]	10 mg/kg PO once or twice	10 mg/kg PO once or twice
Alternative:	Nitazoxanide[7]	500 mg PO bid × 7 days	1-3 yr: 100 mg PO bid 4-11 yr: 200 mg PO bid ≥12 yr: see adult dosing
or	Bithionol[3,7]	30-50 mg/kg PO on alternate days × 10-15 doses	30-50 mg/kg PO on alternate days × 10-15 doses

Fasciolopsis buski, Heterophyes heterophyes, Metagonimus yokogawai (intestinal flukes)

Drug of choice:	Praziquantel[7]	25 mg/kg PO tid × 1 day	25 mg/kg PO tid × 1 day[36]

Metorchis conjunctus (North American liver fluke)[39]

Drug of choice:	Praziquantel[7]	25 mg/kg PO tid × 1 day	25 mg/kg PO tid × 1 day[36]

Nanophyetus salmincola

Drug of choice:	Praziquantel[7]	20 mg/kg PO tid × 1 day	20 mg/kg PO tid × 1 day[36]

Opisthorchis viverrini (Southeast Asian liver fluke), *O. felineus* (cat liver fluke)

Drug of choice:	Praziquantel	25 mg/kg PO tid × 2 days	25 mg/kg PO tid × 2 days[36]
or	Albendazole[7]	10 mg/kg PO × 7 days	<10 kg/2 yr:[11] ≥2 yr: see adult dosing

Paragonimus westermani (lung fluke)

Drug of choice:	Praziquantel[7]	25 mg/kg PO tid × 2 days	25 mg/kg PO tid × 2 days[36]
or	Triclabendazole[7,40]	10 mg/kg PO bid × 1 day or 5 mg/kg daily × 3 days	10 mg/kg PO bid × 1 day or 5 mg/kg daily × 3 days
or	Bithionol[3,7]	30-50 mg/kg PO on alternate days × 10-15 doses	30-50 mg/kg PO on alternate days × 10-15 doses

Giardiasis (*Giardia intestinalis*, also known as *G. duodenalis* or *G. lamblia*)

Drug of choice:	Metronidazole[7]	250 mg PO tid × 5 days	5 mg/kg (max 250 mg) PO tid × 5 days
or	Nitazoxanide[5]	500 mg PO bid × 3 days	1-3 yr: 100 mg PO every 12 hr × 3 days 4-11 yr: 200 mg PO every 12 hr × 3 days 12+ yr: see adult dosing
or	Tinidazole[4]	2 g PO once	50 mg/kg PO once (max 2 g)
Alternative:[41]	Paromomycin[7,42]	25-35 mg/kg/day PO in 3 doses × 7 days	25-35 mg/kg/day PO in 3 doses × 7 days
or	Furazolidone[3]	100 mg PO qid × 7-10 days	6 mg/kg/day PO in 4 doses × 7-10 days
or	Quinacrine[2]	100 mg PO tid × 5 days	2 mg/kg tid PO × 5 days (max 300 mg/day)

[36]Limited safety data in children < 4 yr old but has been used in mass prevention campaigns with no reported adverse effects.

[37]Unlike infections with other flukes, *Fasciola hepatica* infections do not respond to praziquantel. Triclabendazole may be safe and effective, but data are limited (Graham CS, et al: *Clin Infect Dis* 33:1, 2001). In the United States, the drug is not approved by the FDA and is not yet commercially available. However, it is available to U.S.-licensed physicians through the CDC Drug Service, under a special protocol, which requires that both the CDC and FDA agree that the drug is indicated for treatment of a particular patient. Providers should contact the CDC Drug Service, Division of Scientific Resources, at 1-404-639-3670. It is available from Victoria Pharmacy, Zurich, Switzerland (www.pharmaworld.com). The drug should be given with food for better absorption. A single study has found that nitazoxanide has limited efficacy for treating fascioliasis in adults and children (Favennec L, et al: *Aliment Pharmacol Ther* 17:265, 2003).

[38]Richter J, et al: *Curr Treat Options Infect Dis* 4:313, 2002.

[39]MacLean JD, et al: *Lancet* 347:154, 1996.

[40]Triclabendazole may be effective in a dosage of 5 mg/kg once/day × 3 days or 10 mg/kg bid × 1 day (Calvopiña M, et al: *Trans R Soc Trop Med Hyg* 92:566, 1998). In the United States, it is not approved by the FDA and is not yet commercially available. However, it is available to U.S.-licensed physicians through the CDC Drug Service, under a special protocol, which requires both the CDC and FDA to agree that the drug is indicated for treatment of a particular patient. Providers should contact the CDC Drug Service, Division of Scientific Resources, at 1-404-639-3670. The drug is available from Victoria Pharmacy, Zurich, Switzerland; Phone, 41 43 344 60 60; FAX, 41 43 344 60 69; http://www.pharmaworld.com; e-mail, info@pharmaworld.com.

[41]Albendazole 400 mg daily × 5 days alone or in combination with metronidazole may also be effective (Hall A, Nahar Q: *Trans R Soc Trop Med Hyg* 87:84, 1993; Dutta AK, et al: *Indian J Pediatr* 61:689, 1994; Cacopardo B, et al: *Clin Ter* 146:761, 1995). Combination treatment with standard doses of metronidazole and quinacrine given for 3 wk has been effective for a small number of refractory infections (Nash TE, et al: *Clin Infect Dis* 33:22, 2001). In one study, nitazoxanide was used successfully in high doses to treat a case of *Giardia* infection resistant to metronidazole and albendazole (Abboud P, et al: *Clin Infect Dis* 32:1792, 2001).

[42]Not absorbed; may be useful for treatment of giardiasis in pregnancy.

Continued

Table 305.1	Drugs for Parasitic Infections—cont'd		
INFECTION	**DRUG**	**ADULT DOSAGE**	**PEDIATRIC DOSAGE**
Gnathostomiasis (*Gnathostoma spinigerum*)			
Treatment of choice:[43]	Albendazole[7]	400 mg PO bid × 21 days	<10 kg/2 yr:[11] ≥2 yr: see adult dosing
or	Ivermectin[7]	200 µg/kg/day PO × 2 days	<15 kg: not indicated ≥15 kg: see adult dosing
±	Surgical removal		
Gongylonemiasis (*Gongylonema* sp.)[44]			
Treatment of choice:	Surgical removal		
or	Albendazole[7]	400 mg PO daily × 3 days	10 mg/kg/day PO × 3 days
Hookworm infection (*Ancylostoma duodenale, Necator americanus*)			
Drug of choice:	Albendazole[7]	400 mg PO once	<10 kg/2 yr:[11] ≥2 yr: see adult dosing
or	Mebendazole	100 mg PO bid × 3 days or 500 mg once	100 mg PO bid × 3 days or 500 mg once[12]
or	Pyrantel pamoate (OTC)[7]	11 mg/kg (max 1 g) PO × 3 days	11 mg/kg (max 1 g) PO × 3 days
Hydatid cyst, see Tapeworm infection			
***Hymenolepis nana*, see Tapeworm infection**			
***Leishmania* infection[45]**			
Visceral[46]			
Drug of choice:	Liposomal amphotericin B (AmBisome)[47,48]	3 mg/kg/day IV on days 1-5, 14, and 21 (total dose 21 mg/kg)	3 mg/kg/day IV on days 1-5, 14, and 21 (total dose 21 mg/kg)
or	Miltefosine[49]	30-44 kg: 50 mg PO bid × 28 days ≥45 kg: 50 mg PO tid × 28 days	<12 yr: 2.5 mg/kg daily × 28 days[7] 12 yr: see adult dosing
or	Sodium stibogluconate (Pentostam)[27,50]	20 mg/kg/day IV or IM × 28 days	20 mg/kg/day IV or IM × 28 days
or	Amphotericin B deoxycholate[7]	1 mg/kg IV daily or every 2 days for 15-20 doses	1 mg/kg IV daily or every 2 days for 15-20 doses
Alternative:	Meglumine antimoniate[3,50]	20 mg pentavalent antimony/kg/day IV or IM × 28 days	20 mg pentavalent antimony/kg/day IV or IM × 28 days
or	Pentamidine[7]	4 mg/kg IV or IM daily or every 2 days for 15-30 doses	4 mg/kg IV or IM daily or every 2 days for 15-30 doses
Cutaneous[51,52]			
Drug of choice:	Sodium stibogluconate[27,50]	20 mg/kg/day IV or IM × 20 days	20 mg/kg/day IV or IM × 20 days
or	Liposomal amphotericin B (AmBisome)[7]	3 mg/kg/day IV on days 1-5 and 10 or 1-7 (total dose 18-21 mg/kg)	3 mg/kg/day IV on days 1-5 and 10 or 1-7 (total dose 18-21 mg/kg)
or	Amphotericin B deoxycholate[7]	0.5-1 mg/kg IV daily or every 2 days (total dose 15-30 mg/kg)	0.5-1 mg/kg IV daily or every 2 days (total dose 15-30 mg/kg)
or	Miltefosine[49]	30-44 kg: 50 mg PO bid × 28 days ≥45 kg: 50 mg PO tid × 28 days	<12 yr: 2.5 mg/kg daily × 28 days[7] 12 yr: see adult dosing

[43]de Gorgolas M, et al: *J Travel Med* 10:358, 2003. All patients should be treated with a medication regardless of whether surgery is attempted.

[44]Eberhard ML, Busillo C: *Am J Trop Med Hyg* 61:51, 1999; Wilson ME, et al: *Clin Infect Dis* 32:1378, 2001.

[45]Consultation with physicians experienced in management of this disease is recommended. To maximize effectiveness and minimize toxicity, the choice of drug, dosage, and duration of therapy should be individualized based on the region of disease acquisition, likely infecting species, number, significance and location of lesions, and host factors such as immune status (Murray HW: *Lancet* 366:1561, 2005; Aronson N, et al: *Clin Infect Dis* 63:202, 2016). Some of the listed drugs and regimens are effective only against certain *Leishmania* species/strains and only in certain areas of the world (Sundar S, Chakravarty J: *Expert Opin Pharmacother* 14:53, 2013).

[46]Visceral infection is most commonly caused by the Old World species *Leishmania donovani* (kala-azar) and *Leishmania infantum* and the New World species *Leishmania chagasi*. Treatment duration may vary based on symptoms, host immune status, species, and area of the world where infection was acquired. Liposomal amphotericin B is the treatment of choice in the IDSA leishmaniasis guidelines (Aronson N, et al: *Clin Infect Dis* 63:202, 2016).

[47]Three lipid formulations of amphotericin B have been used for treatment of visceral leishmaniasis. Largely based on clinical trials in patients infected with *Leishmania infantum*, the FDA approved liposomal amphotericin B (AmBisome) for treatment of visceral leishmaniasis (Meyerhoff A: *Clin Infect Dis* 28:42, 1999). Amphotericin B lipid complex (Abelcet) and amphotericin B cholesteryl sulfate (Amphotec) have also been used with good results but are considered investigational for this condition by the FDA.

[48]The FDA-approved dosage regimen for immunocompromised patients (e.g., HIV infected) is 4 mg/kg/day on days 1-5 and 4 mg/kg/day on days 10, 17, 24, 31, and 38. The relapse rate is high; maintenance therapy may be indicated, but there is no consensus as to dosage or duration. (Russo R, Nigro LC, Minniti S, et al: Visceral leishmaniasis in HIV infected patients: treatment with high dose liposomal amphotericin B [AmBisome], *J Infect* 32:133-137, 1996).

[49]For treatment of kala-azar in adults in India, oral miltefosine 100 mg/day (~205 mg/kg/day) for 3-4 wk was 97% effective after 6 mo (Jha TK, et al: *N Engl J Med* 341:1795, 1999; Sangraula H, et al: *J Assoc Physicians India* 51:686, 2003). GI adverse effects are common, and the drug is contraindicated in pregnancy. The dose of miltefosine in an open-label trial in children in India was 2.5 mg/kg/day × 28 days (Bhattacharya SK, et al: *Clin Infect Dis* 38:217, 2004). Miltefosine (Impavido) has been FDA approved for treatment of leishmaniasis due to *Leishmania donovani*; cutaneous leishmaniasis due to *L. braziliensis, L. guyanensis,* and *L. panamensis*; and mucosal leishmaniasis due to *L. braziliensis* since 2014 and is now commercially available.

Continued

Table 305.1	Drugs for Parasitic Infections—cont'd		
INFECTION	**DRUG**	**ADULT DOSAGE**	**PEDIATRIC DOSAGE**
Alternatives:	Meglumine antimoniate[3,50]	20 mg pentavalent antimony/kg/day IV or IM × 20 days	20 mg pentavalent antimony/kg/day IV or IM × 20 days
or	Pentamidine[7,53]	3-4 mg/kg IV or IM every 2 days × 3-4 doses	2-3 mg/kg IV or IM daily or every 2 days × 4-7 doses
or	Paromomycin[7,54]	Topically 2x/day × 10-20 days	Topically 2x/day × 10-20 days
or	Ketoconazole[7]	600 mg daily × 28 days	
or	Fluconazole[7]	200 mg daily × 6 wk	
or	Local therapy, including cryotherapy, thermotherapy, intralesional Sb[V], topical paromomycin, photodynamic or laser therapy		
Mucosal[54,55]			
Drug of choice:	Sodium stibogluconate[27,50]	20 mg/kg/day IV or IM × 28 days	20 mg/kg/day IV or IM × 28 days
or	Liposomal amphotericin B (AmBisome)[7]	3 mg/kg/day IV × 10 days or 4 mg/kg on days 1-5, 10, 17, 24, 31, and 38 (total dose 20-60 mg/kg)	2-4 mg/kg/day IV × 10 days or 4 mg/kg on days 1-5, 10, 17, 24, 31, and 38 (total dose 20-60 mg/kg)
or	Amphotericin B deoxycholate[7]	0.5-1 mg/kg IV daily or every 2 days (total dose 20-45 mg/kg)	0.5-1 mg/kg IV daily or every 2 days (total dose 20-45 mg/kg)
or	Miltefosine[49]	30-44 kg: 50 mg PO bid × 28 days ≥45 kg: 50 mg PO tid × 28 days	<12 yr: 2.5 mg/kg daily × 28 days[7] 12 yr: see adult dosing
Alternative:	Meglumine antimoniate[3,50]	20 mg pentavalent antimony/kg/day IV or IM × 28 days	20 mg pentavalent antimony/kg/day IV or IM × 28 days
Lice (head and body) infestation (_Pediculus humanus capitis, Pediculus humanus humanus_)			
Drug of choice:	0.5% Malathion (Ovide)[56]	Topically 2x, 1 wk apart	Topically 2x, 1 wk apart, approved for ≥ 6 yr
or	1% Permethrin (Nix) (OTC)[56]	Topically 2x, 1 wk apart	Topically 2x, 1 wk apart, approved for ≥ 2 mo
or	Pyrethrins with piperonyl butoxide (A-200, Pronto, R&C, Rid, Triple X) (OTC)[57]	Topically 2x, 1 wk apart	Topically 2x, 1 wk, approved for ≥ 2 yr
or	0.5% Ivermectin lotion (Sklice)	Topically, once	Topically once, approved for ≥ 6 mo
or	0.9% Spinosad suspension (Natroba)	Topically once, 2nd dose in 1 wk if live adult lice seen	Topically once, 2nd dose in 1 wk if live adult lice seen, approved for ≥ 6 mo
or	Ivermectin[7,58]	200-400 µg/kg PO 2x, 1 wk apart	<15 kg: not indicated ≥15 kg: see adult dosing
or	5% Benzyl alcohol lotion (Ulesfia)	Topically 2x, 1 wk apart	Topically 2x, 1 wk apart

[50]May be repeated or continued; a longer duration may be needed for some patients (Herwaldt BL: _Lancet_ 354:1191, 1999).

[51]Cutaneous infection is most commonly caused by the Old World species _Leishmania major_ and _Leishmania tropica_ and the New World species _Leishmania mexicana, Leishmania (Viannia) braziliensis_, and others. Treatment duration may vary based on symptoms, host immune status, species, and area of the world where infection was acquired.

[52]In a placebo-controlled trial in patients 12 yr old and older, oral miltefosine was effective for the treatment of cutaneous leishmaniasis caused by _Leishmania (Viannia) panamensis_ in Colombia but not _L. (V.) braziliensis_ in Guatemala at a dosage of about 2.5 mg/kg/day for 28 days. "Motion sickness," nausea, headache, and increased creatinine were the most frequent adverse effects (Soto J, et al: _Clin Infect Dis_ 38:1266, 2004). For treatment of _L. major_ cutaneous lesions, a study in Saudi Arabia found that oral fluconazole, 200 mg once/day × 6 wk, appeared to speed healing (Alrajhi AA, et al: _N Engl J Med_ 346:891, 2002).

[53]At this dosage, pentamidine has been effective against leishmaniasis in Colombia, where the likely organism was _L. (V.) panamensis_ (Soto-Mancipe J, et al: _Clin Infect Dis_ 16:417, 1993; Soto J, et al: _Am J Trop Med Hyg_ 50:107, 1994); its effect against other species is not well established. Updated based on _Leishmania_ practice guidelines (Aronson N, et al: _Clin Infect Dis_ 63:202-264, 2016).

[54]Topical paromomycin should be used only in geographic regions where cutaneous leishmaniasis species have low potential for mucosal spread. A formulation of 15% paromomycin/12% methylbenzethonium chloride (Leshcutan) in soft white paraffin for topical use has been reported to be partially effective in some patients against cutaneous leishmaniasis due to _L. major_ in Israel and against _L. mexicana_ and _L. (V.) braziliensis_ in Guatemala, where mucosal spread is very rare (Arana BA, et al: _Am J Trop Med Hyg_ 65:466, 2001). The methylbenzethonium is irritating to the skin; lesions may worsen before they improve.

[55]Mucosal infection is most commonly due to the New World species _L. (V.) braziliensis, L. (V.) panamensis_, or _L. (V.) guyanensis_. Treatment duration may vary based on symptoms, host immune status, species, and area of the world where infection was acquired

[56]Yoon KS, et al: _Arch Dermatol_ 139:994, 2003.

[57]A second application is recommended 1 wk later to kill hatching progeny. Lice are increasingly demonstrating resistance to pyrethrins and permethrin (Meinking TL, et al: _Arch Dermatol_ 138:220, 2002). Ivermectin lotion 0.5% was approved by the FDA in 2012 for treatment of head lice in persons 6 mo of age and older. It is not ovicidal, but it appears to prevent nymphs from surviving. It is effective in most patients when given as a single application on dry hair without nit combing (www.cdc.gov/parasites/lice/head/treatment.html).

[58]Ivermectin is effective against adult lice but has no effect on nits (Jones KN, English JC III: _Clin Infect Dis_ 36:1355, 2003).

Continued

Table 305.1	Drugs for Parasitic Infections—cont'd		
INFECTION	**DRUG**	**ADULT DOSAGE**	**PEDIATRIC DOSAGE**
Lice (pubic) infestation *(Phthirus pubis)*[59]			
Drug of choice:	1% Permethrin (Nix) (OTC)[56]	Topically 2x, 1 wk apart	Topically 2x, 1 wk apart, approved for ≥ 2 mo
or	Pyrethrins with piperonyl butoxide (A-200, Pronto, R&C, Rid, Triple X) (OTC)[52]	Topically 2x, 1 wk apart	Topically 2x, 1 wk apart, approved for ≥ 2 yr
or	0.5% Malathion (Ovide)[56]	Topically 2x, 1 wk apart	Topically 2x, 1 wk apart, approved for ≥ 6 yr
or	0.5% Ivermectin lotion (Sklice)	Topically, once	Topically once, approved for ≥ 6 mo
or	Ivermectin[7,58]	200-400 μg/kg PO 2x, 1 wk apart	<15 kg: not indicated ≥15 kg: see adult dosing
Loa loa, see Filariasis			
Malaria *(Plasmodium falciparum, Plasmodium ovale, Plasmodium vivax*, and *Plasmodium malariae)* Treatment			
Uncomplicated infection due to *P. falciparum* or species not identified acquired in areas of chloroquine resistance or unknown resistance[60]			
Drug of choice:[61]	Atovaquone/proguanil (Malarone) Adult tablets: 50 mg atovaquone/100 mg proguanil Pediatric tablets: 62.5 mg atovaquone/ 25 mg proguanil[62]	4 adult tablets PO once daily or 2 adult tablets PO bid × 3 days[63]	<5 kg: not indicated 5-8 kg: 2 pediatric tablets PO daily × 3 days 9-10 kg: 3 pediatric tablets PO daily × 3 days 11-20 kg: 1 adult tablet PO daily × 3 days 21-30 kg: 2 adult tablets PO daily × 3 days 31-40 kg: 3 adult tablets PO daily × 3 days >40 kg: 4 adult tablets PO daily × 3 days
or	Coartem (artemether-lumefantrine) Fixed dose of 20 mg artemether and 120 mg lumefantrine per tablet	4 tablets per dose. A 3- day treatment schedule with a total of 6 oral doses is recommended for both adult and pediatric patients based on weight. These 6 doses should be administered over 3 days at 0, 8, 24, 36, 48, and 60 h5.	5 to < 15 kg: 1 tablet PO per dose 15 to < 25 kg: 2 tablets PO per dose 25 to < 35 kg: 3 tablets per dose ≥35 kg: 4 tablets PO per dose
or	Quinine sulfate *plus* Doxycycline[7,16] *or plus* Tetracycline[7,16] *or plus* Clindamycin[7,65]	648 mg salt PO tid × 3-7 days[63] 100 mg PO bid × 7 days 250 mg PO qid × 7 days 20 mg/kg/day PO in 3 divided doses × 7 days[66]	10 mg salt/kg PO tid × 3-7 days[64] 4 mg/kg/day PO in 2 doses × 7 days 6.25 mg/kg PO qid × 7 days 20 mg/kg/day PO in 3 doses × 7 days
Alternative:	Mefloquine[67,68]	750 mg PO followed 12 hr later by 500 mg	15 mg/kg PO followed 12 hr later by 10 mg/kg

[59]For infestation of eyelashes with *Phthirus pubis* lice, use petrolatum; TMP-SMX has also been used (Meinking TL: *Curr Probl Dermatol* 24:157, 1996). For pubic lice, treat with 5% permethrin or ivermectin as for scabies. TMP-SMX has also been effective, together with permethrin for head lice (Hipolito RB, et al: *Pediatrics* 107:E30, 2001).

[60]Chloroquine-resistant *P. falciparum* occurs in all malarious areas except Central America west of the Panama Canal Zone, Mexico, Haiti, the Dominican Republic, and most of the Middle East (chloroquine resistance has been reported in Yemen, Oman, Saudi Arabia, and Iran). For treatment of multidrug-resistant *P. falciparum* in Southeast Asia, especially Thailand, where resistance to mefloquine is frequent, atovaquone/proguanil, artesunate plus mefloquine, or artemether plus mefloquine may be used (Luxemburger JC, et al: *Trans R Soc Trop Med Hyg* 88:213, 1994; Karbwang J, et al: *Trans R Soc Trop Med Hyg* 89:296, 1995).

[61]Uncomplicated or mild malaria may be treated with oral drugs.

[62]To enhance absorption and reduce nausea and vomiting, it should be taken with food or a milky drink. Safety in pregnancy is unknown, and use is generally not recommended. In a few small studies, outcomes were normal in women treated with the combination in the second and third trimesters (Paternak B, et al: *Arch Intern Med* 171:259, 2011; Boggild AK, et al: *Am J Trop Med Hyg* 76:208, 2007). The drug should not be given to patients with severe renal impairment (creatinine clearance < 30 mL/min). There have been isolated case reports of resistance in *P. falciparum* in Africa, but *Medical Letter* consultants do not believe there is a high risk for acquisition of Malarone-resistant disease (Schwartz E, et al: *Clin Infect Dis* 37:450, 2003; Farnert A, et al: *BMJ* 326:628, 2003; Kuhn S, et al: *Am J Trop Med Hyg* 72:407, 2005; Happi C, et al: *Malar J* 5:82, 2006).

[63]Although approved for once-daily dosing, *Medical Letter* consultants usually divide the dose into 2 doses to decrease nausea and vomiting.

[64]In Southeast Asia, relative resistance to quinine has increased and treatment should be continued for 7 days.

[65]For use in pregnancy.

[66]Lell B, Kremsner PG: *Antimicrob Agents Chemother* 46:2315, 2002.

[67]At this dosage, adverse effects, including nausea, vomiting, diarrhea, dizziness, a disturbed sense of balance, toxic psychosis, and seizures can occur. Mefloquine should not be used for treatment of malaria in pregnancy unless there is no other treatment option, because of an increased risk for stillbirth (Nosten F, et al: *Clin Infect Dis* 28:808, 1999). It should be avoided for treatment of malaria in persons with active depression or with a history of psychosis or seizures and should be used with caution in persons with psychiatric illness. Mefloquine can be given to patients taking β blockers if they do not have an underlying arrhythmia; it should not be used in patients with conduction abnormalities. Mefloquine should not be given together with quinine, quinidine, or halofantrine, and caution is required in using quinine, quinidine, or halofantrine to treat patients with malaria who have taken mefloquine for prophylaxis. Resistance to mefloquine has been reported in some areas, such as the Thailand-Myanmar and Thailand-Cambodia borders and in the Amazon basin, where 25 mg/kg should be used. In the United States, a 250 mg tablet of mefloquine contains 228 mg mefloquine base. Outside the United States, each 275 mg tablet contains 250 mg base.

[68]*P. falciparum* with resistance to mefloquine is a significant problem in the malarious areas of Thailand and in areas of Myanmar and Cambodia that border on Thailand. It has also been reported on the borders between Myanmar and China, Laos and Myanmar, and in Southern Vietnam. In the United States, a 250 mg tablet of mefloquine contains 228 mg mefloquine base. Outside the United States, each 275 mg tablet contains 250 mg base.

Continued

Table 305.1	Drugs for Parasitic Infections—cont'd		
INFECTION	**DRUG**	**ADULT DOSAGE**	**PEDIATRIC DOSAGE**
Uncomplicated infection due to *P. falciparum* or species not identified acquired in areas of chloroquine sensitivity or uncomplicated *P. malariae* or *P. knowlesi*			
Drug of choice:	Chloroquine phosphate (Aralen)	600 mg base PO, then 300 mg base PO at 6, 24, and 48 hr	10 mg/kg base PO, then 5 mg/kg base PO at 6, 24, and 48 hr
or	Hydroxychloroquine (Plaquenil)[71]	620 mg base PO, then 310 mg base PO at 6, 24, and 48 hr	10 mg/kg base PO, then 5 mg/kg base PO at 6, 24, and 48 hr
Uncomplicated infection with *P. vivax* acquired in areas of chloroquine resistance[68]			
Drug of choice:	Atovaquone/proguanil (Malarone) Adult tablets: 50 mg atovaquone/100 mg proguanil Pediatric tablets: 62.5 mg atovaquone/ 25 mg proguanil[62]	4 adult tablets PO once daily × 3 days	<5 kg: not indicated 5-8 kg: 2 pediatric tablets PO daily × 3 days 9-10 kg: 3 pediatric tablets PO daily × 3 days 11-20 kg: 1 adult tablet PO daily × 3 days 21-30 kg: 2 adult tablets PO daily × 3 days 31-40 kg: 3 adult tablets PO daily × 3 days >40 kg: 4 adult tablets PO daily × 3 days
	plus Primaquine[70]	30 mg base PO daily × 14 days	0.5 mg/kg/day PO × 14 days
or	Quinine sulfate *plus* Doxycycline[7,16] *or plus* Tetracycline[7,16] *or plus* Clindamycin[7,65]	648 mg salt PO tid × 3-7 days[63] 100 mg PO bid × 7 days 250 mg PO qid × 7 days 20 mg/kg/day PO in 3 divided doses × 7 days[66]	10 mg salt/kg PO tid × 3-7 days[57] 4 mg/kg/day PO in 2 doses × 7 days 6.25 mg/kg PO qid × 7 days 20 mg/kg/day PO in 3 doses × 7 days
	plus Primaquine[69]	30 mg base PO daily × 14 days	0.5 mg/kg/day PO × 14 days
or	Mefloquine[67]	750 mg PO followed 12 hr later by 500 mg PO	15 mg/kg PO followed 12 hr later by 10 mg/kg PO
	plus Primaquine[70]	30 mg base PO daily × 14 days	0.5 mg/kg/day PO × 14 days
Uncomplicated infection with *P. ovale* and *P. vivax* acquired in areas without chloroquine resistance[68]			
Drug of choice:	Chloroquine phosphate (Aralen) *plus* Primaquine[70]	600 mg base PO, then 300 mg base PO at 6, 24, and 48 hr 30 mg base PO daily × 14 days	10 mg/kg base PO, then 5 mg/kg base PO at 6, 24, and 48 hr 0.5 mg/kg/day PO × 14 days
or	Hydroxychloroquine (Plaquenil)[71] *plus* Primaquine[70]	620 mg base PO, then 310 mg base PO at 6, 24, and 48 hr 30 mg base PO daily × 14 days	10 mg/kg base PO, then 5 mg/kg base PO at 6, 24, and 48 hr 0.5 mg/kg/day PO × 14 days
Severe malaria due to all *Plasmodium* spp.			
Drug of choice:[72]	Quinidine gluconate[73]	10 mg salt/kg IV in normal saline loading dose (max 600 mg) over 1-2 hr, followed by continuous infusion of 0.02 mg salt/kg/min until PO therapy can be started	10 mg salt/kg IV in normal saline loading dose (max 600 mg) over 1-2 hr, followed by continuous infusion of 0.02 mg salt/kg/min until PO therapy can be started
	plus Doxycycline[7,16] *or plus* Tetracycline[7,16] *or plus* Clindamycin[7,65]	100 mg PO or IV bid × 7 days 250 mg PO qid × 7 days 20 mg/kg/day PO in 3 divided doses × 7 days or 10 mg/kg IV loading dose, then 5 mg/kg tid until able to take PO[60]	4 mg/kg/day PO or IV in 2 doses × 7 days 6.25 mg/kg PO qid × 7 days 20 mg/kg/day PO in 3 divided doses × 7 days or 10 mg/kg IV loading dose, then 5 mg/kg tid until able to take PO[60]
Alternative: Followed by:	Artesunate[27,74] Atovaquone-proguanil, doxycycline, clindamycin, or mefloquine as above	2.4 mg/kg/dose IV × 3 days, at 0, 12, 24, 48, and 72 hr	2.4 mg/kg/dose IV × 3 days, at 0, 12, 24, 48, and 72 hr

[69]*P. vivax* with decreased susceptibility to chloroquine is a significant problem in Papua New Guinea and Indonesia. There are also a few reports of resistance from Myanmar, India, the Solomon Islands, Vanuatu, Guyana, Brazil, Colombia, and Peru.

[70]Primaquine phosphate can cause hemolytic anemia, especially in patients whose red cells are deficient in glucose-6-phosphate dehydrogenase (G6PD). This deficiency is most common in African, Asian, and Mediterranean peoples. Patients should be screened for G6PD deficiency before treatment. Primaquine should not be used during pregnancy.

[71]If chloroquine phosphate is not available, hydroxychloroquine sulfate is as effective; 400 mg of hydroxychloroquine sulfate is equivalent to 500 mg of chloroquine phosphate.

[72]Exchange transfusion has been helpful for some patients with high-density (>10%) parasitemia, altered mental status, pulmonary edema, or renal complications (Miller KD, et al: *N Engl J Med* 321:65, 1989).

[73]Continuous ECG, blood pressure, and glucose monitoring is recommended, especially in pregnant women and young children. For problems with quinidine availability, call the manufacturer (Eli Lilly, 1-800-545-5979) or the CDC Malaria Hotline (1-770-488-7788). Quinidine may have greater antimalarial activity than quinine. The loading dose should be decreased or omitted in those patients who have received quinine or mefloquine. If more than 48 hr of parenteral treatment is required, the quinine or quinidine dose should be reduced by 30–50%.

[74]Oral artesunate is not available in the United States; the IV formulation is available through the CDC Malaria Branch under an investigational new drug (IND) for patients with severe disease who do not have timely access or cannot tolerate, or fail to respond to, IV quinidine (*Med Lett Drugs Ther* 50:37, 2008). To avoid the development of resistance, adults treated with artesunate must also receive oral treatment doses of either atovaquone/proguanil, doxycycline, clindamycin, or mefloquine; children should take either atovaquone/proguanil, clindamycin, or mefloquine (Nosten F, et al: *Lancet* 356:297, 2000; van Vugt M: *Clin Infect Dis* 35:1498, 2002; Smithuis F, et al: *Trans R Soc Trop Med Hyg* 98:182, 2004). If artesunate is given IV, oral medication should be started when the patient is able to tolerate it (SEAQUAMAT group, *Lancet* 366:717, 2005; Duffy PE, Sibley CH: *Lancet* 366:1908, 2005). Reduced susceptibility to artesunate characterized by slow parasitic clearance has been reported in Cambodia (Rogers WO, et al: *Malar J* 8:10, 2009; Dundorp AM, et al: *N Engl J Med* 361:455, 2009).

Continued

Table 305.1 | Drugs for Parasitic Infections—cont'd

INFECTION	DRUG	ADULT DOSAGE	PEDIATRIC DOSAGE
Prevention of relapses: *P. vivax* and *P. ovale* only			
Drug of choice:	Primaquine phosphate[70]	30 mg base/day PO × 14 days	0.6 mg base/kg/day PO × 14 days
Malaria: Prevention[75]			
Chloroquine-sensitive areas[60]			
Drug of choice	Chloroquine phosphate[76,77,78]	500 mg salt (300 mg base), PO once/wk beginning 1-2 wk before travel to malarious area and 4 wk after leaving	5 mg/kg base once/wk, up to adult dose of 300 mg base beginning 1-2 wk before travel to malarious area and 4 wk after leaving
or	Hydroxychloroquine (Plaquenil)[71]	400 mg (310 mg base) PO once/wk beginning 1-2 wk before travel to malarious area and 4 wk after leaving	5 mg/kg base once/wk, up to adult dose of 310 mg base beginning 1-2 wk before travel to malarious area and 4 wk after leaving
Chloroquine-resistant areas[60]			
Drug of choice:	Atovaquone/proguanil[62,77,79,80]	1 adult tablet PO q day beginning 1-2 days before travel to malarious area and 7 days after leaving	11-20 kg: 1 pediatric tablet PO/day 21-30 kg: 2 pediatric tablets PO/day 31-40 kg: 3 pediatric tablets PO/day >40 kg: 1 adult tablet PO/day
or	Mefloquine[67,77,78,81]	1 adult tablet PO q day beginning 1-2 wk before travel to malarious area and 4 wk after leaving	<9 kg: 5 mg/kg salt once/wk 9-19 kg: ¼ tablet once/wk 19-30 kg: ½ tablet once/wk 31-45 kg: ¾ tablet once/wk >45 kg: 1 tablet once/wk
or	Doxycycline[7,82]	100 mg PO daily	≥8 yr: 2 mg/kg/day, up to 100 mg/day
Alternative for areas with primarily *P. vivax*:	Primaquine[7,83]	30 mg base PO daily beginning 1-2 days before travel to malarious area and 7-14 days after leaving	0.5 mg/kg base (max 30 mg) daily beginning 1-2 days before travel to malarious area and 7-14 days after leaving
Malaria: Presumptive self-treatment[84]			
Drug of choice:	Atovaquone/proguanil (Malarone) Adult tablets: 50 mg atovaquone/100 mg proguanil Pediatric tablets 62.5 mg atovaquone/25 mg proguanil[62]	4 adult tablets PO once daily × 3 days	<5 kg: not indicated 5-8 kg: 2 pediatric tablets PO daily × 3 days 9-10 kg: 3 pediatric tablets PO daily × 3 days 11-20 kg: 1 adult tablet PO daily × 3 days 21-30 kg: 2 adult tablets PO daily × 3 days 31-40 kg: 3 adult tablets PO daily × 3 days >40 kg: 4 adult tablets PO daily × 3 days
or	Quinine sulfate[63] *plus* Doxycycline[7,16]	648 mg salt PO tid × 3-7 days 100 mg PO bid × 7 days	10 mg salt/kg PO tid × 3-7 days 4 mg/kg/day PO in 2 divided doses × 7 days
or	Mefloquine[67,68]	750 mg PO followed 12 hr later by 500 mg	15 mg/kg PO followed 12 hr later by 10 mg/kg

[75]No drug regimen guarantees protection against malaria. If fever develops within a year (particularly within the first 2 mo) after travel to malarious areas, travelers should be advised to seek medical attention. Insect repellents, insecticide-impregnated bed nets, and proper clothing are important adjuncts for malaria prophylaxis (*Med Lett* 45:41, 2003). Malaria in pregnancy is particularly serious for both mother and fetus; therefore, prophylaxis is indicated if exposure cannot be avoided.

[76]In pregnancy, chloroquine prophylaxis has been used extensively and safely.

[77]For prevention of attack after departure from areas where *P. vivax* and *P. ovale* are endemic, which includes almost all areas where malaria is found (except Haiti), some experts prescribe in addition primaquine phosphate 30 mg base/day or, for children, 0.6 mg base/kg/day during the last 2 wk of prophylaxis. Others prefer to avoid the toxicity of primaquine and rely on surveillance to detect cases when they occur, particularly when exposure was limited or doubtful. See also footnote 69.

[78]Beginning 1-2 wk before travel and continuing weekly for the duration of stay and for 4 wk after leaving malarious zone. Most adverse events occur within 3 doses. Some *Medical Letter* consultants favor starting mefloquine 3 wk prior to travel and monitoring the patient for adverse events; this allows time to change to an alternative regimen if mefloquine is not tolerated. Mefloquine should not be taken on an empty stomach; it should be taken with at least 8 oz of water. For pediatric doses less than 1/2 tablet, it is advisable to have a pharmacist crush the tablet, estimate doses by weighing, and package them in gelatin capsules. There are no data for use in children weighing < 5 kg, but based on dosages in other weight groups, a dose of 5 mg/kg can be used.

[79]Beginning 1-2 days before travel and continuing for the duration of stay and for 1 wk after leaving. In one study of malaria prophylaxis, atovaquone/proguanil was better tolerated than mefloquine in nonimmune travelers (Overbosch D, et al: *Clin Infect Dis* 33:1015, 2001).

[80]Beginning 1-2 days before travel and continuing for the duration of stay and for 1 wk after leaving malarious zone. In one study of malaria prophylaxis, atovaquone/proguanil was better tolerated than mefloquine in nonimmune travelers (Overbosch D, et al: *Clin Infect Dis* 33:1015, 2001). The protective efficacy of Malarone against *P. vivax* is variable, ranging from 84% in Indonesian New Guinea (Ling J, et al: *Clin Infect Dis* 35:825, 2002) to 100% in Colombia (Soto J, et al: *Am J Trop Med Hyg* 75:430, 2006). Some *Medical Letter* consultants prefer alternate drugs if traveling to areas where *P. vivax* predominates.

[81]Mefloquine has not been approved for use during pregnancy. However, it has been reported to be safe for prophylactic use during the second or third trimester of pregnancy and possibly during early pregnancy, as well. Mefloquine is not recommended for patients with cardiac conduction abnormalities, and patients with a history of depression, seizures, psychosis, or psychiatric disorders should avoid mefloquine prophylaxis. Resistance to mefloquine has been reported in some areas, such as the Thailand-Myanmar and Thailand-Cambodia borders; in these areas, atovaquone/proguanil or doxycycline should be used for prophylaxis.

[82]Beginning 1-2 days before travel and continuing for the duration of stay and for 4 wk after leaving. Use of tetracyclines is contraindicated in pregnancy and in children younger than 8 yr old. Doxycycline can cause GI disturbances, vaginal moniliasis, and photosensitivity reactions.

[83]Studies have shown that daily primaquine beginning 1 day before departure and continued until 3-7 days after leaving the malaria area provides effective prophylaxis against chloroquine-resistant *P. falciparum* (Baird JK, et al: *Clin Infect Dis* 37:1659, 2003). Some studies have shown less efficacy against *P. vivax*. Nausea and abdominal pain can be diminished by taking with food.

[84]A traveler can be given a course of atovaquone/proguanil, mefloquine, or quinine plus doxycycline for presumptive self-treatment of febrile illness. The drug given for self-treatment should be different from that used for prophylaxis. This approach should be used only in very rare circumstances when a traveler cannot promptly get to medical care.

Continued

Table 305.1	Drugs for Parasitic Infections—cont'd		
INFECTION	**DRUG**	**ADULT DOSAGE**	**PEDIATRIC DOSAGE**
Microsporidiosis			
Ocular (*Encephalitozoon hellem, Encephalitozoon cuniculi, Vittaforma corneae [Nosema corneum]*)			
Drug of choice:	Albendazole[7,85]	400 mg PO bid	<10 kg/2 yr:[11] ≥2 yr: see adult dosing
	plus Fumagillin[86]		
Intestinal (*Enterocytozoon bieneusi, Encephalitozoon [Septata] intestinalis*)			
E. bieneusi[87]			
Drug of choice:	Fumagillin	60 mg/day PO × 14 days in 3 divided doses	
E. intestinalis			
Drug of choice:	Albendazole[7,85]	400 mg PO bid × 21 days	<10 kg/2 yr:[11] ≥2 yr: see adult dosing
Disseminated (*E. hellem, E. cuniculi, E. intestinalis, Pleistophora* sp., *Trachipleistophora* sp., and *Brachiola vesicularum*)			
Drug of choice:[88]	Albendazole[7,85]	400 mg PO bid	<10 kg/2 yr:[11] ≥2 yr: see adult dosing
Mites, see Scabies			
Moniliformis moniliformis infection			
Drug of choice:	Pyrantel pamoate (OTC)[7]	11 mg/kg PO once, repeat twice, 2 wk apart	11 mg/kg PO once, repeat twice, 2 wk apart
Naegleria species, see Amebic meningoencephalitis, primary			
Necator americanus, see Hookworm infection			
Oesophagostomum bifurcum			
Drug of choice:	See footnote 89		
Onchocerca volvulus, see Filariasis			
Opisthorchis viverrini, see Fluke infection			
Paragonimus westermani, see Fluke infection			
Pediculus capitis, Pediculus humanus, Phthirus pubis, see Lice			
Pinworm, see *Enterobius*			
Pneumocystis jiroveci (formerly *Pneumocystis carinii*) pneumonia (PCP)[90]			
Moderate to severe disease			
Drug of choice:	Trimethoprim-sulfamethoxazole (TMP-SMX)	15-20 mg/kg/day TMP component IV in 3-4 divided doses × 21 days (change to PO after clinical improvement)	15-20 mg/kg/day TMP component IV in 3-4 divided doses × 21 days (change to PO after clinical improvement)
Alternative:	Pentamidine	3-4 mg IV daily × 21 days	3-4 mg IV daily × 21 days
or	Primaquine *plus* Clindamycin[7]	30 mg base PO daily × 21 days 600-900 mg IV tid or qid × 21 days, or 300-450 mg PO tid or qid × 21 days (change to PO after clinical improvement)	0.3 mg/kg base PO (max 30 mg) daily × 21 days 15-25 mg/kg IV tid or qid × 21 days, or 10 mg/kg PO tid or qid (max 300-450 mg/dose) × 21 days (change to PO after clinical improvement)

[85]For HIV-infected patients, continue until resolution of ocular symptoms and until CD4 count > 200 cells/μL for > 6 mo after initiation of antiretroviral therapy.

[86]Ocular lesions caused by *E. hellem* in HIV-infected patients have responded to fumagillin eyedrops prepared from Fumidil-B (bicyclohexyl ammonium fumagillin) used to control a microsporidial disease of honey bees (Diesenhouse MC: *Am J Ophthalmol* 115:293, 1993), available from Leiter's Park Avenue Pharmacy (San Jose, CA; 1-800-292-6773; www.leiterrx.com). For lesions caused by *V. corneae*, topical therapy is generally not effective and keratoplasty may be required (Davis RM, et al: *Ophthalmology* 97:953, 1990).

[87]Oral fumagillin (Sanofi Recherche, Gentilly, France) has been effective in treating *E. bieneusi* (Molina J-M, et al: *N Engl J Med* 346:1963, 2002), but it has been associated with thrombocytopenia. HAART may lead to microbiologic and clinical response in HIV-infected patients with microsporidial diarrhea (Benson CA, Kaplan JE, Masur H, et al: Treating opportunistic infections among HIV-infected adults and adolescents: recommendations from CDC, the National Institutes of Health, and the HIV Medicine Association/Infectious Diseases Society of America, *MMWR Recomm Rep* 53([RR-15]:1-112, 2004). Octreotide (Sandostatin) has provided symptomatic relief in some patients with large-volume diarrhea.

[88]Molina J-M, et al: *J Infect Dis* 171:245, 1995. There is no established treatment for *Pleistophora*. For disseminated disease caused by *Trachipleistophora* or *Brachiola*, itraconazole 400 mg PO once/day plus albendazole may also be tried (Coyle CM, et al: *N Engl J Med* 351:42, 2004).

[89]Albendazole or pyrantel pamoate may be effective (Ziem JB, et al: *Ann Trop Med Parasitol* 98:385, 2004).

[90]*Pneumocystis* has been reclassified as a fungus. In severe disease with room air $PO_2 ≤ 70$ mm Hg or $A-aO_2$ gradient ≥ 35 mm Hg, prednisone should also be used (Gagnon S, et al: *N Engl J Med* 323:1444, 1990; Caumes E, et al: *Clin Infect Dis* 18:319, 1994).

Continued

Table 305.1	Drugs for Parasitic Infections—cont'd		
INFECTION	**DRUG**	**ADULT DOSAGE**	**PEDIATRIC DOSAGE**
Mild to moderate disease			
Drug of choice:	Trimethoprim-sulfamethoxazole (TMP-SMX)	320 mg/1600 mg (2 DS tablets) PO tid × 21 days	TMP 15-20 mg/kg/day PO in 3 or 4 doses × 21 days
Alternatives:	Dapsone *plus* Trimethoprim	100 mg PO daily × 21 days 15 mg/kg/day PO in 3 doses	2 mg/kg/day (max 100 mg) PO × 21 days 15 mg/kg/day PO in 3 doses
or	Primaquine *plus* Clindamycin	30 mg base PO daily × 21 days 300-450 mg PO tid or qid × 21 days	0.3 mg/kg base PO daily (max 30 mg) × 21 days 10 mg/kg PO tid or qid (max 300-450 mg/dose) × 21 days
or	Atovaquone	750 mg PO bid × 21 days	1-3 mo: 30 mg/kg/day PO in 2 doses × 21 days
Primary and secondary prophylaxis[91]			
Drug of choice:	Trimethoprim-sulfamethoxazole (TMP-SMX)	1 tablet (single strength or greater) PO daily or 1 DS tablet PO 3 days/wk	TMP 150 mg/m^2 in 1-2 doses daily or on 3 consecutive days per wk[92]
Alternatives:[91]	Dapsone[7]	50 mg PO bid, or 100 mg PO daily	2 mg/kg/day (max 100 mg) PO or 4 mg/kg (max 200 mg) PO each wk
or	Dapsone[7] *plus* Pyrimethamine[93]	50 mg PO daily or 200 mg PO each wk 50 mg PO or 75 mg PO each wk	
or	Pentamidine aerosol	300 mg inhaled monthly via Respirgard II nebulizer	≥5 yr: 300 mg inhaled monthly via Respirgard II nebulizer
or	Atovaquone[7]	1,500 mg/day PO in 1 or 2 doses	1-3 mo: 30 mg/kg/day PO 4-24 mo: 45 mg/kg/day PO in 2 doses × 21 days >24 mo: 30 mg/kg/day PO in 2 doses × 21 days
Roundworm, see Ascariasis			
Sappinia diploidea, see Amebic meningoencephalitis, primary			
Scabies (*Sarcoptes scabiei*)			
Drug of choice:	5% Permethrin[94]	Topically, 2× at least 1 wk apart	Topically 2x, 1 wk apart, approved for ≥ 2 mo
Alternative:[94,95]	Ivermectin[7,94,96]	200 µg/kg PO x2 at least 1 wk apart	<15 kg: not indicated ≥15 kg: see adult dosing
	10% Crotamiton	Topically overnight on days 1, 2, 3, 8	Topically overnight on days 1, 2, 3, 8
Schistosomiasis (*Bilharziasis*)			
Schistosoma haematobium or *S. intercalatum*			
Drug of choice:	Praziquantel	40 mg/kg/day PO in 1 or 2 doses × 1 day	40 mg/kg/day PO in 1 or 2 doses × 1 day[36]
Schistosoma japonicum or *S. mekongi*			
Drug of choice:	Praziquantel	60 mg/kg/day PO in 2 or 3 doses × 1 day	60 mg/kg/day PO in 3 doses × 1 day[36]
Schistosoma mansoni			
Drug of choice:	Praziquantel	40 mg/kg/day PO in 1 or 2 doses × 1 day	40 mg/kg/day PO in 1 or 2 doses × 1 day[36]
Alternative:	Oxamniquine[97,98]	15 mg/kg PO once	20 mg/kg/day PO in 2 doses × 1 day

[91]Primary/secondary prophylaxis in patients with HIV can be discontinued after the CD4 count increases to > 200 × 10^6/L for longer than 3 mo.

[92]An alternative trimethoprim-sulfamethoxazole regimen is 1 DS tablet 3x/wk. Weekly therapy with sulfadoxine 500 mg/pyrimethamine 25 mg/leucovorin 25 mg was effective for *Pneumocystis carinii* pneumonia (PCP) prophylaxis in liver transplant patients (Torre-Cisneros J, et al: *Clin Infect Dis* 29:771, 1999).

[93]Plus leucovorin 25 mg with each dose of pyrimethamine.

[94]In some cases, treatment may need to be repeated in 10-14 days (Currie BJ, McCarthy JS: *N Engl J Med* 362:717, 2010). A second ivermectin dose taken 2 wk later increased the cure rate to 95%, which is equivalent to that of 5% permethrin (Usha V, et al: *J Am Acad Dermatol* 42:236, 2000). Ivermectin, either alone or in combination with a topical scabicide, is the drug of choice for crusted scabies in immunocompromised patients (del Giudice P: *Curr Opin Infect Dis* 15:123, 2004).

[95]Lindane (γ-benzene hexachloride; Kwell) should be reserved as a second-line agent. The FDA has recommended it should not be used for immunocompromised patients, young children, the elderly, and patients who weigh < 50 kg.

[96]Ivermectin, either alone or in combination with a topical scabicide, is the drug of choice for crusted scabies in immunocompromised patients (del Giudice P: *Curr Opin Infect Dis* 15:123, 2004). The safety of oral ivermectin in pregnancy and young children has not been established.

[97]Oxamniquine has been effective in some areas in which praziquantel is less effective (Stelma FF, et al: *J Infect Dis* 176:304, 1997). Oxamniquine is contraindicated in pregnancy.

[98]In East Africa, the dose should be increased to 30 mg/kg, and in Egypt and South Africa to 30 mg/kg/day × 2 days. Some experts recommend 40-60 mg/kg over 2-3 days in all of Africa (Shekhar KC: *Drugs* 42:379, 1991).

Continued

Table 305.1	Drugs for Parasitic Infections—cont'd		
INFECTION	**DRUG**	**ADULT DOSAGE**	**PEDIATRIC DOSAGE**
Sleeping sickness, see Trypanosomiasis			
Strongyloidiasis (*Strongyloides stercoralis*)			
Drug of choice:[99]	Ivermectin	200 µg/kg/day PO × 2 days	<15 kg: not indicated ≥15 kg: see adult dosing
Alternative:	Albendazole[7,100]	400 mg PO bid × 7 days	<10 kg/2 yr:[11] ≥2 yr: see adult dosing
Tapeworm infection			
Adult (intestinal stage)			
Diphyllobothrium latum (fish), ***Taenia saginata*** (beef), ***Taenia solium*** (pork), ***Dipylidium caninum*** (dog)			
Drug of choice:	Praziquantel[7]	5-10 mg/kg PO once	5-10 mg/kg PO once[36]
Alternative:	Niclosamide	2 g PO once	50 mg/kg PO once
Hymenolepis nana (dwarf tapeworm)			
Drug of choice:	Praziquantel[7]	25 mg/kg PO once	25 mg/kg PO once[36]
Alternative:	Niclosamide[101]	2 g PO daily × 7 days	11-34 kg: 1 g PO on day 1, then 500 mg/day PO × 6 days >34 kg: 1.5 g PO on day 1, then 1 g/day PO × 6 days
Larval (tissue stage)			
Echinococcus granulosus (hydatid disease cystic echinococcosis)			
Drug of choice:[102]	Albendazole[7]	400 mg PO bid × 1-6 mo	<10 kg/2 yr: 5-7.5 mg/kg PO bid (max 400 mg)[11] ≥2 yr: 5-7.5 mg/kg PO bid (max 400 mg) × 1-6 mo
Echinococcus multilocularis (alveolar echinococcosis)			
Treatment of choice:	See footnote 103		
Taenia solium (cysticercosis)			
Treatment of choice:[104]	Albendazole	400 mg bid PO × 8-30 days; can be repeated as necessary	<10 kg/2 yr: 7.5 mg/kg PO bid × 8-30 days; can be repeated as necessary[11] ≥2 yr: 7.5 mg/kg PO (max 400 mg) bid × 8-30 days; can be repeated as necessary
	plus Steroids		
Alternative:	Praziquantel[7]	50 mg/kg/day PO in 3 divided doses × 15 days	50 mg/kg/day PO in 3 divided doses × 15 days[36]
or	Surgical removal		

[99]In immunocompromised patients or disseminated disease, it may be necessary to prolong or repeat therapy or to use other agents. Veterinary parenteral and enema formulations of ivermectin have been used in severely ill patients unable to take oral medications (Chiodini PL, et al: *Lancet* 355:43, 2000; Orem J, et al: *Clin Infect Dis* 37:152, 2003; Tarr PE: *Am J Trop Med Hyg* 68:453, 2003).

[100]Albendazole must be taken with food; a fatty meal increases oral bioavailability.

[101]Niclosamide must be thoroughly chewed or crushed and swallowed with a small amount of water. Nitazoxanide may be an alternative (Ortiz JJ, et al: *Trans R Soc Trop Med Hyg* 96:193, 2002; Chero JC, et al: *Trans R Soc Trop Med Hyg* 101:203, 2007; Diaz E, et al: *Am J Trop Med Hyg* 68:384, 2003).

[102]Optimal treatment depends on multiple factors, including size, location, and number of cysts and presence of complications. In some patients, medical therapy alone is preferred, but some patients may benefit from surgical resection or percutaneous drainage of cysts. Praziquantel is useful preoperatively or in case of spillage of cyst contents during surgery. Percutaneous aspiration-injection-reaspiration (PAIR) with ultrasound guidance plus albendazole therapy has been effective for management of hepatic hydatid cyst disease (Smego RA Jr, et al: *Clin Infect Dis* 37:1073, 2003).

[103]Surgical excision is the only reliable means of cure. Reports have suggested that in nonresectable cases, the use of albendazole or mebendazole can stabilize and sometimes cure infection (Craig P: *Curr Opin Infect Dis* 16:437, 2003). Medical treatment is prolonged up to 2 yr or more.

[104]Initial therapy for patients with inflamed parenchymal cysticercosis should focus on symptomatic treatment with antiseizure medication. Treatment of parenchymal cysticerci with albendazole or praziquantel is controversial (Maguire JM: *N Engl J Med* 350:215, 2004). Patients with live parenchymal cysts who have seizures should be treated with albendazole together with steroids (6 mg dexamethasone or 40-60 mg prednisone daily) and an antiseizure medication (Garcia HH, et al: *N Engl J Med* 350:249, 2004). Some recent studies have shown improved outcomes with combination albendazole and praziquantel (Garcia HH, et al: *Lancet Infect Dis* 14:687, 2014). Patients with subarachnoid cysts or giant cysts in the fissures should be treated for at least 30 days (Proaño JV, et al: *N Engl J Med* 345:879, 2001). Surgical intervention or CSF diversion is indicated for obstructive hydrocephalus; prednisone 40 mg/day may be given with surgery. Arachnoiditis, vasculitis, or cerebral edema is treated with prednisone 60 mg/day or dexamethasone 4-6 mg/day together with albendazole or praziquantel (White Jr AC: *Annu Rev Med* 51:187, 2000). Any cysticercocidal drug may cause irreparable damage when used to treat ocular or spinal cysts, even when corticosteroids are used. An ophthalmic exam should always precede treatment to rule out intraocular cysts.

Continued

Table 305.1 | Drugs for Parasitic Infections—cont'd

INFECTION	DRUG	ADULT DOSAGE	PEDIATRIC DOSAGE
Toxocariasis, see Visceral larva migrans			
Toxoplasmosis (Toxoplasma gondii)[105]			
Drug of choice:[106,107]	Pyrimethamine[108]	200 mg PO × 1, then 50-75 mg/day × 3-6 wk	2 mg/kg/day × 3 days, then 1 mg/kg/day (max 25 mg/day) × 3-6 wk[109]
	plus Sulfadiazine	1.5 g PO qid × 3-6 wk	100-200 mg/kg/day in 4 divided doses × 3-6 wk
	or plus Clindamycin	1.8-2.4 g/day IV or PO in 3-4 doses × 3-6 wk	5-7.5 mg/kg IV or PO tid or qid (max 600 mg/dose) × 3-6 wk
	or plus Atovaquone	1,500 mg PO bid	1,500 mg PO bid
Alternative:	Trimethoprim-sulfamethoxazole (TMP-SMX)[7]	15-20 mg/kg/day TMP component PO or IV in 3-4 divided doses × 3-6 wk	15-20 mg/kg TMP component PO or IV in 3 or 4 doses × 3-6 wk
Trichinellosis (Trichinella spiralis)			
Drug of choice:	Steroids for severe symptoms	Prednisone 30-60 mg PO daily × 10-15 days	
	plus Albendazole[7]	400 mg PO bid × 8-14 days	<10 kg/2 yr:[11] ≥2 yr: see adult dosing
Alternative:	Mebendazole[7]	200-400 mg PO tid × 3 days, then 400-500 mg PO tid × 10 days	200-400 mg PO tid × 3 days, then 400-500 mg PO tid × 10 days[12]
Trichomoniasis (Trichomonas vaginalis)			
Drug of choice:[110]	Metronidazole	2 g PO once or 500 mg PO bid × 7 days	15 mg/kg/day PO in 3 doses × 7 days
or	Tinidazole[4]	2 g PO once	50 mg/kg PO once (max 2 g)
Trichostrongylus infection			
Drug of choice:	Pyrantel pamoate[7]	11 mg/kg base PO once (max 1 g)	11 mg/kg PO once (max 1 g)
Alternative:	Mebendazole[7]	100 mg PO bid × 3 days	100 mg PO bid × 3 days[12]
or	Albendazole[7]	400 mg PO once	<10 kg/2 yr:[11] ≥2 yr: 15 mg/kg/day PO (max 800 mg) × 1-6 mo
Trichuriasis (Trichuris trichiura, whipworm)			
Drug of choice:	Mebendazole	100 mg PO bid × 3 days	100 mg PO bid × 3 days[12]
Alternative:	Albendazole[7]	400 mg PO × 3 days	<10 kg/2 yr:[11] ≥2 yr: see adult dosing
or	Ivermectin[7]	200 µg/kg PO daily × 3 days	<15 kg: not indicated ≥15 kg: see adult dosing
Trypanosomiasis[111]			
Trypanosoma cruzi (American trypanosomiasis, Chagas disease)			
Drug of choice:	Benznidazole[27]	5-7 mg/kg/day PO in 2 divided doses × 60 days	≤12 yr: 5-7.5 mg/kg/day PO in 2 divided doses × 60 days >12 yr: see adult dosing
Alternative:	Nifurtimox[27,112]	8-10 mg/kg/day PO in 3-4 doses × 90 days	≤10 yr: 15-20 mg/kg/day PO in 3-4 doses × 90 days 11-16 yr: 12.5-15 mg/kg/day in 3-4 doses × 90 days >16 yr: see adult dosing

[105]In ocular toxoplasmosis with macular involvement, corticosteroids are recommended in addition to antiparasitic therapy for an antiinflammatory effect.

[106]To treat CNS toxoplasmosis in HIV-infected patients, some clinicians have used pyrimethamine 50-100 mg/day (after a loading dose of 200 mg) with sulfadiazine and, when sulfonamide sensitivity developed, have given clindamycin 1.8-2.4 g/day in divided doses instead of the sulfonamide. Atovaquone plus pyrimethamine appears to be an effective alternative in sulfa-intolerant patients (Chirgwin K, et al: Clin Infect Dis 34:1243, 2002). Treatment is followed by chronic suppression with lower-dosage regimens of the same drugs. For primary prophylaxis in HIV patients with < 100 × 10⁶/L CD4 cells, either trimethoprim-sulfamethoxazole, pyrimethamine with dapsone, or atovaquone with or without pyrimethamine can be used. Primary or secondary prophylaxis may be discontinued when the CD4 count increases to > 200 × 10⁶/L for more than 3 mo (Benson CA, Kaplan JE, Masur H, et al: Treating opportunistic infections among HIV-infected adults and adolescents: recommendations from CDC, the National Institutes of Health, and the HIV Medicine Association/Infectious Diseases Society of America, MMWR Recomm Rep 53([RR-15]:1-112, 2004).

[107]Women who develop toxoplasmosis during the first trimester of pregnancy can be treated with spiramycin (3-4 g/day). After the first trimester, if there is no documented transmission to the fetus, spiramycin can be continued until term. If transmission has occurred in utero, therapy with pyrimethamine and sulfadiazine should be started (Montoya JG, Liesenfeld O: Lancet 363:1965, 2004). Pyrimethamine is a potential teratogen and should be used only after the first trimester.

[108]Plus leucovorin 10-25 mg with each dose of pyrimethamine.

[109]Congenitally infected newborns should be treated with pyrimethamine every 2 or 3 days and a sulfonamide daily for about 1 yr (Remington JS, Klein JO, editors: Infectious Disease of the Fetus and Newborn Infant, ed 5, Philadelphia, 2001, WB Saunders, p. 290).

[110]Sexual partners should be treated simultaneously. Metronidazole-resistant strains have been reported and can be treated with higher doses of metronidazole (2-4 g/day × 7-14 days) or with tinidazole (Hager WD: Sex Transm Dis 31:343, 2004).

[111]Barrett MP, et al: Lancet 362:1469, 2003.

[112]The addition of γ-interferon to nifurtimox for 20 days in experimental animals and in a limited number of patients appears to shorten the acute phase of Chagas disease (McCabe RE, et al: J Infect Dis 163:912, 1991).

Continued

Table 305.1	Drugs for Parasitic Infections—cont'd		
INFECTION	**DRUG**	**ADULT DOSAGE**	**PEDIATRIC DOSAGE**
Trypanosoma brucei gambiense (West African trypanosomiasis, sleeping sickness)			
Hemolymphatic stage			
Drug of choice:[113]	Pentamidine isethionate[7]	4 mg/kg/day IM × 7-10 days	4 mg/kg/day IM or IV × 7-10 days
Alternative:	Suramin[27]	100 mg (test dose) IV, then 1 g IV on days 1, 3, 7, 14, and 21	2 mg/kg (test dose) IV, then 20 mg/kg IV on days 1, 3, 7, 14, and 21
Late disease with CNS involvement			
Drug of choice:	Eflornithine[27,114]	100 mg/kg IV qid × 14 days	100 mg/kg IV qid × 14 days
Alternative:	Melarsoprol[27,115]	2-3.6 mg/kg (max 200 mg) daily IV (progressively increased during series) × 3 days. After 7 days, 3.6 mg/kg daily × 3 days. After 7 days, give a 3rd series of 3.6 mg/kg daily × 3 days.	2-3.6 mg/kg (max 200 mg) daily IV (progressively increased during series) × 3 days. After 7 days, 3.6 mg/kg daily × 3 days. After 7 days, give a 3rd series of 3.6 mg/kg daily × 3 days.
Trypanosoma brucei rhodesiense (East African trypanosomiasis, sleeping sickness)			
Hemolymphatic stage			
Drug of choice:	Suramin[27]	100 mg (test dose) IV, then 1 g IV on days 1, 3, 7, 14, and 21	2 mg/kg (test dose), then 20 mg/kg IV on days 1, 3, 7, 14, and 21
Late disease with CNS involvement			
Drug of choice:	Melarsoprol[27,114]	2-3.6 mg/kg (max 200 mg) daily IV (progressively increased during series) × 3 days. After 7 days, 3.6 mg/kg daily × 3 days. After 7 days, give a 3rd series of 3.6 mg/kg daily × 3 days.	2-3.6 mg/kg (max 200 mg) daily IV (progressively increased during series) × 3 days. After 7 days, 3.6 mg/kg daily × 3 days. After 7 days, give a 3rd series of 3.6 mg/kg daily × 3 days.
Visceral larva migrans (Toxocariasis)[116]			
Drugs of choice:	Albendazole[7]	400 mg PO bid × 5 days	<10 kg/2 yr: [11] ≥2 yr: see adult dosing
or	Mebendazole[7]	100-200 mg PO bid × 5 days	100-200 mg PO bid × 5 days[12]
Whipworm, see Trichuriasis			
Wuchereria bancrofti, see Filariasis			

[113]For treatment of *T. b. gambiense,* pentamidine and suramin have equal efficacy but pentamidine is better tolerated.

[114]Eflornithine is highly effective in *T. b. gambiense* but not against *T. b. rhodesiense* infections. It is available in limited supply only from the WHO and the CDC. Eflornithine dose may be reduced to 400 mg/kg IV in 2 doses for 7 days when used in conjunction with nifurtimox at a dose of 5 mg/kg PO tid × 10 days (Priotto G, et al: *Lancet* 374:56, 2009).

[115]In frail patients, begin with as little as 18 mg and increase the dose progressively. Pretreatment with suramin has been advocated for debilitated patients. Corticosteroids have been used to prevent arsenical encephalopathy (Pepin J, et al: *Trans R Soc Trop Med Hyg* 89:92, 1995). Up to 20% of patients with *T. b. gambiense* fail to respond to melarsoprol (Barrett MP: *Lancet* 353:1113, 1999). Consultation with experts at the CDC is recommended.

[116]Optimum duration of therapy is not known; some consultants would treat for 20 days. For severe symptoms or eye involvement, corticosteroids can be used in addition.

CDC, Centers for Disease Control and Prevention; CNS, central nervous system; CSF, cerebrospinal fluid; DS, double strength; ECG, electrocardiography; FDA, U.S. Food and Drug Administration; GI, gastrointestinal; HAART, highly active antiretroviral therapy; SMX, sulfamethoxazole; TMP, trimethoprim; WHO, World Health Organization.

From Drugs for parasitic infection, Med Lett 11(Suppl):e1-e23, 2013. Available at http://www.medicalletter.org.

renal or hepatic function. In addition, no studies have been performed in pregnant or lactating women. Common adverse effects include abdominal pain, diarrhea, nausea, and urine discoloration. Rare side effects include anorexia, flatulence, increased appetite, fever, pruritus, and dizziness. Intriguingly, nitazoxanide has in vitro activity against multiple other pathogens, including influenza virus, rotavirus, and hepatitis C virus, although the clinical use of the agent against these viruses remains investigational.

Tinidazole (Tindamax)

Tinidazole is a synthetic nitroimidazole with a chemical structure similar to metronidazole. It is approved by the Food and Drug Administration (FDA) for patients 3 yr of age and older and for treatment of trichomoniasis, giardiasis, and amebiasis. In the treatment of giardiasis, it has the advantages of very few side effects and only requiring a single dose. It is available as a tablet, which can be crushed and administered with food. Its mechanism of action against *Trichomonas* may be secondary to the generation of free nitro radicals by the **protozoan.** The mechanism

of action against *Giardia lamblia* and *Entamoeba histolytica* is unknown. Like metronidazole, it can cause a disulfiram-like reaction if combined with alcohol. After oral administration, tinidazole is rapidly and completely absorbed and is distributed into almost all tissues and body fluids; it can cross the blood–brain barrier and placental barrier. It is excreted via urine and feces. Hemodialysis increases clearance of the drug. No studies have been performed for patients undergoing peritoneal dialysis or for patients with compromised hepatic function. Tinidazole carries a pregnancy category C classification and can be detected in breast milk. Breastfeeding should be interrupted during treatment and for 3 days after treatment.

Atovaquone/Proguanil (Malarone)

Atovaquone is a hydroxynaphthoquinone and has been used in the past predominantly against *Pneumocystis* pneumonia in AIDS patients. Its mechanism of action is via disruption of the mitochondria membrane potential through interaction with cytochrome B. However, atovaquone can also effectively inhibit liver stages of all *Plasmodium* species, and in

2000 the FDA approved atovaquone/proguanil for the prevention and treatment of acute, uncomplicated *Plasmodium falciparum* malaria in adults and children ≥ 11 kg. Atovaquone alone and in combination with proguanil is the only drug to completely inhibit the liver stage, which provides the advantage of only needing to use the drug for 7 days after departing a malaria-endemic area (compared with several weeks).

Proguanil inhibits the parasite dihydrofolate reductase enzyme by the active form, cycloguanil. When used alone, it has poor efficacy for prophylaxis, but when administered with atovaquone, it acts in synergy on the cytochrome B enzyme in *Plasmodia* mitochondria, though the exact mechanism of synergy is unknown.

Two double-blind, randomized clinical trials assessing malaria prophylaxis demonstrated that atovaquone/proguanil was at least comparable to (and perhaps better than) chloroquine plus proguanil, and that atovaquone/proguanil was comparable to mefloquine. Atovaquone/proguanil was better tolerated than chloroquine plus proguanil and mefloquine. Atovaquone/proguanil treatment of acute uncomplicated *P. falciparum* infection has demonstrated higher or comparable cure rates when compared with other *P. falciparum* treatment drugs. Compared with other antimalarial therapies, atovaquone/proguanil has the highest cost.

Artemisinin Derivatives (Artemether, Artesunate) and Combination Therapies (Artemether/Lumefantrine or Coartem)

Artemisinin is a sesquiterpene lactone isolated from the weed *Artemisia annua*. It was developed in China, where it is known as qinghaosu. Artemisinin and its derivatives act very rapidly against *Plasmodium vivax* as well as chloroquine-sensitive and chloroquine-resistant *P. falciparum*. Artemisinins are also rapidly eliminated. Resistance to artemisinins has been documented in Cambodia, Laos, Myanmar, Thailand, and Vietnam. Coartem is the first artemisinin-containing drug approved for use by the FDA for patients ≥ 5 kg. It is a fixed-dose combination of two novel antimalarials, artemether (20 mg) and lumefantrine (120 mg). It is a highly effective 3-day malaria treatment, with cure rates of > 96%, even in areas of multidrug resistance. Artesunate is available from the CDC through an IND protocol as an intravenous (IV) treatment for severe malaria.

SELECTED ANTIPARASITIC DRUGS FOR HELMINTHS AND ECTOPARASITES
Albendazole (Albenza)
Albendazole is a benzimidazole carbamate structurally related to mebendazole and has similar anthelmintic activity. Its absorption from the gastrointestinal tract is poor but improved with a concomitant high-fat meal. Albendazole sulfoxide, the principal metabolite with anthelmintic activity, has a plasma half-life of 8.5 hr. It is widely distributed in the body, including the bile and cerebrospinal fluid. It is eliminated in bile. Albendazole is FDA approved for treatment of two cestode (tapeworm) infections: neurocysticercosis and hydatid diseases (*Echinococcus granulosus*). It is used off-label for numerous other **helminth** infections, including cutaneous larva migrans (*Ancylostoma caninum* and *Ancylostoma braziliense*), ascariasis (*Ascaris lumbricoides*), Chinese liver fluke (*Clonorchis sinensis*), pinworm (*Enterobius vermicularis*), lymphatic filariasis (*Wuchereria bancrofti, Brugia malayi, Brugia timori*), gnathostomiasis (*Gnathostoma* spp.), hookworms (*Ancylostoma duodenale* and *Necator americanus*), microsporidiosis, and visceral larva migrans (*Toxocara canis* and *Toxocara cati*). Albendazole is generally

well tolerated. Common adverse effects include headache, nausea, vomiting, and abdominal pain. Serious adverse effects include elevated liver enzymes and leukopenia, which have occurred in a few patients with treatment of hydatid disease. Rare adverse effects include acute renal failure, pancytopenia, granulocytopenia, and thrombocytopenia. Despite the fact that albendazole and other antiparasitic drugs, including mebendazole, praziquantel, and pyrimethamine, have been in use for decades, the number of manufacturers is small and costs have risen in recent years.

Ivermectin (Stromectol, Mectizan)
Ivermectin is a semisynthetic derivative of one of the avermectins, which is a group of macrocyclic lactones produced by *Streptomyces avermitilis*. After oral administration, ivermectin has peak plasma concentrations after approximately 4 hr and a plasma elimination half-life of approximately 12 hr. It is excreted as metabolites over a 2-wk period via feces. It is FDA approved for treatment of two nematode (roundworm) infections: onchocerciasis and intestinal strongyloidiasis. It may have some effect in treating a broad range of other **helminths** and **ectoparasites,** including cutaneous larva migrans (*Ancylostoma braziliense*), ascariasis (*Ascaris lumbricoides*), loiasis, pinworm (*Enterobius vermicularis*), whipworm (*Trichuris trichiura*), gnathostomiasis (*Gnathostoma spinigerum*), *Mansonella* infections, lice (*Pediculus humanus* and *Phthirus pubis*), mites (*Demodex* spp.), and scabies. Combination therapies of ivermectin with albendazole or diethylcarbamazine are being used to treat lymphatic filariasis. Combination therapy with albendazole and the off-label use of veterinary injectable formulations have been used to treat complicated *Strongyloides* infections, including disseminated disease and hyperinfection syndrome. Common adverse events include dizziness, headache, pruritus, and gastrointestinal effects. Serious adverse events include **Mazzotti reactions** in patients with onchocerciasis, including arthralgia, synovitis, enlarged lymph nodes, rash, and fever secondary to microfilaria death. A topical formulation is available for treatment of head lice, which are increasingly becoming very resistant to over-the-counter medications such as permethrins.

Praziquantel (Biltricide)
Praziquantel achieves its antiparasitic activity via the pyrazino isoquinoline ring system and was originally synthesized as a potential tranquilizer. After oral administration, praziquantel is rapidly absorbed, with peak levels in 1-2 hr and a plasma half-life of about 1-3 hr. Elimination via the urine and feces is > 80% complete after 24 hr. Praziquantel is metabolized in the liver by the microsomal cytochrome P450 (especially 2B1 and 3A). Bioavailability of praziquantel is increased with concomitant administration of agents that inhibit cytochrome P450. Praziquantel is FDA approved for treatment of several species of trematodes (flatworms) including the Chinese liver fluke (*Clonorchis sinensis*), Southeast Asian liver fluke (*Opisthorchis viverrini*), and schistosomiasis. It is used off-label for treatment of additional trematode pathogens, including the North American liver fluke (*Metorchis conjunctus*), *Nanophyetus salmincola*, intestinal flukes (*Fasciolopsis buski, Heterophyes heterophyes, Metagonimus yokogawai*), and lung flukes (*Paragonimus westermani, Paragonimus kellicotti*). It is also used off-label for multiple cestode (tapeworm) infections. Adverse effects can be seen in 30–60% of patients, although most are mild and disappear within 24 hr. Common adverse effects include headache, abdominal pain, dizziness, and malaise. Serious but rare adverse effects include arrhythmias, heart block, and convulsions.

Section **15**
Protozoan Diseases

第十五篇
原虫疾病

Chapter **306**
Primary Amebic Meningoencephalitis
Matthew D. Eberly

第三百零六章
原发性阿米巴脑膜脑炎

中文导读

本章主要介绍了原发性阿米巴脑膜脑炎病因学、流行病学、发病机制、临床表现、诊断和治疗。引起原发性阿米巴脑膜脑炎的病原包括耐格里阿米巴、棘阿米巴、巴氏阿米巴等。流行病学中，着重阐述了耐格里阿米巴的流行特点。介绍了耐格里阿米巴、棘阿米巴、巴氏阿米巴脑膜脑炎的发病机制。详细介绍了原发性阿米巴脑膜脑炎的临床表现、诊断和治疗。

Naegleria, Acanthamoeba, Balamuthia, and *Sappinia* are small, free-living amebae that cause human amebic meningoencephalitis, which has two distinct clinical presentations. The more common is an acute, fulminant, and usually fatal **primary amebic meningoencephalitis** (PAM) caused by *Naegleria fowleri* that occurs in previously healthy children and young adults. **Granulomatous amebic meningoencephalitis,** which is caused by *Acanthamoeba, Balamuthia,* and *Sappinia,* is a more indolent infection that typically occurs in immunocompromised hosts and may also present with a disseminated form of the disease.

ETIOLOGY

Naegleria is an ameboflagellate that can exist as cysts, trophozoites, and transient flagellate forms. Temperature and environmental nutrient and ion concentrations are the major factors that determine the stage of the ameba. Trophozoites are the only stages that are invasive, although cysts are potentially infective, because they can convert to the vegetative form very quickly under the proper environmental stimuli. Although there are some 30 species of *Naegleria,* only *Naegleria fowleri* has been shown to be pathogenic for humans.

Acanthamoeba exists in cyst and motile trophozoite forms; only the trophozoite form is invasive. Cases of *Acanthamoeba* **keratitis** usually follow incidents of trivial corneal trauma followed by flushing with

contaminated tap water. Infections can also occur among contact lens wearers who come into contact with contaminated water during swimming or use contact lenses cleaned or stored in contaminated tap water. Granulomatous amebic encephalitis from *Acanthamoeba* occurs worldwide and is associated with an immunocompromising condition such as HIV infection, diabetes mellitus, chronic liver disease, renal failure, immunosuppressive therapy, or radiation therapy.

Balamuthia mandrillaris has been implicated as an etiology of granulomatous amebic encephalitis. Although the clinical presentation is similar to infection with *Acanthamoeba,* most patients are not immunocompromised.

Other free-living amebae can also cause infection, as illustrated by a case report of *Sappinia pedata* granulomatous encephalitis.

EPIDEMIOLOGY

The free-living amebae have a worldwide distribution. *Naegleria* species have been isolated from a variety of freshwater sources, including ponds and lakes, domestic water supplies, hot springs and spas, thermal discharge of power plants, groundwater, and, occasionally, from the nasal passages of healthy children. *Acanthamoeba* species have been isolated from soil, mushrooms, vegetables, brackish water, and seawater, as well as most of the freshwater sources for *Naegleria.* It can also be found in tap water, because chlorination does not kill *Acanthamoeba*. *Balamuthia* is present in soil and may be transmitted by inhalation or contamination of preexisting skin lesions.

Naegleria meningoencephalitis has been reported from every continent except Antarctica. Most of the cases occur during the summer months in previously healthy individuals who have a history of swimming in or contact with freshwater lakes and rivers before their illness. Between 1962 and 2017, 143 cases of primary amebic meningoencephalitis (PAM) were reported in the United States. Most of the reports have come from the southern and southwestern states, particularly Florida and Texas, but infections have occurred in Kansas, Indiana, and even Minnesota. Of note, two cases from Louisiana in 2011 were linked to sinus irrigation with neti pots, which contained contaminated tap water. In 2013, a boy also from Louisiana developed PAM from an exposure to a lawn water slide, which derived its tap water from a treated public drinking water system. In 2015, a 21 yr old female developed *N. fowleri* meningoencephalitis possibly from a swimming pool supplied by an overland water pipe.

PATHOGENESIS

The free-living amebae enter the nasal cavity by inhalation or aspiration of dust or water contaminated with trophozoites or cysts. *Naegleria* gains access to the central nervous system through the olfactory epithelium and migrates via the olfactory nerve to the olfactory bulbs located in the subarachnoid space and bathed by the cerebrospinal fluid (CSF). This space is richly vascularized and is the route of spread to other areas of the central nervous system. Grossly, there is widespread cerebral edema and hyperemia of the meninges. The olfactory bulbs are necrotic, hemorrhagic, and surrounded by a purulent exudate. Microscopically, the gray matter is the most severely affected, with severe involvement in all cases. Fibrinopurulent exudate may be found throughout the cerebral hemispheres, brainstem, cerebellum, and upper portions of the spinal cord. Pockets of trophozoites may be seen in necrotic neural tissue, usually in the perivascular spaces of arteries and arterioles.

The route of invasion and penetration in cases of granulomatous amebic meningoencephalitis caused by *Acanthamoeba* and *Balamuthia* may be by direct spread through olfactory epithelium or hematogenous spread from a primary focus in the skin or lungs. Pathologic examination reveals granulomatous encephalitis, with multinucleated giant cells mainly in the posterior fossa structures, basal ganglia, bases of the cerebral hemispheres, and cerebellum. Both trophozoites and cysts may be found in the central nervous system lesions, primarily located in the perivascular spaces and invading blood vessel walls. The olfactory bulbs and spinal cord are usually spared. The single case of *Sappinia* encephalitis

followed a sinus infection, and evaluation revealed a solitary 2 cm temporal lobe mass with mild ring enhancement.

CLINICAL MANIFESTATIONS

The incubation of **Naegleria infection** may be as short as 2 days or as long as 15 days. Symptoms have an acute onset and progress rapidly. Infection is characterized by a sudden onset of severe headache, fever, pharyngitis, nasal congestion or discharge, and nausea and vomiting, followed by altered mental status, nuchal rigidity, photophobia, confusion, somnolence, seizures, and ultimately coma. Most cases end in death within 3-10 days after onset of symptoms.

Granulomatous amebic meningoencephalitis may occur weeks to months after the initial infection. The presenting signs and symptoms are often those of single or multiple central nervous system space-occupying lesions and include hemiparesis, ataxia, personality changes, seizures, and drowsiness. Altered mental status is often a prominent symptom. Headache and fever occur only sporadically, but stiff neck is seen in a majority of cases. Cranial nerve palsies, especially of cranial nerves III and VI, may be present. There is also one report of acute hydrocephalus and fever with *Balamuthia*. Granulomatous amebic meningoencephalitis is usually fatal after 4-6 wk of illness. Results of neuroimaging studies of the brain usually demonstrate multiple low-density lesions resembling infarcts or enhancing lesions of granulomas (Fig. 306.1).

DIAGNOSIS

The CSF in *Naegleria* infection may mimic that of herpes simplex encephalitis early in the disease and that of acute bacterial meningitis later in the disease, with a neutrophilic pleocytosis, elevated protein level, and hypoglycorrhachia. *Motile amebae may be visualized on a wet mount of freshly drawn CSF using Wright or Giemsa stains*, but they are often mistaken for lymphocytes or macrophages. Because *Naegleria* are the only amebae that differentiate into the flagellate state in a hypotonic environment, placing a drop of fresh CSF in 1 mL of distilled water and watching for the development of swimming flagellates after 1-2 hr can confirm the diagnosis of *Naegleria*. *Naegleria* can also be grown on a nonnutrient agar plate coated with *Escherichia coli*, on which they feed.

The diagnosis of granulomatous amebic meningoencephalitis relies on the isolation or histologic identification of *Acanthamoeba* trophozoites or cysts from brain tissue specimens. The CSF findings of granulomatous meningoencephalitis reveal lymphocytic pleocytosis, moderately elevated protein, and low glucose concentrations. However, motile trophozoites of *Acanthamoeba* are more difficult to isolate than *Naegleria*, and the CSF is typically sterile. *Acanthamoeba* may be cultured from the same

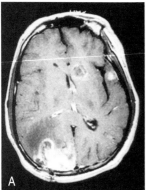 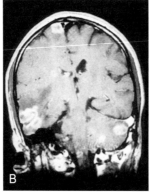 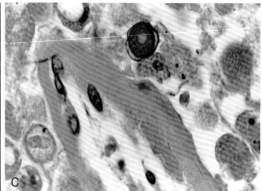

Fig. 306.1 A and **B,** MRIs of the brain of a patient with *Balamuthia mandrillaris* granulomatous amebic encephalitis. Multiple enhancing lesions are seen in the right hemisphere, left cerebellum, midbrain, and brainstem. **C,** Photomicrograph of the brain lesion from the same patient showing perivascular amebic trophozoites. A round amebic cyst with a characteristic double wall is seen in the top center (hematoxylin-and-eosin, original magnification ×100). (*From Deol I, Robledo L, Meza A, et al: Encephalitis due to a free-living amoeba [Balamuthia mandrillaris]: case report with literature review, Surg Neurol 53:611-616, 2000.*)

agar used for growing *Naegleria*, but *Balamuthia* must be grown on mammalian cell cultures. Pediatric cases of *Balamuthia* meningoencephalitis have been diagnosed antemortem by brain biopsy as well as postmortem. Immunofluorescence staining of brain tissue can differentiate *Acanthamoeba* and *Balamuthia*. An indirect fluorescent antibody test from the serum is also available for *Balamuthia*.

TREATMENT

Naegleria infection is nearly always fatal, but early recognition and treatment are crucial to survival. Until 2013, there had been only two known survivors in North America, with treatment regimens of amphotericin B, either alone or in combination with other agents such as rifampin, chloramphenicol, fluconazole, ketoconazole, and dexamethasone. In 2013, however, the U.S. Centers for Disease Control and Prevention (CDC) made available the antileishmanial drug **miltefosine** for the treatment of PAM. That summer, two children who contracted *Naegleria* both survived; both patients received oral miltefosine as part of their treatment, and one underwent external ventricular drain placement and therapeutic hypothermia. The recommended drug treatment for primary amebic meningoencephalitis by the CDC includes intravenous and intrathecal amphotericin B, oral miltefosine, along with azithromycin, fluconazole, rifampin, and dexamethasone. Early identification, early initiation of combination therapy, and aggressive management of increased intracranial pressure remain key elements for a successful outcome. For suspected cases, clinicians should contact the CDC Emergency Operations Center at (770) 488-7100 for assistance.

The optimal therapy for granulomatous amebic meningoencephalitis is uncertain. However, miltefosine has likewise been used to successfully treat patients with *Balamuthia* and disseminated *Acanthamoeba* infections. Strains of *Acanthamoeba* isolated from fatal cases are usually susceptible in vitro to pentamidine, ketoconazole, and flucytosine, and less so to amphotericin B. One patient was successfully treated with sulfadiazine and fluconazole, and another was successfully treated with intravenous pentamidine followed by oral itraconazole. *Acanthamoeba* keratitis responds to long courses of topical propamidine–polymyxin B sulfate or topical polyhexamethylene biguanide or chlorhexidine gluconate, and antifungal azoles plus topical steroids. Limited success has been demonstrated in *Balamuthia* infection with systemic azole therapy combined with flucytosine. More recently, the combination of flucytosine, pentamidine, fluconazole, sulfadiazine, azithromycin, and phenothiazines resulted in the survival of two patients with *Balamuthia* meningoencephalitis, although both were left with mild neuromotor and cognitive impairment. Corticosteroids prior to initiating effective therapy appear to have a detrimental effect, contributing to rapid progression of disease.

Bibliography is available at Expert Consult.

Chapter **307**

Amebiasis

Edsel Maurice T. Salvana
and Robert A. Salata

第三百零七章
阿米巴病

中文导读

　　本章介绍了阿米巴病的病因学、流行病学、发病机制、临床表现、实验室发现、诊断和鉴别诊断、并发症、治疗、预后和预防。其中临床表现部分着重介绍了阿米巴结肠炎和阿米巴肝脓肿的临床表现。在诊断部分提出阿米巴结肠炎的诊断是基于临床表现、粪便中阿米巴抗原或PCR检测以及血清学方法。治疗方面，分别针对侵袭性感染和无症状肠道定植两种情况阐述了相应的药物治疗方案。

Entamoeba species infect or colonize up to 10% of the world's population, particularly in resource-limited settings. In most infected individuals, *Entamoeba histolytica* or a related species parasitizes the lumen of the gastrointestinal tract and causes few symptoms or sequelae. Although *E. histolytica* is the only invasive species, other *Entamoeba* species have been implicated in human disease, and molecular epidemiology is helping to detail the role that these diverse protozoans play in human health. Invasive *E. histolytica* infection can lead to **amebic colitis, amebic liver abscess,** and, less commonly, abscesses in other extraintestinal sites.

ETIOLOGY

Four morphologically identical but genetically distinct species of *Entamoeba* are known to infect humans. *Entamoeba dispar,* the most prevalent species, does not cause symptomatic disease. *Entamoeba moshkovskii,* previously thought to be nonpathogenic, has increasingly been shown to cause diarrhea in infants and children, and asymptomatic infection with *E. moshkovskii* may be as common as *E. dispar* infection in some communities. *E. histolytica,* the main pathogenic species, causes a spectrum of disease and can become invasive in 4–10% of infected patients. Patients previously described as asymptomatic carriers of *E. histolytica* based on microscopy findings were likely harboring *E. dispar* or *E. moshkovskii.* A fourth species, *E. bangladeshi,* was discovered in 2012, but more studies are needed to ascertain its human pathogenicity. Four other species of nonpathogenic *Entamoeba* are known to colonize the human gastrointestinal tract: *E. coli, E. hartmanni, E. gingivalis,* and *E. polecki.*

Infection is usually acquired through the ingestion of parasite cysts, which measure 10-18 μm in diameter and contain four nuclei. Cysts are resistant to harsh environmental conditions, including chlorine concentrations commonly used in water purification, but can be killed by heating to 55°C (131°F). Cysts are resistant to gastric acidity and digestive enzymes and germinate in the small intestine to form trophozoites. These large, actively motile organisms colonize the lumen of the large intestine and may invade the mucosal lining. Some eventually transform to cysts and are passed out in the stool to infect other hosts anew.

EPIDEMIOLOGY

Prevalence of infection with *E. histolytica* varies greatly by region and socioeconomic status. Early prevalence studies did not distinguish between *E. histolytica* and *E. dispar,* but more recent estimates show that infection with *E. histolytica* causes 100 million cases of symptomatic disease and 2,000 to 17,000 deaths annually. Prospective studies have shown that 4–10% of individuals infected with *E. histolytica* develop amebic colitis and that < 1% of infected individuals develop disseminated disease, including amebic liver abscess. These numbers vary by region; for example, in South Africa and Vietnam, liver abscesses form a disproportionately large number of the cases of invasive disease due to *E. histolytica.* Amebic liver abscesses occur equally in male and female children but are generally rare in childhood. Peak abscess formation occurs between 30 to 60 years old and is 10-12 times more prevalent in adult males than females, possibly due to an inhibitory effect of testosterone on innate immune mechanisms.

Amebiasis causes its largest burden of disease in Africa, Southeast Asia, and the Eastern Mediterranean. In the United States, amebiasis is seen most frequently in travelers to and immigrants from developing countries. Residents of mental health institutions and men who have sex with men are at increased risk for invasive amebiasis. Food or drink contaminated with *Entamoeba* cysts and oral-anogenital sex are the most common means of infection. Untreated water and night soil (human feces used as fertilizer) are important sources of infection in resource-limited settings. Food handlers shedding amebic cysts play a role in spreading infection.

PATHOGENESIS

Trophozoites are responsible for tissue invasion and destruction. Hypersecretion of mucus by colonic goblet cells is induced by secreted amebic cysteine protease 5, which eventually leads to degradation of the mucus layer, exposing colonic epithelial cells. Amebae then attach using a galactose and *N*-acetyl-D-galactosamine–specific lectin. This lectin also provides resistance to complement-mediated lysis, and its intermediate subunit has been found to have hemagglutinating, hemolytic, and cytolytic activity. Once attached to the colonic mucosa, trophozoites penetrate the epithelial layer, destroying host cells by cytolysis and induction of apoptosis. Cytolysis is mediated by trophozoite release of amebapores (pore-forming proteins), phospholipases, and hemolysins. Trogocytosis, where amebae ingest pieces of living cells and induce intracellular calcium elevation leading to apoptosis, was recently described as a mechanism for direct host cell killing by amebae.

Once host cells are partially digested by amebic proteases, the degraded material is internalized through phagocytosis. Early invasive amebiasis produces significant inflammation, owing in part to parasite-mediated activation of nuclear factor-κB. Once *E. histolytica* trophozoites invade the intestinal mucosa, the organisms multiply and spread laterally underneath the intestinal epithelium to produce the characteristic *flask-shaped ulcers.* Amebae produce similar lytic lesions if they reach the liver. These lesions are commonly called *abscesses,* although they contain no granulocytes. Well-established ulcers and amebic liver abscesses demonstrate little local inflammatory response.

Immunity to infection is associated with a mucosal secretory IgA response against the galactose/*N*-acetyl-D-galactosaminelectin. Neutrophils appear to be important in the initial host defense, but *E. histolytica*–induced epithelial cell damage releases neutrophil chemoattractants, and *E. histolytica* is able to kill neutrophils, which then release mediators that further damage epithelial cells. The disparity between the extent of tissue destruction by amebae and the absence of a local host inflammatory response in the presence of systemic humoral (antibody) and cell-mediated responses may reflect both parasite-mediated apoptosis and the ability of the trophozoite to kill not only epithelial cells but neutrophils, monocytes, and macrophages. Leptin receptor polymorphisms have been implicated as host genetic factors that affect the susceptibility to infection by *E. histolytica.* The chemotactic effect of leptin is decreased in individuals with an arginine polymorphism in position 223 of the leptin receptor, and this polymorphism also decreases host STAT-3 gene expression leading to enhanced induction of host cell apoptosis by amebae.

The *E. histolytica* genome is functionally tetraploid, and there is evidence of lateral gene transfer from bacteria. The amebapore-A (Ap-A) gene, along with other important genes, can be epigenetically silenced using plasmids with specifically engineered sequences or short hairpin RNAs. Transcriptional profiling using proteomics and microarrays has identified multiple virulence factors, including cysteine proteases, which modulate lysosome and phagosome function, and a total of 219 excretory-secretory proteins. The bacterial microbiome has also been shown to influence *E. histolytica* pathogenicity by affecting lectin expression, with increased *Prevotella copri* populations associated with higher rates of diarrhea in infected children.

CLINICAL MANIFESTATIONS

Clinical presentations range from asymptomatic cyst passage to amebic colitis, amebic dysentery, ameboma, and extraintestinal disease. Up to 10% of infected persons develop invasive disease within a year, and asymptomatic carriers should be treated. Severe disease is more common in young children, pregnant women, malnourished individuals, and persons taking corticosteroids, and invasive disease is more common in men. Extraintestinal disease usually involves the liver, but less common extraintestinal manifestations include amebic brain abscess, pleuropulmonary disease, ulcerative skin, and genitourinary lesions.

Amebic Colitis

Amebic colitis may occur within 2 wk of infection or may be delayed for months. The onset is usually gradual, with colicky abdominal pains and frequent bowel movements (6-8/day). Diarrhea is frequently associated with tenesmus. Almost all stool is heme-positive, but most patients do not present with grossly bloody stools. Generalized constitutional symptoms and signs are characteristically absent, with fever documented in only one third of patients. Amebic colitis affects all age-groups, but its incidence is strikingly common in children 1-5 yr of age. Severe amebic colitis in infants and young children tends to be rapidly progressive, with more frequent extraintestinal involvement and high mortality rates, particularly in tropical countries. Amebic dysentery can result in dehydration and electrolyte disturbances.

Amebic Liver Abscess

Amebic liver abscess, a serious manifestation of disseminated infection, is uncommon in children. Although diffuse liver enlargement has been associated with intestinal amebiasis, liver abscesses occur in < 1% of infected individuals and may appear in patients with no clear history of intestinal disease. Amebic liver abscess may occur months to years after exposure, so obtaining a careful travel history is critical. In children, fever is the hallmark of amebic liver abscess and is frequently associated with abdominal pain, distention, and enlargement and tenderness of the liver. Changes at the base of the right lung, such as elevation of the diaphragm and atelectasis or effusion, may also occur.

LABORATORY FINDINGS

Laboratory examination findings are often unremarkable in uncomplicated amebic colitis. Laboratory findings in amebic liver abscess are a slight leukocytosis, moderate anemia, high erythrocyte sedimentation rate, and elevations of hepatic enzyme (particularly alkaline phosphatase) levels. Stool examination for amebae is negative in more than half of patients with documented amebic liver abscess. Ultrasonography, CT, or MRI can localize and delineate the size of the abscess cavity (Fig. 307.1). The most common finding is a single abscess in the right hepatic lobe.

DIAGNOSIS AND DIFFERENTIAL DIAGNOSIS

A diagnosis of amebic colitis is made in the presence of compatible symptoms with detection of E. histolytica either by stool antigen testing or PCR. This approach has a greater than 95% sensitivity and specificity, and when it is coupled with a positive serology test, it is the most accurate means of diagnosis in developed countries. Several approved stool antigen kits are commercially available in the United States, but most cannot distinguish between E. histolytica and E. dispar. Microscopic examination of stool samples has a sensitivity of 60%. Sensitivity can be increased to 85–95% by examining three stools. Microscopy cannot differentiate between E. histolytica and E. dispar unless phagocytosed erythrocytes (specific for E. histolytica) are seen. Endoscopy and biopsies of suspicious areas should be performed when stool sample results are negative and suspicion remains high.

Various serum antibody tests are available. Serologic results are positive in 70–80% of patients with invasive disease (colitis or liver abscess) at

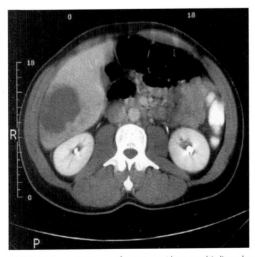

Fig. 307.1 Abdominal CT scan of a patient with an amebic liver abscess. *(From Miller Q, Kenney JM, Cotlar AM: Amebic abscess of the liver presenting as acute cholecystitis, Curr Surg 57:476-479, 2000, Fig. 1, p. 477.)*

presentation and in > 90% of patients after 7 days. The most sensitive serologic test, indirect hemagglutination, yields a positive result years after invasive infection. Therefore, many uninfected adults and children in highly endemic areas demonstrate antibodies to E. histolytica. Conventional and real-time multiplex PCR performed on stool is the most sensitive and preferred method for distinguishing E. histolytica from nonpathogenic E. dispar and E. moshkovskii. Different multiplex formats have also been developed, including enteric pathogen panels with varying sensitivities and specificities. Isothermal nucleic acid methods using recombinase and loop-mediated amplification (LAMP) in point-of-care diagnostics are promising and will greatly facilitate treatment, especially in developing countries.

The **differential diagnosis** for amebic colitis includes colitis due to bacterial, mycobacterial, and viral pathogens, as well as noninfectious causes such as inflammatory bowel disease. Pyogenic liver abscess due to bacterial infection, hepatoma, and echinococcal cysts are in the differential diagnosis for amebic liver abscess. However, echinococcal cysts are rarely associated with systemic symptoms such as fever, unless there is cyst rupture or leakage.

COMPLICATIONS

Complications of amebic colitis include acute necrotizing colitis, ameboma, toxic megacolon, extraintestinal extension, or local perforation and peritonitis. Less commonly, a chronic form of amebic colitis develops, often recurring over several years. Amebomas are nodular foci of proliferative inflammation that sometimes develop in the wall of the colon. Amebiasis should be excluded before initiating corticosteroid treatment for inflammatory bowel disease, because this is associated with high mortality rates.

An amebic liver abscess may rupture into the peritoneum, pleural cavity, skin, and pericardium. Cases of amebic abscesses in extrahepatic sites, including the lung and brain, have been reported.

TREATMENT

Invasive amebiasis is treated with a nitroimidazole such as metronidazole or tinidazole and then a luminal amebicide (Table 307.1). Tinidazole has similar efficacy to metronidazole, with shorter and simpler dosing, and is better tolerated. Adverse effects include nausea, abdominal discomfort, and a metallic taste that disappears after completion of therapy. Therapy with a nitroimidazole should be followed by treatment with a luminal agent, such as paromomycin (which is preferred) or iodoquinol. Diloxanide furoate can also be used in children > 2 yr of age, but it is no longer available in the United States. Paromomycin should not be given concurrently with metronidazole or tinidazole, because diarrhea is a common side effect of paromomycin and may confuse the clinical picture. Asymptomatic intestinal infection with E. histolytica should be treated, preferably with paromomycin or alternatively with either iodoquinol or diloxanide furoate. For fulminant cases of amebic colitis, some experts suggest adding dehydroemetine (1 mg/kg/day subcutaneously or intramuscularly, never intravenously), available only through the Centers for Disease Control and Prevention. Patients should be hospitalized for monitoring if dehydroemetine is administered. Dehydroemetine should be discontinued if tachycardia, T-wave depression, arrhythmia, or proteinuria develops.

Broad-spectrum antibiotic therapy may be indicated in fulminant colitis to cover possible spillage of intestinal bacteria into the peritoneum and translocation into the bloodstream. Intestinal perforation and toxic megacolon are indications for surgery. In amebic liver abscess, image-guided aspiration of large lesions or left lobe abscesses may be necessary if rupture is imminent or if the patient shows a poor clinical response 4-6 days after administration of amebicidal drugs. A Cochrane meta-analysis comparing metronidazole and metronidazole plus aspiration in uncomplicated amebic liver abscess showed that there is insufficient evidence to make any recommendation for or against this approach. Chloroquine, which concentrates in the liver, may also be a useful adjunct to nitroimidazoles in the treatment of amebic liver abscess or in cases of treatment failure or intolerance. To confirm cure, stool examination should be repeated every 2 wk following completion of therapy until clear.

Table 307.1	Drug Treatment for Amebiasis	
MEDICATION	**ADULT DOSAGE (ORAL)**	**PEDIATRIC DOSAGE (ORAL)***
INVASIVE DISEASE		
Metronidazole	Colitis or liver abscess: 750 mg tid for 7-10 days	Colitis or liver abscess: 35-50 mg/kg/day in 3 divided doses for 7-10 days
Or		
Tinidazole	Colitis: 2 g once daily for 3 days	Colitis: 50 mg/kg/day once daily for 3 days
	Liver abscess: 2 g once daily for 3-5 days	Liver abscess: 50 mg/kg/day once daily for 3-5 days
Followed by:		
Paromomycin (preferred)	500 mg tid for 7 days	25-35 mg/kg/day in 3 divided doses for 7 days
Or		
Diloxanide furoate[†]	500 mg tid for 10 days	20 mg/kg/day in 3 divided doses for 7 days
Or		
Iodoquinol	650 mg tid for 20 days	30-40 mg/kg/day in 3 divided doses for 20 days
ASYMPTOMATIC INTESTINAL COLONIZATION		
Paromomycin (preferred)	As for invasive disease	As for invasive disease
Or		
Diloxanide furoate[†]		
Or		
Iodoquinol		

*All pediatric dosages are up to a maximum of the adult dose.
†Not available in the United States.

Auranofin, a gold-containing antirheumatologic drug that inhibits *E. histolytica* thioredoxin reductase, has been shown to be active against amebic trophozoites and shows promise as a broad-spectrum antiparasitic agent. Phase one clinical trials were recently completed.

PROGNOSIS

Most infections evolve to either an asymptomatic carrier state or eradication. Extraintestinal infection carries about a 5% mortality rate.

PREVENTION

Control of amebiasis can be achieved by exercising proper sanitation and hygiene. Regular examination of food handlers and thorough investigation of diarrheal episodes may help identify the source of infection. No prophylactic drug or vaccine is available. Immunization with a combination of galactose/N-acetyl-D-galactosamine lectin and CpG oligodeoxynucleotides has been shown to be protective in animals, and an intranasal galactose-lectin subunit vaccine has been shown to be protective in baboons. Recent work has shown that the C-terminal fragment of the biologically active intermediate subunit of the galactose/N-acetyl-D-galactosamine is a promising vaccine candidate and may also prevent the development of liver abscesses.

Bibliography is available at Expert Consult.

中文导读

本章主要介绍了十二指肠贾第虫（又称蓝氏贾第虫或肠贾第虫）病和小袋虫病。其中在十二指肠贾第虫病部分，详细阐述了十二指肠贾第虫病的病因学、流行病学、临床表现、诊断、治疗、预后和预防。简要介绍了小袋虫病的病原学、临床表现、诊断、治疗和预防。另外还介绍了针对贾第虫病和小袋虫病治疗的药物剂量和疗程。

308.1 Giardia duodenalis

Chandy C. John

Giardia duodenalis is a flagellated protozoan that infects the duodenum and jejunum. Infection results in clinical manifestations that range from asymptomatic colonization to acute or chronic diarrhea and malabsorption. Infection is more prevalent in children than in adults. *Giardia* is endemic in areas of the world with poor levels of sanitation. It is also an important cause of morbidity in developed countries, where it is associated with urban childcare centers, residential institutions for the developmentally delayed, and waterborne and foodborne outbreaks. *Giardia* is a particularly significant pathogen in children with malnutrition and certain immunodeficiencies (IgA deficiency, common variable immunodeficiency, X-linked hypogammaglobulinemia).

ETIOLOGY

The life cycle of *G. duodenalis* (also known as *Giardia lamblia* or *Giardia intestinalis*) is composed of two stages: trophozoites and cysts. *Giardia* infects humans after ingestion of as few as 10-100 cysts, which measure 8-10 μm in diameter. Each ingested cyst produces two trophozoites in the duodenum. After excystation, trophozoites colonize the lumen of the duodenum and proximal jejunum, where they attach to the brush border of the intestinal epithelial cells and multiply by binary fission. The body of the trophozoite is teardrop shaped, measuring 10-20 μm in length and 5-15 μm in width. *Giardia* trophozoites contain two oval nuclei anteriorly, a large ventral disk, a curved median body posteriorly, and four pairs of flagella. As detached trophozoites pass down the intestinal tract, they encyst to form oval cysts that contain four nuclei. Cysts are passed in stools of infected individuals and may remain viable in water for as long as 2 mo. Their viability often is not affected by the usual concentrations of chlorine used to purify water for drinking.

Giardia strains that infect humans are diverse biologically, as shown by differences in antigens, restriction endonuclease patterns, DNA fingerprinting, isoenzyme patterns, and pulsed-field gel electrophoresis. Studies suggest that different *Giardia* genotypes may cause unique clinical manifestations, but these findings appear to vary according to the geographic region tested.

EPIDEMIOLOGY

Giardia occurs worldwide and is the most common intestinal parasite identified in public health laboratories in the United States, where it is estimated that up to 2 million cases of giardiasis occur annually. *Giardia* infection usually occurs sporadically, but *Giardia* is a frequently identified etiologic agent of outbreaks associated with drinking water. The age-specific prevalence of giardiasis is high during childhood and begins to decline after adolescence. The asymptomatic carrier rate of *G. lamblia* in the United States is as high as 20–30% in children younger than 36 mo of age attending childcare centers. Asymptomatic carriage may persist for several months.

Transmission of *Giardia* is common in certain high-risk groups, including children and employees in childcare centers, consumers of contaminated water, travelers to certain areas of the world, men who have sex with men, and persons exposed to certain animals. The major reservoir and vehicle for spread of *Giardia* appears to be water contaminated with *Giardia* cysts, but foodborne transmission occurs. The seasonal peak in age-specific case reports coincides with the summer recreational water season and may be a result of the extensive use of communal swimming venues by young children, the low infectious dose, and the extended periods of cyst shedding that can occur. In addition, *Giardia* cysts are relatively resistant to chlorination and to ultraviolet light irradiation. Boiling is effective for inactivating cysts.

Person-to-person spread also occurs, particularly in areas of low hygiene standards, frequent fecal-oral contact, and crowding. Individual susceptibility, lack of toilet training, crowding, and fecal contamination of the environment all predispose to transmission of enteropathogens, including *Giardia,* in childcare centers. Childcare centers play an important role in transmission of urban giardiasis, with secondary attack rates in families as high as 17–30%. Children in childcare centers may pass cysts for several months. Campers who drink untreated stream or river water, particularly in the western United States, and residents of institutions for the developmentally delayed are also at increased risk for infection.

Humoral immunodeficiencies, including common variable immuno-deficiency and X-linked agammaglobulinemia, predispose humans to chronic symptomatic *Giardia* infection, suggesting the importance of humoral immunity in controlling giardiasis. Selective immunoglobulin A deficiency is also associated with *Giardia* infection. Although many individuals with AIDS have relatively mild *Giardia* infections, *Giardia* infection refractory to treatment may occur in a subset of individuals with AIDS. A higher incidence of *Giardia* infection in patients with cystic fibrosis was reported in 1988, particularly in older children and adults, but there have been no subsequent confirmations of this risk. Human milk contains glycoconjugates and secretory immuno-globulin A antibodies that may provide protection to nursing infants against *Giardia.*

CLINICAL MANIFESTATIONS

The incubation period of *Giardia* infection usually is 1-2 wk but may be longer. A broad spectrum of clinical manifestations occurs, depending on the interaction between *G. lamblia* and the host. Children who are exposed to *G. lamblia* may experience asymptomatic excretion of the organism, acute infectious diarrhea, or chronic diarrhea with persistent gastrointestinal tract signs and symptoms, including failure to thrive and abdominal pain or cramping. *Giardia* was the cause of 15% of nondysenteric diarrheal illnesses in children examined in U.S. outpatient clinics in one study. Most infections in children and adults are asymptomatic. There is usually no extraintestinal spread, but occasionally trophozoites may migrate into bile or pancreatic ducts.

Symptomatic infections occur more frequently in children than in adults. Most symptomatic patients usually have a limited period of acute diarrheal disease with or without low-grade fever, nausea, and anorexia; in a small proportion of patients, an intermittent or more protracted course characterized by diarrhea, abdominal distention and cramps, bloating, malaise, flatulence, nausea, anorexia, and weight loss develops (Table 308.1). Stools initially may be profuse and watery and later become greasy and foul smelling and may float. Stools do not contain blood, mucus, or fecal leukocytes. Varying degrees of malabsorption may occur. Abnormal stool patterns may alternate with periods of constipation and normal bowel movements. Malabsorption of sugars, fats, and fat-soluble vitamins is well documented and may be responsible for substantial weight loss. *Giardia* has been associated with iron deficiency in internationally adopted children. Extraintestinal manifestations of *Giardia* appear to be more common in adults than children and include arthritis and, in one report after an outbreak, chronic fatigue syndrome. Giardiasis in children has been associated with growth stunting, and repeated *Giardia* infections correlate with a decrease in cognitive function in children in endemic areas.

DIAGNOSIS

Giardiasis should be considered in children who have acute nondysenteric diarrhea, persistent diarrhea, intermittent diarrhea and constipation, malabsorption, chronic crampy abdominal pain and bloating, failure to thrive, or weight loss. It should be particularly high in the differential diagnosis of children in child care, children in contact with an index case, children with a history of recent travel to an endemic area, and children with humoral immunodeficiencies. Testing for giardiasis should be standard for internationally adopted children from *Giardia*-endemic areas, and screening for iron deficiency should be considered in internationally adopted children with giardiasis.

Stool enzyme immunoassay (EIA) or direct fluorescent antibody tests for *Giardia* antigens have been tests of choice for giardiasis. EIA is less reader dependent and more sensitive for detection of *Giardia* than microscopy. Some studies report that a single stool is sufficiently sensitive for detection of *Giardia* by EIA, whereas others suggest that sensitivity is increased with testing of two samples. A diagnosis of giardiasis was traditionally established by microscopy documentation of trophozoites or cysts in stool specimens, but three stool specimens are required to achieve a sensitivity of > 90% using this approach. In patients in whom other parasitic intestinal infections are in the differential diagnosis, microscopy examination of stool allows evaluation for these infections in addition to *Giardia.*

Polymerase chain reaction and gene probe–based detection systems specific for *Giardia* have been used in environmental monitoring and clinical testing. Multiplex polymerase chain reaction testing for multiple parasitic pathogens is a viable option for testing.

In patients with chronic symptoms in whom giardiasis is suspected but in whom testing of stool specimens for *Giardia* yields a negative result, aspiration or biopsy of the duodenum or upper jejunum should be considered. In a fresh specimen, trophozoites usually can be visualized by direct wet mount. An alternate method of directly obtaining duodenal fluid is the commercially available Entero-Test (Hedeco Corp, Mountain View, CA), but this method is less sensitive than aspiration or biopsy. The biopsy can be used to make touch preparations and tissue sections for identification of *Giardia* and other enteric pathogens and also to visualize changes in histology. Biopsy of the small intestine should be considered in patients with characteristic clinical symptoms, negative stool and duodenal fluid specimen findings, and one or more of the following: abnormal radiographic findings (such as edema and segmentation in the small intestine); an abnormal lactose tolerance test result; an absent secretory immunoglobulin A level; hypogammaglobulinemia; or achlorhydria. Duodenal biopsy may show findings consistent with chronic inflammation, including eosinophilic infiltration of the lamina propria.

Radiographic contrast studies of the small intestine may show nonspecific findings such as irregular thickening of the mucosal folds. Blood cell counts usually are normal. Giardiasis is not tissue invasive and is not associated with peripheral blood eosinophilia.

TREATMENT

Children with acute diarrhea in whom *Giardia* organisms are identified should receive therapy. In addition, children who manifest failure to thrive or exhibit malabsorption or gastrointestinal tract symptoms such as chronic diarrhea should be treated.

Asymptomatic excreters generally are not treated, except in specific instances such as outbreak control, prevention of household transmission by toddlers to pregnant women and patients with hypogammaglobulinemia or cystic fibrosis, and situations requiring oral antibiotic treatment where *Giardia* may produce malabsorption of the antibiotic.

Table 308.1	Clinical Signs and Symptoms of Giardiasis
SYMPTOM	**FREQUENCY (%)**
Diarrhea	64-100
Malaise, weakness	72-97
Abdominal distention	42-97
Flatulence	35-97
Abdominal cramps	44-81
Nausea	14-79
Foul-smelling, greasy stools	15-79
Anorexia	41-73
Weight loss	53-73
Vomiting	14-35
Fever	0-28
Constipation	0-27

Table 308.2	Drug Treatment for Giardiasis	
MEDICATION	**ADULT DOSAGE (ORAL)**	**PEDIATRIC DOSAGE (ORAL)***
RECOMMENDED		
Tinidazole	2 g once	>3 yr: 50 mg/kg once
Nitazoxanide	500 mg bid for 3 days	1-3 yr: 100 mg (5 mL) bid for 3 days
		4-11 yr: 200 mg (10 mL) bid for 3 days
		>12 yr: 500 mg bid for 3 days
Metronidazole	250 mg tid for 5-7 days	15 mg/kg/day in 3 divided doses for 5-7 days
ALTERNATIVE		
Albendazole	400 mg once a day for 5 days	>6 yr: 400 mg once a day for 5 days
Paromomycin	25-35 mg/kg/day in 3 divided doses for 5-10 days	Not recommended
Quinacrine†	100 mg tid for 5-7 days	6 mg/kg/day in 3 divided doses for 5 days

*All pediatric dosages are up to a maximum of the adult dose.
†Not commercially available. Can be compounded by Medical Center Pharmacy in New Haven, CT (203-688-8970) or Panorama Compounding Pharmacy in Van Nuys, CA (818-988-7979).

The FDA has approved tinidazole and nitazoxanide for the treatment of *Giardia* in the United States. Both medications have been used to treat *Giardia* in thousands of patients in other countries and have excellent safety and efficacy records against *Giardia* (Table 308.2). Tinidazole has the advantage of single-dose treatment and very high efficacy (>90%), while nitazoxanide has the advantage of a suspension form, high efficacy (80–90%), and very few adverse effects. Metronidazole, though never approved by the FDA for treatment of *Giardia*, is also highly effective (80–90% cure rate), and the generic form is considerably less expensive than tinidazole or nitazoxanide. Frequent adverse effects are seen with metronidazole therapy, and it requires 3-times-a-day dosing for 5-7 days. Suspension forms of tinidazole and metronidazole must be compounded by a pharmacy; neither drug is sold in suspension form.

Second-line alternatives for the treatment of patients with giardiasis include albendazole, paromomycin, and quinacrine (see Table 308.2). Albendazole may be of similar efficacy to metronidazole. Albendazole has few adverse effects and is effective against many helminths, making it useful for treatment when multiple intestinal parasites are identified or suspected. Paromomycin is a nonabsorbable aminoglycoside and is less effective than other agents but is recommended for treatment of pregnant women with giardiasis because of the potential teratogenic effects of other agents. Quinacrine is effective and inexpensive but is not available commercially and must be obtained from compounding pharmacies (see Table 308.2). Quinacrine can also rarely have serious side effects, including hallucinations and psychosis. Refractory cases of giardiasis have been successfully treated with a number of regimens including nitazoxanide, prolonged courses of tinidazole, or combination therapy, most commonly a 3 wk course of metronidazole and quinacrine.

PROGNOSIS
Symptoms recur in some patients in whom reinfection cannot be documented and in whom an immune deficiency such as an immunoglobulin abnormality is not present, despite use of appropriate therapy. Several studies have demonstrated that variability in antimicrobial susceptibility exists among strains of *Giardia*, and in some instances resistant strains have been demonstrated. Combined therapy may be useful for infection that persists after single-drug therapy, assuming reinfection has not occurred and the medication was taken as prescribed.

PREVENTION
Infected persons and persons at risk should practice strict handwashing after any contact with feces. This point is especially important for caregivers of diapered infants in childcare centers, where diarrhea is common and *Giardia* organism carriage rates are high.

Methods to purify public water supplies adequately include chlorination, sedimentation, and filtration. Inactivation of *Giardia* cysts by chlorine requires the coordination of multiple variables such as chlorine concentration, water pH, turbidity, temperature, and contact time. These variables cannot be appropriately controlled in all municipalities and are difficult to control in swimming pools. Individuals, especially children in diapers, should avoid swimming if they have diarrhea. Individuals should also avoid swallowing recreational water and drinking untreated water from shallow wells, lakes, springs, ponds, streams, and rivers.

Travelers to endemic areas are advised to avoid uncooked foods that might have been grown, washed, or prepared with water that was potentially contaminated. Purification of drinking water can be achieved by a filter with a pore size of < 1 μm or that has been rated by the National Sanitation Foundation for cyst removal, or by brisk boiling of water for at least 1 min. Treatment of water with chlorine or iodine is less effective but may be used as an alternate method when boiling or filtration is not possible.

Bibliography is available at Expert Consult.

308.2 Balantidiasis
Chandy C. John

Balantidium coli is a ciliated protozoan and is the largest protozoan that parasitizes humans. Both trophozoites and cysts may be identified in feces. Disease caused by this organism is uncommon in the United States and generally is reported where there is a close association of humans with pigs, which are the natural hosts of *B. coli*. Because the organism infects the large intestine, symptoms are consistent with large bowel disease, similar to those associated with amebiasis and trichuriasis, and include nausea, vomiting, lower abdominal pain, tenesmus, and bloody diarrhea. Symptoms associated with chronic infection include abdominal cramps, watery diarrhea with mucus, occasionally bloody diarrhea, and colonic ulcers similar to those associated with *Entamoeba histolytica*. Extraintestinal spread of *B. coli* is rare and usually occurs only in immunocompromised patients. Most infections are asymptomatic.

Diagnosis using direct saline mounts is established by identification of trophozoites (50-100 μm long) or spherical or oval cysts (50-70 μm in diameter) in stool specimens. Trophozoites usually are more numerous than cysts.

The recommended treatment regimen is metronidazole (45 mg/kg/day divided tid PO; maximum: 750 mg/dose) for 5 days, or tetracycline (40 mg/kg/day divided qid PO; maximum: 500 mg/dose) for 10 days for persons older than 8 yr of age. An alternative is iodoquinol (40 mg/kg/day divided tid PO; maximum: 650 mg/dose) for 20 days.

Prevention of contamination of the environment by pig feces is the most important means for control.

Bibliography is available at Expert Consult.

Chapter 309
Cryptosporidium, Cystoisospora, Cyclospora, and Microsporidia

Patricia M. Flynn

第三百零九章

隐孢子虫、囊等孢子虫、环孢子虫和小孢子虫

中文导读

本章主要介绍了隐孢子虫病、囊等孢子虫病、环孢子虫病和小孢子虫病。着重阐述了隐孢子虫病的病原学、流行病学、临床表现、诊断和治疗。简要介绍了囊等孢子虫病、环孢子虫病和小孢子虫病的病原学、流行病学、临床表现、诊断和治疗。

The spore-forming intestinal protozoa *Cryptosporidium, Cystoisospora* (formerly *Isospora*), and *Cyclospora* are important intestinal pathogens in both immunocompetent and immunocompromised hosts. *Cryptosporidium, Cystoisospora,* and *Cyclospora* are coccidian parasites that predominantly infect the epithelial cells lining the digestive tract. Microsporidia were formerly considered spore-forming protozoa but have been reclassified as fungi. Microsporidia are ubiquitous, obligate intracellular parasites that infect many other organ systems in addition to the gastrointestinal tract and cause a broader spectrum of disease.

CRYPTOSPORIDIUM

Cryptosporidium is recognized as a leading protozoal cause of diarrhea in children worldwide and is a common cause of outbreaks in childcare centers; it is also a significant pathogen in immunocompromised patients.

Etiology

Cryptosporidium hominis and *Cryptosporidium parvum* cause most cases of cryptosporidiosis in humans. Disease is initiated by ingestion of infectious oocysts that were excreted in the feces of infected humans and animals. The oocysts are immediately infectious to other hosts or can reinfect the same host. The ingested oocysts release sporozoites that attach to and invade the intestinal epithelial cells.

Epidemiology

Cryptosporidiosis is associated with diarrheal illness worldwide and is more prevalent in developing countries and among children younger than 2 yr of age. It has been implicated as an etiologic agent of persistent diarrhea in the developing world and as a cause of significant morbidity and mortality from malnutrition, including permanent effects on growth.

Transmission of *Cryptosporidium* to humans can occur by close association with infected animals, via person-to-person transmission, or from environmentally contaminated water and food. Although zoonotic transmission, especially from cows, occurs in persons in close association with animals, person-to-person transmission is probably responsible for cryptosporidiosis outbreaks within hospitals and childcare centers, where transmission rates as high as 67% have been reported. Recommendations to prevent outbreaks in childcare centers include exclusion of children with diarrhea from attending, strict handwashing, elimination of water play or swimming activities, use of protective clothes or diapers capable of retaining liquid diarrhea, and separation of diapering and food-handling areas and responsibilities.

Outbreaks of cryptosporidial infection are associated with contaminated community water supplies and recreational waters, including lakes and chlorinated swimming pools. Wastewater in the form of raw sewage and runoff from dairies and grazing lands can contaminate both drinking and recreational water sources. It is estimated that *Cryptosporidium* oocysts are present in 65–97% of the surface water in the United States. The organism's small size (4-6 μm in diameter), resistance to chlorination, and ability to survive for long periods outside a host create problems in public water supplies.

Clinical Manifestations

The incubation period is 2-10 days (average, 7 days) after infection. *Cryptosporidium* infection is associated with profuse, watery, nonbloody diarrhea that can be accompanied by diffuse crampy abdominal pain, nausea, vomiting, and anorexia. Although less common in adults, vomiting occurs in more than 80% of children with cryptosporidiosis. Nonspecific symptoms such as myalgia, weakness, and headache also may occur. Fever occurs in 30–50% of cases. Malabsorption, lactose intolerance, dehydration, weight loss, and malnutrition often occur in severe cases. The clinical spectrum and disease severity have been linked with both the infecting species and host human leukocyte antigen class I and class II alleles.

In immunocompetent persons, the disease is usually self-limiting, typically 5-10 days, although diarrhea may persist for several weeks and oocyst shedding may persist for many weeks after symptoms resolve. Chronic diarrhea is common in individuals with immunodeficiency, such as congenital hypogammaglobulinemia or HIV infection. Symptoms and oocyst shedding can continue indefinitely and may lead to severe malnutrition, wasting, anorexia, and even death.

Cryptosporidiosis in **immunocompromised hosts** is often associated with biliary tract disease, characterized by fever, right upper quadrant pain, nausea, vomiting, and diarrhea. It also is associated with pancreatitis. Respiratory tract disease, with symptoms of cough, shortness of breath, wheezing, croup, and hoarseness, is very rare.

DIAGNOSIS

Infection can be diagnosed by microscopy using modified acid-fast stain or polymerase chain reaction, but immunodetection of antigens on the surface of the organism in stool samples using monoclonal antibody–based assays is the current diagnostic method of choice. Multiplex molecular test panels for gastrointestinal pathogens that include *Cryptosporidium* are available and are a standard test.

In stool, oocysts appear as small, spherical bodies (2-6 μm) and stain red with modified acid-fast staining. Because *Cryptosporidium* does not invade below the epithelial layer of the mucosa, fecal leukocytes are not found in stool specimens. Oocyst shedding in feces can be intermittent, and several fecal specimens (at least three for an immunocompetent host) should be collected for microscopic examination. Serologic diagnosis is not helpful in acute cryptosporidiosis.

In tissue sections, *Cryptosporidium* organisms can be found along the microvillus region of the epithelia that line the gastrointestinal tract. The highest concentration usually is detected in the jejunum. Histologic section results reveal villus atrophy and blunting, epithelial flattening, and inflammation of the lamina propria.

Treatment

Often the diarrheal illness attributable to cryptosporidiosis is self-limited in *immunocompetent* patients and requires no specific antimicrobial therapy. Treatment should focus on supportive care, including rehydration orally or, if fluid losses are severe, intravenously. Nitazoxanide (100 mg bid PO for 3 days for children 1-3 yr of age; 200 mg bid PO for children 4-11 yr of age; 500 mg bid PO for children ≥ 12 yr of age) is approved for treatment of diarrhea caused by *Cryptosporidium.* Clinical studies have not definitively demonstrated that nitazoxanide is superior to placebo in trials of HIV-infected (with low CD4 counts) or immunocompromised patients. However, given the severity of the infection in these populations, nitazoxanide treatment is usually initiated. In patients with HIV infection, treatment with combination antiretroviral therapy should also be administered to improve immune function. Other agents that have been suggested for treatment in clinical reports or small studies include orally administered human serum immunoglobulin or bovine colostrum, paromomycin, spiramycin, azithromycin, and roxithromycin or a combination of antibiotics.

CYSTOISOSPORA

Like *Cryptosporidium, Cystoisospora belli* is implicated as a cause of diarrhea in institutional outbreaks and in travelers and has also been linked with contaminated water and food. *Cystoisospora* appears to be more common in tropical and subtropical climates and in developing areas, including South America, Africa, and Southeast Asia. *Cystoisospora* has not been associated with animal contact. It is also an infrequent cause of diarrhea in patients with AIDS in the United States but may infect up to 15% of AIDS patients in Haiti.

The life cycle and pathogenesis of infection with *Cystoisospora* species are similar to those of *Cryptosporidium* organisms except that oocysts excreted in the stool are not immediately infectious and must undergo further maturation at temperatures below 37°C (98.6°F). Thus, direct person-to-person transmission is unlikely. The most common clinical manifestation is watery, nonbloody diarrhea. Symptoms of infection are indistinguishable from those of cryptosporidiosis, although fever may be a more common finding. Eosinophilia may be present in up to 50% of cases, contrasting with other enteric protozoan infections. The diagnosis is established by detecting the oval, 22- to 33-μm long by 10- to 19-μm wide oocysts by using modified acid-fast staining of the stool. Each oocyst contains two sporocysts, each with four sporozoites. Fecal leukocytes are not detected. Oocysts are shed in low numbers, underscoring the need for repeated stool examinations. The presence of oocysts in the gastrointestinal track is almost always associated with clinical symptoms. The histologic appearance of the gastrointestinal epithelium reveals blunting and atrophy of the villi, acute and chronic inflammation, and crypt hyperplasia.

Isosporiasis responds promptly to treatment with oral trimethoprim-sulfamethoxazole (TMP-SMX: 5 mg TMP and 25 mg SMX/kg/dose; [maximum: 160 mg TMP and 800 mg SMX/dose] bid for 10 days). In patients with AIDS, relapses are common and often necessitate higher doses of TMP/SMX and/or maintenance therapy. Combination antiretroviral therapy associated with immune recovery may also result in improved symptoms. Ciprofloxacin or a regimen of pyrimethamine alone or with folinic acid is effective in patients intolerant of sulfonamide drugs.

CYCLOSPORA

Cyclospora cayetanensis is a coccidian parasite similar to but larger than *Cryptosporidium.* The organism infects both immunocompromised and immunocompetent individuals and is more common in children younger than 18 mo of age. The pathogenesis and pathologic findings of cyclosporiasis are similar to those of isosporiasis. Asymptomatic carriage of the organism has been found, but travelers who harbor the organism almost always have diarrhea. Outbreaks of cyclosporiasis are linked with contaminated food and water. Implicated foods include raspberries, lettuce, snow peas, basil, and other fresh food items. After fecal excretion, the oocysts must sporulate outside the host to become infectious. This finding explains the lack of person-to-person transmission.

The clinical manifestations of cyclosporiasis are similar to those of cryptosporidiosis and isosporiasis and follow an incubation period of approximately 7 days. Moderate *Cyclospora* illness is characterized by a median of 6 stools/day with a median duration of 10 days (range: 3-25 days). The duration of diarrhea in immunocompetent persons is characteristically longer in cyclosporiasis than in the other intestinal protozoan illnesses. Associated symptoms frequently include anorexia; fatigue; abdominal bloating or gas; abdominal cramps or pain; nausea; muscle, joint, or body aches; low-grade fever; chills; headache; and weight loss. Vomiting may occur. Bloody stools are uncommon. Biliary disease has been reported. Intestinal pathology includes inflammation with villus blunting.

The diagnosis is established by identification of oocysts in the stool or molecular diagnostic testing. Oocysts are wrinkled spheres, measure 8-10 μm in diameter, and resemble large *Cryptosporidium* organisms. Each oocyst contains two sporocysts, each with two sporozoites. The organisms can be seen by using modified acid-fast, auramine-phenol, or modified trichrome staining, but stain less consistently than *Cryptosporidium.* They can also be detected with phenosafranin stain and by autofluorescence using strong green or intense blue under ultraviolet epifluorescence. Multiple stool samples enhance identification of the pathogen. Fecal leukocytes are not present. Commercially available multiplex molecular test panels for gastrointestinal pathogens that include *Cyclospora* are now available and may become the new standard.

The treatment of choice for cyclosporiasis is TMP-SMX (5 mg TMP and 25 mg SMX/kg/dose bid PO for 7 days; maximum: 160 mg TMP and 800 mg SMX/dose). Ciprofloxacin or nitazoxanide is effective in patients intolerant of sulfonamide drugs.

MICROSPORIDIA

Microsporidia are ubiquitous and infect most animal groups, including humans. They are classified as fungi, and multiple species of the phylum Microsporidia have been linked with human disease in both immunocompetent and immunocompromised hosts. The species most commonly associated with gastrointestinal disease are *Enterocytozoon bieneusi* and *Encephalitozoon intestinalis*.

Although still not definitive, the source of human infections is likely zoonotic. Like *Cryptosporidium,* there is concern for waterborne transmission through occupational and recreational contact with contaminated water sources. There is also the potential for foodborne outbreaks; the organisms have been identified on vegetables as a consequence of contaminated irrigation water. Vector-borne transmission is hypothesized because one species, *Brachiola algerae,* typically infects mosquitoes. Finally, transplacental transmission has been reported in animals but not in humans. Once infected, intracellular division produces new spores that can spread to nearby cells, disseminate to other host tissues, or be passed into the environment via feces. Spores also have been detected in urine and respiratory epithelium, suggesting that some body fluids may also be infectious. Once in the environment, microsporidial spores remain infectious for up to 4 mo.

Initially, microsporidial intestinal infection had been almost exclusively reported in patients with AIDS, but there is increasing evidence that immunocompetent individuals are also commonly infected. Microsporidia-associated diarrhea is intermittent, copious, watery, and nonbloody. Abdominal cramping and weight loss may be present; fever is unusual. Stromal keratitis and encephalitis may also be associated with microsporidia infections. Disseminated disease involving most organs, including liver, heart, kidney, bladder, biliary tract, lung, bone, skeletal muscle, and sinuses, has been reported.

Microsporidia stain with modified trichrome, hematoxylin-eosin, Giemsa, Gram, periodic acid–Schiff, and acid-fast stains, but are often overlooked because of their small size (1-5 μm) and the absence of associated inflammation in surrounding tissues. Electron microscopy remains the reference method of detection. An immunofluorescence assay is available. The Centers for Disease Control and Prevention offer a molecular identification of *Enterocytozoon bieneusi, Encephalitozoon intestinalis, Encephalitozoon hellem,* and *Encephalitozoon cuniculi* using species-specific polymerase chain reaction (PCR) assays.

There is no proven therapy for microsporidial intestinal infections. Albendazole (adult dose 400 mg bid PO for 3 wk; for children, 7.5 mg/kg body weight [maximum 400 mg/dose] bid PO) is usually effective against *E. intestinalis* infection, but is ineffective against infection caused by some microsporidial species. Fumagillin (adult dose 20 mg tid PO for 2 wk) was effective in a small controlled study of adults with *E. bieneusi* infection, and topical therapy with this agent was also demonstrated to be effective in HIV-infected adults with keratoconjunctivitis. Fumagillin is not currently available in the United States. Supportive care with hydration, correction of electrolyte imbalances, and nutrition should be used in gastrointestinal infection when clinically indicated. Improvement in underlying HIV infection with combination antiretroviral therapy also improves microsporidiosis symptoms.

Bibliography is available at Expert Consult.

Chapter **310**

Trichomoniasis (*Trichomonas vaginalis*)

Edsel Maurice T. Salvana and Robert A. Salata

第三百一十章
滴虫（阴道滴虫）

中文导读

　　本章主要阐述了滴虫病的流行病学、发病机制、临床表现、诊断、并发症、治疗和预防。其中流行病学部分介绍了滴虫病流行现状和传播方式。临床表现部分介绍了滴虫病的不同疾病状态表现，包括症状性感染和无症状感染。治疗部分介绍了成人和儿童滴虫病不同的治疗方案以及治疗失败后的备选方案。

Trichomoniasis is caused by the protozoan *Trichomonas vaginalis*. It is the second most common sexually transmitted infection worldwide. Vulvovaginitis is the symptomatic disease form, but *T. vaginalis* has been implicated in pelvic inflammatory disease, pregnancy loss, chronic prostatitis, and an increased risk of HIV transmission.

EPIDEMIOLOGY

Over 276 million new cases of trichomoniasis occur annually, making it the most common nonviral sexually transmitted infection globally. Most men and up to 30% of women are asymptomatic. Although the disease is easily treated, sequelae of untreated infection remain a significant cause of morbidity because of high reinfection rates from untreated partners, underrecognition of asymptomatic cases, and insensitive diagnostics.

Trichomoniasis is the most common parasitic infection in the United States, with a total of 3.7 million cases and approximately 1.1 million new infections per year. *T. vaginalis* is recovered from > 60% of female partners of infected men and 70% of male sexual partners of infected women. Vaginal trichomoniasis is rare until menarche. Its presence in a younger child should raise the possibility of **sexual abuse.**

Trichomoniasis may be transmitted to neonates during passage through an infected birth canal. Infection in this setting is usually self-limited, but rare cases of neonatal vaginitis and respiratory infection have been reported.

PATHOGENESIS

T. vaginalis is an anaerobic, flagellated protozoan parasite. Infected vaginal secretions contain 10^1 to 10^5 or more protozoa/mL. *T. vaginalis* is pear shaped and exhibits characteristic twitching motility in wet mount (Fig. 310.1). Reproduction is by binary fission. It exists only as vegetative cells; cyst forms have not been described. Many types of adhesion molecules allow attachment of *T. vaginalis* to host cells. Tv lipoglycan is a surface glycoconjugate that binds human galectin-1 and -3 and plays a major role in adhesion, pathogenesis, and immune modulation. In addition, hundreds of putative membrane proteins, BspA proteins, and tetraspanins are involved in cellular attachment. Some of these proteins are contained in exosome vesicles, along with a large concentration of RNA oligonucleotides, which seem to further enhance adhesion. Adhesion is a prerequisite to cytolysis, and once attached the parasite secretes hydrolases, proteases, and cytotoxic molecules that destroy or impair the integrity of host cells. *Trichomonas* is highly dependent on iron for its growth and metabolism, and cysteine proteinase mRNAs have been shown to interact with other parasite proteins for posttranscriptional regulation in the absence of iron-regulatory proteins, which are present in other eukaryotes. This dependence on iron may partially explain the propensity of *T. vaginalis* to infect women due to a higher iron state during menses. The *T. vaginalis* genome is very large, with multiple repetitive sequences and transposable elements making up over 60,000 genes, as well as apparently nonfunctional but transcribed pseudogenes. This unusually large number of genetic elements is thought to have an adaptive function, with differential gene expression occurring in response to differing conditions, giving the organism flexibility for survival.

Macrophage migration and cytokine production have been shown to be downregulated by the parasite in successful infection. Parasite-specific antibodies and lymphocyte priming occur in response to infection, but durable protective immunity does not occur, possibly also owing to degradation of antibodies by parasitic cysteine proteases.

CLINICAL MANIFESTATIONS

The incubation period in females is 5-28 days. Symptoms may begin or worsen with menses. Most infected women eventually develop symptoms, although up to one third remain asymptomatic. Common signs and symptoms include a copious malodorous gray, frothy vaginal discharge, vulvovaginal irritation, dysuria, and dyspareunia. Physical examination may reveal a frothy discharge with vaginal erythema and cervical hemorrhages (strawberry cervix). The discharge usually has a pH of > 4.5. Abdominal discomfort is unusual and should prompt evaluation for pelvic inflammatory disease (see Chapter 146).

Most infections in males are asymptomatic. Symptomatic males usually have dysuria and scant urethral discharge. Trichomonads occasionally cause epididymitis, prostatic involvement, and superficial penile ulceration. Infection is often self-limited, spontaneously resolving in 36% of men. *Trichomonas* has been implicated as a cause of recurrent or relapsing urethritis and can be isolated in 3–20% of men with nongonococcal urethritis. Treatment failures with standard therapy for gonorrhea and *Chlamydia* are frequently treated with antitrichomonal therapy.

DIAGNOSIS

Trichomonads may be recognized in vaginal secretions by wet mount microscopy. This has a sensitivity of approximately 35–60% compared with culture and nucleic acid techniques. Although *Trichomonas* is sometimes seen on Pap smears and urine microscopy, these methods are not considered reliable tests for disease. Culture of the organism used to be the gold standard for detection, but this is increasingly being replaced by nucleic acid amplification tests, which are at least as sensitive. The APTIMA TV (Hologic/Gen-Probe, Inc., Marlborough, MA) assay and the BD Probe Tec TV Q^x Amplified DNA Assay (Becton Dickinson, Franklin Lakes, NJ) are U.S. Food and Drug Administration (FDA) cleared commercial NAATs for testing of samples from men and women. Xpert TV (Cepheid Inc., Sunnyvale, CA) is a cartridge-based nucleic acid test that is FDA-cleared but only for use on urine, endocervical, and vaginal swabs in women. Two point-of-care kits for rapid testing, Affirm VP III (BD Diagnostic Systems, Sparks, MD) and OSOM Trichomonas Rapid Test (Sekisui Diagnostics, Lexington, MA), are also FDA-cleared for use in women and yield results in 45 min and 10 min, respectively. Patients with *T. vaginalis* should be screened for other sexually transmitted infections. Multiplex nucleic acid formats for rapid diagnosis of multiple sexually transmitted diseases including *Trichomonas* have also been developed and are in clinical trials.

COMPLICATIONS

Untreated trichomoniasis has been associated with pelvic inflammatory disease, premature delivery, low birthweight, endometritis, salpingitis, and vaginal cuff cellulitis. The association between trichomoniasis and infertility is relatively weak, but there is some evidence that coinfection with other STIs increases the overall risk of PID. *T. vaginalis* infection increases the risk of acquisition and transmission of HIV. In HIV-infected individuals, trichomoniasis is associated with higher viral loads in cervical secretions and semen, as well as higher levels of infected lymphocytes in urogenital fluids.

TREATMENT

In the United States, metronidazole and tinidazole are used; in other countries, ornidazole is also used. Both metronidazole (single-dose regimen of 2 g orally as a single dose for adolescents and adults; alternative regimen, 500 mg orally bid for 7 days) and tinidazole (single 2 g dose orally in adolescents and adults) are used as first-line treatments.

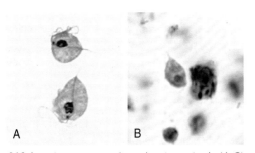

Fig. 310.1 *Trichomonas vaginalis* trophozoites stained with Giemsa **(A)** and iron hematoxylin **(B).** *(From the Centers for Disease Control and Prevention: Laboratory identification of parasites of public health concern. Trichomoniasis (website). https://www.cdc.gov/dpdx/trichomoniasis/index.html.)*

For children infected prior to adolescence, the recommended regimen is metronidazole 15 mg/kg/day divided in 3 doses orally for 7 days; tinidazole is not approved for dosing in younger children. For HIV-infected patients, the 7-day course of metronidazole is superior to and recommended over the single dose regimen. Topical metronidazole gel is not efficacious as monotherapy but may decrease symptoms in severe infection in conjunction with oral therapy. Sexual partners should be treated simultaneously to prevent reinfection. Multiple head-to-head trials comparing the efficacy between single-dose/short courses of metronidazole and single-dose tinidazole have shown either noninferiority or superior efficacy for tinidazole. Tinidazole is more expensive than metronidazole and is generally reserved for treatment failures or intolerance. A small number of patients with severe nitroimidazole hypersensitivity have been treated with intravaginal suppositories of boric acid, nitazoxanide, and paromomycin with varying degrees of success.

Treatment failures have been reported with metronidazole, although a poor response can usually be overcome by higher doses. Second-line treatment is either a 7-day course of metronidazole 500 mg twice daily or a single dose of tinidazole. If this approach fails, either metronidazole or tinidazole at 2 g daily for 5 days is recommended. Further treatment failure should be referred to an infectious diseases specialist and may require susceptibility testing, which is available from the Centers for Disease Control and Prevention. Metronidazole has not been shown to be teratogenic but is currently classified as a category C drug. A Cochrane metanalysis previously showed an association between premature births with metronidazole treatment of asymptomatic *T. vaginalis* infection in pregnancy. Other studies have shown no harm from metronidazole treatment in this setting. Treatment of trichomoniasis in pregnancy should always be considered, especially in symptomatic patients, and may decrease the risk of perinatal transmission.

PREVENTION

Prevention of *T. vaginalis* infection is best accomplished by treatment of all sexual partners of an infected person, and by programs aimed at prevention of all sexually transmitted infections (see Chapter 146). No vaccine is available, and drug prophylaxis is not recommended.

Bibliography available at Expert Consult.

Chapter **311**

Leishmaniasis (Leishmania)

Peter C. Melby

第三百一十一章

利什曼病（利什曼原虫）

中文导读

　　本章主要介绍了利什曼病的病原学、流行病学、病理、临床表现、鉴别诊断、诊断、治疗和预防。以表格形式详细列出了利什曼原虫不同种的临床表现和流行病学特征。在临床表现部分，分别详细阐述了局部皮肤利什曼病、弥漫性皮肤利什曼病、传播利什曼病、黏膜利什曼病、内脏利什曼病的临床表现特点。

The leishmaniases are a diverse group of diseases caused by intracellular protozoan parasites of the genus *Leishmania,* which are transmitted by phlebotomine sandflies. Multiple species of *Leishmania* are known to cause human disease involving the skin and mucosal surfaces and the visceral reticuloendothelial organs (Table 311.1). Cutaneous disease is usually localized and mild but may cause cosmetic disfigurement. Rarely, cutaneous infection can disseminate or involve the skin diffusely. Mucosal and visceral forms of leishmaniasis are associated with significant morbidity and mortality.

ETIOLOGY

Leishmania organisms are members of the Trypanosomatidae family and include 2 subgenera, *Leishmania (Leishmania)* and *Leishmania (Viannia).* The parasite is dimorphic, existing as a flagellate promastigote in the insect vector and as an aflagellate amastigote that resides and replicates within mononuclear phagocytes of the vertebrate host. Within the **sandfly** vector, the promastigote changes from a noninfective procyclic form to an infective metacyclic stage (Fig. 311.1). Fundamental to this transition are changes that take place in the terminal polysaccharides

Table 311.1 Clinical and Epidemiologic Characteristics of Main *Leishmania* spp.

SUBGENUS	CLINICAL FORM	MAIN CLINICAL FEATURES	NATURAL PROGRESSION	RISK GROUPS	MAIN RESERVOIR	HIGH-BURDEN COUNTRIES OR REGIONS	ESTIMATED ANNUAL WORLDWIDE INCIDENCE
*Leishmania donovani** *Leishmania*	VL, PKDL	Persistent fever, splenomegaly, weight loss, and anemia in VL; multiple painless macular, papular, or nodular lesions in PKDL	VL is fatal within 2 yr; PKDL lesions self-heal in up to 85% of cases in Africa but rarely in Asia	Predominantly adolescents and young adults for VL; young children in Sudan and no clearly established risk factors for PKDL	Humans	India, Bangladesh, Ethiopia, Sudan, and South Sudan	50,000-90,000 VL cases; unknown number of PKDL cases
*Leishmania tropica** *Leishmania*	CL, LR, rarely VL	Ulcerating dry lesions, painless, and frequently multiple	CL lesions often self-heal within 1 yr	No well-defined risk groups	Humans, but zoonotic foci exist	Eastern Mediterranean, Middle East, northeastern and southern Africa	200,000-400,000 CL
*Leishmania aethiopica** *Leishmania*	CL, DCL, DsCL, oronasal CL	Localized cutaneous nodular lesions; occasionally oronasal; rarely ulcerates	Self-healing, except for DCL, within 2-5 yr	Limited evidence; adolescents	Hyraxes	Ethiopia, Kenya	20,000-40,000 CL
*Leishmania major** *Leishmania*	CL	Rapid necrosis, multiple wet sores, severe inflammation	Self-healing in >50% of cases within 2-8 mo; multiple lesions slow to heal, and severe scarring	No well-defined risk groups	Rodents	Iran, Saudi Arabia, North Africa, Middle East, Central Asia, West Africa	230,000-430,000 CL
*Leishmania infantum** *Leishmania*	VL, CL	Persistent fever and splenomegaly in VL; typically single nodules and minimal inflammation in CL	VL is fatal within 2 yr; CL lesions self-heal within 1 yr and confers individual immunity	Children <5 yr old and immunocompromised adults for VL; older children and young adults for CL	Dogs, hares, humans	China, southern Europe, Brazil, and South America for VL and CL; Central America for CL	6,200-12,000 cases of Old World VL and 4,500-6,800 cases of New World VL; unknown number of CL cases
Leishmania mexicana† *Leishmania*	CL, DCL, DsCL	Ulcerating lesions, single or multiple	Often self-healing in 3-4 mo	No well-defined risk groups	Rodents, marsupials	South America	Limited number of cases, included in the 187,200-300,000 total cases of New World CL‡
Leishmania amazonensis† *Leishmania*	CL, DCL, DsCL	Ulcerating lesions, single or multiple	Not well described	No well-defined risk groups	Possums, rodents	South America	Limited number of cases, included in the 187,200-300,000 total cases of New World CL‡
Leishmania braziliensis† *Viannia*	CL, MCL, DCL, LR	Ulcerating lesions can progress to mucocutaneous form; local lymph nodes are palpable before and early on in the onset of the lesions	Might self-heal in 6 mo; 2.5% of cases progress to MCL	No well-defined risk groups	Dogs, humans, rodents, horses	South America	Majority of the 187,200-300,000 total cases of New World CL‡
Leishmania guyanensis† *Viannia*	CL, DsCL, MCL	Ulcerating lesions, single or multiple that can progress to mucocutaneous form; palpable lymph nodes	Might self-heal within 6 mo	No well-defined risk groups	Possums, sloths, anteaters	South America	Limited number of cases, included in the 187,200-300,000 total cases of New World CL‡

*Old World leishmaniasis.
†New World leishmaniasis.
‡Estimates are of all New World leishmaniases, with *Leishmania braziliensis* comprising the vast majority of these cases.
CL, Cutaneous leishmaniasis; DCL, diffuse cutaneous leishmaniasis; DsCL, disseminated cutaneous leishmaniasis; LR, leishmaniasis recidivans; MCL, mucocutaneous leishmaniasis; PKDL, post-kala-azar dermal leishmaniasis; VL, visceral leishmaniasis.
Adapted from Burza S, Croft SL, Boelaert ML: Leishmaniasis, *Lancet* 392:951-966, 2018 (Table 1).

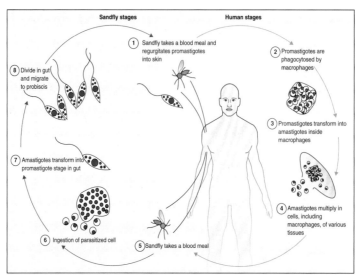

Fig. 311.1 *Leishmania* life cycle. *(From Reithinger R, Dujardin JC, Louzir H, et al: Cutaneous leishmaniasis, Lancet Infect Dis 7:581–596, 2007, Fig 5.)*

of the surface **lipophosphoglycan**, which allow forward migration of the infective parasites to be inoculated in the host skin during a blood meal. Metacyclic lipophosphoglycan also plays an important role in the entry and survival of *Leishmania* in the host cells. Once within the macrophage, the promastigote transforms to an amastigote and resides and replicates within a phagolysosome. The parasite is resistant to the acidic, hostile environment of the macrophage and eventually ruptures the cell and goes on to infect other macrophages. Infected macrophages have a diminished capacity to initiate and respond to an inflammatory response, thus providing a safe haven for the intracellular parasite.

EPIDEMIOLOGY

The leishmaniases are estimated to affect 10-20 million people in endemic tropical and subtropical regions on all continents except Australia and Antarctica. The different forms of the disease are distinct in their causes, epidemiologic characteristics, transmission, and geographic distribution. The leishmaniases may occur sporadically throughout an endemic region or may occur in epidemic waves. With only rare exceptions, the *Leishmania* organisms that primarily cause cutaneous disease do not cause visceral disease.

Localized cutaneous leishmaniasis (**LCL**) in the Old World is caused by *L. (Leishmania) major* and *L. (L.) tropica* in North Africa, the Middle East, Central Asia, and the Indian subcontinent. *L. (L.) aethiopica* is a cause of LCL and **diffuse cutaneous leishmaniasis (DCL)** in Kenya and Ethiopia. In the New World, *L. (L.) mexicana* causes LCL in a region stretching from southern Texas through Central America. *L. (L.) amazonensis, L. (L.) pifanoi, L. (L.) garnhami,* and *L. (L.) venezuelensis* cause LCL in South America, the Amazon basin, and northward. These parasites can also cause DCL. Members of the *Viannia* subgenus (*L. [V.] braziliensis, L. [V.] panamensis, L. [V.] guyanensis,* and *L. [V.] peruviana*) cause LCL and **mucosal leishmaniasis (ML)** from the northern highlands of Argentina northward to Central America. Some species, particularly *L. (V.) braziliensis,* rarely cause **disseminated leishmaniasis (DL)**. **Visceral leishmaniasis (VL)** in the Old World is caused by *L. (L.) donovani* in Kenya, Sudan, India, Pakistan, and China and by *L. (L.) infantum* in the Mediterranean basin, Middle East, and central Asia. *L. tropica* also has been recognized as an uncommon cause of visceral disease in the Middle East and India. VL in the New World is caused by *L. (L.) infantum* (formerly also called *L. chagasi*), which is distributed through Mexico (rare) through Central and South America. *L. infantum* can also cause LCL in the absence of visceral disease in this same geographic distribution.

The maintenance of *Leishmania* in most endemic areas is through a **zoonotic** transmission cycle. In general, the dermotropic strains in both the Old and the New World are maintained in rodent reservoirs, and the domestic dog is the usual reservoir for *L. infantum.* The transmission between reservoir and sandfly is highly adapted to the specific ecologic characteristics of the endemic region. Human infections occur when human activities bring them in contact with the zoonotic cycle. **Anthroponotic** transmission, in which humans are the presumed reservoir for vector-borne transmission, occurs with *L. tropica* in some urban areas of the Middle East and Central Asia, and with *L. donovani* in India and Sudan. Congenital transmission of *L. donovani* or *L. infantum* has been reported.

There is a resurgence of leishmaniasis in long-standing endemic areas as well as in new foci. Tens of thousands of cases of LCL occurred in outbreaks in Syria and Kabul, Afghanistan; severe epidemics with >100,000 deaths from VL have occurred in India and Sudan. VL is most prevalent among the poorest of the poor, with substandard housing contributing to the vector-borne transmission and undernutrition leading to increased host susceptibility. The emergence of the leishmaniases in new areas is the result of (1) movement of a susceptible population into existing endemic areas, usually because of agricultural or industrial development or timber harvesting; (2) increase in vector and/or reservoir populations as a result of agriculture development projects or climate change; (3) increase in anthroponotic transmission resulting from rapid urbanization in some focuses; and (4) increase in sandfly density resulting from a reduction in vector control programs.

PATHOLOGY

Histopathologic analysis of the skin lesions of LCL and DL show intense chronic granulomatous inflammation involving the epidermis and dermis with relatively few amastigotes. Occasionally, neutrophils and even microabscesses can be seen. The lesions of DCL are characterized by dense infiltration with vacuolated macrophages containing abundant amastigotes. ML is characterized by an intense granulomatous reaction with prominent tissue necrosis, which may include adjacent cartilage or bone. In VL there is prominent reticuloendothelial cell hyperplasia in the liver, spleen, bone marrow, and lymph nodes. Amastigotes are abundant in the histiocytes and Kupffer cells. Late in the course of disease, splenic infarcts are common, centrilobular necrosis and fatty infiltration of the liver occur, the normal marrow elements are replaced by parasitized histiocytes, and erythrophagocytosis is present.

PATHOGENESIS

Cellular immune mechanisms determine resistance or susceptibility to infection with *Leishmania*. Resistance is mediated by interleukin (IL)-12–driven generation of a T helper 1 (Th1) cell response, with interferon (IFN)-γ inducing classic macrophage (M1) activation and parasite killing. Susceptibility is associated with expansion of IL-4–producing Th2 cells and/or the production of IL-10 and transforming growth factor (TGF)-β, which are inhibitors of macrophage-mediated parasite killing, and the generation of regulatory T cells and alternatively activated (M2) macrophages. Patients with ML exhibit a hyperresponsive cellular immune reaction that may contribute to the prominent tissue destruction seen in this form of the disease. Patients with DCL or active VL demonstrate reduced or altered *Leishmania*-specific cellular immune responses, with prominent generation of IL-10, but these responses recover after successful therapy.

Within endemic areas, people who have had a subclinical infection can be identified by a positive delayed-type hypersensitivity skin response to leishmanial antigens (**Montenegro skin test**) or by antigen-induced production of IFN-γ in a whole blood assay. Subclinical infection occurs considerably more frequently than does active cutaneous or visceral disease. **Host** factors (genetic background, concomitant disease, nutritional status), **parasite** factors (virulence, size of the inoculum), and possibly **vector**-specific factors (vector genotype, immunomodulatory salivary constituents) influence the expression as either subclinical infection or active disease. Within endemic areas, the prevalence of skin test positivity increases with age, and the incidence of clinical disease decreases with age, indicating that immunity is acquired in the population over time. Individuals with prior active disease or subclinical infection are usually immune to a subsequent clinical infection; however, latent infection can lead to active disease if the patient is immunosuppressed.

CLINICAL MANIFESTATIONS

The different forms of the disease are distinct in their causes, epidemiologic features, transmission, and geographic distribution.

Localized Cutaneous Leishmaniasis

LCL (**Oriental sore**) can affect individuals of any age, but children are the primary victims in many endemic regions. It may present as 1 or a few papular, nodular, plaque-like, or ulcerative lesions that are usually located on exposed skin, such as the face and extremities (Fig. 311.2). Rarely, >100 lesions have been recorded. The lesions typically begin as a small papule at the site of the sandfly bite, which enlarges to 1-3 cm in diameter and may ulcerate over the course of several weeks to months. The shallow ulcer is usually nontender and surrounded by a sharp, indurated, erythematous margin. There is no drainage unless a bacterial superinfection develops. Lesions caused by *L. major* and *L. mexicana* usually heal spontaneously after 3-6 mo, leaving a depressed scar. Lesions on the ear pinna caused by *L. mexicana*, called **chiclero ulcer** because they were common in chicle harvesters in Mexico and Central America, often follow a chronic, destructive course. In general, lesions caused by *L. (Viannia)* species tend to be larger and more chronic. Regional lymphadenopathy and palpable subcutaneous nodules or lymphatic cords, the so-called sporotrichoid appearance, are also more common when the patient is infected with organisms of the *Viannia* subgenus. If lesions do not become secondarily infected, there are usually no complications aside from the residual cutaneous scar.

Diffuse Cutaneous Leishmaniasis

DCL is a rare form of leishmaniasis caused by organisms of the *L. mexicana* complex in the New World and *L. aethiopica* in the Old World. DCL manifests as large, nonulcerating macules, papules, nodules, or plaques that often involve large areas of skin and may resemble lepromatous leprosy. The face and extremities are most often involved. Dissemination from the initial lesion usually takes place over several years. These patients are anergic to the Montenegro skin test, and it is thought that an immunologic defect underlies this severe form of cutaneous leishmaniasis.

Disseminated Leishmaniasis

In rare cases, parasites can spread (likely by the hematogenous route) in an immunocompetent host from a primary lesion to cause DL. This is defined as >10 lesions (usually in the hundreds) involving at least 2 noncontiguous areas of the skin. DL has been most often attributed to *L. (V.) braziliensis*. The lesions are typically inflammatory papules or ulcers, in contrast to the nodular and plaque-like lesions of DCL, and about one third of patients have mucosal involvement.

Mucosal Leishmaniasis

ML (**espundia**) is an uncommon but serious manifestation of leishmanial infection resulting from hematogenous spread of parasites to the nasal or oropharyngeal mucosa from a cutaneous infection. It is usually caused by parasites in the *L. (Viannia)* complex. Approximately half of the patients with mucosal lesions have had active cutaneous lesions within the preceding 2 yr, but ML may not develop until many years after resolution of the primary lesion. ML occurs in <5% of individuals who have, or have had, LCL caused by *L. (V.) braziliensis*. Patients with ML typically have nasal mucosal involvement and present with nasal congestion, discharge, and recurrent epistaxis. Oropharyngeal and laryngeal involvement is less common but associated with severe morbidity. Marked soft tissue, cartilage, and even bone destruction occurs late in the course of disease and may lead to visible deformity of the nose or mouth, nasal septal perforation, and tracheal narrowing with airway obstruction.

Visceral Leishmaniasis

VL (**kala-azar**) typically affects children <5 yr old in the New World and Mediterranean region (*L. infantum*) and older children and young adults in Africa and Asia (*L. donovani*). After inoculation of the organism into the skin by the sandfly, the child may have a completely asymptomatic infection or an oligosymptomatic illness that either resolves spontaneously or evolves into active kala-azar. Children with **asymptomatic** infection are transiently seropositive but show no clinical evidence of disease. Children who are **oligosymptomatic** have mild constitutional symptoms (malaise, intermittent diarrhea, poor activity tolerance) and intermittent fever; most will have a mildly enlarged liver. In most of these children the illness will resolve without therapy, but in approximately 25% it will evolve to active kala-azar within 2-8 mo. Extreme incubation periods of several years have rarely been described. During the 1st few wk to mo of disease evolution, the fever is intermittent, there is weakness and loss of energy, and the spleen begins to enlarge. The classic clinical features of high fever, marked splenomegaly, hepatomegaly, and severe

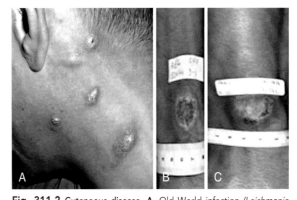

Fig. 311.2 Cutaneous disease. **A,** Old World infection (*Leishmania major*) acquired in Iraq; note 5 papular and nodular lesions on neck. **B,** New World infection (*Leishmania panamensis*) in Colombia; purely ulcerative lesion is characteristic of New World disease. **C,** Healed infection in patient shown in **B** 70 days after 20 days of meglumine antimonate treatment; note paper-thin scar tissue over flat reepithelialized skin. (A, courtesy of P. Weina; B, courtesy of J. Soto. A-C, modified from Murray HW, Berman JD, Davies CR, et al: Advances in leishmaniasis, Lancet 366:1561–1577, 2005.)

cachexia typically develop 3-6 mo after the onset of the illness, but a rapid clinical course over 1 mo has been noted in up to 20% of patients in some series (Fig. 311.3). At the terminal stages of kala-azar, the hepatosplenomegaly is massive, there is gross wasting, the pancytopenia is profound, and jaundice, edema, and ascites may be present. Anemia may be severe enough to precipitate heart failure. Bleeding episodes, especially epistaxis, are frequent. The late stage of the illness is often complicated by secondary bacterial infections, which frequently are a cause of death. A younger age at the time of infection, HIV co-infection, and underlying malnutrition are risk factors for the development and more rapid evolution of active VL. Death occurs in >90% of patients without specific antileishmanial treatment and in 4–10% of treated patients. VL is a known cause of **hemophagocytic lymphohistiocytosis** in endemic areas.

VL is an opportunistic infection associated with **HIV infection**. Most cases have occurred in southern Europe and Brazil, often as a result of needle sharing associated with illicit drug use, with the potential for many more cases as the endemic regions for HIV and VL converge. Leishmaniasis may also result from reactivation of a long-standing subclinical infection. Frequently there is an atypical clinical presentation of VL in HIV-infected individuals with prominent involvement of the gastrointestinal tract and absence of the typical hepatosplenomegaly.

A small percentage of patients previously treated for VL develop diffuse skin lesions, a condition known as **post–kala-azar dermal leishmaniasis.** These lesions may appear during or shortly after therapy (Africa) or up to several years later (India). The lesions of post–kala-azar dermal leishmaniasis are hypopigmented, erythematous, or nodular and usually involve the face and torso. They may persist for several months or for many years.

LABORATORY FINDINGS

Patients with cutaneous leishmaniasis or ML generally do not have abnormal laboratory results unless the lesions are secondarily infected with bacteria. Laboratory findings associated with classic kala-azar include anemia (hemoglobin, 5-8 mg/dL), thrombocytopenia, leukopenia (2,000-3,000 cells/μL), elevated hepatic transaminase levels, and hyperglobulinemia (>5 g/dL) that is mostly immunoglobulin G.

DIFFERENTIAL DIAGNOSIS

Diseases that should be considered in the differential diagnosis of LCL include sporotrichosis, blastomycosis, chromomycosis, lobomycosis, cutaneous tuberculosis, atypical mycobacterial infection, leprosy, ecthyma, syphilis, yaws, and neoplasms. Infections such as syphilis, tertiary yaws, histoplasmosis, and paracoccidioidomycosis, as well as sarcoidosis, granulomatosis with polyangiitis, midline granuloma, and carcinoma, may have clinical features similar to those of ML. VL should be strongly suspected in the patient with prolonged fever, weakness, cachexia, marked splenomegaly, hepatomegaly, cytopenias, and hypergammaglobulinemia who has had potential exposure in an endemic area. The clinical picture may also be consistent with that of malaria, typhoid fever, miliary tuberculosis, schistosomiasis, brucellosis, amebic liver abscess, infectious mononucleosis, lymphoma, and leukemia.

DIAGNOSIS

The development of 1 or several slowly progressive, nontender, nodular, or ulcerative lesions in a patient who had potential exposure in an endemic area should raise suspicion of LCL.

Serologic tests for diagnosis of cutaneous or mucosal disease generally have low sensitivity and specificity and offer little for diagnosis. Serologic testing by enzyme immunoassay, indirect fluorescence assay, or direct agglutination is very useful in VL because of the very high level of antileishmanial antibodies. An immunochromatographic strip test using a recombinant antigen (K39) has a diagnostic sensitivity and specificity for VL of 80–90% and 95%, respectively. Serodiagnostic tests have positive findings in only about half the patients co-infected with HIV.

Definitive diagnosis of leishmaniasis is established by the demonstration of amastigotes in tissue specimens or isolation of the organism by culture. **Amastigotes** can be identified in Giemsa-stained tissue sections, aspirates, or impression smears in about half the cases of LCL but only

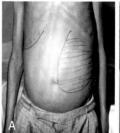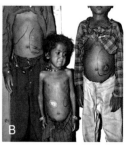

Fig. 311.3 Visceral leishmaniasis *(Leishmania donovani)* in Bihar State, India. **A,** Hepatosplenomegaly and wasting in a young man. **B,** Children with burn marks over enlarged spleen or liver—local shaman's unsuccessful remedy. *(A, Courtesy of D. Sacks; B, courtesy of R. Kenney; A and B, adapted from Murray HW, Berman JD, Davies CR, et al: Advances in leishmaniasis, Lancet 366:1561–1577, 2005.)*

rarely in the lesions of ML. **Culture** of a tissue biopsy or aspirate, best performed by using Novy-McNeal-Nicolle biphasic blood agar medium, yields a positive finding in only approximately 65% of cases of cutaneous leishmaniasis. Identification of parasites in impression smears, histopathologic sections, or culture medium is more readily accomplished in DCL than in LCL. In patients with VL, smears or cultures of material from splenic, bone marrow, or lymph node aspirations are usually diagnostic. In experienced hands, **splenic aspiration** has a higher diagnostic sensitivity, but it is rarely performed in the United States because of the risk for bleeding complications. A positive culture result allows speciation of the parasite, usually by isoenzyme analysis by a reference laboratory, which may have therapeutic and prognostic significance.

TREATMENT

Specific antileishmanial therapy is not routinely indicated for uncomplicated LCL caused by strains that have a high rate of spontaneous resolution and self-healing *(L. major, L. mexicana).* Lesions that are extensive, severely inflamed, or located where a scar would result in disability (near a joint) or cosmetic disfigurement (face or ear), that involve the lymphatics, or that do not begin healing within 3-4 mo should be treated. Cutaneous lesions suspected or known to be caused by members of the *Viannia* subgenus (New World) should be treated because of the low rate of spontaneous healing and the potential risk for development of mucosal or disseminated disease. Similarly, patients with lesions caused by *L. tropica* (Old World), which are typically chronic and nonhealing, should be treated. All patients with VL or ML should receive therapy.

The pentavalent **antimony compounds** (sodium stibogluconate [Pentostam, GlaxoSmithKline, Uxbridge, UK] and **meglumine antimoniate** [Glucantime, Aventis, Strasbourg, France]) have been the mainstay of antileishmanial chemotherapy for >40 yr. These drugs have similar efficacies, toxicities, and treatment regimens. Currently, for **sodium stibogluconate** (available in the United States from the Centers for Disease Control and Prevention, Atlanta, GA), the recommended regimen is 20 mg/kg/day intravenously (IV) or intramuscularly (IM) for 20 days (for LCL and DCL) or 28 days (for ML and VL). Repeated courses of therapy may be necessary in patients with severe cutaneous lesions, ML, DCL, DL, or VL. An initial clinical response to therapy usually occurs in the 1st wk of therapy, but complete clinical healing (reepithelialization and scarring for LCL and ML, and regression of splenomegaly and normalization of cytopenias for VL) is usually not evident for weeks to a few months after completion of therapy. Cure rates with this regimen of 90–100% for LCL, 50–70% for ML, and 80–100% for VL were common in the 1990s, but treatment failures, especially in children, have become common in parts of India, East Africa, and Latin America.

Relapses are common in patients who do not have an effective antileishmanial cellular immune response (DCL or HIV co-infection). Adverse effects of antimony therapy are dose and duration dependent and include fatigue, arthralgias and myalgias (50%), abdominal discomfort (30%), elevated hepatic transaminase level (30–80%), elevated amylase and lipase levels (almost 100%), mild hematologic changes (slightly decreased leukocyte count, hemoglobin level, and platelet count) (10–30%), and nonspecific T-wave changes on electrocardiography (30%). Sudden death from cardiac toxicity has rarely been reported with use of very high doses of pentavalent antimony.

Amphotericin B desoxycholate and the amphotericin lipid formulations are very useful in the treatment of VL, ML or DL, and in some regions have replaced antimony as first-line therapy, especially in HIV-infected patients. However, the prohibitively high cost of these drugs precludes their use in many resource-poor regions of the world. Amphotericin B desoxycholate at doses of 0.5-1.0 mg/kg every day or every other day for 14-20 doses achieved a cure rate for VL of close to 100%, but the renal toxicity associated with amphotericin B was common. The lipid formulations of amphotericin B are especially attractive for treatment of leishmaniasis because the drugs are concentrated in the reticuloendothelial system and are less nephrotoxic. Liposomal amphotericin B is highly effective, with a 90–100% cure rate for VL in immunocompetent children, some of whom were refractory to antimony therapy. **Liposomal amphotericin B** (AmBisome, Gilead Sciences, Foster City, CA) is approved by the U.S. Food and Drug Administration (FDA) for treatment of VL at a recommended dose for *immunocompetent patients* of 3 mg/kg on days 1-5, 14, and 21 (total dose 21 mg/kg) and should be considered for first-line therapy in the United States. Therapy for *immunocompromised patients* should be prolonged (recommended total dose 40 mg/kg). A single high dose of liposomal amphotericin B (10 mg/kg) was found to be effective in India (approximately 95% efficacy) but was less effective in East Africa (58% efficacy).

Parenteral treatment of VL with the aminoglycoside **paromomycin** (aminosidine) has efficacy (95%) similar to that of amphotericin B in India. A dose-sparing regimen of the combination of sodium stibogluconate and paromomycin is effective and used in East Africa. **Miltefosine,** a membrane-activating alkylphospholipid, has been approved as the first oral treatment for VL and has a cure rate of 80–90% in Indian patients with VL when administered orally at 50-100 mg/day (or 2.5 mg/ kg for children <12 yr old) for 28 days. Miltefosine is indicated for cutaneous infection caused by *L. braziliensis, L. guyanensis,* and *L. panamensis*; ML caused by *L. braziliensis*; and VL caused by *L. donovani.* Gastrointestinal adverse effects were frequent but did not require discontinuation of the drug. An increased rate of relapse (up to 20%) has been seen in children treated with miltefosine. Dose-sparing combination regimens are being actively investigated for treatment of VL. Treatment of LCL with oral drugs has had only modest success. Ketoconazole has been effective in treating adults with LCL caused by *L. major, L. mexicana,* and *L. panamensis,* but not *L. tropica* or *L. braziliensis.* Fluconazole in high doses (up to 8 mg/kg/day) for 4-8 wk was demonstrated to be effective in treating LCL in studies in both the Old and New World; however, the experience in young children is limited. Miltefosine, 2.5 mg/kg/day orally for 20-28 days, was effective in 70–90% of patients with LCL in the Americas. Topical treatment of LCL with paromomycin ointment has been effective in selected areas in the both the Old and the New World. Enhanced drug development efforts and clinical trials of new drugs are clearly needed, especially in children.

PREVENTION

Personal protective measures should include avoidance of exposure to the nocturnal sandflies and, when necessary, the use of insect repellent and permethrin-impregnated mosquito netting. Where peridomiciliary transmission is present, community-based residual insecticide spraying has had some success in reducing the prevalence of leishmaniasis, but long-term effects are difficult to maintain. Control or elimination of infected reservoir hosts (e.g., seropositive domestic dogs) has had limited success. Where anthroponotic transmission is thought to occur, as in south Asia, early recognition, diagnosis, and treatment of cases and vector control measures are essential for progress toward elimination. Several vaccines have been demonstrated to have efficacy in experimental models, and vaccination of humans or domestic dogs may have a role in the control of the leishmaniases in the future.

Bibliography is available at Expert Consult.

Chapter **312**
African Trypanosomiasis (Sleeping Sickness; *Trypanosoma brucei* Complex)

Edsel Maurice T. Salvana
and Robert A. Salata

第三百一十二章
非洲锥虫病（睡眠病;布氏锥虫复合体）

中文导读

　　本章主要介绍了非洲锥虫病的病原学、生命周期、流行病学、发病机制、临床表现、诊断、治疗和预防。其中在临床表现部分，分别阐述了锥虫下疳、血液淋巴阶段（第一阶段）、脑膜脑炎阶段（第二阶段）的临床特点。在治疗部分，分别阐述了血液淋巴阶段（第一阶段）和脑膜脑炎阶段（第二阶段）的治疗药物选择和疗程。

Sixty million people in 36 countries are at risk for infection with *Trypanosoma brucei* complex, the causative agent of sleeping sickness. Also known as **human African trypanosomiasis (HAT)**, this disease is restricted to sub-Saharan Africa, the range of the tsetse fly vector. It is a disease of extreme poverty, with the highest disease burden observed in remote rural areas. HAT comes in 2 geographically and clinically distinct forms. *Trypanosoma brucei gambiense* causes a chronic infection and affects people who live in western and central Africa (**West African sleeping sickness, Gambian trypanosomiasis**). *Trypanosoma brucei rhodesiense* is a zoonosis that presents as an acute illness lasting several weeks and usually occurs in residents or travelers from eastern and southern Africa (**East African sleeping sickness, Rhodesian trypanosomiasis**).

ETIOLOGY

HAT is a vector-borne disease caused by parasitic, extracellular, flagellated kinetoplastid protozoans of 2 subspecies of *Trypanosoma brucei*. It is transmitted to humans through the bite of *Glossina*, commonly known as the **tsetse fly**.

Humans usually contract East African HAT when they venture from towns to rural areas to visit woodlands or livestock, highlighting the importance of zoonotic reservoirs in this disease. West African HAT is contracted closer to settlements and only requires a small vector population, making it difficult to eradicate. Animal reservoirs occur, but the main source of infection remains chronically infected human hosts.

LIFE CYCLE

Trypanosoma brucei undergoes several stages of development in the insect and mammalian host. On ingestion with a blood meal, nonproliferative **short stumpy (SS)** forms of the parasite transform into procyclic forms in the insect's midgut. These procyclic forms proliferate and undergo further development into epimastigotes, which then become infective metacyclic forms that migrate to the insect's salivary glands. The life cycle within the tsetse fly takes 15-35 days. On inoculation into the mammalian host, the metacyclic stage transforms into proliferative **long slender (LS)** forms in the bloodstream and the lymphatics, eventually penetrating the central nervous system (CNS). LS forms appear in waves in the peripheral blood, with each wave followed by a febrile crisis and heralding the formation of a new antigenic variant. Once a critical density of LS forms is reached, a quorum-sensing mechanism causes most of these to transform into nonproliferative SS forms that are ingested by *Glossina* and start the cycle anew. Some LS forms remain to maintain the infection in the human host.

Direct transmission to humans has been reported, either vertically to infants or mechanically through contact with tsetse flies with viable LS forms on their mouthparts from a recent blood meal from an infected host.

EPIDEMIOLOGY

HAT remains a major public health problem in sub-Saharan Africa. It occurs in the region between latitudes 14 degrees north and 29 degrees south, where the annual rainfall creates optimal climatic conditions for *Glossina*. In 2009, because of intensive control efforts spearheaded by the World Health Organization (WHO), the number of new HAT cases annually fell below 10,000. In 2015, this further fell to 2,804 cases, with 84% of cases coming from the Democratic Republic of Congo. Gambian trypanosomiasis is targeted for sustainable elimination as a public health problem by 2030.

T. brucei rhodesiense infection is restricted to the eastern third of the endemic area in tropical Africa, stretching from Ethiopia to the northern boundaries of South Africa. *T. brucei gambiense*, which accounts for 98% of HAT cases, occurs mainly in the western half of the continent's endemic region. Rhodesian HAT, which has an acute and often fatal course, greatly reduces chances of transmission to tsetse flies. The ability of *T. brucei rhodesiense* to multiply rapidly in the bloodstream and infect other species of mammals helps maintain its life cycle.

PATHOGENESIS

At the site of the *Glossina* bite, tsetse fly salivary antigens, peptides, and proteins promote an immune-tolerant microenvironment that facilitates parasite invasion. Injected metacyclic parasites transform into LS forms, which rapidly divide by binary fission. The parasites, along with the attendant inflammation, cellular debris, and metabolic products, may give rise to a hard, painful, red nodule known as a **trypanosomal chancre**. Dissemination into the blood and lymphatic systems follows, with subsequent localization to the CNS. Histopathologic findings in the brain are consistent with meningoencephalitis, with lymphocytic infiltration and perivascular cuffing of the membranes. The appearance of **morula** cells of Mott (large, strawberry-like cells, supposedly derived from plasma cells) is a characteristic finding in chronic disease.

Mechanisms underlying virulence in HAT are still incompletely understood but seem to be mediated by a complex interplay of trypanosomal, human, and *Glossina* factors. *T. brucei gambiense* secretes a specific glycoprotein, TgsGP, while *T. brucei rhodesiense* expresses a protein known as serum resistance–associated protein (SRA), which counteracts trypanolytic apolipoprotein L-1 (ApoL1) in human serum. Trypanosomes also secrete a host of biologically active molecules that can dampen immune responses. For example, *T. brucei* adenylate cyclase (TbAdC) is hyperproduced when a trypanosome is phagocytosed by responding macrophages, causing a spike in cyclic adenosine monophosphate (cAMP), which then activates the macrophage's protein kinase and shuts down TNF-α production, acting as a Trojan horse and downregulating the immune response. Another molecule, *T. brucei*–derived kinesin heavy chain (TbKHC1), downregulates host nitrogen oxide production, dampening the proinflammatory response and causing an increase in production of host polyamines, which are essential nutrients for the parasite. Other parasite-derived molecules are involved in modulating B cell and macrophage responses, especially in chronic infection, resulting in an immune-tolerant condition that allows parasite proliferation without killing the host. Although antigenic variation of **variant surface glycoprotein (VSG)** on the trypanosome surface has long been recognized as a major factor in evading acquired immunity during infection, VSG also inhibits complement activation and antibody-mediated aggregation, facilitating establishment and maintenance of infection. Soluble VSG is hypersecreted, especially at the peak of parasitemia, and may serve as a decoy for antibodies and complement factor, diverting immune responses away from trypanosomes.

CLINICAL MANIFESTATIONS

Clinical presentations vary not only because of the 2 subspecies of organisms but also because of differences in host response in the indigenous population of endemic areas and in newcomers or visitors. Visitors usually suffer more from the acute symptoms, but if untreated, death usually follows for natives and visitors alike. Symptoms usually occur within 2-3 wk of infection. The clinical syndromes of HAT are trypanosomal chancre, hemolymphatic stage, and meningoencephalitic stage.

Trypanosomal Chancre

The site of the tsetse fly bite may be the first presenting feature. A nodule

or chancre (3-4 cm) develops in 2-3 days and becomes a painful, hard, red nodule surrounded by an area of erythema and swelling within 1 wk. Nodules are typically seen on the lower limbs and sometimes also on the head. They subside spontaneously in about 2 wk., leaving no permanent scar.

Hemolymphatic Stage (Stage 1)

The most common presenting features of acute HAT occur at the time of invasion of the bloodstream by the parasites, 2-3 wk after infection. Patients usually present with irregular episodes of fever, each lasting up to 7 days, accompanied by headache, sweating, and generalized lymphadenopathy. Attacks may be separated by symptom-free intervals of days or even weeks. Painless, nonmatted **lymphadenopathy**, most often of the posterior cervical and supraclavicular nodes, is one of the most constant signs, particularly in the Gambian form. A common feature of trypanosomiasis in Caucasians is the presence of blotchy, irregular, nonpruritic, erythematous **macules**, which may appear any time after the first febrile episode, usually within 6-8 wk. The majority of macules have a normal central area, giving the rash a circinate outline. This **rash** is seen mainly on the trunk and is evanescent, fading in one place only to appear at another site. Examination of the blood during this stage may show anemia, leukopenia with relative monocytosis, and elevated levels of IgM. Cardiac manifestations of HAT have also been reported but are generally limited to nonspecific ST-T wave electrocardiographic abnormalities. Histopathologic characterization shows a lymphomonohistiocytic infiltrate in the interstitium, with no penetration of the myocardial cells, unlike that for American trypanosomiasis (see Chapter 313). The perimyocarditis is usually self-limited and does not typically progress to congestive heart failure.

Meningoencephalitic Stage (Stage 2)

Neurologic symptoms and signs are nonspecific, including irritability, insomnia, and irrational and inexplicable anxieties with frequent changes in mood and personality. Neurologic symptoms may precede invasion of the CNS by the organisms. In untreated *T. brucei rhodesiense* infections, CNS invasion occurs within 3-6 wk and is associated with recurrent bouts of headache, fever, weakness, and signs of acute toxemia. Death occurs in 6-9 mo as a result of secondary infection or cardiac failure.

In Gambian HAT, cerebral symptoms appear within 2 yr after the acute symptoms. An increase in drowsiness during the day and insomnia at night reflect the continuous progression of infection and may be accompanied by anemia, leukopenia, and muscle wasting. The chronic, diffuse meningoencephalitis without localizing symptoms is the form referred to as **sleeping sickness**. Drowsiness and an uncontrollable urge to sleep are the major features of this stage and become almost continuous in the terminal stages. Tremor or rigidity with stiff and ataxic gait suggest involvement of the basal ganglia. Psychotic changes occur in one third of untreated patients. While most untreated disease is fatal, in rare cases, individuals remain asymptomatic, clear parasitemia, and become seronegative.

DIAGNOSIS

Definitive diagnosis can be established during the early stages by examination of a fresh, thick blood smear, which permits visualization of the motile active forms (Fig. 312.1). HAT can also be detected from blood using a variety of sensitive techniques, such as quantitative buffy coat smears and mini anion exchange resins. The **card agglutination trypanosomiasis test** (CATT) is of value for epidemiologic purposes and for screening for *T. brucei gambiense*. Dried, Giemsa-stained smears should be examined for the detailed morphologic features of the organisms. If a thick blood or buffy coat smear is negative, concentration techniques may help. Aspiration of an enlarged lymph node can also be used to obtain material for parasitologic examination. If positive, cerebrospinal fluid (CSF) should also be examined for the organisms. The presence of trypanosomes, or ≥5 white blood cells (WBCs)/μL, or both, is indicative of stage 2 disease. If trypanosomes are absent in the CSF, some authorities use a count of 10 to 20 WBCs/μL as a cutoff for diagnosing late-stage disease. Polymerase chain reaction–based tests have been shown to be highly sensitive and specific, but these tests

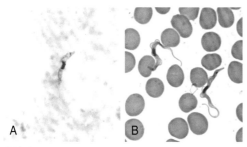

Fig. 312.1 *Trypanosoma brucei* sp. trypomastigotes in thick blood smear stained with Giemsa (**A**) and thin blood smear stained with Wright-Giemsa (**B**). *(From Centers for Disease Control and Prevention: Laboratory identification of parasites of public health concern. Trypanosomiasis, African [website], 2018. https://www.cdc.gov/dpdx/trypanosomiasisafrican/index.html.)*

require advanced laboratory facilities. Field-based loop-mediated isothermal amplification tests have been developed and validated. Low cost, stable, but highly specific rapid tests such as the HAT Sero-Strip and HAT Sero-K-SeT, which detect trypanosome-specific antibodies, have been developed and may prove to be useful for point-of-care diagnosis as the focus shifts from control to elimination. Other areas of active research for diagnostics include new biomarkers, cytokine profiles, proteomics, and polysomnography, which are being used not only to identify disease but to differentiate disease stages.

TREATMENT

The choice of chemotherapeutic agents for treatment depends on the stage of the infection and the causative organisms.

Stage 1 Treatment

Hematogenous forms of both Rhodesian and Gambian HAT can be treated with either suramin or pentamidine, which are better tolerated than drugs for stage 2 or CNS disease but are associated with substantial risks of toxicity. **Suramin** is a polysulphonated symmetric naphthalene derivative given as a 10% solution for intravenous (IV) administration. A **test dose** (10 mg for children; 100-200 mg for adults) is initially administered to detect rare idiosyncratic reactions of shock and collapse. The dose for subsequent IV injections is 20 mg/kg (maximum 1 g) administered on days 1, 3, 7, 14, and 21. Suramin is nephrotoxic, and thus a urinalysis should be performed before each dose. Marked proteinuria, blood, or casts is a contraindication to continuation of suramin. Resistance is rare but has been reported.

Pentamidine isethionate (4 mg/kg/day intramuscularly [IM] daily or on alternate days for 7-10 days) concentrates to high levels in trypanosomes and is highly trypanocidal. It is better tolerated than suramin but carries significant risk of hypoglycemia, nephrotoxicity, hypotension, leukopenia, and liver enzyme elevation. Because of its potency, long half-life, and toxicity, short-course treatment is desirable and is being investigated.

Stage 2 Treatment

The treatment of late-stage *T. brucei gambiense* has substantially changed because of programmatic efforts of the WHO and the donation of large quantities of trypanosomicidal drugs, including eflornithine, pentamidine, suramin, and nifurtimox. Combination **eflornithine and nifurtimox** (NECT) is the treatment of choice for *T. brucei gambiense* CNS infection. This regimen is noninferior to eflornithine monotherapy, and the duration of treatment is shorter. For combination therapy, eflornithine is given at 400 mg/kg/day intravenously (IV) divided every 12 hr for 7 days, along with nifurtimox, 15 mg/kg/day orally divided every 8 hr for 10 days. If nifurtimox is unavailable, eflornithine monotherapy can be given at 400 mg/kg/day IV divided every 6 hr for 14 days. Adverse reactions to these regimens include fever, hypertension, and seizures, with NECT having less frequent events.

Melarsoprol is an arsenical compound and is the only effective treatment for late *T. brucei rhodesiense* disease. Treatment of children is initiated at 0.36 mg/kg IV once daily, with gradually escalating doses every 1-5 days to 3.6 mg/kg once daily; treatment is usually 10 doses (18-25 mg/kg total dose). Treatment of adults is with melarsoprol 2-3.6 mg/kg IV once daily for 3 days; and after 1 wk, 3.6 mg/kg once daily for 3 days, which is repeated after 10-21 days. An alternative regimen is 2.2 mg/kg once daily for 10 days. Guidelines recommend 18-25 mg/kg total over 1 mo. Reactions such as fever, abdominal pain, and chest pain are rare but may occur during or shortly after administration. Serious toxic effects include encephalopathy and exfoliative dermatitis.

Difficulty in administering IV medications, severe side effects, and the emergence of drug resistance have led to the search for better antitrypanosomal agents. Two oral drugs, **fexinidazole** and **benzoxaborole**, are very promising and are currently in clinical trials. Efforts to decrease the toxicity of melarsoprol by making it more water soluble are also being studied.

PREVENTION

A vaccine or consistently effective prophylactic therapy is not available and is particularly challenging because of the antigenic variation caused by VSGs. A single injection of pentamidine (3-4 mg/kg IM) provides protection against Gambian trypanosomiasis for at least 6 mo, but the effectiveness against the Rhodesian form is uncertain.

Vector control programs against *Glossina* have been essential in controlling disease, coupled with the use of screens, traps, insecticides, and sanitary measures. Control of infection in animal reservoirs with mass administration of trypanocidal drugs in cattle has met with some success. Neutral-colored clothing may reduce tsetse fly bites. Mobile medical surveillance of the population at risk by specialized staff has been done, and strong collaboration among WHO, Medecins sans Frontieres, and African governments has shifted the burden of treatment to well-organized and well-funded national control programs. Transgenic techniques, including using **endosymbiotic bacteria** that confer trypanosome resistance to *Glossina*, are being developed and considered.

The full genome of *T. brucei* with about 9,000 genes has been sequenced. Approximately 10% of these genes encode VSGs. This advance has helped identify genes relevant to the disease and its possible prevention, as well as the design of new antitrypanosomal drugs, including those that target specific metabolic pathways.

Bibliography is available at Expert Consult.

Chapter 313

American Trypanosomiasis (Chagas Disease; *Trypanosoma cruzi*)

Edsel Maurice T. Salvana and Robert A. Salata

第三百一十三章

美洲锥虫病（查加斯病；克鲁斯锥虫）

中文导读

　　本章主要介绍了美洲锥虫病的病原学、生命周期、流行病学、发病机制、临床表现、诊断、治疗和预防。以图片形式展现了克鲁斯锥虫的虫媒传播途径和生命周期。在发病机制部分，从急性疾病和慢性疾病两种疾病过程阐述了锥虫病的发病机制。在临床表现部分，分别描述了急性查加斯病、宫内感染、慢性查加斯病的临床特点，并且介绍了免疫低下人群感染克鲁斯锥虫的临床表现特点。

American trypanosomiasis or Chagas disease is caused by the protozoan *Trypanosoma cruzi*. Its natural vectors are the reduviid insects, specifically **triatomines**, variably known as wild bedbugs, assassin bugs, or kissing bugs. It can also be transmitted orally from contaminated food, vertically from mother to child, and through blood transfusion or organ transplantation. Signs and symptoms of acute Chagas disease are usually nonspecific, whereas chronic disease may manifest as cardiomyopathy or severe gastrointestinal (GI) dilation and dysfunction.

ETIOLOGY

American trypanosomiasis is caused by *Trypanosoma cruzi*, a parasitic, flagellated kinetoplastid protozoan. The main vectors for *T. cruzi* are insects of the family Reduviidae, subfamily Triatominae, which includes *Triatoma infestans*, *Rhodnius prolixus*, and *Panstrongylus megistus*.

LIFE CYCLE

T. cruzi has 3 recognizable morphogenetic phases: amastigotes, trypomastigotes, and epimastigotes (Figs. 313.1 and 313.2). **Amastigotes** are intracellular forms found in mammalian tissues that are spherical and have a short flagellum but form clusters of oval shapes (pseudocysts) within infected tissues. **Trypomastigotes** are spindle-shaped, extracellular, nondividing forms that are found in blood and are responsible for both transmission of infection to the insect vector and cell-to-cell spread of infection. **Epimastigotes** are found in the midgut of the vector insect and multiply in the midgut and rectum of arthropods, differentiating into metacyclic forms. **Metacyclic trypomastigotes** are the infectious form for humans and are released onto the skin of a human when the insect defecates close to the site of a bite, entering through the damaged skin or mucous membranes. Once in the host, these multiply intracellularly as amastigotes, which then differentiate into bloodstream trypomastigotes and are released into the circulation when the host cell ruptures. Bloodborne trypomastigotes circulate until they enter another host cell or are taken up by the bite of another insect, completing the life cycle.

EPIDEMIOLOGY

Natural transmission of Chagas disease occurs in North and South America, most frequently in continental Latin America. The disease may arise elsewhere because of migration and transmission through contaminated blood. World Health Organization (WHO) and Pan-American Health Organization–led efforts in large-scale vector control, blood donor screening to prevent transmission through transfusion, and case finding and treatment of chronically infected mothers and newborn infants have effectively halted transmission in a number of areas of South America. The number of cases has dropped from a peak of 24 million in 1984 to a current estimate of 6-7 million, with about 10,000 deaths annually. Overall vectorial transmission continues to drop, although challenges remain, including the emergence of disease in new areas thought to be Chagas free, along with reemergence in previously controlled areas.

Infection is divided into 2 main phases: acute and chronic (Table 313.1). **Acute infection** is asymptomatic in up to 95% of infected individuals, but can manifest as fever, lymphadenopathy, organomegaly, myocarditis, and meningoencephalitis. **Chronic infection** in 60–70% of patients is *indeterminate,* meaning the patient is asymptomatic but has a positive antibody titer. Approximately 30% of infected persons

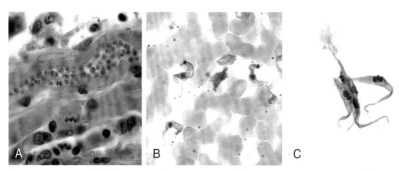

Fig. 313.1 Stages of *Trypanosoma cruzi*. **A,** Amastigote; **B,** trypomastigote; **C,** epimastigote. *(From Centers for Disease Control and Prevention: Laboratory identification of parasites of public health concern. Trypanosomiasis, American [website], 2018.* https://www.cdc.gov/dpdx/trypanoso miasisamerican/index.html.)

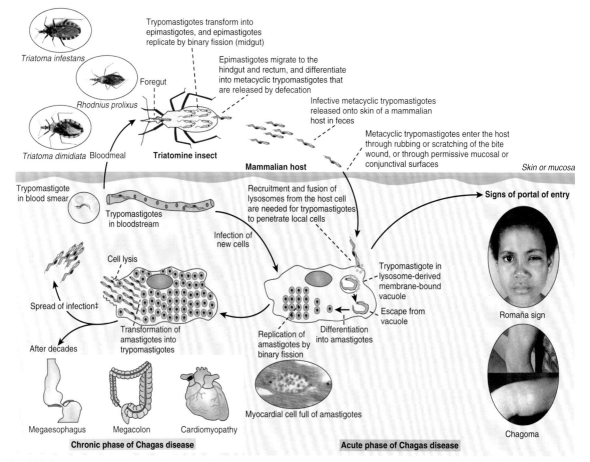

Fig. 313.2 Vector-borne transmission and life cycle of *Trypanosoma cruzi*. *(From Rassi A Jr, Rassi A, Marin-Neto JA: Chagas disease, Lancet 375:1388–1400, 2010, Fig 1.)*

proceed to chronic determinate or symptomatic *T. cruzi* infection. The *T. cruzi* genome has been fully sequenced and contains 12,000 genes, the most widely expanded among trypanosomatids, and may reflect its ability to invade a wide variety of host tissues. Significant variability has been also found, along with extensive epigenetic modification of surface proteins, which may contribute to immune evasion. Six *discrete typing units* (DTUs) are recognized, referred to as TcI to TcVI. A newly described 7th type called Tcbat has recently been identified. DTUs may differ in geographic distribution, predominant vector, and hosts and may also differ in disease manifestations and response to treatment.

T. cruzi infection is primarily a zoonosis, and humans are incidental hosts. *T. cruzi* has a large sylvan reservoir and has been isolated from numerous animal species. The presence of reservoirs and vectors of *T. cruzi* and the socioeconomic and educational levels of the population are the most important risk factors for vector-borne transmission to humans. Insect vectors are found in rural, wooded areas and acquire infection through ingestion of blood from humans or animals with circulating trypomastigotes.

Housing conditions are very important in the transmission chain. Incidence and prevalence of infection depend on the adaptation of the

Table 313.1 Clinical Features and Diagnosis of Chagas Disease

	GEOGRAPHIC DISTRIBUTION	CLINICAL SIGNS/SYMPTOMS	DIAGNOSIS
ACUTE FORMS*			
Vectorial	Endemic countries	Incubation period: 1-2 wk Signs of portal of entry: indurated cutaneous lesion (chagoma) or palpebral edema (Romaña sign) Most cases are mild disease (95–99%) and unrecognized. Persistent fever, fatigue, lymphadenopathy, hepatomegaly, splenomegaly, morbilliform rash, edema In rare cases, myocarditis or meningoencephalitis Anemia, lymphocytosis, elevated AST/ALT concentrations Risk of mortality: 0.2–0.5%	Direct parasitological methods: patent parasitemia up to 90 days Microscopic examination of fresh blood, Giemsa-stained thin and thick blood films, or buffy coat Concentration methods: microhematocrit and Strout method PCR techniques Serology is not useful.
Congenital	Endemic and nonendemic countries	Incubation period: birth to several weeks Most are asymptomatic or have mild disease. Prematurity, low birthweight, neonatal death Fever, jaundice, edema, hepatomegaly, splenomegaly, respiratory distress syndrome, myocarditis, meningoencephalitis Anemia and thrombocytopenia Risk of mortality: <2%	Direct parasitological methods Concentration methods: microhematocrit, Strout method Direct microscopy also useful PCR: most sensitive technique Serology: after 9 mo or later
Oral	Restricted areas of endemic countries (Amazon basin) and local outbreaks	Incubation period: 3-22 days Fever, vomiting, periocular edema, dyspnea, fever, myalgia, prostration, cough, splenomegaly, hepatomegaly, chest pain, abdominal pain, digestive hemorrhage Risk of mortality: 1–35%	Same as for vectorial.
Transfusion and transplant	Endemic and nonendemic countries	Incubation period: 8-160 days; persistent fever Clinical characteristics similar to those of vectorial cases (excluding portal of entry signs) Risk of mortality is variable and depends on the severity of baseline disease.	Same as for vectorial. PCR techniques usually yield positive results days to weeks before trypomastigotes are detectable in blood. Tissue samples are needed in some circumstances.
Reactivation in HIV-infected patients	Endemic and nonendemic countries	Behaves as other opportunistic infections Reactivation with <200 CD4 cells per μL (mostly with <100) Affects CNS (75–90%) as single or multiple space-occupying lesions or as severe necrohemorrhagic meningoencephalitis Cardiac involvement (10–55%): myocarditis, pericardial effusion or worsening of previous cardiomyopathy Risk of mortality: 20%	Direct parasitological methods, as in vectorial cases. Parasite can be found in CSF, other body fluids, and tissue samples. PCR: not useful for diagnosis of reactivation Serology: indicative of chronic infection and helpful in cases of suspected disease
Reactivation in other immunosuppressed patients	Endemic and nonendemic countries	Reactivation after transplantation or in patients with hematologic malignancies Clinical characteristics similar to those of patients who undergo transfusion and those with panniculitis and other skin disorders Risk of mortality is variable and depends on severity of baseline disease and prompt diagnosis.	Direct parasitological methods, as in vectorial cases. Parasite can be found in tissue samples. PCR: increasing parasite load detected with real-time PCR in serial specimens could be indicative of a high risk of reactivation.
CHRONIC FORMS			
Indeterminate	Endemic and nonendemic countries	Asymptomatic Normal chest radiograph and 12-lead ECG.	Serology: detection of IgG PCR: low sensitivity
Cardiac and gastrointestinal	Endemic and nonendemic countries	Cardiac manifestations: fatigue, syncope, palpitations, dizziness, stroke; late manifestations: chest pain (atypical), dyspnea, edema, left ventricular dysfunction, congestive heart failure; alterations in 12-lead ECG, echocardiography, or other heart function tests Gastrointestinal: dysphagia, regurgitation, severe constipation (dilated esophagus or colon); alterations in esophageal manometry, barium swallow, or barium enema	Serology: detection of IgG PCR: low sensitivity

*Including reactivation in immunosuppressed patients.

ALT, Alanine transaminase; AST, aspartate transaminase; CNS, central nervous system; CSF, cerebrospinal fluid; ECG, electrocardiogram; PCR, polymerase chain reaction.

From Pérez-Molina J, Molina I: Chagas disease, *Lancet* 391:82–92, 2018 (Table 2).

triatomines to human dwellings, as well as the vector capacity of the species. Animal reservoirs of reduviid bugs include dogs, cats, rats, opossum, guinea pigs, monkeys, bats, and raccoons. Humans often become infected when land in enzootic areas is developed for agricultural or commercial purposes. An estimated 238,000 immigrants from endemic countries living in the United States are likely infected with *T. cruzi*. Increasing cases of **autochthonous** transmission in the United States have also been reported and confirmed with molecular typing, particularly from California, Louisiana, Texas, and Georgia, although these numbers remain small. One study found that 5.2% of Latin America immigrants in Los Angeles with conduction abnormalities on electrocardiogram (ECG) were seropositive for *T. cruzi*.

Humans can be infected transplacentally, occurring in 10.5% of infected mothers and causing congenital Chagas disease. Transplacental infection is associated with premature birth, fetal wastage, and placentitis. Disease transmission can occur through blood transfusions in endemic areas from asymptomatic blood donors. Seropositivity rates in endemic areas are as high as 20%. The risk for transmission through a single blood transfusion from a chagasic donor is 13–23%. Blood screening for Chagas disease in the United States was started in 2006 and has detected >2,200 seropositive cases since February 2017 (www.aabb.org). Percutaneous injection as a result of laboratory accidents is also a documented mode of transmission. Oral transmission through **contaminated food** is an increasingly important method of transmission as vector transmission is successfully interrupted by control programs. Although breastfeeding is an uncommon mode of transmission, women with acute infections should not nurse until they have been treated.

PATHOGENESIS
Acute Disease
At the site of entry or puncture site, neutrophils, lymphocytes, macrophages, and monocytes infiltrate. *T. cruzi* organisms are engulfed by macrophages and are sequestered in membrane-bound vacuoles. Trypanosomes lyse the phagosomal membrane, escape into the cytoplasm, and replicate. A local tissue reaction, the **chagoma**, develops, and the process extends to a local lymph node (see Fig. 313.2). Blood forms appear, and the process disseminates. Immune evasion and dissemination seem to be facilitated by secretory products from parasite microvesicles and host cell–derived exosomes. These include molecules that facilitate host-parasite adhesion; small tRNAs that increase susceptibility of the host cell to infection; **cruzipain**, which digests human IgG subclasses and facilitates host cell invasion; and other molecules with different functions that make up hundreds of substances found in the microvesicles and exosomes. CCR5 seems to play a dual role in disease severity, helping control infection in the acute phase, but contributing to increased inflammation and myocardial tissue damage when upregulated in chronic infection. The interplay of these cytokines and associated receptors results in a wide variability in disease manifestations and progression to chronic disease. Acute myocarditis likely occurs in all patients with acute disease but is frequently asymptomatic and may only be apparent on biopsy.

Chronic Disease
The pathophysiology of chronic Chagas disease is incompletely understood, but significant progress has recently been made using highly sensitive, quantitative polymerase chain reaction (PCR) methods and real-time bioluminescent markers in animal models. The major driver of cardiac pathology is likely caused by sporadic and repeated bouts of **tissue invasion** from a persistent source, likely the gut, causing lymphocytic infiltration and cumulative fibrosis. Molecular mimicry of host antigens by the parasite and consequent autoimmune stimulation of neurologic receptors were previously thought to be the main driver of cardiomyopathy, but this phenomenon does not seem to occur outside concomitant infection.

T. cruzi demonstrates tropism for certain tissues. It is **myotropic** and invades smooth, skeletal, and heart muscle cells. Attachment is mediated by specific receptors that attach to complementary glycoconjugates on the host cell surface. Attachment to cardiac muscle results in inflammation of the endocardium and myocardium, edema, focal necrosis in the

contractile and conducting systems, periganglionitis, and lymphocytic inflammation. The heart becomes enlarged, and endocardial thrombosis or aneurysm may result. Right bundle branch block (RBBB) is common. Parasites also attach to neural cells and reticuloendothelial cells. In patients with gastrointestinal tract involvement, myenteric plexus destruction leads to pathologic organ dilation. Antibodies involved with resistance to *T. cruzi* are related to the phase of infection. IgG antibodies, probably to several major surface antigens, mediate immunophagocytosis of *T. cruzi* by macrophages. Conditions that depress cell-mediated immunity increase the severity of *T. cruzi* infection. There is increasing evidence that host genetic factors play a significant role in progression and severity of chronic disease.

CLINICAL MANIFESTATIONS
Acute Chagas disease in children is usually asymptomatic or is associated with mild febrile illness characterized by malaise, facial edema, and lymphadenopathy (see Table 313.1). Infants often demonstrate local signs of inflammation at the site of parasite entry, which is then referred to as a **chagoma**. Approximately 50% of children come to medical attention with the **Romaña sign** (unilateral, painless eye swelling), conjunctivitis, and preauricular lymphadenitis. Patients complain of fatigue and headache. Fever can persist for 4-5 wk. More severe systemic presentations can occur in children <2 yr old and may include lymphadenopathy, hepatosplenomegaly, and meningoencephalitis. A cutaneous morbilliform eruption can accompany the acute syndrome. Anemia, lymphocytosis, hepatitis, and thrombocytopenia have also been described.

The heart, central nervous system (CNS), peripheral nerve ganglia, and reticuloendothelial system are often heavily parasitized. The heart is the primary target organ. The intense parasitism can result in acute inflammation and in 4-chamber cardiac dilation. Diffuse myocarditis and inflammation of the conduction system can lead to the development of fibrosis. Histologic examination reveals the characteristic **pseudocysts**, which are the intracellular aggregates of amastigotes.

Intrauterine infection in pregnant women can cause spontaneous abortion or premature birth. In children with congenital infection, severe anemia, hepatosplenomegaly, jaundice, and seizures can mimic congenital cytomegalovirus infection, toxoplasmosis, and erythroblastosis fetalis. *T. cruzi* can be visualized in the cerebrospinal fluid in cases of meningoencephalitis. Children usually undergo spontaneous remission in 8-12 wk and enter indeterminate chronic phase with lifelong low-grade parasitemia and development of antibodies to many *T. cruzi* cell surface antigens. In acute disease, mortality is 5–10%, with deaths caused by acute myocarditis, with resultant heart failure, or meningoencephalitis. Acute Chagas disease should be differentiated from malaria, schistosomiasis, visceral leishmaniasis, brucellosis, typhoid fever, and infectious mononucleosis.

Autonomic dysfunction and peripheral neuropathy can occur. CNS involvement in Chagas disease is uncommon. If granulomatous encephalitis occurs in the acute infection, it is usually fatal.

Chronic Chagas disease may be asymptomatic or symptomatic. The most common presentation of chronic *T. cruzi* infection is **cardiomyopathy**, manifested by congestive heart failure, arrhythmia, and thromboembolic events. ECG abnormalities include partial or complete atrioventricular block and RBBB. Left bundle branch block is unusual. Myocardial infarction has been reported and may be secondary to left apical aneurysm embolization or necrotizing arteriolitis of the microvasculature. Left ventricular apical aneurysms are pathognomonic of chronic chagasic cardiomyopathy.

Gastrointestinal manifestations of chronic Chagas disease occur in 8–10% of patients and involve a diminution in the Auerbach and the Meissner plexus. There are also preganglionic lesions and a reduction in the number of dorsal motor nuclear cells of the vagus nerve. Characteristically, this involvement presents clinically as megaesophagus and megacolon. Sigmoid dilation, volvulus, and fecalomas are often found in **megacolon**. Loss of ganglia in the esophagus results in abnormal dilation; the esophagus can reach up to 26 times its normal weight and hold up to 2 L of excess fluid. **Megaesophagus** presents as dysphagia, odynophagia, and cough. Esophageal body abnormalities occur independently of lower esophageal dysfunction. Megaesophagus can lead to esophagitis and cancer of the esophagus. Aspiration pneumonia and pulmonary tuberculosis are also more common in patients with megaesophagus.

Immunocompromised Persons

T. cruzi infections in immunocompromised persons may be caused by **transmission** from an asymptomatic donor of blood products or **reactivation** of prior infection. Organ donation to allograft recipients can result in a devastating form of the illness. Cardiac transplantation for Chagas cardiomyopathy has resulted in reactivation, despite prophylaxis and postoperative treatment with benznidazole. HIV infection also leads to reactivation in about 20% of cases; cerebral lesions are more common in these patients and can mimic *Toxoplasma* encephalitis. Myocarditis is also frequently observed, and secondary prophylaxis may be of benefit in some HIV–co-infected patients. In immunocompromised patients at risk for reactivation, serologic testing and close monitoring are necessary.

DIAGNOSIS

A careful history with attention to geographic origin and travel is important. A peripheral blood smear or a Giemsa-stained smear during the acute phase of illness may show motile trypanosomes, which is diagnostic for Chagas disease (see Fig. 313.1). These are only seen in the 1st 6-12 wk of illness. Buffy coat smears may improve yield.

Most persons seek medical attention during the chronic phase of the disease, when parasites are not found in the bloodstream and clinical symptoms are not diagnostic. Serologic testing is used for diagnosis, most commonly enzyme-linked immunosorbent assay (ELISA), indirect hemagglutination, and indirect fluorescent antibody testing. No single serology test is sufficiently reliable to make the diagnosis, so repeat or parallel testing using a different method or antigen is required to confirm the result of an initial positive serologic test, and in the case of discordant results, a 3rd test may be employed. Two tests, the Ortho *T. cruzi* ELISA Test System and the Abbott Prism Chagas Assay, are approved by the U.S. Food and Drug Administration (FDA) for screening of blood donors but not for clinical samples. For clinical samples in suspected Chagas cases in the USA, contact the Centers for Disease Control and Prevention (CDC) for further guidance. Confirmatory tests used typically include the radiologic immunoprecipitation assay (Chagas RIPA, used as an unlicensed confirmatory test in U.S. blood donors from 2006 to 2014) and Western blot assays based on trypomastigote excreted-secreted antigens (TESA-WB). Since 2014, the Abbott Enzyme Strip Assay Chagas using recombinant *T. cruzi* antigens has been FDA-approved and used for confirmation in blood donors.

Nonimmunologic methods of diagnosis are available. Mouse inoculation and **xenodiagnosis** (allowing uninfected reduviid bugs to feed on a patient's blood and examining the intestinal contents of those bugs 30 days after the meal) are cumbersome and not routinely performed. Parasites can be cultured in Novy-MacNeal-Nicolle (NNN) media. PCR tests of nuclear and kinetoplast DNA sequences have been developed and can be highly sensitive in acute disease, but are less reliable in chronic disease. PCR is not sufficiently sensitive for blood screening and was positive in only 1 of 22 RIPA-confirmed donors in the United States. Moreover, there is significant variability among methods and parasite strains. Diagnosis of congenital transmission in newborns cannot be made at birth with serology because of the presence of maternal antibodies in the 1st 6 mo of life. Microscopic examination, parasite culture, or PCR can be used. However, a serologic test at 6-12 mo is recommended to exclude infection definitively.

TREATMENT

Biochemical differences between the metabolism of American trypanosomes and that of mammalian hosts have been exploited for chemotherapy. Trypanosomes are very sensitive to oxidative radicals and do not possess catalase or glutathione reductase/glutathione peroxidase, which are key enzymes in scavenging free radicals. All trypanosomes also have an unusual reduced nicotinamide adenine dinucleotide phosphate (NADPH)–dependent disulfide reductase. Drugs that stimulate hydrogen peroxide (H_2O_2) generation or prevent its utilization are

potential trypanosomicidal agents. Other biochemical pathways that have been targeted include ergosterol synthesis using azole compounds and the hypoxanthine-guanine phosphoribosyltransferase pathway using allopurinol.

Drug treatment for T. cruzi infection is currently limited to nifurtimox and benznidazole. Both are effective against trypomastigotes and amastigotes and have been used to eradicate parasites in the acute stages of infection. Treatment responses vary according to the phase of Chagas disease, duration of treatment, dose, age of the patient, and geographic origin of the patient. For acute disease, the average cure rate is about 60–80%. Cure of chronic disease is difficult to assess due to the different definitions of cure, whether with a negative serology or quantitative polymerase chain reaction. In recent trials, benznidazole has shown a cure rate of about 30% using ELISA, and 46–90% using PCR. A trial for chronic disease efficacy with nifurtimox is ongoing. Neither drug is safe in pregnancy. Recent trials with posaconazole, fexinidazole, and E1224 (a prodrug of ravuconazole) for chronic disease have been disappointing.

Benznidazole is a nitroimidazole derivative that may be slightly more effective than nifurtimox. Recent work in metabolomics has shown that benznidazole's primary mechanism of action involves covalent binding with trypanosomal protein thiols and low-molecular-weight thiols, resulting in depletion of these molecules and disruption of the parasite metabolism. The recommended treatment regimen for children <12 yr old is 10 mg/kg/day orally (PO) divided twice daily (bid) for 60 days, and for those >12 yr old, 5-7 mg/kg/day PO bid for 60 days. This drug is associated with significant toxicity, including rash, photosensitivity, peripheral neuritis, granulocytopenia, and thrombocytopenia.

Nifurtimox generates highly toxic oxygen metabolites through the action of nitroreductases, which produce unstable nitroanion radicals, which in turn react with oxygen to produce peroxide and superoxide free radicals. The treatment regimen for children 1-10 yr old is 15-20 mg/kg/day PO divided 4 times daily (qid) for 90 days; for children 11-16 yr, 12.5-15 mg/kg/day PO qid for 90 days; and for children >16 yr, 8-10 mg/kg/day PO divided 3-4 times daily for 90-120 days. Nifurtimox has been associated with weakness, anorexia, gastrointestinal disturbances, toxic hepatitis, tremors, seizures, and hemolysis in patients with glucose-6-phosphate dehydrogenase deficiency.

With the adoption by WHO of control and elimination strategies for Chagas disease, both acute and chronic disease should be treated. Serologic conversion is seen as an appropriate treatment response for chronic disease, although some patients who achieve this still eventually develop symptoms. One study reported cure rates as high as 97% for chronic disease in patients <16 yr old and supports early and aggressive case finding and treatment. Continuing efforts for elimination will necessitate development of more accurate diagnostics and more effective drugs, particularly for chronic disease. Treatment of congestive heart failure is generally in line with recommendations for management of dilated cardiomyopathy from other causes. β-Adrenergic blockers have been validated in the management of these patients. Digitalis toxicity occurs frequently in patients with Chagas cardiomyopathy. Pacemakers may be necessary in cases of severe heart block. Although cardiac transplantation has been used successfully in chagasic patients, it is reserved for those with the most severe disease manifestations. Plasmapheresis to remove antibodies with adrenergic activity has been proposed for refractory patients; this approach has worked in patients with dilated cardiomyopathy from other causes, but its application to Chagas disease is unproved.

A light, balanced diet is recommended for **megaesophagus**. Surgery or dilation of the lower esophageal sphincter treats megaesophagus; pneumatic dilation is the superior mode of therapy. Nitrates and nifedipine have been used to reduce lower esophageal sphincter pressure in patients with megaesophagus. Treatment of **megacolon** is surgical and symptomatic. Treatment of meningoencephalitis is also supportive.

In accidental infection when parasitic penetration is certain, treatment should be immediately initiated and continued for 10-15 days. Blood is usually collected and serologic samples tested for seroconversion at 15, 30, and 60 days.

PREVENTION

Massive coordinated vector control programs under the auspices of WHO and the Pan-American Health Organization and the institution of widespread blood donor screening and targeted surveillance of chronically infected mothers and infants at risk have effectively eliminated or at least drastically reduced transmission in most endemic countries. Chagas disease remains linked to poverty, and thus improvement of living conditions is likewise essential to successful control and eradication. Education of residents in endemic areas, use of bed nets, use of insecticides, and destruction of adobe houses that harbor reduviid bugs are effective methods to control the bug population. Synthetic pyrethroid insecticides help keep houses free of vectors for up to 2 yr and have low toxicity for humans. Paints incorporating insecticides have also been used. A therapeutic vaccine composed of bivalent recombinant *T. cruzi* antigens has been shown to be effective in preclinical proof-of-concept animal models and is currently undergoing further development.

Blood transfusions in endemic areas are a significant risk. **Gentian violet**, an amphophilic cationic agent that acts photodynamically, has been used to kill the parasite in blood. Photoirradiation of blood containing gentian violet and ascorbate generates free radicals and superoxide anions that are trypanosomicidal. **Mepacrine** and **maprotiline** have also been used to eradicate the parasite in blood transfusions.

Because immigrants can carry this disease to nonendemic areas, serologic testing should be performed in blood and organ donors from endemic areas. Potential seropositive donors can be identified by determining whether they have been or have spent extensive time in an endemic area. Questionnaire-based screening of potentially infected blood and organ donors from areas endemic for infection can reduce the risk for transmission. Seropositivity should be considered a contraindication to organ donation, particularly for heart transplantation.

Bibliography is available at Expert Consult.

Chapter **314**

Malaria *(Plasmodium)*

Chandy C. John

第三百一十四章

疟疾（疟原虫）

中文导读

本章主要介绍了疟疾的病原学、流行病学、发病机制、临床表现、诊断、治疗、恶性疟的并发症及预防。在诊断部分，介绍了疟疾的诊断方法，同时强调了疟疾的鉴别诊断。在治疗部分，分别介绍了恶性疟的治疗方案及间日疟、卵形疟、三日疟或诺氏疟的治疗方案，以表格形式展现了美国疾病控制和预防中心（CDC）的疟疾治疗指南。

Malaria is an acute illness characterized by paroxysms of fever, chills, sweats, fatigue, anemia, and splenomegaly. It has played a major role in human history, causing harm to more people than perhaps any other infectious disease. Although substantial progress has been made in combating malaria in endemic areas, with a 37% reduction in malaria incidence and 60% reduction in malaria mortality, malaria remains one of the leading causes of morbidity and mortality worldwide, with an estimated 214 million cases and 438,000 deaths in 2015. Malarial deaths in areas of high malaria transmission occur primarily in children <5 yr of age, but in areas of low transmission, a large percentage of deaths may occur in older children and adults. Although malaria is not endemic in the United States, 1,500-2,000 imported cases are seen in the United States each year. Physicians practicing in nonendemic areas should consider the diagnosis of malaria in any febrile child who has returned from a malaria-endemic area within the previous year, because delay in diagnosis and treatment can result in severe illness or death.

ETIOLOGY

Malaria is caused by intracellular *Plasmodium* protozoa transmitted to humans by female *Anopheles* mosquitoes. Before 2004, only 4 species of *Plasmodium* were known to cause malaria in humans: *P. falciparum*, *P. malariae*, *P. ovale*, and *P. vivax*. In 2004, *P. knowlesi* (a primate malaria species) was also shown to cause human malaria, and cases of *P. knowlesi* infection have been documented in Malaysia, Indonesia, Singapore,

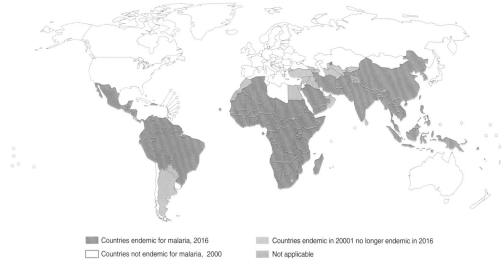

Fig. 314.1 Global spatial distribution of malaria, 2000 compared to 2016. *(From World Malaria Report 2016. Geneva: World Health Organization; 2016. License: CC BY-NC-SA 3.0 IGO.)*

Legend:
- ■ Countries endemic for malaria, 2016
- □ Countries not endemic for malaria, 2000
- ■ Countries endemic in 20001 no longer endemic in 2016
- ▨ Not applicable

and the Philippines. Malaria also can be transmitted through blood transfusion and use of contaminated needles and transplacentally from a pregnant woman to her fetus. The risk for blood transmission is low in the United States, but may occur through transfusion of whole blood, packed red blood cells (RBCs), platelets, and leukocytes and through organ transplantation.

EPIDEMIOLOGY

Malaria is a major worldwide problem, occurring in 95 countries that comprise approximately half the world's population (Fig. 314.1). The principal areas of transmission are Africa, Asia, and South America. *P. falciparum* and *P. malariae* are found in most malarious areas. *P. falciparum* is the predominant species in Africa, Haiti, and New Guinea. *P. vivax* predominates in Bangladesh, Central America, India, Pakistan, and Sri Lanka. *P. vivax* and *P. falciparum* predominate in Southeast Asia, South America, and Oceania. *P. ovale* is the least-common species and is transmitted primarily in Africa. Transmission of malaria has been eliminated in most of North America (including the United States), Europe, and most of the Caribbean, as well as Australia, Chile, Israel, Japan, Lebanon, and Taiwan.

Most cases of malaria in the United States occur among previously infected visitors to the United States from endemic areas and among U.S. citizens who travel to endemic areas without appropriate chemoprophylaxis. The most common regions of acquisition of the approximately 1,700 cases of malaria reported to the Centers for Disease Control and Prevention (CDC) among U.S. citizens in 2013 were Africa (82%), Asia (11%), and the Caribbean and Central or South America (7%). Although only 17% of malaria cases occurred in children (<18 yr old), children <5 yr old were more likely to develop severe malaria (37%) than were persons ≥5 yr old (15%). All the 10 deaths from malaria were caused by *P. falciparum*. Rare cases of apparent locally transmitted malaria have been reported since the 1950s. These cases may result from transmission from untreated and often asymptomatic infected individuals from malaria-endemic countries who travel to the United States and infect local mosquitoes or from infected mosquitoes from malaria-endemic areas that are transported to the United States on airplanes.

PATHOGENESIS

Plasmodium species exist in a variety of forms and have a complex life cycle that enables them to survive in different cellular environments in the human host (asexual phase) and the mosquito (sexual phase) (Fig. 314.2). A marked amplification of *Plasmodium*, from approximately 10^2 to as many as 10^{14} organisms, occurs during a 2-step process in humans, with the 1st phase in hepatic cells (exoerythrocytic phase) and

the 2nd phase in the RBCs (erythrocytic phase). The **exoerythrocytic phase** begins with inoculation of sporozoites into the bloodstream by a female *Anopheles* mosquito. Within minutes, the sporozoites enter the hepatocytes of the liver, where they develop and multiply asexually as a **schizont**. After 1-2 wk, the hepatocytes rupture and release thousands of merozoites into the circulation. The tissue schizonts of *P. falciparum, P. malariae,* and apparently *P. knowlesi* rupture once and do not persist in the liver. There are 2 types of tissue schizonts for *P. ovale* and *P. vivax.* The primary type ruptures in 6-9 days, and the secondary type remains dormant in the liver cell for weeks, months, or as long as 5 yr before releasing merozoites and causing relapse of infection. The **erythrocytic phase** of *Plasmodium* asexual development begins when the merozoites from the liver penetrate erythrocytes. Once inside the erythrocyte, the parasite transforms into the **ring form**, which then enlarges to become a **trophozoite**. These latter 2 forms can be identified with Giemsa stain on blood smear, the primary means of confirming the diagnosis of malaria (Fig. 314.3). The trophozoite multiplies asexually to produce a number of small erythrocytic **merozoites** that are released into the bloodstream when the erythrocyte membrane ruptures, which is associated with fever. Over time, some of the merozoites develop into male and female gametocytes that complete the *Plasmodium* life cycle when they are ingested during a blood meal by the female anopheline mosquito. The male and female gametocytes fuse to form a **zygote** in the stomach cavity of the mosquito. After a series of further transformations, sporozoites enter the salivary gland of the mosquito and are inoculated into a new host with the next blood meal.

Physiology and pathogenesis in malaria differ according to species. Infection with all species leads to **fever**, caused by the host immune response when erythrocytes rupture and release merozoites into the circulation, and **anemia**, caused by hemolysis and bone marrow suppression. Severe malaria is more common in *P. falciparum* because of several process, including higher-density parasitemia, which may lead to excessive production of proinflammatory cytokines; cytoadherence of *P. falciparum*-infected erythrocytes to the vascular endothelium; and polyclonal activation, resulting in both hypergammaglobulinemia and the formation of immune complexes. **Cytoadherence** of infected erythrocytes to vascular endothelium can lead to obstruction of blood flow and capillary damage, with resultant vascular leakage of blood, protein, and fluid and tissue anoxia. Parasite anaerobic metabolism may also lead to hypoglycemia and metabolic acidosis. The cumulative effects of these pathologic processes may lead to cerebral, cardiac, pulmonary, renal, and hepatic failure.

Immunity after *Plasmodium* sp. infection is incomplete, preventing severe disease but still allowing future infection. In some cases, parasites

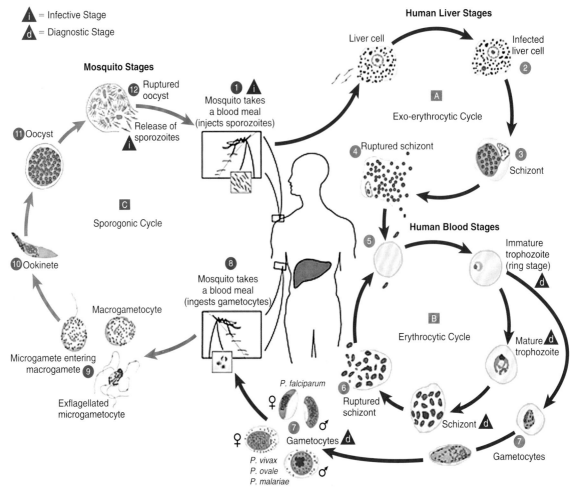

Fig. 314.2 Life cycle of *Plasmodium* spp. *(From Centers for Disease Control and Prevention: Laboratory diagnosis of malaria: Plasmodium spp. https://www.cdc.gov/dpdx/malaria/index.html.)*

circulate in small numbers for a long time but are prevented from rapidly multiplying and causing severe illness. Repeated episodes of infection occur because the parasite has developed a number of immune-evasive strategies, such as intracellular replication, vascular cytoadherence that prevents infected erythrocytes from circulating through the spleen, rapid antigenic variation, and alteration of the host immune system resulting in partial immune suppression. The human host response to *Plasmodium* infection includes natural immune mechanisms that prevent infection by other *Plasmodium* spp., such as those of birds or rodents, as well as several alterations in erythrocyte physiology that prevent or modify malarial infection. Erythrocytes containing **hemoglobin S** (sickle erythrocytes) resist malaria parasite growth, erythrocytes lacking Duffy blood group antigen are relatively resistant to *P. vivax*, and erythrocytes often containing **hemoglobin F** (fetal hemoglobin) and ovalocytes are resistant to *P. falciparum*. In hyperendemic areas, newborns rarely become ill with malaria, in part because of passive maternal antibody and high levels of fetal hemoglobin. Children 3 mo to 2-5 yr of age have little specific immunity to malaria species and therefore suffer yearly attacks of debilitating and potentially fatal disease. Immunity is subsequently acquired, and severe cases of malaria become less common. Severe disease may occur during pregnancy, particularly first pregnancies or after extended residence outside the endemic region. Both T-cell and antibody responses are important in development of biologic and clinical immunity to *Plasmodium* spp.

CLINICAL MANIFESTATIONS

Children and adults are asymptomatic during the initial phase of infection, the incubation period of malaria infection. The usual incubation periods are 9-14 days for *P. falciparum*, 12-17 days for *P. vivax*, 16-18 days for *P. ovale*, and 18-40 days for *P. malariae*. The incubation period can be as long as 6-12 mo for *P. vivax* and can also be prolonged for patients with partial immunity or incomplete chemoprophylaxis. A prodrome lasting 2-3 days is noted in some patients before parasites are detected in the blood. Prodromal symptoms include headache, fatigue, anorexia, myalgia, slight fever, and pain in the chest, abdomen, and joints.

Children with malaria often lack the typical paroxysms in adults (high fever, followed by shaking chills and then diaphoresis) and may have nonspecific symptoms, including fever (may be low-grade but is often >40°C [104°F]), headache, drowsiness, anorexia, nausea, vomiting, and diarrhea. While the rupture of schizonts that occurs every 48 hr with *P. vivax* and *P. ovale* and every 72 hr with *P. malariae* can result in a classic pattern of fevers every other day (*P. vivax* and *P. ovale*) or every 3rd day (*P. malariae*), periodicity is less apparent with *P. falciparum*, and mixed infections and may not be apparent early on in infection, when parasite broods have not yet synchronized. Patients with primary infection, such as travelers from nonendemic regions, also may have irregular symptomatic episodes for 2-3 days before regular paroxysms begin, so most travelers presenting with malaria lack a classic malaria fever pattern. Distinctive physical signs may include splenomegaly (common), hepatomegaly, and

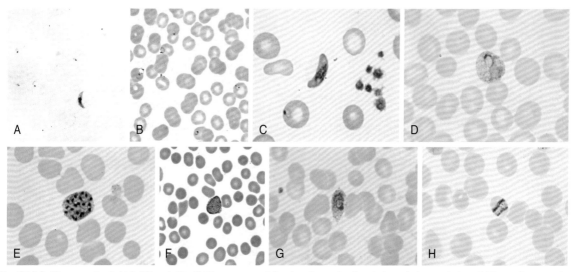

Fig. 314.3 Giemsa-stained thick (**A**) and thin (**B-H**) smears used for the diagnosis of malaria and the speciation of *Plasmodium* parasites. **A,** Multiple signet-ring *Plasmodium falciparum* trophozoites, which are visualized outside erythrocytes. **B,** A multiply infected erythrocyte containing signet-ring *P. falciparum* trophozoites, including an accolade form positioned up against the inner surface of the erythrocyte membrane. **C,** Banana-shaped gametocyte unique to *P. falciparum*. **D,** Ameboid trophozoite characteristic of *Plasmodium vivax*. Both *P. vivax*– and *Plasmodium ovale*–infected erythrocytes exhibit Schüffner dots and tend to be enlarged compared with uninfected erythrocytes. **E,** *P. vivax* schizont. Mature *P. falciparum* parasites, by contrast, are rarely seen on blood smears because they sequester in the systemic microvasculature. **F,** *P. vivax* spherical gametocyte. **G,** *P. ovale* trophozoite. Note Schüffner dots and ovoid shapes of the infected erythrocyte. **H,** Characteristic band-form trophozoite of *Plasmodium malariae*, containing intracellular pigment hemozoin. (*A, B, and F, From Centers for Disease Control and Prevention: DPDx: laboratory identification of parasites of public health concern. https://www.cdc.gov/dpdx/malaria/index.html; C, D, E, G, and H, courtesy of David Wyler, Newton Centre, MA.*)

Table 314.1	World Health Organization Criteria for Severe Malaria, 2000
• Impaired consciousness • Prostration • Respiratory distress • Multiple seizures • Jaundice	• Hemoglobinuria • Abnormal bleeding • Severe anemia • Circulatory collapse • Pulmonary edema

pallor as a consequence of anemia. Typical laboratory findings include anemia, thrombocytopenia, and a normal or low leukocyte count. The erythrocyte sedimentation rate is often elevated.

P. falciparum is the most severe form of malaria and is associated with higher-density parasitemia and a number of complications (Fig. 314.4). The most common serious complication is severe **anemia**, which also is associated with other malaria species. Serious complications that appear unique to *P. falciparum* include cerebral malaria, respiratory distress from metabolic acidosis, acute renal failure, hypotension, and bleeding diatheses (Table 314.1) (see later, Complications of *Plasmodium falciparum* Malaria). The diagnosis of *P. falciparum* malaria in a nonimmune individual constitutes a medical emergency. Severe complications and death can occur if appropriate therapy is not instituted promptly. In contrast to malaria caused by *P. ovale*, *P. vivax*, and *P. malariae*, which usually result in parasitemias of <2%, malaria caused by *P. falciparum* can be associated with parasitemia levels as high as 60%. The differences in parasitemia reflect that *P. falciparum* infects both immature and mature erythrocytes, whereas *P. ovale* and *P. vivax* primarily infect immature erythrocytes and *P. malariae* infects only mature erythrocytes. Like *P. falciparum*, *P. knowlesi* has a 24 hr replication cycle and can also lead to very-high-density parasitemia.

P. vivax malaria has long been considered less severe than *P. falciparum* malaria, but recent reports suggest that in some areas it is as frequent a cause of severe disease and death as *P. falciparum*. Severe disease and death from *P. vivax* are usually caused by severe anemia and sometimes splenic rupture. *P. ovale* malaria is the least common type of malaria. It

is similar to *P. vivax* malaria and usually is found in conjunction with *P. falciparum* malaria. *P. malariae* is the mildest and most chronic of all malaria infections. **Nephrotic syndrome** is a rare complication of *P. malariae* infection that is not observed with any other human malaria species. Nephrotic syndrome associated with *P. malariae* infection is poorly responsive to corticosteroids. Low-level, undetected *P. malariae* infection may be present for years and is sometimes unmasked by immunosuppression or physiologic stress such as splenectomy or corticosteroid treatment. *P. knowlesi* malaria is most often uncomplicated but can lead to severe malaria and death if high-density parasitemia is present.

Recrudescence after a primary attack may occur from the survival of erythrocyte forms in the bloodstream. Long-term relapse is caused by release of merozoites from an exoerythrocytic source in the liver, which occurs with *P. vivax* and *P. ovale*, or from persistence within the erythrocyte, which occurs with *P. malariae* and rarely with *P. falciparum*. A history of typical symptoms in a person >4 wk after return from an endemic area is therefore more likely to be *P. vivax*, *P. ovale*, or *P. malariae* infection than *P. falciparum* infection. In the most recent survey of malaria in the United States (2013) by the CDC, among individuals in whom a malaria species was identified, 61% of cases were caused by *P. falciparum*, 14% by *P. vivax*, 2% by *P. malariae*, 4% by *P. ovale*, and 2% by mixed-species infection; 94% of *P. falciparum* infections were diagnosed within 30 days of arrival in the United States, and 99% within 90 days of arrival. In contrast, 54% of *P. vivax* cases occurred >30 days after arrival in the United States.

Congenital malaria is acquired from the mother prenatally or perinatally but is rarely reported in the United States. Congenital malaria usually occurs in the offspring of a nonimmune mother with *P. vivax* or *P. malariae* infection, although it can be observed with any of the human malaria species. The first sign or symptom typically occurs between 10 and 30 days of age (range: 14 hr to several months of age). Signs and symptoms include fever, restlessness, drowsiness, pallor, jaundice, poor feeding, vomiting, diarrhea, cyanosis, and hepatosplenomegaly. **Malaria in pregnancy** is a major health problem in malaria endemic countries, can be severe, and is associated with adverse outcomes in the fetus or neonate, including intrauterine growth restriction and low birthweight, even in the absence of transmission from mother to child.

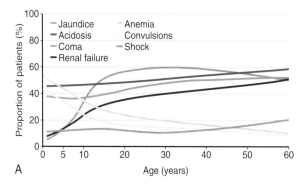

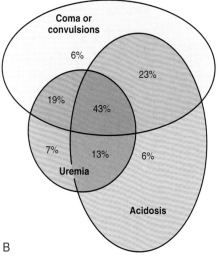

Fig. 314.4 Manifestations of severe falciparum malaria by age (**A**) and mortality in children associated with central nervous system involvement, acidosis, and uremia (**B**). Data from 3,228 prospectively studied African children with severe falciparum malaria. *Uremia* here is defined as a blood urea nitrogen >7.14 mmol/L. Surface areas denote the relative prevalence of the different severity signs, which frequently coexist. The percentages denote the observed mortality associated with the presenting signs. (*From White NJ, Pukrittayakamee S, Hien TT, et al: Malaria, Lancet 383:723–735, 2014; based on data from von Seidlein L, Olaosebikan R, Hendriksen ICE, et al: Predicting the clinical outcome of severe falciparum malaria in African children: findings from a large randomized trial. Clin Infect Dis 54:1080–1090, 2012.*)

DIAGNOSIS

Any child who presents with fever or unexplained systemic illness and has traveled or resided in a malaria-endemic area within the previous year should be evaluated for malaria. Malaria should be considered regardless of the use of chemoprophylaxis. Important criteria that suggest *P. falciparum* malaria include symptoms occurring <1 mo after return from an endemic area, >2% parasitemia, ring forms with double-chromatin dots, and erythrocytes infected with>1 parasite.

The diagnosis of malaria is established by identification of organisms on Giemsa-stained smears of peripheral blood (see Fig. 314.3) or by rapid immunochromatographic assay (rapid diagnostic test). Giemsa stain is superior to Wright stain or Leishman stain. Both thick and thin blood smears should be examined. The concentration of erythrocytes on a **thick smear** is 20-40 times that on a thin smear and is used to quickly scan large numbers of erythrocytes. The **thin smear** allows for positive identification of the malaria species and determination of the percentage of infected erythrocytes and is useful in following the response

to therapy. Identification of the species is best made by an experienced microscopist and checked against color plates of the various *Plasmodium* spp. (see Fig. 314.3). Morphologically, it is impossible to distinguish *P. knowlesi* from *P. malariae*, so polymerase chain reaction (PCR) detection by a reference laboratory or the CDC is required. Although *P. falciparum* is most likely to be identified from blood just after a febrile paroxysm, most children with malaria will have a positive blood smear regardless of the time the smear is obtained. Most guidelines recommend at least 3 negative blood smears to rule out malaria in children in whom malaria is strongly suspected, because low-level parasitemia could potentially go undetected early in the illness. However, few data are available on the utility of repeated blood smears for malaria detection, and most case reports and series document a positive initial smear.

The BinaxNOW Malaria test is approved by the U.S. Food and Drug Administration (FDA) for rapid diagnosis of malaria. This immunochromatographic test for *P. falciparum* histidine-rich protein (HRP2) and aldolase is approved for testing for *P. falciparum* and *P. vivax.* **Aldolase** is present in all 5 of the malaria species that infect humans. Thus, a positive result for *P. vivax* could be because of *P. ovale* or *P. malariae* infection. Sensitivity and specificity for *P. falciparum* (94–99% and 94–99%, respectively) and *P. vivax* (87–93% and 99%, respectively) are good, but sensitivity for *P. ovale* and *P. malariae* is lower. Sensitivity for *P. falciparum* decreases at lower levels of parasitemia, so microscopy is still advised in areas where expert microscopy is available. The test is simple to perform and can be done in the field or laboratory in 10 min. PCR is more sensitive than microscopy but is technically more complex. It is available in some reference laboratories and can be useful for confirmation and for diagnosis of multiple species of malaria, but the time delay in availability of results generally precludes its use for acute diagnosis of malaria. PCR detection may detect asymptomatic parasitemia in children with very-low-level parasitemia (e.g., internationally adopted children from malaria-endemic areas), with greater sensitivity than microscopy, and may be the preferred method of detection in these children, who, since asymptomatic, do not require immediate treatment.

Differential Diagnosis

The differential diagnosis of malaria is broad and includes viral infections such as influenza and hepatitis, sepsis, pneumonia, meningitis, encephalitis, endocarditis, gastroenteritis, pyelonephritis, babesiosis, brucellosis, leptospirosis, tuberculosis, relapsing fever, typhoid fever, yellow fever, viral hemorrhagic fevers, amebic liver abscess, neoplasm, and collagen vascular disease.

TREATMENT

Physicians caring for patients with malaria or traveling to endemic areas need to be aware of current information regarding malaria because resistance to antimalarial drugs has complicated therapy and prophylaxis. The best source for such information is the CDC Malaria webpage (https://www.cdc.gov/malaria/resources/pdf/treatmenttable.pdf),which provides up-to-date guidelines for malaria treatment, and an algorithm for an approach to malaria treatment (Fig. 314.5). In cases where treatment is unclear or complex, the CDC Malaria Hotline is an excellent resource and is available to physicians 24 hr a day (844-856-4713, from 9 AM to 5 PM Eastern Time Monday-Friday, and 770-488-7100 at all other times and on holidays; request to speak to the CDC Malaria Branch Expert).

Fever without an obvious cause in any patient who has left a P. falciparum–endemic area within 30 days and is nonimmune should be considered a medical emergency. Thick and thin blood smears should be obtained immediately, and all children with symptoms of severe disease should be hospitalized. If negative, blood films should be repeated every 12 hr until 3 smears are documented as negative. If the patient is severely ill, antimalarial therapy should be initiated immediately. Outpatient therapy generally is not given to nonimmune children but may be considered in immune or semi-immune children who have low-level parasitemia (<1%), no evidence of complications defined by the World Health Organization (WHO), no vomiting, and a lack of toxic appearance; who are able to contact the physician or emergency department at any time; and in whom follow-up within 24 hr is ensured.

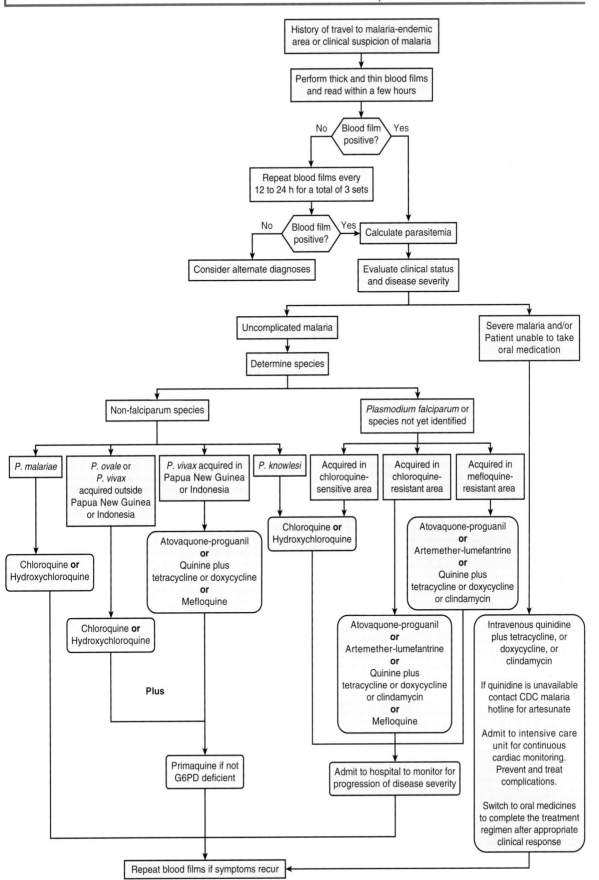

Fig. 314.5 Algorithm for approach to patient with malaria in the United States. (*From Centers for Disease Control and Prevention.* http://www .cdc.gov/malaria/resources/pdf/algorithm.pdf.)

Plasmodium Falciparum Malaria

Malarious regions considered chloroquine-sensitive include Central America west of the Panama Canal, Haiti, the Dominican Republic, and most of the Middle East except Iran, Oman, Saudi Arabia, and Yemen. The CDC website (http://www.cdc.gov/MALARIA/) should be consulted for updated information on chloroquine susceptibility in an area, and current treatment options. Individuals traveling from areas with chloroquine-susceptible *P. falciparum* can be treated with **chloroquine** if they do not have severe malaria. *Malaria acquired in* P. falciparum *areas with chloroquine resistance or where there is any doubt about chloroquine sensitivity after conferring with the CDC should be treated with drugs other than chloroquine.* Trials in Asia and Africa have definitively proved that artesunate treatment of severe malaria is associated with decreased mortality compared to quinine treatment. However, artesunate is still not FDA-approved in the United States for treatment of malaria, or available outside of special-request indications from the CDC, so intravenous (IV) **quinidine gluconate** remains first-line therapy for severe malaria in the United States (Table 314.2). Monotherapy with artesunate agents should never be used because of the development of resistance and treatment failures. Nonetheless, in endemic countries, artesunate derivatives in combination with other antimalarial agents have become the treatment of choice (Tables 314.3 and 314.4). *Children with severe malaria should be admitted to the intensive care unit for monitoring of complications, plasma quinidine levels, and adverse effects during quinidine administration.* During administration of quinidine, blood pressure monitoring for hypotension and cardiac monitoring for widening of the QRS complex or lengthening of the QTc interval should be performed continuously, and blood glucose monitoring for hypoglycemia should be performed periodically. Cardiac adverse events may require temporary discontinuation of the drug or slowing of the IV infusion. *Parenteral therapy should be continued until the parasitemia is <1%, which usually occurs within 48 hr, and the patient can tolerate oral medication.* **Quinidine gluconate** (United States) or **quinine sulfate** (other countries) is administered for a total of 3 days for malaria acquired in Africa or South America and for 7 days for malaria acquired in Southeast Asia. Doxycycline, tetracycline, or clindamycin is then given orally to complete the therapeutic course (see Tables 314.2 and 314.4). Although there are no data to support the use of quinidine followed by **atovaquone-proguanil** or **artemether-lumefantrine**, the difficulty of maintaining compliance with oral quinine has led many clinicians to complete oral therapy after IV quinine with a complete course of atovaquone-proguanil or artemether-lumefantrine.

Parenteral artesunate or artemether can be substituted for quinine for treatment of severe malaria in children and adults (see Table 314.2). **Artesunate** is now available on special request from the CDC (770-488-7788) for treatment of severe malaria but requires a specific indication such as adverse reaction to quinidine, contraindication to quinidine, or lack of availability of quinidine. Empirical therapy should not be delayed while awaiting delivery of artesunate. Children who receive artesunate can follow up with artemether-lumefantrine oral therapy. Oral and rectal administration of these artemisinin-based antimalarial drugs is effective in treatment of malaria, but such formulations are not indicated or approved in the United States.

Patients from areas with chloroquine-resistant *P. falciparum* who have mild infection, parasitemia <1%, no evidence of complications, and no vomiting and who can take oral medication can be considered for oral therapy with either oral atovaquone-proguanil (**Malarone**), oral artemether-lumefantrine (**Coartem**), or oral quinine plus doxycycline, tetracycline, or clindamycin (see Table 314.2). However, as noted in Fig. 314.5, all children with clinical (symptomatic) malaria, even those started on oral therapy, should be admitted to evaluate for progression of disease. Semi-immune children have been treated as outpatients, but there is limited data on the safety of this approach. Coartem is FDA-approved for the treatment of uncomplicated malaria and is an appealing choice because it is highly effective and well-tolerated. Pediatric dosing is well established, but pediatric dispersible tablets, available in some other countries, are not yet available in the United States. Coartem should not be used in children with known QT interval prolongation. Patients who acquire *P. falciparum* in Thailand, Myanmar, or Cambodia

should receive Coartem or Malarone in preference to quinine. **Mefloquine** is contraindicated for use in patients with a known hypersensitivity to mefloquine or with a history of epilepsy or severe psychiatric disorders. Mefloquine is not recommended for persons with cardiac conduction abnormalities but may be administered to persons who are concurrently receiving β-blockers if they have no underlying arrhythmia. Quinidine or quinine may exacerbate the adverse effects of mefloquine and should generally not be given to patients who have received mefloquine unless there are no other alternatives.

Patients with uncomplicated *P. falciparum* malaria acquired in areas without chloroquine resistance should be treated with oral **chloroquine phosphate**. If the parasite count does not drop rapidly (within 24-48 hr) and become negative after 4 days, chloroquine resistance should be assumed, and the patient should be started on a different antimalarial regimen.

Supportive therapy is important and may include RBC transfusion(s) to maintain the hematocrit at >20%, supplemental oxygen and ventilatory support for pulmonary edema or cerebral malaria, careful IV rehydration for severe malaria, IV glucose for hypoglycemia, anticonvulsants for cerebral malaria with seizures, and dialysis for renal failure. Exchange transfusion has been advocated for children and adults with parasitemia >10% and evidence of severe complications (e.g., severe malarial anemia, cerebral malaria), but no randomized clinical trial has been conducted to assess its utility, and some groups, including the CDC, no longer advocate its use for severe malaria. Corticosteroids are not recommended for cerebral malaria because they do not improve outcomes.

Plasmodium Vivax, P. Ovale, P. Malariae, or *P. Knowlesi* Malaria

Uncomplicated infection caused by *P. vivax, P. ovale,* or *P. malariae* can usually be treated with **chloroquine**, except in areas with chloroquine resistance (Papua New Guinea and Indonesia, see Table 314.2). Chloroquine remains the initial drug of choice for *P. vivax* malaria in the absence of good data on drug alternatives. Indications for using alternative therapy are worsening or new symptoms, persistent *P. vivax* parasitemia after 72 hr, and possibly acquisition of infection in Oceania or India. Patients with *P. vivax* or *P. ovale* malaria should also be given **primaquine** once daily for 14 days to prevent relapse from the **hypnozoite** forms that remain dormant in the liver. Some strains may require 2 courses of primaquine. *Testing for glucose-6-phosphate dehydrogenase deficiency must be performed before initiation of primaquine, because it can cause hemolytic anemia in such patients.* Unfortunately, no alternatives to primaquine currently exist for eradication of the hypnozoite forms of *P. vivax* or *P. ovale.* Patients with any type of malaria should be monitored for possible recrudescence because it may occur >90 days after therapy with low-grade resistant organisms. If vomiting precludes oral administration, chloroquine can be given by nasogastric tube. Based on limited evidence, chloroquine plus sulfadoxine-pyrimethamine should be used to treat *P. knowlesi* infections. For cases of severe malaria caused by any *Plasmodium* spp., IV quinidine or quinine with a 2nd drug (clindamycin, doxycycline, or tetracycline) should be used, as for *P. falciparum.* Patients with any type of malaria must be monitored for possible recrudescence with repeat blood smears at the end of therapy, because recrudescence may occur >90 days after therapy with low-grade resistant organisms. For children living in endemic areas, mothers should be encouraged to seek evaluation for malaria any time the child has a fever, because many clinics in endemic areas now have accurate rapid diagnostic tests available. If such children are severely ill, they should be given the same therapy as nonimmune children.

COMPLICATIONS OF *PLASMODIUM FALCIPARUM* MALARIA

WHO has identified 10 complications of *P. falciparum* malaria that define severe malaria (see Table 314.1 and Fig. 314.4). The most common complications in children are severe anemia, impaired consciousness (including cerebral malaria), respiratory distress (a result of metabolic acidosis), multiple seizures, prostration, and jaundice.

Severe malarial anemia (hemoglobin level <5 g/dL) is the most common severe complication of malaria in children and is the leading

Table 314.2	CDC Guidelines for Treatment of Malaria in the United States (Based on Drugs Currently Available for Use in the United States–Updated July 1, 2013)

(CDC Malaria Hotline: [770] 488-7788 or [855] 856-4713 toll-free Monday-Friday 9 AM to 5 PM EST; [770] 488-7100 after hours, weekends, and holidays)

CLINICAL DIAGNOSIS/ *PLASMODIUM* spp.	REGION INFECTION ACQUIRED	RECOMMENDED DRUG AND ADULT DOSE[1]	RECOMMENDED DRUG AND PEDIATRIC DOSE[1]; PEDIATRIC DOSE SHOULD *NEVER* EXCEED ADULT DOSE
Uncomplicated malaria/*P. falciparum* *or* Species not identified If "species not identified" is subsequently diagnosed as *P. vivax* or *P. ovale*: see *P. vivax* and *P. ovale* (below) regarding treatment with primaquine	Chloroquine-resistant or unknown resistance[2] (All malarious regions except those specified as "chloroquine-sensitive," listed below)	Atovaquone-proguanil (Malarone)[3] Adult tab = 250 mg atovaquone/100 mg proguanil 4 adult tabs PO qd × 3 days	Atovaquone-proguanil (Malarone)[3] Adult tab = 250 mg atovaquone/100 mg proguanil Pediatric (ped) tab = 62.5 mg atovaquone/25 mg proguanil 5-8 kg: 2 ped tabs PO qd × 3 days 9-10 kg: 3 ped tabs PO qd × 3 days 11-20 kg: 1 adult tab PO qd × 3 days 21-30 kg: 2 adult tabs PO qd × 3 days 31-40 kg: 3 adult tabs PO qd × 3 days >40 kg: 4 adult tabs PO qd × 3 days
		Artemether-lumefantrine (Coartem)[3] 1 tablet = 20 mg artemether and 120 mg lumefantrine A 3-day treatment schedule with a total of 6 oral doses is recommended for both adult and pediatric patients based on weight. The patient should receive the initial dose, followed by 2nd dose 8 hr later, then 1 dose PO bid for the following 2 days 5-<15 kg: 1 tablet per dose 15-<25 kg: 2 tablets per dose 25-<35 kg: 3 tablets per dose ≥35 kg: 4 tablets per dose	
		Quinine sulfate plus 1 of the following: doxycycline, tetracycline, or clindamycin Quinine sulfate: 542 mg base (=650 mg salt)[4] PO tid × 3 or 7 days[5] Doxycycline: 100 mg PO bid × 7 days Tetracycline: 250 mg PO qid × 7 days Clindamycin: 20 mg base/kg/day PO divided tid × 7 days	Quinine sulfate[4] plus 1 of the following: doxycycline,[6] tetracycline,[6] or clindamycin Quinine sulfate: 8.3 mg base/kg (=10 mg salt/kg) PO tid × 3 or 7 days[5] Doxycycline: 2.2 mg/kg PO every 12 hr × 7 days Tetracycline: 25 mg/kg/day PO divided qid × 7 days Clindamycin: 20 mg base/kg/day PO divided tid × 7 days
		Mefloquine (Lariam and generics)[7] 684 mg base (=750 mg salt) PO as initial dose, followed by 456 mg base (=500 mg salt) PO given 6-12 hr after initial dose Total dose = 1,250 mg salt	Mefloquine (Lariam and generics)[7] 13.7 mg base/kg (=15 mg salt/kg) PO as initial dose, followed by 9.1 mg base/kg (=10 mg salt/kg) PO given 6-12 hr after initial dose. Total dose = 25 mg salt/kg
Uncomplicated malaria/ *P. falciparum* *or* Species not identified	Chloroquine-sensitive (Central America west of Panama Canal; Haiti; the Dominican Republic; and most of the Middle East)	Chloroquine phosphate (Aralen and generics)[8] 600 mg base (=1,000 mg salt) PO immediately, followed by 300 mg base (=500 mg salt) PO at 6, 24, and 48 hr Total dose: 1,500 mg base (=2,500 mg salt) *or* Hydroxychloroquine (Plaquenil and generics) 620 mg base (=800 mg salt) PO immediately, followed by 310 mg base (=400 mg salt) PO at 6, 24, and 48 hr Total dose: 1,550 mg base (=2,000 mg salt)	Chloroquine phosphate (Aralen and generics)[8] 10 mg base/kg PO immediately, followed by 5 mg base/kg PO at 6, 24, and 48 hr Total dose: 25 mg base/kg *or* Hydroxychloroquine (Plaquenil and generics) 10 mg base/kg PO immediately, followed by 5 mg base/kg PO at 6, 24, and 48 hr Total dose: 25 mg base/kg

[1]If a person develops malaria despite taking chemoprophylaxis, that particular medicine should not be used as a part of their treatment regimen. Use 1 of the other options instead.

[2]NOTE: There are 4 options (A, B, C, or D) available for treatment of uncomplicated malaria caused by chloroquine-resistant *P. falciparum*. Options A, B, and C are equally recommended. Because of a higher rate of severe neuropsychiatric reactions seen at treatment doses, we do not recommend option D (mefloquine) unless the other options cannot be used. For option C, because there is more data on the efficacy of quinine in combination with doxycycline or tetracycline, these treatment combinations are generally preferred to quinine in combination with clindamycin.

[3]Take with food or whole milk. If patient vomits within 30 min of taking a dose, patient should repeat the dose.

[4]U.S.-manufactured quinine sulfate capsule is in a 324 mg dosage; therefore 2 capsules should be sufficient for adult dosing. Pediatric dosing may be difficult because of unavailability of noncapsule forms of quinine.

[5]For infections acquired in Southeast Asia, quinine treatment should continue for 7 days. For infections acquired elsewhere, quinine treatment should continue for 3 days.

[6]Doxycycline and tetracycline are not indicated for use in children <8 yr old. For children <8 yr old with chloroquine-resistant *P. falciparum*, atovaquone-proguanil and artemether-lumefantrine are recommended treatment options; mefloquine can be considered if no other options are available. For children <8 yr old with chloroquine-resistant *P. vivax*, mefloquine is the recommended treatment. If it is not available or is not being tolerated and if the treatment benefits outweigh the risks, atovaquone-proguanil or artemether-lumefantrine should be used instead.

[7]Treatment with mefloquine is not recommended in persons who have acquired infections from Southeast Asia as a consequence of drug resistance.

[8]When treating chloroquine-sensitive infections, chloroquine and hydroxychloroquine are recommended options. However, regimens used to treat chloroquine-resistant infections may also be used if available, more convenient, or preferred.

Continued

Table 314.2	CDC Guidelines for Treatment of Malaria in the United States (Based on Drugs Currently Available for Use in the United States–Updated July 1, 2013)—cont'd

CLINICAL DIAGNOSIS/ *PLASMODIUM* spp.	REGION INFECTION ACQUIRED	RECOMMENDED DRUG AND ADULT DOSE[1]	RECOMMENDED DRUG AND PEDIATRIC DOSE[1]; PEDIATRIC DOSE SHOULD *NEVER* EXCEED ADULT DOSE
Uncomplicated malaria/ *P. malariae* or *P. knowlesi*	All regions	Chloroquine phosphate[8]: treatment as above *or* Hydroxychloroquine: treatment as above	Chloroquine phosphate:[8] treatment as above *or* Hydroxychloroquine: treatment as above
Uncomplicated malaria/ *P. vivax* or *P. ovale*	All regions NOTE: for suspected chloroquine-resistant *P. vivax*, see row below	Chloroquine phosphate[8] plus primaquine phosphate[9] Chloroquine phosphate: treatment as above Primaquine phosphate: 30 mg base PO qd × 14 days *or* Hydroxychloroquine plus primaquine phosphate[9] Hydroxychloroquine: treatment as above Primaquine phosphate: 30 mg base PO qd × 14 days	Chloroquine phosphate[8] plus primaquine phosphate[9] Chloroquine phosphate: treatment as above Primaquine: 0.5 mg base/kg PO qd × 14 days *or* Hydroxychloroquine plus primaquine phosphate[9] Hydroxychloroquine: treatment as above Primaquine phosphate: 0.5 mg base/kg PO qd × 14 days
Uncomplicated malaria/ *P. vivax*	Chloroquine-resistant[10] (Papua New Guinea and Indonesia)	Quinine sulfate plus either doxycycline or tetracycline plus primaquine phosphate[9] Quinine sulfate: treatment as above Doxycycline or tetracycline: treatment as above Primaquine phosphate: treatment as above **Atovaquone-proguanil plus primaquine phosphate**[9] **Atovaquone-proguanil:** treatment as above **Primaquine phosphate:** treatment as above **Mefloquine plus primaquine phosphate**[9] **Mefloquine:** treatment as above **Primaquine phosphate:** treatment as above	Quinine sulfate plus either doxycycline[6] or tetracycline[6] plus primaquine phosphate[9] Quinine sulfate: treatment as above Doxycycline or tetracycline: treatment as above Primaquine phosphate: treatment as above **Atovaquone-proguanil plus primaquine phosphate**[9] **Atovaquone-proguanil:** treatment as above **Primaquine phosphate:** treatment as above **Mefloquine plus primaquine phosphate**[9] **Mefloquine:** treatment as above **Primaquine phosphate:** treatment as above
Uncomplicated malaria: alternatives for pregnant women[11-13]	Chloroquine-sensitive (See uncomplicated malaria sections above for chloroquine-sensitive species by region)	Chloroquine phosphate: treatment as above *or* Hydroxychloroquine: treatment as above	Not applicable
	Chloroquine-resistant (See sections above for regions with chloroquine-resistant *P. falciparum* and *P. vivax*)	**Quinine sulfate plus clindamycin** **Quinine sulfate:** treatment as above **Clindamycin:** treatment as above *or* **Mefloquine:** treatment as above	Not applicable

[9]Primaquine is used to eradicate any hypnozoites that may remain dormant in the liver, and thus prevent relapses, in *P. vivax* and *P. ovale* infections. Because primaquine can cause hemolytic anemia in glucose-6-phosphate dehydrogenase (G6PD)-deficient persons, G6PD screening must occur prior to starting treatment with primaquine. For persons with borderline G6PD deficiency or as an alternate to the above regimen, primaquine may be given 45 mg orally 1 time per week for 8 wk; consultation with an expert in infectious disease and/or tropical medicine is advised if this alternative regimen is considered in G6PD-deficient persons. Primaquine must not be used during pregnancy.

[10]NOTE: There are 3 options (A, B, or C) available for treatment of uncomplicated malaria caused by chloroquine-resistant *P. vivax*. High treatment failure rates as a result of chloroquine-resistant *P. vivax* are well documented in Papua New Guinea and Indonesia. Rare case reports of chloroquine-resistant *P. vivax* are also documented in Burma (Myanmar), India, and Central and South America. Persons acquiring *P. vivax* infections outside of Papua New Guinea or Indonesia should be started on chloroquine. If the patient does not respond, the treatment should be changed to a chloroquine-resistant *P. vivax* regimen and CDC should be notified (Malaria Hotline number listed above). For treatment of chloroquine-resistant *P. vivax* infections, options A, B, and C are equally recommended.

[11]For pregnant women diagnosed with uncomplicated malaria caused by chloroquine-resistant *P. falciparum* or chloroquine-resistant *P. vivax* infection, treatment with doxycycline or tetracycline is generally not indicated. However, doxycycline or tetracycline may be used in combination with quinine (as recommended for non-pregnant adults) if other treatment options are not available or are not being tolerated, and the benefit is judged to outweigh the risks.

[12]Atovaquone-proguanil and artemether-lumefantrine are generally not recommended for use in pregnant women, particularly in the 1st trimester because of a lack of sufficient safety data. For pregnant women diagnosed with uncomplicated malaria caused by chloroquine-resistant *P. falciparum* infection, atovaquone-proguanil or artemether-lumefantrine may be used if other treatment options are not available or are not being tolerated, and if the potential benefit is judged to outweigh the potential risks.

[13]For *P. vivax* and *P. ovale* infections, primaquine phosphate for radical treatment of hypnozoites should not be given during pregnancy. Pregnant patients with *P. vivax* and *P. ovale* infections should be maintained on chloroquine prophylaxis for the duration of their pregnancy. The chemoprophylactic dose of chloroquine phosphate is 300 mg base (=500 mg salt) orally once per week. After delivery, pregnant patients who do not have G6PD deficiency should be treated with primaquine.

Continued

Table 314.2	CDC Guidelines for Treatment of Malaria in the United States (Based on Drugs Currently Available for Use in the United States–Updated July 1, 2013)—cont'd

CLINICAL DIAGNOSIS/ PLASMODIUM spp.	REGION INFECTION ACQUIRED	RECOMMENDED DRUG AND ADULT DOSE[1]	RECOMMENDED DRUG AND PEDIATRIC DOSE[1]; PEDIATRIC DOSE SHOULD *NEVER* EXCEED ADULT DOSE
Severe malaria[14-16]	All regions	Quinidine gluconate[14] plus 1 of the following: doxycycline, tetracycline, or clindamycin Quinidine gluconate: 6.25 mg base/kg (=10 mg salt/kg) loading dose IV over 1-2 hr, then 0.0125 mg base/kg/min (=0.02 mg salt/kg/min) continuous infusion for at least 24 hr. An alternative regimen is 15 mg base/kg (=24 mg salt/kg) loading dose IV infused over 4 hr, followed by 7.5 mg base/kg (=12 mg salt/kg) infused over 4 hr every 8 hr, starting 8 hr after the loading dose (see package insert). Once parasite density <1% and patient can take oral medication, complete treatment with oral quinine, dose as above. Quinidine/quinine course = 7 days in Southeast Asia; = 3 days in Africa or South America Doxycycline: treatment as above. If patient not able to take oral medication, give 100 mg IV every 12 hr and then switch to oral doxycycline (as above) as soon as patient can take oral medication. For IV use, avoid rapid administration. Treatment course = 7 days Tetracycline: treatment as above Clindamycin: treatment as above. If patient not able to take oral medication, give 10 mg base/kg loading dose IV followed by 5 mg base/kg IV every 8 hr. Switch to oral clindamycin (oral dose as above) as soon as patient can take oral medication. For IV use, avoid rapid administration. Treatment course = 7 days *Investigational new drug (contact CDC for information):* Artesunate followed by 1 of the following: atovaquone-proguanil (Malarone), doxycycline (clindamycin in pregnant women), or mefloquine. Artemether-lumefantrine is not included in CDC treatment table but may also be given as follow-up drug after artesunate if available.	Quinidine gluconate[14] plus 1 of the following: doxycycline,[4] tetracycline,[4] or clindamycin Quinidine gluconate: same mg/kg dosing and recommendations as for adults Doxycycline: treatment as above. If patient not able to take oral medication, may give IV. For children <45 kg, give 2.2 mg/kg IV every 12 hr and then switch to oral doxycycline (dose as above) as soon as patient can take oral medication. For children >45 kg, use same dosing as for adults. For IV use, avoid rapid administration. Treatment course = 7 days Tetracycline: treatment as above Clindamycin: treatment as above. If patient not able to take oral medication, give 10 mg base/kg loading dose IV followed by 5 mg base/kg IV every 8 hr. Switch to oral clindamycin (oral dose as above) as soon as patient can take oral medication. For IV use, avoid rapid administration. Treatment course = 7 days. *Investigational new drug (contact CDC for information):* Artesunate followed by 1 of the following: atovaquone-proguanil (Malarone), clindamycin, or mefloquine. Artemether-lumefantrine is not included in CDC treatment table but may also be given as follow-up drug after artesunate if available.

[14]Persons with a positive blood smear *or* history of recent possible exposure and no other recognized pathology who have 1 or more of the following clinical criteria (impaired consciousness/coma, severe normocytic anemia, renal failure, pulmonary edema, acute respiratory distress syndrome, circulatory shock, disseminated intravascular coagulation, spontaneous bleeding, acidosis, hemoglobinuria, jaundice, repeated generalized convulsions, and/or parasitemia of >5%) are considered to have manifestations of more severe disease. Severe malaria is most often caused by *P. falciparum.*

[15]Patients diagnosed with severe malaria should be treated aggressively with parenteral antimalarial therapy. Treatment with IV quinidine should be initiated as soon as possible after the diagnosis has been made. Patients with severe malaria should be given an IV loading dose of quinidine unless they have received >40 mg/kg of quinine in the preceding 48 hr or if they have received mefloquine within the preceding 12 hr. Consultation with a cardiologist and a physician with experience treating malaria is advised when treating malaria patients with quinidine. During administration of quinidine, blood pressure monitoring (for hypotension) and cardiac monitoring (for widening of the QRS complex and/or lengthening of the QTc interval) should be monitored continuously and blood glucose (for hypoglycemia) should be monitored periodically. Cardiac complications, if severe, may warrant temporary discontinuation of the drug or slowing of the intravenous infusion.

[16]Pregnant women diagnosed with severe malaria should be treated aggressively with parenteral antimalarial therapy.

IV, Intravenous(ly); PO, orally (by mouth); qd, once daily; bid, twice daily; tid, 3 times daily; qid, 4 times daily.

From US Centers for Disease Control and Prevention. http://www.cdc.gov/malaria/resources/pdf/treatmenttable.pdf.

cause of anemia leading to hospital admission in African children. Anemia is associated with hemolysis, but removal of infected erythrocytes by the spleen and impairment of erythropoiesis likely play a greater role than hemolysis in the pathogenesis of severe malarial anemia. The primary treatment for severe malarial anemia is blood transfusion. With appropriate and timely treatment, severe malarial anemia usually has a relatively low mortality (approximately 1%).

Cerebral malaria is defined as the presence of coma in a child with *P. falciparum* parasitemia and an absence of other reasons for coma.

Children with altered mental status who are not in coma fall into the larger category of *impaired consciousness.* Cerebral malaria is most common in children in areas of midlevel transmission and in adolescents or adults in areas of very low transmission. It is less frequently seen in areas of very high transmission. Cerebral malaria often develops after the patient has been ill for several days but may develop precipitously. Cerebral malaria has a fatality rate of 15–40% and is associated with long-term cognitive impairment in children. Repeated seizures are frequent in children with cerebral malaria. Hypoglycemia is common,

Table 314.3	Treatment of Uncomplicated Malaria in Malaria Endemic Areas

	REGIMENS
All *Plasmodium falciparum* malaria	Artemether-lumefantrine, 1.5 mg/kg–9 mg/kg twice daily for 3 days with food or milk Artesunate, 4 mg/kg daily for 3 days, and mefloquine, 25 mg base per kg (8 mg/kg/daily for 3 days*)[†] Dihydroartemisinin-piperaquine, 2.5 mg/kg–20 mg/kg daily for 3 days
Sensitive *P. falciparum* malaria	Artesunate, 4 mg/kg daily for 3 days, and a single dose of sulfadoxine-pyrimethamine, 25 mg/kg–1.25 mg/kg Artesunate, 4 mg/kg, and amodiaquine,* 10 mg base per kg daily for 3 days
Chloroquine-sensitive *Plasmodium vivax*,[‡] *Plasmodium malariae*,[‡] *Plasmodium ovale*,[‡] *Plasmodium knowlesi*[‡]	Chloroquine, 10 mg base per kg immediately, followed by 10 mg/kg at 24 hr and 5 mg/kg at 48 hr

*World Health Organization prequalified fixed dose formulations are preferable to loose tablets. A taste masked dispersible pediatric tablet formulation of artemether-lumefantrine is available.

[†]High failure rates with artesunate-mefloquine have been reported on the Thailand–Myanmar border.

[‡]Any of the artemisinin combination treatments can be given except for artesunate-sulfadoxine-pyrimethamine where *P. vivax* is resistant. Patients with *P. vivax* or *P. ovale* infections should also be given a 14-day course of primaquine to eradicate hypnozoites (radical cure). However, severe glucose-6-phosphate dehydrogenase deficiency is a contraindication because a 14-day course of primaquine can cause severe hemolytic anemia in this group.

From White NJ, Pukrittayakamee S, Hien TT, et al: Malaria, *Lancet* 383:723–732, 2014.

Table 314.4	Treatment of Severe Malaria in Adults and Children in Malaria-Endemic Areas

- Artesunate, 2.4 mg/kg by intravenous or intramuscular* injection, followed by 2.4 mg/kg at 12 hr and 24 hr; continue injection once daily if necessary[†]
- Artemether, 3.2 mg/kg by immediate intramuscular* injection, followed by 1.6 mg/kg daily
- Quinine dihydrochloride, 20 mg salt per kg infused during 4 hr, followed by maintenance of 10 mg salt per kg infused during 2-8 hr every 8 hr (can also be given by intramuscular injection* when diluted to 60-100 mg/mL)

Artesunate is the treatment of choice. Artemether should only be used if artesunate is unavailable. Quinine dihydrochloride should be given only when artesunate and artemether are unavailable.

*Intramuscular injections should be given to the anterior thigh.

[†]Young children with severe malaria have lower exposure to artesunate and its main biologically active metabolite dihydroartemisinin than do older children and adults. Revised dose regimens to ensure similar drug exposures have been suggested.

From White NJ, Pukrittayakamee S, Hien TT, et al: Malaria, *Lancet* 383:723–732, 2014.

but children with true cerebral malaria fail to arouse from coma even after receiving a dextrose infusion that normalizes their glucose level. Physical findings may include high fever, seizures, muscular twitching, rhythmic movement of the head or extremities, contracted or unequal pupils, retinal hemorrhages, hemiplegia, absent or exaggerated deep tendon reflexes, and a positive Babinski sign. Lumbar puncture reveals increased pressure and mildly increased cerebrospinal fluid protein, typically with no CSF pleocytosis and a normal CSF glucose. Studies suggest that funduscopic findings of **malaria retinopathy** (retinal hemorrhages, peripheral whitening, macular whitening, vessel changes) are relatively specific for cerebral malaria, so children with cerebral malaria who do not have malaria retinopathy should be carefully assessed for other causes of

coma. However, they should still be treated for cerebral malaria because a growing body of evidence suggests that even in these children, *P. falciparum* is a contributor to their comatose state. Treatment of cerebral malaria other than antimalarial medications is largely supportive and includes evaluation of and treatment of seizures and hypoglycemia. A study using MRI to assess children with cerebral malaria documented that cerebral edema with increased intracranial pressure is the leading cause of death in children with cerebral malaria, but treatment with mannitol and corticosteroids has not improved outcomes in these children.

Respiratory distress is a poor prognostic indicator in severe malaria and appears to be caused by **metabolic acidosis** rather than intrinsic pulmonary disease. To date, no successful interventions for treatment of metabolic acidosis in children with severe malaria have been described, and primary therapy of malaria appears to be the most effective way to address acidosis.

Seizures are a common complication of severe malaria, particularly cerebral malaria. Benzodiazepines are first-line therapy for seizures, and intrarectal diazepam has been used successfully in children with malaria and seizures. Many seizures resolve with a single dose of diazepam. For persistent seizures, phenobarbital or phenytoin are the standard medications used. Phenytoin may be preferred for seizure treatment, particularly in hospitals or clinics where ventilatory support is not available. However, no comparative trials of the 2 drugs have been performed. There are currently no drugs recommended for seizure prophylaxis in children with severe malaria. Phenobarbital prophylaxis decreased seizure activity but increased mortality in one major study of children with severe malaria, probably because the respiratory depression associated with phenobarbital may have been exacerbated by benzodiazepine therapy.

Hypoglycemia is a complication of malaria that is more common in children, pregnant women, and patients receiving quinine therapy. Patients may have a decreased level of consciousness that can be confused with cerebral malaria. Any child with impaired consciousness and malaria should have a glucose level checked, and if glucometers are not immediately available, an empirical bolus of dextrose should be given. Hypoglycemia is associated with increased mortality and neurologic sequelae.

Circulatory collapse (**algid malaria**) is a rare complication that manifests as hypotension, hypothermia, rapid weak pulse, shallow breathing, pallor, and vascular collapse. It is most likely caused by bacterial superinfection, since up to 15% of children in endemic areas with severe malaria may have concurrent bacteremia. Death may occur within hours. Any child with severe malaria and hypotension or hypoperfusion should have a blood culture obtained and should be treated empirically for bacterial sepsis.

Long-term cognitive impairment occurs in 25% of children with cerebral malaria and also in children with repeated episodes of uncomplicated disease. Prevention of attacks in these children may improve educational attainment.

Hyperreactive malarial splenomegaly (**HMS**) is a chronic complication of *P. falciparum* malaria in which massive splenomegaly persists after treatment of acute infection. Major criteria include splenomegaly (>10 cm), IgM > 2 SD above local mean, high levels of antibodies to a blood-stage *P. falciparum* antigen, and a clinical response to an antimalarial drug. HMS occurs exclusively in children in endemic areas with repeated exposure to malaria and is thought to be caused by an impaired immune response to *P. falciparum* antigens. Prolonged antimalarial prophylaxis (for at least 1 yr, typically with chloroquine, quinine, or mefloquine) is required to treat this syndrome if the child remains in a malaria-endemic area. Spleen size gradually regresses on antimalarial prophylaxis but often increases again if prophylaxis is stopped.

Other complications in children include **acute kidney injury** and **jaundice**, both of which are associated with a worse outcome and prostration. A growing literature demonstrates that although renal failure requiring dialysis is rare in children with severe malaria, acute kidney injury is common and is associated with increased mortality. **Prostration** is defined as the inability to sit, stand, or eat without support, in the absence of impaired consciousness. Prostration has also been associated with increased mortality in some studies, but the pathophysiology of this process is not well understood. Uncommon complications include hemoglobinuria, abnormal bleeding, and pulmonary edema. Of note, pulmonary edema is more frequent in adolescents and adults.

PREVENTION

Malaria prevention consists of reducing exposure to infected mosquitoes and chemoprophylaxis. The most accurate and current information on areas in the world where malaria risk and drug resistance exist can be obtained by contacting local and state health departments or the CDC or consulting *Health Information for International Travel*, which is published by the U.S. Public Health Service.

Travelers to endemic areas should remain in well-screened areas from dusk to dawn, when the risk for transmission is highest. They should sleep under permethrin-treated mosquito netting and spray insecticides indoors at sundown. During the day, travelers should wear clothing that covers the arms and legs, with trousers tucked into shoes or boots. Mosquito repellent should be applied to thin clothing and exposed areas of the skin, with applications repeated as noted on the repellent instructions, and at least every 4 hr. A child should not be taken outside from

dusk to dawn, but if at risk for exposure, a solution with 25–35% *N,* diethyltoluamide (DEET) (not >40%) should be applied to exposed areas, except for the eyes, mouth, or hands. Hands are excluded because they are often placed in the mouth. DEET should then be washed off as soon as the child comes back inside. The American Academy of Pediatrics recommends that DEET solutions be avoided in children <2 mo old. Adverse reactions to DEET include rashes, toxic encephalopathy, and seizures, but these reactions occur almost exclusively with inappropriate application of high concentrations of DEET. **Picaridin** is an alternative and sometimes better-tolerated repellent. Even with these precautions, a child should be taken to a physician immediately if the child develops illness when traveling to a malarious area.

Chemoprophylaxis is necessary for all visitors to and residents of the tropics who have not lived there since infancy, including children of all ages (Table 314.5). Healthcare providers should consult the latest information on resistance patterns before prescribing prophylaxis for their patients. Chloroquine is given in the few remaining areas of the world free of chloroquine-resistant malaria strains. In areas where chloroquine-resistant *P. falciparum* exists, atovaquone-proguanil, mefloquine, or doxycycline

Table 314.5	Chemoprophylaxis of Malaria for Children				
AREA	**DRUG**	**DOSAGE (ORAL)**	**ADVANTAGES**	**DISADVANTAGES**	**BEST USE**
Chloroquine-resistant area	Mefloquine*†	<10 kg: 4.6 mg base (5 mg salt)/kg/wk 10-19 kg: ¼ tab/wk 20-30 kg: ½ tab/wk 31-45 kg: ¾ tab/wk >45 kg: 1 tab/wk (228 mg base)	Once weekly dosing	Bitter taste No pediatric formulation Side effects of sleep disturbance, vivid dreams	Children going to malaria-endemic area for ≥4 wk Children unlikely to take daily medication
	Doxycycline‡	2 mg/kg daily (max 100 mg)	Inexpensive	Cannot give to children <8 yr Daily dosing Must take with food or causes stomach upset Photosensitivity	Children going to area for <4 wk who cannot take or cannot obtain atovaquone-proguanil
	Atovaquone/proguanil§ (Malarone)	Pediatric tabs: 62.5 mg atovaquone/ 25 mg proguanil Adult tabs: 250 mg proguanil/ 100 mg proguanil 5-8 kg: pediatric tab once daily (off-label) 9-10 kg: pediatric tab once daily (off-label) 11-20 kg: 1 pediatric tab once daily 21-30 kg: 2 pediatric tabs once daily 31-40 kg: 3 pediatric tabs once daily >40 kg: 1 adult tab once daily	Pediatric formulation Generally well tolerated	Daily dosing Expensive Can cause stomach upset	Children going to malaria-endemic area for <4 wk
Chloroquine-susceptible area	Chloroquine phosphate	5 mg base/kg/wk (max: 300 mg base)	Once weekly dosing Inexpensive Generally well tolerated	Bitter taste No pediatric formulation	Best medication for children traveling to areas with *Plasmodium falciparum* or *Plasmodium vivax* that is chloroquine susceptible
	Drugs used for chloroquine-resistant areas can also be used in chloroquine-susceptible areas				

*Chloroquine and mefloquine should be started 1-2 wk prior to departure and continued for 4 wk after last exposure.

†Mefloquine resistance exists in western Cambodia and along the Thailand-Cambodia and Thailand-Myanmar borders. Travelers to these areas should take doxycycline or atovaquone-proguanil. See text for precautions about mefloquine use.

‡Doxycycline should be started 1-2 days prior to departure and continued for 4 wk after last exposure. Do not use in children younger than 8 yr of age or in pregnant women.

§Atovaquone/proguanil (Malarone) should be started 1-2 days prior to departure and continued for 7 days after last exposure. Should be taken with food or a milky drink. Not recommended in pregnant women, children weighing <5 kg, and women breastfeeding infants who weigh <5 kg. Contraindicated in individuals with severe renal impairment (creatinine clearance <30 mL/min).

may be given as chemoprophylaxis. **Atovaquone-proguanil** is generally recommended for shorter trips (up to 2 wk) because it must be taken daily. Pediatric tablets are available and are generally well tolerated, although the taste is sometimes unpleasant to very young children. For longer trips, **mefloquine** is preferred, since it is given only once a week. Mefloquine does not have a pediatric formulation and has an unpleasant taste that usually requires that the cut tablet be disguised in another food, such as chocolate syrup. Mefloquine should not be given to children if they have a known hypersensitivity to mefloquine, are receiving cardiotropic drugs, have a history of convulsive or certain psychiatric disorders, or travel to an area where mefloquine resistance exists (the borders of Thailand with Myanmar and Cambodia, western provinces of Cambodia, and eastern states of Myanmar). Atovaquone-proguanil is started 1-2 days before travel, and mefloquine is started 2 wk before travel. It is important that these doses are given, both to allow therapeutic levels of the drugs to be achieved and to be sure that the drugs are tolerated. **Doxycycline** is an alternative for children >8 yr old. It must be given daily and should be given with food. Side effects of doxycycline include photosensitivity and vaginal yeast infections. **Primaquine** is a daily prophylaxis option for children who cannot tolerate any of the other options, but it should be provided in consultation with a travel medicine specialist if needed, and all children should be checked for glucose-6-phosphate dehydrogenase deficiency before prescribing this medication, because it is contraindicated in children with G6PD deficiency. Provision of medication can be considered in individuals who refuse to take prophylaxis or will be in very remote areas without accessible medical care. Provision of medication for self-treatment of malaria should be done in consultation with a travel medicine specialist, and the medication provided should be different than that used for prophylaxis.

A number of other efforts are currently underway to prevent malaria in malaria-endemic countries. Some have been highly successful, leading to a significant decrease in malaria incidence in many countries in Africa, Asia, and South America in the last decade. These interventions include the use of insecticide-treated bed nets (which have decreased all-cause mortality in children <5 yr old in several highly malaria endemic areas by approximately 20%), indoor residual spraying with long-lasting insecticides, and the use of **artemisinin-combination therapy** for first-line malaria treatment. The first malaria vaccine to have any degree of efficacy is the **RTS,S vaccine**, which is based on the circumsporozoite protein of *P. falciparum*. In various clinical trials, this vaccine has shown an efficacy of 17–56% against uncomplicated malaria and 38–50% against severe malaria in young children in malaria-endemic areas for as long as48 mo after vaccination. Given the relatively low efficacy of this vaccine, it is still unclear if it will be implemented as part of a combination strategy that includes the already successful interventions mentioned. Numerous other vaccines are also in current clinical trials, and it is hoped that future vaccines will improve on the efficacy of the RTS,S vaccine. There is currently no vaccine with sufficient efficacy to be considered for prevention of malaria in travelers.

Intermittent prevention treatment during infancy has been particularly successful in reducing the incidence of malaria in sub Saharan Africa. **Sulfadoxine-pyrimethamine** given to infants at the 2nd and 3rd doses of the diphtheria, tetanus toxoid, and pertussis vaccine is safe and relatively effective. Intermittent prevention treatment has also been given to pregnant women; 3 doses of sulfadoxine-pyrimethamine have resulted in a reduction of low-birthweight infants.

Bibliography is available at Expert Consult.

Chapter **315**
Babesiosis *(Babesia)*
Peter J. Krause

第三百一十五章
巴贝西虫病（巴贝西虫）

中文导读

　　本章主要介绍了巴贝西虫病的病原学、流行病学、发病机制、临床表现、诊断、治疗、预后和预防。在流行病学部分，介绍了巴贝西虫病的感染途径、疾病在全球的分布情况和发病率。在临床表现部分，描述了巴贝西虫病的临床特点，同时指出了引发重症疾病的危险因素。在治疗部分，介绍了巴贝西虫病的药物选择及疗程，同时介绍了换血治疗的适应证。

Babesiosis is a malaria-like disease caused by intraerythrocytic protozoa that are transmitted by hard body (**ixodid**) ticks. The clinical manifestations of babesiosis range from subclinical illness to fulminant disease resulting in death.

ETIOLOGY

More than 100 species of *Babesia* infect a wide variety of wild and domestic animals throughout the world. Only a few of these species have been reported to infect humans, including *Babesia crassa*-like pathogen, *Babesia divergens, Babesia duncani, Babesia microti, Babesia venatorum,* and *Babesia* sp. XXB/HangZhou, and KO1.

EPIDEMIOLOGY

Babesia organisms are transmitted to humans from vertebrate reservoir hosts by the *Ixodes ricinus* family of ticks. *B. microti* is the most common cause of babesiosis in humans. The primary reservoir for *B. microti* in the United States is the white-footed mouse, *Peromyscus leucopus,* and the primary vector is *Ixodes scapularis,* the black-legged tick. *I. scapularis* ticks also transmit the causative agents of **Lyme disease,** human granulocytic anaplasmosis, *Borrelia miyamotoi* infection, *Ehrlichia muris*–like agent ehrlichiosis, and Powassan virus encephalitis and may simultaneously transmit 2 or more microorganisms. White-tailed deer *(Odocoileus virginianus)* serve as the host on which adult ticks most abundantly feed but are incompetent reservoirs. Babesiosis may be transmitted through blood transfusion, and *B. microti* is the most frequently reported transfusion-transmitted microbial agent in the United States. Rarely, babesiosis is acquired by transplacental transmission.

In the United States, human *B. microti* infection is endemic in the Northeast and Upper Midwest (Fig. 315.1). Most cases occur in June, July, and August. *B. duncani* infects humans along the Pacific coast. *B. divergens*–like infections have been described in Kentucky, Missouri, and Washington State. In Europe, human babesiosis caused by *B. divergens, B. microti,* and *B. venatorum* occurs sporadically. In Asia, *B. venatorum* is endemic in northeastern China. Cases of *B. microti* infection have been described in Taiwan, mainland China, and Japan. Cases of *Babesia crassa* and *Babesia* sp. XXB/HangZhou have been reported in China and KO1 in Korea. Human babesiosis also has been documented in Africa, Australia, Canada, India, and South America.

In certain sites and in certain years of high transmission, babesiosis constitutes a significant public health burden. On Nantucket Island, case rates as high as 280 per 100,000 population have been recorded, placing the community burden of disease in a category with gonorrhea as "moderately common." Comparable incidence rates have been described elsewhere on the southern New England coast.

PATHOGENESIS

The pathogenesis of human babesiosis is not well understood. Lysis of infected erythrocytes with resultant anemia and the excessive production of proinflammatory cytokines such as tumor necrosis factor and interleukin-1 may account for most of the clinical manifestations and complications of the disease. The spleen has an important role in clearing parasitemia, as do T and B cells, macrophages, polymorphonuclear leukocytes, cytokines, antibody, and complement.

CLINICAL MANIFESTATIONS

The clinical severity of babesiosis ranges from subclinical infection to fulminant disease and death. In clinically apparent cases, symptoms of babesiosis begin after an incubation period of 1-9 wk from the beginning of tick feeding or 1 wk to 6 mo after transfusion. Typical symptoms in moderate to severe infection include intermittent fever to as high as 40°C (104°F) accompanied by any combination of chills, sweats, headache, and myalgias. Less common are arthralgias, sore throat, abdominal pain, nausea, vomiting, emotional lability, hyperesthesia, conjunctival injection, photophobia, weight loss, and nonproductive cough. The findings on physical examination generally are minimal, often consisting only of fever. Splenomegaly, hepatomegaly, or both are noted occasionally, but rash seldom is reported. Abnormal laboratory findings include moderately severe hemolytic anemia, elevated reticulocyte count, thrombocytopenia, proteinuria, and elevated bilirubin, blood urea nitrogen, and creatinine levels. The leukocyte count is normal to slightly decreased, often with neutropenia. Complications include respiratory failure, disseminated intravascular coagulation, congestive heart failure, renal failure, liver failure, coma, and death. Babesiosis symptoms usually last for 1-2 wk, although prolonged recovery of up to ≥1 yr may occur in highly immunocompromised hosts who experience relapsing infection. Such patients include those with cancer and asplenia, those receiving immunosuppressive therapy, or those with HIV/AIDS, even though they receive multiple courses of antibabesial therapy. More than one fifth of these patients died, while the remainder were cured after an average of 3 mo (range: 1-24 mo) of antibabesial therapy.

Risk factors for severe disease include aging, neonatal prematurity, anatomic or functional asplenia, malignancy, HIV/AIDS, immunosuppressive drugs, acquisition of infection through blood transfusion, or organ transplantation. Concurrent babesiosis and Lyme disease has

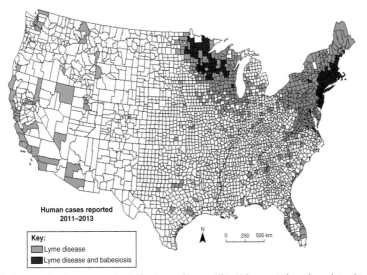

Human cases reported
2011–2013

Key:
☐ Lyme disease
■ Lyme disease and babesiosis

Fig. 315.1 Human babesiosis emerging in areas endemic for Lyme disease. This U.S. map is based on data obtained from the Centers for Disease Control and Prevention that recorded the names of counties that reported cases of Lyme disease and/or babesiosis from 2011 to 2013. Counties with ≥3 cases of Lyme disease but <3 cases of babesiosis are depicted in *green.* Counties with ≥3 cases of Lyme disease and ≥3 cases of babesiosis are depicted in *gray.* No county reported ≥3 cases of babesiosis but <3 cases of Lyme disease. *(Adapted from Diuk-Wasser M, Vannier E, Krause PJ: Coinfection by Ixodes tick-borne pathogens: ecological, epidemiological, and clinical consequences, Trends Parasitol 32:30–42, 2016.)*

been reported in 3–11% of patients experiencing Lyme disease, depending on location in the United States. Such co-infection results in more severe Lyme disease illness. Moderate to severe babesiosis may occur in children, but infection generally is less severe than in adults. About half of infected children are asymptomatic or experience minimal symptoms. Neonates may develop severe illness and usually are infected from blood transfusion.

DIAGNOSIS

Diagnosis of *B. microti* infection in human hosts is confirmed by microscopic demonstration of the organism using Giemsa-stained thin blood films. Parasitemia may be exceedingly low, especially early in the course of illness. Thick blood smears may be examined, but the organisms may be mistaken for stain precipitate or iron inclusion bodies. The polymerase chain reaction is a sensitive and specific test for detection of *Babesia* DNA and can be used in addition to or instead of blood smear to confirm the diagnosis. Subinoculation of blood into hamsters or gerbils and in vitro cultivation are too specialized for all but the most experienced laboratories. Serologic testing is useful, particularly for diagnosing *B. microti* infection. The indirect immunofluorescence serologic assay for both IgG and IgM antibodies is sensitive and specific and can support a diagnosis of babesiosis, although may reflect past infection rather than acute disease. The diagnosis of babesiosis is most reliably made in patients who have lived or traveled in an area where babesiosis is endemic, who experience viral infection–like symptoms, and who have identifiable parasites on blood smear or amplifiable *Babesia* DNA in blood and antibabesial antibody in serum. The diagnosis of active babesial infection based on seropositivity alone is suspect.

TREATMENT

The combination of **clindamycin** (7-10 mg/kg given intravenously [IV] or orally [PO] every 6-8 hr, up to maximum of 600 mg/dose) and **quinine** (8 mg/kg PO every 8 hr, up to maximum of 650 mg/dose) for 7-10 days was the first effective therapeutic combination for the treatment of babesiosis. However, adverse reactions are common, especially tinnitus and abdominal distress. The combination of **atovaquone** (20 mg/kg PO every 12 hr, up to maximum of 750 mg/dose) and **azithromycin**

(10 mg/kg/day PO once on day 1, up to maximum of 500 mg/dose, and 5 mg/kg once daily thereafter, up to maximum of 250 mg/dose) for 7-10 days is as effective as clindamycin and quinine but has far fewer adverse effects. Atovaquone with azithromycin has been used successfully to treat babesiosis in infants and should be used initially in all children experiencing babesiosis. Clindamycin with quinine is an alternative choice. Treatment failure with atovaquone-azithromycin and clindamycin-quinine may occur in highly immunocompromised hosts. Consultation with an infectious diseases expert is recommended in these cases. Exchange blood transfusion can decrease parasitemia rapidly and remove toxic by-products of infection. Partial or complete exchange transfusion is recommended for children with high-grade parasitemia (≥10%), severe anemia (hemoglobin <10 g/dL) or pulmonary, renal, or hepatic compromise.

PROGNOSIS

Moderate to severe disease is frequently observed in some highly endemic areas. The babesiosis case fatality rate was estimated at 5% in a retrospective study of 136 New York cases but may be as high as 21% in immunocompromised hosts and those who acquire babesiosis through blood transfusion. Immunity is sometimes incomplete, with low-level asymptomatic parasitemia persisting for as long as 26 mo after symptoms have resolved, or with relapsing symptomatic disease in immunocompromised hosts.

PREVENTION

Prevention of babesiosis can be accomplished by avoiding areas where ticks, deer, and mice are known to thrive. Use of clothing that covers the lower part of the body and that is sprayed or impregnated with diethyltoluamide (DEET), dimethyl phthalate, or permethrin (Permanone) is recommended for those who travel in the foliage of endemic areas. DEET can be applied directly to the skin. A search for ticks should be carried out and the ticks removed using tweezers. Prospective blood donors with a history of babesiosis are excluded from giving blood to prevent transfusion-related cases.

Bibliography is available at Expert Consult.

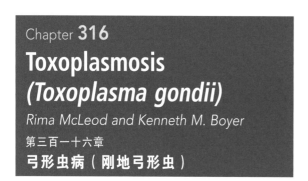

Chapter **316**

Toxoplasmosis (*Toxoplasma gondii*)

Rima McLeod and Kenneth M. Boyer

第三百一十六章
弓形虫病（刚地弓形虫）

中文导读

　　本章主要介绍了弓形虫病的病原学、流行病学、发病机制、临床表现、诊断、治疗、预后和预防。在

流行病学和发病机制部分，特别介绍了先天性弓形虫病的流行病学和发病机制。在临床表现部分，分别描

述了获得性弓形虫病、眼弓形虫病、免疫力低下的人群、先天性弓形虫病的临床特点，特别描述了先天性弓形虫病的各系统征象，包括皮肤、内分泌异常、中枢神经系统、眼、耳的表现。在诊断部分，分别介绍了病原分离、血清学检测方法，同时介绍了获得性弓形虫病、眼弓形虫病、免疫力低下的人群及先天性弓形虫病的诊断方法。在治疗部分，分别阐述了获得性弓形虫病、眼弓形虫病、免疫力低下的人群、先天性弓形虫病及孕妇感染弓形虫的治疗方案。

Toxoplasma gondii, an obligate, intracellular, apicomplexan protozoan, is acquired perorally, transplacentally, or rarely parenterally in laboratory accidents, transfusions, or from a transplanted organ. In immunologically normal children, acute acquired infection most often is asymptomatic or unrecognized, but may cause lymphadenopathy or affect almost any organ. *Once acquired, latent encysted organisms persist in the host throughout life.* In immunocompromised persons, initial acquisition or recrudescence of latent organisms can cause signs or symptoms related to the central nervous system (CNS) or result in systemic disease, as in bone marrow transplant recipients. If untreated, congenital infection usually causes disease that manifests either perinatally or later in life, most frequently chorioretinitis and CNS lesions. Other manifestations, such as intrauterine growth restriction, prematurity, cognitive and motor deficits, fever, lymphadenopathy, rash, hearing loss, pneumonitis, hepatitis, thrombocytopenia, and cerebrospinal fluid (CSF) inflammatory changes may also occur. Unrecognized congenital toxoplasmosis in infants with HIV infection may be fulminant.

ETIOLOGY

Toxoplasma gondii is a coccidian protozoan that multiplies only in living cells. It is descended from an ancient, free-living, single-celled extracellular parasite called *Colpodella* that shares some ultrastructural features with *T. gondii.* Tachyzoites, the pathogenic form of the parasite in active infections, are oval or crescent-like, measuring 2-4 × 4-7 μm. Tissue cysts, which are 10-100 μm in diameter, may contain 1000s of latent parasites called **bradyzoites** and will remain in tissues, especially the CNS and skeletal and heart muscle, for the life of the host. *Toxoplasma* can multiply in all tissues of mammals and birds.

Oocysts, another form of the parasite, are formed in the cat intestine. Newly infected, nonimmune cats and other Felidae species are the definitive hosts of *T. gondii,* in which genetic exchange occurs during a sexual cycle. *Toxoplasma* organisms are transmitted to cats when the cat ingests infected meat containing encysted bradyzoites or ingests oocysts containing sporozoites excreted by other recently infected cats. The parasites then multiply through schizogonic and gametogonic cycles in the distal ileal epithelium of the cat intestine. Oocysts containing 2 sporocysts are excreted, and, under proper conditions of temperature and moisture, each sporocyst matures into 4 sporozoites. For approximately 2 wk the cat excretes 10^5-10^7 oocysts daily, which may retain their viability for >1 yr in a suitable environment. Oocysts sporulate 1-5 days after excretion and are then infectious. Oocysts are killed by drying or boiling but not exposure to bleach. Oocysts have been isolated from soil and sand frequented by cats, and outbreaks associated with contaminated food and water have been reported. Oocysts and tissue cysts are sources of animal and human infections (Fig. 316.1*A* and *B*). There are genetically distinct genetic types of *T. gondii* that have different virulence for mice (and likely for humans) and form different numbers of cysts in the brain of outbred mice. In the United States, there are 4 predominant clonal lineages called **types I, II, III**, and **IV** (haplogroup XII) in addition to atypical, recombinant types (Fig. 316.1*C*). There is 1 predominant clonal type (type II) in France, Austria, and Poland, and nonarchetypal parasites are prevalent in Brazil, Guyana, French Guiana, and Central America (Fig. 316.1*D*). Secreted molecules are primary virulence factors that differ between genetic lineages called **strains** (Fig. 316.1*E*).

EPIDEMIOLOGY

Toxoplasma infection is ubiquitous in animals and is one of the most common latent infections of humans throughout the world, infecting, and remaining in, approximately 2 billion people. Prevalence varies considerably among people and animals in different geographic areas. In different areas of the world, approximately 3–35% of pork, 7–60% of lamb, and 0–9% of beef contain *T. gondii* organisms. Significant antibody titers are detected in 50–80% of residents of some localities, such as France, Brazil, and Central America, and in <5% in other areas. The current prevalence estimate in the United States is 10%, but prevalence varies in differing demographics. For example, in the study of Lancaster County pregnant women in an Amish community, prevalence was 50%. There appears to be a higher prevalence of infection in some warmer, more humid climates. Non type II parasites are more common in mothers of congenitally infected infants in warm, moist southern climates, in rural areas, in those with lower socioeconomic status, and with Hispanic ethnicity in the United States. Non–type II parasites are more often associated with prematurity and severe congenital infection in the United States.

Human infection in older children and adults is usually acquired orally by eating undercooked or raw meat that contains cysts or food (e.g., salad greens) or other material contaminated with oocysts from acutely infected cats. Freezing meat to −20°C (−4°F) or heating meat to 66°C (150.8°F) renders the tissue cysts noninfectious. Outbreaks of acute acquired infection have occurred in families, at social gatherings, and in restaurants where people have consumed the same infected food or water. *Toxoplasma* organisms are not known to be transmitted from person to person except for transplacental infection from mother to fetus and, rarely, by organ transplantation or transfusion. *T. gondii* has been noted in the prostate gland and sperm of nonhuman animals, but no sexual transmission between humans has been proved.

Seronegative transplant recipients who receive an organ or bone marrow from seropositive donors have experienced life-threatening illness requiring therapy. Seropositive recipients who receive an infected donor organ may have increased serologic titers without recognized, associated disease. Laboratory accidents have resulted in infections, including fatalities.

Congenital Toxoplasmosis

Transmission to the fetus usually follows acquisition of primary infection by an immunologically normal pregnant woman during gestation. Congenital transmission from mothers infected before pregnancy is extremely rare except for immunocompromised women who are chronically infected. The estimated incidence of congenital infection in the United States ranges from 1 in 1,000 to 1 in 8,000 live births. An estimated 15 million people are living with congenital toxoplasmosis worldwide. The incidence of infection among pregnant women depends on the general risk for infection in the specific locale and the proportion of the population that has not been infected previously.

PATHOGENESIS

T. gondii is acquired by children and adults from ingesting food that contains cysts or that is contaminated with oocysts from acutely infected cats. Oocysts also may be transported to food by flies and cockroaches.

They may be carried to people on the fur of dogs. When the organism is ingested, bradyzoites are released from cysts or sporozoites from oocysts. The organisms enter gastrointestinal (GI) cells, where they multiply, rupture cells, infect contiguous cells, enter the lymphatics and blood, and disseminate lymphohematogenously throughout the body. **Tachyzoites** proliferate, producing necrotic foci surrounded by a cellular reaction. With development of a normal immune response that is both humoral and cell mediated, tachyzoites disappear from tissues. In immunocompromised persons and also some apparently immunocompetent persons, acute infection progresses and may cause potentially lethal disease, including pneumonitis, myocarditis, or encephalitis.

Alterations of T-lymphocyte populations during acute *T. gondii* infection are common and include lymphocytosis, increased $CD8^+$ T-cell count, and decreased $CD4^+/CD8^+$ ratio. Characteristic histopathologic changes in lymph nodes during acute infection include reactive follicular hyperplasia with irregular clusters of epithelioid histiocytes that encroach on and blur margins of germinal centers, and focal distention of sinuses with monocytoid cells. Depletion of $CD4^+$ T cells in patients with AIDS predisposes to severe manifestations of toxoplasmosis.

Cysts form as early as 7 days after infection and remain for the life of the host. During latent infection they produce little or no inflammatory response but can cause recrudescent disease in immunocompromised persons. **Recrudescent chorioretinitis** can occur in children and adults with postnatally acquired infection and in older children and adults with congenitally acquired infection. Host and parasite genetics influence outcomes.

Congenital Toxoplasmosis

When a mother acquires infection during gestation, organisms may disseminate hematogenously to the placenta. Infection may be transmitted to the fetus transplacentally or during vaginal delivery. Of untreated maternal infections acquired in the first trimester, approximately 17% of fetuses are infected, usually with severe disease. Of untreated maternal infection acquired in the third trimester, approximately 65% of fetuses are infected, usually with disease that is milder or inapparent at birth. These different rates of transmission and outcomes are most likely related to placental blood flow, virulence, inoculum of *T. gondii*, and immunologic capacity of the mother and fetus to limit parasitemia.

Examination of the placenta of infected newborns may reveal chronic inflammation and cysts. Tachyzoites can be seen with Wright or Giemsa stains but are best demonstrated with immunoperoxidase technique. Tissue cysts stain well with periodic acid–Schiff and silver stains as well as with the immunoperoxidase technique. Gross or microscopic areas of necrosis may be present in many tissues, especially the CNS, choroid and retina, heart, lungs, skeletal muscle, liver, and spleen. Areas of calcification occur in the brain.

Almost all congenitally infected individuals who are not treated manifest signs or symptoms of infection, such as chorioretinitis, by adolescence. Some severely involved infants with congenital infection appear to have *Toxoplasma* antigen–specific cell-mediated hyporesponsiveness, which may be important in the pathogenesis of disease.

CLINICAL MANIFESTATIONS

Manifestations of primary infection with *T. gondii* are highly variable and are influenced primarily by host immunocompetence. There may be no signs or symptoms or severe disease. Reactivation of previously asymptomatic congenital toxoplasmosis usually manifests as ocular toxoplasmosis.

Acquired Toxoplasmosis

Immunocompetent children who acquire infection postnatally generally do not have clinically recognizable symptoms. When clinical manifestations are apparent, they may include almost any combination of fever, stiff neck, myalgia, arthralgia, maculopapular rash that spares the palms and soles, localized or generalized lymphadenopathy, hepatomegaly, hepatitis, reactive lymphocytosis, meningitis, brain abscess, encephalitis, confusion, malaise, pneumonia, polymyositis, pericarditis, pericardial effusion, and myocarditis. **Chorioretinitis** occurs in approximately 1% of U.S. cases and in 20% of cases in epidemics in Brazil at 2 years after infection. Approximately 10% of mothers of congenitally infected infants have eye lesions on dilated indirect ophthalmoscopic examinations. Postnatally acquired chorioretinal lesions cannot be distinguished from congenitally acquired lesions based on appearance. In some areas of Brazil, 80% of the population is infected, 20% of whom have retinal involvement, with 50% of those >50 yr old. Symptoms and signs of active ocular infection may be present for a few weeks only or may persist for many months.

The most common manifestation of acute acquired toxoplasmosis is enlargement of 1 or a few cervical lymph nodes. Cases of *Toxoplasma* **lymphadenopathy** can resemble infectious mononucleosis, lymphoma, or other lymphadenopathies (see Chapter 517). Pectoral, mediastinal, mesenteric, and retroperitoneal lymph nodes may be involved. Involvement of intraabdominal lymph nodes may be associated with fever, mimicking appendicitis. Nodes may be tender but do not suppurate. Lymphadenopathy may wax and wane for as long as 1-2 yr. However, almost all patients with lymphadenopathy recover spontaneously without antimicrobial therapy. Significant organ involvement in immunologically normal persons is uncommon, although some individuals have significant morbidity, including rare cases of encephalitis, brain abscesses, hepatitis, myocarditis, pericarditis, and polymyositis. In persons acquiring *T. gondii* in Guyana near the Maroni River, and along Amazon tributaries, a severe form of life-threatening, multivisceral involvement with fever has occurred.

Ocular Toxoplasmosis

In the United States and Western Europe, *T. gondii* is estimated to cause 35% of cases of **chorioretinitis** (Fig. 316.2). In Brazil, *T. gondii* retinal lesions are common. Clinical manifestations include blurred vision, visual floaters, photophobia, epiphora, and, with macular involvement, loss of central vision. Ocular findings of **congenital toxoplasmosis** also include strabismus, microphthalmia, microcornea, cataracts, anisometropia, nystagmus, glaucoma, optic neuritis, and optic atrophy. Episodic recurrences are common, but precipitating factors have not been defined. Recurrent, active disease usually occurs at school-entry age and during adolescence. Anecdotally, stress or trauma seems to precipitate symptoms. Recurrences are most common closest to the time of acquisition of infection, and treatment leads to resolution of activity.

Immunocompromised Persons

Disseminated *T. gondii* infection among older children who are **immunocompromised** by AIDS, malignancy, cytotoxic therapy, corticosteroids, or immunosuppressive drugs given for organ transplantation involves the

---

Fig. 316.1 The parasite: *Toxoplasma* life cycle, ancient ancestor, ultrastructure, life cycle stages affecting humans, genetic variation, and global seroprevalence. **A,** Life cycle of *Toxoplasma gondii* and prevention of toxoplasmosis by interruption of transmission to humans. **B,** Risk of severe neurologic disease or death (SNDD) in children with congenital toxoplasmosis (CT) according to antepartum treatment. Probability of SNDD according to imputed gestational age at seroconversion and 95% bayesian credible limits. *Dotted lines* denote treated pregnancies; *solid lines* denote untreated pregnancies. (SNDD is a composite outcome comprising a pediatric report at any age of microcephaly; insertion of an intraventricular shunt; an abnormal or suspicious neurodevelopmental examination that resulted in referral to a specialist; seizures during infancy or at an older age that required anticonvulsant therapy; severe bilateral visual impairment [visual acuity of Snellen ≤6/60 in both eyes assessed after 3 yr]; cerebral palsy; or death from any cause before age 2 yr, including termination of pregnancy [consistency of SSND findings was checked through multiple assessments].) Severe neurologic sequelae were assessed at a median of 4 yr follow-up, death was assessed by age 2 yr, and severe bilateral visual impairment was included in the composite outcome of severe neurologic sequelae. **C,** Probability of fetal infection according to gestational age at the time of maternal infection before (*n* = 451) and after (*n* = 1624) mid-1992, Lyon cohort (1987–2008). *Continued*

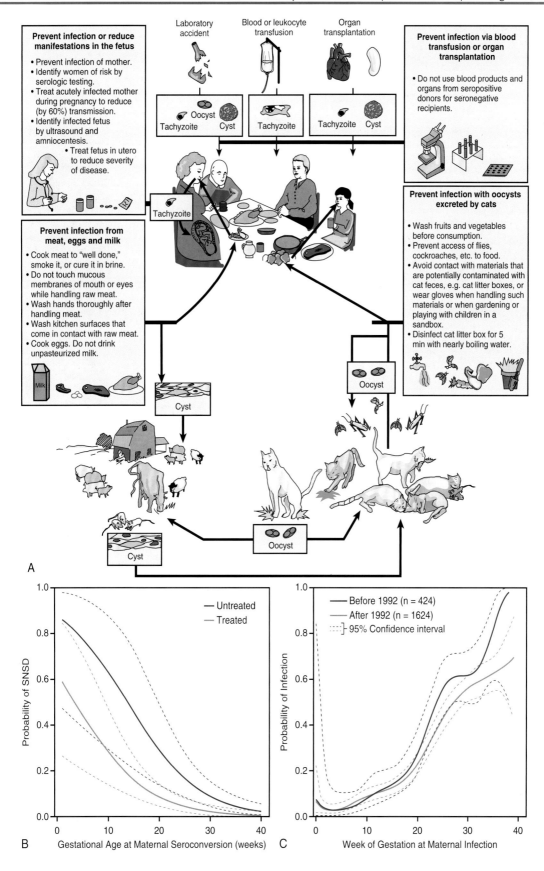

Prevent infection or reduce manifestations in the fetus

- Prevent infection of mother.
- Identify women of risk by serologic testing.
- Treat acutely infected mother during pregnancy to reduce (by 60%) transmission.
- Identify infected fetus by ultrasound and amniocentesis.
  - Treat fetus in utero to reduce severity of disease.

Laboratory accident

Blood or leukocyte transfusion

Organ transplantation

Oocyst
Tachyzoite   Cyst

Tachyzoite

Tachyzoite   Cyst

Tachyzoite

Prevent infection via blood transfusion or organ transplantation

- Do not use blood products and organs from seropositive donors for seronegative recipients.

Prevent infection from meat, eggs and milk

- Cook meat to "well done," smoke it, or cure it in brine.
- Do not touch mucous membranes of mouth or eyes while handling raw meat.
- Wash hands thoroughly after handling meat.
- Wash kitchen surfaces that come in contact with raw meat.
- Cook eggs. Do not drink unpasteurized milk.

Prevent infection with oocysts excreted by cats

- Wash fruits and vegetables before consumption.
- Prevent access of flies, cockroaches, etc. to food.
- Avoid contact with materials that are potentially contaminated with cat feces, e.g. cat litter boxes, or wear gloves when handling such materials or when gardening or playing with children in a sandbox.
- Disinfect cat litter box for 5 min with nearly boiling water.

Milk

Cyst

Oocyst

Cyst

Oocyst

A

B — Probability of SNSD vs Gestational Age at Maternal Seroconversion (weeks)

— Untreated
— Treated

C — Probability of Infection vs Week of Gestation at Maternal Infection

— Before 1992 (n = 424)
— After 1992 (n = 1624)
··· 95% Confidence interval

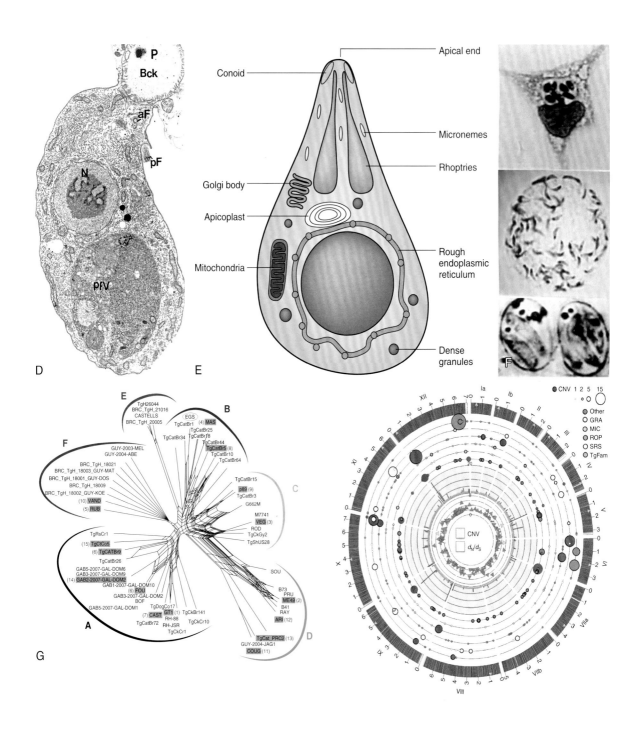

Fig. 316.1, cont'd D, *Colpodella vorax*, an ancient progenitor to the apicomplexans. **E,** Ultrastructure of *T. gondii* tachyzoite. **F,** Light micrographs of *top to bottom*, tachyzoite, bradyzoite, and sporozoite stages of *T. gondii*. **G,** Genetic characterization of EGS strain. Genetic relationship of *T. gondii* isolate strain (*left*) and positions on chromosomes (*right*). (B, *From Cortina-Borja M, Tan HK, Wallon M, et al. Prenatal treatment of serious neurologic sequelae of congenital toxoplasmosis: an observational prospective cohort study, PLoS Med 7:e1000351, 2010; C, from Wallon M, Peyron F, Cornu C, et al: Congenital toxoplasmosis infection: monthly prenatal screening decreases transmission rate and improves clinical outcome at age 3 years, Clin Infect Dis 56:1229, 2013; D, from Brugerolle G: Colpodella vorax: ultrastructure, predation, life-cycle, mitosis, and phylogenetic relationships, Eur J Protistol 38(2):113–125, 2002; E, from Wheeler K: Characterization of* Toxoplasma gondii *dense granule protein 1: genetic, functional, and mechanistic analyses (Undergraduate Honors thesis), Kelsey Wheeler; F, from Dubey JP, Miller N, Frenkel JK: The* Toxoplasma gondii *oocyst from cat feces, J Exp Med 132(4):636-662, 1970; G, from McPhillie M, Zhou Y, El Bissati K, et al: New paradigms for understanding and step changes in treating active and chronic, persistent apicomplexan infections, Sci Rep 6(1), 2016.)*

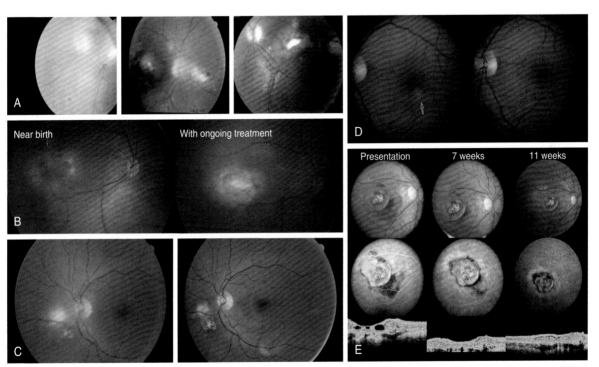

Fig. 316.2 Toxoplasmic chorioretinitis. **A,** Retinal photographs of a child with severe vitreitis that is less intense than the classic "headlight in fog" appearance (*left*). Resolving vitreitis caused by underlying active lesion (*middle*). Resolved healed lesion without vitreitis (*right*). **B,** Retina photographs for a newborn infant with active vitreitis (*left*, "near birth") with clearing of vitreitis and marked, but not complete, resolution of activity of the lesion 3 wk later (*right*, "with ongoing treatment"). **C,** Retinal photographs of a child showing an active lesion at presentation (*left*), and scarred lesion (*right*). **D,** Retinal photographs showing an active retinal lesion before treatment (*left*) and a completely resolved normal appearing retina within 1 mo of initiating treatment (*right*). **E,** Active choroidal neovascular membranes (CNVMs) in a child. Fundus photographs (*top row*), fluorescein angiogram (FA; *middle row*), and ocular coherence tomography (OCT; *bottom row*) of a child at presentation (*first column*), 7 wk after first ranibizumab (Lucentis, antibody to VEGF) injection (*second column*), and 11 wk after first ranibizumab injection (*third column*). (A-D, *Adapted from Delair E, Latkany P, Noble AG, et al: Clinical manifestations of ocular toxoplasmosis, Ocul Immunol Inflamm 19:91–102, 2011; E, adapted from Benevento JD, Jager RD, Noble AG, et al: Toxoplasmosis-associated neovascular lesions treated successfully with ranibizumab and antiparasitic therapy, Arch Ophthalmol 126:1152–1156, 2008.)*

CNS in 50% of cases and may also involve the heart, lungs, and GI tract. Stem cell transplant recipients present a special problem, because active infection is difficult to diagnose serologically. After transplantation, *T. gondii*–specific antibody levels may remain the same, increase, or decrease, and can even become undetectable. Toxoplasmosis in transplantation patients almost always results from transplantation from a seropositive donor to a seronegative recipient. Thus, knowledge of the serologic status of the donor and recipient is essential. Active infection is often fulminant and rapidly fatal without treatment. Following blood PCR can establish diagnosis and monitor efficacy of treatment.

Congenital *T. gondii* infection in infants with HIV infection is rare in the United States but can be a severe and fulminant disease with substantial CNS involvement. Alternatively, it may be more indolent in presentation, with focal neurologic deficits or systemic manifestations such as pneumonitis occurring with progressive CD4 depletion in the highly active antiretroviral therapy (HAART)–untreated infant.

From 25–50% of persons with *T. gondii* antibodies and HIV infection without antiretroviral treatment eventually experience **toxoplasmic encephalitis**, which is fatal if not treated. HAART and trimethoprim-sulfamethoxazole (TMP-SMX) prophylaxis to prevent *Pneumocystis* have diminished the incidence of toxoplasmosis in patients with HIV infection, but toxoplasmic encephalitis remains a presenting manifestation in some adult patients with AIDS. Typical findings include fever, headache, altered mental status, psychosis, cognitive impairment, seizures, and focal neurologic defects, including hemiparesis, aphasia, ataxia, visual field loss, cranial nerve palsies, and dysmetria or movement disorders. In adult patients with AIDS, toxoplasmic retinal lesions are often large with diffuse necrosis and contain many organisms but little inflammatory cellular infiltrate. Diagnosis of presumptive toxoplasmic encephalitis based on neuroradiologic studies in patients with AIDS necessitates a prompt therapeutic trial of medications effective against *T. gondii*. Clear clinical improvement within 7-14 days and improvement of neuroradiologic findings within 3 wk make the presumptive diagnosis almost certain.

Congenital Toxoplasmosis

Congenital toxoplasmosis usually occurs when a woman acquires primary infection while pregnant. Most often, maternal infection is asymptomatic or without specific symptoms or signs. As with other adults with acute toxoplasmosis, lymphadenopathy is the most commonly identified physical finding.

In monozygotic twins the clinical pattern of involvement is most often similar, whereas in dizygotic twins the manifestations often differ, including cases of congenital infection in only 1 twin. The major histocompatibility complex class II gene DQ3 appears to be more common than DQ1 among HIV-infected persons seropositive for *T. gondii* who develop toxoplasmic encephalitis, as well as in children with congenital toxoplasmosis who develop hydrocephalus. These findings suggest that the presence of HLA-DQ3 is a risk factor for severity of toxoplasmosis. Other allelic variants of genes, including *COL2A, ABC4R, P2X7R, NALP1, ALOX12, TLR9*, and *ERAAP*, are also associated with increased susceptibility.

Congenital infection may present as a mild or severe neonatal disease. It may also present with sequelae or relapse of a previously undiagnosed and untreated infection later in infancy or even later in life. There is a wide variety of manifestations of congenital infection, ranging from hydrops fetalis and perinatal death to small size for gestational age, prematurity, peripheral retinal scars, persistent jaundice, mild thrombocytopenia, CSF pleocytosis, and the characteristic triad of chorioretinitis, hydrocephalus, and cerebral calcifications. More than 50% of congenitally infected infants are considered normal in the perinatal period, but almost all such children will develop ocular involvement later in life if they are not treated during infancy. Neurologic signs such as convulsions, setting-sun sign with downward gaze, and hydrocephalus with increased head circumference may be associated with substantial cerebral damage or with relatively mild inflammation obstructing the aqueduct of Sylvius. If affected infants are treated and shunted promptly, signs and symptoms may resolve, and development may be normal.

The spectrum and frequency of neonatal manifestations of 210 newborns with congenital *Toxoplasma* infection identified by a serologic screening program of pregnant women in France were described in 1984. In this study, 10% had severe congenital toxoplasmosis with CNS involvement, eye lesions, and general systemic manifestations; 34% had mild involvement with normal clinical examination results other than retinal scars on dilated indirect exams or isolated intracranial calcifications in brain CT scans; and 55% had no detectable manifestations. These numbers represent an *underestimation* of the incidence of severe congenital infection for several reasons: the most severe cases, including most who died, were not referred; therapeutic abortion sometimes was performed when acute acquired infection of the mother was diagnosed early during pregnancy; in utero **spiramycin** therapy prevented or diminished the severity of infection; only 13 of the 210 congenitally infected newborns had brain CT, and only 77% of these 210 infants had a CSF examination. Routine newborn examinations often yield normal findings for congenitally infected infants, but more careful evaluations may reveal significant abnormalities. A 2012 analysis of the **National Collaborative Chicago-Based Congenital Toxoplasmosis Study** (NCCCTS, 1981–2009) data

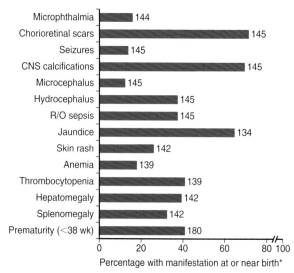

Fig. 316.3 Congenital toxoplasmosis: manifestations at presentation. National Collaborative Chicago-Based Congenital Toxoplasmosis Study (NCCCTS, 1981–2009). *Infants diagnosed with congenital toxoplasmosis in the newborn period and referred to the NCCCTS during the 1st yr of life. Numbers adjacent to histogram bars represent number of infants with this manifestation and is based on information in birth records; R/O, rule out sepsis. Sample size dependent on available birth records/ diagnoses at birth. *(Adapted from McLeod R, Boyer KM, Lee D, et al: Prematurity and severity are associated with* Toxoplasma gondii *alleles [NCCCTS, 1981–2009],* Clin Infect Dis *54:1595–1605, 2012.)*

found that 72% of children at or near birth had chorioretinal scars, 70% had CNS calcifications, 12% microcephaly, 37% hydrocephalus, 41% thrombocytopenia, 39% hepatomegaly, 32% splenomegaly, and 41% were born prematurely (Fig. 316.3). In one study of 28 infants in New England, identified by a universal state-mandated serologic screening program for *T. gondii*–specific IgM, 26 (93%) had normal findings on routine newborn examination, but 14 (50%) had significant abnormalities detected with more careful evaluation. The abnormalities included retinal scars (7 infants), active chorioretinitis (3 infants), and CNS abnormalities (8 infants). In Fiocruz, Belo Horizonte, Brazil, infection is common, affecting 1 in 600 live births. Half these infected infants have active chorioretinitis at birth. When the infection is acquired in utero and the fetus is treated by drug therapy of the pregnant woman with **pyrimethamine**, **sulfadiazine**, and **leucovorin**, signs and symptoms in the infant may be prevented. The newborn infant may appear normal with no CSF abnormalities and no brain or eye disease. In utero therapy initiated rapidly results in a reduction of ocular and neurologic sequelae.

There is also a wide spectrum of symptoms of untreated congenital toxoplasmosis that presents later in the 1st yr of life (Table 316.1). These children may have IQ scores of <70, and have convulsions and severely impaired vision.

SYSTEMIC SIGNS

From 25% to >50% of infants with clinically apparent disease at birth are born prematurely. Parasite clonal types other than type II are more often associated with prematurity and more-severe disease. Intrauterine growth restriction, low Apgar scores, and temperature instability are common. Other manifestations may include lymphadenopathy, hepatosplenomegaly, myocarditis, pneumonitis, nephrotic syndrome, vomiting, diarrhea, and feeding problems. Bands of metaphyseal lucency and irregularity of the line of provisional calcification at the epiphyseal plate may occur without periosteal reaction in the ribs, femurs, and vertebrae. Congenital toxoplasmosis may be confused with erythroblastosis fetalis resulting from isosensitization, although the Coombs test result is usually negative with congenital *T. gondii* infection.

Table 316.1	Signs and Symptoms Occurring Before Diagnosis or During the Course of Untreated Acute Congenital Toxoplasmosis in 152 Infants (A) and in 101 of These Same Children After They Had Been Followed ≥4 Yr (B)

SIGNS AND SYMPTOMS	FREQUENCY OF OCCURRENCE IN PATIENTS WITH	
	"Neurologic" Disease*	"Generalized" Disease†
A. INFANTS	108 PATIENTS (%)	44 PATIENTS (%)
Chorioretinitis	102 (94)	29 (66)
Abnormal cerebrospinal fluid	59 (55)	37 (84)
Anemia	55 (51)	34 (77)
Convulsions	54 (50)	8 (18)
Intracranial calcification	54 (50)	2 (4)
Jaundice	31 (29)	35 (80)
Hydrocephalus	30 (28)	0 (0)
Fever	27 (25)	34 (77)
Splenomegaly	23 (21)	40 (90)
Lymphadenopathy	18 (17)	30 (68)
Hepatomegaly	18 (17)	34 (77)
Vomiting	17 (16)	21 (48)
Microcephaly	14 (13)	0 (0)
Diarrhea	7 (6)	11 (25)
Cataracts	5 (5)	0 (0)
Eosinophilia	6 (4)	8 (18)
Abnormal bleeding	3 (3)	8 (18)
Hypothermia	2 (2)	9 (20)
Glaucoma	2 (2)	0 (0)
Optic atrophy	2 (2)	0 (0)
Microphthalmia	2 (2)	0 (0)
Rash	1 (1)	11 (25)
Pneumonitis	0 (0)	18 (41)
B. CHILDREN ≥4 YR OLD	70 PATIENTS (%)	31 PATIENTS (%)
Intellectual impairment	62 (89)	25 (81)
Convulsions	58 (83)	24 (77)
Spasticity and palsies	53 (76)	18 (58)
Severely impaired vision	48 (69)	13 (42)
Hydrocephalus or microcephaly	31 (44)	2 (6)
Deafness	12 (17)	3 (10)
Normal	6 (9)	5 (16)

*Patients with otherwise undiagnosed central nervous system disease in the 1st yr of life.

†Patients with otherwise undiagnosed nonneurologic diseases during the 1st 2 mo of life.

Adapted from Eichenwald H: A study of congenital toxoplasmosis. In Slim JC, editor: *Human toxoplasmosis,* Copenhagen, 1960, Munksgaard, pp. 41–49. Study performed in 1947. The most severely involved institutionalized patients were not included in the later study of 101 children.

Skin

Cutaneous manifestations among newborn infants with congenital toxoplasmosis include rashes and jaundice and/or petechiae secondary to thrombocytopenia, but ecchymoses and large hemorrhages secondary to thrombocytopenia also occur. Rashes may be fine punctate, diffuse maculopapular, lenticular, deep blue-red, sharply defined macular, or diffuse blue and papular. Macular rashes involving the entire body including the palms and soles, exfoliative dermatitis, and cutaneous calcifications have been described. **Jaundice** with hepatic involvement and/or hemolysis, cyanosis due to interstitial pneumonitis from congenital infection, and edema secondary to myocarditis or nephrotic syndrome may be present. Jaundice and conjugated hyperbilirubinemia may persist for months.

Endocrine Abnormalities

Endocrine abnormalities may occur secondary to hypothalamic or pituitary involvement or end-organ involvement but are not common.

Occasionally reported endocrinopathies include myxedema, persistent hypernatremia with vasopressin-sensitive diabetes insipidus, sexual precocity, and partial anterior hypopituitarism.

Central Nervous System

Neurologic manifestations of congenital toxoplasmosis vary from massive acute encephalopathy to subtle neurologic syndromes. Toxoplasmosis should be considered as a potential cause of any undiagnosed neurologic disease in children <1 yr old, especially if retinal lesions are present.

Hydrocephalus may be the sole clinical neurologic manifestation of congenital toxoplasmosis and almost always requires shunt placement. Hydrocephalus may present prenatally and progress during the perinatal period or, much less often, may present later in life. Patterns of seizures are protean and have included focal motor seizures, petit and grand mal seizures, muscular twitching, opisthotonos, and hypsarrhythmia. Spinal or bulbar involvement may be manifested by paralysis of the extremities, difficulty swallowing, and respiratory distress. **Microcephaly** usually reflects severe brain damage, but some children with microcephaly caused by congenital toxoplasmosis who have been treated have normal or even superior cognitive function. Untreated congenital toxoplasmosis that is symptomatic in the 1st yr of life can cause substantial diminution in cognitive function and developmental delay. Intellectual impairment also occurs in some children with subclinical infection without or despite treatment with pyrimethamine and sulfonamides. Seizures and focal motor defects may become apparent after the newborn period, even when infection is subclinical at birth.

CSF abnormalities occur in at least 50% of infants with congenital toxoplasmosis. A CSF protein level >1 g/dL is characteristic of severe CNS toxoplasmosis and is usually accompanied by hydrocephalus. Local production of *T. gondii*–specific IgG and IgM antibodies may be demonstrated. CT of the brain is useful to detect calcifications, determine ventricular size, and demonstrate porencephalic cystic structures (Fig. 316.4). **Calcifications** occur throughout the brain, but there is a propensity for development of calcifications in the caudate nucleus and basal ganglia, choroid plexus, and subependyma. MRI and contrast-enhanced CT brain scans are useful for detecting active inflammatory lesions. MRI that requires<45 sec or ultrasonography may be useful for following ventricular size. Medical treatment in utero and in the 1st yr of life results in improved neurologic outcomes and, in many cases, diminution or disappearance of calcifications.

Eyes

Almost all untreated congenitally infected infants develop **chorioretinal lesions** by adulthood and may have severe visual impairment. *T. gondii* causes a **focal necrotizing retinitis** in congenitally infected individuals (see Fig. 316.2). Retinal detachment may occur. Any part of the retina may be involved, either unilaterally or bilaterally, including the maculae. The optic nerve may be involved, and toxoplasmic lesions that involve projections of the visual pathways in the brain or the visual cortex also may lead to visual impairment. In association with severe retinal lesions and vitritis, secondary anterior uveitis may develop and occasionally lead to erythema of the external eye. Other ocular findings include cells and protein in the anterior chamber, large keratic precipitates, posterior synechiae, nodules on the iris, and neovascular formation on the surface of the iris, sometimes with increased intraocular pressure and glaucoma. Rarely, the extraocular musculature may also be involved directly. Other manifestations include strabismus, nystagmus, visual impairment, and microphthalmia. Enucleation has been required for a blind, phthisic, painful eye. The **differential diagnosis** of ocular toxoplasmosis includes congenital coloboma and inflammatory lesions caused by cytomegalovirus, lymphocytic choriomeningitis virus, *Bartonella henselae, Toxocara canis, Treponema pallidum, Mycobacterium tuberculosis,* varicella-zoster virus, Zika virus, or vasculitis. Ocular toxoplasmosis may be a recurrent and progressive disease that requires multiple courses of therapy. Limited data suggest that occurrence of lesions in the early years of life may be prevented by instituting **antimicrobial treatment** with pyrimethamine and sulfonamides during the 1st yr of life, and that treatment of the infected fetus in utero followed by treatment in the 1st yr of life with

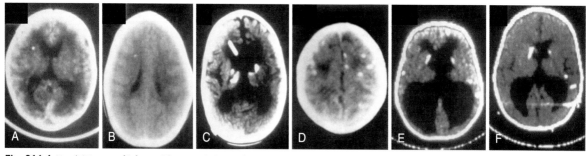

Fig. 316.4 Head CT scans of infants with congenital toxoplasmosis. **A,** CT scan at birth that shows areas of hypolucency, mildly dilated ventricles, and small calcifications. **B,** CT scan of the same child at 1 yr of age (after antimicrobial therapy for 1 yr). This scan is normal with the exception of 2 small calcifications. This child's Mental Development Index (MDI) at 1 yr old was 140 by the Bayley Scale of Infant Development. **C,** CT scan from a 1 yr old infant who was normal at birth. His meningoencephalitis became symptomatic in the 1st few wk of life but was not diagnosed correctly and remained untreated during his 1st 3 mo of life. At 3 mo old, development of hydrocephalus and bilateral macular chorioretinitis led to the diagnosis of congenital toxoplasmosis, and antimicrobial therapy was initiated. This scan shows significant residual atrophy and calcifications. This child had substantial motor dysfunction, development delays, and visual impairment. **D,** CT scan obtained during the 1st mo of life of a microcephalic child. Note the numerous calcifications. This child's IQ scores using the Stanford-Binet Intelligence Scale for children when she was 3 yr old and Wechsler Preschool and Primary Scale Intelligence when 5 yr old were 100 and 102, respectively. She received antimicrobial therapy during her 1st yr of life. **E,** CT scan with hydrocephalus caused by aqueductal obstruction, before shunt. **F,** Scan from the same patient as the scan in **E,** after shunt. This child's IQ scores using the Stanford-Binet Intelligence Scale for children were approximately 100 when she was 3 and 6 yr old. (A-F, Adapted from McAuley J, Boyer K, Patel D, et al: Early and longitudinal evaluations of treated infants and children and untreated historical patients with congenital toxoplasmosis: the Chicago Collaborative Treatment Trial, Clin Infect Dis 18:38–72, 1994.)

pyrimethamine, sulfadiazine, and leucovorin further reduces the incidence and the severity of the retinal disease.

Ears

Sensorineural hearing loss, both mild and severe, may occur. It is not known whether this is a static or progressive disorder. Treatment in the 1st yr of life is associated with decreased frequency of hearing loss.

DIAGNOSIS

Diagnosis of acute *Toxoplasma* infection can be established by a number of methods (Table 316.2): isolation of *T. gondii* from blood or body fluids; identification of tachyzoites in sections or preparations of tissues and body fluids, amniotic fluid, or placenta; identification of cysts in the placenta or tissues of a fetus or newborn; and characteristic lymph node histologic features. Serologic tests are very useful for diagnosis. Polymerase chain reaction (PCR) is useful to identify *T. gondii* DNA in CSF and amniotic fluid and has been reported to be useful with infant peripheral blood and urine to establish the diagnosis definitively and in immunocompromised patients for diagnosis and monitoring treatment.

Isolation

Organisms can be isolated by inoculation of body fluids, leukocytes, or tissue specimens into mice or tissue cultures. Body fluids should be processed and inoculated immediately, but *T. gondii* has been isolated from tissues and blood that have been stored overnight or even for 4-5 days at 4°C (39.2°F). Freezing or treatment of specimens with formalin kills *T. gondii*. From 6-10 days after inoculation into mice, or earlier if mice die, peritoneal fluids should be examined for tachyzoites. If inoculated mice survive for 6 wk and seroconvert, definitive diagnosis is made by visualization of *Toxoplasma* cysts in mouse brain. If cysts are not seen, **subinoculation** of mouse tissue into other mice are performed. Treatment of mice that receive subinoculated tissues with corticosteroid appears to enhance ability to isolate the parasite.

Microscopic examination of tissue culture inoculated with *T. gondii* shows necrotic, heavily infected cells with numerous extracellular tachyzoites. Isolation of *T. gondii* from blood or body fluids reflects acute infection. Except in the fetus or neonate, it is usually not possible to distinguish acute from past infection by isolation of *T. gondii* from tissues (e.g., skeletal muscle, lung, brain, eye) obtained by biopsy or at autopsy.

Diagnosis of acute infection can be established by visualization of tachyzoites in biopsy tissue sections, bone marrow aspirate, or body fluids (e.g., CSF, amniotic fluid). Immunofluorescent antibody and immunoperoxidase staining techniques may be necessary, because it is

often difficult to distinguish the tachyzoite using ordinary stains. Tissue cysts are diagnostic of infection but do not differentiate between acute and chronic infection, although the presence of many cysts suggests recent acute infection. Cysts in the placenta or tissues of the newborn infant establish the diagnosis of congenital infection. Characteristic histologic features strongly suggest the diagnosis of toxoplasmic lymphadenitis.

Serologic Testing

Serologic tests are useful in establishing the diagnosis of congenital or acutely acquired *Toxoplasma* infection. Each laboratory that reports serologic test results must have established values for their tests that diagnose infection in specific clinical settings, provide interpretation of their results, and ensure appropriate quality control before therapy is based on serologic test results. Serologic test results used as the basis for therapy should ideally be confirmed in a reference laboratory.

The **Sabin-Feldman dye test** is sensitive and specific. It measures primarily IgG antibodies. Results should be expressed in international units (IU/mL), based on international standard reference sera available from the World Health Organization (WHO).

The **IgG indirect fluorescent antibody (IgG-IFA) test** measures the same antibodies as the dye test, and the titers tend to be parallel. These antibodies usually appear 1-2 wk after infection, reach high titers ($\geq 1:1,000$) after 6-8 wk, and then decline over months to years. Low titers ($1:4$ to $1:64$) usually persist for life. Antibody titer does not correlate with severity of illness.

An **agglutination test** (Bio-Mérieux, Lyon, France) available commercially in Europe uses formalin-preserved whole parasites to detect IgG antibodies. This test is accurate, simple to perform, and inexpensive.

The **IgM-IFA test** is useful for the diagnosis of acute acquired infection with *T. gondii* in the older child because IgM antibodies appear earlier, often by 5 days after infection, and diminish more quickly than IgG antibodies. In most instances, IgM antibodies rise rapidly ($1:50$ to $<1:1,000$) and then fall to low titers ($1:10$ or $1:20$) or disappear after weeks or months. However, some patients continue to have positive IgM results with low titers for several years. The IgM-IFA test detects *Toxoplasma*-specific IgM in only approximately 25% of congenitally infected infants at birth. IgM antibodies may not be present in sera of immunocompromised patients with acute toxoplasmosis or in patients with reactivation of ocular toxoplasmosis. The IgM-IFA test may yield false-positive results as a result of rheumatoid factor.

The **double-sandwich IgM enzyme-linked immunosorbent assay (IgM-ELISA)** is also useful for detection of *Toxoplasma* IgM antibodies. In the older child, serum IgM-ELISA *Toxoplasma* antibodies of >2 (a

Table 316.2	Generalizations Concerning Clinical Presentations, *Toxoplasma*-Specific Diagnostic Tests, and Treatment												
CLINICAL SETTING & MANIFESTATION	**SAMPLE SOURCE**	**TOXOPLASMA-SPECIFIC DIAGNOSTIC TESTS**								**TREATMENT**				
		G	M	A	E	Av	AC/HS	PCR	Subinoculation	Sp	PSL*	Co	Lu	None
PRENATAL														
Acute infection in pregnant woman ≤18 wk gestation *and* no clinical evidence of fetal infection	Mother	+	+	+	+	L	Acute	AF (17-18 wk)	NS	+	+ †No P 1st trimester			
Acute infection in pregnant woman ≤18 wk gestation *and* signs of fetal infection	Mother	+	+	+	+	L	Acute	AF (may not be necessary)	NS		+ †No P 1st trimester			
Acute infection in pregnant woman at >21 wk gestation	Mother	+	+	+	+	L	Acute	AF	NS		+			
Congenital infection in infant	Infant	+	+	+	+	L	Acute	Placenta/ buffy coat	Placenta/buffy coat		+	‡		
POSTNATAL														
Acute, symptomatic	Child	+	+	+	+	L	Acute	NS	NS		+			+
Acute, self-limited symptoms														
Chronic, asymptomatic	Child	+	–	–	–	H	Chronic	NS	NS					
Acute, severely symptomatic	Child	+	+	+	+	L	Acute	§	Body fluids/ buffy coat		+			
Immune compromised¶	Child	+/–	+/–	+/–	+/–	+/–	+/–	§	Body fluids/ buffy coat					
Laboratory accident‖	Child	+/–	+/–	+/–	+/–	+/–	+/–	NS	NS		+			
Eye Disease														
Quiescent scar**	Child	+	+/–	+/–	+/–	+/–	+/–	NS	NS					+
Active chorioretinitis**	Child	+	+/–	+/–	+/–	+/–	+/–	NS	NS		+		††	
Active CNVM**	Child	+	+/–	+/–	+/–	+/–	+/–	NS	NS		+		††	

*Pyrimethamine and leucovorin should be adjusted for granulocytopenia; complete blood counts, including platelets, should be monitored each Monday and Thursday. If there is sulfonamide allergy, alternative medicines include clindamycin, azithromycin, or clarithromycin in place of sulfadiazine.

†*Do not* use pyrimethamine in the 1st 14 wk of gestation.

‡Occasionally, corticosteroids (prednisone) have been used when CSF protein is ≥1 g/dL or when active chorioretinitis threatens vision and should be continued until signs of inflammation or active chorioretinitis that threatens vision have subsided; then dosage can be tapered and the steroids discontinued.

§Utility of PCR depends on clinical setting. For example, the following may be useful to establish the diagnosis: PCR of body fluids such as amniotic fluid or CSF; cells from bronchoalveolar lavage from a patient with pneumonia; or tissue such as placenta where presence of parasites or parasite DNA would support a diagnosis of infection.

¶In some cases, in immunocompromised persons, there is no detectable serologic response to *T. gondii*. However, if clinical presentation is indicative of infection in the absence of positive serologic results, CSF, buffy coat of peripheral blood, histopathology of tissue samples, or body fluids tested with PCR or subinoculation may be useful. If PCR demonstrates the presence of *T. gondii* DNA in the sample, it is useful for diagnosis. However, the sensitivity of PCR has been variable in this setting. In some circumstances, presumptive treatment may be warranted.

‖Whether a person should be treated for a laboratory accident depends on the nature of the accident, the serology of the person before the accident, and other factors. When there is risk of infection, treatment is given.

**Serologic results depend on whether infection is acute (recently acquired) or chronic. When testing serum from persons with ocular toxoplasmosis, *T. gondii*–specific IgG may be demonstrable only in an undiluted serum sample.

††Corticosteroids (prednisone) are used if inflammation or edema caused by infection threatens vision and should be continued until signs of inflammation or active chorioretinitis that threatens vision have subsided; then dosage can be tapered and the steroids discontinued.

+, Positive; –, negative; +/–, equivocal; A, *T. gondii*–specific IgA; AC/HS, direct agglutination; AF, amniotic fluid; Av, *T. gondii*–specific IgG avidity; CNVM, choroidal neovascular membrane; Co, corticosteroids (prednisone); CSF, cerebrospinal fluid; E, *T. gondii*–specific IgE; G, *T. gondii*–specific IgG; IG, immunoglobulin; Lu, Lucentis (antibody to vascular endothelial growth factor); M, *T. gondii*–specific IgM; NS, not standard to obtain; PCR, polymerase chain reaction; PSL, pyrimethamine, sulfadiazine, leucovorin (folinic acid); Sp, spiramycin.

Adapted from Remington JS, McLeod R, et al: Toxoplasmosis. In Remington JS, Klein JO, editors: *Infectious diseases of the fetus and newborn infant*, ed 6, Philadelphia, 2006, Saunders.

value of one reference laboratory; each laboratory must establish its own value for positive results) indicates that *Toxoplasma* infection most likely has been acquired recently. The IgM-ELISA identifies approximately 50–75% of infants with congenital infection. IgM-ELISA avoids both the false-positive results from rheumatoid factor (RF) and the false-negative results from high levels of passively transferred maternal IgG antibody in fetal serum, as may occur in the IgM-IFA test. Results obtained with commercial kits must be interpreted with caution, because false-positive reactions can occur. Care must also be taken to determine whether kits have been standardized for diagnosis of infection in specific clinical settings, such as in the newborn infant. The **IgA-ELISA** also is a sensitive test for detection of maternal and congenital infection, and results may be positive when those of the IgM-ELISA are not.

The **immunosorbent agglutination assay (ISAGA)** combines trapping of a patient's IgM to a solid surface and use of formalin-fixed organisms or antigen-coated latex particles. It is read as an agglutination test. There are no false-positive results from RF or antinuclear antibodies (ANAs). **IgM-ISAGA** is more sensitive than and may detect specific IgM antibodies before and for longer periods than IgM-ELISA.

At present, IgM-ISAGA and IgA-ELISA are the most useful tests for diagnosis of congenital infection in the newborn but are not positive in all infected infants. The IgE-ELISA and IgE-ISAGA are also sometimes useful in establishing the diagnosis of congenital toxoplasmosis or acute acquired *T. gondii* infection. The presence of IgM antibodies in the older child or adult can never be used alone to diagnose acute acquired infection.

The **differential agglutination test (HS/AC)** compares antibody titers obtained with formalin-fixed tachyzoites (**HS antigen**) with titers obtained using acetone-fixed tachyzoites (**AC antigen**) to differentiate recent and remote infections in adults and older children. This method may be particularly useful in differentiating remote infection in pregnant women, because levels of IgM and IgA antibodies detectable by ELISA or ISAGA may remain elevated for months to years in adults and older children.

The **avidity test** can be helpful to establish time of acquisition of infection. A high-avidity test result indicates that infection began >12-16 wk earlier, which is especially useful in determining time of acquisition of infection in the 1st or final 16 wk of gestation. A low-avidity test result may be present for many months or even years and does not definitively identify recent acquisition of infection.

A relatively higher level of *Toxoplasma* antibody in the aqueous humor or in CSF demonstrates local production of antibody during active ocular or CNS toxoplasmosis. This comparison is performed, and a coefficient [C] is calculated as follows:

$$C = \frac{\text{Antibody titer in body fluid}}{\text{Antibody titer in serum}} \times \frac{\text{Concentration of IgG in serum}}{\text{Concentration of IgG in body fluid}}$$

Significant coefficients [C] are >8 for ocular infection, >4 for CNS for congenital infection, and >1 for CNS infection in patients with AIDS. If the serum dye test titer is >300 IU/mL, it is not possible to demonstrate significant local antibody production using this formula with either the dye test or the IgM-IFA test titer. IgM antibody may be detectable in CSF.

Comparative **Western immunoblot** tests of sera from a mother and infant may detect congenital infection. Infection is suspected when the mother's serum and her infant's serum contain antibodies that react with different *Toxoplasma* antigens.

The **enzyme-linked immunofiltration assay** using micropore membranes permits simultaneous study of antibody specificity by immunoprecipitation and characterization of antibody isotypes by immunofiltration with enzyme-labeled antibodies. This method is able to detect 85% of cases of congenital infection in the 1st few days of life.

Serologic tests in development include multiplex antibody tests for IgG, IgM, and IgA-specific antibodies, as well as point-of-care tests designed to provide accurate and rapid identification of recent infection or seroconversion in pregnant women.

PCR is used to amplify the DNA of *T. gondii*, which then can be detected by using a DNA probe. Detection of repetitive *T. gondii* genes, the B1 or 529 bp, 300 copy gene, in amniotic fluid is the PCR target of choice for establishing the diagnosis of congenital *Toxoplasma* infection in the fetus. Sensitivity and specificity of this test in amniotic fluid obtained to diagnose infections acquired between 17 and 21 wk of gestation are approximately 95%. Before and after that time, PCR with the 529 bp, 300 copy repeat gene as the template is 92% sensitive and 100% specific for detection of congenital infection. PCR of vitreous or aqueous fluids also has been used to diagnose ocular toxoplasmosis. PCR of peripheral white blood cells, CSF, and urine has been reported to detect congenital infection.

Point-of-care tests such as the *Toxoplasma* ICT IgG-IgM test or a nanogold test will lower the cost of and increase the ease of rapid testing.

Lymphocyte blastogenesis to *Toxoplasma* antigens has been used to diagnose congenital toxoplasmosis when the diagnosis is uncertain and other test results are negative. However, a negative result does not exclude the diagnosis because peripheral blood lymphocytes of infected newborns may not respond to *T. gondii* antigens because of immune tolerance testing in specific circumstances.

Acquired Toxoplasmosis

Recent infection is diagnosed by seroconversion from a negative to a positive IgG antibody titer (in the absence of transfusion); a 2-tube increase in *Toxoplasma*-specific IgG titer when serial sera are obtained 3 wk apart and tested in parallel; or the detection of *Toxoplasma*-specific IgM antibody in conjunction with other tests, but never alone.

Ocular Toxoplasmosis

IgG antibody titers of 1:4 to 1:64 are usual in older children with active *Toxoplasma* chorioretinitis. Even the presence of antibodies measurable only when serum is tested undiluted is helpful in establishing the diagnosis. The diagnosis is likely with characteristic retinal lesions and positive serologic tests. PCR of aqueous or vitreous fluid has been used

to diagnose ocular toxoplasmosis but is infrequently performed because of the risks associated with obtaining intraocular fluid.

Immunocompromised Persons

IgG antibody titers may be low, and *Toxoplasma*-specific IgM is often absent in immunocompromised stem cell transplant recipients, but not in kidney or heart transplant recipients with toxoplasmosis. Demonstration of *Toxoplasma* DNA by PCR in serum, blood, and CSF may identify disseminated *Toxoplasma* infection in immunocompromised persons. Resolution of CNS lesions during a therapeutic trial of pyrimethamine and sulfadiazine has been useful to diagnose toxoplasmic encephalitis in patients with AIDS. Brain biopsy has been used to establish the diagnosis if there is no response to a therapeutic trial and to exclude other possible diagnoses such as CNS lymphoma.

Congenital Toxoplasmosis

Fetal ultrasound examination, performed every 2 wk during gestation, beginning at diagnosis of acute acquired infection in a pregnant woman, and PCR analysis of amniotic fluid are used for prenatal diagnosis. *T. gondii* may also be isolated from the placenta at delivery.

Serologic tests are also useful in establishing a diagnosis of congenital toxoplasmosis. Either persistent or rising titers in the dye test or IFA test, or a positive IgM-ELISA or IgM-ISAGA result, is diagnostic of congenital toxoplasmosis. The half-life of IgM is approximately 2 days, so if there is a placental leak, the level of IgM antibodies in the infant's serum decreases significantly, usually within 1 wk. Passively transferred maternal IgG antibodies may require many months to a year to disappear from the infant's serum, depending on the magnitude of the original titer. The half-life of passively transferred maternal IgG is approximately 30 days, so the titer diminishes by half each 30 days. Synthesis of *Toxoplasma* antibody is usually demonstrable by the 3rd mo of life if the infant is untreated, although the rate of IgG synthesis varies considerably in infants <1 yr old. If the infant is treated, synthesis may be delayed for as long as the 9th mo of life and, infrequently, may not occur at all. When an infant begins to synthesize IgG antibody, infection may be documented serologically even without demonstration of IgM antibodies by an increase in the ratio of specific serum IgG antibody titer to the total IgG, whereas the ratio will decrease if the specific IgG antibody has been passively transferred from the mother.

Newborns suspected of having congenital toxoplasmosis should be evaluated by general, ophthalmologic, and neurologic examinations; head CT scan; and some or ideally all of the following tests: an attempt to isolate *T. gondii* from the placenta and infant's leukocytes from peripheral blood buffy coat; measurement of serum *Toxoplasma*-specific IgG, IgM, IgA, and IgE antibodies, and the levels of total serum IgM and IgG; lumbar puncture, including analysis of CSF for cells, glucose, protein, *Toxoplasma*-specific IgG and IgM antibodies, and level of total IgG; and testing of CSF for *T. gondii* by PCR and inoculation into mice. Presence of *Toxoplasma*-specific IgM in CSF that is not contaminated with blood, or confirmation of local antibody production of *Toxoplasma*-specific IgG antibody in CSF, establishes the diagnosis of congenital *Toxoplasma* infection.

Many manifestations of congenital toxoplasmosis are similar to findings that occur in other perinatal infections, especially congenital cytomegalovirus infection. Since neither cerebral calcification nor chorioretinitis is pathognomonic, a negative urine culture or PCR for CMV soon after birth is a useful adjunctive test. The clinical picture in the newborn infant may also be compatible with sepsis, aseptic meningitis, syphilis, or hemolytic disease. Some children <5 yr old with chorioretinitis have postnatally acquired *T. gondii* infection.

TREATMENT

Pyrimethamine and **sulfadiazine** act synergistically against *Toxoplasma*, and combination therapy is indicated for many of the forms of toxoplasmosis. Use of pyrimethamine is contraindicated during the first trimester of pregnancy. **Spiramycin** should be used to attempt to prevent vertical transmission of infection to the fetus of acutely infected pregnant women. Pyrimethamine inhibits the enzyme dihydrofolate reductase, and thus the synthesis of folic acid, and therefore produces a dose-related, reversible, and usually gradual depression of the bone marrow. Neutropenia is most common, but rarely treatment has been reported to result in thrombocytopenia and anemia as well. **Reversible neutropenia** is the most common adverse effect in treated infants. All patients treated with pyrimethamine should have leukocyte counts twice weekly. Seizures may occur with overdosage of pyrimethamine. Potential toxic effects of sulfonamides (e.g., crystalluria, hematuria, rash) should be monitored. Hypersensitivity reactions occur, especially in patients with AIDS. Folinic acid, as calcium **leucovorin**, should always be administered concomitantly and for 1 wk after treatment with pyrimethamine is discontinued to prevent bone marrow suppression.

Acquired Toxoplasmosis

Patients with acquired toxoplasmosis and lymphadenopathy usually do not need specific treatment unless they have severe and persistent symptoms or evidence of damage to vital organs (see Table 316.2). If such signs and symptoms occur, treatment with pyrimethamine, sulfadiazine, and leucovorin should be initiated. Patients who appear to be immunocompetent but have severe and persistent symptoms or damage to vital organs (e.g., chorioretinitis, myocarditis) need specific therapy until these specific symptoms resolve, followed by therapy for an additional 2 wk. Therapy often is administered for at least 4-6 wk. The optimal duration of therapy is unknown. A loading dose of pyrimethamine for older children is 2 mg/kg/day divided twice daily (maximum 50 mg bid), given for the 1st 2 days of treatment. The maintenance dose begins on the 3rd day and is 1 mg/kg/day (maximum 50 mg/day). Sulfadiazine is administered at 100 mg/kg/day bid (maximum 4 g/day). Leucovorin is administered orally (PO) at 5-20 mg 3 times weekly (or even daily depending on the leukocyte count).

Ocular Toxoplasmosis

Patients with active ocular toxoplasmosis are treated with pyrimethamine, sulfadiazine, and leucovorin (see Table 316.2). They are treated while disease is active and then for approximately 1 wk after the lesion has developed a quiescent appearance (i.e., sharp borders, pigmentation at margins of the lesion, and resolution of associated inflammatory cells in the vitreous), which usually occurs in 2-4 wk when treatment is initiated promptly. Within 7-10 days, the borders of the retinal lesions sharpen, and visual acuity usually returns to that noted before development of the acute lesion. Systemic corticosteroids have been administered concomitantly with antimicrobial treatment when lesions involve the macula, optic nerve head, or papillomacular bundle. Corticosteroids must never be given alone but may be initiated after loading doses of pyrimethamine and sulfadiazine have been administered (2 days). With recurrences, new lesions often appear contiguous to old ones. Very rarely, vitrectomy and removal of the lens are needed to restore visual acuity. Active choroidal neovascular membranes as a result of toxoplasmic chorioretinitis have been treated successfully in children with intravitreal injection of antibody to vascular endothelial growth factor in addition to oral anti-*Toxoplasma* medicines. Suppressive treatment has prevented frequent recurrences of vision-threatening lesions.

Immunocompromised Persons

Serologic evidence of acute infection in an immunocompromised patient, regardless of whether signs and symptoms of infection are present or tachyzoites are demonstrated in tissue, are indications for therapy similar to that described for immunocompetent persons with symptoms of organ injury (see Table 316.2). It is important to establish the diagnosis as rapidly as possible and institute treatment early. In immunocompromised patients other than those with AIDS, therapy should be continued for at least 4-6 wk beyond complete resolution of all signs and symptoms of active disease and, if possible, resolution of cause for immune suppression. Careful follow-up of these patients is imperative because relapse may occur, requiring prompt reinstitution of therapy. Relapse was once common in AIDS patients without antiretroviral treatment, and suppressive therapy with pyrimethamine and sulfonamides, or TMP-SMX, was continued for life. Now it is possible to discontinue maintenance therapy when the CD4 count remains at >200 cells/μL for 4 mo and all lesions have resolved. Therapy usually induces a beneficial response clinically but does not eradicate cysts. Treatment of *T. gondii*–seropositive

patients with AIDS should be continued as long as CD4 counts remain at <200/μL. Prophylactic TMP-SMX therapy for *Pneumocystis jirovecii* pneumonia significantly reduces the incidence of toxoplasmosis in AIDS patients.

Congenital Toxoplasmosis

All fetuses and newborns infected with *T. gondii* should be treated regardless of whether they have clinical manifestations of infection, because treatment may be effective in interrupting acute disease that damages vital organs (Fig. 316.5; see Table 316.2). The fetus is treated by treating the pregnant woman with pyrimethamine and sulfadiazine (with leucovorin). Infants should be treated for 1 yr with pyrimethamine (2 mg/kg/day PO bid for 2 days, then beginning on the 3rd day, 1 mg/kg/day for 2 or 6 mo, and then 1 mg/kg given on Monday, Wednesday, and Friday), sulfadiazine (100 mg/kg/day PO bid), and leucovorin (5-10 mg PO given on Monday, Wednesday, and Friday, or more often depending on neutrophil count). The relative efficacy in reducing sequelae of infection and the safety of treatment with 2 mo vs 6 mo of the higher dosage of pyrimethamine are being compared in the U.S. National Collaborative Study. (Updated information about this study and these regimens is available from Dr. Rima McLeod, 773-834-4131.) Pyrimethamine and sulfadiazine are available only in tablet form but can be prepared as suspensions. **Prednisone** (1 mg/kg/day PO bid) has been used in addition when active chorioretinitis involves the macula or otherwise threatens vision, or when the CSF protein is >1,000 mg/dL at birth, but the efficacy of this adjunctive therapy is not established. Prednisone is continued only for as long as the active inflammatory process in the posterior pole of the eye is vision threatening or CSF protein is >1,000 mg/dL, then tapered rapidly if the duration of treatment has been brief.

Pregnant Women With *Toxoplasma gondii* Infection

The immunologically normal pregnant woman who acquired *T. gondii* >6 mo before conception does not need treatment to prevent congenital infection of her fetus. Although data are not available to allow for a definitive time interval, if infection occurs during or shortly before the pregnancy, it is reasonable to evaluate the fetus by PCR with amniotic fluid and ultrasonography and treat to prevent congenital infection in the fetus (see Table 316.2).

Treatment of a pregnant woman who acquires infection at any time during pregnancy reduces the chance of congenital infection in her infant. **Spiramycin** (1 g PO every 8 hr without food) is recommended for prevention of fetal infection if the mother develops acute toxoplasmosis during pregnancy. Spiramycin is available in the United States on an "emergency use" request by a physician through the FDA Division of Anti-Infective Drugs (301-796-1400) after the diagnosis of acute infection is confirmed in a reference laboratory (Palo Alto Medical Facility Toxoplasma Serology Lab, 650-853-4828). With this approval, the physician can then contact the spiramycin manufacturer, Sanofi Pasteur (1-800-822-2463), to obtain spiramycin for the patient. Adverse reactions are infrequent and include paresthesia, rash, nausea, vomiting, and diarrhea.

For treatment of the pregnant woman whose fetus has a confirmed or probable infection, in the second or third trimester, the combination of pyrimethamine, sulfadiazine, and leucovorin is recommended. Following a loading dose of pyrimethamine (50 mg bid) for 2 days, beginning on the 3rd day, pyrimethamine is administered at 50 mg once daily. Beginning on the 1st day of treatment with pyrimethamine, sulfadiazine (1.5-2.0 g PO bid), and leucovorin (10 mg PO once daily) are also given. In the first trimester, when there is definite infection, **sulfadiazine** alone is recommended because pyrimethamine is potentially teratogenic at that time. Spiramycin treatment is used for infection acquired early in gestation when fetal infection is uncertain. Treatment of the mother of an infected fetus with pyrimethamine and sulfadiazine reduces infection in the placenta and the severity of disease in the newborn. Delay in maternal treatment during gestation results in greater brain and eye disease in the infant. Diagnostic amniocentesis should be performed at >17-18 wk of gestation in pregnancies when there is high suspicion of fetal infection. Overall sensitivity of PCR for amniotic fluid is at 85% between 17 and 21 wk of gestation. The sensitivity of PCR using amniotic fluid for diagnosis of fetal infection is 92% in early and late gestation

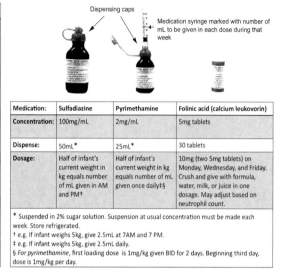

Oral Suspension Formulations	
Sulfadiazine 100mg/mL suspension 1. Crush ten 500mg sulfadiazine tablets in a mortar to a fine powder 2. Add enough sterile water to make a smooth paste 3. Slowly triturate syrup vehicle close to 50mL final volume 4. Transfer mixture to an amber bottle 5. Add enough syrup vehicle to q.s. to 50mL final volume 6. Shake very well. 7. Label and give a 7 day expiration 8. Store refrigerated	**Pyrimethamine** 2mg/mL suspension 1. Crush four 25mg pyrimethamine tablets in a mortar to a fine powder 2. Add 10cc of syrup vehicle 3. Transfer mixture to an amber bottle 4. Rinse motor with 10cc sterile water and transfer to bottle 5. Add enough syrup vehicle to q.s. to 50mL final volume 6. Shake very well. 7. Label and give 7 day expiration 8. Store refrigerated

Medication:	Sulfadiazine	Pyrimethamine	Folinic acid (calcium leukovorin)
Concentration:	100mg/mL	2mg/mL	5mg tablets
Dispense:	50mL*	25mL*	30 tablets
Dosage:	Half of infant's current weight in kg equals number of mL given in AM and PM†	Half of infant's current weight in kg equals number of mL given once daily‡§	10mg (two 5mg tablets) on Monday, Wednesday, and Friday. Crush and give with formula, water, milk, or juice in one dosage. May adjust based on neutrophil count.

* Suspended in 2% sugar solution. Suspension at usual concentration must be made each week. Store refrigerated.
† e.g. If infant weighs 5kg, give 2.5mL at 7AM and 7 PM.
‡ e.g. If infant weighs 5kg, give 2.5mL daily.
§ For pyrimethamine, first loading dose is 1mg/kg given BID for 2 days. Beginning third day, dose is 1mg/kg per day.

Fig. 316.5 Compounding and administration of medications to treat congenital toxoplasmosis in infants. *(Adapted from Remington JS, McLeod R, et al: Toxoplasmosis. In Remington JS, Klein JO, editors: Infectious diseases of the fetus and newborn infant, ed 6, Philadelphia, 2006, Saunders; and McAuley J, Boyer K, Patel D, et al: Early and longitudinal evaluations of treated infants and children and untreated historical patients with congenital toxoplasmosis: the Chicago Collaborative Treatment Trial, Clin Infect Dis 18:38–72, 1994.)*

when amniotic fluid is tested for presence of the 529 bp, 300 copy gene. After 24 wk gestation, incidence of transmission is relatively high, and all pregnant women who are infected acutely after that time are treated with pyrimethamine and sulfadiazine to treat the fetus.

The approach in France to congenital toxoplasmosis includes systematic serologic screening of all women of childbearing age and for those who are sero-negative again intrapartum each month during gestation beginning at ≤11 wk gestational age, at birth, and 1 mo after birth. Mothers with acute infection early in gestation and without evidence of involvement of the fetus are treated with spiramycin, which decreases the transmission. Ultrasonography and amniocentesis for PCR at approximately 17-18 wk of gestation are used for fetal diagnosis and have 97% sensitivity and 100% specificity. Confidence intervals for sensitivity are larger early and late in gestation. Fetal infection is treated with pyrimethamine and sulfadiazine. Termination of pregnancy is very rare at present. Prompt initiation of treatment with pyrimethamine and sulfadiazine during pregnancy usually has an excellent outcome, with normal development of children. Only 19% have subtle findings of congenital infection, including intracranial calcifications (13%) and chorioretinal scars (6%), although 39% may have chorioretinal scars detected at follow-up later in childhood. Several studies have demonstrated improved outcomes with shorter times between diagnosis and initiation of treatment. In Germany, for seroconverting women who are between 15 and 17 weeks' gestation and before amniocentesis, administration of pyrimethamine, sulfadiazine, and leukovorin results in good outcomes for infants but sometimes sulfadiazine hypersensitivity for mothers.

Chronically infected pregnant women who are immunocompromised have transmitted *T. gondii* to their fetuses. Such women should be treated with spiramycin throughout gestation. The optimal management for prevention of congenital toxoplasmosis in the fetus of a pregnant woman with HIV infection, a CD4 count <200 cells/μL, and inactive *T. gondii* infection is unknown. Fortunately, this situation now is rarely encountered in the United States. If the pregnancy is not terminated, some investigators suggest that the mother should be treated with spiramycin or sulfadiazine alone during the 1st 14 wk of gestation and thereafter with pyrimethamine and sulfadiazine until term. There are no universally accepted guidelines at present. In a study of adult patients with AIDS and toxoplasmic encephalitis, pyrimethamine (75 mg PO once daily) combined with high dosages of intravenous clindamycin (1,200 mg every 6 hr) appeared equal in efficacy to sulfadiazine and pyrimethamine in the treatment of the toxoplasmic encephalitis. Other experimental agents include the macrolides clarithromycin and azithromycin.

PROGNOSIS

Early institution of specific treatment for congenitally infected infants usually rapidly controls the active manifestations of toxoplasmosis, including active chorioretinitis, meningitis, encephalitis, hepatitis, splenomegaly, and thrombocytopenia. Rarely, hydrocephalus resulting from aqueductal obstruction may develop or become worse during therapy. Treatment appears to reduce the incidence of some sequelae, such as diminished cognitive and abnormal motor function. Without therapy and in some treated patients as well, chorioretinitis often recurs. Children with extensive involvement at birth may function normally later in life or have mild to severe impairment of vision, hearing, cognitive function, and other neurologic functions. Delays in diagnosis and therapy, perinatal hypoglycemia, hypoxia, hypotension, repeated shunt infections, and severe visual impairment are associated with a poorer prognosis. The prognosis is not necessarily poor for infected babies. Currently available treatments do not eradicate encysted parasites.

Studies in Lyon and Paris, France, demonstrated that outcome of treated fetal toxoplasmosis, even when infection is acquired early in gestation, is usually favorable if no hydrocephalus is detected on ultrasound, and treatment with pyrimethamine and sulfadiazine is initiated promptly. The **Systematic Review on Congenital Toxoplasmosis** (SYROCOT) study in Europe indicated that neurologic outcome is improved with shorter times between diagnosis and initiation of treatment of fetal toxoplasmosis. Work in Lyon has indicated a low incidence of recurrent eye disease in children with congenital toxoplasmosis who had been treated in utero and in their 1st yr of life. The NCCCTS (1981–2004) in the United States found that neurologic, developmental, audiologic, and ophthalmologic outcomes are considerably better for most, but not all, children who were treated in the 1st yr of life with pyrimethamine and sulfadiazine (with leucovorin) compared to children who had not been treated or were treated for only 1 mo in earlier decades described in the literature.

PREVENTION

Counseling pregnant women about the methods of preventing transmission of *T. gondii* (see Fig. 316.1) during pregnancy can reduce acquisition of infection during gestation. Women who do not have specific antibody to *T. gondii* before pregnancy should only eat well-cooked meat during pregnancy and avoid contact with oocysts excreted by cats. Cats that are kept indoors, maintained on prepared food, and not fed fresh, uncooked meat should not contact encysted *T. gondii* or shed oocysts.

Serologic screening, ultrasound monitoring, and treatment of pregnant women during gestation can also reduce the incidence and manifestations of congenital toxoplasmosis. No protective vaccine is yet available for human use.

Point-of-care testing to facilitate gestational screening, recent developments in medicines for treatment of active and chronic infections, and progress toward vaccines to prevent infections in humans and oocyst shedding by cats are all recent advances with promise to prevent or improve outcomes for *Toxoplasma gondii* infections.

ACKNOWLEDGMENT

We gratefully acknowledge the participant families, physicians, and other personnel of the National Collaborative Congenital Toxoplasmosis Study (NCCTS), and colleagues, for helping to create the understanding and knowledge in this chapter; and Cornwell Mann family, Taking out Toxo (TOT), TRI, and NIH, NIAID/DMID ROI AI27530 and RO1 AI071319-01 for support.

Bibliography is available at Expert Consult.

Section 16
Helminthic Diseases
第十六篇
蠕虫病

Chapter 317
Ascariasis (*Ascaris lumbricoides*)

Arlene E. Dent and James W. Kazura

第三百一十七章
蛔虫病（似蚓蛔线虫）

中文导读

本章主要介绍了蛔虫病的病原学、流行病学、发病机制、临床表现、诊断、治疗和预防。在临床表现部分，着重描述了蛔虫引起的肺部疾病和肠或胆道梗阻的相关临床特点。在诊断部分，介绍蛔虫病的病原学诊断和超声检查方法。在治疗部分，介绍了蛔虫病治疗的药物选择及疗程，同时指出部分严重梗阻的患者可能需要外科手术。

ETIOLOGY

Ascariasis is caused by the nematode, or **roundworm**, *Ascaris lumbricoides*. Adult worms of *A. lumbricoides* inhabit the lumen of the small intestine. The reproductive potential of *Ascaris* is prodigious; a gravid female worm produces 200,000 eggs per day. The fertile ova are oval in shape with a thick, mammillated covering measuring 45-70 μm in length and 35-50 μm in breadth (Fig. 317.1). After passage in the feces, the eggs embryonate and become infective in 5-10 days under favorable environmental conditions. Adult worms can live for 12-18 mo (Fig. 317.2).

EPIDEMIOLOGY

Ascariasis occurs globally and is the most prevalent human **helminthiasis** in the world. It is most common in tropical areas (South America, Africa, Asia) where environmental conditions are optimal for maturation of ova in the soil. Approximately 1 billion persons are estimated to be infected. Although the number of cases in the United States is not known precisely, the highest prevalence is thought to be in high-poverty areas of the South and Appalachia. Pig farming in Maine is also associated with *Ascaris* species. Key factors linked with a higher prevalence of

Ascaris lumbricoides

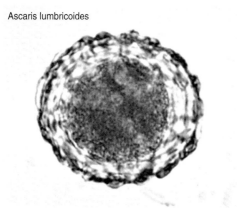

Fig. 317.1 Soil-transmitted helminth eggs *(A. lumbricoides). (From Bethony J, Brooker S, Albonico M, et al: Soil-transmitted helminth infections: ascariasis, trichuriasis, and hookworm, Lancet 367:1521–1532, 2006.)*

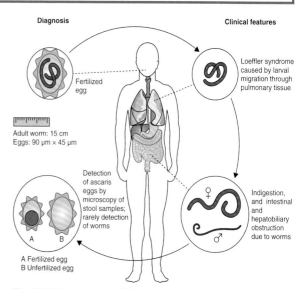

Fig. 317.3 Transmission of *Ascaris lumbricoides*: diagnosis and clinical features. *(From Jourdan PM, Lamberton PHL, Fenwick A, Addiss DG: Soil-transmitted helminth infections, Lancet 391:252–262, 2018, Fig 2A.)*

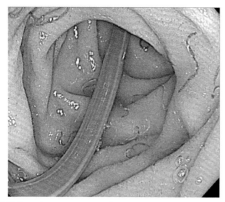

Fig. 317.2 Endoscopic image of intestinal *Ascaris lumbricoides* and hookworm co-infection. The ascaris worm is large in relation to the lumen and multiple blood-filled hookworms. *(Courtesy of Dr. Kunimitsu Inoue, Almeida Hospital, Oita, Japan.)*

infection include poor socioeconomic conditions, use of human feces as fertilizer, and geophagia. Even though infection can occur at any age, the highest rate is in preschool or early school-age children. Transmission is primarily hand to mouth but may also involve ingestion of contaminated raw fruits and vegetables. Transmission is enhanced by the high output of eggs by fecund female worms and resistance of ova to the outside environment. *Ascaris* eggs can remain viable at 5-10°C (41-50°F) for as long as 2 yr.

PATHOGENESIS

Ascaris ova hatch in the small intestine after ingestion by the human host. Larvae are released, penetrate the intestinal wall, and migrate to the lungs by way of the venous circulation. The parasites then cause **pulmonary ascariasis** as they enter into the alveoli and migrate through the bronchi and trachea (Fig. 317.3). They are subsequently swallowed and return to the intestines, where they mature into adult worms. Female *Ascaris* begin depositing eggs in 8-10 wk.

CLINICAL MANIFESTATIONS

The clinical presentation depends on the intensity of infection and the organs involved. Most individuals have low to moderate worm burdens and have no symptoms or signs. The most common clinical problems are from **pulmonary disease** and **obstruction of the intestinal or biliary tract**. Larvae migrating through these tissues may cause allergic symptoms, fever, urticaria, and granulomatous disease. The pulmonary

manifestations resemble Loeffler syndrome and include transient respiratory symptoms such as cough and dyspnea, pulmonary infiltrates, and blood eosinophilia. Larvae may be observed in the sputum. Vague abdominal complaints have been attributed to the presence of adult worms in the small intestine, although the precise contribution of the parasite to these symptoms is difficult to ascertain. A more serious complication occurs when a large mass of worms leads to acute bowel obstruction. Children with heavy infections may present with vomiting, abdominal distention, and cramps. In some cases, worms may be passed in the vomitus or stools. *Ascaris* worms occasionally migrate into the biliary and pancreatic ducts, where they cause cholecystitis or pancreatitis. Worm migration through the intestinal wall can lead to peritonitis. Dead worms can serve as a nidus for stone formation. Studies show that chronic infection with *A. lumbricoides* (often coincident with other helminth infections) impairs growth, physical fitness, and cognitive development.

DIAGNOSIS

Microscopic examination of fecal smears can be used for diagnosis because of the high number of eggs excreted by adult female worms (see Fig. 317.1). A high index of suspicion in the appropriate clinical context is needed to diagnose pulmonary ascariasis or obstruction of the gastrointestinal tract. Ultrasound examination of the abdomen is capable of visualizing intraluminal adult worms.

TREATMENT

Although several chemotherapeutic agents are effective against ascariasis, none has documented utility during the pulmonary phase of infection. Treatment options for gastrointestinal ascariasis include **albendazole** (400 mg orally once, for all ages), **mebendazole** (100 mg orally twice daily for 3 days or 500 mg once, for all ages), or **ivermectin** (150-200 μg/kg orally once). **Piperazine citrate** (75 mg/kg/day for 2 days; maximum dose: 3.5 g/day), which causes neuromuscular paralysis of the parasite and rapid expulsion of the worms, is the treatment of choice for intestinal or biliary obstruction and is administered as syrup through a nasogastric tube. Surgery may be required for cases with severe obstruction. **Nitazoxanide** (100 mg orally twice per day for 3 days for children 1-3 yr old; 200 mg twice per day for 3 days for children 4-11 yr; 500 mg twice per day for 3 days for adolescents and adults) produces cure rates comparable to single-dose albendazole. Drug resistance has not been reported, but repeated treatment for ascariasis may be necessary because reinfection is common.

Table 317.1	Clinical and Public Health Control of Soil-Transmitted Helminthiasis	
	CLINICAL DIAGNOSIS AND MANAGEMENT	**PUBLIC HEALTH CONTROL**
Diagnosis	Individual	Community level (e.g., in select schools)
Diagnostic criteria	Parasitological	Residence in an area with soil-transmitted helminthiasis prevalence >20%
Treatment approach	Single dose or multiple dose	Single-dose periodic mass treatment
Threshold for treatment	Travel history, symptoms and signs, positive laboratory test	Estimated prevalence of infection in target population
Treatment objective	Parasitological cure	Decreased worm burden; reduction in transmission
Ancillary treatment	Based on clinical signs and symptoms	Typically, only if included in mass treatment (e.g., vitamin A supplementation)
Follow-up	Parasitological test of cure; improvement in associated health conditions	Not usually done
Health education (sanitation/hygiene)	Recommended	Recommended

From Jourdan PM, Lamberton PHL, Fenwick A, Addiss DG: Soil-transmitted helminth infections, *Lancet* 391:252–262, 2018 (Table 1).

PREVENTION

Although ascariasis is the most prevalent worm infection in the world, little attention has been given to its control (Table 317.1). **Anthelmintic chemotherapy programs** can be implemented in 1 of 3 ways: (1) offering universal treatment to all individuals in an area of high endemicity; (2) offering treatment targeted to groups with high frequency of infection, such as children attending primary school; or (3) offering individual treatment based on intensity of current or past infection. Improving education about and practices of sanitary conditions and sewage facilities, discontinuing the practice of using human feces as fertilizer, and education are the most effective long-term preventive measures.

Bibliography is available at Expert Consult.

Chapter **318**
Hookworms (*Necator americanus* and *Ancylostoma* spp.)

Peter J. Hotez

第三百一十八章
钩虫病（美洲板口线虫和钩虫属）

中文导读

　　本章主要介绍了钩虫病的病原学、流行病学、发病机制、临床表现、诊断、治疗和预防。在临床表现部分，描述了儿童慢性感染、婴儿钩虫病及嗜酸性肠炎的临床特点。在治疗部分，介绍了钩虫病治疗的药物选择及疗程、儿童钩虫病治疗的注意事项。本章还单独介绍了皮肤幼虫移行症的病原学、流行病学、临床表现、诊断和治疗。

ETIOLOGY

Two major genera of hookworms, which are nematodes, or roundworms, infect humans. *Necator americanus,* the only representative of its genus, is a major **anthropophilic** hookworm and is the most common cause of human hookworm infection. Hookworms of the genus *Ancylostoma* include the anthropophilic hookworm *Ancylostoma duodenale,* which also causes classic hookworm infection, and the less common **zoonotic** species *Ancylostoma ceylanicum* (restricted mostly to Southeast Asia). Human zoonotic infection with the dog hookworm *Ancylostoma caninum* is associated with an eosinophilic enteritis syndrome. The larval stage of *Ancylostoma braziliense,* whose definitive hosts include dogs and cats, is the principal cause of cutaneous larva migrans.

The infective larval stages of the anthropophilic hookworms live in a developmentally arrested state in warm, moist soil. Larvae infect humans either by penetrating through the skin (*N. americanus* and *A. duodenale*) or when they are ingested (*A. duodenale*). Larvae entering the human host by skin penetration undergo **extraintestinal migration** through the venous circulation and lungs before they are swallowed, whereas orally ingested larvae may undergo extraintestinal migration or remain in the gastrointestinal (GI) tract (Figs. 318.1 and 318.2). Larvae returning to the small intestine undergo 2 molts to become adult, sexually mature, male and female worms ranging in length from 5-13 mm. The buccal capsule of the adult hookworm is armed with

cutting plates (*N. americanus*) or teeth (*A. duodenale*) to facilitate attachment to the mucosa and submucosa of the small intestine. Hookworms can remain in the intestine for 1-5 yr, where they mate and produce eggs. Although up to 2 mo is required for the larval stages of hookworms to undergo extraintestinal migration and develop into mature adults, *A. duodenale* larvae may remain developmentally arrested for many months before resuming development in the intestine. Mature *A. duodenale* female worms produce about 30,000 eggs per day; daily egg production by *N. americanus* is <10,000/day (Fig. 318.3). The eggs are thin shelled and ovoid, measuring approximately 40-60 μm. Eggs that are deposited on soil with adequate moisture and shade develop into first-stage larvae and hatch. Over the ensuing several days and under appropriate conditions, the larvae molt twice to the **infective** stage. Infective larvae are developmentally arrested and nonfeeding. They migrate vertically in the soil until they either infect a new host or exhaust their lipid metabolic reserves and die.

EPIDEMIOLOGY

Hookworm infection is one of the most prevalent infectious diseases of humans. The Global Burden of Disease Study 2015 reported that approximately 428 million people are infected with hookworms, with further estimates indicating that hookworm infection globally results in 4.1 million disability-adjusted life-years, possibly leading all **neglected tropical diseases** in years lost through disability. In the case of hookworm infection, all the years lost through disability are attributed to anemia from intestinal blood loss. There is also a massive socioeconomic impact from hookworm infection, with estimates that hookworm can cause up to $139 billion in losses from diminished productivity.

Because of the requirement for adequate soil moisture, shade, and warmth, hookworm infection is usually confined to rural areas, especially where human feces are used for fertilizer or where sanitation is inadequate. Hookworm is an infection associated with *economic underdevelopment and poverty* throughout the tropics and subtropics. Sub-Saharan Africa, East Asia, and tropical regions of the Americas have the highest prevalence of hookworm infection. High rates of infection are often associated with cultivation of certain agricultural products, such as tea in India; sweet potato, corn, cotton, and mulberry trees in China; coffee in Central and South America; and rubber in Africa. It is not uncommon to find dual *N. americanus* and *A. duodenale* infections. *N. americanus* predominates in Central and South America as well as in southern China and Southeast Asia, whereas *A. duodenale* predominates in North Africa, in northern India, in China north of the Yangtze River, and among aboriginal people in Australia. The ability of *A. duodenale* to withstand somewhat harsher environmental and climatic conditions may reflect its ability to undergo arrested development in human tissues. *A. ceylanicum* infection occurs in India and Southeast Asia.

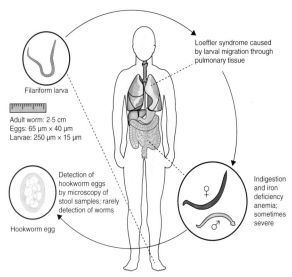

Fig. 318.1 Transmission of hookworm (*Ancylostoma duodenale* and *Necator americanus*): diagnosis and clinical features. *(From Jourdan PM, Lamberton PHL, Fenwick A, Addiss DG: Soil-transmitted helminth infections,* Lancet *391:252–262, 2018, Fig 2C.)*

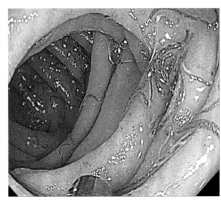

Fig. 318.2 Endoscopic images of intestinal hookworm infection. *(Courtesy of Dr. Kunimitsu Inoue, Almeida Hospital, Oita, Japan.)*

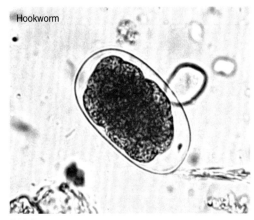

Fig. 318.3 Soil-transmitted hookworm helminth eggs. *(From Bethony J, Brooker S, Albonico M, et al: Soil-transmitted helminth infections: ascariasis, trichuriasis, and hookworm,* Lancet *367:1521–1532, 2006.)*

Eosinophilic enteritis caused by *A. caninum* was first described in Queensland, Australia, with 2 reported cases in the United States. Because of its global distribution in dogs, it was initially anticipated that human *A. caninum* infections would be identified in many locales, but this has not been found.

PATHOGENESIS

The major morbidity of human hookworm infection is a direct result of **intestinal blood loss**. Adult hookworms adhere tenaciously to the mucosa and submucosa of the proximal small intestine by using their cutting plates or teeth and a muscular esophagus that creates negative pressure in their buccal capsules. At the attachment site, host inflammation is downregulated by the release of antiinflammatory polypeptides by the hookworm. Rupture of capillaries in the lamina propria is followed by blood extravasation, with some of the blood ingested directly by the hookworm. After ingestion, the blood is anticoagulated, the red blood cells are lysed, and the hemoglobin released and digested. Each adult *A. duodenale* hookworm causes loss of an estimated 0.2 mL of blood/day; blood loss is less for *N. americanus*. Individuals with light infections have minimal blood loss and thus may have hookworm infection but not hookworm disease. There is a direct correlation between the number of adult hookworms in the gut and the volume of fecal blood loss. Hookworm disease results only when individuals with moderate and heavy infections experience sufficient blood loss to develop iron deficiency and anemia. Hypoalbuminemia and consequent edema and anasarca from the loss of intravascular oncotic pressure can also occur. These features depend heavily on the dietary reserves of the host.

CLINICAL MANIFESTATIONS

Chronically infected children with moderate and heavy hookworm infections suffer from intestinal blood loss that results in **iron deficiency** and can lead to anemia as well as protein malnutrition. Prolonged iron deficiency associated with hookworms in childhood can lead to physical growth retardation and cognitive and intellectual deficits.

Anthropophilic hookworm larvae elicit dermatitis sometimes referred to as **ground itch** when they penetrate human skin. The vesiculation and edema of ground itch are exacerbated by repeated infection. Infection with a zoonotic hookworm, especially *A. braziliense*, can result in lateral migration of the larvae to cause the characteristic cutaneous tracts of **cutaneous larva migrans** (see Chapter 318.1). Cough subsequently occurs in *A. duodenale* and *N. americanus* hookworm infection when larvae migrate through the lungs to cause laryngotracheobronchitis, usually about 1 wk after exposure. Pharyngitis also can occur. The onset of eosinophilia coincides with the entry of hookworm larvae into the GI tract. Upper abdominal pain can occur during this period, but it eventually subsides.

Chronic intestinal hookworm infection is not typically associated with specific GI complaints, although pain, anorexia, and diarrhea have been attributed to the presence of hookworms. The major clinical manifestations are related to intestinal blood loss. Heavily infected children exhibit all the signs and symptoms of **iron-deficiency anemia** and **protein malnutrition**. In some cases, children with chronic hookworm disease acquire a yellow-green pallor known as **chlorosis.**

An infantile form of **ancylostomiasis** resulting from heavy *A. duodenale* infection has been described. Affected infants experience diarrhea, melena, failure to thrive, and profound anemia. Infantile ancylostomiasis has significant mortality.

Eosinophilic enteritis caused by *A. caninum* is associated with colicky abdominal pain that begins in the epigastrium and radiates outward and is usually exacerbated by food. Extreme cases may mimic acute appendicitis.

DIAGNOSIS

Children with hookworm release eggs that can be detected by direct fecal examination (see Fig. 318.3). Quantitative methods are available to determine whether a child has a heavy **worm burden** that can cause hookworm disease. The eggs of *N. americanus* and *A. duodenale* are morphologically indistinguishable. Species identification typically requires

egg hatching and differentiation of third-stage infective larvae; methods using polymerase chain reaction (PCR) methods have been developed but are not generally used in clinical practice.

In contrast, eggs are generally not present in the feces of patients with eosinophilic enteritis caused by *A. caninum*. Eosinophilic enteritis is often diagnosed by demonstrating ileal and colonic ulcerations by colonoscopy in the presence of significant blood eosinophilia. An adult canine hookworm may occasionally be recovered during colonoscopic biopsy. Patients with this syndrome develop IgG and IgE serologic responses.

TREATMENT

The goal of **deworming** is removal of the adult hookworms with an **anthelmintic** drug. The **benzimidazole** anthelmintics, mebendazole and albendazole, are effective at eliminating hookworms from the intestine, although multiple doses are sometimes required. **Albendazole** (400 mg orally [PO] once, for all ages) often results in cure, although *N. americanus* adult hookworms are sometimes more refractory and require additional doses. **Mebendazole** (100 mg PO twice daily [bid] for 3 days, for all ages) is also effective. In many developing countries, mebendazole is administered as a single dose of 500 mg; however, the cure rates with this regimen can be as low as 10% or less. According to the World Health Organization (WHO), children should be encouraged to chew tablets of albendazole or mebendazole, because forcing very young children to swallow large tablets may cause choking or asphyxiation. Mebendazole is recommended for *A. caninum*–associated eosinophilic enteritis, although recurrences are common. Because the benzimidazoles have been reported to be embryotoxic and teratogenic in laboratory animals, their safety during pregnancy and in young children is a potential concern, and the risks vs benefits must be carefully considered. WHO currently supports the use of benzimidazoles in infected children ≥1 yr old but at a reduced dose (200 mg for albendazole) in the youngest age-group (1-2 yr old). In some countries, **pyrantel pamoate** (11 mg/kg PO once daily for 3 days; maximum dose: 1 g) is available in liquid form and is an effective alternative to the benzimidazoles. A newer drug known as **tribendimidine** is still under clinical development and may be available in the future. Replacement therapy with oral iron is not usually required to correct hookworm-associated iron deficiency in children.

PREVENTION

In 2001, the World Health Assembly urged its member states to implement programs of periodic deworming so as to control the morbidity of hookworm and other soil-transmitted helminth infections (see Table 317.1 in Chapter 317). Although anthelmintic drugs are effective at eliminating hookworms from the intestine, the high rates of drug failure from single-dose mebendazole or albendazole and posttreatment reinfection among children suggest that mass drug administration alone is not effective for controlling hookworm in highly endemic areas. Moreover, data suggest that the efficacy of mebendazole decreases with frequent, periodic use, leading to concerns about the possible emergence of **anthelmintic drug resistance**. To reduce the reliance exclusively on anthelmintic drugs, a recombinant human hookworm vaccine has been developed and is undergoing clinical testing. Economic development and associated improvements in sanitation, health education, and avoidance of human feces as fertilizer remain critical for reducing hookworm transmission and endemicity.

Bibliography is available at Expert Consult.

318.1 Cutaneous Larva Migrans

Peter J. Hotez

ETIOLOGY

Cutaneous larva migrans (**creeping eruption**) is caused by the larvae of several nematodes, primarily hookworms, which are not usually parasitic for humans. *A. braziliense*, a hookworm of dogs and cats, is the most common cause, but other animal hookworms may also produce the disease.

EPIDEMIOLOGY

Cutaneous larva migrans is usually caused by *A. braziliense,* which is endemic to the southeastern United States and Puerto Rico. Travelers account for a significant percentage of the cases. Recently, autochthonous cases have been reported from Europe.

CLINICAL MANIFESTATIONS

After penetrating the skin, larvae localize at the epidermal-dermal junction and migrate in this plane, moving at a rate of 1-2 cm/day. The response to the parasite is characterized by raised, erythematous, ser-piginous tracks, which occasionally form bullae (Fig. 318.4). These lesions may be single or numerous and are usually localized to an extremity, although any area of the body may be affected. As the organism migrates, new areas of involvement may appear every few days. Intense localized pruritus, without any systemic symptoms, may be associated with the lesions. Bacterial superinfection can occur.

DIAGNOSIS

Cutaneous larva migrans is diagnosed by clinical examination of the skin. Patients are often able to recall the exact time and location of exposure, because the larvae produce intense itching at the site of penetration. Eosinophilia may occur but is uncommon.

TREATMENT

If left untreated, the larvae die, and the syndrome resolves within a few weeks to several months. Treatment with **ivermectin** (200 μg/kg PO daily for 1-2 days; considered drug of choice by some investigators), **albendazole** (400 mg PO daily for 3 days, for all ages), or topical **thiabendazole** hastens resolution, if symptoms warrant treatment. The U.S. Food and Drug Administration has not approved these drugs for cutaneous larva migrans. The safety of ivermectin in young children

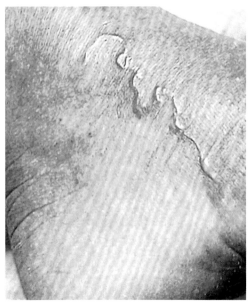

Fig. 318.4 Creeping eruption of cutaneous larva migrans. *(From Korting GW:* Hautkrankheitenbeikindern und jugendlichen, *Stuttgart, Germany, 1969, FK Schattauer Verlag.)*

(weighing <15 kg) and pregnant women remains to be established. Albendazole should be taken with a fatty meal.

Bibliography is available at Expert Consult.

Chapter **319**

Trichuriasis *(Trichuris trichiura)*

Arlene E. Dent and James W. Kazura

第三百一十九章
鞭虫病（毛首鞭形线虫）

中文导读

　　本章主要介绍了鞭虫病的病原学、流行病学、临床表现、诊断、治疗和预防。在流行病学部分，介绍了鞭虫病的全球流行分布、疾病负担、好发年龄及感染途径等相关情况。在临床表现部分，介绍了鞭虫病的无症状感染及症状性感染发生情况，指出儿童更容易出现症状性感染，同时描述了症状性感染的相关临床表现。

ETIOLOGY

Trichuriasis is caused by the **whipworm**, *Trichuris trichiura*, a nematode, or roundworm, that inhabits the cecum and ascending colon. The principal hosts of *T. trichiura* are humans, who acquire infection by ingesting embryonated, barrel-shaped eggs (Fig. 319.1). The larvae escape from the shell in the upper small intestine and penetrate the intestinal villi. The worms slowly move toward the cecum, where the anterior three-quarters whiplike portion remains within the superficial mucosa and the short posterior end is free in the lumen (Fig. 319.2). In 1-3 mo, the adult female worm begins producing 5,000-20,000 eggs per day. After excretion in the feces, embryonic development occurs in 2-4 wk with optimal temperature and soil conditions. The adult worm life span is approximately 2 yr.

EPIDEMIOLOGY

Trichuriasis occurs throughout the world and is especially common in poor rural communities with inadequate sanitary facilities and soil contaminated with human or animal feces. Trichuriasis is one of the most prevalent human helminthiases, with an estimated 1 billion infected individuals worldwide. In many parts of the world, where protein-energy malnutrition and anemia are common, the prevalence of *T. trichiura* infection can be as high as 95%. Although trichuriasis occurs in the rural southeastern United States, its prevalence has not been reported. The highest rate of infection occurs among children 5-15 yr old. Infection develops after ingesting embryonated ova by direct contamination of hands, food (raw fruits and vegetables fertilized with human feces), or drink (Fig. 319.3). Transmission can also occur indirectly through flies or other insects.

CLINICAL MANIFESTATIONS

Most persons harbor low worm burdens and do not have symptoms. Some individuals may have a history of right lower quadrant or vague periumbilical pain. Adult *Trichuris* ingest approximately 0.005 mL of blood per worm per day. Children, who are most likely to be heavily infected, frequently suffer from disease. Clinical manifestations include chronic dysentery, rectal prolapse, anemia, poor growth, as well as developmental and cognitive deficits. There is no significant eosinophilia, even though a portion of the worm is embedded in the mucosa of the large bowel.

DIAGNOSIS

Because egg output is so high, fecal smears frequently reveal the characteristic barrel-shaped ova of *T. trichiura*.

TREATMENT

Albendazole (400 mg orally for 3 days, for all ages) is the drug of choice and is safe and effective, in part because it is poorly absorbed from the gastrointestinal tract. It reduces egg output by 90–99% and has cure rates of 70–90%, although reinfection and resumption of egg production by live worms that presumably survive after treatment may occur. Alternatives include **mebendazole** (100 mg orally twice daily for 3 days) and **ivermectin** (200 µg/kg orally for 3 days). Single-day treatment with albendazole, nitazoxanide, or albendazole plus nitazoxanide lead to cure rates that are low and short-lived. Combination treatment with **oxantel pamoate** (20 mg/kg) plus 400 mg albendazole on consecutive days may have the highest cure rate.

PREVENTION

Disease can be prevented by personal hygiene, improved sanitary conditions, and eliminating the use of human feces as fertilizer (see Table 317.1 in Chapter 317).

Bibliography is available at Expert Consult.

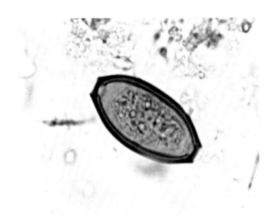

Fig. 319.1 *Trichuris trichiura.* Soil-transmitted helminth eggs. *(From Bethony J, Brooker S, Albonico M, et al: Soil-transmitted helminth infections: ascariasis, trichuriasis, and hookworm, Lancet 367:1521–1532, 2006.)*

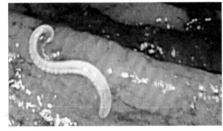

Fig. 319.2 *Trichuris trichiura* infection. *(Courtesy of Dr. Kunimitsu Inoue, Almeida Hospital, Oita, Japan).*

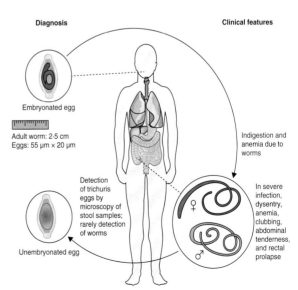

Diagnosis

Embryonated egg

Adult worm: 2·5 cm
Eggs: 55 µm × 20 µm

Detection of trichuris eggs by microscopy of stool samples; rarely detection of worms

Unembryonated egg

Clinical features

Indigestion and anemia due to worms

In severe infection, dysentery, anemia, clubbing, abdominal tenderness, and rectal prolapse

Fig. 319.3 Transmission of *Trichuris trichiura*: diagnosis and clinical features. *(From Jourdan PM, Lamberton PHL, Fenwick A, Addiss DG: Soil-transmitted helminth infections, Lancet 391:252–262, 2018, Fig 2B.)*

Chapter 320
Enterobiasis (Enterobius vermicularis)
Arlene E. Dent and James W. Kazura

第三百二十章
蛲虫病（蠕形住肠线虫）

中文导读

　　本章主要介绍了蛲虫病的病原学、流行病学、临床表现、诊断、治疗和预防。在病原学部分，介绍了蛲虫的生物学特征。在流行病学部分，介绍了蛲虫病全球分布状况、好发年龄及人群流行特征。在临床表现部分，描述了蛲虫病最常表现为瘙痒及由于夜间肛周或会阴瘙痒引起的睡眠不安，偶有因为异位迁移可引起相应的消化系统疾病。在治疗部分，介绍了饶虫病药物治疗方案，并指出勤洗衣物和床单可以减少感染。

ETIOLOGY

The cause of enterobiasis, or **pinworm** infection, is *Enterobius vermicularis,* which is a small (1 cm in length), white, threadlike nematode, or roundworm, that typically inhabits the cecum, appendix, and adjacent areas of the ileum and ascending colon. Gravid females migrate at night to the perianal and perineal regions, where they deposit up to 15,000 eggs. Ova are convex on one side and flattened on the other and have diameters of approximately $30 \times 60\ \mu m$. Eggs embryonate within 6 hr and remain viable for 20 days. Human infection occurs by the fecal-oral route typically by ingestion of embryonated eggs that are carried on fingernails, clothing, bedding, or house dust. After ingestion, the larvae mature to form adult worms in 36-53 days.

EPIDEMIOLOGY

Enterobiasis infection occurs in individuals of all ages and socioeconomic levels. It is prevalent in regions with temperate climates and is the most common helminth infection in the United States. It infects 30% of children worldwide, and humans are the only known host. Infection occurs primarily in institutional or family settings that include children. The prevalence of pinworm infection is highest in children 5-14 yr of age. It is common in areas where children live, play, and sleep close together, thus facilitating egg transmission. Because the life span of the adult worm is short, chronic parasitism is likely caused by repeated cycles of reinfection. **Autoinoculation** can occur in individuals who habitually put their fingers in their mouth.

PATHOGENESIS

Enterobius infection may cause symptoms by mechanical stimulation and irritation, allergic reactions, and migration of the worms to anatomic sites where they become pathogenic. *Enterobius* infection has been associated with concomitant *Dientamoeba fragilis* infection, which causes diarrhea.

CLINICAL MANIFESTATIONS

Pinworm infection is innocuous and rarely causes serious medical problems. The most common complaints include itching and restless sleep secondary to nocturnal perianal or **perineal pruritus**. The precise cause and incidence of pruritus are unknown but may be related to the intensity of infection, psychologic profile of the infected individual and the family, or allergic reactions to the parasite. Eosinophilia is not observed in most cases, because tissue invasion does not occur. Aberrant migration to ectopic sites occasionally may lead to appendicitis, chronic salpingitis, pelvic inflammatory disease, peritonitis, hepatitis, and ulcerative lesions in the large or small bowel.

DIAGNOSIS

A history of nocturnal **perianal pruritus** in children strongly suggests enterobiasis. Definitive diagnosis is established by identification of parasite eggs or worms. Microscopic examination of adhesive cellophane tape pressed against the perianal region early in the morning frequently demonstrates eggs (Fig. 320.1). Repeated examinations increase the chance of detecting ova; 1 examination detects 50% of infections, 3 examinations 90%, and 5 examinations 99%. Worms seen in the perianal region should be removed and preserved in 75% ethyl alcohol until microscopic examination can be performed. Digital rectal examination may also be used to obtain samples for a wet mount. Routine stool samples rarely demonstrate *Enterobius* ova.

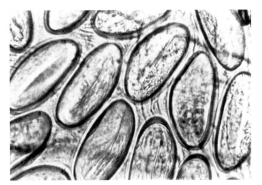

Fig. 320.1 Eggs of *Enterobius vermicularis. (From Guerrant RL, Walker DH, Weller PF, et al: Tropical infectious diseases, Philadelphia, 2006, Churchill Livingstone, p 1248.)*

TREATMENT

Anthelmintic drugs should be administered to infected individuals and their family members. **Albendazole** (400 mg orally with a repeat dose 2 wk later for all age-groups) is the treatment of choice and results in cure rates exceeding 90%. Alternatives include **mebendazole** (100 mg orally with a repeat dose 2 wk later) and **pyrantel pamoate** (11 mg/kg base orally 3 times for 1 day up to a maximum of 1 g; repeat at 2 wk). Morning bathing removes a large portion of eggs. Frequent changing of underclothes, bedclothes, and bedsheets decreases environmental egg contamination and may decrease the risk for autoinfection.

PREVENTION

Household contacts can be treated at the same time as the infected individual. Repeated treatments every 3-4 mo may be required in circumstances with repeated exposure, such as with institutionalized children. Good hand hygiene is the most effective method of prevention.

Bibliography is available at Expert Consult.

Chapter **321**

Strongyloidiasis *(Strongyloides stercoralis)*

Arlene E. Dent and James W. Kazura

第三百二十一章

类圆线虫病（粪类圆线虫）

中文导读

本章主要介绍了类圆线虫病的病原学、流行病学、发病机制、临床表现、诊断、治疗和预防。在病原学部分，描述了类圆线虫生物学特性，同时介绍了过度感染综合征。在流行病学部分，介绍了类圆线虫病全球分布特征、传播方式及易感人群等。在临床表现部分，介绍了类圆线虫病存在无症状感染和症状性感染，症状性感染的临床表现与感染的三个阶段相关，另外描述了过度感染综合征的临床特点。

ETIOLOGY

Strongyloidiasis is caused by the nematode, or roundworm, *Strongyloides stercoralis.* Only adult female worms inhabit the small intestine. The nematode reproduces in the human host by parthenogenesis and releases eggs containing mature larvae into the intestinal lumen. **Rhabditiform** larvae immediately emerge from the ova and are passed in feces, where they can be visualized by stool examination. Rhabditiform larvae either differentiate into free-living adult male and female worms or metamorphose into the infectious **filariform** larvae. Sexual reproduction occurs only in the free-living stage. Humans are usually infected through skin contact with soil contaminated with infectious larvae (Fig. 321.1). Larvae penetrate the skin, enter the venous circulation and then pass to the lungs, break into alveolar spaces, and migrate up the bronchial tree. They are then swallowed and pass through the stomach, and adult female worms develop in the small intestine. Egg deposition begins approximately 28 days after initial infection.

The **hyperinfection syndrome** occurs when large numbers of larvae transform into infective organisms during their passage in feces and then reinfect (**autoinfect**) the host by way of the lower gastrointestinal (GI) tract or perianal region. This cycle may be accelerated in immunocompromised persons, particularly those with depressed T-cell function.

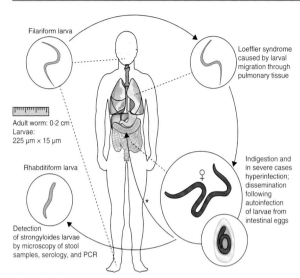

Fig. 321.1 Transmission of *Strongyloides stercoralis*: diagnosis and clinical features. *(From Jourdan PM, Lamberton PHL, Fenwick A, Addiss DG: Soil-transmitted helminth infections, Lancet 391:252–262, 2018, Fig 2D.)*

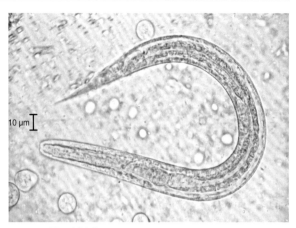

Fig. 321.2 Larvae of intestinal strongyloidiasis.

EPIDEMIOLOGY

S. stercoralis infection is prevalent in tropical and subtropical regions of the world and is endemic in several areas of Europe, the southern United States, and Puerto Rico. Transmission requires appropriate environmental conditions, particularly warm, moist soil. Poor sanitation and crowded living conditions are conducive to high levels of transmission. Dogs and cats can act as reservoirs. The highest prevalence of infection in the United States (4% of the general population) is in impoverished rural areas of Kentucky and Tennessee. Infection may be especially common among residents of mental institutions, veterans who were prisoners of war in areas of high endemicity, and refugees and immigrants. Because of internal autoinfection, individuals may remain infected for decades. Infection may be transmitted by organ transplantation. Individuals with hematologic malignancies, autoimmune diseases, malnutrition, and drug-induced immunosuppression (especially corticosteroids) are at high risk for the hyperinfection syndrome. Patients with AIDS may experience a rapid course of disseminated strongyloidiasis with a fatal outcome.

PATHOGENESIS

The initial host immune response to infection is production of immunoglobulin E and eosinophilia in blood and tissues, which presumably prevents dissemination and hyperinfection in the immunocompetent host. Adult female worms in otherwise healthy and asymptomatic individuals may persist in the GI tract for years. If infected persons become immunocompromised, the reduction in cellular and humoral immunity may lead to an abrupt and dramatic increase in parasite load with systemic dissemination.

CLINICAL MANIFESTATIONS

Approximately 30% of infected individuals are asymptomatic. The remaining patients have symptoms that correlate with the 3 stages of infection: invasion of the skin, migration of larvae through the lungs, and parasitism of the small intestine by adult worms. **Larva currens** is the manifestation of an allergic reaction to filariform larvae that migrate through the skin, where they leave pruritic, tortuous, urticarial tracks. The lesions may recur and are typically found over the lower abdominal wall, buttocks, or thighs, resulting from larval migration from defecated stool. Pulmonary disease secondary to larval migration through the lung rarely occurs and may resemble **Loeffler syndrome** (cough, wheezing, shortness of breath, transient pulmonary infiltrates accompanied

by eosinophilia). GI strongyloidiasis is characterized by indigestion, crampy abdominal pain, vomiting, diarrhea, steatorrhea, protein-losing enteropathy, protein-caloric malnutrition, and weight loss. Edema of the duodenum with irregular mucosal folds, ulcerations, and strictures can be seen radiographically. Infection may be chronic in nature and is associated with **eosinophilia**.

Strongyloidiasis is potentially lethal because of the ability of the parasite to replicate within the host and cause overwhelming hyperinfection in immunocompromised persons. The **hyperinfection syndrome** is characterized by an exaggeration of the clinical features that develop in symptomatic immunocompetent individuals. The onset is usually sudden, with generalized abdominal pain, distention, and fever. Multiple organs can be affected as massive numbers of larvae disseminate throughout the body and introduce bowel flora. The latter may result in bacteremia and septicemia. Cutaneous manifestations may include petechiae and purpura. Cough, wheezing, and hemoptysis are indicative of pulmonary involvement. Whereas eosinophilia is a prominent feature of strongyloidiasis in immunocompetent persons, this sign may be absent in immunocompromised persons. Because of the low incidence of strongyloidiasis in industrialized countries, it is often misdiagnosed, resulting in a significant delay in treatment.

DIAGNOSIS

Intestinal strongyloidiasis is diagnosed by examining feces or duodenal fluid for the characteristic larvae (Fig. 321.2). Several stool samples should be examined by direct smear, the Koga agar plate method, or the Baermann test. Alternatively, duodenal fluid can be sampled by the **enteric string test** (Entero-Test) or aspiration via endoscopy. In children with the hyperinfection syndrome, larvae may be found in sputum, gastric aspirates, and rarely in small intestinal biopsy specimens. An enzyme-linked immunosorbent assay for IgG antibody to *Strongyloides* may be more sensitive than parasitological methods for diagnosing intestinal infection in the immunocompetent host. The utility of the assay in diagnosing infection in immunocompromised patients with the hyperinfection syndrome has not been determined. Eosinophilia is common.

TREATMENT

Treatment is directed at eradication of infection. **Ivermectin** (200 μg/kg/day once daily orally for 2 days) is the drug of choice for uncomplicated strongyloidiasis. Alternatively, **albendazole** (400 mg orally twice daily for 7 days) may be used. Patients with the hyperinfection syndrome should be treated with ivermectin for 7-10 days and may require repeated courses. Reducing the dose of immunosuppressive therapy and treatment of concomitant bacterial infections are essential in the management of the **hyperinfection syndrome**. Close follow-up with repeated stool examination is necessary to ensure complete elimination of the parasite. *Strongyloides* antibodies decrease within 6 mo after successful treatment.

PREVENTION

Sanitary practices designed to prevent soil and person-to-person transmission are the most effective control measures (see Table 317.1). Wearing **shoes** is a main preventive strategy. Reducing transmission in institutional settings can be achieved by decreasing fecal contamination of the environment, such as by the use of clean bedding. Because infection is uncommon in most settings, case detection and treatment are advisable.

Individuals who will be given prolonged high-dose corticosteroids, immunosuppressive drugs before organ transplantation, or cancer chemotherapy should have a screening examination for *S. stercoralis.* If infected, they should be treated before immunosuppression is initiated.

Bibliography is available at Expert Consult.

Chapter 322

Lymphatic Filariasis (*Brugia malayi, Brugia timori,* and *Wuchereria bancrofti*)

Arlene E. Dent and James W. Kazura

第三百二十二章

淋巴丝虫病（马来布鲁线虫、帝汶丝虫和班氏吴策线虫）

中文导读

本章主要介绍了淋巴丝虫病的病原学、流行病学、临床表现、诊断和治疗。在病原学部分，描述了淋巴丝虫的生物学特性及生命周期。在流行病学部分，介绍了淋巴丝虫病全球分布特征。在临床表现部分，介绍了急性淋巴丝虫病和慢性淋巴丝虫病易感年龄及临床表现，对热带肺嗜酸性粒细胞增多症的临床表现作了单独介绍。在治疗部分，介绍了淋巴丝虫病的药物选择及疗程，同时介绍了全球控制和最终根除淋巴丝虫病的药物推荐方案。

ETIOLOGY

The filarial worms *Brugia malayi* (**Malayan filariasis**), *Brugia timori,* and *Wuchereria bancrofti* (**bancroftian filariasis**) are threadlike nematodes that cause similar infections. Infective larvae are introduced into humans during blood feeding by the **mosquito** vector. Over 4-6 mo, the larval forms develop into sexually mature adult worms. Once an adequate number of male and female worms accumulate in the afferent lymphatic vessels, adult female worms release large numbers of microfilariae that circulate in the bloodstream. The life cycle of the parasite is completed when mosquitoes ingest microfilariae in a blood meal, which molt to form infective larvae over 10-14 days. Adult worms have a 5-7 yr life span.

EPIDEMIOLOGY

More than 120 million people living in tropical Africa, Asia, and Latin America are infected; approximately 10–20% of these individuals have clinically significant morbidity attributable to filariasis. *W. bancrofti* is transmitted in Africa, Asia, and Latin America and accounts for 90% of lymphatic filariasis. *B. malayi* is restricted to the South Pacific and Southeast Asia, and *B. timori* is restricted to several islands of Indonesia.

Travelers from nonendemic areas of the world who spend brief periods in endemic areas are rarely infected. Global elimination has been targeted for 2020.

CLINICAL MANIFESTATIONS

The clinical manifestations of *B. malayi*, *B. timori*, and *W. bancrofti* infection are similar; manifestations of acute infection include transient, recurrent lymphadenitis and lymphangitis. The early signs and symptoms include episodic fever, lymphangitis of an extremity, lymphadenitis (especially the inguinal and axillary areas), headaches, and myalgias that last a few days to several weeks. These symptoms are caused by an acute inflammatory response triggered by death of adult worms. Initial damage to lymphatic vessels may remain subclinical for years. The syndrome is most frequently observed in persons 10-20 yr old. Manifestations of chronic lymphatic filariasis occur mostly in adults ≥30 yr old and result from anatomic and functional obstruction to lymph flow. This obstruction results in lymphedema of the legs, arms, breasts, and/or genitalia. Male genital involvement, such as hydrocele, is very common in *W. bancrofti* infection, but uncommon in *Brugia* spp. infection. Chronic lymphedema predisposes affected extremities to bacterial superinfections, sclerosis, and verrucous skin changes, resulting in **elephantiasis**, which may involve 1 or more limbs, the breasts, or genitalia. It is uncommon for children to have overt signs of chronic filariasis.

Tropical Pulmonary Eosinophilia

The presence of microfilariae in the body has no apparent pathologic consequences except in persons with tropical pulmonary eosinophilia, a syndrome of filarial etiology in which microfilariae are found in the lungs and lymph nodes but not the bloodstream. It occurs only in individuals who have lived for years in endemic areas. Men 20-30 yr old are most likely to be affected, although the syndrome occasionally occurs in children. The presentation includes paroxysmal nocturnal cough with dyspnea, fever, weight loss, and fatigue. Rales and rhonchi are found on auscultation of the chest. The x-ray findings may occasionally be normal, but increased bronchovascular markings, discrete

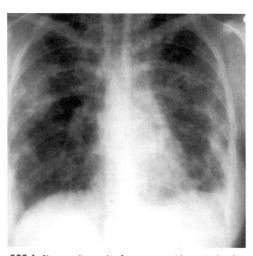

Fig. 322.1 Chest radiograph of a woman with tropical pulmonary eosinophilia. Reticulonodular opacities are scattered throughout both lungs. *(From Mandell GL, Bennett JE, Dolin R, editors: Principles and practice of infectious diseases, ed 6, Philadelphia, 2006, Elsevier, p 3274.)*

opacities in the middle and basal regions of the lung, or diffuse miliary lesions are usually present (Fig. 322.1). Recurrent episodes may result in interstitial fibrosis and chronic respiratory insufficiency in untreated individuals. Hepatosplenomegaly and generalized lymphadenopathy are often seen in children. The **diagnosis** is suggested by residence in a filarial endemic area, eosinophilia (>2,000/μL), compatible clinical symptoms, increased serum IgE (>1,000 IU/mL), and high titers of antimicrofilarial antibodies in the absence of microfilaremia. Although microfilariae may be found in sections of lung or lymph node, biopsy of these tissues is unwarranted in most situations. The clinical response to **diethylcarbamazine** (2 mg/kg/dose orally 3 times daily for 12-21 days) is the final criterion for diagnosis; the majority of patients improve with this therapy. If symptoms recur, a 2nd anthelmintic course should be administered. Patients with chronic symptoms are less likely to show improvement than those who have been ill for a short time.

DIAGNOSIS

Demonstration of microfilariae in the blood is the primary means for confirming the diagnosis of lymphatic filariasis. Because microfilaremia is **nocturnal** in most cases, blood samples should be obtained between 10 PM and 2 AM. Anticoagulated blood is passed through a Nuclepore filter that is stained and examined microscopically for microfilariae. Adult worms or microfilariae can be identified in tissue specimens obtained at biopsy. Infection with *W. bancrofti* in the absence of bloodborne microfilariae may be diagnosed by detection of parasite antigen in the serum. Adult worms in lymphatic vessels can be visualized by ultrasonography.

TREATMENT

The use of antifilarial drugs in the management of acute lymphadenitis and lymphangitis is controversial. No controlled studies demonstrate that administration of drugs such as diethylcarbamazine modifies the course of acute lymphangitis. Diethylcarbamazine may be given to asymptomatic microfilaremic persons to lower the intensity of parasitemia. The drug also kills a proportion of the adult worms. Because treatment-associated complications such as pruritus, fever, generalized body pain, hypotension, and even death may occur, especially with high microfilarial levels, the dose of **diethylcarbamazine** should be increased gradually (*children*: 1 mg/kg orally as a single dose on day 1, 1 mg/kg 3 times daily on day 2, 1-2 mg/kg 3 times daily on day 3, and 2 mg/kg 3 times daily on days 4-14; *adults*: 50 mg orally on day 1, 50 mg 3 times daily on day 2, 100 mg 3 times daily on day 3, and 2 mg/kg 3 times daily on days 4-14). For patients with no microfilaria in the blood, the full dose (2 mg/kg/day orally divided 3 times daily) can be given beginning on day 1. Repeat doses may be necessary to further reduce the microfilaremia and kill lymph-dwelling adult parasites. *W. bancrofti* is more sensitive than *B. malayi* to diethylcarbamazine.

Global programs to control and ultimately eradicate lymphatic filariasis from endemic populations currently recommend a single annual dose of diethylcarbamazine (6 mg/kg orally once) in combination with **albendazole** (400 mg orally once) for 5 yr (mass drug administration). In coendemic areas of filariasis and **onchocerciasis**, mass drug applications with single-dose **ivermectin** (150 μg/kg orally once) and albendazole are used because of severe adverse reactions with diethylcarbamazine in onchocerciasis-infected individuals. Five years of annual mass treatment is thought to be necessary to stop transmission. Adjuvant medicines (e.g., doxycycline) that target endosymbiont bacteria (*Wolbachia*) in filarial parasites may accelerate eradication.

Bibliography is available at Expert Consult.

Chapter **323**
Other Tissue Nematodes
Arlene E. Dent and James W. Kazura
第三百二十三章
其他组织线虫

中文导读

本章介绍了其他组织线虫病，包括盘尾丝虫病、罗阿丝虫病、感染动物丝虫病、广州管圆线虫病、肋管圆线虫病、龙线虫病和棘聘口线虫病等。在各个疾病部分，分别介绍了盘尾丝虫病、罗阿丝虫病、感染

动物丝虫病、广州管圆线虫病、肋管圆线虫病、龙线虫病和棘聘口线虫病的流行区域、感染途径、临床表现、诊断方法、治疗方案及预防。

ONCHOCERCIASIS (ONCHOCERCA VOLVULUS)

Infection with *Onchocerca volvulus* leads to onchocerciasis or **river blindness**. Onchocerciasis occurs primarily in West Africa but also in Central and East Africa and is the world's 2nd leading infectious cause of blindness. There have been scattered foci in Central and South America, but the infection is now thought to be eliminated in the Americas. *O. volvulus* larvae are transmitted to humans by the bite of *Simulium* black flies that breed in fast-flowing streams. The larvae penetrate the skin and migrate through the connective tissue and eventually develop into adult worms that can be found tangled in fibrous tissue. Adult worms can live in the human body for up to 14 yr. Female worms produce large numbers of microfilariae that migrate through the skin, connective tissue, and eye. Most infected individuals are asymptomatic. In heavily infected individuals, clinical manifestations are a result of localized host inflammatory reactions to dead or dying microfilariae and subcutaneous adult worms surrounded by a palpable fibrous capsule. Cutaneous and ocular reactions to microfilariae produce pruritic dermatitis, punctate keratitis, corneal pannus formation, and chorioretinitis. Adult worms in subcutaneous nodules are not painful and tend to occur over bony prominences of the hip. The **diagnosis** can be established by obtaining snips of skin covering the scapulae, iliac crests, buttocks, or calves. The snips are immersed in saline for several hours and examined microscopically for microfilariae that have emerged into the fluid. The diagnosis can also be established by demonstrating microfilariae in the cornea or anterior chamber on slit-lamp examination or finding adult worms on a nodule biopsy specimen. Ophthalmology consultation should be obtained before treatment of eye lesions.

A single dose of **ivermectin** (150 µg/kg orally) is the drug of choice and clears *O. volvulus* microfilariae from the skin for several months but has no effect on the adult worm. Treatment with ivermectin should be repeated every 6-12 mo until the patient is asymptomatic or has no evidence of eye infection. Adverse effects of ivermectin therapy include fever, urticaria, and pruritus, which are more frequent in individuals

not born in endemic areas who acquired the infection following periods of intense exposure, such as Peace Corps volunteers. Patients with concurrent high-density microfilaremia from loiasis may develop potentially fatal encephalopathy with ivermectin therapy. Treatment with ivermectin should be withheld until *Loa loa* microfilaremia can be reduced. **Moxidectin** is a promising new agent. Personal protection includes avoiding areas where biting flies are numerous, wearing protective clothing, and using insect repellent. Programs of mass treatment with ivermectin have been implemented in Africa in an effort to reduce the prevalence of onchocerciasis.

The World Health Organization (WHO) set goals for onchocerciasis elimination by 2020 using mass drug administration with ivermectin. Elimination can be declared only after 3 yr of posttreatment surveillance without microfilaria detection in skin biopsies.

Nodding syndrome, a form of epilepsy in African children living in focal areas of Uganda and South Sudan, was epidemiologically associated with onchocerciasis, but an etiologic link was not established. Recently, researchers identified neurotoxic autoantibodies that cross-react with *O. volvulus* proteins, which were found more frequently in people with nodding syndrome than in those in the same village without the syndrome. Nodding syndrome may be an autoimmune epileptic disorder triggered by *O. volvulus* infection.

LOIASIS (LOA LOA)

Loiasis is caused by infection with the tissue nematode *Loa loa*. The parasite is transmitted to humans by diurnally biting flies *(Chrysops)* that live in the rain forests of West and Central Africa. Migration of adult worms through skin, subcutaneous tissue, and subconjunctival area can lead to transient episodes of pruritus, erythema, and localized edema known as **Calabar swellings**, which are nonerythematous areas of subcutaneous edema 10-20 cm in diameter typically found around joints such as the wrist or the knee (Fig. 323.1). They resolve over several days to weeks and may recur at the same or different sites.

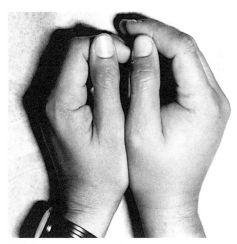

Fig. 323.1 Calabar swelling of the right hand. *(From Guerrant RL, Walker DH, Weller PF, et al: Tropical infectious diseases, Philadelphia, 2006, Churchill Livingstone, p 1165.)*

Lifelong residents of *L. loa*–endemic regions may have microfilaremia and eosinophilia but are often asymptomatic. In contrast, travelers to endemic regions may have a hyperreactive response to *L. loa* infection characterized by frequent recurrences of swelling, high level eosinophilia, debilitation, and serious complications such as glomerulonephritis and encephalitis. **Diagnosis** is usually established on clinical grounds, often assisted by the infected individual reporting a worm being seen crossing the conjunctivae. Microfilariae may be detected in blood smears collected between 10 AM and 2 PM. Adult worms should be surgically excised when possible.

Diethylcarbamazine is the agent of choice for eradication of microfilaremia, but the drug does not kill adult worms. Because treatment-associated complications such as pruritus, fever, generalized body pain, hypertension, and even death may occur, especially with high microfilaria levels, the dose of diethylcarbamazine should be increased gradually in such cases (*children*: 1 mg/kg orally on day 1, 1 mg/kg 3 times daily on day 2, 1-2 mg/kg three times daily on day 3, 2 mg/kg three times daily on days 4-21; *adults*: 50 mg orally on day 1, 50 mg three times daily on day 2, 100 mg three times daily on day 3, 2 mg/kg three times daily on days 4-21). Full doses can be instituted on day 1 in persons without microfilaremia (3 mg/kg orally three times daily for 12 days). A 3 wk course of **albendazole** can also be used to slowly reduce *L. loa* microfilarial levels as a result of embryotoxic effects on the adult worms. Antihistamines or corticosteroids may be used to limit allergic reactions secondary to killing of microfilariae. Personal protective measures include avoiding areas where biting flies are present, wearing protective clothing, and using insect repellents. Diethylcarbamazine (300 mg orally once weekly) prevents infection in travelers who spend prolonged periods in endemic areas. *L. loa* do not harbor *Wolbachia* endosymbionts, and therefore doxycycline has no effect on infection.

INFECTION WITH ANIMAL FILARIAE

The most commonly recognized zoonotic filarial infections are caused by members of the genus *Dirofilaria*. The worms are introduced into humans by the bites of mosquitoes containing third-stage larvae. The most common filarial zoonosis in the United States is *Dirofilaria tenuis*, a parasite of raccoons. In Europe, Africa, and Southeast Asia, infections are usually caused by the dog parasite *Dirofilaria repens*. The **dog heartworm**, *Dirofilaria immitis*, is the second most frequently encountered filarial zoonosis worldwide. Other genera, including *Dipetalonema*-like worms, *Onchocerca*, and *Brugia*, are rare causes of zoonotic filarial infections.

Animal filariae do not undergo normal development in the human host. The clinical manifestations and pathologic findings correspond to the anatomic site of infection and can be categorized into 4 major groups: subcutaneous, lung, eye, and lymphatic. Pathologic examination of affected tissue reveals a localized foreign body reaction around a dead or dying parasite. The lesion consists of granulomas with eosinophils, neutrophils, and tissue necrosis. *D. tenuis* does not leave the subcutaneous tissues, whereas *Brugia beaveri* eventually localizes to superficial lymph nodes. Infections may be present for up to several months. *D. immitis* larvae migrate for several months in subcutaneous tissues and most frequently result in a well-circumscribed, coinlike lesion in a single lobe of the lung. The chest radiograph typically reveals a solitary pulmonary nodule 1-3 cm in diameter. Definitive **diagnosis** and cure depend on surgical excision and identification of the nematode within the surrounding granulomatous response. *D. tenuis* and *B. beaveri* infections present as painful, rubbery, 1-5 cm nodules in the skin of the trunk, of the extremities, and around the orbit. Patients often report having been engaged in activities predisposing to exposure to infected mosquitoes, such as working or hunting in swampy areas. Management is by **surgical excision**.

ANGIOSTRONGYLUS CANTONENSIS

Angiostrongylus cantonensis, the **rat lungworm,** is the most common cause of **eosinophilic meningitis** worldwide. Rats are the definitive host. Human infection follows ingestion of third-stage larvae in raw or undercooked intermediate hosts such as snails and slugs, or transport hosts such as freshwater prawns, frogs, and fish. Most cases are sporadic, but clusters have been reported, including clusters related to consumption of lettuce contaminated with intermediate or transport hosts. Even though most infections have been described in Southeast Asia, the South Pacific, and Taiwan, shipboard travel of infected rats has spread the parasite to Madagascar, Africa, the Caribbean, and most recently Australia and North America. Larvae penetrate the vasculature of the intestinal tract and migrate to the meninges, where they usually die but induce eosinophilic aseptic meningitis. Patients present 2-35 days after ingestion of larvae with severe headache, neck pain or nuchal rigidity, hyperesthesias and paresthesias (often migrating), fatigue, fever, rash, pruritus, nausea, and vomiting. Neurologic involvement varies from asymptomatic to paresthesias, severe pain, weakness, and focal neurologic findings such as cranial nerve palsies. Symptoms can last for several weeks to months, especially headache. Coma and death from hydrocephalus occur rarely in heavy infections. Peripheral blood eosinophilia is not always present on initial examination but peaks about 5 wk after exposure, often when symptoms are improving. Cerebrospinal fluid (CSF) analysis reveals pleocytosis with >10% eosinophils in more than half of patients, with mildly elevated protein, a normal glucose level, and an elevated opening pressure. Head CT or MRI is usually unremarkable. The **diagnosis** is established clinically with supporting travel and diet history. A sensitive and specific enzyme-linked immunosorbent assay (ELISA) is available on a limited basis from the Centers for Disease Control and Prevention (CDC) for testing CSF or serum.

Treatment is primarily supportive because the majority of infections are mild, and most patients recover within 2 mo without neurologic sequelae. Analgesics should be given for headache. Careful, repeated lumbar punctures should be performed to relieve hydrocephalus. Anthelmintic drugs have not been shown to influence the outcome and may exacerbate neurologic symptoms. The use of corticosteroids may shorten the duration of persistent and severe headaches. There is a higher incidence of permanent neurologic sequelae and mortality among children than among adults. Infection can be avoided by not eating raw or undercooked crabs, prawns, or snails.

ANGIOSTRONGYLUS COSTARICENSIS

Angiostrongylus costaricensis is a nematode that infects several species of rodents and causes abdominal **angiostrongyliasis**, which has been described predominantly in Latin America and the Caribbean. The mode of transmission to humans, who are accidental hosts, is unknown. It is speculated that infectious larvae from a molluscan intermediate host, such as the slug *Vaginulus plebeius,* contaminate water or vegetation that is inadvertently consumed (chopped up in salads or on vegetation contaminated with the slug's mucus secretions). Although this slug is not indigenous to the continental United States, it has been found on imported flowers and produce. The incubation period for abdominal angiostrongyliasis is unknown, but limited data suggest that it ranges from 2 wk to several months after ingestion of larvae. Third-stage larvae migrate from the gastrointestinal tract to the mesenteric arteries, where they mature into adults. These eggs degenerate and elicit an eosinophilic granulomatous reaction. The clinical findings of abdominal angiostrongyliasis mimic **appendicitis,** although the former are typically more indolent. Children can have fever, right lower quadrant pain, a tumor-like mass, abdominal rigidity, and a painful rectal examination. Most patients have leukocytosis with eosinophilia. Radiologic examination may show bowel wall edema, spasticity, or filling defects in the ileocecal region and the ascending colon. Examination of stool for ova and parasites is not useful for *A. costaricensis* but is useful for evaluating the presence of other intestinal parasites. An ELISA is available for **diagnosis** on a limited basis from the CDC, but the test has a low specificity and is known to cross react with *Toxocara, Strongyloides,* and *Paragonimus.*

Many patients undergo laparotomy for suspected appendicitis and are found to have a mass in the terminal ileum to the ascending colon. *No specific treatment is known for abdominal angiostrongyliasis.* Even though the use of anthelmintic therapy has not been studied systematically, thiabendazole or diethylcarbamazine has been suggested. The prognosis is generally good. Most cases are self-limited, although surgery may be required in some patients. Cornerstones of **prevention** include avoidance of slugs and not ingesting raw food and water that may be contaminated with imperceptible slugs or slime from slugs. Rat control is also important in preventing the spread of infection.

DRACUNCULIASIS (DRACUNCULUS MEDINENSIS)

Dracunculiasis is caused by the guinea worm, *Dracunculus medinensis.* WHO has targeted dracunculiasis for eradication. As of 2016, the transmission of the infection was confined to Chad, Ethiopia, Mali, and South Sudan. Humans become infected by drinking contaminated stagnant water that contains immature forms of the parasite in the gut of tiny crustaceans (copepods or water fleas). Larvae are released in the stomach, penetrate the mucosa, mature, and mate. Approximately 1 yr later, the adult female worm (1-2 mm in diameter and up to 1 m long) migrates and partially emerges through the human host skin, usually of the legs. Thousands of immature larvae are released when the affected body part is immersed in the water. The cycle is completed when larval forms are ingested by the crustaceans. Infected humans have no symptoms until the worm reaches the subcutaneous tissue, causing a **stinging papule** that may be accompanied by urticaria, nausea, vomiting, diarrhea, and dyspnea. The lesion vesiculates, ruptures, and forms a painful ulcer in which a portion of the worm is visible. **Diagnosis** is established clinically. Larvae can be identified by microscopic examination of the discharge fluid.

Metronidazole (25 mg/kg/day orally divided into 3 doses for 10 days; maximum dose: 750 mg) decreases local inflammation. Although the drug does not kill the worm, it facilitates its removal. The worm must be physically removed by rolling the slowly emerging 1 m–long parasite onto a thin stick over a week. Topical corticosteroids shorten the time to complete healing while topical antibiotics decrease the risk of secondary bacterial infection. Dracunculiasis can be prevented by boiling or chlorinating drinking water or passing the water through a cloth sieve before consumption. Eradication is dependent on behavior modification and education.

GNATHOSTOMA SPINIGERUM

Gnathostoma spinigerum is a dog and cat nematode endemic to Southeast Asia, Japan, China, Bangladesh, and India, but has been identified in Mexico and parts of South America. Infection is acquired by ingesting intermediate hosts containing larvae of the parasite, such as raw or undercooked freshwater fish, chickens, pigs, snails, or frogs. Penetration of the skin by larval forms and prenatal transmission has also been described. Nonspecific signs and symptoms such as generalized malaise, fever, urticaria, anorexia, nausea, vomiting, diarrhea, and epigastric pain develop 24-48 hr after ingestion of *G. spinigerum.* Ingested larvae penetrate the gastric wall and migrate through soft tissue for up to 10 yr. Moderate to severe eosinophilia can develop. Cutaneous **gnathostomiasis** manifests as intermittent episodes of localized, migratory nonpitting edema associated with pain, pruritus, or erythema. Central nervous system involvement in gnathostomiasis is suggested by focal neurologic findings, initially neuralgia followed within a few days by paralysis or changes in mental status. Multiple cranial nerves may be involved, and CSF may be xanthochromic but typically shows an eosinophilic pleocytosis. **Diagnosis** of gnathostomiasis is based on clinical presentation and epidemiologic background. Brain and spinal cord lesions may be seen on CT or MRI. Serologic testing varies in sensitivity and specificity and is available through the CDC.

There is no well-documented effective chemotherapy, although **albendazole** (400 mg orally twice daily for 21 days) as first-line therapy or **ivermectin** (200 µg/kg for 2 days) as an alternative is recommended without or with surgical removal. Multiple courses may be needed. Corticosteroids have been used to relieve focal neurologic deficits. **Surgical resection** of the *Gnathostoma* is the major mode of therapy and the treatment of choice. Blind surgical resection of subcutaneous areas of diffuse swelling is not recommended because the worm can rarely be located. **Prevention** through the avoidance of ingestion of poorly cooked or raw fish, poultry, or pork should be emphasized for individuals living in or visiting endemic areas.

Bibliography is available at Expert Consult.

Chapter **324**
Toxocariasis (Visceral and Ocular Larva Migrans)

Arlene E. Dent and James W. Kazura

第三百二十四章
弓蛔虫病（内脏和眼的幼虫迁移）

中文导读

　　本章主要介绍了弓蛔虫病的病原学、流行病学、发病机制、临床表现、诊断、治疗和预防。在病原学部分，描述了弓蛔虫的生物学特性、生命周期和感染途径。在流行病学部分，介绍了弓蛔虫病全球流行地域特征及易感人群。在临床表现部分，介绍了弓蛔虫病的3种主要临床综合征的表现。在治疗部分，阐明在无症状和轻症病例不需要治疗，介绍了症状性感染的药物治疗方案。

ETIOLOGY

Most cases of human toxocariasis are caused by the **dog roundworm**, *Toxocara canis*. Adult female *T. canis* worms live in the intestinal tracts of young puppies and their lactating mothers. Large numbers of eggs are passed in the feces of dogs and embryonate under optimal soil conditions. *Toxocara* eggs can survive relatively harsh environmental conditions and are resistant to freezing and extremes of moisture and pH. Humans ingest embryonated eggs contaminating soil, hands, or fomites. The larvae hatch and penetrate the intestinal wall and travel via the circulation to the liver, lung, and other tissues. Humans do not excrete *T. canis* eggs because the larvae are unable to complete their maturation to adult worms in the intestine. The **cat roundworm**, *Toxocara cati,* is responsible for far fewer cases of **visceral larva migrans (VLM)** than *T. canis*. Ingestion of infective larvae of the raccoon ascarid *Baylisascaris procyonis* rarely leads to VLM but can cause **neural larva migrans**, resulting in fatal eosinophilic meningitis. Ingestion of larvae from the opossum ascarid *Lagochilascaris minor* leads to VLM rarely.

EPIDEMIOLOGY

Human *T. canis* infections have been reported in almost all parts of the world, primarily in temperate and tropical areas where dogs are popular household pets. Young children are at highest risk because of their unsanitary play habits and tendency to place fingers in the mouth. Other behavioral risk factors include **pica**, contact with puppy litters, and institutionalization. In North America, the highest prevalences of infection are in the southeastern United States and Puerto Rico, particularly among socially disadvantaged African American and Hispanic children. In the United States, serosurveys show that 4.6–7.3% of children are infected. Assuming an unrestrained and untreated dog population, toxocariasis is prevalent in settings where other **geohelminth infections**, such as ascariasis, trichuriasis, and hookworm infections, are common.

PATHOGENESIS

T. canis larvae secrete large amounts of immunogenic glycosylated proteins. These antigens induce immune responses that lead to eosinophilia and polyclonal and antigen-specific immunoglobulin E production. The characteristic histopathologic lesions are granulomas containing eosinophils, multinucleated giant cells (histiocytes), and collagen. Granulomas are typically found in the liver but may also occur in the lungs, central nervous system (CNS), and ocular tissues. Clinical manifestations reflect the intensity and chronicity of infection, anatomic localization of larvae, and host granulomatous responses.

CLINICAL MANIFESTATIONS

Three major clinical syndromes are associated with human toxocariasis: VLM, **ocular larva migrans (OLM)**, and **covert toxocariasis** (Table 324.1). The classic presentation of VLM includes eosinophilia, fever, and hepatomegaly and occurs most often in toddlers with a history of pica and exposure to puppies. The findings include fever, cough, wheezing, bronchopneumonia, anemia, hepatomegaly, leukocytosis, eosinophilia, and positive *Toxocara* serology. Cutaneous manifestations such as pruritus, eczema, and urticaria can be present. OLM tends to occur in older children without signs or symptoms of VLM. Presenting symptoms include unilateral visual loss, eye pain, white pupil, or strabismus that develops over weeks. Granulomas occur on the posterior pole of the retina and may be mistaken for retinoblastoma. Serologic testing for *Toxocara* has allowed the identification of individuals with less obvious or covert symptoms of infection. These children may have nonspecific complaints that do not constitute a recognizable syndrome. Common findings include hepatomegaly, abdominal pain, cough, sleep disturbance, failure to thrive, and headache with elevated *Toxocara* antibody titers. Eosinophilia may be present in 50–75% of cases. The prevalence of positive *Toxocara* serology in the general population supports that most

Table 324.1	Clinical Syndromes of Human Toxocariasis						
SYNDROME	**CLINICAL FINDINGS**	**AVERAGE AGE**	**INFECTIOUS DOSE**	**INCUBATION PERIOD**	**LABORATORY FINDINGS**	**ELISA**	
Visceral larva migrans	Fevers, hepatomegaly, asthma	5 yr	Moderate to high	Weeks to months	Eosinophilia, leukocytosis, elevated IgE	High (≥1:16)	
Ocular larva migrans	Visual disturbances, retinal granulomas, endophthalmitis, peripheral granulomas	12 yr	Low	Months to years	Usually none	Low	
Covert toxocariasis	Abdominal pain, gastrointestinal symptoms, weakness, hepatomegaly, pruritus, rash	School-age to adult	Low to moderate	Weeks to years	± Eosinophilia ± Elevated IgE	Low to moderate	

ELISA, Enzyme-linked immunosorbent assay; IgE, immunoglobulin E; ±, with or without.

Adapted from Liu LX: Toxocariasis and larva migrans syndrome. In Guerrant RL, Walker DH, Weller PF, editors: *Tropical infectious diseases: principles, pathogens & practice*, Philadelphia, 206, Churchill-Livingstone, p 1209.

children with *T. canis* infection are asymptomatic and will not develop overt clinical sequelae over time. A correlation between positive *Toxocara* serology and allergic asthma has also been described.

DIAGNOSIS

A presumptive diagnosis of toxocariasis can be established in a young child with **eosinophilia** (>20%), leukocytosis, hepatomegaly, fevers, wheezing, and a history of geophagia and exposure to puppies or unrestrained dogs. Supportive laboratory findings include hypergammaglobulinemia and elevated isohemagglutinin titers to A and B blood group antigens. Most patients with VLM have an absolute eosinophil count >500/μL. Eosinophilia is less common in patients with OLM. Biopsy confirms the diagnosis. When biopsies cannot be obtained, an enzyme-linked immunosorbent assay using excretory-secretory proteins harvested from *T. canis* larvae maintained in vitro is the standard serologic test used to confirm toxocariasis. A titer of 1:32 is associated with a sensitivity of approximately 78% and a specificity of approximately 92%. The sensitivity for OLM is significantly less. The diagnosis of OLM can be established in patients with typical clinical findings of a retinal or peripheral pole granuloma or endophthalmitis with elevated antibody titers. Vitreous and aqueous humor fluid anti-*Toxocara* titers are usually greater than serum titers. The diagnosis of covert toxocariasis should be considered in individuals with chronic weakness, abdominal pain, or allergic signs with eosinophilia and increased IgE. In temperate regions of the world, nonparasitic causes of eosinophilia that should be considered in the differential diagnosis include allergies, drug hypersensitivity, lymphoma, vasculitis, and **idiopathic hypereosinophilic syndrome** (see Chapter 155).

TREATMENT

Most patients do not require treatment because signs and symptoms are mild and subside over weeks to months. Several anthelmintic drugs have been used for symptomatic cases, often with adjunctive corticosteroids to limit inflammatory responses that presumably result from release of *Toxocara* antigens by dying parasites. **Albendazole** (400 mg orally twice daily for 5 days for all ages) has demonstrated efficacy in both children and adults. **Mebendazole** (100-200 mg PO twice daily for 5 days for all ages) is also useful. Anthelmintic treatment of CNS and ocular disease should be extended (3-4 wk). Even with no clinical trials on OLM therapy, a course of oral corticosteroids such as **prednisone** (1 mg/kg/day PO for 2-4 wk) has been recommended to suppress local inflammation while treatment with anthelmintic agents is initiated.

PREVENTION

Transmission can be minimized by public health measures that prevent dog feces from contaminating the environment. These include keeping dogs on leashes and excluding pets from playgrounds and sandboxes that toddlers use. Children should be discouraged from putting dirty fingers in their mouth and eating dirt. Vinyl covering of sandboxes reduces the viability of *T. canis* eggs. Widespread veterinary use of broad-spectrum anthelmintics effective against *Toxocara* may lead to a decline in parasite transmission to humans.

Bibliography is available at Expert Consult.

Chapter **325**

Trichinellosis (*Trichinella spiralis*)

Arlene E. Dent and James W. Kazura

第三百二十五章
旋毛虫病（旋毛形线虫）

中文导读

　　本章主要介绍了旋毛虫病的病原学、流行病学、发病机制、临床表现、诊断、治疗和预防。在病原学部分，描述了旋毛虫的生物学特性及生命周期。在流行病学部分，介绍了旋毛虫病流行特征及感染途径。

　　在临床表现部分，指出感染后病情表现轻重不一，儿童往往较轻，描述了旋毛虫病的临床表现特点。在治疗部分，介绍了疾病在胃肠道阶段的治疗药物选择，指出疾病在肌肉阶段的治疗尚无共识。

ETIOLOGY

Human trichinellosis (also called **trichinosis**) is caused by consumption of meat containing encysted larvae of *Trichinella spiralis*, a tissue-dwelling nematode with a worldwide distribution. After ingestion of raw or inadequately cooked meat from pigs (or other commercial meat sources such as horses) containing viable *Trichinella* larvae, the organisms are released from the cyst by acid-pepsin digestion of the cyst walls in the stomach and then pass into the small intestine. The larvae invade the small intestine columnar epithelium at the villi base and develop into adult worms. The adult female worm produces about 500 larvae over 2 wk and is then expelled in the feces. The larvae enter the bloodstream and seed striated muscle by burrowing into individual muscle fibers. Over a period of 3 wk, they coil as they increase about 10 times in length and become capable of infecting a new host if ingested. The larvae eventually become encysted and can remain viable for years. **Sylvatic** *Trichinella* spp. (*T. brivoti, T. nativa, T. pseudospiralis,* and *T. murrelli*) present in traditional native foods such as walrus meat, and **game meat** may also cause disease similar to that caused by *T. spiralis*.

EPIDEMIOLOGY

Despite public health efforts to control trichinellosis by eliminating the practice of feeding garbage to domestic swine, epidemics and isolated cases of *Trichinella* spp. infection continue to be a health problem in many areas of the world. It is most common in Asia, Latin America, and Central Europe. Swine fed with garbage may become infected when given uncooked trichinous scraps, usually pig meat, or when the carcasses of infected wild animals such as rats are eaten. Prevalence rates of *T. spiralis* in domestic swine range from 0.001% in the United States to ≥25% in China. The resurgence of this disease can be attributed to translocations of animal populations, human travel, and export of food

as well as ingestion of sylvatic *Trichinella* through game meat. In the United States from 1997 to 2001, wild game meat (especially bear or walrus meat) was the most common source of infection. Most outbreaks occur from the consumption of *T. spiralis*–infected pork (or horse meat in areas of the world where horse is eaten) obtained from a single source.

PATHOGENESIS

During the 1st 2-3 wk after infection, pathologic reactions to infection are limited to the gastrointestinal (GI) tract and include a mild, partial villous atrophy with an inflammatory infiltrate of neutrophils, eosinophils, lymphocytes, and macrophages in the mucosa and submucosa. Larvae are released by female worms and disseminate over the next several weeks. Skeletal muscle fibers show the most striking changes with edema and basophilic degeneration. The muscle fiber may contain the typical coiled worm, the cyst wall derived from the host cell, and the surrounding lymphocytic and eosinophilic infiltrate.

CLINICAL MANIFESTATIONS

The development of symptoms depends on the number of viable larvae ingested. Most infections are asymptomatic or mild, and children often show milder symptoms than adults who consumed the same amount of infected meat. Watery diarrhea is the most common symptom corresponding to maturation of the adult worms in the GI tract, which occurs during the 1st 1-2 wk after ingestion. Patients may also complain of abdominal discomfort and vomiting. Fulminant **enteritis** may develop in individuals with extremely high worm burdens. The classic symptoms of facial and periorbital edema, fever, weakness, malaise, and myalgia peak approximately 2-3 wk after the infected meat is ingested, as the larvae migrate and then encyst in the muscle. Headache, cough, dyspnea, dysphagia, subconjunctival and splinter hemorrhages, and a macular or petechial rash may occur. Patients with high-intensity infection may die from myocarditis, encephalitis, or pneumonia. In symptomatic patients, **eosinophilia** is common and may be dramatic.

DIAGNOSIS

The Centers for Disease Control and Prevention (CDC) diagnostic criteria for trichinellosis require positive serology or muscle biopsy for *Trichinella* with 1 or more compatible clinical symptoms (eosinophilia, fever, myalgia, facial or periorbital edema). To declare a discrete outbreak, at least 1 person must have positive serology or muscle biopsy. Antibodies to *Trichinella* are detectable approximately 3 wk after infection. Severe muscle involvement results in elevated serum creatine phosphokinase and lactic dehydrogenase levels. Muscle biopsy is not usually necessary, but if needed, a sample should be obtained from a tender swollen muscle. A history of eating undercooked meat supports the diagnosis. The cysts may calcify and may be visible on radiograph.

TREATMENT

Recommended treatment of trichinellosis diagnosed at the GI phase is **albendazole** (400 mg orally twice daily for 8-10 days for all ages) to eradicate the adult worms if a patient has ingested contaminated meat within the previous 1 wk. An alternative regimen is mebendazole (200-400 mg PO 3 times daily for 3 days followed by 400-500 mg three times daily for 10 days). There is no consensus for treatment of muscle-stage trichinellosis. Corticosteroids may be used, although evidence for efficacy is anecdotal.

PREVENTION

Trichinella larvae can be killed by cooking meat (≥55°C [131°F]) until there is no trace of pink fluid or flesh, or by storage in a freezer (−15°C [5°F]) for ≥3 wk. Freezing to kill larvae should only be applied to pork meat, because larvae in horse, wild boar, or game meat can remain viable even after 4 wk of freezing. Smoking, salting, and drying meat are unreliable methods of killing *Trichinella*. Strict adherence to public health measures, including garbage feeding regulations, stringent rodent control, prevention of exposure of pigs and other livestock to animal carcasses, constructing barriers between livestock, wild animals, and domestic pets, and proper handling of wild animal carcasses by hunters, can reduce infection with *Trichinella*. Current meat inspection for trichinellosis is by direct digestion and visualization of encysted larvae in meat samples. Serologic testing does not have a role in meat inspection.

Bibliography is available at Expert Consult.

Chapter **326**
Schistosomiasis (*Schistosoma*)

Charles H. King and Amaya L. Bustinduy

第三百二十六章
血吸虫病（血吸虫）

中文导读

　　本章主要介绍了血吸虫病的病原学、流行病学、发病机制、临床表现、诊断、治疗和预防。在病原学部分，指出感染人类的血吸虫病共有5种，介绍了血吸虫生物学特性及生命周期。在流行病学部分，介绍

了血吸虫病流行特征及感染途径。在临床表现部分，描述了慢性感染的临床表现特点，分别介绍了儿童慢性泌尿生殖血吸虫病、女性生殖系统血吸虫病及儿童慢性血吸虫病的临床表现。

The term **schistosomiasis (bilharzia)** encompasses the acute and chronic inflammatory disorders caused by human infection with *Schistosoma* spp. parasites. Disease is related to both the systemic and the focal effects of schistosome infection and its consequent host immune responses triggered by parasite eggs deposited in the tissues. For the affected individuals, this frequently manifests as disabling chronic morbidity.

ETIOLOGY

Schistosoma organisms are the trematodes, or **flukes**, that parasitize the bloodstream. Five schistosome species infect humans: *Schistosoma haematobium, S. mansoni, S. japonicum, S. intercalatum,* and *S. mekongi.* Humans are infected through contact with water contaminated with *cercariae,* the free-living infective stage of the parasite. These motile, forked-tail organisms emerge from infected snails and are capable of penetrating intact human skin. As they reach maturity, adult worms migrate to specific anatomic sites characteristic of each schistosome species: *S. haematobium* adults are found in the perivesical and periureteral venous plexus, *S. mansoni* in the inferior mesenteric veins, and *S. japonicum* in the superior mesenteric veins. *S. intercalatum* and *S. mekongi* are usually found in the mesenteric vessels. Adult schistosome worms (1-2 cm long) are clearly adapted for an intravascular existence. The female accompanies the male in a groove formed by the lateral edges of its body. On fertilization, female worms begin oviposition in the small venous tributaries. The eggs of the 3 main schistosome species have characteristic morphologic features: *S. haematobium* has a terminal spine, *S. mansoni* has a lateral spine, and *S. japonicum* has a smaller size with a short, curved spine (Fig. 326.1). Parasite eggs provoke a significant granulomatous inflammatory response that allows them to ulcerate through host tissues to reach the lumen of the urinary tract or the intestines. They are carried to the outside environment in urine or feces (depending on the species), where they will hatch if deposited in freshwater. Motile miracidia emerge, infect specific freshwater snail intermediate hosts, and divide asexually. After 4-12 wk, the infective cercariae are released by the snails into the contaminated water.

EPIDEMIOLOGY

Schistosomiasis infects more than 300 million people worldwide and puts more than 700 million people at risk, primarily children and young adults. There are 3.3 million disability-adjusted life-years (DALYs) attributed to schistosomiasis, making it the 2nd most disabling parasitic disease after malaria. Prevalence is increasing in many areas as population density increases and new irrigation projects provide broader habitats for vector **snails**. Humans are the main definitive hosts for the 5 clinically important species of schistosomes, although *S. japonicum* is also a zoonosis, infecting animals such as dogs, rats, pigs, and cattle. *S. haematobium* is prevalent in Africa and the Middle East; *S. mansoni* is prevalent in Africa, the Middle East, the Caribbean, and South America; and *S. japonicum* is prevalent in China, the Philippines, and Indonesia, with some sporadic foci in parts of Southeast Asia. The other 2 species are less prevalent. *S. intercalatum* is found in West and Central Africa, and *S. mekongi* is found only along the upper Mekong River in the Far East.

Transmission depends on water contamination by human excreta, the presence of specific intermediate snail hosts, and the patterns of water contact and social habits of the population (Fig. 326.2). The distribution of infection in endemic areas shows that prevalence increases with age, to a peak at 10-20 yr old. Exposure to infected water starts early in life for children living in endemic areas. Passive water contact by infants (accompanying mothers in their daily household activities) evolves to more active water contact as preschool and school-age children pursue recreational activities such as swimming and wading.

Measuring intensity of infection (by quantitative egg count in urine or feces) demonstrates that the heaviest worm loads are found in school-age and adolescent children. Even though schistosomiasis is most prevalent and most severe in older children and young adults, who are at maximal risk for suffering from its acute and chronic sequelae, preschool children can also exhibit significant disease manifestations.

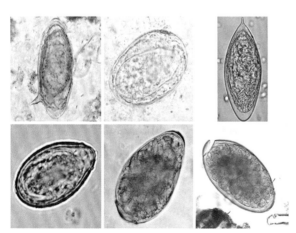

Fig. 326.1 Eggs of common human trematodes. Clockwise from upper left: *Schistosoma mansoni, S. japonicum, S. haematobium, Clonorchis sinensis, Paragonimus westermani,* and *Fasciola hepatica* (note the partially open operculum). *(From Centers for Disease Control and Prevention: DPDx: laboratory identification of parasites of public health concern. http://www.cdc.gov/dpdx/az.html.)*

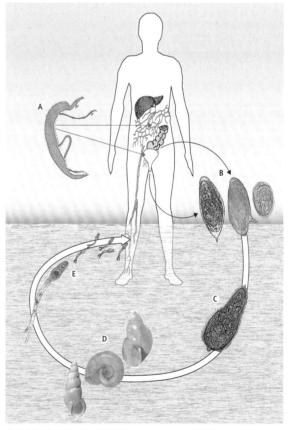

Fig. 326.2 Life cycle of *Schistosoma mansoni, S. haematobium,* and *S. japonicum. A,* Paired adult worms (larger male enfolding slender female). *B,* Eggs (left to right, *S. haematobium, S. mansoni, S. japonicum). C,* Ciliated miracidium. *D,* Intermediate host snails (left to right, *Oncomelania, Biomphalaria, Bulinus). E,* Cercariae. *(From Colley DG, Bustinduy AL, Secor WE, King CH: Human schistosomiasis, Lancet 383:2253–2264, 2014, Fig 1.)*

PATHOGENESIS

Both early and late manifestations of schistosomiasis are immunologically mediated. *Acute* schistosomiasis, known as **snail fever** or **Katayama syndrome**, is a febrile illness that represents an immune complex disease associated with early infection and oviposition. The major pathology of infection occurs later, with *chronic* schistosomiasis, in which retention of eggs in the host tissues is associated with chronic granulomatous injury. Eggs may be trapped at sites of deposition (urinary bladder, ureters, intestine) or may be carried by the bloodstream to other organs, most frequently the liver and less often the lungs and central nervous system (CNS). The host response to these eggs involves local as well as systemic manifestations. The cell-mediated immune response leads to granulomas composed of lymphocytes, macrophages, and eosinophils that surround the trapped eggs and add significantly to the degree of tissue destruction. Granuloma formation in the bladder wall and at the ureterovesical junction results in the major disease manifestations of schistosomiasis haematobia: hematuria, dysuria, and obstructive uropathy. Intestinal as well as hepatic granulomas underlie the pathologic sequelae of the other schistosome infections: ulcerations and fibrosis of intestinal wall, hepatosplenomegaly, and portal hypertension caused by presinusoidal obstruction of blood flow. In terms of systemic disease, antischistosome inflammation increases circulating levels of proinflammatory cytokines such as tumor necrosis factor-α and interleukin-6, associated with elevated levels of C-reactive protein. These responses are associated with hepcidin-mediated inhibition of iron uptake and use, leading to anemia of chronic inflammation. Schistosomiasis-related undernutrition may be the result of similar pathways of chronic inflammation. Acquired partial protective immunity against schistosomiasis has been demonstrated in some animal species and may occur in humans.

CLINICAL MANIFESTATIONS

Two main chronic clinical syndromes arise from *Schistosoma* spp. infection: **urogenital schistosomiasis** caused by *S. haematobium* and **intestinal schistosomiasis** caused by *S. mansoni* or *S. japonicum*. Most chronically infected individuals experience mild symptoms and may not seek medical attention; the more severe symptoms of schistosomiasis occur mainly in those who are heavily infected or who have been infected over longer periods. In addition to organ-specific morbidities, infected patients frequently demonstrate anemia, chronic pain, diarrhea, exercise intolerance, and chronic undernutrition manifesting as growth stunting. Cercarial penetration of human skin may result in a papular pruritic rash known as **schistosomal dermatitis** or **swimmer's itch**. It is more pronounced in previously exposed individuals and is characterized by edema and intense cellular infiltrates in the dermis and epidermis. Acute schistosomiasis (Katayama syndrome) may occur, particularly in heavily infected individuals, 4-8 wk after exposure; this is a serum sickness–like syndrome manifested by the acute onset of fever, cough, chills, sweating, abdominal pain, lymphadenopathy, hepatosplenomegaly, and eosinophilia. Acute schistosomiasis typically presents in first-time visitors to endemic areas who experience primary infection at an older age.

Symptomatic children with chronic urogenital schistosomiasis usually complain of frequency, dysuria, and hematuria. Urine examination shows erythrocytes, parasite eggs, and occasional eosinophiluria. In endemic areas, moderate to severe pathologic lesions have been demonstrated in the urinary tract of >20% of infected children. The extent of disease correlates with the intensity of infection, but significant morbidity can occur even in lightly infected children. The advanced stages of urogenital schistosomiasis are associated with chronic renal failure, secondary infections, and squamous carcinoma of the bladder.

An important complication of *S. haematobium* infection is **female genital schistosomiasis**. Eggs migrate from the vesical plexus to lodge in the female genital tract where they induce a granulomatous inflammatory response that can manifest as contact bleeding, pain, and eventual infertility. Symptoms start as early as 10 yr of age, with an apparent 3-4–fold greater risk of HIV transmission. Pathognomonic lesions can be visualized in the cervix by photocolposcopy. **Male genital schistosomiasis** can also present with hematospermia, pain, and lumpy semen.

Children with chronic schistosomiasis mansoni, japonica, intercalatum, or mekongi may have intestinal symptoms; colicky abdominal pain and bloody diarrhea are the most common. However, the intestinal phase may remain subclinical, and the late syndrome of hepatosplenomegaly, portal hypertension, ascites, and hematemesis may then be the first clinical presentation. Liver disease is caused by granuloma formation and subsequent **periportal fibrosis**; no appreciable liver cell injury occurs, and hepatic function may be preserved for a long time. Schistosome eggs may escape into the lungs, causing **pulmonary hypertension** and cor pulmonale. *S. japonicum* worms may migrate to the brain vasculature and produce localized lesions that cause seizures. **Transverse myelitis**, spinal compression, and other CNS involvement (meningoencephalitis) are rare but well-known complications in children or young adults with either acute or chronic *S. haematobium* or *S. mansoni* infection.

Although end-organ scarring is pathognomonic, affected children may also have persistent long-term systemic effects of infection, including poor growth, anemia, decreased aerobic capacity, and cognitive impairment.

DIAGNOSIS

Schistosome eggs are found in the excreta of infected individuals; quantitative methods should be used to provide an indication of the burden of infection. For diagnosis of *S. haematobium* infection, a volume of 10 mL of urine should be collected around midday, the time of maximal egg excretion, and filtered for microscopic examination. Stool examination by the Kato-Katz thick smear procedure and detection of parasite antigen in patient serum or urine are the methods of choice for diagnosis and quantification of other schistosome infections (*S. mansoni* and *S. japonicum*). The unique schistosome antigens *circulating anodic antigen* (CAA) and *circulating cathodic antigen* (CCA) may also be detected in the urine or plasma.

TREATMENT

Treatment of children with schistosomiasis should be based on an appreciation of the intensity of infection and the extent of disease. The recommended treatment for schistosomiasis is **praziquantel** (40 mg/kg/day orally [PO] divided twice daily [bid] for 1 day for schistosomiasis haematobia, mansoni, and intercalatum; 60 mg/kg/day PO divided 3 times daily [tid] for 1 day for schistosomiasis japonica and mekongi). Children <5 yr old with *S. mansoni* may need up to 60 mg/kg/day PO tid for 1 day to achieve clearance. A 2nd treatment 4-6 wk after the 1st course may help in eliminating residual infection.

PREVENTION

Transmission in endemic areas may be decreased by reducing the parasite load in the human population. The availability of oral, single-dose, effective chemotherapeutic agents may help achieve this goal. When added to national drug-based control programs, other measures such as improved sanitation, antiparasitic treatment given at well-child visits, focal application of molluscicidals, and animal vaccination may prove useful in breaking the cycle of transmission. Ultimately, control of schistosomiasis is closely linked to economic and social development.

Bibliography is available at Expert Consult.

Chapter **327**
Flukes (Liver, Lung, and Intestinal)
Charles H. King and Amaya L. Bustinduy
第三百二十七章
吸虫（肝、肺、肠）

中文导读

本章主要介绍了肝吸虫病、肺吸虫病和肠吸虫病。在肝吸虫病部分，分别介绍了肝片吸虫病、支睾吸虫病及后睾吸虫病的流行特征、感染途径、临床表现和治疗方案。在肺吸虫病部分，着重介绍了并殖吸虫病流行特征、感染途径、临床表现、诊断和治疗方案。在肠吸虫病部分，介绍了肠吸虫的种类、生命周期、临床表现、诊断和治疗方案。

Several different **trematodes,** or flukes, can parasitize humans and cause disease. Flukes are endemic worldwide but are more prevalent in the less developed parts of the world. They include *Schistosoma,* or the blood flukes (see Chapter 326), as well as fluke species that cause infection in the human biliary tree, lung tissue, and intestinal tract. These latter trematodes are characterized by complex life cycles (Fig. 327.1). Sexual reproduction of adult worms in the definitive host produces eggs that are passed in the stool. Larvae, called **miracidia,** develop in freshwater. These in turn infect certain species of mollusks (aquatic snails or clams), in which asexual multiplication by parasite larvae produces cercariae. Cercariae then seek a 2nd intermediate host, such as an insect, crustacean, or fish, or attach to vegetation to produce infectious **metacercariae.** Humans acquire liver, lung, and intestinal fluke infections by eating uncooked, lightly cooked, pickled, or smoked foods containing these infectious parasite cysts. The "alternation of generations" requires that flukes parasitize more than 1 host (often 3) to complete their life cycle. Because parasitic flukes are dependent on these nonhuman species for transmission, the distribution of human fluke infection closely matches the ecologic range of the flukes' intermediate hosts. As a group, these parasites are commonly referred to as **food-borne trematodes.**

LIVER FLUKES
Fascioliasis *(Fasciola hepatica)*
Fasciola hepatica, the sheep liver fluke, infects cattle, other ungulates, and occasionally humans. This infection affects approximately 17 million people worldwide and has been reported in many different parts of the world, particularly South America, Europe, Africa, China, Australia, and Cuba. Although *F. hepatica* is enzootic in North America, reported cases are extremely rare. Humans are infected by ingestion of metacercariae attached to vegetation, especially wild watercress, lettuce, and alfalfa. In the duodenum, the parasites excyst and penetrate the intestinal

wall, liver capsule, and parenchyma. They wander for a few weeks before entering the bile ducts, where they mature. Adult *F. hepatica* (1-2.5 cm) commence oviposition approximately 12 wk after infection; the eggs are large (75-140 μm) and operculated. They pass to the intestines with bile and exit the body in the feces (see Fig. 327.1). On reaching freshwater,

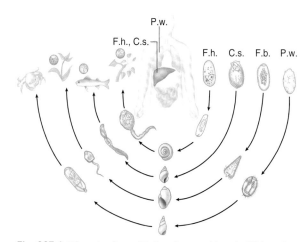

Fig. 327.1 Life cycle of parasitic liver, lung, and intestinal flukes. C.s., *Clonorchis sinensis;* F.b., *Fasciolopsis buski;* F.h., *Fasciola hepatica;* P.w., *Paragonimus westermani. (Adapted from Mandell GL, Bennett JE, Dolin R, editors: Principles and practice of infectious diseases, ed 7, Philadelphia, 2010, Elsevier, Fig 289-2.)*

the eggs mature and hatch into miracidia, which infect specific snail intermediate hosts to multiply into many cercariae. These then emerge from infected snails and encyst on aquatic grasses and plants.

Clinical manifestations usually occur either during the liver migratory phase of the parasites or after their arrival at their final habitat in upper bile ducts. Fever, right upper quadrant pain, and hepatosplenomegaly characterize the 1st phase of illness. Peripheral blood eosinophilia is usually marked. As the worms enter bile ducts, most of the acute symptoms subside. On rare occasions, patients may have obstructive jaundice or biliary cirrhosis, with signs of cholestasis, ascending cholangitis, cholelithiasis and jaundice and increased liver enzymes, direct bilirubin, and γ-glutamyl transpeptidase. *F. hepatica* infection is diagnosed by identifying the characteristic eggs in fecal smears or duodenal aspirates. **Diagnosis** can be suggested by positive serology and imaging that reveals acute, hypodense liver lesions that change over time. Presentation can be dramatic in children, with features including generalized edema, hepatic cirrhosis with esophageal varices, and in severe cases, death from generalized organ failure.

The recommended **treatment** of fascioliasis is triclabendazole (10 mg/kg orally [PO] once or twice) or bithionol (30-50 mg/kg PO once daily on alternate days for a total of 10-15 doses). In the United States, bithionol is not generally available, but may be available from compounding pharmacies.

Clonorchiasis (*Clonorchis sinensis*)
Infection of bile passages with *Clonorchis sinensis,* the Chinese or oriental liver fluke, is endemic in China, South Korea, northern Vietnam, and parts of Russia and Japan, affecting more than 15 million people. Humans acquire infection by ingestion of raw or inadequately cooked freshwater fish carrying the encysted metacercariae of the parasite under their scales or skin. Metacercariae excyst in the duodenum and pass through the ampulla of Vater to the common bile duct and bile capillaries, where they mature into hermaphroditic adult worms (3-15 mm). *C. sinensis* worms deposit small operculated eggs (14-30 μm), which are discharged through the bile duct to the intestine and feces (see Fig. 327.1). The eggs mature and hatch outside the body, releasing motile miracidia into local freshwater streams, rivers, or ponds. If these are taken up by the appropriate snails, they develop into cercariae, which are in turn released from the snail to encyst under the skin or scales of freshwater fish.

Most individuals with *C. sinensis* infection, particularly those with few organisms, are minimally symptomatic. Among heavily infected individuals, who tend to be older (>30 yr), localized obstruction of a bile duct results from repeated local trauma and inflammation. In these patients, cholangitis and cholangiohepatitis may lead to liver enlargement and jaundice. In Hong Kong, Korea, and other parts of Asia, cholangiocarcinoma is associated with chronic *C. sinensis* infection.

Clonorchiasis is diagnosed by examination of feces or duodenal aspirates for the parasite eggs. The recommended **treatment** of clonorchiasis is praziquantel (75 mg/kg/day PO divided 3 times daily [tid] for 2 days). An alternative, used in adults, is albendazole (10 mg/kg once daily PO for 7 days). Tribendimidine (400 mg PO for 3 days) has been recently used in China with good cure rates.

Opisthorchiasis (*Opisthorchis spp.*)
Infections with species of *Opisthorchis* are clinically similar to those caused by *C. sinensis. Opisthorchis felineus* and *Opisthorchis viverrini* are liver flukes of cats and dogs that infect humans through ingestion of metacercariae in freshwater fish. Infection with *O. felineus* is endemic in Eastern Europe and Southeast Asia, and *O. viverrini* is found mainly in Thailand, affecting an estimated 10 million people. Most individuals are minimally symptomatic; liver enlargement, relapsing cholangitis, and jaundice may occur in heavily infected individuals. Diagnosis is

based on recovering eggs from stools or duodenal aspirates. The recommended **treatment** of opisthorchiasis is praziquantel (75 mg/kg/day PO tid for 2 days).

LUNG FLUKES
Paragonimiasis (*Paragonimus spp.*)
Human infection by the lung fluke *Paragonimus westermani,* and less frequently other species of *Paragonimus,* occurs throughout the Far East, in localized areas of West Africa, and in several parts of Central and South America, affecting approximately 20 million people. The highest incidence of paragonimiasis occurs in older children and adolescents 11-15 yr of age. Although *P. westermani* is found in many carnivores, human cases are relatively rare and seem to be associated with specific dietary habits, such as eating raw freshwater crayfish or crabs. These crustaceans contain the infective metacercariae in their tissues. After ingestion, the metacercariae excyst in the duodenum, penetrate the intestinal wall, and migrate to their final habitat in the lungs. Adult worms (5-10 mm) encapsulate within the lung parenchyma and deposit brown operculated eggs (60-100 μm) that pass into the bronchioles and are expectorated by coughing (see Fig. 327.1). Ova can be detected in the sputum of infected individuals or in their feces. If eggs reach freshwater, they hatch and undergo asexual multiplication in specific snails. The cercariae encyst in the muscles and viscera of crayfish and freshwater crabs.

Most individuals infected with *P. westermani* harbor low or moderate worm loads and are minimally symptomatic. The clinical manifestations include cough, production of rust-colored sputum, and hemoptysis (mimicking tuberculosis), which is the principal manifestation and occurs in 98% of symptomatic children. There are no characteristic physical findings, but laboratory examination usually demonstrates marked eosinophilia. Chest radiographs often reveal small, patchy infiltrates or radiolucencies in the middle lung fields; however, radiographs may appear normal in one fifth of infected individuals. In rare circumstances, lung abscess, pleural or pericardial effusion, or bronchiectasis may develop. Extrapulmonary localization of *P. westermani* in the brain, peritoneum, intestines, or pericardium may rarely occur. Cerebral paragonimiasis occurs primarily in heavily infected individuals living in highly endemic areas of the Far East. The clinical presentation resembles jacksonian epilepsy or the symptoms of cerebral tumors.

Definitive diagnosis of paragonimiasis is established by identification of eggs in fecal or sputum smears. The recommended **treatment** of paragonimiasis is praziquantel (75 mg/kg/day PO tid for 2 days). Triclabendazole can also be used (10 mg/kg PO daily for 1-2 days).

INTESTINAL FLUKES
Several wild and domestic animal intestinal flukes, including *Fasciolopsis buski, Nanophyetus salmincola,* and *Heterophyes heterophyes,* may accidentally infect humans who eat uncooked or undercooked fish or water plants. For example, *F. buski* is endemic in the Far East, where humans who ingest metacercariae encysted on aquatic plants become infected. These develop into large flukes (1-5 cm) that inhabit the duodenum and jejunum. Mature worms produce operculated eggs that pass with feces; the organism completes its life cycle through specific snail intermediate hosts. Individuals with *F. buski* infection are usually asymptomatic; heavily infected patients complain of abdominal pain and diarrhea and show signs of malabsorption. Diagnosis of fasciolopsiasis and other intestinal fluke infections is established by fecal examination and identification of the eggs (see Fig. 327.1). As for other fluke infections, praziquantel (75 mg/kg/day PO tid for 2 days) is the drug of choice.

Bibliography is available at Expert Consult.

Chapter **328**
Adult Tapeworm Infections
Philip R. Fischer and A. Clinton White Jr.

第三百二十八章
成年绦虫感染

中文导读

　　本章主要介绍了成年绦虫感染的病原学、流行病学、发病机制、临床表现、诊断、鉴别诊断、治疗和预防。单独介绍了裂头绦虫病的病原学、流行病学、发病机制、临床表现、诊断、鉴别诊断、治疗和预防。另外还简要介绍了膜壳绦虫病和复孔绦虫病的流行特点、感染途径、临床表现及治疗方案。

Tapeworms are adult forms of **cestodes**, multicellular helminth parasites, that live in human intestines and cause non–life-threatening illness. Invasive larval forms of cestodes are associated with cysts that lead to severe human disease such as neurocysticercosis (*Taenia solium*; see Chapter 329) and echinococcosis (mostly *Echinococcus granulosa* and *E. multilocularis*; Chapter 330). The adult worms themselves are flat and multisegmented, varying in length from 8 mm to 10 meters (m). Table 328.1 summarizes the key features of tapeworms that affect children.

ETIOLOGY

The **beef tapeworm** (*Taenia saginata*), the **pork tapeworm** (*T. solium),* and the Asian tapeworm *(Taenia asiatica)* are long worms (4-10 m) named for their intermediate hosts (*T. saginata, T. solium*) or geographic distribution (*T. asiatica*; larval host is the pig). The adult worms are found only in the human intestine. As with the adult stage of all tapeworms, their body is a series of 100s or 1000s of flattened segments (**proglottids**) with an anterior attachment organ (**scolex**) that anchors the parasite to the bowel wall. New segments arise from the distal aspect of the scolex with progressively more mature segments attached distally. The gravid terminal segments contain 50,000-100,000 eggs, and the eggs or even detached intact proglottids pass out of the child through the anus (with or separate from defecation). These tapeworms differ most significantly in that the intermediate stage of the pork tapeworm (**cysticercus**) can also infect humans and cause significant morbidity (see Chapter 329), whereas the larval stage of *T. saginata* does not cause human disease. *T. asiatica* is similar to and often confused with the beef tapeworm.

EPIDEMIOLOGY

The pork and beef tapeworms are distributed worldwide, with the highest risk for infection in Latin America, Africa, India, Southeast Asia, and China, where the relevant intermediate host is raised domestically. The prevalence in adults may not reflect the prevalence in young children, because cultural practices may dictate how well meat is cooked and how much is served to children.

PATHOGENESIS

When children ingest raw or undercooked meat containing larval cysts, gastric acid and bile facilitate release of immature scolices that attach to the lumen of the small intestine. The parasite grows, adding new segments at the base of the scolex. The terminal segments mature and after 2-3 mo produce eggs that are released in stool. The surface of proglottids serves as an absorptive organ to "steal" nutritional elements from the child's small bowel for use by the parasite. There is sometimes a transient eosinophilia before the parasite matures enough to release eggs.

CLINICAL MANIFESTATIONS

Nonspecific abdominal symptoms have been reported with beef and pork tapeworm infections, but the most bothersome symptom is the psychologic distress caused by seeing proglottids in the stool or undergarments. The released segments of the worms are motile (especially those of *T. saginata*) and sometimes lead to anal pruritus. The adult beef and pork tapeworms are only rarely associated with other symptoms.

DIAGNOSIS

Identification of the infecting tapeworm species facilitates understanding of risk for invasive disease. Carriers of adult pork tapeworms are at increased risk for transmitting eggs with the pathogenic intermediate stage (cysticercus) to themselves or others, whereas children infected with the beef tapeworm or *T. asiatica* are a risk only to livestock. Because proglottids are generally passed intact, visual examination for gravid proglottids in the stool is a sensitive test; these segments may be used to identify species. Eggs, by contrast, are often absent from stool and cannot distinguish between *T. saginata* and *T. solium* (Fig. 328.1). If

Table 328.1	Key Features of Common Tapeworms in Children			
PARASITE SPECIES	**GEOGRAPHY**	**SOURCE**	**SYMPTOMS**	**TREATMENT**
Taenia saginata	Asia, Africa, Latin America	Cysts in beef	Abdominal discomfort, motile proglottid migration, passing segments	Praziquantel *or* niclosamide, possibly nitazoxanide
Taenia solium	Asia, Africa, Latin America	Cysticerci in pork	Minimal, proglottids in stool	Praziquantel *or* niclosamide, possibly nitazoxanide
Taenia asiatica	Asia	Pigs	Minimal	Praziquantel *or* niclosamide, possibly nitazoxanide
Diphyllobothrium spp.	Worldwide, often northern areas	Plerocercoid cysts in freshwater fish	Usually minimal; with prolonged or heavy infection with *D. latum*, vitamin B$_{12}$ deficiency	Praziquantel *or* niclosamide
Hymenolepis	Worldwide, often northern areas	Infected humans, rodents	Mild abdominal discomfort	Praziquantel, niclosamide, or nitazoxanide
Dipylidium caninum	Worldwide	Domestic dogs and cats	Proglottids in stool, anal pruritus confused with pinworm	Praziquantel *or* niclosamide

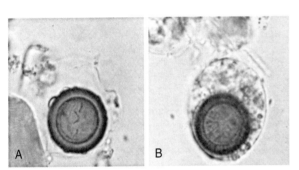

Fig. 328.1 Eggs of *Taenia saginata* recovered from feces (original magnification ×400). **A** and **B,** The eggs are generally bile-stained, dark, and prismatic. There is occasionally some surrounding cellular material from the proglottid in which the egg develops, which is more evident in **B** than in **A.** The larva within the egg shows 3 pairs of hooklets (**A**), which may occasionally be observed in motion.

the parasite is completely expelled, the scolex of each species is diagnostic. The scolex of *T. saginata* has only a set of 4 anteriorly oriented suckers, whereas *T. solium* is armed with a double row of hooks in addition to suckers. The proglottids of *T. saginata* have >20 branches from a central uterine structure, and the proglottids of *T. solium* have ≤10 branches. Expelled proglottid segments are usually approximately 0.5 × 1-2 × 0.1 cm in size. Molecular methods can distinguish *T. saginata* from *T. asiatica.* Antigen detection tests are increasingly available.

Differential Diagnosis
Anal pruritus may mimic symptoms of pinworm (*Enterobius vermicularis*) infection. *Diphyllobothrium latum* and *Ascaris lumbricoides* (a long round worm) may be mistaken for *T. saginata* or *T. solium* in stools.

TREATMENT
Infections with all adult tapeworms respond to praziquantel (25 mg/kg orally [PO] once). When available, an alternative treatment for **taeniasis** is niclosamide (50 mg/kg PO once for children; 2 g PO once for adults). Nitazoxanide is sometimes effective as well. The parasite is usually expelled on the day of administration. Treatment with electrolyte–polyethylene glycol bowel preparations can increase the yield of passage of scolices.

PREVENTION
Prolonged freezing or thorough cooking of beef and pork kills the larval cystic forms of the parasite. Appropriate human sanitation can interrupt transmission by preventing infection in livestock.

DIPHYLLOBOTHRIASIS (*DIPHYLLOBOTHRIUM* SPP.)
Etiology
The **fish tapeworms** of the genus *Diphyllobothrium* are the longest human tapeworms, reaching >10 m in length, and have an anatomic organization similar to that of other adult cestodes. An elongated scolex, equipped with slits (**bothria**) along each side but no suckers or hooks, is followed by 1000s of segments looped in the small bowel. Gravid terminal proglottids detach periodically but tend to disintegrate before expulsion, thus releasing eggs rather than intact worm segments in the feces. In contrast to taeniids, the life cycle of *Diphyllobothrium* spp. requires 2 intermediate hosts. Small, freshwater crustaceans (copepods) take up the larvae that hatch from parasite eggs. The parasite passes up the food chain as small fish eat the copepods and are in turn eaten by larger fish. In this way, the juvenile parasite becomes concentrated in pike, walleye, perch, burbot, and perhaps salmon associated with aquaculture. Consumption of raw or undercooked fish leads to human infection with adult fish tapeworms.

Epidemiology
The fish tapeworm is most prevalent in the temperate climates of Europe, North America, and Asia but may be found along the Pacific coast of South America and in Africa. In North America the prevalence is highest in Alaska, Canada, and northern areas of continental United States. The tapeworm is found in fish from those areas that are then taken to market. Persons who prepare raw fish for home or commercial use or who sample fish before cooking are particularly at risk for infection.

Pathogenesis
The adult worm of *Diphyllobothrium latum* (found in northern Europe) has high-affinity receptors and efficiently scavenges vitamin B$_{12}$ for its own use in the constant production of large numbers of segments and as many as 1 million eggs per day. As a result, diphyllobothriasis causes **megaloblastic anemia** in 2–9% of infections. Interestingly, other *Diphyllobothrium* spp. do not out-compete the host for vitamin B$_{12}$. Children with other causes of vitamin B$_{12}$ or folate deficiency, such as chronic infectious diarrhea, celiac disease, or congenital malabsorption, are more likely to develop symptomatic infection.

Clinical Manifestations
Infection is largely asymptomatic. Segments may be noted in stool. Those who develop vitamin B$_{12}$ or folate deficiency present with megaloblastic anemia with leukopenia, thrombocytopenia, glossitis, and/or signs of spinal cord posterior column dysfunction (loss of vibratory sense, proprioception, and coordination).

Diagnosis
Parasitological examination of the stool is useful because eggs are abundant in the feces and have morphology distinct from that of all other tapeworms. The eggs are ovoid and have an **operculum,** which

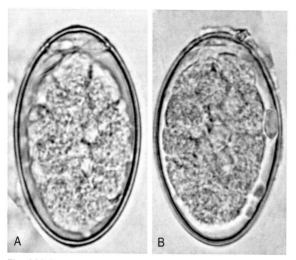

Fig. 328.2 Eggs of *Diphyllobothrium latum* as seen in feces (original magnification ×400). **A** and **B,** The caplike operculum is at the upper end of the eggs here.

is a cap structure at one end that opens to release the embryo (Fig. 328.2). The worm itself has a distinct scolex and proglottid morphology; however, these are not likely to be passed spontaneously.

Differential Diagnosis

A segment or a whole section of the worm might be confused with *Taenia* or *Ascaris* after it is passed. Pernicious anemia, bone marrow toxins, and dietary restriction may contribute to or mimic the nutritional deficiencies associated with diphyllobothriasis.

Treatment

As with all adult tapeworms, *D. latum* infections respond to praziquantel (5-10 mg/kg PO once). Niclosamide (50 mg/kg PO in a single dose) is also effective.

Prevention

The intermediate stage is easily killed by brief cooking or prolonged freezing of fish before ingestion. Because humans are the major reservoir for adult worms, health education is one of the most important tools for preventing transmission, together with improved human sanitation.

HYMENOLEPIASIS *(HYMENOLEPIS)*

Infection with *Hymenolepis nana,* the **dwarf tapeworm,** is very common in developing countries. Most cases are asymptomatic. However, heavy infection has been associated with diarrhea, weight loss, fever, and eosinophilia. The intermediate stage of *Hymenolepis diminuta* develops in various hosts (e.g., rodents, ticks, fleas), but the entire life cycle of *H. nana* is completed in humans. Therefore, hyperinfection with 1000s of small adult worms in a single child may occur. A similar infection may occur less often with *H. diminuta.* Eggs but not segments may be found in the stool. *H. nana* infection responds to praziquantel (25 mg/kg PO once). Nitazoxanide is effective in about three fourths of children (100 mg PO twice daily [bid] for 3 days for children 1-3 yr old, 200 mg bid for 3 days for children 4-11 yr old, and 500 mg bid for 3 days for older children).

DIPYLIDIASIS *(DIPYLIDIUM CANINUM)*

Dipylidium caninum is a common tapeworm of domestic dogs and cats. Human infection is relatively rare. Direct transmission between pets and humans does not occur; human infection requires ingestion of the parasite's intermediate host, the dog or cat flea. Infants and small children are particularly susceptible because of their level of hygiene, generally more intimate contact with pets, and activities in areas where fleas can be encountered. Thus, children are most at risk of inadvertent ingestion of fleas infected with the larvae. The most common symptom is passage of proglottids in stool. The proglottids are similar in size and shape to white rice grains. Anal pruritus, vague abdominal pain, and diarrhea have at times been associated with dipylidiasis, which is thus sometimes confused with pinworm (*E. vermicularis*). Dipylidiasis responds to treatment with praziquantel (5-10 mg/kg PO once) and niclosamide (50 mg/kg PO as a single dose). **Deworming** of pets and **flea control** are the best preventive measures.

Bibliography is available at Expert Consult.

Chapter **329**

Cysticercosis

A. Clinton White Jr. and Philip R. Fischer

第三百二十九章

囊虫病

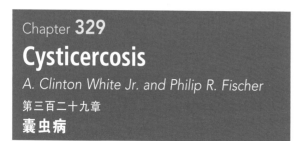

中文导读

　　本章主要介绍了囊虫病的病原学、流行病学、发病机制、临床表现、诊断、治疗和预防。在病原学部分，指出囊虫病在儿童有两种感染形式，介绍了囊虫病在人体内的感染过程。在流行病学部分，介绍了囊虫病的感染途径和流行特征。在临床表现部分，重点阐述了神经系统囊虫病的临床表现。在诊断部分，介绍了影像学检查、血清学检查，指出尚无商业化试剂用于抗原和PCR检测，临床需要与引起抽搐的其他疾病相鉴别。在治疗部分，介绍了药物治疗、超声或CT引导下经皮穿刺抽吸治疗及外科手术治疗等方案。

ETIOLOGY

Taenia solium, also known as the **pork tapeworm**, causes 2 different infections in children. In its normal life cycle, children can acquire the tapeworm form by ingestion of undercooked pork containing the larval cysts (see Chapter 328). In the intestines, the cyst converts into the tapeworm form. Children are also susceptible to infection by the eggs shed by tapeworm carriers. After the eggs are ingested, the larvae are released from the eggs, invade through the intestines, and migrate through the bloodstream to the muscles (and other organs), where they form tissue cysts (0.2-2.0 cm fluid-filled bladders containing a single invaginated **scolex**). Infection with the cystic form is termed **cysticercosis,** and involvement of the central nervous system (CNS) is termed **neurocysticercosis.** The tapeworm form only develops after ingestion of undercooked pork. Ingestion of pork is not necessary to develop cysticercosis, but individuals harboring an adult worm may infect themselves with the eggs by the fecal-oral route.

EPIDEMIOLOGY

The pork tapeworm is widely distributed wherever pigs are raised and have contact with human fecal material. Intense transmission occurs in Central and South America, southern and Southeast Asia, and much of sub-Saharan Africa. In these areas, approximately 30% of cases of seizures may be a result of cysticercosis. Most cases of cysticercosis in the United States are imported; however, local transmission has been documented.

PATHOGENESIS

Living, intact cystic stages usually suppress the host immune and inflammatory responses. Intact cysts can be associated with disease when they obstruct the flow of cerebrospinal fluid. Most cysts remain asymptomatic for a few years. Symptoms typically develop as the cysticerci begin to degenerate, associated with a host inflammatory response. The natural history of cysts is eventually to resolve by complete resorption or calcification, but this process may take years. Cysticerci can also present as subcutaneous nodules, ocular infection, or spinal lesions with myelopathy or radiculopathy.

CLINICAL MANIFESTATIONS

Seizures are the presenting finding in the vast majority of children with neurocysticercosis. Less common manifestations include hydrocephalus, diffuse cerebral edema, or focal neurologic findings. It is important to classify neurocysticercosis as parenchymal, intraventricular, subarachnoid, spinal, or ocular on the basis of anatomic location, clinical presentation, and radiologic appearance, since the prognosis and management vary with location.

Parenchymal neurocysticercosis typically presents with seizures. The seizures are usually focal, but often generalize. Children may present with a single seizure or recurrent epilepsy. Mild neurocognitive defects have been documented from cysticerci alone but are more commonly associated with poorly controlled seizures. A fulminant encephalitis-like presentation may rarely occur after a massive initial infection associated with cerebral edema. **Intraventricular** neurocysticercosis (up to 20% of cases) is associated with obstructive hydrocephalus and acute, subacute, or intermittent signs of increased intracranial pressure, usually without localizing signs. **Subarachnoid** neurocysticercosis is rare in children. It can be associated with basilar arachnoiditis that can present with signs of meningeal irritation, communicating hydrocephalus, cerebral infarction, or **spinal** disease with radiculitis or transverse myelitis. Cysticerci in the tissues may present with focal findings from mass effect. **Ocular** neurocysticercosis causes decreased visual acuity because of cysticerci in the retina or vitreous, retinal detachment, or iridocyclitis.

DIAGNOSIS

Neurocysticercosis should be suspected in a child with onset of seizures or hydrocephalus and who also has a history of residence in an endemic area and/or a care provider from an endemic area. The most useful diagnostic study for parenchymal disease is MRI of the head. MRI provides the most information about cyst location, cyst viability, and associated inflammation. The **protoscolex** is sometimes visible within the cyst, which provides a pathognomonic sign for cysticercosis (Fig. 329.1*A*). The MRI also better detects basilar arachnoiditis (Fig. 329.1*B*), intraventricular cysts (Fig. 329.1*C*), and cysts in the spinal cord. CT is best for identifying calcifications. A solitary parenchymal cyst, with or without contrast enhancement, or CNS calcifications are the most common findings in children (Fig. 329.2). Plain films may reveal calcifications in muscle or brain consistent with cysticercosis. In children from endemic regions, the presentation with a single enhancing lesion that is round and <2 cm in diameter, absence of symptoms or signs of other diseases (e.g., no fever or lymph nodes), no focal findings, and no evidence of increased intracranial pressure is highly specific for neurocysticercosis.

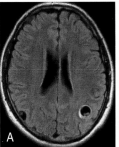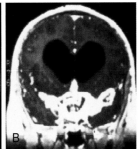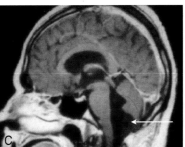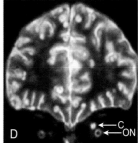

Fig. 329.1 Neurocysticercosis. **A,** MRI (T1 weighted) demonstrating 2 parenchymal cysts with protoscoleces. **B,** MRI (T1 weighted) of cysticercal basilar arachnoiditis. **C,** MRI (T1 weighted) showing a cyst below the fourth ventricle *(arrow).* **D,** MRI (T2 weighted) showing a cysticercus (C) above the optic nerve (ON).

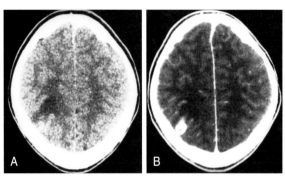

Fig. 329.2 Neurocysticercosis. CT image of a solitary lesion with (**A**) and without (**B**) contrast, showing contrast enhancement. *(Courtesy of Dr. Wendy G. Mitchell and Dr. Marvin D. Nelson, Children's Hospital, Los Angeles.)*

Serologic diagnosis using the enzyme-linked immunotransfer blot is available commercially in the United States and through the Centers for Disease Control and Prevention (CDC). Serum antibody testing is highly specific but is frequently negative in children with single lesions or just calcifications. Antigen-detection assays and polymerase chain reaction assays show promise as diagnostic procedures but currently are not commercially available in the United States.

Differential Diagnosis
Neurocysticercosis is often confused clinically with other seizure disorders. Clinical suspicion is based on travel history, a history of contact with an individual who might carry an adult tapeworm, or suggestive imaging studies. The imaging appearance can be confused with brain abscess, granulomas (including tuberculomas, fungal infections, Langerhans histiocytosis, and toxoplasmosis), and tumors.

TREATMENT
The initial management of cysticercosis should focus on symptomatic therapy for seizures and/or hydrocephalus. Seizures can usually be controlled using standard antiepileptic drugs. If the lesions resolve, antiepileptic drugs can often be tapered and stopped. Frequent seizures or the development of calcified lesions are risk factors for recurrent seizures and indications for prolonged or lifelong antiepileptic therapy.

The natural history of **parenchymal** lesions is to resolve spontaneously, with or without antiparasitic drugs, but this process is often prolonged (months to years). Solitary parenchymal cysts resolve slightly more rapidly with antiparasitic therapy. Antiparasitic drugs also decrease the frequency of recurrent seizures. Other forms of the disease are less common in children. In adults with cystic lesions, randomized controlled trials suggested an overall 2-fold decrease in recurrence of generalized seizures with albendazole treatment. The benefit to children was significantly less, perhaps because most of these infections were with only 1-2 cysts. Corticosteroids likely also decrease seizure frequency.

The most commonly used antiparasitic is **albendazole** (15 mg/kg/day orally [PO] divided twice daily [bid]). It can be taken with a fatty meal to improve absorption. The most common duration of therapy is 7 days for single parenchymal lesions. However, longer duration (months), higher doses (up to 30 mg/kg/day), or combination therapy with praziquantel is often required for multiple lesions or subarachnoid disease. For example, in adults with more than 2 cysticerci, recent trials note improved resolution with combination therapy with albendazole, praziquantel, and corticosteroids. **Praziquantel** (50-100 mg/kg/day PO divided 3 times daily [tid] for 28 days) can be used with albendazole or as an alternative to it. First-pass metabolism is common with corticosteroids or antiepileptic drugs. **Cimetidine** can be used in conjunction with praziquantel to blunt the first-pass metabolism. A worsening of symptoms can follow the use of either drug based on the host's inflammatory response to the dying parasite. Patients should be medicated with prednisone (1-2 mg/kg/day) or oral dexamethasone (0.15 mg/kg/day) beginning before the 1st dose of antiparasitic drugs and continuing for at least 2 wk. **Methotrexate** can be used as a steroid-sparing agent in patients requiring prolonged antiinflammatory therapy.

Most patients with hydrocephalus require neurosurgical interventions. Some cases require emergent placement of a ventriculostomy, but most can be managed by cystectomy alone. For obstructive hydrocephalus caused by ventricular cysticercosis, many patients can be cured by minimally invasive surgery. **Neuroendoscopy** is the preferred approach to cysticerci in the lateral or 3rd ventricle. Cysticerci in the 4th ventricle can be removed by a suboccipital craniotomy. There are also reports of endoscopic removal of 4th ventricular cysticerci using flexible neuroendoscopy. Adherent cysticerci that cannot be removed can be treated by placement of a ventriculoperitoneal shunt (VPS). However, there is a high rate of shunt failure, which can be minimized somewhat by treatment with antiparasitic drugs plus corticosteroids.

Subarachnoid disease has a poor prognosis. The prognosis is much improved by aggressive therapy, including antiparasitic drugs, antiinflammatory treatment, and neurosurgical procedures for hydrocephalus (e.g., VPS placement). However, the duration of antiparasitic and antiinflammatory therapy often needs to be prolonged. **Ocular** cysticercosis is usually treated surgically, although there are reports of cure using medical therapy alone.

PREVENTION
In areas with evolved public health systems, cysticercosis can largely be eliminated by meat inspection, condemnation of infected meat, and thorough cooking of pork. This approach has not worked in countries where most meat is butchered informally. Mass chemotherapy for tapeworm carriers, mass treatment of pigs, and improved personal hygiene have decreased or eliminated transmission in some areas. Screening family members and those preparing food for index cases for cysticercosis has a very low yield, in part because of the poor sensitivity of current tests. Those who have noted passing material consistent with taeniasis should be treated with praziquantel regardless of the results of stool studies. Veterinary vaccines for several cestode infections have a high degree of efficacy and have a potential role in decreasing parasite transmission.

Bibliography is available at Expert Consult.

Chapter **330**

Echinococcosis (*Echinococcus granulosus* and *Echinococcus multilocularis*)

Miguel M. Cabada, Philip R. Fischer, and A. Clinton White Jr.

第三百三十章

棘球蚴病（细粒棘球蚴和多房棘球蚴）

中文导读

　　本章主要介绍了棘球蚴病的病原学、流行病学、发病机制、临床表现、诊断、治疗及预防。在病原学部分，指出棘球蚴的生物学特征、生命周期、感染人体的途径。在临床表现部分，描述了肝包囊、肺包囊等各脏器与包囊相关的临床表现，介绍了泡型棘球蚴病的临床特点。在诊断部分，介绍了影像学检查、血清学检查在棘球蚴病诊断的作用，棘球蚴病需要与良性肝囊肿、细菌性肝脓肿、肝癌及转移性肿瘤相鉴别。指出尚无商业化试剂用于抗原和PCR检测。在治疗部分，介绍了对症抗抽搐治疗和抗寄生虫治疗，指出发生脑积水需要手术治疗。

ETIOLOGY

Echinococcosis (**hydatid disease** or **hydatidosis**) is a widespread, serious human cestode infection (Fig. 330.1). Two major *Echinococcus* groups of species are responsible for distinct clinical presentations. *Echinococcus granulosus* and related species cause **cystic hydatid disease, and** *Echinococcus multilocularis* causes **alveolar hydatid disease**. The adult parasites are small (2-7 mm) tapeworms with only 2-6 segments that inhabit the intestines of canines such as dogs, wolves, dingoes, jackals, coyotes, and foxes. Canines are infected by ingesting contaminated viscera from ungulates (*E. granulosus*) or mice (*E. multilocularis*). These carnivores pass the eggs in their stool, which contaminates the soil, pasture, and water, as well as their own fur. Domestic animals, such as sheep, goats, cattle, and camels, ingest *E. granulosus* complex eggs while grazing. Some species of *E. granulosus* complex have a **sylvatic** cycle involving wild cervids such as moose, elk, and deer. For *E. multilocularis*, the main intermediate hosts are small rodents. Humans are infected by consuming eggs by direct contact with infected canines or from ova in the environment. In Europe, contamination of gardens by fox excrement is a major risk factor for transmission. The larvae hatch, penetrate the gut, and are carried by the vascular or lymphatic systems to the liver, lungs, and less frequently, bones, kidney, brain, or heart in *E. granulosus* infection. *E. multilocularis* larvae infect the liver almost exclusively.

Echinococcus granulosus complex comprises several recognized species previously arranged in genotype groups. These are *E. granulosussensustricto* (G1-G3), *E. equinus* (G4), *E. ortleppi* (G5), and *E. canadensis* (G6-G10). The species within the *E. granulosus* complex show significant variation not only in genetics but also in ecology. While *E. granulosussensustricto* is mainly found in domesticated ovines and dogs around the world, *E. canadensis* is found in a sylvatic wolf/moose cycle in North America and Siberia and has been identified in bovines and swine in South America.

EPIDEMIOLOGY

There is potential for transmission of *E. granulosus* to humans wherever dogs are allowed to ingest the entrails of herd animals. Cysts have been detected in up to 10% of the human population in northern Kenya and western China. Disease is highly endemic in the Middle East and Central Asia. In South America, the disease is prevalent in sheepherding areas of the Andes, the beef-herding areas of the Brazilian/Argentine Pampas, and Uruguay. Among developed countries, the disease is recognized in Italy, Greece, Portugal, Spain, and Australia, and is reemergent in

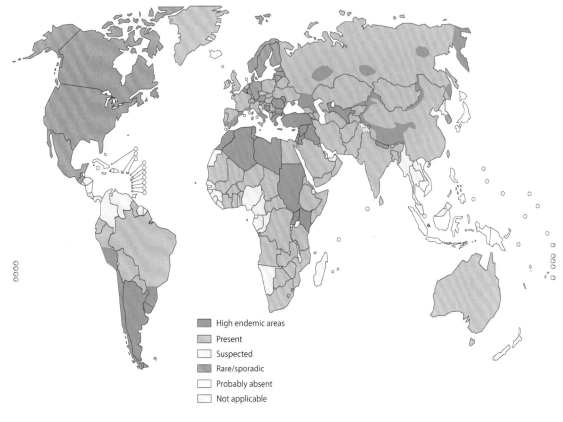

Fig. 330.1 Worldwide distribution of *Echinococcus granulosus* and cystic echinococcosis (hydatidosis), 2009. *(From Control of Neglected Tropical Diseases. © World Health Organization, 2011.* http://gamapserver.who.int/mapLibrary/Files/Maps/Global_echinococcosis_2009.png.)

Legend in figure:
- High endemic areas
- Present
- Suspected
- Rare/sporadic
- Probably absent
- Not applicable

Data Source: World Health Organization
Map Production: Control of Neglected
Tropical Diseases (NTD)
World Health Organization

dogs in Great Britain. In North America, transmission rarely occurs through a sylvatic cycle in the Arctic, as well as in foci of the domestic cycle in sheep-raising areas of western United States.

Transmission of *E. multilocularis* occurs primarily in Western China, Central Europe, Siberia, and Turkey. Transmission is now rare in the Arctic regions of North America. Ingestion of infected rodents by dogs or foxes facilitates transmissions to children. Separate species, *E. vogeli* and *E. oligarthrus*, have mainly a sylvatic cycle involving canines and felines that causes polycystic disease in northern South America.

PATHOGENESIS

E. granulosus complex parasites are often acquired in childhood, but cysts require many years to become large enough to be detected or cause symptoms. In children the lung is a common site, whereas in adults up to 70% of cysts develop in the liver. Cysts can also develop in bone, the genitourinary system, spleen, subcutaneous tissues, and brain. The host surrounds the primary cyst with a tough, fibrous capsule. Inside this capsule, the parasite produces a thick lamellar layer with the consistency of a soft-boiled egg white. Inside the lamellar layer is the thin germinal layer of cells responsible for production of 1000s of protoscoleces that remain attached to the wall or float free in the cyst fluid (Video 330.1). Smaller internal daughter cysts may develop within the primary cyst capsule. The fluid in a healthy cyst is clear, colorless, and watery. Rupture of the cyst, which can occur spontaneously, with trauma, or during surgery, can be associated with immediate hypersensitivity reactions, including anaphylaxis. Protoscoleces released into the tissues can also develop into new cysts.

E. multilocularis almost always involves the liver. The lesions grow very slowly and rarely present in children. The secondary reproductive units bud externally and are not confined within a single, well-defined structure. Thus the lesions are invasive and often confused with a malignancy. Furthermore, the cyst tissues are poorly demarcated from those of the host, making surgical removal difficult. The secondary cysts are also capable of distant metastatic spread. The growing cyst mass eventually replaces a significant portion of the liver and compromises adjacent tissues and structures.

CLINICAL MANIFESTATIONS

In the liver, cysts may remain asymptomatic, may regress spontaneously, or may produce nonspecific symptoms. Symptomatic cysts can cause increased abdominal girth, hepatomegaly, a palpable mass, vomiting, or abdominal pain. In the lung, cysts produce chest pain, chronic cough, or hemoptysis. Expectorated fluid from ruptured lung cysts is often described as "salty." Mass effects can be noted in the brain and bone. Serious complications result from compression of adjacent structures or spillage of cyst contents. **Anaphylaxis** can occur with cyst rupture or spontaneous spillage, from trauma or intraoperatively. Cyst fluid may cause hypersensitivity pneumonitis after rupture. Spillage can also be catastrophic long-term, because each protoscolex can form a new cyst and fill up the abdominal cavity or rarely the pleural space. Jaundice from cystic hydatid disease is rare.

Alveolar hydatid disease may be diagnosed incidentally, but often the proliferating mass may compromise the biliary system and/or hepatic tissue, causing progressive obstructive jaundice and hepatic failure.

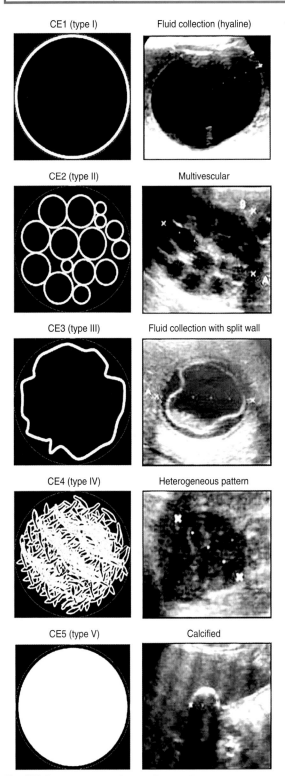

Fig. 330.2 Ultrasound classification of cystic echinococcosis (CE) cysts. The WHO informal working group on echinococcosis classification differs from that of Gharbi and colleagues by the addition of a "cystic lesion" (CL) stage (undifferentiated) *(not shown)*, and by reversing the order of CE types 2 and 3. CE3 transitional cysts may be differentiated into CE3a (with detached endocyst) and CE3b (predominantly solid with daughter vesicles). CE1 and CE3a are early-stage cysts and CE4 and CE5 late-stage cysts. *(From McManus DP, Gray DJ, Zhang W, Yang Y: Diagnosis, treatment, and management of echinococcosis, BMJ 344:e3866, 2012, Fig 4.)*

Symptoms also occur from expansion of extrahepatic foci.

DIAGNOSIS

Ultrasonography is the most valuable tool for both the diagnosis and treatment of cystic hydatid disease of the liver. The World Health Organization (WHO) standardized ultrasound criteria for classification of liver cystic echinococcosis have been shown to be reliable with excellent inter/intraobserver reliability. Ultrasonography staging has a direct use in defining optimal therapy (Fig. 330.2). Chest radiographs frequently reveal characteristic rounded masses in lung hydatid disease (Fig. 330.3). Alveolar disease resembles a diffuse solid tumor. CT findings are similar to those of ultrasonography and may at times be useful in distinguishing alveolar from cystic hydatid disease in geographic regions where both occur (Fig. 330.4). CT or MRI is also important in planning a surgical intervention.

Serologic studies are used to confirm the diagnosis of cystic echinococcosis. However, most of the antibody detection tests available use crude hydatid fluid antigens, which include epitopes that cross-react with other helminths. Cross-reaction has been reported with other noninfectious illness as well. In addition, some children with active cystic echinococcosis may not have circulating levels of specific antibody. Thus the sensitivity and specificity of the enzyme-linked immunosorbent assay to diagnose cystic echinococcosis may vary from 50–100% and 40–100%, respectively, depending on the antigen used and cyst stage, location, number, and viability. The sensitivity is higher for hepatic or bone disease, but the false-negative rate may be >50% with pulmonary or central nervous system (CNS) infection.

Differential Diagnosis

Benign hepatic cysts are common but can be distinguished from cystic hydatid disease by the absence of a distinct 3-layer wall, internal membranes, and hydatid sand. The density of bacterial hepatic abscesses is distinct from the watery cystic fluid characteristic of *E. granulosus* infection, but hydatid cysts may also be complicated by secondary bacterial infection. Alveolar echinococcosis is often confused with hepatoma or metastatic tumor.

TREATMENT

Management of cystic hydatid disease should be individualized and guided by disease stage and location. Approaches range from surgical resection for disease that tends to respond poorly to drugs and complicated cysts to watchful waiting for cysts that have already degenerated. For cystic echinococcosis (**CE**) types 1 or 3a (see Fig. 330.2) that are <5 cm in diameter, **albendazole** chemotherapy alone (15 mg/kg/day orally divided twice daily for 1-6 mo; maximum 800 mg/day) may result in a high rate of cure. Adverse effects include occasional alopecia, mild gastrointestinal disturbance, and elevated transaminases on prolonged use. Because of leukopenia, the U.S. Food and Drug Administration (FDA) recommends that blood counts be monitored at the beginning and every 2 wk during therapy. Medical treatment with albendazole may also be used for cysts that are not suitable for interventions such as **PAIR** (percutaneous, aspiration, instillation, and reaspiration) or surgery, but response rates are low.

For larger CE1 and CE3a lesions, ultrasound- or CT-guided PAIR is the preferred therapy. Compared with surgical treatment alone, PAIR plus albendazole results in similar cyst disappearance with fewer adverse events and fewer days in the hospital. Spillage with PAIR is uncommon, but prophylactic albendazole therapy is routinely administered at least 1 wk before PAIR and 1 mo afterward. PAIR is contraindicated in pregnancy and for bile-stained cysts, which may indicate the presence of a biliary fistula. The scolicidal agents instilled during PAIR may increase risk for biliary complications in these patients. Surgery with albendazole treatment is the recommended approach for CE2 and CE3b cysts of the liver. In experienced centers, cysts with thick internal septation (CE2) can be managed using a trocar to break up the membranes and external drainage. CE4 and CE5 cysts do not require immediate interventions and are followed ultrasonographically for signs of reactivation.

Surgery is the treatment of choice for complicated **cysts**, including

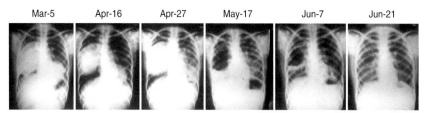

Fig. 330.3 Serial chest radiographs of a young Kenyan woman with bilateral hydatid cysts. *After 2 mo of albendazole therapy, sudden rupture of the right cyst was associated with massive aspiration and acute respiratory distress.*

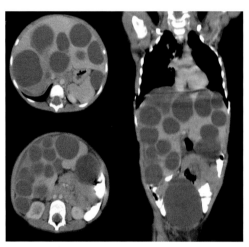

Fig. 330.4 Liver cystic echinococcosis (hydatid disease). Abdominal CT revealed hepatomegaly and multiple (>20) liver cysts. *(From Ben-Shimol S, Zelcer I: Liver hydatid cysts, J Pediatr 163:1792, 2013.)*

ruptured cysts, cysts communicating with the biliary tract, large pulmonary cysts, or cysts of the CNS or bones. Small thoracic cysts may resolve with chemotherapy, but most cysts require operative removal.

For conventional surgery, the inner cyst wall (only laminate and germinal layers are of parasite origin) can be easily peeled from the fibrous layer, although some studies suggest that removal of the whole capsule has a better outcome in terms of recurrent disease. Considerable care must be taken to avoid spillage of cyst contents, and surgical drapes should be soaked in hypertonic saline because cyst fluid contains viable protoscoleces, each capable of producing secondary cysts. An additional risk is anaphylaxis because of spilled cyst fluid, making it useful to employ a surgeon experienced in this surgery. For hepatic cysts, patients should begin therapy with albendazole (ideally in combination with praziquantel) for several days to weeks preoperatively. Antiparasitic drugs should be continued for 4-12 wk postoperatively.

Alveolar hydatidosis frequently requires radical surgery, including partial hepatectomy, lobectomy, or liver transplantation. Medical therapy with albendazole should be continued for 2 yr after presumably curative surgery. In patients who are not operative candidates or whose lesions are not amenable to surgical cure, albendazole long-term suppressive therapy should be used to slow the progression, but the infection generally recurs if albendazole is stopped.

PROGNOSIS

Factors predictive of success with chemotherapy are age of the cyst (<2 yr), low internal complexity of the cyst, and small size. The site of the cyst is not important, although cysts in bone respond poorly. For alveolar hydatidosis, if surgical removal is unsuccessful, the average mortality is 92% by 10 yr after diagnosis.

PREVENTION

Important measures to interrupt transmission include, above all, thorough **handwashing**, avoiding contact with dogs in endemic areas, boiling or filtering water when camping, and proper disposal of animal carcasses. Strict procedures for proper disposal of refuse from slaughterhouses must be instituted and followed so that dogs and wild carnivores do not have access to entrails. Other useful measures are control or treatment of the feral dog population and regular praziquantel treatment of pets and working dogs in endemic areas. Vaccines have been developed to prevent infection in grazing animals but are not widely used.

Bibliography is available at Expert Consult.

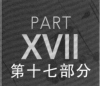
Section **1**
Clinical Manifestations of Gastrointestinal Disease

第一篇
胃肠道疾病的临床表现

Chapter **331**
Normal Digestive Tract Phenomena
Asim Maqbool and Chris A. Liacouras

第三百三十一章
正常消化道现象

中文导读

　　本章主要介绍了吞咽和吸吮出现的时间以及舌系带过短、舌表面的裂纹（地图舌）、腭垂裂、反流、食欲的变化（减少、拒食或贪食）、大便的改变、腹部膨隆、失血和黄疸等常见的症状。具体描述了反流的表现、发病概率和并发症；具体描述了不同时间段中大便的数量、颜色和黏度变化情况；具体描述了间接胆红素症和直接胆红素症的区别。

Gastrointestinal function varies with maturity; what is a physiologic event in a newborn or infant might be a pathologic symptom at an older age. A fetus can swallow amniotic fluid as early as 12 wk of gestation, but nutritive sucking in neonates first develops at about 34 wk of gestation. The coordinated oral and pharyngeal movements necessary for swallowing solids develop within the first few mo of life. Before this time, the tongue thrust is upward and outward to express milk from the nipple, instead of a backward motion, which propels solids toward the esophageal inlet. By 1 mo of age, infants appear to show preferences for sweet and salty foods. Infants' interest in solids increases at approximately 4 mo of age. The recommendation to begin solids at 6 mo of age is based on nutritional and cultural concepts rather than maturation of the swallowing process (see Chapter 56). Infants swallow air during feeding, and burping is encouraged to prevent gaseous distention of the stomach.

A number of normal anatomic variations may be noted in the mouth. A **short lingual frenulum** ("tongue-tie") may be worrisome to parents but only rarely interferes with nursing, bottle feeding, eating, or speech, generally requiring no treatment. **Surface furrowing** of the tongue (a geographic or scrotal tongue) is usually a normal finding. A **bifid uvula** may be isolated or associated with a submucous cleft of the soft palate (Fig. 331.1).

Regurgitation, the result of gastroesophageal reflux, occurs commonly in the 1st yr of life. Effortless regurgitation can dribble out of an infant's mouth but also may be forceful. In an otherwise healthy infant with regurgitation, volumes of emesis are commonly approximately 15-30 mL but occasionally are larger. Most often, the infant remains happy, although possibly hungry, after an episode of regurgitation. Episodes can occur from one to several times per day. Regurgitation gradually resolves in 80% of infants by 6 mo of age and in 90% by 12 mo. If complications develop or regurgitation persists, gastroesophageal reflux is considered pathologic rather than merely developmental and deserves further evaluation and treatment. Complications of gastroesophageal reflux include failure to thrive, pulmonary disease (apnea or aspiration pneumonitis), and esophagitis with its sequelae (see Chapters 349 and 350).

Infants and young children may be erratic eaters; this may be a worry to parents. A toddler might eat insatiably or refuse to consume food during a meal. Toddlers and young children also tend to eat only a limited variety of foods. Parents should be encouraged to view nutritional intake over several days and not be overly concerned about individual meals. Infancy and adolescence are periods of rapid growth; high nutrient requirements for growth may be associated with voracious appetites. The reduced appetite of toddlers and preschool children is often a worry to parents who are used to the relatively greater dietary intake during infancy. Demonstration of age-appropriate growth on a growth curve is reassuring.

The number, color, and consistency of stools can vary greatly in the same infant and between infants of similar age, without apparent explanation. The earliest stools after birth consist of meconium, a dark, viscous material that is normally passed within the 1st 48 hr of life. With the onset of feeding, meconium is replaced by green-brown transition stools, often containing curds, and, after 4-5 days, by yellow-brown milk stools. **Stool frequency** is extremely variable in normal infants and can vary from none to 7 per day. Breastfed infants can have frequent small, loose stools early (transition stools), and then after 2-3 wk

can have very infrequent soft stools. Some nursing infants might not pass any stool for 1-2 wk and then have a normal soft bowel movement. The color of stool has little significance except for the presence of blood or absence of bilirubin products (white-gray rather than yellow-brown). The presence of vegetable matter, such as peas or corn, in the stool of an older infant or toddler ingesting solids is normal and suggests poor chewing and not malabsorption. A pattern of intermittent loose stools, known as **toddler's diarrhea,** occurs commonly between 1 and 3 yr of age. These otherwise healthy growing children often drink excessive carbohydrate-containing beverages. The stools typically occur during the day and not overnight. The volume of fluid intake is often excessive; limiting sugar and unabsorbable carbohydrate-containing beverages and increasing fat in the diet often lead to resolution of the pattern of loose stools.

A protuberant abdomen is often noted in infants and toddlers, especially after large feedings. This can result from the combination of weak abdominal musculature, relatively large abdominal organs, and lordotic stance. In the first yr of life, it is common to palpate the liver 1-2 cm below the right costal margin. The normal liver is soft in consistency and percusses to normal size for age. A Riedel lobe is a thin projection of the right lobe of the liver that may be palpated low in the right lateral abdomen. A soft spleen tip might also be palpable as a normal finding. In thin young children, the vertebral column is easily palpable, and an overlying structure may be mistaken for a mass. Pulsation of the aorta can be appreciated. Normal stool can often be palpated in the left lower quadrant in the descending or sigmoid colon.

Blood loss from the gastrointestinal tract is never normal, but swallowed blood may be misinterpreted as gastrointestinal bleeding. Maternal blood may be ingested at the time of birth or later by a nursing infant if there is bleeding near the mother's nipple. Nasal or oropharyngeal bleeding is occasionally mistaken for gastrointestinal bleeding (see Chapter 124.3). Red dyes in foods or drinks can turn the stool red but do not produce a positive test result for occult blood.

Jaundice is common in neonates, especially among premature infants, and usually results from the inability of an immature liver to conjugate bilirubin, leading to an elevated indirect component (see Chapter 123.3). Persistent elevation of indirect bilirubin levels in nursing infants may be a result of breast milk jaundice, which is usually a benign entity in full-term infants. An elevated direct bilirubin is not normal and suggests liver disease, although in infants it may be a result of extrahepatic infection (urinary tract infection). The direct bilirubin fraction should account for no more than 15–20% of the total serum bilirubin. Elevations in direct bilirubin levels can follow indirect hyperbilirubinemia as the liver converts excessive indirect to direct bilirubin and the rate-limiting step in bilirubin excretion shifts from the glucuronidation of bilirubin to excretion of direct bilirubin into the bile canaliculus. Indirect hyperbilirubinemia, which occurs commonly in normal newborns, tends to tint the sclerae and skin golden yellow, whereas direct hyperbilirubinemia produces a greenish yellow hue. The degree of jaundice does not always directly correlate with serum bilirubin levels. An elevated total serum bilirubin warrants closer examination, fractionation of bilirubin (direct and indirect), and ongoing surveillance. The American Academy of Pediatrics has issued guidelines on the evaluation and management of jaundice in the newborn and on how to follow elevated bilirubin levels, to identify causes of atypical bilirubin elevations, and how to prevent complications. Atypical elevations of unconjugated bilirubin are associated with risk for encephalopathy and kernicterus. Elevations in conjugated bilirubin are reviewed in the chapter on cholestasis (see Chapter 383.1).

Bibliography is available at Expert Consult.

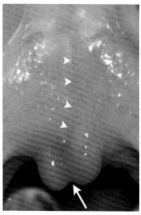 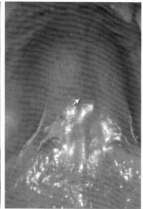

Fig. 331.1 Classic submucous cleft palate with triad of bifid uvula *(large arrow)*, furrow along the midline of the soft palate *(arrowheads)*, and a notch in the posterior margin of the hard palate *(small arrow)*. The midline furrow is sometimes referred to as the zona pellucida, reflecting the translucent nature of this area in some patients. *(From Hasan A, Gardner A, Devlin M, Russell C: Submucous cleft palate with bifid uvula. J Pediatr 165:872, 2014.)*

Chapter **332**

Major Symptoms and Signs of Digestive Tract Disorders

Asim Maqbool and Chris A. Liacouras

第三百三十二章

消化道疾病的主要症状和体征

中文导读

本章主要介绍了吞咽困难、反流、厌食症、呕吐、腹泻、便秘、腹痛、消化道出血及腹胀和腹部肿块等症状。吞咽困难具体描述了吞咽的过程、吞咽困难的分类（分为口咽吞咽困难和食管吞咽困难）、两种吞咽困难的原因；在腹泻部分，具体描述了腹泻的病理生理学、分类及各种类型腹泻的发病机制和特点；腹痛部分具体描述了内脏痛、躯体痛、反射痛的机制和特点；腹胀和腹部肿块部分具体描述了腹水、积气及消化器官的病变。

Disorders of organs outside the gastrointestinal (GI) tract can produce symptoms and signs that mimic digestive tract disorders and should be considered in the differential diagnosis (Table 332.1). In children with normal growth and development, treatment may be initiated without a formal evaluation based on a presumptive diagnosis after taking a history and performing a physical examination. Poor weight gain or weight loss is often associated with a significant pathologic process and usually necessitates a more formal evaluation.

DYSPHAGIA

Difficulty in swallowing is termed *dysphagia*. Painful swallowing is termed **odynophagia**. **Globus** is the sensation of something stuck in the throat without a clear etiology. Swallowing is a complex process that starts in the mouth with mastication and lubrication of food that is formed into a bolus. The bolus is pushed into the pharynx by the tongue. The pharyngeal phase of swallowing is rapid and involves protective mechanisms to prevent food from entering the airway. The epiglottis is lowered over the larynx while the soft palate is elevated against the nasopharyngeal wall; respiration is temporarily arrested while the upper esophageal sphincter opens to allow the bolus to enter the esophagus. In the esophagus, peristaltic coordinated muscular contractions push the food bolus toward the stomach. The lower esophageal sphincter relaxes shortly after the upper esophageal sphincter, so liquids that rapidly clear the esophagus enter the stomach without resistance.

Dysphagia is classified as oropharyngeal dysphagia and esophageal dysphagia. **Oropharyngeal dysphagia** occurs when the transfer of the food bolus from the mouth to the esophagus is impaired (also termed

transfer dysphagia). The striated muscles of the mouth, pharynx, and upper esophageal sphincter are affected in oropharyngeal dysphagia. Neurologic and muscular disorders can give rise to oropharyngeal dysphagia (Table 332.2). Chiari malformations, Russell-Silver syndrome, and cri du chat may present with upper esophageal sphincter dysfunction, manifest by dysphagia with solids. The most serious complication of oropharyngeal dysphagia is life-threatening aspiration.

A complex sequence of neuromuscular events is involved in the transfer of foods to the upper esophagus. Abnormalities of the muscles involved in the ingestion process and their innervation, strength, or coordination are associated with transfer dysphagia in infants and children. In such cases, an oropharyngeal problem is usually part of a more generalized neurologic or muscular problem (botulism, diphtheria, neuromuscular disease). Painful oral lesions, such as acute viral stomatitis or trauma, occasionally interfere with ingestion. If the nasal air passage is seriously obstructed, the need for respiration causes severe distress when suckling. Although severe structural, dental, and salivary abnormalities would be expected to create difficulties, ingestion proceeds relatively well in most affected children if they are hungry.

Esophageal dysphagia occurs when there is difficulty in transporting the food bolus down the esophagus. Esophageal dysphagia can result from neuromuscular disorders or mechanical obstruction (Table 332.3). Primary motility disorders causing impaired peristaltic function and dysphagia are rare in children. Eosinophilic esophagitis can present with esophageal dysphagia. Achalasia is an esophageal motility disorder with associated inability of relaxation of the lower esophageal sphincter, and it rarely occurs in children. Motility of the distal esophagus is disordered

Table 332.1	Some Nondigestive Tract Causes of Gastrointestinal Symptoms in Children

ANOREXIA

Systemic disease: inflammatory, neoplastic
Cardiorespiratory compromise
Iatrogenic: drug therapy, unpalatable therapeutic diets
Depression
Anorexia nervosa

VOMITING

Inborn errors of metabolism
Medications: erythromycin, chemotherapy, nonsteroidal antiinflammatory drugs, marijuana
Increased intracranial pressure
Brain tumor
Infection of the urinary tract
Labyrinthitis
Adrenal insufficiency
Pregnancy
Psychogenic
Abdominal migraine
Poisoning/toxins
Renal disease

DIARRHEA

Infection: otitis media, urinary tract infection
Uremia
Medications: antibiotics, cisapride
Tumors: neuroblastoma
Pericarditis
Adrenal insufficiency

CONSTIPATION

Hypothyroidism
Spina bifida
Developmental delay
Dehydration: diabetes insipidus, renal tubular lesions
Medications: narcotics
Lead poisoning
Infant botulism

ABDOMINAL PAIN

Pyelonephritis, hydronephrosis, renal colic
Pneumonia (lower lobe)
Pelvic inflammatory disease
Porphyria
Fabry disease
Angioedema
Endocarditis
Abdominal migraine
Familial Mediterranean fever
Sexual or physical abuse
Systemic lupus erythematosus
School phobia
Sickle cell crisis
Vertebral disk inflammation
Psoas abscess
Pelvic osteomyelitis or myositis
Medications

ABDOMINAL DISTENTION OR MASS

Ascites: nephrotic syndrome, neoplasm, heart failure
Discrete mass: Wilms tumor, hydronephrosis, neuroblastoma, mesenteric cyst, hepatoblastoma, lymphoma
Pregnancy

JAUNDICE

Hemolytic disease
Urinary tract infection
Sepsis
Hypothyroidism
Panhypopituitarism

Table 332.2	Causes of Oropharyngeal Dysphagia

NEUROMUSCULAR DISORDERS

Cerebral palsy
Brain tumors
Cerebrovascular disease/stroke
Chiari malformation
Polio and postpolio syndromes
Multiple sclerosis
Myositis
Dermatomyositis
Myasthenia gravis
Muscular dystrophies
Acquired or inherited dystonia syndrome
Dysautonomia

METABOLIC AND AUTOIMMUNE DISORDERS

Hyperthyroidism
Systemic lupus erythematosus
Sarcoidosis
Amyloidosis

INFECTIOUS DISEASE

Meningitis
Botulism
Diphtheria
Lyme disease
Neurosyphilis
Viral infection: polio, coxsackievirus, herpes, cytomegalovirus

STRUCTURAL LESIONS

Inflammatory: abscess, pharyngitis
Congenital web
Cricopharyngeal bar
Dental problems
Bullous skin lesions
Plummer-Vinson syndrome
Zenker diverticulum
Extrinsic compression: osteophytes, lymph nodes, thyroid swelling, aberrant
right subclavian artery (dysphagia lusoria)

OTHER

Corrosive injury
Side effects of medications
After surgery
After radiation therapy

Adapted from Gasiorowska A, Faas R: Current approach to dysphagia. *Gastroenterol Hepatol* 5(4):269–279, 2009.

Table 332.3	Causes of Esophageal Dysphagia

NEUROMUSCULAR

Eosinophilic esophagitis
Achalasia cardia
Diffuse esophageal spasm
Scleroderma

GERD

INTRINSIC LESIONS

Foreign bodies including pills
Esophagitis: GERD, eosinophilic esophagitis, infections
Stricture: corrosive injury, pill induced, peptic
Esophageal webs
Esophageal rings
Esophageal diverticula
Neoplasm
Chagas disease

EXTRINSIC LESIONS

Vascular compression
Mediastinal lesion
Cervical osteochondritis
Vertebral abnormalities

GERD, Gastroesophageal reflux disease.
Adapted from Gasiorowska A, Faas R: Current approach to dysphagia. *Gastroenterol Hepatol* 5(4):269–279, 2009.

after surgical repair of tracheoesophageal fistula or achalasia. Abnormal motility can accompany collagen vascular disorders. Mechanical obstruction can be intrinsic or extrinsic. Intrinsic structural defects cause a fixed impediment to the passage of food bolus because of a narrowing within the esophagus, as in a stricture, web, or tumor. Extrinsic obstruction is caused by compression from vascular rings, mediastinal lesions, or vertebral abnormalities. Structural defects typically cause more problems in swallowing solids than liquids. In infants, esophageal web, tracheobronchial remnant, or vascular ring can cause dysphagia. An esophageal stricture secondary to esophagitis (chronic gastroesophageal reflux, eosinophilic esophagitis, chronic infections) occasionally has dysphagia as the first manifestation. An esophageal foreign body or a stricture secondary to a caustic ingestion also causes dysphagia. A Schatzki ring, a thin ring of mucosal tissue near the lower esophageal sphincter, is another mechanical cause of recurrent dysphagia, and again is rare in children.

When dysphagia is associated with a delay in passage through the esophagus, the patient may be able to point to the level of the chest where the delay occurs, but esophageal symptoms are usually referred to the suprasternal notch. When a patient points to the suprasternal notch, the impaction can be found anywhere in the esophagus.

REGURGITATION

Regurgitation is the effortless movement of stomach contents into the esophagus and mouth. It is not associated with distress, and infants with regurgitation are often hungry immediately after an episode. The lower esophageal sphincter prevents reflux of gastric contents into the esophagus. Regurgitation is a result of gastroesophageal reflux through an incompetent or, in infants, immature lower esophageal sphincter. This is often a developmental process, and regurgitation or "spitting" resolves with maturity. Regurgitation should be differentiated from vomiting, which denotes an active reflex process with an extensive differential diagnosis (Table 332.4).

ANOREXIA

Anorexia means prolonged lack of appetite. Hunger and satiety centers are located in the hypothalamus; it seems likely that afferent nerves from the GI tract to these brain centers are important determinants of the anorexia that characterizes many diseases of the stomach and intestine (see Chapter 47). Satiety is stimulated by distention of the stomach or upper small bowel, the signal being transmitted by sensory afferents, which are especially dense in the upper gut. Chemoreceptors in the intestine, influenced by the assimilation of nutrients, also affect afferent flow to the appetite centers. Impulses reach the hypothalamus from higher centers, possibly influenced by pain or the emotional disturbance of an intestinal disease. Other regulatory factors include hormones, ghrelin, leptin, and plasma glucose, which, in turn, reflect intestinal function (see Chapter 47).

VOMITING

Vomiting is a highly coordinated reflex process that may be preceded by increased salivation and begins with involuntary retching. Violent descent of the diaphragm and constriction of the abdominal muscles

Table 332.4	Differential Diagnosis of Emesis During Childhood		
INFANT	**CHILD**		**ADOLESCENT**
COMMON			
Gastroenteritis	Gastroenteritis		Gastroenteritis
Gastroesophageal reflux	Systemic infection		GERD
Overfeeding	Gastritis		Systemic infection
Anatomic obstruction*	Toxic ingestion/poisoning		Toxic ingestion/poisoning/marijuana
Systemic infection[†]	Pertussis syndrome		Gastritis
Pertussis syndrome	Medication		Sinusitis
Otitis media	Reflux (GERD)		Inflammatory bowel disease
	Sinusitis		Appendicitis
	Otitis media		Migraine
	Anatomic obstruction*		Pregnancy
	Eosinophilic esophagitis		Medications
			Ipecac abuse, bulimia
			Concussion
RARE			
Adrenogenital syndrome	Reye syndrome		Reye syndrome
Inborn errors of metabolism	Hepatitis		Hepatitis
Brain tumor (increased intracranial pressure)	Peptic ulcer		Peptic ulcer
Subdural hemorrhage	Pancreatitis		Pancreatitis
Food poisoning	Brain tumor		Cholecystitis
Rumination	Increased intracranial pressure		Brain tumor
Renal tubular acidosis	Middle ear disease/labyrinthitis		Increased intracranial pressure
Ureteropelvic junction obstruction	Chemotherapy		Concussion
Pseudoobstruction	Achalasia		Middle ear disease/labyrinthitis
	Cyclic vomiting (migraine)		Chemotherapy
	Esophageal stricture		Cyclic vomiting (migraine)
	Duodenal hematoma		Biliary colic
	Inborn error of metabolism		Renal colic
	Pseudoobstruction		Porphyria
	Gastroparesis		Diabetic ketoacidosis
			Adrenal insufficiency
			Pseudoobstruction
			Intestinal tumor
			Gastroparesis
			Achalasia
			Superior mesentery artery syndrome
			Distal intestinal obstruction syndrome

*Includes malrotation, pyloric stenosis, intussusception, Hirschsprung disease, adhesions, hernias.
[†]Meningitis, sepsis.
GERD, Gastroesophageal reflux disease, inguinal hernia.

Table 332.5	Causes of Gastrointestinal Obstruction

ESOPHAGUS *Congenital* Esophageal atresia Vascular rings Schatzki ring Tracheobronchial remnant *Acquired* Esophageal stricture Foreign body Achalasia Chagas disease Collagen vascular disease **STOMACH** *Congenital* Antral webs Pyloric stenosis *Acquired* Bezoar, foreign body Pyloric stricture (ulcer) Chronic granulomatous disease of childhood Eosinophilic gastroenteritis Crohn disease Epidermolysis bullosa **SMALL INTESTINE** *Congenital* Duodenal atresia Annular pancreas Malrotation/volvulus Malrotation/Ladd bands	Ileal atresia Meconium ileus Meckel diverticulum with volvulus or intussusception Inguinal hernia Internal hernia Intestinal duplication Pseudoobstruction *Acquired* Postsurgical adhesions Crohn disease Intussusception Distal ileal obstruction syndrome (cystic fibrosis) Duodenal hematoma Superior mesenteric artery syndrome **COLON** *Congenital* Meconium plug Hirschsprung disease Colonic atresia, stenosis Imperforate anus Rectal stenosis Pseudoobstruction Volvulus Colonic duplication *Acquired* Ulcerative colitis (toxic megacolon) Chagas disease Crohn disease Fibrosing colonopathy (cystic fibrosis)

with relaxation of the gastric cardia actively force gastric contents back up the esophagus. This process is coordinated in the medullary vomiting center, which is influenced directly by afferent innervation and indirectly by the chemoreceptor trigger zone and higher central nervous system (CNS) centers. Many acute or chronic processes can cause vomiting (see Tables 332.1 and 332.4).

Vomiting caused by obstruction of the GI tract is probably mediated by intestinal visceral afferent nerves stimulating the vomiting center (Table 332.5). If obstruction occurs below the second part of the duodenum, vomitus is usually bile stained. Emesis can also become bile stained with repeated vomiting in the absence of obstruction when duodenal contents are refluxed into the stomach. Nonobstructive lesions of the digestive tract can also cause vomiting; this includes diseases of the upper bowel, pancreas, liver, or biliary tree. CNS or metabolic derangements and cyclic vomiting syndrome (Table 332.6) can lead to severe, persistent emesis. Marijuana use among teens has also led to cannabis hyperemesis syndrome (see Chapter 140.3).

Potential complications of emesis are noted in Table 332.7. Broad management strategies for vomiting in general and specific causes of emesis are noted in Tables 332.8 and 332.9.

DIARRHEA

Diarrhea is best defined as excessive loss of fluid and electrolyte in the stool. Acute diarrhea is defined as sudden onset of excessively loose stools of >10 mL/kg/day in infants and >200 g/24 hr in older children, which lasts <14 days. When the episode lasts longer than 14 days, it is called *chronic* or *persistent diarrhea.*

Normally, a young infant has approximately 5 mL/kg/day of stool output; the volume increases to 200 g/24 hr in an adult. The greatest volume of intestinal water is absorbed in the small bowel; the colon concentrates intestinal contents against a high osmotic gradient. The small intestine of an adult can absorb 10-11 L/day of a combination of ingested and secreted fluid, whereas the colon absorbs approximately 0.5 L. Disorders that interfere with absorption in the small bowel tend to produce voluminous diarrhea, whereas disorders compromising colonic absorption produce lower-volume diarrhea. **Dysentery**

(small-volume, frequent bloody stools with mucus, tenesmus, and urgency) is the predominant symptom of colitis.

The basis of all diarrheas is disturbed intestinal solute transport and water absorption. Water movement across intestinal membranes is passive and is determined by both active and passive fluxes of solutes, particularly sodium, chloride, and glucose. The pathogenesis of most episodes of diarrhea can be explained by secretory, osmotic, or motility abnormalities or a combination of these (Table 332.10).

Secretory diarrhea occurs when the intestinal epithelial cell solute transport system is in an active state of secretion. It is often caused by a secretagogue, such as cholera toxin, binding to a receptor on the surface epithelium of the bowel and thereby stimulating intracellular accumulation of cyclic adenosine monophosphate or cyclic guanosine monophosphate. Some intraluminal fatty acids and bile salts cause the colonic mucosa to secrete through this mechanism. Diarrhea not associated with an exogenous secretagogue can also have a secretory component (congenital microvillus inclusion disease). Secretory diarrhea is usually of large volume and persists even with fasting. The stool osmolality is predominantly indicated by the electrolytes and the ion

Table 332.6	Criteria for Cyclic Vomiting Syndrome

All of the criteria must be met for the consensus definition of cyclic vomiting syndrome:
- At least 5 attacks in any interval, or a minimum of 3 episodes during a 6-mo period
- Recurrent episodes of intense vomiting and nausea lasting 1 hr to 10 days and occurring at least 1 wk apart
- Stereotypical pattern and symptoms in the individual patient
- Vomiting during episodes occurs ≥4 times/hr for ≥1 hr
- Return to baseline health between episodes
- Not attributed to another disorder

From Li, B UK, Lefevre F, Chelimsky GG, et al: North American Society for Pediatric Gastroenterology, Hepatology, and Nutrition consensus statement on the diagnosis and management of cyclic vomiting syndrome. *J Pediatr Gastroenterol Nutr* 47:379–393, 2008.

Table 332.7	Complications of Vomiting	
COMPLICATION	**PATHOPHYSIOLOGY**	**HISTORY, PHYSICAL EXAMINATION, AND LABORATORY STUDIES**
Metabolic	Fluid loss in emesis HCl loss in emesis Na, K loss in emesis Acidosis	Dehydration Alkalosis; hypochloremia Hyponatremia; hypokalemia Dehydration
Nutritional	Emesis of calories and nutrients Anorexia for calories and nutrients	Malnutrition; "failure to thrive"
Mallory-Weiss tear	Retching → tear at lesser curve of gastroesophageal junction	Forceful emesis → hematemesis
Esophagitis	Chronic vomiting → esophageal acid exposure	Heartburn; Hemoccult + stool
Aspiration	Aspiration of vomitus, especially in context of obtundation	Pneumonia; neurologic dysfunction
Shock	Severe fluid loss in emesis or in accompanying diarrhea	Dehydration (accompanying diarrhea can explain acidosis?)
	Severe blood loss in hematemesis	Blood volume depletion
Pneumomediastinum, pneumothorax	Increased intrathoracic pressure	Chest x-ray
Petechiae, retinal hemorrhages	Increased intrathoracic pressure	Normal platelet count

From Kliegman RM, Greenbaum LA, Lye PS, editors: *Practical strategies in pediatric diagnosis and therapy*, ed 2, Philadelphia, 2004, Elsevier, p 318.

Table 332.8	Pharmacologic Therapies for Vomiting Episodes	
DISORDER/THERAPEUTIC DRUG CLASS	**DRUG**	**DOSAGE**
REFLUX		
Dopamine antagonist	Metoclopramide (Reglan)	0.1-0.2 mg/kg PO or IV qid
GASTROPARESIS		
Dopamine antagonist	Metoclopramide (Reglan)	0.1-0.2 mg/kg PO or IV qid
Motilin agonist	Erythromycin	3-5 mg/kg PO or IV tid-qid
INTESTINAL PSEUDOOBSTRUCTION		
Stimulation of intestinal migratory myoelectric complexes	Octreotide (Sandostatin)	1 µg/kg SC bid-tid
CHEMOTHERAPY		
Dopamine antagonist	Metoclopramide	0.5-1.0 mg/kg IV qid, with antihistamine prophylaxis of extrapyramidal side effects
Serotoninergic 5-HT$_3$ antagonist	Ondansetron (Zofran)	0.15-0.3 mg/kg IV or PO tid
Phenothiazines (extrapyramidal, hematologic side effects)	Prochlorperazine (Compazine) Chlorpromazine (Thorazine)	≈0.3 mg/kg PO bid-tid >6 mo of age: 0.5 mg/kg PO or IV tid-qid
Steroids	Dexamethasone (Decadron)	0.1 mg/kg PO tid
Cannabinoids	Tetrahydrocannabinol (Nabilone)	0.05-0.1 mg/kg PO bid-tid
POSTOPERATIVE		
	Ondansetron, phenothiazines	See under chemotherapy
MOTION SICKNESS, VESTIBULAR DISORDERS		
Antihistamine	Dimenhydrinate (Dramamine)	1 mg/kg PO tid-qid
Anticholinergic	Scopolamine (Transderm Scop)	Adults: 1 patch/3 days
ADRENAL CRISIS		
Steroids	Cortisol	2 mg/kg IV bolus followed by 0.2-0.4 mg/kg/hr IV (±1 mg/kg IM)

ECG, Electrocardiogram; *GI*, gastrointestinal.
From Kliegman RM, Greenbaum LA, Lye PS, editors: *Practical strategies in pediatric diagnosis and therapy*, ed 2, Philadelphia, 2004, Elsevier, p 317.

gap is 100 mOsm/kg or less. The ion gap is calculated by subtracting the concentration of electrolytes from total osmolality:

$$\text{Ion gap} = \text{Stool osmolality} - [(\text{Stool Na} + \text{stool K}) \times 2]$$

Osmotic diarrhea occurs after ingestion of a poorly absorbed solute. The solute may be one that is normally not well absorbed (magnesium, phosphate, lactulose, or sorbitol) or one that is not well absorbed because of a disorder of the small bowel (lactose with lactase deficiency or glucose with rotavirus diarrhea). Malabsorbed carbohydrate is fermented in the colon, and short-chain fatty acids are produced. Although short-chain fatty acids can be absorbed in the colon and used as an energy source, the net effect is increase in the osmotic solute load. This form of diarrhea is usually of lesser volume than a secretory diarrhea and

stops with fasting. The osmolality of the stool will not be explained by the electrolyte content, because another osmotic component is present and so the anion gap is >100 mOsm.

Motility disorders can be associated with rapid or delayed transit and are not generally associated with large-volume diarrhea. Slow motility can be associated with bacterial overgrowth leading to diarrhea. The differential diagnosis of common causes of acute and chronic diarrhea is noted in Table 332.11.

CONSTIPATION

Any definition of constipation is relative and depends on stool consistency, stool frequency, and difficulty in passing the stool. A normal child might have a soft stool only every second or third day without difficulty;

Table 332.9	Supportive and Nonpharmacologic Therapies for Vomiting Episodes
DISEASE	**THERAPY**
All	Treat cause • Obstruction: operate • Allergy: change diet (±steroids) • Metabolic error: Rx defect • Acid peptic disease: H2RAs, PPIs, etc.
COMPLICATIONS	
Dehydration	IV fluids, electrolytes
Hematemesis	Transfuse, correct coagulopathy
Esophagitis	H₂RAs, PPIs
Malnutrition	NG or NJ drip feeding useful for many chronic conditions
Meconium ileus	Gastrografin enema
DIOS	Gastrografin enema; balanced colonic lavage solution (e.g., GoLYTELY)
Intussusception	Barium enema; air reduction enema
Hematemesis	Endoscopic: injection sclerotherapy or banding of esophageal varices; injection therapy, fibrin sealant application, or heater probe electrocautery for selected upper GI tract lesions
Sigmoid volvulus	Colonoscopic decompression
Reflux	Positioning; dietary measures (infants: rice cereal, 1 tbs/oz of formula)
Psychogenic components	Psychotherapy; tricyclic antidepressants; anxiolytics (e.g., diazepam: 0.1 mg/kg PO tid-qid)

DIOS, Distal intestinal obstruction syndrome; *GI,* gastrointestinal; *H₂RA,* H₂-receptor antagonist; *NG,* nasogastric; *NJ,* nasojejunal; *PPIs,* proton pump inhibitors; *tbs,* tablespoon.
From Kliegman RM, Greenbaum LA, Lye PS, editors: *Practical strategies in pediatric diagnosis and therapy,* ed 2, Philadelphia, 2004, Elsevier, p 319.

Table 332.10	Mechanisms of Diarrhea			
PRIMARY MECHANISM	**DEFECT**	**STOOL EXAMINATION**	**EXAMPLES**	**COMMENT**
Secretory	Decreased absorption, increased secretion, electrolyte transport	Watery, normal osmolality with ion gap <100 mOsm/kg	Cholera, toxigenic *Escherichia coli*; carcinoid, VIP, neuroblastoma, congenital chloride diarrhea, *Clostridium difficile*, cryptosporidiosis (AIDS)	Persists during fasting; bile salt malabsorption can also increase intestinal water secretion; no stool leukocytes
Osmotic	Maldigestion, transport defects ingestion of unabsorbable substances	Watery, acidic, and reducing substances; increased osmolality with ion gap >100 mOsm/kg	Lactase deficiency, glucose-galactose malabsorption, lactulose, laxative abuse	Stops with fasting; increased breath hydrogen with carbohydrate malabsorption; no stool leukocytes
Increased motility	Decreased transit time	Loose to normal-appearing stool, stimulated by gastrocolic reflex	Irritable bowel syndrome, thyrotoxicosis, postvagotomy dumping syndrome	Infection can also contribute to increased motility
Decreased motility	Defect in neuromuscular unit(s) stasis (bacterial overgrowth)	Loose to normal-appearing stool	Pseudoobstruction, blind loop	Possible bacterial overgrowth
Decreased surface area (osmotic, motility)	Decreased functional capacity	Watery	Short bowel syndrome, celiac disease, rotavirus enteritis	Might require elemental diet plus parenteral alimentation
Mucosal invasion	Inflammation, decreased colonic reabsorption, increased motility	Blood and increased WBCs in stool	*Salmonella, Shigella* infection; amebiasis; *Yersinia, Campylobacter* infection	Dysentery evident in blood, mucus, and WBCs

VIP, Vasoactive intestinal peptide; *WBC,* white blood cell.
From Kliegman RM, Greenbaum LA, Lye PS, editors: *Practical strategies in pediatric diagnosis and therapy,* ed 2, Philadelphia, 2004, Elsevier, p 274.

this is not constipation. A hard stool passed with difficulty every third day should be treated as constipation. Constipation can arise from defects either in filling or emptying the rectum (Table 332.12).

A nursing infant might have very infrequent stools of normal consistency; this is usually a normal pattern. True constipation in the neonatal period is most likely secondary to Hirschsprung disease, intestinal pseudoobstruction, or hypothyroidism.

Defective rectal filling occurs when colonic peristalsis is ineffective (in cases of hypothyroidism or opiate use and when bowel obstruction is caused either by a structural anomaly or by Hirschsprung disease). The resultant colonic stasis leads to excessive drying of

stool and a failure to initiate reflexes from the rectum that normally trigger evacuation. Emptying the rectum by spontaneous evacuation depends on a defecation reflex initiated by pressure receptors in the rectal muscle. Therefore stool retention can also result from lesions involving these rectal muscles, the sacral spinal cord afferent and efferent fibers, or the muscles of the abdomen and pelvic floor. Disorders of anal sphincter relaxation can also contribute to fecal retention.

Constipation tends to be self-perpetuating, whatever its cause. Hard, large stools in the rectum become difficult and even painful to evacuate; thus more retention occurs and a vicious circle ensues. Distention of

Table 332.11	Differential Diagnosis of Diarrhea

INFANT	CHILD	ADOLESCENT
ACUTE		
Common		
Gastroenteritis (viral > bacterial > protozoal)	Gastroenteritis (viral > bacterial > protozoal)	Gastroenteritis (viral > bacterial > protozoal)
Systemic infection	Food poisoning	Food poisoning
Antibiotic associated	Systemic infection	Antibiotic associated
Overfeeding	Antibiotic associated	
Rare		
Primary disaccharidase deficiency	Toxic ingestion	Hyperthyroidism
Hirschsprung toxic colitis	Hemolytic uremic syndrome	Appendicitis
Adrenogenital syndrome	Intussusception	
Neonatal opiate withdrawal		
CHRONIC		
Common		
Postinfectious secondary lactase deficiency	Postinfectious secondary lactase deficiency	Irritable bowel syndrome
Cow's milk or soy protein intolerance (allergy)	Irritable bowel syndrome	Inflammatory bowel disease
Chronic nonspecific diarrhea of infancy	Celiac disease	Lactose intolerance
Excessive fruit juice (sorbitol) ingestion	Cystic fibrosis	Giardiasis
Celiac disease	Lactose intolerance	Laxative abuse (anorexia nervosa)
Cystic fibrosis	Excessive fruit juice (sorbitol) ingestion	Constipation with encopresis
AIDS enteropathy	Giardiasis	
	Inflammatory bowel disease	
	AIDS enteropathy	
Rare		
Primary immune defects	Primary and acquired immune defects	Secretory tumor
Autoimmune enteropathy	Secretory tumors	Primary bowel tumor
IPEX and IPEX-like syndromes	Pseudoobstruction	Parasitic infections and venereal diseases
Glucose-galactose malabsorption	Sucrase-isomaltase deficiency	Appendiceal abscess
Microvillus inclusion disease (microvillus atrophy)	Eosinophilic gastroenteritis	Addison disease
Congenital transport defects (chloride, sodium)	Secretory tumors	
Primary bile acid malabsorption		
Factitious syndrome by proxy		
Hirschsprung disease		
Shwachman syndrome		
Secretory tumors		
Acrodermatitis enteropathica		
Lymphangiectasia		
Abetalipoproteinemia		
Eosinophilic gastroenteritis		
Short bowel syndrome		

IPEX, Immunodysregulation polyendocrinopathy enteropathy X-linked.
From Kliegman RM, Greenbaum LA, Lye PS, editors: *Practical strategies in pediatric diagnosis and therapy*, ed 2, Philadelphia, 2004, Elsevier, p 272.

Table 332.12	Causes of Constipation

NONORGANIC (FUNCTIONAL)—RETENTIVE	Methylphenidate
Anatomic	Phenytoin
Anal stenosis, atresia with fistula	Antidepressants
Imperforate anus	Chemotherapeutic agents (vincristine)
Anteriorly displaced anus	Pancreatic enzymes (fibrosing colonopathy)
Intestinal stricture (postnecrotizing enterocolitis)	Lead, arsenic, mercury
Anal stricture	Vitamin D intoxication
	Calcium channel blocking agents
Abnormal Musculature	
Prune-belly syndrome	*Metabolic Disorders*
Gastroschisis	Hypokalemia
Down syndrome	Hypercalcemia
Muscular dystrophy	Hypothyroidism
	Diabetes mellitus, diabetes insipidus
Intestinal Nerve or Muscle Abnormalities	Porphyria
Hirschsprung disease	
Pseudoobstruction (visceral myopathy or neuropathy)	*Intestinal Disorders*
Intestinal neuronal dysplasia	Celiac disease
Spinal cord lesions	Cow's milk protein intolerance
Tethered cord	Cystic fibrosis (meconium ileus equivalent)
Autonomic neuropathy	Inflammatory bowel disease (stricture)
Spinal cord trauma	Tumor
Spina bifida	Connective tissue disorders
Chagas disease	Systemic lupus erythematosus
	Scleroderma
Drugs	
Anticholinergics	*Psychiatric Diagnosis*
Narcotics	Anorexia nervosa

the rectum and colon lessens the sensitivity of the defecation reflex and the effectiveness of peristalsis. Fecal impaction is common and leads to other problems. Eventually, watery content from the proximal colon might percolate around hard retained stool and pass per rectum unperceived by the child. This involuntary **encopresis** may be mistaken for diarrhea. Constipation itself does not have deleterious systemic organic effects, but urinary tract stasis with increased risk of urinary tract infections can accompany severe long-standing cases and constipation can generate anxiety, having a marked emotional impact on the patient and family.

ABDOMINAL PAIN

There is considerable variation among children in their perception and tolerance for abdominal pain. This is one reason the evaluation of chronic abdominal pain is difficult. A child with **functional abdominal pain** (no identifiable organic cause) may be as uncomfortable as one with an organic cause. It is very important to distinguish between organic and nonorganic (functional) abdominal pain because the approach for the management is based on this. Normal growth and physical examination (including a rectal examination) and the absence of anemia or hematochezia are reassuring in a child who is suspected of having functional pain.

A specific cause may be difficult to find, but the nature and location of a pain-provoking lesion can usually be determined from the clinical description. Two types of nerve fibers transmit painful stimuli in the abdomen. In skin and muscle, A fibers mediate sharp localized pain; C fibers from viscera, peritoneum, and muscle transmit poorly localized, dull pain. These afferent fibers have cell bodies in the dorsal root ganglia, and some axons cross the midline and ascend to the medulla, midbrain, and thalamus. Pain is perceived in the cortex of the postcentral gyrus, which can receive impulses arising from both sides of the body. In the gut, the usual stimulus provoking pain is tension or stretching. Inflammatory lesions can lower the pain threshold, but the mechanisms producing pain or inflammation are not clear. Tissue metabolites released near nerve endings probably account for the pain caused by ischemia. Perception of these painful stimuli can be modulated by input from both cerebral and peripheral sources. Psychologic factors are particularly important. Tables 332.13 and 332.14 list features of abdominal pain. Pain that suggests a potentially serious organic etiology is associated with age younger than 5 yr; fever; weight loss; bile- or blood-stained emesis; jaundice; hepatosplenomegaly; back or flank pain or pain in a location other than the umbilicus; awakening from sleep in pain; referred pain to shoulder, groin or back; elevated erythrocyte sedimentation rate, white blood cell count, or C-reactive protein; anemia; edema;

Table 332.13	Chronic Abdominal Pain in Children	
DISORDER	**CHARACTERISTICS**	**KEY EVALUATIONS**
NONORGANIC		
Functional abdominal pain	Nonspecific pain, often periumbilical	Hx and PE; tests as indicated
Irritable bowel syndrome	Intermittent cramps, diarrhea, and constipation	Hx and PE
Nonulcer dyspepsia	Peptic ulcer–like symptoms without abnormalities on evaluation of the upper GI tract	Hx; esophagogastroduodenoscopy
GASTROINTESTINAL TRACT		
Chronic constipation	Hx of stool retention, evidence of constipation on examination	Hx and PE; plain x-ray of abdomen
Lactose intolerance	Symptoms may be associated with lactose ingestion; bloating, gas, cramps, and diarrhea	Trial of lactose-free diet; lactose breath hydrogen test
Parasite infection (especially *Giardia*)	Bloating, gas, cramps, and diarrhea	Stool evaluation for O&P; specific immunoassays for *Giardia*
Excess fructose or sorbitol ingestion	Nonspecific abdominal pain, bloating, gas, and diarrhea	Large intake of apples, fruit juice, or candy or chewing gum sweetened with sorbitol
Crohn disease	See Chapter 362	
Peptic ulcer	Burning or gnawing epigastric pain; worse on awakening or before meals; relieved with antacids	Esophagogastroduodenoscopy, upper GI contrast x-rays, or MRI enteroscopy
Esophagitis	Epigastric pain with substernal burning	Esophagogastroduodenoscopy
Meckel diverticulum	Periumbilical or lower abdominal pain; may have blood in stool (usually painless)	Meckel scan or enteroclysis
Recurrent intussusception	Paroxysmal severe cramping abdominal pain; blood may be present in stool with episode	Identify intussusception during episode or lead point in intestine between episodes with contrast studies of GI tract
Internal, inguinal, or abdominal wall hernia	Dull abdomen or abdominal wall pain	PE, CT of abdominal wall
Chronic appendicitis or appendiceal mucocele	Recurrent RLQ pain; often incorrectly diagnosed, may be rare cause of abdominal pain	Barium enema, CT
GALLBLADDER AND PANCREAS		
Cholelithiasis	RUQ pain, might worsen with meals	Ultrasound of gallbladder
Choledochal cyst	RUQ pain, mass ± elevated bilirubin	Ultrasound or CT of RUQ
Recurrent pancreatitis	Persistent boring pain, might radiate to back, vomiting	Serum amylase and lipase ± serum trypsinogen; ultrasound, CT, or MRI-ERCP of pancreas
GENITOURINARY TRACT		
Urinary tract infection	Dull suprapubic pain, flank pain	Urinalysis and urine culture; renal scan
Hydronephrosis	Unilateral abdominal or flank pain	Ultrasound of kidneys
Urolithiasis	Progressive, severe pain; flank to inguinal region to testicle	Urinalysis, ultrasound, IVP, CT
Other genitourinary disorders	Suprapubic or lower abdominal pain; genitourinary symptoms	Ultrasound of kidneys and pelvis; gynecologic evaluation

ERCP, Endoscopic retrograde cholangiopancreatography.

Continued

Table 332.13	Chronic Abdominal Pain in Children—cont'd	
DISORDER	**CHARACTERISTICS**	**KEY EVALUATIONS**
MISCELLANEOUS CAUSES		
Abdominal migraine	See text; nausea, family Hx migraine	Hx
Abdominal epilepsy	Might have seizure prodrome	EEG (can require >1 study, including sleep-deprived EEG)
Gilbert syndrome	Mild abdominal pain (causal or coincidental?); slightly elevated unconjugated bilirubin	Serum bilirubin
Familial Mediterranean fever	Paroxysmal episodes of fever, severe abdominal pain, and tenderness with other evidence of polyserositis	Hx and PE during an episode, DNA diagnosis
Sickle cell crisis	Anemia	Hematologic evaluation
Lead poisoning	Vague abdominal pain ± constipation	Serum lead level
Henoch-Schönlein purpura	Recurrent, severe crampy abdominal pain, occult blood in stool, characteristic rash, arthritis	Hx, PE, urinalysis
Angioneurotic edema	Swelling of face or airway, crampy pain	Hx, PE, upper GI contrast x-rays, serum C1 esterase inhibitor
Acute intermittent porphyria	Severe pain precipitated by drugs, fasting, or infections	Spot urine for porphyrins
Anterior cutaneous nerve entrapment syndrome (ACNES)	Exquisite localized (~2 × 2 cm) tenderness that is replicable, most often right lower quadrant	Pain relief within 15 min of abdominal wall injection of local anesthetic; may need surgery

EEG, Electroencephalogram; *GI,* gastrointestinal; *Hx,* history; *IVP,* intravenous pyelography; *O&P,* ova and parasites; *PE,* physical exam; *RLQ,* right lower quadrant; *RUQ,* right upper quadrant.

Table 332.14	Distinguishing Features of Acute Abdominal Pain in Children				
DISEASE	**ONSET**	**LOCATION**	**REFERRAL**	**QUALITY**	**COMMENTS**
Pancreatitis	Acute	Epigastric, left upper quadrant	Back	Constant, sharp, boring	Nausea, emesis, tenderness
Intestinal obstruction	Acute or gradual	Periumbilical-lower abdomen	Back	Alternating cramping (colic) and painless periods	Distention, obstipation, emesis, increased bowel sounds
Appendicitis	Acute (1-3 days)	Periumbilical, then localized to lower right quadrant; generalized with peritonitis	Back or pelvis if retrocecal	Sharp, steady	Anorexia, nausea, emesis, local tenderness, fever with peritonitis
Intussusception	Acute	Periumbilical-lower abdomen	None	Cramping, with painless periods	Hematochezia, knees in pulled-up position
Urolithiasis	Acute, sudden	Back (unilateral)	Groin	Sharp, intermittent, cramping	Hematuria
Urinary tract infection	Acute	Back	Bladder	Dull to sharp	Fever, costovertebral angle tenderness, dysuria, urinary frequency
Pelvic inflammatory disease	Acute	Pelvis, lower quadrant	Upper thigh	Aching, peritoneal signs	Vaginal discharge, fever
Small bowel obstruction	Acute to subacute	Periumbilical	None	Cramping diffuse	Emesis and obstipation
Ruptured ectopic pregnancy	Acute sudden	Pelvis, lower quadrant	None	Sharp, intense, localized	Vaginal bleeding, shock

hematochezia; or a strong family history of inflammatory bowel disease or celiac disease.

Visceral pain tends to be dull and aching and is experienced in the dermatome from which the affected organ receives innervations. So, most often, the pain and tenderness are not felt over the site of the disease process. Painful stimuli originating in the liver, pancreas, biliary tree, stomach, or upper bowel are felt in the epigastrium; pain from the distal small bowel, cecum, appendix, or proximal colon is felt at the umbilicus; and pain from the distal large bowel, urinary tract, or pelvic organs is usually suprapubic. The pain from the cecum, ascending colon, and descending colon sometimes is felt at the site of the lesion because of the short mesocecum and corresponding mesocolon. The pain caused by appendicitis is initially felt in the periumbilical region, and pain from the transverse colon is usually felt in the supra pubic region. The shifting (localization) of pain is a pointer toward diagnosis; for example, periumbilical pain of a few hours localizing to the right lower quadrant suggests appendicitis. Radiation of pain can be helpful in diagnosis; for example, in biliary colic the radiation of pain is toward the inferior angle of the right scapula, pancreatic pain radiated to the back, and the renal colic pain is radiated to the inguinal region on the same side.

Somatic pain is intense and usually well localized. When the inflamed viscus comes in contact with a somatic organ such as the parietal peritoneum or the abdominal wall, pain is localized to that site. Peritonitis gives rise to generalized abdominal pain with rigidity, involuntary guarding, rebound tenderness, and cutaneous hyperesthesia on physical examination.

Referred pain from extraintestinal locations, from shared central projections with the sensory pathway from the abdominal wall, can give rise to abdominal pain, as in pneumonia when the parietal pleural pain is referred to the abdomen.

GASTROINTESTINAL HEMORRHAGE

Bleeding can occur anywhere along the GI tract, and identification of the site may be challenging (Table 332.15). Bleeding that originates in the esophagus, stomach, or duodenum can cause **hematemesis.** When exposed to gastric or intestinal juices, blood quickly darkens to resemble coffee grounds; massive bleeding is likely to be red. Red or maroon blood in stools, **hematochezia,** signifies either a distal bleeding site or massive hemorrhage above the distal ileum. Moderate to mild bleeding from sites above the distal ileum tends to cause blackened stools of tarry consistency **(melena);** major hemorrhages in the duodenum or above can also cause melena.

Erosive damage to the mucosa of the GI tract is the most common cause of bleeding, although variceal bleeding secondary to portal hypertension occurs often enough to require consideration. Prolapse gastropathy producing subepithelial hemorrhage and Mallory-Weiss lesions secondary to mucosal tears associated with emesis are causes of upper intestinal bleeds. Vascular malformations are a rare cause in children; they are difficult to identify (Figs. 332.1 and 332.2). Upper intestinal bleeding is evaluated with esophagogastroduodenoscopy. Evaluation of the small intestine is facilitated by capsule endoscopy. The capsule-sized imaging device is swallowed in older children or placed endoscopically in younger children. Lower GI bleeding is investigated with a colonoscopy. In brisk intestinal bleeding of unknown location, a tagged red blood cell scan is helpful in locating the site of the bleeding, although CT angiography is usually diagnostic. Occult blood in stool is usually detected by using commercially available fecal occult blood testing cards, which are based on a chemical reaction

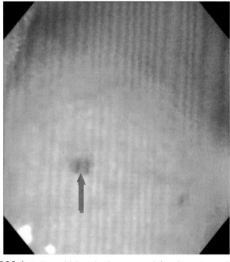

Fig. 332.1 A 7 yr old boy had tarry stool for days. Panendoscopy showed multiple cherry red flat spots in the gastric mucosa, compatible with the findings of angiodysplasia in computed tomographic angiography. *(From Chuang F, Lin JS, Yeung C, et al: Intestinal angiodysplasia: an uncommon cause of gastrointestinal bleeding in children. Pediatr Neonatol 52:214–218, 2011. Fig. 2.)*

Table 332.15	Differential Diagnosis of Gastrointestinal Bleeding in Childhood	
INFANT	**CHILD**	**ADOLESCENT**
COMMON		
Bacterial enteritis	Bacterial enteritis	Bacterial enteritis
Milk protein allergy intolerance	Anal fissure	Inflammatory bowel disease
Intussusception	Colonic polyps	Peptic ulcer/gastritis
Swallowed maternal blood	Intussusception	Prolapse (traumatic) gastropathy secondary
Anal fissure	Peptic ulcer/gastritis	to emesis
Lymphonodular hyperplasia	Swallowed epistaxis	Mallory-Weiss syndrome
	Prolapse (traumatic) gastropathy secondary to emesis	Colonic polyps
	Mallory-Weiss syndrome	Anal fissure
RARE		
Volvulus	Esophageal varices	Hemorrhoids
Necrotizing enterocolitis	Esophagitis	Esophageal varices
Meckel diverticulum	Meckel diverticulum	Esophagitis
Stress ulcer, gastritis	Lymphonodular hyperplasia	Pill ulcer
Coagulation disorder (hemorrhagic	Henoch-Schönlein purpura	Telangiectasia-angiodysplasia
disease of newborn)	Foreign body	Graft versus host disease
Esophagitis	Hemangioma, arteriovenous malformation	Duplication cyst
	Sexual abuse	• Angiodysplasia
	Hemolytic-uremic syndrome	• Angiodysplasia with von Willebrand
	Inflammatory bowel disease	disease
	Coagulopathy	• Blue rubber bleb nevus syndrome
	Duplication cyst	
	• Angiodysplasia	
	• Angiodysplasia with von Willebrand disease	
	• Blue rubber bleb nevus syndrome	

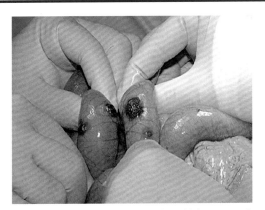

Fig. 332.2 Operative features of blue rubber bleb nevus syndrome: these lesions are similar to cutaneous lesions. *(From Hasosah MY, Abdul-Wahab AA, Bin-Yahab SA, et al: Blue rubber bled nevus syndrome: extensive small bowel vascular lesions responsible for gastrointestinal bleeding. J Pediatr Child Health 46:63–65, 2010. Fig 3.)*

between the chemical guaiac and oxidizing action of a substrate (hemoglobin), giving a blue color. The guaiac test is very sensitive, but random testing can miss chronic blood loss, which can lead to iron-deficiency anemia. GI hemorrhage can produce hypotension and tachycardia but rarely causes GI symptoms; brisk duodenal or gastric bleeding can lead to nausea, vomiting, or diarrhea. The breakdown products of intraluminal blood might tip patients into hepatic coma if liver function is already compromised and can lead to elevation of serum bilirubin.

ABDOMINAL DISTENTION AND ABDOMINAL MASSES

Enlargement of the abdomen can result from diminished tone of the wall musculature or from increased content: fluid, gas, or solid. Ascites, the accumulation of fluid in the peritoneal cavity, distends the abdomen both in the flanks and anteriorly when it is large in volume. This fluid shifts with movement of the patient and conducts a percussion wave. Ascitic fluid is usually a transudate with a low protein concentration resulting from reduced plasma colloid osmotic pressure of hypoalbuminemia and/or from raised portal venous pressure. In cases of portal hypertension, the fluid leak probably occurs from lymphatics on the liver surface and from visceral peritoneal capillaries, but ascites does not usually develop until the serum albumin level falls. Sodium excretion in the urine decreases greatly as the ascitic fluid accumulates, and thus additional dietary sodium goes directly to the peritoneal space, taking with it more water. When ascitic fluid contains a high protein concentration, it is usually an exudate caused by an inflammatory or neoplastic lesion.

When fluid distends the gut, either obstruction or imbalance between absorption and secretion should be suspected. The factors causing fluid accumulation in the bowel lumen often cause gas to accumulate too. The result may be audible gurgling noises. The source of gas is usually swallowed air, but endogenous flora can increase considerably in malabsorptive states and produce excessive gas when substrate reaches the lower intestine. Gas in the peritoneal cavity (pneumoperitoneum) is usually caused by a perforated viscus and can cause abdominal distention depending on the amount of gas leak. A tympanitic percussion note, even over solid organs such as the liver, indicates a large collection of gas in the peritoneum.

An abdominal organ can enlarge diffusely or be affected by a discrete mass. In the digestive tract, such discrete masses can occur in the lumen, wall, omentum, or mesentery. In a constipated child, mobile, nontender fecal masses are often found. Congenital anomalies, cysts, or inflammatory processes can affect the wall of the gut. Gut wall neoplasms are extremely rare in children. The pathologic enlargement of liver, spleen, bladder, and kidneys can give rise to abdominal distention.

Bibliography is available at Expert Consult.

Section **2**

The Oral Cavity

第二篇
口腔

Chapter **333**

Development and Developmental Anomalies of the Teeth

Vineet Dhar

第三百三十三章
牙齿发育和发育异常

中文导读

本章主要介绍了牙齿发育。具体描述了发生、组织分化–形态分化、钙化、萌生和与牙齿发育有关的异常；在萌生部分具体描述了与出牙方式有关的异常、新生牙、脱落失败；与牙齿发育有关的异常内容具体描述了数量的异常（无牙症、多生牙）、大小的异常（双生牙、融合牙、结合牙、巨牙症、小牙症）、形态异常（牙内陷、牙外翻、长冠牙、弯曲牙）、结构异常（牙釉质发育不全、牙本质形成不全、低钙化、发育不全、氟牙症）和颜色的异常（变色牙）及牙病。

Newborn infants do not have teeth for about first 6 mo after birth (predentate period). At this stage, the upper and lower alveolar ridges in the mouth, also known as gum pads, house the primary (deciduous) and some permanent tooth buds. The primary dentition period starts with eruption of the first primary tooth; all 20 primary teeth erupt by 3 yr of age. The permanent teeth start erupting around age of 6 yr, and the transition to full permanent dentition is completed by 13 yr of age. The transition time between primary and permanent dentition, when a mix of primary and permanent teeth are present, is referred to as mixed dentition.

DEVELOPMENT OF TEETH
Initiation
The primary teeth form in dental crypts that arise from a band of epithelial cells incorporated into each developing jaw. By 12 wk of fetal life, each of these epithelial bands (**dental laminae**) has 5 areas of rapid growth on each side of the maxilla and the mandible, seen as rounded, budlike enlargements. Organization of adjacent mesenchyme takes place in each area of epithelial growth, and the 2 elements together are the beginning of a tooth.

After the formation of these crypts for the 20 primary teeth, another generation of tooth buds forms lingually (toward the tongue); these will develop into the succeeding permanent incisors, canines, and premolars that eventually replace the primary teeth. This process takes place from approximately 5 mo of gestation for the central incisors to approximately 10 mo of age for the second premolars. On the other hand, the permanent first, second, and third molars arise from extension of the dental laminae distal to the second primary molars; buds for these teeth develop at approximately 4 mo of gestation, 1 yr of age, and 4-5 yr of age, respectively.

Histodifferentiation–Morphodifferentiation
As the epithelial bud proliferates, the deeper surface invaginates and a mass of mesenchyme becomes partially enclosed. The epithelial cells

differentiate into the ameloblasts that lay down an organic matrix that forms enamel; the mesenchyme forms the dentin and dental pulp.

Calcification

After the organic matrix has been laid down, the deposition of the inorganic mineral crystals takes place from several sites of calcification that later coalesce. The characteristics of the inorganic portions of a tooth can be altered by disturbances in formation of the matrix, decreased availability of minerals, or the incorporation of foreign materials. Such disturbances can affect the color, texture, or thickness of the tooth surface. Calcification of primary teeth begins at 3-4 mo in utero and concludes postnatally at approximately 12 mo, with mineralization of the second primary molars (Table 333.1).

Eruption

At the time of tooth bud formation, each tooth begins a continuous movement toward the oral cavity. Table 333.1 lists the times of eruption of the primary and permanent teeth.

Anomalies Associated With Eruption Pattern: Delayed eruption of the 20 primary teeth can be familial or indicate systemic or nutritional disturbances such as hypopituitarism, hypothyroidism, cleidocranial dysplasia, trisomy 21, and multiple other syndromes. Failure of eruption of single or small groups of teeth can arise from local causes such as malpositioned teeth, supernumerary teeth, cysts, or retained primary teeth. Premature *loss* of primary teeth is most commonly caused by premature *eruption* of the permanent teeth. If the entire dentition is advanced for age and sex, precocious puberty or hyperthyroidism should be considered.

Natal teeth are observed in approximately 1 in 2,000 newborn infants, usually in the position of the mandibular central incisors. Natal teeth are present at birth, whereas **neonatal teeth** erupt in the first mo of life. Attachment of natal and neonatal teeth is generally limited to the gingival margin, with little root formation or bony support. They may be a supernumerary or a prematurely erupted primary tooth. A radiograph can easily differentiate between the 2 conditions. Natal teeth are associated with cleft palate, Pierre Robin syndrome, Ellis-van Creveld syndrome, Hallermann-Streiff syndrome, pachyonychia congenita, and other anomalies. A family history of natal teeth or premature eruption is present in 15–20% of affected children.

Natal or neonatal teeth occasionally result in pain and refusal to feed and can produce maternal discomfort because of abrasion or biting of the nipple during nursing. If the tooth is mobile, there is a danger of detachment, with aspiration of the tooth. Because the tongue lies between the alveolar processes during birth, it can become lacerated (**Riga-Fede disease**). Decisions regarding extraction of prematurely erupted primary teeth must be made on an individual basis.

Exfoliation failure occurs when a primary tooth is not shed before the eruption of its permanent successor. Most often the primary tooth exfoliates eventually, but in some cases the primary tooth needs to be extracted. This occurs most commonly in the mandibular incisor region.

Anomalies Associated With Tooth Development

Both failures and excesses of tooth initiation are observed. Developmentally missing teeth can result from environmental insult, a genetic defect involving only teeth, or the manifestation of a syndrome.

Anomalies of Number: Anodontia, or absence of teeth, occurs when no tooth buds form (ectodermal dysplasia, or familial missing teeth) or when there is a disturbance of a normal site of initiation (the area of a palatal cleft). The teeth that are most commonly absent are the third molars, the maxillary lateral incisors, and the mandibular second premolars.

If the dental lamina produces more than the normal number of buds, **supernumerary teeth** occur, most often in the area between the maxillary central incisors. Because they tend to disrupt the position and eruption of the adjacent normal teeth, their identification by radiographic examination is important. Supernumerary teeth also occur with cleidocranial dysplasia (see Chapter 337) and in the area of cleft palates.

Anomalies of Size: Twinning, in which 2 teeth are joined together, is most often observed in the mandibular incisors of the primary dentition. It can result from gemination, fusion, or concrescence. **Gemination** is the result of the division of one tooth germ to form a bifid crown on a single root with a common pulp canal; an extra tooth appears to be present in the dental arch. **Fusion** is the joining of incompletely developed teeth that, owing to pressure, trauma, or crowding, continue to develop as 1 tooth. Fused teeth are sometimes joined along their entire length; in other cases a single wide crown is supported on 2 roots. **Concrescence** is the attachment of the roots of closely approximated adjacent teeth by an excessive deposit of cementum. This type of twinning, unlike the others, is found most often in the maxillary molar region.

Disturbances during differentiation can result in alterations in dental morphology, such as **macrodontia** (large teeth) or **microdontia** (small teeth). The maxillary lateral incisors can assume a slender, tapering shape (**peg-shaped laterals**).

Anomalies of Shape: Dens in Dente or **Dens Invaginatus** presents as *tooth within tooth* appearance, which results from invagination of inner enamel epithelium caused by disruption during morphodifferentiation,

Dens Evaginatus presents as an extra cusp on anterior or posterior teeth, which contains enamel, dentin, and sometimes even pulp tissue. In the anterior teeth the cusp is talon shaped and presents in the cingulum area.

Taurodontism is more common in permanent molars and is characterized by elongated pulp chamber with short stunted roots due to failure or late invagination of Hertwig epithelial root sheath. It may be associated with several syndromic conditions such as Down syndrome,

Table 333.1	Calcification, Crown Completion, and Eruption		
TOOTH	**FIRST EVIDENCE OF CALCIFICATION**	**CROWN COMPLETED**	**ERUPTION**
PRIMARY DENTITION			
Maxillary			
Central incisor	3-4 mo in utero	4 mo	7.5 mo
Lateral incisor	4.5 mo in utero	5 mo	8 mo
Canine	5.5 mo in utero	9 mo	16-20 mo
First molar	5 mo in utero	6 mo	12-16 mo
Second molar	6 mo in utero	10-12 mo	20-30 mo
Mandibular			
Central incisor	4.5 mo in utero	4 mo	6.5 mo
Lateral incisor	4.5 mo in utero	4¼ mo	7 mo
Canine	5 mo in utero	9 mo	16-20 mo
First molar	5 mo in utero	6 mo	12-16 mo
Second molar	6 mo in utero	10-12 mo	20-30 mo
PERMANENT DENTITION			
Maxillary			
Central incisor	3-4 mo	4-5 yr	7-8 yr
Lateral incisor	10 mo	4-5 yr	8-9 yr
Canine	4-5 mo	6-7 yr	11-12 yr
First premolar	1.5-1¾ yr	5-6 yr	10-11 yr
Second premolar	2-2¼ yr	6-7 yr	10-12 yr
First molar	At birth	2.5-3 yr	6-7 yr
Second molar	2.5-3 yr	7-8 yr	12-13 yr
Third molar	7-9 yr	12-16 yr	17-21 yr
Mandibular			
Central incisor	3-4 mo	4-5 yr	6-7 yr
Lateral incisor	3-4 mo	4-5 yr	7-8 yr
Canine	4-5 mo	6-7 yr	9-10 yr
First premolar	1¾-2 yr	5-6 yr	10-12 yr
Second premolar	2¼-2.5 yr	6-7 yr	11-12 yr
First molar	At birth	2.5-3 yr	6-7 yr
Second molar	2.5-3 yr	7-8 yr	11-13 yr
Third molar	8-10 yr	12-16 yr	17-21 yr

Modified from Logan WHG, Kronfeld R: Development of the human jaws and surrounding structures from birth to age 15 years. *J Am Dent Assoc* 20:379, 1993.

trichodento-osseous syndrome, ectodermal dysplasia (hypohidrotic), and amelogenesis imperfecta (hypomaturation-hypoplastic type).

Dilaceration is an abnormal bend or curve in root possibly due to trauma. It may be subsequent to injury to the primary predecessor tooth.

Anomalies of Structure: Amelogenesis imperfecta represents a group of hereditary conditions that manifest in enamel defects of the primary and permanent teeth without evidence of systemic disorders (Fig. 333.1). The teeth are covered by only a thin layer of abnormally formed enamel through which the yellow underlying dentin is seen. The primary teeth are generally affected more than the permanent teeth. Susceptibility to caries is low, but the enamel is subject to destruction from abrasion. Complete coverage of the crown may be indicated for dentin protection, to reduce tooth sensitivity, and for improved appearance.

Dentinogenesis imperfecta, or hereditary opalescent dentin, is a condition analogous to amelogenesis imperfecta in which the odontoblasts fail to differentiate normally, resulting in poorly calcified dentin (Fig. 333.2). This autosomal dominant disorder can also occur in patients with **osteogenesis imperfecta.** The enamel-dentin junction is altered, causing enamel to break away. The exposed dentin is then susceptible to abrasion, in some cases worn to the gingiva. The teeth are opaque and pearly, and the pulp chambers are generally obliterated by calcification. Both primary and permanent teeth are usually involved. If there is excessive wear of the teeth, selected complete coverage of the teeth may be indicated to prevent further tooth loss and improve appearance.

Localized disturbances of calcification that correlate with periods of illness, malnutrition, premature birth, or birth trauma are common. **Hypocalcification** appears as opaque white patches or horizontal lines on the tooth; **hypoplasia** is more severe and manifests as pitting or areas devoid of enamel. Systemic conditions, such as renal failure and cystic fibrosis, are associated with enamel defects. Local

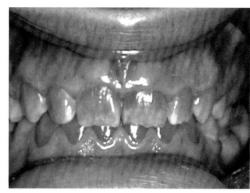

Fig. 333.2 Dentinogenesis imperfecta. The bluish, opalescent sheen on several of these teeth results from genetically defective dentin. This condition may be associated with osteogenesis imperfecta. *(From Nazif MM, Martin BS, McKibben DH, et al: Oral disorders. In Zitelli BJ, Davis HW, editors:* Atlas of pediatric physical diagnosis, *ed 4, Philadelphia, 2002, Mosby, p 703.)*

trauma to the primary incisors can also affect calcification of permanent incisors.

Fluorosis (mottled enamel) can result from systemic fluoride consumption >0.05 mg/kg/day during enamel formation. This high fluoride consumption can be caused by residing in an area of high fluoride content of the drinking water (>2.0 ppm), swallowing excessive fluoridated toothpaste, or inappropriate fluoride prescriptions. Excessive fluoride during enamel formation affects ameloblastic function, resulting in inconspicuous white, lacy patches on the enamel to severe brownish discoloration and hypoplasia. The latter changes are usually seen with fluoride concentrations in the drinking water >5.0 ppm.

Anomalies of Color: Discolored teeth can result from incorporation of foreign substances into developing enamel. Neonatal hyperbilirubinemia can produce blue to black discoloration of the primary teeth. Porphyria produces a red-brown discoloration. Tetracyclines are extensively incorporated into bones and teeth and, if administered during the period of formation of enamel, can result in brown-yellow discoloration and hypoplasia of the enamel. Such teeth fluoresce under ultraviolet light. The period at risk extends from approximately 4 mo of gestation to 7 yr of life. Repeated or prolonged therapy with tetracycline carries the highest risk.

Teething is associated with primary tooth eruption and may manifest with benign symptoms such as gingival hyperemia, irritability, sucking fingers, and drooling; some infants have no symptoms or symptoms not identified by their parents. Low-grade fever is an inconsistent finding. The treatment of symptoms of teething is often unnecessary but could include oral analgesics and iced teething rings. "Natural" (homeopathic) teething remedies may contain toxic additives and should be avoided.

Bibliography is available at Expert Consult.

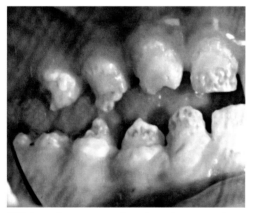

Fig. 333.1 Amelogenesis imperfecta, hypoplastic type. The enamel defect results in areas of missing or thin enamel, as well as grooves and pits.

Chapter 334
Disorders of the Oral Cavity Associated With Other Conditions

Vineet Dhar

第三百三十四章
与其他疾病相关的口腔疾病

中文导读

本章主要介绍了与其他疾病相关的口腔疾病。牙齿和周围结构的紊乱可以单独发生，也可以伴随其他系统性疾病发生，选择性列举了不同疾病状态下相关的牙齿问题。具体描述了唇裂、肾衰竭、囊性纤维化、免疫抑制、低出生体重、细菌性心内膜炎、中性粒细胞趋化性缺乏、1型糖尿病、神经运动功能障碍、牙齿形成期间的长期疾病（全身性）、癫痫发作、产妇感染、维生素D依赖等疾病状态下容易出现的牙齿或口腔问题。

Disorders of the teeth and surrounding structures can occur in isolation or in combination with other systemic conditions (Table 334.1). Most commonly, medical conditions that occur during tooth development can affect tooth formation or appearance. Damage to teeth during their development is permanent.

Table 334.1	Dental Problems Associated With Selected Medical Conditions

MEDICAL CONDITION	COMMON ASSOCIATED DENTAL OR ORAL FINDINGS
Cleft lip and palate	Missing teeth, extra (supernumerary) teeth, shifting of arch segments, feeding difficulties, speech problems
Kidney failure	Mottled enamel (permanent teeth), facial dysmorphology
Cystic fibrosis	Stained teeth with extensive medication, mottled enamel
Immunosuppression	Oral candidiasis with potential for systemic candidiasis, cyclosporine-induced gingival hyperplasia
Low birthweight	Palatal groove, narrow arch with prolonged oral intubation; enamel defects of primary teeth
Heart defects with susceptibility to bacterial endocarditis	Bacteremia from dental procedures or trauma
Neutrophil chemotactic deficiency	Aggressive periodontitis (loss of supporting bone around teeth)
Diabetes mellitus type I (uncontrolled)	Aggressive periodontitis
Neuromotor dysfunction	Oral trauma from falling; malocclusion (open bite); gingivitis from lack of hygiene
Prolonged illness (generalized) during tooth formation	Enamel hypoplasia of crown portions forming during illness
Seizures	Gingival enlargement if phenytoin is used
Maternal infections	Syphilis: abnormally shaped teeth
Vitamin D–dependent rickets	Enamel hypoplasia

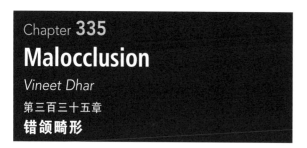

Chapter **335**
Malocclusion
Vineet Dhar
第三百三十五章
错颌畸形

中文导读

本章主要介绍了生长模式的改变、反咬合、开放性咬合和闭合性咬合、牙齿拥挤和吸手指。生长模式的改变部分具体描述了咬合角度的分型和针对不同咬合类型的治疗；反咬合部分具体描述了反咬合的概念和牙齿涉及范围；开放性咬合和闭合性咬合部分具体描述了开放性咬合和闭合性咬合的概念和治疗；牙齿拥挤部分详细描述了牙齿拥挤的发生时间；吸手指部分具体描述了吸手指的后果、患病率和治疗方法。

The oral cavity is essentially a masticatory instrument. The purpose of the anterior teeth is to bite off large portions of food. The posterior teeth reduce foodstuff to a soft, moist bolus. The cheeks and tongue force the food onto the areas of tooth contact. Establishing a proper relationship between the mandibular and maxillary teeth is important for both physiologic and cosmetic reasons.

VARIATIONS IN GROWTH PATTERNS
Growth patterns are classified into 3 main types of occlusion, determined when the jaws are closed and the teeth are held together (Fig. 335.1). According to the Angle classification of malocclusion, in **class I occlusion** (normal), the cusps of the posterior mandibular teeth interdigitate ahead of and inside of the corresponding cusps of the opposing maxillary teeth. This relationship provides a normal facial profile.

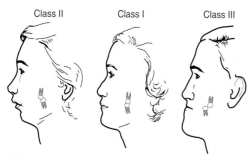

Class II   Class I   Class III

Fig. 335.1 Angle classification of occlusion. The typical correspondence between the facial-jaw profile and molar relationship is shown. *(Data from Borrie FR, Bearn DR, Innes NP, Iheozor-Ejiofor Z: Interventions for the cessation of non-nutritive sucking habits in children.* Cochrane Database Syst Rev 31(3):CD008694, 2015. doi: 10.1002/14651858. CD008694.pub2.)

In **class II malocclusion,** *buck teeth,* the cusps of the posterior mandibular teeth are behind and inside the corresponding cusps of the maxillary teeth. This common occlusal disharmony is found in approximately 45% of the population. The facial profile can give the appearance of a *receding chin* (retrognathia) (mandibular deficiency) or protruding front teeth. The resultant increased space between upper and lower anterior teeth encourage finger sucking and tongue-thrust habits. In addition, children with pronounced class II malocclusions are at greater risks of damage to the incisors as a consequence of trauma. Treatment includes orthodontic retraction of the maxilla or stimulation of the mandible.

In **class III malocclusion,** *underbite,* the cusps of the posterior mandibular teeth interdigitate a tooth or more ahead of their opposing maxillary counterparts. The anterior teeth appear in crossbite with the mandibular incisors protruding beyond the maxillary incisors. The facial profile gives the appearance of a *protruding chin* (**prognathia**) with or without an appearance of maxillary deficiency. If necessary, treatment includes mandibular excess reduction osteotomy or orthodontic maxillary facial protrusion.

CROSSBITE
Normally, the mandibular teeth are in a position just inside the maxillary teeth, so that the outside mandibular cusps or incisal edges meet the central portion of the opposing maxillary teeth. A reversal of this relation is referred to as a crossbite. Crossbites can be anterior, involving the incisors; can be posterior, involving the molars; or can involve single or multiple teeth.

OPEN AND CLOSED BITES
If the posterior mandibular and maxillary teeth make contact with each other, but the anterior teeth are still apart, the condition is called an *open bite.* Open bites can result from skeletal growth pattern or digit sucking. If digit sucking is terminated before skeletal and dental growth

is complete, the open bite might resolve naturally. If mandibular anterior teeth occlude inside the maxillary anterior teeth in an overclosed position, the condition is referred to as a *closed* or *deep bite*.

Treatment of open and closed bites consists of orthodontic correction, generally performed in the preteen or teenage years. Some cases require orthognathic surgery to position the jaws optimally in a vertical direction.

DENTAL CROWDING

Overlap of incisors can result when the jaws are too small or the teeth are too large for adequate alignment of the teeth. Growth of the jaws is mostly in the posterior aspects of the mandible and maxilla, and therefore inadequate space for the teeth at 7 or 8 yr of age will not resolve with growth of the jaws. Spacing in the primary dentition is normal and favorable for adequate alignment of successor teeth.

DIGIT SUCKING

Various and conflicting etiologic theories and recommendations for correction have been proposed for digit sucking in children. Prolonged digit sucking can cause flaring of the maxillary incisor teeth, an open bite, and a posterior crossbite. The prevalence of digit sucking decreases steadily from the age of 2 yr to approximately 10% by the age of 5 yr. The earlier the habit is discontinued after the eruption of the permanent maxillary incisors (age 7-8 yr), the greater the likelihood that there will be lessening effects on the dentition.

A variety of treatments have been suggested, from behavioral modification to insertion of an appliance with extensions that serves as a reminder when the child attempts to insert the digit. Unfortunately, a systematic review has found only low-quality evidence of the effectiveness of interventions such as orthodontic appliances and psychological interventions. The greatest likelihood of success occurs in cases in which the child desires to stop. Stopping of the habit will not rectify a malocclusion caused by a prior deviant growth pattern.

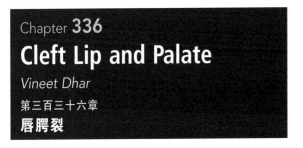

Chapter **336**
Cleft Lip and Palate
Vineet Dhar
第三百三十六章
唇腭裂

中文导读

本章主要介绍了唇腭裂的发病率和流行病学、临床表现、治疗、术后管理、后遗症和腭咽闭合功能障碍。发病率和流行病学中描述了导致唇腭裂发生的可能原因；临床表现中描述了唇腭裂的不同分型；治疗中描述了唇腭裂的婴儿喂养问题、手术治疗适应证和手术目标；后遗症中描述了后遗症的类型和对应的处理。在腭咽闭合功能障碍部分具体描述了腭咽闭合功能障碍的临床表现。

Clefts of the lip and palate are distinct entities which are closely related embryologically, functionally, and genetically. It is thought that cleft of the lip appears because of hypoplasia of the mesenchymal layer, resulting in a failure of the medial nasal and maxillary processes to join. Cleft of the palate results from failure of palatal shelves to approximate or fuse.

INCIDENCE AND EPIDEMIOLOGY

The incidence of cleft lip with or without cleft palate is approximately 1 in 750 white births; the incidence of cleft palate alone is approximately 1 in 2,500 white births. Clefts of the lip are more common in males. Possible causes include maternal drug exposure, a syndrome-malformation complex, or genetic factors. Although clefts of lips and palates appear to occur sporadically, the presence of susceptible genes appears important. There are approximately 400 syndromes associated with cleft lip and palates. There are families in which a cleft lip or palate, or both, is inherited in a dominant fashion (**van der Woude syndrome**), and careful examination of parents is important to distinguish this type from others, because the recurrence risk is 50%. Ethnic factors also affect the incidence of cleft lip and palate; the incidence is highest among Asians (~1 in 500) and Native Americans (~1 in 300) and lowest among blacks (~1 in 2,500). Cleft lip may be associated with other cranial facial anomalies, whereas cleft palate may be associated with central nervous system anomalies.

CLINICAL MANIFESTATIONS

Cleft lip can vary from a small notch in the vermilion border to a complete separation involving skin, muscle, mucosa, tooth, and bone. Clefts of the lip may be unilateral (more often on the left side) or bilateral and can involve the alveolar ridge (Fig. 336.1).

Isolated cleft palate occurs in the midline and might involve only the uvula or can extend into or through the soft and hard palates to the incisive foramen. When associated with cleft lip, the defect can involve the midline of the soft palate and extend into the hard palate on one or both sides, exposing one or both of the nasal cavities as a unilateral or bilateral cleft palate. The palate can also have a **submucosal cleft** indicated by a bifid uvula, partial separation of muscle with intact mucosa, or a palpable notch at the posterior of the palate (see Fig. 336.1).

TREATMENT

A complete program of habilitation for the child with a cleft lip or palate can require years of special treatment by a team consisting of a pediatrician, plastic surgeon, otolaryngologist, oral and maxillofacial surgeon, pediatric dentist, prosthodontist, orthodontist, speech therapist, geneticist, medical social worker, psychologist, and public health nurse.

The immediate problem in an infant born with a cleft lip or palate is feeding. Although some advocate the construction of a plastic obturator to assist in feedings, most believe that, with the use of soft artificial nipples with large openings, a squeezable bottle, and proper instruction, feeding of infants with clefts can be achieved.

Surgical closure of a cleft lip is usually performed by 3 mo of age, when the infant has shown satisfactory weight gain and is free of any oral, respiratory, or systemic infection. Modification of the Millard rotation–advancement technique is the most commonly used technique; a staggered suture line minimizes notching of the lip from retraction of scar tissue. The initial repair may be revised at 4 or 5 yr of age. Corrective surgery on the nose may be delayed until adolescence. Nasal surgery can also be performed at the time of the lip repair. Cosmetic results depend on the extent of the original deformity, healing potential of the individual patient, absence of infection, and the skill of the surgeon.

Because clefts of the palate vary considerably in size, shape, and degree of deformity, the timing of surgical correction should be individualized. Criteria such as width of the cleft, adequacy of the existing palatal segments, morphology of the surrounding areas (width of the oropharynx), and neuromuscular function of the soft palate and pharyngeal walls affect the decision. The goals of surgery are the union of the cleft segments, intelligible and pleasant speech, reduction of nasal regurgitation, and avoidance of injury to the growing maxilla.

In an otherwise healthy child, closure of the palate is usually done before 1 yr of age to enhance normal speech development. When surgical correction is delayed beyond the 3rd yr, a contoured speech bulb can be attached to the posterior of a maxillary denture so that contraction of the pharyngeal and velopharyngeal muscles can bring tissues into contact with the bulb to accomplish occlusion of the nasopharynx and help the child to develop intelligible speech.

A cleft palate usually crosses the alveolar ridge and interferes with the formation of teeth in the maxillary anterior region. Teeth in the cleft area may be displaced, malformed, or missing. Missing teeth or teeth that are nonfunctional are replaced by prosthetic devices.

POSTOPERATIVE MANAGEMENT

During the immediate postoperative period, special nursing care is essential. Gentle aspiration of the nasopharynx minimizes the chances of the common complications of atelectasis or pneumonia. The primary considerations in postoperative care are maintenance of a clean suture line and avoidance of tension on the sutures. The infant is fed with a specially designed bottle and the arms are restrained with elbow cuffs. A fluid or semifluid diet is maintained for 3 wk. The patient's hands, toys, and other foreign bodies must be kept away from the surgical site.

SEQUELAE

Recurrent otitis media and subsequent hearing loss are frequent with cleft palate. Displacement of the maxillary arches and malposition of the teeth usually require orthodontic correction. Misarticulations and velopharyngeal dysfunction are often associated with cleft lip and palate and may be present or persist because of physiologic dysfunction, anatomic insufficiency, malocclusion, or inadequate surgical closure of the palate. Such speech is characterized by the emission of air from the nose and by a hypernasal quality with certain sounds, or by compensatory misarticulations (glottal stops). Before and sometimes after palatal surgery, the speech defect is caused by inadequacies in function of the palatal and pharyngeal muscles. The muscles of the soft palate and the lateral and posterior walls of the nasopharynx constitute a valve that separates the nasopharynx from the oropharynx during swallowing and in the production of certain sounds. If the valve does not function adequately, it is difficult to build up enough pressure in the mouth to make such explosive sounds as p, b, d, t, h, y, or the sibilants s, sh, and ch, and such words as "cats," "boats," and "sisters" are not intelligible. After operation or the insertion of a speech appliance, speech therapy is necessary.

VELOPHARYNGEAL DYSFUNCTION

The speech disturbance characteristic of the child with a cleft palate can also be produced by other osseous or neuromuscular abnormalities where there is an inability to form an effective seal between oropharynx and nasopharynx during swallowing or phonation. In a child who has the potential for abnormal speech, adenoidectomy can precipitate overt hypernasality. If the neuromuscular function is adequate, compensation in palatopharyngeal movement might take place and the speech defect might improve, although speech therapy is necessary. In other cases, slow involution of the adenoids can allow gradual compensation in palatal and pharyngeal muscular function. This might explain why a speech defect does not become apparent in some children who have a submucous cleft palate or similar anomaly predisposing to palatopharyngeal incompetence.

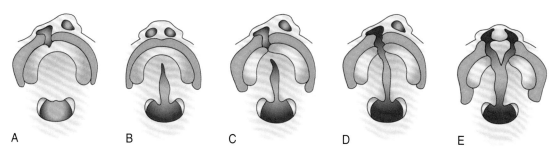

Fig. 336.1 Nonsyndromic orofacial clefts. **A,** Cleft lip and alveolus. **B,** Cleft palate. **C,** Incomplete unilateral cleft lip and palate. **D,** Complete unilateral cleft lip and palate. **E,** Complete bilateral cleft lip and palate. *(From Shaw WC: Orthodontics and occlusal management. Oxford, UK, 1993, Butterworth-Heinemann.)*

Clinical Manifestations

Although clinical signs vary, the symptoms of velopharyngeal dysfunction are similar to those of a cleft palate. There may be hypernasal speech (especially noted in the articulation of pressure consonants such as p, b, d, t, h, v, f, and s); conspicuous constricting movement of the nares during speech; inability to whistle, gargle, blow out a candle, or inflate a balloon; loss of liquid through the nose when drinking with the head down; otitis media; and hearing loss. Oral inspection might reveal a cleft palate or a relatively short palate with a large oropharynx; absent, grossly asymmetric, or minimal muscular activity of the soft palate and pharynx during phonation or gagging; or a submucous cleft.

Velopharyngeal dysfunction may also be demonstrated radiographically. The head should be carefully positioned to obtain a true lateral view; one film is obtained with the patient at rest and another during continuous phonation of the vowel u as in "boom." The soft palate contacts the posterior pharyngeal wall in normal function, whereas in velopharyngeal dysfunction such contact is absent.

In selected cases of velopharyngeal dysfunction, the palate may be retropositioned or pharyngoplasty may be performed using a flap of tissue from the posterior pharyngeal wall. Dental speech appliances have also been used successfully. The type of surgery used is best tailored to the findings on nasoendoscopy.

Bibliography is available at Expert Consult.

Chapter **337**

Syndromes With Oral Manifestations

Vineet Dhar

第三百三十七章

有口腔表现的综合征

中文导读

本章主要介绍了成骨不全、颅骨发育不良、外胚层发育不良、皮罗综合征、Stickler综合征、颌面骨发育不良、半侧颜面发育不全综合征等伴随有口腔表现的综合征。描述了牙本质生成不全的概念和治疗；描述了颅骨发育不良的特征；描述了外胚层发育不良的口腔表现；描述了皮罗综合征的处理措施；描述了Stickler综合征的临床表现；描述了颌面骨发育不良的临床表现。

Many syndromes have distinct or accompanying facial, oral, and dental manifestations (see Apert syndrome, Chapter 609.11; Crouzon disease, Chapter 609.11; Down syndrome, Chapter 98.2).

Osteogenesis imperfecta is often accompanied by effects on the teeth, termed **dentinogenesis imperfecta** (see Chapter 333, Fig. 333.2). Depending on the severity of presentation, treatment of the dentition varies from routine preventive and restorative monitoring to covering affected posterior teeth with stainless steel crowns, to prevent further tooth loss and improve appearance. Dentinogenesis imperfecta can also occur in isolation without the bony effects.

Another syndrome, **cleidocranial dysplasia,** has orofacial features such as frontal bossing, hypoplastic maxilla, and supernumerary teeth. The primary teeth can be overretained, and the permanent teeth remain unerupted. Supernumerary teeth are common, especially in the premolar area. Extensive dental rehabilitation may be needed to correct severe tooth crowding and unerupted and supernumerary teeth.

Ectodermal dysplasias are a heterogeneous group of conditions in which oral manifestations range from little or no involvement (the dentition is completely normal) to cases in which the teeth can be totally or partially absent or malformed (Chapter 668). Because alveolar bone does not develop in the absence of teeth, the alveolar processes can be either totally or partially absent, and the resultant overclosure of the mandible causes the lips to protrude. Facial development is otherwise not disturbed. Teeth, when present, can range from normal to small and conical. If aplasia of the buccal and labial salivary glands is present, dryness and irritation of the oral mucosa can occur. People with ectodermal dysplasia might need partial or full dentures, even at a very young age. The vertical height between the jaws is thus restored, improving the position of the lips and facial contours, as well as restoring masticatory function.

Pierre Robin syndrome consists of micrognathia and is usually accompanied by a high arched or cleft palate (Fig. 337.1). The tongue is usually of normal size, but the floor of the mouth is foreshortened. The air passages can become obstructed, particularly on inspiration, usually requiring treatment to prevent suffocation. The infant should be maintained in a prone or partially prone position so that the tongue falls forward to relieve respiratory obstruction. Some patients require

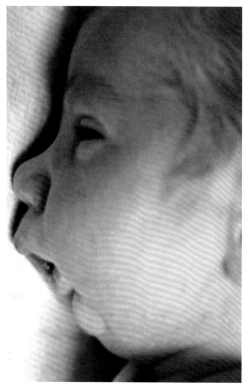

Fig. 337.1 Pierre Robin syndrome. *(From Clark DA: Atlas of neonatology, ed 7, Philadelphia, 2000, WB Saunders, p 144.)*

tracheostomy. Mandibular distraction procedures in the neonate can improve mandibular size, enhance respiration, and facilitate oral feedings.

Sufficient spontaneous mandibular growth can take place within a few months to relieve the potential airway obstruction. Often the growth of the mandible achieves a normal profile in 4-6 yr. Of children with Pierre Robin syndrome, 30–50% have **Stickler syndrome** (types I-VI), an autosomal dominant condition that includes other findings such as prominent joints, arthritis, hypotonia, hypermobile joints, mitral valve prolapse, hearing loss, spine problems (scoliosis, kyphosis, platyspondyly), and ocular problems (high myopia, glaucoma, cataracts, retinal detachment). Symptoms may vary greatly even with a family. Mutations are noted in the genes that produce collagen (*COL2A1* in most; *COL11A1* in others) in many, but not all, patients with Stickler syndrome. Other syndromes are associated with Pierre Robin syndrome, including 22Q11.2 deletion syndrome (velocardiofacial syndrome).

Mandibulofacial dysostosis (Treacher Collins syndrome or Franceschetti syndrome) is an autosomal dominant syndrome that primarily affects the face. The facial appearance varies but is characterized by downward-sloping palpebral fissures, colobomas of the lower eyelids, sunken cheekbones, blind fistulas opening between the angles of the mouth and the ears, deformed pinnae, atypical hair growth extending toward the cheeks, receding chin, and large mouth. Facial clefts, abnormalities of the ears, and deafness are common. The mandible is usually hypoplastic; the ramus may be deficient, and the coronoid and condylar processes are flat or even aplastic. The palatal vault may be either high or cleft. Dental malocclusions are common. The teeth may be missing, hypoplastic, or displaced or be in an open bite position. Initially, the primary concern is breathing and feeding problems. Surgery to restore normal structure of the face can be performed, which may include repair of cleft palate, zygomatic and orbit reconstruction, reconstruction of the lower eyelid, external ear reconstruction, and orthognathic surgery.

Hemifacial microsomia presentation can be quite variable but is usually characterized by unilateral hypoplasia of the mandible and can be associated with partial paralysis of the facial nerve, underdeveloped ear, and blind fistulas between the angles of the mouth and the ears. Severe facial asymmetry and malocclusion can develop because of the absence or hypoplasia of the mandibular condyle on the affected side. Congenital condylar deformity tends to increase with age. Early craniofacial surgery may be indicated to minimize the deformity. This disorder can be associated with ocular and vertebral anomalies (oculoauriculovertebral spectrum, including Goldenhar syndrome); therefore radiographs of the vertebrae and ribs should be considered to determine the extent of skeletal involvement.

Bibliography is available at Expert Consult.

Chapter **338**
Dental Caries
Vineet Dhar
第三百三十八章
龋齿

中文导读

　　本章主要介绍了龋齿的病因学、流行病学、临床表现、并发症、治疗和预防。病因学中描述了龋齿发生的过程；临床表现中描述了不同地区和不同年龄人群的龋齿发生率；并发症中描述了牙髓炎、牙周肿胀和牙齿严重感染的危险信号；治疗中描述了龋齿的修复方法；在预防部分具体描述了应用氟预防龋齿、口腔卫生、饮食和牙齿窝沟封闭等内容。

ETIOLOGY

The development of dental caries depends on interrelationships among the tooth surface, dietary carbohydrates, and specific oral bacteria. Organic acids produced by bacterial fermentation of dietary carbohydrates reduce the pH of dental plaque adjacent to the tooth to a point where demineralization occurs. The initial demineralization appears as an opaque **white spot lesion** on the enamel, and with progressive loss of tooth mineral, cavitation of the tooth occurs (Fig. 338.1).

The group of microorganisms, mutans streptococci, is associated with the development of dental caries. These bacteria have the ability to adhere to enamel, produce abundant acid, and survive at low pH. Once the enamel surface cavitates, other oral bacteria (lactobacilli) can colonize the tooth, produce acid, and foster further tooth demineralization.

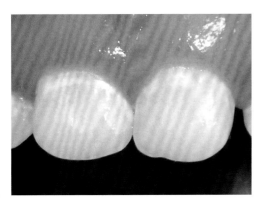

Fig. 338.1 Initial carious lesions (white spot lesions) around the necks of the maxillary central incisors.

Demineralization from bacterial acid production is determined by the frequency of carbohydrate consumption and by the type of carbohydrate. Sucrose is the most cariogenic sugar because one of its by-products during bacterial metabolism is glucan, a polymer that enables bacteria to adhere more readily to tooth structures. Dietary behaviors, such as consuming sweetened beverages in a nursing bottle or frequently consuming sticky candies, increase the cariogenic potential of foods because of the long retention of sugar in the mouth.

EPIDEMIOLOGY

As per the 2011–2012 National Health and Nutrition Examination Survey (NHANES), approximately 15% of children ranging from 2 to 8 yr of age had one or more primary teeth affected by dental caries (Fig. 338.2). In the permanent dentition, over 10% of children aged 12-15 yr had dental caries and one-fourth of children were affected by age 16-19 yr (Fig. 338.3).

CLINICAL MANIFESTATIONS

Dental caries of the primary dentition usually begins in the pits and fissures. Small lesions may be difficult to diagnose by visual inspection, but larger lesions are evident as darkened or cavitated lesions on the tooth surfaces (Fig. 338.4). Rampant dental caries in infants and toddlers, referred to as **early childhood caries**, is the result of early colonization of the child with cariogenic bacteria and the frequent ingestion of sugar, either in the bottle or in solid foods. The carious process in this situation is initiated earlier and consequently can affect the maxillary incisors first and then progress to the molars as they erupt.

The prevalence of untreated caries was significantly higher in children between 3 and 9 yr of age living at or below 100% of federal poverty level compared with those above the poverty level. Besides high frequency of sugar consumption and colonization with cariogenic bacteria, other enabling factors include low socioeconomic status of the family, other

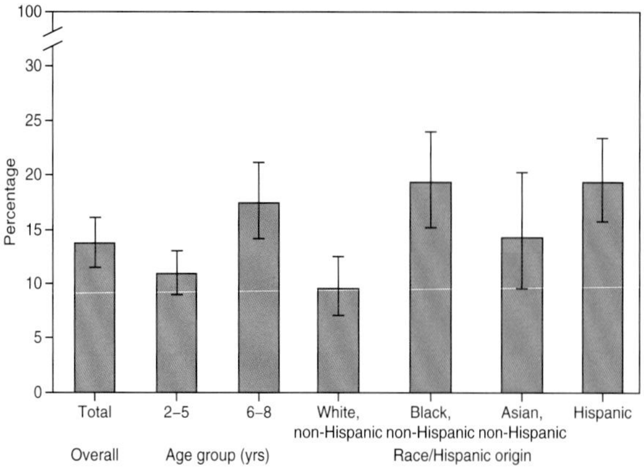

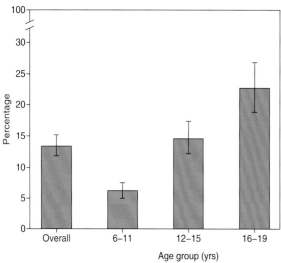

Fig. 338.2 Prevalence* of untreated dental caries† in primary teeth§ among children aged 2-8 yr, by age group and race/Hispanic origin—National Health and Nutrition Examination Survey, 2011-2014. *With 95% confidence intervals indicated with error bars. †Untreated dental caries is defined as tooth decay (dental cavities) that have not received appropriate treatment. Data were collected by dentists in the mobile examination center as part of the oral health component of the National Health and Nutrition Examination Survey. §Primary teeth are the first teeth (baby teeth), which are shed and replaced by permanent teeth. *(From Centers for Disease Control and Prevention: Prevalence of untreated dental caries in primary teeth among children aged 2-8 years, by age group and race/Hispanic origin—National Health and Nutrition Examination Survey, 2011–2014. MMWR 66(9):261, 2017.)*

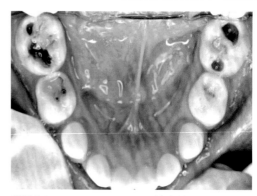

Fig. 338.4 Rampant caries in a 3 yr old child. Note darkened and cavitated lesions on the fissure surfaces of mandibular molars.

family member with carious teeth, recent immigrant status of the child, and the visual presence of dental plaque on the child's teeth. Children who develop caries at a young age are known to be at high risk for developing further caries as they get older. Therefore the appropriate prevention of early childhood caries can result in the elimination of major dental problems in toddlers and less decay in later childhood.

Among adolescents, the prevalence of dental caries experience was higher in age group 16-19 yr (67%) compared with age group 12-15 yr (50%). Overall, the caries experience did not significantly differ by race, Hispanic origin, and poverty levels.

COMPLICATIONS

Left untreated, dental caries usually destroy most of the tooth and invade the dental pulp (Fig. 338.5), leading to an inflammation of the pulp

Fig. 338.3 Prevalence* of untreated dental caries† in permanent teeth among children and adolescents aged 6-19 yr, by age group—National Health and Nutrition Examination Survey, United States, 2011-2014. *With 95% confidence intervals indicated with error bars. †Untreated dental caries (i.e., dental cavities) are defined as tooth decay that has not received appropriate treatment. Data were collected by dentists in the mobile examination center as part of the oral health component of the National Health and Nutrition Examination Survey. *(From Centers for Disease Control and Prevention: Prevalence of untreated dental caries in permanent teeth among children and adolescents aged 6-19 years, by age group—National Health and Nutrition Examination Survey, United States, 2011–2014. MMWR 66(1):36, 2017.)*

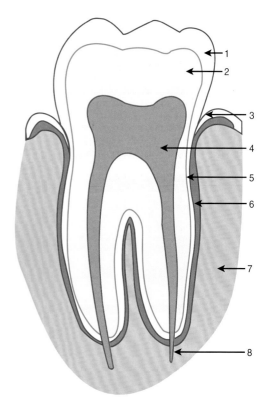

Fig. 338.5 Basic dental anatomy: *1,* enamel; *2,* dentin; *3,* gingival margin; *4,* pulp; *5,* cementum; *6,* periodontal ligament; *7,* alveolar bone; *8,* neurovascular bundle.

(pulpitis) and significant pain. Pulpitis can progress to pulp necrosis, with bacterial invasion of the alveolar bone causing a **dental abscess** (Fig. 338.6). Red flags for serious spreading of dental infection are noted in Table 338.1. Infection of a primary tooth can disrupt normal development of the successor permanent tooth. In some cases, this process leads to spread of infection to other facial spaces (Fig. 338.7).

TREATMENT

The age at which dental caries occurs is important in dental management. Children younger than 3 yr of age lack the developmental ability to

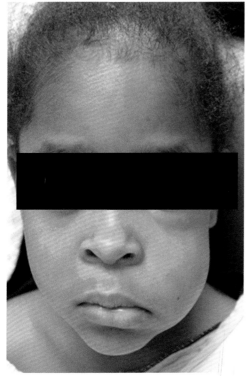

Fig. 338.6 Facial swelling from an abscessed primary molar. Resolution of the inflammation can be achieved by a course of antibiotics, followed by either extraction or root canal of the offending tooth.

Table 338.1	Red Flags Suggestive of a Spreading Dental Infection

- Pyrexia
- Tachycardia or tachypnea
- Trismus; may be relative due to pain or absolute due to a collection within the muscle causing muscle spasm in cases of masticator space involvement
- Raised tongue and floor of mouth, drooling
- Periorbital cellulitis
- Difficulty with speaking, swallowing, and breathing
- Hypotension
- Increased white blood cell count
- Lymphadenopathy
- Dehydration

From Robertson DP, Keys W, Rautemaa-Richardson R, et al: Management of severe acute dental infections. *BMJ* 350:h1300, 2015 (Box 3, p. 151).

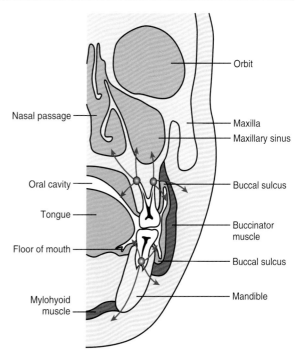

Fig. 338.7 Spread of infection in the maxillofacial region is complicated by the variety of vital structures. Routes of spread are determined by fascial planes and this affects the presentation and management of each subdivision of cervicofacial infection. *(From Robertson DP, Keys W, Rautemaa-Richardson R, et al: Management of severe acute dental infections.* BMJ *350:h1300, 2015. Fig. 3, p. 151.)*

cooperate with dental treatment and often require sedation or general anesthesia to repair carious teeth. After age 4 yr, children can generally cope with dental restorative care with the use of local anesthesia. Children with neurologic impairment or developmental delay may require general anesthesia for dental procedures at older ages.

Dental treatment, using silver amalgam, plastic composite, or stainless-steel crowns, can restore most teeth affected with dental caries. If caries involves the dental pulp, a partial removal of the pulp (pulpotomy) or complete removal of the pulp (pulpectomy) may be required. If a tooth requires extraction, a space maintainer may be indicated to prevent migration of teeth, which subsequently leads to malposition of permanent successor teeth.

Clinical management of the pain and infection associated with untreated dental caries varies with the extent of involvement and the medical status of the patient. Dental infection localized to the dento-alveolar unit can be managed by local measures (extraction, pulpectomy). Oral antibiotics are indicated for dental infections associated with fever, cellulitis, and facial swelling or if it is difficult to anesthetize the tooth in the presence of inflammation. Penicillin is the antibiotic of choice, except in patients with a history of allergy to this agent. Clindamycin and erythromycin are suitable alternatives. Oral analgesics, such as ibuprofen, are usually adequate for pain control.

PREVENTION

Dental caries screening, risk assessment, and preventive management in young children needs to be part of the scope of medical providers because children younger than 3 yr often are not under the care of a dentist. Prevention of early childhood caries is critical because, if primary dental care is not initiated or does not succeed, teeth may develop dental caries requiring restorative care. Dental restorative care to treat caries in young children may require the use of sedation or general anesthesia with its associated high costs and possible health risks, and there is high recurrence of carious lesions once they develop.

Because they are seeing infants and toddlers on a periodicity schedule, physicians have an important role in screening children younger than 3 yr of age for dental caries; providing preventive instructions; applying preventive measures, such as fluoride varnish; and referring the child to a dentist if problems exist.

Fluoride

The most effective preventive measure against dental caries is communal water supplies with optimal fluoride content. Water fluoridation at the level of 0.7-1.2 mg fluoride per liter (ppm F) was introduced in the United States in the 1940s. Because fluoride from water supplies is now one of several sources of fluoride, the Department of Health and Human Services proposes to not have a fluoride range, but instead to limit the recommendation to the lower limit of 0.7 ppm F. The rationale is to balance the benefits of preventing dental caries with reducing the chance of fluorosis. Children who reside in areas with fluoride-deficient water supplies or who consume primarily bottled water, and are at risk for caries, benefit from dietary fluoride supplements (Table 338.2). If the patient uses a private water supply, it is necessary to get the water tested for fluoride levels before prescribing fluoride supplements. To avoid potential overdoses, no fluoride prescription should be written for more than a total of 120 mg of fluoride. However, because of confusion regarding fluoride supplements among practitioners and parents, association of supplements with fluorosis, and lack of parent compliance

Table 338.2	Supplemental Fluoride Dosage Schedule		
	FLUORIDE IN HOME WATER		
AGE	**<0.3 (PPM)**	**0.3-0.6 (PPM)**	**>0.6 (PPM)**
6 mo-3 yr	0.25*	0	0
3-6 yr	0.50	0.25	0
6-16 yr	1.00	0.50	0

*Milligrams of fluoride per day.

with the daily administration, supplements may no longer be the first-line approach for preventing caries in preschool-aged children.

Topical fluoride on a daily basis can be achieved by using fluoridated toothpaste. Supervised use of less than a *pea-sized* amount of toothpaste (approximately 0.25 g) on the toothbrush in children between 3 and 6 yr of age reduces the risk of fluorosis. Children younger than 3 yr of age should brush with less than a *smear or grain-sized* amount of fluoridated toothpaste. Professional topical fluoride applications performed semiannually reportedly reduce caries by approximately 30%. Fluoride varnish is ideal for professional applications in preschool children because of ease of use, even with non–dental health providers, and its safety because of single-dose dispensers. Products that are available come in containers of 0.25, 0.4, or 0.6 mL of varnish, corresponding to 5.6, 9.0, and 13.6 mg fluoride, respectively. Fluoride varnish should be administered twice a year for preschool children at moderate caries risk and 4 times a year for children at high caries risk.

Oral Hygiene

Daily brushing, especially with fluoridated toothpaste, helps to prevent dental caries. Most children younger than 8 yr do not have the coordination required for adequate tooth brushing. Accordingly, parents should assume responsibility for the child's oral hygiene, with the degree of parental involvement appropriate to the child's changing abilities.

Diet

Frequent consumption of sweetened fruit drinks is not generally recognized by parents for its high cariogenic potential. Consuming sweetened beverages in a nursing bottle or sippy cup should be discouraged and special efforts made to instruct parents that their child should consume sweetened beverages only at meal times and not exceed 6 oz/day.

Dental Sealant

Plastic dental sealants have been shown to be effective in preventing caries on the pit and fissure of the primary and permanent molars. Sealants are most effective when placed soon after teeth erupt and used in children with deep grooves and fissures in the molar teeth. Sealants have been shown to reduce caries incidence by 85% over 7 yr.

Bibliography is available at Expert Consult.

Chapter **339**

Periodontal Diseases

Vineet Dhar

第三百三十九章

牙周疾病

中文导读

　　本章主要介绍了牙龈炎、儿童侵袭性牙周炎（青春期前牙周炎）、青少年侵袭性牙周炎、环孢素或苯妥英钠引起的牙龈增生、急性冠周炎和坏死性牙周病（急性坏死性溃疡性牙龈炎）。描述了牙龈炎的临床表现和治疗；描述了儿童侵袭性牙周炎的表现和治疗；描述了青少年侵袭性牙周炎的治疗；描述了环孢素或苯妥英钠引起的牙龈增生的临床表现；描述了急性冠周炎的治疗；描述了坏死性牙周病的临床表现和治疗。

The periodontium includes the gingiva, alveolar bone, cementum, and periodontal ligament (see Fig. 338.5).

GINGIVITIS

Poor oral hygiene results in the accumulation of dental plaque at the tooth-gingival interface that activates an inflammatory response, expressed as localized or generalized reddening and swelling of the gingiva. More than half of American school children experience gingivitis. In severe cases, the gingiva spontaneously bleeds and there is oral malodor. Treatment is proper oral hygiene (careful tooth brushing and flossing); complete resolution can be expected. Fluctuations in hormonal levels during the onset of puberty can increase inflammatory responses to plaque. Gingivitis in healthy children is unlikely to progress to periodontitis (inflammation of the periodontal ligament resulting in loss of alveolar bone).

AGGRESSIVE PERIODONTITIS IN CHILDREN (PREPUBERTAL PERIODONTITIS)

Periodontitis in children before puberty is a rare disease that often begins between the time of eruption of the primary teeth and the age of 4 or 5 yr. The disease occurs in localized and generalized forms. There is rapid bone loss, often leading to premature loss of primary teeth. It is often associated with systemic problems, including neutropenia, leukocyte adhesion or migration defects, hypophosphatasia, Papillon-Lefèvre syndrome, leukemia, and Langerhans cell histiocytosis. However, in many cases, there is no apparent underlying medical problem. Nonetheless, diagnostic workups are necessary to rule out underlying systemic disease.

Treatment includes aggressive professional teeth cleaning, strategic extraction of affected teeth, and antibiotic therapy. There are few reports of long-term successful treatment to reverse bone loss surrounding primary teeth.

AGGRESSIVE PERIODONTITIS IN ADOLESCENTS

Localized aggressive periodontitis (LAgP) in adolescents is characterized by rapid attachment and alveolar bone loss, on at least 2 first molars and incisors. Overall prevalence in the United States is <1%, but the prevalence among African Americans is reportedly 2.5%. This form of periodontitis is associated with a strain of *Aggregatibacter (Actinobacillus)* bacteria. In addition, the neutrophils of patients with aggressive periodontitis can have chemotactic or phagocytic defects. If left untreated, affected teeth lose their attachment and can exfoliate. Treatment varies with the degree of involvement. Patients whose disease is diagnosed at onset are usually managed by surgical or nonsurgical debridement in conjunction with antibiotic therapy. Prognosis depends on the degree of initial involvement and compliance with therapy.

Generalized aggressive periodontitis (GAgP) occurs more in adolescents and young adults and is characterized by generalized interproximal attachment loss and bone loss, including 3 teeth that are not first molars and incisors.

CYCLOSPORINE- OR PHENYTOIN-INDUCED GINGIVAL OVERGROWTH

The use of cyclosporine to suppress organ rejection or phenytoin for anticonvulsant therapy, and in some cases calcium channel blockers, is associated with generalized enlargement of the gingiva. Phenytoin and its metabolites have a direct stimulatory action on gingival fibroblasts, resulting in accelerated synthesis of collagen. Phenytoin induces less gingival hyperplasia in patients who maintain meticulous oral hygiene.

Gingival hyperplasia occurs in 10–30% of patients treated with phenytoin. Severe manifestations can include gross enlargement of the gingiva, sometimes covering the teeth; edema and erythema of the gingiva; secondary infection, resulting in abscess formation; migration of teeth; and inhibition of exfoliation of primary teeth and subsequent impaction of permanent teeth. Treatment should be directed toward prevention and, if possible, discontinuation of cyclosporine or phenytoin. Patients undergoing long-term treatment with these drugs should receive frequent dental examinations and oral hygiene care. Severe forms of gingival overgrowth are treated by gingivectomy, but the lesion recurs if drug use is continued.

ACUTE PERICORONITIS

Acute inflammation of the flap of gingiva that partially covers the crown of an incompletely erupted tooth is common in mandibular permanent molars. Accumulation of debris and bacteria between the gingival flap and tooth precipitates the inflammatory response. A variant of this condition is a gingival abscess caused by entrapment of bacteria because of orthodontic bands or crowns. Trismus and severe pain may be associated with the inflammation. Untreated cases can result in facial space infections and facial cellulitis.

Treatment includes local debridement and irrigation, warm saline rinses, and antibiotic therapy. When the acute phase has subsided, resection of the gingival flap prevents recurrence. Early recognition of the partial impaction of mandibular 3rd molars and their subsequent extraction prevents these areas from developing pericoronitis.

NECROTIZING PERIODONTAL DISEASE (ACUTE NECROTIZING ULCERATIVE GINGIVITIS)

Necrotizing periodontal disease, in the past sometimes referred to as "trench mouth," is a distinct periodontal disease associated with oral spirochetes and fusobacteria. However, it is not clear whether bacteria initiate the disease or are secondary. It rarely develops in healthy children in developed countries, with a prevalence in the United States of <1%, but is seen more often in children and adolescents from developing areas of Africa, Asia, and South America. In certain African countries, where affected children usually have protein malnutrition, the lesion can extend into adjacent tissues, causing necrosis of facial structures (cancrum oris, or noma).

Clinical manifestations of necrotizing periodontal disease include necrosis and ulceration of gingiva between the teeth, an adherent grayish pseudomembrane over the affected gingiva, oral malodor, cervical lymphadenopathy, malaise, and fever. The condition may be mistaken for acute herpetic gingivostomatitis. Dark-field microscopy of debris obtained from necrotizing lesions demonstrates dense spirochete populations.

Treatment of necrotizing periodontal disease is divided into an acute management with local debridement, oxygenating agents (direct application of 10% carbamide peroxide in anhydrous glycerol qid), and analgesics. Dramatic resolution usually occurs within 48 hr. If a patient is febrile, antibiotics (penicillin or metronidazole) may be an important adjunctive therapy. A second phase of treatment may be necessary if the acute phase of the disease has caused irreversible morphologic damage to the periodontium. The disease is not contagious.

Bibliography is available at Expert Consult.

Chapter **340**
Dental Trauma
Vineet Dhar

第三百四十章
牙齿外伤

中文导读

本章主要介绍了牙齿损伤、牙周组织损伤、预防和其他注意事项。在牙齿损伤部分描述了不同年龄段中引起牙齿损伤的常见原因、常见牙齿问题的处理和紧急情况；在牙周组织损伤部分描述了震荡、部分脱位、挫入、移位和脱出，其中具体描述了部分脱位的治疗、挫入的鉴别诊断、移位的特征和治疗、脱出的紧急处理。预防中详细描述了为减少牙齿受伤应该采取的措施。

Traumatic oral injuries may be categorized into 3 groups: injuries to teeth, injuries to soft tissue (contusions, abrasions, lacerations, punctures, avulsions, and burns), and injuries to jaw (mandibular and/or maxillary fractures).

INJURIES TO TEETH

Approximately 10% of children between 18 mo and 18 yr of age sustain significant tooth trauma. Oral injuries are second most common, covering 18% of all somatic injuries in the age group 0-6 yr. Among oral injuries,

injuries to teeth are most common, followed by soft tissue injuries. There appear to be 3 age periods of greatest predilection: toddlers (1-3 yr), usually from falls or child abuse; school-age children (7-10 yr), usually from bicycle and playground accidents; and adolescents (16-18 yr), often the result of fights, athletic injuries, and automobile accidents. Injuries to teeth are more common among children with protruding front teeth. Children with craniofacial abnormalities or neuromuscular deficits are also at increased risk for dental injury. Injuries to teeth can involve the hard dental tissues, the dental pulp (nerve), and injuries to the periodontal structure (surrounding bone and attachment apparatus) (Fig. 340.1; Table 340.1).

Fractures of teeth may be uncomplicated (confined to the hard dental tissues) or complicated (involving the pulp). Exposure of the pulp results in its bacterial contamination, which can lead to infection and pulp necrosis. Such pulp exposure complicates therapy and can lower the likelihood of a favorable outcome.

The teeth most often affected are the maxillary incisors. Uncomplicated crown fractures are treated by covering exposed dentin and by placing an aesthetic restoration. Complicated crown fractures involving the

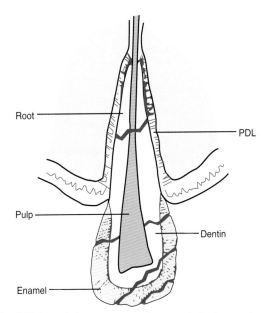

Root

PDL

Pulp

Dentin

Enamel

Fig. 340.1 Tooth fractures can involve enamel, dentin, or pulp and can occur in the crown or root of a tooth. *PDL*, periodontal ligament. *(From Pinkham JR: Pediatric dentistry: infancy through adolescence, Philadelphia, 1988, WB Saunders, p. 172.)*

tooth pulp usually require **endodontic therapy** (root canal). Crown-root fractures and root fractures usually require extensive dental therapy. Such injuries in the primary dentition can interfere with normal development of the permanent dentition, and therefore significant injuries of the primary incisor teeth are usually managed by extraction.

Traumatic oral injuries should be referred to a dentist as soon as possible. Even when the teeth appear intact, a dentist should promptly evaluate the patient. Baseline data (radiographs, mobility patterns, responses to specific stimuli) enable the dentist to assess the likelihood of future complications.

INJURIES TO PERIODONTAL STRUCTURES

Trauma to teeth with associated injury to periodontal structures that hold the teeth usually manifests as mobile or displaced teeth. Such injuries are more common in the primary than in the permanent dentition. Categories of trauma to the periodontium include concussion, subluxation, intrusive luxation, extrusive luxation, and avulsion.

Concussion

Injuries that produce minor damage to the periodontal ligament are termed *concussions*. Teeth sustaining such injuries are not mobile or displaced but react markedly to percussion (gentle hitting of the tooth with an instrument). This type of injury usually requires no therapy and resolves without complication. Primary incisors that sustain concussion can change color, indicating pulpal degeneration, and should be evaluated by a dentist.

Subluxation

Subluxated teeth exhibit mild to moderate horizontal mobility and/or vertical mobility. Hemorrhage is usually evident around the neck of the tooth at the gingival margin. There is no displacement of the tooth. Many subluxated teeth need to be immobilized by splints to ensure adequate repair of the periodontal ligament. Some of these teeth develop pulp necrosis.

Intrusion

Intruded teeth are pushed up into their socket, sometimes to the point where they are not clinically visible. Intruded primary incisors can give the false appearance of being avulsed (knocked out). To rule out avulsion, a dental radiograph is indicated (Figs. 340.2 and 340.3).

Extrusion

Extrusion injury is characterized by displacement of the tooth from its socket. The tooth is usually displaced to the lingual (tongue) side, with fracture of the wall of the alveolar socket. These teeth need immediate treatment; the longer the delay, the more likely the tooth will be fixed in its displaced position. Therapy is directed at reduction (repositioning the tooth) and fixation (splinting). The pulp of such teeth often becomes necrotic and requires endodontic therapy. Extrusive luxation in the

Table 340.1	Injuries to Crowns of Teeth	
TYPE OF TRAUMA	**DESCRIPTION**	**TREATMENT AND REFERRAL**
Enamel infraction (crazing)	Incomplete fracture of enamel without loss of tooth structure	Initially might not require therapy but should be assessed periodically by dentist
Enamel fractures	Fracture of only the tooth enamel	Tooth may be smoothed or treated to replace fragment
Enamel and dentin fracture	Fracture of enamel and dentinal layer of the tooth. Tooth may be sensitive to cold or air. Pulp may become necrotic, leading to periapical abscess	Refer as soon as possible. Area should be treated to preserve the integrity of the underlying pulp
Enamel, dentin fracture involving the pulp	Bacterial contamination can lead to pulpal necrosis and periapical abscess. The tooth might have the appearance of bleeding or might display a small red spot	Refer immediately. The dental therapy of choice depends on the extent of injury, the condition of the pulp, the development of the tooth, time elapsed from injury, and any other injuries to the supporting structures. Therapy is directed toward minimizing contamination in an effort to improve the prognosis

From Josell SD, Abrams RG: Managing common dental problems and emergencies. *Pediatr Clin North Am* 38:1325–1342, 1991.

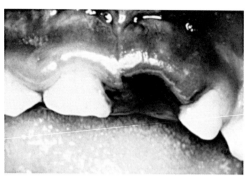

Fig. 340.2 Intruded primary incisor that appears avulsed (knocked out).

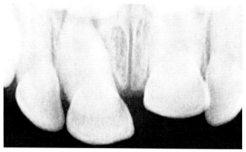

Fig. 340.3 Occlusal radiograph documents intrusion of "missing tooth" presented in Fig. 340.2.

primary dentition is usually managed by extraction because complications of reduction and fixation can result in problems with development of permanent teeth.

Avulsion

If avulsed permanent teeth are replanted as soon as possible after injury, there is a good chance that normal reattachment will follow and the tooth will have a good prognosis. However, if the tooth is in a dry environment for longer than 1 hr, the ligament that holds the tooth in place has little chance for survival and failure (root resorption, ankylosis) is common. Parents confronted with this emergency situation can be instructed to do the following:

◆ Find the tooth.
◆ Briefly rinse the tooth. (Do not scrub the tooth. Do not touch the root. After plugging the sink drain, hold the tooth by the crown and rinse it under running tap water.)
◆ Insert the tooth into the socket. (Gently place it back into its normal position. Do not be concerned if the tooth extrudes slightly. If the parent or child is too apprehensive for replantation of the tooth, the tooth should be placed in cold cow's milk or other cold isotonic solution.)
◆ Go directly to the dentist. (In transit, the child should hold the tooth in its socket with a finger. The parent should place the child in an age-appropriate child seat, buckle a seatbelt around the child, and drive safely.)

After the tooth is replanted, it must be immobilized to facilitate reattachment; endodontic therapy is always required. The initial signs of complications associated with replantation can appear as early as 1 wk after trauma or as late as several years later. Close dental follow-up is indicated for at least 1 yr.

PREVENTION

To minimize the likelihood of dental injuries:

◆ Every child or adolescent who engages in contact sports should wear a **mouth guard**, which may be constructed by a dentist or purchased at any athletic goods store.
◆ Helmets with face guards should be worn by children or adolescents with neuromuscular problems or seizure disorders to protect the head and face during falls.
◆ Helmets should also be used during biking, skiing, skating, and skateboarding.
◆ All children or adolescents with protruding incisors should be evaluated by a pediatric dentist or orthodontist.

ADDITIONAL CONSIDERATIONS

Children who experience dental trauma might also have sustained head or neck trauma, and therefore neurologic assessment is warranted. Tetanus prophylaxis should be considered with any injury that disrupts the integrity of the oral tissues. The possibility of child abuse should always be considered.

Bibliography is available at Expert Consult.

Chapter **341**
Common Lesions of the Oral Soft Tissues
Vineet Dhar

第三百四十一章
口腔软组织常见病变

中文导读

本章主要介绍了口咽念珠菌病、阿弗他溃疡、疱疹性牙龈炎、复发性唇疱疹、牙龈脓肿、唇炎、舌系带过短、地图舌、沟纹舌、发展（正常）变化。描述了口咽念珠菌病的诊断和预防；描述了阿弗他溃疡的病因和特征；描述了疱疹性牙龈炎的临床表现；描述了复发性唇疱疹的表现；描述了牙龈脓肿的治疗；描述了唇炎的诱因和治疗。正常发育部分具体描述了Bohn氏小结、牙板囊肿、Epstein氏小珠和Fordyce颗粒变化。

OROPHARYNGEAL CANDIDIASIS

Oropharyngeal infection with *Candida albicans* (thrush, moniliasis) (see Chapter 261.1) is common in neonates from contact with the organism in the birth canal or contact with the breast during breastfeeding. The lesions of oropharyngeal candidiasis (OPC) appear as white plaques covering all or part of the oropharyngeal mucosa. These plaques are removable from the underlying surface, which is characteristically inflamed and has pinpoint hemorrhages. The diagnosis is confirmed by direct microscopic examination on potassium hydroxide smears and culture of scrapings from lesions. OPC is usually self-limited in the healthy newborn infant, but topical application of nystatin to the oral cavity of the baby and to the nipples of breastfeeding mothers will hasten recovery.

OPC is also a major problem during myelosuppressive therapy. **Systemic candidiasis**, a major cause of morbidity and mortality during myelosuppressive therapy, develops almost exclusively in patients who have had prior oropharyngeal, esophageal, or intestinal candidiasis. This observation implies that prevention of OPC should reduce the incidence of systemic candidiasis. The use of oral rinses of 0.2% chlorhexidine gluconate solution along with systemic antifungals may be effective in preventing OPC, systemic candidiasis, or candidal esophagitis.

APHTHOUS ULCERS

The aphthous ulcer (canker sore) is a distinct oral lesion (Fig. 341.1), prone to recurrence; Table 341.1 notes the differential diagnosis. Aphthous ulcers are reported to develop in 20% of the population. Their etiology is unclear, but allergic or immunologic reactions, emotional stress, genetics, and injury to the soft tissues in the mouth have been implicated. Aphthous-like lesions may be associated with inflammatory bowel disease, Behçet disease, gluten-sensitive enteropathy, periodic fever-aphthae-pharyngitis-adenitis syndrome, Sweet syndrome, HIV infection (especially if ulcers are large and slow to heal), and cyclic neutropenia.

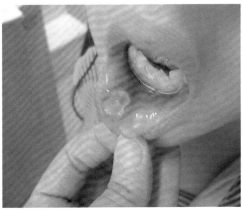

Fig. 341.1 Major aphthous in a child. *(From Gürkan A, Özlü SG, Altiaylik-Özer P, et al: Recurrent aphthous stomatitis in childhood and adolescence: a single-center experience. Pediatr Dermatol 32(4):476–480, 2015. Fig. 1.)*

Table 341.1	Differential Diagnosis of Oral Ulceration
CONDITION	**COMMENT**
COMMON	
Aphthous ulcers (canker sores)	Painful circumscribed lesions; recurrences
Traumatic ulcers	Accidents, chronic cheek biter, after dental local anesthesia
Hand, foot, and mouth disease	Painful; lesions on tongue, anterior oral cavity, hands, and feet
Herpangina	Painful; lesions confined to soft palate and oropharynx
Herpetic gingivostomatitis	Vesicles on mucocutaneous borders; painful, febrile
Recurrent herpes labialis	Vesicles on lips; painful
Chemical burns	Alkali, acid, aspirin; painful
Heat burns	Hot food, electrical
UNCOMMON	
Neutrophil defects	Agranulocytosis, leukemia, cyclic neutropenia; painful
Systemic lupus erythematosus	Recurrent; may be painless
Behçet syndrome	Resembles aphthous lesions; associated with genital ulcers, uveitis
Necrotizing ulcerative gingivostomatitis	Vincent stomatitis; painful
Syphilis	Chancre or gumma; painless
Oral Crohn disease	Aphthous-like; painful
Histoplasmosis	Lingual
Pemphigus	May be isolated to the oral cavity
Stevens-Johnson syndrome	May be isolated to or appear initially in the oral cavity

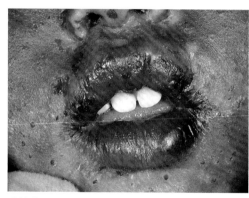

Fig. 341.2 Herpetic gingivostomatitis. Lip erosions with multiple perioral herpetic lesions involving the mucotaneous borders. *(From Paller AS, Mancini AJ, editors: Hurwitz clinical pediatric dermatology, ed 3, Philadelphia, 2006, WB Saunders, p. 398.)*

Clinically, these ulcers are characterized by well-circumscribed, ulcerative lesions with a white necrotic base surrounded by a red halo. The lesions generally last 10-14 days and heal without scarring. Nonprescription palliative therapies, such as benzocaine and topical lidocaine, are effective, as are topical steroids. Tetracycline has benefit with severe outbreaks, but caution is necessary in pregnant women, since it is classified as FDA pregnancy category D. In younger children (≤8 yr), tetracycline can affect developing teeth and cause permanent staining of the teeth.

HERPETIC GINGIVOSTOMATITIS

After an initial incubation period of approximately 1 wk, the primary infection with herpes simplex virus manifests as fever and malaise, usually in a child younger than 5 yr (see Chapter 279). The oral cavity can show various expressions, including the gingiva becoming erythematous, mucosal hemorrhages, and clusters of small vesicles erupting throughout the mouth. There is often involvement of the mucocutaneous margin and perioral skin (Fig. 341.2). The oral symptoms generally are accompanied by fever, lymphadenopathy, and difficulty eating and drinking. The symptoms usually regress within 2 wk without scarring. Fluids should be encouraged because the child may become dehydrated. Analgesics and anesthetic rinses can make the child more comfortable. Oral acyclovir, if taken within the first 3 days of symptoms in immunocompetent patients, is beneficial in shortening the duration of symptoms. Caution should be exercised to prevent autoinoculation, especially of the eyes.

RECURRENT HERPES LABIALIS

Approximately 90% of the worldwide population develops antibodies to herpes simplex virus. In periods of quiescence, the virus is thought to remain latent in sensory neurons. Unlike primary herpetic gingivostomatitis which manifests as multiple painful vesicles on the lips, tongue, palate, gingiva, and mucosa, recurrent herpes is generally limited to the lips. Other than the annoyance of causing pain and being a cosmetic issue, recurrent episodes generally do not involve systemic symptoms. Reactivation of the virus is thought to be the result of exposure to ultraviolet light, tissue trauma, stress, or fevers. There is little advantage of antiviral therapy over palliative therapies in an otherwise healthy patient affected by recurrent herpes.

PARULIS

The parulis (gum boil) is a soft reddish papule located adjacent to the root of a chronically abscessed tooth. It occurs at the end-point of a draining dental sinus tract. Treatment consists of diagnosing which tooth is abscessed and extracting it or performing root canal treatment on the offending tooth.

CHEILITIS

Cheilitis, dryness of the lips followed by scaling and cracking and accompanied by a characteristic burning sensation, is common in children. Cheilitis may be caused by sensitivity to contact substances, lip licking, vitamin deficiency, weakened immune system, or fungal or bacterial infections, and often occurs in association with fever. Treatment may include antifungal or antibacterial agents and frequent application of petroleum jelly.

ANKYLOGLOSSIA

Ankyloglossia, or tongue-tie, is characterized by an abnormally short lingual frenum that can hinder the tongue movement, but rarely interferes with feeding or speech. It is possible that the frenum could spontaneously lengthen as the child gets older. If, in the rare event that the extent of the ankyloglossia is severe, speech may be affected and surgical correction may be indicated.

GEOGRAPHIC TONGUE

Geographic tongue (migratory glossitis) is a benign and asymptomatic lesion that is characterized by one or more smooth bright red patches, often showing a yellow, gray, or white membranous margin on the dorsum of an otherwise normally roughened tongue. The condition has no known cause, and no treatment is indicated (see Chapter 684).

FISSURED TONGUE

The fissured tongue (scrotal tongue) is a malformation manifested clinically by numerous small furrows or grooves on the dorsal surface (see Chapter 684). If the tongue is painful, brushing the tongue or irrigating with water can reduce the bacteria in the fissures.

DEVELOPMENTAL (NORMAL) VARIATIONS
Bohn Nodules

Bohn nodules are small developmental anomalies located along the buccal and lingual aspects of the mandibular and maxillary ridges and in the hard palate of the neonate. These lesions arise from remnants of mucous gland tissue. Treatment is not necessary as the nodules usually disappear within a few weeks.

Dental Lamina Cysts

Dental lamina cysts are small cystic lesions located along the crest of the mandibular and maxillary ridges of the neonate. These lesions arise from epithelial remnants of the dental lamina. Treatment is not necessary; they disappear within a few weeks.

Epstein Pearls

Epstein pearls are small developmental lesions located in the median palatal raphe region due to entrapment of epithelial remnants along the line of fusion of the palatal halves. Treatment is not necessary as these slough off on their own within a few weeks.

Fordyce Granules

Fordyce granules are common and almost 80% of adults have these yellow-white granules in clusters or plaque-like areas on the oral mucosa, most commonly on the buccal mucosa or lips. They are aberrant sebaceous glands. The glands are present at birth, but they can undergo hypertrophy and first appear as discrete yellowish papules during the preadolescent period in approximately 50% of children. No treatment is necessary.

Bibliography is available at Expert Consult.

Chapter **342**
Diseases of the Salivary Glands and Jaws

Vineet Dhar

第三百四十二章
唾液腺和颌骨疾病

中文导读

　　本章主要介绍了腮腺炎、舌下囊肿、黏液囊肿、先天性唇凹、萌出囊肿、口腔干燥、唾液腺肿瘤、组织细胞紊乱和颌骨肿瘤。在腮腺炎部分，具体描述了急性腮腺炎、复发性腮腺炎和化脓性腮腺炎；描述了舌下囊肿的治疗；描述了黏液囊肿的治疗；描述了先天性唇凹的治疗；描述了口腔干燥的致病因素；在颌骨肿瘤部分，具体描述了骨化纤维瘤、中央巨细胞肉芽肿和牙源性囊肿。

With the exception of mumps (see Chapter 275), diseases of the salivary glands are rare in children. Bilateral enlargement of the submaxillary glands can occur in HIV/AIDS, cystic fibrosis, Epstein-Barr virus infection, malnutrition, and transiently during acute asthmatic attacks. Chronic vomiting can be accompanied by enlargement of the parotid glands. Benign salivary gland hypertrophy has been associated with endocrinopathies: thyroid disease, diabetes, and Cushing syndrome. Infiltrative disease or tumors are uncommon; red flags include facial nerve palsy, rapid growth, fixed skin, paresthesias, ulceration, or a history of radiation to the head or neck region.

PAROTITIS

Acute parotitis is often caused by blockage, with further inflammation due to bacterial infection. The blockage may be due to a salivary stone or mucous plug. Stones can be removed by physical manipulation, surgery, or lithotripsy. **Recurrent parotitis** is an idiopathic swelling of the parotid gland that can occur in otherwise healthy children. The swelling is usually unilateral, but both glands can be involved simultaneously or alternately. There is little pain; the swelling is limited to the gland and usually lasts 2-3 wk. Treatment may include local heat, massaging the gland, and antibiotics. **Suppurative parotitis** is usually caused by *Staphylococcus aureus*. It is usually unilateral and may be accompanied by fever. The gland becomes swollen, tender, and painful. Suppurative parotitis responds to antibacterial therapy based on culture obtained from the Stensen duct or by surgical drainage. Viral causes of parotitis include mumps (often in epidemics), Epstein-Barr virus, human herpesvirus 6, enteroviruses, and HIV.

RANULA

A ranula is a cyst associated with a major salivary gland in the sublingual area. It is a large, soft, mucus-containing swelling in the floor of the mouth. It occurs at any age, including infancy. The cyst should be excised, and the severed duct should be exteriorized.

MUCOCELE

Mucocele is a salivary gland lesion caused by a blockage of a salivary gland duct. It is most common on the lower lip and has the appearance of a fluid-filled vesicle, or a fluctuant nodule with the overlying mucosa being normal in color. Treatment is surgical excision, with removal of the involved accessory salivary gland.

CONGENITAL LIP PITS

Congenital lip pits are caused by fistulous tracts that lead to embedded mucous glands in the lower lip. They leak saliva, especially with salivary stimulation. Lip pits can be isolated anomalies, or they can be found in patients with cleft lip or palate. Treatment is surgical excision of the glandular tissue.

ERUPTION CYST

Eruption cyst is a smooth painless swelling over the erupting tooth. If bleeding occurs in the cyst space, it may appear blue or blue-black. In most cases, no treatment is indicated and the cyst resolves with the full eruption of the tooth.

XEROSTOMIA

Also known as dry mouth, xerostomia may be associated with fever, dehydration, anticholinergic drugs, chronic graft-versus-host disease, Mikulicz disease (leukemic infiltrates), Sjögren syndrome, or tumoricidal doses of radiation when the salivary glands are within the field. Long-term xerostomia is a high-risk factor for dental caries.

SALIVARY GLAND TUMORS

See Chapter 527.

HISTIOCYTIC DISORDERS

See Chapter 534.

TUMORS OF THE JAW

Ossifying fibroma is a common benign tumor of the jaw. It is often asymptomatic, being discovered on routine radiographic examinations. Treatment is resection due to the possibility of recurrence. **Central giant cell granuloma** is another common lesion thought to be reactive, rather than neoplastic. Although usually asymptomatic, it can be expansile, with or without resorption of the roots of teeth and perforation of the cortical plate. Treatment is complete curettage or surgical excision. **Dentigerous cysts** are common lesions associated with the crown of an impacted or unerupted tooth. Although usually asymptomatic, they can become large and destructive. Treatment is surgical removal.

The malignant primary tumors of the jaw in children include Burkitt lymphoma, osteogenic sarcoma, lymphosarcoma, ameloblastoma, and, more rarely, fibrosarcoma.

Bibliography is available at Expert Consult.

Chapter **343**

Diagnostic Radiology in Dental Assessment

Vineet Dhar

第三百四十三章
牙科诊断放射学

中文导读

　　本章主要介绍了口腔内牙片、全景射线照相、头颅射线照相和牙锥形束CT扫描。口腔内牙片部分描述了口腔内牙片的功能和应用范围；全景射线照相部分描述了全景射线照相的功能和应用范围；头颅射线照相部分描述了头颅射线照相的概念和功能；牙锥形束CT扫描部分描述了牙锥形束CT扫描的优点和适应证。

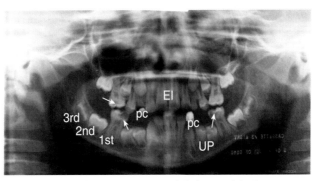

Fig. 343.1 A panoramic radiograph of a 10 yr old child showing extensive dental caries of the 1st permanent molars (*arrows*), as well as normal structures: erupted 1st permanent molar, unerupted 2nd molar, and unerupted 3rd molar; erupted incisors (*EI*), unerupted premolars (*UP*), and erupted primary canines (*pc*).

Diagnostic dental radiology in children follows the As Low As Reasonably Achievable (ALARA) principle. In children, intraoral radiographs such as bitewings and select periapical radiographs are taken during routine dental visits, and repeated every 6 mo to 2 yr based on the caries risk assessment. Additional radiographs such as panoramic views, cephalometric radiographs, and dental cone beam computed tomography (CBCT) are taken when indicated. In general, the cumulative radiation exposure due to routine dental radiographs is minimal. In addition, precautions such as use of high-speed film, collimated beam, protective aprons and thyroid collars, proper technique, and minimizing number of exposures, are all taken to keep radiation exposure minimal.

Intraoral dental radiographs are highly detailed, direct-exposure films that demonstrate sections of the child's teeth and supporting bone structures. The film or image receptor is placed lingual to the teeth, and the x-ray beam is directed through the teeth and supporting structures. The resulting images are used to detect dental caries, loss of alveolar bone (periodontal disease), abscesses at the roots of the teeth, and trauma to the teeth and alveolar bone. These radiographs are also used to demonstrate the developmental status of permanent teeth within the bone.

The **panoramic radiograph** provides a single tomographic image of the upper and lower jaw, including all teeth and supporting structures. The x-ray tube rotates about the patient's head with reciprocal movement of the film or image receptor during the exposure. The panoramic image shows the teeth, mandibular bodies, rami, and condyles; maxillary sinuses; and a majority of the facial buttresses. Such images are used to show abnormalities of tooth number, development and eruption pattern, cystic and neoplastic lesions, bone infections, and fracture, as well as dental caries and periodontal disease (see Fig. 343.1).

Cephalometric radiographs are posteroanterior and lateral skull films that are taken using a **cephalostat** (head positioner) and employ techniques that clearly demonstrate the facial skeleton and soft facial tissues. Similar protocols for positioning children are used throughout the world. From these images, cranial and facial points and planes can be determined and compared with standards derived from thousands of images. A child's facial growth can be assessed serially when cephalometric radiographs are taken sequentially. Relationships among the maxilla, mandible, cranial base, and facial skeleton can be determined in a quantitative manner. Additionally, the alignment of the teeth and the relation of the teeth to the supporting bone can be serially measured.

Dental CBCT is a variation of traditional computed tomography (CT), used mainly to evaluate oral and maxillofacial regions and teeth. Dental CBCT generally delivers lower radiation exposure than traditional CT, but higher than conventional dental radiography. There are several indications for CBCT, such as evaluation of oral-maxillofacial pathologies, diagnosis of dental trauma, endodontic treatment, visualization of abnormal teeth, orthodontic assessment, or cleft palate assessment, among others.

Bibliography is available at Expert Consult.

Section **3**

The Esophagus

第三篇

食管

Chapter **344**

Embryology, Anatomy, and Function of the Esophagus

Seema Khan and Sravan Kumar Reddy Matta

第三百四十四章

食管的胚胎学、解剖学和功能

中文导读

　　本章主要介绍了食管的胚胎学、解剖学和功能，常见的临床症状及辅助诊断。胚胎学部分具体描述了食管形成的过程；解剖学具体描述了食管腔黏膜的组成和变化、食管壁的组成、上下括约肌的结构；功能方面描述了吞咽过程的食管各部分及邻近咽喉部的变化；常见的临床症状包括疼痛、梗阻、吞咽困难、反流、出血；辅助诊断详细阐述了放射照相技术、内镜检查、组织学检查、闪烁照相术、压力测定、pH监测及多通道腔内阻抗测定等方法的优缺点及适应证。

The esophagus is a hollow muscular tube, separated from the pharynx above and the stomach below by two tonically closed sphincters. Its primary function is to convey ingested material from the mouth to the stomach. Largely lacking digestive glands and enzymes, and exposed only briefly to nutrients, it has no active role in digestion.

EMBRYOLOGY

The esophagus develops from the postpharyngeal foregut and can be distinguished from the stomach in the 4 wk old embryo. At the same time, the trachea begins to bud just anterior to the developing esophagus; the resulting laryngotracheal groove extends and becomes the lung. Disturbance of this stage can result in congenital anomalies such as **tracheoesophageal fistula.** The length of the esophagus is 8-10 cm at birth and doubles in the first 2-3 yr of life, reaching approximately 25 cm in the adult. The abdominal portion of the esophagus is as large as the stomach in an 8 wk old fetus but gradually shortens to a few millimeters at birth, attaining a final length of approximately 3 cm by a few years of age. This intraabdominal location of both the distal esophagus and the **lower esophageal sphincter** (LES) is an important antireflux mechanism, because an increase in intraabdominal pressure is also transmitted to the sphincter, augmenting its defense. Swallowing can be seen in utero as early as 16-20 wk of gestation, helping to circulate the amniotic fluid; **polyhydramnios** is a hallmark of lack of normal swallowing or of esophageal or upper gastrointestinal tract obstruction. Sucking and swallowing are not fully coordinated before 34 wk of gestation, a contributing factor for feeding difficulties in premature infants.

ANATOMY

The luminal aspect of the esophagus is covered by thick, protective, nonkeratinized stratified squamous epithelium, which abruptly changes to simple columnar epithelium at the stomach's upper margin at the

gastroesophageal junction (GEJ). This squamous epithelium is relatively resistant to damage by gastric secretions (in contrast to the ciliated columnar epithelium of the respiratory tract), but chronic irritation by gastric contents can result in morphometric changes (thickening of the basal cell layer and lengthening of papillary ingrowth into the epithelium) and subsequent metaplasia of the cells lining the lower esophagus from squamous to columnar. Deeper layers of the esophageal wall are composed successively of lamina propria, muscularis mucosae, submucosa, and the two layers of muscularis propria (circular surrounded by longitudinal). The two delimiting sphincters of the esophagus, the **upper esophageal sphincter (UES)** at the cricopharyngeus muscle and the **LES** at the **GEJ,** constrict the esophageal lumen at its proximal and distal boundaries. The muscularis propria of the upper third of the esophagus is predominantly striated, and that of the lower two-thirds is smooth muscle. Clinical conditions involving striated muscle (cricopharyngeal dysfunction, cerebral palsy) affect the upper esophagus, whereas those involving smooth muscle (achalasia, reflux esophagitis) affect the lower esophagus. The muscular LES and the mucosal "Z-line" of the GEJ may be discrepant up to several centimeters.

FUNCTION

The esophagus can be divided into 3 areas: the UES, the esophageal body, and the LES. At rest, the tonic LES pressure is normally approximately 20 mm Hg; values <10 mm Hg are usually considered abnormal, although it seems that competence against retrograde flow of gastric material is maintained if the LES pressure is >5 mm Hg. The LES pressure rises during intragastric pressure amplifications, whether caused by gastric contractions, abdominal wall muscle contractions ("straining"), or external pressure applied to the abdominal wall. It also rises in response to cholinergic stimuli, gastrin, gastric alkalization, and certain drugs (bethanechol, metoclopramide, cisapride). The UES pressure is more variable and often higher than that of the LES; it decreases almost to zero during deep sleep and it increases markedly during stress and straining. The UES and LES relax briefly to allow material to pass through during swallowing, belching, reflux, and vomiting. They can contract in response to subthreshold levels of reflux (esophagoglottal closure reflex).

Swallowing is initiated by elevation of the tongue, propelling the bolus into the pharynx. The larynx elevates and moves anteriorly, pulling open the relaxing UES, while the opposed aryepiglottic folds close. The epiglottis drops back to cover the larynx and direct the bolus over the larynx and into the UES. The soft palate occludes the nasopharynx. The primary peristalsis thus initiated is a contraction originating in the oropharynx that clears the esophagus aborally (Fig. 344.1). Oropharyngeal swallowing related dysfunction may occur at multiple levels (Table 344.1). The LES, tonically contracted as a barrier against gastroesophageal reflux (GER), relaxes as swallowing is initiated, at nearly the same time as the UES relaxation. The LES relaxation persists considerably longer, until the peristaltic wave traverses it and closes it. The normal esophageal peristaltic speed is approximately 3 cm/sec; the wave takes 4 sec or longer to traverse the 12 cm esophagus of a young infant and considerably longer in a larger child. Facial stimulation by a puff of air can induce swallowing and esophageal peristalsis in healthy young infants, a reflex termed the **Santmyer swallow.**

In addition to relaxing to move swallowed material past the GEJ into the stomach, the LES normally relaxes to vent swallowed air or to allow retrograde expulsion of material from the stomach. Perhaps as an extension of these functions, the normal LES also permits physiologic reflux episodes, brief events that occur approximately 5 times in the first postprandial hour, particularly in the awake state, but are otherwise uncommon. **Transient LES relaxation,** not associated with swallowing, is the major mechanism underlying **pathologic reflux** (see Fig. 344.1).

The close linkage of the anatomy of the upper digestive and respiratory tracts has mandated intricate functional protections of the respiratory tract during retrograde movement of gastric contents as well as during swallowing. The protective functions include the LES tone, the bolstering of the LES by the surrounding diaphragmatic crura, and the *backup protection* of the UES tone. Secondary peristalsis, akin to primary peristalsis but without an oral component, originates in the upper esophagus, triggered mainly by GER, and thereby also clears refluxed

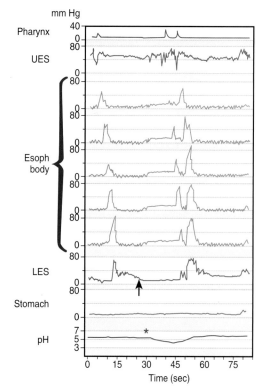

Fig. 344.1 A continuous tracing of esophageal motility showing 2 swallows, as indicated by the pharyngeal contraction associated with relaxation of the upper esophageal sphincter *(UES)* and followed by peristalsis in the body of the esophagus. The lower esophageal sphincter *(LES)* also displays a transient relaxation *(arrow)* unassociated with a swallow. There is an episode of gastroesophageal reflux *(*)* recorded by a *pH* probe at the time of the transient *LES* relaxation. *(Courtesy John Dent, FRACP, PhD and Geoffrey Davidson, MD.)*

Table 344.1	Mechanical Events of the Oropharyngeal Swallow and Evidence of Dysfunction
MECHANICAL EVENT	**EVIDENCE OF DYSFUNCTION**
Nasopharyngeal closure	Nasopharyngeal regurgitation Nasal voice
Laryngeal closure	Aspiration during bolus transit
Upper esophageal sphincter opening	Dysphagia Post-swallow residue/aspiration Diverticulum formation
Tongue loading and bolus propulsion	Sluggish misdirected bolus
Pharyngeal clearance	Post-swallow residue in hypopharynx/aspiration

Modified from Pandolfino JE, Kahrilas PJ: Esophageal neuromuscular function and motility disorders. In Feldman M, Friedman LS, Brandt LJ, editors: *Sleisenger and Fordtran's gastrointestinal and liver disease,* ed 10, New York, 2016, Elsevier (Table 43.1).

gastric contents from the esophagus. Another protective reflex is the *pharyngeal swallow* (initiated above the esophagus, but without lingual participation). Multiple levels of protection against aspiration include the rhythmic coordination of swallowing and breathing and a series of protective reflexes with esophagopharyngeal afferents and efferents that close the UES or larynx. These reflexes include the esophago-UES contractile reflex, the pharyngo-UES contractile reflex, the esophagoglottal closure reflex, and 2 pharyngoglottal adduction reflexes. The last 2 reflexes have chemoreceptors on the laryngeal surface of the epiglottis and mechanoreceptors on the aryepiglottic folds as their sites of stimulus. It is likely that interactions between the esophagus and the respiratory tract, which cause extraesophageal manifestations of gastroesophageal reflux disease (GERD), will be explained by subtle abnormalities in these protective reflexes.

Bibliography is available at Expert Consult.

344.1 Common Clinical Manifestations and Diagnostic Aids

Seema Khan and Sravan Kumar Reddy Matta

Manifestations of esophageal disorders include pain, obstruction or difficulty swallowing, abnormal retrograde movement of gastric contents (reflux, regurgitation, or vomiting), or bleeding; esophageal disease can also engender respiratory symptoms. Pain in the chest unrelated to swallowing (**heartburn**) can be a sign of esophagitis, but similar pain might also represent cardiac, pulmonary, or musculoskeletal disease or visceral hyperalgesia. Pain during swallowing (**odynophagia**) localizes the disease more discretely to the pharynx and esophagus and often represents inflammatory mucosal disease. Complete esophageal obstruction can be produced acutely by esophageal foreign bodies, including food impactions; can be congenital, as in esophageal atresia; or can evolve over time as a peptic stricture occludes the esophagus. Difficulty swallowing (**dysphagia**) can be produced by incompletely occlusive esophageal obstruction (by extrinsic compression, intrinsic narrowing, or foreign bodies) but can also result from dysmotility of the esophagus (whether primary/idiopathic or secondary to systemic disease). Inflammatory lesions of the esophagus without obstruction or dysmotility are a third cause of dysphagia; eosinophilic esophagitis, most often afflicting older boys, is relatively common.

The most common esophageal disorder in children is **GERD,** which is from retrograde return of gastric contents into the esophagus. **Esophagitis** can be caused by GERD, by eosinophilic disease, by infection, or by caustic substances. Esophageal **bleeding** can result from severe esophagitis that produces erosions or ulcerations and can manifest as anemia or Hemoccult-positive stools. More acute or severe bleeding can be from ruptured **esophageal varices.** The resulting hematemesis must be differentiated from more distal bleeding (gastric ulcer) and from more proximal bleeding (a nosebleed or hemoptysis). Respiratory symptoms of esophageal disease can result from luminal contents incorrectly being directed into the respiratory tract or to reflexive respiratory responses to esophageal stimuli.

DIAGNOSTIC AIDS

The esophagus can be evaluated by radiography, endoscopy, histology, scintigraphy, manometry, pH-metry (linked as indicated with other polysomnography), and multichannel intraluminal impedance. Contrast (usually barium) radiographic study of the esophagus usually incorporates fluoroscopic imaging over time so that motility and anatomy can be assessed. Although most often requested to evaluate for GERD, it is neither sensitive nor specific for this purpose; it can detect complications of GERD (stricture) or conditions mimicking GERD (pyloric stenosis or malrotation with intermittent volvulus), or concurrent hiatal hernia complicating GERD.

Barium fluoroscopy is optimal for evaluating for structural anomalies, such as duplications, strictures, hiatal hernia, congenital esophageal stenosis or external esophageal compression by an aberrant blood vessel, or for causes of dysmotility, such as achalasia. Modifications of the routine barium fluoroscopic study are used in special situations. When an *H-type* tracheoesophageal fistula is suspected, the test is most sensitive if the radiologist, with the patient prone, distends the esophagus with barium via a nasogastric tube. The videofluoroscopic evaluation of swallowing performed with varying consistencies of barium (modified barium swallow, oropharyngeal videoesophagram, or cookie swallow) optimally evaluates children with dysphagia by demonstrating incoordination of the pharyngeal and esophageal phases of swallowing and any associated aspiration.

In some centers, fiberoptic endoscopic evaluation of swallowing uses nasopharyngeal endoscopy to visualize the pharynx and larynx during swallowing of dye-enhanced foods when dysphagia, laryngeal penetration, or aspiration is suspected. This is often combined with sensory testing of the laryngeal adductor reflex in response to a calibrated puff of air through the endoscope to the arytenoids, generating the composite fiberoptic endoscopic evaluation of swallowing sensory testing that examines the mechanisms of any aspiration that is present. Endoscopy allows direct visualization of esophageal mucosa and helps therapeutically in the removal of foreign bodies and treatment of esophageal varices. Endoscopy also allows biopsy samples to be taken, thus improving the diagnosis of **endoscopy-negative GERD**, differentiating GERD from eosinophilic esophagitis, and identifying viral or fungal causes of esophagitis.

Radionuclide scintigraphy scans are helpful in evaluating the efficiency of peristalsis and demonstrating reflux episodes. They can be specific, although not very sensitive, for aspiration and can quantify gastric emptying, thus hinting at a cause for GERD. The related radionuclide salivagram can demonstrate aspiration of even minute amounts of saliva.

Esophageal manometry evaluates for dysmotility from the pharynx to the stomach; by synchronized quantitative pressure measurements along the esophagus, it detects and characterizes dysfunctions sometimes missed radiographically. Manometry is often challenging in young infants, and sphincters are optimally evaluated with special Dent sleeves, rather than the simple ports available for the esophageal body. High-resolution esophageal manometry (HRM) along with video fluoroscopic swallowing study (VFSS) to evaluate UES relaxation, pharyngeal and peristaltic pressures is now available at a few centers of expertise.

Extended pH monitoring of the distal esophagus is a sensitive test for acidic GER episodes that can quantify duration and degree of acidity, but not volume, of the reflux episodes. It is linked with polysomnography (a pneumogram) when GER is suspected to cause apnea or similar symptoms. Multichannel intraluminal impedance is a method for pH-independent detection of bolus movements in the esophagus; with a pH probe incorporated, it can distinguish between acid and nonacid liquid and gaseous reflux, the proximal extent of reflux, and several aspects of esophageal function, such as direction of bolus flow, duration of bolus presence, and bolus clearance.

Bibliography is available at Expert Consult.

Chapter **345**
Congenital Anomalies
第三百四十五章
先天畸形

中文导读

本章主要介绍了食管闭锁和气管食管瘘、喉气管食管裂和先天性食管狭窄。食管闭锁和气管食管瘘中具体描述了食管闭锁和气管食管瘘的分型及合并的其他先天性畸形的遗传和基因因素、临床表现、诊断、管理和预后；喉气管食管裂中描述了喉气管食管裂的胚胎学、临床表现、诊断及治疗；先天性食管狭窄中描述了先天性食管狭窄的发病率、分型、临床表现、诊断和治疗等内容。

345.1 Esophageal Atresia and Tracheoesophageal Fistula

Seema Khan and Sravan Kumar Reddy Matta

Esophageal atresia (EA) is the most common congenital anomaly of the esophagus, with a prevalence of 1.7 per 10,000 live births. Of these, >90% have an associated tracheoesophageal fistula (TEF). In the most common form of EA, the upper esophagus ends in a blind pouch and the TEF is connected to the distal esophagus (type C). Fig. 345.1 shows the types of EA and TEF and their relative frequencies. The exact cause is still unknown; associated features include advanced maternal age, European ethnicity, obesity, low socioeconomic status, and tobacco smoking. This defect has survival rates of >90%, owing largely to improved neonatal intensive care, earlier recognition, and appropriate intervention. Infants weighing <1,500 g at birth and those with severe associated cardiac anomalies have the highest risk for mortality. Fifty percent of infants are nonsyndromic without other anomalies, and the rest have associated anomalies, most often associated with the vertebral, anorectal, (cardiac), tracheal, esophageal, renal, radial, (limb) (VACTERL) syndrome. Cardiac and vertebral anomalies are seen in 32% and 24%, respectively. VACTERL is generally associated with normal intelligence. Despite low concordance among twins and the low incidence of familial cases, genetic factors have a role in the pathogenesis of TEF in some patients as suggested by discrete mutations in syndromic cases: Feingold syndrome *(N-MYC)*, CHARGE syndrome (*c*oloboma of the eye; *c*entral nervous system anomalies; *h*eart defects; *a*tresia of the choanae; *r*etardation of growth and/or development; *g*enital and/or urinary defects [hypogonadism]; *e*ar anomalies and/or deafness) *(CHD7)*, and anophthalmia-esophageal-genital syndrome *(SOX2)*.

PRESENTATION

The neonate with EA typically has frothing and bubbling at the mouth and nose after birth as well as episodes of coughing, cyanosis, and respiratory distress. Feeding exacerbates these symptoms, causes regurgitation, and can precipitate aspiration. Aspiration of gastric contents via a distal fistula causes more damaging pneumonitis than aspiration of pharyngeal secretions from the blind upper pouch. The infant with an isolated TEF in the absence of EA ("H-type" fistula) might come to medical attention later in life with chronic respiratory problems, including refractory bronchospasm and recurrent pneumonias.

DIAGNOSIS

In the setting of early-onset respiratory distress, the inability to pass a nasogastric or orogastric tube in the newborn suggests EA. Imaging findings of absence of the fetal stomach bubble and maternal polyhydramnios might alert the physician to EA before birth. Plain radiography in the evaluation of respiratory distress might reveal a coiled feeding tube in the esophageal pouch and/or an air-distended stomach, indicating the presence of a coexisting TEF (Fig. 345.2). Conversely, pure EA can manifest as an airless scaphoid abdomen. In isolated TEF (H type), an esophagogram with contrast medium injected under pressure can demonstrate the defect (Fig. 345.3). Alternatively, the orifice may be detected at bronchoscopy or when methylene blue dye injected into

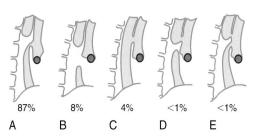

87%	8%	4%	<1%	<1%
A	B	C	D	E

Fig. 345.1 Diagrams of the 5 most commonly encountered forms of esophageal atresia and tracheoesophageal fistula, shown in order of frequency.

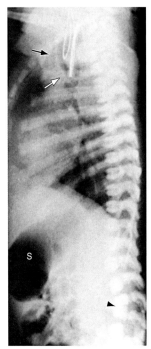

Fig. 345.2 Tracheoesophageal fistula. Lateral radiograph demonstrating a nasogastric tube coiled *(arrows)* in the proximal segment of an atretic esophagus. The distal fistula is suggested by gaseous dilation of the stomach *(S)* and small intestine. The *arrowhead* depicts vertebral fusion, whereas a heart murmur and cardiomegaly suggest the presence of a ventricular septal defect. This patient demonstrated elements of the vertebral, anorectal, tracheal, esophageal, renal, and radial anomalad. *(From Balfe D, Ling D, Siegel M: The esophagus. In Putman CE, Ravin CE, editors:* Textbook of diagnostic imaging, *Philadelphia, 1988, WB Saunders.)*

the endotracheal tube during endoscopy is observed in the esophagus during forced inspiration. The differential diagnosis of congenital esophageal lesions is noted in Table 345.1.

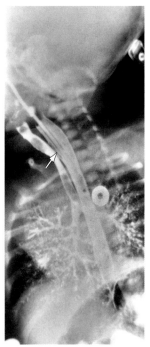

Fig. 345.3 H-type fistula *(arrow)* demonstrated in an infant after barium swallow on frontal-oblique chest x-ray. The tracheal aspect of the fistula is characteristically superior to the esophageal aspect. Barium is seen to outline the tracheobronchial tree. *(From Wyllie R, Hyams JS, editors:* Pediatric gastrointestinal and liver disease, *ed 3, Philadelphia, 2006, Saunders Elsevier, p. 299.)*

MANAGEMENT

Initially, maintaining a patent airway, pre-operative proximal pouch decompression to prevent aspiration of secretions, and use of antibiotics to prevent consequent pneumonia are paramount. Prone positioning

Table 345.1	Clinical Aspects of Esophageal Developmental Anomalies			
ANOMALY	**AGE AT PRESENTATION**	**PREDOMINANT SYMPTOMS**	**DIAGNOSIS**	**TREATMENT**
Isolated atresia	Newborns	Regurgitation of feedings Aspiration	Esophagogram* Plain film: gasless abdomen	Surgery
Atresia + distal TEF	Newborns	Regurgitation of feedings Aspiration	Esophagogram* Plain film: gas-filled abdomen	Surgery
H-type TEF	Infants to adults	Recurrent pneumonia Bronchiectasis	Esophagogram* Bronchoscopy[†]	Surgery
Esophageal stenosis	Infants to adults	Dysphagia Food impaction	Esophagogram* Endoscopy[†]	Dilation[‡] Surgery[§]
Duplication cyst	Infants to adults	Dyspnea, stridor, cough (infants) Dysphagia, chest pain (adults)	EUS* MRI/CT[†]	Surgery
Vascular anomaly	Infants to adults	Dyspnea, stridor, cough (infants) Dysphagia (adults)	Esophagogram* Angiography[†] MRI/CT/EUS	Dietary modification[‡] Surgery[§]
Esophageal ring	Children to adults	Dysphagia	Esophagogram* Endoscopy[†]	Dilation[‡] Endoscopic incision[§]
Esophageal web	Children to adults	Dysphagia	Esophagogram* Endoscopy[†]	Bougienage

TEF, tracheoesophageal fistula.
 *Diagnostic test of choice.
 [†]Confirmatory test.
 [‡]Primary therapeutic approach.
 [§]Secondary therapeutic approach.
 From Madanick R, Orlando RC: Anatomy, histology, embryology, and developmental anomalies of the esophagus. In Feldman M, Friedman LS, Brandt LJ, editors: *Sleisenger and Fordtran's gastrointestinal and liver disease,* ed 10, New York, 2016, Elsevier, Table 42.2.

minimizes movement of gastric secretions into a distal fistula, and esophageal suctioning minimizes aspiration from a blind pouch. Endotracheal intubation with mechanical ventilation is to be avoided if possible because it can worsen distention of the stomach. Surgical ligation of the TEF and primary end-to-end anastomosis of the esophagus via right-sided thoracotomy constitute the current standard surgical approach. In the premature or otherwise complicated infant, a primary closure may be delayed by temporizing with fistula ligation and gastrostomy tube placement. If the gap between the atretic ends of the esophagus is >3 to 4 cm (>3 vertebral bodies), primary repair cannot be done; options include using gastric, jejunal, or colonic segments interposed as a neoesophagus. Careful search must be undertaken for the common associated cardiac and other anomalies. Thoracoscopic surgical repair is feasible and associated with favorable long-term outcomes.

OUTCOME

The majority of children with EA and TEF grow up to lead normal lives, but complications are often challenging, particularly during the first 5 yr of life. Complications of surgery include anastomotic leak, refistulization, and anastomotic stricture. Gastroesophageal reflux disease, resulting from intrinsic abnormalities of esophageal function, often combined with delayed gastric emptying, contributes to management challenges in many cases. Gastroesophageal reflux disease contributes significantly to the respiratory disease (**reactive airway disease**) that often complicates EA and TEF and also worsens the frequent anastomotic strictures after repair of EA.

Many patients have an associated tracheomalacia that improves as the child grows. Hence, it is important to target on prevention of long-term complications using appropriate surveillance techniques (endoscopy, pH-Impedance).

Bibliography is available at Expert Consult.

345.2 Laryngotracheoesophageal Clefts
Seema Khan and Sravan Kumar Reddy Matta

Laryngotracheoesophageal clefts are uncommon anomalies that result when the septum between the esophagus and trachea fails to develop fully, leading to a common channel defect between the pharyngoesophagus and laryngotracheal lumen, thus making the laryngeal closure incompetent during swallowing or reflux. Other developmental anomalies, such as EA and TEF, are seen in 20% of patients with clefts. The severity of presenting symptoms depends on the type of cleft; they are commonly classified as four types (I-IV) according to the inferior extent of the cleft. Early in life, the infant presents with stridor, choking, cyanosis, aspiration of feedings, and recurrent chest infections. The diagnosis is difficult and usually requires direct endoscopic visualization of the larynx and esophagus. When contrast radiography is used, material is often seen in the esophagus and trachea. Treatment is surgical repair, which can be complex if the defects are long.

Bibliography is available at Expert Consult.

345.3 Congenital Esophageal Stenosis
Seema Khan and Sravan Kumar Reddy Matta

Congenital esophageal stenosis (CES) is a rare anomaly of the esophagus with clinical significance. Though the original incidence is not known, it is estimated to affect 1:25,000 to 50,000 live births. The defect results from incomplete separation of respiratory tract from the primitive foregut at 25th day of fetal life. CES is differentiated by histology into 3 types: esophageal membrane/web, total bronchial remnants (TBR), and fibromuscular remnants (FMR). Symptoms vary depending on the location and severity of the defect. Higher lesions present with respiratory symptoms and lower lesions present with dysphagia and vomiting.

Esophagogram (Fig. 345.4), MRI, CT, and endoscopic ultrasound are used for diagnosis. Endoscopy (Fig. 345.5) is done to evaluate mucosal abnormalities like strictures, foreign bodies, and esophagitis. Treatment option (surgical correction, bougie dilation) is chosen based on the location, severity, and type of stenosis.

Bibliography is available at Expert Consult.

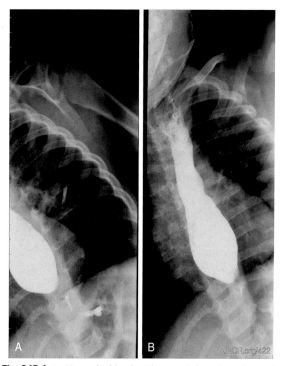

Fig. 345.4 An 18-month-old male with congenital esophageal stenosis. Esophagogram using barium as contrast media, shows an AP projection (**A**) and an unsuccessful attempt to obtain a lateral projection (**B**), due to poor collaboration of the patient. An asymmetric short narrowing of the distal esophagus is observed, as well as proximal dilatation of the esophagus. Gastroesophageal reflux was not identified. *(From Serrao E, Santos, A, Gaivao A: Congenital esophageal stenosis: a rare case of dysphagia, J Radiol Case Rep 4(6):8–14, 2010. Fig. 2).*

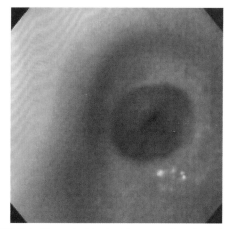

Fig. 345.5 An 18-month-old male with congenital esophageal stenosis. Esophagoscopy showed a circumferential, slightly non-central narrowing at the distal esophagus, 2 cm proximal to the esophagogastric junction. *(From Serrao E, Santos, A, Gaivao A: Congenital esophageal stenosis: a rare case of dysphagia, J Radiol Case Rep 4(6):8–14, 2010. Fig. 3).*

Chapter 346

Obstructing and Motility Disorders of the Esophagus

Seema Khan and
Sravan Kumar Reddy Matta

第三百四十六章

食管梗阻和运动障碍

中文导读

　　本章主要介绍了食管梗阻和运动障碍的外在因素和内在因素。比较了食管梗阻引起的吞咽困难和运动障碍引起的吞咽困难的不同特点；具体描述了外在因素包括食管重复囊肿、神经肠囊肿、纵隔或隆凸下淋巴结肿大、肿瘤、血管畸形等；引起食管腔狭窄的内在因素可能是先天性的或获得性的（溃疡性狭窄、薄膜环、气管食管瘘综合征、反流性食管炎、炎症性狭窄、嗜酸粒细胞性食管炎等）。

Obstructing lesions classically produce **dysphagia** to *solids* earlier and more noticeably than to liquids and can manifest when the infant liquid diet begins to incorporate solids; this contrasts to **dysphagia** from **dysmotility,** in which swallowing of *liquids* is affected as early as, or earlier than, solids. In most instances of dysphagia, evaluation begins with fluoroscopy, which may include videofluoroscopic evaluation of swallowing, particularly if aspiration is a primary symptom. Secondary studies are often endoscopic if intrinsic obstruction is suspected or manometric if dysmotility is suspected; other imaging studies may be used in particular cases. Congenital lesions can require surgery, whereas webs and peptic strictures might respond adequately to endoscopic (or bougie) dilation. Peptic strictures, once dilated, should prompt consideration of fundoplication for ongoing prophylaxis.

EXTRINSIC

Esophageal duplication cysts are the most commonly encountered foregut duplications (see Table 345.1). These cysts are lined by intestinal epithelium, have a well-developed smooth muscle wall, and are attached to the normal gastrointestinal tract. Most of these affect the distal half of the esophagus on the right side. The most common presentation is respiratory distress caused by compression of the adjacent airways. Dysphagia is a common symptom in older children. Upper gastrointestinal bleeding can occur as a result of acid-secreting gastric mucosa in the duplication wall. **Neuroenteric cysts** might contain glial elements and are associated with **vertebral anomalies.** Diagnosis is made using modalities, such as barium swallow, chest CT, and MRI, or endosonography. Treatment is surgical; laparoscopic approach to excision is also possible.

Enlarged mediastinal or subcarinal **lymph nodes,** caused by infection (tuberculosis, histoplasmosis) or neoplasm (lymphoma), are the most common external masses that compress the esophagus and produce obstructive symptoms. **Vascular anomalies** can also compress the esophagus; *dysphagia lusoria* is a term denoting the dysphagia produced by a developmental vascular anomaly, which is often an aberrant right subclavian artery or right-sided or double aortic arch (see Chapter 459.1).

INTRINSIC

Intrinsic narrowing of the esophageal lumen can be congenital or acquired. The etiology is suggested by the location, the character of the lesion, and the clinical situation. The lower esophagus is the most common location for peptic strictures, which are generally somewhat ragged and several cm long. Thin membranous rings, including the **Schatzki ring** at the squamocolumnar junction, can also occlude this area. In the midesophagus, congenital narrowing may be associated with the esophageal atresia–tracheoesophageal fistula complex, in which some of the lesions might incorporate cartilage and might be impossible to dilate safely; alternatively, reflux esophagitis can induce a ragged and extensive narrowing that appears more proximal than the usual peptic stricture, often because of an associated hiatal hernia. Congenital webs or rings can narrow the upper esophagus. The upper esophagus can also be narrowed by an inflammatory stricture occurring after a caustic ingestion or due to epidermolysis bullosa. Cricopharyngeal achalasia can appear radiographically as a cricopharyngeal bar posteriorly in the upper esophagus. **Eosinophilic** esophagitis is one of the most common causes for esophageal obstructive symptoms. Although the pathogenesis of obstructive eosinophilic esophagitis is not yet completely explained and seems to vary among individual patients, endoscopy or radiology demonstrates stricture formation in some children with eosinophilic esophagitis, and in others a noncompliant esophagus is evident, with thickened wall layers demonstrable by ultrasonography.

Bibliography is available at Expert Consult.

Chapter **347**
Dysmotility

Seema Khan and
Sravan Kumar Reddy Matta

第三百四十七章
运动障碍

中文导读

　　本章主要介绍了食管上段和食管上括约肌运动障碍（横纹肌）、食管下段和食管下括约肌运动障碍（平滑肌）。具体描述了环咽失迟缓症的定义以及与环咽肌不协调运动的区别、压力测定是确诊方法、婴儿和儿童环咽失迟缓症治疗的方法、鉴别诊断以及病因等；具体描述引起食管远端运动障碍的原发因素和继发因素、贲门失迟缓的可能原因、病理、临床表现、诊断方法以及治疗等内容。

UPPER ESOPHAGEAL AND UPPER ESOPHAGEAL SPHINCTER DYSMOTILITY (STRIATED MUSCLE)

Cricopharyngeal **achalasia** signifies a failure of complete relaxation of the upper esophageal sphincter (UES), whereas cricopharyngeal **incoordination** implies full relaxation of the UES but incoordination of the relaxation with the pharyngeal contraction. These entities are usually detected on videofluoroscopic evaluation of swallowing (sometimes accompanied by visible cricopharyngeal prominence, termed a *bar*), but often the most precise definition of the dysfunction is obtained with manometry. A self-limited form of cricopharyngeal incoordination occurs in infancy and remits spontaneously in the 1st yr of life if nutrition is maintained despite the dysphagia. In children, treatment options for non-self-limited cricopharyngeal achalasia consist of dilation, Botox injection, and transcervical myotomy. It is important to evaluate such children thoroughly, including cranial MRI to detect **Arnold-Chiari malformations,** which can manifest in this way but are best treated by cranial decompression rather than esophageal surgery. Cricopharyngeal spasm may be severe enough to produce posterior pharyngeal (**Zenker**) **diverticulum** above the obstructive sphincter; this entity occurs rarely in children.

Systemic causes of swallowing dysfunction that can affect the oropharynx, UES, and upper esophagus include cerebral palsy, Arnold-Chiari malformations, syringomyelia, bulbar palsy or cranial nerve defects (Möbius syndrome, transient infantile paralysis of the superior laryngeal nerve), transient pharyngeal muscle dysfunction, spinal muscular atrophy (including Werdnig-Hoffmann disease), muscular dystrophy, multiple sclerosis, infections (botulism, tetanus, poliomyelitis, diphtheria), inflammatory and autoimmune diseases (dermatomyositis, myasthenia gravis, polyneuritis, scleroderma), and familial dysautonomia. All of these can produce dysphagia. Medications (nitrazepam, benzodiazepines) and tracheostomy can adversely affect the function of the UES and thereby produce dysphagia.

LOWER ESOPHAGEAL AND LOWER ESOPHAGEAL SPHINCTER DYSFUNCTION (SMOOTH MUSCLE)

Causes of dysphagia resulting from more distal primary esophageal dysmotility include achalasia, diffuse esophageal spasm, nutcracker esophagus, and hypertensive lower esophageal sphincter (LES); all but achalasia are rare in children. Secondary causes include Hirschsprung disease, pseudoobstruction, inflammatory myopathies, scleroderma, and diabetes.

Achalasia is a primary esophageal motor disorder of unknown etiology characterized by loss of LES relaxation and loss of esophageal peristalsis, both contributing to a functional obstruction of the distal esophagus.

Degenerative, autoimmune (antibodies to Auerbach plexus), and infectious (Chagas disease caused by *Trypanosoma cruzi*) factors are possible causes. In rare cases, achalasia is familial or part of the achalasia, alacrima, and adrenal insufficiency, known as triple A syndrome or **Allgrove syndrome**. *Pseudoachalasia* refers to achalasia caused by various forms of cancer via obstruction of the gastroesophageal junction, infiltration of the submucosa and muscularis of the LES, or as part of the paraneoplastic syndrome with formation of anti-Hu antibodies. Pathologically, in achalasia, inflammation surrounds ganglion cells, which are decreased in number. There is selective loss of postganglionic inhibitory neurons that normally lead to sphincter relaxation, leaving postganglionic cholinergic neurons unopposed. This imbalance produces high basal LES pressures and insufficient LES relaxation. The loss of esophageal peristalsis can be a secondary phenomenon.

Achalasia manifests with regurgitation and dysphagia for solids and liquids and may be accompanied by undernutrition or chronic cough; retained esophageal food can produce esophagitis. *The presentations of chronic regurgitation/vomiting with weight loss, and chronic cough have led to misdiagnoses of anorexia nervosa and asthma, respectively.* The mean age in children is 8.8 yr, with a mean duration of symptoms before diagnosis of 23 mo; it is uncommon before school age. Chest radiograph shows an air–fluid level in a dilated esophagus. **Barium fluoroscopy** reveals a smooth tapering of the lower esophagus leading to the closed LES, resembling a bird's beak (Fig. 347.1). Loss of primary peristalsis in the distal esophagus with retained food and poor emptying are often present. **Manometry** is the most sensitive diagnostic test and helps differentiate the three types of achalasia; it reveals the defining features of aperistalsis in the distal esophageal body and incomplete or absent LES relaxation, often accompanied by high-pressure LES and low-amplitude esophageal body contractions (Fig. 347.2).

The goals of achalasia therapy are relief of symptoms, improvement of esophageal emptying, and prevention of megaesophagus. The two most effective treatment options are pneumatic dilation and laparoscopic or surgical (Heller) myotomy. Pneumatic dilation is the initial treatment of choice and does not preclude a future myotomy. Surgeons often supplement a myotomy with an antireflux procedure to prevent the gastroesophageal reflux disease that otherwise often ensues when the sphincter is rendered less competent. Laparoscopic myotomy is a particularly effective procedure in adolescent and young adult males. Peroral endoscopic myotomy (POEM) may be a feasible, safe, and an effective alternative to the laparoscopic method. Calcium channel blockers (nifedipine) and phosphodiesterase inhibitors offer temporary relief of dysphagia. Endoscopic injection of the LES with **botulinum toxin** counterbalances the selective loss of inhibitory neurotransmitters by inhibiting the release of acetylcholine from

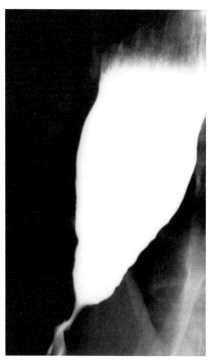

Fig. 347.1 Barium esophagogram of a patient with achalasia demonstrating dilated esophagus and narrowing at the lower esophageal sphincter. Note retained secretions layered on top of barium in the esophagus.

nerve terminals and may be an effective therapy. Botulinum toxin is effective in 50–65% of patients and is expensive; half the patients might require a repeat injection within 1 yr. Most eventually require dilation or surgery.

Diffuse esophageal spasm causes chest pain and dysphagia and affects adolescents and adults. It is diagnosed **manometrically** and can be treated with nitrates or calcium-channel-blocking agents.

Gastroesophageal reflux disease constitutes the most common cause of nonspecific abnormalities of esophageal motor function, probably through the effect of the esophageal inflammation on the musculature.

Bibliography is available at Expert Consult.

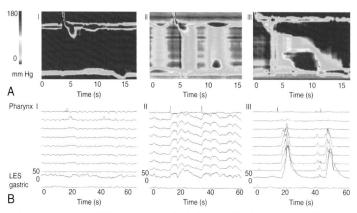

Fig. 347.2 Based on the residual wave type on HRM, 3 subtypes of achalasia can be determined. **A,** No distal pressurization is observed in type I (AI), whereas panesophageal pressurizations and spastic contractions are observed in type II (AII) and type III (AIII), respectively. **B,** A similar classification can be made when conventional manometry is used. Note that pressure recordings in type II achalasia are similar in every line tracing, compatible with panesophageal pressurization. *(From Rohof WO, Salvador R, Annese V: Outcomes of treatment for achalasia depend on manometric subtype. Gastroenterology 144(4): 718–725, 2013. Fig. 1).*

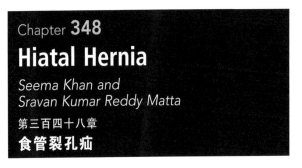

Chapter **348**
Hiatal Hernia
*Seema Khan and
Sravan Kumar Reddy Matta*
第三百四十八章
食管裂孔疝

中文导读

本章主要介绍了食管裂孔疝的分型（Ⅰ型滑动性食管裂孔疝、Ⅱ型食管旁疝、Ⅲ型混合型）、病理，Ⅰ型滑动型食管裂孔疝常合并胃食管反流，上消化道造影及内镜检查等诊断方法以及治疗等内容。描述了Ⅱ型食管旁疝可能是特发性先天异常或跟胃扭转有关，也可见于胃食管反流病胃底折叠术后。餐后饱胀和上腹疼痛是Ⅱ型食管旁疝常见的临床表现。

Herniation of the stomach through the esophageal hiatus can occur as a common sliding hernia (type 1), in which the gastroesophageal junction slides into the thorax, or it can be paraesophageal (type 2), in which a portion of the stomach (usually the fundus) is insinuated next to the esophagus inside the gastroesophageal junction in the hiatus (Figs. 348.1 and 348.2). A combination of sliding and paraesophageal types (type 3) is present in some patients. Sliding hernias are often associated with gastroesophageal reflux, especially in developmentally delayed children. The relationship to hiatal hernias in adults is unclear. Diagnosis is usually made by an upper gastrointestinal series and upper endoscopy. Medical treatment is not directed at the hernia but at the gastroesophageal reflux, unless failure of medical therapy prompts correction of the hernia at the time of fundoplication.

A paraesophageal hernia can be an isolated congenital anomaly or associated with gastric volvulus, or it may be encountered after fundoplication for gastroesophageal reflux, especially if the edges of a dilated esophageal diaphragmatic hiatus have not been approximated. Fullness after eating and upper abdominal pain are the usual symptoms. Infarction of the herniated stomach is rare.

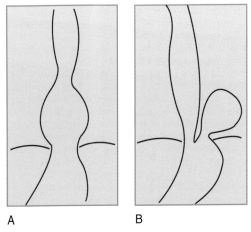

A   B

Fig. 348.1 Types of esophageal hiatal hernia. **A,** Sliding hiatal hernia, the most common type. **B,** Paraesophageal hiatal hernia.

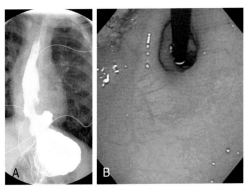

Fig. 348.2 A, An upper gastrointestinal series shows a large hiatal hernia that extends above the diaphragm and impedes the exit of contrast from the esophagus into the stomach. Contrast is also noted to reflux to the upper esophagus. **B,** A retroflexed view of the hernia from the stomach during an upper endoscopy.

Chapter **349**

Gastroesophageal Reflux Disease

Seema Khan and
Sravan Kumar Reddy Matta

第三百四十九章
胃食管反流病

中文导读

　　本章主要介绍了胃食管反流病和并发症。具体描述了胃食管反流病的病理生理学、流行病学和病史、临床表现、诊断和管理；在诊断方面具体描述了钡剂造影、食管远端pH监测、内镜、多通道腔内阻抗、喉气管支气管镜、经验性抗反流治疗等方法；在管理方面具体描述了饮食调整、姿势调整、药物治疗、H₂受体拮抗药、质子泵抑制剂、促动力药及手术治疗等内容。在并发症章节描述了食管并发症（包括食管炎、继发的狭窄、Barrett食管、腺癌）、营养问题、食管外的并发症［如呼吸（非典型）表现］、呼吸暂停和喘鸣。

Gastroesophageal reflux disease (GERD) is the most common esophageal disorder in children of all ages. Gastroesophageal reflux (GER) signifies the retrograde movement of gastric contents across the lower esophageal sphincter (LES) into the esophagus, which occurs physiologically every day in all infants, older children, and adults. Physiologic GER is exemplified by the effortless regurgitation of normal infants. The phenomenon becomes **pathologic GERD** in infants and children who manifest or report bothersome symptoms because of frequent or persistent GER, producing esophagitis-related symptoms, or extra-esophageal presentations, such as respiratory symptoms or nutritional effects.

PATHOPHYSIOLOGY

Factors determining the esophageal manifestations of reflux include the duration of esophageal exposure (a product of the frequency and duration of reflux episodes), the causticity of the refluxate, and the susceptibility of the esophagus to damage. The LES, defined as a high-pressure zone by manometry, is supported by the crura of the diaphragm at the gastroesophageal junction, together with valve-like functions of the esophagogastric junction anatomy, form the antireflux barrier. In the context of even the normal intraabdominal pressure augmentations that occur during daily life, the frequency of reflux episodes is increased by insufficient LES tone, by abnormal frequency of LES relaxations, and by hiatal herniation that prevents the LES pressure from being proportionally augmented by the crura during abdominal straining. Normal intraabdominal pressure augmentations may be further exacerbated by straining or respiratory efforts. The duration of reflux episodes is increased by lack of swallowing (e.g., during sleep) and by defective esophageal peristalsis. Vicious cycles ensue because chronic esophagitis produces esophageal peristaltic dysfunction (low-amplitude waves, propagation disturbances), decreased LES tone, and inflammatory esophageal shortening that induces hiatal herniation, all worsening reflux.

Transient LES relaxation (TLESR) is the primary mechanism allowing reflux to occur, and is defined as simultaneous relaxation of both LES and the surrounding crura. TLESRs occur independent of swallowing, reduce LES pressure to 0-2 mm Hg (above gastric), and last 10-60 sec; they appear by 26 wk of gestation. A vagovagal reflex, composed of afferent mechanoreceptors in the proximal stomach, a brainstem pattern generator, and efferents in the LES, regulates TLESRs. Gastric distention (postprandially, or from abnormal gastric emptying or air swallowing) is the main stimulus for TLESRs. Whether GERD is caused by a higher frequency of TLESRs or by a greater incidence of reflux during TLESRs is debated; each is likely in different persons. Straining during a TLESR makes reflux more likely, as do positions that place the gastroesophageal junction below the air–fluid interface in the stomach. Other factors influencing gastric pressure–volume dynamics, such as increased movement, straining, obesity, large-volume or hyperosmolar meals, gastroparesis, a large sliding hiatal hernia, and increased respiratory effort (coughing, wheezing) can have the same effect.

EPIDEMIOLOGY AND NATURAL HISTORY

Infant reflux becomes evident in the first few mo of life, peaks at 4 mo, and resolves in up to 88% by 12 mo and in nearly all by 24 mo. *Happy* *spitters* are infants who have recurrent regurgitation *without* exhibiting discomfort or refusal to eat and failure to gain weight. Symptoms of GERD in **older children** tend to be chronic, waxing and waning, but completely resolving in no more than half, which resembles adult patterns (Table 349.1). The histologic findings of esophagitis persist in infants who have naturally resolving symptoms of reflux. GERD likely has genetic predispositions: family clustering of GERD symptoms, endoscopic esophagitis, hiatal hernia, Barrett esophagus, and adenocarcinoma have been identified. As a continuously variable and common disorder, complex inheritance involving multiple genes and environmental factors is likely. Genetic linkage is indicated by the strong evidence of GERD in studies with monozygotic twins. A pediatric autosomal dominant form with otolaryngologic and respiratory manifestations has been located to chromosome 13q14, and the locus is termed GERD1.

CLINICAL MANIFESTATIONS

Most of the common clinical manifestations of esophageal disease can signify the presence of GERD and are generally thought to be mediated by the pathogenesis involving acid GER (Table 349.2). Although less noxious for the esophageal mucosa, nonacid reflux events are recognized to play an important role in extraesophageal disease manifestations. **Infantile reflux** manifests more often with regurgitation (especially postprandially), signs of esophagitis (irritability, arching, choking, gagging, feeding aversion), and resulting failure to thrive; symptoms resolve spontaneously in the majority of infants by 12-24 mo. **Older children** can have regurgitation during the preschool years; this complaint diminishes somewhat as children age, and complaints of abdominal and chest pain supervene in later childhood and adolescence. Occasional

Table 349.2	Symptoms and Signs That May Be Associated With Gastroesophageal Reflux

SYMPTOMS
Recurrent regurgitation with or without vomiting
Weight loss or poor weight gain
Irritability in infants
Ruminative behavior
Heartburn or chest pain
Hematemesis
Dysphagia, odynophagia
Wheezing
Stridor
Cough
Hoarseness

SIGNS
Esophagitis
Esophageal stricture
Barrett esophagus
Laryngeal/pharyngeal inflammation
Recurrent pneumonia
Anemia
Dental erosion
Feeding refusal
Dystonic neck posturing (Sandifer syndrome)
Apnea spells
Apparent life-threatening events

From Wyllie R, Hyams JS, Kay M, editors: *Pediatric gastrointestinal and liver disease*, ed 4, Philadelphia, 2011, WB Saunders, Table 22.1, p. 235.

Table 349.1	Symptoms According to Age			
MANIFESTATIONS	**INFANTS**	**CHILDREN**	**ADOLESCENTS AND ADULTS**	
Impaired quality of life	+++	+++	+++	
Regurgitation	++++	+	+	
Excessive crying/irritability	+++	+	−	
Vomiting	++	++	+	
Food refusal/feeding disturbances/anorexia	++	+	+	
Persisting hiccups	++	+	+	
Failure to thrive	++	+	−	
Abnormal posturing/Sandifer syndrome	++	+	−	
Esophagitis	+	++	+++	
Persistent cough/aspiration pneumonia	+	++	+	
Wheezing/laryngitis/ear problems	+	++	+	
Laryngomalacia/stridor/croup	+	++	−	
Sleeping disturbances	+	+	+	
Anemia/melena/hematemesis	+	+	+	
Apnea/BRUE/desaturation	+	−	−	
Bradycardia	+	?	?	
Heartburn/pyrosis	?	++	+++	
Epigastric pain	?	+	++	
Chest pain	?	+	++	
Dysphagia	?	+	++	
Dental erosions/water brush	?	+	+	
Hoarseness/globus pharyngeus	?	+	+	
Chronic asthma/sinusitis	−	++	+	
Laryngostenosis/vocal nodule problems	−	+	+	
Stenosis	−	(+)	+	
Barrett/esophageal adenocarcinoma	−	(+)	+	

+++, Very common; ++ common; + possible; (+) rare; − absent; ? unknown; *BRUE*, brief resolved unexplained event; previously called as *ALTE*, apparent life-threatening event.
From Wyllie R, Hyams JS, Kay M, editors: *Pediatric gastrointestinal and liver disease*, ed 4, Philadelphia, 2011, WB Saunders, Table 22.3, p. 235.

children present with food refusal or neck contortions (arching, turning of head) designated **Sandifer syndrome.** The respiratory presentations are also age dependent: GERD in infants may manifest as obstructive apnea or as stridor or lower airway disease in which reflux complicates primary airway disease such as laryngomalacia or bronchopulmonary dysplasia. Otitis media, sinusitis, lymphoid hyperplasia, hoarseness, vocal cord nodules, and laryngeal edema have all been associated with GERD. Airway manifestations in older children are more commonly related to asthma or to otolaryngologic disease such as laryngitis or sinusitis. Despite the high prevalence of GERD symptoms in asthmatic children, data showing direction of causality are conflicting.

Neurologically challenged children are one group that is recognized to be at an increased risk for GERD. It is not well established if the greater risk is conferred due to inadequate defensive mechanisms and/or inability to express symptoms. A low clinical threshold is important in the early identification and prompt treatment of GERD symptoms in these individuals.

DIAGNOSIS

For most of the typical GERD presentations, particularly in older children, a thorough history and physical examination suffice initially to reach the diagnosis. This initial evaluation aims to identify the pertinent positives in support of GERD and its complications and the negatives that make other diagnoses unlikely. The history may be facilitated and standardized by questionnaires (e.g., the Infant Gastroesophageal Reflux Questionnaire, the I-GERQ, and its derivative, the I-GERQ-R), which also permit quantitative scores to be evaluated for their diagnostic discrimination and for evaluative assessment of improvement or worsening of symptoms. The clinician should be alerted to the possibility of other important diagnoses in the presence of any *alarm or warning signs*: bilious emesis, frequent projectile emesis, gastrointestinal bleeding, lethargy, organomegaly, abdominal distention, micro- or macrocephaly, hepatosplenomegaly, failure to thrive, diarrhea, fever, bulging fontanelle, and seizures. The important differential diagnoses to consider in the evaluation of an infant or a child with chronic vomiting are milk and other food allergies, eosinophilic esophagitis, pyloric stenosis, intestinal obstruction (especially malrotation with intermittent volvulus), nonesophageal inflammatory diseases, infections, inborn errors of metabolism, hydronephrosis, increased intracranial pressure, rumination, and bulimia. Focused diagnostic testing, depending on the presentation and the differential diagnosis, can then supplement the initial examination.

Most of the esophageal tests are of some use in particular patients with suspected GERD. **Contrast (usually barium) radiographic** study of the esophagus and upper gastrointestinal tract is performed in children with vomiting and dysphagia to evaluate for achalasia, esophageal strictures and stenosis, hiatal hernia, and gastric outlet or intestinal obstruction (Fig. 349.1). It has poor sensitivity and specificity in the diagnosis of GERD as a result of its limited duration and the inability to differentiate physiologic GER from GERD. Furthermore, contrast radiography neither accurately assesses mucosal inflammation nor correlates with severity of GERD.

Extended esophageal pH monitoring of the distal esophagus, no longer considered the *sine qua non* of a GERD diagnosis, provides a quantitative and sensitive documentation of acidic reflux episodes, the most important type of reflux episodes for pathologic reflux. The distal esophageal pH probe is placed at a level corresponding to 87% of the nares-LES distance, based on regression equations using the patient's height, on fluoroscopic visualization, or on manometric identification of the LES. Normal values of distal esophageal acid exposure (pH <4) are generally established as <5 to 8% of the total monitored time, but these quantitative normals are insufficient to establish or disprove a diagnosis of pathologic GERD. The most important indications for esophageal pH monitoring are for assessing efficacy of acid suppression during treatment, evaluating apneic episodes in conjunction with a pneumogram and perhaps impedance, and evaluating atypical GERD presentations such as chronic cough, stridor, and asthma. Dual pH probes, adding a proximal esophageal probe to the standard distal one, are used in the diagnosis of extraesopha-

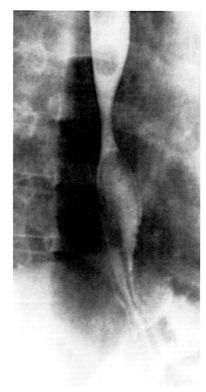

Fig. 349.1 Barium esophagogram demonstrating free gastroesophageal reflux. Note stricture caused by peptic esophagitis. Longitudinal gastric folds above the diaphragm indicate the unusual presence of an associated hiatal hernia.

geal GERD, identifying upper esophageal acid exposure times of 1% of the total time as threshold values for abnormality.

Endoscopy allows diagnosis of erosive esophagitis (Fig. 349.2) and complications such as strictures or Barrett esophagus; esophageal biopsies can diagnose histologic reflux esophagitis in the absence of erosions while simultaneously eliminating allergic and infectious causes. Endoscopy is also used therapeutically to dilate reflux-induced strictures. Radionucleotide scintigraphy using technetium can demonstrate aspiration and delayed gastric emptying when these are suspected.

The multichannel **intraluminal impedance** is a cumbersome test, but with potential applications both for diagnosing GERD and for understanding esophageal function in terms of bolus flow, volume clearance, and (in conjunction with manometry) motor patterns associated with GERD. Owing to the multiple sensors and a distal pH sensor, it is possible to document acidic reflux (pH <4), weakly acidic reflux

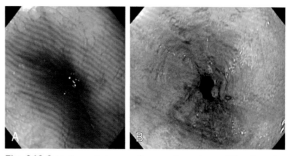

Fig. 349.2 Endoscopic image of a normal esophagus (**A**) and erosive peptic esophagitis (**B**).

(pH 4-7), and weakly alkaline reflux (pH >7) with multichannel intraluminal impedance. It is an important tool in those with respiratory symptoms, particularly for the determination of nonacid reflux, but must be cautiously applied in routine clinical evaluation because of limited evidence-based parameters for GERD diagnosis and symptom association.

Esophageal manometry is not useful in demonstrating gastroesophageal reflux but might be of use to evaluate transient LES relaxations and pressures.

Laryngotracheobronchoscopy evaluates for visible airway signs that are associated with extraesophageal GERD, such as posterior laryngeal inflammation and vocal cord nodules; it can permit diagnosis of silent aspiration (during swallowing or during reflux) by bronchoalveolar lavage with subsequent quantification of lipid-laden macrophages in airway secretions. Detection of pepsin in tracheal fluid is a marker of reflux-associated aspiration of gastric contents. Esophageal manometry permits evaluation for dysmotility, particularly in preparation for antireflux surgery.

Empirical antireflux therapy, using a time-limited trial of high-dose proton pump inhibitor (PPI), is a cost-effective strategy for diagnosis in adults; although not formally evaluated in older children, it has also been applied to this age group. Failure to respond to such empirical treatment, or a requirement for the treatment for prolonged periods, mandates formal diagnostic evaluation.

MANAGEMENT

Conservative therapy and lifestyle modifications that form the foundation of GERD therapy can be effectively implemented through education and reassurance for parents. Dietary measures for infants include normalization of any abnormal feeding techniques, volumes, and frequencies. Thickening of feeds or use of commercially prethickened formulas increases the percentage of infants with no regurgitation, decreases the frequency of daily regurgitation and emesis, and increases the infant's weight gain. However, caution should be exercised when managing preterm infants because of the possible association between xanthan gum-based thickened feeds and necrotizing enterocolitis. The evidence does not clearly favor 1 type of thickener over another; the addition of a Tbsp of rice or oat cereal per oz of formula results in a greater caloric density (30 kcal/oz) and reduced crying time, although it might not modify the number of nonregurgitant reflux episodes. Caution must be exercised while using rice cereal, as studies show increased risk of arsenic exposure in children with rice and rice product consumption. A short trial (2 wk) of a hypoallergenic diet in infants may be used to exclude milk or soy protein allergy before pharmacotherapy. A combination of modified feeding volumes, hydrolyzed infant formulas, proper positioning, and avoidance of smoke exposure satisfactorily improve GERD symptoms in 24–59% of infants with GERD. Older children should be counseled to avoid acidic or reflux-inducing foods (tomatoes, chocolate, mint) and beverages (juices, carbonated and caffeinated drinks, alcohol). Weight reduction for obese patients and elimination of smoke exposure are other crucial measures at all ages.

Positioning measures are particularly important for infants, who cannot control their positions independently. Seated position worsens infant reflux and should be avoided in infants with GERD. Esophageal pH monitoring demonstrates more reflux episodes in infants in supine and side positions compared with the prone position, but evidence that the supine position reduces the risk of sudden infant death syndrome has led the American Academy of Pediatrics and the North American Society of Pediatric Gastroenterology and Nutrition to recommend supine positioning during sleep. When the infant is awake and observed, prone position and upright carried position can be used to minimize reflux. Lying in the flat supine position and semi-seated positions (e.g., car seats, infant carriers) in the postprandial period are considered provocative positions for GER and therefore should be avoided. The efficacy of positioning for older children is unclear, but some evidence suggests a benefit to left side position and head elevation during sleep. The head should be elevated by elevating the head of the bed, rather than using excess pillows, to avoid abdominal flexion and compression that might worsen reflux.

Pharmacotherapy is directed at ameliorating the acidity of the gastric contents or at promoting their aboral movement and should be considered for those symptomatic infants and children who are either highly suspected or proven to have GERD. Antacids are the most commonly used antireflux therapy and are readily available over the counter. They provide rapid but transient relief of symptoms by acid neutralization. The long-term regular use of antacids cannot be recommended because of side effects of diarrhea (magnesium antacids) and constipation (aluminum antacids) and rare reports of more serious side effects of chronic use.

Histamine-2 receptor antagonists (H2RAs: cimetidine, famotidine, nizatidine, and ranitidine) are widely used antisecretory agents that act by selective inhibition of histamine receptors on gastric parietal cells. There is a definite benefit of H2RAs in treatment of mild-to-moderate reflux esophagitis. H2RAs have been recommended as first-line therapy because of their excellent overall safety profile, but they are superseded by PPIs in this role, as increased experience with pediatric use and safety, FDA approval, and pediatric formulations and dosing are available.

PPIs (omeprazole, lansoprazole, pantoprazole, rabeprazole, and esomeprazole) provide the most potent antireflux effect by blocking the hydrogen–potassium adenosine triphosphatase channels of the final common pathway in gastric acid secretion. PPIs are superior to H2RAs in the treatment of severe and erosive esophagitis. Pharmacodynamic studies indicate that children require higher doses of PPIs than adults on a per-weight basis. The use of PPIs to treat infants and children deemed to have GERD on the basis of symptoms is common, however an important systematic review of the efficacy and safety of PPI therapy in pediatric GERD reveals no clear benefit for PPI over placebo use in suspected infantile GERD (crying, arching behavior). Limited pediatric data are available to draw definitive conclusions about potential complications implicated with PPI use, such as respiratory infections, *Clostridium difficile* infection, bone fractures (noted in adults), hypomagnesemia, and kidney damage.

Prokinetic agents available in the United States include metoclopramide (dopamine-2 and 5-HT$_3$ antagonist), bethanechol (cholinergic agonist), and erythromycin (motilin receptor agonist). Most of these increase LES pressure; some improve gastric emptying or esophageal clearance. None affects the frequency of TLESRs. The available controlled trials *have not* demonstrated much efficacy for GERD. In 2009, the FDA announced a black box warning for metoclopramide, linking its chronic use (longer than 3 mo) with tardive dyskinesia, the rarely reversible movement disorder. Baclofen is a centrally acting γ-aminobutyric acid agonist that decreases reflux by decreasing TLESRs in healthy adults and in a small number of neurologically impaired children with GERD. Other agents of interest include peripherally acting γ-aminobutyric acid agonists devoid of central side effects, and metabotropic glutamate receptor 5 antagonists that are reported to reduce TLESRs but are as yet inadequately studied for this indication in children.

Cisapride is a serotonergic-receptor agonist with prokinetic effect that is only available in the United States through a limited access program because of its cardiac side effects (QT prolongation, dysrhythmias).

Surgery, usually **fundoplication,** is effective therapy for intractable GERD in children, particularly those with refractory esophagitis or strictures and those at risk for significant morbidity from chronic pulmonary disease. It may be combined with a gastrostomy for feeding or venting. The availability of potent acid-suppressing medication mandates more-rigorous analysis of the relative risks (or costs) and benefits of this relatively irreversible therapy in comparison to long-term pharmacotherapy. Some of the risks of fundoplication include a wrap that is *too tight* (producing dysphagia or gas-bloat) or *too loose* (and thus incompetent). Surgeons may choose to perform a *tight* (360 degrees, Nissen) or variations of a *loose* (<360 degrees, Thal, Toupet, Boix-Ochoa) wrap, or to add a gastric drainage procedure (pyloroplasty) to improve gastric emptying, based on their experience and the patient's disease. Preoperative accuracy of diagnosis of GERD and the skill of the surgeon are two of the most important predictors of successful outcome. Long-term studies suggest that fundoplications often become incompetent in children, as in adults, with reflux recurrence rates of up to 14% for Nissen and up to 20% for loose wraps (the rates may be highest with laparoscopic procedures); this fact currently combines with the potency of PPI therapy that is available to shift practice toward long-term pharmacotherapy in many cases. Fundoplication procedures may be performed as open operations, by laparoscopy, or by endoluminal (gastroplication) techniques. Pediatric experience is limited with endoscopic application of radiofrequency therapy (Stretta procedure) to a 2-3 cm area of the LES and cardia to create a high-pressure zone to reduce reflux.

Total esophagogastric dissociation is performed in selective neurologically impaired children with repeated failed fundoplications and with severe life-threatening gastroesophageal reflux disease.

Bibliography is available at Expert Consult.

349.1 Complications of Gastroesophageal Reflux Disease
Seema Khan and Sravan Kumar Reddy Matta

ESOPHAGEAL: ESOPHAGITIS AND SEQUELAE—STRICTURE, BARRETT ESOPHAGUS, ADENOCARCINOMA

Esophagitis can manifest as irritability, arching, and feeding aversion in infants; chest or epigastric pain in older children; and, rarely, as hematemesis, anemia, or Sandifer syndrome at any age. Erosive esophagitis is found in approximately 12% of children with GERD symptoms and is more common in boys, older children, neurologically challenged children, children with severe chronic respiratory disease, and in those with hiatal hernia. Prolonged and severe esophagitis leads to formation of strictures, generally located in the distal esophagus, producing dysphagia, and requiring repeated esophageal dilations and often fundoplication. Long-standing esophagitis predisposes to metaplastic transformation of the normal esophageal squamous epithelium into intestinal columnar epithelium, termed **Barrett esophagus,** a precursor of esophageal adenocarcinoma. A large multicenter prospective study of 840 consecutive children who underwent elective endoscopies reported a 25.7% prevalence for reflux esophagitis, and a mere 0.12% for Barrett esophagus in children without neurologic disorders or tracheoesophageal anomalies. Both Barrett esophagus and adenocarcinoma occur more in white males and in those with increased duration, frequency, and severity of reflux symptoms. This transformation increases with age to plateau in the fifth decade; adenocarcinoma is rare in childhood. Barrett esophagus, uncommon in children, warrants periodic surveillance biopsies, aggressive pharmacotherapy, and fundoplication for progressive lesions.

NUTRITIONAL

Esophagitis and regurgitation may be severe enough to induce failure to thrive because of caloric deficits. Enteral (nasogastric or nasojejunal, or percutaneous gastric or jejunal) or parenteral feedings are sometimes required to treat such deficits.

EXTRAESOPHAGEAL: RESPIRATORY ("ATYPICAL") PRESENTATIONS

GERD should be included in the differential diagnosis of children with unexplained or refractory otolaryngologic and respiratory complaints. GERD can produce respiratory symptoms by direct contact of the refluxed gastric contents with the respiratory tract (aspiration, laryngeal penetration, or microaspiration) or by reflexive interactions between the esophagus and respiratory tract (inducing laryngeal closure or bronchospasm). Often, GERD and a primary respiratory disorder, such as asthma, interact and a vicious cycle between them worsens both diseases. Many children with these extraesophageal presentations do not have typical GERD symptoms, making the diagnosis difficult. These atypical GERD presentations require a thoughtful approach to the differential diagnosis that considers a multitude of primary otolaryngologic (infections, allergies, postnasal drip, voice overuse) and pulmonary (asthma,

cystic fibrosis) disorders. Therapy for the GERD must be more intense (usually incorporating a PPI) and prolonged (usually at least 3-6 mo). In these cases a multidisciplinary approach involving otolaryngology, pulmonary for airway disease and gastroenterology for reflux disease is often warranted for specialized diagnostic testing and for optimizing intensive management.

APNEA AND STRIDOR

These upper airway presentations have been linked with GERD in case reports and epidemiologic studies; temporal relationships between them and reflux episodes have been demonstrated in some patients by esophageal pH–multichannel intraluminal impedance studies, and a beneficial response to therapy for GERD provides further support in a number of case series. An evaluation of 1,400 infants with apnea attributed the apnea to GERD in 50%, but other studies have failed to find an association. Apnea and brief resolved unexplained event-like presentation (previously called an "apparent life-threatening event") caused by reflux is generally obstructive, owing to laryngospasm that may be conceived of as an abnormally intense protective reflex. At the time of such apnea, infants have often been provocatively positioned (supine or flexed seated), have been recently fed, and have shown signs of obstructive apnea, with unproductive respiratory efforts. *The evidence suggests that for the large majority of infants presenting with apnea and a brief resolved unexplained event, GERD is not causal.* Stridor triggered by reflux generally occurs in infants anatomically predisposed toward stridor (laryngomalacia, micrognathia). Spasmodic croup, an episodic frightening upper airway obstruction, can be an analogous condition in older children. Esophageal pH probe studies might fail to demonstrate linkage of these manifestations with reflux owing to the buffering of gastric contents by infant formula and the episodic nature of the conditions. Pneumograms can fail to identify apnea if they are not designed to identify obstructive apnea by measuring nasal airflow.

Reflux laryngitis and other otolaryngologic manifestations (also known as laryngopharyngeal reflux) can be attributed to GERD. **Hoarseness,** voice fatigue, throat clearing, chronic cough, pharyngitis, sinusitis, otitis media, and a sensation of globus have been cited. Laryngopharyngeal signs of GERD include edema and hyperemia (of the posterior surface), contact ulcers, granulomas, polyps, subglottic stenosis, and interarytenoid edema. The paucity of well-controlled evaluations of the association contributes to the skepticism with which these associations may be considered. Other risk factors irritating the upper respiratory passages can predispose some patients with GERD to present predominantly with these complaints.

Many studies have reported a strong association between asthma and reflux as determined by history, pH–multichannel intraluminal impedance, endoscopy, and esophageal histology. GERD symptoms are present in an average of 23% (19–80%) of children with asthma as observed in a systematic review of 19 studies examining the prevalence of GERD in asthmatics. The review also reported abnormal pH results in 63%, and esophagitis in 35% of asthmatic children. However, this association does not clarify the direction of causality in individual cases and thus does not indicate which patients with asthma are likely to benefit from anti-GERD therapy. Children with asthma who are particularly likely to have GERD as a provocative factor are those with symptoms of reflux disease, those with refractory or steroid-dependent asthma, and those with nocturnal worsening of asthma. Endoscopic evaluation that discloses esophageal sequelae of GERD provides an impetus to embark on the aggressive (high dose and many months' duration) therapy of GERD.

Dental erosions constitute the most common oral lesion of GERD, the lesions being distinguished by their location on the lingual surface of the teeth. The severity seems to correlate with the presence of reflux symptoms and the presence of an acidic milieu as the result of reflux in the proximal esophagus and oral cavity. The other common factors that can produce similar dental erosions are juice consumption and bulimia.

Bibliography is available at Expert Consult.

Chapter **350**

Eosinophilic Esophagitis, Pill Esophagitis, and Infective Esophagitis

Seema Khan

第三百五十章

嗜酸粒细胞性食管炎、药物性食管炎和感染性食管炎

中文导读

　　本章主要介绍了嗜酸粒细胞性食管炎、感染性食管炎和药物性食管炎。具体描述了嗜酸粒细胞性食管炎的定义、诊断标准、流行病学、临床表现、发病机制、鉴别诊断以及治疗（饮食回避法和激素疗法）；具体描述了感染性食管炎的多发人群、常见的病原、临床表现、内镜下不同病原引起的食管炎的特点及治疗；在药物性食管炎中描述了引起食管炎或造成食管损伤的药物、临床表现及治疗等内容。

EOSINOPHILIC ESOPHAGITIS

Eosinophilic esophagitis (EoE) is a chronic esophageal disorder characterized by esophageal dysfunction and infiltration of the esophageal epithelium by ≥15 eosinophils per high-power field. The diagnostic criteria has recently been updated as a result of the consensus conference on Appraisal of Guidelines for Research and Evaluation (AGREE). The diagnosis of EoE should be considered in the clinical presentation of esophageal dysfunction, associated with esophageal epithelial infiltration of at least 15 eosinophils (eos) per high power field (hpf) or ~60 eos per mm^2, and after a careful evaluation of non-EoE disorders. Proton pump inhibitors should be considered as another treatment option rather than a diagnostic criterion to differentiate from GERD. EoE is a global disease, with incidence and prevalence rates in children 5 and 29.5 per 100,000. While infants and toddlers present commonly with vomiting, feeding problems, and poor weight gain, older children and adolescents usually experience solid food dysphagia with occasional food impactions (Fig. 350.1) or strictures and may complain of heartburn, chest or epigastric pain. Most patients are male. The mean age at diagnosis is 7 yr (range: 1-17 yr), and the duration of symptoms is 3 yr. Many patients have other atopic diseases (or a positive family history) and associated food allergies; laboratory abnormalities can include peripheral eosinophilia and elevated immunoglobulin E (IgE) levels. The pathogenesis involves mainly T-helper type 2 cytokine-mediated (interleukin 5 and 13) pathways leading to production of a potent eosinophil chemoattractant, eotaxin-3, by esophageal epithelium. The eosinophilic esophagitis endoscopic reference score (**EREFS**), based on commonly observed

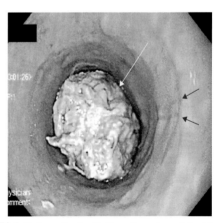

Fig. 350.1 Endoscopic visualization of esophageal food impaction *(yellow arrow)* and mucosal rings *(blue arrows).*

features of edema (E), rings (R; Fig. 350.2), exudates (E; see Fig. 350.2), furrows (F; Fig. 350.3), strictures (S), has utility in diagnosis and monitoring response to treatment. Esophageal histology reveals profound eosinophilia, with a currently acceptable cutoff for diagnosis chosen at ≥15 to 20/high-power field. Up to 30% children with EoE have grossly normal esophageal mucosa. EoE is differentiated from gastroesophageal

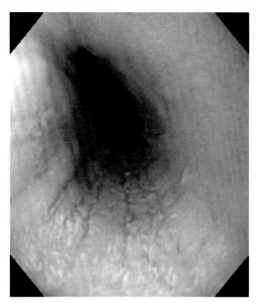

Fig. 350.2 Endoscopic image of eosinophilic esophagitis with characteristic mucosal appearance of furrowing and white specks.

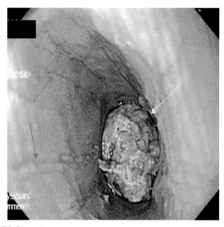

Fig. 350.3 Endoscopy photograph showing mucosal furrowing *(blue arrows)* characteristic of Eosinophilic esophagitis in a patient with food impaction *(yellow arrow).*

reflux disease by concurrent atopic diseases, its general lack of erosive esophagitis, its greater eosinophil density, and its normal esophageal pH-multichannel intraluminal impedance results. A favorable response to proton pump inhibitor therapy should no longer be considered diagnostic of gastroesophageal reflux disease, as approximately two-thirds of children with EoE also demonstrate histologic response and constitute a proton pump inhibitor–responsive EoE (PPI-REF) group. Observations in children and adults with EoE are notable for striking similarities between PPI responders and PPI non-responders with regard to symptoms, histology, molecular signature, and mechanistic features. This response may be because of an acid suppressive action or down regulation of Th-2 allergic cell pathway, an antieosinophil effect of the PPI class that is mediated by inhibition of eotaxin-3 secretion. Evaluation of EoE should include a search for food (aerodigestive) and environmental allergies via skin prick (IgE mediated) and patch (non–IgE mediated) tests to guide decisions regarding dietary elimination and future food challenges.

Treatment involves dietary restrictions that take one of 3 forms: elimination diets guided by circumstantial evidence and food allergy test results; "6 food elimination diet" removing the major food allergens (milk, soy, wheat, egg, peanuts and tree nuts, seafood); and elemental diet composed exclusively of an amino acid-based formula. Elimination diets are generally successful, with highest histologic response observed in nearly 91% on elemental diet and in 72% to empiric dietary elimination. Targeted elimination diets guided by multimodal allergy testing are comparable to empiric food elimination and hence lead to the argument against rigorous testing. The major drawbacks of dietary therapy lie in its cost, difficult access, and lower quality of life, any or all of which influence adherence and outcome.

Topically acting swallowed corticosteroids (fluticasone without spacer, viscous budesonide suspension) have been used successfully for those who refuse, fail to adhere, or have a poor response to restricted diets. Histologic remission is observed in 65-77% children and adults treated with fluticasone for 3 mo. Histologic recurrence after discontinuation of fluticasone is common, and emphasizes the need for maintenance therapy, and an approach that would carefully balance the risks of adrenocortical insufficiency as well as, bone demineralization and fungal infections against the risk of EoE evolution from an inflammatory to fibrostenotic disease producing esophageal stenosis and strictures. Therapies under investigation include anti-interleukin-5 antibodies (mepolizumab, reslizumab). Patients require periodic endoscopy and histologic reassessment for the most reliable monitoring of response to treatment, particularly given a significant disconnect between symptoms and histology in the evolution of the disease. Expert clinical guidelines stress long-term studies to develop systematic treatment and best follow-up protocols.

INFECTIVE ESOPHAGITIS

Uncommon, and most often affecting immunocompromised children, infective esophagitis is caused by fungal agents, such as *Candida* albicans and *Torulopsis glabrata;* viral agents, such as herpes simplex, cytomegalovirus, HIV, and varicella zoster; and, rarely, bacterial infections, including diphtheria and tuberculosis, or parasites. The typical presenting signs and symptoms are odynophagia, dysphagia, and retrosternal or chest pain; there may also be fever, nausea, and vomiting. Candida is the leading cause of infective esophagitis in immunocompetent and immunocompromised children and presents with concurrent oropharyngeal infection in the majority of immunocompromised patients. It may also be an incidental finding in asymptomatic patients, notably in those with EoE receiving topical swallowed corticosteroids. Esophageal viral infections can also manifest in immunocompetent hosts as an acute febrile illness. Infectious esophagitis, like other forms of esophageal inflammation, occasionally progresses to esophageal stricture. Diagnosis of infectious esophagitis is made by endoscopy, usually notable for white plaques in candida, multiple superficial ulcers or *volcano ulcers* in herpes simplex virus, and single deep ulcer in cytomegalovirus. Histopathologic examination solidifies the diagnosis with the detection of yeast and pseudohyphae in Candida; tissue invasion distinguishes esophagitis from mere colonization. Multinucleated giant cells with intranuclear Cowdry type A (eosinophilic) and type B (ground glass appearance) inclusions in HSV, and both intranuclear and intracytoplasmic inclusions producing an *owl's eye* appearance in CMV are typically described. Adding polymerase chain reaction, tissue-viral culture, and immunocytochemistry enhances the diagnostic sensitivity and precision. Treatment is with appropriate antimicrobial agents; azole therapy, particularly oral fluconazole for Candida; oral acyclovir for HSV, and oral valganciclovir for CMV, or alternatively intravenous ganciclovir in severe CMV disease.

PILL ESOPHAGITIS

This acute injury is produced by contact with a damaging agent. Medications implicated in pill esophagitis include tetracycline, doxycycline, potassium chloride, ferrous sulfate, nonsteroidal antiinflammatory medications, cloxacillin, and alendronate (Table 350.1). Most often the offending tablet is ingested at bedtime with inadequate water. This practice often produces acute discomfort followed by progressive

Table 350.1	Medications Commonly Associated With Esophagitis or Esophageal Injury

ANTIBIOTICS
Clindamycin
Doxycycline
Penicillin
Rifampin
Tetracycline

ANTIVIRAL AGENTS
Nelfinavir
Zalcitabine
Zidovudine

BISPHOSPHONATES
Alendronate
Etidronate
Pamidronate

CHEMOTHERAPEUTIC AGENTS
Bleomycin
Cytarabine
Dactinomycin
Daunorubicin
5-Fluorouracil
Methotrexate
Vincristine
NSAIDs
Aspirin
Ibuprofen
Naproxen

OTHER MEDICATIONS
Ascorbic acid
Ferrous sulfate
Lansoprazole
Multivitamins
Potassium chloride
Quinidine
Theophylline

From Katzka DA: Esophageal disorders caused by medications, trauma, and infection. In Feldman M, Friedman LS, Brandt LJ, editors: *Sleisenger and Fordtran's gastrointestinal and liver disease*, ed 10, 2016, Box 46.1.

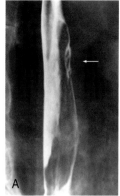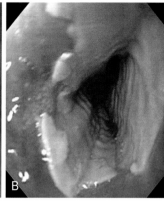

Fig. 350.4 **(A)** Barium esophagogram showing esophageal ulceration secondary to tetracycline, with the *arrow* pointing to an area of ulcerations. **(B)** Endoscopic image of a tetracycline-induced esophageal burn. *(From Katzka DA: Esophageal disorders caused by medications, trauma, and infection. In Feldman M, Friedman LS, Brandt LJ, editors:* Sleisenger and Fordtran's gastrointestinal and liver disease, *ed 10, 2016. Fig. 46.1).*

retrosternal pain, odynophagia, and dysphagia. Endoscopy shows a focal lesion often localized to one of the anatomic narrowed regions of the esophagus or to an unsuspected pathologic narrowing (Fig. 350.4).

Treatment is supportive; lacking much evidence, sucralfate, antacids, topical anesthetics, and bland or liquid diets are often used. The offending pill may be restarted after complete resolution of symptoms, if deemed necessary, though with clear emphasis on ingestion with adequate volume of water, usually at least 4 oz.

Bibliography is available at Expert Consult.

Chapter **351**
Esophageal Perforation
Seema Khan

第三百五十一章
食管穿孔

中文导读

　　本章主要介绍了食管穿孔。具体描述了食管穿孔的原因、特发性食管破裂综合征的好发部位、食管破裂的临床表现、影像学检查方法以及治疗方法等内容。

The majority of esophageal perforations in children are from blunt trauma (automobile injury, gunshot wounds, child abuse) or are iatrogenic. Cardiac massage, the Heimlich maneuver, nasogastric tube placement, traumatic laryngoscopy or endotracheal intubation, excessively vigorous postpartum suctioning of the airway during neonatal resuscitation, difficult upper endoscopy, sclerotherapy of esophageal varices, esophageal compression by a cuffed endotracheal tube, and dilation for therapy of achalasia and strictures have all been implicated. Esophageal rupture has followed forceful vomiting in patients with anorexia and has followed esophageal injury due to caustic ingestion, foreign body ingestion, food impactions, pill esophagitis, or eosinophilic esophagitis. Drinking cold, carbonated beverages rapidly is also known to cause esophageal perforation.

Spontaneous esophageal rupture (**Boerhaave syndrome**) is less common and is associated with sudden increases in intraesophageal pressure wrought by situations such as vomiting, coughing, or straining at stool. Children and adults with eosinophilic esophagitis have also been described with Boerhaave syndrome in the setting of forceful emesis in the aftermath of esophageal food impaction. In older children, as in adults, the tear occurs on the distal left lateral esophageal wall, because the smooth muscle layer here is weakest; in neonates (neonatal Boerhaave syndrome), spontaneous rupture is on the right.

Symptoms of esophageal perforation include pain, neck tenderness, dysphagia, subcutaneous crepitus, fever, and tachycardia; several patients with cervical perforations have displayed cold water polydipsia in an attempt to soothe pain in the throat. Imaging studies are important for a rapid and accurate diagnosis. Perforations in the proximal thoracic esophagus tend to create signs (pneumothorax, effusions) in the left chest, whereas the signs of distal tears are more often on the right. Plain radiography (posteroanterior and lateral views) and computed tomography of the neck and chest are often used, with the latter as more sensitive and accurate in diagnosis. Signs of perforation include pneumomediastinum, mediastinal widening, subcutaneous emphysema, pneumothorax, hydrothorax, pleural effusion, and lung collapse. If these x-rays are normal, an esophagogram using water-soluble contrast media should be performed, but esophagograms miss >30% of cervical perforations. Therefore, a negative water-soluble contrast esophagogram should be followed by a barium study; the greater density of barium can better demonstrate a small defect, although with a higher risk of inflammatory mediastinitis. Endoscopy may also be useful but carries a 30% false-negative rate.

Treatment must be individualized. Small tears in contained perforations with minimal mediastinal contamination in hemodynamically stable patients can be treated conservatively with broad-spectrum antibiotics, nothing given orally, gastric drainage, and parenteral nutrition. Endoscopic techniques, considered less invasive and morbid, are now being used more frequently and include clips for defects <2 cm, and placement of stents and suturing for larger defects. Chest exploration and direct surgical repair is infrequently indicated these days. Mortality rates range between 20% and 28%, with poor prognosis correlated with delayed diagnosis and interventions.

Bibliography is available at Expert Consult.

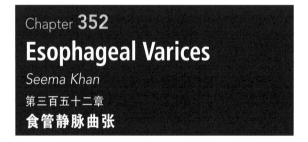

Chapter **352**
Esophageal Varices
Seema Khan

第三百五十二章
食管静脉曲张

中文导读

　　本章主要介绍了食管静脉曲张。具体描述了儿童食管静脉曲张的病因、临床表现、确诊的方法、上消化道内镜检查以及预防措施；在治疗中描述了急性静脉曲张出血的紧急处理，其中包括输血、血管活性药的使用、抗生素的使用、内镜下的套扎和硬化剂治疗等。对于药物和内镜治疗难以处理的难治性静脉曲张出血可采用经颈静脉肝内门体分流术。

Esophageal varices form in adults with portal hypertension with hepatic venous pressure gradient above 10 mm Hg and pose a risk for bleeding at above 12 mm Hg (see Chapter 394). Spontaneous decompression of this hypertension through portosystemic collateral circulation via the coronary vein, in conjunction with the left gastric veins, gives rise to esophageal varices. Most esophageal varices are *uphill varices*;

less commonly, those that arise in the absence of portal hypertension and with superior vena cava obstruction are *downhill varices*. Their treatment is directed at the underlying cause of the superior vena cava abnormality. Hemorrhage from esophageal varices is the major cause of morbidity and mortality from portal hypertension. Presentation is with significant hematemesis and melena; whereas most patients have liver disease, some children with extrahepatic portal venous obstruction might have been previously asymptomatic. Any child with hematemesis and splenomegaly should be presumed to have esophageal variceal bleeding until proved otherwise. The leading causes of pediatric portal hypertension, biliary atresia, and extrahepatic portal vein obstruction are uniquely distinct from diseases encountered in adults. Hence, children tend to tolerate variceal bleeding better due to generally well compensated liver disease, with studies reporting mortality risk <1% after initial variceal bleed.

Upper endoscopy is the preferred diagnostic test for esophageal varices, as it provides definitive diagnosis and delineation of details that aid in predicting the risk for bleeding, as well as enabling therapy for acute bleeding episodes via either sclerotherapy or band ligation. A report comprising a large series of children with biliary atresia and portal hypertension described endoscopic findings of large varices, red marks, and the presence of gastric varices as predictive of bleeding. Noninvasive methods of evaluating varices include barium contrast studies, ultrasound, computerized tomography, magnetic resonance, and elastography, but they are not recommended for routine diagnostic evaluation because of suboptimal accuracy compared to endoscopy.

Primary prophylaxis with the goal of preventing an initial hemorrhage can decrease the incidence of esophageal bleeding; the various modalities used are nonselective β blockade (e.g., propranolol or nadolol), sclerotherapy, ligation, and portosystemic shunt surgery. A recent expert consensus based on a large review of the available evidence has proposed that MesoRex bypass surgery should be offered to children with EHPVO as both primary and secondary prophylaxis in the appropriate context. Due to insufficient evidence, the same cannot be recommended regarding endoscopic therapies and nonselective beta blockers for primary prophylaxis in children. In contrast, adults do have a reduced risk of first-time variceal bleeding with endoscopic variceal ligation when compared with untreated controls as well as patients treated with β blockade; a decrease in mortality is only noted in comparison to the control group (see Chapter 394). The management of acute variceal bleeding must include attention to hemodynamic stability through blood transfusion, vasoactive drugs (e.g., octreotide), short-term antibiotic use, and endoscopy to perform ligation or sclerotherapy, as needed. Transjugular intrahepatic portosystemic shunt should be considered for variceal bleeding refractory to medical and endoscopic therapy. Secondary prophylaxis to reduce recurrence of bleeding uses nonselective β blockade and obliteration of varices through serial treatment via ligation or sclerotherapy. The only randomized controlled pediatric study has shown superiority of ligation over sclerotherapy in reducing the risk for rebleeding and complications.

Bibliography is available at Expert Consult.

Chapter **353**

Ingestions

第三百五十三章

吞入

中文导读

　　本章主要介绍了食管异物和腐蚀性吞入。食管异物部分具体描述了食管异物的好发年龄、常见异物的类型、好发部位、临床表现、影像学检查及针对纽扣电池和硬币等不同类型食管异物的处理措施；腐蚀性吞入部分具体描述了腐蚀性吞入的社会危害性、后遗症、分类（碱性、酸性）、好发人群、临床表现、内镜判断组织损伤程度和治疗方法。

353.1 Foreign Bodies in the Esophagus

Seema Khan

The majority (80%) of accidental foreign-body ingestions occur in children, most of whom are 5 yr of age or younger. Older children and adolescents with developmental delays and those with psychiatric disorders are also at increased risk. The presentation of a foreign body lodged in the esophagus constitutes an emergency and is associated with significant morbidity and mortality because of the potential for perforation and sepsis. Coins are by far the most commonly ingested foreign body, followed by small toy items. Food impactions are less common in children than in adults and usually occur in children in association with eosinophilic esophagitis *(diagnosed in 92% of those presenting with food impactions and dysphagia),* repair of esophageal atresia, and Nissen fundoplication. Most esophageal foreign bodies lodge at the level of the cricopharyngeus (upper esophageal sphincter), the aortic arch, or just superior to the diaphragm at the gastroesophageal junction (lower esophageal sphincter).

At least 30% of children with esophageal foreign bodies may be totally asymptomatic, so any history of foreign body ingestion should be taken seriously and investigated. An initial bout of choking, gagging, and coughing may be followed by excessive salivation, dysphagia, food refusal, emesis, or pain in the neck, throat, or sternal notch regions. Respiratory symptoms such as stridor, wheezing, cyanosis, or dyspnea may be encountered if the esophageal foreign body impinges on the larynx or membranous posterior tracheal wall. Cervical swelling, erythema, or subcutaneous crepitations suggest perforation of the oropharynx or proximal esophagus.

Evaluation of the child with a history of foreign body ingestion starts with plain anteroposterior radiographs of the neck, chest, and abdomen, along with lateral views of the neck and chest. The flat surface of a coin in the esophagus is seen on the anteroposterior view and the edge on the lateral view (Fig. 353.1). The reverse is true for coins lodged in the trachea; here, the edge is seen anteroposteriorly and the flat side is seen laterally. Disk-shaped button batteries can look like coins and be differentiated by the double halo and step-off on anteroposterior and lateral views, respectively (Fig. 353.2). The use of button batteries has been increasingly popular, leading to a sharp rise in accidental ingestions, and critical in the increase in morbidity and mortality. The latter is thought to be due to both an increase in diameter and a change to lithium cells. Children younger than 5 yr of age with ingestion of batteries ≥20 mm are considered to have the highest risk for catastrophic events such as necrosis, tracheoesophageal fistula, perforation, stricture, vocal cord paralysis, mediastinitis, and aortoenteric fistula (Fig. 353.3). Materials such as plastic, wood, glass, aluminum, and bones may be radiolucent; failure to visualize the object with plain films in a symptomatic patient warrants urgent endoscopy. Computed tomography (CT) scan with 3-dimensional reconstruction may increase the sensitivity of imaging a foreign body. Although barium contrast studies may be helpful in the occasional asymptomatic patient with negative plain films, their use is to be discouraged because of the potential of aspiration, as well as making subsequent visualization and object removal more difficult.

In managing the child with an esophageal foreign body, it is important to assess risk for airway compromise and to obtain a chest CT scan and surgical consultation in cases of suspected airway perforation. Treatment of esophageal foreign bodies usually merits endoscopic visualization of the object and underlying mucosa and removal of the object using an appropriately designed foreign body–retrieving accessory instrument through the endoscope and with an endotracheal tube protecting the airway. Sharp objects in the esophagus, multiple magnets or single magnet with a metallic object, or foreign bodies associated with respiratory symptoms mandate urgent removal within 12 hr of presentation. Button batteries, in particular, must be emergently removed within 2 hr of presentation regardless of the timing of patient's last oral intake because they can induce mucosal injury in as little as 1 hr of contact time and involve all esophageal layers within 4 hr (see Figs. 353.3 and 353.4). Asymptomatic blunt objects and coins lodged in the esophagus can be observed for up to 24 hr in anticipation of passage into the stomach. If there are no problems in handling secretions, meat impactions can be observed for up to 24 hr. In patients without prior esophageal surgeries, glucagon (0.05 mg/kg intravenously [IV]) can sometimes be useful in facilitating passage of distal esophageal food boluses by decreasing the lower esophageal sphincter pressure. The use of meat

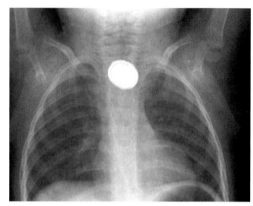

Fig. 353.2 Disk battery impacted in esophagus. Note the double rim. *(From Wyllie R, Hyams JS, editors: Pediatric gastrointestinal and liver disease, ed 3, Philadelphia, 2006, Saunders.)*

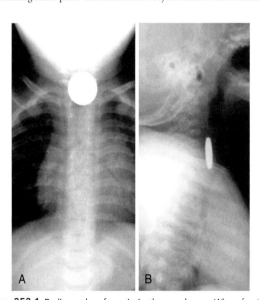

Fig. 353.1 Radiographs of a coin in the esophagus. When foreign bodies lodge in the esophagus, the flat surface of the object is seen in the anteroposterior view **(A)** and the edge is seen in the lateral view **(B)**. The reverse is true for objects in the trachea. *(Courtesy Beverley Newman, MD.)*

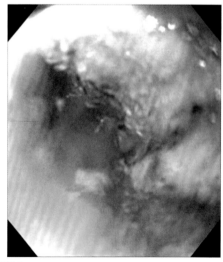

Fig. 353.3 Severe esophageal injury at site of button battery (BB) removal, with necrosis and eschar. *(From Leinwand K, Brumbaugh DE, Kramer RE: Button battery ingestion in children—a paradigm for management of severe pediatric foreign body ingestions, Gastrointest Endoscopy Clin N Am 26:99–118, 2016, Fig. 1.)*

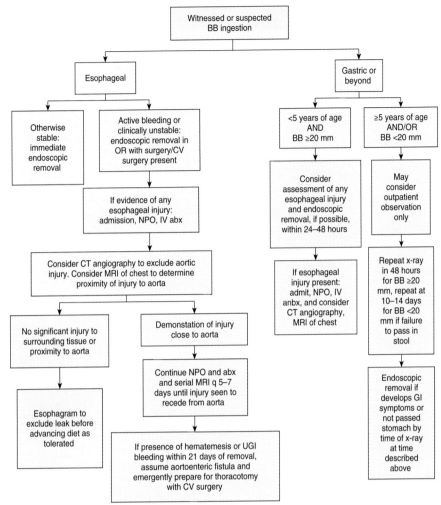

Fig. 353.4 Proposed management algorithm for ingestion of button battery *(BB)* in children. Abx, antibiotics; BB, button battery; CT, computed tomography; CV, cardiovascular; GI, gastrointestinal; IV, intravenous; MRI, magnetic resonance imaging; NPO, nil per os; OR, operating room; Q, every; UGI, upper gastrointestinal series. *(From Kramer RE, Lerner DG, Lin T, et al: Management of ingested foreign bodies in children: a clinical report of the NASPGHAN endoscopy committee, J Pediatr Gastroenterol Nutr 60(4):562–574, 2015, Fig. 1.)*

tenderizers or gas-forming agents can lead to perforation and are not recommended. An alternative technique for removing esophageal coins impacted for <24 hr, performed most safely by experienced radiology personnel, consists of passage of a Foley catheter beyond the coin at fluoroscopy, inflating the balloon, and then pulling the catheter and coin back simultaneously with the patient in a prone oblique position. Concerns about the lack of direct mucosal visualization and, when tracheal intubation is not used, the lack of airway protection prompt caution in the use of this technique. Bougienage of esophageal coins toward the stomach in selected uncomplicated pediatric cases has been suggested to be an effective, safe, and economical modality where endoscopy might not be routinely available.

Bibliography is available at Expert Consult.

353.2 Caustic Ingestions

Seema Khan

Ingestion of caustic substances is a worldwide public health problem accounting for a significant burden on healthcare resources. According to an inpatient database of U.S. pediatric hospital discharges in 2009, the estimated number of caustic ingestions was 807 (95% confidence interval [CI], 731-882) cases, amounting to $22,900,000 in total hospital charges. The medical sequelae of caustic ingestions are esophagitis, necrosis, perforation, and stricture formation (see Chapter 77). Most cases (70%) are accidental ingestions of liquid alkali substances that produce severe, deep liquefaction necrosis; drain decloggers are most common, and because they are tasteless, more is ingested (Table 353.1). **Acidic agents** (20% of cases) are bitter, so less may be consumed; they produce coagulation necrosis and a somewhat protective thick eschar. They can produce severe gastritis, and volatile acids can result in respiratory symptoms. Children younger than 5 yr of age account for half of the cases of caustic ingestions, and boys are far more often involved than girls.

Caustic ingestions produce signs and symptoms such as vomiting, drooling, refusal to drink, oral burns, dysphagia, dyspnea, abdominal pain, hematemesis, and stridor. Twenty percent of patients develop esophageal strictures. Absence of oropharyngeal lesions does not exclude the possibility of significant esophagogastric injury, which can lead to perforation or stricture. The absence of symptoms is usually associated with no or minimal lesions; hematemesis, respiratory distress, or presence of at least 3 symptoms predicts severe lesions. An upper endoscopy is recommended as the most efficient means of rapid identification of tissue damage and must be undertaken in all symptomatic children.

Table 353.1	Ingestible Caustic Materials Around the House	
CATEGORY	**MOST DAMAGING AGENTS**	**OTHER AGENTS**
Alkaline drain cleaners, milking machine pipe cleaners	Sodium or potassium hydroxide	Ammonia Sodium hypochlorite Aluminum particles
Acidic drain openers	Hydrochloric acid Sulfuric acid	
Toilet cleaners	Hydrochloric acid Sulfuric acid Phosphoric acid Other acids	Ammonium chloride Sodium hypochlorite
Oven and grill cleaners	Sodium hydroxide Perborate (borax)	
Denture cleaners	Persulfate (sulfur) Hypochlorite (bleach)	
Dishwasher detergent • Liquid • Powdered • Packaged	Sodium hydroxide Sodium hypochlorite Sodium carbonate	
Bleach	Sodium hypochlorite	Ammonia salt
Swimming pool chemicals	Acids, alkalis, chlorine	
Battery acid (liquid)	Sulfuric acid	
Disk batteries	Electric current	Zinc or other metal salts
Rust remover	Hydrofluoric, phosphoric, oxalic, and other acids	
Household delimers	Phosphoric acid Hydroxyacetic acid Hydrochloric acid	
Barbeque cleaners	Sodium and potassium hydroxide	
Glyphosate surfactant (RoundUp) acid	Glyphosate herbicide	Surfactants
Hair relaxer	Sodium hydroxide	
Weed killer	Dichlorophenoxyacetate, ammonium phosphate, propionic acid	

Source: National Library of Medicine: *Health and safety information on household products* (website). http://householdproducts.nlm.nih.gov/
From Wylie R, Hyams JS, Kay M, editors: *Pediatric gastrointestinal and liver disease*, ed 4, Philadelphia, 2011, WB Saunders, Table 19.1, p. 198.

Dilution by water or milk is recommended as acute treatment, but neutralization, induced emesis, and gastric lavage are contraindicated. Treatment depends on the severity and extent of damage (Table 353.2, Fig. 353.5). Stricture risk is increased by circumferential ulcerations, white plaques, and sloughing of the mucosa and is reported to occur in 70–100% of grade IIB and grade III caustic esophagitis. Strictures can require treatment with dilation, and in some severe cases, surgical resection and colon or small bowel interposition are needed. Silicone stents (self-expanding) placed endoscopically after a dilation procedure can be an alternative and conservative approach to the management of strictures. Rare late cases of superimposed esophageal carcinoma are reported. The role of corticosteroids is controversial; they are not recom-

Table 353.2	Classification of Caustic Injury	
GRADE	**VISIBLE APPEARANCE**	**CLINICAL SIGNIFICANCE**
Grade 0	History of ingestion but no visible damage or symptoms	Able to take fluids immediately
Grade 1	Edema, loss of normal vascular pattern, hyperemia, no transmucosal injury	Temporary dysphagia, able to swallow within 0-2 days, no long-term sequelae
Grade 2a	Transmucosal injury with friability, hemorrhage, blistering, exudate, scattered superficial ulceration	Scarring, no circumferential damage (no stenosis), no long-term sequelae
Grade 2b	Grade 2a plus discrete ulceration and/or circumferential ulceration	Small risk of perforation, scarring that may result in later stenosis
Grade 3a	Scattered deep ulceration with necrosis of the tissue	Risk of perforation, high risk of later stenosis
Grade 3b	Extensive necrotic tissue	High risk of perforation and death, high risk of stenosis

From Wylie R, Hyams JS, Kay M, editors: *Pediatric gastrointestinal and liver disease*, ed 4, Philadelphia, 2011, WB Saunders, Table 19.2, p. 199.

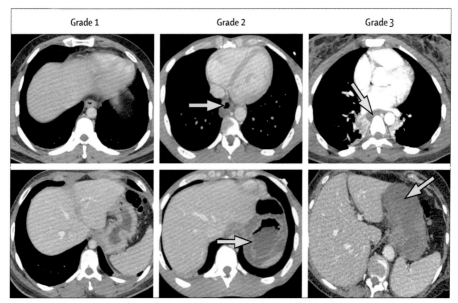

Fig. 353.5 Computed Tomography (CT) Grading of Corrosive Injuries of the Esophagus and the Stomach. Grade 1, normal appearance; grade 2, wall and soft tissue edema, increased wall enhancement *(arrow)*; grade 3, transmural necrosis with absent wall enhancement *(arrow). (From Chirica M, Bonavina L, Kelly MD, et al: Caustic ingestion, Lancet 389:2041–2050, 2017, Fig. 1.)*

mended in grade 1 burns, but they can reduce the risk of strictures in more-advanced caustic esophagitis. Many centers also use proton pump inhibitors as well as antibiotics in the initial treatment of caustic esophagitis on the premise that reducing superinfection in the necrotic tissue bed will, in turn, lower the risk of stricture formation. Studies examining the role of antibiotics in caustic esophagitis have not reported a clinically significant benefit even in those with grade 2 or greater severity of esophagitis.

There may be an increase of esophageal (not gastric) carcinoma following a caustic ingestion.

Bibliography is available at Expert Consult.

Section **4**

Stomach and Intestines

第四篇
胃和肠

Chapter **354**

Normal Development, Structure, and Function of the Stomach and Intestines

Asim Maqbool and Chris A. Liacouras

第三百五十四章
胃和肠的正常发育、结构和功能

中文导读

　　本章主要介绍了消化系统的发育和功能。在发育部分描述了原始肠道在妊娠期可以识别的时间，原始肠道可以分为前肠、中肠和后肠以及各部分所形成的消化器官、肝脏的形成、基因和外在因素的调控以及消化道运动收缩的形式；在消化和吸收功能部分具体描述了碳水化合物的消化、分解和吸收的过程，蛋白的水解、寡肽的分解过程和吸收，脂肪的分解、吸收过程以及影响脂肪吸收的因素、结肠的功能等。

DEVELOPMENT

The primitive gut is recognizable by the 4th wk of gestation and is composed of the foregut, midgut, and hindgut. The **foregut** gives rise to the upper gastrointestinal tract, which includes the esophagus, stomach, and duodenum to the level of the insertion of the common bile duct. The **midgut** gives rise to the rest of the small bowel and the large bowel to the level of the midtransverse colon. The **hindgut** forms the remainder of the colon and upper anal canal. The rapid growth of the midgut causes it to protrude out of the abdominal cavity through the umbilical ring during fetal development. The midgut subsequently returns to the peritoneal cavity and rotates counterclockwise until the cecum lies in the right lower quadrant. The process is normally complete by the 8th wk of gestation.

The liver derives from the hepatic diverticulum that evolves into parenchymal cells, bile ducts, vascular structures, and hematopoietic and Kupffer cells. The extrahepatic bile ducts and gallbladder develop first as solid cords that canalize by the 3rd mo of gestation. The dorsal

and ventral pancreatic buds grow from the foregut by the 4th wk of gestation. The two buds fuse by the 6th wk. Exocrine secretory capacity is present by the 5th mo.

Cis-regulatory genomic sequences govern gene expression during development. Modules of *cis* sequences are linked and allow a cascade of gene regulation that controls functional development. Extrinsic factors have the capacity to influence gene expression. In the gut, several growth factors, including growth factor-β, insulin-like growth factor, and growth factors found in human colostrum (human growth factor and epidermal growth factor), influence gene expression.

Propulsion of food down the gastrointestinal tract relies on the coordinated action of muscles in the bowel wall. The contractions are regulated by the enteric nervous system under the influence of a variety of peptides and hormones. The enteric nervous system is derived from neural crest cells that migrate in a cranial to caudal fashion. Migration of the neural crest tissue is complete by the 24th wk of gestation. Interruption of the migration results in **Hirschsprung disease**. Newborn bowel motor patterns are different from adults. Normal fasting upper gastrointestinal motility is characterized by a triphasic pattern known as the migrating motor complex. Migrating motor complexes occur less often in neonates, and they have more nonmigrating phasic activity. This leads to ineffective propulsion, particularly in premature infants. Motility in the fed state consists of a series of ring contractions that spread caudad over variable distances.

DIGESTION AND ABSORPTION

The wall of the stomach, small bowel, and colon consists of four layers: the mucosa, submucosa, muscularis, and serosa. Eighty-five percent of the gastric mucosa is lined by oxyntic glands containing cells that secrete hydrochloric acid, pepsinogen, and intrinsic factor, and mucous and endocrine cells that secrete peptides having paracrine and endocrine effects. Pepsinogen is a precursor of the proteolytic enzyme pepsin, and intrinsic factor is required for the absorption of vitamin B_{12}. Pyloric glands are located in the antrum and contain gastrin-secreting cells. Acid production and gastrin levels are inversely related to each other except in pathologic secretory states. Acid secretion is low at birth but increases dramatically by 24 hr. Acid and pepsin secretions peak in the first 10 days and decrease from 10 to 30 days after birth. Intrinsic factor secretion rises slowly in the first 2 wk of life.

The small bowel is approximately 270 cm long at birth in a term neonate and grows to an adult length of 450-550 cm by 4 yr of age. The mucosa of the small intestine is composed of villi, which are finger-like projections of the mucosa into the bowel lumen that significantly expand the absorptive surface area. The mucosal surface is further expanded by a brush border containing digestive enzymes and transport mechanisms for monosaccharides, amino acids, dipeptides and tripeptides, and fats. The cells of the villi originate in adjacent crypts and become functional as they migrate from the crypt up the villus. The small bowel mucosa is completely renewed in 4-5 days, providing a mechanism for rapid repair after injury, but in young infants or malnourished children, the process may be delayed. Crypt cells also secrete fluid and electrolytes. The villi are present by 8 wk of gestation in the duodenum and by 11 wk in the ileum.

Disaccharidase activities are measurable at 12 wk, but lactase activity does not reach maximal levels until 36 wk. Even premature infants usually tolerate lactose-containing formulas because of carbohydrate salvage by colonic bacteria. In children of African and Asian ethnicity, lactase levels may begin to fall at 4 yr of age, leading to intolerance to mammalian milk. Mechanisms to digest and absorb protein, including pancreatic enzymes and mucosal mechanisms to transport amino acids, dipeptides, and tripeptides, are in place by the 20th wk of gestation.

Carbohydrates, protein, and fat are normally absorbed by the upper half of the small intestine; the distal segments represent a vast reserve of absorptive capacity. Most of the sodium, potassium, chloride, and water are absorbed in the small bowel. Bile salts and vitamin B_{12} are selectively absorbed in the distal ileum, and iron is absorbed in the duodenum and proximal jejunum. Intraluminal digestion depends on the exocrine pancreas. Secretin and cholecystokinin stimulate synthesis and secretion of bicarbonate and digestive enzymes, which are released by the upper intestinal mucosa in response to various intraluminal stimuli, among them components of the diet.

Carbohydrate digestion is normally an efficient process that is completed in the distal duodenum. Starches are broken down to glucose, oligosaccharides, and disaccharides by pancreatic amylase. Residual glucose polymers are broken down at the mucosal level by glucoamylase. Lactose is broken down at the brush border by lactase, forming glucose and galactose; sucrose is broken down by sucrase-isomaltase to fructose and glucose. Galactose and glucose are primarily transported into the cell by a sodium- and energy-dependent process, whereas fructose is transported by facilitated diffusion.

Proteins are hydrolyzed by pancreatic enzymes, including trypsin, chymotrypsin, elastase, and carboxypeptidases, into individual amino acids and oligopeptides. The pancreatic enzymes are secreted as pro-enzymes, which are activated by release of the mucosal enzyme enterokinase. Oligopeptides are further broken down at the brush border by peptidases into dipeptides, tripeptides, and amino acids. Protein can enter the cell by separate noncompetitive carriers that can transport individual amino acids or dipeptides and tripeptides similar to those in the renal tubule. The human gut is capable of absorbing antigenic intact proteins in the first few wk of life because of *leaky* junctions between enterocytes. Entry of potential protein antigens through the mucosal barrier might have a role in later food- and microbe-induced symptoms.

Fat absorption occurs in two phases. Dietary triglycerides are broken down into monoglycerides and free fatty acids by pancreatic lipase and colipase. The free fatty acids are subsequently emulsified by bile acids, forming micelles with phospholipids and other fat-soluble substances, and are transported to the cell membrane, where they are absorbed. The fats are reesterified in the enterocyte, forming chylomicrons that are transported through the intestinal lymphatics to the thoracic duct. Medium-chain fats are absorbed more efficiently and can directly enter the cell. They are subsequently transported to the liver via the portal system. Fat absorption can be affected at any stage of the digestion and absorption process. Decreased pancreatic enzymes occur in cystic fibrosis, cholestatic liver disease leads to poor bile salt production and micelle formation, celiac disease affects mucosal surface area, abnormal chylomicron formation occurs in abetalipoproteinemia, and intestinal lymphangiectasia affects transport of the chylomicrons.

Fat absorption is less efficient in the neonate compared with adults. Premature infants can lose up to 20% of their fat calories compared with up to 6% in the adult. Decreased synthesis of bile acids and pancreatic lipase and decreased efficiency of ileal absorption are contributing factors. Fat digestion in the neonate is facilitated by lingual and gastric lipases. Bile salt–stimulated lipase in human milk augments the action of pancreatic lipase. Infants with malabsorption of fat are usually fed with formulas that have a greater percentage of medium-chain triglycerides, which are absorbed independently of bile salts.

The colon is a 75-100 cm sacculated tube formed by three strips of longitudinal muscle called *taenia coli* that traverse its length and fold the mucosa into haustra. Haustra and taenia appear by the 12th wk of gestation. The most common motor activity in the colon is nonpropulsive rhythmic segmentation that acts to mix the chyme and expose the contents to the colonic mucosa. Mass movement within the colon typically occurs after a meal. The colon extracts additional water and electrolytes from the luminal contents to render the stools partially or completely solid. The colon also acts to scavenge by-products of bacterial degradation of carbohydrates. Stool is stored in the rectum until distention triggers a defecation reflex that, when assisted by voluntary relaxation of the external sphincter, permits evacuation.

Chapter 355
Pyloric Stenosis and Other Congenital Anomalies of the Stomach

第三百五十五章
幽门狭窄和其他先天性胃畸形

中文导读

本章主要介绍了肥厚性幽门狭窄、先天性胃出口梗阻、胃重复畸形、胃扭转和肥厚性胃病。具体描述了肥厚性幽门狭窄的病因学、临床表现、鉴别诊断和治疗；具体描述了先天性胃出口梗阻的临床表现、诊断要点和治疗；描述了胃重复畸形的定义、好发部位、临床表现、影像学特点和治疗；描述了胃扭转的分类、病因、临床表现、诊断和治疗；描述了肥厚性胃病的发病机制、临床表现、诊断和鉴别诊断以及治疗等内容。

355.1 Hypertrophic Pyloric Stenosis

Asim Maqbool and Chris A. Liacouras

Hypertrophic pyloric stenosis occurs in 1-3/1,000 infants in the United States. It is more common in whites of northern European ancestry, less common in blacks, and rare in Asians. Males (especially firstborns) are affected approximately 4-6 times as often as females. The offspring of a mother and, to a lesser extent, the father who had pyloric stenosis are at higher risk for pyloric stenosis. Pyloric stenosis develops in approximately 20% of the male and 10% of the female descendants of a mother who had pyloric stenosis. The incidence of pyloric stenosis is increased in infants with B and O blood groups. Pyloric stenosis is occasionally associated with other congenital defects, including tracheoesophageal fistula and hypoplasia or agenesis of the inferior labial frenulum.

ETIOLOGY
The cause of pyloric stenosis is unknown, but many factors have been implicated. Pyloric stenosis is usually not present at birth and is more concordant in monozygotic than dizygotic twins. It is unusual in stillbirths and probably develops after birth. Pyloric stenosis has been associated with eosinophilic gastroenteritis, Apert syndrome, Zellweger syndrome, trisomy 18, Smith-Lemli-Opitz syndrome, and Cornelia de Lange syndrome. An association has been found with the use of erythromycin in neonates with highest risk if the medication is given within the first 2 wk of life. There have also been reports of higher incidence of pyloric stenosis among mostly female infants of mothers treated with macrolide antibiotics during pregnancy and breastfeeding. Abnormal muscle innervation, elevated serum levels of prostaglandins, and infant hypergastrinemia have been implicated. Reduced levels of neuronal nitric oxide synthase have been found with altered expression of the neuronal nitric oxide synthase exon 1c regulatory region, which influences the expression of the neuronal nitric oxide synthase gene. Reduced nitric oxide might contribute to the pathogenesis of pyloric stenosis.

CLINICAL MANIFESTATIONS
Non-bilious vomiting is the initial symptom of pyloric stenosis. The vomiting may or may not be projectile initially but is usually progressive, occurring immediately after a feeding. Emesis might follow each feeding, or it may be intermittent. The vomiting usually starts after 3 wk of age, but symptoms can develop as early as the first wk of life and as late as the 5th mo. Approximately 20% have intermittent emesis from birth that then progresses to the classic picture. After vomiting, the infant is hungry and wants to feed again. As vomiting continues, a progressive loss of fluid, hydrogen ion, and chloride leads to *hypochloremic metabolic alkalosis*. Awareness of pyloric stenosis has led to earlier identification of patients with fewer instances of chronic malnutrition and severe dehydration and at times a subclinical self-resolving hypertrophy.

Hyperbilirubinemia is the most common clinical association of pyloric stenosis, also known as *icteropyloric syndrome*. Unconjugated hyperbilirubinemia is more common than conjugated and usually resolves with surgical correction of the pyloric stenosis. It may be associated with a decreased level of glucuronyl transferase as seen in approximately 5% of affected infants; mutations in the bilirubin uridine diphosphate glucuronosyltransferase gene *(UGT1A1)* have also been implicated. If conjugated hyperbilirubinemia is a part of the presentation, other etiologies need to be investigated. Other coexistent clinical diagnoses have been described, including eosinophilic gastroenteritis, hiatal hernia, peptic ulcer, congenital nephrotic syndrome, congenital heart disease, and congenital hypothyroidism.

The diagnosis has traditionally been established by palpating the pyloric mass. The mass is firm, movable, approximately 2 cm in length, olive shaped, hard, best palpated from the left side, and located above and to the right of the umbilicus in the mid epigastrium beneath the liver's edge. The olive is easiest palpated after an episode of vomiting. After feeding, there may be a visible gastric peristaltic wave that progresses across the abdomen (Fig. 355.1).

Two imaging studies are commonly used to establish the diagnosis. Ultrasound examination confirms the diagnosis in the majority of cases. Criteria for diagnosis include pyloric thickness 3-4 mm, an overall pyloric length 15-19 mm, and pyloric diameter of 10-14 mm (Fig. 355.2). Ultrasonography has a sensitivity of approximately 95%. When contrast studies are performed, they demonstrate an elongated pyloric channel (string sign), a bulge of the pyloric muscle into the antrum (shoulder sign), and parallel streaks of barium seen in the narrowed channel, producing a "double tract sign" (Fig. 355.3).

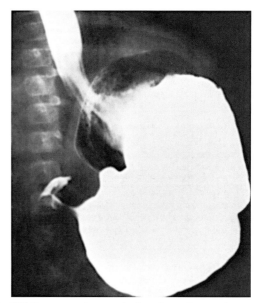

Fig. 355.3 Barium in the stomach of an infant with projectile vomiting. The attenuated pyloric canal is typical of congenital hypertrophic pyloric stenosis.

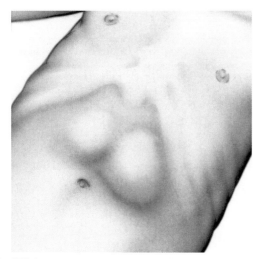

Fig. 355.1 Gastric peristaltic wave in an infant with pyloric stenosis.

DIFFERENTIAL DIAGNOSIS

Gastric waves are occasionally visible in small, emaciated infants who do not have pyloric stenosis. Infrequently, gastroesophageal reflux, with or without a hiatal hernia, may be confused with pyloric stenosis. Gastroesophageal reflux disease can be differentiated from pyloric stenosis by radiographic studies. Adrenal insufficiency from the adrenogenital syndrome can simulate pyloric stenosis, but the absence of a metabolic acidosis and elevated serum potassium and urinary sodium concentrations of adrenal insufficiency aid in differentiation (see Chapter 594). Inborn errors of metabolism can produce recurrent emesis with alkalosis (urea cycle) or acidosis (organic acidemia) and lethargy, coma, or seizures. Vomiting with diarrhea suggests gastroenteritis, but patients with pyloric stenosis occasionally have diarrhea. Rarely, a pyloric membrane or pyloric

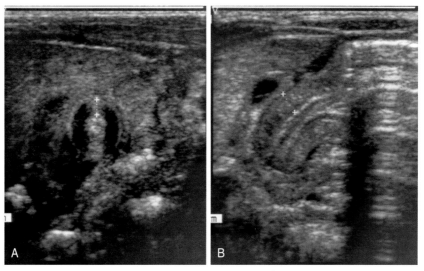

Fig. 355.2 A, Transverse sonogram demonstrating a pyloric muscle wall thickness of >4 mm (distance between *crosses*). **B,** Horizontal image demonstrating a pyloric channel length >14 mm (wall thickness outlined between *crosses*) in an infant with pyloric stenosis.

duplication results in projectile vomiting, visible peristalsis, and, in the case of a duplication, a palpable mass (Table 355.1). Duodenal stenosis proximal to the ampulla of Vater results in the clinical features of pyloric stenosis but can be differentiated by the presence of a pyloric mass on physical examination or ultrasonography.

TREATMENT

The preoperative treatment is directed toward correcting the fluid, acid–base, and electrolyte losses. Correction of the alkalosis is essential to prevent postoperative apnea, which may be associated with anesthesia. Most infants can be successfully rehydrated within 24 hr. Vomiting usually stops when the stomach is empty, and only an occasional infant requires nasogastric suction.

The surgical procedure of choice is pyloromyotomy. The traditional Ramstedt procedure is performed through a short transverse skin incision. The underlying pyloric mass is cut longitudinally to the layer of the submucosa, and the incision is closed. Laparoscopic technique is equally successful and in one study resulted in a shorter time to full feedings and discharge from the hospital as well as greater parental satisfaction. The success of laparoscopy depends on the skill of the surgeon. Postoperative vomiting occurs in half the infants and is thought to be secondary to edema of the pylorus at the incision site. In most infants, feedings can be initiated within 12-24 hr after surgery and advanced to maintenance oral feedings within 36-48 hr after surgery. Persistent vomiting suggests an incomplete pyloromyotomy, gastritis, gastroesophageal reflux disease, or another cause of the obstruction. The surgical treatment of pyloric stenosis is curative, with an operative mortality of 0–0.5%. Endoscopic balloon dilation has been successful in infants with persistent vomiting secondary to incomplete pyloromyotomy.

Conservative management with nasoduodenal feedings is advisable in patients who are not good surgical candidates. Oral and intravenous atropine sulfate (pyloric muscle relaxant) has also been described when surgical expertise is not available with 80% success rate described in some studies. In conservative protocols, atropine is administered intravenously at a dose of 0.01 mg/kg 6 times a day 5 min before feeding. During atropine infusion, the heart rate needs to be continuously monitored by electrocardiography. Oral feeding is started at a volume of 10 mL formula, 6 times a day. The volume is increased day by day until patients tolerate 150 mL/kg/day unless vomiting occurs more than twice a day. When patients are able to tolerate the full volume of formula without vomiting more than twice a day, 0.02 mg/kg atropine is administered orally 6 times a day before feeding. As the conservative

management takes longer and oral feedings may not be tolerated at first, worsening of the nutrition status may occur and total parenteral nutrition may be required. It was also postulated that surgical management is more time and cost effective.

ACKNOWLEDGMENT
Anna K. Hunter, MD contributed to the prior version of this chapter.

Bibliography is available at Expert Consult.

355.2 Congenital Gastric Outlet Obstruction
Asim Maqbool and Chris A. Liacouras

Gastric outlet obstruction resulting from pyloric atresia and antral webs is uncommon and accounts for <1% of all the atresias and diaphragms of the alimentary tract (see Table 355.1). The cause of the defects is unknown. Pyloric atresia has been associated with **epidermolysis bullosa** and usually presents in early infancy. The gender distribution is equal.

CLINICAL MANIFESTATIONS
Infants with pyloric atresia present with nonbilious vomiting, feeding difficulties, and abdominal distention during the first day of life. **Polyhydramnios** occurs in most cases, and low birth weight is common. The gastric aspirate at birth is large (>20 mL fluid) and should be removed to prevent aspiration. Rupture of the stomach may occur as early as the first 12 hr of life. Infants with antral web may present with less dramatic symptoms, depending on the degree of obstruction. Older children with antral webs present with nausea, vomiting, abdominal pain, and weight loss.

DIAGNOSIS
The diagnosis of congenital gastric outlet obstruction is suggested by the finding of a large, dilated stomach on abdominal plain radiographs or in utero ultrasonography. Upper gastrointestinal (GI) contrast series is usually diagnostic and demonstrates a pyloric dimple. When contrast studies are performed, care must be taken to avoid possible aspiration. An antral web may appear as a thin septum near the pyloric channel. In older children, endoscopy has been helpful in identifying antral webs.

Table 355.1	Anomalies of the Stomach			
ANOMALY	**INCIDENCE**	**AGE AT PRESENTATION**	**SYMPTOMS AND SIGNS**	**TREATMENT**
STOMACH				
Gastric, antral, or pyloric atresia	3/100,000, when combined with webs	Infancy	Nonbilious emesis	Gastroduodenostomy, gastrojejunostomy
Pyloric or antral membrane (web)	As above	Any age	Failure to thrive, emesis	Incision or excision, pyloroplasty
Microgastria	Rare	Infancy	Emesis, malnutrition	Continuous-drip feedings or jejunal reservoir pouch
Gastric diverticulum	Rare	Any age	Usually asymptomatic	Usually unnecessary
Gastric duplication	Rare; male:female, 1:2	Any age	Abdominal mass, emesis, hematemesis; peritonitis if ruptured	Excision or partial gastrectomy
Gastric teratoma	Rare	Any age	Upper abdominal mass	Resection
Gastric volvulus	Rare	Any age	Emesis, refusal to feed	Reduction of volvulus, anterior gastropexy
Pyloric stenosis (infantile hypertrophic and adult forms)	United States, 3/1,000 (range, 1-8/1,000 in various regions); male:female, 4:1	Infancy	Non-bilious emesis	Pyloromyotomy
Congenital absence of the pylorus	Rare	Childhood, adulthood	Dyspepsia, if symptomatic	Usually unnecessary

Modified from Semrin MG, Russo MA: Anatomy, histology, and developmental anomalies of the stomach and duodenum. In Feldman M, Friedman LS, Brandt LJ, editors: *Sleisenger and Fordtran's gastrointestinal and liver disease*, ed 10, Philadelphia, Saunders, 2015, Table 48.1.

TREATMENT

The treatment of all causes of gastric outlet obstruction in neonates starts with the correction of dehydration and hypochloremic alkalosis. Persistent vomiting should be relieved with nasogastric decompression. Surgical or endoscopic repair should be undertaken when a patient is stable.

355.3 Gastric Duplication
Asim Maqbool and Chris A. Liacouras

Gastric duplications are uncommon cystic or tubular structures that usually occur within the wall of the stomach (see Table 355.1). They account for 2–7% of all GI duplications. They are most commonly located on the greater curvature. Most are <12 cm in diameter and do not usually communicate with the stomach lumen; however, they do have common blood supply. Associated anomalies occur in as many as 35% of patients. Several hypotheses for the etiology of the duplication cysts have been developed including the splitting notochord theory, diverticulation, canalization defects, and caudal twinning.

The most common clinical manifestations are associated with partial or complete gastric outlet obstruction. In 33% of patients, the cyst may be palpable. Communicating duplications can cause gastric ulceration and be associated with hematemesis or melena.

Radiographic studies usually show a paragastric mass displacing stomach. Ultrasound can show the inner hyperechoic mucosal and outer hypoechoic muscle layers that are typical of GI duplications. Surgical excision is the treatment for symptomatic gastric duplications.

ACKNOWLEDGMENT
Anna K. Hunter, MD contributed to the prior version of this chapter.

Bibliography is available at Expert Consult.

355.4 Gastric Volvulus
Asim Maqbool and Chris A. Liacouras

The stomach is tethered longitudinally by the gastrohepatic, gastrosplenic, and gastrocolic ligaments. In the transverse axis, it is tethered by the gastrophrenic ligament and the retroperitoneal attachment of the duodenum. A volvulus occurs when one of these attachments is absent or elongated, allowing the stomach to rotate around itself. In some children, other associated defects are present, including intestinal malrotation, diaphragmatic defects, hiatal hernia, or adjacent organ abnormalities such as asplenia. Volvulus can occur along the longitudinal axis, producing organoaxial volvulus, or along the transverse axis, producing mesenteroaxial volvulus. Combined volvulus occurs if the stomach rotates around both organoaxial and mesenteroaxial axes.

The clinical presentation of gastric volvulus is nonspecific and suggests high intestinal obstruction. Gastric volvulus in infancy is usually associated with nonbilious vomiting and epigastric distention. It has also been associated with episodes of dyspnea and apnea in this age group. Acute volvulus can advance rapidly to strangulation and perforation. Chronic gastric volvulus is more common in older children; the children present with a history of emesis, abdominal pain and distention, early satiety, and failure to thrive.

The diagnosis is suggested in plain abdominal radiographs by the presence of a dilated stomach. Erect abdominal films demonstrate a double fluid level with a characteristic "beak" near the lower esophageal junction in mesenteroaxial volvulus. The stomach tends to lie in a vertical plane. In organoaxial volvulus, a single air–fluid level is seen without the characteristic beak with stomach lying in a horizontal plane. Upper GI series has also been used to aid the diagnosis.

Treatment of acute gastric volvulus is emergent surgery once a patient is stabilized. Laparoscopic gastropexy is the most common surgical approach. In selected cases of chronic volvulus in older patients, endoscopic correction has been successful.

ACKNOWLEDGMENT
Anna K. Hunter, MD contributed to the prior version of this chapter.

Bibliography is available at Expert Consult.

355.5 Hypertrophic Gastropathy
Asim Maqbool and Chris A. Liacouras

Hypertrophic gastropathy in children is uncommon and, in contrast to that in adults (Ménétrier disease), is usually a transient, benign, and self-limited condition.

PATHOGENESIS
The condition is most often secondary to cytomegalovirus (CMV) infection, but other agents, including herpes simplex virus, *Giardia,* and *Helicobacter pylori,* are also implicated. The pathophysiologic mechanisms underlying the clinical picture are not completely understood but might involve widening of gap junctions between gastric epithelial cells with resultant fluid and protein losses. There is an association with increased expression of transforming growth factor-α in gastric mucosal tissue shown in CMV-induced gastropathy. *H. pylori* infection can cause the elevation of serum glucagon-like peptide-2 levels, a mucosal growth-inducing gut hormone.

CLINICAL MANIFESTATIONS
Clinical manifestations include vomiting, anorexia, upper abdominal pain, diarrhea, edema (hypoproteinemic protein-losing enteropathy), ascites, and, rarely, hematemesis if ulceration occurs.

DIAGNOSIS AND DIFFERENTIAL DIAGNOSIS
The mean age at diagnosis is 5 yr (range: 2 days to 17 yr); the illness usually lasts 2-14 wk. Endoscopy with biopsy and tissue CMV polymerase chain reaction is diagnostic. Endoscopy shows characteristic enlarged gastric folds. The upper GI series might show thickened gastric folds. The differential diagnosis includes eosinophilic gastroenteritis, gastric lymphoma or carcinoma, Crohn disease, and inflammatory pseudotumor.

TREATMENT
Therapy is supportive and should include adequate hydration, antisecretory agents (H_2 receptor blockade, acid suppression with proton pump inhibitors), and albumin replacement if the hypoalbuminemia is symptomatic. When *H. pylori* are detected, appropriate treatment is recommended. Ganciclovir in CMV-positive gastropathy is indicated only in severe cases. There are no official guidelines as far as the length of treatment. In practice, IV therapy is initiated for the 1st 24-48 hr. Treatment is continued with oral valganciclovir for a total of 3 wk. Complete recovery is the rule. Hypertrophic gastropathy should be considered in a previously healthy child with new onset edema and no other causes of protein losses. This is not a chronic condition in children, and the disease tends to have much more severe course in adult patients.

ACKNOWLEDGMENT
Anna K. Hunter, MD contributed to the prior version of this chapter.

Bibliography is available at Expert Consult.

Chapter **356**

Intestinal Atresia, Stenosis, and Malrotation

Asim Maqbool, Christina Bales, and Chris A. Liacouras

第三百五十六章
肠闭锁、狭窄和旋转不良

中文导读

　　本章主要介绍了肠闭锁、狭窄和旋转不良。肠闭锁、狭窄中具体描述了十二指肠梗阻和空肠、回肠闭锁和梗阻；肠旋转不良中详细阐述了肠旋转不良的胚胎发育学、临床表现和治疗。十二指肠梗阻部分具体描述了十二指肠梗阻的临床表现的特点和诊断的要点以及治疗；空肠、回肠闭锁和梗阻具体描述了空肠、回肠闭锁和梗阻的临床表现和诊断以及治疗。

Approximately 1 in 1,500 children is born with intestinal obstruction. Obstruction may be partial or complete, and it may be characterized as simple or strangulating. Luminal contents fails to progress in an aboral direction in simple obstruction, whereas blood flow to the intestine is also impaired in strangulating obstruction. If strangulating obstruction is not promptly relieved, it can lead to bowel infarction and perforation.

Intestinal obstruction can be further classified as either intrinsic or extrinsic based on underlying etiology. Intrinsic causes include inherent abnormalities of intestinal innervation, mucus production, or tubular anatomy. Among these, congenital disruption of the tubular structure is most common and can manifest as obliteration (**atresia**) or narrowing (**stenosis**) of the intestinal lumen. More than 90% of intestinal stenosis and atresia occurs in the duodenum, jejunum, and ileum. Rare cases occur in the colon, and these may be associated with more proximal atresias.

Extrinsic causes of congenital intestinal obstruction involve compression of the bowel by vessels (e.g., preduodenal portal vein), organs (e.g., annular pancreas), and cysts (e.g., duplication, mesenteric). Abnormalities in intestinal rotation during fetal development also represent a unique extrinsic cause of congenital intestinal obstruction. Malrotation is associated with inadequate mesenteric attachment of the intestine to the posterior abdominal wall, which leaves the bowel vulnerable to auto obstruction as a result of intestinal twisting or volvulus. Malrotation is commonly accompanied by congenital adhesions that can compress and obstruct the duodenum as they extend from the cecum to the right upper quadrant.

Obstruction is typically associated with bowel distention, which is caused by an accumulation of ingested food, gas, and intestinal secretions proximal to the point of obstruction. As the bowel dilates, absorption of intestinal fluid is decreased and secretion of fluid and electrolytes is increased. This shift results in isotonic intravascular depletion, which is usually associated with hypokalemia. Bowel distention also results in a decrease in blood flow to the obstructed bowel. As blood flow is shifted away from the intestinal mucosa, there is loss of mucosal integrity. Bacteria proliferate in the stagnant bowel, with a predominance of coliforms and anaerobes. This rapid proliferation of bacteria, coupled with the loss of mucosal integrity, allows bacteria to translocate across the bowel wall and potentially lead to endotoxemia, bacteremia, and sepsis.

The clinical presentation of intestinal obstruction varies with the cause, level of obstruction, and time between the obstructing event and the patient's evaluation. Classic symptoms of obstruction in the neonate include vomiting, abdominal distention, and obstipation. Obstruction high in the intestinal tract results in large-volume, frequent, bilious emesis with little or no abdominal distention. Pain is intermittent and is usually relieved by vomiting. Obstruction in the distal small bowel leads to moderate or marked abdominal distention with emesis that is progressively feculent. Both proximal and distal obstructions are eventually associated with obstipation. However, meconium stools can be passed initially if the obstruction is in the upper part of the intestinal tract or if the obstruction developed late in intrauterine life.

The diagnosis of congenital bowel obstruction relies on a combination of history, physical examination, and radiologic findings. In certain cases, the diagnosis is suggested in the prenatal period. Routine prenatal ultrasound can detect polyhydramnios, which often accompanies high intestinal obstruction. The presence of polyhydramnios should prompt aspiration of the infant's stomach immediately after birth. Aspiration of more than 15-20 mL of fluid, particularly if it is bile stained, is highly indicative of proximal intestinal obstruction.

In the postnatal period, a plain radiograph is the initial diagnostic study and can provide valuable information about potential associated complications. With completely obstructing lesions, plain radiographs reveal bowel distention proximal to the point of obstruction. Upright or crosstable lateral views typically demonstrate a series of air–fluid levels in the distended loops. Caution must be exercised in using plain films to determine the location of intestinal obstruction. Because colonic haustra are not fully developed in the neonate, small and large bowel obstructions may be difficult to distinguish with plain films. In these cases, contrast studies of the bowel or computed tomography images may be indicated. Oral or nasogastric contrast medium may be used to identify obstructing lesions in the proximal bowel, and contrast enemas may be used to diagnose more-distal entities. Indeed, enemas may also play a therapeutic role in relieving distal obstruction caused by meconium ileus or meconium plug syndrome.

Initial treatment of infants and children with bowel obstruction must be directed at fluid resuscitation and stabilizing the patient. Nasogastric decompression usually relieves pain and vomiting. After appropriate cultures, broad-spectrum antibiotics are usually started in ill-appearing neonates with bowel obstruction and those with suspected strangulating infarction. Patients with strangulation must have immediate surgical relief before the bowel infarcts, resulting in gangrene and intestinal perforation. Extensive intestinal necrosis results in short bowel syndrome (see Chapter 364.7). Nonoperative conservative management is usually limited to children with suspected adhesions or inflammatory strictures that might resolve with nasogastric decompression or antiinflammatory medications. If clinical signs of improvement are not evident within 12-24 hr, then operative intervention is usually indicated.

356.1 Duodenal Obstruction

Asim Maqbool and Chris A. Liacouras

Congenital duodenal obstruction occurs in 2.5-10/100,000 live births. In most cases, it is caused by atresia, an intrinsic defect of bowel formation. It can also result from extrinsic compression by abnormal neighboring structures (e.g., annular pancreas, preduodenal portal vein), duplication cysts, or congenital bands associated with malrotation. Although intrinsic and extrinsic causes of duodenal obstruction occur independently, they can also coexist. Thus a high index of suspicion for more than one underlying etiology may be critical to avoiding unnecessary reoperations in these infants.

Duodenal atresia complicates 1/10,000 live births and accounts for 25–40% of all intestinal atresias. In contrast to more-distal atresias, which likely arise from prenatal vascular accidents, duodenal atresia results from failed recanalization of the intestinal lumen during gestation. Throughout the 4th and 5th wk of normal fetal development, the duodenal mucosa exhibits rapid proliferation of epithelial cells. Persistence of these cells, which should degenerate after the 7th wk of gestation, leads to occlusion of the lumen (atresia) in approximately two-thirds of cases and narrowing (stenosis) in the remaining one-third. Duodenal atresia can take several forms, including a thin membrane that occludes the lumen, a short fibrous cord that connects two blind duodenal pouches, or a gap that spans two nonconnecting ends of the duodenum. The membranous form is most common, and it almost invariably occurs near the ampulla of Vater. In rare cases, the membrane is distensible and is referred to as a *windsock web.* This unusual form of duodenal atresia causes obstruction several centimeters distal to the origin of the membrane.

Approximately 50% of infants with duodenal atresia are premature. Concomitant congenital anomalies are common and include congenital heart disease (30%), malrotation (20–30%), annular pancreas (30%), renal anomalies (5–15%), esophageal atresia with or without tracheoesophageal fistula (5–10%), skeletal malformations (5%), and anorectal anomalies (5%). Of these anomalies, only complex congenital heart disease is associated with increased mortality. Annular pancreas is associated with increased late complications, including gastroesophageal reflux disease, peptic ulcer disease, pancreatitis, gastric outlet and recurrent duodenal obstruction, and gastric cancer. Thus long-term follow-up of these patients into adulthood is warranted. Nearly half of

patients with duodenal atresia have chromosome abnormalities; trisomy 21 is identified in up to one-third of patients.

CLINICAL MANIFESTATIONS AND DIAGNOSIS

The hallmark of duodenal obstruction is bilious vomiting without abdominal distention, which is usually noted on the first day of life. Peristaltic waves may be visualized early in the disease process. A history of polyhydramnios is present in half the pregnancies and is caused by inadequate absorption of amniotic fluid in the distal intestine. This fluid may be bile stained because of intrauterine vomiting. Jaundice is present in one-third of the infants.

The diagnosis is suggested by the presence of a *double-bubble* sign on a plain abdominal radiograph (Fig. 356.1). The appearance is caused by a distended and gas-filled stomach and proximal duodenum, which are invariably connected. Contrast studies are occasionally needed to exclude malrotation and volvulus because intestinal infarction can occur within 6-12 hr if the volvulus is not relieved. Contrast studies are generally not necessary and may be associated with aspiration. Prenatal diagnosis of duodenal atresia is readily made by fetal ultrasonography, which reveals a sonographic double-bubble. Prenatal identification of duodenal atresia is associated with decreased morbidity and fewer hospitalization days.

TREATMENT

The initial treatment of infants with duodenal atresia includes nasogastric or orogastric decompression and intravenous fluid replacement. Echocardiography, renal ultrasound, and radiology of the chest and spine should be performed to evaluate for associated anomalies. Definitive correction of the atresia is usually postponed until life-threatening anomalies are evaluated and treated.

The typical surgical repair for duodenal atresia is duodenoduodenostomy. This procedure is also preferred in cases of concomitant or isolated annular pancreas. In these instances, the duodenoduodenostomy is performed without dividing the pancreas. The dilated proximal bowel might have to be tapered to improve peristalsis. Postoperatively, a

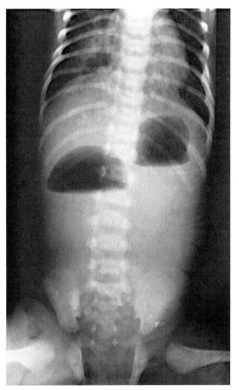

Fig. 356.1 Abdominal radiograph of a newborn infant held upright. Note the "double-bubble" gas shadow above and the absence of gas in the distal bowel in this case of congenital duodenal atresia.

gastrostomy tube can be placed to drain the stomach and protect the airway. Intravenous nutritional support or a transanastomotic jejunal tube is needed until an infant starts to feed orally. Long-term prognosis is excellent, approaching 90% survival in most series.

Bibliography is available at Expert Consult.

356.2 Jejunal and Ileal Atresia and Obstruction

Asim Maqbool and Chris A. Liacouras

The primary etiologies of congenital small bowel obstruction involve intrinsic abnormalities in anatomic development (jejunoileal stenosis and atresia), mucus secretion (meconium ileus), and bowel wall innervation (long-segment Hirschsprung disease).

Jejunoileal atresias are generally attributed to intrauterine vascular accidents, which result in segmental infarction and resorption of the fetal intestine. Underlying events that potentiate vascular compromise include intestinal volvulus, intussusception, meconium ileus, and strangulating herniation through an abdominal wall defect associated with gastroschisis or omphalocele. Maternal behaviors that promote vasoconstriction, such as cigarette smoking and cocaine use, might also have a role. Only a few cases of familial inheritance have been reported. In these families, multiple intestinal atresias have occurred in an autosomal recessive pattern. Jejunoileal atresias have been linked with multiple births, low birthweight, and prematurity. Unlike atresia in the duodenum, they are not commonly associated with extraintestinal anomalies.

Five types of jejunal and ileal atresias are encountered (Fig. 356.2). In type I, a mucosal web occludes the lumen, but continuity is maintained between the proximal and distal bowel. Type II involves a small-diameter solid cord that connects the proximal and distal bowel. Type III is divided into two subtypes. Type IIIa occurs when both ends of the bowel end in blind loops, accompanied by a small mesenteric defect. Type IIIb is similar, but it is associated with an extensive mesenteric defect and a loss of the normal blood supply to the distal bowel. The distal ileum coils around the ileocolic artery, from which it derives its entire blood supply, producing an "apple-peel" appearance. This anomaly is associated with prematurity, an unusually short distal ileum, and significant foreshortening of the bowel. Type IV involves multiple atresias. Types II and IIIa are the most common, each accounting for 30-35% of cases. Type I occurs in approximately 20% of patients. Types IIIb and IV account for the remaining 10–20% of cases, with IIIb being the least-common configuration.

Meconium ileus occurs primarily in newborn infants with cystic fibrosis, an exocrine gland defect of chloride transport that results in abnormally viscous secretions (Chapter 432). Approximately 80–90% of infants with meconium ileus have cystic fibrosis, but only 10–15% of infants with cystic fibrosis present with meconium ileus. In simple cases, the distal 20-30 cm of ileum is collapsed and filled with pellets of pale stool. The proximal bowel is dilated and filled with thick meconium that resembles sticky syrup or glue. Peristalsis fails to propel this viscid material forward, and it becomes impacted in the ileum. In complicated cases, a volvulus of the dilated proximal bowel can occur, resulting in intestinal ischemia, atresia, and/or perforation. Perforation in utero results in meconium peritonitis, which can lead to potentially obstructing adhesions and calcifications.

Both intestinal atresia and meconium ileus must be distinguished from long-segment Hirschsprung disease. This condition involves congenital absence of ganglion cells in the myenteric and submucosal plexuses of the bowel wall. In a small subset (5%) of patients, the aganglionic segment includes the terminal ileum in addition to the entire length of the colon. Infants with long-segment Hirschsprung disease present with a dilated small intestine that is ganglionated but has hypertrophied walls, a funnel-shaped transitional hypoganglionic zone, and a collapsed distal aganglionic bowel.

CLINICAL MANIFESTATION AND DIAGNOSIS

Distal intestinal obstruction is less likely than proximal obstruction to be detected in utero. Polyhydramnios is identified in 20–35% of jejunoileal atresias, and it may be the first sign of intestinal obstruction. Abdominal distention is rarely present at birth, but it develops rapidly after initiation of feeds in the first 12-24 hr. Distention is often accompanied by vomiting, which is often bilious. Up to 80% of infants fail to pass meconium in the first 24 hr of life. Jaundice, associated with unconjugated hyperbilirubinemia, is reported in 20–30% of patients.

In patients with obstruction caused by jejunoileal atresia or long-segment Hirschsprung disease, plain radiographs typically demonstrate multiple air–fluid levels proximal to the obstruction in the upright or lateral decubitus positions (Fig. 356.3). These levels may be absent in patients with meconium ileus because the viscosity of the secretions in the proximal bowel prevents layering. Instead, a typical hazy or ground-glass appearance may be appreciated in the right lower quadrant. This haziness is caused by small bubbles of gas that become trapped in inspissated meconium in the terminal ileal region. If there is meconium peritonitis, patchy calcification may also be noted, particularly in the flanks. Plain films can reveal evidence of pneumoperitoneum due to intestinal perforation. Air may be seen in the subphrenic regions on the upright view and over the liver in the left lateral decubitus position.

Because plain radiographs do not reliably distinguish between small and large bowel in neonates, contrast studies are often required to localize the obstruction. Water-soluble enemas (Gastrografin, Hypaque) are particularly useful in differentiating atresia from meconium ileus and Hirschsprung disease. A small *microcolon* suggests disuse and the presence of obstruction proximal to the ileocecal valve. Abdominal ultrasound may be an important adjunctive study, which can distin-

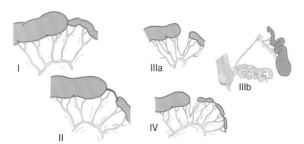

Fig. 356.2 Classification of intestinal atresia. *Type I:* Mucosal obstruction caused by an intraluminal membrane with intact bowel wall and mesentery. *Type II:* Blind ends are separated by a fibrous cord. *Type IIIa:* Blind ends are separated by a V-shaped mesenteric defect. *Type IIIb:* "Apple-peel" appearance. *Type IV:* Multiple atresias. (*From Grosfeld J: Jejunoileal atresia and stenosis. In Welch KJ, Randolph JG, Ravitch MM, editors: Pediatric surgery, ed 4, Chicago, 1986, Year Book Medical Publishers.*)

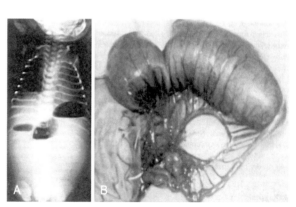

Fig. 356.3 A, Abdominal radiograph in a neonate with bilious vomiting shows a few loops of dilated intestine with air–fluid levels. **B,** At laparotomy, a type I (mucosal) jejunal atresia was observed. (*From O'Neill JA Jr, Grosfeld JL, Fonkalsrud EW, et al, editors: Principles of pediatric surgery, ed 2, St. Louis, 2003, Mosby, p. 493.*)

guish meconium ileus from ileal atresia and also identify concomitant intestinal malrotation.

TREATMENT

Patients with small bowel obstruction should be stable and in adequate fluid and electrolyte balance before operation or radiographic attempts at disimpaction unless volvulus is suspected. Documented infections should be treated with appropriate antibiotics. Prophylactic antibiotics are usually given before surgery.

Ileal or jejunal atresia requires resection of the dilated proximal portion of the bowel followed by end-to-end anastomosis. If a simple mucosal diaphragm is present, jejunoplasty or ileoplasty with partial excision of the web is an acceptable alternative to resection. In uncomplicated meconium ileus, Gastrografin enemas diagnose the obstruction and wash out the inspissated material. Gastrografin is hypertonic, and care must be taken to avoid dehydration, shock, and bowel perforation. The enema may have to be repeated after 8-12 hr. Resection after reduction is not needed if there have been no ischemic complications.

Approximately 50% of patients with simple meconium ileus do not adequately respond to water-soluble enemas and need laparotomy. Operative management is indicated when the obstruction cannot be relieved by repeated attempts at nonoperative management and for infants with complicated meconium ileus. The extent of surgical intervention depends on the degree of pathology. In simple meconium ileus, the plug can be relieved by manipulation or direct enteral irrigation with N-acetylcysteine following an enterotomy. In complicated cases, bowel resection, peritoneal lavage, abdominal drainage, and stoma formation may be necessary. Total parenteral nutrition is generally required.

Bibliography is available at Expert Consult.

356.3 Malrotation

Asim Maqbool and Chris A. Liacouras

Malrotation is incomplete rotation of the intestine during fetal development and involves the intestinal nonrotation or incomplete rotation around the superior mesenteric artery. The gut starts as a straight tube from stomach to rectum. Intestinal rotation and attachment begin in the 5th wk of gestation when the midbowel (distal duodenum to midtransverse colon) begins to elongate and progressively protrudes into the umbilical cord until it lies totally outside the confines of the abdominal cavity. As the developing bowel rotates in and out of the abdominal cavity, the superior mesenteric artery, which supplies blood to this section of gut, acts as an axis. The duodenum, on reentering the abdominal cavity, moves to the region of the ligament of Treitz, and the colon that follows is directed to the left upper quadrant. The cecum subsequently rotates counterclockwise within the abdominal cavity and comes to lie in the right lower quadrant. The duodenum becomes fixed to the posterior abdominal wall before the colon is completely rotated. After rotation, the right and left colon and the mesenteric root become fixed to the posterior abdomen. These attachments provide a broad base of support to the mesentery and the superior mesenteric artery, thus preventing twisting of the mesenteric root and kinking of the vascular supply. Abdominal rotation and attachment are completed by the 12th wk of gestation.

Nonrotation occurs when the bowel fails to rotate after it returns to the abdominal cavity. The first and second portions of the duodenum are in their normal position, but the remainder of the duodenum, jejunum, and ileum occupy the right side of the abdomen and the colon is located on the left. The most common type of malrotation involves failure of the cecum to move into the right lower quadrant (Fig. 356.4). The usual location of the cecum is in the subhepatic area. Failure of the cecum to rotate properly is associated with failure to form the normal broad-based adherence to the posterior abdominal wall. The mesentery, including the superior mesenteric artery, is tethered by a narrow stalk, which can twist around itself and produce a midgut volvulus. Bands of tissue (**Ladd bands**) can extend from the

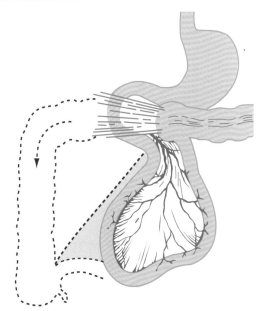

Fig. 356.4 The mechanism of intestinal obstruction with incomplete rotation of the midgut (malrotation). The *dotted lines* show the course the cecum should have taken. Failure to rotate has left obstructing bands across the duodenum and a narrow pedicle for the midgut loop, making it susceptible to volvulus. *(From Nixon HH, O'Donnell B: The essentials of pediatric surgery, Philadelphia, 1961, JB Lippincott.)*

cecum to the right upper quadrant, crossing, and possibly obstructing, the duodenum.

Malrotation and nonrotation are often associated with other anomalies of the abdominal wall such as diaphragmatic hernia, gastroschisis, and omphalocele. Malrotation is also associated with the **heterotaxy syndrome**, which is a complex of congenital anomalies including congenital heart malformations, malrotation, biliary atresia, and either asplenia or polysplenia (see Chapter 458.11).

CLINICAL MANIFESTATIONS

The reported incidence of malrotation is approximately 1 in 500 infants. The majority, about 75–85% of patients, present in the first yr of life, and more than 50% present within the first mo of life, with symptoms of acute or chronic obstruction. Vomiting is the most common symptom in this age group. Infants often present in the first wk of life with **bilious emesis** and acute bowel obstruction. Older infants present with episodes of recurrent abdominal pain that can mimic colic and suggest intermittent volvulus. Malrotation in older children can manifest with recurrent episodes of vomiting and/or abdominal pain. Patients occasionally present with **malabsorption** or **protein-losing enteropathy** associated with bacterial overgrowth. Symptoms are caused by intermittent volvulus or duodenal compression by Ladd bands or other adhesive bands affecting the small and large bowel. Approximately 25–50% of adolescents with malrotation are asymptomatic. Adolescents who become symptomatic present with acute intestinal obstruction or history of recurrent episodes of abdominal pain or postprandial bloating and occasional vomiting. Patients of any age with a rotational anomaly can develop acute bowel-threatening volvulus without preexisting symptoms.

An acute presentation of small bowel obstruction in a patient without previous bowel surgery can be the result of **volvulus** associated with malrotation. This is a life-threatening complication of malrotation, which resembles an acute abdomen or sepsis and is the main reason that symptoms suggesting malrotation should always be investigated. Volvulus occurs when the small bowel twists around the superior mesenteric artery leading to vascular compromise of the bowel. The diagnosis may be suggested by ultrasound but is confirmed by contrast radiographic studies. The abdominal plain film is usually nonspecific but might demonstrate a gasless abdomen or evidence of duodenal obstruction with a double-bubble sign. Upper gastrointestinal series is the imaging test of choice and the gold standard in the evaluation and diagnosis of malrotation and volvulus. Normal rotation is indicated by the duodenal C-loop crossing the midline and a duodenojejunal junction located to the left of the spine. Upper gastrointestinal series is the best exam to visualize the malposition of the ligament of Treitz and can also reveal a corkscrew appearance of the small bowel or a duodenal obstruction with a *bird's beak* appearance of the duodenum. Barium enema usually demonstrates malposition of the cecum but is normal in up to 20% of patients. Ultrasonography can demonstrate the inversion of the superior mesenteric artery and vein. A superior mesenteric vein located to the left of the superior mesenteric artery suggests malrotation. Malrotation with volvulus is suggested by duodenal obstruction, thickened bowel loops to the right of the spine, the superior mesenteric vein coiling around the superior mesenteric artery, and free peritoneal fluid.

TREATMENT

Surgical intervention is recommended for any patient with a significant rotational abnormality, regardless of age. If a volvulus is present, surgery is done immediately as an acute emergency, the volvulus is reduced, and the duodenum and upper jejunum are freed of any bands and remain in the right abdominal cavity. The colon is freed of adhesions and placed in the right abdomen with the cecum in the left lower quadrant, usually accompanied by incidental appendectomy. The Ladd procedure may be done laparoscopically for malrotation without volvulus and if gut ischemia is not present, but it is generally done as an open procedure if volvulus is present. The purpose of surgical intervention is to minimize the risk of subsequent volvulus rather than to return the bowel to a normal anatomic configuration. Extensive intestinal ischemia from volvulus can result in short bowel syndrome (see Chapter 364.7).

ACKNOWLEDGMENT

Melissa Kennedy, MD contributed to the prior version of this chapter.

Bibliography is available at Expert Consult.

Chapter **357**

Intestinal Duplications, Meckel Diverticulum, and Other Remnants of the Omphalomesenteric Duct

第三百五十七章

肠重复畸形、梅克尔憩室和其他卵黄管残余畸形

中文导读

　　本章主要介绍了肠重复畸形、梅克尔憩室和其他卵黄管残余畸形。肠重复畸形部分具体描述肠重复畸形的定义、分类、病因、临床表现、诊断和治疗；梅克尔憩室和其他卵黄管残余畸形部分具体描述了梅克尔憩室形成的胚胎发育学、典型的梅克尔憩室的位置、分型、临床表现及特点（无痛性血便）、梅克尔憩室的诊断方法以及治疗方法等。

357.1 Intestinal Duplication

Asim Maqbool and Chris A. Liacouras

Duplications of the intestinal tract are rare anomalies that consist of well-formed tubular or spherical structures firmly attached to the intestine with a common blood supply. The lining of the duplications resembles that of the gastrointestinal (GI) tract. Duplications are located on the mesenteric border and can communicate with the intestinal lumen. Duplications can be classified into three categories: localized duplications, duplications associated with spinal cord defects and vertebral malformations, and duplications of the colon. Occasionally (10–15% of cases), multiple duplications are found.

Localized duplications can occur in any area of the GI tract but are most common in the ileum and jejunum. They are usually cystic or tubular structures within the wall of the bowel. The cause is unknown, but their development has been attributed to defects in recanalization of the intestinal lumen after the solid stage of embryologic development. Duplication of the intestine occurring in association with **vertebral and spinal cord anomalies** (hemivertebra, anterior spina bifida, band connection between lesion and cervical or thoracic spine) is thought to arise from splitting of the notochord in the developing embryo. **Duplication of the colon** is usually associated with anomalies of the urinary tract and genitals. Duplication of the entire colon, rectum, anus, and terminal ileum can occur. The defects are thought to be secondary to caudal twinning, with duplication of the hindgut, genital, and lower urinary tracts.

CLINICAL MANIFESTATIONS

Symptoms depend on the size, location, and mucosal lining. Duplications can cause bowel obstruction by compressing the adjacent intestinal lumen, or they can act as the lead point of an intussusception or a site for a volvulus. If they are lined by acid-secreting mucosa, they can cause ulceration, perforation, and hemorrhage of or into the adjacent bowel. Patients can present with abdominal pain, vomiting, palpable mass, or acute GI hemorrhage. Intestinal duplications in the thorax (**neuroenteric cysts**) can manifest as respiratory distress. Duplications of the lower bowel can cause constipation or diarrhea or be associated with recurrent prolapse of the rectum.

The diagnosis is suspected on the basis of the history and physical examination. Radiologic studies such as barium studies, ultrasonography, CT, and MRI are helpful but usually nonspecific, demonstrating cystic structures or mass effects. Radioisotope technetium scanning can localize ectopic gastric mucosa. The treatment of duplications is surgical resection and management of associated defects.

357.2 Meckel Diverticulum and Other Remnants of the Omphalomesenteric Duct

Melissa A. Kennedy, Asim Maqbool, and Chris A. Liacouras

Meckel diverticulum is the most common congenital anomaly of the GI tract and is caused by the incomplete obliteration of the omphalomesenteric duct during the 7th wk of gestation. The omphalomesenteric duct connects the yolk sac to the gut in a developing embryo and provides nutrition until the placenta is established. Between the 5th and 7th wk of gestation, the duct attenuates and separates from the intestine. Just before this involution, the epithelium of the yolk sac develops a lining similar to that of the stomach. Partial or complete failure of involution of the omphalomesenteric duct results in various residual structures. Meckel diverticulum is the most common of these structures and is the most common congenital GI anomaly, occurring in 2–3% of all infants. A typical Meckel diverticulum is a 3-6 cm outpouching of the ileum along the antimesenteric border 50-75 cm (approximately 2 feet) from the ileocecal valve (Fig. 357.1). The distance from the ileocecal valve depends on the age of the patient. Meckel diverticulum has been conveniently referred to by the "rule of 2s," which

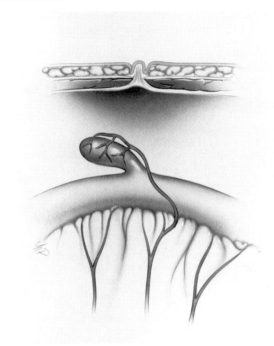

Fig. 357.1 Typical Meckel diverticulum located on the antimesenteric border.

explains the classic presentation of this congenital anomaly. Meckel diverticulum are found in approximately 2% of the general population, are usually located 2 feet proximal to the ileocecal valve and are approximately 2 inches in length, can contain 2 types of ectopic tissue (pancreatic or gastric), generally present before the age of 2 yr, and are found twice as commonly in females. Although intraabdominal in location, a rare presentation of a Meckel diverticulum is entrapment in an inguinal, umbilical, or femoral hernia (Littre hernia). Other omphalomesenteric duct remnants occur infrequently, including a persistently patent duct, a solid cord, or a cord with a central cyst or a diverticulum associated with a persistent cord between the diverticulum and the umbilicus.

CLINICAL MANIFESTATIONS

Symptoms of a Meckel diverticulum usually arise in the first or second yr of life (average: 2.5 yr), but initial symptoms can occur in the first decade. The majority of symptomatic Meckel diverticula are lined by an ectopic mucosa, including an acid-secreting mucosa that causes intermittent painless rectal bleeding by ulceration of the adjacent normal ileal mucosa. This ectopic mucosa is most commonly of gastric origin, but it can also be pancreatic, jejunal, or a combination of these tissues. Unlike the upper duodenal mucosa, the acid is not neutralized by pancreatic bicarbonate.

The stool is typically described as brick colored or currant jelly colored. Bleeding can cause significant anemia but is usually self-limited because of contraction of the splanchnic vessels, as patients become hypovolemic. Bleeding from a Meckel diverticulum can also be less dramatic, with melanotic stools.

Less often, a Meckel diverticulum is associated with partial or complete bowel obstruction. The most common mechanism of obstruction occurs when the diverticulum acts as the lead point of an intussusception. The mean age of onset of obstruction is younger than that for patients presenting with bleeding. Obstruction can also result from intraperitoneal bands connecting residual omphalomesenteric duct remnants to the ileum and umbilicus. These bands cause obstruction by internal herniation or volvulus of the small bowel around the band. A Meckel diverticulum occasionally becomes inflamed (**diverticulitis**) and manifests similarly to acute appendicitis. These children are older, with a mean of 8 yr of age. Diverticulitis can lead to perforation and peritonitis.

DIAGNOSIS

The diagnosis of omphalomesenteric duct remnants depends on the clinical presentation. If an infant or child presents with significant painless rectal bleeding, the presence of a Meckel diverticulum should be suspected because Meckel diverticulum accounts for 50% of all lower GI bleeds in children younger than 2 yr of age.

Confirmation of a Meckel diverticulum can be difficult. Plain abdominal radiographs are of no value, and routine barium studies rarely fill the diverticulum. The most sensitive study is a Meckel radionuclide scan, which is performed after intravenous infusion of technetium-99m pertechnetate. The mucus-secreting cells of the ectopic gastric mucosa take up pertechnetate, permitting visualization of the Meckel diverticulum (Fig. 357.2). The uptake can be enhanced with various agents, including cimetidine, ranitidine, glucagon, and pentagastrin. The sensitivity of the enhanced scan is approximately 85%, with a specificity of approximately 95%. A false-negative scan may be seen in anemic patients; although false-positive results are uncommon, they have been reported with intussusception, appendicitis, duplication cysts, arteriovenous malformations, and tumors. Other methods of detection include radiolabeled tagged red blood cell scan (the patient must be actively bleeding), abdominal ultrasound, superior mesenteric angiography, abdominal CT scan, or exploratory laparoscopy. In patients who present with intestinal obstruction or a picture of appendicitis with omphalomesenteric duct remnants, the diagnosis is rarely made before surgery.

The treatment of a symptomatic Meckel diverticulum is surgical excision. A diverticulectomy can be performed safely as either a laparoscopic or open procedure, although most continue to be performed as open procedures. There is significant debate regarding the proper management of an asymptomatic Meckel diverticulum and whether excision vs observation is appropriate. However, the risk of serious complications does seem to exceed the operative risk in children younger than 8 yr old.

Bibliography is available at Expert Consult.

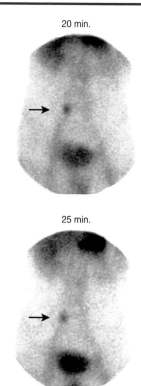

20 min.

25 min.

Fig. 357.2 Meckel scan demonstrating accumulation of technetium in the stomach superior bladder (inferior) and in the acid-secreting mucosa of a Meckel diverticulum.

中文导读

本章主要介绍了慢性假性肠梗阻、线粒体神经胃肠型脑肌病、大便失禁和功能性便秘、先天性无神经节细胞性巨结肠、肠神经元发育不良和肠系膜上动脉综合征。具体描述了慢性假性肠梗阻的临床表现、治疗；具体描述了大便失禁和功能性便秘的临床表现、诊断和治疗；具体描述了先天性无神经节细胞性巨结肠的病理学、临床表现、诊断和治疗等内容。

358.1 Chronic Intestinal Pseudoobstruction

*Asim Maqbool, Kristin N. Fiorino,
and Chris A. Liacouras*

Chronic intestinal pseudoobstruction (CIPO) comprises a group of primary and secondary disorders characterized as a motility disorder with the dominant defect of impaired peristalsis; symptoms are consistent with intestinal obstruction in the absence of mechanical obstruction (Table 358.1). The natural history of primary pseudoobstruction is that of a progressive disorder, although there are occasional cases of secondary pseudoobstruction caused by conditions that can transiently or permanently alter bowel motility. The most common cause of acute pseudoobstruction is Ogilvie syndrome (acute pseudoobstruction of the colon). Pseudoobstruction represents a wide spectrum of pathologic disorders from abnormal myoelectric activity to abnormalities of the nerves (intestinal neuropathy) or musculature (intestinal myopathy) of the gut. The organs involved can include the entire gastrointestinal tract or be limited to certain components, although almost always include the small bowel. The distinctive pathologic abnormalities are considered together because of their clinical similarities. For these reasons, CIPO may be thought of more as a clinical syndrome at times.

Most congenital forms of primary pseudoobstruction occur sporadically, although autosomal dominant *(SOX10)*, autosomal recessive *(RAD21, SGOL1, TYMP, POLG)*, X-linked *(FLNA, L1CAM)*, and familial patterns of inheritance have been identified. Patients with autosomal dominant forms of pseudoobstruction have variable expressions of the disease. Patients with mutations in *TYMP* and *POLG* genes present with mitochondrial neurogastrointestinal encephalomyopathy syndrome (MNGIE); MELAS syndrome is another mitochondrial disorder associated with CIPO. MNGIE is characterized by intestinal dysmotility, abdominal pain and distention, emesis, cachexia, ptosis, leukoencephalopathy, peripheral neuropathy (paresthesia, pain), and myopathy. Sixty percent have symptoms (often subtle) before age 20 yr (see Chapter 358.2). *Acquired* pseudoobstruction can follow episodes of acute gastroenteritis, presumably resulting in injury to the myenteric plexus.

In *congenital* pseudoobstruction, abnormalities of the muscle or nerves can be demonstrated in most cases. In myopathies, the smooth muscle is involved, in which the outer longitudinal muscle layer is replaced by fibrous material. These manifestations of visceral myopathies may be primary or secondary phenomenon. The enteric nervous system is usually altered in neuropathies and may involve disorganized ganglia, hypoganglionosis, or hyperganglionosis. Abnormalities in the interstitial cells of Cajal, the intestinal pacemaker, are classified as mesenchymopathies. In others, mitochondrial defects have been identified.

CLINICAL MANIFESTATIONS

More than half the children with congenital pseudoobstruction experience symptoms in the first few mo of life (Table 358.2). Two-thirds of the infants presenting in the first few days of life are born prematurely, and approximately 40% have malrotation of the intestine. In 75% of all affected children, symptoms occur in the first year of life, while the remainder are usually symptomatic within the next several years. Females present with CIPO more than males do during the first year of life, with equal sex distribution in older children. The most common symptoms are abdominal distention (85–95% of patients) and vomiting (55–90%). Constipation, growth failure, and abdominal pain occur in approximately 60% of patients and diarrhea in 25–30%. The symptoms wax and wane in most patients; poor nutrition, psychologic stress, and intercurrent illness tend to exacerbate symptoms. Urinary tract and bladder involvement occurs in 80% of children with myopathic pseudoobstruction and in 20% of those with neuropathic disease. Symptoms can manifest as recurrent urinary tract infection,

Table 358.1	Causes of Secondary Chronic Intestinal Pseudoobstruction in Children

AUTOIMMUNE
Autoimmune myositis
Autoimmune ganglionitis
Scleroderma

ENDOCRINE
Diabetes mellitus
Hypoparathyroidism
Hypothyroidism

GASTROINTESTINAL
Celiac disease
Eosinophilic gastroenteritis
Inflammatory bowel disease

HEMATOLOGY/ONCOLOGY
Multiple myeloma
Paraneoplastic syndromes
Pheochromocytoma
Sickle cell disease

INFECTION
Chagas disease
Cytomegalovirus
Epstein-Barr virus
Herpes zoster
JC virus
Kawasaki disease
Postviral neuropathy

MEDICATIONS AND TOXINS
Chemotherapy
Cyclopentolate and phenylephrine eye drops
Diltiazem and nifedipine
Fetal alcohol syndrome
Jellyfish envenomation
Opioid medications
Postanesthesia
Radiation injury

MITOCHONDRIAL DISORDERS
Mitochondrial neurogastrointestinal encephalomyopathy

MUSCULOSKELETAL DISORDERS
Ehlers-Danlos syndrome
Myotonic dystrophy
Duchenne muscular dystrophy

RHEUMATOLOGY
Amyloidosis
Dermatomyositis
Polymyositis
Systemic lupus erythematous

From Bitton S, Markowitz JF: Ulcerative colitis in children and adolescents. In Wyllie R, Hyams JS, Kay M, editors: *Pediatric gastrointestinal and liver disease,* 5th ed, Elsevier, 2016, Philadelphia, Box. 44.3, p. 548.

megacystis, or obstructive symptoms. Megacystis-microcolon–intestinal hypoperistalsis syndrome is a prenatal or neonatal manifestation of CIPO.

DIAGNOSIS

The diagnosis of pseudoobstruction is based on the presence of compatible symptoms in the absence of mechanical obstruction (Fig. 358.1). Plain abdominal radiographs demonstrate air-fluid levels in the intestine. Neonates with evidence of obstruction at birth may have a microcolon. Contrast studies demonstrate slow passage of barium; water-soluble agents should be considered. Esophageal motility is abnormal in about half the patients. Antroduodenal (small intestinal) motility and gastric emptying studies have abnormal results if the upper gut is involved

(Table 358.3). The clinical manifestations depend in large part to the areas of the gastrointestinal tract that are involved, with milder forms more common in older children. Although counterintuitive, older children with CIPO may present with both abdominal distention and diarrhea, related to *small bowel bacterial overgrowth* because of altered motility. Other presentations may include constipation and bilious emesis, as well as failure to thrive, as a consequence of decreased enteral feeding tolerance.

The initial focus is to rule out anatomic obstruction and to assess for bladder involvement, because that is a frequent and significant extraintestinal manifestation of concern. Manometric evidence of a normal migrating motor complex and postprandial activity should redirect the diagnostic evaluation. CIPO due to an intestinal myopathy may demonstrate manometry evidence of low-amplitude contractions, whereas CIPO due to enteric neuropathy demonstrates normal amplitude but poorly organized contractions (nonperistaltic or tonic). Anorectal motility is normal and differentiates pseudoobstruction from Hirschsprung disease. Full-thickness intestinal biopsy might show involvement of the muscle layers or abnormalities of the intrinsic intestinal nervous system.

The differential diagnosis is broad and includes such etiologies as Hirschsprung disease, mitochondrial neurogastrointestinal encephalomyopathy, mechanical obstruction, psychogenic constipation, neurogenic bladder, and superior mesenteric artery syndrome. Secondary causes of ileus or pseudoobstruction that should be considered include medication side effects, infectious etiologies, metabolic disturbances, immunologic disorders, oncologic processes, vasculitides, neuropathies, and myopathies (see Table 358.1). Examples include use of opiates hypokalemia, hypothyroidism, hypokalemia, diabetic neuropathy, porphyria, amyloidosis, Chagas disease, scleroderma, hereditary angioedema, mitochondrial disorders, and radiation, and these must be excluded. Other causes of abdominal distention such as small bowel bacterial overgrowth and aerophagia may present similarly and should be considered. *Small bowel bacterial overgrowth is a complication of CIPO.*

TREATMENT

Nutritional support is the mainstay of treatment for pseudoobstruction. Thirty to 50% of patients require partial or complete parenteral nutrition. Some patients can be treated with intermittent enteral supplementation, whereas others can maintain themselves on selective oral diets. Prokinetic drugs are generally used, although studies have not shown definitive evidence of their efficacy. Isolated gastroparesis can follow episodes of viral gastroenteritis and spontaneously resolves, usually in 6-24 mo. Erythromycin, a motilin receptor agonist, and cisapride, a serotonin 5-HT$_4$ receptor agonist, may enhance gastric emptying and proximal small bowel motility and may be useful in this select group of patients. Metoclopramide, a prokinetic and antinausea agent, is effective in gastroparesis, although side effects, such as tardive dyskinesia, limit its use. Domperidone, an antidopaminergic agent, is a prokinetic agent that can be considered. Pain management is difficult and requires a multidisciplinary approach.

Symptomatic small bowel bacterial overgrowth is usually treated with rotated nonabsorbable oral antibiotics and/or probiotics. Bacterial overgrowth can be associated with steatorrhea and malabsorption. Octreotide, a long-acting somatostatin analog, has been used in low doses to treat small bowel bacterial overgrowth. Patients with acid peptic symptoms are generally treated with acid suppression. Many patients with CIPO benefit from a gastrostomy, and some benefit from decompressive enterostomies (Fig. 358.2). Colectomy with ileorectal anastomosis is beneficial if the large bowel is the primary site of the motility abnormality. Bowel transplantation may benefit selected patients with CIPO. The prognosis is better for patients without urinary tract involvement and for those with neuropathic etiologies over myopathic disorders.

Bibliography is available at Expert Consult.

Table 358.2	Main Similarities and Differences in Chronic Intestinal Pseudoobstruction in Children, Adolescents, and Young Adults	
	CHILDREN	**ADOLESCENTS—YOUNG ADULTS**
Etiology	Mainly idiopathic	Half of cases are secondary to acquired diseases
Histopathology	Myopathies and neuropathies	Mainly neuropathies
Symptom onset	In utero, from birth or early infancy with 65–80% of patients symptomatic by 12 mo of age	Median age of onset at 17 yr
Clinical features	Occlusive symptoms at birth and/or chronic symptoms without free intervals Urologic involvement is commonly encountered ranging from 36% to 100% pediatric case series High risk of colonic and small bowel volvulus secondary to severe gut dilation, dysmotility, congenital bridles, or concurrent malrotation	Chronic abdominal pain and distension with superimposed acute episodes of pseudoobstruction Urinary bladder involvement not so often reported
Natural history	Myopathic CIPO, urinary involvement and concurrent intestinal malrotation are poor prognostic factors	The ability to restore oral feeding and the presence of symptoms <20 yr of age is associated with a low mortality; while, systemic sclerosis and severe/diffuse esophageal and intestinal dysmotility are associated with a high mortality
Diagnostic approach	Specialized tests (e.g., intestinal manometry) often difficult to perform; noninvasive, radiation-free imaging tests are warranted	Various methodologic approaches usually starting from endoscopy and radiological tests up to more sophisticated functional exams
Nutritional therapy	To ensure normal growth extensively hydrolyzed and elemental formulas are often empirically used to facilitate intestinal absorption	To improve nutritional status and prevent malnutrition
Pharmacologic therapy	Small number/sample size-controlled trials	Small number/sample-size controlled trials; few conclusions can be drawn for most drugs
Surgical therapy	Venting ostomies (although characterized by high complication rates) possibly helpful; surgery as a "bridge" to transplantation may be indicated in highly selected cases	Venting ostomies can be helpful; resective surgery may be indicated in accurately selected patients (i.e., cases with proven segmental gut dysfunction)

From Di Nardo G, Di Lorenzo C, Lauro A, et al: Chronic intestinal pseudo-obstruction in children and adults: diagnosis and therapeutic options, *Neurogastroenterol Motil* 29:e12945, 2017, Table 2.

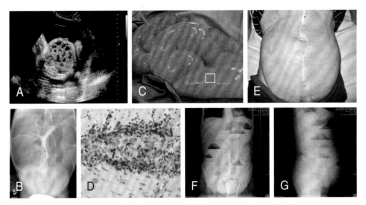

Fig. 358.1 Synoptic view of the chronic intestinal pseudoobstruction (CIPO) spectrum. **A** and **B,** The most severe pediatric cases with antenatal (in utero) evidence of multivisceral dilation—often gut **(B)** and urinary system—commonly associated with an extremely poor prognosis. **C** and **D,** CIPO phenotype with rapid progression to intestinal dilation (± ureter/bladder) and failure, often occurring as a result of an anamnestically reported gastroenteritis. Massive bowel dilation **(C)** and associated histopathology **(D;** corresponds to white squared area in **C)** revealed an intense inflammatory (mainly lymphocytic) neuropathy (hence, myenteric ganglionitis). Alkaline phosphatase antialkaline phosphatase immunohistochemical technique using specific anti-CD8 monoclonal antibodies was used to identify a subset of T lymphocytes. **E** and **G,** Examples of another phenotype of the syndrome that may be seen in patients who have more insidious mild and nonspecific symptoms progressing to a classic CIPO over time. **E,** Markedly distended abdomen of a 32 yr old man who presented with subocclusive episodes after years of unspecific (dyspeptic-/irritable bowel syndrome–like) symptoms. Note the evident air-fluid levels detectable in upright position in anteroposterior **(F)** and laterolateral **(G)** plain abdominal radiographs. (**A,** From Shen O, Schimmel MS, Eitan R, et al: Prenatal diagnosis of intestinal pseudo-obstruction, Ultrasound Obstet Gynecol 29:229–231, 2007. **B–G,** From Di Nardo G, Di Lorenzo C, Lauro A, et al: Chronic intestinal pseudo-obstruction in children and adults: diagnosis and therapeutic options, Neurogastroenterol Motil 29:e12945, 2017.)

Table 358.3	Findings in Pseudoobstruction
GI SEGMENT	**FINDINGS***
Esophageal motility	Abnormalities in approximately half of CIPO, although in some series up to 85% demonstrate abnormalities Decreased LES pressure Failure of LES relaxation Esophageal body: low-amplitude waves, poor propagation, tertiary waves, retrograde peristalsis, occasionally aperistalsis
Gastric emptying	May be delayed
EGG	Tachygastria or bradygastria may be seen
ADM	Postprandial antral hypomotility is seen and correlates with delayed gastric emptying Myopathic subtype: low-amplitude contractions, <10-20 mm Hg Neuropathic subtype: contractions are uncoordinated, disorganized Absence of fed response Fasting MMC is absent, or MMC is abnormally propagated
Colonic	Absence of gastrocolic reflex because there is no increased motility in response to a meal
ARM	Normal rectoanal inhibitory reflex

*Findings can vary according to the segment(s) of the GI tract that are involved.
  ADM, antroduodenal manometry; ARM, anorectal manometry; CIPO, chronic intestinal pseudoobstruction; EGG, electrogastrography; GI, gastrointestinal; LES, lower esophageal sphincter; MMC, migrating motor complex.
  From Steffen R: Gastrointestinal motility. In Wyllie R, Hyams JS, Kay M, editors: *Pediatric gastrointestinal and liver disease*, ed 3, Philadelphia, 2006, WB Saunders, p. 66.

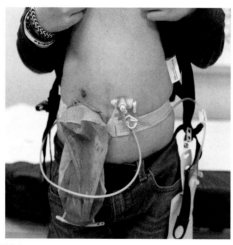

Fig. 358.2 Photograph of a child with chronic intestinal pseudoobstruction who improved clinically after ileostomy creation. He receives enteral feeding through his jejunal feeding tube, whereas his gastrostomy tube remains to straight drain. (*From Bitton S, Markowitz JF: Ulcerative colitis in children and adolescents. In Wyllie R, Hyams JS, Kay M, editors: Pediatric gastrointestinal and liver disease, ed 5, Philadelphia, 2016, Elsevier, Fig. 44.3*).

358.2 Mitochondrial Neurogastrointestinal Encephalomyopathy
Asim Maqbool and Chris A. Liacouras

Mitochondrial neurogastrointestinal encephalomyopathy (MNGIE) is a multisystem autosomal recessive disease that initially presents with

severe gastrointestinal disturbances; the neurologic manifestations usually occur later in the illness and may initially be subtle or asymptomatic.

MNGIE is caused by a mutation in the nuclear DNA *TYMP* gene encoding thymidine phosphorylase that results in abnormalities in intergenomic communication with resulting instability of mitochondrial DNA (some patients have mutations on *POLG1*). There are at least 50 individual mutations with a poor genotype-phenotype correlation and varying manifestations within each family. Consanguinity is present in 30% of families.

MNGIE affects both males and females and is usually diagnosed in the 2nd and 3rd decade (average age: 18 yr; range: 5 mo-35 yr). Onset is usually around age 12 yr, but there is often a 5- to 10-yr delay in the diagnosis.

MNGIE *initially* presents with gastrointestinal symptoms. Severe intestinal dysmotility and gastroparesis are associated with early satiety, postprandial emesis, episodic pseudoobstruction, diarrhea, constipation, and abdominal pain and cramping, which leads to significant cachexia. Because of the age of onset, emesis, early satiety, and cachexia patients are often misdiagnosed with an eating disorder.

Most often, following the onset of gastrointestinal manifestations, ptosis, progressive external ophthalmoplegia, hearing loss, myopathy, and peripheral neuropathy may develop. The neuropathy is either demyelinating or a mixed axonal demyelinating type and manifests as weakness, decreased or absent deep tendon reflexes, and paresthesias. Leukoencephalopathy is initially asymptomatic and noted on MRI as patchy lesions predominantly in the cortex but also in the basal ganglia and brainstem. Eventually the central nervous system lesions become diffuse and confluent. A small number of patients develop cognitive impairment or dementia.

The diagnosis is suggested by the constellation of gastrointestinal and neurologic symptoms, lactic acidosis, ragged red fibers, and cytochrome C oxidase–deficient fibers seen in most patients on muscle biopsy. Reduced activity of thymidine phosphorylase enzyme and elevated plasma levels of thymidine and deoxyuridine are often diagnostic; genetic testing for the mutation or other genes *(POLG1)* is recommended.

Treatment is focused on providing sufficient nutritional support and avoidance of infectious complications and of nutritional deficiencies. Domperidone has been used for nausea and emesis, antibiotics for small bowel bacterial overgrowth, amitriptyline or gabapentin for neuropathic pain, and parenteral alimentation for nutritional support. Opiates and any medications that affect intestinal motility or mitochondrial function must be avoided. Stem cell transplantation has been successful in a small number of patients.

Overall the prognosis is poor, with few surviving into the 4th or 5th decade.

Bibliography is available at Expert Consult.

358.3 Encopresis and Functional Constipation
Asim Maqbool and Chris A. Liacouras

Constipation is defined as a delay or difficulty in defecation present for >1 month and significant enough to cause distress to the patient. Another approach to the definition is the Rome criteria, outlined in Tables 358.4 and 358.5. Functional constipation, also known as idiopathic constipation or fecal withholding, can usually be differentiated from constipation secondary to organic causes based on a history and physical examination. Unlike anorectal malformations and Hirschsprung disease, functional constipation typically starts after the neonatal period. Usually, there is an intentional or subconscious withholding of stool. An acute episode usually precedes the chronic course. This acute event could include a social stressor such as initiation of toilet training, birth of a sibling, starting daycare, or abuse. The acute episode may be a dietary change from human milk to cow's milk, secondary to the change in the protein and carbohydrate ratio or an allergy to cow's milk. Although iron has been suspected of causing issues with cow's milk–related constipation,

Table 358.4	Rome IV Diagnostic Criteria for Defecatory Disorders in Neonates and Toddlers		
FGID	**AGE RANGE**	**CRITERIA REQUIREMENTS**	**CRITERIA ELEMENTS**
Functional constipation	All pediatric age groups	Must include 1 month of ≥2 of the following in infants up to 4 months of age: In toilet trained children, the following additional criteria may be used:	• 2 or fewer defections weekly • History of excessive stool retention • History of hard/painful bowel movements • History of large-diameter stools • Presence of a large fecal mass in the rectum • At least 1 weekly episode of incontinence after being toilet trained • History of large-diameter stools that may clog the toilet

FGID, Functional gastrointestinal disorders.
Modified from Benninga MA, Faure C, Hyman PE, et al. Childhood functional gastrointestinal disorders: neonate/toddler, *Gastroenterology* 150:1443–1455, 2016.

Table 358.5	Rome IV Diagnostic Criteria for Defecatory Disorders in Children and Adolescents		
	AGE RANGE	**CRITERIA REQUIREMENTS**	**CRITERIA ELEMENTS**
Functional Constipation	Developmental age ≥4 yr	Must include ≥2 of the following ≥1/wk for 1 ≥1 mo with insufficient criteria to diagnose irritable bowel syndrome	• ≤ 2 defecations in the toilet per week • ≥1 episode of fecal incontinence per week • History of retentive posturing or excessive volitional stool retention • History of painful or hard bowel movements • Presence of a large fecal mass in the rectum • History of large diameter stools that can obstruct the toilet • After appropriate evaluation, symptoms cannot be fully explained by another medical condition
Nonretentive Fecal Incontinence	developmental age ≥4 yr	≥1-mo history of the following symptoms:	• Defecation into places inappropriate to the sociocultural context • No evidence of fecal retention • After appropriate evaluation, symptoms cannot be fully explained by another medical condition

Modified from Hyams JS, Di Lorenzo C, Saps M, et al. Childhood functional gastrointestinal disorders: child/adolescent, *Gastroenterology* 150:1456–1468, 2016.

this has not been consistently demonstrated or substantiated. The stool becomes firm, smaller, and difficult to pass, resulting in anal irritation and often an anal fissure. In toddlers, coercive or inappropriately early toilet training is a factor that can initiate a pattern of stool retention. In older children, retentive constipation can develop after entering a situation that makes stooling inconvenient such as school. Because the passage of bowel movements is painful, voluntary withholding of feces to avoid the painful stimulus develops.

CLINICAL MANIFESTATIONS
When children have the urge to defecate, typical behaviors include contracting the gluteal muscles by stiffening the legs while lying down, holding onto furniture while standing, or squatting quietly in corners, waiting for the call to stool to pass. The urge to defecate passes as the rectum accommodates to its contents. A vicious cycle of retention develops, as increasingly larger volumes of stool need to be expelled. Caregivers may misinterpret these activities as straining, but it is withholding behavior. There is often a history of blood in the stool noted with the passage of a large bowel movement. Findings suggestive of underlying pathology include failure to thrive, weight loss, abdominal pain, vomiting, or persistent anal fissure or fistula.

In functional constipation, daytime encopresis is common. **Encopresis** is defined as voluntary or involuntary passage of feces into inappropriate places at least once a mo for 3 consecutive months once a chronologic or developmental age of 4 yr has been reached. Encopresis is not diagnosed when the behavior is exclusively the result of the direct effects of a substance (e.g., laxatives) or a general medical condition (except through a mechanism involving constipation). Subtypes include retentive encopresis (with constipation and overflow incontinence), representing 65–95% of cases, and nonretentive encopresis (without constipation and overflow incontinence). **Nonretentive fecal incontinence** is defined as no evidence of fecal retention (impaction), ≥1 episodes per week in the previous 1 mo, or defecation in places inappropriate to the social context in a child who has been previously toilet trained and without

evidence of anatomic, inflammatory, metabolic, endocrine, or neoplastic process that could explain the symptoms. Encopresis can persist from infancy onward (primary) or can appear after successful toilet training (secondary). The updated Rome criteria (IV) differentiate between infants/toddlers and older children who have been toilet trained versus not toilet trained, for practical assessment purposes.

DIAGNOSIS
The physical examination often demonstrates a large volume of stool palpated in the suprapubic area; rectal examination demonstrates a dilated rectal vault filled with guaiac-negative stool. Children with encopresis often present with reports of underwear soiling, and many parents initially presume that diarrhea, rather than constipation, is the cause. In **retentive encopresis**, associated complaints of difficulty with defecation, abdominal or rectal pain, impaired appetite with poor growth, and urinary (day and/or night) incontinence are common. Children often have large bowel movements that obstruct the toilet. There may also be retentive posturing or recurrent urinary tract infections. **Nonretentive encopresis** is more likely to occur as a solitary symptom and have an associated primary underlying psychological etiology. Children with encopresis can present with poor school performance and attendance that is triggered by the scorn and derision from schoolmates because of the child's offensive odor.

The location of the anus relative to perineal anatomic landmarks by sex also needs to be considered. This is expressed as the **anogenital index**, and it can be calculated when necessary. This is determined by the distance in centimeters from the vagina or scrotum to the anus, divided by the distance from the vagina or scrotum to the coccyx. The normal anogenital index in females is 0.39 ± 0.09, whereas 0.56 ± 0.2 is normal for males. The presence of a hair tuft over the spine or spinal dimple, or failure to elicit a cremasteric reflex or anal wink suggests spinal pathology. A tethered cord is suggested by decreased or absent lower leg reflexes. **Spinal cord lesions** can occur with overlying skin anomalies. Urinary tract symptoms include recurrent urinary tract infection and enuresis. Children with no evidence of abnormalities on physical examination rarely require radiologic evaluation.

In refractory patients (intractable constipation), specialized testing should be considered to rule out conditions such as hypothyroidism, hypocalcemia, lead toxicity, celiac disease, and disorders of neuromuscular

Table 358.6	London Classification of Gastrointestinal Neuromuscular Pathology

1. Neuropathies
  1.1 Absent neurons
    1.1.1 Aganglionosis*
  1.2 Decreased numbers of neurons
    1.2.1 Hypoganglionosis
  1.3 Increased numbers of neurons
    1.3.1 Ganglioneuromatosis[†]
    1.3.2 IND, type B[‡]
  1.4 Degenerative neuropathy[§]
  1.5 Inflammatory neuropathies
    1.5.1 Lymphocytic ganglionitis[¶]
    1.5.2 Eosinophilic ganglionitis
  1.6 Abnormal content in neurons
    1.6.1 Intraneuronal nuclear inclusions
    1.6.2 Megamitochondria
  1.7 Abnormal neurochemical coding**
  1.8 Relative immaturity of neurons
  1.9 Abnormal enteric glia
    1.9.1 Increased numbers of enteric glia
2. Myopathies
  2.1 Muscularis propria malformations[††]
  2.2 Muscle cell degeneration
    2.2.1 Degenerative leiomyopathy/[‡‡]
    2.2.2 Inflammatory leiomyopathy
      2.2.2.1 Lymphocytic leiomyositis
      2.2.2.2 Eosinophilic leiomyositis
  2.3 Muscle hyperplasia/hypertrophy
    2.3.1 Muscularis mucosae hyperplasia
  2.4 Abnormal content in myocytes
    2.4.1 Filament protein abnormalities
      2.4.1.1 Alpha-actin myopathy[§§]
      2.4.1.2 Desmin myopathy
    2.4.2 Inclusion bodies
      2.4.2.1 Polyglucosan bodies
      2.4.2.2 Amphophilic
      2.4.2.3 Megamitochondria[¶¶]
  2.5 Abnormal supportive tissue
    2.5.1 Atrophic desmosis***
3. ICC abnormalities (enteric mesenchymopathy)
  3.1 Abnormal ICC networks[†††]

*Can include rare cases of non-Hirschsprung disease severe hypoplastic hypoganglionosis with long interganglionic intervals (zonal aganglionosis).
[†]Although neurons have not been formally quantified, gross increases of disorganized neurons are evident.
[‡]Can include retarded neuronal maturation.
[§]May occur with or without neuronal loss but is best regarded as a separate entity.
[¶]May occur with neuronal degeneration and/or loss; lymphocytic epithelioganglionitis is a variant.
**Includes neurotransmitter loss (e.g., reduced or absent expression) or loss of a neurochemically defined functional subset of nerves (see text).
[††]Includes absence, fusion, or additional muscle coats.
[‡‡]Hollow visceral myopathy may be diagnosed in familial cases with other characteristic phenotypic features; myopathy with autophagic activity and pink blush myopathy with nuclear crowding are rare variants in which degenerative findings are less overt.
[§§]Smooth muscle alpha-actin deficiency is best described, although deficiencies of other proteins related to the contractile apparatus of myocytes have been reported.
[¶¶]Mitochondrial neurogastrointestinal encephalomyopathy causes a degenerative appearance predominantly in the longitudinal muscle.
***Absent connective tissue scaffold has been almost exclusively described in the colon.
[†††]Generally reduced or absent ICC, although abnormal morphology also reported.
ICC, interstitial cells of Cajal; IND, intestinal neuronal dysplasia.
From Knowles CH, De Giorgio R, Kapur RP, et al: The London classification of gastrointestinal neuromuscular pathology: report on behalf of the Gastro 2009 International Working Group, *Gut* 59:882–887, 2010, Table 1, p. 883.

gastrointestinal pathology (Table 358.6). Colonic transit studies using radiopaque markers or scintigraphy techniques may be useful. Selected children can benefit from MRI of the spine to identify an intraspinal process, motility studies to identify underlying myopathic or neuropathic bowel abnormalities, or a contrast enema to identify structural abnormalities. In patients with severe functional constipation, water-soluble contrast enema reveals the presence of a mega rectosigmoid (Fig. 358.3). Anorectal motility studies can demonstrate a pattern of paradoxical contraction of the external anal sphincter during defecation, which can be treated by behavior modification and biofeedback. Colonic motility can guide therapy in refractory cases, demonstrating segmental problems that might require surgical intervention.

Complications of retentive encopresis include day and night urinary incontinence, urinary retention, urinary tract infection, megacystis, and rarely toxic megacolon.

TREATMENT

Therapy for functional constipation and encopresis includes patient education, relief of impaction, and softening of the stool. Caregivers must understand that soiling associated with overflow incontinence is associated with loss of normal sensation and not a willful act. There needs to be a focus on adherence with regular postprandial toilet sitting and adoption of a balanced diet. In addition, caregivers should be instructed not to respond to soiling with retaliatory or punitive measures, because children are likely to become angry, ashamed, and resistant to intervention. From the outset, parents should be actively encouraged to reward the child for adherence to a healthy bowel regimen and to avoid power struggles.

If an impaction is present on the initial physical examination, an enema is usually required to clear the impaction while stool softeners are started as maintenance medications. Typical regimens include the use of polyethylene glycol preparations, lactulose, or mineral oil (Tables 358.7 and 358.8). Prolonged use of stimulants such as senna or bisacodyl should be avoided.

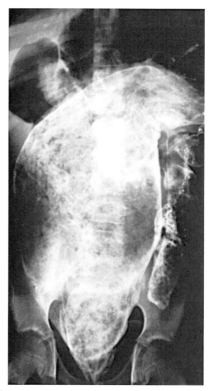

Fig. 358.3 Barium enema in a 14 yr old boy with severe constipation. The enormous dilation of the rectum and distal colon is typical of acquired functional megacolon.

Table 358.7	Suggested Medications and Dosages for Disimpaction	
MEDICATION	**AGE**	**DOSAGE**
RAPID RECTAL DISIMPACTION		
Glycerin suppositories	Infants and toddlers	
Phosphate enema	<1 yr	60 mL
	>1 yr	6 mL/kg body weight, up to 135 mL twice
SLOW ORAL DISIMPACTION IN OLDER CHILDREN		
Over 2-3 Days		
Polyethylene glycol with electrolytes		25 mL/kg body weight/hr, up to 1,000 mL/hr until clear fluid comes from the anus
Over 5-7 Days		
Polyethylene without electrolytes		1.5 g/kg body weight/day for 3 days
Milk of magnesia		2 mL/kg body weight twice/day for 7 days
Mineral oil		3 mL/kg body weight twice/day for 7 days
Lactulose or sorbitol		2 mL/kg body weight twice/day for 7 days

From Loening-Baucke V: Functional constipation with encopresis. In Wyllie R, Hyams JS, Kay M, editors: *Pediatric gastrointestinal and liver disease*, ed 3, Philadelphia, 2006, WB Saunders, p. 183.

Table 358.8	Suggested Medications and Dosages for Maintenance Therapy of Constipation	
MEDICATION	**AGE**	**DOSE**
TYPICAL DOSES FOR LONG-TERM TREATMENT (YEARS)		
Milk of magnesia	>1 mo	1-3 mL/kg body weight/day, divided into 1-2 doses
Mineral oil	>12 mo	1-3 mL/kg body weight/day, divided into 1-2 doses
Lactulose or sorbitol	>1 mo	1-3 mL/kg body weight/day, divided into 1-2 doses
Polyethylene glycol 3350 (MiraLAX)	>1 yr	0.7 g/kg body weight/day (max 17.5 g/day)
FOR SHORT-TERM TREATMENT (MONTHS)		
Senna (Senokot) syrup, tablets	1-5 yr	5 mL (1 tablet) with breakfast, max 15 mL daily
	5-15 yr	2 tablets with breakfast, maximum 3 tablets daily
Glycerin enemas	>10 yr	20-30 mL/day (½ glycerin and ½ normal saline)
Bisacodyl suppositories	>10 yr	10 mg daily

From Loening-Baucke V: Functional constipation with encopresis. In Wyllie R, Hyams JS, Kay M, editors: *Pediatric gastrointestinal and liver disease*, ed 3, Philadelphia, 2006, WB Saunders, p. 185.

Compliance can wane, and failure of this standard treatment approach sometimes requires more intensive intervention. In cases where behavioral or psychiatric problems are evident, involvement of a psychologist or behavioral management (e.g., behavior programs and/or biofeedback) is recommended. Maintenance therapy is generally continued until a regular bowel pattern has been established and the association of pain with the passage of stool is abolished.

For children with chronic diarrhea and/or irritable bowel syndrome where stress and anxiety play a major role, stress reduction and learning effective coping strategies can play an important role in responding to the encopresis. Relaxation training, stress inoculation, assertiveness training, and/or general stress management procedures can be helpful, and the participation of behavioral health specialists is valuable.

Neurostimulation (transcutaneous or sacral implantation) and pelvic physiotherapy are novel approaches used in patients with medication refractory constipation. Children with spinal problems can be successfully managed with low volumes of fluid through a cecostomy or sigmoid tube.

Bibliography is available at Expert Consult.

358.4 Congenital Aganglionic Megacolon (Hirschsprung Disease)

Asim Maqbool and Chris A. Liacouras

Hirschsprung disease, or congenital aganglionic megacolon, is a developmental disorder (neurocristopathy) of the enteric nervous system, characterized by the absence of ganglion cells in the submucosal and myenteric plexus. It is the most common cause of lower intestinal obstruction in neonates, with an overall incidence of 1 in 5,000 live births. The male:female ratio for Hirschsprung disease is 4:1 for short-segment disease and approximately 2:1 with total colonic aganglionosis. Prematurity is uncommon.

There is an increased familial incidence in long-segment disease. Hirschsprung disease may be associated with other congenital defects, including trisomy 21, Joubert syndrome, Goldberg-Shprintzen syndrome, Smith-Lemli-Opitz syndrome, Shah-Waardenburg syndrome, cartilage-hair hypoplasia, multiple endocrine neoplasm 2 syndrome, neurofibromatosis, neuroblastoma, congenital hypoventilation (Ondine's curse), and urogenital or cardiovascular abnormalities. Hirschsprung disease has been seen in association with microcephaly, mental retardation, abnormal facies, autism, cleft palate, hydrocephalus, and micrognathia.

PATHOLOGY

Hirschsprung disease is the result of an absence of ganglion cells in the bowel wall, extending proximally and continuously from the anus for a variable distance. The absence of neural innervation is a consequence of an arrest of neuroblast migration from the proximal to distal bowel. Without the myenteric and submucosal plexus, there is inadequate relaxation of the bowel wall and bowel wall hypertonicity, which can lead to intestinal obstruction.

Hirschsprung disease is usually sporadic, although dominant and recessive patterns of inheritance have been demonstrated in family groups. Genetic defects have been identified in multiple genes that encode proteins of the RET signaling pathway (*RET, GDNF*, and *NTN*) and involved in the endothelin (EDN) type B receptor pathway (*EDNRB, EDN3*, and *EVE-1*). Syndromic forms of Hirschsprung disease have been associated with the *L1CAM, SOX10*, and *ZFHX1B* (formerly *SIP1*) genes.

The aganglionic segment is limited to the rectosigmoid in 80% of patients. Approximately 10–15% of patients have long-segment disease, defined as disease proximal to the sigmoid colon. Total bowel aganglionosis is rare and accounts for approximately 5% of cases. Observed histologically is an absence of Meissner's and Auerbach's plexuses and hypertrophied nerve bundles with high concentrations of acetylcholinesterase between the muscular layers and in the submucosa.

CLINICAL MANIFESTATIONS

Hirschsprung disease is usually diagnosed in the neonatal period secondary to a distended abdomen, failure to pass meconium, and/or bilious emesis or aspirates with feeding intolerance. In 99% of healthy full-term infants, meconium is passed within 48 hr of birth. Hirschsprung disease should be suspected in any full-term infant (the disease is unusual in preterm infants) with delayed passage of stool. Some neonates pass meconium normally but subsequently present with a history of chronic constipation. Failure to thrive with hypoproteinemia from protein-losing enteropathy is a less common presentation because Hirschsprung disease is usually recognized early in the course of the illness but has been known to occur. Breastfed infants might not present as severely as formula-fed infants.

Failure to pass stool leads to dilation of the proximal bowel and abdominal distention. As the bowel dilates, intraluminal pressure increases, resulting in decreased blood flow and deterioration of the mucosal barrier. Stasis allows proliferation of bacteria, which can lead to enterocolitis (*Clostridium difficile, Staphylococcus aureus,* anaerobes, coliforms) with associated diarrhea, abdominal tenderness, sepsis, and signs of bowel obstruction. *Red flags* in the neonatal period then include neonatal intestinal obstruction, bowel perforation, delayed passage of meconium, abdominal distention relieved by digital rectal stimulation or enemas, chronic severe constipation, and enterocolitis. Early recognition of Hirschsprung disease before the onset of enterocolitis is essential in reducing morbidity and mortality.

Hirschsprung disease in older patients must be distinguished from other causes of abdominal distention and chronic constipation (see Tables 358.6 and 358.9 and Figs. 358.4 and 358.5). The history often reveals constipation starting in infancy that has responded poorly to medical management. Failure to thrive is not uncommon. Fecal incontinence, fecal urgency, and stool-withholding behaviors are usually not present. Significant abdominal distention is unusual in non-Hirschsprung related constipation, as is emesis. The abdomen is tympanitic and distended, with a large fecal mass palpable in the left lower abdomen. Rectal examination demonstrates a normally placed anus that easily allows entry of the finger but feels snug. The rectum is usually empty of feces, and when the finger is removed, there may be an explosive discharge of foul-smelling feces and gas. The stools, when passed, can consist of small pellets, be ribbon-like, or have a fluid consistency, unlike

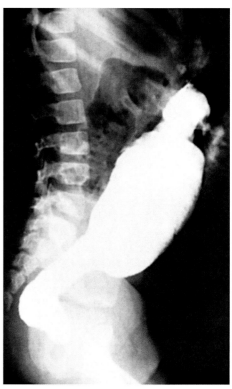

Fig. 358.4 Lateral view of a barium enema in a 3 yr old girl with Hirschsprung disease. The aganglionic distal segment is narrow, with distended normal ganglionic bowel above it.

the large stools seen in patients with functional constipation. Intermittent attacks of intestinal obstruction from retained feces may be associated with pain and fever. Urinary retention with enlarged bladder or hydronephrosis can occur secondary to urinary compression.

In neonates, Hirschsprung disease must be differentiated from meconium plug syndrome, meconium ileus, and intestinal atresia. In older patients, the **Currarino triad** must be considered, which includes anorectal malformations (ectopic anus, anal stenosis, imperforate anus), sacral bone anomalies (hypoplasia, poor segmentation), and presacral

Table 358.9	Distinguishing Features of Hirschsprung Disease and Functional Constipation	
VARIABLE	**FUNCTIONAL**	**HIRSCHSPRUNG DISEASE**
HISTORY		
Onset of constipation	After 2 yr of age	At birth
Encopresis	Common	Very rare
Failure to thrive	Uncommon	Possible
Enterocolitis	None	Possible
Forced bowel training	Usual	None
EXAMINATION		
Abdominal distention	Uncommon	Common
Poor weight gain	Rare	Common
Rectum	Filled with stool	Empty
Rectal examination	Stool in rectum	Explosive passage of stool
Malnutrition	None	Possible
INVESTIGATIONS		
Anorectal manometry	Relaxation of internal anal sphincter	Failure of internal anal sphincter relaxation
Rectal biopsy	Normal	No ganglion cells, increased acetylcholinesterase staining
Barium enema	Massive amounts of stool, no transition zone	Transition zone, delayed evacuation (>24 hr)

From Imseis E, Gariepy C: Hirschsprung disease. In Walker WA, Goulet OJ, Kleinman RE, et al, editors: *Pediatric gastrointestinal disease*, ed 4, Hamilton, ON, 2004, BC Decker, p. 1035.

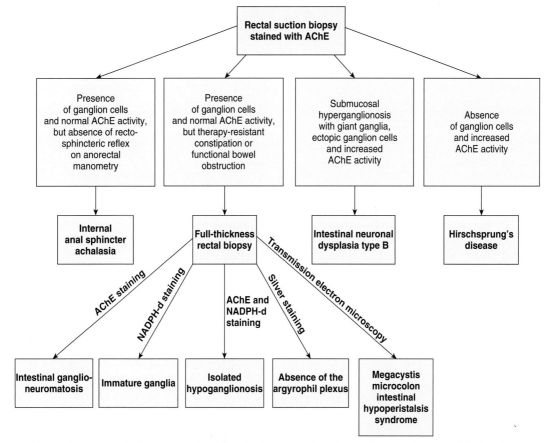

Fig. 358.5 Diagnostic algorithm for investigating chronic constipation and functional bowel obstruction in newborn infants and young children. *AChE*, Acetylcholinesterase; *NADPH-d*, nicotinamide adenine dinucleotide phosphate diaphorase. *(From Friedmacher F, Puri P: Classification and diagnostic criteria of variants of Hirschsprung's disease, Pediatr Surg Int 29:855–872, 2013, Fig. 1.)*

anomaly (anterior meningoceles, teratoma, cyst).

DIAGNOSIS

Rectal suction biopsy is the "gold standard" for diagnosing Hirschsprung disease (see Fig. 358.5). The biopsy material should contain an adequate amount of submucosa to evaluate for the presence of ganglion cells. To avoid obtaining biopsies in the normal area of hypoganglionosis, which ranges from 3 to 17 mm in length, the suction rectal biopsy should be obtained no closer than 2 cm above the dentate line. The biopsy specimen should be stained for acetylcholinesterase to facilitate interpretation. Patients with aganglionosis demonstrate a large number of hypertrophied nerve bundles that stain positively for acetylcholinesterase with an absence of ganglion cells. Calretinin staining may provide a diagnosis of Hirschsprung disease when acetylcholinesterase staining may not be sufficient.

Anorectal manometry evaluates the internal anal sphincter while a balloon is distended in the rectum. In healthy individuals, rectal distention initiates relaxation of the internal anal sphincter in response to rectal distention (known as the rectoanal inhibitory reflux [RAIR]). In patients with Hirschsprung disease, the internal anal sphincter fails to relax in response to rectal distention, and there is absence of the RAIR. Although the sensitivity and specificity can vary widely, in experienced hands, the test can be quite sensitive. However, the test can be technically difficult to perform in young infants. A normal response in the course of manometric evaluation precludes a diagnosis of Hirschsprung disease; an equivocal or paradoxical response requires a repeat motility or rectal biopsy. The sensitivity and specificity of anorectal manometry are both >90%.

An unprepared contrast enema is most likely to aid in the diagnosis in children older than 1 mo of age because the proximal ganglionic segment might not be significantly dilated in the first few wk of life. Classic findings are based on the presence of an abrupt narrow transition zone between the normal dilated proximal colon and a smaller-caliber obstructed distal aganglionic segment. In the absence of this finding, it is imperative to compare the diameter of the rectum to that of the sigmoid colon, because a rectal diameter that is the same as or smaller than the sigmoid colon suggests Hirschsprung disease. Radiologic evaluation should be performed without prior preparation (i.e., *unprepped contrast enema study*) to prevent transient dilation of the aganglionic segment. As many as 10% of newborns with Hirschsprung disease have a normal contrast study. This diagnostic test is most valuable in the disease that involves the distal colon, and specifically, the rectosigmoid. A transition zone may not be readily identifiable in total bowel aganglionosis. Twenty-four-hour delayed films are helpful in showing retained contrast (see Fig. 358.4). If significant barium is still present in the colon, it increases the suspicion of Hirschsprung disease even if a transition zone is not identified. Barium enema examination is useful in determining the extent of aganglionosis before surgery and in evaluating other diseases that manifest as lower bowel obstruction in a neonate. The sensitivity (~70%) and specificity (50–80%) of barium enema studies diagnosing Hirschsprung disease is lower than other methodologies. Full-thickness rectal biopsies can be performed at the time of surgery to confirm the diagnosis, level of involvement and to differentiate other disorders (see Fig. 358.5).

TREATMENT

Once the diagnosis is established, the definitive treatment is operative intervention. Previously, a temporary ostomy was placed, and definitive surgery was delayed until the child was older. Currently, many infants undergo a primary pull-through procedure unless there is associated enterocolitis or other complications, when a decompressing ostomy is usually required.

There are essentially three surgical options. The first successful surgical procedure, described by Swenson, was to excise the aganglionic segment and anastomose the normal proximal bowel to the rectum 1-2 cm above the dentate line. The operation is technically difficult and led to the development of two other procedures. Duhamel described a procedure to create a neorectum, bringing down normally innervated bowel behind the aganglionic rectum. The neorectum created in this procedure has an anterior aganglionic segment with normal sensation and a posterior ganglionic segment with normal propulsion. The endorectal pull-through procedure described by Soave involves stripping the mucosa from the aganglionic rectum and bringing normally innervated colon through the residual muscular cuff, thus bypassing the abnormal bowel from within. Advances in techniques have led to successful laparoscopic single-stage endorectal pull-through procedures, which are the treatment of choice.

In **ultrashort-segment Hirschsprung disease**, also known as **anal achalasia**, the aganglionic segment is limited to the internal sphincter. The clinical symptoms are similar to those of children with functional constipation. Ganglion cells are present on rectal suction biopsy, but the anorectal manometry is abnormal, with failure of relaxation of the internal anal sphincter in response to rectal distention. Current treatment, although controversial, includes anal botulism injection to relax the anal sphincter and anorectal myectomy if indicated.

Long-segment Hirschsprung disease involving the entire colon and, at times, part of the small bowel presents a difficult problem. Anorectal manometry and rectal suction biopsy demonstrate findings of Hirschsprung disease, but radiologic studies are difficult to interpret because a colonic transition zone cannot be identified. The extent of aganglionosis can be determined accurately by biopsy at the time of laparotomy. When the entire colon is aganglionic, often together with a length of terminal ileum, ileal-anal anastomosis is the treatment of choice, preserving part of the aganglionic colon to facilitate water absorption, which helps the stools to become firm.

The prognosis of surgically treated Hirschsprung disease is generally satisfactory; the great majority of patients achieve fecal continence. Long-term postoperative problems include constipation, recurrent enterocolitis, stricture, prolapse, perianal abscesses, and fecal soiling. Some children require myectomy or a redo pull-through procedure.

Hirschsprung disease–associated **enterocolitis** can occur at any time prior to or following surgery and is the leading cause of death in these patients. Dysmotility related to partial obstruction, underlying disease, impaired immune function, and the intestinal microbiome may all contribute to this pathophysiologic process. Explosive, foul-smelling and/or bloody diarrhea, abdominal distention, explosive discharge of rectal contents on digital examination, diminished peripheral perfusion, lethargy, and fever are all ominous signs. Management principles include hydration, decompression from above and below (nasogastric Salem Sump, rectal tube, rectal irrigation), and the use of broad-spectrum antibiotics.

Bibliography is available at Expert Consult.

358.5 Intestinal Neuronal Dysplasia
Asim Maqbool and Chris A. Liacouras

Intestinal neuronal dysplasia (IND) describes different quantitative (hypoganglionosis or hyperganglionosis) and qualitative (immature or heterotropic ganglion cells) abnormalities of the myenteric and/or submucosal plexus. The typical histology is that of hyperganglionosis and giant ganglia. Type A occurs very rarely and is characterized by congenital aplasia or hypoplasia of the sympathetic innervation. Patients present early in the neonatal period with episodes of intestinal obstruction, diarrhea, and bloody stools. This type B, which accounts for more than 95% of cases, is characterized by malformation of the parasympathetic submucous and myenteric plexus with giant ganglia and thickened nerve fibers, increased acetylcholinesterase staining, and isolated ganglion cells in the lamina propria. IND type B mimics Hirschsprung disease, and patients present with chronic constipation (see Table 358.6 and Fig. 358.5). Clinical manifestations include abdominal distention, constipation, and enterocolitis. Various lengths of bowel may be affected from segmental to the entire intestinal tract. IND has been observed in an isolated form and proximal to an aganglionic segment. Other intraintestinal and extraintestinal manifestations are present in patients with IND. It has been reported in all age groups, most commonly in infancy, but is also seen in adults who have had constipation not dating back to childhood.

Associated diseases and conditions include Hirschsprung disease, prematurity, small left colon syndrome, and meconium plug syndrome. Studies have identified a deficiency in substance P in patients with IND. Type A IND may be inherited in a familial, autosomal recessive pattern. Most cases of IND type B are sporadic, with few familial clusters, suggesting autosomal dominant inheritance.

Management includes that for functional constipation, and, if unsuccessful, surgery is indicated.

Bibliography is available at Expert Consult.

358.6 Superior Mesenteric Artery Syndrome (Wilkie Syndrome, Cast Syndrome, Arteriomesenteric Duodenal Compression Syndrome)
Asim Maqbool and Chris A. Liacouras

Superior mesenteric artery syndrome results from compression of the third duodenal segment by the artery against the aorta. Malnutrition or catabolic states may cause mesenteric fat depletion, which collapses the duodenum within a narrowed aortomesenteric angle. Other etiologies include extraabdominal compression (e.g., body cast) and mesenteric tension, as can occur from ileoanal pouch anastomosis. Rapid weight loss and immobilization are risk factors.

Symptoms include intermittent epigastric pain, anorexia, nausea, and vomiting. Risk factors include thin body habitus, prolonged bed rest, abdominal surgery, and exaggerated lumbar lordosis. Onset can be within weeks of a trigger, but some patients have chronic symptoms that evade diagnosis. A classic example is an underweight adolescent who begins vomiting 1-2 wk following scoliosis surgery or spinal fusion. Recognition may be delayed in the context of an eating disorder.

The diagnosis is established radiologically by demonstrating a duodenal cutoff just right of midline along with proximal duodenal dilation, with or without gastric dilation. Although the upper gastrointestinal series remains a mainstay, modalities including CT, MR angiography, or ultrasound may be more appropriate if there is concern for other etiologies such as malignancy. Upper endoscopy should be considered to rule out intraluminal pathology.

Treatment focuses on obstructive relief, nutritional rehabilitation, and correction of associated fluid and electrolyte abnormalities. Lateral or prone positioning can shift the duodenum away from obstructing structures and allow resumption of oral intake. If repositioning is unsuccessful, patients require nasojejunal enteral nutrition past the obstruction or parenteral nutrition if this is not tolerated. This management is successful in the vast majority of cases, with eventual withdrawal of tube feeding once weight has been regained and enteral feeding tolerance orally has been gradually and fully restored. Patients with refractory courses may require surgery to bypass the obstruction.

ACKNOWLEDGMENT
Andrew Chu contributed to the previous version of this chapter.

Bibliography is available at Expert Consult.

Chapter **359**
Ileus, Adhesions, Intussusception, and Closed-Loop Obstructions

第三百五十九章
肠梗阻、肠粘连、肠套叠和闭袢性肠梗阻

中文导读

　　本章主要介绍了肠梗阻、粘连、肠套叠和闭袢性肠梗阻。描述了肠梗阻的定义、原因、伴随的代谢紊乱、临床表现、影像学的特点和治疗；描述了粘连的定义、临床表现和管理措施；详细描述了肠套叠的病因学和流行病学史、病理、临床表现、诊断、鉴别诊断、治疗和预后；描述了闭袢性肠梗阻的定义、病理、危险因素、临床表现、影像学检查和支持治疗等。

359.1 Ileus

Asim Maqbool and Chris A. Liacouras

Ileus is the failure of intestinal peristalsis caused by loss of coordinated gut motility without evidence of mechanical obstruction. In children, it is most often associated with abdominal surgery or infection (gastroenteritis, pneumonia, peritonitis). Ileus also accompanies metabolic abnormalities (e.g., uremia, hypokalemia, hypercalcemia, hypermagnesemia, acidosis) or administration of certain drugs, such as opiates, vincristine, and antimotility agents such as loperamide when used during gastroenteritis.

Ileus manifests with nausea, vomiting, feeding intolerance, abdominal distention with associated pain, and delayed passage of stool and bowel gas. Bowel sounds are minimal or absent, in contrast to early mechanical obstruction, when they are hyperactive. Abdominal radiographs demonstrate multiple air-fluid levels throughout the abdomen. Serial radiographs usually do not show progressive distention as they do in mechanical obstruction. Contrast radiographs, if performed, demonstrate slow movement of barium through a patent lumen. Ileus after abdominal surgery generally resolves in within 72 hr.

Treatment involves correcting the underlying abnormality, supportive care of comorbidities, and mitigation of iatrogenic contributions. Electrolyte abnormalities should be identified and corrected, and narcotic agents, when used, should be weaned as tolerated. Nasogastric decompression can relieve recurrent vomiting or abdominal distention associated with pain; resultant fluid losses should be corrected with isotonic crystalloid solution. Prokinetic agents such as erythromycin are not routinely recommended. Selective peripheral opioid antagonists such as methylnaltrexone hold promise in decreasing postoperative ileus, but pediatric data are lacking.

Bibliography is available at Expert Consult.

359.2 Adhesions

Asim Maqbool and Chris A. Liacouras

Adhesions are fibrous tissue bands that result from peritoneal injury. They can constrict hollow organs and are a major cause of postoperative small bowel obstruction. Most remain asymptomatic, but problems can arise any time after the 2nd postoperative wk to yr after surgery, regardless of surgical extent. In one study, the 5-yr readmission risk because of adhesions varied by operative region (2.1% for colon to 9.2% for ileum) and procedure (0.3% for appendectomy to 25% for ileostomy formation/closure). The overall risk was 5.3% excluding appendectomy and 1.1% when appendectomy was included.

The diagnosis is suspected in patients with abdominal pain, constipation, emesis, and a history of intraperitoneal surgery. Nausea and vomiting quickly follow onset of pain. Initially, bowel sounds are hyperactive, and the abdomen is flat. Subsequently, bowel sounds disappear, and bowel dilation can cause abdominal distention. Fever and leukocytosis suggest bowel necrosis and peritonitis. Plain radiographs demonstrate obstructive features, and a CT scan or contrast studies may be needed to define the etiology.

Management includes nasogastric decompression, intravenous fluid resuscitation, and broad-spectrum antibiotics in preparation for surgery.

Nonoperative intervention is contraindicated unless a patient is stable with obvious clinical improvement. In children with repeated obstruction, fibrin-glued plication of adjacent small bowel loops can reduce the risk of recurrent problems. Long-term complications include female infertility, failure to thrive, and chronic abdominal and/or pelvic pain.

ACKNOWLEDGMENT
Andrew Chu, MD contributed to the prior version of this chapter.

Bibliography is available at Expert Consult.

359.3 Intussusception
Asim Maqbool and Chris A. Liacouras

Intussusception occurs when a portion of the alimentary tract is telescoped into an adjacent segment. It is the most common cause of intestinal obstruction between 5 mo and 3 yr of age and the most common abdominal emergency in children younger than 2 yr of age. Sixty percent of patients are younger than 1 yr of age and 80% of the cases occur before age 24 mo; it is rare in neonates. The incidence varies from 1 to 4 per 1,000 live births. The male:female ratio is 3:1. Many small bowel–small bowel and a few small bowel–colonic intussusceptions reduce spontaneously; if left untreated, ileal-colonic intussusception may lead to intestinal infarction, perforation, peritonitis, and death.

ETIOLOGY AND EPIDEMIOLOGY
Approximately 90% of cases of intussusception in children are idiopathic. The seasonal incidence has peaks in fall and winter. Correlation with prior or concurrent respiratory adenovirus (type C) infection has been noted, and the condition can complicate otitis media, gastroenteritis, Henoch-Schönlein purpura, or other upper respiratory tract infections. A slight increase in intussusception has been noted to occur within 3 wk of the rotavirus vaccine (especially after the first dose), but this is a very rare side effect.

It is postulated that gastrointestinal infection or the introduction of new food proteins results in swollen Peyer patches in the terminal ileum. Lymphoid nodular hyperplasia is another related risk factor. Prominent mounds of lymph tissue lead to mucosal prolapse of the ileum into the colon, thus causing an intussusception. In 2–8% of patients, **recognizable lead points** for the intussusception are found, such as a Meckel diverticulum, intestinal polyp, neurofibroma, intestinal duplication cysts, inverted appendix stump, leiomyomas, hamartomas, ectopic pancreatic tissue, anastomotic suture line, enterostomy tube, posttransplant lymphoproliferative disease, hemangioma, or malignant conditions such as lymphoma or Kaposi sarcoma. Gastrojejunal and jejunostomy tubes can also serve as lead points for intussusception. Lead points are more common in children older than 2 yr of age; the older the child, the higher the risk of a lead point. In adults, lead points are present in 90%. Intussusception can complicate mucosal hemorrhage, as in Henoch-Schönlein purpura, idiopathic thrombocytopenic purpura, or hemophilia. Cystic fibrosis, celiac disease, and Crohn disease are other risk factors. Postoperative intussusception is ileoileal and usually occurs within several days of an abdominal operation. Anterograde intussusception may occur rarely following bariatric surgery with a Roux-en-Y gastric bypass and is noteworthy that there does not seem to be a *lead point* in these cases. Intrauterine intussusception may be associated with the development of intestinal atresia. Intussusception in premature infants is rare.

Ileal-ileal intussusception may be more common than previously believed, is often idiopathic or associated with Henoch-Schönlein purpura, and usually resolves spontaneously.

PATHOLOGY
Intussusceptions are most often ileocolic, less commonly cecocolic, and occasionally ileal. Very rarely, the appendix forms the apex of an intussusception. The upper portion of bowel, the **intussusceptum,** invaginates into the lower, the **intussuscipiens,** pulling its mesentery along with it into the enveloping loop. Constriction of the mesentery obstructs venous return; engorgement of the intussusceptum follows, with edema, and bleeding from the mucosa leads to a bloody stool, sometimes containing mucus. The apex of the intussusception can extend into the transverse, descending, or sigmoid colon, even to and through the anus in neglected cases. This presentation must be distinguished from rectal prolapse. Most intussusceptions do not strangulate the bowel within the first 24 hr but can eventuate in intestinal gangrene and shock.

CLINICAL MANIFESTATIONS
In typical cases, there is sudden onset, in a previously well child, of severe paroxysmal colicky pain that recurs at frequent intervals and is accompanied by straining efforts with legs and knees flexed and loud cries. The infant may initially be comfortable and play normally between the paroxysms of pain, but if the intussusception is not reduced, the infant becomes progressively weaker and lethargic. At times, the **lethargy** is often disproportionate to the abdominal signs. With progression, a shock-like state, with fever and peritonitis, can develop. The pulse becomes weak and thready, the respirations become shallow and grunting, and the pain may be manifested only by moaning sounds. Vomiting occurs in most cases and is usually more frequent in the early phase. In the later phase, the vomitus becomes bile stained. Stools of normal appearance may be evacuated in the first few hr of symptoms. After this time, fecal excretions are small or more often do not occur, and little or no flatus is passed. Blood is generally passed in the first 12 hr but at times not for 1-2 days and infrequently not at all; 60% of infants pass a stool containing red blood and mucus, the currant jelly stool. Some patients have only irritability and alternating or progressive lethargy. The classic triad of pain, a palpable sausage-shaped abdominal mass, and bloody or currant jelly stool is seen in <30% of patients with intussusception. The combination of paroxysmal pain, vomiting, and a palpable abdominal mass has a positive predictive value of >90%; the presence of rectal bleeding increases this to approximately 100%.

Palpation of the abdomen usually reveals a slightly tender sausage-shaped mass, sometimes ill defined, which might increase in size and firmness during a paroxysm of pain and is most often in the right upper abdomen, with its long axis cephalocaudal. If it is felt in the epigastrium, the long axis is transverse. Approximately 30% of patients do not have a palpable mass. The presence of bloody mucus on rectal examination supports the diagnosis of intussusception. Abdominal distention and tenderness develop as intestinal obstruction becomes more acute. On rare occasions, the advancing intestine prolapses through the anus. *This prolapse can be distinguished from prolapse of the rectum by the separation between the protruding intestine and the rectal wall, which does not exist in prolapse of the rectum.*

Ileoileal intussusception in children younger than 2 yr can have a less-typical clinical picture, the symptoms and signs being chiefly those of small intestinal obstruction; these often resolve without treatment. **Recurrent intussusception** is noted in 5–8% and is more common after hydrostatic than surgical reduction. Chronic intussusception, in which the symptoms exist in milder form at recurrent intervals, is more likely to occur with or after acute enteritis and can arise in older children as well as in infants.

DIAGNOSIS
When the clinical history and physical findings suggest intussusception, an ultrasound is typically performed. A plain abdominal radiograph might show a density in the area of the intussusception. Screening ultrasounds for suspected intussusception increases the yield of diagnostic or therapeutic enemas and reduces unnecessary radiation exposure in children with negative ultrasound examinations. The diagnostic findings of intussusception on ultrasound include a tubular mass in longitudinal views and a doughnut or target appearance in transverse images (Fig. 359.1). Ultrasound has a sensitivity of approximately 98–100% and a specificity of approximately 98% in diagnosing intussusception. Air, hydrostatic (saline), and, less often, water-soluble contrast enemas have replaced barium examinations. Contrast enemas demonstrate a filling defect or cupping in the head of the contrast media where its advance is obstructed by the intussusceptum (Fig. 359.2). A central linear column

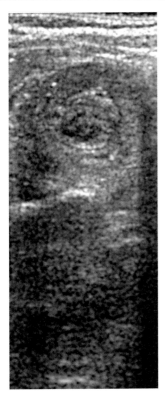

Fig. 359.1 Transverse image of an ileocolic intussusception. Note the loops within the loops of bowel.

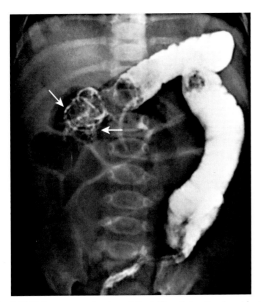

Fig. 359.2 Intussusception in an infant. The obstruction is evident in the proximal transverse colon. Contrast material between the intussusceptum and the intussuscipiens (arrows) is responsible for the coiled-spring appearance.

of contrast media may be visible in the compressed lumen of the intussusceptum, and a thin rim of contrast may be seen trapped around the invaginating intestine in the folds of mucosa within the intussuscipiens (coiled-spring sign), especially after evacuation. Retrogression of the

intussusceptum under pressure and visualized on x-ray or ultrasound documents successful reduction. Air reduction is associated with fewer complications and lower radiation exposure than traditional contrast hydrostatic techniques.

DIFFERENTIAL DIAGNOSIS

It may be particularly difficult to diagnose intussusception in a child who already has gastroenteritis; a change in the pattern of illness, in the character of pain, or in the nature of vomiting or the onset of rectal bleeding should alert the physician. The bloody stools and abdominal cramps that accompany enterocolitis can usually be differentiated from intussusception because in enterocolitis the pain is less severe and less regular, there is diarrhea, and the infant is recognizably ill between pains. Bleeding from a Meckel diverticulum is usually painless. Joint symptoms, purpura, or hematuria usually but not invariably accompany the intestinal hemorrhage of Henoch-Schönlein purpura. Because intussusception can be a complication of this disorder, ultrasonography may be needed to distinguish the conditions.

It is important in patients with cystic fibrosis to distinguish intussusception from distal intestinal obstruction syndrome. Distal intestinal obstruction syndrome requires antegrade treatment, which would be harmful if there was an intussusception.

TREATMENT

Reduction of an acute intussusception is an emergency procedure and should be performed immediately after diagnosis in preparation for possible surgery. In patients with prolonged intussusception and signs of shock, peritoneal irritation, intestinal perforation, or pneumatosis intestinalis, hydrostatic reduction should not be attempted.

The success rate of radiologic hydrostatic reduction under fluoroscopic or ultrasound guidance is approximately 80–95% in patients with ileocolic intussusception. Spontaneous reduction of intussusception occurs in approximately 4–10% of patients. Bowel perforations occur in 0.5–2.5% of attempted barium and hydrostatic (saline) reductions. The perforation rate with air reduction is 0.1–0.2%. Surgical reduction is indicated in the presence of refractory shock, suspected bowel necrosis or perforation, peritonitis, and multiple recurrences (suspected lead point).

An **ileoileal intussusception** is best demonstrated by abdominal ultrasonography. Reduction by instillation of contrast agents, saline, or air might not be possible. Such intussusceptions can develop insidiously after bowel surgery and require reoperation if they do not spontaneously reduce. Ileoileal disease is common with Henoch-Schönlein purpura and other unidentifiable disorders and usually resolves without the need for any specific treatment. If manual operative reduction is impossible or the bowel is not viable, resection of the intussusception is necessary, with end-to-end anastomosis.

PROGNOSIS

Untreated ileal-colonic intussusception in infants is usually fatal; the chances of recovery are directly related to the duration of intussusception before reduction. Most infants recover if the intussusception is reduced in the first 24 hr, but the mortality rate rises rapidly after this time, especially after the 2nd day. Spontaneous reduction during preparation for operation is not uncommon.

The **recurrence rate** after reduction of intussusceptions is approximately 10%, and after surgical reduction it is 2–5%; none has recurred after surgical resection. Most recurrences occur within 72 hr of reduction. Corticosteroids may reduce the frequency of recurrent intussusception but are rarely used for this purpose. Repeated reducible episodes caused by lymphonodular hyperplasia may respond to treatment of identifiable food allergies if present. A single recurrence of intussusception can usually be reduced radiologically. In patients with multiple ileal-colonic recurrences, a lead point should be suspected and laparoscopic surgery considered. It is unlikely that an intussusception caused by a lesion such as lymphosarcoma, polyp, or Meckel diverticulum will be successfully reduced by radiologic intervention. With adequate surgical management, laparoscopic reduction carries a very low mortality.

Bibliography is available at Expert Consult.

359.4 Closed-Loop Obstructions

Asim Maqbool and Chris A. Liacouras

Closed-loop obstructions (i.e., **internal hernia**) result from bowel loops that enter windows created by mesenteric defects or adhesions and become trapped. Vascular engorgement of the strangulated bowel results in intestinal ischemia and necrosis unless promptly relieved. Prior abdominal surgery is an important risk factor. Symptoms include abdominal pain, distention, and bilious emesis. Symptoms can be intermittent if the herniated bowel slides in and out of the defect. Peritoneal signs suggest ischemic bowel. Plain radiographs demonstrate signs of small bowel obstruction or free air if the bowel has perforated. CT scan can identify and delineate internal hernias. Supportive management includes intravenous fluids, antibiotics, and nasogastric decompression. Prompt surgical relief of the obstruction is indicated to prevent bowel necrosis.

Bibliography is available at Expert Consult.

Chapter **360**
Foreign Bodies and Bezoars

第三百六十章
异物和结石

中文导读

　　本章主要介绍了胃肠异物和结石。胃肠异物部分具体描述了胃肠异物的好发年龄、不同年龄段胃肠异物的特点和治疗，治疗中描述了保守治疗、有风险异物的处理（尖锐物体、电池、较大异物、磁珠、含铅异物及吸水聚合物）等；结石部分具体描述了结石的定义、好发人群、结石的分类及各类结石的临床表现、确诊方法、治疗方法等。

360.1 Foreign Bodies in the Stomach and Intestine

Asim Maqbool and Chris A. Liacouras

Once in the stomach, 95% of all ingested objects pass without difficulty through the remainder of the gastrointestinal tract. Perforation after ingestion of a foreign body is estimated to be <1% of all objects ingested. Perforation tends to occur in areas of physiologic sphincters (pylorus, ileocecal valve), acute angulation (duodenal sweep), congenital gut malformations (webs, diaphragms, diverticula), or areas of previous bowel surgery.

Most patients who ingest foreign bodies are between the ages of 6 mo and 6 yr. Coins are the most commonly ingested foreign body in children, and meat or food impactions are the most common accidental foreign body in adolescents and adults. Patients with nonfood foreign bodies often describe a history of ingestion. Young children might have a witness to ingestion. Immediate concerns are what the foreign body is, the location of the foreign body, the size of the foreign body, and the time that the ingestion occurred. Approximately 90% of foreign bodies are opaque. Radiologic examination is routinely performed to determine the type, number, and location of the suspected objects. Contrast radiographs may be necessary to demonstrate some objects, such as plastic parts or toys.

Conservative management is indicated for most foreign bodies that have passed through the esophagus and entered the stomach. Most objects pass though the intestine in 4-6 days, although some take as long as 3-4 wk. While waiting for the object to pass, parents are instructed to continue a regular diet and to observe the stools for the appearance of the ingested object. Cathartics should be avoided. Exceptionally long or sharp objects are usually monitored radiologically. Parents or patients should be instructed to report abdominal pain, vomiting, persistent fever, and hematemesis or melena immediately to their physicians. Failure of the object to progress within 3-4 wk seldom implies an impeding perforation but may be associated with a congenital malformation or acquired bowel abnormality.

Certain objects pose more risk than others. In cases of sharp foreign bodies, such as straight pins, weekly assessments are required. Surgical removal is necessary if the patient develops symptoms or signs of obstruction or perforation or if the foreign body fails to progress for several weeks. Small magnets used to secure earrings or parts of toys are associated with bowel perforation. Whereas a single magnet in the stomach may not require intervention in an asymptomatic child, a magnet in the esophagus requires immediate removal. When the *multiple* magnets disperse after ingestion, they may be attracted to each other across bowel walls, leading to pressure necrosis and perforation (Fig. 360.1). Inexpensive toy medallions containing lead can lead to **lead toxicity.** Newer coins can also decompose when subjected to prolonged acid exposure. Unless multiple coins are ingested, the metals released are unlikely to pose a clinical risk.

Ingestion of batteries rarely leads to problems, but symptoms can arise from leakage of alkali or heavy metal (mercury) from battery degradation in the gastrointestinal tract. Batteries can also generate electrical current and thereby cause low-voltage electrical burns to the intestine. If patients experience symptoms such as vomiting or abdominal pain, if a large-diameter battery (>20 mm in diameter) remains in the stomach for longer than 48 hr, or if a lithium battery is ingested, the battery should be removed. Batteries larger than 15 mm that do not pass the pylorus within 48 hr are less likely to pass spontaneously and generally require removal. In children younger than 6 yr of age, batteries larger than 15 mm are not likely to pass spontaneously and should be removed endoscopically. If the patient develops peritoneal signs, surgical removal is required. Batteries beyond the duodenum pass per rectum in 85% within 72 hr. The battery should be identified by size and imprint code or by evaluation of a duplicate measurement of the battery compartment. The National Button Battery Ingestion Hotline (202-625-3333) can be called for help in identification. The Poison Control Center (800-222-1222) can be called as well for ingestion of batteries and caustic materials. Lithium batteries result in more severe injury than a button alkali battery, with damage occurring in minutes. Button batteries in a symptomatic child should be removed, or if there are multiple batteries, they should be removed.

In older children and adults, oval objects larger than 5 cm in diameter or 2 cm in thickness tend to lodge in the stomach and should be endoscopically retrieved. Thin long objects >6 cm in length fail to negotiate the pylorus or duodenal sweep and should also be removed. In infants and toddlers, objects >3 cm in length or >20 mm in diameter do not usually pass through the pylorus and should be removed. An open safety pin presents a major problem and requires urgent endoscopic removal if within reach. Razor blades can be managed with a rigid endoscope by pulling the blade into instrument. The endoscopist can alternatively use a rubber hood on the head of the endoscope to protect the esophagus. Other sharp objects (needles, bones, pins) usually pass the stomach, but complications may be as high as 35%; if possible, they should be removed by endoscope if in the stomach or proximal duodenum. If sharp objects are not able to be removed but no progress is

observed in location during 3 days, surgical removal is indicated. Drugs (aggregated iron pills, cocaine) may have to be surgically removed; initial management can include oral polyethylene glycol lavage. Drug body packing (heroin, cocaine) is usually seen on kidneys-ureters-bladder or CT imaging and often passes without incident. Endoscopic procedures may rupture the material, causing severe toxicity. Surgery is indicated if toxicity develops, if the packages fail to progress, or if there are signs of obstruction.

Ingestion of magnets poses a danger to children. The number of magnets is thought to be critical. If a single magnet is ingested, there is the least likelihood of complications. If 2 or more magnets are ingested, the magnetic poles are attracted to each other and create the risk of obstruction, fistula development, and perforation. Endoscopic retrieval is emergent after films are taken when multiple magnets are ingested. Abdominal pain or peritoneal signs require urgent surgical intervention. If all magnets are located in the stomach, immediate endoscopic removal is indicated. If the ingestion occurred greater than 12 hr prior to evaluation, or if the magnets are beyond the stomach and the patient is symptomatic, general surgery should be consulted. If the patient is asymptomatic, endoscopic or colonoscopic removal may be considered, along with a surgical evaluation.

Lead-based foreign bodies can cause symptoms from lead intoxication. Early endoscopic removal is indicated of an object suspected to contain lead. A lead level should be obtained.

Water-absorbing polymer balls (beads) can expand to approximately 400 times their starting size and if ingested may produce intestinal obstruction. Initially of a small diameter, they pass the pylorus only to rapidly enlarge in the small intestine. Surgical removal is indicated.

Children occasionally place objects in their rectum. Small blunt objects usually pass spontaneously, but large or sharp objects typically need to be retrieved. Adequate sedation is essential to relax the anal sphincter before attempting endoscopic or speculum removal. If the object is proximal to the rectum, observation for 12-24 hr usually allows the object to descend into the rectum.

Bibliography is available at Expert Consult.

360.2 Bezoars

Asim Maqbool and Chris A. Liacouras

A bezoar is an accumulation of exogenous matter in the stomach or intestine. They are predominantly composed of food or fiber. Most bezoars have been found in females with underlying personality problems or in neurologically impaired persons. Patients who have undergone abdominal surgery are at higher risk for the development of bezoars. The peak age at onset of symptoms is the 2nd decade of life.

Bezoars are classified on the basis of their composition. **Trichobezoars** are composed of the patient's own hair. It is most frequently a complication of the psychiatric disorder trichotillomania, and the most severe form is known as Rapunzel syndrome (hair bezoar extending beyond the stomach to the small intestine). **Phytobezoars** are composed of a combination of plant and animal material, and gastric phytobezoars are the most common in patients with poor motility. **Lactobezoars** were previously found most often in premature infants and can be attributed to the high casein or calcium content of some premature formulas. Swallowed chewing gum can occasionally lead to a bezoar.

Trichobezoars can become large and form casts of the stomach; they can enter into the proximal duodenum. They manifest as symptoms of gastric outlet or partial intestinal obstruction, including vomiting, anorexia, and weight loss. Patients might complain of abdominal pain, distention, and severe halitosis. Physical examination can demonstrate patchy baldness and a firm mass in the left upper quadrant. Patients occasionally have iron-deficiency anemia, hypoproteinemia, or steatorrhea caused by an associated chronic gastritis. Phytobezoars manifest in a similar manner. Detached segments of the bezoar or trichobezoar can migrate to the small intestine as a "satellite masses" and result in small bowel obstruction.

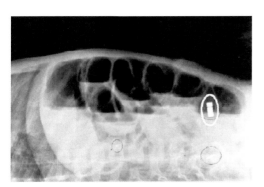

Fig. 360.1 Abdominal radiograph of a boy aged 3 yr, noting three attached magnets that resulted in volvulus (i.e., twisting of the bowel) and multiple bowel perforations. (*Courtesy U.S. Consumer Product Safety Commission. From Centers for Disease Control and Prevention: Gastrointestinal injuries from magnet ingestion in children—United States, 2003–2006. MMWR Morb Mortal Wkly Rep 55:1296–1300, 2006.*)

An abdominal plain film can suggest the presence of a bezoar, which can be confirmed on ultrasound or CT examination. On CT a bezoar appears a nonhomogeneous, nonenhancing mass within the lumen of the stomach or intestine. Oral contrast circumscribes the mass.

Bezoars in the stomach can usually be removed endoscopically. If endoscopy is unsuccessful, surgical intervention may be needed. Lactobezoars usually resolve when feedings are withheld for 24-48 hr. Coca-Cola has been used as a dissolution therapy for gastric phytobezoar

and has been shown to be effective when used with endoscopy. Tricho-bezoars almost always require surgical removal.

Sunflower seed bezoars are reported to cause rectal pain and constipation as a result of the seed shells being associated with fecal impaction. Endoscopic removal is indicated, as these bezoars are refractory to enema or lavage management.

Bibliography is available at Expert Consult.

Chapter 361
Peptic Ulcer Disease in Children
Samra S. Blanchard and Steven J. Czinn

第三百六十一章
儿童消化性溃疡病

中文导读

本章主要介绍了儿童消化性溃疡病的发病机制、临床表现、诊断、治疗，分别介绍了原发性溃疡、继发性溃疡、"应激性"溃疡及胃泌素瘤。发病机制具体描述了酸分泌和黏膜屏障；原发性溃疡具体描述了幽门螺杆菌性胃炎和特发性溃疡；继发性溃疡具体描述了由阿司匹林和其他非甾体抗炎药所致溃疡；介绍了幽门螺杆菌相关性溃疡病的治疗和溃疡的手术治疗。

Peptic ulcer disease, resulting from inflammation caused by an imbalance between cytoprotective and cytotoxic factors in the stomach and duodenum, manifests with varying degrees of gastritis or frank ulceration. The pathogenesis of peptic ulcer disease is multifactorial, but the final common pathway for the development of ulcers is the action of acid and pepsin-laden contents of the stomach on the gastric and duodenal mucosa and the inability of mucosal defense mechanisms to allay those effects. Abnormalities in the gastric and duodenal mucosa can be visualized on endoscopy, with or without histologic changes. Deep mucosal lesions that disrupt the muscularis mucosa of the gastric or duodenal wall define **peptic ulcers.** Gastric ulcers are generally located on the lesser curvature of the stomach, and 90% of duodenal ulcers are found in the duodenal bulb. While there are no large population-based pediatric studies, rates of peptic ulcer disease in childhood appear to be low. Large pediatric centers anecdotally report an incidence of 5-7 children with gastric or duodenal ulcers per 2,500 hospital admissions each year.

Ulcers in children can be classified as **primary** peptic ulcers, which are chronic and more often duodenal, or **secondary,** which are usually

more acute in onset and are more often gastric (Table 361.1). Primary ulcers are most often associated with *Helicobacter pylori* infection; idiopathic primary peptic ulcers account for up to 20% of duodenal ulcers in children. Secondary peptic ulcers can result from stress caused by sepsis, shock, or an intracranial lesion (Cushing ulcer), or in response to a severe burn injury (Curling ulcer). Secondary ulcers are often the result of using aspirin or nonsteroidal antiinflammatory drugs (NSAIDs); hypersecretory states like Zollinger-Ellison syndrome (see Chapter 361.1), short bowel syndrome, and systemic mastocytosis are rare causes of peptic ulceration.

PATHOGENESIS
Acid Secretion
By 3-4 yr of age, gastric acid secretion approximates adult values. Acid initially secreted by the oxyntic cells of the stomach has a pH of approximately 0.8, whereas the pH of the stomach contents is 1-2. Excessive acid secretion is associated with a large parietal cell mass, hypersecretion by antral G cells, and increased vagal tone, resulting in increased or sustained acid secretion in response to meals and increased

Table 361.1	Etiologic Classification of Peptic Ulcers

- Positive for *Helicobacter pylori* infection
- Drug (NSAID)-induced
- *Helicobacter pylori* and NSAID-positive
- *H. pylori* and NSAID-negative*
- Acid hypersecretory state (Zollinger-Ellison syndrome)
- Anastomosis ulcer after subtotal gastric resection
- Tumors (cancer, lymphoma)
- Rare specific causes
- Crohn disease of the stomach or duodenum
- Eosinophilic gastroduodenitis
- Systemic mastocytosis
- Radiation damage
- Viral infections (cytomegalovirus or herpes simplex infection, particularly in immunocompromised patients)
- Colonization of stomach with *Helicobacter heilmannii*
- Severe systemic disease
- Cameron ulcer (gastric ulcer where a hiatal hernia passes through the diaphragmatic hiatus)
- True idiopathic ulcer

*Requires search for other specific causes. *NSAID,* nonsteroidal antiinflammatory drug. (From Vakil N, Megraud F: Eradication therapy for *Helicobacter pylori, Gastroenterology* 133:985–1001, 2007.)

secretion during the night. The secretagogues that promote gastric acid production include acetylcholine released by the vagus nerve, histamine secreted by enterochromaffin cells, and gastrin released by the G cells of the antrum. Mediators that decrease gastric acid secretion and enhance protective mucin production include prostaglandins.

Mucosal Defense

A continuous layer of mucous gel that serves as a diffusion barrier to hydrogen ions and other chemicals covers the gastrointestinal (GI) mucosa. Mucus production and secretion are stimulated by prostaglandin E_2. Underlying the mucous coat, the epithelium forms a second-line barrier, the characteristics of which are determined by the biology of the epithelial cells and their tight junctions. Another important function of epithelial cells is to secrete chemokines when threatened by microbial attack. Secretion of bicarbonate into the mucous coat, which is regulated by prostaglandins, is important for neutralization of hydrogen ions. If mucosal injury occurs, active proliferation and migration of mucosal cells occurs rapidly, driven by epithelial growth factor, transforming growth factor-α, insulin-like growth factor, gastrin, and bombesin, and covers the area of epithelial damage.

CLINICAL MANIFESTATIONS

The presenting symptoms of peptic ulcer disease vary with the age of the patient. Hematemesis or melena is reported in up to half of the patients with peptic ulcer disease. School-age children and adolescents more commonly present with epigastric pain and nausea, similar to the presentation generally seen in adults. Dyspepsia, epigastric abdominal pain, and fullness are also seen in older children. Infants and younger children usually present with feeding difficulty, vomiting, crying episodes, hematemesis, or melena. In the neonatal period, gastric perforation can be the initial presentation.

The classic symptom of peptic ulceration, epigastric pain alleviated by the ingestion of food, is present only in a minority of children. Many pediatric patients present with poorly localized abdominal pain, which may be periumbilical. The vast majority of patients with periumbilical or epigastric pain or discomfort do not have a peptic ulcer, but rather a functional GI disorder, such as irritable bowel syndrome or nonulcer (functional) dyspepsia. Patients with peptic ulceration rarely present with acute abdominal pain from perforation or symptoms and signs of pancreatitis from a posterior penetrating ulcer. Occasionally, bright red blood per rectum may be seen if the rate of bleeding is brisk and the intestinal transit time is short. Vomiting can be a sign of gastric outlet obstruction.

The pain is often described as dull or aching, rather than sharp or burning, as in adults. It can last from minutes to hours; patients have frequent exacerbations and remissions lasting from weeks to months. Nocturnal pain waking the child is common in older children. A history of typical ulcer pain with prompt relief after taking antacids is found in <33% of children. Rarely, in patients with acute or chronic blood loss, penetration of the ulcer into the abdominal cavity or adjacent organs produces shock, anemia, peritonitis, or pancreatitis. If inflammation and edema are extensive, acute or chronic gastric outlet obstruction can occur. *In a child with a normal diet for age, iron deficiency anemia may suggest peptic ulceration.* Other gastric causes of iron deficiency anemia include autoimmune gastritis, gastric hyperplasia, and possible Jervell and Lange-Nielson syndrome (*KCNQ1* mutations).

DIAGNOSIS

Esophagogastroduodenoscopy is the method of choice to establish the diagnosis of peptic ulcer disease. It can be safely performed in all ages by experienced pediatric gastroenterologists. Endoscopy allows the direct visualization of esophagus, stomach, and duodenum, identifying the specific lesions. Biopsy specimens must be obtained from the esophagus, stomach, and duodenum for histologic assessment as well as to screen for the presence of *H. pylori* infection. Endoscopy also provides the opportunity for hemostatic therapy including clipping, injection, and the use of thermal coagulation.

PRIMARY ULCERS
Helicobacter pylori Gastritis

H. pylori is among the most common bacterial infections in humans. *H. pylori* is a Gram-negative, **S**-shaped rod that produces urease, catalase, and oxidase, which might play a role in the pathogenesis of peptic ulcer disease. The mechanism of acquisition and transmission of *H. pylori* is unclear, although the most likely mode of transmission is fecal–oral or oral–oral. Viable *H. pylori* organisms can be cultured from the stool or vomitus of infected patients. Risk factors such as low socioeconomic status in childhood or affected family members also influence the prevalence. All children infected with *H. pylori* develop histologic chronic active gastritis but are often asymptomatic. In children, *H. pylori* infection can manifest with abdominal pain or vomiting and, less often, refractory iron deficiency anemia or growth retardation. *H. pylori* can be associated, though rarely, with chronic autoimmune thrombocytopenia. Chronic colonization with *H. pylori* can predispose children to a significantly increased risk of developing a duodenal ulcer, gastric cancer such as adenocarcinoma, or mucosa-associated lymphoid tissue lymphomas. The relative risk of gastric carcinoma is 2.3-8.7 times greater in infected adults as compared to uninfected subjects. *H. pylori* is classified by the World Health Organization as a group I carcinogen.

Anemia, idiopathic thrombocytopenic purpura, short stature, and sudden infant death syndrome (SIDS) have also been reported as possible extragastric manifestations of *H. pylori* infection. In one published study, *H. pylori* infection has been correlated with cases of SIDS, but there is no evidence to suggest that *H. pylori* plays a role in the pathogenesis of SIDS.

The **diagnosis** of *H. pylori* infection is made histologically by demonstrating the organism in the biopsy specimens (Fig. 361.1). The most recent consensus report recommends against using antibody-based tests (IgG, IgA) for *H pylori* in serum, whole blood, urine, and saliva in the clinical setting.[13] C-urea breath tests and stool antigen tests are reliable noninvasive methods of detecting *H. pylori* infection in patients who do not require endoscopic evaluation. Patients should stop proton pump inhibitor (PPI) therapy 2 wk prior to testing as negative results on therapy may represent false negatives. Nonetheless, for symptomatic children with suspected *H. pylori* infection, an initial upper endoscopy is recommended to evaluate and confirm *H. pylori* disease. The range of endoscopic findings in children with *H. pylori* infection varies from being grossly normal to the presence of nonspecific gastritis with prominent rugal folds, nodularity (Fig. 361.2), or ulcers. Because the antral mucosa appears to be endoscopically normal in a significant number of children with primary *H. pylori* gastritis, gastric biopsies should always be obtained from the body and antrum of the stomach

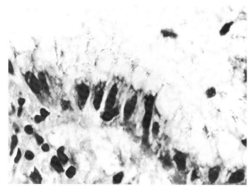

Fig. 361.1 Appearance of *Helicobacter pylori* on the gastric mucosal surface with Giemsa stain (high-power view). *(From Campbell DI, Thomas JE: Helicobacter pylori infection in paediatric practice, Arch Dis Child Educ Pract Ed 90:ep25–ep30, 2005.)*

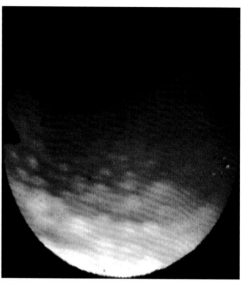

Fig. 361.2 Endoscopic view of lymphoid modular hyperplasia of the gastric antrum. *(From Campbell DI, Thomas JE: Helicobacter pylori infection in paediatric practice, Arch Dis Child Educ Pract Ed 90:ep25–ep30, 2005.)*

regardless of the endoscopic appearance. If *H. pylori* is identified, even in a child with no symptoms, eradication therapy should be offered (Tables 361.2 and 361.3). Successful *H pylori* eradication is associated with cure of peptic ulcer disease and very low risk of relapse. Therefore, monitoring the success of therapy is mandatory in these patients 4-6 wk after stopping antibiotics and at least 2 wk after stopping PPI therapy. Eradication can be tested with the 13C-urea breath (13C-UBT) test or stool antigen test. If there is an eradication failure, the patient should receive rescue therapy (Fig. 361.3). Because of a significant incidence of *H. pylori* resistance to clarithromycin, other treatment options are recommended if the community resistance rate is >15% or if it is unknown.

Idiopathic Ulcers

H. pylori–negative peptic ulcers in children who have no history of taking NSAIDs represent 15–20% of pediatric peptic ulcers. The pathogenesis of idiopathic ulcer remains uncertain. These patients do not have nodularity in the gastric antrum or histologic evidence of gastritis. In idiopathic ulcers, acid suppression *alone* is the preferred effective treatment. Either PPIs or H_2 receptor antagonists may be used. Idiopathic ulcers have a high recurrence rate after discontinuing antisecretory therapy. These children should be followed closely, and if symptoms recur, antisecretory therapy should be restarted. It is also important to consider uncommon but possible conditions like Crohn disease, cytomegalovirus (CMV), and Zollinger-Ellison syndrome.

SECONDARY ULCERS
Aspirin and Other Nonsteroidal Antiinflammatory Drugs

NSAIDs produce mucosal injury by direct local irritation and by inhibiting cyclooxygenase (COX) and prostaglandin formation. Prostaglandins enhance mucosal resistance to injury; therefore a decrease in prostaglandin production increases the risk of mucosal injury. The severe erosive gastropathy produced by NSAIDs can ultimately result in bleeding ulcers or gastric perforations. The location of these ulcers is more common in the stomach than in the duodenum, and usually in the antrum. Use of COX-2-selective NSAIDs can also cause ulcerations in the GI tract.

"STRESS" ULCERATION

Stress ulceration usually occurs within 24 hr of onset of a critical illness in which physiologic stress is present. In many cases, the patients bleed from gastric erosions, rather than ulcers. Approximately 25% of the critically ill children in a pediatric intensive care unit have macroscopic evidence of gastric bleeding. Preterm and term infants

Table 361.2	Recommended Eradication Therapies for *Helicobacter pylori*–Associated Disease in Children		
MEDICATIONS	**DOSE**		**DURATION OF TREATMENT**
Proton pump inhibitor	1 mg/kg/dose twice a day		1 mo
ANTIBIOTICS	**WEIGHT**	**DOSE**	**DURATION OF TREATMENT**
Amoxicillin	15-24 kg 25-34 kg >35 kg	500 mg twice a day 750 mg twice a day 1,000 mg twice a day	14 days
Clarithromycin	15-24 kg 25-34 kg >35 kg	250 mg twice a day 500 mg in AM, 250 mg in PM 500 mg twice a day	14 days
Metronidazole	15-24 kg 25-34 kg >35 kg	250 mg twice a day 500 mg in AM, 250 mg in PM 500 mg twice a day	14 days

Depending on previous antibiotic use history, recommended combinations are Amoxicillin + Clarithromycin + PPI OR Amoxicillin + Metronidazole + PPI OR Clarithromycin + Metronidazole + PPI. (Modified from Jones NL, Koletzko S, Goodman K, et al: Joint ESPGHAN/NASPGHAN Guidelines for the Management of Helicobacter pylori in Children and Adolescents, *J Pediatr Gastroenterol Nutr* 64(6):991–1003, 2017.)

Table 361.3	Antisecretory Therapy With Pediatric Dosages	
MEDICATION	**PEDIATRIC DOSE**	**HOW SUPPLIED**
H₂ RECEPTOR ANTAGONISTS		
Ranitidine	4-10 mg/kg/day Divided 2 or 3 × a day	Syrup: 75 mg/5 mL Tablets: 75, 150, 300 mg
Famotidine	1-2 mg/kg/day Divided twice a day	Syrup: 40 mg/5 mL Tablets: 20, 40 mg
Nizatidine	5-10 mg/kg/day divided twice a day Older than 12 yr: 150 mg twice a day	Solution: 15 mg/mL Capsule 150, 300 Tablet: 75 mg
PROTON PUMP INHIBITORS		
Omeprazole	1.0-3.3 mg/kg/day weigh < 20 kg: 10 mg/day weigh > 20 kg: 20 mg/day Approved for use in those older than 2 yr	Capsules: 10, 20, 40 mg
Lansoprazole	0.8-4 mg/kg/day weigh < 30 kg: 15 mg/day weigh > 30 kg: 30 mg/day Approved for use in those older than 1 yr	Capsules: 15, 30 mg Powder packet: 15, 30 mg SoluTab: 15, 30 mg
Rabeprazole	1-11 yr (weigh < 15 kg): 5 mg/day 1-11 yr (weigh > 15 kg): 10 mg/day >12 yr: 20 mg tablet	Delayed release capsule: 5, 10 mg Delayed release tablet: 20 mg

Pantoprazole	1-5 yr: 0.3-1.2 mg/kg/day (limited data)
	>5 yr of age:
	  weigh > 15 kg to < 40 kg: 20 mg/day
	  weigh > 40 kg: 40 mg/day
		Tablet: 20, 40 mg
		Powder pack: 40 mg

Esomeprazole	1 mo - < 1 yr old
	  weigh 3 kg to 5 kg: 2.5 mg
	  weigh > 5 kg to 7.5 kg: 5 mg
	  weigh > 7.5 kg to 12 kg: 10 mg
	1-11 yr old
	  weigh < 20 kg: 10 mg
	  weigh > 20 kg: 20 mg
	Approved for use 1 mo and older
		Capsules: 20, 40
		Delayed release single dose packs: 2.5, 5,
		  10, 20 mg

Dexlansoprazole	12-17 yr: 30-60 mg Approved for use in 12-17 yr	Capsules: 30, 60
Omeprazole sodium bicarbonate	Not approved for use < 18 yr at time of publication	Capsules: 20, 40 Powder for oral suspension: 20 mg, 40 mg
CYTOPROTECTIVE AGENTS		
Sucralfate	40-80 mg/kg/day	Suspension: 1,000 mg/5 mL Tablet: 1,000 mg

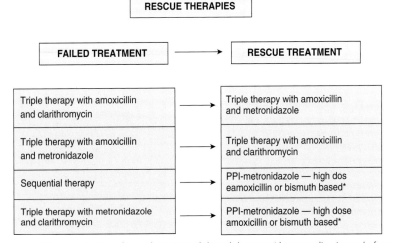

Fig. 361.3 Rescue therapy for failed eradication of *H. pylori.* *Bismuth-based therapy with tetracycline instead of amoxicillin if patients >8 yr. Bismuth dose is 262 mg four times a day for patients 8–10 yr and 524 mg four times a day for those >10 yr. (See Tables 361.2 and 361.3.) In adolescents, levofloxacin or tetracycline can be considered. High-dose amoxicillin ranges from 750 mg twice a day for body weight 15–24 kg, 1000 mg twice a day for 25–34 kg, and 1500 mg twice a day for >35 kg. (*Adapted from Jones NL, Koletzko S, Goodman K, et al: Joint ESPGHAN/ NASPGHAN guidelines for the management of* Helicobacter pylori *in children and adolescents, J Pediatr Gastroenterol Nutr 64:991–1003, 2017.*)

in the neonatal intensive care unit can also develop gastric mucosal lesions and can present with upper GI bleeding or perforated ulcers. Although prophylactic measures to prevent stress ulcers in children are not standardized, drugs that inhibit gastric acid production are often used in the pediatric intensive care unit to reduce the rate of gastric erosions or ulcers.

TREATMENT

The management of acute hemorrhage includes serial monitoring of pulse, blood pressure, and hematocrit to ensure hemodynamic stability and avoid significant hypovolemia and anemia. Normal saline can be used to resuscitate a patient who has poor intravascular volume status. This can be followed by packed red blood cell transfusions for significant symptomatic anemia. The patient's blood should be typed and cross matched, and a large-bore catheter should be placed for fluid or blood replacement. A nasogastric tube should be placed to determine if the bleeding has stopped. Significant anemia can occur after fluid resuscitation as a consequence of equilibration or continued blood loss (which can also cause shock). In adults, a conservative threshold for transfusion (<7 g/dL vs. 9 g hemoglobin) resulted in improved survival and fewer episodes of rebleeding. Fortunately, most acute peptic ulcer bleeding stops spontaneously.

Patients with suspected peptic ulcer hemorrhage should receive high-dose intravenous (IV) PPI therapy, which lowers the risk of rebleeding. Some centers also use octreotide, which lowers splanchnic blood flow and gastric acid production; others use a prokinetic agent to improve endoscopic visualization.

Once the patient is hemodynamically stable, endoscopy within 24 hr is indicated to identify the source of bleeding and to treat a potential bleeding site. Methods used to achieve hemostasis include mechanical devices (clipping), injection therapy (diluted epinephrine 1:10,000), and thermal therapy (heater probe). Ulcer therapy has two goals: ulcer healing and elimination of the primary cause. Other important considerations are relief of symptoms and prevention of complications. The first-line drugs for the treatment of gastritis and peptic ulcer disease in children are PPIs and H_2 receptor antagonists (see Table 361.3). PPIs are more potent in ulcer healing. Cytoprotective agents can also be used as adjunct therapy if mucosal lesions are present. Antibiotics in combination with a PPI must be used for the treatment of *H. pylori*-associated ulcers (see Table 361.2 and Fig. 361.3).

H_2-receptor antagonists (ranitidine, famotidine, nizatidine) competitively inhibit the binding of histamine at the H_2 subtype receptor of the gastric parietal cell. PPIs block the gastric parietal cell H^+/K^+–adenosine triphosphatase pump in a dose-dependent fashion, reducing basal and stimulated gastric acid secretion. Seven PPIs are available in the United States: omeprazole, lansoprazole, pantoprazole, esomeprazole, rabeprazole, dexlansoprazole, and omeprazole/sodium bicarbonate. Apart from the last 2, they are all approved in children and adolescents. They are well tolerated with only minor adverse effects, such as diarrhea (1–4%), headache (1–3%), and nausea (1%). When one considers therapeutic efficacy, the evidence suggests that all PPIs have comparable efficacy in treatment of peptic ulcer disease using standard doses and are superior to H_2-receptor antagonists. PPIs have their greatest effect when given before a meal. Pantoprazole and esomeprazole are the only PPI available in IV form in United States. IV PPI should be used in acute upper GI bleeding. Twice-a-day IV PPI is as effective as continuous infusion and the current recommendation is to start with IV PPI and change to the oral form after evaluating their rebleeding risk at the time of endoscopy. Long-term PPI therapy may result in hypomagnesemia and the risk of QT prolongation, as well as vitamin B12 and iron deficiencies and small bowel bacterial overgrowth. Conflicting results from multiple studies suggest a possible increased risk of community-acquired and ventilator-associated pneumonias as well as *Clostridium difficile* infection.

Treatment of *Helicobacter pylori*–Related Peptic Ulcer Disease

In pediatrics, antibiotics and bismuth salts have been used in combination with PPIs to treat H. pylori infection (see Table 361.2). Eradication rates in children range from 68 to 92% when the dual or triple therapy is used for 4-6 wk. The ulcer healing rate ranges from 91 to 100%. Triple therapy yields a higher cure rate than dual therapy. The optimal regimen for the eradication of *H. pylori* infection in children has yet to be established, but the use of a PPI in combination with clarithromycin and amoxicillin or metronidazole for 2 wk is a well-tolerated and recommended triple therapy (see Table 361.2). Although children younger than 5 yr of age can become reinfected, the most common reason for treatment failure is poor compliance or antibiotic resistance. *H. pylori* has become more resistant to clarithromycin or metronidazole because of the extensive use of these antibiotics for other infections. In the case of resistant *H. pylori* infection, sequential treatment or rescue therapy with different antibiotics are acceptable options (see Fig. 361.3). The sequential treatment regimen is a 10-day treatment consisting of a PPI and amoxicillin (both twice daily) administered for the first 5 days followed by triple therapy consisting of a PPI, clarithromycin, and metronidazole for the remaining 5 days. Levofloxacin, rifabutin, or furazolidone can be used with amoxicillin and bismuth as a rescue therapy depending on the age of the patient. Knowledge of the community's *H. pylori* resistance pattern to clarithromycin or metronidazole might help choose the initial or rescue therapy; if it is unknown, one should assume resistance.

Surgical Therapy

Since the discovery of *H. pylori* and the availability of modern medical management, peptic ulcer disease requiring surgical treatment has become extremely rare. The indications for surgery remain uncontrolled bleeding, perforation, and obstruction. Since the introduction of H_2-receptor antagonists, the recognition and treatment of *H. pylori*, and the use of PPIs, the incidence of surgery for bleeding and perforation has decreased dramatically.

Bibliography is available at Expert Consult.

361.1 Zollinger-Ellison Syndrome

Samra S. Blanchard and Steven J. Czinn

Zollinger-Ellison syndrome is a rare syndrome characterized by refractory, severe peptic ulcer disease caused by gastric hypersecretion due to the autonomous secretion of gastrin by a neuroendocrine tumor, a gastrinoma. Clinical presentations are similar to those of peptic ulcer disease with the addition of diarrhea. The diagnosis is suspected by the presence of recurrent, multiple, or atypically located ulcers. More than 98% of patients have elevated fasting gastrin levels. Zollinger-Ellison syndrome is common in patients with **multiple endocrine neoplasia 1** and rare with **neurofibromatosis** and **tuberous sclerosis**. Prompt and effective management of increased gastric acid secretion is essential in the management. **PPIs are the drug of choice due to their long duration of action and potency.** H_2-receptor antagonists are also effective, but higher doses are required than those used in peptic ulcer disease.

Bibliography is available at Expert Consult.

Chapter **362**

Inflammatory Bowel Disease

Ronen E. Stein and Robert N. Baldassano

第三百六十二章

炎性肠病

中文导读

本章主要介绍炎症性肠病、溃疡性结肠炎、克罗恩病和极早发炎症性肠病。具体描述了炎症性肠病的发病机制、溃疡性结肠炎与克罗恩病的比较以及肠外表现；描述了溃疡性结肠炎和克罗恩病的临床表现及肠外表现、诊断与鉴别诊断、治疗方法及预后；治疗中详细描述了克罗恩病的药物治疗方法（美沙拉秦、抗生素/益生菌、皮质类固醇、免疫调节剂、生物制剂及肠内营养疗法）；在极早发炎症性肠病中详细阐述了炎症性肠病的年龄分型、可能的病因，在诊断时需完善的有关检查，其中包括免疫功能的评估以及治疗等。

The term *inflammatory bowel disease* (IBD) is used to represent 2 distinctive disorders of idiopathic chronic intestinal inflammation: Crohn disease and ulcerative colitis. Their respective etiologies are poorly understood, and both disorders are characterized by unpredictable exacerbations and remissions. The most common time of onset of IBD is during the preadolescent/adolescent era and young adulthood. A bimodal distribution has been shown with an early onset at 10-20 yr of age and a second, smaller peak at 50-80 yr of age. Approximately 25% of patients present before 20 yr of age. IBD may begin as early as the 1st yr of life, and an increased incidence among young children has been observed since the turn of the 20th century. Children with early-onset IBD are more likely to have colonic involvement. In developed countries, these disorders are the major causes of chronic intestinal inflammation in children beyond the first few yr of life. A third, less-common category, *indeterminate colitis*, represents approximately 10% of pediatric patients.

Genetic and environmental influences are involved in the pathogenesis of IBD. The prevalence of Crohn disease in the United States is much lower for Hispanics and Asians than for whites and blacks. The risk of IBD in family members of an affected person has been reported in the range of 7–30%; a child whose parents both have IBD has a >35% chance of acquiring the disorder. Relatives of a patient with ulcerative colitis have a greater risk of acquiring ulcerative colitis than Crohn disease, whereas relatives of a patient with Crohn disease have a greater risk of acquiring this disorder; the 2 diseases can occur in the same family. The risk of occurrence of IBD among relatives of patients with Crohn disease is somewhat greater than for patients with ulcerative colitis.

The importance of genetic factors in the development of IBD is noted by a higher chance that both twins will be affected if they are monozygotic rather than dizygotic. The concordance rate in twins is higher in Crohn disease (36%) than in ulcerative colitis (16%). Genetic disorders that have been associated with IBD include Turner syndrome, the Hermansky-Pudlak syndrome, glycogen storage disease type Ib, and various immunodeficiency disorders. In 2001, the first IBD gene, *NOD2,* was identified through association mapping. A few months later, the IBD 5 risk haplotype was identified. These early successes were followed by a long period without notable risk factor discovery. Since 2006, the year of the first published genome-wide array study on IBD, there has been an exponential growth in the set of validated genetic risk factors for IBD (Table 362.1).

A perinuclear antineutrophil cytoplasmic antibody is found in approximately 70% of patients with ulcerative colitis compared with <20% of those with Crohn disease and is believed to represent a marker of genetically controlled immunoregulatory disturbance. Approximately 55% of those with Crohn disease are positive for anti–*Saccharomyces cerevisiae* antibody. Since the importance of these were first described, multiple other serologic and immune markers of Crohn disease and ulcerative colitis have been recognized.

IBD is caused by dysregulated or inappropriate immune response to environmental factors in a genetically susceptible host. An abnormality in intestinal mucosal immunoregulation may be of primary importance in the pathogenesis of IBD, involving activation of cytokines, triggering a cascade of reactions that results in bowel inflammation. These cytokines are recognized as known or potential targets for IBD therapies.

Table 362.1 | Selection of Most Important Genes Associated With Inflammatory Bowel Disease and the Most Commonly Associated Physiological Functions and Pathways

	GENE NAME	ASSOCIATED DISEASE	GENE FUNCTION AND ASSOCIATED PATHWAYS	PHYSIOLOGICAL FUNCTION
NOD2	Nucleotide-binding oligomerization domain-containing protein 2	Crohn disease	Bacterial recognition and response, NFκB activation and autophagy and apoptosis	Innate mucosal defense
IL10	Interleukin 10	Crohn disease	Antiinflammatory cytokine, NFκB inhibition, JAK-STAT regulation	Immune tolerance
IL10RA	Interleukin 10 receptor A	Crohn disease	Antiinflammatory cytokine receptor, NFκB inhibition, JAK-STAT regulation	Immune tolerance
IL10RB	Interleukin 10 receptor B	Crohn disease	Antiinflammatory cytokine receptor, NFκB inhibition, JAK-STAT regulation	Immune tolerance
IL23R	Interleukin 23 receptor	Crohn disease and ulcerative colitis	Immune regulation, proinflammatory pathways—JAK-STAT regulation	Interleukin 23/T helper 17
TKY2	Tyrosine kinase 2	Crohn disease and ulcerative colitis	Inflammatory pathway signaling (interleukin 10 and 6 etc) through intracellular activity	Interleukin 23/T helper 17
IRGM	Immunity related GTPase M	Crohn disease	Autophagy and apoptosis in cells infected with bacteria	Autophagy
ATG16L1	Autophagy related 16 like 1	Crohn disease	Autophagy and apoptotic pathways	Autophagy
SLC22A4	Solute carrier family 22 member 4	Crohn disease	Cellular antioxidant transporter	Solute transporters
CCL2	C-C motif chemokine ligand 2	Crohn disease	Cytokine involved in chemotaxis for monocytes	Immune cell recruitment
CARD9	Caspase recruitment domain family member 9	Crohn disease and ulcerative colitis	Apoptosis regulation and NFκB pathway activation	Oxidative stress
IL2	Interleukin 2	Ulcerative colitis	Cytokine involved in immune cell activation	T-cell regulation
MUC19	Mucin 19	Crohn disease and ulcerative colitis	Gel-forming mucin protein	Epithelial barrier

JAK-STAT, Janus kinase-signal transducers and activators of transcription; NFκB, nuclear factor κ-light chain enhancer of activated B cells.
From Ashton JJ, Ennis S, Beattie RM: Early-onset paediatric inflammatory bowel disease, Lancet 1:147–158, 2017, Table 1, p 148.

Multiple environmental factors are recognized to be involved in the pathogenesis of IBD, none more critical than the gut microbiota. The increasing incidence of IBD over time is likely in part attributable to alterations in the microbiome. Evidence includes association between IBD and residence in or immigration to industrialized nations, a *Western diet*, increased use of antibiotics at a younger age, high rates of vaccination, and less exposure to microbes at a young age. While gut microbes likely play an important role in the pathogenesis of IBD, the exact mechanism needs to be elucidated further. Some environmental factors are disease specific; for example, cigarette smoking is a risk factor for Crohn disease but paradoxically protects against ulcerative colitis.

It is usually possible to distinguish between ulcerative colitis and Crohn disease by the clinical presentation and radiologic, endoscopic, and histopathologic findings (Table 362.2). It is not possible to make a

Table 362.2 | Comparison of Crohn Disease and Ulcerative Colitis

FEATURE	CROHN DISEASE	ULCERATIVE COLITIS	FEATURE	CROHN DISEASE	ULCERATIVE COLITIS
Rectal bleeding	Sometimes	Common	Strictures	Common	Rare
Diarrhea, mucus, pus	Variable	Common	Fissures	Common	Rare
Abdominal pain	Common	Variable	Fistulas	Common	Rare
Abdominal mass	Common	Not present	Toxic megacolon	None	Present
Growth failure	Common	Variable	Sclerosing cholangitis	Less common	Present
Perianal disease	Common	Rare	Risk for intestinal cancers	Increased	Greatly increased
Rectal involvement	Occasional	Universal	Discontinuous (skip) lesions	Common	Not present
Pyoderma gangrenosum	Rare	Present	Transmural involvement	Common	Unusual
Erythema nodosum	Common	Less common	Crypt abscesses	Less common	Common
Mouth ulceration	Common	Rare	Granulomas	Common	None
Thrombosis	Less common	Present	Linear ulcerations	Uncommon	Common
Colonic disease	50–75%	100%	Perinuclear antineutrophil cytoplasmic antibody–positive	<20%	70%
Ileal disease	Common	None except backwash ileitis			
Stomach–esophageal disease	More common	Chronic gastritis can be seen			

definitive diagnosis in approximately 10% of patients with chronic colitis; this disorder is called *indeterminate colitis*. Occasionally, a child initially believed to have ulcerative colitis on the basis of clinical findings is subsequently found to have Crohn colitis. This is particularly true for the youngest patients, because Crohn disease in this patient population can more often manifest as exclusively colonic inflammation, mimicking ulcerative colitis. The medical treatments of Crohn disease and ulcerative colitis overlap.

Extraintestinal manifestations occur slightly more commonly with Crohn disease than with ulcerative colitis (Table 362.3). Growth retardation is seen in 15–40% of children with Crohn disease at diagnosis. Decrease in height velocity occurs in nearly 90% of patients with Crohn disease diagnosed in childhood or adolescence. Of the extraintestinal manifestations that occur with IBD, joint, skin, eye, mouth, and hepatobiliary involvement tend to be associated with colitis, whether ulcerative or Crohn. The presence of some manifestations, such as peripheral arthritis, erythema nodosum, and anemia, correlates with activity of the bowel disease. Activity of pyoderma gangrenosum correlates less well with activity of the bowel disease, whereas sclerosing cholangitis, ankylosing spondylitis, and sacroiliitis do not correlate with intestinal disease. Arthritis occurs in 3 patterns: migratory peripheral arthritis involving primarily large joints, ankylosing spondylitis, and sacroiliitis. The peripheral arthritis of IBD tends to be nondestructive. Ankylosing spondylitis begins in the 3rd decade and occurs most commonly in patients with ulcerative colitis who have the human leukocyte antigen B27 phenotype. Symptoms include low back pain and morning stiffness; back, hips, shoulders, and sacroiliac joints are typically affected. Isolated sacroiliitis is usually asymptomatic but is common when a careful search is performed. Among the skin manifestations, erythema nodosum is most common. Patients with erythema nodosum or pyoderma gangrenosum have a high likelihood of having arthritis as well. Glomerulonephritis, uveitis, and a hypercoagulable state are other rare manifestations that

Table 362.3	Extraintestinal Complications of Inflammatory Bowel Disease

MUSCULOSKELETAL
Peripheral arthritis
Granulomatous monoarthritis
Granulomatous synovitis
Rheumatoid arthritis
Sacroiliitis
Ankylosing spondylitis
Digital clubbing and hypertrophic osteoarthropathy
Periostitis
Osteoporosis, osteomalacia
Rhabdomyolysis
Pelvic osteomyelitis
Recurrent multifocal osteomyelitis
Relapsing polychondritis

SKIN AND MUCOUS MEMBRANES
Oral lesions
Cheilitis
Aphthous stomatitis, glossitis
Granulomatous oral Crohn disease
Inflammatory hyperplasia fissures and cobblestone mucosa
Peristomatitis vegetans

DERMATOLOGIC
Erythema nodosum
Pyoderma gangrenosum
Sweet syndrome
Metastatic Crohn disease
Psoriasis
Epidermolysis bullosa acquisita
Perianal skin tags
Polyarteritis nodosa
Melanoma and nonmelanoma skin cancers

OCULAR
Conjunctivitis
Uveitis, iritis
Episcleritis
Scleritis
Retrobulbar neuritis
Chorioretinitis with retinal detachment
Crohn keratopathy
Posterior segment abnormalities
Retinal vascular disease

BRONCHOPULMONARY
Chronic bronchitis with bronchiectasis
Chronic bronchitis with neutrophilic infiltrates
Fibrosing alveolitis
Pulmonary vasculitis
Small airway disease and bronchiolitis obliterans
Eosinophilic lung disease
Granulomatous lung disease
Tracheal obstruction

CARDIAC
Pleuropericarditis
Cardiomyopathy
Endocarditis
Myocarditis

MALNUTRITION
Decreased intake of food
• Inflammatory bowel disease
• Dietary restriction
Malabsorption
• Inflammatory bowel disease
• Bowel resection
• Bile salt depletion
• Bacterial overgrowth
Intestinal losses
• Electrolytes
• Minerals
• Nutrients
Increased caloric needs
• Inflammation
• Fever

HEMATOLOGIC/ONCOLOGIC
Anemia: iron deficiency (blood loss)
Vitamin B12 (ileal disease or resection, bacterial overgrowth, folate deficiency)
Anemia of chronic inflammation
Anaphylactoid purpura (Crohn disease)
Hyposplenism
Autoimmune hemolytic anemia
Coagulation abnormalities
Increased activation of coagulation factors
Activated fibrinolysis
Anticardiolipin antibody
Increased risk of arterial and venous thrombosis with cerebrovascular stroke, myocardial infarction, peripheral arterial, and venous occlusions
Systemic lymphoma (nonenteric)

RENAL AND GENITOURINARY
Metabolic
• Urinary crystal formation (nephrolithiasis, uric acid, oxylate)
Hypokalemic nephropathy
Inflammation
• Retroperitoneal abscess
• Fibrosis with ureteral obstruction
• Fistula formation
Glomerulitis
Membrane nephritis
Renal amyloidosis, nephrotic syndrome

Continued

Table 362.3	Extraintestinal Complications of Inflammatory Bowel Disease—cont'd

PANCREATITIS

Secondary to medications (sulfasalazine, 6-mercaptopurine, azathioprine, parenteral nutrition)
Ampullary Crohn disease
Granulomatous pancreatitis
Decreased pancreatic exocrine function
Sclerosing cholangitis with pancreatitis

HEPATOBILIARY

Primary sclerosing cholangitis
Small duct primary sclerosing cholangitis (pericholangitis)
Carcinoma of the bile ducts
Fatty infiltration of the liver
Cholelithiasis
Autoimmune hepatitis

ENDOCRINE AND METABOLIC

Growth failure, delayed sexual maturation
Thyroiditis
Osteoporosis, osteomalacia

NEUROLOGIC

Peripheral neuropathy
Meningitis
Vestibular dysfunction
Pseudotumor cerebri
Cerebral vasculitis
Migraine

Modified from Kugathasan S: Diarrhea. In Kliegman RM, Greenbaum LA, Lye PS, editors: *Practical strategies in pediatric diagnosis and therapy*, ed 2, Philadelphia, 2004, WB Saunders, p 285.

occur in childhood. Cerebral thromboembolic disease has been described in children with IBD.

362.1 Chronic Ulcerative Colitis

Ronen E. Stein and Robert N. Baldassano

Ulcerative colitis, an idiopathic chronic inflammatory disorder, is localized to the colon and spares the upper gastrointestinal (GI) tract. Disease usually begins in the rectum and extends proximally for a variable distance. When it is localized to the rectum, the disease is ulcerative proctitis, whereas disease involving the entire colon is pancolitis. Approximately 50–80% of pediatric patients have extensive colitis, and adults more commonly have distal disease. Ulcerative *proctitis* is less likely to be associated with systemic manifestations, although it may be less responsive to treatment than more-diffuse disease. Approximately 30% of children who present with ulcerative proctitis experience proximal spread of the disease. Ulcerative colitis has rarely been noted to present in infancy. Dietary protein intolerance can easily be misdiagnosed as ulcerative colitis in this age group. Dietary protein intolerance (cow's milk protein) is a transient disorder; symptoms are directly associated with the intake of the offending antigen.

The incidence of ulcerative colitis has increased but not to the extent of the increase in Crohn disease; incidence varies with country of origin. The age-specific incidence rates of pediatric ulcerative colitis in North America is 2/100,000 population. The prevalence of ulcerative colitis in northern European countries and the United States varies from 100 to 200/100,000 population. Men are slightly more likely to acquire ulcerative colitis than are women; the reverse is true for Crohn disease.

Table 362.4	Montreal Classification of Extent and Severity of Ulcerative Colitis

- E1 (proctitis): inflammation limited to the rectum
- E2 (left-sided; distal): inflammation limited to the splenic flexure
- E3 (pancolitis): inflammation extends to the proximal splenic flexure
- S0 (remission): no symptoms
- S1 (mild): 4 or less stools per day (with or without blood), absence of systemic symptoms, normal inflammatory markers
- S2 (moderate): 4 stools per day, minimum signs of systemic symptoms
- S3 (severe): 6 or more bloody stools per day, pulse rate of ≥90 beats/min, temperature ≥37.5°C (99.5°F), hemoglobin concentration <105 g/L, erythrocyte sedimentation rate ≥30 mm/hr

E, extent; *S*, severity.
From Ordàs I, Eckmann L, Talamini M, et al: Ulcerative colitis, *Lancet* 380:1606–1616, 2012, Panel 2, p 1610.

CLINICAL MANIFESTATIONS

Blood, mucus, and pus in the stool as well as diarrhea are the typical presentation of ulcerative colitis. Constipation may be observed in those with proctitis. Symptoms such as tenesmus, urgency, cramping abdominal pain (especially with bowel movements), and nocturnal bowel movements are common. The mode of onset ranges from insidious with gradual progression of symptoms to acute and fulminant (Table 362.4 and Figs. 362.1 and 362.2). Fever, severe anemia, hypoalbuminemia, leukocytosis, and more than 5 bloody stools per day for 5 days define **fulminant**

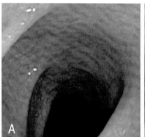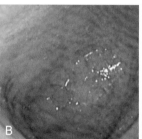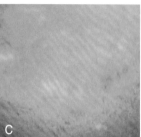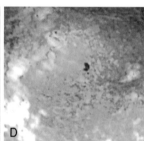

Fig. 362.1 Mayo endoscopic score for ulcerative colitis. **A,** Score 0 = normal; endoscopic remission. **B,** Score 1 = mild; erythema, decreased vascular pattern, mild friability. **C,** Score 2 = moderate; marked erythema, absent vascular pattern, friability, erosions. **D,** Score 3 = severe; spontaneous bleeding, ulceration. *(Images courtesy Elena Ricart. From Ordàs I, Eckmann L, Talamini M, et al: Ulcerative colitis, Lancet 380:1606–1616, 2012, Fig. 2, p 1610.)*

E1: Proctitis	E2: Left-sided Colitis	E3: Extensive (Pan) Colitis
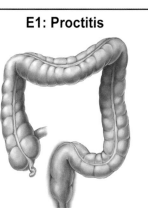	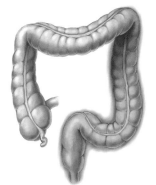	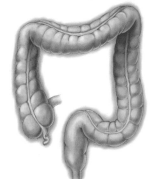
30-60% of Patients	**16-45% of Patients**	**15-35% of Patients**
Symptoms Rectal bleeding, Tenesmus, Urgency	**Symptoms** E1 plus Diarrhea, Abdominal cramping	**Symptoms** E2 plus Constitutional Symptoms (Fatigue, Fever)
General Treatment Strategy Topical +/- Oral 5-ASA or Steroid	**General Treatment Strategy** Oral +/- Topical 5-ASA or Steroid, IMs, Biologics	**General Treatment Strategy** Oral +/- Topical 5-ASA or Steroid, IMs, Biologics

J Gregory ©2016 Mount Sinai Health System

Fig. 362.2 Ulcerative colitis phenotypes by Montreal Classification. Symptoms and treatment strategy can differ based on extent of disease. *(Illustration by Jill Gregory. Printed with permission of ©Mount Sinai Health System.)*

colitis. Chronicity is an important part of the diagnosis; it is difficult to know if a patient has a subacute, transient infectious colitis or ulcerative colitis when a child has had 1-2 wk of symptoms. Symptoms beyond this duration often prove to be secondary to IBD. Anorexia, weight loss, and growth failure may be present, although these complications are more typical of Crohn disease.

Extraintestinal manifestations that tend to occur more commonly with ulcerative colitis than with Crohn disease include pyoderma gangrenosum, sclerosing cholangitis, chronic active hepatitis, and ankylosing spondylitis. Iron deficiency can result from chronic blood loss as well as decreased intake. Folate deficiency is unusual but may be accentuated in children treated with sulfasalazine, which interferes with folate absorption. Chronic inflammation and the elaboration of a variety of inflammatory cytokines can interfere with erythropoiesis and result in the anemia of chronic disease. Secondary amenorrhea is common during periods of active disease.

The clinical course of ulcerative colitis is marked by remission and relapse, often without apparent explanation. After treatment of initial symptoms, approximately 5% of children with ulcerative colitis have a prolonged remission (longer than 3 yr). Approximately 25% of children presenting with severe ulcerative colitis require colectomy within 5 yr of diagnosis, compared with only 5% of those presenting with mild disease. It is important to consider the possibility of enteric infection with recurrent symptoms; these infections can mimic a flare-up or actually provoke a recurrence. The use of nonsteroidal antiinflammatory drugs is considered by some to predispose to exacerbation.

It is generally believed that the risk of colon cancer begins to increase after 8-10 yr of disease and can then increase by 0.5–1% per yr. The risk is delayed by approximately 10 yr in patients with colitis limited to the descending colon. Proctitis alone is associated with virtually no increase in risk over the general population. Because colon cancer is usually preceded by changes of mucosal dysplasia, it is recommended that patients who have had ulcerative colitis for longer than 8-10 yr be screened with colonoscopy and biopsies every 1-2 yr. Although this is the current standard of practice, it is not clear if morbidity and mortality

are changed by this approach. Two competing concerns about this plan of management remain unresolved. The original studies may have overestimated the risk of colon cancer and, therefore, the need for surveillance has been overemphasized; and screening for dysplasia might not be adequate for preventing colon cancer in ulcerative colitis if some cancers are not preceded by dysplasia.

DIFFERENTIAL DIAGNOSIS

The major conditions to exclude are infectious colitis, allergic colitis, and Crohn colitis. Every child with a new diagnosis of ulcerative colitis should have stool cultured for enteric pathogens, stool evaluation for *Clostridium difficile,* ova and parasites, and perhaps serologic studies for amebae (Table 362.5). Cytomegalovirus infection can mimic ulcerative colitis or be associated with an exacerbation of existing disease, usually in immunocompromised patients. The most difficult distinction is from Crohn disease because the colitis of Crohn disease can initially appear identical to that of ulcerative colitis, particularly in younger children. The gross appearance of the colitis or development of small bowel disease eventually leads to the correct diagnosis; this can occur years after the initial presentation.

At the onset, the colitis of hemolytic uremic syndrome may be identical to that of early ulcerative colitis. Ultimately, signs of microangiopathic hemolysis (the presence of schistocytes on blood smear), thrombocytopenia, and subsequent renal failure should confirm the diagnosis of hemolytic-uremic syndrome. Although Henoch-Schönlein purpura can manifest as abdominal pain and bloody stools, it is not usually associated with colitis. Behçet disease can be distinguished by its typical features (see Chapter 186). Other considerations are radiation proctitis, viral colitis in immunocompromised patients, and ischemic colitis (Table 362.6). In infancy, dietary protein intolerance can be confused with ulcerative colitis, although the former is a transient problem that resolves on removal of the offending protein, and ulcerative colitis is extremely rare in this age group. Hirschsprung disease can produce an enterocolitis before or within months after surgical correction; this is unlikely to be confused with ulcerative colitis.

Table 362.5	Infectious Agents Mimicking Inflammatory Bowel Disease		
AGENT	**MANIFESTATIONS**	**DIAGNOSIS**	**COMMENTS**
BACTERIAL			
Campylobacter jejuni	Acute diarrhea, fever, fecal blood, and leukocytes	Culture	Common in adolescents, may relapse
Yersinia enterocolitica	Acute → chronic diarrhea, right lower quadrant pain, mesenteric adenitis–pseudoappendicitis, fecal blood, and leukocytes Extraintestinal manifestations, mimics Crohn disease	Culture	Common in adolescents as fever of unknown origin, weight loss, abdominal pain
Clostridium difficile	Postantibiotic onset, watery → bloody diarrhea, pseudomembrane on sigmoidoscopy	Cytotoxin assay	May be nosocomial Toxic megacolon possible
Escherichia coli O157:H7	Colitis, fecal blood, abdominal pain	Culture and typing	Hemolytic uremic syndrome
Salmonella	Watery → bloody diarrhea, foodborne, fecal leukocytes, fever, pain, cramps	Culture	Usually acute
Shigella	Watery → bloody diarrhea, fecal leukocytes, fever, pain, cramps	Culture	Dysentery symptoms
Edwardsiella tarda	Bloody diarrhea, cramps	Culture	Ulceration on endoscopy
Aeromonas hydrophila	Cramps, diarrhea, fecal blood	Culture	May be chronic Contaminated drinking water
Plesiomonas shigelloides	Diarrhea, cramps	Culture	Shellfish source
Tuberculosis	Rarely bovine, now Mycobacterium tuberculosis Ileocecal area, fistula formation	Culture, purified protein derivative, biopsy	Can mimic Crohn disease
PARASITES			
Entamoeba histolytica	Acute bloody diarrhea and liver abscess, colic	Trophozoite in stool, colonic mucosal flask ulceration, serologic tests	Travel to endemic area
Giardia lamblia	Foul-smelling, watery diarrhea, cramps, flatulence, weight loss; no colonic involvement	"Owl"-like trophozoite and cysts in stool; rarely duodenal intubation	May be chronic
AIDS-ASSOCIATED ENTEROPATHY			
Cryptosporidium	Chronic diarrhea, weight loss	Stool microscopy	Mucosal findings not like inflammatory bowel disease
Isospora belli	As in Cryptosporidium		Tropical location
Cytomegalovirus	Colonic ulceration, pain, bloody diarrhea	Culture, biopsy	More common when on immunosuppressive medications

DIAGNOSIS

The diagnosis of ulcerative colitis or ulcerative proctitis requires a typical presentation in the absence of an identifiable specific cause (see Tables 362.5 and 362.6) and typical endoscopic and histologic findings (see Tables 362.2 and 362.4). One should be hesitant to make a diagnosis of ulcerative colitis in a child who has experienced symptoms for <2-3 wk until infection has been excluded. When the diagnosis is suspected in a child with subacute symptoms, the physician should make a firm diagnosis only when there is evidence of chronicity on colonic biopsy. Laboratory studies can demonstrate evidence of anemia (either iron deficiency or the anemia of chronic disease) or hypoalbuminemia. Although the sedimentation rate and C-reactive protein are often elevated, they may be normal even with fulminant colitis. An elevated white blood cell count is usually seen only with more-severe colitis. Fecal calprotectin levels are usually elevated and are increasingly recognized to be a more sensitive and specific marker of GI inflammation than typical laboratory parameters. Barium enema is suggestive but not diagnostic of acute (Fig. 362.3) or chronic burned-out disease (Fig. 362.4).

The diagnosis of ulcerative colitis must be confirmed by endoscopic and histologic examination of the colon (see Fig. 362.1). Classically, disease starts in the rectum with a gross appearance characterized by erythema, edema, loss of vascular pattern, granularity, and friability. There may be a *cutoff* demarcating the margin between inflammation and normal colon, or the entire colon may be involved. There may be some variability in the intensity of inflammation even in those areas involved. Flexible sigmoidoscopy can confirm the diagnosis; colonoscopy can evaluate the extent of disease and rule out Crohn colitis. A colonoscopy should not be performed when fulminant colitis

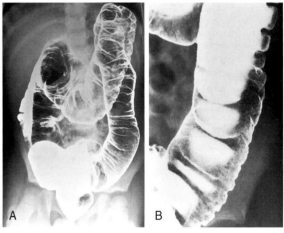

Fig. 362.3 Ulcerative colitis. Double-contrast barium enema in a 5 yr old boy who had had intermittent intestinal and extraintestinal symptoms since the age of 3 yr. **A,** Small ulcerations are distributed uniformly about the colonic circumference and continuously from the rectum to the proximal transverse colon. This pattern of involvement is typical of ulcerative colitis. **B,** In this coned view of the sigmoid in the same patient, small ulcerations are represented by fine spiculation of the colonic contour in tangent and by fine stippling of the colon surface en face. (*From Hoffman AD: The child with diarrhea. In Hilton SW, Edwards DK, editors: Practical pediatric radiology, ed 2, Philadelphia, 1994, WB Saunders, p 260.*)

Table 362.6	Chronic Inflammatory Bowel-Like Intestinal Disorders Including Monogenetic Diseases

INFECTION (SEE Table 362.5)

AIDS-Associated

Toxin

Immune–Inflammatory

Severe combined immunodeficiency diseases
Agammaglobulinemia
Chronic granulomatous disease
Wiskott-Aldrich syndrome
Common variable immunodeficiency diseases
Acquired immunodeficiency states
Dietary protein enterocolitis
Autoimmune polyendocrine syndrome type 1
Behçet disease
Lymphoid nodular hyperplasia
Eosinophilic gastroenteritis
Omenn syndrome
Graft-versus-host disease
IPEX (immune dysfunction, polyendocrinopathy, enteropathy,
  X-linked) syndromes
Interleukin-10 signaling defects
Autoimmune enteropathy*
Microscopic colitis
Hyperimmunoglobulin M syndrome
Hyperimmunoglobulin E syndromes
Mevalonate kinase deficiency
Familial Mediterranean fever
Phospholipase Cγ₂ defects
IL10RA mutation
Familial hemophagocytic lymphohistiocytosis type 5
X-linked lymphoproliferative syndromes types 1, 2 (*XIAP* gene)
Congenital neutropenias
TRIM22 mutation
Leukocyte adhesion deficiency 1

VASCULAR–ISCHEMIC DISORDERS

Systemic vasculitis (systemic lupus erythematosus, dermatomyositis)
Henoch-Schönlein purpura
Hemolytic uremic syndrome
Granulomatosis with angiitis

OTHER

Glycogen storage disease type 1b
Dystrophic epidermolysis bullosa
X-linked ectodermal dysplasia and immunodeficiency
Dyskeratosis congenita
ADAM-17 deficiency
Prestenotic colitis
Diversion colitis
Kindler syndrome
Radiation colitis
Neonatal necrotizing enterocolitis
Typhlitis
Sarcoidosis
Hirschsprung colitis
Intestinal lymphoma
Laxative abuse
Endometriosis
Hermansky-Pudlak syndrome
Trichohepatoenteric syndrome
Phosphatase and tensin homolog (PTEN) hamartoma tumor
  syndrome

*May be the same as IPEX.

is suspected because of the risk of provoking *toxic megacolon* or causing a perforation during the procedure. The degree of colitis can be evaluated by the gross appearance of the mucosa. One does not generally see discrete ulcers, which would be more suggestive of Crohn colitis. The endoscopic findings of ulcerative colitis result from microulcers, which give the appearance of a diffuse abnormality. With very severe chronic colitis, pseudopolyps may be seen. Biopsy of involved bowel demonstrates evidence of acute and chronic mucosal inflammation.

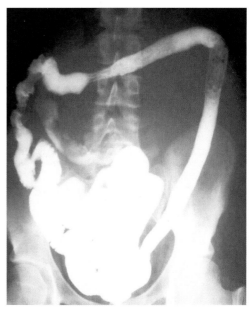

Fig. 362.4 Ulcerative colitis: late changes. This single-contrast barium enema shows the late changes of ulcerative colitis in a 15 yr old girl. The colon is featureless, reduced in caliber, and shortened. Dilation of the terminal ileum (backwash ileitis) is present. *(From The child with diarrhea. In Hoffman AD, Hilton SW, Edwards DK, editors: Practical pediatric radiology, ed 2, Philadelphia, 1994, WB Saunders, p 262.)*

Typical histologic findings are cryptitis, crypt abscesses, separation of crypts by inflammatory cells, foci of acute inflammatory cells, edema, mucus depletion, and branching of crypts. The last finding is not seen in infectious colitis. Granulomas, fissures, or full-thickness involvement of the bowel wall (usually on surgical rather than endoscopic biopsy) suggest Crohn disease.

Perianal disease, except for mild local irritation or anal fissures associated with diarrhea, should make the clinician think of Crohn disease. Plain radiographs of the abdomen might demonstrate loss of haustral markings in an air-filled colon or marked dilation with toxic megacolon. With severe colitis, the colon may become dilated; a diameter of >6 cm, determined radiographically, in an adult suggests toxic megacolon. If it is necessary to examine the colon radiologically in a child with severe colitis (to evaluate the extent of involvement or to try to rule out Crohn disease), it is sometimes helpful to perform an upper GI contrast series with small bowel follow-through and then look at delayed films of the colon. A barium enema is contraindicated in the setting of a potential toxic megacolon.

TREATMENT
Medical

A medical *cure* for ulcerative colitis is not available; treatment is aimed at controlling symptoms and reducing the risk of recurrence, with a secondary goal of minimizing steroid exposure. The intensity of treatment varies with the severity of the symptoms.

The first drug class to be used with mild or mild-to-moderate colitis is an aminosalicylate. Sulfasalazine is composed of a sulfur moiety linked to the active ingredient 5-aminosalicylate (5-ASA). This linkage prevents the premature absorption of the medication in the upper GI tract, allowing it to reach the colon, where the 2 components are separated by bacterial cleavage. The dose of sulfasalazine is 30-100 mg/kg/24 hr (divided in 2-4 doses). Generally, the dose is not more than 2-4 g/24 hr. Hypersensitivity to the sulfa component is the major side effect of sulfasalazine and occurs in 10–20% of patients. Because of poor tolerance, sulfasalazine is used less commonly than other, better tolerated 5-ASA preparations (mesalamine, 50-100 mg/kg/day; balsalazide 2.25-6.75 g/day). Sulfasalazine and the 5-ASA preparations effectively treat active ulcerative colitis and prevent recurrence. It is recommended that the medication be continued even when the disorder is in remission. These medications might also modestly decrease the lifetime risk of colon cancer.

Approximately 5% of patients have an *allergic reaction* to 5-ASA, manifesting as rash, fever, and bloody diarrhea, which can be difficult to distinguish from symptoms of a flare of ulcerative colitis. 5-ASA can also be given in enema or suppository form and is especially useful for proctitis. Hydrocortisone enemas are used to treat proctitis as well, but they are probably not as effective. A combination of oral and rectal 5-ASA as well as monotherapy with rectal preparation has been shown to be more effective than just oral 5-ASA for distal colitis. Extended release budesonide may also induce remission in patients with mild-to-moderate ulcerative colitis.

Probiotics are effective in adults for maintenance of remission for ulcerative colitis, although they do not induce remission during an active flare. The most promising role for probiotics has been to prevent pouchitis, a common complication following colectomy and ileal–pouch anal anastomosis surgery.

Children with moderate to severe pancolitis or colitis that is unresponsive to 5-ASA therapy should be treated with corticosteroids, most commonly prednisone. The usual starting dose of prednisone is 1-2 mg/kg/24 hr (40-60 mg maximum dose). This medication can be given once daily. With severe colitis, the dose can be divided twice daily and can be given intravenously. Steroids are considered an effective medication for acute flares, but they are not appropriate maintenance medications because of loss of effect and side effects, including growth retardation, adrenal suppression, cataracts, osteopenia, aseptic necrosis of the head of the femur, glucose intolerance, risk of infection, mood disturbance, and cosmetic effects.

For a hospitalized patient with persistence of symptoms despite intravenous steroid treatment for 3-5 days, escalation of therapy or surgical options should be considered. The validated pediatric ulcerative colitis activity index can be used to help determine current disease severity based on clinical factors and help determine who is more likely to respond to steroids and those who will likely require escalation of therapy (Table 362.7).

With medical management, most children are in remission within 3 mo; however, 5–10% continue to have symptoms unresponsive to treatment beyond 6 mo. Many children with disease requiring frequent corticosteroid therapy are started on immunomodulators such as azathioprine (2.0-2.5 mg/kg/day) or 6-mercaptopurine (1-1.5 mg/kg/day). Uncontrolled data suggest a corticosteroid-sparing effect in many treated patients. This is not an appropriate choice in a steroid nonresponsive patient with acute severe colitis because of longer onset of action. Lymphoproliferative disorders are associated with thiopurine use. Cyclosporine, which is associated with improvement in some children with severe or fulminant colitis, is rarely used owing to its high side-effect profile, its inability to change the natural history of disease, and the increasing use of infliximab, a chimeric monoclonal antibody to tumor necrosis factor (TNF)-α, which is also effective in cases of fulminant colitis. Infliximab is effective for induction and maintenance therapy in children and adults with moderate to severe disease. TNF blocking agents are associated with an increased risk of infection (particularly tuberculosis) and malignancies (lymphoma, leukemia). Adalimumab is also approved for treatment of moderate to severe ulcerative colitis in adults. Vedolizumab, a humanized monoclonal antibody that inhibits adhesion and migration of leukocytes into the GI tract, is approved for the treatment of ulcerative colitis in adults. Tofacitinib, an oral Janus kinase inhibitor, is also approved for treatment of moderate to severe adult ulcerative colitis. A specific combination of 3-4 wide-spectrum oral antibiotics given over 2-3 wk may be effective in treating severe pediatric ulcerative colitis refractory to other therapies but is being further studied in children.

Surgical

Colectomy is performed for intractable disease, complications of therapy, and fulminant disease that is unresponsive to medical management. No clear benefit of the use of total parenteral nutrition or a continuous

Table 362.7	Pediatric Ulcerative Colitis Activity Index
ITEM	**POINTS**
(1) ABDOMINAL PAIN	
No pain	0
Pain can be ignored	5
Pain cannot be ignored	10
(2) RECTAL BLEEDING	
None	0
Small amount only, in <50% of stools	10
Small amount with most stools	20
Large amount (>50% of the stool content)	30
(3) STOOL CONSISTENCY OF MOST STOOLS	
Formed	0
Partially formed	5
Completely unformed	10
(4) NUMBER OF STOOLS PER 24 HR	
0-2	0
3-5	5
6-8	10
>8	15
(5) NOCTURNAL STOOLS (ANY EPISODE CAUSING WAKENING)	
No	0
Yes	10
(6) ACTIVITY LEVEL	
No limitation of activity	0
Occasional limitation of activity	5
Severe restricted activity	10
Sum of Index (0-85)	

enteral elemental diet in the treatment of severe ulcerative colitis has been noted. Nevertheless, parenteral nutrition is used if oral intake is insufficient so that the patient will be nutritionally ready for surgery if medical management fails. With any medical treatment for ulcerative colitis, the clinician should always weigh the risk of the medication or therapy against the fact that colitis can be successfully treated surgically.

Surgical treatment for intractable or fulminant colitis is total colectomy. The optimal approach is to combine colectomy with an endorectal pull-through, where a segment of distal rectum is retained and the mucosa is stripped from this region. The distal ileum is pulled down and sutured at the internal anus with a J pouch created from ileum immediately above the rectal cuff. This procedure allows the child to maintain continence. Commonly, a temporary ileostomy is created to protect the delicate anastomosis between the sleeve of the pouch and the rectum. The ileostomy is usually closed within several months, restoring bowel continuity. At that time, stool frequency is often increased but may be improved with loperamide. The major complication of this operation is *pouchitis,* which is a chronic inflammatory reaction in the pouch, leading to bloody diarrhea, abdominal pain, and, occasionally, low-grade fever. The cause of this complication is unknown, although it is more common when the ileal pouch has been constructed for ulcerative colitis than for other indications (e.g., familial polyposis coli). Pouchitis is seen in 30–40% of patients who had ulcerative colitis. It commonly responds to treatment with oral metronidazole or ciprofloxacin. Probiotics have also been shown to decrease the rate of pouchitis as well as the recurrence of pouchitis following antibiotic therapy.

Support

Psychosocial support is an important part of therapy for this disorder. This may include adequate discussion of the disease manifestations and management between patient and physician, psychologic counseling for the child when necessary, and family support from a social worker or family counselor. Patient support groups have proved helpful for some families. Children with ulcerative colitis should be encouraged to participate fully in age-appropriate activities; however, activity may need to be reduced during periods of disease exacerbation.

PROGNOSIS

The course of ulcerative colitis is marked by remissions and exacerbations. Most children with this disorder respond initially to medical management. Many children with mild manifestations continue to respond well to medical management and may stay in remission on a prophylactic 5-ASA preparation for long periods. An occasional child with mild onset, however, experiences intractable symptoms later. Beyond the 1st decade of disease, the risk of development of colon cancer begins to increase rapidly. The risk of colon cancer may be diminished with surveillance colonoscopies beginning after 8-10 yr of disease. Detection of significant dysplasia on biopsy would prompt colectomy.

Bibliography is available at Expert Consult.

362.2 Crohn Disease (Regional Enteritis, Regional Ileitis, Granulomatous Colitis)

Ronen E. Stein and Robert N. Baldassano

Crohn disease, an idiopathic, chronic inflammatory disorder of the bowel, involves any region of the alimentary tract from the mouth to the anus. Although there are many similarities between ulcerative colitis and Crohn disease, there are also major differences in the clinical course and distribution of the disease in the GI tract (see Table 362.2). The inflammatory process tends to be eccentric and segmental, often with skip areas (normal regions of bowel between inflamed areas). Although inflammation in ulcerative colitis is limited to the mucosa (except in toxic megacolon), GI involvement in Crohn disease is often *transmural*.

Compared to adult-onset disease, pediatric Crohn disease is more likely to have extensive anatomic involvement. At initial presentation, more than 50% of patients have disease that involves ileum and colon (ileocolitis), 20% have exclusively colonic disease, and upper GI involvement (esophagus, stomach, duodenum) is seen in up to 30% of children. Isolated small bowel disease is much less common in the pediatric population compared to adults. Isolated colonic disease is common in children younger than 8 yr of age and may be indistinguishable from ulcerative colitis. Anatomic location of disease tends to extend over time in children.

Crohn disease tends to have a bimodal age distribution, with the first peak beginning in the teenage years. The incidence of Crohn disease has been increasing. In the United States, the reported incidence of pediatric Crohn disease is 4.56/100,000 and the pediatric prevalence is 43/100,000 children.

CLINICAL MANIFESTATIONS

Crohn disease can be characterized as inflammatory, stricturing, or penetrating. Patients with small bowel disease are more likely to have an obstructive pattern (most commonly with right lower quadrant pain) characterized by fibrostenosis, and those with colonic disease are more likely to have symptoms resulting from inflammation (diarrhea, bleeding, cramping). Disease phenotypes often change as duration of disease lengthens (inflammatory becomes structuring and/or penetrating) (Figs. 362.5 and 362.6).

Systemic signs and symptoms are more common in Crohn disease than with ulcerative colitis. Fever, malaise, and easy fatigability are common. Growth failure with delayed bone maturation and delayed sexual development can precede other symptoms by 1 or 2 yr and is at least twice as likely to occur with Crohn disease as with ulcerative colitis. Children can present with growth failure as the only manifestation of Crohn disease. Decreased height velocity occurs in about 88% of prepubertal patients diagnosed with Crohn disease, and this often precedes GI symptoms. Causes of growth failure include inadequate caloric intake, suboptimal absorption or excessive loss of nutrients, the effects of chronic inflammation on bone metabolism and appetite, and

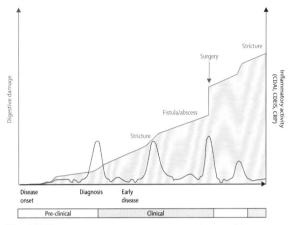

Fig. 362.5 The Lémann Score. Exemplary visualization of the Lémann score, a new technique to score and study intestinal damage in Crohn disease. *CDAI,* Crohn disease activity index; *CDEIS,* Crohn disease of endoscopic severity; *CRP,* C-reactive protein. *(From Baumgart DC, Sandborn WJ: Crohn's disease, Lancet 380:1590–1602, 2012, Fig. 5, p 1596.)*

the use of corticosteroids during treatment. Primary or secondary amenorrhea and pubertal delay are common. In contrast to ulcerative colitis, perianal disease is common (tag, fistula, deep fissure, abscess). Gastric or duodenal involvement may be associated with recurrent vomiting and epigastric pain. Partial small bowel obstruction, usually secondary to narrowing of the bowel lumen from *inflammation* or *stricture*, can cause symptoms of cramping abdominal pain (especially with meals), borborygmus, and intermittent abdominal distention (Figs. 362.7 and 362.8). Stricture should be suspected if the child notes relief of symptoms in association with a sudden sensation of gurgling of intestinal contents through a localized region of the abdomen. Inflammatory obstruction versus fibrotic stricture-induced obstruction may be distinguished by positron emission tomography/magnetic resonance imaging (PET/MRI), which will direct specific therapy (Fig. 362.9).

Penetrating disease is demonstrated by fistula formation. Enteroenteric or enterocolonic fistulas (between segments of bowel) are often asymptomatic but can contribute to malabsorption if they have high output or result in bacterial overgrowth (Fig. 362.10). Enterovesical fistulas (between bowel and urinary bladder) originate from ileum or sigmoid colon and appear as signs of urinary infection, pneumaturia, or fecaluria. Enterovaginal fistulas originate from the rectum, cause feculent vaginal drainage, and are difficult to manage. Enterocutaneous fistulas (between bowel and abdominal skin) often are caused by prior surgical anastomoses with leakage. Intraabdominal abscess may be associated with fever and pain but might have relatively few symptoms. Hepatic or splenic abscess can occur with or without a local fistula. Anorectal abscesses often originate immediately above the anus at the crypts of Morgagni. The patterns of perianal fistulas are complex because of the different tissue planes. Perianal abscess is usually painful, but perianal fistulas tend to produce fewer symptoms than anticipated. Purulent drainage is commonly associated with perianal fistulas. Psoas abscess secondary to intestinal fistula can present as hip pain, decreased hip extension (psoas sign), and fever.

Extraintestinal manifestations occur more commonly with Crohn disease than with ulcerative colitis; those that are especially associated with Crohn disease include oral aphthous ulcers, peripheral arthritis, erythema nodosum, digital clubbing, episcleritis, renal stones (uric acid, oxalate), and gallstones. Any of the extraintestinal disorders described in the section on IBD can occur with Crohn disease (see Table 362.3). The peripheral arthritis is nondeforming. The occurrence of extraintestinal manifestations usually correlates with the presence of colitis.

Extensive involvement of small bowel, especially in association with surgical resection, can lead to short bowel syndrome, which is rare in children. Complications of terminal ileal dysfunction or resection include

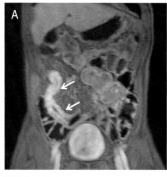

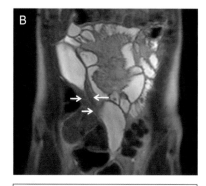

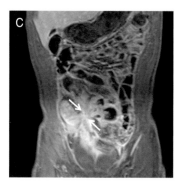

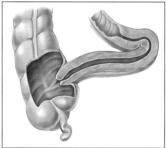

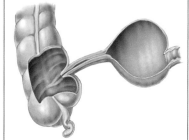

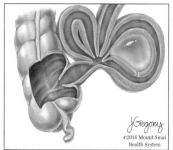

©2016 Mount Sinai
Health System

- Diarrhea
- Abdominal pain
- Weight loss
- Low-grade fever
- Fatigue
- Growth retardation
- Malnourishment

- Postprandial pain
- Bloating
- Nausea and vomiting
- Occlusion/subocclusion

- Symptoms depend on the location of fistulae
- Enterourinary fistula: fecaluria, pneumaturia, recurrent UTI
- Rectovaginal fistula: dispareunia, stool discharge through the vagina
- Enteroenteric fistula: asymptomatic, abdominal abscesses

Fig. 362.6 Behavior of CD as per Montreal classification represented in MRE and illustrated with typical symptoms **A,** T1-weighted MRE imaging with fat saturation after injection of gadolinium chelates shows mural thickening and enhancement in the distal ileum *(arrows)* in a patient with active CD. **B,** T2-weighted MRE imaging shows a narrowed luminal segment with thickened wall and upstream dilation *(arrows)*, suggesting the presence of a stricture. **C,** T1-weighted MRE imaging with fat saturation after injection of gadolinium chelates shows multiple converging enhancing loops of small bowel suggestive of enteroenteric fistulas *(arrows)*. Lower illustration shows a deep and transmural fissure or ulcer leading to the formation of an abscess. *CD,* Crohn disease; *MRE,* magnetic resonance enterography; *UTI,* urinary tract infection. *(Illustration by Jill Gregory. Printed with permission of ©Mount Sinai Health System. From Torres J, Mehandru S, Colombel JF, Peyrin-Biroulet L: Crohn's disease, Lancet 389:1741–1754, 2017, Fig. 1, p 1744.)*

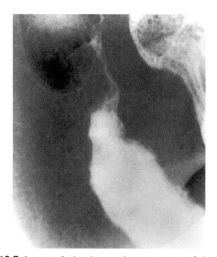

Fig. 362.7 Stenotic Crohn disease. Severe stenosis of the terminal ileum is present in this 16 yr old boy. Inflammatory effacement of the mucosal folds and small ulcerations characterize the proximal nonstenotic segment. *(From Hoffman AD: The child with diarrhea. In Hilton SW, Edwards DK, editors: Practical pediatric radiology, ed 2, Philadelphia, 1994, WB Saunders, p 267.)*

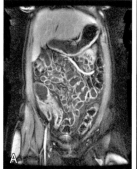

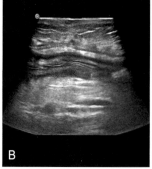

Fig. 362.8 Stenosis in Crohn disease. **A,** Magnetic resonance enterography of Crohn disease restricted to the terminal ileum (Montreal category L1) with inflammatory stenosis. **B,** Ultrasound image of an intestinal stenosis in Crohn disease. *(From Baumgart DC, Sandborn WJ: Crohn's disease, Lancet 380:1590–1602, 2012, Fig. 4, p 1596.)*

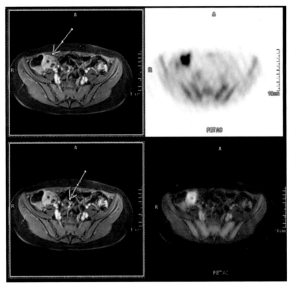

Fig. 362.9 PET/MR (PET, positron emission tomography; MR, magnetic resonance) co-registration and fusion *(right image in the bottom row)* showing a fibrotic stricture of the last bowel loop *(top, arrow)* with active inflammation, and concomitant inflammation of the ileocolic mesentery *(bottom, arrow)*. *(From Pellino G, Nicolai E, Catalano OA, et al: PET/MR versus PET/CT imaging: impact on the clinical management of small-bowel Crohn's disease, J Crohn Colitis 10(3):277–285, 2017, Fig. 3.)*

bile acid malabsorption with secondary diarrhea and vitamin B_{12} malabsorption, with possible resultant deficiency. Chronic steatorrhea can lead to oxaluria with secondary renal stones. Increasing calcium intake can actually decrease the risk of renal stones secondary to ileal inflammation. The risk of cholelithiasis is also increased secondary to bile acid depletion.

A disorder with this diversity of manifestations can have a major impact on an affected child's lifestyle. Fortunately, the majority of children with Crohn disease are able to continue with their normal activities, having to limit activity only during periods of increased symptoms.

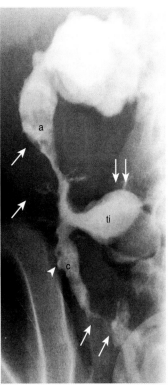

Fig. 362.10 Crohn disease: sinuses and fistula. Severe ileocolitis has resulted in an ileocecal fistula *(single arrows, lower)* and sinus formation in the ascending colon *(a) (arrows on platform)*. *c,* Cecum *(arrowhead); ti,* terminal ileum *(paired arrows)*. *(From The child with diarrhea. In Hoffman AD, Hilton SW, Edwards DK, editors: Practical pediatric radiology, ed 2, Philadelphia, 1994, WB Saunders, p 268.)*

DIFFERENTIAL DIAGNOSIS

The most common diagnoses to be distinguished from Crohn disease are the infectious enteropathies (in the case of Crohn disease: acute terminal ileitis, infectious colitis, enteric parasites, and periappendiceal

Table 362.8	Differential Diagnosis of Presenting Symptoms of Crohn Disease
PRIMARY PRESENTING SYMPTOM	**DIAGNOSTIC CONSIDERATIONS**
Right lower quadrant abdominal pain, with or without mass	Appendicitis, infection (e.g., *Campylobacter, Yersinia* spp.), lymphoma, intussusception, mesenteric adenitis, Meckel diverticulum, ovarian cyst
Chronic periumbilical or epigastric abdominal pain	Irritable bowel syndrome, constipation, lactose intolerance, peptic disease
Rectal bleeding, no diarrhea	Fissure, polyp, Meckel diverticulum, rectal ulcer syndrome
Bloody diarrhea	Infection, hemolytic-uremic syndrome, Henoch-Schönlein purpura, ischemic bowel, radiation colitis
Watery diarrhea	Irritable bowel syndrome, lactose intolerance, giardiasis, *Cryptosporidium* infection, sorbitol, laxatives
Perirectal disease	Fissure, hemorrhoid (rare), streptococcal infection, condyloma (rare)
Growth delay	Endocrinopathy
Anorexia, weight loss	Anorexia nervosa
Arthritis	Collagen vascular disease, infection
Liver abnormalities	Chronic hepatitis

From Kugathasan S: Diarrhea. In Kliegman RM, Greenbaum LA, Lye PS, editors: *Practical strategies in pediatric diagnosis and therapy*, ed 2, Philadelphia, 2004, WB Saunders, p 287.

abscess) (see Tables 362.5, 362.6, and 362.8). *Yersinia* can cause many of the radiologic and endoscopic findings in the distal small bowel that are seen in Crohn disease. The symptoms of bacterial dysentery are more likely to be mistaken for ulcerative colitis than for Crohn disease. Celiac disease and *Giardia* infection have been noted to produce a Crohn-like presentation including diarrhea, weight loss, and protein-losing enteropathy. GI tuberculosis is rare but can mimic Crohn disease. Foreign-body perforation of the bowel (toothpick) can mimic a localized region with Crohn disease. Small bowel lymphoma can mimic Crohn disease but tends to be associated with nodular-filling defects of the bowel without ulceration or narrowing of the lumen. Bowel lymphoma is much less common in children than is Crohn disease. Recurrent functional abdominal pain can mimic the pain of small bowel Crohn disease. *Lymphoid nodular hyperplasia* of the terminal ileum (a normal finding) may be mistaken for Crohn ileitis. Right lower quadrant pain or mass with fever can be the result of periappendiceal abscess. This entity is occasionally associated with diarrhea as well.

Growth failure may be the only manifestation of Crohn disease; other disorders such as growth hormone deficiency, gluten-sensitive enteropathy (celiac disease), Turner syndrome, or anorexia nervosa must be considered. If arthritis precedes the bowel manifestations, an initial diagnosis of juvenile idiopathic arthritis may be made. Refractory anemia may be the presenting feature and may be mistaken for a primary hematologic disorder. Chronic granulomatous disease of childhood can cause inflammatory changes in the bowel as well as perianal disease. Antral narrowing in this disorder may be mistaken for a stricture secondary to Crohn disease. Other immunodeficiencies or autoinflammatory conditions and monogenetic disorders may present with GI symptoms suggestive of IBD, particularly in very early or infant/toddler onset of disease (see Table 362.6).

DIAGNOSIS

Crohn disease can manifest as a variety of symptom combinations (see Fig. 362.6). At the onset, symptoms may be subtle (growth retardation, abdominal pain alone); this explains why the diagnosis might not be made until 1 or 2 yr after the start of symptoms. The diagnosis of Crohn disease depends on finding typical clinical features of the disorder (history, physical examination, laboratory studies, and endoscopic or radiologic findings), ruling out specific entities that mimic Crohn disease, and demonstrating chronicity. The history can include any combination of abdominal pain (especially right lower quadrant), diarrhea, vomiting, anorexia, weight loss, growth retardation, and extraintestinal manifestations. Only 25% initially have the triad of diarrhea, weight loss, and abdominal pain. Most do not have diarrhea, and only 25% have GI bleeding.

Children with Crohn disease often appear chronically ill. They commonly have weight loss and growth failure, and they are often malnourished. The earliest sign of growth failure is decreased height velocity, which can be present in up to 88% of prepubertal patients with Crohn disease and typically precedes symptoms. Children with Crohn disease often appear pale, with decreased energy level and poor appetite; the latter finding sometimes results from an association between meals and abdominal pain or diarrhea. There may be abdominal tenderness that is either diffuse or localized to the right lower quadrant. A tender mass or fullness may be palpable in the right lower quadrant. Perianal disease, when present, may be characteristic. Large anal skin tags (1-3 cm diameter) or perianal fistulas with purulent drainage suggest Crohn disease. Digital clubbing, findings of arthritis, and skin manifestations may be present.

A complete blood cell count commonly demonstrates anemia, often with a component of iron deficiency, as well as thrombocytosis. Although the erythrocyte sedimentation rate and C-reactive protein are often elevated, they may be unremarkable. The serum albumin level may be low, indicating small bowel inflammation or protein-losing enteropathy. Fecal calprotectin and lactoferrin are increasingly being used as more sensitive and specific markers of bowel inflammation as compared to serologic parameters, and these are often elevated. Multiple serologic, immune, and genetic markers can also be abnormal, although the best utilization of these remains to be determined.

The small and large bowel and the upper GI tract should be examined by both endoscopic and radiologic studies in the child with suspected Crohn disease. Esophagogastroduodenoscopy and ileocolonoscopy should be performed to properly assess the upper GI tract, terminal ileum, and entire colon. Findings on colonoscopy can include patchy, nonspecific inflammatory changes (erythema, friability, loss of vascular pattern), aphthous ulcers, linear ulcers, nodularity, and strictures. Findings on biopsy may be only nonspecific chronic inflammatory changes. Noncaseating granulomas, similar to those of sarcoidosis, are the most characteristic histologic findings, although often they are not present. Transmural inflammation is also characteristic but can be identified only in surgical specimens.

Radiologic studies are necessary to assess the entire small bowel and investigate for evidence of structuring or penetrating disease. A variety of findings may be apparent on radiologic studies. Plain films of the abdomen may be normal or might demonstrate findings of partial small bowel obstruction or thumbprinting of the colon wall. An upper GI contrast study with small bowel follow-through might show aphthous ulceration and thickened, nodular folds as well as narrowing or structuring of the lumen. Linear ulcers can give a cobblestone appearance to the mucosal surface. Bowel loops are often separated as a result of thickening of bowel wall and mesentery. Other manifestations on radiographic studies that suggest more-severe Crohn disease are fistulas between bowel (enteroenteric or enterocolonic), sinus tracts, and strictures (see Figs. 362.7, 362.8, and 362.10).

An upper GI contrast examination with small bowel follow-through has typically been the study of choice for imaging of the small bowel, but CT and magnetic resonance (MR) enterography and small bowel ultrasound are increasingly being used. MR and ultrasound have the advantage of not exposing the patient to ionizing radiation. CT and MR enterography can also assess for extraluminal findings such as abscesses and phlegmons. MR of the pelvis is also useful for delineating the extent of perianal involvement. PET/MRI may help define obstructing lesions as either inflammatory or fibrotic (see Fig. 362.9).

Video capsule endoscopy is another modality that allows for evaluation of the small bowel. This study can uncover mucosal inflammation or ulceration that might not have been detected by traditional imaging. However, video capsule endoscopy is contraindicated in the presence of structuring disease, as surgical intervention would be required to remove a video capsule that is unable to pass through the bowel because a stricture. If there is concern for structuring disease, a patency capsule can be swallowed prior to video capsule endoscopy to assess for passage through the GI tract.

TREATMENT

Crohn disease cannot be *cured* by medical or surgical therapy. The aim of treatment is to relieve symptoms and prevent complications of chronic inflammation (anemia, growth failure), prevent relapse, minimize corticosteroid exposure, and, if possible, effect mucosal healing.

Medical

The specific therapeutic modalities used depend on geographic localization of disease, severity of inflammation, age of the patient, and the presence of complications (abscess). Traditionally, a *step-up* treatment paradigm has been used in the treatment of pediatric Crohn disease, whereby early disease is treated with steroids and less immunosuppressive medications. Escalation of therapy would occur if disease severity increased, the patient was refractory to current medications, or for steroid dependence. A *top-down* approach has also been espoused, particularly in adults after multiple studies demonstrated superior efficacy. With this approach, patients with moderate to severe Crohn disease are treated initially with stronger, disease-modifying agents, with the goal of achieving mucosal healing, or deep remission, early in the disease course. This is thought to increase the likelihood of long-term remission while decreasing corticosteroid exposure. Improvements in remission and growth have been shown using a top-down approach in pediatrics and this treatment approach is being increasingly used among children. However, the precise role for this approach in pediatrics is still being determined.

5-Aminosalicylates

For mild terminal ileal disease or mild Crohn disease of the colon, an initial trial of mesalamine (50-100 mg/kg/day, maximum 3-4 g) may be attempted. Specific pharmaceutical preparations have been formulated to release the active 5-ASA compound throughout the small bowel, in the ileum and colon, or exclusively in the colon. Rectal preparations are used for distal colonic inflammation.

Antibiotics/Probiotics

Antibiotics such as metronidazole (10-22.5 mg/kg/day) are used for infectious complications and are first-line therapy for perianal disease (although perianal disease usually recurs when antibiotic is discontinued). Additionally, at low doses antibiotics may be effective for treatment of mild to moderate Crohn disease. To date, probiotics have not been shown to be effective in induction or maintenance of remission for pediatric Crohn disease.

Corticosteroids

Corticosteroids are used for acute exacerbations of pediatric Crohn disease because they effectively suppress acute inflammation, rapidly relieving symptoms (prednisone, 1-2 mg/kg/day, maximum 40-60 mg). The goal is to taper dosing as soon as the disease becomes quiescent. Clinicians vary in their tapering schedules, and the disease can flare during this process. There is no role for continuing corticosteroids as maintenance therapy because, in addition to their side effects, tolerance develops, and steroids do not change disease course or promote healing of mucosa. A special controlled ileal-release formulation of budesonide, a corticosteroid with local antiinflammatory activity on the bowel mucosa and high hepatic first-pass metabolism, is also used for mild to moderate ileal or ileocecal disease (adult dose: 9 mg daily). Ileal-release budesonide appears to be more effective than mesalamine in the treatment of active ileocolonic disease but is less effective than prednisone. Although less effective than traditional corticosteroids, budesonide does cause fewer steroid-related side effects.

Immunomodulators

Approximately 70% of patients require escalation of medical therapy within the 1st yr of pediatric Crohn disease diagnosis. Immunomodulators such as azathioprine (2.0-2.5 mg/kg/day) or 6-mercaptopurine (1.0-1.5 mg/kg/day) may be effective in some children who have a poor response to prednisone or who are steroid dependent. Because a beneficial effect of these drugs can be delayed for 3-4 mo after starting therapy, they are not helpful acutely. The early use of these agents can decrease cumulative prednisone dosages over the first 1-2 yr of therapy. Genetic variations in an enzyme system responsible for metabolism of these agents (thiopurine S-methyltransferase) can affect response rates and potential toxicity. Lymphoproliferative disorders have developed from thiopurine use in patients with IBD. Other common toxicities include hepatitis, pancreatitis, increased risk of skin cancer, increased risk of infection, and slightly increased risk of lymphoma.

Methotrexate is another immunomodulator that is effective in the treatment of active Crohn disease and has been shown to improve height velocity in the 1st yr of administration. The advantages of this medication include once-weekly dosing by either subcutaneous or oral route (15 mg/m², adult dose 25 mg weekly) and a more-rapid onset of action (6-8 wk) than azathioprine or 6-mercaptopurine. Folic acid is usually administered concomitantly to decrease medication side effects. Administration of ondansetron prior to methotrexate has been shown to diminish the risk of the most common side effect of nausea. The most common toxicity is hepatitis. The immunomodulators are effective for the treatment of perianal fistulas.

Biologic Therapy

Therapy with antibodies directed against mediators of inflammation is used for patients with Crohn disease. Infliximab, a chimeric monoclonal antibody to TNF-α, is effective for the induction and maintenance of remission and mucosal healing in chronically active moderate to severe Crohn disease, healing of perianal fistulas, steroid sparing, and preventing postoperative recurrence. Pediatric data additionally support improved

growth with the administration of this medication. The onset of action of infliximab is quite rapid and it is initially given as 3 infusions over a 6 wk period (0, 2, and 6 wk), followed by maintenance dosing beginning every 8 wk. The durability of response to infliximab is variable and dose escalation (higher dose and/or decreased interval) is often necessary. Measurement of serum trough infliximab level prior to an infusion can help guide dosing decisions. Side effects include infusion reactions, increased incidence of infections (especially reactivation of latent tuberculosis), increased risk of lymphoma, and the development of autoantibodies. The development of antibodies to infliximab is associated with an increased incidence of infusion reactions and decreased durability of response. Regularly scheduled dosing of infliximab, as opposed to episodic dosing on an as-needed basis, is associated with decreased levels of antibodies to infliximab. A purified protein derivative test for tuberculosis should be done before starting infliximab.

Adalimumab, a subcutaneously administered, fully humanized monoclonal antibody against TNF-α, is effective for the treatment of chronically active moderate to severe Crohn disease in adults and children. After a loading dose, this is typically administered once every 2 wk, although dose escalation is sometimes required with this medication. Vedolizumab, a humanized monoclonal antibody that inhibits adhesion and migration of leukocytes into the GI tract, is approved for the treatment of Crohn disease in adults. Like infliximab, vedolizumab is initially given as 3 infusions over a 6 wk period followed by maintenance dosing beginning every 8 wk. However, the onset of action for vedolizumab is slower compared to infliximab and adalimumab. Therefore, concomitant therapies may be needed until response is demonstrated. Dose escalation to every 4 wk may be necessary in some patients with loss-of-response but is being further studied. Ustekinumab, a monoclonal antibody against interleukins 12 and 23, was recently approved for treatment of chronically active moderate to severe Crohn disease in adults. A loading dose is given intravenously followed by maintenance dosing administered subcutaneously every 8 wk. New antiselective adhesion molecules and small molecule treatments, such as an oral SMAD7 antisense oligonucleotide that targets TGF-β signaling, are currently being tested.

Enteral Nutritional Therapy

Exclusive enteral nutritional therapy, whereby all of a patient's calories are delivered via formula, is an effective primary as well as adjunctive treatment. The enteral nutritional approach is as rapid in onset of response and as effective as the other treatments. Pediatric studies have suggested similar efficacy to prednisone for improvement in clinical symptoms, but enteral nutritional therapy is superior to steroids for actual healing of mucosa. Because affected patients have poor appetite and these formulas are relatively unpalatable, they are often administered via a nasogastric or gastrostomy infusion, usually overnight. The advantages are that it is relatively free of side effects, avoids the problems associated with corticosteroid therapy, and simultaneously addresses the nutritional rehabilitation. Children can participate in normal daytime activities. A major disadvantage of this approach is that patients are not able to eat a regular diet because they are receiving all of their calories from formula. A novel approach where 80–90% of caloric needs are provided by formula, allowing children to have some food intake, has been successful. For children with growth failure, this approach may be ideal, however.

High-calorie oral supplements, although effective, are often not tolerated because of early satiety or exacerbation of symptoms (abdominal pain, vomiting, or diarrhea). Nonetheless, they should be offered to children whose weight gain is suboptimal even if they are not candidates for exclusive enteral nutritional therapy. The continuous administration of nocturnal nasogastric feedings for chronic malnutrition and growth failure has been effective with a much lower risk of complications than parenteral hyperalimentation.

Surgery

Surgical therapy should be reserved for very specific indications. Recurrence rate after bowel resection is high (>50% by 5 yr); the risk of requiring additional surgery increases with each operation. Potential complications of surgery include development of fistula or stricture, anastomotic leak, postoperative partial small bowel obstruction secondary to adhesions, and short bowel syndrome. Surgery is the treatment of choice for localized disease of small bowel or colon that is unresponsive to medical treatment, bowel perforation, fibrosed stricture with symptomatic partial small bowel obstruction, and intractable bleeding. Intraabdominal or liver abscess sometimes is successfully treated by ultrasonographic or CT-guided catheter drainage and concomitant intravenous antibiotic treatment. Open surgical drainage is necessary if this approach is not successful. Growth retardation was once considered an indication for resection; without other indications, trial of medical and/or nutritional therapy is currently preferred.

Perianal abscess often requires drainage unless it drains spontaneously. In general, perianal fistulas should be managed by a combined medical and surgical approach. Often, the surgeon places a seton through the fistula to keep the tract open and actively draining while medical therapy is administered, to help prevent the formation of a perianal abscess. A severely symptomatic perianal fistula can require fistulotomy, but this procedure should be considered only if the location allows the sphincter to remain undamaged.

The surgical approach for Crohn disease is to remove as limited a length of bowel as possible. There is no evidence that removing bowel up to margins that are free of histologic disease has a better outcome than removing only grossly involved areas. The latter approach reduces the risk of short bowel syndrome. Laparoscopic approach is increasingly being used, with decreased postoperative recovery time. One approach to symptomatic small bowel stricture has been to perform a strictureplasty rather than resection. The surgeon makes a longitudinal incision across the stricture but then closes the incision with sutures in a transverse fashion. This is ideal for short strictures without active disease. The reoperation rate is no higher with this approach than with resection, whereas bowel length is preserved. Postoperative medical therapy with agents such as mesalamine, metronidazole, azathioprine, and, more recently, infliximab, is often given to decrease the likelihood of postoperative recurrence.

Severe perianal disease can be incapacitating and difficult to treat if unresponsive to medical management. Diversion of fecal stream can allow the area to be less active, but on reconnection of the colon, disease activity usually recurs.

Support

Psychosocial issues for the child with Crohn disease include a sense of being different, concerns about body image, difficulty in not participating fully in age-appropriate activities, and family conflict brought on by the added stress of this disease. Social support is an important component of the management of Crohn disease. Parents are often interested in learning about other children with similar problems, but children may be hesitant to participate. Social support and individual psychologic counseling are important in the adjustment to a difficult problem at an age that by itself often has difficult adjustment issues. Patients who are socially "connected" fare better. Ongoing education about the disease is an important aspect of management because children generally fare better if they understand and anticipate problems. The Crohn and Colitis Foundation of America has local chapters throughout the United States and supports several regional 1-wk camps for children with Crohn disease.

PROGNOSIS

Crohn disease is a chronic disorder that is associated with high morbidity but low mortality. Symptoms tend to recur despite treatment and often without apparent explanation. Weight loss and growth failure can usually be improved with treatment and attention to nutritional needs. Up to 15% of patients with early growth retardation secondary to Crohn disease have a permanent decrease in linear growth. Osteopenia is particularly common in those with chronic poor nutrition and frequent exposure to high doses of corticosteroids. Dual energy x-ray absorptiometry can help identify patients at risk for developing osteopenia. Steroid-sparing agents, weight bearing exercise, and improved nutrition, including supplementation with vitamin D and calcium, can improve bone mineralization. Some of the extraintestinal manifestations can, in themselves, be major causes of morbidity, including sclerosing cholangitis, chronic active hepatitis, pyoderma gangrenosum, and ankylosing spondylitis.

The region of bowel-involved and complications of the inflammatory process tend to increase with time and include bowel strictures, fistulas, perianal disease, and intraabdominal or retroperitoneal abscess. Most patients with Crohn disease eventually require surgery for one of its many complications; the rate of reoperation is high. Surgery is unlikely to be curative and should be avoided except for the specific indications noted previously. An earlier, most aggressive medical treatment approach, with the goal of exacting mucosal healing may improve long-term prognosis, and this is an active area of investigation. The risk of colon cancer in patients with long-standing Crohn colitis approaches that associated with ulcerative colitis, and screening colonoscopy after 8-10 yr of colonic disease is indicated.

Despite these complications, most children with Crohn disease lead active, full lives with intermittent flare-up in symptoms.

Bibliography is available at Expert Consult.

362.3 Very Early Onset Inflammatory Bowel Disease

Ronen E. Stein and Robert N. Baldassano

IBD may be classified according to age at onset: pediatric onset (<17 yr), early onset (<10 yr), very early onset (<6 yr), infant/toddler onset (0-2 yr), and neonatal onset IBD (<28 days). The incidence of pediatric IBD is rising with the greatest rates of increase occurring among young children. Very early onset IBD (VEO-IBD) accounts for up to 15% of pediatric onset IBD with an estimated prevalence of 14/100,000 children. Approximately 1% of children with IBD are diagnosed below the age of 2 yr.

Although IBD is a complex disorder with genetics, the immune system, the microbiome, and environmental factors each contributing to its development, children with VEO-IBD are more likely to have a *monogenic* cause for their disease. Advances in genetic testing have led to the identification of novel genetic pathways linked to the development of VEO-IBD. Many of these pathways contain genes associated with primary immunodeficiencies (see Tables 362.1 and 362.6). Family history of IBD among first-degree relatives occurs more frequently in children diagnosed at a younger age. Approximately 44% of children diagnosed with ulcerative colitis under the age of 2 will have a first-degree relative with IBD compared to 19% of older children with IBD.

VEO-IBD has a distinct clinical phenotype characterized by a higher likelihood for extensive colonic involvement and a greater tendency for a more aggressive disease course that is refractory to conventional therapies. However, there is a spectrum of clinical presentations within this population, including patients with milder forms of the disease and a more traditional disease course. Younger patients with IBD can present with any combination of diarrhea, abdominal pain, vomiting, and growth failure. Severe perirectal disease can be present and is often associated with monogenic forms of VEO-IBD, including those caused by interleukin 10 receptor gene mutations.

Diagnosis of IBD is ultimately confirmed by upper endoscopy and ileocolonoscopy. Classic histological findings of IBD can be seen, although atypical findings, such as the presence of extensive epithelial apoptosis, could indicate the presence of monogenic disease. Most children with VEO-IBD will have isolated colonic inflammation on ileocolonoscopy. However, the inflammation can be extensive and involve the entire colon making it challenging to differentiate between Crohn disease and ulcerative colitis; 11–22% of patients with VEO-IBD are diagnosed with *indeterminate colitis* at diagnosis. Additionally, an initial diagnosis of ulcerative colitis occurs in approximately 60% of VEO-IBD patients. However, because children with VEO-IBD are more likely to have disease extension over time, a number of patients felt to have indeterminate colitis or ulcerative colitis at diagnosis may eventually be reclassified as having Crohn disease later in life.

The differential diagnosis of VEO-IBD is similar to older children and adults including infectious and allergic colitis (see Table 362.5). However, primary immunodeficiencies, such as chronic granulomatous disease, common variable immunodeficiency, severe combined immunodeficiency, Wiskott-Aldrich Syndrome and immunodysregulation, polyendocrinopathy, and enteropathy, X-linked are higher on the differential (see Table 362.6). Therefore, immunological evaluation is a critical component of diagnosis and management. History of autoimmunity, atypical infections, recurrent infections, skin disorders, and/or hair abnormalities could indicate an underlying immunodeficiency. Laboratory evaluation could include dihydrorhodamine cytometric testing, quantitative immunoglobulins, vaccine titers, as well as testing of B and T cell function. More targeted immunological testing is guided by clinical history. Genetic testing modalities, such as whole exome sequencing, are helpful in identifying rare monogenic pathways responsible for development of the disease.

There are no official consensus guidelines regarding treatment of children with VEO-IBD. Younger children are more likely to fail conventional therapies, such as 5-ASA, immunomodulators, and biologics, and require surgical intervention. Surgical decisions must be made with caution in very young children as disease extension from the colon to the small intestine can occur with time. More extensive and severe disease at presentation could explain the higher rates of treatment failure among younger children. However, other children may fail conventional therapies if the inflammation is being driven by a monogenic disease process that is not targeted by conventional therapies. Therefore, for children with an underlying primary immunodeficiency or a novel monogenic disease process, the specific disease pathway involved may influence treatment choices. In some cases, bone marrow transplantation may be a necessary treatment for the underlying disease process.

Bibliography is available at Expert Consult.

Chapter **363**

Eosinophilic Gastroenteritis

Ronen E. Stein and Robert N. Baldassano

第三百六十三章

嗜酸粒细胞性胃肠炎

中文导读

本章主要介绍了嗜酸粒细胞性胃肠炎。其中具体描述了嗜酸粒细胞性胃肠炎的定义、常见部位、内镜下的表现以及鉴别诊断的要点；具体描述了嗜酸粒细胞性胃肠炎的血清IgE变化特点、实验室检查异常情况；详细描述了嗜酸粒细胞性胃肠炎的临床表现；治疗中描述了要素饮食、色甘酸钠、孟鲁司特，全身使用糖皮质激素及口服布地奈德等内容。

Eosinophilic gastroenteritis consists of a group of rare and poorly understood disorders that have in common gastric and small intestine infiltration with eosinophils and peripheral eosinophilia. The esophagus and large intestine may also be involved. Tissue eosinophilic infiltration can be seen in mucosa, muscularis, or serosa. The mucosal form is most common and is diagnosed by identifying large numbers of eosinophils in biopsy specimens of gastric antrum or small bowel. Endoscopy may reveal gastritis or colitis, ulceration, and thickened mucosal folds as well as nodules. This condition clinically overlaps the dietary protein hypersensitivity disorders of the small bowel and colon. Peripheral eosinophilia may be absent. The differential diagnosis also includes celiac disease, chronic granulomatous disease, connective tissue disorders and vasculitides (eosinophilic granulomatosis with polyangiitis), multiple infections (particularly parasites), hypereosinophilic syndrome, early inflammatory bowel disease, medications (tacrolimus, enalapril, naproxen, interferon, rifampicin, azathioprine), and rarely malignancy. Many patients have allergies to multiple foods, seasonal allergies, atopy, eczema, and asthma. Serum immunoglobulin E is commonly elevated. Laboratory abnormalities may include hypoalbuminemia, iron deficiency anemia, and elevated liver enzymes.

The presentation of eosinophilic gastroenteritis is nonspecific. Clinical symptoms often correlate with which layers of the gastrointestinal tract are affected. Mucosal involvement can produce nausea, vomiting, diarrhea, abdominal pain, gastrointestinal bleeding, protein-losing enteropathy, or malabsorption. Involvement of the muscularis can produce obstruction (especially of the pylorus) or intussusception, whereas serosal activity produces abdominal distention and eosinophilic ascites. Presentation in infants can be similar to pyloric stenosis. Laboratory testing often reveals peripheral eosinophilia, elevated serum immunoglobulin E levels, hypoalbuminemia, and anemia.

The disease usually runs a chronic, debilitating course with sporadic severe exacerbations. Although almost always effective for the treatment of isolated eosinophilic esophagitis (see Chapter 350), elemental diets are not always successful for the treatment of eosinophilic gastroenteritis. Orally administered cromolyn sodium and montelukast are sometimes successful. Many patients require treatment for acute disease exacerbations with systemic corticosteroids, which are often effective. Systemic corticosteroids may also be needed long-term. Oral budesonide, a corticosteroid with local anti-inflammatory activity on the bowel mucosa and limited systemic absorption due to high hepatic first-pass metabolism, can be attempted for long-term therapy.

Bibliography is available at Expert Consult.

Chapter 364
Disorders of Malabsorption

Raanan Shamir

第三百六十四章
吸收障碍性疾病

中文导读

　　本章主要介绍了儿童吸收障碍性疾病，包括肠黏膜损伤、主要营养物质吸收不良及新生儿期发病的慢性腹泻。具体描述了疑诊小肠吸收不良的疾病，如碳水化合物和脂肪吸收不良、蛋白丢失性肠病、胰腺外分泌功能不全、小肠黏膜功能紊乱等的诊断方法及影像学特点（原文第364.1）。介绍了乳糜泻的病因、流行病学、遗传和免疫机制、临床表现、诊断流程及治疗方法，以及与麸质相关的一些疾病（原文第364.2）。此外还介绍了导致肠吸收不良综合征的疾病谱，包括肠细胞分化及极化异常（如微绒毛包涵体病、簇绒肠病等）、肠内分泌细胞分化缺陷、自身免疫性肠病、蛋白丢失性肠病等（原文第364.3）。简要阐述了与吸收不良有关的小肠感染性疾病，包括感染后腹泻、远端小肠细菌过长、热带菌肠病、Whipple疾病（原文第364.4），以及与肠道吸收不良相关的免疫缺陷疾病（原文第364.5）、小肠免疫增殖性疾病（原文第364.6）。介绍了短肠综合征的病因、临床表现及治疗（原文第364.7）。简要介绍了慢性营养不良疾病（原文第364.8）和与肠吸收不良有关的酶功能缺陷疾病，包括碳水化合物吸收不良（如乳糖、果糖、蔗糖-异麦芽糖、葡萄糖-半乳糖酶功能不良）、胰腺外分泌功能不全、肠激酶缺乏、胰蛋白酶原缺乏等（原文第364.9）。最后简要介绍了引起吸收不良的肝脏和胆道疾病，包括PFIC、Wolman疾病、维生素A缺乏、维生素D缺乏、维生素E缺乏、维生素K缺乏（原文第364.10）和引起吸收不良的罕见先天缺陷病，包括碳水化合物及蛋白质吸收异常，脂肪转运异常，维生素、电解质及矿物质吸收不良引起的先天性疾病（原文第364.11）。

All disorders of malabsorption are associated with diminished intestinal absorption of one or more dietary nutrients. Malabsorption can result from a defect in the nutrient **digestion** in the intestinal lumen or from defective mucosal **absorption.** Malabsorption disorders can be categorized into generalized mucosal abnormalities usually resulting in malabsorption of multiple nutrients (Table 364.1) or malabsorption of specific nutrients (carbohydrate, fat, protein, vitamins, minerals, and trace elements) (Table 364.2). Almost all the malabsorption disorders are accompanied by chronic diarrhea, which further worsens the malabsorption (Chapter 367).

CLINICAL APPROACH

The clinical features depend on the extent and type of the malabsorbed nutrient. The common presenting features, especially in toddlers with malabsorption, are diarrhea, abdominal distention, and failure to gain weight, with a fall in growth chart percentiles. Physical findings include abdominal distention, muscle wasting, and the disappearance of the subcutaneous fat, with subsequent loose skinfolds (Fig. 364.1). The nutritional consequences of malabsorption are more dramatic in toddlers because of the limited energy reserves and higher proportion of calorie intake being used for weight gain and linear growth. In older children, malnutrition can result in growth retardation, as is commonly seen in children with late diagnosis of celiac disease (CD). If malabsorption is

Table 364.1	Malabsorption Disorders and Chronic Diarrhea Associated With Generalized Mucosal Defect

MUCOSAL DISORDERS
Gluten-sensitive enteropathy (celiac disease)
Cow's milk and other protein-sensitive enteropathies
Eosinophilic enteropathy

PROTEIN-LOSING ENTEROPATHY
Lymphangiectasia (congenital and acquired)
Disorders causing bowel mucosal inflammation, Crohn disease

CONGENITAL BOWEL MUCOSAL DEFECTS
Microvillous inclusion disease
Tufting enteropathy
Carbohydrate-deficient glycoprotein syndrome
Enterocyte heparan sulfate deficiency
Enteric anendocrinosis (NEUROG 3, PCSK1 mutations)
Tricho-hepatic-enteric syndrome

IMMUNODEFICIENCY DISORDERS
Congenital immunodeficiency disorders
  Selective immunoglobulin A deficiency (can be associated with celiac disease)
  Severe combined immunodeficiency
  Agammaglobulinemia
  X-linked hypogammaglobulinemia
  Wiskott-Aldrich syndrome
  Common variable immunodeficiency disease
  Chronic granulomatous disease

ACQUIRED IMMUNE DEFICIENCY
HIV infection
Immunosuppressive therapy and post–bone marrow transplantation

AUTOIMMUNE ENTEROPATHY
IPEX (immune dysregulation, polyendocrinopathy, enteropathy, X-linked inheritance)
IPEX-like syndromes
Autoimmune polyglandular syndrome type 1

MISCELLANEOUS
Immunoproliferative small intestinal disease
Short bowel syndrome
Blind loop syndrome
Radiation enteritis
Protein–calorie malnutrition
Crohn disease
Pseudoobstruction

Table 364.2	Classification of Malabsorption Disorders and Chronic Diarrhea Based on the Predominant Nutrient Malabsorbed

CARBOHYDRATE MALABSORPTION
Lactose malabsorption
Congenital lactase deficiency
Hypolactasia (adult type)
Secondary lactase deficiency
Congenital sucrase isomaltase deficiency
Glucose galactose malabsorption

FAT MALABSORPTION
Exocrine pancreatic insufficiency
  Cystic fibrosis
  Shwachman-Diamond syndrome
  Johanson-Blizzard syndrome
  Pearson syndrome
Secondary exocrine pancreatic insufficiency
  Chronic pancreatitis
  Protein–calorie malnutrition
  Decreased pancreozymin/cholecystokinin secretion
Isolated enzyme deficiency
  Enterokinase deficiency
  Trypsinogen deficiency
  Lipase/colipase deficiency
Disrupted enterohepatic circulation of bile salts
  Cholestatic liver disease
  Bile acid synthetic defects
  Deconjugation of bile acids (bacterial overgrowth)
  Bile acid malabsorption (terminal ileal disease)
Intestinal brush border disorders
  Allergic enteropathy
  Autoimmune enteropathy
  Disorders in formation and transport of chylomicrons by enterocytes to the lymphatics
  Abetalipoproteinemia
  Homozygous hypobetalipoproteinemia
  Chylomicron retention disease (Anderson disease)
Disorders of lymph flow
  Lymphangiectasia primary/secondary

PROTEIN/AMINO ACID MALABSORPTION
Lysinuric protein intolerance (defect in dibasic amino acid transport)
Hartnup disease (defect in free neutral amino acids)
Blue diaper syndrome (isolated tryptophan malabsorption)
Oasthouse urine disease (defect in methionine absorption)
Lowe syndrome (lysine and arginine malabsorption)
Enterokinase deficiency
Protein-losing enteropathy
  DGAT1 mutation
  Congenital disorders of glycosylation
  CD55 deficiency

MINERAL AND VITAMIN MALABSORPTION
Congenital chloride diarrhea
Congenital sodium absorption defect
Acrodermatitis enteropathica (zinc malabsorption)
Menkes disease (copper malabsorption)
Vitamin D–dependent rickets
Folate malabsorption
Congenital
Secondary to mucosal damage (celiac disease)
Vitamin B_{12} malabsorption
Autoimmune pernicious anemia
Decreased gastric acid (H_2 blockers or proton pump inhibitors)
Terminal ileal disease (e.g., Crohn disease) or resection
Inborn errors of vitamin B_{12} transport and metabolism
Primary hypomagnesemia

DRUG INDUCED
Sulfasalazine: folic acid malabsorption
Cholestyramine: calcium and fat malabsorption
Anticonvulsant drugs such as phenytoin (causing vitamin D deficiency and folic acid and calcium malabsorption)
Gastric acid suppression: vitamin B_{12}
Methotrexate: mucosal injury

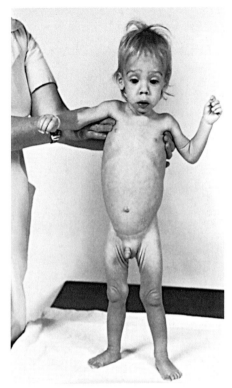

Fig. 364.1 An 18 mo old boy with active celiac disease. Note the loose skinfolds, marked proximal muscle wasting, and distended abdomen. The child looks ill.

left untreated, linear growth slows, and with prolonged malnutrition, death can follow (see Chapter 57). This extreme outcome is usually restricted to children living in the developing world, where resources to provide enteral and parenteral nutrition support may be limited. Nonetheless, monogenetic causes often produce failure to thrive in all countries. Specific findings on examination can guide toward a specific disorder; edema is usually associated with protein-losing enteropathy (PLE), digital clubbing with cystic fibrosis and CD, perianal excoriation and gaseous abdominal distention with carbohydrate malabsorption, perianal and circumoral rash with acrodermatitis enteropathica, abnormal hair with Menkes syndrome, tricho-hepato-enteric syndrome (THE) and the typical facial features diagnostic of the Johanson-Blizzard syndrome.

Many children with malabsorption disorders have a good appetite as they try to compensate for the fecal protein and energy losses. In exocrine pancreatic insufficiency, fecal losses of up to 40% of ingested protein and energy do not lead to malnutrition, as long as they are compensated by an increased appetite. In conditions associated with villous atrophy or inflammation (CD, postinfectious enteropathy), fecal protein and energy losses are usually modest, but associated anorexia and reduced food intake results in malnutrition.

The nutritional assessment is an important part of clinical evaluation in children with malabsorptive disorders (see Chapter 55). Long-term calcium and vitamin D malabsorption can lead to reduced bone mineral density and metabolic bone disease (often resistant to oral vitamin D), with increased risk of bone fractures. Vitamin K malabsorption, irrespective of the underlying mechanism (fat malabsorption, mucosal atrophy), can result in coagulopathy. Severe PLE is often associated with malabsorption syndromes (CD, congenital disorders of glycosylation, intestinal lymphangiectasia) and causes hypoalbuminemia and edema. Other nutrient deficiencies include iron malabsorption causing microcytic anemia and low reticulocyte count, low serum folate levels in conditions associated with mucosal atrophy, especially in the proximal part of the

small intestinal tract and low serum vitamin A and vitamin E concentrations in fat malabsorption.

The evaluation of a child with malabsorption should be proceed in a stepwise manner. Clinical history alone might not be sufficient to make a specific diagnosis, but it can direct the pediatrician toward a more structured and rational investigative approach. Diarrhea is the main clinical expression of malabsorption. The onset of diarrhea in early infancy suggests a congenital defect (Table 364.3). In secretory diarrhea caused by disorders such as congenital chloride diarrhea (CCD) and microvillus inclusion disease (MVID), the stool is watery and voluminous and can be mistaken for urine (see Chapter 367). The onset of symptoms after the introduction of a particular food into a child's diet can provide diagnostic clues, such as with sucrose in sucrase-isomaltase deficiency. The nature of the diarrhea may be helpful: explosive watery diarrhea suggests carbohydrate malabsorption; loose, bulky stools are associated with CD; and pasty and yellowish offensive stools suggest an exocrine pancreatic insufficiency. Stool color is usually not helpful; green stool with undigested "peas and carrots" can suggest rapid intestinal transit in toddler's diarrhea, which by itself is a self-limiting condition unassociated with failure to thrive.

Following medical history, physical examination and laboratory testing (see next Chapter 364.1), intestinal biopsies may assist in the diagnosis. This is usually done for chronic rather than acute diseases (that can be self-limited). Generalized mucosal villous atrophy (flat mucosa) may be associated with malabsorption of multiple *macronutrients* and *micronutrients* and has a wide range of differential diagnoses (see Chapter 364.2).

364.1 Evaluation of Children With Suspected Intestinal Malabsorption

Firas Rinawi and Raanan Shamir

The investigation is guided by the history and physical examination. In a child presenting with chronic or recurrent diarrhea, the initial work-up should include stool cultures and antibody tests for parasites; stool microscopy for ova and parasites such as *Giardia*; and fecal leukocytes and calprotectin or lactoferrin to exclude inflammatory disorders. Stool pH and reducing substances for carbohydrate malabsorption, stool

Table 364.3	Diarrheal Diseases Appearing in the Neonatal Period
CONDITION	**CLINICAL FEATURES**
Congenital enteropathy	
Microvillus inclusion disease	Secretory diarrhea
Tufting enteropathy	Secretory diarrhea
Congenital intestinal transport defect	
Congenital glucose–galactose malabsorption	Acidic diarrhea
Congenital bile acid malabsorption	Steatorrhea
Congenital chloride diarrhea	Secretory diarrhea, metabolic alkalosis
Congenital sodium diarrhea (*GUCY2C* mutation)	Hydramnion, secretory diarrhea
Congenital isolated enzyme deficiency	
Congenital lactase deficiency	Acidic diarrhea
Congenital enterokinase deficiency	Failure to thrive, edema
Congenital trypsinogen deficiency	Failure to thrive, edema
Congenital lipase and/or colipase deficiency	Failure to thrive, oily stool
Enteric anendocrinosis (*NEUROG 3* mutation)	Hyperchloremic acidosis, failure to thrive
Immunodeficiency and autoinflammatory diseases (see Table 362.6)	Failure to thrive, opportunistic infections, eczema

osmolality to differentiate between osmotic and secretory diarrhea and quantitative stool fat examination and α_1-antitrypsin to demonstrate fat and protein malabsorption, respectively, should also be determined. Fecal stool elastase-1 can determine exocrine pancreatic insufficiency.

A complete blood count, including peripheral smear for microcytic anemia, lymphopenia (lymphangiectasia), neutropenia (Shwachman syndrome), and acanthocytosis (abetalipoproteinemia) is useful. If CD is suspected, serum immunoglobulin (Ig) A and tissue transglutaminase (TG2) antibody levels should be determined. Depending on the initial test results, more specific investigations can be planned.

INVESTIGATIONS FOR CARBOHYDRATE MALABSORPTION

The measurement of carbohydrate in the stool for pH and the amount of reducing substances is a simple screening test when available. An acidic stool with >2+ reducing substance suggests carbohydrate malabsorption. Sucrose or starch in the stool is not recognized as a reducing sugar until after hydrolysis with hydrochloric acid, which converts them to reducing sugars.

Breath hydrogen test is used to identify the specific carbohydrate that is malabsorbed. After an overnight fast, the suspected sugar (lactose, sucrose, fructose, or glucose) is administered as an oral solution (carbohydrate load up to 2 g/kg, maximum total of 25 g, depending on the specific carbohydrate type). In malabsorption, the sugar is not digested or absorbed in the small bowel; it passes on to the colon and is metabolized by the normal gut microflora. One of the products of this process is hydrogen gas, which is absorbed through the colon mucosa and excreted in the breath. Increased hydrogen concentration in the breath samples suggests carbohydrate malabsorption. A rise in breath hydrogen of 20 ppm above the baseline preferably with associated symptoms is considered a positive test. The child should not be on antibiotics at the time of the test, because colonic flora is essential for fermenting the sugar.

Small bowel mucosal biopsies can measure mucosal disaccharidase (lactase, sucrase, maltase, palatinase) concentrations directly. In primary enzyme deficiencies the mucosal enzyme levels are low and small bowel mucosal morphology is normal. Primary enzymatic deficiencies can be diagnosed by genetic testing (see Chapters 364. 9 and 367). Partial or total villous atrophy due to disorders such as CD, or following acute rotavirus gastroenteritis can result in secondary disaccharidase deficiency and transient lactose intolerance (see Chapter 364.2 for differential diagnosis of villous atrophy). The disaccharidase levels revert to normal after mucosal healing.

INVESTIGATIONS FOR FAT MALABSORPTION

The presence of fat globules in the stool suggests fat malabsorption. The ability to assimilate fat varies with age; a premature infant can absorb only 65–75% of dietary fat, a full-term infant absorbs almost 90%, and an older child absorbs more than 95% of fat while on a regular diet. Quantitative determination of fat malabsorption requires a 3-day stool collection for evaluation of fat excretion and determination of the coefficient of fat absorption:

$$\text{Coefficient of fat absorption \%} = (\text{fat intake} - \text{fecal fat losses}/\text{fat intake}) \times 100$$

where fat intake and fat losses are in grams. Because fecal fat balance studies are cumbersome, expensive, and unpleasant to perform, simpler tests are often preferred. Among these stool tests, the acid steatocrit test is the most reliable. When BA deficiency is suspected of being the cause of fat malabsorption, the evaluation of BA levels in duodenal fluid aspirate may be useful. Intestinal mucosal abnormalities affect not only fat absorption, but also steatorrhea, and are usually far less severe in intestinal mucosal disorders (CD, cow's milk protein enteropathy) than in exocrine pancreatic insufficiency.

Exocrine pancreatic insufficiency and other fat malabsorption disorders (see Table 364.2) are usually associated with deficiencies of fat-soluble vitamins A, D, E, and K. Serum concentrations of vitamins A, D, and E can be measured. A prolonged prothrombin time is an indirect test to assess vitamin K malabsorption and subsequent deficiency.

INVESTIGATIONS FOR PROTEIN-LOSING ENTEROPATHY

Dietary and endogenous proteins secreted into the bowel are almost completely absorbed and minimal amounts of protein from these sources passes into the colon. The majority of the stool nitrogen is derived from gut bacterial proteins. Excessive bowel protein loss usually manifests as hypoalbuminemia. Because the most common cause of hypoalbuminemia in children is a renal disorder, urinary protein excretion must be determined. Other potential causes of hypoalbuminemia include acute infection, liver disease (reduced production) and inadequate protein intake. Very rarely hypoalbuminemia can result from an extensive skin disorder (burns) causing protein loss via the skin. Measurement of stool α_1-antitrypsin is a useful screening test for PLE. This serum protein has a molecular weight similar to albumin; however, unlike albumin it is resistant to digestion in the gastrointestinal (GI) tract. Excessive α_1-antitrypsin excretion in the stool should prompt further investigations to identify the specific cause of gut or stomach (Menetrier disease) protein loss.

INVESTIGATIONS FOR EXOCRINE PANCREATIC FUNCTION

Cystic fibrosis (Chapter 432) is the most common cause of exocrine pancreatic insufficiency in children; therefore, a sweat chloride test must be performed before embarking on invasive tests to investigate possible exocrine pancreatic insufficiency (Fig. 364.2). Many cases of cystic fibrosis are detected by neonatal genetic screening programs; occasional rare mutations are undetected.

Fecal elastase-1 estimation is a sensitive test to assess exocrine

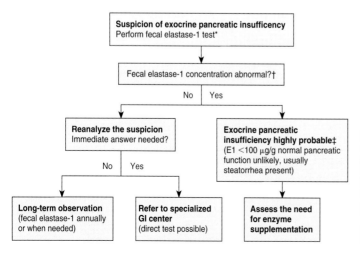

Fig. 364.2 Algorithm for assessment of exocrine pancreatic function. *If not available, use another test. Perform appropriate imaging studies of the pancreas. †In case of borderline values, consider repeating the test with 3 independent samples. ‡Consider differential diagnosis (especially consider mucosal villous atrophy and dilution effect of watery stool). GI, Gastrointestinal. (Modified from Walkowiak J, Nousia-Arvanitakis S, Henker J, et al: Indirect pancreatic function tests in children, J Pediatr Gastroenterol Nutr 40[2]:107–114, 2005.)

pancreatic function in chronic cystic fibrosis and pancreatitis. Elastase-1 is a stable endoprotease unaffected by exogenous pancreatic enzymes. One disadvantage of the fecal elastase-1 test is the lack of full differentiation between primary exocrine pancreatic insufficiency and exocrine pancreatic dysfunction secondary to intestinal villous atrophy. The proximal small bowel is the site for pancreozymin/cholecystokinin production; the latter is the hormone that stimulates enzyme secretion from the exocrine pancreas. Mucosal atrophy can lead to diminished pancreozymin/cholecystokinin secretion and subsequently to exocrine pancreatic insufficiency. Fecal elastase-1 can also give a false-positive result during acute episodes of diarrhea.

Serum trypsinogen concentration can also be used as a screening test for exocrine pancreatic insufficiency. In cystic fibrosis, the levels are greatly elevated early in life, and then they gradually fall, so that by 5-7 yr of age, most patients with cystic fibrosis with pancreatic insufficiency have subnormal levels. Patients with cystic fibrosis and adequate exocrine pancreatic function tend to have normal or elevated levels. In such patients, observing the trend in serial serum trypsinogen estimation may be useful in monitoring exocrine pancreatic function. In Shwachman syndrome, another condition associated with exocrine pancreatic insufficiency, the serum trypsinogen level is low.

Other tests for pancreatic insufficiency (nitroblue tetrazolium–paraaminobenzoic acid test and pancreolauryl test) measure urine or breath concentrations of substances released and absorbed across the mucosal surface following pancreatic digestion. These tests lack specificity and are rarely used in clinical practice.

The gold standard test for exocrine pancreatic function is direct analysis of duodenal aspirate for volume, bicarbonate, trypsin, and lipase upon secretin, and pancreozymin/cholecystokinin stimulation. This involves duodenal intubation (see Chapter 375).

INVESTIGATIONS FOR INTESTINAL MUCOSAL DISORDERS

Establishing a specific diagnosis for malabsorption often requires histologic examination of small bowel mucosal biopsies. These are obtained during endoscopy, which allows multiple biopsies to be performed, because mucosal involvement can be patchy, especially in CD. Periodic acid–Schiff (PAS) staining of mucosal biopsies and electron microscopy are necessary in congenital diarrhea to assess congenital microvillus atrophy. Bowel mucosal lesions can also be segmental in cases of IL. In these situations, radiographic small bowel series, repeated ultrasonographies or lymphoscintigraphy can identify a region of thickened bowel responsible for protein loss. Intestinal biopsies can detect infectious agents such as *Giardia lamblia*. During endoscopy, mucosal biopsies can be obtained to measure mucosal disaccharidase activities. Duodenal aspirates can be performed to measure pancreatic enzyme concentration as well as quantitative bacterial cultures.

IMAGING PROCEDURES

Plain radiographs and barium contrast studies might suggest a site and cause of intestinal motility disorders. Although flocculations of barium and dilated bowel with thickened mucosal folds have been attributed to diffuse malabsorptive lesions such as CD, these abnormalities are nonspecific. Diffuse fluid-filled bowel loops during sonography also suggest malabsorption.

Bibliography is available at Expert Consult.

364.2 Celiac Disease

Riccardo Troncone and Raanan Shamir

ETIOLOGY AND EPIDEMIOLOGY

CD is an immune-mediated systemic disorder elicited by gluten in wheat and related prolamines from rye and barley in genetically susceptible individuals, and is characterized by the presence of a variable combination of gluten-dependent clinical manifestations, CD–specific antibodies, human leukocyte antigen (HLA)-DQ2 or DQ8 haplotypes, and enteropathy. CD–specific antibodies comprise autoantibodies against TG2 including endomysial antibodies (EMAs), and antibodies against deamidated forms of gliadin peptides.

CD is a common disorder with about 1% prevalence of biopsy-proven disease. It is thought to be rare in Central Africa and East Asia. Although CD develops in genetically susceptible individuals, environmental factors might affect the risk of developing CD or the timing of its presentation. Neither breastfeeding during gluten introduction nor any breastfeeding has been shown to reduce the risk of CD. The earlier introduction of gluten is associated with the earlier development of CD autoimmunity (positive serology) and CD, but the cumulative incidence of each in later childhood is not affected. It is advised to introduce gluten into the infant's diet anytime between 4 and 12 mo of age. Infectious agents have been hypothesized to play a causative role as frequent rotavirus infections were shown to be associated with an increased risk of developing CD. It is plausible that the contact with gliadin at a time when there is an ongoing intestinal inflammation alters intestinal permeability, and the enhanced antigen presentation can increase the risk of developing CD, at least in a subset of persons. The mode of delivery, socioeconomic status, season of birth, and the use of drugs have been associated with the risk of developing CD, but the evidence is contradictory.

GENETICS AND PATHOGENESIS

A genetic predisposition is suggested by the family aggregation and the concordance in monozygotic twins, which approaches 100%. The strongest association is with HLA-DQ2.5 (1 or 2 copies encoded by DQA1 *05 [for the alpha] and DQB1*02 genes [for the beta chain]). Such a DQ molecule has been found to be present in more than 90% of CD patients. The highly homologous DQ2.2 molecule confers a much lower risk, while the data available on DQ2-negative CD patients indicate that they almost invariably are HLA-DQ8–positive (DQA1*0301/DQB1*0302). A gene dosage effect has been proved in prospective studies, and a molecular hypothesis for such a phenomenon has been proposed, based on the impact of the number and quality of the HLA-DQ2 molecules on gluten peptide presentation to T cells. The HLA locus is the most significant and dominant gene associated with CD; however, other loci known to contribute to CD have been documented. Most have been found to be associated with other autoimmune diseases such as type 1 diabetes. Interestingly, very few polymorphisms associated with CD are in coding regions, as they often are in binding sites for transcription factors, then affecting gene expression.

CD is a T-cell–mediated chronic inflammatory disorder with an autoimmune component. Altered processing by intraluminal enzymes, changes in intestinal permeability and activation of innate immunity mechanisms precede the activation of the adaptive immune response. Immunodominant epitopes from gliadin are highly resistant to intraluminal and mucosal digestion; incomplete degradation favors the immunostimulatory and toxic effects of these sequences. Some gliadin peptides (p31-43) activate innate immunity, in particular they induce interleukin (IL)-15. The latter, but also type 1 interferons, may alter the tolerogenic phenotype of dendritic cells, resulting in lamina propria T-cell activation by other peptides presented in the context of HLA-DQ2 or HLA-DQ8 molecules. Gliadin-specific T-cell responses are enhanced by the action of TG2: the enzyme converts particular glutamine residues into glutamic acid, which results in higher affinity of these gliadin peptides for HLA-DQ2 or HLA-DQ8. The pattern of cytokines produced following gliadin activation is dominated by interferon-γ (T-helper type 1 skewed); IL-21 is also upregulated. In downstream T-cell activation a complex remodeling of the mucosa takes place, involving increased levels of metalloproteinases and growth factors, which leads to the classical histologic finding of a flat mucosa. A severe impairment of intraepithelial lymphocytes (IELs) homeostasis is present in CD. IL-15 is implicated in the expression of natural killer receptors CD94 and NKG2D, as well as in epithelial expression of stress molecules, thus enhancing cytotoxicity, cell apoptosis, and villous atrophy. The most evident expression of autoimmunity is the presence of serum antibodies to TG2. However, the mechanisms leading to autoimmunity are largely unknown, as well as their pathogenetic significance. *Potential CD*, in which TG2 antibodies can be detected in situ without any histologic abnormality, shows that the production of antibodies does not necessarily lead to intestinal damage. The finding that IgA deposits on extracellular TG2 are not limited to the intestine but can be found in the liver, lymph nodes, and muscles indicates that TG2 is accessible to the gut-derived autoantibodies, turning CD into a systemic disease.

CLINICAL PRESENTATION AND ASSOCIATED DISORDERS

Clinical features of CD vary considerably. Intestinal symptoms are more common in children whose disease is diagnosed *within the first 2 yr of life*; failure to thrive, chronic diarrhea, vomiting, abdominal distention, muscle wasting, anorexia, and irritability are present in most cases (Fig. 364.3). Occasionally there is constipation, with cases presenting with intussusception. As the age at presentation of the disease shifts to later in childhood, and with the more extensive use of serologic screening tests, extraintestinal manifestations, without any accompanying digestive symptoms, have increasingly become recognized, affecting almost all organs (Table 364.4). One of the most common extraintestinal manifestation of CD is iron-deficiency anemia, which is usually unresponsive to iron therapy. Osteoporosis may be present; in contrast to adults, it can be reversed by a gluten-free diet, with restoration of normal peak bone densitometric values. Other extraintestinal manifestations include short stature, delayed puberty, arthritis and arthralgia, epilepsy with bilateral occipital calcifications, peripheral neuropathies, isolated hypertransaminasemia, dental enamel hypoplasia, and aphthous stomatitis. The mechanisms responsible for the severity and the variety of clinical presentations remain obscure. Nutritional deficiencies or abnormal immune responses have been advocated. Silent CD is recognized, mainly in asymptomatic first-degree relatives of CD patients and in subjects affected by diseases associated with CD (Table 364.5). Small bowel biopsy

Table 364.4	Extraintestinal Manifestations of Celiac Disease
MANIFESTATION	**PROBABLE CAUSE(S)**
CUTANEOUS	
Ecchymoses and petechiae	Vitamin K deficiency; rarely, thrombocytopenia
Edema	Hypoproteinemia
Dermatitis herpetiformis	Epidermal (type 3) tTG autoimmunity
Follicular hyperkeratosis and dermatitis	Vitamin A malabsorption, vitamin B complex malabsorption
ENDOCRINOLOGIC	
Amenorrhea, infertility, impotence, delayed puberty	Malnutrition, hypothalamic-pituitary dysfunction, immune dysfunction
Secondary hyperparathyroidism	Calcium and/or vitamin D malabsorption with hypocalcemia
HEMATOLOGIC	
Anemia	Iron, folate, vitamin B_{12}, or pyridoxine deficiency
Hemorrhage	Vitamin K deficiency; rarely, thrombocytopenia due to folate deficiency
Thrombocytosis, Howell-Jolly bodies	Hyposplenism
HEPATIC	
Elevated liver biochemical test levels	Lymphocytic hepatitis
Autoimmune hepatitis	Autoimmunity
MUSCULAR	
Atrophy	Malnutrition due to malabsorption
Tetany	Calcium, vitamin D, and/or magnesium malabsorption
Weakness	Generalized muscle atrophy, hypokalemia
NEUROLOGIC	
Peripheral neuropathy	Deficiencies of vitamin B_{12} and thiamine; immune-based neurologic dysfunction
Ataxia	Cerebellar and posterior column damage
Demyelinating central nervous system lesions	Immune-based neurologic dysfunction
Seizures	Unknown
SKELETAL	
Osteopenia, osteomalacia, and osteoporosis	Malabsorption of calcium and vitamin D, secondary hyperparathyroidism, chronic inflammation
Osteoarthropathy	Unknown
Pathologic fractures	Osteopenia and osteoporosis
OTHER	
Enamel hypoplasia	Vitamin D, calcium malabsorption
Anxiety, schizophrenia	Unknown, uncertain
Pulmonary hemosiderosis	Unknown, uncertain
Aphthous stomatitis	Unknown

tTG, tissue transglutaminase.
Modified from Kelly CP: Celiac disease. In Feldman M, Friedman LS, Brandt LJ, editors: *Sleisenger and Fordtran's gastrointestinal and liver disease,* ed 10, Philadelphia, 2016, Elsevier. Table 107.1.

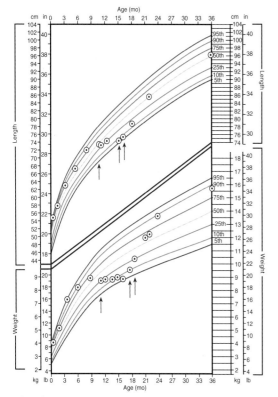

Fig. 364.3 Gluten-sensitive enteropathy. Growth curve demonstrates initial normal growth from 0 to 9 mo, followed by onset of poor appetite with intermittent vomiting and diarrhea after initiation of gluten-containing diet *(single arrow)*. After biopsy conformed diagnosis and treatment with gluten-free diet *(double arrow),* growth improves.

in silent/subclinical CD reveals severe mucosal damage consistent with CD. Potential CD is defined when patients have positive CD–specific antibodies, but without documented small bowel damage (Table 364.6).

Some diseases—many with an autoimmune pathogenesis—are found with a higher-than-normal incidence in CD patients. Among these are type 1 diabetes, autoimmune thyroid disease, Addison disease, Sjögren syndrome, rheumatoid arthritis, autoimmune cholangitis, autoimmune

Table 364.5	National Institute for Health and Care Excellence Guidelines on the Indications That Should Prompt Testing for Celiac Disease

CELIAC TESTING RECOMMENDED
- Persistent unexplained abdominal or gastrointestinal symptoms
- Faltering growth
- Prolonged fatigue
- Unexpected weight loss
- Severe or persistent mouth ulcers
- Unexplained iron, vitamin B12, or folate deficiency
- Type 1 diabetes
- Autoimmune thyroid disease
- Irritable bowel syndrome
- First degree relatives of people with coeliac disease
- Dermatitis herpetiformis

CELIAC TESTING SHOULD BE CONSIDERED
- Metabolic bone disorders (reduced bone mineral density or osteomalacia)
- Unexplained neurological symptoms (particularly peripheral neuropathy or ataxia)
- Unexplained subfertility or recurrent miscarriage
- Persistently increased concentrations of liver enzymes with unknown cause
- Dental enamel defects
- Down syndrome
- Turner syndrome
- William syndrome
- Selective IgA deficiency

IgA, immunoglobulin-A.
From Downey L, Houten R, Murch S, Longson D for the Guideline Development Group: Recognition, assessment, and management of coeliac disease: summary of updated NICE guidance, *BMJ* 351: h4513, 2015.

Table 364.6	Clinical Spectrum of Celiac Disease

SYMPTOMATIC
Frank malabsorption symptoms and signs (e.g., chronic diarrhea, failure to thrive, weight loss)
Extraintestinal symptoms and signs (e.g., anemia, fatigue, hypertransaminasemia, neurologic disorders, short stature, dental enamel defects, arthralgia, aphthous stomatitis)

SILENT
No apparent symptoms in spite of histologic evidence of villous atrophy
In most cases identified by serologic screening in at-risk groups (see Table 364.1)

LATENT
Subjects who have a normal intestinal histology, but at some other time have shown a gluten-dependent enteropathy

POTENTIAL
Subjects with positive celiac disease serology but without evidence of altered intestinal histology. Patients may or may not have symptoms and signs of disease and may or may not develop a gluten-dependent enteropathy later

hepatitis, and primary biliary cholangitis. Such associations have been interpreted as a consequence of the sharing of identical HLA haplotypes, but a direct role of gluten in promoting autoimmunity cannot be excluded. The relation between CD and other autoimmune diseases is poorly defined; once those diseases are established, they are not influenced by a gluten-free diet. Other associated conditions include selective IgA deficiency and Down, Turner, and Williams syndromes.

DIAGNOSIS

The diagnosis of CD is based on a combination of symptoms, antibodies, HLA status, and duodenal histology. The initial approach to symptomatic patients is to test for anti-TG2 IgA antibodies and for total IgA in serum to exclude IgA deficiency. If IgA anti-TG2 antibodies are negative, and serum total IgA is normal for age, CD is unlikely to be the cause of the symptoms. If anti-TG2 antibody testing is positive the patients should be referred to a pediatric gastroenterologist for further diagnostic workup, which depends on the serum antibody levels.

IgA anti-TG2 decline if the patient is on a gluten free diet. In patients with selective IgA deficiency, testing is recommended with IgG antibodies to TG2.

Patients with positive anti-TG2 antibody levels <10 times the upper limit of normal should undergo upper endoscopy with multiple biopsies. In patients with positive anti-TG2 antibody levels at or >10 times the upper limit of normal, blood should be drawn for HLA and EMA testing. If the patient is positive for EMA antibodies and positive for DQ2 or DQ8 HLA testing, the diagnosis of CD is confirmed, a life-long gluten-free diet is started and the patient is followed for the improvement of symptoms and the decline of antibodies. HLA testing is almost always positive; thus, it is possible that HLA testing will not be necessary in the future to establish diagnosis. In the rare case of negative results for HLA and/or anti-EMA in a child with TG2 antibody titers >10 times the upper limits of normal, the diagnostic workup should be extended, including repeated testing and duodenal biopsies (Fig. 364.4). In asymptomatic persons belonging to high-risk groups, CD should always be diagnosed using duodenal biopsies (Fig. 364.5). When biopsies are indicated, at least 4 fragments should be obtained from the descending part of the duodenum and at least 1 from the duodenal bulb. The diagnosis is confirmed by an antibody decline and preferably a clinical response to a gluten-free diet. CD is not the only cause for villous atrophy (Table 364.7). Gluten challenge and biopsies will only be necessary in selected cases in which diagnostic uncertainty remains.

TREATMENT

The only treatment for CD is lifelong strict adherence to a gluten-free diet. This requires a wheat-, barley-, and rye-free diet (Tables 364.8 and 364.9). Despite evidence that oats are safe for most patients with CD, there is concern regarding the possibility of contamination of oats with gluten during harvesting, milling, and shipping. Nevertheless, it seems wise to add oats to the gluten-free diet only when the latter is well established, so that possible adverse reactions can be readily identified. There is a consensus that all CD patients should be treated with a gluten-free diet regardless of the presence of symptoms. However, whereas it is relatively easy to assess the health improvement after treatment of CD in patients with clinical symptoms of the disease, it proves difficult in persons with asymptomatic CD. The nutritional risks, particularly osteopenia and increased risk for other autoimmune disorders, are those mainly feared for subjects who have silent CD and continue on a gluten-containing diet. Little is known about the health risks in untreated patients with potential CD.

Some patients do not respond to a gluten free diet; *refractory or nonresponsive CD* requires a systematic approach to determine the correct diagnosis, compliance, and therapeutic options (Fig. 364.6).

The Codex Alimentarius Guidelines define gluten-free food item for food containing <20 ppm (equivalent to 20 mg gluten in 1 kg of product); however, although analytical methods for gluten detection have reached a satisfactory degree of sensitivity, more information is needed on the daily gluten amount that may be tolerated by CD patients. The data available so far seem to suggest that the threshold should be set to <50 mg/day, although individual variability makes it difficult to set a universal threshold.

It is important that an experienced dietician with specific expertise in CD counseling educates the family and the child about dietary restriction. Compliance with a gluten-free diet can be difficult, especially in adolescents. It is recommended that children with CD be monitored with periodic visits for assessment of symptoms, growth, physical examination, complete blood count, thyroid diseases, and adherence to the gluten-free diet. Periodic measurements of TG2 antibody levels

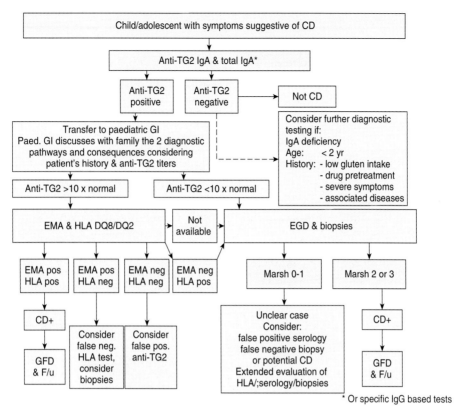

Fig. 364.4 Diagnostic algorithm for celiac disease in symptomatic children/adolescents, according to ESPGHAN. *CD,* Celiac disease; *EGD,* esophagogastroduodenoscopy; *EMA,* endomysial antibodies; *GFD,* gluten-free diet; *GI,* gastrointestinal; *HLA,* human leukocyte antigen; *Ig,* immunoglobulin. (Modified from Husby S, Koletzko S, Korponay-Szabò IR, et al: European Society for Pediatric Gastroenterology, Hepatology and Nutrition Guidelines for the diagnosis of celiac disease, J Pediatr Gastroenterol Nutr 54[1]:136–160, 2012. Fig. 1.)

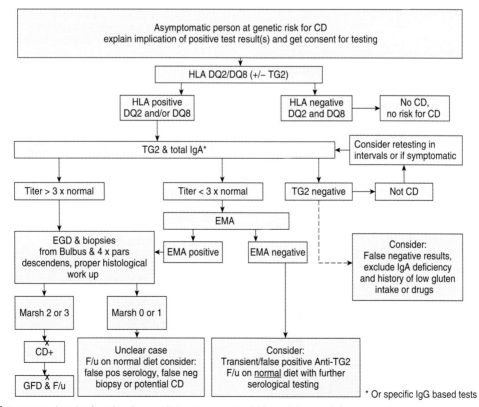

Fig. 364.5 Diagnostic algorithm for celiac disease *(CD)* in asymptomatic children/adolescents belonging to at-risk groups, according to ESPGHAN. *EGD,* Esophagogastroduodenoscopy; *EMA,* endomysial antibodies; *Ig,* immunoglobulin; *HLA,* human leukocyte antigen; *TG2,* transglutaminase. (Modified from Husby S, Koletzko S, Korponay-Szabò IR, et al: European Society for Pediatric Gastroenterology, Hepatology and Nutrition Guidelines for the diagnosis of celiac disease, J Pediatr Gastroenterol Nutr 54[1]:136–160, 2012. Fig. 2.)

Table 364.7	Other Causes of Flat Mucosa

Autoimmune enteropathy
Tropical sprue
Giardiasis
HIV enteropathy
Bacterial overgrowth
Crohn disease
Eosinophilic gastroenteritis
Cow's milk enteropathy
Food allergy
Primary immunodeficiency
Graft-versus-host disease
Chemotherapy and radiation
Protein energy malnutrition

Table 364.8	Principles of Initial Dietary Therapy for Patients With Celiac Disease

Avoid all foods containing wheat, rye, and barley gluten (pure oats usually safe).
Avoid malt unless clearly labeled as derived from corn.
Use only rice, corn, maize, buckwheat, millet, amaranth, quinoa, sorghum, potato or potato starch, soybean, tapioca, and teff, bean, and nut flours.
Wheat starch and products containing wheat starch should only be used if they contain <20 ppm gluten and are marked "gluten free."
Read all labels and study ingredients of processed foods.
Beware of gluten in medications, supplements, food additives, emulsifiers, or stabilizers.
Limit milk and milk products initially if there is evidence of lactose intolerance.
Avoid all beers, lagers, ales, and stouts (unless labeled gluten free).
Wine, most liqueurs, ciders, and spirits, including whiskey and brandy, are allowed.

ppm, Parts per million.

Table 364.9	Some Potential Sources of Hidden Gluten

Beers, ales, other fermented beverages (distilled beverages acceptable)
Bouillon and soups
Candy
Communion wafers
Drink mixes
Gravy and sauces
Herbal tea
Imitation meat and seafood
Nutritional supplements
Play-Doh
Salad dressings and marinades
Self-basting turkeys
Soy sauce

From Kelly CP. Celiac disease. In Feldman M, Friedman LS, Brandt LJ, editors: *Sleisenger and Fordtran's gastrointestinal and liver disease*, ed 10, Philadelphia, Elsevier, 2016. Box 107.3.

to document reduction in antibody titers can be helpful as indirect evidence of adherence to a gluten-free diet, although they are insensitive to slight dietary transgressions. If compliance is uncertain, bone health should be assessed.

THE SPECTRUM OF GLUTEN-RELATED DISORDERS

CD is not the only disorder related to gluten ingestion. Symptoms in IgE-mediated wheat allergy are usually immediate (urticaria, angioedema, asthma, exercise-induced anaphylaxis). Diagnosis is based on dietary challenge, in vitro assay for specific IgE and skin testing.

Non-celiac gluten sensitivity (NCGS) is a poorly understood condition. Diagnosis is suspected in patients who do not have CD or wheat allergy, and yet show GI and non-GI symptoms upon ingestion of gluten- or wheat-containing food. In the general population, the incidence of self-reported gluten avoidance varies from 0.5 to 13%. Similar symptoms are often experienced by patients with irritable bowel syndrome (IBS), and some patients with IBS respond positively to a gluten-free diet.

Bibliography is available at Expert Consult.

364.3 Other Malabsorptive Syndromes
Corina Hartman and Raanan Shamir

DEFECTS OF ENTEROCYTE DIFFERENTIATION AND POLARIZATION

This group mainly includes 2 conditions characterized by typical histological and ultrastructural lesions in the intestinal biopsies, microvillus inclusion disease (MVID) and congenital tufting enteropathy (CTE). Tricho-hepato-enteric syndrome (THE) or syndromic/phenotypic diarrhea is also usually classified in this group.

MICROVILLUS INCLUSION DISEASE (CONGENITAL MICROVILLUS ATROPHY)

MVID is an autosomal recessive disorder, which manifests at birth with profuse watery *secretory diarrhea*. A late-onset variant, with onset 2-3 mo postnatal has also been described. It is the most severe cause of congenital diarrhea involving the development of the intestinal mucosa. Light microscopy of the small bowel mucosa demonstrates diffuse thinning of the mucosa, with hypoplastic villus atrophy and no inflammatory infiltrate. Diagnosis is performed with light microscopy using PAS and CD10 staining, which shows a very thin or absent brush border, together with positive PAS and CD10 intracellular inclusions. Electron microscopy shows enterocytes with absent or sparse microvilli. The apical cytoplasm of the enterocytes contains electron-dense secretory granules; the hallmark is the presence of microvilli with involutions of the apical membrane (Fig. 364.7). Polyhydramnios is observed on prenatal sonography, and neonates usually present very early onset of severe watery diarrhea (up to 200-330 mL/kg/day) causing dehydration and failure to thrive. Despite parenteral nutrition, diarrhea continues, and initial fluid management is difficult. MVID and Fanconi syndrome that have been described in two patients may complicate management because of the additional features of a renal tubular acidosis, phosphaturia, rickets, and renal fluid losses. Mutations of the *MYO5B* gene coding for a nonconventional motor protein, myosin Vb, are associated with MVID in a cohort of patients suffering from early-onset MVID.

MYO5B mutations result in mislocalization of apical proteins and disrupted enterocyte polarization, leading to MVID. Another gene, the t-SNARE syntaxin3 *(STX3)*, has been described in patients with MVID and a milder phenotype. Patients with mutations in the STX3 binding protein *STXBP2/Munc18-2*, causing familial hemophagocytic lymphohistiocytosis type 5, also show microvillus atrophy and histologic findings reminiscent of MVID. Loss of STX3 or Munc18-2 inhibits the fusion of vesicles with the apical membrane, resulting in the intracellular retention of apical proteins. *MYO5B* mutations have also been identified in several patients with progressive familial intrahepatic cholestasis (PFIC)-like phenotype with normal serum gamma-glutamyl transferase activity and without intestinal disease.

TUFTING ENTEROPATHY (CONGENITAL TUFTING ENTEROPATHY)

CTE (intestinal epithelial dysplasia) manifests in the first few weeks of life with persistent watery diarrhea. CTE accounts for a small fraction of infants with *intractable diarrhea of infancy*. The distinctive feature on small intestinal mucosal biopsy is focal epithelial tufts (teardrop-shaped groups of closely packed enterocytes with apical rounding of

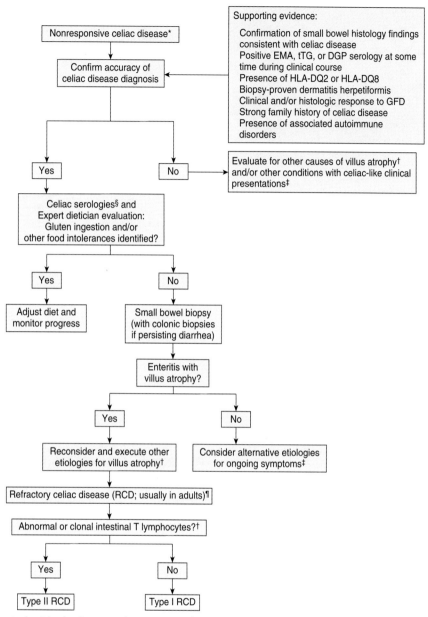

Fig. 364.6 Diagnostic algorithm for the approach to patients with nonresponsive celiac disease. *Nonresponsive celiac disease* may be defined as persistent symptoms and signs despite 6-12 mo of dietary gluten avoidance. Abnormal TTG can last even 2-3 yr. †Causes of non-celiac small intestinal villus atrophy that may be misdiagnosed as celiac disease include autoimmune enteropathy, tropical sprue, SIBO, hypogammaglobulinemia, combined variable immunodeficiency, collagenous sprue, eosinophilic enteritis, Crohn disease, and peptic duodenitis. ‡Conditions that present clinically in a fashion similar to celiac disease but where villus atrophy is not evident include IBS, food intolerances, SIBO, eosinophilic enteritis, Crohn disease, and microscopic colitis. §Positive serologic testing for celiac disease despite 12 mo of treatment with a GFD suggest that there may be ongoing gluten ingestion. ‖*Refractory celiac disease (RCD)* is defined as persistent or recurrent malabsorptive symptoms and signs, with small intestinal villus atrophy despite a strict GFD for more than 12 mo and in the absence of other disorders including overt lymphoma. ¶Abnormal intestinal lymphocytes may be identified by immunohistochemistry of intraepithelial lymphocytes or by flow cytometry showing an increased number of CD3-positive cells that lack CD8 or by the identification of clonal T-cell receptor gene rearrangement by molecular analysis. EMA, Endomysial antibody; DGP, deamidated gliadin peptide; GFD, gluten-free diet; HLA, human leukocyte antigen; tTGA, tissue transglutaminase antibody. (Adapted from Rubio-Tapia A, Murray JA. Classification and management of refractory coeliac disease. Gut 59:547–57, 2010; and Rubio-Tapia A, Hill ID, Kelly CP, et al. ACG clinical guidelines: Diagnosis and management of celiac disease. Am J Gastroenterol 108:656–76, 2013.)

the plasma membrane) involving 80–90% of the epithelial surface. The typical pathology does not appear immediately after birth; other enteropathies may show tufts on the epithelial surface.

CTE is a phenotypic and genetic heterogenous condition. Genetic studies identified mutations in epithelial cell adhesion molecule (*EPCAM*) gene in 73% of patients and mutations in hepatocyte growth factor

activator inhibitor type 2 *SPINT2/HAI2* gene in 21%. No identified mutations are identified in a minority of patients. The phenotype associated with mutations of *EPCAM* is usually an isolated congenital diarrhea without associated extra digestive symptoms, except late-onset arthritis or superficial punctuate keratitis. In the *syndromic* form of CTE, diarrhea is associated with 1 or more of these same anomalies:

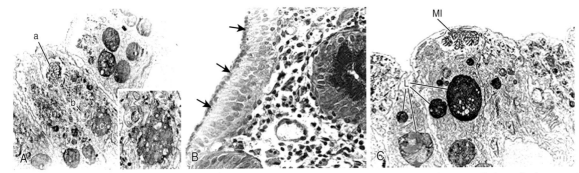

Fig. 364.7 Microvillus inclusion disease. **A,** From top to bottom: microvillus inclusion *(a)*, a granule with few microvilli *(b)*, and a lysosome *(c)* detected in the same enterocyte. *Inset:* Higher magnification of *b* and *c* ×11,000, inset ×21,500. **B,** Microvillus inclusion disease. Periodic acid-Schiff (PAS) staining highlights abundant PAS-positive material *(arrows)* in the apical part of the enterocyte cytoplasm. **C,** Microvillus inclusion disease. The villous enterocyte lack brush-border microvilli, whereas their apical cytoplasm contains a microvillus inclusion *(MI)* and numerous lysosomes *(L)* ×5,500. (A, From Morroni M, Cangiotti AM, Guarino A, et al: Unusual ultrastructural features in microvillous inclusion disease: a report of two cases, Virchows Arch 448[6]:805–810, 2006.)

superficial punctate keratitis (100%), choanal atresia (50%), esophageal or intestinal atresia, anal imperforation, hair dysplasia, skin hyperlaxity, bone abnormalities, hexadactylia, and facial dysmorphism.

No specific treatment exists, thus, as for MVID, management requires permanent parenteral nutrition (PN) with possible intestinal transplantation (see Chapter 365).

TRICHO-HEPATO-ENTERIC SYNDROME (SYNDROMIC DIARRHEA)

THE, also known as *syndromic diarrhea* (SD), is a congenital enteropathy manifesting with early onset of severe diarrhea. Patients are born small for gestational age and present with diarrhea starting in the first 6 mo of life. They have an abnormal phenotype, including facial dysmorphism with prominent forehead, broad nose, and hypertelorism with a distinct abnormality of hair, **trichorrhexis nodosa.** Hairs are woolly, easily removed, and poorly pigmented. Abnormal cutaneous lesions including café-au-lait on the lower limbs may be observed. Liver disease affects about half of the patients with extensive fibrosis or cirrhosis. Cardiac abnormalities and colitis have been reported sporadically, as well as one case involving polyhydramnios, placental abnormalities, and congenital hemochromatosis. Patients may have defective antibody responses despite normal serum Ig levels and defective antigen-specific skin tests despite positive proliferative responses in vitro. Patients with THE can also present as very-early-onset inflammatory bowel disease (IBD). Small bowel biopsies show nonspecific villus atrophy with or without mononuclear cell infiltration of the lamina propria, and without specific histologic abnormalities involving the epithelium. Mutations in either tetratricopeptide repeat domain 37 *(TTC37)* gene (60%) or *SKIV2L* (40%) have been identified as cause of THE syndrome. Enterocytes with *TTC37* mutations, show reduced expression of brush-border-associated NHE-2 and -3, aquaporin-7, the Na+/I- symporter, and the H+/K+-ATPase or mislocalization relative to their normal pattern. Prognosis of this type of intractable diarrhea of infancy is poor. The long-term follow-up of these children reported that at 15 years about 50% of patients were alive or have been weaned off PN. The main complications are liver disease and infections. Most of the children achieve short final stature and half are slightly developmentally delayed.

DEFECTS IN ENTEROENDOCRINE CELLS DIFFERENTIATION

This class of congenital diarrheas is characterized by abnormal enteroendocrine cells development or function. The genes causing these disorders encode either transcription factors essential for the development of all or a subset of enteroendocrine cells, or cellular proteins/endopeptidases that are required for the production of active hormones from prohormones. The conditions manifest with *osmotic* diarrhea and in some, additional systemic endocrine disorders. The treatment is

nutritional support and hormonal replacement if needed. Four genes have been associated with the diseases classified in this group: *NEUROG3, RFX6, ARX,* and *PCSK1.*

ENTERIC ANENDOCRINOSIS

NEUROG3 is a key transcription factor that controls the fate of endocrine cells in both the pancreas and intestine. Mutations of the *NEUROG3* gene produce generalized mucosal malabsorption, vomiting, diarrhea, failure to thrive, dehydration, and a hyperchloremic metabolic acidosis. Oral alimentation with anything other than water produces diarrhea. Villus-crypt architecture in small bowel biopsies is normal, but staining for neuroendocrine cells (e.g., employing antichromogranin antibodies) demonstrates a complete absence of this secretory cell lineage with the preservation of goblet cells and Paneth cells.

PROPROTEIN CONVERTASE 1/3 DEFICIENCY

Autosomal recessive proprotein convertase 1/3 (PC1/3) deficiency, caused by mutations in the *PCSK1* gene, is characterized by severe congenital malabsorptive diarrhea, early-onset obesity, and other endocrine abnormalities. All functional hormones produced by endocrine cells, including those in the gut, are processed by a specific Ca2+-dependent serine endoprotease named proprotein convertase 1/3 (also known as neuroendocrine convertase 1). Chronic watery, neonatal onset diarrhea is described in infants with hyperinsulinism, hypoglycemia, hypogonadism, and hypoadrenalism. A small bowel biopsy reveals a nonspecific enteropathy.

Growth hormone deficiency, adrenal insufficiency, central diabetes insipidus, and hypogonadism are commonly observed.

MITCHELL-RILEY SYNDROME

Mitchell-Riley syndrome is a complex clinical phenotype that includes severe intrauterine growth restriction, neonatal diabetes, GI anomalies (annular pancreas, intestinal malrotation, gallbladder agenesis, abnormal biliary tract) and chronic *osmotic* diarrhea. Several probands previously reported with Mitchell-Riley syndrome had *RFX6* mutations. DNA-binding protein RFX6 (regulatory factor X6; encoded by *RFX6*) is a winged helix transcription factor downstream of neurogenin-3 signal required for islet cell development and enteroendocrine cell function. Immunofluorescence staining in RFX6 knockout mice shows that pancreatic endocrine cells are present, but do not express the islet cell hormones including insulin, glucagon, somatostatin, or ghrelin.

ARISTALESS-RELATED HOMEOBOX GENE MUTATIONS

Aristaless-related homeobox (Arx) gene encodes a homeodomain containing a transcription factor required for the normal development of mouse and human enteroendocrine cells. *Arx* expression is detected in a subset of neurogenin3-positive endocrine progenitors and is also found in a subset of hormone-producing cells. In mice, removal of *Arx* from the developing endoderm results in a decrease of some entero-endocrine cell types, such as gastrin, glucagon/GLP-1, CCK, secretin secreting cells and an increase of somatostatin-expressing cells. Mutations in the *ARX* gene are associated with a complex clinical phenotype of X-linked intellectual disability, seizures, lissencephaly, abnormal genitalia, and occasionally congenital diarrhea.

AUTOIMMUNE ENTEROPATHY

The term autoimmune enteropathy describes a subgroup of infants with severe, protracted diarrhea, no response to dietary restriction, the presence of circulating gut autoantibodies and/or associated autoimmune diseases and the lack of severe immunodeficiency. Symptoms of autoimmune enteropathy usually occur after the first 6 mo of life, presenting with chronic diarrhea, PLE, malabsorption, and failure to thrive. The diagnosis is based on the endoscopic and histologic identification of inflammation mainly of the *small bowel* but also of the colon. Histologic findings in the small bowel include partial or complete villus atrophy, crypt hyperplasia, and an increase in chronic inflammatory cells in the lamina propria. Marked intraepithelial lymphocytosis reminiscent of CD can be present in a subset of patients. Cryptitis and crypt abscesses can also be seen and may obscure the presence of apoptosis. Immunologic analyses indicate the presence of autoantibodies including *anti–enterocyte antibodies (present in ~85% of patients)*, as well as *anti–autoimmune enteropathy-related 75 kDa antigen*.

The differential diagnosis of pediatric autoimmune enteropathy includes other immune-mediated disorders, such as food sensitivity enteropathies (e.g., cow milk intolerance and celiac disease), Crohn disease and graft-versus-host disease. It is essential to exclude an underlying primary immune deficiency, particularly in boys with other autoimmune features because some have **IPEX syndrome** (see Chapter 152.5). Different phenotypes of IPEX syndrome patients, as well as IPEX-like forms of autoimmune enteropathy that are *FOXP3*-independent are described involving females with or without extraintestinal autoimmune disorders.

Treatment options are limited and are based on nutritional support, including parenteral nutrition and glucocorticoids followed by immunosuppressive drugs. Hematopoietic stem cell transplantation is indicated in patients with a known molecular defect, such as IPEX syndrome.

AUTOIMMUNE POLYGLANDULAR SYNDROME TYPE 1

See Chapter 151.

Defects in Lipids Transport and Metabolism

See Chapter 104.3.

After uptake from the lumen, fatty acids and monoacylglycerol are transported to the endoplasmic reticulum (ER). In the ER they are converted to triglycerides in several metabolic steps, the last of which is dependent on acyl CoA:diacylglycerol acyltransferase 1 (DGAT1). Apolipoprotein B (ApoB) and microsomal triglycerides transfer protein (MTTP) act in concert to incorporate triglycerides into chylomicrons. The newly formed chylomicrons bud from the ER in a prechylomicron transport vesicle (PCTV), which subsequently fuses with the Golgi, a process that is dependent on Sar1b. The chylomicron is then transported in a vesicle to the basal membrane, where it exits the cell.

ABETALIPOPROTEINEMIA

Abetalipoproteinemia (Bassen-Kornzweig syndrome) is a rare autosomal recessive disorder of lipoprotein metabolism associated with severe fat malabsorption/steatorrhea from birth (see Chapter 104.3). Children fail to thrive during the 1st yr of life, have stools that are pale, foul smelling, and bulky. The abdomen is distended, and deep tendon reflexes are absent because of peripheral neuropathy, which is secondary to vitamin E deficiency. Intellectual development tends to be slow. After 10 yr of age, intestinal symptoms are less severe, ataxia may develop, with loss of position and vibration sensation, and the onset of intention tremors. These latter symptoms reflect involvement of the posterior

columns, cerebellum, and basal ganglia. In adolescence, in the absence of adequate supplement of vitamin E, atypical retinitis pigmentosa develops.

The diagnosis is suggested by the presence of acanthocytes in the peripheral blood smear and extremely low plasma levels of cholesterol (<50 mg/dL); triglycerides are also very low (<20 mg/dL). Chylomicrons and very-low-density lipoproteins are not detectable, and the low-density lipoprotein (LDL) fraction is virtually absent from the circulation. Marked triglyceride accumulation in villus enterocytes occurs in the duodenal mucosa. Patients with abetalipoproteinemia have mutations of the *MTTP* gene. MTTP catalyzes the transfer of triglycerides to nascent ApoB particles in the ER.

Specific treatment is not available. Nutritional support and large supplements of the fat-soluble vitamins A, D, E, and K should be given. Vitamin E (100-200 mg/kg/24 hr) appears to arrest neurologic and retinal degeneration. Limiting long-chain fat intake can alleviate intestinal symptoms; medium-chain triglycerides (MCTs) can be used to supplement fat intake.

HOMOZYGOUS HYPOBETALIPOPROTEINEMIA

Homozygous hypobetalipoproteinemia (see Chapter 104.3) is a dominantly inherited condition associated with mutations in the *APOB* gene, encoding ApoB, the apolipoprotein of the nascent chylomicron. The homozygous form is indistinguishable from abetalipoproteinemia. The parents of these patients, as heterozygotes, have reduced plasma LDL and apoprotein-B concentrations, whereas the parents of patients with abetalipoproteinemia have normal levels. On transmission electron microscopy of small bowel biopsies, the size of lipid vacuoles in enterocytes differentiates between abetalipoproteinemia and hypobetalipoproteinemia: many small vacuoles are present in hypobetalipoproteinemia, and larger vacuoles are seen in abetalipoproteinemia.

CHYLOMICRON RETENTION DISEASE (ANDERSON DISEASE)

Chylomicron retention disease (CRD) is a rare autosomal recessive disorder caused by mutations in the *SAR1B* gene. *SAR1B* mutations result in defective trafficking of nascent chylomicrons in pre-chylomicron transport vesicles between the ER and the Golgi apparatus, interfering with the successful assembly of chylomicrons and their delivery to the lamina propria. The patients with CRD have steatorrhea, chronic diarrhea, and failure to thrive. Acanthocytosis is rare and neurologic manifestations are less severe than those observed in abetalipoproteinemia. Plasma cholesterol levels are moderately reduced (<75 mg/dL) and fasting triglycerides are normal, but the fat-soluble vitamins, particularly A and E, are very low. Treatment is early aggressive therapy with fat-soluble vitamins and modification of dietary fat intake, as in the treatment of abetalipoproteinemia.

DGAT1 MUTATION

DGAT1 encodes for diacyl CoA:diacylglycerol acyl transferase (DGAT) that converts diacylglycerides to triglycerides by adding an acyl CoA moiety. In the small intestine, DGAT1 helps to reassemble the triglycerides, whereas in the liver it produces triglycerides from fatty acids synthesized de novo or taken up from the circulation. The mechanism by which *DGAT1* mutations causes diarrhea is unclear but is likely to involve the build-up of DGAT1 lipid substrates in the enterocytes or in the gut lumen. Mutations in *DGAT1* gene have been reported in patients presenting with failure to thrive, PLE, hypoalbuminemia, early-onset diarrhea, and oral vitamin D refractory rickets.

WOLMAN DISEASE

Wolman disease is a rare, lethal lipid storage disease that leads to lipid accumulation in multiple organs, including the small intestine. In addition to vomiting, severe diarrhea, and hepatosplenomegaly, patients have steatorrhea as a result of lymphatic obstruction. Insufficient free cholesterol available for steroidogenesis in adrenal glands results in adrenal insufficiency; a characteristic pattern of subcapsular adrenal calcification represents a distinctive marker of disease. Deficiency of lysosomal acid lipase (LAL) is the underlying cause of disease (see Chapter 104.4). LAL is a lysosomal enzyme that hydrolyzes cholesteryl esters and triglycerides within endo-lysosomes. Loss-of-function mutations in the *LIPA* gene are associated with variable phenotypes. Homozygous and compound heterozygous mutations, resulting in complete LAL deficiency, cause Wolman disease. Mutations associated with residual LAL activity cause cholesteryl ester storage disease, a less severe disorder exhibiting a variable phenotype. Common features in infants, children, and adults include elevated serum aminotransferase levels, dyslipidemia, hepatomegaly, liver fibrosis, and cirrhosis. Wolman disease may also present with neonatal cholestasis and severe liver disease as its main feature already in infancy. Hemophagocytic lymphohistiocytosis has been reported in few infants with Wolman disease. The hallmark of the disease is the presence of *adrenal calcification* seen on imaging, and definite diagnosis is done genetically.

Hematopoietic stem cell transplantation has been reported in few patients with variable outcome. A recombinant human enzyme-replacement therapy for LAL deficiency is approved for use in patients suffering from LAL deficiency. This treatment has allowed a small number of infants with Wolman disease to achieve a relatively normal growth rate and to improve survival. In older children and adults, the enzyme has corrected their dyslipidemia and produced significant improvement in markers of hepatic function.

TANGIER DISEASE
See Chapter 104.

Cellular free cholesterol is mobilized, along with phospholipid, through the export pump ABCA1, resulting in the transfer to an extracellular ApoA-I acceptor and the formation of discoidal high-density lipoprotein (HDL) cholesterol. Loss-of-function mutations in *ABCA1*genes in patients with Tangier disease cause cholesterol accumulation in the intestine, spleen, tonsils, relapsing neuropathy, orange-brown spots on the colon and ileum, and diarrhea in association with decreased plasma cholesterol levels (ApoA-I and A-II), with virtually no detectable plasma HDL. Specific therapy for Tangier disease has not yet been established.

SITOSTEROLEMIA
See Chapter 104.4.

Sitosterol and other sterols are preferentially secreted back into the intestinal lumen through the sterol pump, paired half-transporters ABCG5/G8. Mutations of the *ABCG5* (sterolin-1) and *ABCG8* (sterolin-2) transporters result in the defective efflux of sterol and leads to the increased absorption of dietary sterols. The disorder is associated with tendon xanthomas, increased atherosclerosis, and hemolysis. Plasma levels of phytosterols (mainly sitosterol) are typically >10 mg/dL.

BILE ACID MALABSORPTION
Bile acids (BA) are detergent compounds secreted by and excreted from the liver, and are responsible for the solubilization of the dietary lipids, aiding in their digestion and absorption. Approximately 95% of BAs are reabsorbed in the terminal ileum and transported back to the liver, the enterohepatic circulation. The apical Na+-dependent bile salt transporter (ASBT) or ileal BA transporter (IBAT) is responsible for the active reuptake of BAs in the terminal ileum. Mutation in the *ASBT/ SLC10A2* gene are very rare and are responsible for *primary* BA malabsorption, a disease associated with congenital diarrhea, steatorrhea, and reduced plasma cholesterol levels. Unabsorbed BA stimulate chloride excretion in the colon, resulting in diarrhea. *Secondary* BA malabsorption can result from ileal disease, such as in Crohn disease, and following ileal resection. The diagnosis of BA malabsorption is typically based on reduced BA retention of radiolabeled ^{75}Selenium-homocholic acid taurine (^{75}SeHCAT), increased BA synthesis (serum C4) or increased fecal BA loss. In clinical practice, diagnosis is often based on the response to BA sequestrants (e.g., cholestyramine or colesevelam), which are also the treatment of choice for this disorder.

Chronic neonatal-onset diarrhea has also been described in autosomal recessive cerebrotendinous xanthomatosis, which is caused by an inborn error of BA synthesis resulting from 27-hydroxylase deficiency. These children also present with juvenile-onset cataracts and developmental delay. Neonatal cholestasis has also been described as a presenting feature. Tendon xanthomas develop in the 2nd and 3rd decades of life. The diagnosis is important to establish, because treatment is effective when employing oral chenodeoxycholic acid.

PROTEIN-LOSING ENTEROPATHY
PLE is a rare entity caused by a variety of intestinal and extraintestinal disorders and characterized by excessive enteric loss of plasma proteins. The clinical presentation of patients with PLE is variable and depends upon the underlying cause, but generally includes edema and hypoproteinemia. Impaired synthesis (malnutrition, liver disease), protein loss through other organs (kidney or skin) or redistribution (septic states) have to be excluded before considering PLE. The disorders causing PLE can be divided into those due to protein loss from an inflamed or abnormal mucosal surface or from derangements in intestinal lymphatics, such as in primary or secondary **IL** (Table 364.10).

IL is characterized by diffuse or local dilatation of the enteric lymphatics and is located in the mucosa, submucosa, or subserosa. Lymph rich in proteins, lipids, and lymphocytes leak into the bowel lumen, resulting in PLE, steatorrhea, and lymphocyte depletion. Hypoalbuminemia, hypogammaglobulinemia, edema, lymphopenia, malabsorption of fat and fat-soluble vitamins, and chylous ascites often occur. IL can also manifest with ascites, peripheral edema, and a low serum albumin. The etiology of *primary* IL is unknown. Several genes, including vascular endothelial growth factor receptor 3 *(VEGFR3)*, prospero-related homeobox-transcriptional factor *(PROX1)*, forkhead transcriptional factor *(FOXC2)*, and SRY (sex determining region Y)-Box 18 *(SOX18)*, are involved in the development of the lymphatic system and have been shown to have altered expression in the duodenal mucosa in patients with IL. Recently, mutation in CD55, a regulator of complement activation, was described as a cause for primary PLE. The diagnosis of PLE is suggested by the typical clinical and laboratory findings in association with an elevated fecal $α_1$-antitrypsin clearance. Radiologic findings of uniform, symmetric thickening of mucosal folds throughout the small intestine are characteristic but nonspecific. Small bowel mucosal biopsy in patients with IL can show dilated lacteals with distortion of villi and no inflammatory infiltrate. A patchy distribution and deeper mucosal involvement on occasion causes false-negative results on small bowel histology. Video capsule endoscopy may reveal similar lesions (Figs. 364.8 and 364.9).

Treatment of PLE is generally supportive and consists of a low fat and high-protein diet. In patients with IL, a low-fat and high-protein diet supplemented with MCTs is recommended. Besides dietary adjustments, appropriate treatment for the underlying etiology is necessary, as well as supportive care to avoid complications of edema. Rarely, parenteral nutrition is required. If only a portion of the intestine is involved, surgical resection may be considered. Few patients with lymphatic malformation and generalized lymphatic anomalies were successfully treated with propranolol. Successful use of mTOR inhibitor, everolimus, in a patient with primary IL has been reported. Prognosis depends upon the severity and treatment options of the underlying disease.

Bibliography is available at Expert Consult.

364.4 Intestinal Infections and Infestations Associated With Malabsorption
Alfredo Guarino and Raanan Shamir

Malabsorption is a rare consequence of primary intestinal infection and infestation in immunocompetent children, but is relatively common in malnourished children and is associated with significant mortality. Often malabsorption is associated with diarrhea and triggers a vicious circle with wasting and growth failure. For children living in developing countries, malabsorption is associated with long-term growth failure leading to stunting within a peculiar condition defined as environmental enteropathy, in which diarrhea is not always present. Generally, mal-

Table 364.10	Causes of Protein-Losing Enteropathy	
PROTEIN-LOSING ENTEROPATHY		**AGENT, DISEASES (*GENE*)**
Gastrointestinal infections	Viral infections Bacterial and parasitic diseases Gastrointestinal infestations	CMV, rotavirus *Salmonella, Shigella, Campylobacter, Clostridium difficile, Helicobacter pylori, Whipple disease* Small bowel bacterial overgrowth *Giardiasis* *Strongyloides stercoralis*
Gastrointestinal inflammatory disorders	Gastric diseases Gastrointestinal disorders	Menetrier disease Eosinophilic gastroenteropathy Food induced enteropathy Celiac disease, Crohn disease, Ulcerative colitis, Tropical sprue Radiation enteritis GVHD, NEC
Gastrointestinal malignancies	Adenocarcinomas Lymphomas Kaposi sarcoma	Esophageal, gastric, colonic
Vasculitic disorders	Henoch Schönlein purpura Systemic lupus erythematosus	
Drugs	NSAIDs	
Metabolic/genetic	Congenital disorders of glycosylation (CDG) Mutations in *DGAT1* gene Mutations in CD55	CDG-Ib (*MPI*) Congenital enterocyte heparan sulphate deficiency (*ALG6*)
Intestinal lymphangiectasia	Congenital/ Primary IL • Syndromal/genetic/ metabolic	Turner, Noonan, Klippel–Trenaunay–Weber Hennekam syndrome (*CCBE1, FAT4*) PLE with skeletal dysplasia (*FGFR3*) Generalized lymphatic dysplasia (*PIEZO1*)
	Secondary • Infection • Inflammation • Radiotherapy • Neoplastic disorders • Cardiac disorders	Abdominal tuberculosis Crohn disease, sarcoidosis Retroperitoneal fibrosis Retroperitoneal malignancies, lymphoma Constrictive pericarditis, after Fontan operation, congestive heart failure

CDG, Carbohydrate deficient glycoprotein; *CMV,* cytomegalovirus; *GVHD,* graft versus host disease; *IL,* intestinal lymphangiectasia; *NEC, NSAIDs,* nonsteroidal anti-inflammatory drugs; *PLE,* protein-losing enteropathy.

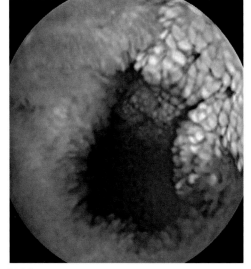

Fig. 364.8 Swollen villi detected by video capsule endoscopy in the proximal ileum. *(From Gortani G, Maschio M, Ventura A: A child with edema, lower limb deformity, and recurrent diarrhea, J Pediatr 161:1177, 2012, Fig. 1.)*

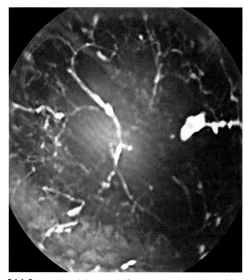

Fig. 364.9 Protein-rich lymphatic fluid aggregates detected by video capsule endoscopy in the intestinal lumen. *(From Gortani G, Maschio M, Ventura A: A child with edema, lower limb deformity, and recurrent diarrhea, J Pediatr 161:1177, 2012, Fig. 2.)*

absorption is associated with a duration of an intestinal infection longer than expected. *Prolonged* diarrhea is an acute-onset diarrhea that lasts >7 days, whereas *chronic* diarrhea lasts >14 days (some use 30 days to define chronic).

POSTINFECTIOUS DIARRHEA

In infants and toddlers, chronic diarrhea can appear following infectious enteritis, regardless of the nature of the pathogen. The pathogenesis of the diarrhea is not always clear and may be related to persistent infection or re-infection, secondary lactase deficiency, food protein allergy, antibiotic-associated diarrhea or a combination of these. In some cases, postinfectious diarrhea may be the initial manifestation of functional diarrhea, in which case is not associated with malabsorption.

Treatment of postinfectious diarrhea is supportive and may include a lactose-free diet in the presence of secondary lactase deficiency; infants might require a semi-elemental diet. The beneficial effect of specific probiotic products may be indicated in selected conditions.

PROXIMAL INTESTINAL BACTERIAL OVERGROWTH

Bacteria are normally present in large numbers in the colon (10^{11}-10^{13} colony-forming units [CFU]/g of feces) and have a symbiotic relationship with the host, providing nutrients and protecting the host from pathogenic organisms. Bacteria are usually present only in a small number in the stomach and small bowel; excessive numbers of bacteria in the stomach or small bowel are harmful. Bacterial overgrowth can result from clinical conditions that alter the gastric pH or small bowel motility, including disorders such as partial bowel obstruction, diverticula, intestinal failure, intestinal duplications, diabetes mellitus, idiopathic intestinal pseudoobstruction syndrome, and scleroderma, as well as proton pump inhibitor use. Prematurity, immunodeficiency, and malnutrition are other factors associated with bacterial overgrowth of the small bowel.

The diagnosis of bacterial overgrowth is often difficult and can be made by culturing small bowel aspirate (>10^5 CFU/mL) or by a lactulose hydrogen breath test. Lactulose is a synthetic disaccharide, which is not digested by mucosal brush border enzymes but can be fermented by bacteria. High baseline breath hydrogen and a quick rise in hydrogen in expired breath samples support the diagnosis of bacterial overgrowth; false-positive tests are common.

Bacterial overgrowth leads to inefficient intraluminal processing of dietary fat with steatorrhea due to bacterial deconjugation of bile salts, vitamin B_{12} malabsorption, and microvillus brush border injury with further malabsorption. Bacterial consumption of vitamin B_{12} and enhanced synthesis of folate result in decreased vitamin B_{12} and increased folate serum levels. Overproduction of D-*lactate* (the isomer of L-lactate) can cause stupor, neurologic dysfunction, and shock from D-lactic acidosis. Lactic acidosis should be suspected in children at risk of bacterial overgrowth, who show signs of neurologic deterioration and a high anion gap metabolic acidosis not explained by measurable acids such as L-lactate. Measurement of D-lactate is required because standard lactate assay only measures the L-isomer.

The treatment of bacterial overgrowth focuses on the correction of underlying causes such as partial obstruction. Oral metronidazole can provide relief for many months, but is not always effective. The cycling of antibiotics, including azithromycin, trimethoprim-sulfamethoxazole, ciprofloxacin, and metronidazole, may be required. Other alternatives are oral nonabsorbable antibiotics such as aminoglycosides, nitazoxanide, or rifaximin. Occasionally, antifungal therapy is required to control fungal overgrowth of the bowel.

ENVIRONMENTAL ENTEROPATHY (TROPICAL SPRUE)

This is the result of the interactions between enteric pathogens, enteropathy, and malnutrition, and is associated with a peculiar intestinal histology (enteropathy) occurring in several developing countries. It is similar or overlaps with tropical sprue and is associated with evident or subclinical malabsorption. It is a frequent cause of death in childhood in endemic regions, particularly in Asian areas, such as south India, and in several African countries. In developing countries selected pathogens including rotavirus, shigella, cryptosporidium, and entero-toxigenic *Escherichia coli* cause the majority of intestinal infections leading to moderate to severe diarrhea and often trigger a vicious circle with malnutrition. This tends to progress to wasting and stunting with or without a clear association with diarrhea.

In addition to a high risk of death, environmental enteropathy impairs normal growth and brain development, and impacts productivity. The etiology of this disorder is unclear because it follows outbreaks of acute diarrheal disease and improves with antibiotic therapy; therefore an infectious etiology is suspected. Nevertheless, environmental enteropathy includes inter-related mechanisms such as intestinal malabsorption, increased permeability, loss of intestinal mass, inflammation, increased bacterial translocation, and impairment of immune response. The incidence is decreasing worldwide, largely because of an improvement in hygiene and access to nutrients. Clinical symptoms include fever and malaise followed by diarrhea. After about a week the acute features subside, and anorexia, intermittent diarrhea, and chronic malabsorption result in severe malnutrition characterized by glossitis, stomatitis, cheilosis, night blindness, hyperpigmentation, and edema, reflecting the various nutrient deficiencies. Muscle wasting is often marked, and the abdomen is often distended. Megaloblastic anemia results from folate and vitamin B_{12} deficiencies.

Diagnosis is made by small bowel biopsy, which shows villous flattening with crypt hyperplasia and mild intestinal inflammation, with lipid accumulation in the surface epithelium.

Treatment requires nutritional supplementation, including supplementation of folate and vitamin B_{12}. To prevent recurrence, 6 mo of therapy with oral folic acid (5 mg) and antibiotics are recommended. Relapses occur in 10–20% of patients who continue to reside in an endemic tropical region. The scale-up of infrastructure, particularly the improvement in hygiene conditions and access to food in association with people empowerment through educational interventions, are the key to prevention rather than medical interventions in individual cases.

WHIPPLE DISEASE

Whipple disease is a chronic systemic infectious disorder. It is a rare disease, especially in childhood caused by *Tropheryma whipplei*, which can be cultured from a lymph node in the involved tissue.

The most common symptoms in Whipple disease are diarrhea, abdominal pain, weight loss, and joint pains. Malabsorption, lymphadenopathy, skin hyperpigmentation, and neurologic symptoms are also common. Involvement of other organs, such as eyes, heart, and kidneys, has been reported.

Diagnosis requires a high index of suspicion and is made upon demonstration of PAS-positive macrophage inclusions in the biopsy material, usually a duodenal biopsy. Positive identification using polymerase chain reaction for *T. whipplei confirms the diagnosis*.

Treatment requires antibiotics, such as trimethoprim sulfamethoxazole, for 1-2 yr. A 2-wk course of intravenous ceftriaxone or meropenem, followed by trimethoprim sulfamethoxazole for 1 yr, is recommended.

Bibliography is available at Expert Consult.

364.5 Immunodeficiency Disorders

Amit Assa and Raanan Shamir

GI disorders are present in 5–50% of patients with primary immune deficiencies driven by the fact that the gut is the largest lymphoid organ in the body. Malabsorption due to either intestinal inflammation or infection is common with primary immunodeficiency disorders; chronic diarrhea with failure to thrive is often the mode of presentation. Defects of humoral and or cellular immunity may be involved, including selective IgA deficiency, agammaglobulinemia, common variable immunodeficiency disease (CVID), severe combined immunodeficiency (SCID), hyper IgM syndrome, Wiskott-Aldrich syndrome, or chronic granulomatous disease. Although most patients with selective IgA deficiency are asymptomatic, malabsorption caused by giardiasis or nonspecific enteropathy with bacterial overgrowth can occur. Malabsorption syndrome or chronic noninfectious diarrhea manifesting as sprue-like enteropathy with villous atrophy has been reported in 60% of children with CVID. Malabsorption has also been reported in approximately 10% of patients with late-onset CVID, often secondary to giardiasis. Malabsorption as a result of infectious diarrhea—most commonly related to giardia, salmonella, campylobacter, cryptosporidium, and enteroviruses—is a well-recognized complication of X-linked agammaglobulinemia. Cryptosporidium is the most common pathogen causing diarrhea and malabsorption in hyper-IgM syndrome patients. SCID-affected children develop severe diarrhea and malabsorption early in life involving viral and opportunistic infections, especially chronic rotavirus infection, cytomegalovirus, and adenovirus. Malabsorption associated with immunodeficiency is exacerbated by villus atrophy and secondary disaccharidase deficiency. In chronic granulomatous disease, phagocytic function is impaired and granulomas develop throughout the GI tract, mimicking Crohn disease. In addition to failure to thrive, it is important to consider that malabsorption associated with immunodeficiency is often complicated by micronutrient deficiencies, including vitamins A, E, and B_{12}, and calcium, zinc, and iron.

Immunodeficiencies in children are more often secondary to other conditions such as cancer and chemotherapy. Malnutrition, diarrhea, and failure to thrive are common in untreated children with HIV infection. The risk of GI infection is related to the depression of the CD4 count. Opportunistic infections include *Cryptosporidium parvum,* cytomegalovirus, *Mycobacterium avium-intracellulare, Isospora belli, Enterocytozoon bieneusi, Candida albicans,* astrovirus, calicivirus, adenovirus, and the usual bacterial enteropathogens. In these patients, *Cryptosporidium* can cause a chronic secretory diarrhea.

Cancer chemotherapy can damage the bowel mucosa, leading to secondary malabsorption of disaccharides such as lactose. After bone marrow transplantation, mucosal damage from graft-versus-host disease can cause diarrhea and malabsorption. Small bowel biopsies show nonspecific villus atrophy, mixed inflammatory cell infiltrates, and increased apoptosis. Cancer chemotherapy and bone marrow transplantation are associated with pancreatic damage, which may lead to exocrine pancreatic insufficiency.

Bibliography is available at Expert Consult.

364.6 Immunoproliferative Small Intestinal Disease

Yael Mozer-Glassberg and Raanan Shamir

Lymphoma (Chapter 523) is the most common small bowel malignancy in the pediatric age group. Malignant lymphomas of the small intestine are categorized into 3 subtypes: Burkitt lymphoma, non-Hodgkin lymphomas, and Mediterranean lymphoma. Burkitt lymphoma, the most common form in children, characteristically involves the terminal ileum with extensive abdominal involvement. The relatively uncommon *Western* type of non-Hodgkin lymphomas (usually large B-cell type), can involve various regions of the small intestine. **Mediterranean lymphoma** (termed by The World Health Organization as *immunoproliferative small intestinal disease [IPSID]* or α-heavy chain disease) is a rare extra-nodal marginal zone B-cell lymphoma occurring primarily in the proximal small intestine. It is a variant of **mucosa-associated lymphoid-tissue lymphoma (MALT)** described in young adults from the developing world, and is characterized by lymphoplasmacytic intestinal infiltrates with monotypic α-heavy chain expression.

IPSID occurs most often in the proximal small intestine in older children and young adults in the Mediterranean basin, Middle East, Asia, and Africa. Poverty and frequent episodes of gastroenteritis during infancy are antecedent risk factors. The initial clinical presentation is intermittent diarrhea and abdominal pain. Later, chronic diarrhea with malabsorption, PLE, weight loss, digital clubbing, and growth failure ensue. Intestinal obstruction, abdominal masses, and ascites are common in advanced stages.

In contrast to primary nonimmunoproliferative small intestinal lymphomas, in which the pathology in the intestine is usually focal, involving specific segments of the intestine and leaving the segments between the involved areas free of disease, the pathology in IPSID is diffuse, with a mucosal cellular infiltrate involving large segments of the intestine and sometimes the entire length of the intestine, thus producing malabsorption. Molecular and immunohistochemical studies demonstrated an association with *Campylobacter jejuni* infection. The differential diagnosis includes chronic enteric infections (parasites, tropical sprue), CD, and other lymphomas. Radiologic findings include multiple filling defects, ulcerations, strictures, and enlarged mesenteric lymph nodes on CT scan.

The diagnosis is usually established by endoscopic biopsies and/or laparotomy. Upper endoscopy shows thickening, erythema, and nodularity of the mucosal folds in the duodenum and proximal jejunum. Capsule endoscopy may be helpful in the diagnosis. As the disease progresses, tumors usually appear in the proximal small intestine and rarely in the stomach. The diagnosis requires multiple duodenal and jejunal mucosal biopsies showing dense mucosal infiltrates, consisting of centrocyte-like and plasma cells. Progression to higher-grade large-cell lymphoplasmacytic and immunoblastic lymphoma is characterized by increased plasmocytic atypia with formation of aggregates and later sheets of dystrophic plasma cells and immunoblasts invading the submucosa and muscularis propria. A serum marker of IgA, a heavy-chain paraprotein, is present in most cases.

Treatment of early-stage IPSID with antibiotics results in complete remission in 30–70% of cases (tetracycline, ampicillin, or metronidazole) and some patients achieving durable remission that may last several years, but they should be monitored closely for relapse. However, the majority of untreated IPSID cases progress to lymphoplasmacytic and immunoblastic lymphoma invading the intestinal wall and mesenteric lymph nodes, which can metastasize to distant organs, requiring aggressive treatment with surgery and/or chemotherapy.

Bibliography is available at Expert Consult.

364.7 Short Bowel Syndrome

Yaron Avitzur and Raanan Shamir

Short bowel (or short gut) syndrome results from congenital malformations or resection of the small bowel (Table 364.11). Its incidence increases with low birth weight and earlier gestational age and is estimated at 7/1,000 live births in U.S. infants with birth weight <1,500 mg. Loss of >50% of the small bowel, with or without a portion of the large intestine, can result in symptoms of generalized malabsorptive disorder or in specific nutrient deficiencies, depending on the region of the bowel resected. At birth, the length of small bowel is 200-250 cm; by adulthood, it grows to 300-800 cm. Bowel resection in an infant has a better prognosis than in an adult because of the potential for intestinal growth and adaptation. An infant with as little as 15 cm of bowel with an ileocecal

Table 364.11	Causes of Short Bowel Syndrome

CONGENITAL
Congenital short bowel syndrome
Intestinal atresia
Gastroschisis

BOWEL RESECTION
Necrotizing enterocolitis
Volvulus with or without malrotation
Long segment Hirschsprung disease
Meconium peritonitis
Crohn disease
Trauma

valve, or 20 cm without, has the potential to survive and be eventually weaned from parenteral nutrition.

In addition to the length of the bowel, the anatomic location of the resection is also important. The proximal 100-200 cm of jejunum is the main site for carbohydrate, protein, iron, and water-soluble vitamin absorption, whereas fat absorption occurs over a longer length of the small bowel. Depending on the region of the bowel resected, specific nutrient malabsorption can result. Vitamin B_{12} and bile salts are only absorbed in the distal ileum (Fig. 364.10). Jejunal resections are generally tolerated better than ileal resections because the ileum, unlike the jejunum, can adapt to absorb nutrients and fluids. Net sodium and water absorption is relatively much higher in the ileum. Ileal resection has a profound effect on fluid and electrolyte absorption due to malabsorption of sodium and water by the remaining ileum; ileal malabsorption of bile salts stimulates increased colonic secretion of fluid and electrolytes. The presence of a colon in continuity is better tolerated and improves absorption and enteral autonomy.

TREATMENT

After bowel resection, treatment of short bowel syndrome is initially focused on repletion of the massive fluid and electrolyte losses while the bowel initially accommodates to absorb these losses. Proton pump inhibitors are usually added to reduce gastric secretions and to improve fluid balance. Nutritional support is often provided via parenteral nutrition. A central venous catheter should be inserted to provide parenteral fluid and nutrition support. The ostomy or stool output should be measured, and fluid and electrolyte losses adequately replaced. Measurement of urinary Na^+ to assess body Na^+ stores is useful to prevent Na^+ depletion. Maintaining urinary Na^+ higher than 20 mmol/L ensures that Na^+ intake is adequate. Early introduction of even a small amount of enteral feeding by mouth or tube feeding is essential and enhances bowel adaptation.

After the initial few weeks following resection, fluid and electrolyte losses stabilize, and the focus of therapy shifts to bowel rehabilitation with a gradual increase in the volume of enteral feeds. Continuous or bolus small-volume enteral feeding should be promoted with an extensively or partially hydrolyzed protein with MCT-enriched formula if the colon is in continuation. Breast milk is preferable over formula and its use should be encouraged as it stimulates gut hormones and promotes mucosal growth. Enteral feeding also increases pancreatobiliary flow and reduces parenteral nutrition-induced hepatotoxicity. Infant should be given a small amount of formula or mother's milk by mouth as early as possible to maintain an interest in oral feeding and to minimize or avoid the development of oral aversion. As intestinal adaptation occurs, enteral feeding increases, and parenteral supplementation decreases. The bowel mucosa proliferates, and the bowel lengthens with growth.

Approximately 60% of patients with short bowel syndrome achieve **enteral autonomy** within 5 yr of bowel resection and the majority achieve it in the first 2-3 yr after resection. In addition to bowel length, the presence of the ileocecal valve, a diagnosis of necrotizing enterocolitis, and care by an intestinal rehabilitation program increase the likelihood of achieving enteral autonomy.

Patients may require repeat surgeries for obstruction or bowel lengthening procedures (longitudinal lengthening, serial transverse enteroplasties or both) to optimize the bowel absorptive capacity. The bowel lengthening procedure is indicated in patients with dilated bowel who are unable to progress towards enteral autonomy or those with refractory bacterial overgrowth.

Vitamin and micronutrient deficiencies are common and worsen over time. The management of specific micronutrient and vitamin deficiencies and the treatment of transient problems, such as postinfectious mucosal malabsorption, are required. GI infections or small bowel bacterial overgrowth can cause setbacks in the progression to full enteral feeding in patients with marginal absorptive function. Marked increase in stool output or evidence of carbohydrate malabsorption (stool pH <5.5 and positive test for reducing substances) contraindicate further increases in enteral feeds. Slow advancement of continuous or bolus enteral feeding rates continues until all nutrients are provided enterally.

In patients with large stool output, the addition of soluble fiber and antidiarrheal agents, such as loperamide and anticholinergics, can be beneficial, although these drugs can increase the risk of bacterial overgrowth. Cholestyramine can be beneficial for patients with distal ileal resection, but its potential depletion of the BA pool can increase steatorrhea. Bacterial overgrowth is common in infants with a short bowel and can delay progression of enteral feedings. Empirical treatment with metronidazole or other antibiotics (nitazoxanide, rifaximin) is often useful. Diets high in fat and without simple sugars may be helpful in reducing bacterial overgrowth as well as enhancing adaptation.

COMPLICATIONS

Long-term complications of short bowel syndrome include those of parenteral nutrition: central catheter infection, thrombosis, intestinal failure associated liver disease (IFALD), and gallstones. Appropriate care of the central line to prevent infection and catheter-related thrombosis is extremely important. Sepsis is a leading cause of death, can occur any time after treatment is initiated (months to years later), and is most often bacterial (single organism more common than polymicrobial), although fungal infection may be noted in 20–25% of septic episodes. The use of an ethanol lock or Taurolidine lock can reduce the incidence of central catheter infections and prevent infections.

Some patients need long-term parenteral nutritional support, and lack of central line access is potentially life threatening; inappropriate removal or frequent changes of central lines in the neonatal period should be avoided. **IFALD** can lead to cholestasis, cirrhosis, and liver failure, and is a common reason for death or need the for transplantation. The incidence and severity of IFALD has significantly reduced over the last decade, probably due to the reduced use of soy-based lipid emulsions and the positive effect of omega–3-based lipid emulsions on cholestasis. Other complications of terminal ileal resection include vitamin B_{12} deficiency, which might not appear until 1-2 yr after parenteral nutrition is withdrawn. Long-term monitoring for deficiencies of vitamin B_{12}, folate, iron, fat-soluble vitamins, and trace minerals, such as zinc and copper, is important. Renal stones can occur as a result of hyperoxaluria secondary to steatorrhea (calcium binds to the excess fat and not to oxalate, so more oxalate is absorbed and excreted in the urine). Venous thrombosis and vitamin deficiency have been associated with hyper-homocysteinemia in short bowel syndrome. Bloody diarrhea secondary

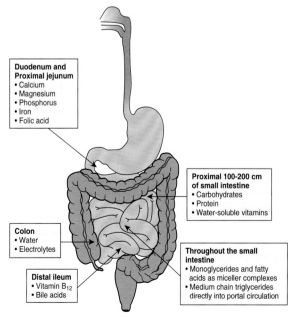

Fig. 364.10 Absorption of nutrients in the small bowel varies with the region.

to patchy, mild colitis can rarely develop during the progression of enteral feedings. The pathogenesis of this *feeding colitis* is unknown, but it is usually benign and can improve with a hypoallergenic diet or treatment with mesalamine.

In some children with life-threatening complications of parenteral nutrition, especially progressive liver failure and loss of vascular access, small intestine and liver transplantation becomes the preferred therapy (see Chapter 365).

Bibliography is available at Expert Consult.

364.8 Chronic Malnutrition
Yaron Avitzur and Raanan Shamir

Primary malnutrition is very common in developing countries and is directly related to increased disease burden and mortality. In developed countries, the etiology, clinical course, and outcomes are different. The American Society for Parenteral and Enteral Nutrition (ASPEN) defined pediatric malnutrition in developed countries as an imbalance between nutrient requirements and intake that results in cumulative deficits of energy, protein, or micronutrients that may negatively affect growth, development, and other relevant outcomes. Malnutrition can be classified as *illness related* (caused by disease/trauma) or *non-illness–related* (caused by environmental/behavioral factors). It can be further classified into *acute* malnutrition (<3 mo; short duration, weight loss without stunting) or *chronic* malnutrition (>3 mo; weight loss and stunting) that may differ in their etiology, growth patterns, and outcome. Chronic malnutrition occurs mainly as a result of decreased food intake, malabsorption syndromes, and increased nutritional needs in children with chronic diseases. Malnutrition is diagnosed in 11–50% of hospitalized children and reports from Europe suggest a prevalence of close to 20% in chronically ill children. Child neglect and improper preparation of formula can result in severe malnutrition. Malnutrition can be identified by evaluating dietary intake, by medical history (anorexia, vomiting, dysphagia, mood and behavioral changes, abdominal pain, diarrhea), by anthropometric measurements (e.g., reduced weight per age and weight per height, body mass index <5th percentile, mid upper arm circumference <−1 z score), by clinical signs of nutrient deficiencies (atrophic tongue in iron deficiency; anemia or alopecia in zinc deficiency) and by laboratory tests assessing vitamin and micronutrient deficiencies. Screening tools for malnutrition are used in adults to provide a simple and fast way of diagnosing those patients at risk for malnutrition. Few such screening tools for the pediatric population were developed to assess children at risk, but their use in clinical practice is still questionable.

Malnourished children suffer from impaired immunity, chronic enteropathy, poor wound healing, muscle weakness, and diminished psychologic drive. Malnutrition has short-term consequences (increased disability, morbidity, and mortality) and long-term consequences (final adult size, developmental deficiencies, economic productivity). Undernutrition in hospitalized children is associated with increased infectious complications, delayed recovery, increased length of stay and costs, increased readmission rate, and increased mortality.

Nutritional rehabilitation in malnourished children is discussed in Chapter 58.

Chronic malnutrition complicated by diarrheal dehydration is a commonly observed phenomenon. Infectious diarrhea is common in tropical and subtropical countries, in the setting of poor hygiene practices and water quality, in immunocompromised hosts (e.g., HIV, congenital immunodeficiency), and when impairment of the immune response is due to chronic malnutrition itself. In children with chronic disorders, diarrhea may be related to the underlying disease that should be sought for. Examples include noncompliance with a gluten-free diet in CD, noncompliance with pancreatic enzyme treatment in cystic fibrosis, and cholestatic liver disease with fat malabsorption. Malnutrition per se can lead to exocrine pancreatic insufficiency, which, in turn, aggravates malabsorption and diarrhea.

In infants and children with severe malnutrition, many of the signs normally used to assess the state of hydration or shock are unreliable. Severe malnutrition might be accompanied by sepsis; thus, children with septic shock might not have diarrhea, thirst, or sunken eyes but may be hypothermic, hypoglycemic, or febrile. Cardiac reserve is lowered, and heart failure is a common complication.

Despite clinical signs of dehydration, urinary osmolality may be low in the chronically malnourished child. Renal acidifying ability is also limited in patients with malnutrition.

Management of the diarrhea in chronically malnourished children is based on 3 principles: oral rehydration to correct dehydration, rapid resumption of feeds with avoidance of periods of nothing by mouth, and treating the etiology of the diarrhea.

When treating the dehydration, it must be remembered that in dehydrated and malnourished infants there appears to be overexpansion of the extracellular space accompanied by extracellular and presumably intracellular hypoosmolality. Thus reduced or hypotonic osmolarity oral rehydration solutions are indicated in this setting. When oral rehydration is not possible, the route of choice is nasogastric, and intravenous therapy should be avoided if possible.

Initial intravenous therapy in profound dehydration is designed to improve the circulation and expand extracellular volume. For patients with edema, the quality of fluid and the rate of administration might need to be readjusted from recommended levels to avoid overhydration and pulmonary edema. Blood should be given if the patient is in shock and severely anemic. Potassium salts can be given early if urine output is good. Clinical improvement may be more rapid with magnesium therapy.

Children with chronic malnutrition are at risk for the refeeding syndrome (see Chapter 58). Therefore initial calorie provision should not exceed the previous daily intake and is usually begun at 50–75% of estimated resting energy expenditure, with rapid increase to caloric goals once there are no severe abnormalities in sodium, potassium, phosphorus, calcium, or magnesium. Correction of malnutrition and catch-up growth are not part of the primary treatment of these children, but a nutrition rehabilitation plan is necessary.

Bibliography is available at Expert Consult.

364.9 Enzyme Deficiencies
Michael J. Lentze and Raanan Shamir

CARBOHYDRATE MALABSORPTION
Symptoms of carbohydrate malabsorption include loose watery diarrhea, flatulence, abdominal distention, and pain. Some children are asymptomatic unless the mal-absorbed carbohydrate is consumed in large amounts. Disaccharidases are present on the brush border membrane of the small bowel. **Disaccharidase deficiency** can be caused by a genetic defect or secondary to damage to the small bowel epithelium, as occurs with infection or inflammatory disorders.

Unabsorbed carbohydrates enter the large bowel and are fermented by intestinal bacteria, producing organic acids and gases such as methane and hydrogen. The gases can cause discomfort and the unabsorbed carbohydrates and the organic acids cause osmotic diarrhea characterized by an acidic pH and the presence of either reducing or nonreducing sugars in the stool. Hydrogen gas can be detected in the breath as a sign of fermentation of unabsorbed **carbohydrates (H_2-breath test).**

LACTASE DEFICIENCY
Congenital lactase deficiency is rare and is associated with symptoms occurring on exposure to lactose in milk. Fewer than 50 cases have been reported worldwide. In patients with congenital lactase deficiency, 5 distinct mutations in the coding region of the *LCT* gene were found. In most patients (84%), homozygosity for a nonsense mutation, 4170T-A (Y1390X; OMIM 223000), designated Fin (major), was found.

Primary adult type-hypolactasia is caused by a physiologic decline in lactase actively that occurs following weaning in most mammals. The brush-border lactase is expressed at low levels during fetal life; activity increases in late fetal life and peaks from term to 3 yr, after which levels gradually decrease with age. This decline in lactase levels varies between ethnic groups. Lactase deficiency occurs in approximately 15% of white adults, 40% of Asian adults, and 85% of African-American adults in the United States. Lactase is encoded by a single gene *(LCT)* of approximately 50 kb located on chromosome 2q21. C/T (−13910) polymorphisms of the *MCM6* gene were found to be related to adult-type hypolactasia in most European populations. In 3 African populations—Tanzanians, Kenyans, and Sudanese—3 single-nucleotide polymorphisms, G/C(−14010), T/G(−13915), and C/G(−13907), were identified with lactase persistence and have derived alleles that significantly enhance transcription from the lactase gene promoter in vitro.

Secondary lactose intolerance follows small bowel mucosal damage (CD, acute severe gastroenteritis) and is usually transient, improving with mucosal healing. Lactase deficiency can be diagnosed by H_2-breath test (2 g/kg up to 25 g) or by measurement of lactase activity in mucosal tissue retrieved by small bowel biopsy. Diagnostic testing is not mandatory, and often simple dietary changes that reduce or eliminate lactose from the diet relieve symptoms.

Treatment of lactase deficiency consists of a milk-free diet. A lactose-free formula (based on either soy or cow's milk) can be used in infants. In older children, low-lactose milk can be consumed. The addition of lactase to dairy products usually abbreviates the symptoms.

Live-culture yogurt contains bacteria that produce lactase enzymes and is therefore tolerated in most patients with lactase deficiency. Hard cheeses and cottage cheeses have a small amount of lactose and are generally well tolerated.

FRUCTOSE MALABSORPTION

Children consuming a large quantity of juice rich in fructose, corn syrup, or natural fructose in fruit juices can present with diarrhea, abdominal distention, and slow weight gain. Restricting the amount of juice in the diet resolves the symptoms and helps avoid unnecessary investigations. A fructose H_2 breath test can be helpful in the diagnosis of fructose malabsorption. The reason for fructose malabsorption is the reduced abundance of GLUT-5 transporter on the surface of the intestinal brush-border membrane, which occurs in approximately 5% of the population.

SUCRASE-ISOMALTASE DEFICIENCY

Sucrase-isomaltase (SI) deficiency is a rare autosomal recessive disorder with a complete absence of sucrase and reduced maltase digestive activity. The SI complex is composed of 1,927 amino acids encoded by a 3,364 bp messenger RNA. The gene locus on chromosome 3 has 30 exons spanning 106.6 kb. The majority of SI mutations result in a lack of enzyme protein synthesis (null mutation). Posttranslational processing defects are also identified.

Approximately 2% of Europeans and Americans are mutant heterozygote. Sucrase deficiency is especially common in indigenous Greenlanders (estimated 5%) in whom it is often accompanied by lactase deficiency. Gene variants of the SI are found to have some implications in IBS, because they were found more often in patients with IBS than in controls.

Symptoms of SI deficiency usually begin when the infant is exposed to sucrose or a glucose polymer diet. This can occur with ingestion of non–lactose-based infant formula or on the introduction of pureed food, especially fruits and sweets. Diarrhea, abdominal pain, and poor growth are observed. Occasionally, patients present with symptoms in late childhood or even adult life, but careful history often indicates that symptoms appeared earlier. Diagnosis of sucrase-isomaltase malabsorption requires acid hydrolysis of stool for reducing substances because sucrase is a nonreducing sugar. Alternatively, a diagnosis can be achieved with a hydrogen breath test, a direct enzyme assay of small bowel biopsy, or genetic testing.

The mainstay of treatment is lifelong dietary restriction of sucrose-containing foods, although symptoms may diminish with age. Enzyme replacement with a purified yeast enzyme, sacrosidase (Sucraid), is a highly effective adjunct to dietary restriction.

GLUCOSE-GALACTOSE MALABSORPTION

More than 30 different mutations of the sodium/glucose cotransporter gene *(SGLT1)* are identified. These mutations cause a rare autosomal recessive disorder of intestinal glucose and galactose/Na^+ cotransport system that leads to osmotic diarrhea. Because most dietary sugars are polysaccharides or disaccharides with glucose or galactose moieties, diarrhea follows the ingestion of glucose, breast milk, or conventional lactose-containing formulas. Dehydration and acidosis can be severe, resulting in death.

The stools are acidic and contain sugar. Patients with the defect have normal absorption of fructose, and their small bowel function and structure are normal in all other aspects. Intermittent or permanent glycosuria after fasting, or after a glucose load, is a common finding because of the transport defect also being present in the kidney. The presence of reducing substances in watery stools and slight glycosuria despite low blood sugar levels is highly suggestive of glucose-galactose malabsorption. Malabsorption of glucose and galactose is easily identified using the breath hydrogen test. It is safe to perform the 1st test with a dose of 0.5 g/kg of glucose; if necessary, a 2nd test can be performed using 2 g/kg. Breath H_2 will rise more than 20 ppm. The small intestinal biopsy is useful to document a normal villous architecture and normal disaccharidase activities. The identification of mutations of *SGLT1* makes it possible to perform prenatal screening in families at risk for the disease.

Treatment consists of rigorous restriction of glucose and galactose. Fructose, the only carbohydrate that can be given safely, should be added to a carbohydrate-free formula at a concentration of 6–8%. Diarrhea immediately ceases when infants are given such a formula. Although the defect is permanent, later in life, limited amounts of glucose, such as starches or sucrose, may be tolerated.

EXOCRINE PANCREATIC INSUFFICIENCY

Chapter 376 discusses disorders of exocrine pancreatic insufficiency. Cystic fibrosis is the most common congenital disorder associated with exocrine pancreatic insufficiency. Although rare, the next most common cause of pancreatic insufficiency in children is Shwachman-Diamond syndrome. Other rare disorders causing exocrine pancreatic insufficiency are Johanson-Blizzard syndrome (severe steatorrhea, aplasia of alae nasi, deafness, hypothyroidism, scalp defects) Pearson bone marrow syndrome (sideroblastic anemia, variable degree of neutropenia, thrombocytopenia), and isolated pancreatic enzyme deficiency (lipase, colipase and lipase-colipase, trypsinogen, amylase). Deficiency of enterokinase—a key enzyme that is produced in the proximal small bowel and is responsible for the activation of trypsinogen to trypsin—manifests clinically as exocrine pancreatic insufficiency.

Autoimmune polyendocrinopathy syndrome type 1, a rare autosomal recessive disorder, is caused by mutation in the autoimmune regulator gene (AIRE). Chronic mucocutaneous candidiasis is associated with failure of the parathyroid gland, adrenal cortex, pancreatic β cells, gonads, gastric parietal cells, and thyroid gland. Pancreatic insufficiency and steatorrhea are associated with this condition.

ENTEROKINASE (ENTEROPEPTIDASE) DEFICIENCY

Enterokinase (enteropeptidase) is a brush-border enzyme of the small intestine. It is responsible for the activation of trypsinogen into trypsin. Deficiency of this enzyme results in severe diarrhea, malabsorption, failure to thrive, and hypoproteinemic edema after birth.

The diagnosis can be established by measuring the enzyme level in intestinal tissue or by genetic testing, as enterokinase deficiency is caused by mutation in the serine protease-7 gene *(PRSS7)* on chromosome 21q21. Treatment of this rare autosomal recessive disorder consists of replacement with pancreatic enzymes and administration of a protein hydrolyzed formula with added MCT oil in infancy.

TREHALASE DEFICIENCY

The disaccharide trehalose is mainly present in mushrooms and has been approved to add to dried food. It is hydrolyzed by the intestinal trehalase into 2 molecules of glucose. Trehalase deficiency has been reported in 8% of Greenlanders, otherwise only 3 cases of this deficiency have been reported elsewhere. In untreated celiac disease the intestinal trehalase activity is reduced as those of other disaccharidases and recovers after introduction of a gluten-free diet.

TRYPSINOGEN DEFICIENCY

Trypsinogen deficiency is a rare syndrome with symptomatology similar to that of enterokinase deficiency. Enterokinase catalyzes the conversion of trypsinogen to trypsin, which, in turn, activates the various pancreatic proenzymes, such as chymotrypsin, procarboxypeptidase, and proelastase, for their active forms. Deficiency of trypsinogen results in severe diarrhea, malabsorption, failure to thrive, and hypoproteinemic edema soon after birth.

The trypsinogen gene is encoded on chromosome 7q35. Treatment is the same as for enterokinase deficiency, with pancreatic enzymes and protein hydrolysate formula with added MCT oil in infancy.

Bibliography is available at Expert Consult.

364.10 Liver and Biliary Disorders Causing Malabsorption

Anil Dhawan and Raanan Shamir

Absorption of lipids and lipid-soluble vitamins depend to a great extent on adequate bile flow delivering BA to the small intestine that help mixed micelle formation of lipid droplets. Most of the liver and biliary disorders lead to impairment of the bile flow, contributing to malabsorption of long-chain fatty acids and vitamins such as A, D, E, and K. Liver disorders that are associated with significant malabsorption and failure to thrive are mainly due to these categories:

PFIC syndromes and BA synthesis defects. PFIC type 1 is also associated with chronic diarrhea caused by bile transport defect in the gut. It is not uncommon for these children to have symptomatic fat-soluble vitamin deficiencies and suffer from pathologic fractures and peripheral neuropathy.

Children with storage disorders (e.g., **Wolman disease**) also manifest with severe failure to thrive and multiple vitamin deficiencies.

Children with biliary disorders such as biliary atresia after porto-enterostomy surgery (Kasai portoenterostomy), cystic fibrosis, neonatal sclerosing cholangitis, Alagille syndrome, and sclerosing cholangitis constitute another major group of disorders with reduced bile flow where malabsorption could be a significant challenge

Chronic liver disease of any etiology could also lead to lipid malabsorption from the above described mechanisms. In addition, severe portal hypertension can lead to portal hypertensive enteropathy, resulting in poor absorption of the nutrients.

Decompensated liver disease leads to anorexia and increased energy expenditures, further widening the gap between calorie intake and net absorption, leading to severe malnutrition. Adequate management of nutrition is essential to improve the outcome with or without liver transplantation. This is usually achieved by using MCT-rich milk formula, supplemental vitamins, and continuous or bolus enteral feed where oral intake is poor.

Vitamin D deficiency is commonly observed on biochemical tests, and children can present with pathologic fractures. Simultaneous administration of vitamin D with the water-soluble vitamin E preparation (TPGS 1,000 succinate) enhances absorption of vitamin D as well. In young infants with **cholestasis**, **oral vitamin D_3 is given** at a dose of 1,000 IU/kg/24 hr. After 1 mo, if the serum 25-hydroxyvitamin D level is low, intramuscular administration of 10,000 units/kg or maximum of 60,000 is recommend. Three 6 mo, 25-hydroxy vitamin D blood level monitoring is suggested in children with severe cholestasis.

Vitamin E deficiency in patients with chronic cholestasis is not usually symptomatic, but it can manifest as a progressive neurologic syndrome, which includes peripheral neuropathy (manifesting as loss of deep tendon reflexes and ophthalmoplegia), cerebellar ataxia, and posterior column dysfunction. Early in the course, findings are partially reversible with treatment; late features might not be reversible. It may be difficult to identify vitamin E deficiency because the elevated blood lipid levels in cholestatic liver disease can falsely elevate the serum vitamin E level. Therefore it is important to measure the ratio of serum vitamin E to total serum lipids; the normal level for patients younger than 12 yr of age is >0.6, and for patients older than 12 yr it is >0.8. The neurologic disease can be prevented with the use of an oral water-soluble vitamin E preparation (TPGS, Liqui-E) at a dose of 25-50 IU/day in neonates and 15-25 IU/kg/day in children.

Vitamin K deficiency can occur as a result of cholestasis and poor fat absorption. In children with liver disease it is very important to differentiate between the coagulopathy related to vitamin K malabsorption and one secondary to the synthetic failure of the liver. A single dose of vitamin K administered intravenously does not correct the prolonged prothrombin time in liver failure, but the deficiency state responds within a few hours. Easy bruising may be the first sign. In neonatal cholestasis, coagulopathy as a result of vitamin K deficiency can manifest with intracranial bleeds with devastating consequences, and prothrombin time should be routinely measured to monitor for deficiency in children with cholestasis. All children with cholestasis should receive regular vitamin K supplementation.

Vitamin A deficiency is rare and is associated with night blindness, xerophthalmia, and increased mortality if patients contract measles. Serum vitamin A levels should be monitored and adequate supplementation considered; caution should be observed as high levels of vitamin A can cause liver damage.

364.11 Rare Inborn Defects Causing Malabsorption

Corina Hartman and Raanan Shamir

Congenital (primary) malabsorption disorders originate from multitude types of defects including structural or functional defects of enterocytes or disorders involving other cellular lineages of the GI tract such as enteroendocrine or immune cells (see Chapter 364.3 and 367). Integral membrane proteins, which fulfill a transport function as receptor or channel across the apical or basolateral membrane of enterocytes for nutritional components, are another class of disorders associated with primary disorders of malabsorption. Histologic examination of the small and large bowel is typically normal. Most of these disorders are inherited in an autosomal recessive pattern. Most are rare, and patients present with a broad phenotypic heterogeneity as a result of modifier genes and nutritional and other secondary factors.

DISORDERS OF CARBOHYDRATE ABSORPTION

These are described in Chapter 364.9.

Patients with **Fanconi-Bickel syndrome** present with tubular nephropathy; rickets; hepatomegaly; glycogen accumulation in liver, kidney, and small bowel; failure to thrive; fasting hypoglycemia and postprandial hyperglycemia. The disorder is caused by homozygous mutations of GLUT2 *(SLC2A2)*, the facilitative monosaccharides transporter at the basolateral membrane of enterocytes, hepatocytes, renal tubules, pancreatic islet cells, and cerebral neurons. The patients exhibit postprandial hyperglycemia secondary to low insulin secretion (impaired glucose-sensing mechanisms in beta-cells) and fasting hypoglycemia due to altered glucose transport out of the liver. The increased intracellular glucose level inhibits glycogen degradation leading to glycogen accumulation and hepatomegaly. Similarly, altered monosaccharides transport out of enterocytes may be responsible for the putative glycogen accumulation and as a consequence, for diarrhea and malabsorption observed in some patients. Therapy includes the substitution of electrolyte losses and vitamin D, and supplying uncooked cornstarch to prevent hypoglycemia. Patients who present in the neonatal period need frequent small meals and galactose-free milk.

DISORDERS OF AMINO ACID AND PEPTIDE ABSORPTION

Protein digestion and absorption in the intestine is accomplished by a combination of proteases, peptidases, and peptide and amino acid transporters. Amino acid transporters are essential for the absorption of amino acids from nutrients, mediate the inter-organ, intercellular transfer of amino acids and the transport of amino acids between cellular compartments. Owing to their ontogenic origins, enterocytes and renal tubules share similar amino acid transporters. Their highest intestinal transporter activity is found in the jejunum. The transporters causing Hartnup disease, cystinuria, iminoglycinuria, and dicarboxylic amino-aciduria are located in the apical membrane, and those causing lysinuric protein intolerance (LPI) and blue diaper syndrome are anchored in the basolateral membrane of the intestinal epithelium.

Dibasic amino acids, including cystine, ornithine, lysine, and arginine are taken up by the Na-independent SLC3A1/SLC7A9, which is defective in cystinuria. Cystinuria is the most common primary inherited ami-noaciduria. This disorder is not associated with any GI or nutritional consequences because of compensation by an alternative transporter. However, hypersecretion of cystine in the urine leads to recurrent cystine stones, which account for up to 6–8% of all urinary tract stones in children. Ample hydration, urine alkalinization, and cystine-binding thiol drugs can increase the solubility of cystine. Cystinuria type I *(SLC3A1)* is inherited as an autosomal recessive trait, whether the transmission of non-type I cystinuria *(SLC7A9)* is autosomal dominant with incomplete penetrance. Cystinuria type I has been described in association with 2p21 deletion syndrome and hypotonia-cystinuria syndrome.

LPI is the second most common disorder of amino acids transport (see Chapter 103.14). LPI is caused by y$^+$LAT-1 (SLC7A7) carrier at the basolateral membrane of the intestinal and renal epithelium and the failure to deliver cytosolic dibasic cationic amino acids into the paracel-lular space. This defect is not compensated by the SLC3A1/SLC7A9 transporter at the apical membrane. The symptoms of LPI, which appear after weaning, include diarrhea, failure to thrive, hepatosplenomegaly, nephritis, respiratory insufficiency, alveolar proteinosis, pulmonary fibrosis, and osteoporosis. Abnormalities of bone marrow have also been described in a subgroup of LPI patients. The disorder is characterized by low plasma concentrations of dibasic amino acids (in contrast to high levels of citrulline, glutamine, and alanine) and massive excretion of lysine (as well as orotic acid, ornithine, and arginine in moderate excess) in the urine. Hyperammonemia and coma usually develop after episodic attacks of vomiting, after fasting, or following the administration of large amounts of protein (or alanine load), possibly because of a deficiency of intramitochondrial ornithine. Some patients show moderate retardation. Cutaneous manifestations can include alopecia, perianal dermatitis, and sparse hair. Some patients avoid protein-containing food. Immune dysfunction potentially attributable to nitric oxide overproduction secondary to arginine intracellular trapping might be the pathophysiological route explaining many LPI complications, including hemophagocytic lymphohistiocytosis, various autoimmune disorders, and an incompletely characterized immune deficiency. Treat-ment includes dietary protein restriction (<1.5 g/kg/day), orally administered citrulline (100 mg/kg/day), which is well absorbed from the intestine and carnitine supplementation.

Hartnup disease is characterized by the malabsorption of all neutral amino acids (except proline), including the essential amino acid tryptophan. It is characterized by aminoaciduria, photosensitive pellagra-like rash, headaches, cerebellar ataxia, delayed intellectual development, and diarrhea. The clinical spectrum ranges from asymptomatic patients to severely affected patients with progressive neurodegeneration leading to death by adolescence. SLC6A19, which is the major luminal sodium-dependent neutral amino acid transporter of small intestine and renal tubules, has been identified as the defective protein. Its association with collectrin and angiotensin-converting enzyme II is likely to be involved in the phenotypic heterogeneity of Hartnup disorder. Tryptophan is a precursor of nicotinamide adenine dinucleotide phosphate biosynthesis; therefore, the disorder can be treated by nicotinamide in addition to a diet of 4 g protein/kg. The use of lipid-soluble esters of amino acids and tryptophan ethyl ester has also been reported.

Defects in specific, basolateral tryptophan transporter (SLC16A10) are the cause of **blue diaper syndrome** (indicanuria, Drummond syndrome). Intestinal bacteria convert the unabsorbed tryptophan to indican, which is responsible for the bluish discoloration of the urine after its hydrolysis and oxidation. Symptoms can include digestive disturbances such as vomiting, constipation, poor appetite, failure to thrive, hypercalcemia,

nephrocalcinosis, fever, irritability, and ocular abnormalities.

The underlying defect of **iminoglycinuria** is the malabsorption of proline, hydroxyproline, and glycine as a consequence of the proton amino acid transporter SLC36A2 defect, with a possible participation of modifier genes, one of which (SLC6A20) is present in the intestinal epithelium. This disorder is usually benign, but sporadic cases with encephalopathy, mental retardation, deafness, blindness, kidney stones, hypertension, and gyrate atrophy have been described.

The neuronal glutamate transporter EAAT3 (SLC1A1) is affected in **dicarboxylic aminoaciduria**. This carrier is present in the small intestine, kidney, and brain, and transports the anionic acids L-glutamate, L- and D-aspartate, and L-cysteine. There are single case reports indicating that this disorder could be associated with hyperprolinemia and neurologic symptoms such as POLIP (polyneuropathy, ophthalmoplegia, leuko-encephalopathy, intestinal pseudoobstruction) syndrome.

DISORDERS OF FAT TRANSPORT
These are described in Chapter 104.3 and 364.3.

DISORDERS OF VITAMIN ABSORPTION
Transporters and receptors of the intestinal epithelium have been described for water-soluble but not fat-soluble vitamins, the latter being absorbed primarily into enterocytes by passive diffusion after the emulsification of fats by bile salts. Transfer proteins (retinol-binding protein, RBP4, and α-tocopherol transfer protein, TTP1) have been involved in deficiency states of vitamins E (spinocerebellar ataxia) and A (ophthalmologic signs), respectively.

Vitamin B$_{12}$ (cobalamin) is synthesized exclusively by microorganisms and is acquired mostly from meat and milk (see Chapter 481.2). Its absorption starts with the removal of cobalamin from dietary protein by gastric acidity and its binding to haptocorrin. In the duodenum, pancreatic proteases hydrolyze the cobalamin-haptocorrin complex, allowing the binding of cobalamin to intrinsic factor (IF), which originates from parietal cells. The receptor of the cobalamin-IF complex (Cbl-IF) is located at the apical membrane of the ileal enterocytes, and represents a heterodimer consisting of cubilin (CUBN) and amnionless (AMN). After endocytic uptake into endosomes, the Cbl-IF and its receptor binds to megalin and forms a cobalamin–transcobalamin-2 complex (after cleavage of IF) for further transcytosis. Vitamin B$_{12}$ exits the lysosome via LMBD1 and ABCD4, and is released to the blood stream most likely through the basolateral transporter multifunctional multidrug resistance protein 1 (MRP1). Biologically available circulating vitamin B$_{12}$ is bound to transcobalamin (TC), a nonglycosylated protein that carries 10–30% of the total vitamin B$_{12}$. TC-vitamin B$_{12}$ complexes enter the cells via 2 members of the LDL receptor gene family, CD320 and renal Lrp2/Megalin. As a cofactor for methionine synthase, cobalamin converts homocysteine to methionine. Cobalamin deficiency can be caused by inadequate intake of the vitamin (e.g., breastfeeding by mothers on a vegan diet), primary or secondary achlorhydria including autoim-mune gastritis, exocrine pancreatic insufficiency, bacterial overgrowth (see Chapter 364.4), ileal disease (Crohn disease, see Chapter 362.2), ileal (or gastric) resection, infections (fish tapeworm), and Whipple disease (see Chapter 367).

Clinical signs of congenital cobalamin malabsorption, which usually appear from a few months to more than 10 yr, are pancytopenia including **megaloblastic anemia**, fatigue, failure to thrive, and neurologic symp-toms, including developmental delay. Recurrent infections and bruising may be present. Laboratory evaluation indicates low serum cobalamin, hyperhomocysteinemia, methylmalonic acidemia, and mild proteinuria. The Schilling test is useful to differentiate between a lack of IF and the malabsorption of cobalamin. Several rare autosomal recessive disorders of congenital cobalamin deficiency affect absorption and transport of cobalamin (in addition to 7 other inherited defects of cobalamin metabolism). These include mutations of the gastric IF *(GIF)* gene with absence of IF (but normal acid secretion and lack of autoantibodies against IF or parietal cells), mutations of the *AMN* and *CUBN* genes subunits of the Cbl-IF receptor in ileum (**Imerslund-Grasbeck syn-drome**), and mutations in the TC 2 cDNA. Two new inborn defects were identified recently in the genes encoding LMBD1 and ABCD4 transporters, and are responsible for the rare Cbl-lF inborn defect resulting in the trapping of free vitamin B_{12} in lysosomes. These disorders require long-term parenteral cobalamin treatment: intramuscular injections of cobalamin. High-dose substitution with oral cyanocobalamin (1 mg biweekly) does not seem to be sufficient for all patients with congenital cobalamin deficiency.

Folate is an essential vitamin required to synthesize methionine from homocysteine. It is found mainly in green leafy vegetables, legumes, and oranges. After its uptake by enterocytes, folate is converted to 5-methyltetrahydrofolate. Secondary folate deficiency is caused by insufficient folate intake, villous atrophy (e.g., CD, IBD), treatment with phenytoin, and trimethoprim, among others (see Chapter 481.1). Several inherited disorders of folate metabolism and transport have been described.

Three mammalian folate transporter systems have been described to date in a variety of tissues: (1) the bidirectional reduced folate carrier 1 (RFC1, SLC19A1), (2) the glycosyl-phosphatidylinositol-anchored folate receptors (FOLR1, FOLR2, and FOLR4) responsible for folate-receptor mediated endocytosis, and (3) the human proton-coupled folate transporter (PCFT). Hereditary **folate malabsorption** is characterized by a defect of the PCFT of the brush-border, leading to impaired absorption of folate in the upper small intestine as well as impaired transport of folate into the central nervous system. Symptoms of congenital folate malabsorption are diarrhea, failure to thrive, megaloblastic anemia (in the first few mo of life), glossitis, infections *(Pneumocystis jiroveci)* with hypoimmunoglobulinemia, and neurologic abnormalities (seizures, intellectual impairment, and basal ganglia calcifications). Macrocytosis, with or without neutropenia, multilobulated polymorphonuclear cells, increased lactate dehydrogenase and bilirubin, increased saturation of transferrin, and decreased cholesterol can be found. Low levels of folate are present in serum and cerebrospinal fluid. Plasma homocysteine concentrations as well as urine excretion of formiminoglutamic acid and orotic acid are elevated. Long-lasting deficiency is best documented using red cell folate. Therapy involves large doses of oral (up to 100 mg/day) or systemic (intrathecal) folate. Sulfasalazine and methotrexate are potent inhibitors of PCFT. Therefore, folate deficiency may develop during treatment with these drugs. Although the RFC1 is ubiquitously expressed, including the brush-border membrane in the small intestine, involvement of RFC1 in intestinal folate uptake has not been confirmed.

The molecular basis of intestinal transport of other water-soluble vitamins such as vitamin C (Na^+-dependent vitamin C transporters 1 and 2), pyridoxine/vitamin B_6, and biotin/vitamin B_5 (Na^+-dependent multivitamin transporter) have been described; congenital defects of these transporter systems have not yet been found in humans. A **thiamine/vitamin B_1-responsive megaloblastic anemia** syndrome, which is associated with early-onset type 1 diabetes mellitus and sensorineural deafness, is caused by mutations of the thiamine transporter protein, THTR-1 (SLC19A2), present in the brush-border.

DISORDERS OF ELECTROLYTE AND MINERAL ABSORPTION

Congenital chloride diarrhea (CCD) belongs to the more common causes of severe congenital diarrhea, with prevalence in Finland of $1:20,000$. It is caused by a defect of the *SLC26A3* gene, which encodes a Na^+-independent Cl^-/HCO_3^- exchanger within the apical membrane of ileal and colonic epithelium. Founder mutations have been described in Finnish, Polish, and Arab patients: V317del, I675-676ins, and G187X, respectively. The Cl^-/HCO_3^- exchanger absorbs chloride originating from gastric acid and the cystic fibrosis transmembrane conductance regulator and secretes bicarbonate into the lumen, neutralizing the acidity of gastric secretion.

Prenatally, CCD is characterized by maternal polyhydramnios, dilated fetal bowel loops and preterm birth. Newborns with CCD present with severe life-threatening *secretory diarrhea* during the first few weeks of life. Volvulus has been reported in few patients with CCD. Laboratory findings are metabolic alkalosis, hypochloremia, hypokalemia, and hyponatremia (with high plasma renin and aldosterone activities). Fecal chloride concentrations are >90 mmol/L and exceed the sum of fecal

sodium and potassium. Early diagnosis and aggressive lifelong enteral substitution of KCl in combination with NaCl (chloride doses of 6-8 mmol/kg/day for infants and 3-4 mmol/kg/day for older patients) prevent mortality and long-term complications (such as urinary infections, hyperuricemia with renal calcifications, renal insufficiency, and hypertension) and allow normal growth and development. Orally administered proton pump inhibitors, cholestyramine, and butyrate can reduce the severity of diarrhea. The diarrheal symptoms usually tend to regress with age. However, febrile diseases are likely to exacerbate symptoms as a consequence of severe dehydration and electrolyte imbalances. (See Chapter 71 for fluid and electrolyte management.)

The classic form of **congenital sodium diarrhea** (CSD) manifests with polyhydramnios, massive *secretory diarrhea*, severe metabolic acidosis, alkaline stools (fecal pH > 7.5) and hyponatremia because of fecal losses of Na^+ (fecal Na^+ > 70 mmol/L). Urinary secretion of sodium is low to normal. CSD is clinically and genetically heterogeneous. A syndromic form of CSD with superficial punctate keratitis, choanal or anal atresia, hypertelorism, and corneal erosions has been related to mutations of *SPINT2,* encoding a serine–protease inhibitor, whose pathophysiologic action on intestinal Na^+ absorption is unclear. This form of CSD is also referred to as **CTE** (intestinal epithelial dysplasia), as it often shows clustered enterocytes that form "tufts" with branching crypts on histology (described in Chapter 364.3). Two genetic defects have been identified so far in several patients with the non-syndromic form of CSD. Dominant activating mutations in receptor guanylate cyclase C *(GUCY2C)* were found to cause a spectrum of secretory diarrheas including nonsyndromic CSD in 4 patients. These mutations were associated with elevated intracellular cyclic guanosine monophosphate (cGMP) levels that induced inhibition of NHE3 exchanger via its phosphorylation by cGMP kinase II. Mutations in *SLC9A3*, the gene encoding the Na^+/H^+ antiporter 3 (NHE3), the major intestinal brush-border Na^+/H^+ exchanger, were identified in 9 patients with non-syndromic CSD. IBD developed in a number of patients with dominant GC-C mutations, and also in 2 of 9 patients with recessive SLC9A3 mutations, implicating NHE3 in the pathogenesis of IBD in a subset of patients. The congenital form of **acrodermatitis enteropathica** manifests with severe deficiency of body zinc soon after birth in bottle-fed children, or after weaning from breastfeeding. Clinical signs of this disorder are anorexia, diarrhea, failure to thrive, humoral and cell-mediated immunodeficiency (poor wound healing, recurrent infections), male hypogonadism, skin lesions (vesicobullous dermatitis on the extremities and perirectal, perigenital, and perioral regions, and alopecia), and neurologic abnormalities (tremor, apathy, depression, irritability, nystagmus, photophobia, night blindness, and hypogeusia). The genetic defect of acrodermatitis enteropathica is caused by a mutation in the Zrt-Irt-like protein 4 (ZIP4, SLC39A4), normally expressed on the apical membrane, which enables the uptake of zinc into the cytosol of enterocytes. The zinc-dependent alkaline phosphatase and plasma zinc levels are low. Paneth cells in the crypt of the small intestinal mucosa show inclusion bodies. Acrodermatitis enteropathica requires long-term treatment with elemental zinc at 1 mg/kg/day. Maternal zinc deficiency impairs embryonic, fetal, and postnatal development. Chapter 67 describes the *acquired* forms of zinc deficiency. Transient neonatal zinc deficiency is an autosomal dominant disorder with similar manifestations as AE. The disease is caused by mutations in ZnT2, the transporter responsible for supplying human milk with zinc.

Menkes disease and **occipital horn syndrome** are both caused by mutations in the gene encoding Cu^{2+} transporting adenosine triphosphatase (ATPase), α-polypeptide (ATP7A), also called Menkes or MNK protein. ATP7A is mainly expressed by enterocytes, placental cells, and the central nervous system, and is localized in the *trans*-Golgi network for copper transfer to enzymes in the secretory pathway or to endosomes to facilitate copper efflux. Copper values in liver and brain are low in contrast to an increase in mucosal cells, including enterocytes and fibroblasts. Plasma copper and ceruloplasmin levels decline postnatally. Clinical features of Menkes disease are progressive cerebral degeneration (convulsions), feeding difficulties, failure to thrive, hypothermia, apnea, infections (urinary tract), peculiar facies, hair abnormalities (kinky hair), hypopigmentation, bone changes, and cutis laxa. Patients with the classic form of Menkes disease usually die before the age of 3 yr. A therapeutic trial with copper-histidinase should start before the age of 6 wk. In contrast to Menkes disease, occipital horn syndrome usually manifests during adolescence with borderline intelligence, craniofacial abnormalities, skeletal dysplasia (short clavicles, pectus excavatum, genu valgum), connective tissue abnormalities, chronic diarrhea, orthostatic hypotension, obstructive uropathy, and osteoporosis. It should be differentiated from Ehlers-Danlos syndrome type V.

Active calcium absorption is mediated by the transient receptor potential channel 6 (TRPV6) at the brush border membrane, calbindin, and the Ca-ATPase, or the Na^+-Ca^{++} exchanger for calcium efflux at the basolateral membrane within the proximal small bowel. A congenital defect of these transporters has not yet been described.

Intestinal absorption of dietary magnesium, which occurs via the transient receptor potential channel TRPM6 at the apical membrane, is impaired in familial **hypomagnesemia with secondary hypocalcemia**, which manifests with neonatal seizures and tetany.

Intestinal iron absorption consists of several complex regulated processes starting with the uptake of heme-containing iron by heme carrier protein 1 (HCP1) and Fe^{2+} (after luminal reduction of oxidized Fe^{3+}) by the divalent metal transporter 1 (DMT1) at the apical membrane, followed by the efflux of Fe^{2+} by ferroportin 1 (also called the iron-regulated transporter) at the basolateral membrane of duodenal enterocytes. Hepatic hormone hepcidin has a key role in iron homeostasis by interacting with ferroportin. When it binds to ferroportin, hepcidin induces phosphorylation of the iron exporter, causing its internalization and degradation. A decrease in the ferroportin protein level on the cell surface inhibits iron export from intracellular pools. Thus, hepcidin controls plasma iron levels by reducing iron absorption in the gut, lowering iron release from hepatocytes, and preventing iron recycling by macrophages Hepcidin deficiency causes iron overload in hereditary hemochromatosis and iron-loading anemias, whereas hepcidin excess causes or contributes to the development of iron-restricted anemia in inflammatory diseases, infections, some cancers, and chronic kidney disease. Mutations of the ferroportin 1 gene have been found in the autosomal dominant form of **hemochromatosis** type 4. Mutations within the hemochromatosis (HFE) gene (Cys282 Tyr, His63Asn, Ser65Cys) of classic hemochromatosis reduce the endocytic uptake of diferric transferrin by the transferrin receptor-1 at the basolateral membrane of the intestinal epithelium. Hepcidin is the defective gene of juvenile hemochromatosis (type 2, subtype B). Elevated hepcidin results in hypoferremia and insufficient supply of iron for erythropoiesis, leading to different types of anemia. The underlying causes of hepcidin elevation in iron-restricted anemias are varied. An example of a genetic cause of hepcidin increase is the familial **iron-refractory iron deficiency anemia** (IRIDA), an autosomal recessive disorder caused by a mutation in matriptase-2 *(TMPRSS6)*, a negative regulator of hepcidin expression. This anemia is characterized by very low plasma iron levels, unresponsiveness to oral iron therapy and partial correction by parenteral iron. Mutations in DMT1 transporter *(SLC11A2)* are another cause of **IRIDA**. The development of severe microcytic, hypochromic anemia typifies these patients; however, surprisingly, some of them load iron in the liver.

Bibliography is available at Expert Consult.

Chapter **365**

Intestinal Transplantation in Children With Intestinal Failure

Jorge D. Reyes and André A.S. Dick

第三百六十五章
儿童小肠衰竭和小肠移植

中文导读

　　本章主要介绍了小肠衰竭肠移植的适应证、手术方式及术后处理。详尽阐述了小肠移植的适应证，包括静脉通路不足、威胁生命的感染及肝脏疾病。详细介绍了肠移植手术的供者选择、肠移植类型及受者手术方法。详尽阐述了移植后的术后处理，包括免疫抑制、同种异体移植后的评估、排异和移植物抗宿主反应的临床表现及处理、感染治疗和小肠移植的预后。

The introduction of tacrolimus and the development of the abdominal multiorgan procurement techniques allowed the tailoring of various types of intestine grafts that can contain other intraabdominal organs, such as the liver, pancreas, and stomach. The understanding that the liver protects the intestine against rejection demonstrates the interaction between recipient and donor immunocytes (host-versus-graft and graft-versus-host) which under the cover of immunosuppression allows varying degrees of graft acceptance and eventual minimization of drug therapy. Over the past several years the number of patients placed on the list for and those undergoing intestinal transplantation has decreased, which may be a result of (1) improvements in the care of patients with intestinal failure under a multidisciplinary intestinal care team management, (2) the introduction of new lipid management strategies for the treatment of cholestatic liver disease, and (3) corrective surgery enhancing absorptive surface and motility, which has led to increased survival and decreased morbidity.

INDICATIONS FOR INTESTINAL TRANSPLANT

Intestinal failure describes a patient who has lost the ability to maintain nutritional support and adequate fluid requirements, needed to sustain growth, with their own intestine and is permanently dependent on total parenteral nutrition (TPN). The majority of these patients have short bowels as a result of a congenital deficiency or acquired condition (see Chapter 364.07). In others, the cause of intestinal failure is a functional disorder of motility or absorption (Table 365.1). Rarely do patients receive intestinal transplants for benign neoplasms. The complications of intestinal failure include loss of venous access, life-threatening infections, and TPN-induced cholestatic liver disease.

Paucity of Venous Access

Administration of TPN requires the insertion of a centrally placed venous catheter, there being only 6 readily accessible sites (bilateral internal jugulars, subclavians, iliac veins). The loss of venous access generally occurs in the setting of recurrent catheter sepsis and thrombosis; clinical convention suggests that loss of 50% of these venous access sites places the patient at risk of not being able to be treated with TPN.

Life-Threatening Infections

Life-threatening infections are usually catheter-related; the absence of significant lengths of intestine may be associated with abnormal motility of the residual bowel (producing both delayed or rapid emptying), with varying degrees of bacterial overgrowth and possible bacterial or fungal translocation as a consequence of loss of intestinal barrier function and/or loss of gut immunity. This situation can produce cholestatic liver disease, multisystem organ failure, and metastatic infectious foci in lungs, kidneys, liver, and the brain.

Table 365.1	Causes of Intestinal Failure in Children Requiring Transplantation

SHORT BOWEL
- Congenital disorders
- Volvulus
- Gastroschisis
- Necrotizing enterocolitis
- Intestinal atresia
- Trauma

INTESTINAL DYSMOTILITY
- Intestinal pseudoobstruction
- Intestinal aganglionosis (Hirschsprung disease)

ENTEROCYTE DYSFUNCTION
- Microvillus inclusion disease
- Tufting enteropathy
- Autoimmune disorders
- Crohn disease

TUMORS
- Familial polyposis
- Inflammatory pseudotumor

Liver Disease

The development of cholestatic liver disease is the most serious complication of intestinal failure and may be a consequence of the toxic drug effects of TPN on hepatocytes, a disruption of bile flow and bile acid metabolism, and the frequent occurrence of bacterial translocation and sepsis with endotoxin release into the portal circulation. This complication varies in frequency depending on the patient's age and the etiology of the intestinal failure; it is most common in neonates with extreme short gut. The effects on the liver include fatty transformation, steatohepatitis and necrosis, fibrosis, and then cholestasis. The development of clinical jaundice (total bilirubin > 3 mg/dL) and thrombocytopenia are significant risk factors for poor outcome, because these changes portend the development of portal hypertensive gastroenteropathy, hypersplenism, coagulopathy, and uncontrollable bleeding.

TRANSPLANTATION OPERATION
Donor Selection

Intestinal grafts are usually procured from hemodynamically stable, ABO-identical brain-dead donors who have minimal clinical or laboratory evidence suggesting intraabdominal ischemia; size matching varies according to age of the recipients; present surgical techniques allow for significant reductions of the graft in order to achieve abdominal closure. Human leukocyte antigen has been random, and cross matching has not been a determinant of graft acceptance. Exclusion criteria include a history of malignancy and intraabdominal evidence of infection; systemic viral or bacterial infections are not excluded. Donor preparation has been limited to the administration of systemic and enteral antibiotics. Prophylaxis for graft-versus-host disease with graft pretreatment using irradiation or a monoclonal antilymphocyte antibody has varied over time. Grafts have been preserved with the University of Wisconsin solution, as is the case with other types of abdominal organs.

Types of Intestinal Grafts

Intestinal allografts are used in various forms, either alone (as an **isolated intestine graft**) or as a composite graft, which can include the liver, duodenum, and pancreas (**liver–intestine graft**); when this composite graft includes the stomach, and the recipient operation requires the removal of all of the patient's gastrointestinal tract (as with intestinal pseudoobstruction) and liver, then this replacement graft is known as a **multivisceral graft**.

The procurement of these various types of grafts focuses on the preservation of the arterial vessels of celiac and/or superior mesenteric arteries, as well as appropriate venous outflow, which would include the superior mesenteric vein or the hepatic veins in the composite grafts. The larger composite grafts inherently retain the celiac and superior mesenteric arteries; this includes multivisceral grafts, liver plus small bowel grafts, and *modified multivisceral grafts* in which the liver is excluded but the entire gastrointestinal tract is replaced, including the stomach. The isolated intestine graft retains the superior mesenteric artery and vein; this graft can be accomplished with preservation of the vessels going to the pancreas, when that organ has been allocated to another recipient. The graft that is to be used in a particular recipient is dissected out in situ and then removed after cardiac arrest of the donor, with core cooling of the organs, using an infusion of preservation solution (Fig. 365.1).

Various modifications in these grafts have included the preservation of visceral ganglia at the base of the arteries, the inclusion of donor duodenum and pancreas for the liver and intestine graft, the inclusion of colon, the reduction of the liver graft (into left or right side) and variable reduction of the intestine graft, and the development of living donor intestine grafts.

The Recipient Operation

Because many children have had multiple previous abdominal operations, intestinal transplantation can be a formidable technical challenge; most children require replacement of the liver because of TPN-induced disease and often present with advanced liver failure. Transplantation of an isolated intestinal allograft involves exposure of the lower abdomen, infrarenal aorta, and inferior vena cava. Placement of vascular homografts

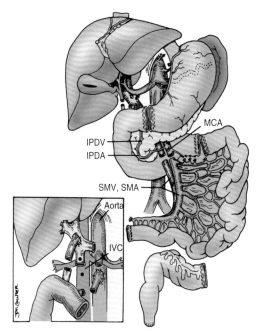

Fig. 365.1 The various abdominal organs can be dissected in situ, providing isolated or composite grafts to fit the individual patient's needs. Separation of intestine and pancreas is feasible, with preservation of the inferior pancreaticoduodenal artery (IPDA) and vein (IPDV). The use of vascular grafts from the donor allow connections to the superior mesenteric pedicle (artery [SMA] and vein [SMV]) to aorta and inferior vena cava (IVC) or portal vein (inset). MCA, Major coronary artery. (From Abu-Elmagd K, Fung J, Bueno J, et al: Logistics and technique for procurement of intestinal, pancreatic and hepatic grafts from the same donor, Ann Surg 232:680–697, 2000.)

using donor iliac artery and vein to these vessels allows arterialization and venous drainage of the intestinal graft. In patients who have retained their intestine and then undergo an enterectomy at the time of transplantation, use of the native superior mesenteric vessels is feasible.

Transplantation of a larger composite graft requires the removal and replacement of the native liver in the liver with intestine transplant, and complete abdominal exenteration in the multivisceral transplant.

In a similar fashion, the infrarenal aorta is exposed for placement of an arterial conduit graft (donor thoracic aorta) for arterialization of the graft. The venous drainage is achieved to the retained hepatic veins, which are fashioned to a single conduit for anastomosis to the allograft liver.

The intestinal anastomosis to native proximal and distal bowel is performed, leaving an enterostomy of distal allograft ileum; this will be used for routine posttransplantation surveillance endoscopy and biopsy. This ostomy is closed 3-6 mo after transplantation (Fig. 365.2).

POSTOPERATIVE MANAGEMENT
Immunosuppression
Successful immunosuppression for intestinal transplantation is initiated with tacrolimus and corticosteroids. This required high levels of tacrolimus (in the nephrotoxic range), and although initial success rates were high they were followed by rejection rates of > 80%, infection, and late drug toxicities, resulting in a gradual loss of grafts and patients. The next generation of protocols incorporated the addition of other agents, such as azathioprine, cyclophosphamide, induction with an interleukin-2 antibody antagonist, mycophenolate mofetil, and rapamycin. This modification resulted in a decreased incidence in the severity of initial rejection; the ability to decrease immunosuppression later did not allow for stabilization of long-term survival. The introduction of *recipient pretreatment* using antilymphocyte antibodies and the elimination of recipient therapy with steroids have resulted in improved transplant survival as a result of a significant decrease in the incidence of rejection and infection, permitting the gradual decrease of immunosuppressive drug therapy within 3 mo, and a decline in drug toxicity events. The most common induction regimen used is T cell depleting agents followed by -2 receptor antagonists (Fig. 365.3). A mainstay of maintenance immunosuppression is tacrolimus and prednisone dual therapy. By 1 yr the majority of patients are on tacrolimus monotherapy (Fig. 365.4).

Allograft Assessment
There are no simple laboratory tools that allow assessment of the intestinal allograft. The gold standard for diagnosis of intestinal allograft rejection has been serial endoscopic surveillance and biopsies through the allograft ileostomy. Clinical signs and symptoms of rejection or infection of the allograft can overlap and mimic each other, producing either rapid diarrhea or complete ileus with pseudoobstruction syndromes, or gastrointestinal bleeding. Any changes in clinical status should warrant thorough evaluation for rejection with endoscopic biopsies and an evaluation for opportunistic infection, malabsorption, and other enteral infections.

Small Bowel Transplantation Surgery

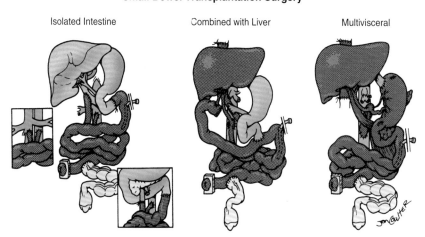

Fig. 365.2 The three basic intestinal transplant procedures (the graft is *shaded*). With the isolated intestine, the venous outflow may be to the recipient portal vein (*main figure*), inferior vena cava (*inset left*), or superior mesenteric vein (*inset right*). With the composite grafts, which include the liver, the arterialization is from the aorta with venous drainage out from the liver graft to the recipient inferior vena cava.

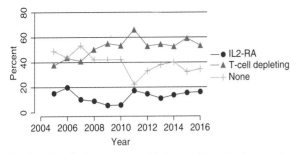

Fig. 365.3 Induction agents used in intestinal transplant recipients. Immunosuppression at transplant reported to the OPTN. *IL2-RA, interleukin-2 receptor antagonist. (From Organ Procurement and Transplantation Network (OPTN) and Scientific Registry of Transplant Recipients (SRTR). OPTN/SRTR 2016 Annual Data Report. Fig IN28. Rockville, MD: Department of Health and Human Services, Health Resources and Services Administration; 2018. Available at https://srtr.transplant.hrsa.gov/annual_reports/Default.aspx)*

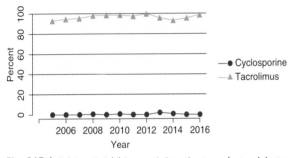

Fig. 365.4 Calcineurin inhibitor use in intestine transplant recipients. Immunosuppression at transplant reported to the OPTN. *(From Organ Procurement and Transplantation Network (OPTN) and Scientific Registry of Transplant Recipients (SRTR). OPTN/SRTR 2016 Annual Data Report. Fig IN29. Rockville, MD: Department of Health and Human Services, Health Resources and Services Administration; 2018. Available at https://srtr.transplant.hrsa.gov/annual_reports/Default.aspx)*

The diagnosis of *acute rejection* is based on seeing destruction of crypt epithelial cells from apoptosis, in association with a mixed lymphocytic infiltrate. These histologic findings may or may not correlate with endoscopic evidence of injury, which varies from diffuse erythema and friability to ulcers and, in cases of severe rejection, exfoliation of the intestinal mucosa. *Chronic rejection* of the allograft can be diagnosed only through full-thickness sampling of the intestine, which shows the typical vasculopathy that can result in progressive ischemia of the allograft.

Rejection and Graft-Versus-Host Disease

Acute rejection rates for the intestinal allograft are significantly higher than with any other organ, in the range of 80–90%, and severe rejection requiring the use of antilymphocyte antibody preparations may be as high as 30%. Triple-drug regimens and the use of interleukin-2 antibody inhibitors have resulted in significant decreases in rejection rates; nonetheless, the amount of immunosuppression was incompatible with improvements in long-term patient and graft survival. Rejection rates of 40% are achievable with the use of antilymphocyte globulin. These protocols induce varying degrees of *proper tolerance*, which can eventually allow for minimization of immunosuppression, thus reducing the risk of drug toxicity and infection. Vascular rejection has been an uncommon

occurrence, and chronic rejection has been seen in approximately 15% of cases.

Graft-versus-host disease is infrequent but potentially life-threatening; the mortality rate exceeds 80% and most recipients die from infectious complications from bone marrow failure. The incidence seen in intestinal transplantation is 5–6%. Although no standard treatment is available, early diagnosis, prevention of infection, and initiation of treatment as soon as possible may improve outcomes.

Infections

Infectious complications are the most significant cause of morbidity and mortality after intestinal transplantation. The most common infections (bacterial, fungal, polymicrobial) occur as a result of the continuing need for venous catheter placement for as long as 1 yr posttransplantation. Infections as a consequence of immunosuppressive drug management are from cytomegalovirus (CMV) infection (22% incidence), Epstein-Barr virus (EBV)–induced infections (21% incidence), and adenovirus enteritis (40% incidence). Despite improvements in monitoring and preventative measures, CMV remains the most common viral infection postintestinal transplantation. CMV may be acquired from blood transfusions, reactivation of endogenous viruses, or the donated allograft. The highest-risk recipients for CMV infection are those who are immunologically naïve and receive an allograft from a donor who is seropositive. The 2 CMV prevention strategies commonly employed are universal prophylaxis and preemptive therapy. Consensus guidelines recommend prophylaxis treatment for high-risk patients (donor+/recipient−). The preferred drugs for CMV prophylaxis are ganciclovir and oral valganciclovir.

Patients at the highest risk for EBV infection are those who are seronegative at the time of transplantation and those requiring a high-burden immunosuppressive therapy to maintain their graft. EBV disease varies from asymptomatic viremia to posttransplant lymphoproliferative disorder (PTLD). The incidence of EBV-related PTLD is highest in patients receiving intestinal allografts compared to liver, heart, or kidney. Children have a higher incidence of PTLD compared to adults, and are most likely to have EBV+PTLD. Early diagnosis and prevention of PTLD is essential and the mainstay of therapy is to reduce immunosuppression, although some patients have required chemotherapy. The use of anti–B-cell monoclonal antibodies, such as the anti-CD20 antibody rituximab, in PTLD has been successful as noted in anecdotal reports. Successful management of these viral infections is achieved through early detection and preemptive therapy, for both CMV and EBV, before the development of a serious life-threatening infection. This approach has improved outcomes for CMV, eliminating the mortality in the pediatric patient population (see Chapters 205, 281, and 282).

Outcomes

Intestinal transplantation is the standard of care for children with intestinal failure who have significant complications of TPN and can no longer tolerate such therapy. Data from the Organ Procurement and Transplantation Network (OPTN)/Scientific Registry of Transplant Recipients (SRTR) Annual Report 2015, and center-specific data reports have documented significant improvements with short- and long-term survivals for transplantations occurring principally in the last 10 yr; isolated intestinal transplantation graft failure rates for deceased donor transplants in 2013-2014 were 24.5% at 1 yr, 42.4% at 3 yr for transplants in 2011-2012, and 54% at 5 yr for transplants in 2009-2010 (Fig. 365.5). For liver-intestine recipients during the same time period graft failure rates were 27% at 1 yr, 33.3% at 3 yr, 48.7% at 5 yr, and 51% at 10 yr for transplants 2003-2004 (Fig. 365.6). It is hoped that with the minimization strategies currently used the long-term survival will plateau as occurs with other organ transplants; rehabilitation and quality-of-life studies have shown that more than 80% of survivors reach total independence from TPN and have meaningful life activities. Consequently, there has been a shift in efforts to improve long-term outcomes and quality of life.

Bibliography is available at Expert Consult.

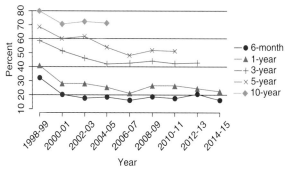

Fig. 365.5 Graft failure among transplant recipients of intestine without liver. All recipients of deceased donor intestines, including multiorgan transplants. Patients are followed until the earliest of retransplant, graft failure, death, or December 31, 2016. Estimates computed with Cox proportional hazards models adjusted for age, sex, and race. *(From Organ Procurement and Transplantation Network (OPTN) and Scientific Registry of Transplant Recipients (SRTR). OPTN/SRTR 2016 Annual Data Report. Fig IN37. Rockville, MD: Department of Health and Human Services, Health Resources and Services Administration; 2018. Available at https://srtr.transplant.hrsa.gov/annual_reports/Default .aspx)*

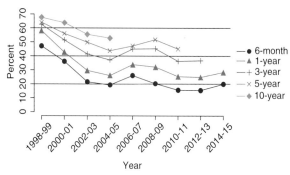

Fig. 365.6 Graft failure among transplant recipients of intestine with liver. All recipients of deceased donor intestines, including multiorgan transplants. Patients are followed until the earliest of retransplant, graft failure, death, or December 31, 2016. Estimates computed with Cox proportional hazards models adjusted for age, sex, and race. *(From Organ Procurement and Transplantation Network (OPTN) and Scientific Registry of Transplant Recipients (SRTR). OPTN/SRTR 2016 Annual Data Report. Fig IN38. Rockville, MD: Department of Health and Human Services, Health Resources and Services Administration; 2018. Available at https://srtr.transplant.hrsa.gov/annual_reports/Default.aspx)*

Chapter 366
Acute Gastroenteritis in Children

Karen L. Kotloff

第三百六十六章
儿童急性胃肠炎

中文导读

　　本章主要介绍了儿童腹泻的危害及相关病原学，详细介绍了美国、中高收入国家和中低收入国家的流行病学特点，以及感染性腹泻的病理生理机制，总结了腹泻的临床表现和肠内肠外并发症，从临床评估及实验室检查方面对腹泻进行鉴别诊断。详细阐述了治疗方案，包括脱水的治疗、喂养及饮食的选择、补锌、抗感染治疗等。介绍了急性腹泻的预防，包括母乳喂养和维生素A的摄入、轮状病毒疫苗以及改善水和卫生条件，提高个人和家庭卫生（原文第366）。简单介绍了旅行者腹泻的治疗及预防（原文第366.1）。

The term *gastroenteritis* denotes inflammation of the gastrointestinal tract, most commonly the result of infections with bacterial, viral, or parasitic pathogens (Tables 366.1 to 366.3). Many of these infections are foodborne illnesses (Table 366.4). Several clinical syndromes are often described because they have different (albeit overlapping) etiologies, outcomes, and treatments. **Acute gastroenteritis** (AGE) captures the bulk of infectious cases of diarrhea. The most common manifestations are diarrhea and vomiting, which can also be associated with systemic features such as abdominal pain and fever. **Dysentery** refers to a syndrome characterized by frequent small stools containing visible blood, often accompanied by fever, tenesmus, and abdominal pain. This should be distinguished from bloody diarrhea (larger volume bloody stools with less systemic illness) because the etiologies may differ. **Prolonged** (lasting 7-13 days) and **persistent diarrhea** (lasting 14 days or longer) are important because of their impact on growth and nutrition.

BURDEN OF CHILDHOOD DIARRHEA

Although global mortality due to diarrheal diseases has declined substantially (39%) during the past 2 decades, it remains unacceptably high. In 2015, diarrheal disease caused an estimated 499,000, or 8.6% of all childhood deaths, making it the 4th most common cause of child mortality worldwide. Over the same period, a smaller decline (10%) was observed in the incidence of diarrhea disease among children younger than 5 yr. Almost 1.0 billion episodes occurred in 2015 worldwide, resulting in an estimated 45 million childhood disability-adjusted life years. Approximately 86% of the episodes occurred in Africa and South Asia (63% and 23%, respectively). The decline in diarrheal mortality, despite the lack of significant changes in incidence, is the result of preventive rotavirus vaccination and improved case management of diarrhea, as well as improved nutrition of infants and children. These interventions have included widespread home- and hospital-based oral rehydration solution (ORS) therapy and improved nutritional management of children with diarrhea.

In addition to the risk of mortality, high rates of diarrhea can be associated with long-term adverse outcomes. Diarrheal illnesses, especially episodes among young children that are recurrent, prolonged, or persistent, can be associated with malnutrition, stunting, micronutrient deficiencies, and significant deficits in psychomotor and cognitive development.

PATHOGENS

Rotavirus is the most common cause of AGE among children throughout the world. Several other viruses occur less frequently. Norovirus and sapovirus are the 2 genera of *Caliciviruses* that cause AGE. Norovirus genogroup II, genotype 4 (GII.4) has predominated globally during the past decade. Among the more than 50 serotypes of adenovirus, 40 and 41 are most often associated with diarrhea. Astroviruses are identified less often (see Table 366.1).

The major bacterial pathogens that cause AGE are nontyphoidal *Salmonella* (NTS), *Shigella*, *Campylobacter*, and *Yersinia* (see Table 366.2). Five pathotypes of *Escherichia coli* infect humans: Shiga toxin–producing (STEC), also known as enterohemorrhagic (EHEC), enterotoxigenic (ETEC), enteropathogenic (EPEC), enteroaggregative (EAEC), and enteroinvasive (EIEC). Two serogroups of *Vibrio cholerae* (O1 and O139) produce epidemic cholera and cause nearly all sporadic cases. *Clostridium difficile* disease can be both nosocomial and community acquired in children. Bacterial pathogens that cause foodborne illness due to their ability to produce emetic and/or enterotoxins include *Bacillus cereus*, *Clostridium perfringens*, and *Staphylococcus aureus*. The significance of isolating *Aeromonas* and *Plesiomonas* in a diarrheal stool remains uncertain.

Giardia intestinalis, *Cryptosporidium* spp., *Cyclospora cayetanensis*, and *Entamoeba histolytica* are the most common parasites that cause diarrhea in the United States (see Table 366.3). At least 13 species of *Cryptosporidium* are associated with human disease, but *C. hominis* and to a less extent *C. parvum* are most common. The genus *Entamoeba* comprises 6 species that colonize humans, but only *E. histolytica* is considered a human pathogen. *G. intestinalis* (formerly *G. lamblia* and *G. duodenalis*) is a flagellate protozoan that infects the small intestine and biliary tract. Other protozoa that uncommonly cause AGE are *Isospora belli* (now designated *Cystoisospora belli*) and *Blastocystic hominis*.

EPIDEMIOLOGY IN THE UNITED STATES AND OTHER MIDDLE- AND HIGH-INCOME COUNTRIES

Risk Factors Related to Economic Development. Insufficient access to adequate hygiene, sanitation, and clean drinking water are the main factors leading to the heavy burden of AGE in developing countries. Nonetheless, infectious AGE remains ubiquitous in middle- and high-income countries, although the severe consequences have become uncommon. In fact, economic development poses its own risks for transmission of enteric pathogens. The ability to mass-produce and widely distribute food has led to large multistate outbreaks of AGE due to NTS, STEC, and other agents. Globalization has cultivated a taste for tropical fruits and vegetables, creating a mechanism for importation of novel pathogens. The increasing frequency of antimicrobial resistance

Text continued on p. 2237

Table 366.1	**Etiologies of Viral Gastroenteritis**					
ETIOLOGY	**INCUBATION PERIOD**	**ACUTE SIGNS AND SYMPTOMS**	**DURATION OF ILLNESS**	**PRINCIPAL VEHICLE AND TRANSMISSION**	**RISK FACTORS**	**COMMERCIALLY AVAILABLE DIAGNOSTIC TEST**
Caliciviruses (including noroviruses and sapoviruses)	12-48 hr	Nausea, vomiting, abdominal cramping, diarrhea, fever, myalgia, and some headache	1-3 days	Person-to-person (fecal-oral and aerosolized vomit), and food, water, and fomites contaminated with human feces.	Very contagious (chlorine and heat resistant); produces large outbreaks in closed settings such as cruise ships, and restaurants.	No. Testing of stool or vomitus using real time reverse transcriptase (RT)-quantitative PCR is the preferred method, available in public health laboratories. Immunoassays for norovirus have poor sensitivity. FDA-cleared multiplex PCR assays are available to detect these organisms. Norovirus genotyping (GI and GII) is performed by CDC.
Rotavirus (groups A-C), astrovirus, and enteric adenovirus (serotypes 40 and 41)	2-4 days	Often begins with vomiting, followed by watery diarrhea, low-grade fever	3-8 days	Person-to-person (fecal-oral), fomites. Aerosol transmission of rotavirus may be possible.	Nearly all infants and children worldwide were infected by 2 yr of age before vaccine introduction.	Yes. Rotavirus: immunoassay (preferred), latex agglutination, and immune-chromatography of stool. Enteric adenovirus: immunoassay. FDA-cleared multiplex PCR assays are available to detect these organisms.

CDC, Centers for Disease Control and Prevention.
Modified from Centers for Disease Control and Prevention: Diagnosis and management of foodborne illnesses, *MMWR* 53(RR-4):1–33, 2004.

Table 366.2	Etiologies of Bacterial Gastroenteritis					
ETIOLOGY	INCUBATION PERIOD	ACUTE SIGNS AND SYMPTOMS	DURATION OF ILLNESS	PRINCIPAL VEHICLE AND TRANSMISSION	RISK FACTORS	COMMERCIALLY AVAILABLE DIAGNOSTIC TEST
Bacillus cereus (preformed emetic toxin)	1-6 hr	Sudden onset of severe nausea and vomiting; diarrhea may be present	24 hr	Soil and water	Improperly refrigerated cooked or fried rice, meats	No. Reference laboratory used for outbreaks.
Bacillus cereus (enterotoxins formed in vivo)	8-16 hr	Abdominal cramps, watery diarrhea; nausea and vomiting may be present	1-2 days	Soil and water	Meats, stews, gravies, vanilla sauce	No. Reference laboratory used for outbreaks.
Campylobacter jejuni	1-5 days	Diarrhea, (10-20% of episodes are prolonged), cramps, fever, and vomiting; bloody diarrhea, bacteremia, extraintestinal infections, severe disease in immunocompromised	5-7 days (sometimes >10 days) usually self-limiting	Wild and domestic animals and animal products, including pets	Raw and undercooked poultry, unpasteurized milk, untreated surface water	Yes. Stool culture (routine in many laboratories, while others require a special request) is preferred; multiplex PCR.
Clostridium difficile toxin	Unknown—can appear weeks after antibiotic cessation	Mild to moderate watery diarrhea that can progress to severe, pseudomembranous colitis with systemic toxicity.	Variable	Person-person (fecal-oral), mostly within healthcare facilities	Immunosuppression, intestinal disease or surgery, prolonged hospitalization, antibiotics	Yes. PCR, immunoassay, tissue cytotoxicity.
Clostridium perfringens toxin	8-16 hr	Watery diarrhea, nausea, abdominal cramps; fever is rare	1-2 days	Environment, human and animal intestines	Meats, poultry, gravy, dried or precooked foods with poor temperature control	No. Reference laboratory used for outbreaks.
Enterohemorrhagic *Escherichia coli* (EHEC) including *E. coli* O157:H7 and other *Shiga* toxin–producing *E. coli* (STEC)	1-9 days (usually 3-4 days)	Watery diarrhea that becomes bloody in 1-4 days in ~40% of infections; in contrast to dysentery, bloody stools are large volume and fever/toxicity are minimal. More common in children <4 yr old.	4-7 days	Food and water contaminated with feces from ruminants; infected people and animals (fecal-oral); predominantly high-resource countries	Undercooked beef especially hamburger, unpasteurized milk and juice, raw fruits and petting zoos, recreational swimming, daycare. Antimotility agents and antibiotics increase risk of hemolytic uremic syndrome	Yes. Culture on sorbitol-MacConkey agar, immunoassay for O157:H7, or Shiga toxin PCR.[†]
Enterotoxigenic *E. coli* (ETEC)	1-5 days	Watery diarrhea, abdominal cramps, some vomiting	3-7 days	Water or food contaminated with human feces	Infants and young children in LMIC and travelers	Yes. Multiplex PCR,[†] or reference laboratory.
Salmonella, nontyphoidal	1-5 days	Diarrhea, (10-20% prolonged), cramps, fever, and vomiting; bloody diarrhea, bacteremia, extraintestinal infections, severe disease in immunocompromised	5-7 days (sometimes >10 days) usually self-limiting	Domestic poultry, cattle, reptiles, amphibians, birds	Ingestion of raw or undercooked food, improper food handling, travelers, immunosuppression, hemolytic anemia, achlorhydria, contact with infected animal	Yes. Routine stool culture (preferred), multiplex PCR.[†]
Shigella spp.	1-5 days (up to 10 days for *S. dysenteriae* type 1)	Abdominal cramps, fever, diarrhea Begins with watery stools that can be the only manifestation or proceed to dysentery.	5-7 days	Infected people or fecally contaminated surfaces (fecal-oral)	Poor hygiene and sanitation, crowding, travelers, daycare, MSM, prisoners	Yes. Routine stool culture (preferred), multiplex PCR[†]

Continued

Organism	Incubation period	Clinical features	Duration	Reservoir	Common food vehicles and other exposures	Available for clinical diagnosis in most clinical laboratories
Staphylococcus aureus (preformed enterotoxin)	1-6 hr	Sudden onset of severe nausea and vomiting. Abdominal cramps. Diarrhea and fever may be present	1-3 days	Birds, mammals, dairy, and environment	Unrefrigerated or improperly refrigerated meats, potato and egg salads, cream pastries	No. Reference laboratory used for outbreaks.
Vibrio cholerae O1 and O139	1-5 days	Watery diarrhea and vomiting, that can be profuse and lead to severe dehydration and death within hours.	3-7 days	Food and water contaminated with human feces	Contaminated water, fish, shellfish, street-vended food from endemic or epidemic settings; blood group O, vitamin A deficiency	Yes. Stool culture (requires special TCBS media so laboratory must be notified). Rapid test is useful in epidemics but does not provide susceptibility or subtype so should not be used for routine diagnosis.
Vibrio parahaemolyticus	2-48 hr	Watery diarrhea, abdominal cramps, nausea, vomiting. Bacteremia and wound infections occur uncommonly, especially in high-risk patients, e.g., with liver disease and diabetes.	2-5 days	Estuaries and marine environments; currently undergoing pandemic spread	Undercooked or raw seafood, such as fish, shellfish	Yes. Stool culture. Requires special TCBS media so laboratory must be notified. Standard culture acceptable for wounds and blood.
Vibrio vulnificus	1-7 days	Vomiting, diarrhea, abdominal pain. Bacteremia and wound infections, particularly in patients with chronic liver disease (presents with septic shock and hemorrhagic bullous skin lesions)	2-8 days	Estuaries and marine environments	Undercooked or raw shellfish, especially oysters, other contaminated seafood, and open wounds exposed to seawater	Yes. Culture of stool requires TCBS agar; alert laboratory if suspected. Standard media acceptable for wound and blood cultures.
Yersinia enterocolitica and *Yersinia pseudotuberculosis*	1-5 days	Diarrhea, (10-20% prolonged), cramps, fever, and vomiting; bloody diarrhea, bacteremia, extraintestinal infections, severe disease in immunocompromised; pseudoappendicitis occurs primarily in older children.	5-7 days (sometimes >10 days) usually self-limiting	Swine products, occasionally person-to-person and animal-to-humans, water-borne, bloodborne (can multiply during refrigeration)	Undercooked pork, improper food handling, unpasteurized milk, tofu, contaminated water, transfusion from a bacteremic person, cirrhosis, chelation therapy.	Yes. Stool culture in special media and temperature. Not performed in many laboratories unless requested. Requires special media to grow. When clinically relevant, can isolate from vomitus, blood, throat, lymph nodes, joint fluid, urine, and bile.

†FDA-cleared multiplex PCR assays are available but generally not recommended for diagnosis in individual patients because of inability to determine antimicrobial susceptibility to guide treatment or speciate the organism for outbreak investigation.

FDA, Food and Drug Administration; *LMIC,* low and middle-income countries; *MSM,* men who have sex with men; *PCR,* polymerase chain reaction; *TCBS,* thiosulfate-citrate-bile salts-sucrose.

Modified from Centers for Disease Control and Prevention: Diagnosis and management of foodborne illnesses, *MMWR* 53(RR-4):1–33, 2004.

Table 366.3 Etiologies of Parasitic Gastroenteritis

ETIOLOGY	INCUBATION PERIOD	ACUTE SIGNS AND SYMPTOMS	DURATION OF ILLNESS	PRINCIPAL VEHICLE AND TRANSMISSION	RISK FACTORS	COMMERCIALLY AVAILABLE DIAGNOSTIC TEST
Cryptosporidium	1-11 days	Diarrhea (usually watery), bloating, flatulence, cramps, malabsorption, weight loss, and fatigue may wax and wane. Persons with AIDS or malnutrition have more severe disease.	1-2 wk; may be remitting and relapsing over weeks to months	Person-to-person (fecal-oral). Contaminated food and water (including municipal and recreational water contaminated with human feces.	Infants 6-18 mo of age living in endemic settings in LMIC, patients with AIDS, childcare settings, drinking unfiltered surface water, MSM, IgA deficiency	Request specific microscopic examination of stool with special stains (direct fluorescent antibody staining is preferable to modified acid fast) for *Cryptosporidium*. Immunoassays and PCR[†] are more sensitive than microscopy.
Cyclospora cayetanensis	1-11 days	Same as *Cryptosporidium*	Same as *Cryptosporidium*	Fresh produce (imported berries, lettuce)	Travelers, consumption of fresh produce imported from the tropics.	Specific microscopic examination of stool for *Cyclospora*; multiplex PCR.[†] May need to examine water or food.
Entamoeba histolytica	2-4 wk	Gradual onset of cramps, watery diarrhea and often dysentery with cramps but rarely fever. Can wax and wane with weight loss. Dissemination to live and other organs can occur.	Variable; may be protracted (several weeks to several months)	Fecal-oral transmission Any uncooked food or food contaminated by an ill food handler after cooking; drinking water	Persons living in or traveling to LMIC, institutionalized persons, MSM.	Microscopy of fresh stool for cysts and parasites on at least 3 samples; immunoassay is more sensitive; multiplex PCR.[†] Serology for extraintestinal infections
Giardia intestinalis	1-4 wk	Diarrhea, stomach cramps, gas, weight loss; symptoms may wax and wane.	2-4 wk	Any uncooked food or food contaminated by an ill food handler after cooking; drinking water	Hikers drinking unfiltered surface water, persons living in or traveling to LMIC, MSM, IgA deficiency	Microscopic examination of stool for ova and parasites; may need at least 3 samples; immunoassay is more sensitive. Multiplex PCR.[†]

[†]FDA-cleared multiplex PCR assays are available.
IgA, immunoglobulin A; LMID, low- and middle-income countries; MSM, men who have sex with men; PCR, polymerase chain reaction.
Modified from Centers for Disease Control and Prevention: Diagnosis and management of foodborne illnesses, *MMWR* 53(RR-4):1–33, 2004.

Table 366.4 Incidence of Bacterial and Parasitic Food-Borne Infections in 2017 and Percentage Change Compared With 2014-2016 Average Annual Incidence by Pathogen FoodNet Sites,* 2014-2017[†]

PATHOGEN	2017		2017 VERSUS 2014-2016	
	NO. OF CASES	INCIDENCE RATE[§]	% CHANGE[¶]	(95% CI)
BACTERIA				
Campylobacter	9,421	19.1	10	(2 to 18)
Salmonella	7,895	16.0	−5	(−11 to 1)
Shigella	2,132	4.3	−3	(−25 to 25)
Shiga toxin-producing *E. coli***	2,050	4.2	28	(9 to 50)
Yersinia	489	1.0	166	(113 to 234)
Vibrio	340	0.7	54	(26 to 87)
Listeria	158	0.3	26	(2 to 55)
PARASITES				
Cryptosporidium	1,836	3.7	10	(−16 to 42)
Cyclospora	163	0.3	489	(253 to 883)

*Connecticut, Georgia, Maryland, Minnesota, New Mexico, Oregon, Tennessee, and selected counties in California, Colorado, and New York.
[†]Data for 2017 are preliminary.
[§]Per 100,000 population.
[¶]Percentage change reported as increase or decrease.
**For Shiga toxin-producing *E. coli*, all serogroups were combined because it is not possible to distinguish between serogroups using culture-independent diagnostic tests. Reports that were only Shiga toxin-positive from clinical laboratories and were Shiga toxin-negative at a public health laboratory were excluded (n = 518). When these were included, the incidence rate was 5.2, which was a 57% increase (CI = 33–85%).
CI, confidence interval; FoodNet, CDC's Foodborne Diseases Active Surveillance Network.
From Marder EP, Griffin PM, Cieslak PR, et al: Preliminary incidence and trends of infections with pathogens transmitted commonly through food—foodborne diseases active surveillance network, 10 U.S. sites, 2006-2017, *MMWR* 67(11):324–328, 2018 (Table 1, p. 325).

among bacteria that causes AGE has been linked to the use of antibiotics as growth-promotors for animals bred for food. Recreational swimming facilities and water treatment systems have provided a vehicle for massive outbreaks of *Cryptosporidium*, a chlorine-resistant organism. Venues serving catered food to large groups of people, such as hotels and cruise ships, are conducive to outbreaks, as are institutions where hygiene is compromised, such as daycare centers, prisons, and nursing homes. Hospitalization and modern medical therapy have created a niche for nosocomial *C. difficile* toxin infection (Table 366.5).

Endemic Diarrhea. In the United States, rotavirus was the most common cause of medically attended AGE among children younger than 5 yr until the introduction of rotavirus vaccine for routine immunization of infants. Annual epidemics swept across the country beginning in the southwest in November and reaching the northeast by May, affecting nearly every child by the age of 2 yr. Since vaccine introduction, healthcare utilization for AGE has decreased markedly. Norovirus is the leading cause of AGE among children in the United States seeking healthcare, followed by sapovirus, adenovirus 40 and 41, and astrovirus (see Table 366.1).

Foodborne Transmission. The most comprehensive resource for describing the burden of bacterial and protozoal diarrhea in the United States is the Foodborne Diseases Active Surveillance Network (FoodNet) maintained by the Centers for Disease Control and Prevention (CDC) (see Table 366.4). FoodNet performs active laboratory-based surveillance

of 9 bacterial and protozoal enteric infections commonly transmitted by food. Among children 0-19 yr of age in 2015, NTS was most common, followed by *Campylobacter* and *Shigella*, then STEC and *Cryptosporidium*. *Vibrio, Yersinia, and Cyclospora* were the least common (see Table 366.5). Children younger than 5 yr have the highest incidence of disease, and the elderly have the highest frequency of hospitalization and death. Only 5% of these infections are associated with recognized outbreaks.

Noninfectious agents may also cause foodborne gastrointestinal symptoms due to a direct toxic effect of the food (mushrooms) or contamination (heavy metals) (Table 366.6).

Diarrhea Outbreaks. The U.S. Foodborne Disease Outbreak Surveillance System quantifies enteric infections associated with foodborne outbreaks. In 2015, among all age groups, norovirus was the most common agent (46%), followed by NTS (23%). Less common are *C. perfringens* (6%), STEC (5%), *Campylobacter* (5%), and *S. aureus* (2%), followed much less often (each 1%) by *B. cereus, Clostridium botulinum, Shigella, Cryptosporidium, Yersinia, Listeria, Vibrio parahaemolyticus,* and *Shigella*. Outbreaks of enteric pathogens propagated by direct person-to-person contact are most often caused by norovirus and *Shigella* species; other pathogens include NTS, rotavirus, *Giardia, Cryptosporidium, C. difficile,* and *C. jejuni.*

Nosocomial Diarrhea. *C. difficile* is the most common cause of healthcare-associated infection in the United States. Severe disease occurs most often in those with predisposing conditions (e.g., recent antibiotics,

Table 366.5	Exposure or Condition Associated With Pathogens Causing Diarrhea
EXPOSURE OR CONDITION	**PATHOGEN(S)**
FOODBORNE	
Foodborne outbreaks in hotels, cruise ships, resorts, restaurants, catered events	Norovirus, nontyphoidal *Salmonella, Clostridium perfringens, Bacillus cereus, Staphylococcus aureus, Campylobacter* spp., ETEC, STEC, *Listeria, Shigella, Cyclospora cayetanensis, Cryptosporidium* spp.
Consumption of unpasteurized milk or dairy products	*Salmonella, Campylobacter, Yersinia enterocolitica, S. aureus* toxin, *Cryptosporidium*, and STEC. *Listeria* is infrequently associated with diarrhea, *Brucella* (goat milk cheese), *Mycobacterium bovis, Coxiella burnetii*
Consumption of raw or undercooked meat or poultry	STEC (beef), *C. perfringens* (beef, poultry), *Salmonella* (poultry), *Campylobacter* (poultry), *Yersinia* (pork, chitterlings), *S. aureus* (poultry), and *Trichinella* spp. (pork, wild game meat)
Consumption of fruits or unpasteurized fruit juices, vegetables, leafy greens, and sprouts	STEC, nontyphoidal *Salmonella, Cyclospora, Cryptosporidium*, norovirus, hepatitis A, and *Listeria monocytogenes*
Consumption of undercooked eggs	*Salmonella, Shigella* (egg salad)
Consumption of raw shellfish	*Vibrio* species, norovirus, hepatitis A, *Plesiomonas*
EXPOSURE OR CONTACT	
Swimming in or drinking untreated fresh water	*Campylobacter, Cryptosporidium, Giardia, Shigella, Salmonella,* STEC, *Plesiomonas shigelloides*
Swimming in recreational water facility with treated water	*Cryptosporidium* and other potentially waterborne pathogens when disinfectant concentrations are inadequately maintained
Healthcare, long-term care, prison exposure, or employment	Norovirus, *Clostridium difficile, Shigella, Cryptosporidium, Giardia,* STEC, rotavirus
Childcare center attendance or employment	Rotavirus, *Cryptosporidium, Giardia, Shigella,* STEC
Recent antimicrobial therapy	*C. difficile*, multidrug-resistant *Salmonella*
Travel to resource-challenged countries	*Escherichia coli* (enteroaggregative, enterotoxigenic, enteroinvasive), *Shigella,* typhi and nontyphoidal *Salmonella, Campylobacter, Vibrio cholerae, Entamoeba histolytica, Giardia, Blastocystis, Cyclospora, Cystoisospora, Cryptosporidium*
Exposure to house pets with diarrhea	*Campylobacter, Yersinia*
Exposure to pig feces in certain parts of the world	*Balantidium coli*
Contact with young poultry or reptiles	Nontyphoidal *Salmonella*
Visiting a farm or petting zoo	STEC, *Cryptosporidium, Campylobacter*
EXPOSURE OR CONDITION	
Age group	Rotavirus (6-18 mo of age), nontyphoidal *Salmonella* (infants from birth to 3 mo of age and adults >50 yr with a history of atherosclerosis), *Shigella* (1-7 yr of age), *Campylobacter* (young adults)
Underlying immunocompromising condition	Nontyphoidal *Salmonella, Cryptosporidium, Campylobacter, Shigella, Yersinia*
Hemochromatosis or hemoglobinopathy	*Y. enterocolitica, Salmonella*
AIDS, immunosuppressive therapies	*Cryptosporidium, Cyclospora, Cystoisospora,* microsporidia, *Mycobacterium avium–intercellulare* complex, cytomegalovirus
Anal-genital, oral-anal, or digital-anal contact	*Shigella, Salmonella, Campylobacter, E. histolytica, Giardia lamblia, Cryptosporidium*

ETEC, enterotoxigenic *Escherichia coli; STEC,* Shiga toxin–producing *Escherichia coli.*
From Shane AL, Mody RK, Crump JA, et al: 2017 Infectious Diseases Society for America clinical practice guidelines for the diagnosis and management of infectious diarrhea, *Clin Infect Dis* 65(12):e45–80, 2017 (Table 2, p. e48).

Table 366.6 Foodborne Noninfectious Illnesses

ETIOLOGY	INCUBATION PERIOD	SIGNS AND SYMPTOMS	DURATION OF ILLNESS	ASSOCIATED FOODS	LABORATORY TESTING	TREATMENT
Antimony	5 min–8 hr usually <1 hr	Vomiting, metallic taste	Usually self-limited	Metallic container	Identification of metal in beverage or food	Supportive care
Arsenic	Few hours	Vomiting, colic, diarrhea	Several days	Contaminated food	Urine Can cause eosinophilia	Gastric lavage, BAL (dimercaprol)
Cadmium	5 min–8 hr usually <1 hr	Nausea, vomiting, myalgia, increase in salivation, stomach pain	Usually self-limited	Seafood, oysters, clams, lobster, grains, peanuts	Identification of metal in food	Supportive care
Ciguatera fish poisoning (ciguatera toxin)	2–6 hr	GI: abdominal pain, nausea, vomiting, diarrhea	Days to weeks to months	A variety of large reef fish: grouper, red snapper, amberjack, and barracuda (most common)	Radioassay for toxin in fish or a consistent history	Supportive care, IV mannitol Children more vulnerable
	3 hr	Neurologic: paresthesias, reversal of hot or cold, pain, weakness				
	2–5 days	Cardiovascular: bradycardia, hypotension, increase in T-wave abnormalities				
Copper	5 min–8 hr usually <1 hr	Nausea, vomiting, blue or green vomitus	Usually self-limited	Metallic container	Identification of metal in beverage or food	Supportive care
Mercury	1 wk or longer	Numbness, weakness of legs, spastic paralysis, impaired vision, blindness, coma Pregnant women and the developing fetus are especially vulnerable	May be protracted	Fish exposed to organic mercury, grains treated with mercury fungicides	Analysis of blood, hair	Supportive care
Mushroom toxins, short-acting (muscimol, muscarine, psilocybin, Coprinus atramentaria, ibotenic acid)	<2 hr	Vomiting, diarrhea, confusion, visual disturbance, salivation, diaphoresis, hallucinations, disulfiram-like reaction, confusion, visual disturbance	Self-limited	Wild mushrooms (cooking might not destroy these toxins)	Typical syndrome and mushroom identified or demonstration of the toxin	Supportive care
Mushroom toxins, long-acting (amanitin)	4–8 hr diarrhea; 24–48 hr liver failure	Diarrhea, abdominal cramps, leading to hepatic and renal failure	Often fatal	Mushrooms	Typical syndrome and mushroom identified and/or demonstration of the toxin	Supportive care, life-threatening, may need life support
Nitrite poisoning	1–2 hr	Nausea, vomiting, cyanosis, headache, dizziness, weakness, loss of consciousness, chocolate-brown blood	Usually self-limited	Cured meats, any contaminated foods, spinach exposed to excessive nitrification	Analysis of the food, blood	Supportive care, methylene blue
Pesticides (organophosphates or carbamates)	Few minutes to few hours	Nausea, vomiting, abdominal cramps, diarrhea, headache, nervousness, blurred vision, twitching, convulsions, salivation, meiosis	Usually self-limited	Any contaminated food	Analysis of the food, blood	Atropine; 2-PAM (pralidoxime) is used when atropine is not able to control symptoms; rarely necessary in carbamate poisoning

Continued

Agent	Incubation period	Signs and symptoms	Duration	Associated foods	Laboratory testing	Treatment
Puffer fish (tetrodotoxin)	<30 min	Paresthesias, vomiting, diarrhea, abdominal pain, ascending paralysis, respiratory failure	Death usually in 4-6 hr	Puffer fish	Detection of tetrodotoxin in fish	Life-threatening, may need respiratory support
Scombroid (histamine)	1 min-3 hr	Flushing, rash, burning sensation of skin, mouth and throat, dizziness, urticaria, paresthesias	3-6 hr	Fish: bluefin, tuna, skipjack, mackerel, marlin, escolar, and mahi	Demonstration of histamine in food or clinical diagnosis	Supportive care, antihistamines
Shellfish toxins (diarrheic, neurotoxic, amnesic)	Diarrheic shellfish poisoning: 30 min-2 hr Neurotoxic shellfish poisoning: few minutes to hours Amnesic shellfish poisoning: 24-48 hr	Nausea, vomiting, diarrhea, and abdominal pain accompanied by chills, headache, and fever Tingling and numbness of lips, tongue, and throat, muscular aches, dizziness, reversal of the sensations of hot and cold, diarrhea, and vomiting Vomiting, diarrhea, abdominal pain and neurologic problems such as confusion, memory loss, disorientation, seizure, coma	Hours to 2-3 days	A variety of shellfish, primarily mussels, oysters, scallops, and shellfish from the Florida coast and the Gulf of Mexico	Detection of the toxin in shellfish; high-pressure liquid chromatography	Supportive care, generally self-limiting Elderly are especially sensitive to amnesic shellfish poisoning
Shellfish toxins (paralytic shellfish poisoning)	30 min-3 hr	Diarrhea, nausea, vomiting leading to paresthesias of mouth and lips, weakness, dysphasia, dysphonia, respiratory paralysis	Days	Scallops, mussels, clams, cockles	Detection of toxin in food or water where fish are located; high-pressure liquid chromatography	Life-threatening, may need respiratory support
Sodium fluoride	Few minutes to 2 hr	Salty or soapy taste, numbness of mouth, vomiting, diarrhea, dilated pupils, spasms, pallor, shock, collapse	Usually self-limited	Dry foods (e.g., dry milk, flour, baking powder, cake mixes) contaminated with NaF-containing insecticides and rodenticides	Testing of vomitus or gastric washings Analysis of the food	Supportive care
Thallium	Few hours	Nausea, vomiting, diarrhea, painful paresthesias, motor polyneuropathy, hair loss	Several days	Contaminated food	Urine, hair	Supportive care
Tin	5 min-8 hr usually <1 hr	Nausea, vomiting, diarrhea	Usually self-limited	Metallic container	Analysis of the food	Supportive care
Vomitoxin	Few minutes to 3 hr	Nausea, headache, abdominal pain, vomiting	Usually self-limited	Grains such as wheat, corn, barley	Analysis of the food	Supportive care
Zinc	Few hours	Stomach cramps, nausea, vomiting, diarrhea, myalgias	Usually self-limited	Metallic container	Analysis of the food, blood and feces, saliva or urine	Supportive care

BAL, bronchoalveolar lavage; GI, gastrointestinal.
From Centers for Disease Control and Prevention: Diagnosis and management of foodborne illnesses, *MMWR* 53(RR-4):1–33, 2004.

gastric acid suppression, immunosuppression, gastrointestinal comorbidities). In contrast to adults, rates of colostomy and in-hospital mortality have not increased in children despite increasing rates of community and hospital-acquired *C. difficile* infection, suggesting that *C. difficile* may be less pathogenic in children. Moreover, high rates of asymptomatic carriage (and presence of toxin) among children younger than 2 yr creates diagnostic uncertainty, so testing and treatment should be reserved for those with supporting clinical evidence (see Table 366.2).

Zoonotic Transmission. Many diarrheal pathogens are acquired from animal reservoirs (see Tables 366.1 to 366.3, 366.5). The ability of NTS to undergo transovarian passage in hens allows infection of intact grade A pasteurized eggs, a source of multiple large outbreaks. Although *Campylobacter* is prevalent in poultry, its lower outbreak potential has been attributed to its lack of transovarian spread in hens and stringent growth requirements, which limit its ability to replicate in foods. On the other hand, *Campylobacter* has an extensive reservoir in domestic and wild animals and remains a major cause of sporadic bacterial foodborne disease in industrialized countries, usually from consumption of contaminated chicken, meat, beef, and milk. Its ubiquitous animal reservoir also has resulted in widespread contamination of surface waters, resulting in diarrhea among hikers and campers who drink from streams, ponds, and lakes in wilderness areas. The predilection for STEC to asymptomatically colonize the intestines of ruminant animals explains

why unpasteurized dairy products, fruits harvested from fields where cattle graze, and undercooked hamburger are common vehicles. The major animal reservoir for *Yersinia* is pigs, so ingestion of raw or undercooked pork products is an important risk factor. Pets can be the source of NTS (asymptomatic young birds, amphibians, and reptiles), *Campylobacter*, and *Yersinia* (puppies and kittens that are usually ill with diarrhea).

Seasonality. Seasonality provides a clue to implicate specific pathogens, although patterns may differ in tropical and temperate climates. Rotavirus and norovirus peak in cool seasons, whereas enteric adenovirus infections occur throughout the year, with some increase in summer. *Salmonella*, *Shigella*, and *Campylobacter* favor warm weather, whereas the tendency for *Yersinia* to tolerate cold manifests as a winter seasonality, with higher prevalence in northern countries, and ability to survive in contaminated blood products during refrigeration.

EPIDEMIOLOGY IN LOW- AND MIDDLE-INCOME COUNTRIES

The Global Enteric Multicenter Study (GEMS) evaluated children younger than 5 yr living in 7 low-income countries in sub-Saharan Africa and South Asia and seeking healthcare for moderate-to-severe diarrhea (Fig. 366.1). Although a broad array of pathogens were identified, most episodes of moderate-to-severe diarrhea were attributed to 4 pathogens:

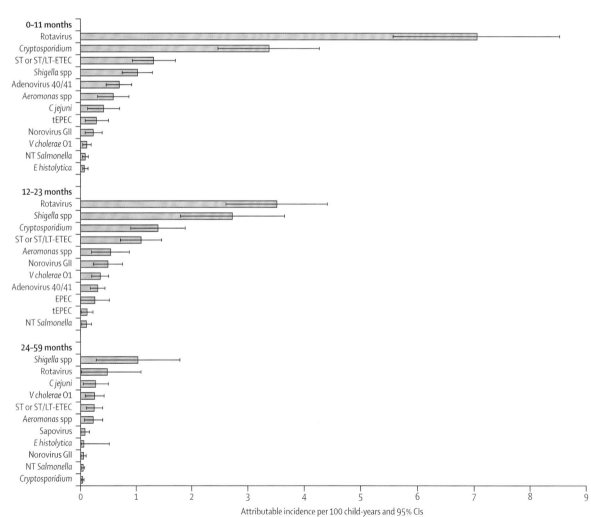

Fig. 366.1 Attributable incidence of pathogen-specific moderate-to-severe diarrhea per 100 child-yr by age stratum, all sites combined. The bars show the incidence rates, and the *error bars* show the 95% confidence intervals. *EPEC*, enteropathogenic; *ETEC*, enterotoxigenic; *LT*, labile toxin; *NT*, Nontyphoidal; *ST*, stable toxin. (Modified from Kotloff KL, Nataro JP, Blackwelder WC, et al: Burden and aetiology of diarrhoeal disease in infants and young children in developing countries [the Global Enteric Multicenter Study, GEMS]: a prospective, case-control study, Lancet 382[9888]:209–222, 2013, Fig. 4.)

rotavirus, *Cryptosporidium, Shigella,* and ETEC producing heat-stable toxin (ST) either alone or in combination with heat-labile toxin (LT), herein termed ST-ETEC, and, to less extent, adenovirus 40 and 41. On the other hand, several etiologic agents that are common causes of AGE in high-resource settings are notable for their low frequency in resource-limited settings: NTS, STEC, norovirus, and *C. difficile* toxin. The 3 agents associated with most deaths among children under 5 yr are rotavirus (29%), *Cryptosporidium* (12%), and *Shigella* (11%). The Etiology, Risk Factors, and Interactions of Enteric Infections and Malnutrition and the Consequences for Child Health and Development Project (MAL-ED) was a study of less severe, community-based diarrhea. Viral causes predominated (36.4% of the overall incidence), but *Shigella* had the single highest attributable incidence (26.1 attributable episodes per 100 child-years).

Host Risk Factors

Most pathogens show an age predilection. The incidence of rotavirus and NTS are highest in infancy. Endemic shigellosis peaks in 1-4 yr olds, whereas *Campylobacter* and *Cryptosporidium* show a bimodal distribution with the greatest number of reported cases in infants and young children and a secondary peak in adolescents and young adults. Pandemic *V. cholerae* and *S. dysenteriae* type 1 produce high attack rates and mortality in all age groups and often afflict displaced persons in emergency settings. Some agents (e.g., NTS, *Shigella, Campylobacter, Yersinia,* and *Cryptosporidium*) are more frequent and more severe when the host is immunocompromised or malnourished.

Additional risks factors for AGE include immunodeficiency, measles, malnutrition, and lack of exclusive or predominant breastfeeding. Malnutrition increases the risk of diarrhea and associated mortality, and moderate to severe stunting increases the odds of diarrhea-associated mortality. The fraction of such infectious diarrhea deaths that are attributable to nutritional deficiencies varies with the prevalence of deficiencies; the highest attributable fractions are in sub-Saharan Africa, South Asia, and Andean Latin America. The risks are particularly high with malnutrition, particularly when associated with micronutrient deficiency. Vitamin A deficiency accounts for 157,000 deaths from diarrhea, measles, and malaria. Zinc deficiency is estimated to cause

116,000 deaths from diarrhea and pneumonia. Table 366.7 summarizes some of the key risk factors associated with childhood diarrhea globally, especially in the presence of micronutrient deficiency.

PATHOGENESIS OF INFECTIOUS DIARRHEA

Intrinsic properties of the organism help to define the mode of transmission and incubation period (Table 366.8). Enteropathogens that are infectious in small inocula (*Shigella,* STEC, norovirus, rotavirus, *G. intestinalis, Cryptosporidium* spp., *C. difficile, E. histolytica*) are readily transmitted by person-to-person contact via the fecal-oral route. Pathogens with larger infectious doses, such as cholera, NTS, ETEC, and *Campylobacter,* generally require food or water vehicles (see Tables 366.1 to 366.3). Pathogens that produce preformed toxins (*S. aureus, B. cereus* emetic toxin) have shorter incubation periods (1-6 hr) compared with 8-16 hr for those that must elaborate enterotoxins in situ (e.g., *C. perfringens* and *B. cereus* enterotoxin). Incubation periods of 1-5 days are seen with pathogens that attach to the epithelium and elaborate enterotoxins (e.g., *V. cholerae,* ETEC) or cytotoxins (e.g., *S. dysenteriae* type 1 and STEC) or those that invade and disrupt the intestinal epithelium (*Shigella,* NTS, *Campylobacter,* and *Yersinia*). The requirement for protozoa to progress through a life cycle to trigger pathogenic processes results in a more extended incubation period. Other properties affecting transmissibility are bioavailability as conferred by a copious and/or prolonged fecal shedding, extended infectivity in the environment, and resistance to disinfection (all exhibited by norovirus and *Cryptosporidium*), or a large environmental or animal reservoir (e.g., *Campylobacter*). The ability to circumvent immune surveillance by frequent antigenic changes resulting from recombinational events (e.g., norovirus) or a large serotype diversity (e.g., *Shigella*) maintains a susceptible host population.

Viral AGE causes a cytolytic infection of the small intestinal villus tips resulting in decreased absorption of water, disaccharide malabsorption, inflammation, and cytokine activation. The rotavirus protein NSP4 acts as a viral enterotoxin that produces secretory diarrhea. In addition, rotavirus activates the enteric nervous system causing decreased gastric emptying and increased intestinal mobility. There is a genetic susceptibility to both rotavirus and norovirus infection that is mediated by histo-blood group antigens on the epithelial cell surface and in mucus

Table 366.7	Proven Risk Factors With Direct Biologic Links to Diarrhea: Relative Risks or Odds Ratios and 95% Confidence Intervals	
	DIARRHEAL MORBIDITY	**DIARRHEAL MORTALITY**
No breastfeeding (0-5 mo)	RR = 2.7 (1.7-4.1) compared with exclusive breastfeeding	RR = 10.5 (2.8-39.6) compared with exclusive breastfeeding
No breastfeeding (6-23 mo)	RR = 1.3 (1.1-1.6) compared with any breastfeeding	RR = 2.2 (1.1-4.2) compared with any breastfeeding
Underweight	(compared with ≥2 WAZ)	(compared with ≥1 WAZ)
–2 to ≤1 WAZ		OR = 2.1 (1.6-2.7)
–3 to ≤2 WAZ	RR = 1.2 (1.1-1.4)	OR = 3.4 (2.7-4.4)
≤3 WAZ		OR = 9.5 (5.5-16.5)
Stunted		
–2 to ≤1 HAZ		OR = 1.2 (0.9-1.7)
–3 to ≤2 HAZ		OR = 1.6 (1.1-2.5)
<–3 HAZ		OR = 4.6 (2.7-14.7)
Wasted		
–2 to ≤1 WHZ		OR = 1.2 (0.7-1.9)
–3 to ≤2 WHZ		OR = 2.9 (1.8-4.5)
≤3 WHZ		OR = 6.3 (2.7-14.7)
Vitamin A deficiency (vs. not deficient)		RR = 1.5 (1.3-1.8)
Zinc deficiency (vs. not deficient)	RR = 1.2 (1.1-1.2)	RR = 1.2 (1.0-1.6)

HAZ, height-for-age Z-score; *OR,* odds ratio; *RR,* relative risk; *WAZ,* weight-for-age Z score; *WHZ,* weight-for-height Z-score.
Modified from Walker CL, Rudan I, Liu L, et al: Global burden of childhood pneumonia and diarrhoea, *Lancet* 381:1405–1416, 2013.

Table 366.8	Comparison of 3 General Pathogenic Mechanisms of Enteric Infection		
	TYPE OF INFECTION		
PARAMETER	**I**	**II**	**III**
Mechanism	Noninflammatory (enterotoxin or adherence/superficial invasion)	Inflammatory, epithelial destruction (invasion, cytotoxin)	Penetrating
Location	Proximal small bowel	Colon	Distal small bowel
Illness	Watery diarrhea	Dysentery	Enteric fever
Stool examination	No fecal leukocytes Mild or no ↑ lactoferrin	Fecal polymorphonuclear leukocytes ↑↑ Lactoferrin	Fecal mononuclear leukocytes
Examples	*Vibrio cholerae* ETEC *Clostridium perfringens* *Bacillus cereus* *Staphylococcus aureus* Also[†]: *Giardia intestinalis* Rotavirus Noroviruses *Cryptosporidium* spp. EPEC, EAEC *Cyclospora cayetanensis*	*Shigella* EIEC STEC NTS *Vibrio parahaemolyticus* *Clostridium difficile* *Campylobacter jejuni* *Entamoeba histolytica**	*Yersinia enterocolitica* *Salmonella* Typhi, *S. Paratyhpi*, and occasionally NTS, *Campylobacter*, and *Yersinia*

*Although amebic dysentery involves tissue inflammation, the leukocytes are characteristically pyknotic or absent, having been destroyed by the virulent amebae.
[†]Although not typically enterotoxic, these pathogens alter bowel physiology via adherence, superficial cell entry, cytokine induction, or toxins that inhibit cell function.
EAEC, enteroaggregative *E. coli*; EIEC, enteroinvasive *E. coli*; EPEC, enteropathogenic *Escherichia coli*; ETEC, enterotoxigenic *Escherichia coli*; NTS, nontyphoidal *Salmonella*; STEC, Shiga toxin–producing *Escherichia coli*.
Modified from Mandell GL, Bennett JE, Dolin R, editors: *Principles and practices of infectious diseases*, ed 7, Philadelphia, 2010, Churchill Livingstone.

secretions (Fig. 366.2).

Pathogens primarily manifesting as secretory diarrhea attach to the surface of the epithelium and stimulate secretion of water and electrolytes by activating adenylate cyclase and raising intracellular cAMP (*V. cholerae* and heat- LT–producing ETEC) and/or cGMP (ETEC producing heat-ST) (Figs. 366.3 and 366.4). The diarrheagenic phenotype of *C. difficile* is attributed to production of toxins A (an enterotoxin) and B (an entero-

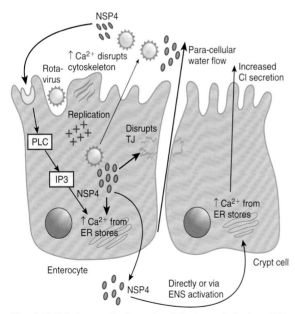

Fig. 366.2 Pathogenesis of rotavirus infection and diarrhea. *ENS,* Enteric nervous system; *ER,* endoplasmic reticulum; *NSP4,* non-structural protein 4; *PLC,* phospholipase C; *TJ,* tight junction. (*Modified from Ramig RF: Pathogenesis of intestinal and systemic rotavirus infection,* J Virol 78:10213–10220, 2004.)

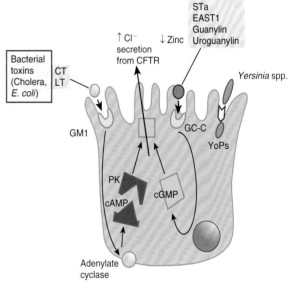

Fig. 366.3 Mechanism of secretory and penetrating diarrhea. *cAMP,* Cyclic adenosine monophosphate; *CFTR,* cystic fibrosis transmembrane conductance regulator through which chloride is secreted; *cGMP,* cyclic guanosine monophosphate; *YoPs,* Yersinia outer proteins that alter host cell functions to promote disease; *CT,* cholera toxin; *EAST 1,* enteroaggregative E. coli ST; *GC-C,* guanylate cyclase, the transmembrane receptor for STa and other toxins; *GM1,* a ganglioside containing one sialic acid residue that serves as the receptor for CT and LT; *LT,* heat labile toxin; *PK,* protein kinase; *STa,* heat stable toxin a. (*Modified from Thapar M, Sanderson IR: Diarrhoea in children: an interface between developing and developed countries,* Lancet 363:641–653, 2004; and Montes M, DuPont HL: Enteritis, enterocolitis and infectious diarrhea syndromes. In Cohen J, Powderly WG, Opal SM, et al, editors: Infectious diseases, ed 2, London, 2004, Mosby, pp. 31–52.)

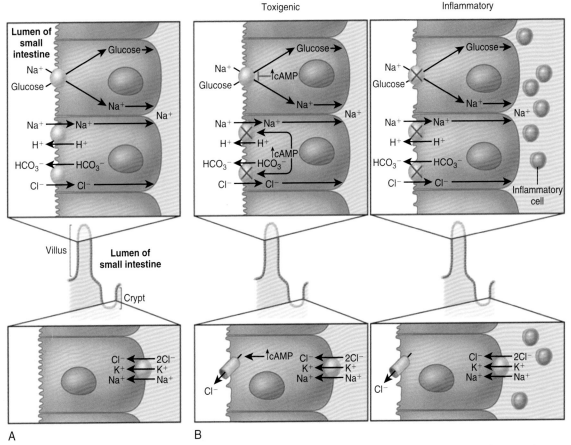

Fig. 366.4 Movement of Na⁺ and Cl⁻ in the small intestine. **A,** Movement in normal subjects. Na⁺ is absorbed by 2 different mechanisms in absorptive cells from villi: glucose-stimulated absorption and electroneutral absorption (which represents the coupling of Na⁺/H⁺ and Cl⁻/HCO₃⁻ exchanges). **B,** Movement during diarrhea caused by a toxin and inflammation. *(From Petri WA, Miller M, Binder HJ, et al: Enteric infections, diarrhea and their impact on function and development,* J Clin Invest *118:1277–1290, 2008.)*

toxin and cytotoxin). The epidemic hypervirulent NAP1 *C. difficile* also makes binary toxin, which may enhance colonization and augment toxin production.

Shigella, NTS, *Campylobacter*, and *Yersinia* all possess an invasive phenotype and elicit diarrhea by a variety of mechanisms that generally involves elicitation of inflammatory cytokines with or without associated toxin production (Fig. 366.5). The pathogenesis of *Shigella*, the most common cause of bacillary dysentery, has been characterized in greatest detail. Following invasion, *Shigella* induces extensive destruction and inflammation of the intestinal epithelium producing ulcers and micro-abscesses that manifest with diarrheal stools containing blood and pus. Production of enterotoxins contributes to secretory diarrhea, which can be seen early in shigellosis or as the sole manifestation. A single serotype of *Shigella*, *S. dysenteriae* type 1, elaborates the Shiga toxin which increases the severity of illness and is responsible for development of hemolytic uremic syndrome (HUS).

Cryptosporidia sporozoites released from ingested cysts penetrate intestinal epithelial cells and develop into trophozoites within the intracellular, but extracytoplasmic, environment. After undergoing asexual multiplication and sexual development, they are released in the colon as infectious oocysts capable of causing autoinfection. Host factors, in particular T-cell function, play a critical role in disease severity. *Cyclospora* cysts are not infectious in freshly passed stools but must sporulate in the environment for 1-2 wk to become infectious; they are usually transmitted in contaminated produce and water (see Table 366.4).

CLINICAL MANIFESTATION OF DIARRHEA

General Findings. Diarrhea is usually defined as the passage of 3 or more abnormally loose or liquid stools per day. Frequent passage of formed stools is not diarrhea, nor is the passing of loose, pasty stools by breastfed babies. Clinical clues to the possible etiology of gastroenteritis are noted in Table 366.9.

In the past, many guidelines divided patients into subgroups for mild (3–5%), moderate (6–9%), and severe (≥10%) dehydration. However, it is difficult to distinguish between mild and moderate dehydration based on clinical signs alone. Therefore most guidelines now combine mild and moderate dehydration and simply use none, some, and severe dehydration. The individual signs that best predict dehydration are prolonged capillary refill time >2 sec, abnormal skin turgor, hyperpnea (deep, rapid breathing suggesting acidosis), dry mucous membranes, absent tears, and general appearance (including activity level and thirst). As the number of signs increases, so does the likelihood of dehydration. Tachycardia, altered level of consciousness, and cold extremities with or without hypotension suggest severe dehydration.

Viral Diarrhea. Symptoms of rotavirus AGE usually begin with vomiting followed by frequent passage of watery nonbloody stools, associated with fever in about half the cases (see Table 366.1). The diarrhea lacks fecal leukocytes, but stools from 20% of cases contain mucus. Recovery with complete resolution of symptoms generally occurs within 7 days. Although disaccharide malabsorption is found in 10–20% of episodes, it is rarely clinically significant.

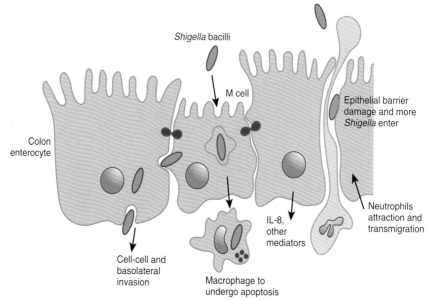

Fig. 366.5 Pathogenesis of shigella infection and diarrhea. *IL-8*, interleukin-8. (*Modified from Opal SM, Keusch GT: Host responses to infection. In Cohen J, Powderly WG, Opal SM, et al, editors: Infectious diseases, ed 2, London, 2004, Mosby, pp. 31–52.*)

Table 366.9	Clinical Presentations Suggestive of Infectious Diarrhea Etiologies

FINDING	LIKELY PATHOGENS
Persistent or chronic diarrhea	*Cryptosporidium* spp., *Giardia lamblia, Cyclospora cayetanensis, Entamoeba histolytica,* non-typhoidal *Salmonella, Yersinia,* and *Campylobacter* spp.
Visible blood in stool	STEC, *Shigella, Salmonella, Campylobacter, Entamoeba histolytica,* noncholera *Vibrio parahaemolyticus, Yersinia, Balantidium coli,* and *Aeromonas*
Fever	Not highly discriminatory—viral, bacterial, and parasitic infections can cause fever. In general, higher temperatures are suggestive of bacterial etiology or *E. histolytica.* Patients infected with STEC usually are not febrile at time of presentation
Abdominal pain	STEC, *Salmonella, Shigella, Campylobacter, Yersinia,* noncholera *Vibrio* species, *Clostridium difficile*
Severe abdominal pain, often grossly bloody stools (occasionally nonbloody), and minimal or no fever	STEC, *Salmonella, Shigella, Campylobacter,* and *Yersinia enterocolitica*
Persistent abdominal pain and fever	*Y. enterocolitica* and *Y. pseudotuberculosis;* may mimic appendicitis
Nausea and vomiting lasting ≤24 hr	Ingestion of *Staphylococcus aureus* enterotoxin or *Bacillus cereus* (short-incubation emetic syndrome)
Diarrhea and abdominal cramping lasting 1-2 days	Ingestion of *Clostridium perfringens* or *Bacillus cereus* (long-incubation emetic syndrome)
Vomiting and nonbloody diarrhea	Norovirus (low-grade fever usually present during the first 24 hr in 40% of infections); diarrhea usually lasts 2-3 days or less; other viral diarrheas (e.g., rotavirus, enteric adenovirus, sapovirus, astrovirus) usually last 3-8 days.
Chronic watery diarrhea, often lasting a year or more	Brainerd diarrhea (epidemic secretory diarrhea, etiologic agent has not been identified); postinfectious irritable bowel syndrome

STEC, Shiga toxin–producing *Escherichia coli.*
From Shane AL, Mody RK, Crump JA, et al: 2017 Infectious Diseases Society for America clinical practice guidelines for the diagnosis and management of infectious diarrhea, *Clin Infect Dis* 65(12):e45–80, 2017 (Table 3, p. e54).

Other viral agents elicit similar symptoms and cannot be distinguished from rotavirus based on clinical findings. In an outbreak setting, the pattern of a brief incubation period (12-48 hr), short duration of illness, and clustering of cases is shared by caliciviruses and preformed bacterial toxin. However, unlike preformed toxins, caliciviruses cause secondary infections, which confirm the contagious nature of the outbreak. Diarrheal illnesses caused by enteric adenovirus infections tend to be more prolonged than rotavirus (7 to 10 days), whereas astroviruses cause a shorter course (~5 days) usually without significant vomiting.

Bacterial Diarrhea. Although there is considerable overlap, fever >40°C, overt fecal blood, abdominal pain, no vomiting before diarrhea onset, and high stool frequency (>10 per day) are more common with bacterial pathogens (see Tables 366.2 and 366.9). Although high fever and overt fecal blood are often absent in bacterial enteritis, when present, there is a high probability of a bacterial etiology. The classical bacterial agents, NTS, *Shigella, Campylobacter,* and *Yersinia,* present with 1 of 5 syndromes.
1. Acute diarrhea, the most common presentation, may be accompanied by fever and vomiting. Clinically silent bacteremia associated with

uncomplicated NTS AGE can be seen among otherwise healthy children younger than 2 yr living in industrialized countries.

2. Bloody diarrhea or frank dysentery is classically caused by *Shigella*. Watery diarrhea typically precedes dysentery and is often the sole clinical manifestation of mild infection. Progression to dysentery indicates colitis and may occur within hours to days. Patients with severe infection may pass more than 20 dysenteric stools in 1 day. Dysenteric illnesses due to *Campylobacter* have been confused with inflammatory bowel disease.

3. Invasive, nonfocal disease (**enteric fever**) is a febrile illness associated with bacteremia without localized infection. Diarrhea may be minimal or absent. Although classically the result of *S.* Typhi or Paratyphi A and B, enteric fever can result from systemic spread of the classical bacterial enteropathogens. Although enteric fever caused by *S.* Typhi or Paratyphi A and B primarily affect preschool and school-age children in endemic countries, other bacterial enteropathogens most often cause disease in infants (particularly <3 mo), the immunocompromised, and children with malnutrition. Additional risk factors include hemolytic anemia and intravascular lesions for NTS, and iron overload, cirrhosis, and chelation therapy for *Yersinia* sepsis. The distinct clones of NTS that have arisen in sub-Saharan Africa described earlier are causing enteric fever–type illnesses often in the absence of AGE. *Shigella* sepsis is rare and is seen most often in malnourished and immunocompromised hosts.

4. Extraintestinal invasive infections can result from either local invasion or bacteremic spread (Table 366.10). Examples of local invasion include mesenteric adenitis, appendicitis, and rarely cholecystitis, mesenteric venous thrombosis, pancreatitis, hepatic, or splenic abscess. Bacteremic spread may result in pneumonia, osteomyelitis, meningitis (3 conditions seen most commonly with NTS), abscesses, cellulitis, septic arthritis, and endocarditis. *Shigella* can cause noninvasive contiguous infections such as vaginitis and urinary tract infections.

5. Vertical transmission of *Shigella*, NTS, and *Campylobacter* can produce perinatal infection resulting in a spectrum of illness from isolated diarrhea or hematochezia to fulminant neonatal sepsis. One species of *Campylobacter*, *C. fetus*, is particularly virulent in pregnant women and can result in chorioamnionitis, abortion, and neonatal sepsis and meningitis.

Crampy abdominal pain and nonbloody diarrhea are the first symptoms of STEC infection, sometimes with vomiting. Within several days, diarrhea becomes bloody and abdominal pain worsens. Bloody diarrhea lasts between 1 and 22 days (median 4 days). In contrast to dysentery, the stools associated with STEC hemorrhagic colitis are large volume and rarely accompanied by high fever. ETEC produce a secretory watery diarrhea that affects infants and young children in developing countries and is the major causative agents of travelers' diarrhea, accounting for about half of all episodes in some studies. EPEC remains a leading cause of persistent diarrhea associated with malnutrition among infants from developing countries. EIEC, which are genetically, biochemically, and clinically nearly identical to *Shigella*, causes rare foodborne outbreaks in industrialized countries. EAEC has been associated with persistent diarrhea in immunocompromised persons and sporadic diarrhea in infants in countries with varying levels of economic development; however, some other studies have not found an association with disease.

C. difficile toxin is associated with several clinical syndromes. The most common is mild to moderate watery diarrhea, low-grade fever, and mild abdominal pain. Occasionally, the illness will progress to full-blown *pseudomembranous colitis* characterized by diarrhea, abdominal cramps, and fever. The colonic mucosa contains 2-5 mm raised, yellowish plaques. Fatal cases are associated with toxic megacolon, systemic toxicity, and multisystem organ failure, possibly related to systemic absorption of toxin. A vomiting illness is associated with *S. aureus* and *B. cereus* emetic toxin, while diarrhea is the major manifesta-

Table 366.10	Intestinal and Extraintestinal Complications of Enteric Infections
COMPLICATION	**ASSOCIATED ENTERIC PATHOGEN(S)**
INTESTINAL COMPLICATIONS	
Persistent diarrhea	All causes
Recurrent diarrhea (usually immunocompromised persons)	*Salmonella, Shigella, Yersinia, Campylobacter, Clostridium difficile, Entamoeba histolytica, Cryptosporidium, Giardia*
Toxic megacolon	*Shigella, C. difficile, E. histolytica*
Intestinal perforation	*Shigella, Yersinia, C. difficile, E. histolytica*
Rectal prolapse	*Shigella*, STEC, *C. difficile*
Enteritis necroticans–jejunal hemorrhagic necrosis	*Clostridium perfringens* type C beta toxin
EXTRAINTESTINAL COMPLICATIONS	
Dehydration, metabolic abnormalities, malnutrition, micronutrient deficiency	All causes
Bacteremia with systemic spread of bacterial pathogens, including endocarditis, osteomyelitis, meningitis, pneumonia, hepatitis, peritonitis, chorioamnionitis, soft tissue infection, and septic thrombophlebitis	Nontyphoidal *Salmonella, Shigella, Yersinia, Campylobacter*
Local spread (e.g., vulvovaginitis and urinary tract infection)	*Shigella*
Pseudoappendicitis	*Yersinia, Campylobacter* (occasionally)
Exudative pharyngitis, cervical adenopathy	*Yersinia*
Rhabdomyolysis and hepatic necrosis	*Bacillus cereus* emetic toxin
POSTINFECTIOUS COMPLICATIONS	
Reactive arthritis	*Salmonella, Shigella, Yersinia, Campylobacter, Cryptosporidium, C. difficile*
Guillain-Barré syndrome	*Campylobacter*
Hemolytic uremic syndrome	STEC, *Shigella dysenteriae* 1
Glomerulonephritis, myocarditis, pericarditis	*Shigella, Campylobacter, Yersinia*
Immunoglobulin A (IgA) nephropathy	*Campylobacter*
Erythema nodosum	*Yersinia, Campylobacter, Salmonella*
Hemolytic anemia	*Campylobacter, Yersinia*
Intestinal perforation	*Salmonella, Shigella, Campylobacter, Yersinia, Entamoeba histolytica*
Osteomyelitis, meningitis, aortitis	*Salmonella, Yersinia, Listeria*

STEC, Shiga toxin–producing *Escherichia coli*.
From Centers for Disease Control and Prevention: Managing acute gastroenteritis among children, *MMWR Recomm Rep* 53:1–33, 2004.

tion of *C. perfringens* and *B. cereus* enterotoxins.

Protozoal Diarrhea. Illnesses due to intestinal protozoa tend to be more prolonged, sometimes for 2 wk or more, but usually self-limited in the otherwise healthy host (see Table 366.3). In general, the duration and severity of *Cryptosporidium* diarrhea is strongly influenced by the immune and nutritional status of the host. A protozoal etiology should be suspected when there is a prolonged diarrheal illness characterized by episodes of sometimes-explosive diarrhea with nausea, abdominal cramps, and abdominal bloating. The stools are usually watery but can be greasy and foul smelling due to concomitant malabsorption of fats, which is more likely to occur if the parasite load is high. Occasionally diarrhea may alternate with constipation.

In addition to diarrhea, *E. histolytica* causes a range of other syndromes. Amebic dysentery is characterized by bloody or mucoid diarrhea, which may be profuse and lead to dehydration or electrolyte imbalances. Hepatic amebiasis is limited to abscess formation in the liver, which may occur with or without intestinal disease.

INTESTINAL AND EXTRAINTESTINAL COMPLICATIONS

The major complications from diarrhea from any cause are dehydration, electrolyte, or acid-base derangements, which can be life-threatening (see Table 366.10). Avoiding delays in diagnosis and treatment, and appropriate supportive care using either oral, enteral, or intravenous hydration can prevent or treat most of these conditions. Children who experience frequent episodes of acute diarrhea or prolonged or persistent episodes (seen especially in low resource settings) are at risk for poor growth and nutrition and complications such as secondary infections and micronutrient deficiencies (iron, zinc, vitamin A). Ensuring continued nutritional support during diarrheal episodes is important because prolonged limitation of the diet may extend diarrheal symptoms. Reestablishing a normal diet generally restores villous anatomy and function with resolution of loose stools.

Viral AGE illnesses are usually self-limited and resolve after several days. Rarely, **intussusception** is triggered by lymphoid hyperplasia associated with viral AGE. Complications of bacterial AGE may be the result of local or systemic spread of the organism; in malnourished children and HIV-infected populations, associated **bacteremia** is well-recognized. Toxic megacolon, intestinal perforation, and rectal prolapse can occur, particularly in association with *Shigella* in developing countries and *C. difficile*. The most dreaded complication of pediatric diarrhea in the United States is **HUS**, the leading cause of acquired renal failure in children, developing in 5–10% of patients infected with STEC. It is usually diagnosed 2-14 days after the onset of diarrhea. HUS is unlikely to occur once diarrhea has remained resolved for 2 or 3 days with no evidence of hemolysis. Risk factors include age 6 mo to 4 yr, bloody diarrhea, fever, elevated leukocyte count, and treatment with antibiotics and antimotility agents. Two-thirds of patients no longer excrete the organism at the time they develop HUS (Chapter 538.5).

Pseudoappendicitis secondary to mesenteric adenitis is a notable complication of *Yersinia*, and sometimes *Campylobacter*. Older children and adolescents are most often affected. It typically presents with fever and abdominal pain with tenderness localized to the right lower quadrant, with or without diarrhea, and can be confused with appendicitis. CT scan or sonogram may be helpful to distinguish true appendicitis.

Immune-mediated complications that are thought to result from immunologic cross reactivity between bacterial antigens and host tissues are more often seen in adults than children. These include reactive arthritis following infection with the classical bacterial enteropathogens and Guillain-Barré syndrome following *Campylobacter* infection.

Protozoan illnesses, when persistent, can lead to poor weight gain in the young and immunocompromised individuals, weight loss, malnutrition, or vitamin deficiencies. Infection with *Entamoeba* can cause severe ulcerating colitis, colonic dilation, and perforation. The parasite may spread systemically, most commonly causing liver abscesses. In high-risk settings, it is critical to exclude *Entamoeba* infection and tuberculosis before initiating corticosteroids for presumed ulcerative colitis.

DIFFERENTIAL DIAGNOSIS

The physician should also consider noninfectious diseases that can present with bright red blood per rectum or hematochezia (Table 366.11). In an infant or young child without systemic symptoms, these may include anal fissures, intermittent intussusception, juvenile polyps, and Meckel diverticulum. Necrotizing enterocolitis can cause lower gastrointestinal bleeding in infants, especially premature neonates. Inflammatory bowel disease should be considered in older children. Examples of noninfectious causes of nonbloody diarrhea include congenital secretory diarrheas, endocrine disorders (hyperthyroidism), neoplasms, food intolerance, and medications (particularly antibiotics). Noninfectious causes of chronic or relapsing diarrhea include cystic fibrosis, celiac disease, milk protein intolerance, and congenital or acquired disaccharidase deficiency. Significant abdominal pain should raise suspicion of other infectious processes in the abdomen such as appendicitis and pelvic inflammatory disease. Prominent vomiting with or without abdominal pain can be a manifestation of pyloric stenosis, intestinal obstruction, pancreatitis, appendicitis, and cholecystitis.

Clinical Evaluation of Diarrhea

In the initial evaluation of all patients with AGE, the physician should focus on the patient's hydration status and electrolyte balance, as well as evidence of sepsis or invasive bacterial infection, which could complicate bacterial AGE (Fig. 366.6). Once the patient is stabilized,

Table 366.11	Differential Diagnosis of Acute Dysentery and Inflammatory Enterocolitis

SPECIFIC INFECTIOUS PROCESSES
- Bacillary dysentery (*Shigella dysenteriae, Shigella flexneri, Shigella sonnei, Shigella boydii; invasive Escherichia coli*)
- Campylobacteriosis (*Campylobacter jejuni*)
- Amebic dysentery (*Entamoeba histolytica*)
- Ciliary dysentery (*Balantidium coli*)
- Bilharzial dysentery (*Schistosoma japonicum, Schistosoma mansoni*)
- Other parasitic infections (*Trichinella spiralis*)
- Vibriosis (*Vibrio parahaemolyticus*)
- Salmonellosis (*Salmonella typhimurium*)
- Typhoid fever (*Salmonella typhi*)
- Enteric fever (*Salmonella choleraesuis, Salmonella paratyphi*)
- Yersiniosis (*Yersinia enterocolitica*)
- Spirillar dysentery (*Spirillum spp.*)

PROCTITIS
- Gonococcal (*Neisseria gonorrhoeae*)
- Herpetic (herpes simplex virus)
- Chlamydial (*Chlamydia trachomatis*)
- Syphilitic (*Treponema pallidum*)

OTHER SYNDROMES
- Necrotizing enterocolitis of the newborn
- Enteritis necroticans
- Pseudomembranous enterocolitis (*Clostridium difficile*)
- Typhlitis

CHRONIC INFLAMMATORY PROCESSES
- Enteropathogenic and enteroaggregative *E. coli*
- Gastrointestinal tuberculosis
- Gastrointestinal mycosis
- Parasitic enteritis

SYNDROMES WITHOUT KNOWN INFECTIOUS CAUSE
- Idiopathic ulcerative colitis
- Celiac disease
- Crohn disease
- Radiation enteritis
- Ischemic colitis
- Immune deficiency including HIV infection
- Allergic enteritis

From Mandell GL, Bennett JE, Dolin R, editors: *Principles and practices of infectious diseases*, ed 7, Philadelphia, 2010, Churchill Livingstone.

the history and physical examination can focus on detecting risk factors and exposures, as well as the clinical features that may suggest specific etiologic agents (see Tables 366.5 and 366.6).

Important elements of the medical history include the duration of diarrhea and a description of stools (frequency, amount, presence of blood or mucus), fever (duration, magnitude), vomiting (onset, amount and frequency), and the amount and type of solid and liquid oral intake.

Clinical signs of dehydration should be evaluated (Table 366.12): urine output (number of wet diapers per day and time since the last urination), whether eyes appear sunken, whether the child is active, whether the child drinks vigorously, and the date and value of the most recent weight measurement. A documented weight loss can be used to calculate the fluid deficit. The past medical history should identify comorbidities that might increase the risk or severity of AGE.

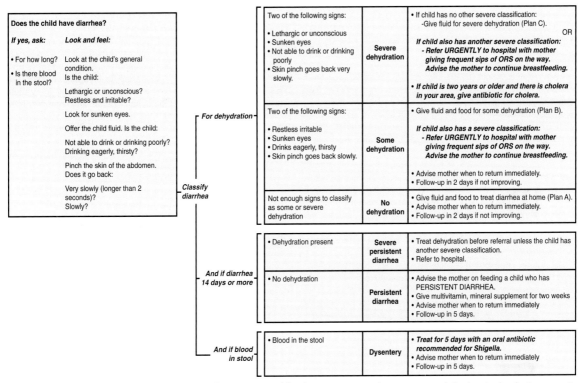

Fig. 366.6 Integrated Management of Childhood Illnesses protocol for the recognition and management of diarrhea in developing countries. *ORS*, oral rehydration solution.

Table 366.12	Clinical Signs Associated With Dehydration		
SYMPTOM	**MINIMAL OR NO DEHYDRATION**	**SOME DEHYDRATION**	**SEVERE DEHYDRATION**
Mental status	Well; alert	Normal, fatigued or restless, irritable	Apathetic, lethargic, unconscious
Thirst	Drinks normally; might refuse liquids	Thirsty; eager to drink	Drinks poorly; unable to drink
Heart rate	Normal	Normal to increased	Tachycardia, with bradycardia in most severe cases
Quality of pulses	Normal	Normal to decreased	Weak, thready, or impalpable
Breathing	Normal	Normal; fast	Deep
Eyes	Normal	Slightly sunken	Deeply sunken
Tears	Present	Decreased	Absent
Mouth and tongue	Moist	Dry	Parched
Skinfold	Instant recoil	Recoil in <2 sec	Recoil in >2 sec
Capillary refill	Normal	Prolonged	Prolonged; minimal
Extremities	Warm	Cool	Cold; mottled; cyanotic
Urine output	Normal to decreased	Decreased	Minimal

Modified from Duggan C, Santosham M, Glass RI: The management of acute diarrhea in children: oral rehydration, maintenance, and nutritional therapy, *MMWR Recomm Rep* 41(RR-16):1–20, 1992; and World Health Organization: *The treatment of diarrhoea: a manual for physicians and other senior health workers*, Geneva, 1995, World Health Organization; and Centers for Disease Control and Prevention: Diagnosis and management of foodborne illnesses, *MMWR* 53(RR-4):1–33, 2004.

Certain physical signs are best assessed before approaching the child directly, so he/she remains calm, including general appearance (activity, response to stimulation) and respiratory patterns. Skin turgor is assessed by pinching a small skin fold on the lateral abdominal wall at the level of the umbilicus. If the fold does not promptly return to normal after release, the recoil time is quantified as delayed slightly or ≥2 sec. Excess subcutaneous tissue and hypernatremia may produce a false negative test and malnutrition can prolong the recoil time. To measure capillary refill time, the palmar surface of the child's distal fingertip is pressed until blanching occurs, with the child's arm at heart level. The time elapsed until restoration of normal color after release usually exceeds 2 sec in the presence of dehydration. Mucous membrane moisture level, presence of tears, and extremity temperature should be assessed.

Laboratory Diagnosis

Most cases of AGE do not require diagnostic laboratory testing. Stool specimens could be examined for mucus, blood, neutrophils or fecal lactoferrin, a neutrophil product. The finding of more than 5 leukocytes per high-power field or a positive lactoferrin assay in an infant not breastfeeding suggests an infection with a classical bacterial entero-pathogen; patients infected with STEC and *E. histolytica* usually have negative tests.

Laboratory diagnosis of viral AGE may be helpful when an outbreak is suspected, cases are linked to a suspected outbreak, or when cohorting of patients is considered to limit the spread of infection. The preferred method of testing norovirus is real-time reverse transcription quantitative polymerase chain reaction (RT-qPCR), available at most public health and virology laboratories. Commercial tests are available for the diagnosis of rotavirus and enteric adenoviruses but not for astrovirus in the United States (see Table 366.1).

Stool cultures for detection of bacterial agents are costly, so requests should be restricted to patients with clinical features predictive of bacterial AGE, have moderate or severe disease, are immunocompromised, in outbreaks with suspected hemolytic-uremic syndrome, or have a highly suggestive epidemiologic history. To optimize recovery of pathogens, stool specimens for culture need to be transported and plated quickly; if the latter is not quickly available, specimens might need to be trans-ported in special transport media. If the child has not passed a stool and antibiotics will be administered, a rectal swab should be collected promptly. After dipping the cotton tip into the medium that will be used for transport, it is gently inserted into the child's rectum and rotated 360 degrees. A properly collected rectal swab is stained or covered with fecal material. Standard stool culture methods performed in clinical microbiology laboratories recover *Shigella* and *Salmonella* species. If *Campylobacter, Yersinia,* or *Vibrio* species are suspected, the laboratory should be notified unless media are routinely used for their detection. All bloody stools should also be inoculated into media specific for detection of *E. coli* 0157:H7 or directly tested for the presence of Shiga-like toxin (or both). Except for *C. difficile,* nosocomial acquisition of a bacterial enteric pathogen is very unlikely. Hence stool microbiologic assays are generally not indicated for patients in whom diarrhea develops more than 3 days after admission unless the patient is immunocom-promised or to investigate a hospital outbreak (see Table 366.2). Stool can also be tested for bacterial pathogens by nucleic acid amplification test (NAAT); if the NAAT is positive, the sample should automatically be cultured to determine antimicrobial sensitivities.

For children older than 2 yr who have recently received antibiotics or have other risk factors, evaluation for *C. difficile* infection may be appropriate. The cytotoxin assay detects toxin B, but testing for toxin A is also available in some laboratories; however, this test is laborious. Several tests are commercially available to detect toxin-producing *C. difficile* in stool, including enzyme immunoassays for toxins A and B, cell culture cytotoxicity assay, and PCR. The sensitivities of cell culture and PCR are superior to that of immunoassay. Testing for *C. difficile* toxin in children younger than 2 yr is discouraged because the organism and its toxins are commonly detected in asymptomatic infants (see Table 366.2).

Evaluation for intestinal protozoa that cause diarrhea is usually indicated in patients who recently traveled to an endemic area, have contact with untreated water, and manifest suggestive symptoms. The most commonly used method is direct microscopy of stool for cysts and trophozoites. However, this approach is time consuming and lacks sensitivity, in part because shedding can be intermittent. Analyzing 3 specimens from separate days is optimal, and fecal concentration techniques provide some benefit. The sensitivity and specificity of micros-copy are substantially improved using immunofluorescence antibodies that are commercially available for visualization of *Cryptosporidium* and *Giardia* cysts. In addition, enzyme immunoassays are available for *Cryptosporidium, Giardia,* and *Entamoeba* that are more sensitive and specific than direct microscopy and provide a useful diagnostic tool (not all commercial kits distinguish between pathogenic *E. histolytica* and nonpathogenic *E. dispar*). Molecular methods (NAAT) are also available.

Several culture-independent *rapid multiplex molecular panels* for detection of viral, bacterial, and protozoal gastrointestinal pathogens directly from stool samples are FDA approved, including xTag GPP (14 pathogens), Verigene EP (9 pathogens), and the FirmArray GI (22 pathogens). These methods offer several advantages over conventional diagnostics, including reduced sample volume requirements, broad coverage without the need to select specific tests, enhanced ability to detect coinfections, increased sensitivity, and rapid turnaround. However, their use is controversial because the available tests do not provide strain specificity or antimicrobial susceptibility testing to assist with outbreak detection and treatment decisions.

Most episodes of diarrheal dehydration are isonatremic and do not warrant serum electrolyte measurements. Electrolyte measurements are most useful in children with severe dehydration, when intravenous fluids are administered, when there is a history of frequent watery stools, yet the skin pinch feels doughy without delayed recoil, which suggests hypernatremia, or when inappropriate rehydration fluids have been administered at home. A suspicion for HUS prompts a complete blood count with review of the peripheral smear, platelets, serum electrolytes, and renal function tests. Patients with shigellosis can demonstrate bandemia or even a leukemoid reaction. Blood culture should be obtained if there is concern for systemic bacterial infection. This includes infants and children with fever and/or blood in the stool who are younger than 3 mo, are immunocompromised, or have hemolytic anemia or other risk factors. If diarrhea persists with no cause identified, endoscopic evaluation may be indicated. Biopsy specimens help in diagnosing inflammatory bowel disease or identifying infecting agents that may mimic it. A sweat test is warranted if cystic fibrosis is suspected.

TREATMENT

The broad principles of management of AGE in children include rehydration and maintenance ORS plus replacement of continued losses in diarrheal stools and vomitus after rehydration, continued breastfeeding, and refeeding with an age-appropriate, unrestricted diet as soon as dehydration is corrected. Zinc supplementation is recommended for children in developing countries.

Hydration

Children, especially infants, are more susceptible than adults to dehydra-tion because of the greater basal fluid and electrolyte requirements per kilogram and because they are dependent on others to meet these demands (Table 366.13). *Dehydration must be evaluated rapidly and corrected in 4-6 hr according to the degree of dehydration and estimated daily requirements.* When there is emesis, small volumes of ORS can be given initially by a dropper, teaspoon, or syringe, beginning with as little as 5 mL at a time. The volume is increased as tolerated. The low-osmolality World Health Organization (WHO) ORS containing 75 mEq of sodium, 64 mEq of chloride, 20 mEq of potassium, and 75 mmol of glucose per liter, with total osmolarity of 245 mOsm/L, is now the global standard of care and more effective than home fluids. Soda beverages, fruit juices, tea, and other home fluids are not suitable for rehydration or maintenance therapy because they have inappropriately high glucose concentration and osmolalities and low sodium concentrations. Tables 366.12 and 366.13 outline a clinical evaluation plan and management strategy for children with moderate to severe diarrhea. Replacement for emesis or stool losses is noted in Table 366.13. Oral rehydration can also be given by a nasogastric tube if needed; this is not the usual route.

Table 366.13	Fluid and Nutritional Management of Diarrhea	
DEGREE OF DEHYDRATION*	**REHYDRATION THERAPY**	**REPLACEMENT OF LOSSES DURING MAINTENANCE†**
Some dehydration	Infants‡ and children: ORS, 50-100 mL/kg over 3-4 hr. Continue breast feeding. After 4 hr, give food every 3-4 hr for children who normally receive solid foods.	Infants and children: <10 kg body weight: 50-100 mL ORS for each diarrheal stool or vomiting episode, up to ~500 mL/day >10 kg body weight: 100-200 mL ORS for each diarrheal stool or vomiting episode; up to ~1 L/day Replace losses as above as long as diarrhea or vomiting continues
Severe dehydration	Malnourished infants may benefit from smaller-volume, frequent boluses of 10 mL/kg body weight due to reduced capacity to increase cardiac output with larger volume resuscitation. Infants (<12 months) and children (12 mo to 5 yr) without malnutrition: Give 20-30 mL/kg boluses of intravenous isotonic crystalloid solution (e.g., normal saline solution) over 30-60 min. Repeat boluses as necessary to restore adequate perfusion. Then give 70 mL/kg over 2.5-5 hr. (Note the slower infusion times are for infants.) Reassess the infant or child frequently and adjust infusion rate if needed. Switch to ORS, breast milk, and feed as described for some dehydration, when the child can drink, perfusion is adequate, and mental status is normal. Adjust electrolytes and administer dextrose based on chemistry values.	Infants and children: <10 kg body weight: 50-100 mL ORS for each diarrheal stool or vomiting episode, up to ~500 mL/day >10 kg body weight: 100-200 mL ORS for each diarrheal stool or vomiting episode; up to ~1 L/day Adolescents and adults: Ad libitum, up to ~2 L/day Replace losses as above as long as diarrhea or vomiting continue. If unable to drink, administer either through a nasogastric tube or give 5% dextrose 0.25 normal saline solution with 20 mEq/L potassium chloride intravenously.

*A variety of scales are available to grade the severity of dehydration in young children, but no single, standard, validated method exists. Note that signs of dehydration may be masked when a child is hypernatremic. The World Health Organization defines some dehydration as the presence of two or more of the following signs: restlessness/irritability, sunken eyes, drinks eagerly, thirsty, and skin pinch goes back slowly. Severe dehydration is defined as two or more of the following signs: lethargy/unconsciousness, sunken eyes, unable to drink/drinks poorly, and skin pinch goes back very slowly (>2 sec).

†After rehydration is complete, maintenance fluids should be resumed along with an age-appropriate normal diet offered every 3-4 hr. Children previously receiving a lactose-containing formula can tolerate the same product in most instances. Diluted formula does not appear to confer any benefit.

‡Breastfed infants should continue nursing throughout the illness.

Low-osmolarity ORS can be given to all age groups, with any cause of diarrhea. It is safe in the presence of hypernatremia, as well as hyponatremia (except when edema is present). Some commercially available formulations that can be used as ORS include Pedialyte Liters (Abbott Nutrition), CeraLyte (Cero Products), and Enfalac Lytren (Mead Johnson). Popular beverages that should not be used for rehydration include apple juice, Gatorade, and commercial soft drinks.

ORS, oral rehydration solution.

Modified from Centers for Disease Control and Prevention: Managing acute gastroenteritis among children: oral rehydration, maintenance, and nutritional therapy. *MMWR Recomm Rep* 52(RR-16):1–16, 2003; and World Health Organization. Pocket book of hospital care for children: Guidelines for the management of common childhood illnesses, ed 2 (http://www.who.int/maternal_child_adolescent/documents/child_hospital_care/en/).

A small minority of children, including those with severe dehydration or unable to tolerate oral fluids, require initial intravenous rehydration, but oral rehydration is the preferred mode of rehydration and replacement of ongoing losses. Signs of severe dehydration that might necessitate intravenous resuscitation are shown in Table 366.13. Limitations to ORS include shock, decreased level of consciousness, an ileus, intussusception, carbohydrate intolerance (rare), severe emesis, and high stool output (>10 mL/kg/hr).

Enteral Feeding and Diet Selection

Continued breastfeeding and refeeding with an age-appropriate, unrestricted diet as soon as dehydration is improving or resolved aids in recovery from the episode. Foods with complex carbohydrates (rice, wheat, potatoes, bread, and cereals), fresh fruits, lean meats, yogurt, and vegetables should be reintroduced while ORS is given to replace ongoing losses from emesis or stools and for maintenance. Fatty foods or foods high in simple sugars (juices, carbonated sodas) should be avoided. The usual energy density of any diet used for the therapy of diarrhea should be around 1 kcal/g, aiming to provide an energy intake of a minimum of 100 kcal/kg/day and a protein intake of 2-3 g/kg/day. In selected circumstances when adequate intake of energy-dense food is problematic, the addition of amylase to the diet through germination techniques can also be helpful.

If the normal diet includes infant formula, it should not be diluted, or changed to a lactose-free preparation unless lactose malabsorption is evident. With the exception of acute lactose intolerance in a small subgroup, most children with diarrhea are able to tolerate milk and lactose-containing diets. *Withdrawal of milk and replacement with specialized lactose-free formulations are unnecessary.* Although children with persistent diarrhea are not lactose intolerant, administration of a lactose load exceeding 5 g/kg/day may be associated with higher purging rates and treatment failure. Alternative strategies for reducing the lactose load while feeding malnourished children who have prolonged diarrhea include addition of milk to cereals and replacement of milk with fermented milk products such as yogurt.

Rarely, when dietary intolerance precludes the administration of cow's milk–based formulations or whole milk, it may be necessary to administer specialized milk-free diets such as a comminuted or blenderized chicken-based diet or an elemental formulation. Although effective in some settings, the latter are unaffordable in most developing countries. In addition to rice-lentil formulations, the addition of green banana or pectin to the diet has also been shown to be effective in the treatment of persistent diarrhea. Fig. 366.7 gives an algorithm for managing children with prolonged diarrhea in developing countries.

Among children in low- and middle-income countries, where the dual burden of diarrhea and malnutrition is greatest and where access to proprietary formulas and specialized ingredients is limited, the use of locally available age-appropriate foods should be promoted for the majority of acute diarrhea cases. Even among those children for whom lactose avoidance may be necessary, nutritionally complete diets composed of locally available ingredients can be used at least as effectively as commercial preparations or specialized ingredients. These same conclusions may also apply to the dietary management of children with persistent diarrhea, but the evidence remains limited.

Zinc Supplementation

Zinc supplementation in children with diarrhea in developing countries leads to reduced duration and severity of diarrhea and could potentially prevent a large proportion of cases from recurring. Zinc administration for diarrhea management can significantly reduce all-cause mortality by 46% and hospital admission by 23%. In addition to improving diarrhea recovery rates, administration of zinc in community settings leads to

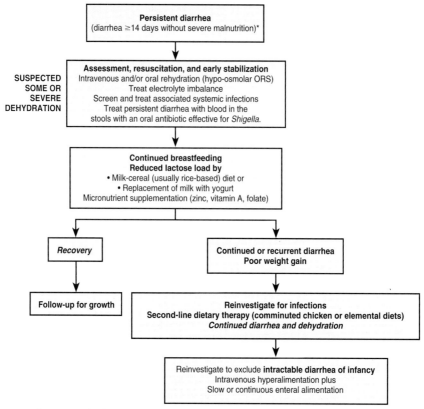

Fig. 366.7 Management of persistent diarrhea. *IV,* intravenous; *NG,* nasogastric tube; *ORS,* oral rehydration solution. *Severely malnourished children require urgent referral for hospitalization and specific treatment.

increased use of ORS and reduction in the inappropriate use of antimicrobials. All children older than 6 mo of age with acute diarrhea in at-risk areas should receive oral zinc (20 mg/day) in some form for 10-14 days during and continued after diarrhea. The role of zinc in well nourished, zinc replete populations in developed countries is less certain.

Additional Therapies

The use of probiotic nonpathogenic bacteria for prevention and therapy of diarrhea has been successful in some settings, although the evidence does not support a recommendation for their use in all settings. A variety of organisms *(Lactobacillus, Bifidobacterium)* have a good safety record; therapy has not been standardized and the most effective (and safe) organism has not been identified. *Saccharomyces boulardii* is effective in antibiotic-associated and in *C. difficile* diarrhea, and there is some evidence that it might prevent diarrhea in daycare centers. Two large randomized placebo-controlled trials evaluating the efficacy of two *Lactobacillus*-based probiotic formulations failed to reduce a clinical severity score in Canadian infants and preschool children with acute gastroenteritis. *Lactobacillus rhamnosus* GG or a combination probiotic product containing *L. rhamnosus* R0011 and *L. helveticus* R0052 is has shown variable efficacy; reduction is more evident in cases of childhood rotavirus diarrhea.

Ondansetron (oral mucosal absorption preparation) reduces the incidence of emesis, thus permitting more effective oral rehydration and is well-established in emergency management of AGE in high-resource settings, reducing intravenous fluid requirements and hospitalization. Because persistent vomiting can limit ORS, a single sublingual dose of an oral dissolvable tablet of ondansetron (4 mg for children 4-11 yr old and 8 mg for children older than 11 yr [generally 0.2 mg/kg]) may be given. However, most children do not require specific antiemetic therapy; careful ORS is usually sufficient. Antimotility agents (loperamide) are contraindicated in children with dysentery and probably

have no role in the management of acute watery diarrhea in otherwise healthy children. Similarly, antiemetic agents, such as the phenothiazines, are of little value and are associated with potentially serious side effects (lethargy, dystonia, malignant hyperpyrexia).

Antibiotic Therapy

Judicious antibiotic therapy for suspected or proven bacterial infections can reduce the duration and severity of illness and prevent complications (Table 366.14). Several factors justify limited use. First, most episodes of AGE are self-limited among otherwise healthy children. Second, the increasing prevalence of antibiotic resistance has prompted restricted use of these drugs. Third, antibiotics may worsen outcome, because some studies have shown that antibiotic therapy of STEC infection increases the risk of HUS and prolongs excretion of NTS without improving clinical outcome. Therefore antibiotics are used primarily to treat severe infections, prevent complications in high-risk hosts, or to limit the spread of infection. Microbiologic (culture) confirmation of the etiology and susceptibility testing should be sought prior to treatment if possible.

Treatment of *C. difficile* infection warrants special consideration. Removal of the offending antibiotic, if possible, is the first step. Antibiotic therapy directed against *C. difficile* should be instituted if the symptoms are severe or persistent. Testing for *C. difficile* is discouraged for children with diarrhea who are <2 yr unless there is strong evidence to implicate *C. difficile* as the etiologic agent. This recommendation is based on the high rates of asymptomatic infection with toxigenic and nontoxigenic strains and the rarity of characteristic clinical manifestations not attributed to other pathogens in this age group. Oral vancomycin and metronidazole for 7-14 days (first line agents) displayed equivalent efficacy in a prospective randomized trial; however, metronidazole is preferred because of lower cost and decreased potential for inducing

Table 366.14	Antibiotic Therapy for Infectious Diarrhea	
ORGANISM	**INDICATION FOR THERAPY**	**DOSAGE AND DURATION OF TREATMENT**
Shigella spp.	In high-income countries, judicious treatment is recommended to curtail growing antibiotic resistance because most shigellosis is self-limited. Treatment should be reserved for moderate to severe disease (require hospitalization, have systemic disease or complications), immunocompromised, or to prevent or mitigate outbreaks in certain settings (e.g., childcare or food handling). Also consider treating patients with significant discomfort, intestinal comorbidities, institutional settings, or household exposure to high-risk individuals. WHO recommends empiric antibiotics for all children in developing countries with dysentery assuming that most cases are caused by *Shigella*.	*First line:* • Ciprofloxacin* 15 mg/kg/day PO bid × 3 days; OR • Ceftriaxone 50-100 mg/kg/day IV or IM, qd × 3 days for severe illness requiring parenteral therapy; OR • Azithromycin* 12 mg/kg once on 1st day, then 6 mg/kg once daily on days 2 through 4 (total course: 4 days) *Second line:* • Cefixime 8 mg/kg once daily for 3 days; OR • Trimethoprim-sulfamethoxazole 4 mg/kg/day of TMP and 20 mg/kg/day SMX twice a day for 5 days (if susceptibility known or likely based on local data)
ETEC	Watery diarrhea in a traveler returning from an endemic area that interferes with planned activities or is persistent.	*First line:* • Azithromycin* 12 mg/kg once on first day, then 6 mg/kg once daily on days 2 and 3 (total course: 3 days) *Second line:* • Ciprofloxacin* 15 mg/kg/day PO bid × 3 days
STEC	Avoid antimicrobials and anti-motility drugs	
Salmonella, non-typhoidal	Antibiotics for uncomplicated gastroenteritis in normal host are ineffective and may prolong excretion and are not recommended Treatment should be reserved for infection in infants younger than 3 mo, and patients with immunocompromise, malignancy, chronic GI disease, severe colitis hemolytic anemia, or HIV infection. Most strains are resistant to multiple antibiotics	See treatment of *Shigella*. Patients without bacteremia can be treated orally for 5-7 days. Patients with bacteremia (proven or until blood culture results are available in a high-risk host) should be treated parenterally for 10-14 days. Focal or disseminated invasive infections (e.g., osteomyelitis, meningitis) and bacteremic patients with HIV/AIDS should be treated parenterally for 4-6 wk.
Yersinia spp.	Antibiotics are not usually required for diarrhea, which is usually self-limited and clinical benefits of antibiotics are not established. Bacteremia and focal invasive infections should be treated. Deferoxamine therapy should be withheld for severe infections or associated bacteremia	For bacteremia or focal invasive infections, use third generation cephalosporins. Can also consider carbapenem, doxycycline (for children ≥8 yr) plus aminoglycoside, TMP-SMX, or fluoroquinolone at doses recommended for sepsis. Begin IV then switch to oral when clinically stable, for a total course of 2-6 wk.
Campylobacter spp.	Dysentery, moderate and severe gastroenteritis or at risk for severe disease (e.g., elderly, pregnant, or immunocompromised), and bacteremia or focal invasive infection should be treated. Treatment of gastroenteritis appears effective if given within 3 days of onset of illness.	*For gastroenteritis or dysentery:* • Erythromycin PO 40 mg/kg/day divided qid × 5 days; OR • Azithromycin PO 10 mg/kg/day × 3 days *For bacteremia or focal invasive infection:* • Consider parenteral macrolides or carbapenems pending susceptibility results. Fluoroquinolone resistance is >50% in some areas of the world.
Clostridium difficile	Colitis • Discontinue inciting antibiotics if possible; • Infectious disease consult suggested if disease is persistent or recurrent.	*First line (mild-moderate colitis):* • Metronidazole PO 30 mg/kg/day divided tid or qid × 10 days; max 500 mg/dose; OR • Vancomycin PO 40 mg/kg/day divided qid × 10 days, max 125 mg/dose *Second line (severe colitis):* • Vancomycin PO 40 mg/kg/day divided qid × 10 days, max 500 mg/dose; OR • If ileus, give same dose PR as 500 mg/100 mL normal saline by retention enema with or without plus metronidazole IV 30 mg/kg/day divided tid × 10 days; max 500 mg/dose • Fidaxomicin not yet approved for children; see text
Entamoeba histolytica	Treat the following conditions: • Asymptomatic cyst excretors • Mild to moderate intestinal disease • Severe intestinal or extraintestinal disease (including liver abscess)	*Asymptomatic cyst excretors:* • Iodoquinol PO 30-40 mg/kg/day, max 2 g, divided tid × 20 days; OR • Paromomycin PO 25-35 mg/kg/d divided tid × 7 days; *Mild to moderate intestinal disease and severe intestinal or extra-intestinal disease:* • Metronidazole PO 30-40 mg/kg/day divided tid × 7-10 days; OR • Tinidazole PO 50 mg/kg, single dose, max 2 g (for children ≥ 3 yr old) × 3 days, OR 5 days for severe disease EITHER FOLLOWED BY (to prevent relapse) • Iodoquinol PO 30-40 mg/kg/day tid × 20 days; OR • Paromomycin PO 25-35 mg/kg/day tid × 7 days

Continued

Table 366.14	Antibiotic Therapy for Infectious Diarrhea—cont'd	
ORGANISM	**INDICATION FOR THERAPY**	**DOSAGE AND DURATION OF TREATMENT**

Giardia intestinalis	Persistent symptoms	• Tinidazole PO 50 mg/kg, single dose, max 2 g (for children ≥ 3 yr old); OR
		• Nitazoxanide PO; OR
		  – Age 1-3 yr: 100 mg bid × 3 days
		  – Age 4-11 yr: 200 mg bid × 3 days
		  – Age over 11 yr: 500 mg bid × 3 days
		• Metronidazole PO 30-40 mg/kg/day divided tid × 7 days (max 250 mg per dose)

Cryptosporidium spp.	Treat immunocompromised and HIV-infected hosts, although efficacy is equivocal Treatment may not be needed in normal hosts	*Immunocompetent children:* • Nitazoxanide, as for *Giardia* *Solid organ transplants:* • Nitazoxanide, as for *Giardia*, × ≥14 days; reduce immunosuppression if possible and consider paromomycin combined with azithromycin for severe symptoms or treatment failure *HIV-infected children:* • Combined antiretroviral therapy is the primary treatment • Nitazoxanide, as for *Giardia*, generally for 3-14 days while awaiting CD4 cell recovery; OR • Consider paromomycin alone or combined with azithromycin in severe disease or treatment failure
Cyclospora spp *Isospora belli* (now designated *Cystoisospora belli*).	All symptomatic children	TMP 5 mg/kg/day and SMX 25 mg/kg/day PO bid × 7-10 days (HIV-infected children may need longer courses)

Blastocystis hominis	The significance of *B. hominis* as a cause of disease is controversial, so treatment should be reserved for those with suggestive symptoms and no other pathogen that could be the cause.	• Metronidazole PO 30-40 mg/kg/day divided tid × 7-10 days; OR
		• Nitazoxanide, as for *Giardia*; OR
		  TMP-SMX as for *Cyclospora*; OR
		  Tinidazole, as for *Giardia*

EIEC, enteroinvasive *Escherichia coli*; *EPEC*, enteropathogenic *E. coli*; *ETEC*, enterotoxigenic *E. coli*; *GI*, gastrointestinal; *IV*, intravenous; *IM*, intramuscular; *max*, maximum; *SMX*, sulfamethoxazole; *TMP*, trimethoprim; *WHO*, World Health Organization.

*Azithromycin and fluoroquinolones should be avoided in patients taking the antimalarial artemether. These drugs can prolong the QT interval on the electrocardiogram and trigger arrhythmias.

vancomycin-resistant enterococci. Twenty percent of adults treated for *C. difficile* diarrhea have a relapse, but the frequency in children is not known. The first relapse should be treated with another course of antibiotics based on severity of illness. For recurrent disease, tapering and/or pulsed regimen of oral vancomycin over a 4- to 6-wk period has been proposed. In the absence of ongoing symptoms, a test of cure is not necessary. The role of probiotics in the prevention of *C. difficile*-associated diarrhea in children has not been established. Fecal transplant is being explored to treat persistent or recurrent *C. difficile* colitis. *Fidaxomicin* is an alternate agent approved for patients ≥18 yr of age; it is recommended for the initial episode (severe and nonsevere) and recurrences. The adult dose is 200 mg BID for 10 days by mouth. *Bezlotoxumab,* a monoclonal antibody against *C. difficile* toxins A and B, has been shown to reduce the recurrence rate.

Antibiotic therapy for parasitic infections is shown in Table 366.14.

PREVENTION
Promotion of Exclusive Breastfeeding and Vitamin A
Exclusive breastfeeding (administration of no other fluids or foods for the first 6 mo of life) protects young infants from diarrheal disease through the promotion of passive immunity and through reduction in the intake of potentially contaminated food and water. In developing countries, exclusive breastfeeding for the first 6 mo of life is widely regarded as one of the most effective interventions to reduce the risk of premature childhood mortality and has the potential to prevent 12% of all deaths of children younger than 5 yr of age. Vitamin A supplementation reduces all-cause childhood mortality by 25% and diarrhea-specific mortality by 30%.

Rotavirus Immunization
Three live oral **rotavirus** vaccines are licensed: the 3-dose pentavalent G1, G2, G3, G4, P[8] human-bovine vaccine (RotaTeq), the 2-dose monovalent human G1P[8] vaccine (ROTARIX), and the 3-dose monovalent human-bovine 116E G6P[11] vaccine (Rotavax). The result has been substantial reductions in rotavirus-associated and all-cause hospitalizations for diarrheal disease in both vaccinated infants (direct protection) and unvaccinated individuals (indirect, or herd protection), as well as reductions in-office visits for less severe rotavirus diarrhea. Reductions in all-cause diarrhea deaths have been demonstrated in some countries.

Programmatic uptake has lagged in low-resource settings where most severe disease and death occurs; however, Gavi, the Vaccine Alliance, has supported introduction of rotavirus vaccine into more than 40 countries to date. Even though vaccine efficacy against severe rotavirus AGE is lower (50–64%) in low- compared with high-resource countries, the number of severe rotavirus AGE prevented per vaccinated child is higher because of the substantially greater baseline rate of severe rotavirus gastroenteritis in developing countries. Vaccine (live virus) associated rotavirus infection has been reported in children with severe combined immunodeficiency disease, but the vaccine has been shown to be safe in HIV-infected populations.

Two licensed, efficacious 2-dose oral inactivated **cholera** vaccines (Dukoral for children 2 yr and older and ShanChol for children 1 yr or older) are available in many countries but currently have no specific indication in endemic and epidemic settings where they could potentially reduce the burden of severe diarrhea and mortality in young children. For travelers, a single-dose live oral cholera vaccine (Vaxchora) was recently licensed for adults in the United States. In addition, 2 forms of typhoid fever vaccine are available: a polysaccharide vaccine delivered intramuscularly that can be administered to children older than 2 yr (Vivotif) and an oral, live attenuated vaccine that can be administered to children over 6 yr of age (Typhim Vi). Conjugate polysaccharide typhoid vaccines that could be used in children younger than 2 yr have recently become available. In 2018, the World Health Organization issued a recommendation for the use of this vaccine in infants and children 6 mo of age or older living in endemic areas, with catch-up vaccination campaigns, if possible, for children up to 15 yr old. The vaccine is not yet available in the United States or Europe.

Improved Water and Sanitary Facilities and Promotion of Personal and Domestic Hygiene

Much of the reduction in diarrhea prevalence in the developed world is the result of improvement in standards of hygiene, sanitation, and water supply. Strikingly, an estimated 88% of all diarrheal deaths worldwide can be attributed to unsafe water, inadequate sanitation, and poor hygiene. Handwashing with soap and safe excreta disposal can reduce the risk of diarrhea by 48% and 36%, respectively, and a 17% reduction is estimated as a result of improvements in water quality.

Bibliography is available at Expert Consult.

366.1 Traveler's Diarrhea
Karen L. Kotloff

Traveler's diarrhea is a common complication of visitors to developing countries and is caused by a variety of pathogens, in part depending on the season and the region visited. It is the most common (28%) travel-associated health problem in children. Traveler's diarrhea can manifest with watery diarrhea or as dysentery. Without treatment, 90% will have resolved within a week and 98% within a month of onset. Some individuals develop more severe or persistent diarrhea and become dehydrated or unwell and may experience complications such as bacteremia and intestinal perforation. Children younger than 2 yr are at higher risk for traveler's diarrhea, as well as more severe disease. According to the FoodNet, the pathogens identified most commonly in travelers in the United States were *Campylobacter* (42%), NTS (32%), and *Shigella* (13%). ETEC and intestinal protozoa (*G. intestinalis* and *E. histolytica*) are also important.

TREATMENT
For infants and children, rehydration, as discussed in Chapter 366, is appropriate, followed by a standard diet. Adolescents and adults should increase their intake of electrolyte-rich fluids. Kaolin-pectin, anticholinergic agents, *Lactobacillus,* and bismuth salicylate are not effective therapies. Loperamide, an antimotility and antisecretory agent, reduces the number of stools in older children with watery diarrhea and improves outcomes when used in combination with antibiotics in traveler's diarrhea. However, loperamide should not be used in febrile or toxic patients with dysentery, in those with bloody diarrhea, and in children younger than 6 yr.

The effectiveness of antibiotics depends on the pathogen and its susceptibility profile. In forming a treatment plan, the potential side effects should be weighed against the treatment need for a short-lasting and self-limiting disease such as traveler's diarrhea. Antibiotics are not recommended for mild diarrhea that is tolerable, is not distressing, and does not interfere with planned activities. When empiric therapy is required abroad, azithromycin is suggested for young children. Fluoroquinolones are recommended for older children and adults and as second line therapy for younger children. Short-duration (3 days) therapy is effective. Travelers should be reminded that diarrhea can be a symptom of other severe diseases, such as malaria. Therefore, if diarrhea persists or additional symptoms such as fever occur, travelers should seek medical advice. For up-to-date information on local pathogens and resistant patterns, see www.cdc.gov/travel.

If the patient has returned home with diarrhea, a microbiologic evaluation can be obtained before initiating antibiotic therapy. Prolonged diarrhea should prompt further investigation into possible parasitic infections or NTS. Prophylactic antibiotics for travelers are not recommended.

PREVENTION
In the pretravel visit, caregivers should be advised about diarrhea prevention, the signs, symptoms, and management of dehydration, and the use of ORS. ORS and age-appropriate antibiotics should be included in a routine health packet. Travelers should drink bottled or canned beverages or boiled water. They should avoid ice, salads, and fruit they did not peel themselves. Food should be eaten hot, if possible. Raw or poorly cooked seafood is a risk, as is eating in a restaurant rather than a private home. Swimming pools and other recreational water sites can also be contaminated.

Chemoprophylaxis is not routinely recommended for previously healthy children or adults. Nonetheless, travelers should bring azithromycin (younger than 16 yr of age) or ciprofloxacin (older than 16 yr of age) and begin antimicrobial therapy if diarrhea develops.

Bibliography is available at Expert Consult.

Chapter **367**

Chronic Diarrhea

Anat Guz-Mark and Raanan Shamir

第三百六十七章
儿童慢性腹泻

中文导读

　　本章主要介绍了慢性腹泻的定义、流行病学，详细介绍了慢性腹泻的病理生理机制，详述了慢性腹泻的常见病因，包括感染、炎症及免疫因素、胰腺功能不全、肝胆疾病、碳水化合物吸收不良、蛋白丢失性肠病、肠动力异常、短肠综合征、非特异性腹泻及先天腹泻性疾病等。详细阐述了慢性腹泻病的评估、检查及治疗方法（原文第367）。简要介绍了神经内分泌肿瘤引起的慢性腹泻（原文第367.1）。

DEFINITION OF EPIDEMIOLOGY

Chronic diarrhea is defined as stool volume of more than 10 g/kg/day in toddlers/infants and greater than 200 g/day in older children that lasts for 4 wk or more. **Persistent** diarrhea began acutely but lasts longer than 14 days. In practice, this usually means having loose or watery stools more than 3 times a day. *Awakening at night to pass stool is often a sign of an organic cause of diarrhea.* The epidemiology has 2 distinct patterns. In *developing* countries, chronic diarrhea is, in many cases, the result of an intestinal infection that persists longer than expected. This syndrome is often defined as **protracted (persistent) diarrhea,** but there is no clear distinction between protracted (persistent) and chronic diarrhea. In countries with higher socioeconomic conditions, chronic diarrhea is less frequent, and the etiology often varies with age. The outcome of diarrhea depends on the cause and ranges from benign, self-limited conditions, such as toddler's diarrhea, to severe congenital diseases, such as microvillus inclusion disease, that may lead to progressive intestinal failure.

PATHOPHYSIOLOGY

The mechanisms of diarrhea are generally divided into **secretory** and **osmotic**, but often diarrhea is a *combination of both mechanisms.* In addition, *inflammation* and *motility disorders* may contribute to diarrhea. Secretory diarrhea is usually associated with large volumes of watery stools and persists when oral feeding is withdrawn. Osmotic diarrhea is dependent on oral feeding, and stool volumes are usually not as massive as in secretory diarrhea (Fig. 367.1).

　　Secretory diarrhea is characterized by active electrolyte and water fluxes toward the intestinal lumen, resulting from either the inhibition of neutral NaCl absorption in villous enterocytes or an increase in electrogenic chloride secretion in secretory crypt cells as a result of the opening of the cystic fibrosis transmembrane regulator (CFTR) chloride channel or both. The result is more secretion from the crypts than absorption in the villous that persists during fasting. The other com-

ponents of the enterocyte ion secretory machinery are (1) the Na-K 2Cl cotransporter for the electroneutral chloride entrance into the enterocyte; (2) the Na-K pump, which decreases the intracellular Na^+ concentration, determining the driving gradient for further Na^+ influx; and (3) the K^+ selective channel, that enables K^+, once it has entered the cell together with Na^+, to return to the extracellular fluid.

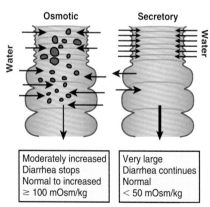

Fig. 367.1 Pathways of osmotic and secretory diarrhea. Osmotic diarrhea is caused by functional or structural damage of intestinal epithelium. Nonabsorbed osmotically active solutes drive water into the lumen. Stool osmolality and ion gap are generally increased. Diarrhea stops in children when not eating. In secretory diarrhea, ions are actively pumped into the intestine by the action of exogenous and endogenous secretagogues. Usually there is no intestinal damage. Osmolality and ion gap are within normal levels. Large volumes of stools are lost independent of food ingestion.

Electrogenic secretion is induced by an increase of intracellular concentration of cyclic adenosine monophosphate, cyclic guanosine monophosphate, or calcium in response to microbial enterotoxins, or to endogenous endocrine or nonendocrine molecules, including inflammatory cytokines. Another mechanism of secretory diarrhea is the inhibition of the electroneutral NaCl-coupled pathway that involves the Na^+/H^+ and the Cl^-/HCO_3^- exchangers. Defects in the genes of the Na^+/H^+ and the Cl^-/HCO_3^- exchangers are responsible for congenital Na^+ and Cl^- diarrhea, respectively.

Osmotic diarrhea is caused by nonabsorbed nutrients in the intestinal lumen as a result of one or more of the following mechanisms: (1) intestinal damage (e.g., enteric infection); (2) reduced absorptive surface area (e.g., active celiac disease); (3) defective digestive enzyme or nutrient carrier (e.g., lactase deficiency); (4) decreased intestinal transit time (e.g., functional diarrhea); and (5) nutrient overload, exceeding the digestive capacity (e.g., overfeeding, sorbitol in fruit juice). Whatever the mechanism, the osmotic force generated by nonabsorbed solutes drives water into the intestinal lumen. A very common example of osmotic diarrhea is lactose intolerance. Lactose, if not absorbed in the small intestine, reaches the colon, where it is fermented to short-chain organic acids, releasing hydrogen that is detected in the lactose breath test, and generating an osmotic overload. Another risk for chronic osmotic diarrhea often noted in patients with diarrhea-associated irritable bowel syndrome are foods containing FODMAPs (fermentable oligo-di-monosaccharides and polyols).

In many children chronic diarrhea may be caused by the combination of multiple mechanisms.

ETIOLOGY

Table 367.1 summarizes the main etiologies of chronic diarrhea in infants and children.

Infectious

Enteric infections are by far the most frequent cause of persistent or chronic diarrhea, both in developing and industrialized countries, however outcomes are often very different. In the former, comorbid conditions, such as HIV/AIDS, malaria, or tuberculosis, result in malnutrition that impairs the child's immune response, thereby potentiating the likelihood of prolonging diarrhea or acquiring another enteric infection. In children with HIV/AIDS, the viral infection itself impairs immune function and may trigger a vicious circle with malnutrition. Sequential infections with the same or different pathogens may also be responsible for chronic diarrhea. In *developing* countries, enteroadherent *Escherichia coli* and *Giardia lamblia* have been implicated in chronic diarrhea, whereas, in *developed* countries, chronic infectious diarrhea usually runs a more benign course and the etiology is often viral, with a major role of rotavirus and norovirus (Table 367.2).

Chronic diarrhea in travelers to or expatriates from developing countries may depend on the country of origin. Nonetheless, common pathogens include giardia, *E. coli*, shigella, campylobacter, salmonella, and enteric viruses. Less common pathogens include amebiasis, strongyloides, and tropical sprue.

Opportunistic microorganisms induce diarrhea exclusively, more severely, or for more prolonged periods, in specific populations, such as immunocompromised children. Specific agents cause chronic diarrhea or exacerbate diarrhea in many chronic diseases. *Clostridium difficile* or cytomegalovirus act as opportunistic agents in oncologic patients as well as in patients with inflammatory bowel diseases. *Cryptosporidium* may induce severe and protracted diarrhea in AIDS patients.

Small intestinal bacterial overgrowth results in chronic diarrhea by either a direct interaction between the microorganism and the enterocyte, or the consequence of deconjugation and dihydroxylation of bile salts and hydroxylation of fatty acids due to an increased proliferation of bacteria in the proximal intestine.

Postenteritis diarrhea syndrome (Chapter 364.4) is a clinicopathologic condition in which small intestinal mucosal damage persists after acute gastroenteritis. Sensitization to food antigens, secondary disaccharidase deficiency, persistent infections, reinfection with an enteric pathogen, or side effects of medication may be responsible for causing postenteritis diarrhea syndrome, thought to be related to dysregulation of the intestinal microbiota. Functional diarrhea which may be related to the pathogenesis of irritable bowel syndrome may be caused by complications of an acute gastroenteritis.

Inflammatory/Immunologic

Celiac disease (Chapter 364.2) is a genetically determined permanent gluten intolerance that affects about 1 in 100 individuals, depending on geographic origin. In the genetically susceptible host, gliadin, the major protein of gluten, reacts with the immune system to cause villous atrophy. A reduction of intestinal absorptive surface is responsible for

Table 367.1	Main Etiologies of Chronic Diarrhea in Children Older and Younger Than 2 Yr of Age	
ETIOLOGY	**YOUNGER THAN 2 YR**	**OLDER THAN 2 YR**
Infections	+++	+++
Postenteritis syndrome	+++	+++
Immune deficiency	++	Rare
Celiac disease	+++ (after gluten introduction)	+++
Food allergy	+++	+
Inflammatory bowel disease	+ (rare)	+++
Pancreatic insufficiency	++	++
Cholestasis and insufficient bile acids	++	++
Cystic fibrosis	++	+
Lactose intolerance	++ (mostly postinfectious)	+++
Intestinal lymphangiectasia	+	+
Motility disorders	++	Rare
Short bowel syndrome	+++	+
Toddler's and functional diarrhea	++	++
Excessive intake of fruit juices and fluids	++	++
Congenital diarrheal disorders, including structural enterocyte defects and enzymatic or transport malabsorption syndromes	++	Unlikely

Table 367.2	A Comparative List of Prevalent Agents and Conditions in Children With Persistent Infectious Diarrhea in Industrialized and Developing Countries

AGENT/DISEASE	
INDUSTRIALIZED COUNTRIES	**DEVELOPING COUNTRIES**
Clostridium difficile	Enteroaggregative *E. coli*
Enteroaggregative *Escherichia coli*	Atypical *E. coli*
	Shigella
	Heat stable/heat labile enterotoxin-producing *E. coli*
Astrovirus	Rotavirus*
Norovirus	Cryptosporidium
Rotavirus*	*Giardia lamblia*
Small intestinal bacterial overgrowth (SIBO)	Tropical sprue
Postenteritis diarrhea syndrome	

*More frequent in industrialized than in developing countries as agent of chronic diarrhea.

the diarrhea in celiac disease, which is reversible upon restriction of gluten from the diet.

Food allergy (mainly cow milk protein allergy Chapter 176) may present during infancy with chronic diarrhea. An abnormal immune response to food proteins can cause a proctitis/colitis or an enteropathy. **Eosinophilic gastroenteritis** is characterized by eosinophilic infiltration of the intestinal wall and is strongly associated with atopy. However, whereas diarrhea in food allergy responds to withdrawal of the responsible food, this does not always occur in eosinophilic gastroenteritis, in which immune suppression may be needed.

Inflammatory bowel diseases, including Crohn disease, ulcerative colitis, and inflammatory bowel disease–undetermined, cause chronic diarrhea that is often associated with abdominal pain, elevated inflammatory markers, and increased concentrations of fecal calprotectin or lactoferrin (see Chapter 362). The age of onset of inflammatory bowel disease is broad, with rare cases described in the 1st few mo of life, but the peak incidence in childhood occurs in adolescence. The severity of the symptoms is highly variable with a pattern characterized by long periods of well-being followed by exacerbations.

Autoimmune processes may target the intestinal epithelium, alone or in association with extraintestinal symptoms. **Autoimmune enteropathy** is associated with the production of antienterocyte and antigoblet cell antibodies, primarily immunoglobulin A, but also immunoglobulin G, directed against components of the enterocyte brush-border or cytoplasm and by a cell-mediated autoimmune response with mucosal T-cell activation. An X-linked immune-dysregulation, polyendocrinopathy, and enteropathy (**IPEX syndrome**) is associated with variable gene mutations and phenotypes of chronic diarrhea (more on autoimmune enteropathy and IPEX syndrome is available on Chapter 364.3).

Immune deficiency can present as chronic diarrhea in children. In these cases (for example, severe combined immunodeficiency or AIDS) the child can be infected by an opportunistic pathogen; can exhibit a persistent diarrhea due to a pathogen usually causing an acute gastroenteritis; or be infected by multiple and recurrent different pathogens causing mucosal damage to the intestines. Other immunoregulatory defects, found in patients with agammaglobulinemia, isolated immunoglobulin A deficiency, and common variable immunodeficiency disorder, may result in mild persistent infectious diarrhea.

Pancreatic Deficiency

Chronic diarrhea may be the manifestation of maldigestion caused by exocrine pancreatic disorders (see Chapters 376 and 378.2). In most patients with **cystic fibrosis**, exocrine pancreatic insufficiency results in steatorrhea and protein malabsorption. In **Shwachman-Diamond syndrome**, exocrine pancreatic hypoplasia may be associated with neutropenia, bone changes, and intestinal protein-losing enteropathy.

Specific isolated pancreatic enzyme defects, such as lipase deficiency, result in fat and/or protein malabsorption. Familial pancreatitis, associated with a mutation in the trypsinogen gene, may be associated with exocrine pancreatic insufficiency and chronic diarrhea. Mutations in *CFTR, CTRC, PRSS1, PRSS2, SPINK 1,* and *SPINK 5* are associated with hereditary pancreatitis.

Liver and Bile Acids Disorders

Liver disorders and **cholestasis** may lead to a reduction in the bile salts pool resulting in fat malabsorption causing chronic diarrhea in the form of steatorrhea. Bile acid loss may be associated with diseases affecting the terminal ileum, such as Crohn disease, or following ileal resection. In **primary bile acid malabsorption**, neonates and young infants present with chronic diarrhea and fat malabsorption caused by mutations of ileal bile transporter. In addition to the fat malabsorption, the bile acid loss from the intestinal lumen is a form of secretory diarrhea by itself (called **cholorrheic diarrhea**, which is usually associated with significant diaper dermatitis).

Carbohydrate Malabsorption

Rare genetic mutations (Chapters 364.9 and 364.11) can cause carbohydrate malabsorption. More commonly, **lactose intolerance** is *secondary* to lactase deficiency caused by intestinal mucosal damage (usually as part of postenteritis syndrome, which is a self-limited process). Depending on ethnicity, a progressive, age-related, loss of lactase activity may begin around 7 yr of age and affects approximately 80% of the non-white population, and acquired hypolactasia may be responsible for chronic diarrhea in older children receiving cow's milk (adult-type lactase deficiency).

Similarly, **fructose malabsorption** is common in Western countries with estimates as high as 40% of the population. These individuals cannot absorb fructose and often develop bloating, abdominal pain, diarrhea, and flatulence. Typically, they do not have liver disease. This is in contrast to **hereditary fructose intolerance**, a rare genetic disorder with incidence estimated to be 1 in 20,000-30,000. This disease is associated with mutations in the *ASDOB* gene that encodes for the aldolase B enzyme that is found primarily in the liver and is involved in the metabolism of fructose. Individuals with hereditary fructose intolerance may have nausea, abdominal pain/bloating, vomiting, diarrhea, and hypoglycemia. Continued ingestion of fructose results in *hepatomegaly* and eventually cirrhosis.

Protein-Losing Enteropathy

Chronic diarrhea can be the manifestation of obstructed intestinal lymphatic drainage, causing protein-losing enteropathy with steatorrhea, diarrhea, and lymphopenia. Besides **intestinal lymphangiectasia**, many diseases that cause intestinal mucosal injury can also result in protein-losing enteropathy, characterized by low serum protein levels and elevated fecal α_1-antitrypsin (see Chapter 364.3).

Motility Disorders

Disorders of intestinal motility include abnormal development and function of the enteric nervous system, such as in **Hirschsprung disease** and **chronic intestinal pseudoobstruction** (which encompass both the neurogenic and the myogenic forms). Other motility disorders may be secondary to extraintestinal disorders, such as in *hyperthyroidism* and *scleroderma*. Motility disorders are associated with either constipation or diarrhea or both, with the former usually dominating the clinical picture.

Short Bowel Syndrome

Short bowel syndrome is the single most frequent etiology of intestinal failure in children (Chapter 364.7). Many intestinal abnormalities such as stenosis, segmental atresia, gastroschisis, and malrotation may require surgical resection, but the most frequent primary cause of short bowel is necrotizing enterocolitis. Rarely, a child can be born with congenitally short small bowel. In these conditions, the residual intestine may be insufficient to carry on its digestive–absorptive functions, resulting in severe chronic diarrhea, malnutrition, and failure to thrive, requiring long-term treatment with parenteral nutrition.

Nonspecific Diarrhea, Including Toddler's Diarrhea

The most benign and common etiology of chronic diarrhea is nonspecific diarrhea that encompasses **functional diarrhea** (or **toddler's diarrhea**) in children younger than 4 yr of age and **irritable bowel syndrome** in those 5 yr of age and older. It is the leading cause of chronic diarrhea in an otherwise well child. Toddler's diarrhea is defined by the daily painless recurrent passage of 4 or more large unformed stools, for 4 or more wk, with onset in infancy or preschool years. Nighttime defecation is usually absent. The child appears unperturbed by the diarrhea, there is no evidence of failure to thrive, and the symptoms resolve spontaneously by school age.

Diarrhea may also be the result of an **excessive intake of fluid and nonabsorbable carbohydrate**. If the child's fluid intake were > 150 mL/kg/24 hr, fluid intake should be reduced not to exceed 90 mL/kg/24 hr in order to decrease the stool frequency and volume. If the dietary history suggests that the child is ingesting significant amounts of fruit juice, especially apple juice, then the consumption of juice should be decreased. *Sorbitol, which is a nonabsorbable sugar, is found in apple, pear, and prune juices, and often causes diarrhea in toddlers.* Moreover, apple and pear juices contain higher amounts of fructose than glucose, a feature postulated to cause diarrhea in toddlers. In older children, irritable bowel syndrome is often associated with abdominal pain and may be related to anxiety, depression, and other psychological disturbances (Chapter 368). When the cause of the diarrhea remains undetermined and the clinical course is inconsistent with organic disorders, **factitious** disorder by proxy should be considered.

Congenital Diarrheal Disorders

The most severe etiology of chronic diarrhea includes a number of heterogeneous congenital conditions leading to syndromes often referred to as **intractable or protracted diarrhea**. This is the result of a permanent defect in the structure or function of the enterocyte, leading to progressive, potentially irreversible intestinal failure. The genetic and molecular basis of many causes of protracted diarrhea has been identified recently and a new classification of **congenital diarrheal disorders (CDDs)** has been proposed (Table 367.3). CDDs are a group of rare but severe enteropathies, with a similar clinical presentation despite a different pathogenesis and outcome. The diarrhea can be either secretory or osmotic, depending on the specific defect. Often severe diarrhea presents at birth or shortly thereafter, but in milder forms diarrhea may go unrecognized for years. CDDs can be classified in 4 groups: defects of digestion, absorption and transport of nutrients and electrolytes; defects of enterocyte differentiation and polarization; defects of enteroendocrine cell differentiation; and defects of modulation of intestinal immune response.

Although CDDs are rare diseases, in most specific disorders the genetic defect and transmission are known. The incidence of genetic disorders associated with CDD can range from 1 in 2,500 for cystic fibrosis, 1 in 5,000 for sucrose-isomaltase deficiency, 1 in 60,000 for congenital lactase deficiency, to 1 in 400,000 for trichohepatoenteric syndrome. For most CDDs, such as IPEX syndrome or autoimmune polyglandular syndrome type 1, the clinical application of exome sequencing is likely to increase identification of more patients with these rare causes of chronic diarrhea. Selected CDDs are more frequent in ethnic groups where consanguineous marriages are common, or in some geographic areas because of founder effects. Congenital lactase deficiency is more common in Finland; lysinuric protein intolerance has a higher incidence either in Finland and in Japan because of founder effect, and a specific mutation is typically found in each of the 2 ethnic groups. A defect in the *DGAT1* gene was identified using whole-exome sequencing in an Ashkenazi Jewish family and associated with the early onset of vomiting and nonbloody diarrhea with protein-losing enteropathy. For specific CDDs see Chapters 364.3 and 364.11.

Most cases of protracted diarrhea syndrome are not easily treated. The natural history of protracted diarrhea is related to the primary intestinal disease and the specific defect in nutrient absorption. Treatment is more favorable for motility disorders and autoimmune enteropathy than for structural enterocyte defects. Children with motility disorders may have persistent symptoms, but they are rarely fatal, whereas children with structural enterocyte defects have a more severe course, poorer prognosis, and are more likely to be candidates for intestinal transplantation (see Chapter 365). Some late-onset CDDs may be relatively mild and are recognized only later in life.

EVALUATION OF PATIENTS

Because of the spectrum of etiologies, the medical approach should be based on diagnostic algorithms that begin with assessment for infectious causes, and then consider the age of the child, growth, and clinical and epidemiologic factors. Early onset in the neonatal period is rare and may suggest a congenital or severe condition (see also Table 364.3), however infections and food allergy are more frequent in this age group, and together with gastrointestinal (GI) malformations should be high on the differential diagnosis. In later infancy and up to 2 yr of age, infections and allergies are the most common; inflammatory diseases are more frequent in older children and adolescents. Celiac disease as well as functional nonspecific diarrhea should always be considered independently of age because of their relatively high frequency at all ages.

Specific clues in the family and personal history may provide useful indications, suggesting a congenital, allergic, or inflammatory etiology. A history of *polyhydramnios* is consistent with congenital chloride-sodium diarrhea (where a typical sonographic finding of dilated fetal bowel loops is present), cystic fibrosis, and other CDDs, as well as a family history of a chronic or intractable diarrhea in a relative presenting in the 1st mo of life, as well as *consanguinity*. An acute onset of diarrhea that runs a protracted course suggests postenteritis diarrhea, secondary lactase deficiency, small intestinal overgrowth, or the onset of chronic nonspecific diarrhea (toddler's diarrhea). The association of diarrhea with specific foods may indicate a nutrient basis, such as intolerance to selected nutrients (fructose). Anthropometric evaluation is essential to understand if diarrhea has affected weight gain and growth, providing estimation of the severity of diarrhea. Normal weight and growth strongly support functional diarrhea that may respond to simple dietary management. It should be noted that a child with functional diarrhea may be inappropriately "treated" with a diluted hypocaloric diet in an effort to reduce the diarrhea, resulting in impaired growth.

Initial clinical examination should include the evaluation of general and nutritional status. Dehydration, marasmus, or kwashiorkor require prompt supportive interventions to stabilize the patient. Nutritional evaluation should start with the evaluation of the weight and height curves, and of the weight-for-height index to determine the impact of diarrhea on growth. Weight is generally impaired before height, but with time, linear growth also becomes affected, and both parameters may be equally abnormal in the long term. Assessment of nutritional status includes a dietary history, physical examination, and biochemical testing including nutritional investigations. Caloric intake should be quantitatively determined, energy requirements determined, and the relationship between weight modifications and energy intake should be carefully considered. Assessment of body composition may be performed by measuring mid-arm circumference and triceps skinfold thickness or by bioelectrical impedance analysis, dual-emission x-ray absorptiometry scans, or air plethysmography. Biochemical markers including albumin, prealbumin, retinol binding protein, serum iron, and transferrin may assist in grading malnutrition, as the half-life of serum proteins may distinguish between short- and long-term malnutrition. Evaluation of micronutrient concentrations should always be considered. Zinc, magnesium, vitamin A, and folate deficiency are associated with chronic diarrhea and should be provided if needed.

In infants with chronic diarrhea, feeding history must be carefully obtained, providing clues for allergy or specific food intolerance, such as cow's-milk protein allergy or sucrose-isomaltase deficiency. Associated symptoms and selected investigations provide important diagnostic clues. Signs of general inflammation such as fever, mucoid or bloody stools, and abdominal pain may suggest inflammatory bowel disease. The presence of eczema or asthma is associated with an allergic disorder, whereas specific extraintestinal manifestations (arthritis, diabetes, thrombocytopenia, etc.) may suggest an autoimmune disease. Specific skin lesions may be suggestive of **acrodermatitis enteropathica** that might respond to zinc supplementation. Typical facial abnormalities and woolly hair are associated with phenotypic diarrhea.

| Table 367.3 | Classification of Congenital Diarrheal Disorders Based on Their Molecular Defect and Their Inheritance |

DEFECTS OF DIGESTION, ABSORPTION, AND TRANSPORT OF NUTRIENTS AND ELECTROLYTES

DISEASE	GENE NAME	GENE LOCATION	TRANSMISSION AND INCIDENCE	MECHANISM
GENES ENCODING BRUSH-BORDER ENZYMES				
Congenital lactase deficiency (LD)	LCT	2q21.3	AR, 1 in 60,000 in Finland; lower in other ethnic groups	Osmotic
Congenital sucrase-isomaltase deficiency (SID)	SI	3q26.1	AR, 1 in 5,000; higher incidence in Greenland, Alaska, and Canada	Osmotic
Congenital maltase-glucoamylase deficiency (MGD)	Not defined	—	Few cases described	Osmotic
GENES ENCODING MEMBRANE CARRIERS				
Glucose-galactose malabsorption (GGM)	SLC5A1	22q13.1	AR, few hundred cases described	Osmotic
Fructose malabsorption (FM)	Not defined	—	Up to 40%	Osmotic
Fanconi-Bickel syndrome (FBS)	SLC2A2	3q26.2	AR, rare, higher frequency in consanguineous	Osmotic
Acrodermatitis enteropathica (ADE)	SLC39A4	8q24.3	AR, 1 in 500,000	Osmotic
Congenital chloride diarrhea (CCD, DIAR 1)	SLC26A3	7q31.1	AR, sporadic; frequent in some ethnicities	Osmotic
Lysinuric protein intolerance (LPI)	SLC7A7	14q11.2	AR, about 1 in 60,000 in Finland and Japan; rare in other ethnic groups	Osmotic
Primary bile acid malabsorption (PBAM)	SLC10A2	13q33.1	AR	Secretory
Cystic fibrosis (CF)	CFTR	7q31.2	AR, 1 in 2,500	Osmotic
GENES ENCODING PANCREATIC ENZYMES				
Enterokinase deficiency (EKD)	PRSS7	21q21	AR	Osmotic
Hereditary pancreatitis (HP)	PRSS1	7q34	AD, cases with compound mutations in different genes; SPINK1 mutations may also cause tropical pancreatitis	Osmotic
	PRSS2	7q34		
	SPINK1	5q32		
	CTRC	1p36.21		
Congenital absence of pancreatic lipase (APL)	PNLIP	10q25.3	AR	Osmotic
GENES ENCODING PROTEINS OF LIPOPROTEIN METABOLISM				
Abetalipoproteinemia (ALP)	MTP	4q27	AR, about 100 cases described; higher frequency among Ashkenazi Jews	Osmotic
Hypobetalipoproteinemia (HLP)	APOB	2p24.1	Autosomal codominant	Osmotic
Chylomicron retention disease (CRD)	SAR1B	5q31.1	AR, about 40 cases described	Osmotic
GENES ENCODING OTHER TYPES OF PROTEINS				
Congenital sodium diarrhea (CSD)	SPINT2 (only syndromic CSD) SLC9A3	19q13.2 5p15.33	AR	Osmotic
Shwachman-Diamond syndrome (SDS)	SBDS	7q11	AR	Osmotic
Activating guanylate cyclase-C mutation	GUCY2C	12p12.3	AD	Secretory
GENES ENCODING FOR OTHER ENZYMES				
Defect in triglyceride synthesis	DGAT1	8q24.3	AR	Protein-losing enteropathy
DEFECTS OF ENTEROCYTE DIFFERENTIATION AND POLARIZATION				
Microvillous inclusion disease (MVID, DIAR 2)	MYO5B	18q21.1	AR; rare; higher frequency among Navajo	Secretory
Congenital tufting enteropathy (CTE, DIAR 5)	EPCAM	2p21	AR; 1 in 50,000-100,000; higher among Arabians	Secretory
Trichohepatoenteric syndrome (THE)	TTC37 SKIV2L	5q15 6p21.33	AR; 1 in 400,000	Secretory
DEFECTS OF ENTEROENDOCRINE CELL DIFFERENTIATION				
Congenital malabsorptive diarrhea (CMD, DIAR 4)	NEUROG3	10q22.1	AR; few cases described	Osmotic
Proprotein convertase 1/3 deficiency (PCD)	PCSK1	5q15	AR	Osmotic
DEFECTS OF MODULATION OF INTESTINAL IMMUNE RESPONSE				
Autoimmune polyglandular syndrome type 1 (APS1)	AIRE	21q22.3	AR; AD (1 family)	Secretory
Immune dysfunction, polyendocrinopathy, X-linked (IPEX)	FOXP3	Xp11.23	X-linked (autosomal cases described), very rare	Secretory
IPEX-like syndrome	Not defined	—	Not X-linked	Secretory

AD, autosomal dominant; AR, autosomal recessive.

INVESTIGATIONS

Microbiologic investigation should include a thorough list of intestinal bacterial, viral, and protozoan pathogens. Proximal intestinal bacterial overgrowth may be determined using the lactulose hydrogen breath test, but false-positive tests are common (see Chapter 364.4).

Initial investigations of a child with chronic diarrhea should always include an assessment of intestinal inflammation using fecal calprotectin or lactoferrin, and serology for celiac disease (see Chapter 364.2). The role of a mucosal biopsy is determined by the noninvasive diagnostic evaluation in consultation with a pediatric gastroenterologist.

Noninvasive assessment of digestive-absorptive function and of intestinal inflammation plays a key role in the diagnostic workup (Table 367.4). Abnormalities in the digestive-absorptive function tests suggest small bowel involvement, whereas intestinal inflammation, as demonstrated by increased fecal calprotectin or lactoferrin, supports colitis.

Determining the osmotic versus secretory nature of the diarrhea in neonates and infants with protracted diarrhea is especially important. The **stool osmolar gap**, sometimes called stool ion gap, is calculated as 290 mOsm/kg (or measured stool osmolality) minus [2 × (stool Na + stool K)]. If the osmolar gap is above 100 mOsm/kg, fecal osmolality is derived from ingested or nonabsorbed osmotically active solutes or nonmeasured ions. In contrast, a low gap (<50 mOsm/kg) is typically observed in secretory diarrhea. It is also important to measure Cl^- concentration in the stool to rule out CCD, which is characterized by low osmolar gap due to high Cl^- fecal loss (>90 mmol/L).

Whereas most etiologies of chronic diarrhea can be exaggerated by feeding and have osmotic or mixed nature to the stool, secretory diarrhea necessitates investigation for congenital defects in enterocytes, defects in the intestinal immune response (IPEX and autoimmune enteropathy), and disorders of bile acid malabsorption. Because of the overlap between secretory and osmotic features of the diarrhea in many diseases, a classification based on the response to bowel rest was also introduced. Severe diarrhea that persists at bowel rest is characteristic of **congenital enteropathies** (microvillous inclusion disease, tufting enteropathy, syndromic diarrhea). Diarrhea that disappears at bowel rest can imply carbohydrate or fat malabsorptive syndromes, as well as defects in enteroendocrine cells. In most other etiologies the diarrhea can decrease significantly, but not disappear, in response to bowel rest, including some congenital diseases as well as acquired inflammatory and other enteropathies.

Histology is important in establishing mucosal involvement, noting changes in the epithelial cells, or in identifying specific intracellular inclusion bodies caused by pathogens, such as cytomegalovirus, or the presence of parasites. Electron microscopy is essential to detect subcellular structural abnormalities such as microvillous inclusion disease. Immunohistochemistry allows the study of mucosal immunity as well as of other cell types (smooth muscle cells and enteric neuronal cells).

Imaging has a major role in the diagnostic approach. Abdominal ultrasound may help in detecting liver and pancreatic abnormalities or an increase in distal ileal wall thickness that suggests inflammatory bowel disease. A preliminary plain abdominal x-ray is useful for detection of abdominal distention, suggestive of intestinal obstruction, or increased retention of colonic feces. Intramural or portal gas may be seen in necrotizing enterocolitis or intussusception. Structural abnormalities such as diverticula, malrotation, stenosis, blind loop, and congenital short bowel, as well as motility disorders, may be investigated through a barium meal and a small bowel follow-through. Capsule endoscopy can be done when the patient weighs more than 10 kg and allows the exploration of the entire intestinal tract searching for structural changes, inflammation, or bleeding; the new SmartPill measures pressure, pH, and temperature as it moves through the GI tract, assessing motility.

Specific investigations should be carried out for specific diagnostic indications. Prick and patch test may support a diagnosis of food allergy. However, an elimination diet with withdrawal of the suspected harmful food from the diet and subsequent challenge is the most reliable strategy by which to establish a diagnosis. Bile malabsorption may be explored by the retention of the bile acid analog ^{75}Se-homocholic acid-taurine (^{75}SeHCAT) in the enterohepatic circulation. A scintigraphic examination, with radio-labeled octreotide is indicated in suspected APUD cell neoplastic proliferation. In other diseases, specific imaging techniques such as computed tomography, or nuclear magnetic resonance endoscopic retrograde cholangiopancreatography and magnetic resonance cholangiopancreatography, may have important diagnostic value.

Once infectious agents have been excluded and nutritional assessment performed, a stepwise approach to the child with chronic diarrhea may be applied. The main causes of chronic diarrhea should be investigated, based on the features of the diarrhea and the specific nutrient(s) that is (are) affected. The use of whole-exome sequencing or specific molecular analysis may be especially essential in children suspected of having CDD. A step-by-step diagnostic approach is important to minimize the unnecessary use of invasive procedures as well as the cost, while optimizing the yield of the diagnostic evaluation (Table 367.5).

TREATMENT

Chronic diarrhea associated with impaired nutritional status should always be considered a serious disease, and therapy should be started promptly. Treatment includes general supportive measures, nutritional rehabilitation, elimination diet, and medications. The latter include therapies for specific etiologies as well as interventions aimed at counteracting fluid secretion and/or promoting restoration of disrupted intestinal epithelium. Because death in most instances is caused by dehydration, replacement of fluid and electrolyte losses is the most important early intervention.

Nutritional rehabilitation is often essential and is based on clinical and biochemical assessment. In moderate to severe malnutrition, caloric intake should be carefully advanced to avoid the development of refeeding syndrome and may be progressively increased to 50% or more above the recommended dietary allowances. The intestinal absorptive capacity should be monitored by digestive function tests. In children with steatorrhea, medium-chain triglycerides may be the main source of lipids. A

Table 367.4	Noninvasive Tests for Intestinal Digestive–Absorptive Function and Inflammation	
TEST	**NORMAL VALUES**	**IMPLICATION**
α_1-Antitripsin concentration	<0.9 mg/g	Increased intestinal permeability/protein loss
Steatocrit	<2.5% (older than 2 yr) fold increase over age-related values (younger than 2 yr)	Fat malabsorption
Fecal-reducing substances	Absent	Carbohydrate malabsorption
Elastase concentration	>200 μg/g	Pancreatic function
Chymotrypsin concentration	>7.5 units/g >375 units/24 hr	Pancreatic function
Fecal occult blood	Absent	Blood loss in the stools/inflammation
Fecal calprotectin concentration	<100 μg/g (in children to 4 yr of age) <50 μg/g (older than 4 yr)	Intestinal inflammation
Fecal leukocytes	<5/microscopic field	Colonic inflammation
Fecal lactoferrin	Absent	Inflammation
Nitric oxide in rectal dialysate	<5 μM of NO_2^-/NO_3^-	Rectal inflammation
Dual sugar (cellobiose/mannitol) absorption test	Urine excretion ratio: 0.010 ± 0.018	Increased intestinal permeability
Xylose oral load	25 mg/dL	Reduced intestinal surface

Table 367.5	Stepwise Diagnostic Approach to Children and Infants With Chronic Diarrhea

INITIAL EVALUATION
- Personal and family history: Prenatal sonography; feeding history; family history of protracted diarrhea; consanguinity
- Physical examination: Dysmorphism; skeletal abnormalities; organomegaly; dermatitis

- Infectious workup: Stool cultures; parasites; viruses
- Allergic workup: Elimination diet trial

⇓

LABORATORY TESTS
- Stool analysis: *Stool volume following fasting; stool electrolytes and ion gap; pH and reducing substances; steatocrit; fecal leukocytes and calprotectin; fecal elastase; α_1-antitrypsin*

- Blood and serum analysis: Serum electrolytes; lipid profile; albumin and pre-albumin; amylase and lipase; inflammatory markers; ammonia; celiac serology

⇓

IMAGING
- Abdominal ultrasound: Bowel wall thickening; liver and bile disorders

- X-ray and contrast studies: Congenital malformation; signs of motility disorders

⇓

ENDOSCOPIES AND INTESTINAL HISTOLOGY
Endoscopy and standard jejunal/colonic histology*; morphometry; PAS staining; intestinal immunohistochemistry; electron microscopy

⇓

GENETIC INVESTIGATION
- Specific molecular analysis

- Whole-exome sequencing

⇓

OTHER SPECIAL INVESTIGATIONS
Sweat test; specific carbohydrates breath tests; ^{75}SeHCAT measurement; antienterocyte antibodies; metabolic diseases workup; motility studies; neuroendocrine tumor markers

*The decision to perform an upper or a lower endoscopy may be supported by noninvasive tests. *PAS,* Periodic acid–Schiff; *75SeHCAT,* ^{75}Se-homocholic acid-taurine.

lactose-free diet should be started in all children with chronic diarrhea and is recommended by the World Health Organization. Lactose is generally replaced by maltodextrin or a combination of complex carbohydrates. A sucrose-free formula is indicated in sucrase-isomaltase deficiency. Semi-elemental or elemental diets have the dual purpose of overcoming food intolerance, which may be the primary cause of chronic diarrhea, particularly in infancy and early childhood, and facilitating nutrient absorption. The sequence of elimination should begin from less to more restricted diets, that is, cow's-milk protein hydrolysate to amino-acid–based formulas, depending on the child's situation. In severely compromised infants, it may be prudent to start with amino-acid–based feeding.

When oral nutrition is not feasible or fails, enteral or parenteral nutrition should be considered. Enteral nutrition may be provided via nasogastric or gastrostomy tube and is indicated in a child who is not able to be fed orally, either because of inability to tolerate nutrient requirements or because of extreme weakness. In extreme wasting and in cases of significant intestinal mucosal damage or dysfunction, enteral nutrition may not be tolerated, and **parenteral nutrition** is required.

Micronutrient and vitamin supplementation are part of nutritional rehabilitation, especially in malnourished children in developing countries. Zinc supplementation is important in both prevention and therapy of chronic diarrhea, since it promotes ion absorption, restores epithelial proliferation, and stimulates immune response. Nutritional rehabilitation has a general beneficial effect on the patient's general condition, intestinal function, and immune response.

Functional diarrhea in children may benefit from a diet based on the "4 F" principles (reduce fructose and fluids, increase fat and fiber). The use of probiotics in persistent infectious and postinfectious diarrhea in children appear to hold promise as adjunctive therapy with reduction in symptom duration, but there is still insufficient evidence to recommend their routine use.

Pharmacologic therapy includes, based on the etiology, anti-infectious drugs, immune suppression, and drugs that may inhibit fluid loss and promote cell growth. If a bacterial agent is detected, specific antibiotics should be prescribed. Empiric antibiotic therapy may be used in children

with either small bowel bacterial overgrowth or with suspected infectious diarrhea. Table 367.6 summarizes the antimicrobial treatment of infectious persistent diarrhea. Immune suppression should be considered in selected conditions such as autoimmune enteropathy and inflammatory bowel disease.

Treatment may be also directed at modifying specific pathophysiologic processes. Secretion of ions may be reduced by antisecretory agents, such as the enkephalinase inhibitor racecadotril. Some benefit from absorbents, such as diosmectite, has been described, with reduction of diarrhea duration in infectious diarrhea. In diarrhea caused by neuroendocrine tumors (NETs), microvillus inclusion disease and enterotoxin-induced severe diarrhea, a trial of somatostatin analog octreotide may be considered. Zinc promotes both enterocyte growth and ion absorption and may be effective when intestinal atrophy and ion secretion are associated. However, when therapeutic attempts and other nutritional support have failed, the only option to treat children with intestinal failure, while maintaining adequate growth and development, may be long-term parenteral nutrition or eventually intestinal transplantation.

Bibliography is available at Expert Consult.

367.1 Diarrhea From Neuroendocrine Tumors

Shimon Reif and Raanan Shamir

The incidence of neuroendocrine tumors (NET) originating in the gastrointestinal (GI) tract is increasing globally. The commonly perceived notion of NETs is of slow-growing malignancies with a benign course. Indeed, well-differentiated GI-NETs may exhibit indolent clinical behavior, but recent studies indicate that they are frequently already metastatic at diagnosis. The most common tumor in children is **carcinoid** and mostly it is a low-grade tumor especially when it is small, that is <1 cm. It is equally distributed between the small and large intestine and can commonly be found in the appendix. Most carcinoids are found

Table 367.6	Antimicrobial Treatment for Persistent Diarrhea			
	DRUG	**INDICATIONS**	**DOSAGE**	**DURATION**
Antibiotics	Trimethoprim-sulfamethoxazole	*Salmonella* spp., *Shigella* spp.	6-12 mg/kg/day (of Trimethoprim) in 2 divided doses–daily os	5-7 days
	Azithromycin	*Shigella* spp., *Campylobacter*	1 day: 12 mg/kg/day once–daily os 2-5 days: 6 mg/kg/day once–daily os *alternative: 10 mg/kg/day once–daily os, for 3 days	5 days
	Ciprofloxacin	*Shigella* spp.	20-30 mg/kg/day in 2 divided doses–os or IV	3 days
	Ceftriaxone	*Shigella* spp.	50-100 mg/kg/day once–IM or IV	2-5 days
	Metronidazole	*Giardia, Amebiasis, Blastocystis, Clostridium difficile*	15-35 mg/kg/day in 2-3 divided doses–os	7-10 days
	Paromomycin	*Amebiasis*	25-35 mg/kg/day in 3 divided doses–os	7 days
	Vancomycin	*Clostridium difficile*	40 mg/kg/day in 4 divided doses–os	10 days
Antiparasitic	Nitazoxanide	*Amebiasis, Giardiasis, Blastocystis, Cryptosporidiosis*	100 mg every 12 hr for children ages 12-47 mo 200 mg every 12 hr for children ages 4-11 yr 500 mg every 12 hr for children older than 11 yr	3 days
	Albendazole	*Ascaris, Hookworm,* and *Pinworm* infection	400 mg	Once

Depends on local susceptibility profile. *IM*, intramuscular; *IV*, intravenous; *os*, by mouth.

incidentally and are asymptomatic, especially those that are located in the appendix. Some NET patients (around 10%) will develop secretory diarrhea requiring symptom control to optimize quality of life and clinical outcomes. Such patients are defined as having carcinoid syndrome, characterized by excessive production of one or more peptides, which, when released into the circulation, exert their endocrine effects and can be measured by radioimmunologic methods (in the plasma or as their urinary metabolites). These peptides therefore also act as tumor markers. In clinically functioning tumors, the secreted peptides cause a recognizable syndrome that can include watery diarrhea. Compared to carcinoid, vasoactive intestinal polypeptide (VIP)omas are much

less frequent. Because it secretes VIP, a more potent vasoactive peptide, it induces more profuse diarrhea, with up to 70% of patients having volumes greater than 3 L/day. Though rare as a cause of watery diarrhea, a NET should be considered in the differential diagnosis when diarrhea is unusually severe or takes a chronic course (resulting in electrolyte and fluid depletion). GI-NETs may be associated with flushing, palpitations, or bronchospasm. Furthermore, patients may have a positive family history of multiple endocrine neoplasia MEN 1 or 2 syndromes. (Table 367.7).

Baseline tests should include plasma chromogranin A and urinary 5-hydroxyindoloacetic acid (metabolite of serotonin) and other specific biochemistry being guided by the suspected syndrome (see Table 367.7).

Table 367.7	Diarrhea Caused by Neuroendocrine Tumors			
TUMOR AND CELL TYPE	**SITE**	**MARKERS**	**SIGNS OF HORMONE HYPERSECRETION**	**THERAPY**
Carcinoid	Intestinal argentaffin cells, typically midgut, also foregut and hindgut, ectopic bronchial tree	**Serotonin (5-HT)**, urine **5-HIAA*** (diagnostic) Also produce substance P, neuropeptide K, somatostatin, VIP Chromogranin A	Secretory diarrhea, crampy abdominal pain, flushing, wheezing (and cardiac valve damage if foregut site)	Resection Somatostatin analog, (palliative) Genetic MEN-1
Gastrinoma, Zollinger-Ellison syndrome	Pancreas, small bowel, liver, and spleen	**Gastrin**	Multiple peptic ulcers, secretory diarrhea	H₂-blockers, PPI, tumor resection, (gastrectomy) Genetic MEN-1
Mastocytoma	Cutaneous, intestine, liver, spleen	**Histamine**, VIP	Pruritus, flushing, apnea If VIP, diarrhea	H₁- and H₂-blockers, steroids, resection if solitary
Medullary carcinoma	Thyroid C-cells	**Calcitonin**, VIP, prostaglandins	Secretory diarrhea	Radical thyroidectomy ± lymphadenectomy (genetic MEN-2A/B, familial MTC)
Ganglioneuroma, pheochromocytoma, ganglioneuroblastoma, neuroblastoma	Chromaffin cells; abdominal > other sites; extraadrenal or adrenal	**Metanephrines** and **catecholamines**, VIP VMA, HMA in neuroblastoma	Hypertension, tachycardia, paroxysmal palpitations, sweating, anxiety, watery diarrhea†	Perioperative α-adrenergic (BP) and β-adrenergic blockade with volume support tumor resection Genetic MEN-2 (*RET* gene), VHL, NF-1, SDH
Somatostatinoma	Pancreas	**Somatostatin**	Secretory diarrhea, steatorrhea, cholelithiasis, diabetes	Resection Genetic MEN-1
VIPoma	Pancreas	**VIP**, prostaglandins	Secretory diarrhea, achlorhydria, hypokalemia	Somatostatin analogs, resection Genetic MEN-1

*Bold indicates major markers.
†Diarrhea has been reported only in adult patients with pheochromocytoma.
BP, blood pressure; *H₁*, histamine receptor type 1; *H₂*, histamine receptor type 2; *HMA*, homovanillic acid; *MEN-1*, multiple endocrine neoplasia type 1; *MTC*, medullary thyroid carcinoma; *NF-1*, neurofibromatosis type 1; *PPI*, proton pump inhibitor; *SDH*, succinate dehydrogenase; *VHL*, von Hippel-Lindau disease; *VIP*, vasoactive intestinal polypeptide; *VMA*, vanillylmandelic acid. (Modified from Spoudeas HA, editor: *Paediatric endocrine tumors. A multidisciplinary consensus statement of best practice from a working group convened under the auspices of the British Society of Paediatric Endocrinology and Diabetes (BSPED) and the United Kingdom Children's Cancer Study Group (UKCCSG)*, Crawley, West Sussex, 2005, Novo Nordisk.)

Localization of any NET is best achieved using a multimodality approach. Whole-body CT, MRI, and somatostatin receptor scintigraphy may be required (because nearly all NETs express membrane receptors for small peptides, e.g., somatostatin), with gallium-68 positron emission tomography. Therapeutic interventions to be considered include surgical, pharmacological, and radioisotope therapy. Details to be considered when making therapeutic decisions include disease extent and location, tumor grade, pace of disease progression, symptoms, and co-morbidities.

Tumor resection is the treatment of choice when the tumor is small and localized. However, resection is potentially hazardous as it can precipitate life-threatening adrenergic crises. When arising in the appendix, carcinoid tumors less than 2 cm in size can be managed by simple appendectomy. When greater than 2 cm in size or arising from the base of the appendix, a right hemicolectomy is indicated. Fortunately, in pediatric patients, metastases (most frequently to the liver) are rare. Tumor histochemistry will confirm the NET type and classification. Pharmacologic treatment may include the use of long-acting somatostatin analogues. This usually results in a pronounced improvement of symptoms including diarrhea. However, the improvement is mostly temporary with many patients becoming resistant to somatostatin. An oral medication, Everolimus, a more specific target of Rapamycin (mTOR)-inhibitor, has been reported as add-on treatment to octreotide mainly in adult patients. Data suggest a positive effect of ondansetron, a serotonin-3-receptor antagonist, on diarrhea. Peptide receptor radioisotope therapy also has been reported as a therapeutic modality.

The diagnosis of NET in children should prompt a genetic referral to exclude a familial tumor predisposition syndrome.

Bibliography is available at Expert Consult.

Chapter 368
Functional Gastrointestinal Disorders
Asim Maqbool and Chris A. Liacouras

第三百六十八章
功能性胃肠病

中文导读

本章详细介绍了婴儿期功能性胃肠病，包括婴儿反刍、婴儿肠绞痛、功能性腹泻及功能性便秘、功能性恶心、功能性呕吐、吞气症等。此外还简要介绍了儿童和青春期功能性胃肠病、功能性腹痛（包括功能性消化不良、儿童肠易激综合征、腹型偏头痛、不能用其他原因解释的功能性腹痛）和肠功能不全疾病（包括功能性便秘及非储留性便失禁）。

Functional gastrointestinal disorders (FGIDs) comprise a group of conditions that relate to the gastrointestinal (GI) tract. These disorders cannot be completely explained by anatomical or biochemical abnormalities (infectious, inflammatory). FGIDs commonly afflict children across a broad range of manifestations and are defined primarily by symptoms. The symptom-based criteria employed to classify FGIDs have been developed by expert consensus and opinion under the auspices of the Rome Foundation, and are referred to as Rome IV Criteria. FGIDs pose diagnostic challenges as there is no anatomical or laboratory-based testing that is used to define them. FGID defining criteria strive not to be entirely based on diagnoses of exclusion, but rather aim to be based on objective, unambiguous, and accurate criteria derived from the presentation as elicited during obtaining the medical history and performing a clinical examination. These criteria strive to be uniform, reliable, reproducible, and to minimize unnecessary evaluations/testing with low diagnostic yield or relevance. FGIDs often coexist across the spectrum of GI disorders, such as inflammatory bowel disease, celiac disease, or irritable bowel syndrome (IBS). FGIDs may be influenced by psychosocial stressors, or a result of an otherwise benign episode of abdominal pain. The brain–gut axis likely plays a prominent role in the pathophysiology of many FGIDs. Some FGID manifestations may relate to dysbiosis and the intestinal microbiota. There may be a genetic basis to some of these disorders as well. Early life physical or psychologic stressors may manifest later as FGID. Maladaptive responses or lack of adequate coping skills may complicate the treatment of FGIDs but may also allow for a valuable approach to management using behavioral therapies.

FGIDs encompass 2 age groups: infants and toddlers or children and adolescents. Aerophagia, functional constipation, and cyclical vomiting span both age groups (Fig. 368.1).

Infant regurgitation implies effortless retrograde and involuntary passage of gastric contents from the stomach cephalad and is more commonly referred to as gastroesophageal reflux (Table 368.1). When refluxate reaches the oropharynx and is visible, it is labelled as regurgitation. This phenomenon is normal for healthy infants, unless there are complications associated with the process, such as esophageal inflammation, dysphagia, feeding difficulties, inadequate oral intake to meet needs leading to failure to thrive, or the inability to protect the airway with risk for aspiration; in this setting gastroesophageal reflux *disease* is the correct designation (Chapter 349). Unlike vomiting, regurgitation does not include the forceful expulsion of gastric contents via the mouth. Rumination is a different phenomenon, in that previously ingested and swallowed food is brought back up to the oral cavity, remasticated and subsequently reswallowed.

Infant rumination is defined as a habitual regurgitation of gastric contents into the oropharynx to allow for remastication and reswallowing (Table 368.2). It is thought to be a form of self-stimulation and may occur in the setting of emotional or sensory deprivation. The regurgitation of gastric contents is effortless and can be remasticated and reswallowed versus expulsion from the oropharynx. Infant rumination occurs between 3 and 8 mo of age and does not respond to measures used to manage regurgitation. This phenomenon does not occur during socialization/interaction with individuals, does not occur during sleep, and is not

associated with distress. Empathy and nurturing lay the foundation for management. Behavior management is important to achieve resolution of this phenomenon.

Infant colic (Chapter 22.1) is a normal developmental process associated with fussiness, irritability, and difficulty consoling the infant (Table 368.3). A trigger is not identifiable. This phenomenon usually occurs between 1 and 4 mo of age. The typical behavior usually leads to consultation with a pediatrician or a pediatric gastroenterologist out of suspicion for abdominal pain. Patients are often unnecessarily treated for gastroesophageal reflux, gas, or suspected cow-milk protein or soy allergy leading to dietary changes and the use of medications for the management of acidity or gas. Probiotics have been investigated as a possible treatment. Probiotics may be more beneficial for breast versus cow-milk-fed infants. Soothing in a quiet, tranquil space may also be effective. Providing reassurance, education, support, and ensuring adequate coping skills and support for family members are key. This is a self-limited phenomenon that resolves on its own.

Functional diarrhea is often also referred to as *toddler's diarrhea* (Table 368.4). This condition excludes steatorrhea. Excessive fruit juice with nonabsorbable carbohydrates (i.e., sorbitol) intake coupled with a low-fat diet drive this osmotic process. An evaluation of the diet for

Table 368.2	Diagnostic Criteria for Infant Rumination Syndrome

Must include all of the following for at least 2 mo:
1. Repetitive contractions of the abdominal muscles, diaphragm, and tongue
2. Effortless regurgitation of gastric contents, which are either expelled from the mouth or rechewed and reswallowed
3. Three or more of the following:
  a. Onset between 3 and 8 mo
  b. Does not respond to management for gastroesophageal reflux disease and regurgitation
  c. Unaccompanied by signs of distress
  d. Does not occur during sleep and when the infant is interacting with individuals in the environment

From Benninga MA, Nurko S, Faure C, et al: Childhood functional gastrointestinal disorders: neonate/toddler, *Gastroenterology* 150(6): 1443–1455.e2, 2016.

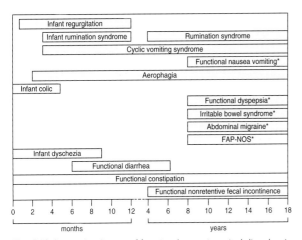

Fig. 368.1 Age distribution of functional gastrointestinal disorders in infants, toddlers, children, and adolescents. *History may not be reliable below this age. *FAP-NOS,* Functional abdominal pain—not otherwise specified. *(Modified from Benninga MA, Nurko S, Faure C, et al: Childhood functional gastrointestinal disorders: neonate/toddler,* Gastroenterology *150[6]:1443–1455.e2, 2016.)*

Table 368.3	Diagnostic Criteria for Infant Colic

For clinical purposes, must include all of the following:
1. An infant who is < 5 mo of age when the symptoms start and stop
2. Recurrent and prolonged periods of infant crying, fussing, or irritability reported by caregivers that occur without obvious cause and cannot be prevented or resolved by caregivers
3. No evidence of infant failure to thrive, fever, or illness

"Fussing" refers to intermittent distressed vocalization and has been defined as "[behavior] that is not quite crying but not awake and content either." Infants often fluctuate between crying and fussing, so that the 2 symptoms are difficult to distinguish in practice.

For clinical research purposes, a diagnosis of infant colic must meet the preceding diagnostic criteria and also include both of the following:
1. Caregiver reports infant has cried or fussed for 3 or more hr per day during 3 or more days in 7 days in a telephone or face-to-face screening interview with a researcher or clinician
2. Total 24-hr crying plus fussing in the selected group of infants is confirmed to be 3 hr or more when measured by at least 1 prospectively kept, 24-hr behavior diary

Table 368.1	Diagnostic Criteria for Infant Regurgitation

Must include both of the following in otherwise healthy infants 3 wk to 12 mo of age:
1. Regurgitation 2 or more times per day for 3 or more wk
2. No retching, hematemesis, aspiration, apnea, failure to thrive, feeding or swallowing difficulties, or abnormal posturing

From Benninga MA, Nurko S, Faure C, et al: Childhood functional gastrointestinal disorders: neonate/toddler, *Gastroenterology* 150(6):1443–1455. e2, 2016.

From Benninga MA, Nurko S, Faure C, et al: Childhood functional gastrointestinal disorders: neonate/toddler, *Gastroenterology* 150(6): 1443–1455.e2, 2016.

Table 368.4	Diagnostic Criteria for Functional Diarrhea

Must include all of the following:
1. Daily painless, recurrent passage of 4 or more large, unformed stools
2. Symptoms last more than 4 wk
3. Onset between 6 and 60 mo of age
4. No failure to thrive if caloric intake is adequate

From Benninga MA, Nurko S, Faure C, et al: Childhood functional gastrointestinal disorders: neonate/toddler, *Gastroenterology* 150(6): 1443–1455.e2, 2016.

possible other etiologies as well as assessment for infections, inflammation, antibiotic, and laxative use is important. In addition, assessments of growth as well as ruling out fecal impaction and encopresis via digital rectal examination are important. The diarrhea is usually stool colored, painless, liquid-watery, and may contain undigested foods. Growth is usually not affected. Dietary changes such as reducing fruit juice intake as well as fructose are helpful in resolving symptoms.

Infant dyschezia is manifested by infants straining prior to defecation associated with visible distress, crying, a red/purple facial discoloration, with symptoms persisting for 10-20 min alleviated by the passage in stools, limited to infants < 9 mo of age. There is no associated obstruction or anal anomaly; stools are passed several times daily and are not associated with other health problems. Dyschezia is thought to represent discoordinated intraabdominal musculature contraction with pelvic floor relaxation. A good medical history and neurological and digital rectal examinations to rule out anatomical or neuromuscular abnormalities are key. Normal growth is to be expected. Reassurance provides the basis of management. Laxative, suppository, or digital manipulation is not required and may be counterproductive.

Functional constipation (Chapter 358.3) is associated with withholding behaviors, which in turn may relate to social stressors or changes in social situations (Table 368.5). These often occur at the time of diet changes in infants and at the initiation of toilet training for toddlers. Painful passage of hard, large caliber stools < 2 times/wk in the setting of withholding behaviors is noted. For those children who have previously been toilet trained, fecal incontinence or encopresis is often observed. Large-caliber stools that obstruct the toilet are also noted frequently. Abdominal examination may reveal a palpable mass, and digital rectal examination may reveal a large rectal stool mass. The differential diagnosis for constipation is extensive, with functional constipation and slow transit constipation common. Dietary factors may play a role. Anorectal malformations, neuromuscular and motility issues may also present as such. Hirschsprung disease is on the differential diagnosis. The evaluation and management are based on a detailed history and thorough physical examination. A defecation history extending to the first 1-2 days of life is particularly important, as almost all children pass

Table 368.5	Diagnostic Criteria for Functional Constipation

Must include 1 mo of at least 2 of the following in infants up to 4 yr of age:
1. Two or fewer defecations per week
2. History of excessive stool retention
3. History of painful or hard bowel movements
4. History of large-diameter stools
5. Presence of a large fecal mass in the rectum

In toilet-trained children, the following additional criteria may be used:
6. At least 1 episode/wk of incontinence after the acquisition of toileting skills
7. History of large-diameter stools that may obstruct the toilet

From Benninga MA, Nurko S, Faure C, et al: Childhood functional gastrointestinal disorders: neonate/toddler, *Gastroenterology* 150(6): 1443–1455.e2, 2016.

their first bowel movement within the first 48 hr of life. Assessment for associated signs and symptoms and growth trends are important. Red flags are noted in Table 368.6. Imaging plays a role, and rectal suction biopsy or even full thickness rectal biopsy may be required to rule out Hirschsprung disease in cases with high index of suspicion. Management encompasses dietary and lifestyle changes, and medications to soften stool with osmotic laxatives over stimulant laxatives. The goal is to achieve painless defecation and resolve fear and withholding revolving around defecation. Behavior modification including reassurance and positive incentive reward systems are useful. Avoidance of toilet training until symptoms resolve and the child shows interest or willingness to proceed are generally advocated.

FUNCTIONAL GASTROINTESTINAL DISORDERS IN CHILDREN AND ADOLESCENTS

Functional nausea and functional vomiting may coexist or may occur independently of one another (Table 368.7). These conditions occur

Table 368.6	Potential Alarm Features in Constipation

Passage of meconium >48 hr in a term newborn

Constipation starting in the 1st mo of life

Family history of Hirschsprung disease

Ribbon stools

Blood in the stools in the absence of anal fissures

Failure to thrive

Bilious vomiting

Severe abdominal distension

Abnormal thyroid gland

Abnormal position of the anus

Absent anal or cremasteric reflex

Decreased lower extremity strength/tone/reflex

Sacral dimple

Tuft of hair on spine

Gluteal cleft deviation

Anal scars

From Hyams JS, Di Lorenzo C, Saps M, et al: Childhood functional gastrointestinal disorders: child/adolescent, *Gastroenterology* 150(6): 1456–1468.e2, 2016 (Table 3, p. 1465).

Table 368.7	Diagnostic Criteria* for Functional Nausea and Functional Vomiting

FUNCTIONAL NAUSEA
Must include all of the following fulfilled for the last 2 mo:
1. Bothersome nausea as the predominant symptom, occurring at least twice per week, and generally not related to meals
2. Not consistently associated with vomiting
3. After appropriate evaluation, the nausea cannot be fully explained by another medical condition

FUNCTIONAL VOMITING
Must include all of the following:
1. On average, 1 or more episodes of vomiting per week
2. Absence of self-induced vomiting or criteria for an eating disorder or rumination
3. After appropriate evaluation, the vomiting cannot be fully explained by another medical condition

*Criteria fulfilled for at least 2 mo before diagnosis.
From Hyams JS, Di Lorenzo C, Saps M, et al: Childhood functional gastrointestinal disorders: child/adolescent, *Gastroenterology* 150(6):1456–1468, 2016 (p. 1457).

without coincident abdominal pain. The presentation may accompany *autonomic symptoms* such as diaphoresis, pallor, tachycardia, and dizziness. The differential diagnosis includes anatomical, inflammatory, infectious, and motility etiologies. Anxiety and other behavioral conditions can be present with these FGIDs and should be evaluated for and managed accordingly. Cyproheptadine may be effective in the management of nausea.

Rumination in *older* children and adolescents may be associated with an unpleasant sensation or discomfort such as abdominal pressure or burning (Table 368.8). Repeated regurgitation and remastication or oral repulsion of regurgitated gastric contents occurs soon after ingesting foodstuffs and does not occur during sleep. It is not preceded by active expulsion of gastric contents/retching and cannot be explained by any other medical condition. *Eating disorders* may also present and must be considered. There is no expectation that older children and adolescents need to be treated for or fail to respond to treatment for gastroesophageal reflux for this diagnosis to be made. A triggering event can be identified prior to symptoms, which may occur following resolution of an infectious illness or with psychosocial stress. Other GI issues to be considered include anatomical, infectious, inflammatory, and motility disorders. An important distinction between rumination and other GI etiologies of emesis includes effortless versus forceful regurgitation, and the time course, which is usually immediately following ingestion of foodstuffs. Given the significant behavioral component in this behavior, psychologic-behavioral therapy is key in management.

Aerophagia is often seen in patients with impairments in neurocognition. Air swallowing is described as excessive, occurring throughout the day with progressive abdominal distention and with repetitive passage of gas via belching and/or flatus. Symptoms may be more severe in those children who cannot belch. Chewing gum and gulping down liquids may be risk factors in cognitively normal children. Symptoms are not attributable to any other causes such as partial obstructions, small bowel bacterial overgrowth, GI dysmotility (pseudoobstruction), or to malabsorptive disorders. Abdominal pain, nausea, and early satiety are reported associated GI symptoms; sleeping difficulty, headaches, and dizziness are also reported. Anxiety is a frequent comorbidity and may contribute to the behavior. Treatment is multidisciplinary and may include behavioral therapy and medications to relieve anxiety.

FUNCTIONAL ABDOMINAL PAIN DISORDERS
Functional Dyspepsia
Functional dyspepsia includes postprandial fullness and early satiety as well as epigastric pain or burning that is exclusive of defecation and not fully explainable by another or an underlying medical condition (Table 368.9). Subtypes may include *postprandial distress syndrome* (symptoms may preclude finishing a meal or be manifest by bloating, nausea, and excessive belching following a meal) as well as *epigastric pain syndrome* (epigastric pain/burning sufficient to preclude or disrupt normal activities, with pain not generalizable or localizable to other abdominal or chest regions, and not relieved by defecation or passage of flatus). An impaired gastric accommodation reflex, food allergy, delayed gastric emptying, or post viral gastroparesis has been implicated.

Increased visceral hypersensitivity has also been suspected. The differential diagnosis includes GI etiologies of epigastric pain. Causes for concern can be guided by the family history and by the nature of symptoms including abdominal pain and other alarm features (Tables 368.10 and 368.11). Evaluation is based on symptoms. Initial treatment measures include a trial of diet (avoiding spicy foods, coffee, NSAID) and lifestyle changes if food triggers can be identified, and gastric acid reduction therapy. Assessment by a pediatric gastroenterologist and upper endoscopy/esophagogastroduodenoscopy are often performed. Further treatment with cyproheptadine to improve gastric accommodation or to decrease visceral hypersensitivity can be attempted. Use of amitriptyline or prokinetic medications can be considered. Electrical stimulation of the stomach (or percutaneous) is a potential option for patients refractory to standard therapy.

Pediatric IBS
Pediatric IBS can be classified into 4 groups: IBS with predominant constipation (IBS-C), IBS with predominant diarrhea (IBS-D), IBS with constipation and diarrhea, and unspecified IBS. IBS includes findings

Table 368.9	Diagnostic Criteria* for Functional Dyspepsia

Must include 1 or more of the following bothersome symptoms at least 4 days/mo:
1. Postprandial fullness
2. Early satiation
3. Epigastric pain or burning not associated with defecation
4. After appropriate evaluation, the symptoms cannot be fully explained by another medical condition.

Within FD, the following subtypes are now adopted:
1. Postprandial distress syndrome includes bothersome postprandial fullness or early satiation that prevents finishing a regular meal. Supportive features include upper abdominal bloating, postprandial nausea, or excessive belching.
2. Epigastric pain syndrome, which includes all of the following: bothersome (severe enough to interfere with normal activities) pain or burning localized to the epigastrium. The pain is not generalized or localized to other abdominal or chest regions and is not relieved by defecation or passage of flatus. Supportive criteria can include (a) burning quality of the pain but without a retrosternal component and (b) the pain commonly induced or relieved by ingestion of a meal but may occur while fasting.

*Criteria fulfilled for at least 2 mo before diagnosis.
From Hyams JS, Di Lorenzo C, Saps M, et al: Childhood functional gastrointestinal disorders: child/adolescent, *Gastroenterology* 150(6):1456–1468, 2016 (p. 1460).

Table 368.10	Alarm Symptoms Usually Needing Further Investigations in Children With Chronic Abdominal Pain

- Pain that wakes up the child from sleep
- Persistent right upper or right lower quadrant pain
- Significant vomiting (bilious vomiting, protracted vomiting, cyclical vomiting, or worrisome pattern to the physician)
- Unexplained fever
- Genitourinary tract symptoms
- Dysphagia
- Odynophagia
- Chronic severe diarrhea or nocturnal diarrhea
- Gastrointestinal blood loss
- Involuntary weight loss
- Deceleration of linear growth
- Delayed puberty
- Family history of inflammatory bowel disease, celiac disease, and peptic ulcer disease

Table 368.8	Diagnostic Criteria* for Rumination Syndrome in Children

Must include all of the following:
1. Repeated regurgitation and rechewing or expulsion of food that:
   a. Begins soon after ingestion of a meal
   b. Does not occur during sleep
2. Not preceded by retching
3. After appropriate evaluation, the symptoms cannot be fully explained by another medical condition. An eating disorder must be ruled out

*Criteria fulfilled for at least 2 mo before diagnosis.From Hyams JS, Di Lorenzo C, Saps M, et al: Childhood functional gastrointestinal disorders: child/adolescent, *Gastroenterology* 150(6):1456–1468, 2016 (p. 1458).)

of abdominal pain ≥ 4 days/mo associated with defecation and/or a change in frequency of stool from baseline and/or a change in form/appearance of stool (Table 368.12). It is noteworthy that pain does not resolve following resolution of constipation; if it does, it is then reclassified as functional constipation. In fact, IBS-C is often confused with functional constipation. IBS cannot be explained by another or underlying medical condition. The pathophysiology of IBS is thought to involve the brain-gut axis and includes a psychosocial stressor component. Visceral hypersensitivity may be attenuated or amplified by psychosocial stressors. Abdominal or rectal pain may occur. A *postinfectious* IBS phenomenon is known to occur in children, adolescents, and adults and may be driven by inflammatory cytokines. Perturbations in the intestinal microbiota or by dysbiosis may be coincident, with causality or consequence not yet established. The GI differential diagnosis includes anatomical, infectious, inflammatory, and motility disorders as well as conditions associated with malabsorption. Differentiation between those GI disorders and IBS is guided by the history and physical, and markers of inflammation particularly in the stool such as fecal calprotectin are clinically useful (see Tables 368.10 and 368.11). Management of symptoms can include dietary modification to reduce or restrict foods that may provoke symptoms or cause gas (see fiber section and FODMAPS [fermentable oligo-di-monosaccharides and polyols] discussion Chapter 55). Altering microbiota by use of probiotics has been effective; drug therapy for IBS is noted in Table 368.13. Peppermint oil has been shown to reduce pain in children with IBS. Cognitive behavioral therapy is important to identify possible psychosocial stressors and to help identify coping mechanisms. Preliminary data suggests that transcutaneous neurostimulation may also be of value.

Abdominal Migraine

Abdominal migraine shares some features with cyclic vomiting syndrome. Stereotypical patterns and symptoms afflict the patient, and are typically of acute onset, intense, lasting for at least an hour, being either periumbilical or generalized, and usually debilitating during a bout (Table 368.14). Episodes can include anorexia, nausea, emesis, headaches, photophobia, and pallor. Episodes are separated by weeks to months, with bouts occurring over at least a 6-mo period. Between bouts, patients return to baseline functioning and are symptom free. *Triggers* include sleep hygiene disruption, fatigue, travel, and are usually alleviated by sleep. The differential diagnosis includes anatomical, infectious, or inflammatory conditions, as well as hepatobiliary and pancreatic disorders, neurological and metabolic conditions, and psychiatric disorders. Anatomical obstruction of the GI or urological tract should be included

Table 368.13	Recommendations for Treatment of Irritable Bowel Syndrome

RECOMMENDATIONS FOR TREATMENT OF IBS
- Mild symptoms often respond to dietary changes.
- Antispasmodics can be used as needed for abdominal pain or postprandial symptoms.
- Antidepressants can improve abdominal pain and global symptoms. They may be considered for patients with moderate to severe symptoms.

IBS WITH CONSTIPATION (IBS-C)
- Fiber may relieve constipation in patients with mild symptoms.
- Polyethylene glycol can increase the frequency of bowel movements, but may not improve overall symptoms or abdominal pain.
- Lubiprostone or linaclotide can be tried in patients whose symptoms have not responded to polyethylene glycol.

IBS WITH DIARRHEA (IBS-D)
- Taken as needed, loperamide can reduce postprandial urgency and stool frequency, but it does not improve global symptoms.
- Rifaximin and eluxadoline have been modestly more effective than placebo in relieving symptoms.
- Alosetron should be reserved for women with severe, chronic IBS-D that is unresponsive to other drugs.

IBS, Irritable bowel syndrome.
From Drugs for irritable bowel syndrome, *The Medical Letter* 58(1504): 121–126, 2016 (p. 121).

Table 368.11	Alarm Signs Usually Needing Further Investigations in Children With Chronic Abdominal Pain

- Localized tenderness in the right *upper* quadrant
- Localized tenderness in the right *lower* quadrant
- Localized fullness or mass
- Hepatomegaly
- Splenomegaly
- Jaundice
- Costovertebral angle tenderness
- Arthritis
- Spinal tenderness
- Perianal disease
- Abnormal or unexplained physical findings
- Hematochezia
- Anemia

Table 368.14	Diagnostic Criteria* for Abdominal Migraine

Must include all of the following occurring at least twice:
1. Paroxysmal episodes of intense, acute periumbilical, midline, or diffuse abdominal pain lasting 1 hr or more (should be the most severe and distressing symptom)
2. Episodes are separated by weeks to months.
3. The pain is incapacitating and interferes with normal activities
4. Stereotypical pattern and symptoms in the individual patient
5. The pain is associated with 2 or more of the following:
   a. Anorexia
   b. Nausea
   c. Vomiting
   d. Headache
   e. Photophobia
   f. Pallor
6. After appropriate evaluation, the symptoms cannot be fully explained by another medical condition.

*Criteria fulfilled for at least 6 mo before diagnosis.
From Hyams JS, Di Lorenzo C, Saps M, et al: Childhood functional gastrointestinal disorders: child/adolescent, *Gastroenterology* 150(6):1456–1468, 2016 (p. 1462).

Table 368.12	Diagnostic Criteria* for Irritable Bowel Syndrome

Must include all of the following:
1. Abdominal pain at least 4 days/mo associated with one or more of the following:
   a. Related to defecation
   b. A change in frequency of stool
   c. A change in form (appearance) of stool
2. In children with constipation, the pain does not resolve with resolution of the constipation (children in whom the pain resolves have functional constipation, not irritable bowel syndrome)
3. After appropriate evaluation, the symptoms cannot be fully explained by another medical condition

*Criteria fulfilled for at least 2 mo before diagnosis.
From Hyams JS, Di Lorenzo C, Saps M, et al: Childhood functional gastrointestinal disorders: child/adolescent, *Gastroenterology* 150(6):1456–1468, 2016 (p. 1461).

in the differential diagnosis. Preventing exposure to known triggers once identified is important. Similar to prophylaxis for cyclic vomiting syndrome, cyproheptadine, propranolol, and amitriptyline may be effective. Oral pizotifen (antiserotonin, antihistamine) is an effective prophylactic agent. Anti-migraine therapies such as triptans may be effective in aborting bouts. This disorder shares many features with both cyclic vomiting syndrome and migraine headaches and may evolve into migraine headaches in adulthood.

Functional Abdominal Pain Not Otherwise Specified

Functional abdominal pain not otherwise specified occurs at least 4 times/mo with either intermittent or continuous abdominal pain not associated with a particular activity or coincident to *another physiologic event* such as menses or eating, cannot be explained by any other or underlying medical condition, and is of ≥2 mo duration. In many ways, it is a FGID of exclusion, as it does not meet criteria for IBS, functional dyspepsia, or abdominal migraine. Psychosocial stressors may play a role. There may be increased coincidence with postural orthostatic hypotension. Behavioral approaches may be helpful to identify and manage stressors and exacerbators.

FUNCTIONAL DEFECATION DISORDERS
Functional Constipation

Functional constipation in children and adolescents may have onset revolving around a social stressor, change in social situation, and peaks at the time of toilet training, when withholding behaviors emerge (Table 368.15). Encopresis may occur without sensation if the rectum is chronically distended sufficiently. Anorexia, abdominal distention, and pain are often coincident. The diagnosis is based on medical history and physical examination, including digital rectal examination. An abdominal x-ray is not required to make the diagnosis if a digital rectal examination can be performed to appreciate the fecal mass. The differential diagnosis for constipation in children and adolescents is similar to that as for infants and toddlers and is the approach to the evaluation and management of constipation (see Table 368.6). Management includes disimpaction followed by dietary and lifestyle approaches, osmotic laxatives to soften stools, and behavioral approaches similar to those employed for younger children discussed previously (Chapter 358.3).

Table 368.15	Diagnostic Criteria for Functional Constipation in Children With Chronic Abdominal Pain

Must include 2 or more of the following occurring at least once per week for a minimum of 1 mo with insufficient criteria for a diagnosis of irritable bowel syndrome:
1. Two or fewer defecations in the toilet per week in a child of a developmental age of at least 4 yr
2. At least 1 episode of fecal incontinence per week
3. History of retentive posturing or excessive volitional stool retention
4. History of painful or hard bowel movements
5. Presence of a large fecal mass in the rectum
6. History of large diameter stools that can obstruct the toilet

After appropriate evaluation, the symptoms cannot be fully explained by another medical condition.

From Hyams JS, Di Lorenzo C, Saps M, et al: Childhood functional gastrointestinal disorders: child/adolescent, *Gastroenterology* 150(6):1456–1468, 2016 (p. 1464).

Nonretentive Fecal Incontinence

Nonretentive fecal incontinence occurs in the setting of not having fecal retention, occurring in inappropriate settings for a specific society and culture, without evidence of another or underlying medical condition, and occurring for ≥1 mo in a child of ≥4 yr of age. These patients otherwise have normal defecatory patterns and function, differentiating and distinguishing them from functional constipation. An emotional disturbance or disorder should be suspected in these cases. A thorough medical history and physical examination are required to fully appreciate what factors are involved in this condition. A rectal examination is important to differentiate this condition from functional constipation and encopresis. Given the significant comorbidity of behavior and emotional axis issues, involvement of behavioral health professionals is essential to the evaluation and management of this condition.

Bibliography is available at Expert Consult.

Chapter 369
Cyclic Vomiting Syndrome

Asim Maqbool, B U.K. Li, and Chris A. Liacouras

第三百六十九章
周期性呕吐综合征

中文导读

本章主要介绍了周期性呕吐的流行病学、一些警惕症状及诊断标准，详细阐述了周期性呕吐的治疗方案，包括支持性治疗（水、电解质平衡，营养支持，止吐镇静治疗，对症治疗以及并发症治疗），生活方式的改变（包括给予患儿安慰及预期指导，避免及控制诱发因素，偏头痛型生活方式干预治疗），周期性呕吐的特殊药物治疗（包括≥5岁和<5岁不同药物组合治疗）和饮食补充（包括补充左卡尼汀和辅酶Q10）。

Cyclic vomiting syndrome (CVS) is an idiopathic disorder manifested as episodic vomiting, usually of sudden onset and high intensity/frequency (4/hr:12-15 episodes/day) of vomiting, with eventual resolution and return to a normal baseline between attacks. Typical bouts last for 24-48 hr, and usually respond promptly to hydration. To meet the criteria for CVS, identifiable organic disorders are excluded following an appropriate workup (Table 369.1).

Table 369.1	Consensus Definition for Diagnostic Criteria and Red Flags for Cyclic Vomiting Syndrome

DIAGNOSTIC CRITERIA
- Episodic (≥2 or more) attacks of intense nausea and paroxysmal vomiting lasting hours to days within a 6-mo period
- Stereotypical pattern and symptoms in the individual patient
- Episodes are separated by weeks to months
- Return to baseline between episodes
- Not attributable to another disorder

RED FLAGS
- Bilious emesis, abdominal tenderness, and/or severe abdominal pain
- Attacks precipitated by an intercurrent illness, fasting, and/or a high protein meal
- Neurological abnormalities (mental status changes, ophthalmic abnormalities asymmetry/focal changes, ataxia)
- Atypical pattern or progression/deterioration from a typical presentation for the individual patient to a more continuous or chronic pattern

Modified from the Rome IV Criteria: Li BU, Lefevre F, Chelimsky GG, et al: North American Society for Pediatric Gastroenterology, Hepatology and Nutrition consensus statement on the diagnosis and management of cyclic vomiting syndrome, *J Pediatr Gastroenterol Nutr* 47(3):379–393, 2008.

The prevalence of CVS in children is estimated at ~2% in predominantly Caucasian populations, although it does occur in those of African or Asian descent, and Hispanic ethnicity. There is a slight female predominance. The median age of onset is 5 yr, but it can begin in infancy and adolescence. Typically, there is a delay of 2.5 yr in making the diagnosis despite multiple episodes and emergency room visits. The natural history of CVS is that most children outgrow it during preadolescence or adolescence, and of those, many will develop migraines. There are also later pediatric-onset (mean age 13) and adult-onset (mean age 32) subgroups indicating that in a minority it can begin or persist in adulthood.

One key clinical feature of CVS is its consistent and stereotypical pattern of presentation within individuals. Typically, symptoms start at the same time, often during early morning hours, lasting the same duration and demonstrating identical autonomic symptoms of pallor and listlessness, unrelenting nausea, abdominal pain, and in less than half, headaches and photophobia. CVS bouts occur at a minimum 5 times, or 3 times over a 6-mo period. About half of cases occur on a cycle as often as monthly; some cycle as infrequently as every 3-4 mo. The other patients have unpredictable sporadic bouts that may be associated with a specific trigger. Potential triggers include infectious illnesses, stress and especially excitement (holidays), sleep deprivation (sleepovers), dietary triggers (chocolate, monosodium glutamate), food allergy, onset of menses, and weather changes. Typically, vomiting bouts are particularly intense, with greater than 4 bouts of emesis per hour at the peak, and can include gastric contents or frequent dry heaves. While most attacks last 2 days, an episode can last anywhere from hours and rarely up to 10 days. CVS attacks are debilitating, often necessitating IV rehydration, and resulting in hospitalization. Seasonal variation apparently occurs in approximately a third of patients, with more attacks in winter, fewer during summer. In some adolescent patients, a *coalescent form* develops with daily nausea between episodes of emesis (which becomes less frequent).

Multiple *comorbid* disorders can further comprise quality of life between episodes; these include anxiety, constipation-predominant irritable bowel syndrome, chronic fatigue or limited stamina, sleep disorders, postural orthostatic tachycardia syndrome, daily nausea, and complex regional pain syndrome.

In all cases of CVS, an underlying causative etiology (anatomical, infectious, inflammatory, neoplastic, and metabolic or endocrine) cannot be identified. There is typically a positive family history of migraines in children with CVS; attacks of both conditions share many clinical features. Although the pathophysiology is not fully known, there is suggestive evidence that an overresponsive hypothalamic-pituitary-adrenal axis (including corticotropin-releasing factor), autonomic nervous system dysregulation (sympathetic predominance), mitochondrial dysfunction (16519T and 3010A), and nuclear mutations *(RYR2)* may play contributory roles. Although the role of cannabis is unknown in CVS, *cannabis-induced hyperemesis syndrome* shares many features with CVS, including the relief of symptoms by hot showers (Chapter 140.3).

Patients with chronic vomiting should always be evaluated for potential etiologies other than CVS. The differential diagnosis includes GI anomalies (malrotation, duplication cysts, choledochal cysts, recurrent intussusceptions), CNS disorders (neoplasm, epilepsy, vestibular pathology), nephrolithiasis, cholelithiasis, hydronephrosis, metabolic-endocrine disorders (urea cycle, mitochondrial disorders, fatty acid metabolism, Addison disease, porphyria, hereditary angioedema, familial Mediterranean fever), chronic appendicitis, and inflammatory bowel disease. Laboratory evaluation is based on a careful history and physical examination and may include, if indicated, endoscopy, contrast GI radiography, brain MRI, and metabolic studies (lactate, organic acids, ammonia). Bilious emesis usually suggests a small bowel obstruction and is considered a red flag; however, children with CVS may have bile stained emesis. A tender abdomen is also unusual for CVS and warrants further workup. Acute and chronic appendicitis can mimic CVS. Prior abdominal surgery may increase risk for adhesion-related partial bowel obstructions (see Table 369.1).

Non-gastrointestinal causes of frequent vomiting include renal, metabolic, endocrine, and neurological disorders. Renal abnormalities to consider include acute or chronic ureteropelvic junction (UPJ) obstruction presenting with hydronephrosis (Dietl crisis) and nephrolithiasis. The clinician must also consider metabolic disorders, especially in the infant or toddler less than 2 yr of age. Fasting or high protein meals that provoke emesis raise a red flag for metabolic disorders, such as disorders of fatty acid oxidation, organic acidemias, or partial ornithine transcarbamylase deficiency. Acute intermittent porphyria can present in the adolescent triggered by alcohol or medications. Endocrine disorders, including diabetic ketoacidosis, Addison disease, and pheochromocytoma, can mimic CVS episodes. Although an atypical presentation, CNS tumors can have episodic vomiting and papilledema; altered mental status and focal neurological findings are red flags requiring neuroimaging. Pregnancy can present with CVS-like symptoms.

Children who meet the diagnostic criteria for CVS and have no red flags should have simple screening tests for electrolyte abnormalities, acidosis, hypoglycemia, and renal dysfunction during episodes, and an UGI radiograph to exclude malrotation. Presenting with gastrointestinal (bilious emesis, abdominal tenderness), metabolic (fasting or meal-induced), and neurological (papilledema, altered mental status) red flags warrants further evaluation (see Table 369.1).

In the management of acute episodes, early and aggressive hydration (especially with dextrose) may shorten episodes in addition to correcting fluid losses. Reducing extraneous sensory stimulation, similar to the management approach for migraines, may also be beneficial (Table 369.2). Regardless of intervention, episodes will eventually spontaneously

Table 369.2	Supportive Care and Abortive Treatment Approaches in Cyclic Vomiting Syndrome		
SUPPORTIVE CARE			
Fluid and electrolyte management		Dextrose containing fluid (D10) and normal saline as a single infusion or as a Y infusion	
Nutrition		• Resume enteral nutrition as soon as possible.	
		• If unable to tolerate enteral nutrition and meets criteria, start parenteral nutrition after 3-4 days.	
Medications	Antiemetics	Ondansetron	
		• 0.3-0.4 mg/kg/dose IV every 4-6 hr (maximum 16 mg/dose)	
		• Side effect: constipation, QTc prolongation	
		Alternative: Granisetron	
	Sedatives	Diphenhydramine	
		• 1-1.25 mg/kg/dose IV every 6 hr	
		Lorazepam 0.05-0.1 mg/kg/dose IV every 6 hr	
		• Side effects: respiratory depression, hallucinations	
		Chlorpromazine 0.5-1 mg/kg/dose every 6-8 hr + diphenhydramine IV	
	Analgesics	Ketorolac 0.5 mg/kg/dose IV every 6 hr (maximum dose 30 mg)	
Treatment of specific signs and symptoms	Epigastric pain		
	• Acid reduction therapy with an H₂RA or a PPI		
	Diarrhea		
	• Antidiarrheals		
	Hypertension		
	• Short-acting ACE inhibitors such as captopril		
Treatment of specific complications	• Dehydration and electrolyte deficits: replace calculated deficits		
	• Metabolic acidosis: determine etiology and rectify		
	• SIADH: restrict free water intake		
	• Hyperemesis: IV acid reduction		
	• Weight loss: enteral or parenteral nutrition		
ABORTIVE CARE			
Antimigraine (triptans)	Sumatriptan		
	• 20 mg intranasally at episode onset		
	• Side effects: neck pain/burning, coronary vasospasm		
	• Contraindications: basilar artery migraine		
RECOVERY AND REFEEDING			
• Feed ad libitum when the child declares that the episode is over			

Medications listed above are for off-label use.

Modified from Li BU, Lefevre F, Chelimsky GG, et al: North American Society for Pediatric Gastroenterology, Hepatology and Nutrition consensus statement on the diagnosis and management of cyclic vomiting syndrome, *J Pediatr Gastroenterol Nutr* 47(3):379–393, 2008.

2270 Part XVII ◆ The Digestive System

resolve with return to a normal baseline. Triptans can be used as an *abortive medication* in patients with a family history of migraines, at the onset of symptoms. Ondansetron may reduce nausea and emesis. Sedation may reduce severity or stop a CVS episode; drugs include antihistamines such as diphenhydramine and promethazine. Lorazepam or rectal diazepam can be also used. These measures are empiric; a lack of evidence base limits our understanding of efficacy. For rare but severe refractory cases, general anesthetics have been used. A dramatic change in presentation of attacks suggests a red flag such as acute hydronephrosis or small bowel obstruction from volvulus.

Prophylactic management begins with lifestyle measures (maintenance fluid intake, adequate calories, sleep hygiene, and exercise), including avoidance of known triggering foods (allergens, chocolate, aged cheese,

monosodium glutamate; Table 369.3). Recommendations for prophylactic regimens include cyproheptadine in patients less than 5 yr of age and amitriptyline in patients ≥5 yr; propranolol serves as a secondary agent in both age groups. Supplements such as coenzyme Q10 and L-carnitine have occasionally been reported to be useful adjuncts. When standard care fails, the addition of anticonvulsants such as topiramate has been implemented. For those with catamenial CVS, low-dose estrogen oral contraceptives or Depo-Provera may prevent episodes. Treatment of *comorbid disorders*, especially anxiety (cognitive behavioral therapy, antianxiety agents) and postural orthostatic tachycardia syndrome (fluids, salt, fludrocortisone), may be needed for effective management of CVS.

Bibliography is available at Expert Consult.

Table 369.3 | Prophylactic Lifestyle Changes and Pharmacological Options for Cyclic Vomiting Syndrome

LIFESTYLE MEASURES

Reassurance and anticipatory Guidance	• Episodes are not intentional. • The natural history of CVS is that it will resolve with time.
Avoidance of triggers	• Identify dietary triggers ("vomit diary") and avoid precipitating factors. • Triggering foods may include chocolate, cheese, monosodium glutamate. • Fasting a common trigger • Excitement a potential trigger • Excessive activity/exhaustion • Avoid sleep deprivation and practice good sleep hygiene
Managing triggers	• Provide supplemental energy as carbohydrates for fasting induced episodes. • Provision of snacks between meals, before sleep and before exertion
Migraine headache type lifestyle interventions	• Aerobic exercise and avoidance of overexertion • Regular mealtime schedule—avoid skipping meals • Avoid/moderate caffeine intake

PROPHYLACTIC PHARMACOLOGICAL APPROACHES

Age <5 yr
Antihistamines:
• Cyproheptadine
  • 0.25-0.5 mg/kg/day in 2 daily divided doses or as a single dose qhs
  • Side effects of increased appetite, weight gain, and sedation
• Pizotifen
β-blockers: (2nd choice)
• Propranolol
  • 0.25-1 mg/kg/day, most often 10 mg 2-3×/day.
  • Side effects include lethargy and reduced exercise tolerance.
  • Contraindicated in asthma, diabetes, heart disease, depression
  • Taper over 1-2 wk to discontinue
	Age ≥5 yr
	Tricyclic antidepressants:
	• Amitriptyline
	  • Begin at 0.25-0.5 mg/kg qhs and increase weekly by 5-10 mg until achieve 1-1.5 mg/kg
	  • Monitor EKG for prolonged QTc interval at baseline before initiation and 10 days after peak dose achieved
	  • Side effects: constipation, sedation, arrhythmias, behavioral changes
	Alternatives: nortriptyline
	β-blockers: (2nd choice):
	• Propranolol
	Other agents:
	Anticonvulsants:
	• Phenobarbital 2 mg/kg qhs
	  • Side effects: sedation, cognitive impairment
	Alternatives:
	• Topiramate, valproic acid, gabapentin, levetiracetam

DIETARY SUPPLEMENTS

• L-Carnitine 50-100 mg/kg/day divided 2-3×/day, maximum dose of 2 g 2×/day
• Coenzyme Q10 200 mg 2×/day divided 2-3×/day, maximum dose 100 mg 3×/day

Medications listed above are for off-label use. *CVS,* cyclic vomiting syndrome.
Modified from Li BU, Lefevre F, Chelimsky GG, et al: North American Society for Pediatric Gastroenterology, Hepatology and Nutrition consensus statement on the diagnosis and management of cyclic vomiting syndrome, *J Pediatr Gastroenterol Nutr* 47(3):379–393, 2008.

Chapter 370
Acute Appendicitis
John J. Aiken

第三百七十章
急性阑尾炎

中文导读

本章主要介绍了急性阑尾炎的流行病学特点、病理生理改变、临床特征及体格检查。介绍了急性阑尾炎危险度评分系统、实验室及影像学检查;详尽阐述了急性阑尾炎X线、超声、CT、MRI及放射性标记的白细胞监测在诊断中的应用。阐述了急性阑尾炎的诊断、鉴别诊断及治疗方法,包括抗生素的使用、手术时机的选择、阑尾穿孔的治疗、单纯阑尾炎的非手术治疗、复发性阑尾炎的治疗等。

Acute appendicitis remains the most common acute surgical condition in children and a major cause of childhood morbidity and health care costs, mostly associated with complicated/perforated appendicitis (PA). The peak incidence of acute appendicitis occurs in children in the second decade, and approximately 100,000 children are treated in children's hospitals for appendicitis each year. The broad spectrum of clinical presentation in acute appendicitis has been associated with significant practice variation in evaluation, diagnostic measures, and treatment of abdominal pain and suspected appendicitis. The traditional strategy of the liberal use of computed tomography (CT) to avoid misdiagnosis and early surgery to avoid progression to perforation has lacked validation in large reviews and resulted in high negative appendectomy rates and excessive radiation exposure. Perforation rates have remained around 40% and negative appendectomy rates as high as 10–20% in the past several decades. In current practice, most centers have adopted clinical practice guidelines (CPGs) combining history, physical examination findings, laboratory data, and appendicitis risk scoring systems to standardize care, improve diagnostic accuracy and outcomes, and direct cost-conscious resource utilization. Appendiceal ultrasound has emerged as a highly sensitive and specific imaging modality for diagnosis and led to a significant decrease in the use of CT and radiation exposure in the initial evaluation of children presenting with abdominal pain and possible suspected appendicitis. While prompt appendectomy remains the standard treatment in acute appendicitis, advances in imaging techniques, improved antibiotic regimens, increased use of percutaneous drainage procedures by interventional radiologists, and emerging data on high success rates with initial antibiotic treatment alone have led to an increase in the initial nonoperative management of both simple and complicated (abscess, phlegmon) appendicitis. Laparoscopic appendectomy (LA, minimally invasive technique) has emerged as the preferred surgical approach for both simple and PA, with an open surgical approach reserved as an alternative for selected cases or when attempted LA is technically difficult and/or deemed unsafe.

EPIDEMIOLOGY

The incidence of acute appendicitis increases with age, from a rate of 1-2 per 10,000 children from birth to 4 yr of age, to a rate of 19-28 per 10,000 children younger than age 14 yr annually. Children have a lifetime risk of 7–9% and appendicitis is diagnosed in 1–8% of children presenting to the emergency department (ED) for evaluation of abdominal pain. Appendicitis is most common in older children, with peak incidence between the ages of 10 and 18 yr; it is rare in children younger than 5 yr of age (<5% of cases) and extremely rare (<1% of cases) in children younger than 3 yr of age.

Infants with appendicitis are often misdiagnosed with sepsis and because of the diagnostic delay, they present in advanced stages of the disease. Most infant cases are primary, but some may be associated with Hirschsprung disease, cystic fibrosis, inguinal hernia, prematurity, meconium plug syndrome, or complex multiorgan syndromes.

Incidence rates for acute appendicitis are higher in males, whites, and Hispanics compared to African Americans and Asians; Hispanics, Asians, and patients with nonprivate insurance have higher odds of perforation. There is a peak incidence of appendicitis in the third quarter between July and September and the incidence is higher in the West and North Central regions compared with the Mid-Atlantic States. The reasons for these ethnic, geographic, and socioeconomic disparities remain unclear with possibilities including cultural differences in interaction with the medical system, limitations in access to care, or differences in disease progression by race.

Mortality is low (<1%), but morbidity remains high, mostly in association with PA. Up to 40% of children have PA at presentation, and perforation rates approach 90% in young children (<3 yr). Children with simple (nonperforated) appendicitis typically recover easily, with a low complication rate and rapid return to premorbid state and full activities. In contrast, PA is associated with substantial postoperative morbidity including readmission rates estimated at 12.8%, postoperative intraabdominal abscess rate ~20%, surgical site infection (SSI) rate ~20%, prolonged length of stay (LOS), need for prolonged antibiotic exposure, increased postoperative use of CT, and significant delay in return to wellness and normal activities. The Healthcare Cost and Utilization Project estimated that appendicitis with peritonitis accounted for 25,410 pediatric hospital admissions in 2012, with a mean LOS of 5.2 days and mean costs of $13,076.

PATHOPHYSIOLOGY

The clinical entity of acute appendiceal inflammation followed by perforation, abscess formation, and peritonitis is most likely a disease of multiple etiologies, the final common pathway of which involves invasion of the appendiceal wall by bacteria. Genetic, environmental, and infectious etiologies (bacterial, viral, fungal, and parasitic) have all been implicated in acute appendicitis. Family history confers a nearly threefold increased risk for appendicitis. One pathway to acute appendicitis begins with luminal obstruction; inspissated fecal material, lymphoid hyperplasia, ingested foreign body, parasites, and tumors have been described. Obstruction of the appendiceal lumen initiates a progressive cascade involving increasing intraluminal pressure, lymphatic and venous congestion and edema, impaired arterial perfusion, ischemia of the appendiceal wall, bacterial proliferation and invasion of the wall, and necrosis. This sequence correlates with the clinical disease progression from simple appendicitis to gangrenous appendicitis and, thereafter, appendiceal perforation.

Because the appendix has the highest concentration of gut-associated lymphoid tissue (GALT) in the intestine, some have hypothesized that the appendix may have an immune function similar to that of the thymus or bursa of Fabricius. Submucosal lymphoid follicles, which can obstruct the appendiceal lumen, are few at birth but multiply steadily during childhood, reaching a peak in number during the teen years, when acute appendicitis is most common.

Enteric infection likely plays a role in many cases of acute appendicitis in association with mucosal ulceration and invasion of the appendiceal wall by bacteria. Bacteria such as *Yersinia, Salmonella,* and *Shigella* spp., and viruses such as infectious mononucleosis, mumps, coxsackievirus B, and adenovirus, are implicated. In addition, case reports demonstrate the occurrence of appendicitis from ingested foreign bodies, in association with carcinoid tumors of the appendix, *Ascaris* infestation and rarely, following blunt abdominal trauma. Children with cystic fibrosis have an increased incidence of appendicitis; the cause is believed to be the abnormal thickened mucus. Appendicitis in neonates is rare and warrants diagnostic evaluation for cystic fibrosis and Hirschsprung disease.

Appendectomy decreases the risk of ulcerative colitis and increases the risk of recurrent *Clostridium difficile-associated colitis*. Appendicoliths and appendicitis are more common in developed countries with refined, low-fiber diets than in developing countries with a high-fiber diet; no causal relationship has been established between lack of dietary fiber and appendicitis. In a large database analysis for genetic inheritability of appendicitis one locus had genome-wide significance, and a candidate gene *(PITX2)* was identified which was associated with a protective risk of appendicitis. A family history is associated with a nearly threefold increased appendicitis risk and genetic factors may account for 30% of appendicitis risk.

Clinical Features

Appendicitis in children has an immensely broad spectrum of clinical presentation; <50% of cases have the classic presentation. The signs and symptoms in acute appendicitis can vary depending on the timing of presentation, patient age, the abdominal/pelvic location of the appendix, and most importantly, individual variability in the evolution of the disease process. Children early in the disease process can appear well and demonstrate mild symptoms, minimal findings on physical examination, and normal laboratory studies, while those with perforation and advanced peritonitis can demonstrate severe illness with bowel obstruction, renal failure, and septic shock. Most patients with appendicitis demonstrate an insidious onset of illness characterized by generalized nonspecific malaise or anorexia in the first 12 hr, and a steady, escalating progression in severity of signs and symptoms over 2-3 days with increasing abdominal pain, vomiting, fever, and tachycardia;

perforation is common beyond 48 hr of illness. Thus, the opportunity for diagnosis before perforation in acute appendicitis in children is most often brief (48-72 hr) and a high percentage of patients are perforated at presentation.

Abdominal pain is consistently the *primary* symptom in acute appendicitis; beginning shortly (hours) after the onset of illness. As with other visceral organs, there are no somatic pain fibers within the appendix; therefore, early appendiceal inflammation results in pain which is vague, poorly localized, unrelated to activity or position, often colicky, and periumbilical in location as a result of visceral inflammation from a distended appendix. Progression of the inflammatory process in the next 24 hr leads to involvement of the adjacent parietal peritoneal surfaces, resulting in somatic pain localized to the right lower quadrant (RLQ); *thus, the classic description of periumbilical mid-abdominal pain migrating to the RLQ. The position of the appendix is a critical factor affecting interpretation of presenting signs and symptoms and accurate diagnosis.* When the appendix is in a retrocecal or pelvic position, a slower progression of illness is typical and clinical presentation is likely to be delayed. Localized pain in the RLQ leads to spasm in the overlying abdominal wall muscles and now the pain is predictably exacerbated by movement. The child often describes marked discomfort with the bumpy car ride to the hospital, moves cautiously, and has difficulty getting onto the examining room stretcher. Nausea and vomiting occur in more than half the patients, and typically *follow* the onset of abdominal pain by several hours. Anorexia is a classic and consistent finding in acute appendicitis, but occasionally affected patients are hungry. Diarrhea and urinary symptoms are also common, particularly in cases of PA when there is likely inflammation near the rectum and possible abscess in the pelvis. Painful voiding may not be from dysuria, but pressure transmitted to an inflamed peritoneum. As it progresses, appendicitis is often associated with adynamic ileus, leading to the complaint of constipation and possible misdiagnosis.

Because enteric infections can cause appendicitis, diarrhea may be a manifestation and gastroenteritis may be the assumed diagnosis. In contrast to gastroenteritis, the abdominal pain in early appendicitis is *constant* (not cramping or relieved by defecation), the emesis may become bile stained and persistent, and the clinical course worsens steadily rather than demonstrating a waxing and waning pattern often seen in viral gastroenteritis. Fever is common in appendicitis and typically low-grade unless perforation has occurred. Most patients demonstrate at least mild tachycardia, likely secondary to pain and dehydration. The temporal progression of symptoms from vague, mild pain, malaise, and anorexia to severe localized pain, fever, and vomiting typically occurs rapidly (24-48 hr) in the majority of cases. If the diagnosis is delayed beyond 48 hr, perforation is likely (>65%). When several days have elapsed in the progression of appendicitis, patients typically develop signs and symptoms evidencing advanced disease, including worsening and diffuse pain, abdominal distension, and bilious emesis suggestive of developing small bowel obstruction. The retrocecal appendix can demonstrate symptoms suggestive of septic arthritis of the hip or a psoas muscle abscess.

A primary focus in the management of appendicitis is the avoidance of sepsis and the infectious complications leading to increased morbidity, mostly seen with PA.

Bacteria can be cultured from the serosal surface of the appendix before microscopic or gross perforation and bacterial invasion of the mesenteric veins (pylephlebitis) can result (rarely) in thrombosis and possible liver abscess or portal hypertension. A period after perforation of lessened abdominal pain and acute symptoms has been described, presumably with the elimination of pressure within the appendix. If, following perforation, the omentum or adjacent intestine is able to wall off the fecal contamination, the evolution of illness is less predictable and delay in presentation is likely. If perforation leads to diffuse peritonitis, the child generally has escalating diffuse abdominal pain and rapid development of toxicity evidenced by dehydration and signs of sepsis including hypotension, oliguria, acidosis, and high-grade fever. Young children have a poorly developed omentum and are often unable to control the spread of infection. Perforation and abscess formation with appendicitis can lead to intestinal fistula formation, scrotal cellulitis and abscess through a patent processus vaginalis (indirect inguinal hernia), or small bowel obstruction. The most likely diagnosis in children who present with signs and symptoms of mechanical small bowel obstruction who have not had prior abdominal surgery is complicated appendicitis.

Physical Examination

Although the hallmark of diagnosing acute appendicitis remains a careful and thorough history and physical examination, all clinicians know the arcane nature of acute appendicitis, the consistent or typical clinical features are not present in all patients, and the diagnosis can be a humbling experience even for the most experienced clinicians. A primary focus of the initial assessment is attention to the *temporal evolution* of the illness in relation to specific presenting signs and symptoms. In some patients, the diagnosis can be made on history and physical examination alone; in current practice the selective use of advanced imaging has improved diagnostic accuracy and resulted in significant progress in lowering of negative appendectomy rates.

Physical examination begins with inspection of the child's demeanor as well as the appearance of the abdomen. Because appendicitis most often has an insidious onset, children rarely present <12 hr from the onset of illness. Children with early appendicitis (18-36 hr) typically appear mildly ill and move tentatively, hunched forward and, often, with a slight limp favoring the right side. Supine, they often lie quietly on their right side with their knees pulled up to relax the abdominal muscles, and when asked to lie flat or sit up, they move cautiously and might use a hand to protect the RLQ. Early in appendicitis, the abdomen is typically flat; abdominal distention suggests more advanced disease characteristic of perforation or developing small bowel obstruction. Auscultation can reveal normal or hyperactive bowel sounds in early appendicitis, which are replaced by hypoactive bowel sounds as the disease progresses to perforation. *The judicious use of morphine analgesia to relieve abdominal pain does not change diagnostic accuracy or interfere with surgical decision making, and patients should receive adequate pain control.* Localized abdominal tenderness is the single most reliable finding in the diagnosis of acute appendicitis. McBurney described the classic point of localized tenderness in acute appendicitis, which is the junction of the lateral and middle thirds of the line joining the right anterior–superior iliac spine and the umbilicus, but the tenderness can also localize to any of the aberrant locations of the appendix. Localized tenderness is a later and less-consistent finding when the appendix is retrocecal in position (>50% of cases). In cases of an appendix localized entirely in the pelvis, tenderness on abdominal examination may be minimal. A gentle touch on the child's arm at the beginning of the examination with the reassurance that the abdominal examination will be similarly gentle can help to establish trust and increase the chance for a reliable and reproducible examination. The examination is best initiated in the left lower abdomen, so that the immediate part of the exam is not uncomfortable and conducted in a counterclockwise direction moving gently to the left upper abdomen, right upper abdomen, and, lastly, the right lower abdomen. This should alleviate anxiety, allow relaxation of the abdominal musculature, and enhance trust. The examiner makes several circles of the abdomen with sequentially more pressure. A soft, compressible, nontender abdominal wall is reassuring. In appendicitis, any abdominal wall movement, including coughing (Dunphy sign), may elicit pain. A consistent finding in acute appendicitis is guarding—rigidity of the overlying abdominal wall muscles in the RLQ. This rigidity may be voluntary, to protect the area of tenderness from the examiner's hand, or involuntary, if the inflammation has progressed to peritonitis causing spasm of the overlying muscle.

Abdominal tenderness may be vague or even absent early in the course of appendicitis and is often diffuse after rupture. Rebound tenderness and referred tenderness (Rovsing sign) are also consistent findings in acute appendicitis, but not always present. Rebound tenderness is elicited by deep palpation of the abdomen followed by the sudden release of the examining hand. This is often very painful to the child and has demonstrated poor correlation with peritonitis, so it should be avoided. Gentle finger percussion is a better test for peritoneal irritation. Similarly, digital rectal examination is uncomfortable and unlikely to contribute to the evaluation of appendicitis in most cases of appendicitis in children. Psoas and obturator internus signs are pain with passive stretch of these muscles. The psoas sign is elicited with active right thigh flexion or passive extension of the hip and typically positive in cases of a retrocecal appendix. The obturator sign is demonstrated by adductor pain after internal rotation of the flexed thigh and typically positive in cases of a pelvic appendix. Physical examination may demonstrate a mass in the RLQ representing an inflammatory mass (phlegmon) around the appendix or a localized intraabdominal abscess (fluid collection).

APPENDICITIS RISK SCORING SYSTEMS

Several risk scoring systems have become commonly used tools to promote standardization of the approach to the child with abdominal pain and suspected appendicitis. The clear aim is to maximize diagnostic accuracy in acute appendicitis, and guide imaging evaluation and resource utilization. They all combine the predictive value of consistent symptoms, physical examination findings, and laboratory data yielding a numerical score. The systems most widely utilized are the Alvarado score and the Pediatric Appendicitis Score (PAS). The PAS combines elements of history (migration of pain, anorexia, nausea, vomiting) with physical examination findings (RLQ tenderness, rebound tenderness, fever) and laboratory data (white blood cell [WBC] >10,000, polymorphonuclear neutrophils >75%) to assign a risk score in the low, intermediate, or high-risk range for acute appendicitis (Table 370.1). Scores of ≤4 suggest a very low likelihood of appendicitis, whereas scores ≥8 are highly sensitive and specific for appendicitis. Intermediate scores, between 4 and 7 on the PAS, are considered inconclusive and typically trigger advanced imaging studies. Targeted (appendiceal) ultrasound has demonstrated high sensitivity and specificity (~90%) in the diagnosis of acute appendicitis in centers experienced with the technique and has become the initial imaging study of choice for suspected appendicitis. The notable benefits of ultrasound compared to CT scan include that it is well-tolerated, non-invasive, and lacks ionizing radiation exposure. CT is reserved for cases of nonvisualization of the appendix on ultrasound, or when the ultrasound findings are inconclusive.

The use of appendicitis risk scoring systems, in conjunction with clinical judgment, have demonstrated high sensitivity and specificity for acute appendicitis (80–90%) and their application has reduced practice variability, improved diagnostic accuracy, decreased preoperative radiation exposure, and enabled efficient resource utilization—all important elements of current quality improvement and safety initiatives. Their greatest value to date appears to be in predicting patients that have a low likelihood of the diagnosis of appendicitis (negative predictive value) and can avoid imaging studies, and particularly ionizing radiation exposure.

Table 370.1	Pediatric Appendicitis Scores	
FEATURE		**SCORE**
Fever > 38°C (100.4°F)		1
Anorexia		1
Nausea/vomiting		1
Cough/percussion/hopping tenderness		2
Right lower quadrant tenderness		2
Migration of pain		1
Leukocytosis > 10,000 (10^9/L)		1
Polymorphonuclear-neutrophilia > 7,500 (10^9/L)		1
Total		10

From Acheson J, Banerjee J: Management of suspected appendicitis in children, *Arch Dis Child Educ Pract Ed.* 95:9–13, 2010.

LABORATORY FINDINGS

A variety of laboratory tests have been used in the evaluation of children with suspected appendicitis. Individually, none are very sensitive or specific for appendicitis, but collectively they can affect the clinician's level of suspicion and decision-making to proceed with pediatric surgery consultation, discharge, or imaging studies.

A complete blood count with differential and urinalysis are obtained. The leukocyte count in early appendicitis may be normal, and typically is only mildly elevated (11,000-16,000/mm^3) with a left shift as the illness progresses in the initial 24-48 hr. Whereas a normal WBC count never completely eliminates appendicitis, a count <8,000/mm^3 in a patient with a history of illness longer than 48 hr should be viewed as highly suspicious for an alternative diagnosis. The leukocyte count may be markedly elevated (>20,000/mm^3) in PA and rarely in nonperforated cases; a markedly elevated WBC count, other than in cases of advanced PA, should raise suspicion of an alternative diagnosis. Urinalysis often demonstrates a few white or red blood cells as a result of the proximity of the inflamed appendix to the ureter or bladder, but it should be free of bacteria. The urine is often concentrated and contains ketones from diminished oral intake and vomiting. Gross hematuria is uncommon, and in association with purpuric skin lesions and arthritis may indicate Henoch-Schönlein purpura.

Electrolytes and liver chemistries are generally normal unless there has been a delay in diagnosis, leading to severe dehydration and/or sepsis. Amylase and liver enzymes are only helpful to exclude alternative diagnoses such as pancreatitis and cholecystitis and are not commonly obtained if appendicitis is the strongly suspected diagnosis. C-reactive protein (CRP) increases in proportion to the degree of appendiceal inflammation. It has not demonstrated high sensitivity or specificity in the diagnosis of appendicitis; some studies have demonstrated an association between disease severity (PA and abscess formation) and elevated CRP levels. In this context, CRP may have a role in identifying patients with complicated appendicitis, which may be managed initially nonoperatively with antibiotics and drainage of fluid collections.

IMAGING STUDIES

Following a thorough initial evaluation including history, physical examination, review of vital signs, and laboratory studies, if the diagnosis is uncertain, radiographic studies can substantially improve diagnostic accuracy.

Plain Radiographs

In the majority of cases, appendiceal ultrasound and CT scan have become the predominant studies in inconclusive cases of acute appendicitis. Plain abdominal radiographs may be helpful in rare select cases of abdominal pain/suspected appendicitis. Plain abdominal x-rays may demonstrate several findings suggestive of acute appendicitis, including sentinel loops of bowel and localized ileus, scoliosis from psoas muscle spasm, a colonic air–fluid level above the right iliac fossa (colon cutoff sign), an RLQ soft tissue mass, or a calcified appendicolith (5–10% of cases); they are normal in 50% of patients, have a low sensitivity, and are not generally recommended (Fig. 370.1). Plain films are most helpful in evaluating complicated cases in which small bowel obstruction or free air is suspected.

Ultrasound

Ultrasound has emerged as the first-choice tool for children requiring an imaging study in the evaluation of suspected acute appendicitis. Ultrasound has demonstrated sensitivity and specificity approaching 90% in pediatric centers experienced with the technique, and has substantial advantages including low cost, ready availability, rapidity, and avoidance of sedation, contrast agents, and radiation exposure. Ultrasound can be particularly helpful in adolescent females, a group with a high negative appendectomy rate (normal appendix found at surgery), because of its ability to evaluate for ovarian pathology without ionizing radiation. Graded abdominal compression is used to displace the cecum and ascending colon and identify the appendix, which has a typical target appearance (Fig. 370.2). The ultrasound criteria for appendicitis include wall thickness ≥6 mm, luminal distention, lack of

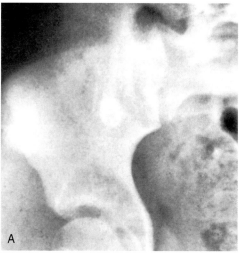

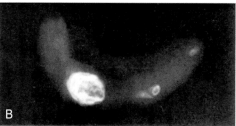

Fig. 370.1 Calcified appendicoliths are seen in a coned-down anteroposterior view of the right lower quadrant (**A**) and in the resected appendix of a 10 yr old girl with acute appendicitis (**B**). *(From Kuhn JP, Slovis TL, Haller JO: Caffrey's pediatric diagnostic imaging, vol 2, ed 10, Philadelphia, 2004, Mosby, p. 1682.)*

compressibility, a complex mass in the RLQ, or an appendicolith. The visualized appendix usually coincides with the site of localized pain and tenderness. In addition, ultrasound may identify PA on *initial evaluation*; initial management of PA has increasingly moved toward percutaneous drainage procedures, broad spectrum antibiotics, and nonoperative treatment. An enlarged appendix (>6 mm), hyperemia, noncompressibility of the appendiceal wall, localized tenderness, and associated mesenteric fat stranding or fluid are all consistent with acute appendicitis. Findings that suggest advanced appendicitis on ultrasound include asymmetric wall thickening, abscess formation, associated free intraabdominal/pelvic fluid, surrounding tissue edema, and decreased local tenderness to compression. *The main limitation of ultrasound is an inability to visualize the appendix, which is reported in 25–60% of cases.* It has been postulated that a normal appendix must be visualized to exclude the diagnosis of appendicitis by ultrasound; however, one report concluded that in patients with a nonvisualized appendix on ultrasound imaging and no evidence of secondary inflammatory changes, the likelihood of appendicitis was <2%. Certain conditions predictably decrease the sensitivity and reliability of ultrasound for appendicitis, including obesity, bowel distention, and uncontrolled pain.

Computed Tomography

CT scan has been the gold standard imaging study for evaluating children with suspected appendicitis, and has sensitivity of 97%, specificity 99%, positive predictive value 98%, and negative predictive value 98% (Figs. 370.3 and 370.4). The advantages of CT imaging include ready availability, rapid acquisition time, and lack of operator dependency. CT carries the significant negative effects of exposure of children to ionizing radiation and increased costs. The exam can be performed using intravenous and enteral (oral or rectal) contrast; however, the administration of enteral contrast has several drawbacks including increasing abdominal

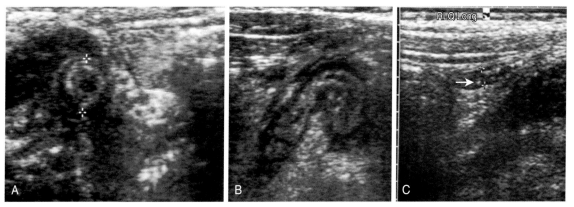

Fig. 370.2 Ultrasound examination of patients with appendicitis. **A,** Transverse ultrasound scan of the appendix demonstrates the characteristic "target sign." In this case, the innermost portion is sonolucent, compatible with fluid or pus. **B,** Longitudinal view of another patient demonstrates the alternating hyperechoic and hypoechoic layers with an outermost hypoechoic layer, suggesting periappendiceal fluid. **C,** Longitudinal ultrasound scan of the right lower quadrant demonstrates a dilated, non-compressible appendix. The bright echo within the appendix represents an appendicolith with acoustic shadowing *(arrow)*. *(From Kuhn JP, Slovis TL, Haller JO: Caffrey's pediatric diagnostic imaging, vol 2, ed 10, Philadelphia, 2004, Mosby, p. 1684.)*

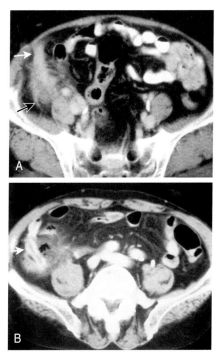

Fig. 370.3 A, Phlegmon *(open arrow)* is noted around the enlarged appendix *(solid arrow)* in perforated appendicitis. **B,** Extraluminal air is shown adjacent to the wall-enhanced appendix *(arrow)* in perforated appendicitis. *(From Yeung KW, Chang MS, Hsiao CP: Evaluation of perforated and non-perforated appendicitis with CT, Clin Imaging 28(6):422–427, 2004.)*

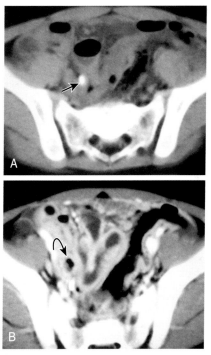

Fig. 370.4 A, Precontrast-enhanced CT reveals an appendicolith *(arrow)* in perforated appendicitis. **B,** Postcontrast-enhanced CT (1 cm below the level in **A**) reveals intraluminal air in the appendix *(curved arrow)* associated with ileal wall enhancement in perforated appendicitis. *(From Yeung KW, Chang MS, Hsiao CP: Evaluation of perforated and non-perforated appendicitis with CT, Clin Imaging 28(6):422–427, 2004.)*

distension, risk of emesis and aspiration, and increasing radiation exposure without demonstrable improvement in accuracy of diagnosis. The use of oral contrast should be reserved for patients in whom alternative diagnoses are suspected, particularly Crohn disease. Because the finding of fat stranding in surrounding tissues is a key component of CT evaluation for appendicitis, CT is less reliable in thin children with minimal body fat.

The avoidance of enteral contrast, targeted CT imaging, and the use of pediatric specific protocols can significantly lower radiation dosages without sacrificing diagnostic accuracy. The use of appendicitis risk scoring systems, in conjunction with CPGs, and increasing experience with appendiceal ultrasound have led to a decreased use of CT scans (<6.6% in most reports), without negatively affecting time to appendectomy or negative appendectomy rates.

Magnetic Resonance Imaging and White Blood Cell Scans

MRI is at least equivalent to CT in diagnostic accuracy for appendicitis and does not involve ionizing radiation; however, its use in the evaluation of appendicitis is limited because it is less available, associated with higher costs, often requires sedation, and does not offer equivalent access for drainage of fluid collections. MRI may prove most useful in adolescent females when ultrasound imaging is equivocal. Radionuclide-labeled WBC scans have also been used in some centers in evaluating atypical cases of possible appendicitis in children and demonstrated a high sensitivity (97%) but only modest specificity (80%).

DIAGNOSIS AND TREATMENT

Acute appendicitis is believed to be a time-sensitive condition, thus, any delay in diagnosis or treatment may lead to an increased risk of perforation and its attendant morbidity. The misdiagnosis of appendicitis is second only to meningitis as a cause of medical malpractice suits in pediatric emergency care. A careful history and physical examination remains primary in the initial assessment of a child presenting with abdominal symptoms. The classic history in acute appendicitis, although possibly not most common, is a 24-hr history of diffuse mid-abdominal pain which migrates and becomes localized to the RLQ. Patients should have a WBC count with differential analysis, as this is a component of most appendicitis risk scoring systems. A urinalysis is also typically obtained and a pregnancy test in appropriately selected patients. CPGs have become common practice in many centers for evaluation of patients with abdominal pain and suspected appendicitis to reduce practice variability and improve diagnostic accuracy and resource utilization. CPGs have been shown to have a high positive and negative predictive value (~95%), and to decrease both LOS and costs without increasing morbidity or complications. These guidelines combine initial history, physical examination, and laboratory data with predictive risk scoring systems to cohort patients into low, intermediate, and high risk for the diagnosis of acute appendicitis. In general, low-risk patients can be discharged without imaging studies, high-risk patients would have pediatric surgical consultation, and the inconclusive or intermediate risk group would most predictably benefit from a period of observation or proceeding with advanced imaging studies. If the initial assessment leads to a high level of suspicion for appendicitis, pediatric surgical consultation should be the next step, with the likelihood of an appendectomy without further studies. In patients with a low concern for appendicitis, the child may be discharged with family education regarding the natural history and progression of acute appendicitis and advice to return for repeat evaluation if the child is not improving on liquids and a bland diet in the next 24 hr. The group of patients with an intermediate risk score would proceed with targeted ultrasound of the appendix if the center has experience with the technique. If the ultrasound study is unable to visualize the appendix, or the appendix is visualized but the findings inconclusive, the next options would include admission for a period of observation and planned reassessment, CT imaging, or diagnostic laparoscopy.

The use of observation units, where the child may be observed with intravenous fluids, serial vital signs, and planned re-examinations is another strategy. At the end of a period of observation, typically 12-24 hr, the clinician decides on discharge based on reassuring clinical status, proceeds to diagnostic laparoscopy and appendectomy, or proceeds with advanced imaging evaluation. The period of observation can occur at home provided the patient is physiologically well; a hospital-based observational unit has the advantage of being able to provide intravenous fluids. An observation strategy seems most useful in patients who present with a brief history of illness (<12 hr) when advanced imaging studies predictably have lower sensitivity and specificity. If observed patients remain equivocal, advanced imaging should be more reliable further into the disease process.

DIFFERENTIAL DIAGNOSIS

The list of illnesses that can mimic acute appendicitis is extensive because many gastrointestinal, gynecologic, and inflammatory disorders can manifest with similar illness history, signs, and symptoms. Differential diagnosis, even limited to common conditions, includes gastroenteritis, mesenteric adenitis, Meckel diverticulitis, intussusception, inflammatory bowel disease, diabetes mellitus, sickle cell disease, streptococcal pharyngitis, lower lobe pneumonia, cholecystitis, pancreatitis, urinary tract infection (UTI), infectious enteritis, and, in females, ovarian torsion, ectopic pregnancy, ruptured/hemorrhagic ovarian cysts, and pelvic inflammatory disease (including tuboovarian abscess). *Epiploic appendagitis*, an inflammation of the fat-filled structures on the antimesenteric surface of the colon, may present with acute lower quadrant abdominal pain after torsion, thrombosis, and ischemic injury to the structure. Viral infections, bacterial infections, and parasitic infections can all closely mimic acute appendicitis. Intestinal tract lymphoma, tumors of the appendix (carcinoid in children), and ovarian tumors are rare but can also masquerade as acute appendicitis. Henoch-Schönlein purpura can initially present as severe abdominal pain. Urinary tract causes of abdominal pain include UTI, nephrolithiasis, and pyelonephritis. In patients with pyelonephritis, the fever and WBC count are likely much higher, symptoms of dysuria will be present, and the tenderness is located more in the flank or costovertebral angle. Rarely, appendicitis may recur in the stump of a previous appendectomy. *Children younger than 3 yr of age and adolescent girls have historically proven to be at particularly high risk for an incorrect diagnosis.*

Viral illnesses are common in children, often are associated with abdominal pain and vomiting, and thus mimic acute appendicitis. The classic patient with acute appendicitis describes abdominal pain as the preeminent symptom, and in general, symptoms of systemic illness such as headache, chills, and myalgias are infrequent in appendicitis and common when viral illness is the correct diagnosis.

The diagnosis of appendicitis in adolescent females is especially challenging, and some series report negative appendectomy rates as high as 30–40%. Ovarian cysts are often acutely painful as a result of rupture, rapid enlargement, or hemorrhage. Rupture of an ovarian follicle associated with ovulation often causes mid-cycle lateralizing pain (mittelschmerz), but there is no progression of symptoms and systemic illness is absent. Ovarian tumors and torsion can also mimic acute appendicitis, although ovarian torsion is typically characterized by the acute onset of severe pain and is associated with more frequent and forceful nausea and vomiting than is typically seen in early appendicitis. In pelvic inflammatory disease, the pain is typically suprapubic, bilateral, and of longer duration. The need for accurate urgent diagnosis in females is influenced by concern that PA can predispose the patient to future ectopic pregnancy or tubal infertility, although data have not consistently demonstrated increased incidence of infertility after PA. For these reasons, adjunct diagnostic studies (ultrasound, CT, MRI, or diagnostic laparoscopy) should be used more liberally in females to keep negative appendectomy rates low.

Torsion of an undescended testis and epididymitis are common but should be discovered on physical exam. Meckel's diverticulitis is an infrequent condition, but the clinical presentation closely mimics appendicitis. The diagnosis is rarely made before surgery. Primary spontaneous peritonitis (PSP) is classically seen in prepubertal females or patients with either nephrotic syndrome or cirrhosis and is frequently mistaken for appendicitis.

Atypical presentations of appendicitis are expected in association with other conditions such as pregnancy, Crohn disease, steroid treatment, and immunosuppressive therapy. Appendicitis in association with Crohn disease often has a protracted presentation with an atypical pattern of recurring but localized abdominal pain. It should be recognized that *missed* appendicitis is the most common cause of small bowel obstruction in children without history of prior abdominal surgery.

ANTIBIOTICS

Antibiotics should be initiated promptly once the diagnosis of appendicitis is made or highly suspected. Antibiotics substantially lower the incidence of postoperative wound infections, SSIs and intraabdominal abscesses—the source of the majority of the substantial morbidity and costs in PA. Many believe the time from onset of illness to the initiation of antibiotics has more impact on postoperative complication rates, LOS, and overall costs than time from diagnosis to surgery.

The antibiotic regimen should be directed against the typical bacterial flora found in the appendix, including anaerobic organisms (*Bacteroides, Clostridia,* and *Peptostreptococcus* spp.) and Gram-negative aerobic bacteria (*Escherichia coli, Pseudomonas aeruginosa, Enterobacter,* and *Klebsiella* spp.). Many antibiotic combinations have demonstrated equivalent efficacy in controlled trials in terms of wound infection rate, resolution of fever, LOS, and incidence of complications. Historically, a triple-antibiotic regimen consisting of ampicillin, gentamicin, and clindamycin was standard. Exhaustive studies of different antibiotic regimens have been performed, mostly aimed at lowering costs and frequency of dosing while maintaining efficacy. Both piperacillin/tazobactam and cefoxitin have demonstrated equivalent effectiveness and may decrease LOS and pharmaceutical costs compared to the triple-antibiotic regimen.

For simple (nonperforated) appendicitis, one preoperative dose of a single broad-spectrum agent (Zosyn) or equivalent is sufficient. In PA, the antibiotic is continued intravenously for 2-3 days postoperatively until the child is afebrile (≥24 hr), tolerating a general diet, and ready for discharge. Some centers prefer to add metronidazole in PA to augment coverage of anaerobes. The decision to discharge patients with PA managed with upfront appendectomy on a course of oral antibiotics (typically 3-5 days) remains controversial. The literature does not support improved outcomes with PA if antibiotics are extended beyond a 4- to 5-day course.

SURGICAL INTERVENTION

Once the diagnosis of appendicitis is confirmed or highly suspected, the standard treatment for acute appendicitis, both simple and complicated, in current practice is most often prompt appendectomy. LA (minimally invasive technique) is the preferred surgical approach (65–70%) in both simple and PA, with open appendectomy markedly declining in the past decade. The laparoscopic approach has demonstrated slight improvement in clinical outcome measures (wound infection rate, intraabdominal abscess, analgesic requirements, wound cosmesis, and return to full activity), however, costs can be higher. The laparoscopic approach (diagnostic laparoscopy/LA) has particular advantages for obese patients, when alternative diagnoses are suspected, and in adolescent females to evaluate for ovarian pathology and alternative diagnoses while avoiding the ionizing radiation associated with CT imaging. The operation should proceed semi-electively within 12-24 hr of diagnosis. Children with appendicitis are typically at least mildly dehydrated and should receive supportive care prior to surgery, including fluid resuscitation to correct hypovolemia and electrolyte abnormalities, antipyretics to lower fever, and broad-spectrum antibiotics. These important fundamentals of care ensure safe anesthesia and optimize outcomes. In most cases, preoperative management can be accomplished during the period of diagnostic evaluation and prompt appendectomy can be performed. Pain management begins even before a definitive diagnosis is made, and consultation of a pain service, if available, is appropriate. Emergency surgery (middle of the night) *is rarely* indicated in acute appendicitis and should only be performed in the rare circumstance when physiologic resuscitation requires urgent control of advanced intraabdominal sepsis not amenable to percutaneous drainage by IR, or when this is not available. No correlation has been demonstrated between timing of surgery and perforation rates or postoperative morbidity when the operation proceeds within 24 hr of diagnosis. When comparing emergent appendectomy (within 5 hr of admission) with urgent appendectomy (within 17 hr of admission), no difference in PA, operative time, readmission rate, postoperative complications, LOS, or hospital charges have been noted. In addition, occasionally unexpected pathology (appendiceal tumors, intestinal lymphoma, congenital renal anomalies, Crohn disease) is discovered at operation, and intraoperative consultation with other specialists and/or frozen section evaluation may be required. The laparoscopic approach, in conjunction with standardized, expedited postoperative recovery protocols, and improved (single drug) and shorter duration antibiotic regimens have led to decreased LOS in both simple and complicated (perforated) appendicitis. The average LOS in most centers is approximately 24 hr for simple appendicitis and 4-5 days for perforated cases that recover without postoperative complications. In simple appendicitis, some centers have initiated same-day discharge.

PERFORATED APPENDICITIS

A major area of focus and challenge in the management of acute appendicitis is the group of patients with delayed presentation (>48 hr of symptoms). In most busy centers, because acute appendicitis often has an insidious onset of generalized malaise, as many as 40–50% of patients have delayed presentation. This cohort of patients has a high incidence of PA at presentation (40–59%) and a 56% greater LOS stay than those presenting within ≤24 hr of the onset of symptoms. The risk for development of postoperative complications (SSI, intraabdominal abscess, small bowel obstruction) approaches 20–30% for children with PA versus an approximately 3% risk of complications in patients with simple appendicitis.

Management options for children presenting with PA include upfront appendectomy following a brief period of stabilization with intravenous fluids and antibiotics, antibiotics alone, and antibiotics in conjunction with percutaneous drainage of intraabdominal fluid collections/abscesses. The past decade has witnessed a substantial trend toward nonoperative management in children with delayed presentation and suspected PA to avoid the high complication rate in these patients and the potential technical challenges of operative treatment in the setting of marked intraabdominal inflammation/peritonitis. Based on patient status, findings on imaging studies, and availability of experienced interventional radiologists, initial nonoperative management of PA with percutaneous drainage of fluid collections, intravenous fluids and broad-spectrum antibiotics has demonstrated success in >80% of patients. Antibiotics are initiated and typically continued intravenously for 1-2 days along with pain control. If the child demonstrates clinical recovery by resolution of fever and pain, and the patient can tolerate a general diet, the child is converted to oral antibiotics and discharged to complete an outpatient antibiotic course (typically 7-10 days of ciprofloxacin/Flagyl). A patient who fails to demonstrate clinical recovery proceeds to prompt appendectomy. This nonoperative management, and particularly the transition to oral antibiotics, has contributed to a decreased LOS and costs in the management of PA. Patients who do not have upfront appendectomy will require a decision regarding interval appendectomy (IA) in 4-6 wk, provided she/he does not fail nonoperative management after discharge by recurrence of pain, fever, or vomiting.

NONOPERATIVE MANAGEMENT OF UNCOMPLICATED APPENDICITIS

Multiple studies in adults have demonstrated highly effective treatment of appendicitis with antibiotics alone. In addition, other conditions similar to appendicitis, such as diverticulitis, intraabdominal abscess in Crohn disease, and tubo-ovarian abscess, are primarily treated with antibiotics alone, with surgery reserved for failures of medical management. These outcomes have led many centers to evaluate initial nonoperative management of acute (simple) appendicitis in children and currently several randomized controlled studies are ongoing. Previous studies demonstrated a success rate for nonoperative management of simple appendicitis in children of 75–80%, with no increased rates of PA in patients who fail initial nonoperative management. Advantages of the antibiotic alone/nonoperative approach in acute appendicitis include avoidance of surgical complications and the risk of general anesthesia, and an operative procedure that may not be necessary. In some children's centers, the nonoperative approach is being offered on experimental protocol. Selection criteria for nonoperative management typically include <48-hr duration of symptoms, age >7 yr, imaging confirmation of acute non-PA, appendiceal diameter <1.2 cm, *absence* of appendicolith, abscess, or phlegmon, WBC >5,000, and <18,000 cells/μL. The clinical pathway for children enrolled consists of an initial 1-2 days of intravenous broad-spectrum antibiotics and pain control. If the child demonstrates clinical recovery by resolution of pain and fever and is tolerating a general diet, he/she is discharged to complete 7-10 days of oral antibiotics. If the child does not demonstrate clinical recovery, prompt appendectomy is performed. Early nonoperative trials found that predictors of failure of nonoperative management included pain >48 hr duration, presence of an appendicolith, inflammatory mass or abscess on imaging, and elevated laboratory values (WBC > 18,000, CRP > 4 mg/dL). Reports of this approach suggest a more rapid return to full activities and lower costs associated with the hospitalization for nonoperative management; however, others have reported that patients with nonoperative management had more subsequent ED visits, advanced imaging studies, and hospitalizations compared with those managed operatively at the first visit.

RECURRENT APPENDICITIS

Prospective studies of the incidence of early recurrent appendicitis (within 1 yr) describe a range between 10 to 20% in patients initially managed nonoperatively. The lifetime risk of recurrent appendicitis in children treated nonoperatively is unknown. Controversies remain in the initial nonoperative management of PA. Most studies have reported significantly fewer overall complications (wound infections, intraabdominal abscesses, bowel obstruction, re-operations) in patients with initial nonoperative management of PA compared to patients with PA managed with upfront appendectomy; other reviews have supported early appendectomy in PA because initial nonoperative management and delayed appendectomy was associated with a significantly longer time to return to normal activities and an adverse event rate of 30% versus 55% in the initial nonoperative cohort. The initial nonoperative management and delayed appendectomy patients also incurred higher costs. Currently under review is the need for delayed appendectomy IA in patients with complicated appendicitis initially managed nonoperatively. While the trend in cases of PA at presentation is toward initial nonoperative management, the data remains uncertain, and there is no convincing data to recommend one approach in all patients.

INTERVAL APPENDECTOMY

In patients with PA initially treated nonoperatively, the decision to proceed with IA, typically in 4-6 wk, is another area of management lacking consensus. Traditionally, most surgeons recommended IA to avoid recurrent appendicitis and to confirm the original diagnosis, citing reports which demonstrated an incidence of unexpected pathology in 30% of IA specimens. This has been questioned with nonoperative management of simple appendicitis gaining acceptance and many debating the risk of recurrent appendicitis (5–20%), believing it to be lower. The lifetime risk of recurrent appendicitis is unknown. Decision-making for IA must be individualized to balance the risks of recurrent appendicitis with the risks of anesthesia and comorbid conditions such as obesity, congenital heart disease, chronic respiratory conditions, and others.

INCIDENTAL APPENDICOLITHS

The question of the incidental appendicolith is an intriguing one for pediatric practitioners. These are patients who do not have appendicitis but are found to have an appendicolith on imaging studies. An appendicolith is defined as a calcification within the appendiceal lumen. In adults, incidental appendicoliths identified by CT scans vary in incidence from <1% to as high as 10%. They have a characteristic dense and laminated appearance when compared to other lower abdominal calcifications, including phleboliths (venous calcifications) and, in females, ovarian calcifications, most commonly seen in ovarian tumors. They can be appreciated on plain film, ultrasound, and CT scan. When an appendicolith is noted in the evaluation of a child with abdominal pain and suspected appendicitis, the finding of the appendicolith confirms the diagnosis; surgical consultation and prompt appendectomy is indicated. Appendicoliths may be noted in the evaluation of patients who have no signs of appendicitis, such as imaging obtained after trauma or for nonspecific abdominal complaints in patients with low likelihood of appendicitis. The concern in this setting is that the appendicolith may increase the eventual development of acute appendicitis. In addition, there is the concern that should appendicitis develop in association with an appendicolith, there may be a rapidly escalating course and early perforation. Some physicians believe that a persistent appendicolith may be associated with recurrent RLQ/iliac fossa pain.

Incidental appendicoliths may be transient and in most short-term follow-up studies have a low risk of subsequent acute appendicitis. In addition, the lifetime risk for the development of appendicitis in patients with an incidental appendicolith is approximately 5%, which is not different from the normal population. The risk of subsequent appendicitis may be higher in those presenting with abdominal pain or those younger than 19 yr of age. Radiographically detected incidental appendicoliths are usually managed with observation, planned follow-up, and patient education for signs of acute appendicitis. After discussing the risks and benefits with the family, and persistence of the appendicolith, an individualized approach is best between the physician and family relative to elective appendectomy.

Bibliography is available at Expert Consult.

中文导读

　　本章详细介绍了肛肠畸形的胚胎学发育及畸形分类。阐述了不同类型病变（低位病变、高位病变、永存泄殖腔、直肠闭锁）的临床表现、诊断及治疗；详细介绍了不同类型病变患者的评估、手术修补的方法及预后（原文第371.1）。此外还分别介绍了肛裂（原文第371.2）、肛周脓肿和瘘管（原文第371.3）、痔疮（原文第371.4）、直肠黏膜脱垂（原文第371.5）、藏毛窦及脓肿（原文第371.6）的临床表现及治疗。

371.1 Anorectal Malformations

Christina M. Shanti

To fully understand the spectrum of anorectal anomalies, it is necessary to consider the importance of the sphincter complex, a mass of muscle fibers surrounding the anorectum (Fig. 371.1). This complex is the combination of the puborectalis, levator ani, external and internal sphincters, and the superficial external sphincter muscles, all meeting at the rectum. Anorectal malformations are defined by the relationship of the rectum to this complex and include varying degrees of stenosis to complete atresia. The incidence is 1/3,000 live births. Significant long-term concerns focus on bowel control and urinary and sexual functions.

EMBRYOLOGY

The hindgut forms early as the part of the primitive gut tube that extends into the tail fold in the 2nd wk of gestation. At about day 13, it develops a ventral diverticulum, the allantois, or primitive bladder. The junction of allantois and hindgut becomes the cloaca, into which the genital, urinary, and intestinal tubes empty. This is covered by a cloacal membrane. The urorectal septum descends to divide this common channel by forming lateral ridges, which grow in and fuse by the middle of the 7th wk. Opening of the posterior portion of the membrane (the anal membrane) occurs in the 8th wk. Failures in any part of these processes can lead to the clinical spectrum of anogenital anomalies.

Imperforate anus can be divided into low lesions, where the rectum has descended through the sphincter complex, and high lesions, where it has not. Most patients with imperforate anus have a fistula. There is a spectrum of malformation in males and females. In males, low lesions usually manifest with meconium staining somewhere on the perineum along the median raphe (Fig. 371.2A). Low lesions in females also manifest as a spectrum from an anus that is only slightly anterior on the perineal body to a fourchette fistula that opens on the moist mucosa of the introitus distal to the hymen (Fig. 371.3A). A high imperforate anus in a male has no apparent cutaneous opening or fistula, but usually has a fistula to the urinary tract, either the urethra or the bladder (see Fig. 371.2B). Although there is occasionally a rectovaginal fistula, in females, high lesions are usually cloacal anomalies in which the rectum, vagina, and urethra all empty into a common channel or cloacal stem of varying length (see Fig. 371.3B). The interesting category of males with imperforate anus and no fistula occurs mainly in children with trisomy 21. The most common lesions are the rectourethral bulbar

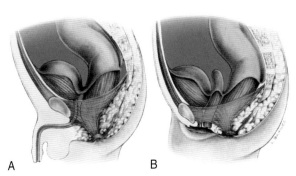

Fig. 371.1 Normal anorectal anatomy in relation to pelvic structures. **A,** Male. **B,** Female. *(From Peña A: Atlas of surgical management of anorectal malformations, New York, 1989, Springer-Verlag, p 3.)*

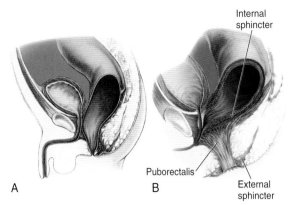

Fig. 371.2 Imperforate anus in males. **A,** Low lesions. **B,** High lesions. *(From Peña A: Atlas of surgical management of anorectal malformations, New York, 1989, Springer-Verlag, pp 7, 26.)*

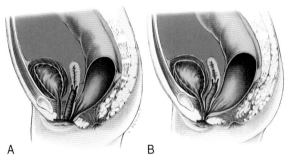

Fig. 371.3 Imperforate anus in females. **A,** Vestibular fistula. **B,** Cloaca. *(From Peña A: Atlas of surgical management of anorectal malformations, New York, 1989, Springer-Verlag, pp 50, 60.)*

fistula in males and the rectovestibular fistula in females; the 2nd most common lesion in both sexes is the perianal fistula (Fig. 371.4).

ASSOCIATED ANOMALIES

There are many anomalies associated with anorectal malformations (Table 371.1). The most common are anomalies of the kidneys and urinary tract in conjunction with abnormalities of the sacrum. This complex is often referred to as *caudal regression syndrome*. Males with a rectovesical fistula and patients with a persistent cloaca have a 90%

| Table 371.1 | Associated Malformations |

GENITOURINARY
- Vesicoureteric reflux
- Renal agenesis
- Renal dysplasia
- Ureteral duplication
- Cryptorchidism
- Hypospadias
- Bicornuate uterus
- Vaginal septa

VERTEBRAL
- Spinal dysraphism
- Tethered chord
- Presacral masses
- Meningocele
- Lipoma
- Dermoid
- Teratoma

CARDIOVASCULAR
- Tetralogy of Fallot
- Ventricular septal defect
- Transposition of the great vessels
- Hypoplastic left-heart syndrome

GASTROINTESTINAL
- Tracheoesophageal fistula
- Duodenal atresia
- Malrotation
- Hirschsprung disease

CENTRAL NERVOUS SYSTEM
- Spina bifida
- Tethered cord

risk of urologic defects. Other common associated anomalies are cardiac anomalies and esophageal atresia with or without tracheoesophageal fistula. These can cluster in any combination in a patient. When combined, they are often accompanied by abnormalities of the radial aspect of the upper extremity and are termed the VACTERL (*v*ertebral, *a*nal, *c*ardiac, *t*racheal, *e*sophageal, *r*enal, *l*imb) anomalad.

Anorectal malformations, particularly anal stenosis and rectal atresia, can also present as Currarino triad, which includes sacral agenesis, presacral mass, and anorectal stenosis. These patients present with a funnel appearing anus, have sacral bony defects on plain x-ray, and have a presacral mass (teratoma, meningocele, dermoid cyst, enteric cyst) on exam or imaging. It is an autosomal dominant disorder due in most patients to a mutation in the *MNX1* gene.

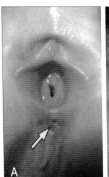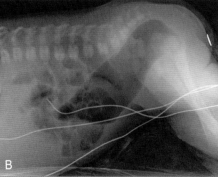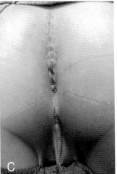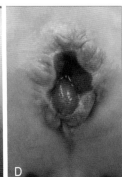

Fig. 371.4 Preoperative and postoperative images of anorectal malformations. **A,** Preoperative rectoperineal fistula. **B,** Radiograph with cross table lateral film showing neonate in prone position and gas below the coccyx. **C,** Postoperative appearance after a posterior sagittal anorectoplasty. **D,** Postoperative large, patulous, and prolapsed anoplasty. *(From Bischoff A, Bealer J, Pená A: Controversies in anorectal malformations, Lancet Child/Adolesc 1:323–330, 2017, Fig. p. 324).*

A good correlation exists between the degree of sacral development and future function. Patients with an absent sacrum usually have permanent fecal and urinary incontinence. Spinal abnormalities and different degrees of dysraphism are often associated with these defects. Tethered cord occurs in approximately 25% of patients with anorectal malformations. Untethering of the cord can lead to improved urinary and rectal continence in some patients, although it seldom reverses established neurologic defects. The diagnosis of spinal defects can be screened for in the first 3 mo of life by spinal ultrasound, although MRI is the imaging method of choice if a lesion is suspected. In older patients, MRI is needed.

MANIFESTATIONS AND DIAGNOSIS
Low Lesions
Examination of a newborn includes the inspection of the perineum. The absence of an anal orifice in the correct position leads to further evaluation. Mild forms of imperforate anus are often called *anal stenosis* or *anterior ectopic anus*. These are typically cases of an imperforate anus with a perineal fistula. The normal position of the anus on the perineum is approximately halfway (0.5 ratio) between the coccyx and the scrotum or introitus. Although symptoms, primarily constipation, have been attributed to anterior ectopic anus (ratio: <0.34 in females, <0.46 in males), many patients have no symptoms.

If no anus or fistula is visible, there may be a low lesion or *covered anus*. In these cases, there are well-formed buttocks and often a thickened raphe or *bucket handle*. After 24 hr, meconium bulging may be seen, creating a blue or black appearance. In these cases, an immediate perineal procedure can often be performed, followed by a dilation program.

In a male, the perineal (cutaneous) fistula can track anteriorly along the median raphe across the scrotum and even down the penile shaft. This is usually a thin track, with a normal rectum often just a few millimeters from the skin. Extraintestinal anomalies are seen in <10% of these patients.

In a female, a low lesion enters the vestibule or fourchette (the moist mucosa outside the hymen but within the introitus). In this case, the rectum has descended through the sphincter complex. Children with a low lesion can usually be treated initially with perineal manipulation and dilation. Visualizing these low fistulas is so important in the evaluation and treatment that one should avoid passing a nasogastric tube for the first 24 hr to allow the abdomen and bowel to distend, pushing meconium down into the distal rectum.

High Lesions
In a male with a high imperforate anus, the perineum appears flat. There may be air or meconium passed via the urethra when the fistula is high, entering the bulbar or prostatic urethra, or even the bladder. In *rectobulbar urethral fistulas* (the most common in males), the sphincter mechanism is satisfactory, the sacrum may be underdeveloped, and an anal dimple is present. In *rectoprostatic urethral fistulas*, the sacrum is poorly developed, the scrotum may be bifid, and the anal dimple is near the scrotum. In *rectovesicular fistulas*, the sphincter mechanism is poorly developed, and the sacrum is hypoplastic or absent. In males with trisomy 21, all the features of a high lesion may be present, but there is no fistula, the sacrum and sphincter mechanisms are usually well developed, and the prognosis is good.

In females with high imperforate anus, there may be the appearance of a rectovaginal fistula. A true rectovaginal fistula is rare. Most are either the fourchette fistulas described earlier or are forms of a cloacal anomaly.

Persistent Cloaca
In persistent cloaca, the embryologic stage persists in which the rectum, urethra, and vagina communicate in a common orifice, the cloaca. It is important to realize this, because the repair often requires repositioning the urethra and vagina as well as the rectum. Children of both sexes with a high lesion require a colostomy before repair.

Rectal Atresia
Rectal atresia is a rare defect occurring in only 1% of anorectal anomalies.

It has the same characteristics in both sexes. The unique feature of this defect is that affected patients have a normal anal canal and a normal anus. The defect is often discovered while rectal temperature is being taken. An obstruction is present approximately 2 cm above the skin level. These patients need a protective colostomy. The functional prognosis is excellent because they have a normal sphincteric mechanism (and normal sensation), which resides in the anal canal.

APPROACH TO THE PATIENT
Evaluation includes identifying associated anomalies (see Table 371.1). Careful inspection of the perineum is important to determine the presence or absence of a fistula. If the fistula can be seen there, it is a low lesion. The invertogram or upside-down x-ray is of little value, but a prone crosstable lateral plain x-ray at 24 hr of life (to allow time for bowel distention from swallowed air) with a radiopaque marker on the perineum can demonstrate a low lesion by showing the rectal gas bubble <1 cm from the perineal skin (see Fig. 371.4). A plain x-ray of the entire sacrum, including both iliac wings, is important to identify sacral anomalies and the adequacy of the sacrum. An abdominal-pelvic ultrasound and voiding cystourethrogram must be performed. The clinician should also pass a nasogastric tube to identify esophageal atresia and should obtain an echocardiogram. In males with a high lesion, the voiding cystourethrogram often identifies the rectourinary fistula. In females with a high lesion, more invasive evaluation, including vaginogram and endoscopy, is often necessary for careful detailing of the cloacal anomaly.

Good clinical evaluation and a urinalysis provide enough data in 80–90% of male patients to determine the need for a colostomy. Voluntary sphincteric muscles surround the most distal part of the bowel in cases of perineal and rectourethral fistulas, and the intraluminal bowel pressure must be sufficiently high to overcome the tone of those muscles before meconium can be seen in the urine or on the perineum. The presence of meconium in the urine and a flat bottom are considered indications for the creation of a colostomy. Clinical findings consistent with the diagnosis of a perineal fistula represent an indication for an anoplasty without a protective colostomy. Ultrasound is valuable not only for the evaluation of the urinary tract, but it can also be used to investigate spinal anomalies in the newborn and to determine how close to the perineum the rectum has descended.

More than 90% of the time, the diagnosis in females can be established on perineal inspection. The presence of a single perineal orifice is a cloaca. A palpable pelvic mass (hydrocolpos) reinforces this diagnosis. A vestibular fistula is diagnosed by careful separation of the labia, exposing the vestibule. The rectal orifice is located immediately in front of the hymen within the female genitalia and in the vestibule. A perineal fistula is easy to diagnose. The rectal orifice is located somewhere between the female genitalia and the center of the sphincter and is surrounded by skin. Less than 10% of these patients fail to pass meconium through the genitalia or perineum after 24 hr of observation. Those patients can require a prone crosstable lateral film.

OPERATIVE REPAIR
Sometimes a perineal fistula, if it opens in good position, can be treated by simple dilation. Hegar dilators are employed, starting with a No. 5 or 6 and letting the baby go home when the mother can use a No. 8. Twice-daily dilatations are done at home, increasing the size every few weeks until a No. 14 is achieved. By 1 yr of age, the stool is usually well formed and further dilation is not necessary. By the time No. 14 is reached, the examiner can usually insert a little finger. If the anal ring is soft and pliable, dilation can be reduced in frequency or discontinued.

Occasionally, there is no visible fistula, but the rectum can be seen to be filled with meconium bulging on the perineum, or a covered anus is otherwise suspected. If confirmed by plain x-ray or ultrasound of the perineum that the rectum is <1 cm from the skin, the clinician can do a minor perineal procedure to perforate the skin and then proceed with dilation or do a simple perineal anoplasty.

When the fistula orifice is very close to the introitus or scrotum, it is often appropriate to move it back surgically. This also requires postoperative dilation to prevent stricture formation. This procedure can be done any time from the newborn period to 1 yr. It is preferable to wait until dilatations have been done for several weeks and the child is bigger. The anorectum is a little easier to dissect at this time. The posterior sagittal approach of Peña is used, making an incision around the fistula and then in the midline to the site of the posterior wall of the new location. The dissection is continued in the midline, using a muscle stimulator to be sure there is adequate muscle on both sides. The fistula must be dissected cephalad for several centimeters to allow posterior positioning without tension. If appropriate, some of the distal fistula is resected before the anastomosis to the perineal skin.

In children with a high lesion, a double-barrel colostomy is performed. This effectively separates the fecal stream from the urinary tract. It also allows the performance of an augmented pressure colostogram before repair to identify the exact position of the distal rectum and the fistula. The definitive repair or posterior sagittal anorectoplasty (PSARP) is performed at about 1 yr of age. A midline incision is made, often splitting the coccyx and even the sacrum. Using a muscle stimulator, the surgeon stays strictly in the midline and divides the sphincter complex and identifies the rectum. The rectum is then opened in the midline and the fistula is identified from within the rectum. This allows a division of the fistula without injury to the urinary tract. The rectum is then dissected proximally until enough length is gained to suture it to an appropriate perineal position. The muscles of the sphincter complex are then sutured around (and especially behind) the rectum.

Other operative approaches (such as an anterior approach) are used, but the most popular procedure is by laparoscopy. This operation allows division of the fistula under direct visualization and identification of the sphincter complex by transillumination of perineum. Other imaging techniques in the management of anorectal malformations include 3D endorectal ultrasound, intraoperative MRI, and colonoscopy-assisted PSARPs, which may help perform a technically better operation. None of these other procedures or innovations has demonstrated improved outcomes.

A similar procedure can be done for female high anomalies with variations to deal with separating the vagina and rectum from within the cloacal stem. When the stem is longer than 3 cm, this is an especially difficult and complex procedure.

Usually the colostomy can be closed 6 wk or more after the PSARP. Two weeks after any anal procedure, twice-daily dilatations are performed by the family. By doing frequent dilatations, each one is not so painful and there is less tissue trauma, inflammation, and scarring.

OUTCOME

The ability to achieve rectal continence depends on both motor and sensory elements. There must be adequate muscle in the sphincter complex and proper positioning of the rectum within the complex. There must also be intact innervation of the complex and of sensory elements, as well as the presence of these sensory elements in the anorectum. Patients with low lesions are more likely to achieve true continence. They are also, however, more prone to constipation, which leads to overflow incontinence. It is very important that all these patients are followed closely, and that the constipation and anal dilation are well managed until toilet training is successful. Tables 371.2 and 371.3 outline the results of continence and constipation in relation to the malformation encountered.

Children with high lesions, especially males with rectoprostatic urethral fistulas and females with cloacal anomalies, have a poorer chance of being continent, but they can usually achieve a socially acceptable defecation (without a colostomy) pattern with a bowel management program. Often, the bowel management program consists of a daily enema to keep the colon empty and the patient clean until the next enema. If this is successful, an *antegrade continence enema* (ACE) procedure, sometimes called the Malone or Malone antegrade continence enema (MACE) procedure, can improve the patient's quality of life. These procedures provide access to the right colon either by bringing the appendix out the umbilicus in a nonrefluxing fashion or by putting a plastic button in the right lower quadrant to access the cecum. The patient can then sit on the toilet and administer the enema through the ACE, thus flushing out the entire colon. Antegrade regimens can

Table 371.2	Types of Anorectal Malformation by Sex

MALE (PERCENTAGE CHANCE OF BOWEL CONTROL*)
- Rectoperineal fistula (100%)
- Rectourethral bulbar fistula (85%)
- Imperforate anus without fistula (90%)
- Rectourethral prostatic fistula (65%)
- Rectobladder neck fistula (15%)

FEMALE (PERCENTAGE CHANCE OF BOWEL CONTROL*)
- Rectoperineal fistula (100%)
- Rectovestibular fistula (95%)
- Imperforate anus without fistula (90%)
- Rectovaginal fistula (rare anomaly)†
- Cloaca (70%)‡

*Provided patients have a normal sacrum, no tethered cord, and they receive a technically correct operation without complications.
†Rectovaginal anomalies are extremely unusual; usually their prognosis is like rectovestibular fistula.
‡Cloaca represents a spectrum; those with a common channel length <3 cm have the best functional prognosis.
From Bischoff A, Bealer J, Peña A: Controversies in anorectal malformations, *Lancet Child/Adolesc* 1:323–330, 2017 (Panel p. 323).

Table 371.3	Constipation and Type of Anogenital Malformation

TYPE	PERCENTAGE
Vestibular fistula	61
Bulbar urethral fistula	64
Rectal atresia/stenosis	50
Imperforate with no fistula	55
Perineal fistula	57
Long cloaca	35
Prostatic fistula	45
Short cloaca	40
Bladder neck fistula	16

Modified from Levitt MA, Peña A: Outcomes from the correction of anorectal malformations, *Curr Opin Pediatr* 17:394–401, 2005.

produce successful 24 hr cleanliness rates of up to 95%. Of special interest is the clinical finding that most patients improve their control with growth. Patients who wore diapers or pull-ups to primary school are often in regular underwear by high school. Some groups have taken advantage of this evidence of psychologic influences to initiate behavior modification early with good results.

Bibliography is available at Expert Consult.

371.2 Anal Fissure

Christina M. Shanti

Anal fissure is a laceration of the anal mucocutaneous junction. It is an acquired lesion of unknown etiology. While likely secondary to the forceful passage of a hard stool, it is mainly seen in infants younger than 1 yr of age when the stool is frequently quite soft. Fissures may be the consequence and not the cause of constipation.

CLINICAL MANIFESTATIONS

A history of constipation is often described, with a recent painful bowel movement corresponding to the fissure formation after passing of hard stool. The patient then voluntarily retains stool to avoid another painful bowel movement, exacerbating the constipation, resulting in harder stools. Complaints of pain on defecation and bright red blood on the surface of the stool are often elicited.

The diagnosis is established by inspection of the perineal area. The infant's hips are held in acute flexion, the buttocks are separated to expand the folds of the perianal skin, and the fissure becomes evident as a minor laceration. Often a small skin appendage is noted peripheral to the lesion. This *skin tag* represents epithelialized granulomatous tissue formed in response to chronic inflammation. Findings on rectal examination can include hard stool in the ampulla and rectal spasm.

TREATMENT

The parents must be counseled as to the origin of the laceration and the mechanism of the cycle of constipation. The goal is to ensure that the patient has soft stools to avoid overstretching the anus. The healing process can take several weeks or even several months. A single episode of impaction with passing of hard stool can exacerbate the problem. Treatment requires that the primary cause of the constipation be identified. The use of dietary and behavioral modification and a stool softener is indicated. Parents should titrate the dose of the stool softener based on the patient's response to treatment. Stool softening is best done by increasing water intake or using an oral polyethylene glycolate such as MiraLAX or GlycoLax. Surgical intervention, including stretching of the anus, "internal" anal sphincterotomy, or excision of the fissure, is not indicated or supported by scientific evidence.

Chronic anal fissures in older patients are associated with constipation, prior rectal surgery, Crohn disease, and chronic diarrhea. They are managed initially like fissures in infants, with stool softeners with the addition of sitz baths. Topical 0.2% glyceryl trinitrate reduces anal spasm and heals fissures, but it is often associated with headaches. Calcium channel blockers, such as 2% diltiazem ointment and 0.5% nifedipine cream, are more effective and cause fewer headaches than glyceryl trinitrate. Injection of botulinum toxin from 1.25 to 25 units is also effective and probably chemically replicates the action of internal sphincterotomy, which is the most effective treatment in adults, although seldom used in children.

Bibliography is available at Expert Consult.

371.3 Perianal Abscess and Fistula
Christina M. Shanti

Perianal abscesses usually manifest in infancy and are of unknown etiology. Fistula appears to be secondary to the abscess rather than a cause. Links to congenitally abnormal crypts of Morgagni have been proposed, suggesting that deeper crypts (3-10 mm rather than the normal 1-2 mm) lead to trapped debris and cryptitis (Fig. 371.5).

Conditions associated with the risk of an anal fistula include Crohn disease, tuberculosis, pilonidal disease, hidradenitis, HIV, trauma, foreign bodies, dermal cysts, sacrococcygeal teratoma, actinomycosis, lymphogranuloma venereum, and radiotherapy.

The most common organisms isolated from perianal abscesses are mixed aerobic *(Escherichia coli, Klebsiella pneumoniae, Staphylococcus aureus)* and anaerobic *(Bacteroides* spp., *Clostridium, Veillonella)* flora. A total of 10–15% yield pure growth of *E. coli, S. aureus,* or *Bacteroides fragilis.* There is a strong male predominance in those affected who are younger than 2 yr of age. This imbalance corrects in older patients, where the etiology shifts to associated conditions such as inflammatory bowel disease, leukemia, or immunocompromised states.

CLINICAL MANIFESTATIONS

In younger patients, symptoms are usually mild and can consist of low-grade fever, mild rectal pain, and an area of perianal cellulitis. Often these spontaneously drain and resolve without treatment. In older patients with underlying predisposing conditions, the clinical course may be more serious. A compromised immune system can mask fever and allow rapid progression to toxicity and sepsis. Abscesses in these patients may be deeper in the ischiorectal fossa or even supralevator

in contrast to those in younger patients, which are usually adjacent to the involved crypt.

Progression to fistula in patients with perianal abscesses occurs in up to 85% of cases and usually manifests with drainage from the perineal skin or multiple recurrences. Similar to abscess formation, fistulas have a strong male predominance. Histologic evaluation of fistula tracts typically reveals an epithelial lining of stratified squamous cells associated with chronic inflammation. It might also reveal an alternative etiology such as the granulomas of Crohn disease or even evidence of tuberculosis.

TREATMENT

Treatment is rarely indicated in infants with no predisposing disease because the condition is often self-limited. Even in cases of fistulization, conservative management (observation) is advocated because the fistula often disappears spontaneously. In one study, 87% of fistulas (in 97/112 infants) closed after a mean of 5 mo of observation and conservative management. Antibiotics are not useful in these patients. When dictated by patient discomfort, abscesses may be drained under local anesthesia. Fistulas requiring surgical intervention may be treated by fistulotomy (unroofing or opening), fistulectomy (excision of the tract leaving it open to heal secondarily), or placement of a seton (heavy suture threaded through the fistula, brought out the anus and tied tightly to itself). In patients with inflammatory bowel disease, topical tacrolimus has been effective.

Older children with predisposing diseases might also do well with minimal intervention. If there is little discomfort and no fever or other sign of systemic illness, local hygiene and antibiotics may be best. The danger of surgical intervention in an immunocompromised patient is the creation of an even larger, nonhealing wound. There certainly are such patients with serious systemic symptoms who require more aggressive intervention along with treatment of the predisposing condition. Broad-spectrum antibiotic coverage must be administered, and wide excision and drainage are mandatory in cases involving sepsis and expanding cellulitis.

Fistulas in older patients are mainly associated with Crohn disease, a history of pull-through surgery for the treatment of Hirschsprung disease, or, in rare cases, tuberculosis. Those fistulas are often resistant to therapy and require treatment of the predisposing condition.

Complications of treatment include recurrence and, rarely, incontinence.

Bibliography is available at Expert Consult.

371.4 Hemorrhoids
Christina M. Shanti

Hemorrhoidal disease occurs in both children and adolescents, often related to a diet deficient in fiber and poor hydration. In younger children,

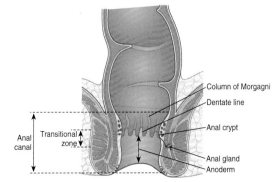

Fig. 371.5 Anatomy of the anal canal. *(Adapted from Brunicardi FC, Anderson DK, Billar TR, et al: Schwartz's principles of surgery, ed 8, New York, 2004, McGraw-Hill.)*

the presence of hemorrhoids should also raise the suspicion of portal hypertension. A third of patients with hemorrhoids require treatment.

CLINICAL MANIFESTATIONS

Presentation depends on the location of the hemorrhoids. External hemorrhoids occur below the dentate line (see Figs. 371.5 and 371.6) and are associated with extreme pain and itching, often due to acute thrombosis. Internal hemorrhoids are located above the dentate line and manifest primarily with bleeding, prolapse, and occasional incarceration.

TREATMENT

In most cases, conservative management with dietary modification, decreased straining, and avoidance of prolonged time spent sitting on the toilet results in resolution of the condition. Discomfort may be treated with topical analgesics or anti-inflammatories such as Anusol (pramoxine) and Anusol-HC (hydrocortisone) and sitz baths. The natural course of thrombosed hemorrhoid involves increasing pain, which peaks at 48-72 hr, with gradual remission as the thrombus organizes and involutes over the next 1-2 wk. In cases where the patient with external hemorrhoids presents with excruciating pain soon after the onset of symptoms, thrombectomy may be indicated. This is best accomplished with local infiltration of bupivacaine 0.25% with epinephrine 1:200,000, followed by incision of the vein or skin tag and extraction of the clot. This provides immediate relief; recurrence is rare and further follow-up is unnecessary.

Internal hemorrhoids can become painful when prolapse leads to incarceration and necrosis. Pain usually resolves with reduction of hemorrhoidal tissue. Surgical treatment is reserved for patients failing conservative management. Techniques described in adults include excision, rubber banding, stapling, and excision using the LigaSure device. Complications are rare (<5%) and include recurrence, bleeding, infection, nonhealing wounds, and fistula formation.

Bibliography is available at Expert Consult.

371.5 Rectal Mucosal Prolapse

Christina M. Shanti

Rectal mucosal prolapse is the exteriorization of the rectal mucosa through the anus. In the unusual occurrence when all the layers of the rectal wall are included, it is called *procidentia* or *rectocele*. Most cases of rectal tissue protruding through the anus are prolapse and not polyps, hemorrhoids, intussusception, or other tissue.

Most cases of prolapse are idiopathic. The onset is often between 1 and 5 yr of age. It usually occurs when the child begins standing and then resolves by approximately 3-5 yr of age when the sacrum has taken its more adult shape and the anal lumen is oriented posteriorly. Thus the entire weight of the abdominal viscera is not pushing down on the rectum, as it is earlier in development.

Other predisposing factors include intestinal parasites (particularly in endemic areas), malnutrition, diarrhea, ulcerative colitis, pertussis, Ehlers-Danlos syndrome, meningocele (more often associated with procidentia owing to the lack of perineal muscle support), cystic fibrosis, and chronic constipation. Patients treated surgically for imperforate anus can also have varying degrees of rectal mucosal prolapse. This is particularly common in patients with poor sphincteric development. Rectal prolapse is also seen with higher incidence in patients with mental issues and behavior problems. These patients are particularly difficult to manage and are more likely to fail medical treatment.

CLINICAL MANIFESTATIONS

Rectal mucosal prolapse usually occurs during defecation, especially during toilet training. Reduction of the prolapse may be spontaneous or accomplished manually by the patient or parent. In severe cases, the prolapsed mucosa becomes congested and edematous, making it more difficult to reduce. Rectal prolapse is usually painless or produces mild discomfort. If the rectum remains prolapsed after defecation, it

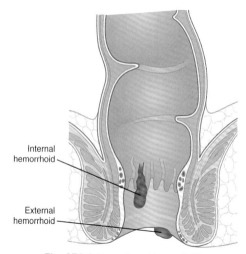

Fig. 371.6 Formation of hemorrhoids.

can be traumatized by friction with undergarments, with resultant bleeding, wetness, and potentially ulceration. The appearance of the prolapse varies from bright red to dark red and resembles a beehive. It can be as long as 10-12 cm. See Chapter 372 for a distinction from a prolapsed polyp.

TREATMENT

Initial evaluation should include tests to rule out any predisposing conditions, especially cystic fibrosis and sacral root lesions. Reduction of protrusion is aided by pressure with warm compresses. An easy method of reduction is to cover the finger with a piece of toilet paper, introduce it into the lumen of the mass, and gently push it into the patient's rectum. The finger is then immediately withdrawn. The toilet paper adheres to the mucous membrane, permitting release of the finger. The paper, when softened, is later expelled.

Conservative treatment consists of careful manual reduction of the prolapse after defecation, attempts to avoid excessive pushing during bowel movements (with patient's feet off the floor), use of laxatives and stool softeners to prevent constipation, avoidance of inflammatory conditions of the rectum, and treatment of intestinal parasitosis when present. If all this fails, surgical treatment may be indicated. Existing surgical options are associated with some morbidity, and therefore medical treatment should always be attempted first.

Sclerosing injections have been associated with complications such as neurogenic bladder. We have found linear cauterization effective and with few complications other than recurrence. In the operating room, the prolapse is recreated by traction on the mucosa. Linear burns are made through nearly the full thickness of the mucosa using electrocautery. One can usually make 8 linear burns on the outside and 4 on the inside of the prolapsed mucosa. In the immediate postoperative period, prolapse can still occur, but in the next several weeks, the burned areas contract and keep the mucosa within the anal canal. The Delorme mucosal sleeve resection addresses mucosal prolapse via a transanal approach by incising, prolapsing, and amputating the redundant mucosa. The resulting mucosal defect is then approximated with absorbable suture.

For patients with procidentia or full-thickness prolapse or intussusception of the rectosigmoid (usually from myelodysplasia or other sacral root lesions), other, more invasive options exist. Those most commonly in use by pediatric surgeons today include the following: A modification of the Thiersch procedure involves placing a subcutaneous suture to narrow the anal opening. Complications include obstruction, fecal impaction, and fistula formation. Laparoscopic rectopexy is effective and can be performed as an outpatient. The Altemeier perineal rectosigmoidectomy is a transanal, full-thickness resection of redundant bowel with a primary anastomosis to the anus.

Bibliography is available at Expert Consult.

371.6 Pilonidal Sinus and Abscess

Christina M. Shanti

The etiology of pilonidal disease remains unknown; 3 hypotheses explaining its origin have been proposed. The first states that trauma, such as can occur with prolonged sitting, impacts hair into the subcutaneous tissue, which serves as a nidus for infection. The second suggests that in some patients, hair follicles exist in the subcutaneous tissues, perhaps the result of some embryologic abnormality, and that they serve as a focal point for infection, especially with secretion of hair oils. The third speculates that motion of the buttocks disturbs a particularly deep midline crease and works bacteria and hair beneath the skin. This theory arises from the apparent improved short-term and long-term results of operations that close the wound off the midline, obliterating the deep natal cleft.

Pilonidal disease usually manifests in adolescents or young adults with significant hair over the midline sacral and coccygeal areas. It can occur as an acute abscess with a tender, warm, flocculent, erythematous swelling or as draining sinus tracts. This disease does not resolve with nonoperative treatment. An acute abscess should be drained and packed open with appropriate anesthesia. Oral broad-spectrum antibiotics covering the usual isolates (*S. aureus* and *Bacteroides* species) are prescribed, and the patient's family withdraws the packing over the course of a week. When the packing has been totally removed, the area can be kept clean by a bath or shower. The wound usually heals completely in 6 wk. Once the wound is healed, most pediatric surgeons feel that elective excision should be scheduled to avoid recurrence. There are some reports, however, this is only necessary if the disease recurs. Usually, patients who present with sinus tracts are managed with a single elective excision.

Most surgeons carefully identify the extent of each sinus tract and excise all skin and subcutaneous tissue involved to the fascia covering the sacrum and coccyx. Some close the wound in the midline; others leave it open and packed for healing by secondary intention. This method has been modified by the application of a vacuum-assisted (VAC sponge) dressing. This is a system that applies continuous suction to a porous dressing. It is usually changed every 3 days and can be done at home with the assistance of a nurse. Some marsupialize the wound by suturing the skin edges down to the exposed fascia covering the sacrum and coccyx. There appears to be improved success with excision and closure in such a way that the suture line is not in the midline. Currently there appears to be enthusiasm for the less radical methods that Bascom has introduced, treating simple sinus tracts with small local procedures and limiting excision to only diseased tissues, while still keeping the incision off the midline. Recurrence or wound-healing problems are relatively common, occurring in 9–27% of cases. The variety of treatments and procedures currently being described indicates that all are associated with significant complications and delays in return to normal activity. Still, it is rare for problems to persist beyond 1-2 yr. Recalcitrant cases are treated by a large, full-thickness gluteal flap or skin grafting.

A simple dimple located in the midline intergluteal cleft, at the level of the coccyx, is seen relatively commonly in normal infants. No evidence indicates that this little sinus provokes any problems for the patient. An open dermal sinus is an asymptomatic, benign condition that does not require operative intervention.

Bibliography is available at Expert Consult.

Chapter **372**
Tumors of the Digestive Tract

Danielle Wendel and Karen F. Murray

第三百七十二章
消化道肿瘤

中文导读

　　最常见的儿童消化道肿瘤是息肉样肿瘤，大多数小肠肿瘤可以分成两组：错构瘤或腺瘤样肿瘤。本章详细介绍了几种错构瘤，包括幼年息肉病综合征、P-J综合征、磷酸酶及张力蛋白同源的错构瘤肿瘤综合征，以及腺瘤样肿瘤中的家族性息肉病（FAP）、MYH相关性息肉病、Gardner综合征、遗传性非息肉样结肠癌等。此外还介绍了其他胃肠道肿瘤，包括淋巴瘤、淋巴组织增生、类癌、平滑肌瘤、胃肠道间质细胞瘤及血管瘤。

Tumors of the digestive tract in children are mostly polypoid. They are also commonly syndromic tumors and tumors with known genetic identification (Table 372.1). They usually manifest as painless rectal bleeding, but when large they can cause obstruction or serve as lead points for intussusception. Most intestinal tumors can be generally classified into 2 groups: hamartomatous or adenomatous.

HAMARTOMATOUS TUMORS

Hamartomas are benign tumors composed of tissues that are normally found in an organ but that are not organized normally. Juvenile, retention, or inflammatory polyps are hamartomatous polyps, which represent the most common intestinal tumors of childhood, occurring in 1–2% of children. Patients generally present in the 1st decade, most often at ages 2-5 yr, and rarely at younger than 1 yr. Polyps may be found anywhere in the gastrointestinal (GI) tract, most commonly in the rectosigmoid colon; they are often solitary but may be multiple.

Histologically, juvenile polyps are composed of hamartomatous collections of mucus-filled glandular and stromal elements with inflammatory infiltrate, covered with a thin layer of epithelium. These polyps are often bulky, vascular, and prone to bleed as their growth exceeds their blood supply with resultant mucosal ulceration, or autoamputation with bleeding from a residual central artery.

Patients often present with painless rectal bleeding after defecation.

Bleeding is generally scant and intermittent; rarely presenting findings can include iron deficiency anemia and/or hypoalbuminemia. Extensive bleeding can occur but is generally self-limited, requiring supportive care until the bleeding stops spontaneously after autoamputation. Occasionally endoscopic polypectomy is required for control of bleeding. Abdominal pain or cramps are uncommon unless associated with intussusception. Patients can present with prolapse, with a dark, edematous, pedunculated mass protruding from the rectum. Mucus discharge and pruritus are associated with prolapse.

Patients presenting with rectal bleeding require a thorough workup; differential diagnosis includes anal fissure, other intestinal polyposis syndromes, Meckel diverticulum, inflammatory bowel disease, intestinal infections, Henoch-Schönlein purpura, or coagulopathy.

Diagnosis and therapy are best accomplished via endoscopy. Polyps may be visualized via ultrasound or cross-sectional imaging, but this provides no therapeutic advantage. Colonoscopy affords opportunity for biopsy, polypectomy by snare cautery, and visualization of synchronous lesions; up to 50% of children have one or more additional polyps, and approximately 20% may have more than 5 polyps. Retrieved polyps should be sent for histologic evaluation for definitive diagnosis.

Juvenile Polyposis Syndrome

Patients with juvenile polyposis syndrome (JPS) present with multiple

Table 372.1	General Features of the Inherited Colorectal Cancer Syndromes					
SYNDROME	**POLYP DISTRIBUTION**	**AGE OF ONSET**	**RISK OF COLON CANCER**	**GENETIC LESION**	**CLINICAL MANIFESTATIONS**	**ASSOCIATED LESIONS**
HAMARTOMATOUS POLYPS						
Juvenile polyposis	Large and small intestine, gastric polyps	1st decade	~10–50%	PTEN, SMAD4, BMPR1A Autosomal dominant	Possible rectal bleeding, abdominal pain, intussusception	Congenital abnormalities in 20% of the nonfamilial type, clubbing, AV malformations
Peutz-Jeghers syndrome	Small and large intestine	1st decade	Increased	LKB1/STK11 Autosomal dominant	Possible rectal bleeding, abdominal pain, intussusception	Orocutaneous melanin pigment spots
Cowden syndrome	Colon	2nd decade	Not increased	PTEN gene	Macrocephaly, breast/thyroid/endometrial cancers, developmental delay	
Bannayan-Riley-Ruvalcaba syndrome	Colon	2nd decade	Not increased	PTEN gene	Macrocephaly, speckled penis, thyroid/breast cancers, hemangiomas, lipomas	
ADENOMATOUS POLYPS						
Familial adenomatous polyposis (FAP)	Large intestine, often >100	16 yr (range: 8-34 yr)	100%	5q (APC gene), autosomal dominant	Rectal bleeding, abdominal pain, bowel obstruction	Desmoids, CHRPE, upper GI polyps, osteoma, hepatoblastoma, thyroid cancer
Attenuated familial adenomatous polyposis (AFAP)	Colon (fewer in number)	>18 yr	Increased	APC gene	Same as FAP	Fewer associated lesions
MYH-associated polyposis	Colon	>20 yr	High risk	MYH autosomal recessive	Same as FAP	May be confused with sporadic FAP or AFAP; few extraintestinal findings
Gardner syndrome	Large and small intestine	16 yr (range: 8-34 yr)	100%	5q (APC gene)	Rectal bleeding, abdominal pain, bowel obstruction	Desmoid tumors, multiple osteomas, fibromas, epidermoid cysts
Hereditary nonpolyposis colon cancer, (Lynch syndrome)	Large intestine	40 yr	30%	DNA mismatch repair genes (MMR) Autosomal dominant	Rectal bleeding, abdominal pain, bowel obstruction	Other tumors (e.g., ovary, ureter, pancreas, stomach)

APC, adenomatous polyposis coli; AV, arteriovenous; CHRPE, congenital hypertrophy of the retinal pigment epithelium; GI, gastrointestinal; PTEN, phosphatase and tensin homolog.

juvenile polyps, ≥5 but typically 50-200. Polyps may be isolated to the colon or distributed throughout the GI tract. There is often a family history (20–50%) with an autosomal dominant pattern of variable penetrance. Alterations in transforming growth factor-β pathways have been identified in some JPS patients and families; mutations in *SMAD4* or *BMPR1A* are found in 50–60% of patients with JPS. Genetic testing is available for both of these mutations. Clinical diagnosis of JPS is established by presence of one of the following: a lifetime total of 5 or more juvenile polyps in the colon, juvenile polyps outside the colon, or any number of juvenile polyps in a patient with a family history of JPS.

Histologically, these polyps are identical to solitary juvenile polyps; however, the GI malignancy risk is greatly increased (10–50%). Most malignancy is colorectal, although gastric, upper GI, and pancreatic tumors have been described. The risk of malignancy is greater in patients with increased polyp burden and a positive family history. These patients should therefore undergo routine esophagogastroduodenoscopy, colonoscopy, and upper GI contrast studies. Serial polypectomy or polyp biopsy should be undertaken if possible. If dysplasia or malignant degeneration is found, a total colectomy is indicated.

Juvenile polyposis of infancy is characterized by early polyp formation (younger than 2 yr of age) and may be associated with protein-losing enteropathy, hypoproteinemia, anemia, failure to thrive, and intussusception. Early endoscopic or surgical intervention may be needed.

Peutz-Jeghers Syndrome

Peutz-Jeghers syndrome (PJS) is a rare autosomal dominant disorder (incidence: ~1:120,000 total population) characterized by mucocutaneous pigmentation and extensive GI hamartomatous polyposis. Macular pigmented lesions may be dark brown to dark blue and are found primarily around the lips and oral mucosa, although these lesions may also be found on the hands, feet, or perineum. Lesions can fade by puberty or adulthood.

Polyps are primarily found in the small intestine (in order of prevalence: jejunum, ileum, duodenum) but may also be colonic or gastric. Histologically, polyps are defined by normal epithelium surrounding bundles of smooth muscle arranged in a branching or frond-like pattern. Symptoms arising from GI polyps in PJS are similar to those of other polyposis syndromes—namely bleeding and abdominal cramping from obstruction or recurrent intussusception. Patients can require repeated laparotomies and intestinal resections.

The diagnosis of PJS is made clinically in patients with histologically proven hamartomatous polyps if 2 of 3 conditions are met: positive family history with an autosomal dominant inheritance pattern, mucocutaneous hyperpigmentation, and small bowel polyposis. Genetic testing can reveal mutations in *LKB1/STK11* (19p13.3), a serine-threonine kinase that acts as a tumor-suppressor gene. Up to 94% of patients with clinical characteristics of PJS have a mutation at this locus. Only 50% of patients with PJS have an affected family member, suggesting a high rate of spontaneous mutations.

Patients with PJS have increased risk of GI and extraintestinal malignancies. Lifetime cancer risk has been reported to be in the range of 47–93%. Colorectal, breast, and reproductive tumors are most common. GI surveillance should begin in childhood (by age 8 yr or when symptoms occur) with upper and lower endoscopy. The small bowel may be evaluated radiographically, with magnetic resonance enterography, endoscopically with balloon or push enteroscopy, or with video capsule endoscopy. Polyps larger than 1.5 cm should be removed, although resection does not lower the cancer risk and is mainly to avoid complications. Screening for breast, gynecologic, and testicular cancers should be routine after age 18 yr.

Phosphatase and Tensin Homolog Hamartoma Tumor Syndromes

Mutations in the tumor-suppressor gene protein tyrosine phosphatase and tensin homolog *(PTEN)* are associated with several rare autosomal dominant syndromes, including Cowden syndrome and Bannayan-Riley-Ruvalcaba syndrome. These patients present with multiple hamartomas in skin (99%), brain, breast, thyroid, endometrium, and GI tract (60%). Other extraintestinal manifestations include macro-

cephaly, developmental delay, lipomas, and genital pigmentation. Patients are at increased risk for breast and thyroid malignancies; the risk of GI cancer does not appear to be elevated.

ADENOMATOUS TUMORS
Adenomatous Polyposis Coli-Associated Polyposis Syndromes

Familial adenomatous polyposis (FAP) is the most common genetic polyposis syndrome (incidence 1:5,000 to 1:17,000 persons) and is characterized by numerous adenomatous polyps throughout the colon, as well as extraintestinal manifestations. FAP and related syndromes (attenuated FAP; Gardner and Turcot syndromes) are linked to mutations in the adenomatous polyposis coli *(APC)* gene, a tumor suppressor mapped to 5q21. *APC* regulates degradation of β-catenin, a protein with roles in regulation of the cytoskeleton, tissue architecture organization, cell migration and adherence, and numerous other functions. Intracellular accumulation of β-catenin may be responsible for colonic epithelial cell proliferation and adenoma formation. More than 400 APC mutations have been described, and up to 30% of patients present with no family history (spontaneous mutations).

Polyps generally develop late in the 1st decade of life or in adolescence (mean age of presentation is 16 yr). At the time of diagnosis, 5 or more adenomatous polyps are present in the colon and rectum. By young adulthood, the number typically increases to hundreds or even thousands. Adenomatous polyps (or adenomas) are precancerous lesions within the surface epithelium of the intestine, displaying various degrees of dysplasia. Without intervention, the risk of developing colon cancer is 100% by the 5th decade of life (average age of cancer diagnosis is 40 yr). Other GI adenomas can develop, particularly in the stomach and duodenum (50–90%). The risk of periampullary or duodenal carcinoma is significantly elevated (4–12% lifetime risk). Extraintestinal malignancies occur at an increased rate in FAP, including hepatoblastoma in young patients (1.6% before age 5 yr) and follicular or papillary thyroid cancer in teens.

Extraintestinal manifestations of FAP may be present from birth or develop in early childhood. Lesions include congenital hypertrophy of retinal pigment epithelium, desmoid tumors, epidermoid cysts, osteomas, fibromas, and lipomas. Many of these benign soft-tissue tumors appear before intestinal polyps develop. Expression of extraintestinal findings can depend on location of mutation on the *APC* gene.

Other syndromes associated with *APC* mutations include *Gardner syndrome*, classically characterized by multiple colorectal polyps, desmoid tumors, and soft-tissue tumors, including fibromas, osteomas (typically mandibular), epidermoid cysts, and lipomas. Once thought to be a distinct clinical entity, Gardner syndrome shares many characteristics with FAP. Up to 20% of FAP patients present with the classic extraintestinal manifestations once associated with Gardner syndrome. Some (but not all) cases of *Turcot syndrome* are also related to *APC*. These patients present with colorectal polyposis and primary brain tumors (medulloblastoma). Attenuated FAP is characterized by a significantly increased risk of colorectal cancer but fewer polyps than classic FAP (average: 30 polyps). The average age of cancer diagnosis in this form of FAP is 50-55 yr. Upper GI tumors and extraintestinal manifestations may be present but are less common.

The clinical presentation of FAP is variable. Polyps are generally sessile, of variable size, and initially asymptomatic. If symptoms develop, they can include rectal bleeding (possibly with secondary anemia), cramping, and diarrhea. The presence of symptoms at presentation does not correlate with malignant changes. Diagnosis should be suspected from family history, and ensuing colonoscopy is confirmatory. Histologic examination of biopsied polyps reveals adenomatous architecture (as opposed to inflammatory or hamartomatous polyps found in other polyposis syndromes) with varying degrees of dysplasia. Genetic testing for *APC* mutations is clinically available, and index patients should be tested. If a mutation is identified, affected family members should be screened and appropriate genetic counseling should be provided. If the index patient does not demonstrate a defined mutation, family members may undergo genetic testing, which might identify novel *APC* mutations. Children with identified *APC* mutations must undergo careful surveillance, with colonoscopy every 1-2 yr. Once polyps are identified, colonoscopy should be performed annually. Patients should also have upper endoscopy after development of colonic polyps to monitor for gastric and especially duodenal lesions.

Treatment of FAP requires prophylactic proctocolectomy to prevent cancer. Ileoanal pull-through procedures restore bowel continuity, with acceptable functional outcomes. Resection should be done once polyposis has become extensive (>20-30) or by the midteens. Nonsteroidal anti-inflammatory agents, such as sulindac, and cyclooxygenase-2 inhibitors, such as celecoxib, might inhibit polyp progression. No guidelines have been established, however, and their efficacy in preventing malignant transformation of existing polyps is unknown.

Carcinoma

Primary carcinomas of the small bowel or colon are extremely rare in children. Development of adenocarcinoma in adolescence or early adulthood may be associated with a genetic predisposition or syndrome such as FAP, hereditary nonpolyposis colon carcinoma, PJS, radiation exposure, or inflammatory bowel disorders such as Crohn disease or ulcerative colitis.

Colorectal carcinoma, though rare (reported incidence of 1 case per 1,000,000 persons younger than 19 yr of age), is the most common primary GI carcinoma in children. Many cases are spontaneous (i.e., not associated with a genetic predisposition or syndrome). Histologically, tumors tend to be poorly differentiated and pathologically aggressive. Patients may be asymptomatic, or they present with nonspecific signs and symptoms such as abdominal pain, constipation, and vomiting. Delay in diagnosis is common. Many patients present with advanced-stage disease, with microscopic or gross metastases at the time of diagnosis. Surgical resection is the primary treatment modality, although with delayed presentation and advanced-stage disease, complete resection may not be possible. Chemotherapy and radiation have a limited role in patients with metastatic disease.

OTHER GASTROINTESTINAL TUMORS
Lymphoma

Lymphoma is the most common GI malignancy in the pediatric population. Approximately 30% of children with non-Hodgkin lymphoma present with abdominal tumors. Immunocompromised patients have an increased incidence of lymphoma. Predisposing conditions include HIV/AIDS, agammaglobulinemia, long-standing celiac disease, and bone marrow or solid-organ transplantation. Lymphoma can occur anywhere in the GI tract, but it most commonly occurs in distal small bowel and ileocecal region. Presenting symptoms include crampy abdominal pain, vomiting, obstruction, bleeding, or palpable mass. Lymphoma should be considered in patients older than 3 yr of age who present with intussusception. Treatment consists of a combination of surgical resection and chemotherapy, depending on the extent of the tumor burden.

Nodular Lymphoid Hyperplasia

Lymphoid follicles in the lamina propria and submucosa of the gut normally aggregate in Peyer patches, most prominently in the distal ileum. These follicles can become hyperplastic, forming nodules that protrude into the lumen of the bowel during times of developmental lymphoid proliferation such as early childhood and adolescence. Some suggested etiologies are infectious (classically *Giardia*), allergic, or immunologic. Nodular lymphoid hyperplasia has been described in infants with enterocolitis secondary to dietary protein sensitivity. This phenomenon has also been described in patients with inflammatory bowel disease and Castleman disease. Patients may be asymptomatic or, especially in cases of immunodeficiency, may present with abdominal pain, rectal bleeding, diarrhea, or intussusception. Nodular lymphoid hyperplasia usually resolves spontaneously. The use of anti-inflammatory medications or elimination diets is unlikely to change the clinical course, although in cases with severe pain or bleeding, corticosteroids may be effective.

Carcinoid Tumor

Carcinoids are neuroendocrine tumors of enterochromaffin cells, which can occur throughout the GI tract, but in children they are typically found in the appendix. This is often an incidental diagnosis at the time of appendectomy. Complete resection of small tumors (<1 cm) with clear surgical margins is curative. Appendiceal tumors >2 cm mandate further bowel resection, typically a right hemicolectomy. Carcinoid tumors outside the appendix (small intestine, rectum, stomach) are more likely to metastasize. Metastatic carcinoid tumor within the liver can give rise to the carcinoid syndrome. Serotonin, 5-hydroxytryptophan, or histamine is elaborated by the tumor, and elevated serum levels cause cramps, diarrhea, vasomotor disturbances (flushing), bronchoconstriction, and right-heart failure. The diagnosis is confirmed by elevated urinary 5-hydroxyindoleacetic acid. Symptomatic relief of carcinoid symptoms may be achieved with administration of somatostatin analogs (octreotide).

Leiomyoma

Leiomyomas are rare benign tumors that can arise anywhere in the GI tract, although most often in the stomach, jejunum, or distal ileum. Age of presentation is variable, from the newborn period through adolescence. Patients may be asymptomatic or can present with an abdominal mass, obstruction, intussusception, volvulus, or pain and bleeding from central necrosis of the tumor. Surgical resection is the treatment of choice. Pathologically, these tumors may be difficult to distinguish from malignant leiomyosarcomas. Smooth muscle tumors occur with increased incidence in children with HIV or those requiring immunosuppression after transplantation.

Gastrointestinal Stromal Cell Tumors

Gastrointestinal stromal cell tumors (GISTs) are intestinal mesenchymal tumors that probably arise from interstitial cells of Cajal or their precursors. Historically, these may have been diagnosed as tumors of smooth muscle or neural cell origin. The World Health Organization recognized GIST in 1990 as a distinct neoplasm. Typically GISTs arise in adults, after the 3rd decade of life. Cases have also been reported in the pediatric population, generally in adolescents with a female predominance. In the pediatric population, tumors are most commonly found in the stomach, though they can occur anywhere in the GI tract or even the mesentery or omentum. Many patients (~45%) present with metastatic disease primarily to the lymph nodes, although metastases to the peritoneum or liver occur as well. Patients may be asymptomatic for years to decades or can present with an abdominal mass, lower GI bleeding, or obstruction. Treatment consists of surgical resection of local disease. Recurrence rates are high, and early postoperative surveillance is recommended. GISTs occurring in adults are typically associated with mutation in the *KIT* oncogene. This mutation is less commonly found in pediatric GISTs (~15%). Adjuvant therapy for *KIT*⁺ lesions is imatinib or sunitinib, tyrosine kinase inhibitors that are available as oral therapy. Patients with persistent disease or metastases might benefit from treatment.

Vascular Tumors

Vascular malformations and hemangiomas are rare in children. The usual presentation is painless rectal bleeding, which may be chronic or acute, with massive or even fatal hemorrhage. There are usually no associated symptoms, although intussusception has been described. Half of patients have associated cutaneous hemangiomas or telangiectasia. These lesions may be associated with blue rubber bleb nevus syndrome, hereditary hemorrhagic telangiectasia, as well as other syndromes. About half of these lesions are in the colon and can be identified on colonoscopy. During acute bleeding episodes, bleeding can be localized via nuclear medicine bleeding scans, mesenteric angiography, or endoscopy. Colonic bleeding may be controlled by endoscopic means. Surgical intervention is required occasionally for isolated lesions.

Bibliography is available at Expert Consult.

Chapter **373**
Inguinal Hernias
John J. Aiken
第三百七十三章
腹股沟疝

中文导读

　　本章主要介绍了腹股沟疝的胚胎学发育及发病机制，以及该病的发病率、临床表现和诊断。详细描述了急性腹股沟–阴囊肿胀、嵌顿疝及两性畸形的评估。详细介绍了腹股沟斜疝的手术指征及手术方式，如开放式及腹腔镜下腹股沟疝修补术、对侧腹股沟探查术。简要介绍了腹股沟直疝及股疝。详细介绍了常见的切口感染、复发及对输精管和男性生殖系统的损伤等并发症的处理。

Inguinal hernias are one of the most common conditions seen in pediatric practice, with an overall incidence of 0.8–4.5% in term infants and children and increasing to nearly 30% in premature and low birthweight (<1 kg) infants. The repair of congenital inguinal hernia is the most common surgical procedure performed in pediatric surgical practice. The frequency of this condition, along with its potential morbidity of ischemic injury to the intestine, testis, or ovary, makes proper diagnosis and management an important aspect of daily practice for pediatric practitioners and pediatric surgeons. Most inguinal hernias in infants and children are **congenital indirect** hernias (99%) because of a patent processus vaginalis (PV), an evagination of peritoneum in the inguinal area important in testicular descent. There is rarely any defect/deficiency in the abdominal wall musculature in congenital indirect inguinal hernia. Inguinal hernias are more common in males compared with females (8:1 ratio), but females have a higher incidence of bilateral inguinal hernias (~25%) compared with males (~12%). Two other types of inguinal hernia are seen rarely in children: **direct** (acquired) hernia (0.5–1.0%) and **femoral** hernia (<0.5%). Femoral hernias are substantially more common in females (2:1 ratio). Approximately 50% of inguinal hernias manifest clinically in the 1st yr of life, most in the first 6 mo. The incidence of incarceration in untreated hernias varies between 6% and 18% across ages. The risk of incarceration is greatest in infancy, with some reports of incarceration rates of 30–40% in the 1st yr of life, mandating prompt identification and operative repair to minimize morbidity and complications related to incarceration and strangulation. Laparoscopic hernia (LH) repair has increasingly emerged in many pediatric centers as an effective alternative to traditional open hernia (OH) repair.

EMBRYOLOGY AND PATHOGENESIS
Indirect inguinal hernias in infants and children are congenital and result from an arrest of embryologic development—failure of obliteration of the PV rather than a weakness in the abdominal wall musculature.

The pertinent developmental anatomy of indirect inguinal hernia relates to development of the gonads and descent of the testis through the inguinal canal and into the scrotum late in gestation. The testes descend from the urogenital ridge in the retroperitoneum to the area of the internal ring by about 28 wk of gestation. The final descent of the testes into the scrotum occurs late in gestation, between weeks 28 and 36, guided by the PV and the gubernaculum. The PV, an outpouching of peritoneum in the inguinal region, is present in the developing fetus at 12 wk gestation. The PV develops lateral to the deep inferior epigastric vessels and descends anteriorly along the spermatic cord within the cremasteric fascia through the internal inguinal ring. The testis accompanies the PV as it exits the abdomen and descends into the scrotum. The gubernaculum testis forms from the mesonephros (developing kidney), attaches to the lower pole of the testis, and directs the testis through the internal ring, inguinal canal and into the scrotum. The testis passes through the inguinal canal in a few days but takes about 4 wk to migrate from the external ring to its final position in the scrotum. The cordlike structures of the gubernaculum occasionally pass to ectopic locations (perineum or femoral region), resulting in ectopic testes.

In the last few weeks of gestation or shortly after birth, the layers of the PV normally fuse together and obliterate the patency from the peritoneal cavity through the inguinal canal to the testis. The PV also obliterates distally just above the testes, and the portion of the PV that envelops the testis becomes the tunica vaginalis. In females, the PV obliterates earlier, at approximately 7 mo of gestation, and may explain why females demonstrate a much lower incidence of inguinal hernia. Proper closure of the PV effectively *seals off* the opening from the abdominal cavity into the inguinal region, containing the abdominal viscera within the abdominal cavity. Failure of the PV to close permits fluid or abdominal viscera to escape the abdominal cavity into the extra-abdominal inguinal canal and accounts for a variety of inguinal–scrotal abnormalities commonly seen in infancy and childhood. Involution of the left-sided PV precedes that of the right, which is consistent with the increased incidence of indirect inguinal hernias on the right side (60%).

The ovaries descend into the pelvis from the urogenital ridge but do not exit from the abdominal cavity. The cranial portion of the gubernaculum in females differentiates into the ovarian ligament, and the inferior aspect of the gubernaculum becomes the round ligament, which passes through the internal ring and terminates in the labia majora. The PV in females is also known as the canal of Nuck.

Androgenic hormones produced by the fetal testis, adequate end-organ receptors, and mechanical factors such as increased intraabdominal pressure combine to regulate complete descent of the testis. The testes and spermatic cord structures (spermatic vessels and vas deferens) are located in the retroperitoneum but are affected by increases in intraabdominal pressure as a consequence of their intimate attachment to the descending PV. The genitofemoral nerve also has an important role: it innervates the cremaster muscle, which develops within the gubernaculum, and experimental division or injury to both nerves in the fetus prevents testicular descent. Failure of regression of smooth muscle (present to provide the force for testicular descent) has also been postulated to play a role in the development of indirect inguinal hernias. Several studies have investigated genes involved in the control of testicular descent for their role in closure of the patent PV—for example, hepatocyte growth factor and calcitonin gene-related peptide. Unlike in adult hernias, there does not appear to be any deficiency in collagen synthesis associated with inguinal hernia in children (Fig. 373.1).

A **direct inguinal hernia** results from a weakness in the abdominal wall musculature in the inguinal region, specifically the transverse abdominis muscle, which forms the floor of the inguinal canal. A direct inguinal hernia originates **medial** to the deep inferior epigastric vessels and is external to the cremasteric fascia; the hernia sac protrudes directly through the posterior wall of the inguinal canal and does not protrude through the external ring. A **femoral hernia** originates medial to the femoral vein and descends inferior to the inguinal ligament along the femoral canal.

Incidence

The incidence of congenital indirect inguinal hernia in full-term newborn infants is estimated at 3.5–5.0%. The incidence of hernia in preterm and low birthweight infants is considerably higher, ranging from 9% to 11%, and approaches 30% in very-low birthweight infants (<1,000 g) and preterm infants (<28 wk of gestation). Inguinal hernia is much more common in males than females, with a male-to-female ratio of approximately 8:1. Approximately 60% of inguinal hernias occur on the right side, 30% are on the left side, and 10% are bilateral. The incidence of bilateral hernias is higher in females (20–40%) and young children (<2 yr). An increased incidence of congenital inguinal hernia has been documented in twins and in family members of patients with inguinal hernia. There is a history of another inguinal hernia in the family in 11.5% of patients. The sisters of affected females are at the highest risk, with a relative risk of 17.8. In general, the risk of brothers of a sibling is approximately 4-5, as is the risk of a sister of an affected brother. Both a multifactorial threshold model and autosomal dominance with incomplete penetrance and sex influence have been suggested as an explanation for this pattern of inheritance.

Inguinal hernia, scrotal hydrocele (communicating and noncommunicating), and hydrocele of the spermatic cord are conditions resulting from varying degrees of failure of closure of the PV. Closure of the PV is often incomplete at birth and continues postnatally; the rate of patency is inversely proportional to the age of the child. It has been estimated that the patency rate of the PV is as high as 80% at birth and decreases to ≈40% during the 1st yr of life, and that ≈20% of males have a persistent patency of the PV at 2 yr of age. Patency of the PV after birth is an opening from the abdominal cavity into the inguinal region and therefore a potential hernia, but not all patients will develop a clinical hernia. An inguinal hernia occurs clinically when intraabdominal contents escape the abdominal cavity and enter the inguinal region through the PV patency. Depending on the extent of patency of the PV, the hernia may be confined to the inguinal region or pass down into the scrotum. Complete failure of obliteration of the PV, mostly seen in infants, predisposes to a complete inguinal hernia characterized by a protrusion of abdominal contents into the inguinal canal and extending into the scrotum. Obliteration of the PV distally (around the testis) with patency proximally results in the classic indirect inguinal hernia with a bulge in the inguinal canal.

A **hydrocele** occurs when only fluid enters the patent PV; the swelling may exist only in the scrotum (scrotal hydrocele), only along the spermatic cord in the inguinal region (hydrocele of the spermatic cord), or extend from the scrotum through the inguinal canal and even into the abdomen (abdominal–scrotal hydrocele). A hydrocele is termed a **communicating hydrocele** if it demonstrates fluctuation in size, often increasing in size after activity and, at other times, being smaller when the fluid decompresses into the peritoneal cavity often after laying recumbent. Occasionally, hydroceles develop in older children following trauma, inflammation, torsion of the appendix testes, or in association with tumors affecting the testis.

Although reasons for failure of closure of the PV are unknown, it is more common in cases of testicular nondescent (cryptorchidism) and prematurity. In addition, persistent patency of the PV is twice as common on the right side, presumably related to later descent of the right testis and interference with obliteration of the PV from the developing inferior vena cava and external iliac vein. Table 373.1 lists the risk factors identified as contributing to failure of closure of the PV and to the development of clinical inguinal hernia. The incidence of inguinal hernia in patients with cystic fibrosis is approximately 15%, believed to be related to an altered embryogenesis of the wolffian duct structures, which leads to an absent vas deferens and infertility in males with this condition. There

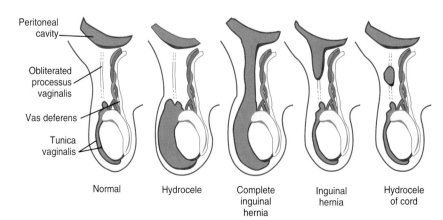

Peritoneal cavity

Obliterated processus vaginalis

Vas deferens

Tunica vaginalis

Normal   Hydrocele   Complete inguinal hernia   Inguinal hernia   Hydrocele of cord

Fig. 373.1 Hernia and hydroceles. *(Modified from Scherer LR III, Grosfeld JL: Inguinal and umbilical anomalies, Pediatr Clin North Am 40: 1121–1131, 1993.)*

Table 373.1	Predisposing Factors for Hernias

- Prematurity
- Urogenital
  - Cryptorchidism
  - Exstrophy of the bladder or cloaca
  - Ambiguous genitalia
  - Hypospadias/epispadias
- Increased peritoneal fluid
  - Ascites
  - Ventriculoperitoneal shunt
  - Peritoneal dialysis catheter
- Increased intraabdominal pressure
  - Repair of abdominal wall defects
  - Severe ascites (chylous)
  - Meconium peritonitis
- Chronic respiratory disease
  - Cystic fibrosis
- Connective tissue disorders
  - Ehlers-Danlos syndrome
  - Hunter-Hurler syndrome
  - Marfan syndrome
  - Mucopolysaccharidosis

is also an increased incidence of inguinal hernia in patients with **testicular feminization syndrome** and other disorders of sexual development. The rate of recurrence after repair of an inguinal hernia in patients with a connective tissue disorder approaches 50%, and often the diagnosis of connective tissue disorders in children results from investigation following development of a recurrent inguinal hernia.

Clinical Presentation and Diagnosis

An inguinal hernia typically appears as an intermittent, asymptomatic bulge or mass in the inguinal region or scrotum, most often noted on routine physical examination or by a parent; after bathing or urination are classic presentations. In females, the mass typically occurs in the upper portion of the labia majora. The bulge or mass is most visible at times of irritability or increased intraabdominal pressure (crying, straining, coughing). Most inguinal hernias present clinically in young children, approximately 50% in the 1st yr, and most are asymptomatic or minimally symptomatic. The classic history from the parents is of intermittent groin, labial, or scrotal swelling that spontaneously reduces but that is gradually enlarging or is more persistent and is becoming more difficult to reduce. The **hallmark signs** of an inguinal hernia on physical examination are a smooth, firm mass that emerges through the external inguinal ring lateral to the pubic tubercle and enlarges with increased intraabdominal pressure. When the child relaxes, the hernia typically reduces spontaneously or can be reduced by gentle pressure, 1st posteriorly to free it from the external ring and then upward toward the peritoneal cavity. In males, the hernia sac contains intestines; female infants often have an ovary and fallopian tube in the hernia sac.

The diagnosis of inguinal hernia is clinical and generally is made by history and physical examination. Methods used to demonstrate the hernia on examination vary depending on the age of the child. A quiet infant can be made to strain the abdominal muscles by stretching the infant out supine on the bed with legs extended and arms held straight above the head. Most infants struggle to get free, thus increasing the intraabdominal pressure and pushing out the hernia. Older children can be asked to perform the Valsalva maneuver by blowing up a balloon or coughing. The older child should be examined while standing, and examination after voiding also can be helpful. With increased intraabdominal pressure, the protruding mass is obvious on inspection of the inguinal region or can be palpated by an examining finger invaginating the scrotum to palpate at the external ring. Another subtle and less definitive test is the *silk glove sign,* which describes the feeling of the layers of the hernia sac as they slide over the spermatic cord structures with rolling of the spermatic cord beneath the index finger at the pubic tubercle. In the absence of a bulge, the finding of increased thickness of the inguinal canal structures on palpation also suggests the diagnosis of an inguinal hernia. It is important on examination to note

the position of the testes because retractile testes are common in infants and young males and can mimic an inguinal hernia with a bulge in the region of the external ring. Because in the female patient approximately 20–25% of inguinal hernias are **sliding** hernias (the contents of the hernia sac are adherent within the sac and therefore not reducible), a fallopian tube or ovary can be palpated in the inguinal canal as a firm, slightly mobile, nontender mass in the labia or inguinal canal. A **femoral** hernia appears as a protrusion on the medial aspect of the thigh, below the inguinal region, and does not enter the scrotum or labia.

Because most young child hernias reduce spontaneously, the physical examination in the office can be equivocal. Infants and children with a strong history suggestive of inguinal hernia and an equivocal clinical examination may be offered ultrasound or referral to a pediatric surgeon. Diagnostic laparoscopy has been increasingly used to evaluate for suspected inguinal hernia; particularly in infants where the risk of incarceration and potential injury to the intestines or testis is high. In an older child with low risk of incarceration, the parents can be reassured and educated relative to the low risk of incarceration and morbidity. If an inguinal hernia is present, it will predictably become increasingly observed. A plan for a period of observation is thoughtful and safe, and the parents can be asked to take a digital image at home if the bulge is noted.

EVALUATION OF ACUTE INGUINAL–SCROTAL SWELLING

Commonly in pediatric practice, an inguinal–scrotal mass appears suddenly in an infant or child and is associated with pain/discomfort. The differential diagnosis includes incarcerated inguinal hernia, acute hydrocele, torsion of an undescended testis, infection (epididymitis/orchitis), and suppurative inguinal lymphadenitis. Differentiating between the incarcerated inguinal hernia and the acute hydrocele is probably the most difficult. The infant or child with an incarcerated inguinal hernia is likely to have associated findings suggesting intestinal obstruction, such as colicky abdominal pain, abdominal distention, vomiting, and cessation of stool, and may appear ill. Plain radiographs, if obtained, typically demonstrate distended intestines with multiple air–fluid levels. The infant with an acute hydrocele may have discomfort but is consolable and tolerates feedings without signs or symptoms suggesting intestinal obstruction.

On examination of the child with the acute scrotal hydrocele, the clinician may note that the mass is somewhat mobile. In addition, the inguinal region is flat and the mass confined to the scrotum. With the incarcerated hernia, there is a lack of mobility of the groin mass and marked swelling or mass extending from the scrotal mass through the inguinal area and up to and including the internal ring. An experienced clinician can selectively use a bimanual examination to help differentiate groin abnormalities. The examiner palpates the internal ring per rectum, with the other hand placing gentle pressure on the inguinal region over the internal ring. In cases of an indirect inguinal hernia, intraabdominal viscera can be palpated extending through the internal ring.

Another method used in diagnostic evaluation is **transillumination** to ascertain if the mass contains only fluid (hydrocele) versus intestine (hernia); however, it must be noted that transillumination can be misleading because the thin wall of the infant's intestine can approximate that of the hydrocele wall and both may transilluminate. This is also the reason aspiration to assess the contents of a groin mass is discouraged. **Ultrasonography** can help distinguish between a hernia, a hydrocele, and lymphadenopathy, and is a simple and well-tolerated test. An expeditious diagnosis is important to avoid the potential complications of an incarcerated hernia, which can develop rapidly. Diagnostic laparoscopy is an effective and reliable tool in this setting by pediatric surgeons but requires general anesthesia.

The occurrence of suppurative adenopathy in the inguinal region can be confused with an incarcerated inguinal hernia. Examination of the watershed area of the inguinal lymph nodes might reveal a superficial infected or crusted skin lesion. In addition, the swelling associated with inguinal lymphadenopathy is typically located more inferior and lateral than the mass of an inguinal hernia, and there may be other associated enlarged nodes in the area. Torsion of an undescended testis can manifest as a painful erythematous mass in the groin. The absence of a gonad in the scrotum on the ipsilateral side should clinch this diagnosis. Infectious etiologies typically demonstrate swelling and tenderness of the testis, but often there is associated urinary symptoms and the swelling is confined to the scrotum and does not extend into the inguinal canal.

Incarcerated Hernia

Incarceration is a common consequence of untreated inguinal hernia in infants and presents as a *nonreducible* mass in the inguinal canal, scrotum, or labia. Contained structures can include small bowel, appendix, omentum, colon, bladder, or, rarely, Meckel diverticulum. In females, the ovary, fallopian tube, or both are commonly incarcerated. Rarely, the uterus in infants can also be pulled into the hernia sac. A **strangulated hernia** is one that is tightly constricted in its passage through the inguinal canal, and as a result, the hernia contents have become ischemic or gangrenous. The incidence of incarceration of an inguinal hernia is between 6% and 18% throughout childhood years, and two thirds of incarcerated hernias occur in the 1st yr of life. The greatest risk is in infants younger than 6 mo of age, with reported incidences of incarceration between 25% and 30%. Reports vary, but many believe a history of prematurity imparts an increased risk of incarceration in the 1st yr of life.

Although incarceration may be tolerated in adults for years, most nonreducible inguinal hernias in children, unless treated, rapidly progress to *strangulation* with potential infarction of the hernia contents or intestinal obstruction. Initially, pressure on the herniated viscera leads to impaired lymphatic and venous drainage. This leads to swelling of the herniated viscera, which further increases the compression in the inguinal canal, ultimately resulting in total occlusion of the arterial supply to the trapped viscera. Progressive ischemic changes take place, culminating in gangrene and/or perforation of the herniated viscera. The testis is at risk of ischemia because of compression of the testicular blood vessels by the strangulated hernia. In females, herniation/incarceration of the ovary places it at risk of torsion with resultant ischemia.

The symptoms of an incarcerated hernia are irritability, feeding intolerance, and abdominal distention in the infant; pain presents in the older child. Within a few hours, the infant becomes inconsolable; lack of flatus or stool signals complete intestinal obstruction. A somewhat tense, nonfluctuant mass is present in the inguinal region and can extend down into the scrotum or labia. The mass is well defined, firm, and does not reduce. With the onset of ischemic changes, the pain intensifies, and the vomiting becomes bilious or feculent. Blood may be noted in the stools. The mass is typically markedly tender, and there is often edema and erythema of the overlying skin. The testes may be normal, demonstrate a reactive hydrocele, or may be swollen and hard on the affected side because of venous congestion resulting from compression of the spermatic veins and lymphatic channels at the inguinal ring by the tightly strangulated hernia mass. Abdominal radiographs demonstrate features of partial or complete intestinal obstruction, and gas within the incarcerated bowel segments may be seen below the inguinal ligament or within the scrotum.

Ambiguous Genitalia

Infants with disorders of sexual development commonly present with inguinal hernias, often containing a gonad, and require special consideration. In female infants with inguinal hernias, particularly if the presentation is bilateral inguinal masses, **testicular feminization syndrome** should be suspected (>50% of patients with testicular feminization have an inguinal hernia; see Chapter 606). Conversely, the true incidence of testicular feminization in all female infants with inguinal hernias is difficult to determine but is approximately 1%. In phenotypic females, if the diagnosis of testicular feminization is suspected preoperatively, the child should be screened with a buccal smear for Barr bodies and appropriate genetic evaluation before proceeding with the hernia repair. The diagnosis of testicular feminization is occasionally made at the time of operation by identifying an abnormal gonad (testis) within the hernia sac or absence of the uterus on laparoscopy or rectal exam. In the normal female infant, the uterus is easily palpated as a distinct midline structure beneath the symphysis pubis on rectal examination. Preoperative diagnosis of testicular feminization syndrome or other disorders of sexual development such as mixed gonadal dysgenesis and selected pseudohermaphrodites enables the family to receive genetic counseling, and gonadectomy can be accomplished at the time of the hernia repair if indicated.

Indications for Surgery

The presence of an inguinal hernia in the pediatric age group constitutes the indication for operative repair. An inguinal hernia does not resolve spontaneously, and prompt repair eliminates the risk of incarceration and the associated potential complications, particularly in the 1st 6-12 mo of life. The timing of operative repair depends on several factors, including age, general condition of the patient, and comorbid conditions. In full-term, healthy infants (younger than 1 yr) with an inguinal hernia, repair should proceed promptly (within 2-3 wk) following diagnosis because as many as 70% of incarcerated inguinal hernias requiring emergency operation occur in infants younger than 11 mo. In addition, the incidence of complications associated with elective hernia repair (intestinal injury, testicular atrophy, recurrent hernia, wound infection) are low (≈1%), but rise to as high as 18–20% when repair is performed emergently at the time of incarceration. The incidence of testicular atrophy after incarceration in infants younger than 3 mo of age has been reported as high as 30%. Therefore, an approach emphasizing prompt elective repair in infants is warranted; anesthetic risks must be considered when determining timing of elective surgery for inguinal hernia repair. The risk factors for apnea following general anesthesia include prematurity, multiple congenital anomalies, history of apnea and bradycardia, chronic lung disease, postconceptual age <60 wk at the time of surgery, and anemia. Unfortunately, while this group of patients would be ideal for inguinal hernia repair under regional (spinal/caudal) anesthesia, inguinal hernia repair in this group is often remarkably technically challenging even for experienced pediatric surgeons, and success is elusive under regional techniques. The outcome advantage of a regional technique is lost if additional intravenous sedation is required. Full-term infants <3 mo of age and preterm infants <60 wk postconceptual age should be observed following repair for a minimum of 12 hr postoperatively and potentially overnight following general anesthesia for the development of apnea and bradycardia.

In children older than 1 yr, the risk of incarceration is less, and the repair can be scheduled with less urgency. For the routine reducible hernia, the operation should be carried out electively shortly after diagnosis. Elective inguinal hernia repair in healthy children can be safely performed in an outpatient setting with an expectation for full recovery within 48 hr. A regional caudal block or local inguinal nerve block using local anesthetic is useful to diminish perioperative pain and optimize recovery. Prophylactic antibiotics are not routinely used except for associated conditions, such as congenital heart disease or the presence of a ventriculoperitoneal shunt. *The operation should be performed at a facility with the ability to admit the patient to an inpatient unit as needed should concerns or complications arise.*

There is controversy as to the optimal timing of inguinal herniorrhaphy in preterm and low-birth-weight infants. In the past 2 decades, most pediatric surgeons have planned hernia repair shortly before discharge from the neonatal intensive care unit. This group has a high rate of incarceration, but also a high risk of anesthesia related postoperative complications with elective surgery, such as apnea, bradycardia, inability to extubate, hemodynamic instability (5–10%), and even cardiopulmonary arrest. In addition, this group also has an increased rate of postoperative surgical-related complications such as wound infection (5–10%) and recurrent hernia (10%). At present, studies to develop evidence-based data for timing of inguinal hernia repair in premature infants are ongoing, but there is a lack of consensus and patients should be individualized, with important consultation with both neonatology and pediatric anesthesia. The operation for inguinal hernia repair is most often performed under general anesthesia, but it can be performed under spinal/caudal anesthesia in selected high-risk infants in whom avoidance of intubation is preferable (e.g., because of chronic lung disease or bronchopulmonary dysplasia). In this setting, open repair (OH) is preferable to the laparoscopic approach, as it can be performed under local/regional techniques.

An incarcerated, irreducible hernia without evidence of strangulation in a clinically stable patient should initially be managed nonoperatively, unless there is evidence of bowel obstruction, peritonitis, or hemodynamic instability, because 70–95% of incarcerated inguinal hernias are successfully reduced. Manual reduction is performed using a surgical technique called taxis, first with traction caudad and posteriorly to free the mass from the external inguinal ring, and then upward to reduce the contents back into the peritoneal cavity. Reduction attempts usually require sedation (intravenous) and analgesics, and thus appropriate experience with monitoring and airway management are critical concerns. In addition, if reduction of the incarcerated hernia is successful, the infant may rapidly become somnolent and apneic, requiring important supportive measures by skilled personnel. Other techniques advocated to assist in the nonoperative reduction of an incarcerated inguinal hernia include elevation of the lower torso and legs. Ice packs should be avoided in infants because of the risk of hypothermia but may be used for brief periods in the older child. If reduction is successful but difficult, the patient should be observed (several hours) to ensure that feedings are tolerated and there is no concern that necrotic intestine was reduced; fortunately, this is an uncommon occurrence. Given the risk of early recurrent incarceration after a successful reduction, it is recommended that herniorrhaphy be performed following a brief period (1-4 days), by which time there is less edema, handling of the sac is easier, and the risk of complications is reduced.

If the inguinal hernia is unable to be reduced, or there is concern for an incomplete reduction, then operative reduction should be performed emergently. In addition, for any patient who presents with a prolonged history of incarceration of an inguinal hernia, signs of peritoneal irritation, or small bowel obstruction, surgery and operative reduction and repair of the hernia should be urgently performed. Initial management includes nasogastric intubation, intravenous fluids, and administration of broad-spectrum antibiotics. When fluid and electrolyte imbalance has been corrected and the child's condition is satisfactory, exploration is undertaken. In current practice, the laparoscopic approach may have advantages, as the abdominal cavity insufflation expands the internal ring, potentially aiding reduction of the incarcerated viscera as well as enabling visualization of the viscera for possible ischemic injury and/or perforation. The risk of postoperative complications such as testicular atrophy, bowel ischemia, wound infections, and recurrence of hernia is increased following emergency inguinal hernia repair, 4.5–33% compared with 1% in elective hernia repairs in healthy, full-term infants.

A common presentation in female patients is an irreducible ovary in the inguinal hernia in an otherwise asymptomatic patient. The inguinal mass is soft and nontender to gentle exam, and there is no swelling or edema; thus there are no findings suggesting strangulation. This represents a *sliding* hernia with the fallopian tube and ovary fused to the wall of the hernia sac preventing reduction to the abdominal cavity. Overzealous attempts to reduce the hernia are unwarranted and potentially harmful to the tube and ovary. The risk that incarceration, most often resulting from torsion of the ovary in this setting, will lead to strangulation is not known. Most pediatric surgeons recommend elective repair of the hernia within 24-48 hr.

The appearance of necrotic ovaries and testes at the time of operation does not consistently evidence irreversible damage or predict future functionality. Multiple studies report that even when ovaries appear persistently ischemic after relief of incarceration and detorsion, most ovaries, if preserved, will recover and demonstrate evidence of follicular development. Similarly, ischemic appearing testes following relief of incarceration survive in as much as 50% of cases. Testicular atrophy occurs in 2.5–15% of incarcerated hernias. Given the potential for retained functionality, the current recommendation is to avoid testicular resection unless there is frank necrosis present.

Open Inguinal Hernia Repair

The open technique for elective inguinal hernia repair in infants and children has been the standard of care since its introduction more than 50 yr ago. The operation is performed through a small (2-3 cm) inguinal skin crease incision. The procedure involves the opening of the inguinal canal, reduction of the contents of the hernia sac if present, careful separation of the hernia sac from the cremasteric muscle fibers, spermatic cord vessels, and vas deferens to avoid injury to these structures in the inguinal canal, division of the hernia sac, and high ligation of the hernia sac at the internal ring, thus preventing protrusion of abdominal contents into the inguinal canal. A communicating hydrocele is approached with the same technique, separation of the spermatic cord structures from the hernia sac, high ligation of the proximal portion of the hernia sac, and opening of the distal sac to relieve the hydrocele. In older children with a noncommunicating hydrocele, the approach may be through a scrotal incision with avoidance of manipulation of the spermatic cord vessels and vas deferens. Open inguinal hernia repair has a low rate of recurrence, vas deferens injury, and testicular atrophy (~1–2%).

In females, surgical repair is technically simpler because the hernia sac and round ligament can be ligated without concern for injury to the ovary and its blood supply, which generally remain within the abdomen. The hernia sac and round ligament are divided from their distal attachment in the labia majora, proximal dissection away from the cremasteric muscle fibers to the internal ring, and high ligation at the internal ring. In female infants, opening of the sac to visualize the ovary and fallopian tube may help avoid injury to these structures during suture ligation of the sac and also rule out testicular feminization syndrome. If the ovary and fallopian tube are within the sac and not reducible, the sac is suture ligated distal to these structures, and the internal ring is closed after reducing the sac and its contents to the abdominal cavity.

Laparoscopic Inguinal Hernia Repair

Although the classic open inguinal hernia repair is most commonly performed, laparoscopic repair (LH) is used by most pediatric surgeons. There are several techniques described, both transperitoneal and preperitoneal, depending on surgeon preference. Like the open technique, the laparoscopic technique is fundamentally a high ligation of the indirect inguinal hernia sac (PV) at the internal ring to prevent protrusion of abdominal viscera into the inguinal canal. The laparoscopic technique affords confirmation of the diagnosis, as well as inspection of the contralateral side for the presence of a hernia or a patent PV (potential hernia). Reported advantages of laparoscopic repair (LR) compared with open repair (OH) include better cosmesis, shorter length of stay (LOS), faster recovery, and greater ability to visualize and repair a contralateral hernia.

In LH, the inguinal canal is not explored, and the spermatic cord structures are not manipulated, which may portend reduced risk to the testicular blood supply or vas deferens, particularly in younger patients. Disadvantages of LH in infants and younger children are the increased risk associated with general anesthesia, the potential hemodynamic effects of abdominal insufflation (acidosis), and technical challenges of the LH technique. Operative times have been similar for the OH and LH approaches; however, there is wide variability with the LH technique based on the experience of the surgeon and surgical team. Laparoscopic procedures in infants should always be performed expeditiously and with low insufflations pressure to avoid the risk of cardiorespiratory compromise and development of acidosis. Postoperative pain in both techniques is managed with oral acetaminophen for 24-48 hr; older children may require a brief period of postoperative narcotics. In a prospective, randomized study, the laparoscopic approach was associated with decreased pain, parental perception of faster recovery, and parental perception of better wound cosmesis. At present, outcomes, recurrence rates, recovery metrics, complications, and family satisfaction appears similar for both approaches (OH and LH), and evidence is lacking to recommend one approach over the other.

Contralateral Inguinal Exploration

Most children (85%) present with a unilateral inguinal hernia. Controversy exists regarding when to proceed with contralateral groin exploration. The only purpose of contralateral exploration is to avoid the occurrence of a hernia on that side at a later date. The advantages of contralateral exploration include avoidance of parental anxiety and possibly a 2nd anesthesia, the cost of additional surgery, and the risk of contralateral incarceration. The disadvantages of exploration include potential injury to the spermatic cord vessels, vas deferens, and testis; increased operative and anesthesia time; and the fact that, in many infants, it is an unnecessary procedure.

With the introduction of minimally invasive techniques and laparoscopy, much of the debate over contralateral inguinal exploration has been resolved, as laparoscopy enables assessment of the contralateral side without risk of injury to the spermatic cord structures or testis. When performing OH repair, the laparoscope can be introduced through an umbilical incision or by passing a 30-degree or 70-degree oblique scope through the OH sac prior to ligation of the hernia sac on the involved side. If patency of the contralateral side is demonstrated, the surgeon can proceed with bilateral hernia repair, and if the contralateral side is properly obliterated, exploration and potential complications are avoided. When performing LH, visualization of the contralateral side is easily performed. The downside of this approach includes the risks associated with laparoscopy, and that laparoscopy cannot differentiate between a patent PV and a true hernia (Figs. 373.2 and 373.3). Infants and children with risk factors for development of an inguinal hernia or with medical conditions that increase the risk of general anesthesia should be approached with a low threshold for routine contralateral exploration.

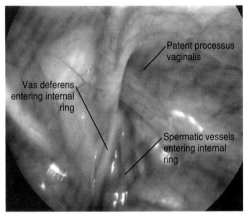

Fig. 373.2 Image on laparoscopy of patent processus vaginalis on right side.

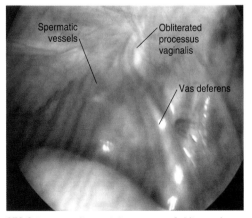

Fig. 373.3 Image on diagnostic laparoscopy of obliterated processus vaginalis on left side.

DIRECT INGUINAL HERNIA

Direct inguinal hernias are rare in children, approximately 0.5–1%. Direct hernias appear as groin masses that extend toward the femoral vessels with exertion or straining. The etiology is from a muscular defect or weakness in the floor of the inguinal canal *medial* to the epigastric vessels. Thus direct inguinal hernias in children are generally considered an acquired problem. In one third of cases, the patient has a history of a prior indirect hernia repair on the side of the direct hernia, which suggests a possible missed direct hernia at the initial surgery, or injury to the floor muscles of the inguinal canal at the time of the 1st herniorrhaphy. Patients with **connective tissue disorders** such as Ehlers-Danlos syndrome or Marfan syndrome and mucopolysaccharidosis such as Hunter-Hurler syndrome are at increased risk for the development of direct inguinal hernias either independently or after indirect inguinal hernia repair.

Operative repair of a direct inguinal hernia involves strengthening of the floor of the inguinal canal, and many standard techniques have been described, similar to repair techniques used in adults. The repair can be performed through a single limited incision, and therefore LR does not offer significant advantage. Recurrence after repair, in contrast to that in adults, is extraordinarily rare. Because typically the area of muscular weakness is small and pediatric tissues have greater elasticity, primary repair is usually possible. Prosthetic material (mesh) for direct hernia repair or other approaches, such as preperitoneal repair, are rarely required in the pediatric age group. The older child with a direct inguinal hernia and a connective tissue disorder may be the exception, and a laparoscopic approach and prosthetic material in such a case can be useful for repair.

FEMORAL HERNIA

Femoral hernias are rare in children (<1% of groin hernias in children). They are more common in females than males, (2 : 1 ratio). They are extremely rare in infancy and occur typically in older children, believed to most often be an acquired defect. Femoral hernias represent a protrusion through the femoral canal. The bulge of a femoral hernia is located below the inguinal ligament and typically projects on the medial aspect of the proximal thigh. Femoral hernias are more often missed clinically than direct hernias on physical examination or at the time of indirect hernia repair. Repair of a femoral hernia involves closure of the defect at the femoral canal, generally suturing the inguinal ligament to the pectineal ligament/fascia.

COMPLICATIONS

Complications after elective inguinal hernia repair are uncommon (≈1.5%) but significantly higher in association with incarceration (≈10%). The major risk of elective inguinal hernia repair in infants and children relates to the need for general anesthesia, and spinal/caudal anesthesia should be considered based on the experience of the surgeon and anesthesia team. Surgical complications can be related to technical factors (recurrence, iatrogenic cryptorchidism or *trapped testicle*, inadvertent injury to the vas deferens or spermatic vessels), or to the underlying process, such as bowel ischemia, gonadal infarction, and testicular atrophy following incarceration. The most critical surgical complication of inguinal hernia repair involves injury to the testicular vessels, vas deferens, testicular atrophy, or iatrogenic cryptorchidism (trapped testicle). Since LH repair generally does not involve inguinal exploration or manipulation of the testicular vessels or vas deferens, the risk of injury is potentially lower, but supportive data are unavailable at present.

Wound Infection

Wound infection occurs in <1% of elective inguinal hernia repairs in infants and children, but the incidence increases to 5–7% in association with incarceration and emergent repair. The patient typically develops fever and irritability 3-5 days after the surgery, and the wound demonstrates warmth, erythema, and fluctuance. Management consists of opening and draining the wound, a short course of antibiotics, and a daily wound dressing. The most common organisms are Gram-positive (*Staphylococcus* and *Streptococcus* spp.), and consideration should be given to coverage of methicillin-resistant *Staphylococcus aureus.* The wound generally heals in 1-2 wk with low morbidity and a good cosmetic result.

Recurrent Hernia

The recurrence rate of inguinal hernias after elective inguinal hernia repairs is generally reported as 0.5–1.0%, with rates as high as 2% for premature infants. The rate of recurrence after emergency repair of an incarcerated hernia is much higher, reported as 3–6% in most large series. The true incidence of recurrence is most certainly even higher, given the problem of accurate long-term follow-up. In the group of patients who develop recurrent inguinal hernia, the recurrence occurs in 50% within 1 yr of the initial repair and in 75% by 2 yr. Recurrence of an indirect hernia may be the result of a technical problem in the original procedure, such as failure to identify the sac properly, failure to perform high ligation of the sac at the level of the internal ring, or a tear in the sac that leaves a strip of peritoneum along the cord structures. Recurrence as a direct hernia can result from injury to the inguinal floor (transversalis fascia) during the original procedure or, more likely, failure to identify a direct hernia during the original exploration. Patients with *connective tissue disorders* (collagen deficiency) or conditions that cause *increased intraabdominal pressure* (ventriculoperitoneal shunts, ascites, chronic lung disease, peritoneal dialysis) are at increased risk for recurrence.

Iatrogenic Cryptorchidism (Trapped Testicle)

Iatrogenic cryptorchidism describes malposition of the testis after inguinal hernia repair. This complication is usually related to disruption of the testicular attachment in the scrotum at the time of hernia repair or failure to recognize an undescended testis during the original procedure, allowing the testes to retract, typically to the region of the external ring. At the completion of inguinal hernia repair, the testis should be placed in a dependent intrascrotal position. If the testis will not remain in this position, proper fixation in the scrotum should be performed at the time of the hernia repair.

Incarceration

Incarceration of an inguinal hernia can result in injury to the intestines, the fallopian tube and ovary, or the ipsilateral testis. The incidence of incarceration of a congenital indirect inguinal hernia is reported as 6–18% throughout childhood and as high as 30% for infants younger than 6 mo of age. Intestinal injury requiring bowel resection is uncommon, occurring in only 1–2% of incarcerated hernias. In cases of incarceration in which the hernia is reduced nonoperatively, the likelihood of intestinal injury is low; however, these patients should be observed closely for 6-12 hr following reduction of the hernia persistent for signs and symptoms of intestinal obstruction, such as fever, vomiting, abdominal distention, or bloody stools. Laparoscopy affords the opportunity to inspect the reduced viscera for injury or necrosis in select cases.

The reported incidence of testicular infarction and subsequent testicular atrophy with incarceration is 4–12%, with higher rates among the irreducible cases requiring emergency operative reduction and repair. The testicular insult can be caused by compression of the gonadal vessels by the incarcerated hernia mass or as a result of damage incurred during operative repair. Young infants are at highest risk, with testicular infarction rates reported as high as 30% in infants younger than 2-3 mo of age. These problems underscore the need for prompt reduction of incarcerated hernias and early repair once the diagnosis is known to avoid repeat episodes of incarceration.

Injury to the Vas Deferens and Male Fertility

Similar to the gonadal vessels, the vas deferens can be injured as a consequence of compression from an incarcerated hernia or during operative repair. This injury is almost certainly underreported because it is unlikely to be recognized until adulthood and, even then, possibly only if the injury is bilateral. Although the vulnerability of the vas deferens has been documented in many studies, no good data exist as to the actual incidence of this complication. One review reported an incidence of injury to the vas deferens of 1.6% based on pathology demonstrating segments of the vas deferens in the hernia sac specimen; this may be overstated, because others have shown that small glandular inclusions found in the hernia sac can represent müllerian duct remnants and are of no clinical importance. The relationship between male fertility and previous inguinal hernia repair is also unknown. There appears to be an association between infertile males with testicular atrophy and abnormal sperm count and a previous hernia repair. A relationship has also been reported between infertile males with spermatic autoagglutinating antibodies and previous inguinal hernia repair. The proposed etiology is that operative injury to the vas deferens during inguinal hernia repair might result in obstruction of the vas with diversion of spermatozoa to the testicular lymphatics, and this breach of the blood–testis barrier produces an antigenic challenge, resulting in formation of spermatic autoagglutinating antibodies.

Bibliography is available at Expert Consult.

Section **5**
Exocrine Pancreas
第五篇
胰腺外分泌部

Chapter **374**

Embryology, Anatomy, and Physiology of the Pancreas

Steven L. Werlin and Michael Wilschanski

第三百七十四章
胰腺的胚胎学、解剖学和生理学

中文导读

本章主要介绍了胰腺解剖异常和胰腺生理学。具体描述了胰腺的解剖和组织学发育过程；描述了胰腺解剖结构特点和毗邻，横卧于上腹部腹膜后，位于十二指肠和脾之间；详细介绍了胰腺发育不全、环状胰腺、异位胰腺、胰腺分裂症、先天性胆总管囊肿、Ivemark综合征和Johanson–Blizzard综合征等导致胰腺发育和解剖异常的疾病；详细阐述了胰腺外分泌功能，包括各种消化酶的分泌与激活、水和碳酸氢盐的分泌及相关的神经–体液调节机制。

The human pancreas develops from the ventral and dorsal domains of the primitive duodenal endoderm beginning at about the 5th wk of gestation (Fig. 374.1). The larger dorsal anlage, which develops into the tail, body, and part of the head of the pancreas, grows directly from the duodenum. The smaller ventral anlage develops as 1 or 2 buds from the primitive liver and eventually forms the major portion of the head of the pancreas. At about the 17th wk of gestation, the dorsal and ventral anlagen fuse as the buds develop and the gut rotates. The ventral duct forms the proximal portion of the major pancreatic duct of Wirsung, which opens into the ampulla of Vater. The dorsal duct forms the distal portion of the duct of Wirsung and the accessory duct of Santorini, which empties independently in approximately 5% of people. Variations in fusion might account for pancreatic developmental anomalies. Pancreatic agenesis has been associated with a base pair deletion in the insulin promoter factor 1-*HOX* gene, *PDX1 (PAGEN1)*, *PTF1A (PAGEN 2), GATA 6 haploinsufficiency* and *FS123TER* genes. Other genes involved in pancreatic organogenesis include the *IHH*, *SHH* or sonic hedgehog

gene, *SMAD2*, and transforming growth factor-1β genes.

The pancreas lies transversely in the upper abdomen between the duodenum and the spleen in the retroperitoneum (Fig. 374.2). The head, which rests on the vena cava and renal vein, is adherent to the C loop of the duodenum and surrounds the distal common bile duct. The tail of the pancreas reaches to the left splenic hilum and passes above the left kidney. The lesser sac separates the tail of the pancreas from the stomach.

By the 13th wk of gestation, exocrine and endocrine cells can be identified. Primitive acini containing immature zymogen granules are found by the 16th wk. Mature zymogen granules containing amylase, trypsinogen, chymotrypsinogen, and lipase are present at the 20th wk. Centroacinar and duct cells, which are responsible for water, electrolyte, and bicarbonate secretion, are also found by the 20th wk. The final 3-dimensional structure of the pancreas consists of a complex series of branching ducts surrounded by grape-like clusters of epithelial cells. Cells containing glucagon are present at the 8th wk. Islets of Langerhans

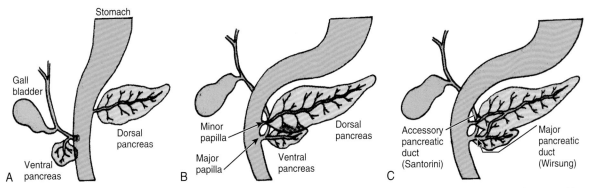

Fig. 374.1 Development of the exocrine pancreas. **A,** Gestational age 6 wk. **B,** Gestational age 7-8 wk. The ventral pancreas has rotated but has not yet fused with the dorsal pancreas. **C,** The ventral and dorsal pancreatic ductal systems have fused. *(From Werlin SL: The exocrine pancreas. In Kelly VC, editor: Practice of pediatrics, vol 3, Hagerstown, MD, 1980, Harper and Row, Fig. 16.1.)*

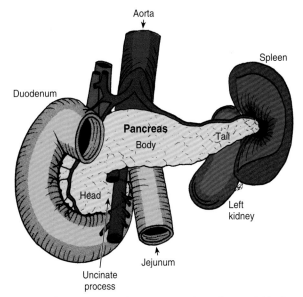

Fig. 374.2 Anterior view of the pancreas: relationship to neighboring structures. *(From Werlin SL: The exocrine pancreas. In Kelly VC, editor: Practice of pediatrics, vol 3, Hagerstown, MD, 1980, Harper and Row, Fig. 16.2.)*

appear between the 12th and 16th wk.

Bibliography is available at Expert Consult.

374.1 Pancreatic Anatomic Abnormalities

Steven L. Werlin and Michael Wilschanski

Complete or partial **pancreatic agenesis** is a rare condition. Complete agenesis is associated with severe neonatal diabetes and usually death at an early age (see Chapter 607). Partial or dorsal pancreatic agenesis is often asymptomatic but may be associated with diabetes, congenital heart disease, polysplenia, and recurrent pancreatitis. Pancreatic agenesis is also associated with malabsorption.

An **annular pancreas** results from incomplete rotation of the left (ventral) pancreatic anlage, which may be a result of recessive mutations in the *IHH* or *SHH* genes. Patients usually present in infancy with symptoms of complete or partial bowel obstruction or in the 4th or 5th decade. There is often a history of maternal polyhydramnios. Other congenital anomalies, such as Down syndrome, tracheoesophageal

fistula, intestinal atresia, imperforate anus, malrotation and cardiorenal abnormalities, and pancreatitis may be associated with annular pancreas. Some children present with chronic vomiting, pancreatitis, or biliary colic. The treatment of choice is duodenojejunostomy. Division of the pancreatic ring is not attempted because a duodenal diaphragm or duodenal stenosis often accompanies annular pancreas.

Ectopic pancreatic rests in the stomach or small intestine occur in approximately 3% of the population. Most cases (70%) are found in the upper intestinal tract. Recognized on barium contrast studies by their typical umbilicated appearance, they are rarely of clinical importance. On endoscopy, they are irregular, yellow nodules 2-4 mm in diameter. A pancreatic rest may rarely be the lead point of an intussusception, produce hemorrhage, or cause bowel obstruction.

Pancreas divisum, which occurs in 5–15% of the population, is the most common pancreatic developmental anomaly. As the result of failure of the dorsal and ventral pancreatic anlagen to fuse, the tail, body, and part of the head of the pancreas drain through the small accessory duct of Santorini rather than the main duct of Wirsung. Some researchers believe that this anomaly may be associated with recurrent pancreatitis when there is relative obstruction of the outflow of the ventral pancreas. Diagnosis is made by endoscopic retrograde cholangiopancreatography or by magnetic resonance cholangiopancreatography. Pancreatitis in patients with pancreas divisum is associated with mutations in the *CFTR* gene. Sphincterotomy is not recommended unless other anomalies are present or the patient has classic pancreatobiliary-type pain, recurrent pancreatitis, or chronic pancreatitis and no other etiology is found.

Choledochal cysts are dilations of the biliary tract and usually cause biliary tract symptoms, such as jaundice, pain, and fever. On occasion, the presentation may be pancreatitis. The diagnosis is usually made with ultrasonography, CT or biliary scanning, or magnetic resonance cholangiopancreatography. Similarly, a choledochocele—an intraduodenal choledochal cyst—may manifest with pancreatitis. The diagnosis can be difficult and require magnetic resonance cholangiopancreatography, endoscopic retrograde cholangiopancreatography, or endoscopic ultrasound.

A number of rare conditions, such as Ivemark (mutation in GDF gene) and Johanson-Blizzard (mutation in UBR1 gene) syndromes, include pancreatic dysgenesis or dysfunction among their features. Many of these syndromes include renal and hepatic dysgenesis along with the pancreatic anomalies.

Bibliography is available at Expert Consult.

374.2 Pancreatic Physiology

Steven L. Werlin and Michael Wilschanski

The acinus is the functional unit of the exocrine pancreas. Acinar cells are arrayed in a semicircle around a lumen. Ducts that drain the acini are lined by centroacinar and ductular cells. This arrangement allows the secretions of the various cell types to mix.

The acinar cell synthesizes, stores, and secretes more than 20 enzymes, which are stored in zymogen granules, some in inactive forms. The relative concentration of the various enzymes in pancreatic juice is affected and perhaps controlled by the diet, probably by regulating the synthesis of specific messenger RNA. The main enzymes involved in digestion include *amylase*, which splits starch into maltose, isomaltose, maltotriose; dextrins; and *trypsin* and *chymotrypsin*, endopeptidases secreted by the pancreas as inactive proenzymes. Trypsinogen is activated in the gut lumen by enterokinase, a brush-border enzyme. Trypsin can then activate trypsinogen, chymotrypsinogen, and procarboxypeptidase into their respective active forms. Pancreatic lipase requires *colipase*, a coenzyme also found in pancreatic fluid, for activity. Lipase liberates fatty acids from the 1 and 3 positions of triglycerides, leaving a monoglyceride.

The stimuli for exocrine pancreatic secretion are neural and hormonal. Acetylcholine mediates the cephalic phase; cholecystokinin (CCK) mediates the intestinal phase. CCK is released from the duodenal mucosa by luminal amino acids and fatty acids. Feedback regulation of pancreatic secretion is mediated by pancreatic proteases in the duodenum. Secretion of CCK is inhibited by the digestion of a trypsin-sensitive, CCK-releasing peptide released in the lumen of the small intestine or by a monitor peptide released in pancreatic fluid.

Centroacinar and duct cells secrete water and bicarbonate. Bicarbonate secretion is under feedback control and is regulated by duodenal intraluminal pH. The stimulus for bicarbonate production is secretin in concert with CCK. Secretin cells are abundant in the duodenum.

Although normal pancreatic function is required for digestion, maldigestion occurs only after considerable reduction in pancreatic function; lipase and colipase secretion must be decreased by 90–98% before fat maldigestion occurs.

Although amylase and lipase are present in the pancreas early in gestation, secretion of both amylase and lipase is low in the infant. Adult levels of these enzymes are not reached in the duodenum until late in the 1st yr of life. Digestion of the starch found in many infant formulas depends in part on the low levels of salivary amylase that reach the duodenum. This explains the diarrhea that may be seen in infants who are fed formulas high in glucose polymers or starch. Neonatal secretion of trypsinogen and chymotrypsinogen is at approximately 70% of the level found in the 1 yr old infant. The low levels of amylase and lipase in duodenal contents of infants may be partially compensated by salivary amylase and lingual lipase. This explains the relative starch and fat intolerance of premature infants.

Bibliography is available at Expert Consult.

Chapter 375

Pancreatic Function Tests

Michael Wilschanski and Steven L. Werlin

第三百七十五章
胰腺功能检查

中文导读

本章主要介绍了胰腺外分泌功能的检测方法，包括直接和间接检测方法两个方面。直接检测方法介绍了3种，目前已少用的是三腔管分离十二指肠胰液并进行碳酸氢盐浓度和酶活性测定，最常用的是肠促胰液素和/或缩胆囊素刺激后内镜下胰液收集，以及作为诊断吸收不良金标准的72小时粪便脂肪含量定量分析。间接检测方法中介绍了粪便弹性蛋白酶测量。

Pancreatic function can be measured by direct and indirect methods. An indirect test, the measurement of *fecal elastase*, which has become the standard screening test for pancreatic insufficiency, has a sensitivity and specificity >90%. When compared to a 72-hr fecal fat content in both pancreatic insufficient and sufficient patients, an elastase value of 100 μg/g stool has a 99% predictive value in ruling out pancreatic insufficiency based on an abnormal fecal fat finding. Falsely abnormal results can occur in many enteropathies and when the stool is very loose. The activity of other pancreatic enzymes in stool is rarely measured.

DIRECT TEST

Classically, a triple-lumen tube was used to isolate the pancreatic secretions in the duodenum. Measurement of bicarbonate concentration and enzyme activity (*trypsin*, *chymotrypsin*, *lipase*, and *amylase*) is performed on the aspirated secretions. This test is cumbersome and infrequently used. The most commonly used direct test is collection of pancreatic juice at endoscopy after stimulation with secretin and/ or cholecystokinin. A 72-hr stool collection for quantitative analysis of fat content is the gold standard for the diagnosis of malabsorption. The collection is usually performed at home, and the parent is asked to keep a careful dietary record, from which fat intake is calculated. A pre-weighed, sealable plastic container is used, which the parent keeps in the freezer. Freezing helps to preserve the specimen and reduce

odor. Infants are dressed in disposable diapers with the plastic side facing the skin so that the complete sample can be transferred to the container. Normal fat absorption is >93% of intake. The presence of fat malabsorption does not differentiate between pancreatic dysfunction and enteropathies, such as celiac disease. Qualitative examination of the stool for microscopic fat globules can give false-positive and false-negative results.

Bibliography is available at Expert Consult.

Chapter **376**
Disorders of the Exocrine Pancreas
Steven L. Werlin and Michael Wilschanski

第三百七十六章
胰腺外分泌疾病

中文导读

　　本章主要介绍了几种与胰腺功能不全相关的疾病，包括囊性纤维化、Shwachman-Diamond综合征、Pearson综合征、Johanson-Blizzard综合征、孤立性胰酶缺乏症和其他与胰腺功能不全有关的综合征［包括IMNEPD（婴儿发病的多系统神经、内分泌和

胰腺疾病）］。其中囊性纤维化是儿童中最常见的导致胰腺功能不全的疾病，其余疾病非常罕见。详细介绍了每种疾病的病因、临床表现，部分疾病提到了分类、遗传方式、辅助检查和治疗等内容。

DISORDERS ASSOCIATED WITH PANCREATIC INSUFFICIENCY

Other than cystic fibrosis (CF), conditions that cause pancreatic insufficiency are very rare in children. They include Shwachman-Diamond syndrome (SDS), Johanson-Blizzard syndrome, Ivemark syndrome, Pearson syndrome, isolated enzyme deficiencies, enterokinase deficiency (see Chapter 364), chronic pancreatitis, protein-calorie malnutrition (see Chapters 57 and 364), and IMNEPD (infantile onset multisystem neurologic, endocrine, and pancreatic disease).

CYSTIC FIBROSIS (see Chapter 432)

By the end of the 1st yr of life, 85–90% of children with CF have pancreatic insufficiency, which, if untreated, will lead to malnutrition. Treatment of the associated pancreatic insufficiency leads to improvement in absorption, better growth, and more normal stools. Pancreatic function can be monitored in children with CF with serial measurements of fecal elastase. Ten to 15% of children present with a neonatal intestinal

obstruction called meconium ileus; in later life a common intestinal complication is distal intestinal obstruction syndrome which is unique to CF. Ten percent of CF patients develop severe liver disease. Ten to 15% of CF patients are pancreatic sufficient and their presentation tends to be later in life, including recurrent pancreatitis, male infertility, and chronic bronchiectasis. CF is part of the newborn screen in every state in the United States and in most countries in the Western world.

SHWACHMAN-DIAMOND SYNDROME (see Chapter 157)

SDS is an autosomal recessive syndrome (1/20,000 births) caused by a mutation of the Shwachman-Bodian-Diamond syndrome *(SBDS)* gene on chromosome 7, which causes ribosomal dysfunction in 90–95% of patients. Signs and symptoms of SDS include pancreatic insufficiency; neutropenia, which may be cyclic; neutrophil chemotaxis defects; metaphyseal dysostosis; failure to thrive; and short stature. Some patients with SDS have liver or kidney involvement, dental disease, or learning difficulty. SDS is a common cause of congenital neutropenia.

Patients typically present in infancy with poor growth and steatorrhea. More varied phenotypes have been described including absence of pancreatic lipomatosis on imaging, normal fecal elastase levels, and normal skeletal survey. These children can be readily differentiated from those with CF by their normal sweat chloride levels, lack of mutations in the CF gene, characteristic metaphyseal lesions, and fatty pancreas characterized by a hypodense appearance on CT and MRI scans (Fig. 376.1).

Despite adequate pancreatic replacement therapy and correction of malabsorption, poor growth commonly continues. Pancreatic insufficiency is often transient, and steatorrhea frequently spontaneously improves with age. Recurrent pyogenic infections (otitis media, pneumonia, osteomyelitis, dermatitis, sepsis) are frequent and are a common cause of death. Thrombocytopenia is found in 70% of patients and anemia in 50%. Development of aplastic anemia or a *myelodysplastic syndrome* can occur, with transformation to *acute myeloid leukemia* in 24%. The pancreatic acini are replaced by fat with little fibrosis. Islet cells and ducts are normal. Bone marrow transplant is the treatment of choice in patients who develop acute myeloid leukemia.

PEARSON SYNDROME

Pearson (marrow-pancreas) syndrome is caused by a contiguous mitochondrial gene depletion involving several mitochondrial genes affecting oxidative phosphorylation, that manifests in infants with severe **macrocytic anemia** and **variable thrombocytopenia**. The bone marrow demonstrates vacuoles in erythroid and myeloid precursors as well as ringed sideroblasts. In addition to its role in severe bone marrow failure, pancreatic insufficiency contributes to growth failure. Mitochondrial DNA mutations are transmitted through maternal inheritance to both sexes or are sporadic.

JOHANSON-BLIZZARD SYNDROME

The features of Johanson-Blizzard syndrome include exocrine pancreatic deficiency, aplasia or hypoplasia of the alae nasi, congenital deafness, hypothyroidism, developmental delay, short stature, ectodermal scalp defects, absence of permanent teeth, urogenital malformations, and imperforate anus. This syndrome is caused by a mutation in the *UBR1* gene found on chromosome 15. The UBR1 protein acts as a ubiquitin ligase.

ISOLATED ENZYME DEFICIENCIES

Isolated deficiencies of trypsinogen, enterokinase, lipase, and colipase have been reported. Although enterokinase is a brush-border enzyme, deficiency causes pancreatic insufficiency because enterokinase is required

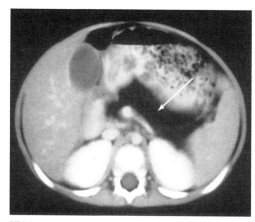

Fig. 376.1 CT appearance of the pancreas in a patient with Shwachman-Diamond syndrome. Note that the pancreas *(arrow)* retains a typical size and shape, but it is highly fatty and therefore appears as a very low-density structure. *(Courtesy Prof. Peter Durie, Hospital for Sick Children, Toronto, Ontario.)*

to activate trypsinogen to trypsin in the duodenum. Deficiencies of trypsinogen or enterokinase manifest with failure to thrive, hypoproteinemia, and edema. Isolated amylase deficiency is typically developmental and resolves by age 2-3 yr.

OTHER SYNDROMES ASSOCIATED WITH PANCREATIC INSUFFICIENCY

Pancreatic agenesis, congenital pancreatic hypoplasia, and congenital rubella are rare causes of pancreatic insufficiency. Pancreatic insufficiency has also been reported in duodenal atresia and stenosis and may also be seen in infants with familial or nonfamilial hyperinsulinemic hypoglycemia, who require 95–100% pancreatectomy to control hypoglycemia. Mutations in at least 6 genes have been described. Pancreatic insufficiency, which may be found in children with celiac disease and undernutrition, recovers with nutritional rehabilitation.

IMNEPD is a rare disease due to mutations in the *PTRH2* gene. Neurologic features dominate the phenotype (microcephaly, intellectual disability, cerebellar atrophy, deafness, and neuropathy), but pancreatic insufficiency is seen in most patients.

Bibliography is available at Expert Consult.

Chapter **377**

Treatment of Pancreatic Insufficiency

Michael Wilschanski and Steven L. Werlin

第三百七十七章

胰腺功能不全的治疗

中文导读

本章主要介绍了胰腺外分泌功能不全的治疗，主要为胰酶替代疗法。具体介绍了几种FDA批准的胰酶替代产品的药物名称、成分和价格；详细介绍了胰酶替代疗法的剂量推荐、剂量监测、调整依据和服用方法；具体介绍了婴儿胰酶制剂的特殊性和使用方法；提到了胰酶替代疗法难以完全纠正脂肪吸收不良的原因和解决方法；以及胰酶替代疗法的不良反应，包括过敏反应、肾结石、纤维性结肠病。

The most important treatment of pancreatic insufficiency (PI) is pancreatic enzyme replacement therapy (PERT). In modern enzyme capsules the enzymes are enterically coated to protect the enzymes from degradation by gastric acid and from autodigestion in the small intestine. It is common for patients to change from one product to another using a 1:1 lipase ratio and then titrating for maximum efficacy (Table 377.1).

The North American CF Foundation has published dosing guidelines based on age and fat ingestion (Table 377.2). Because these products contain excess protease compared with lipase, the dosage is estimated from the lipase requirement. The final dosage of PERT for children is often established by trial and error. An adequate dose is one that is followed by resumption of normal growth and the return of stools to normal fat content, which, when desired, can be verified by a 72-hr fecal fat collection and normalization of stool consistency and color. Because there is no elastase in enzyme preparations, fecal elastase cannot be used to monitor appropriateness of PERT dosage. Enzyme replacement should be divided and given at the beginning of and during the meal. Enzymes should not be chewed, crushed, or dissolved in food, which would allow gastric acid to penetrate the enteric coating and destroy the enzymes. Enzymes must also be given with snacks which contain fat. Increasing enzyme supplements beyond the recommended dose does not improve absorption, might retard growth, and can cause fibrosing colonopathy (see below).

A major concern has been the ingestion of enzymes by infants. The importance of correct enzyme ingestion in infants and children is obvious but there may be difficulty in feeding the infant microspheres however small they may be. Enterically coated microspheres can be mixed with apple sauce for oral use or crushed for use in tube feeding. Patients treated with this approach do achieve growth and weight gain. Pancreatic enzymes specifically prepared for infants and young children with smaller granules have been developed.

Table 377.1	FDA-Approved Pancreatic Enzyme Replacement Products for Exocrine Pancreatic Insufficiency*	
DRUG	**AVAILABLE STRENGTHS**	**COST ($)**[†]
IMMEDIATE-RELEASE–		
Viokace (Allergan)[‡,§,‖]	10,440 or 20,880 units of lipase[¶]	8.80
DELAYED-RELEASE–		
Creon (Abbvie)	3,000, 6,000, 12,000, 24,000, or 36,000 USP units of lipase[¶,**]	8.20
Pancreaze (Janssen)	2,600, 4,200, 10,500, 16,800, or 21,000 units of lipase[¶,**]	8.80
Pertzye (Digestive Care)	4,000, 8,000, 16,000, or 24,000 units of lipase[¶,**]	8.40
Zenpep (Allergan)	3,000, 5,000, 10,000, 15,000, 20,000, 25,000, or 40,000 units of lipase[¶,**]	9.60

*Pancrelipase products are not interchangeable. All of these products contain a combination of porcine-derived lipases, proteases, and amylases.

[†]Approximate WAC for one dose (as close as possible to 35,000 USP units of lipase using available formulations) for a 70-kg patient. WAC is wholesaler acquisition cost, or manufacturer's published price to wholesalers; WAC represents published catalogue or list prices and may not represent an actual transactional price. Source: AnalySource Monthly. September 5, 2017. Reprinted from First Databank, Inc. All rights reserved. ©2017. www.fdbhealth.com/policies/drug-pricing-policy/.

[‡]Viokace is only approved for use in adults.

[§]Should be used in combination with a proton pump inhibitor to maximize absorption in the duodenum.

[‖]FDA-approved only for treatment of adults with EPI due to chronic pancreatitis or pancreatectomy.

[¶]Should not be crushed or chewed.

[**]Capsules can be opened and contents sprinkled on soft acidic food (pH ≤ 4.5) such as applesauce.

From The Medical Letter: Pancreatic enzyme replacement products, *Med Lett* 59(1531):170, 2017.

Table 377.2	Pancreatic Enzyme Replacement Therapy: North American CF Foundation Consensus Statement
Infants (up to 12 mo)	2,000-4,000 U lipase/120 mL breast milk or formula
12 mo to 4 yr	1,000 U lipase/kg/meal initially, then titrate per response
Children >4 yr and adults	500 U lipase/kg/meal initially, up to maximum of 2,500 U lipase/kg/meal or 10,000 U lipase/kg/day or 4,000 U lipase/g fat ingested per day

PLUS: one half the standard meal dose to be given with snacks.

Treatment of exocrine PI by oral enzyme replacement usually corrects protein malabsorption, but steatorrhea is difficult to correct completely. Factors contributing to fat malabsorption include inadequate dosage, incorrect timing of doses in relation to food consumption or gastric emptying, lipase inactivation by gastric acid, and the observation that *chymotrypsin* in the enzyme preparation digests and thus inactivates *lipase*.

When adequate fat absorption is not achieved, gastric acid neutralization with an H_2-receptor antagonist or, more commonly, a proton pump inhibitor, decreases enzyme inactivation by gastric acid and thus improves delivery of lipase into the intestine. Enteric coating also protects lipase from acid inactivation.

Untoward effects secondary to PERT include allergic reactions and kidney stones. Fibrosing colonopathy, consisting of colonic fibrosis and strictures, can occur 7-12 mo after severe overdose of PERT.

Fat-soluble vitamin supplements are required by PI patients due to the ongoing mild to moderate fat malabsorption that occurs despite PERT.

Bibliography is available at Expert Consult.

Chapter 378
Pancreatitis
第三百七十八章
胰腺炎

中文导读

本章主要介绍了急性胰腺炎、急性复发性胰腺炎和慢性胰腺炎。具体介绍了急性胰腺炎的病因、发病机制、病理和正常胰腺的保护机制；详细描述了急性胰腺炎的临床表现、诊断、治疗和预后，其中临床表现包括轻症、中度重症和重症，诊断通常通过血清脂肪酶和淀粉酶活性，治疗目的是缓解疼痛，恢复代谢稳态；详细介绍了急性复发性胰腺炎和慢性胰腺炎的病因、发病机制、慢性胰腺炎的分类，以及相关的辅助检查和可选择的治疗方案。

378.1 Acute Pancreatitis
Steven L. Werlin and Michael Wilschanski

Acute pancreatitis (AP), the most common pancreatic disorder in children, is increasing in incidence, and 50 or more cases are usually seen in major pediatric centers per year. In children, blunt abdominal injuries, multisystem disease such as the hemolytic uremic syndrome and inflammatory bowel disease, biliary stones or microlithiasis (sludging), and drug toxicity are the most common etiologies. Although many drugs and toxins can induce AP in susceptible persons, in children, valproic acid, L-asparaginase, 6-mercaptopurine, and azathioprine are the most common causes of drug-induced pancreatitis. Alcohol should be considered in adolescents. Other cases follow organ transplantation or are caused by infections, metabolic disorders, or mutations in susceptibility genes (see Chapter 378.1). Only 10–20% of cases are idiopathic (Table 378.1).

After an initial insult, such as ductal disruption or obstruction, there is premature activation of trypsinogen to trypsin within the acinar cell. Trypsin then activates other pancreatic proenzymes, leading to autodigestion, further enzyme activation, and release of active proteases. Lysosomal hydrolases colocalize with pancreatic proenzymes within the acinar cell. Pancreastasis (similar in concept to cholestasis) with continued synthesis of enzymes occurs. Lecithin is activated by phospholipase A_2

Table 378.1 | Etiology of Acute and Recurrent Pancreatitis in Children

DRUGS AND TOXINS
- Acetaminophen overdose
- Alcohol
- L-Asparaginase
- Azathioprine
- Cannabis
- Carbamazepine
- Cimetidine
- Corticosteroids
- Cytosine arabinoside
- Dapsone
- Didanosine
- Enalapril
- Erythromycin
- Estrogen
- Furosemide
- Glucagon-like peptide-1 agents
- Interferon α
- Isoniazid
- Lamivudine
- Lisinopril
- 6-Mercaptopurine
- Methyldopa
- Mesalamine
- Metronidazole
- Octreotide
- Organophosphate poisoning
- Pentamidine
- Procainamide
- Retrovirals: DDC (dideoxycytidine), DDI (dideoxyinosine), tenofovir
- Rifampin
- Sulfonamides: mesalamine, 5-aminosalicytates, sulfasalazine, trimethoprim-sulfamethoxazole
- Sulindac
- Tetracycline
- Thiazides
- Valproic acid
- Venom (spider, scorpion, Gila monster lizard)
- Vincristine
- Volatile hydrocarbons

GENETIC
- Cationic trypsinogen gene (PRSS1)
- Chymotrypsin C gene (CTRC)
- Cystic fibrosis gene (CFTR)
- Trypsin inhibitor gene (SPINK1)

INFECTIOUS
- Ascariasis
- Coxsackie B virus
- Echovirus
- Enterovirus
- Epstein-Barr virus
- Hepatitides A, B
- Herpes viruses
- Influenzae A, B
- Leptospirosis
- Malaria
- Measles
- Mumps
- Mycoplasma
- Rabies
- Rubella
- Reye syndrome: varicella, influenza B
- Septic shock
- Thyroid fever

OBSTRUCTIVE
- Ampullary disease
- Ascariasis
- Biliary tract malformations
- Choledochal cyst
- Choledochocele
- Cholelithiasis, microlithiasis, and choledocholithiasis (stones or sludge)
- Duplication cyst
- Endoscopic retrograde cholangiopancreatography (ERCP) complication
- Pancreas divisum
- Pancreatic ductal abnormalities
- Postoperative
- Sphincter of Oddi dysfunction
- Tumor

SYSTEMIC DISEASE
- Autoimmune pancreatitis (IgG$_4$-related systemic disease)
- Brain tumor
- Collagen vascular diseases
- Congenital partial lipodystrophy
- Crohn disease
- Diabetes mellitus (ketoacidosis)
- Head trauma
- Henoch-Schönlein purpura
- Hemochromatosis
- Hemolytic uremic syndrome
- Hyperlipidemia: types I, IV, V
- Hyperparathyroidism/hypercalcemia
- Kawasaki disease
- Malnutrition
- Organic acidemia
- Peptic ulcer
- Periarteritis nodosa
- Renal failure
- Scorpion venom
- Systemic lupus erythematosus
- Transplantation: bone marrow, heart, liver, kidney, pancreas
- Vasculitis

TRAUMATIC
- Blunt injury
- Burns
- Child abuse
- Hypothermia
- Surgical trauma
- Total-body cast

into the toxic lysolecithin. Prophospholipase is unstable and can be activated by minute quantities of trypsin. After the insult, cytokines and other proinflammatory mediators are released.

The healthy pancreas is protected from autodigestion by pancreatic proteases that are synthesized as inactive proenzymes; digestive enzymes that are segregated into secretory granules at pH 6.2 by low calcium concentration, which minimizes trypsin activity; the presence of protease inhibitors both in the cytoplasm and zymogen granules; and enzymes that are secreted directly into the ducts.

Histopathologically, interstitial edema appears early. Later, as the episode of pancreatitis progresses, localized and confluent necrosis, blood vessel disruption leading to hemorrhage, and an inflammatory response in the peritoneum can develop.

The diagnosis of pancreatitis in children is made when 2 of 3 of the following are present: abdominal pain; serum amylase and/or lipase activity at least 3 times greater than the upper limit of normal; and imaging findings characteristic of, or compatible with, AP.

CLINICAL MANIFESTATIONS

The severity of AP in children has been defined by a consensus committee.

Mild Acute Pancreatitis: AP that is not associated with organ failure, local or systemic complications, and usually resolves within the 1st wk after presentation. This is the most common form of pediatric AP.

The patient with mild AP has moderate to severe abdominal pain, persistent vomiting, and possibly fever. The pain is epigastric or in either upper quadrant, steady, often resulting in the child's assuming an antalgic position with hips and knees flexed, sitting upright, or lying on the side. The child is uncomfortable, irritable, and appears acutely ill. The abdomen may be distended and tender and a mass may be palpable. The pain can increase in intensity for 24-48 hr, during which time vomiting may increase and the patient can require hospitalization for fluid and electrolyte therapy and analgesia. There is no organ failure, and imaging does not demonstrate peri- or pancreatic necrosis. The prognosis for complete recovery in the acute uncomplicated case after 4-7 days is excellent.

Moderately Severe Acute Pancreatitis: AP with either transient organ failure/dysfunction (lasting <48 hr) or development of local or systemic complications, such as exacerbation of previously diagnosed comorbid disease (such as lung or kidney disease). Imaging may reveal sterile (peri-) pancreatic necrosis. The prognosis for these patients is also excellent but recovery may be prolonged.

Severe Acute Pancreatitis: AP with development of organ dysfunction that persists longer than 48 hr. Persistent organ failure may be single or multiple. Severe AP is uncommon in children. In this life-threatening condition, the patient is acutely ill with severe nausea, vomiting, and abdominal pain. Shock, high fever, jaundice, ascites, hypocalcemia, and pleural effusions can occur. A bluish discoloration may be seen around the umbilicus (Cullen sign) or in the flanks (Grey Turner sign). The pancreas is necrotic and can be transformed into an inflammatory hemorrhagic mass. The mortality rate, which is approximately 20%, is related to the systemic inflammatory response syndrome with multiple organ dysfunction, shock, renal failure, acute respiratory distress syndrome, disseminated intravascular coagulation, gastrointestinal bleeding, and systemic or intra-abdominal infection. The percentage of necrosis seen on CT and failure of pancreatic tissue to enhance on CT (suggesting necrosis) predicts the severity of the disease.

DIAGNOSIS

AP is usually diagnosed by measurement of serum lipase and amylase activities. Serum lipase is considered the test of choice for AP, as it is more specific than amylase for acute inflammatory pancreatic disease and should be determined when pancreatitis is suspected. The serum lipase rises by 4-8 hr, peaks at 24-48 hr, and remains elevated 8-14 days longer than serum amylase. Serum lipase greater than 7 times the upper limit of normal obtained within 24 hr of presentation may predict a severe course. Serum lipase can be elevated in nonpancreatic diseases. The serum amylase level is typically elevated for up to 4 days. A variety of other conditions can also cause hyperamylasemia

Table 378.2	Differential Diagnosis of Hyperamylasemia

PANCREATIC PATHOLOGY
- Acute or chronic pancreatitis
- Complications of pancreatitis (pseudocyst, ascites, abscess)
- Factitious pancreatitis

SALIVARY GLAND PATHOLOGY
- Parotitis (mumps, *Staphylococcus aureus*, cytomegalovirus, HIV, Epstein-Barr virus)
- Sialadenitis (calculus, radiation)
- Eating disorders (anorexia nervosa, bulimia)

INTRAABDOMINAL PATHOLOGY
- Biliary tract disease (cholelithiasis)
- Peptic ulcer perforation
- Peritonitis
- Intestinal obstruction
- Appendicitis

SYSTEMIC DISEASES
- Metabolic acidosis (diabetes mellitus, shock)
- Renal insufficiency, transplantation
- Burns
- Pregnancy
- Drugs (morphine)
- Head injury
- Cardiopulmonary bypass

without pancreatitis (Table 378.2). Elevation of salivary amylase can mislead the clinician to diagnose pancreatitis in a child with abdominal pain. The laboratory can separate amylase isoenzymes into pancreatic and salivary fractions. Initially serum amylase levels are normal in 10–15% of patients.

Other laboratory abnormalities that may be present in AP include hemoconcentration, coagulopathy, leukocytosis, hyperglycemia, glucosuria, hypocalcemia, elevated γ-glutamyl transpeptidase, and hyperbilirubinemia.

X-ray of the chest and abdomen might demonstrate nonspecific findings such as atelectasis, basilar infiltrates, elevation of the hemidiaphragm, left- (rarely right-) sided pleural effusions, pericardial effusion, and pulmonary edema. Abdominal x-rays might demonstrate a sentinel loop, dilation of the transverse colon (cutoff sign), ileus, pancreatic calcification (if recurrent), blurring of the left psoas margin, a pseudocyst, diffuse abdominal haziness (ascites), and peripancreatic extraluminal gas bubbles.

CT has a major role in the diagnosis and follow-up of children with pancreatitis. Findings can include pancreatic enlargement; a hypoechoic, sonolucent edematous pancreas; pancreatic masses; fluid collections; and abscesses (Fig. 378.1). Normal imaging studies at the time of diagnosis are not uncommon. In adults, CT findings are the basis of a widely accepted prognostic system (Table 378.3). Ultrasonography is more sensitive than CT for the diagnosis of biliary stones. Magnetic resonance cholangiopancreatography and endoscopic retrograde cholangiopancreatography are essential in the investigation of recurrent pancreatitis, nonresolving pancreatitis, and disease associated with gallbladder pathology. Endoscopic ultrasonography also helps visualize the pancreaticobiliary system. Complications of AP are noted in Table 378.4.

TREATMENT

The aims of medical management are to relieve pain and restore metabolic homeostasis. Analgesia should be given in adequate doses. Fluid, electrolyte, and mineral balance should be restored and maintained. Nasogastric suction is useful in patients who are vomiting. Early refeeding decreases the complication rate and length of stay. While he or she is vomiting, the patient should be maintained with nothing by mouth. Recovery is usually complete within 4-5 days.

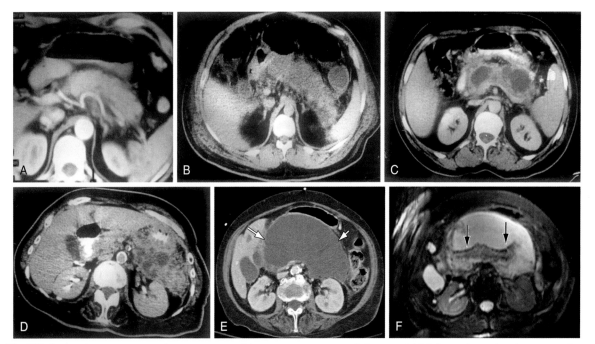

Fig. 378.1 CT and MRI appearance of pancreatitis. **A,** Mild acute pancreatitis. Arterial phase spiral CT. Diffuse enlargement of pancreas without fluid accumulation. **B,** Severe acute pancreatitis. Lack of enhancement of the pancreatic parenchyma due to the necrosis of the entire pancreatic gland. **C,** Pancreatic pseudocyst. A round fluid collection with thin capsule is seen within the lesser sac. **D,** Acute severe pancreatitis and peripancreatic abscess formation. Peripancreatic abscess formation is observed within the peripancreatic and the left anterior pararenal space. **E,** Pancreatic necrosis. A well-defined fluid attenuation collection in the pancreatic bed *(white arrows)* seen on contrast-enhanced CT imaging. **F,** The same collection is more complex appearing on the corresponding T2-weighted MR image. The internal debris and necrotic tissue are better appreciated because of the superior soft-tissue contrast of MRI *(black arrows)*. (A-D, *From Elmas N: The role of diagnostic radiology in pancreatitis,* Eur J Radiol *38[2]:120–132, 2001, Figs. 1, 3b, 4a, and 5. E and F, From Soakar A, Rabinowitz CB, Sahani DV: Cross-sectional imaging in acute pancreatitis,* Radiol Clin North Am *45[3]:447–460, 2007, Fig. 14.)*

Table 378.3	Revised Definitions of Morphologic Features of Acute Pancreatitis

INTERSTITIAL EDEMATOUS PANCREATITIS

Acute inflammation of the pancreatic parenchyma and peripancreatic tissues, but without recognizable tissue necrosis
- CECT criteria
  - Pancreatic parenchyma enhancement by intravenous contrast agent
  - No peripancreatic necrosis

NECROTIZING PANCREATITIS

Inflammation associated with pancreatic parenchymal necrosis and/or peripancreatic necrosis
- CECT criteria
  - Lack of pancreatic parenchymal enhancement by intravenous contrast agent
  - Presence of findings of peripancreatic necrosis

ACUTE PANCREATITIS FLUID COLLECTION

Peripancreatic fluid associated with interstitial edematous pancreatitis with no associated peripancreatic necrosis. Applies only to areas of peripancreatic fluid seen within the first 4 wk after onset of interstitial edematous pancreatitis and without the features of a pseudocyst.
- CECT criteria
  - Occurs in the setting of interstitial edematous pancreatitis
  - Homogeneous collection with fluid density
  - Confined by normal peripancreatic fascial planes
  - No definable wall encapsulating the collection
  - Adjacent to pancreas (no intrapancreatic extension)

PANCREATIC PSEUDOCYST

An encapsulated collection of fluid with a well-defined inflammation wall, usually outside the pancreas, with little or no necrosis. Usually occurs more than 4 wk after onset of interstitial edematous pancreatitis.
- CECT criteria
  - Well circumscribed; usually round or oval
  - Homogeneous fluid density
  - No nonliquid component
  - Well-defined wall that is wholly encapsulated
  - Maturation usually needs >4 wk after onset of acute pancreatitis; occurs after interstitial edematous pancreatitis

ACUTE NECROTIC COLLECTION

A collection containing variable amounts of both fluid and necrosis associated with necrotizing pancreatitis; the necrosis can include the pancreatic parenchyma and/or the peripancreatic tissue.
- CECT criteria
- Occurs only in the setting of acute necrotizing pancreatitis
- Heterogeneous and nonliquid density of varying degrees in different locations (some seem homogeneous early in their course)
- No definable wall encapsulating the collection
- Intrapancreatic and/or extrapancreatic

WALLED-OFF NECROSIS

A mature, encapsulated collection of pancreatic and/or peripancreatic necrosis that has developed a well-defined inflammatory wall. Usually occurs >4 wk after onset of necrotizing pancreatitis.
- CECT criteria
  - Heterogeneous with liquid and nonliquid density, with varying locations (some can seem homogeneous)
  - Well-defined wall that is wholly encapsulated
  - Intrapancreatic and/or extrapancreatic
  - Maturation usually needs 4 wk after onset of acute necrotizing pancreatitis

CECT, contrast-enhanced CT.
From PA Banks, TL Bollen, C Dervenis, et al.; the Acute Pancreatitis Classification Working Group Classification of acute pancreatitis—2012: revision of the Atlanta classification and definitions by international consensus Gut 62:102-111, 2013.

Table 378.4	Complications of Acute Pancreatitis

LOCAL

Pseudocyst
Sterile necrosis
Infected necrosis
Abscess
GI bleeding
- Pancreatitis-related
- Splenic artery or splenic artery pseudoaneurysm rupture
- Splenic vein rupture
- Portal vein rupture
- Splenic vein thrombosis leading to gastroesophageal variceal bleeding
- Pseudocyst or abscess hemorrhage
- Postnecrosectomy bleeding

Nonpancreatitis-related
- Mallory-Weiss tear
- Alcoholic gastropathy
- Stress-related mucosal gastropathy

Splenic complications
- Infarction
- Rupture
- Hematoma
- Splenic vein thrombosis

Fistulization to or obstruction of the small intestine or colon
Hydronephrosis

SYSTEMIC

Respiratory failure
Renal failure
Shock
Hyperglycemia
Hypocalcemia
Disseminated intravascular coagulation
Fat necrosis (subcutaneous nodules)
Retinopathy

PSYCHOSIS

From Tenner S, Steinberg WM: Acute pancreatitis. In Feldman M, Friedman LS, Brandt LJ, editors: *Sleisenger and Fordtran's gastrointestinal and liver disease,* ed 10, Philadelphia, 2016, Elsevier (Box 58.7, p. 991).

Prophylactic antibiotics are not recommended, but antibiotics are used to treat infected necrosis. Gastric acid secretion is suppressed with proton pump inhibitors. Enteral alimentation by mouth, nasogastric tube, or nasojejunal tube (in severe cases or for those intolerant of oral or nasogastric feedings) within 2-3 days of onset reduces the length of hospitalization, complication rate, and survival in patients with severe AP. In children, surgical therapy of nontraumatic AP is rarely required but may include drainage of necrotic material or abscesses. Endotherapy for common bile duct stones, ductal strictures, and for drainage of fluid collections is the standard of care when indicated.

PROGNOSIS

Children with mild AP do well and recover within 4-5 days. When pancreatitis is associated with trauma or systemic disease, the prognosis is typically related to the associated medical conditions.

Bibliography is available at Expert Consult.

378.2 Acute Recurrent and Chronic Pancreatitis

Steven L. Werlin and Michael Wilschanski

Acute recurrent pancreatitis (ARP) is defined as ≥2 distinct episodes of AP with intervening return of enzymes to baseline. Chronic pancreatitis (CP) is defined as the presence of typical abdominal pain plus characteristic imaging findings including pancreatic calcifications, inflammation

and fibrosis, or exocrine insufficiency plus imaging findings, or endocrine insufficiency plus imaging findings. Most children with CP describe a history of ARP and tend to be older at the time of diagnosis compared with children with ARP, suggesting that ARP and CP are a disease continuum.

Table 378.5	Factors Contributing to the Etiology of Chronic Pancreatitis

	No. (%)*
Chronic pancreatitis patients with history of ≥1 episode acute pancreatitis	73 (96)
Risk factors for pancreatitis	
Genetic	51 (67)
PRSS1	33 (43)
SPINK1	14 (19)
CFTR	11 (14)
CTRC	2 (3)
Autoimmune	3 (4)
Obstructive	25 (33)
Pancreas divisum	15 (20)
Sphincter of Oddi dysfunction	1 (1)
Gallstones	3 (4)
Pancreatic duct malunion	2 (3)
Pancreatic duct obstruction	1 (1)
Other	5 (7)
Toxic/metabolic	8 (11)
Alcohol (determined by doctor)	1 (1)
Passive smoking (exposure)	3 (4)
Hyperlipidemia	1 (1)
Medication	1 (1)
Metabolic disease	1 (1)
Other	1 (1)
None cited	8 (11)

*The total exceeds 100% because some children have more than 1 factor.
From Schwarzenberg SJ, Bellin M, Husain SZ, et al: Pediatric chronic pancreatitis is associated with genetic risk factors and substantial disease burden, *J Pediatr* 166:890–896, 2015 (Table II, p. 892).

Table 378.6	Classification of Chronic Pancreatitis

CHRONIC CALCIFYING PANCREATITIS	CHRONIC OBSTRUCTIVE PANCREATITIS	STEROID-RESPONSIVE PANCREATITIS
Alcohol	Stricture	Autoimmune Pancreatitis
Smoking	Blunt trauma	
Genetic	Endoscopic stenting	Type 1
Idiopathic	Acute pancreatitis	Type 2 (IDCP)
Juvenile-onset	Anastomotic stricture	
Tropical	**Tumor**	
	Adenocarcinoma	
	IPMN	
	Serious cystadenoma Islet cell tumor	

IDCP, idiopathic duct-centric pancreatitis; *IPMN,* intraductal papillary mucinous neoplasm.
From Majumder S, Chari ST: Chronic pancreatitis, *Lancet* 387:1957–1966, 2016 (Fig 1, p. 1958).

ARP and CP in children are often due to genetic mutations or due to congenital anomalies of the pancreatic or biliary ductal system (Tables 378.5 and 378.6). Mutations in the *PRSS1* gene (cationic trypsinogen) located on the long arm of chromosome 7, *SPINK1* gene (pancreatic trypsin inhibitor) located on chromosome 5, in the cystic fibrosis gene *(CFTR)*, and chymotrypsin C *(CTRC)* may all lead to CP (Fig. 378.2).

Cationic trypsinogen has a trypsin-sensitive cleavage site. Loss of this cleavage site in the abnormal protein permits uncontrolled activation of trypsinogen to trypsin, which leads to autodigestion of the pancreas. Mutations in *PRSS1* act in an autosomal dominant fashion with incomplete penetrance and variable expressivity. Symptoms often begin in the first decade but are usually mild at the onset. Although spontaneous recovery from each attack occurs in 4-7 days, episodes become progressively more severe. Hereditary pancreatitis may be diagnosed by the presence of the disease in successive generations of a family. An evaluation during symptom-free intervals may be unrewarding until calcifications, pseudocysts, or pancreatic exocrine and endocrine insufficiency develop (Fig. 378.3; see Fig. 378.2). CP is a risk factor for the development of pancreatic cancer. Multiple mutations of the *PRSS1* gene associated with hereditary pancreatitis have been described.

Trypsin inhibitor acts as a fail-safe mechanism to prevent uncontrolled autoactivation of trypsin. Mutations in the *SPINK1* gene have been associated with recurrent or CP. In *SPINK1* mutations, this fail-safe mechanism is lost; this gene may be a modifier gene and not the direct etiologic factor.

Mutations of the cystic fibrosis gene *(CFTR)*, associated with pancreatic sufficiency or which do not typically produce pulmonary disease, can cause CP, possibly due to ductal obstruction. Patients with genotypes associated with mild phenotypic effects have a greater risk of developing pancreatitis than those with genotypes associated with moderate to severe phenotypes.

Mutations in the chymotrypsin C gene, which cause a loss of function, may also cause recurrent pancreatitis. Indications for genetic testing include recurrent episodes of AP, CP, a family history of pancreatitis, or unexplained pancreatitis in children.

Other conditions associated with chronic, relapsing pancreatitis are hyperlipidemia (types I, IV, and V), hyperparathyroidism, and ascariasis. Previously, most cases of recurrent pancreatitis in childhood were considered idiopathic; with the discovery of gene families associated with recurrent pancreatitis, this has changed. Congenital anomalies of the ductal systems, such as pancreas divisum, are more common than previously recognized.

Autoimmune pancreatitis (AIP) typically manifests with jaundice, abdominal pain, and weight loss. The pancreas is typically enlarged and is hypodense on CT. The pathogenesis is unknown. **Type 1** is a systemic disease and is associated with high serum IgG4. In addition to pancreatitis in type 1 disease, the patient may have retroperitoneal fibrosis, orbital inflammation, aortitis, sclerosing cholangitis, cutaneous vasculitis,

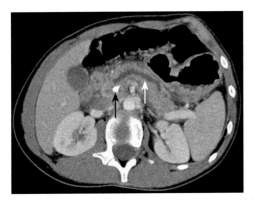

Fig. 378.2 Chronic pancreatitis. Computed tomogram showing calcification in the head of the pancreas *(black arrow)* and dilated pancreatic duct *(white arrow)* in a 12 yr old patient. *(Courtesy Dr. Janet Reid. From Wyllie R, Hyams JS, editors: Pediatric gastrointestinal and liver disease, ed 3, Philadelphia, 2006, WB Saunders.)*

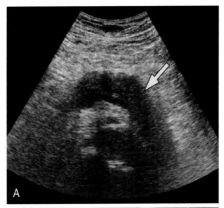

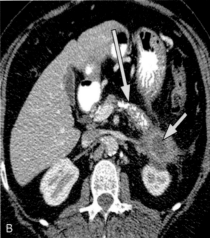

Fig. 378.3 Examples of ultrasound and multidetector images in patients with chronic pancreatitis. **A,** Transabdominal ultrasound scan showing a uniformly swollen, hypoechoic pancreas *(arrow)* typical of autoimmune pancreatitis. **B,** Multidetector CT showing pancreatic calculi in an atrophic pancreas *(long arrow)* and a pseudocyst at the tail of the pancreas *(short arrow)*. *(From Braganza JM, Lee SH, McCloy RF, McMahon MJ: Chronic pancreatitis, Lancet 377:1184–1197, 2011, Fig. 5, p 1191.)*

Table 378.7	Conditions Classification of Chronic Disorders Now Recognized to Be Part of IgG4-Related Disease

Autoimmune pancreatitis (lymphoplasmacytic sclerosing pancreatitis)
Eosinophilic angiocentric fibrosis (affecting the orbits and upper respiratory tract)
Fibrosing mediastinitis
Hypertrophic pachymeningitis
Idiopathic hypocomplementaemic tubulointerstitial nephritis with extensive tubulointerstitial deposits
Inflammatory pseudotumor (affecting the orbits, lungs, kidneys, and other organs)
Küttner tumor (affecting the submandibular glands)
Mikulicz disease (affecting the salivary and lacrimal glands)
Multifocal fibrosclerosis (commonly affecting the orbits, thyroid gland, retroperitoneum, mediastinum, and other tissues and organs)
Periaortitis and periarteritis
Inflammatory aortic aneurysm
Retroperitoneal fibrosis (Ormond disease)
Riedel thyroiditis
Sclerosing mesenteritis
Conditions once regarded as individual disorders now recognized to be part of IgG4-related disease

From Kamisawa T, Zen Y, Pillai S, Stone JH: IgG4-related disease, *Lancet* 385:1460–1471, 2015 (Panel 1, p. 1461).

pulmonary fibrosis, and sialoadenitis. These extrapancreatic features may also be present in the absence of pancreatitis (Table 378.7). Tissue biopsy shows fibrosis, plasmacytosis, and positive staining for IgG4; serum IgG4 levels are not always elevated.

Type 2 is limited to diffuse or focal involvement of just the pancreas. IgG4 levels are normal. *Both types respond to steroids.* Children with AIP typically have type 2.

Juvenile tropical pancreatitis is the most common form of CP in developing equatorial countries. The highest prevalence is in the Indian state of Kerala. Tropical pancreatitis occurs during late childhood or early adulthood, manifesting with abdominal pain and irreversible pancreatic insufficiency followed by diabetes mellitus within 10 years. The pancreatic ducts are obstructed with inspissated secretions, which later calcify. This condition is associated with mutations in the *SPINK* gene in 50% of cases.

A thorough diagnostic evaluation of every child with more than one episode of pancreatitis is indicated. Serum lipid, calcium, and phosphorus levels are determined. Stools are evaluated for ascaris, and a sweat test is performed. Plain abdominal films are evaluated for the presence of pancreatic calcifications. Abdominal ultrasound or CT scanning is performed to detect the presence of a pseudocyst. The biliary tract is evaluated for the presence of stones. After genetic counseling, evaluation of *PRSS1, SPINK1, CFTR,* and *CRTC* genotypes can be measured. Electrophysiologic tests such as nasal potential difference testing may be recommended when the diagnosis of cystic fibrosis (CF) is uncertain.

Magnetic resonance cholangiopancreatography (MRCP) and Endoscopic retrograding cholangiopancreatography (ERCP) are techniques that can be used to define the anatomy of the gland and are mandatory if surgery is considered. MRCP is the test of choice when endotherapy is not being considered and should be performed as part of the evaluation of any child with idiopathic, nonresolving, or recurrent pancreatitis and in patients with a pseudocyst before drainage. In these cases a previously undiagnosed anatomic defect that may be amenable to endoscopic or surgical therapy may be detected. Endoscopic treatments include sphincterotomy, stone extraction, drainage on pseudocysts, and insertion of pancreatic or biliary endoprosthetic stents. These treatments allow the successful nonsurgical management of conditions previously requiring surgical intervention. In patients with intractable pain, total pancreatectomy and islet cell transfusion is performed in specialist centers.

Bibliography is available at Expert Consult.

Chapter **379**
Pancreatic Fluid Collections
Michael Wilschanski and Steven L. Werlin

第三百七十九章
胰液积聚

中文导读

　　本章主要介绍了胰液积聚形成的原因、临床特点、辅助检查以及胰液积聚和胰腺坏死的治疗。具体描述了胰腺假性囊肿的形成原因，是由胰腺酶、血液和坏死组织等物质局部聚集形成，通常是胰腺炎的并发症；临床表现常包括疼痛、恶心、呕吐和腹部包块，要根据病变进行相应的辅助检查；具体介绍了胰液积聚和胰腺坏死的内外科治疗指征和手段。

Pancreatic pseudocyst formation is an uncommon sequela to acute or chronic pancreatitis.

A pancreatic pseudocyst is a circumscribed collection of fluid rich in pancreatic enzymes, blood, and necrotic tissue, typically located in the lesser sac of the abdomen. Pancreatic pseudocysts are usually complications of pancreatitis, although in children they frequently occur following abdominal trauma. They can enlarge or extend in almost any direction, thus producing a wide variety of symptoms (see Fig. 378.1C).

A pancreatic pseudocyst is suggested when an episode of pancreatitis fails to resolve or when a mass develops after an episode of pancreatitis. Clinical features usually include pain, nausea, and vomiting, but many patients are asymptomatic. The most common signs are a palpable mass in 50% of patients and jaundice in 10%. Other findings include ascites and pleural effusions (usually left-sided).

Pancreatic pseudocysts can be detected by transabdominal ultrasonography, CT scanning, magnetic resonance cholangiopancreatography (MRCP), endoscopic retrograde cholangiopancreatography (ERCP), and endoscopic ultrasound (EUS). Because of its ease, availability, and reliability, ultrasonography is the first choice. Sequential ultrasonography studies have demonstrated that most small pseudocysts (<6 cm) resolve spontaneously. It is recommended that the patient with acute pancreatitis undergo an ultrasonographic evaluation 4 wk after resolution of the acute episode for an evaluation of possible pseudocyst formation.

TREATMENT OF FLUID COLLECTIONS AND NECROSIS

Percutaneous and endoscopic drainage of pseudocysts have replaced open surgical drainage, except for complicated or recurrent pseudocysts. Whereas a pseudocyst must be allowed to mature for 4-6 wk before surgical drainage is attempted, percutaneous or endoscopic drainage can be attempted earlier. In some cases, endoscopic creation of a cyst-gastrostomy is performed. When a surgical treatment is planned an MRCP or ERCP is performed to define anatomic abnormalities and aid the surgeon in planning his approach. EUS is helpful when an endoscopic approach is chosen.

Necrotizing pancreatitis includes both pancreatic gland necrosis and peripancreatic fat necrosis. In the initial phases, the necrotic collection is a mix of semisolid and solid tissue. Over a period of 4 wk or longer, the collection becomes more liquid and becomes encapsulated by a visible wall. At this point, the process is termed walled-off pancreatic necrosis. Sterile necrosis does not require therapy except in the rare case of a collection that obstructs a nearby viscus (e.g., duodenal, bile duct, or gastric obstruction).

The development of *infected* necrosis is the main indication for broad-spectrum antibiotic therapy. The development of fever, leukocytosis, and increasing abdominal pain suggests infection of the necrotic tissue. A CT scan may reveal evidence of air bubbles in the necrotic cavity.

Bibliography is available at Expert Consult.

Chapter **380**

Pancreatic Tumors

Meghen B. Browning, Steven L. Werlin, and Michael Wilschanski

第三百八十章

胰腺肿瘤

中文导读

本章主要介绍了内分泌来源和非内分泌来源的胰腺肿瘤，内分泌来源的肿瘤包括胃泌素瘤和胰岛素瘤。详细描述了两种胰腺肿瘤的发病率、其分泌的激素以及导致的相关临床表现，包括症状性低血糖、水样泻–低钾血症–酸中毒综合征等；具体介绍了胰腺肿瘤的治疗方法和预后，治疗为手术切除和药物控制，内分泌肿瘤完全切除后预后良好，但肉瘤和癌预后极差，除一些罕见亚型外。

Pancreatic tumors can be of either endocrine or nonendocrine origin. Tumors of endocrine origin include gastrinomas and insulinomas (Table 380.1). These and other functioning tumors occur in the autosomal dominantly inherited multiple endocrine neoplasia type 1 (MEN-1). Hypoglycemia accompanied by higher-than-expected insulin levels or refractory gastric ulcers (Zollinger-Ellison syndrome) indicates the possibility of a pancreatic tumor (see Chapter 372). Most gastrinomas arise outside of the pancreas. The treatment of choice is surgical removal. If the primary tumor cannot be found, or if it has metastasized, cure might not be possible. Treatment with a high dose of a proton pump inhibitor to inhibit gastric acid secretion is then indicated.

Insulinomas and persistent hyperinsulinemic hypoglycemia of infancy produce symptomatic hypoglycemia caused by mutations in a variety of genes, most commonly *GUUD1* and *KATP*. Massive subtotal or total pancreatectomy is the treatment of choice when medical treatment fails. These children might then develop pancreatic insufficiency and diabetes as a complication of surgery.

Table 380.1	Syndromes Associated With Pancreatic Neuroendocrine Tumors (pNETs)*			
SYNDROME		**INCIDENCE/10⁶/YEAR**	**MALIGNANCY (%)**	**HORMONE**
Insulinoma		1-2	<10	Insulin
Gastrinoma (ZES)		0.5-1.5	60–90	Gastrin
VIPoma (Verner-Morrison syndrome, WDHA, pancreatic cholera)		0.05-0.2	>60	VIP
Glucagonoma		0.01-0.1	50–80	Glucagon
Somatostatinoma		Rare	>70	Somatostatin
GRFoma		Unknown	>30	GH-RF
ACTHoma		Uncommon	>95%	ACTH
pNET secreting PTH-rP		Rare	84%	PTH-rP
Pancreatic carcinoid tumor		Rare (<1% of all carcinoids)	77%	Serotonin, tachykinins
pNET secreting renin		Rare	Unknown	Renin
pNET secreting erythropoietin		Rare	Unknown	Erythropoietin
pNET secreting luteinizing hormone		Rare	Unknown	Luteinizing hormone
pNET secreting cholecystokinin (CCKoma)		Rare	Unknown	CCK

GH-RF, growth hormone–releasing factor; *PP*, pancreatic polypeptide; *PTH-rP*, parathyroid hormone–related protein; *VIP*, vasoactive intestinal polypeptide; *WDHA*, watery diarrhea, hypokalemia, achlorhydria.
    *These syndromes may also be caused by a GI-NET (carcinoid).
    From Jensen RT, Norton JA, Oberg K: Neuroendocrine tumors. In Feldman M, Friedman LS, Brandt LJ, editors: *Sleisenger and Fordtran's gastrointestinal and liver disease*, ed 10, Elsevier, 2016, Philadelphia, Table 33.1.

The **watery diarrhea–hypokalemia–acidosis syndrome** is usually produced by the secretion of vasoactive intestinal peptide by a non–α-cell tumor (VIPoma) (see Table 367.7). Vasoactive intestinal peptide levels are often, but not always, increased in the serum. Treatment is surgical removal of the tumor. When this is not possible, symptoms may be controlled by the use of octreotide acetate (cyclic somatostatin, Sandostatin), a synthetic analog of somatostatin. Pancreatic tumors secreting a variety of hormones, including glucagon, somatostatin, and pancreatic polypeptide, have also been described. The treatment is surgical resection when possible.

Pancreatoblastomas, pancreatic adenocarcinomas, cystadenomas, and sarcomas of the pancreas are rarely encountered. Pancreatoblastoma, a malignant embryonal tumor that secretes α-fetoprotein and can contain both endocrine and exocrine elements, is the most common pancreatic neoplasm in young children. Presurgical chemotherapy should be considered for lesions not primarily resectable. Resection can be curative; adjuvant chemotherapy has been used, but its effectiveness is not established.

Sarcomas are very rarely primary pancreatic but may include Ewing sarcoma, rhabdomyosarcoma, or undifferentiated soft tissue sarcomas. They are treated with multimodal therapy including chemotherapy and either resection or radiation.

Carcinoma of the exocrine pancreas is a major problem in adults, accounting for 2% of diagnoses and 5% of deaths from cancer. It is very rare in childhood. No definite causes are known. Several genetic syndromes including mutations in the *PRSS1* and *MEN-1* genes lead to an increased incidence of pancreatic cancer in adult life. The solid pseudopapillary tumor of the pancreas, also called Frantz tumor, is a more indolent pancreatic carcinoma usually found in adolescent/young adult females. Typical presenting symptoms are abdominal pain, mass, or jaundice. The treatment of choice is total surgical removal. Prognosis is very good.

Pancreatic lesions in **von Hippel-Lindau disease** are usually benign and cystic. Cystadenomas, familial adenocarcinomas, and islet cell tumors are less common. Metastases have been reported, but adjuvant therapy after surgical excision cannot yet be recommended. The diagnosis is suggested by CT scan.

Prognosis is good for completely resected endocrine tumors but very poor for sarcomas and carcinomas, excepting rare subtypes. Children who survive partial or complete pancreatectomy may have decreased pancreatic exocrine and endocrine reserve.

Bibliography is available at Expert Consult.

Section **6**

The Liver and Biliary System

第六篇

肝胆系统

Chapter **381**

Morphogenesis of the Liver and Biliary System

Stacey S. Huppert and William F. Balistreri

第三百八十一章

肝胆系统的形态发生

中文导读

本章主要介绍了肝脏超微结构和肝脏的代谢功能。具体描述了肝胆系统的胚胎形成过程，起源于腹侧前肠内胚层细胞，以及影响胚胎发育的因素；详细描述了反应肝脏生物学功能的肝细胞的超微结构特征；详细介绍了碳水化合物代谢、蛋白质代谢、脂质代谢、生物转化和肝排泄功能。特别指出新生儿肝脏形态形成和功能的不成熟，都会增加婴儿对与肠外营养相关的肝脏疾病的易感性。

During the early embryonic process of gastrulation, the 3 embryonic germ layers (endoderm, mesoderm, and ectoderm) are formed. The liver and biliary system arises from cells of the ventral foregut endoderm; their development can be divided into 3 distinct processes (Fig. 381.1). First, through unknown mechanisms, the ventral foregut endoderm acquires *competence* to receive signals arising from the cardiac mesoderm. These mesodermal signals, in the form of various fibroblast growth factors and bone morphogenetic proteins, lead to *specification* of cells that have the potential to form the liver and activate liver-specific genes. During this period of hepatic fate decision, "pioneer" transcription factors, including *Foxa* and *Gata4*, bind to specific binding sites in compacted chromatin, open the local chromatin structure, and mark genes as competent. However, these will be expressed only if they are correctly induced by additional transcription factors. Newly specified cells then delaminate from the ventral foregut endoderm and migrate in a cranial ventral direction into the septum transversum in the 4th wk of human gestation to initiate liver *morphogenesis*.

The growth and development of the newly budded liver require interactions with endothelial cells. Certain proteins are important for liver development in animal models (Table 381.1). In addition to these proteins, microRNAs, which consist of small noncoding, single-stranded RNAs, have a functional role in the regulation of gene expression and hepatobiliary development in zebrafish and mouse models.

Within the ventral mesentery, proliferation of migrating cells form anastomosing hepatic cords, with the network of primitive liver cells, sinusoids, and septal mesenchyme establishing the basic architectural pattern of liver lobule (Fig. 381.2). The solid *cranial* portion of the hepatic diverticulum (pars hepatis) eventually forms the hepatic parenchyma and the intrahepatic bile ducts. The hepatic lobules are identifiable in the 6th wk of human gestation. The bile canalicular structures, including microvilli and junctional complexes, are specialized loci of the liver cell membrane; these appear very early in gestation, and large canaliculi bounded by several hepatocytes are seen by 6-7 wk.

Hepatocytes and bile duct cells (cholangiocytes) originate from hepatoblasts as common precursors. Notch signaling, which is impaired in Alagille syndrome, promotes hepatoblast differentiation into biliary epithelium, whereas hepatocyte growth factor antagonizes differentiation. The development of the intrahepatic bile ducts is determined by the

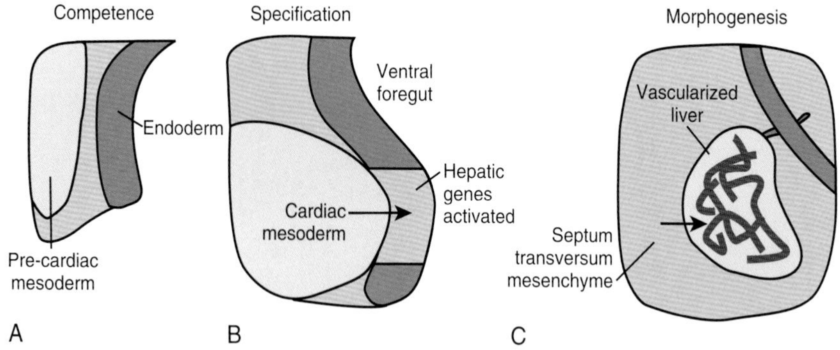

Competence

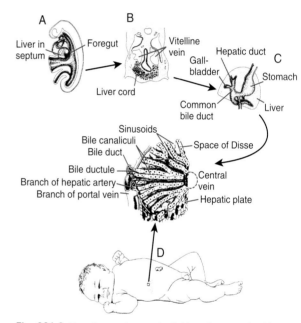

Specification

Morphogenesis

A   B   C

Fig. 381.1 Processes involved in early liver development. **A,** The ventral foregut endoderm acquires *competence* to receive signals arising from the cardiac mesoderm. **B,** Specific cells of the ventral foregut endoderm undergo *specification* and activation of liver-specific genes under the influence of mesodermal signals. **C,** Liver *morphogenesis* is initiated as the newly specified cells migrate into the septum transversum under the influence of signaling molecules and extracellular matrix released by septum transversum mesenchymal cells and of primitive endothelial cells. (*From Zaret K7S: Liver specification and early morphogenesis,* Mech Dev *92:83–88, 2000.*)

Table 381.1	Selected Growth Factors, Receptors, Protein Kinases, and Transcription Factors Required for Normal Liver Development in Animal Models

INDUCTION OF HEPATOCYTE FATE THROUGH CARDIAC MESODERM
- Fibroblast growth factors (FGFs) 1, 2, 8
- FGF receptors 1, 4

INDUCTION OF HEPATOCYTE FATE THROUGH SEPTUM TRANSVERSUM
- Bone morphogenetic proteins 2, 4, 7

STIMULATION OF HEPATOBLAST GROWTH AND PROLIFERATION
- Hepatocyte growth factor (HGF)
- HGF receptor c-met
- "Pioneer" transcription factors Foxa1, Foxa2, and Gata4, Gata6
- Transcription factors Xbp1, Foxm1b, Hlx, Hex, Prox1
- Wnt signaling pathway, β-catenin

SPECIFICATION OF HEPATOCYTE LINEAGE
- HGF
- Transforming growth factor-β and its downstream effectors Smad 2, Smad 3
- Hepatocyte nuclear factors (HNFs) 1α, 4α, 6

SPECIFICATION OF CHOLANGIOCYTE LINEAGE
- Jagged 1 (Notch ligand) and Notch receptors 1, 2
- HNF6, HNF1β
- Wnt signaling pathway, β-catenin
- Vacuolar sorting protein Vps33b

Fig. 381.2 Hepatic morphogenesis. **A,** Ventral outgrowth of hepatic diverticulum from foregut endoderm in the 3.5-wk embryo. **B,** Between the 2 vitelline veins, the enlarging hepatic diverticulum buds off epithelial (liver) cords that become the liver parenchyma, around which the endothelium of capillaries (sinusoids) align (4 wk embryo). **C,** Hemisection of embryo at 7.5 wk. **D,** Three-dimensional representation of the hepatic lobule as present in the newborn. (*From Andres JM, Mathis RK, Walker WA: Liver disease in infants. Part I: developmental hepatology and mechanisms of liver dysfunction,* J Pediatr *90:686–697, 1977.*)

development and branching pattern of the portal vein. Around the 8th wk of gestation, starting at the hilum of the liver, primitive hepatoblasts adjacent to the mesenchyme around the portal vein branches form a cylindrical sleeve, termed the *ductal plate.* From 12 wk of gestation onward, a remodeling of the ductal plate occurs, with some segments of the ductal plate undergoing tubular dilation and excess ductal plate cells gradually disappearing. The ramification of the biliary tree continues throughout human fetal life and at the time of birth the most peripheral branches of the portal veins are still surrounded by ductal plates; these require 4 more wk to develop into definitive portal ducts. Lack of remodeling of the ductal plate results in persistence of primitive ductal plate configurations, an abnormality called *ductal plate malformation.*

This histopathologic lesion has been observed in liver biopsies of a variety of liver conditions, including congenital hepatic fibrosis, Caroli disease, and biliary atresia.

The *caudal* part (pars cystica) of the hepatic diverticulum becomes the gallbladder, cystic duct, and common bile duct. The distal portions of the right and left hepatic ducts develop from the extrahepatic ducts, whereas the proximal portions develop from the first intrahepatic ductal plates. The extrahepatic bile ducts and the developing intrahepatic biliary tree maintain luminal continuity and patency from the beginning of organogenesis (see Fig. 381.2*C*).

Fetal hepatic blood flow is derived from the hepatic artery and from the portal and umbilical veins, which form the portal sinus. The portal venous inflow is directed mainly to the right lobe of the liver and umbilical flow primarily to the left. The ductus venosus shunts blood from the portal and umbilical veins to the hepatic vein, bypassing the sinusoidal network. After birth, the ductus venosus becomes obliterated when oral feedings are initiated. The fetal oxygen saturation is lower in portal than in umbilical venous blood; accordingly, the right hepatic lobe has lower oxygenation and greater hematopoietic activity than the left hepatic lobe.

The transport and metabolic activities of the liver are facilitated by the structural arrangement of liver cell cords, which are formed by rows of hepatocytes, separated by sinusoids that converge toward the tributaries of the hepatic vein (the central vein) located in the center of the lobule (see Fig. 381.2*D*). This establishes the pathways and patterns of flow for substances to and from the liver. In addition to arterial input from the systemic circulation, the liver also receives venous input from the gastrointestinal tract via the portal system. The products of the hepatobiliary system are released by 2 different paths: through the hepatic vein and through the biliary system back into the intestine. Plasma proteins and other plasma components are secreted by the liver. Absorbed and circulating nutrients arrive through the portal vein or the hepatic artery and pass through the sinusoids and past the hepatocytes to the systemic circulation at the central vein. Biliary components are transported via the series of enlarging channels from the bile canaliculi through the bile ductule to the common bile duct.

Bile secretion is first noted at the 12th wk of human gestation. The major components of bile vary with stage of development. Near term, cholesterol and phospholipid content is relatively low. Low concentrations of bile acids, the absence of bacterially derived (secondary) bile acids, and the presence of unusual bile acids reflect low rates of bile flow and immature bile acid synthetic pathways.

The liver reaches a peak relative size of approximately 10% of the fetal weight at the 9th wk. Early in development, the liver is a primary site of hematopoiesis. In the 7th wk, hematopoietic cells outnumber functioning hepatocytes in the hepatic anlage. These early hepatocytes are smaller than at maturity (~20 μm vs. 30-35 μm) and contain less glycogen. Near term, the hepatocyte mass expands to dominate the organ, as cell size and glycogen content increase. Hematopoiesis is virtually absent by the 2nd postnatal mo in full-term infants. As the density of hepatocytes increases with gestational age, the relative volume of the sinusoidal network decreases. The liver constitutes 5% of body weight at birth but only 2% in an adult.

Several metabolic processes are immature in a healthy newborn infant, owing in part to the fetal patterns of activity of various enzymatic processes. Many fetal hepatic functions are carried out by the maternal liver, which provides nutrients and serves as a route of elimination of metabolic end products and toxins. Fetal liver metabolism is devoted primarily to the production of proteins required for growth. Toward term, primary functions become production and storage of essential nutrients, excretion of bile, and establishment of processes of elimination. Extrauterine adaptation requires de novo enzyme synthesis. Modulation of these processes depends on substrate and hormonal input via the placenta and on dietary and hormonal input in the postnatal period.

HEPATIC ULTRASTRUCTURE
Hepatocytes exhibit various ultrastructural features that reflect their biologic functions (Fig. 381.3). Hepatocytes, like other epithelial cells, are polarized, meaning that their structure and function are directionally oriented. One result of this polarity is that various regions of the hepatocyte plasma membrane exhibit specialized functions. Bidirectional transport occurs at the *sinusoidal* surface, where materials reaching the liver via the portal system enter and compounds secreted by the liver leave the hepatocyte. *Canalicular* membranes of adjacent hepatocytes form bile canaliculi, which are bounded by tight junctions, preventing transfer of secreted compounds back into the sinusoid. Within hepatocytes, metabolic and synthetic activities are contained within a number

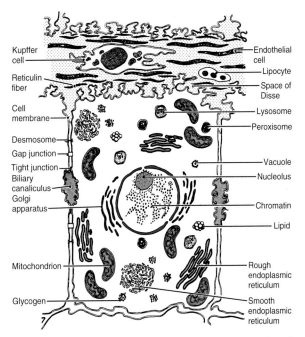

Fig. 381.3 Schematic view of the ultrastructure and organelles of hepatocytes. *(From Sherlock S: Hepatic cell structure. In Sherlock S, editor: Diseases of the liver and biliary system, ed 6. Oxford, 1981, Blackwell Scientific, p. 10, with permission from Blackwell Scientific.)*

of different cell organelles. The oxidation and metabolism of heterogeneous classes of substrates, fatty acid oxidation, key processes in gluconeogenesis, and the storage and release of energy occur in the abundant mitochondria.

The endoplasmic reticulum, a continuous network of rough- and smooth-surfaced tubules and cisternae, is the site of various processes, including protein and triglyceride synthesis and drug metabolism. Low fetal activity of endoplasmic reticulum–bound enzymes accounts for a relative inefficiency of xenobiotic (drug) metabolism. The Golgi apparatus is active in protein packaging and possibly in bile secretion. Hepatocyte peroxisomes are single membrane–limited cytoplasmic organelles that contain enzymes such as oxidases and catalase and those that have a role in lipid and bile acid metabolism. Lysosomes contain numerous hydrolases that have a role in intracellular digestion. The hepatocyte cytoskeleton, composed of actin and other filaments, is distributed throughout the cell and concentrated near the plasma membrane. Microfilaments and microtubules have a role in receptor-mediated endocytosis, in bile secretion, and in maintaining hepatocyte architecture and motility.

METABOLIC FUNCTIONS OF THE LIVER
Carbohydrate Metabolism
The liver regulates serum glucose levels closely via several processes, including storage of excess carbohydrate as glycogen, a polymer of glucose readily hydrolyzed to glucose during fasting. To maintain serum glucose levels, hepatocytes produce free glucose by either glycogenolysis or gluconeogenesis. Immediately after birth, an infant is dependent on hepatic glycogenolysis. Gluconeogenic activity is present at a low level in the fetal liver and increases rapidly after birth. Fetal glycogen synthesis begins at about the 9th wk of gestation, with glycogen stores most rapidly accumulated near term, when the liver contains 2-3 times the amount of glycogen of adult liver. Most of this stored glycogen is used in the immediate postnatal period. Reaccumulation is initiated at about the 2nd wk of postnatal life, and glycogen stores reach adult levels

at approximately the 3rd wk in healthy full-term infants. In preterm infants, serum glucose levels fluctuate in part because efficient regulation of the synthesis, storage, and degradation of glycogen develops only near the end of full-term gestation. Dietary carbohydrates such as galactose are converted to glucose, but there is a substantial dependence on gluconeogenesis for glucose in early life, especially if glycogen stores are limited.

Protein Metabolism

During the rapid fetal growth phase, specific decarboxylases that are rate limiting in the biosynthesis of physiologically important polyamines have higher activities than in the mature liver. The rate of synthesis of albumin and secretory proteins in the developing liver parallels the quantitative changes in endoplasmic reticulum. Synthesis of albumin appears at approximately the 7th-8th wk in the human fetus and increases in inverse proportion to that of α-fetoprotein, which is the dominant fetal protein. By the 3rd-4th mo of gestation, the fetal liver is able to produce fibrinogen, transferrin, and low-density lipoproteins. From this period on, fetal plasma contains each of the major protein classes at concentrations considerably below those achieved at maturity.

The *postnatal* patterns of protein synthesis vary with the class of protein. Lipoproteins of each class rise abruptly in the 1st wk after birth to reach levels that vary little until puberty. Albumin concentrations are low in a neonate (~2.5 g/dL), reaching adult levels (~3.5 g/dL) after several mo. Levels of ceruloplasmin and complement factors increase slowly to adult values in the 1st yr. In contrast, transferrin levels at birth are similar to those of an adult, decline for 3-5 mo, and rise thereafter to achieve their final concentrations. Low levels of activity of specific proteins have implications for the nutrition of an infant. A low level of cystathionine γ-lyase (cystathionase) activity impairs the *trans*-sulfuration pathway by which dietary methionine is converted to cysteine. Consequently, the latter must be supplied in the diet. Similar dietary requirements might exist for other sulfur-containing amino acids, such as taurine.

Lipid Metabolism

Fatty acid oxidation provides a major source of energy in early life, complementing glycogenolysis and gluconeogenesis. Newborn infants are relatively intolerant of prolonged fasting, owing in part to a restricted capacity for hepatic ketogenesis. Rapid maturation of the ability of the liver to oxidize fatty acid occurs in the 1st few days of life. Milk provides the major source of calories in early life; this high-fat, low-carbohydrate diet mandates active gluconeogenesis to maintain blood glucose levels. When the glucose supply is limited, ketone body production from endogenous fatty acids can provide energy for hepatic gluconeogenesis and an alternative fuel for brain metabolism. When carbohydrates are in excess, the liver produces triglycerides. Metabolic processes involving lipids and lipoproteins are predominantly hepatic; liver immaturity or disease affects lipid concentrations and lipoproteins.

Biotransformation

Newborn infants have a decreased capacity to metabolize and detoxify certain drugs, owing to underdevelopment of the hepatic microsomal component that is the site of the specific oxidative, reductive, hydrolytic, and conjugation reactions required for these biotransformations. The major components of the monooxygenase system, such as cytochrome P450, cytochrome-*c* reductase, and the reduced form of nicotinamide-adenine dinucleotide phosphate, are present in low concentrations in fetal microsomal preparations. In full-term infants, hepatic uridine diphosphate glucuronosyltransferase and enzymes involved in the oxidation of polycyclic aromatic hydrocarbons are expressed at very low levels.

Age-related differences in pharmacokinetics vary from compound to compound. The half-life of acetaminophen in a newborn is similar to that of an adult, whereas theophylline has a half-life of approximately 100 hr in a premature infant, as compared with 5-6 hr in an adult. These differences in metabolism, as well as factors such as binding to plasma proteins and renal clearance, determine appropriate drug dosage to maximize effectiveness and to avoid toxicity. Dramatic examples of

the susceptibility of newborn infants to drug toxicity are the responses to chloramphenicol (the *gray baby* syndrome) or to benzoyl alcohol and its metabolic products, which involve ineffective glucuronide and glycine conjugation, respectively. The low concentrations of antioxidants (vitamin E, superoxide dismutase, glutathione peroxidase) in the fetal and early newborn liver lead to increased susceptibility to deleterious effects of oxygen toxicity and oxidant injury through lipid peroxidation.

Conjugation reactions, which convert drugs or metabolites into water-soluble forms that can be eliminated in bile, are also catalyzed by hepatic microsomal enzymes. Newborn infants have decreased activity of hepatic uridine diphosphate glucuronosyltransferase, which converts unconjugated bilirubin to the readily excreted glucuronide conjugate and is the rate-limiting enzyme in the excretion of bilirubin. There is rapid postnatal development of transferase activity irrespective of gestational age, which suggests that birth-related, rather than age-related, factors are of primary importance in the postnatal development of activity of this enzyme. Microsomal activity can be stimulated by administration of phenobarbital, rifampin, or other inducers of cytochrome P450. Alternatively, drugs such as cimetidine can inhibit microsomal P450 activity.

Hepatic Excretory Function

Hepatic excretory function and bile flow are closely related to hepatic *bile acid* excretion and enterohepatic recirculation. Bile acids, the major products of cholesterol degradation, are incorporated into mixed micelles with cholesterol and phospholipid. These micelles act as an efficient vehicle for solubilization and intestinal absorption of lipophilic compounds, such as dietary fats and fat-soluble vitamins. Secretion of bile acids by the liver cells is the major determinant of bile flow in the mature animal. Accordingly, maturity of bile acid metabolic processes affects overall hepatic excretory function, including biliary excretion of endogenous and exogenous compounds.

In humans, the 2 primary bile acids, cholic acid and chenodeoxycholic acid, are synthesized in the liver. Before excretion, they are conjugated with glycine and taurine. In response to a meal, contraction of the gallbladder delivers bile acids to the intestine to assist in fat digestion and absorption. After mediating fat digestion, the bile acids themselves are reabsorbed from the terminal ileum through specific active transport processes. They return to the liver via portal blood, are taken up by liver cells, and are reexcreted in bile. In an adult, this enterohepatic circulation involves 90–95% of the circulating bile acid pool. Bile acids that escape ileal reabsorption reach the colon, where the bacterial flora, through dihydroxylation and deconjugation, produce the secondary bile acids, deoxycholate and lithocholate. In an adult, the composition of bile reflects the excretion of the primary and also the secondary bile acids, which are reabsorbed from the distal intestinal tract.

Intraluminal concentrations of bile acids are low in newborn infants and increase rapidly after birth. The expansion of the bile acid pool is critical because bile acids are required to stimulate bile flow and absorb lipids, a major component of the diet of a newborn. Nuclear receptors, such as farnesoid X receptor, control intrahepatic bile acid homeostasis through several mechanisms, including regulation of expression of the genes encoding 2 key proteins, cholesterol 7α-hydroxylase (CYP7A1) and bile salt export pump (BSEP). These proteins are critical for bile acid synthesis and canalicular secretion, respectively. Neonatal expression of these nuclear receptors varies depending on the studied animal model and is largely unknown for humans.

Because of inefficient ileal reabsorption of bile acids and the low rate of hepatic clearance of bile acids from portal blood, serum concentrations of bile acids are commonly elevated in healthy newborns, often to levels that would suggest liver disease in older persons. Transient phases of physiologic cholestasis and physiologic steatorrhea can often be observed in low birthweight infants and in full-term infants following perinatal stress, such as hypoxia or infection, but are otherwise uncommon in healthy full-term newborns.

Many of the processes related to immaturity of the newborn in liver morphogenesis and function, as discussed earlier, are implied in the increased susceptibility of infants to liver disease associated with parenteral nutrition. The reduced bile salt pool, hepatic glutathione

Table 381.2	Causes of Impaired Bile Acid Metabolism and Enterohepatic Circulation

DEFECTIVE BILE ACID SYNTHESIS OR TRANSPORT
- Inborn errors of bile acid synthesis (reductase deficiency, isomerase deficiency)
- Progressive familial intrahepatic cholestasis (PFIC1, PFIC2, PFIC3)
- Intrahepatic cholestasis (neonatal hepatitis)
- Acquired defects in bile acid synthesis secondary to severe liver disease

ABNORMALITIES OF BILE ACID DELIVERY TO THE BOWEL
- Celiac disease (sluggish gallbladder contraction)
- Extrahepatic bile duct obstruction (e.g., biliary atresia, gallstones)

LOSS OF ENTEROHEPATIC CIRCULATION OF BILE ACIDS
- External bile fistula
- Cystic fibrosis
- Small bowel bacterial overgrowth syndrome (with bile acid precipitation, increased jejunal absorption, and "short-circuiting")
- Drug-induced entrapment of bile acids in intestinal lumen (e.g., cholestyramine)

BILE ACID MALABSORPTION
- Primary bile acid malabsorption (absent or inefficient ileal active transport)
- Secondary bile acid malabsorption
- Ileal disease or resection
- Cystic fibrosis

DEFECTIVE UPTAKE OR ALTERED INTRACELLULAR METABOLISM
- Parenchymal disease (acute hepatitis, cirrhosis)
- Regurgitation from cells
- Portosystemic shunting
- Cholestasis

depletion, and deficient sulfation contribute to production of toxic lithocholic bile acids and cholestasis, whereas deficiencies of essential amino acids, including taurine and cysteine, and excessive lipid infusion can lead to hepatic steatosis in these infants. Beyond the neonatal period, disturbances in bile acid metabolism may be responsible for diverse effects on hepatobiliary and intestinal function (Table 381.2).

Bibliography is available at Expert Consult.

Chapter 382
Manifestations of Liver Disease
James E. Squires and William F. Balistreri

第三百八十二章
肝病表现

中文导读

　　本章主要介绍了肝脏疾病的病理表现和临床表现；具体描述了肝功能不全患者的评价。在临床表现中详细描述了肝大、黄疸、皮肤瘙痒、蜘蛛痣、肝掌、黄色瘤、门静脉高压、腹水、消化道出血、肝性脑病、内分泌紊乱、肾衰竭、肺损伤、复发性胆管炎、肝功能障碍等症状或并发症的形成机制以及评估。在肝功能不全的评估中详细介绍了生化试验、肝活检、肝脏成像和婴儿黄疸的诊断方法。

PATHOLOGIC MANIFESTATIONS

Congenital and acquired alterations in hepatic structure and function (acute or chronic) can be manifest by varying patterns of reaction of the liver to cell injury. Hepatocyte injury can be caused by viral infection, drugs or toxins, hypoxia, immunologic and structural disorders, or inborn errors of metabolism. The injury results in inflammatory cell infiltration and cell death (necrosis), which may be followed by a healing process of scar formation (fibrosis) and, potentially, nodule formation (regeneration). Cirrhosis is the end result of any progressive fibrotic liver disease.

Cholestasis is an alternative or concomitant response to injury caused by extrahepatic or intrahepatic obstruction to bile flow. Substances that are normally excreted in bile, such as bile acids, conjugated bilirubin, cholesterol, and trace elements, accumulate in serum. Bile pigment accumulation in liver parenchyma can be seen in liver biopsy specimens. In *extrahepatic* obstruction, bile pigment may be visible in the intralobular bile ducts or throughout the parenchyma as bile lakes or infarcts. In *intrahepatic* cholestasis, an injury to hepatocytes or an alteration in hepatic physiology leads to a reduction in the rate of secretion of solute and water. Causes include alterations in enzymatic or canalicular transporter activity, permeability of the bile canalicular apparatus, organelles responsible for bile secretion, or ultrastructure of the cytoskeleton of the hepatocyte. The end result may be clinically indistinguishable from obstructive cholestasis.

Cirrhosis, defined histologically by the presence of bands of fibrous tissue that link central and portal areas and form parenchymal nodules, is an end stage of any acute or chronic liver disease. Cirrhosis can be *macronodular*, with nodules of various sizes (up to 5 cm) separated by broad septa, or *micronodular*, with nodules of uniform size (<1 cm) separated by fine septa; mixed forms occur. The progressive scarring results in altered hepatic blood flow, with further impairment of liver cell function. Increased intrahepatic resistance to portal blood flow leads to portal hypertension.

The liver can be secondarily involved in neoplastic (metastatic) and non-neoplastic (storage diseases, fat infiltration) processes, as well as a number of systemic conditions and infectious processes. The liver can be affected by chronic passive congestion (congestive heart failure) or acute hypoxia, with hepatocellular damage.

CLINICAL MANIFESTATIONS
Hepatomegaly

Enlargement of the liver can be caused by several mechanisms (Table 382.1). Normal liver size estimations are based on age-related clinical indices, such as the degree of extension of the liver edge below the costal margin, the span of dullness to percussion, or the length of the vertical axis of the liver, as estimated from imaging techniques. In children, the normal liver edge can be felt up to 2 cm below the right costal margin. In a newborn infant, extension of the liver edge more than 3.5 cm below the costal margin in the right midclavicular line suggests hepatic enlargement. Measurement of liver span is carried out by percussing the upper margin of dullness and by palpating the lower edge in the right midclavicular line. This may be more reliable than an extension of the liver edge alone. The 2 measurements may correlate poorly.

The liver span increases linearly with body weight and age in both sexes, ranging from approximately 4.5-5.0 cm at 1 wk of age to approximately

Table 382.1	Mechanisms of Hepatomegaly
INCREASE IN THE NUMBER OR SIZE OF THE CELLS INTRINSIC TO THE LIVER *Storage* Fat: malnutrition, obesity, metabolic liver disease (diseases of fatty acid oxidation and Reye syndrome–like illnesses), lipid infusion (total parenteral nutrition), cystic fibrosis, medication related, pregnancy Specific lipid storage diseases: Gaucher, Niemann-Pick, Wolman disease Glycogen: glycogen storage diseases (multiple enzyme defects); total parenteral nutrition; infant of diabetic mother, Beckwith syndrome, poorly controlled type 1 diabetes mellitus (Mauriac syndrome) Miscellaneous: α_1-antitrypsin deficiency, Wilson disease, hypervitaminosis A *Inflammation* Hepatocyte enlargement (hepatitis) • Viral: acute and chronic • Bacterial: sepsis, abscess, cholangitis • Toxic: drugs • Autoimmune Kupffer cell enlargement • Sarcoidosis • Systemic lupus erythematosus • Hemophagocytic lymphohistiocytosis • Macrophage activating syndrome **INFILTRATION OF CELLS** *Primary Liver Tumors: Benign* Hepatocellular • Focal nodular hyperplasia • Nodular regenerative hyperplasia • Hepatocellular adenoma Mesodermal • Infantile hemangioendothelioma • Mesenchymal hamartoma Cystic masses • Choledochal cyst • Hepatic cyst • Hematoma • Parasitic cyst • Pyogenic or amebic abscess	*Primary Liver Tumors: Malignant* Hepatocellular • Hepatoblastoma • Hepatocellular carcinoma Mesodermal • Angiosarcoma • Undifferentiated embryonal sarcoma Secondary or metastatic processes • Lymphoma • Leukemia • Lymphoproliferative disease • Langerhans cell histiocytosis • Neuroblastoma • Wilms tumor **INCREASED SIZE OF VASCULAR SPACE** Intrahepatic obstruction to hepatic vein outflow • Venoocclusive disease • Hepatic vein thrombosis (Budd-Chiari syndrome) • Hepatic vein web Suprahepatic • Congestive heart failure Pericardial disease/tamponade/constrictive pericarditis Post-Fontan procedure Hematopoietic: sickle cell anemia, thalassemia **INCREASED SIZE OF BILIARY SPACE** Congenital hepatic fibrosis Caroli disease Extrahepatic obstruction **IDIOPATHIC** Various • Riedel lobe • Normal variant • Downward displacement of diaphragm

7-8 cm in boys and 6.0-6.5 cm in girls by 12 yr of age. The lower edge of the right lobe of the liver extends downward (Riedel lobe) and can normally be palpated as a broad mass in some people. An enlarged left lobe of the liver is palpable in the epigastrium of some patients with cirrhosis. Downward displacement of the liver by the diaphragm (hyperinflation) or thoracic organs can create an erroneous impression of hepatomegaly.

Examination of the liver should note the consistency, contour, tenderness, and presence of any masses or bruits, as well as assessment of spleen size, along with documentation of the presence of ascites and any stigmata of chronic liver disease.

Ultrasound is useful in assessment of liver size and consistency, as well as gallbladder size. Gallbladder length normally varies from 1.5-5.5 cm (average: 3 cm) in infants to 4-8 cm in adolescents; width ranges from 0.5-2.5 cm for all ages. Gallbladder distention may be seen in infants with sepsis. The gallbladder is often absent in infants with biliary atresia.

Jaundice (Icterus)

Yellow discoloration of the sclera, skin, and mucous membranes is a sign of hyperbilirubinemia (see Chapter 123.3). Clinically apparent jaundice in children and adults occurs when the serum concentration of bilirubin reaches 2-3 mg/dL (34-51 μmol/L); the neonate might not appear jaundiced until the bilirubin level is >5 mg/dL (>85 μmol/L). Jaundice may be the earliest and only sign of hepatic dysfunction. Liver disease must be suspected in the infant who appears only mildly jaundiced but has dark urine or acholic (light-colored) stools. Immediate evaluation to establish the cause is required.

Measurement of the total serum bilirubin concentration allows quantitation of jaundice. Bilirubin occurs in plasma in 4 forms: *unconjugated* bilirubin tightly bound to albumin; *free* or *unbound bilirubin* (the form responsible for kernicterus, because it can cross cell membranes); *conjugated bilirubin* (the only fraction to appear in urine); and δ *fraction* (bilirubin covalently bound to albumin), which appears in serum when hepatic excretion of conjugated bilirubin is impaired in patients with hepatobiliary disease. The δ fraction permits conjugated bilirubin to persist in the circulation and delays resolution of jaundice. Although the terms *direct* and *indirect* bilirubin are used equivalently with *conjugated* and *unconjugated* bilirubin, this is not quantitatively correct, because the direct fraction includes both conjugated bilirubin and δ bilirubin.

Investigation of jaundice in an infant or older child must include determination of the accumulation of both unconjugated and conjugated bilirubin. Unconjugated hyperbilirubinemia might indicate increased production, hemolysis, reduced hepatic removal, or altered metabolism of bilirubin (Table 382.2). Conjugated hyperbilirubinemia reflects decreased excretion by damaged hepatic parenchymal cells or disease of the biliary tract, which may be a result of obstruction, sepsis, toxins, inflammation, and genetic or metabolic disease (Table 382.3).

Pruritus

Intense generalized itching can occur in patients with chronic liver disease often in association with cholestasis (conjugated hyperbilirubinemia). Symptoms can be generalized or localized (commonly to palms and soles), are usually worse at night, are exacerbated with stress and heat, and are relieved by cool temperatures. Pruritus is unrelated to the degree of hyperbilirubinemia; deeply jaundiced patients can be asymptomatic.

The pathogenesis of pruritus remains unknown, however, multiple suspected pruritogens have been reported including bile acids, histamine, serotonin, progesterone metabolites, endogenous opioids, the potent neuronal activator lysophosphatidic acid (LPA), and the LPA-forming enzyme, autotaxin (ATX). Ultimately, a multifactorial process is suspected as evidenced by the symptomatic relief of pruritus after administration of various therapeutic agents including bile acid-binding agents (cholestyramine), choleretic agents (ursodeoxycholic acid), opiate antagonists, antihistamines, serotonin reuptake inhibitors (sertraline), and antibiotics. Plasmapheresis, molecular adsorbent recirculating system therapy, and

Table 382.2	Differential Diagnosis of Unconjugated Hyperbilirubinemia

INCREASED PRODUCTION OF UNCONJUGATED BILIRUBIN FROM HEME
Hemolytic Disease (Hereditary or Acquired)
Isoimmune hemolysis (neonatal; acute or delayed transfusion reaction; autoimmune)
• Rh incompatibility
• ABO incompatibility
• Other blood group incompatibilities
Congenital spherocytosis
Hereditary elliptocytosis
Infantile pyknocytosis
Erythrocyte enzyme defects
Hemoglobinopathy
• Sickle cell anemia
• Thalassemia
• Others
Sepsis
Microangiopathy
• Hemolytic-uremic syndrome
• Hemangioma
• Mechanical trauma (heart valve)
Ineffective erythropoiesis
Drugs
Infection
Enclosed hematoma
Polycythemia
• Diabetic mother
• Fetal transfusion (recipient)
• Delayed cord clamping

DECREASED DELIVERY OF UNCONJUGATED BILIRUBIN (IN PLASMA) TO HEPATOCYTE
Right-sided congestive heart failure
Portacaval shunt

DECREASED BILIRUBIN UPTAKE ACROSS HEPATOCYTE MEMBRANE
Presumed enzyme transporter deficiency
Competitive inhibition
• Breast milk jaundice
• Lucey-Driscoll syndrome
• Drug inhibition (radiocontrast material)
Miscellaneous
• Hypothyroidism
• Hypoxia
• Acidosis

DECREASED STORAGE OF UNCONJUGATED BILIRUBIN IN CYTOSOL (DECREASED Y AND Z PROTEINS)
Competitive inhibition
Fever

DECREASED BIOTRANSFORMATION (CONJUGATION)
Neonatal jaundice (physiologic)
Inhibition (drugs)
Hereditary (Crigler-Najjar)
• Type I (complete enzyme deficiency)
• Type II (partial deficiency)
Gilbert disease
Hepatocellular dysfunction

ENTEROHEPATIC RECIRCULATION
Breast milk jaundice
Intestinal obstruction
• Ileal atresia
• Hirschsprung disease
• Cystic fibrosis
• Pyloric stenosis
Antibiotic administration

Table 382.3	Differential Diagnosis of Neonatal and Infantile Cholestasis

INFECTIOUS
Generalized bacterial sepsis
Viral hepatitis
- Hepatitides A, B, C, D, E
- Cytomegalovirus
- Rubella virus
- Herpesviruses: herpes simplex, human herpesvirus 6 and 7
- Varicella virus
- Coxsackievirus
- Echovirus
- Reovirus type 3
- Parvovirus B19
- HIV
- Adenovirus
Others
- Toxoplasmosis
- Syphilis
- Tuberculosis
- Listeriosis
- Urinary tract infection

TOXIC
Sepsis
Parenteral nutrition related
Drug, dietary supplement, herbal related

METABOLIC
Disorders of amino acid metabolism
- Tyrosinemia
Disorders of lipid metabolism
- Wolman disease
- Niemann-Pick disease (type C)
- Gaucher disease
Cholesterol ester storage disease
Disorders of carbohydrate metabolism
- Galactosemia
- Fructosemia
- Glycogenosis IV
Disorders of bile acid biosynthesis
Other metabolic defects
- α_1-Antitrypsin deficiency
- Cystic fibrosis
- Hypopituitarism
- Hypothyroidism
- Zellweger (cerebrohepatorenal) syndrome

- Wilson disease
- Gestational alloimmune liver disease (previously *neonatal iron storage disease*)
- Indian childhood cirrhosis/infantile copper overload
- Congenital disorders of glycosylation
- Mitochondrial hepatopathies
- Citrin deficiency

GENETIC OR CHROMOSOMAL
Trisomies 17, 18, 21

INTRAHEPATIC CHOLESTASIS SYNDROMES
"Idiopathic" neonatal hepatitis
Alagille syndrome
Intrahepatic cholestasis (progressive familial intrahepatic cholestasis [PFIC])
- FIC-1 deficiency
- Bile salt export pump (BSEP) deficiency
- MDR3 deficiency
- Tight junction protein 2 deficiency
- Farnesoid X receptor (FXR) mutations
Familial benign recurrent cholestasis associated with lymphedema (Aagenaes syndrome)
ARC (arthrogryposis, renal dysfunction, and cholestasis) syndrome
Caroli disease (cystic dilation of intrahepatic ducts)

EXTRAHEPATIC DISEASES
Biliary atresia
Sclerosing cholangitis
Bile duct stricture/stenosis
Choledochal–pancreaticoductal junction anomaly
Spontaneous perforation of the bile duct
Choledochal cyst
Mass (neoplasia, stone)
Bile/mucous plug ("inspissated bile")

MISCELLANEOUS
Shock and hypoperfusion
Associated with enteritis
Associated with intestinal obstruction
Neonatal lupus erythematosus
Myeloproliferative disease (trisomy 21)
Hemophagocytic lymphohistiocytosis (HLH)
COACH syndrome (coloboma, oligophrenia, ataxia, cerebellar vermis hypoplasia, hepatic fibrosis)
Cholangiocyte cilia defects

surgical diversion of bile (partial and total biliary diversion) have been used in attempts to provide relief for medically refractory pruritus.

Spider Angiomas

Vascular spiders *(telangiectasias)*, characterized by central pulsating arterioles from which small, wiry venules radiate, may be seen in patients with chronic liver disease. These are usually most prominent in the superior vena cava distribution area (on the face and chest). Their size varies between 1 and 10 mm and they exhibit central clearing with pressure. They presumably reflect altered estrogen metabolism in the presence of hepatic dysfunction.

Palmar Erythema

Blotchy erythema, most noticeable over the thenar and hypothenar eminences and on the tips of the fingers, is also noted in patients with chronic liver disease. Abnormal serum estradiol levels and regional alterations in peripheral circulation have been identified as possible causes.

Xanthomas

The marked elevation of serum cholesterol levels (to >500 mg/dL) associated with some forms of chronic cholestasis, especially Alagille syndrome, can cause the deposition of lipid in the dermis and subcutane-

ous tissue. Brown nodules can develop, first over the extensor surfaces of the extremities; rarely, xanthelasma of the eyelids develops.

Portal Hypertension

Portal hypertension occurs when there is increased portal resistance and/or increased portal flow. The portal system drains the splanchnic area (abdominal portion of the gastrointestinal tract, pancreas, and spleen) into the hepatic sinusoids. Normal portal pressure is between 1 and 5 mm Hg. Portal hypertension is defined as a portal pressure greater than or equal to 6 mm Hg. Clinically significant portal hypertension exists when pressure exceeds a threshold of 10-12 mm Hg. Portal hypertension is the main complication of cirrhosis, directly responsible for 2 of the most common and potentially lethal complications: ascites and variceal hemorrhage.

Ascites

Ascites is a consequence of increased hydrostatic and osmotic pressures within the hepatic and mesenteric capillaries resulting in transfer of fluid from the blood vessels to the lymphatics that overcomes the drainage capacity of the lymphatic system. Ascites can also be associated with nephrotic syndrome and other urinary tract abnormalities, metabolic diseases (such as lysosomal storage diseases), congenital or acquired heart disease, and hydrops fetalis. Factors favoring the intraabdominal accumulation of fluid include decreased plasma colloid (albumin) osmotic pressure, increased capillary hydrostatic pressure, increased ascitic colloid osmotic fluid pressure, and decreased ascitic fluid hydrostatic pressure. Abnormal renal sodium retention plays a central role.

Gastrointestinal Bleeding

Chronic liver disease may manifest as gastrointestinal hemorrhage. Bleeding may result from portal hypertensive gastropathy, gastric antral vascular ectasia, or varix rupture. Variceal hemorrhage is classically from an esophageal origin but may be caused by gastric, duodenal, peristomal, or rectal varices. Variceal hemorrhage results from increased pressure within the varix, which leads to changes in the diameter of the varix and increased wall tension. When the variceal wall strength is exceeded, physical rupture of the varix results. Given the high blood flow and pressure in the portosystemic collateral system, coupled with the lack of a natural mechanism to tamponade variceal bleeding, the rate of hemorrhage can be striking.

Encephalopathy

Hepatic encephalopathy can be manifest as any neurologic dysfunction, but it is most likely to present in subtle forms such as deterioration of school performance, sleep disturbances, depression, or emotional outbursts. It can be recurrent and precipitated by intercurrent illness, drugs, bleeding, or electrolyte and acid-base disturbances. The appearance of hepatic encephalopathy depends on the presence of portosystemic shunting, alterations in the blood–brain barrier, and the interactions of toxic metabolites with the central nervous system. Postulated causes include altered ammonia metabolism, synergistic neurotoxins, decreased cerebral oxygen metabolism and blood flow, or false neurotransmitters with plasma amino acid imbalance.

Endocrine Abnormalities

Endocrine abnormalities are more common in older adolescents and adults with hepatic disease than in children. They reflect alterations in hepatic synthetic, storage, and metabolic functions, including those concerned with hormonal metabolism in the liver. Proteins that bind hormones in plasma are synthesized in the liver, and steroid hormones are conjugated in the liver and excreted in the urine; failure of such functions can have clinical consequences. Endocrine abnormalities can also result from malnutrition or specific deficiencies.

Renal Dysfunction

Systemic disease or toxins can affect the liver and kidneys simultaneously, or parenchymal liver disease can produce secondary impairment of renal function. In hepatobiliary disorders, there may be renal alterations in sodium and water economy, impaired renal concentrating ability, and alterations in potassium metabolism. Ascites in patients with cirrhosis may be related to inappropriate retention of sodium by the kidneys and expansion of plasma volume, or it may be related to sodium retention mediated by diminished effective plasma volume.

Hepatorenal syndrome is defined as functional renal failure in patients with end-stage liver disease. The pathophysiology of hepatorenal syndrome is related to splanchnic vasodilation, mesenteric angiogenesis, and decreased effective blood volume with resulting decreased renal perfusion. The hallmark is intense renal vasoconstriction (mediated by hemodynamic, humoral, or neurogenic mechanisms) with coexistent systemic vasodilation. The diagnosis is supported by the findings of oliguria (<1 mL/kg/day), a characteristic pattern of urine electrolyte abnormalities (urine sodium <10 mEq/L, fractional excretion of sodium of <1%, urine: plasma creatinine ratio <10, and normal urinary sediment), absence of hypovolemia, and exclusion of other kidney pathology. The best treatment of hepatorenal syndrome is timely liver transplantation, with complete renal recovery expected.

Pulmonary Involvement

Hepatopulmonary syndrome (HPS) is characterized by the typical triad of hypoxemia, intrapulmonary vascular dilations, and liver disease. There is intrapulmonic right-to-left shunting of blood resulting from enlarged pulmonary vessels that prevents adequate exposure to oxygen-rich alveoli of red blood cells traveling through the center of the vessel. Shunting of vasodilatory mediators from the mesentery away from the liver is thought to contribute. HPS should be suspected and investigated in the child with chronic liver disease with history of shortness of breath or exercise intolerance and clinical examination findings of cyanosis (particularly of the lips and fingers), digital clubbing, and oxygen saturations <96%, particularly in the upright position. Treatment is timely liver transplantation; resolution of pulmonary involvement usually follows.

Portopulmonary hypertension is a condition characterized by an increase in the resistance to pulmonary arterial blood flow in the setting of portal hypertension. It is defined by a pulmonary arterial pressure >25 mm Hg at rest and above 30 mm Hg with exercise, elevated pulmonary vascular resistance with pulmonary arterial occlusion pressure, or a left-ventricular end-diastolic pressure of <15 mm Hg. Although the pathophysiology is unclear, deficiency in endothelial prostacyclin synthase and increased circulating endothelin-1 have been implicated as a cause for the vasculopathy. Autopsy studies have demonstrated the coexistence of portal hypertension, microscopic pulmonary artery thromboembolism, endothelial and smooth muscle proliferation, and platelet aggregates contributing to portopulmonary hypertension development. Symptoms suggesting a diagnosis include exertional dyspnea, fatigue, syncope, palpitations, and chest pain. Pulmonary artery directed therapy is the cornerstone of management, along with consideration of liver transplant.

Recurrent Cholangitis

Ascending infection of the biliary system is often seen in pediatric cholestatic disorders, most commonly because of Gram-negative enteric organisms such as *Escherichia coli*, *Klebsiella*, *Pseudomonas*, and *Enterococcus*. Liver transplantation is the definitive treatment for recurrent cholangitis, especially when medical therapy is not effective.

Miscellaneous Manifestations of Liver Dysfunction

Nonspecific signs of acute and chronic liver disease include anorexia, which often affects patients with anicteric hepatitis and with cirrhosis associated with chronic cholestasis; abdominal pain or distention resulting from ascites, spontaneous peritonitis, or visceromegaly; malnutrition and growth failure; and bleeding, which may be a result of altered synthesis of coagulation factors (biliary obstruction with vitamin K deficiency or excessive hepatic damage) or to portal hypertension with hypersplenism. In the presence of hypersplenism, there can be decreased synthesis of specific clotting factors, production of qualitatively abnormal proteins, or alterations in platelet number and function. Altered drug metabolism can prolong the biologic half-life of commonly administered medications.

Bibliography is available at Expert Consult.

382.1 Evaluation of Patients With Possible Liver Dysfunction

James E. Squires and William F. Balistreri

Adequate evaluation of an infant, child, or adolescent with suspected liver disease begins with an appropriate and accurate history, a carefully performed physical examination, and skillful interpretation of signs and symptoms. Further evaluation is aided by judicious selection of diagnostic tests, followed by the use of imaging modalities and/or a liver biopsy (Fig. 382.1). Most of the so-called liver "function" tests *do not* measure any specific hepatic function: a rise in serum aminotransferase levels reflects liver cell *injury*, an increase in immunoglobulin levels reflects an immunologic response to injury, or an elevation in serum bilirubin levels can reflect any of several disturbances of bilirubin metabolism (see Table 382.2). Any single biochemical assay provides limited information, which must be placed in the context of the entire clinical picture. The most cost-efficient approach is to become familiar

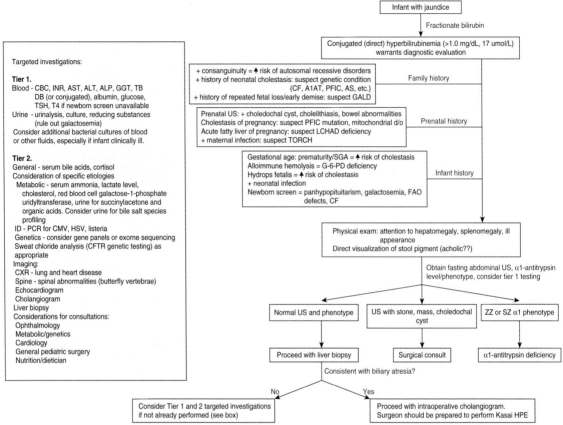

Fig. 382.1 Treatment algorithm for a 2-8 wk-old with cholestasis, based on clinical practice guidelines. *A1AT*, alpha one antitrypsin deficiency; *ALP*, alkaline phosphatase; *ALT*, alanine aminotransferase; *AS*, Alagille syndrome; *AST*, aspartate aminotransferase; *CBC*, complete blood count; *CF*, cystic fibrosis; *CFTR*, cystic fibrosis transmembrane receptor; *CMV*, cytomegalovirus; *CXR*, chest x-ray; *DB*, direct bilirubin; *FAO*, fatty acid oxidation; *GALD*, gestational alloimmune liver disease; *GGT*, gamma glutamyl transpeptidase; *HSV*, herpes simplex virus; *INR*, International normalized ratio; *LCHAD*, long-chain 3-hydroxyacyl-coenzyme A dehydrogenase deficiency; *PCR*, polymerase chain reaction; *PFIC*, progressive familial intrahepatic cholestasis; *SGA*, small for gestational age; *TB*, total bilirubin; *TSH*, thyroid stimulating hormone; *US*, ultrasound. (Data from Fawaz R, Baumann U, Ekong U, et al: Guideline for the evaluation of cholestatic jaundice in infants: joint recommendations of the North American Society for pediatric gastroenterology, hepatology, and nutrition and the European Society for Pediatric Gastroenterology, Hepatology, and Nutrition, J Pediatr Gastroenterol Nutr 64(1):154–168, 2017; and from Feldman AG, Mack CL: Biliary atresia: clinical lessons learned, J Pediatr Gastroenterol Nutr 61(2):167–75, 2015.)

with the rationale, implications, and limitations of a selected group of tests so that specific questions can be answered. Young infants with cholestatic jaundice should be evaluated promptly to identify patients needing specific medical treatment or surgical intervention.

For a patient with suspected liver disease, evaluation addresses the following issues in sequence: Is liver disease present? If so, what is its nature? What is its severity? Is specific treatment available? How can we monitor the response to treatment? What is the prognosis?

BIOCHEMICAL TESTS

Laboratory tests commonly used to screen for or to confirm a suspicion of liver disease include measurements of serum aminotransferase (Table 382.4), bilirubin (total and fractionated), alkaline phosphatase (AP) and gamma glutamyl-transpeptidase (GGT) levels, as well as determinations of prothrombin time (PT) or international normalized ratio (INR) and serum albumin level. These tests are complementary, provide an estimation of synthetic and excretory functions, and might suggest the nature of the disturbance (inflammation or cholestasis).

The severity of the liver disease may be reflected in clinical signs or biochemical alterations. Clinical signs include encephalopathy, variceal hemorrhage, worsening jaundice, apparent shrinkage of liver mass owing to massive necrosis, or onset of ascites. Biochemical alterations reflective of severity include hypoglycemia, acidosis, hyperammonemia, electrolyte

imbalance, continued hyperbilirubinemia, marked hypoalbuminemia, or a prolonged PT or INR that is unresponsive to parenteral administration of vitamin K.

Acute liver cell injury (parenchymal disease) caused by viral hepatitis, drug- or toxin-induced liver disease, shock, hypoxemia, or metabolic disease is best suggested by a marked increase in serum aminotransferase levels. Cholestasis (obstructive disease) involves regurgitation of bile components into serum; the serum levels of total and conjugated bilirubin and serum bile acids are elevated. Elevations in serum AP, 5′ nucleotidase, and GGT levels are also sensitive indicators of obstruction or inflammation of the biliary tract. Fractionation of the total serum bilirubin level into conjugated and unconjugated bilirubin fractions helps to distinguish between elevations caused by processes such as hemolysis and those caused by hepatic dysfunction. A predominant elevation in the conjugated bilirubin level provides a relatively sensitive index of hepatocellular disease or hepatic excretory dysfunction.

Alanine aminotransferase (ALT, serum glutamate pyruvate transaminase) is *liver* specific, whereas aspartate aminotransferase (AST, serum glutamic-oxaloacetic transaminase) is derived from other organs in addition to the liver. The most marked rises of AST and ALT levels can be noted in patients with acute hepatocellular injury; a several thousand–fold elevation can result from acute viral hepatitis, toxic injury (e.g., acetaminophen), hypoxia, or hypoperfusion (see Table 382.4).

Table 382.4	Causes of Elevated Serum Aminotransferase Levels*

CHRONIC, MILD ELEVATIONS, ALT > AST (<150 U/L OR 5 × NORMAL)

Hepatic Causes
α_1-Antitrypsin deficiency
Autoimmune hepatitis
Chronic viral hepatitis (B, C, and D)
Hemochromatosis
Medications and toxins
Steatosis and steatohepatitis
Wilson disease

Nonhepatic Causes
Celiac disease
Hyperthyroidism

SEVERE, ACUTE ELEVATIONS, ALT > AST (>1,000 U/L OR >20-25 × NORMAL)

Hepatic Causes
Acute bile duct obstruction
Acute Budd-Chiari syndrome
Acute viral hepatitis
Autoimmune hepatitis
Drugs and toxins
Hepatic artery ligation
Ischemic hepatitis
Wilson disease

SEVERE, ACUTE ELEVATIONS, AST > ALT (>1,000 U/L OR >20-25 × NORMAL)

Hepatic Cause
Medications or toxins in a patient with underlying alcoholic liver injury

Nonhepatic Cause
Acute rhabdomyolysis

CHRONIC, MILD ELEVATIONS, AST > ALT (<150 U/L, <5 × NORMAL)

Hepatic Causes
Alcohol-related liver injury (AST/ALT > 2:1, AST nearly always <300 U/L)
Cirrhosis

Nonhepatic Causes
Hypothyroidism
Macro-AST
Myopathy
Strenuous exercise

CHRONIC, MILD ELEVATIONS, ALT > AST (<150 U/L OR 5 × NORMAL)

*Virtually any liver disease can cause moderate aminotransferase elevations (5-15 × normal).

After blunt abdominal trauma, parallel elevations in aminotransferase levels can provide an early clue to hepatic injury. A differential rise or fall in AST and ALT levels sometimes provides useful information. In acute hepatitis, the rise in ALT may be greater than the rise in AST. In alcohol-induced liver injury, fulminant echovirus infection, and various metabolic diseases, more predominant rises in the AST level are reported. In chronic liver disease or in intrahepatic and extrahepatic biliary obstruction, AST and ALT elevations may be less marked. Elevated serum aminotransferase levels are seen in patients with nonalcoholic fatty liver disease and nonalcoholic steatohepatitis (NASH).

Hepatic synthetic function is reflected in serum albumin and protein levels and in the PT or INR. Examination of serum globulin concentration and of the relative amounts of the globulin fractions may be helpful. Patients with autoimmune hepatitis often have high γ-globulin levels and increased titers of anti–smooth muscle, antinuclear, and anti–liver-kidney-microsome antibodies. Antimitochondrial antibodies may also be found in patients with autoimmune hepatitis. A resurgence in α-fetoprotein levels can suggest hepatoma, hepatoblastoma, or hereditary

tyrosinemia. Hypoalbuminemia caused by depressed synthesis can complicate severe liver disease and serve as a prognostic factor. Deficiencies of factor V and of the vitamin K–dependent factors (II, VII, IX, and X) can occur in patients with severe liver disease or fulminant hepatic failure. If the PT or INR is prolonged as a result of intestinal malabsorption of vitamin K (resulting from cholestasis) or decreased nutritional intake of vitamin K, parenteral administration of vitamin K should correct the coagulopathy, leading to normalization within 12-24 hr. *Unresponsiveness to parenteral vitamin K suggests severe hepatic disease.* Persistently low levels of factor VII are evidence of a poor prognosis in patients with fulminant liver disease.

Interpretation of results of biochemical tests of hepatic structure and function must be made in the context of age-related changes. The activity of AP varies considerably with age. Normal growing children have significant elevations of serum AP activity originating from influx into serum of the isoenzyme that originates in bone, particularly in rapidly growing adolescents. An isolated increase in AP does not indicate hepatic or biliary disease if other liver tests are normal. Other enzymes such as 5′ nucleotidase and GGT are increased in cholestatic conditions and may be more specific for hepatobiliary disease. 5′ nucleotidase is not found in bone. GGT exhibits high enzyme activity in early life that declines rapidly with age. Cholesterol concentrations increase throughout life but may be markedly elevated in patients with intra- or extrahepatic cholestasis and decreased in severe acute liver disease such as hepatitis.

Interpretation of serum ammonia values must be carried out with caution because of variability in their physiologic determinants and the inherent difficulty in laboratory measurement.

LIVER BIOPSY

Liver biopsy combined with clinical data can suggest a cause for hepatocellular injury or cholestatic disease in most cases. Specimens of liver tissue can be used to determine a precise histologic diagnosis in patients with neonatal cholestasis, chronic hepatitis, nonalcoholic fatty liver disease or NASH, metabolic liver disease, intrahepatic cholestasis, congenital hepatic fibrosis, or undefined portal hypertension. The sample may be subjected to enzyme analysis to detect inborn errors of metabolism and to analysis of stored material such as iron, copper, or specific metabolites. Liver biopsies can monitor responses to therapy or detect complications of treatment with potentially hepatotoxic agents, such as aspirin, antiinfectives (minocycline, ketoconazole, isoniazid), antimetabolites, antineoplastics, or anticonvulsant agents.

In infants and children, needle biopsy of the liver is easily accomplished percutaneously. The amount of tissue obtained, even in small infants, is usually sufficient for histologic interpretation and for biochemical analyses, if the latter are deemed necessary. Percutaneous liver biopsy can be performed safely in infants as young as 1 wk of age. Contraindications to the percutaneous approach include prolonged PT or INR; thrombocytopenia; suspicion of a vascular, cystic, or infectious lesion in the path of the needle; and severe ascites. If administration of fresh-frozen plasma or of platelet transfusions fails to correct a prolonged PT, INR, or thrombocytopenia, a tissue specimen can be obtained via alternative techniques. Considerations include either the open laparotomy (wedge) approach by a general surgeon or the transjugular approach under ultrasound and fluoroscopic guidance by an experienced pediatric interventional radiologist in an appropriately equipped fluoroscopy suite. The risk of development of a complication such as hemorrhage, hematoma, creation of an arteriovenous fistula, pneumothorax, or bile peritonitis is small.

HEPATIC IMAGING PROCEDURES

Various techniques help define the size, shape, and architecture of the liver and the anatomy of the intrahepatic and extrahepatic biliary trees. Although imaging might not provide a precise histologic and biochemical diagnosis, specific questions can be answered, such as whether hepatomegaly is related to accumulation of fat or glycogen or is caused by a tumor or cyst. These studies can direct further evaluation such as percutaneous biopsy and make possible prompt referral of patients with biliary obstruction to a surgeon. Choice of imaging procedure should be part of a carefully formulated diagnostic approach, with avoidance of redundant demonstrations by several techniques.

A *plain x-ray study* can suggest hepatomegaly, but a carefully performed physical examination gives a more reliable assessment of liver size. The liver might appear less dense than normal in patients with fatty infiltration or denser with deposition of heavy metals such as iron. A hepatic or biliary tract mass can displace an air-filled loop of bowel. Calcifications may be evident in the liver (parasitic or neoplastic disease), in the vasculature (portal vein thrombosis), or in the gallbladder or biliary tree (gallstones). Collections of gas may be seen within the liver (abscess), biliary tract, or portal circulation (necrotizing enterocolitis).

Ultrasound provides information about the size, composition, and blood flow to the liver. Increased echogenicity is observed with fatty infiltration; mass lesions as small as 1-2 cm may be shown. Ultrasound has replaced cholangiography in detecting stones in the gallbladder or biliary tree. Even in neonates, ultrasound can accurately assess gallbladder size, detect dilation of the biliary tract, and define a choledochal cyst. In infants with biliary atresia, ultrasound findings might include small or absent gallbladder; nonvisualization of the common duct; and presence of the triangular cord sign, a triangular or tubular-shaped echogenic density in the bifurcation of the portal vein, representing fibrous remnants at the porta hepatis. Hyperechogenic hepatic parenchyma can be seen with metabolic disease (glycogen storage disease) or fatty liver (obesity, malnutrition, parenteral alimentation, corticosteroids). In patients with portal hypertension, Doppler ultrasound can evaluate patency of the portal vein, demonstrate collateral circulation, and assess size of spleen and amount of ascites. Relatively small amounts of *ascitic fluid* can also be detected. The use of Doppler ultrasound has been helpful in determining vascular patency after liver transplantation. In patients with liver lesions, newer intravenous agents consisting of insoluble gas bubbles with a lipoprotein shell have enabled contrast-enhanced ultrasonographic lesion characterization without the associated risks often accompanied by more traditional imaging modalities such as CT scan (radiation, contrast-induced renal injury) and *magnetic resonance imaging* (MRI; sedation).

CT scanning provides information similar to that obtained by ultrasound but is less suitable for use in patients younger than 2 yr of age because of the small size of structures, the paucity of intraabdominal fat for contrast, and the need for heavy sedation or general anesthesia. CT scan may be more accurate than ultrasound in detecting focal lesions such as tumors, cysts, and abscesses. When enhanced by contrast medium, CT scanning can reveal a neoplastic mass density only slightly different from that of a normal liver. When a hepatic tumor is suspected, CT scanning is currently considered the best method to define anatomic extent, solid or cystic nature, and vascularity. CT scanning can also reveal subtle differences in density of liver parenchyma, the average liver attenuation coefficient being reduced with fatty infiltration.

MRI is a useful alternative that limits radiation exposure. Magnetic resonance cholangiography can be of value in differentiating biliary tract lesions. MRI with Eovist (gadoxetate disodium) can assist in the detection and characterization of known or suspected focal liver lesions. In differentiating obstructive from nonobstructive cholestasis, CT scanning or MRI identifies the precise level of obstruction more often than ultrasound. Either CT scanning or ultrasound may be used to guide percutaneously placed fine needles for biopsies, aspiration of specific lesions, or cholangiography.

Elastography is a novel noninvasive method to assess for liver *stiffness*, a measure of the development of hepatic fibrosis in patients with liver disease. Both ultrasound and MR methods have been developed. These noninvasive techniques allow for monitoring fibrosis progression and development of cirrhosis, improved characterization of hepatic tumors, and prognostic stratification of diseases such as nonalcoholic fatty liver disease and NASH.

Radionuclide scanning relies on selective uptake of a radiopharmaceutical agent. Commonly used agents include technetium-99m–labeled sulfur colloid, which undergoes phagocytosis by Kupffer cells; ^{99m}Tc-iminodiacetic acid agents, which are taken up by hepatocytes and excreted into bile in a fashion similar to bilirubin; and gallium-67, which is concentrated in inflammatory and neoplastic cells. The anatomic resolution possible with hepatic scintiscans is generally less than that obtained with CT scanning, MRI, or ultrasound.

The ^{99m}Tc-sulfur colloid scan can detect focal lesions (tumors, cysts, abscesses) >2-3 cm in diameter. This modality can help to evaluate patients with possible cirrhosis and with patchy hepatic uptake and a shift of colloid uptake from liver to bone marrow.

Cholangiography, direct visualization of the intrahepatic and extrahepatic biliary tree after injection of opaque material, may be required in some patients to evaluate the cause, location, or extent of biliary obstruction. Percutaneous transhepatic cholangiography with a fine needle is the technique of choice in infants and young children. The likelihood of opacifying the biliary tract is excellent in patients in whom CT scanning, MRI, or ultrasound demonstrates dilated ducts. Percutaneous transhepatic cholangiography has been used to outline the biliary ductal system.

Endoscopic retrograde cholangiopancreatography is an alternative method of examining the bile ducts in older children. The papilla of Vater is cannulated under direct vision through a fiberoptic endoscope, and contrast material is injected into the biliary and pancreatic ducts to outline the anatomy. The advantage of endoscopic retrograde cholangiopancreatography is that it allows therapeutic interventions of the extrahepatic biliary tree (stone extraction, stent placement).

Selective angiography of the celiac, superior mesenteric, or hepatic artery can be used to visualize the hepatic or portal circulation. Both arterial and venous circulatory systems of the liver can be examined. Angiography is often required to define the blood supply of tumors before surgery and is useful in the study of patients with known or presumed portal hypertension. The patency of the portal system, the extent of collateral circulation, and the caliber of vessels under consideration for a shunting procedure can be evaluated. MRI can provide similar information.

DIAGNOSTIC APPROACH TO INFANTS WITH JAUNDICE

Well-appearing infants can have cholestatic jaundice. Biliary atresia and neonatal hepatitis are the most common causes of cholestasis in early infancy. Biliary atresia portends a poor prognosis unless it is identified early. The best outcome for this disorder is with early surgical reconstruction (45-60 days of age). History, physical examination, and the detection of a conjugated hyperbilirubinemia via examination of total and direct bilirubin are the first steps in evaluating the jaundiced infant (see Fig. 382.1). Consultation with a pediatric gastroenterologist should be sought early in the course of the evaluation.

Bibliography is available at Expert Consult.

Chapter **383**
Cholestasis
第三百八十三章
胆汁淤积

中文导读

本章主要介绍了新生儿胆汁淤积和年长儿童胆汁淤积症。具体描述了新生儿胆汁淤积的发病机制、评估方法、肝内胆汁淤积、胆汁酸辅酶A连接酶缺乏症、胚胎发生障碍、胆道闭锁、慢性胆汁淤积症的治疗和预后；详细阐述了肝内胆汁淤积，其中包括新生儿肝炎以及胆汁酸的运输、分泌、结合和生物合成障碍；详细介绍了胆道闭锁，其中包括新生儿特发性肝炎与胆道闭锁的鉴别诊断和疑似胆道闭锁的处理等内容。

383.1 Neonatal Cholestasis

*H. Hesham Abdel-Kader Hassan
and William F. Balistreri*

Neonatal cholestasis is defined biochemically as prolonged elevation of the serum levels of conjugated bilirubin beyond the first 14 days of life. Jaundice that appears after 2 wk of age, continues to progress, or does not resolve by this age should be evaluated and a conjugated bilirubin level determined.

Cholestasis in a newborn can be caused by infectious, genetic, metabolic, or undefined abnormalities giving rise to *mechanical* obstruction of bile flow or to *functional impairment* of hepatic excretory function and bile secretion (see Table 383.1). Mechanical lesions include stricture or obstruction of the common bile duct; biliary atresia is the prototypic obstructive abnormality. Functional impairment of bile secretion can result from congenital defects or damage to liver cells or to the biliary secretory apparatus.

Neonatal cholestasis can be divided into extrahepatic and intrahepatic disease (Fig. 383.1). The clinical features of any form of cholestasis are similar. In an affected neonate, the diagnosis of certain entities, such as galactosemia, cystic fibrosis, sepsis, or hypothyroidism, is relatively simple and a part of most neonatal screening programs. In most cases, the cause of cholestasis is more obscure. Differentiation among biliary atresia and idiopathic neonatal hepatitis is particularly difficult.

MECHANISMS
Metabolic liver disease caused by inborn errors of bile acid synthesis or transport is associated with accumulation of atypical toxic bile acids and failure to produce normal choleretic and trophic bile acids. The clinical and histologic manifestations are nonspecific and are similar to those noted in other forms of neonatal hepatobiliary injury. Autoimmune mechanisms may also be responsible for some of the enigmatic forms of neonatal liver injury.

Some of the histologic manifestations of hepatic injury in early life are not seen in older patients. Giant cell transformation of hepatocytes occurs commonly in infants with cholestasis and can occur in any form of neonatal liver injury. It is more common and more severe in intrahepatic forms of cholestasis. The clinical and histologic findings of patients with neonatal hepatitis and those with biliary atresia are somewhat similar, but there are distinguishing features. The basic process common to both is an undefined initiating insult causing inflammation of the liver cells or of the cells within the biliary tract. If the bile duct epithelium is the predominant site of disease, cholangitis can result and

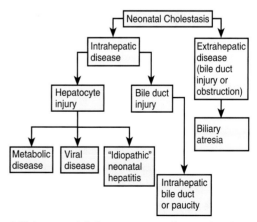

Fig. 383.1 **Neonatal cholestasis.** Conceptual approach to the group of diseases presenting as cholestasis in the neonate. There are areas of overlap. Patients with biliary atresia might have some degree of intrahepatic injury. Patients with "idiopathic" neonatal hepatitis might, in the future, be determined to have a primary metabolic or viral disease.

lead to progressive sclerosis and narrowing of the biliary tree, the ultimate state being complete obliteration *(biliary atresia)*. Injury to liver cells can present the clinical and histologic picture of "neonatal hepatitis." This concept does not account for the precise mechanism, but it offers an explanation for well-documented cases of unexpected postnatal evolution of the disease processes; infants initially considered to have neonatal hepatitis, with a patent biliary system shown on cholangiography, can later manifest biliary atresia.

Functional abnormalities in the generation of bile flow can also cause neonatal cholestasis. Bile flow is directly dependent on effective hepatic bile acid excretion by the hepatocytes. During the phase of relatively inefficient bile acid transport and metabolism by the liver cell in early life, minor degrees of hepatic injury can further decrease bile flow and lead to production of atypical and potentially toxic bile acids. Selective impairment of a single step in the series of events involved in hepatic excretion produces the full expression of a cholestatic syndrome. Specific defects in bile acid synthesis are found in infants with various forms of intrahepatic cholestasis (Table 383.1). Severe forms of familial cholestasis are associated with neonatal hemochromatosis, an alloimmune-mediated gestational (maternal antibodies against fetal hepatocytes) disease responsive to maternal intravenous immunoglobulin. Sepsis is known to cause cholestasis, presumably mediated by an endotoxin produced by *Escherichia coli*.

EVALUATION

Identification of cholestasis warrants a prompt effort to accurately diagnose the cause (Table 383.2). Although cholestasis in the neonate may be the initial manifestation of numerous and potentially serious disorders, the clinical manifestations are usually similar and provide few clues about the etiology. Affected infants have icterus, dark urine, light or acholic stools, and hepatomegaly, all resulting from decreased bile flow as a result of either hepatocyte injury or bile duct obstruction. Hepatic synthetic dysfunction can lead to hypoprothrombinemia and bleeding. Administration of vitamin K should be included in the initial treatment of cholestatic infants to prevent hemorrhage (intracranial).

In contrast to unconjugated hyperbilirubinemia, which can be physiologic, cholestasis (conjugated bilirubin elevation of any degree) in the neonate is **always pathologic** and prompt differentiation of the cause is imperative. The top priority is to recognize conditions that cause cholestasis and for which specific therapy is available to prevent further damage and avoid long-term complications such as sepsis, an endocrinopathy (hypothyroidism, panhypopituitarism), nutritional hepatotoxicity caused by a specific metabolic illness (galactosemia), or other metabolic diseases (tyrosinemia).

Table 383.1	Proposed Subtypes of Intrahepatic Cholestasis

A. Disorders of membrane transport and secretion
   1. Disorders of canalicular secretion
     a. Bile acid transport: BSEP deficiency
       i. Persistent, progressive (PFIC type 2)
       ii. Recurrent, benign (BRIC type 2)
     b. Phospholipid transport: MDR3 deficiency (PFIC type 3)
     c. Ion transport: cystic fibrosis (CFTR)
     d. Tight junction defect (TJP2 deficiency)
   2. Complex or multiorgan disorders
     a. FIC1 deficiency
       i. Persistent, progressive (PFIC type 1, Byler disease)
       ii. Recurrent, benign (BRIC type 1)
     b. Neonatal sclerosing cholangitis *(CLDN1)*
     c. Arthrogryposis-renal dysfunction-cholestasis syndrome *(VPS33B)*
B. Disorders of bile acid biosynthesis, conjugation and regulation
   1. Δ⁴-3-Oxosteroid-5β-reductase deficiency
   2. 3β-hydroxy-5-C27-steroid dehydrogenase/isomerase deficiency
   3. Oxysterol 7α-hydroxylase deficiency
   4. Bile acid-CoA Ligase deficiency
   5. BAAT deficiency (familial hypercholanemia)
   6. Farnesoid X receptor (FXR) deficiency
C. Disorders of embryogenesis
   1. Alagille syndrome (Jagged1 defect, syndromic bile duct paucity)
   2. Ductal plate malformation (ARPKD, ADPLD, Caroli disease)
D. Unclassified (idiopathic "neonatal hepatitis"): mechanism unknown

Note: FIC1 deficiency, BSEP deficiency, and some of the disorders of bile acid biosynthesis are characterized clinically by low levels of serum GGT despite the presence of cholestasis. In all other disorders listed, the serum GGT level is elevated.
   ADPLD, autosomal dominant polycystic liver disease (cysts in liver only); ARPKD, autosomal recessive polycystic kidney disease (cysts in liver and kidney); BAAT, bile acid transporter; BRIC, benign recurrent intrahepatic cholestasis; BSEP, bile salt export pump in; GGT, γ-glutamyl transpeptidase; PFIC, progressive familial intrahepatic cholestasis.
   From Balistreri WF, Bezerra JA, Jansen P, et al: Intrahepatic cholestasis: summary of an American Association for the study of liver diseases single-topic conference, *Hepatology* 42(1):222–235, 2005.

Another potential treatable metabolic disease, lysosomal acid lipase deficiency (LAL-D), is a rare autosomal recessive lysosomal storage disease which results in a mutation in the lysosomal acid lipase *(LIPA)* gene. The mutation creates a decline in the LAL activity, resulting in

Table 383.2	Value of Specific Tests in the Evaluation of Patients With Suspected Neonatal Cholestasis

TEST	RATIONALE
Serum bilirubin fractionation (i.e., assessment of the serum level of conjugated bilirubin)	Indicates cholestasis
Assessment of stool color (does the baby have pigmented or acholic stools?)	Indicates bile flow into intestine
Urine and serum bile acid measurement	Confirms cholestasis; low level indicates inborn error of bile acid biosynthesis
Hepatic synthetic function (albumin, coagulation profile)	Indicates severity of hepatic dysfunction
α₁-Antitrypsin phenotype	Suggests (or excludes) protease inhibitor ZZ phenotype
Thyroxine and thyroid-stimulating hormone	Suggests (or excludes) endocrinopathy
Lysosomal acid lipase enzyme activity	Suggests (or excludes) lysosomal acid lipase deficiency
Sweat chloride and mutation analysis	Suggests (or excludes) cystic fibrosis
Urine and serum amino acids and urine reducing substances	Suggests (or excludes) metabolic liver disease
Ultrasonography	Suggests (or excludes) choledochal cyst; might detect the triangular cord sign, suggesting biliary atresia
Liver biopsy	Distinguishes biliary atresia; suggests alternative diagnosis

accumulation of cholesteryl esters and, to a lesser degree, triglycerides in multiple organs, including the liver, spleen, adrenal glands, lymph nodes, intestinal mucosa, vascular endothelium, and skeletal muscle. Clinically, the disease can present in 2 major phenotypes: infantile-onset Wolman disease (WD) and later-onset cholesterol ester storage disease (CESD). LAL-D usually presents in infants with an acute-severe course progressing to liver failure. Sebelipase Alfa (recombinant human LAL enzyme) is approved for the treatment of patients with LAL-D.

Hepatobiliary disease can be the initial manifestation of homozygous α_1-antitrypsin deficiency or of cystic fibrosis. Neonatal liver disease can also be associated with congenital syphilis and specific viral infections, notably echovirus and herpes viruses including cytomegalovirus. These account for a small percentage of cases of neonatal hepatitis syndrome. The hepatitis viruses (A, B, C) rarely cause neonatal cholestasis.

Mitochondrial disorders may present with acute neonatal hepatic failure, or cholestasis; prominent among these disorders are respiratory chain defects and mitochondrial DNA depletion syndromes (Table 383.3).

The final and critical step in evaluating neonates with cholestasis is to differentiate extrahepatic biliary atresia from neonatal hepatitis.

INTRAHEPATIC CHOLESTASIS
Neonatal Hepatitis
The term *neonatal hepatitis* implies intrahepatic cholestasis (see Fig. 383.1), which has various forms (see Tables 383.1 and 383.4).

Idiopathic neonatal hepatitis, which can occur in either a sporadic or familial form, is a disease of unknown cause. Patients with the sporadic form presumably have a specific yet undefined metabolic or viral disease. Familial forms, on the other hand, presumably reflect a genetic or metabolic aberration; in the past, patients with α-1 antitrypsin deficiency were included in this category.

Aagenaes syndrome is a form of idiopathic familial intrahepatic cholestasis associated with lymphedema of the lower extremities. The relationship between liver disease and lymphedema is not understood and may be attributable to decreased hepatic lymph flow or hepatic

Table 383.3	Phenotypic Classification of Primary Mitochondrial Hepatopathies

RC (electron transport) defects (OXPHOS)
- Neonatal liver failure
  - Complex I deficiency
  - Complex IV deficiency (*SCO1* mutations)
  - Complex III deficiency (*BCS1L* mutations)
  - Co-enzyme Q deficiency
  - Multiple complex deficiencies (transfer and elongation factor mutations)
  - mtDNA depletion syndrome (*DUGOK, MPV17, POLG, SUCLG1, C10orf2/Twinkle* mutations)
- Later-onset liver dysfunction or failure
  - Alpers-Huttenlocher disease (*POLG* mutations)
  - Pearson's marrow pancreas syndrome (mtDNA deletion)
  - Mitochondrial neurogastrointestinal encephalopathy (*TYMP* mutations)
  - NNH (*MPV17* mutations)
Fatty acid oxidation defects
  - Long-chain 3 hydroxyacyl-coenzyme A dehydrogenase
  - Carnitine palmitoyltransferase I and II deficiencies
  - Carnitine-acylcarnitinetranslocase deficiency
Urea cycle enzyme deficiencies
Electron transfer flavoprotein and electron transfer flavoprotein dehydrogenase deficiencies
Phosphoenol pyruvate carboxykinase (mitochondrial) deficiency; nonketotic hyperglycemia
Citrin deficiency; neonatal intrahepatic cholestasis caused by citrin deficiency (*SLC25A13* mutations)

NN, Navajo neurohepatopathy; OXPHOS, oxidative phosphorylation; RC, respiratory chain.

From Lee WS, Sokol RJ: Mitochondrial hepatopathies: advances in genetics, therapeutic approaches, and outcomes, *J Pediatr* 163[4]:942–948, 2013, Table 1, p. 943.

lymphatic hypoplasia. Affected patients usually present with episodic cholestasis with elevation of serum aminotransferase, alkaline phosphatase, and bile acid levels. Between episodes, the patients are usually asymptomatic and biochemical indices improve. Compared to other types of hereditary neonatal cholestasis, patients with Aagenaes syndrome have a relatively good prognosis. The locus for Aagenaes syndrome is mapped to a 6.6 cM interval on chromosome 15q.

Zellweger (cerebrohepatorenal) syndrome is a rare autosomal recessive genetic disorder marked by progressive degeneration of the liver and kidneys. The incidence is estimated to be 1 in 100,000 births; the disease is usually fatal by 6-12 mo of age. Affected infants have severe, generalized hypotonia and markedly impaired neurologic function with psychomotor retardation. Patients have an abnormal head shape and unusual facies, hepatomegaly, renal cortical cysts, stippled calcifications of the patellas and greater trochanter, and ocular abnormalities. Hepatic cells on ultrastructural examination show an absence of peroxisomes. Prenatal diagnosis can be achieved through assays of peroxisomal enzymes activity (dihydroacetone-phosphate acyltransferase), peroxisomal metabolites, or molecular screening techniques. MRI performed in the third trimester can allow analysis of cerebral gyration and myelination, facilitating the prenatal diagnosis of Zellweger syndrome.

Neonatal iron storage disease (neonatal hemochromatosis, gestational alloimmune liver disease) is a rapidly progressive disease characterized by increased iron deposition in the liver, heart, and endocrine organs without increased iron stores in the reticuloendothelial system. Patients have multiorgan failure and shortened survival. Familial cases are reported, and repeated affected neonates in the same family are common. This is an alloimmune disorder with maternal antibodies directed against the fetal liver. Liver injury results in decreased hepatic hepcidin expression and thus dysregulation of placental iron flux. Neonatal hemochromatosis (or fetal loss) seems to be a **gestational alloimmune disease**, and reoccurrence of severe neonatal hemochromatosis in at-risk pregnancies may be reduced by maternal treatment with weekly high-dose intravenous immunoglobulin (1 g/kg) beginning gestational age 18 wk.

Laboratory findings include hypoglycemia, hyperbilirubinemia, hypoalbuminemia, elevated ferritin, and profound hypoprothrombinemia. Serum aminotransferase levels may be high initially but normalize with the progression of the disease. The diagnosis is usually confirmed by buccal mucosal biopsy or MRI demonstrating extrahepatic siderosis. The prognosis is poor; however, liver transplantation can be curative. Although liver transplantation for infants with neonatal hemochromatosis has a high rate of graft loss and death, outcomes are equivalent to the same age-matched recipients with acute liver failure due to other causes. Immune therapy with exchange transfusion and intravenous immunoglobulin has been reported to improve the outcome and reduce the need for liver transplantation in patients with neonatal hemochromatosis. The differential diagnosis includes familial hemophagocytic lymphohistiocytosis.

Disorders of Transport, Secretion, Conjugation, and Biosynthesis of Bile Acids
Progressive familial intrahepatic cholestasis type 1 (PFIC 1) or FIC 1 disease (formerly known as **Byler disease**) is a severe form of intrahepatic cholestasis. The disease was initially described in the Amish kindred of Jacob Byler. Affected patients present with steatorrhea, pruritus, vitamin D-deficient rickets, gradually developing cirrhosis, and low γ-glutamyl transpeptidase (GGT) levels. **PFIC 1** (FIC-1 deficiency) has been mapped to chromosome 18ql2 and results from defect in the gene for FIC-1 (ATP8Bl; see Tables 383.4 and 383.5). FIC-1 is a P-type adenosine triphosphatase that functions as aminophospholipid flippase, facilitating the transfer of phosphatidyl serine and phosphatidyl ethanolamine from the outer to inner hemileaflet of the cellular membrane. FIC-1 might also play a role in intestinal bile acid absorption, as suggested by the high level of expression in the intestine. Defective FIC-1 might also result in another form of intrahepatic cholestasis: **benign recurrent intrahepatic cholestasis (BRIC) type I**. The disease is characterized by recurrent bouts of cholestasis, jaundice, and severe pruritus. The

Table 383.4	Molecular Defects Causing Liver Disease		
GENE	**PROTEIN**	**FUNCTION, SUBSTRATE**	**DISORDER**
ATP8B1	FIC1	P-type ATPase; aminophospholipid translocase that flips phosphatidylserine and phosphatidylethanolamine from the outer to the inner layer of the canalicular membrane	PFIC 1 (Byler disease), BRIC 1, GFC
ABCB11	BSEP	Canalicular protein with ATP-binding cassette (ABC family of proteins); works as a pump transporting bile acids through the canalicular domain	PFIC 2, BRIC 2
ABCB4	MDR3	Canalicular protein with ATP-binding cassette (ABC family of proteins); works as a phospholipid flippase in canalicular membrane	PFIC 3, ICP, cholelithiasis
AKR1D1	5β-Reductase	Δ⁴-3-Oxosteroid 5β-reductase gene; regulates bile acid synthesis	BAS: neonatal cholestasis with giant cell hepatitis
HSD3B7	C27-3β-HSD	3β-Hydroxy-5-C27-steroid oxido-reductase (C27-3β-HSD) gene; regulates bile acid synthesis	BAS: chronic intrahepatic cholestasis
CYP7BI	CYP7BI	Oxysterol 7α-hydroxylase; regulates the acidic pathway of bile acid synthesis	BAS: neonatal cholestasis with giant cell hepatitis
JAG1	JAG1	Transmembrane, cell-surface proteins that interact with Notch receptors to regulate cell fate during embryogenesis	Alagille syndrome
TJP2	Tight junction protein	Belongs to the family of membrane-associated guanylate kinase homologs that are involved in the organization of epithelial and endothelial intercellular junction; regulates paracellular permeability	Intrahepatic cholestasis
NR1H4	Nuclear hormone receptor	Farnesoid X receptor (FXR), a nuclear hormone receptor that regulates bile acid metabolism	Intrahepatic cholestasis
BAAT	BAAT	Enzyme that transfers the bile acid moiety from the acyl coenzyme A thioester to either glycine or taurine	FHC
EPHX1	Epoxide hydrolase	Microsomal epoxide hydrolase regulates the activation and detoxification of exogenous chemicals	FHC
ABCC2	MRP2	Canalicular protein with ATP-binding cassette (ABC family of proteins); regulates canalicular transport of GSH conjugates and arsenic	Dubin-Johnson syndrome
ATP7B	ATP7B	P-type ATPase; function as copper export pump	Wilson disease
CLDN1	Claudin 1	Tight junction protein	NSC
CIRH1A	Cirhin	Cell signaling?	NAICC
CFTR	CFTR	Chloride channel with ATP-binding cassette (ABC family of proteins); regulates chloride transport	Cystic fibrosis
PKHD1	Fibrocystin	Protein involved in ciliary function and tubulogenesis	ARPKD
PRKCSH	Hepatocystin	Assembles with glucosidase II α subunit in endoplasmic reticulum	ADPLD
VPS33B	Vascular protein sorting 33	Regulates fusion of proteins to cellular membrane	ARC

ADPLD, autosomal dominant polycystic liver disease; ARC, arthrogryposis–renal dysfunction–cholestasis syndrome*; ARPKD, autosomal recessive polycystic kidney disease; ATP, adenosine triphosphate; BAAT, bile acid transporter; BAS, bile acid synthetic defect; BRIC, benign recurrent intrahepatic cholestasis; BSEP, bile salt export pump; CFTR, cystic fibrosis transmembrane conductance regulator; FHC, familial hypercholanemia; GFC, Greenland familial cholestasis; GSH, glutathione; ICP, intrahepatic cholestasis of pregnancy; NAICC, North American Indian childhood cirrhosis; NSC, neonatal sclerosing cholangitis with ichthyosis, leukocyte vacuoles, and alopecia; PFIC, progressive familial intrahepatic cholestasis.*

*Low GGT (PFIC types 1 and 2, BRIC types 1 and 2, ARC).

From Balistreri WF, Bezerra JA, Jansen P, et al: Intrahepatic cholestasis: summary of an American Association for the study of liver diseases single-topic conference, *Hepatology* 42(1):222–235, 2005.

episodes vary from few episodes per year to 1 episode per decade but can profoundly affect the quality of life. Nonsense, frame shift, and deletional mutations cause PFIC type I; missense and split-type mutations result in BRIC type I. Typically, patients with BRIC type I have normal serum cholesterol and GGT levels.

PFIC type 2 (BSEP deficiency) is mapped to chromosome 2q24 and is similar to PFIC 1. The disease results from defects in the canalicular adenosine triphosphate -dependent bile acid transporter BSEP (ABCB11). The progressive liver disease results from accumulation of bile acids secondary to reduction in canalicular bile acid secretion. Mutation in ABC11 is also described in another disorder, BRIC type 2, characterized by recurrent bouts of cholestasis.

In contrast to PFIC I and PFIC 2, patients with **PFIC type 3** (*MDR3 disease*) have *high* levels of GGT. The disease results from defects in a canalicular phospholipids flippase, MDR3 (*ABCB4*), which results in deficient translocation of phosphatidylcholine across the canalicular

membrane. Mothers who are heterozygous for this gene can develop intrahepatic cholestasis during pregnancy.

Familial hypercholanemia is characterized by an elevated serum bile acid concentration, pruritus, failure to thrive, and coagulopathy. Familial hypercholanemia is a complex genetic trait associated with mutation of bile acid coenzyme A (CoA), amino acid N-acyltransferase (encoded by bile acid transporter *[BAAT]*) as well as mutations in tight junction protein 2 (encoded by *TJP 2*, also known as *ZO-2*). Mutation of BAAT, which is a bile acid-conjugating enzyme, abrogates the enzyme activity. Patients who are homozygous for this mutation have only unconjugated bile acids in their bile. Mutation of both BAAT and TJP 2 can disrupt bile acid transport and circulation. Patients with familial hypercholanemia usually respond to the administration of ursodeoxycholic acid.

Defective bile acid biosynthesis is postulated to be an initiating or perpetuating factor in neonatal cholestatic disorders; the hypothesis is

| Table 383.5 | Progressive Familial Intrahepatic Cholestasis |

	PFIC1	PFIC2	PFIC3
Transmission	Autosomal recessive	Autosomal recessive	Autosomal recessive
Chromosome	18q21-22	2q24	7q21
Gene	*ATP8B1/F1C1*	*ABCB11/BSEP*	*ABCB4/MDR3*
Protein	FIC1	BSEP	MDR3
Location	Hepatocyte, colon, intestine, pancreas; on apical membranes	Hepatocyte canalicular membrane	Hepatocyte canalicular membrane
Function	ATP-dependent aminophospholipid flippase; unknown effects on intracellular signaling	ATP-dependent bile acid transport	ATP-dependent phosphatidylcholine translocation
Phenotype	Progressive cholestasis, diarrhea, steatorrhea, growth failure, severe pruritus	Rapidly progressive cholestatic giant cell hepatitis, growth failure, pruritus	Later-onset cholestasis, portal hypertension, minimal pruritus, intraductal and gallbladder lithiasis
Histology	Initial bland cholestatic; coarse, granular canalicular bile on EM	Neonatal giant cell hepatitis, amorphous canalicular bile on EM	Proliferation of bile ductules, periportal fibrosis, eventually biliary cirrhosis
Biochemical features	Normal serum γGT; high serum, low biliary bile acid concentrations	Normal serum γGT; high serum, low biliary bile acid concentrations	Elevated serum γGT; low to absent biliary PC; absent serum LPX; normal biliary bile acid concentrations
Treatment	Biliary diversion, ileal exclusion, liver transplantation, but post-OLT diarrhea, steatorrhea, fatty liver	Biliary diversion, liver transplantation	UDCA if residual PC secretion; liver transplantation

ATP, adenosine triphosphate; BCEP, B-cell epitope peptide; BSEP, bile salt export pump; EM, electron microscopy; γGT, γ-glutamyl transpeptidase; LPX, lipoprotein X; OLT, orthotopic liver transplantation; PC, phosphatidylcholine; PFIC, progressive familial intrahepatic cholestasis; UDCA, ursodeoxycholic acid.
From Suchy FJ, Sokol RJ, Balistreri WF, editors: *Liver disease in children*, ed 4, New York, 2014, Cambridge University Press.

that inborn errors in bile acid biosynthesis lead to absence of normal trophic or choleretic primary bile acids and accumulation of atypical (hepatotoxic) metabolites. Inborn errors of bile acid biosynthesis cause acute and chronic liver disease; early recognition allows institution of targeted bile acid replacement, which reverses the hepatic injury. Several specific defects have been described:

- **Deficiency of Δ^4-3-oxosteroid-5β reductase**, the fourth step in the pathway of cholesterol degradation to the primary bile acids, manifests with significant cholestasis and liver failure developing shortly after birth, with coagulopathy and metabolic liver injury resembling tyrosinemia. Hepatic histology is characterized by lobular disarray with giant cells, pseudoacinar transformation, and canalicular bile stasis. Mass spectrometry will display increased urinary bile acid excretion and the predominance of oxo-hydroxy and oxo-dihydroxy cholenoic acids. The diagnosis can be established by screening for mutations in *SRD5B1 (AKR1D1)*, the gene encoding Δ4-3-oxosteroid 5β-reductase. Treatment with cholic acid and ursodeoxycholic acid is associated with normalization of biochemical, histologic, and clinical features.

- **Deficiency of 3β-hydroxy- Δ^5-C^{27}-steroid oxidoreductase (3β-HSD)**, the second step in bile acid biosynthesis from cholesterol, causes PFIC. Affected patients usually have jaundice with increased aminotransferase levels and hepatomegaly; GGT levels and serum cholylglycine levels are *normal*. The histology is variable, ranging from giant cell hepatitis to chronic hepatitis. The diagnosis, suggested by mass spectrometry detection of C^{24} bile acids in urine, which retain the 3β-hydroxy-Δ^5 structure, can be confirmed by genetic screening for mutations in *HSD3B7*, the gene encoding 3β-HSD. Primary bile acid therapy, administered orally to down regulate cholesterol 7α-hydroxylase activity, to limit the production of 3β-hydroxy-Δ^5 bile acids, and to facilitate hepatic clearance, has been effective in reversing hepatic injury.

BILE ACID-COENZYME A LIGASE DEFICIENCY

Conjugation with the amino acids glycine and taurine is the final step in bile acid synthesis. Two enzymes catalyze the amidation of bile acids. In the first reaction, a CoA thioester is formed by the rate-limiting bile acid-CoA ligase. The other reaction involves the coupling of glycine

or taurine and is catalyzed by a cytosolic bile acid-CoA:amino acid N-acyltransferase. Affected patients present with conjugated hyperbilirubinemia, growth failure, or fat-soluble vitamin deficiency, and are identified with mutation of the bile acid-CoA ligase gene. Administration of conjugates of the primary bile acid, glycocholic acid, may be beneficial and can correct the fat-soluble vitamin malabsorption and improve growth.

DISORDERS OF EMBRYOGENESIS

Alagille syndrome (arteriohepatic dysplasia) is the most common syndrome with intrahepatic bile duct paucity. Bile duct *paucity* (often erroneously called *intrahepatic biliary atresia*) designates an absence or marked reduction in the number of interlobular bile ducts in the portal triads, with normal-size branches of portal vein and hepatic arteriole. Biopsy in early life often reveals an inflammatory process involving the bile ducts; subsequent biopsy specimens then show subsidence of the inflammation, with residual reduction in the number and diameter of bile ducts, analogous to the *disappearing bile duct syndrome* noted in adults with immune-mediated disorders. Serial assessment of hepatic histology often suggests progressive destruction of bile ducts.

Clinical manifestations of Alagille syndrome are expressed in various degrees and can be nonspecific; they include unusual facial characteristics (broad forehead; deep-set, widely spaced eyes; long, straight nose; and an underdeveloped mandible). There may also be ocular abnormalities (posterior embryotoxon, microcornea, optic disk drusen, shallow anterior chamber), cardiovascular abnormalities (usually peripheral pulmonic stenosis, sometimes tetralogy of Fallot, pulmonary atresia, ventricular septal defect, atrial septal defect, aortic coarctation), vertebral defects (butterfly vertebrae, fused vertebrae, spina bifida occulta, rib anomalies), and tubulointerstitial nephropathy (Table 383.6, Fig. 383.2–383.3). Other findings such as short stature, pancreatic insufficiency, vasculopathy (Moyamoya syndrome, stroke), and defective spermatogenesis can reflect or produce nutritional deficiency. Patients with Alagille syndrome are likely to have pruritus, xanthomas with markedly elevated serum cholesterol levels, and neurologic complications of vitamin E deficiency if untreated. Mutations in human Jagged l gene *(JAG1)*, which encodes a ligand for the notch receptor, are linked to ~90% of patients with Alagille syndrome. Alagille syndrome type 2 is due to mutations in

Table 383.6	Classic Criteria, Based on 5 Body Systems for a Diagnosis of Alagille Syndrome
SYSTEM/PROBLEM	**DESCRIPTION**
Liver/cholestasis	Usually presenting as jaundice with conjugated hyperbilirubinemia in the neonatal period, often with pale stools
Dysmorphic facies	Broad forehead, deep-set eyes, sometimes with upslanting palpebral fissures, prominent ears, straight nose with bulbous tip, and pointed chin giving the face a somewhat triangular appearance
Congenital heart disease	Most frequently peripheral pulmonary artery stenosis, but also pulmonary atresia, atrial septal defect, ventricular septal defect, and tetralogy of Fallot
Axial skeleton/vertebral anomalies	"Butterfly" vertebrae may be seen on an antero-posterior radiograph, and occasionally hemivertebrae, fusion of adjacent vertebrae, and spina bifida occulta
Eye/posterior embryotoxon	Anterior chamber defects, most commonly posterior embryotoxon, which is prominence of Schwalbe's ring at the junction of the iris and cornea

From Turnpenny PD, Ellard S: Alagille syndrome: pathogenesis, diagnosis and management, *Eur J Hum Genet* 20(3):251–257, 2012, Table 1, p. 252.

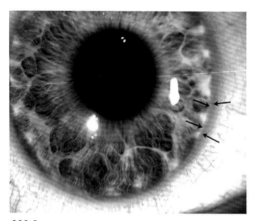

Fig. 383.2 Posterior embryotoxon. *(From Turnpenny PD, Ellard S: Alagille syndrome: pathogenesis, diagnosis and management, Eur J Hum Genet 20[3]:251–257, 2012, Fig. 1.)*

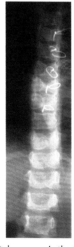

Fig. 383.3 Butterfly vertebrae seen in the thoracic and upper lumbar regions. The child had undergone cardiac surgery, hence the presence of visible wires. *(From Turnpenny PD, Ellard S: Alagille syndrome: pathogenesis, diagnosis and management, Eur J Hum Genet 20[3]: 251–257, 2012, Fig. 2.)*

NOTCH2. Although cirrhosis and manifestations of end-stage liver disease are uncommon early in life, some patients may later develop these complications. Long-term care includes monitoring cardiac and renal function as well as screening for the development of hepatocellular carcinoma.

BILIARY ATRESIA

The term *biliary atresia* is imprecise because the anatomy of abnormal bile ducts in affected patients varies markedly. A more appropriate terminology would reflect the pathophysiology, namely noncystic obliterative cholangiopathy. The term *obliterative cholangiopathy* may be divided into 2 major types: cystic and noncystic. The cystic disorders include the different types of **choledochal cysts** while the noncystic forms are different variants of biliary atresia in addition to neonatal sclerosing cholangitis.

Cystic biliary atresia is an uncommon variant of biliary atresia (about 10–20% of cases) and has a relatively favorable prognosis particularly with early surgery. This disorder is often misdiagnosed as a choledochal cyst. However, it can be differentiated by the absence of epithelial lining in biliary atresia as well as the lack of communication with the intrahepatic bile ducts as seen on intraoperative cholangiography.

There are 3 major variants of **noncystic biliary atresia** (Fig. 383.4). The **first type** (correctable biliary atresia), which presents in only 7% of the cases, is characterized by patency of the proximal extrahepatic bile ducts with atresia of the distal bile duct. In the **second type**, which is seen in 15% of the cases, there is atresia of the common hepatic duct at different levels. Patency of the gallbladder, cystic duct, and the common bile duct can be seen in some cases. The patent gall bladder and bile ducts can be used as biliary conduit. In the **third type** (the most *common* variant) there is nonpatency of the entire extrahepatic biliary system and intrahepatic bile ducts at the hilum.

Biliary atresia can also be classified into 3 categories based on the presence or absence of associated anomalies. The most common type, known as *perinatal* biliary atresia, affecting about 70% of the patients, is not associated with other anomalies or malformations. The patients may not be jaundiced at birth. An evolving process leads to progressive jaundice and acholic stools. Another type, seen in about 15% of the cases, can be associated with heterotaxia malformations including situs inversus, malrotation, polysplenia, interrupted inferior vena cava, and congenital heart disease. This type is also known as **biliary atresia splenic malformation (BASM) syndrome** and usually carries a poor prognosis. Other congenital malformations such as choledochal cysts, kidney anomalies, and cardiac defects can be seen in the third type, which affects the remaining 15% of the cases.

Biliary atresia has been detected in 1 in 10,000-15,000 live births. Biliary atresia is more common in East Asian countries; patients may be born term or preterm. Screening for biliary atresia in infants after birth is not universal, but stool color cards that help detect acholic stools have been used with some success (Fig. 383.5). In addition,

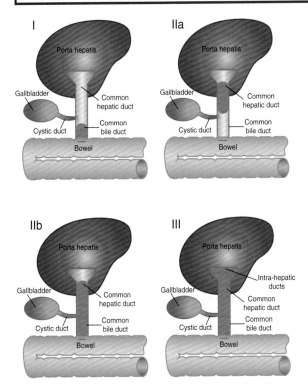

Fig. 383.4 Biliary atresia classified according to the area of involvement *(gray colored).* Type I: Atresia of the distal bile duct with patent proximal extrahepatic bile duct. Type IIa: Atresia of the common hepatic duct. Type IIb: Atresia of the common hepatic duct, cystic duct, and common bile duct. Type III: Nonpatency of the entire extrahepatic biliary system and intrahepatic bile ducts at the hilum. *(Modified from A-Kader HH, Feerick J, Rodriguez-Davalos M: After two centuries biliary atresia remains the darkest chapter in pediatric hepatology, Ann Pediatr Child Health 3[2]:1044, 2015, Fig. 2.)*

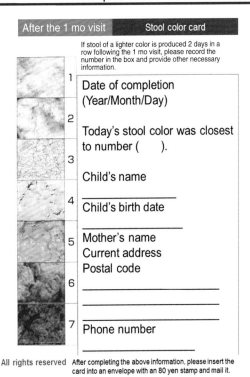

After completing the above information, please insert the card into an envelope with an 80 yen stamp and mail it.

Fig. 383.5 An example of a stool color card used in Tochigi Prefecture from August 1994 to March 2011 consisted of 7 photographic images of stool color taken in both healthy infants and infants with biliary atresia. Images 1-3 denote abnormal stool color, whereas images 4-7 reflect normal stool color. *(From Gu YH, Yokoyama K, Mizuta K, et al: Stool color card screening for early detection of biliary atresia and long-term native liver survival: a 19-year cohort study in Japan, J Pediatr 166[4]: 897–902, 2015, Fig. 2.)*

any infant with new onset or persistent jaundice beyond 2 wk of life should be screened with a total and conjugated bilirubin level to detect cholestasis.

Differentiation of Idiopathic Neonatal Hepatitis From Biliary Atresia

It may be difficult to clearly differentiate infants with biliary atresia who require surgical correction from those with intrahepatic disease (neonatal hepatitis) and patent bile ducts. No single biochemical test or imaging procedure is entirely satisfactory. Diagnostic schemas incorporate clinical, historical, biochemical, and radiologic features.

Idiopathic neonatal hepatitis has a familial incidence of approximately 20%, whereas biliary atresia is unlikely to recur within the same family. A few infants with fetal onset of biliary atresia have an increased incidence of other abnormalities, such as the polysplenia syndrome with abdominal heterotaxia, malrotation, levocardia, and intraabdominal vascular anomalies. Persistently acholic stools suggest biliary obstruction (biliary atresia), but patients with severe idiopathic neonatal hepatitis can have a transient severe impairment of bile excretion. Consistently pigmented stools rule against biliary atresia. Palpation of the liver might find an abnormal size or consistency in patients with biliary atresia; this is less common with idiopathic neonatal hepatitis.

Abdominal ultrasound is a helpful diagnostic tool in evaluating neonatal cholestasis because it identifies choledocholithiasis, perforation of the bile duct, or other structural abnormalities of the biliary tree such as a choledochal cyst. In patients with biliary atresia, ultrasound can detect associated anomalies such as abdominal polysplenia and vascular malformations. The gallbladder either is not visualized or is a microgallbladder in patients with biliary atresia. Children with

intrahepatic cholestasis caused by idiopathic neonatal hepatitis, cystic fibrosis, or total parenteral nutrition can have similar ultrasonographic findings. Ultrasonographic triangular cord sign, which represents a cone-shaped fibrotic mass cranial to the bifurcation of the portal vein, may be seen in patients with biliary atresia (Figs. 383.6 and 383.7). The echogenic density, which represents the fibrous remnants at the porta hepatis of biliary atresia cases at surgery, may be a helpful diagnostic tool in evaluating patients with neonatal cholestasis. High-frequency ultrasonography (HUS) imaging produces much improved spatial resolution by sacrificing the depth of penetration and may prove to be superior to conventional ultrasonography in the diagnostic process of biliary atresia.

Hepatobiliary scintigraphy with technetium-labeled iminodiacetic acid derivatives is a sensitive but not specific test for biliary atresia. It fails to identify other structural abnormalities of the biliary tree or vascular anomalies. The lack of the specificity of the test and the inherent delay (5 days of phenobarbital preloading) makes this procedure impractical and of limited value in the evaluation of children with suspected biliary atresia.

The role of endoscopic retrograde cholangiopancreatography (ERCP) in the diagnostic process of biliary atresia remains indeterminate. Similarly, the value of magnetic resonance cholangiopancreatography (MRCP) in the diagnosis of biliary atresia has not been established.

Percutaneous liver biopsy is the most valuable procedure in the evaluation of neonatal hepatobiliary diseases and provides the most reliable discriminatory evidence. Biliary atresia is characterized by bile ductular proliferation, the presence of bile plugs, and portal or perilobular edema and fibrosis, with the basic hepatic lobular architecture intact. In neonatal hepatitis, there is severe, diffuse hepatocellular disease, with

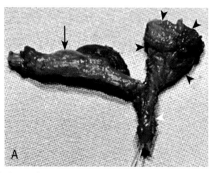 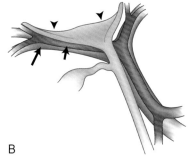

Fig. 383.6 Surgical findings of biliary atresia. **A,** Photograph of surgical specimen of obliterated extrahepatic bile ducts shows the fibrous ductal remnant *(black arrowheads)* in the porta hepatis, atretic gallbladder *(arrow)*, and fibrous common bile duct *(white arrowhead)*. The fibrous ductal remnant is a triangular cone-shaped mass. **B,** Schematic represents the anatomic relationship between the fibrous ductal remnant and blood vessels around the porta hepatis. The triangular, cone-shaped, fibrous ductal remnant *(black arrowheads, green)* is positioned anterior and slightly superior to the portal vein *(long arrow, blue)* and the hepatic artery *(short arrow, red)*. *(**A,** From Park WH, Choi SO, Lee HJ, et al: A new diagnostic approach to biliary atresia with emphasis on the ultrasonographic triangular cord sign: comparison of ultrasonography, hepatobiliary scintigraphy, and liver needle biopsy in the evaluation of infantile cholestasis, J Pediatr Surg 32[11]:1555–1559, 1997.)*

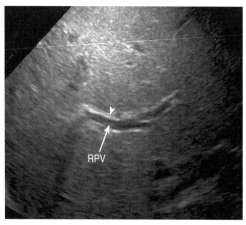

Fig. 383.7 Biliary atresia in an 8 wk old male with elevated conjugated bilirubin. Transverse sonogram shows the triangular cord sign seen as a linear cord of echogenicity *(arrowhead)* along the right portal vein *(RPV)*. *(From Lowe LH: Imaging hepatobiliary disease in children, Semin Roentgenol 43[1]:39–49, 2008, Fig. 1B.)*

distortion of lobular architecture, marked infiltration with inflammatory cells, and focal hepatocellular necrosis; the bile ductules show little alteration. Giant cell transformation is found in infants with either condition and has no diagnostic specificity.

The histologic changes seen in patients with idiopathic neonatal hepatitis can occur in other diseases, including α_1-antitrypsin deficiency, galactosemia, and various forms of intrahepatic cholestasis. Although paucity of intrahepatic bile ducts may be detected on liver biopsy even in the **first** few weeks of life, later biopsies in such patients reveal a more characteristic pattern.

Management of Patients With Suspected Biliary Atresia

All patients with suspected biliary atresia should undergo exploratory laparotomy and direct cholangiography to determine the presence and site of obstruction. Direct drainage can be accomplished in the patients with a correctable lesion. When no correctable lesion is found, an examination of frozen sections obtained from the transected porta hepatis can detect the presence of biliary epithelium and determine the

size and patency of the residual bile ducts. In some cases, the cholangiogram indicates that the biliary tree is patent but of diminished caliber, suggesting that the cholestasis is not due to biliary tract obliteration but to bile duct paucity or markedly diminished flow in the presence of intrahepatic disease. In these cases, transection of or further dissection into the porta hepatis should be avoided.

For patients in whom no correctable lesion is found, the **hepatoportoenterostomy (Kasai) procedure** should be performed. The rationale for this operation is that minute bile duct remnants, representing residual channels, may be present in the fibrous tissue of the porta hepatis; such channels may be in direct continuity with the intrahepatic ductule system. In such cases, transection of the porta hepatis with anastomosis of bowel to the proximal surface of the transection might allow bile drainage. If flow is not rapidly established in the first month of life, progressive obliteration and cirrhosis ensue. If microscopic channels of patency >150 μm in diameter are found, postoperative establishment of bile flow is likely. *The success rate for establishing good bile flow after the Kasai operation is much higher (90%) if performed before 8 wk of life.* Therefore, early referral and prompt evaluation of infants with suspected biliary atresia is important. Educating parents, increased awareness among healthcare providers, and broader implementation of the stool card program are imperative to avoid delayed diagnosis and achieve favorable outcomes.

Some patients with biliary atresia, even of the *noncorrectable* type, derive long-term benefits from interventions such as the Kasai procedure. In most, a degree of hepatic dysfunction persists. Patients with biliary atresia usually have persistent inflammation of the intrahepatic biliary tree, which suggests that biliary atresia reflects a dynamic process involving the entire hepatobiliary system. This might account for the ultimate development of complications such as portal hypertension. The short-term benefit of hepatoportoenterostomy is decompression and drainage sufficient to forestall the onset of cirrhosis and sustain growth until a successful liver transplantation can be done. The use of steroids following the Kasai procedure has not been shown to improve the patient or the native liver survival rates. Similarly, there is no convincing data to support the use of antibiotics or choleretic agents after surgery.

MANAGEMENT OF CHRONIC CHOLESTASIS

With any form of neonatal cholestasis, whether the primary disease is idiopathic neonatal hepatitis, intrahepatic cholestasis, or biliary atresia, affected patients are at increased risk for progression and complications of chronic cholestasis. These reflect various degrees of residual hepatic functional capacity and are due directly or indirectly to diminished bile flow. Any substance normally excreted into bile is retained in the liver, with subsequent accumulation in tissue and in serum. Involved substances include bile acids, bilirubin, cholesterol, and trace elements. Decreased delivery of bile acids to the proximal intestine leads to inadequate digestion and absorption of dietary long-chain triglycerides and fat-soluble vitamins. Impairment of hepatic metabolic function can alter hormonal balance and utilization of nutrients. Progressive liver damage can lead to biliary cirrhosis, portal hypertension, and liver failure.

Treatment of patients with cholestasis is empirical and is guided by careful monitoring (Table 383.7). No therapy is known to be effective in halting the progression of cholestasis or in preventing further hepatocellular damage and cirrhosis. Growth failure is a major concern and is related in part to malabsorption and malnutrition resulting from ineffective digestion and absorption of dietary fat. Use of a medium-chain triglyceride-containing formula can improve caloric balance. With chronic cholestasis and prolonged survival, children with hepatobiliary disease can experience deficiencies of the fat-soluble vitamins (A, D, E, and K). Metabolic bone disease is common. It is essential to monitor the fat-soluble vitamin status in patients.

A **degenerative neuromuscular syndrome** is found in patients with chronic cholestasis, caused by vitamin E deficiency; affected children experience progressive areflexia, cerebellar ataxia, ophthalmoplegia, and decreased vibratory sensation. Specific morphologic lesions were found in the central nervous system, peripheral nerves, and muscles. These lesions are preventable and are not commonly seen today; they were potentially reversible in children younger than 3-4 yr of age. Affected children have low serum vitamin E concentrations, increased hydrogen peroxide hemolysis, and low ratios of serum vitamin E to total serum lipids (<0.6 mg/g for children younger than 12 yr and <0.8 mg/g for older patients). Vitamin E deficiency may be prevented by oral administration of large doses (up to 1,000 IU/day); patients unable to absorb sufficient quantities may require administration of D-α-tocopheryl polyethylene glycol 1,000 succinate orally. Serum levels should be monitored as a guide to efficacy.

Pruritus is a particularly troublesome complication of chronic cholestasis, often with the appearance of xanthomas. Both features seem to be related to the accumulation of cholesterol and bile acids in serum and in tissues. Elimination of these retained compounds is difficult when bile ducts are obstructed, but if there is any degree of bile duct patency, administration of ursodeoxycholic acid can increase bile flow or interrupt the enterohepatic circulation of bile acids and thus decrease the xanthomas and ameliorate the pruritus (see Table 383.7). Ursodeoxycholic acid therapy can also lower serum cholesterol levels. The recommended initial dose is 15 mg/kg/24 hr. Inhibition of the apical sodium dependent bile acid transporter prevents the reabsorption of bile acids in the terminal ileum, is currently under investigation, and may prove to be of therapeutic benefit to relieve pruritus and improve the quality of life.

Partial external biliary diversion (PEBD) is efficacious in managing pruritus refractory to medical therapy and provides a favorable outcome in a select group of patients with chronic cholestasis who have not yet developed cirrhosis. The surgical technique involves resecting a segment of intestine to be used as a biliary conduit. One end of the conduit is attached to the gallbladder and the other end is brought out to the skin, forming a stoma. The main drawback of the procedure is the need to use an ostomy bag. Open button cholecystostomy and laparoscopic PEBD are modified surgical approaches, which have been reported to be efficacious in relieving pruritus. Ileal exclusion has been used successfully but it is less effective compared to PEBD. Unfortunately in some patients who continue to experience excoriating pruritus, liver transplantation is the only remaining consideration.

Progressive fibrosis and cirrhosis lead to the development of portal hypertension and consequently to ascites and variceal hemorrhage. The presence of ascites is a risk factor for the development of spontaneous bacterial peritonitis. *The first step in the management of patients with ascites is to rule out spontaneous bacterial peritonitis and restrict sodium intake to 0.5 g (~1-2 mEq/kg/24 hr).* There is no need for fluid restriction in patients with adequate renal output. Should this be ineffective, diuretics may be helpful. The diuretic of choice is spironolactone (1-3.3 mg/kg/day orally or divided every 12 hr). If spironolactone alone does not control ascites, the addition of another diuretic such as thiazide or furosemide may be beneficial. Patients with ascites but without peripheral edema are at risk for reduced plasma volume and decreased urine output during diuretic therapy. Tense ascites alters renal blood flow and systemic hemodynamics. Paracentesis and intravenous albumin infusion can improve hemodynamics, renal perfusion, and symptoms. Follow-up includes dietary counseling and monitoring of serum and urinary electrolyte concentrations.

In patients with portal hypertension, variceal hemorrhage and the development of hypersplenism are common. It is important to ascertain the cause of bleeding because episodes of gastrointestinal hemorrhage in patients who have chronic liver disease may be from gastritis or peptic ulcer disease. Because the management of these various complications differs, differentiation, perhaps via endoscopy, is necessary before treatment is initiated. If the patient is volume depleted, blood transfusion should be carefully administered, avoiding over transfusion, which can precipitate further bleeding. Balloon tamponade is not recommended in children because it can be associated with significant complications. Sclerotherapy or endoscopic variceal ligation may be useful palliative measures in the management of bleeding varices and may be superior to surgical alternatives.

Table 383.7	Suggested Medical Management of Persistent Cholestasis
CLINICAL IMPAIRMENT	**MANAGEMENT**
Malnutrition resulting from malabsorption of dietary long-chain triglycerides	Replace with dietary formula or supplements containing medium-chain triglycerides
Fat-soluble vitamin malabsorption	
Vitamin A deficiency (night blindness, thick skin)	Replace with 10,000-15,000 IU/day as Aquasol A
Vitamin E deficiency (neuromuscular degeneration)	Replace with 50-400 IU/day as oral α-tocopherol or TPaGS
Vitamin D deficiency (metabolic bone disease)	Replace with 5,000-8,000 IU/day of D_2 or 3-5 µg/kg/day of 25-hydroxycholecalciferol
Vitamin K deficiency (hypoprothrombinemia)	Replace with 2.5-5.0 mg every other day as water-soluble derivative of menadione
Micronutrient deficiency	Calcium, phosphate, or zinc supplementation
Deficiency of water-soluble vitamins	Supplement with twice the recommended daily allowance
Retention of biliary constituents such as cholesterol (itch or xanthomas)	Administer choleretic bile acids (ursodeoxycholic acid, 15-30 mg/kg/day)
Progressive liver disease; portal hypertension (variceal bleeding, ascites, hypersplenism)	Interim management (control bleeding; salt restriction; spironolactone)
End-stage liver disease (liver failure)	Transplantation

TPGS, D-α-tocopherol polyethylene glycol 1000 succinate.

For patients with advanced liver disease, hepatic transplantation has a success rate >90%. If the operation is technically feasible, it will prolong life and might correct the metabolic error in diseases such as α_1-antitrypsin deficiency, tyrosinemia, and Wilson disease. Success depends on adequate intraoperative, preoperative, and postoperative care, and on cautious use of immunosuppressive agents. Scarcity of donors of small livers limits the application of liver transplantation for infants and children. The use of reduced-size transplants and living donors increases the ability to treat small children successfully.

PROGNOSIS

For patients with idiopathic neonatal hepatitis, the variable prognosis might reflect the heterogeneity of the disease. In sporadic cases, 60–70% recover with no evidence of hepatic structural or functional impairment. Approximately 5–10% have persistent fibrosis or inflammation, and a smaller percentage have more severe liver disease, such as cirrhosis. Infants usually die early in the course of the illness, owing to hemorrhage or sepsis. Of infants with idiopathic neonatal hepatitis of the familial variety, only 20–30% recover; 10–15% acquire chronic liver disease with cirrhosis. Liver transplantation may be required.

383.2 Cholestasis in the Older Child

*H. Hesham Abdel-Kader Hassan
and William F. Balistreri*

Cholestasis with onset after the neonatal period is most often caused by acute viral hepatitis or exposure to hepatotoxic drugs. However, many of the conditions causing neonatal cholestasis can also cause chronic cholestasis in older patients. Consequently, older children and adolescents with conjugated hyperbilirubinemia should be evaluated for acute and chronic viral hepatitis, α_1-antitrypsin deficiency, Wilson disease, liver disease associated with inflammatory bowel disease, sclerosing cholangitis, autoimmune hepatitis, drug-induced liver injury and the syndromes of intrahepatic cholestasis. Other causes include obstruction caused by cholelithiasis, abdominal tumors, enlarged lymph nodes, or hepatic inflammation resulting from drug ingestion. Management of cholestasis in the older child is similar to that proposed for neonatal cholestasis (see Table 383.7).

Bibliography is available at Expert Consult.

Chapter 384

Metabolic Diseases of the Liver

Anna L. Peters and William F. Balistreri

第三百八十四章

肝的代谢性疾病

中文导读

　　本章主要介绍了遗传性胆红素结合缺陷、Wilson病、印度儿童肝硬化、妊娠同族免疫性肝病（新生儿铁贮积病）和其他肝脏代谢疾病。详细介绍了属于遗传性胆红素结合缺陷的Crigler-Najjar综合征Ⅰ型、Crigler-Najjar综合征Ⅱ型、遗传性结合高胆红素血症和Dubin-Johnson综合征；具体描述了Wilson病的发病机制、临床表现、病理、诊断、治疗和预后；提到了其他肝脏代谢病包括α1-抗胰蛋白酶缺乏症和Citrin缺乏症。

Metabolic liver diseases in children, although individually rare, altogether represent a significant cause of morbidity and mortality. This is because the liver has a central role in synthetic, degradative, and regulatory pathways involving carbohydrate, protein, lipid, trace element, and vitamin metabolism. Therefore, inborn errors of metabolism will result in metabolic abnormalities, specific enzyme deficiencies or defects, and disorders of protein transport that can have primary or secondary effects on the liver (Table 384.1). Liver disease can arise when absence of an enzyme produces a block in a metabolic pathway, when unmetabolized substrate accumulates proximal to a block, when deficiency of an essential

Table 384.1	Inborn Errors of Metabolism That Affect the Liver

DISORDERS OF CARBOHYDRATE METABOLISM
- Disorders of galactose metabolism
  - Galactosemia (galactose-1-phosphate uridyltransferase deficiency)
- Disorders of fructose metabolism
  - Hereditary fructose intolerance (aldolase deficiency)
  - Fructose-1,6 diphosphatase deficiency
- Glycogen storage diseases
  - Type I
  - Von Gierke Ia (glucose-6-phosphatase deficiency)
  - Type Ib (glucose-6-phosphatase transport defect)
  - Type III Cori/Forbes (glycogen debrancher deficiency)
  - Type IV Andersen (glycogen branching enzyme deficiency)
  - Type VI Hers (liver phosphorylase deficiency)
- Congenital disorders of glycosylation (multiple subtypes)

DISORDERS OF AMINO ACID AND PROTEIN METABOLISM
- Disorders of tyrosine metabolism
  - Hereditary tyrosinemia type I (fumarylacetoacetate deficiency)
  - Tyrosinemia, type II (tyrosine aminotransferase deficiency)
- Inherited urea cycle enzyme defects
  - CPS deficiency (carbamoyl phosphate synthetase I deficiency)
  - OTC deficiency (ornithine transcarbamoylase deficiency)
  - Citrullinemia type I (argininosuccinate synthetase deficiency)
  - Argininosuccinic aciduria (argininosuccinate deficiency)
  - Argininemia (arginase deficiency)
  - N-AGS deficiency (N-acetylglutamate synthetase deficiency)
- Maple serum urine disease (multiple possible defects*)

DISORDERS OF LIPID METABOLISM
- Wolman disease (lysosomal acid lipase deficiency)
- Cholesteryl ester storage disease (lysosomal acid lipase deficiency)
- Homozygous familial hypercholesterolemia (low-density lipoprotein receptor deficiency)
- Gaucher disease type I (β-glucocerebrosidase deficiency)
- Niemann-Pick type C (NPC 1 and 2 mutations)

DISORDERS OF BILE ACID METABOLISM
- Defects in bile acid synthesis (several specific enzyme deficiencies)
- Zellweger syndrome—cerebrohepatorenal (multiple mutations in peroxisome biogenesis genes)

DISORDERS OF METAL METABOLISM
- Wilson disease (ATP7B mutations)
- Hepatic copper overload
- Indian childhood cirrhosis
- Neonatal iron storage disease

DISORDERS OF BILIRUBIN METABOLISM
- Crigler-Najjar (bilirubin-uridine diphosphoglucuronate glucuronosyltransferase mutations)
  - Type I
  - Type II
- Gilbert disease (bilirubin-uridine diphosphoglucuronate glucuronosyltransferase polymorphism)
- Dubin-Johnson syndrome (multiple drug-resistant protein 2 mutation)
- Rotor syndrome

MISCELLANEOUS
- α₁-Antitrypsin deficiency
- Citrullinemia type II (citrin deficiency)
- Cystic fibrosis (cystic fibrosis transmembrane conductance regulator mutations)
- Erythropoietic protoporphyria (ferrochelatase deficiency)
- Polycystic kidney disease
- Mitochondrial hepatopathies (see Table 383.3 and Chapter 388)

*Maple syrup urine disease can be caused by mutations in branched-chain α-keto dehydrogenase, keto acid decarboxylase, lipoamide dehydrogenase, or dihydrolipoamide dehydrogenase.

substance produced distal to an aberrant chemical reaction develops, or when synthesis of an abnormal metabolite occurs. The spectrum of pathologic changes includes **hepatocyte injury,** with subsequent failure of other metabolic functions, often resulting in cirrhosis and/or liver cancer; abnormal **storage** of lipid, glycogen, or other products manifested as hepatomegaly, often with complications specific to deranged metabolism (hypoglycemia with glycogen storage disease); and absence of structural change despite profound **metabolic effects,** as seen in patients with urea cycle defects. Clinical manifestations of metabolic diseases of the liver mimic infections, intoxications, and hematologic and immunologic diseases (Table 384.2).

Many metabolic diseases are detected in expanded newborn metabolic screening programs (see Chapter 102). Clues are provided by family history of a similar illness or by the observation that the onset of symptoms is closely associated with a change in dietary habits; in patients with hereditary fructose intolerance, symptoms follow ingestion of fructose (sucrose). Clinical and laboratory evidence often guides the evaluation. Liver biopsy offers morphologic study and permits enzyme assays, as well as quantitative and qualitative assays of various other constituents (e.g., hepatic copper content in Wilson disease). Genetic/molecular diagnostic approaches are also available. Such studies require cooperation of experienced laboratories and careful attention to collection and handling of specimens. Treatment depends on the specific type of defect and although relatively uncommon, altogether metabolic diseases of the liver account for up to 10% of the indications for liver transplantation in children, a number that may be underestimated given the acute nature of some of these conditions, precluding complete diagnostic investigation prior to transplantation.

384.1 Inherited Deficient Conjugation of Bilirubin (Familial Nonhemolytic Unconjugated Hyperbilirubinemia)
Anna L. Peters and William F. Balistreri

Bilirubin is the metabolic end product of heme. Before excretion into bile, it is first glucuronidated and made water-soluble by the enzyme bilirubin-uridine diphosphoglucuronate glucuronosyltransferase (UDPGT). UDPGT activity is deficient or altered in 3 genetically and functionally distinct disorders (Crigler-Najjar [CN] syndromes type I and II and Gilbert syndrome), producing congenital nonobstructive, nonhemolytic, **unconjugated** hyperbilirubinemia. UGT1A1 is the primary UDPGT isoform needed for bilirubin glucuronidation. Complete absence of UGT1A1 activity causes CN type I, while CN type II is caused by decreased UGT1A1 activity to ~10% of normal.

Gilbert syndrome, the most common hereditary hyperbilirubinemia syndrome, occurs in 5–10% of the white population. Common polymorphisms resulting in a TA insertion in the promoter region of *UGT1A1* lead to decreased binding of the TATA binding protein and decrease

Table 384.2	Clinical Manifestations That Suggest the Possibility of Metabolic Disease

Recurrent vomiting, failure to thrive, short stature
Dysmorphic features
Jaundice, hepatomegaly (±splenomegaly), fulminant hepatic failure, edema/anasarca
Hypoglycemia, organic acidemia, lactic acidemia, hyperammonemia, bleeding (coagulopathy)
Developmental delay/psychomotor retardation, hypotonia, progressive neuromuscular deterioration, seizures, myopathy, neuropathy
Cardiac dysfunction/failure
Unusual odors
Rickets
Cataracts

normal gene activity by ~30%. Snapback primer genotyping can distinguish all *UGT1A1* promoter genotypes and can provide a definitive diagnosis. Unlike the CN syndromes, Gilbert syndrome usually occurs after puberty, is not associated with chronic liver disease, and no treatment is required. Disease manifestations include fluctuating mild elevations in total serum bilirubin concentration from 1 to 6 mg/dL with no evidence of liver injury or hemolysis. Because UGT1A1 catalyzes water-soluble glucuronidation and detoxification of multiple substrates other than bilirubin (i.e., drugs, hormones, environmental toxins, and aromatic hydrocarbons), mutations in the *UGT1A1* gene are implicated in cancer risk and predispose to drug toxicity and episodic jaundice specifically in cancer chemotherapy.

CRIGLER-NAJJAR SYNDROME TYPE I (GLUCURONYL TRANSFERASE DEFICIENCY)

CN type I is a rare, autosomal recessive disease caused by homozygous or compound heterozygous mutations in the *UGT1A1* gene which result in a premature stop codon or frameshift mutation and complete absence of UGT1A1 activity. At least 59 mutations have been identified to date. Parents of affected children have partial defects in conjugation, as determined by hepatic specific enzyme assay or by measurement of glucuronide formation but have normal serum unconjugated bilirubin levels.

Clinical Manifestations

Severe unconjugated hyperbilirubinemia develops in homozygous affected infants in the first 3 days of life. Without treatment, serum unconjugated bilirubin concentrations reach 25-35 mg/dL in the 1st mo, which can cause **kernicterus**. Stools are pale yellow. Persistent unconjugated hyperbilirubinemia at levels >20 mg/dL without hemolysis after the 1st wk of life should suggest the syndrome.

Diagnosis

The diagnosis of CN type I is based on the early age of onset and the extreme level of bilirubin elevation in the absence of hemolysis. In affected infants, bile contains no bilirubin glucuronide and bilirubin concentration in bile is <10 mg/dL compared with normal concentrations of 50-100 mg/dL. The diagnosis is established by measuring hepatic glucuronyl transferase activity in a liver specimen obtained by percutaneous liver biopsy; open liver biopsy should be avoided because surgery and anesthesia can precipitate kernicterus. DNA diagnosis is also available and may be preferable. Identification of the heterozygous state in parents also strongly suggests the diagnosis. The differential diagnosis of unconjugated hyperbilirubinemia is discussed in Chapter 123.3.

Treatment

The serum unconjugated bilirubin concentration should be maintained at <20 mg/dL for the first few weeks of life, and even lower in low birthweight infants. This usually requires repeated exchange transfusions and **phototherapy** in the immediate neonatal period. Oral calcium phosphate supplementation renders phototherapy more effective as it forms complexes with bilirubin in the gut. Phenobarbital therapy, through CYP450 enzyme induction, should be considered to determine responsiveness and differentiation between CN types I and II. In patients with CN type I there is no response to phenobarbital treatment.

The risk of kernicterus persists into adult life, although the serum bilirubin levels required to produce brain injury beyond the neonatal period are considerably higher (usually >35 mg/dL). Therefore, phototherapy is generally continued through the early years of life. In older infants and children, phototherapy is used mainly during sleep so as not to interfere with normal activities. Despite the administration of increasing intensities of light for longer periods, the serum bilirubin response to phototherapy decreases with age. Additional adjuvant therapy using agents that bind photobilirubin products such as cholestyramine or agar can also be used to interfere with the enterohepatic recirculation of bilirubin.

Prompt treatment of intercurrent infections, febrile episodes, and other types of illness might help prevent the later development of

kernicterus, which can occur at bilirubin levels of 45-55 mg/dL. All reported patients with CN type I have eventually experienced severe kernicterus by young adulthood.

Orthotopic liver transplantation cures the disease and has been successful in a small number of patients. Isolated hepatocyte transplantation has been reported as bridge therapy to liver transplantation, with most but not all patients eventually requiring orthotopic transplantation. Other therapeutic modalities have included plasmapheresis and limitation of bilirubin production. The latter option, inhibiting bilirubin generation, is possible via inhibition of heme oxygenase using metalloporphyrin therapy.

CRIGLER-NAJJAR SYNDROME TYPE II (PARTIAL GLUCURONYL TRANSFERASE DEFICIENCY)

CN type II is an autosomal recessive disease caused by homozygous missense mutations in UGT1A1 resulting in reduced (partial) enzymatic activity. More than 45 mutations have been identified to date. Type II disease can be distinguished from type I by the marked decline in serum bilirubin level that occurs in type II disease after treatment with phenobarbital secondary to an inducible phenobarbital response element on the UGT1A1 promoter.

Clinical Manifestations

When this disorder appears in the neonatal period, unconjugated hyperbilirubinemia usually occurs in the first 3 days of life; serum bilirubin concentrations can be in a range compatible with physiologic jaundice or can be at pathologic levels. The concentrations characteristically remain elevated into and after the 3rd wk of life, persisting in a range of 1.5-22 mg/dL; concentrations in the lower part of this range can create uncertainty about whether chronic hyperbilirubinemia is present. Development of kernicterus is unusual. Stool color is normal, and the infants are without clinical signs or symptoms of disease. There is no evidence of hemolysis. Liver enzymes, albumin, and PT/INR are typically normal.

Diagnosis

Concentration of bilirubin in bile is nearly normal in patients with CN type II. Jaundiced infants and young children with CN type II syndrome respond readily to 5 mg/kg/day of oral phenobarbital, with a decrease in serum bilirubin concentration to 2-3 mg/dL in 7-10 days.

Treatment

Long-term reduction in serum bilirubin levels can be achieved with continued administration of phenobarbital at 5 mg/kg/day. Therapy must be lifelong. The cosmetic and psychosocial benefit should be weighed against the risks of an effective dose of the drug because there is a small long-term risk of kernicterus even in the absence of hemolytic disease. Orlistat, an irreversible inhibitor of intestinal lipase, increases fecal fat excretion and may decrease plasma unconjugated bilirubin concentrations (~10%) in patients with CN types I and II.

INHERITED CONJUGATED HYPERBILIRUBINEMIA

Conjugated hyperbilirubinemia can be caused by rare autosomal recessive conditions characterized by asymptomatic mild jaundice. In these conditions, the transfer of bilirubin and other organic anions from the hepatocyte into bile is defective. Chronic mild conjugated hyperbilirubinemia is usually detected during adolescence or early adulthood but can occur as early as 2 yr of age. The results of other routine liver tests are normal. Jaundice can be exacerbated by infection, pregnancy, oral contraceptives, alcohol consumption, and surgery. There is usually no morbidity and life expectancy is normal.

DUBIN-JOHNSON SYNDROME

Dubin-Johnson syndrome is an autosomal recessive inherited defect in hepatocyte secretion of bilirubin glucuronide. The defect in hepatic excretory function is not limited to conjugated bilirubin excretion but also involves several organic anions normally excreted from the liver cell into bile. Disease results from absent function of multiple drug-resistant protein 2 (MRP2, encoded by the gene *ABCC2*), an adenosine triphosphate–dependent canalicular transporter. More than 10 different mutations, including compound heterozygous mutation in the *CMOAT* gene, have been identified and either affect localization of MRP2 with resultant increased degradation or impair MRP2 transporter activity in the canalicular membrane. Bile acid excretion and serum bile acid levels are normal. Total urinary coproporphyrin excretion is normal in quantity but coproporphyrin I excretion increases to approximately 80% with a concomitant decrease in coproporphyrin III excretion. Normally, coproporphyrin III is >75% of the total. Cholangiography fails to visualize the biliary tract and x-ray of the gallbladder is also abnormal. Liver histology demonstrates normal architecture, but hepatocytes contain black pigment similar to melanin. Liver function is normal and prognosis is excellent. The most commonly reported symptoms are abdominal pain and fatigue, jaundice, dark urine, and slight enlargement of the liver. Jaundice fluctuates in intensity and is aggravated by intercurrent disease. Rarely, Dubin-Johnson can present in the neonatal period with severe conjugated hyperbilirubinemia with serum bilirubin >20 mg/dL and hepatosplenomegaly. No treatment is indicated for disease which presents outside of the neonatal period.

Rotor Syndrome

Rotor Syndrome is an autosomal recessive disease resulting from biallelic inactivating mutations in *SLCO1B1* and *SLCO1B3* result in functional deficiencies of both OATP1B1 and OATP1B protein. Importantly, these mutations may confer significant drug toxicity risk. These patients present similarly to Dubin-Johnson syndrome, with asymptomatic mild and fluctuating conjugated hyperbilirubinemia, with total serum bilirubin levels between 2 and 5 mg/dL. Unlike Dubin-Johnson syndrome, total urinary coproporphyrin excretion is elevated with a relative increase in the amount of the coproporphyrin I isomer. If liver biopsy is performed, there is no abnormal pigmentation in contrast to Dubin-Johnson. The gallbladder is normal by roentgenography. Rotor syndrome is benign and no treatment is indicated.

Bibliography is available at Expert Consult.

384.2 Wilson Disease
Anna L. Peters and William F. Balistreri

Wilson disease (hepatolenticular degeneration) is an autosomal recessive disorder that can be associated with liver disease, degenerative changes in the brain, and Kayser-Fleischer (K-F) rings in the cornea (Fig. 384.1). The incidence is approximately 1/30,000 births worldwide. Specific treatment is available; however this disease is progressive and potentially fatal if untreated. Prompt diagnostic evaluation for Wilson disease in all patients over age 5 yr presenting with any form of liver disease facilitates expeditious initiation of treatment of the disease, appropriate genetic counseling, screening of first-degree relatives, and also allows appropriate treatment of non-Wilsonian liver disease once copper toxicosis is ruled out.

PATHOGENESIS

The abnormal gene for Wilson disease is found on chromosome 13 (13q14.3), and encodes *ATP7B*, a copper transporting P-type adenosine triphosphatase (ATPase) which is mainly expressed in hepatocytes and is critical for biliary copper excretion and for copper incorporation into ceruloplasmin. Absence or malfunction of ATP7B results in decreased biliary copper excretion and diffuse accumulation of copper in the cytosol of hepatocytes. With time, liver cells become overloaded and copper is redistributed to other tissues, including the brain and kidneys, causing toxicity, primarily as a potent inhibitor of enzymatic processes. Ionic copper inhibits pyruvate oxidase in brain and ATPase in membranes, leading to decreased adenosine triphosphate-phosphocreatine and potassium content of tissue.

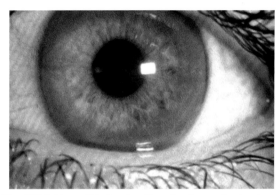

Fig. 384.1 Kayser-Fleischer ring. There is a brown discoloration at the outer margin of the cornea because of the deposition of copper in Descemet's membrane. Here it is clearly seen against the light green iris. Slit-lamp examination is required for secure detection. *(From Ala A, Walker AP, Ashkan K, et al: Wilson's disease, Lancet 369:397–408, 2007.)*

More than 500 mutations have been identified, of which >380 have a confirmed role in disease pathogenesis; genetic testing should be able to identify a pathologic variant. Most patients are compound heterozygotes. Mutations that abolish gene function are associated with an onset of disease symptoms as early as 3 yr of age, when Wilson disease might not typically be considered in the differential diagnosis. Milder mutations can be associated with neurologic symptoms or liver disease as late as 80 yr of age. The most commonly occurring disease-causing *ATP7B* mutations result in a protein which binds copper but is unable to effectively traffic to the apical surface of hepatocytes to perform its copper-exporting function. Pharmacologic inhibition of p38 and Jun N-terminal kinase mitogen-activated protein kinase (JNK MAPK) signaling pathways in vitro can rescue this defect and are potential new therapeutic targets.

CLINICAL MANIFESTATIONS

Forms of Wilsonian hepatic disease include asymptomatic hepatomegaly (with or without splenomegaly), subacute or chronic hepatitis, and acute hepatic failure (with or without hemolytic anemia). Cryptogenic cirrhosis, portal hypertension, ascites, edema, variceal bleeding, or other effects of hepatic dysfunction (delayed puberty, amenorrhea, coagulation defects) can be manifestations of Wilson disease.

Disease presentations are variable, with a tendency to familial patterns. Liver disease is the most common disease manifestation in children and can precede neurologic symptoms by as long as 10 yr. Females are 3 times more likely than males to present with acute hepatic failure. When Wilson disease presents after age 20, *neurologic symptoms* are the most common manifestation.

Neurologic disorders can develop insidiously or precipitously, with intention tremor, dysarthria, rigid dystonia, Parkinsonism, choreiform movements, lack of motor coordination, deterioration in school performance, psychosis, or behavioral changes. K-F rings are absent in young patients with hepatic Wilson disease up to 50% of the time but are present in 95% of patients with neurologic symptoms. **Psychiatric manifestations** include depression, personality changes, anxiety, obsessive-compulsive behavior, or psychosis.

Coombs-negative **hemolytic anemia** may be an initial manifestation, possibly related to the release of large amounts of copper from damaged hepatocytes; this form of Wilson disease is usually fatal without transplantation. During hemolytic episodes, urinary copper excretion and serum free copper levels are markedly elevated. Manifestations of renal Fanconi syndrome and progressive renal failure with alterations in tubular transport of amino acids, glucose, and uric acid may be present. Unusual manifestations include arthritis, pancreatitis, nephrolithiasis, infertility or recurrent miscarriages, cardiomyopathy, and hypoparathyroidism.

PATHOLOGY

All grades of hepatic injury occur in patients with Wilson disease with steatosis, hepatocellular ballooning and degeneration, glycogen granules, minimal inflammation, and enlarged Kupffer cells being most common. The earliest histologic feature of Wilson disease is mild steatosis which may mimic nonalcoholic fatty liver disease or nonalcoholic steatohepatitis. Additionally, the lesion may be indistinguishable from that of autoimmune hepatitis. With progressive parenchymal damage, fibrosis and cirrhosis develop. Ultrastructural changes primarily involve the mitochondria and include increased density of the matrix material, inclusions of lipid and granular material, and increased intracristal space with dilation of the tips of the cristae.

DIAGNOSIS

Wilson disease should be considered in children and teenagers with unexplained acute or chronic liver disease, neurologic symptoms of unknown cause, acute hemolysis, psychiatric illnesses, behavioral changes, Fanconi syndrome, or unexplained bone (osteoporosis, fractures) or muscle disease (myopathy, arthralgia). The clinical suspicion is confirmed by study of indices of copper metabolism.

Most patients with Wilson disease have decreased serum ceruloplasmin levels (<20 mg/dL). The failure of copper to be incorporated into ceruloplasmin leads to a plasma protein with a shorter half-life and, therefore, a reduced steady-state concentration of ceruloplasmin in the circulation. Serum ceruloplasmin levels should be interpreted with caution. Acute inflammatory states and elevated estrogen levels (pregnancy, hormone therapy, or use of oral contraception) can falsely increase ceruloplasmin levels. Additionally, serum ceruloplasmin may be low in autoimmune hepatitis, celiac disease, familial aceruloplasminemia, or in carriers of ATP7B mutations (mild variants of Menkes disease: occipital horn syndrome) who do not show copper overload disease. The serum free copper level may be elevated in early Wilson disease (>1.6 μmol/L), and urinary copper excretion (normally <40 μg/day) is increased to >100 μg/day and often up to 1,000 μg or more per day. Typical urinary copper excretion in patients with untreated Wilson disease is >1.6 μmol/24 hr. in adults and >0.64 μmol/24 hr in children. In equivocal cases, the response of urinary copper output to chelation may be of diagnostic help. Prior to a 24 hr urine collection patients are given 2 500 mg oral doses of D-penicillamine 12 hr apart; affected patients excrete >1,600 μg/24 hr.

Demonstration of K-F rings, which might not be present in younger children, requires a slit-lamp examination by an ophthalmologist. After adequate treatment, K-F rings resolve. Liver biopsy can determine the extent and severity of liver disease and for measuring the hepatic copper content (normally <10 μg/g dry weight) but is only required if clinical signs and noninvasive tests do not allow a final diagnosis or if another liver disorder is suspected. Hepatic copper accumulation is the hallmark of Wilson disease and measurement of hepatic parenchymal copper concentration is the method of choice for diagnosis. Hepatic copper content >250 μg/g dry weight (>4 μmol/g dry weight) is the best biochemical evidence for Wilson disease, but lowering the threshold to 1.2 μmol/g dry weight improves sensitivity without significantly affecting specificity. Intermediate levels of hepatic copper may be present in asymptomatic carriers. In later stages of Wilson disease, hepatic copper content can be unreliable because cirrhosis leads to variable hepatic copper distribution and sampling error.

First-degree relatives of patients with Wilson disease should be screened for presymptomatic disease. This screening should include determination of the serum ceruloplasmin level and 24-hr urinary copper excretion. If these results are abnormal or equivocal, liver biopsy should be carried out to determine morphology and hepatic copper content. Genetic screening by either linkage analysis or direct DNA mutation analysis is possible, especially if the mutation for the proband case is known or the patient is from an area where a specific mutation is prevalent, such as in central and eastern Europe where the H1069Q mutation is present in 50–80% of patients.

TREATMENT

Once the diagnosis of Wilson disease is made, lifelong treatment should be initiated and is focused on limiting copper uptake and promoting copper excretion through dietary and pharmacologic measures. The normal diet contains 2-5 mg of copper per day. For patients with Wilson disease, the dietary intake of copper should be restricted to <1 mg/day. High copper content foods such as liver, shellfish, nuts, and chocolate should be avoided. If the copper content of the drinking water exceeds 0.1 mg/L, it may be necessary to demineralize the water.

The initial treatment in symptomatic patients is the administration of copper-chelating agents, which leads to rapid excretion of excess deposited copper. Chelation therapy is managed with oral administration of D-penicillamine (β,β-dimethylcysteine) in a dose of 1 g/day in 2 doses before meals for adults and 20 mg/kg/day for pediatric patients or triethylene tetramine dihydrochloride (Trien, TETA, trientine) at a dose of 0.5-2.0 g/day for adults and 20 mg/kg/day for children. In response to chelation, urinary copper excretion increases, with marked improvement in hepatic and neurologic function and the disappearance of K-F rings.

Approximately 10–50% of patients initially treated with penicillamine for neurologic symptoms have a worsening of their condition. Toxic effects of penicillamine occur in 10–20% and consist of hypersensitivity reactions (i.e., Goodpasture syndrome, systemic lupus erythematosus, and polymyositis), interaction with collagen and elastin, deficiency of other elements such as zinc, and aplastic anemia and nephrosis. Because penicillamine is an antimetabolite of vitamin B_6, additional amounts of this vitamin are necessary. For these reasons, trientene is the preferred alternative and is considered first-line therapy for some patients. Trientine has few known side effects. Ammonium tetrathiomolybdate is another alternative chelating agent under investigation for patients with neurologic disease; initial results suggest that significantly fewer patients experience neurologic deterioration with this drug compared to penicillamine. The initial dose is 120 mg/day (20 mg between meals 3 times daily and 20 mg with meals 3 times daily). Side effects include anemia, leukopenia, thrombocytopenia, and mild elevations of alanine aminotransferase (ALT) and aspartate aminotransferase (AST). Because of its extensive decoppering effect, ammonium tetrathiomolybdate also has antiangiogenic effects.

Zinc has also been used as adjuvant therapy, maintenance therapy, or primary therapy in presymptomatic patients, owing to its unique ability to impair the gastrointestinal absorption of copper. Zinc acetate can be given (adults) at a dose of 25-50 mg of elemental zinc 3 times a day, and 25 mg 3 times a day in children over age 5 yr. Side effects are predominantly limited to gastric irritation but also include reduced leukocyte chemotaxis and elevations in serum lipase and/or amylase. Current guidelines recommend that all symptomatic patients with Wilson disease receive a chelating agent (penicillamine or trientine). Patients should be counseled not to suddenly stop these medications, since sudden discontinuation of therapy can precipitate fulminant Wilson disease. Zinc may have a role as a first-line therapy in patients with neurologic disease, but exclusive monotherapy with zinc in symptomatic liver disease is controversial and not recommended. Antioxidants (vitamin E and curcumin) and pharmacologic chaperones (4-phenylbutyrate and curcumin) may have a role as adjunctive treatment but more research is needed.

PROGNOSIS

Untreated patients with Wilson disease can die of hepatic, neurologic, renal, or hematologic complications. Medical therapy is rarely effective in those presenting with acute liver failure. The prognosis for patients receiving prompt and continuous penicillamine is variable and depends on the time of initiation of and the individual response to chelation. Liver transplantation should be considered for patients with acute liver failure or decompensated cirrhosis due to Wilson disease. Liver transplantation for progressive neurologic disease remains controversial. Liver transplantation is curative, with a 5-yr survival rate of 85–90%. In asymptomatic siblings of affected patients, early institution of chelation or zinc therapy can prevent disease manifestations.

Bibliography is available at Expert Consult.

384.3 Indian Childhood Cirrhosis

Anna L. Peters and William F. Balistreri

Indian childhood cirrhosis (ICC) is a chronic liver disease of infants and young children unique to the Indian subcontinent, but variants of this syndrome have been described in other populations and have been named accordingly (Tyrolean or North American childhood cirrhosis). ICC-like disease has also been reported in the Middle East, West Africa, and Central America. Affected children present with jaundice, pruritus, lethargy, and hepatosplenomegaly with rapid progression to cirrhosis. Untreated severe ICC has a mortality of 40–50% within 4 wk. Histologically, ICC is characterized by hepatocyte necrosis, Mallory bodies, intralobular fibrosis, inflammation, and excess hepatic copper deposition. Treatment is supportive, especially in the late stages of disease. Copper chelation with D-penicillamine has been beneficial in open-label pre-icteric cases of ICC, however, it is unclear whether these cases were simply less severely affected and would have spontaneously improved without treatment.

The etiology of ICC has remained elusive. It was once believed that excess copper ingestion in the setting of a genetic susceptibility to copper toxicosis was the most likely cause. Epidemiologic data demonstrates that the copper toxicity theory is unlikely. The increased hepatic copper content, usually >700 μg/g dry weight, seen in ICC is only seen in the late stages of disease and is accompanied by even higher levels of zinc, a non-hepatotoxic metal. Furthermore, the copper-contaminated utensils used to feed babies and implicated in excess copper ingestion are found in only 10–15% of all cases. The current hypothesis implicates the postnatal use of local hepatotoxic therapeutic remedies, although the exact causative agent is unknown. North American ICC is due to mutations in the *UTP4* gene.

Over the last few decades, as the awareness of the disease has increased, the incidence of ICC has decreased to the point of being virtually eliminated in some areas of India. However, established and atypical cases are probably being missed because of lack of histologic confirmation and lack of awareness of the protean manifestations and natural history of this disease.

Bibliography is available at Expert Consult.

384.4 Gestational Alloimmune Liver Disease (Neonatal Iron Storage Disease)

Anna L. Peters and William F. Balistreri

Neonatal iron storage disease (NISD), also known as **neonatal hemochromatosis,** is a rare form of fulminant liver disease that manifests in the first few days of life. This disease is unrelated to the familial forms of hereditary hemochromatosis that occur in adulthood. NISD has a high rate of recurrence in families, with approximately 80% probability that subsequent infants will be affected. NISD is postulated to be a gestational alloimmune disease and has also been classified as **gestational alloimmune liver disease**. During gestation, the maternal immune system becomes sensitized to an unknown fetal hepatocyte cell surface antigen. Maternal immunoglobulin G to this fetal antigen then crosses the placenta and induces hepatic injury via immune system activation. The defining feature of gestational alloimmune liver disease is complement-mediated hepatocyte injury, the evidence for which comes from detection of the C5b-9 complex by immunohistochemistry on liver tissue of affected infants. Additional evidence of a gestational insult is given by the fact that affected infants may be born prematurely or with intrauterine growth restriction. Several infants with NISD also have renal dysgenesis.

Excess non-transferrin-bound iron in gestational alloimmune liver disease may result from fetal liver injury that causes reduced synthesis of key iron regulatory and transport proteins. The pattern of extrahepatic siderosis appears to be determined by the normal capacity of various tissues to import non–transferrin-bound iron and not export cellular iron. It is thought that fetal liver injury is the primary event leading to the development of the neonatal hemochromatosis phenotype, providing further evidence that this is not a primary iron overload disease.

NISD is a rapidly fatal, progressive illness characterized by hepatomegaly, hypoglycemia, hypoprothrombinemia, hypoalbuminemia, hyperferritinemia, and hyperbilirubinemia. The coagulopathy is refractory to therapy with vitamin K. Liver biopsy demonstrates severe liver injury with acute and chronic inflammation, fibrosis, and cirrhosis; in some cases there are no surviving hepatocytes. The diagnosis is established in the neonate with severe liver injury and evidence of extrahepatic siderosis either by MRI indicating increased iron deposition in organs such as the pancreas or heart, or by increased iron staining in oral submucosal gland biopsy. The differential diagnosis includes other causes of neonatal hepatic failure such as citrin deficiency, herpes simplex virus (HSV) hepatitis, and familial hemophagocytic lymphohistiocytosis.

The prognosis for affected infants is generally poor. Intravenous immunoglobulin (IVIG) combined with double volume exchange transfusion has been shown to remove the injury-causing maternal IgG and improve outcomes in infants with NISD. Liver transplantation should also be an early consideration. Recurrences of NISD in subsequent pregnancies may be modified with IVIG administered to the mother once weekly from the 14th wk of gestation until delivery. The largest experience reports 48 women with previous infants with NISD who successfully delivered 52 babies after IVIG treatment. The majority of infants had biochemical evidence of liver disease with elevated serum α-fetoprotein and ferritin. All infants survived with medical therapy or no therapy.

Bibliography is available at Expert Consult.

384.5 Miscellaneous Metabolic Diseases of the Liver

Anna L. Peters and William F. Balistreri

α₁-ANTITRYPSIN DEFICIENCY

α_1-Antitrypsin deficiency is an autosomal recessive disorder caused by mutation in the *SERPINA1* gene. α_1-antitrypsin, a protease inhibitor (Pi) synthesized by the liver, protects lung alveolar tissues from destruction by neutrophil elastase (see Chapter 421). α_1-Antitrypsin is present in more than 20 different codominant alleles, only a few of which are associated with defective Pis. The most common allele of the Pi system is M, and the normal phenotype is PiMM. The Z allele predisposes to clinical deficiency; patients with liver disease are usually PiZZ homozygotes and have serum α_1-antitrypsin levels <2 mg/mL (~10–20% of normal). The incidence of the PiZZ genotype in the white population is estimated at 1 in 2,000-4,000 live births. A small percentage of patients homozygous for deficiency of the major serum Pi α_1-antitrypsin develop neonatal cholestasis or later-onset childhood cirrhosis. Compound heterozygotes PiZ-, PiSZ, PiZI are not a cause of liver disease alone but can act as modifier genes, increasing the risk of progression in other liver disease such as nonalcoholic fatty liver disease and hepatitis C. The null phenotype only causes lung disease, and results from either stop codons in the coding exon of the *SERPINA1* gene or complete deletion of *SERPINA1* coding exons leading to the absence of α_1-antitrypsin protein.

Newly formed α_1-antitrypsin polypeptide normally enters the endoplasmic reticulum, where it undergoes enzymatic modification and folding before transport to the plasma membrane, where it is excreted as a 55 kDa glycoprotein. In affected patients with PiZZ, the rate at which the α_1-antitrypsin polypeptide folds is decreased, and this delay allows the formation of polymers that are retained in the endoplasmic reticulum. How the polymers cause liver damage is not completely elucidated, but research indicates that accumulation of abnormally folded protein leads to activation of stress and proinflammatory pathways in the endoplasmic reticulum and hepatocyte programmed cell death. In liver biopsies from patients, polymerized α_1-antitrypsin peptides can be seen by electron microscopy and histochemically as periodic acid–Schiff-positive diastase-resistant globules primarily in periportal hepatocytes, but also in Kupffer cells and biliary epithelial cells. The pattern of neonatal liver injury can be highly variable, and liver biopsies might demonstrate hepatocellular necrosis, inflammatory cell infiltration, bile duct proliferation, periportal fibrosis, or cirrhosis.

The course of liver disease is highly variable in patients with α_1-antitrypsin deficiency. Prospective studies in Sweden have shown that only 10% of patients develop clinically significant liver disease by their fourth decade, indicating that other genetic traits or environmental factors likely influence the development of liver disease. Infants with liver disease are indistinguishable from other infants with "idiopathic" neonatal hepatitis, of whom they constitute approximately 5–10%. Jaundice, acholic stools, and hepatomegaly are present in the 1st wk of life, but the jaundice usually clears by 2-4 mo of age. Complete resolution, persistent liver disease, or the development of cirrhosis can follow. Older children can present with asymptomatic hepatomegaly or manifestations of chronic liver disease or cirrhosis with evidence of portal hypertension. Patients with cirrhosis due to alpha-1 antitrypsin deficiency are at high risk to develop hepatocellular carcinoma. Emphysema is not typically observed in children but an increased risk for developing asthma is reported. Cigarette smoking promotes development of lung disease, so parents should be counseled on smoking cessation and exposure reduction as part of their anticipatory guidance, and older children and adolescents should be advised not to smoke and given cessation counseling if they smoke.

Treatment is supportive, although research is ongoing to develop therapies for α_1-antitrypsin deficiency-associated liver disease which stimulate intracellular degradation of the abnormally folded Z protein polymers. Liver transplantation is indicated for hepatocellular carcinoma or end-stage liver disease with portal hypertension, with survival rates of ~90%.

CITRIN DEFICIENCY

Neonatal intrahepatic cholestasis caused by citrin deficiency (NICCD) presents in the first few months of life with manifestations that initially may be indistinguishable from other causes of neonatal cholestasis, especially biliary atresia. Patients may have jaundice, hepatomegaly, liver dysfunction with coagulopathy, fatty liver infiltration, and hyperammonemia with or without hypoglycemia. Presymptomatic patients may be identified from the newborn metabolic screen with hypergalactosemia, hypermethionemia, and hyperphenylalanemia, but not all patients are identified by newborn screening.

Mutations in the *SLC25A13* gene cause NICCD with an autosomal recessive pattern of inheritance. *SLC25A13* encodes citrin, a mitochondrial carrier protein (calcium binding aspartate-glutamate carrier) involved in the urea cycle, gluconeogenesis and glycolysis. Mutations are more common in those of East Asian descent. Affected infants have hypergalactosemia, elevated bile acids, vitamin K-dependent coagulopathy, and elevated levels of citrulline and methionine. Treatment is supportive in the form of providing fat-soluble vitamin supplementation and dietary feeding with a low-galactose/lactose formula enriched with medium chain triglycerides. More severely affected patients can develop liver failure requiring liver transplantation in the 1st yr of life.

Bibliography is available at Expert Consult.

Chapter **385**
Viral Hepatitis
M. Kyle Jensen and William F. Balistreri

第三百八十五章
病毒性肝炎

中文导读

　　本章主要介绍了各种病毒性肝炎的共同问题以及甲型病毒性肝炎、乙型病毒性肝炎、丙型病毒性肝炎、丁型病毒性肝炎、戊型病毒性肝炎和急性或慢性病毒性肝炎的鉴别方法。详细介绍了病毒性肝炎的鉴别诊断、发病机制、急性期生化特征；具体描述了甲型病毒性肝炎的病因学、流行病学、病原学、临床表现、诊断、并发症、治疗、预防和预后；具体描述了乙型病毒性肝炎的病因学、流行病学、病原学、临床表现、诊断、并发症、治疗、预防和暴露后预防、特殊人群和预后；具体描述了丙型病毒性肝炎、丁型病毒性肝炎、戊型病毒性肝炎的病因学、流行病学、发病机制、临床表现、诊断、并发症、治疗、预防和预后等内容。

Viral hepatitis continues to be a major health problem in both developing and developed countries; there has been significant progress in efforts to recognize and to treat infected subjects. This disorder is caused by the 5 pathogenic hepatotropic viruses recognized to date: hepatitides A (HAV), B (HBV), C (HCV), D (HDV), and E (HEV) viruses (Table 385.1). Many other viruses (and diseases) can cause hepatitis, usually as a component of a multisystem disease. These include herpes simplex virus, cytomegalovirus, Epstein-Barr virus, varicella-zoster virus, HIV, rubella, adenoviruses, enteroviruses, parvovirus B19, and arboviruses (Table 385.2).

The hepatotropic viruses are a heterogeneous group of infectious agents that cause similar acute clinical illness. In most pediatric patients, the acute phase causes no or mild clinical disease. Morbidity is related to rare cases of **acute liver failure (ALF)** in susceptible patients, or to the development of a chronic disease state and attendant complications that several of these viruses (hepatitides B, C, and D) commonly cause.

ISSUES COMMON TO ALL FORMS OF VIRAL HEPATITIS
Differential Diagnosis

Often what brings the patient with hepatitis to medical attention is clinical icterus, with yellow skin and/or mucous membranes. The liver is usually enlarged and tender to palpation and percussion. Splenomegaly and lymphadenopathy may be present. Extrahepatic symptoms (rashes, arthritis) are more commonly seen in HBV and HCV infections. Clinical signs of bleeding, altered sensorium, or hyperreflexia should be carefully sought, because they mark the onset of encephalopathy and ALF.

The differential diagnosis varies with age of presentation. In the newborn period, infection is a common cause of conjugated hyperbilirubinemia; the infectious cause is either a bacterial agent (e.g., *Escherichia coli*, Listeria, syphilis) or a nonhepatotropic virus (e.g., enteroviruses, cytomegalovirus, and herpes simplex virus, which may also cause a nonicteric severe hepatitis). Metabolic diseases (α_1-antitrypsin deficiency,

Table 385.1	Features of the Hepatotropic Viruses				
VIROLOGY	**HAV RNA**	**HBV DNA**	**HCV RNA**	**HDV RNA**	**HEV RNA**
Incubation (days)	15-19	60-180	14-160	21-42	21-63
Transmission					
• Parenteral	Rare	Yes	Yes	Yes	No
• Fecal–oral	Yes	No	No	No	Yes
• Sexual	No	Yes	Rare	Yes	No
• Perinatal	No	Yes	Uncommon (5–15%)	Yes	No
Chronic infection	No	Yes	Yes	Yes	No
Fulminant disease	Rare	Yes	Rare	Yes	Yes

HAV, hepatitis A virus; HBV, hepatitis B virus; HCV, hepatitis C virus; HDV, hepatitis D virus; HEV, hepatitis E virus.

Table 385.2	Causes and Differential Diagnosis of Hepatitis in Children

INFECTIOUS

Hepatotropic viruses
- Hepatitis A virus (HAV)
- Hepatitis B virus (HBV)
- Hepatitis C virus (HCV)
- Hepatitis D virus (HDV)
- Hepatitis E virus (HEV)
- Hepatitis non–A-E viruses

Systemic infection that can include hepatitis
- Adenovirus
- Arbovirus
- Coxsackievirus
- Cytomegalovirus
- Enterovirus
- Epstein-Barr virus
- "Exotic" viruses (e.g., yellow fever)
- Herpes simplex virus
- HIV
- Paramyxovirus
- Rubella
- Varicella zoster

Other

NONVIRAL LIVER INFECTIONS

Abscess
Amebiasis
Bacterial sepsis
Brucellosis
Fitz-Hugh-Curtis syndrome
Histoplasmosis
Leptospirosis
Tuberculosis
Other

AUTOIMMUNE

Autoimmune hepatitis
Sclerosing cholangitis
Other (e.g., systemic lupus erythematosus, juvenile inflammatory arthritis)

METABOLIC

α_1-Antitrypsin deficiency
Tyrosinemia
Wilson disease
Other

TOXIC

Iatrogenic or drug induced (e.g., acetaminophen)
Environmental (e.g., pesticides)

ANATOMIC

Choledochal cyst
Biliary atresia
Other

HEMODYNAMIC

Shock
Congestive heart failure
Budd-Chiari syndrome
Other

NONALCOHOLIC FATTY LIVER DISEASE

Idiopathic
Reye syndrome
Other

From Wyllie R, Hyams JS, editors: *Pediatric gastrointestinal and liver disease*, ed 3, Philadelphia, 2006, WB Saunders.

cystic fibrosis, tyrosinemia), anatomic causes (biliary atresia, choledochal cysts), and inherited forms of intrahepatic cholestasis should always be excluded.

In later childhood, extrahepatic obstruction (gallstones, primary sclerosing cholangitis, pancreatic pathology), inflammatory conditions (autoimmune hepatitis, juvenile inflammatory arthritis, Kawasaki disease), immune dysregulation (hemophagocytic lymphohistiocytosis), infiltrative disorders (malignancies), toxins and medications, metabolic disorders (Wilson disease, cystic fibrosis), and infection (Epstein-Barr virus, varicella, malaria, leptospirosis, syphilis) should be ruled out.

Pathogenesis

The acute response of the liver to hepatotropic viruses involves a direct cytopathic and/or an immune-mediated injury. The entire liver is involved. Necrosis is usually most marked in the centrilobular areas. An acute mixed inflammatory infiltrate predominates in the portal areas but also affects the lobules. The lobular architecture remains intact, although balloon degeneration and necrosis of single or groups of parenchymal cells commonly occur. Fatty change is rare except with HCV infection. Bile duct proliferation, but not bile duct damage, is common. Diffuse Kupffer cell hyperplasia is noticeable in the sinusoids. Neonates often respond to hepatic injury by forming *giant cells*. In fulminant hepatitis, parenchymal collapse occurs on the described background. With recovery, the liver morphology returns to normal within 3 mo of the acute infection. If chronic hepatitis develops, the inflammatory infiltrate settles in the periportal areas and often leads to progressive scarring. Both of these hallmarks of chronic hepatitis are seen in cases of HBV and HCV.

Common Biochemical Profiles in the Acute Infectious Phase

Acute liver injury caused by these viruses manifests in 3 main functional liver biochemical profiles. These serve as an important guide to diagnosis, supportive care, and monitoring in the acute phase of the infection for all viruses. As a reflection of *cytopathic injury* to the hepatocytes, there is a rise in serum levels of alanine aminotransferase (ALT) and aspartate aminotransferase (AST). The magnitude of enzyme elevation does not correlate with the extent of hepatocellular necrosis and has little prognostic value. There is usually slow improvement over several weeks, but AST and ALT levels *lag* the serum bilirubin level, which tends to normalize first. Rapidly falling aminotransferase levels can predict a poor outcome, particularly if their decline occurs in conjunction with a rising bilirubin level and a prolonged prothrombin time (PT); this combination of findings usually indicates that massive hepatic injury has occurred.

Cholestasis, defined by elevated serum conjugated bilirubin levels, results from abnormal bile flow at the canalicular and cellular level because of hepatocyte damage and inflammatory mediators. Elevation of serum alkaline phosphatase, 5′-nucleotidase, and γ-glutamyl transpeptidase levels, mark cholestasis. Absence of cholestatic markers does not rule out progression to chronicity in HCV or HBV infections.

Altered synthetic function is the most important marker of liver injury. Synthetic dysfunction is reflected by a combination of abnormal protein synthesis (prolonged PT, high international normalized ratio [INR], low serum albumin levels), metabolic disturbances (hypoglycemia, lactic acidosis, hyperammonemia), poor clearance of medications dependent on liver function, and altered sensorium with increased deep tendon reflexes (hepatic encephalopathy). Monitoring of synthetic function should be the main focus in clinical follow-up to define the severity of the disease. In the acute phase, the degree of liver synthetic dysfunction guides treatment and helps to establish intervention criteria. *Abnormal liver synthetic function is a marker of liver failure and is an indication for prompt referral to a transplant center.* Serial assessment is necessary because liver dysfunction does not progress linearly.

HEPATITIS A

Hepatitis A is the most prevalent form; this virus is also responsible for most forms of acute and benign hepatitis. Although fulminant hepatic failure due to HAV can occur, it is rare (<1% of cases in the United

States) and occurs more often in adults than in children and in hyperendemic communities.

Etiology

HAV is an RNA virus, a member of the picornavirus family. It is heat stable and has limited host range—namely, the human and other primates.

Epidemiology

HAV infection occurs throughout the world but is most prevalent in developing countries. In the United States, 30–40% of the adult population has evidence of previous HAV infection. Hepatitis A is thought to account for approximately 50% of all clinically apparent acute viral hepatitis in the United States. As a result of aggressive implementation of childhood vaccination programs, the prevalence of symptomatic HAV cases worldwide has declined significantly. However, outbreaks in developing countries and in daycare centers (where the spread of HAV from young, nonicteric, infected children can occur easily) as well as multiple foodborne and waterborne outbreaks have justified the implementation of intensified universal vaccination programs.

HAV is highly contagious. Transmission is almost always by person-to-person contact through the fecal–oral route. Perinatal transmission occurs rarely. No other form of transmission is recognized. HAV infection during pregnancy or at the time of delivery does not appear to result in increased complications of pregnancy or clinical disease in the newborn. In the United States, increased risk of infection is found in contacts with infected persons, childcare centers, and household contacts. Infection is also associated with contact with contaminated food or water and after travel to endemic areas. Common source foodborne and waterborne outbreaks continue to occur, including several caused by contaminated shellfish, frozen berries, and raw vegetables; no known source is found in about half of the cases.

The mean incubation period for HAV is approximately 3 wk. Fecal excretion of the virus starts late in the incubation period, reaches its peak just before the onset of symptoms, and resolves by 2 wk after the onset of jaundice in older subjects. The duration of fecal viral excretion is prolonged in infants. The patient is, therefore, contagious before clinical symptoms are apparent and remains so until viral shedding ceases.

Clinical Manifestations

HAV is responsible for acute hepatitis only. Often, this is an *anicteric* illness, with clinical symptoms indistinguishable from other forms of viral gastroenteritis, particularly in young children.

The illness is more likely to be symptomatic in older adolescents or adults, in patients with underlying liver disorders, and in those who are immunocompromised. It is characteristically an acute febrile illness with an abrupt onset of anorexia, nausea, malaise, vomiting, and jaundice. The typical duration of illness is 7-14 days (Fig. 385.1).

Other organ systems can be affected during acute HAV infection. Regional lymph nodes and the spleen may be enlarged. The bone marrow

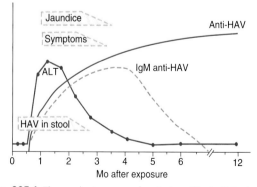

Fig. 385.1 The serologic course of acute hepatitis A. ALT, alanine aminotransferase; HAV, hepatitis A virus; IgM, immunoglobulin class M. *(From Goldman L, Ausiello D: Cecil textbook of medicine, ed 22, Philadelphia, 2004, WB Saunders, p 913.)*

may be moderately hypoplastic, and aplastic anemia has been reported. Tissue in the small intestine might show changes in villous structure, and ulceration of the gastrointestinal tract can occur, especially in fatal cases. Acute pancreatitis and myocarditis have been reported, though rarely, and nephritis, arthritis, leukocytoclastic vasculitis, and cryo-globulinemia can result from circulating immune complexes.

Diagnosis

Acute HAV infection is diagnosed by detecting antibodies to HAV, specifically, anti-HAV (immunoglobulin [Ig] M) by radioimmunoassay or, rarely, by identifying viral particles in stool. A viral polymerase chain reaction (PCR) assay is available for research use (Table 385.3). Anti-HAV is detectable when the symptoms are clinically apparent, and it remains positive for 4-6 mo after the acute infection. A neutralizing anti-HAV (IgG) is usually detected within 8 wk of symptom onset and is measured as part of a total anti-HAV in the serum. Anti-HAV (IgG) confers long-term protection. Rises in serum levels of ALT, AST, bilirubin, alkaline phosphatase, 5′-nucleotidase, and γ-glutamyl transpeptidase are almost universally found and do not help to differentiate the cause of hepatitis.

Complications

Although most patients achieve full recovery, distinct complications can occur. ALF from HAV infection is an infrequent complication of HAV. Those at risk for this complication are adolescents and adults, but also immunocompromised patients or those with underlying liver disorders. The height of HAV viremia may be linked to the severity of hepatitis. In the United States, HAV represents <0.5% of pediatric-age ALF; HAV is responsible for up to 3% mortality in the adult population with ALF. In endemic areas of the world, HAV constitutes up to 40% of all cases of pediatric ALF. HAV can also progress to a *prolonged cholestatic syndrome* that waxes and wanes over several months. Pruritus and fat malabsorption are problematic and require symptomatic support with antipruritic medications and fat-soluble vitamin supplementation. This syndrome occurs in the absence of any liver synthetic dysfunction and resolves without sequelae.

Treatment

There is no specific treatment for hepatitis A. Supportive treatment consists of intravenous hydration as needed, and antipruritic agents and fat-soluble vitamins for the prolonged cholestatic form of disease. Serial monitoring for signs of ALF is prudent and, if ALF is diagnosed, a prompt referral to a transplantation center can be lifesaving.

Prevention

Patients infected with HAV are contagious for 2 wk before and approximately 7 days after the onset of jaundice and should be excluded from school, childcare, or work during this period. Careful hand-washing is necessary, particularly after changing diapers and before preparing or serving food. In hospital settings, contact and standard precautions are recommended for 1 wk after onset of symptoms.

Immunoglobulin

Indications for intramuscular administration of Ig include preexposure and postexposure prophylaxis (Table 385.4). Ig is recommended for *preexposure* prophylaxis for susceptible travelers to countries where HAV is endemic, and it provides effective protection for up to 2 mo. *HAV vaccine* given any time before travel is preferred for *preexposure* prophylaxis in healthy persons, but *Ig* ensures an appropriate prophylaxis in children *younger than 12 mo* old, patients allergic to a vaccine component, or those who elect not to receive the vaccine. If travel is planned in <2 wk, older patients, immunocompromised hosts, and those with chronic liver disease or other medical conditions should receive *both* Ig and the HAV vaccine.

Ig prophylaxis in *postexposure* situations should be used as soon as possible (it is not effective if administered more than 2 wk after exposure). It is exclusively used for children younger than 12 mo old, immuno-compromised hosts, those with chronic liver disease or in whom vaccine

Table 385.4	Indications and Updated Dosage Recommendations for GamaSTAN S/D Human Immune Globulin for Preexposure and Postexposure Prophylaxis Against Hepatitis A Infection

INDICATION	UPDATED DOSAGE RECOMMENDATION
Preexposure prophylaxis	
Up to 1 mo of travel	0.1 mL/kg
Up to 2 mo of travel	0.2 mL/kg
2 mo of travel or longer	0.2 mL/kg (repeat every 2 mo)
Postexposure prophylaxis	0.1 mL/kg

From Nelson NP: Updated dosing instruction for immune globulin (human) gamaSTAN S/D for hepatitis A virus prophylaxis, *MMWR* 66(36):959–960, 2017, Table, p. 959.

Table 385.3	Diagnostic Blood Tests: Serology and Viral Polymerase Chain Reaction

HAV	HBV	HCV	HDV	HEV
ACUTE/ACTIVE INFECTION				
Anti-HAV IgM (+)	Anti-HBc IgM (+)	Anti-HCV (+)	Anti-HDV IgM (+)	Anti-HEV IgM (+)
Blood PCR positive*	HBsAg (+)	HCV RNA (+) (PCR)	Blood PCR positive	Blood PCR positive*
	Anti-HBs (–)		HBsAg (+)	
	HBV DNA (+) (PCR)		Anti-HBs (–)	
PAST INFECTION (RECOVERED)				
Anti-HAV IgG(+)	Anti-HBs (+)	Anti-HCV (+)	Anti-HDV IgG (+)	Anti-HEV IgG (+)
	Anti-HBc IgG (+)†	Blood PCR (–)	Blood PCR (–)	Blood PCR (–)
CHRONIC INFECTION				
N/A	Anti-HBc IgG (+)	Anti-HCV (+)	Anti-HDV IgG (+)	N/A
	HBsAg (+)	Blood PCR (+)	Blood PCR (–)	
	Anti-HBs (–)		HBsAg (+)	
	PCR (+) or (–)		Anti-HBs (–)	
VACCINE RESPONSE				
Anti-HAV IgG (+)	Anti-HBs (+)	N/A	N/A	N/A
	Anti-HBc (–)			

*Research tool.
†Still poses a risk for reactivation.
HAV, hepatitis A virus; HBs, hepatitis B surface; HBsAg, hepatitis B surface antigen; Ig, immunoglobulin; PCR, polymerase chain reaction.

is contraindicated. Ig is preferred in patients older than 40 yr of age, with HAV vaccine preferred in healthy persons 12 mo to 40 yr old. An alternative approach is to immunize previously unvaccinated patients who are 12 *mo* old *or older* with the age-appropriate vaccine dosage as soon as possible. Ig is not routinely recommended for sporadic nonhousehold exposure (e.g., protection of hospital personnel or schoolmates). The vaccine has several advantages over Ig, including long-term protection, availability, and ease of administration, with cost similar to, or less than, that of Ig.

Vaccine

The availability of 2 inactivated, highly immunogenic, and safe HAV vaccines has had a major impact on the prevention of HAV infection. Both vaccines are approved for children older than 12 mo. They are administered intramuscularly in a 2-dose schedule, with the second dose given 6-12 mo after the first dose. Seroconversion rates in children exceed 90% after an initial dose and approach 100% after the second dose; protective antibody titer persists for longer than 10 yr in most patients. The immune response in immunocompromised persons, older patients, and those with chronic illnesses may be suboptimal; in those patients, combining the vaccine with Ig for pre- and postexposure prophylaxis is indicated. HAV vaccine may be administered simultaneously with other vaccines. A combination HAV and HBV vaccine is approved in adults older than age 18 yr. For healthy persons at least 12 mo old, vaccine is preferable to Ig for preexposure and postexposure prophylaxis (see Table 385.3).

In the United States and some other countries, universal vaccination is now recommended for all children older than 12 mo. Nevertheless, studies show <50% of U.S. adolescents have received even a single dose of the vaccine, and <30% have received the complete vaccine series. The vaccine is effective in curbing outbreaks of HAV because of rapid seroconversion and the long incubation period of the disease.

Prognosis

The prognosis for the patient with HAV is excellent, with no long-term sequelae. The only feared complication is ALF. Nevertheless, HAV infection remains a major cause of morbidity; it has a high socioeconomic impact during epidemics and in endemic areas.

HEPATITIS B
Etiology

HBV, a member of the Hepadnaviridae family, has a circular, partially double-stranded DNA genome composed of approximately 3,200 nucleotides. Four constitutive genes have been identified: the S (surface), C (core), X, and P (polymer) genes. The surface of the virus includes particles, designated as the hepatitis B surface antigen (HBsAg), which consist of 22 nm diameter spherical particles and 22 nm wide tubular particles with a variable length of up to 200 nm. The inner portion of the virion contains the hepatitis B core antigen (HBcAg), the nucleocapsid that encodes the viral DNA, and a nonstructural antigen called the hepatitis B e antigen (HBeAg), a nonparticulate soluble antigen derived from HBcAg by proteolytic self-cleavage. HBeAg serves as a marker of active viral replication and usually correlates with the HBV DNA levels. Replication of HBV occurs predominantly in the liver but also occurs in the lymphocytes, spleen, kidney, and pancreas.

Epidemiology

HBV has been detected worldwide, with an estimated 400 million persons chronically infected. The areas of highest prevalence of HBV infection are sub-Saharan Africa, China, parts of the Middle East, the Amazon basin, and the Pacific Islands. In the United States, the native population in Alaska had the highest prevalence rate before the implementation of their universal vaccination programs. An estimated 1.25 million persons in the United States are chronic HBV carriers, with approximately 300,000 new cases of HBV occurring each year, the highest incidence being among adults 20-39 yr of age. One in 4 chronic HBV carriers will develop serious sequelae in their lifetime. The number of new cases in children reported each year is thought to be low but is difficult to estimate because many infections in children are asymptomatic. In the

United States, since 1982 when the first vaccine for HBV was introduced, the overall incidence of HBV infection has been reduced by more than half. Since the implementation of universal vaccination programs in Taiwan and the United States, substantial progress has been made toward eliminating HBV infection in children in these countries. In fact, in Alaska, where HBV neared epidemic proportions, universal newborn vaccination with mass screening and immunization of susceptible Alaska Natives virtually eliminated symptomatic HBV and secondary hepatocellular carcinoma (HCC).

HBV is present in high concentrations in blood, serum, and serous exudates and in moderate concentrations in saliva, vaginal fluid, and semen. Efficient transmission occurs through blood exposure and sexual contact. Risk factors for HBV infection in children and adolescents include acquisition by intravenous drugs or blood products, contaminated needles used for acupuncture or tattoos, sexual contact, institutional care, and intimate contact with carriers. No risk factors are identified in approximately 40% of cases. HBV is not thought to be transmitted via indirect exposure, such as sharing toys. After infection, the incubation period ranges from 45-160 days, with a mean of approximately 120 days. In children, the most important risk factor for acquisition of HBV remains perinatal exposure to an HBsAg-positive mother. The risk of transmission is greatest if the mother is HBeAg-positive; up to 90% of these infants become chronically infected if untreated. Additional risk factors include high maternal HBV viral load (HBeAg/HBV DNA titers) and delivery of a prior infant who developed HBV despite appropriate prophylaxis. In most perinatal cases, serologic markers of infection and antigenemia appear 1-3 mo after birth, suggesting that transmission occurred at the time of delivery. Virus contained in amniotic fluid or in maternal feces or blood may be the source. Immunoprophylaxis with hepatitis B immunoglobulin (HBIG) and the HBV immunization, given within 12 hr of delivery, is highly effective in preventing infection and protects >95% of neonates born to HBsAg-positive mothers. Of the 22,000 infants born each year to HBsAg-positive mothers in the United States, >98% receive immunoprophylaxis and are thus protected. Infants who fail to receive the complete vaccination series (e.g., homeless children, international adoptees, and children born outside the United States) have the highest incidence of developing chronic HBV. These and all infants born to HBsAg-positive mothers should have follow-up HBsAg and anti-HBs tested to determine appropriate follow-up. The mothers (HBeAg positive) of these infants who develop chronic HBV infection should receive antiviral therapy during the third trimester for subsequent pregnancies.

HBsAg is inconsistently recovered in human milk of infected mothers. Breastfeeding of nonimmunized infants by infected mothers does not seem to confer a greater risk of hepatitis than does formula feeding.

The risk of developing chronic HBV infection, defined as being positive for HBsAg for longer than 6 mo, is inversely related to age of acquisition. In the United States, although <10% of infections occur in children, these infections account for 20–30% of all chronic cases. This risk of chronic infection is 90% in children younger than 1 yr; the risk is 30% for those 1-5 yr of age and 2% for adults. Chronic HBV infection is associated with the development of chronic liver disease and HCC. The carcinoma risk is independent of the presence of cirrhosis and was the most prevalent cancer-related death in young adults in Asia where HBV was endemic.

HBV has 10 genotypes (A-J). A is pandemic, B and C are prevalent in Asia, D is seen in Southern Europe, E in Africa, F in the United States, G in the United States and France, H in Central America, I in southeast Asia, and J in Japan. Genetic variants have become resistant to some antiviral agents.

Pathogenesis

The acute response of the liver to HBV is similar to that of other viruses. Persistence of histologic changes in patients with hepatitis B indicates development of chronic liver disease. HBV, unlike the other hepatotropic viruses, is a predominantly noncytopathic virus that causes injury mostly by immune-mediated processes. The severity of hepatocyte injury reflects the degree of the immune response, with the most complete immune response being associated with the greatest likelihood of viral clearance but also the most severe injury to hepatocytes. The first step in the process of acute hepatitis is infection of hepatocytes by HBV, resulting in expression of viral antigens on the cell surface. The most important of these viral antigens may be the nucleocapsid antigens—HBcAg and HBeAg. These antigens, in combination with class I major histocompatibility proteins, make the cell a target for cytotoxic T-cell lysis.

The mechanism for development of chronic hepatitis B is less well understood. To permit hepatocytes to continue to be infected, the core protein or major histocompatibility class I protein might not be recognized, the cytotoxic lymphocytes might not be activated, or some other, yet unknown mechanism might interfere with destruction of hepatocytes. This tolerance phenomenon predominates in the perinatally acquired cases, resulting in a high incidence of persistent HBV infection in children with no or little inflammation in the liver, normal liver enzymes, and markedly elevated HBV viral load. Although end-stage liver disease rarely develops in those patients, the inherent HCC risk is high, possibly related, in part, to uncontrolled viral replication cycles.

ALF has been seen in infants of chronic carrier mothers who have anti-HBe or are infected with a precore-mutant strain. This fact led to the postulate that HBeAg exposure in utero in infants of chronic carriers likely induces tolerance to the virus once infection occurs postnatally. In the absence of this tolerance, the liver is massively attacked by T cells and the patient presents with ALF.

Immune-mediated mechanisms are also involved in the extrahepatic conditions that can be associated with HBV infections. Circulating immune complexes containing HBsAg can result in polyarteritis nodosa, membranous or membranoproliferative glomerulonephritis, polymyalgia rheumatica, leukocytoclastic vasculitis, and Guillain-Barré syndrome.

Clinical Manifestations

Many acute cases of HBV infection in children are asymptomatic, as evidenced by the high carriage rate of serum markers in persons who have no history of acute hepatitis (Table 385.5). The usual acute symptomatic episode is similar to that of HAV and HCV infections but may be more severe and is more likely to include involvement of skin and joints (Fig. 385.2).

The first biochemical evidence of HBV infection is elevation of serum ALT levels, which begin to rise just before development of fatigue, anorexia, and malaise, at approximately 6-7 wk after exposure. The illness is preceded, in a few children, by a serum sickness–like prodrome marked by arthralgia or skin lesions, including urticarial, purpuric, macular, or maculopapular rashes. Papular acrodermatitis, the Gianotti-Crosti syndrome, can also occur. Other extrahepatic conditions associated with HBV infections in children include polyarteritis nodosa, glomeru-

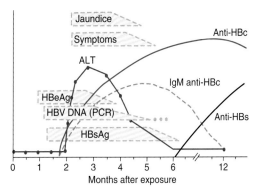

Fig. 385.2 The serologic course of acute hepatitis B. ALT, alanine aminotransferase; HBc, hepatitis B core; HBeAg, hepatitis B e antigen; HBsAg, hepatitis B surface antigen; HBV DNA, hepatitis B virus deoxyribonucleic acid; IgM, immunoglobulin class M; PCR, polymerase chain reaction. (*From Goldman L, Ausiello D: Cecil textbook of medicine, ed 22, Philadelphia, 2004, WB Saunders, p 914.*)

lonephritis, and aplastic anemia. Jaundice is present in approximately 25% of acutely infected patients and usually begins approximately 8 wk after exposure and lasts approximately 4 wk.

In the usual course of resolving HBV infection, symptoms persist for 6-8 wk. The percentage of children in whom clinical evidence of hepatitis develops is higher for HBV than for HAV, and the rate of ALF is also greater. Most patients do recover, but the *chronic carrier state* complicates up to 10% of cases acquired in adulthood. The rate of development of chronic infection depends largely on the mode and age of acquisition and occurs in up to 90% of perinatally-infected cases. Cirrhosis and HCC are only seen with chronic infection. Chronic HBV infection has 3 identified phases: immune tolerant, immune active, and inactive. Most children fall in the *immune-tolerant* phase, against which no effective therapy has been developed. Most treatments target the *immune active* phase of the disease, characterized by active inflammation, elevated ALT/AST levels, and progressive fibrosis. Spontaneous HBeAg seroconversion, defined as the development of anti-HBe and loss of HBeAg, occurs in the immune-tolerant phase, albeit at low rates of 4–5% per year. It is more common in childhood-acquired HBV rather than in perinatally transmitted infections. Seroconversion can occur over many years, during which time significant damage to the liver may take place. There are no large studies that accurately assess the lifetime

| **Table 385.5** | Typical Interpretation of Test Results for Hepatitis B Virus Infection |

HBsAg	TOTAL ANTI-HBc	IgM ANTI-HBc	ANTI-HBs	HBV DNA	INTERPRETATION
–	–	–	–	–	Never infected
+	–	–	–	+ or –	Early acute infection; transient (up to 18 days) after vaccination
+	+	+	–	+	Acute infection
–	+	+	+ or –	+ or –	Acute resolving infection
–	+	–	+	–	Recovered from past infection and immune
+	+	–	–	+	Chronic infection
–	+	–	–	+ or –	False-positive (i.e., susceptible); past infection; "low-level" chronic infection; or passive transfer of anti-HBc to infant born to HBsAg-positive mother
–	–	–	+	–	Immune if anti-HBs concentration is ≥10 mIU/mL after vaccine series completion; passive transfer after hepatitis B immune globulin administration

–, negative; +, positive; anti-HBc, antibody to hepatitis B core antigen; anti-HBs, antibody to hepatitis B surface antigen; HBsAg, hepatitis B surface antigen; HBV DNA, hepatitis B virus deoxyribonucleic acid; IgM, immunoglobulin class M.
From Schillie S, Vellozzi C, Reingold A, et al: Prevention of hepatitis B virus infection in the United States: recommendations of the advisory committee on immunization practices, *MMWR* 67(1):1–29, 2018, Table 1, p. 7.

Table 385.6	Causes of Hepatitis Flares in Patients With Chronic Hepatitis B
CAUSE OF FLARE	**COMMENT**
Spontaneous	Factors that precipitate viral replication are unclear
Immunosuppressive therapy	Flares are often observed during withdrawal of the agent; preemptive antiviral therapy is required
Antiviral therapy for HBV	
Interferon	Flares are often observed during the second to third month of therapy in 30% of patients;
Nucleoside analog	may herald virologic response
During treatment	Flares are no more common than with placebo
Drug-resistant HBV	Severe consequences can occur in patients with advanced liver disease
On withdrawal	Flares are caused by the rapid re-emergence of wild-type HBV; severe consequences can occur in patients with advanced liver disease
HIV treatment	Flares can occur as a result of the direct toxicity of HAART or with immune reconstitution; HBV increases the risk of antiretroviral drug hepatotoxicity
Genotypic variation	
Precore and core promoter mutants	Fluctuations in serum alanine aminotransferase levels are common with precore mutants
Superinfection with other hepatitis viruses	May be associated with suppression of HBV replication

HAART, Highly active antiretroviral therapy; HBV, hepatitis B virus.
From Wells JT, Perillo R: Hepatitis B. In Feldman M, Friedman LS, Brandt LJ, editors: *Sleisenger and Fordtran's gastrointestinal and liver disease*, 10/e, Philadelphia, 2016, Elsevier, Table 79.1.

risks and morbidities of children with chronic HBV infection, making decisions regarding the rationale, efficacy, and timing of still less-than-ideal treatments difficult. Reactivation of chronic infection has been reported in immunosuppressed children treated with chemotherapy, biologic immunomodulators such as infliximab, or T-cell depleting agents, leading to an increased risk of ALF or to rapidly progressing fibrotic liver disease (Table 385.6).

Diagnosis

The serologic profile of HBV infection is more complex than for HAV infection and differs depending on whether the disease is acute or chronic (Fig. 385.3, see Table 385.5). Several antigens and antibodies are used to confirm the diagnosis of acute HBV infection (see Table 385.3). Routine screening for HBV infection requires assay of multiple serologic markers (HBsAg, anti-HBc, anti-HBs). HBsAg is an early serologic marker of infection and is found in almost all infected persons; its rise closely coincides with the onset of symptoms. Persistence of HBsAg beyond 6 mo defines the chronic infection state. During recovery from acute infection, because HBsAg levels fall before symptoms wane, IgM antibody to HBcAg (anti-HBc IgM) might be the only marker of acute infection. Anti-HBc IgM rises early after the infection and remains positive for many months before being replaced by anti-HBc IgG, which then persists for years. Anti-HBs marks serologic recovery and protection. Only anti-HBs is present in persons immunized with hepatitis B vaccine, whereas both anti-HBs and anti-HBc are detected in persons with resolved infection. HBeAg is present in active acute or chronic infection and is a marker of infectivity. The development of anti-HBe, termed seroconversion, marks improvement and is a goal of therapy in chronically infected patients. HBV DNA can be detected in the serum of acutely infected patients and chronic carriers. High DNA titers are seen in patients with HBeAg, and they typically fall once anti-HBe develops.

Complications

ALF with coagulopathy, encephalopathy, and cerebral edema occurs more commonly with HBV than the other hepatotropic viruses. The risk of ALF is further increased when there is coinfection or superinfection with HDV or in an immunosuppressed host. Mortality from ALF is >30%, and liver transplantation is the only effective intervention. Supportive care aimed at sustaining patients and early referral to a liver transplantation center can be lifesaving. As mentioned, HBV infection can also result in chronic hepatitis, which can lead to cirrhosis, end-stage liver disease complications, and HCC. Membranous glomerulonephritis

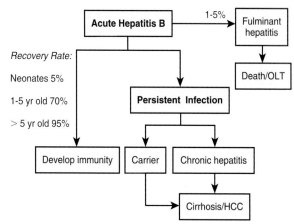

Fig. 385.3 Natural history of hepatitis B virus infection. HCC, hepatocellular carcinoma; OLT, orthotopic liver transplant.

with deposition of complement and HBeAg in glomerular capillaries is a rare complication of HBV infection.

Treatment

Treatment of *acute* HBV infection is largely supportive. Close monitoring for liver failure and extrahepatic morbidities is key. Treatment of *chronic* HBV infection is in evolution; no 1 drug currently achieves consistent, complete eradication of the virus. The natural history of chronic HBV infection in children is complex, and there is a lack of reliable long-term outcome data on which to base treatment recommendations. Treatment of chronic HBV infection in children should be individualized and done under the care of a pediatric hepatologist experienced in treating the disease.

The goal of treatment is to reduce viral replication defined by having undetectable HBV DNA in the serum and development of anti-HBe, termed seroconversion. The development of anti-HBe transforms the disease into an inactive form, thereby decreasing infectivity, active liver injury and inflammation, fibrosis progression, and the risk of HCC. Treatment is only indicated for patients in the immune-active form of the disease, as evidenced by elevated ALT and/or AST, who have fibrosis on liver biopsy, putting the child at higher risk for cirrhosis during childhood.

Treatment Strategies

Interferon-α2b (IFN-α2b) has immunomodulatory and antiviral effects (Table 385.7). It has been used in children, with long-term viral response rates similar to the 25% rate reported in adults. Interferon (IFN) use is limited by its subcutaneous administration, treatment duration of 24 wk, and side effects (flu-like symptoms, marrow suppression, depression, retinal changes, autoimmune disorders). IFN is further contraindicated in decompensated cirrhosis. One advantage of IFN, compared to other treatments, is that viral resistance does not develop with its use.

Lamivudine is an oral synthetic nucleoside analog that inhibits the viral enzyme reverse transcriptase. In children older than 2 yr of age, its use for 52 wk resulted in HBeAg clearance in 34% of patients with an ALT >2 times normal; 88% remained in remission at 1 yr. It has a good safety profile. Lamivudine has to be used for ≥ 6 mo after viral clearance, and the emergence of a mutant viral strain (YMDD) poses a barrier to its long-term use. Combination therapy in children using IFN and lamivudine did not seem to improve the rates of response in most series.

Adefovir (a purine analog that inhibits viral replication) is approved for use in children older than 12 yr of age, in whom a prospective 1-yr study showed 23% seroconversion. No viral resistance was noted in that study but has been reported in adults.

Entecavir (a nucleoside analog that inhibits replication) is currently approved for use in children older than 2 yr of age. Prospective data has shown a 21% seroconversion rate in adults with minimal resistance developing. Patients in whom resistance to lamivudine developed have an increased risk of resistance developing to entecavir.

Tenofovir (a nucleotide analog that inhibits viral replication) is also approved for use in children older than 12 yr of age. Prospective data have shown a 21% seroconversion rate with a very low rate of resistance developing. Patients with lamivudine-resistant mutations do not appear to have an increased rate of resistance. Concern exists over long-term use and bone mineral density.

Peginterferon-α₂ has the same mechanism of action as IFN but is given once weekly. This formulation has not been approved in the United States but is recommended for the treatment of chronic HBV in other countries. Patients most likely to respond to currently available drugs have low serum HBV DNA titers, are HBeAg-positive, have active hepatic inflammation (ALT greater than twice the upper limit of normal for at least 6 mo), and recently acquired disease.

Immune tolerant patients—those with normal ALT and AST, who are HBeAg-positive with elevated viral load—are currently not considered for treatment, although the emergence of new treatment paradigms is promising for this large, yet hard-to-treat, subgroup of patients.

Prevention

The most effective prevention strategies have resulted from the screening of pregnant mothers and the use of HBIG and hepatitis B vaccine in infants (Tables 385.8 to 385.11). In HBsAg-positive and HBeAg-positive mothers, a 10% risk of chronic HBV infection exists compared to 1% in HBeAg-negative mothers. This knowledge offers screening strategies that may affect both mother and infant by using antiviral medications during the third trimester. Guidelines suggest that mothers with an HBV DNA viral load >200,000 IU/mL receive an antiviral such as telbivudine, lamivudine, or tenofovir during the third trimester, especially

Table 385.8	Strategy to Eliminate Hepatitis B Virus Transmission in the United States*

- Screening of all pregnant women for HBsAg

HBV DNA testing for HBsAg-positive pregnant women, with suggestion of maternal antiviral therapy to reduce perinatal transmission when HBV DNA is >200,000 IU/mL

Prophylaxis (HepB vaccine and hepatitis B immunoglobulin) for infants born to HBsAg-positive[†] women

- Universal vaccination of all infants beginning at birth[‡,§] as a safeguard for infants born to HBV-infected mothers not identified prenatally

- Routine vaccination of previously unvaccinated children aged <19 yr

- Vaccination of adults at risk for HBV infection, including those requesting protection from HBV without acknowledgment of a specific risk factor

*Sources: Mast EE, Margolis HS, Fiore AE, et al: A comprehensive immunization strategy to eliminate transmission of hepatitis B virus infection in the United States: recommendations of the Advisory Committee on Immunization Practices (ACIP). Part 1: immunization of infants, children, and adolescents, *MMWR Recomm Rep* 54(No. RR-16):1–31, 2005; Mast EE, Weinbaum CM, Fiore AE, et al: A comprehensive immunization strategy to eliminate transmission of hepatitis B virus infection in the United States: recommendations of the Advisory Committee on Immunization Practices (ACIP). Part II: immunization of adults, *MMWR Recomm Rep* 55(No. RR-16):1–33, 2006.
[†]Refer to Table 385.9 for prophylaxis recommendations for infants born to women with unknown HBsAg status.
[‡]Within 24 hr of birth for medically stable infants weighing ≥2,000 g.
[§]Refer to Table 385.9 for birth dose recommendations for infants weighing <2,000 g.
HBsAg, hepatitis B surface antigen; HBV, hepatitis B virus.
From Schillie S, Vellozzi C, Reingold A, et al: Prevention of hepatitis B virus infection in the United States: recommendations of the advisory committee on immunization practices, *MMWR* 67[1]:1–29, 2018, Box 2, p. 5.

Table 385.7	Positive and Negative Factors to Consider in the Decision to Treat Hepatitis B With Peginterferon or a Nucleoside or Nucleotide Analog	
AGENT	**POSITIVE FACTORS**	**NEGATIVE FACTORS**
Peginterferon	Finite duration of treatment Durable off-treatment response More rapid disappearance of HBsAg Immunostimulatory as well as intrinsically antiviral Better tolerability compared with its use in hepatitis C	Inconvenience of subcutaneous injection Frequent side effects Clearance of HBsAg in a small minority of patients depending on genotype Potential risk of ALT flares in patients with advanced liver fibrosis Relative contraindication in patients older than age 60 or those with comorbid illnesses
Nucleoside or nucleotide analog	Negligible side effects Convenience; ready acceptance by patients Potent inhibition of virus replication Reduced drug resistance with the third-generation nucleoside analogs	Slight risk of nephropathy with nucleotide analogs (adefovir, tenofovir) Drug expense can be considerable during long-term use Long or indefinite treatment needed for both HBeAg-positive and HBeAg-negative patients Access issues in developing nations

HBeAg, hepatitis B e antigen; HBsAg, hepatitis B surface antigen.
From Wells JT, Perillo R: Hepatitis B. In Feldman M, Friedman LS, Brandt LJ, editors: *Sleisenger and Fordtran's gastrointestinal and liver disease*, 10/e, Philadelphia, 2016, Elsevier, Table 79.4.

Table 385.9	Hepatitis B Vaccine Schedules for Infants, by Infant Birthweight and Maternal Hepatitis B Surface Antigen Status

		SINGLE-ANTIGEN VACCINE		SINGLE-ANTIGEN + COMBINATION VACCINE[†]	
BIRTHWEIGHT	MATERNAL HBsAg STATUS	DOSE	AGE	DOSE	AGE
≥2,000 g	Positive	1	Birth (≤12 hr)	1	Birth (≤12 hr)
		HBIG[‡]	Birth (≤12 hr)	HBIG	Birth (≤12 hr)
		2	1-2 mo	2	2 mo
		3	6 mo[§]	3	4 mo
				4	6 mo[§]
	Unknown*	1	Birth (≤12 hr)	1	Birth (≤12 hr)
		2	1-2 mo	2	2 mo
		3	6 mo[§]	3	4 mo
				4	6 mo[§]
	Negative	1	Birth (≤24 hr)	1	Birth (≤24 hr)
		2	1-2 mo	2	2 mo
		3	6-18 mo[§]	3	4 mo
				4	6 mo[§]
<2,000 g	Positive	1	Birth (≤12 hr)	1	Birth (≤12 hr)
		HBIG	Birth (≤12 hr)	HBIG	Birth (≤12 hr)
		2	1 mo	2	2 mo
		3	2-3 mo	3	4 mo
		4	6 mo[§]	4	6 mo[§]
	Unknown	1	Birth (≤12 hr)	1	Birth (≤12 hr)
		HBIG	Birth (≤12 hr)	HBIG	Birth (≤12 hr)
		2	1 mo	2	2 mo
		3	2-3 mo	3	4 mo
		4	6 mo[§]	4	6 mo[§]
	Negative	1	Hospital discharge or age 1 mo	1	Hospital discharge or age 1 mo
		2	2 mo	2	2 mo
		3	6-18 mo[§]	3	4 mo
				4	6 mo[§]

*Mothers should have blood drawn and tested for HBsAg as soon as possible after admission for delivery; if the mother is found to be HBsAg positive, the infant should receive HBIG as soon as possible but no later than age 7 days.
[†]Pediarix should not be administered before age 6 wk.
[‡]HBIG should be administered at a separate anatomical site from vaccine.
[§]The final dose in the vaccine series should not be administered before age 24 wk (164 days).
HBIG, hepatitis B immune globulin; HBsAg, hepatitis B surface antigen.
From Schillie S, Vellozzi C, Reingold A, et al: Prevention of hepatitis B virus infection in the United States: recommendations of the advisory committee on immunization practices, MMWR 67(1):1–29, 2018, Table 3, p. 12.

Table 385.10	Recommended Doses of Hepatitis B Vaccine by Group and Vaccine Type

	SINGLE-ANTIGEN VACCINE				COMBINATION VACCINE			
	RECOMBIVAX		ENGERIX		PEDIARIX*		TWINRIX[†]	
Age Group (yr)	Dose (µg)	Vol (mL)	Dose (µg)	Vol (mL)	Dose (µg)	Vol (mL)	Dose (µg)	Vol (mL)
Birth-10	5	0.5	10	0.5	10*	0.5	N/A	N/A
11-15	10[‡]	1	N/A	N/A	N/A	N/A	N/A	N/A
11-19	5	0.5	10	0.5	N/A	N/A	N/A	N/A
≥20	10	1	20	1	N/A	N/A	20[†]	1
HEMODIALYSIS PATIENTS AND OTHER IMMUNE-COMPROMISED PERSONS								
<20	5	0.5	10	0.5	N/A	N/A	N/A	N/A
≥20	40	1	40	2	N/A	N/A	N/A	N/A

*Pediarix is approved for use in persons aged 6 wk through 6 yr (prior to the 7th birthday).
[†]Twinrix is approved for use in persons aged ≥18 yr.
[‡]Adult formulation administered on a 2-dose schedule.
N/A, not applicable.
From Schillie S, Vellozzi C, Reingold A, et al: Prevention of hepatitis B virus infection in the United States: recommendations of the advisory committee on immunization practices, MMWR 67(1):1–29, 2018, Table 2, p. 10.

if they had a previous child who developed chronic HBV after receiving HBIG and the hepatitis B vaccine. This practice has proven safe with normal growth and development in infants of treated mothers.

Household, sexual, and needle-sharing contacts of patients with chronic HBV infection should be identified and vaccinated if they are susceptible to HBV infection. Patients should be advised about the perinatal and intimate contact risk of transmission of HBV. HBV is not spread by breastfeeding, kissing, hugging, or sharing water or utensils. Children with HBV should not be excluded from school, play, childcare, or work, unless they are prone to biting. A support group might help children to cope better with their disease. Families should not feel obligated to disclose the diagnosis as this information may lead to prejudice or mistreatment of the patient or the patient's family. All patients positive for HBsAg should be reported to the state or local health department, and chronicity is diagnosed if they remain positive past 6 mo HBIG.

HBIG is indicated only for specific *postexposure* circumstances and

Table 385.11	Hepatitis B Vaccine Schedules for Children, Adolescents, and Adults
AGE GROUP	**SCHEDULE* (INTERVAL REPRESENTS TIME IN MONTHS FROM FIRST DOSE)**
Children (1-10 yr)	0, 1, and 6 mo 0, 1, 2, and 12 mo
Adolescents (11-19 yr)	0, 1, and 6 mo 0, 12, and 24 mo 0 and 4-6 mo[†] 0, 1, 2, and 12 mo 0, 7 days, 21-30 days, 12 mo[‡]
Adults (≥20 yr)	0, 1, and 6 mo 0, 1, 2, and 12 mo 0, 1, 2, and 6 mo[§] 0, 7 days, 21-30 days, 12 mo[‡]

*Refer to package inserts for further information. For all ages, when the HepB vaccine schedule is interrupted, the vaccine series does not need to be restarted. If the series is interrupted after the 1st dose, the 2nd dose should be administered as soon as possible, and the 2nd and 3rd doses should be separated by an interval of at least 8 wk. If only the 3rd dose has been delayed, it should be administered as soon as possible. The final dose of vaccine must be administered at least 8 wk after the 2nd dose and should follow the 1st dose by at least 16 wk; the minimum interval between the 1st and 2nd doses is 4 wk. Inadequate doses of hepatitis B vaccine or doses received after a shorter-than-recommended dosing interval should be readministered, using the correct dosage or schedule. Vaccine doses administered ≤ 4 days before the minimum interval or age are considered valid. Because of the unique accelerated schedule for Twinrix, the 4-day guideline does not apply to the 1st 3 doses of this vaccine when administered on a 0-day, 7-day, 21-30-day, and 12-mo schedule (new recommendation).
[†]A 2-dose schedule of Recombivax adult formulation (10 μg) is licensed for adolescents aged 11-15 yr. When scheduled to receive the second dose, adolescents aged >15 yr should be switched to a 3-dose series, with doses 2 and 3 consisting of the pediatric formulation administered on an appropriate schedule.
[‡]Twinrix is approved for use in persons aged ≥ 18 yr and is available on an accelerated schedule with doses administered at 0, 7, 21-30 days, and 12 mo.
[§]A 4-dose schedule of Engerix administered in 2 1 mL doses (40 μg) on a 0-, 1-, 2-, and 6-mo schedule is recommended for adult hemodialysis patients.
From Schillie S, Vellozzi C, Reingold A, et al: Prevention of hepatitis B virus infection in the United States: recommendations of the advisory committee on immunization practices, *MMWR* 67(1):1–29, 2018, Table 4, p. 13.

provides only temporary protection (3-6 mo). It plays a pivotal role in preventing *perinatal* transmission when administered within 12 hr of birth.

Universal Vaccination

Two single-antigen vaccines (Recombivax HB and Engerix-B) are approved for children and are the only preparations approved for infants younger than age 6 mo. Three combination vaccines can be used for subsequent immunization dosing and enable integration of the HBV vaccine into the regular immunization schedule. The safety profile of HBV vaccine is excellent. The most reported side effects are pain at the injection site (up to 29% of cases) and fever (up to 6% of cases). Seropositivity is >95% with all vaccines, achieved after the second dose in most patients. The third dose serves as a booster and may have an effect on maintaining long-term immunity. In immunosuppressed patients and infants whose birthweight is <2,000 g, a fourth dose is recommended (the birth dose does not count as part of the 3-dose series) and these infants should be checked for anti-HBs and HBsAg after completing these shots. In this group of infants, if the anti-HBs level is <10 mIU/mL, they should repeat the 3-dose series. Despite declines in the anti-HBs titer in time, most healthy vaccinated persons remain protected against HBV infection.

Current HBV vaccination recommendations are as noted in Tables 385.9 to 385.11.

Postvaccination testing for HBsAg and anti-HBs should be done at 9-18 mo. If the result is positive for anti-HBs, the child is immune to HBV. If the result is positive for HBsAg only, the parent should be

counseled, and the child evaluated by a pediatric hepatologist. If the result is negative for both HBsAg and anti-HBs, a second complete hepatitis B vaccine series should be administered, followed by testing for anti-HBs to determine if subsequent doses are needed.

Administration of 4 doses of vaccine is permissible when combination vaccines are used after the birth dose; this does not impact vaccine response.

Postexposure Prophylaxis

Recommendations for postexposure prophylaxis for prevention of hepatitis B infection depend on the conditions under which the person is exposed to HBV (see Table 385.11). Vaccination should never be postponed if written records of the exposed person's immunization history are not available, but every effort should still be made to obtain those records.

Special Populations

Patients with cirrhosis may not respond as well to the HBV vaccine and repeating anti-HBs titers should be performed. Adult studies suggest higher dosage or shorter interval between dosages may increase the immunization effectiveness. Patients with inflammatory bowel disease frequently have not been immunized, or did not develop complete immunity to HBV, as demonstrated by inadequate anti-HBs levels. These patients may be at risk for fulminant HBV (reactivation) when immunosuppression is started as part of their treatment regimen, specifically with biologic agents such as infliximab.

Prognosis

In general, the outcome after acute HBV infection is favorable, despite a risk of ALF. The risk of developing chronic infection brings the risks of liver cirrhosis and HCC to the forefront. Perinatal transmission leading to chronicity is responsible for the high incidence of HCC in young adults in endemic areas. Importantly, HBV infection and its complications are effectively controlled and prevented with vaccination and multiple clinical trials are ongoing in an effort to improve and guide treatment regimens.

HEPATITIS C
Etiology

HCV is a single-stranded RNA virus, classified as a separate genus within the Flaviviridae family, with marked genetic heterogeneity. It has 6 major genotypes and numerous subtypes and quasi-species, which permit the virus to escape host immune surveillance. Genotype variation might partially explain the differences in clinical course and response to treatment. Genotype 1b is the most common genotype in the United States and is the least responsive to the approved pediatric medications.

Epidemiology

In the United States, HCV infection, the most common cause of chronic liver disease in adults, is responsible for 8,000-10,000 deaths per year. Approximately 4 million people in the United States and 170 million people worldwide are estimated to be infected with HCV. Approximately 85% of infected adults remain chronically infected. In children, seroprevalence of HCV is 0.2% in those younger than age 11 yr and 0.4% in children age 11 yr or older. However, even more children may be infected as only a small percentage of HCV-infected children are identified, and an even smaller number subsequently receive treatment. Appropriate identification, and screening, for infected individuals should be implemented.

Risk factors for HCV transmission in the United States included blood transfusion before 1992 as the most common route of infection, but, with current blood donor screening practices, the risk of HCV transmission is approximately 0.001% per unit transfused. Illegal drug use with exposure to blood or blood products from HCV-infected persons accounts for more than half of adult cases in the United States. Sexual transmission, especially through multiple sexual partners, is the second most common cause of infection. Other risk factors include occupational exposure, but approximately 10% of new infections have no known transmission source. In children, perinatal transmission is the *most* prevalent mode of transmission (see Table 385.1). Perinatal transmission occurs in up to 5% of infants born to viremic mothers. HIV coinfection and high viremia titers (HCV RNA-positive) in the mother can increase the transmission rate to 20%. The incubation period is 7-9 wk (range: 2-24 wk).

Pathogenesis
The pattern of acute hepatic injury is indistinguishable from that of other hepatotropic viruses. In chronic cases, lymphoid aggregates or follicles in portal tracts are found, either alone or as part of a general inflammatory infiltrate of the portal areas. Steatosis is also often seen in these liver specimens. HCV appears to cause injury primarily by cytopathic mechanisms, but immune-mediated injury can also occur. The cytopathic component appears to be mild because the acute illness is typically the least severe of all hepatotropic virus infections.

Clinical Manifestations
Acute HCV infection tends to be mild and insidious in onset (Fig. 385.4; see also Table 385.1). ALF rarely occurs. HCV is the most likely of all these viruses to cause chronic infection (Fig. 385.5). Of affected adults, <15% clear the virus; the rest develop chronic hepatitis. In pediatric studies, 6–19% of children achieved spontaneous sustained clearance of the virus during a 6-yr follow-up.

Chronic HCV infection is also clinically silent until a complication develops. Serum aminotransferase levels fluctuate and are sometimes normal, but histologic inflammation is universal. Progression of liver fibrosis is slow over several years, unless comorbid factors are present, which can accelerate fibrosis progression. Approximately 25% of infected patients ultimately progress to cirrhosis, liver failure, and, occasionally, primary HCC within 20-30 yr of the acute infection. Although progression is rare within the pediatric age range, cirrhosis and HCC from HCV have been reported in children. The long-term morbidities constitute the rationale for diagnosis and treatment in children with HCV.

Chronic HCV infection can be associated with small vessel vasculitis and is a common cause of essential mixed cryoglobulinemia. Other extrahepatic manifestations, predominantly seen in adults, include cutaneous vasculitis, porphyria cutanea tarda, lichen planus, peripheral neuropathy, cerebritis, polyarthritis, membranoproliferative glomerulonephritis, and nephrotic syndrome. Antibodies to smooth muscle,

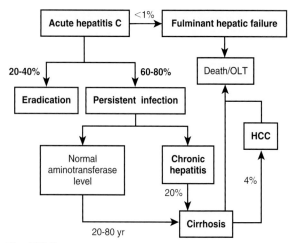

Fig. 385.5 Natural history of hepatitis C virus infection. HCC, hepatocellular carcinoma; OLT, orthotopic liver transplant. *(From Hochman JA, Balistreri WF: Chronic viral hepatitis: always be current! Pediatr Rev 24[12]:399–410, 2003.)*

antinuclear antibodies, and low thyroid hormone levels may also be present.

Diagnosis
Clinically available assays for detection of HCV infection are based on detection of antibodies to HCV antigens or detection of viral RNA (see Table 385.3); neither can predict the severity of liver disease.

The most widely used serologic test is the third-generation enzyme immunoassay to detect anti-HCV. The predictive value of this assay is greatest in high-risk populations, but the false-positive rate can be as high as 50–60% in low-risk populations. False-negative results also occur because antibodies remain negative for as long as 1-3 mo after clinical onset of illness. Anti-HCV is not a protective antibody and does not confer immunity; it is usually present simultaneously with the virus.

The most commonly used virologic assay for HCV is a PCR assay, which permits detection of small amounts of HCV RNA in serum and tissue samples within days of infection. The *qualitative* PCR detection is especially useful in patients with recent or perinatal infection, hypogammaglobulinemia, or immunosuppression and is highly sensitive. The *quantitative* PCR aids in identifying patients who are likely to respond to therapy and in monitoring response to therapy.

Screening for HCV should include all patients with the following risk factors: history of illegal drug use (even if only once), receiving clotting factors made before 1987 (when inactivation procedures were introduced) or blood products before 1992, hemodialysis, idiopathic liver disease, and children born to HCV-infected women (qualitative PCR in infancy and anti-HCV after 12-18 mo of age). In children, it is also important to consider whether the mother has any of the risk factors noted above that would increase her possibility of developing HCV. Routine screening of all pregnant women is currently not recommended. The Centers for Disease Control now recommends that all individuals born between 1945 and 1965 be screened.

Determining HCV genotype is also important, particularly when therapy is considered, because the response to the current therapeutic agents varies greatly. Genotype 1 traditionally responded poorly to therapy while genotypes 2 and 3 had a more favorable response. Newer agents, however, have led to changes in the treatment duration and anticipated outcome (as discussed later).

Aminotransferase levels typically fluctuate during HCV infection and do not correlate with the degree of liver fibrosis. A liver biopsy was previously the only means to assess the presence and extent of hepatic fibrosis, outside of overt signs of chronic liver disease. Newer noninvasive modalities using ultrasound or magnetic resonance elastography, however,

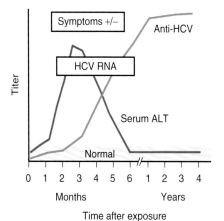

Fig. 385.4 Typical course of acute hepatitis B virus *(HCV)* infection followed by recovery. Symptoms may or may not be present during acute infection. Anti-HCV, antibody to HCV. *ALT,* alanine aminotransferase. *(Modified from the Centers for Disease Control and Prevention, www.cdc.gov/hepatitis/Resources/Professionals/Training/Serology/training.htm#one.)*

are now used to estimate the degree of fibrosis and decrease the need for biopsy. This technology coupled with newer drug regimens have eliminated the need for liver biopsy in many cases of HCV. A liver biopsy is now primarily indicated to rule out other causes of overt liver disease.

Complications

The risk of ALF caused by HCV is low, but the risk of chronic hepatitis is the highest of all the hepatitis viruses. In adults, risk factors for progression to hepatic fibrosis include older age, obesity, male sex, and even moderate alcohol ingestion (two 1 oz. drinks per day). Progression to cirrhosis or HCC is a major cause of morbidity and the most common indication for liver transplantation in adults in the United States.

Treatment

In adults, *peginterferon* (subcutaneous, weekly) combined with ribavirin (oral, daily) was standard therapy until 2012 for genotype 1. Currently recommended first-line adult therapy for HCV includes taking 1 or 2 oral medications with direct-acting antiviral properties, for 12-24 wk dependent on HCV genotype and other clinical factors. Studies show these treatments are more effective and better tolerated, and these same medications are currently being evaluated in children and adolescents.

Traditionally, patients most likely to respond had mild hepatitis, shorter duration of infection, low viral titers, and either genotype 2 or 3 virus. Patients with genotype 1 virus responded poorly. Response to peginterferon alfa/ribavirin may be predicted by single-nucleotide polymorphisms near the interleukin 28B gene, but with these newer treatment regimens excellent response rates are being reported with shorter duration, IFN-free regimens.

The goal of treatment is to achieve a sustained viral response (SVR), as defined by the absence of viremia at a variable period after stopping the medications; SVR is associated with improved histology and decreased risk of morbidities.

The natural history of HCV infection in children is still being defined. It is believed that children have a higher rate of spontaneous clearance than adults (up to 45% by age 19 yr). A multicenter study followed 359 children infected with HCV over 10 yr. Only 7.5% had cleared the virus, and 1.8% progressed to decompensated cirrhosis. Treatment in adults with *acute* HCV in a pilot study showed an 88% SVR in genotype 1 subjects (treated with IFN and ribavirin for 24 wk). Such data, if confirmed, could raise the question whether children, with shorter duration of infection and fewer comorbid conditions than their adult counterparts, could be ideal candidates for treatment. Given the adverse effects of currently available therapy, this strategy is not recommended outside of clinical trials.

Peginterferon (Schering), IFN-α2b, and ribavirin are approved by the Food and Drug Administration (FDA) for use in children older than 3 yr of age with chronic hepatitis C. Studies of IFN monotherapy in children demonstrated a higher SVR than in adults, with better compliance and fewer side effects. An SVR up to 49% for genotype 1 was achieved in multiple studies. Factors associated with a higher likelihood of response are age younger than 12 yr, genotypes 2 and 3, and, in patients with genotype 1b, an RNA titer of <2 million copies/mL of blood, and viral response (PCR at wk 4 and 12 of treatment). Side effects of medications lead to discontinuation of treatment in a high proportion of patients; these include influenza-like symptoms, anemia, and neutropenia. Long-term effects of these medicines also need to be evaluated as significant differences were noted in children's weight, height, body mass index, and body composition. Most of these delays improved following cessation of treatment, but height z-scores continued to lag behind.

Treatment may be considered for children infected with genotypes 2 and 3, because they have an 80–90% response rate to therapy with peginterferon and ribavirin. If the child has genotype 1b virus, the treatment choice remains more controversial as newer regimens are quickly becoming available.

Pediatric guidelines recommend treatment to eradicate HCV infection, prevent progression of liver disease and development of HCC, and to remove the stigma associated with HCV. Treatment should be considered for patients with evidence of advanced fibrosis or injury on liver biopsy. One approved treatment consists of 24-48 wk of peginterferon and ribavirin (therapy should be stopped if still detectable on viral PCR at 24 wk of therapy). In addition, sofosbuvir alone or in combination with ledipasvir has FDA approval for children ages 12-17 yr. The combination is indicated for HCV genotypes 1, 4, 5, and 6, while sofosbuvir with ribavirin is indicated for HCV genotypes 2 or 3; both regimens are used in children with mild or no cirrhosis.

Newer Treatments

Varying IFN-free regimens are now available for adults for all HCV genotypes allowing even greater likelihood of achieving viral eradication, with completely oral medication regimens, and without the use of IFN and its attendant side effects. With the rapid development of new medications and regimens, frequent review of up-to-date resources, such as www.hcvguidelines.org, will be vital to provide optimal care (Table 385.12).

Table 385.12	Ongoing Studies With Direct Acting Antiviral Combinations in Children With Chronic Hepatitis C Virus Infection				
	GENOTYPE	**ESTIMATED ENROLMENT**	**AGE RANGE (YR)**	**IDENTIFIER**	**COMPLETION**
Sofosbuvir + ledipasvir, with or without ribavirin	1,4,5,6	222	3–17	NCT02249182	July 2018
Sofosbuvir + ribavirin	2,3	104	3–17	NCT02175758	April 2018
Ombitasvir + paritaprevir + ritonavir, with or without dasabuvir, with or without ribavirin	1,4	74	3–17	NCT02486406	September 2019
Sofosbuvir + daclatasvir	4	40	8–17	NCT03080415	June 2018
Sofosbuvir + ledipasvir	1,4	40	12–17	NCT02868242	April 2019
Sofosbuvir + velpatasvir	1–6	200	3–17	NCT03022981	December 2019
Glecaprevir + pibrentasvir	1–6	110	3–17	NCT03067129	May 2022
Gratisovir + ribavirin	1–6	41	10–17	NCT02985281	June 2017

From Indolfi G, Serranti D, Resti M: Direct-acting antivirals for children and adolescents with chronic hepatitis C. *Lancet Child Adolesc* 2:298-304, 2018 (Table 1, p. 299).

Prevention

No vaccine is yet available to prevent HCV, although ongoing research suggests this will be possible in the future. Currently available Ig preparations are not beneficial, likely because preparations produced in the United States do not contain antibodies to HCV because blood and plasma donors are screened for anti-HCV and excluded from the donor pool. Broad neutralizing antibodies to HCV were found to be protective and might pave the road for vaccine development.

Once HCV infection is identified, patients should be screened yearly with a liver ultrasound and serum α-fetoprotein for HCC, as well as for any clinical evidence of liver disease. Vaccinating the affected patient against HAV and HBV will prevent superinfection with these viruses and the increased risk of developing severe liver failure.

Prognosis

Viral titers should be checked yearly to document spontaneous remission. Most patients develop chronic hepatitis. Progressive liver damage is higher in those with additional comorbid factors such as alcohol consumption, viral genotypic variations, obesity, and underlying genetic predispositions. Referral to a pediatric hepatologist is strongly advised to take advantage of up-to-date monitoring regimens and to optimize their enrollment in treatment protocols when available.

HEPATITIS D
Etiology

HDV, the smallest known animal virus, is considered defective because it cannot produce infection without concurrent HBV infection. The 36 nm diameter virus is incapable of making its own coat protein; its outer coat is composed of excess HBsAg from HBV. The inner core of the virus is single-stranded circular RNA that expresses the HDV antigen.

Epidemiology

HDV can cause an infection at the same time as the initial HBV infection (coinfection), or HDV can infect a person who is already infected with HBV (superinfection). Transmission usually occurs by intrafamilial or intimate contact in areas of high prevalence, which are primarily developing countries (see Table 385.1). In areas of low prevalence, such as the United States, the parenteral route is far more common. HDV infections are uncommon in children in the United States but must be considered when ALF occurs. The incubation period for HDV superinfection is approximately 2-8 wk; with coinfection, the incubation period is similar to that of HBV infection.

Pathogenesis

Liver pathology in HDV-associated hepatitis has no distinguishing features except that damage is usually severe. In contrast to HBV, HDV causes injury directly by cytopathic mechanisms. The most severe cases of HBV infection appear to result from coinfection of HBV and HDV.

Clinical Manifestations

The symptoms of hepatitis D are similar to, but usually more severe than, those of the other hepatotropic viruses. The clinical outcome for HDV infection depends on the mechanism of infection. In coinfection, *acute* hepatitis, which is much more severe than for HBV alone, is common, but the risk of developing chronic hepatitis is low. In superinfection, acute illness is rare and chronic hepatitis is common. The risk of ALF is highest with superinfection. Hepatitis D should be considered in any child who experiences ALF.

Diagnosis

HDV has not been isolated and no circulating antigen has been identified. The diagnosis is made by detecting IgM antibody to HDV; the antibodies to HDV develop approximately 2-4 wk after coinfection and approximately 10 wk after a superinfection. A test for anti-HDV antibody is commercially available. PCR assays for viral RNA are available as research tools (see Table 385.2).

Treatment

The treatment is based on supportive measures once an infection is identified. There are no specific HDV-targeted treatments to date. The treatment is mostly based on controlling and treating HBV infection, without which HDV cannot induce hepatitis. Small research studies suggest that IFN is the preferred treatment regimen, but ongoing studies still seek the ideal management strategy and the regimen should be personalized for each patient.

Prevention

There is no vaccine for hepatitis D. Because HDV replication cannot occur without hepatitis B coinfection, immunization against HBV also prevents HDV infection. Hepatitis B vaccines and HBIG are used for the same indications as for hepatitis B alone.

HEPATITIS E
Etiology

HEV has been cloned using molecular techniques. This RNA virus has a nonenveloped sphere shape with spikes and is similar in structure to the caliciviruses.

Epidemiology

Hepatitis E is the epidemic form of what was formerly called non-A, non-B hepatitis. Transmission is fecal–oral (often waterborne) and is associated with shedding of 27-34 nm particles in the stool (see Table 385.1). The highest prevalence of HEV infection has been reported in the Indian subcontinent, the Middle East, Southeast Asia, and Mexico, especially in areas with poor sanitation. The prevalence, however, appears to be increasing in the United States and other developed countries and has been postulated to be the most common cause of acute hepatitis and jaundice in the world. The mean incubation period is approximately 40 days (range: 15-60 days).

Pathogenesis

HEV appears to act as a cytopathic virus. The pathologic findings are similar to those of the other hepatitis viruses.

Clinical Manifestations

The clinical illness associated with HEV infection is similar to that of HAV but is often more severe. As with HAV, chronic illness does not occur—the sole exception noted to date is chronic hepatitis E occurring in immunosuppressed patients (e.g., post-transplant). In addition to often causing a more severe episode than HAV, HEV tends to affect older patients, with a peak age between 15 and 34 yr. HEV is a major pathogen in pregnant women, in whom it causes ALF with a high fatality incidence. HEV could also lead to decompensation of preexisting chronic liver disease.

Diagnosis

Recombinant DNA technology has resulted in development of antibodies to HEV particles, and IgM and IgG assays are available to distinguish between acute and resolved infections (see Table 385.3). IgM antibody to viral antigen becomes positive after approximately 1 wk of illness. Viral RNA can be detected in stool and serum by PCR.

Prevention

A recombinant hepatitis E vaccine is highly effective in adults. No evidence suggests that immune-globulin is effective in preventing HEV infections. Ig pooled from patients in endemic areas might prove to be effective.

APPROACH TO ACUTE OR CHRONIC HEPATITIS

Identifying deterioration of the patient with acute hepatitis and the development of ALF is a major contribution of the primary pediatrician (Fig. 385.6). If ALF is identified, the clinician should immediately refer the patient to a transplantation center; this can be lifesaving.

Once chronic infection is identified, close follow-up and referral to a pediatric hepatologist is recommended to enroll the patient in appropri-

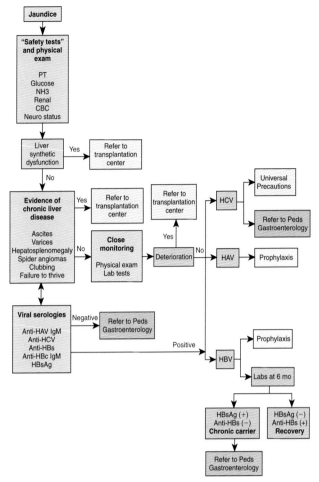

Fig. 385.6 Clinical approach to viral hepatitis. CBC, complete blood count with differential; HAV, hepatitis A virus; HBc, hepatitis B core; HBsAg, hepatitis B surface antigen; HBV, hepatitis B virus; HCV, hepatitis C virus; IgM, immunoglobulin M; NH₃, ammonia; PT, prothrombin time.

ate treatment trials. Treatment of chronic HBV and HCV in children should preferably be delivered within, or using data from, pediatric controlled trials as indications, timing, regimen, and outcomes remain to be defined and cannot be extrapolated from adult data. All patients with chronic viral hepatitis should avoid, as much as possible, further insult to the liver; HAV vaccine is recommended. Patients must avoid alcohol consumption and obesity, and they should exercise care when taking new medications, including nonprescription drugs and herbal medications.

International adoption and ease of travel continue to change the epidemiology of hepatitis viruses. In the United States, chronic HBV and HCV have a high prevalence among international adoptee patients; vigilance is required to establish early diagnosis in order to offer appropriate treatment as well as prophylactic measures to limit viral spread.

Chronic hepatitis can be a stigmatizing disease for children and their families. The pediatrician should offer, with proactive advocacy, appropriate support for them as well as needed education for their social circle. Scientific data and information about support groups are available for families on the websites for the American Liver Foundation (www.liverfoundation.org) and the North American Society for Pediatric Gastroenterology, Hepatology and Nutrition (www.naspghan.org), as well as through pediatric gastroenterology centers.

Bibliography is available at Expert Consult.

Chapter 386
Liver Abscess

Joshua K. Schaffzin and
Robert W. Frenck Jr

第三百八十六章
肝脓肿

中文导读

本章主要介绍了2种感染性病因引起的肝脓肿，即细菌和寄生虫。具体阐述了化脓性肝脓肿的4种感染途径，即通过肝动脉、胆道、门静脉和邻近感染；临床症状及体征具有非特异性；实验室检查最常见炎症标志物升高和低蛋白血症；治疗药物为抗生素。详细介绍了阿米巴肝脓肿的流行病学、临床症状及体征、实验室诊断、治疗和预后，无特异的临床表现，由血清ELISA确诊，有效治疗药物为甲硝唑。

Liver abscesses typically have 1 of 2 infectious etiologies: pyogenic, meaning involving bacteria, or parasitic, such as with amebiasis, ascariasis, or toxocariasis. Liver abscesses are typically difficult to detect due to nonspecific presentation, and diagnosis requires a high index of suspicion. Radiographic diagnosis is often contributory, but further confirmation is often indicated to differentiate infectious abscess from hydatid cyst and noninfectious causes, such as malignancy (primary hepatic or metastasis). The differential diagnosis also includes traumatic injury (including procedural, such as a misplaced vascular catheter).

Pyogenic liver abscesses are uncommon in children but have been reported in all ages. Bacteria can invade the liver through 1 of 4 sources: hematogenously through the hepatic artery (e.g., in the presence of bacteremia), through the biliary tract, through the portal vein (portal sepsis), and directly by contiguous infection. In neonates, a portal vein source can include the umbilical vein (e.g., in the presence of omphalitis or injury caused by an umbilical venous catheter). Pyogenic liver abscesses of unknown source are classified as cryptogenic. Children with chronic granulomatous disease (CGD), hyper–immunoglobulin E (hyper-IgE) syndrome, or malignancies are at increased risk of liver abscess. Pyogenic liver abscesses are also uncommon in adults, although the annual incidence is higher in Southeast Asia (estimated 17.6/100,000 population) than in the United States or Europe (estimated 2-5/100,000 population). They tend to occur more frequently in males, older ages, and in patients with diabetes or a history of liver transplantation or malignancy.

Clinical signs and symptoms of pyogenic liver abscess are nonspecific and can include fever, chills, malaise, fatigue, nausea, abdominal pain (with or without right upper quadrant tenderness), and hepatomegaly; jaundice is uncommon. The most common abnormal laboratory findings are elevated inflammatory markers and hypoalbuminemia. Hepatic function testing is often abnormally elevated, and leukocytosis is common. Radiologic confirmation is often obtained by ultrasound or CT (Fig. 386.1). Chest x-rays may show elevation of the right hemidiaphragm with a right pleural effusion. Solitary lesions of the right hepatic lobe are most common, although solitary abscesses can appear in any hepatic lobe or as multiple disseminated lesions (such as with disseminated candidiasis, bartonellosis, or rarely brucellosis).

Cultures of pyogenic liver abscesses often yield mixed populations. In children, *Staphylococcus aureus*, *Streptococcus* spp., enteric Gram-negative organisms (*Escherichia coli*, *Klebsiella pneumoniae*, and *Serratia* in CGD patients), and anaerobic organisms are most common. Among adults, *K. pneumoniae* predominates, followed by *E. coli*, with less common aerobic Gram-positive and anaerobic organisms. Blood cultures are often positive and may be helpful to determine a therapy plan.

Due to the wide range of causative organisms (i.e., aerobic Gram negative, *S. aureus*, and anaerobic organisms) empiric antimicrobial treatment needs to be broad. Potential empiric antimicrobial choices include; piperacillin-tazobactam, ampicillin-sulbactam, or metronidazole with a 3rd-generation cephalosporin. Depending on local prevalence and degree of suspicion, vancomycin may be added to cover methicillin-resistant *S. aureus*. Therapy can be modified based on culture sensitivities. Treatment duration is not standardized, and should be based on fever resolution, clinical and inflammatory marker improvement, and serial ultrasound monitoring. Many sources recommend completing 4-6 wk of therapy, with the first 2 wk administered parentally. Depending on the size and extent of the lesion(s), percutaneous or surgical drainage may be added to obtain samples for cultures and to shorten illness duration. Percutaneous options include single-pass needle or catheter aspiration, or insertion of a continuously draining catheter. In adults, unless there is evidence of rupture or spread, percutaneous drainage should be attempted first for large lesions (≥5-7 cm in diameter). Numerous case series of pyogenic liver abscess in premature infants described complete resolution with antibiotic therapy alone, and some advocate for this as an initial approach in smaller lesions.

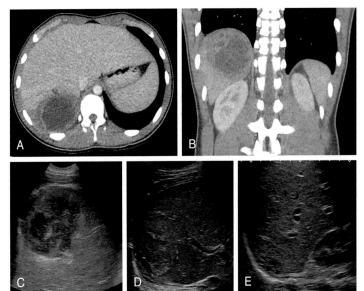

Fig. 386.1 CT (**A** and **B**) and ultrasound (**C**) images of a cryptogenic liver abscess in a 16 yr old male without known risk factors. The lesion was drained percutaneously, and cultures grew multiple anaerobic organisms (*Fusobacterium nucleatum* and *Parvimonas micra*). He was successfully treated with 2 wk of parenteral followed by 4 wk of oral therapy and was followed with serial ultrasounds 5 days (**D**) and 34 days (**E**) after drainage. *(Courtesy Dr. Alexander Towbin, Cincinnati Children's Hospital, Cincinnati, Ohio.)*

Resolution can be monitored by trending inflammatory markers and/or serial imaging.

Amebic liver abscess (ALA) is the most common extraintestinal manifestation of *Entamoeba histolytica* infection. Although more common in endemic areas, cases can be diagnosed in the United States among travelers to, and immigrants from, endemic areas. Presentation can be delayed by mo to yr. ALA is more common among adults aged 18-55, and males predominate. Amoebic trophozoites invade colonic mucosa and reach the liver through the portal circulation. Patients may not have an associated colitis. Fever, right upper quadrant pain, anorexia, and weight loss are often present. Laboratory evaluation typically reveals a leukocytosis without eosinophilia and increased alkaline phosphatase. Ultrasonography or CT demonstrates the abscess (Fig. 386.2).

Diagnosis of ALA is often confirmed by serum ELISA. Serology is considered reliable in nonendemic areas but can be prone to false negatives early in the infection and cannot distinguish active infection from previous exposure. Testing for *E. histolytica* presence in stool is specific but not very sensitive, and patients with ALA may not have detectable organism in their stool. Most sensitive and specific among stool assays is PCR, followed by stool antigen detection, and least reliable is microscopy, because *E. histolytica* cannot easily be distinguished microscopically from its clinically benign relatives *Entamoeba dispar* and *Entamoeba moshkovskii*.

Prior to effective treatment, ALA-associated mortality was high; it has since decreased significantly. Treatment involves 7-10 days of a nitroimidazole (most commonly metronidazole) to kill trophozoites, followed by 7 days of a luminal agent (such as paromomycin) to kill colonic cysts. Patients with large abscesses (≥5-7 cm in diameter) may benefit from percutaneous aspiration in addition to medical therapy.

Bibliography is available at Expert Consult.

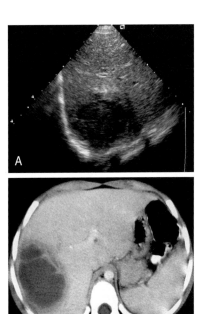

Fig. 386.2 Amebic abscess. **A,** Sonogram demonstrates a hypoechogenic mass in the right lobe of the liver with a more hypoechoic surrounding rim. **B,** CT scan demonstrates a low-attenuation mass in the right lobe of the liver with a prominent halo. *(From Kuhn JP, Slovis TL, Haller JO: Caffrey's pediatric diagnostic imaging, vol 2, ed 10, Philadelphia, 2004, Mosby, p. 1473.)*

Chapter **387**

Liver Disease Associated With Systemic Disorders

Bernadette E. Vitola and
William F. Balistreri

第三百八十七章
肝病和全身性疾病

中文导读

　　本章主要介绍了常见的和肝病相关的全身性疾病以及非酒精性脂肪性肝病；详细介绍了炎症性肠病、细菌性败血症、腹腔疾病、心脏病、慢性完全肠外营养相关的胆汁淤积、囊性纤维化、骨髓移植、血红蛋白病、组织细胞疾病。具体介绍了和炎症性肠病相关的最常见的肝胆疾病为硬化性胆管炎，细菌性败血症最常见病原菌为革兰阴性菌，局灶性胆汁性肝硬化是囊性纤维化中的特征性肝脏病变等内容。非酒精性脂肪性肝病部分详细阐述了流行病学、疾病分型、组织学、临床表现、实验室检查和诊断方法以及治疗手段等内容。

Liver disease is found in a wide variety of systemic illnesses, both as a result of the primary pathologic process and as a secondary complication of the disease or associated therapy.

INFLAMMATORY BOWEL DISEASE

Ulcerative colitis and Crohn disease (Chapter 362) are associated with hepatobiliary disease that includes autoimmune and inflammatory processes related to inflammatory bowel disease (IBD) (sclerosing cholangitis, autoimmune hepatitis [AIH]), drug toxicity (thiopurines, methotrexate, 5-ASA, biologics), malnutrition and disordered physiology (fatty liver, cholelithiasis), bacterial translocation and systemic infections (hepatic abscess, portal vein thrombosis), hypercoagulability (infarction, Budd-Chiari), and long-term complications of these liver diseases, such as ascending cholangitis, cirrhosis, portal hypertension, and biliary carcinoma. Hepatobiliary manifestations may continue to progress even when intestinal symptoms are well-controlled and are unrelated to either the severity or duration of intestinal disease.

Sclerosing cholangitis is the most common hepatobiliary disease associated with IBD, occurring in 2–8% of adult patients with ulcerative colitis and less often in Crohn disease. Conversely, 70–90% of patients with sclerosing cholangitis have ulcerative colitis. In pediatric patients with IBD, the diagnosis typically occurs in the 2nd decade of life, with a median age of 14 yr. Sclerosing cholangitis is characterized by progressive inflammation and fibrosis of segments of the intrahepatic and extrahepatic bile ducts and can progress to complete obliteration. Genetic susceptibility has been demonstrated. Many patients are asymptomatic, and the disease is initially diagnosed by routine liver function testing that reveals elevated serum alkaline phosphatase (ALP), 5′-nucleotidase, or

γ-glutamyl transpeptidase (GGT) activities. Antinuclear or anti–smooth muscle antibodies might also be present in the serum. Ten to 15% of adult patients present with symptoms including anorexia, weight loss, pruritus, fatigue, right upper quadrant pain, and jaundice; intermittent acute cholangitis accompanied by fever, jaundice, and right upper quadrant pain can also occur. Portal hypertension can develop with progressive disease. These symptoms are less common in children, in whom hepatobiliary disease is often recognized by routine screening of liver function tests. In children with sclerosing cholangitis, approximately 11% present initially with hepatic manifestations, and the associated asymptomatic IBD is discovered only on subsequent endoscopy.

Magnetic resonance cholangiography is an established first line diagnostic test for sclerosing cholangitis. Characteristic findings include beading and irregularity of the intrahepatic and extrahepatic bile ducts. Liver biopsy typically reveals periductal fibrosis and inflammation, fibroobliterative cholangitis, and portal fibrosis, but it is not required for the diagnosis in patients with radiologic evidence of sclerosing cholangitis. However, biopsy is required to evaluate for overlap with autoimmune hepatitis or autoimmune sclerosing cholangitis.

Sclerosing cholangitis is strongly associated with hepatobiliary malignancies (cholangiocarcinoma, hepatocellular carcinoma, gallbladder carcinoma) with a reported incidence varying between 9% and 14%. In 1 large series, patients with IBD and sclerosing cholangitis had a 10-fold increased risk of colorectal carcinoma and a 14-fold increased risk of pancreatic cancer compared with the general population. Tumor serology (CA 19-9) and cross-sectional liver imaging may be a useful screening strategy to identify patients with sclerosing cholangitis at increased risk for cholangiocarcinoma.

There is no definitive medical treatment for sclerosing cholangitis; liver transplantation is the only long-term option for progressive cirrhosis, and autoimmune disease can recur in the allograft in 20–25% of patients. Short-term therapy aims at improving biliary drainage and attempting to slow the obliterative process. Ursodeoxycholic acid, at a dose of 15 mg/kg/24 hr, may improve bile flow and laboratory parameters but has not been shown to improve clinical outcome. Dominant extrahepatic biliary strictures may be dilated or endoscopically stented. Immunosuppressive therapy with corticosteroids and/or azathioprine may improve biochemical parameters but has been disappointing in halting long-term histologic progression. Symptomatic therapy should be initiated for pruritus (rifampin, ursodeoxycholic acid, diphenhydramine), malnutrition (enteral supplementation), and ascending cholangitis (antibiotics) as indicated. Total colectomy has not been beneficial in preventing or managing hepatobiliary complications in patients with ulcerative colitis. However, in patients with end-stage liver disease requiring liver transplantation, those with active IBD are 10-fold more likely to lose their grafts.

IBD-associated AIH can closely resemble IBD-associated sclerosing cholangitis, a condition often referred to as **overlap syndrome** or autoimmune sclerosing cholangitis (ASC). These patients typically exhibit hyperglobulinemia (marked increase in serum immunoglobulin [Ig] G levels). In some children the disease is initially diagnosed as AIH and later is found to be sclerosing cholangitis after cholangiography. In other cases, AIH manifests well after diagnosis of IBD-associated sclerosing cholangitis. Liver biopsy in patients with ASC shows interface hepatitis, in addition to the bile duct injury associated with sclerosing cholangitis. Immunosuppressive medication (corticosteroids and/or azathioprine) is the mainstay of therapy for ASC; long-term response does not appear to be as favorable as in AIH alone. Long-term survival in children with ASC appears to be similar to those with sclerosing cholangitis, with an overall median (50%) survival free of liver transplantation of 12.7 yr.

Fatty liver disease might also be more prevalent in adult patients with IBD, ranging from 25% to 40% in 1 large series and often correlates with severity of IBD. Gallstones are more prevalent in those with Crohn disease (11%) than in those with ulcerative colitis (7.5%) and in normal subjects (5%). However, the true prevalence of these IBD-associated liver diseases in pediatric patients is unknown.

BACTERIAL SEPSIS

Sepsis can mimic liver disease and should be excluded in any critically ill patient who develops cholestasis in the absence of markedly elevated serum aminotransferase or AP levels, even when other signs of infection are not evident. Gram-negative organisms are most often isolated from blood cultures, in particular *Escherichia coli, Klebsiella pneumoniae,* and *Pseudomonas aeruginosa.* Lipopolysaccharides and other bacterial endotoxins are thought to interfere with bile secretion by directly altering the structure or function of bile canalicular membrane transport proteins. The serum bilirubin level, predominantly the conjugated fraction, is elevated. Serum AP and aminotransferase activities may also be elevated. Liver biopsy shows intrahepatic cholestasis with little or no hepatocyte necrosis. Kupffer cell hyperplasia and an increase in inflammatory cells are also common. Similar findings can occur with urosepsis.

CELIAC DISEASE

Celiac disease (Chapter 364.2) may present with elevated aminotransferase levels and prolonged prothrombin time, as well as hepatic histologic changes, such as mild periportal and lobular inflammation. These abnormalities typically all improve on a gluten-free diet. Gastrointestinal symptoms may not be present. Other autoimmune liver diseases (AIH, primary sclerosing cholangitis) have also been associated with celiac disease, although they may not respond as well to a gluten-free diet.

CARDIAC DISEASE

Hepatic injury can occur as a complication of severe acute or chronic congestive heart failure (Chapter 469), cyanotic congenital heart disease (Chapters 456 and 457), and acute ischemic shock. In all conditions, passive congestion and reduced cardiac output can contribute to liver damage. Elevated central venous pressure is transmitted to the hepatic veins, smaller venules, and, ultimately, the surrounding hepatocytes, resulting in hepatocellular atrophy in the centrilobular zone of the liver. Owing to decreased cardiac output, there is decreased hepatic arterial blood flow, and centrilobular hypoxia results. Hepatic necrosis leads to lactic acidosis, elevated aminotransferase levels, cholestasis, prolonged prothrombin time, cirrhosis, and possibly hypoglycemia due to impaired hepatocellular metabolism. Jaundice, tender hepatomegaly, and, in some cases, ascites and splenomegaly can occur. However, aminotransferases are often minimally elevated with slowly progressive fibrosis because there is minimal inflammation or cell death.

After acute hypovolemic shock, serum aminotransferase levels can rise to extremely high levels but rapidly return to normal when perfusion and cardiac function improve. Hepatic necrosis or acute liver failure can occur in infants with hypoplastic left heart syndrome and coarctation of the aorta. High systemic venous pressures after Fontan procedures can also lead to hepatic dysfunction, marked by prolonged prothrombin time, and cardiac cirrhosis. The aim of therapy in all causes of cardiac-associated liver disease is to improve cardiac output, reduce systemic venous pressures, and monitor for other signs of hypoperfusion. Even mild liver disease can have an impact on mortality after cardiac surgery, with poorer outcomes with progressively worse liver disease. In adults with cirrhosis undergoing cardiac surgery, overall mortality was 17% but varied significantly from 5% with mild disease to 70% with advanced liver disease.

CHOLESTASIS ASSOCIATED WITH CHRONIC TOTAL PARENTERAL NUTRITION

Total parenteral nutrition (TPN) can cause a variety of liver diseases, including hepatic steatosis, gallbladder and bile duct damage, and cholestasis. Cholestasis is the most severe complication and can lead to progressive fibrosis and cirrhosis. It is the major factor limiting effective long-term use of TPN in children and adults. Risk factors for TPN-associated cholestasis include prolonged duration of TPN (particularly soy-based lipids), prematurity, low birthweight, sepsis, necrotizing enterocolitis, and short bowel syndrome.

The pathogenesis of TPN-associated cholestasis is multifactorial. Sepsis; excess caloric intake; high amounts of protein, fat, or carbohydrate; specific amino acid toxicities; nutrient deficiencies; and toxicities related to components such as manganese, aluminum, and copper can all contribute to hepatic injury. The type (soy based), volume, and frequency of lipid administered may be a significant factor. Prolonged enteral fasting compromises mucosal integrity and increases bacterial mucosal translocation. Fasting also decreases release of cholecystokinin, which promotes bile flow. This leads to biliary stasis, cholestasis, and formation of biliary sludge and gallstones, which exacerbates hepatic dysfunction. Sepsis, in particular due to Gram-negative bacteria and associated endotoxins, can also exacerbate liver damage.

Early histologic findings include macrovesicular steatosis, canalicular cholestasis, and periportal inflammation. These changes can regress after cessation of short-term TPN. Prolonged duration of TPN is marked by bile duct proliferation or ductopenia, portal fibrosis, and expansion of portal triads, and it can progress to cirrhosis and end-stage liver disease.

Clinical onset is typically marked by gradual onset of cholestasis, developing after more than 2 wk of TPN. In low birthweight infants, the onset of jaundice can overlap the phase of physiologic (unconjugated) hyperbilirubinemia. Any icteric infant who has received TPN for more than 1 wk should have bilirubin fractionated. With prolonged duration, hepatic enlargement or splenomegaly can develop. Serum bile acid concentrations can increase. Rises in serum aminotransferase levels may be a late finding. An elevation in serum AP activity may be due to rickets, a common complication of TPN in low birthweight infants.

In addition to cholestasis, biliary complications of intravenous nutrition include cholelithiasis and the development of biliary sludge, associated with thick, inspissated gallbladder contents. These may be asymptomatic. Hepatic steatosis or elevated serum aminotransferase levels can also occur in the absence of cholestasis, particularly in older children. This is generally mild and resolves after TPN is discontinued. Serum bilirubin and bile acid levels remain within the normal range. Other causes of liver disease should also be considered, especially if evidence of hepatic dysfunction persists despite weaning from TPN and initiating enteral feeds. If serum AP or aminotransferase levels remain elevated, liver biopsy may be necessary for accurate diagnosis.

Treatment of TPN-associated cholestasis is focused on avoiding progressive liver injury by limiting the duration of the infusion whenever possible. Enteral feeding should be initiated as soon as tolerated and prolonged fasting should be avoided. Even small volumes of nutrients given by intermittent oral feedings or by continuous nasogastric drip promote bile flow, enterohepatic recirculation of bile acids, and intestinal motility, and they enhance mucosal barrier function, reducing the risk of bacterial translocation. Improved TPN solutions that meet the specific needs of neonates can prevent deficiencies and toxicities. The risk of further hepatic injury should always be considered when weighing the option of continuing TPN indefinitely, and all efforts should be made to try to advance enteral feeds whenever possible. There has been concern that the soy-based lipid infusion provided with TPN may be a significant contributing factor to TPN-associated cholestasis as a result of proinflammatory omega-6 fatty acids. Several strategies have been used to minimize exposure to these fatty acids by limiting total lipid and/or introducing alternate sources of lipid including fish oil and olive oil to provide more omega-3 fatty acids. The long-term effects of these strategies on essential fatty acid deficiency or growth are unclear although there is some evidence that TPN-associated cholestasis may improve.

Ursodeoxycholic acid therapy may be beneficial in improving jaundice and hepatosplenomegaly. Other therapies, such as administration of antibiotics to reduce intraluminal bacterial overgrowth or oral administration of taurine or cholecystokinin, remain experimental.

CYSTIC FIBROSIS

Cystic fibrosis (CF) (Chapter 432) is caused by mutations in the *CFTR* gene, which impair chloride transport across the apical membranes of epithelial cells in numerous organs (including cholangiocytes). Many patients with CF have some evidence of hepatobiliary disease; however, less than one-third of these patients develop clinically significant liver disease. Hepatobiliary complications account for approximately 2.5% of overall mortality in patients with CF. The onset of liver disease occurs at a median age of 10 yr, and >90% occurs by 20 yr.

Focal biliary cirrhosis is the pathognomonic liver lesion in CF and is postulated to result, in part, from impaired secretory function of the bile duct epithelium. Blockage of biliary ductules secondary to viscid secretions results in periductal inflammation, bile duct proliferation, and increased fibrosis within focal portal tracts. Gradual progression to multilobular cirrhosis can occur and result in portal hypertension and end-stage liver disease in 1–8% of patients. Liver disease tends to occur mainly in males with pancreatic insufficiency and requires 2 CFTR mutations without residual function. One candidate gene modifier for clinical phenotypes of CF-related liver disease that shows a strong association is SERPINA1. However, additional study of mutational analysis is necessary before we are able to predict which patients with CF will develop liver disease. Clinical risk factors that may be associated with liver disease include older age, pancreatic insufficiency, male gender, and possibly a history of meconium ileus.

Treatment with oral ursodeoxycholic acid (10-15 mg/kg/day) may be beneficial in improving liver function, presumably by improving bile flow; further research is necessary to determine whether a true long-term benefit exists. Because it is difficult to predict which patients will develop liver disease, prophylactic therapy is not possible. Progression of liver disease is generally slow; the major concern is the development of portal hypertension and the associated complications.

BONE MARROW TRANSPLANTATION

Liver disease is common in patients who have received hematopoietic stem cell transplantation (SCT), whether the cells are harvested from bone marrow or peripheral blood (Chapters 161-165). The pathogenesis is varied and includes infections (viral, bacterial, or fungal); toxicity from parenteral nutrition, chemotherapy, or radiation; venoocclusive disease (VOD); graft versus host disease (GVHD); or hemosiderosis secondary to iron overload from frequent blood transfusions. GVHD,

drug toxicity, and sepsis are the most common causes of liver dysfunction after allogeneic SCT.

Diagnosis is often challenging due to the coexistence of multiple risk factors. Clinical course, symptoms and signs, and biochemical liver function and viral serologic tests must be considered in making the correct diagnosis. Percutaneous liver biopsy may be necessary; histology can show extensive bile duct injury in GVHD, viral inclusions in cytomegalovirus disease, or the characteristic endothelial lesion in VOD. It is important to diagnose the cause accurately, because treatment for GVHD differs markedly from that of other conditions (i.e., initiating immunosuppression for GVHD) and can worsen hepatitis secondary to infections.

GVHD of the liver can be acute or chronic but often occurs with the presence of GVHD in other target organs such as the skin and gut (Chapter 163). Hepatic GVHD is caused by immunologic reaction to bile duct epithelium, leading to a nonsuppurative cholangitis. Histologic features of GVHD include loss of intralobular bile ducts, endothelial injury of hepatic and portal venules, and hepatocellular necrosis.

Onset typically occurs at the time of donor engraftment (days 14-21 after SCT). In acute hepatic GVHD, serum aminotransferase levels can rise markedly in the absence of elevated bilirubin, AP, and GGT levels, mimicking viral hepatitis. Acute hepatic GVHD can manifest both early (days 14-21) and late (>day 70) after allogeneic SCT. In chronic hepatic GVHD, serum aminotransferase levels are not as markedly elevated and cholestasis is more prominent, with marked rises in serum conjugated bilirubin, GGT, and AP levels. Other signs and symptoms can include hepatic tenderness, dark urine, acholic stools, itching, and anorexia.

VOD of the liver usually develops in the first 3 wk after SCT. The incidence ranges from 5% to 39% in pediatric patients, with reported mortality rates varying from 0% to 47%. Risk factors include trauma, high-dose conditioning regimens, coagulopathies, sickle cell anemia, leukemia, polycythemia vera, thalassemia major, hepatic abscesses, irradiation, GVHD, iron overload, preexisting liver disease, and younger age. VOD is caused by fibrous obliteration of the terminal hepatic venules and small lobular veins, with resultant damage to the surrounding hepatocytes and sinusoids. It is not associated with thrombus formation, in contrast with Budd-Chiari syndrome, which involves occlusion of the larger hepatic veins or inferior vena cava by a web, mass, or thrombus.

Pathologic changes in patients with VOD are best demonstrated using special (trichrome) stains to highlight the central veins. The lesions may be patchy. Later in the course, hepatic venules may be completely obliterated.

Symptoms typically include jaundice, painful hepatomegaly, rapid weight gain, and ascites, although jaundice can be absent in nearly a third of pediatric patients with VOD. VOD resolves in the majority of patients but can also lead to multisystem organ failure, hepatic encephalopathy, and fulminant hepatic failure. Less-severe forms may be characterized by jaundice and ascites with a slow resolution; in very mild cases, histologic changes may be the sole manifestation. The diagnosis rests on the exclusion of other diseases, such as GVHD, congestive cardiomyopathy, constrictive pericarditis, and Budd-Chiari syndrome.

Treatment for VOD with defibrotide, an agent with antithrombotic and thrombolytic properties, at doses of 20-40 mg/kg/day, has been successful in multicenter trials in both adult and pediatric patients. Complete response rates vary between 36% and 76% and survival >100 days post SCT of 32–79%, with better outcomes in pediatric patients. Little toxicity has been noted; however, pediatric patients are at a higher risk of bleeding with treatment compared with adults. Oral ursodeoxycholic acid can decrease the incidence of severe liver disease in patients undergoing SCT and has been shown to reduce the incidence of VOD and transplant-related mortality in adults. Supportive management includes maintaining intravenous hydration and renal perfusion.

HEMOGLOBINOPATHIES

Patients with sickle cell anemia (Chapter 489.1) or thalassemia (Chapter 489.10) can have hepatic dysfunction due to acute or chronic viral hepatitis, hemosiderosis from frequent transfusion therapy, hepatic crises related to severe intrahepatic cholestasis, sequestration, or ischemic necrosis. Cholelithiasis and hemosiderosis are both common and treatable. Higher volume of transfusions is associated with both higher hepatic iron content and fibrosis. Chelation therapy for iron overload is usually safe and effective but needs to be properly managed and monitored via imaging and serum ferritin levels.

Hepatic sickle cell crisis or "sickle hepatopathy" occurs in ~10% of patients with sickle cell disease. It manifests with intense RUQ pain and tenderness, fever, leukocytosis, and jaundice. Bilirubin levels may be markedly elevated; serum ALP levels may be only moderately elevated. It can be difficult to distinguish sickle hepatopathy from viral hepatitis, acute cholecystitis, or choledocholithiasis; therefore these conditions should be excluded. In general, hepatic sickle cell crisis is self-limited and symptoms resolve within 1-3 wk. **Sickle cell intrahepatic cholestasis** manifests as hepatomegaly, abdominal pain, hyperbilirubinemia, and coagulopathy and can progress to acute liver failure, leaving transplantation as the only therapeutic option. Transplantation carries a high risk for graft loss due to vascular complications.

On occasion, children with sickle cell disease experience a benign elevation of bilirubin levels >20 mg/dL but unaccompanied by severe pain or fever. There is no change in hematocrit or reticulocyte count nor any association with a hemolytic crisis.

HISTIOCYTIC DISORDERS

Langerhans cell histiocytosis (Chapter 534.1), the most common of the histiocytoses, typically affects the bone and skin. However, it can cause infiltration of high-risk organs such as the liver resulting in periportal inflammation and sclerosing cholangitis. Liver involvement often results in worse outcomes. Hemophagocytic lymphohistiocytosis (HLH) (Chapter 534.2) is a multiorgan, severe, and potentially fatal inflammatory process associated with activation of macrophages that mimics sepsis. The hepatic manifestation of HLH is usually acute liver failure with portal inflammatory infiltrates and hemophagocytosis noted on liver biopsy.

Bibliography is available at Expert Consult.

387.1 Nonalcoholic Fatty Liver Disease

Bernadette E. Vitola and William F. Balistreri

Nonalcoholic fatty liver disease (NAFLD), a spectrum of liver diseases strongly associated with obesity, is the most common chronic liver disease in children. NAFLD can range from fatty liver alone to a triad of fatty infiltration, inflammation, and fibrosis termed **nonalcoholic steatohepatitis (NASH)**, which resembles alcoholic liver disease but occurs with little or no exposure to ethanol. Unlike adults, NASH in children has 2 distinct histologic types. **Type 1 NASH** resembles adult histologic findings with steatosis and balloon degeneration of hepatocytes and/or periportal fibrosis. **Type 2 NASH** includes steatosis and portal inflammation.

Many patients with NAFLD are asymptomatic. Liver histology, obtained from autopsy data, suggest that 10% of children and 38% of obese children aged 2-19 yr old have NAFLD. The risk is lower in African-American children. Elevated serum aminotransferase levels are not sensitive or specific markers for NAFLD. A normal serum ALT level is present in 21–23% of pediatric patients with NAFLD. Although ultrasonography detects NAFLD, no current imaging modalities distinguish between simple steatosis and NASH. A liver biopsy may be required for a delimiting diagnosis. There are no reliable biomarkers available to serve as an alternative to liver biopsy.

The estimated prevalence of fatty liver disease in adults is thought to be as high as 15–20% for NAFLD overall and 2–4% for NASH. Risk factors in pediatric cohorts include obesity, male gender, white or Hispanic ethnicity, hypertriglyceridemia, and insulin resistance. Hepatic steatosis alone may be benign, but up to a quarter of patients with NASH can develop progressive fibrosis with resultant cirrhosis. The long-term prognosis of NASH that has developed in childhood is unknown.

Children diagnosed with NAFLD should be screened for comorbid conditions, including diabetes, hypertension, dyslipidemia, and obstructive sleep apnea. Obese and overweight children with other risk factors >3 yr of age should be screened for NAFLD by checking aminotransferase levels and liver ultrasound, even though neither is highly sensitive or specific. MRI is in use for clinical trials, but further studies are needed prior to its standard use in patient care. **Lysosomal acid lipase deficiency (LAL-D)**, an autosomal recessive disorder due to mutations in *LIPA* may produce a hepatic steatosis like syndrome. In contrast to NAFLD, patients with LAL-D usually demonstrate microvesicular or mixed micro- and macrovesicular steatosis not macrovesicular changes.

Therapeutic trials in children and adolescents with biopsy-proven NAFLD/NASH are rare. Although there is no definitive treatment for NAFLD, gradual weight loss is effective in normalizing serum ALT levels and improving NAFLD. Low glycemic index foods and substituting polyunsaturated fatty acids for saturated fats may help. Vitamin E and vitamin C provide no additional benefit to the efficacy of lifestyle intervention (diet and exercise) in improving steatosis or biochemical abnormalities in pediatric NAFLD. However, vitamin E has been shown to improve balloon degeneration in children with NASH. Metformin has produced mixed results in the treatment of NAFLD. Thiazolidinediones (pioglitazone, rosiglitazone) improve liver histology in adults with NASH but have not been studied in children. In view of the potential role of the gut microbiome in contributing to the pathogenesis of NAFLD, the role of probiotics as an adjunct to lifestyle changes is under investigation. A preliminary study using ω-3 docosahexaenoic acid in children showed improved insulin sensitivity, ALT, triglycerides, BMI, and histology in children with NAFLD. Cysteamine bitartrate (slow release), a potential precursor of glutathione, an antioxidant, may reduce liver enzyme levels, as well as serum leptin and adiponectin levels, and is also a potential candidate for the treatment of NAFLD. GLP-1 is a neuropeptide (incretin) that has an antihyperglycemic effect. A meta-analysis demonstrated decreased ALT and improved imaging findings, as well as histologic features in adults with NAFLD and diabetes treated with GLP-1 agonists. In adults, a fibroblast growth factor 19 (FGF-19)-like agent has shown preliminary positive results. FGF-19 regulates bile acid, carbohydrate and energy metabolism.

Bibliography is available at Expert Consult.

Chapter **388**

Mitochondrial Hepatopathies

Samar H. Ibrahim and William F. Balistreri

第三百八十八章
线粒体肝病

中文导读

本章主要介绍了多种与肝脏疾病有关的线粒体疾病。线粒体疾病可分为原发性和继发性，前者线粒体缺陷是疾病的主要原因，后者线粒体功能受外源性损伤或非线粒体蛋白的基因突变的影响。介绍了线粒体病的流行病学、临床表现、诊断评估及治疗。具体介绍了原发性线粒体肝病中新生儿肝功能衰竭、Alpers综合征、线粒体DNA耗竭综合征、Navajo神经性肝病、皮尔逊综合征、绒毛萎缩综合征、GRACILE综合征、核翻译和延伸因子基因突变等疾病。简要介绍了继发性线粒体肝病。

A wide variety of mitochondrial disorders are associated with liver disease. Hepatocytes contain a high density of mitochondria because the liver, with its biosynthetic and detoxifying functions, is highly dependent on adenosine triphosphate. Defects in mitochondrial function can lead to impaired oxidative phosphorylation, increased generation of reactive oxygen species, impairment of other metabolic pathways, and activation of mechanisms of cellular death.

Mitochondrial disorders can be divided into primary, in which the mitochondrial defect is the primary cause of the disorder, and secondary, in which mitochondrial function is affected by exogenous injury or a genetic mutation that affects nonmitochondrial proteins (see Chapter 105.4). Primary mitochondrial disorders can be caused by mutations affecting mitochondrial DNA (mtDNA) or by nuclear genes that encode mitochondrial proteins or cofactors (see Chapter 383—Table 383.3 and Table 388.1). Specific patterns may be noted (Table 388.2). Secondary mitochondrial disorders include diseases with an uncertain etiology, such as Reye syndrome; disorders caused by endogenous or exogenous toxins, drugs, or metals; and other conditions in which mitochondrial oxidative injury may be involved in the pathogenesis of liver injury.

EPIDEMIOLOGY

Mitochondrial respiratory chain disorders of all types affect 1 in 20,000 children younger than 16 yr of age; liver involvement has been reported in 10–20% of patients with respiratory chain defect. Primary mitochondrial disorders, including mtDNA depletion syndromes (MDSs), occur in 1 in 5,000 live births and are a known cause of acute liver failure in children <2 yr of age.

More than 200 pathogenic point mutations, deletions, insertions, and rearrangements that involve mtDNA and nuclear DNA and encodes mitochondrial proteins are identified. Mitochondrial genetics are unique because mitochondria are able to replicate, transcribe, and translate their mitochondrial-derived DNA independently. A typical hepatocyte contains approximately 1,000 copies of mtDNA. Oxidative phosphorylation (the process of adenosine triphosphate production) occurs in the respiratory chain located in the inner mitochondrial membrane and is divided into 5 multienzyme complexes: reduced nicotinamide adenine dinucleotide coenzyme Q reductase (complex I), succinate–coenzyme Q reductase (complex II), reduced coenzyme Q–cytochrome-*c* reductase (complex III), cytochrome-*c* oxidase (complex IV), and adenosine triphosphate synthase (complex V). The respiratory chain peptide components are encoded by both nuclear and mtDNA genes, hence mutations in either genome can result in disorders of oxidative phosphorylation. Thirteen essential polypeptides are synthesized from the small 16.5-kilobase circular double-stranded mtDNA. mtDNA also encodes the 24 transfer RNAs required for intramitochondrial protein synthesis, whereas nuclear genes encode more than 70 respiratory chain subunits and an array of enzymes and cofactors required to maintain mtDNA, including DNA polymerase-γ (POLG), thymidine kinase 2, and deoxyguanosine kinase.

The expression of mitochondrial disorders is complex, and epidemiologic studies are hampered by technical difficulties in collecting and processing the tissue specimens needed to make accurate diagnoses, the variability in clinical presentation, and the fact that most disorders display maternal inheritance with variable penetrance (see Chapter 97). mtDNA mutates 10 times more often than nuclear DNA due to a lack of introns, protective histones, and an effective repair system in mitochondria. Mitochondrial genetics also displays a threshold effect in that the type and severity of mutation required for clinical expression varies

GENE	RESPIRATORY CHAIN COMPLEX	HEPATIC HISTOLOGY	OTHER ORGANS INVOLVED	CLINICAL FEATURES
Table 388.1				Genotypic Classification of Primary Mitochondrial Hepatopathies and Organ Involvement
Deletion	Multiple (Pearson)	Steatosis, fibrosis	Kidney, heart, CNS, muscle	Sideroblastic anemia, variable thrombocytopenia and neutropenia, persistent diarrhea
MPV17	I, III, IV	Steatosis	CNS, muscle, gastrointestinal tract	Adult-onset multisystemic involvement: myopathy, ophthalmoplegia, severe constipation, parkinsonism
DGUOK	I, III, IV	Steatosis, fibrosis	Kidneys, CNS, muscle	Nystagmus, hypotonia, renal Fanconi syndrome, acidosis
MPV17	I, III, IV	Steatosis, fibrosis	CNS, PNS	Hypotonia
SUCLG1	I, III, IV	Steatosis	Kidneys, CNS, muscle	Myopathy, sensorineural hearing loss, respiratory failure
POLG1	I, III, IV	Steatosis, fibrosis	CNS, muscle	Liver failure preceded by neurologic symptoms, intractable seizures, ataxia, psychomotor regression
C10orf2/Twinkle	I, III, IV	Steatosis	CNS, muscle	Infantile-onset spinocerebellar ataxia, loss of skills
BCS1L	III (GRACILE)		CNS ±, muscle ±, kidneys	Fanconi-type renal tubulopathy
SCO1	IV	Steatosis, fibrosis	Muscle	
TRMU	I, III, IV	Steatosis, fibrosis		Infantile liver failure with subsequent recovery
EFG1	I, III, IV	Steatosis	CNS	Severe, rapidly progressive encephalopathy
EFTu	I, III, IV	Unknown	CNS	Severe lactic acidosis, rapidly fatal encephalopathy

CNS, central nervous system; *GRACILE*, growth restriction, aminoaciduria, cholestasis, iron overload, lactic acidosis, and early death; *PNS*, peripheral nervous system.
From Lee WS, Sokol RJ: Mitochondrial hepatopathies: advances in genetics, therapeutic approaches and outcomes, *J Pediatr* 163:942–948, 2013 (Table 2, p. 944).

Table 388.2	Hepatic Phenotypes of Mitochondrial Cytopathies

- Infantile liver failure
- Neonatal cholestasis
- Pearson syndrome
- Alpers disease
- Chronic liver disease
- Drug-induced mitochondrial toxicity

From Wyllie R, Hyams JS, Kay M, editors: *Pediatric gastrointestinal and liver disease*, ed 5, Philadelphia, 2016, Elsevier (Box 71.2, p. 876).

among people and organ systems; this is explained by the concept of heteroplasmy, in which cells and tissues harbor both normal and mutant mtDNA in various amounts because of random partitioning during cell division. Mutations, deletions, or duplications in either mitochondrial or nuclear genes can cause disease, and mutations in nuclear genes that control mtDNA replication, transcription, and translation may lead to **MDS** or to a translational disorder.

CLINICAL MANIFESTATIONS
Defects in oxidative phosphorylation can affect any tissue to a variable degree, with the most energy-dependent organs being the most vulnerable. One should consider the diagnosis of a mitochondrial disorder in a patient of any age who presents with progressive, multisystem involvement that cannot be explained by a specific diagnosis. Gastrointestinal complaints include vomiting, diarrhea, constipation, failure to thrive, and abdominal pain; certain mitochondrial disorders have characteristic gastrointestinal presentations. Pearson marrow-pancreas syndrome manifests with sideroblastic anemia and exocrine pancreatic insufficiency, whereas mitochondrial neurogastrointestinal encephalomyopathy manifests with chronic intestinal pseudo-obstruction and cachexia. Hepatic presentations range from chronic cholestasis, hepatomegaly, cirrhosis, and steatosis to fulminant hepatic failure and death. Patients with certain mitochondrial diseases may have normal or minimally elevated lactate levels even in the setting of a metabolic crisis. The lactate-to-pyruvate molar ratio (L:P) has been proposed as a screening

test for mitochondrial disorders because it reflects the equilibrium between the product and substrate of the reaction catalyzed by lactase dehydrogenase. An L:P ≥ 25 has been considered to be highly suggestive of respiratory chain dysfunction; however, an elevated lactate or an elevated L:P can also represent secondary mitochondrial dysfunction occurring as a result of severe liver disease.

PRIMARY MITOCHONDRIAL HEPATOPATHIES
Neonatal Liver Failure
A common presentation of respiratory chain defects is severe liver failure manifested as jaundice, hypoglycemia, coagulopathy, renal dysfunction, and hyperammonemia, with onset within the first few weeks to months of life. **Cytochrome-*c* oxidase** (complex IV) is the most common deficiency in these infants, although complexes I and III and MDSs are also implicated (see Tables 388.1 and 383.3). The key biochemical features include a markedly elevated plasma lactate concentration, an elevated molar ratio of plasma lactate to pyruvate (L:P) (>25), and a raised ratio of β-hydroxybutyrate to acetoacetate (>4.0). Symptoms are nonspecific and include lethargy and vomiting. Most patients additionally have neurologic involvement that manifests as a weak suck, recurrent apnea, or myoclonic epilepsy. Liver biopsy shows predominantly microvesicular steatosis, cholestasis, bile duct proliferation, glycogen depletion, and iron overload. With standard therapy the prognosis is poor, and most patients die from liver failure or infection in the first few months of life.

Alpers Syndrome (Alpers-Huttenlocher Syndrome or Alpers Hepatopathic Poliodystrophy)
Diagnostic criteria include refractory mixed-type seizures with a focal component; psychomotor regression that is episodic and triggered by intercurrent infections; and hepatopathy with or without acute liver failure. Alpers syndrome manifests from infancy up to 8 yr of age with seizures, hypotonia, feeding difficulties, psychomotor regression, and ataxia. Patients develop hepatomegaly and jaundice and have a slower progression to liver failure than those with cytochrome-*c* oxidase deficiency. Elevated blood or cerebrospinal fluid lactate and pyruvate levels are supportive of the diagnosis, in addition to characteristic electroencephalographic findings (high-amplitude slow activity with polyspikes), asymmetric abnormal visual evoked responses, and

low-density areas or atrophy in the occipital or temporal lobes on computed tomography scanning of the brain. In some patients complex I deficiency has been found in liver or muscle mitochondria. The disease is inherited in an autosomal recessive fashion; mutations in the catalytic subunit of the nuclear gene mtDNA *POLG* have been identified in multiple families with Alpers syndrome, leading to the advent of molecular diagnosis for Alpers syndrome. Patients with *POLG* mutations are susceptible to *valproate-induced* liver dysfunction.

Mitochondrial DNA Depletion Syndrome

MDS is characterized by a tissue-specific reduction in mtDNA copy number, leading to deficiencies in complexes I, III, and IV. MDS manifests with phenotypic heterogeneity; multisystem and localized disease forms include myopathic, hepatocerebral, and liver-restricted presentations. Infants with the hepatocerebral form present in the neonatal period. The first symptoms are metabolic; these rapidly progress to hepatic failure with hypoglycemia and vomiting. This stage is followed by neurologic involvement affecting the central and peripheral systems. Laboratory studies are characterized by lactic acidosis, hypoglycemia, and markedly elevated α-fetoprotein in plasma. In some patients, iron overload has been found with elevated transferrin saturation, high ferritin levels, and iron accumulation in hepatocytes and Kupffer cells. Death usually occurs by 1 yr of age. Spontaneous recovery has been reported in a patient with liver-restricted disease. Inheritance is autosomal recessive and mutations in the nuclear deoxyguanosine kinase gene *(DGUOK)* have been identified in many patients with hepatocerebral MDS. Thymidine kinase 2 has been implicated in the myopathic form; no known genetic defect has been identified in liver-restricted MDS. Multiple other nuclear genes including *POLG, MPV17,* Twinkle helicase gene, and *SUCLG1* have been implicated in hepatocerebral MDS. Liver biopsies of patients with MDS show microvesicular steatosis, cholestasis, focal cytoplasmic biliary necrosis, and cytosiderosis in hepatocytes and sinusoidal cells. Ultrastructural changes are characteristic, with oncocytic transformation of mitochondria, which is characterized by mitochondria with sparse cristae, granular matrix, and dense or vesicular inclusions. If the native DNA-encoded complex II is normal and the activities of the other complexes are decreased, one should investigate mtDNA copy numbers for a MDS. Diagnosis is established by the demonstration of a low ratio of mtDNA (<10%) to nuclear DNA in affected tissues and/or genetic testing. Importantly, the sequence of the mitochondrial genome is normal.

Navajo Neurohepatopathy

Navajo neurohepatopathy (NNH) is an autosomal recessive sensorimotor neuropathy with progressive liver disease found only in Navajo Indians of the southwestern United States. The incidence is 1 in 1,600 live births. Diagnostic criteria include sensory neuropathy; motor neuropathy; corneal anesthesia; liver disease; metabolic or infectious complications including failure to thrive, short stature, delayed puberty, or systemic infection; and evidence of central nervous system demyelination on radiographic imaging and peripheral nerves biopsies. An *MPV17* gene mutation is implicated in the pathogenesis of NNH. Interestingly, this is the same gene implicated in MDS (see earlier), demonstrating that NNH may be a specific type of MDS found only in Navajos. NNH is divided into three phenotypic variations based on age of presentation and clinical findings.

First, **classic NNH** appears in infancy with severe progressive neurologic deterioration manifesting clinically as weakness, hypotonia, loss of sensation with accompanying acral mutilation, corneal ulcerations, and poor growth. Liver disease, present in the majority of patients, is secondary and variable; it includes asymptomatic elevations of liver function tests, Reye syndrome–like episodes, and hepatocellular carcinoma or cirrhosis. γ-Glutamyl transpeptidase levels tend to be higher than in other forms of NNH. Liver biopsy might show chronic portal tract inflammation and cirrhosis, but there is shows less cholestasis, hepatocyte ballooning, and giant cell transformation than in other forms of NNH.

Infantile NNH manifests between the ages of 1 and 6 mo with jaundice and failure to thrive and progresses to liver failure and death by 2 yr of age. Patients have hepatomegaly with moderate elevations in aspartate aminotransferase, alanine aminotransferase, and γ-glutamyl transpeptidase. Liver biopsy demonstrates pseudoacinar formation, multinucleate giant cells, portal and lobular inflammation, canalicular cholestasis, and microvesicular steatosis. Progressive neurologic symptoms are not usually noticed at presentation but develop later.

Childhood NNH manifests from age 1-5 yr with the acute onset of fulminant hepatic failure leading to death within months. Most patients also have evidence of neuropathy at presentation. Liver biopsies are similar to those in infantile NNH except for significant hepatocyte ballooning and necrosis, bile duct proliferation, and cirrhosis, which are also seen.

There is no effective treatment for any of the forms of NNH, and neurologic symptoms often preclude liver transplantation. The identical *MPV17* mutation is seen in patients with both the infantile and classic forms of NNH, highlighting the clinical heterogeneity of NNH.

Pearson Syndrome

Pearson marrow-pancreas syndrome has a neonatal-onset with severe macrocytic anemia, variable neutropenia and thrombocytopenia, and ringed sideroblasts in the bone marrow. Diarrhea and fat malabsorption develop in early childhood secondary to extensive pancreatic fibrosis, acinar atrophy, and partial villous atrophy of the small intestine. The liver involvement includes hepatomegaly, steatosis, and cirrhosis. Liver failure and death have been reported before the age of 4 yr. Other features of the syndrome include renal tubular disease, photosensitivity, diabetes mellitus, hydrops fetalis, and the late development of visual impairment, tremor, ataxia, proximal muscle weakness, external ophthalmoplegia, and a pigmentary retinopathy. Methylglutaconic aciduria is a useful diagnostic marker. Large deletions of mtDNA are reported in most patients, resulting in deficiency of complexes I and III. mtDNA deletions can be detected in patients' cultured fibroblasts as well as in peripheral blood lymphocytes.

Villous Atrophy Syndrome

Children with this disease present with severe anorexia, vomiting, chronic diarrhea, and villous atrophy in the 1st yr of life. Hepatic involvement includes mild elevation of aminotransferase levels, hepatomegaly, and steatosis. Lactic acidosis is worsened with high-dextrose intravenous infusions or enteral nutrition. Diarrhea improves by 5 yr of age in association with the normalization of intestinal biopsies. Subsequently patients develop retinitis pigmentosa, cerebellar ataxia, sensorineural deafness, and proximal muscle weakness, with eventual death late in the 1st decade of life. The disease is attributed to a mtDNA rearrangement defect. A complex III deficiency was found in the muscle of affected patients.

GRACILE Syndrome

The acronym GRACILE summarizes the most important clinical features, namely fetal growth restriction (birth weight about −4 SD), aminoaciduria (caused by Fanconi-type tubulopathy), cholestasis (with steatosis and cirrhosis), iron overload, severe lactic acidosis, and early death. The syndrome is associated with mutations of the complex III assembly factor BCS1L. The liver histology shows microvesicular steatosis and cholestasis with abundant iron accumulation in hepatocytes and Kupffer cells. The liver iron content decreases slightly with age, concomitantly with increasing fibrosis and cirrhosis. Abnormal aminotransferase levels and coagulation are noted, but the cause of death seems to be related more to energy depletion than to liver failure. About half of these patients die within the first 2 wk of life.

Mutations in Nuclear Translation and Elongation Factor Genes

Mutations in nuclear translation factor genes *(TRMU)* of the respiratory chain enzyme complexes have been identified as the etiology of acute liver failure manifesting at ages 1 day to 6 mo. The respiratory chain deficit was similar to that seen in MDS, where the activity of the native DNA-encoded complex II was normal whereas complexes I, III, and

IV were decreased. The elongation factor EFG1 (gene *GFM1*) mutation was associated with fetal growth restriction, lactic acidosis, liver dysfunction that progresses into liver failure and death. The mutation in the elongation factor EFTu manifests as severe lactic acidosis and lethal encephalopathy with mild hepatic involvement.

Secondary Mitochondrial Hepatopathies

Secondary mitochondrial hepatopathies are caused by exposure to a hepatotoxic metal, drug, toxin, or endogenous metabolite. In the past, the most common secondary mitochondrial hepatopathy was **Reye syndrome,** the prevalence of which peaked in the 1970s and had a mortality rate of >40%. Although mortality has not changed, the prevalence has decreased from >500 cases in 1980 to approximately 35 cases per year since. The decline in the reported incidence of Reye syndrome may be partially related to more accurate modern diagnosis of infectious, metabolic, or toxic disease, thus reducing the percentage of idiopathic or true cases of Reye syndrome. Reye syndrome is precipitated in a genetically susceptible person by the interaction of a viral infection (influenza, varicella) and salicylate and/or antiemetic use. Clinically it is characterized by a preceding viral illness that appears to be resolving and the acute onset of vomiting and encephalopathy (see Table 388.3). Neurologic symptoms can rapidly progress to seizures, coma, and death. Liver dysfunction is invariably present when vomiting develops, with coagulopathy and elevated serum levels of aspartate aminotransferase, alanine aminotransferase, and ammonia. Importantly, patients remain anicteric and serum bilirubin levels are normal. Liver biopsies show microvesicular steatosis without evidence of liver inflammation or necrosis. Death is usually secondary to increased intracranial pressure and cerebral herniation. Patients who survive have full recovery of liver function but should be carefully screened for fatty-acid oxidation and fatty-acid transport defects (Table 388.4).

Acquired abnormalities of mitochondrial function can be caused by several drugs and toxins, including valproic acid, cyanide, amiodarone, chloramphenicol, iron, the emetic toxin of *Bacillus cereus,* and nucleoside analogs. Valproic acid is a branched fatty acid that can be metabolized into the mitochondrial toxin 4-envalproic acid. Children with underlying respiratory chain defects appear more sensitive to the toxic effects of this drug, and valproic acid is reported to precipitate liver failure in patients with **Alpers syndrome** and **cytochrome-*c* oxidase deficiency.** Nucleoside analogs directly inhibit mitochondrial respiratory chain complexes. The reverse transcriptase inhibitors zidovudine, didanosine, stavudine, and zalcitabine—used to treat HIV-infected patients—inhibit DNA POLG of mitochondria and can block elongation of mtDNA, leading to mtDNA depletion. Other conditions that can lead to mitochondrial oxidative stress include cholestasis, nonalcoholic steatohepatitis, α_1-antitrypsin deficiency, and Wilson disease.

DIAGNOSTIC EVALUATION

Screening tests include common biochemical tests (comprehensive metabolic profile, INR, α-fetoprotein, CPK, phosphorus, complete blood cell count, ammonia, lactate, pyruvate, serum ketone bodies:

Table 388.3	Clinical Staging of Reye Syndrome and Reye-Like Diseases

Symptoms at the time of admission:
I. Usually quiet, **lethargic** and sleepy, vomiting, laboratory evidence of liver dysfunction
II. Deep lethargy, **confusion**, delirium, combativeness, hyperventilation, hyperreflexia
III. Obtunded, **light coma** ± seizures, **decorticate** rigidity, intact pupillary light reaction
IV. Seizures, deepening coma, **decerebrate rigidity,** loss of oculocephalic reflexes, fixed pupils
V. Coma, loss of deep tendon reflexes, respiratory arrest, fixed dilated pupils, **flaccidity/decerebration** (intermittent); isoelectric electroencephalogram

Table 388.4	Diseases That Present a Clinical or Pathologic Picture Resembling Reye Syndrome

- Metabolic disease
  - Organic aciduria
  - Disorders of oxidative phosphorylation
  - Urea cycle defects (carbamoyl phosphate synthetase, ornithine transcarbamylase)
  - Defects in fatty acid oxidation metabolism
  - Acyl–coenzyme A dehydrogenase deficiencies
  - Systemic carnitine deficiency
  - Hepatic carnitine palmitoyltransferase deficiency
  - 3-OH, 3-methylglutaryl-coenzyme A lyase deficiency
  - Fructosemia
  - Infantile liver failure syndrome 1. Caused by leucyl-tRNA synthetase (LARS) gene mutations
- Central nervous system infections or intoxications (meningitis), encephalitis, toxic encephalopathy
- Hemorrhagic shock with encephalopathy
- Drug or toxin ingestion (salicylate, valproate)

both quantitative 3-hydroxybutyrate and quantitative acetoacetate, total free fatty acids, serum acylcarnitine profile; serum-free and total carnitines, urine organic acids, and serum amino acids) (Table 388.5). These results will guide subsequent confirmatory testing to establish a molecular diagnosis. Genotyping, including single gene or panel screening for common mitochondrial disease, is used in clinical practice. Whole exome or genome sequencing is also helpful and is replacing single gene or gene panel testing. However, the identification of multiple gene variants of uncertain significance will require detailed clinical and biochemical confirmation for interpretation. Tissue (liver biopsy,

Table 388.5	Tiered Investigations in Suspected Mitochondrial Liver Disease

TIER 1
Pre-/postprandial plasma lactate, glucose, FFA, and 3-OH
Plasma carnitine, acylcarnitines
Plasma amino acids, creatine kinase, thymidine
Urinary organic acids, amino acids, tubular resorption phosphate, albumin/creatinine ratio CSF lactate/protein (if feasible)
Electrocardiography and echocardiography
Electroencephalography and visual-evoked potentials
Common mutations in *POLG, DGUOK, MPV17,* and *TRMU*

TIER 2
Tissue analysis
Liver biopsy: (if feasible). Tissue for light microscopy, electron microscopy, and Oil Red O stain
Frozen tissue for respiratory chain enzyme activity analysis and mtDNA copy number
Muscle biopsy: Tissue for light microscopy, electron microscopy, Oil Red O stain, and histochemistry for respiratory chain complexes
Frozen tissue for respiratory chain enzyme activity analysis and mtDNA copy number
Skin biopsy: set up for fibroblast culture

TIER 3
Cranial MRI/MRS

TIER 4
Extended molecular screening. This will be guided by the clinical phenotype, results of the tissue analysis, and local facilities
Currently suggested genes should include *SUCLG1, BCS1L, SOC1, TFSM, TWINKLE, ACAD9, EARS2, GFM1, RRM2B, TK2,* and *SUCLA2*

From Wyllie R, Hyams JS, Kay M, editors: *Pediatric gastrointestinal and liver disease,* ed 5, Philadelphia, 2016, Elsevier (Box 71-3, p. 876).

skin fibroblast, and muscle biopsy) may be needed to make a specific biochemical diagnosis.

TREATMENT OF MITOCHONDRIAL HEPATOPATHIES

There is no effective therapy for most patients with mitochondrial hepatopathies; neurologic involvement often precludes orthotopic liver transplantation. Patients with mitochondrial disorders remain at risk for transplant-related worsening of their underlying metabolic disease, especially patients with *POLG*-related disease. Several therapeutic drug combinations—including antioxidants, vitamins, cofactors, and electron acceptors—have been proposed, but no randomized controlled trials have been completed to evaluate them. Treatment strategies are supportive and include the infusion of sodium bicarbonate for acute metabolic

acidosis, transfusions for anemia and thrombocytopenia, and exogenous pancreatic enzymes for pancreatic insufficiency. It is important to discontinue or avoid medications that may exacerbate hepatopathy, including sodium valproate, tetracycline, and macrolide antibiotics, azathioprine, chloramphenicol, quinolones, and linezolid. Ringer lactate should be avoided because patients with liver dysfunction may not be able to metabolize lactate. Propofol should be avoided during anesthesia because of potential interference with mitochondrial function. In patients with lactic acidosis, lactate levels should be monitored during procedures. It is important to maintain anabolism using a balanced intake of fat and carbohydrates while avoiding unbalanced intakes (e.g., glucose only at a high intravenous rate) or fasting for >12 hr.

Bibliography is available at Expert Consult.

Chapter **389**
Autoimmune Hepatitis
Benjamin L. Shneider and Frederick J. Suchy

第三百八十九章
自身免疫性肝炎

中文导读

本章主要介绍了自身免疫性肝炎、病因学、病理学、临床表现、实验室发现、诊断、治疗和预后。具体介绍了自身免疫性肝炎中的慢性肝病；病因中详细介绍了T淋巴细胞的作用，其中详细阐述了自身免疫调节基因的作用；临床表现中具体描述了自身免疫性肝病的2种分型；诊断中提到该病无特异性诊断实验，主要依靠排他性诊断；治疗中具体描述了激素及免疫抑制剂的具体剂量及使用注意事项。

AUTOIMMUNE HEPATITIS
Chronic Liver Disease

Autoimmune hepatitis is a chronic hepatic inflammatory process manifested by elevated serum aminotransaminase concentrations, liver-associated serum autoantibodies, and/or hypergammaglobulinemia. The serological autoantibody profile defines 2 main types of autoimmune hepatitis: AIH type 1, with positivity for anti-nuclear antibodies (ANA) and/or anti–smooth muscle antibody (SMA) and AIH type 2, with positivity for anti–liver kidney microsomal type 1 antibody (anti-LKM-1). The targets of the inflammatory process can include hepatocytes and to a lesser extent bile duct epithelium. Chronicity is determined either by duration of liver disease (typically >3-6 mo) or by evidence of chronic hepatic decompensation (hypoalbuminemia, thrombocytopenia) or physical stigmata of chronic liver disease (clubbing, spider telangiectasia, splenomegaly, ascites). The severity is variable; the affected child might

have only biochemical evidence of liver dysfunction, might have stigmata of chronic liver disease, or can present in hepatic failure.

Chronic hepatitis can also be caused by persistent viral infection (see Chapter 358), drugs (see Chapter 363), metabolic diseases (see Chapter 361), fatty liver disease, or idiopathic disorders, which may have features of autoimmunity (Table 389.1). More than 90% of hepatitis B infections in the 1st yr of life become chronic, compared with 5–10% among older children and adults. Chronic hepatitis develops in >50% of acute hepatitis C virus infections. Transmission can occur during the perinatal period from an infected mother or in adolescents from parenteral drug abuse. Hepatitis A does not lead to chronic liver disease. Hepatitis E can become chronic in immunosuppressed patients. **Drugs** commonly used in children that can cause chronic liver injury, which can mimic autoimmune hepatitis, include isoniazid, methyldopa, pemoline, nitrofurantoin, dantrolene, minocycline, pemoline, and the

Table 389.1	Disorders Producing Chronic Hepatitis

- Chronic viral hepatitis
  - Hepatitis B
  - Hepatitis C
  - Hepatitis D
- Autoimmune hepatitis
  - Anti–actin antibody-positive
  - Anti–liver-kidney microsomal antibody-positive
  - Anti–soluble liver antigen antibody-positive
  - Others (includes antibodies to liver-specific lipoproteins or asialoglycoprotein)
  - Overlap syndrome with sclerosing cholangitis and autoantibodies
  - Systemic lupus erythematosus
  - Celiac disease
- Drug-induced hepatitis
- Metabolic disorders associated with chronic liver disease
  - Wilson disease
  - Nonalcoholic steatohepatitis
  - α_1-Antitrypsin deficiency
  - Tyrosinemia
  - Niemann-Pick disease type 2
  - Glycogen storage disease type IV
  - Cystic fibrosis
  - Galactosemia
  - Bile acid biosynthetic abnormalities

sulfonamides. **Metabolic diseases** can lead to chronic hepatitis, including α_1-antitrypsin deficiency, inborn errors of bile acid biosynthesis, and Wilson disease. **Nonalcoholic steatohepatitis,** usually associated with obesity and insulin resistance, is another common cause of chronic hepatitis. It can progress to cirrhosis but responds to weight reduction. In many cases the cause of chronic hepatitis is unknown; in some, an autoimmune mechanism is suggested by the finding of serum antinuclear and anti–SMAs and by multisystem involvement (arthropathy, thyroiditis, rashes, Coombs-positive hemolytic anemia).

Autoimmune hepatitis is a clinical constellation that suggests an immune-mediated process; it is responsive to immunosuppressive therapy

(Table 389.2). Autoimmune hepatitis typically refers to a primarily hepatocyte-specific process, whereas autoimmune cholangiopathy and sclerosing cholangitis predominately involve intrahepatic and extrahepatic bile duct injury. Overlap of the process involving both hepatocyte and bile duct–directed injury may be more common in children. De novo hepatitis can be seen in a subset of liver transplant recipients whose initial disease was not autoimmune.

ETIOLOGY
T Lymphocytes
Autoimmune Regulator Gene
Autoimmune hepatitis arises in a genetically predisposed host after an unknown trigger leads to a T cell–mediated immune response targeting liver autoantigens. A dense portal mononuclear cell infiltrate invades the surrounding parenchyma and comprises T and B lymphocytes, macrophages, and plasma cells. The immunopathogenic mechanisms underlying autoimmune hepatitis are unsettled. Triggering factors can include molecular mimicry, infections, drugs, and the environment (toxins) in a genetically susceptible host. Several human leukocyte antigen class II molecules—particularly DR3, DR4, and DR7 isoforms—confer susceptibility to autoimmune hepatitis. Self-antigenic peptides are processed by populations of antigen-presenting cells and presented to CD4 and CD8 effector T cells. CD4+ T lymphocytes recognizing a self-antigenic liver peptide orchestrate liver injury. Cell-mediated injury by cytokines released by CD8+ cytotoxic T cells and/or antibody-mediated cytotoxicity can be operative. There is also evidence that regulatory T cells from patients with autoimmune hepatitis are impaired in their ability to control the proliferation of CD4 and CD8 effector cells. Cytochrome P450 2D6 is the main autoantigen in type 2 autoimmune hepatitis.

Antibody-coated hepatocytes may be lysed by complement or Fc-bearing natural killer lymphocytes. Heterozygous mutations in the **autoimmune regulator gene (AIRE),** which encodes a transcription factor controlling the negative selection of autoreactive thymocytes, can be found in some children with autoimmune hepatitis types 1 and 2. *AIRE* mutations also cause **autoimmune polyendocrinopathy-candidiasis-ectodermal dystrophy** (also called autoimmune polyendocrinopathy syndrome), in which autoimmune hepatitis occurs in approximately 20% of patients.

Table 389.2	Classification of Autoimmune Hepatitis

VARIABLE	TYPE 1 AUTOIMMUNE HEPATITIS	TYPE 2 AUTOIMMUNE HEPATITIS
Characteristic autoantibodies	Antinuclear antibody* Smooth-muscle antibody* Antiactin antibody[†] Autoantibodies against soluble liver antigen and liver-pancreas antigen[‡] Atypical perinuclear antineutrophil cytoplasmic antibody	Antibody against liver-kidney microsome type 1* Antibody against liver cytosol type 1* Antibody against liver-kidney microsomal type 3
Geographic variation	Worldwide	Worldwide; rare in North America
Age at presentation	Any age	Predominantly childhood and young adulthood
Gender of patients	Female in ~75% of cases	Female in ~95% of cases
Association with other autoimmune diseases	Common	Common[§]
Clinical severity	Broad range, variable	Generally severe
Histopathologic features at presentation	Broad range, mild disease to cirrhosis	Generally advanced
Treatment failure	Infrequent	Frequent
Relapse after drug withdrawal	Variable	Common
Need for long-term maintenance	Variable	~100%

*The conventional method of detection is immunofluorescence.
[†]Tests for this antibody are rarely available in commercial laboratories.
[‡]This antibody is detected by enzyme-linked immunosorbent assay.
[§]Autoimmune polyendocrinopathy-candidiasis-ectodermal dystrophy is seen only in patients with type 2 disease.
Modified from Krawitt EL: Autoimmune hepatitis, *N Engl J Med* 354:54–66, 2006.

PATHOLOGY

The histologic features common to untreated cases include inflammatory infiltrates, consisting of lymphocytes and plasma cells that expand portal areas and often penetrate the lobule (interface hepatitis); moderate to severe piecemeal necrosis of hepatocytes extending outward from the limiting plate; variable necrosis, fibrosis, and zones of parenchymal collapse spanning neighboring portal triads or between a portal triad and central vein (bridging necrosis); and variable degrees of bile duct epithelial injury. Distortion of hepatic architecture can be severe; cirrhosis may be present in children at the time of diagnosis. Histologic features in acute liver failure may be obscured by massive necrosis and multilobular collapse. Other histologic features may suggest an alternative diagnosis: characteristic periodic acid–Schiff-positive, diastase-resistant granules are seen in α_1-antitrypsin deficiency, and macrovesicular and microvesicular steatosis is found in nonalcoholic steatohepatitis and often in Wilson disease. Bile duct injury can suggest an autoimmune cholangiopathy or an overlap syndrome. Ultrastructural analysis might suggest distinct types of storage disorders.

CLINICAL MANIFESTATIONS

The clinical features and course of autoimmune hepatitis are extremely variable. Signs and symptoms at the time of presentation comprise a wide spectrum of disease including a substantial number of asymptomatic patients and some who have an acute, even fulminant, onset. In 25–30% of patients with autoimmune hepatitis, particularly children, the illness mimics acute viral hepatitis. In most the onset is insidious. Patients can be asymptomatic or have fatigue, malaise, behavioral changes, anorexia, and amenorrhea, sometimes for many months before jaundice or stigmata of chronic liver disease are recognized. Extrahepatic manifestations can include arthritis, vasculitis, nephritis, thyroiditis, Coombs-positive anemia, and rash. Some patients' initial clinical features reflect cirrhosis (ascites, hypersplenism, bleeding esophageal varices, or hepatic encephalopathy).

There may be mild to moderate jaundice in severe cases. Spider telangiectasias and palmar erythema may be present. The liver may be tender and slightly enlarged but might not be felt in patients with cirrhosis. The spleen is commonly enlarged. Edema and ascites may be present in advanced cases.

LABORATORY FINDINGS

The findings are related to the severity of presentation. In many asymptomatic cases, serum aminotransferase ranges between 100 and 300 IU/L, whereas levels in excess of 1,000 IU/L can be seen in young symptomatic patients. Serum bilirubin concentrations may be normal in mild cases but are commonly 2-10 mg/dL in more severe cases. Serum alkaline phosphatase and γ-glutamyl transpeptidase activities are normal to slightly increased but may be more significantly elevated in autoimmune cholangiopathy or in the setting of overlap with sclerosing cholangitis. Serum γ-globulin levels can show marked polyclonal elevations. Hypoalbuminemia is common. The prothrombin time is prolonged, most often as a result of vitamin K deficiency but also as a reflection of impaired hepatocellular function. A normochromic normocytic anemia, leukopenia, and thrombocytopenia are present and become more severe with the development of portal hypertension and hypersplenism.

Most patients with autoimmune hepatitis have hypergammaglobulinemia. Serum immunoglobulin G levels usually exceed 16 g/L. Characteristic patterns of serum **autoantibodies** define distinct subgroups of autoimmune hepatitis (see Table 389.2). The most common pattern (type 1) is associated with the formation of non–organ-specific antibodies, such as **antiactin (smooth muscle)** and ANA. Approximately 50% of these patients are 10-20 yr of age. High titers of a **liver-kidney microsomal** antibody are detected in another form (type 2) that usually affects children 2-14 yr of age. A subgroup of primarily young women might demonstrate autoantibodies against a soluble liver antigen but not against nuclear or microsomal proteins. Antineutrophil cytoplasmic antibodies may be seen more commonly in autoimmune cholangiopathy. Autoantibodies are rare in healthy children, so that titers as low as 1:40 may be significant, although nonspecific elevation in autoantibodies can be observed in a variety of liver diseases. Up to 20% of patients with apparent autoimmune hepatitis might not have autoantibodies at presentation but have histological features and clinical course consistent with the disorder. Other, less common autoantibodies include rheumatoid factor, antiparietal cell antibodies, antithyroid antibodies, and anti–liver cytosol type 1 antibody (anti-LC-1). A Coombs-positive hemolytic anemia may be present.

DIAGNOSIS

There is no specific test for autoimmune hepatitis; it is a clinical diagnosis based on certain diagnostic criteria. Diagnostic criteria with scoring systems have been developed for adults and modified slightly for children, although these scoring systems were developed as research rather than diagnostic tools. Important positive features include female gender, primary elevation in transaminases and not alkaline phosphatase (or GGT), elevated γ-globulin levels, the presence of autoantibodies (most commonly antinuclear, smooth muscle, or liver-kidney microsome), and characteristic histologic findings (Fig. 389.1). Important negative features include the absence of viral markers (hepatitides B, C, D) of infection, absence of a history of drug or blood product exposure, and negligible alcohol consumption.

Common conditions that might lead to chronic hepatitis should be excluded (see Table 389.1). The differential diagnosis includes α_1-antitrypsin deficiency (see Chapter 357) and Wilson disease (see Chapter 357.2). The former disorder must be excluded by performing α_1-antitrypsin phenotyping and the latter by measuring serum ceruloplasmin and 24-hr urinary copper excretion and/or hepatic copper levels. Chronic hepatitis may occur in patients with inflammatory bowel disease, but liver dysfunction in such patients is more commonly caused by pericholangitis or sclerosing cholangitis. Celiac disease (see Chapter 338) is associated with liver disease that is akin to autoimmune hepatitis, and appropriate serologic testing should be performed, including assays for anti–tissue transglutaminase antibodies or antiendomysial antibodies. An ultrasonogram should be done to identify a choledochal cyst or other structural disorders of the biliary system. Magnetic resonance (MR) cholangiography may be very useful for screening for evidence of sclerosing cholangitis. An overlap syndrome with features of primary sclerosing cholangitis and autoimmune hepatitis is being increasingly recognized with wider application of MR cholangiography (Table 389.3). Patients with primary sclerosing cholangitis can have elevated γ-globulin levels and autoantibodies; therefore liver biopsy findings in these children may be especially important. Dilated or obliterated veins on ultrasonography suggest the possibility of the Budd-Chiari syndrome. Diagnosis of autoimmune liver disease in the setting of acute liver failure is difficult and care should be taken in applying standardized approaches. "Seronega-

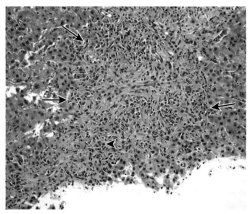

Fig. 389.1 Autoimmune hepatitis. Liver biopsy showing fibrous expansion of the portal tracts with moderate portal lymphocytic infiltrates rich in plasma cells *(arrowhead)*. There is extensive interface hepatitis *(arrows)*. Original magnification ×20. *(Courtesy Margret Magid, Mount Sinai School of Medicine.)*

Table 389.3	Overlap Syndromes of Autoimmune Hepatitis		
	AUTOIMMUNE HEPATITIS WITH OVERLAPPING FEATURES OF:		
	Primary Biliary Cholangitis*	**Primary Sclerosing Cholangitis**	**Cholestasis**
Clinical and laboratory features	AMA + Serum AP frequently > 2-fold ULN	AMA − Serum AP frequently > 2-fold ULN IBD common Abnormal cholangiogram (except in small-duct disease)	AMA − Serum AP frequently > 2-fold ULN No UC Normal cholangiogram
Histology	Destructive cholangitis Ductopenia Cholestasis	Ductopenia Cholangiolar proliferation Swollen fibrotic portal tracts	Lymphoplasmacytic portal and acinar infiltrates Lymphocytic destructive cholangitis Swollen hepatocytes
Treatment	Prednisone (10 mg daily) in combination with azathioprine (50 mg daily) if AP ≤ 2 × ULN Prednisone (10 mg daily) in combination with azathioprine (50 mg daily) and low-dose UDCA (13-15 mg/kg daily) if AP > 2 × ULN and/or florid duct lesions	Prednisone (10 mg daily) in combination with azathioprine (50 mg daily) and low-dose UDCA (13-15 mg/kg daily)	Prednisone (10 mg daily) in combination with azathioprine (50 mg daily) and/or low-dose UDCA (13-15 mg/kg daily) depending on AP level and histologic features

*Primary biliary cholangitis formerly called primary biliary cirrhosis.
  AMA, antimitochondrial antibodies; *AP,* alkaline phosphatase level; *UDCA,* ursodeoxycholic acid; *ULN,* upper limit of normal.
  From Czaja AJ: Autoimmune hepatitis. In Feldman M, Friedman LS, Brandt LJ, editors: *Sleisenger and Fordtran's gastrointestinal and liver disease,* ed 10, Philadelphia, 2016: Elsevier (Table 90.4).

tive" autoimmune hepatitis has been described, so absence of classic autoimmune markers does not exclude this diagnosis.

TREATMENT
Prednisone, with or without azathioprine or 6-mercaptopurine, improves the clinical, biochemical, and histologic features in most patients with autoimmune hepatitis and prolongs survival in most patients with severe disease. The goal is to suppress or eliminate hepatic inflammation with minimal side effects. Prednisone at an initial dose of 1-2 mg/kg/24 hr is continued until aminotransferase values return to less than twice the upper limit of normal. The dose should then be lowered in 5-mg decrements over 2-4 mo until a maintenance dose of 0.1-0.3 mg/kg/24 hr is achieved. In patients who respond poorly, who experience severe side effects, or who cannot be maintained on low-dose steroids, azathioprine (1.5-2.0 mg/kg/24 hr, up to 100 mg/24 hr) can be added, with frequent monitoring for bone marrow suppression. Measurement of thiopurine methyltransferase activity should be done prior to beginning treatment with the thiopurine drugs azathioprine and 6-mercaptopurine. Patients with low activity (10% prevalence) or absent activity (prevalence 0.3%) are at risk for developing severe drug-induced myelotoxicity from accumulation of the unmetabolized drug. Measurement of the drug metabolites, 6-thioguanine nucleotide and 6-methylmercaptopurine, is useful in determining why a patient is not responding to a standard dose of a thiopurine drug and may help in avoiding myelosuppression and hepatotoxicity. Single-agent therapy with alternate-day corticosteroids should be used with great caution, although addition of azathioprine to alternate-day steroids can be an effective approach that minimizes corticosteroid-related toxicity. In patients with a mild and relatively asymptomatic presentation, some favor a lower starting dose of prednisone (10-20 mg) coupled with the simultaneous early administration of either 6-mercaptopurine (1.0-1.5 mg/kg/24 hr) or azathioprine (1.5-2.0 mg/kg/24 hr). Patients with primary sclerosing cholangitis/autoimmune hepatitis overlap syndrome respond similarly to immunosuppressive therapy. Precise diagnostic criteria for autoimmune disease in the setting of sclerosing cholangitis do not exist. Autoimmune markers and immunoglobulin levels are often elevated in children with sclerosing cholangitis and do not necessarily indicate a diagnosis of coincident autoimmune hepatitis. The choleretic agent, ursodeoxycholic acid, is often used in biliary tract disease, but trials in adults with primary sclerosing cholangitis have not shown efficacy, and patients have

experienced toxicity at higher doses. There is a potential role for budesonide combined with azathioprine in treatment of noncirrhotic patients. Budesonide is a corticosteroid with high first-pass clearance by the liver and fewer systemic side effects including suppression of hypothalamic–pituitary axis. Cyclosporine, tacrolimus, mycophenolate mofetil, and sirolimus have been used in the management of cases refractory to standard therapy. Use of these agents should be reserved for practitioners with extensive experience in their administration, because the agents have a more restricted therapeutic to toxic ratio.

Histologic progress does not necessarily need to be assessed by sequential liver biopsies, although biochemical remission does not ensure histologic resolution. Follow-up liver biopsy is an important consideration in patients for whom consideration is given to discontinuing corticosteroid therapy. In patients with disappearance of symptoms and biochemical abnormalities and resolution of the necroinflammatory process on biopsy, an attempt at gradual discontinuation of medication is justified. There is a high rate of relapse after discontinuation of therapy.

Relapse can require reinstitution of induction dosing of immunosuppression to control disease relapse.

PROGNOSIS
The initial response to therapy in autoimmune hepatitis is generally prompt, with a >75% rate of remission. Transaminases and bilirubin fall to near-normal levels, often in the first 1-3 months. When present, abnormalities in serum albumin and prothrombin time respond over a longer period (3-9 mo). In patients meeting the criteria for tapering and then withdrawal of treatment (25–40% of children), 50% are weaned from all medication; in the other 50%, relapse occurs after a variable period. Relapse usually responds to retreatment. Many children will not meet the criteria for an attempt at discontinuation of immunosuppression and should be maintained on the smallest dose of prednisone that minimizes biochemical activity of the disease. A careful balance of the risks of continued immunosuppression and ongoing hepatitis must be continually evaluated. This requires continual screening for complications of medical therapy (monitoring of linear growth velocity, ophthalmologic examination, bone density measurement, blood pressure monitoring). Intermittent flares of hepatitis can occur and can necessitate recycling of prednisone therapy.

Some children have a relatively steroid-resistant form of hepatitis. More extensive evaluations of the etiology of their hepatitis should be undertaken, directed particularly at reassessing for the presence of either sclerosing cholangitis or Wilson disease. Nonadherence to medical therapy is one of the most common causes of "resistance" to medical therapy. Progression to cirrhosis can occur in autoimmune hepatitis despite a good response to drug therapy and prolongation of life. Corticosteroid therapy in fulminant autoimmune disease may be useful, although it should be administered with caution, given the predisposition of these patients to systemic bacterial and fungal infections.

Liver transplantation has been successful in patients with end-stage or fulminant liver disease associated with autoimmune hepatitis (see Chapter 368). Disease recurs after transplantation in approximately 30% of patients and is associated with increased concentrations of serum autoantibodies and interface hepatitis on liver biopsy. Patients generally respond well to an increase in immunosuppression, particularly to the addition of azathioprine.

Bibliography is available at Expert Consult.

Chapter 390

Drug- and Toxin-Induced Liver Injury

Frederick J. Suchy and Amy G. Feldman

第三百九十章

药物和毒素引起的肝损伤

中文导读

本章主要介绍了药物和毒素引起的肝损伤的治疗、预后和预防。具体描述了常见引起肝损伤药物的热门用途、来源、肝毒性成分及不同药物导致的肝损伤的病理类型；详细介绍了肝损伤的发病机制、病理特点、临床表现、实验室检查和鉴别诊断；治疗以支持治疗为主，回避有毒物质；预后取决于其类型和严重程度；预防药物性肝损伤仍具有挑战性。

The liver is the main site of drug metabolism and is particularly susceptible to structural and functional injury after the ingestion, parenteral administration, or inhalation of chemical agents, drugs, plant derivatives (home remedies), herbal or nutritional supplements, or environmental toxins. The possibility of drug use or toxin exposure at home or in the parents' workplace should be explored for every child with liver dysfunction. The clinical spectrum of illness can vary from asymptomatic biochemical abnormalities of liver function to fulminant failure. Liver injury may be the only clinical feature of an adverse drug reaction or may be accompanied by systemic manifestations and damage to other organs. In hospitalized patients, clinical and laboratory findings may be confused with the underlying illness. After acetaminophen, antimicrobials, supplements, and central nervous system agents are the most commonly implicated drug classes causing liver injury in children.

There is growing concern about environmental hepatotoxins that are insidious in their effects. Many environmental toxins—including the plasticizers, biphenyl A, and the phthalates—are ligands for nuclear receptors that transcriptionally activate the promoters of many genes involved in xenobiotic and lipid metabolism and may contribute to obesity and nonalcoholic fatty liver disease. Some herbal, weight loss, and body building supplements have been associated with hepatic injury or even liver failure (Table 390.1) related to their intrinsic toxicity or because of contamination with fungal toxins, pesticides, or heavy metals.

Hepatic metabolism of drugs and toxins is mediated by a sequence of enzymatic reactions that in large part transform hydrophobic, less-soluble molecules into more nontoxic, hydrophilic compounds that can be readily excreted in urine or bile (see Chapter 72). Relative liver size, liver blood flow, and extent of protein binding also influence drug metabolism. Phase 1 of the process involves enzymatic activation of the substrate to reactive intermediates containing a carboxyl, phenol, epoxide, or hydroxyl group. Mixed-function monooxygenase, cytochrome-*c* reductase, various hydrolases, and the cytochrome P450 (CYP) system are involved in this process. Nonspecific induction of these enzymatic pathways, which can occur during intercurrent viral infection, with starvation, and with the administration of certain drugs such as anticonvulsants, can alter drug metabolism and increase the potential for hepatotoxicity. A single agent

Table 390.1	Hepatotoxic Herbal Remedies, Dietary Supplements, and Weight Loss Products

REMEDY	POPULAR USES	SOURCE	HEPATOTOXIC COMPONENT	TYPE OF LIVER INJURY
Ayurvedic herbal medicine	Multiple	Multiple	Uncertain (may contain heavy metal contaminants)	Hepatitis
Barakol	Anxiolytic	*Cassia siamea*	Uncertain	Reversible hepatitis or cholestasis
Black cohosh	Menopausal symptoms	*Cimicifuga racemosa*	Uncertain	Hepatitis (causality uncertain)
"Bush tea"	Fever	*Senecio, Heliotropium, Crotalaria* spp.	Pyrrolizidine alkaloids	SOS
Cascara	Laxative	*Cascara sagrada*	Anthracene glycoside	Cholestatic hepatitis
Chaparral leaf (greasewood, creosote bush)	"Liver tonic," burn salve, weight loss	*Larrea tridenta*	Nordihydroguaiaretic acid	Acute and chronic hepatitis, FHF
Chaso/onshido	Weight loss	—	N-nitro-fenfluramine	Acute hepatitis, FHF
Chinese medicines (traditional)				
Jin bu huan	Sleep aid, analgesic	*Lycopodium serratum*	Levo-tetrahydropalmitine	Acute or chronic hepatitis or cholestasis, steatosis
Ma huang	Weight loss	*Ephedra* spp.	Ephedrine	Severe hepatitis, FHF
Shou-wu-pian	Anti-aging, neuroprotection, laxative	*Polygonum multiflorum* Thunb (fleeceflower root)	Anthraquinone	Acute hepatitis or cholestasis
Syo-saiko-to	Multiple	*Scutellaria* root	Diterpenoids	Hepatocellular necrosis, cholestasis, steatosis, granulomas
Comfrey	Herbal tea	*Symphytum* spp.	Pyrrolizidine alkaloid	Acute SOS, cirrhosis
Germander	Weight loss, fever	*Teucrium chamaedry, T. capitatum, T. polium*	Diterpenoids, epoxides	Acute and chronic hepatitis, FHF, autoimmune injury
Greater celandine	Gallstones, IBS	*Chelidonium majus*	Isoquinoline alkaloids	Cholestatic hepatitis, fibrosis
Green tea leaf extract	Multiple	*Camellia sinensis*	Catechins	Hepatitis (causality questioned)
Herbalife	Nutritional supplement, weight loss	—	Various; ephedra	Severe hepatitis, FHF
Hydroxycut	Weight loss	*Camellia sinensis*, among other constituents	Uncertain	Acute hepatitis, FHF
Impila	Multiple	*Callilepsis laureola*	Potassium atractylate	Hepatic necrosis
Kava	Anxiolytic	*Piper methysticum*	Kava lactone, pipermethystine	Acute hepatitis, cholestasis, FHF
Kombucha	Weight loss	Lichen alkaloid	Usnic acid	Acute hepatitis
Limbrel (Flavocoxid)	Osteoarthritis	Plant bioflavonoids	Baicalin, epicatechin	Acute mixed hepatocellular-cholestatic injury
Lipokinetix	Weight loss	Lichen alkaloid	Usnic acid	Acute hepatitis, jaundice, FHF
Mistletoe	Asthma, infertility	*Viscus album*	Uncertain	Hepatitis (in combination with skullcap)
Oil of cloves	Dental pain	Various foods, oils	Eugenol	Zonal necrosis
Pennyroyal (squawmint oil)	Abortifacient	*Hedeoma pulegoides, Mentha pulegium*	Pulegone, monoterpenes	Severe hepatocellular necrosis
Prostata	Prostatism	Multiple	Uncertain	Chronic cholestasis
Sassafras	Herbal tea	*Sassafras albidum*	Safrole	HCC (in animals)
Senna	Laxative	*Cassia angustifolia*	Sennoside alkaloids; anthrone	Acute hepatitis
Skullcap	Anxiolytic	*Scutellaria*	Diterpenoids	Hepatitis
Valerian	Sedative	*Valeriana officinalis*	Uncertain	Elevated liver enzymes

FHF, fulminant hepatic failure; *HCC,* hepatocellular carcinoma; *SOS,* sinusoidal obstruction syndrome.
From Lewis JH: Liver disease caused by anesthetics, chemicals, toxins, and herbal preparations. In Feldman M, Friedman LS, Brandt LJ, editors: *Sleisenger and Fordtran's gastrointestinal and liver disease,* ed 10, Philadelphia, 2016, Elsevier, (Table 89.6).

can be metabolized by more than 1 biochemical reaction. The reactive intermediates that are potentially damaging to the cell are enzymatically conjugated in phase 2 reactions with glucuronic acid, sulfate, acetate, glycine, or glutathione. Some drugs may be directly metabolized by these conjugating reactions without first undergoing phase 1 activation. Phase 3 is the energy-dependent excretion of drug metabolites and their conjugates by an array of membrane transporters in the liver and kidney such as the multidrug resistant protein 1.

Pathways for biotransformation are expressed early in the fetus and infant, but many phase 1 and phase 2 enzymes are immature, particularly in the 1st yr of life. CYP3A4 is the primary hepatic CYP expressed postnatally and metabolizes more than 75 commonly used therapeutic drugs and several environmental pollutants and procarcinogens. Hepatic CYP3A4 activity is poorly expressed in the fetus but increases after birth to reach 30% of adult values by 1 mo and 50% of adult values between 6 and 12 mo of age. CYP3A4 can be induced by a number of drugs, including phenytoin, phenobarbital, and rifampin. Enhanced production of toxic metabolites can overwhelm the capacity of phase 2 reactions. Conversely, numerous inhibitors of CYP3A4 from several different drug classes, such as erythromycin and cimetidine, can lead to toxic accumulations of CYP3A4 substrates. By contrast, although CYP2D6 is also developmentally regulated (maturation by 10 yr of age), its activity depends more on genetic polymorphisms than on sensitivity to inducers and inhibitors because more than 70 allelic variants of CYP2D6 significantly influence the metabolism of many drugs. Uridine diphosphate glucuronosyltransferase 1A6, a phase 2 enzyme that glucuronidates acetaminophen, is also absent in the human fetus, increases slightly in the neonate, but does not reach adult levels until sometime after 10 yr of age. Mechanisms for the uptake and excretion of organic ions can also be deficient early in life. Impaired drug metabolism via phase 1 and phase 2 reactions present in the 1st few months of life is followed by a period of enhanced metabolism of many drugs in children through 10 yr of age compared with adults.

Genetic polymorphisms in genes encoding enzymes and transporters mediating phases 1, 2, and 3 reactions can also be associated with impaired drug metabolism and an increased risk of hepatotoxicity. Some cases of idiosyncratic hepatotoxicity can occur as a result of aberrations (polymorphisms) in phase 1 drug metabolism, producing intermediates of unusual hepatotoxic potential combined with developmental, acquired, or relative inefficiency of phase 2 conjugating reactions. Genome-wide association studies have identified HLA associations in certain cases of drug- and toxin-induced liver injury (**DILI**). Children may less susceptible than adults to hepatotoxic reactions; liver injury after the use of the anesthetic halothane is rare in children, and acetaminophen toxicity is less common in infants than in adolescents, whereas most cases of fatal hepatotoxicity associated with sodium valproate use have been reported in children. Excessive or prolonged therapeutic administration of acetaminophen combined with reductions in caloric or protein intake can produce hepatotoxicity in children. In this setting, acetaminophen metabolism may be impaired by reduced synthesis of sulfated and glucuronated metabolites and reduced stores of glutathione. Immaturity of hepatic drug metabolic pathways can prevent degradation of a toxic agent; under other circumstances, the same immaturity might limit the formation of toxic metabolites. Severe sodium valproate hepatotoxicity is often associated with an underlying inherited mitochondrial disorder (Alper syndrome).

Chemical hepatotoxicity can be predictable or idiosyncratic. Predictable hepatotoxicity implies a high incidence of hepatic injury in exposed persons depending on dose. It is understandable that only a few drugs in clinical use fall into this category. These agents might damage the hepatocyte directly through alteration of membrane lipids (peroxidation) or through denaturation of proteins; such agents include carbon tetrachloride and trichloroethylene. Indirect injury can occur through interference with metabolic pathways essential for cell integrity or through distortion of cellular constituents by covalent binding of a reactive metabolite; examples include the liver injury produced by acetaminophen or by antimetabolites such as methotrexate or 6-mercaptopurine.

Idiosyncratic hepatotoxicity is unpredictable and accounts for the majority of adverse reactions. In contrast to previous dogma that idiosyncratic reactions are independent of dose, there is new information that higher doses of drugs metabolized in the liver pose a greater risk for hepatotoxicity. Idiosyncratic drug reactions in certain patients can reflect aberrant pathways for drug metabolism, possibly related to genetic polymorphisms, with production of toxic intermediates (isoniazid and sodium valproate can cause liver damage through this mechanism). Duration of drug use before liver injury varies (weeks to ≥1 yr) and the response to reexposure may be delayed.

An idiosyncratic reaction can also be immunologically mediated as a result of prior sensitization (hypersensitivity); extrahepatic manifestations of hypersensitivity can include fever, rash, arthralgia, and eosinophilia. Duration of exposure before reaction is generally 1-4 wk, with prompt recurrence of injury on reexposure. Studies indicate that arene oxides, generated through oxidative (CYP) metabolism of aromatic anticonvulsants (phenytoin, phenobarbital, carbamazepine), can initiate the pathogenesis of some hypersensitivity reactions. Arene oxides, formed in vivo, can bind to cellular macromolecules, thus perturbing cell function and possibly initiating immunologic mechanisms of liver injury.

Although the generation of chemically reactive metabolites has received great attention in the pathogenesis of hepatotoxicity, increasing evidence now exists for the multifactorial nature of the process, in particular the role played by the host immune system. Activation of liver nonparenchymal Kupffer cells and infiltration by neutrophils perpetuate toxic injury by many drugs by release of reactive oxygen and nitrogen species as well as cytokines. Stellate cells can also be activated, potentially leading to hepatic fibrosis and cirrhosis.

The pathologic spectrum of drug-induced liver disease is extremely wide, is rarely specific, and can mimic other liver diseases (Table 390.2). Predictable hepatotoxins, such as acetaminophen, produce centrilobular

Table 390.2	Patterns of Hepatic Drug Injury
DISEASE	**DRUG**
Centrilobular necrosis	Acetaminophen
	Carbon tetrachloride
	Cocaine
	Ecstasy
	Iron
	Halothane
Microvesicular steatosis	Valproic acid
	Tetracycline
	Toluene
	Methotrexate
Acute hepatitis	Isoniazid
	Anti–tumor necrosis factor agents
	Valproic acid
General hypersensitivity	Sulfonamides
	Phenytoin
	Minocycline
Fibrosis	Methotrexate
Cholestasis	Chlorpromazine
	Aniline
	Erythromycin
	Paraquat
	Estrogens
	Sertraline
Sinusoidal obstruction syndrome (venoocclusive disease)	Irradiation plus busulfan
	Arsenic
	Cyclophosphamide
Portal and hepatic vein thrombosis	Estrogens
	Androgens
Biliary sludge	Ceftriaxone
Hepatic adenoma or hepatocellular carcinoma	Oral contraceptives
	Anabolic steroids

necrosis of hepatocytes. Steatosis is an important feature of tetracycline (microvesicular) and ethanol (macrovesicular) toxicities. A cholestatic hepatitis can be observed, with injury caused by erythromycin estolate and chlorpromazine. Cholestasis without inflammation may be a toxic effect of estrogens and anabolic steroids. Use of oral contraceptives and androgens has also been associated with benign and malignant liver tumors. Some idiosyncratic drug reactions can produce mixed patterns of injury, with diffuse cholestasis and cell necrosis. Chronic hepatitis has been associated with the use of methyldopa and nitrofurantoin.

Clinical manifestations can be mild and nonspecific, such as fever and malaise. Fever, rash, and arthralgia may be prominent in cases of hypersensitivity. In ill hospitalized patients, the signs and symptoms of hepatic drug toxicity may be difficult to separate from the underlying illness. The differential diagnosis should include acute and chronic viral hepatitis, biliary tract disease, septicemia, ischemic and hypoxic liver injury, malignant infiltration, and inherited metabolic liver disease.

The laboratory features of drug- or toxin-related liver disease are extremely variable. Hepatocyte damage can lead to elevations of serum aminotransferase activities and serum bilirubin levels and to impaired synthetic function as evidenced by decreased serum coagulation factors and albumin. Hyperammonemia can occur with liver failure or with selective inhibition of the urea cycle (sodium valproate). Toxicologic screening of blood and urine specimens can aid in the detecting drug or toxin exposure. Percutaneous liver biopsy may be necessary to distinguish drug injury from complications of an underlying disorder or from intercurrent infection. Vanishing bile duct syndrome can be seen in a small portion of patients with idiosyncratic DILI.

Slight elevation of serum aminotransferase activities (generally <2-3 times normal) can occur during therapy with drugs, particularly anticonvulsants, capable of inducing microsomal pathways for drug metabolism. Liver biopsy reveals proliferation of smooth endoplasmic reticulum but no significant liver injury. Liver test abnormalities often resolve with continued drug therapy.

TREATMENT

Treatment of drug- or toxin-related liver injury is mainly supportive. Contact with the offending agent should be avoided. Corticosteroids might have a role in immune-mediated disease. Treatment with *n*-acetylcysteine, by stimulating glutathione synthesis, is effective in preventing or attenuating hepatotoxicity when administered within 16 hr after an acute overdose of acetaminophen and appears to improve survival in patients with severe liver injury even up to 36 hr after ingestion (see Chapter 63). Intravenous L-carnitine may be of value in treating valproic acid–induced hepatotoxicity. Orthotopic liver transplantation may be required for treatment of drug- or toxin-induced hepatic failure.

PROGNOSIS

The prognosis of DILI depends on its type and severity. Injury is usually completely reversible when the hepatotoxic factor is withdrawn. The mortality of submassive hepatic necrosis with fulminant liver failure can, however, exceeds 50%. Hyperbilirubinemia, coagulopathy, and elevated serum creatinine are associated with an increased risk of death or need for liver transplantation. With continued use of certain drugs, such as methotrexate, effects of hepatoxicity can proceed insidiously to cirrhosis, even with normal or near normal liver tests. Neoplasia can follow long-term androgen therapy. Rechallenge with a drug suspected of having caused previous liver injury is rarely justified and can result in fatal hepatic necrosis.

PREVENTION

The prevention of drug-induced liver injury remains a challenge. Monitoring of liver biochemical tests may be useful in some cases, but it can prove difficult to sustain for agents used for many years. Such testing may be particularly important in patients with preexisting liver disease. For drugs with hepatotoxic potential, even if episodes are infrequent in children, such as with the use of isoniazid, patients should be advised to immediately stop the medication with onset of nausea, vomiting, abdominal pain, and fatigue until liver damage is excluded. Obvious symptoms of liver disease such as jaundice and dark urine can lag behind severe hepatocellular injury. Monitoring for toxic metabolites and genotyping can be effective in preventing severe toxicity with the use of azathioprine. Advances in pharmacogenomics, such as the use of gene chips to detect variants in some of the CYP enzymes, hold promise of a personalized approach to prevent hepatotoxicity.

Bibliography is available at Expert Consult.

Chapter **391**
Acute Hepatic Failure
Frederick J. Suchy and Amy G. Feldman

第三百九十一章
急性肝衰竭

中文导读

　　本章主要介绍了急性肝衰竭的病因学、病理学、发病机制、临床表现、实验室发现、治疗和预后。具体描述了病因学为感染、自身免疫性肝炎、代谢疾病、感染、肿瘤、妊娠同族免疫性肝病、药物性肝损伤、血管性和特发性急性肝衰竭；具体阐述了临床表现中肝性脑病的四期；具体描述了针对明确病因的治疗方法、婴儿和儿童的治疗特点、注意事项以及进入肝性脑病晚期可考虑肝移植等内容。

Acute liver failure is a clinical syndrome resulting from massive necrosis of hepatocytes or from severe functional impairment of hepatocytes. The synthetic, excretory, and detoxifying functions of the liver are all severely impaired. In adults, hepatic encephalopathy has been an essential diagnostic feature. However, in pediatrics, this narrow definition may be problematic, as early hepatic encephalopathy can be difficult to detect in infants and children, and some children in acute liver failure may not develop encephalopathy. The accepted definition in children includes biochemical evidence of acute liver injury (usually <8 wk duration); no evidence of chronic liver disease; and hepatic-based coagulopathy defined as a prothrombin time (PT) >15 sec or international normalized ratio (INR) >1.5 not corrected by vitamin K in the presence of clinical hepatic encephalopathy, or a PT >20 sec or INR >2 regardless of the presence of clinical hepatic encephalopathy.

Liver failure in the perinatal period can be associated with prenatal liver injury and even cirrhosis. Examples include gestational alloimmune liver disease (GALD), tyrosinemia, familial hemophagocytic lymphohistiocytosis (HLH), and some cases of congenital viral (herpes simplex virus [HSV]) infection. Liver disease may be noticed at birth or after several days of apparent well-being. Fulminant Wilson disease and fulminant autoimmune hepatitis also occurs in older children who were previously asymptomatic but, by definition, have preexisting liver disease. Other forms of acute-on-chronic liver failure can occur when a patient with an underlying liver disease such as biliary atresia develops hepatic decompensation after viral or drug-induced hepatic injury. In some cases of liver failure, particularly in the idiopathic form of acute hepatic failure, the onset of encephalopathy occurs later, from 8 to 28 wk after the onset of jaundice.

ETIOLOGY
Infection
Acute hepatic failure can be a complication of **viral hepatitis** (A, B, D, and rarely E), Epstein-Barr virus, herpes simplex virus, adenovirus, enterovirus, influenza A, cytomegalovirus, parvovirus B19, human herpesvirus-6, varicella zoster infection, parechovirus, and other respiratory illnesses. An unusually high rate of fulminant hepatic failure occurs in young people who have combined infections with the hepatitis B virus (HBV) and hepatitis D. Mutations in the precore and/or promoter region of HBV DNA are associated with fulminant and severe hepatitis. HBV is also responsible for some cases of fulminant liver failure in the absence of serologic markers of HBV infection but with HBV DNA found in the liver. Hepatitis E virus is an uncommon cause of fulminant hepatic failure in the United States, but can occur in pregnant women, in whom mortality rates rise dramatically to up to 25%. Patients with chronic hepatitis C are at risk if they have superinfection with hepatitis A virus.

Autoimmune Hepatitis
Acute hepatic failure is caused by **autoimmune hepatitis** in approximately 5% of cases. Patients have a positive autoimmune marker (e.g., antinuclear antibody, anti–smooth muscle antibody, liver-kidney microsomal antibody, or soluble liver antigen) and possibly an elevated serum immunoglobulin G level. If a biopsy can be performed, liver histology often demonstrates interface hepatitis and a plasma cell infiltrate.

Metabolic Diseases
Metabolic disorders associated with hepatic failure include Wilson disease, acute fatty liver of pregnancy, galactosemia, hereditary tyrosinemia, hereditary fructose intolerance, defects in β-oxidation of fatty acids, and deficiencies of mitochondrial electron transport, in particular mitochondrial DNA depletion disorders. Patients with Wilson disease who present in acute liver failure often have high bilirubin levels, *low* alkaline phosphatase levels, low uric acid levels, aspartate aminotransferase levels that are higher than alanine aminotransferase levels, and a Coombs-negative hemolytic anemia.

Neoplasm

Acute liver failure can occur with malignancies including leukemia, lymphoma, and **familial HLH**. Acute liver failure is a common feature of HLH caused by several gene defects, infections by mostly viruses of the herpes group, and a variety of other conditions including organ transplantation and malignancies. Impaired function of natural killer cells and cytotoxic T-lymphocyte cells with uncontrolled hemophagocytosis and cytokine overproduction is characteristic for genetic and acquired forms of HLH. Patients with HLH present with a combination of fever, splenomegaly, cytopenias, high triglyceride levels, very high ferritin levels, low natural killer cell activity, high soluble CD25 levels; they may also have hemophagocytosis on bone marrow or liver biopsy (see Chapter 534).

Gestational Alloimmune Liver Disease

GALD is the most common cause of acute liver failure in the neonate. In this alloimmune process, maternal immunoglobulin (Ig) G antibodies bind to fetal liver antigens and activate the terminal complement cascade resulting in hepatocyte injury and death. Infants with GALD present with low/normal aminotransferases that are out of proportion to their degree of liver failure. They may have significant hypoglycemia, jaundice, coagulopathy, and hypoalbuminemia. Alpha fetoprotein levels are typically high as are serum ferritin levels.

Drug-Induced Liver Injury

Various hepatotoxic drugs and chemicals can also cause drug-induced liver injury and acute hepatic failure. Predictable liver injury can occur after exposure to carbon tetrachloride, *Amanita phalloides* mushrooms or after acetaminophen overdose. Acetaminophen is the most common identifiable etiology of acute hepatic failure in children and adolescents in the United States and England. In addition to the acute intentional ingestion of a massive dose, a therapeutic misadventure leading to severe liver injury can also occur in ill children given doses of acetaminophen exceeding weight-based recommendations for many days. Such patients can have reduced stores of glutathione after a prolonged illness and a period of poor nutrition. Idiosyncratic damage can follow the use of drugs such as halothane, isoniazid, ecstasy, or sodium valproate. Herbal and weight loss supplements are additional causes of hepatic failure (see Chapter 390).

Vascular

Ischemia and hypoxia resulting from hepatic vascular occlusion, severe heart failure, cyanotic congenital heart disease, or circulatory shock can produce liver failure.

Idiopathic Acute Liver Failure

Idiopathic acute liver failure accounts for 40–50% of acute hepatic failure cases in children. The disease occurs sporadically and usually without the risk factors for common causes of viral hepatitis. It is likely that the etiology of these cases is heterogeneous, including unidentified or variant viruses, excessive immune activation, and undiagnosed genetic or metabolic disorders. There is increasing recognition of some children presenting with indeterminate acute hepatitis or acute liver failure who have evidence of immune activation including markedly elevated sIL-2R levels but never fulfilling diagnostic criteria for HLH.

Recurrent, acute liver failure has been reported with onset in infancy due to mutations of the neuroblastoma amplified sequence gene *(NBAS)*. Episodes are usually precipitated by fever and characterized by bouts of vomiting and lethargy. Massively elevated aminotransferase levels and coagulopathy are present. Microvesicular steatosis is prominent on liver biopsy. Most patients recovered with restoration of normal liver function after control of fever and maintenance of energy balance with the infusion of intravenous glucose. The function of NBAS protein remains uncertain but it appears to be involved in retrograde transport between the endoplasmic reticulum and Golgi apparatus.

PATHOLOGY

Liver biopsy usually reveals patchy or confluent massive necrosis of hepatocytes. Multilobular or bridging necrosis can be associated with collapse of the reticulin framework of the liver. There may be little or no regeneration of hepatocytes. A zonal pattern of necrosis may be observed with certain insults. Centrilobular damage is associated with acetaminophen hepatotoxicity or with circulatory shock. Evidence of severe hepatocyte dysfunction rather than cell necrosis is occasionally the predominant histologic finding (microvesicular fatty infiltrate of hepatocytes is observed in Reye syndrome, β-oxidation defects, and tetracycline toxicity).

PATHOGENESIS

The mechanisms that lead to acute hepatic failure are poorly understood. It is unknown why only approximately 1–2% of patients with viral hepatitis experience liver failure. Massive destruction of hepatocytes might represent both a direct cytotoxic effect of the virus and an immune response to the viral antigens. Of patients with HBV-induced liver failure, $\frac{1}{3}$–$\frac{1}{2}$ become negative for serum hepatitis B surface antigen within a few days of presentation and often have no detectable HBV antigen or HBV DNA in serum. These findings suggest a hyperimmune response to the virus that underlies the massive liver necrosis. Formation of hepatotoxic metabolites that bind covalently to macromolecular cell constituents is involved in the liver injury produced by drugs such as acetaminophen and isoniazid; acute hepatic failure can follow depletion of intracellular substrates involved in detoxification, particularly glutathione. Whatever the initial cause of hepatocyte injury, various factors can contribute to the pathogenesis of liver failure, including impaired hepatocyte regeneration, altered parenchymal perfusion, endotoxemia, and decreased hepatic reticuloendothelial function.

CLINICAL MANIFESTATIONS

Acute hepatic failure can be the presenting feature of liver disease or it can complicate previously known liver disease (acute-on-chronic liver failure). A history of developmental delay and/or neuromuscular dysfunction can indicate an underlying mitochondrial or β-oxidation defect. A child with acute hepatic failure has usually been previously healthy and most often has no risk factors for liver disease such as exposure to toxins or blood products. Progressive jaundice, fetor hepaticus, fever, anorexia, vomiting, and abdominal pain are common. A rapid decrease in liver size without clinical improvement is an ominous sign. A hemorrhagic diathesis and ascites can develop.

Patients should be closely observed for hepatic encephalopathy, which is initially characterized by minor disturbances of consciousness or motor function. Irritability, poor feeding, and a change in sleep rhythm may be the only findings in infants; asterixis may be demonstrable in older children. Patients are often somnolent, confused, or combative on arousal and can eventually become responsive only to painful stimuli. Patients can rapidly progress to deeper stages of coma in which extensor responses and decerebrate and decorticate posturing appear. Respirations are usually increased early, but respiratory failure can occur in stage IV coma (Table 391.1). The pathogenesis of hepatic encephalopathy is likely related to increased serum levels of ammonia, false neurotransmitters, amines, increased γ-aminobutyric acid receptor activity, or increased circulating levels of endogenous benzodiazepine-like compounds. Decreased hepatic clearance of these substances can produce marked central nervous system dysfunction. The mechanisms responsible for cerebral edema and intracranial hypertension in acute liver failure (ALF) suggest both cytotoxic and vasogenic injury. There is increasing evidence for an inflammatory response (synthesis and release of inflammatory factors from activated microglia and endothelial cells) which acts in synergy with hyperammonemia to cause severe astrocyte swelling/brain edema.

LABORATORY FINDINGS

Serum direct and indirect bilirubin levels and serum aminotransferase activities may be markedly elevated. Serum aminotransferase activities do not correlate well with the severity of the illness and can decrease as a patient deteriorates. The blood ammonia concentration is usually increased, but hepatic coma can occur in patients with a normal blood ammonia level. PT and the INR are prolonged and often do not improve after parenteral administration of vitamin K. Hypoglycemia can occur,

Table 391.1	Stages of Hepatic Encephalopathy			
	STAGES			
	I	**II**	**III**	**IV**
Symptoms	Periods of lethargy, euphoria; reversal of day-night sleeping; may be alert	Drowsiness, inappropriate behavior, agitation, wide mood swings, disorientation	Stupor but arousable; confused, incoherent speech	Coma: IVa responds to noxious stimuli; IVb no response
Signs	Trouble drawing figures, performing mental tasks	Asterixis, fetor hepaticus, incontinence	Asterixis, hyperreflexia, extensor reflexes, rigidity	Areflexia, no asterixis, flaccidity
Electroencephalogram	Normal	Generalized slowing, q waves	Markedly abnormal triphasic waves	Markedly abnormal bilateral slowing, d waves, electrocortical silence

particularly in infants. Hypokalemia, hyponatremia, metabolic acidosis, or respiratory alkalosis can also develop.

TREATMENT

Specific therapies for identifiable causes of acute liver failure include *N*-acetylcysteine (acetaminophen), acyclovir (herpes simplex virus), penicillin (*Amanita* mushrooms), nucleos(t)ide analogs such as entecavir (hepatitis B virus [HBV]), and prednisone (autoimmune hepatitis). Immunosuppression with corticosteroids should also be considered in children with the indeterminate form of fulminant hepatic failure with immune activation to avoid progression to liver transplantation or death. However, controlled trials have shown a worse outcome in patients treated with corticosteroids in patients without an immune basis for liver injury. Treatment of GALD involves a combination of double-volume exchange transfusion to remove existing reactive antibody followed immediately by administration of high-dose intravenous immunoglobulin (IVIG) (1 g/kg) to block antibody induced complement activation. Management of other types of acute hepatic failure is supportive. No therapy is known to reverse hepatocyte injury or to promote hepatic regeneration.

An infant or child with acute hepatic failure should be cared for in an institution able to perform a liver transplantation if necessary and managed in an intensive care unit with continuous monitoring of vital functions. Endotracheal intubation may be required to prevent aspiration, to reduce cerebral edema by hyperventilation, and to facilitate pulmonary toilet. Mechanical ventilation and supplemental oxygen are often necessary in advanced coma. Sedatives should be avoided unless needed in the intubated patient because these agents can aggravate or precipitate encephalopathy. Opiates may be better tolerated than benzodiazepines. Prophylactic use of proton pump inhibitors should be considered because of the high risk of gastrointestinal bleeding.

Hypovolemia should be avoided and treated with cautious infusions of *isotonic* fluids and blood products. Renal dysfunction can result from dehydration, acute tubular necrosis, or functional renal failure (hepatorenal syndrome). Electrolyte and glucose solutions should be administered intravenously to maintain urine output, to correct or prevent hypoglycemia, and to maintain normal serum potassium concentrations. Hyponatremia is common and should be avoided; it is usually dilutional and not a result of sodium depletion. Parenteral supplementation with calcium, phosphorus, and magnesium may be required. Hypophosphatemia, probably a reflection of liver regeneration, and early phosphorus administration are associated with a better prognosis in acute liver failure, whereas hyperphosphatemia predicts a failure of spontaneous recovery. Coagulopathy should be treated with parenteral administration of vitamin K. Fresh-frozen plasma, cryoprecipitate, platelets, activated factor VII, or prothrombin complex concentrates can be used to treat clinically significant bleeding or can be given if an invasive procedure such as placement of a central line or an intracranial monitor needs to be performed. Plasmapheresis can permit temporary correction of the bleeding diathesis without resulting in volume overload. Continuous hemofiltration is useful for managing fluid overload, acute renal failure, and hyperammonemia.

Patients should be monitored closely for infection, including sepsis, pneumonia, peritonitis, and urinary tract infections. At least 50% of patients experience serious infection. Gram-positive organisms (*Staphylococcus aureus, Staphylococcus epidermidis*) are the most common pathogens, but Gram-negative and fungal infections are also observed.

Gastrointestinal hemorrhage, infection, constipation, sedatives, electrolyte imbalance, and hypovolemia can precipitate encephalopathy and should be identified and corrected. Protein intake should be initially restricted or eliminated, depending on the degree of encephalopathy. If encephalopathy or hyperammonemia develops, lactulose or rifaximin can be administered. *N*-acetylcysteine is not effective in improving the outcome of patients with acute liver failure not associated with acetaminophen.

Cerebral edema is an extremely serious complication of hepatic encephalopathy that responds poorly to measures such as corticosteroid administration and osmotic diuresis. Monitoring intracranial pressure can be useful in preventing severe cerebral edema, in maintaining cerebral perfusion pressure, and in establishing the suitability of a patient for liver transplantation.

Temporary liver support continues to be evaluated as a bridge for the patient with liver failure to liver transplantation or regeneration. Nonbiologic systems, essentially a form of liver dialysis with an albumin-containing dialysate, and biologic liver support devices that involve perfusion of the patient's blood through a cartridge containing liver cell lines or porcine hepatocytes can remove some toxins, improve serum biochemical abnormalities, and, in some cases, improve neurologic function, but there has been little evidence of improved survival, and few children have been treated.

Orthotopic liver transplantation can be lifesaving in patients who reach advanced stages (III, IV) of hepatic coma. Reduced-size allografts and living donor transplantation have been important advances in the treatment of infants with hepatic failure. Partial auxiliary orthotopic or heterotopic liver transplantation is successful in a small number of children, and in some cases it has allowed regeneration of the native liver and eventual withdrawal of immunosuppression. Orthotopic liver transplantation should not be done in patients with liver failure and neuromuscular dysfunction secondary to a mitochondrial disorder because progressive neurologic deterioration is likely to continue after transplantation.

PROGNOSIS

Children with acute hepatic failure fare better than adults. Improved survival can be attributed to careful intensive care and if necessary liver transplantation. In the largest prospective study from the Pediatric Acute Liver Failure Study Group, 709 children were assessed at 21 days: 50.3% of patients survived with supportive care alone, 36.2% survived after liver transplantation, and 13.4% died. A scoring system based on peak values of total serum bilirubin, PT, and plasma ammonia concentration predicted transplant-free survival. Prognosis varies considerably with the cause of liver failure and stage of hepatic encephalopathy. Survival rates with supportive care may be as high as 90% in acetaminophen overdose and with fulminant hepatitis A. By contrast, spontaneous recovery can be expected in only approximately 40% of patients with liver failure caused by the idiopathic (indeterminate) form of acute liver failure or an acute onset of Wilson disease. Prognosis is also poor for spontaneous recovery in patients with mitochondrial deficits, hemophagocytic syndromes, herpes simplex disease, and idiosyncratic drug reactions. In patients who progress to stage IV coma (see Table 391.1), the prognosis is extremely poor. Brain stem herniation is the most common cause of death. Major complications such as sepsis, severe hemorrhage, or renal failure increase the mortality. The prognosis is particularly poor in patients with liver necrosis and multiorgan failure.

Age <1 yr, stage 4 encephalopathy, an INR >4, PT >90 sec, low factor V levels, and the need for dialysis before transplantation are associated with increased mortality. Pretransplantation serum bilirubin concentration or the height of hepatic enzymes is *not* predictive of posttransplantation survival. A plasma ammonia concentration >200 μmol/L is associated with a 5-fold increased risk of death. Children with acute hepatic failure are more likely to die while on the waiting list compared to children with other liver transplant requiring diagnoses. Owing to the severity of their illness, the 6 mo post–liver transplantation survival of approximately 75% for acute liver failure is significantly lower than the 90% achieved in children with chronic liver disease. Patients who recover from fulminant hepatic failure with only supportive care do not usually develop cirrhosis or chronic liver disease. Aplastic anemia occurs in approximately 10% of children with the idiopathic form of fulminant hepatic failure and is often fatal without bone marrow transplantation. Long-term survivors demonstrate average IQ and visual spatial ability but greater than expected impairments in motor skills, attention, executive function, and health-related quality of life.

Bibliography is available at Expert Consult.

Chapter 392
Cystic Diseases of the Biliary Tract and Liver

Frederick J. Suchy and Amy G. Feldman

第三百九十二章
胆道和肝脏的囊性疾病

中文导读

　　本章主要介绍了胆道和肝脏的囊性疾病。详细介绍了胆总管囊肿、常染色体显性遗传性多囊肾病和常染色体显性遗传性多囊肝病。胆总管囊肿中详细阐述了多囊性肾病、肝内胆管囊性扩张和先天性肝纤维化。具体介绍了几种疾病的病因、病理特点、发病机制、临床表现、实验室检查、治疗和预后。具体描述了病因中家族史和基因的特点，临床表现中多以腹胀、腹痛及右上腹肿块为特点，治疗中具体描述了有明确病因的内科外科的治疗方法。

Cystic lesions of liver may be initially recognized during infancy and childhood. Hepatic fibrosis can also occur as part of an associated developmental defect (Table 392.1). Cystic *renal* disease is usually associated and often determines the clinical presentation and prognosis. Virtually all proteins encoded by genes mutated in combined cystic diseases of the liver and kidney are at least partially localized to primary cilia in renal tubular cells and cholangiocytes.

A solitary, congenital liver cyst (nonparasitic) can occur in childhood and has been identified in some cases on prenatal ultrasound. Abdominal distention and pain may be present, and a poorly defined right-upper-quadrant mass may be palpable. These benign lesions are best left undisturbed unless they compress adjacent structures or a complication occurs, such as hemorrhage into the cyst. Operative management is generally reserved for symptomatic patients and enlarging cysts.

CHOLEDOCHAL CYSTS
Choledochal cysts are congenital dilatations of the common bile duct that can cause progressive biliary obstruction and biliary cirrhosis. Cylindrical (fusiform) and spherical (saccular) cysts of the extrahepatic ducts are the most common types (see Table 392.1). Choledochal cysts

Table 392.1	Syndromes Associated With Congenital Hepatic Fibrosis
DISORDER	**ASSOCIATED FEATURES**
Autosomal recessive polycystic kidney disease	Ductal plate malformation, Caroli syndrome
Autosomal dominant polycystic kidney disease	Ductal plate malformation, Caroli syndrome
Autosomal dominant polycystic liver disease	Rarely, congestive heart failure
Jeune syndrome	Asphyxiating thoracic dystrophy, with cystic renal tubular dysplasia, Caroli syndrome
Joubert syndrome	Central nervous system defects, cardiac malformations
COACH syndrome	Cerebellar vermis hypoplasia, oligophrenia, congenital ataxia, ocular coloboma, hepatic fibrosis
Meckel-Gruber syndrome	Cystic renal dysplasia, abnormal bile duct development with fibrosis, posterior encephalocele, polydactyly
Carbohydrate-deficient glycoprotein syndrome type 1b	Phosphomannose isomerase 1 deficiency chronic diarrhea, protein-losing enteropathy
Ivemark syndrome type 2	Autosomal-recessive renal-hepatic-pancreatic dysplasia
Nephronophthisis type 3	Tapetoretinal degeneration
Bardet-Biedl syndrome	Retinal degeneration, obesity, limb deformities, hypogonadism
Oral-facial-digital syndrome type 1	Oral clefts, hamartomas or cysts of the tongue, digital anomalies pancreatic cysts
Miscellaneous syndromes	Intestinal lymphangiectasia, enterocolitis, cystic short rib (Beemer-Langer) syndrome, osteochondrodysplasia

After Suchy FJ, Sokol RJ, Balistreri WF, editors: *Liver disease in children*, ed 3, New York, 2014, Cambridge University Press, p. 713.

are classified according to the Todani method (Fig. 392.1). Type 1 choledochal cysts, the most common variant, involve a saccular or fusiform dilation of the common bile duct. Type II cysts are congenital diverticula protruding from the common bile duct. Type III cysts or choledochoceles involve a herniation of the intraduodenal segment of the common bile duct into the duodenum. Type IVa cysts or **Caroli disease** involve multiple intrahepatic and extrahepatic cysts. Type IVb cysts involve only the extrahepatic duct. Solitary liver cysts (type V) are very rare.

The pathogenesis of choledochal cysts remains uncertain. Some reports suggest that junction of the common bile duct and the pancreatic duct before their entry into the sphincter of Oddi might allow reflux of pancreatic enzymes into the common bile duct, causing inflammation, localized weakness, and dilation of the duct. It has also been proposed that a distal congenital stenotic segment of the biliary tree leads to increased intraluminal pressure and proximal biliary dilation. Other possibilities are that choledochal cysts represent malformations of the common duct or that they occur as part of the spectrum of an infectious disease that includes neonatal hepatitis and biliary atresia.

Approximately 75% of cases appear during childhood. The infant typically presents with cholestatic jaundice; severe liver dysfunction including ascites and coagulopathy can rapidly evolve if biliary obstruction is not relieved. An abdominal mass is rarely palpable. In an older child, the classic triad of abdominal pain, jaundice, and mass occurs in <33% of patients. Features of acute cholangitis (fever, right-upper-

quadrant tenderness, jaundice, and leukocytosis) may be present. The diagnosis is made by ultrasonography; choledochal cysts have been identified prenatally using this technique. Magnetic resonance cholangiography is useful in the preoperative assessment of choledochal cyst anatomy.

Choledochal cysts have the potential to develop into cholangiocarcinoma; therefore the treatment of choice is primary excision of the cyst and a Roux-en-Y choledochojejunostomy. The postoperative course can be complicated by recurrent cholangitis or stricture at the anastomotic site. Long-term follow-up is necessary to ensure that no malignancy develops.

Autosomal Recessive Polycystic Kidney Disease

Autosomal recessive polycystic kidney disease (ARPKD) manifests predominantly in childhood (see Chapter 541.2). Bilateral enlargement of the kidneys is caused by a generalized dilation of the collecting tubules. The disorder is invariably associated with congenital hepatic fibrosis and various degrees of biliary ductal ectasia, discussed in detail later.

The polycystic kidney and hepatic disease 1 (*PKHD1*) gene, mutated in ARPKD, encodes a protein that is called fibrocystin/polyductin, which is localized to cilia on the apical domain of renal collecting cells and cholangiocytes. The primary defect in ARPKD may be ciliary dysfunction related to the abnormality in this protein. Fibrocystin/polyductin appears to have a role in the regulation of cellular adhesion, repulsion, and proliferation and/or the regulation and maintenance of renal collecting tubules and bile ducts, but its exact role in normal and cystic epithelia remains unknown. Kidney and liver disease are independent and variable in severity; they are not explainable by the type of *PKHD1* mutation. Phenotypic variability among affected siblings suggests the importance of modifier genes as well as possibly environmental influences.

In ARPKD, the cysts arise as ectatic expansions of the collecting tubules and bile ducts, which remain in continuity with their structures of origin. ARPKD normally presents in early life, often shortly after birth, and is generally more severe than autosomal dominant polycystic kidney disease (ADPKD). Fetal ultrasound may visualize large echogenic kidneys, also described as bright, with low or absent amniotic fluid (oligohydramnios). However, in many instances the features of ARPKD are not visualized on sonography until the 3rd trimester or after birth.

Patients with ARPKD can die in the perinatal period owing to renal failure or lung dysgenesis. The kidneys in these patients are usually markedly enlarged and dysfunctional. Respiratory failure can result from compression of the chest by grossly enlarged kidneys, from fluid retention, or from concomitant pulmonary hypoplasia. The clinical pathologic findings within a family tend to breed true, although there has been some variability in the severity of the disease and the time for presentation within the same family. In patients surviving infancy because of a milder renal phenotype, liver disease may be a prominent part of the disorder. The liver disease in ARPKD is related to congenital malformation of the liver with varying degrees of periportal fibrosis, bile ductular hyperplasia, ectasia, and dysgenesis. Initial symptoms are liver related in approximately 26% of patients. This can manifest clinically as variable cystic dilation of the intrahepatic biliary tree with congenital hepatic fibrosis. Congenital hepatic fibrosis and Caroli disease likely result from an abnormality in remodeling of the embryonic ductal plate of the liver. **Ductal plate malformation** refers to the persistence of excess embryonic bile duct structures in the portal tracts. ARPKD patients with recurrent cholangitis or complications of portal hypertension may require combined liver-kidney transplant.

Cystic Dilation of the Intrahepatic Bile Ducts (Caroli Disease/Caroli Syndrome)

In Caroli disease there is isolated ectasia or nonobstructing segmental dilatation of the larger intrahepatic ducts. Caroli syndrome is the more common variant, in which malformations of small bile ducts are associated with congenital hepatic fibrosis. Congenital saccular dilation can affect several segments of the intrahepatic bile ducts; the dilated ducts are lined by cuboidal epithelium and are in continuity with the main duct system, which is usually normal. Choledochal cysts have also been associated with Caroli disease. Bile duct dilation leads to stagnation of

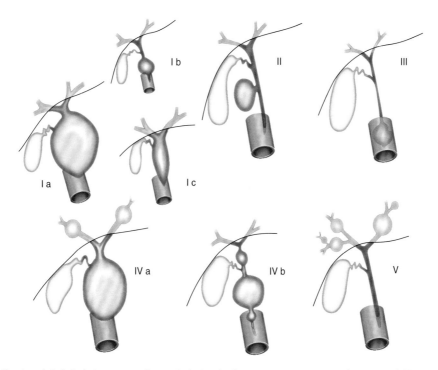

Fig. 392.1 Classification of choledochal cysts according to Todani and colleagues. Ia, common type; Ib, segmental dilation; Ic, diffuse dilation; II, diverticulum; III, choledochocele; IVa, multiple cysts (intra- and extrahepatic); IVb, multiple cysts (extrahepatic); V, single or multiple dilations of the intrahepatic ducts (Caroli disease). *(From Savader SJ, Benenati JF, Venbrux AC, et al. Choledochal cysts: Classification and cholangiographic appearance. AJR Am J Roentgenol 1991;156:327-31.)*

bile and formation of biliary sludge and intraductal lithiasis. There is a marked predisposition to ascending cholangitis, which may be exacerbated by calculus formation within the abnormal bile ducts.

Affected patients usually experience symptoms of acute cholangitis as children or young adults. Fever, abdominal pain, mild jaundice, and pruritus occur, and a slightly enlarged, tender liver is palpable. Elevated alkaline phosphatase activity, direct-reacting bilirubin levels, and leukocytosis may be observed during episodes of acute infection. In patients with Caroli disease, clinical features may be the result of a combination of recurring bouts of cholangitis, reflecting the intrahepatic ductal abnormalities and portal hypertensive bleeding resulting from hepatic fibrosis. Ultrasonography shows the dilated intrahepatic ducts, but definitive diagnosis and extent of disease must be determined by percutaneous transhepatic, endoscopic, or magnetic resonance cholangiography.

Cholangitis and sepsis should be treated with appropriate antibiotics. Calculi can require surgery. Partial hepatectomy may be curative in rare cases in which cystic disease is confined to a single lobe. The prognosis is otherwise guarded, largely owing to difficulties in controlling cholangitis and biliary lithiasis and to a significant risk for developing cholangiocarcinoma.

Congenital Hepatic Fibrosis

Congenital hepatic fibrosis is usually associated with ARPKD and is characterized pathologically by diffuse periportal and perilobular fibrosis in broad bands that contain distorted bile duct–like structures and that often compress or incorporate central or sublobular veins (see Table 392.1). Irregularly shaped islands of liver parenchyma contain normal-appearing hepatocytes. Caroli disease and choledochal cysts are associated. Most patients have renal disease, mostly autosomal recessive polycystic renal disease and rarely nephronophthisis. Congenital hepatic fibrosis also occurs as part of the COACH syndrome (cerebellar vermis hypoplasia, oligophrenia, congenital ataxia, coloboma, and hepatic fibrosis). Congenital hepatic fibrosis has been described in children

with a congenital disorder of glycosylation caused by mutations in the gene encoding phosphomannose isomerase (see Chapter 105.6).

Several different forms of congenital hepatic fibrosis have been defined clinically: portal hypertensive (most common) cholangitic, mixed, and latent. The disorder usually has its onset in childhood, with hepatosplenomegaly or with bleeding secondary to portal hypertension. In a recent study, splenomegaly, as a marker for portal hypertension, developed early in life and was present in 60% of children younger than 5 yr of age.

Cholangitis can occur in these patients, as they have abnormal biliary tracts even without Caroli disease. Hepatocellular function is usually well preserved. Serum aminotransferase activities and bilirubin levels are usually normal in the absence of cholangitis and choledocholithiasis; serum alkaline phosphatase activity may be slightly elevated. The serum albumin level and prothrombin time are normal. Liver biopsy is rarely required for diagnosis, particularly in patients with obvious renal disease.

Treatment of this disorder should focus on control of bleeding from esophageal varices and aggressive antibiotic treatment of cholangitis. Infrequent mild bleeding episodes may be managed by endoscopic sclerotherapy or band ligation of the varices. After more severe hemorrhage, portacaval anastomosis can relieve portal hypertension. The prognosis may be greatly improved by a shunting procedure, but survival in some patients may be limited by renal failure.

AUTOSOMAL DOMINANT POLYCYSTIC KIDNEY DISEASE

ADPKD (see Chapter 541.3), the most commonly inherited cystic kidney disease, affects 1 in 1,000 live births. It is characterized by progressive renal cyst development and cyst enlargement and an array of extrarenal manifestations. There is a high degree of intrafamilial and interfamilial variability in the clinical expression of the disease.

ADPKD is caused by mutation in 1 of 2 genes, *PKD1* or *PKD2*, which account for 85–90% and 10–15% of cases, respectively. The proteins encoded by these genes, polycystin-1 and polycystin-2, are expressed in renal tubule cells and in cholangiocytes. Polycystin-1 functions as a mechanosensor in cilia, detecting the movement of fluid through tubules and transmitting the signal through polycystin-2, which acts as a calcium channel.

Dilated noncommunicating cysts are most commonly observed. Other hepatic lesions are rarely associated with ADPKD, including the ductal plate malformation, congenital hepatic fibrosis, and biliary microhamartomas (the von Meyenburg complexes). Approximately 50% of patients with renal failure have demonstrable hepatic cysts that are derived from the biliary tract but not in continuity with it. The hepatic cysts increase with age. In one study the prevalence of hepatic cysts was 58% in patients 15-24 yr old. Hepatic cystogenesis appears to be influenced by estrogens. Although the frequency of cysts is similar in males and females, the development of large hepatic cysts is mainly a complication in females. Hepatic cysts are often asymptomatic but can cause pain and are occasionally complicated by hemorrhage, infection, jaundice from bile duct compression, portal hypertension with variceal bleeding, or hepatic venous outflow obstruction from mechanical compression of hepatic veins, resulting in tender hepatomegaly and exudative ascites. Cholangiocarcinoma can occur. Subarachnoid hemorrhage can result from the associated cerebral arterial aneurysms.

Selected patients with severe symptomatic polycystic liver disease and favorable anatomy benefit from liver resection or fenestration. Combined liver-kidney transplantation may be required. There is considerable evidence for a role of cyclic adenosine monophosphate in epithelial proliferation and fluid secretion in experimental renal and hepatic cystic disease. Several clinical trials in adults have shown that somatostatin analogs can blunt hepatic cyst expansion by blocking secretin-induced cyclic adenosine monophosphate generation and fluid secretion by cholangiocytes.

AUTOSOMAL DOMINANT POLYCYSTIC LIVER DISEASE

Autosomal dominant polycystic liver disease is a distinct clinical and genetic identity in which multiple cysts develop and are unassociated with cystic kidney disease. Liver cysts arise from but are not in continuity with the biliary tract. Girls are more commonly affected than boys, and the cysts often enlarge during pregnancy. Cysts are rarely identified in children. Cyst complications are related to effects of local compression, infection, hemorrhage, or rupture. The genes associated with autosomal dominant polycystic liver disease are *PRKCSH* and *SEC63*, which encode hepatocystin and Sec63, respectively. Hepatocystin is a protein kinase C substrate adK-H, which is involved in the proper folding and maturation of glycoproteins. It has been localized to the endoplasmic reticulum. *SEC63* encodes the protein SEC63P, which is a component of the protein translocation machinery in the endoplasmic reticulum.

Bibliography is available at Expert Consult.

Chapter 393
Diseases of the Gallbladder
Frederick J. Suchy and Amy G. Feldman

第三百九十三章
胆囊疾病

中文导读

　　本章主要介绍了胆囊疾病的种类、诊断和治疗，包括先天异常、急性水肿、胆囊炎和胆石症以及胆道运动障碍。具体介绍了先天异常的类型，包括胆囊缺如、发育不全、重复、异位和多分隔胆囊；具体描述了胆囊水肿的病因、临床表现和体征、实验室检查和评估、内外科治疗方法；详细阐述了胆囊炎和胆石症的病因、治疗方法；详细描述了胆道运动障碍的病因、临床特征和治疗方法。

The incidence of gallbladder disease, particularly cholelithiasis and biliary dyskinesia, has been increasing in children, and has been associated with a rise in the number of cholecystectomies.

ANOMALIES
The gallbladder is congenitally absent in approximately 0.1% of the population. Hypoplasia or absence of the gallbladder can be associated with extrahepatic biliary atresia or cystic fibrosis. Duplication of the gallbladder occurs rarely. Gallbladder ectopia may occur with a transverse, intrahepatic, left-sided, or retroplaced location. Multiseptate gallbladder, characterized by the presence of multiple septa dividing the gallbladder lumen, is another rare congenital anomaly of the gallbladder.

ACUTE HYDROPS
Table 393.1 lists the conditions associated with hydrops of the gallbladder.

Acute noncalculous, noninflammatory distention of the gallbladder can occur in infants and children. It is defined by the absence of calculi, bacterial infection, or congenital anomalies of the biliary system. The disorder may complicate acute infections and Kawasaki disease, but the cause is often not identified. Hydrops of the gallbladder may also develop in patients receiving long-term parenteral nutrition, presumably because of gallbladder stasis during the period of enteral fasting. Hydrops is distinguished from acalculous cholecystitis by the absence of a significant inflammatory process and is a generally benign prognosis.

Affected patients usually have right upper quadrant pain with a palpable mass. Fever, vomiting, and jaundice may be present and are usually associated with a systemic illness such as streptococcal infection. Ultrasonography shows a markedly distended echo-free gallbladder, without dilation of the biliary tree. Acute hydrops is usually treated conservatively with a focus on supportive care and managing the intercurrent illness; cholecystostomy and drainage are rarely needed. Spontaneous resolution and return of normal gallbladder function usually occur over a period of several weeks. If a laparotomy is required, a large edematous gallbladder is found to contain white, yellow, or green bile. Obstruction of the cystic duct by mesenteric adenopathy is occasionally observed. Cholecystectomy is required if the gallbladder is gangrenous. Pathologic examination of the gallbladder wall shows edema and mild inflammation. Cultures of bile are usually sterile.

CHOLECYSTITIS AND CHOLELITHIASIS
Acute acalculous cholecystitis is uncommon in children and is usually caused by infection. Pathogens include streptococci (groups A and B), Gram-negative organisms—particularly *Salmonella* and *Leptospira interrogans*—and a number of viral infections (hepatitis A, Epstein-Barr [EB] virus, and cytomegalovirus). Parasitic infestation with *Ascaris* or *Giardia lamblia* may be found. Acalculous cholecystitis may be associated with abdominal trauma or burn injury or with a severe systemic illness such as leukemia, end-stage liver disease, and systemic vasculitis.

Clinical features include right upper quadrant or epigastric pain, nausea, vomiting, fever, and jaundice. Right upper quadrant guarding and tenderness are present. Ultrasonography discloses an enlarged, thick-walled gallbladder without calculi. Serum alkaline phosphatase activity and direct-reacting bilirubin levels are elevated. Leukocytosis is usual.

Patients may recover with treatment of systemic and biliary infection. Because the gallbladder can become gangrenous, daily ultrasonography is useful in monitoring gallbladder distention and wall thickness. Cholecystectomy is required in patients who fail to improve with conservative management. Cholecystostomy drainage is an alternative approach in a critically ill patient.

Cholelithiasis is relatively rare in otherwise healthy children, occurring more commonly in patients with various predisposing disorders (Table 393.2). Gallstones are rarely detected by ultrasonography in the fetus, but generally remain asymptomatic and resolve spontaneously during the 1st yr of life. In an ultrasonographic survey of 1570 children (ages 6-19 yr) the overall prevalence of gallstone disease was 0.13% (0.27% in female subjects). Older reports consistently found that >70% of gallstones were the pigment type, 15–20% were cholesterol stones, and the remainder were composed of a mixture of cholesterol, organic matrix, and calcium bilirubinate. Black pigment gallstones, composed mostly of calcium bilirubinate and glycoprotein matrix, are a frequent complication of chronic hemolytic anemias. However, because of obesity, cholesterol gallstones predominate in children, while the number of patients with hemolytic anemia-associated gallstones have remained stable.

Brown pigment stones form mostly in infants as a result of biliary tract infection. Unconjugated bilirubin is the predominant component, formed by the high β-glucuronidase activity of infected bile. Cholesterol gallstones are composed purely of cholesterol or contain >50% cholesterol along with a mucin glycoprotein matrix and calcium bilirubinate. Calcium carbonate stones have also been described in children.

Patients with hemolytic disease (including sickle cell anemia, the thalassemias, and red blood cell enzymopathies) and Wilson disease are at increased risk for black pigment cholelithiasis. In sickle cell disease, pigment gallstones can develop before age 4 yr and have been reported in 17–33% of patients 2-18 yr of age. Genetic variation in the promoter of uridine diphosphate-glucuronosyltransferase 1A1 (the [TA]7/[TA]7 and [TA]7/[TA]8 genotypes) underlies **Gilbert syndrome**, a relatively common, chronic form of unconjugated hyperbilirubinemia, and is a risk factor for pigment gallstone formation in sickle cell disease.

Cirrhosis and chronic cholestasis also increase the risk for pigment gallstones. Sick premature infants may also have gallstones; their treatment is often complicated by such factors as bowel resection, necrotizing enterocolitis, prolonged parenteral nutrition without enteral feeding,

Table 393.1	Conditions Associated With Hydrops of the Gallbladder

Cholelithiasis
Cholecystitis
Kawasaki disease
Streptococcal pharyngitis
Staphylococcal infection
Leptospirosis
Ascariasis
Threadworm
Sickle cell crisis
Typhoid fever
Thalassemia
Total parenteral nutrition
Prolonged fasting
Viral hepatitis
Sepsis
Henoch-Schönlein purpura
Mesenteric adenitis
Necrotizing enterocolitis

Table 393.2	Conditions Associated With Cholelithiasis

Chronic hemolytic disease (sickle cell anemia, spherocytosis, thalassemia, Gilbert disease)
Ileal resection or disease
Cystic fibrosis
Cirrhosis
Cholestasis
Crohn disease
Obesity
Insulin resistance
Prolonged parenteral nutrition
Prematurity with complicated medical or surgical course
Prolonged fasting or rapid weight reduction
Treatment of childhood cancer
Abdominal surgery
Pregnancy
Sepsis
Genetic (*ABCB4, ABCG5/G8*) progressive familial intrahepatic cholestasis
Cephalosporins

cholestasis, frequent blood transfusions, and use of diuretics. Cholelithiasis in premature infants is often asymptomatic and may resolve spontaneously. Brown pigment stones are found in infants with obstructive jaundice and infected intra- and extrahepatic bile ducts. These stones are usually radiolucent, owing to a lower content of calcium phosphate and carbonate and a higher amount of cholesterol than in black pigment stones. MDR3 deficiency caused by *ABCB4* mutations is a cholestatic syndrome related to impaired biliary phospholipid excretion. It is associated with symptomatic and recurring cholelithiasis. Patients may show intrahepatic lithiasis, sludge, or microlithiasis along the biliary tree.

Obesity has assumed an increasingly important role as a risk factor for cholesterol cholelithiasis in children, particularly in adolescent girls. Cholesterol gallstones are also found in children with disturbances of the enterohepatic circulation of bile acids, including patients with ileal disease and bile acid malabsorption, such as those with ileal resection, ileal Crohn disease, and cystic fibrosis. Pigment stones can also occur in these patients.

Cholesterol gallstone formation results from an excess of cholesterol in relation to the cholesterol-carrying capacity of micelles in bile. Supersaturation of bile with cholesterol, leading to crystal and stone formation, could result from decreased bile acid or from an increased cholesterol concentration in bile. Other initiating factors that may be important in stone formation include gallbladder stasis or the presence in bile of abnormal mucoproteins or bile pigments that may serve as a nidus for cholesterol crystallization.

Prolonged use of high-dose ceftriaxone, a 3rd-generation cephalosporin, has been associated with the formation of calcium-ceftriaxone salt precipitates *(biliary pseudolithiasis)* in the gallbladder. Biliary sludge or cholelithiasis can be detected in >40% of children who are treated with ceftriaxone for at least 10 days. In rare cases, children become jaundiced and develop abdominal pain; precipitates usually resolve spontaneously within several months after discontinuation of the drug.

Acute or chronic cholecystitis is often associated with gallstones. The acute form may be precipitated by impaction of a stone in the cystic duct. Proliferation of bacteria within the obstructed gallbladder lumen can contribute to the process and lead to biliary sepsis. Chronic calculous cholecystitis is more common. It can develop insidiously or follow several attacks of acute cholecystitis. The gallbladder epithelium commonly becomes ulcerated and scarred.

More than 50% of patients with gallstones have symptoms, and 18% present with a complication as the first indication of cholelithiasis, such as pancreatitis, choledocholithiasis or acute calculous cholecystitis. The most important clinical feature of cholelithiasis is recurrent abdominal pain, which is often colicky and localized to the right upper quadrant. An older child may have intolerance for fatty foods. Acute cholecystitis is characterized by fever, pain in the right upper quadrant, and often a palpable mass. Jaundice occurs more commonly in children than adults. Pain may radiate to an area just below the right scapula. A plain x-ray of the abdomen may reveal opaque calculi, but radiolucent (cholesterol) stones are not visualized. Accordingly, ultrasonography is the method of choice for gallstone detection. Hepatobiliary scintigraphy is a valuable adjunct in that failure to visualize the gallbladder provides evidence of cholecystitis.

Laboratory evaluation may reveal elevated aminotransferase levels, leukocytosis, and mild hyperbilirubinemia. Marked elevations of the direct bilirubin, alkaline phosphatase, or GGT levels should prompt evaluation for choledocholithiasis.

Patients with cholecystitis and persistent fever or concern for obstruction should be hospitalized and started on antibiotics. Cholecystectomy is curative. Laparoscopic cholecystectomy is routinely performed in symptomatic infants and children with cholelithiasis. Common bile duct stones are unusual in children, occurring in 2–6% of cases with cholelithiasis, often in association with obstructive jaundice and pancreatitis. Operative cholangiography should be done at the time of surgery, however, to detect unsuspected common duct calculi. Endoscopic retrograde cholangiography with extraction of common duct stones is an option before laparoscopic cholecystectomy in older children and adolescents.

Asymptomatic patients with cholelithiasis pose a more difficult management problem. Studies in adults indicate a lag time of more than a decade between initial formation of a gallstone and development of symptoms. Spontaneous resolution of cholelithiasis has been reported in infants and children. However, if surgery is deferred for any patient, parents should be counseled about signs and symptoms consistent with cholecystitis or obstruction of the common bile duct by a gallstone. In patients with chronic hemolysis or ileal disease, cholecystectomy can be carried out at the same time as another surgical procedure. Because laparoscopic surgery can safely be performed in children with sickle cell disease, elective cholecystectomy is being done more frequently at the time of gallstone diagnosis, before symptoms or complications develop. In cases associated with liver disease, severe obesity, or cystic fibrosis, the surgical risk of cholecystectomy may be substantial so that the risks and benefits of the operation need to be carefully considered.

BILIARY DYSKINESIA

Biliary dyskinesia is a motility disorder of the biliary tract that may cause biliary colic in children, often in association with nausea and fatty food intolerance, but symptoms may overlap with functional abdominal pain. There are no gallstones on imaging. Sphincter of Oddi dysfunction may be a variant that can present with chronic abdominal pain and recurrent pancreatitis. The diagnosis is based on a cholecystokinin–diisopropyl iminodiacetic acid scan or an ultrasound done with a fatty meal demonstrating a gallbladder ejection fraction of <35%. Reproduction of pain on cholecystokinin administration may also be seen, as well as the absence of gallbladder filling on an otherwise normal ultrasound examination. Although laparoscopic cholecystectomy is performed for many patients with this disorder, short-term and long-term symptomatic improvement is highly variable.

Bibliography is available at Expert Consult.

Chapter **394**
Portal Hypertension and Varices

Amy G. Feldman and Frederick J. Suchy

第三百九十四章
门静脉高压和静脉曲张

中文导读

　　本章主要介绍了门静脉高压及静脉曲张的病因学、病理生理学、临床表现、诊断、治疗和预后。详细介绍了门静脉高压出现时的临床表现，包括静脉曲张、脾大、腹水和消化道出血。具体介绍了用于诊断的内镜检查、腹部超声、CT等影像学检查；详细介绍了门静脉高压的两种治疗，即对潜在的威胁生命的大出血的急诊治疗和对早期或继发性出血的预防治疗。

Portal hypertension, defined as an elevation of portal pressure >10-12 mm Hg or a hepatic venous pressure gradient >4 mm Hg, is a major cause of morbidity and mortality in children with liver disease. Portal hypertension occurs when there is increased portal resistance or increased blood flow through the portal system. When portal hypertension occurs, children can develop varices, splenomegaly, ascites, and gastrointestinal bleeding.

ETIOLOGY

Portal hypertension can result from obstruction to portal blood flow anywhere along the course of the portal venous system (prehepatic, intrahepatic, or posthepatic). Table 394.1 outlines the various disorders associated with portal hypertension.

Portal vein thrombosis is the most common cause of extrahepatic portal hypertension. The obstruction can occur at any level of the portal vein. In neonates, portal vein thrombosis can occur from umbilical infection (omphalitis) with or without a history of catheterization of the umbilical vein, dehydration, and/or sepsis. Rare developmental anomalies producing extrahepatic portal hypertension include agenesis, atresia, stenosis, or a web of the portal vein. In older children, portal vein thrombosis can occur with intraabdominal infection (appendicitis, peritonitis, pancreatitis), inflammatory bowel disease, primary sclerosing cholangitis, or biliary infection. Portal vein thrombosis is also associated with hypercoagulable states, such as deficiencies of factor V Leiden, protein C, or protein S. The portal vein can be replaced by a fibrous remnant or contain an organized thrombus. At least half of reported cases have no defined cause. Uncommonly, presinusoidal hypertension can be caused by increased flow through the portal system as a result of a congenital or acquired arteriovenous fistula.

The intrahepatic causes of portal hypertension are numerous. The most common cause of portal hypertension in children is **cirrhosis**.

Table 394.1	Causes of Portal Hypertension

EXTRAHEPATIC PORTAL HYPERTENSION
Portal vein agenesis, atresia, stenosis
Portal vein thrombosis or cavernous transformation
Splenic vein thrombosis
Increased portal flow
Arteriovenous fistula

INTRAHEPATIC PORTAL HYPERTENSION
Hepatocellular disease
Acute and chronic viral hepatitis
Cirrhosis
Congenital hepatic fibrosis
Wilson disease
α_1-Antitrypsin deficiency
Glycogen storage disease type IV
Hepatotoxicity
Methotrexate
Parenteral nutrition
Biliary tract disease
Extrahepatic biliary atresia
Cystic fibrosis
Choledochal cyst
Sclerosing cholangitis
Intrahepatic bile duct paucity
Idiopathic portal hypertension
Postsinusoidal obstruction
Budd-Chiari syndrome
Venoocclusive disease

The numerous causes of cirrhosis include recognized disorders such as biliary atresia, autoimmune hepatitis, chronic viral hepatitis, and metabolic liver disease such as α_1-antitrypsin deficiency, Wilson disease, glycogen storage disease type IV, hereditary fructose intolerance, and cystic fibrosis.

Portal infiltration with malignant cells or granulomas can also contribute. An idiopathic form of portal hypertension characterized by splenomegaly, hypersplenism, and portal hypertension without occlusion of portal or splenic veins and with no obvious disease in the liver has been described. In some patients, noncirrhotic portal fibrosis has been observed.

Postsinusoidal causes of portal hypertension are also observed in childhood. **Budd-Chiari syndrome** occurs with obstruction to hepatic veins anywhere between the efferent hepatic veins and the entry of the inferior vena cava into the right atrium. In most cases, no specific cause can be found, but thrombosis can occur from inherited and acquired hypercoagulable states (antithrombin III deficiency, protein C or S deficiency, factor V Leiden or prothrombin mutations, paroxysmal nocturnal hemoglobinemia, pregnancy, oral contraceptives) and can complicate hepatic or metastatic neoplasms, collagen vascular disease, infection, and trauma. Additional causes of the Budd-Chiari syndrome include Behçet syndrome, inflammatory bowel disease, aspergillosis, dacarbazine therapy, autoinflammatory-recurrent fever syndromes, and inferior vena cava webs.

Sinusoidal obstruction syndrome (venoocclusive disease) is the most common cause of hepatic vein obstruction in children. In this disorder, occlusion of the centrilobular venules or sublobular hepatic veins occurs. The disorder most frequently occurs in bone marrow transplant recipients after total body irradiation with or without cytotoxic drug therapy, but can also be seen in patients on azathioprine, mercaptopurine, thioguanine, and those taking herbal remedies that contain pyrrolizidine alkaloids.

PATHOPHYSIOLOGY

The primary hemodynamic abnormality in portal hypertension is increased resistance to portal blood flow. This is the case whether the resistance to portal flow has an intrahepatic cause such as cirrhosis or is due to portal vein obstruction. Portosystemic shunting should decompress the portal system and thus significantly lower portal pressures. However, despite the development of significant collaterals deviating portal blood into systemic veins, portal hypertension is maintained by an overall increase in portal venous flow and thus maintenance of portal hypertension. A hyperdynamic circulation is achieved by tachycardia, an increase in cardiac output, decreased systemic vascular resistance, and increased splanchnic dilation. Overall, the increase in portal flow likely contributes to an increase in variceal transmural pressure. The increase in portal blood flow is related to the contribution of hepatic and collateral flow; the actual portal blood flow reaching the liver is reduced. It is also likely that hepatocellular dysfunction and portosystemic shunting lead to the generation of various humoral factors that cause vasodilation and an increase in plasma volume.

Many complications of portal hypertension can be accounted for by the development of a remarkable collateral circulation. Collateral vessels can form prominently in areas in which absorptive epithelium joins stratified epithelium, particularly in the esophagus or anorectal region. The superficial submucosal collaterals, especially those in the esophagus and stomach, and to a lesser extent, those in the duodenum, colon, or rectum, are prone to rupture and bleeding under increased pressure. In portal hypertension, the vascularity of the stomach is also abnormal and demonstrates prominent submucosal arteriovenous communications between the muscularis mucosa and dilated precapillaries and veins. The resulting lesion, a vascular ectasia, has been called *congestive gastropathy* and contributes to a significant risk of bleeding from the stomach.

CLINICAL MANIFESTATIONS

Bleeding is the most common presentation of portal hypertension in children. In large series of children with portal hypertension, two thirds presented with hematemesis or melena, most commonly from rupture of an esophageal varix. Less commonly, patients bleed from portal gastropathy, gastric antral ectasia, or stomal, intestinal, or anorectal varices. The risk of a first bleed in children with cirrhosis is 22%, but rises to 38% in children with known varices over a 5-yr period. In children with biliary atresia, 15–25% have bleeding on long-term follow-up. The age of first bleed is dependent on the underlying etiology of portal hypertension. Hemorrhage, particularly in children with portal vein obstruction, can be precipitated by minor febrile, intercurrent illness. The mechanism is often unclear; aspirin or other nonsteroidal antiinflammatory drugs may be a contributing factor by damaging the integrity of a congested gastric mucosa or interfering with platelet function. Coughing during a respiratory illness can also increase intravariceal pressure.

Splenomegaly is the second most common finding in children with portal hypertension and may be initially recognized on routine physical examination. As more than half of patients in many series with portal vein obstruction do not experience bleeding until after 6 yr of age, underlying liver disease should be considered in any child with splenomegaly, especially if there is concurrent cytopenias. Most children with splenomegaly are asymptomatic.

Ascites is the presenting sign of portal hypertension in 7–21% of children. Ascites can develop at any time with cirrhosis or if there is new onset portal vein obstruction. Children with portal hypertension can also suffer from growth impairment, minimal hepatic encephalopathy, and impaired quality of life. Some develop **portal hypertensive biliopathy**, where portal vein obstruction occurs as a result of external compression of the bile ducts by cavernous transformation of the portal vein.

Children with portal hypertension may also develop pulmonary complications, including **hepatopulmonary syndrome** (HPS) and **portopulmonary hypertension** (PP-HTN). HPS is defined as an arterial oxygenation defect induced by intrapulmonary microvascular dilation, resulting from release of a number of endogenous vasoactive molecules, including endothelin-1 and nitric oxide into the venous circulation. HPS develops in ≥10% of patients with portal hypertension. Patients with HPS may present with dyspnea, cyanosis, clubbing, and spider nevi. PP-HTN is defined by a pulmonary arterial pressure greater than 25 mm Hg at rest or a left-ventricular end-diastolic pressure of less than 15 mm Hg. Patients with PP-HTN most commonly present with exertional dyspnea. Histologically, these patients have pulmonary arteriopathy with laminar intimal fibrosis.

DIAGNOSIS

In patients with established chronic liver disease or in those in whom portal vein obstruction is suspected, an experienced ultrasonographer should be able to demonstrate the patency of the portal vein, and Doppler flow ultrasonography can demonstrate the direction of flow within the portal system. The pattern of flow correlates with the severity of cirrhosis and encephalopathy. Reversal of portal vein blood flow (hepatofugal flow) is more likely to be associated with variceal bleeding. Ultrasonography is also effective in detecting the presence of esophageal varices. Another important feature of extrahepatic portal vein obstruction is cavernous transformation of the portal vein, in which an extensive complex of small collateral vessels forms in the paracholedochal and epicholedochal venous system to bypass the obstruction. Other imaging techniques also contribute to further definition of the portal vein anatomy but are required less often; contrast-enhanced CT and magnetic resonance angiography provide information similar to ultrasonography. Selective arteriography of the celiac axis, superior mesenteric artery, and splenic vein may be useful in precise mapping of the extrahepatic vascular anatomy. This is not required to establish a diagnosis but can prove valuable in planning surgical decompression of portal hypertension. The platelet count, spleen length measured by ultrasonography, and serum albumin are the best noninvasive predictors of portal hypertension in children.

In a patient with hypoxia (HPS), intrapulmonary microvascular dilation is demonstrated with contrast-enhanced bubble echocardiography that shows delayed appearance in the left heart of microbubbles from a saline bolus injected into a peripheral vein.

Endoscopy is the most reliable method for detecting esophageal varices and for identifying the source of gastrointestinal bleeding. Although bleeding from esophageal or gastric varices is most common in children with portal hypertension, up to one third of patients, particularly those with cirrhosis, have bleeding from some other source, such as portal hypertensive gastropathy or gastric or duodenal ulcerations. There is a strong correlation between variceal size as assessed endoscopically and the probability of hemorrhage. Red spots apparent over varices at the time of endoscopy are a strong predictor of imminent hemorrhage.

TREATMENT

The therapy of portal hypertension can be divided into emergency treatment of potentially life-threatening hemorrhage and prophylaxis directed at prevention of initial or subsequent bleeding. It must be emphasized that the use of many therapies is based on experience in adults with portal hypertension; there are few randomized trials of therapies for portal hypertension in the pediatric population.

Treatment of patients with acute variceal hemorrhage must focus on stabilization of the patient. Fluid resuscitation should be administered, initially in the form of crystalloid infusion, followed by the replacement of red blood cells. Care should be taken to avoid overtransfusing children with portal hypertension-induced bleeding, as this can result in overfilling the intravascular space and increasing portal pressure. A reasonable goal hemoglobin level after variceal bleed is between 7 and 9 g/dL. Correction of coagulopathy by administration of vitamin K and/or infusion of platelets or fresh-frozen plasma may be required. A nasogastric tube should be placed to document the presence of blood within the stomach and to monitor for ongoing bleeding. An H_2-receptor blocker or proton pump inhibitor should be given intravenously to reduce the risk of bleeding from gastric erosions. Intravenous antibiotics should be considered, as there is high risk of infectious complications during variceal bleeding.

Pharmacologic therapy to decrease portal pressure should be initiated in patients with continued bleeding. Vasopressin or one of its analogs is commonly used and is thought to act by increasing splanchnic vascular tone and thus decreasing portal blood flow. Vasopressin is administered initially with a bolus of 0.33 units/kg over 20 min, followed by a continued infusion of the same dose on an hourly basis or a continuous infusion of 0.2 units/1.73 m²/min. The drug has a half-life of approximately 30 min. Its use may be limited by the side effects of vasoconstriction, which can impair cardiac function and perfusion to the heart, bowel, and kidneys and can also, as a result, exacerbate fluid retention. More commonly, the somatostatin analog, octreotide, is used, as it decreases splanchnic blood flow with few side effects. Octreotide is initially administered with a bolus of 1 µg/kg followed by a continuous intravenous infusion of 1.0-5.0 µg/kg/hr. A total of 15% of children with a portal hypertensive bleed will have persistent hemorrhage despite initiation of some form of splanchnic vasoconstriction.

After an episode of variceal hemorrhage or in patients in whom bleeding cannot be controlled with pharmacologic therapy, endoscopy with variceal band ligation or variceal sclerotherapy should be performed. Endoscopic band ligation is preferred, as it has been shown in adults to be more effective and has fewer side effects. For smaller children in whom the banding device cannot be used, sclerosants can be injected either intra- or paravariceal until bleeding has stopped. Sclerotherapy treatments may be associated with bleeding, bacteremia, esophageal ulceration, and stricture formation. After band ligation or sclerosis, repeat endoscopy should be performed until varices are obliterated.

In patients who continue to bleed despite pharmacologic and endoscopic methods to control hemorrhage, a Sengstaken-Blakemore tube may be emergently placed to stop hemorrhage by mechanically compressing esophageal and gastric varices. The device is rarely used now, but it may be the only option to control life-threatening hemorrhage until a more definite procedure can be performed. It carries a significant rate of complications and a high rate of bleeding when the device is removed, and it poses a particularly high risk for pulmonary aspiration. The tube is not well tolerated in children without significant sedation and intubation.

Various surgical procedures have been devised to divert portal blood flow and to decrease portal pressure. A portacaval shunt diverts nearly all of the portal blood flow into the subhepatic inferior right vena cava. Although portal pressure is significantly reduced, because of the significant diversion of blood from the liver, patients with parenchymal liver disease have a marked risk for hepatic encephalopathy. Even mild hepatic encephalopathy can impair cognitive function, including school performance. More selective shunting procedures, such as mesocaval or distal splenorenal shunt, can effectively decompress the portal system while allowing a greater amount of portal blood flow to the liver. The small size of the vessels makes these operations technically challenging in infants and small children, and there is a significant risk of failure as a result of shunt thrombosis. A shunt may be good option for a child with relatively well-preserved liver function, as sometimes occurs in patients with biliary atresia, congenital hepatic fibrosis, or cystic fibrosis. For children with an extrahepatic portal vein thrombosis, a Meso-Rex shunt (superior mesenteric vein to left portal vein bypass) may successfully restore physiologic portal blood flow and inflow of hepatotrophic factors. In one large single-center experience, 84% of children with idiopathic extrahepatic portal vein thrombosis were successfully treated with a Meso-Rex shunt. Growth and cognitive function improve after this procedure.

A transjugular intrahepatic portosystemic shunt, in which a stent is placed by an interventional radiologist between the right hepatic vein and the right or left branch of the portal vein, can aid in the management of portal hypertension in children, especially in those needing temporary relief before liver transplantation. The transjugular intrahepatic portosystemic shunt procedure can precipitate hepatic encephalopathy and is prone to thrombosis.

Orthotopic liver transplantation represents a much better therapy for portal hypertension resulting from intrahepatic disease and cirrhosis. A prior portosystemic shunting operation does not preclude a successful liver transplantation but makes the operation technically more difficult.

Long-term treatment with nonspecific β-blockers, such as propranolol, has been used extensively in adults with portal hypertension. These agents might act by lowering cardiac output and inducing splanchnic vasoconstriction. Evidence in adult patients shows that β-blockers can reduce the incidence of variceal hemorrhage and improve long-term survival. A therapeutic effect is thought to result when the pulse rate is reduced by ≥25%. There is limited published experience with the use of this therapy in children.

PROGNOSIS

Portal hypertension secondary to intrahepatic disease has a poor prognosis. Portal hypertension is usually progressive in these patients and is often associated with deteriorating liver function. Efforts should be directed toward prompt treatment of acute bleeding and prevention of recurrent hemorrhage with available methods. Patients with progressive liver disease and significant esophageal varices ultimately require orthotopic liver transplantation. Liver transplantation is the only effective therapy for HPS and should also be considered for patients with portal hypertension secondary to hepatic vein obstruction or resulting from severe venoocclusive disease.

Bibliography is available at Expert Consult.

Chapter 395
Liver Transplantation
Jorge D. Reyes and Evelyn Hsu
第三百九十五章
肝移植

中文导读

本章主要介绍了肝移植的适应证、技术新进展、肝移植后的免疫抑制及肝移植的并发症和预后。详细介绍了肝移植在胆道闭锁、先天性代谢性肝病、急性坏死性肝病、原发性恶性肝肿瘤、慢性肝病中的应用。技术新进展部分详细介绍了部分肝脏移植及自身肝脏的切除方法；具体描述了肝脏移植后如何抑制免疫反应；详细阐述了肝脏移植后并发症产生的原因、常见的并发症及处理方法。

Survival rates for pediatric liver transplantation are now >90% in the United States, in large part to refinements made in the critical care management of children with liver failure and advances in perioperative care and immunosuppression management. Protocols for immune suppression withdrawal enhancing tolerance have introduced the possibility of transplantation without the need for long-term immunosuppression. In the United States, a national allocation system matches donor organs with wait-list candidates (the Organ Procurement and Transplantation Network and the United Network for Organ Sharing [UNOS]); this organization has been given the responsibility of allocating scarce organs to the neediest patients and has undergone continuous revisions with this goal in mind—the most significant in 2002, with the adoption of the Pediatric End-Stage Liver Disease and Medical End-Stage Liver Disease (for adolescents) illness severity scoring system.

INDICATIONS

The diseases for which liver transplantation is indicated can be categorized into the following groups:
- *Obstructive biliary tract disease:* biliary atresia, sclerosing cholangitis, traumatic or postsurgical injury
- *Metabolic disorders with liver parenchymal disease:* α_1-antitrypsin deficiency, tyrosinemia type I, glycogen storage disease type IV, Wilson disease, gestational alloimmune liver disease (GALD, previously known as neonatal hemochromatosis), cystic fibrosis
- *Metabolic disorders without liver parenchymal disease:* Crigler-Najjar type I, familial hypercholesterolemia, primary oxalosis (with kidney), organic acidemia, urea cycle defects
- *Acute hepatitis:* fulminant hepatic failure, viral, toxin, or drug-induced
- *Chronic hepatitis with cirrhosis:* hepatitis B or C, autoimmune
- *Intrahepatic cholestasis:* idiopathic neonatal hepatitis, Alagille syndrome, progressive familial intrahepatic cholestasis, bile acid synthetic disorders
- *Primary liver tumors:* benign tumors (hamartomas, hemangioendothelioma), unresectable hepatoblastoma, and hepatocellular carcinoma
- *Miscellaneous:* cryptogenic cirrhosis, congenital hepatic fibrosis, Caroli disease, polycystic kidney and liver disease, cirrhosis induced by total parenteral nutrition
- *Emerging indications:* graft-versus-host disease (a complication of bone marrow transplantation), hemophilia, and portosystemic shunts

Biliary atresia is the most common indication for liver transplantation in children, accounting for more than half of all pediatric liver transplants performed in the United States, followed by metabolic liver disease and inborn errors of metabolism, autoimmune and familial cholestatic disorders, and acute hepatic necrosis. Biliary atresia may present with 2 clinical patterns: an acquired form for which there may be nonrandom clustering of potential etiologies (80% of cases), and a syndromic/embryonic form that includes other anomalies, such as polysplenia preduodenal portal vein, intestinal malrotation, situs anomalies, and absence of the retrohepatic vena cava. Hepatoportoenterostomy benefits survival if performed within the first 60 days of life; however, some patients with successful drainage later develop cirrhosis with portal hypertension (variceal bleeding and ascites). Children with biliary atresia (or any other obstructive biliary disorder) who do not achieve successful drainage will experience continued decline and end-stage liver disease, usually requiring liver transplantation within the 1st yr of life.

Inborn errors of metabolism result from a single enzyme deficiency that results in alteration of synthesis, breakdown, transport, or function of carbohydrate, fat, or protein. These disorders can be grouped into those diseases that cause liver parenchymal disease and eventual cirrhosis with end-stage liver disease, as well as liver cancer (i.e., α_1-antitrypsin deficiency, Wilson disease, cystic fibrosis, progressive familial intrahepatic cholestasis), and those inborn errors that manifest principally by their hepatic enzyme deficiency with no hepatocellular injury; complications occur in "satellite" systems such as the brain (hyperammonemic conditions), the kidney (hyperoxaluria type 1), or heart (familial hypercholesterolemia). Some metabolic disorders place patients at risk for decompensation throughout their entire lives, and others manifest principally after adolescence. Liver transplantation is a form of enzyme replacement; the value and risk benefit of doing so in the absence of cirrhosis has prompted the pursuit of gene therapy and hepatocyte transplantation as possible alternatives, but the therapeutic benefit of these modalities of treatment is as yet equivocal.

Although a proportion of children with **acute hepatic necrosis** will survive without transplant, it accounts for approximately 13% of pediatric liver transplantation and requires the most intense concentration of multimodal management/support yet devised. This diagnosis lacks clear etiology in the majority of cases, and posttransplantation survival varies but is worse than the general population, likely due to multifactorial issues related to comorbidities and listing/transplantation graft option availability.

Primary hepatic malignancies in children are rare (<2% of all pediatric malignancies) and account for a fewer than 5% of pediatric transplants. Hepatoblastoma accounts for the majority of cases (75% of primary liver tumors in childhood) and usually presents in an advanced stage; adjuvant chemotherapy and total hepatectomy with transplantation provide cure and long-term survival for the majority of these children. Survival of >85% has been reported by the International Society of Pediatric Oncology and several American centers.

The impact of chronic liver disease and its impact on growth, development, and quality of life of children can be devastating. Liver transplantation is a valid therapy and cure. The allocation of deceased donor livers in the United States follows guidelines based on severity of liver disease as reflected in the Pediatric End-Stage Liver Disease/Model for End-Stage Liver Disease (PELD/MELD) scoring system implemented in 2002, which is calculated from the measurable values of bilirubin, albumin or creatinine (depending upon age), and international normalization ratio. The PELD scoring system was initially modeled from a cohort of 884 children on the pediatric liver transplant wait list, and is intended to predict death, decompensation, or transplantation within 3 mo. Since 2002 the number of liver transplants performed in children in the United States has remained relatively stable, while the number of liver transplants performed in adults has steadily increased by approximately 10% per year. Due to an allocation algorithm that prioritizes local adults over critically ill children nationally, a significant proportion of livers from pediatric deceased donors have been transplanted into adults without ever being offered to a child. This and other issues highlight the importance of advocacy on behalf of children in this growing field.

Contraindications to liver transplantation include uncontrolled infection of extrahepatic origin, extrahepatic malignancies, and severely disabling and uncorrectable disease in other organ systems, principally the brain, heart, and lungs. Although combined liver and heart or lung transplantation has been performed in adults and children, such cases require special consideration and centers dedicated to the complexities of posttransplantation management.

TECHNICAL INNOVATIONS

There are no limitations on age or weight for liver transplantation; to enhance the availability of liver grafts to children and optimize the timing of transplantation, techniques allowing the use of reduced-size or segmental grafts (a right or left lobe of liver, or the left lateral segment of the left lobe) were developed; this allows a liver from a larger donor to be implanted into a child, overcoming the barrier of size mismatch. In the same era, techniques were developed for the use of segments from living donors (usually the left lateral segment for small pediatric recipients), and then split-liver grafts from deceased donors where the left lateral segment is transplanted into a child and the remaining segments of right lobe and medial segment of left lobe transplanted

into an adult, allowing increased utilization of deceased donor grafts without affecting adult wait-list mortality. Reduction of a liver graft is performed ex vivo (i.e., outside of the body); split-liver procurement surgery can be performed either ex vivo or in situ (in the hemodynamically stable brain-dead donor). Donors suitable for aforementioned graft variants should ideally be young (younger than 45 yr of age), healthy, and nonobese; however, variations are guided by the severity of illness and urgency for transplantation of the recipient. Not all centers have the degree of surgical expertise required to perform these more complex surgeries; thus options may be limited for children at centers that only accept size-matched organs.

The implantation of a liver (either whole organ or segment) involves removal of the native liver and encompasses 4 anastomoses: the suprahepatic vena cava, the portal vein, the hepatic artery, and the bile duct. Modifications of the procedure generally involve retaining (or not) of the retrohepatic vena cava, the performance (or not) of a temporary portocaval shunt to decompress the splanchnic venous system during the anhepatic phase, and the use of vascular homografts of donor iliac vein or artery to replace the native inflow (guided by the presence of recipient anomalies or thrombosis of native vessels). The donor bile duct may be connected to a loop of recipient intestine (Roux-en-Y limb) or the native bile duct. UNOS reported outcomes analyzing graft types, and outcomes have shown improved graft survival in children younger than 3 yr of age for live donor grafts when compared with deceased donor whole, split, and reduced grafts. After the 1st yr, however, patient and allograft survivals were similar, independent of graft type.

IMMUNOSUPPRESSION

The long-term goal of effective clinical immunosuppression after solid-organ transplantation is to inhibit antigen-induced T-lymphocyte activation and cytokine production, and to interrupt alloimmune–major histocompatibility complex recognition. To prevent weakening the host response to infection, this goal should be achieved while preserving host immunocompetence. A major emphasis is on the prevention of acute and chronic rejection and preserving the ability to reverse refractory acute rejection. These efforts have been successful; the challenge for the future of pediatric liver transplantation is achieving long-term survival and improved quality of life; this inherently involves strategies to minimize the long-term toxicity of immunosuppressive drug therapy, which can include renal dysfunction, cardiovascular complications, and infections. Strategies of drug minimization, steroid free therapy, and complete withdrawal of drugs have been accomplished in select patients and under careful medical supervision.

Immediately peri- or posttransplantation induction immunosuppressive therapy can involve antilymphocyte antibody induction with depleting antibodies (monoclonal or polyclonal), such as antithymocyte globulin antibody, or the use of a chimeric mouse–human antibody that blocks the interleukin-2 receptor of the T cell, thus preventing activation and replication of antigen-selected T cells. Corticosteroids act through the suppression of antibody production and cytokine synthesis (interleukin-2, and interferon-γ), decreasing proliferation of T cells (helper, suppressor, and cytotoxic), B cells, and neutrophils. Maintenance immunosuppression is achieved by using calcineurin phosphatase inhibitor (cyclosporine or tacrolimus); these drugs interfere with the production and release of interleukin-2, a critical factor in the cytotoxic T-cell response. Calcineurin phosphatase inhibitors are most effectively directed toward inhibiting T-cell–mediated acute cellular rejection. Tacrolimus is the mainstay of most immunosuppressive regimens, and its ability to progress or initiate maintenance immunosuppression in the absence of corticosteroids is of particular benefit in the children. Adjuvant immunosuppression, such as azathioprine or mycophenolate mofetil, which inhibits the synthesis of purine nucleosides and subsequently the proliferation of T and B lymphocytes as well as antibody formation, may be added to enhance the antirejection profile, allow for decrease in the calcineurin dosage, or manage chronic rejection. Rapamycin, a macrolide that binds its molecular target of mammalian target of rapamycin receptor, decreases interleukin-2 production, and in turn T- and B-cell activation and proliferation.

COMPLICATIONS

Posttransplantation complications can be related to the pretransplantation condition of the recipient and the donor match and type, immunologic responses to the graft and the need for enhanced immunosuppressive drug therapy, and toxicity effects of these drugs or infections from over-immunosuppression. Posttransplant complications can occur at varying specific frequencies over a fairly well-defined time course (early, late, remote).

The most anticipated early complications involve those inherent to the transplantation operation: primary nonfunction of the graft, hepatic artery thrombosis, portal/hepatic venous strictures or occlusions, and biliary strictures. Primary nonfunction of the graft is rare in pediatric recipients given the selection criteria of potential donors. Hepatic artery thrombosis is the most frequent and early vascular complication; it occurs in 5–10% of recipients and can have devastating consequences on the graft (acute necrosis and gangrene, biliary leaks/stricture/bilomas) and may require urgent retransplantation. Portal vein or hepatic vein strictures/occlusions are rare and generally occur later posttransplantation. Biliary strictures are the most frequent surgical complication (10–30%) after liver transplantation and should be included in the differential diagnosis of any posttransplantation liver allograft dysfunction. Management of these complications varies and may include interventional radiologic procedures, reoperation, or retransplantation. Advancements in interventional radiology technique have allowed for a less invasive and equally efficacious approach to resolving these complications.

Rejection usually occurs after the first 2 wk after transplantation, with the highest incidence (30–60%) within the first 90 days. Diagnosis of rejection is suspected based on abnormal liver function studies; rarely are there systemic signs such as fever, abdominal pain, new-onset ascites, or hydrothorax. Diagnosing rejection requires biopsy confirmation; treatment algorithms include high doses of corticosteroids and anti-lymphocyte antibodies. Chronic rejection is less frequent (5–10%) and is characterized by progressive damage and loss of bile ductules with consequent cholestasis; treatment involves long-term enhancement of maintenance immunosuppression with corticosteroids and other agents.

The need to treat rejection can place the patient at a higher risk of drug toxicity or infection. The most common transplantation-related infections are cytomegalovirus and Epstein-Barr virus infections, for which there are well-developed algorithms of prophylaxis and screening. Epstein-Barr virus–induced **posttransplant lymphoproliferative disease** (PTLD) represents a unique complication of over-immunosuppression and infection occurring in approximately 10% of patients. It is managed primarily by withdrawal of immunosuppression and antiviral therapy; some patients require chemotherapy.

OUTCOMES

The clinical, surgical, and immunosuppressive drug therapy advances since the 1990s have dramatically improved survival of liver transplantation in children. UNOS data reveal a 1 yr patient and graft survival for biliary atresia of 95% and 87%, respectively. Examination of 461 5-yr survivors of pediatric liver transplantation in a North American registry found a 1st graft survival of 88%, with 12% requiring a 2nd graft and 2% requiring a 3rd transplant. The same investigators published a study of 167 10-yr survivors and found that only 30% of the group had an "ideal outcome" of normal liver-associated enzymes, no retransplant, and no evidence of PTLD, chronic rejection, hypertension, or renal disease. Longer-term survival is inherently dependent on adequacy of long term immunosuppression management, adherence to care protocols, and prevention of infection/toxicities/chronic rejection.

Pediatric liver recipients have excellent and sustained survival following childhood transplantation. With improved survival, the new frontier of care needs to battle the issues of growth, patient loss with a functioning graft, cognitive functioning, and quality of life. The goals of the field have been reset to discovery of the induction protocols and long-term strategies that can foster minimization of drug therapy, and even the induction of tolerance and a life free of the burden of immunosuppression.

Bibliography is available at Expert Consult.

Section **7**

Peritoneum

第七篇

腹膜

Chapter **396**
Peritoneal Malformations
Asim Maqbool and Chris A. Liacouras
第三百九十六章
腹膜畸形

中文导读

本章主要介绍了先天性腹膜带和肠系膜囊肿两种腹膜畸形。详细介绍了先天性腹膜带产生的解剖学原因、常见的解剖部位，并提到该病为良性疾病但可导致肠梗阻及肠坏死等严重并发症；同时介绍了大网膜缺乏或重复畸形、网膜囊肿这两种先天性腹膜带畸形。详细介绍了肠系膜囊肿常见的解剖部位、临床表现、并发症、需要进行的辅助检查，可通过腹腔镜单纯切除治疗囊肿，预后良好。

Congenital peritoneal bands represent anatomically unabsorbed portions of omentum and mesentery, and most commonly occur in the regions of the duodenum, duodenojejunal flexure, ileocecal junction, and ascending colon. Although usually benign, they may be responsible for intestinal obstruction or midgut volvulus and resulting intestinal necrosis. Intraabdominal herniations infrequently occur through ringlike formations produced by anomalous peritoneal bands. Numerous other anomalies can occur in the course of the development of the peritoneum but are rarely of clinical importance. Absence of the omentum or its duplication occurs rarely. Omental cysts arise in obstructed lymphatic channels within the omentum. They may be congenital or can result from trauma and are usually asymptomatic. Abdominal pain or partial small bowel obstruction can result from compression or torsion of the small bowel from traction on the omentum.

Mesenteric cysts are also rare and may co-exist with omental cysts. They may arise from the retroperitoneum, the small bowel mesentery, or even the sigmoid colon. Mesenteric cysts involve the small bowel most frequently but are also reported in association with the colon. Cysts can be single or multiple and are often large. Presentation varies, but most frequently involves abdominal pain and appreciation of an abdominal mass on examination. Gastrointestinal symptoms may also include nausea, emesis, constipation, or loose stools. Mesenteric cysts are mostly benign lesions but may act as lead points for torsion and intussusception. Cysts are usually well defined and identified on imaging via ultrasound or CT scan. Treatment is with simple excision, which can be performed laparoscopically in most cases, with excellent results and generally good prognosis.

ACKNOWLEDGMENT
Melissa Kennedy, MD contributed to the prior version of this chapter.

Bibliography is available at Expert Consult.

Chapter **397**
Ascites

Asim Maqbool, Jessica W. Wen, and Chris A. Liacouras

第三百九十七章
腹水

中文导读

　　本章主要介绍了不同年龄段儿童腹水形成的原因、腹水的临床表现、腹腔穿刺在腹水诊断和治疗中的作用、腹水的治疗及决定。重点介绍了儿童乳糜性腹水，详细阐述了乳糜性腹水的定义、形成的原因、临床表现、诊断和治疗方法。儿童中最常见的病因是淋巴畸形（淋巴管扩张），最常见的表现是无痛性腹胀，诊断主要依靠在喂养含有脂肪的食物后进行腹腔穿刺，在治疗中介绍了营养治疗、药物治疗、腹腔穿刺及手术治疗的适应证。

Ascites is the pathologic accumulation of fluid within the peritoneal cavity. Multiple causes of ascites have been described in different age groups (Tables 397.1 to 397.3). In children, hepatic and renal disease are the most common causes, but ascites can also be caused by cardiac disease, trauma, infection, or neoplasia.

The clinical hallmark of ascites is abdominal distention. Early satiety and dyspnea can occur with a moderate amount of ascites. Considerable intraperitoneal fluid can accumulate before ascites is detectable by the classic physical signs: bulging flanks, dullness to percussion, shifting dullness, a fluid wave, and the *puddle sign* (percussion of a supine person's abdomen over the umbilicus becomes dull as the patient is moved to a prone position and ascitic fluid puddles in dependent regions). Umbilical herniation can be associated with tense ascites. Ultrasound examination is useful for detecting small amounts of ascites.

Abdominal paracentesis can provide symptomatic relief and may be diagnostic of the cause of the ascites. Determining the serum-ascites albumin gradient can help determine the cause of ascites. A gradient greater than 1.1 g/dL (high-gradient ascites) is consistent with ascites caused by portal hypertension, whereas a gradient <1.1 g/dL (low-gradient ascites) indicates ascites of non-portal-hypertensive etiology.

The course, prognosis, and treatment of ascites depend entirely on the cause. For most patients, treatment consists of dietary sodium restriction and diuretic therapy with spironolactone, with the addition of furosemide in more severe cases. Supplemental albumin can also aid in ascitic fluid mobilization. Refractory cases may require large volume paracentesis or transjugular intrahepatic portosystemic shunting. Patients with any type of ascites are at increased risk for spontaneous bacterial peritonitis.

Bibliography is available at Expert Consult.

Table 397.1	Causes of Fetal Ascites
Gastrointestinal disorders 　Meconium peritonitis 　Intestinal malrotation 　Small intestinal or colonic 　　atresia 　Intussusception 　Volvulus 　Cystic fibrosis 　Biliary atresia 　Portal venous malformations Infection 　Parvovirus 　Syphilis 　Cytomegalovirus 　Toxoplasmosis 　Acute maternal hepatitis Genitourinary disorders 　Hydronephrosis 　Polycystic kidney disease 　Urinary obstruction 　Ovarian cyst 　Persistent cloaca	Chylous ascites Cardiac disorders 　Arrhythmia 　Heart failure Chromosomal abnormalities 　Trisomy 　Turner syndrome Neoplasm Hematologic 　Hemolytic anemia 　Neonatal hemochromatosis Metabolic disease 　Niemann-Pick type C 　Congenital disorders of 　　glycosylation 　Wolman disease 　Lysosomal storage disease Other 　Maternal/fetal abuse 　Idiopathic

From Giefer MJ, Murray KF, Colletti RB: Pathophysiology, diagnosis, and management of pediatric ascites, *J Pediatr Gastroenterol Nutr* 52(5):503–513, 2011 (Table 1).

Table 397.2	Causes of Neonatal Ascites

Hepatobiliary disorders
  Cirrhosis
  Alpha-1-antitrypsin deficiency
  Congenital hepatic fibrosis
  Viral hepatitis
  Budd-Chiari syndrome
  Biliary atresia
  Bile duct perforation
  Portal venous malformation
  Ruptured mesenchymal
    hamartoma
Gastrointestinal disorders
  Intestinal malrotation
  Intestinal perforation
  Acute appendicitis
  Intestinal atresia
  Pancreatitis
Chylous ascites
  Intestinal lymphangiectasia
  Lymphatic duct obstruction
  Lymphatic duct trauma
Parenteral nutrition extravasation
Metabolic disease
	Genitourinary disorders
	  Obstructive uropathy
	    Posterior urethral valves
	    Ureterocele
	    Lower ureteral stenosis
	    Ureteral atresia
	    Imperforate hymen
	    Bladder rupture
	    Bladder injury from umbilical
	      artery catheterization
	  Nephrotic syndrome
	  Ruptured corpus luteum cyst
	Cardiac
	  Arrhythmia
	  Heart failure
	Hematologic
	  Neonatal hemochromatosis
	Other
	  Cutis marmorata
	    telangiectatica congenita
	  Intravenous vitamin E
	  Pseudo-ascites
	    Small bowel duplication
	    Abdominal trauma
	    Idiopathic

From Giefer MJ, Murray KF, Colletti RB: Pathophysiology, diagnosis, and management of pediatric ascites, *J Pediatr Gastroenterol Nutr* 52(5):503–513, 2011 (Table 2).

Table 397.3	Causes of Ascites in Infants and Children

Hepatobiliary disorders
  Neoplasm
  Cirrhosis
  Congenital hepatic fibrosis
  Acute hepatitis
  Budd-Chiari syndrome
  Bile duct perforation
  Liver transplantation
Gastrointestinal disorders
  Acute appendicitis
  Intestinal atresia
  Pancreatitis
  Pyloric duplication
Serositis
  Crohn disease
  Eosinophilic enteropathy
  Henoch-Schönlein purpura
Chylous ascites
  Intestinal lymphangiectasia
  Lymphatic duct obstruction
  Lymphatic duct trauma
Parenteral nutrition
  extravasation
Infectious
  Tuberculosis
  Abscess
  Schistosomiasis
	Neoplasm
	  Lymphoma
	  Wilms tumor
	  Clear cell renal sarcoma
	  Glioma
	  Germ cell tumor
	  Ovarian tumor
	  Mesothelioma
	  Neuroblastoma
	Metabolic disease
	Genitourinary disorders
	  Nephrotic syndrome
	  Peritoneal dialysis
	Cardiac
	  Heart failure
	Pseudo-ascites
	  Celiac disease
	  Cystic mesothelioma
	  Omental cyst
	  Ovarian cyst
	Other
	  Systemic lupus erythematosus
	  Ventriculoperitoneal shunt
	  Vitamin A toxicity
	  Chronic granulomatous disease
	  Nonaccidental trauma
	  Protein losing enteropathy
	  Idiopathic

Modified from Giefer MJ, Murray KF, Colletti RB: Pathophysiology, diagnosis, and management of pediatric ascites, *J Pediatr Gastroenterol Nutr* 52(5):503–513, 2011 (Table 3).

397.1 Chylous Ascites

Asim Maqbool, Jessica W. Wen,
and Chris A. Liacouras

Chylous ascites refers to peritoneal fluid that contains lymphatic drainage with a characteristic milky appearance that is rich in triglycerides. Chylous ascites can result from congenital anomaly, injury, or obstruction of the intraabdominal portion of the thoracic duct. Although uncommon, it can occur at any age. In the pediatric population, the most common cause is lymphatic malformation (lymphangiectasia). Other causes include surgical injury to the lymphatics, trauma, cirrhosis, peritoneal bands, generalized lymphangiomatosis, chronic inflammatory processes of the bowel, and mycobacterial infection. Malignancy is a common cause in the adult population but uncommon in pediatrics. Congenital anomalies of the lymphatic system can be associated with Turner, Noonan, yellow nail, and Klippel-Trenaunay-Weber syndromes. Other etiologies include nephrotic syndrome, familial visceral myopathy, sarcoidosis, intestinal malrotation and volvulus, pancreatitis, constrictive pericarditis, Behcet disease, and after appendectomy.

The most common presentation is painless abdominal distention, and it may be accompanied by poor weight gain and loose stools. Peripheral edema is common. Massive chylous ascites can result in scrotal edema, inguinal and umbilical herniation, and respiratory difficulties.

Diagnosis of chylous ascites depends on the demonstration of milky ascitic fluid obtained via paracentesis after a fat-containing feeding. Ascites fluid analysis reveals high protein content, elevated triglycerides, and lymphocytosis. If the patient has had nothing by mouth, the fluid may appear serous. Hypoalbuminemia, hypogammaglobulinemia, and lymphopenia are common in these patients.

Treatment includes a high-protein, low-fat diet supplemented with medium-chain triglycerides that are absorbed directly into the portal circulation and decrease lymph production. Parenteral alimentation may be necessary if nutrition remains impaired on oral feedings; this may also significantly decrease lymph flow and facilitate sealing at the point of lymph leakage. Octreotide, a somatostatin analog, has been used subcutaneously in chylous ascites. The mechanism is not clearly understood; however, it decreases intestinal blood flow, leading to decreased portal pressure, and it also inhibits lymphatic secretion through somatostatin receptors in the intestinal wall. Paracentesis should be repeated only if abdominal distention causes respiratory distress. Lymphangiography with adjunctive embolization may be very successful in treating chylous ascites with identified site of leakage. Finally, laparotomy may be indicated if conservative management has been unsuccessful for potential surgical ligation of lymphatics.

Bibliography is available at Expert Consult.

Chapter **398**
Peritonitis
*Asim Maqbool, Jessica W. Wen,
and Chris A. Liacouras*
第三百九十八章
腹膜炎

中文导读

　　本章主要介绍了感染性腹膜炎的具体分类，包括急性原发性腹膜炎、急性继发性腹膜炎和急性继发性局限性腹膜炎。详细介绍了急性原发性腹膜炎的病原学和流行病学、临床表现及诊断和治疗，最常见的细菌是肺炎链球菌，以发热、腹痛和中毒表现为特征，治疗包括腹腔穿刺和抗生素治疗；具体描述了急性继发性腹膜炎的临床表现和治疗，治疗包括积极支持治疗和抗生素应用；详细介绍了急性继发性局限性腹膜炎的病因学、临床表现和治疗，最常见的是阑尾穿孔引起的阑尾周围脓肿及盆腔的脓肿，脓肿应引流并给予合适的抗生素治疗。

Inflammation of the peritoneal lining of the abdominal cavity can result from infectious, autoimmune, neoplastic, and chemical processes. Infectious peritonitis is usually defined as primary (spontaneous) or secondary. In primary peritonitis, the source of infection originates outside the abdomen and seeds the peritoneal cavity via hematogenous, lymphatic, or transmural spread. Secondary peritonitis arises from the abdominal cavity itself through extension from or rupture of an intraabdominal viscus or an abscess within an organ. Tertiary peritonitis refers to recurrent diffuse or localized disease and is associated with poorer outcomes than secondary peritonitis.

Clinically, patients have abdominal pain, abdominal tenderness, and rigidity on exam. Peritonitis can result from rupture of a hollow viscus, such as the appendix or a Meckel diverticulum; disruption of the peritoneum from trauma or peritoneal dialysis catheter; chemical peritonitis from other bodily fluid, including bile and urine; and infection. Meconium peritonitis is described in Chapter 123.1. Peritonitis is considered a surgical emergency and requires exploration and lavage of the abdomen, except in spontaneous bacterial peritonitis.

Bibliography is available at Expert Consult.

398.1 Acute Primary Peritonitis
*Asim Maqbool, Jessica W. Wen,
and Chris A. Liacouras*

ETIOLOGY AND EPIDEMIOLOGY
Primary peritonitis usually refers to bacterial infection of the peritoneal cavity without a demonstrable intraabdominal source. Most cases occur in children with ascites resulting from cirrhosis and nephrotic syndrome. Infection can result from translocation of gut bacteria as well as immune dysfunction. Rarely, primary peritonitis occurs in previously healthy children. Pneumococci (most common), group A streptococci, enterococci, staphylococci, and Gram-negative enteric bacteria, especially *Escherichia coli* and *Klebsiella pneumoniae*, are most commonly found. *Mycobacterium tuberculosis*, *Neisseria meningitidis*, and *Mycobacterium bovis* are rare causes.

CLINICAL MANIFESTATIONS
Onset may be insidious or rapid and is characterized by fever, abdominal pain, and a toxic appearance. Vomiting and diarrhea may be present. Hypotension and tachycardia are common, along with shallow, rapid respirations because of discomfort associated with breathing. Abdominal palpation might demonstrate rebound tenderness and rigidity. Bowel sounds are hypoactive or absent. However, signs and symptoms may be subtle at times, and increased vigilance is needed in cirrhotic patients who have ascites and present with unexplained leukocytosis, azotemia, or metabolic acidosis.

DIAGNOSIS AND TREATMENT
Peripheral leukocytosis with a marked predominance of polymorphonuclear cells is common, although the white blood cell (WBC) count can be affected by preexisting hypersplenism in patients with cirrhosis. Patients with nephrotic syndrome generally have proteinuria, and low serum albumin in these patients is associated with an

increased risk of peritonitis. X-ray examination of the abdomen reveals dilation of the large and small intestines, with increased separation of loops secondary to bowel wall thickening. Distinguishing primary peritonitis from appendicitis may be impossible in patients without a history of nephrotic syndrome or cirrhosis; accordingly, the diagnosis of primary peritonitis is made by CT scan, laparoscopy, or laparotomy. In a child with known renal or hepatic disease and ascites, the presence of peritoneal signs should prompt diagnostic paracentesis. Infected fluid usually reveals a WBC count of ≥250 cells/mm³, with >50% polymorphonuclear cells.

Primary peritonitis is usually monomicrobial. The presence of mixed bacterial flora on ascitic fluid examination or free air on abdominal roentgenogram in children with presumed peritonitis mandates laparotomy to localize a perforation as a likely intraabdominal source of the infection. Inoculation of ascitic fluid obtained at paracentesis directly into blood culture bottles increases the yield of positive cultures. Parenteral antibiotic therapy with broad spectrum coverage, such as cefotaxime, should be started promptly, with subsequent changes dependent on sensitivity testing (vancomycin for resistant pneumococci). Therapy should be continued for 10-14 days.

Culture-negative neutrocytic ascites is a variant of primary peritonitis with an ascitic fluid WBC count of >500 cells/mm³, a negative culture, no intraabdominal source of infection, and no prior treatment with antibiotics. It should be treated in a similar manner as primary peritonitis.

Bibliography is available at Expert Consult.

398.2 Acute Secondary Peritonitis

Asim Maqbool, Jessica W. Wen, and Chris A. Liacouras

Acute secondary peritonitis most often results from entry of enteric bacteria into the peritoneal cavity through a necrotic defect in the wall of the intestines or other viscus as a result of obstruction or infarction or after rupture of an intraabdominal visceral abscess. It most commonly follows perforation of the appendix. Other causes include incarcerated hernias, rupture of a Meckel diverticulum, midgut volvulus, intussusception, hemolytic uremic syndrome, peptic ulceration, inflammatory bowel disease, necrotizing cholecystitis, necrotizing enterocolitis, typhlitis, and traumatic perforation.

Peritonitis in the neonatal period most often occurs as a complication of necrotizing enterocolitis but may be associated with meconium ileus or spontaneous (or indomethacin-induced) rupture of the stomach or intestines. In postpubertal girls, bacteria from the genital tract *(Neisseria gonorrhoeae, Chlamydia trachomatis)* can gain access to the peritoneal cavity via the fallopian tubes, causing secondary peritonitis. The presence of a foreign body, such as a ventriculoperitoneal catheter or peritoneal dialysis catheter, can predispose to peritonitis, with skin microorganisms, such as *Staphylococcus epidermidis, Staphylococcus aureus,* and *Candida albicans,* contaminating the shunt. Secondary peritonitis results from direct toxic effects of bacteria as well as local and systemic release of inflammatory mediators in response to organisms and their products (lipopolysaccharide endotoxin). The development of sepsis depends on various host and disease factors, as well as promptness of antimicrobial and surgical intervention.

CLINICAL MANIFESTATIONS
Similar to primary peritonitis, characteristic symptoms include fever, diffuse abdominal pain, nausea, and vomiting. Physical findings of peritoneal inflammation include rebound tenderness, abdominal wall rigidity, a paucity of body motion (lying still), and decreased or absent bowel sounds from paralytic ileus. Massive exudation of fluid into the peritoneal cavity, along with the systemic release of vasodilative substances, can lead to the rapid development of shock. A toxic appearance, irritability, and restlessness are common. Basilar atelectasis as well as intrapulmonary shunting can develop, with progression to acute respira-

tory distress syndrome.

Laboratory studies reveal a peripheral WBC count >12,000 cells/mm³, with a marked predominance of polymorphonuclear forms. X-rays of the abdomen can reveal free air in the peritoneal cavity, evidence of ileus or obstruction, peritoneal fluid, and obliteration of the psoas shadow. Other peritoneal fluid findings suggestive of secondary peritonitis include elevated total protein (>1 g/dL), and low glucose (<50 mg/dL).

TREATMENT
Aggressive fluid resuscitation and support of cardiovascular function should begin immediately. Stabilization of the patient before surgical intervention is mandatory. Antibiotic therapy must provide coverage for organisms that predominate at the site of presumed origin of the infection. In contrast to primary peritonitis, secondary peritonitis is typically polymicrobial. For perforation of the lower gastrointestinal tract, a regimen of ampicillin, gentamicin, and clindamycin or metronidazole will adequately address infection by *E. coli, Klebsiella,* and *Bacteroides* spp. and enterococci. Alternative therapy could include piperacillin/tazobactam or a carbapenem (imipenem-cilastatin, meropenem, ertapenem or doripenem). Surgery to repair a perforated viscus should proceed after the patient is stabilized and antibiotic therapy is initiated. Intraoperative peritoneal fluid cultures will indicate whether a change in the antibiotic regimen is warranted. Empirical treatment for peritoneal dialysis catheter–related peritonitis may include intraperitoneal cefepime or cefazolin plus ceftazidime. Serious infection from peritoneal dialysis catheters can generally be prevented with good catheter hygiene and prompt removal and replacement with signs of progressive infection.

Bibliography is available at Expert Consult.

398.3 Acute Secondary Localized Peritonitis (Peritoneal Abscess)

Asim Maqbool, Jessica W. Wen, and Chris A. Liacouras

ETIOLOGY
Intraabdominal abscesses occur less commonly in children and infants than in adults, but can develop in visceral intraabdominal organs (hepatic, splenic, renal, pancreatic, tubo-ovarian abscesses) or in the interintestinal, periappendiceal, subdiaphragmatic, subhepatic, pelvic, or retroperitoneal spaces. Most commonly, periappendiceal and pelvic abscesses arise from a perforation of the appendix. Transmural inflammation with fistula formation can result in intraabdominal abscess formation in children with inflammatory bowel disease.

CLINICAL MANIFESTATIONS
Prolonged fever, anorexia, vomiting, and lassitude suggest the development of an intraabdominal abscess. The peripheral WBC count is elevated, as is the erythrocyte sedimentation rate. With an appendiceal abscess, there is localized tenderness and a palpable mass in the right lower quadrant. A pelvic abscess is suggested by abdominal distention, rectal tenesmus with or without the passage of small-volume mucous stools, and bladder irritability. Rectal examination might reveal a tender mass anteriorly. Subphrenic gas collection, basal atelectasis, elevated hemidiaphragm, and pleural effusion may be present with a subdiaphragmatic abscess. Psoas abscess can develop from extension of infection from a retroperitoneal appendicitis, Crohn disease, or perirenal or intrarenal abscess. Abdominal findings may be minimal, and presentation can include a limp, hip pain, and fever. Ultrasound examination, CT scanning, and MRI may be used to localize intraabdominal abscesses; MRI gives the best resolution of disease involvement.

TREATMENT
An abscess should be drained, and appropriate antibiotic therapy provided. Drainage can be performed under radiologic control (ultrasonogram or CT guidance) and an indwelling drainage catheter left in

place, or surgically depending on location of abscess. Initial broad-spectrum antibiotic coverage such as a combination of ampicillin, gentamicin, and clindamycin or ciprofloxacin and metronidazole should be started and can be modified, depending on the results of sensitivity testing. The treatment of appendiceal rupture complicated by abscess formation may be problematic because intestinal phlegmon formation can make surgical resection more difficult. Intensive antibiotic therapy for 4-6 wk followed by an interval appendectomy is often the treatment course followed.

Bibliography is available at Expert Consult.

Chapter 399
Epigastric Hernia
John J. Aiken

第三百九十九章
上腹部疝

中文导读

本章主要介绍了上腹部疝，详细介绍了切口疝。具体介绍了上腹部疝的定义、病因，详细描述了临床表现、诊断及治疗方法，病因中提到血管腔隙假说和肌腱纤维分解假说，临床表现为肿块、疼痛，体格检查即可诊断，影像学检查可作为辅助，需要及时手术修补治疗。具体描述了出现切口疝的高危因素，包括腹内压升高、伤口感染和中线切口；详细说明了切口疝的手术时机，应推迟到1岁以后，以及嵌顿作为急诊手术指征。

Epigastric hernias in children are ventral hernias in the midline of the abdominal wall between the xiphoid process of the sternum and the umbilicus. Epigastric hernias are more likely congenital than acquired. The defect typically contains only preperitoneal fat without a peritoneal sac or abdominal viscera. Because most epigastric hernias are small and asymptomatic, the true incidence is unknown, but the reported incidence in childhood varies from <1% to as high as 5%. The etiology of epigastric hernia is unknown. The 2 main hypotheses are the vascular lacunae hypothesis and the tendinous fiber decussation hypothesis: the former proposes that the protrusion is through small spaces created where the vascular lacunae penetrate the linea alba, and the latter that epigastric hernia occurs exclusively at sites where affected patients do not have triple lines of decussation. In addition, undiagnosed collagen disorders, increased intraabdominal pressure, and in older patients, previous midline incision may play a role in the development of epigastric hernia. Epigastric hernias may be single or multiple and are 2-3 times more common in males than females. Through the small midline defect there is often herniation of preperitoneal fat into the superficial abdominal wall, although as the defect becomes progressively larger, the rare possibility exists of herniation of intraabdominal contents. Epigastric (incisional) hernias can occur in a previous incision site or be associated with ventricular-peritoneal shunts.

CLINICAL PRESENTATION
Epigastric hernias typically appear in young children as a visible or palpable mass in the midline, between the umbilicus and the xiphoid process of the sternum, noted by the parents or primary care practitioner. The mass is almost always small (<1 cm), asymptomatic, and typically reported as always present, but most apparent at times of irritability or straining. Occasionally the mass is intermittent, and the child relates pain localized to the site. Physical examination demonstrates a firm mass, directly in the midline, anywhere between the umbilicus and the xiphoid process. The mass may be intermittent if the fat reduces with relaxation of the abdominal muscles. Epigastric hernias typically contain only preperitoneal fat, and most are not reducible because of the small size of the fascial defect. Rarely, a fascial defect is noted without a

palpable mass. Herniation of intestines or abdominal viscera in an epigastric hernia would be exceptionally rare, if the defect enlarges over time. The mass may be tender to examination, but strangulation of the hernia contents is uncommon. Physical examination is almost always diagnostic, and imaging studies are generally unnecessary. If the diagnosis is unclear, imaging may be useful. Ultrasound typically shows a small mass that is isoechoic to the adjacent subcutaneous fat and possibly connection through a small fascial defect with the preperitoneal fat. MRI imaging might be helpful in diagnosis but is not routinely used.

The natural history of epigastric hernia is for gradual enlargement over time as intermittently more preperitoneal fat is extruded through the defect at times of straining or increased intraabdominal pressure. Left untreated, the defect can enlarge and allow herniation of intraabdominal viscera within a peritoneal sac, mostly seen in adults. Epigastric hernias do not resolve spontaneously, and therefore operative repair is the recommended treatment. The site should be carefully marked preoperatively because the mass and defect can be difficult to localize in a relaxed abdominal wall after induction of anesthesia. A limited transverse incision is made over the mass, and dissection is performed to delineate the edges of the fascial defect. If herniated fat is present, it is dissected free of the subcutaneous tissues and can be reduced or ligated and excised. The defect is closed using absorbable suture. The skin is closed with an absorbable subcuticular suture. Postoperative complications are rare, and the recurrence rate is low.

399.1 Incisional Hernia

John J. Aiken

Hernia formation in the site of a previous laparotomy is uncommon in childhood. Incisional hernias can also occur at the incision sites for the laparoscopic ports used in minimally invasive surgery. Factors associated with an increased risk of incisional hernia include increased intraabdominal pressure, wound infection, and midline incision. The laparoscopic ports sites pose a technical challenge to visualize the fascia in a small incision. Transverse abdominal incisions are favored because of their increased strength and blood supply, which reduces the likelihood of wound infection and incisional hernia. Although most incisional hernias require repair, operation should be deferred until the child is in optimal medical condition. Some incisional hernias resolve, especially those occurring in infants. Some recommend elastic bandaging to discourage enlargement of the hernia and to promote spontaneous healing. Initial management should be conservative, with repair deferred until around 1 yr of age. Incarceration is very uncommon in incisional hernias but is an indication for prompt repair. Newborns with abdominal wall defects represent the largest group of children with incisional hernias.

Bibliography is available at Expert Consult.

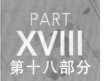

The Respiratory System
呼吸系统

PART XVIII
第十八部分

Section 1
Development and Function
第一篇
发育与功能

Chapter 400
Diagnostic Approach to Respiratory Disease
Julie Ryu, James S. Hagood, and Gabriel G. Haddad
第四百章
呼吸系统疾病的诊断方法

中文导读

　　本章主要介绍了病史采集、体格检查、血气分析、胸部透视法、放射线照相技术、肺功能检查、微生物学［肺部分泌物检测、微生物群（见第一百九十六章）］以及基于气道可视化和肺标本的诊断检测。具体描述了放射线照相技术的胸部X线、上呼吸道平片、鼻窦影像、胸部CT和MRI、透视、钡剂吞咽检查、肺动脉造影和主动脉造影以及通气-灌注扫描和放射性核素肺扫描；具体描述了微生物检测（见第一百九十六章）、运动激发试验以及睡眠监测；基于气道可视化和肺标本的诊断检测中具体描述了喉镜检查、支气管镜检查和支气管肺泡灌洗术、胸腔镜检查、胸腔穿刺、肺穿刺、肺活检以及发汗试验。

HISTORY

The history begins with a narrative provided by the parent/caretaker with input from the patient. It should include questions about respiratory symptoms (dyspnea, cough, pain, wheezing, snoring, apnea, cyanosis, exercise intolerance), as well as their chronicity, timing during day or night, and associations with activities including exercise or food intake. The respiratory system interacts with a number of other systems, and questions related to cardiac, gastrointestinal, central nervous, hematologic, and immune systems may be relevant. Questions related to gastrointestinal reflux, congenital abnormalities (airway anomalies, ciliary dyskinesia), or immune status may be important in a patient with repeated pneumonia. The family history is essential and should include inquiries about siblings and other close relatives with similar symptoms, or any chronic disease with respiratory components.

PHYSICAL EXAMINATION

Respiratory dysfunction usually produces detectable alterations in the pattern of breathing. Values for normal respiratory rates are presented in Table 81.1 and depend on many factors—most importantly, age. Repeated respiratory rate measurements are necessary because respiratory rates, especially in the young, are exquisitely sensitive to extraneous stimuli. Sleeping respiratory rates are more reproducible in infants than those obtained during feeding or activity. These rates vary among infants but average 40-50 breaths/min in the 1st few wk of life and usually <60 breaths/min in the 1st few days of life.

Respiratory control abnormalities can cause the child to breathe at a low rate or periodically. Mechanical abnormalities produce compensatory changes that are generally directed at altering minute ventilation to maintain alveolar ventilation. Decreases in lung compliance require increases in muscular force and breathing rate, leading to variable increases in chest wall retractions and nasal flaring. The respiratory excursions of children with restrictive disease are shallow. An expiratory grunt is common as the child attempts to raise the **functional residual capacity (FRC)** by closing the glottis at the end of expiration. The FRC is the amount of air left in the lungs after tidal expiration. Children with obstructive disease might take slower, deeper breaths. When the obstruction is **extrathoracic** (from the nose to the mid-trachea), inspiration is more prolonged than expiration, and an inspiratory stridor (a predominant inspiratory monophonic noise) can usually be heard (Fig. 400.1). When the obstruction is **intrathoracic**, expiration is more prolonged than inspiration, and the patient often has to make use of accessory expiratory muscles. Intrathoracic obstruction results in air trapping and, therefore, a larger residual volume, as well as a possible increase in FRC (Fig. 400.2).

Lung percussion has limited value in small infants because it cannot discriminate between noises originating from tissues that are close to each other. In adolescents and adults, percussion is usually dull in restrictive

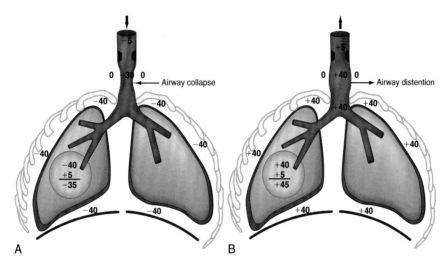

Fig. 400.1 A, In extrathoracic airway obstruction, the increased negative pressure during inspiration is transmitted up to the site of obstruction. This results in collapse of the extrathoracic airway below the site of obstruction, making the obstruction worse during inspiration. Note that the pressures are compared with the atmospheric pressure, which is traditionally represented as 0 cm. Terminal airway pressure is calculated as intrapleural pressure plus lung recoil pressure. Lung recoil pressure is arbitrarily chosen as 5 cm for the sake of simplicity. **B,** During expiration, the positive pressure below the site of obstruction results in distention of extrathoracic airway and amelioration of symptoms. *(Courtesy of Dr. Ashok Sarnaik.)*

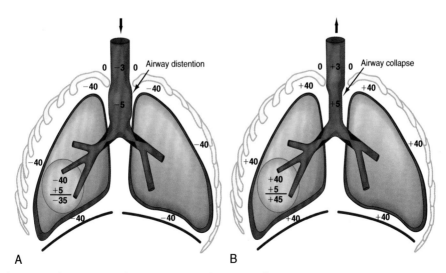

Fig. 400.2 A and **B,** In intrapulmonary airway obstruction, even a wider segment of intrathoracic airway is subjected to pressure changes compared with those observed in intrathoracic-extrapulmonary airway obstruction. Such lesions are associated with marked increase in airway obstruction during expiration. *(Courtesy of Dr. Ashok Sarnaik.)*

lung disease, with a pleural effusion, pneumonia, and atelectasis, but it is tympanitic in obstructive disease (asthma, pneumothorax).

Auscultation confirms the presence of inspiratory or expiratory prolongation and provides information about the symmetry and quality of air movement. In addition, it often detects abnormal or adventitious sounds such as **stridor**; **crackles** or **rales**, high-pitched, interrupted sounds found during inspiration and more rarely during early expiration, which denote opening of previously closed air spaces; or **wheezes**, musical, continuous sounds usually caused by the development of turbulent flow in narrow airways (Table 400.1). **Digital clubbing** is a sign of chronic hypoxia and chronic lung disease (Fig. 400.3) but may be a result of nonpulmonary etiologies (Table 400.2).

BLOOD GAS ANALYSIS

The main function of the respiratory system is to remove carbon dioxide from and add oxygen to the systemic venous blood brought to the lung. The composition of the inspired gas, ventilation, perfusion, diffusion, and tissue metabolism has a significant influence on the arterial blood gases.

The total pressure of the atmosphere at sea level is 760 torr. With increasing altitude, the atmospheric pressure decreases. The total atmospheric pressure is equal to the sum of partial pressures exerted by each of its component gases. Alveolar air is 100% humidified, so in alveolar gas calculations, the inspired gas is also presumed to be 100% humidified. At a temperature of 37°C (98.6°F) and 100% humidity, water vapor exerts pressure of 47 torr, regardless of altitude. In a natural setting, the atmosphere consists of 20.93% oxygen. **Partial pressure of oxygen in inspired gas (Pio$_2$)** at sea level is therefore $(760 - 47) \times 20.93\% = 149$ torr. When breathing 40% oxygen at sea level, Pio$_2$ is $(760 - 47) \times 40\% = 285$ torr. At higher altitudes, breathing different concentrations of oxygen, Pio$_2$ is less than at sea level, depending on the prevalent atmospheric pressures. In Denver (altitude of 5,000 feet and barometric pressure of 632 torr), Pio$_2$ in room air is $(632 - 47) \times 20.93\% = 122$ torr, and in 40% oxygen, it is $(632 - 47) \times 40\% = 234$ torr.

Minute volume is a product of V$_T$ and respiratory rate. Part of the V$_T$ occupies the conducting airways (anatomic dead space), which does not contribute to gas exchange in the alveoli. **Alveolar ventilation** is the volume of atmospheric air entering the alveoli and is calculated as (V$_T$ − dead space) × respiratory rate. Alveolar ventilation is inversely proportional to arterial Pco$_2$ (Paco$_2$). When alveolar ventilation is halved, Paco$_2$ is doubled. Conversely, doubling of alveolar ventilation decreases Paco$_2$ by 50%. **Alveolar Po$_2$ (Pao$_2$)** is calculated by the **alveolar air equation** as follows, where R is the respiratory quotient. For practical purposes, Paco$_2$ is substituted by **arterial Pco$_2$ (Paco$_2$)**, and R is assumed to be 0.8. According to the alveolar air equation, for a given Pio$_2$, a rise in Paco$_2$ of 10 torr results in a decrease in Pao$_2$ by 10 ÷ 0.8, or 10 × 1.25, or 12.5 torr. Thus proportionately inverse changes in Pao$_2$ occur to the extent of 1.25× the changes in Paco$_2$ (or Paco$_2$).

After the alveolar gas composition is determined by the inspired gas conditions and process of ventilation, gas exchange occurs by the process

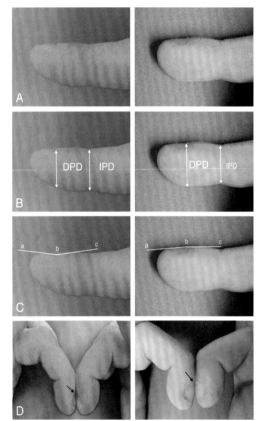

Fig. 400.3 A, Normal and clubbed finger viewed in profile. **B,** The normal finger demonstrates a distal phalangeal finger depth *(DPD)/* interphalangeal finger depth *(IPD)* ratio <1. The clubbed finger demonstrates a DPD/IPD ratio >1. **C,** The normal finger on the left demonstrates a normal profile *(abc)* with angle less than 180 degrees. The clubbed finger demonstrates a profile angle >180 degrees. **D,** Schamroth sign is demonstrated in the clubbed finger with the loss of diamond shape window in between finger beds *(arrow)* that is demonstrated in the normal finger. *(From Wilmott RW, Bush A, Deterding RR, et al: Kendig's disorders of the respiratory tract in children, ed 9, Philadelphia, 2019, Elsevier [Fig. 1.14, p. 20].)*

of diffusion and equilibration of alveolar gas with pulmonary capillary blood. Diffusion depends on the alveolar capillary barrier and the amount of available time for equilibration. In health, the equilibration of alveolar gas and pulmonary capillary blood is complete for both oxygen and carbon dioxide. In diseases in which the alveolar capillary barrier is

Table 400.1	Respiratory Sounds			
BASIC SOUNDS	**MECHANISMS**	**ORIGIN**	**ACOUSTICS**	**RELEVANCE**
Lung	Turbulent flow, vortices, other	Central (expiration), lobar to segmental airways (inspiration)	Low pass filtered noise (<100 to >1,000 Hz)	Regional ventilation, airway caliber
Tracheal	Turbulent flow, flow impinging on airway walls	Pharynx, larynx, trachea, large airways	Noise with resonances (<100 to >3,000 Hz)	Upper airway configuration
ADVENTITIOUS SOUNDS				
Wheezes	Airway wall flutter, vortex shedding, other	Central and lower airways	Sinusoidal (<100 to >1,000 Hz, duration typically >80 msec)	Airway obstruction, flow limitation
Rhonchi	Rupture of fluid films, airway wall vibration	Larger airways	Series of rapidly dampened sinusoids (typically <300 Hz and duration <100 msec)	Secretions, abnormal airway collapsibility
Crackles	Airway wall stress-relaxation	Central and lower airways	Rapidly dampened wave deflections (duration typically <20 msec)	Airway closure, secretions

Modified from Pasterkamp H, Kraman SS, Wodicka GR: Respiratory sounds. Advances beyond the stethoscope, *Am J Respir Crit Care Med* 156[3]:974–987, 1997.

Table 400.2	Nonpulmonary Diseases Associated With Clubbing

CARDIAC
Cyanotic congenital heart disease
Bacterial endocarditis
Chronic heart failure

HEMATOLOGIC
Thalassemia
Congenital methemoglobinemia (rare)

GASTROINTESTINAL
Crohn disease
Ulcerative colitis
Celiac disease
Chronic dysentery, sprue
Polyposis coli
Severe gastrointestinal hemorrhage
Small bowel lymphoma
Liver cirrhosis (including α_1-antitrypsin deficiency)
Chronic active hepatitis

OTHER
Thyroid deficiency (thyroid acropachy)
Thyrotoxicosis
Chronic pyelonephritis (rare)
Toxic (e.g., arsenic, mercury, beryllium)
Lymphomatoid granulomatosis
Fabry disease
Raynaud disease, scleroderma
Hodgkin disease
Familial

UNILATERAL CLUBBING
Vascular disorders (e.g., subclavian arterial aneurysm, brachial arteriovenous fistula)
Subluxation of shoulder
Median nerve injury
Local trauma

From Pasterkamp H: The history and physical examination. In Wilmott RW, Boat TF, Bush A, et al, editors: *Kendig and Chernick's disorders of the respiratory tract in children*, ed 8, Philadelphia, 2012, Elsevier.

abnormally increased (alveolar interstitial diseases) and/or when the time available for equilibration is decreased (increased blood flow velocity), diffusion is incomplete. Because of its greater solubility in liquid medium, carbon dioxide is 20 times more diffusible than oxygen. Therefore, diseases with diffusion defects are characterized by marked **alveolar-arterial oxygen (A-aO_2)** gradients and hypoxemia. Significant elevation of CO_2 does not occur as a result of a diffusion defect unless there is coexistent hypoventilation.

Venous blood brought to the lungs is "arterialized" after diffusion is complete. After complete arterialization, the pulmonary capillary blood should have the same PO_2 and PCO_2 as in the alveoli. The arterial blood gas composition is different from that in the alveoli, even in normal conditions, because there is a certain amount of dead space ventilation as well as venous admixture in a normal lung. Dead space ventilation results in a higher $PaCO_2$ than $PACO_2$, whereas venous admixture or right-to-left shunting results in a lower PaO_2 compared with the alveolar gas composition (Fig. 400.4). PaO_2 is a reflection of the amount of oxygen dissolved in blood, which is a relatively minor component of total blood oxygen content. For every 100 torr PO_2, there is 0.3 mL of dissolved O_2 in 100 mL of blood. The total blood oxygen content is composed of the dissolved oxygen and the oxygen bound to hemoglobin (Hb). Each gram of Hb carries 1.34 mL of O_2 when 100% saturated with oxygen. Thus 15 g of Hb carries 20.1 mL of oxygen. **Arterial oxygen content (CaO_2)**, expressed as mL O_2/dL blood, can be calculated as ($PaO_2 \times 0.003$) + (Hb $\times$ 1.34 $\times$ SO_2), where Hb is grams of Hb per deciliter of blood and SO_2 is percentage of oxyhemoglobin saturation. The relationship of PO_2 and the amount of oxygen carried by the Hb

is the basis of the O_2-Hb dissociation curve (Fig. 400.5). The PO_2 at which Hb is 50% saturated is referred to as P_{50}. At a normal pH, Hb is 94% saturated at PO_2 of 70, and little further gain in saturation is accomplished at a higher PO_2. At PO_2 <50, there is a steep decline in saturation and therefore the oxygen content.

Oxygen delivery to tissues is a product of oxygen content and cardiac output. When Hb is near 100% saturated, blood contains approximately 20 mL oxygen per 100 mL or 200 mL/L. In a healthy adult, cardiac output is approximately 5 L/min, oxygen delivery 1,000 mL/min, and oxygen consumption 250 mL/min. Mixed venous blood returning to the heart has a PO_2 of 40 torr and is 75% saturated with oxygen. Blood oxygen content, cardiac output, and oxygen consumption are important determinants of mixed venous oxygen saturation. Given a steady-state blood oxygen content and oxygen consumption, the mixed venous saturation is an important indicator of cardiac output. A declining mixed venous saturation in such a state indicates decreasing cardiac output.

Clinical observations and interpretation of blood gas values are critical in localizing the site of the lesion and estimating its severity (Table 400.3). In airway obstruction above the carina (subglottic stenosis, vascular ring), blood gases reflect overall alveolar hypoventilation. This is manifested by an elevated $PACO_2$ and a proportionate decrease in PaO_2 as determined by the alveolar air equation. A rise in $PaCO_2$ of 20 torr decreases PaO_2 by 20×1.25 or 25 torr. In the absence of significant parenchymal disease and intrapulmonary shunting, such lesions respond very well to supplemental oxygen in reversing hypoxemia. Similar blood gas values, demonstrating alveolar hypoventilation and response to supplemental oxygen, are observed in patients with a depressed respiratory center and ineffective neuromuscular function, resulting in respiratory insufficiency. Such patients can be easily distinguished from those with airway obstruction by their poor respiratory effort.

In intrapulmonary airway obstruction (asthma, bronchiolitis), blood gases reflect ventilation-perfusion imbalance and venous admixture. In these diseases, the obstruction is not uniform throughout the lungs, resulting in areas that are hyperventilated and others that are hypoventilated. Pulmonary capillary blood coming from hyperventilated areas has a higher PO_2 and lower PCO_2, whereas that coming from hypoventilated regions has a lower PO_2 and higher PCO_2. A lower blood PCO_2 can compensate for the higher PCO_2 because the Hb-CO_2 dissociation curve is relatively linear. In mild disease, the hyperventilated areas predominate, resulting in hypocarbia. An elevated PaO_2 in hyperventilated areas cannot compensate for the decreased PaO_2 in hypoventilated areas because of the shape of the O_2-Hb dissociation curve. This results in venous admixture, arterial desaturation, and decreased PaO_2 (see Fig. 400.4). With increasing disease severity, more areas become hypoventilated, resulting in normalization of $PaCO_2$ with a further decrease in PaO_2. A normal or slightly elevated $PaCO_2$ in asthma should be viewed with concern as a potential indicator of impending respiratory failure. In severe intrapulmonary airway obstruction, hypoventilated areas predominate, leading to hypercarbia, respiratory acidosis, and hypoxemia. The degree to which supplemental oxygenation raises PaO_2 depends on the severity of the illness and the degree of venous admixture.

In alveolar and interstitial diseases, blood gas values reflect both intrapulmonary right-to-left shunting and a diffusion barrier. Hypoxemia is a hallmark of such conditions occurring early in the disease process. $PaCO_2$ is either normal or decreased. An increase in $PaCO_2$ is observed only later in the course, as muscle fatigue and exhaustion result in hypoventilation. Response to supplemental oxygen is relatively poor with shunting and diffusion disorders compared with other lesions.

Most clinical entities present with mixed lesions. A child with a vascular ring might also have an area of atelectasis; the arterial blood gas reflects both processes. The blood gas values reflect the more dominant lesion.

An arterial blood gas analysis is probably the single most useful rapid test of pulmonary function. Although this analysis does not specify the cause of the condition or the specific nature of the disease process, it can give an overall assessment of the functional state of the respiratory system and clues about the pathogenesis of the disease. Because the detection of cyanosis is influenced by skin color, perfusion, and blood Hb concentration, the clinical detection by inspection is an unreliable

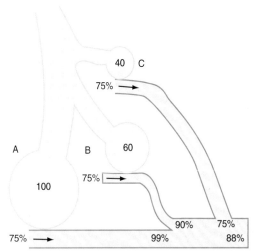

Fig. 400.4 Diagram demonstrating the effects of decreased ventilation–perfusion ratios on arterial oxygenation in the lungs. Three alveolar–capillary units are illustrated. Unit *A* has normal ventilation and an alveolar PO_2 of 100 mm Hg (shown by the number in the middle of the space). The blood that circulates through this unit raises its oxygen saturation from 75% (the saturation of mixed venous blood) to 99%. Unit *B* has a lower ventilation–perfusion ratio and a lower alveolar PO_2 of 60 mm Hg. The blood that circulates through this unit reaches a saturation of only 90%. Finally, unit *C* is not ventilated at all. Its alveolar PO_2 is equivalent to that of the venous blood, which travels through the unit unaltered. The oxygen saturation of the arterial blood reflects the weighted contributions of these 3 units. If it is assumed that each unit has the same blood flow, the arterial blood would have a saturation of only 88%. Ventilation–perfusion mismatch is the most common mechanism of arterial hypoxemia in lung disease. Supplemental oxygen increases the arterial PO_2 by raising the alveolar PO_2 in lung units that, like B, have a ventilation–perfusion ratio >0.

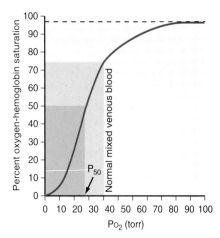

Fig. 400.5 Oxygen-hemoglobin dissociation curve. P_{50} of adult blood is around 27 torr. Under basal conditions, mixed venous blood has PO_2 of 40 torr and oxygen-hemoglobin saturation of 75%. In arterial blood, these values are 100 torr and 97.5%, respectively. Note that there is a steep decline in oxygen-hemoglobin saturation at PaO_2 <50 torr, but relatively little increase in saturation is gained at PO_2 >70 torr. *(Courtesy of Dr. Ashok Sarnaik.)*

sign of hypoxemia. Arterial hypertension, tachycardia, and diaphoresis are late, and not exclusive, signs of hypoventilation.

Blood gas exchange is evaluated most accurately by the direct measurement of arterial pressure of oxygen (PO_2), pressure of carbon dioxide (PCO_2), and pH. The blood specimen is best collected anaerobically in a heparinized syringe containing only enough heparin solution to displace the air from the syringe. The syringe should be sealed, placed in ice, and analyzed immediately. Although these measurements have no substitute in many conditions, they require arterial puncture and have been replaced to a great extent by noninvasive monitoring, such as capillary samples and/or oxygen saturation.

The age and clinical condition of the patient need to be taken into account when interpreting blood gas tensions. With the exception of

neonates, values of arterial PO_2 <85 mm Hg are usually abnormal for a child breathing room air at sea level. Calculation of the alveolar–arterial oxygen gradient is useful in the analysis of arterial oxygenation, particularly when the patient is not breathing room air or in the presence of hypercarbia. Values of arterial PCO_2 >45 mm Hg usually indicate hypoventilation or a severe ventilation–perfusion mismatch, unless they reflect respiratory compensation for metabolic alkalosis (see Chapter 68).

TRANSILLUMINATION OF THE CHEST
In infants up to at least 6 mo of age, a pneumothorax (see Chapter 122.14) can often be diagnosed by transilluminating the chest wall using a fiberoptic light probe. Free air in the pleural space often results in an unusually large halo of light in the skin surrounding the probe. Comparison with the contralateral chest is often very helpful in interpreting findings. This test is unreliable in older patients and in those with subcutaneous emphysema or atelectasis.

RADIOGRAPHIC TECHNIQUES
Chest X-Rays
A posteroanterior and a lateral view (upright and in full inspiration) should be obtained, except in situations in which the child is medically unstable (Fig. 400.6). Portable images although useful in the latter situation, can give a somewhat distorted image. Expiratory images can be misinterpreted, although a comparison of expiratory and inspiratory images may be useful in evaluating a child with a suspected foreign

Table 400.3	Interpretation of Arterial Blood Gas Values	
LESION	**EFFECT**	**TYPICAL ABG**
Central (above the carina) airway obstruction, or Depressed respiratory center, or Ineffective neuromuscular function	Uniform alveolar hypoventilation	Early increase in PCO_2. Proportionate decrease in PO_2 depending on alveolar air equation Response to supplemental oxygen: Excellent
Intrapulmonary airway obstruction	Venous admixture mismatch	Mild: ↓ PCO_2, ↓ PO_2. Moderate: "normal" PCO_2, ↓↓ PO_2. Severe: ↑↑ PCO_2, ↓↓↓ PO_2. Response to supplemental oxygen: good
Alveolar–interstitial pathology	Diffusion defect R → L shunt	Early decrease in PO_2 depending on severity Normal or low PCO_2, ↑ PCO_2 if fatigue develops Response to supplemental oxygen: fair to poor

ABG, Arterial blood gas.
(Courtesy of Dr. Ashok Sarnaik.)

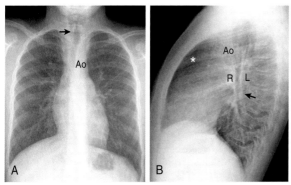

Fig. 400.6 Normal appearance of the trachea and lungs on chest radiography. **A,** On the frontal view, there is normal shouldering of the subglottic trachea *(arrow)*. The trachea courses inferiorly with a fairly uniform diameter to the level of the carina apart from a mild, smooth indentation at the level of the aortic arch *(Ao)*. The lungs are symmetrically inflated, with normal arborization of the vasculature. The hemidiaphragms are domed, not flattened. The normal heart size is less than 50% the transverse dimension of the chest. **B,** On the lateral view, the trachea is of uniform diameter to the level of the aortic arch, with the exception of a mild, smooth impression from the aortic arch anteriorly *(Ao)*. The hemidiaphragms are domed. The heart occupies less than 50% of the anteroposterior dimension of the chest and should not fill the retrosternal clear space *(asterisk)*. The bronchus intermedius *(arrow)* courses posterior to the right pulmonary artery *(R)*, and the arch of the left pulmonary artery *(L)* projects posterior to the carina. *(From Walters MM, Robertson RL, editors: Pediatric radiology—The requisites, ed 4, Philadelphia, 2017, Elsevier [Fig. 2.11].)*

body (localized failure of the lung to empty reflects bronchial obstruction: Chapter 414). Although images taken in a recumbent position are difficult to interpret when there is fluid within the pleural space or a cavity, if pleural fluid is suspected (see Chapter 429), decubitus images are indicated.

Upper Airway Film
A lateral view of the neck can yield invaluable information about upper airway obstruction (see Chapter 412) and particularly about the condition of the retropharyngeal, supraglottic, and subglottic spaces (which should also be viewed in an anteroposterior projection) (Fig. 400.7). Knowing the phase of respiration during which the film was taken is often essential for accurate interpretation. Magnified airway images are often helpful

in delineating the upper airways. Patients with suggested obstruction should not be unattended in the radiology department.

Sinus and Nasal Images
The general utility of radiologic examination of the sinuses is uncertain because a large number of images have positive findings (low sensitivity and specificity). Imaging studies are not necessary to confirm the diagnosis of sinusitis in children younger than age 6 yr. CT scans are indicated if surgery is required, in cases of complications caused by sinus infection, in immunodeficient patients, and for recurrent infections that are not responsive to medical management.

Chest Computed Tomography and Magnetic Resonance Imaging
Chest CT and MRI can potentially provide images of higher quality and sensitivity than is possible with other imaging modalities. Chest CT identifies early abnormalities in young children with cystic fibrosis before pathologic changes are detectable by either plain chest radiographs or pulmonary function testing. However, several caveats must be noted. Conventional chest CT involves considerably higher radiation doses than plain images (see Chapter 736). The time required to perform chest CT examinations and the complications of respiratory and body motion mandates the use of sedation for this procedure in many infants and young children. However, improvements in imaging hardware and software have drastically reduced required radiation doses as well as imaging time, obviating the need for sedation in many patients. Chest CT is particularly useful in evaluating very small lesions (e.g., early metastases, mediastinal and pleural lesions, solid or cystic parenchymal lesions, pulmonary embolism, and bronchiectasis). The use of intravenous contrast material during CT imaging enhances vascular structures, distinguishing vessels from other soft-tissue densities. MRI does not involve ionizing radiation, but long imaging times are still involved, and sedation will be necessary to limit spontaneous movement. The utility of MRI of the chest is largely limited to the analysis of mediastinal, hilar, and vascular anatomy. Parenchymal structures and lesions are not well evaluated by MRI.

Fluoroscopy
Fluoroscopy is especially useful for evaluating stridor and abnormal movement of the diaphragm or mediastinum. Many procedures, such as needle aspiration or biopsy of a peripheral lesion, are also best accomplished with the aid of fluoroscopy, CT, or ultrasonography. Videotape recording, which does not increase radiation exposure, can allow detailed study during a brief exposure to fluoroscopy, through its replay capabilities.

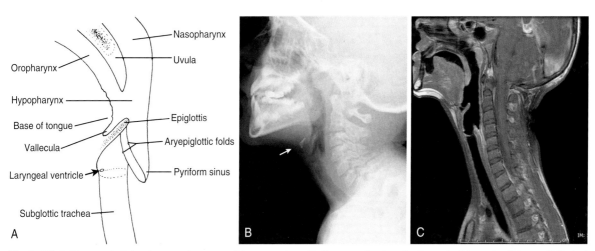

Fig. 400.7 A, Diagram depicting the normal anatomy of the upper airway. **B,** Corresponding lateral radiograph of the neck soft tissues. **C,** Sagittal T1-weighted magnetic resonance image. The hyoid bone "points to" the epiglottis on the radiograph *(arrow)*. *(From Walters MM, Robertson RL editors: Pediatric radiology—The requisites, ed 4, Philadelphia, 2017, Elsevier [Fig. 2.5].)*

Barium Swallow

A barium swallow study, performed with fluoroscopy and spot images is indicated in the evaluation of patients with recurrent pneumonia, persistent cough of undetermined cause, stridor, or persistent wheezing. The technique can be modified by using barium of different textures and thicknesses, ranging from thin liquid to solids, to evaluate swallowing mechanics, the presence of vascular rings (see Chapter 413), and tracheoesophageal fistulas (see Chapter 345), especially when aspiration is suspected. A contrast esophagram has been used in evaluating newborns with suggested esophageal atresia, but this procedure entails a high risk of pulmonary aspiration and is not usually recommended. Barium swallows are useful in evaluating suggested gastroesophageal reflux (see Chapter 349), but because of the high incidence of asymptomatic reflux in infants, the applicability of the findings to the clinical problem may be complicated.

Pulmonary Arteriography and Aortograms
Pulmonary arteriography has been used to allow detailed evaluation of the pulmonary vasculature. This imaging technique has also been helpful in assessing pulmonary blood flow and in diagnosing congenital anomalies, such as lobar agenesis, unilateral hyperlucent lung, vascular rings, and arteriovenous malformations. In addition, pulmonary arteriography is sometimes useful in evaluating solid or cystic lesions. Thoracic aortograms demonstrate the aortic arch, its major vessels, and the systemic (bronchial) pulmonary circulation. They are useful in evaluating vascular rings and suspected pulmonary sequestration. Although most hemoptysis is from the bronchial arteries, bronchial arteriography is seldom helpful in diagnosing or treating intrapulmonary bleeding in children. Real-time and Doppler echocardiography, as well as thoracic CT with contrast, are 2 noninvasive methods that often reveal similar information; therefore arteriography is now rarely performed.

Ventilation-Perfusion Relation and Radionuclide Lung Scans
Gravitational force pulls the lung away from the nondependent part of the parietal pleura. Consequently, alveoli and airways in the nondependent parts (the upper lobes in upright position) of the lung are subjected to greater negative intrapleural pressure during tidal respiration and are kept relatively more inflated compared with the dependent alveoli and airways (the lower lobes in upright position). The nondependent alveoli are less compliant because they are already more inflated. Ventilation therefore occurs preferentially in the dependent portions of the lung that are more amenable to expansion during tidal inspiration. Although perfusion is also greater in the dependent portions of the lung because of greater pulmonary arterial hydrostatic pressure from gravity, the increase in perfusion is greater than the increase in ventilation

in the dependent portions of the lung. Thus the ratios favor ventilation in the nondependent portions and perfusion in the dependent portions. Because the airways in the dependent portion of the lung are narrower, they close earlier during expiration. The lung volume at which the dependent airways start to close is referred to as the **closing capacity**. In normal children, the FRC is greater than the closing capacity. During tidal respiration, airways remain patent both in the dependent and the nondependent portions of the lung. In newborns, the closing capacity is greater than the FRC, resulting in perfusion of poorly ventilated alveoli during tidal respiration. Therefore, normal neonates have a lower PaO_2 compared with older children.

The relationship is adversely affected in a variety of pathophysiologic states. Air movement in areas that are poorly perfused is referred to as **dead space ventilation**. Examples of dead space ventilation include pulmonary thromboembolism and hypovolemia. Perfusion of poorly ventilated alveoli is referred to as **intrapulmonary right-to-left shunting** or **venous admixture**. Examples include pneumonia, asthma, and hyaline membrane disease. In intrapulmonary airway obstruction, the closing capacity is abnormally increased and can exceed the FRC. In such situations, perfusion of poorly ventilated alveoli during tidal respiration results in venous admixture.

The usual scan uses intravenous injection of material (macroaggregated human serum albumin labeled with ^{99m}Tc) that will be trapped in the pulmonary capillary bed. The distribution of radioactivity, proportional to pulmonary capillary blood flow, is useful in evaluating pulmonary embolism, as well as congenital cardiovascular and pulmonary defects. Acute changes in the distribution of pulmonary perfusion can reflect alterations of pulmonary ventilation.

The distribution of pulmonary ventilation can also be determined by scanning after the patient inhales a radioactive gas such as xenon-133. After the intravenous injection of xenon-133 dissolved in saline, pulmonary perfusion and ventilation can be evaluated by continuous recording of the rate of appearance and disappearance of the xenon over the lung. Appearance of xenon early after injection is a measure of perfusion, and the rate of washout during breathing is a measure of ventilation in the pediatric population. The most important indication for this test is the demonstration of defects in the pulmonary arterial distribution that can occur with congenital malformations or pulmonary embolism. **Spiral reconstruction CT** with contrast medium enhancement is very helpful in evaluating pulmonary thrombi and emboli. Abnormalities in regional ventilation are also easily demonstrable in congenital lobar emphysema, cystic fibrosis, and asthma.

PULMONARY FUNCTION TESTING
Traditionally, lung volumes are measured with a spirogram (Fig. 400.8). **Tidal volume (V_T)** is the amount of air moved in and out of the lungs during each breath; at rest, V_T is normally 6-7 mL/kg body weight.

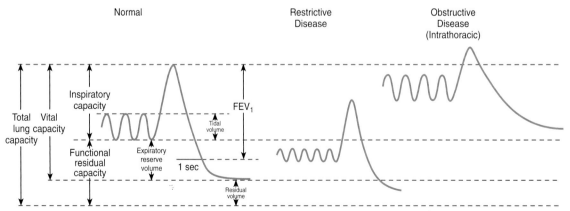

Fig. 400.8 Spirogram showing lung volumes and capacities. Forced expiratory volume 1 (*FEV₁*) is the maximum volume exhaled in 1 sec after maximum inspiration. Restrictive diseases are usually associated with decreased lung volumes and capacities. Intrathoracic airway obstruction is associated with air trapping and abnormally high functional residual capacity and residual volume. FEV₁ and vital capacity are decreased in both restrictive and obstructive diseases. The ratio of FEV₁ to vital capacity is normal in restrictive disease but decreased in obstructive disease.

Inspiratory capacity is the amount of air inspired by maximum inspiratory effort after tidal expiration. **Expiratory reserve volume** is the amount of air exhaled by maximum expiratory effort after tidal expiration. The volume of gas remaining in the lungs after maximum expiration is **residual volume. Vital capacity (VC)** is defined as the amount of air moved in and out of the lungs through maximum inspiration and expiration. VC, inspiratory capacity, and expiratory reserve volume are decreased in lung pathology but are also effort dependent. **Total lung capacity (TLC)** is the volume of gas occupying the lungs after maximum inhalation.

The **flow volume relationship** offers a valuable means at the bedside or in an office setting to detect abnormal pulmonary mechanics and response to therapy with relatively inexpensive and easy-to-use devices. After maximum inhalation, the patient forcefully exhales through a mouthpiece into the device until residual volume is reached, followed by maximum inhalation (Fig. 400.9). Flow is plotted against volume. **Maximum forced expiratory flow (FEF$_{max}$)** is generated in the early part of exhalation, and it is a commonly used indicator of airway obstruction in asthma and other obstructive lesions. Provided maximum pressure is generated consistently during exhalation, a decrease in flow is a reflection of increased airway resistance (R$_{AW}$). The total volume exhaled during this maneuver is **forced vital capacity (FVC). Volume exhaled in 1 sec** is referred to as **forced expiratory volume 1 (FEV$_1$).** FEV$_1$/FVC is expressed as a percentage of FVC. FEF$_{25-75\%}$ is the mean flow between 25% and 75% of FVC, and is considered relatively effort independent. Individual values and shapes of flow-volume curves show characteristic changes in obstructive and restrictive respiratory disorders (Fig. 400.10). In intrapulmonary airway obstruction such as asthma or cystic fibrosis, there is a reduction of FEF$_{max}$, FEF$_{25-75\%}$, FVC, and FEV$_1$/FVC. Also, there is a characteristic concavity in the middle part of the expiratory curve. In restrictive lung disease such as interstitial pneumonia (see Chapter 327.5) and kyphoscoliosis (see Chapter 445.5), FVC is decreased with relative preservation of airflow and FEV$_1$/FVC. The flow volume curve assumes a vertically oblong shape compared with normal. Changes in shape of the flow volume loop and individual values depend on the type of disease and the extent of severity. Serial determinations provide valuable information regarding disease evolution and response to therapy.

FRC has important pathophysiologic implications. Chest wall compliance is a major determinant of FRC. Because the chest wall and the lungs recoil in opposite directions at rest, FRC is reached at the point where the outward elastic recoil of the thoracic cage counterbalances the inward lung recoil. This balance is attained at a lower lung volume in a young infant's ribs because they are oriented much more horizontally and the diaphragm is flatter and less domed. Consequently, the infant is unable to duplicate the efficiency of upward and outward movement of obliquely oriented ribs or the downward displacement of a domed diaphragm in an adult to expand the thoracic capacity. This creates an extremely high thoracic compliance compared with older children and adults (Fig. 400.11). The measured FRC in infants is higher than expected because infant respiratory muscles maintain the thoracic cage in an inspiratory position at all times. In addition, young infants experience some amount of air trapping during expiration.

Alveolar gas composition changes during inspiration and expiration. **Alveolar PO$_2$ (PAO$_2$)** increases and **alveolar PCO$_2$ (PACO$_2$)** decreases during inspiration as fresh atmospheric gas enters the lungs. During exhalation, PAO$_2$ decreases and PACO$_2$ increases as pulmonary capillary blood continues to remove oxygen from and add CO$_2$ into the alveoli (Fig. 400.12). FRC acts as a buffer, minimizing the changes in PAO$_2$ and PACO$_2$ during inspiration and expiration. FRC represents the environment available for pulmonary capillary blood for gas exchange at all times.

A decrease in FRC is often encountered in alveolar interstitial diseases and thoracic deformities. The major pathophysiologic consequence of decreased FRC is **hypoxemia**. Reduced FRC results in a sharp decline in PAO$_2$ during exhalation because a limited volume is available for gas exchange. PO$_2$ of pulmonary capillary blood therefore falls excessively during exhalation, leading to a decline in **arterial PO$_2$ (PaO$_2$).** Any increase in PAO$_2$ (and therefore PaO$_2$) during inspiration cannot

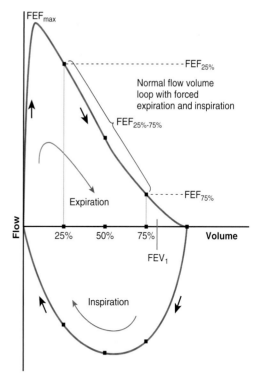

Fig. 400.9 Flow volume loop in a normal person performed after maximal inspiration followed by forced complete expiration and forced complete inhalation. Maximum expiratory flow *(FEF$_{max}$)* represents maximum flow during expiration. This is attained soon after initiation of the expiration. Fall in expiratory flow is gradual until it reaches zero after exhalation is complete. FEF$_{25-75\%}$ represents mean flow from 25% (FEF$_{25\%}$) to 75% (FEF$_{75\%}$) of exhaled forced expiratory volume *(FEV)*, also termed *forced vital capacity* (FVC). FEV$_1$ is amount of volume after 1 sec of forced exhalation. Normally FEV$_1$ is around 80% of FVC. *(Courtesy of Dr. Ashok Sarnaik.)*

compensate for the decreased PaO$_2$ during expiration. The explanation for this lies in the shape of O$_2$-Hb dissociation curve, which is sigmoid shaped (see Fig. 400.5). Because most of the oxygen in blood is combined with Hb, it is the percentage of **oxyhemoglobin (SO$_2$)** that gets averaged rather than the PO$_2$. Although an increase in arterial PO$_2$ cannot increase O$_2$-Hb saturation >100%, there is a steep desaturation of Hb below a PO$_2$ of 50 torr; thus decreased SO$_2$ during exhalation as a result of low FRC leads to overall arterial desaturation and hypoxemia. The adverse pathophysiologic consequences of decreased FRC are ameliorated by applying **positive end-expiratory pressure (PEEP)** and increasing the inspiratory time during mechanical ventilation.

The lung pressure–volume relationship is markedly influenced by FRC (Fig. 400.13). Pulmonary compliance is decreased at abnormally low or high FRC.

FRC is abnormally increased in intrathoracic airway obstruction, which results in incomplete exhalation, and abnormally decreased in alveolar-interstitial diseases. At excessively low or high FRC, tidal respiration requires higher inflation pressures compared to normal FRC. Abnormalities of FRC result in increased work of breathing with spontaneous respiration and increased barotrauma in mechanical ventilation.

The measurement of respiratory function in infants and young children can be difficult because of the lack of cooperation. Attempts have been made to overcome this limitation by creating standard tests that do not require the patient's active participation. Respiratory function tests still provide only a partial insight into the mechanisms of respiratory disease at early ages.

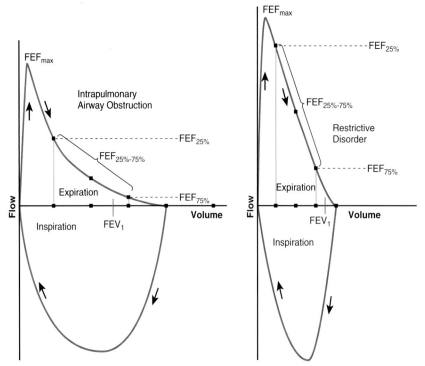

Fig. 400.10 Flow volume loops in intrapulmonary airway obstruction and restrictive disorders. Note that in intrapulmonary airway obstruction, there is a decrease in maximum forced expiratory flow (*FEF*$_{max}$), FEF$_{25-75\%}$, and forced expiratory volume 1/forced vital capacity (*FEV*$_1$/FVC%). The middle part of expiratory loop appears concave. In restrictive disorder, the flow volume loop assumes a more vertically oblong shape with reduction in FVC but not the FEV$_1$/FVC%. Expiratory and inspiratory flow rates are relatively unaffected. *(Courtesy of Dr. Ashok Sarnaik.)*

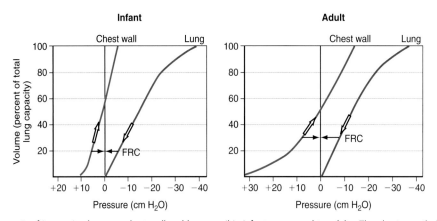

Fig. 400.11 Schematic of interaction between chest wall and lung recoil in infants compared to adults. The elastic recoil of a relatively more compliant chest wall is balanced by the lung recoil at a lower volume functional residual capacity (*FRC*) in infants compared to adults. *(Courtesy of Dr. Ashok Sarnaik.)*

Whether restrictive or obstructive, most forms of respiratory disease cause alterations in lung volume and its subdivisions. Restrictive diseases typically decrease **TLC**. TLC includes residual volume, which is not accessible to direct determinations. It must therefore be measured indirectly by gas dilution methods or, preferably, by **plethysmography**. Restrictive disease also decreases **VC**. Obstructive diseases produce gas trapping and thus increase residual volume and FRC, particularly when these measurements are considered with respect to TLC.

Airway obstruction is most commonly evaluated from determinations of gas flow in the course of a forced expiratory maneuver. The **peak expiratory flow** is reduced in advanced obstructive disease. The wide availability of simple devices that perform this measurement at the bedside makes it useful for assessing children who have airway obstruction. Evaluation of peak flows requires a voluntary effort, and peak flows may not be altered when the obstruction is moderate or mild. Other gas flow measurements require that the child inhale to TLC and then exhale as far and as fast as possible for several seconds. Cooperation and good muscle strength are therefore necessary for the measurements to be reproducible. FEV$_1$ correlates well with the severity of obstructive diseases. The **maximal midexpiratory flow rate**, the average flow during the middle 50% of the forced VC, is a more reliable indicator of mild airway obstruction. Its sensitivity to changes in residual volume and VC, however, limits its use in children with more severe disease. The construction of flow-volume relationships during the forced VC maneuvers overcomes some of these limitations by expressing expiratory flows as a function of lung volume.

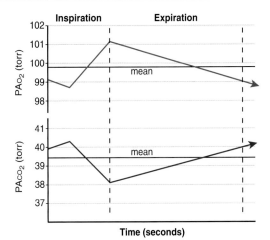

Fig. 400.12 Alveolar PO_2 rises and PCO_2 falls during inspiration as fresh atmospheric gas is brought into the lungs. During expiration, the opposite changes occur as pulmonary capillary blood continues to remove O_2 and add CO_2 from the alveoli without atmospheric enrichment. Note that during the early part of inspiration, alveolar PO_2 continues to fall and PCO_2 continues to rise because of inspiration of the dead space that is occupied by the previously exhaled gas. *(Modified from Comroe JH:* Physiology of respiration, *ed 2, Chicago, 1974, Year Book Medical Publishers, p 12.). (Courtesy of Dr. Ashok Sarnaik.)*

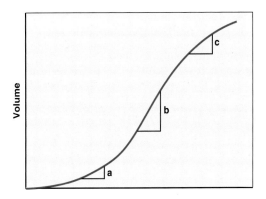

Fig. 400.13 Lung compliance is significantly influenced by the functional residual capacity (FRC). The same change in pressure is associated with less change in volume when FRC is abnormally decreased *(a)* or abnormally increased *(c)* compared to the normal state *(b)*. *(Courtesy of Dr. Ashok Sarnaik.)*

A **spirometer** is used to measure VC and its subdivisions and expiratory (or inspiratory) flow rates (see Fig. 400.8). A simple manometer can measure the maximal inspiratory and expiratory force a subject generates, normally at least 30 cm H_2O. This is useful in evaluating the neuromuscular component of ventilation. Expected normal values for VC, FRC, TLC, and residual volume are obtained from prediction equations based on body height.

Flow rates measured by spirometry usually include the FEV_1 and the **maximal midexpiratory flow rate**. More information results from a maximal expiratory flow-volume curve, in which expiratory flow rate is plotted against expired lung volume (expressed in terms of either VC or TLC). Flow rates at lung volumes less than approximately 75% VC are relatively independent of effort. Expiratory flow rates at low lung volumes (<50% VC) are influenced much more by small airways than flow rates at high lung volumes (FEV_1). The flow rate at 25% VC is a useful index of small airway function. Low flow rates at high lung

volumes associated with normal flow at low lung volumes suggest upper airway obstruction.

Airway resistance (R_{AW}) is measured in a plethysmograph, or alternatively, the reciprocal of R_{AW}, **airway conductance**, may be used. Because R_{AW} measurements vary with the lung volume at which they are taken, it is convenient to use **specific airway resistance**, SR_{AW} (SR_{AW} = R_{AW}/lung volume), which is nearly constant in subjects older than age 6 yr (normally <7 sec/cm H_2O).

The **diffusing capacity for carbon monoxide** is related to oxygen diffusion and is measured by rebreathing from a container having a known initial concentration of carbon monoxide or by using a single-breath technique. Decreases in diffusing capacity for carbon monoxide reflect decreases in effective alveolar capillary surface area or decreases in diffusibility of the gas across the alveolar-capillary membrane. Primary diffusion abnormalities are unusual in children; therefore, this test is most commonly employed in children with rheumatologic or autoimmune diseases and in children exposed to toxic drugs to the lungs (e.g., oncology patients) or chest wall radiation. Regional gas exchange can be conveniently estimated with the perfusion-ventilation xenon scan. Determining arterial blood gas levels also discloses the effectiveness of alveolar gas exchange.

Pulmonary function testing, although rarely resulting in a diagnosis, is helpful in defining the type of process (obstruction, restriction) and the degree of functional impairment, in following the course and treatment of disease, and in estimating the prognosis. It is also useful in preoperative evaluation and in confirmation of functional impairment in patients having subjective complaints but a normal physical examination. In most patients with obstructive disease, a repeat test after administering a bronchodilator is warranted.

Most tests require some cooperation and understanding by the patient. Interpretation is greatly facilitated if the test conditions and the patient's behavior during the test are known. Infants and young children who cannot or will not cooperate with test procedures can be studied in a limited number of ways, which often require sedation. Flow rates and pressures during tidal breathing, with or without transient interruption of the flow, may be useful to assess some aspects of R_{AW} or obstruction and to measure compliance of the lungs and thorax. Expiratory flow rates can be studied in sedated infants with passive compression of the chest and abdomen using a rapidly inflatable jacket. Gas dilution or plethysmographic methods can also be used in sedated infants to measure FRC and R_{AW}.

The measurement of **fractional exhaled nitric oxide** (FENO) is used as a surrogate measure for eosinophilic inflammation of the lower airways. It can be used as a part of a diagnostic evaluation for asthma, a tool for predicting or assessing an individual's response to antiinflammatory therapy, and in monitoring adherence to treatment. There are a number of commercially available devices for measurement of FENO. Some degree of cooperation is required, but FENO has been measured in preschool-aged children. Normal cutoff values vary by age and device. FENO has been used to distinguish asthma (particularly allergic asthma) from other wheezing phenotypes. FENO achieves moderate diagnostic performance for the detection of asthma in children, with sensitivity, specificity, and diagnostic odds ratios of 0.79, 0.81, and 16.52, respectively. Children managed using FENO may have fewer asthma exacerbations. A decrease of FENO by 20% is considered indicative of a positive response to antiinflammatory therapy. Some studies using FENO have contradictory results, and it is likely that FENO may be more useful in some asthma phenotypes than others.

The measurement of **nasal nitric oxide** (nNO) is accomplished by collecting exhaled gas from a nostril during glottic closure, and correlates to nasal mucosal inflammation. There is a great deal of interest in use of nNO to diagnose **primary ciliary dyskinesia** (PCD, see Chapter 404), because of challenges diagnosing PCD with currently available techniques. A cutoff value of less than or equal to 77 nL/min showed excellent sensitivity and specificity using a standardized technique at multiple centers. The sensitivity and specificity of 0.95 and 0.94 is excellent. Equipment for measurement of nNO is not yet FDA-approved in the USA.

MICROBIOLOGY: EXAMINATION OF LUNG SECRETIONS

The specific diagnosis of infection in the lower respiratory tract depends on the proper handling of an adequate specimen obtained in an appropriate fashion. Nasopharyngeal or throat cultures are often used but might not correlate with cultures obtained by more direct techniques from the lower airways. Sputum specimens are preferred and are often obtained from patients who do not expectorate by deep throat swab immediately after coughing or by saline nebulization. Specimens can also be obtained directly from the tracheobronchial tree by nasotracheal aspiration (usually heavily contaminated), by transtracheal aspiration through the cricothyroid membrane (useful in adults and adolescents but hazardous in children), and in infants and children by a sterile catheter inserted into the trachea either during direct laryngoscopy or through a freshly inserted endotracheal tube. A specimen can also be obtained at bronchoscopy. A percutaneous lung tap or an open biopsy is the only way to obtain a specimen absolutely free of oral flora.

A specimen obtained by direct expectoration is usually assumed to be of tracheobronchial origin, but often, especially in children, it is not from this source. The presence of alveolar macrophages (large mononuclear cells) is the hallmark of tracheobronchial secretions. Nasopharyngeal and tracheobronchial secretions can contain ciliated epithelial cells, which are more commonly found in sputum. Nasopharyngeal and oral secretions often contain large numbers of squamous epithelial cells. Sputum can contain both ciliated and squamous epithelial cells.

During sleep, mucociliary transport continually brings tracheobronchial secretions to the pharynx, where they are swallowed. An early-morning fasting gastric aspirate often contains material from the tracheobronchial tract that is suitable for culture for acid-fast bacilli.

The absence of polymorphonuclear leukocytes in a Wright-stained smear of sputum or **bronchoalveolar lavage** (BAL) fluid containing adequate numbers of macrophages may be significant evidence against a bacterial infectious process in the lower respiratory tract, assuming that the patient has normal neutrophil counts and function. Eosinophils suggest allergic disease. Iron stains can reveal hemosiderin granules within macrophages, suggesting pulmonary hemosiderosis. Specimens should also be examined by Gram stain. Bacteria within or near macrophages and neutrophils can be significant. Viral pneumonia may be accompanied by intranuclear or cytoplasmic inclusion bodies visible on Wright-stained smears, and fungal forms may be identifiable on Gram or silver stains.

With advances in the area of genomics and the speed with which it is possible to identify microbes, microbiologic analysis has been expanded. Specific bacteria in the lungs of children with cystic fibrosis (see Chapter 432) are linked to morbidity and mortality. There is a correlation between patient age and morbidity and mortality (as expected), but that there are important microbes that are correlated either negatively or positively with early or late pathogenic processes. *Haemophilus influenzae* (see Chapter 221) is negatively correlated, and *Pseudomonas aeruginosa* and *Stenotrophomonas maltophilia* (see Chapter 232.3) have a strong positive correlation with patient age in cystic fibrosis. The microbiota diversity is much broader in those who are healthier individuals or those who are younger patients with cystic fibrosis than the older and sicker population.

In addition, the microbiomes (see Chapter 196) in the respiratory tract of smokers and nonsmokers differ substantially. In all patients, most of the bacteria found in the lungs are also present in the oral cavity, but some bacteria, such as *Haemophilus* and enterobacteria, are much more represented in the lungs than in the mouth. Principal differences in microbiome composition between smokers and nonsmokers are found in the mouth. For example, *Neisseria* levels are much lower in smokers as compared with nonsmokers.

THE MICROBIOME (see Chapter 196)
Exercise Testing
Exercise testing (see Chapter 450.5) is a more-direct approach for detecting diffusion impairment and other forms of respiratory disease. Exercise is a strong provocateur of bronchospasm in susceptible patients, so exercise testing can be useful in the diagnosis of patients with asthma

that is only apparent with activity. Measurements of heart and respiratory rate, minute ventilation, oxygen consumption, carbon dioxide production, and arterial blood gases during incremental exercise loads often provide invaluable information about the functional nature of the disease. Often a simple assessment of the patient's exercise tolerance in conjunction with other, more static forms of respiratory function testing can allow a distinction between respiratory and nonrespiratory disease in children.

Sleep Studies
See Chapter 31.

AIRWAY VISUALIZATION AND LUNG SPECIMEN–BASED DIAGNOSTIC TESTS
Laryngoscopy
The evaluation of stridor, problems with vocalization, and other upper airway abnormalities usually requires direct inspection. Although indirect (mirror) laryngoscopy may be reasonable in older children and adults, it is rarely feasible in infants and small children. Direct laryngoscopy may be performed with either a rigid or a flexible instrument. The safe use of the rigid scope for examining the upper airway requires topical anesthesia and either sedation or general anesthesia, whereas the flexible laryngoscope can often be used in the office setting with or without sedation. Further advantages to the flexible scope include the ability to assess the airway without the distortion that may be introduced by the use of the rigid scope and the ability to assess airway dynamics more accurately. Because there is a relatively high incidence of concomitant lesions in the upper and lower airways, it is often prudent to examine the airways above and below the glottis, even when the primary indication is in the upper airway (stridor).

Bronchoscopy and Bronchoalveolar Lavage
Bronchoscopy is the inspection of the airways. Flexible bronchoscopy is commonly used in pediatrics to visualize the airways. There are several sizes of scopes that enable visualization of the proximal and distal airways. Many fiberoptic bronchoscopes also have a channel that allows for the collection of fluids, or in larger scopes allows for the insertion of tools such as forceps, baskets, or brushes. The smallest scope is a 2.2 mm outer diameter bronchoscope that does not have a channel; therefore only visualization of the airways is possible. The smallest bronchoscope with a channel is a 2.8 mm outer diameter scope, which has a 1.2 mm working channel. This scope is commonly used in pediatrics and is predominately used to visualize the airways and to collect a lavage sample. In larger "adult" scopes (4.9-5.5 mm outer diameter and 2.0 mm working channel), small instruments such as forceps can be inserted. Therapeutic bronchoscopes require an even larger channel (2.8 mm working channel, which requires a larger outer diameter of 6.0-6.3 mm), so they are not used often in the pediatric population. A smaller scope (4.1 mm outer diameter) with a larger working channel (2.0 mm) has become available and may make interventional pediatric bronchoscopy more common in the future.

Visualization of the airway has improved through new advances in optics and insertable tools. **Narrow-band imaging** and **autofluorescence** imaging bronchoscopes are 2 types of bronchoscopes that can aid in the detection of airway lesions. These scopes appear no different than the conventional bronchoscope but utilize different bandwidths of lights to highlight mucosal and submucosal vasculature. These bronchoscopes allow the operator to see airway mucosal lesions that would be difficult or not seen under normal white light. The autofluorescence imaging bronchoscope uses the fluorophores, such as tryptophan, collagen, elastin and porphyrins, within the airway tissue to emit fluorescence when irradiated with a light source. Changes in concentrations of the fluorophores in bronchial mucosa would appear as an irregular lesion when viewed with an autofluorescence imaging bronchoscope. The narrow-band imaging bronchoscope also uses light absorption characteristics of Hb to enhance images of blood vessels. This bronchoscope uses blue wavelengths in the range of 390-445 nm to visualize the mucosal layer capillaries and green wavelengths at 530 and 550 nm to detect deeper submucosal thick blood vessels. Both types of bronchoscopes allow the operator to detect findings that would not be seen under normal white light. These scopes are being used more often in adults where lesions are biopsied to detect premalignant and malignant lesions. These scopes are noninvasive and would be well tolerated in children, but are currently only available in larger "adult" sizes.

The **EBUS, endobronchial ultrasound**, is a scope that allows ultrasound images to be captured from the tip of the scope and also contains a working channel to collect a needle biopsy. This technology is particularly useful in the evaluation of mediastinal lymph nodes. This scope may be useful in the diagnosis of other conditions such as sarcoidosis, tuberculosis, and the staging of lung cancers. The EBUS is currently being investigated in older pediatric patients as an alternative to CT-guided transthoracic fine needle aspiration for the evaluation of mediastinal lymph nodes. EBUS has the benefit of no radiation, but has not been extensively studied in pediatrics.

Bronchial thermoplasty (BT) is a technology that can be used to treat patients with severe asthma. This technique uses the working channel of a fiberoptic bronchoscope to deliver targeted thermal energy to the airways to ablate the airway smooth muscle (ASM). The ablation of ASM may reduce the ability to bronchoconstrict. It may also impact the ASM's role in immunomodulation, ultimately altering the pathophysiology of asthma. BT requires a minimum of a 2.0 mm working channel, which limits this technology to bronchoscopes of at least an outer diameter of 4.1 mm. In general, BT is performed over 3 bronchoscopy sessions to ablate different sections of the lung: right lower lobe, left lower lobe, and bilateral upper lobes. The right middle lobe is usually not ablated for the potential risk of stenosis. The treatments are divided into 3 separate procedures to allow for shorter procedure times (30-60 min per session) and decrease the risk of widespread irritation. Patients are also given oral steroids for 3 days prior to the procedure to decrease airway inflammation associated with the ablation procedure. While BT is gaining momentum in the treatment of severe asthma in the adult population, the long-term ramifications of airway smooth muscle ablation in a child are still unknown. In adult studies that investigated BT as a therapeutic tool for asthma, small studies demonstrated an improvement in clinical symptoms, and in a smaller cohort of patients (12 patients), no significant structural abnormalities were seen on chest radiographs 5 yr after the procedure.

The most common diagnostic tool used in conjunction with fiberoptic bronchoscopy is **bronchoalveolar lavage (BAL)**. BAL is a method used to obtain a representative specimen of fluid and secretions from the lower respiratory tract, which is useful for the cytologic and microbiologic diagnosis of lung diseases, especially in those who are unable to expectorate sputum. BAL is performed after the general inspection of the airways and before tissue sampling with a brush or biopsy forceps. It is accomplished by gently wedging the scope into a lobar, segmental, or subsegmental bronchus, and sequentially instilling and withdrawing sterile nonbacteriostatic saline in a volume sufficient to ensure that some of the aspirated fluid contains material that originated from the alveolar space. Nonbronchoscopic BAL can be performed in intubated patients by instilling and withdrawing saline through a catheter passed though the artificial airway and blindly wedged into a distal airway, although nonbronchoscopic BAL is less accurate and therefore has less-reliable results. In either case, the presence of alveolar macrophages documents that an alveolar sample has been obtained. Because the methods used to perform BAL involve passage of the equipment through the upper airway, there is a risk of contamination of the specimen by upper airway secretions. Careful cytologic examination and quantitative microbiologic cultures are important for correct interpretation of the data. BAL can often obviate the need for more-invasive procedures such as open lung biopsy, especially in immunocompromised patients.

Indications for diagnostic bronchoscopy and BAL include recurrent or persistent pneumonia or atelectasis, unexplained or localized and persistent wheeze, the suspected presence of a foreign body, hemoptysis, suspected congenital anomalies, mass lesions, interstitial disease, and pneumonia in the immunocompromised host. Indications for therapeutic bronchoscopy and BAL include bronchial obstruction by mass lesions, foreign bodies or mucus plugs, and general bronchial toilet and bronchopulmonary lavage. The patient undergoing bronchoscopy ventilates around the flexible scope, whereas with the rigid scope, ventilation is accomplished through the scope. Rigid bronchoscopy is preferentially indicated for extracting foreign bodies and removing tissue masses. It is also indicated in patients with massive hemoptysis. In other cases, the flexible scope has multiple advantages: it can be passed through endotracheal or tracheostomy tubes, can be introduced into bronchi that come off the airway at acute angles, and can be safely and effectively inserted with topical anesthesia and conscious sedation.

Regardless of the instrument used, the procedure performed, or the resulting indications, the most common complications are related to sedation. The relatively more common complications related to the bronchoscopy itself include transient hypoxemia, laryngospasm, bronchospasm, and cardiac arrhythmias. Iatrogenic infection, bleeding, pneumothorax, and pneumomediastinum are rare but reported complications of bronchoscopy or BAL. Bronchoscopy in the setting of possible pulmonary abscess or hemoptysis must be undertaken with advance preparations for definitive airway control, mindful of the possibility that pus or blood might flood the airway. Subglottic edema is a more common complication of rigid bronchoscopy than of flexible procedures, in which the scopes are smaller and less likely to traumatize the mucosa. Postbronchoscopy croup is treated with oxygen, mist, vasoconstrictor aerosols, and corticosteroids as necessary.

Thoracoscopy

The pleural cavity can be examined through a thoracoscope, which is similar to a rigid bronchoscope. The thoracoscope is inserted through an intercostal space and the lung is partially deflated, allowing the operator to view the surface of the lung, the pleural surface of the mediastinum and the diaphragm, and the parietal pleura. Multiple thoracoscopic instruments can be inserted, allowing endoscopic biopsy of the lung or pleura, resection of blebs, abrasion of the pleura, and ligation of vascular rings.

Thoracentesis

For diagnostic or therapeutic purposes, fluid can be removed from the pleural space by needle. In general, as much fluid as possible should be withdrawn, and an upright chest roentgenogram should be obtained after the procedure. Complications of thoracentesis include infection, pneumothorax, and bleeding. Thoracentesis on the right may be complicated by puncture or laceration of the capsule of the liver and, on the left, by puncture or laceration of the capsule of the spleen. Specimens obtained should always be cultured, examined microscopically for evidence of bacterial infection, and evaluated for total protein and total differential cell counts. Lactic acid dehydrogenase, glucose, cholesterol, triglyceride (chylous), and amylase determinations may also be useful. If malignancy is suspected, cytologic examination is imperative.

Transudates result from mechanical factors influencing the rate of formation or reabsorption of pleural fluid and generally require no further diagnostic evaluation. Exudates result from inflammation or other disease of the pleural surface and underlying lung, so they require a more complete diagnostic evaluation. In general, transudates have a total protein of <3 g/dL or a ratio of pleural protein to serum protein <0.5, a total leukocyte count of fewer than 2,000/mm³ with a predominance of mononuclear cells, and low lactate dehydrogenase levels. Exudates have high protein levels and a predominance of polymorphonuclear cells (although malignant or tuberculous effusions can have a higher percentage of mononuclear cells). Complicated exudates often require continuous chest tube drainage and have a pH <7.2. Tuberculous effusions can have low glucose and high cholesterol content.

Lung Tap

Using a technique similar to that used for thoracentesis, a percutaneous lung tap is the most direct method of obtaining bacteriologic specimens from the pulmonary parenchyma and is the only technique other than open lung biopsy not associated with at least some risk of contamination by oral flora. After local anesthesia, a needle attached to a syringe containing nonbacteriostatic sterile saline is inserted using aseptic technique through the inferior aspect of an intercostal space in the area of interest. The needle is rapidly advanced into the lung; the saline is injected and reaspirated, and the needle is withdrawn. These actions are performed as quickly as possible. This procedure usually yields a few drops of fluid from the lung, which should be cultured and examined microscopically.

Major indications for a lung tap are infiltrates of undetermined cause, especially those unresponsive to therapy in immunosuppressed patients who are susceptible to unusual organisms. Complications are the same as for thoracentesis, but the incidence of pneumothorax is higher and somewhat dependent on the nature of the underlying disease process. In patients with poor pulmonary compliance, such as children with *Pneumocystis* pneumonia, the rate can approach 30%, with 5% requiring chest tubes. Bronchopulmonary lavage has replaced lung taps for most purposes.

Lung Biopsy

Lung biopsy may be the only way to establish a diagnosis, especially in protracted, noninfectious disease. In infants and small children, thoracoscopic or open surgical biopsies are the procedures of choice, and in expert hands there is low morbidity. Biopsy through the 3.5 mm diameter pediatric bronchoscopes limits the sample size and diagnostic abilities. In addition to ensuring that an adequate specimen is obtained, the surgeon can inspect the lung surface and choose the site of biopsy. In older children, transbronchial biopsies can be performed using flexible forceps through a bronchoscope, an endotracheal tube, a rigid bronchoscope, or an endotracheal tube, usually with fluoroscopic guidance. This technique is most appropriately used when the disease is diffuse, as in the case of *Pneumocystis* pneumonia, or after rejection of a transplanted lung. The diagnostic limitations related to the small size of the biopsy specimens can be mitigated by the ability to obtain several samples. The risk of pneumothorax related to bronchoscopy is increased when transbronchial biopsies are part of the procedure; however, the ability to obtain biopsy specimens in a procedure performed with topical anesthesia and conscious sedation offers is advantageous.

Sweat Testing
See Chapter 432.

Portions of this chapter, written by Dr. Ashok Sarnaik, were carried over from the previous edition.

Bibliography is available at Expert Consult.

Chapter 401
Chronic or Recurrent Respiratory Symptoms

Anne G. Griffiths

第四百零一章
慢性或反复呼吸系统症状

中文导读

本章主要介绍了慢性呼吸系统疾病严重程度的判断、反复或持续性咳嗽、反复或持续性哮鸣、反复或持续性喘息以及反复和持续性肺浸润的诊治。反复或持续性咳嗽主要包括病因、体格检查、实验室及其他检查、痉挛性咳嗽或躯体性咳嗽障碍（心因性咳嗽或习惯性咳嗽）。反复或持续性哮鸣包括哮鸣的概念、伴随症状以及体格检查。反复或持续性喘息主要包括病因以及辅助检查。反复和持续性肺浸润主要包括慢性肺浸润、反复肺浸润以及相关的辅助检查。详细阐述了肺外疾病伴肺部表现，其中包括肺外疾病伴肺部表现的评估。

Respiratory tract symptoms, including cough, wheeze, and stridor, occur frequently or persist for long periods in a substantial number of children; other children have persistent or recurring lung infiltrates with or without symptoms. Determining the cause of these chronic findings can be difficult because symptoms can be caused by a close succession of unrelated acute respiratory tract infections or by a single pathophysiologic process. Specific and easily performed diagnostic tests do not exist for many acute and chronic respiratory conditions. Pressure from the affected child's family for a quick remedy because of concern over symptoms related to breathing may complicate diagnostic and therapeutic efforts.

A systematic approach to the diagnosis and treatment of these children consists of assessing whether the symptoms are the manifestation of a minor problem or a life-threatening process; determining the most likely underlying pathogenic mechanism; selecting the simplest effective therapy for the underlying process, which often is only symptomatic therapy; and carefully evaluating the effect of therapy. Failure of this approach to identify the process responsible or to effect improvement signals the need for more extensive and perhaps invasive diagnostic efforts, including bronchoscopy.

JUDGING THE SERIOUSNESS OF CHRONIC RESPIRATORY COMPLAINTS

Clinical manifestations suggesting that a respiratory tract illness may be life-threatening or associated with the potential for chronic disability are listed in Table 401.1. If none of these findings is detected, the chronic respiratory process is likely to be benign. Active, well-nourished, and appropriately growing infants who present with intermittent noisy breathing but no other physical or laboratory abnormalities require only symptomatic treatment and parental reassurance. Benign-appearing but persistent symptoms are occasionally the harbinger of a serious lower respiratory tract problem. By contrast, occasionally children (e.g., with infection-related asthma) have recurrent life-threatening episodes but few or no symptoms in the intervals. Repeated examinations over an extended period, both when the child appears healthy and when the child is symptomatic, may be helpful in sorting out the severity and chronicity of lung disease.

RECURRENT OR PERSISTENT COUGH

Cough is a reflex response of the lower respiratory tract to stimulation of irritant or cough receptors in the airways' mucosa. The most common cause of recurrent or persistent cough in children is airway reactivity (asthma). Because cough receptors also reside in the pharynx, paranasal sinuses, stomach, and external auditory canal, the source of a persistent cough may need to be sought beyond the lungs. Specific lower respiratory stimuli include excessive secretions, aspirated foreign material, inhaled dust particles or noxious gases, cold or dry air, and an inflammatory response to infectious agents or allergic processes. Table 401.2 lists some of the conditions responsible for chronic cough. Table 401.3 presents characteristics of cough that can aid in distinguishing a cough's origin. Additional useful information can include a history of atopic conditions (asthma, eczema, urticaria, allergic rhinitis), a seasonal or environmental variation in frequency or intensity of cough, and a strong family history of atopic conditions, all suggesting an allergic cause; symptoms of malabsorption or family history indicating cystic fibrosis; symptoms related to feeding, suggesting aspiration or gastroesophageal reflux; a choking episode, suggesting foreign-body aspiration; headache or facial edema associated with sinusitis; and a smoking history in older children and adolescents or the presence of a smoker in the home (Table 401.4).

The physical examination can provide much information pertaining to the cause of chronic cough. Posterior pharyngeal drainage combined with a nighttime cough suggests chronic upper airway disease such as sinusitis. An overinflated chest suggests chronic airway obstruction, as in asthma or cystic fibrosis. An expiratory wheeze, with or without diminished intensity of breath sounds, strongly suggests asthma or asthmatic bronchitis, but may also be consistent with a diagnosis of cystic fibrosis, bronchomalacia, vascular ring, aspiration of foreign material, or pulmonary hemosiderosis. Careful auscultation during forced expiration may reveal expiratory wheezes that are otherwise undetectable and that are the only indication of underlying reactive airways. Coarse crackles suggest bronchiectasis, including cystic fibrosis, but can also occur with an acute or subacute exacerbation of asthma. Clubbing of the digits is seen in most patients with bronchiectasis but in only a few other respiratory conditions with chronic cough (see Table 401.2). Tracheal deviation suggests foreign body aspiration, pleural effusion, or a mediastinal mass.

Allowing sufficient examination time to detect a spontaneous cough is important. If a spontaneous cough does not occur, asking the child to take a maximal breath and forcefully exhale repeatedly usually induces

a cough reflex. Most children can cough on request by 4-5 yr of age. Children who cough as often as several times a minute with regularity are likely to have a habit (tic) cough (see Chapter 37). If the cough is loose, every effort should be made to obtain sputum; many older children can comply. It is sometimes possible to pick up small bits of sputum with a throat swab quickly inserted into the lower pharynx while the child coughs with the tongue protruding. Clear mucoid sputum is most often associated with an allergic reaction or asthmatic bronchitis. Cloudy (purulent) sputum suggests a respiratory tract infection but can also reflect increased cellularity (eosinophilia) from an asthmatic process. Very purulent sputum is characteristic of bronchiectasis (see Chapter 430). Malodorous expectorations suggest anaerobic infection of the

Table 401.1	Indicators of Serious Chronic Lower Respiratory Tract Disease in Children

Persistent fever
Ongoing limitation of activity
Failure to grow
Failure to gain weight appropriately
Clubbing of the digits
Persistent tachypnea and labored ventilation
Shortness of breath and exercise intolerance
Chronic purulent sputum
Persistent hyperinflation
Substantial and sustained hypoxemia
Refractory infiltrates on chest x-ray
Persistent pulmonary function abnormalities
Hemoptysis
Family history of heritable lung disease
Cyanosis and hypercarbia
Unusual (opportunistic) or recurrent nonpulmonary infections

Table 401.2	Differential Diagnosis of Recurrent and Persistent Cough in Children

RECURRENT COUGH
Reactive airway disease (asthma)
Drainage from upper airways
Aspiration
Frequently recurring respiratory tract infections in immunocompetent or immunodeficient patients
Symptomatic Chiari malformation
Idiopathic pulmonary hemosiderosis
Hypersensitivity (allergic) pneumonitis

PERSISTENT COUGH
Hypersensitivity of cough receptors after infection
Reactive airway disease (asthma)
Chronic sinusitis
Chronic rhinitis (allergic or nonallergic)
Bronchitis or tracheitis caused by infection or smoke exposure
Bronchiectasis, including cystic fibrosis, primary ciliary dyskinesia, immunodeficiency
Habit cough
Foreign-body aspiration
Recurrent aspiration owing to pharyngeal incompetence, tracheolaryngoesophageal cleft, or tracheoesophageal fistula
Gastroesophageal reflux, with or without aspiration
Pertussis
Extrinsic compression of the tracheobronchial tract (vascular ring, neoplasm, lymph node, lung cyst)
Tracheomalacia, bronchomalacia
Endobronchial or endotracheal tumors
Endobronchial tuberculosis
Hypersensitivity pneumonitis
Fungal infections
Inhaled irritants, including tobacco smoke
Irritation of external auditory canal
Angiotensin-converting enzyme inhibitors

Table 401.3	Characteristics of Cough and Other Clinical Features and Possible Causes
SYMPTOMS AND SIGNS	**POSSIBLE UNDERLYING ETIOLOGY***
Auscultatory findings (wheeze, crepitations/crackles, differential breath sounds)	Asthma, bronchitis, pneumonia, congenital lung disease, foreign body aspiration, airway abnormality
Cough characteristics (e.g., cough with choking, cough quality, cough starting from birth)	Congenital airway or lung abnormalities
Cardiac abnormalities (including murmurs)	Any cardiac illness
Chest pain	Asthma, functional, pleuritis
Chest wall deformity	Any chronic lung disease, neuromuscular disorders
Daily moist or productive cough	Chronic bronchitis, suppurative lung disease
Digital clubbing	Suppurative lung disease, arteriovenous shunt
Dyspnea (exertional or at rest)	Compromised lung function of any chronic lung or cardiac disease
Failure to thrive	Compromised lung function, immunodeficiency, cystic fibrosis
Feeding difficulties (including choking and vomiting)	Compromised lung function, aspiration, anatomic disorders
Hemoptysis	Bronchitis, foreign body aspiration, suctioning trauma, pulmonary hemorrhage
Immune deficiency	Atypical and typical recurrent respiratory or nonrespiratory infections
Medications or drugs	Angiotensin-converting enzyme inhibitors, puffers, illicit drug use
Neurodevelopmental abnormality	Aspiration
Recurrent pneumonia	Immunodeficiency, congenital lung problem, airway abnormality
Symptoms of upper respiratory tract infection	Can coexist or be a trigger for an underlying problem

*This is not an exhaustive list; only the more common respiratory diseases are mentioned.
  Modified from Chang AB, Landau LI, Van Asperen PP, et al: Cough in children: definitions and clinical evaluation. Thoracic Society of Australia and New Zealand, *Med J Aust* 184(8):398–403, 2006, Table 2, p. 399.

Table 401.4	Clinical Clues About Cough
CHARACTERISTIC	**THINK OF**
Staccato, paroxysmal	Pertussis, cystic fibrosis, foreign body, *Chlamydia* spp., *Mycoplasma* spp.
Followed by "whoop"	Pertussis
All day, never during sleep	Habit cough
Barking, brassy	Croup, habit cough, tracheomalacia, tracheitis, epiglottitis
Hoarseness	Laryngeal involvement (croup, recurrent laryngeal nerve involvement), papillomatosis
Abrupt onset	Foreign body, pulmonary embolism
During or following exercise	Reactive airway disease
Accompanies eating, drinking	Aspiration, gastroesophageal reflux, tracheoesophageal fistula
Throat clearing	Postnasal drip, vocal tic
Productive (sputum)	Infection, cystic fibrosis, bronchiectasis
Night cough	Sinusitis, reactive airway disease, gastroesophageal reflux
Seasonal	Allergic rhinitis, reactive airway disease
Immunosuppressed patient	Bacterial pneumonia, *Pneumocystis jiroveci*, *Mycobacterium tuberculosis*, *Mycobacterium avium-intracellulare*, cytomegalovirus, fungi
Dyspnea	Hypoxia, hypercarbia
Animal exposure	*Chlamydia psittaci* (birds), *Yersinia pestis* (rodents), *Francisella tularensis* (rabbits), Q fever (sheep, cattle), hantavirus (rodents), histoplasmosis (pigeons)
Geographic	Histoplasmosis (Mississippi, Missouri, Ohio River Valley), coccidioidomycosis (Southwest), blastomycosis (North and Midwest)
Workdays with clearing on days off	Occupational exposure

From Kliegman RM, Greenbaum LA, Lyle PS: *Practical strategies in pediatric diagnosis and therapy*, ed 2, Philadelphia, 2004, WB Saunders, p. 19.

lungs. In cystic fibrosis (see Chapter 432), the sputum, even when purulent, is rarely foul smelling.

Laboratory tests can help in the evaluation of a chronic cough. Only sputum specimens containing alveolar macrophages should be interpreted as reflecting lower respiratory tract processes. Sputum eosinophilia suggests asthma, asthmatic bronchitis, or hypersensitivity reactions of the lung (see Chapter 418), but a polymorphonuclear cell response suggests infection; if sputum is unavailable, the presence of eosinophilia in nasal secretions also suggests atopic disease. If most of the cells in sputum are macrophages, postinfectious hypersensitivity of cough receptors should be suspected. Sputum macrophages can be stained for hemosiderin content, which is diagnostic of pulmonary hemosiderosis (see Chapter 435), or for lipid content, which in large amounts suggests, but is not specific for, repeated aspiration. Rarely, children may

expectorate partial casts of the airway, which can be characterized in investigating causes of plastic bronchitis. Children whose coughs persist for more than 6 wk should be tested for cystic fibrosis regardless of their race or ethnicity (see Chapter 432). Sputum culture is helpful in evaluation of cystic fibrosis, but less so for other conditions because throat flora can contaminate the sample.

Hematologic assessment can reveal a microcytic anemia that is the result of pulmonary hemosiderosis (see Chapter 435) or hemoptysis, or eosinophilia that accompanies asthma and other hypersensitivity reactions of the lung. Infiltrates on the chest radiograph suggest cystic fibrosis, bronchiectasis, foreign body, hypersensitivity pneumonitis, tuberculosis, or other infection. When asthma-equivalent cough is suggested, a trial of bronchodilator therapy may be diagnostic. If the cough does not respond to initial therapeutic efforts, more-specific diagnostic procedures may be warranted, including an immunologic or allergic evaluation, chest and paranasal sinus imaging, esophagograms, tests for gastroesophageal reflux (see Chapter 349), and special microbiologic studies including rapid viral testing. Evaluation of ciliary morphology, nasal endoscopy, laryngoscopy, and bronchoscopy may also be indicated.

Tic cough or somatic cough disorder (psychogenic cough or habit cough) must be considered in any child with a cough that has lasted for weeks or months, that has been refractory to treatment, and that disappears with sleep or with distraction. Typically, the cough is abrupt and loud, and has a harsh, honking, or barking quality. A disassociation between the intensity of the cough and the child's affect is typically striking. This cough may be absent if the physician listens outside the examination room, but it will reliably appear immediately on direct attention to the child and the symptom. It typically begins with an upper respiratory infection but then lingers. The child misses many days of school because the cough disrupts the classroom. This disorder accounts for many unnecessary medical procedures and courses of medication. It is treatable with assurance that a pathologic lung condition is absent and that the child should resume full activity, including school. This assurance, together with speech therapy techniques that allow the child to reduce musculoskeletal tension in the neck and chest and that increase the child's awareness of the initial sensations that trigger cough, has been very successful. Self-hypnosis is another successful therapy, often effective with 1 session. The designation "tic cough" or "somatic cough disorder" is preferable to "habit cough" or "psychogenic cough" because it carries no stigma and because most of these children do not have significant emotional problems. When the cough disappears, it does not reemerge as another symptom. Nonetheless, other symptoms such as irritable bowel syndrome may be present in the patient or family.

FREQUENTLY RECURRING OR PERSISTENT STRIDOR

Stridor, a harsh, medium-pitched, inspiratory sound associated with obstruction of the laryngeal area or the extrathoracic trachea, is often accompanied by a croupy cough and hoarse voice. Stridor is most commonly observed in children with croup (see Chapter 412); foreign bodies and trauma can also cause acute stridor. A few children, however, acquire recurrent stridor or have persistent stridor from the 1st days or weeks of life (Table 401.5). Most congenital anomalies of large airways that produce stridor become symptomatic soon after birth. Increase of stridor when a child is supine suggests **airway malacia**, such as laryngomalacia or tracheomalacia. It is important to note that when evaluating for a specific anatomic cause of abnormal breath sounds, it is not uncommon to identify additional congenital anomalies of the airway. An accompanying history of hoarseness or aphonia suggests involvement of the vocal cords. Associated dysphagia may also suggest a vascular ring. In a child with intermittent stridor (with wheezing) that accompanies physical activity and is not responsive to asthma therapies, **paradoxical vocal cord dysfunction** may be of consideration. Paradoxical vocal cord dysfunction may be highly supported by history and confirmed by laryngoscopy during an exercise challenge test if symptoms are successfully elicited. Speech therapy and behavior modification may be therapeutic.

Physical examination for recurrent or persistent stridor is usually unrewarding, although changes in its severity and intensity due to changes of body position should be assessed. Anteroposterior and lateral radiographs, contrast esophagography, fluoroscopy, computed tomography (CT), and magnetic resonance imaging (MRI) are potentially useful diagnostic tools. In most cases, direct observation by laryngoscopy is necessary for definitive diagnosis. Undistorted views of the larynx are best obtained with fiberoptic laryngoscopy.

RECURRENT OR PERSISTENT WHEEZE

See also Chapter 418.

Parents often complain that their child wheezes, when, in fact, they are reporting respiratory sounds that are audible without a stethoscope, produce palpable resonance throughout the chest, and occur most prominently in inspiration. Some of these children have stridor, although many have audible sounds when the supraglottic airway is incompletely cleared of feedings or secretions.

True wheezing is a relatively common and particularly troublesome manifestation of obstructive *lower* respiratory tract disease in children. The site of obstruction may be anywhere from the intrathoracic trachea to the small bronchi or large bronchioles, but the sound is generated

Table 401.5	Causes of Recurrent or Persistent Stridor in Children

RECURRENT
Allergic (spasmodic) croup
Respiratory infections in a child with otherwise asymptomatic anatomic narrowing of the large airways
Laryngomalacia

PERSISTENT
Laryngeal obstruction
- Laryngomalacia
- Papillomas, hemangiomas, other tumors
- Cysts and laryngoceles
- Laryngeal webs
- Bilateral abductor paralysis of the cords
- Foreign body
Tracheobronchial disease
- Tracheomalacia
- Subglottic tracheal webs
- Endobronchial, endotracheal tumors
- Subglottic tracheal stenosis, congenital or acquired
Extrinsic masses
- Mediastinal masses
- Vascular ring
- Lobar emphysema
- Bronchogenic cysts
- Thyroid enlargement
- Esophageal foreign body
Tracheoesophageal fistula

OTHER
Gastroesophageal reflux
Macroglossia, Pierre Robin syndrome
Cri-du-chat syndrome
Paradoxical vocal cord dysfunction
Hypocalcemia
Vocal cord paralysis
Chiari crisis
Severe neonatal episodic laryngospasm caused by *SCN4A* mutation

by turbulence in larger airways that collapse with forced expiration (see Chapter 400). Children younger than 2-3 yr are especially prone to wheezing, because bronchospasm, mucosal edema, and accumulation of excessive secretions have a relatively greater obstructive effect on their smaller airways. In addition, the compliant airways in young children collapse more readily with active expiration. Isolated episodes of acute wheezing, such as can occur with bronchiolitis, are not uncommon, but wheezing that recurs or persists for more than 4 wk suggests other diagnoses (see Table 418.1 in Chapter 418). Most recurrent or persistent wheezing in children is the result of airway reactivity. Nonspecific environmental factors such as cigarette smoke may be important contributors.

Frequently recurring or persistent wheezing starting at or soon after birth suggests a variety of other diagnoses, including congenital structural abnormalities involving the lower respiratory tract or tracheobronchomalacia (see Chapter 413). Wheezing that attends cystic fibrosis is most common in the 1st yr of life. Sudden onset of severe wheezing in a previously healthy child should suggest foreign-body aspiration.

Either wheezing or coughing when associated with tachypnea and hypoxemia may be suggestive of **interstitial lung disease** (see Chapter 427.5). However, many patients with interstitial lung disease demonstrate no symptoms other than rapid breathing on initial physical examination. Although chest roentgenograms may be normal in interstitial lung disease, diffuse abnormalities on chest X-ray may support further evaluation in patients suspected to have interstitial lung disease with characteristic findings described on high-resolution CT scan and lung biopsy.

Repeated examination may be required to verify a history of wheezing in a child with episodic symptoms and should be directed toward assessing air movement, ventilatory adequacy, and evidence of chronic lung disease, such as fixed overinflation of the chest, growth failure, and digital clubbing. Patients should be assessed for oropharyngeal dysphagia in cases of suspected recurrent aspiration. Clubbing suggests chronic lung infection and is rarely prominent in uncomplicated asthma. Tracheal deviation from foreign body aspiration should be sought. It is essential to rule out wheezing secondary to congestive heart failure. Allergic rhinitis, urticaria, eczema, or evidence of ichthyosis vulgaris suggests asthma or asthmatic bronchitis. The nose should be examined for polyps, which can exist with allergic conditions or cystic fibrosis.

Sputum eosinophilia and elevated serum immunoglobulin E levels suggest allergic reactions. A forced expiratory volume in 1 sec increase of 15% in response to bronchodilators confirms reactive airways. Specific microbiologic studies, special imaging studies of the airways and cardiovascular structures, diagnostic studies for cystic fibrosis, and bronchoscopy should be considered if the response is unsatisfactory.

RECURRENT AND PERSISTENT LUNG INFILTRATES

Radiographic lung infiltrates resulting from acute pneumonia usually resolve within 1-3 wk, but a substantial number of children, particularly infants, fail to completely clear infiltrates within a 4 wk period. These children may be febrile or afebrile, and may display a wide range of respiratory symptoms and signs. Persistent or recurring infiltrates present a diagnostic challenge (Table 401.6).

Symptoms associated with chronic lung infiltrates in the 1st several weeks of life (but not related to neonatal respiratory distress syndrome) suggest infection acquired in utero or during descent through the birth canal. Early appearance of chronic infiltrates can also be associated with cystic fibrosis or congenital anomalies that result in aspiration or airway obstruction. A history of recurrent infiltrates such as in **middle lobe syndrome** (see Chapters 430 and 437), wheezing, and cough may reflect asthma, even in the 1st yr of life.

A controversial association has been posed regarding recurrent lung infiltrates in pulmonary hemosiderosis related to cow's milk hypersensitivity or unknown causes appearing in the 1st yr of life. Children with a history of bronchopulmonary dysplasia often have episodes of respiratory distress attended by wheezing and new lung infiltrates. **Recurrent pneumonia** in a child with frequent otitis media, nasopharyngitis, adenitis, or dermatologic manifestations suggests an immunodeficiency state, complement deficiency, or phagocytic defect (see Chapters 148, 156, and 160). Primary ciliary dyskinesia is also of consideration in patients with frequent otitis media and suppurative sinopulmonary disease, with or without accompanying heterotaxy, or history of neonatal respiratory distress (see Chapter 433). Pulmonary sequestration may be suspected in patients with recurrent findings on radiograph that occur in the same location, both during illness and when well (see Chapter 423). Traction bronchiectasis may also be suggested on radiography with persistent findings in a given region of the film following a history of respiratory infection. Particular attention must be directed to the possibility that the infiltrates represent lymphocytic interstitial pneumonitis or opportunistic infection associated with HIV infection (see Chapter 302). A history of paroxysmal coughing in an infant suggests pertussis syndrome or cystic fibrosis. Persistent infiltrates, especially with loss of volume, in a toddler may suggest foreign-body aspiration.

Overinflation and infiltrates suggest cystic fibrosis or chronic asthma. A silent chest with infiltrates should arouse suspicion of alveolar proteinosis (see Chapter 434), *Pneumocystis jiroveci* infection (see Chapter 271), genetic disorders of surfactant synthesis and secretion causing interstitial pneumonitis, or tumors. Growth should be carefully assessed to determine whether the lung process has had systemic effects, indicating substantial severity and chronicity as in cystic fibrosis or alveolar proteinosis. Cataracts, retinopathy, or microcephaly suggest in utero infection. Chronic rhinorrhea can be associated with atopic disease, cow's milk intolerance, cystic fibrosis, primary ciliary dyskinesia, or congenital syphilis. The absence of tonsils and cervical lymph nodes suggests an immunodeficiency state.

Table 401.6	Diseases Associated With Recurrent, Persistent, or Migrating Lung Infiltrates Beyond the Neonatal Period

Aspiration
 Pharyngeal incompetence (e.g., cleft palate)
 Laryngotracheoesophageal cleft
 Tracheoesophageal fistula
 Gastroesophageal reflux
 Lipid aspiration
 Neurologic dysphagia
 Developmental dysphagia
Congenital anomalies
 Lung cysts (cystic adenomatoid malformation)
 Pulmonary sequestration
 Bronchial stenosis or aberrant bronchus
 Vascular ring
 Congenital heart disease with large left-to-right shunt
 Pulmonary lymphangiectasia
Genetic conditions
 α_1-Antitrypsin deficiency
 Cystic fibrosis
 Primary ciliary dyskinesia (including Kartagener syndrome)
 Sickle cell disease (acute chest syndrome)
Immunodeficiency, phagocytic deficiency
 Humoral, cellular, combined immunodeficiency states
 Chronic granulomatous disease and related phagocytic defects
 Hyper immunoglobulin E syndromes
 Complement deficiency states
Immunologic and autoimmune diseases
 Asthma
 Allergic bronchopulmonary aspergillosis
 Hypersensitivity pneumonitis
 Pulmonary hemosiderosis
 Collagen-vascular diseases
Infection, congenital
 Cytomegalovirus
 Rubella
 Syphilis
Infection, acquired
 Cytomegalovirus
 Tuberculosis
 HIV
 Other viruses
 Chlamydia
 Mycoplasma, Ureaplasma
 Pertussis
 Fungal organisms
 Pneumocystis jiroveci
 Visceral larva migrans
 Inadequately treated bacterial infection
Interstitial pneumonitis and fibrosis
 Usual interstitial pneumonitis
 Lymphoid (AIDS)
 Genetic disorders of surfactant synthesis, secretion
 Desquamative
 Acute (Hamman-Rich)
 Alveolar proteinosis
 Drug-induced, radiation-induced inflammation and fibrosis
Neoplasms and neoplastic-like conditions
 Primary or metastatic pulmonary tumors
 Leukemia
 Histiocytosis
 Eosinophilic pneumonias
Other etiologies
 Bronchiectasis
  Congenital
  Postinfectious
 Sarcoidosis

Diagnostic studies should be performed selectively, based on information obtained from history and physical examination and on a thorough understanding of the conditions listed in Table 401.6. Cytologic evaluation of sputum, if available, may be helpful. Chest CT often provides more precise anatomic detail concerning the infiltrate or further characterizes a region of anatomic abnormality. Bronchoscopy is indicated for detecting foreign bodies, congenital or acquired anomalies of the tracheobronchial tract, and obstruction by endobronchial or extrinsic masses (see Chapters 413–417). Bronchoscopy provides access to secretions that can be studied cytologically and microbiologically. Alveolar lavage fluid is diagnostic for alveolar proteinosis and persistent pulmonary hemosiderosis, and can suggest aspiration syndromes. Ciliary biopsy may be obtained from the inferior epithelial surface of nasal turbinates or from the lower airway during bronchoscopy. If all appropriate studies have been completed and the condition remains undiagnosed, lung biopsy might yield a definitive diagnosis, such as in interstitial lung disease or in fungal disease.

Optimal medical or surgical treatment of chronic lung infiltrates often depends on a specific diagnosis, but chronic conditions may be self-limiting (severe and prolonged viral infections in infants); in these cases, symptomatic therapy can maintain adequate lung function until spontaneous improvement occurs. Helpful measures include inhalation and physical therapy for excessive secretions, antibiotics for bacterial infections, supplementary oxygen for hypoxemia, and maintenance of adequate nutrition. Because the lung of a young child has remarkable recuperative potential, normal lung function may ultimately be achieved with treatment despite the severity of pulmonary insult occurring in infancy or early childhood.

Bibliography is available at Expert Consult.

401.1 Extrapulmonary Diseases With Pulmonary Manifestations
Susanna A. McColley

Respiratory symptoms commonly originate from extrapulmonary processes. The respiratory system adapts to metabolic demands and is exquisitely responsive to cortical input; therefore, **tachypnea** is common in the presence of metabolic stress such as fever, whereas dyspnea may be related to anxiety. **Cough** most commonly arises from upper or lower respiratory tract disorders, but it can originate from the central nervous system, as with cough tic or psychogenic cough, and it can be a prominent symptom in children with gastroesophageal reflux disease. **Chest pain** does not commonly arise from pulmonary processes in otherwise healthy children but more often has a neuromuscular or inflammatory etiology. **Cyanosis** can be caused by cardiac or hematologic disorders, and **dyspnea** and **exercise intolerance** can have a number of extrapulmonary causes. These disorders may be suspected on the basis of the history and physical examination, or they may be considered in children in whom diagnostic studies have atypical findings or who show poor response to usual therapy. Table 401.7 lists more common causes of such symptoms.

EVALUATION
In the evaluation of a child or adolescent with respiratory symptoms, it is important to obtain a detailed past medical history, family history,

Table 401.7	Respiratory Signs and Symptoms Originating From Outside the Respiratory Tract		
SIGN OR SYMPTOM	**NONRESPIRATORY CAUSE(S)**	**PATHOPHYSIOLOGY**	**CLUES TO DIAGNOSIS**
Chest pain	Cardiac disease	Inflammation (pericarditis), ischemia (anomalous coronary artery, vascular disease)	Precordial pain, friction rub on examination; exertional pain, radiation to arm or neck
Chest pain	Gastroesophageal reflux disease	Esophageal inflammation and/or spasm	Heartburn, abdominal pain
Cyanosis	Congenital heart disease	Right-to-left shunt	Neonatal onset, lack of response to oxygen
	Methemoglobinemia	Increased levels of methemoglobin interfere with delivery of oxygen to tissues	Drug or toxin exposure, lack of response to oxygen
Dyspnea	Toxin exposure, drug side effect, or overdose	Variable, but often metabolic acidosis	Drug or toxin exposure confirmed by history or toxicology screen, normal oxygen saturation measured by pulse oximetry
	Anxiety, panic disorder	Increased respiratory drive and increased perception of respiratory efforts	Occurs during stressful situation, other symptoms of anxiety or depression
Exercise intolerance	Anemia	Inadequate oxygen delivery to tissues	Pallor, tachycardia, history of bleeding, history of inadequate diet
Exercise intolerance	Deconditioning	Self-explanatory	History of inactivity, obesity
Hemoptysis	Nasal bleeding	Posterior flow of bleeding causes appearance of pulmonary origin	History and physical findings suggest nasal source; normal chest examination and chest radiography
	Upper gastrointestinal tract bleeding	Hematemesis mimics hemoptysis	History and physical examination suggest gastrointestinal source; normal chest examination and chest radiography
Wheezing, cough, dyspnea	Congenital or acquired cardiac disease	Pulmonary overcirculation (atrioseptal defect, ventriculoseptal defect, patent ductus arteriosus), left ventricular dysfunction	Murmur Refractory to bronchodilators Radiographic changes (prominent pulmonary vasculature, pulmonary edema)
Wheezing, cough	Gastroesophageal reflux disease	Laryngeal and bronchial response to stomach contents Vagally mediated bronchoconstriction	Emesis, pain, heartburn Refractory to bronchodilators

Table 401.8	Disorders With Frequent Respiratory Tract Complications	
UNDERLYING DISORDER(S)	**RESPIRATORY COMPLICATIONS**	**DIAGNOSTIC TESTS**
Autoimmune disorders	Pulmonary vascular disease, restrictive lung disease, pleural effusion (especially systemic lupus erythematosus), upper airway disease (Wegener granulomatosis)	Spirometry, lung volume determination, oximetry, diffusing capacity of the lung for carbon monoxide, chest radiography, upper airway endoscopy, and/or CT
Central nervous system disease (static or progressive)	Aspiration of oral or gastric contents	Chest radiography, videofluoroscopic swallowing study, esophageal pH probe, fiberoptic bronchoscopy
Immunodeficiency	Infection, bronchiectasis	Chest radiography, fiberoptic bronchoscopy, chest CT
Liver disease	Pleural effusion, hepatopulmonary syndrome	Chest radiography, assessment of orthodeoxia
Malignancy and its therapies	Infiltration, metastasis, malignant or infectious effusion, parenchymal infection, graft versus host disease (bone marrow transplant)	Chest radiography, chest CT, fiberoptic bronchoscopy, lung biopsy
Neuromuscular disease	Hypoventilation, atelectasis, pneumonia	Spirometry, lung volume determination, respiratory muscle force measurements
Obesity	Restrictive lung disease, obstructive sleep apnea syndrome, asthma	Spirometry, lung volume determination, nocturnal polysomnography

CT, Computed tomography.

and review of systems to evaluate the possibility of extrapulmonary origin. A comprehensive physical examination is also essential in obtaining clues as to extrapulmonary disease.

Disorders of other organ systems, and many systemic diseases, can have significant respiratory system involvement. Although it is most common to encounter these complications in patients with known diagnoses, respiratory system disease is sometimes the sole or most prominent symptom at the time of presentation. Acute aspiration during feeding can be the presentation of neuromuscular disease in an infant who initially appears to have normal muscle tone and development. Complications can be life-threatening, particularly in immunocompromised patients. The onset of respiratory findings may be insidious; for example, pulmonary vascular involvement in patients with systemic vasculitis may appear as an abnormality in diffusing capacity of the lung for carbon monoxide before the onset of symptoms. Table 401.8 lists disorders that commonly have respiratory complications.

Bibliography is available at Expert Consult.

Chapter 402
Sudden Infant Death Syndrome

Fern R. Hauck, Rebecca F. Carlin, Rachel Y. Moon, and Carl E. Hunt

第四百零二章
婴儿猝死综合征

中文导读

　　本章主要介绍了婴儿猝死综合征的流行病学、病理学、环境危险因素、遗传危险因素、基因–环境相互作用，婴儿猝死综合征风险增加的婴儿群体以及临床策略。环境危险因素中具体描述了不可控的环境风险因素以及可控的环境危险因素；婴儿猝死综合征风险增加的婴儿群体中具体包括因婴儿猝死综合征而死亡的婴儿家庭随后出生的孩子、早产儿以及生理学异常的孩子；临床策略中具体描述了家庭监测以及如何降低婴儿猝死综合征发生风险；详细阐述了新生儿出生后突发脏器功能衰竭，其中包括流行病学、发病机制、危险因素、诊断和鉴别诊断、预后、治疗以及预防等内容。

Sudden infant death syndrome (SIDS) is defined as the sudden, unexpected death of an infant that is unexplained by a thorough postmortem examination, which includes a complete autopsy, investigation of the scene of death, and review of the medical history. An autopsy is essential to identify possible natural explanations for sudden unexpected death such as congenital anomalies or infection and to diagnose traumatic child abuse (Tables 402.1 to 402.3; see Chapter 16). The autopsy typically cannot distinguish between SIDS and intentional suffocation, but the scene investigation and medical history may be of help if inconsistencies are evident. **Sudden unexpected infant death (SUID)** is a term that generally encompasses all SUIDs that occur during sleep, including SIDS (ICD-10 R95), accidental suffocation and strangulation in bed (ICD-10 W75), and ill-defined deaths, also known as undetermined (ICD-10 R99).

EPIDEMIOLOGY
SIDS is the 3rd leading cause of infant mortality in the United States, accounting for approximately 7% of all infant deaths. It is the most common cause of postneonatal infant mortality, accounting for 21% of all deaths between 1 mo and 1 yr of age. The annual rate of SIDS in the United States was stable at 1.3-1.4 per 1,000 live births (approximately 7,000 infants per year) before 1992, when it was recommended that infants sleep nonprone as a way to reduce the risk for SIDS. Since then, particularly after initiation of the national Back to Sleep campaign in 1994, the rate of SIDS progressively declined and then leveled off in 2001 at 0.55 per 1,000 live births (2,234 infants). There has been a slower rate of decline since that time; in 2015 the rate was 0.39 per 1,000 live births (1,568 infants). The decline in the number of SIDS deaths in the United States and other countries has been attributed to increasing use of the supine position for sleep. In 1992, 82% of sampled infants in the United States were placed prone for sleep. Although several other countries have decreased prone sleeping prevalence to ≤2%, in the United States in 2010 (the last year for which these data were collected by the National Infant Sleep Position study), 13.5% of infants were still being placed prone for sleep and 11.9% were being placed in the side position. Among black infants, these rates were even higher: 27.6% prone and 16.1% side in 2010.

There is increasing evidence that infant deaths previously classified as SIDS are now being classified by medical examiners and coroners as due to other causes, notably **accidental suffocation and strangulation in bed** and **ill-defined deaths**. Between 1994 and 2013, there has been a 7-fold increase in the rate of accidental suffocation and strangulation in bed, from 0.03 to 0.21 deaths per 1,000 live births. There has also been an increase in the rate of ill-defined deaths between 1995 and 2013, from 0.21 to 0.28 deaths per 1,000 live births. These sudden and unexpected infant deaths are primarily associated with unsafe sleeping environments, including prone positioning, sharing a sleep surface with others, and soft bedding in the sleep environment. Based on these trends and the commonality of many of the sleep environment risk factors that are associated with both SIDS and other sleep-related SUID, risk reduction measures that will be later described are applicable to all sleep-related SUID.

PATHOLOGY
Although there are no autopsy findings pathognomonic for SIDS and no findings are required for the diagnosis, there are some that are

Table 402.1	Differential Diagnosis of Sudden Unexpected Infant Death		
CAUSE OF DEATH	**PRIMARY DIAGNOSTIC CRITERIA**	**POTENTIAL CONFOUNDING DIAGNOSES**	**FREQUENCY DISTRIBUTION (%)**
EXPLAINED AT AUTOPSY			
Natural			18–20*
Infections	History, autopsy, and cultures	If minimal findings: SIDS	35–46†
Congenital anomaly	History and autopsy	If minimal findings: SIDS	14–24†
Unintentional injury	History, scene investigation, autopsy	Traumatic child abuse	15*
Traumatic child abuse	Autopsy and scene investigation	Unintentional injury	13–24*
Other natural causes	History and autopsy	If minimal findings: SIDS, or intentional suffocation	12–17*
UNEXPLAINED AT AUTOPSY			
SIDS	History, scene investigation, absence of explainable cause at autopsy	Intentional suffocation	80–82
Intentional suffocation (filicide)	Perpetrator confession, absence of explainable cause at autopsy	SIDS	Unknown, but <5% of all SUID
Accidental suffocation or strangulation in bed (ASSB)	History and scene investigation, ideally including doll re-enactment	Assigned to ICD-10 code (SIDS) for US vital statistics database Unexplained Undetermined	Varies with individual medical examiners and coroners
Genetic mutations	*SCN5A, SCN1B-4B, SCN4A*, long QT syndromes, plus Table 402.4	May have negative family history secondary to recessive mutations, de novo mutation, or incomplete penetrance	Unknown, perhaps <10%

*As a percentage of all sudden unexpected infant deaths explained at autopsy.
†As a percentage of all natural causes of sudden unexpected infant deaths explained at autopsy.
ICD-10, International Classification of Diseases, Version 10; *SIDS,* sudden infant death syndrome; *SUID,* sudden unexpected infant death.
Modified from Hunt CE: Sudden infant death syndrome and other causes of infant mortality: diagnosis, mechanisms and risk for recurrence in siblings, *Am J Respir Crit Care Med* 164(3):346–357, 2001.

Table 402.2	Conditions That Can Cause Apparent Life-Threatening Events* or Sudden Unexpected Infant Death

CENTRAL NERVOUS SYSTEM
Arteriovenous malformation
Subdural hematoma
Seizures
Congenital central hypoventilation
Neuromuscular disorders (Werdnig-Hoffmann disease)
Chiari crisis
Leigh syndrome

CARDIAC
Subendocardial fibroelastosis
Aortic stenosis
Anomalous coronary artery
Myocarditis
Cardiomyopathy
Arrhythmias (prolonged QT syndrome, Wolff-Parkinson-White syndrome, congenital heart block)

PULMONARY
Pulmonary hypertension
Vocal cord paralysis
Aspiration
Laryngotracheal disease

GASTROINTESTINAL
Diarrhea and/or dehydration
Gastroesophageal reflux
Volvulus

ENDOCRINE–METABOLIC
Congenital adrenal hyperplasia
Malignant hyperpyrexia
Long- or medium-chain acyl coenzyme A deficiency
Hyperammonemias (urea cycle enzyme deficiencies)

Glutaric aciduria
Carnitine deficiency (systemic or secondary)
Glycogen storage disease type I
Maple syrup urine disease
Congenital lactic acidosis
Biotinidase deficiency

INFECTION
Sepsis
Meningitis
Encephalitis
Brain abscess
Pyelonephritis
Bronchiolitis (respiratory syncytial virus)
Infant botulism
Pertussis

TRAUMA
Child abuse
Accidental or intentional suffocation
Physical trauma
Factitious syndrome (formerly Munchausen syndrome) by proxy

POISONING (INTENTIONAL OR UNINTENTIONAL)
Boric acid
Carbon monoxide
Salicylates
Barbiturates
Ipecac
Cocaine
Insulin
Others

*Recommended terminology now is "brief resolved unexplained events."
From Kliegman RM, Greenbaum LA, Lye PS: *Practical strategies in pediatric diagnosis and therapy*, ed 2, Philadelphia, 2004, Elsevier Saunders, p. 98.

Table 402.3	Differential Diagnosis of Recurrent Sudden Infant Death in a Sibling

IDIOPATHIC
Recurrent sudden infant death syndrome

CENTRAL NERVOUS SYSTEM
Congenital central hypoventilation
Neuromuscular disorders
Leigh syndrome

CARDIAC
Endocardial fibroelastosis
Wolff-Parkinson-White syndrome
Prolonged QT syndrome or other cardiac channelopathy
Congenital heart block

PULMONARY
Pulmonary hypertension

ENDOCRINE–METABOLIC
See Table 402.2

INFECTION
Disorders of immune host defense

CHILD ABUSE
Filicide or infanticide
Factitious syndrome (formerly Munchausen syndrome) by proxy

From Kliegman RM, Greenbaum LA, Lye PS: *Practical strategies in pediatric diagnosis and therapy*, ed 2, Philadelphia, 2004, Elsevier Saunders, p 101.

commonly seen on postmortem examination. Petechial hemorrhages are found in 68–95% of infants who died of SIDS and are more extensive than in explained causes of infant mortality. Pulmonary edema is often present and may be substantial. The reasons for these findings are unknown. Infants who died of SIDS have higher levels of vascular endothelial growth factor (VEGF) in the cerebrospinal fluid. These increases may be related to VEGF polymorphisms (see "Genetic Risk Factors" later and Table 402.4) or might indicate recent hypoxemic events because VEGF is upregulated by hypoxia.

SIDS infants have several identifiable changes in the lungs and other organs. Nearly 65% of these infants have structural evidence of preexisting, chronic, low-grade asphyxia, and other studies have identified biochemical markers of asphyxia. Some studies have shown carotid body abnormalities, consistent with a role for impaired peripheral arterial chemoreceptor function in SIDS. Numerous studies have shown brain abnormalities that could cause or contribute to an impaired autonomic response to an exogenous stressor, including in the hippocampus and brainstem, the latter being the major area responsible for respiratory and autonomic regulation. The affected brainstem nuclei include the retrotrapezoid nucleus and the dorsal motor nucleus of the vagus, primary sites of central chemoreception and respiratory drive. Abnormalities in both the structure and expression of the *PHOX2B* gene, which is involved in neuronal maturation, have also been reported in significantly more SIDS infants than controls.

The ventral medulla has been a particular focus for studies in infants who died of SIDS. It is an integrative area for vital autonomic functions including breathing, arousal, and chemosensory function. Some SIDS infants have hypoplasia of the arcuate nucleus and up to 60% have histopathologic evidence of less-extensive bilateral or unilateral hypoplasia. Consistent with the apparent overlap between putative mechanisms for SIDS and for unexpected late fetal deaths, approximately 30% of sudden intrauterine unexplained deaths also have hypoplasia of the arcuate nucleus. Imaging mass spectroscopy of postmortem medullary tissue has identified abnormal expression of 41 peptides, especially in the raphe, hypoglossal, and pyramidal nuclei that include components

Table 402.4	Identified Genes for Which the Distribution of Polymorphisms Differs in Sudden Infant Death Syndrome Infants Compared With Control Infants

CARDIAC CHANNELOPATHIES
Potassium ion channel genes (KCNE2, KCNH2, KCNQ1, KCNJ8)
Sodium ion channel gene (SCN5A) (long QT syndrome 3, Brugada syndrome)
GPD1-L-encoded connexin43 (Brugada syndrome)
SCN3B (Brugada syndrome)
CAV3 (long QT syndrome 9)
SCN4B (long QT syndrome 10)
SNTA-1 (long QT syndrome 11)
RyR2 (catecholaminergic polymorphic ventricular tachycardia)

SEROTONIN (5-HT)
5-HT transporter protein (5-HTT)
Intron 2 of SLC6A4 (variable number tandem repeat [VNTR] polymorphism)
5-HT fifth Ewing variant (FEV) gene

GENES PERTINENT TO DEVELOPMENT OF AUTONOMIC NERVOUS SYSTEM
Paired-like homeobox 2a (PHOX2A)
PHOX2B
Rearranged during transfection factor (RET)
Endothelin converting enzyme-1 (ECE1)
T-cell leukemia homeobox (TLX3)
Engrailed-1 (EN1)
Tyrosine hydroxylase (THO1)
Monamine oxidase A (MAOA)
Sodium/proton exchanger 3 (NHE3) (medullary respiratory control)

INFECTION AND INFLAMMATION
Complement C4A
Complement C4B
Interleukin-1RN (gene encoding IL-1 receptor antagonist [ra]; proinflammatory)
Interleukin-6 (IL-6; proinflammatory)
Interleukin-8 (IL-8; proinflammatory; associated with prone sleeping position)
Interleukin-10 (IL-10)
Vascular endothelial growth factor (VEGF) (proinflammatory)
Tumor necrosis factor (TNF)- α (proinflammatory)

OTHER
Mitochondrial DNA (mtDNA) polymorphisms (energy production)
Flavin-monooxygenase 3 (FMO3) (enzyme metabolizes nicotine; risk factor with smoking mothers)
Aquaporin-4 (T allele and CT/TT genotype associated with maternal smoking and with increased brain/body weight ratio in SIDS infants)
SCN4A (nondystrophic myotonia, laryngospasm)

Modified from Hunt CE, Hauck FR: Sudden infant death syndrome: gene-environment interactions. In Brugada R, Brugada J, Brugada P, editors: *Clinical care in inherited cardiac syndromes*, Guildford, UK, 2009, Springer-Verlag London.

for developmental neuronal/glial/axonal growth, cell metabolism, cytoarchitecture, and apoptosis. These findings suggest that SIDS infants have abnormal neurologic development contributing to pathogenesis, with the impairments suggesting delayed neurologic maturation.

Neurotransmitter studies of the arcuate nucleus have also identified several receptor abnormalities relevant to state-dependent autonomic control overall and to ventilatory and arousal responsiveness in particular. These deficits include significant decreases in binding to kainate, muscarinic cholinergic, and serotonin (5-HT) receptors. Studies of the ventral medulla have identified morphologic and biochemical deficits in 5-HT neurons and decreased γ-aminobutyric acid receptor A receptor binding in the medullary serotonergic system. Immunohistochemical analyses reveal an increased number of 5-HT neurons and an increase in the fraction of 5-HT neurons showing an immature morphology,

suggesting a failure or delay in the maturation of these neurons. High neuronal levels of interleukin (IL)-1β are present in the arcuate and dorsal vagal nuclei in SIDS infants compared with controls, perhaps contributing to molecular interactions affecting cardiorespiratory and arousal responses.

The neuropathologic data provide compelling evidence for altered 5-HT homeostasis, creating an underlying vulnerability contributing to SIDS. 5-HT is an important neurotransmitter, and the 5-HT neurons in the medulla project extensively to neurons in the brainstem and spinal cord that influence respiratory drive and arousal, cardiovascular control including blood pressure, circadian regulation, and non–rapid eye movement (REM) sleep, thermoregulation, and upper airway reflexes. Decreases in 5-HT_{1A} and 5-HT_{2A} receptor immunoreactivity have been observed in the dorsal nucleus of the vagus, solitary nucleus, and ventrolateral medulla. There are extensive serotoninergic brainstem abnormalities in SIDS infants, including increased 5-HT neuronal count, a lower density of 5-HT_{1A} receptor-binding sites in regions of the medulla involved in homeostatic function, and a lower ratio of 5-HT transporter (5-HTT) binding density to 5-HT neuronal count in the medulla. Male SIDS infants have lower receptor-binding density than do female SIDS infants. Overall, these 5-HT–related studies suggest that the synthesis and availability of 5-HT are decreased within 5-HT pathways, and medullary tissue levels of 5-HT and its primary biosynthetic enzyme (tryptophan hydroxylase) are lower in SIDS infants compared with age-matched controls.

ENVIRONMENTAL RISK FACTORS
Declines of 50% or more in rates of SIDS in the United States and around the world have occurred following national education campaigns directed at reducing risk factors associated with SIDS (Table 402.5). Although many risk factors are nonmodifiable and most of the modifiable factors have not changed appreciably, self-reported maternal smoking prevalence during pregnancy has decreased by 25% in the past decade in the United States.

Table 402.5	Risk Factors Associated With Sudden Infant Death Syndrome

MATERNAL AND ANTENATAL RISK FACTORS
Elevated 2nd trimester serum α-fetoprotein
Smoking
Alcohol use
Drug use (cocaine, heroin)
Nutritional deficiency
Inadequate prenatal care
Low socioeconomic status
Younger age
Lower education
Single marital status
Shorter interpregnancy interval
Intrauterine hypoxia
Fetal growth restriction

INFANT RISK FACTORS
Age (peak 1-4 mo)
Male gender
Race and ethnicity (African American, American Indian, Alaska Native, other minorities)
Growth failure
No breastfeeding
No pacifier (dummy)
Prematurity
Prone and side sleep position
Recent febrile illness (mild infections)
Inadequate immunizations
Smoking exposure (prenatal and postnatal)
Soft sleeping surface, soft bedding
Bed sharing with parent(s) or other children
Thermal stress, overheating
Colder season, no central heating

Nonmodifiable Environmental Risk Factors

Lower socioeconomic status has consistently been associated with higher risk, although SIDS affects infants from all social strata. In the United States, African-American, American Indian, and Alaska Native infants are 2-3 times more likely than white infants to die of SIDS, whereas Asian, Pacific Islander, and Hispanic infants have the lowest incidence. Some of this disparity may be related to the higher concentration of poverty and other adverse environmental factors found within some, but not all, of the communities with higher incidence.

Infants are at greatest risk of SIDS at 1-4 mo of age, with most deaths having occurred by 6 mo. This characteristic age has decreased in some countries as the SIDS incidence has declined, with deaths occurring at earlier ages and with a flattening of the peak age incidence. Similarly, the commonly observed winter seasonal predominance of SIDS has declined or disappeared in some countries as prone prevalence has decreased, supporting prior findings of an interaction between sleep position and factors more common in colder months (overheating as a consequence of elevated interior temperatures or bundling with blankets and heavy clothing, or infection). Male infants are 30–50% more likely to be affected by SIDS than are female infants.

Modifiable Environmental Risk Factors
Pregnancy-Related Factors

An increased SIDS risk is associated with numerous obstetric factors, suggesting that the in utero environment of future SIDS infants is suboptimal. SIDS infants are more commonly of higher birth order, independent of maternal age, and of gestations after shorter interpregnancy intervals. Mothers of SIDS infants generally receive less prenatal care and initiate care later in pregnancy. In addition, low birthweight, preterm birth, and slower intrauterine and postnatal growth rates are risk factors.

Cigarette Smoking

There is a major association between **intrauterine exposure to cigarette smoking** and risk for SIDS. The incidence of SIDS was 2-3 times greater among infants of mothers who smoked in studies conducted before SIDS risk-reduction campaigns and 4 times higher in studies after implementation of risk-reduction campaigns. The risk of death is progressively greater as daily cigarette use increases. The effects of smoking by the infant's father and other household members are more difficult to interpret because they are highly correlated with maternal smoking. There appears to be a small independent effect of paternal smoking, but data on other household members have been inconsistent. The effect of prenatal smoking on SIDS risk is not believed to be caused by lower birthweight, which is often found among infants of smoking mothers.

It is very difficult to assess the independent effect of infant exposure to **environmental tobacco smoke** because parental smoking behaviors during and after pregnancy are also highly correlated. However, a 2-fold increased risk of SIDS is found for infants exposed only to postnatal maternal environmental tobacco smoke. There is a dose-response for the number of household smokers, number of people smoking in the same room as the infant, and the number of cigarettes smoked. These data suggest that keeping the infant free of environmental tobacco smoke can further reduce an infant's risk of SIDS.

Drug and Alcohol Use

Most studies link maternal prenatal drug use, especially opiates, with an increased risk of SIDS, ranging from a 2- to 15-fold increased risk. Studies looking at the association between maternal alcohol use prenatally or postnatally and SIDS have conflicting results. In one study of Northern Plains Indians, periconceptional alcohol use and binge drinking in the 1st trimester were associated with a 6-fold and an 8-fold increased risk of SIDS, respectively. A Danish cohort study found that mothers admitted to the hospital for an alcohol- or a drug-related disorder at any time before or after the birth of their infants had a 3-time higher risk of their infant dying from SIDS, and a Dutch study reported that maternal alcohol consumption in the 24 hr before the infant died carried an 8-fold increased risk of SIDS. Siblings of infants with fetal alcohol syndrome have a 10-fold increased risk of SIDS compared with controls. Although there are conflicting reports of illicit drug use and SIDS overall, prenatal drug use, especially opiates, is associated with an increased risk of SIDS, ranging from 2- to 15-fold. Data on cannabis use and SIDS are extremely limited, with only one study from New Zealand reporting results for postpartum maternal use. This study found that nighttime cannabis use was associated with a 2-fold increased risk of SIDS, whereas daytime use was not associated with increased risk.

Infant Sleep Environment

Sleeping prone has consistently been shown to increase the risk of SIDS. As rates of prone positioning have decreased in the general population, the odds ratios for SIDS in infants still sleeping prone have increased. *The highest risk of SIDS occurs in infants who are usually placed nonprone but placed prone for last sleep ("unaccustomed prone") or found prone ("secondary prone").* The "unaccustomed prone" position may be more likely to occur in daycare or other settings outside the home and highlights the need for all infant caretakers to be educated about appropriate sleep positioning.

Side-Sleeping: Significant Risk Factor. The initial SIDS risk-reduction campaign recommendations considered side-sleeping to be nearly equivalent to the supine position in reducing the risk of SIDS. Subsequent studies documented that side-sleeping infants were twice as likely to die of SIDS as infants sleeping supine. This increased risk may be related to the relative instability of the position. Infants who are placed on their side and roll to prone are at exceptional risk, with one study finding they are almost 9 times more likely to die of SIDS than those placed supine. Although the majority of SIDS occurrences are still associated with infants being found prone, a higher proportion of SIDS is now attributed to being placed on the side for sleeping than for being placed prone. The current recommendations call for supine position for sleeping for all infants except those few with specific medical conditions for which recommending a different position may be justified, in infants with anatomic or functional upper airway compromise.

Many parents and healthcare providers were initially concerned that supine sleeping would be associated with an increase in adverse consequences, such as difficulty sleeping, vomiting, or aspiration. However, evidence suggests that the risk of regurgitation and choking is highest for prone-sleeping infants. Some newborn nursery staff still tend to favor side positioning, which models inappropriate infant care practice to parents. Infants sleeping on their backs do not have more episodes of cyanosis or apnea, and reports of apparent life-threatening events actually decreased in Scandinavia after increased use of the supine position. Among infants in the United States who maintained the same sleep position at 1, 3, and 6 mo of age, no clinical symptoms or reasons for outpatient visits (including fever, cough, wheezing, trouble breathing or sleeping, vomiting, diarrhea, or respiratory illness) were more common in infants sleeping supine or on their sides compared with infants sleeping prone. Three symptoms were actually less common in infants sleeping supine or on their sides: fever at 1 mo, stuffy nose at 6 mo, and trouble sleeping at 6 mo. Outpatient visits for ear infection were less common at 3 and 6 mo for infants sleeping supine and also less common at 3 mo for infants sleeping on their side. These results provide reassurance for parents and healthcare providers and should contribute to universal acceptance of supine as the safest and optimal sleep position for infants.

Soft Sleep Surfaces and Soft or Loose Bedding. Soft sleep surfaces and soft or loose bedding, including comforters, pillows, bumper pads, stuffed animals, mattress toppers, pillow-top mattresses, sheepskins, polystyrene bean pillows, and old or soft mattresses, are associated with increased risk of SIDS. Infant sleep positioners, including pillows and wedges, which are often marketed to hold infants on their side or at an angle to help with reflux, are also not recommended. Based on available research, **swaddling infants**, or wrapping them in a blanket, is not recommended as a strategy to reduce SIDS. Infants who roll to the prone position while swaddled are at particularly high risk of SIDS. Wearable blankets, which may have a built-in swaddle, are an acceptable alternative.

Overheating. **Overheating,** based on indicators such as higher room temperature, a history of fever, sweating, and excessive clothing or bedding, has been associated with increased risk of SIDS. Some studies have identified an interaction between overheating and prone sleeping, with overheating increasing the risk of SIDS only when infants are sleeping prone. Higher external environmental temperatures have not been associated with increased SIDS incidence in the United States.

Bed Sharing. Several studies have implicated **bed sharing** as a risk factor for SIDS. Bed sharing is particularly hazardous when other children are in the same bed, when the parent is sleeping with an infant on a couch, sofa, or other soft or confining sleeping surface, when the mother is a smoker, and when the bed sharer has used alcohol or arousal-altering drugs or medications. Infants younger than 4 mo of age are at increased risk even when mothers are nonsmokers. A meta-analysis of 19 studies found that low-risk infants (i.e., those who were breastfed and never exposed to cigarette smoke in utero or after birth) still had a 5-fold increased risk of SIDS until the age of 3 mo if bed sharing. Risk is also increased with longer duration of bed sharing during the night, whereas returning the infant to the infant's own crib has not been associated with increased risk. Room sharing without bed sharing is associated with lower SIDS rates and is therefore recommended.

Infant Feeding Care Practices and Exposures

Breastfeeding is Associated With a Lower Risk of Sudden Infant Death Syndrome. A meta-analysis found that breastfeeding was associated with a 45% reduction in SIDS after adjusting for confounding variables and that this protective effect increased for exclusive breastfeeding compared with partial breastfeeding.

Pacifier (dummy) use is associated with a lower risk of SIDS in the majority of studies. Although it is not known if this is a direct effect of the pacifier itself or from associated infant or parental behaviors, use of the pacifier is protective even if it is dislodged during sleep. Concerns have been expressed about recommending pacifiers as a means of reducing the risk of SIDS for fear of adverse consequences, particularly interference with breastfeeding. However, well-designed clinical trials have found no association between pacifiers and breastfeeding duration.

Upper respiratory tract infections have generally not been found to be an independent risk factor for SIDS, but these and other minor infections may still have a role in the causal pathway of SIDS when other risk factors are present. Risk for SIDS has been found to be increased after illness among prone sleepers, those who were heavily wrapped, and those whose heads were covered during sleep.

No adverse association between immunizations and SIDS has been found. Indeed, SIDS infants are less likely to be immunized than control infants, and, in immunized infants, no temporal relationship between vaccine administration and death has been identified. In a meta-analysis of case-control studies that adjusted for potentially confounding factors, the risk of SIDS for infants immunized with diphtheria, tetanus, and pertussis was half that for nonimmunized infants.

Sudden Infant Death Syndrome Rates Remain Higher Among American Indians, Alaska Natives, and African Americans. This may be due, in part, to group differences in adopting supine sleeping or other risk-reduction practices. Greater efforts are needed to address this persistent disparity and to ensure that SIDS risk-reduction education reaches all parents and other care providers, including other family members and personnel at daycare centers.

GENETIC RISK FACTORS

As summarized in Table 402.4, there are numerous genetic differences identified in infants who died of SIDS compared with healthy infants and to infants dying from other causes. Polymorphisms occurring at higher incidence in SIDS infants compared with controls include multiple cardiac ion channelopathy genes that are proarrhythmic, autonomic nervous system development genes, proinflammatory genes related to infection and immunity, and several 5-HT genes.

Multiple studies have established the importance of a pathway to SIDS that involves cardiac sodium or potassium channel dysfunction resulting in **either long QT syndrome (LQTS)** or other proarrhythmic conditions. LQTS is a known cause of sudden unexpected death in children and adults as the result of a prolonged cardiac action potential causing either increased depolarization or decreased repolarization current (Fig. 402.1). The first evidence supporting a causal role for LQTS in SIDS was a large Italian study in which a corrected QT interval >440 msec on an electrocardiogram performed on days 3-4 of life was associated with an odds ratio of 41 for SIDS. Several case reports have subsequently provided proof of concept that cardiac channelopathy polymorphisms are associated with SIDS. LQTS is associated with polymorphisms related mainly to gain-of-function mutations in the

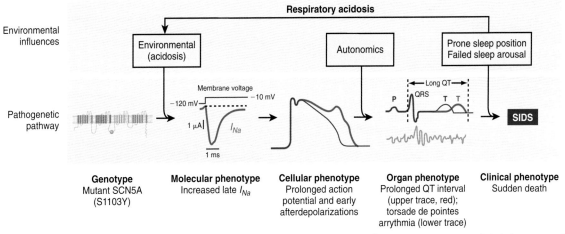

Fig. 402.1 A proarrhythmic pathogenetic pathway for sudden infant death syndrome *(SIDS)* from patient genotype to clinical phenotype, with environmental influences noted. The genetic abnormality—in this instance, a polymorphism in the cardiac Na⁺ channel SCN5A—causes a molecular phenotype of increased late Na⁺ current (I_{Na}) under the influence of environmental factors such as acidosis. Interacting with other ion currents that may themselves be altered by genetic and environmental factors, the late Na⁺ current causes a cellular phenotype of prolonged action potential duration, as well as early afterdepolarizations. Prolonged action potential in the cells of the ventricular myocardium and further interaction with environmental factors such as autonomic innervation, which, in turn, may be affected by genetic factors, produce a tissue-organ phenotype of a prolonged QT interval on the electrocardiogram (ECG) and torsades de pointes arrhythmia in the whole heart. If this is sustained or degenerates to ventricular fibrillation, the clinical phenotype of SIDS results. Environmental and multiple genetic factors can interact at many different levels to produce the characteristic phenotypes at the molecular, cellular, tissue, organ, and clinical levels. *(From Makielski JC: SIDS: genetic and environmental influences may cause arrhythmia in this silent killer, J Clin Invest 116(2):297–299, 2006.)*

sodium channel gene *(SCN5A)* that encode critical channel pore-forming α subunits or essential channel-interacting proteins. LQTS also is associated with mainly loss-of-function polymorphisms in potassium channel genes. **Short QT syndrome (SQTS)** is more recently recognized as another cause of life-threatening arrhythmia or sudden death, often during rest or sleep. Gain-of-function mutations in genes including *KCNH2* and *KCNQ1* have been causally linked to SQTS, and some of these deaths have occurred in infants, suggesting that SQTS may also be causally linked to SIDS.

In addition to LQTS and SQTS, the other cardiac ion-related channelopathy polymorphisms are also proarrhythmic, including Brugada syndrome *(BrS1, BrS2)* and catecholaminergic paroxysmal ventricular tachycardia *(CPVT1)*. Collectively, these mutations in cardiac ion channels provide a lethal proarrhythmic substrate in some infants (see Fig. 402.1) and may account for 10% or more of SIDS cases.

Impaired central respiratory regulation is an important biologic abnormality in SIDS, and genetic polymorphisms have been identified in SIDS infants that affect both serotonergic and adrenergic neurons. Monoamine oxidase A metabolizes both of these neurotransmitters, and a recent study has observed a high association between SIDS and low expressing alleles in males, perhaps contributing to the higher incidence of SIDS in males. Many genes are involved in the control of 5-HT synthesis, storage, membrane uptake, and metabolism. Polymorphisms in the promoter region of the 5-HTT protein gene occur with greater frequency in SIDS than control infants. The long "L" allele increases effectiveness of the promoter and reduces extracellular 5-HT concentrations at nerve endings, compared with the short "S" allele. White, African-American, and Japanese SIDS infants were more likely than ethnicity-matched controls to have the "L" (long) allele, and there was also a negative association between SIDS and the S/S genotype. The L/L genotype was associated with increased 5-HT transporters on neuroimaging and postmortem binding studies. However, in a large San Diego dataset of SIDS infants, no relationship was found between SIDS and the L allele or the LL genotype.

An association has also been observed between SIDS and a 5-HTT intron 2 polymorphism, which differentially regulates *5-HTT* expression. There were positive associations between SIDS and the intron 2 genotype distributions in African-American infants who died of SIDS, compared with African-American controls. The human *FEV* gene is specifically expressed in central 5-HT neurons in the brain, with a predicted role in specification and maintenance of the serotoninergic neuronal phenotype. An insertion mutation has been identified in intron 2 of the *FEV* gene, and the distribution of this mutation differs significantly in SIDS compared with control infants.

Molecular genetic studies in SIDS victims have also identified mutations pertinent to early embryologic development of the autonomic nervous system (see Table 402.4). Protein-changing mutations related to the *PHOX2a, RET, ECE1, TLX3,* and *EN1* genes have been identified, particularly in African-American infants who died of SIDS. Eight polymorphisms in the *PHOX2B* gene occurred significantly more frequently in SIDS compared with control infants. One study has reported an association between SIDS and a distinct tyrosine hydroxylase gene *(THO1)* allele, which regulates gene expression and catecholamine production.

Multiple studies have observed altered expression of genes involved in the inflammatory process and immune system regulation. Differences in SIDS infants, compared with controls, have been reported for 2 complement *C4* genes. Some SIDS infants have loss-of-function polymorphisms in the gene promoter region for IL-10, another antiinflammatory cytokine. IL-10 polymorphisms associated with decreased IL-10 levels could contribute to SIDS by delaying initiation of protective antibody production or reducing capacity to inhibit inflammatory cytokine production. However, other studies have not found differences in IL-10 genes in SIDS infants compared with age-matched controls.

An association has been reported between single nucleotide polymorphisms in the proinflammatory gene encoding IL-8 and SIDS infants found prone, compared with SIDS infants found in other sleep positions. IL-1 is another proinflammatory gene, and a higher prevalence of the IL-1 receptor antagonist, which would predispose to higher risk for

infection, has been reported in infants who died of SIDS. Significant associations with SIDS are also reported for polymorphisms in VEGF, IL-6, and tumor necrosis factor-α (TNFα). These 3 cytokines are proinflammatory, and these gain-of-function polymorphisms would result in increased inflammatory response to infectious or inflammatory stimuli and hence contribute to an adverse imbalance between proinflammatory and antiinflammatory cytokines. As apparent proof of principle, elevated levels of IL-6 and VEGF have been reported from cerebrospinal fluid in SIDS infants. There were no group differences in the IL6-174G/C polymorphism in a Norwegian SIDS study, but the aggregate evidence nevertheless suggested an activated immune system in SIDS and implicated genes involved in the immune system. Almost all SIDS infants in one study had positive histories for prone sleeping and fever prior to death and positive HLA-DR expression in laryngeal mucosa, and high HLA-DR expression was associated with high levels of IL-6 in cerebrospinal fluid.

GENE-ENVIRONMENT INTERACTIONS

Interactions between genetic and environmental risk factors determine the actual risk for SIDS in individual infants (Fig. 402.2). Equally important, there is a dynamic interaction between genetic or intrinsic vulnerability and the sleep environment (Fig. 402.3). There appears to be an interaction between prone sleep position and impaired ventilatory and arousal responsiveness. Facedown or nearly facedown sleeping does occasionally occur in prone-sleeping infants, but normal healthy infants arouse before such episodes become life-threatening. However, infants with insufficient arousal responsiveness to hypoxia may be at risk for sudden death from resulting episodes of airway obstruction and asphyxia. There may also be links between modifiable risk factors (such as soft bedding, prone sleep position, and thermal stress) and genetic risk factors, such as ventilatory and arousal abnormalities and temperature or metabolic regulation deficits. Cardiorespiratory control deficits could be related to 5-HTT polymorphisms, for example, or to polymorphisms in genes pertinent to autonomic nervous system development. Affected infants could be at increased risk for sleep-related hypoxemia and hence more susceptible to adverse effects associated with unsafe sleep position or bedding. Infants at increased risk for sleep-related hypoxemia could also be at greater risk for fatal arrhythmias in the presence of a cardiac ion channelopathy polymorphism.

In >50% of SIDS victims, recent febrile illnesses, often related to upper respiratory infection, have been documented (see Table 402.5). Benign infections might increase risk for SIDS if interacting with genetically determined proinflammatory or impaired immune responses. Deficient inflammatory responsiveness can also occur as a result of mast cell degranulation, which has been reported in SIDS infants. This is consistent with an anaphylactic reaction to a bacterial toxin, and some family members of SIDS infants also have mast cell hyperreleasability and degranulation, suggesting that increased susceptibility to an anaphylactic reaction is another genetic factor influencing fatal outcomes to otherwise minor infections. Interactions between upper respiratory infections or other minor illnesses and factors such as prone sleeping might also play a role in the pathogenesis of SIDS.

The increased risk of SIDS associated with fetal and postnatal exposure to cigarette smoke may be related at least in part to genetic or epigenetic factors, including those affecting brainstem autonomic control. Infant studies document decreased ventilatory and arousal responsiveness to hypoxia following fetal nicotine exposure, and impaired autoresuscitation after apnea has been associated with postnatal nicotine exposure. Decreased brainstem immunoreactivity to selected protein kinase C and neuronal nitric oxide synthase isoforms occurs in rats exposed to cigarette smoke prenatally, another potential cause of impaired hypoxic responsiveness. Smoking exposure also increases susceptibility to viral and bacterial infections and increases bacterial binding after passive coating of mucosal surfaces with smoke components, implicating interactions between smoking, cardiorespiratory control, and immune status. Flavin-monooxygenase 3 *(FMO3)* is one of the enzymes that metabolizes nicotine, and a polymorphism has recently been identified that occurs more frequently in SIDS infants compared with controls and more frequently in infants whose mothers reported heavy smoking (see Table 402.4). This polymorphism would result in increased nicotine levels and hence is a potential genetic risk factor for SIDS in infants exposed to cigarette smoke.

In infants with a cardiac ion channelopathy, risk for a fatal arrhythmia during sleep may be substantially enhanced by predisposing perturbations that increase electrical instability. These perturbations could include REM sleep with bursts of vagal and sympathetic activation, minor respiratory infections, or any other cause of sleep-related hypoxemia or hypercarbia, especially those resulting in acidosis. The prone sleeping position is associated with increased sympathetic activity.

INFANT GROUPS AT INCREASED RISK FOR SUDDEN INFANT DEATH SYNDROME

Subsequent Siblings of an Infant who Died of Sudden Infant Death Syndrome

The next-born siblings of first-born infants dying of any noninfectious natural cause are at significantly increased risk for infant death from the same cause, including SIDS. The relative risk is 9.1 for the same cause of recurrent death versus 1.6 for a different cause of death. The relative risk for recurrent SIDS (range: 5.4-5.8) is similar to the relative risk for non-SIDS causes of recurrent death (range: 4.6-12.5). The risk for recurrent infant mortality from the same cause as in the index sibling thus appears to be increased to a similar degree in subsequent siblings for both explained causes and for SIDS. This increased risk for recurrent SIDS in families is consistent with genetic risk factors interacting with environmental risk factors (see Tables 402.4 and 402.5 and Figs. 402.2 and 402.3). However, recurrent SIDS in a family should also alert the clinician to consider other causes of sudden and unexpected death (see Table 402.2).

Prematurity

Despite reductions of more than 50% in SIDS and SUID among infants born preterm since initiation of the Back to Sleep campaign in the United States in 1994, the risk of death remains significantly higher for these infants than for those born full term. The risk increases as gestational age decreases. Compared with infants born at 37-42 wk, the odds ratio for SIDS is greatest for infants born at 24-28 wk gestation (2.57, 95% confidence interval 2.08, 3.17). Even at 33-36 wk gestational age at birth, the risk of SIDS remains significantly increased compared with infants born at term. The peak chronologic age for SIDS is later in infants born preterm; chronologic age at death is inversely proportional to gestational age at birth.

Although infants born preterm are at increased risk for apnea, apnea of prematurity per se *does not* seem to be related to the increased SIDS

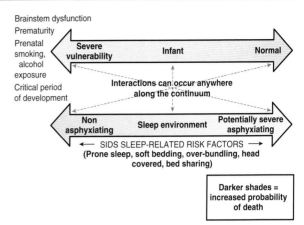

Fig. 402.3 Dynamic interactions between intrinsic vulnerability to sudden infant death syndrome (SIDS) and degree of risk of the sleep environment, ranging from nonasphyxiating (completely safe) to potentially severe asphyxiating (very unsafe). Intrinsic vulnerability could be related to genetic risk factors, fetal or early infant exposures, or other factors. (Modified from Hunt CE, Darnall RA, McEntire BL, Hyma BA: Assigning cause for sudden unexpected infant death, Forensic Sci Med Pathol 11(2):283–288, 2015.)

risk. This increased risk is instead likely related in part to immaturity of brainstem responses; physiologic studies have found impaired cortical arousals, lower baroreflex sensitivity, and impaired autonomic control. Sociodemographic and environmental risk are also important. Infants born preterm have more sociodemographic risk factors overall than infants born at term. In addition, infants born preterm are more likely to be placed prone at home; this may be in part because these infants are often placed prone while mechanically ventilated in the neonatal intensive care unit, and safe sleep practices are often not well-modeled during the remainder of the NICU admission. The association between prone position and SIDS in preterm and low birthweight infants is equal or greater than this association in infants born full term.

Physiologic Studies

Physiologic studies have been performed in healthy infants in early infancy, a few of whom later died of SIDS. Physiologic studies have also been performed on infant groups who were believed to be at increased risk for SIDS, especially those with brief resolved unexplained events (BRUE; formerly known as apparent life-threatening events; Chapter 403) and subsequent siblings of infants who died of SIDS. In the aggregate, these studies have indicated brainstem abnormalities in the neuroregulation of cardiorespiratory control or other autonomic functions and are consistent with the autopsy findings and genetic studies in infants who died of SIDS (see "Pathology" and "Genetic Risk Factors"). In addition to physiologic abnormalities in chemoreceptor sensitivity, other observed physiologic abnormalities have been found in respiratory pattern, control of heart and respiratory rate or variability, and asphyxic arousal responsiveness. A deficit in arousal responsiveness may be a necessary prerequisite for SIDS to occur but may be insufficient to cause SIDS in the absence of other genetic or environmental risk factors. **Autoresuscitation (gasping)** is a critical component of the asphyxic arousal response, and a failure of autoresuscitation in SIDS infants may be the final and most devastating physiologic failure. In one study, most normal full-term infants younger than 9 postnatal wk of age aroused in response to mild hypoxia, whereas only 10–15% of infants older than 9 wk of age aroused. These data suggest that ability to arouse to mild to moderate hypoxic stimuli may be at a nadir at the age range of greatest risk for SIDS.

The ability to shorten the QT interval as heart rate increases appears to be impaired in some infants who died of SIDS, suggesting that such infants may be predisposed to ventricular arrhythmia. Although this

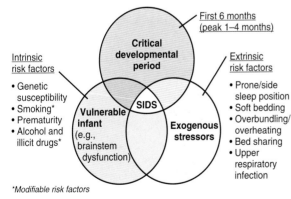

Fig. 402.2 Schematic of the triple-risk model for sudden infant death syndrome (SIDS) showing the critical interactions between intrinsic risk factors (including genetic risk factors) resulting in a vulnerable infant, a critical developmental period or age, and exogenous stressors or extrinsic risk factors. (Modified from Filiano JJ, Kinney HC: A perspective on the neuropathologic findings in victims of the sudden infant death syndrome: the triple risk model, Biol Neonate 65(3–4):194–197, 1994.)

is consistent with the observations of cardiac ion channel gene polymorphisms in some SIDS infants (see Table 402.4), there are no antemortem QT interval data for these infants that confirm the importance of this finding. Infants who were studied physiologically and then died of SIDS a few weeks later had higher heart rates and lower heart rate variability in all sleep–wake states and diminished heart rate variability during wakefulness. These SIDS infants also had longer QT intervals than control infants during both REM and non-REM sleep, especially in the late hours of the night when most SIDS likely occurs. However, the QT interval exceeded 440 msec in only one of these SIDS infants.

It has been postulated that the decreased heart rate variability and increased heart rate observed in infants who later died of SIDS may in part be related to decreased vagal tone, perhaps from vagal neuropathy or brainstem damage in areas responsible for parasympathetic cardiac control. Power spectrum analysis of heart rate variability is 1 way to assess sympathetic and parasympathetic cardiac control. In a comparison of heart rate power spectra before and after obstructive apneas in clinically asymptomatic infants, infants later dying of SIDS did not have the decreases in low-frequency to high-frequency power ratios observed in infants who survived. Some infants may thus have different autonomic responsiveness to obstructive apnea, perhaps indicating impaired autonomic nervous system control associated with higher vulnerability to external or endogenous stresses, and hence reduced electrical stability of the heart; this may create a vulnerability for SIDS.

Home cardiorespiratory monitors with memory capability have recorded the terminal events in some infants who died of SIDS. However, these recordings did not include pulse oximetry and could not identify obstructed breaths due to reliance on transthoracic impedance for breath detection. In most instances, there was sudden and rapid progression of severe bradycardia that was either unassociated with central apnea or appeared to occur too soon to be explained by the central apnea. These observations are consistent with an abnormality in autonomic control of heart rate variability or with obstructed breaths resulting in bradycardia or hypoxemia and associated with impaired autoresuscitation or arousal.

CLINICAL STRATEGIES
Home Monitoring
SIDS cannot be *prevented* in individual infants because it is not possible to identify prospective SIDS infants, and no effective intervention has been established even if infants at risk could be prospectively identified. Studies of cardiorespiratory pattern or other autonomic abnormalities do not have sufficient sensitivity and specificity to be clinically useful as screening tests. Home electronic surveillance using existing technology *does not* reduce the risk of SIDS. Although a prolonged QT interval in an infant may be treated if diagnosed, neither the role of routine postnatal electrocardiographic screening, the cost-effectiveness of diagnosis and treatment, nor the safety of treatment in infants has been established (see Chapter 456). Parental electrocardiographic screening is not helpful, in part because spontaneous mutations are common.

Reducing the Risk of Sudden Infant Death Syndrome
Reducing risk behaviors and increasing protective behaviors among infant caregivers to achieve further reductions and eventual elimination of SIDS is a critical goal. Recent plateaus in placing infants supine for sleep in the United States at approximately 75% for all races and only 56% for African Americans are cause for concern and require renewed educational efforts. The American Academy of Pediatrics (AAP) guidelines to reduce the risk of SIDS were updated in 2016 and are aimed at reducing the risk of all sudden and unexpected sleep-related infant deaths. The guidelines are appropriate for most infants, but physicians and other healthcare providers might, on occasion, need to consider alternative approaches. The major components of the AAP guidelines are:

- Full-term and premature infants should be placed for sleep in the supine position. There are no adverse health outcomes from supine sleeping. Side-sleeping is not recommended.

- Infants should be put to sleep on a firm mattress. Waterbeds, sofas, soft mattresses, or other soft surfaces should not be used. In addition, car seats, strollers, swings, and other sitting devices should not be used for sleeping. Sleeping in an upright position can lead to gastroesophageal reflux or upper airway obstruction from head flexion.

- Breastfeeding is recommended. If possible, mothers should exclusively breastfeed or feed with expressed human milk until the infant is 6 mo of age.

- It is recommended that infants sleep in the same room as their parents but in their own crib or bassinet that conforms to the safety standards of the Consumer Product Safety Commission. Placing the crib or bassinet near the mother's bed facilitates nursing and contact. If parents bring the infant into the adult bed for feeding or comforting, the infant should be returned to a separate sleep surface when the parents are ready for sleep.

- Soft materials and loose bedding in the infant's sleep environment—over, under, or near the infant—should be avoided. These include pillows, comforters, quilts, sheepskins, bumper pads, and stuffed toys. Sleep clothing, such as a wearable blanket, can be used in place of blankets.

- Consider offering a pacifier at bedtime and naptime. The pacifier should be used when placing the infant down for sleep and need not be reinserted once it falls out. For breastfed infants, delay introduction of the pacifier until breastfeeding is well established.

- Mothers should not smoke during pregnancy or after birth, and infants should not be exposed to second-hand smoke.

- Mothers should avoid alcohol and illicit drug use during pregnancy and after birth.

- Avoid overheating and overbundling. The infant should be lightly clothed for sleep and the thermostat set at a comfortable temperature.

- Pregnant women should obtain regular prenatal care, following guidelines for prenatal visits.

- Infants should be immunized in accordance with recommendations of the AAP and the Centers for Disease Control and Prevention. There is no evidence that immunizations increase the risk of SIDS. Indeed, recent evidence suggests that immunizations may have a protective effect against SIDS.

- Avoid the use of commercial devices that are inconsistent with safe sleep recommendations. Devices advertised to maintain sleep position, "protect" a bed sharing infant, or reduce the risk of rebreathing are not recommended because there is no evidence to support their safety or efficacy.

- Home cardiorespiratory and/or O_2 saturation monitoring may be of value for selected infants who have extreme instability, but there is no evidence that monitoring decreases the incidence of SIDS, and it is therefore not recommended for this purpose.

- Infants should have some time in the prone position (tummy time) while awake and observed. Alternating the placement of the infant's head, as well as orientation in the crib, can also minimize the risk of head flattening from supine sleeping (positional plagiocephaly).

- Swaddling cannot be recommended as a strategy to reduce SIDS. If infants are placed in a swaddle it should be using a light blanket that is snug around the shoulders but looser around the hips to avoid hip dysplasia. Swaddled infants should always be placed supine, and once infants can roll to the prone position all swaddling should be discontinued.

- Healthcare professionals, staff in newborn nurseries and neonatal intensive care units, and child care providers should adopt the SIDS reduction recommendations beginning at birth to model safe sleep for caregivers.

- Media and manufacturers should follow safe sleep guidelines in their messaging and advertising.

- The national "Safe to Sleep" campaign should be continued with additional emphasis placed on strategies to increase breastfeeding while decreasing bed sharing and tobacco smoke exposure. The campaign should continue to have a special focus on the groups with higher rates of SIDS, including educational strategies tailored to individual racial-ethnic groups. Secondary care providers need to be targeted to receive these educational messages, including daycare providers, grandparents, foster parents, and baby sitters. Efforts should also be made to introduce sleep recommendations before pregnancy and ideally in secondary school curricula.

- Research and surveillance should be continued on the risk factors, causes, and pathophysiologic mechanisms of SIDS and other sleep-related SUID, with the ultimate goal of preventing these deaths entirely. Federal and private funding agencies need to remain committed to this research.

Bibliography is available at Expert Consult.

402.1 Sudden Unexpected Postnatal Collapse

Sarah Vepraskas

EPIDEMIOLOGY

Sudden unexplained postnatal collapse (SUPC) is a rare but potentially fatal event in an otherwise healthy term newborn that includes any condition resulting in temporary or permanent cessation of breathing or cardiorespiratory failure. SUPC results in death in about half of the infants and significant impairment in many survivors.

SUPC, in some definitions, includes both severe apparent life-threatening events (currently referred to as BRUE) and SUID, occurring within the 1st *postnatal week* of life. In general, SUID is a term that encompasses all SUIDs. Some BRUEs may be low risk and require simple interventions such as positional changes, brief stimulation, or procedures to resolve the airway obstruction; these seemingly more benign events are in contrast to SUPC, which can be potentially fatal.

The definition of SUPC used in the AAP report on safe sleep and skin-to-skin care is by the British Association of Perinatal Medicine and includes any term or near-term (defined as >35 wk gestation) infant who meets the following criteria: (1) is well at birth (normal 5-min Apgar and deemed well enough for routine care), (2) collapses unexpectedly in a state of cardiorespiratory extremis such that resuscitation with intermittent positive-pressure ventilation is required, (3) collapses within the 1st 7 days of life, and (4) either dies, goes on to require intensive care, or develops encephalopathy. A majority of reported events occur within 2 hr after birth, often at the time of the 1st breastfeeding attempt. Other potential medical conditions that place infants at higher risk, such as prematurity (<35 wk gestation), perinatal asphyxia, sepsis, or congenital malformations, should be excluded for SUPC to be diagnosed.

The incidence of SUPC is estimated to be 2.6-133 per 100,000 live births. However, the incidence varies widely because there is a lack of consensus on the definition, differing inclusion and exclusion criteria exist, and no standardized reporting system. In addition, a consensus for coding SUPC has not been established, which likely contributes to it being underreported.

The published estimations of SUPC are lower than what occur in the hospital and reflect only the critical events. When a defined time for the SUPC event is described, approximately one third of reported events occur during the 1st 2 hr, another one third between 2 and 24 hr, and another one third between 1 and 7 days after birth.

PATHOGENESIS

The mechanism for SUPC is not completely known. Many of the events may be related to suffocation or entrapment. It is also hypothesized that the transition from fetal to extrauterine life could make the newborn more vulnerable during the 1st hr of life. During birth there is an initial surge of adenosine and prostaglandins, followed by a postnatal surge of catecholamines. A healthy newborn baby is aroused and awake after birth and starts continuous breathing movements. Shortly after birth, there is a rapid decrease in the inhibitory neuromodulator adenosine as the partial pressure of oxygen in the arterial blood rapidly increases and contributes to the increased activity in the newborn infant compared

with the fetus. Following the hormone surges, there is a period of diminished responsiveness to external stimuli and increased vagal tone; it is possible that autonomic instability could make infants vulnerable during this transitioning period.

It is also possible that impaired cardiorespiratory control due to hypoxic ischemic injury occurring days before birth could contribute to fatal cases of SUPC. Mild gliosis in brainstem areas involved in cardiorespiratory control was found at autopsy of 7 infants with SUPC. However, there are insufficient data to support an association between in utero hypoxic events and SUPC.

RISK FACTORS

Many of reported SUPC cases occur while the infant is in prone position, during skin-to-skin contact (SSC) with their mothers. SSC is traditionally defined as beginning at birth and lasting continually until the end of the first breastfeeding.

Additional risk factors for SUPC include the first breastfeeding attempt, cosleeping, a mother in the episiotomy position, a primiparous mother, and parents left alone with baby during the 1st hr after birth.

SSC and rooming-in have become common practice for healthy newborns and align with Baby-Friendly Hospital Initiative (BFHI), a global program launched by the World Health Organization (WHO) and the United Nations Children's Fund (UNICEF) to encourage and recognize hospitals and birthing centers that promote the optimal level of care for infant feeding and mother/baby bonding. The BFHI recognizes and awards birthing facilities that successfully implement the "Ten Steps to Successful Breastfeeding," with step 4 being to initiate breastfeeding within 1 hr of birth and step 7 recommending the practice of rooming-in. The AAP clinical report on safe sleep and SSC in the newborn period both reviews the evidence supporting SSC and rooming-in during the newborn period, while addressing the safety concerns and providing suggestions to improve safety after delivery. The literature supporting SSC also emphasizes the importance that mother and baby should not be left unattended during this early period.

DIAGNOSIS AND DIFFERENTIAL DIAGNOSIS

The diagnosis of SUPC should be made only after other pathologic causes are excluded. One study consisting of 45 cases of unexpected collapse in newborns found that one third of infants had an underlying pathologic or clinical condition, such as sepsis, ductal dependent congenital heart disease, congenital diaphragmatic hernia, intracranial hemorrhage, or a metabolic disorder (1 infant with Zellweger syndrome and another infant with an unidentified metabolic disorder). Additional etiologies to consider include airway obstruction, pneumonia, respiratory distress syndrome, hypoglycemia, vascular thrombosis or embolism, and pulmonary hypertension of the newborn. The differential diagnosis of SUPC is broad, and many conditions overlap with the differential diagnoses for BRUE (Chapter 403), SUID, and SIDS.

For those infants who survive the event, testing to screen for an underlying pathology should be performed and tailored to the specific details of each case. A thorough history and physical exam should be performed prior to initiating the diagnostic workup to assist one in focusing the evaluation. Laboratory tests to consider include electrolytes; metabolic evaluation including glucose, ammonia, and lactate; an infectious evaluation including blood cultures, urinalysis, and urine cultures; and CSF analysis with CSF culture. Chest radiography, neuroimaging, echocardiogram, electrocardiogram, and comprehensive metabolic screening (included as part of the newborn screen in most states) could also be useful diagnostic tools. Postmortem examination in the case of death from presumed SUPC should also be considered because underlying etiology of the event may be discovered during autopsy.

OUTCOME

Approximately half of SUPC cases are thought to result in death. A review of 17 and 45 SUPC cases in Germany and United Kingdom showed a mortality rate of 42% and 27%, respectively. In the German study, almost two-thirds of the surviving cases had neurologic deficits, and in the United Kingdom study, one third of infants either died or had residual neurologic deficits. Rates of death and neurologic abnormalities reported in the 2 aforementioned studies are comparable with other available case reports.

TREATMENT

There are data suggesting that hypothermia treatment may improve neurologic outcomes after a SUPC event that results in hypoxic-ischemic encephalopathy (HIE) (see Chapter 120.4). The hypothermia treatment of 4 patients with HIE after SUPC were deemed successful, with follow-up at 24 mo having 3 children being developmentally normal and 1 child having mild cerebral palsy.

PREVENTION

The known risk factors for SUPC can be used to aid in preventive efforts. Specifically, safety during SSC and rooming-in should be emphasized.

Initiatives developed to standardize the procedure for immediate postnatal SSC have not proven to reduce the risk of SUPC. Frequent assessments of newborns should be performed, including observation of breathing, activity, color, tone, and position, to ensure they are in a position to avoid obstructive breathing or events leading to SUPC. It has also been suggested that continuous monitoring by trained staff members be done during SSC. However, that may be obtrusive to mother-infant bonding. Some have suggested continuous pulse oximetry during this period, but there is no evidence to support this practice and this overmonitoring could lead to unnecessary parental concern. Because many cases of SUPC occur within the 1st few hr of life, the delivery unit should be staffed to permit frequent newborn assessments, while preserving the developing mother-child bond.

Many of the same safety concerns that occur during SSC immediately after birth continue to be a concern during rooming-in, if mother is not given guidance on the safe rooming-in practices. Cosleeping should not be permitted on the postpartum unit. Mothers and families need to be informed of the risks of cosleeping. Staffing ratios should be determined to meet the needs of both mother and infant to allow for frequent assessments, rapid response time to call lights, and time for maternal education.

Bibliography is available at Expert Consult.

Chapter **403**

Brief Resolved Unexplained Events and Other Acute Events in Infants

Joel S. Tieder

第四百零三章
短暂且已解决的婴儿不明原因事件和其他婴儿急性事件

中文导读

本章主要介绍了婴儿不明原因事件和其他婴儿急性事件的背景、定义、流行病学以及初始病史。定义主要包括短暂且已解决的婴儿不明原因事件表现以及低风险婴儿的概念。流行病学主要包括发病率、死亡率以及发病风险。阐述了病史、体格检查、筛查以及管理等内容。病史主要包括其他临床症状、生长史、喂养史、家族史、社交经历、感染接触史等。筛查主要包括对低风险人群的筛查，高风险人群需要进一步检查。

BACKGROUND

Infants commonly experience acute, self-resolving changes in their breathing, tone, mental status, and skin color. Usually these events are normal manifestations of developmental immaturity. Nonetheless, caregivers may worry that the acute event could have been life-threatening or is a sign of an undiagnosed medical problem and seek medical attention. In most cases, after a comprehensive history and physical examination, a clinician will determine the event to have been a benign or normal process, such as gastroesophageal reflux (GER) or periodic breathing of the newborn. At times, however, the event defies a simple explanation and drives uncertainty about risk from a serious underlying cause or a future event. This situation poses a diagnostic and management challenge for both the family and the clinician.

Historically, these events were feared as precursors to sudden infant death syndrome (SIDS) and were referred to as *near-miss SIDS, aborted crib deaths*, or *apparent life-threatening events (ALTEs)*. These terms have been replaced because we now know that these events are not associated with SIDS and are rarely life-threatening. Clinical use of ALTE as a diagnostic term is additionally problematic because it relies on the subjective interpretation of the caregiver and includes a nonspecific constellation of symptoms. It also does not distinguish well-appearing patients from those with symptoms.

Most of these acute events in infants are best described as brief resolved unexplained events (BRUEs). A BRUE is a diagnosis of exclusion and should be used only when the event is transient and remains unexplained after an appropriate medical evaluation.

DEFINITION

A BRUE (pronounced *brew*) is an event that occurs in an infant younger than 1 yr that typically lasts less than 30 sec and is described by the observer as a sudden, brief, and now-resolved episode that involved at least one of the following:
- cyanosis or pallor
- absent, decreased, or irregular breathing
- marked change in tone, either hyper- or hypotonia
- altered level of responsiveness

The diagnosis of BRUE applies only to infants who were asymptomatic prior to the event and during evaluation, and when no explanation for the event is found through appropriate history and physical examination.

Infants who experience a BRUE are categorized as either lower or higher risk for a subsequent event or a serious underlying disorder based on patient factors, characterization of the event, additional historical factors, and the physical examination.

A lower-risk infant is defined as
- age >60 days
- gestational age ≥32 wk and postconceptional age ≥45 wk
- occurrence of only 1 BRUE (no prior BRUE ever and not occurring in a cluster)
- duration of event <1 min
- no cardiopulmonary resuscitation (CPR) by trained medical provider required
- no concerning historical features
- no concerning physical examination finding

EPIDEMIOLOGY

The incidence of BRUEs is unknown. However, studies of ALTE patients provide some insight because BRUEs are a subset of what had been considered ALTEs. Hospitalization for an ALTE was common; 1 out of every 2.5-9.4/1,000 infants was hospitalized for an ALTE. Acute events that do not lead to hospitalization are even more common according to large epidemiologic studies of healthy infants. Of normal infants followed longitudinally with home monitoring, up to 43% had a 20-sec apnea episode over a 3-mo period. Of parents asked when their infant was 1 yr of age, 5% recalled an apneic event.

BRUEs are not precursors to SIDS. The incidence of mortality after a BRUE from an underlying cause is unknown but is also likely to be extremely uncommon. The few reports of mortality in studies of ALTE are limited to patients who would not qualify as a BRUE because of the presence of other symptoms or an explanatory diagnosis.

However, for patients presenting with a BRUE, numerous risks must be considered. First is the risk of an underlying serious diagnosis. Although each is rare, clinicians must consider a wide variety of illnesses, such as cardiac arrhythmias, metabolic disorders, and brain injury (Table 403.1). The risk for an underlying serious diagnosis in patients with a BRUE is much lower than the rate reported in ALTE research, where many of the patients had underlying conditions or ongoing symptoms (e.g., lower respiratory tract infection). In infants meeting lower-risk criteria, the likelihood of an underlying serious cause is extremely low. In higher-risk infants, the likelihood is unknown but probably much lower than suggested by research on ALTEs. Second is the risk of a recurrent event, which is currently unknown. These events can be stressful for caregivers, particularly when the cause is unknown. Third is the risk that the caregivers become unnecessarily concerned about their healthy child. Clinicians should be aware the challenges caregivers face when perceiving a threat of losing their child, there is medical uncertainty, or when their child is hospitalized. Fourth are the risks associated with medical care, such as nosocomial infections and inaccurate testing.

INITIAL HISTORY

An appropriate history and physical examination are key to evaluating an infant who has experienced an acute event (Table 403.2). Attention should be given to characterizing the event and interpreting the subjective experience of the caregiver to provide an objective description. The following questions can guide this process:

What was the infant doing before, during, and after the event? An event occurring during or after feeding will likely have a different explanation than one occurring during sleep or after crying. The sequence of events can also be diagnostic. A **breath holding spell** begins with crying, followed by a period of apnea, perioral cyanosis, change of consciousness, and return to baseline.

Did the infant change color? It is often normal for infants to have blueish discoloration (**perioral cyanosis or acrocyanosis**) around the lips or hands because of circulatory immaturity. Turning red or purple is also common when infants cry or become upset. The clinician's goal is to distinguish less concerning color change from **central cyanosis**, which is blue discoloration of the face, trunk, gums, or tongue that can indicate hypoxemia.

Did the infant experience central or obstructive apnea, or just choking or gagging? It is normal for infants to exhibit respiratory pauses of up to 20 sec while awake and asleep. These can reflect **periodic breathing of the newborn** or normal REM sleep. Much more concerning are periods of no air movement that last longer than 20 sec. **Obstructive apnea** results in paradoxical movement of the diaphragm and upper airway. In infants, this is most commonly caused by upper and lower respiratory tract infections (e.g., bronchiolitis) and may precede the recognition of symptoms typically seen in viral respiratory infections. Infants also commonly gag or choke briefly during or shortly after feeds or with GER or vomiting. The resulting reflexive pause in respiration to protect the airway is sometimes referred to as **laryngospasm**. **Central apnea** is always concerning and occurs when the brainstem does not properly control the respiratory muscles. This may be seen in brain trauma from **non-accidental trauma** and in rare disorders such as **congenital central hypoventilation syndrome**.

Was there a concerning change in muscle tone? Seizures in infants are concerning and difficult to diagnose, and they rarely present as typical seizure activity. They can present as staring spells, periods of episodic increased or decreased tone, or **infantile spasms**. It is normal for infants to have rapid jerking movements because of neurological immaturity and infant reflexes (e.g., Moro, startle, and fencing reflex), and sometimes these can appear similar to seizures. One of the most serious and time-sensitive causes of seizures or central apnea is undiagnosed brain trauma from non-accidental trauma, which may result in no other symptoms or physical examination findings upon presentation.

Was there an altered level of responsiveness? Episodic changes in consciousness and mental status can be difficult to assess in infants because of neurological immaturity and variability in sleep-wake cycles.

| Table 403.1 | Symptom-Based Approach to BRUEs: Possible and Other Conditions That Might Be Confused With BRUE |

DIAGNOSTIC CATEGORIES	COMMON AND/OR CONCERNING CAUSES TO CONSIDER	SUGGESTIVE HISTORICAL FINDINGS	SUGGESTIVE PHYSICAL EXAMINATION FINDINGS	TESTING TO CONSIDER
Gastrointestinal	GER Intussusception Volvulus Oropharyngeal dysphagia	Coughing, vomiting, choking, gasping temporally related to feeds or regurgitation of gastric contents Feeding difficulties Recent preceding feed Irritability following feeds Milk in mouth/nose Bilious emesis Pulling legs to chest Bloody/mucousy stool Lethargy following event	Gastric contents in the nose and mouth Choking, gagging, or oxygen desaturation temporally related to feeding or regurgitation of gastric contents	Upper GI to assess for anatomic anomalies Clinical swallow evaluation Abdominal ultrasound pH probe
Infectious	Upper and lower respiratory tract infection (RSV, pertussis, pneumonia) Bacteremia Meningitis Urinary tract infection	Preceding URI symptoms Multiple events on the day of presentation Sick exposures Foul-smelling urine	Fever/hypothermia Lethargy Ill appearance Coryza Cough Wheeze Tachypnea	NP swab for RSV, pertussis Chest radiograph CBC and blood culture Cerebrospinal fluid analysis and culture Urinalysis and culture
Neurologic	Seizures Breath holding spells Congenital central hypoventilation syndrome Neuromuscular disorders Congenital malformations of the brain and brainstem Malignancy Intracranial hemorrhage	Multiple events Loss of consciousness Change in tone Abnormal muscular movements Eye deviation Preceding triggers	Papilledema Abnormal muscular movements Hypertonicity or flaccidity Abnormal reflexes Micro- or macrocephaly Dysmorphic features Signs of trauma or poisoning (see "Child maltreatment" below)	EEG Neuroimaging
Respiratory/ENT	Apnea of prematurity Apnea of infancy Periodic breathing Airway anomaly Aspiration Foreign body Obstructive sleep apnea	Prematurity Foreign body Aspiration Noisy breathing	Wheezing Stridor Crackles Rhonchi Tachypnea	Chest radiograph Neck radiograph Laryngoscopy Bronchoscopy Esophagoscopy Polysomnography
Child maltreatment	Nonaccidental head trauma Smothering Poisoning Factitious syndrome (formerly Munchausen syndrome) by proxy	Multiple events Unexplained vomiting or irritability Recurrent BRUEs Historical discrepancies Family history of unexplained death, SIDS, or BRUEs Single witness of event Delay in seeking care	Bruising (especially in a nonmobile child) Ear trauma, hemotympanum Acute abdomen Painful extremities Oral bleeding/trauma Frenulum tears Unexplained irritability Retinal hemorrhages Depressed mental status	Skeletal survey Computed tomography/MRI of the head Dilated funduscopic examination if head imaging concerning for trauma Toxicology screen Social work evaluation
Cardiac	Dysrhythmia (prolonged QT syndrome, Wolff-Parkinson-White syndrome) Cardiomyopathy Congenital heart disease Myocarditis	Feeding difficulties Growth difficulties Diaphoresis Prematurity	Abnormal heart rate/rhythm Murmur Decreased femoral pulses	Four-extremity blood pressure Pre- and postductal oxygen saturation measurements ECG Echocardiogram Serum electrolytes, calcium, magnesium
Metabolic/genetic	Hypoglycemia Inborn errors of metabolism Electrolyte abnormalities Genetic syndromes including those with craniofacial malformations	Severe initial event Multiple events Event associated with period of stress or fasting Developmental delay Associated anomalies Growth difficulties Severe/frequent illnesses Family history of BRUE, consanguinity, seizure disorder, or SIDS	Dysmorphic features Microcephaly Hepatomegaly	Serum electrolytes; glucose, calcium, and magnesium levels Lactate Ammonia Pyruvate Urine organic and serum amino acids Newborn screen

BRUE, Brief resolved unexplained event; *ECG*, electrocardiogram; *EEG*, electroencephalogram; *ENT*, ear, nose, and throat; *GER*, gastroesophageal reflux; *GI*, gastrointestinal; *NP*, nasopharyngeal; *RSV*, respiratory syncytial virus; *SIDS*, sudden infant death syndrome; *URI*, upper respiratory infection.
From Kliegman RK, Lye PS, Bordini BJ, et al: *Nelson pediatric symptom-based diagnosis*, Philadelphia, 2018, Elsevier. Table 5.3.

Table 403.2	Important Historical Features of a BRUE
PREEVENT	
Condition of child	Awake vs. asleep
Location of child	Prone vs. supine, flat or upright, in crib/car seat, with pillows, blankets
Activity	Feeding, crying, sleeping
EVENT	
Respiratory effort	None, shallow, gasping, increased
	Duration of respiratory pauses
Color	Pallor, red, cyanotic
	Peripheral, whole body, circumoral, lighting of room
Tone/movement	Rigid, tonic-clonic, decreased, floppy
	Focal vs. diffuse
	Ability to suppress movements
Level of consciousness	Alert, interactive, sleepy, nonresponsive
Duration	Time until normal breathing, normal tone, normal behavior
	Detailed history of caregiver actions during event to aid in defining time course
Associated symptoms	Vomiting, sputum production, blood in mouth/nose, eye rolling
POSTEVENT	
Condition	Back to baseline, sleepy, postictal, crying
	If altered after event, duration of time until back to baseline
INTERVENTIONS	
What was performed	Gentle stimulation, blowing in face, mouth-to-mouth, cardiopulmonary resuscitation
Who performed intervention	Medical professional vs. caregiver
Response to intervention	Resolution of event vs. self-resolving
Duration of intervention	How long was intervention performed
MEDICAL HISTORY	
History of present illness	Preceding illnesses, fever, rash, irritability, sick contacts
Past medical history	Prematurity, prenatal exposures, gestational age, birth trauma
	Noisy breathing since birth
	Any medical problems, prior medical conditions, prior hospitalizations
	Developmental delay
	Medications
Feeding history	Gagging, coughing with feeds, poor weight gain
Family history	Neurologic problems
	Cardiac arrhythmias
	Sudden death, childhood deaths, BRUEs
	Neonatal problems
	Consanguinity
Social history	Home situation
	Caregivers
	Smoke exposure
	Medications in the home

BRUE, Brief resolved unexplained event.
From Kliegman RK, Lye PS, Bordini BJ, et al: *Nelson pediatric symptom-based diagnosis*, Philadelphia, 2018, Elsevier. Table 5.4.

However, abrupt changes where the infant appears to lose consciousness after episodes of apnea or color change can be concerning for hypoxemia, hypoglycemia, or seizures.

Did the event self-resolve, or was an intervention required? Infants with choking from GER, vomit, or feeding difficulties generally improve spontaneously or with help clearing the airway. A serious underlying cause is more likely if CPR was indicated and then provided, though

this may be difficult to assess if no medically trained individuals witnessed the event.

Additional History

A careful, detailed history can lead to an explanation; the key elements are summarized in Tables 403.1 and 403.2. A clinician should inquire about other symptoms (e.g., fever, upper respiratory infection [URI] symptoms, spitting up). A history of breathing problems, prenatal or perinatal concerns, prematurity, and growth and developmental problems is important. Premature infants, particularly those still under 43 wk after correcting for gestational age, are at higher risk for underlying causes, such as apnea of prematurity. A careful feeding history can detect oropharyngeal dysphagia or GER-related problems (i.e., laryngospasm).

A targeted family history can reveal risk for sudden death, cardiac arrhythmias, and metabolic, genetic, and neurologic disease.

A social history, particularly by someone trained to detect non-accidental trauma, can reveal recent trauma, prior child welfare involvement, substance abuse, poisoning or misuse of medications, and environmental exposures (e.g., second-hand smoke and mold). It is important to understand who observed the event, who normally takes care of the infant, and if there are any discrepancies in the explanation of the event.

Consider infectious exposures. Infants exposed to underimmunized family members are at risk for pertussis. Respiratory syncytial virus (RSV) and other respiratory viruses, as well as pertussis, and can present with apnea prior to the onset of URI symptoms.

Physical Examination

A careful physical examination may reveal a causative or underlying diagnosis. Abnormal growth and head circumference may reflect feeding, developmental, and neurological problems. Abnormal vital signs and pulse oximetry can suggest infectious, cardiac, and neurological abnormalities. A careful skin and mouth examination can reveal subtle signs. For example, child abuse should be suspected in infants with bruises, petechiae, or a torn frenulum. Signs of airway abnormalities, such as inspiratory or expiratory stridor or stertor, can lead to diagnosis of respiratory infections, vascular rings, hemangioma, laryngomalacia, tracheomalacia, or facial dysmorphism.

Testing

In the past, it was common for clinicians to routinely test infants presenting with such events using complete blood counts (CBC), appropriate cultures, and GER testing. However, it is known that these tests are unlikely to reveal a cause and even more likely to lead to a false positive result. False positives can, in turn, contribute to missed diagnoses, additional unnecessary testing, patient harm, greater parental concern, and increased costs.

In lower-risk infants, routine laboratory testing and diagnostic imaging (CBC, bacterial cultures, blood gas and glucose, metabolic panels, urinalysis, GER testing, chest radiograph, neuroimaging, electroencephalogram [EEG], sleep study) is not recommended. *The few situations where testing may be considered in the lower-risk population include:*

- *Pertussis* testing in underimmunized or exposed individuals
- ECG may reveal a prolonged QtC syndrome, particularly when there is a concerning family history.
- Rapid viral testing can help diagnose subclinical viral causes, but these tests can be positive from recent past infections that may not be the cause of the concerning event.
- A brief period of continuous pulse oximetry and serial observations to detect hypoxemia and apnea

In higher-risk infants, routine screening tests may not be needed. Testing should be done due to concerns from the history and physical, or to further characterize repeat BRUEs.

- Continuous pulse oximetry or cardiorespiratory monitoring under a period of observation may help characterize repeat events.
- A swallow evaluation by a trained feeding expert might reveal oropharyngeal dysphagia in premature or young infants.

- Head imaging with CT or MRI is indicated when there is suspicion of non-accidental trauma due to bruising in nonambulatory infants, concerning bruising patterns, history of unexplained death in a sibling, or inconsistent history of event.
- Neurology consult or EEG or head imaging may lead to a diagnosis of epilepsy if there is a concern for seizure. However, it is reasonable to perform this consultation and testing as an outpatient in well-appearing infants.
- Otolaryngology consultation to detect anatomic disorders of the airway (e.g., laryngomalacia, tracheomalacia, and tracheoesophageal fistula)
- Pulmonary/sleep medicine consultation to detect disordered breathing (e.g., central apnea and obstructive sleep apnea)

Management

Although the value of hospital admission is debatable, lower-risk infants are much less likely to benefit from admission compared to higher-risk infants. For all BRUEs, it is uncommon for a hospital admission to lead to a diagnosis of a serious underlying disorder. Sometimes, however, a longer period of observation than is practical in a clinic or emergency department can help characterize repeat events, should they recur, and reduce the uncertainty of a recurrent event for parents. Additional benefits of hospitalization include serial assessments of feeding, breathing, sleep, and social patterns. *The decision for hospital admission should incorporate the needs and preferences of the family and patient, and the ability to follow-up closely with a primary care physician.* In weighing the risks and benefits of this decision, it is important to recognize that hospitalization can unnecessarily increase stress for the family and patient through false alarms and iatrogenic complications. CPR education should be considered for all families. Home apnea monitoring should not be done. Close outpatient follow-up with a primary care physician is important to monitor for repeat events and caregiver support.

Bibliography is available at Expert Consult.

Section 2
Disorders of the Respiratory Tract

第二篇
呼吸道疾病

Chapter 404
Congenital Disorders of the Nose

Joseph Haddad Jr and Sonam N. Dodhia

第四百零四章
先天性鼻部疾病

中文导读

　　本章主要介绍了正常新生儿的鼻部生理学、先天性疾病、后鼻孔闭锁、先天性鼻中隔缺损、梨状孔狭窄、先天性鼻中线肿块以及诊断和治疗。鼻部的生理学主要包括前鼻腔和鼻甲区的功能、鼻黏膜和鼻部分泌物的作用。后鼻孔闭锁具体阐述了临床表现、诊断以及治疗等内容。先天性鼻中隔缺损主要包括鼻中隔穿孔和轻度鼻中隔偏曲。先天性鼻中线肿块主要包括皮样囊肿、神经胶质瘤以及其他鼻部肿块。

NORMAL NEWBORN NOSE

In contrast to children and adults who preferentially breathe through their nose unless nasal obstruction interferes, most newborn infants are obligate nasal breathers. Significant nasal obstruction presenting at birth, such as choanal atresia, may be a life-threatening situation for the infant unless an alternative to the nasal airway is established. Nasal congestion with obstruction is common in the 1st year of life and can affect the quality of breathing during sleep; it may be associated with a narrow nasal airway, viral or bacterial infection, enlarged adenoids, or maternal estrogenic stimuli similar to rhinitis of pregnancy. The internal nasal airway doubles in size in the 1st 6 mo of life, leading to resolution of symptoms in many infants. Supportive care with a bulb syringe and saline nose drops, topical nasal decongestants, and antibiotics, when indicated, improve symptoms in affected infants.

PHYSIOLOGY

The nose is responsible for the initial warming and humidification of inspired air and olfaction. In the anterior nasal cavity, turbulent airflow and coarse hairs enhance the deposition of large particulate matter; the remaining nasal airways filter out particles as small as 6 μm in diameter. In the turbinate region, the airflow becomes laminar and the airstream is narrowed and directed superiorly, enhancing particle deposition, warming, and humidification. Nasal passages contribute as much as 50% of the total resistance of normal breathing. Nasal flaring, a sign of respiratory distress, reduces the resistance to inspiratory airflow through the nose and can improve ventilation (see Chapter 400).

Although the nasal mucosa is more vascular (especially in the turbinate region) than in the lower airways, the surface epithelium is similar, with ciliated cells, goblet cells, submucosal glands, and a covering blanket of mucus. The nasal secretions contain lysozyme and secretory immunoglobulin A (IgA), both of which have antimicrobial activity, and IgG, IgE, albumin, histamine, bacteria, lactoferrin, and cellular debris, as well as mucous glycoproteins, which provide viscoelastic properties. Aided by the ciliated cells, mucus flows toward the nasopharynx, where the airstream widens, the epithelium becomes squamous, and secretions are wiped away by swallowing. Replacement of the mucous layers occurs about every 10-20 min. Estimates of daily mucus production vary from 0.1 to 0.3 mg/kg/24 hr, with most of the mucus being produced by the submucosal glands.

CONGENITAL DISORDERS

Congenital *structural nasal malformations* are uncommon compared with acquired abnormalities. The nasal bones can be congenitally absent so that the bridge of the nose fails to develop, resulting in *nasal hypoplasia.* Congenital absence of the nose *(arhinia),* complete or partial duplication, or a single centrally placed nostril can occur in isolation but is usually part of a malformation syndrome. Rarely, *supernumerary teeth* are found in the nose, or teeth grow into it from the maxilla.

Nasal bones can be sufficiently malformed to produce severe narrowing of the nasal passages. Often, such narrowing is associated with a high and narrow hard palate. Children with these defects can have significant obstruction to airflow during infections of the upper airways and are more susceptible to the development of chronic or recurrent hypoventilation (see Chapter 31). Rarely, the alae nasi are sufficiently thin and poorly supported to result in inspiratory obstruction, or there may be congenital nasolacrimal duct obstruction with cystic extension into the nasopharynx, causing respiratory distress.

CHOANAL ATRESIA

This is the most common congenital anomaly of the nose and has a frequency of approximately 1 in 7,000 live births. It consists of a unilateral or bilateral bony (90%) or membranous (10%) septum between the nose and the pharynx; most cases are a combination of bony and membranous atresia. The pathogenesis is unknown, but theories include persistence of the buccopharyngeal membranes or failure of the oronasal membrane to rupture. The unilateral defect is more common and the female:male ratio is approximately 2:1. Approximately 50–70% of affected infants have other congenital anomalies (CHARGE syndrome [see later], Treacher-Collins, Kallmann syndrome, VATER [vertebral defects, imperforate anus, tracheoesophageal fistula, and renal defects] association, Pfeiffer syndrome), with the anomalies occurring more often in bilateral cases.

The **CHARGE syndrome** (*c*oloboma, *h*eart disease, *a*tresia or stenosis of the choanae, *r*etarded growth and development or central nervous system (CNS) anomalies or both, *g*enital anomalies or hypogonadism or both, and *e*ar [external, middle, inner ear] anomalies or deafness or both) is one of the more common anomalies associated with choanal atresia—approximately 10–20% of patients with choanal atresia have it. The CNS involvement (~90%) includes reduced function of cranial nerves I, V, VII, VIII, IX, and X, as well as vision and hearing deficits. Most (~90%) patients with CHARGE syndrome have autosomal dominant de novo mutations in the *CHD7* gene, which is involved in chromatin organization. Immunologic deficiencies may be noted that overlap with the 22q11.2 deletion syndrome.

Clinical Manifestations

Newborn infants have a variable ability to breathe through their mouths, so nasal obstruction does not produce the same symptoms in every infant. When the obstruction is unilateral, the infant may be asymptomatic for a prolonged period, often until the first respiratory infection, when unilateral nasal discharge or persistent nasal obstruction can suggest the diagnosis. Infants with bilateral choanal atresia who have difficulty with mouth breathing make vigorous attempts to inspire, often suck in their lips, and develop cyanosis. Distressed children then cry (which relieves the cyanosis) and become calmer, with normal skin color, only to repeat the cycle after closing their mouths. Those who are able to breathe through their mouths at once experience difficulty when sucking and swallowing, becoming cyanotic when they attempt to feed.

Diagnosis

Diagnosis is established by the inability to pass a firm catheter through each nostril 3-4 cm into the nasopharynx. The atretic plate may be seen directly with fiberoptic rhinoscopy. The anatomy is best evaluated by using high-resolution CT (Fig. 404.1).

Treatment

Initial treatment consists of prompt placement of an oral airway, maintaining the mouth in an open position, or intubation. A standard oral airway (such as that used in anesthesia) can be used, or a feeding nipple can be fashioned with large holes at the tip to facilitate air passage. Once an oral airway is established, the infant can be fed by gavage until breathing and eating without the assisted airway is possible. In bilateral cases, intubation or, less often, tracheotomy may be indicated. If the child is free of other serious medical problems, operative intervention is considered in the neonate; transnasal repair is the treatment of choice, with the introduction of small magnifying endoscopes and smaller surgical instruments and drills. Stents are usually left in place for weeks after the repair to prevent closure or stenosis, although a large meta-analysis demonstrated that there is no benefit to stenting. Another option is a transpalatal repair, and this is done when a transnasal endoscope cannot be placed through the nose due to thick bony atresia or stenosis. Tracheotomy should be considered in cases of bilateral atresia in which the child has other potentially life-threatening problems and in whom early surgical repair of the choanal atresia may not be appropriate or feasible. Operative correction of unilateral obstruction may be deferred for several years. In both unilateral and bilateral cases, restenosis necessitating dilation or reoperation, or both, is common. Mitomycin C has been used to help prevent the development of granulation tissue and stenosis, although its efficacy is questionable.

CONGENITAL DEFECTS OF THE NASAL SEPTUM

Perforation of the septum is most commonly acquired after birth secondary to infection, such as syphilis or tuberculosis, or trauma; rarely, it is developmental. Continuous positive airway pressure cannulas are a cause of iatrogenic perforation. Trauma from delivery is the most common cause of septal deviation noted at birth. When recognized early, it can be corrected with immediate realignment using blunt probes, cotton

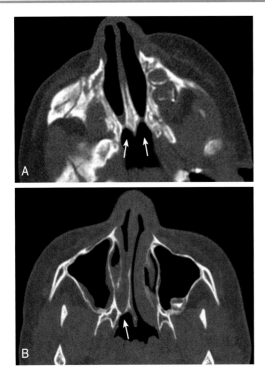

Fig. 404.1 Choanal atresia. **A,** Axial CT image in a 1 day old neonate with severe respiratory distress shows bilateral bony choanal atresia with retained fluid in the right nasal cavity, medial bowing of the lateral nasal wall, and a thickened vomer *(arrows)*. **B,** Axial CT image in a 12 yr old child with chronic nasal obstruction and purulent rhinorrhea shows unilateral *(right)* bony atresia with fluid in the nasal cavity *(arrow)*. *(From Coley BD (ed): Caffey's pediatric diagnostic imaging, ed 12,vol 1, Philadelphia, 2013, Saunders, Fig. 8.13.)*

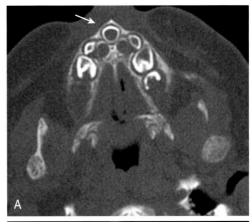

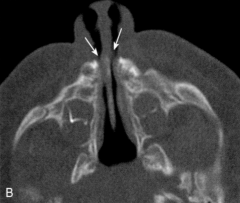

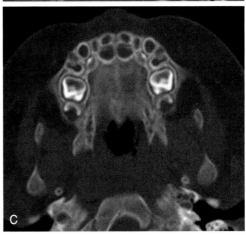

Fig. 404.2 Congenital nasal pyriform aperture stenosis in a 1½ mo old infant with episodes of respiratory distress during breastfeeding. **A,** Axial CT image shows a triangular hard palate and solitary central maxillary mega-incisor *(arrow)*. **B,** An axial CT image shows narrowing of the anterior and inferior nasal passages *(arrows)*. **C,** Normal infant maxilla for comparison. *(From Coley BD (ed): Caffey's pediatric diagnostic imaging, ed 12, vol 1, Philadelphia, 2013, Saunders, Fig. 8.14.)*

applicators, and topical anesthesia. Formal surgical correction, when required, is usually postponed to avoid disturbance of midface growth.

Mild septal deviations are common and usually asymptomatic; abnormal formation of the septum is uncommon unless other malformations are present, such as cleft lip or palate.

Congenital isolated absence of a membranous nasal septum has also been reported.

PYRIFORM APERTURE STENOSIS

Infants with this bony abnormality of the anterior nasal aperture present at birth or shortly thereafter with severe nasal obstruction leading to noisy breathing and respiratory distress that worsen with feeding and improve with crying. It can occur in isolation or in association with other malformations including holoprosencephaly, hypopituitarism, and cardiac and urogenital malformations. Diagnosis is made by CT of the nose (Fig. 404.2) with a pyriform aperture width less than ~11 mm. Medical management (nasal decongestants, humidification, nasopharyngeal airway insertion, management of reflux) is typically attempted for about 2 wk; if the child still cannot feed or breathe without difficulty, then surgical repair by means of an anterior, sublabial approach may be needed. A drill is used to enlarge the stenotic anterior bone apertures.

CONGENITAL MIDLINE NASAL MASSES

Dermoids, gliomas, and *encephaloceles* (in descending order of frequency) occur intranasally or extranasally and can have intracranial connections or extend intracranially with communication to the subarachnoid space. The theory for the embryologic development of congenital midline nasal masses is faulty retraction of the dural diverticulum. Dermoids and epidermoids are the most common type of congenital midline nasal mass and have been reported to represent up to 61% of lesions. Nasal

dermoids are firm, noncompressible, and painless, and often have a dimple or pit on the nasal dorsum (sometimes with hair being present). They can predispose to intracranial infections if an intracranial fistula or sinus is present, although recurrent infection of the dermoid itself is more common; given the risk for serious infection, surgical excision is always indicated for nasal dermoids. Gliomas or heterotopic brain tissue are firm, whereas encephaloceles are soft and enlarge with crying or the Valsalva maneuver. Diagnosis is based on physical examination findings and results from imaging studies. CT provides the best bony detail, but magnetic resonance imaging (MRI) is also helpful because of its superior ability to define intracranial extension (Fig. 404.3). Surgical excision of these masses is generally required, with the extent and surgical approach based on the type and size of the mass.

Other nasal masses include *hemangiomas, congenital nasolacrimal duct obstruction* (which can occur as an intranasal mass) (Fig. 404.4), nasal polyps, and tumors such as rhabdomyosarcoma (see Chapter 527). Nasal polyps are rarely present at birth, but the other masses often present at birth or in early infancy (see Chapter 406).

Poor development of the paranasal sinuses and a narrow nasal airway are associated with recurrent or chronic upper airway infection in Down syndrome (see Chapter 98.2).

DIAGNOSIS AND TREATMENT

In children with congenital nasal disorders, supportive care of the airway is given until the diagnosis is established. Diagnosis is made through a combination of flexible scoping and imaging studies, primarily CT scan. In the case of surgically correctable congenital problems such as choanal atresia, surgery is performed after the child is deemed healthy and free of life-threatening problems such as congenital heart disease.

Bibliography is available at Expert Consult.

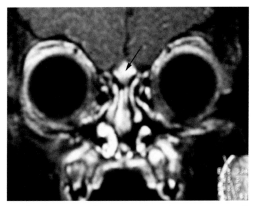

Fig. 404.3 Coronal CT scan of nasal dermoid with intracranial extension *(arrow)*. *(From Manning SC, Bloom DC, Perkins JA, et al: Diagnostic and surgical challenges in the pediatric skull base, Otolaryngol Clin North Am 38:773–794, 2005, Fig. 2.)*

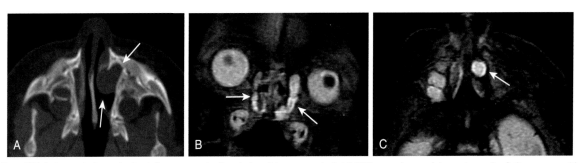

Fig. 404.4 Congenital nasolacrimal duct mucoceles in a 1 day old neonate. **A,** Axial CT image shows a left nasal round soft tissue mass with enlargement of the ipsilateral nasolacrimal duct and canal *(arrows)*. **B** and **C,** Coronal and axial fast spin echo inversion recovery MR images show bilateral cystic enlargement of the nasolacrimal sacs and ducts *(arrows)*. *(From Coley BD (ed): Caffey's pediatric diagnostic imaging, ed 12, vol 1, Philadelphia, 2013, Saunders, Fig. 8.15, p. 78.)*

Chapter **405**
Acquired Disorders of the Nose

Joseph Haddad Jr and Sonam N. Dodhia

第四百零五章
鼻部获得性疾病

中文导读

本章详细阐述了鼻异物和鼻出血，包括鼻异物的病因、诊断、治疗、并发症和预防；鼻出血的解剖、病因、临床表现、治疗和预防。鼻异物的病因为食物、珠子等小物件的吸入，诊断包括鼻和/或耳镜检查、头颅侧位X线片协助诊断，治疗为异物清除，并发症包括异物吸入、创伤、感染、后鼻孔狭窄，预防需将物品远离儿童或在成人监督下使用。鼻出血常见出血部位是Kiesselbach丛，病因主要为原发性或继发性，临床表现为无预兆的单侧或双侧鼻出血，治疗为一般治疗、药物治疗、手术治疗等，预防包括防止鼻腔干燥、注意手部卫生、及时停用使鼻腔出血的药物。

Tumors, septal perforations, and other acquired abnormalities of the nose and paranasal sinuses can manifest with epistaxis. Midface trauma with a nasal or facial fracture may also be accompanied by epistaxis. Trauma to the nose can cause a *septal hematoma;* if treatment is delayed, this can lead to necrosis of septal cartilage and a resultant *saddle nose deformity.* Other abnormalities that can cause a change in the shape of the nose and paranasal bones, with obstruction but few other symptoms, include *fibroosseous lesions* (ossifying fibroma, fibrous dysplasia, cementifying fibroma) and *mucoceles of the paranasal sinuses.* These conditions may be suspected on physical examination and confirmed by CT scan and biopsy. Although these are considered benign lesions, they can all greatly change the anatomy of surrounding bony structures and often require surgical intervention for management.

405.1 Nasal Foreign Bodies

Joseph Haddad Jr and Sonam N. Dodhia

ETIOLOGY

Foreign bodies (food, beads, crayons, small toys, erasers, paper wads, buttons, batteries, beans, stones, pieces of sponge, and other small objects) are often placed in the nose by young or developmentally delayed children and constitute ≤1% of pediatric emergency department visits. Nasal foreign bodies can go unrecognized for long periods of time because they initially produce few symptoms and are difficult to visualize. First symptoms include unilateral obstruction, sneezing, relatively mild discomfort, and, rarely, pain. Presenting clinical symptoms include history of insertion of foreign bodies (86%), mucopurulent nasal discharge (24%), foul nasal odor (9%), epistaxis (6%), nasal obstruction (3%), and mouth breathing (2%). Irrigation results in mucosal swelling because some foreign bodies are hygroscopic and increase in size as water is absorbed; signs of local obstruction and discomfort can increase with time. The patient might also present with a generalized body odor known as *bromhidrosis.*

DIAGNOSIS

Unilateral nasal discharge and obstruction should suggest the presence of a foreign body, which can often be seen on examination with a nasal speculum or wide otoscope placed in the nose. Purulent secretions may have to be cleared so that the foreign object can actually be seen; a headlight, suction, and topical decongestants are often needed. The object is usually situated anteriorly, but unskilled attempts at removal can force the object deeper into the nose. A long-standing foreign body can become embedded in granulation tissue or mucosa and appear as a nasal mass. A lateral skull radiograph assists in diagnosis if the foreign body is metallic or radiopaque or if foreign body is suspected but physical exam with sinus endoscopy or anterior rhinoscopy is negative.

TREATMENT

An initial examination of the nose is made to determine if a foreign body is present and whether it needs to be removed emergently. Planning is then made for office or operating room extrication of the foreign body. Prompt removal minimizes the danger of aspiration and local tissue necrosis, and this can usually be performed with the aid of topical anesthesia, with forceps or nasal suction. Common noninvasive techniques include simple nose blowing and the "mother's kiss" technique. The "mother's kiss" approach has been successful in acute situations where a person occludes the unaffected nostril and then, with a complete seal over the child's mouth, attempts to dislodge the foreign body by blowing into the mouth. A similar approach uses an Ambu bag over the mouth with the unaffected nostril occluded. Other noninvasive options include blowing air into a drinking straw in a child's mouth and applying high flow oxygen (10-15 L/min) to the unaffected nostril. Alternatively, a Katz catheter (made specifically for the removal of foreign bodies from the nose and ear) can be inserted above and distal to the object, inflated, and drawn back with gentle traction. If there is marked swelling, bleeding, or tissue overgrowth, general anesthesia may be needed to remove the object. Infection usually clears promptly after the removal of the object, and generally no further therapy is necessary. Magnets can be used to extract metal foreign bodies, 2% lidocaine can be used to kill live insects before removal, and irrigation should be avoided with vegetable matter or sponges because of the risk of foreign body swelling. Age (>5) and disk-shaped foreign body are predictors for operating room removal of foreign body.

COMPLICATIONS

Serious complications include posterior dislodgement and aspiration, trauma caused by the object itself or removal attempts, infection, and choanal stenosis. Infection is common and gives rise to a purulent, malodorous, or bloody discharge. Local tissue damage from long-standing foreign body, or alkaline injury from a disk battery, can lead to local tissue loss and cartilage destruction. A synechia or scar band can then form, causing nasal obstruction. Loss of septal mucosa and cartilage can cause a septal perforation or saddle nose. Disk batteries are especially dangerous when placed in the nose; they leach base, which causes pain and local tissue destruction in a matter of hours. Magnets also carry a risk of septal perforation and necrosis.

Tetanus is a rare complication of long-standing nasal foreign bodies in nonimmunized children (see Chapter 238). Toxic shock syndrome is also rare and most commonly occurs from nasal surgical packing (see Chapter 208.2); oral antibiotics should be administered when nasal surgical packing is placed.

PREVENTION

Tempting objects, such as round, shiny beads, should be used only under adult supervision. Disk batteries should be stored away from the reach of small children.

Bibliography is available at Expert Consult.

405.2 Epistaxis

Joseph Haddad Jr and Sonam N. Dodhia

Although rare in infancy, nosebleeds are common in children between the ages of 3 and 8, then decline in incidence after puberty. They are also more common during winter months. Diagnosis and treatment depend on the location and cause of the bleeding.

ANATOMY

The most common site of bleeding is the Kiesselbach plexus, an area in the anterior septum where vessels from both the internal carotid (anterior and posterior ethmoid arteries) and external carotid (sphenopalatine and terminal branches of the internal maxillary arteries) converge. The thin mucosa in this area, as well as the anterior location, make it prone to exposure to dry air and trauma.

ETIOLOGY

Epistaxis can be classified as primary (idiopathic; majority of cases) or secondary based on cause, and this has implications for diagnosis and management. Common causes of secondary nosebleeds from the anterior septum include digital trauma, foreign bodies, dry air, and inflammation, including upper respiratory tract infections, sinusitis, and allergic rhinitis (Table 405.1). There is often a family history of childhood epistaxis. Nasal steroid sprays are commonly used in children, and their chronic use may be associated with nasal mucosal bleeding. Young infants with significant gastroesophageal reflux into the nose rarely present with epistaxis secondary to mucosal inflammation. Susceptibility is increased during respiratory infections and in the winter when dry air irritates the nasal mucosa, resulting in formation of fissures and crusting. Severe bleeding may be encountered with congenital vascular abnormalities, such as *hereditary hemorrhagic telangiectasia* (see Chapter 459.3), varicosities, hemangiomas, and, in children with thrombocytopenia, deficiency of clotting factors, particularly von Willebrand disease (see Chapter 504), hypertension, renal failure, or venous congestion. Recurrent epistaxis despite cauterization is associated with mild coagulation disorders. The family history may be positive for abnormal bleeding (epistaxis or other sites); specific testing for von Willebrand disease is indicated because the prothrombin time or partial thromboplastin time may be normal despite having a bleeding disorder. Nasal polyps or other intranasal growths may be associated with epistaxis. Recurrent, and often severe, unilateral nosebleeds may be the initial presenting symptom in **juvenile nasal angiofibroma,** which occurs in adolescent males.

CLINICAL MANIFESTATIONS

Epistaxis usually occurs without warning, with blood flowing slowly but freely from 1 nostril or occasionally from both. In children with nasal lesions, bleeding might follow physical exercise. When bleeding occurs at night, the blood may be swallowed and become apparent only when the child vomits or passes blood in the stools. Posterior epistaxis can manifest as anterior nasal bleeding, or, if bleeding is copious, the patient might vomit blood as the initial symptom.

TREATMENT

Most nosebleeds stop spontaneously in a few minutes. The nares should be compressed and the child kept as quiet as possible, in an upright position with the head tilted forward to avoid blood trickling back into the throat. Cold compresses applied to the nose can also help. If these measures do not stop the bleeding, local application of a solution of oxymetazoline (Afrin) or phenylephrine (Neo-Synephrine) (0.25–1%) may be useful. If bleeding persists, an anterior nasal pack may need to be inserted; if bleeding originates in the posterior nasal cavity, combined anterior and posterior packing is necessary. After bleeding is under control, and if a bleeding site is identified, its obliteration by cautery

Table 405.1	Possible Causes of Epistaxis

Epistaxis digitorum (nose picking)
Rhinitis (allergic or viral)
Chronic sinusitis
Foreign bodies
Intranasal neoplasm or polyps
Irritants (e.g., cigarette smoke)
Septal deviation
Septal perforation
Trauma including child abuse
Vascular malformation or telangiectasia (hereditary hemorrhage telangiectasia)
Hemophilia
von Willebrand disease
Platelet dysfunction
Thrombocytopenia
Hypertension
Leukemia
Liver disease (e.g., cirrhosis)
Medications (e.g., aspirin, anticoagulants, nonsteroidal antiinflammatory drugs, topical corticosteroids)
Cocaine abuse

From Kucik CJ, Clenney T: Management of epistaxis, *Am Fam Physician* 71(2):305–311, 2005.

with silver nitrate may prevent further difficulties. Because the septal cartilage derives its nutrition from the overlying mucoperichondrium, only one side of the septum should be cauterized at a time to reduce the chance of a septal perforation. During the winter, or in a dry environment, a room humidifier, saline drops, and petrolatum (Vaseline) applied to the septum can help to prevent epistaxis. Ointments prevent infection, increase moisture, decrease bleeding, and are commonly used in clinical practice. Antiseptic cream (e.g., mupirocin) has been used for epistaxis because it has been found that many patients with idiopathic epistaxis have nasal bacterial colonization with subsequent inflammation, new vessel formation, and irritation, likely leading to epistaxis. However, studies showing the efficacy of antiseptics in epistaxis are equivocal. Patients with severe epistaxis despite conservative medical measures should be considered for surgical ligation techniques or embolization. In patients with severe or repeated epistaxis, blood transfusions may be necessary. Otolaryngologic evaluation is indicated for these children and for those with bilateral bleeding or with hemorrhage that does not arise from the Kiesselbach plexus. For those with recurrent epistaxis, there may be short-term benefits to using bipolar electrocautery over silver nitrate chemical cautery, although treatments were equivocal after 2 yr. Secondary epistaxis should be managed by identification of the cause, application of appropriate nasal therapy, and correct systemic medical management. Hematologic evaluation (for coagulopathy and anemia), along with nasal endoscopy and diagnostic imaging, may be needed to make a definitive diagnosis in cases of severe recurrent epistaxis. Replacement of deficient clotting factors may be required for patients who have an underlying hematologic disorder (see Chapter 503). Profuse unilateral epistaxis associated with a nasal mass in an adolescent boy near puberty might signal a **juvenile nasopharyngeal angiofibroma.** This unusual tumor has also been reported in a 2 yr old and in 30-40 yr olds, but the incidence peaks in adolescent and pre-adolescent boys. CT with contrast medium enhancement and magnetic resonance imaging (MRI) are part of the initial evaluation; arteriography, embolization, and extensive surgery may be needed.

Surgical intervention may also be needed for bleeding from the internal maxillary artery or other vessels that can cause bleeding in the posterior nasal cavity.

PREVENTION
The discouragement of nose picking and attention to proper humidification of the bedroom during dry winter months help to prevent many nosebleeds. Prompt attention to nasal infections and allergies is beneficial to nasal hygiene. Prompt cessation of nasal steroid sprays prevents ongoing bleeding.

Bibliography is available at Expert Consult.

Chapter **406**
Nasal Polyps
Joseph Haddad Jr and Sonam N. Dodhia

第四百零六章
鼻息肉

中文导读

本章主要介绍了鼻息肉的病因、临床表现、诊断和鉴别诊断以及治疗。其中病因主要包括囊性纤维化、慢性鼻窦炎、变应性鼻炎等，临床表现主要包括鼻腔阻塞伴闭塞性鼻音和张口呼吸、鼻腔分泌物增多，诊断和鉴别诊断主要包括进行外鼻检查和鼻镜检查，以及面中部CT检查为诊疗关键，治疗主要包括鼻内类固醇喷雾剂药物治疗、手术治疗。

ETIOLOGY
Nasal polyps are benign pedunculated tumors formed from edematous, usually chronically inflamed nasal mucosa. They commonly arise from the ethmoidal sinus and occur in the middle meatus. Occasionally they appear within the maxillary antrum and can extend to the nasopharynx (antrochoanal polyp).

It is estimated that between 1% and 4% of the population will develop nasal polyps at some point; the incidence of nasal polyps increases with age. Antrochoanal polyps represent only 4–6% of all nasal polyps in the general population but account for approximately one third of polyps in the pediatric population. Large or multiple polyps can completely obstruct the nasal passage. The polyps originating from the ethmoidal sinus are usually smaller and multiple, as compared with the large and usually single antrochoanal polyp.

Cystic fibrosis (CF; see Chapter 432) is the most common childhood cause of nasal polyposis, and up to 50% of CF patients experience obstructing nasal polyposis, which is rare in non-CF children. Therefore, CF should be suspected in any child younger than 12 yr old with nasal polyps, even in the absence of typical respiratory and digestive symptoms. Nasal polyposis is also associated with chronic sinusitis (see Chapter 408) and allergic rhinitis. Large population studies have noted a significant familial risk in having chronic rhinosinusitis with polyposis. Furthermore, it has been noted in a substantial number of studies that low vitamin D levels are correlated with polypoid chronic rhinosinusitis, likely related to the role vitamin D plays as an immunomodulator in the respiratory epithelium. In the *Samter triad*, nasal polyps are associated with aspirin sensitivity and asthma; this condition is rare in children.

CLINICAL MANIFESTATIONS

Obstruction of nasal passages is prominent, with associated hyponasal speech and mouth breathing. Profuse unilateral mucoid or mucopurulent rhinorrhea may also be present. An examination of the nasal passages shows glistening, gray, grape-like masses squeezed between the nasal turbinates and the septum.

DIAGNOSIS AND DIFFERENTIAL DIAGNOSIS

Examination of the external nose and rhinoscopy should be performed. Ethmoidal polyps can be readily distinguished from the well-vascularized turbinate tissue, which is pink or red; antrochoanal polyps may have a more fleshy appearance (Fig. 406.1). Antrochoanal polyps may prolapse into the nasopharynx; flexible nasopharyngoscopy can assist in making this diagnosis. Prolonged presence of ethmoidal polyps in a child can widen the bridge of the nose and erode adjacent osseous structures.

Tumors of the nose cause more local destruction and distortion of the anatomy. CT scan of the midface is key to diagnosis and planning for surgical treatment (Fig. 406.2).

TREATMENT

Local or systemic decongestants are not usually effective in shrinking the polyps, although they may provide symptomatic relief from the associated mucosal edema. Intranasal steroid sprays, and sometimes systemic steroids, can provide some shrinkage of nasal polyps with symptomatic relief and have proved useful in children with CF and adults with nasal polyps. Topical nasal steroid therapy, fluticasone, mometasone, and budesonide appears to result in nasal symptom improvement, but were found to have no effect on those with CF. Doxycycline (100 mg daily) has a significant effect on the size of nasal polyps, nasal symptoms, and mucosal and systemic markers of inflammation. Polyps should be removed surgically if complete obstruction, uncontrolled rhinorrhea, or deformity of the nose appears. If the underlying pathogenic mechanism cannot be eliminated (such as CF), the polyps may soon return. Functional endoscopic sinus surgery provides more complete polyp removal and treatment of other associated nasal disease; in some cases, this has reduced the need for frequent surgeries. Nasal steroid sprays should also be started preventively, once postsurgical healing occurs.

Antrochoanal polyps do not respond to medical measures and must be removed surgically, typically via endoscopic sinus surgery, or alternatively with a mini-Caldwell procedure. Since these types of polyps are not associated with any underlying disease process, the recurrence rate is much less than for other types of polyps.

Bibliography is available at Expert Consult.

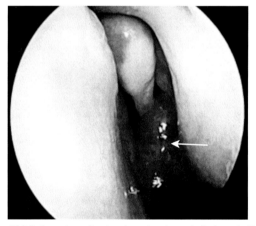

Fig. 406.1 Antrochoanal polyp viewed endoscopically *(arrow)*. *(From Basak S, Karaman CZ, Akdilli A, et al: Surgical approaches to antrochoanal polyps in children,* Int J Pediatr Otorhinolaryngol *46:197–205, 1998.)*

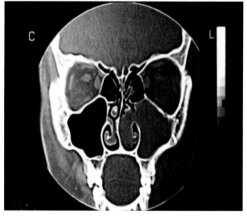

Fig. 406.2 A typical CT image of an isolated antrochoanal polyp on the left side. *(From Basak S, Karaman CZ, Akdilli A, et al: Surgical approaches to antrochoanal polyps in children,* Int J Pediatr Otorhinolaryngol *46:197–205, 1998.)*

Chapter **407**

The Common Cold

Santiago M.C. Lopez and John V. Williams

第四百零七章
普通感冒

中文导读

本章主要介绍了普通感冒的病因、流行病学、发病机制、临床表现、诊断、实验室检查、治疗、并发症以及预防。病因包括人类鼻病毒、呼吸道合胞病毒等，流行病学涉及季节性、年龄因素与病毒流行的关系，发病机制主要包括传播途径、病毒逃避宿主防御机制、鼻上皮感染机制、宿主免疫防御系统的反应，临床表现依赖于年龄和病毒种类，常表现为上呼吸道相关体征，诊断主要为鉴别非传染性疾病和其他上呼吸道感染，治疗中具体描述了抗病毒治疗、支持性护理与对症治疗并提及了常用的但实际上并无效果的治疗，并发症主要包括急性中耳炎、鼻窦炎、哮喘。

The common cold is an acute viral infection of the upper respiratory tract in which the symptoms of rhinorrhea and nasal obstruction are prominent. Systemic symptoms and signs such as headache, myalgia, and fever are absent or mild. The common cold is frequently referred to as *infectious rhinitis* but may also include self-limited involvement of the sinus mucosa and is more correctly termed *rhinosinusitis*.

ETIOLOGY

The most common pathogens associated with the common cold are the more than 200 types of human rhinoviruses (see Chapter 290), but the syndrome can be caused by many different virus families (Table 407.1). Rhinoviruses (HRV) are associated with more than 50% of colds in adults and children. In young children, other viral etiologies of the common cold include respiratory syncytial virus (RSV; see Chapter 287), human metapneumovirus (MPV; see Chapter 288), parainfluenza viruses (PIVs; see Chapter 286), and adenoviruses (see Chapter 289). Common cold symptoms may also be caused by influenza viruses, nonpolio enteroviruses, and human coronaviruses. Many viruses that cause rhinitis are also associated with other symptoms and signs such as cough, wheezing, and fever.

EPIDEMIOLOGY

Colds occur year-round, but the incidence is greatest from the early fall until the late spring, reflecting the seasonal prevalence of the viral

Table 407.1	Pathogens Associated With the Common Cold		
ASSOCIATION	**PATHOGEN**	**RELATIVE FREQUENCY***	**OTHER COMMON SYMPTOMS AND SIGNS**
Agents primarily associated with the common cold	Human rhinoviruses Coronaviruses	Frequent Frequent	Wheezing/bronchiolitis
Agents primarily associated with other clinical syndromes that also cause common cold symptoms	Respiratory syncytial virus Human metapneumovirus Influenza viruses Parainfluenza viruses Adenoviruses	Occasional Occasional Uncommon Uncommon Uncommon	Bronchiolitis in children <2 yr of age Pneumonia and bronchiolitis Influenza, pneumonia, croup Croup, bronchiolitis Pharyngoconjunctival fever (palpebral conjunctivitis, watery eye discharge, pharyngeal erythema)
	Enteroviruses Coxsackievirus A Other nonpolio enteroviruses	Uncommon	Herpangina (fever and ulcerated papules on posterior oropharynx) Aseptic meningitis

*Relative frequency of colds caused by the agent.

pathogens associated with cold symptoms. In the northern hemisphere, the highest incidence of HRV infection occurs in the early fall (August–October) and in the late spring (April–May). The seasonal incidence for PIV usually peaks in the late fall and late spring and is highest between December and April for RSV, influenza viruses, MPV, and coronaviruses. Adenoviruses are detected at a low prevalence throughout the cold season, and enteroviruses may also be detected during summer months or throughout the year.

Young children have an average of 6-8 colds per yr, but 10–15% of children have at least 12 infections per yr. The incidence of illness decreases with increasing age, with 2-3 illnesses per yr by adulthood. The incidence of infection is primarily a function of exposure to the virus. Children in out-of-home daycare centers during the 1st yr of life have 50% more colds than children cared for only at home. The difference in the incidence of illness between these groups of children decreases as the length of time spent in daycare increases, although the incidence of illness remains higher in the daycare group through at least the 1st 3 yr of life. When they begin primary school, children who attended daycare have less frequent colds than those who did not. Mannose-binding lectin deficiency with impaired innate immunity may be associated with an increased incidence of colds in children.

PATHOGENESIS

Viruses that cause the common cold are spread by three mechanisms: direct hand contact (self-inoculation of one's own nasal mucosa or conjunctivae after touching a contaminated person or object), inhalation of small-particle aerosols that are airborne from coughing, or deposition of large-particle aerosols that are expelled during a sneeze and land on nasal or conjunctival mucosa. Although the different common cold pathogens could be spread by any of these mechanisms, some routes of transmission appear to be more efficient than others for particular viruses. Studies of HRV and RSV indicate that direct contact is an efficient mechanism of transmission of these viruses, although transmission by large-particle aerosols can also occur. By contrast, influenza viruses and coronaviruses appear to be most efficiently spread by small-particle aerosols.

The respiratory viruses have evolved different mechanisms to avoid host defenses. Infections with HRV and adenoviruses result in the development of serotype-specific protective immunity. Repeated infections with these pathogens occur because there are a large number of distinct serotypes of each virus. Influenza viruses change the antigens presented on the surface of the virus due to genetic drift and thus behave as though there were multiple viral serotypes. The interaction of coronaviruses (see Chapter 291) with host immunity is not well defined, but it appears that multiple distinct strains of coronaviruses are capable of inducing at least short-term protective immunity. There are four types of PIV, 2 antigenic subgroups of RSV, and 4 genotypes of MPV. In addition to antigenic diversity, many of these viruses are able to reinfect the upper airway because mucosal immunoglobulin A (IgA) induced by previous infection is short lived, and the brief incubation period of these viruses allows the establishment of infection before immune memory responses. Although reinfection is not completely prevented by the adaptive host response to these viruses, the severity of illness is moderated by preexisting immunity.

Viral infection of the nasal epithelium can be associated with destruction of the epithelial lining, as with influenza viruses and adenoviruses, or there can be no apparent histologic damage, as with HRV, coronaviruses, and RSV. Regardless of the histopathologic findings, infection of the nasal epithelium is associated with an acute inflammatory response characterized by release of a variety of inflammatory cytokines and infiltration of the mucosa by inflammatory cells. This acute inflammatory response appears to be partially or largely responsible for many of the symptoms associated with the common cold. Viral shedding of most respiratory viruses peaks 3-5 days after inoculation, often coinciding with symptom onset; low levels of viral shedding may persist for up to 2 wk in the otherwise recovering healthy host. Inflammation can obstruct the sinus ostia or eustachian tube, predisposing to bacterial sinusitis or otitis media, respectively.

The host immune system is responsible for most cold symptoms, rather than direct damage to the respiratory tract. Infected cells release cytokines, such as interleukin-8, that attract polymorphonuclear cells into the nasal submucosa and epithelium. HRV also increases vascular permeability in the nasal submucosa, releasing albumin and bradykinin, which may contribute to symptoms.

CLINICAL MANIFESTATIONS

Symptoms of the common cold vary by age and virus. In infants, fever and nasal discharge may predominate. Fever is uncommon in older children and adults. The onset of common cold symptoms typically occurs 1-3 days after viral infection. The first symptom noted is often sore or scratchy throat, followed closely by nasal obstruction and rhinorrhea. The sore throat usually resolves quickly, and, by the 2nd and 3rd day of illness, nasal symptoms predominate. Cough is associated with two-thirds of colds in children and usually begins after the onset of nasal symptoms. Cough may persist for an additional 1-2 wk after resolution of other symptoms. Influenza viruses, RSV, MPV, and adenoviruses are more likely than HRV or coronaviruses to be associated with fever and other constitutional symptoms. Other symptoms of a cold may include headache, hoarseness, irritability, difficulty sleeping, or decreased appetite. Vomiting and diarrhea are uncommon. The usual cold persists for approximately 1 wk, although 10% last for 2 wk.

The physical findings of the common cold are limited to the upper respiratory tract. Increased nasal secretion is usually obvious; a change in the color or consistency of the secretions is common during the course of the illness and does not indicate sinusitis or bacterial superinfection but may indicate accumulation of polymorphonuclear cells. Examination of the nasal cavity might reveal swollen, erythematous nasal turbinates, although this finding is nonspecific and of limited diagnostic value. Abnormal middle ear pressure is common during the course of a cold. Anterior cervical lymphadenopathy or conjunctival injection may also be noted on exam.

DIAGNOSIS

The most important task of the physician caring for a patient with a cold is to exclude other conditions that are potentially more serious or treatable. The differential diagnosis of the common cold includes noninfectious disorders and other upper respiratory tract infections (Table 407.2).

LABORATORY FINDINGS

Routine laboratory studies are not helpful for the diagnosis and management of the common cold. A nasal smear for eosinophils (Hansel stain) may

Table 407.2	Conditions That Can Mimic the Common Cold
CONDITION	**DIFFERENTIATING FEATURES**
Allergic rhinitis	Prominent itching and sneezing, nasal eosinophils. Hansel stain can aid diagnosis
Vasomotor rhinitis	May be triggered by irritants, weather changes, spicy foods, etc.
Rhinitis medicamentosa	History of nasal decongestant use
Foreign body	Unilateral, foul-smelling secretions Bloody nasal secretions
Sinusitis	Presence of fever, headache or facial pain, or periorbital edema or persistence of rhinorrhea or cough for longer than 10-14 days
Streptococcosis	Mucopurulent nasal discharge that excoriates the nares, no cough
Pertussis	Onset of persistent or severe paroxysmal cough
Congenital syphilis	Persistent rhinorrhea with onset in the 1st 3 mo of life

be useful if allergic rhinitis is suspected (see Chapter 168). A predominance of polymorphonuclear cells in the nasal secretions is characteristic of uncomplicated colds and *does not* indicate bacterial superinfection. Self-limited radiographic abnormalities of the paranasal sinuses are common during an uncomplicated cold; imaging *is not* indicated for most children with simple rhinitis.

The viral pathogens associated with the common cold can be detected by polymerase chain reaction (PCR), culture, antigen detection, or serologic methods. These studies are generally not indicated in patients with colds, because a specific etiologic diagnosis is useful only when treatment with an antiviral agent is contemplated, such as for influenza viruses. Bacterial cultures, PCR, or antigen detection are useful only when group A streptococcus (see Chapter 210) or *Bordetella pertussis* (see Chapter 224) is suspected. The isolation of other bacterial pathogens from nasopharyngeal specimens is not an indication of bacterial nasal infection and is not a specific predictor of the etiologic agent in sinusitis.

TREATMENT

The management of the common cold consists primarily of supportive care and anticipatory guidance as recommended by American Academy of Pediatrics and United Kingdom National Institute for Health and Clinical Excellence guidelines.

Antiviral Treatment

Specific antiviral therapy is not available for HRV infections. Ribavirin, which is approved for treatment of severe RSV infections, has no role in the treatment of the common cold. The neuraminidase inhibitors oseltamivir and zanamivir have a modest effect on the duration of symptoms associated with influenza viral infections in children. Oseltamivir also reduces the frequency of influenza-associated otitis media. The difficulty of distinguishing influenza from other common cold pathogens and the necessity that therapy be started early in the illness (within 48 hr of onset of symptoms) to be beneficial are practical limitations to the use of these agents for mild upper respiratory tract infections. *Antibacterial therapy is of no benefit in the treatment of the common cold and should be avoided to minimize possible adverse effects and the development of antibiotic resistance.*

Supportive Care and Symptomatic Treatment

Supportive interventions are frequently recommended by providers. Maintaining adequate oral hydration may help to prevent dehydration and to thin secretions and soothe respiratory mucosa. The common home remedy of ingesting warm fluids may soothe mucosa, increase nasal mucous flow, or loosen respiratory secretions. Topical nasal saline may temporarily remove secretions, and saline nasal irrigation may reduce symptoms. Cool, humidified air has not been well studied but may loosen nasal secretions; however, cool-mist humidifiers and vaporizers must be cleaned after each use. The World Health Organization suggests that neither steam nor cool-mist therapy be used in treatment of a cold.

The use of oral **nonprescription** therapies (often containing antihistamines, antitussives, and decongestants) for cold symptoms in children is controversial. Although some of these medications are effective in adults, no study demonstrates a significant effect in children, and there may be serious side effects. Young children cannot participate in the assessment of symptom severity, so studies of these treatments in children have generally been based on observations by parents or other observers, a method that is likely to be insensitive for detection of treatment effects. Because of the lack of direct evidence for effectiveness and the potential for unwanted side effects, it is recommended that nonprescription cough and cold products *not* be used for infants and children younger than 6 yr of age. A decision whether to use these medications in older children must consider the likelihood of clinical benefit compared with the potential adverse effects of these drugs. The prominent or most bothersome symptoms of colds vary in the course of the illness. If symptomatic treatments are used, it is reasonable to target therapy to specific bothersome symptoms and care should be taken to ensure that caregivers understand the intended effect and can determine the proper dosage of the medications.

Zinc, given as oral lozenges to previously healthy patients, reduces the duration but not the severity of symptoms of a common cold if begun within 24 hr of symptoms. The function of the HRV 3C protease, an essential enzyme for HRV replication, is inhibited by zinc, but there has been no evidence of an antiviral effect of zinc *in vivo*. The effect of zinc on symptoms has been inconsistent, with some studies reporting dramatic treatment effects (in adults), whereas other studies find no benefit. Side effects are common and include decreased taste, bad taste, and nausea.

Fever

Fever is not usually associated with an uncomplicated common cold, and antipyretic treatment is generally not indicated. NSAIDs may decrease discomfort from cold related headache or myalgias.

Nasal Obstruction

Either topical or oral adrenergic agents may be used as nasal decongestants in older children and adults. Effective topical adrenergic agents such as xylometazoline, oxymetazoline, or phenylephrine are available as either intranasal drops or nasal sprays. Reduced-strength formulations of these medications are available for use in younger children, although they are not recommended for use in children younger than 6 yr old. Systemic absorption of the imidazolines (oxymetazoline, xylometazoline) has very rarely been associated with bradycardia, hypotension, and coma. Prolonged use of the topical adrenergic agents should be avoided to prevent the development of **rhinitis medicamentosa**, an apparent rebound effect that causes the sensation of nasal obstruction when the drug is discontinued. The oral adrenergic agents are less effective than the topical preparations and are occasionally associated with systemic effects such as central nervous system stimulation, hypertension, and palpitations. Pseudoephedrine may be more effective than phenylephrine as an oral agent to treat nasal congestion. Aromatic vapors (such as menthol) for external rub may improve perception of nasal patency but do not affect spirometry.

Saline nose drops (wash, irrigation) can improve nasal symptoms and may be used in all age groups.

Rhinorrhea

The 1st-generation antihistamines may reduce rhinorrhea by 25–30%. The effect of the antihistamines on rhinorrhea appears to be related to the anticholinergic rather than the antihistaminic properties of these drugs, and therefore the 2nd-generation or nonsedating antihistamines have no effect on common cold symptoms. The major adverse effects associated with the use of the antihistamines are sedation or paradoxical hyperactivity. Overdose may be associated with respiratory depression or hallucinations. Rhinorrhea may also be treated with ipratropium bromide, a topical anticholinergic agent. This drug produces an effect comparable to the antihistamines but is not associated with sedation. The most common side effects of ipratropium are nasal irritation and bleeding.

Sore Throat

The sore throat associated with colds is generally not severe, but treatment with mild analgesics is occasionally indicated, particularly if there is associated myalgia or headache. The use of acetaminophen during HRV infection is associated with suppression of neutralizing antibody responses, but this observation has no apparent clinical significance. Aspirin *should not* be given to children with respiratory infections, because of the risk of Reye syndrome in children with influenza (see Chapter 388). **Nonsteroidal antiinflammatory drugs** are somewhat effective in relieving discomfort caused by a cold, but there is no clear evidence of an effect on respiratory symptoms.

Cough

Cough suppression is generally not necessary in patients with colds. Cough in some patients appears to be from upper respiratory tract irritation associated with postnasal drip. Cough in these patients is most prominent during the time of greatest nasal symptoms, and treatment with a 1st-generation antihistamine may be helpful. Cough lozenges or hard candy may be temporarily effective and are unlikely to be harmful in children for whom they do not pose risk of aspiration (older than age 6 yr). **Honey** (5-10 mL in children ≥1 yr old) has a modest effect on relieving nocturnal cough and is unlikely to be harmful in children older than 1 yr of age. Honey should be avoided in children younger than 1 yr of age because of the risk for botulism (see Chapter 237).

In some patients, cough may be a result of **virus-induced reactive airways disease**. These patients can have cough that persists for days to weeks after the acute illness and might benefit from bronchodilator or other therapy. Codeine or dextromethorphan hydrobromide has no effect on cough from colds and has potential enhanced toxicity. Expectorants such as guaifenesin are not effective antitussive agents. The combination of camphor, menthol, and eucalyptus oils may relieve nocturnal cough, but studies of their effectiveness are limited.

Ineffective Treatments
Vitamin C, guaifenesin, and inhalation of warm, humidified air are no more effective than placebo for the treatment of cold symptoms.

Echinacea is a popular herbal treatment for the common cold. Although echinacea extracts have biologic effects, echinacea is not effective as a common cold treatment. The lack of standardization of commercial products containing echinacea also presents a formidable obstacle to the rational evaluation or use of this therapy.

There is no evidence that the common cold or persistent acute purulent rhinitis of less than 10 days in duration benefits from antibiotics. In fact, there is evidence that antibiotics cause significant adverse effects when given for acute purulent rhinitis.

COMPLICATIONS
The most common complication of a cold is **acute otitis media (AOM;** see Chapter 658), which may be indicated by new-onset fever and earache after the 1st few days of cold symptoms. AOM is reported in 5–30% of children who have a cold, with the higher incidence occurring in young infants and in children cared for in a group daycare setting. Symptomatic treatment of the common cold symptoms has no effect on the subsequent development of AOM.

Sinusitis is another complication of the common cold (see Chapter 408). Self-limited sinus inflammation is a part of the pathophysiology of the common cold, but 0.5–2% of viral upper respiratory tract infections in adults, and 5–13% in children, are complicated by acute bacterial sinusitis. The differentiation of common cold symptoms from bacterial sinusitis may be difficult. The diagnosis of bacterial sinusitis should be considered if rhinorrhea or daytime cough persists without improvement for at least 10-14 days, if acute symptoms worsen over time, or if acute signs of more severe sinus involvement such as fever, facial pain, or facial swelling develop. There is no evidence that symptomatic treatment of the common cold alters the frequency of development of bacterial sinusitis. Bacterial pneumonia is an uncommon complication of the common cold.

Exacerbation of **asthma** is a potentially serious complication of colds. The majority of asthma exacerbations in children are associated with common cold viruses. There is no evidence that treatment of common cold symptoms prevents this complication; however, studies are underway in patients with underlying asthma to determine effectiveness of preventive or acute treatment at the onset of upper respiratory tract infection symptoms.

Although not a complication, another important consequence of the common cold is the inappropriate use of antibiotics for these illnesses and the associated contribution to the problem of increasing antibiotic resistance of pathogenic respiratory bacteria, as well as adverse effects from antibiotics.

PREVENTION
Chemoprophylaxis or immunoprophylaxis is generally not available for the common cold. Immunization or chemoprophylaxis against influenza can prevent colds caused by this pathogen, but influenza is responsible for only a small proportion of all colds. Palivizumab is recommended to prevent RSV lower respiratory infection in high-risk infants but does not prevent upper respiratory infections from this virus. Vitamin C, garlic, or echinacea do not prevent the common cold. Vitamin C prophylaxis may shorten the duration of cold symptoms. Vitamin D deficiency is associated with increased risk of viral respiratory tract infection in some studies; nonetheless, vitamin D prophylaxis does not reduce incidence or severity of the common cold in adults; studies in children are lacking. Zinc sulfate taken for a minimum of 5 mo may reduce the rate of cold development. However, because of duration of use and adverse effects of bad taste and nausea, this is not a recommended prevention modality in children.

Hand-to-hand transmission of HRV followed by self-inoculation may be prevented by frequent handwashing and avoiding touching one's mouth, nose, and eyes. Some studies report the use of alcohol-based hand sanitizers and virucidal hand treatments were associated with decreased transmission. In the experimental setting, virucidal disinfectants or virucidal-impregnated tissues also reduce transmission of cold viruses; under natural conditions none of these interventions prevents common colds.

Bibliography is available at Expert Consult.

Chapter **408**

Sinusitis

Diane E. Pappas and J. Owen Hendley†

第四百零八章

鼻窦炎

中文导读

　　本章主要介绍了鼻窦炎的病因、流行病学、发病机制、临床表现、诊断、治疗、并发症以及预防。其中病因主要为肺炎链球菌、不可分型流感嗜血杆菌和卡他莫拉菌引起的急性细菌性鼻窦炎，流行病学包括疾病易感因素，发病机制为急性细菌性鼻窦炎，通常发生在病毒性上呼吸道感染之后，临床表现主要为非特异性症状、少见症状、其他症状、体征以及区别细菌性鼻窦炎和感冒的症状，诊断主要基于病史采集、鼻窦抽吸培养以及鉴别诊断，治疗主要为对抗感染药治疗和其他疗法的探讨，并发症主要包括颅内并发症，预防措施为经常洗手、避免接触患有感冒的人群。

Sinusitis is a common illness of childhood and adolescence. There are 2 common types of acute sinusitis—viral and bacterial—with significant acute and chronic morbidity as well as the potential for serious complications. Fungal sinusitis is rare in immunocompetent patients but can also occur. The common cold produces a viral, self-limited *rhinosinusitis* (see Chapter 407). Approximately 0.5–2% of viral upper respiratory tract infections in children and adolescents are complicated by acute symptomatic bacterial sinusitis. Some children with underlying predisposing conditions have chronic sinus disease that does not appear to be infectious. The means for appropriate diagnosis and optimal treatment of sinusitis remain controversial.

Typically, the ethmoidal and maxillary sinuses are present at birth, but only the ethmoidal sinuses are pneumatized. The maxillary sinuses are not pneumatized until 4 yr of age. The sphenoidal sinuses are present by 5 yr of age, whereas the frontal sinuses begin development at age 7-8 yr and are not completely developed until adolescence. The ostia draining the sinuses are narrow (1-3 mm) and drain into the ostiomeatal complex in the middle meatus. The paranasal sinuses are normally sterile, maintained by the mucociliary clearance system.

ETIOLOGY

The bacterial pathogens causing **acute bacterial sinusitis** in children and adolescents include *Streptococcus pneumoniae* (~30%; see Chapter 209), nontypeable *Haemophilus influenzae* (~30%; see Chapter 221), and *Moraxella catarrhalis* (~10%; see Chapter 223). Approximately 50% of *H. influenzae* and 100% of *M. catarrhalis* are β-lactamase positive. Approximately 25% of *S. pneumoniae* may be penicillin resistant. *Staphylococcus aureus,* other streptococci, and anaerobes are uncommon causes of *acute* bacterial sinusitis in children. Although *S. aureus* (see Chapter 208.1) is an uncommon pathogen for acute sinusitis in children,

the increasing prevalence of methicillin-resistant *S. aureus* is a significant concern. *H. influenzae,* α- and β-hemolytic streptococci, *M. catarrhalis,* *S. pneumoniae,* and coagulase-negative staphylococci are commonly recovered from children with *chronic* sinus disease.

EPIDEMIOLOGY

Acute bacterial sinusitis can occur at any age. Predisposing conditions include viral upper respiratory tract infections (associated with out-of-home daycare or a school-age sibling), allergic rhinitis, and tobacco smoke exposure. Children with immune deficiencies, particularly of antibody production (immunoglobulin (Ig)G, IgG subclasses, IgA; see Chapter 150), cystic fibrosis (see Chapter 432), ciliary dysfunction (see Chapter 433), abnormalities of phagocyte function, gastroesophageal reflux, anatomic defects (cleft palate), nasal polyps, cocaine abuse, and nasal foreign bodies (including nasogastric tubes), can develop chronic or recurrent sinus disease. Immunosuppression for bone marrow transplantation or malignancy with profound neutropenia and lymphopenia predisposes to severe fungal (aspergillus, mucor) sinusitis, often with intracranial extension. Patients with nasotracheal intubation or nasogastric tubes may have obstruction of the sinus ostia and develop sinusitis with the multiple-drug resistant organisms of the intensive care unit.

Acute sinusitis is defined by a duration of <30 days, subacute by a duration of 1-3 mo, and chronic by a duration of longer than 3 mo.

PATHOGENESIS

Acute bacterial sinusitis typically follows a viral upper respiratory tract infection. Initially, the viral infection produces a viral rhinosinusitis;

---

†Deceased.

magnetic resonance imaging (MRI) evaluation of the paranasal sinuses demonstrates abnormalities (mucosal thickening, edema, inflammation) of the paranasal sinuses in 68% of healthy children in the normal course of the common cold. Nose blowing has been demonstrated to generate sufficient force to propel nasal secretions into the sinus cavities. Bacteria from the nasopharynx that enter the sinuses are normally cleared readily, but during viral rhinosinusitis, inflammation and edema can block sinus drainage and impair mucociliary clearance of bacteria. The growth conditions are favorable, and high titers of bacteria are produced.

CLINICAL MANIFESTATIONS

Children and adolescents with sinusitis can present with nonspecific complaints, including nasal congestion, purulent nasal discharge (unilateral or bilateral), fever, and cough. Less-common symptoms include bad breath (halitosis), a decreased sense of smell (hyposmia), and periorbital edema (Table 408.1). Complaints of headache and facial pain are rare in children. Additional symptoms include maxillary tooth discomfort and pain or pressure exacerbated by bending forward. Physical examination might reveal erythema and swelling of the nasal mucosa with purulent nasal discharge. Sinus tenderness may be detectable in adolescents and adults. Transillumination reveals an opaque sinus that transmits light poorly.

Differentiating bacterial sinusitis from a cold may be difficult, but certain patterns suggestive of sinusitis have been identified. These include

Table 408.1	Conventional Criteria for the Diagnosis of Sinusitis Based on the Presence of at Least 2 Major or 1 Major and ≥2 Minor Symptoms

MAJOR SYMPTOMS	MINOR SYMPTOMS
• Purulent anterior nasal discharge • Purulent or discolored posterior nasal discharge • Nasal congestion or obstruction • Facial congestion or fullness • Facial pain or pressure • Hyposmia or anosmia • Fever (for acute sinusitis only)	• Headache • Ear pain, pressure, or fullness • Halitosis • Dental pain • Cough • Fever (for subacute or chronic sinusitis) • Fatigue

From Chow AW, Benninger MS, Brook I, et al: IDSA clinical practice guideline for acute bacterial rhinosinusitis in children and adults. *CID* 54:e72–e112, 2012, Table 2, p. e78.

persistence of nasal congestion, rhinorrhea (of any quality), and daytime cough ≥10 days without improvement; *severe symptoms* of temperature ≥39°C (102°F) with purulent nasal discharge for 3 days or longer; and *worsening symptoms* either by recurrence of symptoms after an initial improvement or new symptoms of fever, nasal discharge, and daytime cough (double sickening; Fig. 408.1).

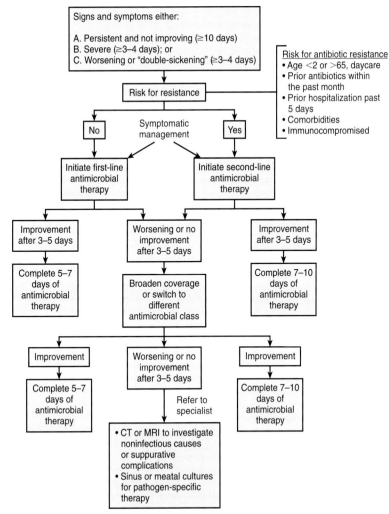

Fig. 408.1 Algorithm for the management of acute bacterial rhinosinusitis. (*From Chow AW, Benninger MS, Brook I, et al: Infectious Diseases Society of America. IDSA clinical practice guideline for acute bacterial rhinosinusitis in children and adults. Clin Infect Dis 54(8):e72–e112, 2012, Fig. 1.)*

DIAGNOSIS

The clinical diagnosis of *acute* bacterial sinusitis is based on history. Persistent symptoms of upper respiratory tract infection, including nasal discharge and cough, for longer than 10 days without improvement, or severe respiratory symptoms, including temperature of at least 39°C (102°F) and purulent nasal discharge for 3-4 consecutive days, suggest a complicating acute bacterial sinusitis. Bacteria are recovered from maxillary sinus aspirates in 70% of children with such persistent or severe symptoms studied. Children with *chronic* sinusitis have a history of persistent respiratory symptoms, including cough, nasal discharge, or nasal congestion, lasting longer than 90 days.

Sinus aspirate culture is the only accurate method of diagnosis but is not practical for routine use for immunocompetent patients. It may be a necessary procedure for immunosuppressed patients with suspected fungal sinusitis. In adults, *rigid nasal endoscopy* is a less-invasive method for obtaining culture material from the sinus but detects a great excess of positive cultures compared with aspirates. Findings on radiographic studies (sinus plain films, computed tomography [CT] scans), including opacification, mucosal thickening, or presence of an air-fluid level, are not diagnostic and are not recommended in otherwise healthy children. Such findings can confirm the presence of sinus inflammation but cannot be used to differentiate among viral, bacterial, or allergic causes of inflammation.

Given the nonspecific clinical picture, differential diagnostic considerations include viral upper respiratory tract infection, allergic rhinitis, nonallergic rhinitis, and nasal foreign body. Viral upper respiratory tract infections are characterized by clear and usually nonpurulent nasal discharge, cough, and initial fever; symptoms do not usually persist beyond 10-14 days, although a few children (10%) have persistent symptoms even at 14 days. In a recent study using nasal sampling, new viruses were present in 29% of sinusitis episodes in children, suggesting sequential URIs as the cause of persistent symptoms in many cases. Allergic rhinitis can be seasonal; evaluation of nasal secretions should reveal significant eosinophilia.

TREATMENT

It is unclear whether antimicrobial treatment of clinically diagnosed acute bacterial sinusitis offers any substantial benefit. A randomized, placebo-controlled trial comparing 14-day treatment of children with clinically diagnosed sinusitis with amoxicillin, amoxicillin-clavulanate, or placebo found that antimicrobial therapy did not affect resolution of symptoms, duration of symptoms, or days missed from school. A similar study in adults demonstrated improved symptoms at day 7 but not day 10 of treatment. Major guidelines recommend antimicrobial treatment for acute bacterial sinusitis with severe onset or a worsening course to promote resolution of symptoms and prevent suppurative complications, although 50–60% of children with acute bacterial sinusitis may recover without antimicrobial therapy.

Initial therapy with amoxicillin (45 mg/kg/day divided bid) is adequate for most children with uncomplicated mild to moderate severity acute bacterial sinusitis (Table 408.2). Alternative treatments for the penicillin-allergic patient include cefdinir, cefuroxime axetil, cefpodoxime, or cefixime. In older children, levofloxacin is an alternative antibiotic. *Azithromycin and trimethoprim-sulfamethoxazole are no longer indicated because of a high prevalence of antibiotic resistance.* For children with risk factors (antibiotic treatment in the preceding 1-3 mo, daycare attendance, or age younger than 2 yr) for the presence of resistant bacterial species, and for children who fail to respond to initial therapy with amoxicillin within 72 hr, or with severe sinusitis, treatment with high-dose amoxicillin-clavulanate (80-90 mg/kg/day of amoxicillin) should be initiated. Ceftriaxone (50 mg/kg, IV or IM) may be given to children who are vomiting or who are at risk for poor compliance; it should be followed by a course of oral antibiotics. Failure to respond to these regimens necessitates referral to an otolaryngologist for further evaluation because maxillary sinus aspiration for culture and susceptibility testing may be necessary (Table 408.3). The appropriate duration of therapy for sinusitis has yet to be determined; individualization of therapy is a reasonable approach, with treatment recommended for a minimum of 10 days or 7 days after resolution of symptoms (see Fig. 408.1).

Frontal sinusitis can rapidly progress to serious intracranial complications and necessitates initiation of parenteral ceftriaxone until substantial clinical improvement is achieved (Figs. 408.2 and 408.3). Treatment is then completed with oral antibiotic therapy.

The use of decongestants, antihistamines, mucolytics, and intranasal corticosteroids has not been adequately studied in children and is not recommended for the treatment of acute uncomplicated bacterial sinusitis. Likewise, saline nasal washes or nasal sprays can help liquefy secretions and act as a mild vasoconstrictor, but the effects have not been systematically evaluated in children.

COMPLICATIONS

Because of the close proximity of the paranasal sinuses to the brain and eyes, serious orbital and/or **intracranial complications** can result from acute bacterial sinusitis and progress rapidly. Orbital complications, including *periorbital cellulitis* and more often *orbital cellulitis* (see Chapter 652), are most often secondary to acute bacterial ethmoiditis. Infection can spread directly through the lamina papyracea, the thin bone that forms the lateral wall of the ethmoidal sinus. Periorbital cellulitis produces erythema and swelling of the tissues surrounding the globe, whereas orbital cellulitis involves the intraorbital structures and produces proptosis, chemosis, decreased visual acuity, double vision and impaired extraocular movements, and eye pain (Fig. 408.4). Evaluation should

Table 408.2	Antimicrobial Regimens for Acute Bacterial Rhinosinusitis in Children	
INDICATION	**FIRST-LINE (DAILY DOSE)**	**SECOND-LINE (DAILY DOSE)**
Initial empirical therapy	Amoxicillin-clavulanate (45 mg/kg/day PO bid)	• Amoxicillin-clavulanate (90 mg/kg/day PO bid)
β-LACTAM ALLERGY		
Type I hypersensitivity		• Levofloxacin (10-20 mg/kg/day PO every 12-24 h)
Non-type I hypersensitivity		• Clindamycin* (30-40 mg/kg/day PO tid) plus cefixime (8 mg/kg/day PO bid) or cefpodoxime (10 mg/kg/day PO bid)
Risk for antibiotic resistance or failed initial therapy		• Amoxicillin-clavulanate (90 mg/kg/day PO bid)
		• Clindamycin* (30-40 mg/kg/day PO tid) plus cefixime (8 mg/kg/day PO bid) or cefpodoxime (10 mg/kg/day PO bid)
		• Levofloxacin (10-20 mg/kg/day PO every 12-24 h)
Severe infection requiring hospitalization		• Ampicillin/sulbactam (200-400 mg/kg/day IV every 6 h)
		• Ceftriaxone (50 mg/kg/day IV every 12 h)
		• Cefotaxime (100-200 mg/kg/day IV every 6 h)
		• Levofloxacin (10-20 mg/kg/day IV every 12-24 h)

*Resistance to clindamycin (~31%) is found frequently among *Streptococcus pneumoniae* serotype 19A isolates in different regions of the United States.
bid, 2 times daily; IV, intravenously; PO, orally; qd, daily; tid, 3 times a day.
From Chow AW, Benninger MS, Brook I, et al: IDSA clinical practice guideline for acute bacterial rhinosinusitis in children and adults. *CID* 54:e72–e112, 2012, Table 9, p. e94.

Table 408.3	Indications for Referral to a Specialist

• Severe infection (high persistent fever with temperature >39°C [>102°F]; orbital edema; severe headache, visual disturbance, altered mental status, meningeal signs) • Recalcitrant infection with failure to respond to extended courses of antimicrobial therapy • Immunocompromised host • Multiple medical problems that might compromise response to treatment (e.g., hepatic or renal impairment, hypersensitivity to antimicrobial agents, organ transplant) • Unusual or resistant pathogens	• Fungal sinusitis or granulomatous disease • Nosocomial infection • Anatomic defects causing obstruction and requiring surgical intervention • Multiple recurrent episodes of acute bacterial rhinosinusitis (3-4 episodes per year) suggesting chronic sinusitis • Chronic rhinosinusitis (with or without polyps or asthma) with recurrent ABRS exacerbations • Evaluation of immunotherapy for allergic rhinitis

From Chow AW, Benninger MS, Brook I, et al: IDSA clinical practice guideline for acute bacterial rhinosinusitis in children and adults. *CID* 54:e72–e112, 2012, Table 14, p. e106.

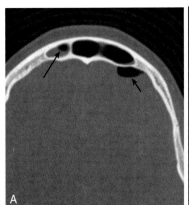 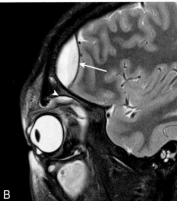 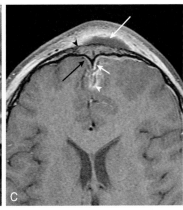

Fig. 408.2 **Acute complicated sinusitis. A,** Frontal sinusitis and epidural abscess. Axial computed tomography image shows a frontal sinus air–fluid level *(long arrow)*. There is also an intracranial air–fluid level associated with an epidural abscess *(short arrow)*. **B,** Frontal sinusitis, epidural abscess, and orbital abscess. Sagittal fat-suppressed (FS) T2-weighted magnetic resonance (MR) image demonstrates a biconvex epidural abscess *(arrow)* containing a sediment level. There is also a small superior extraconal subperiosteal abscess *(arrowhead)*. Periorbital STS is present, and there are secretions within the maxillary antrum. **C,** Pott puffy tumor, frontal osteomyelitis, and subdural empyema. Axial gadolinium-enhanced FS T1-weighted MR image shows frontal scalp swelling ventral to an elliptical low signal intensity, peripherally enhancing, frontal subperiosteal abscess *(long white arrow)*. There is enhancement of the subjacent frontal bone, consistent with osteomyelitis *(black arrowhead)*. There is also dural enhancement *(black arrow)* and a small left frontal interhemispheric subdural empyema *(short white arrow)* with subtle enhancement of the adjacent frontal leptomeninges and cortex caused by meningitis and cerebritis *(white arrowhead)*. *(From Walters MM, Robertson RL, editors: Pediatric radiology, the requisites, ed 4, Philadelphia, 2017, Elsevier, Fig. 10.40.)*

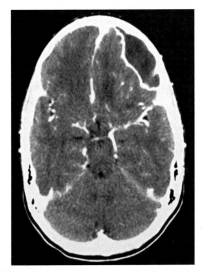

Fig. 408.3 Axial plane contrast-enhanced CT scan of an 11 yr old obtunded girl with a subfrontal lobe abscess secondary to frontal sinusitis. The CT scan demonstrates an eliptiform ring-enhancing fluid-filled cavity adjacent to the frontal lobe with contralateral shift of the midline. *(From Parikh SR, Brown SM: Image-guided frontal sinus surgery in children, Operative Tech Otolaryngol Head Neck Surg 15:37–41, 2004.)*

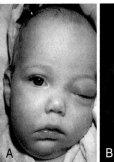 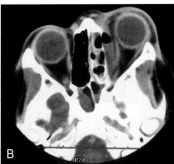

Fig. 408.4 Orbital complications of acute sinusitis. **A,** An 11 mo old infant with a swollen left eye and limited ocular movement. **B,** Axial CT shows opacification of sinuses and an inflammatory mass with an air–fluid level displacing the medial rectus laterally. *(From Cooper, ML, Slovis T: The sinuses. In Slovis T, editor: Caffey's pediatric diagnostic imaging, ed 11, Philadelphia, 2008, Mosby, Fig. 43-7, p. 573.)*

include CT scan of the orbits and sinuses with ophthalmology and otolaryngology consultations. Treatment with intravenous antibiotics should be initiated. Orbital cellulitis may require surgical drainage of the ethmoidal sinuses or orbit.

Intracranial complications can include epidural abscess, meningitis, cavernous sinus thrombosis, subdural empyema, and brain abscess (see

Chapter 622). Children with altered mental status, nuchal rigidity, severe headache, focal neurologic findings, or signs of increased intracranial pressure (headache, vomiting) require immediate CT scan of the brain, orbits, and sinuses to evaluate for the presence of intracranial complications of acute bacterial sinusitis. Black children and males are at increased risk, but there is no evidence of increased risk due to socioeconomic status. Treatment with broad-spectrum intravenous antibiotics (usually cefotaxime or ceftriaxone combined with vancomycin) should be initiated immediately, pending culture and susceptibility results. In 50% the abscess is a polymicrobial infection. Abscesses can require surgical drainage. Other complications include osteomyelitis of the frontal bone (**Pott puffy tumor**), which is characterized by edema and swelling of the forehead (see Fig. 408.2), and **mucoceles**, which are chronic inflammatory lesions commonly located in the frontal sinuses that can expand, causing displacement of the eye with resultant diplopia. Surgical drainage is usually required.

PREVENTION
Prevention is best accomplished by frequent handwashing and avoiding persons with colds. Because acute bacterial sinusitis can complicate influenza infection, prevention of influenza infection by yearly influenza vaccine will prevent some cases of complicating sinusitis. Immunization or chemoprophylaxis against influenza with oseltamivir or zanamivir may be useful for prevention of colds caused by this pathogen and the associated complications; influenza is responsible for only a small proportion of all colds.

Bibliography is available at Expert Consult.

Chapter **409**
Acute Pharyngitis
Robert R. Tanz

第四百零九章
急性咽炎

中文导读

　　本章主要介绍了急性咽炎的病原、诊断、治疗、慢性A组链球菌携带者、复发性咽炎、并发症和预后以及预防。病原中具体描述了病毒、A组链球菌以外的细菌、A组链球菌相关内容，诊断主要包括Mc-Isaac评分、咽喉培养和快速抗原检测试验、A组链球菌分子检测，治疗包括病毒性咽炎非特异性症状治疗、细菌性咽炎抗生素治疗。介绍了慢性A组链球菌携带者的发病风险、检测方法、诊疗建议，复发性咽炎的病因、诊疗建议，并发症和预后包括细菌性中耳炎、鼻窦炎、局部化脓性并发症等，预防包括预防疫苗和其他预防措施。

Pharyngitis refers to inflammation of the pharynx, including erythema, edema, exudates, or an enanthem (ulcers, vesicles). Pharyngeal inflammation can be related to environmental exposures, such as tobacco smoke, air pollutants, and allergens; from contact with caustic substances, hot food, and liquids; and from infectious agents. The pharynx and mouth can be involved in various inflammatory conditions such as the periodic fever, aphthous stomatitis, pharyngitis, adenitis (PFAPA) syndrome, Kawasaki disease, inflammatory bowel disease (IBD), Stevens-Johnson syndrome, and systemic lupus erythematous (SLE). Noninfectious etiologies are typically evident from history and physical exam, but it can be more challenging to distinguish from among the numerous infectious causes of acute pharyngitis.

Acute infections of the upper respiratory tract account for a substantial number of visits to pediatricians and many feature sore throat as a symptom or evidence of pharyngitis on physical examination. The usual clinical task is to distinguish important, potentially serious, and treatable causes of acute pharyngitis from those that are self-limited and require no specific treatment or follow-up. Specifically, identifying patients who have **group A streptococcus** (GAS; *Streptococcus pyogenes*; see Chapter 210) pharyngitis and treating them with antibiotics forms the core of the management paradigm.

INFECTIOUS ETIOLOGIES
Viruses
In North America and most industrialized countries, GAS is the most important bacterial cause of acute pharyngitis, but viruses predominate

as acute infectious causes of pharyngitis. Viral upper respiratory tract infections are typically spread by contact with oral or respiratory secretions and occur most commonly in fall, winter, and spring—that is, the respiratory season. Important viruses that cause pharyngitis include influenza, parainfluenza, adenoviruses, coronaviruses, enteroviruses, rhinoviruses, respiratory syncytial virus (RSV), cytomegalovirus, Epstein-Barr virus (EBV), herpes simplex virus (HSV), and human metapneumovirus (HMPV) (Table 409.1). Most viral pharyngitis, except mononucleosis, is mild. Common nonspecific symptoms such as rhinorrhea and cough develop gradually before they become prominent. However, specific findings are sometimes helpful in identifying the infectious viral agent (Table 409.2).

Gingivostomatitis and ulcerating vesicles throughout the anterior pharynx and on the lips and perioral skin are seen in primary oral HSV infection. High fever and difficulty taking oral fluids are common. This infection can last for 14 days.

Discrete **papulovesicular** lesions or **ulcerations** in the posterior oropharynx, severe throat pain, and fever are characteristic of **herpangina**, caused by various enteroviruses. In **hand-foot-mouth disease**, there are vesicles or ulcers throughout the oropharynx, vesicles on the palms and soles, and sometimes on the trunk and extremities. Coxsackie A16 is the most common agent, but Enterovirus 71 and Coxsackie A6 can also cause this syndrome. Enteroviral infections are most common in the summer.

Various adenoviruses cause pharyngitis. When there is concurrent **conjunctivitis**, the syndrome is called *pharyngoconjunctival fever*. The pharyngitis tends to resolve within 7 days but conjunctivitis may persist for up to 14 days. Pharyngoconjunctival fever can be epidemic or sporadic; outbreaks have been associated with exposure in swimming pools.

Intense, diffuse pharyngeal erythema and Koplik spots, the pathognomonic enanthem, occur in advance of the characteristic rash of measles. Splenomegaly, lymphadenopathy, or hepatomegaly may be the clue to EBV infectious mononucleosis in an adolescent with exudative tonsillitis. Primary infection with HIV can manifest as the **acute retroviral syndrome**, with non-exudative pharyngitis, fever, arthralgia, myalgia, adenopathy, and often a maculopapular rash.

Bacteria Other Than Group A Streptococcus

In addition to GAS, bacteria that cause pharyngitis include group C and group G streptococcus, *Arcanobacterium haemolyticum*, *Francisella tularensis*, *Neisseria gonorrhoeae*, *Mycoplasma pneumoniae*, *Chlamydophila* (formerly *Chlamydia*) *pneumoniae*, *Chlamydia trachomatis*, *Fusobacterium necrophorum*, and *Corynebacterium diphtheriae*. *Haemophilus influenzae* and *Streptococcus pneumoniae* may be cultured from the throats of children with pharyngitis, but their role in causing pharyngitis has not been established.

Group C and Group G streptococcus and *A. haemolyticum* pharyngitis have been diagnosed most commonly in adolescents and adults. They resemble group A β-hemolytic streptococcus (GAS) pharyngitis. A scarlet fever–like rash may be present with *A. haemolyticum* infections.

F. necrophorum has been suggested to be a fairly common cause of pharyngitis in older adolescents and adults (15-30 yr old). Prevalence in studies has varied from 10% to 48% of patients with non-GABHS pharyngitis, but large surveillance studies have not been performed. *F. necrophorum* was detected by PCR in 20.5% of patients with pharyngitis in a study based in a university health clinic and in 9.4% of an asymptomatic convenience sample; some patients had more than 1 bacterial species detected by PCR. Pharyngitis patients with *F. necrophorum* had signs and symptoms similar to GAS pharyngitis: about one third had fever, one third had tonsillar exudates, two thirds had anterior cervical adenopathy, and most did not have cough. This organism is difficult to culture from the throat, and diagnostic testing with PCR is not generally available. *F. necrophorum* pharyngitis is associated with the development of **Lemierre syndrome** (see Chapter 410), internal jugular vein septic thrombophlebitis. Approximately 80% of cases of Lemierre syndrome are caused by this bacterium. Patients present initially with fever, sore throat, exudative pharyngitis, and/or peritonsillar abscess. The symptoms may persist, neck pain and swelling develop, and the patient appears toxic. Septic shock may ensue, along with metastatic complications from septic emboli that can involve the lungs, bones and joints, central nervous system, abdominal organs, and soft tissues. The case fatality rate is 4–9%.

Gonococcal pharyngeal infections are usually asymptomatic but can cause acute ulcerative or exudative pharyngitis with fever and cervical lymphadenitis. Young children with proven gonococcal disease should be evaluated for sexual abuse.

Diphtheria is extremely rare in most developed countries due to extensive immunization with diphtheria toxoid. However, it remains endemic in many areas of the world, including the former Soviet bloc countries, Africa, Asia, the Middle East, and Latin America. It can be considered in patients with recent travel to or from these areas and in unimmunized patients. Key physical findings are bull neck (extreme neck swelling) and a gray pharyngeal pseudomembrane that can cause respiratory obstruction.

Ingestion of water, milk, or undercooked meat contaminated by *F. tularensis* can lead to oropharyngeal tularemia. Severe throat pain, tonsillitis, cervical adenitis, oral ulcerations, and a pseudomembrane

Table 409.1	Infectious Agents That Cause Pharyngitis

VIRUSES	BACTERIA
Adenovirus	*Streptococcus pyogenes* (Group A streptococcus)
Coronavirus	
Cytomegalovirus	*Arcanobacterium haemolyticum*
Epstein-Barr virus	*Fusobacterium necrophorum*
Enteroviruses	*Corynebacterium diphtheriae*
Herpes simplex virus (1 and 2)	*Neisseria gonorrhoeae*
Human immunodeficiency virus	Group C streptococci
Human metapneumovirus	Group G streptococci
Influenza viruses (A and B)	*Francisella tularensis*
Measles virus	*Yersinia pestis*
Parainfluenza viruses	*Chlamydophila pneumoniae*
Respiratory syncytial virus	*Chlamydia trachomatis*
Rhinoviruses	*Mycoplasma pneumoniae*
	Mixed anaerobes (Vincent angina)

Table 409.2	Epidemiologic and Clinical Features Suggestive of Group A Streptococcal and Viral Pharyngitis

FEATURE, BY SUSPECTED ETIOLOGIC AGENT

Group A Streptococcal
- Sudden onset of sore throat
- Age 5-15 yr
- Fever
- Headache
- Nausea, vomiting, abdominal pain
- Tonsillopharyngeal inflammation
- Patchy tonsillopharyngeal exudates
- Palatal petechiae
- Anterior cervical adenitis (tender nodes)
- Winter and early spring presentation
- History of exposure to strep pharyngitis
- Scarlatiniform rash

Viral
- Conjunctivitis
- Coryza
- Cough
- Diarrhea
- Hoarseness
- Discrete ulcerative stomatitis
- Viral exanthema

From Shulman ST, Bisno AL, Clegg HW, et al: Clinical practice guideline for the diagnosis and management of group A streptococcal pharyngitis: 2012 update by the Infectious Diseases Society of America. *Clin Infect Dis* 55(10):e86–e102, 2012, Table 4, p. e91.

(as in diphtheria) may be present. *M. pneumoniae* and *C. pneumoniae* cause pharyngitis, but other upper and lower respiratory infections are more important and more readily recognized. Development of a severe or persistent cough subsequent to pharyngitis may be the clue to infection with 1 of these organisms.

Group A Streptococcus

Streptococcal pharyngitis is relatively uncommon before 2-3 yr of age, is quite common among children 5-15 yr old, and declines in frequency in late adolescence and adulthood. Illness occurs throughout the year but is most prevalent in winter and spring. It is readily spread among siblings and schoolmates. GAS causes 15–30% of pharyngitis in school-age children.

Colonization of the pharynx by GAS can result in either asymptomatic carriage or acute infection. After an incubation period of 2-5 days, pharyngeal infection with GAS classically presents as rapid onset of significant sore throat and fever (see Table 409.2). The pharynx is red, the tonsils are enlarged and often covered with a white, grayish, or yellow exudate that may be blood-tinged. There may be petechiae or doughnut lesions on the soft palate and posterior pharynx, and the uvula may be red and swollen (see Fig. 411.1). The surface of the tongue can resemble a strawberry when the papillae are inflamed and prominent (strawberry tongue). Initially, the tongue is often coated white, and with the swollen papillae it is called a *white strawberry tongue* (see Fig. 210.1*B*). When the white coating is gone after a few days, the tongue is often quite red, and is called a *red strawberry tongue* (see Fig. 210.1*C*). Enlarged and tender anterior cervical lymph nodes are frequently present. Headache, abdominal pain, and vomiting are frequently associated with the infection, but in the absence of clinical pharyngitis, gastrointestinal signs and symptoms should not be attributed to GAS. Ear pain is a frequent complaint, but the tympanic membranes are usually normal. Diarrhea, cough, coryza, ulcerations, croup/laryngitis/hoarseness, and conjunctivitis *are not* associated with GAS pharyngitis and increase the likelihood of a viral etiology (see Table 409.2).

Patients infected with GAS that produce streptococcal pyrogenic exotoxin A, B, or C may demonstrate the fine red, papular (sandpaper) rash of **scarlet fever** (see Fig. 210.1*A*). It begins on the face and then becomes generalized. The cheeks are red, and the area around the mouth is less intensely red (more pale), giving the appearance of circumoral pallor. The rash blanches with pressure, and it may be more intense in skin creases, especially in the antecubital fossae, axillae, and inguinal creases (Pastia lines or sign). Pastia lines are sometimes petechial or slightly hemorrhagic. Capillary fragility can cause petechiae distal to a tourniquet or constriction from clothing, a positive tourniquet test or Rumpel-Leeds phenomenon. Erythema fades in a few days, and when the rash resolves, it typically peels like a mild sunburn. Sometimes there is sheet-like desquamation around the free margins of the finger nails. Streptococcal pyrogenic exotoxin A, encoded by the gene *spe A*, is the exotoxin most commonly associated with scarlet fever.

The M protein is an important GAS virulence factor that facilitates resistance to phagocytosis. The M protein is encoded by the *emm* gene and determines the M type (or *emm* type). Molecular methods have identified more than 200 *emm* genes (*emm* types, M types). The M protein is immunogenic and protects against reinfection with the homologous M type; an individual can experience multiple episodes of GAS pharyngitis in a lifetime because natural immunity is M type–specific and does not prevent infection with a new M type. Numerous GAS M types can circulate in a community simultaneously, and they enter and leave communities unpredictably and for unknown reasons.

DIAGNOSIS

The clinical presentations of streptococcal and viral pharyngitis often overlap. In particular, the pharyngitis of mononucleosis can be difficult to distinguish from GAS pharyngitis. Physicians relying solely on clinical judgment often overestimate the likelihood of a streptococcal etiology. Various clinical scoring systems have been described to assist in identifying patients who are likely to have GAS pharyngitis. Criteria developed for adults by Centor and modified for children by McIsaac give 1 point for each of the following criteria: history of temperature >38°C (100.4°F), absence of cough, tender anterior cervical adenopathy, tonsillar swelling or exudates, and age 3-14 yr. It subtracts a point for age ≥45 yr. At best, a McIsaac score ≥4 is associated with a positive laboratory test for GAS in less than 70% of children with pharyngitis (Table 409.3), so it, too, overestimates the likelihood of GAS. *Consequently, laboratory testing is essential for accurate diagnosis.* Clinical findings and/or scoring systems can best be used to assist the clinician in identifying patients in need of testing. Evaluating patients indiscriminately can lead to overdiagnosis and overtreatment. Streptococcal antibody tests are not useful in assessing patients with acute pharyngitis.

Throat culture and rapid antigen-detection tests (RADTs) are the diagnostic tests for GAS most available in routine clinical care. Throat culture plated on blood agar remains the gold standard for diagnosing streptococcal pharyngitis. There are both false-negative cultures as a consequence of sampling errors or prior antibiotic treatment and false-positive cultures as a consequence of misidentification of other bacteria as GAS. Streptococcal RADTs detect the group A carbohydrate of GAS. They are used by the vast majority of office-based pediatricians. All RADTs have very high specificity, generally ≥95%, so when a RADT is positive it is assumed to be accurate and throat culture is unnecessary. Because RADTs are generally much less sensitive than culture, confirming a negative rapid test with a throat culture is recommended. RADTs and throat culture exhibit spectrum bias: they are more sensitive when the pretest probability of GAS is high (signs and symptoms are typical of GAS infection, higher McIsaac scores) and less sensitive when the pretest probability is low. Avoidance of testing when patients have signs and symptoms more suggestive of a viral infection is recommended by expert guidelines.

Many laboratories have replaced throat culture with one of the highly sensitive and specific **GAS molecular tests**. A variety of methods are available to amplify the DNA of a specific GAS gene from a throat swab in less than 1 hr. In studies both sensitivity and specificity are reported

Table 409.3	Positive Predictive Value of McIsaac Score in Children in Clinical Studies*			
SCORE	McISAAC, 2004 (N = 454) (%)	EDMONSON, 2005 (N = 1184) (%)	TANZ, 2009 (N = 1848) (%)	FINE, 2012 (N = 64,789) (%)
0	—	—	7	17
1	—	0.5	19	23
2	20.5	8.9	20	34
3	27.5	42.4	29	50
≥4	67.8	48.2	49	68
GAS prevalence	34	38	30	37

*One point is given for each of the following criteria: history of temperature >38°C (100.4°F); absence of cough; tender anterior cervical adenopathy; tonsillar swelling or exudates; and age 3-14 yr. Note that the Centor score lacks only the age criterion. Positive predictive value refers to the proportion of patients with documented GAS by rapid antigen-detection test and/or throat culture.

to be ≥98% when compared with standard throat culture. Polymerase chain reaction (PCR) usually matches the molecular test when used to adjudicate discrepancies between the culture and molecular test results. Some of these nucleic acid amplification tests are approved by the FDA for use in physician office laboratories and can be used as the initial test for GAS or as a confirmatory test when the RADT is negative. Unlike throat culture and RADTs, molecular tests may not exhibit spectrum bias—that is, although test sensitivity is extremely high, it is independent of the pretest probability that GAS are the cause of illness (using signs and symptoms, McIsaac score), thus increasing the potential to identify a chronic GAS carrier who actually has an intercurrent illness not due to GAS (discussed later). However, the ability of these stand-alone tests to deliver a definitive result in less than 1 hr makes them attractive (there is one test that takes 15 min)—the potential to swab symptomatic children, have them wait or send them home, and electronically prescribe an antibiotic when the test is positive can speed initiation of therapy and subsequent return to school and activities. The role of molecular tests in diagnosis of GAS pharyngitis is currently unclear because of 3 concerns: (1) they are so sensitive they may cause unnecessary treatment of more patients who are carriers than would ordinarily occur with RADT and/or culture; (2) unless rigorous technique is followed, they may be prone to contamination with exogenous GAS DNA from other swabs, a particular concern in physician offices when performed by staff who are not trained laboratory technologists; and (3) they are much more expensive than throat culture.

Testing for bacteria other than GAS is performed infrequently, and should be reserved for patients with persistent symptoms and symptoms suggestive of a specific non-GAS bacterial pharyngitis—for example, when there is concern for gonococcal infection or sexual abuse. Special culture media and a prolonged incubation are required to detect *A. haemolyticum*. A complete blood cell count showing many atypical lymphocytes and a positive mononucleosis slide agglutination test can help confirm a clinical suspicion of EBV infectious mononucleosis. Viral cultures are often unavailable and are generally too expensive and slow to be clinically useful. PCR is more rapid and multiplex PCR (respiratory viral panel) testing for respiratory pathogens can identify a variety of viral and bacterial agents within a few hours. This may be useful in determining the isolation needs of hospitalized patients, assisting in patient prognosis, and epidemiology, but in the absence of specific treatment for most viral infections such testing is usually not necessary or useful. In fact, interpreting such tests can be difficult unless the patient has signs or symptoms characteristic of a specific pathogen.

TREATMENT

Specific therapy is unavailable for most viral pharyngitis. However, nonspecific, symptomatic therapy can be an important part of the overall treatment plan. An oral antipyretic/analgesic agent (acetaminophen or ibuprofen) can relieve fever and sore throat pain. Anesthetic sprays and lozenges (often containing benzocaine, phenol, or menthol) can provide local relief in children who are developmentally appropriate to use them. Systemic corticosteroids are sometimes used in children who have evidence of upper airway compromise due to mononucleosis. Although corticosteroids are used commonly in adults with pharyngitis, large-scale studies capable of providing safety and efficacy data are lacking in children. *Corticosteroids cannot be recommended for treatment of most pediatric pharyngitis.*

Antibiotic therapy of bacterial pharyngitis depends on the organism identified. On the basis of in vitro susceptibility data, oral penicillin is often suggested for patients with group C streptococcal isolates, and oral erythromycin is recommended for patients with *A. haemolyticum*, but the clinical benefit of such treatment is uncertain.

Most untreated episodes of GAS pharyngitis resolve uneventfully within a few days, but early antibiotic therapy hastens clinical recovery by 12-24 hr and also reduces suppurative complications of GAS pharyngitis such as peritonsillar abscess and cervical adenitis. *The primary benefit and intent of antibiotic treatment is the prevention of acute rheumatic fever (ARF)*; it is highly effective when started within 9 days of onset of illness. Antibiotic therapy does not prevent acute poststreptococcal glomerulonephritis (APSGN). Antibiotic treatment should not be delayed for children with symptomatic pharyngitis and a positive test for GAS. Presumptive antibiotic treatment can be started when there is a clinical diagnosis of scarlet fever, a symptomatic child has a household contact with documented streptococcal pharyngitis, or there is a history of ARF in the patient or a family member, but a diagnostic test should be performed to confirm the presence of GAS and antibiotics should be discontinued if GAS are not identified.

A variety of antimicrobial agents are effective for GAS pharyngitis (Table 409.4). Group A streptococci are universally susceptible to penicillin and all other β-lactam antibiotics. Penicillin is inexpensive, has a narrow spectrum of activity, and has few adverse effects. Amoxicillin

Table 409.4	Recommended Treatment for Acute Streptococcal Pharyngitis				
MOST PATIENTS					
	WEIGHT <27 kg		**WEIGHT ≥27 kg**	**ROUTE**	**DURATION**
Amoxicillin	50 mg/kg once daily (maximum 1,000 mg)			Oral	10 days
Penicillin V	250 mg bid		500 mg bid	Oral	10 days
Benzathine penicillin G	600,000 units		1.2 million units	IM	Once
Benzathine penicillin G + procaine penicillin G	900,000 units + 300,000 units		900,000 units + 300,000 units	IM	Once

PENICILLIN-ALLERGIC PATIENTS			
	ORAL DOSE	**FREQUENCY**	**DURATION**
Cephalosporins*	Varies with agent chosen		10 days
Erythromycins			
Ethylsuccinate	40 mg/kg/day up to 1,000 mg/day	bid	10 days
Estolate	20-40 mg/kg/day up to 1,000 mg/day	bid	10 days
Clarithromycin	15 mg/kg/day up to 500 mg/day	bid	10 days
Azithromycin†	12 mg/kg day 1; 6 mg/kg days 2-5	qd	5 days
Clindamycin	20 mg/kg/day up to 1.8 g/day	tid	10 days

*First-generation cephalosporins are preferred; dosage and frequency vary among agents. Do not use in patients with history of immediate (anaphylactic) hypersensitivity to penicillin or other β-lactam antibiotics.
†Maximum dose is 500 mg the 1st day, 250 mg subsequent days.

is often preferred for children because of taste, availability as chewable tablets and liquid, and the convenience of once-daily dosing. The duration of oral penicillin and amoxicillin therapy is 10 days. A single intramuscular dose of benzathine penicillin or a benzathine-procaine penicillin G combination is effective and ensures compliance. Follow-up testing for GAS is unnecessary after completion of therapy and is not recommended unless symptoms recur.

Patients allergic to the penicillins can be treated with a 10-day course of a narrow-spectrum, 1st-generation cephalosporin (cephalexin or cefadroxil) if the previous reaction to penicillin was not an immediate, type I hypersensitivity reaction. Frequently, penicillin-allergic patients are treated for 10 days with erythromycin, clarithromycin, or clindamycin, or for 5 days with azithromycin.

The increased use of macrolides and related antibiotics for a variety of infections, especially the azalide, azithromycin, is associated with increased rates of resistance to these drugs among GAS in many countries. Approximately 5% of GAS in the United States and more than 10% in Canada are macrolide-resistant (macrolide resistance includes azalide resistance), but there is considerable local variation in both countries. Rates are much higher in many European and Asian countries. Some macrolide-resistant GAS isolates are also resistant to clindamycin. Although not a major hindrance for treatment of pharyngitis, clindamycin resistance may be important in management of invasive GAS infections. The use of macrolides and related antibiotics should be restricted to patients who cannot safely receive a β-lactam drug for GAS pharyngitis. Tetracyclines, fluoroquinolones, or sulfonamides should *not* be used to treat GAS pharyngitis.

CHRONIC GROUP A STREPTOCOCCUS CARRIERS

Streptococcal carriers are patients who continue to harbor GAS in the pharynx despite appropriate antibiotic therapy or when they are well. They have little or no evidence of an inflammatory response to the organism. The pathogenesis of chronic carriage is not known; it is assuredly not related to penicillin resistance or nonadherence to therapy, and there is little direct evidence to support the concept of co-pathogenicity (presence of β-lactamase-producing organisms in the pharynx). Carriage generally poses little risk to patients and their contacts, but it can confound testing in subsequent episodes of sore throat. A child who is chronically colonized with GAS (streptococcal carrier) can have a positive test for GAS if it is obtained when the child is evaluated for pharyngitis that is actually caused by a viral infection. Patients with repeated test-positive pharyngitis create anxiety among their families and physicians. It is usually unnecessary to attempt to eliminate chronic carriage. Instead, evaluation and treatment of clinical pharyngitis should be undertaken without regard for chronic carriage, using clinical criteria to determine the need for testing, treating test-positive patients in routine fashion, and avoiding antibiotics in patients who have negative tests. This approach often requires considerable effort to reassure the patient and family that chronic carriage is not a significant health risk. Expert opinion suggests that eradication might be attempted in select circumstances: a community outbreak of ARF or APSGN; personal or family history of ARF; an outbreak of GAS pharyngitis in a closed or semiclosed community, nursing home, or healthcare facility; repeated episodes of symptomatic GAS pharyngitis in a family with ping pong spread among family members despite adequate therapy; when tonsillectomy is being considered because of chronic carriage or recurrent streptococcal pharyngitis; and extreme, unmanageable anxiety related to GAS carriage ("streptophobia") among family members. Clindamycin given by mouth for 10 days is effective therapy (20 mg/kg/day divided in 3 doses; adult dose 150-450 mg tid). Amoxicillin-clavulanate (40 mg amoxicillin/kg/day up to 2,000 mg amoxicillin/day divided tid for 10 days), and 4 days of oral rifampin (20 mg/kg/day up to 600 mg divided in 2 doses) plus either intramuscular benzathine penicillin given once or oral penicillin given for 10 days have

also been used (rifampin is started on the 1st day of penicillin therapy).

RECURRENT PHARYNGITIS

True recurrent GAS pharyngitis can occur for several reasons: reinfection with the same M type if type-specific antibody has not developed; poor compliance with oral antibiotic therapy; macrolide resistance if a macrolide was used for treatment; and infection with a new M type. Unfortunately, determining the GAS M type in an acute infection is not available to the clinician. Treatment with intramuscular benzathine penicillin eliminates nonadherence to therapy. Apparent recurrences can represent pharyngitis of another cause in the presence of streptococcal carriage. Chronic GAS carriage is particularly likely if the illnesses are mild and otherwise atypical for GAS pharyngitis.

Tonsillectomy may lower the incidence of pharyngitis for 1-2 yr among children with frequent episodes of documented pharyngitis (≥7 episodes in the previous year or ≥5 in each of the preceding 2 yr, or ≥3 in each of the previous 3 yr). However, the frequency of pharyngitis (GAS and non-GAS) generally declines over time. By 2 yr posttonsillectomy, the incidence of pharyngitis in severely affected children is similar among those who have tonsillectomy and those who do not. Few children are so severely affected, and the limited clinical benefit of tonsillectomy for most must be balanced against the risks of anesthesia and surgery. *Undocumented history of recurrent pharyngitis is an inadequate basis for recommending tonsillectomy.*

Recurrent GAS pharyngitis is rarely, if ever, a sign of an immune disorder. However, recurrent pharyngitis can be part of a recurrent fever or autoinflammatory syndrome such as PFAPA syndrome. Prolonged pharyngitis (>1 wk) can occur in infectious mononucleosis and Lemierre syndrome, but it also suggests the possibility of another disorder such as neutropenia, a recurrent fever syndrome, or an autoimmune disease such as SLE or IBD. In such instances, pharyngitis would be 1 of a number of clinical findings that together should suggest the underlying diagnosis.

COMPLICATIONS AND PROGNOSIS

Viral respiratory tract infections can predispose to bacterial middle ear infections and bacterial sinusitis. The complications of GAS pharyngitis include local suppurative complications, such as parapharyngeal abscess, and subsequent nonsuppurative illnesses, such as ARF, APSGN, poststreptococcal reactive arthritis, and possibly PANDAS (pediatric autoimmune neuropsychiatric disorders associated with streptococci) (sometimes referred to as CANS [childhood acute neuropsychiatric symptoms] or PANS [pediatric acute-onset neuropsychiatric syndrome], recognizing that many infections other than GAS may predispose to these syndromes).

PREVENTION

Vaccines intended to prevent infection with various viruses (e.g., RSV) and GAS are being developed. A recombinant multivalent GAS M-type vaccine uses the terminal portions of various M proteins to take advantage of their immunogenicity. Other GAS vaccines are based on more conserved epitopes in order to avoid the necessity of matching the vaccine with the M types prevalent in a community or target population. None of the investigational GAS vaccines are near licensing for use. A recent comprehensive study of the immune response to childhood GAS pharyngeal acquisition raises questions about how to best design effective vaccines. This is complicated by the variety of clinical scenarios and clinical syndromes associated with GAS and the need to determine the intended clinical benefit(s) of vaccination. Antimicrobial prophylaxis with daily oral penicillin prevents recurrent GAS infections but is recommended only to prevent recurrences of ARF.

Bibliography is available at Expert Consult.

Chapter 410

Retropharyngeal Abscess, Lateral Pharyngeal (Parapharyngeal) Abscess, and Peritonsillar Cellulitis/Abscess

Diane E. Pappas and J. Owen Hendley[†]

第四百一十章

咽后脓肿、咽侧（咽旁）脓肿和扁桃体周围蜂窝织炎/脓肿

中文导读

　　本章主要介绍了咽后脓肿和咽旁脓肿、扁桃体周围蜂窝织炎和/或脓肿。其中咽后脓肿和咽旁脓肿主要包括咽后脓肿的流行病学特征、临床症状和体征，咽旁脓肿的临床表现、鉴别诊断、CT检查特征，咽后和咽旁脓肿感染的常见病原体、药物治疗和手术引流等治疗方法。扁桃体周围蜂窝织炎和/或脓肿主要包括其流行病学特征、临床表现、体格检查、影像学检查、常见病原体、药物和手术治疗方法以及预后。

The *retropharyngeal* and the *lateral pharyngeal lymph nodes* that drain the mucosal surfaces of the upper airway and digestive tracts are located in the neck within the *retropharyngeal space* (located between the pharynx and the cervical vertebrae and extending down into the superior mediastinum) and the *lateral pharyngeal space* (bounded by the pharynx medially, the carotid sheath posteriorly, and the muscles of the styloid process laterally). The lymph nodes in these deep neck spaces communicate with each other, allowing bacteria from either cellulitis or node abscess to spread to other nodes. Infection of the nodes usually occurs as a result of extension from a localized infection of the oropharynx. A **retropharyngeal abscess** can also result from penetrating trauma to the oropharynx, dental infection, and vertebral osteomyelitis. Once infected, the nodes may progress through 3 stages: *cellulitis, phlegmon,* and *abscess.* Infection in the retropharyngeal and lateral pharyngeal spaces can result in airway compromise or posterior mediastinitis, making timely diagnosis important. Incidence based on analysis of a 2009 national database is estimated to be 4.6 per 100,000 children in the United States.

RETROPHARYNGEAL AND LATERAL PHARYNGEAL ABSCESS

Retropharyngeal abscess occurs most commonly in children younger than 3-4 yr of age; as the retropharyngeal nodes involute after 5 yr of age, infection in older children and adults is much less common. In the United States, abscess formation occurs most commonly in winter and early spring. Males are affected more often than females and approximately two-thirds of patients have a history of recent ear, nose, or throat infection.

Clinical manifestations of retropharyngeal abscess are nonspecific and include fever, irritability, decreased oral intake, and drooling. Neck stiffness, torticollis, and refusal to move the neck may also be present. The verbal child might complain of sore throat and neck pain. Other signs can include muffled voice, stridor, respiratory distress, or even obstructive sleep apnea. Physical examination can reveal bulging of the posterior pharyngeal wall, although this is present in <50% of infants with retropharyngeal abscess. Cervical lymphadenopathy may also be present.

Lateral pharyngeal abscess commonly presents as fever, dysphagia, and a prominent bulge of the lateral pharyngeal wall, sometimes with medial displacement of the tonsil.

The differential diagnosis includes acute epiglottitis and foreign body aspiration. In the young child with limited neck mobility, meningitis

---

[†]Deceased

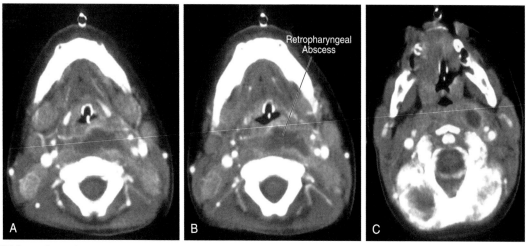

Fig. 410.1 CT of retropharyngeal abscess. **A,** CT image at level of epiglottis. **B,** Sequential CT slice exhibiting ring-enhancing lesion. **C,** Further sequential CT slice demonstrating inferior extent of lesion. *(From Philpott CM, Selvadurai D, Banerjee AR: Paediatric retropharyngeal abscess, J Laryngol Otol 118:925, 2004.)*

must also be considered. Other possibilities include lymphoma, hematoma, and vertebral osteomyelitis.

Incision and drainage and culture of an abscessed node provides the definitive diagnosis, but CT can be useful in identifying the presence of a retropharyngeal, lateral pharyngeal, or parapharyngeal abscess (Figs. 410.1 and 410.2). Deep neck infections can be accurately identified and localized with CT scans, but CT accurately identifies abscess formation in only 63% of patients. Soft-tissue neck films taken during inspiration with the neck extended might show increased width or an air–fluid level in the retropharyngeal space. CT with contrast medium enhancement can reveal central lucency, ring enhancement, or scalloping of the walls of a lymph node. Scalloping of the abscess wall is thought to be a late finding and predicts abscess formation.

Retropharyngeal and lateral pharyngeal infections are most often polymicrobial; the usual pathogens include group A streptococcus (see Chapter 210), oropharyngeal anaerobic bacteria (see Chapter 240), and *Staphylococcus aureus* (see Chapter 208.1). In children younger than age 2 yr, there has been an increase in the incidence of retropharyngeal abscess, particularly with *S. aureus,* including methicillin-resistant strains. Mediastinitis may be identified on CT in some of these patients. Other pathogens can include *Haemophilus influenzae, Klebsiella,* and *Mycobacterium avium-intracellulare.*

Treatment options include intravenous antibiotics with or without surgical drainage. A third-generation cephalosporin combined with ampicillin-sulbactam or clindamycin to provide anaerobic coverage is effective. The increasing prevalence of methicillin-resistant *S. aureus* can influence empiric antibiotic therapy. Studies show that >50% of children with retropharyngeal or lateral pharyngeal abscess as identified by CT can be successfully treated without surgical drainage; the older the child, the more likely it is that antimicrobial treatment alone will be successful. Drainage is necessary in the patient with respiratory distress or failure to improve with intravenous antibiotic treatment. The optimal duration of treatment is unknown; the typical treatment course is intravenous antibiotic therapy for several days until the patient has begun to improve, followed by a course of oral antibiotics.

Complications of retropharyngeal or lateral pharyngeal **abscess** include significant upper airway obstruction, rupture leading to aspiration pneumonia, and extension to the mediastinum. Thrombophlebitis of the internal jugular vein and erosion of the carotid artery sheath can also occur.

An uncommon but characteristic infection of the parapharyngeal space is **Lemierre disease,** in which infection from the oropharynx extends to cause septic thrombophlebitis of the internal jugular vein and embolic abscesses in the lungs (Fig. 410.3). The causative pathogen is *Fusobacterium necrophorum,* an anaerobic bacterial constituent of

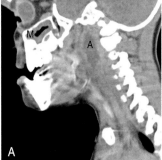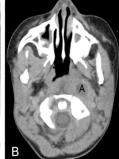

Fig. 410.2 CT of parapharyngeal abscess in a 3 yr old child. **A,** Sagittal section demonstrating parapharyngeal abscess *(A)* and mucosal swelling *(M)* in the maxillary sinus. **B,** Coronal section of parapharyngeal abscess *(A).*

the oropharyngeal flora. The typical presentation is that of a previously healthy adolescent or young adult with a history of recent pharyngitis who becomes acutely ill with fever, hypoxia, tachypnea, and respiratory distress. Chest radiography demonstrates multiple cavitary nodules, often bilateral and often accompanied by pleural effusion. Blood culture may be positive. Treatment involves prolonged intravenous antibiotic therapy with penicillin or cefoxitin; surgical drainage of extrapulmonary metastatic abscesses may be necessary (see Chapters 409 and 411).

PERITONSILLAR CELLULITIS AND/OR ABSCESS
Peritonsillar cellulitis and/or abscess, which is relatively common compared to the deep neck infections, is caused by bacterial invasion through the capsule of the tonsil, leading to cellulitis and/or abscess formation in the surrounding tissues. The typical patient with a peritonsillar abscess is an adolescent with a recent history of acute pharyngotonsillitis. Clinical manifestations include sore throat, fever, trismus, muffled or garbled voice, and dysphagia. Physical examination reveals an asymmetric tonsillar bulge with displacement of the uvula. An asymmetric tonsillar bulge is diagnostic, but it may be poorly visualized because of trismus. CT is helpful for revealing the abscess, but recent small studies in adults and children have demonstrated that ultrasound may be used to differentiate peritonsillar abscess from peritonsillar cellulitis and avoids radiation exposure, as well as the need for sedation that CT often necessitates in children. Group A streptococci and mixed oropharyngeal anaerobes are the most common pathogens, with more than four bacterial isolates per abscess typically recovered by needle aspiration.

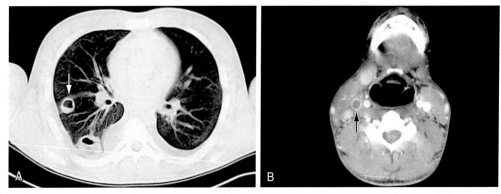

Fig. 410.3 CT of Lemierre disease. **A,** CT demonstrating nodular appearance of pulmonary infiltrates *(arrow)*. **B,** CT of neck demonstrating thrombosis of right internal jugular vein *(arrow)*. *(From Plymyer MR, Zoccola DC, Tallarita G: An 18 year old man presenting with sepsis following a recent pharyngeal infection,* Arch Pathol Lab Med *128:813, 2004. Reprinted with permission from Archives of Pathology & Laboratory Medicine. Copyright 2004. College of American Pathologists.)*

Treatment includes surgical drainage and antibiotic therapy effective against group A streptococci and anaerobes. Surgical drainage may be accomplished through needle aspiration, incision and drainage, or tonsillectomy. Needle aspiration can involve aspiration of the superior, middle, and inferior aspects of the tonsil to locate the abscess. Intraoral ultrasound can be used to diagnose and guide needle aspiration of a peritonsillar abscess. General anesthesia may be required for the uncooperative patient. Approximately 95% of peritonsillar abscesses resolve after needle aspiration and antibiotic therapy. A small percentage of these patients require a repeat needle aspiration. The 5% with infections that fail to resolve after needle aspiration require incision and drainage. Tonsillectomy should be considered if there is failure to improve within 24 hr of antibiotic therapy and needle aspiration, history of recurrent peritonsillar abscess or recurrent tonsillitis, or complications from peritonsillar abscess. The feared, albeit rare, complication is rupture of the abscess, with resultant aspiration pneumonitis. There is a 10% recurrence risk for peritonsillar abscess.

Bibliography is available at Expert Consult.

Chapter **411**
Tonsils and Adenoids
Ralph F. Wetmore
第四百一十一章
扁桃体和腺样体

中文导读

　　本章主要介绍了扁桃体和腺样体的解剖、正常功能、病理表现、临床表现、治疗、并发症及慢性气道阻塞；具体描述了腺样体扁桃体的急性感染、慢性感染、上呼吸道阻塞和扁桃体肿瘤的病理表现和临床表现；治疗中描述了药物治疗、扁桃体切除术、腺样体切除术、腺样体扁桃体切除术；并发症中描述了A组乙型溶血性链球菌感染后的扁桃体炎，可能并发链球菌感染后肾小球肾炎及急性风湿热、扁桃体周围感染、咽后间隙感染、咽旁间隙感染、复发性或慢性咽扁桃体炎，介绍了出现慢性气道阻塞时采用腺样体扁桃体切除术的利弊等内容。

ANATOMY

The *Waldeyer ring* (the lymphoid tissue surrounding the opening of the oral and nasal cavities into the pharynx) comprises the palatine tonsils, the pharyngeal tonsil or adenoid, lymphoid tissue surrounding the eustachian tube orifice in the lateral walls of the nasopharynx, the lingual tonsil at the base of the tongue, and scattered lymphoid tissue throughout the remainder of the pharynx, particularly behind the posterior pharyngeal pillars and along the posterior pharyngeal wall. The *palatine tonsil* consists of lymphoid tissue located between the palatoglossal fold (anterior tonsillar pillar) and the palatopharyngeal fold (posterior tonsillar pillar) forms. This lymphoid tissue is separated from the surrounding pharyngeal musculature by a thick fibrous capsule. The *adenoid* is a single aggregation of lymphoid tissue that occupies the space between the nasal septum and the posterior pharyngeal wall. A thin fibrous capsule separates it from the underlying structures; the adenoid does not contain the complex crypts that are found in the palatine tonsils but rather more simple crypts. Lymphoid tissue at the base of the tongue forms the *lingual tonsil* that also contains simple tonsillar crypts.

NORMAL FUNCTION

Located at the opening of the pharynx to the external environment, the tonsils and adenoid are well situated to provide primary defense against foreign matter. The immunologic role of the tonsils and adenoids is to induce secretory immunity and to regulate the production of the secretory immunoglobulins. Deep crevices within tonsillar tissue form tonsillar crypts that are lined with squamous epithelium and host a concentration of lymphocytes at their bases. The lymphoid tissue of the Waldeyer ring is most immunologically active between 4 and 10 yr of age, with a decrease after puberty. Adenotonsillar hypertrophy is greatest between ages 3 and 6 yr; in most children tonsils begin to involute after age 8 yr. No major immunologic deficiency has been demonstrated after removal of either or both of the tonsils and adenoid.

PATHOLOGY
Acute Infection

Most episodes of acute pharyngotonsillitis are caused by viruses (see Chapter 409). Group A β-hemolytic streptococcus (GABHS) is the most common cause of bacterial infection in the pharynx (see Chapter 210).

Chronic Infection

The tonsils and adenoids can be chronically infected by multiple microbes, which can include a high incidence of β-lactamase–producing organisms. Both aerobic species, such as streptococci and *Haemophilus influenzae,* and anaerobic species, such as *Peptostreptococcus, Prevotella,* and *Fusobacterium,* contribute. The tonsillar crypts can accumulate desquamated epithelial cells, lymphocytes, bacteria, and other debris, causing cryptic tonsillitis. With time, these cryptic plugs can calcify into tonsillar concretions or tonsillolith. Biofilms appear to play a role in chronic inflammation of the tonsils.

Airway Obstruction

Both the tonsils and adenoids are a major cause of upper airway obstruction in children. Airway obstruction in children is typically manifested in sleep-disordered breathing, including obstructive sleep apnea, obstructive sleep hypopnea, and upper airway resistance syndrome (see Chapter 31). Sleep-disordered breathing secondary to adenotonsillar breathing is a cause of growth failure (see Chapter 59).

Tonsillar Neoplasm

Rapid enlargement of one tonsil is highly suggestive of a tonsillar malignancy, typically lymphoma in children.

CLINICAL MANIFESTATIONS
Acute Infection

Symptoms of GABHS infection include odynophagia, dry throat, malaise, fever and chills, dysphagia, referred otalgia, headache, muscular aches, and enlarged cervical nodes. Signs include dry tongue, erythematous enlarged tonsils, tonsillar or pharyngeal exudate, palatine petechiae, and enlargement and tenderness of the jugulodigastric lymph nodes (Fig. 411.1; see Chapter 210).

Chronic Infection

Children with chronic or cryptic tonsillitis often present with halitosis, chronic sore throats, foreign-body sensation, or a history of expelling foul-tasting and foul-smelling cheesy lumps. Examination reveals tonsils of a range of sizes, often containing copious debris within the crypts. The offending organism is not usually GABHS.

Airway Obstruction

The diagnosis of airway obstruction (see Chapter 31) can frequently be made by history and physical examination. Daytime symptoms of airway obstruction, secondary to adenotonsillar hypertrophy, include chronic mouth breathing, nasal obstruction, hyponasal speech, hyposmia, decreased appetite, poor school performance, and, rarely, symptoms of right-sided heart failure. Nighttime symptoms consist of loud snoring, choking, gasping, frank apnea, restless sleep, abnormal sleep positions, somnambulism, night terrors, diaphoresis, enuresis, and sleep talking. Large tonsils are typically seen on examination, although the absolute size might not indicate the degree of obstruction. The size of the adenoid tissue can be demonstrated on a lateral neck radiograph or with flexible endoscopy. Other signs that can contribute to airway obstruction include

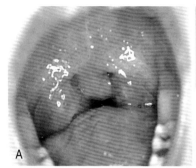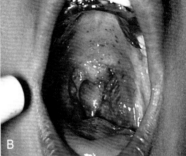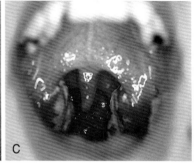

Fig. 411.1 **Pharyngotonsillitis.** This common syndrome has a number of causative pathogens and a wide spectrum of severity. **A,** The diffuse tonsillar and pharyngeal erythema seen here is a nonspecific finding that can be produced by a variety of pathogens. **B,** This intense erythema, seen in association with acute tonsillar enlargement and palatal petechiae, is highly suggestive of group A β-streptococcal infection, though other pathogens can produce these findings. **C,** This picture of exudative tonsillitis is most commonly seen with either group A streptococcal or Epstein-Barr virus infection. (*B, Courtesy Michael Sherlock, MD, Lutherville, MD. From Yellon RF, McBride TP, Davis HW: Otolaryngology. In Zitelli BJ, Davis HW, editors:* Atlas of pediatric physical diagnosis, *ed 4, Philadelphia, 2002, Mosby, p. 852.*)

the presence of a craniofacial syndrome or hypotonia.

Tonsillar Neoplasm

The rapid unilateral enlargement of a tonsil, especially if accompanied by systemic signs of night sweats, fever, weight loss, and lymphadenopathy, is highly suggestive of a tonsillar malignancy. The diagnosis of a tonsillar malignancy should also be entertained if the tonsil appears grossly abnormal. Among 54,901 patients undergoing tonsillectomy, 54 malignancies were identified (0.087% prevalence); all but 6 malignancies had been suspected based on suspicious anatomic features preoperatively.

TREATMENT
Medical Management

The treatment of acute pharyngotonsillitis is discussed in Chapter 409 and antibiotic treatment of GABHS in Chapter 210. Because copathogens such as staphylococci or anaerobes can produce β-lactamase that can inactivate penicillin, the use of cephalosporins or clindamycin may be more efficacious in the treatment of chronic throat infections. Tonsillolith or debris may be expressed manually with either a cotton-tipped applicator or a water jet. Chronically infected tonsillar crypts can be cauterized using silver nitrate.

Tonsillectomy

Tonsillectomy alone is most commonly performed for recurrent or chronic pharyngotonsillitis. Tonsillectomy has been shown to be effective in reducing the number of infections and the symptoms of chronic tonsillitis such as halitosis, persistent or recurrent sore throats, and recurrent cervical adenitis in severely affected patients. In resistant cases of cryptic tonsillitis, tonsillectomy may be curative. Rarely in children, tonsillectomy is indicated for biopsy of a unilaterally enlarged tonsil to exclude a neoplasm or to treat recurrent hemorrhage from superficial tonsillar blood vessels. Tonsillectomy has not been shown to offer clinical benefit over conservative treatment in children with mild symptoms or in those with severe infections 2 yr after surgery.

There are large variations in surgical rates among children across countries: 144 in 10,000 in Italy; 115 in 10,000 in the Netherlands; 65 in 10,000 in England; and 50 in 10,000 in the United States. Rates are generally higher in boys. With the issuance of practice guidelines, these variations may decrease. The American Academy of Otolaryngology (AAO)–Head and Neck Surgery *Taskforce on Clinical Practice Guidelines: Tonsillectomy in Children* issued evidence-based guidelines in 2019 (Table 411.1). Table 411.2 illustrates the differences and similarities between these guidelines with those of the other major professional groups across the globe. The 2019 guidelines recommend watchful waiting for recurrent throat infections if there has been <7 episodes in the past year, <5 episodes/yr in the past 2 yr, or <3 episodes/yr in the past 3 yr.

Adenoidectomy

Adenoidectomy alone may be indicated for the treatment of chronic nasal infection (chronic adenoiditis), chronic sinus infections that have failed medical management, and recurrent bouts of acute otitis media, including those in children with tympanostomy tubes who suffer from recurrent otorrhea. Adenoidectomy may be helpful in children with chronic or recurrent otitis media with effusion. Adenoidectomy alone may be curative in the management of patients with nasal obstruction, chronic mouth breathing, and loud snoring suggesting sleep-disordered breathing. Adenoidectomy may also be indicated for children in whom upper airway obstruction is suspected of causing craniofacial or occlusive developmental abnormalities.

Tonsillectomy and Adenoidectomy

The criteria for both tonsillectomy and adenoidectomy for recurrent infection are the same as those for tonsillectomy alone. The other major indication for performing both procedures together is upper airway obstruction secondary to adenotonsillar hypertrophy that results in sleep-disordered breathing, failure to thrive, craniofacial or occlusive developmental abnormalities, speech abnormalities, or, rarely, cor pulmonale. A high proportion of children with failure to thrive in the context of adenotonsillar hypertrophy resulting in sleep disorder experi-

Table 411.1	Paradise Criteria for Tonsillectomy
CRITERION	**DEFINITION**
Minimum frequency of sore throat episodes	At least 7 episodes in the previous year, at least 5 episodes in each of the previous 2 yr, or at least 3 episodes in each of the previous 3 yr
Clinical features	• Sore throat plus at least 1 of the following features qualifies as a counting episode: • Temperature of greater than 38.3°C (100.9°F) • Cervical adenopathy (tender lymph nodes or lymph node size >2 cm) • Tonsillar exudate • Culture positive for group A β-hemolytic streptococcus
Treatment	Antibiotics administered in the conventional dosage for proved or suspected streptococcal episodes
Documentation	Each episode of throat infection and its qualifying features substantiated by contemporaneous notation in a medical record If the episodes are not fully documented, subsequent observance by the physician of 2 episodes of throat infection with patterns of frequency and clinical features consistent with the initial history*

*Allows for tonsillectomy in patients who meet all but the documentation criterion. A 12 mo observation period is usually recommended before consideration of tonsillectomy.

Adapted from Baugh RF, Archer SM, Mitchell RB, et al: American Academy of Otolaryngology–Head and Neck Surgery Foundation. Clinical practice guideline: tonsillectomy in children. *Otolaryngol Head Neck Surg* 144(1 Suppl):S8, 2011, Table 5.

ence significant growth acceleration after adenotonsillectomy.

COMPLICATIONS
Poststreptococcal Glomerulonephritis and Acute Rheumatic Fever

The two major complications of untreated GABHS infection are poststreptococcal glomerulonephritis and acute rheumatic fever (see Chapters 537.4 and 210).

Peritonsillar Infection

Peritonsillar infection can occur as either cellulitis or a frank abscess in the region superior and lateral to the tonsillar capsule (see Chapter 409). These infections usually occur in children with a history of recurrent tonsillar infection and are polymicrobial, including both aerobes and anaerobes. Unilateral throat pain, referred otalgia, drooling, and trismus are presenting symptoms. The affected tonsil is displaced down and medial by swelling of the anterior tonsillar pillar and palate. The diagnosis of an abscess can be confirmed by CT or by needle aspiration, the contents of which should be sent for culture.

Retropharyngeal Space Infection

Infections in the retropharyngeal space develop in the lymph nodes that drain the oropharynx, nose, and nasopharynx (see Chapter 410).

Parapharyngeal Space Infection

Tonsillar infection can extend into the parapharyngeal space, causing symptoms of fever, neck pain and stiffness, and signs of swelling of the lateral pharyngeal wall and neck on the affected side. The diagnosis is confirmed by contrast medium-enhanced CT, and treatment includes intravenous antibiotics and external incision and drainage if an abscess is demonstrated on CT (see Chapter 410). Septic thrombophlebitis of the jugular vein, **Lemierre syndrome,** manifests with fever, toxicity, neck pain and stiffness, and respiratory distress as a result of multiple

Table 411.2	Comparison of American, Italian, and Scottish Guidelines for Tonsillectomy in Children and Adolescents		
PARAMETER	**AAO-HNS GUIDELINES**	**ITALIAN GUIDELINES**	**SCOTTISH GUIDELINES**
Audience	Multidisciplinary	Multidisciplinary	Multidisciplinary
Target population	Children and adolescents 1-18 yr of age	Children and adults	Children 4-16 yr of age and adults
Scope	Treatment of children who are candidates for tonsillectomy	Appropriateness and safety of tonsillectomy	Management of sore throat and indications for tonsillectomy
Methods	Based on a priori protocol, systematic literature review, American Academy of Pediatrics scale of evidence quality	Systematic literature review, Italian National Program Guidelines scale of evidence quality	Based on a priori protocol, systematic literature review, Scottish Intercollegiate Guidelines Network scale of evidence quality
Recommendations			
Recurrent infection	Tonsillectomy is an option for children with recurrent throat infection that meets the Paradise criteria (see Table 411.1) for frequency, severity, treatment, and documentation of illness	Tonsillectomy is indicated in patients with at least 1 yr of recurrent tonsillitis (5 or more episodes per year) that is disabling and impairs normal activities, but only after an additional 6 mo of watchful waiting to assess the pattern of symptoms using a clinical diary	Tonsillectomy should be considered for recurrent, disabling sore throat caused by acute tonsillitis when the episodes are well documented, are adequately treated, and meet the Paradise criteria (see Table 411.1) for frequency of illness
Pain control	Recommendation to advocate for pain relief (e.g., provide information, prescribe) and educate caregivers about the importance of managing and reassessing pain	Recommendation for acetaminophen before and after surgery	Recommendation for adequate dose of acetaminophen for pain relief in children
Antibiotic use	Recommendation against perioperative antibiotics	Recommendation for short-term perioperative antibiotics*	NA
Steroid use	Recommendation for a single intraoperative dose of dexamethasone	Recommendation for a single intraoperative dose of dexamethasone	Recommendation for a single intraoperative dose of dexamethasone
Sleep-disordered breathing	Recommendation to counsel caregivers about tonsillectomy as a means to improve health in children with sleep-disordered breathing and comorbid conditions	Recommendation for diagnostic testing in children with suspected sleep respiratory disorders	NA
Polysomnography	Recommendation to counsel caregivers about tonsillectomy as a means to improve health in children with abnormal polysomnography	Recommendation for polysomnography when pulse oximetry results are not conclusive in agreement with Brouillette criteria	NA
Surgical technique	NA	Recommendation for "cold" technique	NA
Hemorrhage	Recommendation that the surgeon document primary and secondary hemorrhage after tonsillectomy at least annually	NA	NA
Adjunctive therapy	NA	NA	Recommendation against *Echinacea purpurea* for treatment of sore throat
			Recommendation for acupuncture in patients at risk of postoperative nausea and vomiting who cannot take antiemetic drugs

*Statement made prior to most recent Cochrane review.

AAO-HNS, American Academy of Otolaryngology–Head and Neck Surgery; NA, not applicable.

Adapted with permission from Baugh RF, Archer SM, Mitchell RB, et al: American Academy of Otolaryngology–Head and Neck Surgery Foundation. Clinical practice guideline: tonsillectomy in children. *Otolaryngol Head Neck Surg* 144(1 Suppl):S23, 2011, Table 9.

septic pulmonary emboli and is a complication of a parapharyngeal space or odontogenic infection from *Fusobacterium necrophorum.* Concurrent Epstein-Barr virus mononucleosis (see Chapter 281) can be a predisposing event before the sudden onset of fever, chills, and respiratory distress in an adolescent patient. Treatment includes high-dose intravenous antibiotics (ampicillin-sulbactam, clindamycin, penicillin, or ciprofloxacin) and heparinization.

Recurrent or Chronic Pharyngotonsillitis
See Chapter 409.

CHRONIC AIRWAY OBSTRUCTION
Although rare, children with chronic airway obstruction from enlarged tonsils and adenoids can present with cor pulmonale.

The effects of chronic airway obstruction and mouth breathing on facial growth remain a subject of controversy. Studies of chronic mouth breathing, both in humans and animals, have shown changes in facial development, including prolongation of the total anterior facial height and a tendency toward a retrognathic mandible, the so-called adenoid facies. Adenotonsillectomy can reverse some of these abnormalities. Other studies have disputed these findings.

Tonsillectomy and Adenoidectomy
The risks and potential benefits of surgery must be considered (Table 411.3). Bleeding can occur in the immediate postoperative period or be delayed (consider von Willebrand disease) after separation of the eschar. The Clinical Guidelines for Tonsillectomy include a recommendation for a single intravenous dose of intraoperative dexamethasone (0.5 mg/kg), which decreases postoperative nausea and vomiting and reduces swelling. There is no evidence that use of dexamethasone in postoperative tonsillectomy patients results in an increased risk of postoperative bleeding. Routine use of antibiotics in the postoperative period is ineffective and thus the AAO Clinical Practice Guidelines advise against its use, although this recommendation is not consistent among the major professional organizations who have issued guidelines (see Table 411.2). Codeine is associated with excessive sedation and fatalities and is not recommended.

Swelling of the tongue and soft palate can lead to acute airway obstruction in the first few hours after surgery. Children with underlying hypotonia or craniofacial anomalies are at greater risk for suffering this complication. Dehydration from odynophagia is not uncommon in the first postoperative week. Rare complications include velopharyngeal insufficiency, nasopharyngeal or oropharyngeal stenosis, and psychologic problems.

Bibliography is available at Expert Consult.

Table 411.3	Risks and Potential Benefits of Tonsillectomy or Adenoidectomy or Both

RISKS
- Cost*
- Risk of anesthetic accidents
  - Malignant hyperthermia
  - Cardiac arrhythmia
  - Vocal cord trauma
  - Aspiration with resulting bronchopulmonary obstruction or infection
- Risk of miscellaneous surgical or postoperative complications
  - Hemorrhage
  - Airway obstruction from edema of tongue, palate, or nasopharynx, or retropharyngeal hematoma
  - Central apnea
  - Prolonged muscular paralysis
  - Dehydration
  - Palatopharyngeal insufficiency
  - Otitis media
  - Nasopharyngeal stenosis
  - Refractory torticollis
  - Facial edema
  - Emotional upset
- Unknown risks

POTENTIAL BENEFITS
- Reduction in frequency of ear, nose, throat illness, and thus in
  - Discomfort
  - Inconvenience
  - School absence
  - Parental anxiety
  - Work missed by parents
  - Costs of physician visits and drugs
- Reduction in nasal obstruction with improved
  - Respiratory function
  - Comfort
  - Sleep
  - Craniofacial growth and development
  - Appearance
- Reduction in hearing impairment
- Improved growth and overall well-being
- Reduction in long-term parental anxiety

*Cost for tonsillectomy alone and adenoidectomy alone are somewhat lower.
Modified from Bluestone CD, editor: *Pediatric otolaryngology*, ed 4, Philadelphia, 2003, WB Saunders, p. 1213.

Chapter 412

Acute Inflammatory Upper Airway Obstruction (Croup, Epiglottitis, Laryngitis, and Bacterial Tracheitis)

Kristine Knuti Rodrigues and Genie E. Roosevelt

第四百一十二章

急性上呼吸道阻塞性炎症（哮吼、会厌炎、喉炎、细菌性气管炎）

中文导读

　　本章主要介绍了感染性上呼吸道阻塞和细菌性气管炎；具体介绍了感染性上呼吸道阻塞性疾病的发病原因及流行病学，详细描述其临床表现为哮吼（喉气管支气管炎）、急性会厌炎（声门上喉炎）、急性感染性喉炎、痉挛性哮吼，具体介绍了感染性上呼吸道阻塞的鉴别诊断、并发症、治疗和预后；介绍了细菌性气管炎的临床表现、诊断、并发症、治疗和预后等内容。

Airway resistance is inversely proportional to the 4th power of the radius (see Chapter 400). Because the lumen of an infant's or child's airway is narrow, minor reductions in cross-sectional area as a result of mucosal edema or other inflammatory processes cause an exponential increase in airway resistance and a significant increase in the work of breathing. The larynx is composed of 4 major cartilages (epiglottic, arytenoid, thyroid, and cricoid cartilages, ordered from superior to inferior) and the soft tissues that surround them. The cricoid cartilage encircles the airway just below the vocal cords and defines the narrowest portion of the upper airway in children younger than 10 yr of age.

Inflammation involving the vocal cords and structures inferior to the cords is called **laryngitis**, **laryngotracheitis**, or **laryngotracheobronchitis**, and inflammation of the structures superior to the cords (i.e., arytenoids, aryepiglottic folds ["false cords"], epiglottis) is called **supraglottitis**. The term **croup** refers to a heterogeneous group of mainly acute and infectious processes that are characterized by a bark-like or brassy cough and may be associated with hoarseness, inspiratory stridor, and respiratory distress. **Stridor** is a harsh, high-pitched respiratory sound that is usually inspiratory but can be biphasic and is produced by turbulent airflow; it is not a diagnosis but a sign of upper airway obstruction (see Chapter 400). Croup typically affects the larynx, trachea, and bronchi. When the involvement of the larynx is sufficient to produce symptoms, these symptoms dominate the clinical picture more so than the tracheal and bronchial signs. A distinction has been made between spasmodic or recurrent croup and laryngotracheobronchitis. Some clinicians believe that spasmodic croup might have an allergic component and improves rapidly without treatment, whereas laryngotracheobronchitis is always associated with a viral infection of the respiratory tract. Others believe that the signs and symptoms are similar enough to consider them within the spectrum of a single disease, in part because studies have documented viral etiologies in both acute and recurrent croup.

412.1 Infectious Upper Airway Obstruction

Kristine Knuti Rodrigues and Genie E. Roosevelt

ETIOLOGY AND EPIDEMIOLOGY

With the exceptions of diphtheria (see Chapter 214), bacterial tracheitis, and epiglottitis, most acute infections of the upper airway are caused by viruses. The parainfluenza viruses (types 1, 2, and 3; see Chapter 286) account for approximately 75% of cases; other viruses associated with croup include influenza A and B, adenovirus, respiratory syncytial virus, and measles. Influenza A is associated with severe laryngotracheobronchitis. *Mycoplasma pneumoniae* has rarely been isolated from children with croup and causes mild disease (see Chapter 250). Most patients with croup are between the ages of 3 mo and 5 yr, with the peak in the 2nd yr of life. The incidence of croup is higher in boys. It occurs most commonly in the late fall and winter but can occur throughout the year. Approximately 15% of patients have a strong family history of croup. Recurrences are frequent from 3 to 6 yr of age and decrease with growth of the airway. Recurrent croup is defined as 2 or more croup-like episodes. Patients with recurrent croup have a higher incidence of asthma, allergies, and gastroesophageal reflux; less than 9% of patients with recurrent croup demonstrate clinically significant findings on bronchoscopy (e.g., subglottic stenosis, reflux changes, broncho/tracheomalacia).

In the past, *Haemophilus influenzae* type b was the most commonly identified etiology of **acute epiglottitis**. Since the widespread use of the *H. influenzae* type b vaccine, invasive disease caused by *H. influenzae* type b in pediatric patients has been reduced by 99% (see Chapter 221). Therefore, other agents, such as *Streptococcus pyogenes, Streptococcus pneumoniae*, nontypeable *H. influenzae*, and *Staphylococcus aureus*, represent a larger portion of pediatric cases of epiglottitis in vaccinated children. In the prevaccine era, the typical patient with epiglottitis caused by *H. influenzae* type b was 2-4 yr of age, although cases were seen in the 1st yr of life and in patients as old as 7 yr of age. Currently, the most common presentation of epiglottitis is an adult with a sore throat, although cases still do occur in underimmunized children; vaccine failures have rarely been reported.

CLINICAL MANIFESTATIONS
Croup (Laryngotracheobronchitis)
Viruses typically cause croup, the most common form of acute upper respiratory obstruction. The term laryngotracheobronchitis refers to viral infection of the glottic and subglottic regions. Some clinicians use the term *laryngotracheitis* for the most common and most typical form of croup and reserve the term *laryngotracheobronchitis* for the more severe form that is considered an extension of laryngotracheitis associated with bacterial superinfection that occurs 5-7 days into the clinical course.

Most patients have an upper respiratory tract infection with some combination of rhinorrhea, pharyngitis, mild cough, and low-grade fever for 1-3 days before the signs and symptoms of upper airway obstruction become apparent. The child then develops the characteristic barking cough, hoarseness, and inspiratory stridor. The low-grade fever can persist, although temperatures may occasionally reach 39-40°C (102.2-104°F); some children are afebrile. Symptoms are characteristically worse at night and often recur with decreasing intensity for several days and resolve completely within a week. Agitation and crying greatly aggravate the symptoms and signs. The child may prefer to sit up in bed or be held upright. Other family members might have mild respiratory illnesses with laryngitis. Most young patients with croup progress only as far as stridor and slight dyspnea before they start to recover.

Physical examination can reveal a hoarse voice, coryza, normal to moderately inflamed pharynx, and a slightly increased respiratory rate. Patients vary substantially in their degrees of respiratory distress. Rarely, the upper airway obstruction progresses and is accompanied by an increasing respiratory rate; nasal flaring; suprasternal, infrasternal, and intercostal retractions; and continuous stridor. Croup is a disease of the upper airway, and alveolar gas exchange is usually normal. Hypoxia and low oxygen saturation are seen only when complete airway obstruction is imminent. *The child who is hypoxic, cyanotic, pale, or obtunded needs immediate airway management.* Occasionally, the pattern of severe laryngotracheobronchitis is difficult to differentiate from epiglottitis, despite the usually more acute onset and rapid course of the latter.

Croup is a clinical diagnosis and does not require a radiograph of the neck. Radiographs of the neck can show the typical subglottic

narrowing, or steeple sign, of croup on the posteroanterior view (Fig. 412.1). However, the steeple sign may be absent in patients with croup, may be present in patients without croup as a normal variant, and may rarely be present in patients with epiglottitis. The radiographs do not correlate well with disease severity. Radiographs should be considered only after airway stabilization in children who have an atypical presentation or clinical course. Radiographs may be helpful in distinguishing between severe laryngotracheobronchitis and epiglottitis, but airway management should always take priority.

Acute Epiglottitis (Supraglottitis)
This now rare, but still dramatic and potentially lethal, condition is characterized by an acute rapidly progressive and potentially fulminating course of high fever, sore throat, dyspnea, and rapidly progressing respiratory obstruction. The degree of respiratory distress at presentation is variable. The initial lack of respiratory distress can deceive the unwary clinician; respiratory distress can also be the 1st manifestation. Often, the otherwise healthy child suddenly develops a sore throat and fever. Within a matter of hours, the patient appears toxic, swallowing is difficult, and breathing is labored. Drooling is usually present, and the neck is hyperextended in an attempt to maintain the airway. The child may assume the tripod position, sitting upright and leaning forward with the chin up and mouth open while bracing on the arms. A brief period of air hunger with restlessness may be followed by rapidly increasing cyanosis and coma. Stridor is a late finding and suggests near-complete airway obstruction. Complete obstruction of the airway and death can ensue unless adequate treatment is provided. *The barking cough typical of croup is rare.* Usually no other family members are ill with acute respiratory symptoms.

The diagnosis requires visualization under controlled circumstances of a large, cherry red, swollen epiglottis by laryngoscopy. Occasionally, the other supraglottic structures, especially the aryepiglottic folds, are more involved than the epiglottis itself. In a patient in whom the diagnosis is certain or probable based on clinical grounds, laryngoscopy should be performed expeditiously in a controlled environment such as an operating room or intensive care unit. Anxiety-provoking interventions such as phlebotomy, intravenous line placement, placing the child supine, or direct inspection of the oral cavity should be avoided until the airway is secure. If epiglottitis is thought to be possible but not certain in a patient with acute upper airway obstruction, the patient may undergo lateral radiographs of the upper airway 1st. Classic radiographs of a child who has epiglottitis show the thumb sign (Fig. 412.2). Proper positioning of the patient for the lateral neck radiograph is crucial in

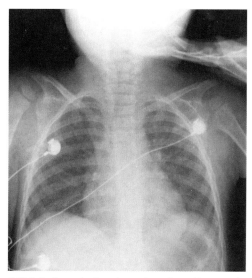

Fig. 412.1 Radiograph of an airway of a patient with croup, showing typical subglottic narrowing (steeple sign).

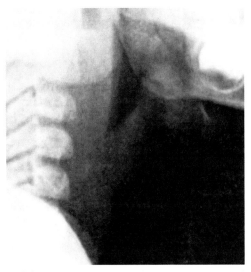

Fig. 412.2 Lateral roentgenogram of the upper airway reveals the swollen epiglottis (thumb sign).

order to avoid some of the pitfalls associated with interpretation of the film. Adequate hyperextension of the head and neck is necessary. In addition, the epiglottis can appear to be round if the lateral neck is taken at an oblique angle. If the concern for epiglottitis still exists after the radiographs, direct visualization should be performed. A physician skilled in airway management and use of intubation equipment should accompany patients with suspected epiglottitis at all times. An older cooperative child might voluntarily open the mouth wide enough for a direct view of the inflamed epiglottis.

Establishing an airway by endotracheal or nasotracheal intubation or, less often, by tracheostomy is indicated in patients with epiglottitis, regardless of the degree of apparent respiratory distress, because as many as 6% of children with epiglottitis without an artificial airway die, compared with <1% of those with an artificial airway. No clinical features have been recognized that predict mortality. Pulmonary edema can be associated with acute airway obstruction. The duration of intubation depends on the clinical course of the patient and the duration of epiglottic swelling, as determined by frequent examination using direct laryngoscopy or flexible fiberoptic laryngoscopy. In general, children with acute epiglottitis are intubated for 2-3 days, because the response to antibiotics is usually rapid. Most patients have concomitant bacteremia; occasionally, other infections are present, such as pneumonia, cervical adenopathy, or otitis media. Meningitis, arthritis, and other invasive infections with *H. influenzae* type b are rarely found in conjunction with epiglottitis.

Acute Infectious Laryngitis

Laryngitis is a common illness. Viruses cause most cases; diphtheria is an exception but is extremely rare in industrialized countries (see Chapter 214). The onset is usually characterized by an upper respiratory tract infection during which sore throat, cough, and hoarseness appear. The illness is generally mild; respiratory distress is unusual except in the young infant. Hoarseness and loss of voice may be out of proportion to systemic signs and symptoms. The physical examination is usually not remarkable except for evidence of pharyngeal inflammation. Inflammatory edema of the vocal cords and subglottic tissue may be demonstrated laryngoscopically. The principal site of obstruction is usually the subglottic area.

Spasmodic Croup

Spasmodic croup occurs most often in children 1-3 yr of age and is clinically similar to acute laryngotracheobronchitis, except that the history of a viral prodrome and fever in the patient and family are often

absent. The cause is viral in some cases, but allergic and other factors may also contribute.

Occurring most commonly in the evening or nighttime, spasmodic croup begins with a sudden onset that may be preceded by mild to moderate coryza and hoarseness. The child awakens with a characteristic barking, metallic cough, noisy inspiration, and respiratory distress, and appears anxious and frightened. The patient is usually afebrile. The severity of the symptoms generally diminishes within several hours, and the following day, the patient often appears well except for slight hoarseness and cough. Similar, but usually less severe, attacks without extreme respiratory distress can occur for another night or 2. Such episodes often recur several times. Spasmodic croup might represent more of an allergic reaction to viral antigens than direct infection, although the pathogenesis is unknown.

DIFFERENTIAL DIAGNOSIS

These 4 syndromes must be differentiated from one another and from a variety of other entities that can present as upper airway obstruction. **Bacterial tracheitis** is the most important differential diagnostic consideration and has a high risk of airway obstruction. Diphtheritic croup is extremely rare in North America, although a major epidemic of diphtheria occurred in countries of the former Soviet Union beginning in 1990 from the lack of routine immunization. Early symptoms of **diphtheria** include malaise, sore throat, anorexia, and low-grade fever. Within 2-3 days, pharyngeal examination reveals the typical gray-white membrane, which can vary in size from covering a small patch on the tonsils to covering most of the soft palate. The membrane is adherent to the tissue, and forcible attempts to remove it cause bleeding. The course is usually insidious, but respiratory obstruction can occur suddenly. **Measles** croup almost always coincides with the full manifestations of systemic disease, and the course may be fulminant (see Chapter 273).

Sudden onset of respiratory obstruction can be caused by aspiration of a **foreign body** (see Chapter 405.1). The child is usually 6 mo to 3 yr of age. Choking and coughing occur suddenly, usually without prodromal signs of infection, although children with a viral infection can also aspirate a foreign body. A **retropharyngeal** or **peritonsillar abscess** can mimic respiratory obstruction (see Chapter 410). CT scans of the upper airway are helpful in evaluating the possibility of a retropharyngeal abscess. A peritonsillar abscess is a clinical diagnosis. Other possible causes of upper airway obstruction include extrinsic compression of the airway (laryngeal web, vascular ring) and intraluminal obstruction from masses (laryngeal papilloma, subglottic hemangioma); these tend to have chronic or recurrent symptoms.

Upper airway obstruction is occasionally associated with **angioedema** of the subglottic areas as part of anaphylaxis and generalized allergic reactions, edema after endotracheal intubation for general anesthesia or respiratory failure, hypocalcemic tetany, infectious mononucleosis, trauma, and tumors or malformations of the larynx. A croupy cough may be an early sign of asthma. Vocal cord dysfunction can also occur. Epiglottitis, with the characteristic manifestations of drooling or dysphagia and stridor, can also result from the accidental ingestion of very hot liquid.

COMPLICATIONS

Complications occur in approximately 15% of patients with viral croup. The most common is extension of the infectious process to involve other regions of the respiratory tract, such as the middle ear, the terminal bronchioles, or the pulmonary parenchyma. Bacterial tracheitis may be a complication of viral croup rather than a distinct disease. If associated with toxin producing *S. aureus* or *S. pyogenes*, toxic shock syndrome can develop. **Bacterial tracheitis** may have a 2-phased illness, with the 2nd phase after a croup-like illness associated with high fever, toxicity, and airway obstruction. Alternatively, the onset of tracheitis occurs without a 2nd phase and appears as a continuation of the initial croup-like illness, but with higher fever and worsening respiratory distress rather than the usual recovery after 2-3 days of viral croup. Pneumonia, cervical lymphadenitis, otitis media, or, rarely, meningitis or septic arthritis can occur in the course of epiglottitis. Pneumomediastinum and pneumothorax are the most common complications of tracheotomy.

TREATMENT

The mainstay of treatment for children with **croup** is airway management and treatment of hypoxia. Treatment of the respiratory distress should take priority over any testing. Most children with either acute spasmodic croup or infectious croup can be managed safely at home. Despite the observation that cold night air is beneficial, a Cochrane review has found no evidence supporting the use of cool mist in the emergency department for the treatment of croup.

Nebulized racemic epinephrine is the established treatment for moderate or severe croup. The mechanism of action is believed to be constriction of the precapillary arterioles through the β-adrenergic receptors, causing fluid resorption from the interstitial space and a decrease in the laryngeal mucosal edema. Traditionally, racemic epinephrine, a 1:1 mixture of the D- and L-isomers of epinephrine, has been administered. A dose of 0.25-0.5 mL of 2.25% racemic epinephrine in 3 mL of normal saline can be used as often as every 20 min. Racemic epinephrine was initially chosen over the more active and more readily available L-epinephrine to minimize anticipated cardiovascular side effects such as tachycardia and hypertension. Current evidence does not favor racemic epinephrine over L-epinephrine (5 mL of 1:1,000 solution) in terms of efficacy or safety.

The indications for the administration of nebulized epinephrine include moderate to severe stridor at rest, the possible need for intubation, respiratory distress, and hypoxia. The duration of activity of racemic epinephrine is <2 hr. Consequently, observation is mandated. The symptoms of croup might reappear, but racemic epinephrine does not cause rebound worsening of the obstruction. Patients can be safely discharged home after a 2-3 hr period of observation provided they have no stridor at rest; have normal air entry, normal pulse oximetry, and normal level of consciousness; and have received steroids. Nebulized epinephrine should still be used cautiously in patients with tachycardia, heart conditions such as tetralogy of Fallot, or ventricular outlet obstruction because of possible side effects.

The effectiveness of oral corticosteroids in viral croup is well established. Corticosteroids decrease the edema in the laryngeal mucosa through their antiinflammatory action. Oral steroids are beneficial, even in mild croup, as measured by reduced hospitalization, shorter duration of hospitalization, and reduced need for subsequent interventions such as epinephrine administration. Most studies that demonstrated the efficacy of oral dexamethasone used a single dose of 0.6 mg/kg, a dose as low as 0.15 mg/kg may be just as effective. Intramuscular dexamethasone and nebulized budesonide have an equivalent clinical effect; oral dosing of dexamethasone is as effective as intramuscular administration. A single dose of oral prednisolone is less effective; 1 randomized controlled trial found no difference in the effectiveness of prednisolone 2 mg/kg/day for 3 days versus 1 dose of dexamethasone 0.6 mg/kg. The only adverse effect in the treatment of croup with corticosteroids is the development of *Candida albicans* laryngotracheitis in a patient who received dexamethasone, 1 mg/kg/24 hr, for 8 days. Corticosteroids should not be administered to children with varicella or tuberculosis (unless the patient is receiving appropriate antituberculosis therapy) because they worsen the clinical course.

Antibiotics are not indicated in croup. Nonprescription cough and cold medications should not be used in children younger than 6 yr of age. A helium-oxygen mixture (heliox) may be considered in the treatment of children with severe croup for whom intubation is being considered, although the evidence is inconclusive. Children with croup should be hospitalized for any of the following: progressive stridor, severe stridor at rest, respiratory distress, hypoxia, cyanosis, depressed mental status, poor oral intake, or the need for reliable observation.

Epiglottitis is a medical emergency and warrants immediate treatment with an artificial airway placed under controlled conditions, either in an operating room or intensive care unit. All patients should receive oxygen en route unless the mask causes excessive agitation. Racemic epinephrine and corticosteroids are ineffective. Cultures of blood, epiglottic surface, and, in selected cases, cerebrospinal fluid should be collected after the airway is stabilized. Ceftriaxone, cefepime, or meropenem should be given parenterally, pending culture and susceptibility reports, because 10–40% of *H. influenzae* type b cases are resistant to ampicillin. After insertion of the artificial airway, the patient should improve immediately, and respiratory distress and cyanosis should disappear. Epiglottitis resolves after a few days of antibiotics, and the patient may be extubated; antibiotics should be continued for at least 10 days. Chemoprophylaxis is not routinely recommended for household, childcare, or nursery contacts of patients with invasive *H. influenzae* type b infections, but careful observation is mandatory, with prompt medical evaluation when exposed children develop a febrile illness. **Indications for rifampin prophylaxis** (20 mg/kg orally once a day for 4 days; maximum dose: 600 mg) for all household members include a child within the home who is younger than 4 yr of age and incompletely immunized, younger than 12 mo of age and has not completed the primary vaccination series, or immunocompromised.

Acute laryngeal swelling on an **allergic basis** responds to epinephrine (1:1,000 dilution in dosage of 0.01 mL/kg to a maximum of 0.5 mL/dose) administered intramuscularly, or racemic epinephrine (dose of 0.5 mL of 2.25% racemic epinephrine in 3 mL of normal saline) (see Chapter 174). Corticosteroids are often required (1-2 mg/kg/24 hr of prednisone for 3-5 days). After recovery, the patient and parents should be discharged with a preloaded syringe of epinephrine to be used in emergencies. Reactive mucosal swelling, severe stridor, and respiratory distress unresponsive to mist therapy may follow endotracheal intubation for general anesthesia in children. Racemic epinephrine and corticosteroids are helpful.

Endotracheal/Nasotracheal Intubation and Tracheotomy

With the introduction of routine intubation or, less often, tracheotomy for epiglottitis, the mortality rate for epiglottis has decreased to almost zero. These procedures should always be performed in an operating room or intensive care unit if time permits; prior intubation and general anesthesia greatly facilitate performing a tracheotomy without complications. The use of an endotracheal or nasotracheal tube that is 0.5-1.0 mm smaller than estimated by age or height is recommended to facilitate intubation and reduce long-term sequelae. The choice of procedure should be based on the local expertise and experience with the procedure and postoperative care.

Intubation or less often tracheotomy is required for most patients with bacterial tracheitis and all young patients with epiglottitis. It is rarely required for patients with laryngotracheobronchitis, spasmodic croup, or laryngitis. Severe forms of laryngotracheobronchitis that require intubation in a high proportion of patients have been reported during severe measles and influenza A virus epidemics. Assessing the need for these procedures requires experience and judgment because they should not be delayed until cyanosis and extreme restlessness have developed (see Chapter 89). An endotracheal or nasotracheal tube that is 0.5-1.0 mm smaller than estimated by age or height is recommended.

The endotracheal tube or tracheostomy must remain in place until edema and spasm have subsided and the patient is able to handle secretions satisfactorily. It should be removed as soon as possible, usually within a few days. Adequate resolution of epiglottic inflammation that has been accurately confirmed by fiberoptic laryngoscopy, permitting much more rapid extubation, often occurs within 24 hr. Racemic epinephrine and dexamethasone (0.5 mg/kg/dose 6-12 hr prior to extubation then every 6 hr for 6 doses with a maximum dose of 10 mg) may be useful in the treatment of upper airway edema seen postintubation.

PROGNOSIS

In general, the length of hospitalization and the mortality rate for cases of acute infectious upper airway obstruction increase as the infection extends to involve a greater portion of the respiratory tract, except in epiglottitis, in which the localized infection itself can prove to be fatal. Most deaths from croup are caused by a laryngeal obstruction or by the complications of tracheotomy. Rarely, fatal out-of-hospital arrests caused by viral laryngotracheobronchitis have been reported, particularly in infants and in patients whose course has been complicated by bacterial tracheitis. Untreated epiglottitis has a mortality rate of 6% in some series, but if the diagnosis is made and appropriate treatment is initiated before the patient is moribund, the prognosis is excellent. The outcome of acute laryngotracheobronchitis, laryngitis, and spasmodic croup is also excellent.

Bibliography is available at Expert Consult.

412.2 Bacterial Tracheitis

Kristine Knuti Rodrigues and Genie E. Roosevelt

Bacterial tracheitis is an acute bacterial infection of the upper airway that is potentially life-threatening. *S. aureus* (see Chapter 208.1) is the most commonly isolated pathogen, with isolated reports of methicillin-resistant *S. aureus*. *S. pneumoniae, S. pyogenes, Moraxella catarrhalis,* nontypeable *H. influenzae*; anaerobic organisms have also been implicated. The mean age is between 5 and 7 yr. There is a slight male predominance. Bacterial tracheitis often follows a viral respiratory infection (especially laryngotracheitis), so it may be considered a bacterial complication of a viral disease, rather than a primary bacterial illness. This life-threatening entity is more common than epiglottitis in vaccinated populations.

CLINICAL MANIFESTATIONS
Typically the child has a brassy cough, apparently as part of a viral laryngotracheobronchitis. High fever and toxicity with respiratory distress can occur immediately or after a few days of apparent improvement. The patient can lie flat, does not drool, and does not have the dysphagia associated with epiglottitis. The usual treatment for croup (racemic epinephrine) is ineffective. Intubation or tracheostomy may be necessary, but only 50–60% of patients require intubation for management; younger patients are more likely to need intubation. The major pathologic feature appears to be mucosal swelling at the level of the cricoid cartilage, complicated by copious, thick, purulent secretions, sometimes causing pseudomembranes. Suctioning these secretions, although occasionally affording temporary relief, usually does not sufficiently obviate the need for an artificial airway.

DIAGNOSIS
The diagnosis is based on evidence of bacterial upper airway disease, which includes high fever, purulent airway secretions, and an absence of the classic findings of epiglottitis. X-rays are not needed but can show the classic findings (Fig. 412.3); purulent material is noted below the cords during endotracheal intubation (Fig. 412.4).

TREATMENT
Appropriate antimicrobial therapy, which usually includes antistaphylococcal agents, should be instituted in any patient whose course suggests bacterial tracheitis. Empiric therapy recommendations for bacterial tracheitis include vancomycin or clindamycin and a 3rd-generation cephalosporin (e.g., ceftriaxone or cefepime). When bacterial tracheitis is diagnosed by direct laryngoscopy or is strongly suspected on clinical grounds, an artificial airway should be strongly considered. Supplemental oxygen is usually necessary.

COMPLICATIONS
Chest radiographs often show patchy infiltrates and may show focal densities. Subglottic narrowing and a rough and ragged tracheal air column can often be demonstrated radiographically. If airway management is not optimal, cardiorespiratory arrest can occur. Toxic shock syndrome has been associated with staphylococcal and group A streptococcal tracheitis (see Chapter 208.2).

PROGNOSIS
The prognosis for most patients is excellent. Patients usually become

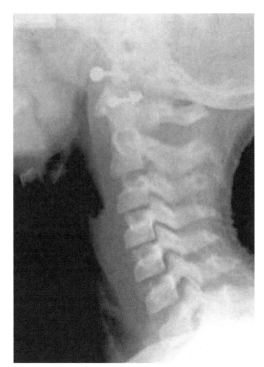

Fig. 412.3 Lateral radiograph of the neck of a patient with bacterial tracheitis, showing pseudomembrane detachment in the trachea. *(From Stroud RH, Friedman NR: An update on inflammatory disorders of the pediatric airway: epiglottitis, croup, and tracheitis, Am J Otolaryngol 22:268–275, 2001. Photo courtesy of the Department of Radiology, University of Texas Medical Branch at Galveston.)*

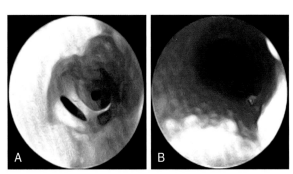

Fig. 412.4 Thick tracheal membranes seen on rigid bronchoscopy. The supraglottis was normal. **A,** Thick adherent membranous secretions. **B,** The distal tracheobronchial tree is unremarkable. In contrast to croup, tenacious secretions are seen throughout the trachea, and in contrast to bronchitis, the bronchi are not affected. *(From Salamone FN, Bobbitt DB, Myer CM, et al: Bacterial tracheitis reexamined: is there a less severe manifestation? Otolaryngol Head Neck Surg 131:871–876, 2004. © 2004 American Academy of Otolaryngology–Head and Neck Surgery Foundation, Inc.)*

afebrile within 2-3 days of the institution of appropriate antimicrobial therapy, but prolonged hospitalization may be necessary. In recent years, there appears to be a trend toward a less-morbid condition. With a decrease in mucosal edema and purulent secretions, extubation can be accomplished safely, and the patient should be observed carefully while antibiotics and oxygen therapy are continued.

Bibliography is available at Expert Consult.

Chapter **413**

Congenital Anomalies of the Larynx, Trachea, and Bronchi

Jill N. D'Souza and James W. Schroeder Jr

第四百一十三章

喉、气管和支气管的先天畸形

中文导读

本章主要介绍了喉软化病的临床表现、诊断和治疗；先天性声门下狭窄的临床表现及诊断；声带麻痹的诊断和治疗；先天性喉蹼和喉闭锁；先天性声门下血管瘤；喉气囊肿和囊状囊肿；喉后裂及喉气管食管裂；血管和心脏异常；气管狭窄、气管蹼及气管闭锁；前肠囊肿；气管软化和支气管软化等内容。

The larynx functions as a breathing passage, a valve to protect the lungs, and the primary organ of communication; symptoms of laryngeal anomalies are those of airway obstruction, noisy breathing, difficulty feeding, and abnormalities of phonation (see Chapter 400). Obstructive congenital lesions of the upper airway produce turbulent airflow according to the laws of fluid dynamics. This rapid, turbulent airflow across a narrowed segment of respiratory tract produces distinctive sounds that are diagnostically useful. The location of the obstruction produces characteristic changes in the sound of inspiration and/or expiration. Intrathoracic lesions typically cause expiratory wheezing and stridor, often masquerading as asthma. The expiratory wheezing contrasts to the inspiratory stridor caused by the extrathoracic lesions of congenital laryngeal anomalies, specifically laryngomalacia and bilateral vocal cord paralysis. Stertor describes the low-pitched inspiratory snoring sound typically produced by nasal or nasopharyngeal obstruction.

The timing of noisy breathing in relation to the sleep–wake cycle is important. Obstruction of the pharyngeal airway (by enlarged tonsils, adenoids, tongue, or syndromes with midface hypoplasia) typically produces worse obstruction during sleep than during waking. Obstruction that is worse when awake is typically laryngeal, tracheal, or bronchial and is exacerbated by exertion. The location of the obstruction dictates the respiratory phase, tone, and nature of the sound, and these qualities direct the differential diagnosis.

With airway obstruction, the severity of the obstructing lesion, the work of breathing, determines the necessity for diagnostic procedures and surgical intervention. Obstructive symptoms vary from mild to severe stridor with episodes of apnea, cyanosis, suprasternal (tracheal tugging) and subcostal retractions, dyspnea, and tachypnea. Congenital anomalies of the trachea and bronchi can create serious respiratory difficulties from the 1st min of life and may sometimes be diagnosed in the prenatal period. If a severe obstruction is suspected prenatally, an airway birth plan should be developed by a high-risk maternal fetal medicine expert, a neonatologist, and a pediatric airway surgeon. *Congenital high airway obstruction syndrome*, or *CHAOS*, can lead to immediate postnatal distress. Chronic obstruction can cause failure to thrive and chronic hypoxemia and may have long-term effects on growth and development.

Bibliography is available at Expert Consult.

413.1 Laryngomalacia

Jill N. D'Souza and James W. Schroeder Jr

CLINICAL MANIFESTATIONS

Laryngomalacia accounts for 45% to 75% of congenital laryngeal anomalies in children with stridor. Stridor is inspiratory, low-pitched, and exacerbated by any exertion: crying, agitation, or feeding. The stridor is caused, in part, by decreased laryngeal tone leading to supraglottic collapse during inspiration. Symptoms usually appear within the 1st 2 wk and increase in severity for up to 6 mo, although gradual improvement can begin at any time. Gastroesophageal reflux disease, laryngopharyngeal reflux disease, and neurologic disease influence the severity of the disease and thereby the clinical course.

DIAGNOSIS

The diagnosis is made primarily based on symptoms. The diagnosis is confirmed by outpatient flexible laryngoscopy (Fig. 413.1). When the work of breathing is moderate to severe, airway films and chest radiographs are indicated. Laryngomalacia can contribute to feeding difficulties and dysphagia in some children because of decreased laryngeal sensation and poor suck-swallow-breath coordination. When the inspiratory stridor sounds wet or is associated with a cough or when there is a history of repeat upper respiratory illness or pneumonia, dysphagia should be considered. When dysphagia is suspected, a contrast swallow study and/or a fiberoptic endoscopic evaluation of swallowing (FEES) may be considered. Because 15–60% of infants with laryngomalacia have synchronous airway anomalies, complete bronchoscopy is undertaken for patients with moderate to severe obstruction.

TREATMENT

Expectant observation is suitable for most infants because most symptoms resolve spontaneously as the child and airway grow. Laryngopharyngeal reflux is managed aggressively with antireflux medications, such as histamine H2 receptor antagonists (H2RAs) or proton pump inhibitors (PPIs). Risk:benefit ratio should be assessed in each patient because these medications, particularly PPIs, have been associated with iron-deficiency anemia, increased incidence of pneumonia, gastroenteritis, and *Clostridium difficile* infections, among others. In 15–20% of patients, symptoms are severe enough to cause progressive respiratory distress, cyanosis, failure to thrive, or cor pulmonale. In these patients, surgical intervention via supraglottoplasty is considered. Supraglottoplasty is 90% successful in relieving upper airway obstruction caused by laryngomalacia. Some comorbidities, such as cardiac disease, neurologic disease, pulmonary disorders, or craniofacial anomalies may be poor prognostic indicators that would suggest earlier intervention.

Bibliography is available at Expert Consult.

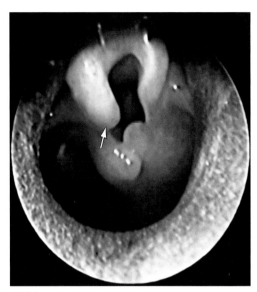

Fig. 413.1 Endoscopic example of laryngomalacia. On inspiration, the epiglottic folds collapse into the airway. The lateral tips of the epiglottis are also collapsing inward *(arrow)*. *(From Slovis TL, editor: Caffey's pediatric diagnostic imaging, ed 11, Philadelphia, 2008, Mosby.)*

413.2 Congenital Subglottic Stenosis

Jill N. D'Souza and James W. Schroeder Jr

CLINICAL MANIFESTATIONS

Congenital subglottic stenosis is the second most common cause of stridor. The subglottis is the narrowest part of the upper airway in a child and is located in the space extending from the undersurface of the true vocal folds to the inferior margin of the cricoid cartilage. Subglottic stenosis is a narrowing of the subglottic larynx and manifests in the infant with respiratory distress and biphasic or primarily inspiratory stridor. It may be congenital or acquired. Symptoms often occur with a respiratory tract infection as the edema and thickened secretions of a common cold narrow an already compromised airway leading to recurrent or persistent croup-like symptoms.

Biphasic or primarily inspiratory stridor is the typical presenting symptom for congenital subglottic stenosis. The edema and thickened secretions of the common cold further narrow an already marginal airway that leads to croup-like symptoms. In a child with recurrent bronchiolitis, diagnosis of congenital subglottic stenosis should be considered. The stenosis can be caused by an abnormally shaped cricoid cartilage; by a tracheal ring that becomes trapped underneath the cricoid cartilage; or by soft tissue thickening caused by ductal cysts, submucosal gland hyperplasia, or fibrosis. Acquired subglottic stenosis refers to stenosis caused by extrinsic factors, most commonly resulting from prolonged intubation, and is discussed in further detail in Chapter 415.

DIAGNOSIS

The diagnosis made by airway radiographs is confirmed by direct laryngoscopy. During diagnostic laryngoscopy the subglottic larynx is visualized directly and sized objectively using endotracheal tubes (Fig. 413.2). The percentage of stenosis is determined by comparing the size of the patients' larynx to a standard of laryngeal dimensions based on age. Stenosis >50% is usually symptomatic and often requires treatment.

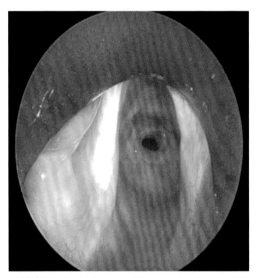

Fig. 413.2 Subglottic stenosis. *(Courtesy Rn Cantab, Wikipedia Commons.)*

As with all cases of upper airway obstruction, tracheostomy is avoided when possible. Subglottic stenosis is typically measured using the Myer-Cotton system, with grade I through grade IV subglottic stenosis indicating the severity of narrowing. Dilation and endoscopic laser surgery can be attempted in grade I and II, although they may not be effective because most congenital stenoses are cartilaginous. Anterior cricoid split or laryngotracheal reconstruction with cartilage graft augmentation is typically used in grade III and IV subglottic stenosis. The differential diagnosis includes other anatomic anomalies, as well as a hemangioma or papillomatosis.

Bibliography is available at Expert Consult.

413.3 Vocal Cord Paralysis
Jill N. D'Souza and James W. Schroeder Jr

Vocal cord paralysis is the third most common congenital laryngeal anomaly that produces stridor in infants and children. Congenital central nervous system lesions such as Chiari malformation, myelomeningocele, and hydrocephalus or birth trauma may be associated with bilateral paralysis. Bilateral vocal cord paralysis produces airway obstruction manifested by respiratory distress and high-pitched inspiratory stridor, aphonatory or dysphonic sound, or inspiratory weak cry.

Unilateral vocal cord paralysis is most often iatrogenic, as a result of surgical treatment for aerodigestive (tracheoesophageal fistula) and cardiovascular (patent ductus arteriosus repair) anomalies, although they may also be idiopathic. Unilateral paralysis causes aspiration, coughing, and choking; the cry is weak and breathy, but stridor and other symptoms of airway obstruction are less common. Vocal cord paralysis in older children may be due to a Chiari malformation or tumors compressing the vagus or recurrent laryngeal nerve.

DIAGNOSIS
The diagnosis of vocal cord paralysis is made by awake flexible laryngoscopy. The examination will demonstrate an inability or weakness to abduct the involved vocal cord. A thorough investigation for the underlying primary cause is indicated. Because of the association with other congenital lesions, evaluation includes neurology and cardiology consultations, imaging of the course of the recurrent laryngeal nerve, and diagnostic endoscopy of the larynx, trachea, and bronchi.

TREATMENT
Treatment is based on the severity of the symptoms. Idiopathic vocal cord paralysis in infants usually resolves spontaneously within 6-12 mo. If it is not resolved by 2-3 yr of age, function typically does not recover.

For unilateral vocal cord paralysis, injection laterally to the paralyzed vocal cord moves it medially to reduce aspiration and related complications. Reinnervation procedures using the ansa cervicalis have been successful in regaining some function of unilateral vocal cord.

Bilateral paralysis may require temporary tracheotomy in 50% of patients. Airway augmentation procedures in bilateral vocal cord paralysis typically focus on widening the posterior glottis, such as an endoscopically placed or open posterior glottis cartilage graft, arytenoidectomy, or arytenoid lateralization. These procedures are generally successful in reducing the obstruction; however, they may result in dysphagia and aspiration.

Bibliography is available at Expert Consult.

413.4 Congenital Laryngeal Webs and Atresia
Jill N. D'Souza and James W. Schroeder Jr

Congenital laryngeal webs are typically located in the anterior glottis with subglottic extension and associated subglottic stenosis, and they result from incomplete recanalization of the laryngotracheal tube. They may be asymptomatic. Thick webs may be suspected in lateral radiographs of the airway. Chromosomal and cardiovascular anomalies, as well as chromosome 22q11 deletion, are common in patients with congenital laryngeal web. Diagnosis is made by direct laryngoscopy (Fig. 413.3). Treatment might require only incision or dilation. Webs with associated subglottic stenosis are likely to require cartilage augmentation of the cricoid cartilage (laryngotracheal reconstruction). Laryngeal atresia occurs as a complete glottic web due to failure of laryngeal and tracheal recanalization and may be associated with tracheal agenesis and tracheoesophageal fistula. Laryngeal atresia may be detected in the prenatal period, and preparations should be made for establishment of definitive airway at birth. Other times, congenital laryngeal atresia is a cause of respiratory distress in the newborn and is diagnosed only upon initial

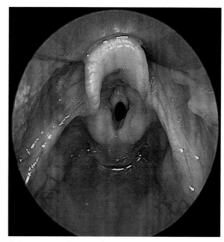

Fig. 413.3 Anterior glottic web, endoscopic view. *(Courtesy Dr. Jeff Rastatter, Division of Pediatric Otolaryngology, Lurie Children's Hospital, Chicago, IL.)*

direct laryngoscopy.

Bibliography is available at Expert Consult.

413.5 Congenital Subglottic Hemangioma
Jill N. D'Souza and James W. Schroeder Jr

Subglottic hemangioma is a rare cause of early infancy respiratory distress. Symptoms typically present within the 1st 2-6 mo of life. The most common presenting symptom is biphasic stridor, somewhat more prominent during inspiration. This is exacerbated by crying and acute viral illnesses. A barking cough, hoarseness, and symptoms of recurrent or persistent croup are typical. Only 1% of children who have cutaneous hemangiomas will have a subglottic hemangioma. However, 50% of those with a subglottic hemangioma will have a cutaneous hemangioma. A facial hemangioma is not always present, but when it is evident, it is in the beard distribution, and thus, respiratory distress in a child with a vascular lesion in this area should prompt further investigation. Chest and neck radiographs can show the characteristic asymmetric narrowing of the subglottic larynx. Airway vascular lesions may also be associated with **PHACES syndrome**, characterized by Posterior Fossa Malformations, Hemangioma, Arterial lesions of head and neck, Cardiac anomalies, Eye Anomalies, and Sternal cleft. More than 50% of children with PHACES syndrome have an airway vascular lesion. Treatment options range from conservative monitoring, steroid injection to tracheotomy and airway reconstruction. Propranolol has become a mainstay in initial therapy of subglottic hemangioma; however, it is estimated that up to 50% of patients with subglottic hemangioma may not have a long-term response to propranolol, indicating a need for close airway monitoring in these patients (Fig. 413.4). Treatment is further discussed in Chapter 417.3.

Bibliography is available at Expert Consult.

413.6 Laryngoceles and Saccular Cysts
Jill N. D'Souza and James W. Schroeder Jr

A laryngocele is an abnormal air-filled dilation of the laryngeal saccule that arises vertically between the false vocal cord, the base of the epiglottis,

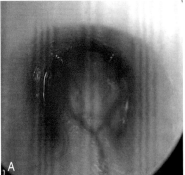
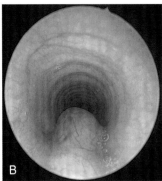

Fig. 413.4 A and **B,** Case of tracheal hemangioma prepropranolol and postpropranolol therapy (pictures 2 wk apart). *(From Bush A, Abel R, Chitty L, et al: Congenital lung disease. In Wilmott RW, Deterding R, Li A, et al, editors: Kendig's disorders of the respiratory tract in children, ed 9, Philadelphia, 2019, Elsevier, Fig. 18.18, p. 308.)*

and the inner surface of the thyroid cartilage. It communicates with the laryngeal lumen and, when intermittently filled with air, causes hoarseness and dyspnea. A saccular cyst (congenital cyst of the larynx) is distinguished from the laryngocele in that its lumen is isolated from the interior of the larynx and it contains mucus, not air. In infants and children, laryngoceles cause hoarseness and dyspnea that may increase with crying. Saccular cysts may cause respiratory distress and stridor at birth and may require early airway intervention. Intubation can be challenging because the supraglottic and laryngeal anatomy may be distorted. In addition, complete airway obstruction may occur on induction with neuromuscular blockade acting on laryngeal tone. A saccular cyst may be visible on radiography, but the diagnosis is made by laryngoscopy (Fig. 413.5). Needle aspiration of the cyst confirms the diagnosis but rarely provides a cure. Surgical excision is the therapy of choice for management of saccular cysts and laryngoceles. Approaches include endoscopic CO_2 laser excision, endoscopic extended ventriculotomy (marsupialization or unroofing), or, traditionally, external excision.

Bibliography is available at Expert Consult.

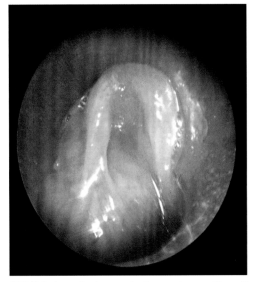

Fig. 413.5 Endoscopic photograph of a saccular cyst. *(From Ahmad SM, Soliman AMS: Congenital anomalies of the larynx, Otolaryngol Clin North Am 40:177–191, 2007, Fig. 3.)*

413.7 Posterior Laryngeal Cleft and Laryngotracheoesophageal Cleft
Jill N. D'Souza and James W. Schroeder Jr

The posterior laryngeal cleft is characterized by aspiration and is the result of a deficiency in the midline of the posterior larynx. Posterior laryngeal clefts are categorized into 4 types. Type 1 clefts are mild and the interarytenoid notch extends only down to the level of the true vocal cords; 60% of these will cause no symptoms and will not require surgical repair. In severe cases, the cleft (type 4) extends inferiorly into the cervical or thoracic trachea so there is no separation between the trachea and esophagus, creating a laryngotracheoesophageal cleft. Laryngeal clefts can occur in families and are likely to be associated with tracheal agenesis, tracheoesophageal fistula, and multiple congenital anomalies, as with G syndrome, Opitz-Frias syndrome, and Pallister-Hall syndrome.

Initial symptoms are those of aspiration and recurrent respiratory infections. Esophagogram is undertaken to evaluate presence of aspiration or laryngeal penetration of ingested contrast material. A FEES exam may be undertaken by an otolaryngologist with assistance of a speech language and pathology team to observe pattern of liquid spillage during swallow and may identify a cleft. However, the gold standard of diagnosis remains operative laryngoscopy and bronchoscopy with palpation of the posterior larynx. This assists in determining length of the cleft and guides treatment options. A type I cleft extends to, but not beyond, the vocal cords. A type II cleft extends beyond the vocal cords to, but not through, the cricoid cartilage. A type III cleft extends through cricoid into cervical trachea. A type IV cleft extends into thoracic trachea. Treatment is based on the cleft type and the symptoms; in general, a type I cleft may be managed endoscopically, whereas higher grades may require an open procedure. Stabilization of the airway is the first priority. Gastroesophageal reflux must be controlled and a careful assessment for other congenital anomalies is undertaken before repair. Several endoscopic and open cervical and transthoracic surgical repairs have been described.

Bibliography is available at Expert Consult.

413.8 Vascular and Cardiac Anomalies
Jill N. D'Souza and James W. Schroeder Jr

Aberrant cardiopulmonary vascular anatomy may directly impact the trachea and bronchi. The aberrant innominate artery is the most common cause of secondary tracheomalacia (see Chapter 459). It may be asymptomatic and discovered incidentally, or it may cause severe symptoms. Expiratory wheezing and cough occur and, rarely, reflex apnea or "dying spells." Surgical intervention is rarely necessary. Infants are most commonly treated expectantly because the problem is often self-limited.

The term *vascular ring* is used to describe vascular anomalies that result from abnormal development of the aortic arch complex. The double aortic arch is the most common complete vascular ring, encircling both the trachea and esophagus, compressing both. With few exceptions, these patients are symptomatic by 3 mo of age. Respiratory symptoms predominate, but dysphagia may be present. The diagnosis is established by barium esophagogram that shows a posterior indentation of the esophagus by the vascular ring (see Fig. 459.2 in Chapter 459). CT or MRI with angiography provides the surgeon the information needed.

Other vascular anomalies include the pulmonary artery sling, which also requires surgical correction. The most common open (incomplete) vascular ring is the left aortic arch with aberrant right subclavian artery. Although common, it is usually asymptomatic, although dysphagia lusoria may be described. This is characterized as dysphagia caused by an aberrant subclavian coursing behind the esophagus, leading to esophageal compression and difficulty with bolus transit.

Congenital cardiac defects are likely to compress the left main bronchus or lower trachea. Any condition that produces significant pulmonary hypertension increases the size of the pulmonary arteries, which in turn cause compression of the left main bronchus. Surgical correction of the underlying pathology to relieve pulmonary hypertension relieves the airway compression.

Bibliography is available at Expert Consult.

413.9 Tracheal Stenoses, Webs, and Atresia
Jill N. D'Souza and James W. Schroeder Jr

Long segment congenital tracheal stenosis with complete tracheal rings typically occurs within the 1st yr of life, usually after a crisis has been precipitated by an acute respiratory illness. The diagnosis may be suggested by plain radiographs. CT with contrast delineates associated intrathoracic anomalies such as the pulmonary artery sling, which occurs in one third of patients; one-fourth have associated cardiac anomalies. Bronchoscopy is the best method to define the degree and extent of the stenosis and the associated abnormal bronchial branching pattern. Treatment of clinically significant stenosis involves tracheal resection of short segment stenosis, slide tracheoplasty for long segment stenosis or tracheal rings. Congenital soft tissue stenosis and thin webs are rare. Dilation may be all that is required.

Bibliography is available at Expert Consult.

413.10 Foregut Cysts
Jill N. D'Souza and James W. Schroeder Jr

The embryologic foregut gives rise to the pharynx, lower respiratory tract, esophagus, stomach, duodenum, and hepatobiliary tract, and duplication cysts can occur anywhere along this tract. Foregut duplications account for approximately one third of all duplications. The bronchogenic cyst, intramural esophageal cyst (esophageal duplication), and enteric cyst can all produce symptoms of respiratory obstruction and dysphagia. The diagnosis is suspected when chest radiographs or CT scan delineate the mass and, in the case of enteric cyst, the associated vertebral anomaly. The treatment of all foregut cysts is surgical excision.

Bibliography is available at Expert Consult.

413.11 Tracheomalacia and Bronchomalacia

See Chapter 416.

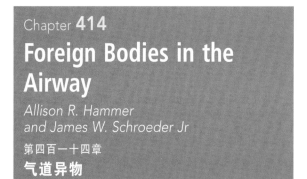

Chapter **414**
Foreign Bodies in the Airway
Allison R. Hammer and James W. Schroeder Jr

第四百一十四章
气道异物

中文导读

　　本章主要介绍了气道异物的流行病学及病因、临床表现、诊断和治疗；分别介绍了喉异物、气管异物、支气管异物等内容。流行病学包括导致儿童窒息最常见物体是食物，年幼的儿童吸入大量异物的风险更大（原文414.1）。临床表现为咳嗽、窒息、气道阻塞、异物滞留、侵蚀或感染等（原文414.2）。诊断包括病史采集、体格检查、支气管镜及影像学检查（原文414.3）。治疗主要由专家用器械迅速在内镜下取出，加强预防、教育意识（原文414.4）。

EPIDEMIOLOGY AND ETIOLOGY

Choking is a leading cause of morbidity and mortality among children, especially those younger than 4 yr of age. Most victims of foreign body aspiration are older infants and toddlers (Fig. 414.1); males have been found to be victims up to 1.7 times more likely than females. Studies show that children younger than 4 yr of age account for 61.7–70% of airway foreign body cases. The most common objects on which children choke are food items (59.5–81% of all choking cases). Nuts, seeds, hot dogs, hard candy, gum, bones, and raw fruits and vegetables are the most frequently aspirated food items. From 2001 to 2009, an average of 12,435 children ages 0-14 yr in the United States were treated in emergency departments for choking on food without fatality. Common inorganic objects on which children choke include coins, latex balloons, pins, jewelry, magnets, pen caps, and toys. Globular, compressible, or round objects such as hot dogs, grapes, nuts, balloons, marshmallows, meats, and candies are particularly hazardous due to their ability to completely occlude the airway.

Young children are more at risk to aspirate a foreign body largely because of their developmental vulnerabilities and their underdeveloped ability to swallow food. Infants and toddlers often use their mouths to explore their surroundings, and children generally are more likely to be distracted, playing, or ambulatory while eating. An infant is able to suck and swallow and is equipped with involuntary reflexes (gag, cough, and glottis closure) that help to protect against aspiration during swallowing. Dentition develops at approximately 6 mo of age with the eruption of the incisors. Molars do not erupt until approximately 1.5 yr of age; mature mastication takes longer to develop. Despite a strong gag reflex, a child's airway is more vulnerable to obstruction than an adult's airway. Young children are more likely to experience significant blockage by small foreign bodies due to their smaller airway diameter. Mucus and secretions may form a seal around the foreign body, making it more difficult to dislodge by forced air. In addition, the force of air generated by an infant or young child's cough is less effective in dislodging an airway obstruction. It is recommended that children younger than 5 yr of age should avoid hard candy and chewing gum and that raw fruits and vegetables be cut into small pieces. Other factors, such as developmental delays or disorders causing neurologic or muscular issues, can also put children at higher risk for foreign body aspiration.

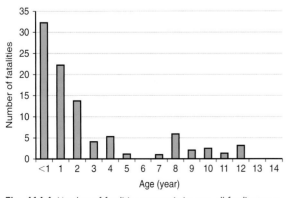

Fig. 414.1 Number of fatalities versus victim age, all fatality types. *(From Milkovich SM, Altkorn R, Chen X, et al: Development of the small parts cylinder: lessons learned, Laryngoscope 118[11]:2082–2086, 2008.)*

CLINICAL MANIFESTATIONS

Foreign bodies of the airway have variable presentations and complications, depending on the characteristics, duration, and location of the foreign body. The clinical manifestations range from an asymptomatic state to severe respiratory distress. The most serious complication of foreign body aspiration is complete obstruction of the airway, which may be recognized in the conscious child as sudden respiratory distress followed by an inability to speak or cough.

There are typically three stages of symptoms that result from aspiration of an object into the airway:
1. **Initial event:** Paroxysms of coughing, choking, gagging, and possibly airway obstruction occur immediately after aspiration of the foreign body. The child is sometimes able to expel the foreign body during this stage.
2. **Asymptomatic interval:** The foreign body becomes lodged, reflexes fatigue, and the immediate irritating symptoms subside. *The lack of symptoms can be particularly misleading to the provider when a child presents in this stage and accounts for a large percentage of delayed diagnoses and overlooked foreign bodies.* A large meta-analysis of more than 30,000 patients showed that diagnosis is delayed more than 25 hr in almost 40% of airway foreign body cases.
3. **Complications:** Obstruction, erosion, or infection develops, which again directs attention to the presence of a foreign body. In this third stage, complications include fever, cough, hemoptysis, pneumonia, and atelectasis. Acute or chronic complications have been reported in almost 15% of cases of foreign bodies of the airway.

DIAGNOSIS

History is the most important factor in determining the need for bronchoscopy. A positive history must never be ignored, but a negative history can be misleading. Because nuts and seeds are the most common bronchial foreign bodies, the physician should specifically question the child's parents about these items, and bronchoscopy should be carried out promptly. A comprehensive physical exam is also essential, including examination of the nose, oral cavity, pharynx, neck, and lungs. Choking or coughing episodes accompanied by new-onset wheezing and asymmetric breath sounds are highly suggestive of foreign body in the airway. In addition to history and physical examination, radiology studies have an important role in diagnosing foreign bodies in the airway. Plain films are typically recommended first, although many foreign bodies are radiolucent (80–96%), and therefore providers often must rely on secondary findings (such as air trapping, asymmetric hyperinflation, obstructive emphysema, atelectasis, mediastinal shift, and consolidation) to indicate suspicion of a foreign body. Expiratory or lateral decubitus films can assist in revealing these suggestive secondary findings. The indication for computed tomography of the chest is currently being explored due to its high sensitivity and specificity, its ability to detect radiolucent objects, and its potential to eliminate the need for an anesthesia and procedure. However, the known risks of radiation must certainly be considered. If there is a high index of suspicion despite negative or inconclusive imaging, bronchoscopy should be performed.

TREATMENT

The treatment of choice for airway foreign bodies is prompt endoscopic removal with rigid instruments by a specialist (otolaryngologist or pulmonologist). Bronchoscopy is deferred only until providers have obtained preoperative studies and the patient has been prepared by

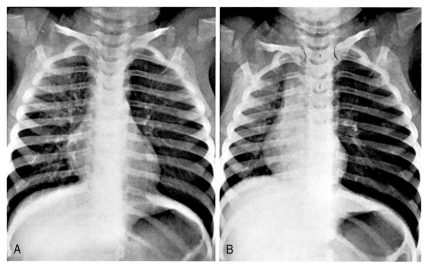

Fig. 414.2 A, Normal inspiratory chest radiograph in a toddler with a peanut fragment in the left main bronchus. **B,** Expiratory radiograph of the same child showing the classic obstructive emphysema (air trapping) on the involved *(left)* side. Air leaves the normal right side allowing, the lung to deflate. The medium shifts toward the unobstructed side.

adequate hydration and emptying of the stomach. Airway foreign bodies are usually removed the same day the diagnosis is first considered. As with any treatment modality, providers must give careful consideration to the risks and benefits of the bronchoscopy procedure when diagnosis is unclear. Potential complications of rigid bronchoscopy include bronchospasm, desaturation, bleeding, and airway edema, in addition to the inherent risks of anesthesia.

Beyond the understanding of diagnosis and management of airway foreign bodies, there is a strong need and push for awareness, education, and prevention among caregivers, healthcare providers, and manufacturers of food and toys.

414.1 Laryngeal Foreign Bodies
Allison R. Hammer and James W. Schroeder Jr

Although laryngeal foreign bodies are less common (2–12% of cases) than bronchial or tracheal foreign bodies, they are particularly dangerous due to risk of complete laryngeal obstruction, which can asphyxiate the child unless it is promptly relieved with the Heimlich maneuver (see Chapter 81 and Figs. 81.6 and 81.7). Objects that are partially obstructive of the larynx are usually flat and thin and lodge between the vocal cords in the sagittal plane, causing symptoms of croup, hoarseness, cough, stridor, and dyspnea.

414.2 Tracheal Foreign Bodies
Allison R. Hammer and James W. Schroeder Jr

Tracheal foreign bodies account for 3–12% of airway foreign body

cases. Children who have tracheal foreign bodies can present with dysphonia, dysphagia, dry cough, or biphasic stridor. Posteroanterior and lateral soft tissue neck radiographs (airway films) are abnormal in 92% of children, whereas chest radiographs are abnormal in only 58% of these cases.

414.3 Bronchial Foreign Bodies
Allison R. Hammer and James W. Schroeder Jr

Most airway foreign bodies lodge in a bronchus (80–90% of cases). Occasionally, fragments of a foreign body may produce bilateral involvement or shifting infiltrates if they move from lobe to lobe. Some children with bronchial foreign bodies present asymptomatically, whereas others have asymmetric breath sounds, coughing, and wheezing. Posteroanterior and lateral chest radiographs (including the abdomen) are standard in the assessment of infants and children suspected of having aspirated a foreign object. An expiratory posteroanterior chest film is most helpful. During expiration, the bronchial foreign body obstructs the exit of air from the obstructed lung, producing obstructive emphysema and air trapping. The persistent inflation of the obstructed lung causes shift of the mediastinum toward the opposite side (Fig. 414.2). Air trapping is an immediate complication, whereas atelectasis is a late finding. Lateral decubitus chest films or fluoroscopy can provide the same information as expiratory films but are often unnecessary. History and physical examination, not radiographs, determine the indication for bronchoscopy.

Bibliography is available at Expert Consult.

Chapter 415
Laryngotracheal Stenosis and Subglottic Stenosis

Taher Valika and James W. Schroeder Jr

第四百一十五章
喉气管狭窄和声门下狭窄

中文导读

本章主要介绍了先天性声门下狭窄和继发性喉气管狭窄；具体介绍了继发性喉气管狭窄的临床表现、诊断和治疗。继发性喉气管狭窄90%继发于气管内插管，也包括胃酸反流等（原文415.2），临床表现为痉挛性哮吼，多次拔管失败的新生儿也可表现为痉挛性哮吼，以及患有永久性呼吸困难、喘鸣或发声困难的儿童（原文415.2）。诊断可通过后前位和侧位气道X线片，金标准是直接用喉镜和支气管镜检查。狭窄的严重程度、位置和类型（软骨或软组织）决定了治疗措施（原文415.3）。

Laryngotracheal stenosis is the second most common cause of stridor in neonates and is the most common cause of airway obstruction requiring tracheostomy in infants. The glottis (vocal cords) and the upper trachea are compromised in most laryngeal stenosis, particularly those that develop following endotracheal intubation. Subglottic stenosis is a narrowing of the subglottic larynx, which is the space extending from the undersurface of the true vocal cords to the inferior margin of the cricoid cartilage. **Subglottic stenosis** is considered congenital when there is no other apparent cause such as a history of laryngeal trauma or intubation. Approximately 90% of cases manifest in the 1st yr of life. Management relies on fine-tuning the airway, while ensuring the patient continues to grow. Knowledge of preventative measures is imperative to all healthcare members.

415.1 Congenital Subglottic Stenosis

See Chapter 413.2.

415.2 Acquired Laryngotracheal Stenosis

Taher Valika and James W. Schroeder Jr

Ninety percent of acquired stenoses are a result of endotracheal intubation. The narrowest portion of the pediatric larynx is the subglottic region due to the narrow cricoid cartilage. When the pressure of the endotracheal tube against the cricoid mucosa is greater than the capillary pressure, ischemia occurs, followed by necrosis and ulceration. Secondary infection and perichondritis develop with exposure of cartilage (Fig. 415.1). Granulation tissue forms around the ulcerations. These changes

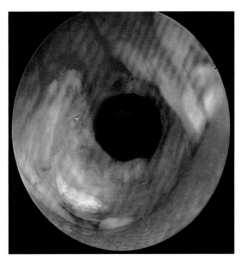

Fig. 415.1 Bronchoscopy in a 2 mo old infant showing mucosal erosion and cartilage exposure in the subglottic region. Child was intubated with an age-appropriate tube but with an excess of air in cuff. *(Courtesy Dr. Taher Valika, Division of Pediatric Otolaryngology, Ann & Robert H. Lurie Children's Hospital of Chicago.)*

and edema throughout the larynx usually resolve spontaneously after extubation. Chronic edema and fibrous stenosis develop in only a small percentage of cases.

A number of factors predispose to the development of laryngeal stenosis. Laryngopharyngeal reflux of acid and pepsin from the stomach is known to exacerbate endotracheal tube trauma. More damage is caused in areas left unprotected, owing to loss of mucosa. Congenital subglottic stenosis narrows the larynx which makes the patient more likely to develop acquired subglottic stenosis because significant injury is more likely to occur with use of an endotracheal tube of age-appropriate size. Other risk factors for the development of acquired subglottic stenosis include sepsis, malnutrition, chronic inflammatory disorders, and immunosuppression. An oversized endotracheal tube is the most common factor contributing to laryngeal injury. A tube that allows a small air leak at the end of the inspiratory cycle minimizes potential trauma. Other extrinsic factors—traumatic intubation, multiple reintubations, movement of the endotracheal tube, and duration of intubation—can contribute to varying degrees in individual patients.

CLINICAL MANIFESTATIONS

Symptoms of acquired and congenital stenosis are similar. Spasmodic croup, the sudden onset of severe croup in the early morning hours, is usually caused by laryngopharyngeal reflux with transient laryngospasm and subsequent laryngeal edema. These frightening episodes resolve rapidly, often before the family and child reach the emergency department. Other presentations can also involve neonates who fail extubation, despite multiple attempts, and children with permanent dyspnea, stridor, or dysphonia.

DIAGNOSIS

The diagnosis can be made by posteroanterior and lateral airway radiographs. The gold standard to confirm the diagnosis is via direct laryngoscopy and bronchoscopy in the operating room. High-resolution CT imaging and ultrasonography are of limited value. This is similar to the workup associated with congenital subglottic stenosis.

TREATMENT

The severity, location, and type (cartilaginous or soft tissue) of the stenosis determine the treatment. Mild cases can be managed without operative intervention because the airway will improve as the child grows. Moderate soft tissue stenosis is treated by endoscopy using gentle dilations or CO_2 laser. Severe laryngotracheal stenosis is likely to require laryngotracheal reconstructive (expansion) surgery or resection of the narrowed portion of the laryngeal and tracheal airway (cricotracheal resection). Every effort is made to avoid tracheotomy using endoscopic techniques or open surgical procedures.

Fundamental knowledge of the airway can help to reduce the incidence of stenoses. The use of age-appropriate tubes and cuffless tubes, treatment of gastroesophageal reflux, and reducing the duration of mechanical ventilation have led to an overall decrease in laryngotracheal stenoses in the past decade.

Bibliography is available at Expert Consult.

Chapter **416**

Bronchomalacia and Tracheomalacia

Jonathan D. Finder

第四百一十六章

气管软化症和支气管软化症

中文导读

本章主要介绍了气管软化症和支气管软化症的临床表现、诊断、治疗及预后。其中，临床表现包括呼气像低音调的喘鸣音；诊断方法包括支气管镜检查、胸部平片、透视、肺功能检查、MRI、CT和磁共振血管造影；治疗包括体位引流、异丙托溴铵雾化、支气管内支架、经气管切开进行持续气道正压通气、外科手术以及气管支气管外支架。原发性气管、支气管软化症预后较好，继发性和获得性气管、支气管软化预后因病因而异。

Tracheomalacia and bronchomalacia refer to chondromalacia of a central airway, leading to insufficient cartilage to maintain airway patency throughout the respiratory cycle. These are common causes of persistent wheezing in infancy. Tracheomalacia and bronchomalacia can be either primary or secondary (Table 416.1). Primary tracheomalacia and bronchomalacia are often seen in premature infants, although most affected patients are born at term. Secondary tracheomalacia and bronchomalacia refer to the situation in which the central airway is compressed by an adjacent structure (e.g., vascular ring; see Chapter 345) or deficient in cartilage because of tracheoesophageal fistula (see Chapter 345). Bronchomalacia is common following lung transplantation, assumed to be secondary to the loss of bronchial artery supply leading to ischemia of the bronchial cartilage. This form of bronchomalacia may take months to present following transplantation. Laryngomalacia can accompany primary bronchomalacia or tracheomalacia. Involvement of the entire central airway (laryngotracheobronchomalacia) is also seen.

CLINICAL MANIFESTATIONS

Primary tracheomalacia and bronchomalacia are principally disorders of infants, with a male:female ratio of 2:1. The dominant finding, low-pitched monophonic wheezing heard predominantly during expiration, is most prominent over the central airways. Parents often describe persistent respiratory congestion even in the absence of a viral respiratory infection. When the lesion involves only one main bronchus (more commonly the left), the wheezing is louder on that side and there may be unilateral palpable fremitus. In cases of tracheomalacia, the wheeze is loudest over the trachea. Hyperinflation and/or subcostal retractions do not occur unless the patient also has concurrent asthma, viral bronchiolitis, or other causes of peripheral airways obstruction. In the absence of asthma, patients with tracheomalacia and bronchomalacia are not helped by administration of a bronchodilator. Acquired tracheomalacia and bronchomalacia are seen in association with vascular compression (vascular rings, slings, and innominate artery compression)

Table 416.1 | Classification of Tracheomalacia

PRIMARY TRACHEOMALACIA
Congenital absence of tracheal-supporting cartilages

SECONDARY TRACHEOMALACIA
Esophageal atresia, tracheoesophageal fistula
Vascular rings (double aortic arch)
Tracheal compression from an aberrant innominate artery
Tracheal compression from mediastinal masses
Abnormally soft tracheal cartilages associated with connective tissue disorders
Prolonged mechanical ventilation, chronic lung disease

From McNamara VM, Crabbe DC: Tracheomalacia, *Paediatr Respir Rev* 5:147–154, 2004.

---

or in association with the loss of bronchial artery supply in lung transplantation. Tracheomalacia is the rule following correction of tracheoesophageal fistula. Other causes of acquired tracheomalacia, which may persist after surgical correction include cardiomegaly. The importance of the physical exam cannot be understated; one study found that pediatric pulmonologists made a correct assessment of malacia based on symptoms, history, and lung function prior to bronchoscopy in 74% of cases.

DIAGNOSIS

Definitive diagnoses of tracheomalacia and bronchomalacia are established by flexible or rigid bronchoscopy (Fig. 416.1). The lesion is difficult to detect on plain radiographs. Although fluoroscopy can demonstrate dynamic collapse and avoid the need for invasive diagnostic techniques, it is poorly sensitive. Pulmonary function testing can show a pattern of decreased peak flow and flattening of the flow-volume loop. Other important diagnostic modalities include MRI and CT scanning. MRI with angiography is especially useful when there is a possibility of vascular ring and should be performed when a right aortic arch is seen on plain film radiography.

TREATMENT

Postural drainage can help with clearance of secretions. β-Adrenergic agents should be avoided in the absence of asthma because they can exacerbate loss of airway patency due to decreased airway tone. Nebulized ipratropium bromide may be useful. Endobronchial stents have been used in severely affected patients but have a high incidence of complications, ranging from airway obstruction due to granulation tissue to erosion into adjacent vascular structures. Continuous positive airway pressure via tracheostomy may be indicated for severe cases. A surgical approach (aortopexy and bronchopexy) is rarely required and only for patients who have life-threatening apnea, cyanosis, and bradycardia (cyanotic spells) from airway obstruction and/or who demonstrated vascular compression. Reports of creation and use of 3-dimensional (3D) printed, bioresorbable external tracheobronchial stents in pediatric patients with life-threatening tracheobronchomalacia have shown great promise.

PROGNOSIS

Primary bronchomalacia and tracheomalacia have excellent prognoses because airflow improves as the child and the airways grow. Patients with primary airway malacia usually take longer to recover from common respiratory infections. Wheezing at rest usually resolves by age 3 yr. Prolonged bacterial bronchitis has been reported as a complication of bronchomalacia. Prognosis in secondary and acquired forms varies with cause. Patients with concurrent asthma need considerable supportive treatment and careful monitoring of respiratory status.

Bibliography is available at Expert Consult.

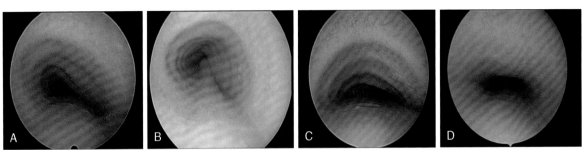

Fig. 416.1 Four examples of tracheomalacia appearances. **A,** Comma-shaped trachea caused by innominate artery compression requiring aortopexy. **B,** Bunched-up trachealis muscle and compressed trachea caused by a double aortic arch. **C,** Flattened trachea and increased trachealis diameter with a tracheoesophageal fistula in the posterior wall. **D,** Ovoid-shaped trachea from external compression by innominate artery. *(From Deacon JWF, Widger J, Soma MA: Paediatric tracheomalacia—A review of clinical features and comparison of diagnostic imaging techniques, Int J Pediatr Otorhinolaryngol 98:75–81, 2017.)*

Chapter **417**
Neoplasms of the Larynx, Trachea, and Bronchi

Saied Ghadersohi
and James W. Schroeder Jr

第四百一十七章
喉、气管和支气管肿瘤

中文导读

本章介绍了声带结节、复发性呼吸道乳头状瘤病、先天性声门下血管瘤、血管发育异常、其他喉部肿瘤、气管及支气管肿瘤。本章描述了声带结节的病因、鉴别诊断及治疗方法；描述了复发性呼吸道乳头状瘤的病因、病变部位、临床表现、治疗及预防方法；描述了先天性声门下血管瘤的临床表现、诊断及治疗方法；血管发育异常部分描述了分类、检查及治疗方法；其他喉部肿瘤部分介绍了神经纤维瘤病、横纹肌肉瘤及其他喉部恶性肿瘤的临床表现；气管肿瘤中描述了最常见的良性气管肿瘤，包括炎性假瘤和错构瘤的临床表现；支气管肿瘤部分介绍了类癌、黏液表皮样癌等肿瘤的临床表现。

417.1 Vocal Nodules
Saied Ghadersohi and James W. Schroeder Jr

Vocal nodules, which are not true neoplasms, are the most common cause of chronic hoarseness in children. Chronic vocal abuse or misuse (i.e., frequent yelling and screaming) produces localized vascular congestion, edema, hyalinization, and epithelial thickening in the bilateral vocal cords. This grossly appears as nodules that disrupt the normal vibration of the cords during phonation. **Vocal abuse** is the main factor, and the voice is worse in the evenings. Differential can include unilateral lesions such as **vocal cord cysts and polyps;** however, these usually have an acute inciting event and are rarer in children.

Treatment is primarily nonsurgical with voice therapy used in children >4 yr of age who can participate in therapy, and clinical monitoring with behavioral therapy in younger children or those with developmental delay. In addition, laryngopharyngeal reflux commonly exacerbates vocal abuse–induced irritation of the cord, Therefore antireflux therapy can also be implemented (see Chapter 349). Surgical excision of vocal cord lesions in children is controversial and is rarely indicated but may be necessary if the child is unable to communicate adequately, becomes aphonic, or requires tension and straining to make any utterance whatsoever.

417.2 Recurrent Respiratory Papillomatosis
Saied Ghadersohi and James W. Schroeder Jr

Papillomas are the most common respiratory tract neoplasms in children, occurring in 4.3 in 100,000. They are simply warts—benign tumors—caused by the human papillomavirus (HPV), most commonly types 6 and 11 (see Chapter 293). Seventy-five percent of recurrent respiratory papilloma cases occur in children younger than age 5 yr, but the diagnosis may be made at any age. In general, neonatal-onset disease is a negative prognostic factor with higher mortality and need for tracheostomy. Sixty-seven percent of children with RRP are born to mothers who had condylomas during pregnancy or parturition. The mode of HPV transmission is still not clear. Neonates have been reported to have RRP, suggesting intrauterine transmission of HPV. Despite close association with vaginal condylomata, only 1 in 231 to 400 vaginal births go on to develop respiratory papillomatosis. Therefore other risk factors contribute to transmission, and C-section delivery for prevention cannot be recommended. However, preventive measures can include the prospective widespread use of the quadrivalent HPV vaccine to help eliminate maternal and paternal HPV reservoirs and possibly decrease cases of RRP caused by HPV 6 and 11.

CLINICAL MANIFESTATIONS

The clinical course involves remissions and exacerbations of recurrent papillomas most commonly on the larynx (usually the vocal cords), causing progressively worsening hoarseness, sleep-disordered breathing, exertional dyspnea, stridor, and, if left untreated, eventually severe airway obstruction (Fig. 417.1). Although it is a benign disease, lesions can spread throughout the aerodigestive tract in 31% of patients, most commonly the oral cavity, trachea, and bronchi. Rarely these lesions can undergo malignant conversion (1.6%); however, some patients may have spontaneous remission. Patients may be initially diagnosed with asthma, croup, vocal nodules, or allergies.

TREATMENT

The treatment of RRP is endoscopic surgical removal with three goals. First, debulking/complete removal of the lesions, secondly, preservation of normal structures, and finally, prevention of scar formation in the affected areas. Most surgeons in North America prefer the microdebrider, although microsurgery, CO_2, and KTP laser techniques have been described. Despite these techniques, some form of adjunct therapy may be needed in up to 20% of cases. The most widely accepted indications for adjunct therapy are a need for more than four surgical procedures per year, rapid regrowth of papillomata with airway compromise, or distal multisite spread of disease. Adjunct therapies can be inhaled or administered intralesionally or systemically and include antiviral modalities (interferon, ribavirin, acyclovir, cidofovir), antiangiogenic agents such as bevacizumab (Avastin), photodynamic therapy, dietary supplement (indole-3-carbinol), nonsteroidal antiinflammatory drugs (COX2 inhibitors, Celebrex), retinoids, and mumps vaccination.

Bibliography is available at Expert Consult.

417.3 Congenital Subglottic Hemangioma
Saied Ghadersohi and James W. Schroeder Jr

CLINICAL MANIFESTATIONS

Typically, congenital subglottic hemangiomas are symptomatic within the first 2 mo of life, almost all occurring before 6 mo of age. Much like the cutaneous infantile hemangiomas, these lesions have 2 phases: a **proliferative phase** with rapid growth in the first 6 mo of life, then they stabilize by 1 yr, and a slow **involution phase** typically by age 3. Patients present with usually inspiratory but sometimes biphasic stridor. The infant can have a barking cough and temporarily respond to steroids,

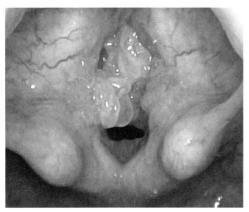

Fig. 417.1 Laryngoscopic view of respiratory papillomas causing near complete obstruction at glottic level. *(From Derkay CS, Wiatrak B: Recurrent respiratory papillomatosis: a review, Laryngoscope 118:1236–1245, 2008.)*

similar to persistent croup. Fifty percent of congenital subglottic hemangiomas are associated with facial lesions, but the converse is not true. Radiographs classically delineate an asymmetric subglottic narrowing. The diagnosis is made by direct laryngoscopy.

TREATMENT

The medical treatment of hemangiomas traditionally was with long-term systemic steroids, which often had severe side effects, including growth retardation and adrenal suppression. Prednisone 2-4 mg/kg/day is given orally for 4-6 wk, typically with partial regression of the lesion. The dosage is then tapered. If there is no response, the drug is discontinued. Propranolol was introduced in 2008 and rapidly became the first-line treatment of infantile and subglottic hemangiomas, including in a recent randomized clinical trial comparing it with systemic steroids. The mechanism is thought to be through VEGF or adrenergic vasoconstriction pathways and can involute the lesion in a few days. Typically, treatment is with 1-3 mg/kg/day of propranolol for 4-12 mo, based on clinical monitoring as noted in a 2011 consensus guideline. Prescreening patients with cardiology workup (i.e., electrocardiogram) is advised. Side effects include hypotension, bradycardia, bronchospasm, and hypoglycemia; children treated with propranolol need to be monitored closely.

Surgical management can range from intralesional steroid injection to avoid systemic steroid side effects, CO_2, or KTP laser endoscopic excision, and ultimately as a last resort tracheostomy can establish a safe airway, allowing time for the lesion to involute per its natural course.

Bibliography is available at Expert Consult.

417.4 Vascular Anomalies
Saied Ghadersohi and James W. Schroeder Jr

Based on the International Society for the Study of Vascular Anomalies classification system, these lesions can be classified into vascular malformations and vascular tumors. The most common vascular tumors are infantile/subglottic hemangiomas and were previously discussed. Vascular malformations are not true neoplastic lesions. They have a normal rate of endothelial turnover and various channel abnormalities. They are subcategorized based on high or low flow and by their predominant type (capillary, venous, arterial, lymphatic, or a combination thereof). Overall, vascular malformations are uncommon, and they rarely occur in the larynx and airway. When they do occur, they are often an extension from elsewhere in the head and neck. It should be noted that these lesions can expand with a viral upper respiratory infection. They can be diagnosed with direct visualization during laryngoscopy or bronchoscopy or seen on CT/MRI imaging. Treatment usually entails a multidisciplinary team approach with early surgical or laser resection or sclerotherapy.

Bibliography is available at Expert Consult.

417.5 Other Laryngeal Neoplasms
James W. Schroeder Jr and Lauren D. Holinger

Neurofibromatosis (see Chapter 614.1) rarely involves the larynx. When children are affected, limited local resection is undertaken to maintain an airway and optimize the voice. Complete surgical extirpation is virtually impossible without debilitating resection of vital laryngeal structures. Most surgeons select the option of less-aggressive symptomatic surgery because of the poorly circumscribed and infiltrative nature of these fibromas. **Rhabdomyosarcoma** (see Chapter 527) and other malignant tumors of the larynx are rare. Symptoms of hoarseness and progressive airway obstruction prompt initial evaluation by flexible laryngoscopy in the office.

417.6 Tracheal Neoplasms

Saied Ghadersohi, James W. Schroeder Jr, and Lauren D. Holinger

Tracheal tumors are extremely rare and include malignant and benign neoplasms; they may initially be misdiagnosed as asthma. The 2 most common benign tumors are inflammatory pseudotumor and hamartoma. The **inflammatory pseudotumor** is probably a reaction to a previous bronchial infection or traumatic insult. Growth is slow, and the tumor may be locally invasive. Hamartomas are tumors of primary tissue elements that are abnormal in proportion and arrangement.

Tracheal neoplasms manifest with stridor, wheezing, cough, or pneumonia and are rarely diagnosed until 75% of the lumen has been obstructed (Fig. 417.2). Chest radiographs or airway films can identify the obstruction. Pulmonary function studies demonstrate an abnormal flow-volume loop. A mild response to bronchodilator therapy may be misleading. Treatment is based upon the histopathology.

Bibliography is available at Expert Consult.

417.7 Bronchial Tumors

Saied Ghadersohi and James W. Schroeder Jr

Bronchial tumors are rare. In 1 series, carcinoid tumors were the most common, followed by mucoepidermoid and pseudotumors. These patients

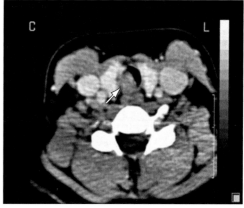

Fig. 417.2 A CT scan of the trachea with a circumscribed intraluminal tracheal mass *(arrow)* in the tracheal wall. *(From Venizelos I, Papathomas T, Anagnostou E, et al: Pediatric inflammatory myofibroblastic tumor of the trachea: a case report and review of the literature, Pediatr Pulmonol 43:831–835, 2008.)*

can present with persistent pneumonia despite adequate treatment. The diagnosis is confirmed at bronchoscopy and biopsy; treatment depends on the histopathology.

Bibliography is available at Expert Consult.

Chapter 418

Wheezing, Bronchiolitis, and Bronchitis

第四百一十八章
喘息、毛细支气管炎和支气管炎

中文导读

　　本章介绍了婴儿喘息、毛细支气管炎及支气管炎。本章介绍了婴儿喘息的病理生理机制、临床表现、病史采集和体格检查要点、诊断评估等；描述了婴儿期喘息的3种类型，以及婴儿期喘息日后发展为哮喘的危险因素；详细描述了急性毛细支气管炎的病理生理学特征、病原学、流行病学情况、临床特征、诊断评估、治疗、预后及预防等；支气管炎部分介绍了急性支气管炎、慢性支气管炎，以及吸烟和空气污染；急性支气管炎部分描述了临床表现、鉴别诊断及治疗方法。

418.1 Wheezing in Infants: Bronchiolitis

Samantha A. House and Shawn L. Ralston

GENERAL PATHOPHYSIOLOGY OF WHEEZING IN INFANTS

Wheezing, the production of a musical continuous sound that originates in narrowed airways, is heard on expiration as a result of airway obstruction. Infants are more likely to wheeze than are older children, as a result of differing lung mechanics. Obstruction of airflow is affected by both airway size and compliance of the infant lung. Resistance to airflow through a tube is inversely related to the radius of the tube to the 4th power. In children younger than 5 yr, small-caliber peripheral airways can contribute up to 50% of the total airway resistance. Marginal additional narrowing, such as that caused by inflammation related to viral infection, is then more likely to result in wheezing.

Infant chest wall compliance is also quite high, thus the inward pressure produced in normal expiration subjects the intrathoracic airways to collapse. Differences in tracheal cartilage and airway smooth muscle tone increase the collapsibility of the infant airways in comparison with older children. These mechanisms combine to make the infant more susceptible to airway obstruction, increased resistance, and subsequent wheezing. The mechanical portion of the infant propensity to wheeze resolves with normal growth and muscular development.

Although wheezing in infants most frequently results from inflammation due to acute viral infections, there are many potential causes of wheezing (Table 418.1).

Acute Bronchiolitis

Acute bronchiolitis is a diagnostic term used to describe the clinical picture produced by several different viral lower respiratory tract infections in infants and very young children. The respiratory findings observed in bronchiolitis include tachypnea, wheezing, crackles, and rhonchi which result from inflammation of the small airways (Fig. 418.1). Despite its commonality, a universal set of diagnostic criteria for bronchiolitis does not exist, with significant disagreement about the upper age limit for appropriate use of the diagnosis. Some clinicians restrict the term to children younger than 1 yr, and others extend it to the age of 2 yr or beyond.

The pathophysiology of acute bronchiolitis is characterized by bronchiolar obstruction with edema, mucus, and cellular debris (see Fig. 418.1). Resistance in the small air passages is increased during both inspiration and exhalation, but because the radius of an airway is smaller during expiration, the resultant respiratory obstruction leads to expiratory wheezing, air trapping, and lung hyperinflation. If obstruction becomes complete, trapped distal air will be resorbed and the child will develop atelectasis. Hypoxemia is a consequence of ventilation-perfusion mismatch. With severe obstructive disease hypercapnia can develop.

Respiratory syncytial virus (RSV) is responsible for more than 50% of cases of bronchiolitis in most reports. Other agents include human metapneumovirus, rhinovirus, parainfluenza, influenza, bocavirus, and adenovirus. Viral coinfection is reported to impact severity and clinical manifestations, although its significance remains contested. Respiratory viruses can be identified in more than one third of asymptomatic patients younger than the age of 1 yr, calling into question the specificity of current tests for active infection. Although bacterial pneumonia is sometimes confused clinically with bronchiolitis, viral bronchiolitis is rarely followed by bacterial superinfection.

Well over 100,000 young children are hospitalized annually in the United States with the diagnosis of bronchiolitis, making it the most common diagnosis resulting in hospitalization for children younger than 1 yr of age in the United States over the past several decades. The increasing rates of hospitalization for bronchiolitis observed from 1980 to 1996 (thought to reflect increased attendance of infants in daycare centers, changes in criteria for hospital admission linked to pulse oximetry use, and/or improved survival of premature infants and other children at risk for severe disease) have not continued. Hospitalization rates have been stable in subsequent years despite introduction and routine use of RSV immunoprophylaxis in high-risk populations.

Table 418.1	Differential Diagnosis of Wheezing in Infancy

INFECTION
Viral
Respiratory syncytial virus
Human metapneumovirus
Parainfluenza
Adenovirus
Influenza
Rhinovirus
Bocavirus
Coronavirus
Enterovirus
Other
Chlamydia trachomatis
Tuberculosis
Histoplasmosis
Papillomatosis

ASTHMA

ANATOMIC ABNORMALITIES
Central Airway Abnormalities
Malacia of the larynx, trachea, and/or bronchi
Laryngeal or tracheal web
Tracheoesophageal fistula (specifically H-type fistula)
Laryngeal cleft (resulting in aspiration)
Extrinsic Airway Anomalies Resulting in Airway Compression
Vascular ring or sling
Mediastinal lymphadenopathy from infection or tumor
Mediastinal mass or tumor
Esophageal foreign body
Intrinsic Airway Anomalies
Airway hemangioma, other tumor
Congenital pulmonary airway malformation (cystic adenomatoid malformation)
Bronchial or lung cyst
Congenital lobar emphysema
Aberrant tracheal bronchus
Sequestration
Congenital heart disease with left-to-right shunt (increased pulmonary edema)
Foreign body
Immunodeficiency States
Immunoglobulin A deficiency
B-cell deficiencies
AIDS
Bronchiectasis

MUCOCILIARY CLEARANCE DISORDERS
Cystic fibrosis
Primary ciliary dyskinesia
Bronchiectasis

ASPIRATION SYNDROMES
Gastroesophageal reflux disease
Pharyngeal/swallow dysfunction

OTHER
Bronchopulmonary dysplasia
Eosinophilic granulomatosis with polyangiitis
Interstitial lung disease, including bronchiolitis obliterans
Heart failure
Anaphylaxis
Inhalation injury—burns

Bronchiolitis is more common in males, those exposed to second-hand tobacco smoke, those who have not been breastfed, and those living in crowded conditions. Risk is also higher for infants with mothers who smoked during pregnancy. Older family members, including older siblings, are a common source of infection; they might experience only minor upper respiratory symptoms (colds) given that bronchiolar edema may be less clinically apparent as airway size increases.

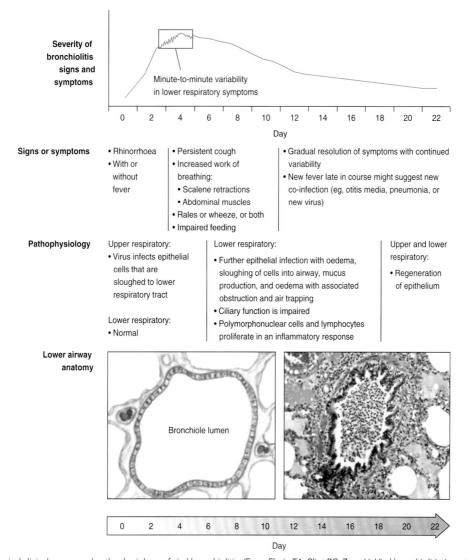

Fig. 418.1 Typical clinical course and pathophysiology of viral bronchiolitis. *(From Florin TA, Plint PC, Zorc JJ: Viral bronchiolitis*, Lancet *389:211–224, 2017 [Fig. 1, p. 212]).*

Asthma (see Chapter 169) is another important cause of wheezing, and the possibility of this diagnosis complicates the treatment of young children with bronchiolitis, although accurate diagnosis of asthma in the very young can be difficult. In prospective, longitudinal population cohort studies of infants, up to half of the cohort experienced a wheezing illness prior to school age, although when followed into adulthood only about 5–8% of patients prove to have asthma. In the largest U.S. cohort, 3 patterns of infant wheezing were proposed: transient early wheezing, comprising about 20% of the cohort, characterized by lower lung function at birth which improves with growth resulting in resolution of wheezing by age 3; persistent wheezing, comprising about 14% of the cohort, characterized by declining lung function and wheezing before and after age 3; and late-onset wheezing, comprising 15% of the cohort, characterized by relatively stable lung function and wheezing that does not begin until after age 3. The remaining 50% of the population did not suffer a wheezing illness. Following the cohort into adulthood revealed continued declines in the rates of persistent symptoms. Similar patterns are also seen in birth cohort studies in other countries.

Multiple studies attempting to predict which infants suffering from early wheezing illnesses will go on to have asthma in later life have failed to achieve discriminant validity. Interestingly, in both U.S. and U.K. prospective cohorts, wheezing with an onset *after* the first 18-36 mo of life is one of the strongest predictors of eventual asthma in both cohorts. Other proposed risk factors for persistent wheezing include parental history of asthma and allergies, maternal smoking, persistent rhinitis (apart from acute upper respiratory tract infections), allergen sensitization, eczema, and peripheral eosinophilia, although no single factor is strongly discriminative. Despite several randomized trials, there is no evidence that early administration of inhaled corticosteroids to high-risk populations can prevent the development of asthma.

CLINICAL MANIFESTATIONS
History and Physical Examination
The initial history of a wheezing infant should describe the recent event including onset, duration, and associated factors (Table 418.2). *Birth history* includes weeks of gestation, neonatal complications including history of intubation or oxygen requirement, maternal complications, and prenatal smoke exposure. Past medical history includes any comorbid conditions. *Family history* of cystic fibrosis, immunodeficiencies, asthma in a first-degree relative, or any other recurrent respiratory conditions

in children should be obtained. *Social history* should include any second-hand tobacco or other smoke exposure, daycare exposure, number of siblings, pets, and concerns regarding home environment (e.g., dust mites, construction dust, heating and cooling techniques, mold, cockroaches). The patient's growth chart should be reviewed for signs of failure to thrive.

Acute bronchiolitis is usually preceded by exposure to contacts with a minor respiratory illness within the previous week (see Fig. 418.1). The infant first develops signs of upper respiratory tract infection with sneezing and clear rhinorrhea. This may be accompanied by diminished appetite and fever. Gradually, respiratory distress ensues, with paroxysmal cough, dyspnea, and irritability. The infant is often tachypneic, which can interfere with feeding. Apnea may precede lower respiratory signs early in the disease, particularly with very young infants. Term infants at a postconceptual age of <44 wk and preterm infants at postconceptual age <48 wk are at highest risk for *apneic* events.

On physical examination, evaluation of the patient's vital signs with special attention to the respiratory rate and oxygen saturation is an important initial step. The exam is often dominated by wheezing and crackles. Expiratory time may be prolonged. Work of breathing may be markedly increased, with nasal flaring and retractions. *Complete obstruction to airflow can eliminate the turbulence that causes wheezing; thus the lack of audible wheezing is not reassuring if the infant shows other signs of respiratory distress.* Poorly audible breath sounds suggest severe disease with nearly complete bronchiolar obstruction.

Diagnostic Evaluation

Evaluation of wheezing in infancy and early childhood depends on suspected etiology. The diagnosis of **acute bronchiolitis** is clinical, particularly in a previously healthy infant presenting with a first episode of wheezing following a period of upper respiratory symptoms. Chest radiography is not routinely indicated in children with suspected bronchiolitis. Areas of atelectasis associated with bronchiolitis are often observed on chest radiographs and may be difficult to distinguish from bacterial pneumonia; as a result, obtaining chest radiography in a patient whose clinical course and exam are consistent with bronchiolitis may encourage unnecessary antibiotic use. Laboratory testing is also not routinely indicated; the white blood cell and differential counts are

Table 418.2	Pertinent Medical History in the Wheezing Infant

Did the onset of symptoms begin at birth or thereafter?
Is the infant a noisy breather, and when is it most prominent?
Is the noisy breathing present on inspiration, expiration, or both?
Is there a history of cough apart from wheezing?
Was there an earlier lower respiratory tract infection?
Is there a history of recurrent upper or lower respiratory tract infections?
Have there been any emergency department visits, hospitalizations, or intensive care unit admissions for respiratory distress?
Is there a history of eczema?
Does the infant cough after crying or cough at night?
How is the infant growing and developing?
Is there associated failure to thrive?
Is there a history of electrolyte abnormalities?
Are there signs of intestinal malabsorption including frequent, greasy, or oily stools?
Is there a maternal history of genital herpes simplex virus infection?
What was the gestational age at delivery?
Was the patient intubated as a neonate?
Does the infant bottle-feed in the bed or the crib, especially in a propped position?
Are there any feeding difficulties including choking, gagging, arching, or vomiting with feeds?
Is there any new food exposure?
Is there a toddler in the home or lapse in supervision in which foreign body aspiration could have occurred?
Change in caregivers or chance of nonaccidental trauma?

usually normal and are not predictive of bacterial superinfection. Viral testing (polymerase chain reaction, or rapid immunofluorescence) is not routinely recommended in the diagnosis of bronchiolitis but may be helpful if such testing prevents more invasive evaluations. Concurrent serious bacterial infection (sepsis, pneumonia, meningitis) is unlikely, although confirmation of viral bronchiolitis may obviate the need for a sepsis evaluation in the young febrile infant. Otitis media may complicate bronchiolitis.

For young children with wheezing in whom the presentation does not clinically fit with the diagnosis of viral infection, including those without other signs of viral infection, with very severe presentation, or complicated clinical course, further workup should be considered and should be dictated by individual clinical context. Children with recurrent or refractory episodes of wheezing in infancy, particularly if associated with failure to thrive, may require evaluation for chronic disorders such as cystic fibrosis or immunodeficiency.

Treatment

The treatment of children with viral **bronchiolitis** is supportive management. Those who are experiencing respiratory distress (hypoxia, inability to feed, apnea, extreme tachypnea) should be hospitalized. Risk factors for severe disease include younger age, preterm birth, or underlying comorbidity such as cardiovascular, pulmonary, neurologic, or immunologic disease. Hypoxemic children should receive supplemental oxygen. There is a developing consensus surrounding target oxygen saturations; national guidelines in the United States propose a threshold of 90%. Oxygen can be administered via a number of delivery devices, and some children with severe disease may require positive pressure ventilation. High-flow nasal cannula is a noninvasive mode of oxygen delivery capable of providing some positive end expiratory pressure, particularly in young children. Some use high flow as rescue therapy in patients who do not respond to standard care. The utility of high-flow nasal cannula in avoiding intubation in some children and reducing the duration of required supplemental oxygen is being actively explored because current data are mixed.

Some children may also require support with supplemental hydration. Fluid can be administered intravenously or enterally via nasogastric tube, with some preference given to the latter due to an association between better outcomes and continued provision of enteral nutrition. If intravenous fluids are administered, care should be taken to use isotonic fluids due to risk of hyponatremia. Frequent suctioning of nasal and oral secretions often provides relief of distress and improves work of breathing and ability to feed, although this should be limited to the nares or oropharynx because deep tracheal suctioning does not provide additional benefit. Chest physiotherapy has been extensively evaluated and provides *no benefit* to children with bronchiolitis.

Pharmacologic agents have largely proven *ineffective* in the management of bronchiolitis. Cochrane reviews have failed to demonstrate any impact on clinical outcomes with use of albuterol or corticosteroids in bronchiolitis; neither are currently recommended for management. Response to bronchodilators is unlikely and unpredictable in children younger than 1 yr, and there is no validated method of assessing response in the clinical setting. The use of inhaled or oral steroids in very young children with wheezing has not been shown to prevent the progression of childhood wheezing or development of asthma. There is debate over the use of hypertonic saline in children with bronchiolitis, although most studies and meta-analyses fail to demonstrate any benefit. Racemic epinephrine has not been found to improve length of stay or clinical outcomes among inpatients with bronchiolitis, although there is some evidence to suggest that it may reduce risk of hospitalization when used in the outpatient setting. Ribavirin, the only currently available antiviral medication targeting RSV, is also *not* currently recommended, because of minimal impact on disease outcomes, and because it is costly, difficulty to administer, and associated with important toxicities.

PROGNOSIS

Infants with **acute bronchiolitis** are at highest risk for further respiratory compromise in the first 72 hours after onset of cough and dyspnea. The case fatality rate is <1% in developed countries, with death attributable to respiratory arrest and/or failure or severe dehydration and electrolyte disturbances. *A majority of deaths due to bronchiolitis occur in children with complex medical conditions or comorbidities such as bronchopulmonary dysplasia, congenital heart disease, or immunodeficiency. The* median duration of symptoms in ambulatory patients is approximately 14 days; 10% may be symptomatic for 3 wk. Severe lower respiratory tract infection at an early age has been identified as a possible risk factor for the development of asthma, although most children with early childhood wheezing will not go on to suffer from asthma. It is unclear whether viral infections causing bronchiolitis incite an immune response that manifests as asthma later in life or whether those infants have an inherent predilection for asthma that is first manifested as viral bronchiolitis.

PREVENTION

Meticulous hand hygiene is the best measure to prevent transmission of the viruses responsible for bronchiolitis. For high-risk populations, **palivizumab**, an intramuscular monoclonal antibody to the RSV F protein, may be given as a prophylactic agent. Palivizumab has been demonstrated to reduce risk of hospitalization due to RSV bronchiolitis in certain populations. It has not been shown to decrease mortality and does not protect against bronchiolitis caused by other viruses and is also quite costly. As a result, there is some controversy surrounding which populations should receive palivizumab. U.S. guidelines suggest use for children born at <29-wk completed gestation or those with significant heart disease or chronic lung disease of prematurity, through the 1st or 2nd (for those with persistent chronic lung disease of prematurity) yr of life. Prophylaxis may be considered in infants with neuromuscular disease and immunocompromised states. The development of an effective preventive strategy available at a lower cost would be particularly advantageous in developing nations, where access to care and intervention for severe bronchiolitis are more limited.

Bibliography is available at Expert Consult.

418.2 Bronchitis

Lauren E. Camarda and Denise M. Goodman

Nonspecific bronchial inflammation is termed bronchitis and occurs in multiple childhood conditions. Acute bronchitis is a syndrome, usually viral in origin, with cough as a prominent feature.

Acute tracheobronchitis is a term used when the trachea is prominently involved. Nasopharyngitis may also be present, and a variety of viral and bacterial agents, such as those causing influenza, pertussis, and diphtheria, may be responsible. Isolation of common bacteria such as *Staphylococcus aureus* and *Streptococcus pneumoniae* from the sputum might not imply a bacterial cause that requires antibiotic therapy.

ACUTE BRONCHITIS
Clinical Manifestations

Acute bronchitis often follows a viral upper respiratory tract infection. It is more common in the winter when respiratory viral syndromes predominate. The tracheobronchial epithelium is invaded by the infectious agent, leading to activation of inflammatory cells and release of cytokines. Constitutional symptoms including fever and malaise follow. The tracheobronchial epithelium can become significantly damaged or hypersensitized, leading to a protracted cough lasting 1-3 wk.

The child first presents with nonspecific upper respiratory infectious symptoms, such as rhinitis. Three to 4 days later, a frequent, dry, hacking cough develops, which may or may not be productive. After several days, the sputum can become purulent, indicating leukocyte migration but not necessarily bacterial infection. Many children swallow their sputum which can produce emesis. Chest pain may be a prominent complaint in older children and is exacerbated by coughing. The mucus gradually thins, usually within 5-10 days, and then the cough gradually abates. The entire episode usually lasts about 2 wk and seldom longer than 3 wk.

Findings on physical examination vary with the age of the patient and stage of the disease. Early findings include no or low-grade fever and upper respiratory signs such as nasopharyngitis, conjunctivitis, and rhinitis. Auscultation of the chest may be unremarkable at this early phase. As the syndrome progresses and cough worsens, breath sounds become coarse, with coarse and fine crackles and scattered high-pitched wheezing. Chest radiographs are normal or can have increased bronchial markings.

The principal objective of the clinician is to exclude pertussis and pneumonia, which is more likely caused by bacterial agents requiring antibiotic therapy. Absence of abnormality of vital signs (tachycardia, tachypnea, fever) and a normal physical examination of the chest reduce the likelihood of pneumonia.

Differential Diagnosis

Persistent or recurrent symptoms should lead the clinician to consider entities other than acute bronchitis. Many entities manifest with cough as a prominent symptom (Table 418.3).

Treatment

There is no specific therapy for acute bronchitis. The disease is self-limited, and antibiotics, although often prescribed, do not hasten improvement. Frequent shifts in position can facilitate pulmonary drainage in infants. Older children are sometimes more comfortable with humidity, but this does not shorten the disease course. Cough suppressants can relieve symptoms but can also increase the risk of suppuration and inspissated secretions and therefore should be used judiciously. Antihistamines dry secretions and are not helpful; expectorants are likewise not indicated. Nonprescription cough and cold medicines should not be used in children younger than 4 yr of age, and their use is cautioned in children age 4-11 yr.

CHRONIC BRONCHITIS

Chronic bronchitis is well recognized in adults, formally defined as 3 mo or longer of productive cough each year for 2 or more yr. The disease can develop insidiously, with episodes of acute obstruction alternating with quiescent periods. Some predisposing conditions can lead to progression of airflow obstruction or chronic obstructive pulmonary disease, with

Table 418.3	Disorders With Cough as a Prominent Finding
CATEGORY	**DIAGNOSES**
Inflammatory	Asthma
Chronic pulmonary processes	Bronchopulmonary dysplasia Postinfectious bronchiectasis Cystic fibrosis Tracheomalacia or bronchomalacia Ciliary abnormalities Other chronic lung diseases
Other chronic disease or congenital disorders	Laryngeal cleft Swallowing disorders Gastroesophageal reflux Airway compression (such as a vascular ring or hemangioma) Congenital heart disease
Infectious or immune disorders	Immunodeficiency Eosinophilic lung disease Tuberculosis Allergy Sinusitis Tonsillitis or adenoiditis *Chlamydia, Ureaplasma* (infants) *Bordetella pertussis* *Mycoplasma pneumoniae*
Acquired	Foreign body aspiration, tracheal or esophageal

smoking as the major factor (up to 80% of patients have a smoking history). Other conditions include air pollution, occupational exposures, and repeated infections. In children, cystic fibrosis, bronchopulmonary dysplasia, and bronchiectasis must be ruled out.

The applicability of this definition to children is unclear. The existence of chronic bronchitis as a distinct entity in children is controversial. Like adults, children with chronic inflammatory diseases or those with toxic exposures can develop damaged pulmonary epithelium. Thus chronic or recurring cough in children should lead the clinician to search for underlying pulmonary or systemic disorders (see Table 418.3). One proposed entity that shares characteristics with asthma and other forms of suppurative lung disease is persistent or protracted bacterial bronchitis. Protracted bacterial bronchitis is defined as a chronic (>3 wk) wet cough, characterized by bacterial counts of 10^4 colony-forming units/mL or greater from bronchoalveolar lavage and resolution of cough within 2 wk of treatment with antimicrobial therapy.

CIGARETTE SMOKING AND AIR POLLUTION

Exposure to environmental irritants, such as tobacco smoke and air pollution, can incite or aggravate cough. There is a well-established association between tobacco exposure and pulmonary disease, including bronchitis and wheezing. This can occur through cigarette smoking or by exposure to passive smoke. Marijuana smoke and inhalants are other irritants sometimes overlooked when eliciting a history.

A number of pollutants compromise lung development and likely precipitate lung disease, including particulate matter, ozone, acid vapor, and nitrogen dioxide. Proximity to motor vehicle traffic is an important source of these pollutants. Because these substances coexist in the atmosphere, the relative contribution of any one to pulmonary symptoms is difficult to discern.

Bibliography is available at Expert Consult.

Chapter **419**
Plastic Bronchitis
Brett J. Bordini

第四百一十九章
塑型性支气管炎

中文导读

本章介绍了塑型性支气管炎的流行病学特点、发病机制、临床表现、诊断、治疗方法、并发症和预后情况。介绍了引起塑型性支气管炎的相关疾病。塑型性支气管炎有两种病理类型：1型为炎症性塑型，与炎症及肺部感染性疾病有关；2型为无细胞性塑型，与结构性心脏病手术有关。塑型性支气管炎的临床表现包括咳嗽、呼吸困难、喘息、胸膜炎样胸痛、低氧血症、呼吸窘迫。诊断包括咯出或内镜下发现较大的气管支气管塑型、相关疾病史、体格检查异常、胸片、支气管镜检查、塑型的组织学。治疗包括取出塑型、减轻气道炎症、降低复杂先天性心脏病患者的中心静脉压、选择性淋巴管栓堵及心脏移植。

Plastic bronchitis is a rare condition characterized by recurrent episodes of airway obstruction secondary to the formation of large proteinaceous branching casts that take on the shape of and obstruct the tracheobronchial tree. It is not a single disease entity, but rather represents a state of altered respiratory epithelial function and is most frequently encountered in the setting of underlying pulmonary or cardiac disease, although plastic bronchitis may also arise in lymphatic disorders, pulmonary infections, and the acute chest syndrome of sickle cell disease (Table 419.1). In comparison with the smaller bronchial and bronchiolar casts seen with mucus plugging, the lesions of plastic bronchitis are more extensive, with casts that can outline large segments of the airway to the level of the terminal bronchioles (Fig. 419.1). These casts may be spontaneously expectorated or may require bronchoscopic removal for relief of potentially fatal airway obstruction. Cast composition varies, although it typically consists of either a fibrin-predominant or mucin-predominant laminated matrix with or without inflammatory cell infiltration. Plastic bronchitis may be classified according to an associated disease, the cast histology, or a combination.

Table 419.1	Conditions Associated With Plastic Bronchitis

PROVEN CONDITIONS
Congenital heart disease with Fontan physiology
Pulmonary lymphatic anomalies
Influenza A pulmonary infection

POSSIBLE CONDITIONS
Toxic inhalation
Sickle cell acute chest syndrome
Hypersecretory and near-fatal asthma (eosinophilic casts)

UNLIKELY AND UNPROVEN CONDITIONS
Cystic fibrosis
Chronic obstructive pulmonary disease
Bronchiectasis
Bacterial pneumonia

From Rubin BK: Plastic bronchitis, *Clin Chest Med* 37:405–408, 2016 (Box 1, p. 406).

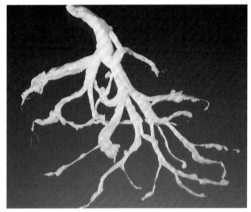

Fig. 419.1 Tracheobronchial casts following bronchoscopic extraction. Casts show branched architecture corresponding to the bronchial tree. *(From Corrin B, Nicholson AG: Pathology of the lungs, ed 3, London, 2011, Churchill Livingstone. Fig 3.20.)*

EPIDEMIOLOGY

Plastic bronchitis is rare, and its true prevalence in the pediatric population is not known but is estimated to be 6.8 cases per 100,000 patients. Prevalence does vary in relation to the underlying associated disease state, with rates as high as 4–14% estimated in patients who have undergone staged palliation of complex congenital heart disease and much lower rates seen complicating asthma and atopic disease. A slight male predominance exists for cast formation in the setting of structural heart disease, whereas cast formation in the setting of asthma and atopic disease demonstrates a female predominance. Children with single-ventricle Fontan physiology are at high risk for developing plastic bronchitis.

PATHOGENESIS

The mechanism of cast formation is unclear, although it is believed to vary based on the underlying disease association and cast type. One classification system differentiates type 1 inflammatory casts, composed primarily of fibrin with neutrophilic or more often eosinophilic infiltration, and type 2 acellular casts, composed primarily of mucin with little to no cellular infiltration. Type 1 casts tend to be associated with inflammatory and infectious disorders of the lung, whereas type 2 casts tend to be associated with surgically palliated structural heart disease, particularly single ventricle lesions. However, these distinctions are not absolute; patients with structural heart disease can have fibrin-predominant casts, and patients with asthma or atopic disease can have mucin-predominant casts, with both mucin casts and fibrin casts demonstrating various degrees of cellular infiltration.

Cast formation in the setting of structural heart disease may result from alterations in pulmonary blood flow or lymphatic drainage, particularly following staged surgical palliation. Under these circumstances, increased central venous pressure is believed to compromise the integrity of the bronchial mucosa, impeding lymphatic flow and resulting in the development of collateral lymphatic vessels and potentially of lymphoalveolar fistulae that may exude proteinaceous material into the airway lumen.

CLINICAL MANIFESTATIONS

Patients with plastic bronchitis may present with cough, dyspnea, wheeze, or pleuritic chest pain. Depending on the degree of airway obstruction, patients may be hypoxemic or in severe respiratory distress. The expectoration of large, branched casts that are often tan in color and rubbery in consistency is pathognomonic for plastic bronchitis. Lung examination may reveal diminished breath sounds or wheezing in the affected area. Rarely, auscultation may reveal a sound similar to a flag flapping in the wind *(bruit de drapeau)*, believed to be related to the free end of a cast striking the bronchial wall during inspiration or expiration. Further examination may provide clues to underlying comorbidities.

DIAGNOSIS

The expectoration or endoscopic discovery of large tracheobronchial casts is pathognomonic for plastic bronchitis. History should be directed at assessing for conditions known to have an associated risk of tracheobronchial cast formation, such as uncorrected or surgically palliated complex congenital heart disease (Fontan physiology); a history of atopic disease or asthma; lymphatic disorders such as Noonan syndrome, Turner syndrome, lymphangiectasia, and yellow nail syndrome; sickle cell disease; and infectious exposures, particularly to tuberculosis or atypical mycobacteria. Other predisposing conditions include cystic fibrosis, allergic bronchopulmonary aspergillosis, bronchiectasis, toxic inhalants, and granulomatous lung diseases.

Physical examination may provide indications of an underlying diagnosis. Digital clubbing of the fingers or toes may suggest long-standing hypoxemia associated with cardiac or pulmonary disease. Cardiac examination may provide information suggesting the presence of unrecognized structural heart disease.

Chest radiography may demonstrate collapse of the involved areas of the lung or areas of bronchiectasis distal to sites of long-standing obstruction.

There should be a high index of suspicion for plastic bronchitis in patients with known comorbidities who present with sudden respiratory decompensation. In the absence of cast expectoration, direct visualization of casts via bronchoscopy is required for diagnosis and is potentially therapeutic in relieving airway obstruction. Cast histology should be defined so as to allow for specific therapies directed at alleviating residual obstruction or preventing recurrence. In particular, the predominant component of the cast's laminated matrix—either fibrin or mucin—should be defined, and signs of inflammation or infiltration, such as the presence of neutrophils, eosinophils, or Charcot-Leyden crystals, should be documented.

TREATMENT

Treatment is directed at correcting the underlying condition associated with the development of plastic bronchitis, at relieving acute airway obstruction secondary to the presence of casts, and at preventing the development of further casts. Rigid or flexible bronchoscopy is typically required for cast removal, and if the predominant content of the cast is known, therapy with either fibrinolytics such as tissue plasminogen activator or mucolytics such as *N*-acetylcysteine or deoxyribonuclease may be considered as an adjunct to direct removal. Aerosolized heparin or mucolytics have also been used for treatment or prevention of recurrence, with varying success.

In the setting of inflammatory airway disease, additional preventive measures include the appropriate use of bronchodilators as indicated, as well as inhaled or systemic corticosteroids, low-dose azithromycin, and leukotriene inhibitors to minimize airway inflammation.

In patients with surgically palliated complex congenital heart disease, measures aimed at decreasing central venous pressure, such as sildenafil or Fontan conduit fenestration, have had varied success. Lymphangi-ography may be undertaken to identify aberrant lymphatic vessels contributing to plastic bronchitis in the setting of congenital heart disease or lymphangitic disorders, and MRI-guided selective lymphatic emboliza-tion of these channels has led to resolution of plastic bronchitis while preserving central lymphatic flow. Cardiac transplantation typically results in resolution of plastic bronchitis in the setting of repaired complex congenital heart disease.

COMPLICATIONS AND PROGNOSIS

Prognosis is related primarily to the underlying condition associated with the development of plastic bronchitis. Patients whose plastic bronchitis is related to surgically palliated complex congenital heart disease are at high risk for plastic bronchitis-related mortality. Mortality can be high if casts obstruct significant portions of the airway, regardless of underlying etiology. Mortality estimates vary from 6% to 50% in the setting of asthma or atopic disease and from 14% to 50% in the setting of complex congenital heart disease, with central airway obstruction leading to death in the majority of patients.

Bibliography is available at Expert Consult.

Chapter 420
Emphysema and Overinflation

Steven R. Boas and Glenna B. Winnie

第四百二十章
肺气肿和肺过度充气

中文导读

　　本章介绍了肺局部阻塞性过度充气及广泛阻塞性过度充气。详细描述了肺气肿及过度充气的病理生理机制；局部阻塞性过度充气部分描述了单侧透明肺、Swyer-James综合征或Macleod综合征、先天性大叶性肺气肿及肺血管发育异常，介绍了不同疾病的病因、临床表现、影像学异常表现及治疗方法；介绍了广泛阻塞性过度充气的病因、病理学、临床特点及诊断方法，具体描述了肺大疱的病因、病理机制及治疗原则，描述了皮下气肿的病因、临床表现及治疗原则。

Pulmonary emphysema consists of distention of air spaces with irrevers-ible disruption of the alveolar septa. It can involve part or all of a lung. **Overinflation** is distention with or without alveolar rupture and is often reversible. **Compensatory overinflation** can be acute or chronic and occurs in normally functioning pulmonary tissue when, for any reason, a sizable portion of the lung is removed or becomes partially or completely airless, which can occur with pneumonia, atelectasis, empyema, and pneumothorax. **Obstructive overinflation** results from partial obstruction of a bronchus or bronchiole, when it becomes more difficult for air to leave the alveoli than to enter. Air gradually accumulates distal to the obstruction, the so-called bypass, ball-valve, or check-valve type of obstruction.

LOCALIZED OBSTRUCTIVE OVERINFLATION

When a ball-valve type of obstruction partially occludes the main stem bronchus, the entire lung becomes overinflated; individual lobes are affected when the obstruction is in lobar bronchi. Segments or subseg-ments are affected when their individual bronchi are blocked. When most or all of a lobe is involved, the percussion note is hyperresonant over the area and the breath sounds are decreased in intensity. The distended lung can extend across the mediastinum into the opposite hemithorax. Under fluoroscopic scrutiny during exhalation, the over-inflated area does not decrease and the heart and the mediastinum shift to the opposite side because the unobstructed lung empties normally.

Unilateral Hyperlucent Lung

The differential diagnosis for this resultant **unilateral hyperlucent lung** is quite broad and can involve the lung parenchyma, airways, pulmonary vasculature, chest wall (see Chapter 445), and mediastinum. Localized obstructions that can be responsible for overinflation include airway foreign bodies and the inflammatory reaction to them (see Chapter 414), abnormally thick mucus (cystic fibrosis, Chapter 432), endobron-chial tuberculosis or tuberculosis of the tracheobronchial lymph nodes (see Chapter 242), and endobronchial or mediastinal tumors.

Patients with unilateral hyperlucent lung can present with clinical manifestations of pneumonia, but in some patients the condition is discovered only when a chest radiograph is obtained for an unrelated reason. A few patients have hemoptysis. Physical findings can include hyperresonance and a small lung with the mediastinum shifted toward the more abnormal lung.

Swyer-James or Macleod Syndrome

The condition is thought to result from an insult to the lower respiratory tract following most commonly adenovirus (see Chapter 289) or respira-tory syncytial virus (see Chapter 287), *Mycoplasma pneumoniae* (see Chapter 250), or measles (see Chapter 273). The infection can cause pulmonary vascular hypoplasia with resultant hypoperfusion leading to unilateral hyperlucent lung (underdevelopment). Clinically, children with this condition often have chronic cough, recurrent pneumonia, hemoptysis, and wheezing, although some are asymptomatic. Some patients show a classic mediastinal shift away from the lesion with exhalation. CT scanning or bronchography can often demonstrate bronchiectasis. Thorascopic evaluation may be useful. The triad of unilateral hyperlucent lung, diffusely decreased ventilation, and matching decreased perfusion of the affected lung supports the diagnosis. In some patients, previous chest radiographs have been normal or have shown only an acute pneumonia, suggesting that a hyperlucent lung is an acquired lesion. For those with recurrent infection or severe lung destruction, treatment may include immunization with influenza and pneumococcal vaccines, as well as surgical resection. However, without treatment, some individuals may become less symptomatic with time.

Congenital Lobar Emphysema (Congenital Large Hyperlucent Lobe)

Congenital lobar emphysema (CLE) can result in severe respiratory distress in early infancy and can be caused by localized obstruction. Familial occurrence has been reported. In 50% of cases, a cause of CLE can be identified. Congenital deficiency of the bronchial cartilage, external compression by aberrant vessels, bronchial stenosis, redundant bronchial mucosal flaps, and kinking of the bronchus caused by herniation into the mediastinum have been described as leading to bronchial obstruction and subsequent CLE and commonly affect the left upper lobe.

Clinical manifestations usually become apparent in the neonatal period but are delayed for as long as 5-6 yr in 5% of patients. Many cases are diagnosed by antenatal ultrasonography. Infants with prenatally diagnosed cases are not always symptomatic at birth. In some patients, CLE remains undiagnosed until school age or beyond. Clinical signs range from mild tachypnea and wheeze to severe dyspnea with cyanosis. CLE can affect one or more lobes; it affects the upper and middle lobes, and the left upper lobe is the most common site. The affected lobe is essentially nonfunctional because of the overdistention, and atelectasis of the ipsilateral normal lung can ensue. With further distention, the mediastinum is shifted to the contralateral side, with impaired function seen as well (Fig. 420.1). A radiolucent lobe and a mediastinal shift are often revealed by radiographic examination. A CT scan can demonstrate the aberrant anatomy of the lesion, and MRI or MR angiography can demonstrate any vascular lesions, which might be causing extraluminal compression. Nuclear imaging studies are useful to demonstrate perfusion defects in the affected lobe. Fig. 420.2 outlines evaluation of an infant

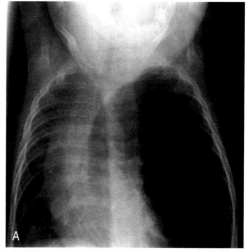
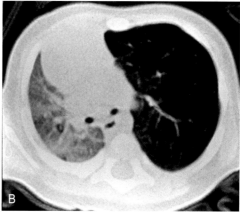

Fig. 420.1 (A) Chest x-ray and (B) computed tomography scan of a congenital large hyperlucent lobe (congenital lobar emphysema). *(From Bush A, Abel R, Chitty L, et al: Congenital lung disease. In Wilmott RW, Deterding R, Li A, et al., editors: Kendig's disorders of the respiratory tract in children, 9th ed. Elsevier, Philadelphia, 2019. Fig. 18.32.)*

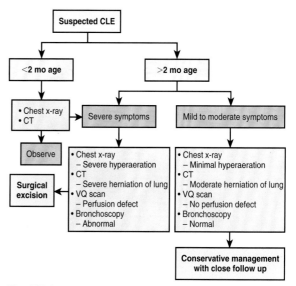

Fig. 420.2 Algorithm for evaluation and treatment of congenital lobar emphysema *(CLE). (Adapted from Karnak I, Senocak ME, Ciftci AO, et al: Congenital lobar emphysema: diagnostic and therapeutic consid-erations, J Pediatr Surg 34:1347–1351, 1999, Fig. 4.)*

presenting with suspected CLE. The differential diagnosis includes pneumonia with or without an effusion, pneumothorax, and cystic adenomatoid malformation.

Treatment by immediate surgery and excision of the lobe may be lifesaving when cyanosis and severe respiratory distress are present, but some patients respond to medical treatment. Selective intubation of the unaffected lung may be of value. Some children with apparent CLE have reversible overinflation, without the classic alveolar septal rupture implied in the term *emphysema*. Bronchoscopy can reveal an endobronchial lesion.

Pulmonary Vascular Abnormalities

Unilateral hyperlucency may result from **unilateral pulmonary agenesis** (see Chapter 423) that typically presents in the neonatal period. Volume loss of the affected lung results in a mediastinal shift with hyperinflation of the contralateral lung. An **anomalous origin of the left pulmonary artery** (see Chapter 459), also known as a *pulmonary artery sling*, can impinge the right mainstem bronchus with resultant right-sided hyperinflation or atelectasis producing hyperlucency on either the ipsilateral or contralateral side. **Pulmonary venolobar syndrome** (see Chapter 453), also known as **scimitar syndrome**, can also result in a hyperlucent contralateral lung dependent on the extent of hypoplasia of the right lung.

GENERALIZED OBSTRUCTIVE OVERINFLATION

Acute generalized overinflation of the lung results from widespread involvement of the bronchioles and is usually reversible. It occurs more commonly in infants than in children and may be secondary to a number of clinical conditions including asthma, cystic fibrosis, acute bronchiolitis, interstitial pneumonitis, atypical forms of acute laryngotracheobronchitis, aspiration of zinc stearate powder, chronic passive congestion secondary to a congenital cardiac lesion, and miliary tuberculosis.

Pathology

In chronic overinflation, many of the alveoli are ruptured and communicate with one another, producing distended saccules. Air can also enter the interstitial tissue (i.e., interstitial emphysema), resulting in pneumothorax and pneumomediastinum (see Chapters 439 and 440).

Clinical Manifestations

Generalized obstructive overinflation is characterized by dyspnea, with difficulty in exhaling. The lungs become increasingly overdistended, and the chest remains expanded during exhalation. An increased respiratory rate and decreased respiratory excursion result from the overdistention of the alveoli and their inability to be emptied normally through the narrowed bronchioles. Air hunger is responsible for forced respiratory movements. Overaction of the accessory muscles of respiration results in retractions at the suprasternal notch, the supraclavicular spaces, the lower margin of the thorax, and the intercostal spaces. Unlike the flattened chest during inspiration and exhalation in cases of laryngeal obstruction, minimal reduction in the size of the overdistended chest during exhalation is observed. The percussion note is hyperresonant. On auscultation, the inspiratory phase is usually less prominent than the expiratory phase, which is prolonged and roughened. Fine or medium crackles may be heard. Cyanosis is more common in the severe cases.

Diagnosis

Radiographic and fluoroscopic examinations of the chest assist in establishing the diagnosis. Both leaves of the diaphragm are low and flattened, the ribs are farther apart than usual, and the lung fields are less dense. The movement of the diaphragm during exhalation is decreased, and the excursion of the low, flattened diaphragm in severe cases is barely discernible. The anteroposterior diameter of the chest is increased, and the sternum may be bowed outward.

Bullous Emphysema

Bullous emphysematous blebs or cysts (pneumatoceles) result from overdistention and rupture of alveoli during birth or shortly thereafter, or they may be sequelae of pneumonia and other infections. They have been observed in tuberculosis lesions during specific antibacterial therapy and in end stage cystic fibrosis lung disease. These emphysematous areas presumably result from rupture of distended alveoli, forming a single or multiloculated cavity. The cysts can become large and might contain some fluid; an air-fluid level may be demonstrated on the radiograph (Fig. 420.3). The cysts should be differentiated from pulmonary abscesses. In most cases, treatment is not required as the cysts disappear spontaneously within a few months, although they can persist for a yr or more. Aspiration or surgery is not indicated except in cases of severe respiratory and cardiac compromise.

Subcutaneous Emphysema

Subcutaneous emphysema results from any process that allows free air to enter into the subcutaneous tissue (Fig. 420.4). The most common causes include pneumothorax or pneumomediastinum (see Chapters

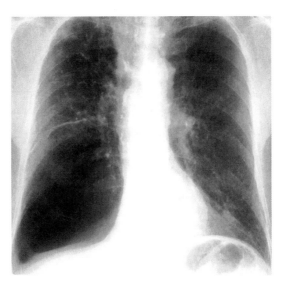

Fig. 420.3 Increased transradiancy in the right lower zone. A large emphysematous bulla occupies the lower half of the right lung, and the apical changes are in keeping with previous tuberculosis. *(From Padley SPG, Hansell DM: Imaging techniques. In Albert RK, Spiro SG, Jett JR, editors: Clinical respiratory medicine, ed 3, Philadelphia, 2008, Mosby, Fig. 1.48.)*

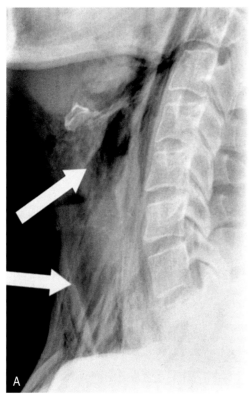
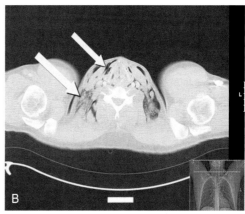

Fig. 420.4 A, Lateral X-ray of neck showing subcutaneous emphysema. **B,** Axial section CT neck/thorax showing subcutaneous emphysema and pneumomediastinum. *(From Zakaria R, Khwaja H: Subcutaneous emphysema in a case of infective sinusitis: a case report,* J Med Case Rep 4:235, *2010, Figs, 1 and 2.)*

439 and 440). In addition, it can be a complication of fracture of the orbit, which permits free air to escape from the nasal sinuses. In the neck and thorax, subcutaneous emphysema can follow tracheotomy, deep ulceration in the pharyngeal region, esophageal wounds, or any perforating lesion of the larynx or trachea. It is occasionally a complication of thoracentesis, asthma, or abdominal surgery. Rarely, air is formed in the subcutaneous tissues by gas-producing bacteria.

Tenderness over the site of emphysema and a crepitant quality on palpation of the skin are classic manifestations. Subcutaneous emphysema is usually a self-limited process and requires no specific treatment. Minimization of activities that can increase airway pressure (cough, performance of high-pressure pulmonary function testing maneuvers) is recommended. Resolution occurs by resorption of subcutaneous air after elimination of its source. Rarely, dangerous compression of the trachea by air in the surrounding soft tissue requires surgical intervention.

Bibliography is available at Expert Consult.

Chapter **421**
α₁-Antitrypsin Deficiency and Emphysema

Glenna B. Winnie and Steven R. Boas

第四百二十一章
α₁-抗胰蛋白酶缺乏症和肺气肿

中文导读

　　本章介绍了α₁-抗胰蛋白酶缺乏症的发病机制、临床表现、实验室检查、替代治疗及支持治疗方法。α₁-抗胰蛋白酶缺乏症的临床表现包括呼吸困难、喘息、咳嗽等慢性肺部症状，肺活检证实广泛的全小叶肺气肿，体格检查可见生长落后、胸廓前后径增宽、叩诊过清音、感染时出现爆裂音、杵状指/趾等；实验室检查包括血清免疫学α₁-抗胰蛋白酶水平测定、基因检测、胸片、肺部CT、肺功能检测；本病的治疗方法包括静脉注射和吸入α₁-抗胰蛋白酶替代物、肺移植及基因治疗；支持治疗包括积极治疗肺部感染、常规使用肺炎链球菌疫苗和流感疫苗、支气管舒张剂及避免吸烟等。

Homozygous deficiency of α₁-antitrypsin (α₁-AT) rarely produces lung disease in children, but it is an important cause of early-onset severe panacinar pulmonary emphysema in adults in the 3rd and 4th decades of life and a significant cause of liver disease in children (see Chapter 384.5). It is associated with panniculitis and vasculitis in adults.

PATHOGENESIS

The type and concentration of α₁-AT are inherited as a series of codominant alleles on chromosomal segment 14q31-32.3. (See Chapter 384.5 for a discussion of genotypes and liver disease.) The autosomal recessive deficiency affects 1 in 1,600-2,500 people, but it remains underdiagnosed. The highest risk for α₁-AT deficiency is found in whites, followed by Hispanics and blacks, with the lowest prevalence among Mexican Americans and little to no risk for Asians. Worldwide there are an estimated 116,000,000 carriers and 1,100,000 subjects with severe α₁-AT deficiency. The normal α₁-AT PiM protein is secreted by the liver into the circulation at a rate of approximately 34 mg/kg/day; it is also produced by lung epithelial cells and monocytes. Mutant protein is not produced (null) or is misfolded (PiZ and others); it can polymerize in the endoplasmic reticulum or be degraded, with subsequent low serum levels. Early adult-onset emphysema associated with α₁-AT deficiency occurs most commonly with PiZZ (mutation in *SERPINA1* gene), although Pi (null) (null) and, to less extent, other mutant Pi types such as SZ have been associated with emphysema.

α₁-AT and other serum antiproteases help to inactivate proteolytic enzymes released from dead bacteria or leukocytes in the lung. Deficiency of these antiproteases leads to an accumulation of proteolytic enzymes in the lung, resulting in destruction of pulmonary tissue with subsequent development of emphysema. Polymerized mutant protein in the lungs may also be proinflammatory, and there is evidence of increased oxidative stress. The concentration of proteases (elastase) in an individual's leukocytes may also be an important factor in determining the severity of clinical pulmonary disease with a given level of α₁-AT.

CLINICAL MANIFESTATIONS

Most patients who have the PiZZ defect have little or no detectable pulmonary disease during childhood. A few have early onset of chronic pulmonary symptoms, including dyspnea, wheezing, and cough, and panacinar emphysema has been documented by lung biopsy; it is probable that these findings occur secondarily to infection which caused inflammation with consequent early disease. Smoking increases the risk of emphysema in patients with mutant Pi types. Although newborn screening to identify children with PiZZ phenotype does not affect parental smoking habits, it does decrease smoking rates among affected adolescents.

Physical examination in *childhood* is usually normal. Affected children very rarely have growth failure, an increased anteroposterior diameter of the chest with a hyperresonant percussion note, crackles if there is active infection, and clubbing. Severe emphysema can depress the diaphragm, making the liver and spleen more easily palpable.

LABORATORY FINDINGS

Serum immunoassay measures low levels of α₁-AT; normal serum levels are ~80-220 mg/dL. Serum electrophoresis reveals the phenotype, and genotype is determined by polymerase chain reaction; whole gene sequencing is possible. In the rare patient with lung disease in adolescence, chest radiograph reveals overinflation with depressed diaphragms. Chest CT can show more hyperexpansion in the lower lung zones, with occasional bronchiectasis; CT densitometry can be a sensitive method to follow changes in lung disease. Lung function testing is usually normal in children, but it can show airflow obstruction and increased lung volumes, particularly in adolescents who smoke.

TREATMENT

Therapy for α_1-AT deficiency is intravenous replacement (augmentation) with enzyme derived from pooled human plasma. A level of 80 mg/dL is protective for emphysema. This target level for augmentation therapy is usually achieved with initial doses of 60 mg/kg IV weekly and results in the appearance of the transfused antiprotease in pulmonary lavage fluid. The Food and Drug Administration has approved the use of purified blood-derived human enzyme for ZZ and null-null patients. Replacement therapy is indicated for those with moderately severe obstructive lung disease (forced expiratory volume in 1 sec is 30–65% of predicted) or those with mild lung disease experiencing a rapid decline in lung function. Augmentation therapy is not indicated for persons with the PiMZ type who have pulmonary disease, because their disease is not from enzyme deficiency. Recombinant sources of α_1-AT are under development, but current products are rapidly cleared from the circulation when given intravenously; they may be useful for inhalation therapy. Inhalation of the plasma-derived product is under evaluation. Lung transplantation has been performed for end-stage disease. Multiple strategies for gene therapy are under development.

SUPPORTIVE THERAPY

Standard supportive therapy for chronic lung disease includes aggressive treatment of pulmonary infection, routine use of pneumococcal and influenza vaccines, bronchodilators, and advice about the serious risks of smoking. Such treatment is also indicated for asymptomatic family members found to have PiZZ or null-null phenotypes but not those with PiMZ type. The clinical significance of the PiSZ type is unclear, but nonspecific treatment is reasonable. All persons with low levels of serum antiprotease should be warned that the development of emphysema is partially mediated by environmental factors and that cigarette smoking is particularly deleterious. Although early identification of affected persons could help to prevent development of obstructive lung disease, population screening programs are being considered but are currently suspended.

Bibliography is available at Expert Consult.

Chapter **422**
Other Distal Airway Diseases
第四百二十二章
其他远端气道疾病

中文导读

本章主要介绍了闭塞性细支气管炎、滤泡性支气管炎和肺泡微石症。具体描述了闭塞性细支气管炎的流行病学、发病机制、临床表现、诊断、治疗和预后，介绍了闭塞性细支气管炎综合征的特点；描述了滤泡性支气管炎的临床特点、诊断、治疗和预后；描述了肺泡微石症的流行病学及病因、病理表现、临床特点、诊断、治疗和预后。

422.1 Bronchiolitis Obliterans
Steven R. Boas

EPIDEMIOLOGY

Bronchiolitis obliterans (BO) is a histopathologic diagnosis characterized by chronic obstructive lung disease of the bronchioles and smaller airways, resulting from an insult to the lower respiratory tract leading to inflammation and fibrosis of the small airways. In the nontransplant patient, BO most commonly occurs in the pediatric population after respiratory infections, particularly adenovirus (see Chapter 289), but also *Mycoplasma pneumoniae* (see Chapter 250), measles (see Chapter

273), *Legionella pneumophila* (see Chapter 235), influenza (see Chapter 285), and pertussis (see Chapter 224); other causes include inflammatory diseases (juvenile idiopathic arthritis, systemic lupus erythematosus [see Chapter 183], scleroderma [see Chapter 185], Stevens-Johnson syndrome [see Chapter 177]), and inhalation of toxic fumes or particulate exposure (NO_2, incinerator fly ash, NH_3, diacetyl flavorings from microwave popcorn, papaverine, fiberglass) (Table 422.1). Postinfection obliterans may be more common in the southern hemisphere and among persons of Asian descent. BO is also commonly seen in post lung or bone marrow transplant recipients.

Bronchiolitis obliterans syndrome (BOS) is a clinical diagnosis related to graft deterioration after transplantation defined as a progressive decline in lung function based on FEV1. The airway obstruction is generally irreversible. BOS is considered once other causes of airway obstruction are excluded. BOS is recognized as a long-term complication of both lung and bone marrow transplantation with more than one third of survivors of lung transplantation developing this disorder. Risk factors for the development of BOS include the presence of CMV pneumonitis, aspergillus colonization, primary graft dysfunction, gastroesophageal reflux, and community-acquired respiratory viruses, as well as prolonged transplantation ischemic time.

PATHOGENESIS

After the initial insult, inflammation affecting terminal bronchioles, respiratory bronchioles, and alveolar ducts can result in the obliteration of the airway lumen (Fig. 422.1). Epithelial damage resulting in abnormal repair is characteristic of BO. Complete or partial obstruction of the airway lumen can result in air trapping or atelectasis. Parenchymal

Table 422.1	Etiology of Bronchiolitis Obliterans

POSTINFECTION
Adenovirus types 3, 7, and 21
Influenza
Parainfluenza
Measles
Respiratory syncytial virus
Varicella
Mycoplasma pneumoniae

POSTTRANSPLANTATION
Chronic rejection of lung or heart/lung transplantation
Graft versus host disease associated with bone marrow
  transplantation

CONNECTIVE TISSUE DISEASE
Juvenile idiopathic arthritis
Sjögren syndrome
Systemic lupus erythematosus

TOXIC FUME INHALATION
NO_2
NH_3
Diacetyl flavorings (microwave popcorn)

CHRONIC HYPERSENSITIVITY PNEUMONITIS
Avian antigens
Mold

ASPIRATION
Stomach contents: gastroesophageal reflux
Foreign bodies

DRUGS
Penicillamine
Cocaine

STEVENS-JOHNSON SYNDROME
Idiopathic
Drug induced
Infection related

From Moonnumakal SP, Fan LL: Bronchiolitis obliterans in children, *Curr Opin Pediatr* 20:272–278, 2008.

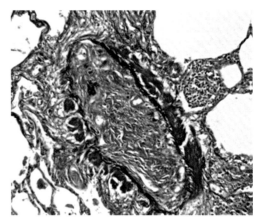

Fig. 422.1 Complete obliteration of airway lumen with fibromyxoid tissue in lung transplant recipient with bronchiolitis obliterans. *(From Kurland G, Michelson P: Bronchiolitis obliterans in children,* Pediatr Pulmonol *39:193–208, 2005.)*

involvement is not seen. **Bronchiolitis obliterans organizing pneumonia (BOOP)** or what has also been termed **cryptogenic organizing pneumonia** is a histopathologic diagnosis. Although it is similar to many of the histologic features of BO, BOOP is also characterized by extension of the inflammatory process from distal alveolar ducts into alveoli with proliferation of fibroblasts (parenchymal involvement).

CLINICAL MANIFESTATIONS AND DIAGNOSIS

Cough, fever, cyanosis, dyspnea, chest pain, and respiratory distress followed by initial improvement may be the initial signs of BO. In this phase, BO is easily confused with pneumonia, bronchitis, or bronchiolitis. Progression of the disease can ensue, with increasing dyspnea, chronic cough, sputum production, and wheezing. Physical examination findings are usually nonspecific and can include wheezing, hypoxemia, and crackles. Chest radiographs may be relatively normal compared with the extent of physical findings but can demonstrate hyperlucency and patchy infiltrates. Occasionally, a Swyer-James syndrome (unilateral hyperlucent lung; see Chapter 420) develops. Pulmonary function tests demonstrate variable findings but typically show signs of airway obstruction with a variable degree of bronchodilator response although more commonly irreversible. Exercise testing shows reduced exercise capacity and impaired oxygen consumption. Ventilation-perfusion scans reveal a typical moth-eaten appearance of multiple matched defects in ventilation and perfusion. High-resolution chest CT often demonstrates patchy areas or a mosaic pattern of hyperlucency, air trapping, and bronchiectasis (Fig. 422.2). Table 422.2 provides an overview of CT findings of BO and related disorders. Physical and radiologic signs can wax and wane over weeks or months. Open lung biopsy or transbronchial biopsy remains the best means of establishing the diagnosis of BO or BOOP.

TREATMENT

No definitive therapy exists for BO. Administration of corticosteroids may be beneficial. Immunomodulatory agents, such as sirolimus, tacrolimus, aerosolized cyclosporine, hydroxychloroquine, and macrolide antibiotics, have been used in post–lung transplantation recipients with BO with variable success. Supportive measures with oxygen, antibiotics for secondary infections, and bronchodilators are adjunct therapies. The role of gastroesophageal reflux and its association with BO has been raised, with treatment suggested whenever the diagnosis is made. Azithromycin may be effective in patients with BOS. For BOOP, use of oral corticosteroids for up to 1 yr has been advocated as first-line therapy for symptomatic and progressive disease. Patients with asymptomatic or nonprogressive BOOP can be observed.

PROGNOSIS

Some patients with BO experience rapid deterioration in their condition and die within weeks of the initial symptoms; most nontransplant patients

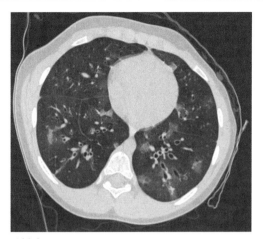

Fig. 422.2 High-resolution CT scan of the chest of a child with bronchiolitis obliterans demonstrating mosaic perfusion and vascular attenuation. Air-trapping is demonstrated by lack of increase in attention or decrease in lung volume in dependent lung. *(Image courtesy Alan Brody, MD, Cincinnati Children's Hospital Medical Center, Ohio.)*

survive with chronic disability. BO tends to be severe once progression ensues. In contrast to BO, a better prognosis exists for patients with BOOP, with complete recovery seen in many patients, although outcome depends on the underlying systemic disease. BOOP can relapse, especially if treatment duration is <1 yr; BOOP is amenable to repeat courses of oral corticosteroids. Unlike the more common idiopathic BOOP, progressive BOOP characterized by acute respiratory distress syndrome is rare but is aggressive in its clinical course, leading to death.

Bibliography is available at Expert Consult.

422.2 Follicular Bronchitis

Steven R. Boas

Follicular bronchitis is a lymphoproliferative lung disorder characterized by the presence of lymphoid follicles alongside the airways (bronchi or bronchioles) and infiltration of the walls of bronchi and bronchioles. Although the cause is unknown, an infectious etiology (viral, *L. pneumophila*; see Chapter 235) has been proposed. This disorder has been reported following lung transplant and in an HIV-positive child. It can occur in adults and children; in children, onset of symptoms generally occurs by 6 wk of age and peaks between 6 and 18 mo. Cough, moderate respiratory distress, fever, and fine crackles are common clinical findings. Fine crackles generally persist over time, and recurrence of symptoms is common. Chest radiographs may be relatively benign initially (air trapping, peribronchial thickening) but evolve into the typical interstitial pattern. Chest CT can show a fine reticular pattern, as well as bronchiectasis and centrilobular branching, but can also appear normal (see Table 422.2). Definitive diagnosis is made by open lung biopsy (Fig. 422.3). Treatment is limited, although some patients with follicular bronchitis respond to corticosteroid therapy. Prognosis is variable, with some patients having significant progression of pulmonary disease and others developing only mild obstructive airway disease. In children, it is generally associated with immunodeficiency; the differential diagnosis includes the pulmonary complications of HIV infection (see Chapter 302).

Bibliography is available at Expert Consult.

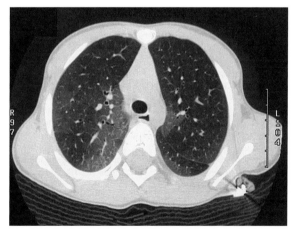

Fig. 422.3 Follicular bronchiolitis in a 3 yr old girl with mosaic attenuation and cylindrical bronchiectasis. CT findings suggested bronchiolitis obliterans, but a biopsy documented the presence of follicular bronchiolitis. *(From Long FR, Druhan SM, Kuhn JP: Diseases of the bronchi and pulmonary aeration. In Slovis TL, editor:* Caffey's pediatric diagnostic imaging, *ed 11, Philadelphia, 2008, Mosby, Fig. 73.71.)*

Table 422.2	High-Resolution CT Patterns in Child With Interstitial Lung Disease					
	STUDIES (N)	**GROUND-GLASS OPACITY**	**THICK SEPTA**	**NODULES**	**MOSAIC PATTERN**	**HONEYCOMBING**
Bronchiolitis obliterans	4	—	—	—	X	—
Nonspecific interstitial pneumonitis	6	X	—	—	—	X
Desquamative interstitial pneumonitis	4	X	—	—	—	X
Follicular bronchitis or neuroendocrine cell hyperplasia of infancy	4	X	—	—	X	—
Lymphocytic interstitial pneumonitis	4	—	—	X	—	—
Lymphangiomatosis	2	—	X	—	—	—
Lymphangiectasia	2	—	X	—	—	—
Pulmonary alveolar proteinosis	2	X	X	—	—	—

From Long FR: Interstitial lung disease. In Slovis TL, editor: *Caffey's pediatric diagnostic imaging*, ed 11, Philadelphia, 2008, Mosby, Table 74.1; original data from Lynch DA, Hay T, Newell JD Jr, et al: Pediatric diffuse lung disease: diagnosis and classification using high-resolution CT, *AJR Am J Roentgenol* 173:713–718, 1999, and Copley SJ, Coren M, Nicholson AG, et al: Diagnostic accuracy of thin-section CT and chest radiography of pediatric interstitial lung disease, *AJR Am J Roentgenol* 174:549–554, 2000.

422.3 Pulmonary Alveolar Microlithiasis

Steven R. Boas

Pulmonary alveolar microlithiasis (PAM) is a rare disease characterized by the formation of lamellar concretions of calcium phosphate or "microliths" within the alveoli, creating a classic pattern on the radiograph (Fig. 422.4).

EPIDEMIOLOGY AND ETIOLOGY

Although the mean age at time of diagnosis is in the mid-30s, the onset of the disease can occur in childhood and in newborns. PAM is inherited in an autosomal recessive disorder and is caused by a mutation in the type II sodium phosphate cotransporter NPT2b *(SCL34A2)*. There are more than 15 mutations. This gene is expressed in high levels in the lungs, predominantly on the surface of alveolar type II cells. Although the precise role of this protein is unknown, it is speculated that it helps to remove phosphate generated from surfactant metabolism in the alveolar space, as well as functioning as a phosphate regulator in other organs.

In some families, progression of disease is rapid. An equal male and female incidence is noted. Although PAM is found throughout the world, there is a high incidence in Turkey and a lesser incidence in Italy, Japan, and India.

CLINICAL MANIFESTATIONS

In early stages of the disease, patients are usually asymptomatic. When symptomatic, patients with PAM usually complain of dyspnea on exertion and nonproductive cough. Physical examination of the lungs can reveal fine inspiratory crackles and diminished breath sounds. Clubbing occurs, although this is usually a more advanced sign. Discordance between the clinical and radiographic manifestations is common. Many children are often asymptomatic on initial presentation and present with symptoms during adulthood. Complications of pneumothorax, pleural adhesions and calcifications, pleural fibrosis, apical bullae, and extrapulmonary sites of microliths have been reported (kidneys, prostate, sympathetic chain, and testes).

DIAGNOSIS

Chest radiography typically reveals bilateral infiltrates with a fine micronodular appearance or sandstorm appearance with greater density in the lower and middle lung fields (see Fig. 422.4). CT of the chest shows diffuse micronodular calcified densities, with thickening of the microliths along the septa and around distal bronchioles, especially in the inferior and posterior regions (see Table 422.2). Diffuse uptake of technetium-99 methylene diphosphonate by nuclear scan has been reported. Open lung and transbronchial lung biopsy reveal 0.1- to 0.3-mm laminated calcific concretions within the alveoli. Although the alveoli are often normal initially, progression to pulmonary fibrosis with advancing disease usually ensues. Sputum expectoration might reveal small microliths, although this finding is not diagnostic for PAM and is not typically seen in children. Detection of calcium deposits in bronchoalveolar lavage (BAL) fluid on bronchoscopy supports the diagnosis. Pulmonary function testing reveals restrictive lung disease with impaired diffusing capacity as the disease progresses, whereas exercise testing demonstrates arterial oxygen desaturation. The diagnosis can usually be established radiographically. However, lung tissue biopsy, BAL, and detection of a mutation in the *SCL34A2* gene can also be used to help confirm the diagnosis. The differential diagnosis includes sarcoidosis,

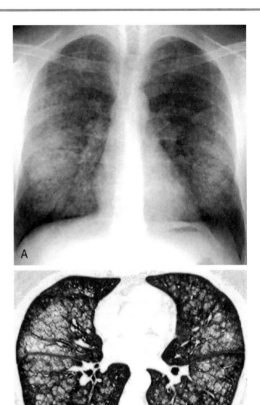

Fig. 422.4 Radiographic features of pulmonary alveolar microlithiasis. **A,** Posteroanterior chest radiograph showing the classic "sandstorm" appearance of pulmonary alveolar microlithiasis, including diffuse, patchy, bilateral sharp micronodular disease. **B,** High-resolution CT scan of the chest showing micronodular densities. *(From Brandenburg VM, Schubert H: Images in clinical medicine. Pulmonary alveolar microlithiasis, N Engl J Med 348:1555, 2003.)*

miliary tuberculosis, hemosiderosis, healed disseminated histoplasmosis, pulmonary calcinosis, and metastatic pulmonary calcifications.

TREATMENT

No specific treatment is effective, although some clinicians have used glucocorticosteroids, etidronate disodium, and bronchopulmonary lavage with limited success. Lung transplantation has been performed for this condition without recurrence in the transplanted lung.

PROGNOSIS

Progressive cardiopulmonary disease can ensue, leading to cor pulmonale, superimposed infections, and subsequent death in mid-adulthood. Because of the familial nature of this disease, counseling and chest radiographs of family members are indicated.

Bibliography is available at Expert Consult.

Chapter **423**

Congenital Disorders of the Lung

第四百二十三章
先天性肺疾病

中文导读

本章主要介绍了肺未发生及肺未发育、肺发育不良、先天性囊性腺瘤样畸形（先天性肺气道畸形）、肺隔离症、支气管囊肿、先天性肺淋巴管扩张症、肺疝和其他先天性肺发育畸形。具体描述了肺未发生及肺未发育、肺发育不良及先天性囊性腺瘤样畸形的病因学和病理学、临床表现、诊断治疗及预后；具体描述了肺隔离症的病理生理学、临床表现、诊断和治疗；具体描述了支气管囊肿、先天性肺淋巴管扩张症、肺疝的病理学、病因学、临床表现和治疗；介绍了支气管胆道瘘的临床表现及治疗方法。

423.1 Pulmonary Agenesis and Aplasia

Joshua A. Blatter and Jonathan D. Finder

ETIOLOGY AND PATHOLOGY

Pulmonary agenesis differs from hypoplasia in that agenesis entails the complete absence of a lung. Agenesis differs from aplasia by the absence of a bronchial stump or carina that is seen in aplasia. Bilateral pulmonary agenesis is incompatible with life, manifesting as severe respiratory distress and failure. Pulmonary agenesis is thought to be an autosomal recessive trait, with an estimated incidence of 1 in 10,000-15,000 births.

CLINICAL MANIFESTATIONS AND PROGNOSIS

Unilateral agenesis or hypoplasia can have few symptoms and nonspecific findings, resulting in only 33% of the cases being diagnosed while the patient is living. Symptoms tend to be associated with central airway complications of compression, stenosis, and/or tracheobronchomalacia. In patients in whom the right lung is absent, the aorta can compress the trachea and lead to symptoms of central airway compression. Right lung agenesis has a higher morbidity and mortality than left lung agenesis. Pulmonary agenesis is often seen in association with other congenital anomalies such as the **VACTERL sequence** (*v*ertebral anomalies, *a*nal atresia, *c*ongenital heart disease, *t*racheoesophageal fistula, *r*enal anomalies, and *l*imb anomalies), ipsilateral facial and skeletal malformations, and central nervous system and cardiac malformations. Compensatory growth of the remaining lung allows improved gas exchange, but the mediastinal shift can lead to scoliosis and airway compression. Scoliosis can result from unequal thoracic growth.

DIAGNOSIS AND TREATMENT

Chest radiographic findings of unilateral lung or lobar collapse with a shift of mediastinal structures toward the affected side can prompt referral for suspected foreign body aspiration, mucous plug occlusion, or other bronchial mass lesions. The diagnosis requires a high index of suspicion to avoid the unnecessary risks of bronchoscopy, including potential perforation of the rudimentary bronchus. CT of the chest is diagnostic, although the diagnosis may be suggested by chronic changes in the contralateral aspect of the chest wall and lung expansion on chest radiographs. Because pulmonary agenesis can be associated with a wide variety of congenital lesions, whole body MRI can be useful to determine whether other systems (e.g., cardiac, gastrointestinal) are affected. Conservative treatment is usually recommended, although surgery has offered benefit in selected cases.

Bibliography is available at Expert Consult.

423.2 Pulmonary Hypoplasia

Joshua A. Blatter and Jonathan D. Finder

ETIOLOGY AND PATHOLOGY

Pulmonary hypoplasia involves a decrease in both the number of alveoli and the number of airway generations. The hypoplasia may be bilateral in the setting of bilateral lung constraint, as in oligohydramnios or thoracic dystrophy. Pulmonary hypoplasia is usually secondary to other intrauterine disorders that produce an impairment of normal lung development (see Chapter 122). Conditions such as deformities of the thoracic spine and rib cage (thoracic dystrophy), pleural effusions with fetal hydrops, congenital pulmonary airway malformation, and congenital diaphragmatic hernia physically constrain the developing lung. Any condition that produces oligohydramnios (fetal renal insufficiency or prolonged premature rupture of membranes) can also lead to diminished lung growth. In these conditions, airway and arterial branching are inhibited, thereby limiting the capillary surface area. Large unilateral lesions, such as congenital diaphragmatic hernia or pulmonary airway malformation, can displace the mediastinum and thereby produce a contralateral hypoplasia, although usually not as severe as that seen on the ipsilateral side.

CLINICAL MANIFESTATIONS

Pulmonary hypoplasia is usually recognized in the newborn period, owing to either the respiratory insufficiency or the presentation of persistent pulmonary hypertension (see Chapter 122.7). Later presentation (tachypnea) with stress or respiratory viral infection can be seen in infants with mild pulmonary hypoplasia.

DIAGNOSIS AND TREATMENT

A variety of imaging techniques, including MRI and ultrasound, with estimation of oligohydramnios, can be helpful to identify hypoplasia but not to predict pulmonary function. Mechanical ventilation and oxygen may be required to support gas exchange. Specific therapy to control associated pulmonary hypertension, such as inhaled nitric oxide, may be useful. In cases of severe hypoplasia, the limited capacity of the lung for gas exchange may be inadequate to sustain life. Extracorporeal membrane oxygenation can provide gas exchange for a critical period of time and permit survival. Rib-expanding devices (vertically expansible prosthetic titanium ribs) can improve the survival of patients with thoracic dystrophies (see Chapter 720).

Bibliography is available at Expert Consult.

423.3 Congenital Cystic Malformation (Congenital Pulmonary Airway Malformation)

Joshua A. Blatter and Jonathan D. Finder

PATHOLOGY

Congenital pulmonary airway malformation (**CPAM**), formerly known as cystic adenomatoid malformation, consists of hamartomatous or dysplastic lung tissue mixed with more normal lung, generally confined to 1 lobe. This congenital pulmonary disorder occurs in approximately 1-4 in 100,000 births. Prenatal ultrasonographic findings are classified as **macrocystic** (single or multiple cysts >5 mm) or **microcystic** (echogenic cysts <5 mm). Five histologic patterns have been described. **Type 0** (acinar dysplasia) is least common (<3%) and consists of microcystic disease throughout the lungs. The prognosis is poorest for this type, and infants die at birth. **Type 1** (60%) is macrocystic and consists of a single or several large (>2 cm in diameter) cysts lined with ciliated pseudostratified epithelium; the lesion is localized involving only a part of 1 lobe. One third of cases have mucus-secreting cells. Presentation is in utero or in the newborn period. Cartilage is rarely seen in the wall of the cyst. This type has a good prognosis for survival. **Type 2** (20%) is microcystic and consists of multiple small cysts with histology similar to that of the type 1 lesion. Type 2 is associated with other serious congenital anomalies (renal, cardiac, diaphragmatic hernia) and carries a poor prognosis. **Type 3** (<10%) is seen mostly in males; the lesion is a mixture of microcysts and solid tissue with bronchiole-like structures lined with cuboidal ciliated epithelium and separated by areas of nonciliated cuboidal epithelium. The prognosis for this type, like type 0, is poor. **Type 4** (10%) is commonly macrocystic and lacks mucus cells. It is associated with malignancy (pleuropulmonary blastoma) and can present either in childhood or in asymptomatic adults.

ETIOLOGY

The lesion probably results from an embryologic injury before the 35th day of gestation, with maldevelopment of terminal bronchiolar structures. Histologic examination reveals little normal lung and many glandular elements. Cysts are very common; cartilage is rare. The presence of cartilage might indicate a somewhat later embryologic insult, perhaps extending into the 10th-24th wk. Although growth factor interactions and signaling mechanisms have been implicated in altered lung-branching morphogenesis, the exact roles in the maldevelopment seen here remain obscure.

DIAGNOSIS

Cystic airway malformations can be diagnosed in utero by ultrasonography (Fig. 423.1). Fetal cystic lung abnormalities can include CPAM (40%), pulmonary sequestration (14%) (see Chapter 423.4), or both (26%); the median age at diagnosis is usually 21 wk of gestation. In one series, only 7% had severe signs of fetal distress including hydrops, pleural effusion, polyhydramnios, ascites, or severe facial edema; 96% of the fetuses were born alive, 2 of whom died in the neonatal period. CPAM volume (i.e., CPAM volume ratio [CVR]) can be used to predict risk of hydrops. Lesions causing fetal hydrops have a poor prognosis.

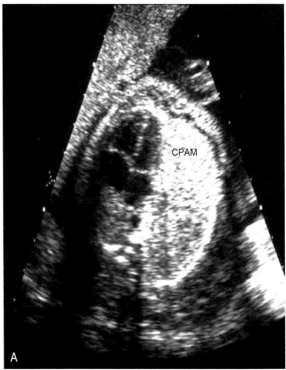

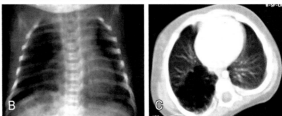

Fig. 423.1 Imaging of congenital pulmonary airway malformation of the lung *(CPAM)* on the same patient with prenatal ultrasound scan **(A)**, chest radiograph **(B)**, and CT scan **(C)**. Note that the lesion is not visible on the chest radiograph. *(From Lakhoo K: Management of congenital cystic adenomatous malformations of the lung, Arch Dis Child Fetal Neonatal Ed 94:F73–F76, 2009.)*

Large lesions, by compressing adjacent lung, can produce pulmonary hypoplasia in nonaffected lobes (see Chapter 423.2). Even lesions that appear large in early gestation can regress considerably or decrease in relative size and be associated with good pulmonary function in childhood. CT allows accurate diagnosis and sizing of the lesion and is indicated even in asymptomatic neonates.

CLINICAL MANIFESTATIONS

Patients can present in the newborn period or early infancy with respiratory distress, recurrent respiratory infection, and pneumothorax. The lesion may be confused with a diaphragmatic hernia (see Chapter 122.10). Patients with smaller lesions are usually asymptomatic until mid-childhood, when episodes of recurrent or persistent pulmonary infection or chest pain occur. Breath sounds may be diminished, with mediastinal shift away from the lesion on physical examination. Chest radiographs reveal a cystic mass, sometimes with mediastinal shift (Fig. 423.2). Occasionally, an air-fluid level suggests a lung abscess (see Chapter 431).

TREATMENT

Antenatal intervention in severely affected infants is controversial but can include excision of the affected lobe for microcystic lesions, aspiration of macrocystic lesions, and, rarely, open fetal surgery. In the postnatal period, surgery is indicated for symptomatic patients. Although surgery may be delayed for asymptomatic infants because postnatal resolution has been reported, true resolution appears to be very rare in that abnormalities usually remain detectable on CT or MRI. Sarcomatous and carcinomatous degeneration have been described in patients with CPAM, so surgical resection by 1 yr of age is recommended to limit malignant potential. The mortality rate is <10%. Another indication for surgery is to rule out **pleuropulmonary blastoma (PPB)**, a malignancy that can appear radiographically similar to type 1 CPAM. PPB is associated with germline mutations in *DICER1*. In addition to the risk of malignancy, "asymptomatic" patients may have chronic inflammation with subtle systemic manifestations, which parents report resolves after the lesion is resected.

Bibliography is available at Expert Consult.

423.4 Pulmonary Sequestration
Joshua A. Blatter and Jonathan D. Finder

Pulmonary sequestration is a congenital anomaly of lung development that can be intrapulmonary or extrapulmonary, according to the location within the visceral pleura. The majority of sequestrations are intrapulmonary.

PATHOPHYSIOLOGY

The lung tissue in a sequestration does not connect to a bronchus and receives its arterial supply from the systemic arteries (commonly off the aorta) and returns its venous blood to the right side of the heart through the inferior vena cava (**extralobar**) or pulmonary veins (**intralobar**). The sequestration functions as a space-occupying lesion within the chest; it does not participate in gas exchange and does not lead to a left-to-right shunt or alveolar dead space. Communication with the airway can occur as the result of rupture of infected material into an adjacent airway. Collateral ventilation within intrapulmonary lesions via pores of Kohn can occur. Pulmonary sequestrations can arise through the same pathoembryologic mechanism as a remnant of a diverticular outgrowth of the esophagus. Some propose that intrapulmonary sequestration is an acquired lesion primarily caused by infection and inflammation; inflammation leads to cystic changes and hypertrophy of a feeding systemic artery. This is consistent with the rarity of this lesion in autopsy series of newborns. Gastric or pancreatic tissue may be found within the sequestration. Cysts also may be present. Other associated congenital anomalies, including CPAM (see Chapter 423.3), diaphragmatic hernia (see Chapter 122.10), and esophageal cysts, are not uncommon. Some believe that intrapulmonary sequestration is often a manifestation of CPAM and have questioned the existence of intrapulmonary sequestration as a separate entity.

CLINICAL MANIFESTATIONS AND DIAGNOSIS

Physical findings in patients with sequestration include an area of dullness to percussion and decreased breath sounds over the lesion. During infection, crackles may also be present. A continuous or purely systolic murmur may be heard over the back. If findings on routine chest radiographs are consistent with the diagnosis, further delineation is indicated before surgical intervention (Fig. 423.3). CT with contrast can demonstrate both the extent of the lesion and its vascular supply. MR angiography is also useful. Ultrasonography can help to rule out a diaphragmatic hernia and demonstrate the systemic artery. Surgical removal is recommended. Identifying the blood supply before surgery avoids inadvertently severing its systemic artery. Coil embolization (transumbilical in neonates; arterial in older patients) has been successful in treating patients with sequestration.

Intrapulmonary sequestration is generally found in a lower lobe and does not have its own pleura. Patients usually present with infection. In older patients, hemoptysis is common. A chest radiograph during a period when there is no active infection reveals a mass lesion; an air-fluid level may be present. During infection, the margins of the lesion may be blurred. There is no difference in the incidence of this lesion in each lung.

Extrapulmonary sequestration is much more common in boys and almost always involves the left lung. This lesion is enveloped by a pleural covering and is associated with diaphragmatic hernia and other abnormalities such as colonic duplication, vertebral abnormalities, and pulmonary hypoplasia. Many of these patients are asymptomatic when the mass is discovered by routine chest radiography. Other patients present with respiratory symptoms or heart failure. Subdiaphragmatic extrapulmonary sequestration can manifest as an abdominal mass on prenatal ultrasonography. The advent of prenatal ultrasonography has also enabled evidence that fetal pulmonary sequestrations can spontaneously regress.

TREATMENT

Treatment of intrapulmonary sequestration is surgical removal of the lesion, a procedure that usually requires excision of the entire involved lobe. Segmental resection occasionally suffices. Surgical resection of the involved area is often recommended for extrapulmonary sequestration as well, but observation can be considered for asymptomatic patients with small lesions. Coil embolization of the feeding artery has also been successful.

Bibliography is available at Expert Consult.

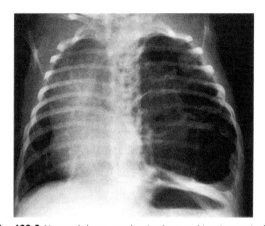

Fig. 423.2 Neonatal chest x-ray showing large multicystic mass in the left hemithorax with mediastinal shift as a result of congenital pulmonary airway malformation. *(From Williams HJ, Johnson KJ: Imaging of congenital cystic lung lesions, Paediatr Respir Rev 3:120–127, 2002.)*

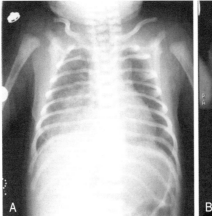
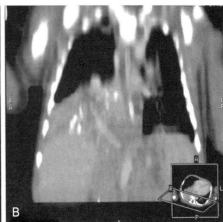

Fig. 423.3 A, Plain chest x-ray showing changes in the region of the right lower/middle lobe of the lung. **B,** CT showing parenchymal changes in the right lower lobe of the lung in keeping with a sequestration. *(From Corbett HJ, Humphrey GME: Pulmonary sequestration, Paediatr Respir Rev 5:59–68, 2004.)*

423.5 Bronchogenic Cysts

Joshua A. Blatter and Jonathan D. Finder

ETIOLOGY AND PATHOLOGY

Bronchogenic cysts arise from abnormal budding of the tracheal diverticulum of the foregut before the 16th wk of gestation and are originally lined with ciliated epithelium. They are more commonly found on the right and near a midline structure (trachea, esophagus, carina), but peripheral lower lobe and perihilar intrapulmonary cysts are not infrequent. Diagnosis may be precipitated by enlargement of the cyst, which causes symptoms by pressure on an adjacent airway. When the diagnosis is delayed until an infection occurs, the ciliated epithelium may be lost, and accurate pathologic diagnosis is then impossible. Cysts are rarely demonstrable at birth. Later, some cysts become symptomatic by becoming infected or by enlarging and compromising the function of an adjacent airway.

CLINICAL MANIFESTATIONS AND TREATMENT

Fever, chest pain, and productive cough are the most common presenting symptoms. Dysphagia may be present; some bronchogenic cysts are asymptomatic. A chest radiograph reveals the cyst, which can contain an air-fluid level (Fig. 423.4). CT scan or MRI is obtained in most cases to better demonstrate anatomy and extent of lesion before surgical resection. Treatment of symptomatic cysts is surgical excision after appropriate antibiotic management. Asymptomatic cysts are generally excised in view of the high rate of infection.

Bibliography is available at Expert Consult.

423.6 Congenital Pulmonary Lymphangiectasia

Joshua A. Blatter and Jonathan D. Finder

ETIOLOGY AND PATHOLOGY

Congenital pulmonary lymphangiectasia is characterized by greatly dilated lymphatic ducts throughout the lung. It can occur in three pathologic circumstances: **pulmonary venous obstruction** that produces an elevated transvascular pressure and engorges the pulmonary lymphatics; **generalized lymphangiectasia**, as a generalized disease of several organ systems, including lymphedema, lungs, and the intestines either associated with other syndromes (Noonan, Hennekam, yellow nail, trisomy 21) or nonsyndromic. Gorham-Stout disease (vanishing bone disease) presents with pulmonary and abdominal chylous effusions, destructive bone cysts, and multiple lymphangiomas; and **primary**

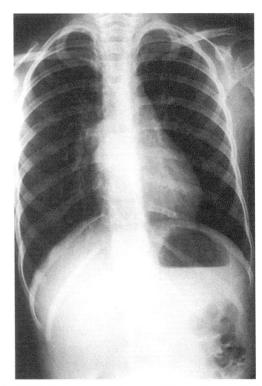

Fig. 423.4 Chest x-ray showing an ovoid, well-defined, soft tissue density causing splaying of the carina due to bronchogenic cyst. *(From Williams HJ, Johnson KJ: Imaging of congenital cystic lung lesions, Paediatr Respir Rev 3:120–127, 2002.)*

lymphangiectasia limited to the lung as a manifestation of an abnormality in lymphatic development.

CLINICAL MANIFESTATIONS AND TREATMENT

Children with pulmonary venous obstruction or severe pulmonary lymphangiectasia present with dyspnea and cyanosis in the newborn period. Hydrops fetalis may be diagnosed antenatally. Chest radiographs reveal diffuse, dense, reticular densities with prominence of Kerley B lines. Pleural effusions are common; thoracentesis will reveal **chylothorax** in this setting. If the lung is not completely involved, the spared areas appear hyperlucent. Respiration is compromised because of impaired diffusion and decreased pulmonary compliance. The diagnosis can be suggested by CT scan and/or cardiac catheterization; definitive diagnosis requires lymphangiography or lung biopsy (either thoracoscopic or open) (Fig. 423.5).

Treatment is supportive and includes administration of oxygen, mechanical ventilation, nutritional support (including gastrostomy placement and use of feedings containing medium-chain triglycerides), and careful fluid management with diuretics. Octreotide, the somatostatin analog, can reduce chylous effusion in some patients. Primary pulmonary lymphangiectasia in the neonate can produce severe pulmonary dysfunction that can require long-term mechanical ventilation; long-term survival and resolution of respiratory insufficiency are possible even in severe cases, especially if the chylous effusions can be managed. Occasionally, the pulmonary venous obstruction is secondary to left-sided cardiac lesions; relief of the latter can produce improvement in pulmonary dysfunction. Generalized lymphangiectasia produces milder pulmonary dysfunction, and survival to mid-childhood and beyond is not unusual.

Bibliography is available at Expert Consult.

423.7 Lung Hernia

Joshua A. Blatter and Jonathan D. Finder

ETIOLOGY AND PATHOLOGY

A lung hernia is a protrusion of the lung beyond its normal thoracic boundaries. Approximately 20% are congenital, with the remainder being noted after chest trauma or thoracic surgery or in patients with pulmonary diseases such as cystic fibrosis (see Chapter 432) or asthma (see Chapter 169), which cause frequent cough and generate high intrathoracic pressure. A congenital weakness of the suprapleural membrane (Sibson fascia) or musculature of the neck can play a role in the appearance of a lung hernia. More than half of congenital lung

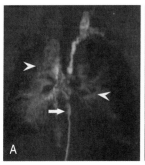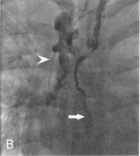

Fig. 423.5 A, Dynamic contrast MR lymphangiogram (DCMRL) in a patient with pulmonary lymphangiectasia demonstrating dilated thoracic duct (TD) *(white arrow)* and abnormal pulmonary lymphatic perfusion in the lung hilum *(white arrowheads)*. **B,** Corresponding fluoroscopy image of the TD of the same patient, following injection of contrast material through the microcatheter positioned in proximal part of TD, confirms the dilation of the TD *(white arrow)* and retrograde flow of the contrast in the mediastinal lymphatic ducts *(white arrowhead)*. *(From Itkin M, McCormack FX: Nonmalignant adult thoracic lymphatic disorders, Clin Chest Med 37:409–420, 2016. Fig 7.)*

hernias and almost all acquired hernias are cervical. Congenital cervical hernias usually occur anteriorly through a gap between the scalenus anterior and sternocleidomastoid muscles. Cervical herniation is usually prevented by the trapezius muscle (posteriorly, at the thoracic inlet) and by the 3 scalene muscles (laterally).

CLINICAL MANIFESTATIONS AND TREATMENT

The presenting sign of a cervical hernia (Sibson hernia) is usually a neck mass noticed while straining or coughing. Some lesions are asymptomatic and detected only when a chest film is taken for another reason. Findings on physical examination are normal except during Valsalva maneuver, when a soft bulge may be noticed in the neck. In most cases, no treatment is necessary, although these hernias can cause problems during attempts to place a central venous catheter through the jugular or subclavian veins. They can resolve spontaneously.

Paravertebral or parasternal hernias are usually associated with rib anomalies. Intercostal hernias usually occur parasternally, where the external intercostal muscle is absent. Posteriorly, despite the seemingly inadequate internal intercostal muscle, the paraspinal muscles usually prevent herniation. Straining, coughing, or playing a musical instrument can have a role in causing intercostal hernias, but in most cases, there is probably a preexisting defect in the thoracic wall.

Surgical treatment for lung hernia is occasionally justified for cosmetic reasons. In patients with severe chronic pulmonary disease and chronic cough and for whom cough suppression is contraindicated, permanent correction might not be achieved.

Bibliography is available at Expert Consult.

423.8 Other Congenital Malformations of the Lung

Joshua A. Blatter and Jonathan D. Finder

CONGENITAL LOBAR EMPHYSEMA AND PULMONARY CYSTS
See Chapter 420.

PULMONARY ARTERIOVENOUS MALFORMATION
See Chapters 459 and 471.

BRONCHOBILIARY FISTULA
A bronchobiliary fistula consists of a fistulous connection between the right middle lobe bronchus and the left hepatic ductal system. Although diagnosis can be delayed until adulthood, this rare anomaly typically manifests with life-threatening bronchopulmonary infections in early infancy. Girls are more commonly affected. Definitive diagnosis requires endoscopy or exploratory surgery. Treatment includes surgical excision of the entire intrathoracic portion of the fistula. If the hepatic portion of the fistula does not communicate with the biliary system or duodenum, the involved segment might also have to be resected. Bronchobiliary communications also occur as acquired lesions resulting from hepatic disease complicated by infection.

Bibliography is available at Expert Consult.

Chapter **424**

Pulmonary Edema

Brandon T. Woods and Robert L. Mazor

第四百二十四章

肺水肿

中文导读

　　本章主要介绍了肺水肿的病理生理学、病因学、临床特点和治疗。肺水肿可分为心源性肺水肿和非心源性肺水肿，病理生理学均为肺泡腔和肺间质液体的积聚；肺水肿的病因包括引起肺毛细血管压力升高、血管渗透性增加、淋巴管功能障碍、胶体渗透压降低、组织间隙负压增高的疾病，也包括多种病因共同致病或其他未知病因；其临床特点包括呼吸次数增加、呼吸急促和呼吸困难，听诊可闻及细湿啰音和喘鸣音，胸片可见肺水肿改变；治疗方法包括吸氧、利尿药、正性肌力药、全身血管舒张剂及气道正压通气等。

Pulmonary edema is an abnormal fluid collection in the interstitium and air spaces of the lung resulting in oxygen desaturation, decreased lung compliance, and respiratory distress. The condition is common in the acutely ill child.

PATHOPHYSIOLOGY

Although pulmonary edema is traditionally separated into two categories according to cause (*cardiogenic* and *noncardiogenic*), the end result of both processes is a net fluid accumulation within the interstitial and alveolar spaces. Noncardiogenic pulmonary edema, in its most severe state, is also known as acute respiratory distress syndrome (see Chapters 89 and 400).

The *hydrostatic pressure* and colloid *osmotic (oncotic) pressure* on either side of a pulmonary vascular wall, along with vascular permeability, are the forces and physical factors that determine fluid movement through the vessel wall. Baseline conditions lead to a net filtration of fluid from the intravascular space into the interstitium. This extra interstitial fluid is usually rapidly reabsorbed by pulmonary lymphatics. Conditions that lead to altered vascular permeability, increased pulmonary vascular pressure, and decreased intravascular oncotic pressure increase the net flow of fluid out of the vessel (Table 424.1). Once the capacity of the lymphatics for fluid removal is exceeded, water accumulates in the lung.

To understand the sequence of lung water accumulation, it is helpful to consider its distribution among four distinct compartments, as follows:

◆ *Vascular compartment:* This compartment consists of all blood vessels that participate in fluid exchange with the interstitium. The vascular compartment is separated from the interstitium by capillary endothelial cells. Several endogenous inflammatory mediators, as well as exogenous toxins, are implicated in the pathogenesis of pulmonary capillary endothelial damage, leading to the leakiness seen in several systemic processes.

◆ *Interstitial compartment:* The importance of this space lies in its interposition between the alveolar and vascular compartments. As fluid leaves the vascular compartment, it collects in the interstitium before overflowing into the air spaces of the alveolar compartment.

◆ *Alveolar compartment:* This compartment is lined with type 1 and type 2 epithelial cells. These epithelial cells have a role in active fluid transport from the alveolar space, and they act as a barrier to exclude fluid from the alveolar space. The potential fluid volume of the alveolar compartment is many times greater than that of the interstitial space, perhaps providing another reason that alveolar edema clears more slowly than interstitial edema.

◆ *Pulmonary lymphatic compartment:* There is an extensive network of pulmonary lymphatics. Excess fluid present in the alveolar and interstitial compartments is drained via the lymphatic system. When the capacity for drainage of the lymphatics is surpassed, fluid accumulation occurs.

ETIOLOGY

The specific clinical findings vary according to the underlying mechanism (see Table 424.1).

Transudation of fluid as a result of increased pulmonary vascular pressure *(capillary hydrostatic pressure)* occurs in several cardiac processes. A significant left-to-right shunting lesion, such as a septal defect, leads to a pressure and volume load on the pulmonary vasculature. The resultant pulmonary edema is one of the hallmarks of congestive heart failure. Left ventricular failure, mitral valve disease, and pulmonary venous obstructive lesions cause increased backpressure in the pulmonary vasculature. This results in an increase in pulmonary capillary pressure.

Increased capillary permeability is usually secondary to endothelial damage. Such damage can occur secondary to direct injury to the alveolar epithelium or indirectly through systemic processes that deliver circulating inflammatory mediators or toxins to the lung. Inflammatory mediators

Table 424.1	Etiology of Pulmonary Edema

INCREASED PULMONARY CAPILLARY PRESSURE
Cardiogenic, such as left ventricular failure
Noncardiogenic, as in pulmonary venoocclusive disease, pulmonary venous fibrosis, mediastinal tumors

INCREASED CAPILLARY PERMEABILITY
Bacterial and viral pneumonia
Acute respiratory distress syndrome
Inhaled toxic agents
Circulating toxins
Vasoactive substances such as histamine, leukotrienes, thromboxanes
Diffuse capillary leak syndrome, as in sepsis
Immunologic reactions, such as transfusion reactions
Smoke inhalation
Aspiration pneumonia/pneumonitis
Drowning and near drowning
Radiation pneumonia
Uremia

LYMPHATIC INSUFFICIENCY
Congenital and acquired

DECREASED ONCOTIC PRESSURE
Hypoalbuminemia, as in renal and hepatic diseases, protein-losing states, and malnutrition

INCREASED NEGATIVE INTERSTITIAL PRESSURE
Upper airway obstructive lesions, such as croup and epiglottitis
Reexpansion pulmonary edema

MIXED OR UNKNOWN CAUSES
Neurogenic pulmonary edema
High-altitude pulmonary edema
Eclampsia
Pancreatitis
Pulmonary embolism
Heroin (narcotic) pulmonary edema

Modified from Robin E, Carroll C, Zelis R: Pulmonary edema, *N Engl J Med* 288:239, 292, 1973; and Desphande J, Wetzel R, Rogers M: In Rogers M, editor: *Textbook of pediatric intensive care*, ed 3, Baltimore, 1996, Williams & Wilkins, pp. 432–442.

(tumor necrosis factor, leukotrienes, thromboxanes) and vasoactive agents (nitric oxide, histamine) formed during pulmonary and systemic processes potentiate the altered capillary permeability that occurs in many disease processes, with sepsis being a common cause.

Fluid homeostasis in the lung largely depends on drainage via the lymphatics. Experimentally, pulmonary edema occurs with obstruction of the lymphatic system. Increased lymph flow and dilation of lymphatic vessels occur in chronic edematous states.

A decrease in intravascular oncotic pressure leads to pulmonary edema by altering the forces promoting fluid reentry into the vascular space. This occurs in dilutional disorders, such as fluid overload with hypotonic solutions, and in protein-losing states, such as nephrotic syndrome and malnutrition.

The **excessive negative interstitial pressure** seen in upper airway diseases, such as croup and laryngospasm, may promote pulmonary edema. Aside from the physical forces present in these diseases, other mechanisms may also be involved. Theories implicate an increase in CO_2 tension, decreased O_2 tension, and extreme increases in cardiac afterload, leading to transient cardiac insufficiency.

The mechanism causing **neurogenic pulmonary edema** is not clear. A massive sympathetic discharge secondary to a cerebral injury may produce increased pulmonary and systemic vasoconstriction, resulting in a shift of blood to the pulmonary vasculature, an increase in capillary pressure, and edema formation. Inflammatory mechanisms may also play a role by increasing capillary permeability.

The mechanism responsible for **high-altitude pulmonary edema** is unclear, but it may also be related to sympathetic outflow, increased

pulmonary vascular pressures, and hypoxia-induced increases in capillary permeability (see Chapter 90).

Active ion transport followed by passive, osmotic water movement is important in clearing the alveolar space of fluid. There are some experimental data that β-agonists and growth factors increase alveolar fluid removal. Interindividual genetic differences in the rates of these transport processes may be important in determining which individuals are susceptible to altitude-related pulmonary edema. Although the existence of these mechanisms suggests that therapeutic interventions may be developed to promote resolution of pulmonary edema, no such therapies currently exist.

CLINICAL MANIFESTATIONS

The clinical features depend on the mechanism of edema formation. In general, interstitial edema and alveolar edema prevent the inflation of alveoli, leading to atelectasis and decreased surfactant production. This results in diminished pulmonary compliance and tidal volume. The patient must increase respiratory effort and/or the respiratory rate so as to maintain minute ventilation. The earliest clinical signs of pulmonary edema include increased work of breathing, tachypnea, and dyspnea. As fluid accumulates in the alveolar space, auscultation reveals fine crackles and wheezing, especially in dependent lung fields. In cardiogenic pulmonary edema, a gallop may be present, as well as peripheral edema and jugular venous distention.

Chest radiographs can provide useful ancillary data, although findings of initial radiographs may be normal. Early radiographic signs that represent accumulation of interstitial edema include peribronchial and perivascular cuffing. Diffuse streakiness reflects interlobular edema and distended pulmonary lymphatics. Diffuse, patchy densities, the so-called butterfly pattern, represent bilateral interstitial or alveolar infiltrates and are a late sign. Cardiomegaly is often seen with cardiogenic causes of pulmonary edema. Heart size is usually normal in noncardiogenic pulmonary edema (Table 424.2). Chest tomography demonstrates edema accumulation in the dependent areas of the lung. As a result, changing the patient's position can alter regional differences in lung compliance, functional residual capacity, and alveolar ventilation.

Measurement of brain natriuretic peptide, often elevated in heart disease, can help to differentiate cardiac from pulmonary causes of

| Table 424.2 | Radiographic Features That May Help Differentiate Cardiogenic From Noncardiogenic Pulmonary Edema |

RADIOGRAPHIC FEATURE	CARDIOGENIC EDEMA	NONCARDIOGENIC EDEMA
Heart size	Normal or greater than normal	Usually normal
Width of the vascular pedicle*	Normal or greater than normal	Usually normal or less than normal
Vascular distribution	Balanced or inverted	Normal or balanced
Distribution of edema	Even or central	Patchy or peripheral
Pleural effusions	Present	Not usually present
Peribronchial cuffing	Present	Not usually present
Septal lines	Present	Not usually present
Air bronchograms	Not usually present	Usually present

*The width of the vascular pedicle in adults is determined by dropping a perpendicular line from the point at which the left subclavian artery exits the aortic arch and measuring across to the point at which the superior vena cava crosses the right mainstem bronchus. A vascular pedicle width >70 mm on a portable digital anteroposterior radiograph of the chest obtained when the patient is supine is optimal for differentiating high from normal-to-low intravascular volume.
From Ware LB, Matthay MA: Acute pulmonary edema, *N Engl J Med* 353:2788–2796, 2005.

pulmonary edema. A brain natriuretic peptide level >500 pg/mL suggests heart disease; a level <100 pg/mL suggests lung disease.

TREATMENT

The treatment of a patient with noncardiogenic pulmonary edema is largely supportive, with the primary goal to ensure adequate ventilation and oxygenation. Additional therapy is directed toward the underlying cause. Patients should receive supplemental oxygen to increase alveolar oxygen tension and pulmonary vasodilation. Patients with pulmonary edema of cardiogenic causes should be managed with diuretics, inotropic agents, and systemic vasodilators to reduce left ventricular afterload (see Chapter 442). Diuretics are also valuable in the treatment of pulmonary edema associated with total body fluid overload (sepsis, renal insufficiency). Morphine is often helpful as a vasodilator and a mild sedative.

Positive airway pressure improves gas exchange in patients with pulmonary edema. In tracheally intubated patients, positive end-expiratory pressure can be used to optimize pulmonary mechanics. Noninvasive forms of ventilation, such as mask or nasal prong continuous positive airway pressure, are also effective. The mechanism by which positive airway pressure improves pulmonary edema is not entirely clear but is not associated with decreasing lung water. Rather, continuous positive airway pressure prevents complete closure of alveoli at the low lung volumes present at the end of expiration. It may also recruit already collapsed alveolar units. This leads to increased functional residual capacity and improved pulmonary compliance, improved surfactant function, and decreased pulmonary vascular resistance. The net effect is to decrease the work of breathing, improve oxygenation, and decrease cardiac afterload.

When mechanical ventilation becomes necessary, especially in noncardiogenic pulmonary edema, care must be taken to minimize the risk of development of complications from volutrauma or barotrauma, including pneumothorax, pneumomediastinum, and primary alveolar damage (see Chapter 89.1). Lung protective strategies include setting low tidal volumes, relatively high positive end-expiratory pressure, and allowing for permissive hypercapnia.

High-altitude pulmonary edema should be managed with altitude descent and supplemental oxygen. Portable continuous positive airway pressure or a portable hyperbaric chamber is also helpful. Nifedipine (10 mg initially, and then 20-30 mg by slow release every 12-24 hr) in adults is also helpful. If there is a history of high-altitude pulmonary edema, nifedipine and β-adrenergic agonists (inhaled) may prevent recurrence (see Chapter 90).

Bibliography is available at Expert Consult.

Chapter **425**
Aspiration Syndromes
John L. Colombo

第四百二十五章
吸入综合征

中文导读

　　本章主要介绍了吸入综合征、胃内容物吸入、碳氢化合物吸入。胃内容物吸入的治疗包括建立人工气道、吸出分泌物、支气管镜检查、医学观察、合理的抗生素使用等；预防胃内容物吸入包括气管内插管、喂养管留置位置穿过幽门、抬高床头、减少镇静药的使用、监测胃内残留物和抑制胃酸等。碳氢化合物吸入的临床特点包括咳嗽、发热、胸凹陷、嗓子呼噜、肺气肿、胸腔积液、肺功能异常和其他器官损害，碳氢化合物吸入的治疗包括给氧、液体支持和通气支持等。

ASPIRATION SYNDROMES

Aspiration of material that is foreign to the lower airway produces a varied clinical spectrum ranging from an asymptomatic condition to acute life-threatening events, such as occur with massive aspiration of gastric contents or hydrocarbon products. Other chapters discuss mechanical obstruction of large- or intermediate-size airways as occurs with foreign bodies (see Chapter 414) and infectious complications of aspiration and recurrent microaspiration (see Chapter 426), such as may occur with gastroesophageal reflux (see Chapter 349.1) or dysphagia (see Chapter 332). Occult aspiration of nasopharyngeal secretions into the lower respiratory tract is a normal event in healthy people, usually without apparent clinical significance.

GASTRIC CONTENTS

Aspiration of substantial amounts of gastric contents typically occurs in the context of vomiting. It is an infrequent complication of general anesthesia, gastroenteritis, or altered level of consciousness. Among 63,180 pediatric patients undergoing general anesthesia, 24 cases of aspiration occurred, but symptoms developed in only 9. Pathophysiologic consequences can vary, depending primarily on the pH and volume of the aspirate and the amount of particulate material. Increased clinical severity is noted with volumes greater than approximately 0.8 mL/kg and/or pH < 2.5. Hypoxemia, hemorrhagic pneumonitis, atelectasis, intravascular fluid shifts, and pulmonary edema all occur rapidly after massive aspiration. These occur earlier, become more severe, and last longer with acid aspiration. Most clinical changes are present within minutes to 1-2 hr after the aspiration event. In the next 24-48 hr, there is a marked increase in lung parenchymal neutrophil infiltrations, mucosal sloughing, and alveolar consolidation that often correlates with increasing infiltrates on chest radiographs. These changes tend to occur significantly later and are more prolonged after aspiration of particulate material. Although infection usually does not have a role in initial lung injury after aspiration of gastric contents, aspiration may impair pulmonary defenses, predisposing the patient to secondary bacterial pneumonia. In the patient who has shown clinical improvement but then demonstrates clinical worsening, especially with fever and leukocytosis, secondary bacterial pneumonia should be suspected.

Treatment

If large-volume or highly toxic substance aspiration occurs in a patient who already has an artificial airway in place, it is important to perform immediate suctioning of the airway. If immediate suctioning cannot be performed, later suctioning or bronchoscopy is usually of limited therapeutic value except when there is suspicion of significant particulate aspiration. Attempts at acid neutralization are not warranted because acid is rapidly neutralized by the respiratory epithelium. Patients in whom large-volume or toxic aspiration is suspected should be observed, should undergo oxygenation measurement by oximetry or blood gas analysis, and should undergo a chest radiograph, even if they are asymptomatic. If the chest radiograph findings and oxygen saturation are normal, and the patient remains asymptomatic, home observation, after a period of observation in the hospital or office, is adequate. No treatment is indicated at that time, but the caregivers should be instructed to bring the child back in for medical attention should respiratory symptoms or fever develop. For patients who present with abnormal findings or in whom such findings develop during observation, oxygen therapy is given to correct hypoxemia. Endotracheal intubation and mechanical ventilation are often necessary for more severe cases. Bronchodilators may be tried, although they are usually of limited benefit. Animal studies indicate that treatment with corticosteroids does not provide benefit, unless given nearly simultaneously with the aspiration event; use of these agents may increase the risk of secondary infection. Prophylactic antibiotics are not indicated, although in the patient with limited reserve, early antibiotic coverage may be appropriate. If used, antibiotics that cover for anaerobic microbes should be considered. If the aspiration event occurs in a hospitalized or chronically ill patient, coverage of *Pseudomonas, Staphylococcus aureus,* and enteric Gram-negative organisms should also be considered. Various antibiotic choices have included clindamycin plus ampicillin-sulbactam or a carbapenem or a respiratory fluoroquinolone. If empiric antibiotics are given, they should be discontinued when cultures and course warrant. A mortality rate of ≤ 5% is seen if 3 or fewer lobes are involved. Unless complications develop, such as infection or barotrauma, most patients recover in 2-3 wk. Prolonged lung damage may persist, including scarring, bronchiolitis obliterans, and bronchiectasis.

Prevention

Prevention of aspiration should always be the goal when airway manipulation is necessary for intubation or other invasive procedures. Feeding with enteral tubes passed beyond the pylorus, elevating the head of the bed 30-45 degrees in mechanically ventilated patients, and oral decontamination reduce the incidence of aspiration complications in the intensive care unit. Minimizing use of sedation, monitoring for gastric residuals, and gastric acid suppression may all help prevent aspiration. However, the latter is not without some controversy. Any patient with altered consciousness, especially one who is receiving tube feedings, should be considered at high risk for aspiration. Preoperative restriction of oral fluids to otherwise normal children for 6 hr does not appear to provide benefit compared to restriction for only 2 hr in terms of risk for aspiration.

HYDROCARBON ASPIRATION

Aspiration and resulting pneumonitis are typically the most dangerous consequences of acute hydrocarbon ingestion (see Chapter 77). Although significant pneumonitis occurs in <2% of all hydrocarbon ingestions, an estimated 20 deaths occur annually from hydrocarbon aspiration in both children and adults. Some of these deaths represent suicides. Hydrocarbons with lower surface tensions (gasoline, turpentine, naphthalene) have more potential for aspiration toxicity than heavier mineral or fuel oils. Ingestion of >30 mL (approximate volume of an adult swallow) of hydrocarbon is associated with an increased risk of severe pneumonitis. Clinical findings including chest retractions, grunting, cough, and fever may occur as soon as 30 min after aspiration or may be delayed for several hours. Lung radiographic changes usually occur within 2-8 hr, peaking in 48-72 hr (Fig. 425.1). Pneumatoceles and pleural effusions may occur. Patients initially presenting with cough, shortness of breath, or hypoxemia are at high risk for pneumonitis. Persistent pulmonary function abnormalities can be present many years after hydrocarbon aspiration. Other organ systems, especially the liver, central nervous system, and heart, may suffer serious injury. Cardiac dysrhythmias may occur and may be exacerbated by hypoxia and acid–base or electrolyte disturbances.

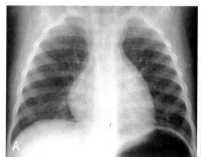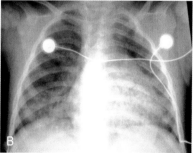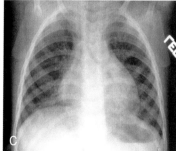

Fig. 425.1 Chest radiographs of a 17 mo old who ingested furniture polish. **A,** Three hours after ingestion, the lungs are clear. **B,** At 24 hr, there are bibasilar coalescing nodular opacities. **C,** Three days later there is much clearing. *(From Slovis TL, editor: Caffey's pediatric diagnostic imaging, ed 11, Philadelphia, 2008, Mosby, p. 1287.)*

Treatment

Gastric emptying is contraindicated in nearly all situations because the risk of aspiration is greater than any systemic toxicity. Treatment is generally supportive, consisting of oxygen, fluids, and ventilatory support, and rarely extracorporeal membrane oxygenation, as necessary. Exogenous surfactant administration has been described as helpful in case reports. The child who has no symptoms and normal chest radiograph findings should be observed for 6-8 hr to ensure safe discharge.

Certain hydrocarbons have more inherent systemic toxicity. The mnemonic **CHAMP** refers collectively to the following hydrocarbons: **c**amphor, **h**alogenated carbons, **a**romatic hydrocarbons, and those associated with **m**etals and **p**esticides. Patients who ingest these compounds in volumes > 30 mL, such as might occur with intentional overdose, *may* benefit from gastric emptying. This is still a high-risk procedure that can result in further aspiration. If a cuffed endotracheal tube can be placed without inducing vomiting, this procedure should be considered, especially in the presence of altered mental status. Treatment of each case should be considered individually, with guidance from a poison control center.

Other substances that are particularly toxic and cause significant lung injury when aspirated or inhaled include baby powder, chlorine, shellac, beryllium, and mercury vapors. Repeated exposure to low concentrations of these agents can lead to chronic lung disease, such as interstitial pneumonitis and granuloma formation. Corticosteroids may help reduce fibrosis development and improve pulmonary function, although the evidence for this benefit is limited.

Bibliography is available at Expert Consult.

Chapter 426
Chronic Recurrent Aspiration

John L. Colombo

第四百二十六章
慢性反复吸入

中文导读

本章主要介绍了慢性反复吸入的病因学、诊断及治疗。慢性反复吸入的病因包括解剖学结构异常、神经肌肉系统异常及其他多因素异常；慢性反复吸入的诊断包括详细询问病史、体格检查、辅助检查等。诊断吸入的相关检查包括胸片、高分辨CT、吞咽功能评估、食管pH监测、食管阻力监测、放射性核素检查以及染料检测等；慢性反复吸入的治疗包括治疗原发病、改变喂养体位、限制单次喂养量、抗胆碱药以及手术治疗等。

ETIOLOGY

Repeated aspiration of even small quantities of gastric, nasal, or oral contents can lead to recurrent bronchitis or bronchiolitis, recurrent pneumonia, atelectasis, wheezing, cough, apnea, and/or laryngospasm. Pathologic outcomes include granulomatous inflammation, interstitial inflammation, fibrosis, lipoid pneumonia, and bronchiolitis obliterans. Most cases clinically manifest as airway inflammation and are rarely associated with significant morbidity. Table 426.1 lists underlying disorders that are frequently associated with recurrent aspiration. Oropharyngeal incoordination is reportedly the most common underlying problem associated with recurrent pneumonias in hospitalized children. In 2 reports, between 26% and 48% of such children were found to have dysphagia with aspiration as the underlying problem. Lipoid

pneumonia may occur after the use of home/folk remedies involving oral or nasal administration of animal or vegetable oils to treat various childhood illnesses. Lipoid pneumonia has been reported as a complication of these practices in the Middle East, Asia, India, Brazil, and Mexico. The initial underlying disease, language barriers, and a belief that these are not medications may delay the diagnosis (see Chapter 11).

Gastroesophageal reflux disease (**GERD**; see Chapter 349) is also a common underlying finding that may predispose to recurrent respiratory disease, but it is less frequently associated with recurrent pneumonia than is dysphagia (see Chapter 349). GERD is associated with microaspiration and bronchiolitis obliterans in lung transplant recipients. Aspiration has also been observed in infants with respiratory symptoms but no other apparent abnormalities. Recurrent microaspiration has been

Table 426.1	Conditions Predisposing to Aspiration Lung Injury in Children

ANATOMICAL AND MECHANICAL
Tracheoesophageal fistula
Laryngeal cleft
Vascular ring
Cleft palate
Micrognathia
Macroglossia
Cysts, tumors
Achalasia
Esophageal foreign body
Tracheostomy
Endotracheal tube
Nasal or oral feeding tube
Collagen vascular disease (scleroderma, dermatomyositis)
Gastroesophageal reflux disease
Obesity

NEUROMUSCULAR
Altered consciousness
Immaturity of swallowing/Prematurity
Dysautonomia
Increased intracranial pressure
Hydrocephalus
Vocal cord paralysis
Cerebral palsy
Muscular dystrophy
Hypotonia
Myasthenia gravis
Guillain-Barré syndrome
Spinal muscular atrophy
Ataxia-telangiectasia
Cerebral vascular accident

MISCELLANEOUS
Poor oral hygiene
Gingivitis
Prolonged hospitalization
Gastric outlet or intestinal obstruction
Poor feeding techniques (bottle propping, overfeeding, inappropriate foods for toddlers)
Bronchopulmonary dysplasia
Viral infection/bronchiolitis

reported in otherwise apparently normal newborns, especially premature infants. Aspiration is also a risk in patients suffering from acute respiratory illness from other causes, such as respiratory syncytial virus infection (see Chapter 287). Modified barium swallow and videofluoroscopy may reveal silent aspiration in these patients. This finding emphasizes the need for a high degree of clinical suspicion for ongoing aspiration in a child with an acute respiratory illness, being fed enterally, who deteriorates unexpectedly.

DIAGNOSIS

Some underlying predisposing factors (see Table 426.1) are frequently clinically apparent but may require specific further evaluation. Initial assessment begins with a detailed history and physical examination. The caregiver should be asked about spitting, vomiting, arching, or epigastric discomfort in an older child; the timing of symptoms in relation to feedings; positional changes; and nocturnal symptoms, such as coughing and wheezing. It is important to remember that coughing or gagging may be minimal or absent in a child with a depressed cough or gag reflex. Observation of a feeding is an essential part of the exam when a diagnosis of recurrent aspiration is being considered. Particular attention should be given to nasopharyngeal reflux, difficulty with sucking or swallowing, and associated coughing and choking. Voice changes (wet voice) and noisy (wet) breathing should be noted. The oral cavity should be inspected for gross abnormalities and stimulated to assess the gag reflex. Drooling or excessive accumulation of secretions in the

mouth suggests dysphagia. Lung auscultation may reveal transient crackles or wheezes after feeding, particularly in the dependent lung segments.

The diagnosis of recurrent microaspiration is challenging because of the lack of highly specific and sensitive tests (Table 426.2). A plain chest radiograph is the usual initial study for a child in whom recurrent aspiration is suspected. The classic findings of segmental or lobar infiltrates localized to dependent areas may be found (Fig. 426.1A), but there are a wide variety of radiographic findings. These findings include diffuse infiltrates, lobar infiltrates, bronchial wall thickening, hyperinflation, and even no detectable abnormalities. CT scans, though generally not indicated to establish a diagnosis of aspiration, may show infiltrates with decreased attenuation suggestive of lipoid pneumonia (see Fig. 426.1B). A carefully performed barium esophagram is useful in looking for anatomic abnormalities such as vascular ring, stricture, hiatal hernia, and tracheoesophageal fistula. It also yields qualitative information about esophageal motility and, when extended, of gastric emptying. However, primarily because of the very short viewing time, the esophagram is quite insensitive and nonspecific for aspiration or GERD. A modified barium swallow study with videofluoroscopy (videofluoroscopic swallowing study) is generally considered the gold standard for evaluating the swallowing mechanism. This study is preferably done with the assistance of a pediatric feeding specialist and a caregiver in the attempt to simulate the usual feeding technique of the child. The child is seated in normal eating position, and various consistencies of barium or

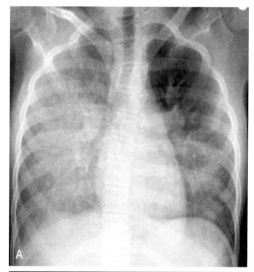
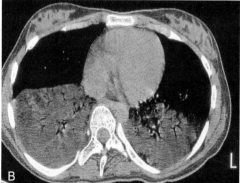

Fig. 426.1 A, Chest radiograph of a developmentally delayed 15 yr old with chronic aspiration of oral formula. Note posterior (dependent areas) distribution with sparing of heart borders. **B,** Chest CT scan of same patient. Note lung consolidation in dependent regions is of similar density to subcutaneous fat.

| Table 426.2 | Summary of Diagnostic Tests of Aspiration |

EVALUATION	BENEFITS	LIMITATIONS
Chest radiograph	Inexpensive and widely available Assesses accumulation of injury over time	Insensitive to early subtle changes of lung injury
High-resolution CT	Sensitive in detecting lung injury, such as bronchiectasis, tree-in-bud opacities, and bronchial thickening Less radiation than conventional CT Assesses accumulation of injury over time	More radiation exposure than plain radiograph Expensive
Video swallow study	Evaluates all phases of swallowing Evaluates multiple consistencies Feeding recommendations made at time of study	Information limited if child consumes only small quantities Difficult to perform in child who has not been feeding by mouth Radiation exposure proportional to study duration Cannot be performed at bedside Limited evaluation of anatomy Evaluates 1 moment in time Expensive
FEES/with sensory testing	Ability to thoroughly evaluate functional anatomy Evaluates multiple consistencies Can assess risk of aspiration in non-orally feeding child; airway protective reflexes can be assessed Feeding recommendations made at time of study Visual feedback for caregivers Can be performed at bedside No radiation exposure	Blind to esophageal phase and actual swallow Invasive and may not represent physiological swallowing conditions Evaluates 1 moment in time Not widely available Expensive
BAL	Evaluates anatomy of entire upper and lower airways Samples the end-organ of damage Sample available for multiple cytological and microbiologic tests Widely available	Uncertainty regarding interpretation of lipid-laden macrophage index Index cumbersome to calculate Requires sedation or anesthesia Invasive Expensive
Esophageal pH monitoring	Current gold standard for diagnosis of acid gastroesophageal reflux Established normative data in children	Blind to majority of reflux (nonacid) events Difficult to establish causal relationship between gastroesophageal reflux and aspiration Somewhat invasive Evaluates short time interval
Esophageal impedance monitoring	Likely gold standard for diagnosis of GERD with supraesophageal manifestations Able to detect acid and nonacid reflux events Detects proximal reflux events Able to evaluate for GERD without stopping medications	Lack of normative data for children Somewhat invasive Expensive and cumbersome to interpret Not widely available Evaluates short time interval
Gastroesophageal scintigraphy	Performed under physiologic conditions Low radiation exposure	Poor sensitivity May not differentiate between aspiration from dysphagia or GERD
Radionuclide salivagram	Child does not have to be challenged with food bolus Low radiation exposure	Unknown sensitivity Unknown relationship to disease outcomes Evaluates 1 moment in time
Dye studies	Can be constructed as screening test or confirmatory test Can evaluate aspiration of secretions or feeds Repeating over time allows for broader evaluation	Uncertainty in interpretation owing to variability of technique Can only be performed in children with tracheostomies
Other biomarkers (pepsin, bile acids) milk protein	Theoretical high specificity and sensitivity	Limited availability and standardization Variable results to date

BAL, bronchoalveolar lavage; FEES, fiberoptic-endoscopic evaluation of swallowing; GERD, gastroesophageal reflux disease.
Modified from Boesch RP, Daines C, Willging JP, et al: Advances in the diagnosis and management of chronic pulmonary aspiration in children, *Eur Respir J* 28:847–861, 2006; and Tutor JD, Gosa MM: Dysphagia and aspiration in children, *Pediatr Pulmonol* 47(4):321–337, 2012.

barium-impregnated foods are offered. This study is more sensitive for demonstrating aspiration than bedside assessment or a traditional barium swallow study. The sensitivity of the modified barium swallow study is such that it occasionally detects aspiration in patients without apparent respiratory abnormalities.

A gastroesophageal milk scintiscan offers theoretical advantages over a barium swallow in being more physiologic and giving a longer window of viewing than the barium esophagram for detecting aspiration and GERD. However, this study has been found to have a low sensitivity and provides relatively little anatomic detail. Another radionuclide scan

termed the salivagram may also be useful to assess aspiration of esophageal contents. When this scan is performed by experienced personnel, its sensitivity appears to be comparable to that of the modified barium swallow study. The use of fiberoptic endoscopic evaluation of swallowing has been found useful in adult and some pediatric patients, to observe swallowing directly without radiation exposure. The child's reaction to placement of the endoscope may alter the assessment of function, depending on level of comfort and cooperation.

Tracheobronchial aspirates can be examined for numerous entities to evaluate for aspiration. For patients with artificial airways, the use of an oral dye and visual examination of tracheal secretions is useful. This test should not be done on a chronic basis, such as in tube feedings, because of possible dye toxicity. In using this test acutely, the best method is to place a few drops of dye on the patient's tongue and perform subsequent suctioning of the airway over the next several minutes. Quantitation of lipid-laden alveolar macrophages from bronchial aspirates has been shown to be a sensitive test for aspiration in children, but false-positive tests occur, especially with endobronchial obstruction, use of intravenous lipids, sepsis, and pulmonary bleeding. Bronchial washings may also be examined for various food substances, including lactose, glucose, food fibers, and milk antigens, as well as pepsin. Specificity and sensitivity of these tests have not been well studied.

TREATMENT

If chronic aspiration is associated with another underlying medical condition, treatment should be directed toward that problem. The level of morbidity from respiratory problems should determine the level of intervention. Often milder dysphagia can be treated with alteration of feeding position, limiting texture of foods to those best tolerated on modified barium esophagram (usually thicker foods), or limiting quantity per feeding. Currently evidence is lacking regarding the advisability of restricting oral intake of water by children whose aspiration is largely

of thin fluids. Nasogastric tube feedings can be utilized temporarily during periods of transient vocal cord dysfunction or other dysphagia. Postpyloric feedings may also be helpful, especially if gastroesophageal reflux is present, although this does not eliminate reflux. There are several surgical procedures that may be considered. Tracheostomy, although sometimes predisposing to aspiration, may provide overall benefit from improved bronchial hygiene and the ability to suction aspirated material. Use of a one-way (Passy-Muir) valve on a tracheostomy tube has been shown to improve swallowing. Fundoplication with gastrostomy or jejunostomy feeding tube will reduce the probability of gastroesophageal reflux-induced aspiration, but recurrent pneumonias often persist because of dysphagia and presumed aspiration of upper airway secretions. Medical treatment with anticholinergics, such as glycopyrrolate or scopolamine, may significantly reduce morbidity from salivary aspiration but often has side effects. Aggressive surgical intervention with salivary gland excision, ductal ligation, laryngotracheal separation, or esophagogastric disconnection can be considered in severe, unresponsive cases. Although usually reserved for the most severe cases, surgical therapy may significantly improve quality of life and ease of care for some patients.

Bibliography is available at Expert Consult.

Chapter **427**
Immune and Inflammatory Lung Disease

第四百二十七章
免疫和炎症性肺疾病

中文导读

　　本章主要介绍了过敏性肺炎、职业性和环境性肺疾病、肉芽肿性肺疾病、嗜酸细胞性肺疾病、间质性肺疾病、婴儿神经内分泌细胞增生症和纤维化性肺疾病。描述了过敏性肺炎的病因学和病理学、临床特点、分类、辅助检查（包括影像学、肺组织活检、吸入抗原激发试验等）和治疗；职业性和环境性肺疾病的分类、发病机制和治疗；肉芽肿性多血管炎、结节病、铍中毒、原发性免疫缺陷相关肉芽肿性肺疾病的发病机制、临床特点、辅助检查和治疗；介绍了嗜酸

细胞性肺疾病、间质性肺疾病、婴儿神经内分泌细胞增生症的发病机制、临床特点、诊断和治疗等；其中嗜酸细胞性肺疾病包括LÖFFLER综合征、急性嗜酸细胞性肺炎、慢性嗜酸细胞性肺炎、嗜酸细胞性肉芽肿伴多血管炎（Churg-Strauss综合征）、变应性支气管肺曲霉菌病及高嗜酸细胞综合征；间质性肺疾病中主要介绍了肺泡表面活性物质代谢异常、系统性疾病所致的间质性肺疾病以及抗肾小球基底膜病。纤维化性肺疾病的临床特点、评估，以及治疗。

427.1 Hypersensitivity Pneumonia

Kevin J. Kelly and Michelle L. Hernandez

Hypersensitivity pneumonia (HP), aptly called *extrinsic allergic alveolitis* because the inciting agent is almost uniformly inhaled from the environment, is a complex immunologic-mediated syndrome of the pulmonary alveoli and interstitium. There are numerous specific disease names based on the origin of the inhaled offending antigen to describe HP. Prompt recognition of the signs and symptoms allows for complete reversal of the disease without long-term adverse consequences if the source of the exposure is recognized and abated. Failure to recognize the disease early may lead to chronic irreversible lung changes with persistent symptoms in the patient.

ETIOLOGY

The most common sources of offending agents that cause HP include agricultural aerosols, inhaled protein antigens from animals, antigens from microorganisms of bacteria, fungi, or protozoan origin, as well as chemicals of low and high molecular weight (Table 427.1). Many inciting agents are associated with *occupational diseases* in which children do not regularly work. However, the same diseases can occur in children due to exposures to similar antigen sources in nonoccupational environments, or in occupational environments with teenage workers. In addition to HP, the same antigens may lead to allergic asthma or chronic bronchitis as seen with animal proteins, contaminated metal working fluids, and other inhaled antigens.

More than 300 antigens have been associated with HP. In children, primary sources of HP have been the result of exposure to pet birds (or feathers in bedding and pillows) such as parakeets, canaries, cockatiels, or cockatoos. Aerosol spread of bird droppings can also occur by clothes dryer vents or by heating vents from a garage where the pet birds were housed. Humidifiers and hot tubs are notorious for contamination with thermophilic organisms (bacteria and mold) as well as *Mycobacterium avium* complex. Buildings with inadequate ventilation and insufficient air turnover present an increased risk of mold exposure from prior flooding or damp condensation. Despite exposures to the same antigen sources, members of the same family may exhibit different presentations of allergic disease. Some family members may have symptoms of asthma or rhinitis, while another may have HP.

PATHOGENESIS

HP has been traditionally classified as acute, subacute, or chronic. During the acute phase, the offending antigen triggers an inflammatory response promoting the development of immune complexes. These immune complexes activate the complement pathway, ultimately resulting in the accumulation of neutrophils in the airway that release enzymes such as neutrophil elastase, that damage surrounding lung tissue. Activated macrophages in the lung promote recruitment of lymphocytes into the tissues. Pathology shows alveolitis with a mixed cellular infiltration comprised of lymphocytes, macrophage, plasma cells, and neutrophils. Continued exposure to the offending antigen will lead to subacute or chronic HP. This chronic exposure results in the formation of loose, noncaseating granulomas located near the respiratory or terminal bronchioles. It is critical when a biopsy is being performed (transbronchial or surgical) that the pathologist knows that HP is being considered as there are other interstitial lung diseases (ILDs) that produce similar granulomas with subtle location differences depending on their origin.

CLINICAL MANIFESTATIONS AND CLASSIFICATION

Acute HP is typically caused by heavy exposure to an offending antigen. This is the most common form of exposure but is frequently not recognized. Symptoms are confused with bacterial or viral disease leading to treatment with antibiotics. Four to 8 hr after exposure, patients can present with the abrupt onset of cough, chest tightness, dyspnea, fever, chills, and fatigue (Table 427.2). Rarely, findings of wheezing are present on the initial examination. Rather, tachypnea with fine crackles may be heard by auscultation in the lung bases. However, auscultation

may be normal at this stage. After cessation of exposure, symptoms may subside after 24-48 hr.

When **recurrent subacute HP** is present, the symptoms become progressive with shortness of breath and cough (productive), weight loss, malaise, and loss of appetite. When HP becomes chronic and *progressive*, the patient is hypoxic, and clubbing of the fingers is evident. If the disease progresses to interstitial fibrosis, the symptoms tend to not respond to therapy and mortality risk is increased. Histology is hard to distinguish from **idiopathic pulmonary fibrosis** at this stage.

Distinguishing chronic disease from subacute disease is difficult without clear differentiating criteria, but a diagnosis of HP at any stage results in the clinician recommending very specific interventions for improvement. HP is characterized as (1) acute nonprogressive and intermittent, (2) acute progressive and intermittent, (3) chronic nonprogressive, and (4) chronic progressive (Table 427.3). A diagnosis of HP is certain when the known exposure with immune response to the offending antigen is identified; the medical history and physical finding are abnormal on examination; **bronchoalveolar lavage (BAL)** and lung biopsy are abnormal. Some clinicians have foregone the lung biopsy when a cluster of cases occurs and 1 patient biopsy is already abnormal.

LABORATORY

Most of the abnormal laboratory findings in HP are not specific and represent evidence of activated inflammatory markers or lung injury. Nonspecific elevation of immune globulins or the erythrocyte sedimentation rate and C-reactive protein may also be found. Circulating immune complexes may be detected. Lactate dehydrogenase may be elevated in the presence of lung inflammation and normalizes with response to therapy.

Serum IgG precipitins to the offending agent are frequently positive and have a poor positive predictive value for disease. Among asymptomatic pigeon breeders, precipitating antibodies are nearly universal. False negatives can also be seen due to fluctuating serum antibody levels over time, and lack of standardized commercial antigens and reagents available for laboratory testing. It is critical that laboratories familiar with the performance of these tests be utilized. Those laboratories often recognize the value of processing antigens for precipitation from the *environmental source directly* as the test substrate with patient serum. Skin testing for IgE-mediated disease is not warranted unless there is evidence of mixed lung pathology such as asthma and interstitial lung opacities.

Radiology

Chest radiograph almost always precedes the use of high-resolution computerized tomography (HRCT) of the chest in children because of the need for sedation and concerns regarding risk of irradiation dose from HRCT. The plain radiograph will often demonstrate a ground-glass appearance, interstitial prominence, with a predominant location in the upper and middle lung fields. It is common for a chest radiograph to be considered normal by a radiologist early in the disease progression. Late in the disease, interstitial fibrosis may become prominent in the presence of increasing dyspnea, hypoxemia on room air, and clubbing of the fingers. Mediastinum widening from lymphadenopathy is *not* usually present; when present, the lymph nodes are prominent along the airway near the carina, suggesting that the antigen source is inhaled and being responded to by the immune system.

Classical findings of mid zone and upper zone opacities with ground-glass appearance and nodularity on HRCT in the presence of typical clinical exam HP findings (lung crackles, cough, dyspnea) and lymphocytosis on BAL are almost sufficient to make a diagnosis (Fig. 427.1). These findings must prompt the clinician to identify the exposure in order to secure the diagnosis and eliminate the offending antigen. Without therapy, the progressive inflammatory response leads to air trapping, honeycombing, emphysema, and mild fibrosis in the chronic state. It is in this latter stage that idiopathic pulmonary fibrosis and nonspecific interstitial fibrosis are hard to differentiate. Whether true idiopathic pulmonary fibrosis exists in children where fibroblast foci are found on biopsy with usual interstitial fibrosis has been questioned.

Table 427.1 | Antigen Sources Associated with Specific Causes of Hypersensitivity Pneumonitis

HYPERSENSITIVITY PNEUMONITIS	ANTIGEN SOURCE	HYPERSENSITIVITY PNEUMONITIS	ANTIGEN SOURCE
Bagassosis (mold on pressed sugar cane)	*Thermoactinomyces sacchari* *Thermoactinomyces vulgaris*	Maple bark disease (moldy maple bark)	*Cryptostroma corticale*
Bat lung (bat droppings)	Bat serum protein	Miller's lung (dust-contaminated grain)	*Sitophilus granarius* (i.e., wheat weevil)
Bible printer's lung	Moldy typesetting water	Moldy hay, grain, silage (farmer's lung)	Thermophilic actinomycetes Fungi (e.g., *Aspergillus umbrosus*)
Bird fancier's lung (parakeets, budgerigars, pigeons)	Droppings, feathers, serum proteins	Mollusk shell hypersensitivity pneumonitis	Sea-snail shell
Byssinosis ("brown lung") (unclear if a true cause of hypersensitivity pneumonitis; asthma is common)	Cotton mill dust (carding and spinning areas of cotton, flax, and soft-hemp)	Mushroom worker's lung	Mushroom spores Thermophilic actinomycetes
Canary fancier's lung	Serum proteins	Paprika slicer's lung (moldy paprika pods)	*Mucor stolonifer*
Cheese washer's lung (moldy cheese)	*Penicillium casei* *Aspergillus clavatus*	Pauli's reagent alveolitis	Sodium diazobenzene sulfate
Chemical hypersensitivity pneumonitis	Diphenylmethane diisocyanate (MDI) Toluene diisocyanate (TDI)	Pearl oyster shell pneumonitis	Oyster shells
Coffee worker's lung	Coffee-bean dust	Pituitary snuff taker's disease	Dried, powdered cattle or pig pituitary proteins
Composter's lung	*T. vulgaris* *Aspergillus* species	Potato riddler's lung (moldy hay around potatoes)	Thermophilic actinomycetes *T. vulgaris* *Faenia rectivirgula* *Aspergillus* spp.
Contaminated basement (sewage) pneumonitis	*Cephalosporium*		
Coptic lung (mummy handler's lung)	Cloth wrappings of mummies	Poultry worker's lung (feather plucker's disease)	Serum proteins (chicken products)
Detergent worker's lung (washing powder lung)	*Bacillus subtilis* enzymes	Pyrethrum (pesticide)	Pyrethrum
Dry rot lung	*Merulius lacrymans*	Sauna taker's lung	*Aureobasidium* spp., other sources
Duck fever	Feathers, serum proteins	Sequoiosis (moldy wood dust)	*Graphium* *Pullularia* *Trichoderma* spp. *Aureobasidium pullulans*
Epoxy resin lung	Phthalic anhydride (heated epoxy resin)		
Esparto dust (mold in plaster dust)	*Aspergillus fumigatus* Thermophilic actinomycetes	Suberosis (moldy cork dust)	*Thermoactinomyces viridis* *Penicillium glabrum* *Aspergillus conidia*
Farm worker lung	Thermophilic actinomycetes plus others	Summer-type pneumonitis	*Trichosporon cutaneum*
Feather duvet (pillow) lung	Goose or duck feathers	Tea grower's lung	Tea plants
Fish meal worker's lung	Fish meal	Thatched-roof lung (huts in New Guinea)	*Saccharomonospora viridis* (dead grasses and leaves)
Furrier's lung (sewing furs; animal fur dust)	Animal pelts	Tobacco grower's lung	*Aspergillus* spp. *Scopulariopsis brevicaulis*
Grain measurer's lung	Cereal grain (*Sporobolomyces*) Grain dust (mixture of dust, silica, fungi, insects, and mites)	Turkey handling disease	Serum proteins (turkey products)
		Unventilated shower	*Epicoccum nigrum*
Hot-tub lung (mists; mold on ceiling and around tub)	*Cladosporium* spp. *Mycobacterium avium* complex	Upholstery fabric (nylon filament, cotton/polyester, and latex adhesive)	Aflatoxin-producing fungus, *Fusarium* spp.
Humidifier fever	*Thermoactinomyces* (*T. vulgaris, T. sacchari, T. candidus*) *Klebsiella oxytoca* *Naegleria gruberi* *Acanthamoeba polyphaga* *Acanthamoeba castellani*	Velvet worker's lung	Unknown (? nylon velvet fiber, tannic acid, potato starch)
		Vineyard sprayer's lung	Copper sulfate (bordeaux mixture)
		Wind instrument lung	Bacteria or mold contamination of instrument
Laboratory worker's lung (rats, gerbils)	Urine, serum, pelts, proteins	Wine maker's lung (mold on grapes)	*Botrytis cinerea*
Lifeguard lung	Aerosolized endotoxin from pool-water sprays and fountains	Wood dust pneumonitis (oak, cedar, and mahogany dust, pine and spruce pulp)	*Alternaria* spp. *Bacillus subtilis*
Lycoperdonosis (*Lycoperdon* puffballs)	Puffball spores		
Machine operator's lung	*Pseudomonas fluorescens* Aerosolized metal working fluid	Wood pulp worker's disease (oak and maple trees)	*Penicillium* spp.
Malt worker's disease (moldy barley)	*Aspergillus fumigatus, Aspergillus clavatus*	Wood trimmer's disease (contaminated wood trimmings)	*Rhizopus* spp., *Mucor* spp.

Table 427.2	Clinical History Clues Leading to a Diagnosis of Hypersensitivity Pneumonitis

Recurrent pneumonia
Pneumonia after repeat exposures (week, season, situation)
Cough, fever, and chest symptoms after making a job change or home change
Cough, fever, wheezing after return to school or only at school
Pet exposure (especially birds that shed dust such as pigeons, canaries, cockatiels, cockatoos)
Bird contaminant exposure (e.g., pigeon infestation)
Farm exposure to birds and hay
History of water damage despite typical cleaning
Use of hot tub, sauna, swimming pool
Other family members or workers with similar recurrent symptoms
Improvement after temporary environment change (e.g., vacation)

Table 427.3	Criteria Used in the Diagnosis of Hypersensitivity Pneumonitis

1. Identified exposure to offending antigen(s) by:
   - Medical history of exposure to suspected antigen in the patient's living environment
   - Investigations of the environment confirm the presence of an inciting antigen
   - Identification of specific immune responses (immunoglobulin G serum precipitin antibodies against the identified antigen) are suggestive of the potential etiology but are insufficient in isolation to confirm a diagnosis
2. Clinical, radiographic, or physiologic findings compatible with hypersensitivity pneumonitis:
   - Respiratory and often constitutional signs and symptoms
   - Crackles on auscultation of the chest
   - Weight loss
   - Cough
   - Breathlessness
   - Episodic fever
   - Wheezing
   - Fatigue
   NOTE: These findings are especially suggestive of hypersensitivity pneumonitis when they appear or worsen several hours after antigen exposure.
   - A reticular, nodular, or ground-glass opacities on chest radiograph or high-resolution CT
   - Abnormalities in the following pulmonary function tests
   - Spirometry (restrictive, obstructive, or mixed patterns)
   - Lung volumes (low or high)
   - Reduced diffusion capacity by carbon monoxide
   - Altered gas exchange either at rest or with exercise (reduced partial pressure of arterial oxygen by blood gas or pulse oximeter testing)
3. Bronchoalveolar lavage with lymphocytosis:
   - Usually with low CD4:CD8 ratio (i.e., CD8 is higher than normal)
   - Lymphocyte stimulation by offending antigen results in proliferation and cytokine production
4. Abnormal response to inhalation challenge testing to the offending antigen:
   - Reexposure to the environment
   - Inhalation challenge to the suspected antigen (rarely done now because of the risk of exacerbating the disease)
5. Histopathology showing compatible changes with hypersensitivity pneumonitis by 1 of these findings:
   - Poorly formed, noncaseating granulomas (most often found closer to the respiratory epithelium where deposition of the offending antigen occurs)
   - Mononuclear cell infiltrate in the pulmonary interstitium

Bronchoalveolar Lavage

BAL is one of the most sensitive tests and very helpful to the clinician in supporting the diagnosis of HP. Lymphocytosis frequently exceeding 50% of the recovered cells is seen on the BAL and should alert the clinician to the possibility of HP. Sarcoid, idiopathic pulmonary fibrosis,

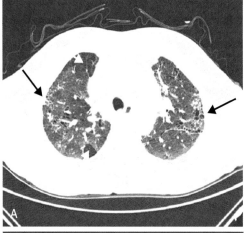

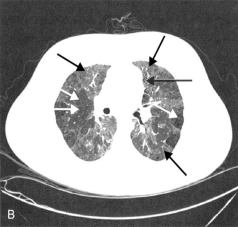

Fig. 427.1 Radiologic findings in subacute (A) and chronic (B) hypersensitivity pneumonitis. **A,** Interstitial fibrosis *(black arrows)* and emphysematous changes *(white arrows)* in chronic HP with superimposed subacute HP. **B,** Ground-glass opacities *(black arrows),* mosaic perfusion *(white arrows),* and fibrosis *(red arrow)* in chronic HP caused by pigeon exposure. *(From Douglass JA, Sandrini A, Holgate ST, O'Hehir RE: Allergic bronchopulmonary aspergillosis and hypersensitivity pneumonitis. In Adkinson AF, editor: Middleton's allergy principles and practice, Philadelphia, 2014, Elsevier, Fig. 61.5.)*

cryptogenic organizing pneumonia, berylliosis, granite workers lung disease, amiodarone pneumonia, lymphoma, and Langerhans cell histiocytosis may demonstrate lymphocytosis on BAL. All BAL specimens should have flow cytometry measurements of T-cell markers (CD3, CD4, and CD8 at a minimum). The predominant phenotype of the lymphocytosis is CD3+/CD8+/CD56+/CD57+/CD10−. In the normal circulation, lymphocytes with CD4 markers predominate at a ratio of approximately 2:1 compared to CD8 lymphocytes. *In the lung compartment with HP, this ratio becomes approximately equal to or less than 1 (CD4:CD8 ≤ 1) with either an increase in CD8 lymphocytes or a decline in CD4 lymphocytes.* This ratio assists the clinician in making a diagnosis of HP. This is in sharp contrast to other lymphocytic granulomatous diseases, like sarcoidosis, where the CD4:CD8 is ≥ 2, or pulmonary fibrosis associated with connective tissue disease. Cryptogenic organizing pneumonia, a rare disease in children, also may present with BAL where the CD4:CD8 is ≤ 1 and may be confused initially with HP.

Lung Biopsy

Lung biopsy is necessary to confirm a diagnosis of HP in the absence of critical elements like antigen exposure, typical medical history, characteristic physical exam, and CD8+ lymphocytes in the BAL. Open lung biopsy is often the route of choice in young children because of the difficulty in safely obtaining satisfactory amounts of tissue by transbronchial biopsy. Lack of positive serum precipitins to offending antigen and exposure history are common reasons for obtaining lung biopsies. It is crucial to inform the pathologist about the suspicion of HP so that the findings can be interpreted appropriately.

Histological examination shows poorly formed, noncaseating granulomas near the respiratory and terminal bronchioles and multinucleated giant cells. This is in sharp contrast to the well-formed granulomas seen in sarcoidosis. Lymphocytes and plasma cells infiltrate the alveolar walls predominantly in a bronchocentric pattern. Fibrosis in the peribronchial region supports a diagnosis of HP. Foamy cytoplasm accompanying large histiocytes in the alveoli and interstitium may be characteristically found.

Antigen Challenge by Inhalation
Inhalation challenge can support the diagnosis of HP by demonstrating a causal relationship between environmental exposure and symptoms. Inhalation challenge can be performed by 2 methods: (1) reexposure of the patient to the environment where the suspected antigen is present and (2) direct inhalation challenge at the hospital to material collected from the suspected source of the antigen. As the second method has resulted in severe exacerbation of disease in some individuals, its use is discouraged.

Two abnormal response patterns may be seen. Most commonly, where there is HP without asthma, symptoms occur 8-12 hr after direct challenge in the hospital or reexposure at the source of the antigen. The challenges replicate some or all the symptoms observed in the acute syndrome with fever, dyspnea, fatigue, and crackles on lung auscultation. Blood drawn prior to challenge and then repeated during these symptoms often demonstrates an increased neutrophil count compared to baseline. Pulmonary function tests demonstrate a fall in forced vital capacity (FVC) and often a concurrent fall in the forced expiratory volume at 1 sec (FEV_1) with a stable or increasing ratio of FEV_1:FVC percentage reflecting a restrictive defect. Hypoxemia may accompany this decline in pulmonary function as well as a fall in the diffusion capacity of carbon monoxide (DLCO). To see the complete effect, exercise during this period may show a considerable fall in oxygenation despite normal arterial blood gas oxygen tension and normal pulse oximetry at rest. This finding denotes the onset of worsening restrictive lung disease.

Atopic patients may experience a biphasic response to inhalation challenge. These patients may develop an early reduction in FEV_1, followed 4 to 6 hr by a second drop in FEV_1 accompanied by decreased FEV_1 and FVC, fever, and leukocytosis.

TREATMENT
The control of environmental exposure to the offending antigen is a key to curing HP and remains the ideal method of treatment and prevention of recurrence. The clinical and pathologic manifestations of acute and subacute HP are reversible with removal of the offending antigen. Counseling about the risk to children of exposure to birds and feathered bedding, or other environmental antigens, biologic aerosols, or agricultural dusts that are known to induce HP are important. Certainly, the source of the antigen and type of antigen appears to affect the response to treatment and long-term prognosis. Older individuals who contract farmer's lung are likely to recover with minimal permanent residual effect, whereas individuals with bird fancier's lungs from antigens produced by pigeons have a poorer prognosis, especially if fibrosis is detected on lung biopsy. The pediatrician should advise—in the strongest terms—removal of the antigen source from the affected child's environment. This may be an extraordinary challenge given various children's living circumstances and lack of independent control of the environment in which they live.

In addition, pediatricians should be familiar with recommendations about the maintenance of heating, ventilation, and air conditioning systems, as well as of humidifiers and vaporizers. Daily drainage, cleansing of residue, and routine cleaning with hydrogen peroxide or bleach help rid humidifiers and vaporizers of harmful pathogens such as thermophiles that cause HP.

Glucocorticoids at a dose of 0.5 mg/kg/day of prednisolone or equivalent (up to a maximum dose of 60 mg prednisolone daily) will reduce the immune inflammatory response in the lungs. In some cases, high dose pulse intravenous methylprednisolone is required, supplemented by treatment with oral prednisolone or other immunosuppressive therapies including cyclosporine or azathioprine. Comparative trials in adults demonstrate that the use of 4 wk of therapy is as effective as 12 wk of therapy. Removal of antigen alone is sufficient to normalize lung function in most patients, but symptoms and pulmonary functions return to normal faster with the use of glucocorticoids. Because of the rapid reversal of symptoms, successful abatement of the environment is sometimes compromised when the family sees improvement prior to the antigen source removal.

Bibliography is available at Expert Consult.

427.2 Occupational and Environmental Lung Disease
Kevin J. Kelly and Michelle L. Hernandez

Occupational and environmental lung diseases constitute a larger part of primary care pediatrics, pediatric emergency medicine, and other pediatric subspecialties than most pediatric practitioners expect or realize. Although occupational and environmental lung diseases include **occupational asthma**, **reactive airways dysfunction syndrome (RADS)**, HP, hard metal inhalation lung disease, berylliosis, and air pollution, this chapter focuses on occupational asthma and RADS. Berylliosis has a propensity to form granulomas (see Chapter 427.3). Although some diseases will be seen with regularity, the important role that a part-time workplace, school, daycare, neighbors' housing, multiple family housing, and indoor and outdoor environments may have in the causation of signs and symptoms in the patient is not always considered by the clinician.

The vast array of exposures shown to cause disease of the lungs is daunting, such as the inhalation of baking flour or household cleaning fluids causing asthma, microwave popcorn exposure to diacetyl resulting in bronchiolitis obliterans, and exposure to thermophilic organisms or mold resulting in hypersensitivity pneumonitis. The acute eosinophilic pneumonias associated with new onset of smoking and chemical inhalation of 1,1,1-trichloroethane (Scotchgard) require a high index of suspicion and unique lines of questioning. The same antigen encountered in a work, school, home, or outdoor environment may result in a different disease presentation because of host factors, dose exposure, and genetic susceptibility. One of the most prominent examples is an investigation of workers who inhaled metal working fluid. Despite similar exposures, some developed HP, others developed asthma, and some displayed no symptoms at all. Immunologic evaluation in some exposures has shown similar immune responses in different individuals, but a wide range of disease provocation. When high molecular weight proteins cause asthma, symptoms of rhinoconjunctivitis frequently precede the onset of pulmonary symptoms. The medical history of occupational and environmental lung diseases has used an expanded construct with a simple acronym, **WHACOS** (Table 427.4).

It is important to remember that in patients with occupational- or environmental-induced disease, the onset of symptoms has a lag time between exposure and symptoms. In **occupational asthma**, there may be an immediate response within 1-2 hr of exposure, demonstrated as a decline in pulmonary function, specifically the FEV_1. Usually, lung function returns to normal spontaneously unless persistent exposure occurs. Some patients demonstrate no immediate reduction in lung function, but rather experience a delayed response, 4-6 hr after the exposure. Treating physicians can take advantage of this physiology in occupational and environmental asthma by use of spirometry before and after work or school, or peak flow measurements hourly during exposure and after leaving the exposure. Because workers and schoolchildren have prolonged periods of exposure followed by a number of days without exposure, the use of pulmonary function plus bronchial

Table 427.4	A Construct (WHACOS) That Has Been Used in Medical Interviewing of Patients, Coworkers, and Family Members When Environmental or Occupational Lung Disease Is Being Considered
W	*W*hat do you do?
H	*H*ow do you do what you do?
A	Are symptoms *A*cute or are they *Chronic*?
C	Do any *C*oworkers, family, classmates, or friends have the same symptoms?
O	Do you have any hobbies, travel, or animal/pet exposures *O*utside of school or work?
S	Are you *S*atisfied with work or school?

hyperresponsiveness (e.g., methacholine) testing is helpful. Pulmonary function tests prior to starting work on a Monday of a typical work week may be normal. By Friday of a typical work or school week, the baseline pulmonary functions may have fallen, and bronchial responsiveness may have become more sensitive to a lower concentration of histamine, methacholine, or mannitol. By the following Monday, the tests may have returned to normal or near normal with no change other than reduced exposure.

In the case of HP, a lag of 4-8 hr between the time of exposure and the onset of fever, cough, and dyspnea is common. Unfortunately, the return home from hospitalization for culture-negative pneumonia to a source of antigen-causing HP often results in complete reoccurrence of symptoms. Clinicians must have a high index of suspicion for HP with reoccurrence of pulmonary infiltrates shortly after reexposure (see Chapter 427.1).

CLASSIFICATION AND PATHOGENESIS

Occupational and environmental lung diseases include numerous syndromes of human lung disease such as **occupational asthma**, **RADS (reactive upper airway disease syndrome)**, hypersensitivity pneumonitis (see Chapter 427.1), air pollution–induced disease, hard metal inhalation lung disease, berylliosis, occupation-induced lung cancer (e.g., mesothelioma from asbestosis), and chronic obstructive pulmonary disease without smoking. Most of these diseases are not problematic for children, but adolescents may be exposed through part-time work or by single exposures as seen in RADS.

Occupational and Environmental Asthma

The general principles of diagnosis, clinical signs and symptoms, treatment, and causes of asthma are discussed in Chapter 169. *High molecular weight* causes of occupational and environmental asthma can be characterized as allergens, which are normally proteins and enzymes, inhaled from multiple sources (Table 427.5). These include various animals, shellfish, fish, enzymes (e.g., *Bacillus subtilis* in laundry detergent), and flour or cereals. Occupational and environmental asthma is also caused by a number of low molecular weight agents including reactive chemicals, transition metals, and wood dusts (Table 427.6). These *low molecular weight agents* are sufficient to induce an immune response, but often not by an IgE-mediated mechanism. These low molecular weight chemicals appear to act as haptens that bind directly to human proteins, causing an immune response in the human host.

The pathogenesis of asthma in patients exposed to high molecular weight antigens follows the experience of nonoccupational asthma in patients where atopy, gender, genetics, concentration of antigen, duration of exposure, and other individual factors all contribute to the development of disease. Most individuals require a concentration and duration of exposure sufficient to cause IgE antibody sensitization to the offending allergen with development of bronchial hyperresponsiveness and airway inflammatory disease upon reexposure. If the allergen exposure is sufficient, these proteins can drive the immune response to a T-lymphocyte type 2 phenotype (Th2), even in patients without prior atopic disposition. This occurred in the case of latex allergy, where many nonatopic individuals and patients exposed to allergen in their personal healthcare developed occupational allergy to multiple proteins from natural rubber latex. Atopic individuals are at the highest risk of developing latex allergy. A longitudinal study demonstrated that powdered latex gloves with high allergen content were the reason for the epidemic of latex allergy and occupational asthma. Unfortunately, despite primary removal of the offending sensitizing agent, asthma symptoms and bronchial hyperresponsiveness induced from multiple causes persist in approximately 70% of individuals with occupational asthma.

Reactive Airways Disease Syndrome and Irritant-Induced Asthma

RADS presents with acute respiratory symptoms within minutes or hours following a single inhalation of a *high concentration* of irritant gas, aerosol, or smoke. The clinical manifestations and pathophysiology of RADS have been studied through experimental design or epidemiology studies following exposure to chlorine gas, acetic acid, dimethylaminoethanol, chlorofluorocarbons, epichlorohydrin, and diisocyanates.

Table 427.7 lists the criteria for diagnosis of RADS. Asthma-like symptoms and airway hyperresponsiveness then ensue, which often persist for prolonged periods. Unlike typical asthma, RADS is often not reversible by use of a bronchodilator. This is probably a consequence of the direct injury to the epithelium and subsequent submucosal fibrosis.

Irritant-induced asthma is a closely related form of asthma resulting from nonimmunologic provocation of bronchial hyperresponsiveness with airflow obstruction. In contrast to RADS, irritant-induced asthma occurs after single or multiple exposures to irritant chemicals in *low concentration*. If the resultant pulmonary symptoms occur after multiple exposures at a plant, it is termed *nonimmunologic-induced asthma*.

Predisposing factors for the development of RADS are not well characterized. Atopy and cigarette smoking may increase the risk of developing RADS when exposure through inhalation of irritant chemicals occurs. In addition to host factors, the type of chemical appears to be important. Higher concentrations of chemicals, the type of chemical (vapor or wet aerosols), and bleaching agents are the most offending agents to cause RADS. Dry particle aerosols are less likely to cause RADS. Analysis of the World Trade Center firefighters indicates that the presence of bronchial hyperresponsiveness prior to a chemical exposure *does not* increase the risk for an individual to develop RADS.

Pathogenesis of RADS follows a typical pattern, driven by the initial injury to the airway epithelium. Initial histology demonstrates rapid denudation of the mucosa accompanied by a submucosal fibrinous, hemorrhagic exudate. Subepithelial edema subsequently occurs with some regeneration of the epithelial layer, proliferation of basal and parabasal cells, and eventually areas of fibrosis. The desquamation, subepithelial fibrosis, thickening of the basement membrane, and regeneration of basal cells are all more prominent in RADS than in occupational asthma. This may explain the limited response to bronchodilator therapy in this syndrome compared to asthma.

The clinical manifestations of RADS and irritant-induced asthma are different from each other mostly in the onset of symptoms. Patients with RADS typically can pinpoint the exact time of onset of symptoms as well as the exact number of hours post exposure. The symptoms are so severe that nearly 80% of subjects in one study presented to an emergency department for care. The lower airway symptoms of cough, dyspnea, chest tightness, and wheezing are prominent features in RADS, with cough being most prevalent. Because of the toxic nature of the inhaled chemical, it is predictable that an upper airway syndrome of throat and nose burning will often accompany the lower airway symptoms. This part of the complex has been referred to as **respiratory upper airway dysfunction syndrome.**

Individuals with **irritant-induced asthma** present with a more insidious onset of symptoms. Because of the recurrent nature of the low concentration of chemical, patients may not be able to identify the underlying trigger initially. Similar to allergic rhinitis, patients may describe nasal congestion, rhinorrhea, sneezing, postnasal drip, ocular

Table 427.5	High Molecular Weight Antigens Known to Induce Occupational or Environmental Asthma

OCCUPATION OR ENVIRONMENT	SOURCE	OCCUPATION OR ENVIRONMENT	SOURCE
ANIMAL-DERIVED ANTIGENS		**ACARIANS**	
Agricultural worker	Cow dander	Apple grower	Fruit tree red spider mite (*Panonychus ulmi*)
Bakery	Lactalbumin		
Butcher	Cow bone dust, pig, goat dander	Citrus farmer	Citrus red mite (*Panonychus citri*)
Cook	Raw beef	Farmer	Barn mite, two-spotted spider mite (*Tetranychus urticae*), grain mite
Dairy industry	Lactoserum, lactalbumin		
Egg producer	Egg protein	Flour handler	Mites and parasites
Farmer	Deer dander, mink urine	Grain-store worker	Grain mite
Frog catcher	Frog	Horticulturist	*Amblyseius cucumeris*
Hairdresser	Sericin	Poultry worker	Fowl mite
Ivory worker	Ivory dust	Vine grower	McDaniel spider mite (*Tetranychus mcdanieli*)
Laboratory technician	Bovine serum albumin, laboratory animal, monkey dander		
Nacre buttons	Nacre dust	**MOLDS**	
Pharmacist	Endocrine glands	Agriculture	*Plasmopara viticola*
Pork producer	Pig gut (vapor from soaking water)	Baker	*Alternaria, Aspergillus* (unspecified)
Poultry worker	Chicken	Beet sugar worker	*Aspergillus* (unspecified)
Tanner	Casein (cow's milk)	Coal miner	*Rhizopus nigricans*
Various	Bat guano	Coffee maker	*Chrysonilia sitophila*
Veterinarian	Goat dander	Laborer	Sooty molds (*Ascomycetes, deuteromycetes*)
Zookeeper	Birds		
		Logging worker	*Chrysonilia sitophila*
CRUSTACEANS, SEAFOOD, FISH		Plywood factory worker	*Neurospora*
Canning factory	Octopus	Sausage processing	*Penicillium nalgiovense*
Diet product	Shark cartilage	Sawmill worker	*Trichoderma koningii*
Fish food factory	Gammarus shrimp	Stucco worker	*Mucor* spp. (contaminating esparto fibers)
Fish processor	Clam, shrimp, crab, prawn, salmon, trout, lobster, turbot, various fishes	Technician	*Dictyostelium discoideum* (mold), *Aspergillus niger*
Fisherman	Red soft coral, cuttlefish		
Jewelry polisher	Cuttlefish bone	**MUSHROOMS**	
Laboratory grinder	Marine sponge	Agriculture	*Agaricus bisporus* (white mushroom)
Oyster farm	Hoya (oyster farm prawn or sea-squirt)	Baker	Baker's yeast (*Saccharomyces cerevisiae*), *Boletus edulis*
Restaurant seafood handler	Scallop and shrimp		
Scallop plant processor	King scallop and queen scallop	Greenhouse worker	Sweet pea (*Lathyrus odoratus*)
Technician	Shrimp meal (*Artemia salina*)	Hotel manager	*Boletus edulis*
		Mushroom producer	*Pleurotus cornucopiae*
ARTHROPODS		Mushroom soup processor	Mushroom unspecified
Agronomist	*Bruchus lentis*	Office worker	*Boletus edulis*
Bottling	Ground bug	Seller	*Pleurotus ostreatus* (spores of white spongy rot)
Chicken breeder	Herring worm (*Anisakis simplex*)		
Engineer at electric power plant	Caddis flies (*Phryganeidae*)	**ALGAE**	
		Pharmacist	Chlorella
Entomologist	Lesser mealworm (*Alphitobius diaperinus* Panzer), moth, butterfly	Thalassotherapist	Algae (species unspecified)
		FLOURS	
Farmer	Grain pests (*Eurygaster* and *Pyrale*)	Animal fodder	Marigold flour (*Tagetes erecta*)
Fish bait handler	Insect larvae (*Galleria mellonella*), mealworm larvae (*Tenebrio molitor*), green bottle fly larvae (*Lucila caesar*), daphnia, fish-feed Echinodorus larva (*Echinodorus plasmosus*), Chiromids midge (*Chironomus thummi thummi*)	Baker	Wheat, rye, soya, and buckwheat flour; Konjac flour; white pea flour (*Lathyrus sativus*)
		Food processing	White Lupin flour (*Lupinus albus*)
		POLLENS	
Fish processing	Herring worm (*Anisakis simplex*)	Florist	Cyclamen, rose
Flight crew	Screw worm fly (*Cochliomyia hominivorax*)	Gardener	Canary island date palm (*Phoenix canariensis*), Bell of Ireland (*Moluccella laevis*), Bell pepper, chrysanthemum, eggplant (*Solanum melongena*), *Brassica oleracea* (cauliflower and broccoli)
Honey processors	Honeybee		
Laboratory worker	Cricket, fruit fly, grasshopper (*Locusta migratoria*), locust		
Mechanic in a rye plant	Confused flour beetle (*Tribolium confusum*)	Laboratory worker	Sunflower (*Helianthus* spp.), thale cress (*Arabidopsis thaliana*)
Museum curator	Beetles (Coleoptera)	Olive farmer	White mustard (*Sinapis alba*)
Seed house	Mexican bean weevil (*Zabrotes subfasciatus*)	Processing worker	*Helianthus annuus*
Sericulture	Silkworm, larva of silkworm		
Sewage plant worker	Sewer fly (*Psychoda alternata*)		
Technician	Arthropods (*Chrysoperla carnea, Leptinotarsa decemlineata, Ostrinia nubilalis,* and *Ephestia kuehniella*), sheep blowfly (*Lucilia cuprina*)		
Wool worker	*Dermestidae* spp.		

Continued

Table 427.5	High Molecular Weight Antigens Known to Induce Occupational or Environmental Asthma—cont'd		

OCCUPATION OR ENVIRONMENT	SOURCE	OCCUPATION OR ENVIRONMENT	SOURCE
PLANTS		Horticulture	Freesia (Freesia hybrida), paprika (Capsicum annuum), Brazil ginseng (Pfaffia paniculata)
Brewery chemist	Hops		
Brush-maker	Tampico fiber in agave leaves	Laborer	Citrus food handling (dl-limonene, l-citronellol, and dichlorophen)
Butcher	Aromatic herb		
Chemist	Linseed oilcake, Voacanga africana seed dust	Oil industry	Castor bean, olive oilcake
		Pharmaceutical	Rose hip, passion flower (Passiflora alata), cascara sagrada (Rhamnus purshiana)
Cosmetics	Dusts from seeds of Sacha Inchi (Plukenetia volubilis), chamomile (unspecified)	Powder	Lycopodium powder
		Sewer	Kapok
Decorator	Cacoon seed (Entage gigas)	Sheller	Almond shell dust
Floral worker	Decorative flower, safflower (Carthamus tinctorius) and yarrow (Achillea millefolium), spathe flower, statice (Limonium tataricum), baby's breath (Gypsophila paniculata), ivy (Hedera helix), flower (various), sea lavender (Limonium sinuatum)	Stucco handler	Esparto (Stipa tenacissima and Lygeum spartum)
		Tobacco manufacturer	Tobacco leaf
		PLANT-DERIVED NATURAL PRODUCTS	
		Baker	Gluten, soybean lecithin
		Candy maker	Pectin
Food industry	Aniseed, fenugreek, peach, garlic dust, asparagus, coffee bean, sesame seed, grain dust, carrot (Daucus carota L.), green bean (Phaseolus multiflorus), lima bean (Phaseolus lunatus), onion, potato, swiss chard (Beta vulgaris L.), courgette, carob bean, spinach powder, cauliflower, cabbage, chicory, fennel seed, onion seeds (Allium cepa, red onion), rice, saffron (Crocus sativus), spices, grain dust	Glove manufacturer	Latex
		Health professional	Latex
		Rose extraction	Rose oil
		BIOLOGIC ENZYMES	
		Baker	Fungal amylase, fungal amyloglucosidase and hemicellulase
		Cheese producer	Various enzymes in rennet production (proteases, pepsine, chymosins)
		Detergent industry	Esterase, Bacillus subtilis
		Factory worker	Bacillus subtilis
		Fruit processor	Pectinase and glucanase
Gardener	Copperleaf (Acalypha wilkesiana), grass juice, weeping fig (Ficus benjamina), umbrella tree (Schefflera spp.), amaryllis (Hippeastrum spp.), Madagascar jasmine sap (Stephanotis floribunda), vetch (Vicia sativa)	Hospital personnel	Empynase (pronase B)
		Laboratory worker	Xylanase, phytase from Aspergillus niger
		Pharmaceutical	Bromelin, flaviastase, lactase, pancreatin, papain, pepsin, serratia peptidase, and lysozyme chloride; egg lysozyme, trypsin
Hairdresser	Henna (unspecified)	Plastic	Trypsin
Herbal tea processor	Herbal tea, sarsaparilla root, sanyak (Dioscorea batatas), Korean ginseng (Panax ginseng), tea plant dust (Camellia sinensis), chamomile (unspecified)	**VEGETABLE GUMS**	
		Carpet manufacturing	Guar
		Dental hygienist	Gutta-percha
		Gum importer	Tragacanth
Herbalist	Licorice roots (Glycyrrhiza spp.), wonji (Polygala tenuifolia), herb material	Hairdresser	Karaya
		Printer	Acacia

Table 427.6	Low Molecular Weight Chemicals Known to Induce Occupational or Environmental Asthma		

CHEMICALS	OCCUPATION OR ENVIRONMENT SOURCE	CHEMICALS	OCCUPATION OR ENVIRONMENT SOURCE
Diisocyanates • Diphenylmethane • Hexamethylene • Naphthalene • Toluene	• Polyurethane • Roofing materials • Insulations • Paint	Metals • Chromic acid • Potassium dichromate • Nickel sulfate • Vanadium • Platinum salts	Metal work • Plating • Welding
Anhydrides • Trimellitic • Phthalic	Manufacturers or users • Paint • Plastics • Epoxy resins	Drugs • β-Lactams • Opioids • Other	Exposure to drugs in environment • Pharmaceutical workers • Farmers • Healthcare workers
Dyes • Anthraquinone • Carmine • Henna • Persulfate	Personal or business use of dyes • Hair dye • Fur dye • Fabric dye	Chemicals • Formaldehyde • Glutaraldehyde • Ethylene oxide	Exposure in the healthcare field • Laboratory work • Healthcare professionals
Glue or resin • Methacrylate • Acrylates • Epoxy	Plastic • Manufacturers • Healthcare professionals • Orthopedic specialists	Wood dust • Western red cedar (plicatic acid) • Exotic woods • Maple • Oak	Workers/hobbyists • Sawmill • Carpentry • Woodworking

Table 427.7	Criteria for the Diagnosis of Reactive Airways Disease Syndrome

- Absence of previous documented respiratory symptom
- Onset of symptoms most often occur after a single specific exposure
- Exposure is most often to a high concentration of gas, smoke, fume, or vapor with irritant qualities
- Symptoms occur within 24 hr of exposure and persist for 3 mo or longer
- Symptoms mimic asthma with cough, wheezing, shortness of breath, and/or dyspnea
- Pulmonary function tests may demonstrate airflow obstruction but not always
- Bronchial hyperresponsiveness is documented by methacholine challenge
- Alternative pulmonary diseases are not able to be found

irritation, and conjunctival injection. Pulmonary symptoms include those typically seen with asthma exacerbations.

Initial evaluation of the patient with RADS or irritant-induced asthma usually includes the medical history, physical examination, and pulse oximetry. Because of the acute nature of RADS, a chest radiograph is obtained in order to rule out other acute causes of dyspnea including pneumonia or pulmonary edema. In patients with RADS and irritant-induced asthma, the chest radiograph is frequently normal or may show hyperinflation. Ideally, if the patient is not in significant distress, complete pulmonary function testing with spirometry, lung volumes, and diffusion capacity are very helpful in the initial evaluation. The lack of abnormality on initial chest radiograph reassures the clinician that HRCT is not indicated.

TREATMENT

Treatment of RADS and irritant-induced asthma focuses on prevention of exposure. Because the exposure in RADS is often associated with a single known exposure, this task is readily accomplished. The low, persistent exposures are more challenging to identify and remove.

Implementing treatment guidelines for asthma from all causes is recommended when intervention is required beyond antigen removal. The management of an acute presentation of RADS is essentially the same as the treatment of an acute asthma exacerbation. Short-acting beta-agonist treatment may not be effective in most patients; a trial of inhaled ipratropium may add benefit in the short term. For moderate to severe symptoms and FEV_1 less than 70% of predicted, administration of systemic glucocorticoids (2 mg/kg prednisone equivalent, up to 60 mg daily) can be beneficial based on some clinical case studies and animal studies. Unlike the typical 5-day courses of systemic glucocorticoids for asthma exacerbations, many patients remain symptomatic beyond 5 days due to the extent of the airway epithelial injury. Steroid treatment may be prolonged through 10-15 days after the onset of symptoms, accomplished through a slow taper of corticosteroids. High-dose inhaled corticosteroids (ICS) may be added while the systemic steroids are being tapered. The initial dose of ICS is based on the National Asthma Education and Prevention Program (NAEPP) and the Global Initiative for Asthma (GINA) guidelines. For patients whose initial symptoms are less severe and/or spirometry demonstrates milder airway obstruction (FEV_1 greater than 70% of predicted), high-dose ICS therapy alone can be started without requiring systemic corticosteroid treatment. Once patients' asthma symptoms are improved, ICS doses can be tapered by 25–50% increments over a period of up to 6 mo in some case series based on patient symptoms. However, prolonged ICS treatment beyond 6 mo has also been noted.

Bibliography is available at Expert Consult.

427.3 Granulomatous Lung Disease
Kevin J. Kelly and Timothy J. Vece

GRANULOMATOSIS WITH POLYANGIITIS

Granulomatosis with polyangiitis (GPA) is a disease that involves both the lower and upper respiratory tracts with granulomatous inflammation of small vessels; formerly it was known as *Wegener granulomatosis* (see Chapter 192). The pulmonary disease is frequently associated with glomerulonephritis. The simultaneous presence of pulmonary and renal disease should immediately raise the suspicion that either GPA, microscopic polyangiitis, or anti-glomerular basement membrane (anti-GBM) disease (see Chapter 427.5) may be causing the disease.

Etiology and Epidemiology

The prevalence of GPA disease appears to be increasing by up to 4-fold in the last 2 decades, but without male or female predominance. Improved diagnostic tests, such as antineutrophil antibodies, may explain some of this increased prevalence.

Pathogenesis

Clinically, the development of both upper and lower airway disease with granulomas in GPA implies that exposure to antigen in the airway of endogenous or exogenous source is involved with aberrant cell-mediated immune response. Cytokine expression by peripheral blood CD4+ lymphocytes and cells collected by BAL indicate there is a predominantly T-lymphocyte type 1 response with overexpression of interferon-γ (IFN-γ) and tumor necrosis factor (TNF). In vitro studies demonstrate a skewed T-lymphocyte type 17 response by blood CD4+ T cells in GPA, suggesting there is an immune regulatory defect that leads to excessive production of T-lymphocyte type 1/T-lymphocyte type 17 cytokines (interleukin [IL]-17, TNF, and IFN-γ) presumed to be from the environment or autoantigens. Such an inflammatory response may be sufficient to induce and sustain granuloma formation.

Detection of *autoantibodies reactive against proteins in the cytoplasmic granules of neutrophils and monocytes (antineutrophil cytoplasmic antibodies [ANCAs])* are found in 90% of the patients with GPA. The first major type of ANCA is directed against cytoplasmic proteinase-3 and is frequently named **c-ANCA**. The second major type of ANCA recognizes the enzyme myeloperoxidase. It is found in a small number (<10%) of patients with GPA but is frequent in *microscopic polyangiitis*. Anti-myeloperoxidase antibodies fluoresce in a perinuclear pattern and are often referred to as perinuclear or **p-ANCA**. In contrast, some patients develop the clinical phenotype of GPA in the absence of detectable ANCA.

Clinical Manifestations

Children with GPA present with respiratory complaints accompanied by fever, loss of energy, and vague joint complaints. Some may present with severe nasal disease manifested as ulceration, septal perforation, pain, sinusitis, and/or epistaxis. The septal perforation may lead to deformation of the nasal bridge from erosion of the underlying cartilage but is more common in adults. Pulmonary disease occurs in the majority of patients as noted above. Symptoms range from cough, hemoptysis (seen in less than 50% of patients), dyspnea, and chest discomfort to asymptomatic infiltrates on chest radiography. Occasionally, patients with GPA will present with hemoptysis or recurrent fleeting infiltrates from *pulmonary hemorrhage*. The pathology is confusing because granulomatous disease may be difficult to demonstrate, and *pulmonary capillaritis*, the other main component seen on histology, can be seen in other disorders including anti-GBM disease, microscopic polyangiitis, idiopathic pulmonary capillaritis, and Henoch-Schönlein purpura. Distinguishing GPA from other pulmonary renal syndromes is easiest when there are classical symptoms of upper airway disease (nasal/sinus), lower airway disease with necrosis, granulomas on biopsy of the lung with vasculitis, and renal disease consistent with glomerulonephritis.

As many as 20% of patients with GPA will present with subglottic or endobronchial stenosis from scarring and inflammatory changes. Although it may be the presenting symptom, it often occurs in conjunction with other disease manifestations. Dyspnea and voice changes are common complaints from the patients.

Skin, ocular (uveitis), and joint symptoms are common in GPA and have been found to accompany the lung and renal disease in most series 50% or more of the time. Biopsy of the skin may show nonspecific leukocytoclastic vasculitis, venulitis, or capillaritis.

Laboratory and Pathology
c-ANCA or anti–proteinase-3 antibodies are found in 90% of patients with GPA. However, they are also found in other types of vasculitis and are not sufficient in themselves to make a diagnosis without a tissue biopsy (see Chapter 192). Because of the necrotizing nature of the vasculitis, lung tissue is required for definitive diagnosis of pulmonary disease. Biopsy of the upper airway may demonstrate evidence of granulomatous disease, but it is uncommon to find evidence of vasculitis therefore lung biopsy is warranted. Usual pathology demonstrates multiple parenchymal nodules that may be located in either the bronchial, vascular, or interstitial tissues (Fig. 427.2). The granulomatous inflammation is often found in areas of necrosis and/or vasculitis.

Renal biopsy rarely demonstrates granulomas or vasculitis. Rather, kidney tissues may show focal, segmental, or necrotizing glomerulonephritis without deposits of immune complexes. When the tissues fail to demonstrate classical findings, a variety of diseases (e.g., tuberculosis, sarcoid, microscopic polyangiitis, malignancy, and other autoimmune disorders) must be considered in the evaluation.

Radiology
Chest radiography in GPA will show multiple infiltrates, nodules, cavitary lesions, or ILD. Fleeting infiltrates may be seen when recurrent hemorrhage is a part of the clinical manifestation. HRCT often demonstrates more extensive lung disease and the cavitation associated with the necrotizing nature of the disease (Fig. 427.3).

Treatment
Rapidly progressive, debilitating disease may occur when failure to diagnose GPA leads to inadequate treatment. One series of patients showed death occurred in 90% of patients within 2 yr of diagnosis. Glucocorticoid therapy alone resulted in relapses and inadequate control of disease in many subjects.

Therapy is divided into *induction* and *maintenance* phases. Systemic corticosteroids, while ineffective as monotherapy, are a mainstay of therapy in conjunction with other immune suppressive agents. Prednisone can be given orally at a dosage of 1-2 mg/kg/day (max 60 mg). Alternatively, intravenous methylprednisolone may be used at a dosage of 10-30 mg/kg (max 1 gram) given either weekly or for 3 consecutive days monthly. Combination therapy traditionally included cyclophosphamide given either orally at 2 mg/kg/day or intravenous dosing at 15 mg/kg monthly. Rituximab, an anti-CD20 antibody, is as effective as cyclophosphamide in inducing remission of the GPA. Rituximab dosing is either 350 mg/m^2 given weekly for the first 4 wk or 500 mg/m^2 given on initiation of therapy and 2 wk after initiation. A second dose of 500 mg/m^2 is often given 6 mo after the first dosage of rituximab. Induction therapy should be continued for 3-6 mo.

Continued therapy is required past the initial induction phase to maintain remission, however, due to the toxicity of cyclophosphamide, other immune-suppressive agents are preferred. Both methotrexate and azathioprine have been shown to be equally effective as cyclophosphamide in maintaining remission. Mycophenolate mofetil, in contrast, has higher relapse rates than azathioprine and should be avoided in ANCA-associated vasculitis. Systemic steroid dosages should be progressively weaned at the beginning of the maintenance phase of therapy to a dosage of 5-10 mg/day. Therapy should be continued for an additional 1.5-2 yr. Rituximab, given every 6 mo for 2 yr, is at least as effective in maintaining remission as other regimens.

Adjuvant therapy with plasma exchange may be considered when life-threatening GPA disease presents. This is advocated on the premise that ANCAs are inducing disease and will be removed from the circulation with this intervention; its use has been favorably evaluated in GPA-induced renal disease. Adjuvant plasma exchange has been studied

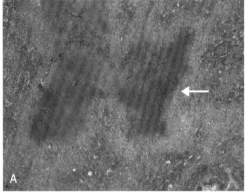

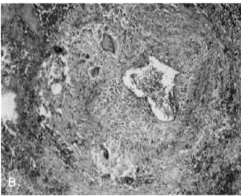

Fig. 427.2 A, Low-power view of granulomatous inflammation and geographic necrosis *(arrow)* in a lung biopsy from a patient with GPA. **B,** Granulomatous vasculitis involving a small pulmonary artery in the lung of a patient with GPA. The vessel wall is markedly thickened with an inflammatory infiltrate that includes multinucleated giant cells. *(From Sneller MC, Fontana JR, Shelhamer JH: Immunologic nonasthmatic diseases of the lung. In Adkinson AF, editor: Middleton's allergy principles and practice, Philadelphia, 2014, Elsevier, Fig. 61.1B and C.)*

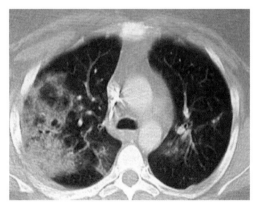

Fig. 427.3 Chest CT scan of a patient with granulomatosis with polyangiitis shows typical nodular lung infiltrate with cavitation. *(From Sneller MC, Fontana JR, Shelhamer JH: Immunologic nonasthmatic diseases of the lung. In Adkinson AF, editor: Middleton's allergy principles and practice, Philadelphia, 2014, Elsevier, Fig. 61.1A.)*

mainly in patients with severe renal vasculitis, but there are also reports of success in severe pulmonary hemorrhage. The results of a meta-analysis of patients with renal vasculitis in 9 trials suggest that adjuvant plasma exchange may be associated with improved renal outcome.

Recurrent disease remains a major problem with relapse rates of up to 50% reported in most studies. ANCA levels have not been shown to correlate with activity of disease or severity. Patients with isolated disease of the sinuses and nose may not warrant such toxic therapy. Therapy with topical corticosteroid and antibiotics for infection appear to be warranted. If unsuccessful, steroid with methotrexate appears to be an effective therapy.

The development of subglottic stenosis requires specific treatment. Use of cyclophosphamide with oral corticosteroid may have an incomplete or no response in the airway. Local injection of a prolonged acting corticosteroid locally appears to be indicated to reduce the inflammation and prevent further scarring. If this complication is found at presentation, simultaneous airway intervention with induction of corticosteroid and cyclophosphamide is warranted and encouraged.

SARCOIDOSIS

Sarcoidosis is an idiopathic inflammatory disease involving multiple organ systems, with characteristic histology of noncaseating granulomas (see Chapter 190). It has been postulated that sarcoidosis represents an immune response to a yet-to-be-identified agent from the environment that is likely inhaled in a susceptible host. It remains a diagnosis of exclusion from other diseases with granuloma formation on histology, such as immune deficiency of chronic granulomatous disease (CGD), granulomatous lymphocytic ILD associated with common variable immune deficiency (CVID), HP associated with some drugs and inhalation agents, granuloma with polyangiitis, typical and atypical *Mycobacterium*, *Pneumocystis jiroveci*, and malignancy.

Epidemiology and Pathogenesis

African-American females are disproportionately affected by sarcoidosis; however, it can present in any group. Because an asymptomatic sarcoid-like distribution of noncaseating granulomas may be frequently found at autopsy, the contribution of the granulomas to the disease is not always clear. Some countries do mass chest radiograph screening for multiple diseases. In that setting, up to 50% of diagnosed sarcoidosis is asymptomatic. The severity of the disease appears to be worse in African-Americans who tend to have acute illness, whereas white subjects are more likely to be asymptomatic with a more chronic disease. There have been clusters of disease in families and genetic testing suggests that MHC linkage on the short arm of chromosome 6 is most likely to be observed.

Sarcoidosis is rarely found in children younger than the age of 8 yr; those of African descent are most affected. The disease presentation is similar to adults with multisystem disease being the most common. Skin rash, iridocyclitis, and arthritis are seen most often without pulmonary symptoms. In northern Europe, erythema nodosum with the ocular involvement of iridocyclitis is seen most frequently. Despite the lack of symptoms, chest radiography may be abnormal in approximately 90% of children. The pulmonary disease appears to be less progressive compared to adults and patients recover spontaneously without corticosteroids. Rarely, pulmonary disease may progress to fibrosis. Ocular disease is more likely to be progressive and warrant intervention as the inflammatory response may lead to blindness from complications of iritis.

Unrecognized infection or inhalation of an immune response–inducing antigen continues to be at the forefront of consideration as a cause of the disease. Clusters of sarcoidosis in small populations, variable prevalence by geography and race, transfer of disease by organ transplant, and the reproducible granuloma formation only in patients with sarcoidosis in the skin when homogenized lymph node tissue from patients with sarcoid is injected intradermally (Kveim-Siltzbach test) have supported this hypothesis.

Clinical Manifestations

Patients with lung disease are more likely to be asymptomatic as the presentation often may be an abnormal chest radiograph. When symptomatic, patients demonstrate shortness of breath, cough, and dyspnea. Children are more likely to manifest the disease as iridocyclitis, skin rash, and arthritis. African-American children appear to have more frequent lymph node involvement, nonspecific elevations of gamma globulin,

erythema nodosum, and hypercalcemia. Physical exam may reveal only an elevated respiratory rate without crackles or rales by auscultation. Pleural involvement has been seen but is uncommon. When present, a lymphocytic predominant exudate may be observed with laboratory evaluation of the pleural fluid. Unusual but reported findings include cases of pneumothorax, hemothorax, and chylothorax. One specific syndrome, **Lofgren syndrome**, with hilar lymphadenopathy, erythema nodosum, and migratory polyarthralgias, is almost exclusively seen in females. This syndrome has a strong association with HLA-DQB1*0201 and polymorphisms in the C-C chemokine receptor 2 (CCR2); these genetic markers are a predictor of a good outcome.

Although almost 90% of patients with sarcoidosis demonstrate parenchymal or mediastinal disease on chest radiography, there are many who have minimal to no symptoms. Approximately 40% of adults with stage 1 disease have endobronchial involvement found at bronchoscopy. The higher the staging level of disease, the more likely patients are to have airway involvement.

Diagnostic Laboratory Testing

The most common but nonspecific findings are hypergammaglobulinemia, hypercalciuria, hypercalcemia, elevated alkaline phosphatase when liver disease is present, and, occasionally, anemia of chronic disease. Serum angiotensin-converting enzyme may be elevated in 75% of patients with untreated sarcoid. False-positive tests occur from other diseases so that it is not considered a diagnostic test but rather a test that strongly supports the diagnosis.

Pulmonary function tests can be performed accurately in most children older than the age of 4 yr. There are no specific diagnostic findings of spirometry, lung volumes, or diffusion capacity in sarcoidosis. Exercise coupled with pulmonary function tests may demonstrate a decline in diffusion capacity when alveolitis is present in hypersensitivity pneumonitis and could add diagnostic help to the clinician when attempting to differentiate sarcoidosis from HP prior to biopsy.

BAL is of great help when differentiating HP from sarcoid. BAL in sarcoid shows a marked predominance of CD4 cells. *A lymphocyte percentage > 16% on BAL, a CD4:CD8 ratio > 4, and noncaseating granulomas on bronchial biopsy in the presence of abnormal angiotensin-converting enzyme levels are nearly completely diagnostic for sarcoid.* In addition, T cells are activated on BAL. BAL in HP shows a significant change in the balance of CD4 to CD8 cells with the 2 cell types being nearly equal compared to the normal mild predominance of CD4 cells in the circulation. A ratio of CD4:CD8 of <1 predicts 100% of patients with BAL lymphocytosis to *not* have sarcoidosis. Neutrophil counts >2% and/or eosinophil counts >1% exclude the diagnosis of sarcoidosis.

The analysis of D-dimers in BAL fluid from subjects with sarcoidosis demonstrates an elevation in 80% of patients compared to no detectable D-dimers in unaffected control.

Histopathology

The characteristic feature of sarcoidosis is the noncaseating granuloma formation in the lung (Fig. 427.4). These granulomas are found in the bronchial walls, alveolar septa, and vascular walls of pulmonary arteries and veins. The formation of noncaseating granulomas is likely preceded by alveolitis involving the interstitium more than the alveolar spaces. There is accumulation of inflammatory cells, including monocytes, macrophages, and lymphocytes that accompany the granulomas. Multinucleated giant cells are frequently found among the epithelioid cells within the granuloma follicle. These may show cytoplasmic inclusions (e.g., asteroid bodies and Schaumann bodies) as well as some birefringent crystalline particles made of calcium oxalate and other calcium salts. These are most often identified in the upper lobes of the lungs which may lead to confusion with diseases such as hypersensitivity pneumonitis, eosinophilic granuloma, collagen vascular disease, pneumoconiosis, berylliosis, and infectious disease such as tuberculosis or histoplasmosis.

Radiology

Pulmonary imaging in sarcoid has included plain chest radiography, HRCT, positron emission tomography using fluorine-18-fluorodeoxyglucose, and radiotracer using gallium-67. The staging of sarcoid is

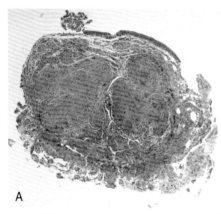 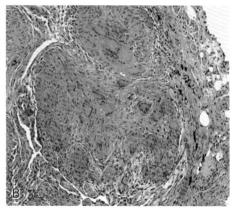

Fig. 427.4 Transbronchial biopsy specimen showing a sarcoid granuloma. **A,** The granulomas are located below the bronchiolar epithelial layer that appears at the top of the frame. **B,** A higher-power view of the same biopsy specimen. The epithelioid granuloma is tightly packed and contains multiple multinucleated giant cells. There is no caseous necrosis. Special stains for acid-fast bacilli and fungi were negative. *(From Sneller MC, Fontana JR, Shelhamer JH: Immunologic nonasthmatic diseases of the lung. In Adkinson AF, editor: Middleton's allergy principles and practice, Philadelphia, 2014, Elsevier, Fig. 61.6.)*

performed using plain radiography and is outlined as follows:

- Stage I—Bilateral hilar lymphadenopathy accompanied by right paratracheal lymphadenopathy
- Stage II—Bilateral hilar lymphadenopathy accompanied by reticular opacities are present. If symptomatic, patients have cough and dyspnea. Occasional fever and fatigue accompany the respiratory symptoms.
- Stage III—Reticular opacities are found predominantly in the upper lobes with regression of hilar lymphadenopathy.
- Stage IV—Reticular opacities start to coalesce and lead to volume loss in the lung fields, traction bronchiectasis from conglomeration of the inflamed tissues. Extensive calcium deposits may be seen at this stage.

HRCT may be helpful in further staging of the disease, as well as in revealing abnormalities not appreciated on chest radiography. Findings in patients with sarcoidosis by HRCT include hilar lymphadenopathy, paratracheal nodules, middle to upper lung parenchymal ground-glass appearance, bronchial wall thickening, bronchiectasis, cystic changes, and fibrosis. The ground-glass appearance suggests that alveolitis, as seen in hypersensitivity pneumonitis, may be present. Biopsy has usually shown granuloma formation as the predominant histologic finding.

Treatment

Because pulmonary sarcoidosis spontaneously resolves without therapy in almost 75% of patients, clear guidelines for treatment focused on minimizing side effects of therapy is required. Glucocorticosteroids (GCSs) have long been the mainstay of therapy in sarcoid and are often used because of extra pulmonary disease. When pulmonary disease is progressive, GCS therapy is aimed at prevention of fibrosis, honeycombing, and irreversible lung disease. Assuring that disseminated infections, heart failure, thromboembolism, or pulmonary hypertension are not present is important. In addition to HRCT of the chest, performance of pulmonary function tests, electrocardiogram, and echocardiogram should be considered prior to starting GCS therapy.

GCS therapy is often not started when stage I or II is present without symptoms. This scrutiny of the benefit of therapy was highlighted when prospective evaluation of GCS therapy for pulmonary disease found that nearly 50% of patients receiving GCSs had active or relapsing disease 2 yr later. In contrast, 90% of patients who did not receive GCSs had spontaneous remission of disease with the other 10% needing intervention 2 yr later. Absolute indications include progressive stage III disease with symptoms of shortness of breath, cough, or other chest symptoms such as pain. Progressive restriction shown on pulmonary function testing is an indication for therapy. Specific pulmonary function changes where lung capacity declines a total of 10% or greater, FVC declines

15% or more, or diffusion capacity degradation is seen of 20% or more are all indications for GCS intervention.

Dosage with oral prednisone at 0.3-0.5 mg/kg is a reasonable starting point depending on the severity of symptoms. Stability is usually achieved within 6-8 wk, after which slow progressive tapering of GCS may occur every 4-8 wk. Many favor the use of alternate-day steroids to reduce the side effects of GCSs, but little data exist to show efficacy.

For patients who do not tolerate GCSs or develop progressive disease, alternative immunosuppressive agents may add benefit to the regimen. Progressive disease also is a reminder for the clinician to reassess the diagnosis of sarcoid and review the chance that beryllium may have been the underlying reason for the progressive disease.

Inhaled GCSs have been evaluated in patients with stage I disease with variable results. Evaluation of therapy with pulmonary function testing and symptoms are the best methods to judge responsiveness to this therapy. Persistent symptoms after 4-8 wk of therapy suggest that systemic GCSs may be indicated.

BERYLLIOSIS

Chronic beryllium disease or berylliosis is an example of environmental exposure and unique granulomatous response in the lungs. Beryllium is an alkaline metal that is used in a number of industrial settings.

A diagnosis of berylliosis requires 3 criteria: (1) history of beryllium exposure; (2) positive response to lymphocyte proliferation tests to beryllium in lymphocytes obtained by BAL or blood test; and (3) noncaseating granulomas on lung biopsy. Exposure to beryllium may occur in industries such as automotive, ceramic, aerospace, metal extraction, electronics, computer, jewelry making, and dental alloys. Teenagers working summer jobs in machine work, ceramics, or wire production may be exposed. Sensitization is associated with dose and duration of exposure and has been seen to be as high as 20% in certain industries. Secretaries working in buildings where manufacturing with beryllium is active have developed berylliosis.

Pathogenesis

Genetic susceptibility coupled with immunologic response to beryllium are the 2 key contributors to the development of disease. A T-lymphocyte cell–mediated delayed hypersensitivity response to beryllium appears to be the mechanism involved with granuloma formation in the lung. The lymphocyte proliferation by T cells to beryllium is specific and does not occur in reaction to other metals. Similar to sarcoidosis, CD4+ T cells predominate on bronchoalveolar response. Beryllium appears to be inhaled and then couple with proteins in the lung or can be ingested by antigen-presenting cells. The cytokines elicited and granuloma formation suggests that sensitization is primarily a T-lymphocyte type 1 response with elevated IFN-γ and IL-2 production.

Clinical Manifestations

The clinical manifestations of berylliosis are not specific. Dry cough, fever, fatigue, weight loss, and shortness of breath all may be present. Although symptoms may occur within 3 mo, new disease has been detected up to 3 decades after exposure. Physical examination is somewhat different than the HPs and sarcoid with bibasilar crackles found on auscultation. The other mentioned diseases are more prominent in the upper lobes. Small nodules on exposed skin may also be present.

Laboratory Testing

Suspicion of berylliosis should prompt the clinician to have a blood beryllium lymphocyte proliferation test and complete pulmonary function tests performed. These tests need to be sent to a special center where multiple tests are run with comparison to proper positive and negative controls. When positive, the test has very high specificity for defining the presence of berylliosis at approximately 96%. However, sensitivity of the test hovers at <70%, suggesting that approximately 30% who have the disease may have a negative test.

Similar to other pulmonary granulomatous diseases, increased production of calcitriol is commonly found. The source of this active form of vitamin D is from activated pulmonary macrophages, which may result in hypercalciuria and hypercalcemia.

Radiography

Chest radiographs should be obtained on all patients suspected of having berylliosis. The chest radiograph may be normal, show hilar lymphadenopathy, pulmonary nodules, ground-glass, or alveolar opacities. The parenchymal abnormalities may be diffuse or may be more prominent in the upper lobes. These findings are dependent upon the stage of the disease.

HRCT is the most sensitive test in the identification of chronic berylliosis. Almost 25% of the HRCT exams in patients with biopsy-proven berylliosis are found to be normal. Similar to other granulomatous and HPs of the lungs, HRCT findings include parenchymal nodules of varying size, thick septal lines, ground-glass opacities, cystic cavitation, and lymphadenopathy in the hilum or mediastinum. Pleural abnormalities are less common, but thickening may be observed in proximity to parenchymal nodules.

Treatment

Managing berylliosis involves avoiding further exposure and therapy with glucocorticoids or other immunosuppressive agents. A decision to intervene depends on the severity of symptoms, physiologic impairment based on pulmonary function tests, and extent of radiographic changes. Treatment is usually started when the patient has dyspnea or cough, >10% decline in lung volumes or gas exchange, or abnormal pulmonary function tests at baseline.

Small case series have demonstrated efficacy of steroids judged by improvement of clinical symptoms, radiographic clearing of disease, and improvement in pulmonary functions, including diffusion capacity. Some patients despite improved symptoms have recurrence which may progress to fibrosis and persistent lung disease.

The differentiation between berylliosis and sarcoidosis appears to be important for long-term outcomes. It appears that the longer the delay in prescribing GCSs to patients with berylliosis may lead to a state where the lung disease is unresponsive to therapy. In contrast, use of steroids in sarcoidosis may lead to a higher rate of recurrent disease. What makes the 2 responses different is not known.

Dosing of steroids is similar to sarcoid with a starting dose of 0.5 mg/kg/day of prednisone for a duration of 6-12 wk. Once a response is established, conversion to every-other-day corticosteroid use at the same dose followed by tapering should be attempted until the lowest dose is achieved that controls the disease. Patients may require persistent therapy for the rest of their life. Genetic susceptibility to the disease may predict relapse of disease. Mutations in the HLA-DPB1 gene (homozygous for glutamate substitution at the β69 position) appear to predict specific patients who are susceptible to relapse of symptoms.

When patients fail to respond or experience recurrent relapse, methotrexate in low dose has conferred a favorable response in some patients as has been seen with sarcoidosis. Azathioprine may also be considered since sarcoidosis has responded favorably, however there are no published trials using this immunosuppressive agent. A small number of cases have also shown promise with TNF-α inhibitors both in sarcoid and beryllium-induced disease.

GRANULOMATOUS LUNG DISEASE IN PRIMARY IMMUNE DEFICIENCY

Primary immune deficiency (PID) often presents with recurrent or persistent pulmonary symptoms of recurrent infections, pneumonia, bronchiectasis, and ILD with or without fibrosis. Immune dysregulation occurs in many of the PIDs with the development of granulomatous lung disease and autoimmune disease. Most effort is focused on the discovery of infectious pathogens in the PID causing pulmonary disturbance, but immune dysregulation may be the primary problem causing symptoms and disease progression. This requires counterintuitive therapies with suppression of the immune system concurrently with immune deficiency therapy. The 2 most prominent PIDs associated with granulomatous lung disease are **chronic granulomatous disease** (see Chapter 156) and **common variable immune deficiency** (see Chapter 150).

The prototype organism causing granuloma formation in the lung is *Mycobacterium tuberculosis*. Nontuberculous mycobacterial infections also can cause granulomas in the presence of specific PID. These have been seen in impaired IL-12/IL-23/ IFN-γ signaling, or the presence of **autoantibodies to IFN-γ**. Patients with defective regulation of nuclear factor-kappa B (**nuclear factor-kappa B essential modifier defects**) have also been described as well with nontuberculous mycobacteria. The clinician must be certain that this low-virulence organism is not causing disease before therapy for immune dysregulation is considered.

Pathogenesis

CGD is a PID involving multiple defects in the phagocyte nicotinamide adenine dinucleotide phosphate oxidase system, which impairs the respiratory burst capacity to generate reactive species of oxygen (see Chapter 156).

Up to 25% of patients with **CVID** develop lung disease (see Chapter 150). These pulmonary changes include organizing pneumonia, ILD, mucosa-associated lymphoid tissue lymphoma, and noncaseating granulomas in granulomatous and lymphocytic interstitial lung disease (GLILD). Elevated levels of TNF from TNF polymorphisms have been implicated as a possible mechanism. GLILD is becoming recognized more frequently in CVID. It is defined by the presence of granulomatous and a lymphocytic proliferative pattern in the lung. Granulomas may be found in other organs including bone marrow, spleen, gastrointestinal tract, skin, and liver.

The etiology of GLILD is unknown. In a case cohort study, a majority of subjects with pathology diagnostic of GLILD were found to have human herpesvirus 8 infection of the lung. These may represent a subgroup of patients with GLILD which may point to a mechanism underlying the development of pulmonary granulomas.

GLILD is sometimes misdiagnosed as sarcoidosis initially because both involve pulmonary granuloma, often accompanied by hilar and/or mediastinal lymphadenopathy. Sarcoidosis has several features that distinguish it from GLILD, such as normal or elevated serum immunoglobulin levels and frequent spontaneous remissions.

Clinical Manifestations of Granulomatous Lung Disease in Primary Immune Deficiency

Chronic respiratory disease as a result of recurrent infections is common in CGD. This is accompanied by clubbing in some patients and the other organ manifestations in the skin, liver, and genitourinary and gastrointestinal tracts. Granulomas are especially problematic in the gastrointestinal and genitourinary tracts. The inhalation of fungal spores and hyphae has led to acute pneumonia in CGD with rapid progression to respiratory failure with hypoxemia, dyspnea, and fever. This entity, characterized as *mulch pneumonia*, appears to be best treated with antifungal medications and corticosteroids.

Radiography

Hilar and/or mediastinal lymphadenopathy occur with granulomatous lung involvement. These may manifest as parenchymal nodules and/or ground-glass abnormalities and can be seen commonly in CVID and CGD. Differentiating infectious causes of pulmonary infiltration in PID is often difficult on chest radiography; HRCT is often mandatory in the initial evaluation of the patients with CVID.

Laboratory and Pulmonary Function Testing

Definitive diagnosis is made by lung biopsy. Transbronchial biopsy in children is often insufficient and lung biopsy by video-assisted thoracoscopy or open biopsy is preferred. Unless the patient's underlying immune deficiency is unknown, other laboratory testing except for infectious organisms does not contribute significantly to the diagnosis. When the child is old enough, complete pulmonary functions with spirometry, flow volume loop, lung volumes, and diffusion capacity should be obtained at baseline and then followed serially for response to therapy or progression of disease.

Therapy

The presence of GLILD in CVID can be associated with significant morbidity and possibly death. Without therapy, progressive pulmonary fibrosis and respiratory failure may occur in GLILD. The parenchymal disease may not always be controlled or relieved by glucocorticoid treatment. Other treatments include TNF antagonists, cyclosporine, or a combination therapy with rituximab and azathioprine. Response to therapy is monitored clinically and by interval HRCT of the chest, and pulmonary function testing, including spirometry, lung volumes, and diffusing capacity.

Bibliography is available at Expert Consult.

427.4 Eosinophilic Lung Disease
Kevin J. Kelly and Timothy J. Vece

The eosinophilic lung diseases are a group of heterogeneous pulmonary disorders with a predominant diffuse infiltration of eosinophils in the alveolar spaces or interstitial pulmonary spaces. Lung architecture is well preserved throughout the inflammatory response, often with complete reversal of the inflammation without long-term sequelae in the majority of cases. The peripheral white blood count often (but not always) reveals elevated eosinophils. Prompt recognition of the nature of these diseases allows for lifesaving interventions in the idiopathic **acute eosinophilic pneumonia (AEP) syndrome** or resolution of persistent symptoms in the patients with chronic disease.

ETIOLOGY

Eosinophilic lung diseases are often classified under 2 subheadings: idiopathic disease and known causation (Tables 427.8–427.10). They are frequently further subdivided as acute and chronic or infectious and noninfectious. The division of acute or chronic is arbitrary based on the length of symptoms present but is relevant to the clinician in determining the etiology of the symptoms in the differential diagnosis (Table 427.11). Löffler eosinophilic pneumonia, induced by *Ascaris lumbricoides* and other ascarids, produces transient symptoms that self-resolve and is classified as neither acute nor chronic. Löffler syndrome has been more correctly termed **pulmonary infiltrates with eosinophilia syndrome** and is the most common eosinophilic infiltrative disease in children.

PATHOLOGY AND PATHOGENESIS

Eosinophilic lung disease, regardless of the stage of disease or etiology, shows mixed cellular infiltration of the alveoli and interstitial spaces with a predominance of eosinophils when transbronchial biopsy or

Table 427.8	Key Elements in the Medical History and Physical Exam to Raise Clinical Suspicion for Diagnostic Testing to Confirm Eosinophilic Lung Disease

Medical history and examination
- Drug exposure (especially antibiotics, NSAIDs, antiepileptics, antileukotriene modifiers in EGPA) (see Table 478.10)
- Environmental inhalation exposures to dust or inhaled chemicals
- New onset of smoking cigarettes
- Travel or immigration status from areas endemic with various parasites or coccidioidomycosis
- Asthma (may be severe or poorly controlled with ABPA, CSS, or is relatively new in onset with IAEP)
- ABPA concurrent in 7–10% of patients with cystic fibrosis
- Extrapulmonary symptoms suggestive of vasculitis, neuropathy, heart failure, or neoplasm
- Rash (creeping eruption in visceral larval migrans disease or ulceration in EGPA)

Diagnostic imaging and testing
- Radiography helpful in AEP, CEP, and ABPA
- Radiography not diagnostic in EGPA or drug-induced eosinophilic disease of the lung
- Simple chest radiography findings
- Nonlobar infiltrate
- Classic description as mirror image of pulmonary edema with peripheral infiltrates
- Bilateral pleural effusion in AEP
- Central bronchiectasis in ABPA
- High-resolution computerized tomography of the chest
- Middle and upper lobe nonlobar infiltrates with areas of ground-glass appearance
- Mucous plugging in ABPA
- Central bronchiectasis in ABPA (confused with cystic fibrosis)
- Blood eosinophil count
- Elevated in many eosinophilic lung diseases
- Magnitude of eosinophil blood count does not distinguish different pulmonary diseases
- Usually not elevated in AEP (eosinophilic disease compartmentalized to lungs)
- May occasionally not be elevated in CEP or after use of corticosteroids
- Total serum IgE elevated in ABPA but not always in patients with cystic fibrosis with ABPA
- Serology for helminthic infections or parasites may be diagnostic but are usually not available acutely
- P-ANCA (MPO ANCA) is positive in 40–70% of EGPA (CSS)
- BAL eosinophil percentage
- ≥25% eosinophils diagnostic in AEP
- ≥40% eosinophils diagnostic in CEP or tropical pulmonary eosinophilia
- Eosinophil percentages below these criteria may require lung biopsy
- <25% eosinophils seen in connective tissue disease, sarcoid, drug-induced disease, histiocytosis X of pulmonary Langerhans cells, and interstitial pulmonary fibrosis
- Lung biopsy
- Open lung biopsy or video-assisted thoracoscopic surgery when BAL nondiagnostic
- Transbronchial biopsy is usually insufficient with peripheral infiltrative disease
- Histology with alveolar and interstitial infiltrates of eosinophils, non-necrotizing non-granulomatous vasculitis, multinucleated giant cells without granuloma
- EGPA shows eosinophil rich small to medium vessel, necrotizing, granulomatous vasculitis

ABPA, Allergic bronchopulmonary aspergillosis; *AEP*, acute eosinophilic pneumonia; *BAL*, bronchoalveolar lavage; *CEP*, chronic eosinophilic pneumonia; *CSS*, Churg-Strauss syndrome; *EGPA*, eosinophilic granulomatosis with polyangiitis; *IAEP*, idiopathic acute eosinophilic pneumonia; *MPO ANCA*, myeloperoxidase antineutrophil cytoplasmic antibody; *NSAID*, nonsteroidal antiinflammatory drug; *P-ANCA*, perinuclear antineutrophil cytoplasmic antibody.

Table 427.9	Classification of the Eosinophilic Pneumonias in Clinical Practice

Eosinophilic pneumonias of unknown cause
Solitary idiopathic eosinophilic pneumonias
  Idiopathic chronic eosinophilic pneumonia
  Idiopathic acute eosinophilic pneumonia
Eosinophilic pneumonia in systemic syndromes
  Eosinophilic granulomatosis with polyangiitis
  Idiopathic hypereosinophilic syndromes (lymphocytic or
    myeloproliferative variant)
Eosinophilic pneumonias of known cause
Allergic bronchopulmonary aspergillosis and related syndromes
  (including bronchocentric granulomatosis)
Eosinophilic pneumonias of parasitic origin
Eosinophilic pneumonias of other infectious causes
Drug-induced eosinophilic pneumonias
Eosinophilic airways diseases
Eosinophilic asthma
Hypereosinophilic asthma
Idiopathic hypereosinophilic constrictive bronchitis
Other pulmonary syndromes with possible usually mild eosinophilia
Organizing pneumonia, asthma, idiopathic pulmonary fibrosis,
  Langerhans cell histiocytosis, malignancies, and so forth

From Cottin V: Eosinophilic lung diseases, *Clin Chest Med* 37:535–556, 2016 (Box 1, p. 536).

Table 427.10	Drugs Commonly Causing Eosinophilic Pneumonia

Antiinflammatory drugs and related drugs: acetylsalicylic acid, diclofenac, ibuprofen, naproxen, phenylbutazone, piroxicam, sulindac, and tolfenamic acid
Antibiotics: ethambutol, fenbufen, minocycline, nitrofurantoin, penicillins, pyrimethamine, sulfamides, sulfonamides, and trimethoprim-sulfamethoxazole
Other drugs: captopril, carbamazepine, and GM-CSF
A more extensive list of drugs reported to cause eosinophilic pneumonia may be found at www.pneumotox.com.

From Cottin V, Cordier JF: Eosinophilic lung diseases, *Immunol Allergy Clin North Am* 32(4):557–586, 2012 (Box 6, p. 575).

Table 427.11	Diagnostic Criteria for Idiopathic Chronic Eosinophilic Pneumonia and for Idiopathic Acute Eosinophilic Pneumonia

IDIOPATHIC CHRONIC EOSINOPHILIC PNEUMONIA
1. Diffuse pulmonary alveolar consolidation with air bronchogram and/or ground-glass opacities at chest imaging, especially with peripheral predominance.
2. Eosinophilia at bronchoalveolar lavage differential cell count ≥ 40% (or peripheral blood eosinophils ≥ 1,000/mm³).
3. Respiratory symptoms present for at least 2 to 4 wk.
4. Absence of other known causes of eosinophilic lung disease (especially exposure to drug susceptible to induce pulmonary eosinophilia).

IDIOPATHIC ACUTE EOSINOPHILIC PNEUMONIA
1. Acute onset with febrile respiratory manifestations (≤1 mo, and especially ≤ 7 days duration before medical examination).
2. Bilateral diffuse infiltrates on imaging.
3. PaO_2 on room air ≤ 60 mm Hg (8 kPa), or PaO_2/FIO_2 ≤ 300 mm Hg (40 kPa), or oxygen saturation on room air < 90%.
4. Lung eosinophilia, with ≥ 25% eosinophils at BAL differential cell count (or eosinophilic pneumonia at lung biopsy when done).
5. Absence of determined cause of acute eosinophilic pneumonia (including infection or exposure to drugs known to induce pulmonary eosinophilia). Recent onset of tobacco smoking or exposure to inhaled dusts may be present.

BAL, Bronchoalveolar lavage.
  From Cottin V: Eosinophilic lung diseases, *Clin Chest Med* 37:535–556, 2016 (Box 2, p. 538).

open lung biopsy is performed. This may be accompanied by a fibrinous exudate with intact lung architecture. Other findings include eosinophilic microabscesses, a nonnecrotizing nongranulomatous vasculitis, and occasional multinucleated giant cells again without granuloma formation. BAL is the diagnostic procedure of choice, especially with the acute types of eosinophilic pneumonia where peripheral eosinophilia is often absent; the differential cell count on the BAL is ≥ 25% eosinophils and is often more than 40%. This highly sensitive and specific test has allowed clinicians to forego lung biopsy.

Eosinophils are filled with numerous toxic granules. Evidence of eosinophil degranulation may be found by electron microscopy, biopsy, urine excretion, and BAL fluid. Most commonly, eosinophil-derived neurotoxin, leukotriene E_4, other granule proteins, such as major basic protein, Charcot Leyden crystals, or proinflammatory cytokines, are identified and support the evidence that eosinophils are not only present but contributing to the disease process.

CLINICAL MANIFESTATIONS
Specific eosinophilic lung diseases present with a variable clinical picture; however, there are some common findings across many of the eosinophilic diseases. Dyspnea is the most common and prevalent symptom in patients with acute or chronic eosinophilic pneumonia and is accompanied by cough in the majority of patients (90%). Rhinitis and sinusitis symptoms are of lower prevalence with wide variability in children with eosinophilic pulmonary disease. **Acute eosinophilic pneumonia** often presents with respiratory failure and the requirement for mechanical ventilation at high levels of positive end expiratory pressure and high concentrations of oxygen, whereas chronic eosinophilic pneumonia has a more indolent presentation (see Table 427.11). Although malignancy (e.g., eosinophilic leukemia) and organizing pneumonia may present with need for mechanical ventilation, they are less common. A history of asthma is common in the chronic eosinophilic pneumonias and in allergic bronchopulmonary aspergillosis (**ABPA**); it often precedes the diagnosis of these 2 conditions.

Other symptoms of fever, myalgia, fatigue, weight loss, poor appetite, and night sweats may accompany the acute or chronic eosinophilic pneumonias. When abnormalities of the liver are detected, or if arthralgia, skin changes, pericardial effusion, or peripheral neuropathy accompany the disease presentation, a diagnosis of **eosinophilic granulomatosis with polyangiitis (EGPA)** (formerly known as the Churg-Strauss syndrome) or the **hypereosinophilic syndrome** (HES) should be aggressively investigated.

Chest Imaging
The chest radiograph is one of the most helpful tests for evaluating the child with dyspnea. The characteristic feature of fluffy alveolar infiltrates in the peripheral lung field is classic (Fig. 427.5). The images may be easily recognizable by astute clinicians who have identified the etiology of the disease without eosinophil counts or BAL.

HRCT is the best advanced imaging modality for eosinophilic lung disease. Spontaneous migration of lung opacities is commonly seen in the chronic pneumonias. Most often HRCT shows simultaneous evidence of bilateral alveolar infiltrates with both confluent consolidations and ground-glass appearance. The most prominent areas of abnormality are visualized in the upper lobes and subpleural regions. Specific diseases have unique findings, such as *proximal bronchiectasis* in **ABPA** and pleural effusion in acute eosinophilic pneumonia. HRCT is most sensitive in identifying the correct etiology of disease when chest radiographic findings are nonspecific.

LÖFFLER SYNDROME
The **transient pulmonary infiltrates with eosinophilia syndrome** that is most often seen in children (formerly known as Löffler syndrome) is characterized by migrating pulmonary infiltrates with peripheral blood eosinophilia caused by the helminthic infections. *A. lumbricoides* or roundworm is the most common parasite causing this disease in the United States. When a fertilized egg is ingested from contaminated food, it becomes a larval worm that can penetrate the duodenum of the small intestine and migrate in the circulation to the liver, heart,

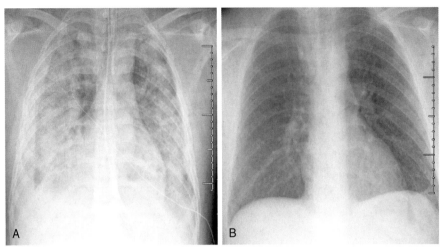

Fig. 427.5 Acute eosinophilic pneumonia demonstrating the mirror image **(A)** pulmonary edema with a right pleural effusion on admission and **(B)** complete clearing upon discharge from the hospital after corticosteroid usage.

and lungs. In the pulmonary venous circulation, the larvae can break through the interstitial space to the alveoli. The juvenile larva may subsequently migrate to the trachea where they are coughed up and swallowed. The cycle may then recur with subsequent absorption of eggs that are produced in the intestinal track. Other nematodes cannot mature in the intestinal tract so their disease is limited to a single passage into the lungs.

Visceral larva migrans from multiple nematodes may cause this disease. The most common cause of these includes the dog roundworm, *Toxocara canis*, while *Toxocara cati, Strongyloides stercoralis, Baylisascaris procyonis,* and *Lagochilascaris minor* can all produce visceral larva migrans. Outside the United States, the common lung fluke, *Paragonimus westermani,* may cause a similar pulmonary disease in older children and adolescents. Western Africa, Central and South America, and the Far East are regions that paragonimiasis may be found, especially in those who eat raw crabs or crawfish. Many other parasites may have a transient pulmonary syndrome, but their diseases are most commonly manifested in other organs.

The pulmonary syndrome is classic with cough, dyspnea, migratory peripheral pulmonary infiltrates, and blood eosinophilia that is self-limited. Young children most often have a history of pica and eating dirt that is contaminated with the eggs. Because the larva can migrate to other organs as well as multiply in the intestinal and biliary tract, symptoms of abdominal pain, vomiting, rarely obstruction, cholecystitis, and pancreatitis may be found. Diagnosis is frequently made by examination of the stool where the eggs may be detected microscopically. Treatment is aimed at the intestinal disease and not the pulmonary disease per se. It is possible that anthelminthic treatment of other organ disease during the pulmonary phase of the disease will increase the inflammatory response in the lung and may require corticosteroid therapy.

ACUTE EOSINOPHILIC PNEUMONIA

A unique and dramatic presentation of the eosinophilic pneumonias is **AEP** (see Table 427.11). AEP mimics infectious pneumonia or acute respiratory distress syndrome with its rapid onset and marked hypoxemia. In pediatrics, this disease most frequently occurs in the teenage population. Overall, young adults most commonly contract this idiopathic disease. Essentially all patients present within 7 days of symptom onset with dyspnea, fever, and cough, and more than 50% have chest pain. Myalgia and abdominal pain also frequently accompany this disease. Rarely, patients have presented up to 4-5 wk after onset of symptoms. Physical exam demonstrates tachypnea, tachycardia, and crackles in the lung fields on physical exam. Many patients rapidly deteriorate and require mechanical ventilation.

There is an *absence* of circulating eosinophilia, which contrasts the dramatic number of eosinophils seen in the BAL representing at least 25% of the inflammatory cells (often 40–55%) (Fig. 427.6). This feature helps distinguish it from the chronic pulmonary disease of eosinophilic origin.

Although this disease has been labeled as idiopathic, there have been identifiable exposures (e.g., 1,1,1-trichloroethane or Scotchgard). Numerous reports link the onset of smoking tobacco, change in smoking frequency, reinitiation of smoking in young male adolescents or adults, and even massive secondary smoke exposure as critical associations with onset of AEP. World Trade Center dust is associated with development of AEP. A single smoke challenge study is associated with recurrence. Some medications are also linked to the onset of AEP. The most complete and current resource for medications linked to pulmonary disease is "The Drug-Induced Respiratory Disease Website" (http://www.pneumotox.com). When AEP is identified in a patient, the pediatrician should educate the patient and family about the link to smoking exposure and risk of AEP upon reexposure.

In addition to smoke exposure, AEP has been reported after smoking cocaine; typically, within hours to days after use. Whether this is a unique eosinophilic response to cocaine that represents 1 manifestation of *crack lung* or is a separate disease is unknown. Crack lung refers to diffuse alveolitis with pulmonary hemorrhage from an unknown mechanism that occurs within 48 hr of cocaine smoke inhalation.

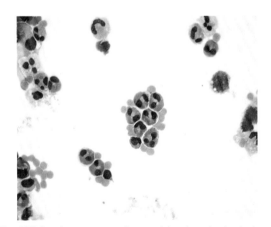

Fig. 427.6 Light microscopy of eosinophils in bronchoalveolar lavage fluid.

Lung function has not been measured frequently in the disease because the patients have proceeded rapidly to the ICU and need for mechanical ventilation. When measured, a restrictive pattern of lung disease and reduced diffusion capacity is the usual finding. Arterial blood gases will also show a significant increase in the alveolar–arterial gradient.

The criteria for diagnosis include the acute onset of disease, bilateral pulmonary infiltrates, reduced oxygen saturation or $PaO_2 \leq 60$ mm Hg, BAL of $\geq 25\%$, and absence of a determined cause of eosinophilia (see Table 427.11). The recent onset of tobacco exposure, dust, or chemical inhalation are supporting factors in confirming a diagnosis.

Treatment has uniformly been the use of a corticosteroid (e.g., methylprednisolone 1-2 mg/kg/day) either intravenously or orally for 2-4 wk. A minimum or maximum treatment time has not been determined. Rare fatalities have been reported. Complete recovery has been seen in days with resolution of pleural effusions within the 4 wk treatment time. Most important, relapse and persistent symptoms are rare, which sharply contrasts the idiopathic chronic eosinophilic pneumonias. Follow-up testing of pulmonary function is usually normal which supports the contention that lung parenchyma heals without evidence of compromise or fibrosis.

CHRONIC EOSINOPHILIC PNEUMONIA
Chronic eosinophilic pneumonia is another idiopathic pulmonary condition without a known exposure to toxin, dust, or chemical inhalation. Eosinophils infiltrate the lung parenchyma resulting in dyspnea, cough, fever, and weight loss. It is primarily a problem for adults, with a female predominance (2:1 female:male ratio) usually in patients who are nonsmokers. Chest examination reveals tachypnea, crackles, and occasional wheezing as preceding asthma is a common finding. The classic finding on chest x-ray of the *radiographic negative of pulmonary edema* is found in these patients: central clear lung fields but fluffy, patchy peripheral infiltrates of the lung parenchyma.

When compared to AEP, the onset of disease is indolent and subtle, but the accompanying fever and weight loss may lead the clinician to a concern for an underlying malignancy prior to chest radiograph and laboratory investigation. *Peripheral* blood eosinophilia is commonly as high as 5,000/mm³ or greater, accompanied by BAL eosinophilia >40% on the differential count (see Table 427.11). The peripheral eosinophilia sharply contrasts the lack of eosinophils seen in the blood in AEP. HRCT scan contrasts the AEP with pleural effusion as a rare finding, as well as rare cavitation.

In contrast to AEP, pulmonary function testing shows a mixed obstructive and restrictive pattern when asthma occurs concurrently with pneumonia.

Inflammatory markers associated with migration and activation of eosinophils are predictably found in BAL and the urine. These include the T-lymphocyte type 2 cytokines of IL-4, IL-5, IL-6, IL-10, IL-13, and IL-18. However, T-lymphocyte type 1 cytokines of IL-2 and IL-12 are also present with many of the potent eosinophilic chemoattractants such as CCL5 (RANTES [regulated upon activation, normal T cell expressed and secreted]) and CCL11 (eotaxin-1). Toxic granule proteins of major basic protein, eosinophil-derived neurotoxin, and eosinophil cationic protein are frequently present. Unfortunately, these important molecules help confirm the eosinophilic nature of the disease, but their presence adds no additional sensitivity or specificity over the presence of eosinophils on BAL.

Treatment is similar to most eosinophilic lung syndromes where corticosteroids (oral) are the mainstay of treatment. The minimum dose of steroid needed to induce remission is not known, but most clinicians recommend prednisone (or equivalent) at 0.5 mg/kg/day for 2 wk. The dose is reduced to half (0.025 mg/kg/day) for an additional 2 wk if symptoms have abated. The remaining dose of steroid may need to be weaned over 6 mo. Symptoms and pulmonary infiltrates rapidly disappear after initiation of this treatment but frequently recur with tapering of the steroid. Asthma concurrently in patients with chronic eosinophilic pneumonia identifies a phenotype of the disease that appears to have lower relapse risk yet up to 50% of all identified patients with chronic eosinophilic pneumonia relapse during or after corticosteroid taper.

Many believe that this disease is a precursor to the development of EGPA (formerly Churg-Strauss syndrome). The utility of ICS in chronic eosinophilic pneumonia is unknown but is warranted for the persistent asthma phenotype of disease. A subset of patients develops permanent lower airway obstruction without reversibility, which requires patients with this disease to have close follow-up and monitoring of pulmonary function tests routinely.

EOSINOPHILIC GRANULOMATOSIS WITH POLYANGIITIS (THE CHURG-STRAUSS SYNDROME)
The EGPA syndrome is a systemic disease involving multiple organs but most prominently the lung. Patients present with difficult to control asthma, allergic rhinitis, and peripheral eosinophilia (>10% or >1,500 cells/μL) in the blood. Evidence of vasculitis on clinical grounds must be present in at least 2 organs. The polyangiitis appears later in the disease process with asthma being the precursor symptom in more than 90% of the cases reported. EGPA affects multiple organs including the skin, heart, gastrointestinal tract, kidneys, and central nervous system (Table 427.12). Rhinitis is present in 75% of the patients but is not specific. Symptom complexes of fever, weight loss, fatigue, arthralgia, and myalgia may be seen in approximately two-thirds of patients. Cardiac and renal involvement is insidious in onset and should be screened for. It is the multiple organ involvement that results in the morbidity and mortality of this disease. The typical progression of the disease is in 3 phases: rhinitis and asthma first, tissue eosinophilia second, and, finally, systemic vasculitis.

The pathogenesis of EGPA is still unknown but several factors are suspected to contribute to the development of the disease. The possible link between leukotriene-receptor antagonists (zafirlukast, montelukast, or pranlukast) is controversial but still considered possible. It is suspected that use of this class of adjunctive medications in severe asthma allows for the reduction in use of corticosteroid leading to the full-blown (unmasking) manifestation of EGPA. Isolated use of leukotriene-receptor antagonists may induce disease, lead to remission with cessation of leukotriene-receptor antagonists, and cause recurrence of EGPA upon reintroduction of this class of medications. Many refrain from use of leukotriene-receptor antagonists when the EGPA syndrome has been diagnosed.

Clinical and laboratory findings pinpoint the diagnosis with high specificity (99.7%) and sensitivity (85%) when 4 of 6 criteria are met (asthma, eosinophilia >10%, mononeuropathy or polyneuropathy, nonfixed pulmonary infiltrates, paranasal sinus abnormalities, and biopsy findings of extravascular eosinophil infiltrates). In contrast to GPA,

Table 427.12	Eosinophilic Granulomatosis With Polyangiitis	
	VASCULITIC PHENOTYPE	**EOSINOPHILIC TISSULAR DISEASE PHENOTYPE**
Respective frequency	~40%	~60%
ANCA	Present (mostly perinuclear-ANCA with anti-MPO specificity)	Absent
Predominant manifestations	Glomerular renal disease Peripheral neuropathy Purpura Biopsy-proven vasculitis	Cardiac involvement (eosinophilic myocarditis) Eosinophilic pneumonia Fever

ANCA, Antineutrophil cytoplasmic antibody; *MPO*, myeloperoxidase.
Data from Sablé-Fourtassou R, Cohen P, Mahr A, et al: Antineutrophil cytoplasmic antibodies and the Churg-Strauss syndrome, *Ann Intern Med* 2005;143:632–638; and Sinico RA, Di Toma L, Maggiore U, et al: Prevalence and clinical significance of antineutrophil cytoplasmic antibodies in Churg-Strauss syndrome, *Arthritis Rheum* 2005;52:2926–2935.
From Cottin V, Cordier JF: Eosinophilic lung diseases, *Immunol Allergy Clin North Am* 32(4):557–586, 2012 (Table 2, p. 569).

the rhinitis is not destructive and nasal septal perforation does not occur in EGPA.

Radiography of the chest by plain radiography or HRCT demonstrates the migratory, peripheral predominant opacities with ground-glass appearance to full consolidation. Bronchiectasis and bronchial wall thickening are reported. Pleural effusion should raise suspicion for the presence of heart failure from **cardiomyopathy**.

Laboratory findings include striking eosinophilia with values generally between 5,000 and 20,000/mm³ at the time of diagnosis. These counts often parallel vasculitis activity. The BAL shows striking eosinophilia with differential counts of >60%. Other organ system levels reflect activity of eosinophils and are not specific for the EGPA diagnosis.

ANCAs may be present in the EGPA syndrome. The perinuclear-ANCA targeting myeloperoxidase is specifically found in EGPA in approximately 40% of the patients; the absence of myeloperoxidase-ANCA does not exclude the diagnosis. Those patients with eosinophilic pneumonia, fever, and cardiac involvement are less likely to have myeloperoxidase-ANCA detected. Those with peripheral neuropathy, renal glomerular disease, and skin purpura usually have detectable myeloperoxidase-ANCAs (see Table 427.12).

Pulmonary function tests while on bronchodilators and ICS for asthma show an obstructive pattern. The pulmonary obstruction is responsive to oral corticosteroid use but often has mild persistence of obstruction.

Treatment of EGPA with systemic oral corticosteroid remains the mainstay of therapy at a starting dose of 1 mg/kg/day for 4 wk. This therapy is often required for up to 12 mo or longer with a steady taper in dosage over that time. EGPA resistant to corticosteroid has responded to cyclophosphamide, IFN-α, cyclosporine, intravenous immunoglobulin, and plasmapheresis. The use of anti–IL-5 (mepolizumab) has been encouraging and may be used as a steroid-sparing agent in the future.

ALLERGIC BRONCHOPULMONARY ASPERGILLOSIS

ABPA is a complex mixed immunologic hypersensitivity reaction in the lungs and bronchi in response to exposure and colonization of *Aspergillus* species (usually *Aspergillus fumigatus*; see Chapter 264). This disease almost exclusively occurs in patients with preexisting asthma and up to 15% of patients with cystic fibrosis (see Chapter 432). The quantity of *Aspergillus* exposure does not correlate with the severity of disease.

The clinical pattern of disease (Table 427.13) is remarkably similar with a clinical presentation of difficult-to-treat asthma, periods of acute obstructive lung disease with bronchial mucous plugs, elevated total IgE antibody, elevated specific IgE and IgG anti-*Aspergillus* antibodies, skin prick test reactions to *Aspergillus* species, precipitating antibody to *Aspergillus* species, as well as proximal bronchiectasis. Other clinical

manifestations include dyspnea, cough, shortness of breath, and peripheral eosinophilia, as well as pulmonary eosinophilia with infiltration of the parenchyma. The use of systemic corticosteroid may lower the total IgE antibody levels such that a diagnosis may be in question when the first tests are performed at that time.

ABPA should be considered in patients with cystic fibrosis when clinical deterioration occurs without evidence of an identifiable cause. Symptoms heralding such deterioration include increasing cough, wheezing, loss of exercise tolerance, worsening exercise-induced asthma, reduction of pulmonary function, or increased sputum production without another discernible reason. Clinical findings of elevated total IgE antibody, anti-*Aspergillus* IgE, precipitating antibodies to *A. fumigatus*, and/or new abnormalities on chest radiography that fail to clear with antibiotics should alert the clinician to the possibility of ABPA.

When evaluating a child with asthma symptoms, the clinician must distinguish asthma from ABPA. If the diagnosis is suspected, skin prick test for evidence of IgE-specific antibody directed against *A. fumigatus* is essential. Intradermal skin testing when the skin prick test is negative, although not routinely performed because of poor specificity, may be performed. The absence of a positive skin prick test and intradermal test to *A. fumigatus* virtually excludes the diagnosis of ABPA. The prevalence of ABPA in patients with an existing diagnosis of asthma and an abnormal immediate skin prick test response to *A. fumigatus* has been evaluated. Between 2% and 32% of patients with asthma with concurrent skin prick test–positive reactions to *Aspergillus* have evidence of ABPA.

It is uncommon for the patient with cystic fibrosis to develop ABPA before the age of 6 yr. When the total IgE antibody in patients with cystic fibrosis exceeds 500 IU/mL (1,200 ng/mL), a strong clinical suspicion of ABPA is necessary.

ABPA pathology has characteristic findings of mucoid bronchi impaction, eosinophilic pneumonia, and bronchocentric granulomas in addition to the typical histologic features of asthma. Septated hyphae are often found in the mucus-filled bronchial tree. However, the fungi do not invade the mucosa in this unique disease. *Aspergillus* may be cultured from sputum in more than 60% of ABPA patients. Interestingly, hyphae may not always be seen on microscopy.

Staging of the disease (Table 427.14) represents distinct phases of the disease but do not necessarily progress in sequence from stage 1 to stage 5. Staging of ABPA is important for treatment considerations. In many hypersensitivity diseases where IgE antibody contributes to the pathogenesis (e.g., asthma), total IgE is often used for screening for an atopic state but is not a test that helps the clinician with serial measures. In sharp contrast, the measurement of IgE during acute exacerbations, remission, and recurrent ABPA disease is helpful in identifying the activity of disease and may herald the recurrence. During stage 1 disease, the level of IgE antibody is often very high. During stage 2 remission, a fall in the levels may be as much as 35% or more. Recurrence of activity may result in a marked rise of total IgE with a doubling of the baseline level seen during remission. During the use of glucocorticoid therapy, monthly or bimonthly levels of IgE are followed serially to

Table 427.13	Criteria for the Diagnosis of Allergic Bronchopulmonary Aspergillosis

Allergic bronchopulmonary aspergillosis–central bronchiectasis
- Medical history of asthma*
- Immediate skin prick test reaction to *Aspergillus* antigens*
- Precipitating (IgG) serum antibodies to *Aspergillus fumigatus**
- Total IgE concentration > 417 IU/mL (>1,000 ng/mL)*
- Central bronchiectasis on chest CT*
- Peripheral blood eosinophilia >500/mm³
- Lung infiltrates on chest x-ray or chest HRCT
- Elevated specific serum IgE and IgG to *A. fumigatus*

Allergic bronchopulmonary aspergillosis seropositive†
- Medical history of asthma†
- Immediate skin prick test reaction to *A. fumigatus* antigens†
- Precipitating (IgG) serum antibodies to *A. fumigatus†*
- Total IgE concentration > 417 IU/mL (>1,000 ng/mL)†

*The criteria required for diagnosis of ABPA with central bronchiectasis.
†The first 4 criteria are required for a diagnosis of seropositive ABPA.
ABPA, Allergic bronchopulmonary aspergillosis; *CSD*, corticosteroid dependent; *HRCT*, high-resolution computerized tomography.

Table 427.14	Staging of Allergic Bronchopulmonary Aspergillosis		
Staging of allergic bronchopulmonary aspergillosis			
Stage 1	Acute	Upper and middle lobe infiltration	High IgE
Stage 2	Remission	No infiltrate off steroids >6 mo	Normal to high IgE
Stage 3	Exacerbation	Upper and middle lobe infiltration	High IgE
Stage 4	CSD asthma	Minimal infiltrate	Normal to high IgE
Stage 5	End stage	Fibrosis and/or bullae	Normal

CSD, Corticosteroid dependent.

assist the clinician in tapering therapy. Because exacerbations of ABPA are asymptomatic to the patient in approximately 25% of the recurrences, serial IgE accompanied by chest radiography are helpful to the clinician to guide therapy.

Radiography

Plain chest X-ray shows evidence of infiltrates especially in the upper lobes and the classic findings of bronchiectasis (Fig. 427.7). The use of HRCT demonstrates central bronchiectasis in the central regions of the lung (Fig. 427.8). HRCT may add value, for the patient with a positive skin prick test and normal chest radiograph, to detecting characteristic abnormalities of ABPA.

Treatment

The mainstay of therapy for ABPA has been systemic glucocorticoids with adjunct therapy, antifungal medications, and anti-IgE therapy with omalizumab. Exacerbations in stages 1 and 3 are treated for 14 days with 0.5-1 mg/kg of glucocorticoid followed by every-other-day usage

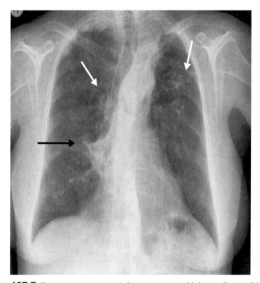

Fig. 427.7 Transitory opacities *(white arrows)* and lobar collapse *(black arrow)* in patient with allergic bronchopulmonary aspergillosis. *(From Douglass JA, Sandrini A, Holgate ST, O'Hehir RE: Allergic bronchopulmonary aspergillosis and hypersensitivity pneumonitis. In Adkinson AF, editor: Middleton's allergy principles and practice, Philadelphia, 2014, Elsevier, Fig. 61.2.)*

and tapering over 3 mo or as long as 6 mo. Stage 2 remission phase and stage 5 where fibrosis has occurred do not require glucocorticoid therapy. Stage 4 denotes a state where glucocorticoid weaning has not been successful and continued long-term therapy is required.

Antifungal therapy with a 16-wk course of itraconazole improves the response rate during exacerbations allowing the reduction of glucocorticoid dosage by 50% and resulting in a reduction of total serum IgE of 25% or more. The proposed mechanisms of action have been to either reduce the antigen load driving the immune response or possibly raising the corticosteroid serum levels by slowing the metabolism of the steroid. This latter mechanism would be true for prednisone, which is methylated in the liver, but not for methylprednisolone, which does not require methylation.

The adult dosage recommendation for itraconazole is 200 mg 3 times per day for 3 days followed by 200 mg twice daily for the remainder of the 16 wk. Children should receive 5 mg/kg/day in a single dose. If the proper calculated dose exceeds 200 mg, then the total dose should be divided equally and given twice daily. Serum levels of itraconazole are necessary to ensure proper absorption of the drug is occurring from the capsule form. The liquid form is more readily absorbed and has achieved substantially higher levels. The use of proton pump inhibitors and histamine 2 antagonists may reduce absorption by blocking acid production. Voriconazole has been used as a substitute antifungal medication. Proper dosing has been established for invasive *Aspergillus* disease, but not for ABPA. Typical dosage regimen in children of 7 mg/kg/day may cause hepatotoxicity so liver function must be monitored.

Omalizumab, an anti-IgE humanized monoclonal antibody, has been used in case series of patients with cystic fibrosis and ABPA as well as a small cohort of adults without cystic fibrosis but with ABPA. Both case series demonstrated significant reductions in asthma exacerbations, ABPA exacerbations, and glucocorticoid usage. The dose prescribed has been 300-375 mg every 2 wk by subcutaneous injection.

HYPEREOSINOPHILIC SYNDROME

See Chapter 155.

The HES is a descriptive name of a group of disorders that are characterized by the persistent overproduction of eosinophils accompanied by eosinophil infiltration in multiple organs with end-organ damage from mediator release. The term HES should only be used when there is eosinophilia with end-organ damage from the eosinophils and not from another cause. The discovery of underlying genetic, biochemical, or neoplastic reasons for HES has led to the classification of primary, secondary, and idiopathic HES (Table 427.15). Specific syndromes such as EGPA have eosinophilia but the contribution of eosinophils to the organ damage is incompletely understood.

Some variants of HES have genetic mutations in tyrosine kinase receptor platelet-derived growth factor receptor-α (*PDGFRA*); males

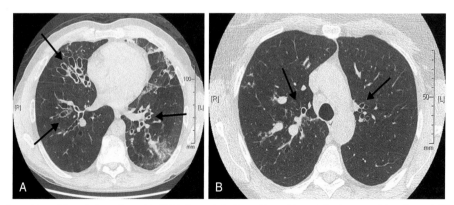

Fig. 427.8 A, Central bronchiectasis in patient with ABPA *(arrows).* **B,** Central bronchiectasis in the upper lobes *(arrows). (From Douglass JA, Sandrini A, Holgate ST, O'Hehir RE: Allergic bronchopulmonary aspergillosis and hypersensitivity pneumonitis. In Adkinson AF, editor: Middleton's allergy principles and practice, Philadelphia, 2014, Elsevier, Fig. 61.3.)*

Table 427.15	Hypereosinophilic Syndrome Variants
Myeloproliferative	Nonclonal Clonal–F1P1L1/PDGFRA-positive chronic eosinophilic leukemia
Lymphocytic	Nonclonal T cells Clonal T-cell expansion with T-cell activation
Overlap	Organ restricted
Familial	Family history of eosinophilia without known cause
Associated	Eosinophilia in chronic disease like inflammatory bowel disease or EGPA (Churg-Strauss syndrome)
Undefined	Asymptomatic Cyclic angioedema with eosinophilia (Gleich syndrome) Symptomatic without myeloproliferation or lymphocytic form

EGPA, Eosinophilic granulomatosis with polyangiitis; PDGFRA, platelet-derived growth factor receptor-α.

are almost exclusively affected. Otherwise, HES appears to be distributed equally among females and males.

Hypereosinophilia is defined as an absolute eosinophil number in the blood that exceeds 1.5×10^9 eosinophils on 2 separate occasions separated by at least 1 mo. Tissues are abnormal when more than 20% of nucleated cells in the bone marrow are of eosinophil origin, a pathologist determines the presence of eosinophilia, or the presence of extensive eosinophilic granule proteins are determined on biopsy to be deposited in large quantities. These disorders can be subclassified into primary (neoplastic), secondary (reactive), and idiopathic (Fig. 427.9).

Clinical manifestations of the HES include organ involvement of the heart (5%), gastrointestinal (14%), skin (37%), and pulmonary (25–63%).

The HES is complicated by thrombosis and/or neurologic disease in many patients, although the exact prevalence of this problem is incompletely categorized. Peripheral neuropathy, encephalopathy, transverse sinus thrombosis, or cerebral emboli are the most common neurologic complications. The exact mechanism of the manifestations is unclear especially in major artery thrombosis such as the femoral artery.

The most frequent pulmonary symptoms include cough and dyspnea. Many patients have obstructive lung disease with clinical wheezing. Evidence of pulmonary fibrosis and pulmonary emboli are seen with regularity. Because biopsy shows eosinophilic infiltrates similar to other pulmonary eosinophilic diseases of the lung, it is the constellation of other organ involvement or thromboembolic phenomena and other organs that must lead the clinician to a high index of suspicion for the HES.

Laboratory evaluation should include evaluation of liver enzymes, kidney function tests, creatine kinase, and troponin. The extent of cardiac involvement should be evaluated by electrocardiogram and echocardiogram. Some unique biomarkers may be tested when evaluating the myeloproliferative and T-lymphocyte HES diagnoses. Vitamin B_{12} and serum tryptase may be elevated, especially the latter, when the myeloproliferative disease is accompanied by mastocytosis. These 2 biomarkers are most frequently elevated when the mutation is present or fusion in the FIP1L1/PDGFRA sites.

Because of the extensive pulmonary disease that is seen in the HES, pulmonary function tests should be performed at diagnosis when possible to include spirometry and lung volumes. Dead space ventilation may be significantly elevated in the patients with pulmonary emboli. Pulse oximetry may be very helpful in the evaluation as well.

Chest radiography and CT are very helpful in the evaluation. Spiral chest CT should also be performed when pulmonary emboli are being considered. In 1 series of patients, nearly half of the patients with HES had evidence of pulmonary abnormalities including ground-glass appearing infiltrates, pulmonary emboli, mediastinal lymphadenopathy, and/or pleural effusion.

Treatment of HES depends on the type of variant (myeloproliferative, lymphocytic forms, undefined, associated with systemic diseases such as EGPA, or familial). Rarely, some patients present with marked

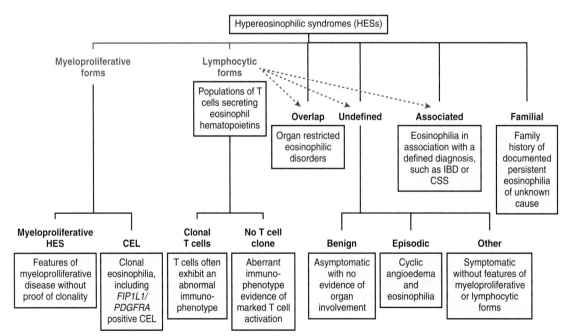

Fig. 427.9 A revised classification of hypereosinophilic syndrome *(HES)*. Changes from the previous classification are indicated in red. *Dashed arrows* identify HES forms in some patients that have T-cell–driven disease. Classification of myeloproliferative forms has been simplified, and patients with HES and eosinophil hematopoietin-producing T cells in the absence of a T-cell clone are included in the lymphocytic forms of HES. CSS, Churg-Strauss syndrome; IBD, inflammatory bowel disease. *(From Simon H, Rothenberg ME, Bochner BS, et al: Refining the definition of hypereosinophilic syndrome, J Allergy Clin Immunol 126:45–49, 2010, Fig. 1.)*

eosinophilia, where the total count exceeds 100,000 cells/μL, and vascular insufficiency symptoms. Prednisone at 15 mg/kg is indicated to acutely reduce the eosinophil count after diagnostic tests are performed and when safe. If the patient is unstable, the glucocorticoid should be administered to prevent progression of symptoms. Other acute therapies aimed at reduction of eosinophil counts include vincristine, imatinib mesylate, or even leukophoresis.

When eosinophil counts are not as dramatically elevated, therapy begins with glucocorticoids at 1 mg/kg for patients who do not have the FIP1L1/PDGFRA mutation. Patients with this mutation are resistant to glucocorticoids and initial treatment should begin with imatinib, a tyrosine kinase inhibitor. Because this genetic test is often not readily available, surrogate markers for the presence of this mutation are vitamin B_{12} levels > 2,000 pg/mL or serum tryptase >11.5 ng/mL. It denotes the presence of resistant disease that should initially be treated with imatinib. The goal of therapy is to reduce and maintain eosinophil counts below 1.5×10^9 at the lowest dose of prednisone possible to reduce or avoid corticosteroid side effects. If corticosteroid doses cannot be lowered below 10 mg/day, then imatinib can be added as combination therapy in order to spare the dose of steroid. Caution must be used in the presence of cardiac disease as introduction of imatinib has precipitated left ventricular failure.

Additional or alternative adjunct therapies that have shown promise include hydroxyurea, interferon α, anti–IL-5 monoclonal antibody therapy, and a monoclonal antibody directed against CD52. Failure of the above modalities may signal a need for hematopoietic stem cell transplantation. This therapy has been successful in some patients.

Bibliography is available at Expert Consult.

427.5 Interstitial Lung Disease
Kevin J. Kelly and Timothy J. Vece

ILD in children is caused by a large group of rare, heterogeneous, familial, or sporadic diseases that involve the pulmonary parenchyma and cause significant impairment of gas exchange (Tables 427.16 and 427.17). While there are some shared diseases, ILD in children is often different than ILD in adults, especially notable for the absence of idiopathic pulmonary fibrosis in children. Despite wide variations in cause, these disorders are classified together because of the similar clinical, physiologic, radiographic, and pathologic processes involving disruption of alveolar interstitium and airways. Prevalence estimates vary widely with a range of 0.13-16.2 cases/100,000 children, likely due to the lack of standardization of diseases included in the definition of ILD in children. The pathophysiology is believed to be more complex than that of adult disease because pulmonary injury occurs during the process of lung

Table 427.16	The Pediatric Interstitial Lung Diseases in Children Under 2 Yr of Age

AGE-RELATED INTERSTITIAL LUNG DISEASES IN INFANCY AND EARLY CHILDHOOD
Diffuse developmental disorders
  Acinar dysplasia
  Congenital alveolar dysplasia
  Alveolar capillary dysplasia with misalignment of pulmonary veins (some due to *FOXF1* mutation)
Growth abnormalities reflecting deficient alveolarization
  Pulmonary hypoplasia
  Chronic neonatal lung disease
  Chromosomal disorders
  Congenital heart disease
Neuroendocrine cell hyperplasia of infancy
  Pulmonary interstitial glycogenosis (infantile cellular interstitial pneumonia)
  Surfactant dysfunction disorders (pulmonary alveolar proteinosis)
  Surfactant protein–B mutation
  Surfactant protein–C mutation
  ABCA3 mutation
  Granulocyte-macrophage colony-stimulating factor receptor (*CSF2RA*) mutation
  NKX2.1 (transcription factor for SP-B, SPC, ABCA3)
 	
INTERSTITIAL LUNG DISEASE DISORDERS WITH KNOWN ASSOCIATIONS
Infectious/postinfectious processes
  Adenovirus viruses
  Influenza viruses
  Chlamydia pneumoniae
  Mycoplasma pneumoniae
Environmental agents
  Hypersensitivity pneumonitis
  Toxic inhalation
Aspiration syndromes
 	
PULMONARY DISEASES ASSOCIATED WITH PRIMARY AND SECONDARY IMMUNE DEFICIENCY
Opportunistic infections
Granulomatous lymphocytic interstitial lung disease associated with common variable immunodeficiency syndrome
Lymphoid intestinal pneumonia (HIV infection)
Therapeutic interventions: chemotherapy, radiation, transplantation, and rejection
	IDIOPATHIC INTERSTITIAL LUNG DISEASES
	Usual interstitial pneumonitis
	Desquamative interstitial pneumonitis
	Lymphocytic interstitial pneumonitis and related disorders
	Nonspecific interstitial pneumonitis (cellular/fibrotic)
	Eosinophilic pneumonia
	Bronchiolitis obliterans syndrome
	Pulmonary hemosiderosis and acute idiopathic pulmonary hemorrhage of infancy
	Pulmonary alveolar proteinosis
	Pulmonary vascular disorders
	Pulmonary lymphatic disorders
	Pulmonary microlithiasis
	Persistent tachypnea of infancy
	Brain-thyroid-lung syndrome
	
	SYSTEMIC DISORDERS WITH PULMONARY MANIFESTATIONS
	Anti-GBM disease
	Gaucher disease and other storage diseases
	Malignant infiltrates
	Hemophagocytic lymphohistiocytosis
	Langerhans cell histiocytosis
	Sarcoidosis
	Systemic sclerosis
	Polymyositis/dermatomyositis
	Systemic lupus erythematosus
	Rheumatoid arthritis
	Lymphangioleiomyomatosis
	Pulmonary hemangiomatosis
	Neurocutaneous syndromes
	Hermansky-Pudlak syndrome

Modified from Deutsch GH, Young LR, Deterding RR, et al: diffuse lung disease in young children: application of a novel classification scheme, *Am J Respir Crit Care Med* 176:1120–1128, 2007.

Table 427.17	The Pediatric Interstitial Lung Diseases in Children Over 2 Yr of Age

DISORDERS OF THE IMMUNOCOMPETENT HOST

Disorders of Infancy
- Growth abnormalities
- NEHI
- Disorders of surfactant metabolism

Systemic Disease
- Immune mediated disorders
  - Connective tissue disease related lung disease
  - Pulmonary hemorrhage syndromes
- Storage diseases
- Sarcoidosis

DISORDERS OF THE IMMUNOCOMPROMISED HOST
- Opportunistic infections
- Related to treatment
- Chemotherapy
- Radiation
- Drug hypersensitivity
- Related to transplantation
- Rejection
- GVHD
- PTLD
- Lymphoid Infiltrates

GVHD, Graft-versus-host disease; *NEHI*, neuroendocrine cell hyperplasia of infancy; *PTLD*, post-transplant lymphoproliferative disease.
   Modified from Fan LL, Dishop MK, Galambos C, et al: Diffuse lung disease in biopsied children 2 to 18 years of age. Application of the chILD Classification Scheme, *Ann Am Thorac Soc* 2015;12(10):1498–1505.

Table 427.18	Clinical Features, Age, and Onset of Surfactant Protein Dysfunction Syndromes (SPDS)

SPDS	CLINICAL FEATURES	AGE AND ONSET
SFTPB	Neonatal ‣ Respiratory distress	Neonate, acute
ABCA3	Neonatal ‣ Respiratory distress Infancy ‣ Cough ‣ Tachypnoea, hypoxemia ‣ Failure to thrive Childhood ‣ Wheeze, crackles ‣ Exercise intolerance ‣ Dyspnea ‣ Retractions, crackles, digital clubbing ‣ Low body weight	Neonate, acute Infancy and childhood, subacute Late childhood and adulthood, chronic
SFTPC	Neonatal ‣ Respiratory distress Childhood ‣ Cough ‣ Tachypnoea, hypoxemia	Neonate, acute (infrequent) Infancy and childhood, subacute Late childhood and adulthood, chronic
NKX2.1	Respiratory ‣ Neonatal respiratory distress ‣ Recurrent infections ‣ Chronic interstitial lung disease Neurological ‣ Chorea ‣ Ataxia ‣ Developmental delay ‣ Hypotonia Hypothyroidism	Any age Acute or chronic

ABCA3, ATP binding cassette number A3.
   From Gupta A, Zheng SL: Genetic disorders of surfactant protein dysfunction: when to consider and how to investigate, *Arch Dis Child* 102:84–90, 2017 (Table 2, p. 86).

growth and differentiation. In ILD, the initial injury causes damage to the alveolar epithelium and capillary endothelium. Abnormal healing of injured tissue may be more prominent than inflammation in the initial steps of the development of chronic ILD. Genetic causes of ILD are becoming increasingly important, especially disorders of surfactant metabolism (DSM) and immune dysregulatory disorders.

CLASSIFICATION AND PATHOLOGY
Through the work of both the children's ILD research network in the United States and the children's ILD-European Union group in Europe, consensus on a classification scheme has been reached. The classification is broken down by age with 2 yr of age serving as a cut-off, and by histologic pattern. The classification scheme was first applied to biopsies from children under 2 and was extended to children over 2 yr of age (see Tables 427.16 and 427.17). Growth disorders such as alveolar simplification, unique diseases of infants such as neuroendocrine cell hyperplasia of infancy (**NEHI**), and **DSM** were common in children under 2. In contrast, disorders of the immunocompromised host such as ILD related to immune deficiency, and disorders of systemic diseases such as the collagen vascular disorders, were much more common in older children.

Neuroendocrine Cell Hyperplasia of Infancy
See Chapter 427.6.

Disorders of Surfactant Metabolism
One of the more important groups of disorders in pediatric ILD is the **DSM** (Table 427.18). These disorders likely account for previously unknown cases of neonatal respiratory distress in full-term infants. Surfactant protein B deficiency, caused by mutations in the surfactant protein B gene, is a cause of severe neonatal respiratory distress. Chest CT often has a pattern of diffuse ground-glass opacities with septal thickening. Histopathology reveals alveolar proteinosis with interstitial widening, and electron microscopy shows disorganized lamellar bodies. Most children die within the first 2 mo of life without a lung transplant. Surfactant protein C deficiency can cause disease in older infants, children, or adults. Chest CT can show diffuse ground-glass opacities with septal thickening early in the disease or significant fibrosis and

honeycombing in more advanced disease. Histopathologic findings vary with age, with alveolar proteinosis and interstitial widening seen in young children, and fibrosis seen in older children and adults. Electron microscopy reveals normal lamellar bodies. ABCA3 mutations cause variable lung disease in children with some having severe disease similar to surfactant protein B deficiency, while other children have less severe disease similar to surfactant protein C. Chest CT most often shows diffuse ground-glass opacities with septal thickening early in the disease (Fig. 427.10). Histopathology depends on the age of the child similar to surfactant protein C, however, electron microscopy shows characteristic changes in the lamellar bodies with an eccentric electron dense body without the characteristic concentric circles—the so-called fried egg appearance. **DSM** due to mutations in the gene NKX2.1 has also been described. NKX2.1 encodes for thyroid transcription factor 1 (TTF-1), which is a major regulator or surfactant protein transcription. Mutations in NKX2.1 cause variable disease in the lungs, brain, and thyroid (see Table 427.18). Lung disease is variable and can present similar to surfactant protein B deficiency, or as recurrent pulmonary infections. Finally, mutations in the alpha and beta subunits of the granulocyte-macrophage colony-stimulating factor (GM-CSF) receptor cause failure of response to GM-CSF by the pulmonary alveolar macrophages. This leads to an inability to recycle surfactant with subsequent accumulation of proteinaceous material and pulmonary alveolar proteinosis.

Interstitial Lung Disease Due to Systemic Disease
ILD due to systemic disease is more common in older children with diffuse lung disease. The most common lung disease seen on biopsy is nonspecific interstitial pneumonia, however, other patterns are seen depending on the

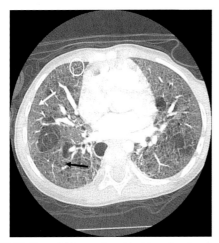

Fig. 427.10 Chest CT from a 2 yr old with a disorder of surfactant metabolism from mutations in ABCA3. Note the ground-glass opacities *(white arrow)* and septal thickening *(white circle)* and early cyst formation *(black arrow)*. *(Courtesy R. Paul Guillerman, MD.)*

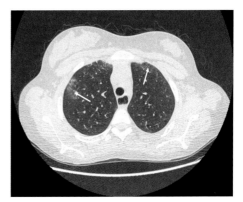

Fig. 427.11 Chest CT from a 11 yr old patient with systemic sclerosis and cellular nonspecific interstitial pneumonia. Note the areas of ground-glass opacities in the periphery *(white arrow)*. *(Courtesy R. Paul Guillerman, MD.)*

underlying disorder, such as lymphocytic interstitial pneumonia in Sjögren syndrome or cryptogenic organizing pneumonia in dermatomyositis. CT scans depend on the underlying ILD with nonspecific interstitial pneumonia having areas of ground-glass opacities and septal thickening in the early cellular phase of the disease (Fig. 427.11), progressing to diffuse fibrosis with traction bronchiectasis and peripheral cysts in the later fibrotic stage of the disease. The exact mechanism for disease is unknown but likely is due to auto-antibodies to respiratory tissue.

Pulmonary vasculitis, either due to GPA, microscopic polyangiitis, idiopathic pulmonary capillaritis, or anti-glomerular basement membrane syndrome (formerly Goodpasture disease) is another common manifestation of systemic diseases. Disease is likely due to auto-antibody stimulation of lymphocytes with resultant inflammation of pulmonary endothelium causing interstitial changes and pulmonary hemorrhage. Histopathology reveals diffuse alveolar hemorrhage, interstitial widening, and with the exception of anti-glomerular basement membrane disease, neutrophilic inflammation of the pulmonary vasculature.

Genetic causes of immune dysregulation may also be responsible for ILD in children. Mutations in both *STAT3b* and *LRBA* have been shown to cause lymphocytic interstitial pneumonia and lymphoproliferative disease. Mutations in *COPA*, a protein involved in ER to Golgi transport, cause familial pulmonary hemorrhage and/or ILD.

Persistent pulmonary symptoms can occur after **respiratory infections** caused by adenoviruses, influenza viruses, *Chlamydia pneumoniae*, and *Mycoplasma pneumoniae*. The resultant pulmonary disease is called **bronchiolitis obliterans** and is characterized by obstructive lung disease and obliteration or constriction of the bronchioles on lung biopsy. There is a characteristic appearance on HRCT with mosaicism, vascular attenuation, and central bronchiectasis, which if present, can obviate the need for lung biopsy (Fig. 427.12). **Aspiration** is a frequent cause of chronic lung disease in childhood and can mimic ILD. Children with developmental delay or neuromuscular weakness are at an increased risk for aspiration of food, saliva, or foreign matter, secondary to swallowing dysfunction and/or gastroesophageal reflux (GER). An undiagnosed tracheoesophageal fistula can also result in pulmonary complications related to aspiration of gastric contents and interstitial pneumonia.

Children experiencing an exaggerated immunologic response to organic dust, molds, or bird antigens may demonstrate hypersensitivity pneumonitis. Children with malignancies may have ILD related to the primary malignancy, an opportunistic infection, or chemotherapy or radiation treatment.

CLINICAL MANIFESTATIONS
A detailed history is needed to assess the severity of symptoms and the possibility of an underlying systemic disease in a patient with suspected

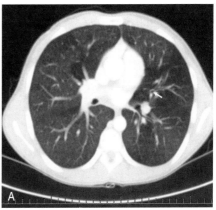

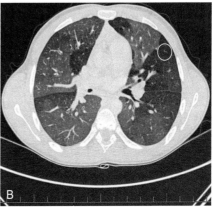

Fig. 427.12 Chest CT from an 11 yr old patient with bronchiolitis obliterans after Stevens-Johnson syndrome. **A,** Volumetric scan at full inspiration shows central bronchiectasis *(arrow)* and mosaic attenuation. **B,** High-resolution image taken in exhalation better highlights the mosaic attenuation, as well as vascular attenuation *(circle)*.

ILD as well as any family history of lung disease. Identification of precipitating factors, such as exposure to molds or birds and a severe lower respiratory infection, is important in establishing the diagnosis and instituting avoidance measures. Most patients develop hypoxia and hypercarbia, usually a late and ominous complication. Symptoms are usually insidious and occur in a continuous, not episodic, pattern. Tachypnea, crackles on auscultation, and retractions are noted on physical examination in children with ILD, but chest physical examination findings can be normal. Wheezing and fever are uncommon findings in pediatric ILD. Cyanosis accompanied by a prominent P2 heart sound is indicative of severe disease with the development of secondary pulmonary hypertension. Anemia or hemoptysis suggests a pulmonary vascular disease or pulmonary hemosiderosis. Rashes or joint complaints are consistent with an underlying connective tissue disease.

DIAGNOSIS
Radiography
Chest radiographic abnormalities can be classified as interstitial, reticular, nodular, reticulonodular, or honeycombed. The chest radiographic appearance may also be normal despite significant clinical impairment and may correlate poorly with the extent of disease. HRCT of the chest better defines the extent and distribution of disease and can provide specific information for selection of a biopsy site. Volume-controlled full-inspiratory and end-expiratory protocols used during HRCT can provide more information. These protocols may show air trapping, ground-glass patterns, mosaic patterns of attenuation, hyperinflation, bronchiectasis, cysts, and/or nodular opacities. Serial HRCT scans have been beneficial in monitoring disease progression and severity.

Pulmonary Function Tests
Pulmonary function tests are important in defining the degree of pulmonary dysfunction and in following the response to treatment. In ILD, pulmonary function abnormalities demonstrate a restrictive ventilatory deficit with decreased lung volumes and reduced lung compliance. The functional residual capacity is often reduced but is usually less affected than vital capacity and total lung capacity (TLC). The residual volume (RV) is usually maintained; therefore, ratios of functional residual capacity:TLC and RV:TLC are increased. Diffusion capacity of the lung is often reduced. Exercise testing may detect pulmonary dysfunction, even in the early stage of ILD with a decline in oxygen saturation.

Bronchoalveolar Lavage
BAL may provide helpful information regarding secondary infection, bleeding, and aspiration and allows cytology and molecular analyses. Evaluation of cell counts, differential, and lymphocyte markers may be helpful in determining the presence of hypersensitivity pneumonitis or sarcoid. Although BAL does not usually determine the exact diagnosis, it can be diagnostic for disorders such as pulmonary alveolar proteinosis.

Lung Biopsy
Lung biopsy for histopathology by conventional thoracotomy or video-assisted thoracoscopy *is usually the final step and is often necessary for a diagnosis*, except in **NEHI** and bronchiolitis obliterans. Biopsy yields a diagnosis in greater than 80% of patients. Due to the small size of biopsies obtained and low diagnostic yield, transbronchial biopsies are not recommended for the evaluation of ILD in children. Genetic testing for surfactant dysfunction mutational analysis is available. Evaluation for possible systemic disease may also be necessary.

TREATMENT
Supportive care of patients with ILD is essential and includes supplemental oxygen for hypoxia and adequate nutrition for growth failure. Antimicrobial treatment may be necessary for secondary infections. Some children may receive symptomatic relief from the use of bronchodilators. Antiinflammatory treatment with corticosteroids remains the initial treatment of choice. Controlled trials in children are lacking, however, and the clinical responses reported in case studies are variable. The usual dose of prednisone is 1-2 mg/kg/24 hr or 10-30 mg/kg of IV methylprednisolone given either weekly or for 3 consecutive days per month. Treatment length varies but is often initially given for 3-6 mo with tapering of dosage dictated by clinical response. Alternative, but not adequately evaluated, agents include hydroxychloroquine, azathioprine, cyclophosphamide, cyclosporine, methotrexate, and intravenous immunoglobulin. Investigational approaches involve specific agents directed against the action of cytokines, growth factors, or oxidants. Lung transplantation for progressive or end-stage ILD is used and outcomes are similar to other end-stage lung diseases in children such as cystic fibrosis. Appropriate treatment for underlying systemic disease is indicated. Preventive measures include avoidance of all inhalation irritants, such as tobacco smoke and, when appropriate, molds and bird antigens. Supervised pulmonary rehabilitation programs may be helpful.

Genetic Counseling
A high incidence of ILD in some families suggests a genetic predisposition to either development of the disease or severity of the disorder. Genetic counseling may be beneficial if a positive familial history is obtained.

PROGNOSIS
The overall mortality of ILD is variable and depends on specific diagnosis. Some children recover spontaneously without treatment, but other children steadily progress to death. Pulmonary hypertension, failure to thrive, and severe fibrosis are considered poor prognostic indicators.

ANTI-GLOMERULAR BASEMENT MEMBRANE DISEASE (ANTI-GBM DISEASE)
Anti-glomerular basement membrane disease, (**anti-GBM disease**) formerly known as Goodpasture disease, is the prototypical immunologic mediated ILD (see Chapter 538.4). Because of the concurrent presentation of renal and pulmonary disease, the differential diagnosis focuses on distinguishing anti-GBM disease from GPA, microscopic polyangiitis, Henoch-Schönlein purpura, and idiopathic pulmonary hemorrhage syndromes.

Pathophysiology
Immunology Factors
The development of anti-GBM antibodies directly correlates with the development of pulmonary and renal disease. Removal of such antibodies by plasmapheresis results in improvement of the disease process in some patients but not in all. The anti-GBM antibodies are IgG_1 and IgG_4 complement-binding subclasses of IgG which activate complement. Complement fragments signal the recruitment of neutrophils and macrophage in both the lung and kidney basement membranes resulting in damage and capillaritis.

Genetic Factors
Genetics appears to contribute strongly to the development of this disease with the presence of major histocompatibility complex class II alleles DR15, DR4, DRB1*1501, DRB1*04, and DRB1*03 predisposing to disease.

Environmental Factors
Exposure to smoke appears to be a strong factor in the development anti-GBM disease. Whether smoking alters the ultrastructure of the basement membrane or exogenous particles or noxious substances in smoke alter the type IV collagen is unknown. Smokers are more likely to develop pulmonary hemorrhage than non-smokers who have anti-GBM disease. Other injuries to the alveoli from infection, hydrocarbon inhalation, or cocaine inhalation have been reported as associated events prior to development of anti-GBM disease.

Clinical Manifestations
The majority of patients present with many days or weeks of cough, dyspnea, fatigue, and sometimes hemoptysis. Young children tend to swallow small amounts of blood from hemoptysis and may present with vomiting blood. Occasionally, the hemoptysis is large and resultant anemia is a consequence of large quantities of blood loss. Renal compromise is found with abnormal renal function tests. Younger patients tend to present with both the pulmonary and renal syndrome concurrently. Adults are less likely to develop pulmonary disease.

Laboratory
Serologic detection of anti-GBM antibodies is positive in more than 90% of patients with anti-GBM disease. A complete blood count will show anemia that is normocytic and normochromic as seen in chronic inflammatory disease. Urinalysis may reveal hematuria and proteinuria, while blood tests demonstrate renal compromise with elevated blood urea nitrogen and creatinine.

Studies for pANCA (antimyeloperoxidase ANCA) should also be performed and are positive in approximately 25–30% of patients concurrently with anti-GBM antibodies. Clinical disease may be more difficult to treat, and the presence of these antibodies may herald a more severe form of disease.

Chest Radiography

Chest radiography in anti-GBM disease will often show widely scattered patches of pulmonary infiltrates. If these infiltrates are in the periphery of the lung, they may be difficult to distinguish from the eosinophilic lung diseases. Interstitial patterns of thickening may be found as well. HRCT is usually not performed in this disease as the constellation of pulmonary hemorrhage, renal compromise, and positive serologic tests with anti-GBM antibodies detected often preclude the need for this test.

Pulmonary Function Testing

Pulmonary spirometry often reveals a restrictive defect with reduction in FVC and FEV_1. DLCO is a valuable test when pulmonary hemorrhage is a strong consideration. The intent of this test is to measure the ability of the lung to transfer inhaled gas to the red blood cell in the pulmonary capillary bed. This takes advantage of the hemoglobin's high affinity to bind carbon monoxide. It was once thought that reduction of DLCO was a measure of reduced surface area of the alveoli. Current data suggests that it directly correlates with the volume of blood in the pulmonary capillary bed. In pulmonary hemorrhage syndromes, blood in the alveoli plus the blood in the capillary bed increase the DLCO significantly and should alert the clinician to the possibility of pulmonary hemorrhage.

Bronchoscopy and Bronchoalveolar Lavage

Pulmonary abnormalities can often be best assessed by a bronchoscopy with BAL. The visual presence of blood on inspection as well as BAL will be obvious. Infections must be ruled out in many cases, and this technique adds significant value. BAL cell count will show hemosiderin-laden macrophages that have engulfed and broken down the red blood cells, leaving iron in these cells.

Lung Biopsy

Lung biopsy in patients with active disease reveals capillaritis from neutrophils, hemosiderin-laden macrophages, type II pneumocyte hyperplasia, and interstitial thickening at the level of the alveolus. Staining for IgG and complement is found by immunofluorescence along the basement membrane in a linear pattern. This antibody deposition pattern led to the investigation of endogenous antigens in the basement membrane.

Treatment

More than half of patients with anti-GBM disease who forego treatment die within 2 yr from either respiratory failure, renal failure, or both. After a diagnosis is made, therapy with corticosteroids (e.g., prednisone, 1 mg/kg/day) coupled with oral cyclophosphamide (2.5 mg/kg/day) is begun. The addition of daily plasmapheresis for 2 wk may accelerate improvement. Cyclophosphamide may be discontinued after 2-3 mo. Steroids are often weaned over a 6-9 mo period. Survival is affected by the need for ongoing dialysis. Patients who do not require persistent dialysis have a survival rate at 1 yr of 80% or more.

Bibliography is available at Expert Consult.

427.6 Neuroendocrine Cell Hyperplasia of Infancy
W. Adam Gower

BACKGROUND/SUMMARY

Neuroendocrine cell hyperplasia of Infancy (NEHI) (previously called persistent tachypnea of infancy) is an idiopathic form of diffuse lung disease that typically presents within the 1st yr of life with persistent tachypnea, retractions, hypoxemia, crackles, failure to thrive, and characteristic findings on chest imaging studies and lung histopathology. Pulmonary function studies typically demonstrate an obstructive picture with air trapping. There are no effective specific therapies for NEHI, and the usual approach is supportive care. The natural course is typically one of gradual improvement of symptoms, although exacerbations may occur throughout childhood. The long-term consequences of this disorder are not entirely known.

EPIDEMIOLOGY

The prevalence of NEHI is not known, but it is generally regarded to be a rare lung disease. Children with NEHI have accounted for around 10% of children who had lung biopsies in previous multicenter case series. There does not appear to be a clear racial or gender predisposition, and no other maternal or patient-level risk factors have been identified. Cases of NEHI have been reported in the literature from North and South America, Europe, Asia, and Australia.

PATHOPHYSIOLOGY

The primary clue to the pathophysiology of NEHI is increased numbers of airway neuroendocrine cells (NEC) in the airways of affected children. These cells are normally found in the airways, where they exist as innervated clusters known as NEB and secrete factors such as bombesin and serotonin (5-HT). They are thought to be involved in local oxygen sensing and may transmit neuroendocrine signals to other cells. Increases in NECs are seen in other respiratory disorders of childhood, usually with other additional findings. It is unclear whether their presence in increased numbers in NEHI causes the clinical picture, or is the result of abnormal pulmonary physiology secondary to some other primary factor. Increased numbers of NECs seem to be associated with increased small airways obstruction.

Although most cases appear to be sporadic, familial NEHI has been described, suggesting a possible inherited mechanism and/or shared environmental influences. The association of NEHI with heterozygosity for a variant in the gene *Nkx2.1*, which encodes the protein TTF-1, has been described in one kindred. Variants in this gene are also known to cause a wide spectrum of disorders, including more severe forms of diffuse lung disease (see Chapter 427.5).

CLINICAL PRESENTATION

The symptoms of NEHI characteristically appear during infancy, although the diagnosis may be delayed until after the 1st yr of life. The typical presentation includes persistent tachypnea, hypoxemia, retractions, and poor weight gain in an otherwise healthy infant. The exam usually reveals crackles or clear lung sounds, while cough and wheezing are uncommon. Typically, affected infants do not have a history of premature delivery. Echocardiograms usually show absence of structural heart disease or pulmonary hypertension.

DIAGNOSIS

The diagnosis of NEHI requires that other more common causes of the presenting symptoms are ruled out. Although children with NEHI may have GER and/or swallowing dysfunction, this is not thought to be sufficient to cause all of the findings, and may be secondary to tachypnea and increased work of breathing. Plain chest films may show hyperinflation. When biopsy material from the lung is stained with bombesin, increased numbers of positive-staining cells are noted in the airways. In general, biopsies from children with NEHI are remarkably void of fibrosis, inflammation, or signs of airway or parenchymal injury (Fig. 427.13).

Although the pattern of NEC hyperplasia seen in histopathology has classically been the gold standard for diagnosis of NEHI, high-resolution chest computed tomography (CT) has a high specificity, such that biopsy may be avoided in most cases. The classic pattern seen on chest CT is ground-glass opacities in the lingula, right middle lobe, and perihilar regions, with air trapping on expiratory images. The lungs otherwise appear normal (Fig. 427.14). Some designate a diagnosis made clinically without biopsy as **NEHI syndrome** and reserve the term NEHI for a diagnosis made by biopsy. If a patient with clinically diagnosed NEHI

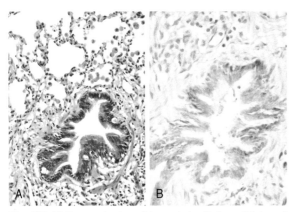

Fig. 427.13 Neuroendocrine cell hyperplasia of infancy. **(A)** A small airway showing only minimal chronic inflammation on routine staining but **(B)** staining for bombesin shows increased numbers of neuroendocrine cells within the surface epithelium. *(From Corrin B, Nicholson AG: Pathology of the lungs, ed 3, Churchill Livingstone, 2011. Fig. 2.19.)*

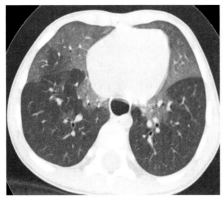

Fig. 427.14 2 yr old boy with neuroendocrine cell hyperplasia of infancy. CT shows well-defined areas of ground-glass opacity seen centrally and in the right middle lobe and lingula. *(From Brody AS: Imaging considerations: interstitial lung disease in children, Radiol Clin North Amer 43:391–403, 2005. Fig. 4.)*

syndrome has a more severe clinical course than expected, biopsy may be helpful to rule out other pathology.

The diagnosis of NEHI may be supported by an obstructive pattern that does not reverse with bronchodilators, on either infant pulmonary function testing (iPFT) or standard spirometry. Static lung volumes may show air trapping with increased RV relative to the TLC. BAL findings are notable for lack of inflammatory markers, as compared to other pulmonary diseases of infancy.

Genetic testing may be useful to rule out DSM and other causes of infant diffuse lung disease. Targeted testing for variants in *Nkx2.1* can be considered, but as this association has been found in only one kindred thus far, the predictive value of such testing is limited.

NATURAL COURSE AND TREATMENT
As the symptoms of NEHI typically improve and eventually largely resolve over the first few years of life, the standard approach to treatment of NEHI is supportive. The time frame for clinical improvement in NEHI is variable, and symptoms with rest may improve while those on exertion or with sleep persist. Until this occurs, affected children may require supplemental oxygen to maintain normal saturations, sometimes only with sleep or illnesses, but often at all times. The degree of obstruction on iPFTs may be somewhat predictive of degree of desaturation and obstruction in the future.

Because they may expend more energy to breathe, children with NEHI may have difficulty gaining weight, and often require supplemental nutrition. This is often delivered by gastrostomy tube. Management of GER when present may be helpful. When the disease improves, the need for supplemental oxygen and/or nutritional support typically decreases. *Inhaled or systemic corticosteroids are generally not thought to be helpful in treating the primary manifestations of NEHI.* Children with NEHI, whose symptoms have shown improvement, may experience exacerbations later in childhood. These episodes are associated with increased air trapping.

Although the symptoms of NEHI typically resolve during childhood, limited data suggest that some symptoms may persist into the adult years. This may manifest as exercise intolerance, or an asthma-like picture. Obstruction with air trapping may be seen on PFT and persistent abnormalities may be identified on chest imaging. No cases of respiratory failure, need for lung transplantation, or death associated with NEHI have been reported. **Diffuse idiopathic neuroendocrine epithelial cell hyperplasia** may be a related disorder but is seen predominantly in adult females who have diffuse pulmonary nodules and fixed obstruction or obstructive/restrictive lung disease on pulmonary function testing.

Bibliography is available at Expert Consult.

427.7 Fibrotic Lung Disease
Deborah R. Liptzin, Jason P. Weinman,
and Robin R. Deterding

Pulmonary fibrosis is scarring in the lung parenchyma (as opposed to bronchiectasis which is scarring of the airways). Idiopathic pulmonary fibrosis is a common form of fibrotic lung disease in adults. This presents with usual interstitial pneumonia (a pathologic finding with patchy interstitial fibrosis, fibroblastic foci, and honeycomb change) (see Chapter 427.5). Additional adult fibrotic lung diseases include sarcoidosis, silicosis, coal workers pneumoconiosis and hypersensitivity pneumonitis (e.g., farmer's lung). In children, fibrotic lung disease is rare, and *idiopathic* pulmonary fibrosis has not been described. The differential diagnosis of *fibrotic* lung disease includes surfactant dysfunction mutations (Chapter 423), radiation-induced fibrosis, bronchiolitis obliterans (Chapter 422.1), nonspecific interstitial pneumonia (connective tissue disorders) (Chapter 427), hypersensitivity pneumonitis (Chapter 427.1), and aspiration (Chapter 425) (Tables 427.19–427.21).

Table 427.19	Diseases Associated With Pulmonary Fibrosis

- Idiopathic pulmonary fibrosis / nonspecific interstitial pneumonia
- Familial pulmonary fibrosis / familial interstitial pneumonia
- Hypersensitivity pneumonitis (many agents)
- Cryptogenic organizing pneumonia
- Adverse reaction to therapy (drugs, radiation)
- Pleuroparenchymal fibroelastosis
- Hermansky–Pudlak syndrome
- Sarcoidosis
- Eosinophilic pneumonia (primary or parasitic)
- Langerhans cell histiocytosis
- Dyskeratosis congenita
- Tuberous sclerosis
- Neurofibromatosis
- Erdheim–Chester disease
- Gaucher disease
- Niemann–Pick disease
- Familial hypocalciuric hypercalcemia
- Lysinuric protein intolerance
- IgG4 mediated immune disorder
- Myelodysplastic syndrome
- Progressive systemic sclerosis
- Other connective tissue diseases (SLE, dermatomyositis)
- Granulomatosis with polyangiitis
- Eosinophilic granulomatosis with polyangiitis

Table 427.20	Pediatric Fibrotic Lung Diseases

DISEASES	CT FINDINGS	PATHOLOGY FINDINGS	ADDITIONAL EVALUATION	TREATMENT
Surfactant dysfunction	**Early:** Diffuse ground glass, septal thickening (crazy paving) **Chronic:** See NSIP	Variable: fibrosis, honeycomb cysts at end stage, NSIP, CPI, few globules of pulmonary alveolar proteinosis, foamy macrophages and cholesterol clefts (endogenous lipoid pneumonia)	Genetic testing	Hydroxychloroquine, azithromycin, high-dose intravenous steroids. Genetic counseling
Aspiration	**Acute:** Consolidation and centrilobular (tree in bud) nodules with a dependent distribution. **Chronic:** possible UIP with honeycombing	Airway-centered lesions/bronchiolitis, food particles with or without granulomas, foamy macrophages (endogenous lipoid pneumonia), organizing pneumonia	Video fluoroscopic swallow evaluation	Stop aspiration through thickening feeds, gastric feeds, cleft repair
Radiation fibrosis	Architectural distortion, volume loss, traction bronchiectasis. Often with geometric distribution related to radiation field	Pleural, septal, and paraseptal fibrosis; reactive atypia of alveolar epithelium and endothelium		
Bronchopulmonary dysplasia	Hyperlucent regions, architectural distortion (linear and subpleural triangular opacities)	Alveolar simplification and enlargement. Patchy hyperinflation. Interstitial fibrosis, with or without interlobular septal fibrosis.		Supportive care. Consider inhaled corticosteroids
Nonspecific interstitial pneumonia (NSIP)	Basilar predominant findings of ground-glass opacities (often with subpleural sparing), reticulation, architectural distortion, and traction bronchiectasis	Interstitial lymphocytic inflammation and fibrosis with homogenous distribution		
Hypersensitivity pneumonitis (chronic)	Patchy and often parahilar reticulation, ground glass, centrilobular nodules. Honeycombing (rare)	Airway-centered small non-caseating granulomas, multinucleated giant cells, lymphocytic bronchiolitis and peribronchiolitis, airway fibrosis, organizing pneumonia	Lymphocytosis in bronchoalveolar lavage, precipitins to specific antigen	Remove trigger, intravenous steroids
Autoimmune connective tissue disorders (collagen vascular disease)	See NSIP. Honeycombing (rare)	NSIP. Lymphoid hyperplasia. Fibrosis and cystic change. Pleuritis and pleural fibrosis (variable). Chronic vasculopathy (variable). Airway fibrosis (variable).	Serologic studies	Disease-specific immune modulation
Drug reactions	Peripheral predominant consolidation or ground glass. Reverse halo sign. See NSIP. Honeycombing (rare)	Variable: organizing pneumonia, NSIP, UIP, DAD, pulmonary hemorrhage, eosinophilic pneumonia		Drug avoidance
Infection	**Acute:** Consolidation and centrilobular (tree in bud) nodules. Appearance and distribution varies with type of infection. **Chronic:** May progress to IPF/UIP with honeycombing	**Acute:** Neutrophilic alveolitis (bacterial) or lymphocytic bronchiolitis (viral). **Chronic:** Variable airway fibrosis (constrictive/ obliterative bronchiolitis) and interstitial fibrosis.		Antimicrobials
Immunodeficiency	Bronchiectasis, consolidation, centrilobular nodules	Follicular bronchiolitis or diffuse lymphoid hyperplasia. NSIP. LIP. GLILD	Immunologic and genetic testing	Treat underlying immunodeficiency
Usual interstitial pneumonia (UIP)	Honeycombing, reticulation, traction bronchiectasis, ground glass (less prominent than NSIP)	Fibroblast foci. Interstitial, septal, and pleural fibrosis with heterogenous distribution. Minimal to absent inflammation.	Genetic testing	

CLINICAL PRESENTATION

Patients with pulmonary fibrosis will typically present with nonspecific respiratory symptoms such as cough, crackles, wheezes, prolonged expiratory phase, exercise intolerance, and hypoxemia, especially at nighttime. Symptom onset can be insidious or rapid.

EVALUATION

Pulmonary function tests typically show restriction and reduced diffusion capacity. Air trapping can also be seen. Patients may desaturate with exercise challenges or 6-min walks.

There are a variety of findings on computed tomography scan that suggest pulmonary fibrosis. These include reticular opacities, architectural distortion, traction bronchiectasis, and honeycomb cysts. A common late finding in several etiologies of fibrotic lung disease in children is nonspecific interstitial pneumonia: subpleural sparing, ground-glass opacities, reticular change, and bronchiectasis. Typical CT findings in

Table 427.21	Genes Associated With Familial* or Idiopathic Pulmonary Fibrosis
GENE	**GENE FUNCTION**
IL1RN	Inhibitor of pro-inflammatory effect of IL-1alpha and IL-1beta
IL8	Pro-inflammatory cytokine
FAM13A	Signal transduction
TLR3	Pathogen recognition and activation of innate immunity
TERT	Enzyme in telomerase complex maintaining telomere length
HLA-DRB1	Major histocompatibility complex—immune system
DSP	Tightly links adjacent cells
OBFC1	Stimulates the activity of DNA polymerase-alpha-primase
MUC5B	Influence on rheological properties of airway mucus, mucociliary transport, and airway defense
MUC2	Mucin production
TOLLIP	Regulator of innate immune responses mediated by toll-like receptor and the transforming growth factor β signaling pathway
ATP11A	Phospholipid translocation
MDGA2	Cell–cell interaction
MAPT	Promotes microtubule assembly and stability
SPPL2C	Protein cleavage
DPP9	Cell–cell adhesion
TGFB1	Set of peptides that controls proliferation, differentiation, and other functions in many cell types
SFTPC[†]	Component of surfactant fluid
SFTPA2[†]	To modulate innate and adaptive immunity
ABCA3[†]	Transport of lipids across plasma membrane
TERC[†]	Template in telomerase complex
DKC1[†]	Stabilization of the template in telomerase complex
TINF2[†]	Telomere maintenance
RTEL1[†]	DNA helicase
PARN[†]	mRNA stability

*Also called familial interstitial pneumonia.
[†]Rarer variant.
Adapted from Kaur A, Mathai SK, Schwartz DA: Genetics in idiopathic pulmonary fibrosis pathogenesis, prognosis, and treatment. *Frontiers Med* 4:154, 2017. Tables 1 and 2.

pediatric patients with nonspecific interstitial pneumonia include basilar predominant ground-glass opacities, reticulation, mild cystic change, and bronchiectasis (Fig. 427.15).

In certain disease processes such as surfactant dysfunction mutations (positive genetic testing) or bronchiolitis obliterans (decline in lung function and typical computed tomography scan), biopsy is not necessary for diagnosis. In the absence of a definitive diagnosis, a thoracoscopic wedge biopsy is necessary for diagnosis and to guide treatment. Transthoracic biopsies in pediatrics are of limited utility because the small instruments typically obtain inadequate tissue specimens; transthoracic biopsies in pediatrics are limited to monitoring post-lung transplantation and for diagnosis of sarcoidosis. Pathologic findings in pulmonary fibrosis are variable, depending on duration and etiology of disease (see Table 427.20), but typically include a component

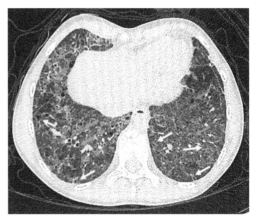

Fig. 427.15 Chest CT demonstrates typical CT findings in a pediatric patient with nonspecific interstitial pneumonia including basilar-predominant ground-glass opacities (blue arrows), reticulation (yellow arrows), mild cystic change (green arrows) and bronchiectasis (orange arrow).

of interstitial inflammation, interstitial expansion by dense collagen, and lobular remodeling (parenchymal architectural distortion and honeycomb cysts). Interlobular septal fibrosis, pleural fibrosis, and chronic pulmonary arteriopathy are common associated findings. Rare dense globules of pulmonary alveolar proteinosis material may indicate a genetic disorder of surfactant metabolism. Reactive lymphoid follicles suggest an immunologic process, such as autoimmune disease or immunodeficiency. Organizing pneumonia (polypoid aggregates of fibroblasts, *Masson bodies*) is a common feature in hypersensitivity pneumonitis and autoimmune diseases. The usual interstitial pneumonia pattern is signaled by fibroblast foci arising within a background of dense interstitial fibrosis and is a rare pattern of disease in children. Connective tissue stains, such as Masson trichrome, Elastic Verhoff von Giesen, and Movat pentachrome, aid in determining the severity and distribution of collagen deposition.

TREATMENT
Treatment varies based on disease process (see Tables 427.19–427.21). Due to the nature of rare disease, treatment regimens are largely based on expert opinion as controlled clinical trials are challenging to perform. Antifibrotic agents approved in adults with idiopathic pulmonary fibrosis (pirfenidone and nintedanib) are not approved for use in children.

Patients with fibrotic lung disease should be closely followed by pediatric pulmonary specialists for disease and comorbidity monitoring. Monitoring may include evaluation of pulmonary function (spirometry, lung volumes, and diffusion capacity), functional evaluation of exercise (6-min walk), and screening for comorbidities such as pulmonary hypertension, aspiration, and sleep disordered breathing. Treatment is disease specific but should also include nutritional support secondary to increased metabolic demands. Respiratory support varies depending on each patient's needs, from no support to oxygen via nasal cannula while asleep only, oxygen via nasal cannula all the time, or with ventilation (noninvasive or invasive). Comorbidities should be treated appropriately. Genetic counseling and recurrence risk should be provided with genetic forms of fibrotic lung disease. Patients should be counseled about preventing further lung damage from air pollution, smoking (cigarette, electronic cigarettes, hookah, water pipe, marijuana, etc.), and secondhand smoke exposure.

OUTCOMES
Outcomes vary depending on the underlying disease process.

Bibliography is available at Expert Consult.

Chapter **428**
Community-Acquired Pneumonia

Matthew S. Kelly and Thomas J. Sandora

第四百二十八章
社区获得性肺炎

中文导读

本章主要介绍了社区获得性肺炎的流行病学、病原学、发病机制、临床表现、诊断、治疗、预后、并发症以及预防。其中病原学部分列举了部分导致社区获得性肺炎的病原体，并归纳了常见和不常见的病原体以及不同年龄和暴露病史提示的病原体；具体描述了病毒性肺炎、细菌性肺炎、反复肺炎的发病机制及社区获得性肺炎的症状和体征；详细阐述了胸片、超声检查、白细胞计数、病原学检查等辅助检查在诊断和鉴别诊断方面的意义，并给出了针对细菌性肺炎、病毒性肺炎等的治疗原则、经验用药和抗生素等药物的使用建议。

EPIDEMIOLOGY

Pneumonia, defined as inflammation of the lung parenchyma, is the leading infectious cause of death globally among children younger than 5 yr, accounting for an estimated 920,000 deaths each year (Fig. 428.1). Pneumonia mortality is closely linked to poverty. More than 99% of pneumonia deaths are in low- and middle-income countries, with the highest pneumonia mortality rate occurring in poorly developed countries in Africa and South Asia (Table 428.1).

In the United States, mortality from pneumonia in children declined by 97% between 1939 and 1996. This decline likely resulted from the development of antibiotics and vaccines and the expansion of medical insurance coverage for children. Effective vaccines against measles (see Chapter 273) and pertussis (see Chapter 224) contributed to the decline in pneumonia-related mortality during the 20th century. *Haemophilus influenzae* type b (see Chapter 221) was also an important cause of bacterial pneumonia in young children but became uncommon following licensure of a conjugate vaccine in 1987. The introduction of pneumococcal conjugate vaccines (PCVs) (see Chapter 209) has been an important contributor to the further reductions in pneumonia-related mortality achieved over the past 15 yr.

ETIOLOGY

Although most cases of pneumonia are caused by microorganisms, noninfectious causes include aspiration (of food or gastric acid, foreign bodies, hydrocarbons, and lipoid substances), hypersensitivity reactions, and drug- or radiation-induced pneumonitis (see Chapter 427). The cause of pneumonia in an individual patient is often difficult to determine

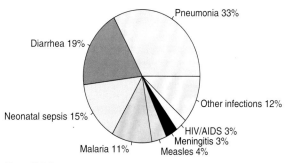

Fig. 428.1 Pneumonia is the leading infectious killer of children worldwide, as shown by this illustration of global distribution of cause-specific infectious mortality among children younger than age 5 yr in 2015. Pneumonia causes one-third of all under-5 deaths from infection. *(From World Health Organization and Maternal and Child Epidemiology Estimation Group estimates, 2015.)*

because direct sampling of lung tissue is invasive and rarely performed. Bacterial cultures of sputum or upper respiratory tract samples from children typically do not accurately reflect the cause of lower respiratory tract infection. *Streptococcus pneumoniae* (pneumococcus) is the most common bacterial pathogen in children 3 wk to 4 yr of age, whereas

Table 428.1	Pneumonia Cases and Mortality Rate in Children Younger Than Age 5 Yr by UNICEF Region, 2015	
UNICEF REGIONS	**PNEUMONIA CASES IN CHILDREN YOUNGER THAN 5 YR OF AGE**	**PNEUMONIA MORTALITY RATE (UNDER-5 DEATHS PER 1,000 LIVE BIRTHS)**
West and Central Africa	298,000	16.2
Sub-Saharan Africa	490,000	13.7
Eastern and Southern Africa	177,000	10.9
South Asia	282,000	7.9
Middle East and North Africa	46,000	4.1
East Asia and the Pacific	81,000	2.7
Latin America and the Caribbean	23,000	2.1
Least Developed Countries	363,000	12.0
World	920,000	6.6

From United Nations Children's Fund: One is too many—ending child deaths from pneumonia and diarrhoea. https://data.unicef.org/resources/one-many-ending-child-deaths-pneumonia-diarrhoea/. Accessed January 21, 2017.

Mycoplasma pneumoniae and *Chlamydophila pneumoniae* are the most frequent bacterial pathogens in children age 5 yr and older. In addition to pneumococcus, other bacterial causes of pneumonia in previously healthy children in the United States include group A streptococcus (*Streptococcus pyogenes*; see Chapter 210) and *Staphylococcus aureus* (see Chapter 208.1) (Tables 428.2, 428.3, and 428.4). *S. aureus* pneumonia often complicates an illness caused by influenza viruses.

S. pneumoniae, H. influenzae, and *S. aureus* are the major causes of hospitalization and death from bacterial pneumonia among children in developing countries, although in children with HIV infection, *Mycobacterium tuberculosis* (see Chapter 242), non-tuberculous mycobacteria (see Chapter 244), *Salmonella* (see Chapter 225), *Escherichia coli* (see Chapter 227), *Pneumocystis jiroveci* (see Chapter 271), and cytomegalovirus (see Chapter 282) must be considered. The incidence of pneumonia caused by *H. influenzae* or *S. pneumoniae* has been significantly reduced in areas where routine immunization has been implemented.

Viral pathogens are the most common causes of lower respiratory tract infections in infants and children older than 1 mo but younger than 5 yr of age. Viruses can be detected in 40–80% of children with pneumonia using molecular diagnostic methods (e.g., polymerase chain reaction [PCR]). Of the respiratory viruses, respiratory syncytial virus (RSV; see Chapter 287) and rhinoviruses (see Chapter 290) are the most commonly identified pathogens, especially in children younger than 2 yr of age. However, the role of rhinoviruses in severe lower respiratory tract infection remains unclear as these viruses are frequently detected with co-infecting pathogens and among asymptomatic children. Other common viruses causing pneumonia include influenza viruses (see Chapter 285), human metapneumovirus (see Chapter 288), parainfluenza viruses (see Chapter 286), adenoviruses (see Chapter 289), and enteroviruses (see Chapter 277). Infection with more than one respiratory virus occurs in up to 20% of cases. The age of the patient can suggest the likely pathogens (see Table 428.3).

Lower respiratory tract viral infections are much more common in the fall and winter in both the northern and southern hemispheres in relation to the seasonal epidemics of respiratory viruses that occur each year. The typical pattern of these epidemics usually begins in the fall, when parainfluenza virus infections appear and most often manifest as croup. Later in winter, RSV, human metapneumovirus, and influenza viruses cause widespread infection, including upper respiratory tract infections, bronchiolitis, and pneumonia. RSV is particularly severe among infants and young children, whereas influenza viruses cause disease and excess hospitalization for acute respiratory illness in all age groups. Knowledge of the prevailing viruses circulating in the community may lead to a presumptive initial diagnosis.

Immunization status is relevant because children fully immunized against *H. influenzae* type b and *S. pneumoniae* are less likely to have pneumonia caused by these pathogens. Children who are immunocompromised or who have certain medical comorbidities may be at risk for specific pathogens, such as *Pseudomonas* spp. in patients with cystic fibrosis (see Chapter 432).

PATHOGENESIS

The lower respiratory tract possesses a number of defense mechanisms against infection, including mucociliary clearance, macrophages and secretory immunoglobulin A, and clearing of the airways by coughing. Previously, it was believed that the lower respiratory tract was—in the absence of infection—kept sterile by these mechanisms, supported primarily by culture-based studies. However, recent use of culture-independent techniques, including high-throughput sequencing methods, suggests that the lower respiratory tract contains diverse microbial communities. These data have challenged the traditional model of pneumonia pathogenesis that maintained that pneumonia was the result of invasion of the sterile lower respiratory tract by a single pathogen. More recent conceptual models postulate that pneumonia results from disruption of a complex lower respiratory ecosystem that is the site of dynamic interactions between potential pneumonia pathogens, resident microbial communities, and host immune defenses.

Viral pneumonia usually results from spread of infection along the airways, accompanied by direct injury of the respiratory epithelium, which results in airway obstruction from swelling, abnormal secretions, and cellular debris. The small caliber of airways in young infants makes such patients particularly susceptible to severe infection. Atelectasis, interstitial edema, and hypoxemia from ventilation–perfusion mismatch often accompany airway obstruction. Viral infection of the respiratory tract can also predispose to secondary bacterial infection by disturbing normal host defense mechanisms, altering secretions, and through disruptions in the respiratory microbiota.

Bacterial pneumonia most often occurs when respiratory tract organisms colonize the trachea and subsequently gain access to the lungs, but pneumonia may also result from direct seeding of lung tissue after bacteremia. When bacterial infection is established in the lung parenchyma, the pathologic process varies according to the invading organism. *M. pneumoniae* (see Chapter 250) attaches to the respiratory epithelium, inhibits ciliary action, and leads to cellular destruction and an inflammatory response in the submucosa. As the infection progresses, sloughed cellular debris, inflammatory cells, and mucus cause airway obstruction, with spread of infection occurring along the bronchial tree, as is seen in viral pneumonia. *S. pneumoniae* produces local edema that aids in the proliferation of organisms and their spread into adjacent portions of lung, often resulting in the characteristic focal lobar involvement. Group A streptococcus lower respiratory tract infection typically results in more diffuse lung involvement with interstitial pneumonia. The pathology includes necrosis of tracheobronchial mucosa; formation of large amounts of exudate, edema, and local hemorrhage, with extension into the interalveolar septa; and involvement of lymphatic vessels with frequent pleural involvement. *S. aureus* pneumonia manifests as confluent bronchopneumonia, which is often unilateral and characterized by the presence of extensive areas of hemorrhagic necrosis and irregular areas of cavitation of the lung parenchyma, resulting in pneumatoceles, empyema, and, at times, bronchopulmonary fistulas.

Recurrent pneumonia is defined *as 2 or more* episodes in a single year *or 3 or more* episodes ever, with radiographic clearing between occurrences. An underlying disorder should be considered if a child experiences recurrent pneumonia (Table 428.5).

Table 428.2	Causes of Infectious Pneumonia

BACTERIAL		**VIRAL**	
COMMON		Measles	Rash, coryza, conjunctivitis
Streptococcus pneumoniae	Consolidation, empyema	Varicella	Unimmunized; immunocompromised persons
Group B streptococci	Neonates		
Group A streptococci	Empyema	*Hantavirus*	Southwestern United States, rodents
Staphylococcus aureus	Pneumatoceles, empyema; infants; nosocomial pneumonia	Coronaviruses [severe acute respiratory syndrome (SARS), Middle East respiratory syndrome (MERS)]	Asia, Arabian Peninsula
*Mycoplasma pneumoniae**	Adolescents; summer–fall epidemics		
*Chlamydophila pneumoniae**	Adolescents	**FUNGAL**	
Chlamydia trachomatis	Infants	*Histoplasma capsulatum*	Ohio/Mississippi River valley; bird, bat contact
Mixed anaerobes	Aspiration pneumonia		
Gram-negative enterics	Nosocomial pneumonia	*Blastomyces dermatitidis*	Ohio/Mississippi River valley
UNCOMMON		*Coccidioides immitis*	Southwestern United States, Great Lakes states
Haemophilus influenzae type b	Unimmunized	*Cryptococcus neoformans* and *C. gattii*	Bird contact; immunocompromised; Northwestern United States (*C. gattii*)
Moraxella catarrhalis			
Neisseria meningitidis			
Francisella tularensis	Animal, tick, fly contact; bioterrorism	*Aspergillus* species	Immunocompromised persons; nodular lung infection
Nocardia species	Immunocompromised patients		
*Chlamydophila psittaci**	Bird contact (especially parakeets)	Mucormycosis	Immunocompromised persons
Yersinia pestis (plague)	Rat contact; bioterrorism	*Pneumocystis jiroveci*	Immunocompromised persons (particularly HIV-infected infants); steroids
Legionella species*	Exposure to contaminated water; nosocomial		
*Coxiella burnetii** (Q fever)	Animal (goat, sheep, cattle) exposure		
VIRAL		**RICKETTSIAL**	
COMMON		*Rickettsia rickettsiae*	Tick bite
Respiratory syncytial virus	Bronchiolitis	**MYCOBACTERIAL**	
Parainfluenza types 1-4	Croup	*Mycobacterium tuberculosis*	Travel to endemic region; exposure to high-risk persons
Influenza A, B	High fever; winter months		
Adenovirus	Can be severe; often occurs between January and April	*Mycobacterium avium* complex	Immunocompromised (particularly HIV-infected) persons
Human metapneumovirus	Similar to respiratory syncytial virus	Other non-tuberculous mycobacteria	Immunocompromised persons; cystic fibrosis
UNCOMMON			
Rhinovirus	Rhinorrhea	**PARASITIC**	
Enterovirus	Neonates	Various parasites (e.g., *Ascaris*, *Strongyloides* species)	Eosinophilic pneumonia
Herpes simplex	Neonates, immunocompromised persons		
Cytomegalovirus	Infants; immunocompromised persons (particularly HIV-infected infants)		

*Atypical pneumonia syndrome; may have extrapulmonary manifestations, low-grade fever, patchy diffuse infiltrates, and poor response to β-lactam antibiotics.
Adapted from Kliegman RM, Greenbaum LA, Lye PS: *Practical strategies in pediatric diagnosis & therapy*, ed 2, Philadelphia, 2004, Elsevier, p. 29.

Table 428.3	Pneumonia Etiologies Grouped by Age of the Patient

AGE GROUP	**FREQUENT PATHOGENS (IN ORDER OF FREQUENCY)**
Neonates (<3 wk)	Group B streptococcus, *Escherichia coli*, other Gram-negative bacilli, *Streptococcus pneumoniae*, *Haemophilus influenzae* (type b,* nontypeable)
3 wk-3 mo	Respiratory syncytial virus, other respiratory viruses (rhinoviruses, parainfluenza viruses, influenza viruses, human metapneumovirus, adenovirus), *S. pneumoniae*, *H. influenzae* (type b,* nontypeable); if patient is afebrile, consider *Chlamydia trachomatis*
4 mo-4 yr	Respiratory syncytial virus, other respiratory viruses (rhinoviruses, parainfluenza viruses, influenza viruses, human metapneumovirus, adenovirus), *S. pneumoniae*, *H. influenzae* (type b,* nontypeable), *Mycoplasma pneumoniae*, group A streptococcus
≥5 yr	*M. pneumoniae*, *S. pneumoniae*, *Chlamydophila pneumoniae*, *H. influenzae* (type b,* nontypeable), influenza viruses, adenovirus, other respiratory viruses, *Legionella pneumophila*

*H. influenzae type b is uncommon with routine immunization.
Adapted from Kliegman RM, Marcdante KJ, Jenson HJ, et al: *Nelson essentials of pediatrics*, ed 5, Philadelphia, 2006, Elsevier, p. 507.

CLINICAL MANIFESTATIONS

Pneumonia is frequently preceded by several days of symptoms of an upper respiratory tract infection, typically rhinitis and cough. In viral pneumonia, fever is usually present but temperatures are generally lower than in bacterial pneumonia. Tachypnea is the most consistent clinical manifestation of pneumonia. Increased work of breathing accompanied by intercostal, subcostal, and suprasternal retractions, nasal flaring, and use of accessory muscles is common. Severe infection may be accompanied by cyanosis and lethargy, especially in infants. Auscultation of the chest may reveal crackles and wheezing, but it is often difficult to

Table 428.4	Pneumonia: Etiology Suggested by Exposure History

EXPOSURE HISTORY	INFECTIOUS AGENT
Exposure to concurrent illness in school dormitory or household setting	*Neisseria meningitidis, Mycoplasma pneumoniae*
ENVIRONMENTAL EXPOSURES	
Exposure to contaminated aerosols (e.g., air coolers, hospital water supply)	Legionnaires' disease
Exposure to goat hair, raw wool, animal hides	Anthrax
Ingestion of unpasteurized milk	Brucellosis
Exposure to bat droppings (caving) or dust from soil enriched with bird droppings	Histoplasmosis
Exposure to water contaminated with animal urine	Leptospirosis
Exposure to rodent droppings, urine, saliva	Hantavirus
Potential bioterrorism exposure	Anthrax, plague, tularemia
ZOONOTIC EXPOSURES	
Employment as abattoir work or veterinarian	Brucellosis
Exposure to cattle, goats, pigs	Anthrax, brucellosis
Exposure to ground squirrels, chipmunks, rabbits, prairie dogs, rats in Africa or southwestern United States	Plague
Hunting or exposure to rabbits, foxes, squirrels	Tularemia
Bites from flies or ticks	Tularemia
Exposure to birds (parrots, budgerigars, cockatoos, pigeons, turkeys)	Psittacosis
Exposure to infected dogs and cats	*Pasteurella multocida*, Q fever (*Coxiella burnetii*)
Exposure to infected goats, cattle, sheep, domestic animals, and their secretions (milk, amniotic fluid, placenta, feces)	Q fever (*C. burnetii*)
TRAVEL EXPOSURES	
Residence in or travel to San Joaquin Valley, southern California, southwestern Texas, southern Arizona, New Mexico	Coccidioidomycosis
Residence in or travel to Mississippi or Ohio river valleys, Great Lakes States, Caribbean, Central America, or Africa	Histoplasmosis, blastomycosis
Residence in or travel to southern China	SARS, avian influenza
Residence in or travel to Arabian peninsula	MERS-CoV
Residence in or travel to Southeast Asia	Paragonimiasis, melioidosis
Residence in or travel to West Indies, Australia, or Guam	Melioidosis

MERS-CoV, Middle East respiratory syndrome coronavirus; SARS, severe acute respiratory syndrome.

From Ellison RT III, Donowitz GR: Acute pneumonia, In Bennett JE, Dolin R, Blaser MJ, editors: *Mandell, Douglas, and Bennett's principles and practice of infectious diseases*, ed 8, vol 1, Philadelphia, 2015, Elsevier, Table 69.3, p. 828.

localize the source of these adventitious sounds in very young children with hyperresonant chests. It is often not possible to distinguish viral pneumonia (especially adenovirus) clinically from disease caused by *Mycoplasma* and other bacterial pathogens.

Bacterial pneumonia in adults and older children typically begins suddenly with high fever, cough, and chest pain. Other symptoms that may be seen include drowsiness with intermittent periods of restlessness;

Table 428.5	Differential Diagnosis of Recurrent Pneumonia

HEREDITARY DISORDERS
Cystic fibrosis
Sickle cell disease

DISORDERS OF IMMUNITY
HIV/AIDS
Bruton agammaglobulinemia
Selective immunoglobulin G subclass deficiencies
Common variable immunodeficiency syndrome
Severe combined immunodeficiency syndrome
Chronic granulomatous disease
Hyperimmunoglobulin E syndromes
Leukocyte adhesion defect

DISORDERS OF CILIA
Primary ciliary dyskinesia
Kartagener syndrome

ANATOMIC DISORDERS
Pulmonary sequestration
Lobar emphysema
Congenital cystic adenomatoid malformation
Gastroesophageal reflux
Foreign body
Tracheoesophageal fistula (H type)
Bronchiectasis
Aspiration (oropharyngeal incoordination)
Aberrant bronchus

Adapted from Kliegman RM, Marcdante KJ, Jenson HJ, et al: *Nelson essentials of pediatrics*, ed 5, Philadelphia, 2006, Elsevier, p. 507.

rapid respirations; anxiety; and, occasionally, delirium. In many children, splinting on the affected side to minimize pleuritic pain and improve ventilation is noted; such children may lie on one side with the knees drawn up to the chest.

Physical findings depend on the stage of pneumonia. Early in the course of illness, diminished breath sounds, scattered crackles, and rhonchi are commonly heard over the affected lung field. With the development of increasing consolidation or complications of pneumonia such as pleural effusion or empyema, dullness on percussion is noted and breath sounds may be diminished. A lag in respiratory excursion often occurs on the affected side. Abdominal distention may be prominent because of gastric dilation from swallowed air or ileus. Abdominal pain is common in lower-lobe pneumonia. The liver may seem enlarged because of downward displacement of the diaphragm secondary to hyperinflation of the lungs or superimposed congestive heart failure.

Symptoms described in adults with pneumococcal pneumonia may be noted in older children but are rarely observed in infants and young children, in whom the clinical pattern is considerably more variable. In infants, there may be a prodrome of upper respiratory tract infection and poor feeding, leading to the abrupt onset of fever, restlessness, apprehension, and respiratory distress. These infants typically appear ill, with respiratory distress manifested as grunting; nasal flaring; retractions of the supraclavicular, intercostal, and subcostal areas; tachypnea; tachycardia; air hunger; and often cyanosis. Auscultation may be misleading, particularly in young infants, with meager findings disproportionate to the degree of tachypnea. Some infants with bacterial pneumonia may have associated gastrointestinal disturbances characterized by vomiting, anorexia, diarrhea, and abdominal distention secondary to a paralytic ileus. Rapid progression of symptoms is characteristic in the most severe cases of bacterial pneumonia.

DIAGNOSIS

In 2011, the Pediatric Infectious Diseases Society (PIDS) and the Infectious Diseases Society of America (IDSA) published clinical practice guidelines for community-acquired pneumonia in children older than 3 mo of age. These evidence-based guidelines provide recommendations for diagnostic testing and treatment of previously healthy children with pneumonia in both outpatient and inpatient settings.

An infiltrate on chest radiograph (posteroanterior and lateral views) supports the diagnosis of pneumonia; images may also identify a complication such as a pleural effusion or empyema. Viral pneumonia is usually characterized by hyperinflation with bilateral interstitial infiltrates and peribronchial cuffing (Fig. 428.2). Confluent lobar consolidation is typically seen with pneumococcal pneumonia (Fig. 428.3). The radiographic appearance alone does not accurately identify pneumonia etiology, and other clinical features of the illness must be considered. Repeat chest radiographs are not required for proof of cure for patients with uncomplicated pneumonia. Moreover, current PIDS–IDSA guidelines do not recommend that a chest radiograph be performed for children with suspected pneumonia (cough, fever, localized crackles, or decreased breath sounds) who are well enough to be managed as outpatients because imaging in this context only rarely changes management.

Point-of-care use of portable or handheld ultrasonography is highly sensitive and specific in diagnosing pneumonia in children by determining lung consolidations and air bronchograms or effusions (Fig. 428.4). However, the reliability of this imaging modality for pneumonia diagnosis is highly user-dependent, which has limited its widespread use.

The peripheral white blood cell (WBC) count can be useful in differentiating viral from bacterial pneumonia. In viral pneumonia, the WBC count can be normal or elevated but is usually not higher than 20,000/mm³, with a lymphocyte predominance. Bacterial pneumonia is often associated with an elevated WBC count, in the range of

15,000-40,000/mm³, and a predominance of polymorphonuclear leukocytes. A large pleural effusion, lobar consolidation, and a high fever at the onset of the illness are also suggestive of a bacterial etiology. Atypical pneumonia caused by *C. pneumoniae* or *M. pneumoniae* is difficult to distinguish from pneumococcal pneumonia on the basis of radiographic and laboratory findings; although pneumococcal pneumonia

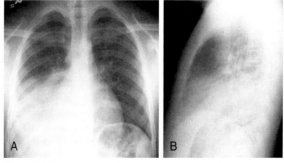

Fig. 428.3 Radiographic findings characteristic of pneumococcal pneumonia in a 14 yr old boy with cough and fever. Posteroanterior **(A)** and lateral **(B)** chest radiographs reveal consolidation in the right lower lobe, strongly suggesting bacterial pneumonia.

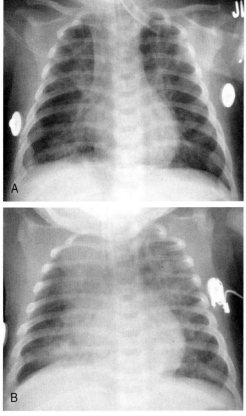

Fig. 428.2 A, Radiographic findings characteristic of respiratory syncytial virus pneumonia in a 6 mo old infant with rapid respirations and fever. Anteroposterior radiograph of the chest shows hyperexpansion of the lungs with bilateral fine air space disease and streaks of density, indicating the presence of both pneumonia and atelectasis. An endotracheal tube is in place. **B,** One day later, the anteroposterior radiograph of the chest shows increased bilateral pneumonia.

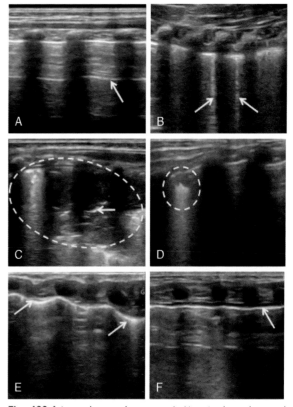

Fig. 428.4 Lung ultrasound patterns. **A,** Negative lung ultrasound pattern with A-line *(arrow)* and no other findings. Positive lung ultrasound patterns with **(B)** B-lines *(arrows)*; **(C)** large consolidation (>1 cm) with tissue-like echo-texture *(circle)* and ultrasonographic bronchograms *(arrow)*; **(D)** small consolidation (<1 cm; *circle*); **(E)** pleural line abnormality with thickening and irregularity (arrows); and **(F)** pleural effusion *(arrow)*. *(From Varshney T, Mok E, Shapiro AJ, et al: Point-of-care lung ultrasound in young children with respiratory tract infections and wheeze, Emerg Med J 33(9):603–610, 2016, Fig. 1, p. 604.)*

is associated with a higher WBC count, erythrocyte sedimentation rate, procalcitonin, and C-reactive protein level, there is considerable overlap.

The definitive diagnosis of a viral infection rests on the detection of the viral genome or antigen in respiratory tract secretions. Reliable PCR assays are widely available for the rapid detection of many respiratory viruses, including RSV, parainfluenza, influenza, human metapneumovirus, adenovirus, enterovirus, and rhinovirus. Serologic techniques can also be used to diagnose a recent respiratory viral infection but generally require testing of acute and convalescent serum samples for a rise in antibodies to a specific virus. This diagnostic technique is laborious, slow, and not generally clinically useful because the infection usually has resolved by the time it is confirmed serologically. Serologic testing may be valuable as an epidemiologic tool to define the incidence and prevalence of the various respiratory viral pathogens.

The definitive diagnosis of a typical bacterial infection requires isolation of an organism from the blood, pleural fluid, or lung. Culture of sputum is of little value in the diagnosis of pneumonia in young children, while percutaneous lung aspiration is invasive and not routinely performed. Blood culture is positive in only 10% of children with pneumococcal pneumonia and is not recommended for nontoxic-appearing children treated as outpatients. Blood cultures are recommended for children who fail to improve or have clinical deterioration, have complicated pneumonia (Table 428.6), or require hospitalization. Urinary antigen tests should not be used to diagnose pneumonia caused by *S. pneumoniae* in children because of a high rate of false positives resulting from nasopharyngeal carriage. Pertussis infection can be diagnosed by PCR or culture of a nasopharyngeal specimen; although culture is considered the gold standard for pertussis diagnosis, it is less sensitive than the available PCR assays. Acute infection caused by *M. pneumoniae* can be diagnosed on the basis of a PCR test result from a respiratory specimen or seroconversion in an immunoglobulin G assay. Cold agglutinins at titers > 1:64 are also found in the blood of roughly half of patients with *M. pneumoniae* infections; however, cold agglutinins are nonspecific because other pathogens such as influenza viruses may also cause increases. Serologic evidence, such as antistreptolysin O and anti-DNase B titers, may also be useful in the diagnosis of group A streptococcal pneumonia.

There is a great deal of interest in developing a non-invasive diagnostic test that can accurately differentiate children with bacterial versus viral causes of pneumonia. Various biomarkers, including C-reactive protein, procalcitonin, lipocalin-2, and tumor necrosis factor-related apoptosis-inducing ligand, have been evaluated for their ability to differentiate these pneumonia etiologies. For many of these biomarkers, values differ in children with bacterial compared with viral causes of pneumonia, but the reliability of these tests is not sufficiently high to justify routine

use. Studies of these biomarkers have also been hampered by the lack of a gold standard for determining pneumonia etiology and the relatively frequent occurrence of viral–bacterial co-infections. Patient peripheral cell gene expression patterns determined by microarray reverse transcription PCR is an emerging technology that may help differentiate bacterial from viral causes of pneumonia, although further study is needed.

TREATMENT

Treatment of suspected bacterial pneumonia is based on the presumptive cause and the age and clinical appearance of the child. For mildly ill children who do not require hospitalization, amoxicillin is recommended. With the emergence of penicillin-resistant pneumococci, high doses of amoxicillin (90 mg/kg/day orally divided twice daily) should be prescribed unless local data indicate a low prevalence of resistance (Table 428.7). Therapeutic alternatives include cefuroxime and amoxicillin/clavulanate. For school-aged children and adolescents or when infection with *M. pneumoniae* or *C. pneumoniae* is suspected, a macrolide antibiotic is an appropriate choice for outpatient management. Azithromycin is generally preferred, while clarithromycin or doxycycline (for children 8 yr or older) are alternatives. For adolescents, a respiratory fluoroquinolone (levofloxacin, moxifloxacin) may also be considered as an alternative if there are contraindications to other agents.

The empiric treatment of suspected bacterial pneumonia in a hospitalized child requires an approach based on local epidemiology, the immunization status of the child, and the clinical manifestations at the time of presentation. In areas without substantial high-level penicillin resistance among *S. pneumoniae*, children who are fully immunized against *H. influenzae* type b and *S. pneumoniae* and are not severely ill should receive ampicillin or penicillin G. For children who do not meet these criteria, ceftriaxone or cefotaxime may be used. If clinical features suggest staphylococcal pneumonia (pneumatoceles, empyema), initial antimicrobial therapy should also include vancomycin or clindamycin. Moreover, if infection with *M. pneumoniae* or *C. pneumoniae* is suspected, a macrolide antibiotic should be included in the treatment regimen.

If viral pneumonia is suspected, it is reasonable to withhold antibiotic therapy, especially for preschool-aged patients who are mildly ill, have clinical evidence suggesting viral infection, and are in no respiratory distress. However, up to 30% of patients with known viral infection, particularly influenza viruses, may have coexisting bacterial pathogens. Therefore, if the decision is made to withhold antibiotic therapy on the basis of presumptive diagnosis of a viral infection, deterioration in clinical status should signal the possibility of superimposed bacterial infection, and antibiotic therapy should be initiated.

Table 428.7 notes the indications for admission to a hospital. Hospitalized children should receive supportive care and may require intravenous fluids; respiratory support, including supplemental oxygen, continuous positive airway pressure (CPAP), or mechanical ventilation; or vasoactive medications for hypotension or sepsis physiology.

The optimal duration of antibiotic treatment for pneumonia has not been well-established in controlled studies. However, antibiotics should generally be continued until the patient has been afebrile for 72 hr, and the total duration should be not less than 10 days (or 5 days if azithromycin is used). Shorter courses (5-7 days) may also be effective, particularly for children managed on an outpatient basis, but further study is needed. Available data do not support prolonged courses of treatment for uncomplicated pneumonia. Preliminary studies suggest that a reduction of previously elevated serum procalcitonin levels to an absolute level (0.1-0.25 µg/L) may help determine when to stop treatment.

Despite substantial gains over the past 15 yr, in developing countries less than two-thirds of children with symptoms of pneumonia are taken to an appropriate caregiver, and fewer than half receive antibiotics. The World Health Organization and other international groups have developed systems to train mothers and local healthcare providers in the recognition and appropriate antibiotic treatment of pneumonia. In addition to antibiotics, oral zinc (10 mg/day for < 12 mo, 20 mg/day for ≥ 12 mo given for 7 days) may reduce mortality among children in developing countries with clinically defined severe pneumonia. Bubble CPAP improves mortality from pneumonia with hypoxemia compared

Table 428.6	Factors Suggesting Need for Hospitalization of Children With Pneumonia

Age <6 mo
Immunocompromised state
Toxic appearance
Moderate to severe respiratory distress
Hypoxemia (oxygen saturation <90% breathing room air, sea level)
Complicated pneumonia*
Sickle cell anemia with acute chest syndrome
Vomiting or inability to tolerate oral fluids or medications
Severe dehydration
No response to appropriate oral antibiotic therapy
Social factors (e.g., inability of caregivers to administer medications at home or follow-up appropriately)

*Pleural effusion, empyema, abscess, bronchopleural fistula, necrotizing pneumonia, acute respiratory distress syndrome, extrapulmonary infection (meningitis, arthritis, pericarditis, osteomyelitis, endocarditis), hemolytic uremic syndrome, or sepsis.
  Adapted from Baltimore RS: Pneumonia. In Jenson HB, Baltimore RS, editors: *Pediatric infectious diseases: principles and practice*, Philadelphia, 2002, WB Saunders, p. 801.

with standard oxygen therapy in settings without access to ventilator-derived CPAP or mechanical ventilation.

PROGNOSIS

Typically, patients with uncomplicated community-acquired bacterial pneumonia show response to therapy, with improvement in clinical symptoms (fever, cough, tachypnea, chest pain), within 48-72 hr of initiation of antibiotics. Radiographic evidence of improvement lags substantially behind clinical improvement. A number of possibilities must be considered when a patient does not improve with appropriate antibiotic therapy: (1) complications, such as pleural effusion or empyema (see Table 428.6); (2) bacterial resistance; (3) nonbacterial etiologies

Table 428.7	Selection of Antimicrobial Therapy for Specific Pathogens	
PATHOGEN	**PARENTERAL THERAPY**	**ORAL THERAPY (STEP-DOWN THERAPY OR MILD INFECTION)**
Streptococcus pneumoniae with MICs for penicillin ≤ 2.0 μg/mL	Preferred: ampicillin (150-200 mg/kg/day every 6 hr) or penicillin (200,000-250,000 U/kg/day every 4-6 hr); Alternatives: ceftriaxone (50-100 mg/kg/day every 12-24 hr) (preferred for parenteral outpatient therapy); may also be effective: clindamycin (40 mg/kg/day every 6-8 hr) or vancomycin (40-60 mg/kg/day every 6-8 hr)	Preferred: amoxicillin (90 mg/kg/day in 2 doses or 45 mg/kg/day in 3 doses); Alternatives: second- or third-generation cephalosporin (cefpodoxime, cefixime, cefprozil); oral levofloxacin, if susceptible (16-20 mg/kg/day in 2 doses for children 6 mo to 5 yr old and 8-10 mg/kg/day once daily for children 5-16 yr old; maximum daily dose, 750 mg) or oral linezolid (30 mg/kg/day in 3 doses for children <12 yr old and 20 mg/kg/day in 2 doses for children ≥12 yr old)
S. pneumoniae resistant to penicillin, with MICs ≥ 4.0 μg/mL	Preferred: ceftriaxone (100 mg/kg/day every 12-24 hr); Alternatives: ampicillin (300-400 mg/kg/day every 6 hr), levofloxacin (16-20 mg/kg/day every 12 hr for children 6 mo to 5 yr old and 8-10 mg/kg/day once daily for children 5-16 yr old; maximum daily dose, 750 mg), or linezolid (30 mg/kg/day every 8 hr for children <12 yr old and 20 mg/kg/day every 12 hr for children ≥12 yr old); may also be effective: clindamycin (40 mg/kg/day every 6-8 hr) or vancomycin (40-60 mg/kg/day every 6-8 hr)	Preferred: oral levofloxacin (16-20 mg/kg/day in 2 doses for children 6 mo to 5 yr and 8-10 mg/kg/day once daily for children 5-16 yr, maximum daily dose, 750 mg), if susceptible, or oral linezolid (30 mg/kg/day in 3 doses for children <12 yr and 20 mg/kg/day in 2 doses for children ≥12 yr); Alternative: oral clindamycin (30-40 mg/kg/day in 3 doses)
Group A streptococcus	Preferred: intravenous penicillin (100,000–250,000 U/kg/day every 4-6 hr) or ampicillin (200 mg/kg/day every 6 hr); Alternatives: ceftriaxone (50-100 mg/kg/day every 12-24 hr); may also be effective: clindamycin, if susceptible (40 mg/kg/day every 6-8 hr) or vancomycin (40-60 mg/kg/day every 6-8 hr)	Preferred: amoxicillin (50-75 mg/kg/day in 2 doses), or penicillin V (50-75 mg/kg/day in 3 or 4 doses); Alternative: oral clindamycin (40 mg/kg/day in 3 doses)
Staphylococcus aureus, methicillin susceptible (combination therapy not well studied)	Preferred: cefazolin (150 mg/kg/day every 8 hr) or semisynthetic penicillin, e.g., oxacillin (150-200 mg/kg/day every 6-8 hr); Alternatives: clindamycin (40 mg/kg/day every 6-8 hr) or vancomycin (40-60 mg/kg/day every 6-8 hr)	Preferred: oral cephalexin (75-100 mg/kg/day in 3 or 4 doses); Alternative: oral clindamycin (30-40 mg/kg/day in 3 or 4 doses)
S. aureus, methicillin resistant, susceptible to clindamycin (combination therapy not well-studied)	Preferred: vancomycin (40-60 mg/kg/day every 6-8 hr or dosing to achieve an AUC/MIC ratio of >400) or clindamycin (40 mg/kg/day every 6-8 hr); Alternatives: linezolid (30 mg/kg/day every 8 hr for children <12 yr old and 20 mg/kg/day every 12 hr for children ≥ 12 yr old)	Preferred: oral clindamycin (30-40 mg/kg/day in 3 or 4 doses); Alternatives: oral linezolid (30 mg/kg/day in 3 doses for children <12 yr and 20 mg/kg/day in 2 doses for children ≥12 yr)
S. aureus, methicillin resistant, resistant to clindamycin (combination therapy not well studied)	Preferred: vancomycin (40-60 mg/kg/day every 6-8 hr or dosing to achieve an AUC/MIC ratio of >400); Alternatives: linezolid (30 mg/kg/day every 8 hr for children <12 yr old and 20 mg/kg/day every 12 hr for children ≥12 yr old)	Preferred: oral linezolid (30 mg/kg/day in 3 doses for children <12 yr and 20 mg/kg/day in 2 doses for children ≥12 yr old); Alternatives: none; entire treatment course with parenteral therapy may be required
Haemophilus influenza, typeable (A-F) or nontypeable	Preferred: intravenous ampicillin (150-200 mg/kg/day every 6 hr) if β-lactamase negative, ceftriaxone (50-100 mg/kg/day every 12-24 hr) if β-lactamase producing; Alternatives: intravenous ciprofloxacin (30 mg/kg/day every 12 hr) or intravenous levofloxacin (16-20 mg/kg/day every 12 hr for children 6 mo to 5 yr old and 8-10 mg/kg/day once daily for children 5-16 yr old; maximum daily dose, 750 mg)	Preferred: amoxicillin (75-100 mg/kg/day in 3 doses) if β-lactamase negative, or amoxicillin clavulanate (amoxicillin component, 45 mg/kg/day in 3 doses or 90 mg/kg/day in 2 doses) if β-lactamase producing; Alternatives: cefdinir, cefixime, cefpodoxime, or ceftibuten
Mycoplasma pneumoniae	Preferred: intravenous azithromycin (10 mg/kg on days 1 and 2 of therapy; transition to oral therapy if possible); Alternatives: intravenous erythromycin lactobionate (20 mg/kg/day every 6 hr) or levofloxacin (16-20 mg/kg/day every 12 hr; maximum daily dose, 750 mg)	Preferred: azithromycin (10 mg/kg on day 1, followed by 5 mg/kg/day once daily on days 2-5); Alternatives: clarithromycin (15 mg/kg/day in 2 doses) or oral erythromycin (40 mg/kg/day in 4 doses); for children >7 yr old, doxycycline (2-4 mg/kg/day in 2 doses; for adolescents with skeletal maturity, levofloxacin (500 mg once daily) or moxifloxacin (400 mg once daily)

Continued

Table 428.7	Selection of Antimicrobial Therapy for Specific Pathogens—cont'd	
PATHOGEN	**PARENTERAL THERAPY**	**ORAL THERAPY (STEP-DOWN THERAPY OR MILD INFECTION)**
Chlamydia trachomatis or *Chlamydophila pneumoniae*	Preferred: intravenous azithromycin (10 mg/kg on days 1 and 2 of therapy; transition to oral therapy if possible); Alternatives: intravenous erythromycin lactobionate (20 mg/kg/day every 6 hr) or levofloxacin (16-20 mg/kg/day in 2 doses for children 6 mo to 5 yr old and 8-10 mg/kg/day once daily for children 5-16 yr old; maximum daily dose, 750 mg)	Preferred: azithromycin (10 mg/kg on day 1, followed by 5 mg/kg/day once daily days 2-5); Alternatives: clarithromycin (15 mg/kg/day in 2 doses) or oral erythromycin (40 mg/kg/day in 4 doses); for children >7 yr old, doxycycline (2-4 mg/kg/day in 2 doses); for adolescents with skeletal maturity, levofloxacin (500 mg once daily) or moxifloxacin (400 mg once daily)

Doses for oral therapy should not exceed adult doses.
[a]Clindamycin resistance appears to be increasing in certain geographic areas among *S. pneumoniae* and *S. aureus* infections.
[b]For β-lactam–allergic children.
AUC, area under the time vs. serum concentration curve; MIC, minimum inhibitory concentration.
From Bradley JS, Byington CL, Shah SS, et al: The management of community-acquired pneumonia in infants and children older than 3 months of age: clinical practice guidelines by the Pediatric Infectious Diseases Society and the Infectious Diseases Society of America, *Clin Infect Dis* 53(7):617–630, 2011, Table 5, pp. 623–624.

such as viruses or fungi and aspiration of foreign bodies or food; (4) bronchial obstruction from endobronchial lesions, foreign body, or mucous plugs; (5) preexisting diseases such as immunodeficiencies, ciliary dyskinesia, cystic fibrosis, pulmonary sequestration, or congenital pulmonary airway malformation; and (6) other noninfectious causes (including bronchiolitis obliterans, hypersensitivity pneumonitis, eosinophilic pneumonia, and granulomatosis with polyangiitis, formerly called Wegener granulomatosis). A chest radiograph is the first step in determining the reason for a lack of response to initial treatment. Bronchoalveolar lavage may be indicated in children with respiratory failure; high-resolution CT scans may better identify complications or an anatomic reason for a poor response to therapy.

Mortality from community-acquired pneumonia in developed countries is rare, and most children with pneumonia do not experience long-term pulmonary sequelae. Some data suggest that up to 45% of children have symptoms of asthma 5 yr after hospitalization for pneumonia; this finding may reflect either undiagnosed asthma at the time of presentation or a propensity for development of asthma after pneumonia.

COMPLICATIONS

Complications of pneumonia (see Table 428.6) are usually the result of direct spread of bacterial infection within the thoracic cavity (pleural effusion, empyema, and pericarditis) or bacteremia and hematologic spread (Fig. 428.5). Meningitis, endocarditis, suppurative arthritis, and osteomyelitis are rare complications of hematologic spread of pneumococcal or *H. influenzae* type b infection.

S. aureus, *S. pneumoniae*, and *S. pyogenes* are the most common causes of parapneumonic effusions and empyema. Nonetheless many effusions that complicate bacterial pneumonia are sterile. Analysis of pleural fluid parameters, including pH, glucose, protein, and lactate dehydrogenase, can differentiate transudative from exudative effusions (Table 428.8). However, current PIDS–IDSA guidelines do not recommend that these tests be performed because this distinction rarely changes management. Pleural fluid should be sent for Gram stain, and bacterial culture as this may identify the bacterial cause of pneumonia. Molecular methods, including bacterial species-specific PCR assays or sequencing of the bacterial 16S ribosomal RNA gene, detect bacterial DNA and can often determine the bacterial etiology of the effusion if the culture is negative, particularly if the pleural fluid sample was obtained after initiation of antibiotics. A pleural fluid WBC count with differential may be helpful if there is suspicion for pulmonary tuberculosis or a noninfectious etiology for the pleural effusion, such as malignancy.

Small (<1 cm on lateral decubitus radiograph), free-flowing parapneumonic effusions often do not require drainage but respond to appropriate antibiotic therapy. Larger effusions should typically be drained, particularly if the effusion is purulent (empyema) or associated with respiratory distress. Chest ultrasound, or alternatively CT, may be helpful in determining whether loculations are present. The mainstays

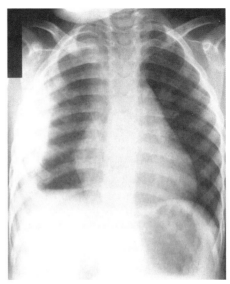

Fig. 428.5 Pneumococcal empyema on the chest radiography of a 3 yr old child who has had upper respiratory symptoms and fever for 3 days. A pleural fluid collection can be seen on the right side. The patient had a positive pleural tap and blood culture result for pneumococci. The child recovered completely within 3 wk. (*From Kuhn JP, Slovis TL, Haller JO, editors: Caffrey's pediatric diagnostic imaging, ed 10, Philadelphia, 2004, Mosby, p. 1002.*)

Table 428.8	Features Differentiating Exudative From Transudative Pleural Effusion	
FEATURE	**TRANSUDATE**	**EXUDATE**
Appearance	Serous	Cloudy
Leukocyte count	<10,000/mm³	>50,000/mm³
pH	>7.2	<7.2
Protein	<3.0 g/dL	>3.0 g/dL
Ratio of pleural fluid protein to serum	<0.5	>0.5
LDH	<200 IU/L	>200 IU/L
Ratio of pleural fluid LDH to serum	<0.6	>0.6
Glucose	≥60 mg/dL	<60 mg/dL

LDH, lactate dehydrogenase.
From Septimus EJ: Pleural effusion and empyema, In Bennett JE, Dolin R, Blaser MJ, editors: *Mandell, Douglas, and Bennett's principles and practice of infectious diseases*, ed 8, vol 1, Philadelphia, 2015, Elsevier, Table 70-1, p. 851.

of therapy include antibiotic therapy and drainage by tube thoracostomy with the instillation of fibrinolytic agents (urokinase, streptokinase, tissue plasminogen activator). Video-assisted thoracoscopy is a less often employed alternative that enables debridement or lysis of adhesions and drainage of loculated areas of pus. Early diagnosis and intervention, particularly with fibrinolysis or less often video-assisted thoracoscopy, may obviate the need for thoracotomy and open debridement.

PREVENTION

The introduction of PCVs resulted in a substantial reduction in the incidence of pneumonia hospitalizations among children. The annual rate of all-cause pneumonia hospitalization among children younger than 2 yr of age in the United States was 12.5 per 1,000 children during the period from 1997 to 1999. In 2000, 7-valent pneumococcal conjugate vaccine (PCV7) was licensed and recommended. In 2006, the pneumonia hospitalization rate in this age group was 8.1 per 1,000 children, a 35%

decrease from the pre-vaccine rate. In 2010, 13-valent pneumococcal conjugate vaccine (PCV13) was licensed in the United States. Early data indicate that introduction of this vaccine resulted in a 16–27% further reduction in pneumonia hospitalizations among children relative to the post-PCV7 era.

Influenza vaccine may also prevent pneumonia hospitalizations among children and should be administered to all children >6 mo of age. For infants <6 mo of age, household contacts and other primary caregivers should be immunized. Maintaining high rates of vaccination for *H. influenzae* type b, pertussis, and measles remains important for the prevention of pneumonia from these causes. Several RSV vaccines are currently under development; introduction of an effective vaccine against RSV would be anticipated to substantially reduce pneumonia incidence among children, particularly young infants.

Bibliography is available at Expert Consult.

Chapter **429**
Pleurisy, Pleural Effusions, and Empyema

Glenna B. Winnie, Aarthi P. Vemana, Suraiya K. Haider, and Steven V. Lossef

第四百二十九章
胸膜炎、胸腔积液和脓胸

中文导读

本章主要介绍了干性胸膜炎、浆液纤维素性（或称浆液性）胸膜炎伴胸腔积液以及脓胸。并分别从病原学、发病机制、临床表现、实验室检查、诊断及鉴别诊断、并发症以及治疗等方面进行阐述。其中重点阐述了胸腔积液的产生和吸收机制以及渗出性和漏出性胸腔积液的区别，并进一步描述了不同量的胸腔积液引起的不同症状和体征；具体说明了胸部影像学检查、超声检查、胸腔穿刺等的诊断和鉴别诊断意义；治疗中介绍了胸腔穿刺、胸膜腔闭式引流、纤溶疗法、电视胸腔镜手术等。

Pleurisy is the inflammation of the pleura; it may be accompanied by an effusion. The most common cause of pleural effusion in children is bacterial pneumonia (see Chapter 428); heart failure (see Chapter 469), rheumatologic causes, and metastatic intrathoracic malignancy are also common causes. A variety of other diseases account for the remaining cases, including tuberculosis (see Chapter 242), lupus erythematosus

(see Chapter 183), aspiration pneumonitis (see Chapter 425), uremia, pancreatitis, subdiaphragmatic abscess, and rheumatoid arthritis.

Inflammatory processes in the pleura are usually divided into 3 types: dry pleurisy, serofibrinous or serosanguineous, and purulent pleurisy or empyema.

429.1 Dry Pleurisy

Glenna B. Winnie, Aarthi P. Vemana,
Suraiya K. Haider, and Steven V. Lossef

ETIOLOGY

Dry pleurisy, formerly called plastic pleurisy, may be associated with acute bacterial or viral pulmonary infections or may develop during the course of an acute upper respiratory tract illness. The condition is also associated with tuberculosis and autoimmune diseases such as systemic lupus erythematosus.

PATHOLOGY AND PATHOGENESIS

The process is usually limited to the visceral pleura, with small amounts of yellow serous fluid and adhesions between the pleural surfaces. In tuberculosis, pleurisy can be caused by a severe delayed-type hypersensitivity reaction to *Mycobacterium tuberculosis*; the adhesions develop rapidly, and the pleura are often thickened. Occasionally, fibrin deposition and adhesions are severe enough to produce a fibrothorax that markedly inhibits the excursions of the lung.

CLINICAL MANIFESTATIONS

The primary disease often overshadows signs and symptoms of pleurisy. Pain, the principal symptom, is exaggerated by deep breathing, coughing, and straining. Occasionally, pleural pain is described as a dull ache, which is less likely to vary with breathing. The pain is often localized over the chest wall and is referred to the shoulder or the back. Pain with breathing is responsible for grunting and guarding of respirations, and the child often lies on the affected side in an attempt to decrease respiratory excursions. Early in the illness, a leathery, rough, inspiratory and expiratory friction rub may be audible, but it usually disappears rapidly. If the layer of exudate is thick, increased dullness to percussion and decreased breath sounds may be heard. Pleurisy may

be asymptomatic. Chronic pleurisy is occasionally encountered with conditions such as atelectasis, pulmonary abscess, connective tissue diseases, and tuberculosis.

LABORATORY FINDINGS

Dry pleurisy may be detected on radiographs as a diffuse haziness at the pleural surface or a dense, sharply demarcated shadow (Figs. 429.1 and 429.2). The latter finding may be indistinguishable from small amounts of pleural exudate. Chest radiographic findings may be normal, but ultrasonography or CT findings will be positive.

DIFFERENTIAL DIAGNOSIS

Pleurisy must be distinguished from other diseases, such as epidemic pleurodynia, trauma to the rib cage (rib fracture), lesions of the dorsal root ganglia, tumors of the spinal cord, herpes zoster, gallbladder disease, and trichinosis. Even if evidence of pleural fluid is not found on physical or radiographic examination, a CT- or ultrasound-guided pleural tap in suspected cases often results in the recovery of a small amount of exudate, which when cultured may reveal the underlying bacterial cause in patients with an acute pneumonia. Patients with pleurisy and pneumonia should always be screened for tuberculosis.

TREATMENT

Therapy should be aimed at the underlying disease. When pneumonia is present, neither immobilization of the chest with adhesive plaster nor therapy with drugs capable of suppressing the cough reflex is indicated. If pneumonia is not present or is under good therapeutic control, strapping of the chest to restrict expansion may afford relief from pain. Analgesia with nonsteroidal antiinflammatory agents may be helpful.

Bibliography is available at Expert Consult.

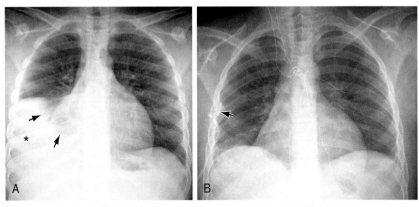

Fig. 429.1 A, Right pleural effusion *(asterisk)* caused by lupus erythematosus in a 12 yr old child. Note compressed middle and lower lobes of the right lung *(arrows)*. **B,** The effusion was evacuated and the right lung was completely reexpanded after insertion of the pigtail chest tube *(arrow)*.

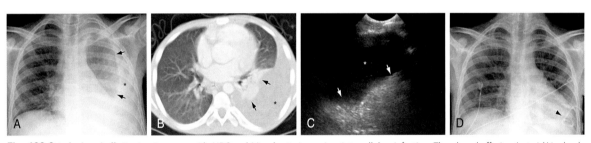

Fig. 429.2 Left pleural effusion in a teenager with AIDS and *Mycobacterium avium-intracellulare* infection. The pleural effusion *(asterisk)* is clearly seen on the chest radiograph **(A)**, CT scan **(B)**, and ultrasonogram **(C)** of the left chest. *Arrows* point to the compressed and atelectatic left lung. **D,** A pigtail chest tube *(arrowhead)* was inserted, resulting in reexpansion of the left lung.

429.2 Serofibrinous or Serosanguineous Pleurisy With Pleural Effusion

Glenna B. Winnie, Aarthi P. Vemana, Suraiya K. Haider, and Steven V. Lossef

ETIOLOGY

Serofibrinous pleurisy is defined by a fibrinous exudate on the pleural surface and an exudative effusion of serous fluid into the pleural cavity. In general, it is associated with infections of the lung or with inflammatory conditions of the abdomen or mediastinum; occasionally, it is found with connective tissue diseases such as lupus erythematosus, periarteritis, and rheumatoid arthritis, and it may be seen with primary or metastatic neoplasms of the lung, pleura, or mediastinum. Tumors are commonly associated with a hemorrhagic pleurisy.

PATHOGENESIS

Pleural fluid originates from the capillaries of the parietal pleura and is absorbed from the pleural space via pleural stomas and the lymphatics of the parietal pleura. The rate of fluid formation is dictated by the Starling law, by which fluid movement is determined by the balance of hydrostatic and osmotic pressures in the pleural space and pulmonary capillary bed, and the permeability of the pleural membrane. Normally, approximately 10 mL of fluid is present in the pleural space, but if formation exceeds clearance, fluid accumulates. Pleural inflammation increases the permeability of the plural surface, with increased protein-aceous fluid formation; there may also be some obstruction to lymphatic absorption.

CLINICAL MANIFESTATIONS

Because serofibrinous pleurisy is often preceded by the dry type, early signs and symptoms may be those of dry pleurisy. As fluid accumulates, pleuritic pain may disappear. The patient may become asymptomatic if the effusion remains small, or there may be only signs and symptoms of the underlying disease. Large fluid collections can produce cough, dyspnea, retractions, tachypnea, orthopnea, or cyanosis.

Physical findings depend on the amount of effusion. Dullness to flatness may be found on percussion. Breath sounds are decreased or absent, and there is a diminution in tactile fremitus, a shift of the mediastinum away from the affected side, and, occasionally, fullness of the intercostal spaces. If the fluid is not loculated, these signs may shift with changes in position. If extensive pneumonia is present, crackles and rhonchi may also be audible. Friction rubs are usually detected only during the early or late plastic stage. In infants, physical signs are less definite, and bronchial breathing may be heard instead of decreased breath sounds.

LABORATORY FINDINGS

Radiographic examination shows a generally homogeneous density obliterating the normal markings of the underlying lung. Small effusions may cause obliteration of only the costophrenic or cardiophrenic angles or a widening of the interlobar septa. Examinations should be performed with the patient both supine and upright, to demonstrate a shift of the effusion with a change in position; the decubitus position may be helpful. Ultrasonographic examinations are useful and may guide thoracentesis if the effusion is loculated. Examination of the fluid is essential to differentiate **exudates** from **transudates** and to determine the type of exudate (see Table 428.8). Depending on the clinical scenario, pleural fluid is sent for culture for bacterial, fungal, and mycobacterial cultures; antigen testing; Gram staining; and chemical evaluation of content, including protein, lactic dehydrogenase and glucose, amylase, specific gravity, total cell count and differential, cytologic examination, and pH. Complete blood count and serum chemistry analysis should be obtained; hypoalbuminemia is often present. **Exudates** usually have at least 1 of the following features: protein level >3.0 g/dL, with pleural fluid:serum protein ratio >0.5; pleural fluid lactic dehydrogenase values >200 IU/L; or fluid:serum lactic dehydrogenase ratio >0.6. Although systemic acidosis reduces the usefulness of pleural fluid pH measurements, pH < 7.20 suggests an exudate (see Chapter 400). Glucose is usually <60 mg/dL in malignancy, rheumatoid disease, and tuberculosis; the finding of many small lymphocytes and a pH < 7.20 suggest tuberculosis. The fluid of serofibrinous pleurisy is clear or slightly cloudy and contains relatively few leukocytes and, occasionally, some erythrocytes. Gram staining may occasionally show bacteria; however, acid-fast staining rarely demonstrates tubercle bacilli.

DIAGNOSIS AND DIFFERENTIAL DIAGNOSIS

Thoracentesis should be performed when pleural fluid is present or is suggested, unless the effusion is small, and the patient has a classic-appearing lobar pneumococcal pneumonia. Thoracentesis can differentiate serofibrinous pleurisy, empyema, hydrothorax, hemothorax, and chylothorax. Exudates are usually associated with an infectious process. In hydrothorax, the fluid has a specific gravity <1.015, and evaluation reveals only a few mesothelial cells rather than leukocytes. Chylothorax and hemothorax usually have fluid with a distinctive appearance, but differentiating serofibrinous from purulent pleurisy is impossible without microscopic examination of the fluid. Cytologic examination may reveal malignant cells. Serofibrinous fluid may rapidly become purulent.

COMPLICATIONS

Unless the fluid becomes purulent, it usually disappears relatively rapidly, particularly with appropriate treatment of bacterial pneumonia. It persists somewhat longer if a result of tuberculosis or a connective tissue disease and may recur or remain for a long time if caused by a neoplasm. As the effusion is absorbed, adhesions often develop between the 2 layers of the pleura, but usually little or no functional impairment results. Pleural thickening may develop and is occasionally mistaken for small quantities of fluid or for persistent pulmonary infiltrates. Pleural thickening may persist for months, but the process usually disappears, leaving no residua.

TREATMENT

Therapy should address the underlying disease. If the effusion is less than 10 mm in size on a chest x-ray, then there is no need for drainage. With a large effusion, draining the fluid makes the patient more comfortable. When a diagnostic thoracentesis is performed, as much fluid as possible should be removed for therapeutic purposes. Rapid removal of ≥1 L of pleural fluid may be associated with the development of reexpansion pulmonary edema (see Chapter 396). If the underlying disease is adequately treated, further drainage is usually unnecessary, but if sufficient fluid reaccumulates to cause respiratory embarrassment, chest tube drainage should be performed. In older children with suspected parapneumonic effusion, tube thoracostomy is considered necessary if the pleural fluid pH is <7.20 or the pleural fluid glucose level is <50 mg/dL. If the fluid is thick, loculated, or clearly purulent, tube drainage with fibrinolytic therapy or less often video-assisted thoracoscopic surgery (VATS) is indicated. Patients with pleural effusions may need analgesia, particularly after thoracentesis or insertion of a chest tube. Those with acute pneumonia may need supplemental oxygen in addition to specific antibiotic treatment. Studies in adults suggest that dexamethasone may be beneficial in addition to antibiotics and drainage in patients with parapneumonic effusions.

Bibliography is available at Expert Consult.

429.3 Empyema

Glenna B. Winnie, Aarthi P. Vemana, Suraiya K. Haider, and Steven V. Lossef

ETIOLOGY

Empyema is an accumulation of pus in the pleural space. It is most often associated with pneumonia (see Chapter 428) caused by *Streptococcus pneumoniae* (see Chapter 209), although *Staphylococcus aureus* (see Chapter 208.1) is most common in developing nations and Asia, as well as in posttraumatic empyema. The relative incidence of *Haemophilus influenzae* (see Chapter 221) empyema has decreased since the introduction of the *H. influenzae* type b vaccination. Group A streptococcus, Gram-negative organisms, tuberculosis, fungi, viruses, and malignancy are less common causes. The disease can also be produced by rupture of a lung abscess into the pleural space, by contamination introduced from trauma or thoracic surgery, or, rarely, by mediastinitis or the extension of intraabdominal abscesses.

EPIDEMIOLOGY
Empyema is most frequently encountered in infants and preschool children. Although rates of bacterial pneumonia have decreased, the incidence of parapneumonic effusions has increased. This may be related to a shift towards more virulent organisms after the introduction of the heptavalent pneumococcal vaccine with a trend towards serotypes not covered by the vaccine. It occurs in 5–10% of children with bacterial pneumonia and in up to 86% of children with necrotizing pneumonia.

PATHOLOGY
Empyema has 3 stages: exudative, fibrinopurulent, and organizational. During the exudative stage, fibrinous exudate forms on the pleural surfaces. In the fibrinopurulent stage, fibrinous septa form, causing loculation of the fluid and thickening of the parietal pleura. If the pus is not drained, it may dissect through the pleura into lung parenchyma, producing bronchopleural fistulas and pyopneumothorax, or into the abdominal cavity. Rarely, the pus dissects through the chest wall (i.e., empyema necessitatis). During the organizational stage, there is fibroblast proliferation; pockets of loculated pus may develop into thick-walled abscess cavities or the lung may collapse and become surrounded by a thick, inelastic envelope (peel).

CLINICAL MANIFESTATIONS
The initial signs and symptoms are primarily those of bacterial pneumonia. Children treated with antibiotic agents may have an interval of a few days between the clinical pneumonia phase and the evidence of empyema. Most patients are febrile, develop increased work of breathing or respiratory distress, and often appear more ill. Physical findings are identical to those described for serofibrinous pleurisy, and the 2 conditions are differentiated only by thoracentesis, which should always be performed when empyema is suspected.

LABORATORY FINDINGS
Radiographically, all pleural effusions appear similar, but the absence of a shift of the fluid with a change of position indicates a loculated empyema (Figs. 429.3 to 429.5). Although on an ultrasound a lenticular shape may indicate the presence of loculated fluid, septa are better visualized by CT. The maximal amount of fluid obtainable should be withdrawn by thoracentesis and studied as described in Chapter 429.2. The effusion is an empyema if bacteria are present on Gram staining, the pH is <7.20, and there are >100,000 neutrophils/μL (see Chapter 428). Cultures of the fluid must always be performed to help identify the causal organism. Using standard culture methods, the organism can be identified in up to 60% of cases. The yield improves significantly with concomitant use of nucleic acid amplification techniques. Blood cultures may be positive and have a higher yield than cultures of the pleural fluid. Leukocytosis and an elevated sedimentation rate may be found.

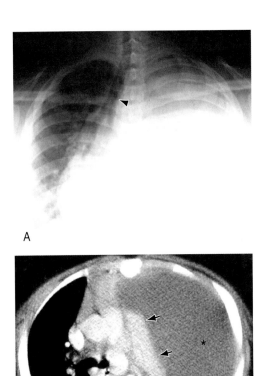

Fig. 429.3 Empyema and pneumonia in a teenager. **A,** Chest radiograph shows opacification of the left thorax. Note shift of mediastinum and trachea (*arrowhead*) to right. **B,** Thoracic CT scan shows massive left pleural effusion (*asterisk*). Note the compression and atelectasis of the left lung (*arrows*) and shift of the mediastinum to the right.

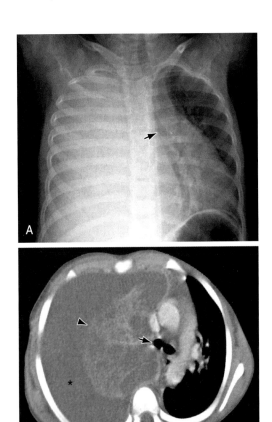

Fig. 429.4 Pneumonia and parapneumonic effusion in a 4 yr old child. **A,** Chest radiograph shows complete opacification of the right thorax as a result of a large pleural effusion. Note the shift of the mediastinum and trachea (*arrow*) to the left. **B,** Thoracic CT scan shows a large right pleural effusion (*asterisk*) surrounding and compressing the consolidated right lung (*arrowhead*). Note the shift of the mediastinum and tracheal carina (*arrow*) to the left.

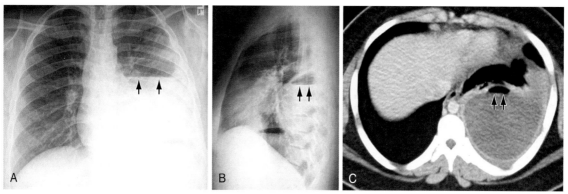

Fig. 429.5 Loculated hydropneumothorax. Frontal **(A)** and lateral **(B)** chest radiographs show loculated hydropneumothorax that complicated pneumonia in a 14 yr old child. *Arrows* point to the horizontal air-fluid level at the interface between the intrapleural effusion and air. **C,** Thoracic CT scan helps to localize the loculated hydropneumothorax, with its air-fluid level *(arrows).*

COMPLICATIONS

With staphylococcal infections, bronchopleural fistulas and pyopneumo-thorax commonly develop. Other local complications include purulent pericarditis, pulmonary abscesses, peritonitis from extension through the diaphragm, and osteomyelitis of the ribs. Septic complications such as meningitis, arthritis, and osteomyelitis may also occur. Septicemia is often encountered in *H. influenzae* and pneumococcal infections. The effusion may organize into a thick "peel," which may restrict lung expansion and may be associated with persistent fever and temporary scoliosis.

TREATMENT

The aim of empyema treatment is to sterilize pleural fluid and restore normal lung function. Treatment includes systemic antibiotics and thoracentesis and chest tube drainage initially with a fibrinolytic agent; if no improvement occurs, VATS is indicated. Open decortication is indicated if fibrinolysis and VATS are ineffective (see Chapter 439). If empyema is diagnosed early, antibiotic treatment plus thoracentesis achieves a complete cure. The selection of antibiotic should be based on the in vitro sensitivities of the responsible organism. See Chapters 208, 209, and 221 for treatment of infections by *Staphylococcus, S. pneumoniae,* and *H. influenzae,* respectively. Clinical response in empyema is slow, and systemic antibiotics may be needed for up to 4 wk. Instillation of antibiotics into the pleural cavity does not improve results.

When pus is obtained by thoracentesis or pleural fluid septation is detected on radiographic studies, closed-chest tube drainage with fibrolytics is the initial procedure, followed by VATS if there is no improvement. Multiple aspirations of the pleural cavity should not be attempted. Closed-chest tube drainage is controlled by an underwater seal or continuous suction; sometimes more than 1 tube is required to drain loculated areas. Closed drainage is usually continued for 5-7 days. Chest tubes that are no longer draining are removed.

Instillation of fibrinolytic agents into the pleural cavity via the chest tube often promotes drainage, decreases the length of time a chest tube is in place, decreases fever, lessens need for surgical intervention, and shortens hospitalization. The optimal fibrinolytic drug and dosages have not been determined. Streptokinase 15,000 units/kg in 50 mL of 0.9% saline, urokinase 40,000 units in 40 mL saline, and alteplase (tPA) 4 mg in 40 mL of saline have been used in the pediatric population. The combination of fibrinolytic therapy with DNAse is superior to the use of fibrinolytics alone to promote chest tube drainage. There is a risk of anaphylaxis with streptokinase, and all 3 drugs can be associated with hemorrhage and other complications.

Extensive fibrinous changes may take place over the surface of the lungs owing to empyema, but they eventually resolve. In the child who remains febrile and dyspneic for more than 72 hr after initiation of therapy with intravenous antibiotics and thoracostomy tube drainage, surgical decortication via VATS or, less often, open thoracotomy may speed recovery. If pneumatoceles form, no attempt should be made to treat them surgically or by aspiration, unless they reach sufficient size to cause respiratory compromise or become secondarily infected. Pneumatoceles usually resolve spontaneously with time. The long-term clinical prognosis for adequately treated empyema is excellent, and follow-up pulmonary function studies suggest that residual restrictive disease is uncommon, with or without surgical intervention.

Bibliography is available at Expert Consult.

Chapter 430
Bronchiectasis
Oren J. Lakser

第四百三十章
支气管扩张症

中文导读

本章主要介绍了支气管扩张症的病理生理学、发病机制、临床表现、诊断、治疗以及预后。详细描述了支气管扩张症的三个发病机制分别为阻塞、感染和慢性炎症，介绍了柱状支气管扩张、曲张型支气管扩张和囊状支气管扩张三种病理类型；强调了高分辨CT

对于支气管扩张症的诊断及鉴别诊断意义；支气管扩张症急性加重期的诊断依据及处理原则。治疗中描述了气道廓清技术、湿化气道、手术切除和肺移植等方法，着重阐述了抗生素的应用原则。

Bronchiectasis is characterized by irreversible abnormal dilation and anatomic distortion of the bronchial tree and represents the common end stage of many nonspecific and unrelated antecedent events. Its incidence has been decreasing overall in industrialized countries, but it persists as a problem in lower- and middle-income countries and among some ethnic groups in industrialized nations (particularly in aboriginal children). Females are afflicted more frequently than males.

PATHOPHYSIOLOGY AND PATHOGENESIS

In industrialized nations, cystic fibrosis (see Chapter 432) is the most common cause of clinically significant bronchiectasis. Other conditions associated with bronchiectasis include primary ciliary dyskinesia (see Chapter 433), foreign body aspiration (see Chapter 405), aspiration of gastric contents, immune deficiency syndromes (especially humoral immunity), and infection, especially pertussis, measles, and tuberculosis (Table 430.1). Bronchiectasis can also be congenital, as in **Williams-Campbell syndrome**, in which there is an absence of annular bronchial cartilage, and **Marnier-Kuhn syndrome** (congenital tracheobronchomegaly), in which there is a connective tissue disorder. Other disease entities associated with bronchiectasis are **yellow nail syndrome** (pleural effusion, lymphedema, discolored nails) and **right middle lobe syndrome**. The right middle lobe syndrome is mostly associated with other generalized causes of bronchiectasis including asthma, cystic fibrosis, primary ciliary dyskinesia, severe pneumonia, aspiration pneumonia, foreign bodies, and immune deficient states. Early phases of the right middle lobe syndrome manifest as persistent or recurrent right middle lobe infiltrates (pneumonia). The right middle lobe syndrome may be classified as intrinsic or extrinsic obstructive (tumors, granulomas, lymphadenopathy) and nonobstructive (aspiration, asthma, cystic fibrosis).

Three basic mechanisms are involved in the pathogenesis of bronchiectasis. **Obstruction** can occur because of tumor, foreign body,

Table 430.1	Conditions That Predispose to Bronchiectasis in Children

PROXIMAL AIRWAY NARROWING

Airway wall compression (i.e., vascular ring, adenopathy impinging on airways)

Airway intraluminal obstruction (e.g., inhaled foreign body, granulation tissue)

Airway stenosis and malacia

AIRWAY INJURY

Bronchiolitis obliterans (e.g., postviral, after lung transplantation)

Recurrent pneumonitis or pneumonia (e.g., pneumococcal pneumonia, aspiration pneumonia)

ALTERED PULMONARY HOST DEFENSES

Cystic fibrosis

Ciliary dyskinesia

Impaired cough (e.g., neuromuscular weakness conditions)

ALTERED IMMUNE STATES

Primary abnormalities (e.g., hypogammaglobulinemia, common variable immune deficiency)

Secondary abnormalities (e.g., HIV infection, immunosuppressive agents)

OTHER

Allergic bronchopulmonary aspergillosis

Plastic bronchitis

Right middle lobe syndrome

From Redding GJ: Bronchiectasis in children, *Pediatr Clin North Am* 56:157–171, 2009, Box 1, p. 158.

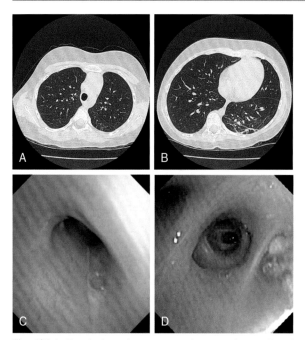

Fig. 430.1 Chest high-resolution computed tomography scan (**A** and **B**) and bronchoscopy (**C** and **D**) in a child with bronchiectasis. (**C** and **D**) Bronchoscopy findings. Images from a chest high-resolution computed tomography (cHRCT) scan (**A** and **B**) in a 10 yr old girl who presented with a chronic wet cough. The child was treated with a 2-wk course of IV antibiotics (after failing oral antibiotic treatment). The scan was reported as having no evidence of bronchiectasis by pediatric radiologists. At bronchoscopy thick mucopus was seen in the trachea (**C**) and the right lower lobe (**D**). The case highlights the need to consider the diagnosis of bronchiectasis on the basis of history, examination findings and using the pediatric cutoff (bronchoarterial ratio >0.8) 104 for defining bronchiectasis on the cHRCT scan. *(From Goyal V, Grimwood K, Marchant J, et al: Pediatric bronchiectasis: no longer an orphan disease, Pediatr Pulmonol 51:450–469, 2016.)*

impacted mucus because of poor mucociliary clearance, external compression, bronchial webs, and atresia. **Infections** caused by *Bordetella pertussis*, measles, rubella, togavirus, respiratory syncytial virus, adenovirus, and *Mycobacterium tuberculosis* induce chronic inflammation, progressive bronchial wall damage, and dilation. More recently,

nontypeable *Haemophilus influenzae* seems to be a common cause of infection in adults and children with bronchiectasis. *Streptococcus pneumoniae* and *Moraxella catarrhalis* are more common in children with bronchiectasis than in adult patients. **Chronic inflammation** similarly contributes to the mechanism by which obstruction leads to bronchiectasis. Both inadequate and exaggerated/dysregulated immune responses may play a role in the development of bronchiectasis. Activation of Toll-like receptors results in the activation of nuclear factor κB and the release of proinflammatory cytokines interleukin (IL)-1β, IL-8, and tumor necrosis factor-α. IL-8 is a chemoattractant for neutrophils, which are the main inflammatory cell involved in the pathogenesis of bronchiectasis. Once activated, neutrophils produce neutrophil elastase and matrix metalloproteinases, MMP-8 and MMP-9. IL-6, IL-8, and tumor necrosis factor-α are elevated in the airways of patients with bronchiectasis. Eosinophils are also elevated in airways of indigenous children with bronchiectasis which promote neutrophil recruitment, goblet cell hyperplasia, and airway destruction. There is an increase in proinflammatory cytotoxic T lymphocytes in peripheral blood of children with bronchiectasis. The mechanism by which bronchiectasis occurs in congenital forms is likely related to abnormal cartilage formation. The common thread in the pathogenesis of bronchiectasis consists of difficulty clearing secretions and recurrent infections with a "vicious cycle" of infection and inflammation resulting in airway injury and remodeling (Fig. 430.1). In early stages, bronchiectasis consists primarily of bronchiolar wall thickening and destruction of elastin resulting in bronchial dilation. In later stages, the bronchial walls develop cartilage destruction with associated pulmonary artery/arteriole vascular remodeling, resulting in pulmonary hypertension.

Bronchiectasis can manifest in any combination of 3 pathologic forms, best defined by high-resolution CT (HRCT) scan (Fig. 430.2). In **cylindrical** bronchiectasis, the bronchial outlines are regular, but there is diffuse dilation of the bronchial unit. The bronchial lumen ends abruptly because of mucous plugging. In **varicose** bronchiectasis, the degree of dilation is greater, and local constrictions cause an irregularity of outline resembling that of varicose veins. There may also be small sacculations. In **saccular** (cystic) bronchiectasis, bronchial dilation progresses and results in ballooning of bronchi that end in fluid- or mucus-filled sacs. This is the most severe form of bronchiectasis. Bronchiectasis lies within a disease spectrum of chronic pediatric suppurative lung disease. The following definitions have been proposed: **prebronchiectasis** (chronic or recurrent endobronchial infection with nonspecific HRCT changes; may be reversible); **HRCT bronchiectasis** (clinical symptoms with HRCT evidence of bronchial dilation; may persist, progress, or improve and resolve); **established bronchiectasis** (like the previous but with no resolution within 2 yr). Early diagnosis and aggressive therapy are important to prevent the development of established bronchiectasis.

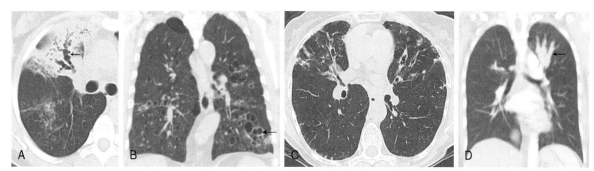

Fig. 430.2 Bronchiectasis. **A,** Axial CT image demonstrates a beaded appearance of dilated bronchi *(arrow)* in the right upper lobe, consistent with varicoid bronchiectasis. **B,** Coronal reformation CT image shows multiple foci of cystic bronchiectasis, with a few air-fluid levels *(arrow)*. Also note paraseptal emphysema, most marked at the right apex. **C,** Bronchiectatic form of chronic atypical mycobacterial infection. Axial CT scan shows extensive bronchiectasis, bronchial wall thickening, and centrilobular nodules, most severe in the middle lobe and lingula. **D,** Allergic bronchopulmonary aspergillosis. Coronal reformation CT image demonstrates impacted bronchi in the left upper lobe *(arrow)* producing a "gloved finger" appearance. *(From Boiselle PM: Airway. In Haaga JR, Boll DT: CT and MRI of the whole body, ed 6, Philadelphia, 2017, Elsevier, Figs 40-30, 32-34.)*

CLINICAL MANIFESTATIONS

The most common complaints in patients with bronchiectasis are cough and production of copious purulent sputum. Younger children may swallow the sputum. Hemoptysis is seen with some frequency. Fever can occur with infectious exacerbations. Anorexia and poor weight gain may occur as time passes. Physical examination typically reveals crackles localized to the affected area but wheezing as well as digital clubbing may also occur. In severe cases, dyspnea and hypoxemia can occur. Pulmonary function studies may demonstrate an obstructive, restrictive, or mixed pattern. Typically, impaired diffusion capacity is a late finding.

DIAGNOSIS

Conditions that can be associated with bronchiectasis should be ruled out by appropriate investigations (e.g., sweat test, immunologic workup). Chest radiographs of patients with bronchiectasis tend to be nonspecific. Typical findings can include increase in size and loss of definition of bronchovascular markings, crowding of bronchi, and loss of lung volume. In more severe forms, cystic spaces, occasionally with air-fluid levels and honeycombing, may occur. Compensatory overinflation of unaffected lung may be seen. Thin-section HRCT scanning is the gold standard because it has excellent sensitivity and specificity. CT provides further information on disease location, presence of mediastinal lesions, and the extent of segmental involvement. The addition of radiolabeled aerosol inhalation to CT scanning can provide even more information. The CT findings in patients with bronchiectasis typically include cylindrical ("tram lines," "signet ring appearance"), varicose (bronchi with "beaded contour"), cystic (cysts in "strings and clusters"), or mixed forms (see Fig. 430.2). The lower lobes are most commonly affected.

TREATMENT

The initial therapy for patients with bronchiectasis is medical and aims at decreasing airway obstruction and controlling infection. Airway clearance techniques (e.g., gravity-assisted drainage, active cycle of breathing, positive expiratory pressure [PEP], acapella, high-frequency chest wall oscillation), antibiotics, and bronchodilators are essential. Two to 4 wk of parenteral antibiotics is often necessary to manage acute exacerbations adequately. Exacerbations can be defined as the presence of 1 major criteria (wet cough enduring longer than 72 hr, increased cough frequency over 72 hr) plus 1 laboratory criteria (C-reactive protein >3 mg/L, serum

IL-6 >2 ng/L, serum amyloid A >5 mg/L, elevated neutrophil percentage), 2 major criteria, or 1 major criteria plus 2 minor criteria (change in sputum color, breathlessness, chest pain, crackles/crepitations, wheeze). Antibiotic choice is dictated by the identification and sensitivity of organisms found on deep throat, sputum (induced or spontaneous), or bronchoalveolar lavage fluid cultures. The most common organisms found in children with bronchiectasis include S. pneumoniae, H. influenzae non–type b, M. catarrhalis, and Mycoplasma pneumoniae. Amoxicillin/clavulanic acid (22.5 mg/kg/dose twice daily) has been particularly successful at treating most pulmonary exacerbations. Viruses (most commonly human rhinovirus) are often found in children with bronchiectasis suffering from an exacerbation. Long-term prophylactic macrolide antibiotics or nebulized antibiotics (e.g., tobramycin, colistin, aztreonam) may be beneficial (reduced exacerbations and hospitalizations, improved lung function) but may also increase antibiotic resistance. Airway hydration (inhaled hypertonic saline or mannitol) also improves quality of life in adults with bronchiectasis. Any underlying disorder (immunodeficiency, aspiration) that may be contributing must be addressed. When localized bronchiectasis becomes more severe or resistant to medical management, segmental or lobar resection may be warranted. Lung transplantation can also be performed in patients with bronchiectasis. A review of randomized trials among children and adult patients with bronchiectasis did not find strong evidence to support the routine use of inhaled corticosteroids, although some studies demonstrate improved quality of life and reduced exacerbations in patients with bronchiectasis treated with inhaled corticosteroids. Although preventative strategies, including immunization against typical respiratory pathogens (influenza, pneumococci), are generally recommended, no studies have been conducted to date to address the efficacy of these recommendations.

PROGNOSIS

Children with bronchiectasis often suffer from recurrent pulmonary illnesses, resulting in missed school days, stunted growth, osteopenia, and osteoporosis. The prognosis for patients with bronchiectasis has improved considerably in the past few decades. Earlier recognition or prevention of predisposing conditions, specialist multidisciplinary management, more powerful and broad-spectrum antibiotics, and improved surgical outcomes are likely reasons.

Bibliography is available at Expert Consult.

Chapter **431**
Pulmonary Abscess
Oren J. Lakser

第四百三十一章
肺脓肿

中文导读

　　本章主要介绍了肺脓肿的病理学、发病机制、临床表现、诊断、治疗以及预后。描述了包括误吸、肺炎、囊性纤维化等易导致儿童发生肺脓肿的诸多因素；列举了肺脓肿常见病原菌，包括多种厌氧菌和需氧菌；诊断中详细描述了肺脓肿在胸片上的表现，并

与肺囊肿进行鉴别，同时介绍了直接肺穿刺和支气管肺泡灌洗等可以明确肺脓肿病原学的临床手段；治疗中详细介绍了抗生素的应用原则并提出对于重症患者可应用手术等治疗手段。

Lung infection that destroys the lung parenchyma, resulting in cavitations and central necrosis, can result in localized areas composed of thick-walled purulent material, called lung abscesses. Primary lung abscesses occur in previously healthy patients with no underlying medical disorders and are usually solitary. Secondary lung abscesses occur in patients with underlying or predisposing conditions and may be multiple. Lung abscesses are much less common in children (estimated at 0.7 per 100,000 admissions per year) than in adults.

PATHOLOGY AND PATHOGENESIS

A number of conditions predispose children to the development of pulmonary abscesses, including aspiration, pneumonia, cystic fibrosis (see Chapter 432), gastroesophageal reflux (see Chapter 349), tracheo-esophageal fistula (see Chapter 345), immunodeficiencies, postoperative complications of tonsillectomy and adenoidectomy, seizures, a variety of neurologic diseases, and other conditions associated with impaired mucociliary defense. In children, aspiration of infected materials or a foreign body is the predominant source of the organisms causing abscesses. Initially, pneumonitis impairs drainage of fluid or the aspirated material. Inflammatory vascular obstruction occurs, leading to tissue necrosis, liquefaction, and abscess formation. Abscess can also occur as a result of pneumonia and hematogenous seeding from another site.

If the aspiration event occurred while the child was recumbent, the right and left upper lobes and apical segment of the right lower lobes are the dependent areas most likely to be affected. In a child who was upright, the posterior segments of the upper lobes were dependent and therefore are most likely to be affected. Primary abscesses are found most often on the right side, whereas secondary lung abscesses, particularly in immunocompromised patients, have a predilection for the left side.

Both anaerobic and aerobic organisms can cause lung abscesses. Common anaerobic bacteria that can cause a pulmonary abscess include *Bacteroides* spp., *Fusobacterium* spp., and *Peptostreptococcus* spp. Abscesses can be caused by aerobic organisms such as *Streptococcus* spp., *Staphylococcus aureus*, *Escherichia coli*, *Klebsiella pneumoniae*, *Pseudomonas aeruginosa*, and very rarely *Mycoplasma pneumoniae*. Aerobic and anaerobic cultures should be part of the workup for all patients with lung abscess. Occasionally, concomitant viral-bacterial infection can be detected. Fungi can also cause lung abscesses, particularly in immunocompromised patients.

CLINICAL MANIFESTATIONS

The most common symptoms of pulmonary abscess in the pediatric population are fever, cough, and emesis. Other common symptoms include tachypnea, dyspnea, chest pain, sputum production, weight loss, and hemoptysis. Physical examination typically reveals tachypnea, dyspnea, retractions with accessory muscle use, decreased breath sounds, and dullness to percussion in the affected area. Crackles and occasionally a prolonged expiratory phase may be heard on lung examination.

DIAGNOSIS

Diagnosis is most commonly made on the basis of chest radiography. Classically, the chest radiograph shows a parenchymal inflammation with a cavity containing an air-fluid level (Fig. 431.1). A chest CT scan can provide better anatomic definition of an abscess, including location and size (Fig. 431.2).

An abscess is usually a thick-walled lesion with a low-density center progressing to an air-fluid level. Abscesses should be distinguished from pneumatoceles, which often complicate severe bacterial pneumonias and are characterized by thin- and smooth-walled, localized air

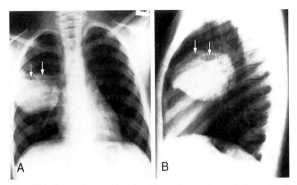

Fig. 431.1 A and **B,** Multiloculated lung abscess *(arrows). (From Brook I: Lung abscess and pulmonary infections due to anaerobic bacteria. In Chernick V, Boat TF, Wilmott RW, et al, editors: Kendig's disorders of the respiratory tract in children, ed 7, Philadelphia, 2006, WB Saunders, p. 482.)*

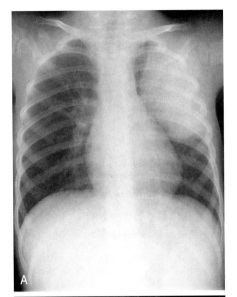

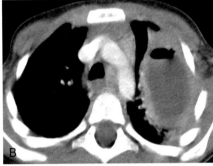

Fig. 431.2 Pulmonary abscess in a 2 yr old boy with persistent cough. **A,** Chest radiograph shows large oval mass in the left upper lobe. **B,** CT scan demonstrates an abscess with a thick enhancing wall that contains both air and fluid. *(From Slovis TL, editor: Caffey's pediatric diagnostic imaging, ed 11, Philadelphia, 2008, Mosby, Fig. 78-3, p. 1297.)*

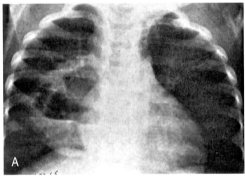

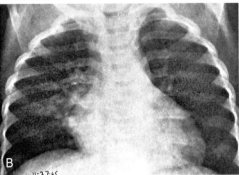

Fig. 431.3 Appearance over a period of 5 days of a large multiloculated pneumonocele in a segment of alveolar consolidation. **A,** There is a large cavity with 2 air-fluid levels in a segment of alveolar pneumonia in the right upper lobe. **B,** Five days later, the cavity and most of the pneumonic consolidation have disappeared. *(From Silverman FN, Kuhn JP: Essentials of Caffey's pediatric x-ray diagnosis, Chicago, 1990, Year Book, p. 303.)*

collections with or without air-fluid level (Fig. 431.3). Pneumatoceles often resolve spontaneously with the treatment of the specific cause of the pneumonia.

The determination of the etiologic bacteria in a lung abscess can be very helpful in guiding antibiotic choice. Although Gram stain of sputum can provide an early clue as to the class of bacteria involved, sputum cultures typically yield mixed bacteria and therefore are not always reliable. Attempts to avoid contamination from oral flora include direct lung puncture, percutaneous (aided by CT guidance) or transtracheal aspiration, and bronchoalveolar lavage specimens obtained bronchoscopically. Bronchoscopic aspiration should be avoided because it can be complicated by massive intrabronchial aspiration, and great care should therefore be taken during the procedure. To avoid invasive procedures in previously normal hosts, empiric therapy can be initiated in the absence of culturable material.

TREATMENT

Conservative management is recommended for pulmonary abscess. Most experts advocate a 2- to 3-wk course of parenteral antibiotics for uncomplicated cases, followed by a course of oral antibiotics to complete a total of 4-6 wk. Antibiotic choice should be guided by results of Gram stain and culture but initially should include agents with aerobic and anaerobic coverage. Treatment regimens should include a penicillinase-resistant agent active against *S. aureus* and anaerobic coverage, typically with clindamycin or ticarcillin/clavulanic acid. If gram-negative bacteria are suspected or isolated, an aminoglycoside should be added. Early CT-guided percutaneous aspiration or drainage has been advocated because it can hasten the recovery and shorten the course of parenteral antibiotic therapy needed.

For severely ill patients, patients with larger abscess, or those whose status fails to improve after 7-10 days of appropriate antimicrobial therapy, surgical intervention should be considered. Minimally invasive percutaneous aspiration techniques, often with CT guidance, are the initial and, often, only intervention required. Thorascopic drainage has also been successfully used with minimal complications. In rare complicated cases, thoracotomy with surgical drainage or lobectomy and/

or decortication may be necessary. Abscess drainage is reportedly required in ~20% of cases of pulmonary abscess in children.

PROGNOSIS

Overall, prognosis for children with primary pulmonary abscesses is excellent. The presence of aerobic organisms may be a negative prognostic indicator, particularly in those with secondary lung abscesses. Most children become asymptomatic within 7-10 days, although the fever can persist for as long as 3 wk. Radiologic abnormalities usually resolve in 1-3 mo but can persist for years.

Bibliography is available at Expert Consult.

Chapter **432**
Cystic Fibrosis
Marie E. Egan, Michael S. Schechter, and Judith A. Voynow

第四百三十二章
囊性纤维化

中文导读

本章主要介绍了囊性纤维化的遗传学、发病机制、病理学、临床表现、诊断和评估、治疗、各种并发症、治疗以及预后。其中临床表现部分详细描述了囊性纤维化对呼吸道、肠道、胆道、囊性纤维化相关的糖尿病、胰腺炎、泌尿生殖道和汗腺的影响；诊断和评估部分介绍了汗液检测、DNA检测、胰腺功能测定等；治疗中详细阐述了一般护理、肺部治疗、支气管舒张剂治疗、抗炎治疗等；针对肺部并发症的治疗重点介绍了对肺不张、咯血、气胸、变应性支气管肺曲霉病、非结核分支杆菌感染、骨关节病、睡眠呼吸紊乱、急慢性呼吸衰竭、肺动脉高压及肺源性心脏病、营养不良等的治疗；介绍了肠道并发症的胎粪性肠梗阻、远端肠梗阻综合征等的治疗；以及其他并发症的治疗，如鼻息肉、鼻窦炎、失盐综合征等。

Cystic fibrosis (CF) is an inherited multisystem disorder of children and adults; it is the most common life-limiting recessive genetic trait among whites. Dysfunction of the cystic fibrosis transmembrane conductance regulator (CFTR) protein, the primary defect, leads to a wide and variable array of presenting manifestations and complications.

CF is responsible for most cases of exocrine pancreatic insufficiency in early life and is the major cause of severe chronic lung disease in children. It is also responsible for many cases of hyponatremic salt depletion, nasal polyposis, pansinusitis, rectal prolapse, pancreatitis, cholelithiasis, and nonautoimmune insulin-dependent hyperglycemia. Because CF may manifest as failure to thrive and hepatic dysfunction, including cirrhosis, this disorder enters into the differential diagnosis of many pediatric conditions (Table 432.1).

GENETICS

CF occurs most frequently in white populations of northern Europe, North America, and Australia/New Zealand. The prevalence in these populations varies but approximates 1 in 3,500 live births (1 in 9,200 individuals of Hispanic descent and 1 in 15,000 African Americans). Although less frequent in African, Hispanic, Middle Eastern, South Asian, and eastern Asian populations, the disorder does exist in these populations as well (Fig. 432.1).

CF is inherited as an autosomal recessive trait. The CF gene codes for the CFTR protein, which is 1,480 amino acids. CFTR is expressed largely in epithelial cells of airways, the gastrointestinal tract (including the pancreas and biliary system), the sweat glands, and the genitourinary system. CFTR is a member of the adenosine triphosphate–binding cassette superfamily of proteins. It functions as a chloride channel and has other regulatory functions that are perturbed variably by the different mutations. More than 1,900 *CFTR* polymorphisms have been described, many of which are not clearly of clinical significance. Those that are associated with clinical manifestations may be grouped into 6 main classes based upon how they impact upon protein structure and function (Table 432.2; Fig. 432.2). Mutation class I-III are generally considered to

Table 432.1	Complications of Cystic Fibrosis

RESPIRATORY
Bronchiectasis, bronchitis, bronchiolitis, pneumonia
Atelectasis
Hemoptysis
Pneumothorax
Nasal polyps
Sinusitis
Reactive airway disease
Mucoid impaction of the bronchi
Allergic bronchopulmonary aspergillosis
Cor pulmonale
Respiratory failure

GASTROINTESTINAL
Meconium ileus, meconium plug (neonate)
Meconium peritonitis (neonate)
Distal intestinal obstruction syndrome (non-neonatal obstruction)
Rectal prolapse
Intussusception
Volvulus
Fibrosing colonopathy (strictures)
Appendicitis
Intestinal atresia
Pancreatitis
Biliary cirrhosis (portal hypertension: esophageal varices, hypersplenism)
Neonatal obstructive jaundice
Hepatic steatosis
Gastroesophageal reflux
Cholelithiasis
Inguinal hernia
Growth failure (malabsorption)
Vitamin deficiency states (vitamins A, K, E, D)
Insulin deficiency, symptomatic hyperglycemia, diabetes
Malignancy (rare)

OTHER
Infertility
Delayed puberty
Edema-hypoproteinemia
Dehydration–heat exhaustion
Hypertrophic osteoarthropathy-arthritis
Clubbing
Amyloidosis
Diabetes mellitus
Aquagenic palmoplantar keratoderma (skin wrinkling)

Adapted from Silverman FN, Kuhn JP: *Essentials of Caffey's pediatric x-ray diagnosis*, Chicago, 1990, Year Book, p. 649.

be *severe* mutations in that they lead to a complete or nearly complete absence of CFTR function, whereas class IV-VI mutations are associated with some residual functional protein. The most prevalent mutation of *CFTR* is the deletion of a single phenylalanine residue at amino acid 508 (F508del). This mutation is responsible for the high incidence of CF in northern European populations and is considerably less frequent in other populations, such as those of southern Europe and Israel. Nearly 50% of individuals with CF in the United States Cystic Fibrosis Foundation (CFF) Patient Registry are homozygous for F508del, and approximately 87% carry at least 1 F508del gene. Remaining patients have an extensive array of mutations, none of which has a prevalence of more than several percentage points, except in certain populations; for example, the W1282X mutation occurs in 60% of Ashkenazi Jews with CF. Through the use of probes for 40 of the most common mutations, the genotype of 80–90% of Americans with CF can be ascertained. Genotyping using a discreet panel of mutation probes is quick and less costly than more comprehensive sequencing and is the approach typically used in state newborn screening programs. In remaining patients, sequencing the entire *CFTR* gene and looking for deletions and duplications are necessary

to establish the genotype. As sequencing technologies evolve and costs decrease, sequencing the entire *CFTR* gene may become mainstream for all patients.

The relationship between CFTR genotype and clinical phenotype is highly complex. CFTR mutation class is strongly associated with pancreatic dysfunction and will usually predict this manifestation in any given patient. Respiratory complications and lung function decline are also correlated with mutation class severity but with greater variation due to the influence of non-CFTR modifier gene polymorphisms and environmental influences on the manifestations of lung disease in any one individual. Studies have identified specific non-CFTR modifier genes of importance; genome-wide association studies identified a polymorphism on chromosome 11 in the intergenic region between *EHF* (an epithelial transcription factor) and *APIP* (an inhibitor of apoptosis) that is associated with lung disease severity and may influence the expression of *EHF* and *APIP*, as well as other genes in the region, including *PDHX, CD44,* and *ELF5*. A region on chromosome 20 may also be found to relate to lung disease severity. This region encompasses several genes *(MC3R, CASS4, AURKA)* that may play a role in lung host defense involving neutrophil function, apoptosis, and phagocytosis. Genome-wide association studies analysis also identified genetic regions that predispose to risk for liver disease, CF-related diabetes, and meconium ileus.

The high-frequency of *CFTR* mutations has been ascribed to resistance to the morbidity and mortality associated with infectious dysenteries through the ages. Cultured CF intestinal epithelial cells homozygous for the F508del mutation are unresponsive to the secretory effects of cholera toxin. CFTR heterozygous mice experience less mortality when treated with cholera toxin than their unaffected wild-type littermates.

PATHOGENESIS
A number of long-standing observations of CF are of fundamental pathophysiologic importance; they include failure to clear mucous secretions, a paucity of water in mucous secretions, an elevated salt content of sweat and other serous secretions, and chronic infection limited to the respiratory tract. In addition, there is a greater negative potential difference across the respiratory epithelia of patients with CF than across the respiratory epithelia of control subjects. Aberrant electrical properties are also demonstrated for CF sweat gland duct and rectal epithelia. The membranes of CF epithelial cells are unable to secrete chloride or bicarbonate in response to cyclic adenosine monophosphate–mediated signals, and at least in the respiratory epithelial cells, excessive amounts of sodium are absorbed through these membranes. These defects can be traced to a dysfunction of CFTR. CFTR function is highly regulated and energy dependent; it requires both cyclic adenosine monophosphate–stimulated protein kinase A phosphorylation of the regulatory domain and ATP binding and hydrolysis at the nucleotide binding domains. CFTR also interacts with other ion channels, signal transduction proteins, and the cytoskeleton (Fig. 432.3 and see Fig. 432.2).

Many hypotheses have been postulated to explain how CFTR dysfunction results in the clinical phenotype (Fig. 432.4). It is likely that no one hypothesis explains the full spectrum of disease. One model is that airway hydration homeostasis requires both CFTR and P2Y$_2$-regulated calcium-activated chloride secretion. When extracellular ATP is depleted such as after viral infections, calcium-activated chloride secretion is not activated and the failure of mutant CFTR chloride secretion results in dehydrated airway secretions, increased concentration of mucin solids, and more viscoelastic mucus that is not cleared by normal mucociliary transport. Another mechanism that is supported by both primary human airway studies and investigations in the CF pig is that mutant CFTR causes failure of HCO_3^- secretion and a more acidic airway surface liquid, which increases mucous viscoelasticity resulting in poor mucociliary clearance. Mucous secretions are tethered to submucosal gland ducts and are retained and obstruct airways, starting with those of the smallest caliber, the bronchioles. Airflow obstruction at the level of small airways is the earliest observable physiologic abnormality of the respiratory system. CFTR dysfunction in airway smooth muscle has been implicated in tracheal and airway abnormalities in humans and in animal models

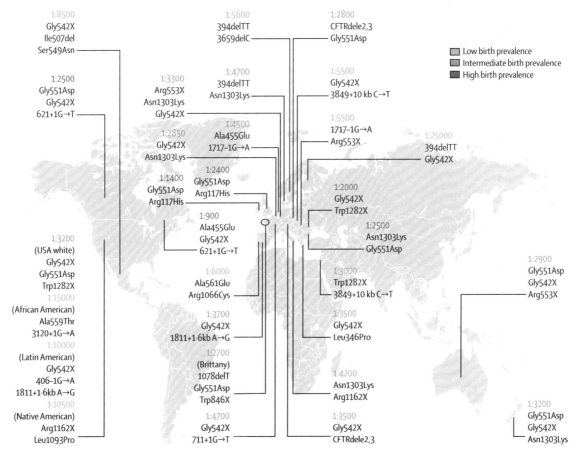

Fig. 432.1 Approximate cystic fibrosis birth prevalence and common mutations for selected countries. Birth prevalence is reported as number of live births per case of cystic fibrosis. Common/important mutations in each region are listed below the prevalence figures. The birth prevalence can vary greatly among ethnic groups in a country. *(From O'Sullivan BP, Freedman SD: Cystic fibrosis,* Lancet *373:1891–1902, 2009.)*

Table 432.2	One Proposed Classification of Cystic Fibrosis Transmembrane Conductance Regulator (CFTR) Mutations		
CLASS	**EFFECT ON CFTR**	**FUNCTIONAL CFTR PRESENT?**	**SAMPLE MUTATIONS**
I	Lack of protein production	No	Stop codons (designation in X; e.g., Trp1282X, Gly542X); splicing defects with no protein production (e.g., 711+1G→T, 1717-1G→A)
II	Defect in protein trafficking with ubiquitination and degradation in endoplasmic reticulum/ Golgi body	No/substantially reduced	Phe508del, Asn1303Lys, Gly85Gly, leu1065Pro, Asp507, Ser549Arg
III	Defective regulation; CFTR not activated by adenosine triphosphate or cyclic adenosine monophosphate	No (nonfunction CFTR present in apical membrane)	Gly551Asp, Ser492Phe, Val520Phe, Arg553Gly, Arg560Thr, Arg560Ser
IV	Reduced chloride transport through CFTR at the apical membrane	Yes	Ala455Glu, Arg117Cys, Asp1152His, Leu227Arg, Arg334Trp, Arg117His*
V	Splicing defect with reduced production of CFTR	Yes	3849+10kbC→T, 1811+16kbA→G, IVS8-5T, 2789+5G→A

*Function of Arg117His depends on the length of the polythymidine track on the same chromosome in intron 8 (IVS8): 5T, 7T, or 9T. There is more normal CFTR function with a longer polythymidine track.
From O'Sullivan BP, Freedman SD: Cystic fibrosis, *Lancet* 373:1891–1902, 2009.

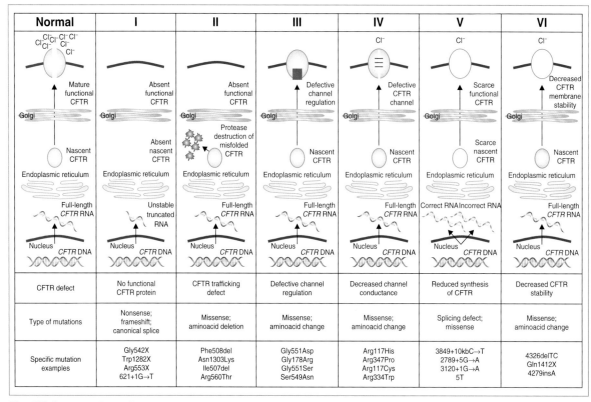

Fig. 432.2 Classes of cystic fibrosis transmembrane conductance regulator *(CFTR)* mutations. Mutations in the *CFTR* gene can be divided into 6 classes. Class I mutations result in no protein production. Class II mutations (including the most prevalent, Phe508del) cause retention of a misfolded protein at the endoplasmic reticulum and subsequent degradation in the proteasome. Class III mutations affect channel regulation, impairing channel opening (e.g., Gly551Asp). Class IV mutants show reduced conduction—that is, decreased flow of ions (e.g., Arg117His). Class V mutations cause substantial reduction in mRNA or protein, or both, Class VI mutations cause substantial plasma membrane instability and include Phe508del when rescued by most correctors (rPhe508del). *(From Boyle MP, De Boeck K: A new era in the treatment of cystic fibrosis: correction of the underlying CFTR defect,* Lancet Respir Med *1:158–63, 2013.)*

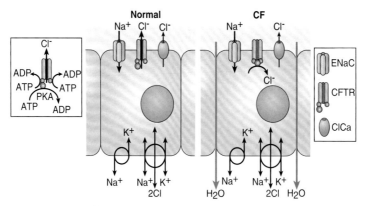

Fig. 432.3 Schematic diagram depicting cystic fibrosis *(CF)* epithelial channel defects, characterized by impaired chloride secretion, massive sodium absorption, and movement of water through the epithelium, leading to a dehydrated airway surface. *ADP,* Adenosine diphosphate; *ATP,* adenosine triphosphate; *CFTR,* cystic fibrosis transmembrane conductance regulator; *ClCa,* alternative chloride channel; *ENaC,* epithelium sodium channel; *PKA,* protein kinase A. *(From Michelson P, Faro A, Ferkol T: Pulmonary disease in cystic fibrosis. In Kendig's Disorders of the Respiratory Tract in Children, ed 9, Philadelphia, 2019, Elsevier, [Fig. 51.1, p. 778].)*

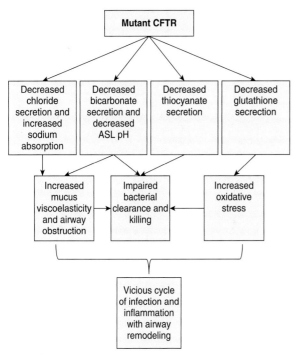

Fig. 432.4 Schema of mutant cystic fibrosis transmembrane conductance regulator (CFTR) mechanisms of chronic airway disease. CFTR conducts several anions including chloride, bicarbonate, thiocyanate, and gluta-thione. The loss of CFTR function impacts critical airway epithelial functions: (1) It increases the risk for dehydration of airway surface liquid (ASL) with loss of chloride efflux and associated increased sodium channel activity. (2) The loss of secreted bicarbonate and/or acidic pH of the ASL increases mucous viscoelasticity resulting in failure of mucociliary transport. (3) Acidic pH in the ASL impairs normal innate immune clearance of bacteria. (4) Loss of thiocyanate impairs lactoperoxidase bacterial killing. (5) Loss of glutathione secretion depletes the antioxidant capacity of the airway resulting in increased inflammation, increased mucous secretion, and increased mucous viscoelasticity. These factors lead to a vicious cycle of infection and inflammation that is progressive.

of the disease (pig and mice). These data suggest that CFTR expression in this nonepithelial tissue contributes to airway constriction.

It is plausible that similar pathophysiologic events take place in the pancreatic and biliary ducts (and in the vas deferens), leading to desiccation of proteinaceous secretions and obstruction. Because the function of sweat gland duct cells is to absorb rather than secrete chloride, salt is not retrieved from the isotonic primary sweat as it is transported to the skin surface; chloride and sodium levels are consequently elevated.

Chronic infection in CF is limited to the airways. One explanation for infection is a sequence of events starting with failure to clear inhaled bacteria promptly and then proceeding to persistent infection and an inflammatory response in airway walls. Another explanation for early infection is the failure of innate immune proteins to kill bacteria in an abnormally acidic airway milieu. In addition, it has been proposed that abnormal CFTR creates a proinflammatory state or amplifies the inflammatory response to initial infections (viral or bacterial). Some investigators have identified primary differences in CF-affected immune cells (including macrophage, neutrophils, lymphocytes, and dendritic cells) and have suggested that these alterations contribute to this proinflammatory state as well as a dysregulated immune response. It appears that inflammatory events occur first in small airways, perhaps because it is more difficult to clear altered secretions and microorganisms from these regions. The agents of airway injury include neutrophil products, such as oxidative radicals and proteases, and immune reaction products. These inflammatory products further aggravate airway obstruction by increasing mucin secretion and altering

mucin structure to promote both intramolecular and intermolecular interactions. Excessive inflammatory cell polymers in CF sputum, including DNA, filamentous actin, and glycosaminoglycans, further contribute to abnormal mucous viscoelastic properties and airway obstruction. Chronic bronchiolitis and bronchitis are the initial lung manifestations (see Chapter 418), but after months to years, structural changes in airway walls produce bronchiolectasis and **bronchiectasis**. With advanced lung disease, infection may extend to peribronchial lung parenchyma.

A central feature of lung disease in patients with CF is the high prevalence of airway infection with **Staphylococcus aureus** (see Chapter 208.1), **Pseudomonas aeruginosa** (see Chapter 232.1), and **Burkholderia cepacia complex** (see Chapter 232.2), organisms that rarely infect the lungs of other individuals. It has been postulated that the CF airway epithelial cells or surface liquids may provide a favorable environment for harboring these organisms. CF airway epithelium may be compromised in its innate defenses against these organisms, through either acquired or genetic alterations. Antimicrobial activity is diminished in CF secretions; this diminution may be related to hyperacidic surface liquids or other effects on innate immunity. Another puzzle is the propensity for P. aeruginosa to undergo mucoid transformation in the CF airways. The complex polysaccharide produced by these organisms generates a biofilm that provides a hypoxic environment and thereby protects Pseudomonas against antimicrobial agents.

Altered lipid homeostasis has been implicated as a predisposing factor for respiratory tract infection and inflammation. Concentrations of lipoxins—molecules that suppress neutrophilic inflammation—are suppressed in CF airways. There is an imbalance of lipids with increased arachidonic acid and decreased docosahexaenoic acid, which promotes inflammation. There is also an imbalance of ceramide in the CF airway that is proinflammatory. Supporting the idea that altered lipid uptake affects infection and inflammation is the observation that the 10–15% of individuals with CF who retain substantial exocrine pancreatic function have delayed acquisition of P. aeruginosa and slower deterioration of lung function. However, it appears that nutritional factors are contributory only because preservation of pancreatic function does not preclude development of typical lung disease.

The variation in progression of lung disease seen in patients with CF is largely influenced by social and physical environment factors, whose impact matches that of CFTR genotype. Exposure to environmental tobacco smoke and outdoor air pollutants, and early acquisition of respiratory virus infections, as well as pathogenic organisms like P. aeruginosa and methicillin-resistant S. aureus, have been implicated as causes of worsening disease. Sex/gender disparities also seem to exist, with females having a poorer prognosis. Although studies have suggested that estrogen may influence disease exacerbations, the gap seems to be narrowing in the past decade.

Although most CF care is delivered at specialty centers and is broadly influenced by current clinical guidelines, there is enough variability in treatment approaches to cause large variation in respiratory and nutritional outcomes across the care networks in both North America and Europe. Social determinants of health are associated with significant disparities in outcome; socioeconomic status has been shown to be a strong predictor of mortality, as well as both nutritional status and lung function on both sides of the Atlantic. The specific mechanism of effect is unclear, but evidence suggests a role for socioeconomic status–related differences in health behaviors and disease self-management practices, stress and mental health issues, and environmental tobacco smoke exposure. Differential access to specialty care and medications is not a major factor in North American children (lack of insurance in some adults is a problem); however, differences in disease outcomes across European countries of varying wealth are quite clear.

PATHOLOGY

The earliest pathologic lesion in the lung is that of **bronchiolitis** (mucous plugging and an inflammatory response in the walls of the small airways); with time, mucous accumulation and inflammation extend to the larger airways (**bronchitis**) (see Chapter 418.2). Goblet cell hyperplasia and submucosal gland hypertrophy become prominent pathologic findings, which is most likely a response to chronic airway infection. Organisms appear to be confined to the endobronchial space; invasive bacterial infection is not characteristic. With long-standing disease, evidence of airway destruction such as **bronchiolar obliteration, bronchiolectasis**, and **bronchiectasis** (see Chapter 430) becomes prominent. Imaging modalities demonstrate both increased airway wall thickness and luminal cross-sectional area relatively early in lung disease evaluation. Bronchiectatic cysts and emphysematous bullae or subpleural blebs are frequent with advanced lung disease, the upper lobes being most commonly involved. These enlarged air spaces may rupture and cause pneumothorax. Interstitial disease is not a prominent feature, although areas of fibrosis appear eventually. Bronchial arteries are enlarged and tortuous, contributing to a propensity for hemoptysis in bronchiectatic airways. Small pulmonary arteries eventually display medial hypertrophy, which would be expected in secondary pulmonary hypertension.

The **paranasal sinuses** are uniformly filled with secretions containing inflammatory products, and the epithelial lining displays hyperplastic and hypertrophied secretory elements (see Chapter 408). Polypoid lesions within the sinuses and erosion of bone have been reported. The nasal mucosa may form large or multiple **polyps**, usually from a base surrounding the ostia of the maxillary and ethmoidal sinuses.

The **pancreas** is usually small, occasionally cystic, and often difficult to find at postmortem examination. The extent of involvement varies at birth. In infants, the acini and ducts are often distended and filled with eosinophilic material. In 85–90% of patients, the lesion progresses to complete or almost complete disruption of acini and replacement with fibrous tissue and fat. Infrequently, foci of calcification may be seen on radiographs of the abdomen. The islets of Langerhans contain normal-appearing β cells, although they may begin to show architectural disruption by fibrous tissue in the 2nd decade of life.

The **intestinal tract** shows only minimal changes. Esophageal and duodenal glands are often distended with mucous secretions. Concretions may form in the appendiceal lumen or cecum. Crypts of the appendix and rectum may be dilated and filled with secretions.

Focal biliary cirrhosis secondary to blockage of intrahepatic bile ducts is uncommon in early life, although it is responsible for occasional cases of prolonged neonatal jaundice. This lesion becomes much more prevalent and extensive with age and is found in 70% of patients at postmortem examination. This process can proceed to symptomatic multilobular biliary cirrhosis that has a distinctive pattern of large irregular parenchymal nodules and interspersed bands of fibrous tissue. Approximately 30–70% of patients have fatty infiltration of the liver, in some cases despite apparently adequate nutrition. At autopsy, hepatic congestion secondary to cor pulmonale is frequently observed. The gallbladder may be hypoplastic and filled with mucoid material and often contains stones. The epithelial lining often displays extensive mucous metaplasia. Atresia of the cystic duct and stenosis of the distal common bile duct have been observed.

Glands of the **uterine cervix** are distended with mucus, copious amounts of which collect in the cervical canal. In >95% of males, the body and tail of the epididymis, the vas deferens, and the seminal vesicles are obliterated or atretic, resulting in male infertility.

CLINICAL MANIFESTATIONS
Since the universal adoption of CF newborn screening in the United States and overseas, as well as the evolution of aggressive and proactive treatment approaches, the clinical face of CF is very different from what it was in earlier decades. Diagnosis is typically accomplished before 1 mo of age, prior to any obvious clinical symptoms or signs, and treatment is targeted on immediately correcting nutritional deficiencies and delaying the respiratory complications of the disease. The interaction of mutational heterogeneity and environmental factors leads to highly variable involvement of the lungs, pancreas, and other organs. A summary of the time course of potential development of clinical manifestations is shown in Fig. 432.5.

Respiratory Tract
Infants diagnosed by CF newborn screening are generally asymptomatic from a respiratory standpoint. Nonetheless, the majority are infected with *S. aureus*, *Haemophilus influenza*, or even *P. aeruginosa* within the 1st mo of life, and chest CT scans show characteristic heterogeneous air trapping in ⅔ of infants by their first birthday, and bronchiectasis is found in more than 10% of 1 yr olds and ~60% of 5 yr olds. The earliest symptom is usually cough that may begin with a viral respiratory tract infection but then persists unless treated with antibiotics. With treatment, the generally realized goal is for patients to remain asymptomatic throughout childhood, except for the periodic development of cough, chest congestion, sputum production, and/or wheezing that define a *pulmonary exacerbation*.

The rate of progression of lung disease is the chief determinant of morbidity and mortality. As lung disease slowly progresses, chronic cough, sputum production, exercise intolerance, shortness of breath,

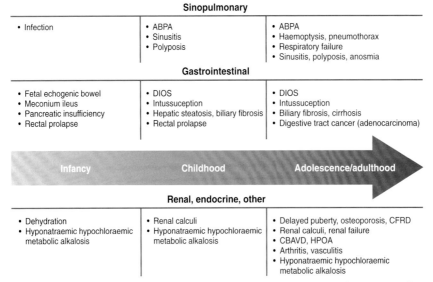

Fig. 432.5 Approximate age of onset of clinical manifestations of cystic fibrosis. *ABPA*, Allergic bronchopulmonary aspergillosis; *CBAVD*, congenital bilateral absence of the vas deferens; *CFRD*, cystic fibrosis–related diabetes mellitus; *DIOS*, distal intestinal obstruction syndrome; *HPOA*, hypertrophic pulmonary osteoarthritis. *(From O'Sullivan BP, Freedman SD: Cystic fibrosis, Lancet 373:1891–1902, 2009.)*

and failure to thrive are noted. Cor pulmonale, respiratory failure, and death eventually supervene unless lung transplantation is accomplished; this has become increasingly uncommon in childhood. Infection with certain strains of *B. cepacia* and other multidrug-resistant organisms may be associated with particularly rapid pulmonary deterioration and death.

Eventual physical findings include increased anteroposterior diameter of the chest, generalized hyperresonance, scattered or localized coarse crackles, and digital clubbing. Expiratory wheezes may be heard, a manifestation of airway inflammation and edema that may or may not be associated with bronchodilator responsiveness. Cyanosis is a late sign. Common pulmonary complications include atelectasis, hemoptysis, pneumothorax, and cor pulmonale; these usually appear in late adolescence or beyond.

Even though the paranasal sinuses are virtually always opacified radiographically, acute sinusitis is infrequent. Nasal obstruction and rhinorrhea are common, caused by inflamed, swollen mucous membranes or, in some cases, nasal polyposis. Nasal polyps are most troublesome between 5 and 20 yr of age.

Intestinal Tract
In 15–20% of newborn infants with CF, the ileum is completely obstructed by meconium (**meconium ileus**). The frequency is greater among siblings born subsequent to a child with meconium ileus and is particularly striking in monozygotic twins, reflecting a genetic contribution from one or more unknown modifying genes. Abdominal distention, emesis, and failure to pass meconium appear in the first 24-48 hr of life (see Chapters 123.1 and 356.2) and often requires surgical intervention. Abdominal radiographs (Fig. 432.6) show dilated loops of bowel with air-fluid levels and, frequently, a collection of granular, "ground-glass" material in the lower central abdomen. Rarely, **meconium peritonitis** results from intrauterine rupture of the bowel wall and can be detected radiographically as the presence of peritoneal or scrotal calcifications.

Ileal obstruction with fecal material (**distal intestinal obstruction syndrome [DIOS]**) occurs in older children, causing cramping abdominal pain, abdominal distention, and obstruction that can be treated with medical approaches to bowel evacuation.

More than 85% of children with CF have *exocrine* pancreatic insufficiency, causing protein and fat malabsorption. Symptoms, if untreated, include frequent, bulky, greasy stools and failure to gain weight even when food intake appears to be large. Weight gain can be challenging, but attainment of normal growth and development is an expectation of treatment. A protuberant abdomen, decreased muscle mass, poor growth, and delayed maturation are classic and rarely seen physical signs. Excessive flatus may be a problem. Supplementation with fat-soluble vitamin preparations has made deficiencies of vitamin A, E, and K unusual, but vitamin D deficiency continues to be prevalent and, although

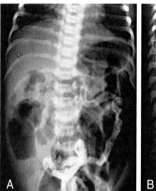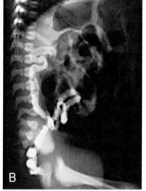

Fig. 432.6 A and **B,** Contrast enema study in a newborn infant with abdominal distention and failure to pass meconium. Notice the small diameter of the sigmoid and ascending colon and dilated, air-filled loops of small intestine. Several air-fluid levels in the small bowel are visible on the upright lateral view.

rickets is rare, osteoporosis is common, especially in older patients and those with more severe lung disease. Class IV-VI mutations are associated with pancreatic sufficiency, but patients with these mutations are prone to pancreatitis when they reach adolescence.

Historically a relatively common event, **rectal prolapse** occurs much less frequently as the result of earlier diagnosis and initiation of pancreatic enzyme replacement therapy.

Biliary Tract
Infants may occasionally present with **neonatal jaundice** suggestive of biliary obstruction. Evidence for liver dysfunction is most often detected in the first 15 yr of life and can be found in up to 30% of individuals. **Biliary cirrhosis** becomes symptomatic in only 5–7% of patients. Manifestations can include icterus, ascites, hematemesis from esophageal varices, and evidence of hypersplenism. Biliary colic secondary to cholelithiasis may occur in the 2nd decade or later. Liver disease occurs independent of genotype but is associated with meconium ileus and pancreatic insufficiency.

Cystic Fibrosis–Related Diabetes and Pancreatitis
Endocrine pancreatic insufficiency tends to develop in the 2nd decade and beyond and is more common in patients with a family history of type II diabetes mellitus. It most commonly begins with postprandial hyperglycemia and may or may not be accompanied by weight loss or flattening weight gain. Fasting hyperglycemia and elevated hemoglobin A_{1c} are later manifestations. Ketoacidosis usually does not occur, but eye, kidney, and other vascular complications have been noted in patients living ≥10 yr after the onset of hyperglycemia. Recurrent, acute pancreatitis occurs occasionally in individuals who have residual exocrine pancreatic function and may be the sole manifestation of homozygotic *CFTR* mutations.

Genitourinary Tract
Virtually all males are **azoospermic** because of failure of development of wolffian duct structures, but sexual function is generally unimpaired. The female fertility rate is diminished, especially in women who have poor nutrition or advanced lung disease. Pregnancy is generally tolerated well by women with good pulmonary function but may accelerate pulmonary progression in those with advanced lung problems and may lead to glucose intolerance. Urinary incontinence associated with cough occurs in 18–47% of female children and adolescents.

Sweat Glands
Excessive loss of salt in the sweat predisposes young children to salt depletion episodes, especially during episodes of gastroenteritis and during warm weather. These children may present with **hypochloremic alkalosis.** Hyponatremia is a risk particularly in warm climates. Frequently, parents notice salt *frosting* of the skin or a salty taste when they kiss the child. A few genotypes are associated with normal sweat chloride values.

DIAGNOSIS AND ASSESSMENT
The diagnosis of CF has been based on a positive quantitative sweat test ($Cl^- \geq 60$ mEq/L) in conjunction with one or more of the following features: identification of 2 CFTR mutations, typical chronic obstructive pulmonary disease, documented exocrine pancreatic insufficiency, and a positive family history. With newborn screening, diagnosis is often made prior to obvious clinical manifestations such as failure to thrive and chronic cough. Diagnostic criteria have been recommended to include additional testing procedures (Table 432.3).

Sweat Testing
The sweat test, which involves using pilocarpine iontophoresis to collect sweat and performing chemical analysis of its chloride content, is the standard approach to diagnosis of CF. The procedure requires care and accuracy. An electric current is used to carry pilocarpine into the skin of the forearm and locally stimulate the sweat glands. If an adequate amount of sweat is collected, the specimens are analyzed for chloride concentration. Infants with a positive newborn screen for CF should

Table 432.3	Diagnostic Criteria for Cystic Fibrosis (CF)

Presence of typical clinical features (respiratory, gastrointestinal, or genitourinary)
or
A history of CF in a sibling
or
A positive newborn screening test
plus
Laboratory evidence for CFTR (CF transmembrane regulator) dysfunction:
  Two elevated sweat chloride concentrations obtained on separate days
  or
  Identification of two CF mutations
  or
  An abnormal nasal potential difference measurement

have the sweat chloride testing performed after 36-wk corrected gestational age and at a weight greater than 2 kg and at age greater than 10 days to increase the likelihood of sufficient sweat collection for an accurate study. Positive results should be confirmed; for a negative result, the test should be repeated if suspicion of the diagnosis remains.

More than 60 mmol/L of chloride in sweat is diagnostic of CF when one or more other criteria are present. In individuals with a positive newborn screen, a sweat chloride level less than 30 mmol/L indicates that CF is unlikely. Borderline (or intermediate) values of 30-59 mmol/L have been reported in patients of all ages who have CF with atypical involvement and require further testing. Table 432.4 lists the conditions associated with false-negative and false-positive sweat test results.

DNA Testing

Several commercial laboratories test for 30-96 of the most common *CFTR* mutations. This testing identifies ≥90% of individuals who carry 2 CF mutations. Some children with typical CF manifestations are found to have 1 or no detectable mutations by this methodology. Some laboratories perform comprehensive mutation analysis screening for all the >1,900 identified mutations.

Table 432.4	Conditions Associated With False-Positive and False-Negative Sweat Test Results

WITH FALSE-POSITIVE RESULTS
Eczema (atopic dermatitis)
Ectodermal dysplasia
Malnutrition/failure to thrive/deprivation
Anorexia nervosa
Congenital adrenal hyperplasia
Adrenal insufficiency
Glucose-6-phosphatase deficiency
Mauriac syndrome
Fucosidosis
Familial hypoparathyroidism
Hypothyroidism
Nephrogenic diabetes insipidus
Pseudohypoaldosteronism
Klinefelter syndrome
Familial cholestasis syndrome
Autonomic dysfunction
Prostaglandin E infusions
Munchausen syndrome by proxy

WITH FALSE-NEGATIVE RESULTS
Dilution
Malnutrition
Edema
Insufficient sweat quantity
Hyponatremia
Cystic fibrosis transmembrane conductance regulator mutations with preserved sweat duct function

Other Diagnostic Tests

The finding of increased potential differences across nasal epithelium (nasal potential difference) that is the increased voltage response to topical amiloride application, followed by the absence of a voltage response to a β-adrenergic agonist, has been used to confirm the diagnosis of CF in patients with equivocal or frankly normal sweat chloride values. This testing is primarily used in research applications and has never undergone extensive validation as a clinical tool.

Pancreatic Function

The diagnosis of pancreatic malabsorption can be made by the quantification of *elastase-1 activity* in a fresh stool sample by an enzyme-linked immunosorbent assay specific for human elastase. The quantification of fat malabsorption with a 72-hr stool collection is rarely necessary in the clinical setting. CF-related diabetes affects approximately 20% of adolescents and 40-50% of adults, and clinical guidelines recommend yearly oral glucose tolerance testing (OGTT) after age 10. OGTT may sometimes be clinically indicated at an earlier age. Spot testing of blood and urine glucose levels and glycosylated hemoglobin levels are not sufficiently sensitive.

Radiology

Hyperinflation of lungs occurs early and is often accompanied by nonspecific peribronchial thickening (Fig. 432.7). Bronchial thickening and plugging and ring shadows suggesting bronchiectasis usually appear first in the upper lobes. Nodular densities, patchy atelectasis, and confluent infiltrate follow. Hilar lymph nodes may be prominent. With advanced disease, impressive hyperinflation with markedly depressed diaphragms, anterior bowing of the sternum, and a narrow cardiac shadow are noted. Cyst formation, extensive bronchiectasis, dilated pulmonary artery segments, and segmental or lobar atelectasis is often apparent with advanced disease. Most CF centers obtain chest radiographs (posteroanterior [PA] and lateral) at least annually. Standardized scoring of radiologic changes has been used to follow progression of lung disease. CT of the chest can detect heterogeneous hyperinflation and localized thickening of bronchial airway walls, mucous plugging, focal hyperinflation, and early bronchiectasis (Fig. 432.8). CT abnormalities are commonly seen at a young age, even in asymptomatic children with normal lung function.

Radiographs of paranasal sinuses reveal panopacification and, often, failure of frontal sinus development. CT provides better resolution of sinus changes if this information is required clinically. Fetal ultrasonography may show pancreatic changes indicative of CF and suggest ileal obstruction with meconium early in the second trimester, but this finding is not predictive of meconium ileus at birth.

Pulmonary Function

Infant pulmonary function testing is done routinely for clinical evaluation at a few CF centers but, given its complexity and the need for sedation, for the most part it is reserved for research protocols. Lung clearance index (LCI) measured by multiple breath washout can be done in infants and young children and is a sensitive measure of ventilation inhomogeneity caused by small airways disease. Currently it is primarily used for research, but given its ease and applicability it may be adopted as a standard monitoring tool in the future as CF care centers become more accustomed to its use.

Standard pulmonary function studies are usually obtained starting at about 4 yr of age and are routinely done by age 6. **Forced expiratory volume in 1 sec** (FEV_1) is the measurement that has been shown to correlate most closely with mortality and shows a gradual decline averaging 2-3% per year throughout childhood. Although a small number of children may already show evidence of airway obstruction by age 6, trends over the past several decades, as reported by the CFF patient registry, show a steady improvement in average FEV1 of the CF population, and as of 2015 ~75% had normal or near-normal lung function at age 18 yr. Residual volume and functional residual capacity are increased early in the course of lung disease and are the cause of decreasing forced vital capacity (FVC) measurement. Restrictive changes, characterized by declining total lung capacity and vital capacity, correlate

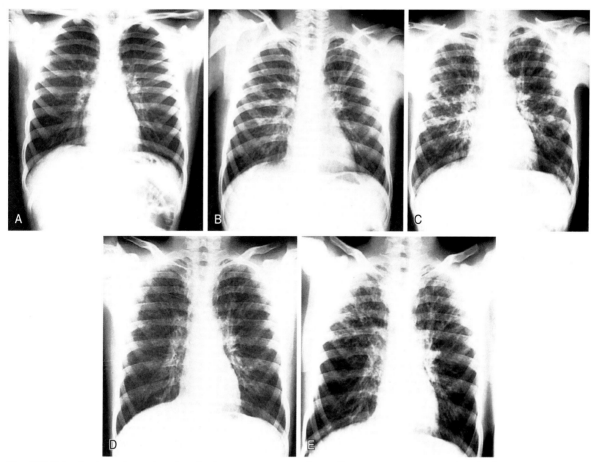

Fig. 432.7 Serial radiographs in a boy show the changing appearance of cystic fibrosis over 6 yr. **A,** At 9 yr, frontal radiograph shows minimal peribronchial thickening and hyperaerated lungs indistinguishable from asthma. **B,** Nineteen mo later, the radiographic picture has worsened considerably. Extensive peribronchial thickening is now noted. Mucoid impaction of the bronchus is seen in the left upper lobe and hilar shadows have become abnormally prominent. **C,** Ten mo later, further deterioration is obvious. Widespread typical changes of cystic fibrosis (CF) are noted throughout both lungs. **D,** Follow-up studies show considerable improvement, which suggested that some of the changes evident on **C** were from superimposed infection. **E,** One yr later, note the progressive changes of CF—most severe in the upper lobes bilaterally. *(From Long FR, Druhan SM, Kuhn JP. Diseases of the bronchi and pulmonary aeration. In Slovis TL, editor: Caffey's pediatric diagnostic imaging, ed 11, Philadelphia, 2008, Mosby, Fig. 73-54.)*

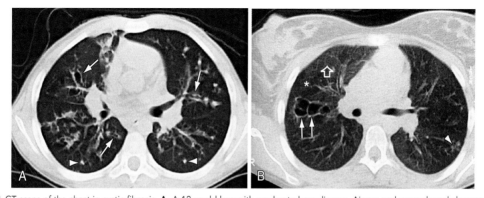

Fig. 432.8 CT scans of the chest in cystic fibrosis. **A,** A 12 yr old boy with moderate lung disease. Airway and parenchymal changes are present throughout both lungs. Multiple areas of bronchiectasis *(arrows)* and mucous plugging *(arrowheads)* can be seen. **B,** A 19 yr old girl has mostly normal lung with 1 area of saccular bronchiectasis in the right upper lobe *(arrows)* and a focal area of peripheral mucous plugging in the right lower lobe *(arrowhead)*. Lung density is heterogeneous with areas of normal lung *(open arrow)* and areas of low attenuation reflecting segmental and subsegmental air trapping *(asterisk)*.

with extensive lung injury and fibrosis and are a late finding. Testing at each clinic visit is recommended to evaluate the course of the pulmonary involvement and allow for early intervention when clinically significant decrements are documented—this is probably the most sensitive indicator of a pulmonary exacerbation that should be treated with systemic antibiotics.

Microbiologic Studies

H. influenza and *S. aureus* are the most common organisms recovered in young children (Fig. 432.9). *Pseudomonas* may be acquired early and is eventually an organism of key significance. *P. aeruginosa* appears to have a special propensity for the CF airway and over time characteristically develops a biofilm associated with a mucoid appearance in the microbiology lab and which correlates with more rapid progression of lung disease. Once *P. aeruginosa* develops a mucoid phenotype, it is extremely difficult to eradicate from the airway. A wide range of other organisms are frequently recovered, particularly in advanced lung disease; they include a variety of Gram-negative rods including the *Burkholderia cepacia* complex, which may be associated with a fulminant downhill course (the cepacia syndrome); *Stenotrophomonas maltophilia*, and *Achromobacter xylosoxidans*; assorted fungi, especially *Aspergillus fumigatus*, which is most important due to the relatively common development of **allergic bronchopulmonary aspergillosis**; and nontuberculous mycobacterial species, especially *Mycobacterium avium* complex and *Mycobacterium abscessus*. Airway cultures are obtained regularly, most typically using oropharyngeal swabs in young children, and then sputum (which may be induced) in older children capable of expectoration. Oropharyngeal swabs typically give a good indication of the lower airway flora, but fiberoptic bronchoscopy may be used to gather lower respiratory tract secretions of infants and young children who do not expectorate if there is a concern for false-negative cultures, especially regarding the presence of *P. aeruginosa*.

The CF airway microbiome consists of a large number of additional organisms, especially anaerobes that are identified through antigen detection but not culture methods. The significance of this finding and its therapeutic implications remain somewhat unclear, but it has long been appreciated that response to antibiotic treatment of pulmonary exacerbations is not always predictable based upon culture and sensitivity of airway cultures.

Newborn Screening

Newborn screening for CF is mandated in all 50 states and is the most common way that CF is diagnosed. A variety of newborn screening algorithms are in place to identify infants with CF. Most algorithms use a combination of immunoreactive trypsinogen (IRT) results and limited DNA testing on blood spots; because not all mutations can be found using this approach, babies with an elevated IRT and a single detected mutation are considered a positive screen, and all positive

screens are followed by a confirmatory sweat analysis. Depending upon race and ethnicity, about 10–15% of infants with a positive screen based on the finding of only 1 CF mutation will be found to have CF. This screening test is ≈95% sensitive and should result in a median age at diagnosis of less than 1 mo. Newborn diagnoses can prevent early nutritional deficiencies and improve long-term growth and may improve cognitive function. Importantly, good nutritional status (50 percentile weight for length or 50 percentile body mass index) is associated with better lung function at 6 yr of age.

An occasional patient may be missed by newborn screening, and those caring for adolescents and adults need to be aware that most of those older patients were not screened at birth and may present at later ages, into late adulthood. Prior to the advent of newborn screening, infants and children commonly presented with malabsorption and failure to thrive, in addition to respiratory symptoms. Most older patients whose diagnosis was missed early in life will have unusual class IV, V, or VI mutations and therefore *normal* pancreatic function. They will more typically present with chronic productive cough due to either bronchitis or chronic sinusitis and may have nasal polyps or allergic bronchopulmonary aspergillosis or unexplained bronchiectasis. The most common nonrespiratory manifestations will be congenital bilateral absence of the vas deferens (CBAVD) (in males) or recurrent pancreatitis. It is important to recognize that sweat testing at an adept lab (typically limited to CF Foundation accredited care centers) is the most accurate way to diagnose CF in this group. CFTR mutation testing with standard panels is never as sensitive as sweat testing and will frequently miss the unusual mutations that are seen more commonly in people who present late in this manner.

There is a subset of infants with a positive newborn screen for CF who have a nondiagnostic sweat chloride (30-59 mmol/L) and/or 1 or 2 CFTR mutations that is not clearly disease causing. These infants have **CFTR-related metabolic syndrome (CRMS)** (also called CFTR-related disease) and should be followed in a CF center closely through the 1st yr and then annually to evaluate them for the development of CF symptoms. Indeed, in some (~10%) patients, the sweat test becomes clearly abnormal over time and they can be diagnosed as having CF. Because CRMS is a condition defined by asymptomatic detection in the context of newborn screening and CF newborn screening has been commonly performed only in the past decade or so, it is not clear whether some children in this group will eventually develop manifestations of CFTR-related disorder, such as CBAVD, chronic sinusitis, recurrent pancreatitis, or even bronchiectasis. An approach to the evaluation of patients with CRMS is seen in Fig. 432.10.

TREATMENT
General Approach to Care

Initial efforts after diagnosis should be intensive and should include baseline assessment, initiation of treatment to prevent pulmonary

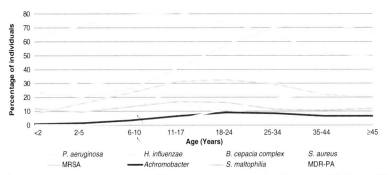

Fig. 432.9 Prevalence of respiratory microorganisms by age cohort. In young patients, early colonization with *Haemophilus influenza* and *Staphylococcus aureus* take place. Over time, *Pseudomonas aeruginosa* is detected in respiratory cultures and may become chronic. *P. aeruginosa* may change over time to become mucoidy, and *P. aeruginosa* is at risk for becoming multidrug resistant *(MDR)*. Other organisms may infect the CF airway including methicillin-resistant *S. aureus (MRSA)*, *Achromobacter*, *Burkholderia cepacia* complex, and *Stenotrophomonas maltophilia*. (From the Cystic Fibrosis Foundation Patient Registry 2015. Annual Data Report. ©2016 Cystic Fibrosis Foundation, Bethesda, Maryland.)

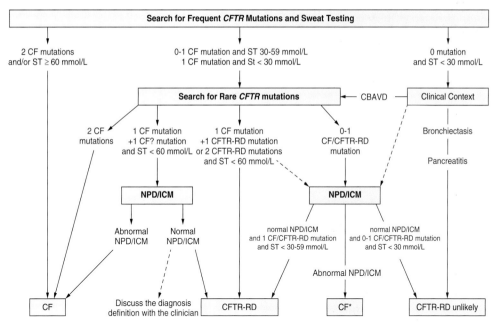

Fig. 432.10 2015 European Cystic Fibrosis Society recommended process for diagnosis of CFTR-RD. Global diagnostic algorithm for CF and CFTR-RD. A global flow-chart of genetic and functional diagnostic testing in CF and CFTR-RD is presented. *CBAVD*, congenital bilateral absence of the vas deferens; *CF*, cystic fibrosis; *CF? mutation*, mutation of unproven or uncertain clinical significance; *CF**, diagnosis of CF or consider this diagnosis; *CFTR*, cystic fibrosis transmembrane conductance regulator; *CFTR-RD*, CFTR-related disorders; *ICM*, intestinal current measurement; *NPD*, nasal potential difference; *ST*, sweat test (repeated; false positive should be excluded/sought in a specialized center). *(From Bombieri C, Claustres M, De Boeck K, Derichs N, Dodge J, Girodon E, et al. Recommendations for the classification of diseases as CFTR-related disorders, J Cyst Fibros 10(Suppl 2):S86–102, 2011. Fig 1.)*

involvement in young infants or reverse it in those diagnosed later, nutritional maintenance or remediation, and education of the patient and parents. Follow-up evaluations are scheduled every 1-3 mo, depending on the age at diagnosis, because many aspects of the condition require careful monitoring. An interval history and physical examination should be obtained at each visit. A sputum sample or, if that is not available, a lower pharyngeal swab taken during or after a forced cough is obtained for culture and antibiotic susceptibility studies. Because irreversible loss of pulmonary function from low-grade infection can occur gradually and without acute symptoms, emphasis is placed on a thorough pulmonary history and physical exam and routine pulmonary function testing. Table 432.5 lists symptoms and signs that suggest the need for more intensive antibiotic and physical therapy (PT). Protection against exposure to methicillin-resistant *S. aureus, P. aeruginosa, B. cepacia,* and other resistant Gram-negative organisms is essential, including contact isolation procedures and careful attention to cleaning of inhalation therapy equipment. A nurse, physical therapist, respiratory therapist, social worker, and dietitian, as members of the multidisciplinary care team, should evaluate children regularly and contribute to the development of a comprehensive daily care plan. Considerable education and programs to empower families and older children to take responsibility for care are likely to result in the best adherence to daily care programs. Screening patients and caregivers for anxiety and depression annually is expected to identify issues that can interfere with adherence to daily care. Standardization of practice, on the part of both caregivers and families, as well as close monitoring and early intervention for new or increasing symptoms appears to result in the best long-term outcomes.

Because secretions of CF patients are not adequately hydrated, attention in early childhood to oral hydration, especially during warm weather or with acute gastroenteritis, may minimize complications associated with impaired mucous clearance. Intravenous therapy for dehydration should be initiated early.

The goal of therapy is to maintain a stable condition for prolonged periods. This can be accomplished for most patients by interval evaluation and adjustments of the home treatment program. Some children have

Table 432.5	Symptoms and Signs Associated With Exacerbation of Pulmonary Infection in Patients With Cystic Fibrosis

SYMPTOMS

Increased frequency and duration of cough
Increased sputum production
Change in appearance of sputum
Increased shortness of breath
Decreased exercise tolerance
Decreased appetite
Feeling of increased congestion in the chest

SIGNS

Increased respiratory rate
Use of accessory muscles for breathing
Intercostal retractions
Change in results of auscultatory examination of chest
Decline in measures of pulmonary function consistent with the presence of obstructive airway disease
Fever and leukocytosis
Weight loss
New infiltrate on chest radiograph

From Ramsey B: Management of pulmonary disease in patients with cystic fibrosis, *N Engl J Med* 335:179, 1996.

episodic acute or low-grade chronic lung infection that progresses. For these patients, intensive inhalation and airway clearance and intravenous antibiotics are indicated. Improvement is most reliably accomplished in a hospital setting; selected patients have demonstrated successful outcomes while completing these treatments at home. Intravenous antibiotics may be required infrequently or as often as every 2-3 mo. The goal of treatment is to return patients to their previous pulmonary and functional status.

The basic daily care program varies according to the age of the child, the degree of pulmonary involvement, other system involvement, and the time available for therapy. The major components of this care are pulmonary and nutritional therapies. Because therapy is medication intensive, iatrogenic problems frequently arise. Monitoring for complications is also an important part of management

Pulmonary Therapy
The object of pulmonary therapy is to clear secretions from airways and to control infection. When a child is not doing well, every potentially useful aspect of therapy should be reconsidered.

Inhalation Therapy
Human recombinant DNase (2.5 mg) enzymatically dissolves extracellular DNA released by neutrophils, a major contributor to the characteristically sticky and viscous CF airway secretions. It is usually given as a single daily aerosol dose, improves pulmonary function, decreases the number of pulmonary exacerbations, and promotes a sense of well-being. Benefit for those with mild, moderate, and severe lung disease has been documented. Improvement is sustained for 12 mo or longer with continuous therapy.

Nebulized hypertonic saline, acting as a hyperosmolar agent, is believed to draw water into the airway and rehydrate mucus and the periciliary fluid layer, resulting in improved mucociliary clearance. Seven percent hypertonic saline nebulized 2-4 times daily increases mucous clearance and reduces pulmonary exacerbation, with only a slight short-term improvement in pulmonary function.

Airway Clearance Therapy
Airway clearance treatment begins in infancy with chest percussion (with or without postural drainage) and derives its rationale from the idea that cough clears mucus from large airways, but chest vibrations are required to shear secretions for the airway wall and move secretions from small airways, where expiratory flow rates are low. **Chest PT** can be particularly useful for patients with CF because they accumulate secretions in small airways first, even before the onset of symptoms. Cessation of chest PT in children with mild to moderate airflow limitation results in deterioration of lung function within 3 wk, and prompt improvement of function occurs when therapy is resumed, but it is less clear which available modality is best. Airway clearance therapy is recommended 2-4 times a day, depending on the severity of lung dysfunction, and usually increased during acute exacerbations. Cough, huffing, or forced expirations are encouraged intermittently throughout the session. Vest-type mechanical percussors *(high-frequency chest wall oscillation)* are commonly used past infancy due to their convenience, as are a variety of oscillatory positive expiratory pressure devices (such as Acapella and Aerobika) and other controlled breathing techniques (e.g., *autogenic drainage*). Routine aerobic exercise appears to slow the rate of decline of pulmonary function, and benefit has also been documented with weight training. No one airway clearance technique can be shown to be superior to any other, so all modes should be considered in the development of an airway clearance prescription. Adherence to daily therapy is important but rarely achieved; therefore airway clearance technique plans are individualized for each patient.

Antibiotic Therapy
Antibiotics are the mainstay of therapy designed to control progression of lung infection. The goal is to reduce the intensity of endobronchial infection and to delay progressive lung damage. The usual guidelines for acute chest infections, such as fever, tachypnea, or chest pain, are often absent. Consequently, all aspects of the patient's history and examination, including anorexia, weight loss, and diminished activity, must be used to guide the frequency and duration of therapy. Antibiotic treatment varies from intermittent short courses of 1 antibiotic to nearly continuous treatment with 1 or more antibiotics. Dosages for some antibiotics are often 2-3 times the amount recommended for minor infections because patients with CF have proportionately more lean body mass and higher clearance rates for many antibiotics than other

individuals. In addition, it is difficult to achieve effective drug levels of many antimicrobials in respiratory tract secretions.

Oral Antibiotic Therapy
Indications for oral antibiotic therapy in a patient with CF include the presence of respiratory tract symptoms, physical signs, or changes in pulmonary function testing or chest x-ray. Treatment is guided by identification of pathogenic organisms in respiratory tract cultures and in vitro sensitivity testing. Common organisms, including *S. aureus (MRSA or MSSA),* nontypeable *H. influenzae, P. aeruginosa; B. cepacia* and other Gram-negative rods, are encountered with increasing frequency. The usual course of therapy is 2 wk, and maximal doses are recommended. Table 432.6 lists useful oral antibiotics. The quinolones are the only broadly effective oral antibiotics for *Pseudomonas* infection, but resistance against these agents may emerge. Macrolides may reduce the virulence properties of *P. aeruginosa,* such as biofilm production, and contribute antiinflammatory effects. Long-term therapy with azithromycin 3 times a week improves lung function in patients with chronic *P. aeruginosa* infection.

Aerosolized Antibiotic Therapy
Aerosolized antibiotics are often used as part of daily therapy when the airways are infected with *P. aeruginosa.* Aerosolized tobramycin inhalation solution or powder, or aztreonam inhalation solution used as a suppressive therapy (on 1 mo, off 1 mo), may reduce symptoms, improve pulmonary function, and decrease the occurrence of pulmonary exacerbations. Although these therapies are sometimes used in acute pulmonary exacerbations, the evidence to support this application is limited.

Another important indication for aerosolized antibiotic therapy is to eradicate *P. aeruginosa* in the airways after initial detection. Early infection may be cleared for mo to several yr in this way, although eventual reinfection is common. Other antibiotics have been used via inhalation, including liposomal amikacin and levofloxacin for *P. aeruginosa,* and there was no inferiority of efficacy compared with inhaled tobramycin.

Intravenous Antibiotic Therapy
For the patient who has not responded to oral antibiotics and intensive home measures with return of signs, symptoms, and FEV_1 to baseline, intravenous antibiotic therapy is indicated. This therapy is usually initiated in the hospital but is sometimes completed on an ambulatory basis if the likelihood of complete adherence to the therapeutic regimen is good. The ideal duration of treatment is unknown; although many patients show improvement within 7 days, many CF physicians believe that it is usually advisable to extend the period of treatment to at least 14 days. Permanent intravenous access can be provided for long-term or frequent courses of therapy in the hospital or at home. Thrombophilia screening should be considered before the use of totally implantable intravenous devices or for recurring problems with venous catheters.

Table 432.6 lists commonly used intravenous antibiotics. In general, treatment of *Pseudomonas* infection is thought to require 2-drug therapy. A 3rd agent may be given for optimal coverage of *S. aureus* or other organisms. Aminoglycosides are usually effective when given every 24 hr to minimize toxicity and optimize convenience. Some CF physicians use peak and trough levels to guide dosing, but most clinical pharmacists recommend measuring levels at other times, commonly 2 and 12 hr, to use pharmacokinetic calculations to guide dosing. Changes in therapy should be guided by lack of improvement more than by culture results; sensitivities do not always predict response to therapy, and this may be due to the presence of other organisms that are not detected by culture methods. If patients do not show improvement, complications such as right heart failure, asthma, or infection with viruses, *A. fumigatus* (especially ABPA) (see Chapter 237), nontuberculous mycobacteria (see Chapters 217 and 399), or other unusual organisms should be considered. *B. cepacia* complex and acinetobacter are Gram-negative rods that may be particularly refractory to antimicrobial therapy. Infection control in both the outpatient and inpatient medical setting is critically important

Table 432.6	Antimicrobial Agents for Cystic Fibrosis Lung Infection			
ROUTE	**ORGANISMS**	**AGENTS**	**DOSAGE (mg/kg/24 hr)**	**NO. DOSES/24 hr**
Oral	Staphylococcus aureus	Dicloxacillin	25-50	4
		Linezolid	20	2
		Cephalexin	50	4
		Clindamycin	10-30	3-4
		Amoxicillin-clavulanate	25-45	2-3
	Haemophilus influenzae	Amoxicillin	50-100	2-3
	Pseudomonas aeruginosa	Ciprofloxacin	20-30	2-3
	Burkholderia cepacia	Trimethoprim-sulfamethoxazole	8-10*	2-4
	Empirical	Azithromycin	10, day 1; 5, days 2-5	1
		Erythromycin	30-50	3-4
Intravenous	S. aureus	Nafcillin	100-200	4-6
		Vancomycin	40	3-4
	P. aeruginosa	Tobramycin	8-12	1-3
		Amikacin	15-30	2-3
		Ticarcillin	400	4
		Piperacillin	300-400	4
		Ticarcillin-clavulanate	400†	4
		Piperacillin-tazobactam	240-400‡	3
		Meropenem	60-120	3
		Imipenem-cilastatin	45-100	3-4
		Ceftazidime	150	3
		Aztreonam	150-200	4
	B. cepacia	Chloramphenicol	50-100	4
		Meropenem	60-120	3
Aerosol		Tobramycin (inhaled)	300§	2
		Aztreonam (inhaled)	75	3

*Quantity of trimethoprim.
†Quantity of ticarcillin.
‡Quantity of piperacillin.
§In mg per dose.

to prevent nosocomial spread of resistant bacterial organisms between patients.

Bronchodilator Therapy

Reversible airway obstruction occurs in many children with CF, sometimes in conjunction with frank asthma or allergic bronchopulmonary aspergillosis. Reversible obstruction is conventionally defined as improvement of ≥12% in FEV_1 or FVC after inhalation of a bronchodilator. In many patients with CF, these may improve by only 5–10% (physiologic response), but subjects may report subjective benefit.

Antiinflammatory Agents

Corticosteroids are useful for the treatment of allergic bronchopulmonary aspergillosis and severe asthma occasionally encountered in children with CF. Prolonged systemic corticosteroid treatment of CF lung disease reduces the decline in lung function modestly but causes predictably prohibitive side effects. Inhaled corticosteroids have theoretical appeal, but there are contradictory and weak data regarding efficacy unless the patient has clinically diagnosable asthma. Ibuprofen, given chronically in high doses adjusted to achieve a peak serum concentration of 50-100 µg/mL, is associated with a slowing of disease progression, particularly in younger patients with mild lung disease. However, there are concerns regarding side effects of nonsteroidal antiinflammatory drugs, so this therapy has not gained broad acceptance. Macrolide antibiotics have an antiinflammatory effect, and 3 days/wk azithromycin has been shown to reduce the likelihood of development of pulmonary exacerbations, especially in patients with chronic *Pseudomonas* airway infection, so this is a commonly used therapy.

Cystic Fibrosis Transmembrane Conductance Regulator Modulator Therapies

A major breakthrough in CF therapy is ivacaftor, a small molecule potentiator of the CFTR mutation, G551D (present in ~5% of patients). Ivacaftor activates the CFTR-G551D mutant protein, a class III CFTR mutation that results in protein localized to the plasma membrane but

loss of chloride channel function (Fig. 432.11). Ivacaftor therapy resulted in improvement in FEV_1 by an average of 10.6%, decreased the frequency of pulmonary exacerbations by 55%, decreased sweat chloride by an average of 48 mEq/L, and increased weight gain by an average of 2.7 kg. Ivacaftor is approved for patients older than 2 yr of age with class III and class IV mutations.

The combination of ivacaftor with lumacaftor, a corrector that stabilizes misfolded F508del and enables trafficking of the mutant molecule to the apical cell membrane where it is potentiated by ivacaftor, is available for patients older than 6 yr of age who are homozygous for the F508del mutation (see Fig. 432.11). This medication is associated with smaller increments in pulmonary and nutritional outcomes but is an important proof-of-concept treatment.

Tezacaftor and ivacaftor is another combination indicated for patients ≥ 12 yr with 1 or 2 Phe508del alleles. This combination improves predicted FEV_1 and overall well-being (Table 432.7). VX-445 combined with tezacaftor-ivacaftor adds another CFTR correction agent; the triple combination improves predicted FEV_1 and reduces sweat chloride levels.

Other Therapies

Attempts to clear recalcitrant atelectasis and airway plugging with bronchopulmonary lavage and direct installation of various medications are sometimes used in exceptional cases; there is no evidence for sustained benefit from repeated procedures. Expectorants such as iodides and guaifenesin do not effectively assist with the removal of secretions from the respiratory tract. Inspiratory muscle training can enhance maximum oxygen consumption during exercise, as well as FEV_1.

TREATMENT OF PULMONARY COMPLICATIONS
Atelectasis

Lobar atelectasis occurs relatively infrequently; it may be asymptomatic and noted only at the time of a routine chest radiograph. Aggressive intravenous therapy with antibiotics and increased chest PT directed at the affected lobe may be effective. If there is no improvement in 5-7 days, bronchoscopic examination of the airways may be indicated. If

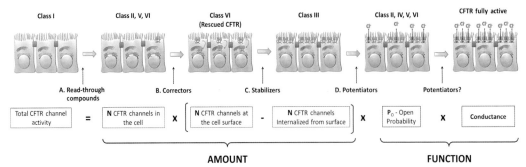

Fig. 432.11 Cystic fibrosis transmembrane conductance regulator *(CFTR)* pharmacologic modulators have different modes of action. **A,** Read-through compounds which include aminoglycoside antibiotics (e.g., gentamicin, tobramycin) act by suppressing premature termination codons (PTCs), thus permitting translation to continue to the normal termination of the transcript and thus increasing the total amount of complete CFTR being produced in the cell. **B,** Correctors (e.g., VX-809 also known as lumacaftor; VX-661) potentially promote folding of mutant CFTR protein, allowing it to escape ER degradation and reach the cell surface, thus increasing the number of channels present at the plasma membrane. **C,** Stabilizers include compounds (e.g., hepatocyte growth factor) that enhance CFTR retention/anchoring at the cell surface, thus also contributing to increase the number of channels present at the cell surface. **D,** Potentiators (e.g., VX-770 also known as ivacaftor) activate CFTR, that is, increase the open probability *(P_o)* of the channel by regulating its gating and possibly also the conductance. *(From Bell SC, De Boeck K, Amaral MD: New pharmacological approaches for cystic fibrosis: promises, progress, pitfalls, Pharmacol Therapeu 145:19–34, 2015 [Fig. 4, p. 26].)*

Table 432.7	Cystic Fibrosis Transmembrane Regulator Modulators for Cystic Fibrosis		
DRUG	**FDA-APPROVED INDICATION**	**FORMULATIONS**	**USUAL DOSAGE**
Ivacaftor	≥ 12 mo with a responsive mutation[1]	150 mg tabs; 50, 75 mg granule packets[2]	≥ 6 years: 150 mg q12 hr[3]
Lumacaftor/ivacaftor	≥ 2 yr, F508del-homozygous	100/125, 200/125 mg tabs; 100/125, 150/188 mg granule packets[2]	6-11 yr: 200/250 mg q12 hr ≥ 12 yr: 400/250 mg q12 hr[4]
Tezacaftor/ivacaftor	≥ 12 yr, F508del-homozygous or F508del-heterozygous with another responsive mutation[1]	100/150 mg tabs co-packaged with ivacaftor 150 mg tabs	≥ 12 yr: 100/150 mg tab qAM, then 150 mg ivacaftor qPM

[1]Responsive mutations are those in which chloride transport is expected to increase to at least 10% of untreated normal over baseline with drug therapy, based on clinical or in vitro data.
[2]The granules should be mixed with 5 mL of room-temperature or cold soft food or liquid and consumed within 1 hr.
[3]In patients 12 mo to 6 yr old, the recommended dosage is 50 mg every 12 hr for those weighing <14 kg, and 75 mg every 12 hr for those weighing ≥ 14 kg.
[4]In patients 2-5 yr old, the recommended dosage is 100/125 mg every 12 hr for those weighing <14 kg, and 150/188 mg every 12 hr for those weighing ≥ 14 kg.
Modified from The Medical Letter on Drugs and Therapeutics: Tezacaftor/Ivacaftor (Symdeko) for cystic fibrosis; *Med Lett* 60(1558):174–176, 2018 (Table 3, p. 175).

the atelectasis does not resolve, continued intensive home therapy is indicated because atelectasis may resolve during a period of wk or mo.

Hemoptysis

Endobronchial bleeding usually reflects airway wall erosion into hypertrophied bronchial vessels secondary to infection. Although more common in patients with advanced disease, it is sometimes seen in adolescents with relatively mild lung disease. Blood streaking of sputum is particularly common. Small-volume hemoptysis (<20 mL) is usually viewed as a need for intensified antimicrobial therapy and chest PT. **Massive hemoptysis,** defined as total blood loss of ≥250 mL in a 24-hr period, is rare in the 1st decade and occurs in <1% of adolescents, but it requires close monitoring and the capability to replace blood losses rapidly. Bronchoscopy rarely reveals the site of bleeding. Bronchial artery embolization can be useful to control persistent, significant hemoptysis.

Pneumothorax

Pneumothorax (see Chapter 439) is encountered uncommonly in children and teenagers with CF, although it may lead to significant compromise in lung function and occasionally may be life threatening. The episode may be asymptomatic but is often attended by chest and shoulder pain, shortness of breath, or hemoptysis. A small air collection that does not grow can be observed closely. Chest tube placement with or without pleurodesis is often the initial therapy. Intravenous antibiotics are also begun on admission. Video-assisted thoracoscopic surgery (VATS) with plication of blebs, apical pleural stripping, and basal pleural abrasion should be considered if the air leak persists. Surgical intervention is usually well tolerated even in cases of advanced lung disease. The

thoracotomy tube is removed as soon as possible. Previous pneumothorax with or without pleurodesis is not a contraindication to subsequent lung transplantation.

Allergic Bronchopulmonary Aspergillosis

Allergic bronchopulmonary aspergillosis occurs in 5–10% of patients with CF and may manifest as wheezing, increased cough, shortness of breath, and marked hyperinflation, or most commonly, a decrease in FEV$_1$ that does not respond to antibiotic therapy (see Chapters 237 and 399). In some patients, a chest radiograph shows new, focal infiltrates. A very elevated total serum immunoglobulin E (IgE) level (>1,000) is usually the initial indication of the diagnosis. The presence of rust-colored sputum, the recovery of *Aspergillus* organisms from the sputum, a positive skin test for *A. fumigatus,* the demonstration of specific IgE and IgG antibodies against *A. fumigatus,* or the presence of eosinophils in a fresh sputum sample supports the diagnosis. Treatment is directed at controlling the inflammatory reaction with oral corticosteroids. Oral antifungals are usually reserved for patients who relapse after initial steroid treatment. For refractory cases, omalizumab, humanized monoclonal anti-IgE, has been effective.

Nontuberculous Mycobacteria Infection
See Chapter 244.

Injured airways with poor clearance may be colonized by *Mycobacterium avium*-complex but also *Mycobacterium abscessus, Mycobacterium chelonae,* and *Mycobacterium kansasii.* Distinguishing endobronchial colonization (frequent) from invasive infection (infrequent) is challenging. Persistent fevers and new infiltrates or cystic lesions coupled with the finding of acid-fast organisms on sputum smear suggest infection. Infection with these organisms, or at least its recognition, had become increasing common. Treatment is prolonged and requires multiple antimicrobial agents. Symptoms may improve, but the nontuberculous mycobacteria are not usually cleared from the lungs.

Bone and Joint Complications

Hypertrophic osteoarthropathy causes elevation of the periosteum over the distal portions of long bones and bone pain, overlying edema, and joint effusions. Acetaminophen or ibuprofen may provide relief. Control of lung infection usually reduces symptoms. Intermittent arthropathy unrelated to other rheumatologic disorders occurs occasionally, has no recognized pathogenesis, and usually responds to nonsteroidal antiinflammatory agents. Back pain or rib fractures from vigorous coughing may require pain management to permit adequate airway clearance. These and other fractures may stem from diminished bone mineralization, the result of reduced vitamin D absorption, corticosteroid therapy, diminished weight-bearing exercises, and perhaps other factors. There may be a bone phenotype in CF that is unrelated to therapies or nutritional status and may be due to CFTR dysfunction.

Sleep-Disordered Breathing

Particularly with advanced pulmonary disease and during chest exacerbations, individuals with CF may experience more sleep arousals, less time in rapid eye movement sleep, nocturnal hypoxemia, hypercapnia, and associated neurobehavioral impairment. Nocturnal hypoxemia may hasten the onset of pulmonary hypertension and right-sided heart failure. Efficacy of specific interventions for this complication of CF has not been systematically assessed. Prompt treatment of airway symptoms and nocturnal oxygen supplementation or bilevel positive airway pressure support should be considered in selected cases, especially in patients with advanced lung disease.

Acute Respiratory Failure

Acute respiratory failure (see Chapter 89) rarely occurs in patients with mild to moderate lung disease and is usually the result of a severe viral or other infectious illness. Because patients with this complication can regain their previous status, intensive therapy is indicated. In addition to aerosol, postural drainage, and intravenous antibiotic treatment, oxygen is required to raise the arterial PaO_2. An increasing PCO_2 may require ventilatory assistance. Endotracheal or bronchoscopic suction may be necessary to clear airway inspissated secretions and can be repeated daily. Right-sided heart failure should be treated vigorously. High-dose steroids have been anecdotally reported to be of benefit in this setting. Recovery is often slow. Intensive intravenous antibiotic therapy and postural drainage should be continued for 1-2 wk after the patient has regained baseline status.

Chronic Respiratory Failure

Patients with CF acquire chronic respiratory failure after prolonged deterioration of lung function. Although this complication can occur at any age, it is seen most frequently in adult patients. Because a long-standing PaO_2 <50 mm Hg promotes the development of right-sided heart failure, patients usually benefit from low-flow oxygen to raise arterial PO_2 to ≥55 mm Hg. Increasing hypercapnia may prevent the use of optimal fraction of inspired oxygen. Most patients improve somewhat with intensive antibiotic and pulmonary therapy measures and can be discharged from the hospital. Low-flow oxygen therapy is needed at home, especially with sleep. Noninvasive ventilatory support can improve gas exchange and has been documented to enhance quality of life. Ventilatory support may be particularly useful for patients awaiting lung transplantation. These patients usually display pulmonary hypertension and cor pulmonale, and this complication should be treated. Caution should be exercised to avoid ventilation-suppressing metabolic alkalosis that results from CF-related chloride depletion and, in many cases, from diuretic-induced bicarbonate retention. Chronic pain (headache, chest pain, abdominal pain, and limb pain) is frequent at the end of life and responds to judicious use of analgesics, including opioids. Dyspnea has been ameliorated with nebulized fentanyl.

Lung transplantation is an option for end-stage lung disease that is increasingly offered (see Chapter 470). Criteria for referral continue to be a subject of investigation and ideally include estimates of longevity with and without transplant based on lung function and exercise tolerance data. Survival and quality of life after lung transplantation is better in patients with CF than other chronic lung diseases, probably due to the relatively younger age of recipients with CF, but the current estimated 5-yr survival is about 50%, somewhat reduced compared with that of other solid organ transplants. Because of bronchiolitis obliterans (see Chapter 422.1) and other complications, transplanted lungs cannot be expected to function for the lifetime of a recipient, and repeat transplantation is increasingly common. The demand for donor lungs exceeds the supply, and waiting lists and duration of waits continue to be a problem.

Pulmonary Hypertension and Cor Pulmonale

Individuals with long-standing, advanced pulmonary disease, especially those with severe hypoxemia (PaO_2 < 50 mm Hg), often acquire pulmonary hypertension and chronic right-sided heart failure. Evidence for concomitant left ventricular dysfunction is often found. The arterial PO_2 should be maintained at >50 mm Hg, if possible, and hypercarbia corrected with noninvasive ventilation or intubation if necessary. Intensive pulmonary therapy, including intravenous antibiotics, is most important. Adjunctive therapy with salt restriction, diuretics, and pulmonary vasodilators may be indicated. The prognosis for heart failure is poor, but a number of patients survive for ≥5 yr after the appearance of heart failure. Heart-lung transplantation may be an option (see preceding section).

Nutritional Therapy

Up to 90% of patients with CF have loss of exocrine pancreatic function leading to inadequate digestion and absorption of fats and proteins. They require dietary adjustment and augmentation, pancreatic enzyme replacement, and supplementary vitamins. In general, children with CF need to exceed the usual required daily caloric intake to grow. Daily supplements of the fat-soluble vitamins are required.

Diet

Historically, at the time of diagnosis, many infants presented with nutritional deficits; this situation has changed because of newborn screening, but even at 2-4 wk it is not uncommon to see that weight gain has begun to fall off the standard curve.

Most children with CF have a higher-than-normal caloric need because of malabsorption despite the use of pancreatic enzyme supplementation. Encouragement to eat high-calorie foods is important and often begins with more concentrated, high-calorie formulas in the 1st yr. Even so, most mothers can breastfeed successfully. It is vitally important to promote adequate weight gain in the early years, both because of a clear relationship to later lung function and also because early deficiencies make later catch up growth more difficult. Not infrequently, parent–child interactions at feeding time are maladaptive, and behavioral interventions can improve caloric intake. The liberal use of appetite stimulants, especially cyproheptadine, in early childhood, makes the struggle a bit easier. Poorly controlled lung disease increases metabolism and decreases appetite and needs to be considered when efforts to improve weight gain are unsuccessful.

Maintenance of good weight gain and body mass index in the 1st yr of life leads to better long-term preservation of lung function, but there is a strong correlation between body mass index and FEV_1 that persists through all ages in people with CF. Better nutrition also leads to improved quality of life and psychologic well-being and provides better reserves when weight loss occurs in association with intermittent acute pulmonary exacerbations.

Malabsorption is an important contributor to nutritional deficiencies, and it is important to ensure that pancreatic enzyme dosing is adequate and consistently being taken correctly with all meals and feedings. Appetite stimulants when cyproheptadine is not successful may include megestrol, oxandrolone, dronabinol, antidepressants such as mirtazaoine, and even growth hormone. CF-related diabetes needs to be ruled out.

When all these therapies fail, weight stabilization or gain can be achieved with nocturnal feeding via nasogastric tube or gastrostomy tube. These are most commonly resorted to in infants and adolescents, the 2 age groups that have the most difficulty with weight gain due to high normal demands.

Pancreatic Enzyme Replacement

Pancreatic exocrine replacement therapy given with ingested food reduces but does not fully correct stool fat and nitrogen losses. Current products are enteric-coated, pH-sensitive enzyme microspheres that come in capsules and given to children before they can swallow by opening the capsule and mixing the beads in small amounts of acidic foods such as applesauce. Strengths ranging from 3 to 40,000 IU of lipase/capsule are available. Administration of excessive doses has been linked to fibrosing colonopathy and **colonic strictures,** so recommendations are for enzyme dosing to stay below 2,500 lipase units/kg/meal in most circumstances. Snacks should also be covered. Some individuals require proton pump inhibitor therapy to correct acid pH in the duodenum which is due to lack of exocrine pancreatic secretions; neutralization of duodenal pH permits activation of enteric-coated pancreatic exocrine replacement therapy granules.

Vitamin and Mineral Supplements

Because pancreatic insufficiency results in malabsorption of fat-soluble vitamins (A, D, E, K), vitamin supplementation is recommended. Several vitamin preparations containing all 4 vitamins for patients with CF are available. They should be taken daily. Despite this supplementation, vitamin D deficiency is common and should be treated with doses of cholecalciferol (vitamin D3) rather than ergocalciferol (vitamin D2) in the range of 1,000 units/kg/wk. Salt supplementation is also needed during infancy and is started at the time of diagnosis.

TREATMENT OF INTESTINAL COMPLICATIONS
Meconium Ileus

When meconium ileus (see Chapter 102) is suspected, diatrizoate (Gastrografin) enemas with reflux of contrast material into the ileum not only confirm the diagnosis but may also result in the passage of meconium and clearing of the obstruction. Children in whom this procedure fails require operative intervention. Children who have had meconium ileus are at greater risk for nutritional deficiency and more likely to develop problems with DIOS when older. Infants with meconium ileus should be assumed to have CF unless proven otherwise.

Distal Intestinal Obstruction Syndrome and Other Causes of Abdominal Symptoms

Despite appropriate pancreatic enzyme replacement, a number of patients accumulate fecal material in the terminal portion of the ileum and in the cecum, which may result in partial or complete obstruction. For intermittent symptoms, pancreatic enzyme replacement should be continued or even increased, and stool hydrators such as polyethylene glycol (MiraLAX) should be given. If this fails or symptoms are more severe, large-volume bowel lavage with a balanced salt solution containing polyethylene glycol may be taken by mouth or by nasogastric tube. When there is complete obstruction, a diatrizoate enema, accompanied by large amounts of intravenous fluids, can be therapeutic.

Rectal Prolapse

See Chapter 371.5.

Although uncommon, rectal prolapse occurs most often in infants with CF and less frequently in older children with the disease. It was much more frequently seen in the past among undiagnosed young children with steatorrhea, malnutrition, and repetitive cough. The prolapsed rectum can usually be replaced manually by continuous gentle pressure with the patient in the knee-chest position. Sedation may be helpful. To prevent an immediate recurrence, the buttocks can be temporally taped closed. Adequate pancreatic enzymes, stool softener, and control of pulmonary infection result in improvement. Occasionally, a patient may continue to have rectal prolapse and may require sclerotherapy or surgery.

Hepatobiliary Disease

Liver function abnormalities associated with biliary cirrhosis can be improved by treatment with ursodeoxycholic acid. The ability of bile acids to prevent progression of cirrhosis has not been clearly documented. Portal hypertension with esophageal varices, hypersplenism, or ascites occurs in ≤8% of children with CF (see Chapter 394).

Obstructive jaundice in newborns with CF needs no specific therapy once the etiology has been established. End-stage liver disease is an indication for liver transplantation in children with CF (see Chapter 395).

Pancreatitis

Recurrent pancreatitis is seen primarily in patients with pancreatic sufficiency, and it can lead to the development of pancreatic insufficiency. Patients can be treated with pancreatic enzyme therapy and a low-fat diet (in well-nourished patients) to rest the pancreas. Further treatment of this disorder is discussed in Chapter 378.

Cystic Fibrosis-Related Hyperglycemia and Diabetes

Onset of hyperglycemia occurs most frequently *after* the 1st decade. Approximately 20% of young adults are treated for hyperglycemia, although the incidence of CF-related diabetes may be up to 50% in CF adults. Ketoacidosis is rarely encountered. The pathogenesis includes both impaired insulin secretion and insulin resistance. Routine screening consisting of an annual 2-hr oral glucose tolerance test is recommended in children older than 10 yr of age, although some cases may begin earlier. Glucose intolerance with blood sugars that remain less than 200 is usually not treated unless nutrition is compromised or lung function seems affected. When treatment is indicated, insulin treatment should be instituted. The development of significant hyperglycemia favors acquisition of *P. aeruginosa* and *B. cepacia* in the airways and may adversely affect pulmonary function, especially in women. Thus careful control of blood glucose level is an important goal. Long-term vascular complications of diabetes can occur, providing an additional rationale for good control of blood glucose levels.

OTHER COMPLICATIONS
Nasal Polyps

Nasal polyps (see Chapter 406) occur in 15–20% of patients with CF and are most prevalent in the 2nd decade of life. Local corticosteroids and nasal decongestants occasionally provide some relief. When the polyps completely obstruct the nasal airway, rhinorrhea becomes constant or widening of the nasal bridge is noticed, surgical removal of the polyps is indicated; polyps may recur promptly or after a symptom-free interval of months to years. Polyps inexplicably stop developing in many adults.

Rhinosinusitis

Opacification of paranasal sinuses is universal in CF and is not an indication for intervention. Acute or chronic sinus-related symptoms are treated initially with antimicrobials, with or without maxillary sinus aspiration for culture. Functional endoscopic sinus surgery has anecdotally provided benefit.

Salt Depletion

Salt losses from sweat in patients with CF can be high, especially in warm arid climates. Children should have free access to salt, especially when thirsty in hot weather. Salt supplements are often prescribed to newborns and to children who live in hot weather climates. Hypochloremic alkalosis should be suspected in any patient who feels unwell in hot weather or who has had symptoms of gastroenteritis, and prompt fluid and electrolyte therapy should be instituted as needed.

Surgery

Patients with good or excellent pulmonary status can tolerate general anesthesia without any intensive pulmonary measures before the procedure but should be adherent to their usual prescribed airway clearance therapy. Those with moderate or severe pulmonary infection usually do better with a 1- to 2-wk course of intensive antibiotic treatment and increased airway clearance before surgery. If this approach is impossible, prompt intravenous antibiotic therapy is indicated once it is recognized that major surgery is required. General anesthesia may provide an opportunity to perform bronchoscopy to evaluate the airway and obtain good cultures, and this should be considered in any child with CF who will undergo surgery for any indication.

After major surgery, cough should be encouraged, and airway clearance treatments should be reinstituted as soon as possible, usually within 24 hr.

PROGNOSIS

CF remains a life-limiting disorder, although survival has dramatically improved (Fig. 432.12). With exceptions, most children remain relatively healthy into adolescence or adulthood. The slow progression of lung disease eventually does reach disabling proportions. Life table data indicate a median cumulative survival of more than 40 yr, and the expectation is younger children with the disease have a life expectancy far in excess of this estimate. Outcomes are variable and related to CFTR mutation class, modifier genes, biologic and chemical exposures, disease management, and socioeconomic status.

Children with CF should not be restricted in their activities. A high percentage eventually attend and graduate from college. Most adults with CF find satisfactory employment, and an increasing number marry. Transitioning care from pediatric to adult care centers by 21 yr of age is an important objective and requires a thoughtful, supportive approach involving both the pediatric and internal medicine specialists.

With increasing life span for patients with CF, a new set of psychosocial considerations has emerged, including dependence-independence issues, self-care, peer relationships, sexuality, reproduction, substance abuse, educational and vocational planning, medical care costs and other financial burdens, and anxiety concerning health and prognosis. Anxiety and depression are prevalent, as in any other chronic disease, and impact quality of life and disease self-management; screening for both is now part of comprehensive care. Many of these issues are best addressed in an anticipatory fashion, before the onset of psychosocial dysfunction. With appropriate medical and psychosocial support, children and adolescents with CF generally cope well. Achievement of an independent and productive adulthood is a realistic goal for many.

Bibliography is available at Expert Consult.

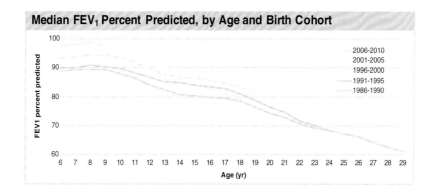

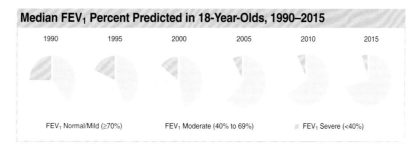

Fig. 432.12 Forced expiratory volume in 1 sec (FEV₁) percent predicted is steadily improving and currently is greater than 90% predicted into early adolescence. The proportion of people with CF age 18 yr who are in the normal/mild category (FEV1 ≥ 70% predicted) has increased from 39.9% in 1990 to 72.1% in 2015, whereas the proportion in the severe category (FEV1 < 40% predicted) has decreased from 24.9% to 5.3%. *(From the Cystic Fibrosis Foundation Patient Registry 2015. Annual Data Report. ©2016 Cystic Fibrosis Foundation, Bethesda, Maryland.)*

Chapter **433**

Primary Ciliary Dyskinesia (Immotile Cilia Syndrome, Kartagener Syndrome)

Thomas W. Ferkol Jr

第四百三十三章

原发性纤毛运动障碍（不动纤毛综合征、Kartagener综合征）

中文导读

　　本章主要介绍了正常纤毛的超微结构和功能，原发性纤毛运动障碍的遗传学、临床表现、诊断、治疗以及预后。分别描述了运动纤毛、初级（感觉）纤毛和结纤毛的结构、分布和功能等；阐述了原发性纤毛运动障碍的遗传方式、致病基因以及相应的致病机制；详细介绍了新生儿呼吸窘迫、长期湿咳、支气管扩张、持续性鼻塞和鼻炎等特征性临床表现；提供了基于年龄的诊断标准，并着重阐述了基因检测和透射电子显微镜对诊断的价值；治疗中描述了提高黏液纤毛清除率、治疗感染、手术切除和肺移植等方法，并在预后部分推荐了需常规监测的项目。

Primary ciliary dyskinesia (PCD) is an inherited disorder characterized by impaired ciliary function leading to diverse clinical manifestations, including chronic sinopulmonary disease, persistent middle ear effusions, laterality defects, and infertility. The estimated frequency of PCD is 1 in 12,000 to 1 in 20,000 live births, but its prevalence in children with repeated respiratory infections has been estimated to be as high as 5%.

NORMAL CILIARY ULTRASTRUCTURE AND FUNCTION

Three types of cilia exist in humans: motile cilia, primary (sensory) cilia, and nodal cilia. The respiratory epithelium in the nasopharynx, middle ear, paranasal sinuses, and larger airways are lined by a ciliated, pseudostratified columnar epithelium that is essential for mucociliary clearance. A mature ciliated epithelial cell has approximately 200 uniform **motile cilia**, hair-like organelles that move fluids, mucus, and inhaled particulates vectorially from conducting airways (Fig. 433.1). Motor cilia are anatomically and functionally oriented in the same direction, moving with intracellular and intercellular synchrony. Anchored by a basal body to the apical cytoplasm and extending from the apical cell surface into the airway lumen, each cilium is a complex, specialized structure, composed of hundreds of proteins. It contains a cylinder of microtubule doublets organized around a central pair of microtubules

(Fig. 433.2), leading to the characteristic "9+2" arrangement seen on cross-sectional views on transmission electron microscopy. A membrane continuous with the plasma membrane covers the central fibrillar structure, or axoneme. The ciliary axoneme is highly conserved across species, and the structural elements of simple algal flagella and the mammalian cilium are similar. Attached to the A microtubules as distinct

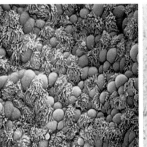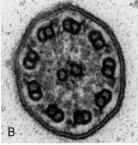

Fig. 433.1 Electron photomicrographs showing **(A)** an airway epithelium grown in primary culture, showing ciliated and nonciliated cells and **(B)** a normal motor cilium.

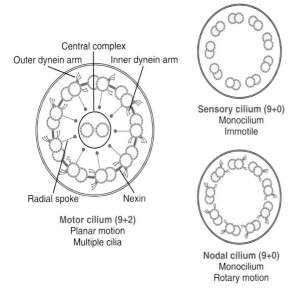

Fig. 433.2 Schemata showing the 3 general classes of normal cilia (motile "9+2," motile "9+0," and nonmotile "9+0"), which demonstrate the complex structure and arrangement of the ciliary axoneme.

inner and outer dynein arms, multiple adenosine triphosphatases, called dyneins, serve as motors of the cilium and promote microtubule sliding, which is converted into bending. Each dynein arm is a multimer with heavy, intermediate, and light chains, with each dynein protein encoded by a different gene. The inner dynein arm influences the bend shape of the cilium, whereas the outer dynein arm controls beat force and frequency. The inner dynein arm and radial spokes are also parts of the dynein regulatory complex, a key regulator of motor activity. Nexin links connecting adjacent outer microtubular doublets limit the degree of sliding between microtubules. All these structures lead to synchronized ciliary beating, resulting in a ciliary stroke and coordinated beating at a frequency constant throughout the airway, 8-20 beats/sec, but can be negatively affected by several factors, such as anesthetics and dehydration. Alternatively, beat frequency may be accelerated by exposure to irritants or bioactive molecules, including β-adrenergic agents, acetylcholine, and serotonin. Cilia beat frequency can be increased through the activity of nitric oxide synthases that are localized in the apical cytoplasm. The coordinated wavelike pattern of ciliary motion has important functions in fluid and cell movement, and any disturbance in the precise, orchestrated movement of the cilia can lead to disease.

Primary (sensory) cilia are solitary organelles present during interphase on most cell types. These cilia lack a central microtubule doublet and dynein arms, thus creating a "9+0" arrangement and leaving them immotile (see Fig. 433.2). These structures were once considered nonfunctional vestigial remnants, but primary cilia are important signaling organelles that sense the extracellular environment. They are mechanoreceptors, chemosensors, and osmosensors and, in specialized cases, detect changes in light, temperature, and gravity. Defects (ciliopathies) are linked to wide-ranging pediatric conditions, such as various polycystic kidney diseases, nephronophthisis, Bardet-Biedl syndrome, Meckel-Gruber syndrome, Joubert syndrome, Alström syndrome, Ellis-van Creveld syndrome, and Jeune thoracic dystrophy.

The third type of cilia exists only during a brief period of embryonic development. **Nodal cilia** have a "9+0" microtubule arrangement similar to that of primary cilia, but they exhibit a whirling, rotational movement (see Fig. 433.2), resulting in leftward flow of extracellular fluid that establishes body sidedness. Nodal cilia defects result in body orientation abnormalities, such as **situs inversus totalis**, **situs ambiguus**, and **heterotaxy** associated with congenital heart disease, asplenia, and polysplenia (see Chapter 458.11).

GENETICS OF PRIMARY CILIARY DYSKINESIA

PCD typically has autosomal recessive patterns of inheritance, although X-linked inheritance has been reported. PCD is a genetically heterogeneous disorder involving multiple genes; mutations in any protein that is involved in ciliary assembly, structure, or function could theoretically cause disease. Early linkage studies showed substantial locus heterogeneity, which made correlations between ciliary defects and the underlying mutations difficult. Mutations in 40 different genes have been linked to PCD (Fig. 433.3), including those that encode proteins integral to the outer dynein arm: *DNAH5, DNAH1, DNAI1, DNAL1, DNAI2, TXNDC3, CCDC114, CCDC151, ARMC4,* and *TTC25;* dynein regulatory complex and nexin components: *CCDC39, CCDC40,* and *GAS8;* and radial spoke and central apparatus proteins: *RSPH1, RSPH3, RSPH4A, RSPH9, HYDIN,* and *DNAJB13.* Mutations in genes coding several cytoplasmic proteins, not part of the cilia axoneme, have also been identified and appear to have roles in cilia assembly or protein transport, including: *HEATR2, DNAAF1, DNAAF2, DNAAF3, CCDC103, LRRC6, DYX1C1, SPAG1, ZMYND10,* and an open reading frame sequence, *C21orf59.* Not all patients with PCD have an identifiable genetic mutation.

The genetic bases of ciliopathies have yielded greater understanding of genotype-phenotype relationships in PCD. Mutations in nexin-dynein regulatory complex proteins create inconsistent ultrastructural abnormalities characterized by absent inner dynein arms in all axonemes, but misplaced radial spokes and microtubular disorganization in only some cilia. A cross-sectional study showed that children who had microtubular disorganization, primarily due to biallelic mutations in *CCDC39* or *CCDC40,* had more severe lung disease. In contrast, patients with mutations in *RSPH1* appear to have milder respiratory phenotypes.

CLINICAL MANIFESTATIONS OF PRIMARY CILIARY DYSKINESIA

See Table 433.1.

PCD has several characteristic clinical features. Neonatal respiratory distress (NRD) is a common feature, and most affected term newborns develop increased work of breathing, tachypnea, and upper and middle lobe atelectasis on chest radiographs. The association of respiratory distress in *term neonates* with PCD has been underappreciated. Often diagnosed with transient tachypnea of the newborn or pneumonia, PCD infants frequently require supplemental oxygen flow for days to weeks. When NRD occurs in infants with situs anomalies, PCD is highly likely.

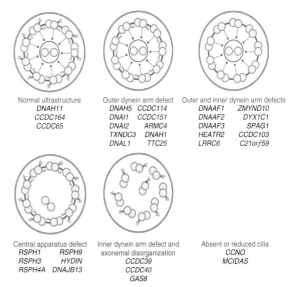

Fig. 433.3 Classification of genes mutated in primary ciliary dyskinesia based on ultrastructural findings.

Table 433.1	Clinical Manifestations of Primary Ciliary Dyskinesia

RESPIRATORY
- Unexplained respiratory distress in term neonate
- Daily productive (wet) cough since early infancy
- Daily, nonseasonal rhinosinusitis since early infancy
- Chronic otitis media and persistent middle ear effusions
- Digital clubbing (rare in children)
- Atypical asthma unresponsive to therapy
- Recurrent pneumonias
- Bronchiectasis

LEFT-RIGHT LATERALITY DEFECTS
- Situs inversus totalis
- Heterotaxy with or without complex congenital heart disease

MISCELLANEOUS
- Male infertility, immotile sperm
- Female subfertility, ectopic pregnancy
- Hydrocephalus (rare)

Table 433.2	New Consensus-Based Primary Ciliary Dyskinesia (PCD) Diagnostic Criteria by Age

NEWBORNS (0–1 MO OF AGE)
Situs inversus totalis and unexplained neonatal respiratory distress (NRD) at term birth, plus at least one of the following:
- Diagnostic ciliary ultrastructure on electron micrographs or 2 mutations in PCD-associated gene

CHILDREN (1 MO TO 5 YR)
2 or more major PCD clinical criteria (NRD,* daily wet cough, persistent nasal congestion, laterality defect), plus at least one of the following (nasal nitric oxide not included in this age group because it is not yet sufficiently tested):
- Diagnostic ciliary ultrastructure on electron micrographs
- 2 mutations in 1 PCD-associated gene
- Persistent and diagnostic ciliary waveform abnormalities on high-speed videomicroscopy, on multiple occasions

CHILDREN (5–18 YR OF AGE) AND ADULTS
2 or more PCD clinical criteria (NRD,* daily productive cough or bronchiectasis, persistent nasal congestion, laterality defect), plus at least one of the following:
- Nasal nitric oxide during plateau <77 nL/min on 2 occasions, >2 mo apart (with CF excluded)
- Diagnostic ciliary ultrastructure on electron micrographs
- Two mutations in 1 PCD-associated gene
- Persistent and diagnostic ciliary waveform abnormalities on high-speed videomicroscopy, on multiple occasions

*In term neonates.

Chronic, year-round productive (wet) cough that begins in infancy is an almost universal feature of PCD. Bacterial cultures of sputum or lavage fluid frequently yield nontypeable *Haemophilus influenzae* (see Chapter 221), *Staphylococcus aureus* (see Chapter 208.1), *Streptococcus pneumoniae* (see Chapter 209), and *Pseudomonas aeruginosa* (see Chapter 232.1). Persistent airway infection and inflammation lead to **bronchiectasis**, even in preschool children. Clubbing is a sign of long-standing pulmonary disease.

Persistent nasal congestion and rhinitis is common, typically presenting in early infancy with little to no seasonal variation. Most patients describe chronic mucopurulent nasal drainage. Inadequate innate mucous clearance leads to chronic sinusitis (see Chapter 408) and nasal polyposis. Middle ear disease occurs in nearly all children with PCD, with varying degrees of **chronic otitis media** leading to conductive hearing loss and requiring myringotomy tube placement, which is often complicated by intractable otorrhea. Middle ear findings may be most helpful in distinguishing PCD from cystic fibrosis or other causes of chronic lung disease.

Left-right laterality defects (e.g., *situs inversus totalis*) are found in half of all children with PCD. Without functional nodal cilia in the embryonic period, thoracoabdominal orientation is random. Approximately 25% of patients who have *situs inversus totalis* have PCD; therefore *situs inversus totalis* alone does not establish the diagnosis. Other laterality defects, such as heterotaxy, are also associated with PCD and may coexist with congenital cardiac defects, asplenia, or polysplenia.

Most men with PCD have dysmotile spermatozoa because flagellar and ciliary ultrastructure is similar. Male infertility is typical but not always found in this disease. Subfertility has also been reported in affected women and may be due to ciliary dysfunction in the fallopian tubes.

A few case reports have associated **neonatal hydrocephalus** with PCD. The ependyma of the brain ventricles are lined by ciliated epithelium and are important for cerebrospinal fluid flow through the ventricles and aqueduct of Sylvius. The finding of enlarged brain ventricles on sonograms, when linked with *situs inversus totalis,* has been proposed as a prenatal diagnostic marker for PCD. X-linked retinitis pigmentosa has been associated with recurrent respiratory infections in families with *RPGR* gene mutations. Intraflagellar transport proteins are essential for photoreceptor assembly and, when mutated, lead to apoptosis of the retinal pigment epithelium (see Chapter 648).

DIAGNOSIS OF PRIMARY CILIARY DYSKINESIA

The diagnosis of PCD should be suspected in children with chronic or recurring upper and lower respiratory tract symptoms that begin in early infancy and is currently based on the presence of characteristic clinical phenotype and ultrastructural defects of cilia, though this approach will miss affected individuals (Table 433.2). The diagnosis is often delayed, even in children who have classic clinical features, such as *situs inversus totalis.* A high index of suspicion is necessary. The

diagnosis should be entertained in infants and children with unexplained NRD in term newborns, daily year-round productive (wet) cough that begins in infancy, persistent rhinosinusitis, and left-right laterality defects.

Imaging studies show extensive involvement of the paranasal sinuses. Chest radiographs frequently demonstrate bilateral lung overinflation, peribronchial infiltrates, and lobar atelectasis. Computed x-ray tomography of the chest often reveals bronchiectasis, often involving the anatomic right middle lobe or lingula, even in young children. *Situs inversus totalis* in a child who has chronic respiratory tract symptoms is highly suggestive of PCD, but this configuration occurs in only half of patients with PCD. Pulmonary function tests may be normal early but demonstrate obstructive airway disease as the disease progresses. Typical findings include decreased expiratory flow rates and increased residual volume. Bronchodilator responsiveness is variable. Longitudinal analyses of children with PCD show wide variation in intrathoracic airway obstruction.

Transmission electron microscopy is the current gold standard to assess structural defects within the cilium. These ultrastructural defects are found in cilia throughout the upper and lower airways and oviduct, as well as in sperm flagella. Curettage from the nasal epithelium or endobronchial brushing can provide an adequate specimen for review. Identification of a discrete, consistent defect in any aspect of the ciliary structure with concurrent phenotypic features is sufficient to make the diagnosis. There are several characteristic ciliary abnormalities: outer dynein arm defects, combined inner and outer dynein arm defects, central apparatus defects, and inner dynein arm defects with microtubular disorganization. Inner dynein arm defects alone are uncommon. Ultrastructural examination of cilia as a diagnostic test for PCD has limitations. First, the absence of axonemal defects does not exclude PCD; nearly 30% of all affected individuals have normal ciliary ultrastructure. Other patients with symptoms consistent with PCD have been found to have ciliary aplasia or few motor cilia on the epithelial surface (Table 433.3).

Careful interpretation of the ultrastructural findings is necessary because nonspecific changes may be seen in relation to exposure to environmental pollutants or infection. Ciliary defects can be acquired. Acute airway infection or inflammation can result in structural changes (e.g., compound cilia or blebs). Ciliary disorientation has been proposed as a form of PCD, but this phenomenon is the result of airway injury. Frequently, the diagnosis of PCD can be delayed or

Table 433.3	Electron Microscopic Findings in Primary Ciliary Dyskinesia

DYNEIN ARM DEFECTS
- Total or partial absence of outer dynein arms
- Total or partial absence of inner and outer dynein arms
- Total or partial absence of inner dynein arms alone (rare)

RADIAL SPOKE DEFECTS
- Total absence of radial spokes
- Absence of radial spoke heads

MICROTUBULAR TRANSPOSITION DEFECTS
- Inner dynein arm defect with microtubular derangement (in some axonemes)
- Absent central pair of tubules with outer doublet transposition

OTHER
- Central microtubular agenesis
- Ciliary aplasia or reduced cilia numbers
- Normal ultrastructure

missed because of inadequate tissue collection or sample processing, or misinterpretation of ciliary defects. Some investigators have advocated culturing of airway epithelial cells and allowing the secondary changes to resolve.

Qualitative tests to assess ciliary function have been used to screen for PCD. Ciliary beat frequency measurements that use conventional microscopic techniques have been used as a screen, but this method alone will miss cases of PCD. Cilia inspection using standard light microscopy is insufficient to support or exclude the diagnosis. High-resolution, high-speed, digital imaging of ciliary motion in multiple planes permits comprehensive analysis of cilia beating, which has shown that certain beat patterns are associated with specific ultrastructural defects. This approach is available only at a limited number of clinical centers, primarily in Europe, and requires sophisticated software and expertise. Immunofluorescent staining for ciliary proteins is a newer approach that holds promise and may address some limitations of transmission electron microscopy. This approach is currently a research tool and not widely available.

Another promising approach has exploited the observation that nasal nitric oxide concentrations are reduced in subjects with PCD. Because nasal nitric oxide measurements are relatively easy to perform and noninvasive, this method is a promising screen and potentially a diagnostic test for PCD, provided that cystic fibrosis has been excluded (see Chapter 432). Few studies in children <5 yr have been reported, and the accuracy of nasal nitric oxide measurements in infants has not been established.

PCD is highly heterogenic owing to the large number of proteins involved in cilia assembly and function. Recent advances in gene sequencing techniques have led to the identification of a growing number of PCD-associated genes. Biallelic, disease-causing mutations have been found in more than 70% of known cases.

There are limitations in traditional diagnostic approaches. For instance, *DNAH11* mutations have been shown to cause typical clinical phenotypes without ultrastructural defects or reduced ciliary beat frequency. Children with mutations in cyclin O (CCNO) and multiciliate differentiation and DNA synthesis–associated cell cycle protein (MCIDAS) have symptoms consistent with PCD with only rare cilia on the epithelial surface. Thus genetic testing has become an important diagnostic tool for PCD.

TREATMENT
No therapies have been shown to correct ciliary dysfunction in PCD. Many of the treatments applied to PCD patients are similar to those used in other chronic suppurative lung diseases characterized by impaired airway clearance and bronchiectasis, such as cystic fibrosis, but none has been adequately studied to demonstrate efficacy in PCD.

Strategies to enhance mucociliary clearance are central to PCD therapy, and routine airway clearance techniques using postural drainage, percussion vests, positive expiratory pressure devices, or other techniques should be instituted daily. Because ciliary function is impaired, cough becomes a critical mechanism for mucous clearance and should not be suppressed. Exercise can enhance airway clearance in patients with PCD and should be encouraged. Inhaled mucolytic agents are often used in cystic fibrosis care, but only a few case reports have shown improvement in lung function in patients with PCD after treatment.

When children with PCD develop increasing respiratory symptoms consistent with infection, antimicrobial therapy should be instituted based on respiratory culture results and bacterial sensitivities. Early eradication strategies to clear bacteria from the PCD lung have not been studied. Maintenance therapy with inhaled or oral antibiotics can be used cautiously in patients with PCD who have bronchiectasis or frequent exacerbations, though current literature lacks evidence supporting long-term antimicrobial therapy. Immunizations against pertussis, influenza, and pneumococci are cornerstones of care. Additional preventive measures include avoidance of cigarette smoke and other airway irritants.

Although β-adrenergic agonists increase ciliary beat frequency in normal epithelial cells, data are lacking that show these agents improve function of dyskinetic cilia. Moreover, they do not necessarily provide bronchodilation in patients with PCD and obstructive airway disease.

Surgical resection of bronchiectatic lung has been performed on patients with PCD, typically in cases of localized disease with severe hemoptysis or intractable infections. It is unclear whether surgical interventions provide reduction in symptoms or survival benefit.

Progression to end-stage lung disease and respiratory failure has been reported in patients with PCD. Adult patients have undergone successful heart-lung, double lung, or living donor lobar lung transplantation. *Situs inversus totalis* complicates the procedure, owing to anatomic considerations. Otherwise, survival is similar to that for other transplant recipients.

Treatment of chronic otitis media and middle ear effusions in patients with PCD is controversial. Myringotomy tubes are frequently placed in affected children, but they are not without complications because they may lead to chronic mucoid otorrhea, tympanosclerosis, and permanent membrane perforation. Myringotomy tubes have not measurably improved hearing acuity. While hearing tends to improve with time, patients should be routinely screened and hearing aids used when necessary.

Chronic rhinitis and sinusitis are frequent clinical manifestations of PCD. No treatments have been shown to be effective, although patients are often treated with nasal washes, paranasal sinus lavage, and systemic antibiotics when they are symptomatic. As with any overuse of antimicrobial agents, the development of resistant organisms is a concern. When nasal symptoms are severe or refractory to medical management, endoscopic sinus surgery can be used to promote drainage or local delivery of medications, but the benefit may be short lived.

PROGNOSIS
Although signs and symptoms related to upper respiratory involvement predominate early in PCD, clinical manifestations of lower respiratory tract disease tend to increase with age and become the leading cause of morbidity and mortality in PCD patients. It is believed that progression and extent of lung disease can be slowed with early diagnosis and therapy. Thus routine surveillance studies recommended for the care of children with PCD include (1) regular spirometry to monitor pulmonary function, (2) chest imaging, and (3) sputum or oropharyngeal cultures to assess respiratory flora.

Patients with PCD typically have slower decline in pulmonary function than those with cystic fibrosis. Its prognosis and long-term survival are better. Many patients have a normal or near-normal life span, while others can experience progressive bronchiectasis and respiratory deterioration at a younger age.

Bibliography is available at Expert Consult.

Chapter **434**
Diffuse Lung Diseases in Childhood
第四百三十四章
儿童期弥漫性肺部疾病

中文导读

本章主要介绍了遗传性表面活性物质代谢异常疾病和肺泡蛋白沉积症。遗传性表面活性物质代谢异常疾病中具体描述了其病理学以及肺泡表面活性蛋白B缺乏、肺泡表面活性蛋白C基因变异、ABCA3基因突变相关疾病、NKX1-2基因突变相关疾病的遗传学、

临床表现及诊断，并介绍了表面活性物质功能障碍的治疗；肺泡蛋白沉积症中具体描述了原发性肺泡蛋白沉积症和继发性肺泡蛋白沉积症的病因学与病理生理学、临床表现、诊断以及治疗。

See also Chapter 427.

434.1 Inherited Disorders of Surfactant Metabolism

Jennifer A. Wambach, Lawrence M. Nogee, F. Sessions Cole III, and Aaron Hamvas

Pulmonary surfactant is a mixture of phospholipids and proteins synthesized, packaged, and secreted by alveolar type II pneumocytes (AEC2s) that line the distal air spaces. This mixture forms a monolayer at the air–liquid interface that lowers surface tension at end-expiration of the respiratory cycle, preventing atelectasis and ventilation–perfusion mismatch. Four surfactant-associated proteins have been characterized: surfactant proteins A and D (SP-A, SP-D) participate in host defense in the lung, whereas surfactant proteins B and C (SP-B, SP-C) contribute to the surface tension–lowering activity of pulmonary surfactant. The adenosine triphosphate–binding cassette protein member A3, ABCA3, is a transporter located on the limiting membrane of lamellar bodies, the storage organelle for surfactant within alveolar type II cells, and has an essential role in surfactant phospholipid metabolism. The proper expression of the surfactant proteins and ABCA3 is dependent on a number of transcription factors, particularly thyroid transcription factor 1 (TTF-1). Two genes for SP-A (*SFTPA1, SFTPA2*) and 1 gene for SP-D (*SFTPD*) are located on human chromosome 10, whereas single genes encode SP-B (*SFTPB*), SP-C (*SFTPC*), TTF-1 (*NKX2-1*), and ABCA3 (*ABCA3*), which are located on human chromosomes 2, 8, 14, and 16, respectively. Inherited disorders of SP-B, SP-C, ABCA3, and TTF-1

have been recognized in humans and are collectively termed **surfactant dysfunction disorders** (Table 434.1).

PATHOLOGY

Histopathologically, these disorders share a unique constellation of features, including AEC2 hyperplasia, alveolar macrophage accumulation, interstitial thickening and inflammation, and alveolar proteinosis. A number of different descriptive terms have historically been applied to these disorders, including ones borrowed from adult forms of interstitial lung disease (**desquamative interstitial pneumonia**, nonspecific interstitial pneumonia) as well as a disorder unique to infancy (**chronic pneumonitis of infancy**). These diagnoses in infants and children are strongly indicative of surfactant dysfunction disorders but do not distinguish which gene is responsible. As the prognosis and inheritance patterns differ depending upon the gene involved, genetic testing should be offered when one of these conditions is reported in the lung biopsy or autopsy of a child.

DEFICIENCY OF SURFACTANT PROTEIN B (SURFACTANT METABOLISM DYSFUNCTION, PULMONARY, 1; SMDP1; OMIM #265120)
Clinical Manifestations

Infants with an inherited deficiency of SP-B present in the *immediate* neonatal period with respiratory failure. This autosomal recessive disorder is clinically and radiographically similar to the respiratory distress syndrome (RDS) of premature infants (see Chapter 122.3) but typically affects full-term infants. The initial degree of respiratory distress is variable, but the disease is progressive and is refractory to mechanical ventilation, surfactant replacement therapy, and glucocorticoid

Table 434.1	Comparison of Surfactant Dysfunction Disorders			
	SP-B DEFICIENCY	**SP-C DISEASE**	**ABCA3 DEFICIENCY**	**TTF-1 DISORDERS**
Gene name	*SFTPB*	*SFTPC*	*ABCA3*	*NKX2-1*
Age of onset	Birth	Birth–adulthood	Birth–childhood; rarely adult	Birth–childhood
Inheritance	Recessive	Dominant/sporadic	Recessive	Sporadic/dominant
Mechanism	Loss of function	Gain of toxic function or dominant negative	Loss of function	Loss of function Gain of function
Natural history	Lethal	Variable	Generally lethal, may be chronic	Variable
DIAGNOSIS				
Biochemical (tracheal aspirate)	Absence of SP-B and presence of incompletely processed proSP-C	None	None	None
Genetic (DNA)	Sequence SFTPB	Sequence SFTPC	Sequence ABCA3	Sequence NKX2-1; deletion analysis
Ultrastructural (lung biopsy–electron microscopy)	Disorganized lamellar bodies	Not specific; may have dense aggregates	Small dense lamellar bodies with eccentrically placed dense cores	Variable
Treatment	Lung transplantation or compassionate care	Supportive care, lung transplantation if progressing	Lung transplantation or compassionate care for infants with biallelic null mutations; lung transplantation for other mutations if progressing	Supportive care; treat coexisting conditions (hypothyroidism)

SP, Surfactant protein.

administration. SP-B deficiency is observed in diverse racial and ethnic groups. Almost all affected patients have died without lung transplantation, but prolonged survival is possible in cases of partial deficiency of SP-B. Humans heterozygous for loss-of-function mutations in *SFTPB* are clinically normal as adults but may be at increased risk for obstructive lung disease if they also have a history of smoking.

Genetics
Multiple loss-of-function mutations in *SFTPB* have been identified. The most common is a net 2 base-pair insertion in codon 133 (originally termed "121ins2", currently termed c.397delCinsGAA, p.Pro133Glu*fs**95) that results in a frameshift, an unstable SP-B transcript, and absence of SP-B protein production. This mutation has accounted for 60–70% of the alleles found to date in infants identified with SP-B deficiency and is present in approximately 0.07% of European-descent individuals in large-scale sequencing projects. Most other mutations have been family-specific. A large deletion encompassing 2 exons of the SP-B gene has also been reported.

Diagnosis
A rapid, definitive diagnosis can be established with sequence analysis of *SFTPB,* which is available through clinical laboratories (http://www.genetests.org). While sequencing of *SFTPB* alone is available, as the phenotype of SP-B deficiency overlaps that of other surfactant dysfunction disorders, multi-gene panels using next generation sequencing (NGS) methods are supplanting sequencing of single genes. For families in which *SFTPB* mutations were previously identified, antenatal diagnosis can be established by preimplantation genetic diagnosis or molecular assays of DNA from chorionic villous biopsy or amniocytes, which permits advanced planning of a therapeutic regimen. Other laboratory tests remain investigational, including analysis of tracheal aspirate (effluent) for the presence or absence of SP-B protein and for incompletely processed precursor proSP-C peptides that have been identified in SP-B–deficient human infants. Immunostaining of lung biopsy tissue for the surfactant proteins can also support the diagnosis, although immunohistochemical assays for SP-B and SP-C are also generally available only on a research basis. Staining for SP-B is usually absent, but robust extracellular staining for proSP-C because of incompletely processed proSP-C peptides is observed and is diagnostic for SP-B deficiency. Such studies require a lung biopsy in a critically ill child but may be performed on lung blocks acquired at the time of autopsy, allowing for retrospective diagnosis. With electron microscopy, a lack of tubular myelin, disorganized lamellar bodies, and an accumulation of abnormal-appearing multivesicular bodies suggest abnormal lipid packaging and secretion.

SURFACTANT PROTEIN C GENE ABNORMALITIES (SURFACTANT METABOLISM DYSFUNCTION, PULMONARY, 2; SMDP2; OMIM #610913)
SP-C is a very low molecular weight, extremely hydrophobic protein that, along with SP-B, enhances the surface tension–lowering properties of surfactant phospholipids. It is derived from proteolytic processing of a larger precursor protein (proSP-C).

Clinical Manifestations
The clinical presentation of patients with *SFTPC* mutations is quite variable. Some patients present at birth with symptoms, signs, and radiographic findings typical of RDS. Others present later in life, *ranging from early infancy until well into adulthood*, with gradual onset of respiratory insufficiency, hypoxemia, failure to thrive, and chest radiograph demonstration of interstitial lung disease, or, in the 5th or 6th decade of life, as **pulmonary fibrosis**. The age and severity of disease vary even within families with the same mutation. The natural history is also quite variable, with some patients improving either spontaneously or as the result of therapy or prolonged mechanical ventilation, some with persistent respiratory insufficiency, and some progressing to the point of requiring lung transplantation. This variability in severity and course of the disease does not appear to correlate with the specific mutation and also hinders accurate assessment of prognosis.

Genetics
Multiple mutations in *SFTPC* have been identified in association with acute and chronic lung disease in patients ranging in age from newborn to adult. A mutation on only *one SFTPC* allele is sufficient to cause disease. Approximately half of these mutations arise spontaneously, resulting in sporadic disease, but the remainder are inherited as a *dominant trait*. A threonine substitution for isoleucine in codon 73 (termed p.I73T or p.Ile73Thr) has accounted for 25–35% of the cases identified to date but is rare (not identified in gnomAD ~123,000 individuals). *SFTPC* mutations have been identified in diverse racial

and ethnic groups. Mutations in *SFTPC* are thought to result in production of misfolded proSP-C that accumulates within the alveolar type II cell and causes cellular injury, or alters the normal intracellular routing of proSP-C.

Diagnosis

Sequencing of *SFTPC,* the only definitive diagnostic test, is available in clinical laboratories. The relatively small size of the gene facilitates such analyses, which are quite sensitive, but because most *SFTPC* mutations are missense mutations, distinguishing true disease-causing mutations from rare yet benign sequence variants may be difficult. Immunostaining of lung tissue may demonstrate proSP-C aggregates but is available only on a research basis.

DISEASE CAUSED BY MUTATIONS IN ABCA3 (SURFACTANT METABOLISM DYSFUNCTION, PULMONARY, 3; SMDP3; OMIM #610921)
Clinical Manifestations

Lung disease caused by mutations in *ABCA3* generally presents as either a severe, lethal form that manifests in the *immediate newborn period* clinically similar to SP-B deficiency, or a chronic form that appears most typically in the 1st yr of life with **interstitial lung disease** similar to SP-C–associated disease. Infants who are homozygous or compound heterozygous for null mutations, that is, the mutation is predicted to result in absence of protein expression (i.e., nonsense or frameshift mutations), typically present with lethal neonatal respiratory failure, whereas infants with other types of mutations have more variable age of onset and outcomes. Heterozygosity for an *ABCA3* mutation may contribute to the risk for RDS in late preterm and term infants, who, in contrast to ABCA3-deficient infants with mutations on both alleles, may eventually completely recover from their initial lung disease.

Genetics

Recessive mutations in *ABCA3* were first described among infants who presented with lethal RDS in the newborn period, but now have been identified in older infants and children with interstitial lung disease. There is considerable allelic heterogeneity: more than 400 mutations scattered throughout the gene have been identified, most of which are family-specific. The presence of null mutations on both alleles that are predicted to preclude any ABCA3 production has been associated with early-onset disease and a uniformly fatal prognosis. A missense mutation that results in a valine substitution for glutamine in codon 292 (p.E292V or p.Glu292Val) in association with a 2nd *ABCA3* mutation has been found in children with severe neonatal respiratory failure and in older children with interstitial lung disease and is present in approximately 0.7% of European-descent individuals. *ABCA3* mutations have been identified in diverse racial and ethnic groups. The precise frequency of disease is unknown, but large-scale sequencing projects indicate that the overall carrier rate for *ABCA3* mutations may be as high as 1 in 50 to 1 in 70 individuals. ABCA3 deficiency may thus contribute to a substantial proportion of *unexplained fatal lung disease* in term infants and of *interstitial lung disease* in older children.

Diagnosis

Sequence analysis of *ABCA3* is available in clinical laboratories and is the most definitive approach for diagnosis. Considerable variation in *ABCA3* necessitates careful interpretation regarding the functionality of an individual variant and its contribution to the clinical presentation. Additionally, *sequence analysis is not 100% sensitive* as functionally significant mutations may exist in untranslated regions that are not generally analyzed. In these situations, lung biopsy with electron microscopy to examine lamellar body morphology may be a useful adjunct to the diagnostic approach. Small lamellar bodies that contain electron-dense inclusions may be observed in association with *ABCA3* mutations. These findings support the hypothesis that ABCA3 function is necessary for lamellar body biogenesis. There are no biochemical markers to establish the diagnosis.

DISEASE CAUSED BY MUTATIONS IN *NKX2-1* (THYROID TRANSCRIPTION FACTOR 1, CHOREOATHETOSIS, HYPOTHYROIDISM, AND NEONATAL RESPIRATORY DISTRESS, OMIM #600635)
Clinical Manifestations

A large deletion of the region of chromosome 14 (14q13.3) encompassing the *NKX2-1* locus was first recognized in an infant with hypothyroidism and neonatal RDS. Since then, multiple large deletions involving the *NKX2-1* locus and contiguous genes as well as missense, frameshift, nonsense, and small insertion or deletion mutations scattered throughout the gene have been reported in individuals with hypothyroidism, lung disease, and neurologic symptoms, including benign familial chorea. Manifestation of dysfunction in all 3 organ systems has been referred to as **brain-thyroid-lung syndrome**, but disease may manifest in only 1 or 2 organ systems. The lung disease can range from severe and eventually *lethal neonatal respiratory distress* to *chronic lung disease in childhood and adulthood*. Recurrent pulmonary infections have been reported, likely caused by reduced expression of the pulmonary collectins, SP-A and SP-D, but could also result from decreased expression of other proteins. No clear genotype–phenotype correlations have emerged, but children harboring complete gene deletions have tended to have more severe and earlier-onset disease. This observation could also be related to the deletion of other adjacent genes. While limited data are available, the pulmonary phenotype may depend upon the expression of which *NKX2-1* target genes are most affected. Children with decreased SP-B or ABCA3 expression may present with acute neonatal respiratory failure whereas those with decreased SP-C or pulmonary collectin expression are more likely to have chronic lung disease.

Genetics

The gene is small, spanning < 3,000 bases, with only 3 exons. TTF-1 is expressed not only in the lung but also in the thyroid gland, as well as in the central nervous system. In the lung it is important for the expression of a wide variety of proteins, including the surfactant proteins, ABCA3, club cell secretory protein, and many others. Two transcripts that differ depending upon whether the transcriptional start site is in the 1st or 2nd exon have been recognized, although the shorter transcript is the predominant transcript in the lung. Most mutations are thought to result in a loss of function, with the mechanism of disease thus being haploinsufficiency, but discordant effects on different target genes have been reported. Loss of function mutations in *NKX2-1* are rare in large sequencing projects, but the prevalence of disease is unknown. Mutations in diverse ethnic groups have been recognized. Most reported mutations and deletions have occurred *de novo* resulting in sporadic disease, but familial disease transmitted in a dominant manner has been recognized.

Diagnosis

Sequence analysis of the *NKX2-1* gene is available through clinical laboratories and is the preferred method for diagnosis. As deletions comprise a significant fraction of reported mutant alleles, specific methods to look for such deletions should also be performed, such as a comparative genomic hybridization assay, a multiplex ligation-dependent probe amplification assay, or utilizing NGS methodology. A mutation on 1 allele is sufficient to cause disease. While isolated pulmonary disease has been recognized, the majority of reported affected individuals have manifestations in 2 or more other organ systems. Thus the presence of **hypothyroidism** or neurologic abnormality in a proband or a family history of chorea should prompt consideration of the diagnosis. The most specific neurologic finding is **chorea**, but hypotonia, developmental delay, ataxia, and dysarthria have been reported. In very young, non-ambulatory infants the neurologic symptoms may not be evident, or muscle weakness or hypotonia may be attributed to the severity of lung disease or a result of the hypothyroidism. Affected individuals may not be overtly hypothyroid but have compensated hypothyroidism with borderline low T4 (thyroxine) and high thyroid-stimulating hormone levels. The lung pathology associated with *NKX2-1* mutations may be typical of that of other surfactant dysfunction disorders, but because *NKX2-1* is important for lung development, growth abnormalities and arrested pulmonary development also may be seen. Immunostaining studies of surfactant protein expression have yielded variable results, with decreased expression of one or more surfactant-related proteins observed in some patients. No characteristic electron microscopy findings have been identified.

TREATMENT OF SURFACTANT DYSFUNCTION DISORDERS

Virtually all patients with SP-B deficiency die within the 1st yr of life. Conventional neonatal intensive care interventions can maintain extrapulmonary organ function for a limited time (weeks to months). Replacement therapy with commercially available surfactants is ineffective. Lung transplantation has been successful, but the pretransplantation, transplantation, and posttransplantation medical and surgical care is highly specialized and available only at pediatric pulmonary transplantation centers; prompt recognition is critical if patients are to be considered for lung transplantation. Palliative care consultation is helpful.

No specific treatment is available for patients with lung disease caused by mutations in *SFTPC* or *ABCA3*. Therapeutic approaches used for interstitial lung diseases, such as the use of corticosteroids, quinolones, and macrolide antibiotics have been reported but not systematically evaluated (Fig. 434.1). Infants with severe and progressive respiratory failure attributable to ABCA3 deficiency may be candidates for lung transplantation. The variable natural history of patients with *SFTPC* mutations and older children with ABCA3 deficiency makes predictions of prognosis difficult. Lung transplantation is reserved for patients with progressive and refractory respiratory failure who would otherwise qualify for transplantation irrespective of their diagnosis.

Treatment for patients with *NKX2-1* mutations is largely supportive. Hypothyroidism if present should be treated with thyroid replacement. Corticosteroids and other agents used for other types of surfactant dysfunction have not been formally evaluated. Some individuals have progressive lung disease and have undergone lung transplantation. The variable progression of disease and presence of extrapulmonary disease may make evaluation and selection of subjects for transplantation particularly difficult.

Parents of children with surfactant dysfunction disorders should be offered genetic counseling to inform recurrence risk for future pregnancies, to present antenatal diagnostic options and offer delivery at a center with neonatal intensive care, and to facilitate discussions regarding whether testing should be offered to other family members who may not be symptomatic.

Bibliography is available at Expert Consult.

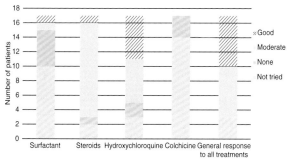

Fig. 434.1 Response to therapies for 17 patients with SFTPC mutations. (*Data from Kröner C, Reu S, Teusch V, et al: Genotype alone does not predict the clinical course of SFTPC deficiency in paediatric patients,* Eur Respir J 46:197–206, 2015.)

434.2 Pulmonary Alveolar Proteinosis

Jennifer A. Wambach, Lawrence M. Nogee, F. Sessions Cole III, and Aaron Hamvas

Pulmonary alveolar proteinosis (PAP) is a rare syndrome characterized by the intra-alveolar and terminal airway accumulation of surfactant leading to progressive hypoxemic respiratory failure. PAP can result from abnormalities in surfactant production or surfactant clearance. Histopathologic examination shows distal air spaces are filled with a granular, eosinophilic material that stains positively with periodic acid–Schiff reagent and is diastase resistant. This material contains large amounts of surfactant proteins and lipids and the primary mechanism for its accumulation is impaired catabolism by alveolar macrophages. PAP is classified as either *primary* due to disruption of granulocyte-macrophage colony-stimulating factor (GM-CSF) signaling or *secondary* due to several different diseases that reduce alveolar macrophage number or function (Table 434.2). A fulminant, usually lethal form of PAP

	AUTOIMMUNE	GM-CSF RECEPTOR DEFICIENCY	LYSINURIC PROTEIN INTOLERANCE	MARS DEFICIENCY	GATA2 DEFICIENCY
Gene(s)		*CSFR2A, CSFR2B*	*SLC7A7*	*MARS*	*GATA2*
Age of onset	Adult > child	Childhood to adult	Childhood	Childhood to adult	Childhood to adult
Inheritance	N.A.	Recessive	Recessive	Recessive	Sporadic/dominant
Mechanism	Neutralizing antibodies to GM-CSF	Loss of function	Loss of function	Loss of function	Loss of function; haploinsufficiency
Other manifestations			Emesis; failure to thrive	Liver disease; hypothyroidism	Immune deficiency; myelodysplasia
DIAGNOSIS					
Biochemical	Detection of serum GM-CSF autoantibody	Elevated serum GM-CSF levels	Increased cationic amino acids in urine, especially lysine	None	None
Genetic (*DNA*)	N.A.	Sequence *CSFR2A, CSFR2B*	Sequence *SLC7A7*	Sequence *MARS*	Sequence *GATA2*
Treatment	Whole lung lavage; inhaled GM-CSF	Whole lung lavage; bone marrow transplantation	Whole lung lavage, dietary protein restriction, administration of citrulline and nitrogen scavenging drugs	Whole lung lavage	Whole lung lavage; bone marrow transplantation

Table 434.2 | Comparison of Pulmonary Alveolar Proteinosis Syndromes

GM-CSF, Granulocyte-macrophage colony-stimulating factor.

manifesting shortly after birth has been termed **congenital alveolar proteinosis**, but because this condition is caused by disrupted surfactant metabolism or surfactant dysfunction within alveolar type II cells, the disease is included under "Inherited Disorders of Surfactant Metabolism," above (see Chapter 434.1).

ETIOLOGY AND PATHOPHYSIOLOGY
Primary Alveolar Proteinosis
Disordered signaling of GM-CSF leading to impaired alveolar macrophage maturation is the major underlying cause of primary PAP in children and adults. Most cases of primary PAP in older children and adults are mediated by neutralizing autoantibodies directed against GM-CSF, which can be detected in serum and bronchoalveolar lavage (BAL) fluid. These autoantibodies block binding of GM-CSF to its receptor, thereby inhibiting alveolar macrophage maturation and function and surfactant clearance. Mutations in the genes encoding both the α and β subunits of the GM-CSF receptor *(CSF2RA, CSFR2B)* in children with primary alveolar proteinosis account for a genetic basis for some cases of primary PAP in childhood.

Secondary Alveolar Proteinosis
Alveolar proteinosis has also been reported in children, including young infants, with lysinuric protein intolerance, a rare autosomal recessive disorder caused by mutations in the cationic amino acid transporter SLC7A7 (see Chapter 103.14). These children generally present with vomiting, hyperammonemia, and failure to thrive, although their pulmonary disease may prove fatal. Defective macrophage function has been demonstrated in lysinuric protein intolerance and a case of *recurrence* of the disease after lung transplantation also supports a primary role for alveolar macrophage dysfunction in the pathogenesis of PAP associated with lysinuric protein intolerance. PAP is also a prominent feature in patients with biallelic mutations in the gene encoding methionyl tRNA synthetase *(MARS)*, who have a multi-organ phenotype that also includes liver disease as a prominent feature, and is prevalent among individuals on Reunion Island. The mechanism for PAP in patients with *MARS* mutations is unknown. Heterozygous mutations in the gene encoding the transcription factor GATA2 have also been associated with a phenotype that includes PAP, as well as immune deficiencies, myelodysplasia, and lymphatic abnormalities. The mechanism for PAP in patients with such mutations is likely related to GATA2's role in alveolar macrophage development. PAP may also be associated with some subtypes of Niemann-Pick disease (see Chapter 104.4).

Secondary alveolar proteinosis also may occur in association with *infection*, particularly in immunocompromised individuals. However, because the same pathologic process occurs in severely immunodeficient mice raised in a pathogen-free environment, it is not clear whether this phenotype results from a secondary infection or the underlying immunodeficiency. Environmental exposures to dust, silica, and chemicals and chemotherapeutic agents, hematologic disorders (esp. myelodysplastic syndrome), and non-hematologic malignancies have also been associated with the development of secondary alveolar proteinosis.

CLINICAL MANIFESTATIONS
Infants and children with PAP present with dyspnea, fatigue, cough, weight loss, chest pain, or hemoptysis. In the later stages, cyanosis and digital clubbing may be seen. Pulmonary function changes include decreased diffusing capacity of carbon monoxide, lung volumes with a restrictive abnormality, and arterial blood gas values indicating marked hypoxemia and/or chronic respiratory acidosis. Alveolar proteinosis in infants and children is rare and males are affected 3 times as often as females.

DIAGNOSIS
Histopathologic examination of lung biopsy specimens currently remains the gold standard for diagnosis of PAP in children, although this is likely to change as molecular tests become available. Immunohistochemi-

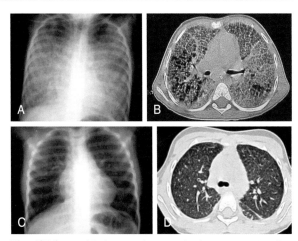

Fig. 434.2 A and **B,** Severe pulmonary alveolar proteinosis in a 5 yr old boy before therapeutic lung lavage. **A,** Chest radiograph shows diffuse alveolointerstitial infiltrates. **B,** CT scan demonstrates major air-space opacities and crazy-paving pattern. **C** and **D,** Same patient after 12 therapeutic lung lavages. **C,** Chest radiograph demonstrates improvement of alveolointerstitial infiltrates. **D,** CT scan shows regression of the air-space opacities with a residual micronodular pattern. *(From De Blic J: Pulmonary alveolar proteinosis in children,* Paediatr Respir Rev *5:316–322, 2004.)*

cal staining reveals abundant quantities of alveolar and intracellular surfactant proteins A, B, and D. Latex agglutination tests for the presence of anti–GM-CSF antibodies in BAL fluid or blood are highly sensitive and specific for the autoimmune forms of alveolar proteinosis. Elevations of GM-CSF in peripheral blood suggest a GM-CSF receptor defect, and molecular analysis of these genes should be pursued. The examination of sputum or BAL fluid for surfactant components has been used diagnostically in adults, but these methods have not been validated in children. Examination of peripheral blood and/or bone marrow for clonogenic stimulation of monocyte-macrophage precursors, GM-CSF receptor and ligand expression, and GM-CSF binding and signaling studies are available through research protocols.

TREATMENT
The natural history of primary PAP is highly variable, making prognostic and therapeutic decisions difficult. Total lung lavage has been associated with prolonged remissions of PAP in adults and remains a therapeutic option for patients with childhood PAP (Fig. 434.2). Younger infants with PAP may be more likely to have genetic mechanisms underlying their disease, and the role of repeated BAL in children has not been well studied, nor is it likely to be effective. It may provide a temporizing measure in some circumstances and may benefit patients with autoimmune or secondary PAP. Subcutaneous or inhaled administration of recombinant GM-CSF may improve pulmonary function in some adults with later-onset PAP. The role of exogenous GM-CSF treatment in children has not been well studied, although successful treatment has been reported in an adolescent with autoimmune-mediated PAP. Because children with GM-CSF receptor defects generally have high serum levels of GM-CSF, exogenous GM-CSF seems unlikely to be effective in most such cases. Depending upon the nature of the mutation(s) responsible for the deficiency, some responsiveness of the receptor may be retained such that a response to exogenous GM-CSF is possible. As the primary defect for PAP resides in the alveolar macrophage, which is a bone marrow–derived cell, lung transplantation would not be expected to correct primary PAP.

Bibliography is available at Expert Consult.

Chapter 435
Pulmonary Hemosiderosis
Mary A. Nevin

第四百三十五章
肺含铁血黄素沉着症

中文导读

　　本章主要介绍了肺含铁血黄素沉着症。介绍了该病的病因学、流行病学、病理学、病理生理学、临床表现、实验室检查和诊断、治疗以及预后。其中病因学方面对可能表现为复发性或慢性弥漫性肺泡出血的病因进行了总结和分类；病理生理学方面详细阐述了肺毛细血管炎相关性弥漫性肺泡出血，如肉芽肿性多血管炎、显微镜下血管炎、肺出血肾炎综合征等，以及非肺毛细血管相关性弥漫性肺泡出血，如牛奶过敏、乳糜泻以及移植物抗宿主病等相关的弥漫性肺泡出血。

Pulmonary hemorrhage may be characterized as focal or diffuse based on the location(s) of bleeding. A detailed review of pulmonary hemorrhage is in Chapter 436.2. The diagnosis of pulmonary hemosiderosis refers to the subset of patients with **diffuse alveolar hemorrhage (DAH)**. Bleeding in DAH occurs as a result of injury to the microvasculature of the lung and may be slow and insidious due to the low-pressure pulmonary circulation. Pulmonary hemosiderosis has classically been characterized by the triad of iron-deficiency anemia, hemoptysis, and radiographic evidence of alveolar infiltration. However, many of those affected, particularly young patients, are likely to present atypically and a high index of suspicion for this condition must be maintained. Pulmonary hemosiderosis can exist in isolation, but more commonly occurs in association with an underlying condition. A precise etiology for hemorrhage may not always be found. A diagnosis of **idiopathic pulmonary hemosiderosis (IPH)** is made when DAH occurs in isolation and an exhaustive evaluation for an underlying pathologic etiology is found to be unrevealing or nondiagnostic.

ETIOLOGY
The varied etiologies of pulmonary hemosiderosis are classified on the basis of the presence or absence of pulmonary **capillaritis**, a pathologic process that is characterized by inflammation and cellular disruption of the alveolar interstitium and capillary bed. Although the finding of pulmonary capillaritis is nonspecific with regard to underlying diagnosis, its presence appears to be an important negative prognostic factor in DAH and may indicate an underlying systemic vasculitic process or collagen vascular disease.

Disorders associated with pulmonary capillaritis may include systemic lupus erythematosus (SLE; see Chapter 183), drug-induced capillaritis, granulomatosis with polyangiitis (previously Wegener granulomatosis),

Goodpasture syndrome, and Henoch-Schönlein purpura (see Chapter 192). The finding of DAH in patients with granulomatosis with polyangiitis and microscopic polyangiitis (MPA; see Chapter 192) is frequently associated with pathologic evidence of pulmonary capillaritis. In patients with Goodpasture syndrome or SLE, DAH has been reported both with and without the associated finding of capillaritis. A number of systemic autoimmune and inflammatory disorders may predispose a host to DAH with pulmonary capillaritis. Similarly, a variety of drugs have been associated with the finding of pulmonary capillaritis but mechanisms of cellular derangement are as yet unidentified.

These disorders are distinguished from those without pulmonary capillaritis. Those disorders in which the pathologic finding of capillary network disruption is absent are further divided into cardiac (pulmonary hypertension, mitral stenosis) and noncardiac (immunodeficiency, Heiner syndrome, coagulopathies, IPH) etiologies. Table 435.1 provides a summary and classification of the diagnoses that may manifest as recurrent or chronic pulmonary bleeding.

EPIDEMIOLOGY
Disorders that present as DAH are highly variable in their severity, as well as in their associated symptomatology and identifiable abnormalities in laboratory testing; the diagnosis may be significantly delayed, making frequency estimates unreliable. Similarly, the prevalence of IPH is largely unknown. Of the children and young adults diagnosed with IPH in the past, it has been postulated that the etiology of the hemorrhage might have been discovered if they had been studied with the newer and more advanced diagnostics available today; specific serologic testing has vastly improved our ability to appreciate immune mediated disease. Estimates of prevalence obtained from Swedish and Japanese retrospective case analyses vary from 0.24 to 1.23 cases per million. Children and ado-

Table 435.1	Diffuse Alveolar Hemorrhage Syndromes

CLASSIFICATION	SYNDROME
DISORDERS WITH PULMONARY CAPILLARITIS	
	Idiopathic (isolated) pulmonary capillaritis (ANCA positive or negative)
	Granulomatosis with polyangiitis (Wegener granulomatosis)
	Microscopic polyangiitis
	Systemic lupus erythematosus (SLE)
	Scleroderma
	Polymyositis
	Goodpasture syndrome
	Antiphospholipid antibody syndrome
	Henoch-Schönlein purpura
	Immunoglobulin A nephropathy
	Behçet syndrome
	Cryoglobulinemia
	Drug-induced capillaritis (phenytoin, retinoic acid, propylthiouracil)
	Idiopathic pulmonary-renal syndrome
	Acute lung transplant rejection
	Eosinophilic granulomatosis angiitis (Churg-Strauss syndrome)
	Idiopathic pulmonary fibrosis
DISORDERS WITHOUT PULMONARY CAPILLARITIS	
Noncardiovascular causes	Idiopathic pulmonary hemosiderosis
	Heiner syndrome
	Acute idiopathic pulmonary hemorrhage of infancy
	Bone marrow transplantation
	Immunodeficiency
	Coagulation disorders
	Hemolytic uremic syndromes
	Celiac disease (Lane-Hamilton syndrome)
	SLE
	Non-accidental trauma
	Radiation therapy
	Infection (HIV, cryptococcosis, Legionnaires disease)
	Drugs—toxins
Cardiovascular causes	Mitral stenosis
	Pulmonary venoocclusive disease
	Arteriovenous malformations
	Pulmonary lymphangioleiomyomatosis
	Pulmonary hypertension
	Pulmonary capillary hemangiomatosis
	Chronic heart failure
	Vascular thrombosis with infarction
	Endocarditis

Modified from Susarla SC, Fan LL: Diffuse alveolar hemorrhage syndromes in children, *Curr Opin Pediatr* 19:314–320, 2007.

lescents account for 30% of cases. The ratio of affected males:females is 1:1 in the childhood diagnosis group, and men are only slightly more affected in the group diagnosed as young adults.

PATHOLOGY

In pulmonary capillaritis, key histologic features include (1) fibrin thrombi, which occlude capillaries, (2) fibrin clots adherent to interalveolar septae, (3) fibrinoid necrosis of capillary walls, and (4) interstitial erythrocytes and hemosiderin. Illustrative but nonspecific pathologic findings, such as vascular smooth muscle hypertrophy (pulmonary hypertension), edema (mitral stenosis), or thrombosis (vascular thrombosis with infarction), may be found in those disorders that cause DAH without pulmonary capillaritis. The finding of blood in the airways or alveoli is representative of a recent hemorrhage. With repeated episodes of pulmonary hemorrhage, lung tissue appears brown secondary to this

presence of hemosiderin. *Hemosiderin-laden macrophages (HLMs)* are seen with recovering, recurrent, or chronic pulmonary hemorrhage and are identifiable both in bronchoalveolar lavage fluid and in pathologic specimens of lung tissue. It takes 48-72 hr for the alveolar macrophages to convert iron from erythrocytes into hemosiderin. In a murine model, HLMs appear 3 days after a single episode of pulmonary hemorrhage and peak at 7-10 days. HLMs may be detectable for weeks to months after a hemorrhagic event. Other nonspecific pathologic findings include thickening of alveolar septa, goblet cell hyperplasia, and hypertrophy of type II pneumocytes. Fibrosis may be seen with chronic disease.

PATHOPHYSIOLOGY

Diffuse Alveolar Hemorrhage Associated With Pulmonary Capillaritis

Granulomatosis with polyangiitis is a recognized etiology for DAH in children. This disease is classically characterized by necrotizing granuloma formation (with or without cavitation) of the upper and lower respiratory tract and by a necrotizing glomerulonephritis and small vessel vasculitis. In children, presentations attributable to the upper airway, including subglottic stenosis, may suggest the diagnosis. The presence of antineutrophil cytoplasmic antibodies (ANCAs) may be helpful in diagnosis and management, but the clinician must be aware that other ANCA-positive vasculitides, such as MPA and Churg-Strauss syndrome, may share this nonspecific laboratory finding. In small-vessel vasculitides, ANCAs cause an inflammatory reaction that results in injury to the microvasculature. Antiproteinase-3 antibodies (cANCA) are classically associated with granulomatosis with polyangiitis whereas antimyeloperoxidase antibodies (pANCA) are typically found in patients with MPA.

Patients with **MPA** (previously the microscopic variant of polyarteritis nodosa) demonstrate a systemic necrotizing vasculitis with a predilection for small vessels (venules, arterioles, capillaries) but without necrotizing granuloma formation. This diagnosis is precluded by the finding of immune complex deposition in order to differentiate MPA from other diseases (Henoch-Schönlein purpura, cryoglobulinemic vasculitis) that are associated with immune complex–mediated small-vessel vasculitis.

Goodpasture syndrome is an immune complex–mediated disease in which anti–glomerular basement membrane (GBM) antibody binds to the basement membrane of both the alveolus and the glomerulus. GBM antibodies attach to type IV collagen contained in the vascular endothelium. At the alveolar level, immunoglobulin (Ig) G, IgM, and complement are deposited at alveolar septa. Electron microscopy shows disruption of basement membranes and vascular integrity, which allows blood to escape into alveolar spaces.

Although alveolar hemorrhage is not commonly encountered in association with SLE, its occurrence is often severe and potentially life-threatening; mortality rates exceed 50%. Pathologic vasculitic features may be absent. Some immunofluorescent studies have revealed IgG and C3 deposits at the alveolar septa. However, a clear link between immune complex formation and alveolar hemorrhage has not been established.

In **Henoch-Schönlein purpura,** pulmonary hemorrhage is a rare but recognized complication. Pathologic findings have included transmural neutrophilic infiltration of small vessels, alveolar septal inflammation, and intra-alveolar hemorrhage. Vasculitis is the proposed mechanism for hemorrhage.

Pulmonary renal syndromes are defined as those where pulmonary and renal disease manifestations are predominant. These include the aforementioned granulomatosis with polyangiitis, Goodpasture syndrome, SLE, and MPA. As Henoch-Schönlein purpura may also have renal involvement, it has been suggested for inclusion as a pulmonary renal syndrome.

Diffuse Alveolar Hemorrhage Not Associated With Pulmonary Capillaritis

A premature infant's neonatal course can be complicated by pulmonary hemorrhage. The alveolar and vascular networks are immature and particularly prone to inflammation and damage by ventilator mechanics, barotrauma, oxidative stress, and infection. Pulmonary hemorrhage may be unrecognized if the volume of blood is insufficient to reach the proximal airways. The chest radiographic findings in pulmonary hemorrhage may be appreciated instead as a worsening picture of respiratory distress syndrome, edema, or infection.

Pulmonary hemosiderosis in association with **cow's milk hypersensitivity** was first reported by Heiner in 1962. This condition is characterized by variable symptoms of milk intolerance. Symptoms can include grossly bloody or occult heme-positive stools, vomiting, failure to thrive, symptoms of gastroesophageal reflux, and/or upper airway congestion. Pathologic findings have included elevations of IgE and peripheral eosinophilia, as well as alveolar deposits of IgG, IgA, and C3. Association with pulmonary hemorrhage has remained controversial, but multiple case series have provided support for the anecdotal association. In one series, infants presenting with recurrent respiratory symptoms and iron-deficiency anemia; all infants improved with elimination of cow's milk from their diets and a subset thereafter had a recurrence of pulmonary disease with a cow's milk challenge. However, many patients with milk precipitins did not have symptoms of hemosiderosis and patients with hemosiderosis did not always have milk precipitins; the relationship may be an association rather than causal in nature.

A number of case reports and case series have suggested an association between **celiac disease** (see Chapter 364.2) and DAH. In these reports, a resolution of intestinal and pulmonary symptoms along with resolution of radiographic disease has been seen after the adoption of a gluten-free diet. Consideration of testing for celiac disease in those patients with pulmonary hemorrhage and suggestive gastrointestinal symptomatology may be warranted.

A number of additional associated conditions and exposures exist as causes for DAH. These are typically noninflammatory in nature and may be diversely attributable to cardiac, vascular, lymphatic, or hematologic etiologies. **Graft-versus-host disease** has been implicated in transplant recipients and DAH may rarely be attributable to nonaccidental trauma. These etiologies for DAH occur relatively infrequently in the pediatric population, and suggested mechanisms for hemorrhage are variable.

The diagnosis of IPH is a diagnosis of exclusion and is only made when there is evidence of chronic or recurrent DAH and when exhaustive evaluations for primary or secondary etiologies have negative results. Renal and systemic involvement should be absent and a biopsy specimen should not reveal any evidence of granulomatous disease, vasculitis, infection, infarction, immune complex deposition, or malignancy. Some patients initially diagnosed with IPH will later be found to have Goodpasture syndrome, SLE, or MPA; therefore some cases of IPH may represent unrecognized immune-mediated disorders.

CLINICAL MANIFESTATIONS

The clinical presentation of pulmonary hemosiderosis is highly variable. In most symptomatic cases, DAH is heralded by symptoms of hemoptysis and dyspnea with associated hypoxemia and the finding of alveolar infiltration on chest radiograph. The diagnosis may be problematic as young children often lack the ability to effectively expectorate and may not present with hemoptysis. As the presence of blood in the lung is a trigger for airway irritation and inflammation, the patient may present after an episode of hemorrhage with wheezing, cough, dyspnea, and alterations in gas exchange, reflecting bronchospasm, edema, mucus plugging, and inflammation; this presentation may result in an incorrect diagnosis of asthma or bronchiolitis. A lack of pulmonary symptoms does not preclude the diagnosis of DAH and children may present only with chronic fatigue or pallor. In particular, young infants and children with DAH may come to attention with entirely nonspecific and nonpulmonary symptomatology such as failure to thrive or jaundice.

Primary or reported symptoms may reflect an underlying and associated disease process or comorbid condition. Presentations can vary widely from a relative lack of symptoms to shock or sudden death. Bleeding may occasionally be recognized from the presence of alveolar infiltrates on a chest radiograph alone. It should be noted, however, that the absence of an infiltrate does not rule out an ongoing hemorrhagic process.

On physical examination, the patient may be pale with tachycardia and tachypnea. During an acute exacerbation, children are frequently febrile. Examination of the chest may reveal retractions and differential or decreased aeration, with crackles or wheezes. The patient may present in shock with respiratory failure from massive hemoptysis.

LABORATORY FINDINGS AND DIAGNOSIS

Pulmonary hemorrhage is classically associated with a microcytic, hypochromic anemia. Reductions of serum iron levels, decreased or normal total iron-binding capacity, and normal to increased ferritin levels may be found with chronic disease. An elevated erythrocyte sedimentation rate is a nonspecific finding. The reticulocyte count is frequently elevated. Patients with pulmonary capillaritis have lower hematocrits and higher erythrocyte sedimentation rates. The anemia of IPH can mimic a hemolytic anemia. Elevations of plasma bilirubin are caused by absorption and breakdown of hemoglobin in the alveoli. Any or all of these hematologic manifestations may be absent in the presence of recent hemorrhage.

White blood cell count and differential should be evaluated for evidence of infection and eosinophilia. A peripheral smear and direct Coombs test may suggest a vasculitic process. A stool specimen positive for occult blood may suggest associated gastrointestinal disease but can also reflect swallowed blood. Renal and liver functions should be reviewed. A urinalysis should be obtained to assess for evidence of a pulmonary–renal syndrome. A coagulation profile, quantitative immunoglobulins (including IgE), and complement studies are recommended. Testing for von Willebrand disease is also indicated.

Testing for ANCA (cANCA, pANCA), antinuclear antibody, double-stranded DNA, rheumatoid factor, antiphospholipid antibody, and GBM antibody evaluates for a number of immune-mediated and vasculitic processes that may be associated with pulmonary capillaritis.

Sputum or pulmonary secretions should be analyzed for significant evidence of blood or HLMs and may provide supportive evidence in a patient who is able to adequately expectorate secretions from the lower airway. Gastric secretions may also reveal HLMs. Flexible bronchoscopy provides visualization of any areas of active bleeding. With bronchoalveolar lavage, pulmonary secretions may be sent for pathologic review and culture analysis. The ability to perform flexible bronchoscopy will be limited if there are large amounts of blood or clots in the airway. Active bleeding may be exacerbated by airway occlusion with a bronchoscope and by installation of fluid. A patient with respiratory failure can be ventilated more effectively through a rigid bronchoscope.

Chest x-rays may reveal evidence of acute or chronic disease. Hyperaeration is frequently seen, especially during an acute hemorrhage. Infiltrates are typically symmetric and may spare the apices of the lung. Atelectasis may also be appreciated. With chronic disease, fibrosis, lymphadenopathy, and nodularity may be seen. CT findings may demonstrate a subclinical and contributory disease process. The presence of a cardiac murmur, cardiomegaly on X-ray, or a clinical suspicion for left-sided heart lesion suggests the need for a complete cardiac evaluation, including electrocardiogram and echocardiogram.

Pulmonary function testing will likely reveal primarily obstructive disease in the acute period. With more chronic disease, fibrosis and restrictive disease tend to predominate. Oxygen saturation levels may be decreased. Lung volumes may reveal air trapping acutely and decreases in total lung capacity chronically. The diffusing capacity of carbon monoxide may be low or normal in the chronic phase but is likely to be elevated in the setting of an acute hemorrhage, because carbon monoxide binds to the hemoglobin in extravasated red blood cells.

Lung biopsy is warranted when DAH occurs without discernible etiology, extrapulmonary disease, or circulating GBM antibodies. When surgically obtained, pulmonary tissue should be evaluated for evidence of vasculitis, immune complex deposition, and granulomatous disease.

Many have supported a diagnosis of IPH without lung biopsy if the patient has a typical presentation with diffuse infiltration on radiography, anemia, HLMs in bronchoalveolar lavage, sputum or gastric aspirate, absence of systemic disease, and negative serology for immune-mediated disease. However, a number of patients meeting these criteria have been proven to have pulmonary capillaritis on review of pathologic lung tissue specimens. Therefore, a lung biopsy is recommended in any child presenting with DAH of uncertain etiology.

TREATMENT

Supportive therapy, including volume resuscitation, ventilatory support, supplemental oxygen, and transfusion of blood products, may be warranted in the patient presenting acutely with pulmonary hemorrhage. Surgical or medical therapy should be directed at any treatable underlying condition. In IPH, systemic corticosteroids are frequently utilized as first-line treatment and are expected to be of particular benefit in the setting of immune-mediated disease. Steroids modulate neutrophil influx and the inflammation associated with hemorrhage; consequently, they may decrease progression toward fibrotic disease.

Medication dosing may vary with regard to primary diagnosis, age, comorbidities, and other factors. Clinical-pharmacologic correlation is advocated. Treatment may be provided in the form of methylprednisolone 2-4 mg/kg/day divided every 6 hr or in the form of prednisone 0.5-1 mg/kg daily and decreased to every other day after resolution of acute symptoms. Successful treatment is also associated with the use of pulse steroid therapy; methylprednisolone may be given at a dose of 10-30 mg/kg (maximum 1 g) infused over 1 hr for 3 consecutive days and repeated weekly or monthly. Early treatment with corticosteroids appears to decrease episodes of hemorrhage. Steroid therapy is associated with improved survival and may be tapered as tolerated with disease remission or chronically maintained.

A variety of steroid-sparing and alternative immunosuppressive agents, including cyclophosphamide, cytoxan, azathioprine, hydroxychloroquine, methotrexate, rituximab, 6-mercaptopurine, and intravenous Ig, have all been successfully used anecdotally as adjunctive therapy in patients with severe, chronic, unremitting, or recurrent hemorrhage. Maintenance therapy with 6-mercaptopurine may produce favorable results in achieving long-term remission.

Plasmapheresis is a recognized therapy for anti-GBM antibody disease. Intravenous Ig has been used in immune complex–mediated disease.

In the most critically ill children, additional life-sustaining interventions may be required; extracorporeal membrane oxygenation (ECMO) combined with immunosuppression was reported to be successful in allowing recovery from a severe hemorrhage with hypoxemic respiratory failure in the setting of p-ANCA positive MPA. In neonatal and infantile pulmonary hemorrhage, clinical improvement in blood gas and ventilatory requirements have been described with intrapulmonary administration of exogenous surfactant.

The potential adverse effects of these pharmacologic and therapeutic interventions should be recognized and treated patients must be closely monitored for drug-related complications. Cushing syndrome is a well-recognized complication of chronic steroid therapy. Thrombocytopenia in association with low-dose cyclophosphamide has also been reported. Chronically immunosuppressed patients are at risk for opportunistic infection; *Legionella* pneumonia infection has been described in a survivor of IPH.

In chronic disease, progression to debilitating pulmonary fibrosis has been described. Lung transplantation has been performed in patients with IPH refractory to immunosuppressive therapy. In one reported case study, IPH recurred in the transplanted lung.

Many patients (~50%) are diagnosed with IPH 2 mo after presentation. Additionally ~15% are diagnosed after a period of 6 mo.

PROGNOSIS

The outcome of patients suffering from DAH is largely dependent on the underlying disease process. Some conditions respond well to immunosuppressive therapies and remissions of disease are well documented. Other syndromes, especially those associated with pulmonary capillaritis, carry a poorer prognosis. In IPH, mortality is usually attributable to massive hemorrhage or, alternatively, to progressive fibrosis, respiratory insufficiency, and right-sided heart failure.

Long-term prognosis in patients with IPH varies among studies. Initial case study reviews suggested an average survival after symptom onset of only 2.5 yr. In this early review, a minority of patients were treated with steroids. Newer reviews have demonstrated vastly improved 5 yr (86%) and 8 yr (93%) survival in association with the use of immunosuppressive therapies. To date, specific immunosuppressive treatment regimens have not been studied in a prospective manner.

Bibliography is available at Expert Consult.

Chapter **436**

Pulmonary Embolism, Infarction, and Hemorrhage

第四百三十六章
肺栓塞、肺梗死和肺出血

中文导读

　　本章第1节介绍了肺栓塞和肺梗死，第2节介绍了肺出血和咯血。肺栓塞和肺梗死中具体描述了病因学、流行病学、病理生理学、临床表现、实验室检查和诊断、治疗及预后，其中病因学方面，详细阐述了儿童肺栓塞的危险因素，治疗方面详细阐述了深静脉血栓形成和肺栓塞的抗凝治疗；肺出血和咯血中具体描述了病因学、流行病学、病理生理学、临床表现、实验室检查、诊断及治疗。

436.1 Pulmonary Embolus and Infarction

Mary A. Nevin

Venous thromboembolic disease (VTE) has become an increasingly recognized critical problem in children and adolescents with chronic disease, as well as in patients without identifiable risk factors (Table 436.1). Improvements in survival with chronic illness have likely contributed to the larger number of children presenting with these thromboembolic events; they are a significant source of morbidity and mortality and may only be recognized on postmortem examination. A high level of clinical suspicion and appropriate identification of at-risk individuals is therefore recommended.

ETIOLOGY

A number of risk factors may be identified in children and adolescents; the presence of immobility, malignancy, pregnancy, infection, indwelling central venous catheters, and a number of inherited and acquired thrombophilic conditions have all been identified as placing an individual at risk. In children, a significantly greater percentage of VTEs are risk associated as compared with their adult counterparts. Children with **deep venous thrombosis (DVT)** and **pulmonary embolism (PE)** are much more likely to have one or more identifiable conditions or circumstances placing them at risk. In contrast to adults, idiopathic thrombosis is a rare occurrence in the pediatric population. In a retrospective cohort of patients with VTE in U.S. children's hospitals from 2001 to 2007, the majority (63%) of affected children were found to have one or more chronic medical comorbidities. In a large Canadian registry, 96% of pediatric patients were found to have one risk factor and 90% had two or more risk factors. In contrast, approximately 60% of adults with this disorder have an identifiable risk factor (see Table 436.1). The most common identified risk factors in children include infection, congenital heart disease, and the presence of an indwelling central venous catheter.

Embolic disease in children is varied in its origin. An embolus can contain thrombus, air, amniotic fluid, septic material, or metastatic neoplastic tissue. Thromboemboli are the type most commonly encountered. A commonly encountered risk factor for DVT and PE in the pediatric population is the presence of a central venous catheter. More than 50% of DVTs in children and more than 80% in newborns are found in patients with indwelling central venous lines. The presence of a catheter in a vessel lumen, as well as instilled medications, can induce endothelial damage and favor thrombus formation.

Children with malignancies are also at considerable risk. Although PE has been described in children with leukemia, the risk of PE is more significant in children with solid rather than hematologic malignancies. A child with malignancy may have numerous risk factors related to the primary disease process and the therapeutic interventions. Infection from chronic immunosuppression may interact with hypercoagulability of malignancy and chemotherapeutic effects on the endothelium. In a retrospective cohort of patients with VTE from 2001 to 2007, pediatric malignancy was the medical condition most strongly associated with recurrent VTE.

In the neonatal period, thromboembolic disease and PE may be related to indwelling catheters used for parenteral nutrition and medication delivery. Pulmonary thromboemboli in neonates generally occurs as a complication of underlying disease; the most common associated diagnosis is congenital heart disease, but sepsis and birth asphyxia are also notable associated conditions. Other risk factors include a relative immaturity of newborn infants' coagulation; plasma concentrations of

Table 436.1	Risk Factors for Pulmonary Embolism

ENVIRONMENTAL
Long-haul air travel (>4 hr)
Obesity
Cigarette smoking
Hypertension
Immobility

WOMEN'S HEALTH
Oral contraceptives, including progesterone-only and, especially, third-generation pills
Pregnancy or puerperium
Hormone replacement therapy
Septic abortion

MEDICAL ILLNESS
Personal or family history of prior pulmonary embolism or deep venous thrombosis
Cancer
Heart failure
Chronic obstructive pulmonary disease
Diabetes mellitus
Inflammatory bowel disease
Antipsychotic drug use
Long-term indwelling central venous catheter
Permanent pacemaker
Internal cardiac defibrillator
Stroke with limb paresis
Spinal cord injury
Nursing home confinement or current or repeated hospital admission

SURGICAL
Trauma
Orthopedic surgery
General surgery
Neurosurgery, especially craniotomy for brain tumor
Vascular anomalies
May-Turner syndrome

THROMBOPHILIA
Factor V Leiden mutation
Prothrombin gene (20210G A) mutation
Hyperhomocysteinemia (including mutation in methylenetetrahydrofolate reductase)
Antiphospholipid antibody syndrome
Deficiency of antithrombin III, protein C, or protein S
High concentrations of factor VIII or XI
Increased lipoprotein (a)

NONTHROMBOTIC
Air
Foreign particles (e.g., hair, talc, as a consequence of intravenous drug misuse)
Amniotic fluid
Bone fragments, bone marrow
Fat
Tumors (Wilms tumor)

Modified from Goldhaber SZ: Pulmonary embolism, *Lancet* 363:1295–1305, 2004.

vitamin K-dependent coagulation factors (II, VII, IX, X); factors XII, XI, and prekallikrein and high molecular weight kininogen are only approximately half of adult levels (see Chapter 502). PE in neonates may occasionally reflect maternal risk factors, such as diabetes and toxemia of pregnancy. Infants with congenitally acquired homozygous deficiencies of antithrombin, protein C, and protein S are also more likely to present with thromboembolic disease in the neonatal period (see Chapter 505).

Pulmonary air embolism is a defined entity in the newborn or young infant and is attributed to the conventional ventilation of critically ill (and generally premature) infants with severe pulmonary disease. In the majority of instances, the pulmonary air embolism is preceded by an air-leak syndrome. Infants may become symptomatic and critically compromised by as little as 0.4 mL/kg of intravascular air; these physiologic derangements are thought to be secondary to the effects of nitrogen.

Prothrombotic disease can also manifest in older infants and children. Disease can be congenital or acquired. **Inherited thrombophilic** conditions include deficiencies of antithrombin, protein C, and protein S, as well as mutations of factor V Leiden (G1691A) (see Chapter 505) and prothrombin (factor II 20210A mutation) (see Chapter 505), and elevated values of lipoprotein A. In addition, multiple acquired thrombophilic conditions exist; these include the presence of lupus anticoagulant (may be present without the diagnosis of systemic lupus erythematosus), anticardiolipin antibody, and anti-β_2-glycoprotein 1 antibody. Finally, conditions such as hyperhomocysteinemia (see Chapter 104) may have both inheritable and dietary determinants. All have all been linked to thromboembolic disease. DVT/PE may be the initial presentation.

Children with sickle cell disease are also at high risk for pulmonary embolus and infarction. Acquired prothrombotic disease is seen in conditions such as nephrotic syndrome (see Chapter 545) and antiphospholipid antibody syndrome. From one-quarter to one-half of children with systemic lupus erythematosus (see Chapter 183) have thromboembolic disease. There is a significant association with VTE onset in children for each inherited thrombophilic trait evaluated, thereby illuminating the importance of screening for thrombophilic conditions for those at risk for VTE. Septic emboli are rare in children but may be caused by osteomyelitis, jugular vein or umbilical thrombophlebitis, cellulitis, urinary tract infection, and right-sided endocarditis.

Other risk factors include infection, cardiac disease, recent surgery, and trauma. Surgical risk is thought to be more significant when immobility will be a prominent feature of the recovery. Use of oral contraceptives confers additional risk, although the level of risk in patients taking these medications appears to be decreasing, perhaps because of the lower amounts of estrogen in current formulations. In a previously healthy adolescent patient, the risk factors are often unknown or are similar to adults (see Tables 436.1 and 436.2).

EPIDEMIOLOGY

A retrospective cohort study was performed with patients younger than 18 yr of age, discharged from 35 to 40 children's hospitals across the United States from 2001 to 2007. During this time, a dramatic increase was noted in the incidence of VTE; the annual rate of VTE increased by 70% from 34 to 58 cases per 10,000 hospital admissions. Although this increased incidence was noted in all age groups, a bimodal distribution of patient ages was found, consistent with prior studies; infants younger than 1 yr of age and adolescents made up the majority of admissions with VTE, but neonates continue to be at greatest risk. The peak incidence for VTE in childhood appears to occur in the 1st mo of life. It is in this neonatal period that thromboembolic events are more problematic, likely as a result of an imbalance between procoagulant factors and fibrinolysis. The yearly incidence of venous events was estimated at 5.3/10,000 hospital admissions in children and 24/10,000 in the neonatal intensive care.

Pediatric autopsy reviews have estimated the incidence of thromboembolic disease in children as between 1% and 4%, although not all were clinically significant. Thromboembolic pulmonary disease is often unrecognized, and antemortem studies may underestimate the true incidence. Pediatric deaths from isolated pulmonary emboli are rare. Most thromboemboli are related to central venous catheters. The source of the emboli may be lower or upper extremity veins as well as the pelvis and right heart. In adults, the most common location for DVT

Table 436.2	Clinical Decision Rules for Deep Vein Thrombosis and Pulmonary Embolism

WELLS' SCORE FOR DEEP VEIN THROMBOSIS*		
Active cancer	+1	NA
Paralysis, paresis, or recent plaster cast on lower extremities	+1	NA
Recent immobilization >3 days or major surgery within the past 4 wk	+1	NA
Localized tenderness of deep venous system	+1	NA
Swelling of entire leg	+1	NA
Calf swelling >3 cm compared to asymptomatic side	+1	NA
Unilateral pitting edema	+1	NA
Collateral superficial veins	+1	NA
Previously documented deep vein thrombosis	+1	NA
Alternative diagnosis at least as likely as deep vein thrombosis	−2	NA

WELLS' SCORE FOR PULMONARY EMBOLISM[†,‡]		
Alternative diagnosis less likely than pulmonary embolism	+3	+1
Clinical signs and symptoms of deep vein thrombosis	+3	+1
Heart rate >100 beats/min	+1·5	+1
Previous deep vein thrombosis or pulmonary embolism	+1·5	+1
Immobilization or surgery within the past 4 wk	+1·5	+1
Active cancer	+1	+1
Hemoptysis	+1	+1

REVISED GENEVA SCORE FOR PULMONARY EMBOLISM[§,‖]		
Heart rate ≥95 beats/min	+5	+2
Heart rate 75–94 beats/min	+3	+1
Pain on lower-limb deep venous palpation and unilateral edema	+4	+1
Unilateral lower-limb pain	+3	+1
Previous deep vein thrombosis or pulmonary embolism	+3	+1
Active cancer	+2	+1
Hemoptysis	+2	+1
Surgery or fracture within the past 4 wk	+2	+1
Age >65 yr	+1	+1

*Classification for original Wells' score for deep vein thrombosis: deep vein thrombosis unlikely if score ≤2; deep vein thrombosis likely if score >2.

[†]Classification for original Wells' score for pulmonary embolism: pulmonary embolism unlikely if score ≤4; pulmonary embolism likely if score >4.

[‡]Classification for simplified Wells' score for pulmonary embolism: pulmonary embolism unlikely if score ≤1; pulmonary embolism likely if score >1.

[§]Classification for original revised Geneva score for pulmonary embolism: non-high probability of pulmonary embolism if score ≤10; high probability of pulmonary embolism if score >10.

[‖]Classification for simplified revised Geneva score for pulmonary embolism: non-high probability of pulmonary embolism if score ≤4; high probability of pulmonary embolism if score >4.

From Di Nisio M, van Es N, Büller HR: Deep vein thrombosis and pulmonary embolism, *Lancet* 388:3060–3069, 2016 (Table 1, p. 3062).

is the lower leg. However, one of the largest pediatric VTE/PE registries found two-thirds of DVTs occurring in the upper extremity.

PATHOPHYSIOLOGY

Favorable conditions for thrombus formation include injury to the vessel endothelium, hemostasis, and hypercoagulability. In the case of PE, a thrombus is dislodged from a vein, travels through the right atrium, and lodges within the pulmonary arteries. In children, emboli that obstruct <50% of the pulmonary circulation are generally clinically silent unless there is significant coexistent cardiopulmonary disease. In severe disease, right ventricular afterload is increased with resultant right ventricular dilation and increases in right ventricular and pulmonary arterial pressures. In severe cases, a reduction of cardiac output and hypotension may result from concomitant decreases in left ventricular filling. In rare instances of death from massive pulmonary embolus, marked increases in pulmonary vascular resistance and heart failure are usually present.

Arterial hypoxemia results from unequal ventilation and perfusion; the occlusion of the involved vessel prevents perfusion of distal alveolar units, thereby creating an increase in dead space and hypoxia with an elevated alveolar–arterial oxygen tension difference (see Chapter 400). Most patients are hypocarbic secondary to hyperventilation, which often persists even when oxygenation is optimized. Abnormalities of oxygenation and ventilation are likely to be less significant in the pediatric population, possibly owing to less underlying cardiopulmonary disease and greater reserve. The vascular supply to lung tissue is abundant, and pulmonary infarction is unusual with pulmonary embolus but may result from distal arterial occlusion and alveolar hemorrhage.

CLINICAL MANIFESTATIONS

Presentation is variable, and many pulmonary emboli are silent. Rarely, a massive PE may manifest as cardiopulmonary failure. Children are more likely to have underlying disease processes or risk factors but might still present asymptomatically with small emboli. Common symptoms and signs of PE caused by larger emboli include hypoxia (cyanosis), dyspnea, tachycardia, cough, pleuritic chest pain, and hemoptysis. Pleuritic chest pain is the most common presenting symptom in adolescents (84%), whereas unexplained and persistent tachypnea may suggest PE in all pediatric patients. Localized crackles may occasionally be appreciated on examination. A high level of clinical suspicion is required because a variety of diagnoses may cause similar symptoms; nonspecific complaints may frequently be attributed to an underlying disease process or an unrelated/incorrect diagnosis. Confirmatory testing should follow a clinical suspicion for PE. In older adolescents and adults, clinical prediction rules have been published and are based on risk factors, clinical signs, and symptoms (see Table 436.2). No such clinical prediction rules have been validated in the pediatric population.

LABORATORY FINDINGS AND DIAGNOSIS

The electrocardiogram, arterial blood gas, and chest radiograph may be used to rule out contributing or comorbid disease but are not sensitive or specific in the diagnosis of PE. Electrocardiographs may reveal ST-segment changes or evidence of pulmonary hypertension with right ventricular failure (cor pulmonale); such changes are nonspecific and nondiagnostic. Radiographic images of the chest are often normal in a child with PE and any abnormalities are likely to be nonspecific. Patients with septic emboli may have multiple areas of nodularity and cavitation, which are typically located peripherally in both lung fields. Many patients with PE have hypoxemia. The alveolar–arterial oxygen tension difference gradient is more sensitive in detecting gas exchange derangements.

A review of results of a complete blood count, urinalysis, and coagulation profile is warranted. Prothrombotic diseases should be highly suspected on the basis of past medical or family history; additional laboratory evaluations include fibringen assays, protein C, protein S, and antithrombin III studies, and analysis for factor V Leiden mutation, as well as evaluation for lupus anticoagulant and anticardiolipin antibodies.

Echocardiograms may be warranted to assess ventricular size and function. An echocardiogram is required if there is any suspicion of intracardiac thrombi or endocarditis.

Noninvasive venous ultrasound testing with Doppler flow can be used to confirm DVT in the lower extremities; ultrasonography may not detect thrombi in the upper extremities or pelvis (Fig. 436.1A). In patients with significant venous thrombosis, D dimers are usually elevated. It is a sensitive but nonspecific test for venous thrombosis. The D dimer may not be clinically relevant in the children with PE as this group is more likely to have an underlying comorbid condition that is also associated with an increased level of D dimers. When a high level of suspicion exists, confirmatory testing with venography should be pursued. DVT can be recurrent and multifocal and may lead to repeated episodes of PE.

Although much more commonly encountered in the adult population, thrombus migration to the pulmonary circulation in children and adolescents may be prevented through surgical placement of an inferior vena cava (IVC) filter. This may be considered when DVT is detected and risk of pulmonary thrombus is high or when there is a medical contraindication to or intolerance for anticoagulant therapy. IVC filter may also be considered prophylactically in the setting of trauma.

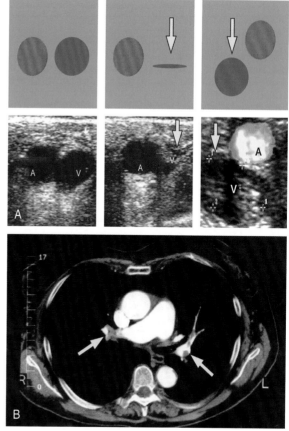

Fig. 436.1 A, Compression ultrasound. Upper series, from left to right, representation of vein and artery without and with *(arrow)* gentle compression with the echocardiographic probe; lower series, corresponding echocardiographic findings. The third image from the left shows a thrombus in the vein (vein not compressible by the probe). **B,** CT angiography. CT angiography showing several emboli *(arrows)* in the main right pulmonary artery and in left lobar and segmental arteries. *A,* Artery; *V,* vein. *(From Goldhaber SZ, Bounameaux H: Pulmonary embolism and deep vein thrombosis, Lancet 379:1835–1844, 2012, Fig. 2, p. 1838.)*

Although a ventilation–perfusion ($\dot{V} - \dot{Q}$) radionuclide scan is a noninvasive and potentially sensitive method of pulmonary embolus detection, the interpretation of $\dot{V} - \dot{Q}$ scans can be problematic. *Helical or spiral CT with an intravenous contrast agent is valuable and the diagnostic test of choice to detect a PE* (see Fig. 436.1B). CT studies detect emboli in lobar and segmental vessels with acceptable sensitivities. Poorer sensitivities may be encountered in the evaluation of the subsegmental pulmonary vasculature. Pulmonary angiography is the gold standard for diagnosis of PE, but with availability of multidetector spiral CT angiography, it is not necessary except in unusual cases.

MRI may be emerging as a diagnostic option for patients with VTE. The accuracy of this method is similar to that of multidetector CT. It may be preferable in patients with allergic reactions to contrast material and in pediatric patients in whom the risk of early exposure to ionizing radiation has been established.

TREATMENT

Initial treatment should always be directed toward stabilization of the patient. Careful approaches to ventilation, fluid resuscitation, and inotropic support are always indicated, because improvement in one area of decompensation can often exacerbate coexisting pathology.

After the patient with a PE has been stabilized, the next therapeutic step is anticoagulation. Evaluations for prothrombotic disease must precede anticoagulation. Acute-phase anticoagulation therapy may be provided with unfractionated heparin (UFH) or low molecular weight heparin (LMWH). Heparins act by enhancing the activity of antithrombin. LMWH is generally preferred in children; this drug can be administered subcutaneously and the need for serum monitoring is decreased. The risk of heparin-induced thrombocytopenia is also decreased with LMWH as compared to UFH. Alternatively, UFH is preferred with patients who have an elevated risk of bleeding as UFH has a shorter half-life than LMWH. UFH is also used preferentially in patients with compromised renal function. In monitoring of drug levels, laboratories must be aware of the drug chosen in order to use the appropriate assay. For UFH, the therapeutic range is 0.3-0.7 anti-Xa activity units/mL. In LMWH, the therapeutic range is 0.5-1.0 units/mL. When the anti-Xa assay is not available, the activated partial thromboplastin time may be used with a goal of 60-85 sec or approximately 1.5-2 times the upper limit of age appropriate normal values. The recommended duration of heparinization during acute treatment is 5-10 days; this length of therapy has been extrapolated from adult data. Long-term therapy with heparin should be avoided whenever possible. Side effects include the aforementioned heparin-induced thrombocytopenia as well as bleeding and osteoporosis.

Extension of anticoagulation therapy occurs in the subacute phase and may utilize LMWH or warfarin. Warfarin is generally initiated after establishing effective anticoagulation with heparin because severe congenital deficiencies of protein C may be associated with warfarin skin necrosis. When the international normalized ratio (INR) is measured between 1.0 and 1.3, the starting dose for warfarin in children is recommended as 0.2-0.3 mg/kg administered orally once daily. Titration of dosing may be needed to achieve a therapeutic INR of 2 to 3. Dosing requirements may vary and clinical pharmacologic correlation is required. The INR is generally monitored 5 days after initiating therapy or a similar period after dose changes and weekly thereafter until stable.

The INR should be obtained with any evidence of abnormal bleeding and should be discontinued at least 5 days prior to invasive procedures. The utilization of an anticoagulation team and/or established treatment algorithms is recommended in order to optimize patient safety. With a first occurrence of VTE, anticoagulation is recommended for 3-6 mo in the setting of an identifiable, reversible, and resolved risk factor (e.g., postoperative state). Longer treatment is indicated in patients with idiopathic VTE (6-12 mo) and in those with chronic clinical risk factors (12 mo-lifelong). In the setting of a congenital thrombophilic condition, the duration of therapy is often indefinite. Inhibitors of factor Xa (rivaroxaban, etc.) may become an alternate therapy for both acute PE and long-term treatment (Table 436.3).

Thrombolytic agents such as recombinant tissue plasminogen activator, may be utilized in combination with anticoagulants in the early stages of treatment; their use is most likely to be considered in children with hemodynamically significant PE (echocardiogram evidence of right ventricular dysfunction) or other severe potential clinical sequelae of VTE. Combined therapy may reduce the incidences of progressive thromboembolism, pulmonary embolus, and postthrombotic syndrome. Mortality rate appears to be unaffected by additional therapies; nonetheless, the additional theoretic risk of hemorrhage limits the use of combination therapy in all but the most compromised patients. The use of thrombolytic agents in patients with active bleeding, recent cerebrovascular accidents, or trauma is contraindicated.

Surgical embolectomy is invasive and is associated with significant mortality. Its application should be limited to those with large emboli that result in persistent hemodynamic compromise refractory to standard therapy.

PROGNOSIS

Mortality in pediatric patients with PE is likely to be attributable to an underlying disease process rather than to the embolus itself. Short-term

Table 436.3	Anticoagulant Therapies for Deep Vein Thrombosis and Pulmonary Embolism					
	ROUTE OF ADMINISTRATION	**RENAL CLEARANCE (%)**	**HALF-LIFE**	**INITIAL TREATMENT DOSING**	**MAINTENANCE TREATMENT DOSING**	**EXTENDED TREATMENT DOSING**
Unfractionated heparin (UFH)	Intravenous	~30	~1.5 hr	Maintain aPTT 1.5-times upper limit of normal		
Low molecular weight heparin (LMWH)	Subcutaneous	~80	3-4 hr	Weight-based dosing	Weight-based dosing*	
Fondaparinux	Subcutaneous	100	17-21 hr	Weight-based dosing	Weight-based dosing	
Vitamin K antagonists	Oral	Negligible	Acenocoumarol 8-11 hr; warfarin 36 hr; phenprocoumon 160 hr	Target at INR at 2.0-3.0 and give parallel heparin treatment for at least 5 days	Maintain INR at 2.0-3.0	Maintain INR at 2.0-3.0
Dabigatran	Oral	~80[†]	14-17 hr	Requires at least 5 days heparin lead-in	150 mg twice a day	150 mg twice a day
Rivaroxaban	Oral	~33[‡]	7-11 hr	15 mg twice a day for 3 wk	20 mg once a day	20 mg once a day
Apixaban	Oral	~25[‡]	8-12 hr	10 mg twice a day for 1 wk	5 mg twice a day	2.5 mg twice a day
Edoxaban	Oral	~35[‡]	6-11 hr	Requires at least 5 days heparin lead-in	60 mg once a day[§]	60 mg once a day[§]
Aspirin	Oral	~10	15 min			80–100 mg once a day

Medication dosing may vary with regard to primary diagnosis, age, comorbidities, and other factors. Clinical-pharmacologic correlation is advocated.
*Treatment with low molecular weight heparin is recommended for patients with active cancer and pregnant women.
[†]Dabigatran is contraindicated in patients with a creatinine clearance below 30 mL/min.
[‡]Apixaban, edoxaban, and rivaroxaban are contraindicated in patients with a creatinine clearance below 15 mL/min.
[§]The recommended edoxaban dose is 30 mg once a day for patients with a creatinine clearance of 30–50 mL/min, a bodyweight less than or equal to 60 kg, or for those on certain strong P-glycoprotein inhibitors.
aPTT, activated partial thromboplastin time; *INR*, international normalized ratio.
From Di Nisio M, van Es N, Büller HR: Deep vein thrombosis and pulmonary embolism, *Lancet* 388:3060–3069, 2016 (Table 2, p. 3065).

complications include major hemorrhage (either due to the thrombosis or secondary to anticoagulation). Conditions associated with a poorer prognosis include malignancy, infection, and cardiac disease. The mortality rate in children from PE is 2.2%. Recurrent thromboembolic disease may complicate recovery. The practitioner must conduct an extensive evaluation for underlying pathology so as to prevent progressive disease. Postthrombotic syndrome is another recognized complication of pediatric thrombotic disease. Venous valvular damage can be initiated by the presence of DVT, leading to persistent venous hypertension with ambulation and valvular reflux. Symptoms include edema, pain, increases in pigmentation, and ulcerations. Affected pediatric patients may suffer lifelong disability.

Bibliography is available at Expert Consult.

436.2 Pulmonary Hemorrhage and Hemoptysis

Mary A. Nevin

Pulmonary hemorrhage is relatively uncommon but a potentially fatal occurrence in children. The patient with suspected hemoptysis may present acutely or subacutely and to a variety of different practitioners with distinct areas of specialty. Diffuse, slow bleeding in the lower airways may become severe and manifest as anemia, fatigue, or respiratory compromise without the patient ever experiencing episodes of hemoptysis. Hemoptysis must also be separated from episodes of hematemesis or epistaxis, each of which may have indistinguishable presentations in the young patient.

ETIOLOGY

Table 436.4 and Table 435.1 (in Chapter 435) present conditions that can manifest as pulmonary hemorrhage or hemoptysis in children. The chronic (opposed to an acute) presence of a foreign body can lead to inflammation and/or infection, thereby inducing hemorrhage. Bleeding is more likely to occur in association with a chronically retained foreign body of vegetable origin.

Hemorrhage most commonly reflects chronic inflammation and infection such as that seen with bronchiectasis due to cystic fibrosis or with cavitary disease in association with infectious tuberculosis. Hemoptysis may occasionally reflect an acute and intense infectious condition such as bronchitis or bronchopneumonia.

Other relatively common etiologies are congenital heart disease and trauma. Pulmonary hypertension secondary to cardiac disease is a prominent etiology for hemoptysis in those patients without cystic fibrosis. Traumatic irritation or damage in the airway may be accidental in nature. Traumatic injury to the airway and pulmonary contusion may result from motor vehicle crashes or other direct force injuries. Bleeding can also be related to instrumentation or iatrogenic irritation of the airway as is commonly seen in a child with a tracheostomy or a child with repeated suction trauma to the upper airway. Children who have been victims of nonaccidental trauma or deliberate suffocation can also be found to have blood in the mouth or airway (see Chapter 16). Factitious hemoptysis may rarely be encountered in the setting of Factitious Disorder by Proxy (formerly Munchausen's by proxy; see Chapter 16.2).

Rare causes for hemoptysis include tumors and vascular anomalies such as arteriovenous malformations (Fig. 436.2). Congenital vascular malformations in the lung may also be associated with **hereditary hemorrhagic telangiectasia**. Tumors must be cautiously investigated when encountered with a flexible fiberoptic bronchoscope as bleeding may be massive and difficult to control.

Syndromes associated with vasculitic, autoimmune, and idiopathic disorders can be associated with diffuse alveolar hemorrhage (see Chapter 435).

Acute idiopathic pulmonary hemorrhage of infancy is a distinct entity and is described as an episode of pulmonary hemorrhage in a previously healthy infant born at greater than 32 wk of gestation and

Table 436.4	Etiology of Pulmonary Hemorrhage (Hemoptysis)

FOCAL HEMORRHAGE
Bronchitis and bronchiectasis (especially cystic fibrosis–related)
Infection (acute or chronic), pneumonia, abscess
Tuberculosis
Trauma
Pulmonary arteriovenous malformation (with or without hereditary hemorrhagic telangiectasia)
Foreign body (chronic)
Neoplasm including hemangioma
Pulmonary embolus with or without infarction
Bronchogenic cysts

DIFFUSE HEMORRHAGE
Idiopathic of infancy
Congenital heart disease (including pulmonary hypertension, venooclusive disease, congestive heart failure)
Prematurity
Cow's milk hyperreactivity (Heiner syndrome)
Goodpasture syndrome
Collagen vascular diseases (systemic lupus erythematosus, rheumatoid arthritis)
Henoch-Schönlein purpura and vasculitic disorders
Granulomatous disease (granulomatosis with polyangiitis)
Celiac disease
Coagulopathy (congenital or acquired)
Malignancy
Immunodeficiency
Exogenous toxins, especially inhaled
Hyperammonemia
Pulmonary hypertension
Pulmonary alveolar proteinosis
Idiopathic pulmonary hemosiderosis
Tuberous sclerosis
Lymphangiomyomatosis or lymphangioleiomyomatosis
Physical injury or abuse
Catamenial

See also Table 435.1.

whose age is less than 1 yr with the following: (1) abrupt or sudden onset of overt bleeding or frank evidence of blood in the airway, (2) severe presentation leading to acute respiratory distress or failure and requiring intensive care and invasive ventilatory support, and (3) diffuse bilateral infiltration on chest radiographs or computed tomography. Prior suggestions of an association between acute idiopathic pulmonary hemorrhage of infancy and toxic mold exposure have not been supported on subsequent review.

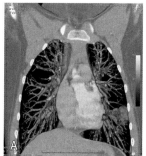 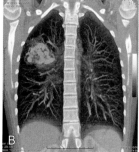

Fig. 436.2 A, Volume-rendering reconstruction of the contrast-enhanced spiral CT showing a large arteriovenous fistula in the left upper lobe (lingula). **B,** Volume-rendering reconstruction of the contrast-enhanced spiral CT showing an arteriovenous fistula in the right upper lobe. *(From Grzela K, Krenke K, Kulus M: Pulmonary arteriovenous malformations: clinical and radiological presentation, J Pediatr 158:856, 2011, Figs. 1 and 2, p. 856.)*

EPIDEMIOLOGY

The frequency with which pulmonary hemorrhage occurs in the pediatric population is difficult to define. This difficulty is largely related to the variability in disease presentation. Chronic bronchiectasis as seen in cystic fibrosis (see Chapter 432) or ciliary dyskinesia (see Chapter 433) can cause hemoptysis, but usually occurs in children older than 10 yr of age. The incidence of pulmonary hemorrhage may be significantly underestimated because many children and young adults swallow rather than expectorate mucus, a behavior that may prevent recognition of hemoptysis, the primary presenting symptom of the disorder.

PATHOPHYSIOLOGY

Pulmonary hemorrhage can be localized or diffuse. Focal hemorrhage from an isolated bronchial lesion is often secondary to infection or chronic inflammation. Erosion through a chronically inflamed airway into the adjacent bronchial artery is a mechanism for potentially massive hemorrhage. Bleeding from such a lesion is more likely to be bright red, brisk, and secondary to enlarged bronchial arteries and systemic arterial pressures. The severity of more diffuse hemorrhage can be difficult to ascertain. The rate of blood loss may be insufficient to reach the proximal airways. Therefore, the patient may present without hemoptysis. The diagnosis of pulmonary hemorrhage is generally achieved by finding evidence of blood or hemosiderin in the lung. Within 48-72 hr of an episode of bleeding, alveolar macrophages convert the iron from erythrocytes into hemosiderin. It may take weeks to clear these hemosiderin-laden macrophages completely from the alveolar spaces. This fact may allow differentiation between acute and chronic hemorrhage. Hemorrhage is often followed by the influx of neutrophils and other proinflammatory mediators. With repeated or chronic hemorrhage, pulmonary fibrosis can become a prominent pathologic finding.

CLINICAL MANIFESTATIONS

The severity of presentation in patients with hemoptysis and pulmonary hemorrhage is highly variable. Older children and young adults with a focal hemorrhage may complain of warmth or a "bubbling" sensation in the chest wall. This can occasionally aid the clinician in locating the area involved. Rapid and large-volume blood loss manifests as symptoms of cyanosis, respiratory distress, and shock. Chronic, subclinical blood loss may manifest as anemia, fatigue, dyspnea, or altered activity tolerance. Less commonly, patients present with persistent infiltrates on chest radiograph or symptoms of chronic illness such as failure to thrive. Pulmonary arteriovenous malformations may present with hemoptysis, hemothorax, a round localized mass on x-ray or CT, clubbing, cyanosis, or embolic phenomenon (central nervous system).

LABORATORY FINDINGS AND DIAGNOSIS

A patient with suspected hemorrhage should have a laboratory evaluation with complete blood count and coagulation studies. The complete blood count result may demonstrate a microcytic, hypochromic anemia but may be normal early in an acute bleeding episode. If iron stores are sufficient, a reticulocytosis may be present. Other laboratory findings are highly dependent on the underlying diagnosis. A urinalysis may show evidence of nephritis in patients with a comorbid pulmonary renal syndrome. The classic and definitive finding in pulmonary hemorrhage is that of **hemosiderin-laden macrophages** in pulmonary secretions. Hemosiderin-laden macrophages may be detected by sputum analysis with Prussian blue staining when a patient is able to successfully expectorate sputum from the lower airways. In younger children, or in weak or neurodevelopmentally compromised patients unable to expectorate sputum, induced sputum may provide an acceptable specimen; alternatively, a flexible bronchoscopy with **bronchoalveolar lavage** may be required for specimen retrieval.

Chest radiographs may demonstrate fluffy bilateral densities, as seen in acute idiopathic pulmonary hemorrhage of infancy (Fig. 436.3) or the patchy consolidation seen in idiopathic pulmonary hemosiderosis (Fig. 436.4). Alveolar infiltrates seen on chest radiograph may be regarded as a representation of recent bleeding, but their absence does not rule out the occurrence of pulmonary hemorrhage. Infiltrates, when present,

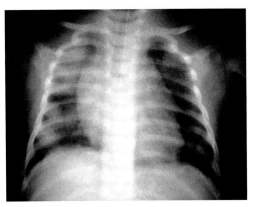

Fig. 436.3 Radiographic appearance of acute idiopathic pulmonary hemorrhage in infancy. *(From Brown CM, Redd SC, Damon SA, Centers for Disease Control and Prevention [CDC]: Acute idiopathic pulmonary hemorrhage among infants: recommendations from the Working Group for Investigation and Surveillance, MMWR Recomm Rep 53:1–12, 2004.)*

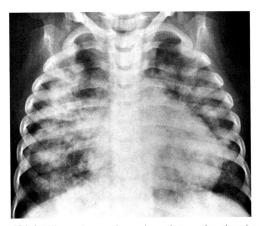

Fig. 436.4 Diffuse pulmonary hemorrhage that was thought to be the result of idiopathic pulmonary hemosiderosis in a 3 yr old boy. Frontal radiograph reveals bilateral airspace consolidation that is patchy. Tracheal washing contained large numbers of macrophages filled with hemosiderin. Ten days later, most of the consolidative changes in the lungs had cleared. The patient's anemia was successfully treated with blood transfusion. *(From Slovis T, editor: Caffey's pediatric diagnostic imaging, ed 11, Philadelphia, 2008, Mosby/Elsevier; courtesy of Bertram Girdany, MD, Pittsburgh, PA.)*

are often symmetric and diffuse and may be preferentially located in the perihilar regions and lower lobes. The costophrenic angles and lung apices are frequently spared. CT may be indicated to assess for underlying disease processes.

Lung biopsy is rarely necessary unless bleeding is chronic or an etiology cannot be determined with other methods. Pulmonary function testing, including a determination of gas exchange, is important to assess the severity of the ventilatory defect. In older children, spirometry may demonstrate evidence of predominantly obstructive disease in the acute period. Restrictive disease secondary to fibrosis is typically seen with more chronic disease. Diffusion capacity of carbon monoxide measurements are typically elevated in the setting of pulmonary hemorrhage because of the strong affinity of the intra-alveolar hemoglobin for carbon monoxide.

TREATMENT

In the setting of massive blood loss, volume resuscitation and transfusion of blood products are necessary. Maintenance of adequate ventilation and circulatory function is crucial. Rigid bronchoscopy may be utilized for localization of bleeding and for removal of debris, but active bleeding may be exacerbated by airway manipulation. Flexible bronchoscopy and bronchoalveolar lavage may be required for diagnosis. Ideally, treatment is directed at the specific pathologic process responsible for the hemorrhage. When bronchiectasis is a known entity and a damaged artery can be localized, bronchial artery embolization is often the therapy of choice. If embolization fails, total or partial lobectomy may be required. Embolization is the initial treatment of choice for an arteriovenous malformation. In circumstances of diffuse hemorrhage, corticosteroids and other immunosuppressive agents have been shown to be of benefit. Transcatheter vaso-occlusive embolotherapy with detachable stainless-steel coils or other occlusive devices is the treatment of choice for pulmonary arteriovenous malformation (pulmonary AVM). Prognosis depends largely on the underlying disease process and the chronicity of bleeding.

Bibliography is available at Expert Consult.

Chapter **437**
Atelectasis

Ranna A. Rozenfeld

第四百三十七章
肺不张

中文导读

本章主要介绍了肺不张。具体描述了肺不张的病理生理学、临床表现、诊断及治疗，其中病理生理学方面详细阐述了肺不张的多种病因，如感染、张力性气胸、异物吸入等；肺不张的临床表现与病因及肺不张程度有关；通常可以通过胸部影像学得以诊断；治疗方面详细阐述了针对不同病因导致肺不张的不同治疗方法，如针对胸腔积液或气胸、黏液栓、异物、哮喘、神经肌肉病及囊性纤维化等的治疗方法。

Atelectasis is the incomplete expansion or complete collapse of air-bearing tissue, resulting from obstruction of air intake into the alveolar sacs. Segmental, lobar, or whole lung collapse is associated with the absorption of air contained in the alveoli, which are no longer ventilated.

PATHOPHYSIOLOGY

The causes of atelectasis can be divided into 5 groups (Table 437.1). Respiratory syncytial virus (see Chapter 287) and other viral infections, including influenza viruses in young children can cause multiple areas of atelectasis. Mucous plugs are a common predisposing factor to atelectasis. Massive collapse of one or both lungs is most often a postoperative complication but occasionally results from other causes, such as trauma, asthma, pneumonia, tension pneumothorax (see Chapter 439), aspiration of foreign material (see Chapters 414 and 425), paralysis, or after extubation. Massive atelectasis is usually produced by a combination of factors, including immobilization or decreased use of the diaphragm and the respiratory muscles, obstruction of the bronchial tree, and abolition of the cough reflex.

CLINICAL MANIFESTATIONS

Symptoms vary with the cause and extent of the atelectasis. A small area is likely to be asymptomatic. When a large area of previously normal lung becomes atelectatic, especially when it does so suddenly, dyspnea accompanied by rapid shallow respirations, tachycardia, cough, and often cyanosis occurs. If the obstruction is removed, the symptoms disappear rapidly. Although it was once believed that atelectasis alone can cause fever, studies have shown no association between atelectasis and fever. Physical findings include limitation of chest excursion, decreased breath sound intensity, and coarse crackles. Breath sounds are decreased or absent over extensive atelectatic areas.

Massive pulmonary atelectasis usually presents with dyspnea, cyanosis, and tachycardia. An affected child is extremely anxious and, if old enough, complains of chest pain. The chest appears flat on the affected side, where decreased respiratory excursion, dullness to percussion, and feeble or absent breath sounds are also noted. Postoperative atelectasis usually manifests within 24 hr of operation but may not occur for several days.

Acute lobar collapse is a frequent occurrence in patients receiving intensive care. If undetected, it can lead to impaired gas exchange, secondary infection, and subsequent pulmonary fibrosis. Initially, hypoxemia may result from ventilation-perfusion mismatch. In contrast to atelectasis in adult patients, in whom the lower lobes and, in particular, the left lower lobe are most often involved, 90% of cases in children involve the upper lobes and 63% involve the right upper lobe.

Table 437.1	Anatomic Causes of Atelectasis
CAUSE	**CLINICAL EXAMPLES**
External compression on the pulmonary parenchyma	Pleural effusion, pneumothorax, intrathoracic tumors, diaphragmatic hernia
Endobronchial obstruction completely obstructing the ingress of air	Enlarged lymph node, tumor, cardiac enlargement, foreign body, mucoid plug, broncholithiasis
Intraluminal obstruction of a bronchus	Foreign body, asthma, granulomatous tissue, tumor, secretions including mucous plugs, bronchiectasis, pulmonary abscess, chronic bronchitis, acute laryngotracheobronchitis, plastic bronchitis
Intrabronchiolar obstruction	Bronchiolitis, interstitial pneumonitis, asthma
Respiratory compromise or paralysis	Neuromuscular abnormalities, osseous deformities, overly restrictive casts and surgical dressings, defective movement of the diaphragm, or restriction of respiratory effort

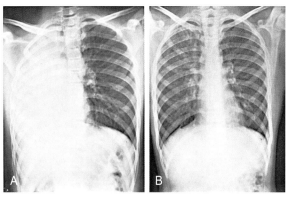

Fig. 437.1 **A,** Massive atelectasis of the right lung. The patient has asthma. The heart and other mediastinal structures shift to the right during the atelectatic phase. **B,** Comparison study after reaeration subsequent to bronchoscopic removal of a mucous plug from the right mainstem bronchus.

Table 437.2	Treatment for Atelectasis
CAUSE OF ATELECTASIS	**TREATMENT**
Pleural effusion or pneumothorax	Relieve compression
Mucus plug	Tracheal or bronchoscopic aspiration Continuous positive airway pressure
Foreign body	Bronchoscopic examination
Asthma	Bronchodilator and corticosteroid treatment Recombinant human deoxyribonuclease (off label use) Hypertonic saline with or without bronchodilator
Neuromuscular diseases	Intermittent positive pressure breathing Mechanical insufflator–exsufflator Noninvasive bi-level positive pressure ventilation
Cystic fibrosis	Airway clearance therapies Hypertonic saline with or without bronchodilator

There is also a high incidence of upper lobe atelectasis and, especially, right upper lobe collapse in patients with atelectasis being treated in neonatal intensive care units. This high incidence may be a result of movement of the endotracheal tube into the right mainstem bronchus, where it obstructs or causes inflammation of the bronchus to the right upper lobe.

DIAGNOSIS

The diagnosis of atelectasis can usually be established by chest radiograph. Typical findings include volume loss and displacement of fissures. Atypical presentations include atelectasis manifesting as a mass-like opacity and atelectasis in an unusual location. Lobar atelectasis may be associated with pneumothorax.

In asthmatic children, chest radiography demonstrates an abnormality rate of 44%, compared with a thorax high-resolution CT scan abnormality rate of 75%. Children with asthma and atelectasis have an increased incidence of right middle lobe syndrome, acute asthma exacerbations, pneumonia, and upper airway infections.

In foreign-body aspiration, atelectasis is one of the most common radiographic findings. The site of atelectasis usually indicates the site of the foreign body (see Chapter 405.1). Atelectasis is more common when diagnosis of foreign-body aspiration is delayed for greater than 2 wk. Bronchoscopic examination reveals a collapsed main bronchus when the obstruction is at the tracheobronchial junction and may also disclose the nature of the obstruction.

Massive pulmonary atelectasis is generally diagnosed on chest radiograph. Typical findings include elevation of the diaphragm, narrowing of the intercostal spaces, and displacement of the mediastinal structures and heart toward the affected side (Fig. 437.1).

TREATMENT

Treatment depends on the cause of the collapse (Table 437.2). If effusion or pneumothorax is responsible, the external compression must first be removed. Often vigorous efforts at cough, deep breathing, and percussion will facilitate expansion. Aspiration with sterile tracheal catheters may facilitate removal of mucous plugs. Continuous positive airway pressure may improve atelectasis.

Bronchoscopic examination is immediately indicated if atelectasis is the result of a foreign body or any other bronchial obstruction that can be relieved. For bilateral atelectasis, bronchoscopic aspiration should also be performed immediately. It is also indicated when an isolated area of atelectasis persists for several weeks. If no anatomic basis for atelectasis is found and no material can be obtained by suctioning, the introduction of a small amount of saline followed by suctioning allows recovery of bronchial secretions for culture and, possibly, for cytologic examination. Frequent changes in the child's position, deep breathing, and chest physiotherapy may be beneficial. Intrapulmonary percussive ventilation is a chest physiotherapy technique that is safe and effective. Oxygen therapy is indicated when there is dyspnea or desaturation. Intermittent positive-pressure breathing and incentive spirometry are recommended when atelectasis does not improve after chest physiotherapy.

In some conditions, such as asthma, bronchodilator and corticosteroid treatment may accelerate atelectasis clearance. Recombinant human deoxyribonuclease, which is approved only for the treatment of cystic fibrosis, has been used off-label for patients without cystic fibrosis who have persistent atelectasis. This product reduces the viscosity of purulent bronchial debris. In patients with acute severe asthma, diffuse airway plugging with thick viscous secretions frequently occurs, with the resulting atelectasis often refractory to conventional therapy. Recombinant human deoxyribonuclease is used in both nebulized form for nonintubated patients with acute asthma as well as intratracheally for atelectasis in intubated asthmatics, with resolution of atelectasis unresponsive to conventional asthma therapies. Recombinant human deoxyribonuclease is also used in ventilated infants and children with atelectasis not caused by asthma.

Hypertonic saline solution increases mucociliary clearance in patients with asthma, bronchiectasis, and cystic fibrosis and infants with acute bronchiolitis. It is delivered via nebulization either via face mask or endotracheal tube. It can be delivered alone or in combination with a bronchodilator. This therapy is being used in the outpatient and inpatient setting, as well as in both the neonatal intensive care unit and the pediatric intensive care unit, to help facilitate airway clearance, though studies of its use in bronchiolitis have had mixed results (see Chapter 418.1).

Lobar atelectasis in cystic fibrosis is discussed in Chapter 432.

Atelectasis can occur in patients with neuromuscular diseases. These patients tend to have ineffective cough and difficulty expelling respiratory tract secretions, which lead to pneumonia and atelectasis. Several devices and treatments are available to assist these patients, including intermittent positive-pressure breathing, a mechanical insufflator–exsufflator, and noninvasive bi-level positive-pressure ventilation via nasal mask or full-face mask. Patients with neuromuscular disease who have undergone

surgery are at substantial risk for postoperative atelectasis and subsequent pneumonia. Migrating atelectasis in the newborn infant, a rare and unique presentation, may be secondary to neuromuscular disease.

There is an association between the development of lobar collapse and the requirement for mechanical ventilation. Although lobar collapse is rarely a cause of long-term morbidity, its occurrence may necessitate the prolongation of mechanical ventilation or re-intubation. In ventilated patients, positive-end expiratory pressure or continuous positive airway pressure is generally indicated.

Airway clearance therapies used for adults are often recommended and/or used in pediatric populations. However, given the differences in respiratory physiology and anatomy between children and adults, practices applicable to one may or may not apply to the other. Atelectasis caused by cystic fibrosis is the only pediatric entity that clearly benefits from airway clearance therapy, although atelectasis caused by neuromuscular disease, cerebral palsy, or mechanical ventilation probably benefits from such therapy. Thus far no specific airway clearance therapy has been demonstrated to be superior.

Bibliography is available at Expert Consult.

Chapter **438**
Pulmonary Tumors
Susanna A. McColley

第四百三十八章
肺部肿瘤

中文导读

本章主要介绍了肺部肿瘤。具体描述了肺部肿瘤的病因学、临床表现及评估。原发性肺部肿瘤在儿童及青少年中罕见，支气管腺瘤（支气管类癌、腺样囊性癌以及黏液表皮样癌）是最常见的原发性肿瘤，其中支气管类癌约占80%，儿童最常见的肺部恶性肿瘤是转移瘤，包括Wilms瘤、骨肉瘤、肝母细胞瘤等；肺部肿瘤可表现为发热、咯血、喘息、咳嗽、胸痛、呼吸困难、反复或持续肺炎或肺不张等；胸部CT检查是必要的，手术切除肿瘤前应对患者进行仔细的评估。

ETIOLOGY

Primary tumors of the lung are rare in children and adolescents. An accurate estimate of frequency is currently not possible because the literature is composed of case reports and case series. A high incidence of "inflammatory pseudotumors" further clouds the statistics. Bronchial adenomas (including bronchial carcinoid, adenoid cystic carcinoma, and mucoepidermoid carcinomas) are the most common primary tumors;

bronchial carcinoid tumors represent ~80%. Carcinoids are low-grade malignancies; carcinoid syndrome is rare in children. Metastatic lesions are the most common forms of pulmonary malignancy in children; primary processes include Wilms tumor, osteogenic sarcoma, and hepatoblastoma (see Part XXI: Cancer and Benign Tumors). Adeno-carcinoma and undifferentiated histology are the most common pathologic findings in primary lung cancer; pulmonary blastoma is rarer and frequently occurs in the setting of cystic lung disease. Mediastinal involvement with lymphoma is more common than primary pulmonary malignancies.

CLINICAL MANIFESTATIONS AND EVALUATION

Pulmonary tumors may manifest as fever, hemoptysis, wheezing, cough, pleural effusion, chest pain, dyspnea, or recurrent or persistent pneumonia or atelectasis. Localized wheezing, and wheezing unresponsive to bronchodilators, can occur with bronchial tumors. Tumors may be suspected from plain chest radiographs; CT scanning of the chest is necessary for precise anatomic definition (Fig. 438.1). Depending on the tumor size and location, pulmonary function tests may be normal or show an obstructive, restrictive, or mixed pattern; as with the physical exam, there is no responsiveness to bronchodilators. Bronchial tumors are occasionally diagnosed during fiberoptic bronchoscopy performed for persistent or recurrent pulmonary infiltrates or for hemoptysis.

Patients with symptoms or with radiographic or other laboratory findings suggesting pulmonary malignancy should be evaluated carefully for a tumor at another site before surgical excision is carried out. Isolated primary lesions and isolated metastatic lesions discovered long after the primary tumor has been removed are best treated by excision. The prognosis varies and depends on the type of tumor involved; outcomes for inflammatory pseudotumors and primary pulmonary carcinoid tumors treated with resection are good.

Bibliography is available at Expert Consult.

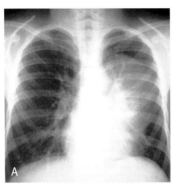 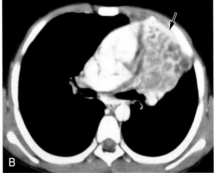

Fig. 438.1 Endobronchial mucoepidermoid carcinoma in a 10 yr old boy who presented with cough and fever. **A,** The chest radiograph shows a left upper lobe mass, a hyperinflated left lower lobe, and a prominent left hilum. **B,** The CT scan shows complete obstruction of the left upper lobe bronchus by a low-attenuation mass *(arrow)* that extends into the left mainstem bronchus. *(From Slovis TL, editor: Caffey's pediatric diagnostic imaging, ed 11, Philadelphia, 2008, Mosby, Fig. 78-20.)*

Chapter **439**

Pneumothorax

Glenna B. Winnie, Suraiya K. Haider, Aarthi P. Vemana, and Steven V. Lossef

第四百三十九章

气胸

中文导读

　　本章主要介绍了气胸。具体描述了气胸的病因学和流行病学、发病机制、临床表现、诊断、鉴别诊断以及治疗。其中病因学和流行病学详细地从自发性气胸和创伤性气胸两个方面进行阐述；诊断中具体介绍了对气胸量的评估，以及如何识别张力性气胸；对于气胸的治疗选择取决于肺压缩的程度、潜在疾病的性质和严重程度，包括保守观察、吸氧、胸腔穿刺、胸膜腔闭式引流等。

Pneumothorax is the accumulation of extrapulmonary air within the chest, most commonly from leakage of air from within the lung. Air leaks can be primary or secondary and can be spontaneous, traumatic, iatrogenic, or catamenial (Table 439.1). Pneumothorax in the neonatal period is also discussed in Chapter 122.1.

ETIOLOGY AND EPIDEMIOLOGY

A **primary spontaneous pneumothorax** occurs without trauma or underlying lung disease. Spontaneous pneumothorax with or without exertion occurs occasionally in teenagers and young adults, most frequently in males who are tall, thin, and thought to have subpleural blebs. Smoking and asthma are also risk factors for developing pneumothorax. Familial cases of spontaneous pneumothorax occur and have been associated with mutations in the folliculin gene *(FCLN)*. Over 150 unique *FCLN* mutations have been associated in the Birt-Hogg-Dube syndrome (skin fibrofolliculomas, multiple basal lung cysts, renal malignancies) or in patients with familial or recurrent spontaneous pneumothoraces. Individuals with other inherited disorders such as α_1-antitrypsin (see Chapter 421) and homocystinuria are also predisposed to pneumothorax. Patients with collagen synthesis defects such as Ehlers-Danlos disease (see Chapter 678) and Marfan syndrome (see Chapter 722) are at increased risk for the development of pneumothorax.

Table 439.1	Causes of Pneumothorax in Children

SPONTANEOUS
Primary Idiopathic (no underlying lung disease)
Spontaneous rupture of subpleural blebs
Secondary (underlying lung disease)
Congenital lung disease
- Congenital cystic adenomatoid malformation
- Bronchogenic cysts
- Pulmonary hypoplasia
- Birt-Hogg-Dube syndrome

Conditions associated with increased intrathoracic pressure
- Asthma
- Bronchiolitis
- Cystic fibrosis
- Airway foreign body
- Smoking (cigarettes, marijuana, crack cocaine)

Infection
- Tuberculosis
- *Pneumocystis carinii (jirovecii)*
- Echinococcosis
- Pneumatocele
- Lung abscess
- Bronchopleural fistula

Lung disease
- Langerhans cell histiocytosis
- Tuberous sclerosis
- Marfan syndrome
- Ehlers-Danlos syndrome
- Pulmonary fibrosis
- Sarcoidosis
- Rheumatoid arthritis, scleroderma, ankylosing spondylitis
- Metastatic neoplasm—usually osteosarcoma (rare)
- Pulmonary blastoma

TRAUMATIC
Non-iatrogenic
- Penetrating trauma
- Blunt trauma

Iatrogenic
- Thoracotomy
- Thoracoscopy, thoracentesis
- Tracheostomy
- Tube or needle puncture
- Mechanical ventilation
- High-flow therapy (moved from non-iatrogenic)

Adapted from Noppen M. Spontaneous pneumothorax:epidemiology, pathophysiology and cause. *Eur Respir Rev* 19:117, 217–219, 2010 (Table 1, 2, p 218).

A pneumothorax arising as a complication of an underlying lung disorder but without trauma is a **secondary spontaneous pneumothorax.** Pneumothorax can occur in pneumonia, usually with empyema; it can also be secondary to pulmonary abscess, gangrene, infarct, rupture of a cyst or an emphysematous bleb (in asthma), or foreign bodies in the lung. In infants with staphylococcal pneumonia, the incidence of pneumothorax is relatively high. It can be found in children hospitalized with asthma exacerbations, and usually resolves without treatment. Pneumothorax is a serious complication in cystic fibrosis (see Chapter 432). Pneumothorax also occurs in patients with lymphoma or other malignancies, and in graft-versus-host disease with bronchiolitis obliterans.

External chest or abdominal blunt or penetrating trauma can tear a bronchus or abdominal viscus, with leakage of air into the pleural space. Ecstasy (methylenedioxymethamphetamine), crack cocaine, and marijuana abuse are associated with pneumothorax.

Iatrogenic pneumothorax can complicate transthoracic needle aspiration, tracheotomy, subclavian line placement, thoracentesis, or transbronchial biopsy. It may occur during mechanical or noninvasive ventilation, high-flow nasal cannula therapy, acupuncture, and other diagnostic or therapeutic procedures.

Catamenial pneumothorax, an unusual condition that is related to menses, is associated with diaphragmatic defects and pleural blebs.

Pneumothorax can be associated with a serous effusion (hydropneumothorax), a purulent effusion (pyopneumothorax), or blood (hemopneumothorax). Bilateral pneumothorax is rare after the neonatal period but has been reported after lung transplantation and with *Mycoplasma pneumoniae* infection and tuberculosis.

PATHOGENESIS

The tendency of the lung to collapse, or elastic recoil, is balanced in the normal resting state by the inherent tendency of the chest wall to expand outward, creating negative pressure in the intrapleural space. When air enters the pleural space, the lung collapses. Hypoxemia occurs because of alveolar hypoventilation, ventilation–perfusion mismatch, and intrapulmonary shunt. In simple pneumothorax, intrapleural pressure is atmospheric, and the lung collapses up to 30%. In **tension pneumothorax**, continuing leak causes increasing positive pressure in the pleural space, with further compression of the lung, shift of mediastinal structures toward the contralateral side, and decreases in venous return and cardiac output causing hemodynamic instability.

CLINICAL MANIFESTATIONS

The onset of pneumothorax is usually abrupt, and the severity of symptoms depends on the extent of the lung collapse and on the amount of preexisting lung disease. Pneumothorax may cause dyspnea, chest pain, and cyanosis. When it occurs in infancy, symptoms and physical signs may be difficult to recognize. Moderate pneumothorax may cause little displacement of the intrathoracic organs and few or no symptoms. The severity of pain usually does not directly reflect the extent of the collapse.

Usually, there is respiratory distress, with retractions, markedly decreased breath sounds, and a tympanitic percussion note over the involved hemithorax. The larynx, trachea, and heart may be shifted toward the unaffected side. When fluid is present, there is usually a sharply limited area of tympany above a level of flatness to percussion. The presence of bronchial breath sounds or, when fluid is present in the pleural cavity, of gurgling sounds synchronous with respirations suggests an open fistula connecting with air-containing tissues.

DIAGNOSIS AND DIFFERENTIAL DIAGNOSIS

The diagnosis of pneumothorax is usually established by radiographic examination (Figs. 439.1 to 439.6). The amount of air outside the lung varies with time. A radiograph that is taken early shows less lung collapse than one taken later if the leak continues. Expiratory views accentuate the contrast between lung markings and the clear area of the pneumothorax (see Fig. 439.1). Variations exist in the measurement techniques defining the size of a pneumothorax. A large pneumothorax is measured by The American College of Chest Physicians as ≥3 cm from the lung apex to the thoracic cupola, and by the British Thoracic

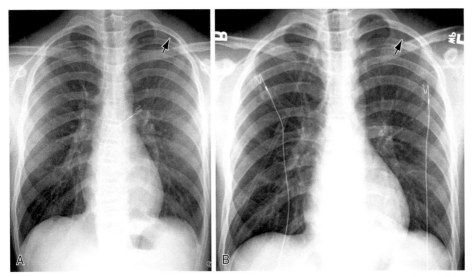

Fig. 439.1 Utility of an expiratory film in detection of a small pneumothorax. **A,** Teenage boy with stab wound and subtle radiolucency in the left apical region *(arrow)* on inspiratory chest radiograph. The margin of the visceral pleura is very faintly visible. **B,** On an expiratory film, the pneumothorax *(arrow)* is more obvious as the right lung has deflated and become more opaque, providing better contrast with the air in the pleural space.

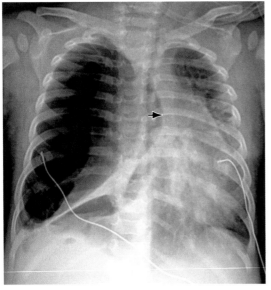

Fig. 439.2 Right pneumothorax, with lung collapse of a compliant lung. Shift of the mediastinum to the left *(arrow)* indicates that this is a tension pneumothorax.

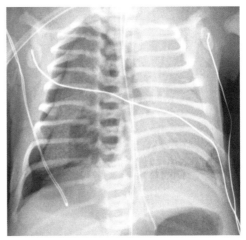

Fig. 439.3 Right pneumothorax, with only limited collapse of a poorly compliant lung.

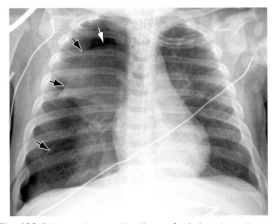

Fig. 439.4 Pneumothorax, with collapse of right lung *(arrows)* caused by barotrauma in a 7 mo old child who was intubated for respiratory failure.

Society as ≥2 cm from the lung margin to the chest wall at the level of the hilum.

It may be difficult to determine whether a pneumothorax is under tension. Tension pneumothorax is present when there is a shift of mediastinal structures away from the side of the air leak. A shift may be absent in situations in which the other hemithorax resists the shift, such as in the case of bilateral pneumothorax. On occasion, the diagnosis of tension pneumothorax is made only on the basis of evidence of circulatory compromise or on hearing a "hiss" of rapid exit of air under tension with the insertion of the thoracostomy tube. When the lungs are both stiff, such as in cystic fibrosis or respiratory distress syndrome, the unaffected lung may not collapse easily, and shift may not occur (see Fig. 439.3).

Pneumothorax must be differentiated from localized or generalized emphysema, an extensive emphysematous bleb, large pulmonary

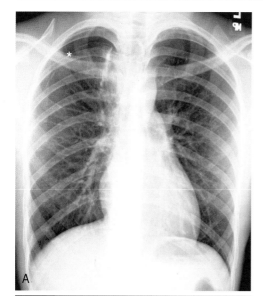

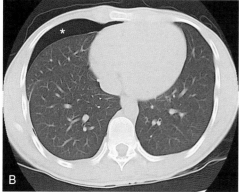

Fig. 439.5 Teenager in whom a spontaneous right pneumothorax developed because of a bleb. He had a persistent air leak despite recent surgical resection of the causative apical bleb. Chest radiograph **(A)** and CT scan **(B)** clearly show the persistent pneumothorax *(asterisk)*.

cavities or other cystic formations, diaphragmatic hernia, compensatory overexpansion with contralateral atelectasis, and gaseous distention of the stomach. In most cases, chest radiography or CT differentiates among these possibilities. In addition, CT may identify underlying pathology such as blebs (Fig. 439.7). Further evaluation to determine if a diaphragmatic hernia is present should include a barium swallow with a small amount of barium to demonstrate that it is not free air but is a portion of the gastrointestinal tract that is in the thoracic cavity (Chapter 122.10). Ultrasound can also be used to establish the diagnosis.

TREATMENT

Therapy varies with the extent of the collapse and the nature and severity of the underlying disease. A small or even moderate-sized pneumothorax in an otherwise normal child may resolve without specific treatment, usually within 1 wk. A small pneumothorax complicating asthma may also resolve spontaneously. Administering 100% oxygen may hasten resolution, but patients with chronic hypoxemia should be monitored closely during administration of supplemental oxygen. Pleural pain deserves analgesic treatment. Needle aspiration into the second intercostal space in the midclavicular line may be required on an emergency basis for tension pneumothorax and is as effective as tube thoracostomy in the emergency room management of primary spontaneous pneumothorax. If the pneumothorax is recurrent, secondary, or under tension, or there is more than a small collapse, chest tube drainage may be necessary. Pneumothorax-complicating cystic fibrosis frequently recurs, and definitive treatment may be justified with the first episode. Similarly, if pneumothorax complicating malignancy does not improve rapidly with observation, chemical pleurodesis or surgical thoracotomy is often necessary. In cases with severe air leak or bronchopleural fistula, occlusion with an endobronchial balloon has been successful.

Closed thoracotomy (simple insertion of a chest tube) and drainage of the trapped air through a catheter, the external opening of which is kept in a dependent position under water, is adequate to reexpand the lung in most patients; pigtail catheters are frequently used. In the case of recurrent pneumothorax, a sclerosing procedure may be indicated to induce the formation of strong adhesions between the lung and chest wall with the introduction of talc, doxycycline, or iodopovidone into the pleural space (chemical pleurodesis). Open thoracotomy through a limited incision, with plication of blebs, closure of fistula, stripping of the pleura (usually in the apical lung, where the surgeon has direct vision), and basilar pleural abrasion is also an effective treatment for recurrent pneumothorax. Stripping and abrading the pleura leaves raw, inflamed surfaces that heal with sealing adhesions. Postoperative pain is comparable to that with chemical pleurodesis, but the chest tube can usually be removed in 24-48 hr, compared with the usual 72 hr minimum

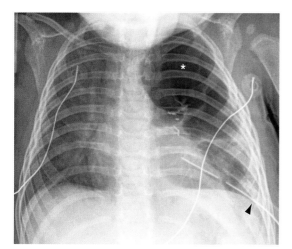

Fig. 439.6 Bronchopleural fistula following surgical resection of the left upper lobe as a result of congenital lobar emphysema. Chest radiograph shows localized pneumothorax *(asterisk)* that persisted despite prior insertion of a large-bore chest tube *(arrowhead)*.

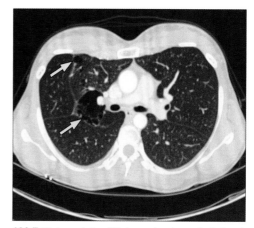

Fig. 439.7 High-resolution CT thorax showing multiple basal cysts. *(From Hopkins TG, Maher ER, Reid E, Marciniak S: Recurrent pneumothorax, Lancet 377:1624, 2011, Fig. 1, p. 1624.)*

for closed thoracotomy and pleurodesis. Video-assisted thoracoscopic surgery (VATS) is a preferred therapy for blebectomy, pleural stripping, pleural brushing, and instillation of sclerosing agents, with less morbidity than occurs with traditional open thoracotomy. There is risk of recurrence after VATS in the pediatric population, although this is often not related to surgical failure, but rather associated with the formation of new bullae.

Pleural adhesions help prevent recurrent pneumothorax, but they also make subsequent thoracic surgery difficult. When lung transplanta-tion may be a future consideration (e.g., in cystic fibrosis), steps should be taken to avoid, if at all possible, chemical or mechanical pleurodesis. It should also be kept in mind that the longer a chest tube is in place, the greater the chance of pulmonary deterioration, particularly in a patient with cystic fibrosis, in whom strong coughing, deep breathing, and postural drainage are important. These are all difficult to accomplish with a chest tube in place.

Bibliography is available at Expert Consult.

Chapter **440**
Pneumomediastinum
Glenna B. Winnie, Aarthi P. Vemana, and Suraiya K. Haider

第四百四十章
纵隔气肿

中文导读

　　本章主要介绍了纵隔气肿。具体描述了纵隔气肿的病因学、发病机制、实验室检查、临床表现及并发症。纵隔气肿可以为自发性或由创伤引起，下呼吸道感染及哮喘急性发作是常见继发性纵隔气肿的病因；呼吸困难及短暂胸痛是纵隔气肿的主要临床症状；胸部影像学检查可发现纵隔气肿；纵隔气肿的治疗主要针对潜在的阻塞性肺疾病或其他诱发因素。

Air or gas in the mediastinum is called **pneumomediastinum.**

ETIOLOGY
Pneumomediastinum is typically caused by alveolar rupture which can be due to either a spontaneous or traumatic cause. A spontaneous pneumomediastinum can either be primary without an underlying etiology or can occur secondary to an underlying cause. Primary pneumomediastinum can be due to increases in intrathoracic pressure as is seen with a Valsalva maneuver, vomiting, Boerhaave syndrome (esophageal perforation), weightlifting, and choking events. Common causes of secondary pneumomediastinum in children younger than age 7 years are lower respiratory tract infections and asthma exacerbations. Simultaneous pneumothorax is unusual in these patients. Other causes of secondary pneumomediastinum are anorexia nervosa, normal menses, and diabetes mellitus with ketoacidosis. Traumatic causes of pneumo-mediastinum include both iatrogenic (dental extractions, adenotonsil-lectomy, high flow nasal cannula therapy, esophageal perforation, and inhalation of helium gas), and non-iatrogenic (inhaled foreign body, penetrating chest trauma, and illicit drug use).

PATHOGENESIS
According to the **Macklin effect**, after an intrapulmonary alveolar rupture, air dissects along the pressure gradient through the perivascular sheaths and other soft tissue planes toward the hilum and enters the mediastinum.

CLINICAL MANIFESTATIONS
Dyspnea and transient stabbing chest pain that may radiate to the neck are the principal features of pneumomediastinum. Other symptoms may be present and may include globus pharyngeus, abdominal pain, cough, chest tightness, facial swelling, choking, tachypnea, fever, stridor, and sore throat. Pneumomediastinum is difficult to detect by physical examination alone. Subcutaneous emphysema is present in the majority of patients. When present, **Hamman sign** (a mediastinal "crunch") is nearly pathognomonic for pneumomediastinum. Cardiac dullness to percussion may be decreased, but the chests of many patients with pneumomediastinum are chronically overinflated and it is unlikely that the clinician can be sure of this finding.

LABORATORY FINDINGS
Chest radiography reveals mediastinal air, with a more distinct cardiac

border than normal (Figs. 440.1 and 440.2). A "spinnaker sail sign" or "angel wing sign" occurs when air deviates the thymus upward and outward, which is seen more often in pediatric patients. On the lateral projection, the posterior mediastinal structures are clearly defined, there may be a lucent ring ("ring sign") around the right pulmonary artery, and retrosternal air can usually be seen. Vertical streaks of air in the mediastinum and subcutaneous air are often observed (see Fig. 440.1). If a pneumomediastinum is clinically suspected, but is not visualized on a chest x-ray, a chest CT can be performed to provide further radiologic evidence.

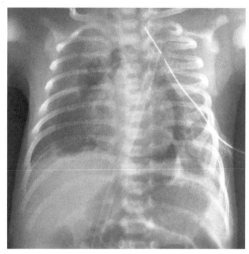

Fig. 440.2 Sail sign—thymic elevation. *(From Clark DA: Atlas of neonatology, ed 7, Philadelphia, 2000, WB Saunders, p. 94.)*

TREATMENT

Treatment is directed primarily at the underlying obstructive pulmonary disease or other precipitating condition. Children who have had pneumomediastinum should be screened for asthma. Analgesics are occasionally needed for chest pain. Children can be observed in the emergency room and discharged if stable. They should be cautioned to avoid heavy lifting and the Valsalva maneuver. Hospital admission with supplemental oxygen administration is more common for patients with secondary pneumomediastinum. Rarely, subcutaneous emphysema can cause sufficient tracheal compression to justify tracheotomy; the tracheotomy also decompresses the mediastinum.

COMPLICATIONS

Pneumomediastinum is rarely a major problem in older children because the mediastinum can be depressurized by escape of air into the neck or abdomen. In the newborn, however, the rate at which air can leave the mediastinum is limited, and pneumomediastinum can lead to dangerous cardiovascular compromise or pneumothorax (see Chapters 122.14 and 439).

Bibliography is available at Expert Consult.

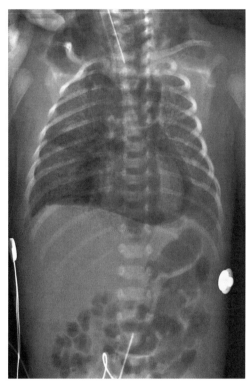

Fig. 440.1 Large pneumomediastinum surrounding the heart and dissecting into the neck. *(From Clark DA: Atlas of neonatology, ed 7, Philadelphia, 2000, WB Saunders.)*

Chapter **441**
Hydrothorax

Glenna B. Winnie, Aarthi P. Vemana, and Suraiya K. Haider

第四百四十一章
胸腔积液（漏出性）

中文导读

　　本章主要介绍了漏出性胸腔积液的病因、临床表现、实验室检查和治疗。病因包括心脏、肾脏或肝脏疾病、严重营养不良性水肿和低蛋白血症、肿瘤、淋巴结肿大、肺栓塞或粘连导致的上腔静脉阻塞。临床表现中介绍了漏出性胸腔积液通常是双侧的，在心脏或肝脏疾病中，可局限于右侧或右侧多于左侧。实验室检查包括积液的性质、相对密度、胸腔积液与血清总蛋白比值、胸腔积液与血清乳酸脱氢酶比值等。治疗针对基础疾病。

Hydrothorax is a transudative pleural effusion; typically, it is caused by abnormal pressure gradients in the lung.

ETIOLOGY
Hydrothorax is most often associated with cardiac, renal, or hepatic disease. It can also be a manifestation of severe nutritional edema and hypoalbuminemia. Rarely, it results from superior vena cava obstruction by neoplasms, enlarged lymph nodes, pulmonary embolism, or adhesions. It may occur from a ventriculoperitoneal shunt, central venous catheter, or peritoneal dialysis.

CLINICAL MANIFESTATIONS
Hydrothorax is usually bilateral, but in cardiac or hepatic disease it can be limited to the right side or greater on the right than on the left side. The physical signs are the same as those described for serofibrinous pleurisy (see Chapter 429.2), but in hydrothorax there is more rapid shifting of the level of dullness with changes of position. Depending on the etiology, it can be associated with an accumulation of fluid in other parts of the body.

LABORATORY FINDINGS
The fluid is **transudative**, noninflammatory, has few cells, and has a lower specific gravity (<1.015) than that of a serofibrinous exudate (see Chapters 428 and 429). The ratio of pleural fluid to serum total protein is <0.5, the ratio of pleural fluid to serum lactic dehydrogenase is <0.6, and the pleural fluid lactic dehydrogenase value is less than 66% of the upper limit of the normal serum lactic dehydrogenase range. In a patient with a VP shunt, B-transferrin assays and radionuclide tracer shunt series may be helpful for diagnosis. Peritoneal scintigraphy may be considered to evaluate for a peritoneal-pleural leak. In hepatic hydrothorax, the pleural fluid resembles spontaneous bacterial peritonitis, with positive bacterial cultures and polymorphonuclear leukocyte counts >250 cell/mm^3.

TREATMENT
Therapy is directed at the underlying disorder. If a transudative fluid is clinically suspected, aspiration may not be needed unless pressure symptoms are noted or there are atypical symptoms such as fever, pleuritic pain, or asymmetric effusions.

Bibliography is available at Expert Consult.

Chapter **442**

Hemothorax

Glenna B. Winnie, Suraiya K. Haider,
Aarthi P. Vemana, and Steven V. Lossef

第四百四十二章

血胸

中文导读

　　本章主要介绍了血胸的病因、临床表现、诊断和治疗。病因包括胸部外伤、医源性创伤、炎症侵蚀血管、先天畸形、胸腔内肿瘤等，自发性血胸十分罕见。临床上，除胸腔积液的症状及体征外，还偶表现出与出血量及出血速度相关的血流动力学改变以及通气功能障碍。诊断包括X线片、CT、胸腔穿刺，必须积极查找血胸的原因。治疗包括氧疗、液体复苏、胸腔穿刺术、电视胸腔镜手术（VATS）、开胸手术、纤溶治疗及栓堵治疗等。

Hemothorax, an accumulation of blood in the pleural cavity, is rare in children.

ETIOLOGY

Bleeding into the chest cavity most commonly occurs after chest trauma, either blunt or penetrating. It can be the result of iatrogenic trauma, including surgical procedures and venous line insertion. Hemothorax can also result from erosion of a blood vessel in association with inflammatory processes such as tuberculosis and empyema. It may complicate a variety of congenital anomalies including sequestration, patent ductus arteriosus, and pulmonary arteriovenous malformation (see Fig. 436.2 in Chapter 436). It is also an occasional manifestation of intrathoracic neoplasms, costal exostoses, blood dyscrasias, bleeding diatheses, or thrombolytic therapy. Rupture of an aneurysm is unlikely during childhood. Hemothorax may occur spontaneously in neonates and older children but is very rare. A pleural hemorrhage associated with a pneumothorax is a *hemopneumothorax*; it is usually the result of a ruptured bulla with lung volume loss causing a torn pleural adhesion.

CLINICAL MANIFESTATIONS

In addition to the symptoms and signs of pleural effusion (see Chapter 429.2), hemothorax is associated with hemodynamic compromise related to the amount and rapidity of bleeding, with ventilatory collapse. Spontaneous hemothorax presents with sudden onset of chest or back pain or dyspnea and can progress rapidly to hemorrhagic shock.

DIAGNOSIS

The diagnosis of a hemothorax is initially suspected from radiographs or CT scans but can be made definitively with thoracentesis (Fig. 442.1).

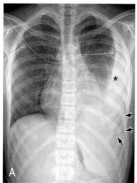
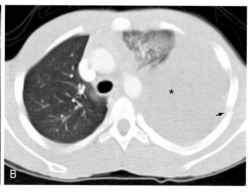

Fig. 442.1 Hemothorax *(asterisk)* and associated rib fractures *(arrows)* in a teenager involved in a motor vehicle accident. **A,** Chest radiograph. **B,** CT scan.

In every case, an effort must be made to determine and treat the cause.

TREATMENT

Therapy includes supplemental oxygen, fluid resuscitation (including possible blood transfusion), and tube thoracostomy. Video-assisted thorascopic surgery (VATS) can be considered in most patients with stable vital signs to visualize the source of bleeding, remove blood clots, resect bullae or blebs, and to perform pleurodesis. An open thoracotomy may be indicated if there is uncontrolled bleeding or in a hemodynami-cally compromised patient. Inadequate removal of blood in extensive hemothorax leading to a retained hemothorax can increase the risk for development of pneumonia, empyema, or substantial restrictive disease secondary to organization of fibrin. Fibrinolytic therapy or a decortication may then be necessary. Embolization is the treatment of choice for an arteriovenous malformation.

Bibliography is available at Expert Consult.

Chapter **443**

Chylothorax

Glenna B. Winnie, Suraiya K. Haider, Aarthi P. Vemana, and Steven V. Lossef

第四百四十三章
乳糜胸

中文导读

　　本章主要介绍了乳糜胸的病因、临床表现、实验室检查、治疗和并发症。病因包括心脏外科手术引起的胸导管损伤、体外膜肺治疗、胸腔恶性肿瘤、胸部外伤、新生儿娩出时静脉压迅速升高所致的胸导管破裂、唐氏综合征、Noonan综合征、Turner综合征等，少见原因包括淋巴管瘤病、限制性肺疾病、上下腔静脉血栓形成、结核或组织胞浆菌病以及淋巴系统先天畸形等。胎儿期难治性乳糜胸与整合素α₉β1基因错义突变有关。临床表现包括咳嗽、胸部不适和呼吸困难。实验室检查包括胸片、CT、胸腔穿刺等检查。治疗包括低脂肪或中链甘油三酯的肠内喂养、高蛋白饮食、全肠外营养、胸腔穿刺减压、奥曲肽等治疗、手术治疗和介入治疗。并发症包括营养不良、免疫缺陷等。

Chylothorax is a pleural collection of fluid formed by the escape of chyle from the thoracic duct or lymphatics into the thoracic cavity.

ETIOLOGY

Chylothorax in children occurs most frequently because of thoracic duct injury as a complication of cardiothoracic surgery (post Fontan surgery) (Fig. 443.1). Other cases are associated with chest injury (Fig. 443.2), extracorporeal membrane oxygenation, or with primary or metastatic intrathoracic malignancy, particularly lymphoma. In newborns, rapidly increased venous pressure during delivery may lead to thoracic duct rupture. Chylothorax has also been associated with Down syndrome, Noonan syndrome, and Turner syndrome. Less common causes include lymphangiomatosis (Fig. 443.3); restrictive pulmonary diseases; thrombosis of the duct, superior vena cava, or subclavian vein; tuberculosis or histoplasmosis; and congenital anomalies of the lymphatic system (Fig. 443.4). Refractory chylothorax in the fetus has been associated with a missense mutation in integrin α₉β1 gene. Chylothorax can occur in trauma and child abuse (see Chapter 16). It is important to establish the etiology because treatment varies with the cause. In some patients no specific cause is identified.

CLINICAL MANIFESTATIONS

The signs and symptoms of chylothorax are the same as those from pleural effusion of similar size including cough, chest discomfort, and dyspnea. **Chyle** is not irritating, so pleuritic pain is uncommon. Onset is often gradual. However, after trauma to the thoracic duct chyle may accumulate in the posterior mediastinum for days and then rupture into the pleural space with sudden onset of dyspnea, hypotension, and

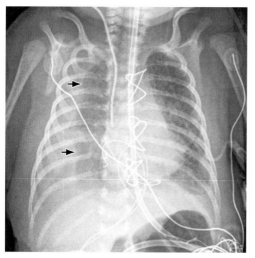

Fig. 443.1 Chylothorax *(arrows)* following cardiac surgery in a 2 wk old infant.

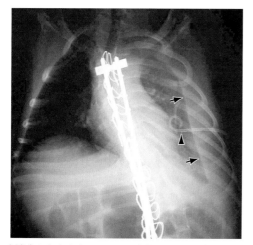

Fig. 443.2 Left chylothorax *(arrows)* following spinal fusion with Harrington rods. It is postulated that the thoracic duct was injured during spine surgery. The pigtail chest tube *(arrowhead)* needed to be retracted to better drain the effusion.

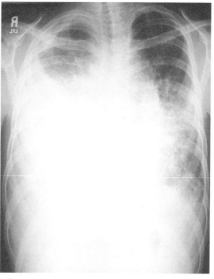

Fig. 443.3 Large right chylous effusion opacifying much of the right thorax in a teenager with pulmonary lymphangiomatosis and hemangiomatosis. Note the associated interstitial lung disease.

hypoxemia. Approximately 50% of newborns with chylothorax present with respiratory distress in the 1st day of life. Chylothorax is rarely bilateral and usually occurs on the right side.

LABORATORY FINDINGS

Chest radiographs can help to delineate the location of an effusion; CT scans show normal pleural thickness and may demonstrate a mediastinal mass such as a lymphoma as the etiology of the chylothorax. Thoracentesis demonstrates a chylous effusion, a milky fluid containing triglycerides, protein, lymphocytes, and other constituents of chyle; fluid may be yellow or bloody. In newborn infants or those who are not ingesting food, the fluid may be clear. A pseudochylous milky fluid may be present in chronic serous effusion, in which fatty material arises from degenerative changes in the fluid and not from lymph. In chylothorax, the fluid triglyceride level is >110 mg/dL, the pleural fluid:serum triglyceride ratio is >1.0, and pleural fluid:serum cholesterol ratio is <1.0; lipoprotein analysis reveals chylomicrons. Fluid immunoglobulin levels are elevated. The cells are primarily (~90%) T lymphocytes and often exceed 1,000 cells per mm^3. After diagnosing chylothorax, a lymphangiogram can

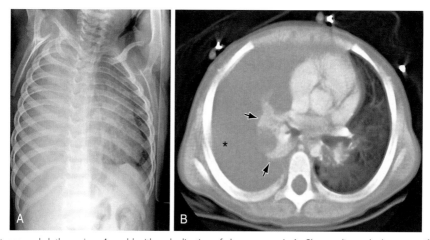

Fig. 443.4 Spontaneous chylothorax in a 4 yr old with a duplication of chromosome 6. **A,** Chest radiograph shows opacification of the right thorax. **B,** CT scan shows the chylous pleural effusion *(asterisk)* compressing the atelectatic right lung *(arrows)*.

localize the site of the leak, and lymphoscintigraphy may demonstrate abnormalities of the lymphatic trunks and peripheral lymphatics.

TREATMENT

Spontaneous recovery occurs in >50% of cases of neonatal chylothorax. Therapy includes enteral feedings with a low-fat or medium-chain triglyceride, high-protein diet, and total parenteral nutrition. Thoracentesis is repeated as needed to relieve pressure symptoms; tube thoracostomy is often performed. Somatostatin and octreotide have been used to manage chylothorax. Various octreotide dosages have been described in the literature including 1-4 µg/kg/hr intravenously and 10 µg/kg/day subcutaneously; however, the optimal dose is not known and further study is needed. Other therapeutic approaches include percutaneous thoracic duct embolization, pressure control ventilation with positive end-expiratory pressure, and inhalation of nitric oxide. If medical management is unsuccessful, surgical options should be considered and can include a pleuroperitoneal shunt, thoracic duct ligation, and pleurodesis with the use of a sclerosing agent such as fibrin glue, talc, or iodopovidone. Treatment is similar for traumatic chylothorax. Chemical pleurodesis or irradiation is used in malignant chylothorax. OK432 (picibanil) has been used to treat fetal and newborn

chylothorax. Etilefrine, a sympathomimetic agent with both α- and β-adrenergic activity, has been successfully used in a few patients. Constriction of the thoracic duct by this drug may reduce pleural chyle accumulation. Percutaneous thoracic duct embolization or treatment of other lymphatic vessels is a highly successful interventional radiology strategy. Surgery should be considered earlier in neonates with massive chylothorax and chyle output of > 50 mL/kg/day despite maximum medical therapy for 3 days.

COMPLICATIONS

If repeated thoracenteses are required due to the rapid reaccumulation of chyle, malnutrition may occur with significant loss of calories, protein, and electrolytes. Immunodeficiencies, including hypogammaglobulinemia and abnormal cell-mediated immune responses, have been associated with repeated and chronic thoracenteses for chylothorax. The loss of T lymphocytes is associated with increased risk of infection in neonates; otherwise, infection is uncommon, but patients should not receive live virus vaccines. Lack of resolution of chylothorax can lead to malnutrition, infection, and death.

Bibliography is available at Expert Consult.

Chapter **444**

Bronchopulmonary Dysplasia

Sharon A. McGrath-Morrow and J. Michael Collaco

第四百四十四章
支气管肺发育不良

中文导读

　　本章阐述了支气管肺发育不良的概念，介绍了支气管肺发育不良的临床表现、治疗和预后。支气管肺发育不良的严重程度不同，临床表现也不同，重症者可有慢性呼吸功能不全表现。治疗中介绍了出院后的

治疗和护理要点，并具体描述了支气管肺发育不良合并肺动脉高压的病因、危险因素、筛查和治疗等。此病预后通常较好，幼年期可有哮喘样表现。

BRONCHOPULMONARY DYSPLASIA

Bronchopulmonary dysplasia (BPD) is a chronic lung disease of infancy and childhood that occurs primarily in preterm infants born at less than 32 wk gestation. BPD is characterized by alveolar hypoplasia, often with concomitant small airway dysfunction and impaired pulmonary

vascular growth. Contributing factors to the development of BPD may include early gestational age, low birth weight, lung barotrauma, exposure to hyperoxia, lung inflammation, and pre- and postnatal infections, as well as potential modifier genes and epigenetic factors. The currently accepted definition includes an oxygen requirement for 28 days

Table 444.1	Definitions of Bronchopulmonary Dysplasia		
FEATURES OF ALL BPD	**ADDITIONAL FEATURES OF MILD BPD**	**ADDITIONAL FEATURES OF MODERATE BPD**	**ADDITIONAL FEATURES OF SEVERE BPD**
<32 wk gestational age at birth Oxygen requirement for at least 28 days	Breathing room air at 36 wk PMA or at discharge, whichever comes first	<30% supplemental oxygen at 36 wk PMA or at discharge, whichever comes first	>30% supplemental oxygen and/or positive pressure ventilation at 36 wk PMA or at discharge, whichever comes first
>32 wk gestational age at birth Oxygen requirement for at least 28 days	Breathing room air at 56 days of life or at discharge, whichever comes first	<30% supplemental oxygen at 56 days of life or at discharge, whichever comes first	>30% supplemental oxygen and/or positive pressure ventilation at 56 days of life or at discharge, whichever comes first

BPD, bronchopulmonary dysplasia; PMA, postmenstrual age.

postnatally, and the disorder is graded as mild, moderate, or severe on the basis of supplemental oxygen and ventilation requirements at specific timepoints (Table 444.1). For initial inpatient presentation and management, see Chapter 122.

CLINICAL MANIFESTATIONS

Physical findings of the pulmonary exam vary with the severity of disease and with respiratory illnesses. Although some patients may appear to be comfortably breathing when well, they can experience significant deterioration when ill or with periods of stress due to decreased pulmonary reserve secondary to alveolar hypoplasia and small airway disease. Children with BPD may exhibit tachypnea, head bobbing, and retractions when ill or at baseline depending on the severity of disease. Although breath sounds may be clear, many patients have baseline wheeze or coarse crackles. A persistent fixed wheeze or stridor suggests subglottic stenosis (see Chapter 415) or large airway malacia. Fine crackles may be present in patients prone to fluid overload. Chest radiographs may demonstrate air trapping, focal atelectasis, interstitial changes, and/or peribronchial thickening.

The most severely affected patients may require respiratory support to achieve adequate gas exchange. Supplemental oxygen may be required to maintain acceptable oxygen saturations and often is needed to minimize the work of breathing. Chronic respiratory insufficiency may be evidenced as elevation of serum bicarbonate, elevated carbon dioxide on blood gas analysis, hypoxemia, or polycythemia; the most severe cases may require tracheostomy and ventilation to achieve long-term respiratory stability. Patients must be monitored for the development of pulmonary hypertension, especially if they require supplemental oxygen and have chronic respiratory insufficiency.

Aspiration from dysphagia and/or gastroesophageal reflux (GERD) (see Chapter 349) can compromise pulmonary status. The risk of aspiration may increase during periods of illness due to worsening tachypnea and air trapping. Other comorbidities resulting from premature birth that complicate the management of BPD include fixed and functional upper airway obstruction, CNS injuries leading to abnormal control of breathing, abnormal airway tone, increased aspiration risk, gastrointestinal dysmotility, systemic hypertension, and poor growth. Of note, infants with significant lung disease can exhibit growth failure from the elevated energy expenditure essential to maintain the increased metabolic demands of respiration and/or ongoing hypoxia.

A *pulmonary exacerbation* in a child with BPD is typically triggered during viral respiratory infections. Other frequent risk factors for pulmonary exacerbations may include weather changes, exposure to cigarette smoke, attending daycare, and aspiration. During an exacerbation, the infant may exhibit increased work of breathing, crackles, and wheezing, with tachypnea and retractions becoming more prominent. Underlying pulmonary hypertension may worsen with pulmonary exacerbations as well.

TREATMENT

Treatment is directed toward decreasing the work of breathing and normalizing gas exchange, to allow for optimal growth and neurodevelopment. After initial hospital discharge, infants and children with BPD are at high risk for rehospitalization. Up to 50% of infants with BPD

are readmitted for acute respiratory illnesses within the first 2 yr of life. These children also may require multiple daily medications, supplemental oxygen, and/or chronic ventilation.

Adherence to prescribed daily medication regimens may decrease the risk of acute care use and chronic respiratory symptoms; however, there are no standard guidelines for management of BPD with regard to post-NICU care. Although commonly used, there are limited data regarding the efficacy of diuretics in the outpatient setting.

With regard to respiratory support, targeted oxygen saturations should be ≥92% outside of the NICU to ensure adequate growth and neurocognitive development. Pulse-oximetry and polysomnography may be helpful for titration purposes. Prior to initial hospital discharge, infants and children who require chronic ventilatory support have been shown to benefit from standardized protocols to determine medical readiness, assess familial proficiency in respiratory cares, and establish adequate support in an outpatient setting. After discharge, these patients will require close follow-up from pulmonologists and otolaryngologists to manage ventilator titration and weaning, and tracheostomy cares and decannulation, respectively. As infants and children with tracheostomies are at high risk for adverse events, including death, an awake and alert trained caregiver is recommended at all times.

Pulmonary function testing in children with a history of BPD has consistently demonstrated obstructive small airway disease. Small airway disease in this population may be partially responsive to bronchodilators, but may also have a fixed obstructive component. Inhaled corticosteroids and β-agonists may be effective in treating symptoms, such as wheezing or chronic cough. Leukotriene-modifying agents may be a useful adjunct therapy.

Adequate caloric intake is important to ensure catch-up lung growth. Some children may require fortified breast milk or formula to achieve adequate growth. Patients at risk for aspiration and those with inadequate oral intake may require tube feeding to meet nutritional goals. Placement of a gastrostomy tube should be considered prior to discharge to home to avoid inadvertent dislodgement. Aspiration secondary to dysphagia and/or gastroesophageal reflux should be considered in patients with recurrent respiratory symptoms or pneumonia without obvious infectious etiologies. Due to their tenuous respiratory status, some infants and children with BPD may not be able to tolerate even minimal amounts of aspiration from gastroesophageal reflux. There are limited data regarding risks and benefits of anti-reflux medications in infants with BPD, such has histamine-2 blockers, proton pump inhibitors, and motility agents. Medications that reduce gastric acidity may increase the risk of pneumonia in some children. Consideration for either Nissen fundoplication or gastrojejunostomy tubes may be required in cases of failure of anti-reflux medical therapy.

Up to 15–25% of infants with severe BPD will be diagnosed with **pulmonary hypertension**, which may be secondary to decreased pulmonary vascular growth and/or a reactive vascular bed. Other risk factors for developing pulmonary hypertension may include extreme prematurity and decreased intrauterine growth; recurrent aspiration, hypoxia, and hypercarbia may worsen severity. Pulmonary hypertension is associated with increased morbidity and mortality compared to infants without pulmonary hypertension. Although definitive diagnosis of pulmonary hypertension requires cardiac catheterization, in practice transthoracic echocardiography provides a low-risk screening tool. Screening should also attempt to identify potential structural causes of pulmonary hypertension such as pulmonary vein stenosis. Serum biomarkers, such as brain natriuretic protein, may be useful in tracking response to therapy. Abrupt worsening of pulmonary hypertension (*pulmonary hypertensive crises*) can occur in the context of illnesses and with anesthesia. Crises can occur even in stable children with a history of pulmonary hypertension who become acutely ill. Although pulmonary hypertension that is associated with BPD can improve with adequate lung growth, therapies such as sildenafil and other anti-pulmonary hypertensive agents have been used in management.

Prevention of respiratory viral illness is vitally important; frequent handwashing by caregivers (especially before they handle the baby) and avoidance of contact with children and adults with current respiratory symptoms are essential. Respiratory syncytial virus (see Chapter 260) immunoprophylaxis should be considered on the basis of the severity of lung disease, as well as the patient's gestational age and current age. Another environmental factor that can worsen respiratory symptoms is exposure to secondhand tobacco smoke (see Chapter 737.1).

PROGNOSIS
The prognosis for infants with BPD is generally good, although the presence of BPD may result in a longer initial hospitalization compared to preterm infants without BPD. Most infants are weaned off of oxygen during the 1st yr of life, and those requiring home mechanical ventilation are often weaned from this support during toddlerhood. Many children exhibit an asthma-like phenotype during early childhood, characterized by episodes of wheezing or coughing triggered by upper respiratory tract infections, exertion, allergens, etc. For some of these children symptoms improve by school age; others may continue to have asthma-like exacerbations with viral illnesses and exercise throughout childhood, which may persist into adulthood. Even asymptomatic patients with a history of BPD can continue to demonstrate small airway flow limitations by spirometry.

Bibliography is available at Expert Consult.

Chapter 445
Skeletal Diseases Influencing Pulmonary Function

Steven R. Boas

第四百四十五章
影响肺功能的骨骼疾病

中文导读

本章介绍了各类影响肺功能的骨骼疾病，主要介绍了胸廓凹陷（漏斗胸）的病因、流行病学、临床表现、实验室检查和治疗；鸡胸和胸骨裂的病因、流行病学、临床表现及治疗；窒息性胸廓发育不良（胸廓–骨盆–指趾骨发育不良）的病因、临床表现、诊断、治疗和预后；软骨发育不全的病因、临床表现、诊断、治疗和预后；脊柱后侧凸（青少年特发性脊柱侧凸和先天性脊柱侧凸）的病因、临床表现、诊断和治疗；以及先天性肋骨发育异常的临床表现、诊断和治疗。

Pulmonary function is influenced by the structure of the chest wall (see Chapter 400). Chest wall abnormalities can lead to restrictive or obstructive pulmonary disease, impaired respiratory muscle strength, and decreased ventilatory performance in response to physical stress.

The congenital chest wall deformities include *pectus excavatum, pectus carinatum, sternal clefts, Poland syndrome,* and skeletal and *cartilage dysplasias.* Vertebral anomalies such as kyphoscoliosis can alter pulmonary function in children and adolescents.

445.1 Pectus Excavatum (Funnel Chest)

Steven R. Boas

ETIOLOGY

Pectus excavatum—midline narrowing of the thoracic cavity—is usually an isolated skeletal abnormality. The cause is unknown. Pectus excavatum can occur in isolation or it may be associated with a connective tissue disorder (Marfan [see Chapter 722] or Ehlers-Danlos syndrome [see Chapter 678]). It may be acquired secondarily to chronic lung disease, neuromuscular disease, or trauma.

EPIDEMIOLOGY

Pectus excavatum occurs in 1 in 400 births with a 9:1 male preponderance and accounts for >90% of congenital chest wall anomalies. There is a positive family history in one-third of cases.

CLINICAL MANIFESTATIONS

The deformity is present at or shortly after birth in one-third of cases but is usually not associated with any symptoms at that time. In time, fatigue, chest pain, palpitations, recurrent respiratory infections, wheezing, stridor, and cough may be present. Decreased exercise tolerance is one of the most common symptoms. Because of the cosmetic nature of this deformity, children may experience significant psychologic stress. Physical examination may reveal sternal depression, protracted shoulders, kyphoscoliosis, dorsal lordosis, inferior rib flares, rib cage rigidity, forward head tilt, scapular winging, and loss of vertebral contours (Fig. 445.1). Patients exhibit paroxysmal sternal motion and a shift of point of maximal impulse to the left. Innocent systolic murmurs may be heard.

LABORATORY FINDINGS

Lateral chest radiograms demonstrate the sternal depression. The Haller index on chest CT (maximal internal transverse diameter of the chest divided by the minimal anteroposterior diameter at the same level) in comparison with age- and gender-appropriate normative values have been used historically to help determine the extent of the anatomic abnormality. However, the correlation of the Haller index with the physiologic compromise or associated systems appears suboptimal. Use of 3D chest optical imaging or "surface scan" is gaining popularity in the evaluation. An electrocardiogram may show a right-axis deviation or Wolff-Parkinson-White syndrome (see Chapter 463); an echocardiogram may demonstrate mitral valve prolapse (see Chapter 455.3) and ventricular compression. Results of static pulmonary function tests may be normal but commonly show an obstructive defect in the lower airways and, less commonly, a restrictive defect as the result of abnormal chest wall mechanics. Exercise testing may demonstrate either normal tolerance or limitations from underlying cardiopulmonary dysfunction that are associated with the severity of the defect. Pulmonary limitations such as ventilatory limitations and associated flow volume loop abnormalities are commonly seen in younger children and adolescents, whereas

additional cardiac limitations secondary to stroke volume impairments are more commonly seen in older adolescents and young adults.

TREATMENT

Treatment is based on the severity of the deformity and the extent of physiologic compromise as defined by physical examination and physiologic assessment of cardiopulmonary function (lung function and exercise tolerance assessment). Therapeutic options include careful observation, use of physical therapy to address musculoskeletal compromise, corrective surgery, cosmetic surgery, and noninvasive thorascopic techniques. For patients with significant physiologic compromise, surgical correction may improve the cosmetic deformity and may help minimize progression or even improve the cardiopulmonary compromise. The 2 main surgical interventions are the Ravitch and Nuss procedures. Superiority of one approach has not been established. The extent of the anatomic defect including the degree of asymmetry may help determine the appropriate surgical approach. While surgical repair may result in improved exercise tolerance for some individuals, usually observed at submaximal exercise intensities, many patients do not show improvement in either respiratory or cardiac function. Normalization of lung perfusion scans and maximal voluntary ventilation have also been observed after surgery. Utilization of a magnetic brace with gradual remodeling (Magnetic Mini Mover procedure) of the pectus deformity is under clinical investigation. The use of surgically placed silicone implants for cosmetic appearance has also been utilized with high patient satisfaction. For selected patients, the use of a more noninvasive approach (i.e., cup suction) has been gaining popularity. Regardless of the treatment approach, addressing the secondary musculoskeletal findings is commonly employed before and after any intervention.

Bibliography is available at Expert Consult.

445.2 Pectus Carinatum and Sternal Clefts

Steven R. Boas

PECTUS CARINATUM

Etiology and Epidemiology

Pectus carinatum is a sternal deformity accounting for 5–15% of congenital chest wall anomalies. Anterior displacements of the mid and lower sternum and adjacent costal cartilages are the most common types. They are most commonly associated with protrusion of the upper sternum; depression of the lower sternum occurs in only 15% of patients. Asymmetry of the sternum is common, and localized depression of the lower anterolateral chest is also often observed. Males are affected 4 times more often than females. There is a high familial occurrence and a common association of mild to moderate scoliosis. Mitral valve disease and coarctation of the aorta are associated with this anomaly. Three types of anatomic deformity occur (upper, lower, and lateral pectus carinatum), with corresponding physiologic changes and treatment algorithms.

Clinical Manifestations

In early childhood, symptoms appear minimal. School-age children and adolescents commonly complain of dyspnea with mild exertion, decreased endurance with exercise, and exercise-induced wheezing. The incidence of increased respiratory infections and use of asthma medication is higher than in nonaffected individuals. On physical examination, a marked increase in the anteroposterior chest diameter is seen, with resultant reduction in chest excursion and expansion (Fig. 445.2). Spirometry has demonstrated both restrictive and obstructive patterns, although the majority of individuals have normal values. Increases in residual volume are often present and result in tachypnea and diaphragmatic respirations. Exercise testing shows variable results. Chest radiographs show an increased anteroposterior diameter of the chest wall, emphysematous-appearing lungs, and a narrow cardiac shadow. The pectus severity score (width of chest divided by distance between sternum and spine; analogous to the Haller index)

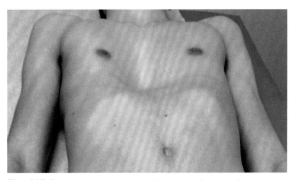

Fig. 445.1 Pectus excavatum in a 15 yr old male. Note the presence of protracted shoulders, inferior rib flares, and sternal depression.

is reduced.

TREATMENT
For symptomatic patients with pectus carinatum, minimally invasive surgical correction procedures may result in improvement of the clinical symptoms. Many surgeons prefer to use bracing techniques as a first-line treatment. Although surgery is performed for some individuals who are symptomatic, it is often performed for cosmetic and psychological reasons.

STERNAL CLEFTS
Sternal clefts are rare congenital malformations that result from the failure of the fusion of the sternum during the 8th wk of gestation. No familial predisposition has been described. Sternal clefts occur in less than 1% of all chest wall deformities. Sternal clefts are classified as partial or complete. Partial sternal clefts are more common and may involve the superior sternum in association with other lesions, such as vascular dysplasias and supraumbilical raphe, or the inferior sternal clefts, which are often associated with other midline defects (pentalogy of Cantrell). Complete sternal clefts with complete failure of sternal fusion are rare. These disorders may also occur in isolation. The paradoxic movement of thoracic organs with respiration may alter pulmonary mechanics. Rarely, respiratory infections and even significant compromise result. Surgery is required early in life, before fixation and immobility occur.

Bibliography is available at Expert Consult.

445.3 Asphyxiating Thoracic Dystrophy (Thoracic-Pelvic-Phalangeal Dystrophy)
Steven R. Boas

ETIOLOGY
A multisystem autosomal recessive disorder, asphyxiating thoracic dystrophy results in a constricted and narrow rib cage. Also known as *Jeune syndrome*, the disorder is associated with characteristic skeletal abnormalities as well as variable involvement of other systems, including

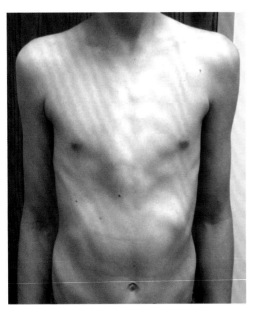

Fig. 445.2 Pectus carinatum in a 13 yr old male. Note the central sternal prominence.

renal, hepatic, neurologic, pancreatic, and retinal abnormalities (see Chapter 720).

CLINICAL MANIFESTATIONS
Most patients with this disorder die shortly after birth from respiratory failure, although less-aggressive forms have been reported in older children. For those who survive the neonatal period, progressive respiratory failure often ensues, owing to impaired lung growth, recurrent pneumonia, and atelectasis originating from the rigid chest wall.

DIAGNOSIS
Physical examination reveals a narrowed thorax that, at birth, is much smaller than the head circumference. The ribs are horizontal, and the child has short extremities. Chest radiographs demonstrate a bell-shaped chest cage with short, horizontal, flaring ribs and high clavicles.

TREATMENT
No specific treatment exists, although thoracoplasty to enlarge the chest wall and long-term mechanical ventilation has been tried. Rib-expanding (vertical expandable prosthetic titanium rib/[VEPTR]) procedures have resulted in improved survival (Fig. 445.3).

PROGNOSIS
For some children with asphyxiating thoracic dystrophy, improvement in the bony abnormalities occurs with age. However, children younger than age 1 yr often succumb to respiratory infection and failure. Progressive renal disease often occurs with older children. Use of vaccines for influenza and other respiratory pathogens is warranted, as is aggressive use of antibiotics for respiratory infections.

Bibliography is available at Expert Consult.

445.4 Achondroplasia
Steven R. Boas

ETIOLOGY
Achondroplasia is the most common condition characterized by disproportionate short stature (see Chapter 716). This condition is inherited as an autosomal dominant disorder that results in disordered growth. Much has been learned about this disorder, including its genetic origins (95% of cases caused by mutations in the gene coding for fibroblast growth factor receptor type 3) and how to minimize its serious complications.

CLINICAL MANIFESTATIONS
Restrictive pulmonary disease, affecting <5% of children with achondroplasia who are younger than 3 yr, is more likely at high elevation. Recurrent infections, cor pulmonale, and dyspnea are commonly associated. There is an increased risk of obstructive sleep apnea or hypopneas. Hypoxemia during sleep is a common feature. Onset of restrictive lung disease can begin at a very young age. On examination, the breathing pattern is rapid and shallow, with associated abdominal breathing. The anteroposterior diameter of the thorax is reduced. Special growth curves for chest circumference of patients with achondroplasia from birth to 7 yr are available. Three distinct phenotypes exist: phenotypic group 1 patients possess relative adenotonsillar hypertrophy, group 2 patients have muscular upper airway obstruction and progressive hydrocephalus, and group 3 patients have upper airway obstruction without hydrocephalus. Kyphoscoliosis may develop during infancy.

DIAGNOSIS
Pulmonary function tests reveal a reduced vital capacity that is more pronounced in males. The lungs are small but functionally normal. Sleep studies are recommended due to the high prevalence of sleep-disordered breathing. Chest radiographs demonstrate the decreased anteroposterior diameter along with anterior cupping of the ribs. The

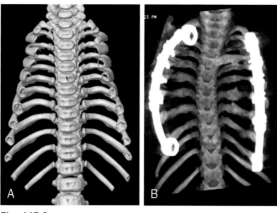

Fig. 445.3 A, Seven month old with Jeune syndrome preoperatively. **B,** 18 mo post-VEPTR insertion. *(From Mayer OH: Chest wall hypoplasia—principles and treatment. Pediatr Respir Rev 16:30–34, 2015, Fig. 3, p. 34.)*

degree of foramen magnum involvement correlates with the extent of respiratory dysfunction.

TREATMENT
Treatment of sleep apnea, if present, is supportive (see Chapter 31). Physiotherapy and bracing may minimize the complications of both kyphosis and severe lordosis. Aggressive treatment of respiratory infections and scoliosis is warranted.

PROGNOSIS
The life span is normal for most children with this condition, except for the phenotypic groups with hydrocephalus or with severe cervical or lumbar spinal compression.

Bibliography is available at Expert Consult.

445.5 Kyphoscoliosis: Adolescent Idiopathic Scoliosis and Congenital Scoliosis
Steven R. Boas

ETIOLOGY
Adolescent idiopathic scoliosis (AIS) is characterized by lateral bending of the spine (see Chapter 699). It commonly affects children during their teen years, as well as during periods of rapid growth. The cause is unknown. Congenital scoliosis is uncommon, affecting females more than males, and is apparent in the 1st yr of life (see Chapter 699.2).

CLINICAL MANIFESTATIONS
The pulmonary manifestations of scoliosis may include chest wall restriction, leading to a reduction in total lung capacity, abnormal gas exchange, airway obstruction, and hypoinflation with associated atelectasis. The angle of scoliosis deformity has been correlated with the degree of lung impairment only for patients with thoracic curves. Vital capacity, forced expiratory volume in 1 sec (FEV_1), work capacity, oxygen consumption, diffusion capacity, chest wall compliance, and partial pressure of arterial oxygen decrease as the severity of thoracic curve increases. These findings can be seen in even mild to moderate AIS (Cobb angle <30 degrees) but generally do not occur in other, nonthoracic curves. Respiratory compromise is often more severe in children younger than 5 yr of age with large scoliotic curves. Reduction in peripheral muscle function is associated with AIS through either intrinsic mechanisms or deconditioning. Severe impairment can lead to cor pulmonale or respiratory failure and can occur before age 20 yr. Children with severe scoliosis (Cobb's angle >70 degrees), especially males, may have abnormalities of breathing during sleep, and the resultant periods of

hypoxemia may contribute to the eventual development of pulmonary hypertension.

DIAGNOSIS
Physical examination and an upright, posteroanterior radiograph with subsequent measurement of the angle of curvature (Cobb technique) remain the gold standard for assessment of scoliosis. Curves >10 degrees define the presence of scoliosis. Lung volume, respiratory muscle strength, and exercise capacity determination are essential in assessing the degree of respiratory compromise associated with scoliosis.

TREATMENT
Depending on the extent of the curve and the degree of skeletal maturation, treatment options include reassurance, observation, bracing, and surgery (spinal fusion). Influenza vaccine should be administered, given the extent of pulmonary compromise that may coexist. Because vital capacity is a strong predictor for the development of respiratory failure in untreated AIS, surgical goals are to diminish the scoliotic curve, maintain the correction, and prevent deterioration in pulmonary function. Abnormalities of vital capacity and total lung capacity, exercise intolerance, and the rate of change of these variables over time should be taken into consideration for the timing of surgical correction. Preoperative assessment of lung function (i.e., lung volumes, oxygen consumption, muscle strength, ventilation/perfusion) may assist in predicting postsurgical pulmonary difficulties. Many patients undergoing surgical correction may be managed postoperatively without mechanical ventilation. Even patients with mild scoliosis may have pulmonary compromise immediately after spinal fusion, secondary to pain and a body cast that may restrict breathing and interfere with coughing. Children with a preoperative $FEV_1 < 40\%$ predicted are at risk for requiring prolonged postoperative mechanical ventilation. Rib-expanding procedures have been successful in severe cases of congenital scoliosis. Choice of surgical approach may also impact lung function postoperatively.

Bibliography is available at Expert Consult.

445.6 Congenital Rib Anomalies
Steven R. Boas

CLINICAL MANIFESTATIONS
Isolated defects of the highest and lowest ribs have minimal clinical pulmonary consequences. Missing midthoracic ribs are associated with the absence of the pectoralis muscle (Poland syndrome), and lung function can become compromised. Associated kyphoscoliosis and hemivertebrae may accompany this defect. If the rib defect is small, no significant sequelae ensue. When the 2nd to 5th ribs are absent anteriorly, lung herniation and significant abnormal respiration ensue. The lung is soft and nontender and may be easily reducible on examination. Complicating sequelae include severe lung restriction (secondary to scoliosis), cor pulmonale, and congestive heart failure. Symptoms are often minimal but can cause dyspnea. Respiratory distress is rare in infancy.

DIAGNOSIS
Chest radiographs demonstrate the deformation and absence of ribs with secondary scoliosis. Most rib abnormalities are discovered as incidental findings on a chest film.

TREATMENT
If symptoms are severe enough to cause clinical compromise or significant lung herniation, then homologous rib grafting can be performed. Rib-expanding procedures are also of great value. A modified Nuss procedure has been used to correct associated chest wall anomalies with rib abnormalities. Adolescent girls with congenital rib anomalies may require cosmetic breast surgery.

Bibliography is available at Expert Consult.

Chapter **446**
Chronic Respiratory Insufficiency

第四百四十六章
慢性呼吸功能不全

中文导读

　　本章主要介绍了慢性呼吸衰竭的流行病学、呼吸支持模式及其他管理措施（包括气道廓清、吸入治疗、黏液溶解剂及抗胆碱药治疗、监测、氧气治疗、营养支持、物理治疗、职业训练以及语言训练）、撤机准备、感染管理、社会心理问题以及如何向成人过渡等问题。还介绍了先天性中枢性低通气综合征的遗传学、临床表现、鉴别诊断和管理。其他影响呼吸的疾病包括脊髓脊膜膨出伴Arnold-Chiari Ⅱ型畸形、快速肥胖、下丘脑功能障碍和自主神经失调、肥胖低通气综合征、获得性肺泡通气不足、阻塞性睡眠呼吸暂停、脊髓损伤和代谢性疾病，介绍了这些疾病的流行病学、病理生理、临床表现及治疗等。本章进一步介绍了长期机械通气的目标和如何制定通气决策、无创通气和经气管有创呼吸支持的优缺点、长期机械通气对呼吸和消化系统的影响、气体交换目标及呼吸机策略、心肺相互作用、长期机械通气对胸壁结构、营养状况和增加体重的影响、对生长发育的影响、如何转诊至康复机构或社区、常规保持健康状况、逐渐降低呼吸机条件并撤出气管内插管等。

446.1 Chronic Respiratory Failure and Long-Term Mechanical Ventilation

Denise M. Goodman and Steven O. Lestrud

EPIDEMIOLOGY

There are continual improvements in invasive (ventilation through a tracheostomy) and noninvasive (mask ventilation) devices and management to care for those conditions predisposing to the need for chronic ventilation, such as acute respiratory failure, prematurity, and neuromuscular disease. Although difficult to determine the prevalence of chronic ventilation, estimates range from approximately 4 to 6/100,000 children. With a US Census estimate of 73,604,909 children under 18 in 2015 [https://www.census.gov/quickfacts/table/PST045216/00. Accessed January 17, 2017] this would mean that 3,000-4,000 children are currently receiving home ventilation. This number may be much higher, as studies rarely focus on children alone (a Canadian study found a prevalence of 12.9/100,000 general population) and studies may report invasive, noninvasive, or total ventilation. There may be approximately 3 times more children receiving mask ventilation than invasive mechanical ventilation. One study using the Kids' Inpatient Database reported that there were 7,812 discharges in 2006 of children on either invasive or noninvasive long-term ventilation. The conditions leading to the need for home ventilation are diverse. Most literature focuses on single-center experience, but broad themes emerge. About two-thirds of children have a primary neurologic indication, including neuromuscular weakness or abnormal ventilatory control, and about one-third have chronic lung disease (Table 446.1).

Patients with primarily pulmonary indications have a greater likelihood of ultimately being weaned from the need for ventilation than do those with neuromuscular or central nervous system disease. Mortality for patients requiring chronic ventilation is reported to be approximately 12–34% depending on underlying disease. The lower mortality range is for children with neonatal lung disease, with the higher value for children with congenital heart disease. An overall mortality rate of 20% is common. Approximately 12–40% of children are eventually weaned from ventilation and decannulated, again reflecting the underlying cause for which ventilation is required. This can usually be accomplished within the first 5 yr of life. Nonetheless, the care of these children can be challenging. One study reported that up to 40% of chronically ventilated children are readmitted within the 1st yr of discharge, usually within the first 3 mo. Children requiring long-term mechanical ventilation

Table 446.1	Indications for Long-Term Mechanical Ventilation

PULMONARY/ALVEOLAR
BRONCHOPULMONARY DYSPLASIA (BPD)
PARDS (Severe acquired lung disease, such as after pediatric acute
respiratory distress syndrome)
Pulmonary fibrosis syndromes

AIRWAY
Severe tracheomalacia
Severe bronchomalacia
Obstructive sleep apnea
Storage diseases

CHEST (SEE CHAPTER 445)
Kyphoscoliosis
Skeletal dysplasias
Obesity

NEUROMUSCULAR
Spinal muscular atrophy
Spinal cord injury
Diaphragmatic dysfunction
Mitochondrial diseases

CNS
Congenital central hypoventilation syndrome (CCHS)
Rapid-onset obesity with hypothalamic dysregulation,
hypoventilation, and autonomic dysfunction (ROHHAD)
Severe ischemic brain injury
Myelomeningocele with Arnold-Chiari type II malformation
Acquired hypoventilation syndromes

(LMV) benefit from comprehensive care coordination incorporating generalists, specialists, home nursing, therapies, and a durable medical equipment (DME) resource.

MODALITIES FOR RESPIRATORY SUPPORT
The goals of home mechanical ventilation are to maintain appropriate oxygenation and ventilation, minimizing metabolic demands of chronic respiratory failure to ensure adequate somatic growth and optimal developmental gains (see Chapter 446.4).

Invasive Positive Pressure Ventilation
The term *invasive* designates ventilation through a tracheostomy. Some devices are suitable for both noninvasive positive pressure ventilation (NPPV) and invasive ventilation, while other devices are suitable for only one approach. The ideal home ventilator is lightweight, portable, and quiet. All home ventilators differ from hospital-based ventilators in that air movement is affected either by a piston or turbine that is electrically controlled. This contrasts with hospital ventilators which are often gas-driven. A home ventilator should be able to provide continuous flow and have a wide range of settings (particularly for pressure, volume, pressure support, and rate) that allows ventilatory support from infancy to adulthood. Battery power for the ventilator, both internal and external, should be sufficient to permit unrestricted portability in the home and community. The equipment must also be impervious to electromagnetic interference and must be relatively easy to understand and troubleshoot. A variety of ventilators that are approved for home use are available, and familiarity with these devices is necessary to choose the best option for the individual child.

While families and care teams may at first resist placement, a tracheostomy has several advantages. It provides a secure and stable airway, a standardized interface for attaching the ventilator circuit to the patient, and the ability to easily remove airway secretions and deliver inhaled medications. Pediatric tracheostomy tubes typically have a single lumen and may have an inflatable cuff. Tracheostomy tubes with/without cuff inflation should be sized to control the air leak around the tube and promote adequate gas exchange, yet allow enough space around the tube to facilitate vocalization and prevent tracheal irritation and erosion

from the tube. The child's caregivers need to learn stoma care, elective and emergent tracheostomy changes, proper securing of the tube, suctioning of secretions, and recognition of emergencies such as tube obstruction or decannulation.

Optimal Ventilator Support
Factors such as underlying neuromuscular disease; medications such as sedatives, analgesics, steroids, and muscle relaxants; and prolonged immobility, as well as utilization of mechanical ventilation, may decondition the respiratory muscles, and more so the diaphragm, resulting in muscle weakness. Consequently, it is important to avoid 24 hr/day patient synchrony with ventilation and titrate the amount of ventilator support to prevent fatigue, yet facilitate spontaneous breathing. While assessing ventilator needs frequent evaluation of gas exchange is needed, but can usually be done noninvasively. Ventilator settings should be stable for a period of time, dictated by severity of pulmonary disease, before discharge home.

OTHER MANAGEMENT CONSIDERATIONS
Airway Clearance
One of the most important considerations is maintenance of airway patency. Adequate removal of secretions may minimize intercurrent pulmonary infections. In turn, infections may cause a transient increase in secretions requiring an escalation of clearance strategies. If the child has an adequate cough, periodic suctioning may be all that is needed. Some children, however, need additional help mobilizing and clearing secretions. This becomes particularly important in children with neuromuscular disease, for whom regularly scheduled clearance therapies are an imperative. There are 2 main types of devices that are used. **Vest therapy** (high frequency chest wall oscillation) uses an inflatable vest that encircles the chest. Air inflates and deflates the vest with phasic pulses against the chest wall, loosening secretions. This device still requires a preserved and strong enough cough to expel secretions. The **cough assist** device provides more active airway clearance, delivering a forceful positive pressure adjunct during inspiration and active negative pressure during expiration. Thus, the cough is more effective due to the rapid pressure changes. The cough assist can be used with an artificial airway or mask. Controls will set the inspiratory and expiratory pressures and periods.

Inhalation Medications
Clearance of secretions may be promoted with delivery of hypertonic (3% saline) nebulizations. These are often timed to cough assist sessions to maximize the clearance benefits of both. Children requiring ventilation also commonly need bronchodilators.

Mucolytics and Anticholinergics
Some patients may need additional interventions due to excess secretions. Anticholinergic drugs, principally glycopyrrolate, are often effective, but must be dosed carefully to avoid thickening secretions excessively, which can lead to inspissated secretions and life-threatening plugging of the airway. Oral secretions are sometimes amenable to localized injection of botulinum toxin, or select surgical ligation of salivary ducts. It is also wise to ensure that the patient is adequately hydrated as dehydration may produce thick tenacious secretions. At times a mucolytic may be used. Hypertonic saline is the most common mucolytic, but a number of other agents have been tried, such as dornase alfa and N-acetylcysteine.

Monitoring
A patient who is ventilated in the home must be electronically and/or physically monitored at all times. Infants and young children, children who are cognitively impaired, and children who are completely tracheostomy dependent for airway patency because of suprastomal obstruction must be under direct observation of the caregivers at all times. Caregivers should also closely monitor children whose pulmonary status is fragile or fluctuant. Continuous monitoring of O_2 saturation and heart rate is recommended during sleep, and either continuous or intermittent monitoring during the daytime, depending on patient stability. Patients with congenital central hypoventilation syndrome (CCHS) or pulmonary hypertension are particularly vulnerable to episodes of hypoxemia and/

or hypercarbia, and those with pulmonary hypertension are particularly susceptible to rapid drops in O_2 saturation.

Supplemental Oxygen

Supplemental oxygen may be delivered from a tank or concentrator. Whether on room air or oxygen at baseline, even mild intercurrent infections may lead to an increase in oxygen requirement. In these situations, the child should be evaluated in person rather than over the phone to ensure that a more serious illness is not developing.

Nutrition

Ventilated patients may have nutritional needs that are equal to, greater, or lesser than those of comparably aged well children. Growth should be tracked at each well-child and subspecialty visit. Excessive growth is as harmful as inadequate growth, and excess calories may lead to increased carbon dioxide (CO_2) production. Anthropometry or measured energy expenditure may be needed to assure a more precise prescription of nutritional support. Many children with tracheostomies have oral aversion and/or dyscoordination of swallowing, with resultant risk for aspiration. In these children a gastrostomy tube may ensure adequate nutrition in the interim while ongoing speech therapy promotes oral feeding.

Physical, Occupational, Speech Therapy

The technology needed to support physical well-being should not overshadow the inherent developmental needs common to all children—to play, grow, develop, and interact. Ongoing physical therapy, occupational therapy, and speech therapy can help a child reach full potential, and many achieve complete catch-up development. Early intervention programs and access to play groups are important factors to attaining cognitive and social milestones. When normal development is not attainable, therapies can improve mobilization and muscle strength. Core trunk and abdominal strength is particularly important for pulmonary rehabilitation and essential for successful weaning off ventilation. Other important skills include oromotor skills for feeding and communication. Evaluation of swallow is a key component of therapy for children with chronic respiratory failure. Sign language is frequently used for communication because of delayed speech or hearing loss. Audiology specialists should be involved in the assessment of hearing because there is a higher incidence of hearing loss in patients undergoing long-term ventilation.

PREPARING FOR DISCHARGE

A number of components need to come together for a safe and effective discharge, including medical stability, family education, financial support (insurance or a state waiver program), availability of a DME company, and, when appropriate, home private-duty nursing. A poor outcome may occur with any of the many medical or process factors, or family factors including not only education but also home readiness and psychosocial supports. A standardized discharge process can ensure that all details are addressed, minimizing length of stay and improving safety. An awake and attentive trained caregiver should be in the home of a child with invasive ventilation at all times; this expectation may differ for those receiving NPPV depending on clinical circumstance. For those receiving invasive ventilation, the caregiver may be a nurse, but nursing resources are often scarce, so many programs require 2 trained family caregivers. The training given to the family includes tracheostomy stoma care, suctioning, equipment expertise, administration of medications, and facility with other devices, such as gastrostomy tubes. In addition, the family is instructed in emergency preparedness, including what to do for acute changes in clinical status, desaturation, or airway obstruction or decannulation. Cardiopulmonary resuscitation training is essential. Parents also need to be able to travel portably with the child and equipment. A standardized emergency bag containing critical tracheostomy and ventilator supplies should accompany the child at all times. Other preparations center around home readiness, including accessibility (number of stairs if any, members of the household, assuring no smoking in the home) and notification of utility companies such as the electric or heating company to ensure the home is serviced quickly in the event of power interruption. The family must also have

a functioning telephone to ensure adequate accessibility and communication between the family and care team. For those going home with invasive mechanical ventilation, both a primary and back-up ventilator may be needed, as well as batteries, a self-inflating bag and mask, suctioning equipment, supplemental oxygen, and appropriate monitoring including a pulse oximeter. Family training often culminates in an autonomous 24 hr stay *in the hospital* during which time 1 caregiver must continuously remain awake, and all cares including ventilator checks, suctioning, tracheostomy tube changes, medications, and the like are provided by the family.

CARE BY THE GENERAL PEDIATRICIAN
See Chapters 446.4 and 734.1.

Infections

Tracheitis (see Chapter 412.2), bronchitis (see Chapter 418.2), and pneumonia (see Chapters 426 and 428) are common in patients with chronic respiratory failure. Infections may be caused by community-acquired viruses (adenovirus, influenza, respiratory syncytial virus, parainfluenza, rhinovirus) or community- or hospital-acquired bacteria. Common pathogens are Gram-negative, highly antimicrobial-resistant pathogens that may cause further deterioration in pulmonary function. Bacterial infection is most likely in the presence of fever, deteriorating lung function (hypoxia, hypercarbia, tachypnea, and retractions), leukocytosis, and mucopurulent sputum. The presence of leukocytes and organisms on Gram stain of tracheal aspirate, as well as the visualization of new infiltrates on radiographs, may be consistent with bacterial infection.

Infection must be distinguished from tracheal *colonization* of bacteria, which is asymptomatic and associated with normal amounts of clear tracheal secretions. Colonization may also be distinguished from infection in that colonization usually has few, if any, white blood cells on Gram stain of tracheal secretions. If infection is suspected, it must be treated with antibiotics, based on the culture and sensitivities of organisms recovered from the tracheal aspirate. At times inhaled antibiotic such as tobramycin might avert progression of infection. Antibiotics should be used judiciously to prevent further colonization with drug-resistant organisms. However, some patients who have recurrent infections may benefit from prophylaxis with inhaled antibiotics. Clinical decisions will be based on the child's appearance, any increased need for ventilation or supplemental oxygen, and consultation with the subspecialist. A final caveat is that, if a respiratory viral panel is desired, this must be obtained from nasal secretions similar to a well child; tracheal aspirate does not provide an appropriate specimen.

CARE BY THE SUBSPECIALTY TEAM
See Chapter 734.1.

WEANING OFF THE VENTILATOR

A substantial number of children are eventually weaned from mechanical ventilation. Typically the ventilator settings are reduced minimizing ventilator parameters to achieve physiologic respiratory rates and 6-8 mL/kg tidal volumes. Subsequent maneuvers will evaluate the patient free breathing, initially with simple observed transition times of 5-10 min, extending time off as clinically indicated. This can be done in the outpatient setting during visits with the pulmonologist or other subspecialist responsible for ventilator management. Additional factors that reflect tolerance of increased work of breathing, including weight gain, energy levels, general behavior, and sleep patterns, are also monitored carefully. When the child has completely weaned off ventilator support while awake and is only on the ventilator approximately 6 hr nightly during sleep, a polysomnogram study performed off the ventilator may be considered prior to complete liberation from the mechanical ventilation device. Successful liberation from mechanical ventilation, if it occurs, often takes place between the ages of 2 and 5 yr. One thought is that with ambulation and development of core strength, respiratory reserve improves, facilitating weaning. Even so, residual lung disease is common. Children with a history of bronchopulmonary dysplasia (BPD) and previous ventilator dependence often have significant airway obstruction on pulmonary function testing.

PSYCHOSOCIAL CONSIDERATIONS

Caring for a child on long-term ventilatory support in the home is a complex, physically demanding, emotionally taxing, and expensive process for the family. It changes the family routines, priorities, and overall lifestyle, and may adversely affect relationships both within the family and with extended family and friends. Practical considerations include loss of spontaneity in family outings, sleep disturbance, extra expenses, having strangers in the house providing care, and adhering to medical regimens and follow-up visits. Intangible stresses are also prominent, including disruption in the usual parent-child caregiving roles, and stresses between parent partners and with other children. The loss of normality, sense of isolation, and concerns regarding what is best for the child are additional sources of distress. For children with a life-limiting condition, there is the additional need to periodically revisit the child's current medical state, sense of well-being, and trajectory of illness, as critical decisions will eventually arise regarding end-of-life care. The general pediatrician can often be a familiar and comfortable safe place to explore these issues, as parents may be conflicted in wanting to be a good parent while feeling guilty about their own needs and vulnerabilities.

ADULT TRANSITION

There are a growing number of children surviving into adulthood who require chronic ventilation. There is little empiric data regarding this transition, including identifying patients for whom transition is appropriate, implementing a standardized transition process, partnering with adult pulmonologists, or replicating in an adult environment the care coordination provided by the pediatric care team. The pulmonary team ideally initiates ongoing discussions regarding self-care responsibilities and transitioning of medical care to adult providers with the adolescent and his/her parents when the patient reaches the early teens. Discussion about self-care should take into consideration realistic expectations about the adolescent's physical and cognitive capabilities. The actual transition of care occurs for most young adults at age 18-21 yr, and includes referral to an internist as well as an adult pulmonologist. Transition of medical care also includes transition from pediatric to adult support services for funding sources and nursing care. Ideally, an outpatient visit that includes current and future adult medical providers together is completed to facilitate communication and formally transition care.

Bibliography is available at Expert Consult.

446.2 Congenital Central Hypoventilation Syndrome

Debra E. Weese-Mayer, Casey M. Rand, Amy Zhou, and Michael S. Carroll

CCHS is a clinically complex *neurocristopathy* that includes a variable severity of respiratory and autonomic dysregulation, as well as Hirschsprung disease and neural crest tumors in a subset of patients. In the classic CCHS presentation, symptoms of alveolar hypoventilation manifest in the newborn period and during sleep only—with diminished tidal volume and a typically monotonous respiratory rate leading to cyanosis and hypercarbia. In more severe cases of CCHS, the hypoventilation manifests during wakefulness and sleep. In the later-onset cases of CCHS (LO-CCHS), symptoms appear after 1 mo of age and older (often into childhood and adulthood). Hypoventilation is typically during sleep only and usually milder in later-onset cases than in patients who present in the neonatal period. CCHS and LO-CCHS are further characterized by partial to complete peripheral and central chemoreceptor failure to properly respond to hypercarbia and hypoxemia during wakefulness and sleep, coupled with physiologic and/or anatomic autonomic nervous system (ANS) dysregulation (ANSD). Physiologic dysregulation may include all organ systems affected by the ANS, specifically the respiratory, cardiac, sudomotor, vasomotor, ophthalmologic, neurologic, and enteric systems (Table 446.2). The anatomic or structural

Table 446.2	Congenital Central Hypoventilation Syndrome-Related Symptoms
THE SYMPTOMS EMERGE FROM DIFFERENT ORGAN SYSTEMS AND COULD BE OVERLOOKED BY THE CLINICIANS	
Respiratory symptoms	Nocturnal hypoventilation and possible daytime hypoventilation
	Ability to hold breath for a long period of time and absence of air hunger afterwards
Cardiovascular symptoms	Arrhythmias
	Reduced heart rate variability
	Vasovagal syncope
	Syncope
	Cold extremities
	Postural hypotension
Neurologic symptoms	Developmental delay
	Seizures (primarily during infancy)
	Motor and speech delay
	Learning disabilities
	Altered perception of pain
Gastrointestinal symptoms	Hirschsprung disease-related symptoms: dysphagia, constipation, and gastroesophageal reflux
Ophthalmologic symptoms	Nonreactive/sluggish pupils
	Altered lacrimation and near response
	Anisocoria, miosis, and ptosis
	Strabismus
Temperature instability	Altered perspiring
	Absence of fever with infections
Malignancies	Tumors of neural crest origin
Psychological	Decreased anxiety

From Lijubić K, Fister I Jr, Fister I: Congenital central hypoventilation syndrome: a comprehensive review and future challenges, *J Respir Med* 856149:1–8, 2014 (Table 1, p. 3).

ANSD includes Hirschsprung disease and tumors of neural crest origin (neuroblastoma, ganglioneuroma, or ganglioneuroblastoma).

GENETICS

The paired-like homeobox 2B *(PHOX2B)* gene is the disease-defining gene for CCHS. *PHOX2B* encodes a highly conserved homeodomain transcription factor, is essential to the embryologic development of the ANS from the neural crest, and is expressed in key regions and systems that explain much of the CCHS phenotype. Individuals with CCHS are **heterozygous** for either a *polyalanine repeat expansion mutation (PARM)* in exon 3 of the *PHOX2B* gene (normal number of alanines is 20 with normal genotype 20/20), such that individuals with CCHS have 24-33 alanines on the affected allele (genotype range is 20/24-20/33), or a *non-polyalanine repeat expansion mutation (NPARM)* resulting from a missense, nonsense, frameshift, stop codon, or splice site mutation. Approximately 90–92% of the cases of CCHS have PARMs and the remaining 8–10% of cases have NPARMs.

LO-CCHS cases have consistently had short PARMs (primarily 20/25 genotype but 20/24 genotype also presents as LO-CCHS), or occasionally very mild NPARMs. The specific type of *PHOX2B* mutation is clinically significant because it can help with anticipatory guidance in patient management. Less than 1% of CCHS cases will have a deletion of a majority of exon 3 or the entire *PHOX2B* gene, although the specific phenotype related to these large deletion mutations is not entirely clear. Step-wise clinical *PHOX2B* testing for probands with the CCHS phenotype is advised—step 1: *PHOX2B* Screening Test (fragment analysis), then if negative, step 2: sequel *PHOX2B* Sequencing Test, then if negative, step 3: *PHOX2B* Multiplex Ligation-dependent Probe Amplification (MLPA) Test to minimize expenses and expedite confirmation of the diagnosis.

The majority of CCHS cases occur because of a de novo *PHOX2B* mutation, but up to 35% of children with CCHS inherit the mutation in an autosomal dominant manner from a seemingly asymptomatic parent who is mosaic for the *PHOX2B* mutation. An individual with CCHS has a 50% chance of transmitting the mutation, and resulting disease phenotype, to each offspring. Mosaic parents have up to a 50% chance of transmitting the *PHOX2B* mutation to each successive offspring, with risk related to the percent of mosaicism. Genetic counseling is essential for family planning and for delivery room preparation in anticipation of a CCHS birth. *PHOX2B* testing is also advised for both parents of a child with CCHS to anticipate risk of recurrence in subsequent pregnancies (if mosaic) and to determine if a parent has yet undiagnosed LO-CCHS. Fragment analysis *PHOX2B* testing (also known as the Screening Test) will best identify low-level somatic mosaicism. Prenatal testing for *PHOX2B* mutation is clinically available (www.genetests.org) for families with a known *PHOX2B* mutation.

Ventilator Dependence and Control of Breathing
Patients with CCHS have deficient CO_2 sensitivity during wakefulness and sleep such that they do not respond with a normal increase in ventilation in either state nor do they arouse in response to hypercarbia and/or hypoxemia during sleep. During wakefulness, a subset of patients may respond sufficiently to avoid significant hypercarbia, but most individuals with CCHS have hypoventilation that is severe enough that hypercarbia is apparent in the resting *awake* state. Children with CCHS also have altered sensitivity to hypoxia while awake and asleep. A key feature of CCHS is the lack of respiratory distress or sense of asphyxia with physiologic compromise (hypercarbia and/or hypoxia). This lack of responsiveness to hypercarbia and/or hypoxemia, which can result in respiratory failure, does not consistently improve with advancing age. A subset of older children with CCHS may show an increase in ventilation (specifically increase in respiratory rate rather than increase in tidal volume) when they are exercised at various work rates. This response is possibly secondary to neural reflexes from rhythmic limb movements, although an increase in minute ventilation is often insufficient to avoid physiologic compromise. Report of oral contraceptives improving awake CO_2 chemosensitivity in 2 adult women suggests need for further exploration.

The greater the number of extra alanines, the more likely the need for continuous ventilatory support, at least among the most common *PHOX2B* PARM genotypes (20/25, 20/26, 20/27). Thus, patients with the 20/25 genotype seldom require awake ventilatory support, although they do require artificial ventilation during sleep. Patients with the 20/26 genotype have variable awake support needs, but all require artificial ventilation during sleep. Patients with the 20/27 genotype and those with NPARMs are likely to need continuous ventilatory support. Although *PHOX2B* genotype seems to anticipate severity of hypoventilation, it does not correlate with exogenous ventilatory challenge responses. Infants and young children as a group have improved ventilatory response slopes while awake, but this advantage seems to vanish by school age.

Hirschsprung Disease (Chapter 358)
Overall, 20% of children with CCHS also have Hirschsprung disease (HSCR), and any infant or child with CCHS or LO-CCHS who presents with constipation should undergo rectal biopsy to screen for absence of ganglion cells. The frequency of Hirschsprung disease seems to increase with the longer polyalanine repeat tracts (genotypes 20/27-20/33) and in those with NPARMs. Thus far, only 1 infant with the 20/25 genotype has ever been reported to have Hirschsprung disease. Even in cases without frank HSCR disease, individuals with CCHS may display symptoms of gastrointestinal abnormalities such as severe constipation and abnormal esophageal motility, suggesting ganglion cell dysfunction.

Tumors of Neural Crest Origin (Chapter 525)
Tumors of neural crest origin are more frequent in patients with NPARMs (50%) than in those with PARMs (1%). These extracranial tumors are more often neuroblastomas in individuals with NPARMs, but ganglioneuromas and ganglioneuroblastomas in a small subset of patients with longer PARMs (20/29, 20/30, and 20/33 genotype only). Thus far, only 1 infant with a PARM (20/33 genotype) has been reported to have a neuroblastoma.

Cardiac Asystole
Transient, abrupt, and prolonged sinus pauses have been identified in patients with CCHS, necessitating implantation of cardiac pacemakers when the pauses are ≥3 sec. Among patients with the most common *PHOX2B* genotypes, 19% of those with the 20/26 genotype and 83% of those with the 20/27 genotype have cardiac pauses of 3 sec or longer. Children with the 20/25 genotype have not been noted to have prolonged asystole, although 2 adults diagnosed with LO-CCHS have demonstrated prolonged asystoles of 4-8 sec duration. Risk for sinus pauses among children with NPARMs is unknown at present.

Heart rate variability is characteristically decreased in CCHS due to a decrease in cardiac baroreflex sensitivity and blunted sympathetic response. A recent report demonstrated a genotype-phenotype relationship for heart rate variability during exogenous ventilatory response testing, prompting assessment of risk for sinus pauses. Introduction of 72-hr Holter recordings every 12 mo at a minimum has allowed for early identification of these sinus pauses, permitting timely cardiac pacemaker implantation.

Autonomic Nervous System Dysregulation
A higher number of polyalanine repeats on the affected allele among patients with a PARM is associated with an increased number of physiologic symptoms of ANSD. In addition, there is a spectrum of physiologic ANSD symptoms, including decreased heart rate variability, esophageal/gastric/colonic dysmotility, decreased pupillary response to light, reduced basal body temperature, altered distribution and amount of diaphoresis, altered vasomotor tone, and altered pain and anxiety perception.

Neuropathology
Brain imaging studies and functional MRI (fMRI) responses have identified structural deficiencies in CCHS cases which may contribute to the observed respiratory and autonomic phenotypes. These findings may be primarily due to *PHOX2B* mutation-induced failure of neurogenesis in the human embryo, but a significant contribution from postnatal hypoxic, hypercarbic, or perfusion damage cannot be excluded. The neuroanatomic defects in CCHS are likely the result of focal *PHOX2B* (mis)expression coupled with sequelae of recurrent hypoxemia/hypercarbia in the subset of suboptimally managed patients. On the basis of rodent studies and fMRI studies in humans, the following regions pertinent to respiratory control in the pons and medulla of the brainstem show *PHOX2B* expression: locus coeruleus, dorsal respiratory group, nucleus ambiguus, parafacial respiratory group, among other areas. Physiologic evidence suggests that the respiratory failure in these children is mostly based on defects in central mechanisms, but peripheral mechanisms (mainly carotid bodies) may also be important.

CLINICAL MANIFESTATIONS
Patients with CCHS usually present with symptoms in the first few hours after birth. Most children are the products of uneventful pregnancies and are term infants with appropriate weight for gestational age. Variable Apgar scores have been reported. The affected infants do not show signs of respiratory distress, but their shallow respirations and respiratory pauses (apnea) usually evolve to respiratory failure with apparent cyanosis in the 1st days of life. In neonates with CCHS, $PaCO_2$ accumulates during sleep to very high levels, sometimes >90 mm Hg, and may decline to normal levels after the infants awaken. This problem becomes most apparent when multiple attempts at extubation fail in an intubated neonate, who appears well with ventilatory support but develops respiratory failure after removal of the support. However, more severely affected infants hypoventilate awake and asleep; thus, the previously described difference in $PaCO_2$ between states may not be apparent. Often, the respiratory rate is higher in rapid eye movement (REM) sleep than in non-REM sleep in individuals with CCHS, and in general, respiratory rates are higher in infants and children with CCHS than peers with intact control of breathing.

LO-CCHS should be suspected in infants, children, and adults who have unexplained centrally mediated hypoventilation and/or seizures or cyanosis, especially subsequent to the use of anesthetic agents and/or sedation, acute respiratory illness or recurrent severe respiratory illness with difficulty weaning from ventilator support (and failed extubations), and potentially obstructive sleep apnea (OSA) unresponsive to traditional intervention. These individuals may have other evidence of chronic hypoventilation, including pulmonary hypertension, polycythemia, elevated bicarbonate concentration, difficulty concentrating, and mild unexplained neurocognitive impairment. A heightened level of suspicion has led to increasing numbers of older children and adults diagnosed with LO-CCHS receiving proper treatment. This later presentation reflects the variable penetrance of a subset of *PHOX2B* mutations and potential role of an environmental cofactor.

In addition to treatment for the alveolar hypoventilation, children with CCHS require comprehensive physiologic evaluation during sleep and wakefulness, including activities of daily living such as eating, as their hypoxemia and hypercarbia from insufficient artificial ventilation may go unnoticed. It is necessary to provide coordinated care to optimally manage associated, multisystem abnormalities such as Hirschsprung disease, tumors of neural crest origin, and symptoms of physiologic ANSD including cardiac asystole, among other findings (details provided in American Thoracic Society 2010 Statement on CCHS).

DIFFERENTIAL DIAGNOSIS
Testing should be performed to rule out primary neuromuscular, lung, and cardiac disease as well as an identifiable brainstem lesion that could account for the full constellation of symptoms characteristic of CCHS. The availability of clinical *PHOX2B* genetic testing allows for early and definitive diagnosis of CCHS (Table 446.3). Because individual features of CCHS mimics many treatable and/or genetic diseases, the following disorders should also be considered: altered airway or intrathoracic anatomy (diagnosis made with bronchoscopy and chest CT), diaphragm dysfunction (diagnosis made with diaphragm fluoroscopy), a structural hindbrain or brainstem abnormality (diagnosis made with MRI of the brain and brainstem), Möbius syndrome (diagnosis made with MRI of the brain and brainstem and neurologic examination), and specific metabolic diseases, such as Leigh syndrome, pyruvate dehydrogenase deficiency, and discrete carnitine deficiency. However, profound hypercarbia without respiratory distress during sleep will quickly lead the clinician to consider the diagnosis of CCHS or LO-CCHS.

MANAGEMENT
Supported Ventilation—Diaphragm Pacing
Depending on the severity of the hypoventilation, the individual with

Table 446.3	Differential Diagnoses of Congenital Central Hypoventilation Syndrome

METABOLIC
Mitochondrial defects, e.g., Leigh disease
Pyruvate dehydrogenase deficiency
Hypothyroidism

NEUROLOGIC
Structural central nervous system abnormalities, e.g., Arnold Chiari malformation, Moebius syndrome
Vascular injury, e.g., central nervous system (CNS) hemorrhage, infarct
Trauma
Tumor

PULMONARY
Primary lung disease
Respiratory muscle weakness, e.g., diaphragm paralysis, congenital myopathy

GENETIC
Prader Willi syndrome
Familial dysautonomia

SEDATIVE DRUGS

OTHER
Rapid-onset obesity, hypothalamic dysregulation hypoventilation, autonomic dysregulation (ROHHAD)

Modified from Healy F, Marcus CL: Congenital central hypoventilation syndrome in children, *Pediatr Respir Rev* 12:253–263, 2011 (Table 1, p. 258).

CCHS can have various options for artificial ventilation: positive pressure ventilation (noninvasive via mask or via tracheostomy) or negative pressure ventilation (pneumosuit, chest cuirass, or diaphragm pacing). Chronic mechanical ventilation is addressed in Chapters 446.1 and 446.4. Diaphragm pacing offers another mode of supported ventilation, involving bilateral surgical implantation of electrodes beneath the phrenic nerves, with connecting wires to subcutaneously implanted receivers. The external transmitter, which is much smaller and lighter in weight than a ventilator, sends a signal to flat donut-shaped antennae that are placed on the skin over the subcutaneously implanted receivers. A signal travels from the external transmitter to the phrenic nerve to stimulate contraction of the diaphragm. A tracheostomy is typically required, because the pacers induce a negative pressure on inspiration as a result of the contraction of the diaphragm being unopposed by pharyngeal dilatation, resulting in airway obstruction with paced breaths. Individuals with CCHS who are ventilator-dependent for 24 hr a day are ideal candidates for diaphragm pacing to provide increased ambulatory freedom (without the ventilator tether) while they are awake; however, they still require mechanical ventilator support while they are asleep. This balance between awake pacing and asleep mechanical ventilation allows for a rest from phrenic nerve stimulation at night. In addition, a growing number of children and adults who require artificial ventilatory support only during sleep are now using diaphragm pacing. This is likely because of the introduction of thoracoscopic diaphragm pacer implantation and shortened postoperative recovery time. However, in the absence of a tracheostomy, diaphragm pacing during sleep may cause airway obstruction at varied levels of the airway depending on the specific patient. The potential for these obstructions needs to be carefully considered before diaphragm pacer implantation, and definitely before tracheal decannulation.

Monitoring in the Home
Home monitoring for individuals with CCHS and LO-CCHS is distinctly different from and more conservative than that for other children requiring long-term ventilation, because CCHS individuals lack innate ventilatory and arousal responses to hypoxemia and hypercarbia. In the event of physiologic compromise, other children will show clinical signs of respiratory distress. By contrast, for children and adults with CCHS and LO-CCHS, the only means of determining adequate ventilation and oxygenation is with objective measures from a pulse oximeter, end-tidal CO_2 monitor, and close supervision of these values by a highly trained registered nurse (RN) in the home and at school. While awake, patients with CCHS themselves are unable to sense or adequately respond to a respiratory challenge that may occur with ensuing respiratory illness, increased exertion, or even the simple activity of eating. At a minimum, it is essential that individuals with CCHS have continuous monitoring with pulse oximetry and end-tidal CO_2 with RN supervision during all sleep time, but ideally 24 hr/day. These recommendations apply to all CCHS and LO-CCHS patients regardless of the nature of their artificial ventilatory support, but especially those with diaphragm pacers as they have no intrinsic alarms in the diaphragm pacer device.

Noninvasive Equipment
Supplemental oxygen with positive pressure support can be administered by nasal cannulae. The nasal cannula system has the ability to deliver heated, supersaturated, high-flow gases. There are a number of mechanical devices available for the delivery of bi-level ventilation via an actual ventilator, but this is suitable only for children with milder hypoventilation during sleep only. Long-term use of mask ventilation in small children may result in mid-face dysplasia or pressure wounds.

Positive Pressure Ventilators
Ideally, a ventilator intended for home use is lightweight and small, quiet so it does not interfere with activities of daily living or sleep, is able to entrain room air, preferably has continuous flow, and has a wide range of settings (particularly for pressure support, pressure, volume, and rate) that allows ventilatory support from infancy to adulthood. Battery power for the ventilator, both internal and external, should be sufficient to permit unrestricted portability in the home and community.

The equipment must also be impervious to electromagnetic interference and must be relatively easy to understand and troubleshoot. A variety of ventilators that are approved for home use are available, and familiarity with these devices is necessary to choose the best option for the individual child. Children who are chronically ventilated via positive pressure ventilation will require surgical placement of a tracheostomy tube. The tracheostomy tube provides stable access to the airway, a standardized interface for attaching the ventilator circuit to the patient, and the ability to easily remove airway secretions or deliver inhaled medications. Pediatric tracheostomy tubes typically have a single lumen and may have an inflatable cuff. Tracheostomy tubes with/without cuff inflation should be sized to control the air leak around the tube and promote adequate gas exchange, yet allow enough space around the tube to facilitate vocalization and prevent tracheal irritation and erosion from the tube.

When a tracheostomy tube is surgically placed, a slit opening is made in the trachea between the cartilaginous rings. Stay sutures are attached to the margins of the incision to facilitate emergent tube replacement prior to healing of the stoma tract. The tracheostomy tube is often electively changed by ENT about 1 wk after initial placement, and the child is subsequently cleared for tracheostomy tube changes by the nursing staff. The child's caregivers, usually parents or family members and home nursing staff, are instructed in all aspects of tracheostomy care: stoma care, elective and emergent tracheostomy change, proper securing of the tracheostomy tube, suctioning of secretions, and recognition of tube obstruction or decannulation. The child's caregivers have to demonstrate competency with all the tasks, and with cardiopulmonary resuscitation, prior to home discharge.

Optimizing Neurocognitive Performance
Impaired oxygen delivery to the brain, whether acute or chronic, can have detrimental effects on neurocognitive development. The ATS statement recommends positive pressure ventilation via tracheostomy in the first several years of life to ensure optimal oxygenation and ventilation. The method of choice in later years will depend on a variety of factors including severity of disease, patient age, level of patient and family cooperation, and availability and quality of home health care, among other factors. The level of oxygen stability obtained with each varies. Thus, the method of respiratory assistance, especially in infancy and early childhood, is likely to play a factor in neurocognitive outcome.

Past literature has indicated deficiencies of mental abilities in school-age children with CCHS. Even in preschool years, children with CCHS demonstrate reduced neurocognitive performance. In these cases, *PHOX2B* genotype is clearly associated with both mental and motor outcomes. This association is also found with CCHS-related features such as severe cyanotic breath holding spells, sinus pauses, seizures, and severity of hypoventilation. It is unclear if this association is intrinsic to the specific mutation, the phenotypes associated with the mutation, or most likely both. Despite observed delays, 29% of preschool subjects had mid-average mental development scores, and 13% performed above that level. These findings suggest the potential for excellent neurocognitive outcome. This potential appears greatest in individuals with a 20/25 genotype (Bayley mental scores over the population mean of 100). However, a 2015 report identified remarkably low IQs in a cohort of 19 Japanese children with the 20/25 genotype, with 42% of these cases reported as having displayed cognitive impairment. Many of these 20/25 genotype Japanese patients were diagnosed after the 1st mo of life and some were managed with minimal support including home oxygen only, despite clear recommendations against such support. These contrasting results indicating disparity within the same genotype emphasizes need for early recognition and conservative management to insure optimized neurocognitive outcome. Recognizing this, neurodevelopmental monitoring would be most beneficial beginning in early infancy.

Efforts are underway to evaluate and characterize the CCHS phenotype longitudinally through the International CCHS Registry (https://clinicaltrials.gov/show/NCT03088020) (Northwestern University). Delineating markers of disease progression and understanding the clinical manifestations of CCHS with advancing age will provide more accurate guidelines to healthcare providers, allowing physicians, families, and patients to better anticipate healthcare needs of affected individuals.

Bibliography is available at Expert Consult.

446.3 Other Conditions Affecting Respiration
Zehava L. Noah and Cynthia Etzler Budek

MYELOMENINGOCELE WITH ARNOLD-CHIARI TYPE II MALFORMATION
Arnold-Chiari type II malformation (see Chapter 609) is associated with myelomeningocele, hydrocephalus, and herniation of the cerebellar tonsils, caudal brainstem, and the 4th ventricle through the foramen magnum. Sleep-disordered breathing, including OSA and hypoventilation, has been reported. Direct pressure on the respiratory centers or brainstem nuclei or increased intracranial pressure because of the hydrocephalus may be responsible. Vocal cord paralysis, apnea, hypoventilation, and bradyarrhythmias have also been reported. Patients with Arnold-Chiari type II malformation have blunted responses to hypercapnia, and, to a lesser degree, hypoxia.

MANAGEMENT
An acute change in the ventilatory state of a patient with this malformation requires immediate evaluation. Consideration must be given to posterior fossa decompression and/or treatment of the hydrocephalus. If this treatment is unsuccessful in resolving central hypoventilation or apnea, tracheostomy and LMV should be considered.

RAPID-ONSET OBESITY, HYPOTHALAMIC DYSFUNCTION, AND AUTONOMIC DYSREGULATION
See Chapter 60.1.

OBESITY HYPOVENTILATION SYNDROME
As its name implies, obesity hypoventilation syndrome is a syndrome of central hypoventilation during wakefulness in obese patients with sleep-disordered breathing. Although it was initially described mainly in adult obese patients, obese children have also demonstrated the syndrome. Sleep-disordered breathing is a combination of OSA, hypopnea, and/or sleep hypoventilation syndrome. Patients are hypercapnic with cognitive impairment, morning headache, and hypersomnolence during the day. Chronic hypoxemia may lead to pulmonary hypertension and cor pulmonale.

Obesity is associated with reduced respiratory system compliance, increased airway resistance, reduced functional residual capacity, and increased work of breathing. Affected patients are unable to increase their respiratory drive in response to hypercapnia. Leptin may have a role in this syndrome. The sleep-disordered breathing leads to compensatory metabolic alkalosis. Because of the long half-life of bicarbonate, its elevation causes compensatory respiratory acidosis during wakefulness with elevated $PaCO_2$.

MANAGEMENT
The use of **CPAP** during sleep may be sufficient for many patients. Patients with hypoxemia may require **BiPAP** and supplemental oxygen. Tracheostomy may be considered for patients who do not tolerate mask ventilation.

ACQUIRED ALVEOLAR HYPOVENTILATION
Traumatic, ischemic, and inflammatory injuries to the brainstem, brainstem infarction, brain tumors, bulbar polio, and viral paraneoplastic encephalitis may also result in central hypoventilation.

OBSTRUCTIVE SLEEP APNEA
Epidemiology
Habitual snoring during sleep is extremely common during childhood. As many as 27% of children who snore are affected by **OSA**. The current obesity epidemic has affected the epidemiology of this condition. Peak

prevalence is at 2-8 yr of age. The ratio between habitual snoring and OSA is 4:1 to 6:1.

Pathophysiology

OSA occurs when the luminal cross-sectional area of the upper airway is significantly reduced during inspiration. With increased airway resistance and reduced activation of pharyngeal dilators, negative pressure leads to upper airway collapse. The site of upper airway closure in children with OSA is at the level of tonsils and adenoids. The size of tonsils and adenoids increases throughout childhood up to 12 yr of age. Environmental irritants such as cigarette smoke or allergic rhinitis may accelerate the process. Reports suggest that early viral infections may affect adenotonsillar proliferation.

Clinical Presentation

Snoring during sleep, behavioral disturbances, learning difficulties, excessive daytime sleepiness, metabolic issues, and cardiovascular morbidity may alert the parent or physician to the presence of OSA. Diagnosis is made with the help of airway radiograms and a polysomnogram.

Treatment

When adenotonsillar hypertrophy is suspected, a consultation with an ear, nose, and throat specialist for adenoidectomy and/or tonsillectomy may be indicated. For patients who are not candidates for surgical intervention or persist with OSA despite adenoidectomy and/or tonsillectomy, CPAP or BiPAP during sleep may alleviate the obstruction (see Chapter 31).

SPINAL CORD INJURY

Epidemiology

There are an estimated 11,000 new spinal cord injuries (**SCIs**) annually in the United States, with more than 50% resulting in quadriplegia. SCI is relatively rare in pediatric patients, with an incidence of 1–13% of all SCI patients. The incidence in infancy and early childhood is similar for boys and girls. The preponderance of SCI in adolescents is in males. Motor vehicle accidents, falls, sports injuries, and assaults are the main causes. SCI usually leads to lifelong disability.

Pathophysiology

Children with SCI have a disproportionately higher involvement of the upper cervical spine, high frequency of SCI without radiographic abnormality, delayed onset of neurologic deficits, and higher proportion of complete injury. Thus, there is a high likelihood in pediatric SCI of quadriplegia with intercostal muscle and/or diaphragmatic paralysis leading to respiratory failure.

Management

Immobilization and stabilization of the spine must be accomplished simultaneously with initial patient resuscitation. Children with high SCI typically require lifelong ventilation, so the decision to place a tracheostomy for chronic ventilatory support is usually made early in their course of treatment. Depending on the child's age and general condition, diaphragmatic pacing may be considered. Often patients with diaphragmatic pacing need tracheostomy placement if there is dyscoordination between pacing and glottal opening. Muscle spasms occur frequently in the SCI patient and are treated with muscle relaxants. Occasionally the muscle spasms involve the chest and present a serious impediment to ventilation. Continuous intrathecal infusion of muscle relaxant via an implanted subcutaneous pump may be indicated (see Chapter 83).

METABOLIC DISEASE

Mucopolysaccharidoses

See Chapter 107.

Mucopolysaccharidoses are a group of progressive hereditary disorders that lack the lysosomal enzymes that degrade glycosaminoglycans. Incompletely catabolized mucopolysaccharides accumulate in connective tissue throughout the body. The inheritance is autosomal recessive except

for Hunt syndrome, which is X-linked. The diagnosis is suggested by the presence of glycosaminuria and is confirmed by a lysosomal enzyme assay. I-cell disease mucolipidosis type II is an inherited lysosomal disorder with accumulation of mucolipids. Phenotypically, it is similar to mucopolysaccharidoses, but the age of onset is earlier and there is no mucopolysacchariduria. Mucopolysaccharide deposits are frequently found in the head and neck and cause airway obstruction. Typically, the affected child has a coarse face and large tongue. Significant deposits are found in the adenoids, tonsils, and cartilage. Airway radiograms and a polysomnogram may help define the severity of the upper airway obstruction.

Treatment options have included enzyme replacement therapy and stem cell transplantation with limited success. Adenoidectomy and/or tonsillectomy may be indicated but surgery alone seldom solves the problem of airway obstruction. Noninvasive CPAP or BiPAP, or tracheostomy with ventilatory support may be helpful.

Dysplasias

Campomelic dysplasia (see Chapter 718) and thanatophoric dysplasia (see Chapter 716) affect rib cage size, shape, and compliance, leading to respiratory failure. Most patients with these disorders do not survive beyond early infancy. Tracheostomy and ventilation may prolong life.

Glycogenosis Type II

See Chapter 105.1.

Glycogenosis type II is an autosomal recessive disorder. Clinical manifestations include cardiomyopathy and generalized muscle weakness. Cardiac issues may include heart failure and arrhythmias. Muscle weakness leads to respiratory insufficiency and sleep-disordered breathing. Treatment includes emerging therapies such as enzyme replacement therapy, chaperone molecules, and gene therapy. Supportive therapy may consist of either noninvasive ventilation, or tracheostomy and mechanical ventilation. Cardiac medications, protein-rich nutrition, and judicious physical therapy are additional measures that can be utilized.

Severe Tracheomalacia and/or Bronchomalacia (Airway Malacia)

Conditions associated with airway malacia include tracheoesophageal fistula, innominate artery compression, and pulmonary artery sling after surgical repair (see Chapter 416). Patients with tracheobronchomalacia present with cough, lower airway obstruction, and wheezing. Diagnosis is made via bronchoscopy, preferably with the patient breathing spontaneously in order to evaluate dynamic airway function. Positive end-expiratory pressure titration during the bronchoscopy helps identify the ideal airway pressure required to maintain airway patency and prevent tracheobronchial collapse.

Neuropathy of Severe Illness

Children recuperating from severe illness in the intensive care unit often have neuromuscular weakness from suboptimal nutrition. This neuromuscular weakness can be devastating when coupled with the catabolic effects of severe illness and the residual effects of sedatives, analgesics, and muscle relaxants, particularly if corticosteroids were administered. Children with neuromuscular compromise have limited ability to increase ventilation and usually do so by increasing respiratory rate. Because of weakness, costal and sternal retractions may not be observed. Children with severe neuromyopathy may respond to increased respiratory load by becoming apneic. A look of panic, a change in vital signs such as significant tachycardia or bradycardia, and cyanosis may be the only signs of impending respiratory failure.

Mitochondrial Diseases

See Chapter 106.

Mitochondria are primarily responsible for the production of adenosine triphosphate. Mitochondrial diseases are a heterogeneous group of diseases in which adenosine triphosphate production is disrupted. Mitochondrial diseases are increasingly recognized and diagnosed in the pediatric population. Organs with high-energy requirements such as the neurons, and skeletal and cardiac muscles are particularly vulnerable. Although myopathy is the most frequently recognized presentation of mitochondrial disease, it is often part of a multisystem disease process. Neurologic complications include progressive proximal myopathy, kyphoscoliosis, dyskinesia, dystonia and spasticity, stroke, epilepsy, and visual and hearing impairment. Nonneurologic manifestations include cardiomyopathy, gastrointestinal dysmotility, gastroesophageal reflux, delayed gastric emptying, and pseudoobstruction.

Respiratory complications of mitochondrial disease are multi-factorial. Muscle weakness, kyphoscoliosis, muscle spasms, and movement disorders may result in a restrictive pattern, and respiratory compromise. Additionally, dyscoordinated swallow and reflux may result in aspiration. In some mitochondrial diseases such as Leigh syndrome (see Chapter 106), central hypoventilation is an integral part of the disease. Supportive care for these patients may include noninvasive or invasive ventilation, tracheostomy placement, diuretics, appropriate nutrition, and dietary supplements.

446.4 Long-Term Mechanical Ventilation
Robert J. Graham

See also Chapter 734.1.

GOALS AND DECISION-MAKING
The decision to implement LMV has many challenges stemming from a diversity of underlying pathophysiology, uncertain disease trajectories, the development of new condition-specific therapies, personal experiences, and values held by providers, patients, parents, and the broader community, variability in resources, and lack of standards. While optimizing gas exchange (i.e., oxygenation and CO_2 removal) remains a primary objective, it represents a tool for the comprehensive care of children with complex needs (see Chapters 446.1 and 734.1).

LMV has a role within the spectrum of palliative care. It is used proactively to attenuate cumulative morbidities (respiratory and cardiac) associated with progressive neuromuscular conditions, such as Duchenne muscular dystrophy. LMV is also used reactively when acute illness (e.g., acute respiratory distress syndrome) does not resolve. In infants with premature lung disease or complex airway anomalies, LMV may be implemented as a temporary measure, as these conditions may resolve with maturity or surgical interventions. LMV can also represent a bridge to lung transplant for those with intrinsic pulmonary or pulmonary vascular disease. LMV has become a destination therapy to optimize symptom management and prolong life in complex conditions. Etiology of the respiratory insufficiency includes, but is not limited to, congenital anomalies (e.g., complex cardiac conditions, central nervous system disorders, interruptions in aerodigestive morphogenesis, and skeletal dysplasias), acquired central neurological injuries from perinatal, infectious, traumatic, and hypoxic-ischemic events, metabolic disorders, or progressive neuromuscular conditions. Progress in other areas of medicine, such as gene-targeted therapy in spinal muscular atrophy and myotubular myopathy, may alter the LMV decision-making landscape as families foresee the prospect of improvement.

NONINVASIVE AND TRANSTRACHEAL SUPPORTS
The essential modalities for LMV include negative pressure, noninvasive positive pressure ventilation (NIPPV with either continuous or biphasic support provided through an occlusive mask interface), or transtracheal positive pressure. Considerations for a given patient should include, but are not limited to, anatomic factors, physiologic goals, long-term care goals, comfort, tolerability/compliance, and safety (mobility/portability, monitoring, device availability and back-up, training capacity).

Negative pressure devices, such as the cuirass ventilator, do not require any interface with the face or trachea and are more *natural* from a mechanical perspective. *NIPPV* can address dynamic upper airway obstruction as well as augment respiratory mechanics and gas-exchange. This modality may, however, have limitations if upper airway obstruction is severe or fixed or the need for oxygen supplementation is high. Masks,

prongs, and pillows of varying sizes are available for nasal, oral, combination, and full interface, including those for infants. Mouthpiece interface has also been demonstrated to be effective and feasible. The choice of continuous positive airway pressure (CPAP) versus biphasic positive airway pressure (BiPAP) is dependent upon the underlying pathophysiology. Conceptually, CPAP can overcome a dynamic upper airway obstruction and allow for spontaneous ventilation, while BiPAP is more versatile in compensating for upper airway obstruction and supporting lung recruitment and gas-exchange. In practice, CPAP is limited to management of mild OSA. While NIPPV can be maintained 24 hr/day, efficacy of ventilation, difficult airway considerations (i.e., Can the child be intubated?), developmental needs, implications for midface hypoplasia, and secretion clearance are among factors that impact the decision to pursue tracheostomy placement and invasive LMV.

Transtracheal LMV provides the most secure and effective respiratory support. Fixed and dynamic upper airway obstruction are bypassed with tracheostomy tube placement. Secretions are more readily cleared from the lower airway. Positive pressure and oxygen delivery via a tracheostomy tube more consistently address primary impairments in gas exchange (within limits) as well as mechanical disadvantages from neuromuscular insufficiency and restrictive disease. When possible, placement of a tracheostomy tube in a child should be coordinated at an institution with pediatric expertise, because the short-term morbidities and, potentially, mortality are not insignificant.

Individuals using NIPPV are at risk for pressure ulcerations on the face as well as on the scalp. Proper fit of the interface must be assured since a tighter fit is not necessarily commensurate with better support. Alternating masks on a regular basis may alleviate pressure on a given site. Additional non-adhesive dressings can also be used to facilitate mask seal and minimize skin breakdown. For those with a tracheostomy tube in place, care of tracheostomy ties and regular assessment of the stoma is required. Moisture-wicking dressings can attenuate risk of maceration, but their use should be balanced against the value of exposure to air for drying. Stomal assessment should include evaluation of granulation, fissures, and traction created by additional torque from ventilator tubing, which should be maintained midline and without weight displacement on the tracheostomy tube itself. Any areas of integument interruption are potential niduses for infection and of great concern for immunocompromised hosts.

AUGMENTED SECRETION CLEARANCE
(See Chapter 446.1).

AERODIGESTIVE AND COMMUNICATION CONSIDERATIONS
Assessment of swallowing and speaking capacity should be part of an assessment for LMV and may help guide the modality. In general, implementation of noninvasive or transtracheal supports will not further impair either of these functions. Rather, the underlying condition is the primary determinant. This consideration is most notable in patients with neurologic injury or neuromuscular conditions. Decision-making around placement of a transabdominal gastric or gastrojejunal enteral feeding tube, if not already in place, should coincide with decisions around LMV. Nasogastric tubes, it should be appreciated, may impair NIPPV mask seal as well as cause laryngeal irritation in the long-term.

Use of NIPPV must be approached cautiously in those with impaired swallowing as positive pressure will increase the risk of macro- and micro-aspiration. Individuals using NIPPV can eat and drink while on support with risk versus benefit determination and quality of life. Aerophagia on NIPPV is also problematic, regardless of bulbar function and swallowing capacity; abdominal distention is uncomfortable, contributes to satiety as well as vomiting risk, and further impairs respiratory mechanics with decreased functional residual capacity and increased inspiratory workload. If a gastrostomy is present, active evacuation of swallowed air and use of passive *venting* tubes can be helpful.

Children with swallowing capacity can continue to eat and drink by mouth with a tracheostomy tube in place on LMV. The presence of a cuffed tracheostomy tube does not prevent aspiration if swallowing is impaired. Speaking may be facilitated by LMV, as settings can be increased or a speaking valve utilized to increased airflow across the vocal cords. Regardless, multidisciplinary care with a speech language pathologist, feeding specialist, and augmented communication services can be helpful for many children and their families utilizing LMV. Conditioned aversions to oral stimulation can be challenging for infants but developmental gains should not be impeded by LMV.

GAS-EXCHANGE GOALS AND VENTILATOR STRATEGIES

Pressure- or volume-regulated modes, spontaneous or controlled settings, and mixed modes are all feasible for NIPPV and transtracheal supports with new devices. The appropriate support should coincide with oxygenation and ventilation goals on a case-by-case basis. Consideration, however, should be given to the site of care and contingencies for presentation to acute cure during intercurrent illness or emergency. Providers should assess limitations in oxygen supplementation outside of the hospital; measured or estimated delivered fractional inspired oxygen (FIO_2) will inform families and providers of capacity when adding oxygen in liters/minute flow to the ventilator circuit; dilution can have a dramatic effect and achieving $FIO_2 > 0.60$ may be difficult when oxygen is added to a home ventilator circuit. Safety allowances should also account for the duration of portable oxygen provision, which is based upon liter flow and tank/reservoir volume.

Monitoring of CO_2 in the homecare setting is not usual, although portable end-tidal CO_2 devices are available. Conditions such as congenital central hypoventilation syndrome warrant vigilance, and parameters for implementation, or titration, of mechanical ventilation should be discussed with families. Recognition that significant and indolent hypercapnia can precede hypoxia is necessary, and long-term effects on cerebral and pulmonary vasculature should be considered. In the absence of direct CO_2 monitoring, periodic measurement of serum bicarbonate may be helpful to assess for renal compensation for altered CO_2 clearance; interpretation, however, may be altered in the presence of diuretic therapy, metabolic disease, or ketogenic diets.

CARDIOPULMONARY INTERACTIONS

Closely linked to the gas-exchange goals are considerations for cardiopulmonary interactions. While there are subtle implications for systemic venous return of any form of positive pressure ventilation, LMV can be used to decrease transmural myocardial load as well as optimize right ventricular afterload through lung recruitment and pulmonary vascular reactivity. The prolonged survival of young males with Duchenne muscular dystrophy is in part due to consistent respiratory support to optimize lung health as well as attenuate myocardial dysfunction. Primary or secondary pulmonary hypertension, whether overt or indolent, requires consideration of oxygenation and ventilation goals. Echocardiograms are not required for all patients with LMV, but this modality may be helpful to guide management in cohorts with congenital heart lesions, cardiomyopathies, severe obstructive pulmonary disease, significant central dysregulation, and on a case-by-case basis.

When considering gas-change goals and cardiopulmonary interactions, providers must also consider daytime and nocturnal differences. Neuromuscular-derived hypoventilation is more prominent at night as is upper airway obstructive disease; the latter is more important for those using noninvasive LMV. Daytime support provision must account for increased oxygen consumption and demand based upon variable activity as well as stressors, including environmental temperature. Providers and families must factor in mobility, behavioral tolerance, and quality of life.

CHEST WALL/THORACIC CONFIGURATION

Positive pressure through LMV in early childhood for children with neuromuscular conditions and/or restrictive lung disease is also used to improve thoracic compliance and configuration. Lung inflation can be used to attenuate the impact of thoracic asphyxiation as well as progressive parasol chest deformation in diaphragm-dependent conditions, such spinal muscular atrophy. This use has implications for atelectasis and secretion inspissation, associated pulmonary vasoconstriction, and

cumulative restrictive or asymmetric pulmonary mechanics.

NUTRITION AND WEIGHT GAIN

See Chapter 446.1.

DEVELOPMENTAL CONSIDERATIONS

Decisions regarding the LMV modality, noninvasive or transtracheal, requires consideration of development as well. Beyond safety factors, tolerance of interventions, availability of appropriate sized interfaces, and portability, there remains substantial subjectivity with respect to perspective on the implication for social interactions (i.e., devices covering the face versus a device in the neck). While there are no published series, long-term or near-continuous NIV also has implications for midface hypoplasia and potentially compounds upper airway obstructive symptoms, as is evident by images of *BiPAP faces*. Swallowing and speech capacity primarily reflect the child's underlying condition rather than the LMV.

PROJECTED INTERVENTIONS AND NEEDS

Trajectory and management of the underlying disease as well as symptom management are primary drivers in determining the need and duration of LMV. Stakeholders should also consider future interventions, specifically surgical procedures. LMV, noninvasive or transtracheal, can be utilized to optimize perioperative standing and facilitate recovery and provision of opiate-based analgesia that could alter respiratory drive. The maintenance of a tracheostomy tube in anticipation of sequential surgeries (e.g., spinal instrumentation, craniofacial and airway reconstruction, or serial cardiac interventions) may be required for practical reasons, but also minimizes the need for repeated intubation.

MONITORING

Conceptually, monitoring is used to detect early physiologic changes and determine adequacy of LMV to minimize cumulative morbidities and risk of mortality. Recommendations for monitoring children and young adults on LMV vary based upon underlying vulnerability, care setting, and activity (e.g., home, long-term care facility, school, or in transport via car), and adjuvant supports (e.g., home nursing or personal care assistant). Pulse oximetry can be used intermittently or on a continuous basis with oxygen and heart rate parameters determined on a case-by-case basis. Internal ventilator alarm settings, for both NIV and transtracheal ventilators, are utilized to monitor high- and low-pressure parameters and minute ventilation. Stakeholders must acknowledge, however, that internal alarms may be insufficient in the setting of a large mask or peri-tracheal leak or in the event of a device malfunction. There are also pragmatic considerations of signal-to-noise when determining monitoring parameters; recurrent false alarms will desensitize providers and may disturb a child's sleep; conversely, wide alarm parameters circumvent early warning systems with significant consequences.

TRANSITIONING FROM ACUTE CARE TO REHABILITATION OR COMMUNITY SETTING

Disposition of children and young adults with LMV will vary based upon their relative stability, local support services, and goals of care. A proactive, comprehensive care model is required to assure safe and effective provision. The impact of care needs on the child and family are inextricably linked.

ROUTINE HEALTH MAINTENANCE
Airway Evaluation

There is no standard for regular airway assessment for children with LMV, specifically those with transtracheal support, but annual evaluation should represent the minimum. Office-based transtracheal tube endoscopy can facilitate assessment of tube upsizing for linear growth, presence of granulation tissue, airway inflammation, and general mucosal integrity. Formal diagnostic laryngoscopy and bronchoscopy under general anesthesia is required to assess for suprastomal and laryngeal level pathology as well as the rare, acquired trachea-esophageal fistulae. Of note, independent of routine evaluation, recurrent or unexpected tracheal bleeding may warrant evaluation for a trachea-vascular fistula via CT angiogram and bronchoscopy.

Bacterial Colonization

Chronic respiratory failure lends itself to airway bacterial colonization due to alterations in secretion clearance, aerodigestive interactions, the presence of artificial airways with the development of biofilms, and other factors. Hydrophilic and Gram-negative bacteria (e.g., *Pseudomonas, Serratia,* and *Stenotrophomonas*) are not uncommon. There is no standard of care for determining pathogenicity versus colonization. Use of systemic or inhaled antibacterial agents to decrease colonization load, frequency of tracheostomy tube exchanges to reduce biofilm accumulation, utility of viral screening, and threshold for treatment of an acute lower airway process or tracheitis is provider and case dependent. Providers should appreciate that recurrent empiric antibacterial treatment may select for resistant bacterial strains and has implications for enteric bacterial colonization.

Dental Care

Routine daily and office-based dental care should follow standard recommendations for all children. Extrapolation from the acute care setting and general population would suggest that oropharyngeal care and minimization of bacterial overgrowth would impact the risk of superimposed respiratory illness in LMV and long-term cardiovascular outcomes, respectively. Special consideration with respect to aspiration risk, developmental tolerance, and prophylaxis and procedural sedation for intervention may require engagement of specialty providers.

Immunizations

There are no immunizations specifically indicated for individuals receiving LMV. Routine provision is recommended, including seasonal vaccinations for viral pathogens.

Radiography, Laboratory Evaluation, Polysomnography, and Pulmonary Function Testing

There are no recommendations for routine chest radiography, standard or cross-sectional, in the context of LMV. The cumulative radiation exposure would need to be considered. Gas exchange adequacy can often be assessed noninvasively. Venous, capillary, or arterial puncture for determining resting and long-term oxygenation and ventilation status may be of limited utility and validity, as intercurrent illness, technique with tourniquet, and associated agitation will alter results. Condition-specific (e.g., muscular dystrophy, polysomnography, spirometry, or pulmonary function) testing recommendations have been established. Regular assessment may also be helpful when gauging disease trajectory, LMV titration, safety parameters, and weaning potential.

LONG-TERM MECHANICAL VENTILATION WEANING AND TRACHEAL DECANNULATION

Reassessment of the role of LMV should be part of routine and family-centered care. Determination should include, but is not limited to, the factors described above with open discussion of goals of care, developmental appropriateness, physiologic and anatomic consideration, growth implications, and contingencies. As there are no definitive conditioning regimens or LMV weaning strategies, providers can determine the value of time off versus decreased level of supports as well as pragmatic considerations for the child and family. Continuity of care, however, holds implicit value. Monitoring provision may need to be increased during weaning. If tracheal decannulation is required, a formal diagnostic laryngoscopy and bronchoscopy should be considered to rule out granulation (supra and infrastomal) as well as dynamic airway collapse that may prohibit immediate tracheostomy tube removal. If positive pressure or oxygen supplementation will still be required after decannulation, determination of the child's tolerance of NIV or other interventions (e.g., cough assist) should be determined in advance. Desensitization may be required.

Ultimately, LMV has an increasing role in the support of children and young adults with chronic respiratory failure. Transition from pediatric to adult services should be anticipated as this population ages. Additional research is required to inform all stakeholders regarding daily management decisions as well as healthcare resource utilization and long-term patient-centered outcomes.

Bibliography is available at Expert Consult.

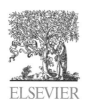

ELSEVIER

Elsevier (Singapore) Pte Ltd.
3 Killiney Road, #08-01 Winsland House I, Singapore 239519
Tel: (65) 6349-0200; Fax: (65) 6733-1817

This English Adaptation of Nelson Textbook of Pediatrics, 21E by Robert M. Kliegman,
Joseph W. St. Geme Ⅲ, Nathan J. Blum, Samir S. Shah, Robert C. Tasker, Karen M. Wilson
was undertaken by Hunan Science & Technology Press and is published by arrangement with
Elsevier (Singapore) Pte Ltd.

Nelson Textbook of Pediatrics, 21E by Robert M. Kliegman, Joseph W. St. Geme Ⅲ, Nathan
J. Blum, Samir S. Shah, Robert C. Tasker, Karen M. Wilson 由湖南科学技术出版社进行改
编影印，并根据湖南科学技术出版社与爱思唯尔（新加坡）私人有限公司的协议约定出版。

尼尔森儿科学Nelson Textbook of Pediatrics, 影印中文导读版,（张金哲，王天有等改编）
ISBN：978-7-5710-0730-0

Notices
The adaptation has been undertaken by Hunan Science & Technology Press at its sole
responsibility. Practitioners and researchers must always rely on their own experience and
knowledge in evaluating and using any information, methods, compounds or experiments
described herein. Because of rapid advances in the medical sciences, in particular,
independent verification of diagnoses and drug dosages should be made. To the fullest extent
of the law, no responsibility is assumed by Elsevier, authors, editors or contributors in
relation to the adaptation or for any injury and/or damage to persons or property as a matter
of products liability, negligence or otherwise, or from any use or operation of any methods,
products, instructions, or ideas contained in the material herein.

图书在版编目（ＣＩＰ）数据

尼尔森儿科学 : 第 21 版 : 影印中文导读版 : 汉、英文 中册 ／（美）罗伯特 M. 克利格曼（Robert M. Kliegman）等主编 ; 张金哲, 王天有等编译. — 长沙 : 湖南科学技术出版社, 2020.10

（西医经典名著集成）

ISBN 978-7-5710-0730-0

Ⅰ．①尼… Ⅱ．①罗… ②张… ③王… Ⅲ．①儿科学－汉、英文 Ⅳ．①R72

中国版本图书馆 CIP 数据核字(2020)第 157308 号

著作权合同登记号 18-2020-187

西医经典名著集成

NIERSHEN ERKEXUE

尼尔森儿科学 第 21 版 影印中文导读版 中册

主　　编：[美]罗伯特 M. 克利格曼（Robert M. Kliegman），[美]约瑟夫 W. St. 盖门（Joseph W. St. Geme III），

　　　　　[美]内森 J. 布卢姆（Nathan J. Blum），[美]萨米尔 S. 沙阿（Samir S. Shah），

　　　　　[美]罗伯特 C. 塔斯克（Robert C. Tasker），[美]凯伦 M. 威尔逊（Karen M. Wilson）

编 译 者：张金哲，王天有等

责任编辑：李　忠

出版发行：湖南科学技术出版社

社　　址：长沙市湘雅路 276 号

　　　　　http://www.hnstp.com

印　　刷：长沙德三印刷有限公司

　　　　　（印装质量问题请直接与本厂联系）

厂　　址：宁乡市城郊乡东沩社区东沩北路 192 号

邮　　编：410600

版　　次：2020 年 10 月第 1 版

印　　次：2020 年 10 月第 1 次印刷

开　　本：787mm×1092mm　1/16

印　　张：86.25

字　　数：5100 千字

书　　号：ISBN 978-7-5710-0730-0

定　　价：1100.00 元（上、中、下册）